# Textbook of Rheumatology

VOLUME 1    SECOND EDITION

**WILLIAM N. KELLEY, M.D.**

John G. Searle Professor and Chairman,
Department of Internal Medicine, and
Professor, Department of Biological Chemistry,
University of Michigan Medical Center,
Ann Arbor, Michigan

**EDWARD D. HARRIS, JR., M.D.**

Professor and Chairman, Department of Medicine,
UMDNJ - Rutgers Medical School,
New Brunswick, New Jersey

**SHAUN RUDDY, M.D.**

Professor of Medicine, Microbiology and Immunology,
Chairman, Division of Immunology and
Connective Tissue Diseases,
Medical College of Virginia, Health Sciences Division,
Virginia Commonwealth University,
Richmond, Virginia

**CLEMENT B. SLEDGE, M.D.**

John B. and Buckminster Brown Professor
of Orthopedic Surgery, Harvard Medical School,
Orthopedic Surgeon-in-Chief,
Brigham and Women's Hospital,
Boston, Massachusetts

W.B. SAUNDERS COMPANY

Philadelphia □ London □ Toronto □ Mexico City □ Rio de Janeiro □ Sydney □ Tokyo

W. B. Saunders Company: West Washington Square
Philadelphia, PA 19105

1 St. Anne's Road
Eastbourne, East Sussex BN21 3UN, England

1 Goldthorne Avenue
Toronto, Ontario M8Z 5T9, Canada

Apartado 26370–Cedro 512
Mexico 4, D.F., Mexico

Rua Coronel Cabrita, 8
Sao Cristovao Caixa Postal 21176
Rio de Janeiro, Brazil

9 Waltham Street
Artarmon, N.S.W. 2064, Australia

Ichibancho, Central Bldg., 22-1 Ichibancho
Chiyoda-Ku, Tokyo 102, Japan

**Library of Congress Cataloging in Publication Data**
Main entry under title:

Textbook of rheumatology.

1. Rheumatism. 2. Collagen diseases. I. Kelley, William N. [DNLM: 1. Arthritis. 2. Rheumatism. WE 544 T355]
RC927.T49 1985 616.7'23 83-20114
ISBN 0-7216-5362-6

Textbook of Rheumatology

Single Volume ISBN 0-7216-5362-6
Volume I ISBN 0-7216-5363-4
Volume II ISBN 0-7216-5364-2
Two Volume Set ISBN 0-7216-5365-0



Last digit is the print number: 9 8 7 6 5 4 3

We wish to dedicate this edition of the
Textbook of Rheumatology to our wives and children.

Lois Kelley and children:
Paige Kelley, Ginger Kelley, Lori Kelley and Mark Kelley.

Mary Ann Harris and children:
Ned Harris, Tom Harris, and Chandler Harris.

Millicent Ruddy and children:
Christi Ruddy and Candace Ruddy.

Georgia Sledge and children:
Mego Sledge, John Sledge, Matthew Sledge, and Claire Sledge.

# Contributors

**Margaret A. Alspaugh, Ph.D.**
Associate Professor of Medicine and Pathology, University of Missouri; Associate Scientist, Cancer Research Center, Columbus, Missouri
*Sjögren's Syndrome*

**Roy D. Altman, M.D.**
Professor of Medicine, University of Miami School of Medicine; Chief, Arthritis Division, Miami Veterans Administration Medical Center, Miami, Florida
*Hypertrophic Osteoarthropathy*

**Ronald J. Anderson, M.D.**
Associate Professor of Medicine, Harvard Medical School; Director of Clinical Training, Department of Rheumatology and Immunology, Brigham and Women's Hospital, Boston, Massachusetts
*Polyarticular Arthritis*

**William J. Arnold, M.D., F.A.C.P.**
Clinical Associate Professor of Medicine, Abraham Lincoln School of Medicine, University of Illinois at The Medical Center; Director, Section of Rheumatology, Lutheran General Hospital, Park Ridge, Illinois
*The Rheumatic Manifestations of Sarcoidosis*

**Dianna Ausprunk, Ph.D.**
Assistant Professor, Department of Anatomy, Harvard Medical School; Research Associate, Children's Hospital Medical Center, Boston, Massachusetts
*Connective Tissue: Small Blood Vessels and Capillaries*

**Lloyd Axelrod, M.D.**
Associate Professor of Medicine, Harvard Medical School; Associate Physician, Massachusetts General Hospital; Chief, Medical Unit, Massachusetts Eye and Ear Infirmary, Boston, Massachusetts
*Glucocorticoids*

**Barbara Figley Banwell, M.A., P.T.**
Program Leader in Physical Therapy, University of Michigan Multipurpose Arthritis Center, University Medical Center, Ann Arbor, Michigan
*Psychological and Sexual Health in Rheumatic Disease*

**Alan J. Barrett, Ph.D., Sc.D.**
Head of Department of Biochemistry, Strangeways Laboratory, Cambridge, England
*Proteinases in Joint Disease*

**J. Claude Bennett, M.D.**
Professor and Chairman, Department of Medicine, and Director, Multipurpose Arthritis Center, University of Alabama in Birmingham; Physician, University of Alabama Hospitals, Birmingham, Alabama
*The Etiology of Rheumatoid Arthritis*

**Robert M. Bennett, M.D., M.R.C.P., F.A.C.P.**
Professor of Medicine, Oregon Health Sciences University; Head, Division of Rheumatic Diseases, Oregon Health Sciences University Hospital and Clinics; Consultant, Portland Veterans Administration Medical Center, Portland, Oregon
*Mixed Connective Tissue Disease and Other Overlap Syndromes*

**A.G. Björkengren, M.D.**
New York, New York
*Surgery for Arthritis of the Cervical Spine*

**George L. Blackburn, M.D., Ph.D.**
Associate Professor of Surgery, Harvard Medical School; Director, Nutrition Support Service, New England Deaconess Hospital, Boston, Massachusetts
*Nutrition and Rheumatic Diseases*

**R. Michael Blaese, M.D.**
Chief, Cellular Immunology Section, Metabolism Branch, National Cancer Institute, National Institutes of Health; Attending Physician, Clinical Center, National Institutes of Health, Bethesda, Maryland
*Immunodeficiency Diseases*

**Arthur L. Boland, Jr., M.D.**
Assistant Clinical Professor of Orthopedic Surgery, Harvard Medical School; Associate in Orthopedic Surgery, Brigham and Women's Hospital; Staff Orthopedic Surgery, New England Baptist Hospital; Staff Orthopedic Surgery, Harvard Community Health Plan Hospital, Boston, Massachusetts
*Recreational Musculoskeletal Injuries*

**Alfred Jay Bollet, M.D.**
Clinical Professor of Medicine, Yale University School of Medicine New Haven, Connecticut; Adjunct Professor of Medicine, New York Medical College; Chairman, Department of Medicine, Danbury Hospital, Danbury, Connecticut
*Nonsteroidal Anti-inflammatory Drugs*

**Walter G. Bradley, D.M., F.R.C.P.**
Professor and Chairman, Department of Neurology, University of Vermont College of Medicine and Medical Center Hospital of Vermont, Burlington, Vermont
*Structure and Function of the Motor Unit; Muscle Weakness; Diagnostic Tests in Neuromuscular Diseases; Inflammatory Diseases of Muscle*

**Kenneth D. Brandt, M.D.**
Professor of Medicine and Chief, Rheumatology Division, Indiana University School of Medicine; Attending Physician, University Hospital, Indiana University Medical Center; Consulting Physician, Richard L. Roudebush Veterans Administration Medical Center, Indianapolis, Indiana
*Glycosaminoglycans; Pathogenesis of Osteoarthritis; Osteoarthritis: Clinical Patterns and Pathology; Management of Osteoarthritis*

**Joel N. Buxbaum, M.D.**
Professor of Medicine, New York University Medical Center; Chief, Rheumatology Section, Department of Medicine, New York Veterans Administration Medical Center, New York, New York
*Immunoglobulins and Their Genes*

**David S. Caldwell, M.D.**
Assistant Professor of Medicine, Duke University School of Medicine; Attending Rheumatologist, Duke University Hospital, Durham, North Carolina, Consulting Rheumatologist, Fayetteville Veterans Administration Hospital, Fayetteville, North Carolina; Consulting Rheumatologist, The Memorial Hospital, Danville, Virginia
*Musculoskeletal Syndromes Associated with Malignancy*

**Andrei Calin, M.D., M.R.C.P.**
Consultant Rheumatologist, Royal National Hospital for Rheumatic Diseases, Bath, England
*Ankylosing Spondylitis; Reiter's Syndrome*

**Dennis A. Carson, M.D.**
Associate Member, Department of Basic and Clinical Research, Scripps Clinic and Research Foundation, La Jolla, California
*Rheumatoid Factor*

**James T. Cassidy, M.D.**
Professor and Chairman, Department of Pediatrics, Creighton University School of Medicine, Omaha, Nebraska
*Juvenile Rheumatoid Arthritis*

**John E. Castaldo, M.D.**
Instructor of Clinical Medicine, Section of Neurology, Dartmouth Medical School, Hanover, New Hampshire; Attending Neurologist, Lehigh Valley Hospital Center, Allentown, Pennsylvania
*Peripheral Nerve: Structure, Function, and Dysfunction*

**Edgar S. Cathcart, M.D., D.Sc.**
Professor of Medicine, Boston University School of Medicine, Boston; Chief, Arthritis Gerontology Center, Edith Nourse Rogers Memorial Veterans Administration Hospital, Bedford, Massachusetts
*Amyloidosis*

**Zanvil A. Cohn, M.D.**
Professor and Senior Physician, Laboratory of Cellular Physiology and Immunology, The Rockefeller University; Senior Physician, The Rockefeller University Hospital, New York, New York
*Cellular Components of Inflammation: Monocytes and Macrophages*

**Robert O. Cone, III, M.D.**
Assistant Professor, Department of Radiology, University of Texas Health Science Center, and Medical Center Hospital, San Antonio, Texas
*Radiographic Evaluation of Articular Disorders*

**Doyt L. Conn, M.D.**
Professor of Medicine, Mayo Medical School; Chairman, Division of Rheumatology, and Consultant in Rheumatology and Internal Medicine, Mayo Clinic, Rochester, Minnesota
*Necrotizing Vasculitis; Giant Cell Arteritis and Polymyalgia Rheumatica*

**E. Dayer, M.D.**
Research Associate, Transfusion Center, Department of Medicine, Hôpital Cantonal Universitaire, Genève, Switzerland
*Immune Complexes*

**Frederick C. Ewald, M.D.**
Associate Clinical Professor, Orthopedic Surgery, Harvard Medical School; Orthopedic Surgeon, Brigham and Women's Hospital; Consultant, West Roxbury Veterans Administration Hospital and New England Baptist Hospital, Boston, Massachusetts
*Reconstructive Surgery and Rehabilitation of the Elbow*

**Anthony S. Fauci, M.D.**
Chief, Laboratory of Immunoregulation, National Institute of Allergy and Infectious Diseases, National Institutes of Health, Bethesda, Maryland
*Cytotoxic and Other Immunoregulatory Agents*

**Andrew P. Ferry, M.D., F.A.C.S.**
Professor and Chairman, Department of Ophthalmology, and Professor of Pathology, Medical College of Virginia of Virginia Commonwealth University; Ophthalmic Surgeon-in-Chief, Medical College of Virginia Hospitals; Consultant, Veterans Administration Hospital, Richmond, Virginia
*Ocular Manifestations of Rheumatic Diseases*

**J. William Fielding, M.D., F.R.C.S.(C.)**
Clinical Professor of Orthopaedic Surgery, Columbia University College of Physicians and Surgeons; Clinical Professor of Orthopaedic Surgery, New York University School of Medicine; Attending Orthopaedic Surgeon, New York University Medical Center and Bellevue Hospital; Director, Department of Orthopaedic Surgery, St. Luke's–Roosevelt Center Hospital, New York, New York
*Surgery for Arthritis of the Cervical Spine*

**Judah Folkman, M.D.**
Julia Dyckman Andrus Professor of Pediatric Surgery and Professor of Anatomy, Harvard Medical School; Director of The Surgical Research Laboratories, Children's Hospital, Boston, Massachusetts
*Connective Tissue: Small Blood Vessels and Capillaries*

**Irving H. Fox, M.D., C.M.**
Professor, Department of Internal Medicine, and Associate Professor, Department of Biological Chemistry, University of Michigan; Director, Clinical Research Center, University Hospital, Ann Arbor, Michigan
*Gout and Related Disorders of Purine Metabolism; Arthropathy with Iron Storage Disease*

**Blas Frangione, M.D., Ph.D.**
Professor of Pathology, New York University Medical Center, New York, New York
*Immunoglobulins and Their Genes*

**James F. Fries, M.D.**
Associate Professor of Medicine, Stanford University School of Medicine and Stanford University Hospital, Palo Alto; Attending Physician, Palo Alto Veterans Administration Hospital, Palo Alto, and Santa Clara Valley Medical Center, Santa Clara, California
*General Approach to the Rheumatic Disease Patient*

**Lynn H. Gerber, M.D.**
Chief, Department of Rehabilitation Medicine, National Institutes of Health; Adjunct Associate Professor of Medicine, George Washington University; Physician, Arthritis and Rheumatism Branch, NIADDK, National Institutes of Health, Bethesda, Maryland
*Rehabilitation of Patients with Rheumatic Diseases*

**William W. Ginsburg, M.D.**
Assistant Professor of Internal Medicine, Mayo Foundation; Consultant, Rochester Methodist Hospital and St. Marys Hospital, Rochester, Minnesota
*Multicentric Reticulohistiocytosis*

**Edward J. Goetzl, M.D.**
Professor of Medicine, University of California, San Francisco; Director, Division of Allergy and Immunology, Moffitt-Long Hospitals of the University of California, San Francisco, California
*Cellular Components of Inflammation: Granulocytes*

**Ira M. Goldstein, M.D.**
Professor of Medicine, University of California, San Francisco; Chief, Division of Rheumatology, San Francisco General Hospital, San Francisco, California
*Cellular Components of Inflammation: Granulocytes*

**Armin E. Good, M.D.**
Professor of Medicine, University of Michigan; Chief, Arthritis Section, Ann Arbor Veterans Administration Medical Center, Ann Arbor, Michigan
*Enteropathic Arthritis*

**Paul F. Good**
Research Technologist, Department of Pathology, University of Vermont College of Medicine, Burlington, Vermont
*Structure and Function of the Motor Unit*

**John L. Gordon, Ph.D.**
Head of Vascular Biology, Clinical Research Centre, Medical Research Council; Head of Vascular Biology, Northwick Park Hospital, Harrow, England
*Cellular Components of Inflammation: Platelets*

**Norman L. Gottlieb, M.D.**
Professor of Medicine, University of Miami School of Medicine, Miami, Florida
*Gold Compounds*

**Norbert Gschwend, Prof. Dr. Med.**
Medical Faculty, University of Zürich; Chief Orthopaedic Surgeon, Klinik Wilhelm Schulthess, Zürich, Switzerland
*Synovectomy*

**Virgil Hanson, M.D.**
Professor of Pediatrics, University of Southern California, School of Medicine; Head, Division of Rheumatology, Childrens Hospital of Los Angeles, Los Angeles, California
*Systemic Lupus Erythematosus, Dermatomyositis, Scleroderma, and Vasculitides in Childhood*

**Edward D. Harris, Jr., M.D.**
Professor and Chairman, Department of Medicine, UMDNJ–Rutgers Medical School;

Chief of Medical Services, Middlesex General–University Hospital, New Brunswick, New Jersey
*Biology of the Joint; Pathogenesis of Rheumatoid Arthritis; Rheumatoid Arthritis: The Clinical Spectrum*

**Brian L. Hazleman, M.B.**
Associate Lecturer, Faculty of Clinical Medicine, University of Cambridge; Consultant Physician, Department of Rheumatology, Addenbrooke's Hospital, Cambridge, England
*Giant Cell Arteritis and Polymyalgia*

**Peter M. Henson, D.V.M., Ph.D.**
Professor, Department of Pathology and Medicine, University of Colorado School of Medicine; Vice-President for Biomedical Affairs, National Jewish Hospital and Research Center/National Asthma Center, Denver, Colorado
*Cellular Components of Inflammation: Platelets*

**Jerome H. Herman, M.D.**
Professor of Medicine, University of Cincinnati, College of Medicine; Attending Physician, University Hospital and Holmes Division of the University of Cincinnati; Consultant (Immunology/Rheumatology), Veterans Administration Hospital, Cincinnati, Ohio
*Polychondritis*

**Gary S. Hoffman, M.D., F.A.C.P.**
Associate Professor of Clinical Medicine, Columbia University College of Physicians and Surgeons, New York; Attending Physician, The Mary Imogene Bassett Hospital, Cooperstown, New York
*Mycobacterial and Fungal Infections of Bones and Joints*

**Edward W. Holmes, M.D.**
Professor of Medicine, Duke University School of Medicine; Chief, Division of Metabolism, Endocrinology, and Genetics, Duke University Medical Center, Durham, North Carolina
*Antihyperuricemic Drugs*

**David S. Howell, M.D.**
Professor of Medicine, and Director, Arthritis Division, Department of Medicine, University of Miami School of Medicine; Attending Staff, Veterans Administration Medical Center and Jackson Memorial Hospital, Miami, Florida
*Diseases Due to the Deposition of Calcium Pyrophosphate and Hydroxyopatite*

**Gene G. Hunder, M.D.**
Professor of Medicine, Mayo Medical School; Consultant in Rheumatology and Internal Medicine, Mayo Clinic, Rochester, Minnesota
*Examination of the Joints; Giant Cell Arteritis and Polymyalgia; Necrotizing Vasculitis*

**David S. Hungerford, M.D.**
Associate Professor of Orthopaedics, The Johns Hopkins University School of Medicine; Chief, Orthopaedic Surgery, Good Samaritan Hospital, Baltimore, Maryland
*Osteonecrosis*

**Thomas F. Ignaczak, M.D.**
Memphis, Tennessee
*Amyloidosis*

**John N. Insall, M.D.**
Professor of Orthopaedic Surgery, Cornell University Medical College, Ithaca; Attending Orthopaedic Surgeon, Hospital for Special Surgery and New York Hospital; Chief of Knee Service, Hospital for Special Surgery, New York, New York
*Reconstructive Surgery and Rehabilitation of the Knee*

**Israeli A. Jaffe, M.D.**
Professor of Clinical Medicine, Columbia University College of Physicians and Surgeons; Attending Physician, The Presbyterian Hospital, New York, New York
*D-Penicillamine*

**Andrew H. Kang, M.D.**
Professor and Chairman, Department of Medicine, University of Tennessee College of Medicine; Physician-in-Chief, Regional Medical Center of Memphis; Staff Physician, Veterans Administration Medical Center, Memphis, Tennessee
*Structural Proteins: Collagen, Elastin, and Fibronectin; Localized Fibrotic Disorders*

**Allen P. Kaplan, M.D.**
Professor of Medicine and Head, Division of Allergy, Rheumatology, and Clinical Immunology, State University of New York at Stony Brook; Attending Physician, SUNY–Stony Brook Hospital, Veterans Administration Medical Center, Stony Brook, New York
*The Intrinsic Coagulation, Fibrinolytic, and Kinin–Forming Pathways of Man*

**William N. Kelley, M.D.**
John G. Searle Professor and Chairman, Department of Internal Medicine, Professor, Department of Biological Chemistry, University of Michigan Medical Center, Ann Arbor, Michigan
*Purine and Deoxypurine Metabolism; Approach to the Patient with Hyperuricemia; Antihyperuricemic Drugs; Gout and Related Disorders of Purine Metabolism*

**William J. Koopman, M.D.**
Professor of Medicine and Director, Division of Clinical Immunology and Rheumatology, University of Alabama in Birmingham Medical School; Attending Physician, University of Alabama in Birmingham Hospitals, Birmingham, Alabama
*Genetic Control of Immune Responses*

**Brian L. Kotzin, M.D.**
Assistant Professor of Medicine, University of Colorado Health Sciences Center; Chief, Rheumatology Section, Veterans Administration Medical Center, Denver, Colorado
*Immunologic Aspects of Inflammation: Lymphocyte Populations*

**Irving Kushner, M.D.**
Professor of Medicine, Case Western Reserve University; Director, Division of Rheumatology, and Associate Director, Department of Medicine, Cleveland Metropolitan General Hospital, Cleveland, Ohio
*The Acute Phase Reactants*

**P.H. Lambert, M.D.**
Head, World Health Organization/Immunology Research and Training Center, Lausanne and Geneva; Blood Transfusion Center, Hôpital Cantonal Universitaire, Genève Switzerland
*Immune Complexes*

**Robert Langer, Sc.D.**
Dorothy Poitras Associate Professor of Biochemical Engineering, Massachusetts In-

stitute of Technology, Cambridge; Research Associate in Surgery, Children's Hospital, Boston, Massachusetts
*Connective Tissue: Small Blood Vessels and Capillaries*

**E. Carwile LeRoy, M.D.**
Professor of Medicine, Professor of Physical Medicine and Rehabilitation, and Professor of Basic and Clinical Immunology and Microbiology, Medical University of South Carolina; Attending Physician, Medical University Hospital, Veterans Administration Medical Center, St. Francis Hospital, and Charleston Memorial Hospital, Charleston, South Carolina
*Scleroderma (Systemic Sclerosis)*

**Peter H. Levine, M.D.**
Professor of Medicine, University of Massachusetts Medical School; Chief of Medicine, Worcester Memorial Hospital, Worcester, Massachusetts
*Hemophilia and Arthritis*

**Robert W. Lightfoot, Jr., M.D., F.A.C.P.**
Associate Professor of Medicine and Chief, Rheumatology Section, Medical College of Wisconsin; Director, Rheumatology Service, and Senior Attending Physician, Milwaukee County Medical Complex; Director, Veterans Administration Pilot Rheumatology Program, Wood Veterans Administration Medical Center, Milwaukee, Wisconsin
*Cryoglobulinemia and Other Dysproteinemias*

**Stephen J. Lipson, M.D.**
Assistant Professor of Orthopedic Surgery, Harvard Medical School; Orthopedic Surgeon, Brigham and Women's Hospital, Boston, Massachusetts
*Low Back Pain*

**Carlo L. Mainardi, M.D.**
Associate Professor of Medicine and Chief, Rheumatology Division, UMDNJ–Rutgers Medical School, University of Medicine and Dentistry of New Jersey; Physician, Middlesex General–University Hospital, New Brunswick, New Jersey
*Localized Fibrotic Disorders; Hemophilia and Arthritis*

**Stephen E. Malawista, M.D.**
Professor of Medicine, Department of Internal Medicine, and Chief, Section of Rheumatology, Yale University School of Medicine, New Haven, Connecticut
*Lyme Disease*

**Edward A. Mascioli, M.D.**
Clinical Fellow in Medicine, Harvard Medical School; Nutrition Support Service, New England Deaconess Hospital, Boston, Massachusetts
*Nutrition and Rheumatic Diseases*

**John B. McGinty, M.D.**
Clinical Professor of Orthopaedic Surgery, Tufts University School of Medicine, Boston; Chief of Orthopaedic Surgery, Newton-Wellesley Hospital, Newton, Massachusetts
*Arthroscopy*

**James L. McGuire, M.D.**
Assistant Professor of Medicine, University of Massachusetts Medical School, Worcester, Massachusetts
*Arthropathies Associated with Endocrine Disorders*

**Clement J. Michet, M.D., M.P.H.**
Assistant Professor of Medicine, Mayo Medical School, Division of Rheumatology, Department of Internal Medicine, Mayo Clinic, Rochester, Minnesota
*Examination of the Joints*

**Lewis H. Millender, M.D.**
Clinical Professor of Orthopedic Surgery, Tufts University School of Medicine; Assistant Chief, Hand Surgery Service, New England Baptist Hospital, Boston, Massachusetts
*Reconstructive Surgery and Rehabilitation of the Hand*

**G. James Morgan, Jr., M.D., F.A.C.P.**
Assistant Professor of Clinical Medicine, Dartmouth Medical School; Acting Chief, Section of Rheumatology, and Staff Rheumatologist, Mary Hitchcock Memorial Hospital, Hanover, New Hampshire
*Panniculitis and Erythema Nodosum*

**Allen R. Myers, M.D.**
Professor and Acting Chairman, Department of Medicine, Temple University School of Medicine, Philadelphia, Pennsylvania
*Septic Arthritis Caused by Bacteria*

**Kenneth K. Nakano, M.D., M.P.H., S.M., F.R.C.P.(C.), F.A.A.N.A.O.S.-C.**
Former Assistant Professor of Neurology, Harvard Medical School; Neurologist, Straub Clinic and Hospital, Honolulu, Hawaii
*Neck Pain; Entrapment Neuropathies*

**Edward A. Nalebuff, M.D.**
Clinical Professor of Orthopedic Surgery, Tufts University School of Medicine; Chief, Hand Surgery Service, New England Baptist Hospital, Boston, Massachusetts
*Reconstructive Surgery and Rehabilitation of the Hand*

**Thomas C. Namey, M.D., F.A.C.P.**
Associate Professor of Medicine and Radiology and Chief, Division of Rheumatology, Medical College of Ohio; Adjunct Professor, Department of Electrical Engineering, University of Toledo; Attending Physician and Director of Rheumatology Clinics, Medical College of Ohio Hospital, Toledo, Ohio
*Nuclear Medicine and Special Radiologic Imaging and Technique in the Diagnosis of Rheumatic Diseases*

**Carl F. Nathan, M.D.**
Associate Professor, Rockefeller University; Adjunct Associate Professor, Cornell University Medical Center, Ithaca, New York
*Cellular Components of Inflammation: Monocytes and Macrophages*

**Charles S. Neer, II, M.D.**
Professor of Clinical Orthopaedic Surgery, College of Physicians and Surgeons, Columbia University; Attending Orthopaedic Surgeon and Chief of Adult Reconstruction Service, New York Orthopaedic Hospital–Columbia-Presbyterian Medical Center; Chief of Shoulder and Elbow Clinic, New York Orthopaedic Hospital–Columbia-Presbyterian Medical Center, New York, New York
*Reconstructive Surgery and Rehabilitation of the Shoulder*

**Jose L. Ochoa, M.D., D.Sc.**
Professor of Neurology, University of Wisconsin-Madison; Neurologist, University Hospital and Clinics, Madison, Wisconsin
*Peripheral Nerve: Structure, Function, and Dysfunction*

**J. Desmond O'Duffy, M.D.**
Professor of Medicine, Mayo Medical School; Consultant in Medicine, Mayo Clinic; Staff, Methodist Hospital and St. Marys Hospital, Rochester, Minnesota
*Behçet's Disease; Multicentric Reticulohistiocytosis*

**Duncan S. Owen, Jr., M.D.**
Professor of Medicine, Medical College of Virginia, Virginia Commonwealth University; Attending Physician, Medical College of Virginia Hospitals and McGuire Veterans Administration Hospital, Richmond, Virginia
*Aspiration and Injection of Joints and Soft Tissues*

**Thomas D. Palella, M.D.**
Assistant Professor of Internal Medicine, University of Michigan Medical School; Director of Education and Evaluation, Multipurpose Arthritis Center, University Medical Center, Ann Arbor, Michigan
*Purine and Deoxypurine Metabolism*

**Robert S. Pinals, M.D.**
Professor of Medicine and Director, Division of Connective Tissue Diseases, University of Tennessee Center for the Health Sciences; Attending Physician, University of Tennessee Hospital, Veterans Administration Medical Center, Regional Medical Center, and Le Bonheur Childrens Medical Center, Memphis, Tennessee
*Felty's Syndrome*

**Paul H. Plotz, M.D.**
Chief, Connective Tissue Diseases Section, Arthritis and Rheumatism Branch National Institute of Arthritis, Diabetes, Digestive, and Kidney Diseases, National Institutes of Health, Bethesda, Maryland
*Aspirin and Salicylate*

**Robert Poss, M.D.**
Associate Professor, Orthopedic Surgery, Harvard Medical School; Orthopedic Surgeon, Brigham and Women's Hospital, Boston, Massachusetts
*Surgery of the Hip in Rheumatoid Arthritis and Ankylosing Spondylitis*

**Morris Reichcin, M.D.**
Member and Head, Arthritis and Immunology Laboratory, Oklahoma Medical Research Foundation; Professor and Chief, Combined Immunology Section, Department of Medicine, University of Oklahoma Health Sciences Center, Oklahoma City, Oklahoma
*Antinuclear Antibodies*

**Donald Resnick, M.D.**
Professor, University of California, San Diego, School of Medicine; Chief of Radiology, San Diego Veterans Administration Hospital; Staff, University Hospital, San Diego, California
*Radiographic Evaluation of Articular Disorders*

**Donald S. Robinson, M.D.**
Professor of Pharmacology and Medicine and Chairman, Department of Pharmacology, Marshall University School of Medicine; Attending Physician, Veterans Administration Hospital, Cabell-Huntington Hospital and St. Mary's Hospital, Huntington, West Virginia
*Principles of Pharmacodynamics and Pharmacokinetics*

**Dwight R. Robinson, M.D.**
Associate Professor of Medicine, Harvard Medical School; Physician, Massachusetts General Hospital, Boston, Massachusetts
*Low Molecular Weight Mediators of Inflammation: Prostaglandins, Leukotrienes, and Cyclic Nucleotides*

**Naomi Rothfield, M.D.**
Professor of Medicine and Chief, Division of Rheumatic Diseases, University of Connecticut School of Medicine; Attending Physician, University Hospital, Farmington, and Veterans Administration Hospital, Newington, Connecticut
*Clinical Features of Systemic Lupus Erythematosus*

**David W. Rowe, M.D.**
Associate Professor of Pediatrics, University of Connecticut School of Medicine; Attending Pediatrician, John Dempsey Hospital, University of Connecticut Health Center, Farmington, Connecticut
*Heritable Disorders of Connective Tissue*

**Shaun Ruddy, M.D.**
Professor of Medicine, Microbiology and Immunology, and Chairman, Division of Immunology and Connective Tissue Diseases, Medical College of Virginia, Virginia Commonwealth University, Richmond, Virginia
*Process and Principles of Inflammation; Plasma Effectors of Inflammation: Complement; The Management of Rheumatoid Arthritis; Complement Deficiencies and the Rheumatic Diseases*

**Richard I. Rynes, M.D.**
Professor of Medicine, Albany Medical College; Attending Physician, Albany Medical Center Hospital, Albany, New York
*Antimalarials*

**Jeremy Saklatvala, Ph.D.**
Strangeways Laboratory, Cambridge, England
*Proteinases in Joint Disease*

**Alan L. Schiller, M.D.**
Associate Professor of Pathology, Harvard Medical School; Chief, Autopsy, Pathology, and Bone Laboratory, Massachusetts General Hospital; Consultant Pathologist, Brigham and Women's Hospital; Visiting Assistant in Orthopedic Surgery, Children's Hospital Medical Center, Boston, Massachusetts
*Tumors and Tumor-like Lesions Involving Joints*

**Frank R. Schmid, M.D.**
Professor of Medicine and Chief, Section of Arthritis–Connective Tissue Diseases, Northwestern University Medical School; Attending Physician, Northwestern Memorial Hospital; Consultant, Rehabilitation Institute of Chicago, Veterans Administration Lakeside Medical Center, and Children's Memorial Hospital, Chicago, Illinois
*Approach to Monarticular Arthritis*

**Thomas J. Schnitzer, M.D., Ph.D.**
Associate Professor, University of Michigan Medical School; Attending Physician, University Hospital, Ann Arbor, Michigan
*Viral Arthritis*

**H. Ralph Schumacher, Jr., M.D.**
Professor of Medicine, University of Pennsylvania School of Medicine; Director, Rheumatology–Immunology Center, Veterans Administration Medical Center; Staff Rheumatologist, Hospital of the University of Pennsylvania, Philadelphia, Pennsylvania
*Synovial Fluid Analysis; Synovial Biopsy and Pathology; Arthritis Associated with Sickle Cell Disease and Other Hemoglobinopathies*

**Richard D. Scott, M.D.**
Assistant Clinical Professor of Orthopedic Surgery, Harvard Medical School; Surgeon, Brigham and Women's Hospital, New England Baptist Hospital, Children's Hospital Medical Center, Boston, Massachusetts
*The Surgery of Juvenile Rheumatoid Arthritis*

**Jerome M. Seyer, Ph.D.**
Professor of Biochemistry, University of Tennessee Center for the Health Sciences, Memphis, Tennessee
*Structural Proteins: Collagen*

**Jay R. Shapiro, M.D.**
Director, Pratt Diagnostics, Tufts University Medical Center, Boston, Massachusetts; Consultant in Endocrinology, Washington Hospital Center, Seattle, Washington
*Heritable Disorders of Connective Tissue*

**Sheldon R. Simon, M.D.**
Associate Professor of Orthopaedics, Harvard Medical School; Director, Rehabilitation Service, Brigham and Women's Hospital; Associate in Orthopedic Surgery, Brigham and Women's Hospital and Children's Hospital; Director, Gait Analysis Laboratory, Children's Hospital, Boston, Massachusetts
*Biomechanics of Joints*

**Frederick R. Singer, M.D.**
Professor of Medicine and Orthopaedic Surgery, University of Southern California School of Medicine; Associate Program Director, USPHS General Clinical Research Center, Los Angeles County/University of Southern California Medical Center; Director, Endocrine Laboratory, Orthopaedic Hospital/University of Southern California Bone and Connective Laboratories, Los Angeles, California
*Metabolic Bone Disease*

**Clement B. Sledge, M.D.**
John B. and Buckminster Brown Professor of Orthopedic Surgery, Harvard Medical School; Orthopedic Surgeon-in-Chief, Brigham and Women's Hospital, Boston, Massachusetts
*Formation and Resorption of Bone; Introduction to the Surgical Management of Arthritis; The Surgery of Juvenile Rheumatoid Arthritis; Surgery of the Hip in Rheumatoid Arthritis and Ankylosing Spondylitis*

**Hugh A. Smythe, M.D., F.R.C.P.(C.)**
Professor and Director, Division of Rheumatology, University of Toronto; Director, Rheumatic Disease Unit, Wellesley Hospital, Toronto, Ontario, Canada
*"Fibrositis" and Other Diffuse Musculoskeletal Syndromes*

**Nicholas A. Soter, M.D.**
Professor of Dermatology, New York University School of Medicine; Medical Director, Skin and Cancer Unit, and Attending Physician, University Hospital, New York University Medical Center, New York, New York
*Cutaneous Manifestations of Rheumatic Disorders*

**Steven K. Spencer, M.D.**
Associate Professor of Clinical Medicine (Dermatology), Dartmouth Medical School; Staff Physician, Mary Hitchcock Memorial Hospital, Hanover, New Hampshire; Consulting Staff, Veterans Administration Medical Center, White River Junction, and Gifford Memorial Hospital, Randolph, Vermont
*Localized Scleroderma–Morphea*

**Allen C. Steere, M.D.**
Associate Professor of Medicine, Department of Internal Medicine, Yale University School of Medicine, New Haven, Connecticut
*Lyme Disease*

**Alfred D. Steinberg, M.D.**
Chief, Cellular Immunology Section, Arthritis and Rheumatism Branch, NIADDK, National Institutes of Health, Bethesda, Maryland
*Management of Systemic Lupus Erythematosus*

**Gene H. Stollerman, M.D.**
Professor of Medicine, Boston University School of Medicine; Chief, Section of General Medicine, University Hospital, Boston, Massachusetts
*Rheumatic Fever*

**Samuel Strober, M.D.**
Professor of Medicine and Chief, Division of Clinical Immunology, Stanford University School of Medicine, Palo Alto, California
*Immunologic Aspects of Inflammation: Lymphocyte Populations*

**Jerry Tenenbaum, M.D. F.R.C.P. (C.), F.A.C.P.**
Assistant Professor, University of Toronto Faculty of Medicine; Consultant Rheumatologist, Mount Sinai Hospital, Baycrest Geriatric Centre, and Toronto General Hospital, Toronto, Ontario
*Hypertrophic Osteoarthropathy*

**William H. Thomas, M.D.**
Associate Clinical Professor of Orthopedic Surgery, Harvard Medical School; Orthopedic Surgeon, Brigham and Women's Hospital; Consultant Orthopedic Surgeon, New England Baptist Hospital, Boston, Massachusetts
*Reconstructive Surgery and Rehabilitation of the Ankle and Foot*

**Thomas S. Thornhill, M.D.**
Assistant Clinical Professor, Harvard Medical School; Orthopedic Surgeon, Brigham and Women's Hospital and New England Baptist Hospital, Boston, Massachusetts
*The Painful Shoulder*

**Peter D. Utsinger, M.D.**
Professor of Clinical Medicine, Temple University School of Medicine; Chief, Immunology, and Director, Research and Development, Germantown Hospital and Medical Center, Philadelphia, Pennsylvania
*Enteropathic Arthritis*

**Stanley L. Wallace, M.D.**
Professor of Medicine and Director of the Division of Internal Medicine, State University of New York Downstate Medical Center; Attending Physician, Kings County Hospital and State University Hospital; Rheumatology Consultant, Brooklyn Veterans Administration Hospital, Brooklyn, New York
*Colchicine*

**Barbara N.W. Weissman, M.D.**
Associate Professor of Radiology, Harvard Medical School; Director, Bone Radiology Service, Brigham and Women's Hospital, Boston, Massachusetts
*Radiographic Evaluation of Total Joint Replacement*

**Keith Whaley, M.D., Ph.D., F.R.C.P., M.R.C. Path.**
Professor of Immunopathology, Department of Pathology, University of Glasgow; Honorary Consultant in Immunopathology, Western Infirmary, Glasgow, Scotland
*Sjögren's Syndrome*

**Robert J. Winchester, M.D.**
Professor of Medicine, Mount Sinai School of Medicine, City University of New York; Director, Department of Rheumatic Diseases, Hospital for Joint Diseases, Orthopaedic Institute, New York, New York
*The Major Histocompatibility Complex*

**Bruce Wood, D.P.M.**
Associate in Orthopedics (Podiatry), Harvard Medical School; Associate in Orthopedics (Podiatry), Brigham and Women's Hospital; Staff Podiatrist, New England Deaconess Hospital, Boston, Massachusetts
*The Painful Foot*

**Virgil L. Woods, Jr., M.D.**
Assistant Professor of Medicine in Residence, School of Medicine, University of California, San Diego; Physician, University of California Medical Center, San Diego, California
*Etiology and Pathogenesis of Systemic Lupus Erythematosus*

**V. Wright, M.D., F.R.C.P.**
Professor of Rheumatology, University of Leeds Medical School; Consultant Physician in Rheumatology, Leeds Area Health Authority and Yorkshire Regional Health Authority, Harrogate, England
*Psoriatic Arthritis*

**Beth Ziebell, Ph.D.**
Tucson, Arizona
*Psychological and Sexual Health in Rheumatic Disease*

**Thomas M. Zizic, M.D.**
Associate Professor of Medicine, The Johns Hopkins University School of Medicine; Associate Director, NIADDK Multipurpose Arthritis Center, The Johns Hopkins University; Assistant Professor of Medicine, Department of Medicine, University of Maryland; Physician, The Johns Hopkins Hospital and University of Maryland; Associate Director, Rheumatic Disease Unit, The Good Samaritan Hospital; Rheumatology Consultant, Loch Raven Veteran's Administration Hospital and United States Public Health Service Hospital, Baltimore, Maryland
*Osteonecrosis*

**Nathan J. Zvaifler, M.D.**
Professor of Medicine, School of Medicine, University of California, San Diego; Physician, University of California Medical Center, San Diego, California
*Etiology and Pathogenesis of Systemic Lupus Erythematosus*

# Preface

The field of rheumatology continues to show remarkable progress. An impressive transition has occurred from the empiric approach practiced in spas of the nineteenth century to the multidisciplinary specialty of today. Indeed, the discipline spans the monumental advances in immunogenetics and immunoregulation to the modern miracle of total joint replacement. There are many critical elements in this evolutionary process. Pathologists and orthopedic surgeons such as Goldthwaite, Smith-Peterson, and Wilson began their important work early in this century. In the 1930s, internists such as Bauer, Cecil, Hench, Holbrooke, and Pemberton contributed their creative, scientific, and organizational skills to the embryonic discipline. Societies were created to stimulate the exchange of ideas. The explosion of federal funding for research and the resultant expansion of new scientific information began; remarkable progress occurred.

Over the past three decades, consolidation of efforts in diverse disciplines has provided a truly scientific basis for rheumatology. The basic structure and function of immunoglobulins is now clarified, not only at the protein but also at the gene level. Highly sophisticated techniques have allowed the careful study of specific lymphocyte subpopulations and their role in control of the immune response. A multitude of effectors and the target cells that respond to them as part of the inflammatory process have been defined. The genes coding for these effectors are now being cloned, as are the genes for the receptors on the target cells. Such studies will allow not only an improved understanding of their specific structure but may also eventually allow for the production of effectors in pharmacologic quantities. The relevance of the biochemistry of connective tissue, proteolytic enzymes, glycosaminoglycans, and purines to rheumatology has become increasingly apparent. Critical breakthroughs in bioengineering, matched with sophisticated surgical approaches, have made use of metal and polymer prostheses as replacements for destroyed joints a major factor in reduction of morbidity of these diseases. The exciting breakthroughs in molecular biology highlight the possibility that many of the lymphokines will be available for therapeutic purposes at some point in the near future. Finally, we have come to understand the epidemiology, pathogenesis, and in some cases, etiology of certain connective tissue diseases; the outlook for progress is bright.

In the first edition, the editors paid particularly careful attention to the organization and content. The principal goal was to include a complete spectrum of information necessary for the understanding, differential diagnosis, and management of the patient with the rheumatic complaint. This led to the inclusion of chapters in areas not covered by existing reference books in rheumatology such as the scientific basis of rheumatology, a large section on the general approach to the patient, a full evaluation of the diagnostic tests utilized in the evaluation of patients with rheumatic diseases, as well as extensive coverage of rehabilitation and reconstructive surgery as they relate to rheumatology.

The overall organization of the second edition is very similar to the first in terms of the major sections in the Textbook. The first section deals with the scientific basis of rheumatology and includes a detailed consideration of immunology, immunogenetics, the inflammatory process, the structure and function of connective tissue, the physiology of bones and joints, and purine and deoxypurine metabolism. The second section describes the approach to the patient presenting with rheumatic complaints or with a problem possibly related to an underlying rheumatic disease. Although chapters dealing with this subject matter are difficult to write, they are especially useful to the clinician. In the third section, we review the more important diagnostic tests used in the evaluation of the patient with rheumatic complaints. The clinical pharmacology of the drugs used most often in rheumatology is provided in section four. The next seventeen sections deal with specific diseases. The last three sections of the book focus on medical orthopedics, rehabilitation, and reconstructive surgery. In these latter chapters we have chosen to cover not only the current indications for the various surgical procedures but a brief description of the relevant surgical techniques, potential complications, and appropriate postoperative rehabilitation.

The editors continue to be well aware that the quality of a book such as this relates to the quality of the contributions and, hence, the contributors. We also recognize the importance of a regular turnover of contributors for a book such as this to ensure over a period of several editions that even the best chapters will be updated extensively. In the second edition, we strictly follow this deliberate policy of asking new authors to contribute a substantial fraction of the chapters in the book. This allowed us to cover certain areas with a different approach, including immunogenetics, the biology of inflammation, the major histocompatibility complex, the use of cytotoxic agents, and the understanding of immune complex diseases. In addition, we were able to consolidate several areas of cellular physiology to improve the flow of the text. Even in those chapters where new authors were not selected, we were pleased to see a substantial updating and, where possible, on improvement in quality. The editors are highly pleased with the final product.

The expertise of the professionals with whom we worked at W. B. Saunders throughout the preparation of this book continued to be impressive to us. We benefited from the assistance of Mr. Jack Hanley, who as President and Publisher helped us to conceive of the second edition aboard the sloop Windlove off the Maine coast near Damariscove during the summer of 1982. Subsequently we worked closely with Mr. Dereck Jeffers. Further work on the book required several site visits to places such as the "R Lazy S" Dude Ranch in Jackson Hole, Wyoming. Others of considerable help to us included Mr. Robert Butler, Production Supervisor, and Mr. William Donnelly, Designer. Their help was obviously necessary and deeply appreciated. We also wish to express our thanks to our teachers and to our students from whom we have learned as well as to our colleagues at our institutions for their patience and understanding with respect to the time demands that the development of this textbook placed upon us. Finally, we wish to thank our secretaries and editorial assistants, including Candace Johnson, Linda Newman, Ollie May Lee, and Phyllis White, who have been of unmeasurable value.

William N. Kelley, M.D.
Edward D. Harris, Jr., M.D.
Shaun Ruddy, M.D.
Clement B. Sledge, M.D.

# Contents


**Section I**
**SCIENTIFIC BASES OF RHEUMATOLOGY**

Chapter 1
PROCESS AND PRINCIPLES OF INFLAMMATION .......... 1
*Shaun Ruddy*
Introduction .......... 1
The Process of Inflammation .......... 1
Common Themes in the Inflammatory Process .......... 4

Chapter 2
IMMUNOGLOBULINS AND THEIR GENES .......... 5
*Blas Frangione and Joel N. Buxbaum*
Introduction .......... 5
Human Immunoglobulins: Nomenclature and Classification .......... 5
Variable and Constant Regions .......... 7
Immunoglobulin G .......... 8
Immunoglobulin M .......... 9
Immunoglobulin A .......... 10
Immunoglobulin D .......... 11
Immunoglobulin E .......... 11
Genetic Polymorphism or Allotypes .......... 12
Idiotypes and the Combining Site .......... 12
Immunoglobulin Genes .......... 13
B Lymphocyte Differentiation .......... 16
Antibody Diversity .......... 18
Evolutionary Considerations .......... 18
Implications for Disease .......... 19

Chapter 3
IMMUNOLOGIC ASPECTS OF INFLAMMATION: LYMPHOCYTE POPULATIONS .......... 22
*Brian L. Kotzin and Samuel Strober*
Introduction .......... 22
Two Types of Immunity .......... 22
Lymphocyte Migration and Homing .......... 23
T Lymphocytes .......... 25
B Lymphocytes .......... 30
Null Lymphocytes .......... 32
Experimental Methods for Studying Human Lymphocyte Subpopulations .......... 32
Conclusions .......... 33

Chapter 4
THE MAJOR HISTOCOMPATIBILITY COMPLEX .......... 36
*R. J. Winchester*
Introduction .......... 36
Historical Orientation .......... 37
Genetic Principles .......... 38
Nomenclature of Relationships .......... 40
Serologic Analysis of MHC Antigens .......... 40
Determinants Defined by Lymphocyte Responses .......... 42
The IA System .......... 45
Disease Associations .......... 49
Conclusion .......... 53

Chapter 5
GENETIC CONTROL OF IMMUNE RESPONSES .......... 54
*William J. Koopman*
Genes Regulate Immune Responses at Several Levels—An Overview .......... 54
Genes of the Major Histocompatibility Complex .......... 55
Immunoglobulin Genes .......... 61
Conclusions .......... 66

Chapter 6
LOW MOLECULAR WEIGHT MEDIATORS OF INFLAMMATION: PROSTAGLANDINS, LEUKOTRIENES, AND CYCLIC NUCLEOTIDES .......... 71
*Dwight R. Robinson*
Introduction .......... 71
Prostaglandin Biochemistry .......... 71
Metabolism .......... 72
Cyclic Nucleotide Biochemistry .......... 72
Functions of Cyclic Nucleotides .......... 74
Leukotrienes and Other Lipoxygenase Products .......... 74
Functions of Prostaglandins and Leukotrienes .......... 75
Inflammation .......... 76
Anti-Inflammatory Drugs .......... 78
Mechanisms of PG Synthesis Inhibition .......... 79
Prostaglandins and Bone Resorption .......... 80
An Experimental Nutritional Approach to Modification of PG Synthesis .......... 80

Chapter 7
PLASMA PROTEIN EFFECTORS OF INFLAMMATION: COMPLEMENT........ 83
*Shaun Ruddy*
Introduction ................................ 83
Chemistry and Reaction Mechanisms....... 84
The Terminal Sequence...................... 88
Biologic Consequences of Complement Activation ................................ 89
Metabolism of Complement Proteins........ 90
Clinical Significance of Complement Measurements ............................ 90

Chapter 8
THE INTRINSIC COAGULATION, FIBRINOLYTIC, AND KININ-FORMING PATHWAYS OF MAN....................... 95
*Allen P. Kaplan*
Introduction ................................ 95
Hageman Factor............................ 97
Prekallikrein ................................ 101
HMW Kininogen........................... 103
Factor XI.................................... 105
The Role of the Early Steps of the Intrinsic Coagulation Pathway in Fibrinolysis ..... 106
Control Mechanisms....................... 107
Effects of the Hageman Factor Dependent Pathways Upon Other Systems and Their Potential Role in Rheumatic Diseases ................................ 108

Chapter 9
CELLULAR COMPONENTS OF INFLAMMATION: GRANULOCYTES
*Edward J. Goetzl and Ira M. Goldstein*
Introduction ................................ 115
The Origin, Distribution, and Fate of Granulocytes ............................. 116
Cellular Functions of Granulocytes ......... 116
Characteristics of Granulocyte Interactions with Particulate Stimuli .................. 119
Oxidative Metabolism ...................... 124
Granulocytes as Sources of Peptide and Lipid Mediators of Inflammation......... 128
Generation and Release of Chemical Mediators of the Basophil ............... 129
Abnormalities of Neutrophil Function in Human Disease.......................... 130
Abnormal Neutrophil Functions Associated with Rheumatic Diseases................. 131
Other Rheumatic Syndromes and Inflammatory States Associated with Abnormalities of Neutrophil Function.... 133
Specific Chemotactic Factors in Rheumatic Disorders ................................ 135
Special Functions of the Eosinophil and the Spectrum of Hypereosinophilic Diseases.. 135

Chapter 10
CELLULAR COMPONENTS OF INFLAMMATION: MONOCYTES AND MACROPHAGES............................ 144
*Carl F. Nathan and Zanvil A. Cohn*
Introduction ................................ 144
The Life Cycle of Mononuclear Phagocytes 145
The Congregation of Macrophages in Inflammatory Sites ....................... 150
Intake: Endocytosis......................... 152
Output: The Secretions of Macrophages .... 153
Antimicrobial Functions.................... 158
Antitumor Function ........................ 159
Immunoregulatory Functions............... 160
Selective Removal of Autologous Cells ..... 160
Effects of Anti-Inflammatory Drugs on Macrophages ............................. 161
An Overview: Macrophage Activation ...... 162

Chapter 11
CELLULAR COMPONENTS OF INFLAMMATION: PLATELETS
*Peter M. Henson and John L. Gordon*
Introduction ................................ 169
Platelet Biology ............................ 170
Platelet Products with Potential Inflammatory Actions.................... 174
Interaction of Platelets with Components of the Inflammatory System ............. 175
The Inflammatory Process—A Role for Platelets?................................. 179
Summary.................................... 179

Chapter 12
PROTEINASES IN JOINT DISEASE ....... 182
*Alan J. Barrett and Jeremy Saklatvala*
Introduction ................................ 182
The Proteinases of the Joint................ 182
Endogenous Proteinase Inhibitors........... 187
Articular Tissue Damage: The Molecular Processes ................................ 188
Degradative Proteinases in Joint Disease: Their Cellular Origins and Control Processes ................................ 190
Control Processes........................... 192
Conclusions................................. 192

Chapter 13
CONNECTIVE TISSUE: SMALL BLOOD VESSELS AND CAPILLARIES............. 197
*Judah Folkman, Dianna Ausprunk, and Robert Langer*

Introduction ... 197
Embryology ... 197
Maintenance of Normal Vascular Endothelium During Adult Life ... 197
Neovascularization ... 198

Chapter 14
STRUCTURAL PROTEINS: COLLAGEN, ELASTIN, AND FIBRONECTIN ... 211
*Jerome M. Seyer and Andrew H. Kang*
Introduction ... 211
Collagen ... 211
Elastin ... 228
Fibronectin ... 230

Chapter 15
GLYCOSAMINOGLYCANS ... 237
*Kenneth D. Brandt*
Nomenclature ... 237
GAG Composition and Structure ... 237
Linkage of GAGs to Protein ... 240
GAG Biosynthesis ... 243
GAG Degradation ... 244
GAGs In the Genetic Mucopolysaccharidoses ... 245
Physical Properties of GAGs in Relation to their Structure ... 247
Role of Hyaluronate in Skeletal Morphogenesis ... 247
GAGs as Regulators of Cartilage Mineralization ... 248
Binding of GAGs to Lysosomal Enzymes ... 248
Function of GAGs in the Clotting of Blood ... 249
Possible Role of Heparin in Inflammation ... 250
Heparin-Induced Osteoporosis ... 250

Chapter 16
BIOLOGY OF THE JOINT ... 254
*Edward D. Harris, Jr.*
Introduction ... 254
Classification of Joints ... 254
Developmental Biology of the Diarthrodial Joint ... 254
Organization of the Mature Joint ... 257
Organization of Articular Cartilage ... 260
Synovium ... 265

Chapter 17
FORMATION AND RESORPTION OF BONE ... 271
*Clement B. Sledge*
Introduction ... 271
Bone as a Tissue ... 271
Bones as Organs ... 280

Chapter 18
STRUCTURE AND FUNCTION OF THE MOTOR UNIT ... 287
*Walter G. Bradley and Paul F. Good*
Introduction ... 287
Anatomy ... 287
Contractile Proteins ... 287
Excitation-Contraction Coupling ... 292
The Biochemistry of Contraction ... 292
Muscle Energy Metabolism ... 293
The Pharmacology of the Motor Unit ... 294

Chapter 19
PERIPHERAL NERVE: STRUCTURE, FUNCTION, AND DYSFUNCTION ... 295
*John E. Castaldo and Jose Ochoa*
Introduction ... 295
General Organization of the Peripheral Nervous System ... 295
Gross Structure of Nerve Trunks ... 295
Nerve Fiber Populations and Some of Their Selective Disorders ... 297
Axons and Axoplasm ... 297
The Clinical Syndrome of Peripheral Neuropathy ... 303
Neuropathies of Special Interest to Rheumatologists ... 306
Peripheral Neuropathy and Dysimmunoglobulinemia ... 307
Mechanical Injuries of Nerve ... 310
Aging of the Peripheral Nervous System ... 313
Laboratory Investigations ... 313

Chapter 20
BIOMECHANICS OF JOINTS ... 317
*Sheldon R. Simon*
Introduction ... 317
Biomechanics of Normal Joints ... 317
Biomechanics of Joint Degeneration ... 328

Chapter 21
PURINE AND DEOXYPURINE METABOLISM ... 337
*Thomas D. Palella and William N. Kelley*
Biochemistry of Purine Compounds ... 337
Regulation of Purine Metabolism ... 342
Origin of Uric Acid in Man ... 343
Extrarenal Disposition of Uric Acid ... 343
Renal Handling of Uric Acid in Normal Man ... 343

Chapter 22
NUTRITION AND RHEUMATIC DISEASES ... 352
*Edward A. Mascioli and George L. Blackburn*

Introduction ............ 352
Nutrition Assessment and Body Composition ............ 352
Metabolic Response to Inflammation ............ 354
Surveys of Malnutrition ............ 355
Nutritional Requirements ............ 356
Nutritional Therapy Approaches ............ 357
Further Nutritional Considerations ............ 358
Prostaglandins and Dietary Fatty Acids ............ 358
Obesity ............ 359

**Section II**
**GENERAL APPROACH TO THE PATIENT ............ 361**

Chapter 23
GENERAL APPROACH TO THE RHEUMATIC DISEASE PATIENT ............ 361
*James F. Fries*
Introduction ............ 361
What Is Wrong with This Patient? ............ 361
What Investigations, If Any, Are Required? ............ 363
What Are the Goals of Management for This Patient? ............ 364
Over What Time Period Should the Goals Be Achieved? ............ 365
What Therapeutic Strategy Is Most Likely to Achieve the Goals? ............ 365
Does the Patient Understand Enough to Achieve the Goals? ............ 365

Chapter 24
EXAMINATION OF THE JOINTS ............ 369
*Clement J. Michet and Gene G. Hunder*
History in the Patient with Musculoskeletal Disease ............ 369
Classification of the Joints ............ 370
Systemic Method of Examination ............ 371
Examination of Specific Joints ............ 372

Chapter 25
APPROACH TO MONARTICULAR ARTHRITIS ............ 391
*Frank R. Schmid*
General Considerations ............ 391
Initial History and Examination ............ 392
Immediate Laboratory Studies ............ 395
Immediate Management ............ 395
Reassessment ............ 398
The Undiagnosed Monarticular Arthritis ............ 398

Chapter 26
POLYARTICULAR ARTHRITIS ............ 401
*Ronald J. Anderson*
The Differential Diagnosis of Polyarticular Symptoms ............ 401
Multiple Structural Lesions ............ 401
Features of Benign Myalgias ............ 402
The Diagnosis of Synovitis ............ 402
The Differential Diagnosis of Polyarthritis ............ 406
Patterns of Therapeutic Response ............ 408
Systemic Associations with Polyarticular Arthritis ............ 408

Chapter 27
MUSCLE WEAKNESS ............ 410
*Walter G. Bradley*
Introduction ............ 410
History of the Present Illness ............ 411
Systematic Inquiry ............ 411
Past History ............ 411
Family History ............ 412
Examination ............ 412
Summary and Conclusions ............ 415

Chapter 28
NECK PAIN ............ 416
*Kenneth K. Nakano*
Introduction ............ 416
Anatomy and Biomechanics ............ 417
Clinical Evaluation ............ 421
Differential Diagnosis ............ 429
Treatment ............ 434
Summary ............ 435

Chapter 29
THE PAINFUL SHOULDER ............ 435
*Thomas S. Thornhill*
Introduction ............ 435
Diagnostic Aids ............ 435
Periarticular Disorders ............ 439
Glenohumeral Disorders ............ 443
Regional Disorders ............ 445

Chapter 30
LOW BACK PAIN ............ 448
*Stephen J. Lipson*
Incidence and Disability ............ 448
Overall Advances ............ 448
Back Pain and Clinical Evaluation ............ 449
Disease States ............ 458

Chapter 31
THE PAINFUL FOOT ............ 469
*Bruce Wood*

The Normal Foot .......................... 469
Osteoarthritis–Degenerative Joint Disease... 469
Neuropathic Arthropathy–Charcot's Joint .. 471
Rheumatoid Arthritis ...................... 471
Juvenile Rheumatoid Arthritis ............. 480
Summary ................................... 480

Chapter 32
"FIBROSITIS" AND OTHER DIFFUSE MUSCULOSKELETAL SYNDROMES...... 481
*Hugh Smythe*
Introduction .............................. 481
The Point Count ........................... 483
The "Fibrositis" Syndrome ................. 483
Psychogenic Musculoskeletal Pain Syndromes ... 486
Psychogenic Regional Pain or Hysteria ..... 487
Other Soft Tissue Pain Syndromes .......... 487
Problems in Therapy ....................... 487

Chapter 33
APPROACH TO THE PATIENT WITH HYPERURICEMIA ........................ 489
*William N. Kelley*
What is Hyperuricemia and Does the Patient Have It? ........................ 489
Has Tissue or Organ Damage Occurred Owing to the Hyperuricemia? ............ 490
Are Associated Findings Present? .......... 492
What is the Cause of Hyperuricemia? ....... 492
The General Workup ........................ 492
Management of Hyperuricemia ............... 495

Chapter 34
PSYCHOLOGICAL AND SEXUAL HEALTH IN RHEUMATIC DISEASES .... 497
*Barbara Figley Banwell and Beth Ziebell*
Introduction .............................. 497
Features of Rheumatic Diseases That Evoke Psychological Responses ........... 498
Psychological Responses Common to Rheumatic Diseases ...................... 499
Management of Psychological Issues in Rheumatic Diseases ...................... 500
Behavioral Aspects of Pain ................ 501
Sexual Health and Rheumatic Disease ...... 503
Psychosocial Research in Rheumatic Diseases; Methodology and Results ...... 505
Psychological Factors in Juvenile Arthritis . 507
A View to the Future ...................... 508
Conclusion ................................ 509

Chapter 35
OCULAR MANIFESTATIONS OF RHEUMATIC DISEASES .................... 511
*Andrew P. Ferry*
Introduction .............................. 511
Rheumatic Fever ........................... 512
Rheumatoid Arthritis ...................... 512
Juvenile Rheumatoid Arthritis (Still's Disease) ................................ 517
Ankylosing Spondylitis (Marie-Strümpell Disease) ................................ 521
Systemic Lupus Erythematosus .............. 521
Connective Tissue Diseases Other Than Rheumatoid Arthritis and Lupus Erythematosus ........................... 523
Giant Cell Arteritis (Temporal Arteritis, Cranial Arteritis) and Polymyalgia Rheumatica ............................. 524
Wegener's Granulomatosis .................. 526
Relapsing Polychondritis .................. 526
Enteropathic Arthropathy .................. 526
Sarcoidosis ............................... 529
Amyloidosis ............................... 531
Gout ...................................... 531

Chapter 36
CUTANEOUS MANIFESTATIONS OF RHEUMATIC DISORDERS ................ 533
*Nicholas A. Soter*
Introduction .............................. 533
Interpretation of Alterations in the Skin .... 533
Cutaneous Manifestations of Certain Rheumatologic Disorders ................ 534

**Section III**
**DIAGNOSTIC TESTS ...................... 546**

Chapter 37
ASPIRATION AND INJECTION OF JOINTS AND SOFT TISSUES ............... 546
*Duncan S. Owen, Jr.*
Introduction .............................. 546
Mechanism(s) of Action of Intrasynovial Corticosteroids ........................... 546
Potential Sequelae ........................ 547
Precautions ............................... 548
Efficacy of Injections .................... 548
Types of Preparations ..................... 549
Indications ............................... 550
Contraindications to Intra-articular Corticosteroid Injections ................ 553
Anesthesia ................................ 553
Techniques ................................ 554

Chapter 38
SYNOVIAL FLUID ANALYSIS ............ 561
*H. Ralph Schumacher*
Introduction ............ 561
Technique for Arthrocentesis ............ 562
Gross Examination ............ 562
Leukocyte Count ............ 563
Microscopic Studies ............ 564
Special Tests ............ 567

Chapter 39
RADIOGRAPHIC EVALUATION OF ARTICULAR DISORDERS ............ 569
*Robert O. Cone, III, and Donald Resnick*
Introduction ............ 569
Radiographic Techniques and Modalities ............ 569
Rheumatoid Arthritis ............ 570
Juvenile Arthritis ............ 576
The Seronegative Spondyloarthropathies ............ 578
Connective Tissue Diseases ............ 584
Degenerative Joint Disease ............ 587
Neuroarthropathy ............ 594
Crystal-Related Arthropathies ............ 595
Septic Arthritis ............ 600
Miscellaneous Arthropathies ............ 602

Chapter 40
NUCLEAR MEDICINE, AND SPECIAL RADIOLOGIC IMAGING AND TECHNIQUE IN THE DIAGNOSIS OF RHEUMATIC DISEASES ............ 608
*Thomas C. Namey*
Introduction ............ 608
Nuclear Imaging ............ 609
Imaging Methods and Devices ............ 611
Peripheral Joint Scintigraphy in Inflammatory Arthritis ............ 611
Arthrography ............ 624
Ultrasound ............ 629
Thermography ............ 630
Computed Tomography ............ 631
*Donald Resnick, M.D.*

Chapter 41
ARTHROSCOPY ............ 640
*John B. McGinty*
Introduction ............ 640
Technique of Arthroscopy ............ 643
Intra-articular Pathology ............ 645
Accuracy of Arthroscopy ............ 646
Documentation in Arthroscopy ............ 646
Future of Arthroscopy ............ 647

Chapter 42
SYNOVIAL BIOPSY AND PATHOLOGY ............ 648
*H. Ralph Schumacher*
Introduction ............ 648
Methods for Obtaining Synovium ............ 648
Methods of Handling Tissue ............ 649
Findings of Light Microscopic Examination of Synovial Biopsies ............ 650
Conclusions ............ 652

Chapter 43
THE ACUTE PHASE REACTANTS ............ 653
*Irving Kushner*
The Acute Phase Response in Man ............ 653
Erythrocyte Sedimentation Rate ............ 654
C-Reactive Protein ............ 657
Other Acute Phase Reactants ............ 659
Clinical Value of Assessment of Acute Phase Reactants ............ 659

Chapter 44
RHEUMATOID FACTOR ............ 664
*Dennis A. Carson*
Introduction ............ 664
Assay Methods ............ 664
Incidence of Rheumatoid Factor ............ 667
Etiology of Rheumatoid Factor ............ 669
Immunochemical Properties of Rheumatoid Factor ............ 672
Role of Rheumatoid Factor in Rheumatoid Arthritis ............ 673
Summary ............ 676

Chapter 45
IMMUNE COMPLEXES ............ 680
*E. Dayer and P. H. Lambert*
Introduction ............ 680
Generation of Immune Complexes ............ 680
Principles of the Methods for Detection of Immune Complexes in Serum and Synovial Fluid ............ 682
Evaluation of Immune Complex Detection in Rheumatic Disease ............ 686

Chapter 46
ANTINUCLEAR ANTIBODIES ............ 690
*Morris Reichlin*
Introduction ............ 690
History ............ 690
ANA Classification ............ 690
Detection of Antinuclear Antigens ............ 691
Identification of Individual Antigen-Antibody Reactions ............ 694

Specific Autoantibodies Characteristic of Rheumatic Diseases ........ 696
Molecular Specificities of ANA ........ 703
Summary ........ 704

Chapter 47
DIAGNOSTIC TESTS IN NEUROMUSCULAR DISEASES ........ 707
*Walter G. Bradley*
Introduction ........ 707
Screening Tests for Muscle Damage ........ 708
Electrophysiologic Studies of Neuromuscular Function ........ 709
Pathological Studies ........ 712
Summary and Conclusions ........ 715

**SECTION IV**
**CLINICAL PHARMACOLOGY ........ 717**

Chapter 48
PRINCIPLES OF PHARMACODYNAMICS AND PHARMACOKINETICS ........ 717
*Donald S. Robinson*
Factors Influencing Drug Pharmacodynamics and Clinical Effects ........ 717
Effects of Ionization on Drug Behavior ........ 718
Drug Absorption ........ 718
Drug Distribution, Plasma Levels, and Drug Binding Interactions ........ 719
Drug Biotransformation ........ 720
Renal Function and Drug Pharmacokinetics ........ 721
Pharmacokinetics and Drug Dosing Strategies ........ 722

Chapter 49
ASPIRIN AND SALICYLATE ........ 725
*Paul H. Plotz*
Introduction ........ 725
Structure, Absorption, and Metabolism ........ 725
Major Therapeutic Actions ........ 727
The Clinical Use of Aspirin and Salicylates in the Rheumatic Diseases ........ 731
Interactions with Other Drugs ........ 733
Aspirin and Salicylates in Pregnancy ........ 735
Side Effects and Toxicities ........ 735
Conclusion ........ 745

Chapter 50
NONSTEROIDAL ANTI-INFLAMMATORY DRUGS ........ 752
*Alfred Jay Bollet*
Introduction ........ 752
Mechanisms of Action ........ 752
Pharmacokinetics of the Nonsteroidal Anti-Inflammatory Drugs ........ 757
Clinical Effects of Nonsteroidal Anti-Inflammatory Agents ........ 759
Comments About Individual Agents ........ 764
Clinical Usefulness of the Nonsteroidal Anti-Inflammatory Agents ........ 769

Chapter 51
ANTIMALARIALS ........ 774
*Richard I. Rynes*
Historical Perspective ........ 774
Definition and Structure ........ 775
Pharmacokinetics ........ 776
Possible Mechanisms of Therapeutic Action ........ 776
Therapeutic Effectiveness ........ 778
Side Effects and Toxicity ........ 782
Guidelines for Use of Antimalarials ........ 785

Chapter 52
GOLD COMPOUNDS ........ 789
*Norman L. Gottlieb*
History of Gold Treatment ........ 789
Indications and Patient Selection ........ 789
Efficacy ........ 790
Gold Preparations ........ 792
Dosage Schedules ........ 794
Gold Distribution ........ 795
Pharmacokinetics ........ 796
Clinical-Pharmacologic Correlates ........ 798
Mechanisms of Action ........ 798
Precautions, Contraindications and Costs ........ 800
Gold Toxicity ........ 802
Treatment of Gold Toxicity ........ 805
Selection of Gold Compound: Oral or Intramuscular? ........ 805

Chapter 53
D-PENICILLAMINE ........ 809
*Israeli A. Jaffe*
Chemistry ........ 809
Metabolism ........ 809
Clinical Pharmacology ........ 809
Indications ........ 810
Dosage ........ 810
Response Pattern ........ 810
Side Effects and Toxicity ........ 811
Indications, Contraindications, and Precautions ........ 812
Mechanism of Action ........ 813

Chapter 54
GLUCOCORTICOIDS........................ 815
*Lloyd Axelrod*
Introduction ................................ 815
Structure of Commonly Used Glucocorticoids........................... 816
Physiology: The Regulation of Cortisol Secretion................................. 816
Pharmacodynamics .......................... 816
Considerations Prior to the Use of Glucocorticoids as Pharmacologic Agents................................... 819
Effects of Exogenous Glucocorticoids....... 820
Suppression of the Hypothalmic-Pituitary-Adrenal (HPA) System .................. 824
Withdrawal of Patients from Glucocorticoids........................... 825
Alternate-Day Glucocorticoid Therapy ..... 825
Daily Single-Dose Glucocorticoid Therapy . 828
Glucocorticoids or ACTH?................. 828

Chapter 55
CYTOTOXIC AND OTHER IMMUNOREGULATORY AGENTS........ 833
*Anthony S. Fauci*
Introduction ............................... 833
The Immune System and Its Regulation.... 833
Aberrancies of Immune Reactivity .......... 834
Potential Areas of Modification of Immune Responses by Therapeutic Agents ........ 835
Cytotoxic Agents ........................... 836
Theoretical and Practical Considerations in the Use of Cytotoxic Agents for the Treatment of Non-Neoplastic Diseases ... 843
Therapeutic Apheresis ...................... 845
Ionizing Radiation.......................... 846
Total Lymph Node Irradiation............. 847
Antilymphocyte Antibodies ................ 847
Steroid Hormones .......................... 848
Other Agents ............................... 849
Conclusions................................. 853

Chapter 56
ANTIHYPERURICEMIC DRUGS .......... 857
*William N. Kelley and Edward W. Holmes*
Uricosuric Drugs ........................... 857
Xanthine Oxidase Inhibitors................ 861
Other Therapeutic Agents .................. 867

Chapter 57
COLCHICINE................................ 871
*Stanley L. Wallace*
Introduction ................................ 871
Structure-Function Relationships........... 872
Mechanism of Action........................ 873
Colchicine-cAMP ........................... 874
Colchicine Metabolism ...................... 875
Toxicology ................................. 875

**Section V**
**RHEUMATOID ARTHRITIS .............. 879**

Chapter 58
THE ETIOLOGY OF RHEUMATOID ARTHRITIS................................. 879
*J. Claude Bennett*
Introduction ............................... 879
The Link to Genetically Controlled Host Response Factors......................... 880
Immune Complexes and Induction of the Inflammatory Process.................... 880
Organisms Implicated in the Initiation of the Rheumatoid Process ................. 881
Animal Models ............................ 883
Summary.................................. 885

Chapter 59
PATHOGENESIS OF RHEUMATOID ARTHRITIS................................. 886
*Edward D. Harris, Jr.*
Introduction ............................... 886
A Working Scheme for the Pathogenesis of Rheumatoid Arthritis ................... 886
Details of Pathogenesis..................... 888
The Early Lesion in a Rheumatoid Arthritis: Immune Processing and New Blood Vessel Formation................. 889
Acute Inflammation: A Phenomenon in Rheumatoid Synovial Fluid But Not Synovium................................ 890
The Chronic Immunoproliferative Reaction in Synovium............................. 894
The Synovial Cells in Rheumatoid Arthritis 898
The Biochemistry of Tissue Destruction in Rheumatoid Arthritis ................... 901
Pathology of Rheumatoid Arthritis ......... 903

Chapter 60
RHEUMATOID ARTHRITIS: THE CLINICAL SPECTRUM..................... 915
*Edward D. Harris, Jr.*
Introduction ............................... 915
Epidemiology and Diagnosis ............... 916
Early Rheumatoid Arthritis ................ 918
Established Rheumatoid Arthritis: Its Course and Complications ............... 927
Prognosis in Rheumatoid Arthritis.......... 942

Chapter 61
FELTY'S SYNDROME 950
*Robert Pinals*
Introduction 950
Clinical Features 950
Hematologic Features 952
Serologic Features 952
Pathogenesis 952
Splenectomy 954
Other Treatments 954

Chapter 62
SJÖGREN'S SYNDROME 956
*Keith Whaley and Margaret A. Alspaugh*
Introduction: Definition and Historical Aspects 956
Incidence and Prevalence 956
Clinical Features 956
Laboratory Findings 965
Animal Models of Sjögren's Syndrome 972
Treatment 973

Chapter 63
THE MANAGEMENT OF RHEUMATOID ARTHRITIS 979
*Shaun Ruddy*
Introduction 979
Goals of Management 980
Supportive Measures 981
Relief of Pain 985
Anti-Inflammatory Drugs 985
Remission-Inducing Agents 987
Experimental Treatments 989
Surgery 990

**Section VI**
**SPONDYLARTHROPATHIES 993**

Chapter 64
ANKYLOSING SPONDYLITIS 993
*Andrei Calin*
Introduction 993
Diagnostic Criteria 994
Epidemiology 995
Pathology 996
Clinical Features 997
Physical Examination 999
Radiologic Evaluation 999
Laboratory Abnormalities 1002
Ankylosing Spondylitis and Women 1002
Etiology 1003
Prognosis 1004
Management 1004
Summary 1005

Chapter 65
REITER'S SYNDROME 1007
*Andrei Calin*
Introduction 1007
Definition 1007
Historical Review 1008
Etiology 1008
Incidence and Prevalence 1009
Geographic Distribution 1010
Sex Distribution 1010
Age Distribution 1010
Clinical Features 1010
Late Sequelae 1014
Radiologic Evaluation 1015
Laboratory Evaluation 1015
HLA-B27 1015
Pathology 1016
Reiter's Syndrome in Females and Children 1016
Differential Diagnosis 1016
The Relationship of Reiter's Syndrome to Ankylosing Spondylitis 1017
Natural History and Prognosis 1017
Management 1018

Chapter 66
PSORIATIC ARTHRITIS 1021
*V. Wright*
Definition 1021
Prevalence 1021
Etiology 1021
Pathology 1022
Clinical Features 1022
Radiologic Features 1026
Differential Diagnosis 1028
Treatment 1028

Chapter 67
ENTEROPATHIC ARTHRITIS 1031
*Armin E. Good and Peter D. Utsinger*
Introduction 1031
Bacteriology 1031
Immunology 1032
Arthropathy with Inflammatory Bowel Disease 1032
Reactive Arthritis Following Enteric Infection 1036
Bypass Disease 1037
Whipple's Disease 1038

**Section VII**
**SYSTEMIC LUPUS ERYTHEMATOSUS AND OVERLAP SYNDROMES 1042**

Chapter 68
ETIOLOGY AND PATHOGENESIS OF SYSTEMIC LUPUS ERYTHEMATOSUS ... 1042
*Nathan J. Zvaifler and Virgil L. Woods, Jr.*
Etiology of Systemic Lupus Erythematosus 1042
Pathogenesis of Systemic Lupus Erythematosus ... 1052

Chapter 69
CLINICAL FEATURES OF SYSTEMIC LUPUS ERYTHEMATOSUS ... 1070
*Naomi Rothfield*
Introduction ... 1070
Incidence and Prevalence ... 1070
General Systemic Symptoms ... 1071
Cutaneous Lesions ... 1073
Renal Disease ... 1077
Vascular Manifestations ... 1080
Gastrointestinal Manifestations ... 1081
Liver Disease ... 1082
Spleen ... 1082
Lymph Nodes ... 1083
Thymus ... 1083
Ocular Manifestations ... 1083
Parotid Glands ... 1083
Nervous System Manifestations ... 1083
Cardiac Manifestations ... 1087
Pleuropulmonary Manifestations ... 1088
Menstrual Abnormalities and Pregnancy ... 1090
Hematologic Abnormalities ... 1090
Precipitating Factors ... 1091
Diagnosis and Differential Diagnosis ... 1093

Chapter 70
MANAGEMENT OF SYSTEMIC LUPUS ERYTHEMATOSUS ... 1098
*Alfred D. Steinberg*
Introduction ... 1098
Major Organ Involvement Versus Nonmajor Organ Involvement ... 1099
Treatment of Nonmajor Organ Symptoms ... 1100
Measures of Disease Activity and Prognostic Factors—A Guide to Therapy? 1101
Infections ... 1103
Treatment of Major Organ Involvement in SLE ... 1103
Marriage and Pregnancy ... 1107
Use of Specific Drugs in SLE ... 1108
Systemic Lupus Erythematosus in Children 1111
Immunizations ... 1112
Use of Drugs Associated with Injection of SLE-Like Illness in Normals ... 1112
Experimental Forms of Therapy ... 1112
Concluding Remarks ... 1113

Chapter 71
MIXED CONNECTIVE TISSUE DISEASE AND OTHER OVERLAP SYNDROMES ... 1115
*Robert M. Bennett*
Introduction ... 1115
The Overlap Syndromes ... 1116
Mixed Connective Tissue Disease ... 1116
Immunopathology ... 1127
The Antigen for Anti-RNP Antibodies ... 1127
Immunoregulatory Dysfunction ... 1128
Reticuloendothelial Dysfunction ... 1129
Histologic Microvascular Abnormalities ... 1129
Treatment ... 1132

**Section VIII**
**VASCULITIC SYNDROMES ... 1137**

Chapter 72
NECROTIZING VASCULITIS ... 1137
*Doyt L. Conn and Gene G. Hunder*
Introduction ... 1137
Classification ... 1137
Pathogenesis of Vasculitis ... 1139
Polyarteritis ... 1142
Vasculitis Associated with Rheumatic Diseases ... 1148
Hypersensitivity Vasculitis (Leukocytoclastic Vasculitis) ... 1149
Allergic Angiitis and Granulomatosis (Churg-Strauss Vasculitis) ... 1153
Wegener's Granulomatosis ... 1155
Lymphomatoid Granulomatosis ... 1158
Takayasu's Arteritis ... 1159
Kawasaki's Disease (Mucocutaneous Lymph Node Syndrome) ... 1161

Chapter 73
GIANT CELL ARTERITIS AND POLYMYALGIA RHEUMATICA ... 1166
*Gene G. Hunder and Brian L. Hazleman*
Introduction ... 1166
Definitions ... 1166
Epidemiology ... 1166
Etiology and Pathogenesis ... 1167
Pathology ... 1167
Clinical Features ... 1168
Relationship Between Polymyalgia Rheumatica and Giant Cell Arteritis ... 1170
Laboratory Studies ... 1171
Diagnosis ... 1171
Treatment and Course ... 1172

Chapter 74
BEHÇET'S DISEASE ........................ 1174
*J. Desmond O'Duffy*
Introduction ................................ 1174
Diagnostic Criteria.......................... 1174
Clinical Features ........................... 1174
Pathology .................................. 1175
Immunopathogenesis......................... 1176
Treatment .................................. 1176

Chapter 75
PANNICULITIS AND ERYTHEMA NODOSUM................................ 1178
*G. James Morgan, Jr.*
Introduction ................................ 1178
Septal Panniculitis .......................... 1178
Lobular Panniculitis ......................... 1180
Malignancy and Infection .................... 1181

**Section IX**
**CONNECTIVE TISSUE DISEASES CHARACTERIZED BY FIBROSIS ........ 1183**

Chapter 76
SCLERODERMA (SYSTEMIC SCLEROSIS)................................ 1183
*E. Carwile LeRoy*
Introduction ................................ 1183
Definition and Classification ............... 1183
The Clinical Setting......................... 1184
The Early Diagnosis ......................... 1184
Microvascular Abnormalities ................ 1187
Clinical Characteristics ..................... 1190
Scleroderma Variants ........................ 1195
Pathogenesis ................................ 1197
Therapy ..................................... 1198
Summary .................................... 1201

Chapter 77
LOCALIZED SCLERODERMA–MORPHEA ................................ 1206
*Steven K. Spencer*
Definition .................................. 1206
Epidemiology ................................ 1206
Clinical Manifestations ..................... 1206
Histopathology.............................. 1206
Etiology and Pathogenesis................... 1207
Relationship of Morphea to Systemic Sclerosis ................................ 1207
Differential Diagnosis....................... 1208
Management ................................ 1208

Chapter 78
LOCALIZED FIBROTIC DISORDERS..... 1209
*Carlo L. Mainardi and Andrew H. Kang*
Introduction ................................ 1209
Mechanisms of Pathogenesis of Fibrosis .... 1209
Fibroblast Function.......................... 1211
Proteolytic Enzymes in the Fibrotic Process 1215
An Overview ................................ 1216
Fibrotic Pulmonary Disease ................ 1216
Fibrotic Liver Disease ...................... 1218
Dupuytren's Contracture .................... 1218
Keloids...................................... 1219
Retroperitoneal Fibrosis .................... 1219
Other Localized Fibroses ................... 1219

**Section X**
**INFLAMMATORY DISEASES OF MUSCLE .................................... 1225**

Chapter 79
INFLAMMATORY DISEASES OF MUSCLE.................................... 1225
*Walter G. Bradley*
Introduction ................................ 1225
Classification............................... 1225
Incidence of Inflammatory Diseases of Muscle.................................... 1226
Primary Idiopathic Adult Polymyositis ..... 1227
Primary Idiopathic Adult Dermatomyositis 1234
Dermatomyositis-Polymyositis with Neoplasia .................................. 1235
Dermatomyositis-Polymyositis of Childhood ................................. 1236
The Dermatomyositis-Polymyositis Overlap Group .................................... 1236
Other Types of Polymyositis ............... 1238
The Heart and Lungs In Dermatomyositis-Polymyositis............................. 1240
Etiology of Dermatomyositis-Polymyositis.. 1240
Treatment and Prognosis of Dermatomyositis and Polymyositis ...... 1241

**Section XI**
**RHEUMATIC DISEASES OF CHILDHOOD.............................. 1247**

Chapter 80
JUVENILE RHEUMATOID ARTHRITIS.. 1247
*James T. Cassidy*
Introduction ................................ 1247
Historical Review........................... 1247
Epidemiology ............................... 1247

Etiology and Pathogenesis .................. 1247
Clincal Manifestations .................. 1248
Pathology .................. 1254
Laboratory Examinations .................. 1256
Radiologic Examination .................. 1258
Diagnosis .................. 1259
Treatment .................. 1265
Coure of Disease and Prognosis .................. 1269

Chapter 81
RHEUMATIC FEVER .................. 1277
*Gene H. Stollerman*
Definition .................. 1277
Etiology and Pathogenesis .................. 1277
Pathogenesis .................. 1278
Epidemiology .................. 1279
Pathology .................. 1280
Clinical Manifestations .................. 1281
Laboratory Findings .................. 1285
Diagnosis .................. 1286
Course, Prognosis, and Natural History .................. 1287
Treatment and Management .................. 1288
Prevention of Rheumatic Fever .................. 1290

Chapter 82
SYSTEMIC LUPUS ERYTHEMATOSUS, DERMATOMYOSITIS, SCLERODERMA, AND VASCULITIDES IN CHILDHOOD .................. 1293
*Virgil Hanson*
Introduction .................. 1293
Systemic Lupus Erythematosus (SLE) .................. 1293
Dermatomyositis and Polymyositis .................. 1298
Scleroderma .................. 1303
Vasculitis .................. 1306

**Section XII**
**PRIMARY DISORDERS OF IMMUNE FUNCTION .................. 1315**

Chapter 83
IMMUNODEFICIENCY DISEASES .................. 1315
*R. Michael Blaese*
Introduction .................. 1315
Patient Evaluation, History, and Physical Examination .................. 1315
Laboratory Evaluation: Screening Work-Up 1318
Ontogeny and Organization of the Immune System .................. 1319
Specific Immunodeficiency Diseases .................. 1320
Conclusions .................. 1333

Chapter 84
CRYOGLOBULINEMIA AND OTHER DYSPROTEINEMIAS .................. 1337
*Robert W. Lightfoot, Jr.*
Introduction .................. 1337
The Monoclonal Dysproteinemias—Multiple Myeloma .................. 1338
The Monoclonal Dysproteinemias—Waldenström's Macroglobulinemia .................. 1340
The Monoclonal Dysproteinemias—Heavy-Chain Diseases .................. 1341
The Monoclonal Dysproteinemias—Idiopathic Monoclonal Gammopathy .................. 1342
Cryoglobulinemias .................. 1343
Pathogenetic Mechanisms and Symptomatology in Cryoglobulin-Induced Disease .................. 1347
Treatment of the Cryoglobulinemia Syndromes .................. 1349

Chapter 85
COMPLEMENT DEFICIENCIES AND THE RHEUMATIC DISEASES .................. 1351
*Shaun Ruddy*
Introduction .................. 1351
Methods of Measuring Complement .................. 1351
Specific Deficiency States Found with Rheumatic Diseases .................. 1352
Recurrent Neisserial Infections in Deficiency of Membrane Attack Components .................. 1355
Summary and Conclusions .................. 1356

**Section XIII**
**CRYSTAL-INDUCED SYNOVITIS .................. 1359**

Chapter 86
GOUT AND RELATED DISORDERS OF PURINE METABOLISM .................. 1359
*William N. Kelley and Irving H. Fox*
Introduction .................. 1359
History .................. 1359
Epidemiology .................. 1359
Clinical Features .................. 1359
Classification and Pathogenesis of Hyperuricemia and Gout .................. 1371
Genetics of Gout .................. 1378
Acute Gouty Arthritis .................. 1378
Treatment of Gout .................. 1382
Other Related Disorders of Purine Metabolism .................. 1390

Chapter 87
DISEASES DUE TO THE DEPOSITION OF CALCIUM PYROPHOSPHATE AND HYDROXYAPATITE........................ 1398
*David S. Howell*
Clinical Features of Calcium Pyrophosphate Deposition Disease (CPDD)................................. 1398
Pathogenesis................................ 1406
Etiological Considerations.................. 1412
Management of CPDD ..................... 1413
Hydroxyapatite Arthropathy .............. 1413

**Section XIV**
**DEGENERATIVE JOINT DISEASE AND OTHER PRIMARY DISEASES OF CARTILAGE ................................ 1417**

Chapter 88
PATHOGENESIS OF OSTEOARTHRITIS . 1417
*Kenneth D. Brandt*
Normal Articular Cartilage................. 1417
Osteoarthritic Cartilage...................... 1421

Chapter 89
OSTEOARTHRITIS: CLINICAL PATTERNS AND PATHOLOGY........... 1432
*Kenneth D. Brandt*
Introduction ............................... 1432
Clinical Features of Osteoarthritis........... 1433
Primary Osteoarthritis ...................... 1436
Osteoarthritis of Specific Sites.............. 1439
Secondary Osteoarthritis.................... 1441

Chapter 90
MANAGEMENT OF OSTEOARTHRITIS.. 1448
*Kenneth D. Brandt*
The Correct Diagnosis...................... 1448
Components and Goals of the Treatment Program ................................. 1448
Attention to Factors Causing Excessive Joint Loading ........................... 1449
Diet ........................................ 1450
Psychological Coping ....................... 1450
Sexuality ................................... 1451
Physical Therapy............................ 1451
Drug Therapy............................... 1452
Orthopedic Surgery ......................... 1454
Treatment of Osteoarthritis at Specific Sites 1455
Vocational Rehabilitation.................... 1456
Social Security Disability ................... 1456

Chapter 91
POLYCHONDRITIS.......................... 1458
*Jerome H. Herman*
Characterization of Disease................. 1458
Pathology .................................. 1462
Etiologic and Pathophysiologic Considerations............................ 1463
Clinical Course, Prognosis, and Treatment . 1465

**Section XV**
**INFILTRATIVE SYSTEMIC DISEASES... 1469**

Chapter 92
AMYLOIDOSIS ............................. 1469
*Edgar S. Cathcart and Thomas F. Ignaczak*
Introduction ............................... 1469
Amyloid Deposits........................... 1470
Clinical Amyloidosis Syndromes ........... 1474
Amyloid Infiltration of Organ Systems ..... 1477
Diagnosis of Amyloidosis .................. 1481
Treatment of Amyloidosis.................. 1482

Chapter 93
THE RHEUMATIC MANIFESTATIONS OF SARCOIDOSIS........................... 1488
*William J. Arnold*
Introduction ............................... 1488
Clinical Features............................ 1488
Immunology and Biochemistry............. 1488
Rheumatic Manifestations ................. 1490

Chapter 94
ARTHROPATHY WITH IRON STORAGE DISEASE................................... 1494
*Irving H. Fox*
Introduction ............................... 1494
Etiology.................................... 1494
Iron Deposition and Musculoskeletal Disease ................................. 1495
Clinical Features............................ 1496
Laboratory Features ........................ 1498
Diagnosis................................... 1499
Treatment .................................. 1499

Chapter 95
MULTICENTRIC RETICULOHISTIOCYTOSIS ............... 1502
*William W. Ginsburg and J. Desmond O'Duffy*
Introduction ............................... 1502
Clinical Features and Course............... 1502
Laboratory and Roentgenographic Features 1502

Associated Disorders ........................ 1502
Pathology and Etiology..................... 1504
Differential Diagnosis........................ 1504
Treatment.................................. 1504

**Section XVI**
**ARTHRITIS ASSOCIATED WITH RECOGNIZED INFECTIOUS DISEASE... 1507**

Chapter 96
SEPTIC ARTHRITIS CAUSED BY BACTERIA.................................. 1507
*Allen R. Myers*
Introduction ............................... 1507
Predisposing Factors........................ 1507
Pathogenesis of Acute Infectious Arthritis.. 1509
Clinical Features........................... 1512
Diagnostic Studies .......................... 1512
Specific Infectious Agents in Septic Arthritis Caused by Bacteria............. 1515
Disseminated Infection By *N. gonorrhoeae*.. 1516
Management of Acute Infectious Arthritis.. 1519
Special Problems............................ 1522

Chapter 97
MYCOBACTERIAL AND FUNGAL INFECTIONS OF BONES AND JOINTS... 1527
*Gary S. Hoffman*
Introduction ............................... 1527
Tuberculous Skeletal Disease............... 1527
Musculoskeletal Infections Due to Atypical Mycobacteria............................ 1530
Mycotic Infections of Bones and Joints..... 1532
Therapy ................................... 1537

Chapter 98
VIRAL ARTHRITIS......................... 1540
*Thomas J. Schnitzer*
Introduction ............................... 1540
Hepatitis B Virus .......................... 1542
Rubella.................................... 1545
Rubella Vaccine Virus...................... 1546
Alphaviruses ............................... 1547
Mumps..................................... 1548
Enteroviruses: Coxsackievirus and Echovirus................................ 1550
Smallpox and Vaccinia ..................... 1550
Adenovirus................................. 1551
Varicella-Zoster Virus ...................... 1551
Epstein-Barr Virus......................... 1552
Herpes Simplex Virus....................... 1552
Cytomegalovirus............................ 1552
Erythema Infectiosum ...................... 1552

Chapter 99
LYME DISEASE............................ 1557
*Allen C. Steere and Stephen E. Malawista*
Introduction ............................... 1557
Clinical Characteristics ..................... 1557
Laboratory Findings........................ 1559
Epidemiology .............................. 1560
Other Spirochetal Diseases ................. 1561
Differential Diagnosis....................... 1562
Treatment.................................. 1562

**Section XVII**
**ARTHRITIS AS A MANIFESTATION OF OTHER SYSTEMIC DISEASES ........... 1564**

Chapter 100
HEMOPHILIA AND ARTHRITIS.......... 1564
*Carlo L. Mainardi and Peter H. Levine*
Introduction ............................... 1564
Clinical Features........................... 1564
Roentgenographic Features................. 1565
Pathologic Features......................... 1565
Pathogenesis ............................... 1566
Laboratory Diagnosis....................... 1567
Therapy of Hemarthrosis.................... 1567

Chapter 101
ARTHRITIS ASSOCIATED WITH SICKLE CELL DISEASE AND OTHER HEMOGLOBINOPATHIES ................. 1573
*H. Ralph Schumacher, Jr.*
Introduction ............................... 1573
Sickle Cell Disease......................... 1573
Thalassemia................................ 1578

Chapter 102
ARTHROPATHIES ASSOCIATED WITH ENDOCRINE DISORDERS................. 1579
*James L. McGuire*
Introduction ............................... 1579
Diabetes Mellitus ........................... 1580
Hyperparathyroidism ....................... 1581
Hypoparathyroidism........................ 1583
Hyperthyroidism (Graves' Disease) ........ 1585
Hypothyroidism............................ 1587
Cushing's Syndrome ........................ 1587
Acromegaly ................................ 1588
Pregnancy.................................. 1590
Summary................................... 1591

Chapter 103
HYPERTROPHIC OSTEOARTHROPATHY.................... 1594
*Roy D. Altman and Jerry Tenenbaum*
Introduction ................................ 1594
Classification................................ 1594
Clinical Syndromes .......................... 1594
Laboratory Findings.......................... 1598
Radiographs and Radionuclide Scanning ... 1598
Pathology ................................... 1599
Differential Diagnosis........................ 1600
Etiology and Pathogenesis................... 1601
Management ................................. 1601
Course and Prognosis........................ 1601

Chapter 104
MUSCULOSKELETAL SYNDROMES ASSOCIATED WITH MALIGNANCY ..... 1603
*David S. Caldwell*
Introduction ................................ 1603
Direct Associations Between Musculoskeletal Syndromes and Malignancy................................ 1604
Indirect Associations Between Musculoskeletal Syndromes and Malignancy................................ 1605
Pre-Existing Connective Tissue Disease ..... 1609
Malignancy as a Complication of Treatment ................................ 1614

**Section XVIII**
**DISEASES ASSOCIATED WITH ABNORMALITIES OF STRUCTURAL PROTEINS.................................. 1621**

Chapter 105
DISEASES ASSOCIATED WITH ABNORMALITIES OF STRUCTURAL PROTEINS .................................. 1621
*David W. Rowe and Jay R. Shapiro*
Introduction ................................ 1621
Biochemical and Molecular Aspects of Heritable Disorders of Connective Tissue 1621
Clinical Evaluation of Heritable Connective Tissue Disorders.......................... 1624

**Section XIX**
**METABOLIC BONE DISEASE ............ 1645**

Chapter 106
METABOLIC BONE DISEASE............. 1645
*Frederick R. Singer*
Introduction ................................ 1645
Clinical Evaluation .......................... 1645
Primary Hyperparathyroidism.............. 1649
Osteoporosis ................................ 1657
Miscellaneous ............................... 1662
Osteomalacia................................ 1662
Renal Osteodystrophy ...................... 1670
Osteopetrosis................................ 1673
Fibrous Dysplasia........................... 1674
Hereditary Hyperphosphatasia .............. 1675
Paget's Disease of Bone .................... 1676

**Section XX**
**DISORDERS OF BONE OF UNCERTAIN ETIOLOGY.................................. 1689**

Chapter 107
AVASCULAR NECROSIS OF BONE....... 1689
*Thomas M. Zizic and David S. Hungerford*
Introduction ................................ 1689
Epidemiology ............................... 1689
Disease Entities Associated with Development of AVN and Pathogenesis of AVN................................. 1689
Pathogenesis ............................... 1693
Pathology ................................... 1695
Clinical Symptoms and Signs............... 1696
Diagnosis.................................... 1698
Treatment................................... 1704

**Section XXI**
**TUMORS INVOLVING JOINTS........... 1713**

Chapter 108
TUMORS AND TUMOR-LIKE LESIONS INVOLVING JOINTS ....................... 1713
*Alan L. Schiller*
Introduction ................................ 1713
Fatty Lesions of the Synovium............. 1713
Vascular Lesions of Synovium.............. 1713
Intra-Articular Ossicles..................... 1715
Synovial Chondromatosis................... 1716
Intracapsular or Periarticular Chondroma .. 1720
Villonodular Synovitis ...................... 1720
Tenosynovial Sarcoma ...................... 1726
Synovial Sarcoma ........................... 1728
Clear Cell Sarcoma ......................... 1731
Epithelioid Sarcoma ........................ 1732
Secondary Tumors of Synovium and "Pseudotumors".......................... 1733

**Section XXII**
**MEDICAL ORTHOPEDICS ................. 1733**

Chapter 109
RECREATIONAL MUSCULOSKELETAL INJURIES ................................... 1733
*Arthur L. Boland*
Introduction ................................ 1733
General Anatomical Considerations......... 1733
The Shoulder................................ 1734
The Elbow .................................. 1738
The Hip..................................... 1740
The Knee ................................... 1741
Lower Leg Pain.............................. 1748
Ankle Sprains............................... 1749

Chapter 110
ENTRAPMENT NEUROPATHIES.......... 1754
*Kenneth K. Nakano*
Introduction ................................ 1754
Interpretation of Electrodiagnostic Studies.. 1754
Upper Limbs................................. 1754
Lower Limbs................................. 1762
Compartment Syndromes.................... 1767
Conclusion .................................. 1767

**Section XXIII**
**REHABILITATION ......................... 1769**

Chapter 111
REHABILITATION OF PATIENTS WITH RHEUMATIC DISEASES.................... 1769
*Lynn H. Gerber*
Introduction ................................ 1769
Evaluation .................................. 1769
Treatment................................... 1772
Management of Specific Diseases........... 1780
Appendix I: Financial and Vocational Resources for Handicapped Persons...... 1786

**Section XXIV**
**RECONSTRUCTIVE SURGERY ........... 1787**

Chapter 112
INTRODUCTION TO THE SURGICAL MANAGEMENT OF ARTHRITIS.......... 1787
*Clement B. Sledge*
Introduction ................................ 1787
Preoperative Evaluation .................... 1788
Choice of Procedure—Operative Versus Nonoperative Treatment .................. 1790
Postoperative Management .................. 1791
Conclusion .................................. 1791

Chapter 113
SYNOVECTOMY ............................ 1793
*Norbert Gschwend*
Historical ................................... 1793
Theoretical Basis............................ 1793
Indications and Contraindications for Synovectomy ............................ 1793
Contraindications ........................... 1795
Joint Synovectomies on the Lower Extremity................................ 1795
Joint Synovectomies of the Upper Extremity................................ 1798
Results of Joint Synovectomy ............... 1805
Recurrent Synovitis.......................... 1810
Chemical and Radioisotope Synovectomy... 1810
Treatment of Tenosynovitis.................. 1812
Synovectomy in Nonrheumatic Conditions . 1814

Chapter 114
RECONSTRUCTIVE SURGERY AND REHABILITATION OF THE HAND....... 1818
*Edward A. Nalebuff and Lewis H. Millender*
Introduction ................................ 1818
Nonsurgical Treatment ...................... 1818
Preventive and Therapeutic Surgery......... 1819
Reconstructive and Salvage Surgery......... 1824
Osteoarthritis .............................. 1832
Lupus Erythematosus........................ 1833

Chapter 115
RECONSTRUCTIVE SURGERY AND REHABILITATION OF THE ELBOW...... 1838
*Frederick C. Ewald*
Function and Disease........................ 1838
Biomechanics................................ 1838
Arthroplasty ................................ 1839
Surgical Technique.......................... 1849
Team Approach to Postoperative Rehabilitation ........................... 1852
Surgical Indications for Various Procedures 1853

Chapter 116
RECONSTRUCTIVE SURGERY AND REHABILITATION OF THE SHOULDER 1855
*Charles S. Neer II*
How the Shoulder is Unique ................ 1855
Clinical Aspects of the Rheumatoid Shoulder................................... 1856
Conservative Treatment .................... 1861

Indications for Surgery ...................... 1861
Surgical Technique........................... 1865
Result to Be Expected....................... 1868

Chapter 117
RECONSTRUCTIVE SURGERY AND REHABILITATION OF THE KNEE........ 1870
*John N. Insall*
Introduction ................................ 1870
Indications.................................. 1870
Pathology ................................... 1872
Types of Prostheses......................... 1874
Indications for Total Knee Replacement.... 1878
Contraindications to Knee Replacement .... 1878
Surgical Technique.......................... 1880
Management of Instability, Deformity, and Contracture.............................. 1882
Varus Deformity ............................ 1883
Valgus Deformity ........................... 1884
Flexion Contracture ........................ 1884
Complications of Knee Replacement........ 1887
Results of Total Knee Arthroplasty......... 1892
Summary..................................... 1895

Chapter 118
RECONSTRUCTIVE SURGERY AND REHABILITATION OF THE ANKLE AND FOOT ................................. 1896
*William H. Thomas*
Ankle ....................................... 1896
Hindfoot .................................... 1899
Forefoot..................................... 1902
Conclusion .................................. 1909

Chapter 119
THE SURGERY OF JUVENILE RHEUMATOID ARTHRITIS............... 1910
*Richard D. Scott and Clement B. Sledge*
Introduction ................................ 1910
Synovectomy................................. 1911
Epiphysiodesis .............................. 1911
Arthroplasty of the Hip and Knee.......... 1912

Chapter 120
SURGERY OF THE HIP IN RHEUMATOID ARTHRITIS AND ANKYLOSING SPONDYLITIS............. 1916
*Robert Poss and Clement B. Sledge*
Introduction ................................ 1916
Evaluation of the Patient with A Painful Hip ...................................... 1916
Nonsurgical Therapy ....................... 1917
The Rheumatoid Patient as a Candidate for Surgery .................................. 1917
Assessment of Status of Other Joints ....... 1918
Profile of Patients with Rheumatoid Arthritis Undergoing Total Hip Arthroplasty............................. 1918
Previous Surgical Alternatives to Total Hip Replacement.............................. 1918
Biomechanics of the Hip .................... 1919
Total Hip Replacement (Low Friction Arthroplasty)............................. 1921
Complications............................... 1923
Results of Revision Total Hip Replacement 1925
Total Hip Replacement in Ankylosing Spondylitis............................... 1925
Current Surgical Alternatives to Conventional Total Hip Replacement .... 1925
Current State of Surgery of the Hip for Arthritis .................................. 1927

Chapter 121
SURGERY FOR ARTHRITIS OF THE CERVICAL SPINE........................... 1929
*J. William Fielding and A. G. Björkengren*
Introduction ................................ 1929
Ankylosing Spondylitis...................... 1935

Chapter 122
RADIOGRAPHIC EVALUATION OF TOTAL JOINT REPLACEMENT ........... 1938
*Barbara N. W. Weissman*
Introduction ................................ 1938
Total Hip Joint Replacement................ 1938
Total Knee Replacement .................... 1956
Total Shoulder Replacement ................ 1964
Total Elbow Prostheses...................... 1965
Total Ankle Prostheses ..................... 1965
Hand Prostheses ............................ 1968

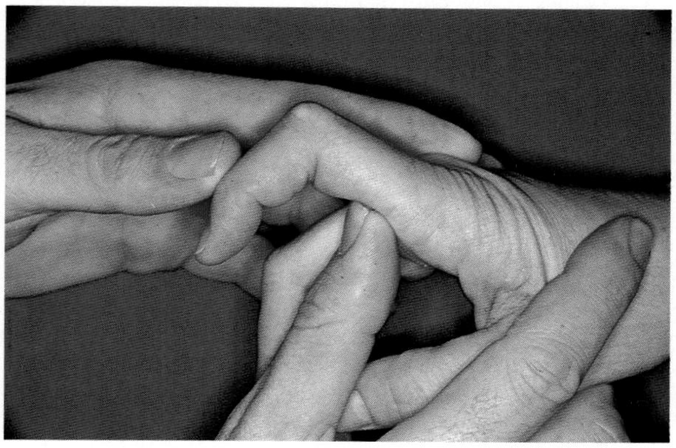

Figure 26–1*A*

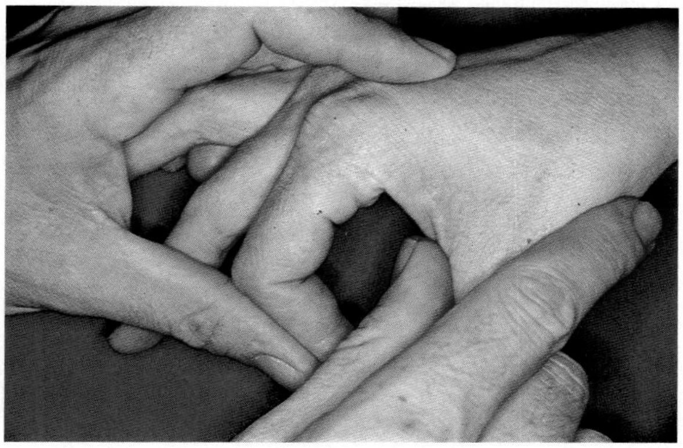

Figure 26–1*B*

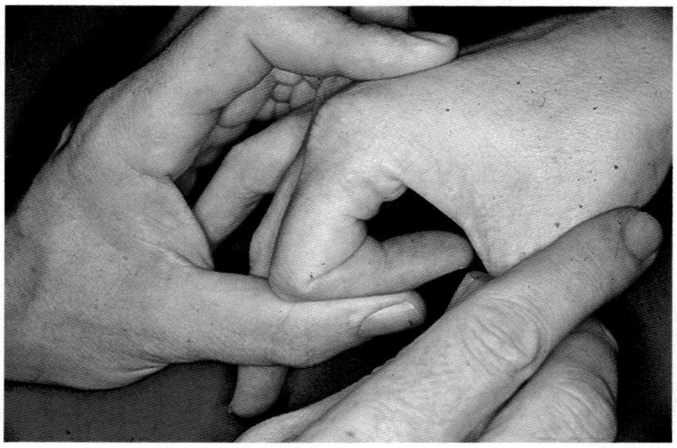

Figure 26–1*C*

**PLATE 1**

**Figure 26–1.** Bunnel's sign. This sign is used to distinguish synovitis of the proximal interphalangeal joint from spasm of the intrinsic muscles due to metacarpophalangeal synovitis as the cause of decreased motion of the proximal interphalangeal joint. *A*, With the metacarpophalangeal joint extended, decreased flexion of the proximal interphalangeal joint is noted. If normal flexion is noted (i.e., the tip of the finger can touch the volar pad), then involvement of all three joints (metacarpophalangeal, proximal interphalangeal, and distal intraphalangeal) is excluded. *B*, With the metacarpophalangeal joint flexed, the contracted intrinsic muscles are relaxed. Restricted motion with the metacarpophalangeals flexed therefore is indicative of proximal interphalangeal involvement. *C*, Normal proximal interphalangeal motion when the metacarpophalangeal joints are flexed indicates that the prior proximal interphalangeal restriction was due to intrinsic muscle contracture, presumably caused by metacarpophalangeal synovitis.

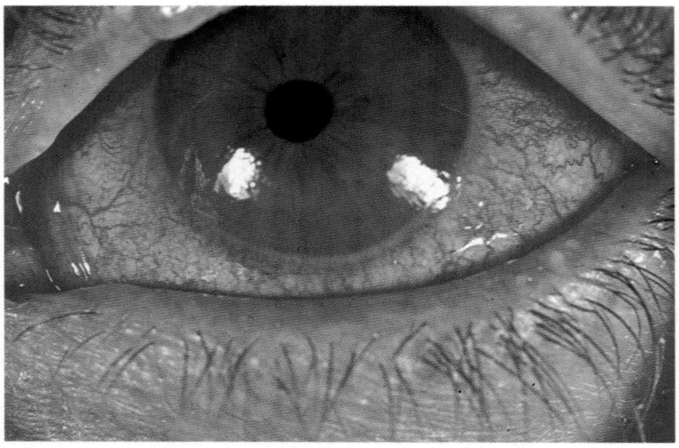

Figure 35–1

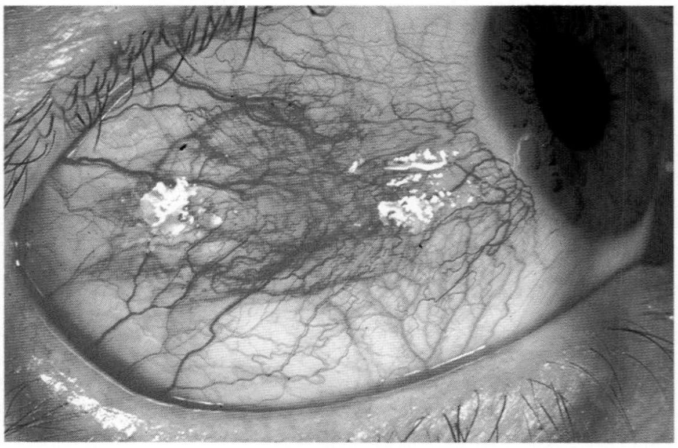

Figure 35–4

**Figure 35–1.** Keratoconjunctivitis sicca. Intense hyperemia of the conjunctival vessels accounts for the prominent redness. Dryness of the corneal epithelium causes the reflection from the photographic flash to be dull and irregular rather than normally sharp and highly polished.

**Figure 35–4.** Severe episcleritis involving the temporal aspect of the right eye in the region of the interpalpebral fissure. Congestion of the episcleral vessels accounts for the bright red appearance.

**Figure 35–5.** Necrotizing scleritis. *B*, Same patient as shown in *A* (p. 516), 2 weeks later. The eye is adducted and slightly elevated. Further destruction of sclera has rendered visible the underlying ciliary body, which has a bluish-gray color.

**Figure 35–15.** Wegener's granulomatosis. Deep ring ulcer in corneal periphery supratemporally in patient with previously undiagnosed Wegener's granulomatosis. Note also the episcleritis adjacent to the corneal lesion. Necrotizing scleritis developed in this area within several weeks after the photograph was made.

**Figure 35–20.** Amyloidosis of the vitreous body. On ophthalmoscopic examination the retina inferonasal to the left optic nerve head is partially obscured by a grayish-white, veil-like, opaque accumulation of amyloid in the vitreous body.

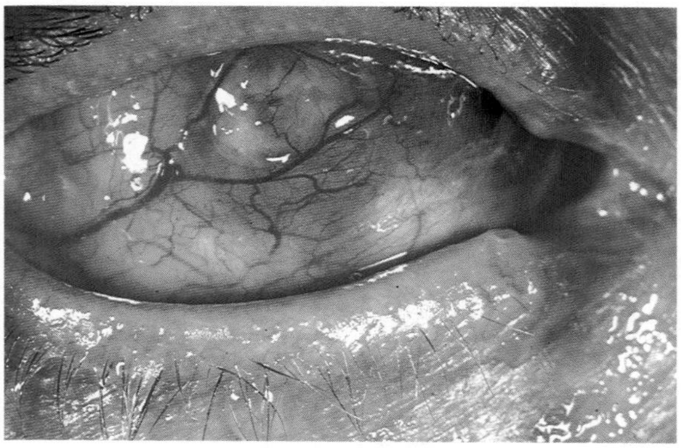

Figure 35–5*B*

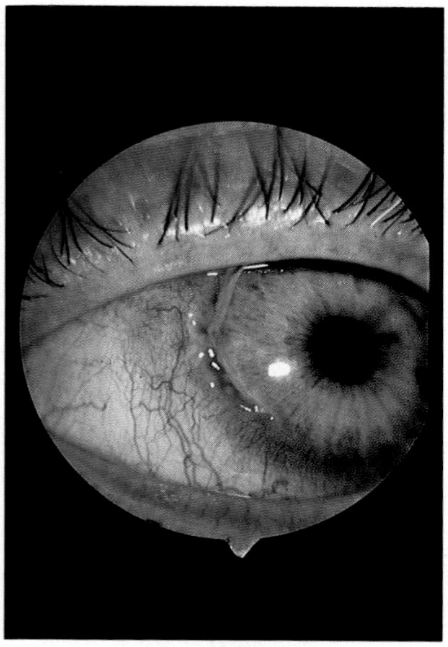

Figure 35–15

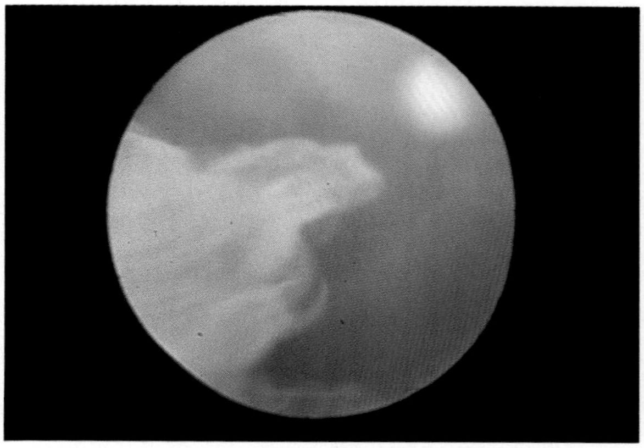

Figure 35–20

PLATE 2

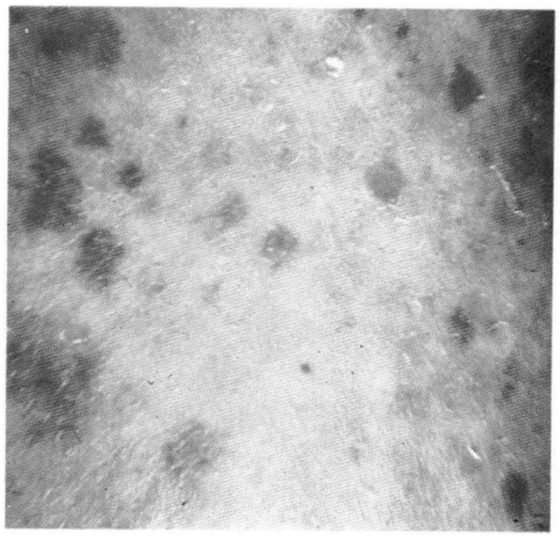

Figure 36–10*B*

Figure 36–11

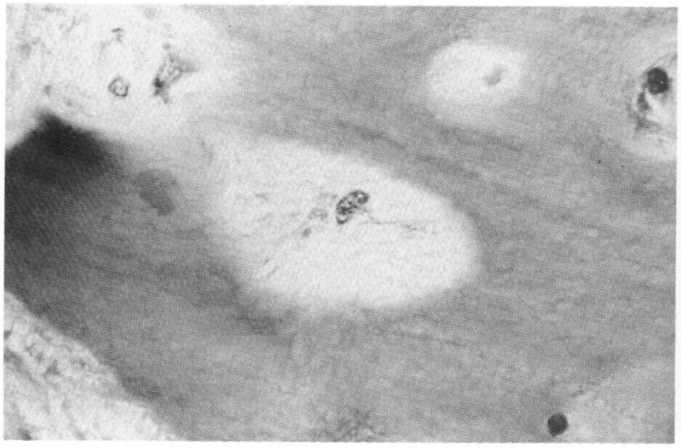

Figure 59–16

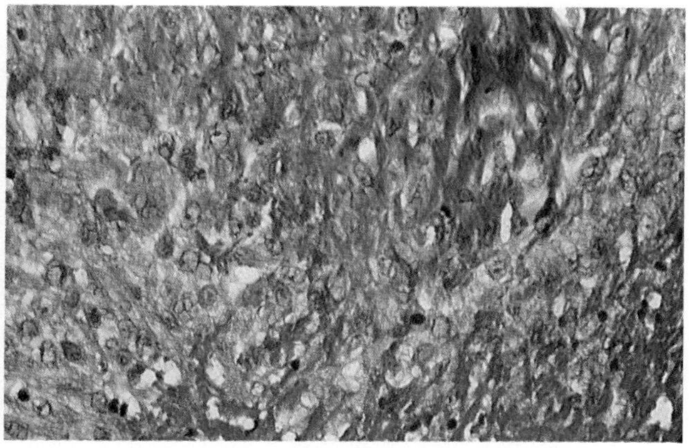

Figure 59–23

**PLATE 3**

**Figure 36–10.** Necrotizing venulitis. *B.* Close-up view of the lesions.

**Figure 36–11.** Necrotizing venulitis. Circumscribed area of edema (urticaria).

**Figure 59–16.** The collagen matrix of cartilage at this pannus/cartilage junction stains darkly. The pale area represents destroyed cartilage in the perimeter around an invasive cell which has many thin cell processes (accentuated by a modification of a trichrome stain), which may be the "in vivo equivalent" of stellate cells seen on cell cultures of dissociated rheumatoid synovial tissue. (Courtesy of Fred Meyer, M.D.)

**Figure 59–23.** Trichrome stain of a micronodule within a larger rheumatoid nodule. Radially arranged strands of collagen separate large histiocytes. The central necrotic area is composed of cellular debris, fibrin, and collagen fragments.

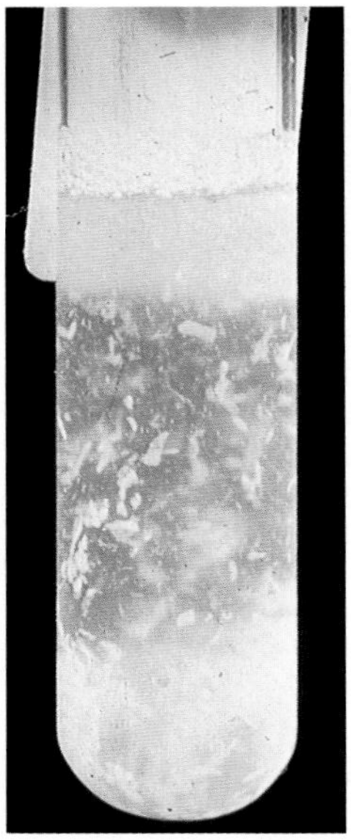

Figure 38–2

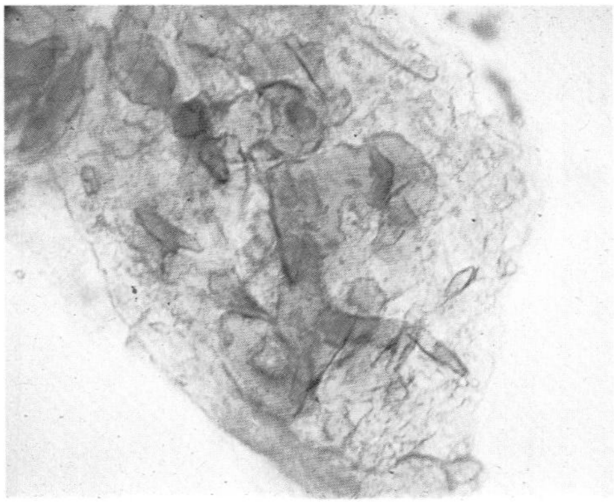

Figure 38–4

Figure 38–2. Synovial fluid rice bodies containing fibrin and debris from degenerated villi are especially common in rheumatoid arthritis but can also be seen in other conditions such as tuberculous arthritis.

Figure 38–4. Shards of golden or ochre cartilage fragments embedded in detached synovium found floating in synovial fluid in a patient with ochronotic arthropathy.

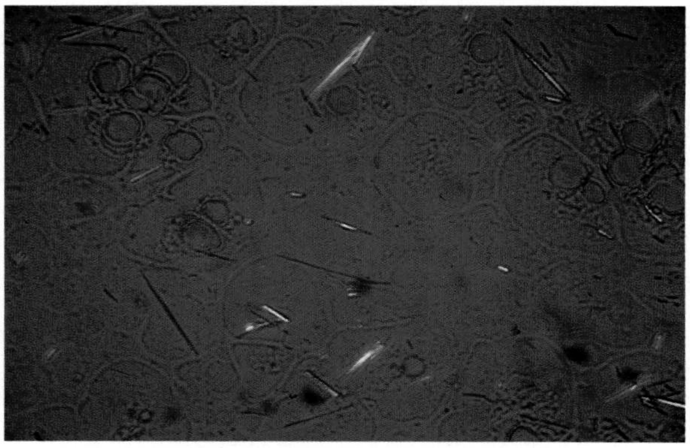

Figure 38–5

Figure 38–5. Monosodium urate crystals from a gouty synovial fluid as viewed with compensated polarized light. The crystals are yellow parallel to the axis of slow vibration marked on the compensator (negative birefringence).

Figure 38–6. CPPD crystals can be needle, rod, or rhomboid shaped but usually have blunt ends (*A*). They often have fainter birefringence than is seen with urates (*B*). CPPD are blue when aligned longitudinally with the axis of slow vibration of the compensator (positive birefringence).

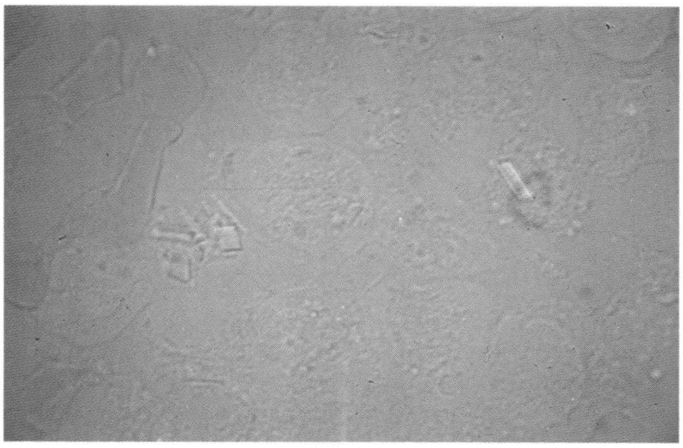

Figure 38–6 A

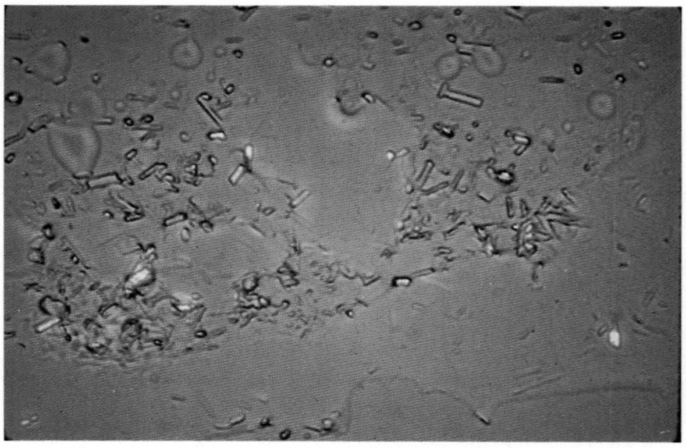

Figure 38–6 B

PLATE 4

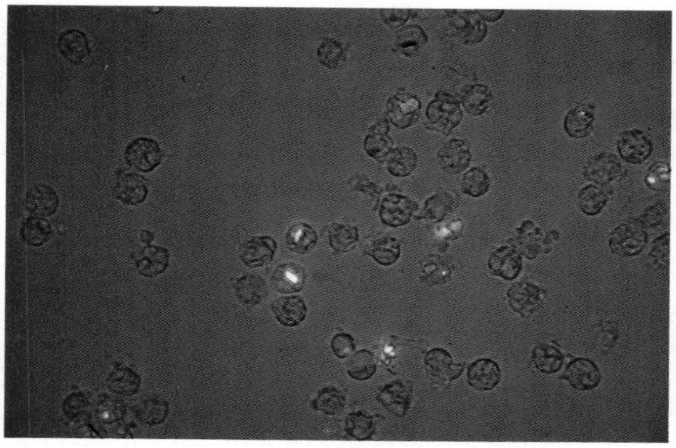

Figure 38–7

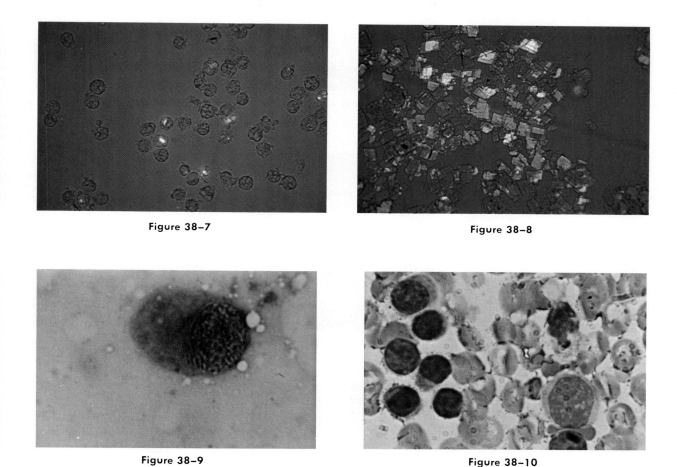

Figure 38–8

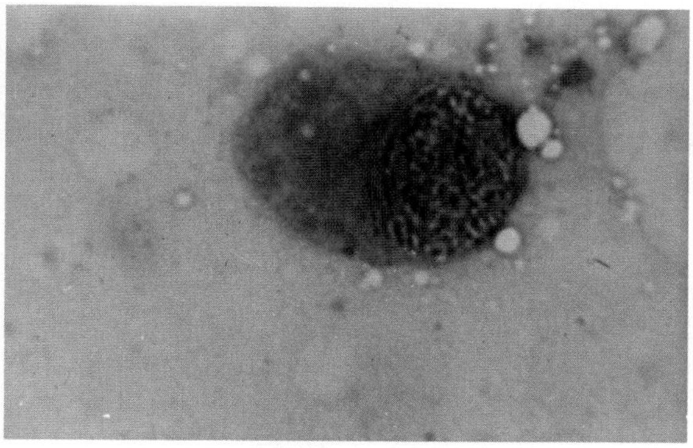

Figure 38–9

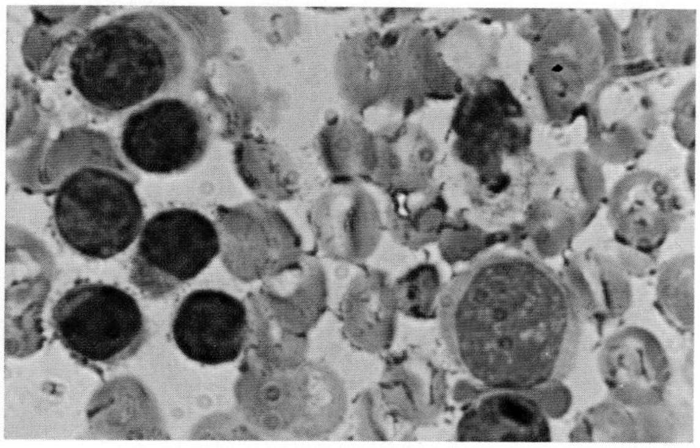

Figure 38–10

PLATE 5

**Figure 38–7.** Triamcinolone acetonide (Aristospan) crystals phagocytized by synovial fluid cells after intra-articular injection.

**Figure 38–8.** Cholesterol crystals from a chronic rheumatoid olecranon bursal effusion. These are most often flat plates with notched corners.

**Figure 38–9.** Synovial lining cell. The prominent homogeneous blue cytoplasm is typical of type B or synthetic cells. Other large cells with nucleus:cytoplasm ratio of less than 50 percent have vacuolated cytoplasm and are either phagocytic lining cells or large monocytes (macrophages).

**Figure 38–10.** Synovial fluid small lymphocytes with one activated lymphocyte, the larger cell with nucleus filling most of the cytoplasm.

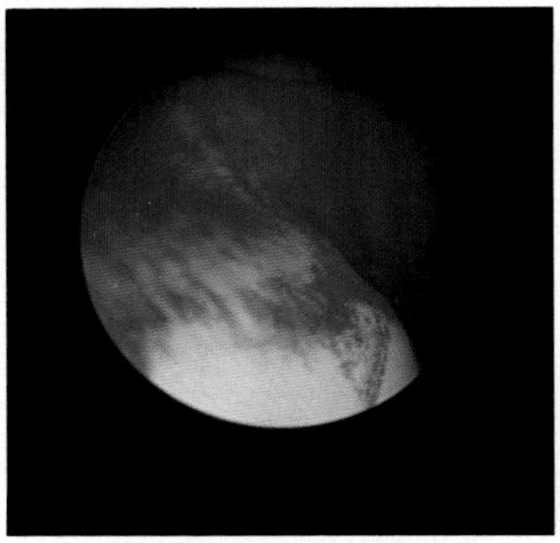

Figure 41–4

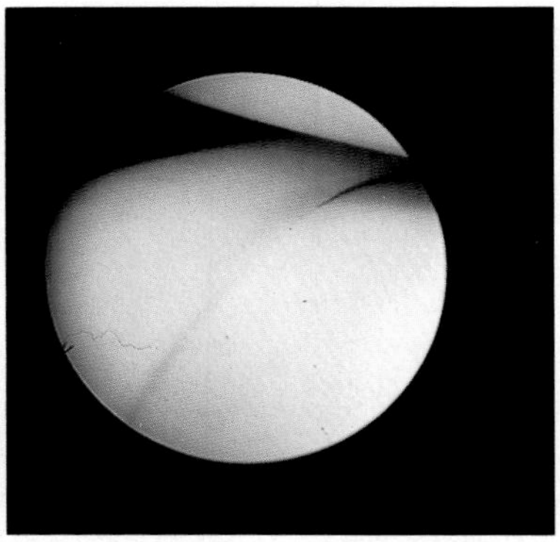

Figure 41–6

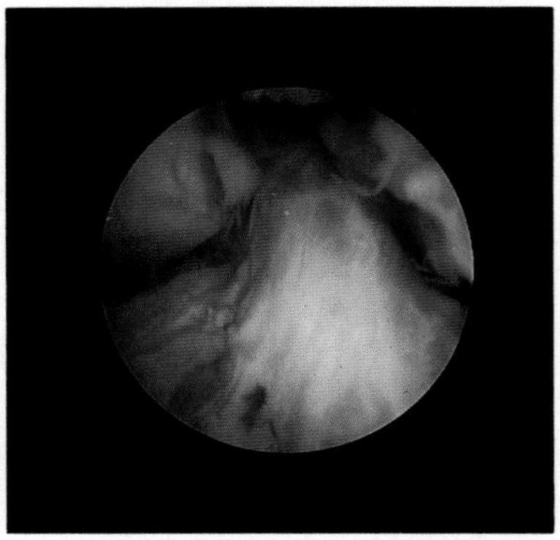

Figure 41–7

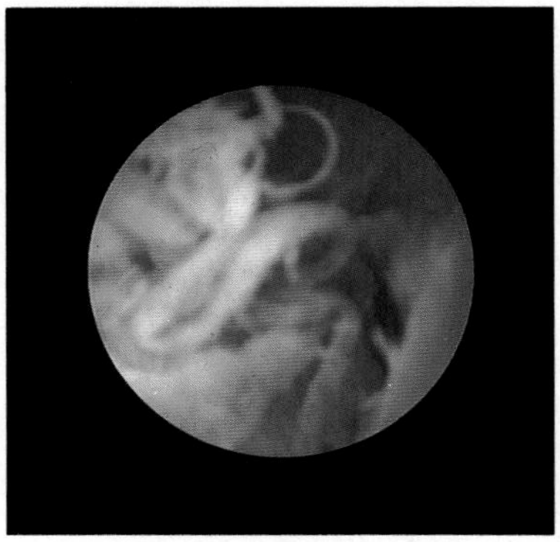

Figure 41–9

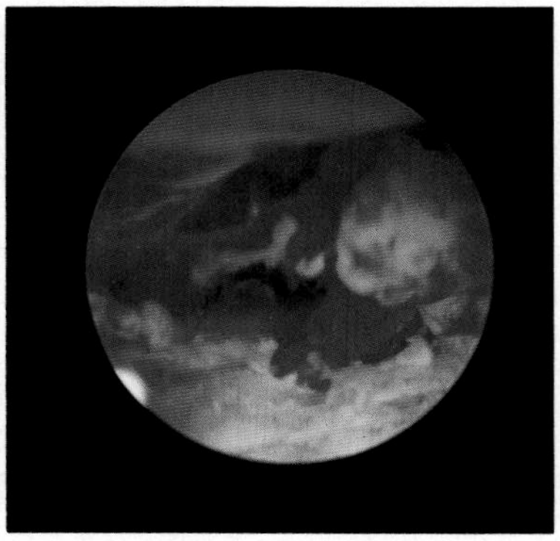

Figure 41–10

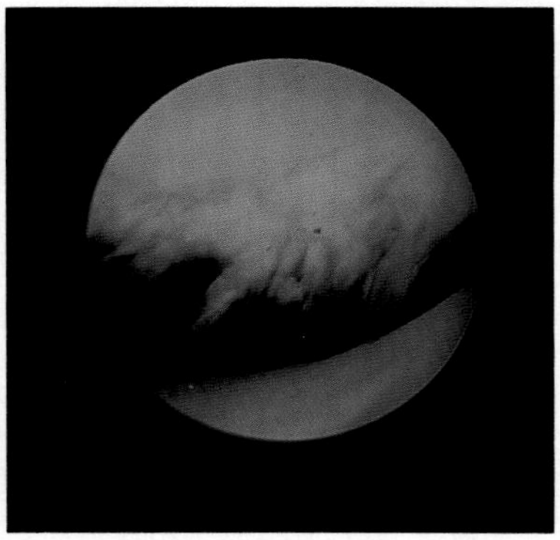

Figure 41–11

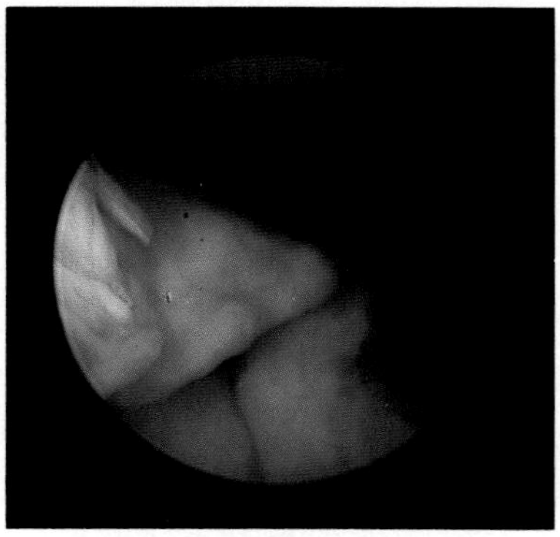

Figure 41–12

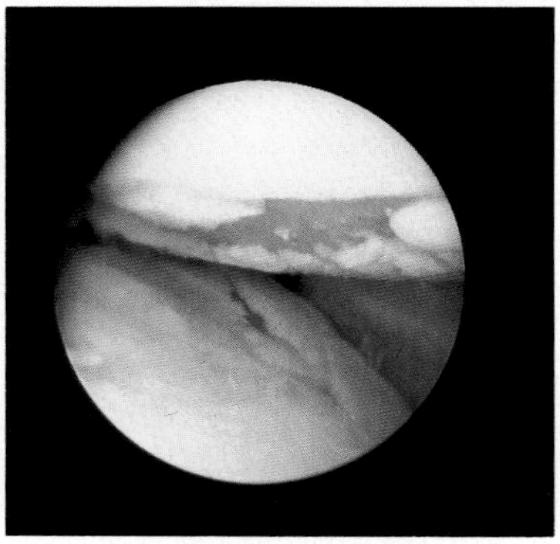

Figure 41–13

**PLATE 6**

**Figure 41–4.** Normal synovium. Note details of vascular pattern.

**Figure 41–6.** Normal medial meniscus, left knee. Femoral condyle above, tibia below.

**Figure 41–7.** Anterior cruciate ligament in intercondylar notch, proximal attachment above.

**Figure 41–9.** Rheumatoid arthritis with proliferative, injected synovial villi.

**Figure 41–10.** Acute pyogenic arthritis with fibrous debris, granular exudate in superior surface of meniscus, and loss of articular cartilage on femur.

**Figure 41–11.** Chondromalacia patellae.

**Figure 41–12.** Bucket handle tear of medial meniscus looking into apex of tear where torn fragment leaves rim.

**Figure 41–13.** Chondromalacia. Medial femoral condyle with exposed subchondral bone. Note changes on tibia. These changes represent a postmeniscectomy degenerative change in the medial compartment.

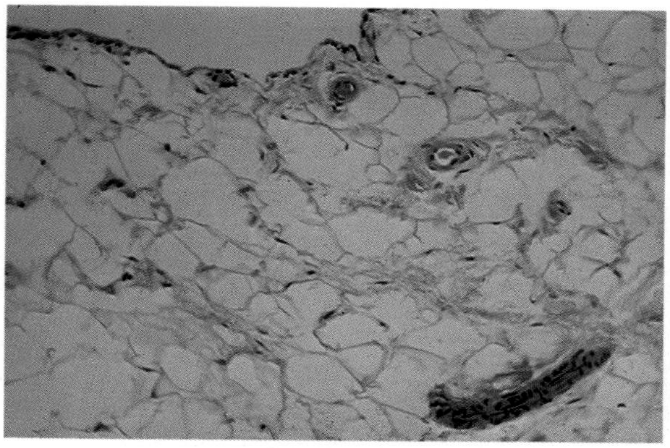

Figure 42–4

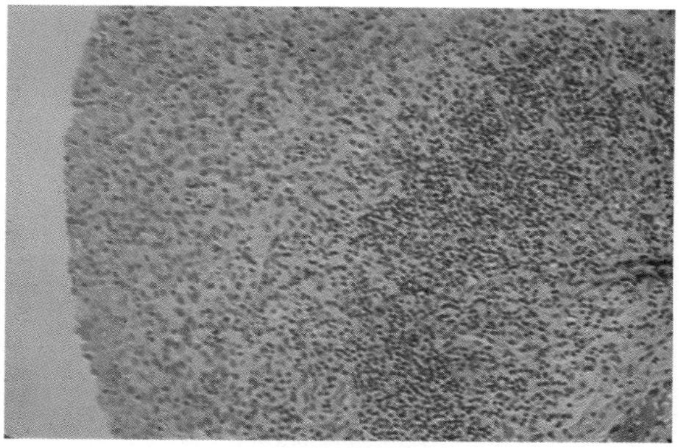

Figure 42–5

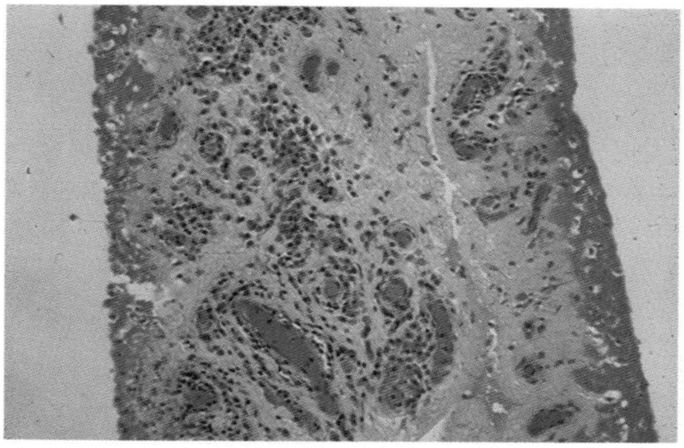

Figure 42–6

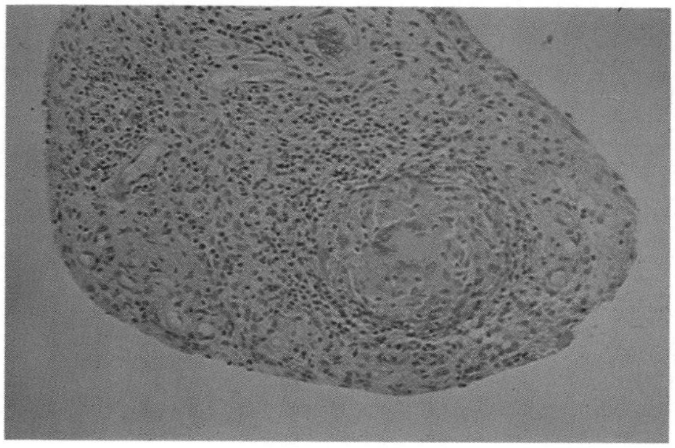

Figure 42–8

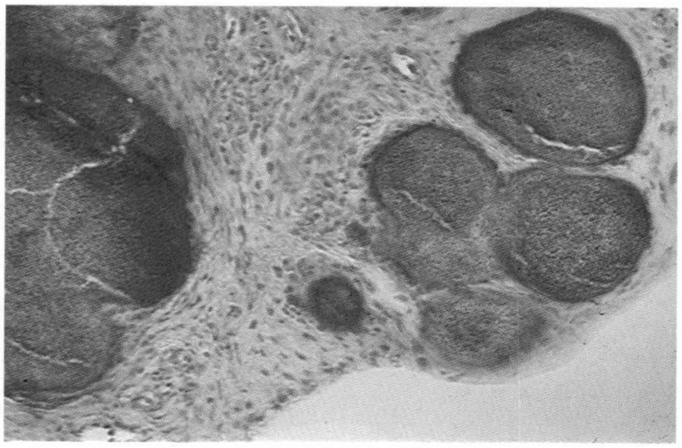

Figure 42–9

PLATE 7

**Figure 42–4.** Normal synovial membrane of the knee. There is a single layer of flattened synovial cells overlying areolar connective tissue. Note the small synovial vessels immediately under the lining layer and the larger vessel in the lower right corner. × 100. Hematoxylin and eosin stain.

**Figure 42–5.** Rheumatoid arthritis synovium showing many layers of synovial lining cells on the left and infiltration of lymphocytes and plasm cells on the right. × 100. Hematoxylin and eosin stain.

**Figure 42–6.** Synovial membrane in early scleroderma shows massive superficial fibrin, loss of lining cells, and infiltration with lymphocytes and plasma cells. × 100. Hematoxylin and eosin stain.

**Figure 42–8.** Granuloma in superficial synovium in tuberculous arthritis. Some superficial granulomas such as this one do not show caseation. There is also scattered chronic inflammatory cell infiltration. × 100. Hematoxylin and eosin stain.

**Figure 42–9.** Tophus-like deposits in synovium containing positively birefringent crystals in pseudogout. × 100. Hematoxylin and eosin stain.

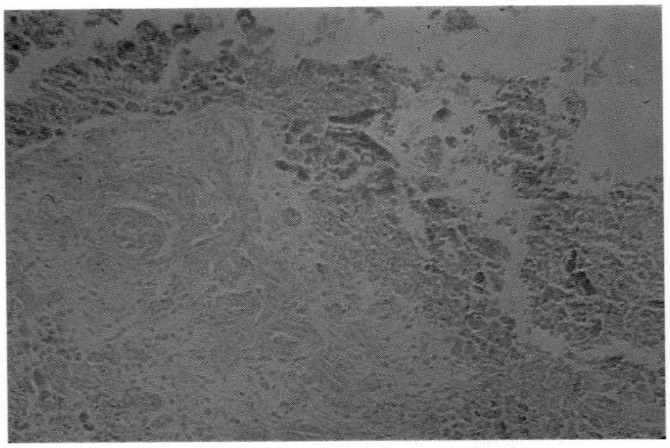

Figure 42–10

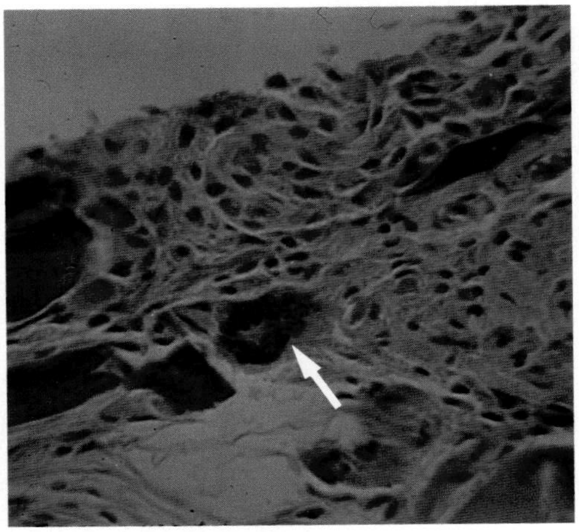

Figure 42–11

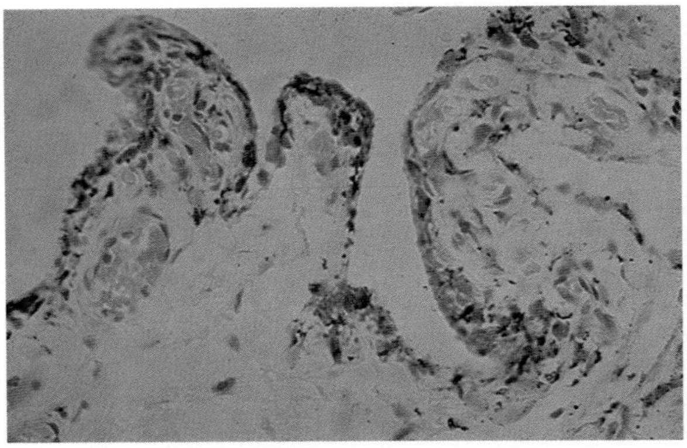

Figure 42–12

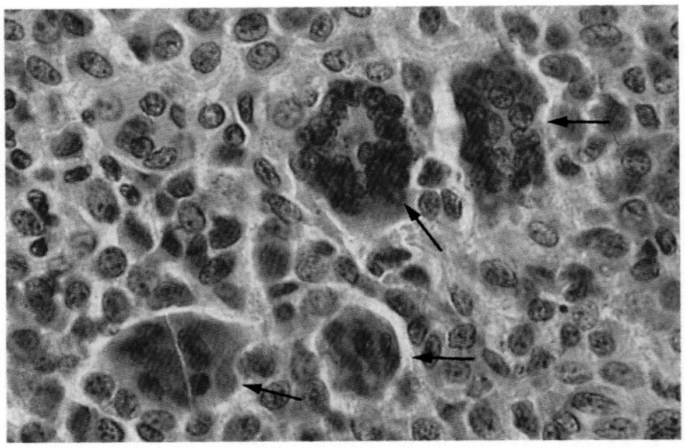

Figure 42–13

## PLATE 8

**Figure 42–10.** Amyloid arthritis as seen here in a patient with multiple myeloma is characterized by Congo red staining on the surface and sparing the synovial vessels (V). $\times$ 100. Congo red stain.

**Figure 42–11.** Dark, angular cartilage shards pigmented brown with homogentisic acid polymer are embedded in ochronotic synovium. Note also a giant cell (arrow) and mild proliferation of synovial lining cells. $\times$ 400. Hematoxylin and eosin stain.

**Figure 42–12.** Iron stain of synovial membrane in idiopathic hemochromatosis shows blue (dark) staining predominantly in the lining cells. $\times$ 100. Prussian blue stain.

**Figure 42–13.** Pigmented villonodular synovitis is characterized by golden brown hemosiderin in deep macrophages, giant cells (marked by arrows), monotonous proliferation of deep cells with pale nuclei, and, not illustrated here, foam cells, lining cell hyperplasia (dark), and villous proliferation. $\times$ 400. Hematoxylin and eosin stain. (Courtesy of Schumacher, H.R.: Sem. Arthritis Rheum. 12:32, 1982.)

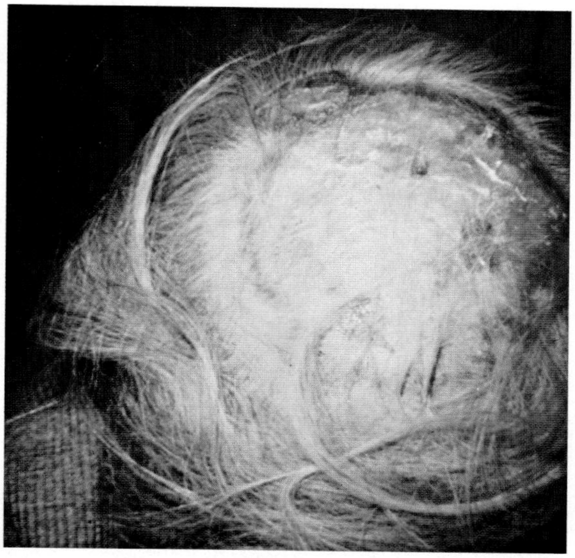

Figure 69–2

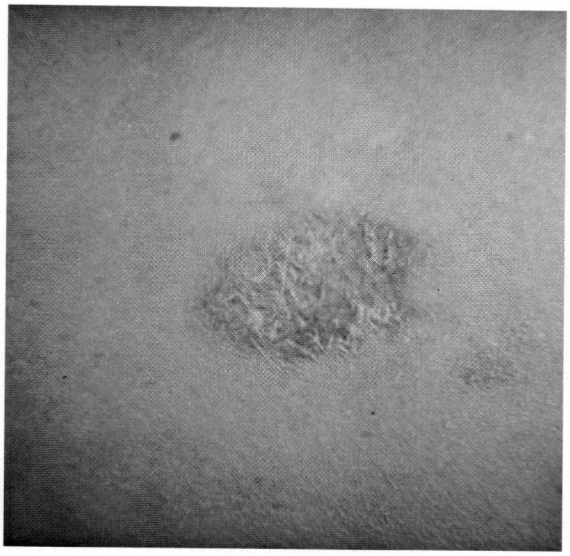

Figure 69–3

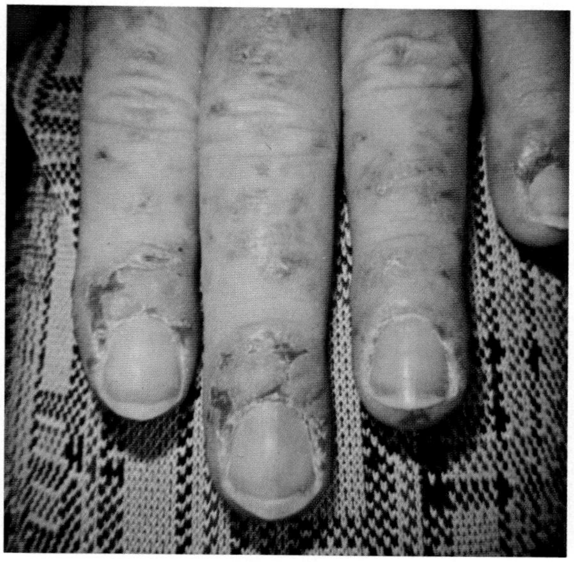

Figure 69–5

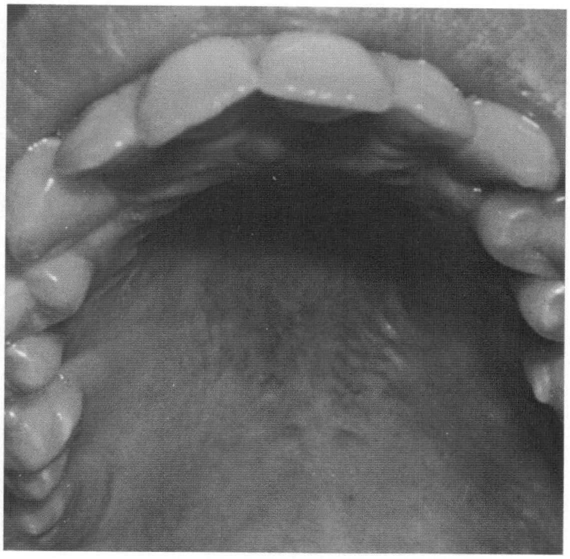

Figure 69–9

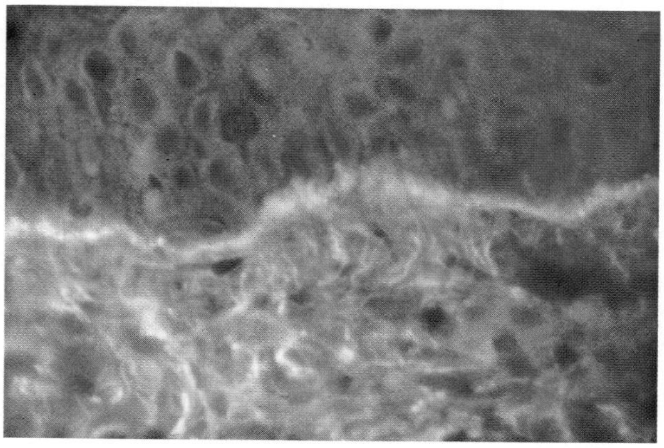

Figure 69–12

**Figure 69–2.** Extensive discoid lesion in the scalp. The lesion is inactive. Note hyperpigmented margins.

**Figure 69–3.** Active hyperkeratotic discoid lesion, which may be confused with hypertrophic psoriasis or lichen planus.

**Figure 69–5.** Vasculitic lesions. Note periungual involvement and vasculitic lesions on tip of the fourth finger.

**Figure 69–9.** Large superficial mucosal ulcer on hard palate.

**Figure 69–12.** Green granules in the dermal-epidermal junction of nonlesional skin from an SLE patient, stained with anti-IgG conjugated to fluorescein isothiocyanate. Dermis (top) has pinkish autofluorescence.

**PLATE 9**

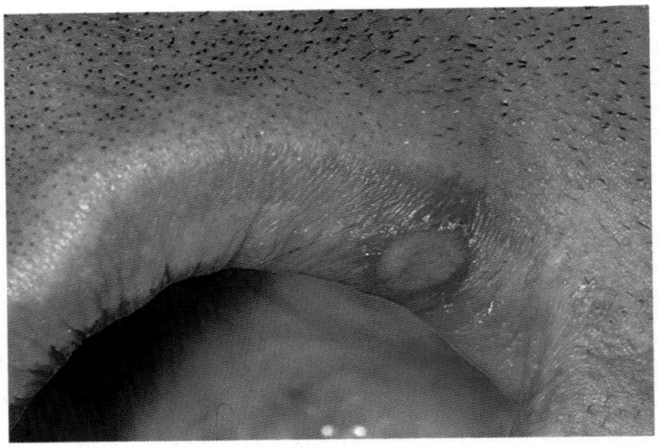

Figure 74–1

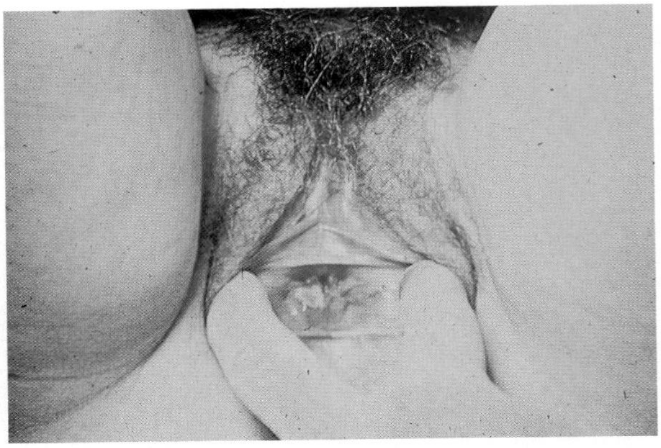

Figure 74–2

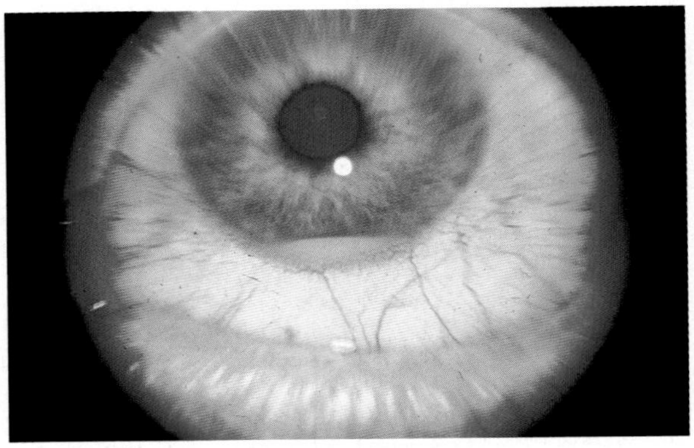

Figure 74–3

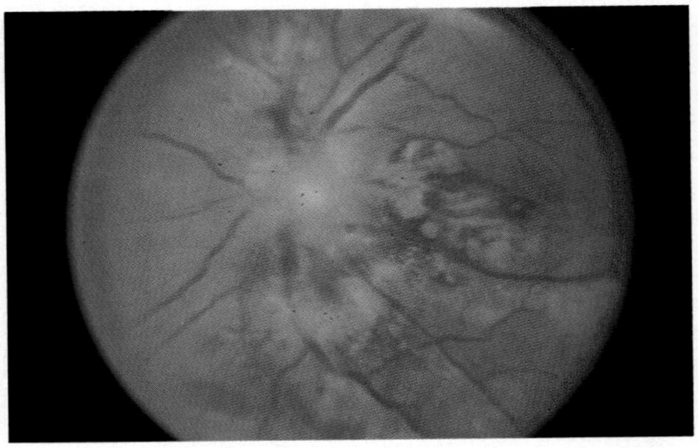

Figure 74–4

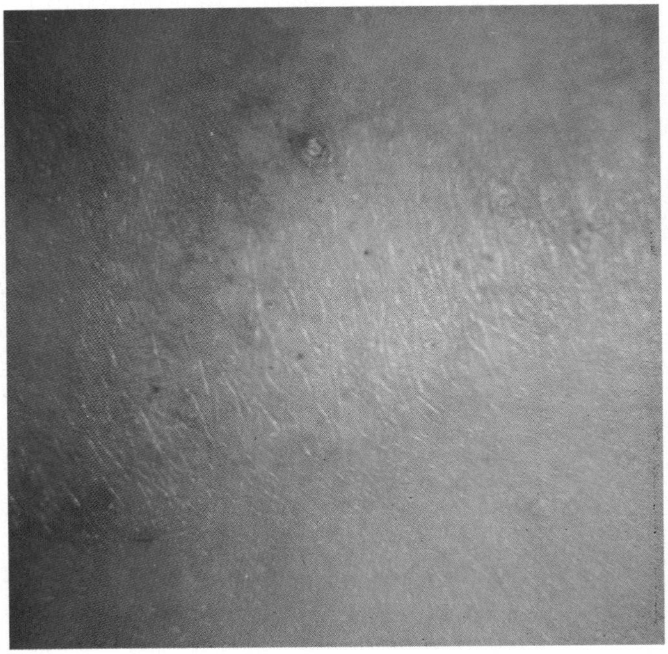

Figure 77–1

**Figure 74–1.** Painful oral aphtha of the upper lip; an erythematous border surrounds a necrotic yellow ulcer. (Photo provided by Dr. R. Rogers III.)

**Figure 74–2.** Vaginal aphthous ulcer. This asymptomatic vaginal ulcer was discovered on routine pelvic examination of a patient presenting with polyarthritis, oral aphthae, and visual symptoms. (From O'Duffy, J.D., et al.: Ann. Intern. Med. 75:561, 1971.)

**Figure 74–3.** Hypopyon, or pus in the anterior chamber, is clearly shown as a yellow segment in front of the iris at 6 o'clock. Previously common in Behçet's disease, anterior uveitis of this severity is now uncommon. (Courtesy of Dr. Dennis Robertson.)

**Figure 74–4.** Ocular fundus demonstrating inflammation of the optic nerve head with retinal infarction and hemorrhage. The medium is cloudy because of vitreous cellular infiltration associated with posterior uveitis. (Courtesy of Dr. M. Colvard.)

**Figure 77–1.** Localized plaque of morphea, showing ivory-colored center with wrinkled surface and surrounding telangiectasia and hyperpigmentation.

**PLATE 10**

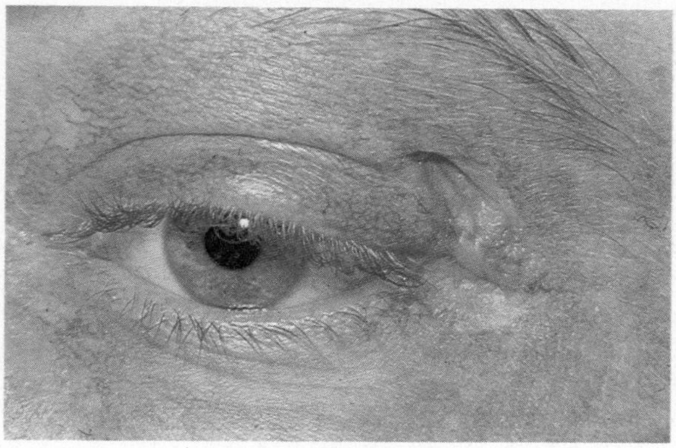

Figure 79–8

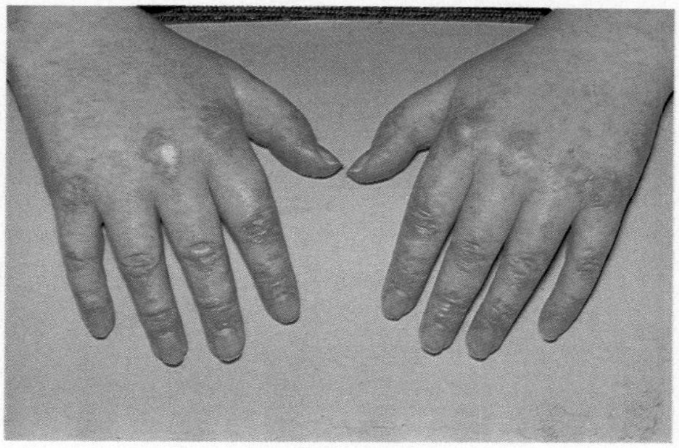

Figure 79–9C

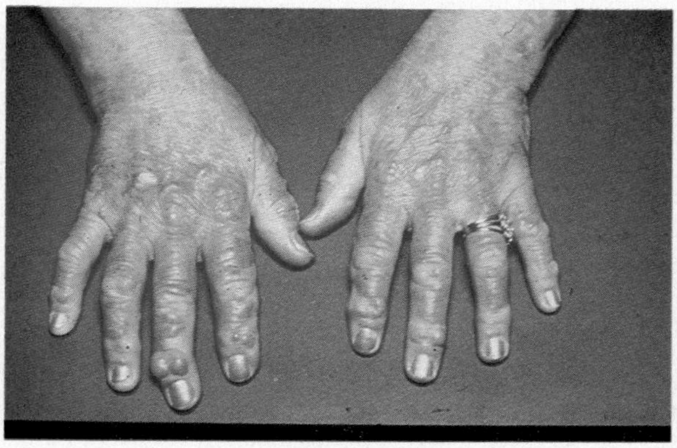

Figure 95–1

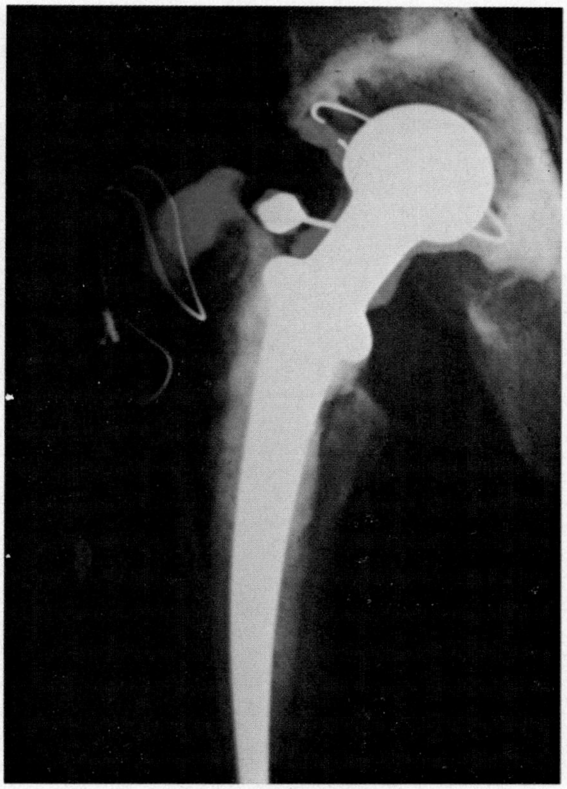

Figure 122–14C

**Figure 79–8.** The eye of the patient in Figure 79–7 (p. 1235) 2½ years after the previous photograph, showing a severe relapse of the skin rash and ulceration of the skin.

**Figure 79–9.** *C,* View of a 15-year-old boy with severe dermatomyositis, showing a very extensive skin rash of the knuckles in the characteristic distribution despite 3 months of treatment with prednisone.

**Figure 95–1.** Reddish-brown nodules on dorsum of hands and around nail folds.

**Figure 122–14.** Subtraction technique. *C,* Color subtraction (different patient from *A* and *B* (p. 1952)). Contrast fills a normal pseudocapsule. Filling of the trochanteric bursa suggests trochanteric bursitis. There is no evidence of component loosening.

PLATE 11

# Section I
# Scientific Bases of Rheumatology

## Chapter 1
# Process and Principles of Inflammation

*Shaun Ruddy*

### INTRODUCTION

Although rheumatologists are occupied with lessening the redness, heat, pain, and swelling of inflammation, the ability of an organism to recognize a foreign or injurious stimulus and to defend against it is essential to survival. As every physician quickly learns, the more aggressive and potent is the pharmacologic attempt to suppress this reaction, the more defenseless is the resulting host. The widespread prescription of nonspecific anti-inflammatory agents substitutes for the use of specific remedies based on knowledge of the proximate or ultimate causes of rheumatic diseases. The availability of antimicrobials significantly diminished the fervor with which antipyretics were administered to patients with pneumonia. As knowledge about the etiologies of the rheumatic diseases increases and specific treatments directed at the causes are developed, the use of nonspecific anti-inflammatory agents will also wane.

Different kinds of inflammation and repair produce widely disparate manifestations. Time courses range from the few hours required for the development of florid acute gouty or septic arthritis to the many years involved in the chronic progressive fibrosis of scleroderma. Distribution in space may range from the single distal interphalangeal joint involved in psoriatic arthritis to the life-threatening multisystem involvement with which systemic lupus erythematosus may present. While it might be argued that such variations and complexities preclude any useful summary of inflammation, the process may be subjected to systematic analysis. This chapter will provide that analysis, a framework within which to place the detailed descriptions of the components of inflammation contained in the next 20 chapters.

### THE PROCESS OF INFLAMMATION

The components of the inflammatory process are diagrammed in Figure 1–1. These include the *selectors,* which serve to locate the abnormal area of injury or invasion, and the *detectors,* which transduce the signal from a selector to one or more *delivery* vehicles. *Effector* systems delivered to the selected area catalyze reactions that are almost exclusively hydrolytic in nature—the addition of a water molecule to a covalent bond such as the peptide of a protein (Fig. 1–2), the ester of a lipid (Fig. 1–3), or glycoside of a polysaccharide (Fig. 1–4).[1] Though not central to the process of inflammation, inhibiting or *controlling* factors that retard the rate and extent of the process[2] are of sufficient importance to warrant being shown in Figure 1–1. Similarly, the *resynthesis* phase, in which the hydrolyzed materials are replaced either appropriately (repair) or inappropriately (fibrosis), is not integral to inflammation but an important consequence. Since the final effectors are chiefly enzymes that catalyze hydrolytic reactions, an energy source for the process is also required. Normal body heat, which is often increased locally in the area of inflammation due to increased rate of blood flow, is one energy source. Mechanical pressure in tissues, also increased because of loss of vascular integrity with flow of water, proteins, and other solutes into the extravascular space in the area of tissue inflammation, is another potential source. Finally, nutrients and oxygen, normally used by cells that localize to the inflamed area, are most important. Inflammatory cells require energy for locomotion, phagocytosis, and synthesis of reactive metabolites.[3] In some instances, especially in body cavities not adequately supplied with blood vessels, evidence of anaerobiosis, such as increased lactate and reduced pH, or evidence of nutrient depletion, such as low glucose levels, may be found.[4]

**Selectors.** These elements specify the area in which the inflammation will occur. Some examples are listed in Table 1–1. While the most obviously specific are antibody, or the antibody-like antigen-binding sites on the surface of T lymphocytes (see Chapters 2 and 3), a number of nonimmunologic elements may select the area of inflammation. Contact of the plasma protein Hageman factor with negatively charged surfaces initiates the

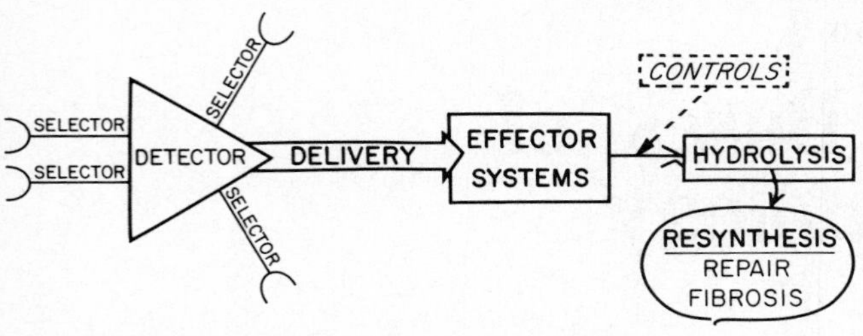

**Figure 1–1.** The inflammatory process.

kinin-forming, coagulation, and fibrinolytic cascades (see Chapter 8). Recognition by the alternative pathway for complement activation of bacterial polysaccharides or other foreign materials involves assembly of the complement enzymes on the activating surface so that they are protected from dissociation by the control protein, Factor H (see Chapter 7). Mechanical or ischemic damage may specify the locale for inflammation by releasing materials from cells resident in the damaged area. Degranulation of tissue mast cells with release of low molecular weight mediators into the surrounding area is responsible for the wheal and flare that follows stroking of the skin. Intracellular proteases liberated following ischemic death of myocardial cells are capable of acting on plasma substrates, e.g., the fifth complement component, to form chemotactic factors.[5] Although inflammation may occur in a totally denervated extremity or organ, areas of inflammation may be specified by neurologic control, perhaps by regulating or perturbating vascular dynamics or by altering chemical or electrical potentials.

Antibodies or other immunologic selectors may specify not only the locale but also the character of the reaction that ensues. Union of antigen with IgE antibody molecules bound to the surface of a basophil results in the secretion of mediators of the immediate allergic reaction. Union of antigen with IgG or IgM antibody to form immune complexes may trigger the complement system and cause the changes of subacute tissue damage and vasculitis. Union of antigen with antibody-like antigen-binding sites on the surface of T lymphocytes initiates the formation and secretion of lymphokines, which signal the development of a delayed hypersensitivity reaction. Similar effects of the selector on the nature of the inflammation that follows seem likely for the nonimmunologic selecting elements, but these have not been as thoroughly studied.

**Detectors.** These elements monitor the status of the selectors—which may be viewed as a set of switches—

detect those that are "turned on," and transduce this signal to the delivery system. A clear example of a detector is the C1q subunit of the first complement component. This protein has six sites which are capable of weak interactions with native IgG or IgM; such binding has no effect on the remainder of the C1 complex or the complement system.[6] If the IgG or IgM is combined with antigen or in an aggregated state, however, then the multivalent binding of the C1q subunit results in the internal proteolysis of C1 and activation of the remaining components.[7] Receptors for plasma proteins or their fragments present on cell membranes constitute a large class of detectors.[8] Only recently have some of the mechanisms by which these membrane proteins function been elucidated. For example, the receptor sites on mast cells for IgE antibodies signal the "triggered" state when they are aggregated. Usually this occurs when antibody molecules occupying the receptor sites are bridged by antigen, but direct cross-linking of the detectors by antireceptor antibody also opens a calcium channel and results in mediator secretion.[9] Other cell membrane receptors that serve as detectors are those for the Fc end of IgG and for fragments of complement proteins. There must also be proteins in the membranes of lymphocytes that detect the union of antigen with specific binding sites on these cells and trigger the release of lymphokines or other events. Finally, plasma protein substrates of such activatable selectors as Hageman factor may transduce the signal to the delivery system (Chapter 8).[10]

**Delivery.** Ultimately the means of delivery of the effectors of inflammation is the vasculature (Chapter 13). Avascular tissues such as cornea, sclera, or articular cartilage do not manifest florid inflammatory reactions until they have been invaded by vascular granulation tissue. Locally, delivery involves the movement of cells and plasma proteins or other solutes from within the intravascular compartment into the extravascular one. A large number of parallel mechanisms have evolved for accomplishing these movements into areas specified by the selectors. The mechanisms are triggered by the detectors.

Observations of the microvasculature identify alterations in blood flow through an inflamed area as one of the earliest changes.[11] The total blood flow through the tissue is increased, chiefly owing to opening of preferential channels connecting arterioles and venules. Flow through the capillaries, however, becomes stagnated, owing to a generalized relaxation of capillary sphincters. Normal laminar streaming is disrupted and leukocytes that usually roll along the endothelium slow down, so that the vessel wall becomes coated with these cells, thus further slowing capillary flow. Simultaneous with these changes, increased permeability of the vessels occurs, allowing egress of plasma proteins and resulting in the loss of oncotic pressure within the vessel lumen due to the normal intravascular location of these proteins; egress of water and other solutes also ensues.[12] These initial steps in delivery are usually attributed to the low molecular weight mediators of inflammation, including histamine, serotonin (in some species), bradykinin, and

PROTEOLYSIS

$$(a.a._n)-NHCHC-NHCHC-(a.a._n) \xrightarrow[\text{PROTEASE}]{\text{HOH}} (a.a._n)-NHCHC-OH + HNHCHC-(a.a._n)$$

PROTEIN          POLYPEPTIDE #1   POLYPEPTIDE #2

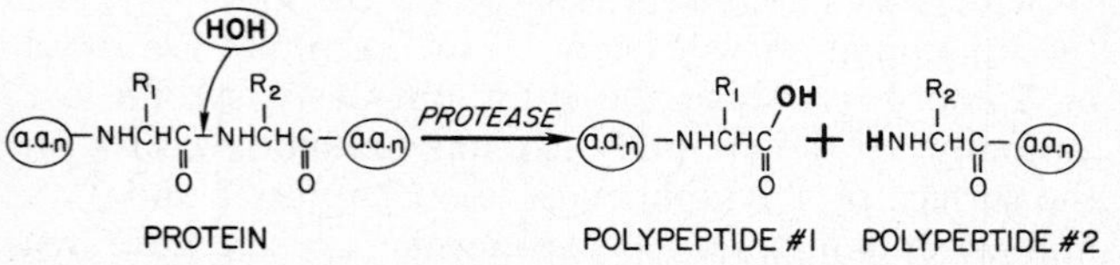

**Figure 1–2.** A general equation for the hydrolysis of peptide bonds.

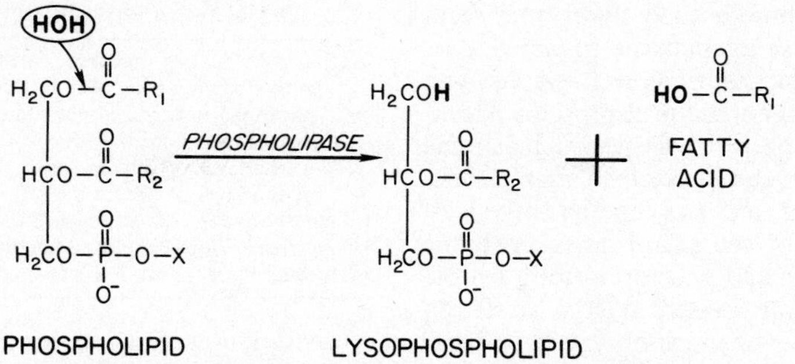


**Figure 1–3.** An example of lipolysis: the hydrolysis of phospholipid.

**Table 1–1.** Selectors of the Inflammatory Process

| | |
|---|---|
| Immunologic | |
| | Antibody (IgG, IgM, IgA, or IgE) |
| | Antigen-binding sites on surfaces of cells |
| Nonimmunologic | |
| | Hageman factor |
| | $\beta$1H globulin |
| | Tissue cells which secrete mediators |
| | Tissue cells which release proteases |
| | Nerve cells or smooth muscle of vasculature(?) |

arachidonate metabolites, including prostaglandins and leukotrienes.[13] The primary site of action of many of these materials within the vasculature appears to be the small venule. Sequential action of these mediators appears likely, since in many experimental models antihistaminics block permeability changes seen within the first few minutes, whereas inhibitors of prostaglandin synthesis suppress changes observed from 1 to 24 hours later.

The same opening-up of clefts between endothelial cells that allows escape of plasma proteins, water, and solutes also permits the delivery of leukocytes into the inflamed area.[14] In contrast to the egress of proteins, which may be viewed as a passive phenomenon consequent to change in pore size and pressure, the emigration of leukocytes is an active process. A variety of chemotactic factors (Chapter 9) attract leukocytes into the area. These include bacterial products, active enzymes of the complement and kinin-forming systems, fragments of complement components, and peptides released by mast cells or lymphocytes. Some of these factors attract a number of different types of cells, whereas others tend to specify a particular type, such as eosinophils.[16] All have in common the property of inducing migration of their target cells in the direction of the chemical gradient of the chemotactic factor. Once located in the area of inflammation, the cells may be induced to remain there either by the absence of any further chemotactic factor gradient or by other proteins, such as macrophage migration inhibition factor,[17] which actively reduce their mobility.

**Effectors.** With the exception of the amphipathic terminal complement component complex[18] and reactive oxygen metabolites, which can cause damage by nonenzymatic means, all effects of inflammation can be reduced to hydrolysis of proteins, lipids, or carbohydrates. An example of each of these is diagrammed in Figures 1–2, 1–3, and 1–4. The enzymes that catalyze these reactions are usually brought to the inflammatory site

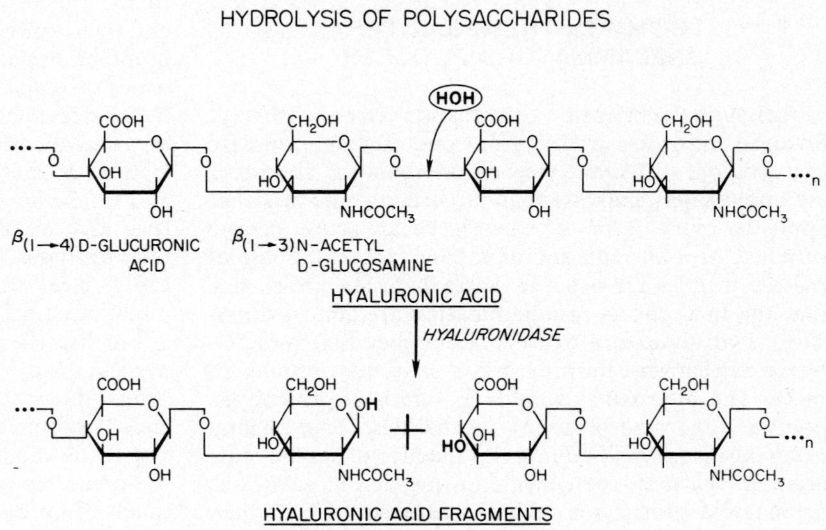


**Figure 1–4.** An example of the hydrolysis of glycosidic bonds: hyaluronic acid digestion by hyaluronidase.

packaged within cells. Although such hydrolytic reactions are effective in defense against the invading parasite, they may destroy host tissues as well. Proteolysis of collagen, elastin, and other structural proteins is central to the destruction of supporting tissues such as bone cartilage and basement membrane seen in many rheumatic diseases (Chapters 12 and 14). The hydrolysis of lipids, e.g., phospholipids of cell membranes, with the mobilization of arachidonic acid and formation of prostaglandins, leukotrienes, and related agents, is clearly important to the destructive changes observed with inflammation. Secondary damage mediated by lysophosphatides formed during the process of lipolysis may also contribute. Finally, disruption of glycosidic linkages, which contributes to the destruction of cartilage, may also have direct effects on cell function when the carbohydrates being hydrolyzed are parts of membrane glycoproteins.

All the hydrolyses catalyzed by the effector enzymes are essentially irreversible; proteins, for example, are not reassembled by condensation reactions among the polypeptides into which they have been hydrolyzed. The same is true of the lipids and carbohydrates. De novo resynthesis of the hydrolyzed molecule is, therefore, required for repair of tissue damage consequent to inflammation. The extent of the damage in part governs the success of the reparative resynthesis in reproducing the original tissue. In particular, loss of framework or structural molecules appears important. In viral hepatitis, for example, extensive hepatocellular necrosis may occur, but complete repair ensues provided the underlying reticulin and collagen framework of the lobules has not been destroyed. Once collapse of the framework has occurred, the disorganized and fibrotic reaction of postnecrotic cirrhosis is the consequence.[19] Similarly, once the hyaline cartilage lining a joint is lost, "resynthesis" implies replacement by fibrocartilage. In some diseases, such as scleroderma, an uncontrolled or exuberant fibrotic reparative process appears to be the major pathogenic feature.

## COMMON THEMES IN THE INFLAMMATORY PROCESS

Although the intensity, extent, and even the pathways involved may vary greatly from one rheumatic disease to another, a systematic view of inflammation as a process immediately makes apparent certain principles that apply to every form, whether it be an acute allergic response or a chronic granulomatous process. Some of these principles are listed in Table 1–2. The knowledge that the final effects of inflammation are almost exclusively hydrolytic and irreversible implies that these effector mechanisms must exist in a *precursor or protected form.* The alternative would be rampant proteolysis, lipolysis, and hydrolysis of saccharides. Two general mechanisms for maintaining this inactive precursor state exist. In the first, the enzyme in question circulates as an inactive proenzyme which is cleaved by a limited proteolytic reaction to form an active protease. This mechanism is especially prevalent in delivery cascades such as complement, kinin-forming, and coagulation systems. The second, and more common, involves the "packaging" of hydrolytic enzymes within intracellular vesicles, or lysosomes (Chapter 9).[20]

**Table 1–2.** General Principles of Inflammation

| | |
|---|---|
| 1. | Effectors exist in precursor form—<br>activated by proteolysis in fluid phase<br>packaged in intracellular vesicles and released |
| 2. | Controls modulate the process—<br>at the level of delivery mechanisms<br>at the level of effectors |
| 3. | Alternative pathways reach the same biologic end (redundancy) |
| 4. | Feedback loops amplify detection or delivery |
| 5. | Interactive network is representative |

A second principle implicit in effector function is the existence of *controlling or modulating influences,* which serve to dampen the inflammatory effects and to limit their extent. A number of different plasma proteins that inhibit the delivery cascades have been described.[21] Not infrequently deficiency of such a protein leads to undesirable spontaneous activation of the delivery system. Other plasma proteins inhibit the hydrolytic effector proteolytic enzymes. Deficiency of alpha-1 antitrypsin, the plasma protein effective in inhibiting leukocyte elastase, is associated with premature pulmonary emphysema and other effects that have been attributed to uncontrolled digestion of the structural protein elastin.[22]

The existence of multiple factors, all of which attract leukocytes, is an excellent example of the *multiplicity of pathways* leading to a common biologic event. There are many others, such as the duplicate pathways leading to activation of the coagulation cascade, or the two pathways, classic and alternative, leading to activation of the terminal complement sequence. The survival value of such duplication is readily apparent, and the existence of apparently healthy individuals with isolated deficiencies of a single pathway constituent bears witness to its usefulness (Chapter 85).

The existence of *feedback loops* is by no means unique to the process of inflammation, but their multiplicity and their tendency to have a positive or amplifying effect in inflammation are remarkable. At the level of the delivery systems, the feedback effects within the Hageman factor-dependent systems are extremely complex. The alternative complement pathway is primarily an amplification loop.[23] Interactions between cellular products and fluid-phase constituents also frequently have positive feedback effects. The number and variety of amplifying loops in the inflammatory process make especially clear the importance of the controlling or modulating influences mentioned above.

Finally, the foregoing analysis of the inflammatory process (Fig. 1–1) tends to give the impression of a simple linear system with a beginning, a middle, and an end. It should already be clear from the multiple pathways, the modulation by controls, the feedbacks, and the precursor forms that the process of inflammation is much more correctly represented by a complex interactive multilevel network. Although many of these interactions have been defined, the rate constants or other parameters allowing quantification or precise representation of the most important interactions are not yet available, even for a single segment of the system. The complexities of this interactive network will become readily apparent as the next 20 chapters are read.

## References


1. Weissmann, G., Serhan, C., Korchak, H.M., and Smolen, J.E.: Neutrophils: Release of mediators of inflammation with special reference to rheumatoid arthritis. Ann. N.Y. Acad. Sci. 389:11, 1982.
2. Ruddy, S.: Function of the control proteins of the classical and alternative complement activation pathways. *In* Thompson, R.A. (ed.): Recent Advances in Clinical Immunology. London, Churchill Livingstone, 1980, pp. 91–111.
3. Weisdorf, D.S., Craddock, P.R., and Jacob, H.S.: Granulocytes utilize different energy sources for movement and phagocytosis. Inflammation 6:245, 1982.
4. Falchuk, K.H., Goetzl, E.J., and Kulka, J.P.: Respiratory gases of synovial fluids. Am. J. Med. 49:223, 1970.
5. Hugli, T.E.: The structural basis for anaphylatoxin and chemotactic functions of C3a, C4a, and C5a C.R.C. Crit. Rev. Immunol. 1:321, 1981.
6. Reid, K.B.M.: Proteins involved in the activation and control of the two pathways of human complement. Biochem. Soc. Trans. 11:1, 1983.
7. Ziccardi, R.J., and Cooper, N.R.: Activation of C1r by proteolytic cleavage. J. Immunol. 116:504, 1976.
8. Bianco, C., and Nussenzweig, V.: Complement receptors. Contemp. Top. Mol. Immunol. 68:145, 1977.
9. Ishizaka, T., Ishizaka, K., Conrad, D.H., and Froese, A.H.: A new concept of triggering mechanisms of IgE-mediated histamine release. J. Allergy Clin. Immunol. 61:320, 1978.
10. Kaplan, A.P., Silverberg, M., Dunn, J.P., and Ghebrehiwet, B.: Interaction of the clotting, kinin-forming, complement and fibrinolytic pathways in inflammation. Ann. N.Y. Acad. Sci. 389:25, 1982.
11. Cotran, R.S., and Majno, G.: A light and electron microscopic analysis of vascular injury. Ann. N.Y. Acad. Sci. 116:750, 1964.
12. Intaglietta, M., Pawula, R.F., and Tompkins, W.R.: Pressure measurements in the mammalian microvasculature. Microvasc. Res. 2:212, 1970.
13. Samuelsson, B.: Leukotrienes: mediators of allergic reactions and inflammation. Int. Arch. Allergy Appl. Immunol. 66(Suppl. 1):98, 1981.
14. Marchesi, V.T., and Florey, H.W.: Electron microscopic observations on the emigration of leukocytes. Quart. J. Exp. Physiol. 45:343, 1960.
15. Ward, P.A.: Leukotactic factors in health and disease. Am. J. Pathol. 64:521, 1971.
16. Kay, A.B., Stechschulte, D.J., and Austen, K.F.: An eosinophil leukocyte chemotactic factor of anaphylaxis. J. Exp. Med. 133:602, 1971.
17. David, J.R.: Lymphocyte mediators and cellular hypersensitivity. N. Engl. J. Med. 288:143, 1973.
18. Mayer, M.M., Hammer, C.H., Michaels, D.W., and Shin, M.I.: Immunologically mediated membrane damage: The mechanism of complement action and the similarity of lymphocyte-mediated cytotoxicity. Immunochemistry 15:813, 1978.
19. Boyer, J.L., and Klatskin, G.: Pattern of necrosis in acute viral hepatitis: Prognostic value of bridging (subacute hepatic necrosis). N. Engl. J. Med. 283:1063, 1970.
20. Goldstein, I.: Lysosomal hydrolases and inflammatory materials. *In* Weissman, G. (ed.): The Plasma Proteins. New York, Academic Press, 1975, p. 51.
21. Laurell, C.B., and Jeppsson, J.: Protease inhibitors in plasma. *In* Putnam, F.W. (ed.): The Plasma Proteins. New York, Academic Press, 1975, p. 229.
22. Janoff, A., and Carp, H.: Proteases, antiproteases and oxidants: Pathways of tissue injury during inflammation. Monogr. Pathol. 23:163, 1982.
23. Kazatchkine, M.D., and Nydegger, U.E.: The human alternative complement pathway: Biology and immunopathology of activation and regulation. Prog. Allergy 30:193, 1982.


# Chapter 2
# Immunoglobulins and Their Genes

*Blas Frangione and Joel N. Buxbaum*

## INTRODUCTION

The elucidation of the molecular mechanisms responsible for the origin of antibody diversity has been a scientific challenge of long standing. The answer to this problem resides in the genes that code for the polypeptide chains of which antibody molecules are composed. For many years scientists who were looking for the answer had to examine the structure of a large number of myeloma proteins and then reason backward to work out the genetic arrangements that could best explain the structures. In the last few years, as a result of the development of techniques for probing genes, nucleotide sequence analysis, and more efficient determination and comparison of the amino acid sequence of proteins, investigators are acquiring the kind of information they need to unravel the mystery of antibody diversity: how is a single animal able to make more than a million different antibodies. This chapter discusses the structure and function of immunoglobulin molecules and explains how antibody diversity is generated.

## HUMAN IMMUNOGLOBULINS: NOMENCLATURE AND CLASSIFICATION

The symbol Ig is used to designate immunoglobulins. There are five classes of immunoglobulin molecules in man (Table 2–1): IgG, IgA, IgM, IgD, and IgE. They have the same basic four-chain structure: two heavy (H) and two light (L) chains ($H_2L_2$). The H chain in each immunoglobulin is class specific, and it is designated by the corresponding Greek letter, as shown in Table 2–1. They differ in length, disulfide bridge pattern, number of domains, degree of polymerization, amino acid sequence, and number and kind of oligosaccharides. IgG and IgA can be further divided into subclasses based on specific antigenic determinants present on the H chains. Subclasses are indicated by arabic numerals following the letter denoting the class. The corresponding H chains are named $\gamma_1$, $\gamma_2$, $\gamma_3$, $\gamma_4$, and $\alpha_1$ and $\alpha_2$, respectively.

**Table 2–1.** Human Immunoglobulins

| Isotypes | Molecular Weight | Serum Level (mg/ml) | Carbohydrate (%) | Half-life (days) | L Chain (common) | H Chain (unique) | Subclasses of H Chain | Genetic Markers (alleles)* C+ | N, M |
|---|---|---|---|---|---|---|---|---|---|
| IgG | 150,000 | 12 | 2.5 | 25 | κ or λ | γ(gamma) | γ1<br>γ2<br>γ3<br>γ4 | Za · fa⁻<br>n⁻· n<br>g · b<br>4a · 4b | Za<br>n⁻<br>b<br>4a |
| IgA | 160,000–350,000 | 2 | 8 | 6 | κ or λ | α(alpha) | α1<br>α2 | A2m(1) · A2m(2) | A2m(2) |
| IgM | 900,000 | 1 | 10 | 5 | κ or λ | μ(mu) | | | |
| IgD | 160,000 | 0.03 | 10 | 3 | κ or λ | δ(delta) | | | |
| IgE | 180,000 | 0.0003 | 12 | 2 | κ or λ | ε(epsilon) | | | |

+C: Caucasian; N: Negro; M: Mongoloid

*Alternative nomenclature (1,2)

| | | | |
|---|---|---|---|
| Gm z,a | = G1m (17,1) | Gm fa⁻ | = G1m (3,N1) |
| Gm n | = G2m (23) | | |
| Gm g | = G3m (21) | Gmb | = G3n (5) |
| Gm 4a | = G4m (N4a) | Gm4b | = G4m (N4b) |

L chains exist in two different types, kappa (κ ) and lambda (λ), which can be readily distinguished immunologically. They are not class specific, and both types occur in all classes. In human serum, the number of immunoglobulins containing κ chains is approximately twice that of those bearing λ chains. Subclasses have been found only for the λ type, and at present they are identified in terms of the specific markers that distinguish them.[1,2]

The different classes, subclasses, and types of immunoglobulin polypeptide chains are called *isotypes.* They are present in all individuals, and they are the products of different structural genes. Two of the Ig classes contain other nonhomologous chains. IgA in external secretions is dimeric and contains a chain not present in serum IgA. The additional polypeptide chain is called secretory component (SC), and the entire molecule is termed secretory IgA (sIgA).[3] Furthermore, polymeric immunoglobulins (IgM, IgA, and sIgA molecules) contain an antigenically and physicochemically distinctive polypeptide termed the J chain.[4]

## VARIABLE AND CONSTANT REGIONS

Each immunoglobulin chain consists of two regions. One is designated the variable (V) region; the other, the constant (C) region. The V region is the amino terminal portion of the L and H chain (about 110 to 120 residues) and is made up of many different amino acid sequences, even within one class or subclass. On the other hand, the C region is the carboxyl terminal portion of the chain and has the same primary structure as all other chains of the same class, subclass, and type. The particular immunoglobulin chain in which these regions are studied is designated by subscripts, e.g., $V_L$, $C_L$, $V_H$, $C_H$. The C regions of κ and λ chains contain 110 residues; the C regions of γ, α, and δ chains are three times larger; and the C regions of μ and ϵ chains are four times larger. The various V and C regions are homologous in structure and evolutionarily related. Owing to their amino acid sequence and the presence of one intrachain disulfide bond, each homology region folds in a somewhat similar conformation, a compact globular domain. The average amount of homology of all domains is about 25 percent, although the degree of homology varies from domain to domain. This shows that individual domains of L and H chains evolved with different mutation rates from a common primordial gene.

### $\beta_2$ Microglobulin

$\beta_2$Microglobulin ($\beta_2$M) is a protein of low molecular weight (11,800 daltons) present in small amounts in normal urine, serum, and other biological fluids. It is synthesized by all nucleated cells and is present on their surfaces. Its biological role remains unclear. Several reports indicate that in patients with a variety of malignant tumors, serum $\beta_2$M levels may be abnormally elevated[5] when compared with controls (normal values range from 900 to 2800 μg per liter[6]). The elevation of serum $\beta_2$M in malignancies of the B lymphocyte type has helped to differentiate idiopathic benign monoclonal gammopathies from B lymphocyte neoplasms.[5] Certain inflammatory diseases involving polyclonal lymphocyte activation are also associated with increased $\beta_2$M synthesis. Elevated serum $\beta_2$M levels have been reported in rheumatoid arthritis, Sjögren's syndrome, systemic lupus erythematosus, sarcoidosis, Crohn's disease, and angioimmunoblastic lymphadenopathy.[7] $\beta_2$M was the first nonantibody molecule that could be shown to be homologous with immunoglobulins. The $\beta_2$M protein can be readily aligned with a single Ig domain.[8] $\beta_2$M was subsequently found to be the smaller of two noncovalently associated polypeptides that constitute the class I major histocompatibility antigens (HLA-A, B, and C antigens).[9] The H chain of the HLA-A, B, and C antigens contains two disulfide bonded loops, each of which shows homology with C domains.[10] Very recently, two other molecules, class II histocompatibility antigens (or D antigens) and Thy-1 antigen, a surface glycoprotein characteristic of murine T lymphocytes, have also been shown to be homologous to Ig, although less so (Fig. 2–1). These findings have led to a provocative hypothesis about the genetics and evolution of Ig superfamily genes.[11–12]

V regions sharing certain similarities in their amino acid sequence can be classified as belonging to a single

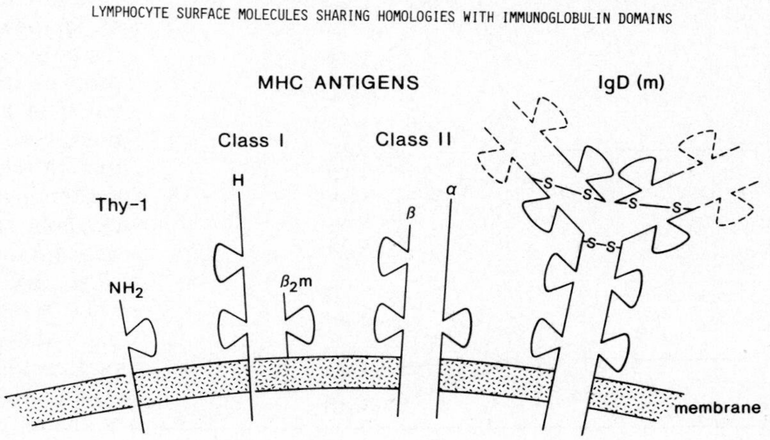


**Figure 2–1.** Lymphocyte surface molecules sharing homologies with Ig domains (represented by loops). IgD (m); MHC, major histocompatibility complex, class I antigens consist of a heavy (H) variable chain and a light chain, $\beta_2$ microglobulin. MHC class II antigens are composed of two chains, α and β. Thy-1 antigen is a surface glycoprotein characteristic of T lymphocytes.

subgroup (Table 2–2). Within a subgroup, a number of subdivisions can be made such that V regions of any one subgroup resemble one another more closely than they do members of other subgroups. Four subgroups of κ chains and six subgroups of λ chains are identified. The V regions of H chains also can be classified into at least three subgroups, which are not class specific, i.e., they can be expressed in any of the Ig classes. Certain positions in the variable region are highly conserved; in fact, 65 percent of this region shows limited sequence variation. Within a subgroup, most variations involve amino acid interchanges due to single base replacements in the corresponding codons. Other V region positions vary to a greater extent. These are clustered in three areas of both chains (amino acids 24–34, 50–56, and 89–97 in the light chains and residues 31–35, 50–65, and 95–102 in the heavy chains), which are called the hypervariable or complementarity-determining regions (CDR). These broad regions of sequence hypervariability are believed to be related to the antigen-binding site.[13,14] They are surrounded by relatively invariant framework (FR) regions.

## IMMUNOGLOBULIN G

IgG molecules consist of identical pairs of H and L chains (MW = 50,000 and 25,000, respectively) linked by disulfide bridges (Fig. 2–2). A proteolytic enzyme (papain) splits IgG into three fragments, which retain biologic activity: two Fab (for antigen binding) fragments and one Fc (for crystallizable).[15] Each Fab fragment contains one antigen-combining site and consists of one L chain and the amino terminal half of the H chain, termed the Fd fragment. The remaining carboxy-terminal halves of the two H chains, including the inter-H chain disulfide bonds (or hinge region), are the Fc fragment, which contains the sites responsible for the mediation of most biologic functions (Table 2–3). Pepsin cleaves the basic unit at the carboxyl end of the hinge region and thus liberates a bivalent section comparable to two papain-derived Fab fragments termed $F(ab')_2$ and a smaller Fc fragment (pFc′), which contains the $C_H3$ domain.[14]

**Table 2–2.** Subgroups of the Light Chain ($V_L$) and Heavy Chain ($V_H$) Variable Regions

| Chain | Variable Region | Subgroup |
|---|---|---|
| L | $V_L$ → $V_\kappa$ | $V_\kappa I$ |
| | | $V_\kappa II$ |
| | | $V_\kappa III$ |
| | | $V_\kappa IV$ |
| | $V_L$ → $V_\lambda$ | $V_\lambda I$ |
| | | $V_\lambda II$ |
| | | $V_\lambda III$ |
| | | $V_\lambda IV$ |
| | | $V_\lambda V$ |
| | | $V_\lambda VI$ |
| H | $V_H$ | $V_H I$ |
| | | $V_H II$ |
| | | $V_H III$ |

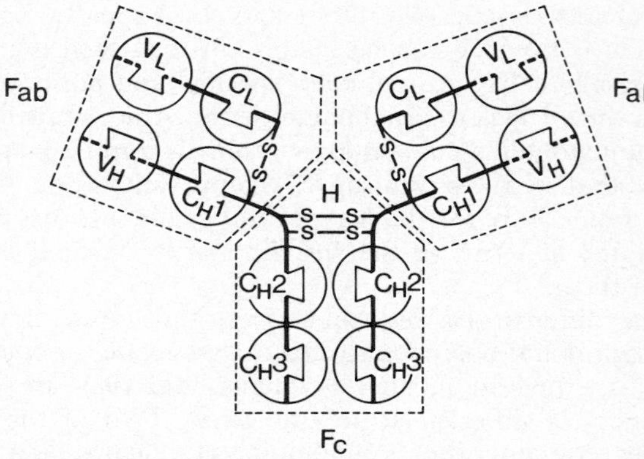


**Figure 2–2.** Diagram of a human IgG molecule. The L chains are divided into two domains, $V_L$ and $C_L$. The H chains are divided into four domains, $V_H$, $C_H1$, $C_H2$, and $C_H3$. The heavy chains are joined by disulfide bridges in the hinge region (H). Cleavage of IgG by papain generates Fab fragments and an Fc fragment.

In 1969, the first complete amino acid sequence of a human $IgG_{1\kappa}$ myeloma protein was reported.[16] One of the most striking features of the immunoglobulin molecule was the demarcation of its chains into connected regions that are associated with different biological functions.[17]

Normal human IgG contains a mixture of different subclasses of H chains: $\gamma_1$, $\gamma_2$, $\gamma_3$, and $\gamma_4$. IgG activates complement by the classic pathway, with $IgG_1$ and $IgG_3$ subclasses being most effective (Table 2–3). $IgG_4$ does not fix complement in the native state but does so after proteolytic cleavage. This property appears to be associated primarily with the $C_H2$ domain. IgG is the only class of immunoglobulin that provides passive immunity to the newborn, since the four gamma subclasses are the only immunoglobulins that cross the placenta. IgG proteins also interact with cell receptors for the Fc fragment on polymorphonuclear cells, monocytes, macrophages, and platelets. This property is important in initiating the inflammatory response, and it is associated predominantly with the $C_H3$ domain. IgG has a slow catabolic rate; its half-life is approximately 3 weeks, with only $IgG_3$ being degraded more rapidly. However, the rates vary directly with the serum concentration.

In most species immunologic memory resides primarily in the IgG fraction, with certain antigens eliciting preferential responses of one or another of the subclasses. Amino acid sequence studies of different subclasses of γ chains provide additional evidence that the immu-

**Table 2–3.** Biological Properties (Effector Functions) of Human Immunoglobulins

| Property | IgG 1 | IgG 2 | IgG 3 | IgG 4 | IgM | IgA | IgE | Domain Localization |
|---|---|---|---|---|---|---|---|---|
| *Antigen-Dependent* | | | | | | | | |
| Complement Fixation — Classical Pathway | + | + | + | | + | | | $C_H2$(IgG) $C_H4$(IgM) |
| Complement Fixation — Alternate Pathway | | | | | | + | + | |
| Opsonic Activity (neutrophils and monocytes) | + | | + | | | + | | |
| *Antigen-Independent* | | | | | | | | |
| Mast Cell and Basophil Binding | | | | | | | + | |
| Macrophage Binding | + | | + | | | | | $C_H3$ |
| Lymphocyte Binding | + | | + | | + | | | $C_H3$ |
| Placental Passage | + | + | + | + | | | | Fc |
| Immunoglobulin Catabolism | + | + | + | + | + | + | + | $C_H2$ |
| Passive Cutaneous Anaphylaxis | + | | + | + | | | | $C_H3$ |
| Interaction with Protein "A" | + | + | | + | | | | $C_H2$, $C_H3$ |
| Antigenic Target for Rheumatoid Factor | + | + | + | + | + | + | + | Fc |

noglobulin molecule evolved by the successive duplication of a precursor gene of about 300 nucleotides and that a loop of approximately 60 residues is a fundamental subunit that is repeated 12 times in an IgG molecule. The $\gamma$ subclasses are almost identical in this primary structure (over 95 percent amino acid sequence homology). The main subclass-related differences are in the hinge segment.[18] The hinge region varies from 15 to 60 residues; it is rich in proline and cysteine residues. The latter are involved in the disulfide bridges linking both H chains.

$IgG_1$ and $IgG_4$ proteins contain four interchain bridges. Two such bonds join the H chains to each other, and two bonds join H to L chains. $IgG_2$ proteins are crosslinked by six interchain bonds, two joining H to L chains and the other four binding both H chains. It has recently become evident that human $IgG_3$ has structural and biologic features not shared by the other three subclasses. $IgG_3$ does not bind to staphylococcal protein A, which tightly binds the other subclasses; it has a more rapid turnover; and it is the most potent subclass in activating the first component of complement. Structurally, the $\gamma_3$ chain has a higher molecular weight than other human chains, owing to an extended hinge region. This region is four times larger than the same region in the three other subclasses. This is due to a quadruplication of a 45-nucleotide DNA segment, resulting in a $\gamma_3$ hinge region that is 62 amino acid residues long and consists of an $NH_2$-terminal 17-residue segment followed by a 15-residue segment, which is identically and consecutively repeated three times.[19] Very recently, an $IgG_3$ protein carrying a rare allotype G3m (s,t) has been shown to bind staphylococcal protein A.[20] A histidine residue at the carboxyl end of the H chain (position 435) has been implicated in the binding of the protein.[21] It has been suggested that protein-A-binding $IgG_3$-like molecules comprise a fifth subclass of IgG, since they appear to be present in normal sera.[20]

## IMMUNOGLOBULIN M

The IgM molecule is a pentamer composed of five identical subunits and one nonimmunoglobulin chain, the J chain. The J chain and a disulfide interchanging enzyme facilitate the formation of the polymer.[4,22] IgM appears to fill a special role in the primary immune response, and certain antigens such as the I antigen, aggregated immunoglobulins, and other red cell antigens stimulate a persistent IgM response. However, most antigenic stimuli result in a switch to other immunoglobulins after the initial burst of IgM. IgM is located predominantly in the intravascular space; its turnover is fast; and it cannot cross the placenta. It can however, initiate complement activation. While the valence of the IgM pentamer is 10 for small antigens, it may not exceed 5 for larger antigens, presumably as a consequence of steric hindrance.

Of great interest is the finding in recent years that the monomer of an IgM appears to be, together with IgD, the major protein on the surface of B lymphocytes. The V regions of both surface H chains ($\mu$ and $\delta$) appear to be identical on the same cell. It has been suggested that both molecules act as receptors for antigens.[23,24]

Structural analyses of IgM were performed primarily with proteins obtained from patients suffering from Waldenström's macroglobulinemia. The availability of these homogeneous products of monoclonal lymphoid populations allowed the detailed study of IgM, just as myeloma proteins and Bence Jones proteins served as models for IgG antibodies and light chains, respectively. A disulfide-bonded model for human IgM is shown in Figure 2–3. Four bonds are interchain; ten, intrachain. The interchain disulfide bridges are arranged as follows: one joins H to L; one joins H to H in the monomer subunit; one is intersubunit; and the fourth cysteine apparently joins either the J chain or the homologous cysteine of the next monomer subunit, that is, it behaves as a J

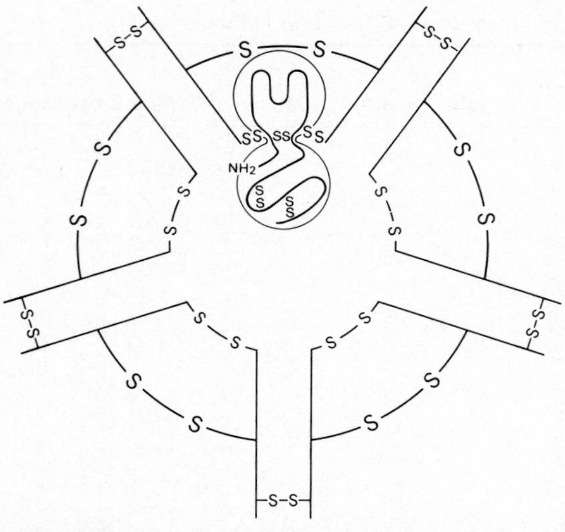

**Figure 2–3.** Schematic diagram of the pentameric structure of the Fc fragment of human IgM. A two-domain structure for J chain is indicated.[37] One J chain is attached per pentameric IgM, through the C-terminal cysteine of $\mu$ chains and the amino terminal domain of the J chain.

bond or as a second intersubunit bond. The $\mu$ chain (MW = 70,000) contains five domains instead of the four present in $\gamma$ chains: $V_H$, $C_\mu 1$, $C_\mu 2$, $C_\mu 3$, and $C_\mu 4$. Most of $C_\mu 2$ is degraded to peptides after trypsin digestion, suggesting that there is an exposed and flexible region resembling the hinge region in other Ig molecules.[25]

B lymphocyte membranes contain immunoglobulins that act as receptors for antigen. Membrane-bound IgM ($IgM_m$) is present as a four-chain monomer and differs from the secreted molecule ($IgM_s$) only near the C-terminal end of the $\mu$ chain. The last 20 amino acid residues of the secreted chain ($\mu_s$) are missing from $\mu_m$ and are replaced by a different sequence of 41 residues (21 residues longer than $\mu_s$). The extended $\mu_m$ includes a stretch of about 26 hydrophobic residues which is responsible for the insertion of IgM into the cell membrane.[26] A hydrophobic C-terminal region is present in the membrane-bound forms of all immunoglobulin H chains.

## IMMUNOGLOBULIN A

In lower vertebrates, including fish, reptiles, and amphibians, IgM in tetrameric and pentameric configurations, represents the predominant immunoglobulin in serum as well as external secretions.[27] IgA first appears in birds and mammals, and secretory IgM is replaced by polymeric secretory IgA (sIgA). In man, IgA is produced in large quantities in areas adjacent to secretory surfaces. Mucosal B lymphocyte follicles in the intestinal and respiratory tracts have been implicated in the generation of cells enriched in precursors for IgA plasma cells. The precursors of the IgA plasma cells are first recognizable as bone-marrow-derived B lymphocytes in the Peyer's patches (PP), where they can encounter antigens entering from the gut by way of epithelial cells. The precursors may initiate DNA synthesis in the PP, but eventually they leave by way of lymphatics draining into the mesenteric lymph nodes (MLN) where they proliferate further and eventually mature into IgA-containing blast cells. These blasts are capable of leaving the MLN and migrating to the small intestine and by the afferent and thoracic duct lymph entering into the bloodstream, from which they emerge at mucosal sites. This process is called the IgA-cell cycle.[28-32] Polymeric IgA interacts specifically with epithelial cells by means of the membrane glycoprotein secretory component (SC), which acts as a receptor and mediates its selective transport into secretions.

Unlike the other classes of immunoglobulins, IgA tends to be polydisperse in size. In normal human sera most of the IgA is monomeric, i.e., composed of a single four-chain unit, $\alpha_2 L_2$; about 10 percent consists of dimer or higher oligomers. Recognition of antigenic heterogeneity among IgA myelomas has led to the detection of two subclasses, $IgA_1$ and $IgA_2$. The genetic locus coding for $IgA_2$ heavy-chain constant region ($\alpha_2$) has two allelic forms, $A_2m(_1)$ and $A_2m(_2)$, with some linkage to the Gm system of IgG. Unlike other immunoglobulins, $A_2m(_1)$ molecules lack covalent links between H and L chains, and their L chains are instead covalently linked to one another. In the $\alpha_1$ and $\alpha_2$ chains the major chemical differences lie in the hinge region and in the number, locations, and types of oligosaccharides. The hinge region of the $\alpha_1$ chain contains a triplicated octapeptide that is lacking in $\alpha_2$ chains; instead $\alpha_2$ chains have a deletion and an unusual pentaproline sequence. In addition, there are a number of other amino acid substitutions that correlate with subclass or allotype. About 90 percent of the IgA in serum is $IgA_1$; but external secretions contain a more equal division.[34]

**Secretory Component.** sIgA is a special form of IgA, found predominantly in gastrointestinal and respiratory secretions, and represents a first line of local defense against environmental pathogens.[33] Its consists of two monomeric IgA subunits, a J chain and the SC, or transport piece, which has a molecular weight of approximately 70,000 daltons. SC is synthesized by the epithelial cells of the glands that secrete IgA polymer. More than 85 percent of the plasma cells in the intestinal lamina propria elaborate IgA, and there are high concentrations of sIgA in all secretions. In addition to the functions it shares with serum IgA (such as complement activation by the alternative pathway and viral neutralization), sIgA appears to prevent bacterial adherence to the intestinal mucosal surface and inhibits uptake of some proteins by the gut and other surfaces.

Oral immunization produces higher levels of sIgA antibodies. This reaction is of great practical significance, as orally administered polio vaccines are more effective than systemic vaccines, which fail to induce production of IgA antipoliovirus antibodies. After local stimulation, lymphocytes of the lamina propria of the intestines and other secretory organs develop into mature plasma cells and synthesize IgA molecules, which are dimerized by the presence of J chain on lymphocyte membranes. The SC synthesized by the epithelial cells combines with IgA antibodies and facilitates the entrance of the complete sIgA molecule into the intracellular space and secretion into intestinal lumen. The precise site and the mechanism by which SC accomplishes this function are not known.

The SC is linked to the H chains of one IgA subunit by a disulfide bridge,[34] which appears to protect it against proteolytic digestion. Normal feces contain a proteolytic enzyme that cleaves serum and sIgA to yield Fab and Fc fragments. The enzyme was termed IgA protease because enzymatic activity has thus far been found only against IgA. IgA protease can be obtained from centrifuged suspensions of feces or from culture fluids of *Streptococcus sanguis, Neisseria gonorrhoeae, N. meningitidis,* and *Haemophilus influenzae.* The specificity of the enzyme is quite restricted. It cleaves the Pro-Thr or Pro-Ser peptide bond in the hinge region of $IgA_1$. It does not cleave $IgA_2$, since the target dipeptide is absent in this class. The presence of $\alpha_1$ Fc fragments in normal feces suggests a role for this enzyme in the secretory immune system. Of considerable interest is the observation that the enzyme is produced in those regions of the alimentary tract populated by bacteria, mainly the mouth and the colon. The increased ratio of $IgA_2$:$IgA_1$ detected in secretions may represent an evolutionary adaptation of man to what has become the normal flora of the gastrointestinal tract.[35,36]

**J Chain.** J chain is structurally unrelated to L and H chains and evolved independently of them. It combines covalently with the H chains of IgA and IgM in the unusual stoichiometric proportion of one J chain per polymeric molecule regardless of the size of the polymer. J chain is linked by the disulfide bond to a cysteine that is the penultimate residue in human $\mu$ and $\alpha$ chains. The similarity in location is not surprising because the carboxyl terminal ends of $\mu$ and $\alpha$ chains are homologous. J chain is thought to initiate polymerization by sequential disulfide exchange with the C-terminal intrachain S–S bond of monomeric IgA or IgM. Because the stoichiometry indicates one J chain per polymer, the mode of attachment poses a problem. Recent results favor the "clasp" model, in which the J chain acts as a disulfide clasp between two monomers and the polymer is closed by disulfide bonds between the other monomer units (Fig. 2–3). Human J chain consists of a single polypeptide chain, with a molecular weight of 15,000, and a single oligosaccharide. Unlike L and H chains, J chain appears to have a unique sequence; there is no evidence for variation, and $J_\alpha$ and $J_\mu$ appear to be identical both chemically and antigenically. Little progress has been made in correlating the structure and function of the J chain, owing to the lack of mutant forms of J chain with altered function. It has also been difficult to isolate sufficient J chain for detailed chemical analysis, sinceJ chain is highly susceptible to enzymatic degradation. Very recently, comparison of the primary structure of the human polypeptide with the murine J chain sequence deduced from nucleotide analysis of cloned cDNA suggested that the J chain possesses two domains having different characteristics. It would appear that the polymerization function resides in its amino terminal half.[37]

## IMMUNOGLOBULIN D

IgD was described 20 years ago; nonetheless a distinct functional role for this class remains an enigma.[38] The most striking aspect of IgD is its distribution. It is present in normal serum in very low quantities and yet is found on the surface of most B lymphocytes as a membrane Ig, usually in association with another Ig class (most frequently IgM), sharing the same $V_H$-$V_L$ regions.[39] Early findings, not surprisingly therefore, focused on the possibility that IgD might be the antigen receptor for B cells. A wealth of evidence now suggests that IgD is not the sole Ig serving a receptor function.

Structural studies of the IgD protein were greatly hindered by several factors. First, concentrations of normal serum IgD are low, and IgD myeloma proteins are rare. Second, IgD is very susceptible to spontaneous enzymatic degradation either in serum or during preparation. The antigenic distinctiveness of IgD, as in other immunoglobulins, lies in its $\delta$ chain. Human IgD myeloma proteins are predominantly of $\lambda$ chain type, although this is not true of cells expressing surface IgD. IgD has a molecular weight of approximately 160,000 and contains about 10 percent carbohydrate, all bound to the $\delta$ chain. The complex sugars consist of three large glucosamine oligosaccharides linked to the Fc region and four or five galactosamine trisaccharides in close proximity in the hinge. The glucosamine is always N-linked to an asparagine in the obligatory tripeptide acceptor sequence Asn-*X*-Thr/Ser, where *X* may be any amino acid.[40] In the serum the protein may be degraded almost completely to fragments similar to Fc and Fab in several days, even at 4°C. This may be retarded by addition of $\epsilon$-aminocaproic acid (EACA) at a final concentration of 0.02M immediately after the plasma is collected. IgD is crosslinked by three interchain bridges, two H-L and one H-H. The presence of only a single inter-H chain bond is unique among human immunoglobulins, although it has also been found in rabbit IgG. IgD from lymphocyte membranes has an apparently higher molecular weight (a property shared with membrane IgM). There has also been a suggestion of different subclasses of IgD; however, in view of the lack of any chemical evidence, it would be premature to conclude that such is the case.

## IMMUNOGLOBULIN E

This quantitatively minor class of Ig contains most of the molecules bearing the biologic and immunochemical characteristics of reaginic antibodies. IgE antibodies have the ability to bind reversibly with high affinity to specific membrane receptors on basophils and mast cells. The combination of specific cell-bound antibody with antigens triggers a series of events that ultimately lead to the release of vasoactive amines and other pharmacologically active substances responsible for the clinical manifestations of hypersensitivity. One can confidently state that without myeloma proteins much of the information we now have about IgE would not exist. This is because the level of IgE, even in the most severely allergic individual, seldom exceeds 1 $\mu$g per ml. Myeloma protein IgE has been used to prepare radiolabeled anti-IgE; and together with allergen coupled to an insoluble adsorbent it is used in the radioallergosorbent test (RAST) to measure antibodies to a specific allergen in the serum of atopic patients. It also seems possible that IgE antibodies play a protective role in parasitic infections, perhaps by increasing vascular permeability and thus allowing other antibodies to arrive at the site of inflammation.

IgE has a molecular weight of 180,000, of which approximately 12 percent is accounted for by carbohydrate. The molecule has the same basic four-chain structure found in other immunoglobulins. A comparison of the molecular size of the H chain ($\epsilon$) with that of the H chains of the other classes shows it to be greater (11,000 daltons greater) than $\gamma$, $\delta$, or $\alpha$ but about the same as $\mu$. The $\epsilon$ chain consists of 547 amino acid residues, organized into the V region, and four constant homology regions ($C_\epsilon 1$, $C_\epsilon 2$, $C_\epsilon 3$, and $C_\epsilon 4$). Thus, both IgE and IgM possess an extra domain and lack a hinge region. Of the 15 half-cystine residues present on the $\epsilon$ chain, 10 participate in the formation of intrachain disulfide bridges, one in each of the five homology regions. Only three interchain bonds are present: one inter-H-L chain bond and two inter-H chain bonds. The two remaining half-cystines are engaged in the formation of an additional intrachain bond located in the $C_H 1$ region. The high carbohydrate content in IgE is explained by the presence of six oligosaccharide chains attached to the $\epsilon$ chain. The ability of IgE to bind to specific receptors is mediated through sites localized within the Fc region. Thermal inactivation of IgE is correlated with structural changes involving both the $C_\epsilon 3$ and $C_\epsilon 4$ domains, but not the $C_\epsilon 2$ region; on the other hand the loss of cytotropic activity accompanying reduction of IgE seems to correlate with the cleavage of one interchain disulfide bond between the paired $C_H 2$ domains. The current interpretation is that reduction of this bond alters the quaternary structure of Fc, leading to inactivation.[41-43]

## GENETIC POLYMORPHISM OR ALLOTYPES

Allotypes are genetic variants of immunoglobulins and are inherited according to simple Mendelian laws. These genetic markers are detected by intraspecies antisera, as obtained in humans after inadvertent immunization by transfusion of whole blood or after pregnancy. In humans, allotypes appear to be the product of a single autosomal codominant gene.[44] Three sets of allotypic markers are recognized in human immunoglobulins, the closely linked Gm and Am factors and the independently inherited km system. Genetic markers have been shown to reside mainly in the constant region of human H chain (Table 2–1). So far, no clear cut allotypic differences have been demonstrated for the $\mu$, $\delta$, and $\epsilon$ chains. The km factors are associated with $\kappa$ type Bence Jones proteins and L chains. Since L chains are common to all classes of Ig, km antigens can be found in IgG, A, M, D, and E proteins.

Km markers are inherited through a series of three alleles $km^{1,2}$, $km^1$, and $km^3$. The serologic allotypic specificities are due to amino acid sequence differences that involve interchanges at one or two contiguous positions that are not critical to the overall structure of function of the antibody molecule. $Km^{1,2}$ is associated with a leucine residue in the C region of $\kappa$ chain (position 191), and $km^3$ is associated with a valine at the same position. When the rare antigen $km^1$ is present, valine is in position 153 instead of alanine. Gm factors are associated with IgG molecules and are located on the $C_\gamma$ region. Some of them have been structurally defined.[44] The A2m(2) allotype is predominant in the human $A_2$ subclass and is characterized by the absence of the H-L interchain disulfide bonds. Studies of allotypic markers in the constant and variable regions in conjunction with amino acid sequence data have been of major importance in the understanding of the polygenic control of immunoglobulin polypeptide synthesis. These genetic differences have also proved to be of use in serology, rheumatology, and forensic medicine.

## IDIOTYPES AND THE COMBINING SITE

Idiotypes are antigenic determinants localized on the V region and correspond to the antigen-binding specificity of a given antibody molecule. Antibody specificity results from the molecular complementarity between determinant groups on the antigen molecule and amino acid residues in the active site. H and L chains contribute to the combining site, as shown by reassociation experiments. In general, most studies have come to the same general conclusion, namely that both H and L chains can bind specifically to the antigen to which the antibody is directed, although binding to the H chain is invariably stronger.

Antigen binding by antibodies involves weak noncovalent associations, including electrostatic bonding, hydrogen bonding, and van der Waals interactions. The specific sites are predominantly nonpolar niches. Evidence obtained from amino acid sequence analysis and affinity labeling studies has been used to identify the segments of polypeptide chains involved in the antibody combining sites (hypervariable regions, or CDRs). These findings led to the hypothesis that CDRs contributed in some way to the conformation of the antibody active sites. Definitive evidence was obtained by x-ray crystallographic studies of Fab fragments obtained from two myeloma proteins.[45,46] Their combining sites extended over a large area surrounding a central groove or pocket, which was 15 Å long, 6 Å wide, and 6 Å deep, the walls of which were composed of hypervariable segments. CDRs contain insertions, deletions, and amino acid substitutions. Sequence modifications of this type have a very significant effect on the size and shape of the combining site and consequently on the specificity. Moreover, extensive binding-site diversity can be generated by the combinatorial properties of L-H chain association. It is further increased by the ability of a single antibody molecule to combine with a spectrum of different antigens (multispecificity). Thus, every antibody will react with the inducing antigen, but each antibody will differ in the spectrum of disparate antigens it can bind (crossreactivity).

## IMMUNOGLOBULIN GENES

The structures we recognize as immunoglobulin heavy and light chains are the products of genes organized into three discrete families, each located on a separate chromosome. One of the major insights into the structure of Ig genes was the demonstration that the elements coding for the variable and constant regions of the heavy and light polypeptides were not contiguous on their respective chromosomes. In the germ line, V and C gene families are separated by many thousands of nucleotides, although the distance has not yet been defined.[47]

**Kappa Chain Germ Line Genes.** In man the kappa gene family has been localized to chromosome 2.[48] The variable region complex is the most 5′ of the elements (Fig. 2–4). It appears that there are between 15 and 30 $V_\kappa$ genes in humans, which is about 10 percent of the number found in mouse DNA, an observation consistent with amino acid sequence data showing that there are four human kappa subgroups compared to many in the mouse.[49]

The genes are generally homologous in the two species, with DNA segments from human easily hybridizable with mouse and vice versa.[50] Each of the $V_\kappa$ genes examined has a fairly well conserved 5′ sequence which contains a promoter site and a CAP (or ribosome-binding) site.[51] The spatial relationships between these two functionally important regions and the initiation codon (ATG) seem to be well preserved and analogous to those found in most eukaryotic proteins. The initiation codon is followed by a run of some 45 to 75 bases, which code for a hydrophobic amino acid sequence. This structure has been shown to play a role in the binding of the polyribosomes synthesizing immunoglobulins to the endoplasmic reticulum.[52] After most of the polypeptide has been synthesized, these N-terminal residues are proteolytically cleaved and are not found on the mature cytoplasmic or secreted immunoglobulin.[53] Immediately 3′ (or downstream) from the leader exon (or coding sequence) is an intervening sequence (intron), which varies from 85 to 105 base pairs. The major single exon of the V region follows, with the bases specifying the last 4 or 5 amino acids of the leader and the 95 amino acids coded by the $V_\kappa$ gene. The V gene terminates with a sequence CACAGTG, a heptamer, followed by a 12-base spacer, TTACACACCCGA, followed by a nanomer, ACATAAACC. These sequences and their spatial configuration have a functional importance in the recombinations between gene segments.

Within the coding sequence, the greatest differences among members of the same family of V sequences are found in those regions coding for the CDRs 1, 2, and 3. Amino acid residues 89 to 95 represent most of CDR 3. The remaining residues in the expressed light chain are not encoded in the V region exon per se but are derived from one of four $J_\kappa$ (or joining) segments, each of 85 bases separated one from the other by 300 base-

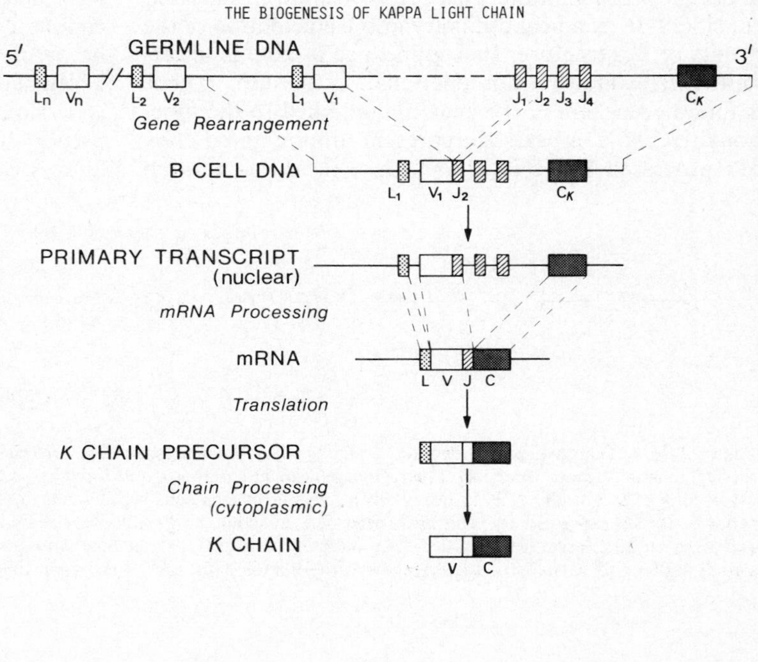


**Figure 2–4.** The biogenesis of a kappa light chain. The transition from germ line to B-lymphocyte configuration is accomplished by translocation and deletion (see text). Nuclear processing removes the transcribed introns to generate a mature mRNa.

intervening sequences.[54] The amount of germ line DNA between the Vs and the Js is not known. The single kappa constant region exon is located 2.5 kilobases (kb) 3′ to the 4th $J_\kappa$ segment. Each $J_\kappa$ contains the 39 nucleotides sufficient to code for the amino acids comprising the c-terminal portion of CDR 3, framework region 4, and some 30 nucleotides of flanking sequence on either side. The constant region segment codes for the remaining amino acids (109–214), the termination codon, and a 3′ untranslated region of 180 bases followed by a polyadenylation signal AATAAA.[55] This germ line organization of the kappa locus is found in the DNA of sperm, oocytes, and all nonlymphoid tissues (Fig. 2–4). The changes that occur in the course of B lymphocyte differentiation will be described below.

**Lambda Chain Germ Line Genes.** The lambda chain locus on chromosome 22 has a similar general configuration in the germ line but has certain attributes that are distinct.[56] First, its constellation of V genes is uniquely its own. Amino acid sequence analysis has indicated that there are at least six $V_\lambda$ subgroups[57] (versus four $V_\kappa$ subgroups). It is likely that the greatest differences between human and mouse Ig genes will be found at this locus, since λ-chain-containing molecules comprise only 5 percent of the total murine antibody population but 30 to 40 percent of human immunoglobulins. There is little experimental data currently available concerning the makeup of the $V_\lambda$ complex in humans. The $J_\lambda$ constant region segment has been the subject of intense investigation in both species. In contrast to the $C_\kappa$ locus, which contains only one gene, the human $C_\lambda$ locus contains at least six nonallelic genes, which are spread over approximately 50 kb of DNA.[58] One of these genes has been shown to have its own J segment, a feature likely to be shared by all the functional $C_\lambda$ genes.[59] This structural feature has also been noted in murine lambda genes. Thus, in contrast to the kappa locus, there is no discrete $J_\lambda$ cluster. In the center of the $C_\lambda$ cluster is a region that seems to be particularly predisposed to undergo recombination. This predisposition has created considerable technical difficulty in the elucidation of the details of $C_\lambda$ structure. Its significance in vivo is uncertain. Interestingly, a nonfunctional, or pseudo, λ gene is found elsewhere in the genome, unlinked to the functional locus. It appears to represent an integrated copy of a processed λ mRNA.[60] As with κ, the differentiation of a cell along the B lymphocyte pathway to become a λ-expressing lymphocyte or plasma cell is associated with alterations in the germ line gene configuration.

**Heavy Chain Germ Line Genes.** The heavy chain locus on chromosome 14 exhibits a germ line composition similar to, but more complex than, those coding for the two light chain classes[61] (Fig. 2–5). Again, the most 5′ portion of the heavy chain complex is the V region cluster. Protein sequence data have suggested that there are three $V_H$ subgroups, hence three $V_H$ gene families. There is considerable homology between human and mouse $V_H$ gene families; the same DNA probes have been used to determine the size of particular $V_H$ groups in both species.[62] These experiments suggested that there might be 2- to 3-fold more members of the human $V_{HIII}$ gene subgroup.[63] Additional studies in the mouse have indicated that the $V_H$ genes of different subgroups were not intermingled. Within the subgroups it has been found that $V_H$ genes may be separated from each other by 8 to 16 kb of noncoding sequence.[64]

The structure of individual $V_H$ genes is quite similar to that of $V_L$. There is an exon that codes for most of the hydrophobic signal sequence followed by an intron of 84 ($V_{HI}$) or 104 ($V_{HIII}$) base pairs (depending on the particular $V_H$ subgroup). This is followed by an exon containing the remainder (usually four or five amino acids) of the leader sequence and V region amino acids 1 to 94, followed by two base pairs, then the consensus recombination sequence CACAGTG–21 base pair spacer–GACACAAACC.

The first major organizational departure of the heavy chain locus from that of the light chains is the presence of a region containing at least three and perhaps more families of D (diversity) segments.[65] To date, families have been described which contain from 2 to 9 D segments. The segments themselves contain about 30 nucleotides and are flanked on both sides by the heptamer–12 or 13 base pair spacer–nanomer consensus recombination signal. The families thus far described have been spread over 30 to 60 kb of sequence. These codons contribute to the amino acids comprising the heavy chain CDR 3 (vide infra).[66] 3′ to the bulk of the D segment region is the $J_H$ cluster. Included in the cluster is a single, presumably functional D segment, three pseudo $J_H$ genes, and six bona fide $J_H$ segments[67] (Fig. 2–5). Each functional J is comprised of the nanomer-

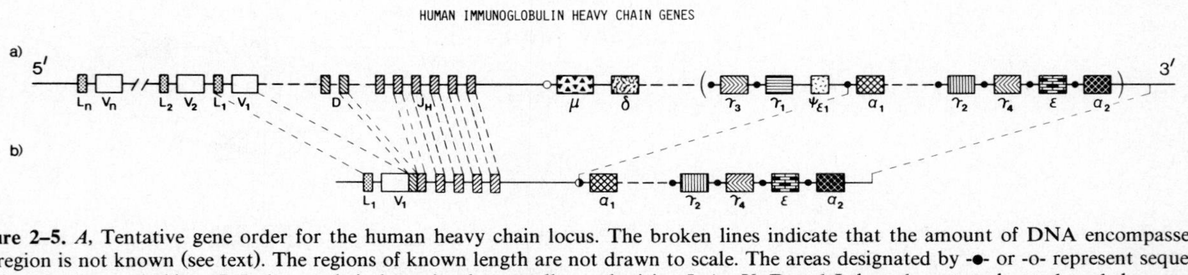


**Figure 2–5.** *A*, Tentative gene order for the human heavy chain locus. The broken lines indicate that the amount of DNA encompassed by the region is not known (see text). The regions of known length are not drawn to scale. The areas designated by -●- or -o- represent sequences involved in class switching. *B*, Ig heavy chain locus in plasma cells synthesizing $IgA_1$. V, D and $J_H$ have been translocated, and the germ line genes 5′ to the expressed $\alpha_1$ gene have been deleted from the productively rearranged chromosome. The constant region genes 3′ to the expressed $\alpha_1$ gene have been retained. The intron 5′ to the $C_\alpha 1$ exon now contains a switch region comprised partially of the germ line μ switch region and partially of sequences from the homologous area of the germ line $\alpha_1$ gene (-◑-).

21-23 base pair spacer-heptamer, 45 to 60 base pairs of coding sequence followed by a consensus splice site (vide infra). From the 3′ end of $J_H6$ is a region of 2000 base pairs extending approximately 3 kb that is involved in the class switch. It consists of multiple tandem repeats of the sequence GGCCTGAGCTGAGCTGAACT, with some variation in the repeats, and is 90 percent homologous with the murine sequence that has been demonstrated to be utilized in the switching of the cell from the synthesis of one class of Ig to another, e.g., from IgM to IgG (vide infra).[68]

Approximately 1.5 kb further downstream is the first exon of the $\mu$ constant region gene.[67–70] The $C_\mu$ gene is the most 5′ of the heavy chain constant region genes. It contains 5 exons. The first four of these code for the four $\mu$ chain domains found in serum IgM. $C_\mu1$ contains *306* bases; it is followed by an intron of 130 bases, $C_\mu2$ (330 bases), an intervening sequence (IVS) of 242 bases, $C_\mu3$ (317 bases), an IVS of approximately 150 nucleotides, and $C_\mu4$, 387 bases coding for the carboxy-terminal domain of the $\mu$ chain. This is followed by 101 bases of 3′ untranslated DNA and the polyadenylation signal (AATAAA). At 1.9 kb 3′ to the end of $C_\mu4$ are 2 exons separated by a small intron. They encode a protein segment of 39 amino acids that is hydrophobic and represents the portion of the $\mu$ chain that is anchored in the cell membrane when the cell expresses IgM as a cell-bound receptor[68,71] (Fig. 2–6).

The general structure, comprising separate exons coding for each protein domain with consensus splice signals at the 5′ and 3′ termini of each exon, is characteristic of all the human heavy chain genes. Further, the presence of small "membrane" exons at a distance 3′ to the carboxy-terminal coding exon has been demonstrated to be characteristic of each $\gamma$ class in the mouse and is probably true in humans.[72] $C_\mu$ and $C_\epsilon$ have four relatively equally sized exons, while the $C_\delta$, $C_\gamma$, and $C_\alpha$ genes have three similar exons coding for $C_H1$, $C_H2$, and $C_H3$ but, between the first and second domains, we find a small separate exon coding for the hinge segment[73] (Fig. 2–7). The exons in all the genes are separated by introns. The intron sequences, apart from the intron-exon borders, show much less conservation of sequence than the exons.

In humans, $C_\delta$ is located some 5000 bases 3′ to the end of $C_\mu4$ and approximately 3000 nucleotides 3′ to $C_{\mu m}$, a spacing quite similar to that in the mouse. The human and mouse IgD heavy chains vary considerably, and little more is known about the human genes. The murine $\delta$ gene has been fully sequenced.[74] It is likely that the human gene will share some but not all of its features. All of the intron-exon borders in both are marked by consensus splice sequences.[75] The distance between the $\delta$ gene and the next heavy chain gene in the human genome is not known, while in the mouse, $\delta$ and $C_\gamma3$ have been linked with an intervening segment of 55,000 bases.[76] Although the general structure of the remaining individual heavy chain constant region genes is similar in the two species, their organization and number appear to differ. Hence, the distances between the $\mu$ and $\delta$ genes and the $\gamma$, $\epsilon$, $\alpha$ complex may not be comparable.

The available data suggest that in the human genome the presently identified heavy chain genes 3′ of $\mu$ and $\delta$ exist as two separate clusters.[77] The most 5′ of the clusters consists of $C_\gamma3$, 26 kb of intervening sequence; $C_\gamma1$, a 19-kb IVS; a pseudo-$\epsilon$ gene; a 13-kb IVS; and the $\alpha_1$ gene. The cluster is separated by an undetermined interval from a second homologous cluster containing $C_\gamma2$, an 18-kb intron; $C_\gamma4$, 23 kb of intervening DNA; $C_\epsilon$, a 10-kb IVS, followed by $C_\alpha2$ (Fig. 2–5). This type of genomic structure, deduced in part from the analysis of the DNA of individuals showing a germ line deletion of the $\gamma_1$, $\gamma_2$, $\gamma_4$, and $\alpha$ genes, suggests that not only did the individual Ig genes evolve by duplication of an original domain-sized unit but that an entire cluster of relatively mature constant region genes may have duplicated in the period after the primate and murine lineages separated.[78]

Each of the genes in the two human clusters exhibit the prototypic exon-intron structure plus the presence of a region 5′ to the $C_H1$ exon which participates in the class switching process. It comprises approximately 2.7 kb located about 2 kb 5′ to the $C_H1$ exon, which is homologous to a similar region 5′ to $C_\mu1$ and highly conserved between mouse and human. Similar sequences have been identified 5′ to the constant region genes for

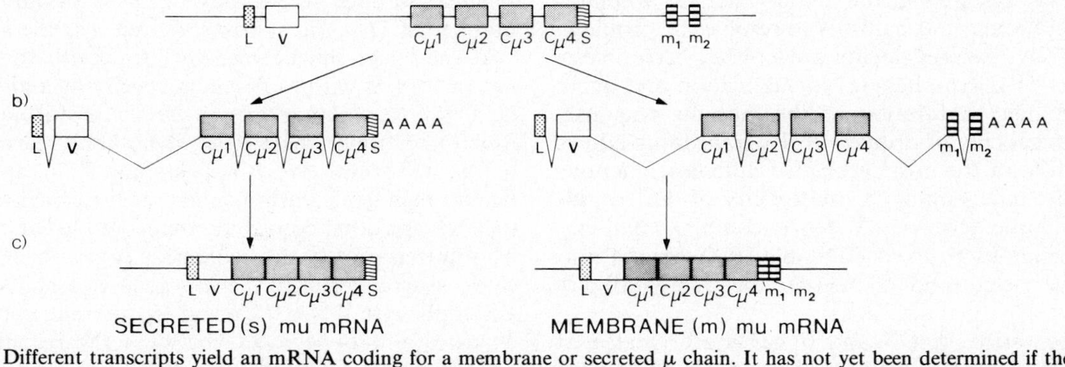


**Figure 2–6.** Different transcripts yield an mRNA coding for a membrane or secreted $\mu$ chain. It has not yet been determined if the transcript coding for $\mu_s$ results from termination at the first polyadenylation signal or from alternative processing of a single transcript extending from V to $\mu_m$.

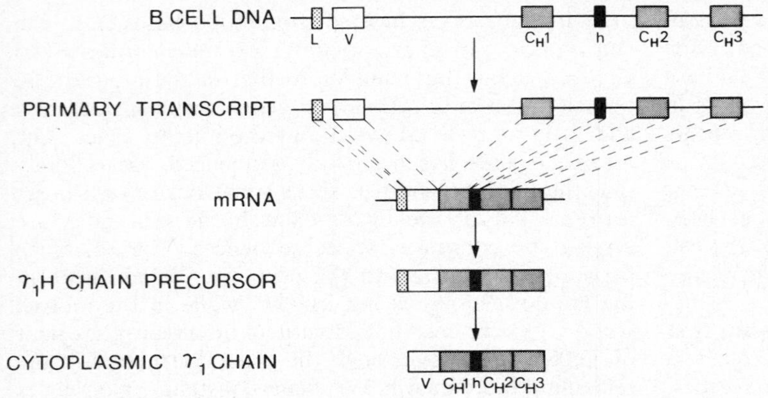


**Figure 2–7.** The exon-intron structure of a rearranged $\gamma_1$ heavy chain gene. Each domain is coded by a single exon. The introns are removed from the primary transcript in the nucleus. Splice junctions, sites from which introns have been removed, generally have the dinucleotide GT on the 5′ (donor) side and AG on the 3′ (acceptor) side. The rearranged heavy chain gene contains six exons derived from two genes.

the remaining $\gamma$, $\epsilon$, and $\alpha$ heavy chains. The pseudo-$\epsilon$ gene between $C_\gamma 1$ and $C_\alpha 1$ lacks sequences coding for $C_H1$ and $C_H2$ and cannot be expressed.[79] A second human pseudo-$\epsilon$ gene has been identified unlinked to either cluster and localized to chromosome 9.[80]

As expected, all four identified $C_\gamma$ genes have similar structures. $C_\gamma 3$ shows the only departure in that its hinge region is coded by four exons of 59 bases (H1) and 53 bases (H2, H3, H4) separated by IVS (not shown).[81] Such a structure was predicted on the basis of amino acid sequence analysis of human heavy chain disease proteins in which the heavy chain deletions seemed to end at hinge segment borders.[82] A pseudo-$\gamma_1$ gene has also been identified, but its location in the cluster has not been established.[81] The presence of at least one additional gamma gene has been hypothesized on the basis of amino acid sequence data; however, since it has not yet been isolated, its existence remains putative.[83]

## B LYMPHOCYTE DIFFERENTIATION

Given these gene structures, which are present in all cells, how do B lymphocytes manage to produce up to $10^6$ different antibody specificities, which can be expressed either on the cell surface or as secreted molecules with different biologic functions, without totally reconstructing the system in every generation? Evolution appears to have resulted in the employment of a combination of molecular mechanisms to resolve the problem. Specific DNA rearrangements are utilized early in the preparation of B lymphocytes for activation and again in the serologic maturation of the immune response. Differential splicing of primary RNA transcripts allows the utilization of the same genes for different functions at the same time. Finally, a multiplicity of devices, including multiple germ line V genes, complex combinatorial associations to form CDR 3′s, and somatic mutation have been used to insure adequate antibody diversity.

The observation that V and C genes are located at an enormous distance from each other in embryonic DNA was followed by experiments indicating that the distance is much smaller in immunoglobulin-expressing lymphocytes and plasma cells.[84] T lymphocyte DNA in general, with some exceptions, and the DNA of non-lymphoid organs are maintained in the germ line configuration with respect to immunoglobulin genes.[85]

**Gene Rearrangements.** It appears that the first recognizable event occurring in the Ig genes of a cell of B lineage is the rearrangement of a D segment to a $J_H$ segment.[67] The coupling is mediated by the heptamer-spacer-nanomer sequences. It has been established that the spacer length is critical, in that an element with a 12 base pair (bp) spacer can only recombine with an element containing a 23–25 base pair spacer.[86] Hence, the 5′ spacer sequence of each $J_H$ has a 25 bp sequence while the D segment has a 12 bp spacer on both the 3′ and 5′ sides. The DNA between the recombining D and J segments may be deleted during the process, while the DNA between the utilized J and $C_\mu$ is retained. The recombined D still has a free recombination site with a 12 bp spacer present on its 5′ side. This site is now available for recombination with a $V_H$ gene. All the $V_H$ genes have a recombination signal with a 23–25 bp spacer at their 3′ termini; therefore, VDJ–$\mu$ joining can readily occur. The VDJ junction is reflected in the amino acid sequence of CDR 3. Hence, the protein product of the same germ line $V_H$ gene can vary in its CDR 3 depending upon which D and J are involved in the recombination. Further, there is imprecision in the D segment joining, which may result in variability in the number of D segment bases included in the site.

If the bases can be read in frame with the $V_H$ gene, i.e., in triplets with each codon specifying a given amino acid, the recombination will be successful and yield a functional heavy chain gene; if not, the rearrangement will be nonproductive. It appears that if a nonproductive heavy chain gene rearrangement occurs, the heavy chain locus on the other copy of chromosome 14 can rearrange. The presence of both a successfully and a nonproductively rearranged heavy chain gene is very common in B lymphocyte DNA.[87] During $V_H$ rearrangement all the V genes and D segments between the recombining V and D may be deleted from that chromosome. A cell that has successfully rearranged its heavy chain genes may also be identified as a pre-B lymphocyte by the presence of $\mu$ or, less commonly, other heavy chain polypeptide chains in the cytoplasm.[88]

Light chain gene rearrangement appears to follow successful heavy chain rearrangement, although it is not clear what signals the light chain chromosome to rearrange. The process is simpler, since only $V_L$ and $J_L$ have to recombine. Again the process is mediated by the consensus recombination sequence, with V carrying a 12 bp spacer and J a 23 bp spacer. The intervening DNA between the rearranging V and J is deleted.[89] The third CDR varies with the choice of J segment utilized in the recombination.

In most B lymphocytes, from data obtained in normal and leukemic human lymphocytes, it appears that after H chain rearrangement, $\kappa$ chain genes rearrange first; if neither of the $\kappa$ chromosomes is successfully rearranged, $\lambda$ genes are free to rearrange until a successful event occurs.[85-87,89-91] At present, the data suggest that the apparent $\kappa$, $\lambda$ hierarchy is stochastic rather than mechanistic, reflecting the larger $V_\kappa$ repertoire.[87] In either case the biologic signals that initiate and control the process have not been identified.

**Allelic Exclusion.** It has been noted for many years that immunoglobulin-producing cells exhibit what has been termed allelic exclusion. Each B lymphocyte expresses the immunoglobulin genes coded by only one of the pair of parental chromosomes. The term "allelic exclusion" implied a positive genetic mechanism controlling the utilization of only one of two available alleles. From the foregoing, it appears that allelic exclusion is a result, rather than a cause, of a mechanism giving each B lymphocyte precursor the greatest possible chance to express its V region repertoire. It is evident on all three Ig-coding chromosomes and implies that there must be regulatory elements that can sense when successful rearrangements have occurred. The first productive heavy chain gene rearrangement should turn off the translocation mechanism at the allelic locus. The evidence to date suggests that it also initiates rearrangement of one copy of the $\kappa$ locus (chromosome 2) without activating the other copy or the similar $\lambda$ locus on chromosome 22. The stimulus to each of these events may be the protein product itself (i.e., the synthesized $\mu$ chain), its mRNA, the conformation of the rearranged gene, or some other molecule, either protein or nucleic acid, coded by the rearranged gene.

**Differential Processing of Immunoglobulin Gene Transcripts.** The successfully rearranged heavy and light chain genes must be transcribed and translated in order to be expressed as proteins. The primary transcripts include both the exons and the intervening sequences. Processing then occurs that utilizes consensus splice sequences found at each intron–exon border to remove the nonstructural RNA[75] (Figs. 2–4 and 2–5). This process is not specific for immunoglobulin molecules, since almost all eukaryotic protein coding genes contain introns that must be spliced out after transcription. All the intron sequences are removed, leaving only coding sequences in the final cytoplasmic mRNA. Similarly, the transcription termination signal for all genes appears to be the AATAA site, which specifies that adenylic acid residues (poly-A) should be added to the transcript within 20 to 30 bases downstream.[55]

The B lymphocyte uses these mechanisms in the same way as other cells; however, it also uses them to segregate heavy chains within the cell (Fig. 2–6). Studies utilizing murine B lymphocyte tumors indicate that if the $\mu$ chain is to be expressed on the cell surface, the transcript includes the large intervening sequence 3′ to $C_\mu 4$ and the two membrane exons and recognizes the polyadenylation site 3′ to the gene segment encoding the hydrophobic membrane insertion site. During processing, the usual introns are excised, as is the sequence between $C_\mu 4$ and $C_{\mu m}$, and a protein with a carboxy terminus appropriate to interact with the cell membrane is available. If a cytoplasmic or secreted type $\mu$ chain is to be produced, an mRNA with a poly-A tail just 3′ to the end of the $C_\mu 4$ exon is found in the cytoplasm.[92,93] No explanation was given as to how the differential polyadenylation would be controlled, but the fact is that the same specificity can be expressed on both the cell surface and as secreted antibody. The signals that allow cells to choose between membrane and secreted transcripts are not understood; however, it is likely that cells producing other immunoglobulin classes utilize the same scheme to produce membrane and secreted molecules.

The successful rearrangement of the heavy and light chain loci identify a B lymphocyte as having specificity and as being capable of responding to the appropriate antigen. Many early B lymphocytes express both IgM and IgD of the same specificity on the cell surface. If only IgM is synthesized, the $C_\delta$ gene is fully methylated.[94] In the mouse, and presumably the human, if both chains are to be expressed, neither is methylated and a single long transcript encompassing VDJ–$C_\mu$, the IVS between the $\mu$ and $\delta$ genes, and the VDJ–$C_\delta$ introns and exons is produced. The expressed proteins reflect the differential splicing patterns. A cell expressing both $\mu$ and $\delta$ on the cell surface will have processed transcripts encompassing VDJ–$C_{\mu m}$ and some encompassing VDJ–$C_{\delta m}$, each of which has the introns and inappropriate exons spliced out. The primary transcript will also include the exons coding for the secretory c-termini of both proteins. If only SIgD is expressed, then the VDJ–$C_{\delta s}$ will be dominant. Differential processing is thus utilized to express a new class of immunoglobulin bearing the same antigen-binding specificity in its V region.[74] It is possible that the simultaneous expression of two other classes of Ig heavy chains (e.g., $\alpha$ and $\gamma$) on the surface of small numbers of normal human B lymphocytes may reflect the use of differential splicing of a long transcript.[95] However, this hypothesis has not been tested.

**Heavy Chain Class Switching.** The maturation of the immune response is characterized by the expression of the same binding specificity on immunoglobulins of different heavy chain classes with a variety of biologic effector functions. Murine myeloma cells synthesizing a given Ig heavy chain, e.g., $\gamma_{2b}$, were found to have one chromosome unrearranged or with its $J_H$ nonproductively rearranged and the other missing its $\mu$ and some $\gamma$ genes.[96] When the germ line genes were cloned and placed in order on the chromosome, it was found that on the productively rearranged chromosome the heavy chain genes 5′ to the expressed gene were deleted up to the switch sequences adjacent to that constant region gene.[97] Observations in human lymphoid cells are consistent with those in the mouse. Further analysis of rearranged genes showed that the intervening sequence between the rearranged VDJ and $C_H1$ contained some sequences derived from the germ line $\mu$ gene, i.e., those 3′ to the J, including the region of tandem repeats, and some from the similar sequences 5′ to the germ line $C_H1$ sequence. A model was proposed suggesting that heavy chain class switching was accomplished by recombination between switch sites with deletion of the intervening DNA[96] (Fig. 2–7). It implied that switching should occur in a 5′ to 3′ order and could never go 3′ to 5′. However, one or two instances of the latter have been reported (e.g., murine $\gamma_{2b}$ to $\gamma_{2a}$), resulting in the further proposal that sister chromatid exchange might be a mechanism whereby switching could go in either direction with or without deletion, but with the 5′ to 3′ direction dominant.[98]

It is not clear whether the development of each B lymphocyte is characterized by a phase in which each heavy chain class is transiently expressed. It is also unclear what makes the switching stop, or whether potential sequences can be skipped (i.e., can a cell go directly from $\mu$ to $\alpha$?).

Phenotypic analysis indicates that switching does not take place prior to exposure to antigen and that it may be under specific T lymphocyte control.[99] Other studies, analyzing Ig class expression in human pre-B lymphocyte leukemias, suggest that switching is stochastic, a hypothesis based on the fact that the frequency of expression of the heavy chains roughly corresponds to the 5′ to 3′ order of the genes.[88] The latter type of argument is weakened by the necessarily limited sample size from which the frequency distribution was determined.

**Isotype Exclusion.** It has thus emerged that the general observations that each antibody-producing cell expresses only one heavy chain and one light chain bearing specificity for only one antigen (apart from considerations of crossreactivity) have a basis in the DNA coding for the polypeptides. The cell does not choose to express $\kappa$ or $\lambda$. It can only rearrange a $\lambda$ gene if it has failed to successfully activate $\kappa$.

With respect to the heavy chain chromosome, it is apparent that the deletional mechanism precludes cellular expression of two heavy chains simultaneously. Genes coding for $\mu$ and $\delta$ may be a special case because of their proximity and their relatively specialized function on the cell surface. However, it appears that when IgD is expressed as a secreted protein, as in IgD myeloma, the 5′ $\mu$ gene is deleted.[100] Recent data in the mouse have also suggested that IgE-bearing cells have not deleted their 5′ genes.[101] Hence, it may be that the deletional mechanism is active in all Ig secretory plasma cells but not necessarily in B lymphocytes with primarily surface Ig expression. The cloned or single human B lymphocytes that have been reported to express two classes of Ig other than IgM and IgD on the cell surface may be the result of differential splicing of long transcripts.[95]

## ANTIBODY DIVERSITY

The immune system is capable of expressing the same antigen-binding specificity coded in the V region as an antibody of any heavy chain class expressed either as a membrane or secreted molecule. Much of the diversity found in the V-region repertoire can be accounted for by a large number of germ line $V_H$ and $V_L$ genes coupled with the enormous variability in CDR3 generated by the various types of combinatorial joining, i.e., $V_LJ_L$ and $V_HDJ_H$. However, there are two other mechanisms utilized to expand the variability of response. One is the selection of different pairs of activated heavy and light chains, which may generate diversity in the tertiary structure of the binding site. While there is much circumstantial evidence suggesting specific interactions between heavy and light chain coding genes, particularly in the regulation of rearrangement and synthesis, there is little knowledge of how these events take place.

Recent data, obtained primarily in the mouse, have clearly demonstrated that somatic mutation in rearranged heavy and light chain V region genes can add substantially to the diversity of the antibody response.[102,103] Much of the mutational activity seems to localize to CDRs 1 and 2, although some has also been noted in CDR3. It has been suggested that somatic mutation in $V_H$ regions is more likely to occur in $\gamma$ and $\alpha$ proteins than in IgM antibodies, i.e., after the class switch.[104]

A small number of germ line V genes have now been subjected to nucleotide sequencing, and it is striking that almost 40 percent of the analyzed genes appear to be pseudogenes, that is, incapable of coding for a functional V gene.[63] Nonetheless, some of them may be available for recombination events and could be responsible for some of the nonproductive gene rearrangements noted so frequently.

## EVOLUTIONARY CONSIDERATIONS

DNA analysis has added substantially to our concepts of how the Ig loci have evolved. While protein sequences certainly indicate that the basic unit of evolution was the single protein domain, nucleic acid studies have shown unequivocally that even in the heavy chain polypeptides, which are the result of multiple duplications, a domain-sized unit, the exon, is retained as the basic genomic structure. The conservation of regions, not expressed at the protein level, which are required for the expression of complete functional immunoglobulins, e.g., 5′ regulatory sequences, switch sequences, and splice junctions, suggests that polymorphism is poorly tolerated at some sites.

The phenomenon of gene conversion among tandemly arranged homologous Ig genes has only been appreciated recently with the observations that different alleles at the murine $IgG_{2a}$ locus differ not only by mutation but by the substitution of an exon-length segment from the adjacent $IgG_{2b}$ gene for the original $IgG_{2a}$ exon.[105] A similar process has been suggested for the genesis of the human $\gamma_3$ gene.[81] While the mechanism of gene conversion is not understood, the ability of tandem genes, each bearing regions of homology, to recombine in a variety of locations with either its paired chromosome, its sister chromatid, or even itself can allow for both expansion and contraction of the size of a gene family and yet retain the structural features necessary for the protein products of the locus.[106]

A good example of this phenomenon, with respect to immunoglobulins, are the $\gamma$ chain subclasses. The mouse and human both have four $\gamma$ subclasses identified to date. In each species the homology among the classes is greater than that between any combination of human and mouse subclasses, suggesting that in each species the four classes arose independently, yet the complex appears to have evolved similarly in the two species. The analyses above imply that gene conversion has occurred between members of the group in both man and mouse, presumably responding to the same evolutionary pressures.

## IMPLICATIONS FOR DISEASE

Humans, as an outbred experimental species, would be expected to show substantial polymorphism. Many of the analyses of human Ig genes have noted so-called restriction enzyme polymorphism in the human Ig loci. These are characterized by the presence of differently sized pieces of DNA carrying identifiable Ig genes when germ line (unrearranged) DNA is digested by a given enzyme. Some of these have been noted around the switch site of the $\mu$ gene and appear to be inherited in a Mendelian fashion linked to Gm loci.[107] In addition, recent data from experiments utilizing inbred mouse strains strongly suggest that $V_H$ gene families may be inherited linked to heavy chain loci.[108] None of this should be terribly surprising, since the linkage analysis confirms what we already know from looking at the DNA of the chromosome. However, if specific human $V_H$ families containing the structural genes for certain antibodies are either increased or diminished in some individuals, they may be at greater or lesser risk for disease states characterized by enhanced or reduced production of those antibodies.

While most of the markers that have shown increased associations with rheumatic diseases have been on chromosome 6, i.e., the MHC locus (see Chapters 4 and 5), it is possible that investigations of the Ig loci may prove fruitful and that analysis of $V_H$ polymorphic profiles may be informative with respect to the pathogenesis of rheumatic diseases.[109]

The genetic mechanisms responsible for retaining the structural features of the immunoglobulin proteins over the centuries have managed to amplify a relatively limited amount of genetic information by employing recombinational events among various elements, post-transcriptional differential processing, somatic mutation, and combinatorial association between gene products to simultaneously generate common structures with enormous variation in specificity and families of proteins with the same or similar specificities and multiple biologic effector functions. The present Ig genes represent one set of constraints under which the B-lymphocyte arm of the immune response operates. The role of these genes in T lymphocyte function has not been established. While there is much circumstantial evidence indicating that Ig $V_H$ gene products function in T lymphocytes, attempts to demonstrate functional rearrangements of Ig genes in these cells have failed. Recently, work from several laboratories has established that the T-lymphocyte antigen receptor is composed of two nonimmunoglobulin polypeptide chains.[110-113] The gene family coding for one of these chains has been identified and shown to have a structure similar to that coding for Ig heavy chains with V, D, J, and C segments, which appear to rearrange by translocation to yield the active genes. Hence the generation of T-lymphocyte specificity seems to involve the same general process as does that of B lymphocytes but an independent set of similar gene segments carried on different chromosomes.

## References


1. World Health Organization: WHO Bul. J. Immunol. 35:953, 1966; 38:151, 1968; 41:975, 1969; 108:1733, 1972. Eur. J. Immunol. 6:599, 1976.
2. Natvig, J.B., and Kunkel, H.G.: Human immunoglobulins: Classes, subclasses, genetic variants, and idiotypes. Adv. Immunol. 16:1, 1973.
3. Lamm, M.D.: Cellular aspects of immunoglobulin A. Adv. Immunol. 22:223, 1976.
4. Koshland, M.E.: Structure and function of the J chain. Adv. Immuno. 20:41, 1975.
5. Caserto, J.P., and Kress, B.P.: $\beta_2$M, a tumor marker of lymphoproliferative disorders. Lancet 2:108, 1978.
6. Ervin, P.E., and Wibell, L.: The serum levels and urinary excretion of $\beta_2$-microglobulin in apparently healthy subjects. Scand. J. Clin. Lab. Invest. 29:69, 1982.
7. Poulik, M.D., and Reisfeld, R.A.: $\beta_2$-Microglobulins. *In* Inman, F.P., and Mandy, W.J. (eds.): Contemporary Topics in Molecular Immunology. Vol. 4. New York, Plenum Press, 1975.
8. Peterson, P.A., Cunningham, B.A., Berggard, I., and Edelman, G.M.: $\beta_2$-microglobulin: A free immunoglobulin domain. Proc. Natl. Acad. Sci. (USA) 69:1697, 1972.
9. Snell, G.D., Dausset, J., and Nathenson, S.G.: Histocompatibility. New York, Academic Press, 1976.
10. Ploegh, H.L., Orr, H.T., and Strominger, J.L.: Major histocompatibility antigens: The human (HLA-A, -B, -C) and murine (H-2K, H-2D) class I molecules. Cell 24:287, 1981.
11. Klein, J., Juretic, A., Baxevanis, C.N., and Nagy, Z.A.: The traditional and a new version of the mouse H-2 complex. Nature 291:455, 1981.
12. Williams, A.F., and Gagnon, J.: Neuronal cell Thy-l glycoprotein: Homology with immunoglobulins. Science 216:696, 1982.
13. Kabat, E.A., Wu, T.T., and Bilofsky, H.: Variable regions of immunoglobulin chains. Tabulations and analyses of amino acid sequence. Bethesda, Maryland, National Institutes of Health, 1983.
14. Capra, J.D., and Kehoe, J.M.: Hypervariable regions, idiotype and the antibody combining site. Adv. Immunol. 20:1, 1975.
15. Porter, R.R.: The combining sites of antibodies. Harvey Lect. 65:157, 1971.
16. Edelman, G.M., Cunningham, W.E., Gall, P.D., Gottlieb, H., Rutishau-

ser, U., and Waxdal, M.J.: The covalent structure of entire $IgG_1$ immunoglobulin molecule. Proc. Natl. Acad. Sci. (USA) 63:78, 1969.
17. Spiegelberg, H.: Biological activities of immunoglobulins of different classes and subclasses. Adv. Immunol. 19:259, 1974.
18. Frangione, B., Milstein, C., and Franklin, E.C.: Chemical typing of immunoglobulins. Nature 221:149, 1969.
19. Michaelsen, T.E., Frangione, B., and Franklin, E.C.: Primary structure of the "hinge" region of human IgG3. J. Biol. Chem. 253:883, 1977.
20. Recht, B., Frangione, B., Franklin, E.C., and van Loghem, E.: Structural studies of a human $\gamma_3$myeloma protein (GOE) that binds staph protein A. J. Immunol. 127:917, 1981.
21. Haake, D.A., Franklin, E.C., and Frangione, B.: The modification of human immunoglobulin binding to staphylococcal protein A using diethylpyrocarbonate. J. Immunol. 129:190, 1982.
22. Mestecky, J., and Schrohenloher, R.E.: Site of attachment of J chain to human immunoglobulin M. Nature 249:650, 1974.
23. Fu, S.M., Winchester, R.J., and Kunkel, H.G.: Occurrence of surface IgM, IgD, and free light chains on human lymphocytes. J. Exp. Med. 139:1451, 1974.
24. Vitetta, E.A., and Uhr, J.W.: Immunoglobulin-receptors revisited. A model for the differentiation of bone marrow-derived lymphocytes is described. Science 189:964, 1975.
25. Putnam, F.: Immunoglobulins. I. Structure. *In* Putnam, F.W. (ed.): The Plasma Proteins: Structure, Function and Genetic Control. New York, Academic Press, 1977.
26. Rogers, J., Early, P., Carter, C., Calame, K., Bond, M., Hood, L., and Wall, R.: Two mRNA's with different 3' ends encode membrane-bound and secreted forms of immunoglobulin $\mu$ chain. Cell 20:303, 1980.
27. Lobb, C.J., and Clem, L.W.: Phylogeny of immunoglobulin structure and function XII. Secretory immunoglobulins in the bile of the marine teleost *Archosargus probatocephalus.* Mol. Immunol. 18:615, 1981.
28. Gowans, J.L., and Knight, E.J.: The route of recirculating lymphocytes in the rat. Proc. Royal Soc. (Series B) 159:257, 1964.
29. Craig, S.W., and Cebra, J.J.: Rabbits' Peyer's patches, appendix and popliteal lymph node lymphocytes: A comparative analysis of their membrane immunoglobulin components and plasma cell precursor potential. J. Immunol. 114:492, 1975.
30. McWilliams, M., Phillips-Quagliata, J., and Lamm, M.E.: Mesenteric node B lymphoblasts which home to the small intestine are precommitted to IgA synthesis. J. Exp. Med. 145:866, 1977.
31. McDermott, M.R., and Bienenstock, J.: Evidence for a common mucosal immunological system. I. Migration of B immunoblasts into intestinal, respiratory and genital tissues. J. Immunol. 122:1892, 1979.
32. Roux, M.E., McWilliams, M., Phillips-Quagliata, J., and Lamm, M.E.: Differentiation pathway of Peyer's patch precursors of IgA plasma cells in the secretory immune system. Cell. Immunol. 61:141, 1981.
33. Tomasi, T.B., Jr.: The gamma A globulins. First line of defense. *In* Good, R.A., and Fisher, D.W. (eds.): Immunobiology. Stamford, Connecticut, Sinauer, 1971.
34. Garcia-Pardo, A., Lamm, M.E., Plaut, A.G., and Frangione, B.: Secretory component is covalently bound to a single subunit in human secretory IgA. Immunochemistry 16:477, 1979.
35. Plaut, A.G., Genco, R.J., and Tomasi, T.B., Jr.: Isolation of an enzyme from Streptococcus sanguis which specifically cleaves IgA. J. Immunol. 113:289, 1974.
36. Mulks, M.H., Plaut, A.G., Feldman, H.A., and Frangione, B.: IgA proteases of two distinct specificities are released by Neiseria Meningitidis. J. Exp. Med. 152:1442, 1980.
37. Cann, G.M., Zaritsky, A., and Koshland, M.E.: Primary structure of the immunoglobulin J chain from the mouse. Proc. Natl. Acad. Sci. (USA) 79:6656, 1982.
38. Rowe, D.S., and Fahey, J.L.: A new class of human immunoglobulins. I. A unique myeloma protein. J. Exp. Med. 121:171, 1965.
39. Rowe, D.S., Hug, K., Forni, L., and Pernis, B.: Immunoglobulin D as a lymphocyte receptor. J. Exp. Med. 138:965, 1973.
40. Takahashi, N., Tetaert, D., Debuire, B., Lin, L.C., and Putnam, F.W.: Complete amino acid sequence of the heavy chain of human immunoglobulin D. Proc. Natl. Acad. Sci. (USA) 79:2850, 1982.
41. Ishizaka, K., Ishizaka, T., and Lee, E.H.: Biologic function of the Fc fragments of E myeloma protein. Immunochemistry 7:687, 1970.
42. Dorrington, K.J., and Bennich, H.: Structure-function relationship in human immunoglobulin E. Immunol. Rev. 41:3, 978.
43. Holowka, D., and Metzger, H.: Further characterization of the B-component of the receptor for immunoglobulin E. Molec. Immunol. 19:219, 1982.
44. Kunkel, H.G., and Kindt, T.: Allotypes and idiotypes. *In* Benaceraff, B. (ed.): Immunogenetics and Immunodeficiency. Lancaster, England, Medical and Technical Publishing Company, 1975.
45. Poljak, R.J., Amzel, L.M., Avey, H.P., Chen, B.L., Phizackerley, R.P., and Saul, F.: Three-dimensional structure of the Fab' fragment of a human immunoglobulin at 2.8Å resolution. Proc. Natl. Acad. Sci. (USA) 70:3305, 1973.
46. Davies, D.R., Padlan, E.A., and Segal, D.M.: Immunoglobulin structures at high resolution. *In* Inman, F.P., and Mandy, W.J. (eds.): Contemporary Topics in Molecular Immunology. Vol. 4. New York, Plenum Press, 1975.
47. Hozumi, N., and Tonegawa, S.: Evidence for somatic rearrangement of immunoglobulin genes coding for variable and constant region. Proc. Natl. Acad. Sci. (USA) 73:3628, 1976.
48. Malcolm, S., Barton, P., Murphy, C., Ferguson-Smith, M.A., Bentley, D.L., and Rabbitts, T.H.: Localization of human immunoglobulin $\kappa$ light gene variable region genes to the short arm of chromosome 2 by in situ hybridization. Proc. Natl. Acad. Sci. (USA) 79:4957, 1982.
49. Bentley, D.L., and Rabbitts, T.H.: Human $V_\kappa$immunoglobulin gene number: Implications for the origin of antibody diversity. Cell 24:613, 1981.
50. Rabbitts, T.H., Matthyssens, G., and Hamlyn, P.H.: Contribution of immunoglobulin heavy-chain variable region genes to antibody diversity. Nature 284:238, 1980.
51. Bentley, D.L., and Rabbitts, T.H.: Human immunoglobulin variable region genes: DNA sequences of two $V_\kappa$ genes and a pseudogene. Nature 288:730, 1980.
52. Blobel, G., and Dobberstein, B.: Transfer of proteins across membranes. I. Presence of proteolytically processed and unprocessed mascent immunoglobulin light chains on membrane-bound ribosomes of murine myeloma. J. Cell Biol. 67:834, 1975.
53. Milstein, C., Brownlee, G.G., Harrison, T.M., Mathews, M.B.: A possible precursor of immunoglobulin light chains. Nature (New Biol.) 239:117, 1972.
54. Hieter, P.A., Max, E.E., Seidman, J.G., Maizel, J.V., Jr., Leder, P.: Cloned human and mouse kappa immunoglobulin constant and J region genes conserve homology in functional segments. Cell 22:197, 1980.
55. Proudfoot, N.J., and Brownlee, G.G.: 3' Non-coding region sequences in eukaryotic messenger RNA. Nature 263:211, 1976.
56. Erikson, J., Martinis, J., and Croce, C.M.: Assignment of the genes for human $\lambda$ immunoglobulin chains to chromosome 22. Nature 294:173, 1981.
57. Kabat, E.A., Wu, T.T., Bilofsky, H., Reid-Miller, M., Perry, H.: Sequences of proteins of immunological interest. U.S. Dept. of Health and Human Services, Public Health Service, National Institutes of Health, p. 14, 1983.
58. Hieter, P.A., Hollis, G.F., Korsmeyer, S.J., Waldmann, T.A., Leder, P.: Clustered arrangement of immunoglobulin $\lambda$ constant region genes in man. Nature 294:536, 1981.
59. Taub, R.A., Hollis, G.F., Hieter, P.A., Korsmeyer, S., Waldmann, T.A., and Leder, P.: Variable amplification of immunoglobulin $\lambda$ light chain genes in human populations. Nature 304:172, 1983.
60. Hollis, G.F., Hieter, P.A., McBride, O.W., Sloan, D., Leder, P.: Processed genes: A dispersed human immunoglobulin gene bearing evidence of RNA-type processing. Nature 296:321, 1982.
61. Croce, C.M., Shander, M., Martinis, J., Cicurel, L., D'Ancona, G., Dolby, T.W., and Koprowski, H.: Chromosomal location of the genes for human immunoglobulin heavy chain. Proc. Natl. Acad. Sci. (USA) 76:3416, 1979.
62. Matthyssens, G., and Rabbitts, T.H.: Structure and multiplicity of genes for the human immunoglobulin heavy chain variable region. Proc. Natl. Acad. Sci. (USA) 77:6561, 1980.
63. Rechavi, G., Bienz, B., Ram, D., Ben-Neriah, Y., Cohen, J.B., Zakut, R., and Givol, D.: Organization and evolution of immunoglobulin $V_H$ subgroups. Proc. Natl. Acad. Sci. (USA) 79:4405, 1982.
64. Rechavi, G., Ram, D., Glazer, L., Zakut, R., Givol, D.: Evolutionary aspects of immunoglobulin heavy chain variable region ($V_H$) gene subgroups. Proc. Natl. Acad. Sci. (USA) 80:855, 1983.
65. Siebenlist, U., Ravetch, J.V., Korsmeyer, S., Waldmann, T., and Leder, P.: Human immunoglobulin D-segments encoded in tandem multigenic families. Nature 294:631, 1981.
66. Schilling, J., Clevinger, B., Davie, J.M., and Hood, L.: Amino acid sequence of homogeneous antibodies to dextran and DNA rearrangements in heavy chain V-region gene segments. Nature 283:35, 1980.
67. Ravetch, J.V., Siebenlist, U., Korsmeyer, S., Waldmann, T., and Leder, P.: Structure of the human immunoglobulin $\mu$ locus: Characterization of embryonic and rearranged J and D genes. Cell 27:583, 1981.
68. Rabbitts, T.H., Forster, A., and Milstein, C.P.: Human immunoglobulin heavy chain genes: Evolutionary comparisons of $C_\mu$, $C_\delta$, and $C_\gamma$ genes and associated switch sequences. Nucleic Acids Res. 9:4509, 1981.
69. Ravetch, J.V., Kirsch, I.R., and Leder, P.: Evolutionary approach to the question of immunoglobulin heavy chain switching. Evidence from cloned human and mouse genes. Proc. Natl. Acad. Sci. (USA) 77:6734, 1980.
70. Takahashi, N., Nakai, S., Honjo, T.: Cloning of human immunoglobulin $\mu$ gene and comparison with mouse $\mu$ gene. Nucleic Acids Res. 8:5983, 1980.
71. Williams, P.B., Kubo, R.T., and Grey, H.M.: $\mu$-Chains from a nonsecretor B-cell line differ from secreted $\mu$ chains at the C-terminal end. J. Immunol. 121:2435, 1978.

72. Rogers, J., Choi, E., Souza, L., Carter, C., Word, C., Kuehl, M., Eisenberg, D., and Wall, R.: Gene segments encoding transmembrane carboxy termini of immunoglobulin $\gamma_1$ chains. Cell 26:19, 1981.
73. Ellison, J., Buxbaum, J., and Hood, L.: The nucleotide sequence of a human immunoglobulin gamma 4 constant region gene. DNA 1:11, 1981.
74. Cheng, H.L., Blattner, F.R., Fitzmaurice, L., Mushinski, J.F., and Tucker, P.W.: Structure of genes for membrane and secreted murine IgD heavy chains. Nature 296:410, 1982.
75. Breathnach, R., and Chambon, P.: Organization and expression of eukaryotic split genes coding for proteins. Ann. Rev. Biochem. 50:349, 1981.
76. Shimizu, A., Takahashi, N., Yaoita, Y., and Honjo, T.: Organization of the constant-region gene family of the mouse immunoglobulin heavy chain. Cell 28:499, 1982.
77. Flanagan, J.G., and Rabbitts, T.H.: Arrangement of human immunoglobulin heavy chain constant region genes implies evolutionary duplication of a segment containing $\gamma$, $\epsilon$ and $\alpha$ genes. Nature 300:709, 1982.
78. Lefranc, M., Lefranc, G., and Rabbitts, T.H.: Inherited deletion of immunoglobulin heavy chain constant region genes in normal human individuals. Nature 300:760, 1982.
79. Max, E.E., Battey, J., Neu, R., Kirsch, I.R., and Leder, P.: Duplication and deletion in the human immunoglobulin $\epsilon$ genes. Cell 29:691, 1982.
80. Battey, J., Max, E.E., McBride, W.O., Swan, D., and Leder, P.: A processed human immunoglobulin $\epsilon$ gene has moved to chromosome 9. Proc. Natl. Acad. Sci. (USA) 79:5956, 1982.
81. Takahashi, N., Ueda, S., Obata, M., Nikaido, T., Nakai, S., and Honjo, T.: Structure of human immunoglobulin gamma genes: Implications for evolution of a gene family. Cell 29:671, 1982.
82. Franklin, E.C., and Frangione, B.: Structural variants of human and murine immunoglobulins. *In* Inman, F.P., and Mandy, W.J. (eds.): Contemporary Topics in Molecular Immunology, Vol. 4, New York, Plenum Press, 1975.
83. Alexander, A., Steinmetz, M., Barritault, D., Frangione, B., Franklin, E.C., Hood, L., and Buxbaum, J.: Gamma heavy chain disease in man: cDNA sequence supports partial gene deletion model. Proc. Natl. Acad. Sci. (USA) 79:3260, 1982.
84. Matthyssens, G., and Tonegawa, S.: V and C parts of immunoglobulin $\kappa$-chain genes are separate in myeloma. Nature 273:763, 1978.
85. Korsmeyer, S.J., Hieter, P.A., Sharrow, S.O., Goldman, C.K., Leder, P., and Waldmann, T.: Normal human B cells display ordered light chain gene rearrangements and deletions. J. Exp. Med. 156:975, 1982.
86. Early, P., Huang, H., Davis, M., Calame, K., and Hood, L.: An immunoglobulin heavy chain variable region gene is generated from three segments of DNA: $V_H$, D and $J_H$. Cell 19:981, 1980.
87. Coleclough, C., Perry, R.P., Karjalainen, K., and Weigert, M.: Aberrant rearrangements contribute significantly to the allelic exclusion of immunoglobulin gene expression. Nature 290:372, 1981.
88. Kubagawa, H., Mayumi, M., Crist, W.M., and Cooper, M.D.: Immunoglobulin heavy-chain switching in pre-B leukemias. Nature 301:340, 1983.
89. Sakano, H., Hüppi, K., Heinrich, G., and Tonegawa, S.: Sequences at the somatic recombination sites of immunoglobulin light chains. Nature 280:288, 1979.
90. Korsmeyer, S.J., Hieter, P.A., Ravetch, J.V., Poplack, D.G., Waldmann, T.A., and Leder, P.: Developmental hierarchy of immunoglobulin gene arrangements in human leukemic pre-B cells. Proc. Natl. Acad. Sci. (USA) 78:7096, 1981.
91. Hieter, P.A., Korsmeyer, S.J., Waldmann, T.A., and Leder, P.: Human immunoglobulin $\kappa$ light chain genes are deleted or rearranged in $\lambda$-producing B-cells. Nature 290:368, 1981.
92. Early, P., Rogers, J., Davis, M., Calame, K., Bond, M., Wall, R., and Hood, L.: Two mRNA's can be producing from a single immunoglobulin $\mu$ gene by alternative RNA processing pathways. Cell 20:313, 1980.
93. Kemp, D.J., Morahan, G., Cowman, A.F., and Harris, A.W.: Production of RNA for secreted immunoglobulin $\mu$ chains does not require transcriptional termination 5′ to the $\mu_M$ exons. Nature 301:84, 1983.
94. Rogers, J., and Wall, R.: Immunoglobulin heavy chain genes: Demethylation accompanies class switching. Proc. Natl. Acad. Sci. (USA) 78:7497, 1981.
95. Vessiere-Louveaux, F.M.Y.R., Hijmans, W., and Schuit, H.R.E.: Multiple heavy chain isotypes on the membrane of the small B-lymphocytes in human blood. Clin. Exp. Immunol. 43:149, 1981.
96. Honjo, T., and Kataoka, T.: Organization of immunoglobulin heavy chain genes and allelic deletion model. Proc. Natl. Acad. Sci. (USA) 75:2140, 1978.
97. Yaoita, Y., and Honjo, T.: Deletion of immunoglobulin heavy chain genes from expressed allelic chromosome. Nature 286:850, 1980.
98. Obata, M., Kataoka, T., Nakai, S., Yamagishi, H., Takahashi, N., Yamawaki-Kataoka, Y., Nikaido, T., Shimizu, A., and Honjo, T.: Structure of a rearranged $\gamma_1$ chain gene and its implication to immunoglobulin class-switch mechanism. Proc. Natl. Acad. Sci. (USA) 78:2437, 1981.
99. Isakson, P.C., Pure, E., Vitetta, E.A., and Kramer, P.H.: T-cell derived B-cell differentiation factors. J. Exp. Med. 155:734, 1982.
100. Moore, K.W., Rogers, J., Hunkapiller, T., Early, P., Nottenburg, C., Weissman, I., Bazin, H., Wall, R., and Hood, L.E.: Expression of IgD may use both DNA rearrangement and RNA splicing mechanisms. Proc. Natl. Acad. Sci. (USA) 78:1800, 981.
101. Yaoita, Y., Kimagai, Y., Okumura, J., and Honjo, T.: Expression of lymphocyte surface IgE does not require switch recombination. Nature 297:697, 1982.
102. Selsing, E., and Storb, U.: Somatic mutation of immunoglobulin light chain variable region genes. Cell 25:47, 1981.
103. Crews, S., Griffin, J., Huang, H., Calame, K., and Hood, L.: A single $V_H$ gene segment encodes the immune response to phosphoryl choline: Somatic mutation is correlated with the class of antibody. Cell 25:59, 1981.
104. Kim, S., Davis, M., Sinn, E., Patten, P., and Hood, L.: Antibody diversity: Somatic hypermutation of rearranged $V_H$ genes. Cell 27:573, 1981.
105. Ollo, R., and Rougeon, F.: Gene conversion and polymorphism: Generation of mouse immunoglobulin $\gamma_{2a}$ chain alleles by differential gene conversion by $\gamma_{2b}$ chain gene. Cell 32:515, 1983.
106. Baltimore, D.: Gene conversion: Some implications for immunoglobulin genes. Cell 24:592, 1981.
107. Migone, N., Feder, J., Cann, H., van West, B., Hwang, H., Takahashi, N., Honjo, T., Piazza, A., and Cavalli-Sforza, L.L.: Multiple DNA fragment polymorphisms associated with immunoglobulin $\mu$ chain switch-like regions in man. Proc. Natl. Acad. Sci. (USA) 80:467, 1983.
108. Ben-Neriah, Y., Cohen, J.B., Rechavi, G., Zakut, R., Givol, D.: Polymorphism of germline immunoglobulin $V_H$ genes correlates with allotype and idiotype markers. Eur. J. Immunol. 11:1017.
109. Rechavi, G., Givol, D., and Geltner, D.: Human $V_H$ restriction length polymorphism: A possible association with autoimmune disease. Arth. Rheum. 26:S23, 1983.
110. Yanagi, Y., Yasunobo, Y., Leggett, K., Clark, S.P., Aleksander, I., and Mak, T.W.: A human T-cell specific cDNA clone encodes a protein having extensive homology to immunoglobulin chains. Nature 308:145, 1984.
111. Hedrick, S.M., Nielsen, E.A., Kavaler, J., Cohen, D.I., and Davis, M.M.: Sequence relationships between putative T-cell receptor polypeptides and immunoglobulins. Nature 308:153, 1984.
112. Chien, Y., Gascoigne, N.R.J., Kavaler, J., Lee, N.E., and Davis, M.M.: Somatic recombination in a murine T-cell receptor gene. Nature 309:322, 1984.
113. Siu, G., Clark, S.P., Yoshikai, Y., Malissen, M., Yanagi, Y., Strauss, E., Mak, T.W., and Hood, L.: The human T-cell antigen receptor is encoded by variable, diversity and joining gene segments that rearrange to generate a complete V-gene. Cell 37:393, 1984.

## *Acknowledgments*

The authors gratefully acknowledge the secretarial expertise of Beverly Coopersmith, Randi Klein, and Carol O'Brien. Work from the authors' laboratories was supported by NIH grants AM01431, AM02594 and research funds from the Veterans Administration.

# Chapter 3

# Immunologic Aspects of Inflammation: Lymphocyte Populations

*Brian L. Kotzin and Samuel Strober*

## INTRODUCTION

Although a variety of cell populations participate in the inflammatory response, the specificity of the immune response for antigen resides within the lymphocytes. Only lymphocytes have surface receptors that allow specific recognition of foreign substances and the development of antigen-specific immunologic memory. Differences in lymphocyte populations were initially defined by differences in function and organs of origin. Recently major technological advances have allowed the development of specific reagents (including monoclonal antibodies) that identify surface markers on distinct lymphocyte subpopulations. There has ensued a rapid accumulation of experimental data. Events in lymphocyte differentiation before and after antigen stimulation have been further clarified, and in addition, a series of complex lymphocyte interactions that control the immune response have been defined.

## TWO SYSTEMS OF IMMUNITY

Studies of immunity in chickens demonstrated a clear dichotomy in the immune system.[1-3] Removal of the thymus gland shortly after hatching resulted in the elimination of immune responses mediated by cells but, not those mediated by serum antibodies in irradiated birds. On the other hand, neonatal removal of the bursa of Fabricius rendered the birds agammaglobulinemic and unable to develop serum antibody responses after antigenic challenge. Cell-mediated immune responses in these bursectomized birds remained intact.

This dichotomy is also seen in two congenital immunodeficiency syndromes in humans (Table 3–1). Children with X-linked agammaglobulinemia (Bruton's syndrome) appear to have deficits similar to those of bursectomized chickens. Humoral immunity is lacking, as judged by the marked reduction in the concentration of serum immunoglobulins (~1 percent of normals), by the absence of isohemagglutinins, and by the inability to make serum antibodies to the usual vaccines (e.g., DPT vaccine). However, cell-mediated immunity is intact in these patients, as judged by the ability to reject skin allografts and to mediate delayed hypersensitivity responses to the intradermal injection of certain antigens (e.g., dinitrochlorobenzene [DNCB], streptokinase-streptodornase [SKSD], and tuberculin [PPD]). Children with Bruton's syndrome become increasingly susceptible to bacterial infections (i.e., sinusitis, pneumonia, furunculosis, meningitis) after 6 months of age when maternal antibodies begin to disappear. Viral exanthems and superficial fungal infections are generally not major threats to these children.

Children born without a thymus gland, resulting from improper development of the fourth pharyngeal pouch during embryogenesis (DiGeorge syndrome), show immune deficits similar to those of thymectomized birds. Thus, allograft rejection and delayed hypersensitivity reactions are absent, but the concentration of serum immunoglobulins is near normal. These children frequently succumb to viral infection and can develop disseminated fungal infections after superficial skin involvement.

The two systems of immunity were subsequently shown to be mediated by two different lines of lymphocytes.[4-6] Thus, B ("bursa-equivalent") lymphocytes are capable of developing from cells in the bone marrow independent of the influence of the thymus, and give rise to antibody-producing cells. The other line of cells, which requires the thymus for development, is called T (thymus-derived) lymphocytes. T and B lymphocytes are morphologically similar, although some differences have been described by electron microscopy. With the development of reagents that identify surface markers, B lymphocytes were shown to carry immunoglobulin on the cell surface. This appears to be true for all mammals studied thus far. The mouse was the first animal to be extensively studied for T lymphocyte surface antigens. Raff and his colleagues showed that nearly all cells in the thymus and the progeny of thymus cells in peripheral lymphoid tissues (spleen and lymph nodes) could be identified by antisera directed against $\theta$ (Thy-1) antigen.[5] This antigen is the product of a single genetic locus called the Thy-1 locus, which is known to have different alleles. Although all mouse T lymphocytes are recognized by anti-Thy-1 antisera, this antigen is not expressed on B lymphocytes or other hematolymphoid cells. There is no crossreactivity of this antisera with human T lymphocytes, which are recognized by their surface receptors for sheep red blood cells and more recently by surface determinants recognized by a variety of monoclonal antibodies (see below).[6]

**Table 3–1.** Dichotomy of the Immune System

| | Humoral Immunity | Cellular Immunity |
|---|---|---|
| *Effector Cell:* | B lymphocyte | T lymphocyte |
| *Defense Against:* | Extracellular organisms (e.g., pyogenic bacterial infections) | Intracellular organisms (e.g., viral, fungal, and opportunistic bacterial infections) |
| *Examples of Immuno-deficiency:* | X-linked agammaglobulinemia (Bruton's syndrome) | Congenital thymic aplasia (DiGeorge syndrome) |
| | Acquired hypogammaglobulinemia | Acquired immunodeficiency syndrome (AIDS) |
| *Laboratory Findings:* | Decreased serum Ig levels | Decreased delayed hypersensitivity reaction (e.g., PPD, SKSD, DNCB) |
| | Low to absent isohemagglutinins | |
| | Decreased antibody response to injected antigens (e.g., DPT vaccine) | Decreased allograft rejection |
| | Decreased Ig production by peripheral blood cells after in vitro stimulation (e.g., with pokeweed mitogen) | Decreased proliferative response of peripheral blood cells to mitogens (e.g., phytohemmagglutin [PHA] and conanavalin A [ConA]) |

## LYMPHOCYTE MIGRATION AND HOMING

Studies by Everett and his co-workers[7] suggested that small lymphocytes in mammals could be divided into two major categories: long-lived cells with a life span greater than 2 weeks and short-lived cells with a life span of less than 2 weeks (usually a few days). Their work showed that small lymphocytes in the thymus and bone marrow had a life span of approximately 48 hours, and that these cells were probably renewed in these organs from rapidly dividing precursors. On the other hand, over 90 percent of thoracic duct and lymph node cells had a life span measured in weeks to months. Gowans showed that the long-lived cells in the thoracic duct continually recirculate from the blood to the lymph (Fig. 3–1) and that small lymphocytes from thymus and bone marrow are not members of the recirculating pool.[8] These findings indicated that the physiologic characteristics of small lymphocytes could be used to divide them into two major categories—(1) recirculating long-lived cells and (2) nonrecirculating short-lived cells.

Speculation that the recirculating long-lived cells were T lymphocytes and that the nonrecirculating short-lived cells were B lymphocytes was proved incorrect. Experiments clearly demonstrated that B lymphocytes can recirculate in rats and that a portion of B lymphocytes had a life span of at least several weeks.[9,10] Several studies using both surface markers and immune function to identify T and B lymphocytes indicated that both populations contain mixtures of long- and short-lived cells and that these mixtures depend upon the lymphoid tissue investigated.[11] The thymus and bone marrow contain almost exclusively short-lived T and B lymphocytes, respectively, and the thoracic duct lymph contains mainly long-lived T and B lymphocytes.

Studies of the relationship between nonrecirculating, short-lived B lymphocytes and recirculating, long-lived B lymphocytes suggested that antigen is the signal that transforms the former cells into the latter. Strober and colleagues showed that B lymphocytes that have not seen antigen previously ("virgin B lymphocytes") are unable to recirculate from the blood to the lymph and are replaced through cell division approximately every 48 hours.[9] On the other hand, B lymphocytes that have encountered antigen previously ("memory B lymphocytes") continuously recirculate and have a long life span.[9] Thus virgin B lymphocytes are ordinarily destined

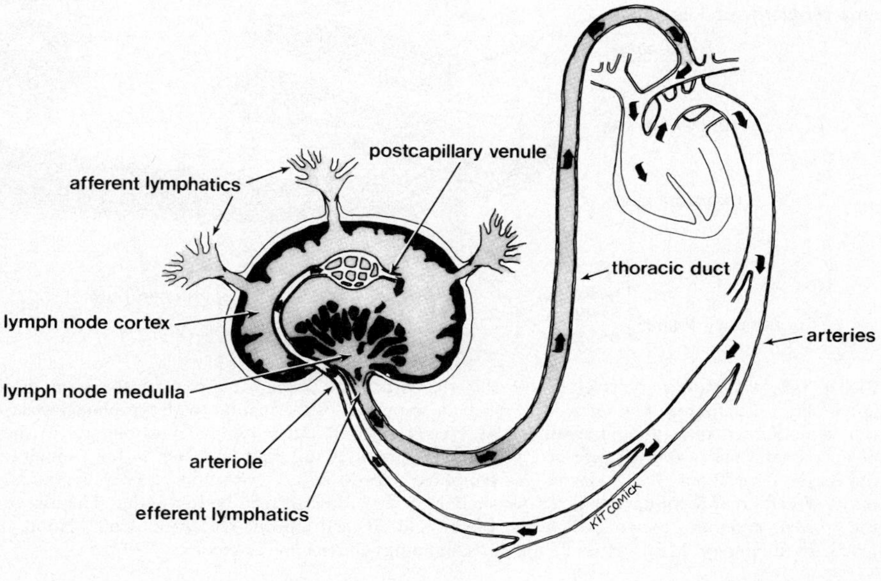


**Figure 3–1.** Lymphocyte recirculation. Arrows indicate pathway of lymphocyte migration through arterial system, postcapillary venule, lymph node cortex and medulla, efferent lymphatics, thoracic duct, and major veins leading back to the heart. (Adapted from Douglas, S.D.: Development and structure of cells in the immune system. *In* Fudenberg, H.H., Stites, D.P., Caldwell, J.L., and Wells, J.V. (eds.): Basic and Clinical Immunology. 3rd ed. Los Altos, Lange Medical Publications, 1980.)

for a short life in the peripheral lymphoid tissues, unless their lives are "saved" by the chance encounter with antigen, which transforms them into memory cells.

A similar transformation may occur with T lymphocytes. The earliest migrants to arrive in the peripheral lymphoid tissues from the thymus appear to be short-lived T lymphocytes. On the other hand, memory T lymphocytes have been shown to be recirculating, long-lived cells.[12] It is possible that antigen is the signal that triggers this transformation. However, it is not clear that antigen is the only signal that mediates this process, since there are instances in which T lymphocytes recirculate without obvious prior exposure to antigen.

Although T and B lymphocytes are similar in some of the physiologic characteristics discussed above, they differ in their migratory and homing characteristics within the peripheral lymphoid tissues.[13] T lymphocytes injected intravenously into laboratory animals home to the periarteriolar sheaths in the splenic white pulp and to the paracortex of lymph nodes (Fig. 3–2). The latter are "T lymphocyte areas" of the lymphoid tissues. B lymphocytes take the same initial migration pathway as T lymphocytes in leaving the central arterioles of the spleen and postcapillary venules of the lymph nodes. However, they eventually home to the primary follicles or mantle areas near the germinal centers in the spleen and to the primary follicles in the nodes (Fig. 3–2). The latter are "B lymphocyte areas" of the lymphoid tissues and are thus compartmentalized by virtue of splenic and lymph node architecture from the "T lymphocyte areas." Germinal centers contain both T and B lymphocytes and are thought to contain recently activated cells from both populations which may contribute to the memory cell pool.

There is also evidence for organ specificity of lymphocyte migration.[14-16] For example, lymphocytes isolated from intestinal lymphoid tissues (Peyer's patches) will migrate back to intestinal lymphoid tissues, while lymphocytes isolated from peripheral lymph nodes return preferentially to the peripheral nodes. This organ

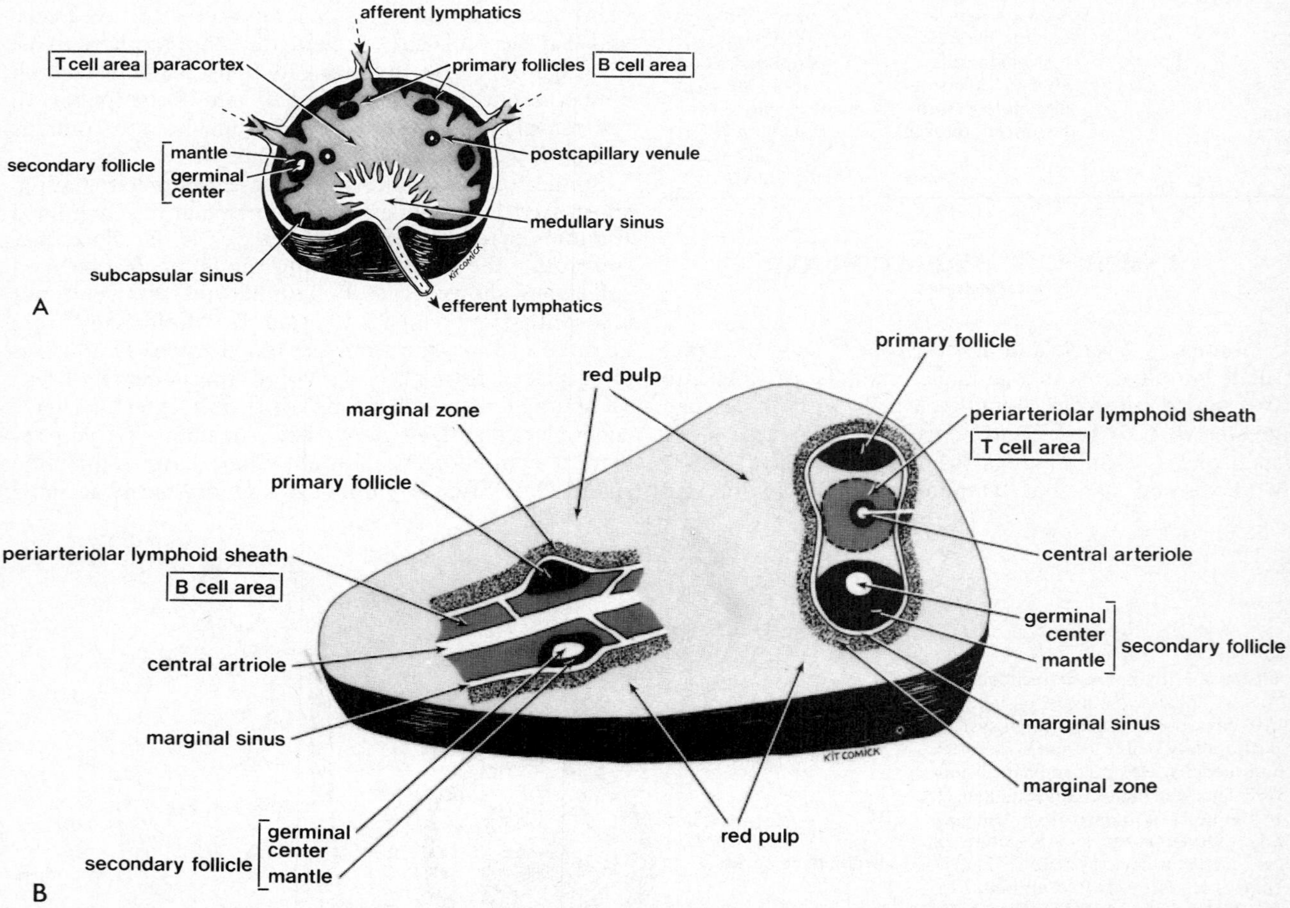


**Figure 3–2.** *A*, Lymph node structure. Within the cortex, the primary follicles are the major B cell area while the paracortex (diffuse cortex) is the major T cell area. The secondary follicle is composed of the mantle (with lymphocytes similar to the primary follicle) and the germinal center, composed of large and small B and T cells. Both T and B lymphocytes migrate to their respective domains after exiting from the postcapillary venule. *B*, Structure of a segment of spleen. White pulp is shown in both longitudinal and cross section. Primary follicles are the major B cell area. The periarteriolar lymphoid sheath, an accumulation of small lymphocytes surrounding the central arteriole, is the major T cell area. Secondary follicles are similar to those described in lymph nodes. The marginal areas receive much of the blood entering the spleen and are the major areas of T and B cell entry. (Adapted from Hood, L.E., Weissman, I.L., and Wood, W.B. (eds.): Immunology. Menlo Park, Benjamin/Cummings Publishing Company; 1978.)

specificity of lymphocyte migration seems to be determined by a selective interaction of lymphocytes with the specialized endothelial cells of the postcapillary high endothelial venules in lymph nodes (Fig. 3–2).[16] When in lymphocyte development organ specificity develops is unclear. Selective migration to different lymphoid organs occurs in the absence of antigenic stimulation, and may determine the distribution of functionally distinct lymphocyte populations (i.e., B versus T lymphocytes) in mucosal versus nonmucosal lymphoid tissues. Blast cells (i.e., after antigenic stimulation) initially lose the ability to migrate but may demonstrate homing specificity later after a period of local proliferation and differentiation.

## T LYMPHOCYTES

**Maturation of T Lymphocytes.** As noted above, neonatal thymectomy results in the failure of T lymphocyte surface markers and T lymphocyte function to develop.[17] The cellular deficits can be restored by transplantation of a thymus gland. Surprisingly the cells repopulating the thymus graft and the T lymphocytes repopulating the peripheral lymphoid tissues after thymic transplantation are of host rather than donor origin.[18] This suggests that cells that migrate from the thymus to the T lymphocyte areas of the peripheral lymphoid tissues are not generated de novo in the thymus. Instead, it appears that there is a traffic of cells that enter and then leave the thymus. More recent chromosomal marker studies indicate that the bone marrow is the source of cells entering the thymus. These cells are called pre-T lymphocytes, since they do not have the surface or functional characteristics of mature T lymphocytes but are thought to be the precursors of the latter cells.[19]

The actual conversion of pre-T into T lymphocytes appears to occur in the thymus by virtue of interactions between the former cells and the thymic epithelial cells.[19] The contribution of thymic hormones to T lymphocyte maturation in mammals remains controversial (reviewed in ref. 20). It is not clear to what extent maturation of T lymphocytes occurs within the thymus and to what extent maturation occurs after T lymphocytes migrate out of the thymus and into the peripheral tissues. Furthermore, it is uncertain that the in-migration of bone marrow cells to the thymus contributes significantly to the out-migration of thymus cells in the adult, since the thymus may develop the capacity for self-renewal after it is initially populated by pre-T lymphocytes from the marrow. The precise role of the thymus and thymus cell maturation in adult animals remains to be elucidated, since adult thymectomy produces few acute changes in the number and function of T lymphocytes in the peripheral tissues. The lack of reported immunologic deficits after removal of the thymus gland during open heart surgery in children suggests that the role of the thymus gland in the maintenance of cellular immunity in man may be minimal after the first few years of life. This may be due in part to the long life span of mature T lymphocytes, to the self-renewing capacity of T lymphocytes in the periphery, and possibly to the extrathymic maturation of some T lymphocyte precursors (i.e., without physically entering the thymus).[21]

Profound changes in cell surface antigens mark the various stages of T lymphocyte maturation in both mouse and man (Fig. 3–3).[22-25] In the differentiation of mouse T lymphocytes, pre-T lymphocytes do not express the membrane glycoprotein Thy-1 antigen but do have surface major histocompatibility (H-2) antigens (which continue to be expressed during cell differentiation). These cells are induced in the thymus to express Thy-1 as well as TL and Lyt antigens. The TL antigen is expressed on greater than 95 percent of normal thymocytes and is present on most thymic leukemia (TL) cell lines.[23,26] However, nearly all peripheral T lymphocytes are Thy-1+ but TL negative. Thus, TL is an example of a surface antigen that defines an intrathymic differentiation stage. Lyt antigens (Lyt-1, 2, and 3) are *all* expressed on greater than 90 percent of thymocytes and on less than 50 percent of peripheral T lymphocytes.[22-24] Cytotoxic depletion studies suggested that the majority of peripheral T lymphocytes carry either the Lyt-1 antigen alone (Lyt-1$^+$,23$^-$) or a combination of the Lyt-2 and Lyt-3 antigens without the Lyt-1 antigen (Lyt-1$^-$,23$^+$). The two different phenotypes define functionally distinct peripheral T lymphocyte subsets (see below). More sensitive immunofluorescence techniques have shown that Lyt-1 is found on all peripheral T lymphocytes but is present in lower levels on those cells previously identified as Lyt-1$^-$,23$^+$.[27]

A series of monoclonal antibodies have been developed that are reactive with human thymocyte and/or peripheral T lymphocyte cell surface antigens. As proposed by Reinherz and Schlossman (Fig. 3–3),[25] using the OKT series of monoclonal antibodies, the earliest thymocytes bear OKT9 and OKT10, and this stage defines the minority (10 percent) of thymocytes. With further maturation, human thymocytes concurrently express OKT6, OKT4, OKT5, and OKT8 (accounting for more than 70 percent of the thymic population). With further maturation, thymocytes lose OKT6 reactivity, acquire OKT3 and OKT1, and segregate into OKT4 and OKT5/T8 subsets. As the thymocyte is exported into the peripheral T lymphocyte compartment, it loses the T10 marker. The OKT4 (or Leu-3, using the analagous Leu series of monoclonal antibodies) and OKT5/OKT8 (or Leu-2) subsets appear to be nonoverlapping, relatively functionally distinct populations in the peripheral lymphoid tissues (see below).

**T Lymphocyte Subpopulations.** Table 3–2 summarizes some distinctive surface markers present on two major peripheral lymphoid T lymphocyte subpopulations in mice and humans.[22-25,28-38] Included in the "helper/inducer" subset are T lymphocytes that help in the differentiation of B lymphocytes into immunoglobulin-secreting cells (help antibody production), T lymphocytes that help in the development of cell-mediated lymphocytotoxicity (CML), and T lymphocytes that are effectors for delayed hypersensitivity. The other major subset

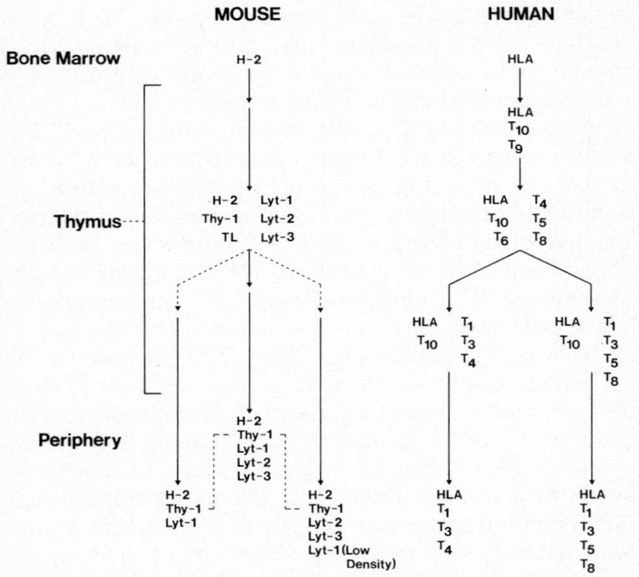


**Figure 3–3.** Differentiation of mouse and human T lymphoctytes showing acquisition of cell surface antigens within the thymus. (Adapted from Hood, L.E., Weissman, I.L., and Wood, W.B. (eds.): Immunology. Menlo Park, Benjamin/Cummings Publishing Company, 1978; and Reinherz, E.L., and Schlossman, S.F.: The differentiation and function of human T lymphoctytes. Cell 19:821, 1980.)

contains T lymphocytes that suppress B lymphocyte differentiation and other T lymphocyte functions, as well as those that mediate CML (T cytotoxic cells). Monoclonal antibodies to all of the surface determinants in Table 3–2 now exist. The Leu-1 (OKT1) antigen is present on nearly all human peripheral blood T lymphocytes but is present in lower amounts on those 20 to 30 percent of T lymphocytes that carry Leu-2a and Leu-2b (OKT5) antigens. Leu-3 (or OKT4) antigens are present on 60 percent of peripheral blood T lymphocytes.

The human T lymphocyte antigens Leu-1, Leu-2a, and Leu-2b appear to have strong analogies to the mouse Lyt-1, Lyt-2, and Lyt-3 antigens, respectively.[38] This is based on studies of tissue distribution, molecular weight, subunit composition, and sensitivity to proteolysis of the respective cell surface antigens. Although these similarities exist, there is no crossreactivity between the murine and human T lymphocyte antigens when staining with either anti-Leu or anti-Lyt antibodies. The maintenance of these surface structures through evolution suggests that these molecules perform essential functions for the cells on which they are found. Some evidence for this has been provided in studies showing that both anti-Leu-2 and anti-Lyt-2 (in the absence of complement) can block cell-mediated cytotoxicity.[35,39] This observed blocking, however, could also be due to a tendency for the Leu or Lyt molecules to associate with other molecules relevant to the killing activity.

Some differences in function of the two major human T lymphocyte subsets are presented in Table 3–3.[25,32-37] Some of these are discussed below. It should be emphasized that the broad classification of lymphocyte subsets by surface phenotype does not imply that all lymphocytes with a given surface phenotype have the same function. Indeed, examples of OKT4 cells with suppressor or cytotoxic functions exist.[40,41] However, when OKT4 (Leu-3) lymphocytes are isolated from peripheral blood, they mediate predominantly helper/inducer functions in a variety of assay systems, and similarly, when OKT5 or OKT8 (Leu-2) cells are isolated, they mediate predominantly suppressor or cytotoxic functions. Recently, it has been suggested that these surface markers primarily determine the class of major histocompatibility antigens that are recognized (especially in association with antigens) rather than function.[37,41] Leu-3 (OKT4) cells recognize class II HLA antigens, whereas Leu-2 (OKT8) cells recognize class I HLA antigens (in association with antigen).

The mature T lymphocyte populations can be further divided into functional subpopulations based on differences in the display of major histocompatibility (MHC)-encoded determinants. This has allowed further delineation of T lymphocyte interactions in immunoregulatory circuits (see below).

Human T lymphocytes have also been separated into functionally distinct subsets by the specificity of their Fc receptors for either IgG (T$\gamma$ cells) or IgM (T$\mu$ cells).[42-45] T$\gamma$ lymphocytes mediate suppression of in vitro immunoglobulin production while T$\mu$ lymphocytes

**Table 3–2.** Surface Determinants of the Major T Lymphocyte Subpopulations in Mouse and Man

| | Human Surface Ag | Murine Surface Ag |
|---|---|---|
| *All T Lymphocytes* | SRBC Receptor | |
| | OKT1, OKT3 | Thy-1 |
| | Leu-1, Leu-4 | Lyt-1* |
| *Suppressor/Cytotoxic Lymphocytes* | OKT5, OKT8 | Lyt-2, 3 |
| | Leu-2a, Leu-2b | |
| *Helper/Inducer Lymphocytes* | OKT4 | L3T4* |
| | Leu-3 | (Lyt-1$^{+}$,23$^{-}$)* |

*By immunofluorescence techniques, the Lyt-1 antigen is present on all mature mouse T lymphocytes, although present in lower density on suppressor/cytotoxic cells. By cytotoxic depletion techniques, the Lyt-1 antigen is present on the the helper/inducer subset but not on the suppressor/cytotoxic subset. The murine helper/inducer subset can be recognized by the *absence* of Lyt-2 and Lyt-3 antigens. The L3T4 antigen has been recently described as the murine homologue of the human Leu-3/OKT4 molecule.[124]

**Table 3–3.** Immunologic Functions of the Two Major Human T Lymphocyte Subsets

| | Leu-3 OKT4 | Leu-2 OKT5, OKT8 |
|---|---|---|
| *Proliferative Responses (In Vitro)* | | |
| To Phytohemagglutin | + | + |
| Concanavalin A (ConA) | + | + |
| Allogeneic non-T cells | + | + |
| Autologous non-T cells | + | — |
| Soluble Antigens | + | — |
| *Helper/Inducer Function (T-T, T-B,)* | + | — |
| *Delayed Hypersensitivity* | + | — |
| *Cytotoxic Effector Function* | — | + |
| *Suppressor Function (T-T, T-B)* | — | + |

mediate helper function. Unlike the subsets identified by monoclonal antibodies, Tγ lymphocytes may not maintain cell surface phenotype stability. For example, after incubation with immune complexes, the Fc-IgG receptor can be irreversibly lost and later Fc-IgM expression has been observed.[44,45] Some groups have compared T lymphocyte subsets defined by Fc receptors and by reactivity with monoclonal antibodies, and suggest that all Tγ lymphocytes may not even be of the T lymphocyte lineage (i.e., carry the OKT3 or Leu-1 antigens).[46,47] Other studies concluded that the majority of Tγ lymphocytes are T lymphocytes but that correlation with the OKT8 or Leu-2 subset (suppressor/cytotoxic cells by monoclonal antibodies) was poor.[48] Unlike subsets defined by monoclonal antibodies, subsets defined by Fc receptors are not analogous to functionally distinct murine T lymphocyte subsets. Thus, the Fc receptor T lymphocyte classification system has considerable disadvantages compared with the monoclonal antibody classification scheme defined above, especially in the study of autoimmune diseases such as SLE.

**T Helper ($T_H$)–T Cytotoxic ($T_c$) Cell Interactions.** In the allogeneic mixed leukocyte reaction (MLR), T lymphocytes are stimulated in vitro to proliferate by the MHC determinants on stimulator non-T cells. In addition, T lymphocytes are induced to differentiate into cytotoxic cells ($T_c$ cells), which are capable of lysing allogeneic target cells without added antibody or complement.[23] It was demonstrated in murine MLR systems that the T lymphocytes mediating cytotoxicity were surface Lyt-1$^-$,23$^+$ (determined by cytotoxic depletion studies). However, collaboration between an Lyt-1$^+$,23$^-$ (T helper/inducer cell) subset and the Lyt-1$^-$,23$^+$ subset was necessary for optimum development of cytotoxicity (Fig. 3–4).[28,29] In the absence of Lyt-1$^+$ cells ($T_H$ cells), little cytotoxicity was generated. Interestingly these $T_H$ lymphocytes were shown to recognize predominantly antigens on the surface of the stimulatory cells coded for by the I gene region of the H-2 locus (analogous to the D region in man; class II MHC antigens). In contrast, the $T_c$ lymphocytes recognized target cell antigens coded for by K and D gene regions of H-2 (analogous to A and B regions in man, class I MHC antigens).[23,29,49,50] Thus, two stimulatory signals are required for the most efficient development of cytotoxicity. As shown in Figure 3–4, there is now evidence that the helper effect is mediated in large part by a soluble T lymphocyte product, T lymphocyte growth factor (interleukin II).[51,52]

The above in vitro system may relate to immune events that occur in tissue transplantation such as graft rejection or the graft-versus-host reaction. However, the

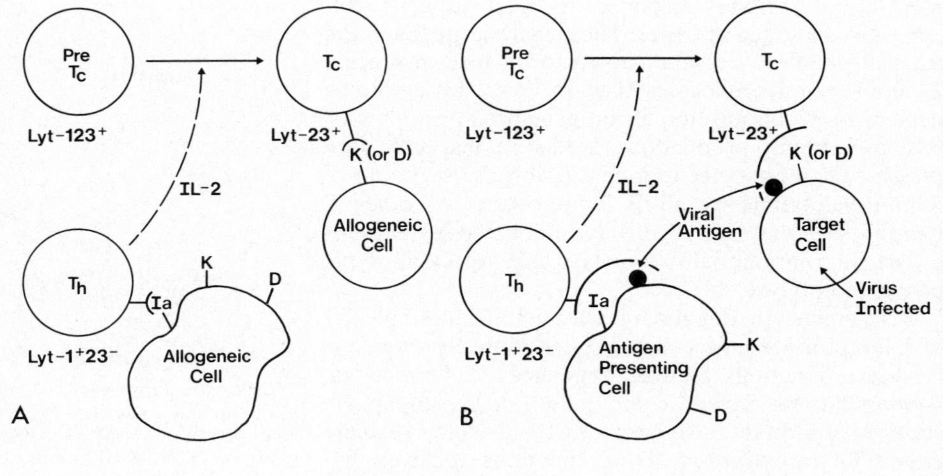


**Figure 3–4.** Cellular interactions involved in the generation of cell-mediated cytotoxicity both for allogeneic cells and virus infected cells. $T_h$, T helper cell; $T_c$, T cytotoxic cell; Pre-$T_c$, precursor of the T cytotoxic cell; *IL-2*, interleukin 2 or T cell growth factor. *A*, In the generation of cytotoxicity for allogeneic cells, $T_h$ cells recognize allogeneic I region determinants, whereas $T_c$ cells recognize allogeneic K or D region determinants. *B*, In the generation of cytotoxicity for virus-infected cells, all cells depicted are autologous, and $T_h$ cells recognize viral antigens in the context of *self* I region determinants, whereas $T_c$ cells recognize viral antigens in the context of *self* K or D region determinants (see text for details).

response to allogeneic cells is not likely to be required during everyday living. The allogeneic system does have strong analogies to the T lymphocyte interactions required to kill virus-infected cells (Fig. 3–4).[23,53-55] Thus, in the mouse, $T_H$(Lyt-1+,23−) lymphocytes can only recognize viral or virus-encoded surface antigens when presented on cells that express *self* I region determinants. The $T_H$ lymphocyte must therefore recognize both viral antigens *and* I region cell surface products, and the $T_H$ response is said to be restricted for I region determinants. The $T_c$ cell (Lyt-1−,23+) recognizes viral antigens in association with *self* K and D antigens (restricted to K and D). Although $T_H$–$T_c$ cooperation in man has not been elucidated in the same detail as in mice, studies suggest that similar mechanisms are operative.

**T Suppressor ($T_s$) Lymphocytes**. The preceding discussion focused on the $T_H$–$T_c$ interaction. The systems that induce cell-mediated cytotoxicity are also regulated by suppressor T lymphocytes ($T_s$ cells). These cells have a function opposite that of the helper cells and therefore decrease the amount of cytotoxicity generated. Different types of suppressor T lymphocytes have been described in the MLR-CML system.[23,56-63] For example, some suppressor cells suppress responder cell proliferation while others suppress only the development of cytotoxicity. Suppressor cells can function at the level of $T_c$ precursor at initiation of cytotoxicity (afferent suppressor cell) or at the level of cytotoxic effector events (efferent suppressor cell). Suppressor cells can also be specific for the alloantigen stimulating cell (antigen specific) or suppress any MLR combination (antigen nonspecific).

The existence of suppressor T lymphocytes was actually first shown for antibody production by Gershon and his colleagues.[28] These investigators induced tolerance to sheep red blood cells (SRBC) in mice. Thus, these mice were unable to generate a normal antibody response after immunization with SRBC. The tolerant state was then passed to other mice by transferring lymphoid cells from the tolerant donors to otherwise immunocompetent recipients. The recipients of the tolerant cells became tolerant themselves and were unable to mount an immune response to SRBC. However, they had normal antibody responses to other antigens (tolerance was antigen specific). The cells that mediated the transfer of tolerance were shown to be antigen-specific T suppressor lymphocytes (Lyt-1−,23+) (by cytotoxic depletion).[28,31] In addition to antigen-specific suppressor cells of antibody production, there are nonspecific suppressor T lymphocytes that can inhibit the secretion of immuno-globulins by all B lymphocytes, or other T lymphocytes that can selectively inhibit the secretion of a particular immunoglobulin class (e.g., IgA), allotype, or even idiotype.[23,64-67]

**T Lymphocyte Regulatory Circuits.** The complexity of T lymphocyte subsets increases enormously when one studies interactions between regulatory T lymphocyte subpopulations. Several complex murine T lymphocyte suppressor circuits have been described which regulate either T-lymphocyte-mediated functions (delayed hypersensitivity) or B-lymphocyte-mediated functions (antibody production).[68] These amplification circuits have numerous similarities and apparently serve to maintain a finely balanced expression of immunity. In these circuits, surface markers that have additionally helped in determining subsets of functional T lymphocytes are related to the expression of determinants encoded by the MHC (e.g., I-J locus) and closely related loci (e.g., Qa).

Figure 3–5 depicts a suppressor pathway that is activated concomitantly with normal immunization to the T-lymphocyte-dependent antigen SRBC.[68-71] If Lyt-1+, 23− T lymphocytes are isolated from a mouse previously immunized to SRBC and then combined in vitro with B lymphocytes in the presence of SRBC, an in vitro anti-SRBC antibody response can be measured. Immunization also activates an inducer cell (Lyt-1+,23−, Qa-1+,I-J+), which acts on a nonprimed (no previous antigen stimulation required) Lyt-123+, I-J+, Qa-1+ target cell (feedback suppressor cell), which eventually results in an Lyt-1−,23+ suppressor effector cell. The suppressor effector cell mediates suppression of anti-SRBC antibody production in an antigen (SRBC)-specific, MHC-restricted fashion at the level of the $T_H$ lymphocyte. This suppression has been known to be mediated by suppressor factors. Another T lymphocyte circuit is also induced, which actually decreases the amount of feedback suppression (contrasuppression) (not shown in Fig. 3–5).[72]

Analogous but less detailed "suppressor amplifier" circuits have been described using human peripheral

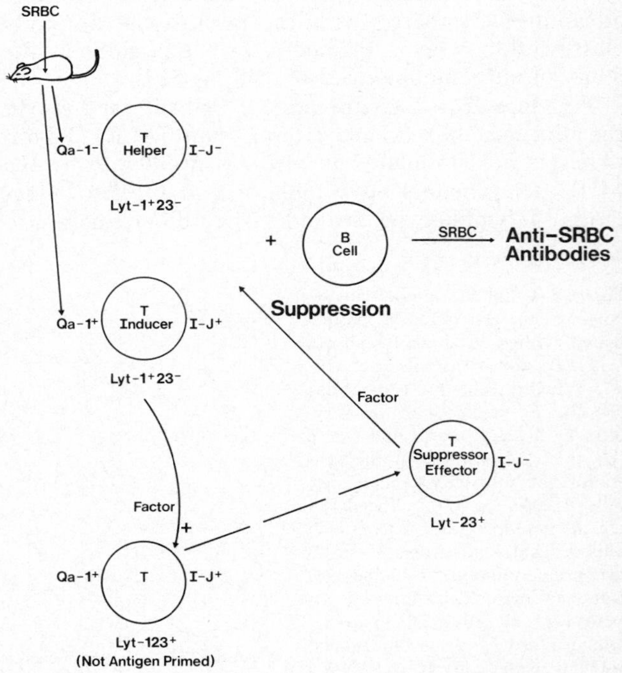


**Figure 3–5.** Suppressor pathway activation when mice are immunized with an antigen such as sheep red blood cells (SRBC). The resulting generation of "feedback suppression" negatively regulates the production of anti-SRBC antibodies (see text for details).

blood lymphocytes.[73-76] Various methods of in vitro B lymphocyte activation that are $T_H$ lymphocyte dependent (require Leu-3 [OKT4] cells for antibody production) have been employed. In these systems, activation of the Leu-2 (OKT8) (suppressor amplifier) cell requires a Leu-3 (OKT4) inducer cell.

**T Lymphocyte Clones and the Nature of the T Lymphocyte Receptor.** The functions of the different T lymphocyte subpopulations described in the preceding section were studied using whole lymphocyte populations isolated by their respective surface markers. The heterogeneity of these populations must be continually emphasized. The ability to obtain pure populations of immunocompetent T lymphocytes (T lymphocyte clones) in vitro has been a recent major advance in the study of T lymphocytes. One technique of T lymphocyte cloning takes advantage of the lymphokine T lymphocyte growth factor (interleukin II), which causes the continued in vitro proliferation of activated T lymphocytes.[77-79] Thus, cells from an immunized animal with a particular antigen specificity and function (e.g., T helper, T delayed hypersensitivity, T cytotoxic, or T suppressor) can be propagated as cell lines and then cloned at the single cell level. Another technique is analogous to that used to produce monoclonal antibodies. However, instead of fusing antigen-stimulated B lymphocytes to malignant myeloma cells to "immortalize" cells secreting the desired antibody, immunocompetent T lymphocytes are fused to malignant thymoma cell lines.[79,80] The T lymphocyte hybridomas that result are screened for the desired antigen specificity and functions and then expanded into large numbers from a single cell.

T lymphocyte cloning has considerably increased our understanding of the molecular nature of the T lymphocyte receptor.[78-83] As alluded to previously, observations suggest that during antigen presentation, most T lymphocytes recognize both the antigen and the MHC region gene products expressed by the antigen-presenting cell. $T_H$ lymphocytes and those lymphocytes that mediate delayed hypersensitivity recognize antigen in the context of I region (class II) gene products. $T_H$ lymphocytes do not bind soluble antigens nor do they bind to I region determinants alone. $T_c$ lymphocytes recognize antigen in the context of class I MHC determinants. In contrast to $T_H$ and $T_c$ lymphocytes, T suppressor lymphocytes have been noted to bind free antigen and thus might be activated by free antigen alone. This might have important consequences in those situations in which Ia-positive antigen-presenting cells are absent (e.g., in the early neonatal period), blocked (e.g., by anti-Ia antisera), or saturated (e.g., by high concentrations of antigen). The result might be selective suppressor cell activation with net immunologic unresponsiveness. Some T lymphocyte receptors have been noted to bear crossreactive idiotypes with antibodies directed at thesame antigenic determinants.[78-86] However, studies have demonstrated that T lymphocyte receptors do not carry conventional immunoglobulin light chains nor immunoglobulin heavy chain constant region determinants.

**T Lymphocyte Soluble Mediators—Lymphokines.** T lymphocytes and especially activated T lymphocytes produce a wide variety of soluble mediators called lymphokines. These lymphokines are critically important for T lymphocyte communication with other cell types and for the generation and amplification of the inflammatory response. For example, it is thought that much of the recruitment of immunologically uncommitted cells in the delayed hypersensitivity reaction is mediated by lymphokines. A partial list of lymphokines with their functions is shown in Table 3–4.[87-93] While these substances exert marked biologic effects, they are produced in only minute quantities by activated lymphocytes. Some of the mediators have been purified sufficiently for determination of their structure, but most have not been, and

**Table 3–4.** T Lymphocyte Lymphokines

| Lymphokine | Function |
|---|---|
| *Affecting Macrophages* | |
| Macrophage activation factor (MAF) | Activates macrophage to increase bacteriocidal and tumorcidal activity |
| Migration inhibition factor (MIF) | Inhibits macrophage movement; localizes macrophages in area of antigen-lymphocyte interaction |
| Macrophage chemotactic factor | Attracts macrophages and monocytes to site of inflammation |
| Macrophage Ia-Inducing Factor | Induces and increases expression of Ia on macrophage cell surface; important for antigen presenting function |
| *Affecting Polymorphonuclear Leukocytes* | |
| Leukocyte inhibitory factor (LIF) | Analagous to MIF |
| Chemotactic factor | Analagous to macrophage chemotactic factor |
| *Affecting T Lymphocytes* | |
| T Cell Growth factor (interleukin II) | Induces stimulated T cells to proliferate |
| Other mitogen factors | Induce T cells to proliferate |
| Gamma interferon | Inhibits viral replication; increases T cell cytotoxicity; suppresses lymphocyte proliferation induced by alloantigens and mitogens; enhances natural killer function; regulates antibody production |
| Transfer factor | Induces lymphocytes to become antigen specific effector cells in delayed hypersensitivity reactions |
| *Affecting B Lymphocytes* | |
| B cell growth factor (BCGF) | Induces B cells to proliferate after initial stimulation |
| T cell replacing factor | Induces B cells to differentiate into antibody producing cells after initial stimulation |
| Gamma interferon | See above |
| *Affecting Other Cell Types* | |
| Lymphotoxin (LT) | Cytotoxin released in area of antigen-lymphocyte interactions |

they are identified by their different biologic functions. The number of chemically distinct humoral substances is not known, and one molecule may serve more than one function.

## B LYMPHOCYTES

**Maturation of B Lymphocytes.** Early work in chickens showed that the first B lymphocytes appear in the bursa of Fabricius at about the time of hatching.[23,94] After hatching, the bursa involutes, and B lymphocyte precursors are thought to leave the bursa to populate the bone marrow and perhaps other lymphoid tissues. A bursalike organ has not been found in mammals. However, the mammalian fetal liver may have a function similar to that of the bursa, since pre-B lymphocytes and B lymphocytes appear first in this organ during embryogenesis.[95,96]

Maturation of B lymphocytes continues after embryogenesis and throughout the life of the adult. The continuous generation of B lymphocytes from precursors in the adult bone marrow is similar to that of the other blood elements. Indeed, B lymphocytes are derived from the same pluripotent hematopoietic stem cells in the marrow that generate erythrocytes, granulocytes, megakaryocytes, and monocytes.[97] Similarly, B lymphocytes are constantly replaced through cell division from precursor cells in the marrow every few days.[98] Many of the small lymphocytes produced in the marrow are immature cells of the B lymphocyte lineage. The maturation of B lymphocytes differs from that of the other blood elements in that the B lymphocytes have an antigen-independent and an antigen-dependent maturation scheme (Fig. 3–6).

Pre-B lymphocytes in the marrow are identified by cytoplasmic immunoglobulin without surface immunoglobulin expression.[98,99] The heavy chain of IgM is the first immunoglobulin molecule to appear in the cytoplasm, followed later by light chain expression. The first surface immunoglobulin to appear on the developing B lymphocyte is also IgM (Fig. 3–6).[98] Unlike secreted IgM, surface IgM is monomeric and has an additional hydrophobic addition on the carboxy-terminal portion of the $\mu$ chain, which apparently allows for insertion into the membrane.[100] After surface IgM expression, the B lymphocyte acquires other surface markers, including Ia antigens and both surface receptors for complement and the Fc region of immunoglobulin (not shown in Fig. 3–6).[23,101,102] Subsequently, the cell acquires surface IgD or other immunoglobulin isotypes, or both, and can be identified as the mature virgin B lymphocyte.[98,103]

Although Ig-bearing small lymphocytes are constantly generated in the marrow from rapidly dividing cells that bear no surface immunoglobulin, the last part of the antigen-independent maturation sequence may take place after B lymphocytes have migrated to the periphery. Surface IgD may be gained after migration to the periphery (i.e., to lymph nodes or spleen), since almost

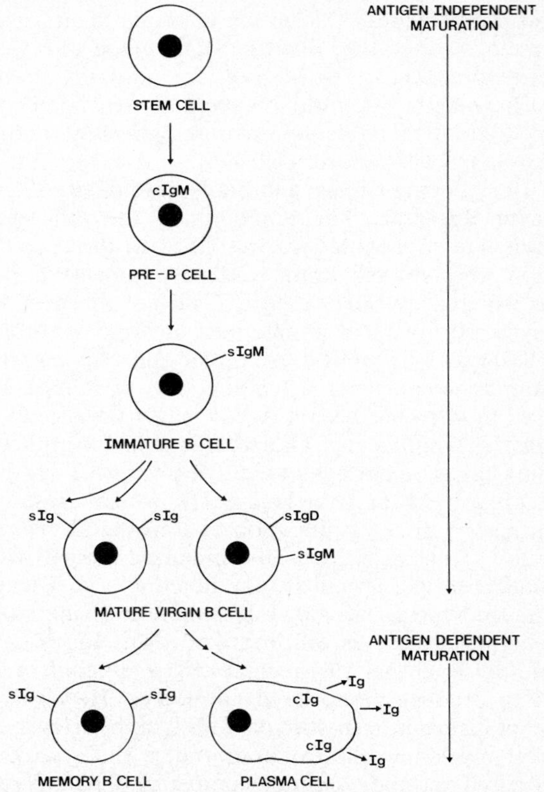


**Figure 3–6.** *B* lymphocyte development and differentiation. The maturation from stem cell through pre-B cell (recognized by cytoplasmic IgM without surface immunoglobulin) to mature virgin *B* cell occurs without interaction with antigen. The differentiation of the virgin *B* cell to either memory *B* cell or immunoglobulin-producing cell requires activation by antigen (see text for details).

all B lymphocytes in the marrow express surface IgM without IgD, but the majority of IgM-bearing cells in the periphery also express IgD.[103] The marrow thus contains few mature virgin B lymphocytes. The weight of evidence favors the notion that the diversity of Ig classes found on the B lymphocyte surface (i.e., IgM, IgD, IgG, IgA) is gained during antigen-independent maturation. Although individual B lymphocytes can express more than one Ig heavy chain isotype, they express only one Ig heavy chain variable region and one light chain, and thus only one idiotype.

The antigen-dependent scheme includes those differentiation steps after the virgin B lymphocyte is stimulated by antigen to give rise to (1) antibody-secreting cells or to (2) memory B cells or to (3) both (Fig. 3–6). The memory B lymphocytes differ from the virgin B lymphocytes in several important ways, including their migration pattern and life span.[9] The former cells are nonrecirculating, short-lived cells and are found in highest concentrations in the thoracic duct lymph. The marrow contains few memory B lymphocytes.

Recently, B lymphocyte differentiation antigens were described as a result of studies of mice with an X-linked immunodeficiency syndrome (CBA/N mice).[104-110] These mice are unable to generate an antibody response to one group of thymic-independent antigens (T lymphocyte help not required for the antibody response). These mice do produce antibodies to other thymic-independent antigens and to thymic-dependent antigens. The defect appears to result from the absence of a particular subset of B lymphocytes, and alloantisera were prepared that recognized distinct antigens on this subset, including the Lyb-5 antigen. The Lyb-5$^+$ B lymphocytes, which are absent in these defective mice, appear later in ontogeny, are not present in high numbers in bone marrow, have a high density of surface IgD, are difficult to tolerize, and are responsible for the antibody response to the thymic-independent antigens to which CBA/N mice cannot respond. The B lymphocytes that do not bear Lyb-5 appear early in ontogeny, are the predominant B lymphocytes in adult bone marrow, have a high density of surface IgM with little surface IgD, and are easy to tolerize. Both subsets are found in the adult spleen, although Lyb-5$^+$ B lymphocytes predominate. Interestingly, although both subsets can produce antibody to T-dependent antigens, the T lymphocyte–B lymphocyte interactions appear to be different. Thus, T lymphocyte help for the Lyb-5$^-$ B lymphocytes is MHC (I region) restricted for both the accessory (antigen-presenting) cell and B cell, while help for the Lyb-5$^+$ B cells is only MHC restricted for the accessory cell. Furthermore the Lyb-5$^+$ but not the Lyb-5$^-$ subset can be activated by soluble products from activated T helper cells. It is as yet unclear whether the Lyb-5$^+$ and Lyb-5$^-$ subsets represent further differentiation of the same B lymphocyte line, or two separate B lymphocyte lineages.

**B Lymphocyte Subpopulations.** B lymphocytes exist as a heterogeneous population in the peripheral lymphoid tissues, which includes cells at distinct stages of development. For example, peripheral blood B lymphocytes appear to be a variable mixture of early marrow migrants, mature virgin B lymphocytes, and memory B lymphocytes, which enter from the lymph. Studies of B lymphocyte subpopulations have been hampered by the relative lack of reagents (compared with those for T lymphocytes) that detect surface markers on functionally distinct subsets. For example, there continue to be no surface markers that easily distinguish virgin and memory B lymphocytes.

Subpopulations of B lymphocytes can, of course, be recognized by their different expression of surface immunoglobulin. The majority of B lymphocytes in mouse and man express both IgM and IgD on the cell surface.[103,107,111] The minority of cells express surface IgG.[112] Most of the IgG-bearing cells in the mouse spleen express an additional class of surface immunoglobulin (either IgM or IgD). The functional significance of having the same antigen-combining site (idiotype) associated with more than one immunoglobulin heavy chain on the surface of a single B lymphocyte is not well understood at present. However, some investigators have theorized that IgM receptors on the cell surface bind antigen and provide a tolerizing or "off" signal and that antigen interaction with IgD receptors provides a triggering or "on" signal.[112-115] Thus, the first B lymphocytes to appear during embryogenesis bear only IgM and are tolerized after antigenic challenge. More mature B lymphocytes, which have acquired IgD receptors, are stimulated to give rise to antibody-forming cells after antigenic challenge. This may play an important role in eliminating B lymphocyte clones that recognize "self" antigens, since all young B lymphocytes come in contact with the latter antigens during early stages of differentiation.

There is evidence that the subpopulation of IgG-bearing cells contains memory cells that give rise to a rapid secondary IgG antibody response after rechallenge with antigen.[116,117] However, there appears to be no simple correlation between memory cells and surface IgG. In addition, there is no clear correlation between the expression of a given class of Ig on the surface of a B lymphocyte and the class of antibody secreted by its progeny. For example, Strober and his colleagues have shown that virgin and memory B lymphocytes bearing surface IgM but little or no IgG give rise to an early IgM antibody response followed by an IgG response.[118] This "switching" of immunoglobulin classes by B lymphocyte clones has been shown to take place during the secretory phase of immunoglobulin synthesis.

B lymphocytes have been commonly identified by other surface markers in addition to immunoglobulins. These include the receptor for the Fc piece of immunoglobulins, the receptor for the C3 component of complement, and surface antigens coded for by the I gene region in the mouse (D region in man).[23,101,102] These other B lymphocyte markers (Fc receptor, C3 receptor, Ia antigen) are present on the majority of, but not all, mature B lymphocytes. The subpopulations of B lymphocytes carrying these markers may differ in their function from those which do not. However, the role of these markers or receptors in the function of B lymphocytes in the immune response is unclear.

**B Lymphocyte Activation.** Studies suggest that for T lymphocyte dependent antibody production, B lymphocytes require at least two signals to become antibody-secreting cells.[23,89,92,93,119,120] One signal involves the interaction between antigen and B lymphocyte immunoglobulin receptors. Another signal is provided by the T helper lymphocyte and B lymphocyte interaction. As emphasized above, T helper lymphocytes require the presence of accessory cells (antigen-presenting cells) in order to augment the triggering of B lymphocytes into antibody-forming cells. While the T helper and accessory cell interaction is restricted to the I region, the T helper restriction for B lymphocytes may vary (see previous discussion of Lyb-5 antigen). T helper lymphocytes also elaborate factors necessary for B lymphocyte activation. After antigen exposure or appropriate initial stimulus, B lymphocytes express receptors for a B lymphocyte growth factor. This factor seems capable of maintaining proliferation of activated B lymphocytes in the absence of differentiation. These cells go on to express receptors for another T lymphocyte factor (T lymphocyte replacing factor or B lymphocyte differentiation factor), which drives B lymphocytes to terminal differentiation.

## NULL LYMPHOCYTES

A small proportion of lymphocytes (~10 percent) in the peripheral tissues bear no surface markers for either T lymphocytes or B lymphocytes and are referred to as null lymphocytes. Two in vitro functions mediated by subpopulations of these cells have gained widespread interest and have been extensively studied.[121,122] Natural killer (NK) cells kill certain cell targets, especially tumor cells, in the absence of antibodies to the target cells and without prior immunization. The cells that mediate antibody-dependent cellular cytotoxicity (ADCC) are able to kill target cells that are coated with specific antibody. Again, no prior immunization of the effector cell is necessary. Thus, these null-cell-mediated functions show no recognition of specific antigens. Although the in vitro assays of natural killing generally use tumor cell targets, NK cells may also be involved in killing of virus-infected cells, foreign tissue, altered cellular self-antigens, or even other normal lymphoid cells. It has been theorized that NK cells may be involved in a primitive host defense and may perhaps be the front line of defense against malignancy.

Recent evidence has demonstrated that human null cells that mediate natural killing activity and ADCC against tumor target cells are large granular lymphocytes.[121,122] These cells are morphologically distinct from most T and B lymphocytes. The cells that mediate natural killing appear to be quite heterogeneous with regard to surface markers, and the exact lineage of these cells is still controversial. Most, but not all, carry the Fc receptor for the heavy chain of IgG. Although large granular lymphocytes do not carry the usual array of pan-T surface markers, and NK cells are actually increased in thymectomized animals, NK cells share characteristics of some T lymphocytes, such as reactivity with certain monoclonal anti-T lymphocyte antibodies. Some investigators have also noted the presence of surface markers characteristic of monocytes-macrophages. However, NK cells are nonphagocytic and nonadherent, and their enzyme pattern is in line with that of lymphoid cells. Recently, several reagents (including monoclonal antibodies) have become available for identifying major subpopulations of NK cells, and cell clones with natural killing activity have been developed. These studies should greatly increase our understanding of the NK cell.

## EXPERIMENTAL METHODS FOR STUDYING HUMAN LYMPHOCYTE SUBPOPULATIONS

**Assays for Enumeration and Separation of B and T Lymphocytes.** Assays for B and T lymphocytes in man are generally confined to those contained in peripheral blood lymphocytes. Peripheral blood mononuclear leukocytes (PBL), which include both lymphocytes and monocytes, are separated from red blood cells and granulocytes on the basis of buoyant density (Table 3–5). The most commonly used technique is the Ficoll-Hypaque separation procedure.

Human B lymphocytes are most often identified by the presence of cell surface immunoglobulin. Heterologous antisera made against whole human immunoglobulin molecules or purified light chains can be used to detect all B lymphocytes. Antisera (heterologous or monoclonal) directed against the heavy chains of purified myeloma proteins can be used to detect only those B lymphocytes that bear $\mu$, $\delta$, $\gamma$, or $\alpha$ heavy chains. These antisera are generally used in direct or indirect immunofluorescence assays. In the former assay, the antihuman antisera is directly conjugated with a fluorochrome (i.e., fluorescein). PBL are incubated with this reagent and then the number of fluorescent-positive cells are counted. In the latter assay, PBL are first incubated with the appropriate antihuman antisera (unconjugated), washed, and then reacted with a fluorochrome-conjugated antibody directed against the first step reagent (i.e., a fluorescein conjugated goat antirabbit immunoglobulin if the first step antisera was raised in rabbits, or a fluorescein conjugated antimouse immunoglobulin if the first reagent was a mouse monoclonal antibody).

The number of positively staining cells can be determined by fluorescence microscopy or by cytofluorograph machines such as the fluorescence-activated cell sorter (FACS).[123] These machines have become powerful tools for the immunologist in both enumerating and separating lymphocyte subpopulations. After cells are stained as described above, the machine can arrange them as single cells in a row, each enclosed within a microdroplet. The cells are then passed in front of a laser beam, and those cells that fluoresce are recognized by photoelectric receivers. The number of positive-staining cells and the intensity of fluorescence, as well as

**Table 3–5.** Approximate Percentage of T and B Lymphocytes in Normal Human Peripheral Blood Mononuclear Cells Purified on a Ficoll-Hypaque Gradient

| | T Lymphocytes | B Lymphocytes | Null (Non-T,Non-B) Lymphocytes | Monocytes and Myeloid Cells |
|---|---|---|---|---|
| *% Lymphocytes* | 77 | 11 | 12 | – |
| *% Total Cells* | 64 | 9 | 10 | 17 |

other cellular parameters, are electronically recorded. The machine can routinely count $10^4$ cells in a few seconds, separate live from dead cells, accurately and quantitatively determine the intensity of fluorescence, and separate the positive cells from the negative cells (see below).

Human T lymphocytes and their subsets can be identified by distinct surface markers using several techniques. A commonly used method for enumerating all T lymphocytes is based on the ability of human peripheral blood T lymphocytes to bind to sheep red blood cells. These erythrocyte-rosette-forming cells are counted in a standard hematocytometer. More recently, T lymphocytes and T lymphocyte subpopulations have been identified using monoclonal antibodies that recognize all T lymphocytes or a particular T lymphocyte subset. Generally, indirect immunofluorescence techniques are employed (as described above) using a second step fluorochrome-conjugated antimouse immunoglobulin reagent. Positively stained cells are enumerated as described above. T lymphocytes can also be enumerated by complement-dependent cytotoxicity methods using the same monoclonal antihuman antibodies (provided they are complement fixing). Cells are incubated with antibody and complement, and the percentage of dead cells is determined.

Similar techniques can be used to separate B and T lymphocytes from human PBL. T lymphocytes are generally isolated by their ability to bind to sheep red blood cells. After the formation of T lymphocyte-erythrocyte rosettes, the T lymphocytes can be separated from other nonrosetting mononuclear cells by buoyant density. After lysis of the attached sheep red blood cells, nearly pure T lymphocytes are obtained. The non-T (nonrosetting) cells contain a mixture of B lymphocytes, null lymphocytes, and monocytes. The monocytes can be removed by a variety of techniques (e.g., plastic or glass adherence), resulting in a greatly enriched B lymphocyte population.

B lymphocytes can also be "positively" isolated by using antisera directed against surface immunoglobulin, and either adherence or immunofluorescence techniques.

## CONCLUSIONS

A striking variety of lymphocyte subpopulations have been detected during the past several years. Each population appears to play an important function in the ever increasing complexity of control of the immune system. There are cells that augment the immune response, those that suppress it, those that specialize in antibody secretion, those that specialize in killing, and those that specialize in the production of different lymphokines. Given the complexity of cell populations, it is not surprising that there is a wide variety of congenital and acquired defects in the immune system in man. Elucidation of the characteristics and function of these cell populations in health and disease continues to provide a firm scientific basis for the diagnosis and treatment of both immunodeficiency and autoimmune diseases.

## References


1. Szenberg, A., and Warner, N.L.: Immunological function of thymus and bursa of Fabricius. Dissociation of immunological responsiveness in fowls with a hormonally arrested development of lymphoid tissues. Nature 194:145, 1962.
2. Cooper, M.D., Peterson, R.D.A., and Good, R.A.: Delineation of thymic and bursal lymphoid systems in the chicken. Nature 205:143, 1965.
3. Cooper, M.D., Peterson, R.D.A., South, M.A. and Good, R.A.: The functions of the thymus system and the bursa system in the chicken. J. Exp. Med. 123:75, 1966.
4. Miller, J.F.A.P., and Mitchell, G.F.: Thymus and antigen-reactive cells. Transplant. Rev. 1:3, 1969.
5. Raff, M.C.: Surface antigenic markers for distinguishing T and B lymphocytes in mice. Transplant. Rev. 6:52, 1971.
6. Moller, G.(ed.): T and B Lymphocytes in Humans. Transplant Rev. 15:1, 1973 (entire volume).
7. Everett, N.B., and Tyler, R.W.: Lymphopoiesis in the thymus and other tissues: Functional implications. Int. Rev. Cytol. 22:205, 1967.
8. Gowans, J.L., and McGregor, D.D.: The immunological activities of lymphocytes. Prog. Allergy 9:1, 1965.
9. Strober, S.: Immune function, cell surface characteristics, and maturation of B cell subpopulations. Transplant. Rev. 24:84, 1975.
10. Howard, J.C., Hunt, S.V., and Gowans, J.L.: Identification of marrow-derived and thymus-derived small lymphocytes in the lymphoid tissue and thoracic duct lymph of normal rats. J. Exp. Med. 135:200, 1972.
11. Sprent, J., and Basten, A.: Circulating T and B lymphocytes of the mouse. II. Lifespan. Cell. Immunol. 7:40, 1973.
12. Strober, S., and Dilley, J.: Biological characteristics of T and B memory lymphocytes in the rat. J. Exp. Med. 137:1275, 1973.
13. Weissman, I.L., Gutman, G.A., and Friedberg, S.H.: Tissue localization of lymphoid cells. Ser. Haematol. 7:482, 1974.
14. Guy-Grand, D., Griscelli, C., and Vassalli, P.: The mouse gut T lymphocyte, a novel type of T cell. Nature, origin, and traffic in mice in normal and graft-versus-host conditions. J. Exp. Med. 148:1661, 1978.
15. Hall, J.G., Hopkins, J., and Orlans, E.: Studies on the lymphocytes of sheep. III. Destination of lymph born immunoblasts in relation to their tissue of origin. Eur. J. Immunol. 7:30, 1979.
16. Butcher, E.C., Scollay, R.G., and Weissman, I.L.: Organ specificity of lymphocyte migration: Mediation by highly selective lymphocyte interaction with organ-specific determinants on high endothelial venules. Eur. J. Immunol. 10:556, 1980.
17. Miller, J.F.A.P.: Role of the thymus in transplantation immunity. Ann. N.Y. Acad. Sci. 99:340, 1962.
18. Haris, J.E., and Ford, C.E.: Cellular traffic of the thymus: Experiments with chromosome markers. Nature 201:884, 1964.
19. Cantor, H., and Weissman, I.L.: Development and function of subpopulations of thymocytes and T lymphocytes. Prog. Allergy 20:1, 1976.
20. Freidman, H.(ed.): Thymus factors in immunity. Ann. N.Y. Acad. Sci. 249:1, 1975.
21. Kruisbeek, A.M., Sharrow, S.O., and Singer, A.: Differences in the MHC-restricted self-recognition repertoire of intrathymic and extra-thymic cytotoxic T lymphocyte precursors. J. Immunol. 130:1027, 1983.
22. Cantor, H., and Boyse, E.A.: Functional subclasses of T lymphocytes bearing different Ly antigens 1. The generation of functionally distinct T-cell subclasses is a differentiative process independent of antigen. J. Exp. Med. 141:1376, 1975.
23. Katz, D.A.: Lymphocyte Differentiation Recognition, and Regulation. Academic Press, New York, 1977.
24. Hood, L.E., Weissman, I.L., Wood, W.B. (eds.): Immunology. Menlo Park, California, Benjamin/Cummings Pub. Co., Menlo Park, 1978, p. 13.
25. Reinherz, E.L., and Schlossman, S.F.: The differentiation and function of human T lymphocytes. Cell 19:821, 1980.
26. Boyse, E.A., Old, L.J., and Stockert, E.: The TL (thymus leukemia) antigen: A review. *In* Grabar, P., and Miescher, P.A. (eds.): Immunopathology. IV. International Symposium. Basel, Switzerland, Schwabe and Co., 1967, p. 23.
27. Ledbetter, J.A., Rouse, R.V., Micklem, H.S., and Herzenberg, L.A.: T cell subsets defined by expression of Lyt-1, 2, 3 and Thy-1 antigens. Two-parameter immunofluorescence and cytotoxicity analysis with monoclonal antibodies modifies current views. J. Exp. Med. 152:280, 1980.

28. Gershon, R.K.: T cell suppression. Contemp Top. Immunobiol. 3:1, 1974.
29. Cantor, H., and Boyse, E.A.: Functional subclasses of T lymphocytes bearing different Ly antigens. II. Cooperation between subclasses of Ly+ cells in the generation of killer activity. J. Exp. Med. 141:1390, 1975.
30. Jandinski, J., Cantor, H., Tadakuma, T., Peavy, D.L., and Pierce, C.W.: Separation of helper T cells from suppressor T cells expressing different Ly components. 1. Polyclonal activation: suppressor and helper activities are inherent properties of distinct T-cell subclasses. J. Exp. Med. 143:1382, 1976.
31. Cantor, H., Shen, F.W., and Boyse, E.A.: Separation of helper T cells from suppressor T cells expressing different Ly components. II. Activation by antigen: after immunization, antigen-specific suppressor and helper activities are mediated by distinct T-cell subclasses. J. Exp. Med. 143:1391, 1976.
32. Reinherz, E.L., Kung, P.C., Goldstein, G., and Schlossman, S.F.: Further characterization of the human inducer T cell subset defined by monoclonal antibody. J. Immunol. 123:2894, 1979.
33. Reinherz, E.L., Kung, P.C., Goldstein, G., and Schlossman, S.F.: A monoclonal antibody reactive with the human cytotoxic suppressor T cell subset previously defined by a heteroantiserum termed $TH_2$. J. Immunol. 124:1301, 1980.
34. Reinherz, E.L., Morimoto, C., Penta, A.C., and Schlossman, S.F.: Regulation of B cell immunoglobulin secretion by functional subsets of T lymphocytes in man. Eur. J. Immunol. 10:570, 1980.
35. Evans, R.L., Wall, D.W., Platsoucas, C.D., Siegal, F.P., Fikrig, S.M., Testa, C.M., and Good, R.A.: Thymus-dependent membrane antigens in man: Inhibition of cell-mediated lympholysis by monoclonal antibodies to the $TH_2$ antigen. Proc. Natl. Acad. Sci. (USA) 78:544, 1981.
36. Kotzin, B.L., Benike, C.J., and Engleman, E.G.: Induction of immunoglobulin-secreting cells in the allogeneic mixed leukocyte reaction: regulation by helper and suppressor lymphocyte subsets in man. J. Immunol. 127:931, 1981.
37. Engleman, E.G., Benike, C.J., Grumet, F.C., and Evans, R.L.: Activation of human T lymphocyte subsets: Helper and suppressor/cytotoxic T cells recognize and respond to distinct histocompatibility antigens. J. Immunol. 127:2124, 1981.
38. Ledbetter, J.A., Evans, R.L., Lipinski, M., Cunningham-Rundles, C., Good, R.A., and Herzenberg, L.A.: Evolutionary conservation of surface molecules that distinguish T lymphocyte helper/inducer and T cytotoxic/suppressor subpopulations in mouse and man. J. Exp. Med. 153:310, 1981.
39. Moller, G. (ed.): Effects of anti-membrane antibodies on killer T cells. Immunol. Rev. 68:1, 1982 (entire volume).
40. Thomas, Y., Rogozinski, L., Irigoyen, O., Friedman, M., Kung, P.C., Goldstein, G., and Chess, L.: Functional analysis of human T cell subsets defined by monoclonal antibodies. IV. Induction of suppressor cells within the $OKT4^+$ population. J. Exp. Med. 154:459, 1981.
41. Krensky, A.M., Clayberger, C., Reiss, C.S., Strominger, J.L., and Burakoff, S.J.: Specificity of $OKT4^+$ cytotoxic T lymphocyte clones. J. Immunol. 129:2001, 1982.
42. Moretta, L., Ferrarini, M., Mingari, M.C., Moretta, A., and Webb, S.R.: Subpopulations of human T cells identified by receptors for immunoglobulins and mitogen responsiveness. J. Immunol. 117:2171, 1976.
43. Moretta, L., Webb, S.R., Grossi, C.E., Lydyard, P.M., and Cooper, M.D.: Functional analysis of two human T-cell subpopulations: Help and suppression of B-cell responses by T cells bearing receptors for IgM or IgG. J. Exp. Med. 146:184, 1977.
44. Moretta, L., Moretta, A., Canonica, G.W., Bacigalupo, A., Mingari, M.C., and Cerottini, J-C.: Receptors for immunoglobulins on resting and activated human T cells. Immunol. Rev. 56:141, 1981.
45. Pichler, W.J., and Broder, S.: In vitro functions of human T cells expressing Fc-IgG or Fc-IgM receptors. Immunol. Rev. 56:163, 1981.
46. Reinherz, E.L., Moretta, L., Roper, M., Breard, J.M., Mingari, M.C., Cooper, M.D., and Schlossman, S.F.: Human T lymphocyte subpopulations defined by Fc receptors and monoclonal antibodies: A comparison. J. Exp. Med. 151:969, 1980.
47. Kay, H.D., and Horwitz, D.A.: Evidence by reactivity with hybridoma antibodies for a probable myeloid origin of peripheral blood cells active in natural cytotoxicity and antibody dependent cell mediated cytotoxicity. J. Clin. Invest. 66:847, 1980.
48. Fox, R.I., Thompson, L.F., and Huddlestone, J.F.: $T\gamma$ cells express T-lymphocyte-associated antigens. J. Immunol. 126:2062, 1981.
49. Alter, B.J., Schendel, D.J., Bach, M.L., Bach, F.J., Klein, J., and Stimpfling, J.H.: Cell-mediated lympholysis: Importance of serologically defined H-2 regions. J. Exp. Med. 137:1303, 1973.
50. Bach, F.H., Bach, M.L., and Sondel, P.M.: Differential function of major histocompatibility complex antigens in T-lymphocyte activation. Nature 259:273, 1976.
51. Plate, J.M.D. Soluble factors substitute for T-T cell collaboration in generation of T killer lymphocytes. Nature 260:329, 1976.
52. Wagner, H., Hardt, C., Heeg, K., Pfizenmaier, K., Solbach, W., Bartlett, R., Stockinger, H., and Rollinghoff, M.: T-T cell interactions during cytotoxic T lymphocyte (CTL) responses: T cell-derived helper factor (Interleukin 2) as a probe to analyze CTL responsiveness and thymic maturation of CTL progenitors. Immunol. Rev. 51:215, 1980.
53. Zinkernagel, R.M., and Doherty, P.C.: MHC-restricted cytotoxic T cells: Studies on the biological role of polymorphic major transplantation antigens determining T-cell restriction-specificity, function, and responsiveness. Adv. Immunol. 27:51, 1979.
54. Finberg, R., and Benacerraf, B.: Induction, control, and consequences of virus specific cytotoxic T cells. Immunol. Rev. 58:157, 1981.
55. Reiss, C.S., and Burakoff, S.J.: Specificity of the helper T cell for the cytolytic T lymphocyte response to influenza viruses. J. Exp. Med. 154:541, 1981.
56. Gershon, R.K.: Suppressive interactions between different MLR loci. *In* Katz, D.H., and Benacerraf, B. (eds.): The Role of Products of the Histocompatibility Gene Complex in Immune Responses. New York, Academic Press, 1976, p. 193.
57. Rich, S.S., and Rich, R.R.: Regulatory mechanisms in cell-mediated immune responses. 1. Regulation of mixed lymphocyte reactions by alloantigen-activated thymus-derived lymphocytes. J. Exp. Med. 140:1588, 1974.
58. Nadler, L.M., and Hodes, R.J.: Regulatory mechanisms in cell-mediated immune responses. II. Comparison of culture-induced and alloantigen-induced suppressor cells in MLR and CML. J. Immunol. 118:1886, 1977.
59. Truitt, G.A., Dennison, D.K., Rich, R.R., and Rich, S.S.: Interaction between T cells and non-T cells in suppression of cytotoxic lymphocyte responses. J. Immunol. 123:745, 1979.
60. Sasportes, M., Wollman, E., Cohen, D., Carosella, E., Bensussan, A., Fradelizi, D., and Dausset, J.: Suppression of the human allogeneic response in vitro with primed lymphocytes and suppressor supernates. J. Exp. Med. 152:270S, 1980.
61. Chaout, G., Mathieson, B.J., and Asofsky, R.: Regulatory mechanisms in the mixed lymphocyte reaction: evidence for the requirement of two T cells to interact in the generation of effective suppression. J. Immunol. 129:502, 1982.
62. Okada, S., and Strober, S.: Spleen cells from adult mice given total lymphoid irradiation or from newborn mice have similar regulatory effects in the mixed leukocyte reaction. 1. Generation of antigen-specific suppressor cells in the mixed leukocyte reaction after the addition of spleen cells from adult mice given total lymphoid irradiation. J. Exp. Med. 156:522, 1982.
63. Susskind, B.M., Merluzzi, V.J., Faanes, R.B., Palladino, M.A., and Choi, Y.S.: Regulatory mechanisms in cytotoxic T lymphocyte development. 1. A suppressor T cell subset that regulates the proliferative stage of CTL development. J. Immunol. 130:527, 1983.
64. Waldman, T.A., Blaese, R.M., Broder, S., and Krakauer, R.S.: Disorders of suppressor immunoregulatory cells in the pathogenesis of immunodeficiency and autoimmunity. Ann. Intern. Med. 88:226, 1978.
65. Herzenberg, L.A., Okumura, K., and Metzler, C.M.: Regulation of immunoglobulin and antibody production by allotype suppressor T cells in mice. Transplant. Rev. 27:57, 1975.
66. Eichmann, K.: Idiotype suppression. II. Amplification of a suppressor T cell with anti-idiotypic activity. Eur. J. Immunol 5:511, 1975.
67. Bona, C., and Paul, W.E.: Cellular basis of regulation of expression of idiotype. I. T-suppressor cells specific for MOPC 460 idiotype regulate the expression of cells secreting anti-TNP antibodies bearing 460 idiotype. J. Exp. Med. 149:592, 1979.
68. Germain, R.N., and Benacerraf, B.: A single major pathway of T-lymphocyte interactions in antigen specific immune suppression. Scand. J. Immunol. 13:1, 1981.
69. Gershon, R.K.: Immunoregulation circa 1980: Some comments on the state of the art. J. Allergy Clin. Immunol. 66:18, 1980.
70. Cantor, H., Hugenberger, J., McVay-Boudreau, L., Eardley, D.D., Kemp, J., Shen, F.W., and Gershon, R.K.: Immunoregulatory circuits among T-cell subsets: Identification of a subpopulation of T-helper cells that induces feedback inhibition. J. Exp. Med. 148:871, 1979.
71. Eardley, D.D., Murphy, D.B., Kemp, J.D., Shen, F.W., Cantor, H., and Gershon, R.K.: Ly-1 inducer and Ly-1,2 acceptor T cells in the feedback suppression circuit bear an I-J-subregion controlled determinant. Immunogenetics 11:549, 1980.
72. Gershon, R.K., Eardley, D.D., Durum, S., Green, D.R., Shen, F,W., Yamauchi, K., Cantor, H., and Murphy, D.B.: Contrasuppression: A novel immunoregulatory activity. J. Exp. Med. 153:1533, 1981.
73. Thomas, Y., Sosman, J., Origoyen, O., Friedman, S.M., Kung, P.C., Goldstein, G., and Chess, L.: Functional analysis of human T cell subsets defined by monoclonal antibodies. 1. Collaborative T-T interactions in the immunoregulation of B cell differentiation. J. Immunol. 125:2402, 1980.
74. Gatenby, P.A., Kotzin, B.L., Kansas, G.S., and Engleman, E.G.: Immunoglobulin secretion in the human autologous mixed leukocyte reaction. Definition of a suppressor-amplifier circuit using monoclonal antibodies. J. Exp. Med. 156:55, 1982.
75. Morimoto, C., Distaso, J.A., Borel, Y., Schlossman, S.F., and Reinherz,

E.L.: Communicative interactions between subpopulations of human T lymphocytes required for generation of suppressor effector function in a primary antibody response. J. Immunol. 128:1645, 1982.
76. Yachie, A., Miyawaki, T., Yokoi, T., Nagaoki, T., and Taniguchi, N.: Ia-positive cells generated by PWM-stimulation within OKT4+ subset interact with OKT8+ cells for inducing active suppression on B cell differentiation in vitro. J. Immunol. 129:103, 1982.
77. Gillis, S., and Smith, K.A.: Long-term culture of tumor-specific cytotoxic T cells. Nature 268:154, 1977.
78. Moller, G. (ed.): T cell clones. Immunol. Rev. 54:1, 1981 (entire volume).
79. Fitch, F., and Fathman, C.G. (eds.): Isolation, Characterization, and Utilization of T Lymphocyte Clones. Academic Press, New York, 1982.
80. Kappler, J.W., Skidmore, B., White, J., and Marrack, P.: Antigen-inducible, H-2 restricted, interleukin-2-producing T cell hybridomas. Lack of independent antigen and H-2 recognition. J. Exp. Med. 153:1198, 1981.
81. Infante, A.J., Infante, P.D., Gillis, S., and Fathman, C.G.: Definition of T cell idiotypes using anti-idiotypic antisera produced by immunization with T cell clones. J. Exp. Med. 155:1100, 1982.
82. Marrack, P., and Kappler, J.: Use of somatic cell genetics to study chromosomes contributing to antigen plus I recognition by T cell hybridomas. J. Exp. Med. 147:404, 1983.
83. Haskins, K., Kubo, R., White, J., Pigeon, M., Kappler, J., Marrack P.: The major histocompatibility restricted antigen receptor on T cells. 1. Isolation with a monoclonal antibody. J. Exp. Med. 157:1149, 1983.
84. Eichmann, K.: Expression and function of idiotypes on lymphocytes. Adv. Immunol. 26:195, 1978.
85. Binz, H., and Wigzell, H.: Idiotypic, alloantigen-reactive T lymphocyte receptors and their use to induce specific transplantation tolerance. Prog. Allergy 23:154, 1977.
86. Germain, R.N., Ju, S-T., Kipps, T.J., Benacerraf, B., and Dorf, M.E.: Shared idiotypic determinants on antibodies and T-cell-derived suppressor factor specific for the random terpolymer L-glutamic acid-L-alanine-L-tyrosine. J. Exp. Med. 149:613, 1979.
87. Rocklin, R.E., Bendtzen, K., and Greineder, D.: Mediators of immunity: Lymphokines and monokines. Adv. Immunol. 29:55, 1980.
88. Smith, K.A., and Ruscetti, F.W.: T cell growth factor and the culture of cloned functional T cells. Adv. Immunol. 31:137, 1981.
89. Moller, G. (ed.): Interleukins and lymphocyte activation. Immunol. Rev. 63:1, 1982 (entire volume).
90. Beller, D.I., and Ho, K.: Regulation of macrophage populations V. Evaluation of the control of macrophage Ia expression in vitro. J. Immunol. 129:971, 1982.
91. Fleisher, T.A., Attallah, A.M., Tosato, G., Blaese, R.M., and Greene, W.C.: Interferon-medicated inhibition of human polyclonal immunoglobulin synthesis. J. Immunol. 129:1099, 1982.
92. Muraguchi, A., and Fauci, A.S.: Proliferative responses of normal human B lymphocytes. Development of an assay system for human B cell growth factor (BCGF). J. Immunol. 129:1104, 1982.
93. Okada, M., Sakaguchi, N., Yoshimura, N., Hara, H., Shimizu, K., Yoshida, N., Yoshizaki, K., Kishimoto, S., Yamamura, Y., and Kishimoto, T.: B cell growth factors and B cell differentiation factor from human T hybridomas: Two distinct kinds of B cell growth factor and their synergism in B cell proliferation. J. Exp. Med. 157:583, 1983.
94. Kincade, P.W., and Cooper, M.D.: Development and distribution of immunoglobulin-containing cells in the chicken: An immunofluorescent analysis using purified antibodies to $\mu$, $\gamma$, and light chains. J. Immunol. 106:371, 1971.
95. Owen, J.J.T., Cooper, M.D., and Raff, M.C.: In vitro generation of B lymphocytes in mouse foetal liver, a mammalian bursa equivalent. Nature 249:361, 1974.
96. Melchers, F., Von Boehmer, H., and Phillips, R.A.: B lymphocyte subpopulations in the mouse: Organ distribution and ontogeny of immunoglobulin-synthesizing and of mitogen sensitive cells. Transplant. Rev. 25:26, 1975.
97. Abramson, S., Miller, R.G., and Phillips, R.A.: The identification in adult bone marrow of pluripotent and restricted stem cells of the myeloid and lymphoid systems. J. Exp. Med. 145:1567, 1977.
98. Cooper, M.D.: Ontogeny and differentiation of B cells. *In* Cooper, M.D., Mosier, D.E., Scher, I., and Vitetta, E.S. (eds.): B Lymphocytes in the Immune Response. New York, Elsevier/North-Holland, 1979, p. 61.
99. Raff, M.C., Megson, M., Owen, J.J.T., and Cooper, M.D.: Early production of intracellular IgM by B lymphocyte precursors in mouse. Nature (Lond.) 259:224, 1975.
100. Grey, H.: Surface markers on B cells. *In* Cooper, M.D., Mosier, D.E., Scher, I., and Vitetta, E.S. (eds.): B Lymphocytes in the Immune Response. New York, Elsevier/North-Holland, 1979, p. 1.
101. Kearney, J.F., Cooper, M.D., Klein, J., Abney, E.R., Parkhouse, R.M.E., and Lawton, A.R.: Ontogeny of Ia and IgD on IgM-bearing B lymphocytes in mice. J. Exp. Med. 146:297, 1977.
102. Rosenberg, Y.J., and Parish, C.R.: Ontogeny of the antibody-forming cell line in mice. IV. Appearance of cells bearing Fc receptors, complement receptors, and surface immunoglobulin. J. Immunol. 118:612, 1977.
103. Vitetta, E.S., Melcher, U., McWilliams, M., Lamm, M.E., Phillips-Quagliata, J.M., and Uhr, J.W.: Cell surface immunoglobulin. XI. The appearance of an IgD-like molecule on murine lymphoid cells during ontogeny. J. Exp. Med. 141:206, 1975.
104. Scher, I., Ahmed, A., Strong, D.M., Steinberg, A.D., and Paul, W.E.: X-linked B lymphocyte immune defect in CBA/N mice. 1. Studies of the function and composition of spleen cells. J. Exp. Med. 141:788, 1975.
105. Scher, I., Steinberg, A.D., Berning, A.K., and Paul, W.E.: X-linked B lymphocyte immune defect in CBA/N mice. II. Studies of the mechanisms underlying the immune defect. J. Exp. Med. 142:637, 1975.
106. Ahmed, A., Scher, I., Sharrow, S.O., Smith, A.H., Paul, W.E., Sachs, D.H., and Sell, K.W.: B lymphocyte heterogeneity: Development and characterization of an alloantiserum which distinguishes B lymphocyte differentiation alloantigens. J. Exp. Med. 145:101, 1977.
107. Scher, I., Titus, J.A., and Finkelman, F.D.: The ontogeny and distribution of B cells in normal and mutant immunedefective CBA/N mice: Two-parameter analysis of surface IgM and IgD. J. Immunol. 130:619, 1983.
108. Singer, A., Morrissey, J., Hathcock, K.S., Ahmed, A., Scher, I., and Hodes, R.J.: Role of the major histocompatibility complex (MHC) in T cell activation of B cell subpopulations. Lyb5− and Lyb5+ B cell subpopulations differ in their requirement for MHC restricted T cell recognition. J. Exp. Med. 145:501, 1977.
109. Klinman, N., Mosier, D.E., Scher, I., and Vitetta, E.S. (eds.): B Lymphocytes in the Immune Response: Functional, Developmental, and Interactive Properties. New York, Elsevier/North-Holland, 1981, p. 295.
110. Moller, G. (ed.): Genetic models of B cell differentiation. Immunol. Rev. 64:1, 1982 (entire volume).
111. Gathings, W.E., Lawton, A.R., and Cooper, M.D.: Immunofluorescent studies of the development of pre-B cells, B lymphocytes, and immunoglobulin isotype diversity in humans. Eur. J. Immunol. 7:804, 1977.
112. Vitetta, E.S., and Uhr, J.W.: Immunoglobulin-receptors revisited: A model for the differentiation of bone marrow-derived lymphocyte is described. Science 189:964, 1975.
113. Metcalf, E.S., and Klinman, N.R.: In vitro tolerance induction of neonatal murine B cells. J. Exp. Med. 143:1327, 1976.
114. Raff, M.C., Owen, J.J.T., Cooper, M.D., Lawton, A.R., Megson, M., and Gathings, W.E.: Differences in susceptibility of mature and immature mouse B lymphocytes to anti-immunoglobulin-induced immunoglobulin suppression in vitro: Possible implications for B-cell tolerance to self. J. Exp. Med. 142:1052, 1975.
115. Vitetta, E.S., Cambier, J.C., Ligler, F.L., Kettman, J.R., Zan-Bar, I., Strober, S., and Uhr, J.W.: The role of surface immunoglobulins in triggering and tolerance of B cells. *In* Cooper, M.D., Mosier, D.E., Scher, I., Vitetta, E.S. (eds.): B Lymphocytes in the Immune Response. New York, Elsevier/North-Holland, 1979, p. 233.
116. Okumura, K., Julius, M.H., Tsu, T., Herzenberg, L.A., and Herzenberg, L.A.: Demonstration that IgG memory is carried by IgG-bearing cells. Eur. J. Immunol. 6:467, 1976.
117. Mason, D.W.: The class of surface immunoglobulin on cells carrying IgG memory in rat thoracic duct lymph: The size of the subpopulation mediating IgG memory. J. Exp. Med. 143:1122, 1976.
118. Zan-Bar, I., Vitetta, E.S., Assisi, F., and Strober, S.: The relationship between surface immunoglobulin isotype and immune function of murine B lymphocytes. III. Expression of a single predominant isotype on primed and unprimed B cells. J. Exp. Med. 147:1374, 1978.
119. Moller, G. (ed.): Concepts of B lymphocyte activation. Immunol. Rev. 23:1, 1975 (entire volume).
120. Falkoff, R.J., Zhu, L.P., and Fauci, A.S.: Separate signals for human B cell proliferation and differentiation in response to Staphylococcus aureus: evidence for a two-signal model of B cell activation. J. Immunol. 129:97, 1982.
121. Herberman, R.B., (ed.): Natural Cell-Mediated Immunity Against Tumors. Academic Press, New York, 1980.
122. Moller, G. (ed.): Natural killer cells. Immunol. Rev. 44:1, 1979 (entire volume).
123. Herzenberg, L.A., and Herzenberg, L.A.: Analysis and separation using the fluorescence activated cell sorter (FACS). *In* Weir, D.M. (ed.): Handbook of Experimental Immunology. 3rd ed. Oxford, Blackwell, 1978, p. 22.1.
124. Dialynas, D.P., Wilde, D.B., Marrack, P., Pierres, A., Wall, K.A., Havran, W., Otten, G., Loken,, M.R., Pierres, M., Kappler, J., and Fitch, F.W.: Characterization of the murine antigenic determinant, designated L3T4a, recognized by monoclonal antibody GK1.5: Expression of L3T4a by functional T cell clones appears to correlate primarily with class II MHC antigen-reactivity. Immunol. Rev. 74:29, 1983.

# Chapter 4
# The Major Histocompatibility Complex

*R. J. Winchester*

## INTRODUCTION

The segment on the short arm of the sixth chromosome that is usually termed the major histocompatibility complex (MHC) contains the genetic determinants for a number of characteristics that have regulation of the immune response as their principal focal point. These gene products achieve this regulation in part by controlling the differentiation and proliferation of T lymphocytes and B lymphocytes induced by contact with antigen.

One of the most interesting aspects of this control is that recognition of conventional antigens by T lymphocytes occurs in a context of "self" that is provided by the MHC molecules. This molecular definition of biologic individuality derives from the products of the extremely large number of alternative MHC genes found in the population. A second aspect of control is that the functional capabilities of the immune response differ according to the MHC alleles an individual inherits. As a consequence of this variation, the MHC genes have a profound influence on resistance or susceptibility to certain diseases, particularly a number of those that are rheumatic in character. The survival of allografts is also determined by this variation because the different alternative molecules are in themselves intensely antigenic. Indeed it was this property of histocompatibility that first directed attention to the existence of the MHC long before its central role in immune regulation was known. Understanding the basis of the biologic impetus to development of this genetic diversity is one of the tantalizing challenges in the study of the MHC.

A distinctive feature of many genes of the MHC is that their products are expressed on the cell membrane and appear to mediate cell-to-cell interactions. These cell surface molecules occur in two entirely distinct varieties. The first class, sometimes designated class I, consists of the HLA-A, B, and C molecules (Table 4–1). These molecules are encoded by genes located at the most distal position of the MHC (Fig. 4–1). The genes encoding the class II products, or Ia/DR molecules, are present at the centromeric end of the major histocompatibility complex. There are two additional classes of MHC gene products: the class III molecules, which comprise the C3 convertase systems of the classic and alternative complement pathways, and are located between the class I and class II genes; and the class IV cytoplasmic molecules, about which relatively little is known in the human. The class III complement component molecules will be discussed in Chapter 7.

The basic structure of the class I molecule consists of two chains. One chain, the heavy or $\alpha$ chain is an intrinsic membrane component of several distinct regions or domains. The molecule extends across the entire membrane (Fig. 4–2). The much smaller light or $\beta$ chain is $\beta^2$ microglobulin and is an extrinsic membrane component and is present only on the exterior of the membrane. It is shown as a shaded structure associated by noncovalent interactions with the $\alpha$-2 and $\alpha$-3 domains. The gene encoding the $\beta$ chain is located on chromosome 15.

The basic structure of the class II or Ia molecules consists of two different chains more nearly equivalent in size that are both intrinsic membrane components (Fig. 4–2). Both chains are encoded by genes that are located in the same region of chromosome 6, designated "class II" in Fig. 4–1. Each chain is organized into two intracellular domains, a transmembrane portion and a small intercellular portion.

The total size of the MHC is considerable, and it has been calculated that there is sufficient space for several hundred genes. Thus, to the dismay of some but the joy of others, it is evident that there are large areas of ignorance despite the fact that the MHC is perhaps the most intricate biologic response to have been analyzed in man. In this context the disease associations may result in the appreciation of entirely unsuspected elements in the MHC.

Because of the astonishing rapidity with which knowledge concerning disease associations is unfolding, coupled with the promise of its immediate practical application, the content of this chapter has been oriented to provide much of the background that is necessary to gain access to the current literature, with primary emphasis on the markers that constitute the reference points for these disease associations.

## HISTORICAL ORIENTATION

Knowledge regarding the human MHC spans a period of less than three decades. The early history was dominated by the clinical problem of transplantation and aimed at defining the population genetics of the allodeterminants. The initial studies began with the observation that sera from multiply transfused patients contained antibodies termed "leukoagglutinins," which agglutinated a suspension of donor leukocytes.[1,2] Subsequently, pregnancy sera were found to be a source of

**Table 4–1.** Comparison of the Two Classes of Cell Surface Glycoproteins Encoded by Genes of the Major Histocompatibility Complex

| | Class I | Class II |
|---|---|---|
| Terminology | HLA-A, B, C | Ia(DR) |
| Expression | Essentially all cells except mature RBC trophoblast, early embryonic tissue (?) | Certain cells of immune system B, monocyte, dendritic stimulated T cells plus a few other cell types |
| Structure | | |
| α chain | 44 kD | 34 kD |
| β chain | 11.5 kD | 29 kD |
| Membrane Relationship | | |
| α chain | intrinsic | intrinsic |
| β chain | extrinsic | intrinsic |
| Location of polymorphisms | | |
| α chain | α1 and α2 domains | α1 domains of DS and SB |
| β chain | – | β1 domains of DR, DS, and SB |
| Site of gene | | |
| α chain | chromosome 6 | chromosome 6 |
| β chain | chromosome 15 | chromosome 6 |
| Number of loci | | |
| α chain | 3 (HLA-A, B, C) | 1DR, 2DS, 2SB |
| β chain | 1(?) | 3DR, 2DS, 2SB |

the leukoagglutinins. This finding simplifed the recognition of discrete alloantigen specificities because of the more limited antigenic challenge provided by the paternal MHC antigens expressed in the fetus. The delineation of specificities in these reagent sera for various leukocyte antigens was further assisted by the introduction of analytic approaches that enabled clusters of related specificities to be recognized.[3] In 1964, the complement-mediated cytotoxic assay using lymphocytes was introduced, and its superiority over the agglutination technique was clearly demonstrated.[4] By the end of the first decade of studies, two leukocyte antigen segregant series, now designated HLA-A and B, were characterized. Furthermore, an international collaborative arrangement for assigning specificities was established. At that time all observations were concerned with the class I MHC molecules.

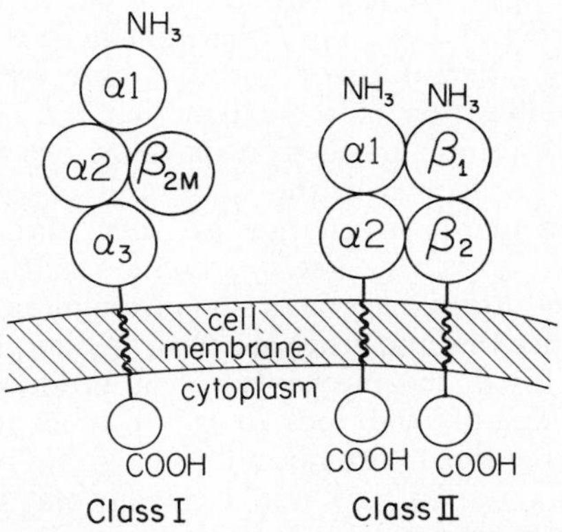


**Figure 4–2.** Domain structure of class I and class II MHC molecules.

Subsequent progress has moved in three main directions. First, there has been continual refinement of the A and B locus specificities, especially among non-Caucasian populations. In addition, a third locus, C, was also described. Secondly, one of the biologic roles of the class I molecules was found to be participation as a component of the structures recognized by cytotoxic T lymphocytes when they attack target cells expressing viral antigens.[5] Thirdly, the entry of this field of knowledge into the mainstream of internal medicine began in 1973 with the observations on the association between the HLA-B27 allele and susceptibility to ankylosing spondylitis.[6,7]

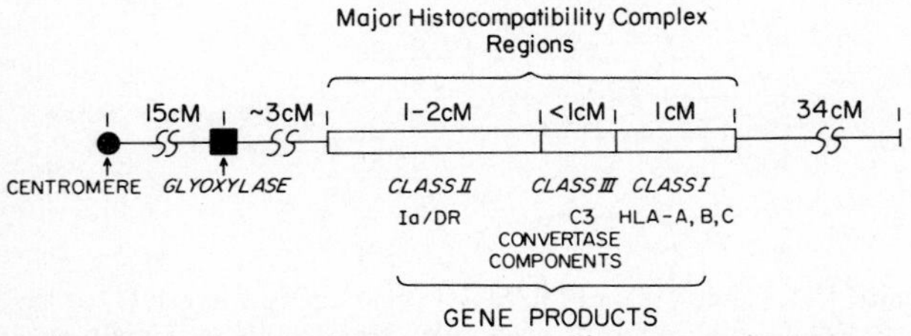


**Figure 4–1.** Schematic representation of the short arm of the 6th chromosome illustrating the location of the major histocompatibility complex.

The focus of the field shifted further from histocompatibility to the significance of these gene products in the biology of the individual during the mid 1970s with the recognition of the class II molecules and their central role of regulating the immune response. Indeed, some emphasize this change in perspective by referring to the MHC as the MIC, the *major immunogene complex.* In the latter years of the 1970s the importance of the class II or IA/DR alleles in influencing susceptibility to nearly all rheumatic diseases with immunologic features provided a further dimension of clinical significance to the biology of the MHC. Lastly, the concept of the MHC as the site of other loci was expanded by the finding that genes for the complement component C2 mapped within it.

A dominant characteristic of all research on the MHC has been the interchange of information between investigators primarily concerned with different species, particularly research performed using the mouse.[8] Insights obtained in one species can often be readily transferred to another because of the intriguing biologic fact that the MHC of each species is organized in a homologous manner.

## GENETIC PRINCIPLES

**Terminology.** The basic unit of genetic information is the *gene.* The segment of chromosome that contains the gene and codes for all or part of a specific single polypeptide chain is a *locus.* A *region* is the portion of the chromosome where the locus is situated. Other *traits* can map in this region without necessarily inferring that they are specified by the same locus or gene. Alternative forms of genes are termed *alleles.* These arise by mutation. An individual with different alleles ($A_1$ and $A_2$) of the same gene is a *heterozygote,* with each allelic gene on a different homologous chromosome of either maternal or paternal origin. The offspring of this individual illustrate Mendel's first law that these alleles will segregate. Mendel's second law—that nonallelic traits, determined by different genes, will sort independently—requires modification to the extent that the genes are located close to one another on the same chromosome in *linkage.* Or, defined in the reciprocal sense, linkage is the degree to which genes on the same chromosome are inherited together. *Recombination* resulting from crossing over during meiosis occurs in rough proportion to the distance that the genes are separated on the chromosome. This is the mechanism that produces independent sorting of genes located at a distance from one another on the same chromosome. The group of linked alleles of loci located on a single chromosome of either maternal or paternal origin is a *haplotype.* The concept of haplotype is important because the haploid chromosome is the vehicle of inheritance of the genome, and thus the haplotype represents the basic unit of inheritance. The various genes under consideration define the *genotype* of an individual. The expression of the genotype is the *phenotype* of an individual. This can take the form of a trait or of a specific structurally defined component. The Mendelian concepts of *dominance* and *recessivity* primarily apply to the expression of traits. In contrast, the genes of each haplotype that have structurally recognized products are almost always both expressed, and this pattern of gene expression is termed *codominance.*

Usually, as a result of natural selection, the number of alleles in a population is limited and mutant forms are present at low frequencies. For certain loci, an unusual situation exists in which there are two or more alleles that are each present at a frequency higher than can be accounted for by mutation. This state of multiple allelic forms is a *polymorphism,* and most of the loci of the MHC are composed of highly polymorphic series.[9,10]

The term *complex* refers to two or more loci. The "complexity" of the MHC is very real, but progress can be materially aided by always recalling there are only two families or classes of MHC molecules and that each family varies in only two ways. One dimension of this variation consists of duplicated genes, by which an individual is endowed with several loci on one chromosome that encode similar but not identical gene products, each with somewhat different functions. For example, there are three loci on each chromosome 6 that encode slightly different types of class I molecules (Fig. 4–3). This can be thought of as complexity or diversity at the level of the *locus.* It presumably serves to multiply the roles of the MHC molecules within an individual, since the independently segregating genes of each locus can undergo separate evolutionary routes. The second dimension of this variation is evident in the species but not necessarily in all individuals. It involves the development of alternative gene forms for each of the duplicated loci. These new alleles become the property of the species, endowing different individuals with regulatory molecules that have different properties. This second dimension of *allele diversity* results in a biologic individuality that presumably is the substrate for fitness to a particular environment. This strategy is unlike that found in the immunoglobulin system, where each individual is provided with an immense repertoire of alternative variable regions and there is very little difference among individuals. The existence of the MHC gene cluster on one chromosome in all higher species suggests that in some way the products interact to maintain this association. Most duplicated genes, such as the hemoglobin $\alpha$ and $\beta$ genes, are not located in proximity to one another.

**Genetic Relationships Within a Family.** In the case of a typical polymorphic MHC gene with a product that is codominantly expressed on the cell surface, a situation would frequently be found in which each parent will not share any MHC gene product with the other parent. If the alleles, or their haplotypes that result from meiotic division in the parent, are designated a, b, c, d, the kinds of genotypes found in the family and their interrelationships can be designated as in Figure 4–4. If the genotypes of the father and mother are a/b and c/d, respectively, the children, according to Mendel's first law, will be a/c, a/d, b/c, or b/d. Thus, a total of six genotypes are present in such a family (Fig.4–4). Note that individuals II-1 and II-5 are identical.

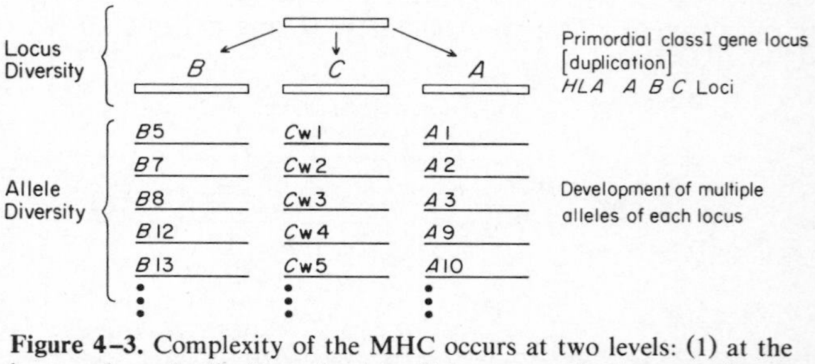


**Figure 4–3.** Complexity of the MHC occurs at two levels: (1) at the locus, where duplication of primordial gene results in a multi-gene family and (2) at the generation of a family of alleles for each locus by mutation, conversion, and so on.

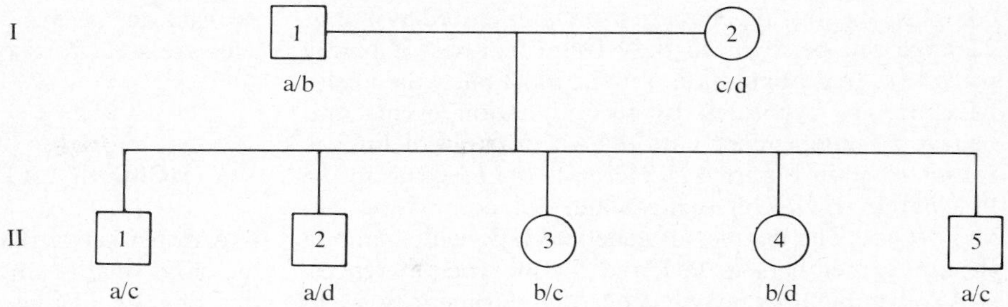


**Figure 4–4.** Genotype of idealized family illustrating inheritance of a polymorphic gene with four alleles: a, b, c, and. d.

There are three types of genetic relationship among various members of the family: (1) identity (0 haplotype difference), (2) complete dissimilarity (2 haplotype difference), and (3) partial sharing or haplo-identity (1 haplotype difference). Among the siblings of a sufficiently large family, all three relationships will be found. The relationship of parent to child, however, always involves a one allele difference.

**Genes in a Population.** The task of measuring gene frequency is simplified in the case of class I and class II molecules to counting alternative gene products in a population because of the codominant expression of all the products encoded by genes at each locus of each chromosome 6. This works particularly well in families in which haplotypes are easily defined. Since the unit of inheritance is the haploid chromosome, it is convenient to approach the idea of studying the gene pool by considering first the frequency of genes on gametes. For example, if the frequency of the HLA-A1 allotype in a population is $p$ and the frequency of the HLA-A3 allotype is $q$, then among individuals of the entire population, $p$ gametes will contain the HLA-A1 gene and $q$ gametes will contain the HLA-A3 gene. If there are no restrictions on mating choice, and the presence of the gene is neutral with respect to survival, the combination of male and female gametes in the fertilized zygote will occur in the proportions of $(p + q) \times (p + q)$ or $p^2$, $2pq$, and $q^2$. These describe the expected frequencies of homozygotes for HLA-A1, heterozygotes expressing HLA-A1 and HLA-A2, and homozygotes for HLA-A3 (Table 4–2). Again assuming random mating generation, since there has not been any change in the frequency of gametes bearing the A1 or A3 alleles, the same proportion of individuals heterozygous or homozygous for A1 or A3 will result. This is the basic concept of Hardy-Weinberg equilibrium.

By rearranging terms, a useful expression for calculating gene frequency can be derived as follows:

$$\text{Gene frequency} = 1 - \sqrt{1 - \text{phenotype frequency}}$$

where the phenotype frequency is expressed as a decimal fraction. Although these concepts are widely used in this field, in a strict sense it is not likely that the genes of the human MHC are in perfect Hardy-Weinberg equilibrium, because certain combinations confer a selective advantage or disadvantage on individuals.

The observed frequencies and proportions of heterozygotes and homozygotes would be tested against those expected on the basis of genetic theory, assuming that the population is at equilibrium. This test would support the hypothesis that the measurement of the allelic products was exact and unbiased from a genetic view. The reader is referred to the field of population genetics for a full treatment of this area.[9]

A bias is particularly likely for genes determining disease susceptibility because of the problem in deciding whether an affected individual is homozygous or heterozygous. Therefore, in practice, it is usually best to estimate gene frequency directly by counting haplotypes in families.

**Linkage and Recombination.** When two loci are located close together, as within the histocompatibility

**Table 4–2.** Terminology*

| Prefix | Meaning | Noun | Adjective | Immunogenetic Relationship |
|---|---|---|---|---|
| Auto- | Self | Autoantigen<br>Autoantibody | Autologous<br>Autochthonous | Self to self |
| Iso-(syn-) | Same | Isograft<br>Isotype† | Syngeneic<br>Isogeneic | Same species, genetically identical |
| Allo-(homo) | Other | Allotype<br>Alloantigen<br>Alloantibody | Allogeneic | Same species, genetically different |
| Hetero-(xeno-) | Foreign | Heteroantigen<br>Heteroantibody | Heterologous<br>Xenogeneic | Different species |

*After Cunningham, A.J.: Understanding Immunology, New York, Academic Press, 1978.

†In certain situations, blood group antibodies have been termed "isoantibodies." The term isotype is also applied to the different classes of immunoglobulin present in an individual.

complex, the linked genes are usually inherited as a unit. Linkage can be deduced only from analyses of family pedigrees. In a population, for the most part, the alleles have become separated by recombination events and behave as independent entities. An example of linkage is illustrated in Figure 4–5. Here the linked genes in the first parent are designated a-b and c-d, comprising two haplotypes. The degrees of genetic relationships among the family members are 0, 1, and 2 haplotype differences.

A recombination event occurring during meiosis in the father gave rise to the recombinant haplotype a-d seen in the fifth child. This occurs in about 1 percent of families. Recombination ultimately leads to genetic equilibrium, where the expected frequency of finding a and b on the same haplotype is simply the product of the frequencies of the a and the b gene in the population.

$$p(a,b) = p(a) \cdot p(b)$$

It is a matter of very great interest, however, that among unrelated individuals certain alleles of one locus are found together on a haplotype with particular alleles of a second locus much more frequently than expected. This indicates that for this pair of alleles, normal recombination has not occurred and a state of non-or disequilibrium exists. The two alleles are said to be in positive *linkage disequilibrium.* This is measured mathematically by the following formula:

$$\text{Observed frequency} - \text{expected frequency} = \Delta$$

Since the value of Δ is the difference between two frequencies, it is expressed either as a decimal or, more conveniently, as an integer after multiplication by 1000. If the sign of Δ is positive, the alleles occur together more frequently than expected by chance, and the linkage disequilibrium is said to be positive. If the alleles are encountered together less frequently than expected, the linkage disequilibrium is negative. It should be stressed that the nonrandom recombination evident as linkage disequilibrium is only a property of pairs of alleles in a haplotype and not a general property of the locus. The origin of this disequilibrium results either from the recent introduction into the gene pool of particular gene combinations from genetically isolated individuals or from a selective advantage resulting from the presence of the two alleles in one individual. An alternative designation for this phenomenon is gametic association, because it appears that certain pairs of alleles are seen in association at high frequency.

## NOMENCLATURE OF RELATIONSHIPS

Another set of distinctions and terms arises through the close relationship of transplantation to the topic of this chapter. Table 4–2 summarizes the categories of relationship that one's "self" can have, and the terms that describe and name them.

Perhaps the most important set of these terms derives from the concept of an allele. Allotype refers to the genetically determined alternative form of the same molecule. Most commonly, these structural differences are demonstrated as allotypic antigenic determinants or simply alloantigens that are recognized by alloantibodies. Classically, an alloserum is prepared by immunizing one member of a species with cells from another. This occurs during pregnancy or transplantation. More recently, monoclonal antibodies obtained from mice immunized with human materials have begun to replace the human antihuman alloreagents. It should be stressed that the distinction between allele and allotype, one between gene and gene product, should be carefully maintained. By convention, when one refers to the locus or allotypic gene, the term is italicized or underlined.

## SEROLOGIC ANALYSIS OF MHC ANTIGENS

**Serologic Specificity.** The delineation of an alloantigen through the use of a reagent serum containing alloantibodies is a central theme in analysis of the histocompatibility complex. The use of an alloantiserum implicitly assumes that a genetic difference is responsible for the recognition of the alternative form of the products of one locus. The origin of this immunogenetic approach came from observations on blood groups, and the basic principles established apply to histocompatibility testing. The primary sources of reagent sera are from pregnant women, organ transplant and transfusion recipients, and, less commonly, intentionally immunized normal donors. In each instance, the alloantiserum recognizes foreign histocompatibility determinants on the

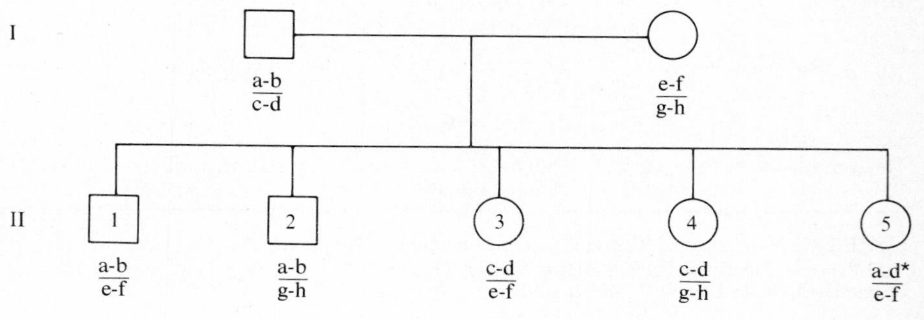


**Figure 4–5.** Genotype of a family illustrating linkage and recombination. Two loci are depicted: the first with alleles a, c, e, and g; the second with alleles b, d, f, and h. The pairs of alleles form haplotypes a-b and c-d in the father, and e-f and g-h in the mother. In all but one of the offspring the linked genes (haplotypes) are inherited as a unit. In individual II-5, the paternal haplotype (a-d) reflects a recombination occurring during meiosis.

immunizing cells that, in the case of the fetus, are of paternal origin.

**HLA Specificities.** The path taken in serologic analysis involves first, the recognition that various allosera define a HLA specificity, and second, the application of these sera to determine whether an individual has the particular specificity. An example of the approach used in establishing serologic specificity of a system is illustrated in Table 4–3. The situation involves a family similar to that of Figure 4–4 in which an alloantibody appeared after the birth of a third child. The antibody reacts with lymphocytes from the father and the third and fourth children, suggesting it detects antigen b.

In practice the events would occur in opposite sequence: the serum typing reaction would be performed first and the phenotype of the individual would be thereby assigned. Then by consideration of the pattern of antigens in the family that reflects the genotype of the individuals, the haplotype assignments would be made.

The central problem in serologic analysis is the development of methods to arrive at the conclusion that a discrete and generally testable specificity is being detected. The first step in this process could be the demonstration that a number of different alloantisera recognize the same determinants. To return to the example, further testing of this serum with a panel of 100 unrelated individuals yields a 20 percent frequency of positive reactions. Testing of a second serum on the same 100 individuals reveals a 24 percent frequency of positive reactions. The relationship of the specificities of the two sera can be seen in a 2 × 2 table in which each of the 100 individuals is scored as positive or negative for the presence of the alloantigen (Fig. 4–6). The use of a 2 × 2 table is an important analytic tool because through the comparison, reagent sera with similar but not precisely identical specificities can be identified. In this example 20 individuals expressed an antigen detected by both sera, and 76 lacked these determinants. There were no individuals positive for serum 1 who were not also positive for serum 2, but the reciprocal case was different. Four persons bore an antigen detected only by serum 2. These are "extra" reactions; however, serum 2 might still be useful for indicating the presence of the antigen detected by both sera.

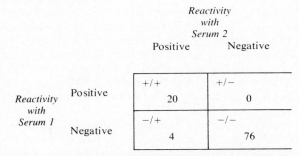

| | | *Reactivity with Serum 2* Positive | *Reactivity with Serum 2* Negative |
|---|---|---|---|
| *Reactivity with Serum 1* | Positive | +/+ 20 | +/− 0 |
| | Negative | −/+ 4 | −/− 76 |

**Figure 4–6.** 2 × 2 table illustrating analysis of a serum cluster for coincidence of reactivity of 100 patients. Chi square = 79,167. Chi square (Yates = 74.044; p < <0.001 that the sera have unrelated specificities.

**Statistical Analysis.** The statistic applied to testing the hypothesis that the two sera react with the same determinant is the chi square ($\chi^2$).[9] If the sample size were smaller, a modification of the chi square statistic, such as the Yates correction for continuity, should be used. For still smaller samples, the exact probability can be calculated by the method of Fisher. In the case of the example given for serum 1 and serum 2, the $\chi^2$ is 79.167 and the corrected $\chi^2$ (Yates) is 74.044. Since the degree of freedom is one, reference to $\chi^2$ tables shows the probability that serum 1 and serum 2 react with independent antigens to be very much less than 1 in 1000. This suggests the interpretation that the two sera detect the same or closely related specificities.

A further refinement is the calculation of a modified coefficient of correlation, usually designated "r", by the formula $r = \sqrt{\chi^2/N}$. This provides an index that is independent of the sample size. This statistic in effect measures the extent of the similarity between the two sera, and is 0.89 in this example. The sign of r is obtained by comparing the products of the two diagonals. It is taken as positive when (+/+) (−/−) exceeds (+/−) (−/+). It is evident that other sera, when tested on the same 100 individuals, can have one of three categories of relationship that reflect the value and sign of the coefficient of correlation. A high positive value indicates similar specificities; a value near zero indicates a lack of relationship; a negative number is interpreted as describing a reciprocal repulsion relationship between the specificities such as would exist for an allelic alloantigen.

For statistical analyses it is necessary that the immunization event that yields the alloantiserum be between two "outbred" individuals who might potentially differ for many alloantigens. This would result in a reagent that contains minor interfering specificities. At early stages in the delineation of an alloantigenic system, the reagents have frequently been complex, and the mathematical treatments were essential.

The same mathematical analysis can be applied to the situation in which other facts are known about the mem-

**Table 4–3.** Relation of Genotype to Phenotype: Detection of Phenotypes by Alloantibodies Appearing in Pregnancy Serum Induced by Paternal MHC Antigens

| | | Lymphocytes Killed After Addition of Complement (%) | | |
|---|---|---|---|---|
| **Lymphocyte Source** | **Genotype** | *Control Serum* | *Mother I-2 Pregnancy Serum* | *Presumed Phenotype* |
| Sib 1 II-1 | a/c | <5 | <5 | — |
| Sib 2 II-2 | a/d | <5 | <5 | — |
| Sib 3 II-3 | b/c | <5 | 100 | b |
| Sib 4 II-4 | b/d | <5 | 100 | b |
| Father I-1 | a/b | <5 | 100 | b |
| Mother I-2 | c/d | <5 | <5 | — |

bers of the panel. If it were known that 18 individuals were of the HLA type B7, it could be determined whether or not sera 1 and 2 detected HLA-B7 (Fig. 4–7). It would be concluded that both sera have, as their major specificity, alloantibodies that react with the HLA-B7 alloantigen but that both sera have extra reactions that presumably reflect minor contaminant specificities.

**Practical Aspects of Serologic Typing.** Each specificity is determined by several different sera to assure accurate typing results. Sometimes, combinations of sera, each with more than one specificity, must be used to detect certain antigens. In practice a large number of sera are used in HLA typing because of the great variety of MHC alloantigens (Table 4–4). Usually 120 sera or more are used for typing an individual. In order to conserve lymphocytes and reagent sera, each reaction is performed with 0.001 ml volumes of serum and cells. Binding of antibodies is most commonly detected by complement-dependent cytotoxicity, and dyes are used to determine cell death. The entire reaction is performed on a 60-well "Terasaki tray" filled with oil to prevent evaporation.

**Typing for Class I or Class II Alloantigens.** The evaluation of the two classes of MHC molecules is simply performed by taking advantage of the fact that class I molecules are expressed on all lymphocytes and monocytes, while class II molecules are usually restricted to B lymphocytes and monocytes. The analysis of alleles of the class I loci is carried out using whole mononuclear cell preparations, while the class II Ia allodeterminants are defined with mononuclear cells that have been depleted of T lymphocytes, yielding a "B cell" preparation that contains some monocytes and various other cells. Since B lymphocytes also contain class I molecules the reagent allosera that define Ia allodeterminants must be freed of antibodies to class I molecules by absorption. Platelets, since they only express class I alloantigens, are usually used for this purpose.

**Class I Allodeterminants.** The class I alloantigens form three segregant series designated HLA-A, HLA-B, and HLA-C, and the respective genetic loci receive the same designation but are italicized.[11–13] The alloantigens of the *HLA-A, B,* and *C* series are highly polymorphic.[11–13] This is illustrated in Table 4–4. There are at least 18 distinct alloantigenic forms comprising HLA-A and 24 comprising HLA-B. The *C* locus is less well defined, and considerably fewer alleles are known. The terminology that refers to the different alloantigens reflects an extensive international collaborative effort. The first term is a letter referring to the locus; the second, a number that is simply assigned when the specificity is delineated. The prefix "w" before a number signifies that the specificity is recognized but still requires additional definition. In general, typing results include the alloantigen phenotype of the HLA-A and B segregant series as well as the specification of the individual as Bw4 or Bw6. *C* locus typing is not as advanced, in part because of the difficulty of obtaining good typing sera. This is so because the antigens appear to be poorly immunogenic, and the problem is compounded by the tight linkage with the HLA-B locus.

The specificities previously termed "4a" and "4b" and now designated "Bw4" and "Bw6" are an incompletely understood alloantigenic system. Recent chemical evidence supports the prevailing view that these are "supratypic specificities" of various HLA-B antigens. They have practical value in permitting the assignment of certain difficult HLA specificities because of characteristics in their association, and their matching is reported to be relevant to renal transplant survival.

The interpretation of the results of HLA typing should be made with attention to class, locus or allelic series, and particular allele. For example, a report of *HLA-A1-B8 and B7* signifies that all three alleles are of class I, and that for the *A* locus only one allelic product is detected. This could mean that the individual is homozygous for the *A1* allele or that an uncharacterized allelic product is encoded by the *A* locus gene of one chromosome 6. The two *B* locus alleles are located on the two different 6 chromosomes. If the individual were Caucasian, it would be likely that the *A1* and the *B8* alleles were present on the same chromosome by virtue of their linkage disequilibrium.

Certain *A* and *B* locus alleles are found together on the same chromosome more frequently than would be expected by the product of their respective gene frequencies. This nonrandom distribution of certain alleles is an example of linkage disequilibrium (Table 4–5).[9,14]

| | | *SERUM 1* Positive + | *SERUM 1* Negative − |
|---|---|---|---|
| *Anti-HLA-B7* | Positive | +/+ 17 | +/− 0 |
| | Negative | −/+ 3 | −/− 80 |

**Figure 4–7.** Identification of specificity of serum 1 as related to HLA-B7. Chi square=81,928. Chi square (Yates) = 76.014; p< <0.001 that serum 1 and an anti-HLA-B7 serum have unrelated specificities.

## DETERMINANTS DEFINED BY LYMPHOCYTE RESPONSES

In contrast to the antigens detected by serologic means, there is another category of MHC determinants that are recognized directly by lymphocytes. The recognition event is detected either by killing of the target cell by a lymphocyte, e.g., cell-mediated lympholysis (CML), or by proliferation of the responding lymphocyte, e.g., mixed lymphocyte culture (MLC) or primed lymphocyte test (PLT). Proliferation is usually assayed by incorporation of radiolabeled thymidine into the newly synthesized DNA.[15–17]

The MHC determinants recognized by these lymphocyte responses are relatively restricted to class I molecules in the case of cell-mediated lympholysis and to class II molecules for the MLC and PLT reaction. This restriction is paralleled by the fact that T lymphocytes belonging to different T lymphocyte lineages primarily mediate either reactivity to class I molecules, the Leu 2+,T8+ suppressor-cytotoxic cell or reactivity to class II molecules, the Leu 3+,T4+ helper-inducer cell. Exceptions to this generalization exist, such as Leu 3+,T4+ cells that have class II antigens as the target of their cytotoxicity.

The MLC reaction is of special historical interest because it was used to define the existence of the class II gene products. As a practical test for typing an individual it has been supplanted by the simpler serologic determination of Ia allotype. However, the reaction still is of very considerable importance in defining subspecificities among Ia allodeterminants and in situations such as transplantation, where histocompatibility is critical.

**Table 4–4.** HLA Gene Frequencies in Different Populations*

| | North American Caucasoids | American Blacks | African Blacks | Japanese | American Indians |
|---|---|---|---|---|---|
| *A Locus Alleles:* | | | | | |
| A1 | 16.1 | 8.1 | 3.9 | 1.2 | 2.5 |
| A2 | 28.0 | 16.3 | 9.4 | 25.3 | 45.3 |
| A3 | 14.1 | 7.0 | 6.4 | 0.7 | 0.6 |
| A9 { Aw23 | 1.9 | 10.6 | 10.8 | 37.2 | 23.2 |
| A9 { Aw24 | 7.3 | 5.1 | 2.4 | | |
| A10 { Aw25 | 2.6 | 0.4 | 3.5 | 12.7 | 0.6 |
| A10 { Aw26 | 3.4 | 2.3 | 4.5 | | |
| A11 | 5.1 | 2.8 | — | 6.7 | — |
| A28 | 4.2 | 5.8 | 8.9 | — | 2.8 |
| A29 | 3.6 | 2.3 | 6.4 | 0.2 | 0.6 |
| Aw30 | 2.9 | 13.0 | 22.1 | 0.5 | 1.1 |
| Aw31 | 4.5 | 2.8 | 4.2 | 8.7 | 19.9 |
| Aw32 | 3.7 | 1.9 | 1.5 | 0.5 | 1.1 |
| Aw33 | 1.2 | 5.1 | 1.0 | 2.0 | 0.6 |
| Aw43 | — | — | 4.0 | — | — |
| Blank | 1.3 | 16.5 | 11.0 | 4.2 | 1.8 |
| *B Locus Alleles:* | | | | | |
| B5 | 5.9 | 4.9 | 3.0 | 20.9 | 14.0 |
| B7 | 10.5 | 12.6 | 7.3 | 7.1 | 0.6 |
| B8 | 10.4 | 5.5 | 7.1 | 0.2 | 1.7 |
| B12 — Bw6 | 13.8 | 14.0 | 12.7 | 6.5 | 1.7 |
| B13 | 2.6 | 0.4 | 1.5 | 0.8 | — |
| Bw4 — B14 | 5.1 | 4.6 | 3.6 | 0.5 | — |
| B15 | 5.9 | 4.7 | 3.0 | 9.3 | 13.7 |
| Bw16 { Bw38 | 2.5 | 0.4 | — | 1.8 | 14.5 |
| Bw16 { Bw39 | 1.4 | 0.4 | 1.5 | 4.7 | |
| B17 | 4.9 | 11.2 | 16.1 | 0.6 | — |
| B18 | 3.1 | 3.6 | 2.0 | — | 0.6 |
| Bw21 | 3.8 | 4.4 | 1.5 | 1.5 | |
| Bw22 | 2.3 | 3.9 | — | 6.5 | 0.6 |
| B27 | 5.6 | 0.8 | — | 0.3 | 6.2 |
| Bw35 | 8.6 | 12.5 | 7.2 | 9.4 | 22.1 |
| B37 | 1.7 | 1.2 | — | 0.8 | — |
| B40 | 9.2 | 3.9 | 2.0 | 21.8 | 16.6 |
| Bw41 | — | — | 1.5 | — | — |
| Bw42 | — | — | 12.3 | — | — |
| Blank | 2.8 | 11.0 | 17.9 | 7.6 | 7.8 |
| *C Locus Alleles:* | | | | | |
| Cw1 | 3.7 | 1.9 | — | 11.1 | 10.1 |
| Cw2 | 6.0 | 9.2 | 11.4 | 1.4 | 4.6 |
| Cw3 | 11.4 | 8.8 | 5.5 | 26.3 | 16.6 |
| Cw4 | 10.2 | 12.9 | 14.2 | 4.3 | 23.4 |
| Cw5 | 5.2 | 1.4 | 1.0 | 1.2 | 1.1 |
| Cw6 | 11.3 | — | 17.7 | 2.1 | — |
| Blank | 52.1 | 65.8 | 50.2 | 53.5 | 44.2 |

Alleles marked with a minus sign (—) are not present in this population.

*From data of the VII Workshop on histocompatibility testing. *In* Bodmer, W.F., et al. (eds.): Histocompatibility Testing 1977. Copenhagen, Munksgaard, 1978.

**Table 4–5.** Some Haplotypes in Different Populations*

| | | | Linkage Disequilibrium | Haplotype Frequency |
|---|---|---|---|---|
| **HLA-A, B Haplotypes:** | | | | |
| *North American Caucasoid* | | | | |
| | A1 | B8 | 59.2 | 67.9 |
| | A3 | B7 | 27.6 | 38.0 |
| | A3 | B14 | 14.5 | 19.3 |
| | A28 | B14 | 12.7 | 13.3 |
| | A26 | B38 | 9.2 | 10.0 |
| | A26 | B5 | 8.8 | 9.7 |
| | A25 | B18 | 7.5 | 8.3 |
| *Japanese* | | | | |
| | Aw24 | B7 | 34.9 | 55.1 |
| | A26 | Bw35 | 16.6 | 25.8 |
| | Aw33 | B12 | 11.5 | 11.5 |
| | A1 | B37 | 7.6 | 7.7 |
| *American Indian* | | | | |
| | Aw24 | Bw35 | 69.2 | 103.2 |
| | A1 | B8 | 10.8 | 11.3 |
| *African Black* | | | | |
| | Aw30 | Bw42 | 44.6 | 61.6 |
| | Aw32 | Bw35 | 13.0 | 13.5 |
| **HLA-B, D Haplotypes:** | | | | |
| *North American Caucasoid* | | | | |
| | B27 | Dw1 | 8.4 | 11.4 |
| | Bw35 | Dw1 | 13.4 | 20.4 |
| | B12 | Dw2 | 30.0 | 41.1 |
| | B7 | Dw2 | 23.2 | 30.9 |
| | B8 | Dw3 | 56.9 | 57.6 |
| | Bw44 | Dw4 | 19.4 | 24.4 |
| | B12 | Dw4 | 19.0 | 22.4 |
| | B15 | Dw4 | 9.3 | 13.1 |
| | B14 | Dw5 | 15.3 | 16.5 |
| | Bw51 | Dw5 | 10.6 | 12.9 |
| | B5 | Dw5 | 9.7 | 12.6 |
| | Bw22 | Dw6 | 11.7 | 12.9 |

*From data of the VII Workshop on histocompatibility testing. *In* Bodmer, W.F., et al. (eds.): Histocompatibility Testing 1977. Copenhagen, Munksgaard, 1978.

**The Mixed Lymphocyte Culture Reaction.** The basic elements of the MLC are the co-culture of responder lymphocytes from one individual with stimulator lymphocytes from another. The stimulator lymphocytes are treated by γ-irradiation or alkylating agents, rendering them incapable of DNA synthesis. This reaction is a one-way MLC. By the fifth day of culture, a vigorous proliferative response of the responder cells in the culture indicates that foreign histocompatibility determinants are present. Conversely, compatibility or "MLC identity" is signaled by the absence of a significant response. This implies that the stimulator and responder cells share certain genetic markers.

The components in the cell membrane responsible for inducing stimulation are not yet precisely defined on a molecular basis. They clearly involve the class II or Ia/DR allodeterminants. For this reason B lymphocytes, dendritic cells, and monocytes are considered to be the principal stimulators in the MLC. Conversely, the responding lymphocytes are T cells.

The mixed lymphocyte culture reaction has deeper biologic aspects that are only beginning to be understood. Several distinctive features of the reaction are as follows: The number of T lymphocytes that respond is greater than the response to conventional antigens such as tetanus toxoid. Furthermore, the response to allodeterminants is greater than that to heterodeterminants on lymphocytes from other species, a pattern that contrasts with antibody responses. Lastly, the responding T lymphocytes elaborate factors that interact with autologous B lymphocytes and provide a supplemental stimulus to the B lymphocytes' response to an antigen.

A curious phenomenon that may be of considerable biologic significance is termed the autologous MLC. This proliferative response of T lymphocytes is initiated by *isolated* autologous cells that bear class II molecules.[19]

However, B lymphocytes and monocytes are relatively inefficient as stimulators in the autologous reaction, reflecting an interesting divergence between cells capable of presenting antigen and those most capable of initiation in an autologous MLC.

**Genetic Control of the Mixed Lymphocyte Culture Response.** The major genetic control of the stimulating determinants in the classic allogeneic MLC maps at one locus, termed *HLA-D.*[17] This locus is located very near *HLA-B.* Evidence exists for a second minor locus near *HLA-A,* but less information is available about this.

A representative experiment illustrating the relationships among family members as revealed by the MLC reaction is given in Figure 4–8. The results of this experiment demonstrate that the two siblings that share the same haplotype are compatible, as is indicated by the absence of a mixed lymphocyte culture response. In about 1 to 2 percent of HLA-A and B identical individuals the expected compatibility is not observed. This is due to recombination, and these results provide the evidence that the *D* locus is distinct from the *B* locus.

**Homozygous Typing Cells.** The fact that compatibility requires identity between heterozygous individuals necessarily limited the application of MLC analysis as a tool of genetic analysis. The solution to the use of MLC reaction as a practical analytic method was the introduction of homozygous stimulator lymphocytes as a typing reagent. A MLC homozygous individual must fulfill the criterion that neither parent be significantly stimulated by their child.

Table 4–6 illustrates the typing of the individuals of the family illustrated in Figure 4–8 using homozygous typing cells. The presence of compatibility of stimulator and responder cells is illustrated by a low level of DNA synthesis. This implies that the individual shares the MHC-stimulating determinants with the cells of the homozygous stimulator.

Through the identification of a number of different homozygous individuals in an extensive international effort, a series of lymphocyte-defined allodeterminants that comprise a segregant series were found. These alleles are designated HLA-D1, 2, and so on. Certain of these *D* locus alleles exhibit linkage disequilibrium forming haplotypes; for example, A1-B8-D3 and A3-B7-D2.[11-13]

Newer approaches using lymphocytes primed to respond in an enhanced secondary manner (PLT) to determinants involving HLA-D components appear to offer considerable simplification in regard to performance. The reader is referred to the histocompatability literature for a detailed explanation.[11-13,17]

## THE IA SYSTEM

The genes encoding the class II gene products form a chromosomal region, the presumed organization of which was summarized in Figure 4–1. The $\beta$ chains are of special interest because they appear to contain the determinants responsible for all of the allo variation of the molecules. In addition to the $\beta$ chain polymorphisms the $\alpha$ chain genes of the DS and SB molecules are polymorphic. In recognition of the terminology initially developed in the murine system that names homologous molecules with emphasis on their role in regulating the immune response, the general designation of the class II gene products used in this chapter will be "Ia antigens" or "Ia molecules."

**The DR Allotypes.** A relatively imperfect relationship

Pedigree (same as in Fig. 4–4):

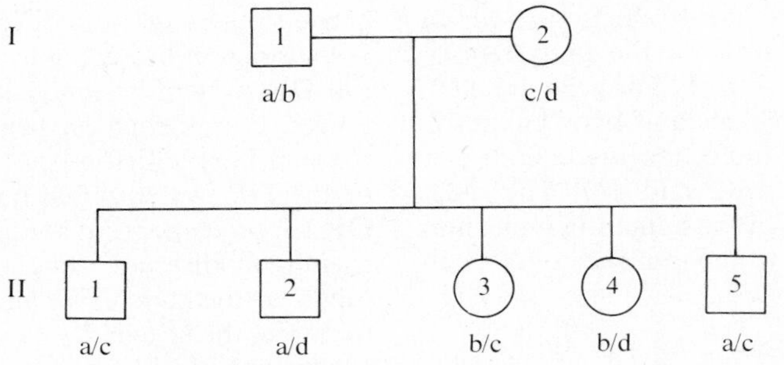


*Representative MHC Testing Results:*

| Haplotype Difference | Stimulator (Irradiated) | Responder | Stimulation DNA Synthesis cpm $^3$H Thymidine Incorporated |
|---|---|---|---|
| 2 | I: 1 (a/b) | I: 2 (c/d) | 45,000 |
| 2 | II: 1 (a/c) | II: 4 (b/d) | 42,000 |
| 1 | II: 1 (a/c) | II: 2 (a/d) | 30,000 |
| 0 | II: 1 (a/c) | II: 5 (a/c) | 300 |

**Figure 4–8.** Relationships among family members revealed by MHC testing.

**Table 4–6.** MHC Results Using a Homozygous Typing Cell (in Family of Fig. 4–8)

| Stimulator (Irradiated) | Responder | Stimulation DNA Synthesis CPM 3H Thymidine Incorporated | Interpretations |
|---|---|---|---|
| a/a | I 1 (a/b) | 400 | Type a |
| a/a | I 2 (c/d) | 41,000 | |
| a/a | II 1 (a/c) | 450 | Type a |
| a/a | II 3 (b/c) | 39,000 | |

between certain allospecificities of the class II molecules and particular MLC determinants resulted in the designation of certain of the class II alloantigens as "DR" (*D* Related antigens).[19] Evidence has been gathered that at least 10 serologically Ia allospecificities form a segregant series that has been assumed to map to a single locus designated *DR.* Table 4–7 lists the frequencies of the major DR specificities in different populations. The population variation is of great interest and will be discussed later. These DR specificities are, however, still in the process of being defined, and the use of DR to designate a segregant series is only an operational one, since tests, such as the existence of a Hardy-Weinberg equilibrium, are not met for this series of alloantigens; moreover, there is chemical evidence of increased complexity. This chemical evidence has revealed, for example, that the serologic specificity $DR^4$ is present on five molecularly differentiable species that are each a distinct allele. Since the Ia molecule consists of two chains, then according to this greatly oversimplied early model, there was a single MHC locus that encoded $\alpha$ chains and a second locus for the multiple alternative $\beta$ chain alleles, one for each DR specificity.

This simple model serves as an introduction to the Ia system but is not at all accurate. In the Ia system of the mouse, the two main types of Ia antigens are each composed of two types of $\alpha$ chains and two types of $\beta$ chains, and all four types of molecules are encoded in two subregions designated *I-E/C* and *I-A.* The most frequent amino acid structure of the human Ia molecules was found to be homologous to the sequence of $\alpha$ chain

**Table 4–7.** Frequencies of Some Major Ia Alleles in Different Races*

| Designation | Phenotype (Alloantigen) Frequency (%) | | |
|---|---|---|---|
| | *Caucasoid* | *Negroid* | *Mongoloid* |
| DR1 | 16 | 13 | 12 |
| DR2 | 25 | 32 | 36 |
| DR3 | 21 | 32 | 3 |
| DR4 | 21 | 10 | 41 |
| DR5 | 20 | 28 | 4 |
| DR7 | 24 | 20 | 1 |
| DR8 | 4 | 8 | 9 |

*VIII Workshop Data.[13]

and $\beta$ chain molecules encoded by the murine *I-E/C* subregion (Table 4–8).[20-22] For this reason the structure of the DR allodeterminants are referred to as *I-E/C*-like.

However, biochemical and immunologic studies have demonstrated that in man there are three DR $\beta$ chains that have a very similar but not identical *I-E/C*-like amino acid sequence.[21-23] The inter-relationships of these gene products are illustrated in Figure 4–9, which emphasizes the distinctness of each of the Ia species on the cell surface. These new data raise two challenging problems. The first is the nature of the basis of the DR specificities in terms of the multiple $\beta$ chains. Are the polyclonal anti-DR allosera actually directed to a number of distinct but generally similar gene products that are too closely linked to be separated by recombination? Secondly, what is the genetic basis of these molecules and allospecificities? The conventional view might be summarized as "one distinct alloantigen implies one molecule under the control of one gene." Alternatively, in view of the revolution in eukaryotic molecular biology, there could be a more intricate system involving lateral gene transfer and movable genetic elements such as "mini genes" that encode only the particular segment of the allodeterminant. These genes would be inserted into one or several basic $\beta$ chain genes to result in a large variety of molecules bearing distinct allodeterminants. Furthermore, there is the potential for additional diversity being generated by post-translational events such as $\alpha$ and $\beta$ chain combination or modification by the addition of complex carbohydrates. Of course, the resolution of these questions is of critical importance in determining the precise genetic basis of disease susceptibility influenced by these gene products. The resolution of this will have to await further studies involving monoclonal allotypic reagents or recombinant DNA technology.

**The DS/DC System of Non-DR Ia Specificities.** Evidence for a second major locus analogous to the murine *I-A* subregion has come forward (Fig. 4–9). Well before the DR system assumed its present degree of characterization, information began to accumulate about additional Ia specificities that were not able to be included in the DR system. The initial evidence for these non-DR Ia loci came from studies on susceptibility to certain rheumatic diseases: Sjögren's syndrome and systemic lupus erythematosus[24,25] and rheumatoid arthritis.[26] For example, the specificity Ia 4×7×10 that would now be designated MT3 was shown, by co-capping studies and segregation analysis, to be distinct from the allele of the DR series DR4.[19,26]

More recently a number of the non-DR allospecificities of the Ia system were grouped into DC, MB, and MT and other related segregant series.[27-29] The relationship of these newer specificities to those of the DR system is summarized in Table 4–9. There were two contradictory views of the nature of this relationship. In one view, for example, the sera defining the MB3 specificity would be considered to recognize a "public" or supratypic antigen expressed on the DR4 and DR5

**Table 4–8.** Amino Acid Sequence Comparison of Murine I-E, I-A, and Human DR, DS, and IVD12 Allodeterminants

**Alpha Chains**

| *Position:* | 1 | 3 | 4 | 6 | 7 | 8 | 1 | 12 | 13 | 14 | 15 | 16 | 19 | 22 | 24 | 29 |
|---|---|---|---|---|---|---|---|---|---|---|---|---|---|---|---|---|
| I-E | Ilu | – | – | – | Ilu | Ilu | – | Phe | Tyr | – | – | – | – | Phe | Phe | – |
| DR | Ilu | – | – | Val | Ilu | Ilu | – | Phe | Tyr | Leu | – | – | – | Phe | Phe | – |
| I-A | – | Ilu | – | – | – | Val | Tyr | | – | – | Val | Tyr | – | – | – | – |
| DS | – | Ilu | Val | – | – | Val | Tyr | | Val | – | Leu | Tyr | Tyr | – | – | Phe |
| IVD12 | – | Ilu | Val | – | – | Val | Tyr | – | Val | – | Leu | Tyr | Tyr | – | – | Phe |

**Beta Chains**

| *Position:* | 7 | 8 | 9 | 10 | 11 | 14 | 16 | 17 | 18 | 24 | 26 | 27 | 30 | 31 | 32 |
|---|---|---|---|---|---|---|---|---|---|---|---|---|---|---|---|
| I-E | Phe | Leu | – | Tyr • | Val | – | – | Phe | Tyr | – | Phe | Leu | Phe | – | – |
| DR | Phe | Leu | – | – | – | – | – | Phe | Phe | Val | Phe | Leu | Tyr | Phe | Tyr |
| I-A | Phe | Val | Tyr | Tyr | Phe | Phe | Tyr | Phe | – | – | Tyr | – | Tyr | – | – |
| DS | Phe | Val | – | – | Phe | – | Tyr | Phe | – | – | – | – | – | – | – |
| IVD12 | Phe | Val | Tyr | – | Phe | – | Tyr | Phe | – | Val | – | Val | Tyr | – | Tyr |

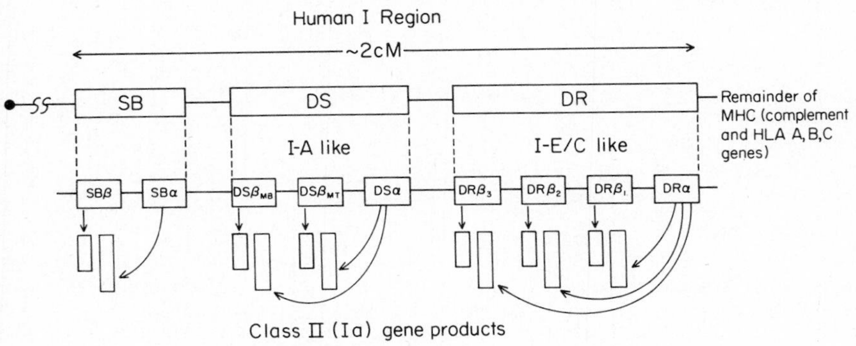


**Figure 4–9.** Working model of chromosomal region coding for Ia antigens. Based on analysis of known gene products, recent advances in molecular biology reveal an additional β and α gene in the SB region and another α gene in the DS region.

β chains. This supratypic antigen would signify an evolutionary relationship of these two alleles to a common ancestral antecedent. For example, the presence of the MB3 specificity might be taken as an indication that the genes encoding DR4 and DR5 arose by mutation from an MB3+ precursor. Immediately, however, it is evident that the MT3 specificity would argue for a different ancestry. No simple scheme was advanced to explain the systems in this way.

In another view, for which considerable evidence is emerging, the non-DR specificities of the Ia system belong to entirely distinct molecules and hence define alleles of a new segregant series, tentatively designated DS,[23,28,30-33] that involves the MB and possibly some of the MT specificities. The MT determinants are primarily expressed on one or two of the DR β chains. The amino acid sequence of the Ia molecules bearing MB determinants resembles that of the murine I-A molecules[34] (Table 4–8). These data, along with those derived from recombinant DNA technology, provide firm evidence for the existence of a second Ia locus entirely unrelated to DR. These other loci presumably arose by gene duplication of an original Ia locus, giving daughter loci that developed their separate allelic series by further mutational events. The alleles of this locus are still under investigation.

The current view of the DS region is that it contains two genes encoding α chains and two genes encoding β chains, all of which are polymorphic. The possibility of 16 different combinational products arising from trans and cis interactions emphasizes the complexity of the resulting determinants.

**Table 4–9.** DR Specificity Associations

| DR: | 1 | 2 | 3 | 4 | 5 | 6 | 7 | 6Y | 8 | 9 |
|---|---|---|---|---|---|---|---|---|---|---|
| MT 1 | x | x | | | | | | x | | |
| MT 2 | | | x | | x | x | | | x | |
| MT 3 | | | | x | | | x | | | x |
| MT 4 | | | | x | x | | | | x | |
| MT 5 | x | x | | | | | | | | |
| MT 6 | | | x | | | x | | | | |
| MB 1 | x | x | | | | x | | | x | |
| MB 2 | | | x | | | x | | | | |
| MB 3 | | | | x | x | x | | | | x |
| TE 21 | x | x | | | | | | | | |
| TE 22 | | | | x | x | | | | | |
| TE 23 | x | | | x | | | | | | |
| TE 24 | | | x | | | x | | | | |

The amino acid sequence of the MT system is at present difficult to harmonize with a simple origin at either an *I-A* or *I-E/C*-like locus. Even with the use of monoclonal antibodies the MT specificities are present on molecules that have curious mixtures of amino acid sequences resembling both DR and DS molecules. This latter fact adds support to the nonclassical genetic mechanisms involving gene transfer. The evidence that the β chains of the MT and MB specificities are encoded by different genes, at least in the DR4 haplotype, is provided by co-capping experiments.

***Monoclonal Antibodies.*** An important methodologic advance that is revolutionizing this field has been the application of monoclonal antibody technology to the problem of detecting alloantigens. Until this advance, polyclonal human alloantisera were used which, although they were operationally monospecific typing reagents, contained a variety of alloantibodies resulting from the immune response to closely linked genes encoding the foreign histocompatibility antigens. Monoclonal antibodies, in contrast, can be selected so that they can be used as probes for the presence of a single alloantigenic determinant.

**The SB Subregion.** The third well-documented subregion of the human Ia system is termed SB and encodes α and β chains that are distinct from both DS and DR α and β chains.[35] The recognition of the alleles of this locus is made largely by primed lymphocyte typing, and these alleles are not related to any of the DR, MT, or MB specificities. The genetic organization here resembles that of DS with two α and two β chains. There is no homologue of this subregion in the mouse. Monoclonal antibodies have been identified that react with the SB molecules.

**Ia Antigens as Markers of Differentiation.** The Ia alloantigen-bearing molecules have been most extensively studied, in part because of the simplicity with which heteroantisera can be raised to isolated preparations of the Ia molecules.[19] These antisera are of considerable value in the examination of the distribution of the Ia molecule on different cell types.

Within the B lymphocyte lineage, Ia molecules, while present on the earliest recognizable stage, are progressively lost from the B lymphocyte when entering the terminal phase of differentiation as plasma cells. While all but a few percent of unstimulated T lymphocytes lack detectable Ia antigens, after mitogen or antigen stimulation a major proportion of the T lymphocytes can be found to express Ia antigen determinants. This implies a considerable degree of control over the activation of genes that specify the Ia molecules.

The monocyte is the most frequent cell in the blood that expresses Ia antigens. The level of Ia antigens is independently controlled on monocytes. One example of this is that in most individuals the incubation of monocytes with lipopolysaccharide-endotoxin preparations results in suppression of Ia synthesis and expression. Monocytes are also distinctive in that certain Ia antigens primarily associated with the MT specificities are found at higher levels on monocytes compared with B cells. This lack of coordinate expression of different Ia species is another example of the special control of Ia synthesis and expression on this lineage that perhaps relates to the role of these cells in antigen presentation to T lymphocytes.

Among other Ia antigen-bearing cells are the dendritic cells. These cells lack detectable membrane antigens of the monocyte lineage and are highly efficient stimulators in the autologous MLC. The dendritic cells also appear to be capable of presenting soluble protein antigens. Similarly present in the blood are small numbers of committed hematopoietic progenitor cells that are Ia(+).

Ia antigens are also found as a major cell membrane glycoprotein during the early stages of differentiation in each of the principal hematopoietic cell lineages. In the granulocyte series, Ia molecues are demonstrable on the committed progenitor cell through the myeloblast stage. In the erythrocyte series, the erythropoietin sensitive burst and colony forming progenitor cells, as well as pronormoblasts, have readily demonstrable Ia antigens. In both these lineages, the disappearance of Ia at an early stage contrasts with the persistence of this molecule on the surface membrane of B lymphocytes and monocytes until a more terminal stage.[19]

The presence of Ia antigens on analogous stages of murine hematopoietic cells has not been identified, and this fact suggests that in man Ia molecules serve an additional function outside that of the immune system. Possibly this function relates to the control of proliferative hematopoietic differentiation.

**Function.** The functions of the class I and II molecules are known only to a limited degree. Both classes of molecules have central roles in controlling immunologic defense mechanisms. The class I molecules have their best defined function in the effector phase of T lymphocyte cytotoxic reactions. Antigen recognition and killing of the target cell is restricted to T lymphocyte–target cell systems that are compatible for specific class I locus alleles. The functions of the class II molecules that have been recognized are primarily in the afferent limits of the immune response. Through antigen presentation to T lymphocytes, the specific immume response to T-lymphocyte-dependent antigens is controlled by the class II molecules. It appears that the T lymphocyte by itself is incapable of responding to an antigen unless the antigen is presented to the T lymphocyte in the context of class II molecules on the surface of a monocyte or dendritic cell. A second element of the function of class II molecules is apparent in the various antigen-dependent interactions among cell subpopulations during the immune response. This is especially evident in circuits involving suppressor cells and their factors. Other kinds of class II molecule functions suggest that they have a direct role in determining cellular interactions. In terms of the Niels Jerne view of clonal selection, the particular MHC allodeterminants also influence the T lymphocyte antigen receptor repertoire by causing the elimination of any strongly autoreactive T cell clones. These deleted T lymphocyte clones leave gaps in the recognition of certain antigens. Each of these functions, along with those to be discovered, are relevant for their potential derangement and subsequent role in influencing susceptibility to disease.

## DISEASE ASSOCIATIONS

With the emerging knowledge concerning the association of certain diseases with genes that map in the MHC, the MHC has acquired a relevance to the practice of medicine that will be substantial in its implications.[19,36] This is particularly the case in the rheumatic diseases, of which a number have been demonstrated to have this association. Among the implications of these associations are the following: (1) the potential for improved diagnostic accuracy, (2) an enhanced knowledge of the pathogenetic mechanisms through which a genetic predisposition is turned into a disease process, (3) an improvement in the nosologic classifications of the rheumatic diseases as an outgrowth of the increase in knowledge, and (4) perhaps the most novel, the ability to define in precise terms who is at risk for the development of a disease. Here there is the potential for a new area of specific preventative medical therapy directed to altering the disease predisposition state.

**Background.** The initial assertion of an association between the MHC and human disease was made in patients with Hodgkin's disease. While the exact nature of this particular relationship has remained difficult to characterize until very recently, the subsequent finding that HLA-B27 was associated with axial arthropathies has galvanized attention to this area of investigation. The presence or absence of HLA-B27 has proved itself to be an important practical diagnostic test in the evaluation of a patient with perplexing back pain or rheumatoid factor-negative arthritis, and the application of the test facilitated an enlargement of the concept of a family of axial arthropathies and their extra-articular manifestations. Furthermore, the puzzling limited inheritance of ankylosing spondylitis was clarified by the ability to identify the haplotype that conferred susceptibility.

While other diseases were found that had associations to particular HLA-A or B alleles, notably Behçet's syndrome and psoriasis (see Chapters 66 and 74), the emphasis has switched to studies on diseases primarily associated with the more newly described determinants of histocompatibility, including those relating to the HLA-D alleles. Studies on multiple sclerosis led this line of investigation when in 1973 the strong association with HLA-D2 was reported and in 1975 when the first association of a B lympocyte alloantigen with disease was made in patients with multiple sclerosis. The previously reported weak association of multiple sclerosis with HLA-A3 and B7 was shown to be simply a reflection of the linkage disequilibrium of these determinants with the B lymphocyte alloantigens associated with the DR2 specificity.[19]

More recently, a number of rheumatic diseases have been found that are associated with B lymphocyte alloantigens or, to a slightly lesser extent, with HLA-D alleles. In these diseases, the linkage disequilibrium with the HLA-A and B alloantigens was usually insufficient to provide a clue to the presence of the disease association. Thus, there now exist two main categories of MHC disease associations within the rheumatic diseases: (1) The constellations of arthritides associated with HLA-B27 and other alleles involved in susceptibility to psoriasis. These will be discussed in detail elsewhere in this book. (2) Those that are related to the B lymphocyte alloantigens, including, in part, rheumatoid arthritis,[26,37-40] systemic lupus erythematosus,[39,41,42] Sjögren's syndrome,[43] and rheumatic fever.[44]

**Genetics.** From the perspective of genetics, the acquisition of one of these diseases can be considered as a trait determined by a polymorphic gene mapping within the MHC. However, the common denominator in all these associations is that the MHC phenotype associated with a disease does not automatically confer the disease on all individuals who receive the particular allele. It is, rather, susceptibility or predisposition that is inherited, and it is evident that some additional factors—either inherited or acquired from the environment—are necessary in order to result in the disease.

Mendelian inheritance of a disease is readily recognized by the simple patterns of dominance or recessivity of either autosomal or sex chromosome genes. In contrast, the diseases under discussion are characterized by a more elusive mode of inheritance in which the disease, while occasionally appearing to be familial, lacks a well-defined genetic pattern (Fig. 4–10).

*NUMBER OF INDIVIDUALS (2 × 2 TABLE)*

| | | Diagnosis: RA | Diagnosis: Normal |
|---|---|---|---|
| Alloantigen delected by serum 1038 | + | 36 | 11 |
| | − | 9 | 29 |

$$\text{Relative risk} = \frac{\dfrac{\text{Patients positive}}{\text{Patients negative}}}{\dfrac{\text{Controls positive}}{\text{Controls negative}}} \quad \frac{\dfrac{36}{9}}{\dfrac{11}{29}} = 9.1$$

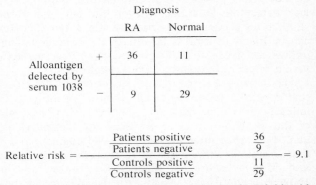

**Figure 4–10.** Calculation of association of rheumatoid arthritis with presence of an alloantigen detected by a B cell alloantiserum. Chi square (Yates) = 18.9. $p < 0.001$.

In general, a number of distinct events can account for non-Mendelian inheritance. These include a basic heterogeneity in the disease under study, reflecting several distinct types of disease, each with a separate gene. Alternatively, the disease can vary in detectability so that subclinical cases go unnoticed and obscure proper patient ascertainment. Lastly, the occurrence of the disease may be the result of the action of two independent events, with the second event being either the presence of a second gene or a particular environmental circumstance. This latter situation is referred to as incomplete penetrance. In each of these explanations of non-Mendelian inheritance, the existence of a genetic marker that characterized the individual at risk for development of the disease would provide a method for deciding among the possibilities.

**Methods of Procedure.** In practice, the determination that a gene mapping within the MHC determines susceptibility to a particular disease involves two levels of investigation. In the first, a significant association with an allele of the MHC is determined. In the second, the mode of inheritance of the disease trait in relation to the locus of the MHC allele is defined by examination of family pedigrees.

Two statistics are used to determine the association between the MHC allele and disease. The intensity of the association is measured by the relative risk.[45,46] This is simply calculated by the formula:

$$RR = \frac{\text{Patients positive for allele}}{\text{Patients negative for allele}} \times \frac{\text{Controls negative for allele}}{\text{Controls positive for allele}}$$

The ratio has an expectation of 1 if there is no association between the presence of the allele and the occurrence of the disease. A positive association results in an increasing positive number that is the ratio of the odds of developing the illness if the particular allele is present compared with its likelihood when the allele is absent. Because a negative association or protection from acquiring the disease has an expectation of less than 1, it is difficult to compare values ranging between 0 and 1 with those that range above 1 without limit. These fractional or protective relative risks are frequently represented as the reciprocal of the relative risk preceded by a negative sign. For smaller samples the calculation recommended by Haldane is preferable and results in a less biased value.[46] Independent of the RR, which measures the intensity of the disease association, the standard $\chi^2$ statistic is used to determine the significance of the association. Both RR and $\chi^2$ can be conveniently calculated from a simple 2 × 2 tabular presentation of data (Fig. 4–11).

An idea of the intensity of the association of certain diseases with particular alleles depicted in Table 4–10 can be obtained by considering that the classic relative

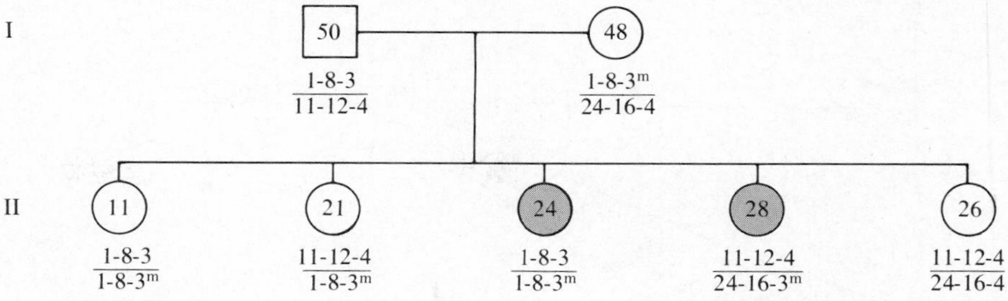

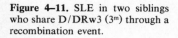

**Figure 4–11.** SLE in two siblings who share D/DRw3 ($3^m$) through a recombination event.

risk of the association between blood group O and duodenal ulcer disease was only 1.3.[45] It is obvious that the percentage of patients expressing the marker is also of major importance. A significant association with a marker that is present on only a proportion of patients implies either that the disease is heterogeneous with only one form associated with a MHC determinant or, alternatively, that the MHC determinant identified is a clue to the presence of an allele of another locus with which the disease has a more complete and perhaps mechanistic relation.

**Ethnic Relationships of MHC Alleles.** It is of very considerable interest that different races and ethnic groups vary markedly with respect to the composition of their pools of MHC alleles (Tables 4–4, 4–5, and 4–7). For example, *DR3* is infrequent among Mongoloids yet common among central and northern European Caucasians, where it is often present as a haplotype, *HLA A1-B8-DR3.* A second haplotype found in this same region, and especially in the North, is the haplotype *HLA-A3-B7-DR2.* Neither of these haplotypes is frequent among other populations. Among Caucasians they are uncommon among those of the Mediterranean basin. *HLA-B27* is distributed more evenly among all Caucasians, achieving its greatest frequency among some American Indian tribes, yet it is rare among the Mongoloid races from which these Indians were derived.

In a practical sense the calculation of a relative risk requires that the control population and the disease population be identical with respect to their ethnic composition. For example, there would be a major bias in such data derived from a disease associated with Mediterranean origin, such as familial Mediterranean fever if the control group were composed of randomly selected North American Caucasians.

The origins of the ethnic differences are still not well understood. Certain ones reflect relatively recent migrations: The *HLA-A3-B7-DR2* haplotype is Nordic in origin, and its presence correlates well with the extent of the Viking sphere of influence approximately 1000 years ago. Similarly, the distribution of the *HLA-A1-B8-DR3* haplotype suggests that it is Indo-European in origin, possibly having been introduced into Europe by invasions along this route (Fig. 4–12).

However, if mixing of populations were the only factor responsible for the linkage disequilibrium, one should not encounter the high values for $\Delta$ in the outbred human population. A difference in gene frequency of $\Delta = 0.1$ would take approximately 200 generations or 4000 years to fall to the insignificant value of 0.02. The presence of the elevated $\Delta$ values suggests that a positive survival value could be associated with certain haplotypes. Similarly, the associations of disease with haplotypes or allotypes appear to reflect a much more fundamental event than a historical accident. Certain diseases, such as the spondyloarthropathies, are closely associated with HLA-B27 in all populations. Other categories of diseases shift their associations even within

**Table 4–10.** Contrasting Activities of B Lymphocyte Alloantisera in Patients with Systemic Lupus Erythematosus, Rheumatic Fever, or Rheumatoid Arthritis

| | | Normal (n = 40) | Systemic Lupus Erythematosus (n = 24) | | | Rheumatic Fever (n = 21) | | | Rheumatoid Arthritis (n = 45) | | |
|---|---|---|---|---|---|---|---|---|---|---|---|
| **Reagent** | **HLA-DR Specificity** | % | % | *p** | *RR*† | % | *p* | *RR* | % | *p* | *RR* |
| 7AO | 1 | 28 | 28 | 0.55 | 1.0 | 26 | 0.50 | −1.1 | 9 | 0.02 | −3.6 |
| 1239 | 2 | 28 | 46 | 0.11 | 2.0 | | | | 13 | 0.09 | −2.5 |
| 1146 | 2 | 26 | 50 | 0.04 | 2.8 | 25 | 0.59 | −1.1 | 12 | 0.08 | −2.5 |
| CH | 2 + 3 + ? | 40 | 72 | 0.02 | 3.7 | | | | 34 | 0.34 | −1.3 |
| 1033 | 3 | 24 | 55 | 0.02 | 3.7 | 20 | 0.43 | −1.2 | 14 | 0.14 | −1.9 |
| 2134 | 3 | 26 | 56 | 0.02 | 3.5 | | | | 14 | 0.14 | −2.1 |
| 1283 | 4 × 7 × 10 (MT3) | 28 | 12 | 0.14 | −2.6 | | | | 80 | $<1\times10^{-5}$ | 9.6 |
| 1038 | 4 × 7 × 10 (MT3) | 24 | 6 | 0.03 | −3.9 | 24 | 0.59 | 1.0 | 76 | $<1\times10^{-5}$ | 9.4 |
| 191 | 4 × 10 (DR4) | 22 | 4 | 0.049 | −4.8 | 26 | 0.57 | 1.3 | 60 | $4.6\times10^{-4}$ | 5.1 |
| 1995 | 5 | 12 | 8 | 0.47 | −1.4 | 11 | 0.54 | −1.0 | 4 | 0.17 | −2.8 |
| 883 | Undefined | 17 | 0 | 0.03 | −10.6 | 71 | $5\times10^{-5}$ | 10.8 | 4 | 0.054 | −4.1 |

**p* = Fisher exact probability.
†RR = relative risk (defined in text), calculated, according to Haldane.

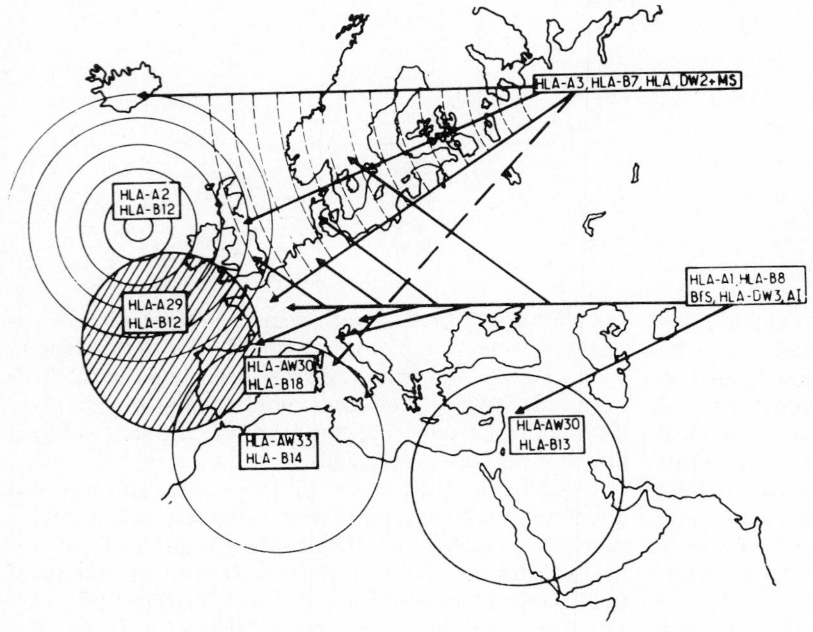


**Figure 4–12** A map of Europe with the circles illustrating the basic geographic distribution of MHC haplotypes, presumably established at the time when agriculture stablized the peoples of this area. Two subsequent major migrations are illustrated by the branching lines with arrows. The "Nordic" haplotype HLA-A3-B7-DR2 and the "Indo-European" haplotype HLA-A1-B8-DR3 may have been introduced by military conquest. (Courtesy of Professor J. Dausset.)

different Caucasian ethnic subsets. For example, among Eastern Mediterraneans the Ia alloantigen associations of multiple sclerosis and rheumatoid arthritis are different from those in the main Caucasian population. An explanation of these associations is one of the challenges of current medical research.

**Rheumatic Disease Associations.** The analysis of B lymphocyte alloantigens in patients with rheumatoid arthritis or systemic lupus erythematosus, summarized in Table 4–10, demonstrates that both diseases are related to B cell alloantigens; however, the profile of alloantigens in each disease is entirely different. This indicates that while there are certain autoimmune features in common between these two diseases, the MHC determinants for susceptibility to either one are entirely contrasting.

The fact that patients with systemic lupus erythematosus have two DR allospecificities has several interpretations, and it is not yet possible to choose among them: (1) That there are two clinically similar but pathogenetically distinct categories of patients. (2) That the primary association is with disease resistance, e.g., possibly mediated by the allele bearing MT3. (3) That susceptibility is associated with an as yet unrecognized allele that occurs most commonly with DR2 and DR3.

Of further interest in regard to the presence of DR2 in patients with systemic lupus erythematosus is the presence of DR2 in two disease states usually considered to have some interrelationship: the atypical lupus like syndrome associated with C2 deficiency, and idiopathic thrombocytopenic purpura.[47] In the case of C2 deficiency, the association is most frequently with a special haplotype—A10, B18, D2, DR2.[48] These observations suggest that the findings of an association with DR2 could be considered as evidence that these diseases have a nosologic relationship.

Family studies are the most reliable method of defining the relationship of disease susceptibility to genetic factors. The study illustrated in Figure 4–11 serves to illustrate several aspects of this approach. Two siblings, aged 24 and 28, presented with classic SLE. Conventional HLA testing of A, B, and C alleles revealed that they appeared not to share any haplotype. MHC studies and typing for B lymphocyte alloantigens, however, cast a different perspective on the family. Both siblings typed for the presence of D/DR3. Since the assignment of D/DR could be verified among other family members not illustrated, it appears that a maternal recombination occurred, with the major portion of the sixth chromosome bearing *HLA A1, B8, D/DR3* losing its distal short arm between *HLA B* and *HLA D* and exchanging this segment for one bearing HLA A24,B16, manifested as the haplotype 24-16-$3^{m}$. The susceptibility to disease presumably maps in the vicinity of the D/DR locus in association with the D/DR3 specificity. A similar association with the *HLA-A1-B8-DR3* haplotype in families with multiple instances of males with lupus erythematosus has been reported.[49]

**Hypothetical Mechanisms of Disease Associations.** If indeed the association of the B27 arthropathy complex remains maximal with the B locus and is not related to another determinant of histocompatibility that maps at a nearby locus, then the disease mechanisms of this group would most likely relate to the specific functions of the class I MHC antigens. These relate to the recognition phase in cytotoxic effector functions and could include B locus allele linked differences in the efficiency of eliminating particular targets. The concept of a mimetic relationship between pathogen and cell receptor is also an attractive one. Alternatively, the role of the MHC in immune functions may not be involved, and it is possible that other aspects of MHC function, such as cell interactions or differentiation, could result in the disease state.

The second category of diseases that relate to alleles of class II molecules raises an entirely different spectrum of possibilities, as a reflection of the presumed functions of genes in this region. The dominant hypotheses would relate to the role of these gene products in the positive or negative control of the immune response. These take two general forms: one in which the determinants controlling the selective response to a pathogenic agent such as a virus are absent or abnormal; and the other in which the immune system is disregulated because of imperfect receptor-acceptor interactions, without any particular pathogen or inciting organism. The influence of the MHC alloantigens on the T cell antigen repertoire could also result in a deficiency of T cell clones necessary to recognize an antigen on a pathogenic organism. Here, as in the previous HLA-B locus mechanisms, an excessive reliance on immune phenomena may be unwarranted. The fact that the same diseases in different ethnic groups are stongly associated with entirely distinct MHC specificities, depending on the ethnic group,[19] serves to highlight the challenge of understanding the biologic significance of the disease associations and their potential role in determining human evolution. A recent survey of some aspects of disease associations provides additional access to the current literature.[50]

## CONCLUSION

The manner in which the MHC is intertwined with many of the rheumatic diseases is a logical reflection of the participation of the immune system in their pathogenesis, as well as the multiple organ involvement that characterizes them. Mastery of this aspect of basic rheumatology is complicated by the inherent intricacy of the subject matter, as well as its dependence upon genetics and a basically subtle methodology. This difficulty is tempered by the potential for imminent application of this knowledge. Already, assays for B27 have been of practical diagnostic assistance in patients and have served to enhance the understanding of several categories of arthritic disease. Very much the same is now occurring in the area of B lymphocyte alloantigen measurements for a larger sphere of diseases. At the next level of application, the ability of the MHC determinants to identify individuals at risk for these diseases should serve as an additional stimulus for the development of preventive measures. Finally, it is very likely that the study of mechanisms of these diseases will contribute major insights into the basic biologic knowledge of what is an extraordinary adaptive mechanism.[51]

## References

1. Payne, R.: The association of febrile transfusion reactions with leuko-agglutinins. Vox Sang. 2:233, 957.
2. Dausset, J.: Iso-leuco-corps. Acta Haematol. 20:156, 1958.
3. Van Rood, J.J., and van Leeuwen, A.: Leukocyte grouping: A method and its application. J. Clin. Invest. 42:1382, 1963.
4. Terasaki, P.I., and McClelland, J.D.: Microdroplet assay of human serum cytotoxins. Nature 204:998, 1964.
5. Zinkernagel, R.M., and Doherty, P.C.: Major transplantation antigens, viruses, and specificity of surveillance T-cells: The "altered self" hypothesis. Contemp. Topics Immunobiol. 7:179, 1977.
6. Brewerton D.A., Hart, F.D., Nicholls, A., Caffrey, M., James, D.C.O., and Sturrock, R.D.: Ankylosing spondylitis and HL-A 27. Lancet 1:904, 1973.
7. Schlosstein, L., Terasaki, P.I., Bluestone, R., and Pearson, C. M.: High association of an HLA antigen, W27, with ankylosing spondylitis. N. Engl. J. Med. 288:704, 1973.
8. Klein, J.: Biology of the Mouse Histocompatibility-2 Complex. New York, Springer, 1975.
9. Cavalli-Sforza, L.L., and Bodmer, W.F.: The Genetics of Human Populations. San Francisco, W.H. Freeman, 1971.
10. Bodmer, W.F.: Evolutionary significance of the HL-A system. Nature 237:139, 1972.
11. Kissmeyer-Nielsen, F.: Histocompatibility Testing, 1975. Copenhagen, Munksgaard, 1975.
12. Bodmer, W.F., Batchelor, J.R., Bodmer, J.G., Festenstein, H., and Morris, P.J.: Histocompatibility Testing, 1977 Copenhagen, Munksgaard, 1978.
13. Terasaki, P.I. (ed.): Histocompatibility Testing. Los Angeles, UCLA Press, 980.
14. Albert, E.D.: The major histocompatibility complex (MHC) in man. Clin. Rheum. Dis. 3:175, 1977.
15. van Rood, J.J., de Vries, R.P., Bradley, B.A.: Genetics and biology of the HLA System. *In* Dorf, M.E. (ed.): The Role of the Major Histocompatibility Complex in Immunology. New York, Garland Press, 1981, p. 59.
16. Bruakoff, S.J.: Specificity of cytolytic T-cell responses. *In* Dorf, M.E. (ed.): The Role of the Major Histocompatibility Complex in Immunology. New York, Garland Press, 1981, p. 343.
17. Bach, F.H., and van Rood, J.J.: The major histocompatibility complex. Genetics and biology. N. Engl. J. Med. 295:806, 872, 927, 1976.
18. Green, S.S., and Sell, K.W.: Mixed leukocyte stimulation of normal peripheral leukocytes by autologous lymphoblastoid cells. Science 170:989, 1970.
19. Winchester, R., and Kunkel, H.G.: The human Ia system. Advances in Immunology. New York, Academic Press, 1979, p. 221.
20. Korman, A.J., Auffray, C., Schamboeck, A., and Strominger, J.L.: The amino acid sequence and gene organization of the heavy chain of the HLA-DR antigen: Homology to immunoglobulins. Proc. Natl. Acad. Sci. USA 79:6013, 1982.
21. Kratzin, H., Yang, C., Gotz, H., Pauly, E., Kolbel, S., Egert, G., Thinnes, F.P., Wernet, P., Altevogt, P., and Hilschmann, N.: Primärstruktur menschlicher Histokompatibilitätsantigene der Klasse II. I. Mitteilung: Aminosäuresequenz der N-terminalen 198 Reste der beta-Kette des HLA-Dw2,2; DR2,2-Alloantigens. Hoppe Seylers Z. Physiol. Chem. 362:1665, 1981 (English Abstr.).
22. Hurley, C.K., Nunez, G., Winchester, R., Finn, O.J., Levy, R., and Capra, J.D.: The human HLA-DR antigens are encoded by multiple beta chain loci. J. Immunol 129:2103, 1982.
23. Karr, W.R., Kannapell, C.C., Stein, J.A, Fuller, T.C., Duquesnoy, R.J., Rodey, G.E., Mann, D.L., Gebel, H.M. and Schwartz, B.D.: Demonstration of a third structurally distinct human Ia beta chain by two dimensional gel electrophoresis. J. Exp. Med. 156:652, 1982.
24. Moutsopoulos, H.M., Mann, D.L., Johnson, A.H., and Chused, T.M.: Genetic differences between primary and secondary sicca syndrome. N. Engl. J. Med. 302:761, 1979.
25. Reinertsen, J.L., Klippel, J.H., Johnson, A.H., Steinberg, A.D., Decker, J.L., and Mann, D.L.: B-lymphocyte alloantigens associated with systemic lupus erythematosus. N. Engl. J. Med. 299:515, 1978.
26. Gibofsky, A., Winchester, R., Hansen, J., Patarroyo, M., Dupont, B., Paget, S., Lahita, R., Halper, J., Fotino, M., Yunis, E., and Kunkel, H.G.: Contrasting patterns of newer histocompatibility determinants in patients with rheumatoid arthritis and systemic lupus erythematosus. Arthritis Rheum. 21:S123, 1978.
27. Duquesnoy, R.J., Marrari, M., and Annen, K.: Identification of an HLA-DR associated system of B cell alloantigens. Trans. Proc. 11:1757, 1979.
28. Corte, G., Calabi, F., Damiani, G., Bargellesi, A., Tosi, R., and Sorrentino, R.: Human Ia molecules carrying DC1 determinants differ in both A- and B-subunits from Ia molecules carrying DR determinants. Nature 292:357, 1981.
29. Park, M.S., Teresaki, P.I., Nakata, S., and Adki, D.: Supertypic DR groups: MT1, MT2 and MT3. In Teraski, P.I. (ed.): Histocompatibility Testing 1980. Los Angeles, UCLA Press, 1980, p. 854.
30. Goyert, S.M., Shively, J.E., and Silver J.: Biochemical characterization of a second family of human Ia molecules, HLA-DS, equivalent to murine I-A subregion molecules. J. Exp. Med. 156:550, 1982.
31. Bona, M.R., and Strominger, J.L.: Direct evidence of homology between human DC-1 antigen and murine I-A molecules. Nature 299:836, 1982.

32. Tanigaki, N., and Tosi, R.: The genetic control of human Ia alloantigens: A three-locus model derived from the immunochemical analysis of "supertypic specificities. Immunol. Rev. 66:5, 1982.
33. Schackelford, D.A., Kaufman, J.F., Korman, A.J. and Strominger, J.L., HLA-DR antigens: structure, separation of subpopulations, gene and cloning and function. Immunol. Rev. 66:133, 1982.
34. Giles, R.C., Nunez, G., Hurley, C.K., Nunez-Roldan, A., Winchester, R., Stastny, P., and Capra, J.D.: Structural analysis of a human I-A homologue using a monoclonal antibody which recognizes an MB3-like specificity. J. Exp. Med. 157:1461, 1981.
35. Shaw, S., Kavathas, P., Pollack, M.S., Charmot, D., and Mawas, C.: Family studies define a new histocompatibility locus, *SB*, between *HLA-DR* and *GLO*. Nature (Lond.) 293:745, 1981.
36. Sasazuki, T., McDevitt, H.O., and Grumet, F.C.: The association between genes in the major histocompatibility complex and disease susceptibility. Ann Rev. Med. 28:425, 1977.
37. Winchester, R.J.: B-lymphocyte allo-antigens, cellular expression, and disease significance with special reference to rheumatoid arthritis. Arthritis Rheum. 20:159s, 1977.
38. Stastny, P.: Association of the B-cell alloantigen DRw4 with rheumatoid arthritis. N. Engl. J. Med. 298:869, 1978.
39. Gibofsky, A., Winchester, R.J., Patarroyo, M., Fotino, M., and Kunkel, H.G.: Disease associations of the Ia like human alloantigens. Contrasting patterns in rheumatoid arthritis and systemic lupus erythematosus. J. Exp. Med. 148:1728, 1978.
40. Winchester, R.J.: Genetic aspects of rheumatoid arthritis, Springer Semin. Immunopathol. (Springer-Verlag) 4:89, 1981.
41. Ahearn, J.M., Provost, T.T., Dorsch, C.A., Stevens, M.B., Bias, W.B. and Arnett, F.C.: Interrelationships of HLA-DR, MB, and MT phenotypes, autoantibody expression, and clinical features in systemic lupus erythematosus. Arthritis Rheum. 25:1031, 1982.
42. Winchester, R.J., and Nunez-Roldan, A.: Some genetic aspects of systemic lupus erythematosus. Arthritis Rheum. 25:833, 1982.
43. Chused, T.M., Kassan, S.S., and Opelz, G.: Sjögren's syndrome associated with HLA-Dw3. N. Engl. J. Med. 296:895, 977.
44. Patarroyo, M.E., Winchester, R.J., Veherano, A., Gibofsky, A., Chalem, F., Zabriskie, J.B., and Kunkel, H.G.: Association of a particular B cell alloantigen with susceptibility to rheumatic fever. Nature 278:173, 1979.
45. Woolf, B.: On estimating the relation between blood group and disease. Ann. Hum. Genet. 19:251, 1955.
46. Haldane, J.B.S.: The estimation and significance of the logarithm of a ratio of frequencies. Ann. Hum. Genet. 20:309, 1955.
47. Karpatkin, S., Fotino, M., Gibofsky, A., and Winchester, R.J.: Association of HLA DRw2 with auto-immune thrombocytopenic purpura. J. Clin. Invest. 63:1085, 1979.
48. Fu, S.M., Kunkel, H.G., Brussman, H.P., Allen, F.H., Jr., and Fotino, M.: Evidence for linkage between HL-A histocompatibility genes and those involved in the synthesis of the second component of complement. J. Exp. Med. 140:1108, 1974.
49. Lahita, R.G., Chiorazzi, N., Gibofsky, A., Winchester, R.J., and Kunkel, H.G.: Familial SLE in males. Arthritis Rheum. 26:39, 1983.
50. Moller, G. (ed.): HLA and disease susceptibility. Immunol. Rev. 70:1, 1983.
51. Bodmer, W.F.: Evolution and function of the HLA system. Br. Med. Bull. 34:309, 1978.

# Chapter 5
# Genetic Control of Immune Responses

*William J. Koopman*

## GENES REGULATE IMMUNE RESPONSES AT SEVERAL LEVELS—AN OVERVIEW

It has long been recognized that individual animal strains differ considerably in their capacity to mount specific humoral and/or cellular immune responses against a variety of immunogens. More recently, genetically related differences in immune response characteristics have also been documented in man. While the precise mechanism(s) underlying genetically determined immune response characteristics has not yet been elucidated, it has become increasingly clear that distinct genetic loci are capable of influencing specific immune responses. A major role(s) for genes residing within the major histocompatibility complex (MHC) and for genes linked to immunoglobulin (Ig) structural genes, particularly immunoglobulin heavy chains (IgH), has been well established for responses to several immunogens. That other loci also influence responses to particular antigens seems certain; however, the nature of these loci is less well defined at this time.

More generalized effects of certain genetic factors on immune responses have also been identified. In this regard genetically determined cell surface differentiation antigens (markers) have facilitated identification of functionally (and antigenically) distinct lymphoid cell subpopulations. The interactions among these distinct cell types play a critical role in determining the quality and quantity of an ensuing immune response. In several instances, these genetically determined differentiation markers have been implicated as contributing to the functional properties of these distinct cell populations.

In discussing the influence of genetic factors on immune responses, it seems appropriate to focus on two distinct groups of genes: (1) major histocompatibility complex (MHC) genes and (2) Ig-linked genes. Interest in genes that influence immune responses has been heightened by increasing evidence that closely related, if not identical, genes also influence susceptibility to a variety of diseases in which immune events appear to play a critical role. Most striking in this regard is the significant association of enhanced susceptibility to several rheumatic diseases with genes residing within the MHC. An important role(s) for genes associated with immune response characteristics is further suggested by studies in which genes linked to Ig structural loci, particularly IgH loci, have been demonstrated to associate with an increased prevalence of several autoimmune diseases. Moreover, parallel analysis of MHC and IgH genetic markers has convincingly established that these genetic loci situated on separate chromosomes exert more than additive effects with regard to susceptibility to some of these diseases. Taken together, these observations suggest that genes regulating immune responses concurrently influence predisposition to certain diseases.

In approaching the subject of genetic control of immune responses, familiarity with basic genetic concepts is helpful. A glossary of relevant terms is provided in Table 5–1.

## GENES OF THE MAJOR HISTOCOMPATIBILITY COMPLEX

The MHC consists of a cluster of genes residing on the short arm of the human chromosome 6 (chromosome 17 in the mouse) that encodes three distinct classes of proteins of immunologic importance (Fig. 5–1). Class I MHC proteins are heterodimers consisting of a highly polymorphic heavy chain (MW ~ 45,000) encoded by MHC genes which is noncovalently associated with $\beta_2$ microglobulin ($\beta_2$M, MW ~ 12,000), an essentially invariant polypeptide encoded by a non-MHC locus.[1-3] These antigens are expressed on the cell surfaces of all nucleated cells and platelets and serve as restriction elements in the recognition of target cells by cytotoxic T lymphocytes.[4] HLA-A, HLA-B, and HLA-C antigens in man[3] and H-2K, H-2L, and H-2D antigens in the mouse[5] are class I MHC proteins. Class II MHC molecules are polymorphic bimolecular complexes consisting of an $\alpha$ heavy chain and a smaller $\beta$ polypeptide chain, with the $\beta$ chains accounting for most of the polymorphism of these antigens.[6-10] These antigens, also referred to as Ia antigens, are encoded by I region genes of the mouse and the corresponding D region genes of man. Ia antigens have a more restricted tissue distribution than class I antigens and are found on B lymphocytes, monocyte/macrophages, activated T lymphocytes, Langerhans' cells, dendritic cells, some endothelial cells, sperm, and a population of thymic epithelial cells. Class II antigens function as restriction elements in the recognition of antigen on monocyte/macrophages of B lymphocytes by T lymphocytes.[11] Furthermore, genes controlling the magnitude of immune responses to a variety of antigens (immune response (Ir) genes)[12] have been mapped to the I region of the mouse, specifically the I-A and I-E subregions.[13] Ia antigens appear to be equivalent to Ir gene products.[14] Finally, class III proteins constitute complement components encoded by genes residing within the MHC (C4, C2, and B in man). A detailed discussion of the MHC is presented in Chapter 4. Attention in this chapter is directed primarily toward the Ir genes of the MHC, in view of their evident role in regulation of immune responses.

**Table 5–1.** Glossary of Genetic Terms

| | |
|---|---|
| **Gene** | a segment of DNA (the basic unit of inheritance) that directs the transcription of a specific messenger RNA, which directs the translation of a specific polypeptide chain. |
| **Locus** | the location of a gene on a chromosome. |
| **Allele** | alternative forms of the same gene, having usually arisen by some mutational event. Within the major histocompatibility complex (MHC) each locus possesses multiple alleles. When this occurs with considerable frequency within a given population, it is said to represent polymorphism. |
| **Genotype** | the description of the combination of genes inherited by an individual from both parents. |
| **Phenotype** | the genetically determined expressed characteristics of an individual, which reflect the summation of all of his genes and thereby give him a descriptive identity. |
| **Haplotype** | a combination of closely linked genes on the same chromosome. |
| **Linkage** | the tendancy of genes located near each other on the same chromosome to segregate together. |
| **Allogeneic** | a description for the genetic relationship of two individuals from the same species possessing different allelic forms of a particular gene. |
| **Syngeneic** | a description for the genetic relationship of two individuals from the same species possessing the same allelic forms of a particular gene. |
| **Congenic** | two strains bred in such a way that they differ genetically only at a particular locus (and generally at a segment of the chromosome surrounding or adjacent to that particular locus). |

### Immune Response (Ir) Genes

**Location of Ir Genes in the MHC.** ***Murine Ir Genes.*** As previously mentioned, experimental data strongly suggest that Ir genes reside within the I region of the mouse. The murine I region has been subdivided into five subregions on the basis of recombinational analysis: I-A, I-B, I-J, I-E, and I-C.[15,16] In mice, two well characterized groups of Ia antigens (the putative products of Ir genes) have been identified: I-A and I-E. I-A subregion molecules consist of an A$\alpha$ and A$\beta$ bimolecular complex with both $\alpha$ and $\beta$ chains encoded by genes residing entirely within the I-A subregion. In contrast, I-E antigens consist of an E$\alpha$ polypeptide chain encoded within the I-E subregion and an E$\beta$ chain derived from the I-A subregion[17] (Fig. 5–2). The I-J subregion was initially defined by antisera that recognized determinants on suppressor T cells[18] and soluble antigen-specific suppressor factors.[19] Although characterization studies are in progress,[20-22] the structure of I-J molecules remains considerably less certain than that of I-A and I-E antigens. The precise location of the I-J subregion is also unclear at present in view of recent observation of Steinmetz and colleagues.[23] These workers have analyzed segments of DNA totaling 200 kilobases in the I region, and their results limit the I-B and I-J subregions to a segment of DNA no longer than 3.4 kilobases in length, raising the possibility that I-J products may be encoded by genes located outside the I region. The status of I-B also appears to be uncertain, since no Ia specificity has been exclusively localized to I-B.[24]

***Human Ir Genes.*** Although evidence for specific immune response genes in man is less substantial than in the mouse, there is, nonetheless, strong evidence indicating that the D region in man is equivalent to the

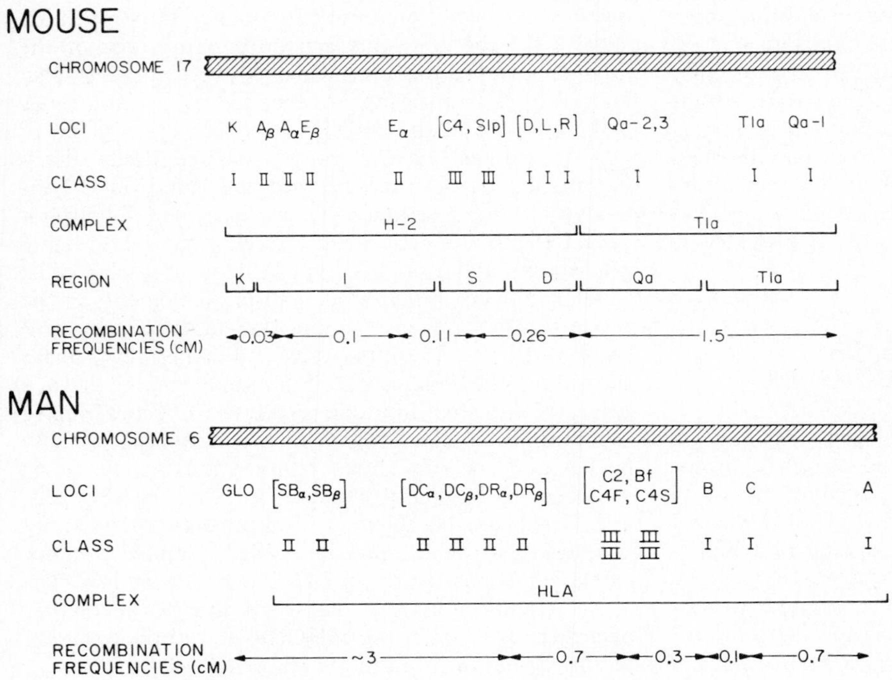


**Figure 5–1.** Comparison of the major histocompatibility complex (MHC) of mouse and man. (Reproduced, with permission, from the Annual Review of Immunology, Volume 1. ©1983 by Annual Reviews Inc.)

murine I region, including (1) comparable structure of protein products encoded by the two regions,[6] (2) homology of amino acid sequence between human D and murine I region products,[25] and (3) homology in sequences between human D and murine I region genes.[23]

**Structure of Ir Gene Products.** *Murine Ia Antigens.* As alluded to previously, two groups of murine Ia molecules encoded by genes located within the I region have been identified and characterized, the I-A and I-E molecules. These molecules have both been demonstrated to be integral cell membrane glycoproteins[26] and can be

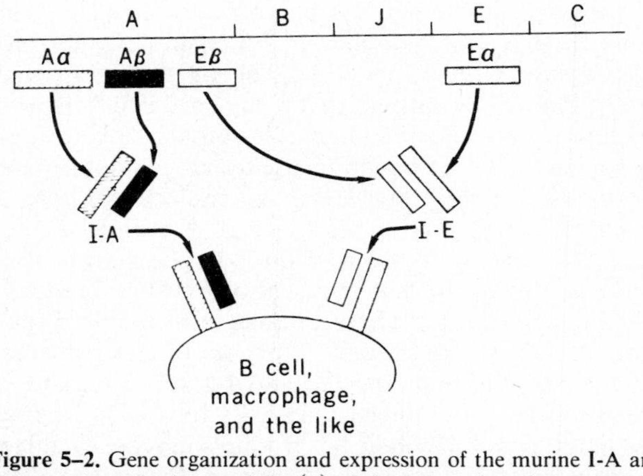


**Figure 5–2.** Gene organization and expression of the murine I-A and I-E antigens. The heavy chain (α) of the I-A antigen is encoded by the gene Aa, whereas the polymorphic β chain is encoded by the gene Aβ. Both I-A chains are therefore encoded for by genes residing in the I-A subregion of the MHC. In contrast, the α heavy chain of the I-E antigen is encoded by the Ea gene, which resides in the I-E (or I-C) subregion, while the lighter β chain is encoded by the Eβ gene, which resides in the I-A subregion. (From Uhr, J.W., et al.: Science 206:292, 1979, Copyright 1979 by the AAAS.)

immunoprecipitated from solubilized membrane preparations utilizing antibodies generated by immunizing mice with cells from congenic strains of mice differing only at the I-A or I-E subregion of the MHC.[27] I-A antigens consist of a disulfide-bonded αβ dimer with an approximate molecular weight of 55,000. Under reducing conditions, the Aα and Aβ chains can be separated and demonstrate apparent molecular weights of 35,000 and 26,000, respectively.[25] Similarly, I-E antigens also consist of two polypeptide chains designated Eα and Eβ of approximate molecular weights of 32,000 and 29,000, respectively.[6] Also associated with both I-A and I-E molecules is a third polypeptide (Mr ~ 31,000), designated (Ii), that is not encoded by MHC genes and appears to be invariant in structure.[28] Although I-A and I-E molecules are both heterodimers of similar molecular size, finer structural analysis has clearly demonstrated the two molecules to be distinct. In this regard, differences between the α and β chains of the two groups of molecules have been identified utilizing both N-terminal amino acid sequencing[29-31] and peptide mapping[32,17] techniques. Since the Ia molecules are obviously quite polymorphic[33] it has been important to delineate the structural basis of this polymorphism. Comparison of Ia molecules isolated from different congenic strains differing only at the I region has clearly demonstrated that the β chain is highly polymorphic whereas the α chain is more conserved.[6,34,35] Further heterogeneity may be introduced as a result of differences in glycosylation.[10] Heterogeneity may also result from the random association of Aα and Aβ chains in heterozygotes.[6] Furthermore, expression of Eα and Eβ chains has also been demonstrated in situations in which the genes are trans to each other.[36]

It should be stressed that other murine Ia antigens may exist. Utilizing E$\alpha$ and human DC$\beta$ cDNA probes, Southern blot analyses of the murine I region suggest the existence of at least two $\alpha$ and four to six $\beta$ genes.[23] The existence of additional class II genes, which may not be sufficiently homologous to the probes to be identified, cannot be excluded.

Progress has been made in the analysis of the structure of murine class II genes. Analyses of cDNA and genomic clones of the A$\alpha$ and E$\alpha$ genes have been reported.[37,38] Interestingly, the exon-intron organization of the E$\alpha$ gene appears quite similar to the human DR$\alpha$ gene.[39-41] Furthermore, the deduced amino acid sequence of E$\alpha$ exhibits 76 percent homology with DR$\alpha$,[38] thus confirming the earlier hypothesis that DR$\alpha$ and E$\alpha$ are homologous genes.[25] The exon organization of the E$\alpha$ gene corresponds with the domains of the protein product. Specifically, two external domains (N-terminal and membrane proximal) and the transmembrane and cytoplasmic domains are encoded by four distinct exons. The second external domain (i.e., membrane proximal) of both E$\alpha$ and A$\alpha$ exhibits strong homology with immunoglobulin constant regions.[37]

***Human Ia Antigens.*** Serologic analysis of human Ia antigens has been pursued utilizing heteroantisera, alloantisera, and, more recently, monoclonal reagents. At least three groups of human Ia antigens have been identified utilizing these serologic reagents in conjunction with mixed leukocyte reaction testing or discriminatory recognition of the antigens utilizing cytotoxic T lymphocytes. Human DR antigens consist of a bimolecular complex of $\alpha$ "heavy chain" of approximately 34,000 molecular weight associated with a $\beta$ "light chain" of molecular weight 29,000.[6] A third polypeptide, the Ia-associated invariant chain (Ii), has also been identified in immunoprecipitates containing human DR antigens.[42] N-terminal amino acid analysis indicates close homology between DR$\alpha$ and murine E$\alpha$ chains and between DR$\beta$ and murine E$\beta$ chains.[25] The polymorphism of human DR antigens is predominantly determined by the $\beta$ chain subunit.[8,6,10,9,43] Shaw and colleagues have identified another group of Ia molecules, designated SB,[44,45] which consists of two chains that resemble the $\alpha$ and $\beta$ chains of DR antigens with regard to molecular weight.[46] This set of antigens is encoded by an HLA-D subregion distinct from DR. While limited N-terminal sequence data indicate that SB$\alpha$ and SB$\beta$ chains differ from DR$\alpha$ and DR$\beta$ chains,[47] SB$\alpha$ appears to be related to murine E$\alpha$, suggesting that SB antigen may also be homologous to murine I-E molecules.[47]

A third group of polymorphic Ia molecules, termed DC antigens, has been identified. It differs from DR molecules in both $\alpha$ and $\beta$ subunits by two-dimensional gel analysis[48] and by peptide mapping.[49] Amino acid sequence analysis suggests that DC antigens are homologous to murine I-A molecules.[50] The DS molecules described by Goyert and colleagues[51] appear to belong to the DC Ia group, and, indeed, limited sequence analysis of these molecules indicates homology with the murine I-A group. The SB locus appears to be localized centromeric to the DR locus in the D region on the basis of recombinational analysis[45] and study of deletion mutants.[52] The precise location of the DC locus has not been determined.

Human class II $\alpha$ and $\beta$ genes have recently been cloned and characterized; sequencing has provided important insights into the structure of the corresponding protein products.[39,53-56] The predicted amino acid sequence of DR$\alpha$ chains suggests that $\alpha$ chains consist of two external domains similar to murine E$\alpha$ chains; moreover, sequence homology between immunoglobulin constant regions and the second external domain (membrane proximal) of the $\alpha$ chain has been identified.[39,57] Partial DR$\beta$ chain amino acid sequence data indicate that the membrane proximal external domain of these chains is also homologous to immunoglobulin constant regions.[58-60] As mentioned previously, the homology between DR$\alpha$ and E$\alpha$ genes is supported by the similar exon-intron structure of the two genes in addition to the deduced amino acid sequences of the two $\alpha$ chains.[38]

**Ir Genes Regulate Immune Responses to Antigens.** ***Animal Studies.*** Although individual differences in immune responses to particular antigens had been previously recognized by immunologists, Levine and colleagues first demonstrated genetic control of such responses. These workers observed that humoral and cellular immune responses by outbred guinea pigs to the antigen DNP-poly-L-lysine (DNP-PLL) were controlled by a single autosomal dominant gene.[61,62] "Responders" possessed the gene that was therefore designated an immune response or Ir gene. Ir genes were subsequently demonstrated in inbred strains of guinea pigs for several synthetic antigens[63] and for conventional antigens, particularly at low concentrations (presumably related to selection for response to a limited number of dominant determinants).[64,65] Moreover, Ir genes were documented in several other species, including mice,[66] rats,[67] and monkeys.[68] The availability of inbred strains of mice permitted rapid progress in the localization of Ir genes in the genome. These genes were shown to map to the murine MHC (H-2 complex).[69,70] Similar linkage of Ir genes with the MHC was subsequently demonstrated in other species, including guinea pigs,[71] rats,[67] and monkeys.[68] Analysis of immune response characteristics of recombinant and congenic strains of mice permitted more precise localization of Ir genes to the I region of the murine MHC.[72] Additional studies indicated that Ir genes for some antigens mapped strictly to the I-A subregion of the I region whereas others mapped to both the I-A and I-E subregions.[73,74] The latter Ir genes were of considerable interest, since "responder" status for these antigens was dependent upon inheritance of both I-A and I-E-linked Ir genes (termed $\alpha$ and $\beta$, respectively) located either cis or trans to each other.[73,74] Referred to as gene complementation, this phenomenon later facilitated identification of cell surface Ia antigens as the likely products of Ir genes.

Immunization of mice with lymphoid cells from strains differing only at the I region elicits production of antibodies in the recipient strain that recognize characteristic cell surface glycoproteins (Ia antigens) expressed particularly on B lymphocytes, macrophages, dendritic cells, and activated T lymphocytes. Considerable evidence suggests that these Ia antigens are the products of Ir genes: (1) Ia molecules are encoded by genes residing in the same location of the I region as Ir genes; (2) antibodies directed against I-A molecules are able to block specific immune responses governed by Ir genes mapping to the same I-A subregion;[75] (3) antibodies directed against either I-A or I-E products block immune responses to antigens under dual Ir gene control in which the two genes map to the I-A and I-E subregions;[75] (4) the dual genetic control of expression of I-E antigens by genes residing in the I-A subregion (E$\beta$) and I-E subregion (E$\alpha$) correlates with the dual Ir gene complementation observed for certain antigens; (5) response to antigens under dual Ir gene control correlates with cell surface levels of relevant E$\alpha\beta$ complexes,[76,77] and (6) the predicted amino acid sequence of protein products encoded by genes residing in the I region agrees with limited sequence data obtained for isolated Ia molecules[57] (Table 5–2). Taken together, these observations provide convincing evidence that Ia antigens are encoded by structural genes located within the I region and are indistinguishable from Ir genes.

In contrast to the positive influence of Ir genes on immune responses to several antigens, unresponsiveness to some antigens appears to be related to negative influences of immune suppressor (Is) gene(s) residing in the I region. For example, the synthetic terpolymer GAT (poly[L-glu$^{60}$-L-ala$^{30}$-L-tyr$^{10}$])[78] and hen egg lysozyme[79] elicit predominantly T suppressor cell responses when injected into certain nonresponder strains of mice. The

**Table 5–2.** Evidence That ρDR-α-1 Is the Structural Gene of the HLA-DR α Chain*

| | |
|---|---|
| ρDR-α-1 | Ile-Ile-Gln-Ala- |
| | 5 10 |
| Raji α chain | Ile-Lys-Glu-Asp-His-Val-Ile-Ile-Gln-Ala- |
| ρDR-α-1 | Glu-Phe-Tyr-Leu-Asn-Pro-Asp-Gln-Ser-Gly- |
| | 15 20 |
| Raji α chain | Glu-Phe-Tyr-Leu-Asn-Pro-Asp-Gln-Ser-Gly- |
| ρDR-α-1 | Glu-Phe-Met-Phe-Asp-Phe-Asp-Gly-Asp-Glu- |
| | 25 30 |
| Raji α chain | Glu-Phe-Met-Phe-Asp-Phe-Asp-Gly-Asp-Glu- |
| ρDR-α-1 | Ile-Phe-His-Val-Asp- |
| | 35 |
| Raji α chain | Ile-Phe-His-Val-Asp- |

*adapted from Larhammar, D., et al.: Cell 30:153, 1982, Copyright MIT Press. Comparison of the predicted amino acid sequence obtained from the 5′ end of the coding strand of the cDNA clone ρDR-α-1 and the actual amino-terminal amino acid sequence of the alpha chain (Raji) of the HLA-DR antigen. Since the latter contained more than one amino acid at some positions, only the dominant amino acid obtained at any position is indicated.

Is genes have not yet been precisely localized in the I region, and the relationship of these genes to the I-J subregion has not been determined. Genes tentatively assigned to the I-J subregion had been previously demonstrated to direct the expression of I-J antigens present on the cell surface of T suppressor lymphocytes[18,19] and on antigen-specific suppressor factors produced by T suppressor lymphocytes.[19,80] The precise localization of these putative I-J subregion genes is uncertain at present in view of difficulties in identifying a corresponding suitable length of DNA in the I region for the postulated I-J subregion.[23]

***Human Studies.*** Demonstration of specific Ir genes in man has been predictably more difficult to achieve than in animal models. Several studies have established a statistical association between the presence of particular HLA antigens and immune responsiveness (or unresponsiveness) to specific antigens, including ragweed allergen Ra5,[81,82] collagen,[83] streptococcal antigens,[84] influenza A antigens,[85] vaccinia virus,[86] and tetanus toxoid.[87] In some cases antigen responsiveness was shown to associate with particular D region specificities.[81-83] Such an association would, of course, be expected in view of overwhelming evidence demonstrating homology between the murine I region and the human D region. Mechanisms underlying the association of HLA antigens and immune responsiveness have received limited attention. Responsiveness to collagen in vitro was shown to correlate with HLA-DR4 positivity and was attributed to absence of OKT $8^+$ suppressor T lymphocyte activity for collagen otherwise present in DR4 negative individuals.[88]

While these studies have provided circumstantial evidence of MHC-linked Ir (or Is) genes in man, family studies are clearly required to establish linkage between particular HLA antigens and immune responsiveness and to determine the mode of inheritance of these gene(s). Toward this end, Sasazuki and colleagues[89,90] have analyzed T lymphocyte proliferative responses to streptococcal cell wall (SCW) antigen(s) in Japanese families and have reported evidence for a single dominant immune suppression gene for SCW linked to HLA in these families. Thus, despite the experimental constraints of analyzing antigen specific responses in man, the available data strongly supports the existence of MHC-linked Ir (or Is) genes in man. With the recent development of serologic reagents for the detection of distinct Ia antigen groups in man (e.g., DC, DR, and SB), additional progress is anticipated in the precise localization of Ir genes in the human D region.

**Association of Ir Genes with Disease Susceptibility.** In recent years many human diseases have been demonstrated to associate with the presence of particular HLA specificities (see Chapter 4). For several of these diseases the primary association appears to be with D region antigens[91] (Table 5–3). Although family studies are required to determine the precise location of susceptibility gene(s) for these diseases, it is tempting to speculate that diseases associated with class II MHC (i.e., D region) antigens reflect the inheritance of specific

**Table 5–3.** Associations of Some Diseases with HLA-D/DR Antigens*

| Disease | Race | HLA-D/DR | Relative Risk† |
|---|---|---|---|
| Grave's disease | Cau | DR3 | 5.5–4.1 |
| Hashimoto's with goiter | Cau | DR5 | 3.7–3.2 |
| Multiple sclerosis | Cau | DR2 | 4.8 |
| Giant cell arteritis | Cau | DR4 | 8.2 |
| Rheumatoid arthritis | Cau | DR4 | 6.0 |
| Juvenile arthritis, systemic | Cau | DR2 | 3.6 |
| Systemic lupus erythematosus | Cau | DR3 | 5.7–3.0 |
| | | DR2 | 3.6 |
| Subacute cutaneous lupus erythematosus | Cau | DR3 | 11.8 |
| Dermatomyositis | Cau | DR3 | 3.9 |
| Scleroderma | Cau | DR5 | 5.0 |
| CREST syndrome | Cau | DR3 | 6.2 |
| Sjögren's syndrome, primary | Cau | DR3 | 3.9 |
| Sjögren's syndrome with arthritis | Cau | DR4 | 4.7 |

*Adapted from Stastny, P., et al.: Immunol. Rev. 70:113, 1983.
†Where appropriate, the range of published values is indicated.

Ir (or Is) genes that predispose an individual to disease development. Recent evidence indicating that expression of certain autoantibodies correlates with D region specificities strengthens this possibility. In this regard, previous studies have demonstrated an association between susceptibility to systemic lupus erythematosus (SLE) and D region antigens, particularly DR3.[92-95] It is therefore of interest that the presence of anti-native DNA antibodies also significantly associates with DR3 not only in patients with SLE but also in patients with other diagnoses.[96] A similar association between DR3 and anti-Ro (SS-A) antibodies has been demonstrated by Bell and Maddison.[97]

In view of evidence that distinct profiles of autoantibodies characterize various rheumatic diseases,[99] these data raise the possibility that expression of particular autoantibodies is regulated by Ir genes residing in the D region and that acquisition of such gene(s) constitutes one mechanism underlying disease susceptibility. Genetic studies of inbred autoimmune strains of mice have provided some support for this possibility. For example, at least six genes appear to be responsible for the SLE syndrome manifested by the autoimmune NZB mouse strain,[99] and some of these genes appear to govern expression of specific autoantibodies (e.g., anti-nDNA).[100] Although genes associated with specific autoantibody expression have been localized to the murine chromosome 17, linkage of these genes with the MHC (H-2) region has not been demonstrable with recombinant inbred lines.[101] It is evident that further studies are required to determine whether Ir (or Is) genes contribute to autoantibody expression in murine or human autoimmune disease.

**Theories of Ir Gene Function.** Considerable progress has been achieved in the elucidation of mechanisms underlying Ir gene regulation of immune responses. These genes have been demonstrated to regulate T lymphocyte dependent responses to a variety of antigens, including T lymphocyte dependent antibody responses, delayed hypersensitivity reactions, lymphokine production, and antigen-induced T lymphocyte proliferation. An initial dilemma concerning Ir gene function related to the cell types involved. Specifically, it was difficult to reconcile the influence of Ir genes on T lymphocyte responses with the restricted cellular distribution of Ia antigens, the apparent products of Ir genes. These antigens could be easily identified on the surfaces of B lymphocytes, macrophage/monocytes, and dendritic cells but were generally present on only a small fraction of T lymphocytes. The initial observation that T lymphocyte activation required simultaneous recognition of antigen and MHC-encoded products suggested an explanation for how Ia antigens present on antigen-presenting cells (APC) might influence subsequent T lymphocyte responses. It was clearly demonstrated that antigen-primed T lymphocytes from guinea pigs[102] and mice[103] proliferated in response to antigen presented on syngeneic but not allogeneic APC. These studies established that the presence of antigen on APC was not sufficient for T lymphocyte activation but that genetic restrictions also existed. Shevach and Rosenthal extended these observations by demonstrating that T lymphocytes from (nonresponder $\times$ responder)$F_1$ guinea pigs only responded to antigen when presented on $F_1$ or responder APC but not on nonresponder APC.[104] Evidence that Ia antigens on APC were the restricting genetic elements in these T lymphocyte responses included the demonstration that APC possessing I-A and I-E antigens were required for murine T lymphocyte proliferation[105] and that function of APC could be blocked by treatment with appropriate anti-Ia antisera.[106] Taken together with evidence that I antigens are the products of Ir genes, these observations provided strong support for the view that Ir genes are expressed on APC and that activation of T lymphocytes by antigen requires co-recognition of antigen and the Ir gene product (Ia antigen) on the APC by the responding T lymphocyte. It should be stressed that the responding T lymphocytes in these Ia-restricted responses bear the Lyl+ phenotype.[107] Similarly, cytotoxic T lymphocytes that bear the Ly2+ phenotype also exhibit MHC restrictions in their recognition of antigen on target cells, but in this case class I MHC gene products (K or D antigens) are generally the responsible restricting elements(s).[4,108,109] Thus, cytotoxic T lymphocyte recognition of antigen is blocked by appropriate anti-K or anti-D reagents but not anti-Ia antisera.

Less extensive studies in man have strongly suggested that the HLA-D region encoded antigens present on APC restrict antigen-specific human T lymphocyte responses also. Antigen-induced T lymphocyte proliferative responses have been demonstrated to require HLA-DR compatible APC.[110] Similar requirements for antigen presentation by HLA-D compatible APC for long-term proliferation of antigen-specific T lymphocytes have been observed.[111] Further evidence indicating that HLA-D-antigen-bearing APC are involved in T lymphocyte activation comes from experiments indicating that cytolytic treatment of APC with anti-Ia antisera eliminated the capacity of these cells to support antigen-specific T lymphocyte proliferation.[112] More recently, antigen-specific human T lymphocyte clones have been generated that recognize specific antigen only in the context of HLA-DR compatible APC.[113]

The precise nature of the HLA-D encoded restriction elements required for antigen recognition by T lymphocytes has not been fully elucidated. In this regard, tetanus-toxoid-induced T lymphocyte proliferative responses were prevented by treatment of APC with monoclonal anti-DR but not anti-DC antibodies.[114] Interestingly, anti-DC antibody did block generation of cytotoxic effector T lymphocytes in MLC reactions despite having no effect on antigen-specific (tetanus toxoid) T lymphocyte proliferative responses.[114] In view of evidence that both I-A and I-E antigens may serve as restriction elements for antigen-induced murine T lymphocyte responses,[75] it would be anticipated that human antigens homologous to murine I-A antigens (e.g., DC [DS] molecules) are also involved in T lymphocyte recognition for at least some antigens. Recent studies have suggested that this is indeed the case. Using antigen-primed T lymphocyte blasts, Berle and Thorsby have provided evidence that DC antigens may function as restriction elements in T lymphocyte responses to herpes simplex virus.[115] Furthermore, APC bearing both DR and DS (i.e., DC) antigens were shown to be necessary for induction of antigen-induced (*Candida albicans*) T lymphocyte proliferation whereas macrophages bearing DR antigens alone were ineffective.[116] In this system monoclonal anti-DS antibody also effectively blocked T lymphocyte proliferation in response to *Candida,* further suggesting a role for these class II molecules as restriction elements in T lymphocyte antigen recognition.[116] These observations closely parallel previously discussed observations in the mouse and suggest that: (1) Ir genes in man are expressed at the APC level; (2) class II antigens homologous to murine I-E and I-A antigens are products of Ir genes; and (3) these Ia antigens function by serving as restriction elements for T lymphocyte recognition of antigen.

While evidence for MHC-restricted antigen recognition by T lymphocytes has been well established, the mechanism(s) underlying actual antigen recognition by T cells has not been elucidated. Specifically, do T lymphocytes possess distinct receptors for Ia antigens and nominal antigen (dual receptor recognition), or does a single receptor recognize an Ia antigen-nominal antigen complex on the APC surface? Conclusive evidence for physical linkage of Ia antigens and nominal antigen has not yet been obtained. Nonetheless, the elegant somatic cell hybridization experiments of Kappler and colleagues indicate that recognition of Ia and antigen could not be dissociated, suggesting that antigen recognition was mediated either by linked receptors for Ia and antigen or by a single receptor recognizing the Ia antigen-nominal antigen complex.[117] Regardless of the precise mechanism(s) underlying antigen recognition by T lymphocytes (dual receptor recognition versus single receptor recognition), the basis of Ir-gene-controlled immune responsiveness remains unclear. Several hypotheses have been advanced; however, current evidence suggests that two theories are most plausible: (1) the determinant selection hypothesis[118,119] and (2) the clonal deletion theory.[120,121]

***The Determinant Selection Hypothesis of Ir Gene Function.*** The determinant selection theory of Ir gene function provides that antigen processing by the APC results in selective display of restricted portions of the nominal antigen to the responding T lymphocyte. Presumably, Ia antigens on the APC interact with the nominal antigen such that a specific orientation of the antigen on the cell surface of the APC ensues. Ir gene-linked unresponsiveness would presumably result either from failure of the nominal antigen to associate with APC Ia molecules or because of failure of Ia-antigen interaction to result in display of a particular antigenic determinant. Thus, this theory attributes Ir-linked unresponsiveness to inability of the APC to present the antigen (determinants) to responding cells.

Recent studies that suggest an important role for the T lymphocyte in Ir gene function have provided strong evidence against this theory. After depleting alloreactive T lymphocytes, Ishii and colleagues were able to induce T lymphocyte responses to poly($glu^{40}ala^{60}$) (GA) and poly($glu^{51}lys^{34}tyr^{15}$) (GLT) despite presentation of the antigens on nonresponder APC.[122] Clark and Shevach were able to generate antigen-specific guinea pig strain 2 T lymphocyte colonies capable of proliferating to the synthetic copolymer L-glutamic acid, L-lysine when it was presented by APC from nonresponder strain 13 guinea pigs.[123] More recently, APC from strain 2 guinea pigs (bovine insulin B chain nonresponders) were clearly shown to be capable of displaying the B chain of bovine insulin to T lymphocytes derived from strain 13 guinea pigs, which are normally responsive to the insulin B chain.[124] Taken together, these results cast doubt on the determinant selection theory and suggest that APC per se are not solely responsible for Ir gene-linked antigen unresponsiveness.

***Clonal Deletion Model of Ir Gene Function.*** According to this theory, T lymphocyte unresponsiveness to a particular antigen mediated by Ir genes is attributable to the deletion of T lymphocyte clones reactive with complexes of self Ia molecules and the specific antigen.[120] This "hole" in the T lymphocyte repertoire results from the elimination of T lymphocytes strongly reactive with self Ia molecules and/or complexes of self Ia with self antigens. Presumably, antigen unresponsiveness occurs in situations in which the Ia antigen-nominal antigen complex mimics self closely enough such that T lymphocytes that might have been capable of recognizing the complex have previously been eliminated during development because of their strong reactivity to self (Fig. 5–3). While the clonal deletion theory places the expression of Ir gene products at the APC level, responsiveness ultimately reflects the presence (or absence) of T lymphocytes capable of recognizing the complex of self Ia and nominal antigen presented on the APC surface. Thus, the Ia-negative T lymphocyte plays a critical role in Ir gene-linked antigen unresponsiveness according to this theory.

Emerging evidence that antigen presented by nonresponder haplotype APC is capable of triggering T lymphocyte responses by allogeneic responder T lymphocytes is compatible with this view. Furthermore, the observation that autologous insulin presented on allogeneic APC but not autologous APC is capable of eliciting T lymphocyte responses against autologous insulin further supports this model[124] (Table 5–4). Evidence that self antigens presented in the context of foreign (or altered) Ia molecules are capable of inducing "anti-self" responses is particularly provocative and raises the possibility that alterations of self Ia antigens could trigger responses to a variety of self antigens by virtue of activation of autologous T lymphocytes capable of reacting with altered Ia antigen–self antigen complexes present on APC.

In summary, strong evidence suggests that Ir gene expression occurs at the APC level. Ir gene-linked antigen responsiveness does not appear to be solely attributable to the APC, since nonresponder APC are capable of presenting the relevant antigen to allogeneic T lymphocytes. Considerable evidence indicates that T lymphocytes must recognize both Ia antigen and nominal antigen on the APC (either separately or as a complex) in order to respond to the particular antigen. The hypothesis that Ir gene-linked unresponsiveness reflects the deletion of T lymphocytes capable of reacting with a particular Ia antigen–nominal antigen complex is compatible with the available data, but further studies to test this model are clearly required.

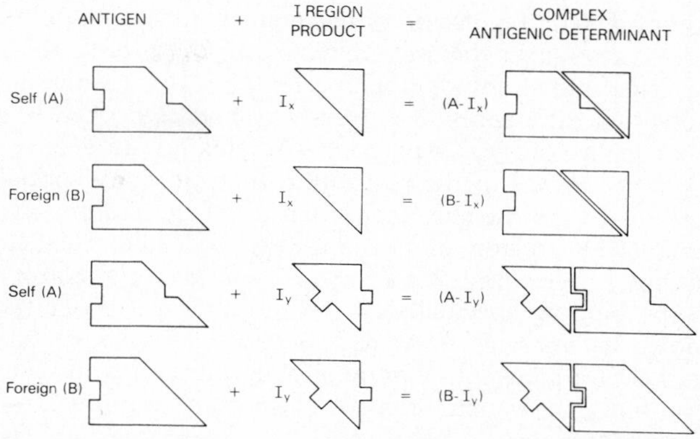


**Figure 5–3.** Schematic diagram of the type of complex antigenic determinants that might be formed as a result of interaction of a self antigen (A) or foreign antigen (B) with an I region product of the haplotype x(Ix) or y(Iy). The interaction of the self antigen A or foreign antigen B with the Ix product results in complex antigenic determinants, which have identical shape. In this case, the deletion of T cells reactive with the self-Ix complex would be associated with unresponsiveness to the foreign antigen B. In contrast, interaction of self antigen A and foreign antigen B with the Iy product leads to the formation of complexes with differing shapes. In this case, deletion of T cells reactive with the A-Iy complex would not be associated with lack of response to B-Iy. (From Schwartz, R.H.: Scand. J. Immunol. 7:3, 1978.)

## IMMUNOGLOBULIN GENES

### Introduction

A fundamental characteristic of the vertebrate immune system is the capacity for discriminant recognition of the incredible array of different molecules (antigens) routinely encountered in the environment by the host. It is therefore not surprising that this requirement for diverse (but specific) immune recognition is reflected at the B lymphocyte level by the capacity of an individual to elaborate an estimated $10^6$ to $10^8$ different antibody molecules. Genes responsible for the generation of antibody diversity clearly must be considered in a discus-

**Table 5–4.** Strain 13 T Lymphocyte Colonies Recognize a Determinant Present on the Autologous Guinea Pig Insulin B Chain (5–16) Peptide Sequence Presented by Strain 2 Accessory Cells*

| T Lymphocyte Stimulation By | ($^3$H)TdR Incorporation by Colony *I-30-D4* | *I-32-F5* | *I-32-D8* | *I-32-D9* |
|---|---|---|---|---|
| Strain 13 accessory cells alone (peritoneal exudate cells) | 628 | 330 | 340 | 573 |
| Strain 13 accessory cells + guinea pig insulin B chain (5–16) | 228 | 550 | 531 | 442 |
| Strain 2 accessory cells alone | 1,496 | 1,012 | 644 | 638 |
| Strain 2 accessory cells + guinea pig insulin B chain (5–16) | 16,546 | 6,242 | 4,115 | 4,342 |

*Adapted from Dos Reis, G.A., and Shevach, E.M.: J. Exp. Med. 157:1287, 1983, by copyright permission of the Rockefeller University Press.

sion of genetic regulation of immune responses. An obvious question in this regard relates to the precise role that inherited immunoglobulin genes play in determining individual differences in antibody responses evoked by a particular antigen. Approaches to this question have taken advantage of the realization that antibody specificity is due to the chemical structure of the binding or variable (V) region of the antibody molecule. Hence, antibody molecules bear antigenic determinants related to the binding specificity of the molecules, a property known as *idiotypy.* Idiotypes therefore serve as useful markers for analyzing immunoglobulin diversity and for examining the genetic control of specific immunoglobulin expression.

In this section we briefly discuss the genetic mechanisms underlying expression of the antibody repertoire (see Chapter 2 for additional details) and consider the evidence that inherited immunoglobulin genes influence specific immune responses. It should be stressed that specific recognition structures are also clearly expressed at the T lymphocyte level and that genes governing expression of these T lymphocyte recognition structures appear to be distinct from immunoglobulin heavy chain variable region ($V_H$) genes. Unfortunately these genes have yet to be identified, and, therefore, the genetic mechanisms contributing to establishment of the T lymphocyte repertoire are not yet clear.

## Organization of Immunoglobulin Genes

The structure of the immunoglobulin protein provided important clues with regard to genetic mechanisms underlying the generation of antibody diversity. Specifically, both heavy (H) and light (L) chains possessed constant region domains that were identical for all antibody molecules of the same isotype, subclass, and light chain type present in the same individual. Moreover, H and L chains also contained a variable region domain that varied among different antibody molecules and therefore accounted for the tremendous diversity of immunoglobulins encountered in each individual. These properties led Dreyer and Bennett[125] to postulate that multiple genes contributed to the expression of variable region diversity whereas only single genes were necessary for the expression of constant regions of light chains ($C_L$) or of each heavy chain isotype ($C_H$). This radical "two gene–one polypeptide" hypothesis predicted that joining between a constant region gene ($C_L$ or $C_H$) and one of many available variable region genes ($V_H$ or $V_L$) accounted for the peculiar structural features of the immunoglobulin molecule. Subsequent studies in several laboratories have confirmed and amplified this hypothesis such that the tremendous diversity of the B lymphocyte repertoire is now understandable at a molecular level.

**Heavy Chain Genes.** Located on chromosome 14 in humans,[126] immunoglobulin heavy (H) chain genes in the germ line consist of four linked multigene families arranged sequentially in the following order on the chromosome (5′end → 3′end): variable ($V_H$), diversity (D), joining ($J_H$) and constant ($C_H$) gene segments (Fig. 5–4). While the precise number of $V_H$ gene segments remains to be elucidated, there appear to be several groups of $V_H$ genes, with the members of each group exhibiting homologous sequences. Although presumably closely related, the members of each $V_H$ group do not necessarily encode for the same antigen-binding specificity. This has been demonstrated in the antiphosphorylcholine antibody system in the mouse in which only one of the four members of the so-called T15 group of $V_H$ genes is used for antiphosphorylcholine antibody.[127] Multiple D gene segments are located in clusters close to the 5′ end of $J_H$ genes. Although the precise location of these gene segments is under investigation, a germ line D gene segment has been identified 750 nucleotide base pairs (bp) to the 5′ end of the initial mouse $J_H$ segment.[128] D region gene segments vary in both base sequence and length (18 to 41 bp in the mouse).[129,130] Situated approximately 8 kilobases (kb) to the 5′ side of $C\mu$, the $J_H$ group of genes in humans consists of a 3.2 kb nucleotide segment that contains six complete $J_H$ genes and three incomplete (or pseudo) $J_H$ genes.[131] The last group of H genes are the $C_H$ genes, which determine the class of the H-chain polypeptide. Five classes of H chain ($\alpha$, $\delta$, $\epsilon$, $\gamma$, and $\mu$), four $\gamma$ subclasses ($\gamma_1$, $\gamma_2$, $\gamma_3$, and $\gamma_4$), and two $\alpha$ subclasses ($\alpha_1$ and $\alpha_2$) occur in humans. The

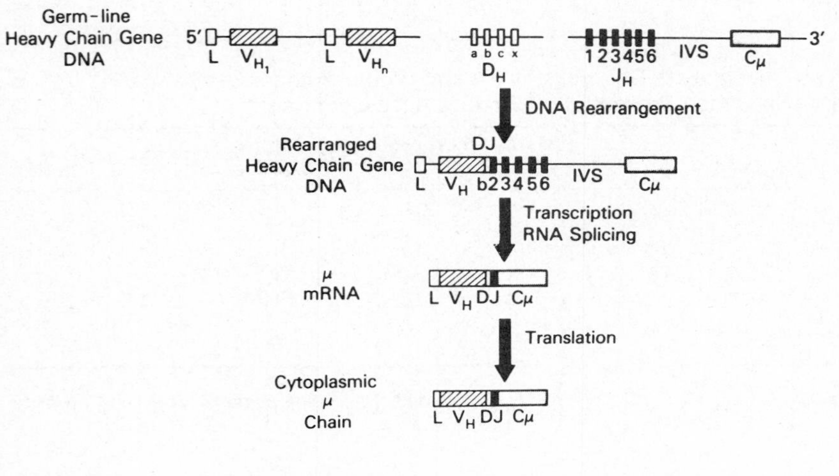


**Figure 5–4.** A schematic diagram of the germ-line organization and subsequent assembly of the human immunolglobulin heavy chain gene. The immunoglobulin heavy chain genes consist of multiple $V_H$ regions, each preceded by its own leader (L) sequence; six functional $J_H$ segments; families of D segments; and one constant $C\mu$ gene per chromosome. Initially, a single $V_H$, D, $J_H$ region must be successfully recombined at the DNA level to form an active gene. The remaining intervening sequence (IVS) is then removed at the RNA level by splicing, thereby producing a complete $\mu$-mRNA, which is subsequently translated to a complete $\mu$ heavy chain. (From Korsmeyer, S.J., et al.: J. Clin. Invest. 71:301, 1983, by copyright permission of The American Society for Clinical Investigation.)

order of these $C_H$ genes has recently been determined in man to be 5′end→$J_H$→8kb→ Cμ→5kb→ Cδ→ Cγ3→26kb→ Cγ1→19kb→ pseudoCε→13kb→ Cα1→ Cγ2→18kb→ Cγ4→23kb→ Cε→10kb→ Cα2→3′ end.[132] This arrangement of human $C_H$ genes suggests a duplication of a γ-γ-ε-α multigene segment.[132]

**Light Chain Genes.** Genes for human κ and λ light (L) chains are located on chromosomes 2 and 22, respectively.[132] L chain genes consist of three multigene families ($V_L$, $J_L$, and $C_L$). In the case of κ chain genes, 15 to 20 Vκ genes have been estimated to be present in the human germ line, situated in a cluster 5′ to the Jκ gene family.[134] The human Jκ gene family consists of five complete Jκ genes located in a cluster approximately 2.5 kb 5′ to the single Cκ gene.[135] Lambda chain genes are arranged differently then κ chain genes. The precise number of Vλ genes has not been determined, but several are assumed to exist.[136] In contrast to the single Cκ gene in man, at least six human Cλ genes have been identified.[137] As demonstrated in the mouse, each human Cλ gene is assumed to be associated with its own Jλ segment.[138,139]

**Assembly of Variable Region Gene Segments—the Generation of Variable Region Diversity.** The complete variable region of the immunoglobulin H polypeptide chain is encoded by a DNA segment created by the recombinational joining of a $V_H$, D, and $J_H$ gene with associated deletion of the DNA previously separating these segments in the germ line gene configuration (Fig. 5–4). In the case of L chains, a $V_L$ and a $J_L$ gene segment are joined. Investigation of DNA rearrangement mechanisms underlying V-(D)-J joining have yielded important insights into the generation of immunoglobulin variable region diversity. At least five mechanisms contribute to the generation of antibody diversity:[136] (1) the large number of germ line $V_H$ and $V_L$ genes; (2) random joining of V, (D), and J genes; (3) imprecisions (flexibility) in the precise site of recombination of these gene segments; (4) somatic mutations arising in V genes; and (5) random association of H and L chains. Further studies are required to delineate the precise relative contributions of each of these mechanisms to variable region diversity; however, theoretical calculations of the possibilities arising from these processes indicate that one need not invoke additional explanations.

It should be noted that the occurrence of V-(D)-J joining at the pre-B lymphocyte level implies that the generation of antibody diversity largely occurs independent of antigen stimulation, since these immature cells do not exhibit surface Ig. On the other hand, observations that somatic mutation is frequently expressed in the variable regions (H or L) of IgA or IgG molecules, but not IgM molecules, raises the possibility that isotype switching may trigger somatic mutational processes.[140,141] A role for antigen in influencing somatic mutation (perhaps via triggering B lymphocyte proliferation and differentiation) cannot be excluded at this time.

**Genetic Basis of Heavy Chain "Switching"—the Generation of Isotype Diversity.** The formation of a particular $V_H$-D-$J_H$ combination at the pre-B lymphocyte level is necessary before the expression of μ heavy chains in the cytoplasm of the cell.[142,143] This is accomplished by the transcription of an RNA segment containing the $V_HDJ_H$ segment and the Cμ gene followed by deletion of the intervening RNA (RNA splicing) resulting in μ mRNA (Fig. 5–4). The $V_HDJ_H$ may be subsequently expressed in combination with a different $C_H$ gene, a process referred to as "switching."

Pre-B lymphocytes, the earliest recognizable stage of B lymphocyte differentiation, are characterized by the expression of cytoplasmic μ heavy chains without light chains. At the DNA level, these cells exhibit a productive arrangement of heavy chain gene segments (V-D-J joining). Combination of this V-D-J segment with Cμ at the mRNA level as a result of RNA splicing events results in a μ polypeptide H chain being translated (Figs. 5–4 and 5–5). It is now clear that subsequent differentiation of the pre-B cell is associated with an orderly sequence of immunoglobulin L chain rearrangements.[143,145] Initially a rearrangement of κ genes occurs on one chromosome 2, with resultant joining of a $V_κ$ and $J_κ$ gene and subsequent formation of a κ chain mRNA with synthesis of intact κ chains. However, the flexibility or imprecision of V-J joining events leads to frequent nonproductive arrangements (null genes), which are excluded from expression and which may actually be deleted at the DNA level (Fig. 5–6). In this case, rearrangement of κ chain genes on the other chromosome 2 occurs. Should this also prove to be ineffective, rearrangements of λ chain genes are then attempted on one chromosome 22, followed by DNA rearrangements on the other chromosome 22 if the first try also proves unproductive. This model of B lymphocyte differentiation in which H chain rearrangements are followed by κ gene rearrangements and then, if necessary, by λ gene recombinations has been observed in both transformed and normal human B lymphocytes.[144,145]

In addition to intact surface IgM molecules, B lymphocytes may also express other surface immunoglobulins. At least two mechanisms for the expression of

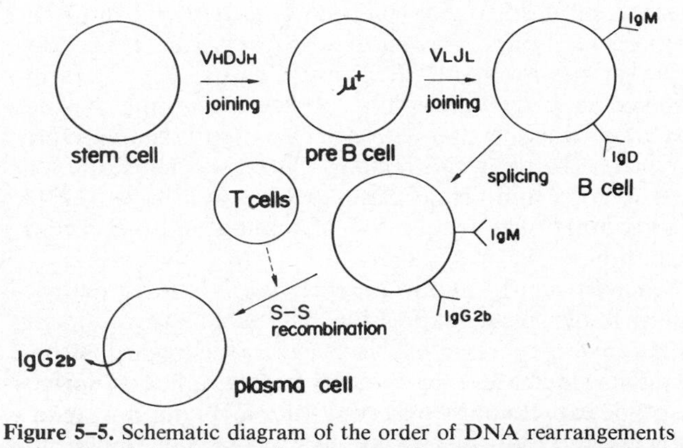


**Figure 5–5.** Schematic diagram of the order of DNA rearrangements during B cell development from the pre-B to the plasma cell level. (Reproduced, with permission, from the Annual Review of Immunology, Volume 1. ©1983 by Annual Reviews Inc.)

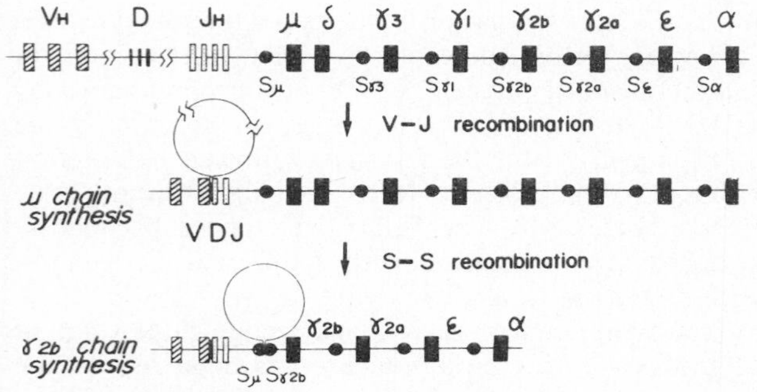


**Figure 5–6.** Diagram of the two types of DNA rearrangements that occur in the H chain gene locus. In V-J recombination, $V_H$, D, and $J_H$ segments are joined together at the DNA level and the intervening sequence between the active $V_HDJ_H$ gene and the Cμ gene is removed at the RNA level by splicing. In S-S recombination, DNA between two switch (S) sites is deleted, with subsequent movement of the Cγ2b gene adjacent to the $V_HDJ_H$ complex. (From Honjo, T., et al.: Immunol. Rev. 59:33, 1981.)

immunoglobulin isotypes other than μ have been delineated. In the case of lymphocytes expressing both IgM and IgD on the surface, Cμ and Cδ genes appear not to be rearranged, suggesting that RNA splicing mechanisms account for the dual expression of IgM and IgD.[146,147] Presumably, a large RNA transcript containing a V-D-J sequence in addition to Cμ and Cδ would be variably spliced in such a way that mRNAs for both μ and δ could be produced. A similar mechanism has been proposed to account for lymphocytes co-expressing IgM and IgE in the absence of demonstrable $C_H$ gene rearrangements.[148] On the basis of such observations it has been postulated that class switching may be initially accomplished by RNA splicing mechanisms before $C_H$ gene rearrangements occur.[148,136] Direct evidence for the existence of the large RNA transcripts predicted by this theory has not yet been obtained.

The second mechanism responsible for isotype switching involves rearrangement of $C_H$ genes at the DNA level. Sequencing studies of the $C_H$ genes have revealed the presence of long stretches of homologous nucleotide sequences (S regions), which are repeated in tandem and located to the 5′ of each $C_H$ gene.[149-152] Interestingly, the length of the S region preceding each $C_H$ gene in the mouse varies and correlates with the serum concentration of the isotype.[150] Rearrangement of $C_H$ genes involved in isotype switching observed in some plasmacytomas is associated with deletion of intervening DNA sequence between S-S regions (Fig. 5–7). Thus, the formation of a complete H chain involves at least two DNA recombinational events: V-D-J joining and S-S recombination.

A particularly important question relates to the regulation of isotype expression, i.e., what are the forces that govern expression of isotype? In this regard, strong evidence indicates that diversity of B lymphocyte surface isotype expression is observed during B lymphocyte ontogeny and that this isotype switching occurs independently of antigen and T lymphocyte influence.[153] Indeed, heavy chain switching has been observed at the pre-B lymphocyte level preceding the expression of surface Ig.[154] On the other hand, additional evidence suggests that isotype diversity can be influenced by T lymphocytes. Cloned T lymphocyte lines obtained from murine Peyer's patches, a rich source of IgA-committed B lymphocytes,[155] have been demonstrated to induce isotype switching in B lymphocytes from surface IgM+ to surface IgA+ cells. Moreover, soluble factors released by T lymphocyte hybridomas have been shown to influence the subclass of IgG produced by lipopolysaccharide (LPS)-stimulated B lymphocytes.[157] Pure and coworkers have been able to separate two soluble B lymphocyte differentiation factors (BCDF): a high molecular weight BCDFμ (MW 30,000 to 60,000), which

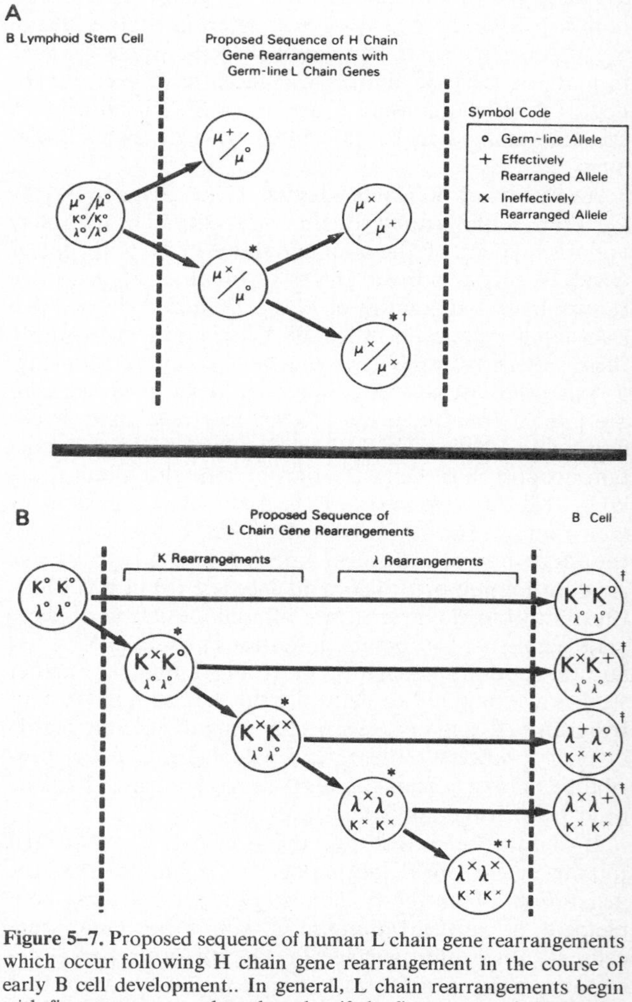


**Figure 5–7.** Proposed sequence of human L chain gene rearrangements which occur following H chain gene rearrangement in the course of early B cell development.. In general, L chain rearrangements begin with first one κ gene, then the other if the first attempt is ineffective (x). If both κ gene rearrangement attempts are unsuccessful, then λ rearrangements would follow. Cells with effectively rearranged κ or λ genes could become mature B cells (‡) if prior H chain rearrangements were successful. Cells with ineffectively rearranged L chain genes (*) would lack L chain production and therefore be unable to synthesize intact immunoglobulin molecules. Theoretically, a population of B cells with totally ineffective κ and λ gene rearrangements (†) could exist. (From Korsmeyer, S.J., et al.: J. Clin. Invest. 71:301, 1983, by copyright permission of The American Society for Clinical Investigation.)

preferentially induces IgM secretion by B cells, and a smaller BCDFγ (MW < 20,000), which induces predominant IgG1 secretion in LPS-stimulated B lymphocytes.[158] Further evidence for T lymphocyte regulation 41of isotype expression has come from studies in mice indicating that T lymphocytes are capable of enhancing IgG2 responses to the type 2 T-independent antigens TNP-Ficoll and TNP-Levan.[159] Certainly these data strongly suggest a role for T lymphocytes in regulation of the isotype profile of specific immune responses. Whether this is accomplished by means of triggering of switching events or through selective amplification of already committed ("preswitched") B lymphocytes has not been unequivocally established.

**The T Lymphocyte Antigen Receptor and Immunoglobulin Heavy Chain Genes.** The structural basis for T lymphocyte antigen specificity remains uncertain. Observations that anti-idiotypic and anti-$V_H$ framework reagents were capable of interfering with T lymphocyte function and binding to soluble antigen by specific T lymphocyte factors suggested that $V_H$ genes encoded for at least a portion of the T lymphocyte antigen receptor.[160-162] Linkage of these serologically recognized T lymphocyte receptor determinants to immunoglobulin H chain genes supported this view.[163-166] Moreover, the identification of T lymphocyte surface alloantigens and mapping of the responsible genes to murine chromosome 12 between the $C_H$ gene cluster and the prealbumin gene (Pre-1)[167-169] raised the possibility that these structures represented the constant region portion of the T lymphocyte antigen receptor. Evidence for this association was obtained from studies in which anti-T lymphocyte allotype reagents blocked the binding of idiotypic-specific suppressor T lymphocytes to idiotype-bearing Ig.[169] More recently Tokuhisa and colleagues have successfuly raised monoclonal antibodies that recognize constant region determinants present on both antigen-specific helper and suppressor T lymphocyte factors.[170] Taken together, these observations suggest that the T lymphocyte antigen receptor consists of a constant region encoded by $C_H$-linked genes and an antigen-binding variable region encoded by $V_H$-like genes. Efforts to directly demonstrate a role for $V_H$ genes in determining the variable region portion of the T lymphocyte receptor, however, have been unsuccessful. Indeed, Kronenberg and colleagues were unable to find evidence of RNA transcripts in three T lymphocyte hybridomas (one helper; two suppressor) that contained $V_H$ gene sequences.[171] Analysis of B and T lymphocytes sharing the same antigen-binding specificity and cell surface idiotypic determinants revealed that the T lymphocytes did not transcribe the same $V_H$ gene segment as the B lymphocytes.[172] The evidence indicates therefore that the antigen-binding variable region of the T lymphocyte receptor is encoded by V genes distinct from the $V_H$ genes.

**Relationship of Immunoglobulin Genes to Immune Response Characteristics.** Since Ig genes determine the potential for variable region diversity expressed in antibody molecules, it is not surprising that these genes have been demonstrated to control specific immune responses. Two Ig gene markers have been primarily utilized to investigate the relationship between immune responses and inherited Ig genes: *allotypes* and *idiotypes.*

Immunoglobulin allotypes are genetic variants of immunoglobulins and are inherited by simple Mendelian genetics. These variants reflect the presence of alleles for $C_H$ and $C_L$ genes. In man, alleles for $V_H$ or $V_L$ genes have not been clearly demonstrated (although this does occur in the rabbit). Allotypic differences resulting from slight amino acid sequence differences in the constant regions of H or L chains can be recognized by serologic reagents. Utilizing this approach, allotypes for κ light chains and for IgG and IgA heavy chains have been identified in man (Table 5–5). These allotype-specific reagents have provided useful tools for analyzing the relationship between immune response characteristics and inherited Ig genes.

While allotypes reflect allelic heterogeneity of $C_H$ and $C_L$ genes, idiotypes are encoded by V region genes. Idiotypes can be defined as a group of determinants (idiotopes) expressed in the V region of an antibody or in the V regions of antibodies with similar specificity.[173,174] Serologic reagents reactive with particular idiotypes (anti-idiotypes) can be prepared and have been quite helpful in examining genetic mechanisms underlying antibody diversity. Idiotypes shared by antibodies (or T lymphocyte receptors) possessing similar antigen-binding specificity are referred to as crossreactive idiotypes. The structural basis of idiotype expression is under intense investigation. Current evidence indicates that im-

**Table 5–5.** Human Immunoglobulin Allotypes*

| Class and Subclass or Light Chain Type | Allotype (Numerical Designation) | Location of Determinant |
|---|---|---|
| IgG1 | G1m (1) | $C_H3$ |
| | (2) | $C_H3$ |
| | (3) | $C_H1$ |
| | (17) | $C_H1$ |
| IgG2 | G2m (23) | $C_H2$ |
| IgG3 | G3m (11) | $C_H3$ |
| | (5) | $C_H2$ |
| | (13) | $C_H3$ |
| | (14) | $C_H2$ |
| | (10) | $C_H3$ |
| | (6) | |
| | (24) | |
| | (21) | |
| | (15) | |
| | (16) | |
| | (26) | |
| | (27) | |
| IgA2 | A2m (1) | |
| | A2m (2) | |
| κ | Km (1) | |
| | (2) | |
| | (3) | |

*Adapted from WHO Committee Report: J. Immunogenet. 3:357, 1976.

munoglobulin idiotypes generally reflect amino acid sequences of immunoglobulin complementarity-determining regions (CDR). Thus, sequences determined by V, D, and J genes appear to be responsible for the expression of idiotypic determinants in immunoglobulin molecules.

It has become evident that the expression of a particular idiotype is under genetic control. This has been clearly shown in mice responding to $\alpha$(1-3) dextran (DEX), in which the expression of a dominant idiotype (IdX) on anti-DEX antibodies correlates with the inherited allotype of the strain.[175,176] Mice bearing the Igh-$C^a$ allotype are high IdX responders to DEX whereas mice of the Igh-$C^b$ allotype do not produce detectible concentrations of IdX in response to DEX. Molecular analysis of specific immune responses dominated by a particular IdX has revealed that these responses are associated with inheritance of a single (or few) relevant $V_H$ and $V_L$ genes in the germ line. Examples of this phenomenon include the responses to arsonate,[177] phosphorylcholine,[178,179] and (4-hydroxy-3-nitrophenyl) acetyl groups (NP).[180,181] Thus, the responses to these particular antigens appear to be restricted because of the limited number of relevant or expressible V genes available in the germ line. A critical question then relates to whether the expressed idiotype repertoire is entirely dependent upon the nature of inherited V genes or whether other genetically determined influences are operative.

Linkage of IdX responses with particular IgH genes (allotypes) has been interpreted as evidence for the former hypothesis. In this regard, recent studies in normal mice and T lymphocyte deficient nude mice have shown linkage between allotype background and the frequency of $IdX^+$ precursor B lymphocytes.[182] These data appear to support the view that selection and maintenance of the B lymphocyte V region repertoire is encoded by germ line genes and that its expression is independent of T lymphocytes. However, several investigators have succeeded in inducing expression of IdX-bearing antibodies of desired antigenic specificites in mice of "nonresponder" allotypes by administration of anti-idiotypic antibodies.[183-186] These results suggest that regulatory influences contribute to the expression of particular idiotypes, and, indeed, evidence for suppressor T cell participation in idiotype expression is convincing in some systems.[187,184] A role for helper T lymphocytes in governing idiotype expression is also suggested by other studies.[188,186,189] Presumably these regulatory influences are heavily dependent upon idiotype–anti-idiotype interactions, the so-called "network theory" of immune regulation initially proposed by Jerne.[190] The precise role of $V_H$ genes and T lymphocyte V genes in these complementary interactions is not clear.

Taken together, these results indicate that the expressed V region repertoire is restricted by the inherited germ line V gene repertoire. In addition, regulatory influences (T lymphocyte and ?other) contribute to the pattern of immunoglobulin V region determinants (idiotypes) expressed in response to a particular antigen. The well-documented linkage of allotype background with idiotype expression could reflect an association of allotype with a particular set of germ line V region genes and/or linkage of IgH genes with regulatory genes that restrict the pattern of V gene expression (through T lymphocytes or other mechanisms).

**Immunoglobulin Genes and Disease Susceptibility.** Evidence for an association between immunoglobulin genes (allotype) and responsiveness to specific antigens in man has been obtained for some antigens, including bacterial flagellin[191,192] and various bacterial polysaccharides.[193,194] That certain diseases are also associated with inheritance patterns of immunoglobulin genes is not surprising in view of the apparent relationship of these genes to immune response characteristics of the individual. These associations have most frequently been established through an analysis of immunoglobulin allotype patterns. Associations of particular Gm allotypes with several diseases have been recently identified, including myasthenia gravis,[195] chronic active hepatitis,[196] Grave's disease,[195,197] SLE[195,198] multiple sclerosis,[199] and Hashimoto's thyroiditis.[195] In each of these diseases it appears that both MHC-linked and immunoglobulin-linked genes contribute to disease susceptibility. The precise mechanisms underlying apparent dual gene control of disease susceptibility remain uncertain. Recent evidence that MHC-linked genes are capable of influencing idiotypic interactions suggests at least one mechanism underlying interaction between MHC-linked and Ig-linked genes.[200]

## CONCLUSIONS

Immune responses to specific antigens are controlled by several distinct genetic loci. Moreover, genes residing in (or near) these loci also appear to influence susceptibility to a variety of diseases in which immune mechanisms have been implicated. Presumably, at least some of these putative disease susceptibility genes function through regulation of specific immune responses critical to expression of the disease in question. Elucidation of mechanisms underlying gene regulation of immune response characteristics should furnish important insights into pathogenetic mechanisms operative in these diseases.

Two major gene groups, MHC and Ig, have been clearly implicated in the regulation of specific immune responsiveness. The available evidence suggests that MHC genes operate at the level of antigen recognition by T lymphocytes. Thus, MHC-linked unresponsiveness to a particular antigen appears to result from the inability of T lymphocytes to recognize the antigen presented in the context of self MHC antigens. In some cases, suppressor T lymphocytes, which contribute to the lack of antigen responsiveness, may be preferentially induced. Evidence that modification of self MHC antigens may promote development of enhanced reactivity to self antigens is provocative and clearly warrants further investigation as a plausible mechanism underlying susceptibility to autoimmune conditions. Moreover, reversal of antigen unresponsive states by alteration of relevant self MHC antigens may prove to be feasible.

The role(s) of Ig genes in controlling specific immune responses appears to be complex. The pattern of inherited immunoglobulin V region genes restricts the potential repertoire of the antibody response; however, closely linked genes also appear to regulate the pattern of immunoglobulin V region products ultimately expressed. The precise identity of these putative regulatory genes is unclear but there is reason to suspect that T lymphocyte V genes, which appear to be distinct from B lymphocyte $V_H$ genes, are likely to be involved. Indeed, immunoregulatory T lymphocyte circuits that modulate B lymphocyte function have been demonstrated to be dependent upon genes closely linked to IgH genes for their function. The availability of techniques for cloning human T lymphocytes of desired specificity should provide opportunities for in vivo manipulation of immune responses. The implications with regard to interruption of potentially harmful immune responses (e.g., autoimmune phenomena) are clear.

## References


1. Vitetta, E.S., and Capra, J.D.: The protein products of the murine 17th chromosome. Genetics and structure. Adv. Immunol. 26:147, 1978.
2. Klein, J., Figueroa, F., and Nagy, Z.A.: Genetics of the major histocompatibility complex: The final act. Ann. Rev. Immunol. 1:119, 1983.
3. Ploegh, H.L., Orr, H.T., and Strominger, J.L.: Major histocompatibility antigens: The human (HLA-A,-B,-C) and murine (H-2K, H-2D) class I molecules. Cell 24:287, 1981.
4. Zinkernagel, R.M., and Doherty, P.C.: Immunological surveillance against altered self components by sensitized T lymphocytes in lymphocytic choriomeningitis. Nature 251:547, 1974.
5. Klein, J.: Biology of the Mouse Histocompatibility-2 Complex. New York, Springer, 1975.
6. Silver, J., Walker, L.E., Reisfield, R.A., Pellegrino, M.A., and Ferrone, S.: Structural studies of murine I-E and human DR antigens. Mol. Immunol. 16:37, 1979.
7. Ferrone, S., Allison, J.P., and Pellegrino, M.A.: Human DR (Ia-like) antigens: Biological and molecular profile. Contemp. Top. Mol. Immunol. 7:239, 1978.
8. Tosi, R., Tanigaki, N., Centis, G., Ferrara, D.B., and Pressman, D.: Immunological dissection of human Ia molecules. J. Exp. Med. 148:1592, 1978.
9. Charron, D.J., and McDevitt, H.O.: Characterization of HLA-D region antigens by two-dimensional gel electrophoresis. J. Exp. Med. 152:18s, 1980.
10. Shackelford, D.A., and Strominger, J.L.: Demonstration of structural polymorphism among HLA-DR light chains by two-dimensional gel electrophoresis. J. Exp. Med. 151:144, 1980.
11. Nagy, Z., Baxevanis, C., Ishii, N., and Klein, J.: Ia antigens as restriction molecules in Ir-gene controlled T cell proliferation. Immunol. Rev. 60:59, 1981.
12. McDevitt, H.O., and Benacerraf, B.: Genetic control of specific immune response. Adv. Immunol. 11:31, 1969.
13. Shreffler, D., David, C., Cullen, S., Frelinger, J., and Niederhuber, J.: Serological and functional evidence for further subdivision of the I regions of the H-2 gene complex. Cold Spring Harbor Symp. Quant. Biol. 41:477, 1976.
14. Klein, J., Juretic, A., Baxevanis, C.N., and Nagy, Z.A.: The traditional and the new version of the mouse H-2 complex. Nature 291:455, 1981.
15. Dorf, M.E.: The Role of the Major Histocompatibility Complex in Immunobiology. New York, Garland Publishing, 1980.
16. Shreffler, D.C., and David, C.S.: The H-2 major histocompatibility complex and the I immune response region. Genetic variation, function and organization. Adv. Immunol. 20:125, 1975.
17. Silver, J.: Genetic and structural organization of murine Ia and human DR antigens. CRC Crit. Rev. Immunol. 2:225, 1981.
18. Murphy, D.B., Herzenberg, L.A., Okumura, K., and McDevitt, H.O.: A new I subregion (I-J) marked by a locus (Ia-4) controlling surface determinants on suppressor lymphocytes. J. Exp. Med. 144:699, 1976.
19. Tada, T., Taniguchi, M., and David, C.S.: Properties of the antigen specific suppressive T cell factor in the regulation of antibody response in the mouse. IV. Special subregion assignment of the gene(s) that code for the suppressive T cell factor in the H-2 histocompatibility complex. J. Exp. Med. 144:713, 1976.
20. Taniguchi, M., Tokuhisa, T., Kanno, M., Yaoita, Y., Shimizu, A., and Honjo, T.: Reconstitution of antigen-specific suppressor activity with translation products of mRNA. Nature 298:172, 1982.
21. Krupen, K., Araneo, B.A., and Brink, L.: Purification and characterization of a monoclonal T cell suppressor factor specific for poly(L-Glu[60]L-Ala[30]L-Tyr[10]). Proc. Natl. Acad. Sci. USA 79:1254, 1982.
22. Wieder, K.J., Araneo, B.A., Kapp, J.A., and Webb, D.R.: Cell-free translation of a biological active, antigen-specific suppressor T cell factor. Proc. Natl. Acad. Sci. USA 79:3599, 1982.
23. Steinmetz, M., Minard, K., Horvath, S., McNicholas, J., Frelinger, J., Wake, C., Long, E., Mach, B., and Hood, L.: A molecular map of the immune response region from the major histocompatibility complex of the mouse. Nature 300:35, 1982.
24. McKenzie, I.F.C., and Potter, T.: Murine lymphocyte surface antigens. Adv. Immunol. 27:179, 1979.
25. Allison, J.P., Walker, L.E., Russell, W.A., Pellegrino, M.A., Ferrone, S., Reisfield, R.A., Frelinger, J.A., and Silver, J.: Murine Ia and DR antigens. Homology of amino terminal sequences. Proc. Natl. Acad. Sci. USA 75:3953, 1978.
26. Cullen, S.E., Freed, J.H., and Nathenson, S.G.: Structural and serological properties of murine Ia alloantigens. Transplant. Rev. 30:236, 1976.
27. Cullen, S.E., Kindle, C.S., and Littman, D.R.: Structural comparison of murine Ia antigens determined by the I-A and I-E subregions. J. Immunol. 122:855, 1979.
28. Jones, P., Murphy, D., Hewgill, D., and McDevitt, H.O.: Detection of a common polypeptide chain in I-A and I-E subregion immunoprecipitates. Immunochemistry 16:51, 1978.
29. Cecka, J., McMillon, M., Murphy, D., McDevitt, H.O., and Hood, L.: Partial N-terminal amino acid sequence analyses and comparative tryptic peptide maps of murine Ia molecules encoded by the I-A subregion. Eur. J. Immunol. 9:955, 1979.
30. Cook, R.G., Siegelman, M.H., Capra, J.D., Uhr, J.W., and Vitetta, E.S.: Structural studies on the murine Ia alloantigens. IV. $NH_2$-terminal sequence analysis of allelic products of the I-A and E/C subregions. J. Immunol. 122:2232, 1979.
31. Uhr, J.W., Capra, J.D., Vitetta, E.S. and Cook, R.G.: Organization of the immune response genes. Science 206:292, 1979.
32. Freed, J.H., David, C.S., Shreffler, D.C., and Nathenson, S.G.: Structural studies of the protein portion of the H-2-linked Ia glycoprotein antigens of the mouse. Tryptic peptide comparison of products from the I-A and I-C subregions of B10.HTT. J. Immunol. 121:91, 1978.
33. Klein, J., and Figueroa, F.: Polymorphism of the mouse H-2 loci. Immunol. Rev. 60:23, 1981.
34. Silver, J., and Russell, W.A.: Genetic mapping of the component chains of Ia molecules. Immunogenetics 8:339, 1979.
35. Cook, R.G., Vitetta, E.S., Uhr, J.W., and Capra, J.D.: Structural studies on the murine Ia alloantigens. V. Evidence that the structural gene for the E/C $\beta$ polypeptide is encoded within the I-A subregion. J. Exp. Med. 149:981, 1979.
36. Silver, J.: Transgene complementation of I-E subregion antigens. J. Immunol. 123:1423, 1979.
37. Benoist, C.O., Mathis, D.J., Kanter, M.R., Williams, V.E., and McDevitt, H.O.: The murine Ia $\alpha$ chains, E$\alpha$ and A$\alpha$, show a surprising degree of sequence homology. Proc. Natl. Acad. Sci. USA 80:534, 1983.
38. Mathis, D.J., Benoist, C.O., Williams, V.E., Kanter, M.R., and McDevitt, H.O.: The murine E$\alpha$ immune response gene. Cell 32:745, 1983.
39. Lee, J., Trowsdale, J., Travers, P., Carey, J., Grosveld, F., Jenkins, J., and Bodmer, W.: Sequence of an HLA-DR $\alpha$ chain cDNA clone and intron-exon organization of the corresponding gene. Nature 299:750, 1982.
40. Korman, A., Auffray, C., Schamboeck, A., and Strominger, J.: The amino acid sequence and gene organization of the heavy chain of the HLA-DR antigens. Homology to immunoglobulins. Proc. Natl. Acad. Sci. USA 79:6013, 1982.
41. Das, H., Lawrance, S., and Weissman, S.: The structure and nucleotide sequence of the heavy chain gene of HLA-DR. Proc. Natl. Acad. Sci. USA, in press.
42. Charron, D.J., and McDevitt, H.O.: Analysis of HLA-D region-associated molecules with monoclonal antibody. Proc. Natl. Acad. Sci. USA 76:6567, 1979.
43. Corte, G., Damiani, G., Calabi, F., Fabbi, M., and Bargellesi, A.: Analysis of HLA-DR polymorphism by two-dimensional peptide mapping. Proc. Natl. Acad. Sci. USA 78:534, 1981.
44. Shaw, S., Johnson, A.H., and Shearer, G.M.: Evidence for a new segregant series of B cell antigens which are encoded in the HLA-D region and stimulate secondary allogeneic proliferative and cytotoxic responses. J. Exp. Med. 152:565, 1980.
45. Shaw, S., Kavathas, P., Pollack, M.S., Charmot, D., and Mawas, C.:

Family studies define a new histocompatibility locus, SB, between HLA-DR and GLO. Nature 293:745, 1981.
46. Nadler, L.M., Stashenko, P., Hardy, R., Tomaselli, K.J., Yunis, E.J., Schlossman, S.F., and Pesando, J.M.: Monoclonal antibody identifies a new Ia-like (p29,34) polymorphic system linked to the HLA-D/DR region. Nature 290:591, 1981.
47. Hurley, C.K., Shaw, S., Nadler, L., Schlossman, S., and Capra, J.D.: Alpha and beta chains of SB and DR antigens are structurally distinct. J. Exp. Med. 156:1557, 1982.
48. Shackelford, D.A., Mann, D.C., van Rood, J.J., Ferrara, G.B., and Strominger, J.L.: Human B cell alloantigens DC1, MT1 and LB12 are identical to each other but distinct from the HLA-DR antigens. Proc. Natl. Acad. Sci. USA 78:4566, 1981.
49. Corte, G., Calabi, F., Damiani, G., Bargellesi, A., Tosi, R., and Sorrentino, R.: Human Ia molecules carrying DC1 determinants differ in both alpha and beta subunits from Ia molecules carrying DR determinants. Nature 292:357, 1981.
50. Bono, R., and Strominger, J.L.: Direct evidence of homology between DC-1 antigen and murine I-A molecules. Nature 299:836, 1982.
51. Goyert, S.M., Shively, J.E., and Silver, J.: Biochemical characterization of a second family of human Ia molecules, HLA-DS, equivalent to murine I-A subregion molecules. J. Exp. Med. 156:550, 1982.
52. Kavathas, P., Demars, R., Bach, F.H., and Shaw, S.: SB: A new HLA-linked human histocompatibility gene defined using HLA-mutant cell lines. Nature 293:747, 1981.
53. Korman, A., Knudsen, P.J., Kaufman, J.F., and Strominger, J.L.: cDNA clones for the heavy chain of HLA-DR antigens obtained after immunization of polysomes by monoclonal antibody. Proc. Natl. Acad. Sci. USA 79:1844, 1982.
54. Larhammar, D., Schenning, L., Gustafsson, K., Wiman, K., Claesson, L., Rask, L., and Peterson, P.A.: The complete amino acid sequence of an HLA-DR antigen-like $\beta$ chain as predicted from the nucleotide sequence. Similarities with immunoglobulins and HLA-A,B,C antigens. Proc. Natl. Acad. Sci. USA 79:3687, 1982.
55. Stetler, D., Das, H., Nunberg, J., Saiki, R., Shen-Dong, R., Mullis, K.B., Weissman, S.M., and Erlich, H.A.: Isolation of a cDNA clone for the human HLA-DR antigen $\alpha$ chain by using a synthetic oligonucleotide as a hybridization probe. Proc. Natl. Acad. Sci. USA 79:5966, 1982.
56. Wiman, K., Larhammar, D., Claesson, L., Gustafsson, K., Schenning, L., Bill, P., Bohme, J., Denaro, M., Dobberstein, B., Hammerling, U., Kvist, S., Servenius, B., Sundelin, J., Peterson, P.A., and Rask, L.: Isolation and identification of a cDNA clone corresponding to an HLA-DR antigen $\beta$ chain. Proc. Natl. Acad. Sci. USA 79:1703, 1982.
57. Larhammer, D., Gustafsson, K., Claesson, L., Bill, P., Wiman, K., Schenning, L., Sundelin, J., Widmark, E., Peterson, P.A., and Rask, L.: Alpha chain of HLA-DR transplantation antigens is a member of the same protein superfamily as the immunoglobulins. Cell 30:153, 1982.
58. Kratzin, H., Yang, C.-Y., Götz, H., Pauly, E., Kölbel, S., Egert, G., Thinnes, F.P., Wernet, P., Altevogt, P., and Hilschmann, N.: Primary structure of class II human histocompatibility antigens. Hoppe-Seyler's Z. Physiol. Chem. 362:1665, 1981.
59. Larhammar, D., Wiman, K., Schenning, L., Claesson, L., Gustafsson, K., Peterson, P.A., and Rask, L.: Evolutionary relationship between HLA-DR antigen $\beta$ chains, HLA-A,B,C antigen subunits and immunoglobulin chains. Scand. J. Immunol. 14:617, 1981.
60. Kaufman, J.F., and Strominger, J.L.: HLA-DR light chain has a polymorphic N-terminal region and a conserved Ig-like C-terminal region. Nature 297:694, 1982.
61. Levine, B.B., Ojeda, A., and Benacerraf, B.: Studies on artificial antigens. III. The genetic control of the immune response to hapten poly-L-lysine conjugates in guinea pigs. J. Exp. Med. 118:953, 1963.
62. Levine, B.B., and Benacerraf, B.: The genetic control of the immune response to hapten polylysine conjugates in guinea pigs. Science 147:517, 1965.
63. Bluestein, H.G., Green, I., and Benacerraf, B.: Specific immune response genes of the guinea pig. I. Dominant genetic control of immune responsiveness to co-polymers of L-glutamic acid and L-alanine and L-glutamic acid and L-tyrosine. J. Exp. Med. 134:458, 1971.
64. Vaz, N.M., deSouza, C.M., and Maia, L.C.S.: Genetic control of immune responsiveness in mice. Responsiveness to ovalbumin in (C57BL x DBA/2)$F_1$ mice. Int. Arch. Allergy 46:275, 1974.
65. Green, I., and Benacerraf, B.: Genetic control of immune responsiveness to limiting doses of proteins and hapten protein conjugates in guinea pigs. J. Immunol. 107:374, 1971.
66. McDevitt, H.O., and Sela, M.: Genetic control of the antibody response. I. Demonstration of determinant-specific differences in response to synthetic polypeptide antigens in two strains of inbred mice. J. Exp. Med. 122:517, 1965.
67. Günther, R., Rüde, E., and Stark, O.: Antibody response in rats to the synthetic polypeptide (T,G)-A–L genetically linked to the major histocompatibility system. Eur. J. Immunol. 2:151, 1972.
68. Dorf, M.E., Balner, H., and Benacerraf, B.: Mapping of the immune response genes in the major histocompatibility complex of the rhesus monkey. J. Exp. Med. 142:673, 1975.
69. McDevitt, H.O., and Benacerraf, B.: Genetic control of specific immune response. Adv. Immunol. 11:31, 1969.
70. Benacerraf, B., and McDevitt, H.O.: The histocompatibility-linked immune response genes. Science 175:273, 1972.
71. Ellman, L., Green, I., Martin, W.J., and Benacerraf, B.: Linkage between the PLL gene and the locus controlling the major histocompatibility antigens in strain 2 guinea pigs. Proc. Natl. Acad. Sci. USA 66:322, 1970.
72. McDevitt, H.O., Deak, B.D., Shreffler, D.C., Klein, J., Stimpfling, J.H., and Snell, G.D.: Genetic control of the immune response. Mapping of the Ir.1 locus. J. Exp. Med. 135:1259, 1972.
73. Dorf, M.E., and Benacerraf, B.: Complementation of H-2 linked Ir genes in the mouse. Proc. Natl. Acad. Sci. USA 72:3671, 1975.
74. Benacerraf, B., and Germain, R.N.: The immune response genes of the major histocompatibility complex. Immunol. Rev. 38:70, 1978.
75. Schwartz, R.H., David, C.S., Dorf, M.E., Benacerraf, B., and Paul, W.E.: Inhibition of dual Ir gene-controlled T-lymphocyte proliferative response to poly($Glu^{56}Lys^{35}Phe^{9}$)n with anti-Ia antisera directed against products of either I-A or I-C subregion. Proc. Natl. Acad. Sci. USA 75:2387, 1978.
76. McNicholas, J.M., Murphy, D.B., Matis, L.A., Schwartz, R.H., Lerner, E.A., Janeway, C.A., and Jones, P.P.: Immune response gene function correlates with the expression of an Ia antigen. I. Preferential association of certain Ae and E$\alpha$ chains results in a quantitative deficiency in expression of an Ae:E$\alpha$ complex. J. Exp. Med. 155:490, 1982.
77. Matis, L.A., Jones, P.P., Murphy, D.B., Hedrick, S.M., Lerner, E.A., Janeway, C.A., McNicholas, J.M., and Schwartz, R.H.: Immune response gene function correlates with the expression of an Ia antigen. II. A quantitative deficiency in Ae:E$\alpha$ complex expression causes a corresponding defect in antigen-presenting cell function. J. Exp. Med. 155:508, 1982.
78. Kapp, J.A., Pierce, C.W., Schlossman, S., and Benacerraf, B.: Genetic control of immune responses in vitro. V. Stimulation of suppressor T cells in nonresponder mice by the terpolymer L-glutamic acid$^{60}$-L-alanine$^{30}$-L-tyrosine$^{10}$ (GAT). J. Exp. Med. 140:648, 1974.
79. Adorini, L., Miller, A., and Sercarz, E.E.: The fine specificity of regulatory cells. I. Hen-egg-white lysozyme-induced suppressor T cells in a genetically non-responder mouse strain do not recognize a closely related immunogeneic lysozyme. J. Immunol. 122:871, 1979.
80. Theze, J., Waltenbaugh, C., Dorf, M.E., and Benacerraf, B.: Immunosuppressive factors specific for L-glutamic acid$^{50}$-L-tyrosine$^{50}$(GT). II. Presence of I-J determinants on the GT suppressive factor. J. Exp. Med. 146:287, 1977.
81. Marsh, D.G., Hsu, S.H., Roebber, M., Ehrlich-Kautsky, E., Freidhoff, L.R., Meyers, D.A., Pollard, M.K., and Bias, W.B.: HLA-Dw2: A genetic marker for human immune response to short ragweed pollen allergen Ra5. I. Response resulting primarily from natural antigenic exposure. J. Exp. Med. 155:1439, 1982.
82. Marsh, D.G., Meyers, D.A., Freidhoff, L.R., Erhlich-Kautzky, E., Roebber, M., Norman, P.S., Hsu, S.H., and Bias, W.B.: HLA-Dw2: A genetic marker for human immune response to short ragweed pollen allergen Ra5. II. Response after ragweed immunotherapy. J. Exp. Med. 155:1452, 1982.
83. Solinger, A.M., Bhatnagar, R., and Stobo, J.D.: Cellular, molecular, and genetic characteristics of T cell reactivity to collagen in man. Proc. Natl. Acad. Sci. USA 78:3877, 1981.
84. Greenberg, L.J., Gray, E.D., and Yunis, E.J.: Association of HLA-5 and immune responsiveness in vitro to streptoccocal antigens. J. Exp. Med. 141:953, 1975.
85. Spencer, M.J., Cherry, J.D., and Terasaki, P.I.: HL-A antigens and antibody response after influenza A vaccination. Decreased response associated with HL-A type w/6. N. Engl. J. Med. 294:13, 1976.
86. DeVries, R.R.P., Kreeftenberg, H.G., Loggen, H.G., and van Rood, J.J.: In vitro immune responsiveness to vaccinia virus and HLA. N. Engl. J. Med. 297:692, 1977.
87. Sasazuki, T., Kohno, Y., Iwamoto, I., Tanimuro, M., and Naito, S.: Association between an HLA haplotype and low responsiveness to tetanus toxoid in man. Nature 272:359, 1978.
88. Solinger, A.M., and Stobo, J.D.: Immune response gene control of collagen reactivity in man. Collagen unresponsiveness in HLA-DR4 negative nonresponders is due to the presence of T-dependent suppressive influences. J. Immunol. 129:1915, 1982.
89. Sasazuki, T., Kaneoka, H., Nishimura, Y., Kaneoka, R., Hayama, M., and Ohkuni, H.: An HLA-linked immune suppression gene in man. J. Exp. Med. 152:297s, 1980.
90. Sasazuki, T., Nishimura, Y., Muto, M., and Ohta, N.: HLA-linked genes controlling immune response and disease susceptibility. Immunol. Rev. 70:51, 1983.
91. Stastny, P., Ball, E.J., Dry, P.J., and Nunez, G.: The human immune response region (HLA-D) and disease susceptibility. Immunol. Rev. 70:113, 1983.

92. Reinertsen, J.L., Klippel, J.H., Johnson, A.H., Steinberg, A.D., Decker, J.L., and Mann, D.L.: Lymphocyte alloantigens associated with systemic lupus erythematosus. N. Engl. J. Med. 299:515, 1978.
93. Gibofsky, A., Winchester, R.J., Patarroyo, M., Fotino, M., and Kunkel, H.G.: Disease associations of the Ia-like human alloantigens. Contrasting patterns in rheumatoid arthritis and systemic lupus erythematosus. J. Exp. Med. 148:1728, 1978.
94. Celada, A., Barras, C., Benzonana, G., and Jeannet, M.: Increased frequency of HLA-DR3 in systemic lupus erythematosus. New Engl. J. Med. 301:1398, 1979.
95. Scherak, O., Smolen, J.S., and Mayr, W.R.: HLA-DRw3 and systemic lupus erythematosus. Arth. Rheum. 23:954, 1980.
96. Griffing, W.L., Moore, S.B., Luthra, H.S., McKenna, C.H., and Fathman, C.G.: Associations of antibodies to native DNA with HLA-DRw3. A possible major histocompatibility complex-linked human immune response gene. J. Exp. Med. 152:319s, 1980.
97. Bell, D.A., and Maddison, P.J.: Serologic subsets in systemic lupus erythematosus: An examination of autoantibodies in relationship to clinical features of disease and HLA antigens. Arth. Rheum. 23:1268, 1980.
98. Notman, D.D., Kurata, N., and Tan, E.M.: Profiles of antinuclear antibodies in systemic rheumatic diseases. Ann. Intern. Med. 83:464, 1975.
99. Raveche, E.S., Novotny, E.A., Hansen, C.T., Tjio, J.H., and Steinberg, A.D.: Genetic studies in NZB mice. V. Recombinant inbred lines demonstrate that separate genes control autoimmune phenotype. J. Exp. Med. 153:1187, 1981.
100. Shirai, T.: The genetic basis of autoimmunity in murine lupus. Immunol. Today 3:187, 1982.
101. Bocchieri, M.H., Cooke, A., Smith, J.B., Weigert, M., and Riblet, R.J.: Independent segregation of NZB autoimmune abnormalities in NZBxC58 recombinant inbred mice. Eur. J. Immunol. 12:349, 1982.
102. Rosenthal, A.S., and Shevach, E.M.: Function of macrophages in antigen recognition by guinea pig T lymphocytes. I. Requirements for histocompatible macrophages and lymphocytes. J. Exp. Med. 138:1194, 1973.
103. Yano, A., Schwartz, R.H., and Paul, W.E.: Antigen presentation in the murine T-lymphocyte proliferative response. I. Requirements for genetic identity at the major histocompatibility complex. J. Exp. Med. 146:828, 1977.
104. Shevach, E.M., and Rosenthal, A.S.: Function of macrophages in antigen recognition by guinea pig T lymphocytes. II. Role of the macrophage in the regulation of genetic control of the immune response. J. Exp. Med. 138:1213, 1973.
105. Cowing, C., Pincus, S.H., Sachs, D.H., and Dickler, H.B.: A subpopulation of adherent accessory cells bearing both I-A and I-E or C subregion antigens is required for antigen specific murine T lymphocyte proliferation. J. Immunol. 121:1680, 1978.
106. Schwartz, R.H., David, C.S., Sachs, D.H., and Paul, W.E.: T lymphocyte-enriched murine peritoneal exudate cells. III. Inhibition of antigen-induced T lymphocyte proliferation with anti-Ia antisera. J. Immunol. 117:531, 1976.
107. Cantor, H., and Boyse, E.A.: Functional subclasses of T lymphocytes bearing different Ly antigens. J. Exp. Med. 141:1376, 1975.
108. Shearer, G.M.: Cell mediated cytotoxicity to trinitrophenyl modified syngeneic lymphocytes. Eur. J. Immunol. 4:527, 1974.
109. Bevan, M.J.: The major histocompatibility complex determines susceptibility to cytotoxic T-cells directed against minor histocompatibility antigens. J. Exp. Med. 142:1349, 1975.
110. Bergholtz, B.O., and Thorsby, E.: HLA-D restriction of the macrophage-dependent response of immune human T lymphocytes to PPD in vitro. Inhibition by anti-HLA-DR antisera. Scand. J. Immunol. 8:63, 1978.
111. Kurnick, J.T., Altevogt, P., Lindblom, J., Sjöberg, O., Danneus, A., and Wigzell, H.: Long-term maintainance of HLA-D restricted T cells specific for soluble antigens. Scand. J. Immunol. 11:131, 1980.
112. Breard, J., Fuks, A., Friedman, S.M., Schlossman, S.F., and Chess, L.: The role of p23,30 bearing human macrophages in antigen induced T lymphocyte responses. Cell. Immunol. 45:108, 1979.
113. Sredni, B., Volkman, D., Schwartz, R.H., and Fauci, A.S.: Antigen-specific human T-cell clones. Development of clones requiring HLA-DR-compatible presenting cells for stimulation in presence of antigen. Proc. Natl. Acad. Sci. USA 78:1858, 1981.
114. Corte, G., Moretta, A., Cosulich, M.E., Ramarli, D., and Bargellesi, A.: A monoclonal anti-DC1 antibody selectively inhibits the generation of effector T cells mediating specific cytolytic activity. J. Exp. Med. 156:1539, 1982.
115. Berle, E.J., and Thorsby, E.: Both DR and MT class II HLA molecules may restrict proliferative T-lymphocyte responses to antigen. Scand. J. Immunol. 16:543, 1982.
116. Gonwa, T.A., Picker, L.J., Raff, H.V., Goyert, S.M., Silver, J., and Stobo, J.: Antigen-presenting capabilities of human monocytes correlates with their expression of HLA-DS, an Ia-determinant distinct from HLA-DR. J. Immunol. 130:706, 1983.
117. Kappler, J.W., Skidmore, B., White, J., and Marrack, P.: Antigen-inducible, H-2 restricted, IL-2-producing T cell hybridomas. Lack of independent antigen and H-2 recognition. J. Exp. Med. 153:1198, 1981.
118. Rosenthal, A.S.: Determinant selection and macrophage function in genetic control of the immune response. Immunol. Rev. 40:136, 1978.
119. Benacerraf, B.: A hypothesis to relate the specificity of T-lymphocytes and the activity of I region-specific Ir genes in macrophages and B lymphocytes. J. Immunol. 120:1809, 1978.
120. Schwartz, R.H.: A clonal deletion model for Ir gene control of the immune response. Scand. J. Immunol. 7:3, 1978.
121. Singer, A., Hathcock, K.S., and Hodes, R.J.: Self recognition in allogeneic radiation bone marrow chimeras. A radiation-resistant host element dictates the self specificity and immune response gene phenotype of T-helper cells J. Exp. Med. 153:1286, 1981.
122. Ishii, N., Baxevanis, C.N., Nagy, Z.A., and Klein, J.: Responder T cells depleted of alloreactive cells react to antigen presented on allogeneic macrophages from nonresponder strains. J. Exp. Med. 154:978, 1981.
123. Clark, R.B., and Shevach, E.M.: Generation of T cell colonies from responder strain 2 guinea pigs that recognize the copolymer L-glutamic acid, L-lysine in association with nonresponder strain 13 Ia antigens. J. Exp. Med. 155:635, 1982.
124. Dos Reis, G.A., and Shevach, E.M.: Antigen-presenting cells from nonresponder strain 2 guinea pigs are fully competent to present bovine insulin B chain to responder strain 13 T cells. Evidence against a determinant selection model and in favor of a clonal deletion model of immune response gene function. J. Exp. Med. 157:1287, 1983.
125. Dreyer, W.J., and Bennett, J.C.: The molecular basis of antibody formation. A paradox. Proc. Natl. Acad. Sci. USA 54:854, 1965.
126. Croce, C.M., Shandler, M., Martinis, J., Cicurel, L., D'Ancona, G.G., Dolby, T.W., and Koprowski, H.: Chromosomal location of the genes for human immunoglobulin heavy chains. Proc. Natl. Acad. Sci. USA 76:3416, 1979.
127. Crews, S., Griffin, J., Huang, H., Calame, K., and Hood, L.: A single $V_H$ gene segment encodes the immune response to phosphorylcholine: Somatic mutation is correlated with the class of the antibody. Cell 25:59, 1981.
128. Sakano, H., Kurosawa, Y., Weigert, M., and Tonegawa, S.: Identification and nucleotide sequence of a diversity DNA segment (D) of immunoglobulin heavy-chain genes. Nature 290:562, 1981.
129. Kurosawa, Y., von Boehmer, H., Haas, W., Sakano, H., Trauneker, A., and Tonegawa, S.: Identification of D segments of immunoglobulin heavy-chain genes and their rearrangement in T lymphocytes. Nature 290:565, 1981.
130. Kurosawa, Y., and Tonegawa, S.: Organization, structure, and assembly of immunoglobulin heavy chain diversity DNA segments. J. Exp. Med. 155:201, 1982.
131. Ravetch, J.V., Siebenlist, U., Korsmeyer, S., Waldmann, T., and Leder, P.: Structure of the human immunoglobulin $\mu$ locus. Characterization of embryonic and rearranged J and D genes. Cell 27:583, 1981.
132. Flanagan, J.G., and Rabbitts, T.H.: Arrangement of human immunoglobulin heavy chain constant region genes implies evolutionary duplication of a segment containing $\gamma$, $\epsilon$ and $\alpha$ genes. Nature 300:709, 1982.
133. McBride, O.W., Hieter, P.A., Hollis, G.F., Swan, D., Otey, M.C., and Leder, P.: Chromosomal location of human kappa and lambda immunoglobulin light chain constant region genes. J. Exp. Med. 155:1480, 1982.
134. Bentley, D.L., and Rabbitts, T.H.: Human $V_K$ immunoglobulin gene number. Implication for the origin of antibody diversity. Cell 24:613, 1981.
135. Hieter, P.A., Maizel, J.V., and Leder, P.: Evolution of human immunoglobulin $\kappa$ J region genes. J. Biol. Chem. 257:1516, 1982.
136. Honjo, T.: Immunoglobulin genes. Ann. Rev. Immunol. 1:499, 1983.
137. Hieter, P.A., Hollis, G.F., Korsmeyer, S.J., Waldmann, T.A., and Leder, P.: Clustered arrangement of immunoglobulin $\lambda$ constant region genes in man. Nature 294:536, 1981.
138. Miller, J., Selsing, E., and Storb, U.: Structural alterations in J regions of mouse immunoglobulin $\lambda$ genes are associated with differential gene expression. Nature 295:428, 1982.
139. Blomberg, B., and Tonegawa, S.: DNA sequences of the joining regions of mouse $\lambda$ light chain immunoglobulin genes. Proc. Natl. Acad. Sci. USA 79:530, 1982.
140. Gearhart, P.J.: Generation of immunoglobulin variable region diversity. Immunol. Today 3:107, 1982.
141. Bothwell, A.L.M., Paskind, M., Reth, M., Imanishi-Kari, T., Rajewsky, K., and Baltimore, D.: Somatic variants of murine immunoglobulin $\lambda$ light chains. Nature 298:380, 1982.
142. Early, P., Huang, H., Davis, M., Calame, K., and Hood, L.: An immunoglobulin heavy chain variable region gene is generated from three segments of DNA: $V_H$, D and $J_H$. Cell 19:981, 1980.
143. Korsmeyer, S.J., Hieter, P.A., Ravetch, J.V., Poplack, D.G., Waldmann, T.A., and Leder, P.: Developmental hierarchy of immunoglobulin gene

rearrangements in human leukemic pre-B-cells. Proc. Natl. Acad. Sci. USA 78:7096, 1981.
144. Hieter, P.A., Korsmeyer, S.J., Waldmann, T.A., and Leder, P.: Human immunoglobulin κ light-chain genes are deleted or rearranged in λ-producing B cells. Nature 290:368, 1981.
145. Korsmeyer, S.J., Arnold, A., Bakhshi, A., Ravetch, J.V., Siebenlist, U., Hieter, P., Sharrow, S.O., LeBien, T.W., Kersey, J.H., Poplack, D.G., Leder, P., and Waldmann, T.A.: Immunoglobulin gene rearrangement and cell surface antigen expression in acute lymphocytic leukemias of T cell and B cell precursor origins. J. Clin. Invest. 71:301, 1983.
146. Moore, K.W., Rogers, J., Hunkapiller, T., Early, P., Nottenburg, C., Weissman, I., Bazir, H., Wall, R., and Hood, L.E.: Expression of IgD may use both DNA rearrangement and RNA splicing mechanisms. Proc. Natl. Acad. Sci. USA 78:1800, 1981.
147. Maki, R., Roeder, W., Traunecker, A., Sidman, C., Wabl, M., Rasehke, W., and Tonegawa, S.: The role of DNA rearrangement and alternative RNA processing in the expression of immunoglobulin delta genes. Cell 24:353, 1981.
148. Yaoita, Y., Kumagai, Y., Okumura, K., and Honjo, T.: Expression of lymphocyte surface IgE does not require switch recombination. Nature 297:697, 1982.
149. Nikaido, T., Nakai, S., and Honjo, T.: The switch (S) region of the immunoglobulin Cμ gene is composed of simple tandem repetitive sequences. Nature 292:845, 1981.
150. Nakaido, T., Yamawaki-Kataoka, Y., and Honjo, T.: Nucleotide sequences of switch regions of immunoglobulin Cε and Cγ genes and their comparison. J. Biol. Chem. 257:7322, 1982.
151. Kataoka, T., Miyata, T., and Honjo, T.: Repetitive sequences in class-switch recombination regions of immunoglobulin heavy chain genes. Cell 23:357, 1981.
152. Dunnick, W., Rabbitts, T.H., and Milstein, C.: An immunoglobulin deletion mutant with implications for the heavy chain switch and RNA splicing. Nature 286:669, 1980.
153. Kincade, P.W., and Cooper, M.D.: Development and distribution of immunoglobulin-containing cells in the chicken. An immunofluorescent analysis using purified antibodies to μ, γ and light chains. J. Immunol. 106:371, 1971.
154. Vogler, L.B., Gathings, W.E., Preud'homme, J.L., Bollum, F.J., Crist, W.M., Seligmann, M., and Cooper, M.D.: Diversity of immunoglobulin expression in leukaemic cells resembling B lymphocyte precursors. Nature 290:339, 1981.
155. Craig, S.W., and Cebra, J.J.: Peyer's patches. An enriched source of precursors for IgA-producing immunocytes in the rabbit. J. Exp. Med. 134:188, 1971.
156. Kawanishi, H., Saltzman, L.E., and Strober, W.: Mechanisms regulating IgA class-specific immunoglobulin production in murine gut-associated lymphoid tissues. I. T cells derived from Peyer's patches that switch sIgM B cells to sIgA B cells in vitro. J. Exp. Med. 157:433, 1983.
157. Isakson, P.C., Pure, E., Vitetta, E.S., and Krammer, P.H.: T cell derived B cell differentiation factor(s). Effect on the isotype switch of murine B cells. J. Exp. Med. 155:734, 1982.
158. Pure, E., Isakson, P.C., Kappler, J.W., Marrack, P., Krammer, P.H., and Vitetta, E.S.: T cell derived B cell growth and differentiation factors. Dichotomy between the responsiveness of B cells from adult and neonatal mice. J. Exp. Med. 157:600, 1983.
159. Mongini, P.K., Paul, W.E., and Metcalf, E.S.: T cell regulation of immunoglobulin class expression in the antibody response to trinitrophenyl-Ficoll. Evidence for T cell enhancement of the immunoglobulin class switch. J. Exp. Med. 155:884, 1982.
160. Binz, H., and Wigzell, H.: Antigen-binding, idiotypic T-lymphocyte receptors. Contemp. Top. Immunobiol. 7:113, 1977.
161. Rajewski, K.: Genetics, expression, and function of idiotypes. Ann. Rev. Immunol. 1:569, 1983.
162. Krammer, P.H.: The T cell receptor problem. Curr. Top. Microbiol. 91:179, 1981.
163. Binz, H., Wigzell, H., and Bazin, H.: T-cell idiotypes are linked to immunoglobulin heavy chain genes. Nature 264:639, 1976.
164. Bach, B.A., Greene, M.I., Benacerraf, B., and Nisonoff, A.: Mechanisms of regulation of cell-mediated immunity. IV. Azobenzenearsonate-specific suppressor factor(s) bear cross-reactive idiotypic determinants the expression of which is linked to the heavy-chain allotype linkage group of genes. J. Exp. Med. 149:1084, 1979.
165. Mozes, E., and Haimovich, J.: Antigen specific T-cell helper factor cross reacts idiotypically with antibodies of the same specificity. Nature 278:56, 1979.
166. Suzan, M., Boned, A., Lieberkind, J., Valsted, F., and Rubin, B.: The 5936 Ig-idiotype(s): Genetic linkage to Ig-$C_H$ loci, T cell-dependence of synthesis and possible specificities. Scand. J. Immunol. 14:673, 1981.
167. Owen, F.L., Finnergar, A., Gates, E.R., and Gottlieb, P.D.: A mature T lymphocyte subpopulation marker closely linked to the Igh-1 allotype $C_H$ locus. Eur. J. Immunol. 9:948, 1979.
168. Spurll, G.M., and Owen, F.L.: A family of T cell alloantigens linked to Igh-1. Nature 293:742, 1981.
169. Owen, F.L., Riblet, R., and Taylor, B.A.: The T suppressor cell alloantigen $Tsu^d$ maps near immunoglobulin allotype genes and may be a heavy chain constant region marker on a T cell receptor. J. Exp. Med. 153:801, 1981.
170. Tokuhisa, T., Komatsu, Y., Uchida, Y., and Taniguchi, M.: Monoclonal alloantibodies specific for the constant region of T cell antigen receptors. J. Exp. Med. 156:888, 1982.
171. Kronenberg, M., Kraig, E., Siu, G., Kappa, J.A., Kappler, J., Marrack, P., Pierce, C.W., and Hood, L.: Three T-cell hybridomas do not contain detectable heavy chain variable gene transcripts. J. Exp. Med., in press.
172. Kraig, E., Kronenberg, M., Kapp, J.A., Pierce, C.W., Abruzzini, A.F., Sorensen, C.M., Samelson, L.E., Schwartz, R.H., and Hood, L.E.: GAT-specific T and B cells do not transcribe similar heavy chain variable region gene segments. J. Exp. Med., in press.
173. Kunkel, H.G., Mannik, M., and Williams, R.C.: Individual antigenic specificity of isolated antibodies. Science 140:1218, 1963.
174. Oudin, J., and Michel, M.: Une nouvelle forme d'allotypie des globulines du sérum de lapin, apparemment liée à la fonction et la spécifité anticorps. Compt. Rend. Acad. Sci. 257:805, 1963.
175. Blomberg, B., Geckelev, W.R., and Weigert, M.: Genetics of the antibody response to dextran in mice. Science 177:178, 1972.
176. Riblet, R., Blomberg, B., Weigert, M., Lieberman, R., Taylor, B.A., and Potter, M.: Genetics of mouse antibodies. I. Linkage of the dextran response locus, $V_H$-Dex, to allotype. Eur. J. Immunol. 5:775, 1975.
177. Nisonoff, A., Ju, S.-T., and Owen, F.L.: Studies of structure and immunosuppression of a cross-reactive idiotype in strain A mice. Immunol. Rev. 34:89, 1977.
178. Lieberman, R., Potter, M., Mushinski, E.B., Humphrey, W. Jr., and Rudikoff, S.: Genetics of a new $IgV_H$ (T15 idiotype) marker in the mouse regulating natural antibody to phosphorylcholine. J. Exp. Med. 139:983, 1974.
179. Cosenza, H., Julius, M.H., and Augustin, A.A.: Idiotypes as variable region markers: Analogies between receptors on phosphorylcholine-specific T and B lymphocytes. Immunol. Rev. 34:3, 1977.
180. Jack, R.S., Imanishi-Kari, T., and Rajewsky, K.: Idiotypic analysis of the response of C57BL/6 mice to the (4-hydroxy-3-nitrophenyl) acetyl group. Eur. J. Immunol. 7:559, 1977.
181. Mäkelä, O., and Karjalainen, K.: Inherited immunoglobulin idiotypes of the mouse. Immunol. Rev. 34:119, 1977.
182. Juy, D., Primi, D., Sanchez, P., and Cazenave, P.-A.: The selection and maintenance of the V region determinant repertoire is germ-line encoded and T cell-independent. Eur. J. Immunol. 13:326, 1983.
183. LeGuern, C., BenAissa, F., Juy, D., Mariamé, B., Buttin, G., and Cazenzve, P.A.: Expression and induction of MOPC-460 idiotypes in different strains of mice. Ann. Immunol. (Paris) 130C:193, 1979.
184. Bona, C., Hooghe, R., Cazenave, P.A., LeGuern, C., and Paul, W.E.: Cellular basis of regulation of expression of idiotype. II. Immunity to anti-MOPC-460 idiotype antibodies increases the level of anti-trinitrophenyl antibodies bearing 460 idiotypes. J. Exp. Med. 149:815, 1979.
185. Bona, C., Heber-Katz, E., and Paul, W.E.: Idiotype-anti-idiotype regulation. I. Immunization with a levan-binding myeloma protein leads to the appearance of auto-anti-(anti-idiotype) antibodies and to the activation of silent clones. J. Exp. Med. 153:951, 1981.
186. Miller, G.G., Nadler, P.I., Hodes, R.J., and Sachs, D.H.: Modification of T cell antinuclease idiotype expression by in vivo administration of anti-idiotype. J. Exp. Med. 155:190, 1982.
187. Juy, D., Primi, D., Sanchez, P., and Cazenave, P.A.: Idiotype regulation. Evidence for the involvement of Igh-C-restricted T cells in the M-460 idiotype suppressive pathway. Eur. J. Immunol. 12:24, 1982.
188. Rubinstein, L.J., Yeh, M., and Bona, C.: Idiotype-anti-idiotype network. II. Activation of silent clones by treatment at birth with idiotypes is associated with the expansion of idiotype specific helper T-cells. J. Exp. Med. 156:506, 1982.
189. Eichmann, K., Falk, I., and Rajewsky, K.: Recognition of idiotypes in lymphocyte interactions. II. Antigen-dependent cooperation between T-and B-lymphocytes that possess similar and complementary idiotypes. Eur. J. Immunol. 8:853, 1978.
190. Jerne, N.K.: Towards a network theory of the immune response. Ann. Immunol. (Paris) 125C:373, 1974.
191. Wells, J.V., Fudenberg, H.H., and MacKay, I.R.: Relation of the human antibody response to flagellin to Gm genotype. J. Immunol. 107:1505, 1971.
192. Whittingham, S., Mathews, J.D., Schanfield, M.S., Matthews, J.V., Tait, B.D., Morris, P.J., and MacKay, I.R.: Interactive effect of Gm allotypes and HLA-B locus antigens on the human antibody response to a bacterial antigen. Clin. Exp. Immunol. 40:8, 1980.
193. Pandey, J.P., Fudenberg, H.H., Virella, G., Kyong, C.U., Loadholt, C.B., Galbraith, R.M., Gotschlich, E.C., and Parke, J.C.: Association between immunoglobulin allotypes and immune responses to *Haemophilus influenza* and meningococcus polysaccharides. Lancet I:190, 1979.
194. Pandey, J.P., Zollinger, W.D., Fudenberg, H.H., and Loadholt, C.B.:

Immunoglobulin allotypes and immune responses to meningococcal group B polysaccharide. J. Clin. Invest. 68:1378, 1981.
195. Nakao, Y., Matsumoto, H., Miyazaki, T., Nishitani, H., Takatsuki, K., Kasukawa, R., Nakayama, S., Izumi, S., Fujita, T., and Tsuji, K.: IgG heavy chain allotypes (Gm) in autoimmune diseases. Clin. Exp. Immunol. 42:20, 1980.
196. Whittingham, S., Mathews, J.D., Schanfield, M.S., Tait, B.D., and MacKay, I.R.: Interaction of HLA and Gm in autoimmune chronic active hepatitis. Clin. Exp. Immunol. 43:80, 1980.
197. Uno, H., Sasazuki, T., Tamai, H., and Matsumoto, H.: Two major genes, linked to HLA and Gm, control susceptibility to Grave's disease. Nature 292:768, 1981.
198. Whittingham, S., Mathews, J.D., Schanfield, M.S., Tait, B.D., and MacKay, I.R.: HLA and Gm genes in systemic lupus erythematosus. Tissue Antigens 21:50, 1983.
199. Pandey, J.P., Goust, J.-M., Salier, J.-P., and Fudenberg, H.H.: Immunoglobulin G heavy chain (Gm) allotypes in multiple sclerosis. J. Clin. Invest. 67:1797, 1981.
200. Holmberg, D., Ivars, F., and Coutinho, A.: An example of major histocompatibility complex-linked control of idiotype interactions. Eur. J. Immunol. 13:82, 1983.

# Chapter 6
# Low Molecular Weight Mediators of Inflammation: Prostaglandins, Leukotrienes, and Cyclic Nucleotides

*Dwight R. Robinson*

## INTRODUCTION

The numerous and varied events that constitute an inflammatory reaction involve several soluble mediators influencing cellular activity. Vasodilatation, vascular permeability, chemotaxis, cell proliferation, phagocytosis, and other functions may be modified by a number of chemical and hormonal agents or messengers. In any particular inflammatory reaction, however, it may be difficult to determine the relative importance of any given agent acting as a mediator or regulator. It becomes important to know which mediators are of greatest significance, since the inhibition or stimulation of these agents may provide a basis for the rational design or choice of anti-inflammatory drugs. Prostaglandins, leukotrienes, and cyclic nucleotides have a wide variety of physiologic effects involving essentially all human tissues. Some of these effects appear to be important factors in the development of inflammatory reactions and in the mechanisms of action of anti-inflammatory drugs. In this chapter we will briefly review certain aspects of prostaglandin, leukotriene, and cyclic nucleotide biochemistry and physiology and their possible contributions to the pathogenesis of the inflammatory rheumatic diseases.

## PROSTAGLANDIN BIOCHEMISTRY

Prostaglandins (PGs) and thromboxanes and their metabolites comprise a large number of compounds, and only a few of the most important of these will be considered here (Fig. 6–1). The prostaglandins are 20-carbon fatty acid derivatives characterized by a 5-membered ring. They are designated alphabetically (e.g., PGE and PGF) depending upon the structure and substituents on the 5-membered ring and further by numerical subscripts (e.g., $PGE_1$, $PGE_2$), which refer to the number of double bonds in the aliphatic limbs of each compound. The compounds shown in Figure 6–1 are all of the 2 series, containing two double bonds in their aliphatic side chains, and these appear to be the most important, although compounds of the 1 and 3 series also occur in nature. Thromboxane $A_2$ differs from prostaglandins by possessing a 6-membered ring structure. The subscript $\alpha$, in $PGF_{2\alpha}$, refers to the steric configuration of the two hydroxy substituents on the 5-membered ring.[1-3]

The pathway of synthesis of PGs is also briefly outlined in Figure 6–1. Prostaglandins are not stored in tissues to any appreciable extent. Their precursors, arachidonic acid in the case of compounds of the 2 series, are stored in cell membranes in the form of complex lipids, primarily phospholipids (I). Under the

$$\begin{array}{c} H_2COOCR_1 \\ | \\ HCOOCR_2 \\ | \\ H_2COPO_3R_3 \end{array}$$

I

influence of certain stimuli, such as tissue injury, activation of the phospholipase enzymes occurs, hydrolyzing

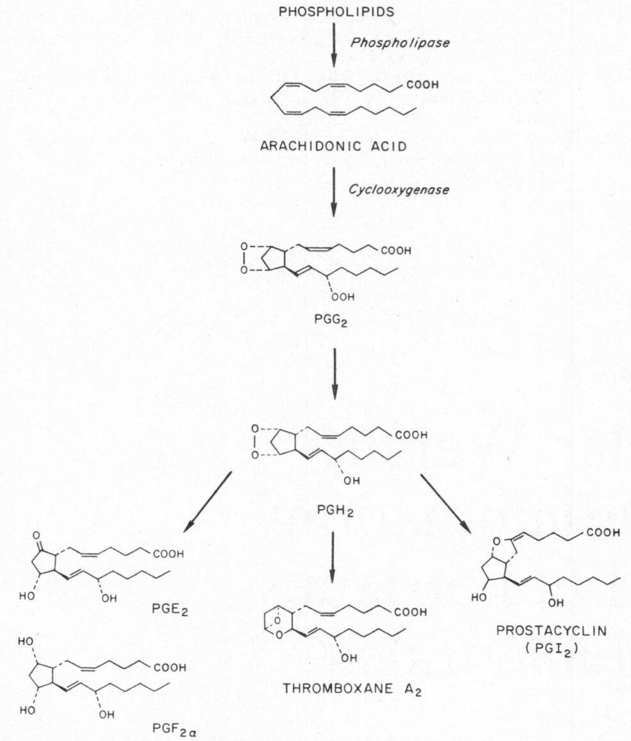


**Figure 6–1.** Formation of prostaglandins and thromboxane $A_2$ from arachidonic acid in phospholipids.

arachidonic acid from its ester linkage, on the two position of glycerol in phospholipids (I,$R_2$).

Having been released from phospholipids through the action of phospholipase, arachidonic acid becomes available for the first reaction on the pathway of PG and thromboxane synthesis, catalyzed by the enzyme cyclooxygenase. This is a complex reaction involving the addition of two molecules of oxygen to arachidonic acid, with closure of the 5-membered ring to form $PGG_2$. Subsequently the peroxy group at the 15 position is reduced to the 15 hydroxy group to form $PGH_2$.[1-3]

The endoperoxide $PGH_2$ is a key intermediate in PG synthesis because the other prostaglandins arise from $PGH_2$ by the action of enzymes generally termed isomerases. The amount of each PG or thromboxane produced is determined by the activities of these different isomerase enzymes present in each tissue. For example, platelets produce primarily thromboxane $A_2$ and only small quantities of the classic prostaglandins $PGE_2$ and $PGF_{2\alpha}$; vascular tissues, predominantly $PGI_2$ (prostacyclin);[4] and rheumatoid synovial tissue, mainly $PGE_2$.[5]

## METABOLISM

Prostaglandins are generally labile in tissues. Some, such as the classic PGs, $PGE_2$ and $PGF_{2\alpha}$, are chemically stable but are rapidly hydrolyzed to inactive metabolites in the circulation. Others, including the prostaglandin endoperoxides, thromboxane $A_2$ and prostacyclin, are chemically labile, with half-lives ranging from about 30 seconds to a few minutes under physiologic conditions.[6-8] In addition, the breakdown of these labile compounds to inactive metabolites may be further accelerated by enzyme action.

The classic PGs are metabolized rapidly, having a half-life in the circulation of less than 30 seconds. Some of the major metabolites of $PGE_2$ are shown in Figure 6–2, and similar products are formed from metabolism of $PGF_{2\alpha}$. Most of the biological activities of $PGE_2$ are reduced or eliminated by the first metabolic step, the formation of 15-keto-$PGE_2$ by the oxidation of the 15-hydroxy group of $PGE_2$ catalyzed by the enzyme 15-hydroxy-prostanoate dehydrogenase utilizing NAD or NADH coenzymes. This compound is reduced by the $\Delta_{13}$-reductase to form 13,14-dihydro-15-keto-$PGE_2$. After several steps a major portion of $PGE_2$ released into the blood is converted to the 16-carbon decarboxylic acid PGE-M and excreted in the urine. Several other compounds are formed in smaller amounts and will not be considered here. Measurements of the PGE-M levels in urine have been used as a measure of total PGE synthesis. Measurements of the 13,14-dihydro-15-keto metabolites of $PGF_{2\alpha}$ and $PGE_2$ in blood have similarly been used as a measure of PG synthesis, since these compounds are more stable than their parent PGs and are not formed artifactually during sampling of blood.[3,9]

Thromboxane $A_2$ is rapidly hydrolyzed to thromboxane $B_2$, giving a half-life of thromboxane $A_2$ of about 30 seconds under physiologic conditions. Thromboxane $B_2$ is reasonably stable in biologic fluids, and its levels may provide a good estimate of thromboxane $A_2$ production. Finally, prostacyclin ($PGI_2$) is also labile, with a half-life of about 2 minutes under physiologic conditions. It is hydrolyzed to 6-keto-$PGF_{1\alpha}$ in an acid-catalyzed reaction with loss of most biologic activity.[3,9]

These and other observations of the synthesis and metabolism of PGs lead to some general conclusions relating to the functions of these compounds in tissues. Nearly all cells and tissues are capable of synthesizing PGs. They are not stored in tissues but are synthesized in response to certain stimuli. The PGs synthesized are released to interact with neighboring cells, possibly through contact with specific PG receptors on cell surfaces. Because of the lability of PGs it seems unlikely that they often have effects at sites distant from their cells of origin, especially by way of the circulation.

## CYCLIC NUCLEOTIDE BIOCHEMISTRY

The cyclic nucleotides also have a widespread distribution throughout the animal kingdom and are present in nearly all human tissues. They have a wide variety of physiologic effects and are regulated by a large number of hormones and other agents. Two cyclic nucleotides are important in human biology, adenosine 3′,5′-cyclic monophosphate (cAMP) and guanosine 3′,5′-cyclic monophosphate (cGMP).

The levels of cyclic nucleotides in tissues are regulated

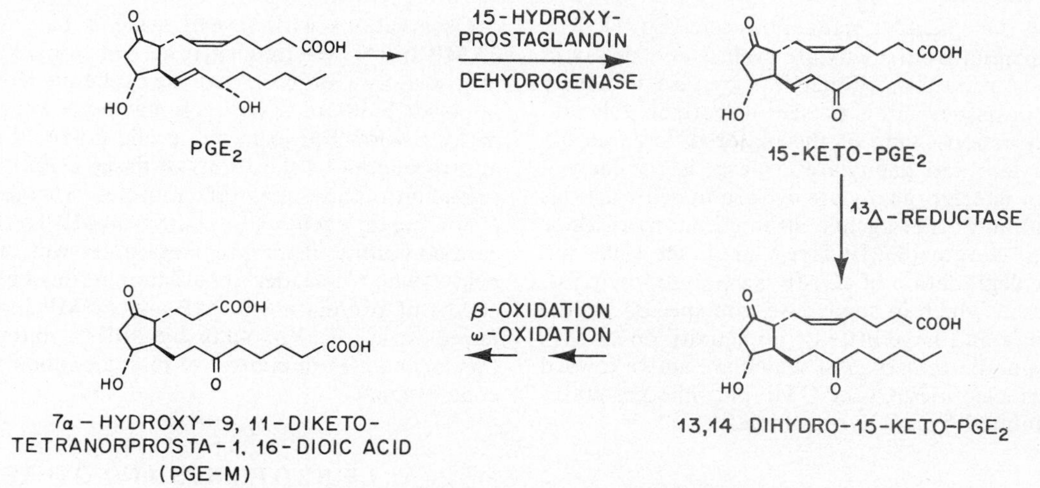


**Figure 6–2.** Major metabolic products of prostaglandin $E_2$.

by their rates of synthesis and degradation. Cyclic AMP is synthesized from adenosine triphosphate by the enzyme adenylate cyclase (Fig. 6–3). This enzyme consists of regulatory and catalytic subunits and is located within the plasma membrane of cells. The regulatory subunit is exposed to the cell surface and contains receptors for several different hormones. Interaction of hormones at the cell surface with receptors on the regulatory subunit modulates the activity of the catalytic subunit near the interior of the plasma membrane. Adenylate cyclase is subject to multivalent regulation by many hormones, but the specificity for the hormones recognized varies with different tissues.[10]

Degradation of cAMP is accomplished by phosphodiesterases catalyzing the hydrolysis of the cyclic phosphate diester linkage of cAMP to form 5′-adenosine monophosphate (5′-AMP).[11] These enzymes are also widely distributed in human tissues and are present in both soluble and membrane fractions of cells. Regulation of cAMP levels in cells could result from control of either synthesis or degradation steps. In general, regulation of cAMP levels by hormones is accomplished primarily by changes in adenylate cyclase activity rather than by changes in phosphodiesterase. Changes in phosphodiesterase activity may also be responsible for changes in cAMP levels. For example, many of the effects of methylxanthines such as theophylline have been attributed to inhibition of phosphodiesterase, leading to elevations in tissue levels of cAMP.[11]

The other cyclic nucleotide of importance is cyclic GMP, although its biological functions are not well established at present. It has effects on tissues which are often opposite or antagonistic to those of cAMP. Cyclic GMP is synthesized from guanosine triphosphate in a reaction resembling the synthesis of cAMP. The reaction is catalyzed by the enzyme guanylate

$$\text{GTP} \xrightarrow[\text{Mn}^{++}]{\text{Guanylate cyclase}} \text{cGMP} \xrightarrow{\text{Phospho-diesterase}} 5'\text{-GMP} \quad (1)$$
$$+ \text{ pyrophosphate}$$

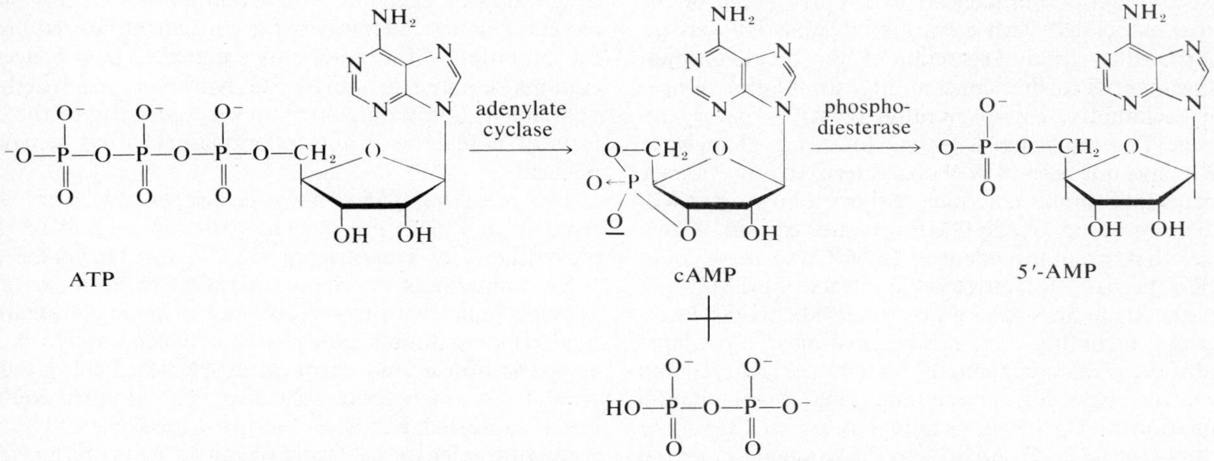


**Figure 6–3.** Synthesis and degradation of adenosine 3′,5′-cyclic monophosphate (cAMP).

cyclase with the cofactor, manganous ion (Eq. 1). The enzyme is distinct from adenylate cyclase and differs in several of its properties. Guanylate cyclase is widely distributed in tissues and is present in both soluble and membrane fractions. One of the major differences between adenylate and guanylate cyclases is the lack of sensitivity of isolated guanylate cyclase in cell fractions to hormonal and other agents, although many of these same agents elevate cGMP levels in intact cells and tissues. The degradation of cGMP is catalyzed by phosphodiesterases, which in some cases are specific for the guanyl moiety and have little or no activity on cAMP. Other phosphodiesterases exist which are active toward both cyclic nucleotides. Cyclic GMP phosphodiesterases are also inhibited by methylxanthines.[11]

## FUNCTIONS OF CYCLIC NUCLEOTIDES

Cyclic AMP probably acts as a mediator of the actions of a wide variety of hormones and other agents in essentially all tissues. A few of these hormonal agents are adrenergic agents, glucagon, parathyroid hormone, ACTH, prostaglandins $E_1$, $E_2$, $D_2$, $I_2$, and the PG endoperoxides. $PGF_{2\alpha}$ is essentially inactive toward adenylate cyclase. The specificity of hormone effects appears to be related to the presence of specific hormone receptors on the regulatory subunits of adenylate cyclase in the cell membranes of appropriate tissues, leading to activation of cell functions in response to adenylate cyclase activation and elevation of cellular cAMP levels. There may be multivalent regulation of adenylate cyclase brought about by receptors for several hormones on each adenylate cyclase enzyme, at least in some tissues.[10]

The biologic effects of changes in cAMP levels in cells are thought to be a consequence of the activation of various cyclic AMP dependent protein kinases, leading in turn to specific protein phosphorylation. The formation of these phosphoproteins may be the basis for the physiologic effects of cAMP.[10,12]

Many tissue functions have been associated with changes in levels of cGMP, although they are not as varied as functions influenced by cAMP. Some of the changes associated with elevations of cGMP levels include the stimulation of secretion of lysosomal enzymes, enhancement of cardiac contractility, stimulation of neuronal excitability, and promotion of inflammatory responses. The biochemical events following changes in cGMP have not been as well characterized, but evidence indicates that similar reactions to those following cAMP stimulation occur. Cyclic GMP activates certain protein kinases that are independent of cAMP, and these could provide the basis for physiologic effects of cGMP.[13,14]

Numerous factors are known to elevate cGMP levels in tissues, including certain hormonal agents, oxidants or substances with oxidizing potential, free radicals, and fatty acids, especially arachidonic acid. Prostaglandin stimulation of cGMP is usually limited to $PGF_{2\alpha}$, or possibly also to $PGG_2$ because of the oxidizing potential of the latter. The E prostaglandins are ineffective toward cGMP.[14]

Observations with several systems have shown that cAMP and cGMP frequently act antagonistically. It was proposed by Goldberg that the cyclic nucleotides act as opposite limbs of a bidirectional regulatory system in many tissues. For example, cyclic GMP or cholinergic agents leading to elevations of tissue cGMP levels suppress contraction of cardiac muscles, whereas cAMP or $\beta$-adrenergic agents stimulating cAMP levels augment cardiac contractility. Other examples will be described below when considering inflammation. The opposing effects of stimulating cAMP and cGMP have been referred to as the Yin-Yang hypothesis, but the role of this mechanism of control of biologic functions remains controversial.[14]

## LEUKOTRIENES AND OTHER LIPOXYGENASE PRODUCTS

Several other products besides PGs are formed from reactions of polyunsaturated fatty acids with oxygen. Molecular oxygen may react at one of several positions of arachidonic acid to form hydroperoxy- and hydroxy-derivatives, catalyzed by lipoxygenase enzymes. An example is the reaction shown in Figure 6–4, in which oxygen reacts at the 12 position of arachidonic acid to form 12-hydroperoxyeicosatetraenoic acid (HPETE). A subsequent peroxidase-catalyzed reaction reduces HPETE to 12-hydroxytetraenoic acid (HETE), and as a by-product forms an oxygen free radical, most likely a hydroxyl radical. Oxygen-free radicals are highly reactive and have been postulated to contribute to tissue injury during inflammatory reactions.[15] A similar peroxidase reaction occurs on the pathway of PG synthesis during the conversion of $PGG_2$ to $PGH_2$ (Fig. 6–1). Therefore some contributions to events occurring in inflammatory reactions may be mediated by free radical by-products as well as by the PGs and LTs themselves.

Inhibition of the peroxidase reaction converting 12-HPETE to 12-HETE (Fig. 6–4) has been described for aspirin, indomethacin, and sodium salicylate, and it was suggested that the anti-inflammatory effects of these drugs may be accounted for by inhibition of this peroxidase reaction.[16] However, the concentrations required for inhibition of this reaction were greater than concentrations required to inhibit PG synthesis, and whether peroxidase inhibition contributes significantly to the effects of nonsteroidal anti-inflammatory drugs remains unclear.

The most important lipoxygenase products are derived from the 5-lipoxygenase pathway leading to the biosynthesis of leukotrienes (Fig. 6–5). The name of these compounds is related to their synthesis by leukocytes (leuko) and to the presence of three conjugated or alternating double bonds (triene), which leads to characteristic optical and chemical properties. Each LT derived from arachidonic acid also has a fourth double bond, indicated by the subscript 4, and the letters A through E refer to the nature of substituents on the fatty acid backbone. The first LT on the 5-lipoxygenase pathway is $LTA_4$. It contains a reactive three-member ring,

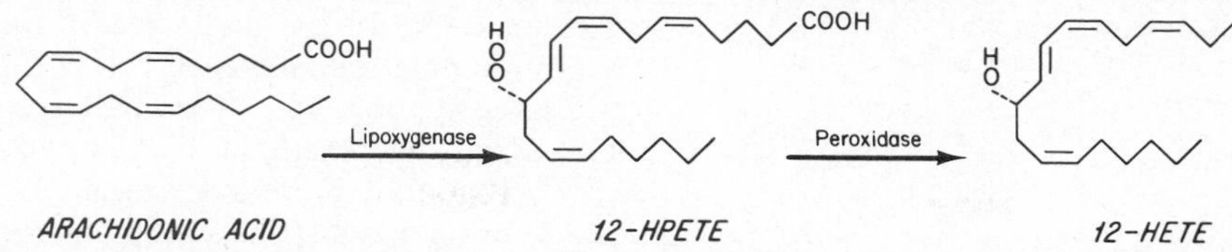


**Figure 6–4.** Formation of 12-hydroperoxyeicosatetraenoic acid (HPETE) and 12-hydroxyeicosatetraenoic acid. These compounds are representative of several hydroperoxy and hydroxy derivatives of arachidonic acid.

an epoxide, which may react either with water at the 12 position to give $LTB_4$, a potent chemotactic agent, or with glutathione at the 6 position, leading to three thionylpeptide derivatives, $LTC_4$, $LTD_4$, and $LTE_4$. The latter three compounds account for the activity of slow-reacting substance of anaphylaxis (SRS-A) and are therefore important mediators of immediate hypersensitivity reactions and other inflammatory processes.[17]

Although the PGs and LTs described thus far have been derived from AA and are quantitatively the most important of these compounds, two other polyunsaturated fatty acids give rise to PGs and lipoxygenase products. These are 20-carbon fatty acids differing from AA in the number of double bonds they possess (Fig. 6–6). Production of the 1 series of PGs (e.g., $PGE_1$) is quantitatively unimportant compared with the 2 series, probably because of the small amounts of its precursor, dihomo-γ-linolenic acid, in tissues. Furthermore, the absence of the double bond in the 5 position of dihomo-γ-linolenic acid eliminates the possibility of forming 5-lipoxygenase products, and for the same reason a prostacyclin analogue cannot be formed. On the other hand, eicosapentaenoic acid, a fatty acid plentiful in marine animals, gives rise to PGs and LTs that are analogues of the AA products but contain an additional double bond at the 17 position (3 carbon atoms from the methyl terminal end of the molecule) (Fig. 6–6). Some of these compounds have been examined and found to be biologically active, e.g. $PGE_3$, $PGI_3$, $TBX_3$, and $LTD_5$, although usually less active than their AA analogues. These considerations are of some importance in view of recent studies demonstrating that alterations in dietary fatty acids may lead to changes in tissue fatty acid composition and in the biosynthesis of eicosanoids (vide infra).

## FUNCTIONS OF PROSTAGLANDINS AND LEUKOTRIENES

The properties and functions of most PGs are well known, although their role in inflammation is incompletely understood. The LTs and HETEs have for the most part been studied recently, and while they have several more potent biologic effects, much remains to be learned about the functions of many of these compounds. The PGs are ubiquitous compounds, produced by every tissue and every cell with the exception of erythrocytes. LTs have been less extensively studied, but are also widespread. Neither class of compounds is stored in cells but is rapidly synthesized and released following appropriate stimuli, including certain hormones, drugs, and cell injury. The life span of most PGs is transient in the circulation. They are rapidly converted

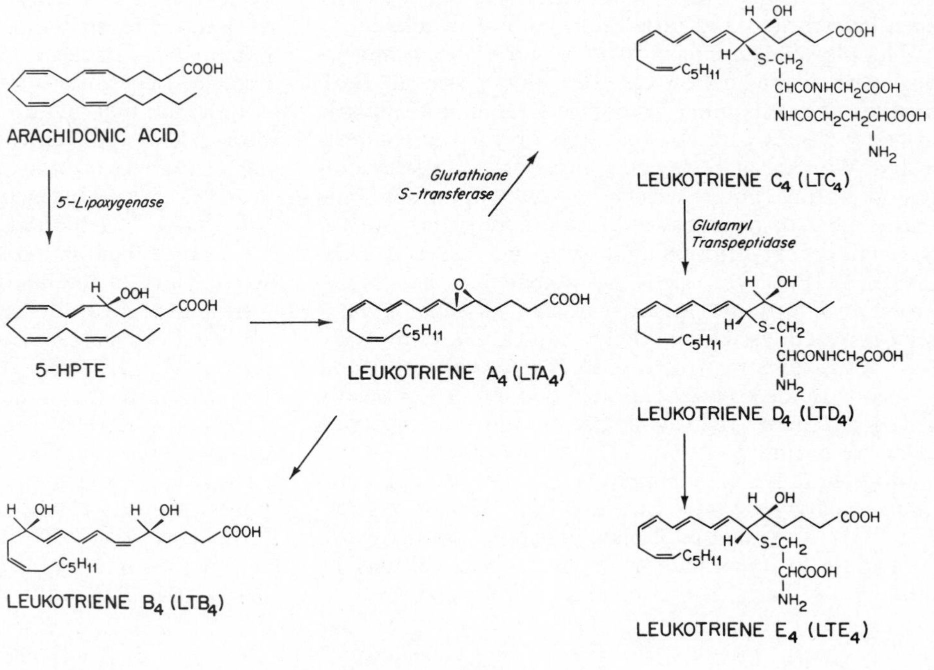


**Figure 6–5.** The 5-lipoxygenase pathway leading to formation of leukotrienes (LTs). $LTA_4$ reacts with glutathione to form $LTC_4$, $LTD_4$ and $LTE_4$. These three LTs account for the activity of slow-reacting substance of anaphylaxis (SRS-A). Reaction of $LTA_4$ with water forms $LTB_4$, an active chemotactic factor.

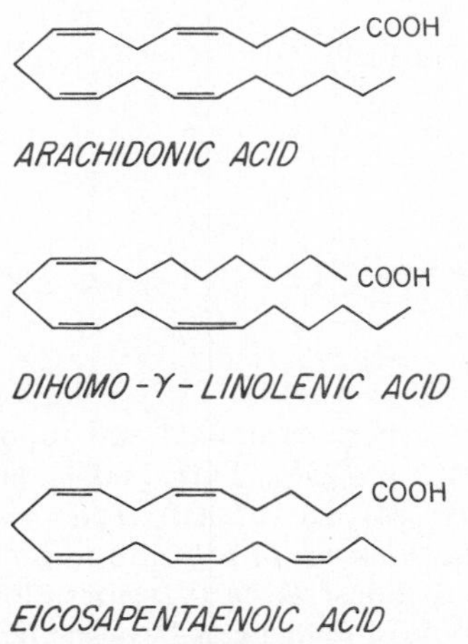


**Figure 6–6.** Structures of all-*cis* polyunsaturated fatty acids which are precursors of prostaglandins and leukotrienes.

to inactive metabolites by dehydrogenase and reductase enzymes, leading to almost complete inactivation, for example, of $PGE_2$ during one passage through the pulmonary vascular bed.[6] Prostacyclin and thromboxane $A_2$ are labile compounds and decompose, with half-lives ranging from 30 seconds to a few minutes, respectively, under physiologic conditions.[6-8] However, prostacyclin is not readily inactivated in the pulmonary circulation, in contrast to other PGs.[18] It was thus postulated that prostacyclin may act as a circulating hormone and maintain a continuous antithrombotic effect, but more recent studies have shown that circulating levels of $PGE_1$ are below the range capable of significant effects on platelet aggregation.[19] It has been difficult to measure PGs by assays of body fluids or tissues. Circulating levels of some PGs have been estimated to be extremely low, on the order of $10^{-11}$ M, generally below the range of convenient analytical techniques such as radioimmunoassay. Levels of LTs and their metabolites have only recently been investigated and little information is available.

The physiologic effects of PGs and LTs are numerous, with potent action on every organ system. Both families of compounds have effects on smooth muscle in many tissues, and different PGs may act antagonistically. We cannot review the functions of these compounds in any comprehensive way but will outline some that appear to be important for inflammation and for the actions of anti-inflammatory drugs. Several PGs, ($PGE_2$, $PGE_1$, $PGD_2$, $PGI_2$) are potent vasodilators and probably contribute to the vascular phase of inflammatory reactions. Others, $PGF_{2\alpha}$ and the thromboxane $A_2$, are vasoconstrictors, the latter being the most potent vasoconstrictor known. The vasodilator PGs, especially $PGE_2$, potentiate the vasodilatation and increased vascular permeability produced by other mediators, including bradykinin, histamine, the complement component anaphylatoxin, C5a, and $LTB_4$.[20] Effects of $TBA_2$ and $PGI_2$ as regulators of platelet aggregation may also contribute to inflammation under some conditions by modulating the release of mediators from platelets.

The leukotrienes are undoubtedly important mediators of inflammation, and their roles are currently under active investigation. It is clear that the LTs are highly potent agents; for example, $LTC_4$ aerosol was found to be over 1000-fold more active than histamine in promoting bronchoconstriction in human volunteers.[21] $LTC_4$, $LTD_4$, and $LTE_4$ produce vasoconstriction of small arterioles but are more potent than histamine in increasing permeability of capillaries and venules.[17] The latter property may contribute to the edema of inflammation. Inflammatory cells are the major sources of LTs. Neutrophils produce large quantities of $LTB_4$, whereas monocyte/macrophages produce large quantities of $LTC_4$, $LTD_4$, and $LTE_4$.[22,23] Many other lipoxygenase products, especially hydroxyl and hydroperoxyl derivatives of arachidonic acid, are produced in tissues, but little is known of their functions at this time.

## INFLAMMATION

The arachidonate metabolites and cyclic nucleotides are potentially capable of participating in the pathogenesis of inflammatory reactions of various types, but the actual functions of these substances in inflammation have not been resolved. Several lines of evidence have indicated that prostaglandins, primarily $PGE_2$ and $PGI_2$, may act as mediators of inflammatory processes.[24-28] (1) These PGs cause inflammation on injection. They are vasodilators in most systems, and they potentiate the formation of edema induced by other agents. They sensitize tissue to stimulation of pain. They cause fever when injected into the central nervous system of experimental animals. (2) As implied above, the prostaglandins not only act by themselves to produce inflammation but also potentiate several effects of other mediators of inflammation such as bradykinin and histamine.[20] (3) Prostaglandins $E_1$, $E_2$, and $I_2$ have been found in elevated concentrations in inflammatory exudates. (4) The biosynthesis of prostaglandins is strongly inhibited by anti-inflammatory drugs.

Leukotrienes may also contribute to the pathogenesis of inflammation. $LTB_4$ is a potent chemotactic agent toward leukocytes, including neutrophils, eosinophils, and monocytes. It may act synergistically with vasodilator PGs to increase vascular permeability.[20] The SRS-A LTs ($LTC_4$, $LTD_4$, and $LTE_4$) may contribute to the edema of inflammation by their ability to increase the permeability of the microvascular bed.[17]

In spite of the evidence that certain PGs may promote inflammatory reactions, other evidence indicates that the E prostaglandins may have anti-inflammatory properties. This has most often been proposed for immune reactions and their regulation by cyclic nucleotides. Many immune reactions are suppressed by cAMP or its derivatives, or by agents that elevate levels of cAMP in tissues, such as $\beta$-adrenergic agents, methylxanthines, $PGE_1$, or $PGE_2$.[29] We will briefly review some of the evidence, examining the effects of cyclic nucleotides and their interactions with PGs on immune reactions and immune-induced inflammation. At the outset it might be noted that many of the effects of PGs may be mediated by their effects on cyclic nucleotides, especially cAMP, since $PGE_1$ and $PGE_2$ stimulate adenylate cyclase in many systems. However, it does not necessarily follow that all effects of PGs are mediated through effects on cyclic nucleotides, and in fact, examples have been described in which alterations in cell functions by PGE are not accompanied by changes in cAMP levels.[30,31] Even in systems in which exposure to PGE leads to elevations in cAMP levels, it may be hard to prove (or disprove) that the PG effects are mediated by changes in the cyclic nucleotide.

Several classes of immune reactions are influenced by PGs and/or cyclic nucleotides. Certain reactions of immediate hypersensitivity are suppressed by cAMP derivatives or agents, leading to elevation of cAMP levels in intact animals and in tissue preparation. Antigen-induced histamine and SRS-A release from sensitized human leukocytes and lung preparations are inhibited by cAMP.[29]

A large number of investigations have been carried out examining the effects of PGs and cyclic nucleotides on various aspects of cellular immunity. Elevation of levels of cyclic AMP invariably suppresses in vitro manifestations of cellular immunity.[29] In some systems elevation of cGMP has been shown to augment these reactions.[13] Prostaglandin $E_1$ or $E_2$ generally suppresses cellular immunity, often in association with elevation of cAMP.[29] Some of the systems demonstrating these effects are briefly summarized here.

Antibody-dependent lymphocyte-mediated cytotoxicity (K cells) is suppressed by $PGE_1$ and other agents associated with increased levels of cAMP. A derivative of cGMP augmented this cytotoxic effect.[32] Another form of cellular cytotoxicity, lymphocyte(T cell)-mediated cytotoxicity toward alloantigen-bearing target cells, was inhibited by agents leading to elevation of cAMP and augmented by agents elevating cGMP.[33] Lymphocyte proliferation induced by lectin stimulation is modified by cyclic nucleotides. The effects on B cell mitogenesis in mixed populations of mononuclear cells are indirect, apparently mediated through macrophages. Macrophage-rich preparations release a nondialyzable factor (lymphocyte-activating factor or interleukin 1) that stimulates mitogenesis in the presence of lectins. The release of the lymphocyte-activating factor is suppressed by cAMP and enhanced by cGMP.[34,35] Prostaglandins $E_1$ and $E_2$ reduced the antigen-stimulated secretion of macrophage inhibitory factor by lymphocytes. It was not determined whether these effects were associated with changes in cyclic nucleotides.[36]

Several investigators have reported studies of PGs (and cyclic nucleotides) on T lymphocyte mitogenesis. In the studies of Goodwin and colleagues on suppression of lectin-induced mitogenesis of human peripheral blood mononuclear cells, the T lymphocyte mitogen phytohemagglutinin induced mitogenesis, which was suppressed by added $PGE_2$ at concentrations as low as $10^{-8}$M.[37] It was also demonstrated that other mononuclear cells in these preparations secreted sufficient $PGE_2$ to partially inhibit lectin-induced mitogenesis. Other studies by these investigators have demonstrated a higher degree of suppression of T cell mitogenesis in vitro by the population of prostaglandin $E_2$-producing mononuclear cells in the peripheral blood of patients with Hodgkin's disease. It was suggested that the deficiency of cellular immunity in patients with Hodgkin's disease may be related to increased activity of $PGE_2$-producing suppressor cells.[38]

It is not clear whether or not these effects of $PGE_2$ are mediated through changes in cAMP, since nucleotide levels in these cells were not determined. Earlier work in similar systems has shown that cyclic AMP levels in human lymphocytes are elevated after exposure to phytohemagglutinin, so it is possible that cAMP elevation is associated with $PGE_2$-induced suppression of lymphocyte mitogenesis in the previous experiments.[39]

Studies directed toward the regulation of antibody production have led to the conclusion that B lymphocyte mitogenesis and antibody production may be regulated by cyclic nucleotides, with cAMP suppression and cGMP stimulation. The effects of B lymphocyte mitogens may be inhibited directly by cyclic AMP elevation in B lymphocytes, whereas B lymphocyte stimulation by antigens may involve T lymphocyte regulation, which is in turn influenced by cyclic nucleotides.[40]

On the other hand, T lymphocyte reactivity may be enhanced by $PGE_1$, as measured by enhanced production of the lymphokine, osteoclast-activating factor,[41] and by enhanced blastogenic responses of a certain subpopulation of T lymphocytes exposed to $PGE_1$.[42] Since T lymphocyte subpopulations may either augment (helper-inducer) or inhibit (suppressor) immune reactions, the consequence of an overall suppression of T lymphocyte function on any given immune reaction may be difficult to predict. Recently others have shown that IgM rheumatoid factor production in vitro is inhibited by nonsteroidal anti-inflammatory drugs (NSAIDs), an effect attributed to the reduction of $PGE_2$-inhibited T helper cell influence on rheumatoid-factor-producing B lymphocytes.[43] Whether this mechanism is important in vivo is unknown at the present time.

There are other in vitro phenomena influenced by PGs and cyclic nucleotides, and these effects may contribute to modification of immune-induced as well as other forms of inflammation. It has been demonstrated that lysosomal enzyme release from polymorphonuclear leukocytes undergoing phagocytosis is influenced by these agents. Elevation of cAMP associated with exposure of cells to $PGE_1$ or other agents is accompanied by significant reduction in the release of lysosomal enzymes, and cholinergic stimulation leads to elevation of cGMP and augmentation of lysosomal enzyme release.[44,45] Another system is the chemotactic response of polymorphonuclear leukocytes. These cells exposed to chemotactic stimuli have their responsiveness inhibited by cAMP and augmented by cGMP.[46] It is also of interest that the opposite responses are observed with human monocytes; cAMP stimulates chemotaxis and cGMP is inhibitory. The differences between the influences of cyclic nucleotides on the responses of polymorphonuclear leukocytes and monocytes to chemotactic stimuli have been suggested to account for the sequential accumulation of these cell types at sites of inflammation.[47]

It is obvious from even a brief review that there are a large number of laboratory observations indicating that cyclic nucleotides may modulate the inflammatory response. In addition, the consistent observations that the E prostaglandins stimulate cAMP in many (but not all) systems suggest that $PGE_1$ and $PGE_2$ may inhibit inflammatory responses under some circumstances. This may seem contradictory to the observations previously described indicating that the E prostaglandins act to promote inflammation. It is possible that PGs may have opposing effects on inflammation under different circumstances or at different times during an inflammatory response.[48,49] It has also been shown that certain forms of inflammation in experimental animals are suppressed by injection of $PGE_1$. Both adjuvant arthritis in rats and the glomerulonephritis of NZB/NZW hybrid mice are suppressed by repeated injections of $PGE_1$. Although the mechanisms of these effects are not known, Zurier and co-workers have suggested the hypothesis that in the NZB/NZW mice adenylate cyclase stimulation by $PGE_1$ may promote thymocyte maturation and thereby relieve a deficiency of suppressor T lymphocytes in these animals.[50-52]

It should be pointed out that most if not all of the experiments discussed here pertaining to effects of cyclic nucleotides on immune and other systems have utilized concentrations of PGs which are pharmacologic, certainly greatly exceeding concentrations of PGs achieved in biologic fluids. It is possible, therefore, that many of the observed phenomena in vitro are irrelevant to events that occur in vivo. At present it is not possible to *prove* that PGs have a role in the pathogenesis of any form of clinical inflammation. While it seems likely that PGs do modulate inflammatory reactions, their functions may be varied and complex.

## ANTI-INFLAMMATORY DRUGS

**Nonsteroidal Compounds.** In 1971 it was first reported that aspirin and related drugs inhibited the synthesis of PGs.[53-55] Since that time a large body of evidence has accumulated in support of the hypothesis of Vane and co-workers that the major effects of these drugs can be accounted for by PG synthesis inhibition.[56] This hypothesis largely rests on correlations that have been established in many tissues between the relative potency of series of compounds as anti-inflammatory agents and their potency as inhibitors of PG synthesis. An example of this kind of correlation is shown in Table 6–1. Here, the relative effectiveness of three drugs on four different forms of experimental inflammation is compared with a microsomal prostaglandin synthesizing system from bovine seminal vesicle. Although the correlation is not exact, the order of effectiveness of the three anti-inflammatory drugs on experimental inflammation and on in vitro $PGE_2$ synthesis is the same. Furthermore, the specificity of these effects is demonstrated by the lack of effectiveness of the 1-stereoisomer of naproxen either on inflammation or on PG synthesis.[57] Many other similar correlations have been made utilizing a wide variety of tissues with similar results.[58]

Other evidence that PG synthesis inhibition may account for the pharmacologic effects of anti-inflammatory drugs is that the concentrations of these drugs that inhibit PG synthesis are similar to concentrations achieved in plasma during therapy. An example is given in Table 6–2. Rheumatoid synovial fragments in tissue culture produce large quantities of PG, primarily $PGE_2$, and many anti-inflammatory drugs have been shown to strongly inhibit PG synthesis. The data in Table 6–2 compare concentrations of the drugs required to suppress rheumatoid synovial $PGE_2$ synthesis by 50 percent ($IC_{50}$) with plasma concentrations of the same drugs achieved in patients taking therapeutic doses. The total drug concentrations have been corrected for plasma protein binding to give peak free drug concentrations. The concentrations of drugs giving 50 percent inhibition of $PGE_2$ synthesis by rheumatoid synovium in tissue culture is similar to or lower than the levels of these drugs achieved in plasma.[5] Therefore, it is reasonable to assume that therapeutic doses of these drugs actually inhibit $PGE_2$ in urine (see Metabolism, above).[59]

Finally, it is worth noting that there is no other persuasive explanation for the mechanism of action of these anti-inflammatory drugs. At present, the most reasonable mechanism appears to be their suppression of PG synthesis, although it is possible that other as yet undiscovered mechanisms may exist.[56]

It has also been found that certain other drugs used for their anti-inflammatory effects in treatment of rheu-

**Table 6–1.** Pharmacologic Effects of Anti-Inflammatory Drugs Compared with Prostaglandin Synthesis Inhibition*

| Compound | Adjuvant Arthritis | Carrageenan | Antipyretic | Analgesic | $PGE_2$ Synthesis Inhibition BSVM |
|---|---|---|---|---|---|
| Indomethacin | 2000 | 48 | 18 | 58 | 2140 |
| Naproxen(d) | 200 | 33 | 22 | 7 | 150 |
| Naproxen(1) (inactive enantiomer) | – | ≥1.5 | 1.5 | ≥0.5 | 2 |
| Aspirin | 1 | 1 | 1 | 1 | 1 |

*From Tomlinson, R. W., et al.: Biochem. Biophys. Res. Commun. 46:552, 1972. Relative activity of aspirin set at 1.

**Table 6–2.** Comparison of Plasma Concentrations of Anti-Inflammatory Drugs During Therapy with Concentrations Inhibiting Prostaglandin Synthesis by Rheumatoid Synovial Cultures*

| | Approximate Peak Plasma Concentration In Man (μM) | Plasma Protein Binding (%) | Peak Free Plasma Concentration (μM) | $IC_{50}$† (μM) |
|---|---|---|---|---|
| Indomethacin | 5.0 | 90 | 0.5 | 0.005 |
| Flufenamic acid | 53.0 | 90 | 5.3 | 0.2 |
| Ibuprofen | 155.0 | 99 | 1.6 | 2.0 |
| D-Naproxen | 305.0 | 99.4 | 1.8 | 6.0 |
| Phenylbutazone | 320.0 | 98.0 | 6.4 | 10.0 |
| Acetylsalicylic acid | 110.0 | 0 | 110.0 | 20.0 |

*From Robinson, D.R., et al.: Prostaglandins and Medicine 1:461, 1978.

†$IC_{50}$ is the concentration of drug giving 50 percent reduction of $PGE_2$ production by rheumatoid synovial organ cultures.

matic diseases have weak or absent effects on rheumatoid synovial tissue in culture and on other in vitro systems. These drugs include antimalarials, gold, sodium thiomalate, penicillamine, and colchicine. These drugs are relatively specific and have clinical properties differing from the nonsteroidal drugs considered in Table 6–2 and related compounds. These differences suggest that the previous group of drugs acts by different mechanisms, and their lack of potent effects on PG synthesis indicates that PGs are not involved in their mechanisms of action.[5]

Thus far, it can be concluded that NSAIDs have no important effects on LT biosynthesis in the low concentration ranges at which PG synthesis inhibition is observed. The development of effective LT synthesis inhibitors should yield agents with important clinical usefulness in inflammatory, allergic, and other disease states.

**Corticosteroids.** Recently it has been discovered that anti-inflammatory corticosteroids are also potent inhibitors of PG synthesis in many cells and tissues.[60-63] Effects of corticosteroids on $PGE_2$ synthesis by rheumatoid synovial tissue culture are summarized in Table 6–3. The inhibitory effects of glucocorticoids are potent, with $IC_{50}$ values in the range of $10^{-8}$ M. The order of effectiveness in inhibiting $PGE_2$ synthesis—dexamethasone > prednisolone > hydrocortisone—is the same as the relative anti-inflammatory potency of these drugs. The ability to inhibit PG synthesis is limited to glucocorticoids, since the two mineralocorticoids are inactive, in parallel with their lack of anti-inflammatory effects. While glucocorticoids have many biologic effects that might be related to their anti-inflammatory properties, it seems likely that their ability to inhibit PG synthesis may contribute to their anti-inflammatory effects.

## MECHANISMS OF PG SYNTHESIS INHIBITION

It is well established that aspirin and other nonsteroidal anti-inflammatory drugs inhibit PG synthesis by interacting with the enzyme cyclooxygenase.[64,65] Aspirin has been found to irreversibly inactivate cyclooxygenase in human platelets by acetylating a serine residue of the enzyme.[66] The platelet enzyme is sensitive to low doses of aspirin; as little as 160 mg per day is sufficient to inactivate essentially all platelet enzyme in man.[67,68] Other nonsteroidal drugs have been shown also to act by a direct interaction with cyclo-oxygenase, although the mechanism of inhibition is unclear. A variety of chemical structures are active inhibitors, including indomethacin, phenylbutazone, fenamates, and the phenylalkanoic acid derivatives such as ibuprofen, naproxen, tolmetin, and many others. Although the activity includes a wide variety of different chemical structures, the interaction is also specific in that many similar structures, including stereoisomers of these compounds (lacking anti-inflammatory effects), are inactive as inhibitors of cyclo-oxygenase.[58,69] The mechanism of inhibition of PG synthesis by corticosteroids is less clear than the mechanism of nonsteroidal drugs. It seems clear that in some tissues, including rheumatoid synovia, the steroids actually inhibit synthesis rather than accelerate PG catabolism or modify transport of PGs from cells.[61-63] However, there is no direct effect of steroids on isolated subcellular preparations of cyclo-oxygenase enzyme.[53-55] Evidence in some systems suggests that steroids inhibit the release of the precursor of PGs, arachidonic acid, from phospholipids by inhibiting the enzyme phospholipase.[70-72] In both cases, the steroids as well as nonsteroidal drugs inhibit at an early step in PG synthesis, and therefore the formation of all cyclo-oxygenase products is reduced. If glucocorticoids inhibit the release of arachidonic acid from phospholipids, it might be expected that these steroids would also inhibit the synthesis of lipoxygenase products, HETEs and leukotrienes. This possibility has not yet been studied in detail.

**Table 6–3.** Effects of Corticosteroids on Prostaglandin $E_2$ Synthesis by Rheumatoid Synovial Cultures

| Steroid | $IC_{50}$ (μM) |
|---|---|
| Dexamethasone | 0.0030 |
| Prednisolone | 0.010 |
| Hydrocortisone | 0.030 |
| Deoxycorticosterone | >1.0 |
| Aldosterone | >1.0 |

## PROSTAGLANDINS AND BONE RESORPTION

Prostaglandins $E_1$ and $E_2$ stimulate osteoclastic activity and resorption of bone when added in vitro to bone culture systems. Other PGs have negligible activity, with the exception of moderate activity of a $PGE_2$ metabolite.[73-76] It was found by Tashjian and co-workers, and later by others, that two experimental transplantable tumors, a mouse fibrosarcoma and the rabbit $VX_2$ carcinoma, cause hypercalcemia in tumor-bearing animals on the basis of secretion of large quantities of $PGE_2$ by the tumor cells. The $PGE_2$ secreted from the implanted tumors appears to cause hypercalcemia on a humoral basis, with stimulation of osteoclast activity by circulating $PGE_2$.[74,77,78] It remains possible that a metabolite of $PGE_2$ retains some ability to stimulate bone resorption, since $PGE_2$ is rapidly metabolized in the circulation, but this possibility has not been resolved.[77]

A similar role for $PGE_2$ has been postulated in hypercalcemia associated with human neoplastic disease. A group of patients has been described with hypercalcemia that returned to or toward normal on treatment with aspirin or indomethacin. Hypercalcemia was associated with elevated excretion of a major metabolite of the E prostaglandins, PGE-M, in the urine, a measure of total production of the E prostaglandins, PGE, by these individuals. Levels of PGE-M were markedly reduced in association with aspirin or indomethacin therapy. Levels of parathyroid hormone in plasma were normal by radioimmunoassay. This study and similar observations by others suggest that hypercalcemia associated with malignancy in some patients may develop because of excessive circulating PGE produced by the neoplasm. In particular, this mechanism may account for the hypercalcemia in the absence of demonstrable bone metastases.[79,80]

Prostaglandin-induced bone resorption has also been postulated to be of significance in rheumatoid arthritis. Explants of rheumatoid synovium and isolated synovial cells in tissue culture produce large quantities of $PGE_2$.[81] It was demonstrated that rheumatoid synovial tissue also releases potent bone resorption stimulating activity in tissue culture media. In a model system utilizing mouse calvarial bone cultures, potent bone resorption stimulating activity was found secreted into culture media by rheumatoid synovial tissue. As shown in Figure 6–7, stimulation of osteoclastic bone resorption in culture was detected by release of bone calcium into culture medium. Addition of small volumes of rheumatoid synovial culture media caused maximal release of bone calcium, shown in the cross-hatched bars. Evidence that this bone resorption stimulating activity is prostaglandin induced includes the following points: (1) The activity is completely recovered in an ether extract of the rheumatoid synovial culture media (clear bars). (2) The activity is completely suppressed by indomethacin in doses shown to completely (> 99 percent) suppress $PGE_2$ synthesis. (3) The concentration of $PGE_2$ in several rheumatoid synovial cultures determined by radioimmunoassay was sufficient to account for the observed effects, based on the known response of the bone cultures to $PGE_2$.[82,83]

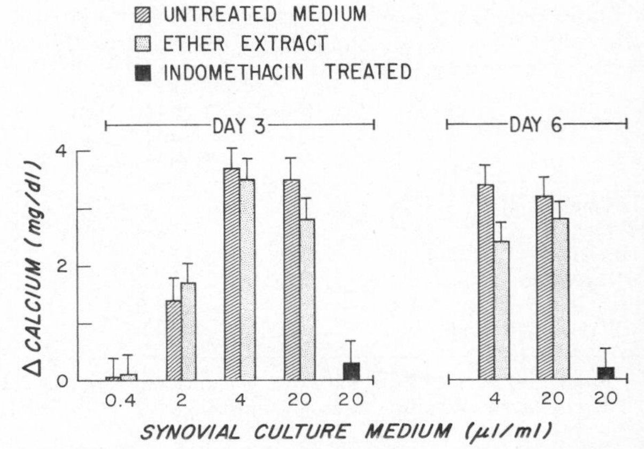


**Figure 6–7.** Bone resorption stimulating activity in rheumatoid synovial culture media (tissue R37). Aliquots of synovial culture media were added to groups of three or four bone cultures at each dosage level. The elevation in medium calcium concentrations from treated bone cultures above that obtained in control bones is the calcium concentration. A portion of the synovial culture media was extracted with ether, and the reconstituted ether extracts were also assayed (▩) and compared to unextracted media (▨). Each bar represents the mean calcium elevation from duplicate synovial cultures (six to eight bones), with standard errrors. Replicate synovial cultures were treated with indomethacin (5 μg per milliliter), which reduced $PGE_2$ levels to < 1 percent of controls. (From Robinson, D. R., et al.: Trans. Assoc. Am. Physicians 88:146, 1975. Reproduced with the permission of the publisher.)

We have suggested, based on this model system, that $PGE_2$ secreted by the invading rheumatoid synovial pannus may stimulate osteoclastic bone resorption, leading to erosions of juxta-articular bone. Because of the close proximity of the synovial pannus to subchondral bone and the localization of bone destruction to areas of pannus invasion, the $PGE_2$ may be released from the pannus in close apposition to bone. It may therefore escape exposure to degradative enzymes as it passes from synovial cells to osteoclasts, or their precursors. The model system further suggests that adequate therapy with anti-inflammatory drugs that inhibit $PGE_2$ synthesis should prevent or retard the development of juxta-articular bone erosions in rheumatoid arthritis.

## AN EXPERIMENTAL NUTRITIONAL APPROACH TO MODIFICATION OF PG SYNTHESIS

Since PGs and related compounds are derived from polyunsaturated fatty acids in tissues, it may seem reasonable that PG and LT production may be manipulated by changing the fatty acid composition of tissues. Long chain fatty acids may be synthesized from fatty acid precursors or may be directly incorporated into tissues from dietary sources. Epidemiologic studies have demonstrated that, in fact, the fatty acid composition of the diet is capable of altering tissue fatty acid composition in man, and subsequent experimental studies have provided further confirmation. Eskimos in northwestern Greenland ingest a diet almost completely derived from marine sources, which contain a high content of ω3 fatty acids, which are compounds each having a double bond between carbons 17 and 18, near the methyl end of the molecule. Analyses of serum and platelet lipids have shown that Greenland Eskimos have high levels of ω3 fatty acids, primarily eicosapentaenoic (EPA) acid (C20:5), an analogue of arachidonic acid, and docosahexaenoic acid (C22:6).[84,85] Studies of Greenland Eskimos, as well as short-term (2 to 3 weeks) feeding of fish oil to human volunteers, have demonstrated that there is a mild bleeding time prolongation and defective platelet aggregation accompanying the ingestion of a marine diet and associated with alterations in PG synthesis and changes in fatty acid composition in tissues.[85-88]

Although EPA may be converted to cyclo-oxygenase products, including thromboxane $A_3$, which may have some effects similar to the AA product thromboxane $A_2$, many studies have demonstrated that EPA is a poor substrate for cyclo-oxygenase in cells and therefore the end result of enrichment of tissue lipids with EPA is an inhibition of AA-derived cyclo-oxygenase products, without formation of significant quantities of products derived from EPA.[89] Ingestion of diets containing a high content of fish oils then may lead to inhibition of the usual PGs formed from AA, and marine diets may thus provide a form of cyclo-oxygenase inhibition. The effects of marine diets on lipoxygenase products, including leukotrienes, have not been studied extensively, but initial investigations indicate that marine diets may lead to production of lipoxygenase products derived from EPA.[90-92] It has been suggested that the marine diet–induced antiplatelet effect may be responsible, at least in part, for the reduced incidence of coronary thrombosis in Greenland Eskimos, although these diets are also associated with lower levels of serum cholesterol and triglycerides than are Western diets.[84,85]

The ability of dietary lipids to alter PG formation and induce abnormal platelet functions suggested to us that similar dietary programs could alter other functions attributed to PGs, especially in inflammatory reactions. Studies investigating the effects of dietary fish oils on inflammatory states in experimental animals have demonstrated a striking protection from glomerulonephritis in the New Zealand black-white hybrid mouse (NZB × NZW)$F_1$ or (NZB/W), a model for human systemic lupus erythematosus.[93] Previous work by other investigators had demonstrated that essential fatty acid deficiency prolonged the life span of these animals.[94] Other investigators had also shown that essential fatty acid deficiency could reduce the intensity of certain inflammatory reactions, and this anti-inflammatory effect has been postulated to be secondary to inhibition of PG synthesis, due to reduction of fatty acid precursors of PGs in tissues.[95] Another series of experiments initially carried out by Zurier and colleagues and subsequently confirmed in several laboratories demonstrated that the NZB/W mouse and other strains developing murine lupus could also be protected by daily injections of the E PGs.[51,52]

It may seem paradoxical at first that essential fatty acid deficiency, a disorder leading to deficiency of polyunsaturated fatty acids and PGs derived from these substances, should lead to protection from renal disease in NZB/W mice, and at the same time, that administration of PGs should also lead to similar beneficial effects. One possible explanation is that protection from murine lupus by administration of PGs requires large doses of PGs. Furthermore, the parenteral administration of PGs requires absorption and transport of the PGs to sites through the circulation, whereas endogenous PGs and LTs exert their physiologic effects on tissues near their sites of synthesis rather than at distant sites via the circulation. Therefore it is possible that repeated administration of large doses of PGs may produce effects that differ from effects of endogenously synthesized PGs. Of course, it is also possible that essential fatty acid deficiency or other alterations in tissue fatty acid composition may produce effects that are mediated by factors independent of PGs or related compounds.

The mechanism of the protective effect of essential fatty acid deficiency or a fish oil-containing diet on murine lupus glomerulonephritis is unknown. These diets could produce alterations in PG and LT synthesis that might change the course of the disease, but other possibilities exist. Alterations in cell fatty acid composition itself could affect cell functions in many ways. Regardless of the mechanisms involved, these experiments suggest that dietary approaches may be effective therapy for renal disease in human systemic lupus and possibly in other inflammatory diseases. Manipulation of tissue fatty acid by dietary means, referred to as polyenoic acid competition by Lands, and its effect on human disease are in the early stages of investigation.[96] Preliminary indications suggest that ω3 fatty acid substitution may hold promise as a therapeutic approach to some inflammatory disease states as well as in vascular diseases. We may speculate that many diseases in which PGs and/or LTs are involved may be influenced by suitable alterations in ingested lipids, but the clinical usefulness of this approach remains to be determined.

## References


1. Adv. Prostaglandin, Thromboxane, Leukotriene Res. 1976–1983. Volumes 1–12. New York, Raven Press.
2. Nelson N.A., Kelly R.C., and Johnson R.A.: Prostaglandins and the arachidonic acid cascade. Chem. Eng. News (August 16):30, 1982.
3. Samuelsson, B., Goldyne, M., Granstrom, E., Hamberg, M., Hammarström, S., and Malmsten, C.: Prostaglandins and thromboxanes. Ann. Rev. Biochem. 47:997, 1978.
4. Bunting, S., Gryglewski, R., Moncado, S., and Vane, J.R.: Arterial walls generate from prostaglandin endoperoxides a substance (prostaglandin X) which relaxes strips of mesenteric and coeliac arteries and inhibits platelet aggregation. Prostaglandins 12:897, 1976.
5. Robinson, D.R., McGuire, M.B., Bastian, D., Kantrowitz, F., and Levine, L.: The effects of anti-inflammatory drugs on prostaglandin production by rheumatoid synovial tissue. Prostaglandins and Medicine 1:461, 1978.
6. Ferreira, S.H., and Vane, J.R.: Prostaglandins: Their disappearance from and release into the circulation. Nature (Lond.) 216:868, 1967.
7. Johnson, R.A., Morton, D.R., Kinner, J.H., Gorman, R.R., McGuire,

J.C., and Sun, F.F.: The chemical structure of prostaglandin X (prostacyclin). Prostaglandins 12:915, 1976.
8. Hamberg, M., Svensson, J., and Samuelsson, B.: Thromboxanes: a new group of biologically active compounds derived from prostaglandin endoperoxides. Proc. Natl. Acad. Sci. USA 72:2994, 1975.
9. Samuelsson, B., Granstrom, E., Green, K., Hamberg, M., and Hammarström, S.: Prostaglandins. Ann. Rev. Biochem. 44:669, 1975.
10. Perkins, J.P.: Adenyl cyclase. *In* Greengard, P., and Robison, G.A. (eds.): Advances in Cyclic Nucleotide Research. Vol. 3. New York, Raven Press, 1973.
11. Appleman, M.M., Thompson, W.J., and Russell, T.R.: Cyclic nucleotide phosphodiesterases. *In* Greengard, P., and Robison, G.A. (eds.): Advances in Cyclic Nucleotide Research. Vol. 3. New York, Raven Press, 1973.
12. Ingebritsen, T.S., and Cohen, P.: Protein phosphatases: Properties and role in cellular regulation. Science 221:331, 1983.
13. Goldberg, N.D., O'Dea, R.F., and Haddox, M.K.: Cyclic GMP. *In* Greengard, P., and Robison, G.A. (eds.): Advances in Cyclic Nucleotide Research. Vol. 3. New York, Raven Press, 1973.
14. Goldberg, N.D., and Haddox, M.K.: Cyclic GMP metabolism and involvement in biological regulation. Ann. Rev. Biochem. 46:823, 1977.
15. Fridovich, I.: The biology of oxygen radicals. Science 201:875, 1978.
16. Siegel, M.I., McConnell, R.T., and Cuatrecasas, P.: Aspirin-like drugs interfere with arachidonate metabolism by inhibition of the 12-hydroperoxy-5,8,10,14-eicosatetraenoic acid peroxidase activity of the lipoxygenase pathway. Proc. Natl. Acad. Sci. USA 76:3774, 1979.
17. Lewis, R.A., and Austen, K.F.: Mediation of local homeostasis and inflammation by leukotrienes and other mast cell-dependent compounds. Nature 293:103, 108, 1981.
18. Armstrong, J.M., Lattimer, N., Moncada, S., and Vane, J.R.: Comparison of the vasodepressor effects of prostacyclin and 6-oxo-prostaglandin $F_{1\alpha}$ with those of prostaglandin $E_2$ in rats and rabbits. Br. J. Pharmacol. 62:125, 1978.
19. Fitzgerald, G.A., Brash, A.R., Falardeau, P., and Oates, J.A.: Estimated rate of prostacyclin secretion into the circulation of normal man. J. Clin. Invest. 68:1272, 1981.
20. Wedmore, C.V., and Williams, T.J.: Control of vascular permeability by polymorphonuclear leukocytes in inflammation. Nature 289:646, 1981.
21. Weiss, J.W., Drazen, J.M., Coles, N., McFadden, E.R., Jr., Weller, P.F., Corey, E.J., Lewis, R.A., and Austen, K.F.: Bronchoconstrictor effects of leukotriene C in humans. Science 216:196, 1982.
22. Borgeat, P., and Samuelsson, B.: Arachidonic acid metabolism in polymorphonuclear leukocytes: effects of ionophore A23187. Proc. Natl. Acad. Sci. USA 76:2148, 1979.
23. Scott, W.A., Pawlowski, N.A., Murray, H.W., Andreach, M., Zrike, J., and Cohn, Z.: Regulation of arachidonic acid metabolism by macrophage activation. J. Exp. Med. 155:1148, 1982.
24. Vane, J.R.: Prostaglandins as mediators of inflammation. *In* Samuellson, B., and Paoletti, R. (eds.): Advances in Prostaglandin and Thromboxane Research. Vol. 2. New York, Raven Press, 1976.
25. Komoriya, K., Ohmori, H., Azuma, A., Kurozumi, S., and Hashimoto, Y.: Prostaglandin $I_2$ as a potentiator of acute inflammation in rats. Prostaglandins 15:557, 1978.
26. Ferreria, S.H., Nakamura, M., and deAbreu Castro, M.S.: The hyperalgesic effects of prostacyclin and prostaglandin $E_2$. Prostaglandins 16:31, 1978.
27. Ford-Hutchinson, A.W., Walker, J.R., Davidson, E.M., and Smith, M.J.H.: $PGI_2$: A potential mediator of inflammation. Prostaglandins 16:253, 1978.
28. Higgs, E.A., Moncada, S., and Vane, J.R.: Inflammatory effects of prostacyclin ($PGI_2$) and 6-OXO-$PGF_{1\alpha}$ in the rat paw. Prostaglandins 16:153, 1978.
29. Bourne, H.R., Lichtenstein, L.M., Melmon, K.L., Henney, C.S., Weinstein, Y., and Shearer, G.M.: Modulation of inflammation and immunity by cyclic AMP. Science 184:19, 1974.
30. Polgar, P., and Taylor, L.: Effects of prostaglandin on substrate uptake and cell division in human diploid fibroblasts. Biochem. J. 162:1, 1977.
31. Feher, I., and Gidaili, J.: Prostaglandin $E_2$ as a stimulator of haemopoietic stem cell proliferation. Nature 247:550, 1974.
32. Garavoy, M.R., Strom, B.T., Kaliner, M., and Carpenter, C.B.: Antibody-dependent lymphocyte mediated cytotoxicity mechanism and modulation by cyclic nucleotides. Cell. Immunol. 20:197, 1975.
33. Strom, T., Deisseroth, A., Morganroth, J., Carpenter, C., and Merriel, J.: Alteration of the cytotoxic action of sensitized lymphocytes by cholinergic agents and activators of adenylate cyclase. Proc. Natl. Acad. Sci. USA 69:2995, 1972.
34. Diamantstein, T., and Ulmer, A.: Stimulation by cyclic AMP of lymphocytes mediated by soluble factor released from adherent cells. Nature 256:418, 1975.
35. Diamantstein, T., and Ulmer, A.: The antagonistic action of cGMP and cAMP on proliferation of B and T lymphocytes. Immunology 28:113, 1975.
36. Gordon, D., Bray, M.A., and Morley, J.: Control of lymphokine secretion by prostaglandins. Nature 262:401, 1976.
37. Goodwin, J.S., Bankhurst, A.D., and Messner, R.P.: Suppression of human T-cell mitogenesis by prostaglandin: Existence of a prostaglandin-producing suppressor cell. J. Exp. Med. 146:1719, 1977.
38. Goodwin, J.S., Messner, R.P., Bankhurst, A.D., Peake, G.T., Saiki, J.H., and Williams, R.G.: Prostaglandin producing suppressor cells in Hodgkin's disease. N. Engl. J. Med. 297:963, 1977.
39. Smith, J.W., Steiner, A.L., Newberry, W., Jr., and Parker, C. W.: Cyclic adenosine 3'5'-monophosphate in human lymphocytes. Alterations after phytohemagglutinin stimulation. J. Clin. Invest. 60:432, 1971.
40. Watson J.: Cyclic nucleotides as intracellular mediators of B cell activation. Transplant. Rev. 23:223, 1975.
41. Yoneda, T., and Mundy, G.R.: Monocytes regulate osteoclast activating factor production by releasing prostaglandin. J. Exp. Med. 150:338, 1979.
42. Stobo, J.D., Kennedy, M.S., and Goldyne, M.E.: Prostaglandin E modulation of the mitogenic response of human T cells. J. Clin. Invest. 64:1188, 1979.
43. Ceuppens, J.L., Rodriguez, M.A., and Goodwin, J.S.: Non-steroidal anti-inflammatory agents inhibit the synthesis of IgM rheumatoid factor in vitro. Lancet I:528, 1982.
44. Weissmann, G., Goldstein, I., Hoffstein, S., Chauvet, G., and Robineaux, R.: Yin/Yang modulation of lysosomal enzyme release from polymorphonuclear leukocytes by cyclic nucleotides. Ann. N.Y. Acad. Sci. 256:222, 1975.
45. Weissmann, G., Goldstein, I., Hoffstein, S., and Tsung, P.K.: Reciprocal effects of cAMP and cGMP on microtubule-dependent release of lysosomal enzymes. Ann. N.Y. Acad. Sci. 253:750, 1975.
46. Hill, H.R., Estensen, R.D., Quie, P.G., Hogan, N.A., and Goldberg, N.D.: Modulation of human neutrophil chemotactic responses by cyclic 3',5'-guanosine monophosphate and cyclic 3',5'-adenosine monophosphate. Metabolism 24:447, 1975.
47. Genta, G.E., and Hill, H.R.: Paradoxical influence of cyclic AMP on human monocyte chemotactic responses. Clin. Res. 24:180A, 1976.
48. Bonta, I.L., Parnham, M.J., and Van Vliet, L.: Combination of theophylline and prostaglandin $E_1$ as inhibitors of the adjuvant-induced arthritis syndrome of rats. Ann. Rheum. Dis. 37:212, 1978.
49. Parnham, M.J., Bonta, I.L., and Adolfs, M.J.P.: Cyclic AMP and prostaglandin E in perfusates of rat hind paws during the development of adjuvant arthritis. Ann. Rheum. Dis. 37:218, 1978.
50. Zurier, R.B., and Quagliata, F.: Effect of prostaglandin $E_1$ on adjuvant arthritis. Nature 234:304, 1971.
51. Zurier, R.B., Sayadoff, D.M., Torrey, S.B., and Rothfield, N.F.: Prostaglandin $E_1$ treatment of NZB/W mice. I. Prolonged survival of female mice. Arthritis Rheum. 20:723, 1977.
52. Zurier, R.B., Damjanov, I., Sayadoff, D.M., and Rothfield, N.F.: Prostaglandin $E_1$ treatment of NZB/W mice. II. Prevention of glomerulonephritis. Arthritis Rheum. 20:1449, 1977.
53. Vane, J.R.: Inhibition of prostaglandin synthesis as a mechanism of action for aspirin-like drugs. Nature New Biol. 231:232, 1971.
54. Smith J.B., and Willis, A.L.: Aspirin selectively inhibits prostaglandin production in human platelets. Nature New Biol. 231:235, 1971.
55. Ferreira, S.H., Moncada, S., and Vane J.R.: Indomethacin and aspirin abolish prostaglandin release from the spleen. Nature New Biol. 231:237, 1971.
56. Ferreira, S.H., and Vane, J.R.: New aspects of the mode of action of nonsteroid anti-inflammatory drugs. Ann. Rev. Pharmacol. 14:57, 1974.
57. Tomlinson, R.W., Ringold, H.J., Qureshi, M.C., and Forchielli, E.: Relationship between inhibition of prostaglandin synthesis and drug efficacy: Support for the current theory on mode of action of aspirin-like drugs. Biochem. Biophys. Res. Commun. 46:552, 1972.
58. Flower, R.J.: Drugs which inhibit prostaglandin biosynthesis. Pharmacol. Rev. 26:33, 1974.
59. Hamberg, M.: Inhibition of prostaglandin synthesis in man. Biochem. Biophys. Res. Commun. 49:720, 1972.
60. Lewis, G.P., and Piper, P.J.: Inhibition of release of prostaglandins as an explanation of some of the actions of anti-inflammatory corticosteroids. Nature 254:308, 1975.
61. Gryglewski, R.J., Panczenko, B., Korbut, R., Grodzinska, L., and Ocetkiewcz, A.: Corticosteroids inhibit prostaglandin release from perfused mesenteric blood vessels of rabbit and from perfused lungs of sensitized guinea pig. Prostaglandins 10:343, 1975.
62. Kantrowitz, F., Robinson, D.R., McGuire, M.B., and Levine, L.: Corticosteroids inhibit prostaglandin production by rheumatoid synovia. Nature 258:737, 1975.
63. Tashjian, A.H., Jr., Voelkel, E.F., McDonough, J., and Levine, L.: Hydrocortisone inhibits prostaglandin production by mouse fibrosarcoma cells. Nature 258:739, 1975.
64. Roth, G.J., Stanford, N., and Majerus, P.W.: Acetylation of prostaglandin synthase by aspirin. Proc. Natl. Acad. Sci. USA 72:3073, 1975.

65. Roth, G.J., and Majerus, P.W.: The mechanism of the effect of aspirin on human platelets. I. Acetylation of a particulate fraction protein. J. Clin. Invest. 56:624, 1975.
66. Van Der Ouderaa, F.J., Buytenhek, M., Nugeren, D.H., and Van Dorp, D.A.: Acetylation of prostaglandin endoperoxide synthetase with acetylsalicyclic acid. Eur. J. Biochem. 109:1, 1980.
67. Patrignani, P., Filabozzi, P., and Patrono, C.: Selective cumulative inhibition of platelet thromboxane production by low-dose aspirin in healthy subjects. J. Clin. Invest. 69:1366, 1982.
68. Weksler, B.B., Pett, S.B., Alonso, D., Richter, R.C., Stelzer, P., Subramanian, V., Tack-Goldman, K., and Gay, W.A., Jr.: Differential inhibition by aspirin of vascular and platelet prostaglandin synthesis in atherosclerotic patients. N. Engl. J. Med. 308:800, 1083.
69. Rome, L.H., and Lands, W.E.: Structural requirements for time-dependent inhibition of prostaglandin biosynthesis by anti-inflammatory drugs. Proc. Natl. Acad. Sci. USA 72:4863, 1975.
70. Hong, S.-C., and Levine, L.: Inhibition of arachidonic acid release from cells as the biochemical action of anti-inflammatory corticosteroids. Proc. Natl. Acad. Sci. USA 73:1730, 1976.
71. Blackwell, G.J., Carnuccio, R., DiRosa, M., Flower, R.J., Parente, L., and Persico, P.: Macrocortin: a polypeptide causing the anti-phospholipase effect of glucocorticoids. Nature 287:147, 1980.
72. Hirata, F.: The regulation of lipomodulin, a phospholipase inhibitory protein, in rabbit neutrophils by phosphorylation. J. Biol. Chem. 256:7730, 1981.
73. Klein, D.C., and Raisz, L.G.: Prostaglandins: Stimulation of bone resorption in tissue culture. Endocrinology 86:1436, 1970.
74. Tashjian, A.H., Jr., Voelkel, E.F., Levine, L., and Goldhaber, P.: Evidence that the bone resorption stimulating factor produced by mouse fibrosarcoma cells is prostaglandin $E_2$. J. Exp. Med. 36:1329, 1972.
75. Dietrich, J.W., Goodson, J.M., and Raisz, L.G.: Stimulation of bone resorption by various prostaglandins in organ culture. Prostaglandins 10:231, 1975.
76. Tashjian, A.H., Jr., Tice, J.E., and Sides, K.: Biological activities of prostaglandin analogs and metabolites on bone in organ culture. Nature 266:645, 1977.
77. Seyberth, H.W., Hubbard, W.C., Oelz, O., Sweetman, B.J., Watson, J.T., and Oates, J.A.: Prostaglandin-mediated hypercalcemia in the $VX_2$ carcinoma-bearing rabbit. Prostaglandins 14:319, 1977.
78. Tashjian, A.H., Jr., Voelkel, E.F., and Levine, L.: Plasma concentrations of 13,14-dihydro-15-keto-prostaglandin $E_2$ in rabbits bearing the $VX_2$ carcinoma: Effects of hydrocortisone and indomethacin. Prostaglandins 14:309, 1977.
79. Seyberth, H.W., Segre, G.V., Morgan, J.L., Sweetman, B.J., Potts, J.T., Jr., and Oates, J.A.: Prostaglandins as mediators of hypercalcemia associated with certain types of cancer. N. Engl. J. Med. 293:1278, 1975.
80. Seyberth, H.W., Segre, G.V., Hamet, P., Sweetman, G.J., Potts, J.T., Jr., and Oates, J.A.: Characterization of the group of patients with the hypercalcemia of cancer who respond to treatment with prostaglandin synthesis inhibitors. Trans. Assoc. Am. Physicians 89:93, 1976.
81. Robinson, D.R., and McGuire, M.B.: Prostaglandins in the rheumatic diseases. Ann. N.Y. Acad. Sci. 256:318, 1975.
82. Robinson, D.R., Tashjian, A.H., Jr., and Levine, L.: Prostaglandin-induced bone resorption by rheumatoid synovia. Trans. Assoc. Am. Physicians 88:146, 1975.
83. Robinson, D.R., Tashjian, A.H., Jr., and Levine, L.: Prostaglandin-stimulated bone resorption by rheumatoid synovia. J. Clin. Invest. 56:1181, 1975.
84. Dyerberg, J., Bang, H.O., and Hjorne, N.: Fatty acid composition of the plasma lipids in Greenland Eskimos. Am. J. Clin. Nutr. 28:958, 1975.
85. Dyerberg, J., Bang, H.O., Stoffersen, E., Moncada, S., and Vane, J.R.: Eicosapentaenoic acid and prevention of thrombosis and atherosclerosis? Lancet II:117, 1978.
86. Goodnight, S.H., Jr., Harris, W.S., and Connor, W.E.: The effects of dietary $\omega$3 fatty acids on platelet composition and function in man: A prospective, controlled study. Blood 58:880, 1981.
87. Thorngren, M., and Gustafson, A.: Effects of 11-week increase in dietary eicosapentaenoic acid on bleeding time, lipids, and platelet aggregation. Lancet II:1190, 1981.
88. Hay, C.R.M., Saynor, R., and Durber, A.P.: Effect of fish oil on platelet kinetics in patients with ischaemic heart disease. Lancet I:1269, 1982.
89. Whitaker, M.O., Wyche, A., Fitzpatrick, F., Sprecher, H., and Needleman, P.: Triene prostaglandins: prostaglandin $D_3$ and eicosapentaenoic acid as potential antithrombotic substances. Proc. Natl. Acad. Sci. USA 76:5919, 1979.
90. Hammarström, S.: Conversion of $^{14}$C-labeled eicosapentaenoic acid (n-3) to leukotriene $C_5$. Biochim. Biophys. Acta 663:575, 1981.
91. Murphy, R.C., Pickett, W.C., Culp, B.R., and Lands, W.E.M.: Tetraene and pentaene leukotrienes: selective production from murine mastocytoma cells after dietary manipulation. Prostaglandins 22:613, 1981.
92. Hammarström, S.: Conversion of 5,8,11-eicosatrienoic acid to leukotrienes $C_3$ and $D_3$. J. Biol. Chem. 256:2275, 1981.
93. Prickett, J.D., Robinson, D.R., and Steinberg, A.D.: Effects of dietary enrichment with eicosapentaenoic acid upon autoimmune nephritis in female NZB × NZW/$F_1$ mice. Arthritis Rheum. 26:133, 1983.
94. Hurd, E.R., Johnston, J.M., Okita, J.R., MacDonald, P.C., Ziff, M., and Gilliam, J.N.: Prevention of glomerulonephritis and prolonged survival in New Zealand black/New Zealand white $F_1$ hybrid mice fed an essential fatty acid-deficient diet. J. Clin. Invest. 67:476, 1981.
95. Bonta, I.L., Bult, H., Vincent, J.E., and Zijlstra, F.J.: Acute anti-inflammatory effects of aspirin and dexamethasone in rats deprived of endogenous prostaglandin precursors. J. Pharm. Pharmacol. 29:1, 1977.
96. Lands, W.E.M.: manuscript in preparation.

# Chapter 7

# Plasma Protein Effectors of Inflammation: Complement

*Shaun Ruddy*

## INTRODUCTION

Originally defined as the heat-labile serum factor required to "complete" the killing of bacteria coated with antibody, complement is now known to be a system of 18 plasma proteins that act together to mediate many inflammatory effects.[1-4] Like the other groups of plasma proteins that deliver inflammatory effects—the coagulation, kinin-forming, and fibrinolytic sequences (Chapter 8)—complement is characterized by the underlying principle of latent, recurrent, limited proteolysis. At several steps in the sequence a precursor or zymogen is activated to a protease, which cleaves a plasma protein substrate. This liberates an activation peptide and generates a new protease or modifies the specificity of an already active protease. In its turn, this new proteolytic enzyme cleaves yet another plasma protein, forming a new proteolytic activity, and the process recurs in cascade fashion. Products of the proteolysis have biologic activities, including the alteration of vascular permeability, the attraction of leukocytes and enhancement of their ability to ingest coated particles, the immobilization of these cells at the site of inflammation, and the assembly in cell membranes of the cytolytic membrane attack complex. Binding of complement cleavage products to specific receptors on the surface of erythrocytes, mast cells, macrophages or monocytes, lymphocytes, and platelets triggers additional biologic effects. Included among these may be the facilitation of cell-cell interactions required for the processing of antigen, for the initiation of an immune response, or for the control of an effective response.

All the complement proteins have been obtained in chemically homogeneous form (Table 7–1), and their functions are now well understood. Recognition of activating agents by either of two proteolytic pathways leads to a final common pathway, which assembles the membrane attack complex. The "classic" pathway for activation is so named because it was discovered first, but phylogenetic studies indicate that the "alternative" activation pathway is probably the older and more primitive.[5] The classic pathway is triggered by immune complexes formed from the union of IgG or IgM antibodies with their antigens, and such antibodies are found later in evolution than are analogues of alternative pathway factors. Animals without antibodies have plasma proteins that can be activated by repeating polysaccharides or other polymeric structures in the absence of specific antibody. Activation by either pathway generates endopeptidases with identical specificity: Both the alternative and classic pathway enzymes cleave the third complement component, C3, at arginine number 77 on the $\alpha$-chain. The events that follow—assembly of the membrane attack complex—are also identical.

Proteins of the classic activation pathway and the terminal sequence are called "components" and are symbolized by the letter "C" followed by a number, e.g., C1, C4, C2, C3, C5, C6, C7, C8, and C9. Proteins of the alternative activation pathway are termed "factors" and are symbolized by letters, e.g., B, D, and P. Enzymatically active forms are indicated by a bar over the letter or number, e.g., C$\overline{1}$, $\overline{D}$; and cleavage fragments are denoted with suffixed lower case letters, e.g., C3a, C3b, C3c, and C3d. Polypeptide subunit chains are suffixed with Greek letters, starting with the largest chain, e.g., C3$\alpha$, C3$\beta$. Control proteins are symbolized with contractions of their trivial names, e.g., C$\overline{1}$ inhibitor (C$\overline{1}$ INH), C3b inactivator (I), $\beta$1H globulin (H), C4 binding protein (C4BP).

## CHEMISTRY AND REACTION MECHANISMS

**Classic Activation Pathway** (Fig. 7–1). Immune complexes containing antibodies of either the IgG or IgM class induce the internal proteolysis of C1 and thereby convert the precursor form of C1 to an active enzyme, C$\overline{1}$.[6-8] The first component comprises three glycoprotein molecules, C1q, C1r, and C1s, held together in a calcium-dependent complex.[9] In normal human serum these three subunits are present in equimolar concentrations.[10] The C1q subunit contains the binding site for immunoglobulins, and the C1r and C1s subunits are proteases. In agreement with physical measurements indicating that the valence of C1q for IgG is 6, electron microscopic studies of C1q find a hexamer structure with six globular "heads" joined together by fibrillar "stalks" (Fig. 7–2).[7,11] The heads interact with immunoglobulin; and the "stalks," which resemble collagen in their content of repeating glycines, hydroxylated lysines and prolines, and glucosylgalactose disaccharide, bind to C1r and C1s.

**Table 7–1.** Physicochemical Characteristics of Proteins of the Complement System

| | Molecular Weight | Electrophoretic Mobility | Serum Concentration ($\mu$g/ml) | Cleavage Fragments |
|---|---|---|---|---|
| Classic activation pathway | | | | |
| C1q | 385,000 | $\gamma_2$ | 70 | |
| C1r | 190,000 | $\beta$ | 34 | |
| C1s | 174,000 | $\alpha_2$ | 31 | |
| C4 | 209,000 | $\beta_1$ | 430 | C4a, C4b, C4c, C4d |
| C2 | 117,000 | $\beta_2$ | 30 | C2a, C2b |
| Alternative activation pathway | | | | |
| Properdin | 220,000 | $\gamma_2$ | 25 | |
| $\overline{D}$ | 23,500 | $\alpha$ | 2 | |
| B | 100,000 | $\beta_2$ | 240 | Bb, Ba |
| C3 | 180,000 | $\beta_1$ | 1300 | C3a, C3b, C3c, C3d, C3g |
| Terminal sequence | | | | |
| C5 | 206,000 | $\beta_1$ | 75 | C5a, C5b |
| C6 | 128,000 | $\beta_2$ | 60 | |
| C7 | 121,000 | $\beta_2$ | 55 | |
| C8 | 153,000 | $\gamma$ | 80 | |
| C9 | 79,000 | $\alpha$ | 160 | |
| Combined proteins | | | | |
| C$\overline{1}$INH | 105,000 | $\alpha_2$ | 150 | |
| I | 88,000 | $\beta_2$ | 35 | |
| H | 150,000 | $\beta_1$ | 360 | |
| C4BP | 590,000 | $\beta_2$ | 400 | |

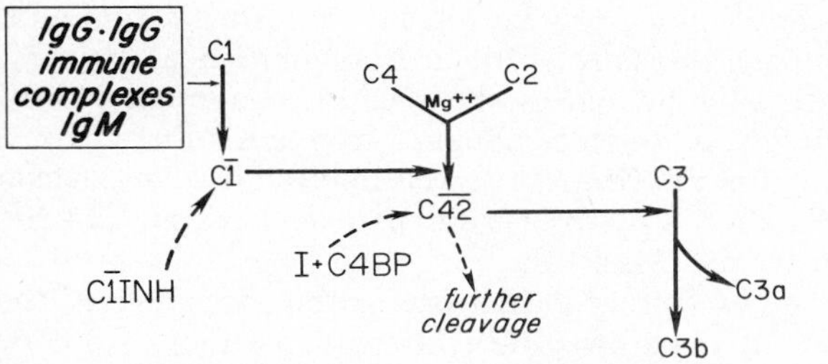


**Figure 7–1.** The classic pathway for complement activation.

C1q binds to immunoglobulins in the Fc region; $F(ab')_2$ fragments prepared by pepsin digestion do not interact with C1q (although they activate complement via the alternative pathway). Multivalent interaction of C1q with IgG is required for activation, since monomeric IgG has no effect, but IgG that has been aggregated either artificially or in an immune complex does activate. Complexes of polycations with polyanions such as protamine with heparin, or C polysaccharide with C-reactive protein are also capable of binding C1q and activating C1.[12]

C1r and C1s are both serine proteases with very similar structures and mechanisms of action. Both are non-covalently linked dimers of two identical polypeptide chains.[13,14] C1r binds to C1q in the presence of calcium and forms a physical link between C1q and C1s. During activation both polypeptide chains of C1r and C1s are cleaved one third of the way from the N-terminus, and the resulting two pieces of each chain remain linked by disulfide bonds. The active proteolytic sites on both molecules are on the lighter of the two pieces, as judged by the binding of diisopropylfluorophosphidate, which reacts with a serine in the active site and blocks further enzymatic activity. Amino acid sequences of peptides containing the reactive serine residue in C1s are closely homologous with those in C1r as well with other serine

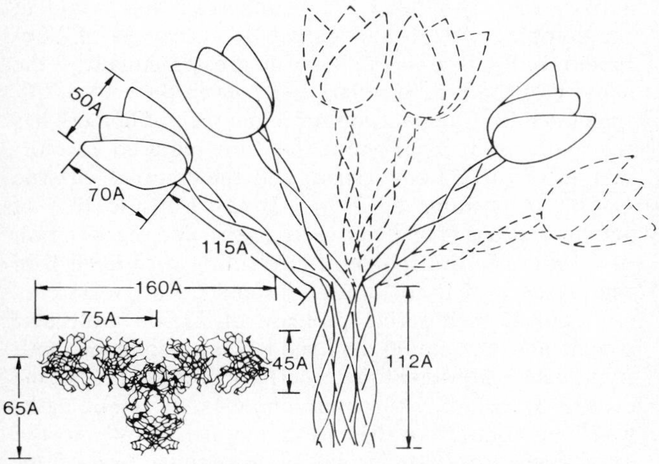


**Figure 7–2.** Comparison of the C1q model proposed by Reid and Porter with the three-dimensional structure of an IgG protein as determined by x-ray crystallography. (Courtesy of Dr. Manuel Navia, National Institutes of Health.)

proteases such as trypsin, thrombin, plasmin, and factor $\overline{D}$.[7] Activation involves the apposition of one chain of the C1r protease to the other chain and internal proteolysis. Subsequent cleavage of C1s by C1r is highly specific; thus far no other protein substrates for this protease have been found.

The fourth component is a glycoprotein of 209,000 molecular weight composed of three polypeptide chains of 90,000, 80,000 and 30,000 each.[15] C1s, whether bound to immune complexes in intact C$\overline{1}$ or free in solution, cleaves a peptide bond in the $\alpha$-chain, releasing a 6000 molecular weight activation peptide, C4a. The remaining fragment, C4b, is transiently able to bind covalently to immune complexes or other acceptors. Another more stable site on the C4b molecule allows its interaction in a magnesium-dependent complex with C2a.[8] A third site binds C4b to complement receptors on a variety of cell types.[16]

The presence of C4b greatly enhances the rate at which C$\overline{1s}$ cleaves its other natural substrate, C2.[17] This component, a glycoprotein of 117,000 molecular weight, is split into a catalytically active fragment, C2a, of 85,000 molecular weight and an activation peptide, C2b, of 35,000 molecular weight.[18] C2a becomes incorporated in a magnesium-dependent complex with C4b, forming C$\overline{42}$, the classic pathway C3 convertase. C$\overline{42}$ is unstable: At 37° C it decays with a half-life of a few minutes, losing C3 convertase activity and leaving C4b, which is capable of regenerating active C$\overline{42}$ in the presence of fresh C2. A glycoprotein in the membranes of human erythrocytes accelerates this decay rate.[19]

***Inhibition of C$\overline{1}$.*** Normal serum contains an $\alpha$-2 neuraminoglycoprotein of 105,000 molecular weight that forms an equimolar complex with both C$\overline{1s}$ and C$\overline{1r}$, irreversibly blocking the activities of these proteases and preventing activation of C1s or cleavage of C4 and C2.[20-22] This C$\overline{1}$ inhibitor functions as a "false substrate," entering the active site of the protease, forming an acyl intermediate, but then failing to be cleaved and to dissociate out of the active site. Direct binding studies have shown that the interaction between C$\overline{1s}$ and C$\overline{1}$INH occurs on the light peptide chain of C$\overline{1s}$, which contains the active proteolytic site. The complex thus formed is stable under conditions that normally dissociate non-covalent bonds.[22] C$\overline{1}$INH also inhibits the activity of kallikrein in the kinin-forming system, factor XI of the intrinsic clotting pathway, plasmin of the fibrinolytic pathway, and activated Hageman factor or its fragments. Plasmin cleaves C$\overline{1}$INH, producing lower molecular weight fragments, which retain the ability to interact with C$\overline{1s}$.[22] Individuals with congenital partial deficiency of C$\overline{1}$INH experience unopposed spontaneous activation of C1 with consequent hypercatabolism of C4 and C2; clinically, they have the syndrome of hereditary angioedema (Chapter 85).[23]

***Degradation of C4b.*** Control of the assembly of active C$\overline{42}$ is effected by the further cleavage of C4b into two inactive fragments, C4c and C4d, with molecular weights of approximately 150,000 and 47,000, respectively. This is the result of the cooperative effect of two plasma proteins: the C4 binding protein (C4BP)[24] and the C3b inactivator (I).[25] C4BP is a glycoprotein that consists of six to eight identical subunits of 70,000 daltons linked by disulfide bridges. Binding of C4b to C4BP renders it susceptible to attack by I. Proteolysis at two points in the $\alpha$-chain of C4b yields three peptides with molecular weights of 47,000, 25,000, and 17,000. The first of these is C4d, which is released from the molecule; the other two remain bridged by disulfide linkages to the intact $\beta$- and $\gamma$-chains in the form of C4c. In the case of C4b bound to complexes, C4c is released into the fluid phase, indicating that the site by which C4b binds covalently is located on the C4d portion of the $\alpha$-chain. C4b that has been degraded by I in the presence of C4BP is incapable of interacting with C2 to form active $\mathrm{C\overline{42}}$. Complexes bearing only C4d on their surfaces do not react in immune adherence with C4b receptors present on human erythrocytes or leukocytes.[26]

**The Alternative Pathway: Activation and Amplification** (Fig. 7–3). The addition of polysaccharides such as yeast cell wall zymosan or gram-negative bacterial endotoxin to the serum of animals congenitally deficient in either C4 or C2 leads to cleavage of C3 and assembly of the membrane attack complex by a mechanism that is independent of the classic activation pathway. The reaction sequence resembles that of the classic pathway, with factor $\overline{\mathrm{D}}$ functioning as the homologous protein for $\mathrm{C\overline{1s}}$, C3 for C4, and factor B for C2. An extra protein, properdin, serves to stablilize the magnesium-dependent complex enzyme C3 convertase, $\mathrm{\overline{C3bBb}}$, which like its classic homologue, $\mathrm{C\overline{42}}$, decays rapidly at 37° C. Like the classic pathway, activation of the alternative pathway produces an enzyme that cleaves C3 and C5 and initiates the terminal sequence.

A pathway for C3 inactivation that was independent of antibody and the early classic components was attributed to a single isolatable nonspecific substance termed "properdin."[27] This material was thought to be involved in numerous biologic systems, including the killing of gram-negative bacteria, the neutralization of certain viruses, the lysis of erythrocytes in paroxysmal nocturnal hemoglobinuria, and protection against the lethal effects of whole-body radiation.[28] As evidence for specificity of the system appeared, and its effects were reproduced by small amounts of antibody and the early complement components,[29] the entire properdin system was discredited. The important report that properdin was a unique protein present in normal serum and immunochemically distinct from immunoglobulin[30] was virtually ignored by the scientific community. Only the weight of evidence obtained from a number of converging lines of research served to establish the existence of the alternative (properdin) pathway separate and distinct from the classic one.

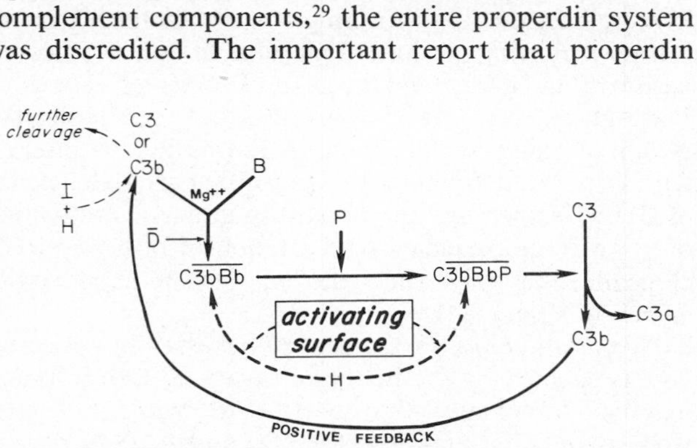


**Figure 7–3.** The alternative pathway for complement activation.

Four factors participate in the formation of the alternative pathway C3 convertase. Of these, C3 is by far the most important, since it serves as a link between the classic, alternative, and terminal pathways and is involved in the positive feedback or amplification loop. C3 is a glycoprotein composed of two polypeptide chains of 115,000 and 75,000 molecular weight linked by disulfide bridges.[31] With a plasma concentration of 1 mg per ml, it is also the most plentiful of the complement proteins. Cleavage of the $\alpha$-chain of C3 at arginine 77 by either the classic or alternative pathway C3 convertases releases an 8000 molecular weight activation peptide, C3a, and exposes a labile internal thioester bond on the $\alpha$-chain formed between the gamma carboxyl group of a glutamic acid residue and the thiol group on a neighboring cysteine. The resulting activated carbonyl on the major fragment, C3b, forms covalent ester or amide linkages with appropriate acceptors, such as sugar residues on polysaccharides or immunoglobulin oligosaccharides.[32] As in the case of C4b, failure to react promptly with an appropriate acceptor surface results in irreversible inactivation of the C3b in the fluid phase, presumably by reaction of the carbonyl group with water. Just as cleavage of C4 to C4b reveals a stable site for interaction with C2, cleavage of C3 to C3b permits C3b to develop the ability to participate in a magnesium-dependent complex with factor B.[33-36]

Factor B is the alternative pathway homologue of C2. Linkage studies locate C2 and B in the major histocompatibility complex in such close proximity that gene duplication is virtually certain.[37] B is a single polypeptide chain of 102,000 molecular weight. The catalytic site of B is present on the native form as judged by its esterase activity and by weak C3 convertase activity found in the complex of C3b and native B.[38] Cleavage of C3b-bound B by $\overline{\mathrm{D}}$ to form $\mathrm{\overline{C3bBb}}$ greatly enhances the activity of the B-derived enzyme.[39] As in the case of C2, the major Bb fragment, of molecular weight 65,000, has the active site; magnesium ions are required for formation of the C3 convertase; and the complex enzyme $\mathrm{\overline{C3bBb}}$ is unstable at 37° C. Decay leads to loss of activity, release of an inactive fragment, and regeneration of C3b in a form capable of interacting with fresh B in the presence of $\overline{\mathrm{D}}$ to form additional C3 convertase.

Factor $\overline{\mathrm{D}}$ is a serine protease of 23,500 molecular weight and has amino acid sequence homologies, both in the active site and at the N-terminus, with other serine proteases, including thrombin and C1s, its classic pathway homologue.[40] In the case of factor $\overline{\mathrm{D}}$, however, the enzyme already exists in plasma in its active form. Control of proteolysis is exerted by the limited availability of substrate: $\overline{\mathrm{D}}$ acts only on B that has complexed with C3b, and not on free or unbound B.[41]

Properdin is not required for alternative pathway activation, but it increases the efficiency of the other proteins in the system. Properdin is a 220,000 molecular weight gamma globulin consisting of four identical subunits of 53,000 each.[42,43] In free solution it binds to polymeric C3b. Interaction of properdin with surface-bound C3b probably involves more than one molecule of C3b in close proximity.[44] Following binding, there occurs a reversible conformational change from native P to an activated form, which binds much more avidly to C3.[45] The function of properdin appears to be that of stabilizing the $\overline{C3bBb}$ interaction; a dose-dependent increase in the half-life of this enzyme occurs upon the introduction of properdin.[46]

An autoantibody with specificity for antigenic determinants unique to the assembled alternative pathway C3 convertase ($\overline{C3bBb}$) appears in the serum of patients with membranoproliferative glomerulonephritis and mimics the action of properdin.[47-49] The immunoglobulin nature of C3 nephritic factor (C2NeF) was confirmed when a mother with nephritis and C3NeF in her plasma gave birth to an infant with C3NeF in his plasma as well.[50] Like properdin, C3NeF functions by binding to the $\overline{C3bBb}$ enzyme and stabilizing it.[51] Although C3NeFs may be of any IgG subclass and either light chain type, and are usually heterogeneous in these attributes,[52] some C3NeF proteins have restricted heterogeneity and abnormal heavy chains.[53] Like properdin, C3NeF greatly increases the efficiency of the alternative pathway proteins, and it is not absolutely required for alternative pathway activation.

***Control Proteins of the Alternative Pathway.*** Agents that trigger the alternative pathway do so by protecting the newly formed $\overline{C3bBb}$ enzyme from dissociation and degradation by the control proteins, H and I. Activators shift the proteolytic activity from the fluid phase to the solid state and accelerate the assembly of the particle-bound C3 and C5 convertases. Factor I was initially recognized by its ability to inhibit the reactivity of C3b-coated erythrocytes with cells bearing receptors for them in the immune adherence phenomenon.[54] Subsequently, the proteolytic activity of I for C3b was identified, and cleavage of C3b into C3c and C3d was recognized.[55] Later studies have shown that the degradation of C3b occurs in several steps and involves the action of other proteins in addition to I.

The first protein shown to cooperate in the inactivation of C3b was Factor H, a 150,000 molecular weight glycoprotein that physically binds to C3b and thereby greatly increases its susceptibility to cleavage by I.[56-58] H is required for the cleavage of fluid phase C3b by I,[59] but surface-bound C3b is susceptible to slow digestion by I alone.[57] The first cleavage of the $\alpha'$-chain of C3b by factor I results in $NH_2$-terminal 68,000-dalton and COOH-terminal 46,000-dalton peptides. A second cleavage releases a 3000-dalton peptide from the 46,000-dalton fragment.[60] The product C3bi consists of the two major $\alpha$-chain fragments, which remain disulfide-bonded to the intact $\beta$-chain. It has no activity in binding to C3b receptors on human erythrocytes but does adhere to C3bi receptors on the surfaces of glomerular epithelial cells and certain leukocytes.[61] C3bi has no activity in continuing the cytolytic sequence by modifying the C3 convertases so that they can attack C5, nor can it complex with B to form an alternative pathway convertase.

The third cleavage of the $\alpha'$-chain of C3bi occurs at a site 27,000 daltons from the amino terminus and yields C3c (140,000 daltons) and C3dg (40,000 daltons).[60] The latter fragment contains the thioester region by which C3b is covalently linked to acceptors, so that if acceptor-bound C3bi is being cleaved, C3dg remains bound and C3c is released into the fluid phase. The cofactor for factor I in production of C3c and C3dg is the C3b receptor present on the surface of human erythrocytes.[62] Elastase purified from human polymorphonuclear leukocytes is active at nanogram concentrations and also fragments the $\alpha'$-chain of C3b.[63]

In addition to its ability to enhance the rate at which I digests C3b, H physically binds to C3b, competes with B for binding to C3b, and accelerates decay of the $\overline{C3bBb}$ and $\overline{C3bBbP}$ enzymes.[64] Once the B has been stripped from the complex by accelerated decay-dissociation induced by H, the C3b becomes available for cleavage by I. As will be seen below, the "activating" capacity of polysaccharides and certain cell membranes reflects the extent to which they provide a microenvironment that protects the complexed $\overline{C3bBb}$ from this action of H.

***Mechanism of Activation: Solid-State Amplification.*** Since a role for immunoglobulins as an enhancing factor is demonstrable for activation of the alternative pathway under certain circumstances, and activation by polysaccharides clearly occurs independently of antibody, it is likely that there is more than one set of events leading to such activation. Activating agents increase the formation of alternative pathway convertase by transforming an inefficient fluid phase reaction into a fruitful solid-state assembly of the enzyme complex. In the fluid phase a small amount of C3 is continuously being hydrolyzed at its internal thioester bond, permitting B to complex with it and become susceptible to cleavage by $\overline{D}$.[65] This generates small amounts of C3 convertase and produces small amounts of C3b. In the fluid phase, these small amounts of C3b are effectively controlled by I and H before the C3b fragment can cycle through the positive feedback loop and result in the amplification phase whereby a product of C3 cleavage induces the formation of more C3-cleaving enzyme. Surfaces that activate the alternative pathway provide a haven for the small amount of C3b produced by the fluid phase reactions, where it can be deposited and be protected from the action of the control proteins. Such surface-bound C3b is, however, capable of interacting with B in the presence of $\overline{D}$ to form $\overline{C3bBb}$ and with properdin to form $\overline{C3bBbP}$, both of which are also protected from the control proteins. The slow fluid phase reaction is thus shifted to an amplified solid state cleavage. "Activators" thus exist in name only; initiation is a spontaneous event occurring continuously in the fluid phase. The "activating" surfaces might better be termed "protectors," since their function appears to be one of affording a microenvironment in which C3b and complex enzymes containing C3b are protected from inactivation by I and decay dissociation by H.[66]

At least one chemical characteristic of the protecting surface has been identified: sialic acid content.[67,68] Cells that do not normally provide surfaces for alternative pathway amplification acquire this capacity after membrane sialic acid residues have been removed by treatment with sialidase or modified by chemical treatment. Among inbred strains of mice, there is an inverse relationship between the capacity to activate the human alternative complement pathway and membrane sialic acid content.[69] Comparative binding studies with radiolabeled B and H indicate that these two proteins compete for a single binding site on C3b. Decreases in sialic acid content do not affect the ability of B to bind to C3b located on the particle surface, but they greatly reduce the number and affinity of C3b sites available for binding and inhibition by H.

## THE TERMINAL SEQUENCE (Fig. 7–4)

Cleavage of additional C3 by either the C$\overline{42}$ or C$\overline{3bBb}$ convertases results in the development of C5 convertase activity. While the C3b was once thought to be incorporated into the enzyme complex, thereby modifying its substrate specificity, more recent data indicate that C3b provides a binding site for native C5 and makes it susceptible to the action of the convertase.[70] Only surface-bound C3b functions to promote C5 cleavage, and the C3b molecule that is involved in C5 binding and subsequent cleavage must be free of other ligands such as B, P, or H. In the case of the alternative pathway, therefore, this means that at least two molecules of C3b are involved in C5 cleavage: one to interact with B and form the cleaving enzyme and another to interact with C5 and support the cleavage reaction.[71]

C5 is remarkably similar both in structure and reaction mechanism to C3.[72] It is a $\beta$-glycoprotein of 206,000 molecular weight, consisting of two nonidentical peptide chains of 80,000 and 130,000 daltons. Cleavage

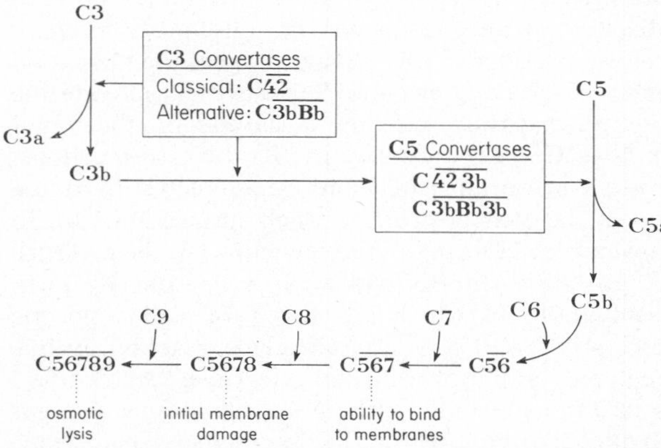


**Figure 7–4.** The terminal sequence leading to membrane damage.

of C5 by its convertase occurs at an argininyl-leucine bond between residues 74 and 75 on the $\alpha$-chain (versus arginine 77 for C3 cleavage), releasing an 11,000-dalton peptide, C5a.[73] C5a and C3a, which represent the N-terminal ends of the $\alpha$-chains of the corresponding parent molecules, have extensive sequence homology, including the conservation of three disulfide bridges,[72] and nearly equal contents of regular secondary structure as judged by circular dichroism studies. A major difference is the carbohydrate (25 percent) present in C5a but not in C3a.[73]

Both C6 and C7 are single polypeptide chains, with molecular weights of 128,000 and 121,000 daltons, respectively, and both have identical electrophoretic mobilities.[74] Both show genetic polymorphism, and the loci for these are closely linked.[75] An individual with combined deficiency of C6 and C7 has been found, and inheritance of these two deficiencies within his family behaves as a single genetic characteristic.[76] It seems likely that C6 and C7 are, like C2 and B, products of tandem gene duplication.

C8 has an unusual structure: It contains three polypeptide chains of 77,000, 63,000, and 13,700 daltons, termed $\alpha$, $\beta$, and $\gamma$. These subunits occur as a disulfide-linked $\alpha$-$\gamma$ dimer which is noncovalently associated with $\beta$. Interaction of C8 with C5b-7 complexes is mediated through $\beta$, whereas interaction with the membrane bilayer occurs primarily through the $\alpha$-chain of $\alpha$-$\gamma$. Failure of the $\alpha$-chain to label with radioactive iodine suggests that it may be relatively hydrophobic and sequestered within the interior of the molecule, a formulation that is attractive in view of the function of C8 within the C5-9 cytolytic complex.[77] The last component to react, C9, is an $\alpha$-globulin of 79,000 molecular weight.

**Assembly of the Membrane-Damaging C5b-9 Complex.** Activated C5b has a specific metastable binding site for C6, as well as exposed hydrophobic sites. It combines with C6 in a reversible complex[78,79] to form C56, which reacts with C7. The product is the highly labile C5b,6,7 complex, which, if generated in the fluid phase, is capable of reacting with lipid membranes in its immediate vicinity. If the interaction occurs between C7 and C5b,6 bound to a cell membrane (favored by interaction of C5b with binding sites provided by C3b), more efficient binding of the C5b,6,7 complex to the target membrane occurs. In either case, binding of the C5b,6,7 complex to the membrane is the first step in assembling the membrane attack complex. It has been shown to occur on the membranes of bacteria and nucleated cells as well as on the sheep erythrocytes usually used in model systems. Even liposomes, synthetic vesicles prepared from mixtures of phospholipid and cholesterol, have been shown to bind C5b,6,7. Reaction with C8 initiates membrane damage, and C5b-8 complexes have been shown to penetrate membranes of about 6 nm thickness.[80] A stable transmembrane channel is formed by the addition of multiple molecules of C9, possibly in polymeric form, to the complex. Evidence obtained from enzymatic stripping experiments, from studies of planar lipid concentration, from electron microscopy, and from the structure of the C5b-9 complex itself supports the notion that the complex forms a tunnel or channel inserted through the lipid bilayer, with hydrophobic residues on the exterior in contact with the lipid bilayer and a hydrophilic interior allowing the passage of ions and water.[81-84] The loss of control over ion flux dooms the cell to the imbibition of water from isosmotic media with eventual swelling and rupture of the cell.

## BIOLOGIC CONSEQUENCES OF COMPLEMENT ACTIVATION (Table 7–2)

Although assembly of the C5b-9 complex and membrane damage is the most well known effect of complement activation, a variety of other inflammatory events also ensue. Changes in vascular permeability have been attributed to the cleavage of C4 and C2 by $\overline{\text{C1}}$ and may explain the pathogenesis of the angioedema associated with $\overline{\text{C1}}$INH deficiency,[85] but the peptide(s) responsible for inducing the permeability change have not yet been fully characterized, and even the existence of a kinin-like fragment derived from C2 is in doubt.[86] Biologic activities have been identified for products of the alternative activation pathway. Specifically, the active enzyme $\overline{\text{C3bBb}}$ is chemotactic for polymorphonuclear neutrophils.[87] The Bb fragment of factor B induces rapid spreading and increase in surface area of unstimulated

**Table 7–2.** Biologic Activities of the Products of Complement Activation

| Product | Activity |
|---|---|
| C4, C2 kinin | Increase in vascular permeability; putative mediator of edema in hereditary angioedema |
| $\overline{\text{C3bBb}}$ | Chemotaxis of polymorphonuclear leukocytes |
| Bb | Spreading of monocytes |
| C3a | Anaphylatoxin; releases histamine from basophils and mast cells, serotonin from platelets, possibly direct cytotoxic effect, possibly chemotactic, suppresses lymphocytes |
| C5a | Anaphylatoxin; same activities as C3a on mast cells, marked chemotactic effect for monocytes and polymorphonuclear leukocytes |
| C3b | Multiple effects, depending on cell-bearing receptor: phagocytosis enhancement, triggers cycling of alternative pathway amplification loop (Fig. 7–3) |
| C3bi | Binding to glomerular, monocyte complement receptors |
| C3d | Binding to lymphocyte complement receptors |
| $\overline{\text{C567}}$ | Active complex capable of binding to "innocent bystander" cell membranes and initiating formation of C5b-9 |
| C5b-9 | Membrane attack complex: forms transmembrane channels leading to cytolysis |

peritoneal macrophages[88] and inhibits their migration in the capillary tube assay used to measure macrophage migration inhibitory factor.[89] The enzymatic site on Bb is required for these activities, since they are inhibited by chemicals or monoclonal antibodies that react with the active site. Since macrophages can synthesize C3, factor B and factor $\overline{\text{D}}$,[90] the relation of these factors to migration inhibition observed following antigen stimulation of mixed mononuclear cells requires further investigation.

The activation peptides C3a and C5a are anaphylatoxins capable of inducing the secretion of histamine by mast cells and basophils.[91-93] The degranulating effects on skin mast cells are observable at a concentration of $10^{-12}$ and $10^{-15}$ M for C3a and C5a, respectively. Both peptides also possess some smooth muscle contractile activity that is independent of histamine release. The anaphylatoxic activities are blocked by scission of the terminal arginine from either C3a or C5a by carboxypeptidase N, a magnesium-dependent enzyme, which also has been termed the anaphylatoxin inactivator.[94]

C5a is responsible for most of the chemotactic activity in plasma after activation of the complement system.[95] It attracts neutrophils, eosinophils, and monocytes and also releases lysosomal enzymes of polymorphonuclear neutrophils into phagocytic vacuoles or the surrounding medium.[96] Aggregation of granulocytes is observable after exposure to C5a.[97] Unlike the anaphylatoxic activity, which requires the terminal arginine, these other activities of C5a persist following its removal, so that $C5a_{des\ arg}$ is fully chemotactic.[98] C3a does not appear to have chemotactic activity,[99] but C3e, a polypeptide derived from the α-chain of C3, produces an initial leukopenia followed by a leukocytosis.[100] C3e also causes release of leukocytes from the perfused rat femur and has been termed leukocyte-mobilizing factor.[101]

The fragment C3b has several different biologic activities, specified by the type of cell bearing the C3b receptor to which it binds. Perhaps the most important of these, judging from the clinical features of C3 deficiency in which sepsis with pyogenic organisms is prominent,[102] is the enhancement of phagocytosis by polymorphonuclear neutrophils and monocytes. Binding of C3b-coated immune complexes to polymorphonuclear leukocytes enhances phagocytosis of the complexes by these cells, provided the complexes contain IgG antibody that interacts with the Fc receptors also present on the polys; C3b by itself promotes adherence but not ingestion. A marked synergy between the effects of IgG and C3b on phagocytosis has been demonstrated.[103] In contrast, "activated" macrophages elicited by intraperitoneal injection of thioglycollate or bacterial endotoxin or by antigen in the sensitized animal both bind *and* ingest complexes coated only with C3b; unstimulated monocytes are not active in this regard and require IgG, as do neutrophils.[104] Receptors for both C3b and for C3bi are present in the renal glomerulus and on the Kupffer cells of the hepatic sinusoids.[105,106] Receptors for C3d are present on some human lymphocytes and lymphoblastoid cell lines.[106,107] Although a close association between the presence of C3d receptors and receptors for the Epstein-Barr virus was described,[108] this was found to be due to co-selection of the two receptors, and they are separate and distinct entities.[109]

Although the existence of C3bi or C3d receptors on monocytes or B lymphocytes has been known for a long time, the functional significance of these receptors remains incompletely understood. Interpretation of some experiments may be confused by the capacity of these cells to synthesize C3 and other complement proteins during the course of the culture experiment. C3 has been implicated in such functions as lymphokine production,[110] lymphocyte proliferation,[111] and prostaglandin release from monocytes.[112] In vivo, depletion of C3 prevents the development of a primary antibody response to T-dependent antigens[113] but not a secondary response. The failure of this response and the generation of B memory cells have been attributed to the role of activated C3 in binding antigen-containing complexes to dendritic antigen-processing cells in the lymphoid follicle. In the absence of C3 there is a failure of normal interaction between the antigen-processing cells and virgin B lymphocytes.[114] Experiments demonstrating that the lymphocyte response to antigens or mitogens is inhibited by other fragments of C3 may indicate direct effects on lymphocytes as well.[115]

## METABOLISM OF COMPLEMENT PROTEINS

In vitro culture studies have detected synthesis of C4, C2,[116] C3, B, D, and P by peritoneal macrophages[90] and synthesis of C3, C5, and C9 by hepatoma cells.[116] By contrast, in vivo studies have tended to identify the liver as the primary, if not sole, source of synthesis. Patients with severe hepatic failure have marked depressions of the serum levels of C4 and C3, and impaired synthesis of C3 has been measured directly in metabolic turnover studies.[117] Following hepatic allografting, the electrophoretic polymorphic types of C3 and C6 change from that of the recipient to those of the donor.[118] Although immunofluorescent studies indicate synthesis of C3 by hepatic parenchymal cells, examination of inflammatory synovium from rheumatoid arthritis identifies cells in this tissue that appear to be synthesizing C3.[119] Explants of inflamed rheumatoid synovial tissue incorporate $^{14}C$-amino acids into complement protein.[119] Such complement synthesis during immune inflammation may be induced by the lymphokine, monocyte complement stimulator. This substance, produced by sensitized T lymphocytes when exposed to antigen, stimulates the synthesis of C2 by human peripheral blood monocytes.[120]

Measurements of the fractional catabolic rates of C4, C3, C5, and B from the turnover of purified and radiolabeled proteins indicate that complement proteins are among the most rapidly metabolized of all plasma proteins.[121] The mean fractional catabolic rates in normals are in the range of 50 percent of the plasma pool per 24 hours. Synthetic rates are significantly correlated with serum levels, indicating that in normal individuals the rate of synthesis is the major determinant of plasma concentration. Considering the highly positive correlation between levels of C3, B, and P and those of the two proteins that control their interaction, I and H,[122] it is possible that normal catabolism of the alternative pathway proteins is accounted for by their participation in continuous low level activation of the pathway, much as the catabolic route of fibrinogen may involve normal in vivo activation of the coagulation sequence.

Biosynthetic studies in cell-free systems indicate that both C4 and C3 are synthesized as single polypeptide chains and post-translationally cleaved into the three and two polypeptide chains, respectively, in which they appear in plasma.[123,124] Small amounts of the single chain precursor molecules may be found in normal plasma.[125] Genomic clones coding for the major portions of C3, C4, and factor B have been isolated and partly sequenced (Chapter 85).

## CLINICAL SIGNIFICANCE OF COMPLEMENT MEASUREMENTS

**Methods of Measurement.** Since the complement proteins have hemolytic activity, assays based on the ability of a test specimen to lyse cells afford a sensitive assay technique. The traditional method for the determination of complement in serum or other body fluids measures the ability of the test specimen to lyse 50 percent of a standard suspension of sheep erythrocytes coated with rabbit antibody in a reaction that includes the entire classic reaction sequence.[126] This test, the "CH50" (for "complement hemolytic 50 percent") is widely available and has been in use for more than 30 years, so that it has the advantage that many of the observations relating complement levels to human disease are based on it. The CH50 continues to be a useful screening procedure, particularly when deficiency states are suspected or when the measurement is performed on a body fluid, e.g., synovial or pleural fluid, where failure of normal clearance mechanisms may have allowed the persistence of hemolytically inactive but immunoreactive complement protein. Specific hemolytic assays for each of the classic and alternative pathways and the terminal sequence are available, but their difficulty of performance has restricted them to the research laboratory.[127]

Concentrations of complement proteins may also be measured by their reactivities in immunoassays based on reaction with antibody specific for the protein in question.[128] These are the most inexpensive and widely available of assays because materials required for their performance are offered by commercial suppliers in the form of kits for use in the clinical pathology laboratory. Physicians interpreting the results of tests should keep in mind the following caveats:

1. Under the best conditions, the coefficient of variation of immunoassays such as the commonly available

radial immunodiffusion is likely to be of the order of 8 percent, well above that which applies to most other results obtained from the clinical pathology laboratory.

2. There are no agreed-upon international standards, so that considerable variation in absolute values obtained by kits from different suppliers or even in lots of kits from the same supplier may be observed. The clinical pathology laboratory must maintain independent checks of the "range of normal" and of the lot-to-lot variation rather than uncritically accepting the standards and normal ranges provided by the supplier. This "normal range" should be provided with the test result.

3. As is the case for other plasma proteins, the range of normal for complement proteins is quite broad, often of the order of ± 50 percent of the mean value for the population. Thus, serial changes in levels for a given patient over a period of time may often be more informative than comparison with an absolute range of normal. Furthermore, since plasma levels of many of the complement proteins tend to rise during acute inflammation, a "normal" value may actually reflect a marked fall from a previous level and indicate an active disease process. A striking example of this occurs in systemic lupus erythematosus, in which levels of C9 in patients with relatively quiescent disease are two to three times the normal mean; with activity, levels fall dramatically by 50 or 75 percent—into the "normal" range.[129]

4. The most widely available test for a complement component (C3) is not necessarily the most useful. Because C3 is the most plentiful of the complement components, it was the first to be purified and measured in immunoassays. Measurements of C4 are more sensitive to minor episodes of in vivo complement activation. Most workers agree that a useful routine complement screen includes measurements of C4 and C3 by immunoassay and total hemolytic activity by CH50.

**Interpretation of Complement Abnormalities.** As a consequence of their participation in complement activation, the complement proteins become recognizable as "altered" and are rapidly cleared from the plasma space.[130] Clearance from extravascular spaces such as pleural, synovial, or cerebrospinal proceeds more slowly.[131] Although some compensatory increases in synthesis may occur, the result is usually a fall in the plasma level of one or more of the complement proteins. In reverse fashion, as the complement-activating stimulus or disease abates, there may be a parallel return of the complement level toward normal. Virtually any disease that gives rise to circulating immune complexes may result in hypocomplementia, provided the complexes contain IgG or IgM antibodies capable of activating complement. A list of such diseases is contained in Table 7–3. In systemic lupus erythematosus, complement depressions are associated with increased severity of disease, and particularly with renal involvement.[132] Serial observations have revealed decreased levels in advance of clinical exacerbations; reductions in C4 usually precede those of C3 or CH50.[129] As attacks subside, levels return toward normal in reverse order. Discoid lupus or drug-induced lupus is not ordinarily associated with hypocomplementemia.

**Table 7–3.** Hypocomplementemic States

| |
|---|
| Hyposynthesis |
| Congenital deficiencies (see Chapter 85) |
| Severe hepatic failure |
| Severe malnutrition |
| Glomerulonephritis* |
| Systemic lupus erythematosus* |
| Hypercatabolism |
| Deficiency of control proteins |
| $C\bar{1}$ inhibitor deficiency: Hereditary angioedema |
| C3b inactivator deficiency |
| Rheumatic diseases with immune complexes |
| Systemic lupus erythematosus |
| Rheumatoid arthritis (with extra-articular disease) |
| Systemic vasculitis |
| Essential mixed cryoglobulinemia |
| Infectious diseases |
| Subacute bacterial endocarditis |
| Infected atrioventricular shunts |
| Pneumococcal sepsis |
| Gram-negative sepsis |
| Viremias, e.g., hepatitis B surface antigenemia, measles, dengue |
| Parasitemias, e.g., trypanosomiasis, malaria, babesiosis |
| Glomerulonephritis |
| Post-streptococcal |
| Membranoproliferative |
| Idiopathic proliferative or focal sclerosing |

*Usually associated with simultaneous and marked hypercatabolism.

Any cause of chronic antigenemia is likely to be associated with acquired hypocomplementemia, including, for example, subacute bacterial endocarditis,[133] hepatitis B surface antigenemia,[134] pneumococcal infections,[135] gram-negative sepsis,[136] viremias such as measles,[137] or recurrent parasitemias such as malaria.[138] Other diseases of unknown etiology may be associated with hypocomplementemia, such as essential mixed cryoglobulinemia[139] or certain kinds of nephritis.[140] In contrast to all the diseases mentioned previously, which usually have evidences of classic pathway activation such as low C4, type II membranoproliferative glomerulonephritis patients usually have only low C3, indicating direct activation of the alternative pathway, perhaps as a consequence of circulating C3NeF, which stabilizes the $\overline{C3bBb}$ enzymes and favors positive feedback into the amplification loop[141] (Fig. 7–3).

Inactive complement fragments may persist in joint or pleural spaces, so that radial immunodiffusion determinations of C3 or C4 in synovial or pleural fluid detect only spent fragments. Functional assays such as CH50 are required to detect evidence of local complement activation in diseases such as rheumatoid arthritis.[142,143] Although one report has indicated that depressed levels of C4 in cerebrospinal fluid correlated with central nervous system involvement,[144] another study has failed to confirm these findings, except in patients from whom serial specimens of cerebrospinal fluid are analyzed in a prospective fashion.[145]

Serum complement levels are elevated in rheumatoid arthritis, except in patients with systemic rheumatoid vasculitis, which usually is accompanied by a high titer of rheumatoid factor and the clinical finding of multiple subcutaneous nodules. Synovial fluid levels are frequently profoundly depressed, especially in patients with positive tests for rheumatoid factor.[142,143] Although both functional and immunodiffusion tests have demonstrated depressions of C1 in some patients and marked reductions in C4 and C2 in most, immunodiffusion results may not be reliable, because they detect complement protein that has already participated in an ongoing in vivo complement activation process but that has not yet been cleared from the joint space. An additional source of confusion arises from the local synthesis of complement proteins occurring in or near the joint space.[119] Thus, the abundant evidence for intra-articular activation of the complement system in rheumatoid arthritis is helpful in understanding the pathogenesis of the disease process, but it is rarely of value as a discriminating diagnostic test.

## References

1. Atkinson, J.P., and Frank, M.M.: Complement. In Parker, C.W. (ed.): Clinical Immunology. Philadelphia, W.B. Saunders Co., 1980. p. 219.
2. Ruddy, S., Gigli, I., and Austen, K.F.: The complement system of man. N. Engl. J. Med. 287:489, 545, 592, 642, 1972.
3. Mayer, M.M.: The complement system. Sci. Am. 229:54, 1973.
4. Müller-Eberhard, H.I.: Chemistry and function of the complement system. Hosp. Pract. 12:33, 1978.
5. Colten, H.R., and Goldberger, G.: Ontogeny of serum complement proteins. Pediatrics 64(5 Pt. 2 Suppl.):775, 1979.
6. Reid, K.B., and Porter, R.R.: The proteolytic activation systems of complement. Ann. Rev. Biochem. 50:433, 1981.
7. Porter, R.R.: The Croonian Lecture, 1980. The complex proteases of the complement system. Proc. R. Soc. Lond. (Biol.) 210:477, 1980.
8. Kerr, M.A.: The human complement system: Assembly of the classical pathway C3 convertase. Biochem. J. 189:173, 1980.
9. Ziccardi, R.J.: Nature of the metal ion requirement for assembly and function of the first component of human complement. J. Biol. Chem. 258:6187, 1983.
10. Ziccardi, R.J., and Cooper, N.R.: The subunit composition and sedimentation properties of human C1. J. Immunol. 118:2047, 1977.
11. Knobel, H.R., Villiger, W., and Isliker, H.: Chemical analysis and electron microscopy studies of human C1q prepared by different methods. Eur. J. Immunol. 5:78, 1975.
12. Claus, D.R., Siegel, J., Petras, K., Skor, D., Osmand, A.P., and Gewurz, H.: Complement activation by interaction of polyanions and polycations. III. Complement activation by interaction of multiple polyanions and polycations in the presence of C-reactive protein. J. Immunol. 118:83, 1977.
13. Valet, G., and Cooper, N.R.: Isolation and characterization of the proenzyme form of the C1s subunit of the first complement component. J. Immunol. 112:339, 1974.
14. Ziccardi, R.J., and Cooper, N.R.: Physiochemical and functional characterization of the C1r subunit of the first complement component. J. Immunol. 116:496, 1976.
15. Schreiber, R.D., and Müller-Eberhard, H.J.: Fourth component of human complement. Description of a three polypeptide chain structure. J. Exp. Med. 140:1324, 1974.
16. Dykman, T.R., Cole, J.L., Iida, K., and Atkinson, J.P.: Polymorphism of human erythrocyte C3b/C4b receptor. Proc. Natl. Acad. Sci. USA 80:1698, 1983.
17. Gigli, I., and Austen, K.F.: Fluid phase destruction of $C2^{hu}$ by $C1^{hu}$. II. Unmasking by $C4i^{hu}$ of $C1^{-hu}$ specificity for $C2.^{hu}$ J. Exp. Med. 130:833, 1969.
18. Polley, M.J., and Müller-Eberhard, H.J.: The second component of human complement: Its isolation, fragmentation by C'1 esterase, and incorporation into C'3 convertase. J. Exp. Med. 128:533, 1968.
19. Nicholson-Weller, A., Burge, J., Fearon, D.T., Weller, P.F., Austen, K.F.: Isolation of a human erythrocyte membrane glycoprotein with decay-accelerating activity for C3 convertases of the complement system. J. Immunol. 129:184, 1982.
20. Pensky, J., Levy, L.R., and Lepow, I.H.: Partial purification of a serum inhibitor of C'1-esterase. J. Biol. Chem. 236:1674, 1961.
21. Sim, R.B., and Reboul, A.: Preparation and properties of human C1 inhibitor. Methods Enzymol. 80:43, 1981.
22. Harpel, P.C., and Cooper, N.R.: Studies on human plasma C1 inactivator enzyme interactions. I. Mechanisms of interaction with C1s, plasmin, and trypsin. J. Clin. Invest. 55:593, 1975.
23. Donaldson, V.H., and Evans, R.R.: A biochemical abnormality in hereditary angioneurotic edema. Absence of serum inhibitor of C'1-esterase. Am. J. Med. 35:37, 1963.
24. Scharfstein, J., Ferreira, A., Gigli, I., and Nussenzweig, V.: Human C4-binding protein. I. Isolation and characterization. J. Exp. Med. 147:207, 1978.
25. Cooper, N. R.: Isolation and analysis of the mechanism of action of an inactivator of C4b in normal human serum. J. Exp. Med. 141:890, 1975.
26. Dobson, N.J., Lambris, J.D., Ross, G.D.: Characteristics of isolated erythrocyte complement receptor type one (CR1, C4b-C3b receptor) and CR1-specific antibodies. J. Immunol. 126:693, 1981.
27. Pillemer, L., Blum, L., Lepow, I.H., Ross, D.A., Todd, E.W., and Wardlaw, A.C.: The properdin system and immunity: I. Demonstration and isolation of a new serum protein, properdin, and its role in immune phenomena. Science 120:279, 1954.
28. Pillemer, I.: The nature of the properdin system and its interactions with polysaccharide complexes. Ann. N.Y. Acad. Sci. 66:233, 1956.
29. Nelson, R.A., Jr.: Alternative mechanism for properdin system. J. Exp. Med. 108:515, 1958.
30. Pensky, J., Hinz, C.F., Jr., Todd, E.W., Wedgwood, R.J., Boyer, J.T., and Lepow, I.H.: Properties of highly purified human properdin. J. Immunol. 100:142, 1968.
31. Bokisch, V.A., Dierich, M.P., and Müller-Eberhard, H.J.: Third component of complement (C3): Structural properties in relation to functions. Proc. Natl. Acad. Sci. 72:1989, 1975.
32. Law, S.K., and Levine, R.P.: Interaction between the third complement protein and cell surface macromolecules. Proc. Natl. Acad. Sci. 74:2701, 1977.
33. Müller-Eberhard, H.J., and Götze, O.: C3 proactivator convertase and its mode of action. J. Exp. Med. 135:1003, 1972.
34. Fearon, D.T., and Austen, K.F.: Properdin: Initiation of alternative complement pathway. Proc. Natl. Acad. Sci. 72:3220, 1975.
35. Schreiber, R.D., Medicus, R.G., Götze, O., and Müller-Eberhard, H.J.: Properdin- and nephritic factor-dependent C3 convertases: Requirement of native C3 for enzyme formation and the function of bound C3b as properdin receptor. J. Exp. Med. 142:760, 1975.
36. Schreiber, R.D., Pangburn, M.K., Lesavre, P.H., and Müller-Eberhard, H.J.: Initiation of the alternative pathway of complement: Recognition of activators by bound C3b and assembly of the entire pathway from six isolated proteins. Proc. Natl. Acad. Sci. 75:3848, 1978.
37. Raum, D., Glass, D., Carpenter, C.B., Alper, C.A., and Schur, P.H.: The chromosomal order of genes controlling the major histocompatibility complex, properdin factor B, and deficiency of the second component of complement. J. Clin. Invest. 58:1240, 1976.
38. Medicus, R.G., Götze, O., and Müller-Eberhard, H.J.: The serine protease nature of the C3 and C5 convertases of the classical and alternative complement pathways. Scand. J. Immunol. 5:1049, 1976.
39. Fearon, D.T., Austen, K.F., and Ruddy, S.: Formation of a hemolytically active cellular intermediate by the interaction between properdin factors B and D and the activated third component of complement. J. Exp. Med. 138:1305, 1973.
40. Davis, A.E., III: Active site amino acid sequence of human factor D. Proc. Natl. Acad. Sci. USA 77:4938, 1980.
41. Lesavre, P.H., and Müller-Eberhard, H.J.: Mechanism of action of factor D of the alternative complement pathway. J. Exp. Med. 148:1498, 1978.
42. Götze, O., and Müller-Eberhard, H.J.: The role of properdin in the alternate pathway of complement activation. J. Exp. Med. 139:44, 1974.
43. Müller-Eberhard, H.J., and Schreiber, R.D.: Molecular biology and chemistry of the alternative pathway of complement. Adv. Immunol. 29:1, 1980.
44. Chapitis, J., and Lepow, I.H.: Multiple sedimenting species of properdin in human serum and interaction of purified properdin with the third component of complement. J. Exp. Med. 143:241, 1976.
45. Götze, O., Medicus, R.G., and Müller-Eberhard, H.J.: Alternative pathway of complement: Non-enzymatic reversible transition of precursor to active properdin. J. Immunol. 118:525, 1977.
46. Fearon, D.T., and Austen, K.F.: Properdin: Binding to C3b and stabilization of the C3b-dependent C3 convertase. J. Exp. Med. 142:856, 1975.
47. Spitzer, R.E., Vallota, E.H., Forristal, J., Sudora, E., Stitzel, A., Davis, N.C., and West, C.D.: Serum C'3 lytic system in patients with glomerulonephritis. Science 164:436, 1969.
48. Thompson, R.A.: C3 inactivating factor in the serum of a patient with

chronic hypocomplementemic proliferative glomerulonephritis. Immunology 22:147, 1972.
49. Whaley, K., Ward, D., and Ruddy, S.: Modulation of the properdin amplification loop in membranoproliferative and other forms of glomerulonephritis. Clin. Exp. Immunol. 35:101, 1979.
50. Davis, A.E., III, Arnaout, M.A., Alper, C.A., and Rosen, F.S.: Transfer of C3 nephritic factor from mother to fetus. N. Engl. J. Med. 297:144, 1977.
51. Daha, M.R., Fearon, D.T., and Austen, K.F.: Isolation of alternative pathway C3 convertase containing uncleaved B and formed in the presence of C3 nephritic factor (C3NeF). J. Immunol. 116:568, 1976.
52. Daha, M.R., Austen, K.F., and Fearon, D.T.: Heterogeneity, polypeptide chain composition and antigenic reactivity of C3 nephritic factor. J. Immunol. 120:1389, 1978.
53. Scott, D.M., Amos, N., Sissons, J.G.P., Lachmann, P.J., and Peters, D.K.: The immunoglobulin nature of nephritis factor (NeF). Clin. Exp. Immunol. 32:12, 1978.
54. Tamura, N., and Nelson, R.A., Jr.: Three naturally occurring inhibitors of components of complement in guinea pig and rabbit serum. J. Immunol. 99:582, 1967.
55. Ruddy, S., and Austen, K.F.: C3b inactivator of man. II. Fragments produced by C3b inactivator cleavage of cell-bound or fluid phase C3b. J. Immunol. 107:742, 1971.
56. Whaley, K., and Ruddy, S.: Modulation of C3b hemolytic activity by a plasma protein distinct from C3b inactivator. Science 193:1011, 1976.
57. Whaley, K., and Ruddy, S.: Modulation of the alternative complement pathway by $\beta$1H globulin. J. Exp. Med. 144:1147, 1977.
58. Weiler, J.M., Daha, M.D., Austen, K.F., and Fearon, D.T.: Control of the amplification convertase of complement by the plasma protein $\beta$1H. Proc. Natl. Acad. Sci. 73:3268, 1976.
59. Pangburn, M.K., Schreiber, R.D., and Müller-Eberhard, H.J.: Human complement C3b inactivator: Isolation, characterization, and demonstration of an absolute requirement for the serum protein $\beta$1H for cleavage of C3b and C4b in solution. J. Exp. Med. 146:257, 1977.
60. Law, S.K., Fearon, D.T., and Levine, R.P.: Action of the C3b inactivator on cell bound C3b. J. Immunol. 122:759, 1979.
61. Carlo, J., Conrad, D.H., and Ruddy, S.: Complement receptor binding of C3b-coated cells treated with C3b inactivator, $\beta$IH globulin and trypsin. J. Immunol. 123:523, 1979.
62. Medicus, R.G., Melamed, J., and Arnaout, M.A.: Role of human factor I and C3b receptor in the cleavage of surface-bound C3bi molecules. Eur. J. Immunol. 13:465, 1983.
63. Carlo, J.R., Spitznagel, J.K., Studer, E.J., Conrad, D.H., and Ruddy, S.: Cleavage of membrane bound C3bi, an intermediate of the third component of complement, to C3c and C3d-like fragments by crude leucocyte lysosomal lysates and purified leucocyte elastase. Immunology 44:381, 1981.
64. Conrad, D.H., Carlo, J.R., and Ruddy, S.: Interaction of $\beta$1H-globulin with cell-bound C3b: Quantitative analysis of binding and influence of alternative pathway components on binding. J. Exp. Med. 122:523, 1978.
65. Pangburn, M.K., Schreiber, R.D., and Müller-Eberhard, H.J.: Formation of the initial C3 convertase of the alternative complement pathway. Acquisition of C3b-like activities by spontaneous hydrolysis of the putative thioester in native C3. J. Exp. Med. 154:856, 1981.
66. Fearon, D.T., and Austen, K.F.: Activation of the alternative complement pathway due to resistance of zymosan-bound amplification convertase to endogenous regulatory mechanisms. Proc. Nat. Acad. Sci. 74:1683, 1977.
67. Fearon, D.T.: Regulation by membrane sialic acid of $\beta$1H-dependent decay-dissociation of amplification C3 convertase of the alternative complement pathway. Proc. Natl. Acad. Sci. 75:1971, 1978.
68. Kazatchkine, M.D., Fearon, D.T., and Austen, K.F.: Human alternative complement pathway: Membrane-associated sialic acid regulates the competition between B and $\beta$1H for cell bound C36. J. Immunol. 122:75, 1979.
69. Nydegger, U.E., Fearon, D.T., and Austen, K.F.: Autosomal locus regulates inverse relationship between sialic acid content and capacity of mouse erythrocytes to activate human alternative complement pathway. Proc. Natl. Acad. Sci. 75:6078, 1978.
70. Vogt, W., Schmidt, G., von Buttlar, B., and Dieminger, L.: A new function of the activated third component of complement: Binding to C5, an essential step for C5 activation. Immunology 34:29, 1978.
71. Daha, M.R., Fearon, D.T., and Austen, K.F.: C3 requirements for formation of alternative pathway C5 convertase. J. Immunol. 117:630, 1976.
72. Fernandez, H.N., and Hugli, T.E.: Chemical evidence for common genetic ancestry of complement components C3 and C5. J. Biol. Chem. 252:1826, 1977.
73. Fernandez, H.N., and Hugli, T.E.: Partial characterization of human C5a anaphylatoxin. I. Chemical description of the carbohydrate and polypeptide portions of human C5a. J. Immunol. 117:1688, 1976.
74. Podack, E.R., Kolb, W.P., and Müller-Eberhard, H.J.: Purification of the sixth and seventh component of human complement without loss of hemolytic activity. J. Immunol. 116:263, 1976.
75. Hobart, M.J., Joysey, V., and Lachmann, P.J.: Inherited structural variation and linkage relationships of C7. J. Immunogenet. 5:157, 1978.
76. Lachmann, P.J., Hobart, M.J., and Woo, P.: Combined genetic deficiency of C6 and C7 in man. Clin. Exp. Immunol. 33:193, 1978.
77. Kolb, W.P., and Müller-Eberhard, H.J.: The membrane attack mechanism of complement: The three polypeptide chain structure of the eighth component (C8). J. Exp. Med. 143:1131, 1976.
78. Thompson, R.A., and Lachmann, P.J.: Reactive lysis: The complement-mediated lysis of unsensitized cells. I. The characterization of the indicator factors and its identification as C7. J. Exp. Med. 131:629, 1970.
79. Goldman, J.N., Ruddy, S., and Austen, K.F.: Reaction mechanisms of nascent C567 (reactive lysis). I. Reaction characteristics for production of EC567 and lysis by C8 and C9. J. Immunol. 109:353, 1972.
80. Mayer, M.M., Hammer, C.H., Michaels, D.W., and Shin, M.L.: Immunologically mediated membrane damage: The mechanism of complement action and the similarity of lymphocyte-mediated cytotoxicity. Immunochemistry 15:813, 1978.
81. Green, H., Barrow, P., and Goldberg, B.: Effect of antibody and complement on permeability control in ascites tumor cells and erythrocytes. J. Exp. Med. 110:699, 1959.
82. Podack, E.R., Kolb, W.P., and Müller-Eberhard, H.J.: The C5b-9 complex: Subunit composition of the classical and alternative pathway-generated complex. J. Immunol. 116:1431, 1976.
83. Bhakdi, S., and Tranum-Jensen, J.: Membrane damage by complement. Biochim. Biophys. Acta. 737:343, 1983.
84. Steckel, E.W., Welbaum, B.E., and Sodetz, J.M.: Evidence of direct insertion of terminal complement proteins into cell membrane bilayers during cytolysis. Labeling by a photosensitive membrane probe reveals a major role for the eighth and ninth components. J. Biol. Chem. 258:4318, 1983.
85. Donaldson, V.H., Ratnoff, O.D., Dias da Silva, W., and Rosen, F.S.: Permeability-increasing activity in hereditary angioneurotic edema plasma. II. Mechanism of formation and partial characterization. J. Clin. Invest. 48:642, 1969.
86. Fields, T., Ghebrehiwet, B., and Kaplan, A.P.: Kinin formation in hereditary angioedema plasma: Evidence against kinin derivation from C2 and in support of "spontaneous" formation of bradykinin. J. Allergy Clin. Immunol. 72:54, 1983.
87. Ruddy, S., Austen, K.F., and Goetzl, E.J.: Chemotactic activity derived from interaction of factors D and B of the properdin pathway with cobra venom factor or C3b. J. Clin. Invest. 55:587, 1975.
88. Götze, O., Bianco, C., and Cohn, Z.A.: The induction of macrophage spreading by factor B of the properdin system. J. Exp. Med. 149:372, 1979.
89. Bianco, C., Götze, O., and Cohn, Z.A.: Regulation of macrophage migration by products of the complement system. Proc. Natl. Acad. Sci. 76:888, 1979.
90. Bentley, C., Fries, W., and Brade, V.: Synthesis of factors D, B and P of the alternative pathway of complement activation, as well as of C3, by guinea-pig peritoneal macrophages in vitro. Immunology 35:971, 1978.
91. Cochrane, C.G., and Müller-Eberhard, H.J.: The derivation of two distinct anaphylatoxin activities from the third and fifth components of human complement. J. Exp. Med. 122:99, 1968.
92. Becker, S., Meuer, S., Hadding, U., and Bitter-Suermann, D: Platelet activation: A new biological activity of guinea-pig C3a anaphylatoxin. Scand. J. Immunol. 7:173, 1978.
93. Ferluga, L., Schorlemmer, H., Baptista, L.C., and Allison, A.C.: Cytolytic effects of the complement cleavage product, C3a. Br. J. Cancer 34:626, 1976.
94. Bokisch, V.A., Müller-Eberhard, H.J., and Cochrane, C.G.: Isolation of a fragment (C3a) of the third component of human complement containing anaphylatoxin and chemotactic activity and description of an anaphylatoxin inactivator of human serum. J. Exp. Med. 129:1109, 1969.
95. Ward, P.A., and Newman. L.J.: A neutrophil chemotactic factor from human C'5. J. Immunol. 102:93, 1969.
96. Goldstein, I.M., and Weissmann, G.: Generation of C5-derived lysosomal enzyme-releasing activity (C5a) by lysates of leukocyte lysosomes. J. Immunol. 113:1583, 1974.
97. Craddock, P.R., Hammerschmidt, D., White, J.G., Dalmasso, A.P., and Jacob, H.S.: Complement (C5a)-induced granulocyte aggregation in vitro. J. Clin. Invest. 60:260, 1977.
98. Fernandez, H.N., Henson, P.M., Otani, A., and Hugli, T.E.: Chemotactic response to human C3a and C5a anaphylatoxins. I. Evaluation of C3a and C5a leukotaxis in vitro and under simulated in vivo conditions. J. Immunol. 120:109, 1978.
99. Damerau, B., Grünefeld, E., and Vogt, W.: Chemotactic effects of the complement derived peptides C3a, $C3a_i$ and C5a (classical anaphyla-

toxin) on rabbit and guinea pig polymorphonuclear leukocytes. Arch. Pharmacol. 305:181, 1978.
100. McCall, C.E., de Chatelet, L.R., Brown, D., and Lachmann, P.: New biological activity following intravascular activation of the complement cascade. Nature 249:841, 1974.
101. Rother, K.: Leukocyte mobilizing factor: A new biological activity derived from the third component of complement. Eur. J. Immunol. 2:550, 1972.
102. Alper, C.A., Propp, R.P., Klemperer, M.R., and Rosen, F.S.: Inherited deficiency of the third component of human complement (C'3). J. Clin. Invest. 48:533, 1969.
103. Ehlenberger, A.G., and Nussenzweig, V.: The role of membrane receptors for C3b and C3d in phagocytosis. J. Exp. Med. 145:357, 1977.
104. Bianco, C., Griffin, F.M., and Silverstein, S.C.: Studies of the macrophage complement receptor. Alteration of receptor function upon macrophage activation. J. Exp. Med. 141:1278, 1975.
105. Shin, M.L., Gelfand, M.C., Nagle, R.B., Carlo, J.R., Green, I., and Frank, M.M.: Localization of receptors for activator complement on visceral epithelial cells of the human renal glomerulus. J. Immunol. 118:869, 1977.
106. Inada, S., Brown, E.J., Gaither, T.A., Hammer, C.H., Takahaski, T., and Frank, M.M.: C3d receptors are expressed on human monocytes after in vitro activation. Proc. Nat. Acad. Sci. 80:2351, 1983.
107. Lay, W.H., and Nussenzweig, V.: Receptors for complement on leukocytes. J. Exp. Med. 128:991, 1968.
108. Jondal, M., Klein, G., Oldstone, M.B.A., Bokish, V., and Yefenof, E.: Surface markers on human B and T lymphocytes: VIII. Association between complement and Epstein-Barr virus receptors on human lymphoid cells. Scand. J. Immunol. 5:401, 1976.
109. Hutt-Fletcher, L.M., Fowler, E., Lambris, J.D., Feighny, R.J., Simmons, J.G., and Ross, G.D.: Studies of the Epstein-Barr virus receptor found on Raji cells. II. A comparison of lymphocyte binding studies for Epstein-Barr virus and C3d. J. Immunol. 130:1309, 1983.
110. Sandberg, A.L., Wahl, S.M., and Mergenhagen, S.E.: Lymphokine production by C3b-stimulated B cells. J. Immunol. 116:139, 1975.
111. Hartman, K-V, and Bokisch, V.A.: Stimulation of murine B lymphocytes by isolated C3b. J. Exp. Med. 145:600, 1975.
112. Rutherford, B., and Schenkein, H.: C3 cleavage products stimulate release of prostaglandins by human mononuclear cells in vitro. J. Immunol. 130:874, 1983.
113. Pepys, M.B.: Role of complement in the induction of the immunological responses. Transplant. Rev. 32:157, 1976.
114. Klaus, G.G.B., and Humphrey, J.H.: The generation of memory cells. I. The role of C3 in the generation of B memory cells. Immunology 33:31, 1977.
115. Ballas, Z.K., Feldbush, T.L., Needleman, B.W., and Weiler, J.M.: Complement inhibits immune responses: C3 preparations inhibit the generation of human cytotoxic T lymphocytes. Eur. J. Immunol. 13:274, 1983.
116. Colten, H.R.: Biosynthesis of complement. Adv. Immunol. 22:67, 1976.
117. Petz, L.D.: Variable mechanisms for low serum complement in liver disease. Lancet 2:1033, 1971.
118. Alper, C.A., Johnson, A.M., Birtch, A.G., and Moore, F.D.: Human C'3: Evidence for the liver as the primary site of synthesis. Science 163:286, 1969.
119. Ruddy, S., and Colten, H.R.: Rheumatoid arthritis: Biosynthesis of complement proteins by synovial tissues. N. Engl. J. Med. 290:1284, 1974.
120. Littman, B.H., and Ruddy, S.: Production of the second component of complement by human monocytes: Stimulation by antigen-activated lymphocytes or lymphokines. J. Exp. Med. 145:1344, 1977.
121. Ruddy, S., Carpenter, C.B., Chin, K.W., Knostman, J.N., Soter, N.A., Götze, O., Müller-Eberhard, H.J., and Austen, K.F.: Human complement metabolism: An analysis of 144 studies. Medicine 54:165, 1975.
122. Whaley, K., Widener, H., and Ruddy, S.: Modulation of the alternative pathway amplification loop in rheumatic diseases. *In* Opferkuch, W., Rother, K., and Schultz, D.R. (eds.): Clinical Aspects of the Complement System, Proceedings of an International Symposium held in Bochum, Germany. Stuttgart, George Thieme Publishers, 1978, p. 99.
123. Sakiyama, U., Hall, R.E., and Colten, H.R.: Translation of precursors of C4 and albumin by isolated guinea pig M-RNA. J. Immunol. 120:1795, 1978.
124. Patel, F., and Minta, J.O.: In vitro studies on the biosynthesis of rabbit C3: Evidence for the synthesis of a nascent single chain precursor C3. J. Immunol. 122:1582, 1979.
125. Gorski, J.P., and Müller-Eberhard, H.J.: Single-chain C4 from human plasma. J. Immunol. 120:1775, 1978.
126. Mayer, M.M.: Complement and complement fixation. *In* Kabat, E.A., and Mayer, M.M. (eds.): Experimental Immunochemistry. Springfield, Ill., Charles C Thomas, 1961, p. 133.
127. Ruddy, S., and Austen, K.F.: Complement and its components. *In* Cohen, A. (ed.): Laboratory Diagnostic Procedures in the Rheumatic Diseases. 2nd ed. Boston, Little, Brown & Company, 1975, p. 131.
128. Ruddy, S., Carpenter, C.B., Müller-Eberhard, H.J., and Austen, K.F.: Complement component levels in hereditary angioneurotic edema and isolated C'2 deficiency in man. *In* Miescher, P.A., and Grabar, P. (eds.): Mechanisms of Inflammation Induced by Immune Reactions. Vth International Immunopathology Symposium. Basel, Schwabe and Company, 1968, p. 231.
129. Ruddy, S., Everson, L.K., Schur, P.H., and Austen, K.F.: Hemolytic assay of the ninth complement component: Elevation and depletion in rheumatic diseases. J. Exp. Med. 134:259S, 1971.
130. Alper, C.A., and Rosen, F.S.: Studies in the in vivo behavior of human C'3 in normal subjects and patients. J. Clin. Invest. 46:2021, 1967.
131. Rynes, R.I., Ruddy, S., Schur, P.H., Spragg, J., and Austen, K.F.: Levels of complement components, properdin factors, and kininogen in patients with inflammatory arthritides. J. Rheumatol. 1:413, 1974.
132. Schur, P.H.: Complement studies of sera and other biologic fluids. Hum. Pathol. 14:338, 1983.
133. Williams, R.C., Jr., and Kunkel, H.G.: Rheumatoid factor, complement and conglutinin aberrations in patients with subacute bacterial endocarditis. J. Clin. Invest. 41:666, 1962.
134. Alpert, E., Isselbacher, K.J., and Schur, P.H.: Pathogenesis of arthritis associated with viral hepatitis. N. Engl. J. Med. 285:185, 1971.
135. Reed, W.P., Davidson, M.S., and Williams, R.C., Jr.: Complement system in pneumococcal infections. Infect. Immun. 13:1120, 1976.
136. Fearon, D.T., Ruddy, S., Schur, P.H., and McCabe, W.R.: Activation of the properdin pathway of complement in patients with gram-negative bacteremia. N. Engl. J. Med. 292:937, 1975.
137. Charlesworth, J.A., Pussell, B.A., Roy, L.P., Robertson, M.R., and Beveridge, J.: Measles infection: Involvement of the complement system. Clin. Exp. Immunol. 24:401, 1976.
138. Ward, P.A., and Kibukamusoke, J.W.: Evidence for soluble immune complexes in the pathogenesis of the glomerulonephritis of quartan malaria. Lancet 1:283, 1969.
139. Riethmuller, G., Meltzer, M., Franklin, E., and Miescher, P.A.: Serum complement levels in patients with mixed (IgM-IgG) cryoglobulinemia. Clin. Exp. Immunol. 1:337, 1966.
140. West, C.D., Northway, J.D., and Davis, N.C.: Serum levels of $\beta_{1c}$ globulin, a complement component, in the nephritides, lipoid nephrosis and other conditions. J. Clin. Invest. 43:1507, 1964.
141. Hunsicker, L.G., Ruddy, S., Carpenter, C.B., Schur, P.H., Merrill, J.P., Müller-Eberhard, H.J., and Austen, K.F.: Metabolism of third complement component (C3) in nephritis involvement of the classic and alternate (properdin) pathways for complement activation. N. Engl. J. Med. 287:835, 1972.
142. Pekin, T.J., Jr., and Zvaifler, N.J.: Hemolytic complement in synovial fluid. J. Clin. Invest. 43:1372, 1964.
143. Ruddy, S., and Austen, K.F.: Activation of the complement system in rheumatoid synovitis. Fed. Proc. 32:134, 1973.
144. Petz, L.D., Sharp, G.C., Cooper, N.R., et al.: Serum and cerebrospinal fluid complement and serum autoantibodies in systemic lupus erythematosus. Medicine 50:259, 1971.
145. Hadler, N.M., Gerwin, R.D., Frank, M.M., Whitaker, J.N., Baker, M., and Decker, J.L.: The fourth component of complement in the cerebrospinal fluid in systemic lupus erythematosus. Arthritis Rheum. 16:507, 1973.

# Chapter 8

# The Intrinsic Coagulation, Fibrinolytic, and Kinin-Forming Pathways of Man

*Allen P. Kaplan*

## INTRODUCTION

During the past decade, considerable progress has been made in understanding the mechanism by which the intrinsic coagulation and fibrinolytic pathways are activated and defining their relationship to the generation of the vasoactive peptide, bradykinin.

In Figure 8–1 is shown a simplified section scheme for bradykinin formation which subdivides it into three critical steps. First, Hageman factor is activated, a reaction dependent upon interaction with certain negatively charged surfaces. Next, activated Hageman factor converts prekallikrein to kallikrein, and then kallikrein digests high molecular weight (HMW) kininogen to generate bradykinin. In addition, activated Hageman factor also converts coagulation factor XI to factor XIa, and factor XIa then continues the intrinsic coagulation pathway. Although this scheme is technically correct, it does not indicate the complex manner in which those proteins interact so as to link the initiation of coagulation with kinin formation. In fact, the three proteins of the plasma kinin-forming system, Hageman factor, prekallikrein, and HMW kininogen, are all required for contact activation of plasma. In addition, we have learned that prekallikrein and factor XI each circulate as a complex with HMW kininogen and are bound to surfaces where they then interact with surface-bound Hageman factor. Methods have been developed for the purification of each of these reactants; their mechanism of activation has been determined; and considerable progress has been made in understanding their interactions. In this review I will present a detailed analysis of our present concept of the early events of these pathways and attempt to relate such events to the inflammatory reactions that are characteristic of connective tissue disorders.

**Identification of the Factors Required for Contact Activation of Plasma.** The intrinsic coagulation pathway is initiated by interaction of plasma with certain negatively charged surfaces;[1-4] thus activation proceeds upon contact with glass or kaolin when a clotting time or partial thromboplastin time (PTT) is determined. In 1955, Ratnoff and Colopy described a patient named Hageman[5] who had a markedly prolonged PTT and appeared to lack a plasma factor, designated Hageman factor, which bound to the surface and was active at the initiating step of the coagulation cascade.[6] The protein was partially purified from normal plasma[7,8] and was found to be a $\beta$ globulin with a sedimentation coefficient of approximately 5S.[9] In addition, Hageman factor deficient plasma was subsequently shown to possess a profound abnormality of surface-dependent fibrinolysis[10,11] and generated no bradykinin upon incubation with glass beads or kaolin.[12-15]

In 1965, a new coagulation abnormality was discovered in a family named Fletcher,[16] which was characterized as having a prolonged PTT that autocorrected as the time of incubation with surfaces was increased.[16,17] This latter property suggested that it possessed an abnormal *rate* of contact activation. In addition, the abnormality could be corrected upon addition of small quantities of normal plasma, and the corrective factor was partially purified.[18] It was clearly distinguishable from Hageman factor, and, although it appeared in fractions containing factor XI, chromatographic separation of the Fletcher factor from factor XI was achieved.[18] Subsequently Wuepper identified the Fletcher factor to be prekallikrein.[19] A detailed analysis of the functional abnormalities associated with prekallikrein deficiency revealed a diminished rate of Hageman factor dependent fibrinolysis,[20-22] which was corrected upon prolonged incubation with surfaces,[21] and an inability to generate any bradykinin regardless of the incubation time.[20-22] Fletcher trait plasma not only lacked functional prekallikrein, but possessed no detectable antigenic prekallikrein.[18-22] Weiss and colleagues[21] observed that the addition of preparations of activated Hageman factor to prekallikrein deficient plasma corrected the diminished rate of intrinsic coagulation and fibrinolysis but not the inability to generate bradykinin. These data suggested that the plasma possessed an abnormal rate of formation of activated Hageman factor and thereby implicated prekallikrein as a factor required for contact activation. The autocorrection with time, in the absence of prekallikrein, suggested that a slower, alternative mechanism existed that could also lead to the formation of activated Hageman factor. Reconstitution with prekallikrein, however, was an absolute requirement for kinin generation, as suggested by earlier work in which kallikrein was identified to be the plasma enzyme that digests kininogen to generate bradykinin (Fig. 8–1).

The next development in the identification of the plasma factors required for contact activation was ob-

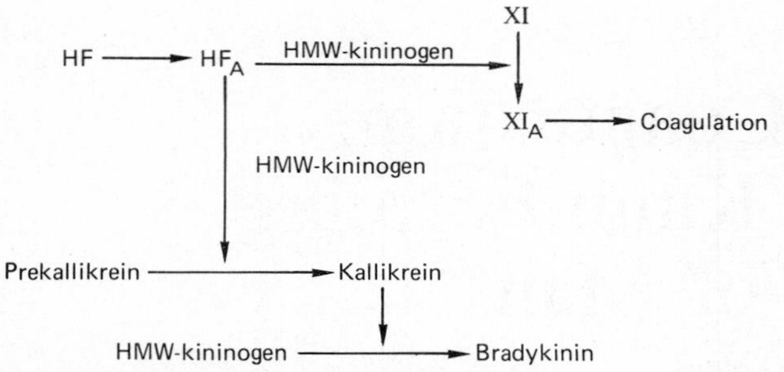


**Figure 8–1.** Scheme indicating those proteins required for initiation of the coagulation-kinin forming system.

servations by Webster and Pierce[24] and by Schiffman and Lee[25] indicating that the combination of a surface, Hageman factor, and prekallikrein was not sufficient to initiate kinin generation or factor XI activation. Evidence that an additional plasma factor is required for contact activation was presented, and the latter workers called it the "contact activation cofactor." Soon thereafter, three different patients possessing unique abnormalities of contact activation were reported; two of these patients, named Williams and Fitzgerald, were reported at an international "kallikrein-kinin" meeting,[26,27] and the third patient, named Flaujeac, was reported at a coagulation meeting in France.[28] Each plasma was shown to possess a markedly prolonged PTT that did not autocorrect with time, diminished surface-dependent fibrinolysis, and absent kinin formation.[26,28-30] Flaujeac trait plasma was then shown to possess only 8 percent of normal plasma kininogen, and the functional abnormalities were each corrected upon addition of plasma fractions containing HMW kininogen.[31,32] Williams trait plasma was found to be completely devoid of functional or antigenic kininogen,[26,33] and the abnormality was attributed to a new coagulation factor[33] that was also identified to be HMW kininogen.[34] These observations were confirmed when Fitzgerald trait was identified as HMW kininogen deficiency in a fourth patient (Washington) possessing the identical functional abnormalities.[35] HMW kininogen was also shown to be the same protein whose function had been observed using partially purified plasma fractions,[24,25] and the contact activation cofactor was shown to be lacking in Fitzgerald trait plasma[36] and then to be identical to HMW kininogen.[37,38]

The triad of abnormal coagulation, fibrinolysis, and kinin generation appears to be a property of each abnormal plasma that functions at the initial step of the cascade. Thus, although factor XI was shown to be a substrate of Hageman factor,[39] factor XI deficient plasma has a normal initial rate of kaolin-activatable fibrinolysis and normal kinin generation. Factor XI deficient plasma does not, therefore, possess an abnormal rate of Hageman factor activation or function. A time course of surface dependent activation of the intrinsic coagulation pathway is shown in Figure 8–2 and demonstrates the marked abnormality present in both Hageman factor deficient plasma and HMW kininogen deficient plasma as well as the abnormal rate of activation of prekallikrein deficient plasma.

**Interaction of Prekallikrein, Factor XI, and HMW Kininogen in Plasma.** It is clear that Hageman factor, prekallikrein, HMW kininogen, factor XI, and plasminogen are intimately related functionally, but they clearly represent different plasma proteins that are antigenically unrelated and are represented in the genome by distinct structural genes. However, reports suggesting that kallikrein can be purified as a complex with another plasma protein[40] and that prekallikrein appears to circulate in plasma as a complex[41] prompted the studies of Mandle and colleagues[42] and Thompson and associates,[43] in which prekallikrein and factor XI were each shown to circulate bound to HMW kininogen.

When normal human plasma was fractionated on Sephadex G-200, the apparent molecular weight of each of the aforementioned proteins could be determined. Factor XI was found at a molecular weight of 380,000, prekallikrein was found at 260,000, Hageman factor fractionated at 115,000, and plasminogen was located at 95,000. However, when the molecular weights of purified factor XI and prekallikrein were assessed by gel filtration, values of 175,000 and 100,000, respectively, were obtained, a discrepancy of approximately 200,000. Purified Hageman factor and plasminogen fractionated at the same position as they did when whole plasma was assessed, and therefore did not appear to circulate as part of a complex. When the molecular weight of prekallikrein and factor XI was determined in plasma that was deficient in HMW kininogen, factor XI was found at 175,000 and prekallikrein was found at 100,000, suggesting that each protein normally circulates bound to HMW kininogen. Reconstitution of HMW kininogen deficient plasma with purified HMW kininogen followed by fractionation by Sephadex G-200 gel filtration reproduced the chromatographic pattern of factor XI and prekallikrein in normal plasma.[42,43] In addition, direct binding of purified prekallikrein to HMW kininogen[42] and direct binding of partially purified factor XI to HMW kininogen[43] have been demonstrated. Normal plasma contains approximately twice the concentration of HMW kininogen as the sum of the factor XI and prekallikrein concentrations; thus complete binding of

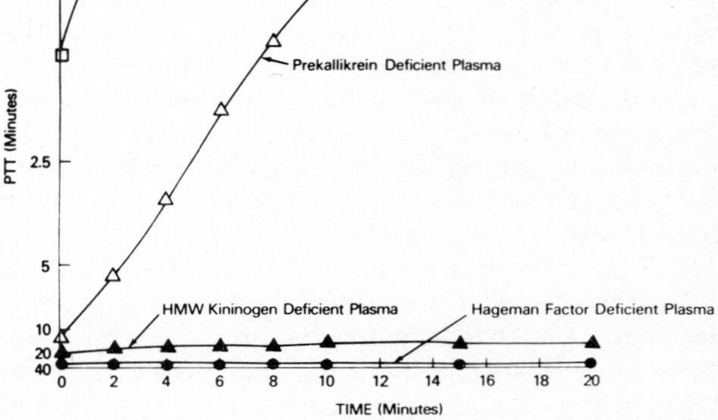

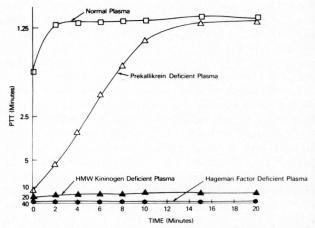


**Figure 8–2.** Time course of activation of the Hageman factor–dependent coagulation pathway.

factor XI and prekallikrein results, and the major peak of HMW kininogen seen represents uncomplexed protein.[43] No complex has been observed containing prekallikrein, factor XI, and HMW kininogen as a single entity; prekallikrein and factor XI appear to circulate bound to different molecules of HMW kininogen. Binding to HMW kininogen also appears to be a specific property of the Hageman factor substrates, and the complexes of prekallikrein–HMW kininogen and factor XI–HMW kininogen are each adsorbed to surfaces where they then interact with surface-bound Hageman factor. A schematic diagram showing the critical constituents bound to the surface is shown in Figure 8–3.

**Identification of Surfaces upon Which Activation Can Proceed.** The materials that serve as initiators of the intrinsic coagulation pathway include a diverse array of substances, such as silicon dioxide, glass, kaolin, talc, diatomaceous earth, celite, supercel, barium carbonate, cellulose sulfate, dextran sulfate (molecular weight 500,000), carrageenan, and ellagic acid.[15,44-49] In addition certain biologic materials can initiate the cascade; for example, crystals of sodium urate,[50] calcium pyrophosphate,[50] or L-homocysteine,[51] which are produced by patients with gout, pseudogout, and homocystinuria, respectively, may act as appropriate surfaces. Exposure of human plasma to articular cartilage also yields kininlike activity that appears to be Hageman factor dependent,[52] while skin contact[53] and interaction with fatty acids[54-56] may also lead to Hageman factor activation. Activation of Hageman factor has been reported to occur upon contact with certain bacterial lipopolysaccharides[57] in which the lipid A fraction containing negatively charged phosphate groups appears to be the functional moiety. Evidence of Hageman factor activation during episodes of endotoxic shock has been reported,[58-64] and the products of this reaction may contribute to the intravascular coagulation and hypotension seen. Of particular interest is the observation that endotoxic shock in monkeys was not inhibited by prior complement depletion, although much of the tissue inflammatory reaction was diminished.[63] It is possible that the generation of vasoactive peptides such as bradykinin is responsible for the vasodilatation and pooling of fluid into tissues that is characteristic of endotoxic shock. Immune complexes have been thought to be capable of initiating the Hageman factor dependent pathways.[64-70] However, incubation of purified Hageman factor with immune complexes or aggregated immunoglobulins did not lead to activation of Hageman factor, and binding of Hageman factor to the complexes was not observed.[71] It is possible that the positive results reported may have been attributable to traces of kallikrein contaminating immunoglobulin preparations, or that activation was observed by a pathway independent of Hageman factor.

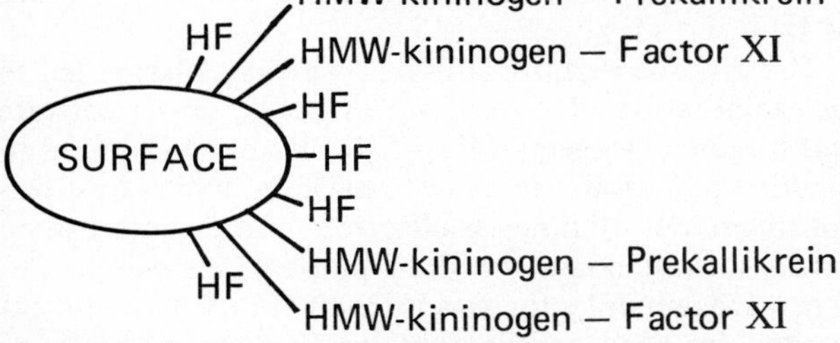


**Figure 8–3.** Schematic diagram depicting the interaction of surface-bound Hageman factor (HF) with complexes of HMW kininogen and prekallikrein and complexes of HMW kininogen and factor XI.

It would be of obvious interest and importance to identify connective tissue components that can act as appropriate surfaces for binding the critical reactants in order to initiate the Hageman factor dependent pathways. Crude preparations of collagen[72-74] or vascular basement membrane[74] appear to be capable of initiating the cascade, and the carboxyl groups of collagen have been reported to be required for the reaction to proceed. In addition, insoluble bovine collagen preparations have been shown to bind kallikrein, and such binding was dependent upon the availability of both carboxyl and amino groups.[75] However, one study reported no activation of Hageman factor when purified Hageman factor was incubated with purified triple helical soluble collagen.[76] In addition, Meier and Kaplan[77] have reported that preparation of purified type I, II, and III collagens, chondroitin sulfates A and C, dermatan sulfate, bovine nasal cartilage proteoglycans, and collagen fibrils formed with incorporated proteoglycans all failed to initiate kinin formation when incubated with normal plasma. Thus we have not yet been able to identify the specific component or combination of components present in connective tissue that can initiate Hageman factor dependent coagulation, fibrinolysis, and kinin formation.

## HAGEMAN FACTOR

**Properties of Human Hageman Factor.** Hageman factor was found to be a single chain $\beta$ globulin of molecular weight 80,000 and was present in plasma at concentrations ranging from 23 to 47 $\mu$g per milliliter (mean, 29 $\mu$g per milliliter).[78] The peak isoelectric point of human Hageman factor was reported to be between 6.1 and 6.5; however, considerable charge heterogeneity was observed with a pH range of 5.9 to 7.0.[71]

**Assays of Unactivated and Activated Hageman Factor.** Hageman factor can be assayed by a modification of the PTT,[79] utilizing Hageman factor deficient plasma as the substrate. This method is routinely utilized in coagulation laboratories and consists of an initial incubation of the deficient plasma with the Hageman factor source, kaolin, and cephalin for 2 minutes at 37° C. Calcium is added, and the time of formation of a clot is recorded. A 1:10 dilution of pooled normal human plasma is serially diluted, each dilution is assayed for Hageman factor, and a standard dose-response curve is constructed. The Hageman factor content of samples can then be expressed as a percentage of normal plasma Hageman factor or in units per milliliter if 1 unit represents the quantity of Hageman factor in pooled plasma. This method is reliable only for the determination of unactivated Hageman factor. Upon activation,

Hageman factor readily fragments, resulting in considerable loss of coagulant activity.[80,81] The presence of activated Hageman factor can be detected using a coagulation assay by clotting the sample in the absence of kaolin.[81] If a sample shortens the PTT of Hageman factor deficient plasma but has no effect upon factor XI deficient plasma, it is likely to contain activated Hageman factor. However, the assay does not distinguish the particular form of activated Hageman factor present; e.g., one might have an active but nonfragmented form of Hageman factor or one or more active fragments of Hageman factor. Since the various fragments differ in specific activity, the assay cannot be used in a quantitative fashion.

A sensitive, specific, primary assay for activated Hageman factor is not available; thus most assays require at least one incubation with a second plasma protein. Activated Hageman factor has been shown to digest D-pro-phe-arg-*p*-nitro-anilide[82] and this is particularly useful when assaying the purified protein. It does not distinguish the various activated forms of Hageman factor (all are equally reactive), and it cannot be used in plasma, since this substrate is cleaved by a variety of proteases, particularly kallikrein. Utilizing a very different approach we have recently developed a double antibody ELISA assay which measures the circulating complex of activated HF and its inhibitor, $C\bar{1}$ INH.[82a] In this assay IgG antihuman HFa is bound to a microtiter plate, and the sample is added, incubated, and washed. We then incubate with $(Fab')_2$ antihuman $C\bar{1}$ INH to which alkaline phosphatase is covalently coupled. *p*-Nitrophenyl phosphate is then added as an alkaline phosphatase substrate, which when cleaved, yields *p*-nitrophenol, a yellow component whose absorbance is read at O.D.405 nm. The color formation is dependent upon reaction with bound $C\bar{1}$ INH, which in turn is directly proportional to the amount of activated HF present. The assay does not distinguish HFa from HFf but does detect both since the antibody to HFa also detects HFf. This assay is presently being utilized as a sensitive and specific measure of initiation of the Hageman factor dependent pathways, but there are no data available as yet for specific disease entities. Similar assays are now available for the determination of kallikrein[83] and plasmin.[84]

Activated Hageman factor can also be determined by its ability to convert prekallikrein to kallikrein. This approach has the advantage of detecting all the various forms of activated Hageman factor (although it does not distinguish one from the other), and the kallikrein generated can be accurately determined. A purified "standard" prekallikrein preparation can be used and its rate of conversion to kallikrein determined. Alternatively, the Hageman factor sample can be added directly to normal plasma anticoagulated with EDTA and the kallikrein generated assayed, using synthetic substrates that are specific for kallikrein[85] (see Prekallikrein, below, for details of these assays). A major limitation of such assays is that activated Hageman factor exists for only a short period of time and it is inactivated by binding to $C\bar{1}$ INH. Thus the aforementioned assay for the activated Hageman factor-$C\bar{1}$ INH complex is a more reliable assessment of activation.

Hageman factor protein can be assayed immunologically using monospecific antisera. By radial immunodiffusion, its concentration in plasma has been estimated to be 27 to 45 $\mu$g per milliliter,[74] and a sensitive radioimmunoassay for Hageman factor has been reported.[86] Immunologic assays do not, of course, give any information regarding the state of activation of the protein and can yield erroneous results if the Hageman factor is fragmented. For example, if an antiserum is reactive with the Hageman factor fragments, the more rapid diffusion of the fragments can yield falsely elevated results by immunodiffusion. A radioimmunoassay may also give spurious results, depending upon the relative ability of the Hageman factor fragments and the standard Hageman factor preparation to compete for binding to the antiserum.

**Activation and Fragmentation of Hageman Factor: The Role of the Surface, HMW Kininogen, and Prekallikrein.** The activation of Hageman factor differs from that observed with the other proenzymes to be described herein because two different proteolytic steps are involved; the first consists of a cleavage without obvious fragmentation, and the second, a cleavage that liberates one or more active fragments. The discovery of the active fragments of Hageman factor by Kaplan and Austen[80] provided the first evidence that activation could be performed enzymatically.[81] The final product, a prealbumin fragment observed as two closely migrating bands upon alkaline disc gel electrophoresis, functioned as a potent prekallikrein activator but retained only 2 to 5 percent of the coagulant activity of the unfragmented Hageman factor. These fragments are designated HFf. Subsequently, plasmin was shown to be capable of directly digesting Hageman factor to yield these fragments.[81] Similar prealbumin activities described in the rabbit,[86] guinea pig,[87] and man[88,89] were subsequently shown to be derived from Hageman factor,[90,91] and the ability of plasmin to activate and fragment Hageman factor was confirmed.[92] Although not purified, an activated preparation of Hageman factor was also described whose molecular weight upon gel filtration was identical to that of unactivated Hageman factor, yet it readily clotted Hageman factor deficient plasma in the absence of kaolin. This preparation was designated intact activated Hageman factor or HFa.[81] In addition, at least two active fragments were described whose molecular weight was intermediate between that of HFf and HFa.

The discovery of prekallikrein deficient plasma led to an examination of the ability of kallikrein to activate and fragment Hageman factor. Kallikrein was found to function in a similar manner to plasmin; however, it was approximately 10 times as effective[94] and could act upon either surface bound or fluid phase Hageman factor. When Hageman factor was iodinated, digested, and examined by SDS gel electrophoresis, trypsin, plasmin, and kallikrein were found to yield similar patterns.[78] The molecular weight of Hageman factor was 90,000 in unreduced gels and 80,000 after reduction; upon digestion it was converted to HFf, and a 50,000-dalton fragment remained. Further digestion converted the 50,000-dalton fragment to fragments of 40,000 and 10,000. However, the formation of HFa was not detected. The 50,000-dalton fragment was subsequently shown to be the portion of the molecule that binds to surfaces.[95]

These studies suggested that activated Hageman factor converts prekallikrein to kallikrein and kallikrein enzymatically activates Hageman factor, i.e., they activate each other. With the discovery of HMW kininogen deficiency, it became clear that such a reciprocal mechanism was an oversimplification. For example, addition of HFa to Hageman factor deficient plasma causes coagulation in the absence of kaolin by activation of factor XI. Addition of factor XIa to factor XI deficient plasma causes coagulation in the absence of kaolin by activation of factor IX. However, addition of kallikrein to prekallikrein deficient plasma, in the absence of a surface, did not result in appreciable coagulation.[96] Thus the surface appeared to be required for this function of kallikrein to be expressed. Furthermore, the addition of activated Hageman factor to HMW kininogen deficient plasma, even in the presence of a surface, did not significantly shorten its partial thromboplastin time.[97,98] HMW kininogen therefore appeared to be required for the activation of Hageman factor and/or the expression of Hageman factor activity. When the role of HMW kininogen was further examined, it was found to enhance both the function of activated Hageman factor and the formation of activated Hageman factor.[97–101] For a fixed amount of surface-bound Hageman factor, the subsequent activation of prekallikrein and factor XI appeared proportional to the quantity of HMW-kininogen added.[97,101] Such an experiment could be performed utilizing HFf in the absence of a surface[100] or limited trypsin treatment of surface-bound Hageman factor (presumably HFa),[97] indicating that the effect of HMW kininogen observed was upon the function of activated Hageman factor, i.e., it facilitated its ability to activate prekallikrein and factor XI. However, these observations do not preclude an effect upon the activation of Hageman factor. Griffin and Cochrane reported that the rate of cleavage of Hageman factor by kallikrein appeared to be enhanced by HMW kininogen,[97] suggesting an effect upon Hageman factor activation. Meier and colleagues assessed this reaction functionally and demonstrated that the ability of kallikrein to activate Hageman factor was markedly augmented by HMW kininogen.[101] When the presence of activated Hageman factor was assessed functionally, formation of new active sites was determined by incorporation of $^{3}$H-DFP.[101] In the presence of HMW kininogen, the function of each of these sites could then be fully expressed. Figure 8–4 is a schematic diagram of this reciprocal interaction of surface-bound Hageman factor and prekallikrein, indicating that the reaction rate in each direction is augmented by HMW kininogen.

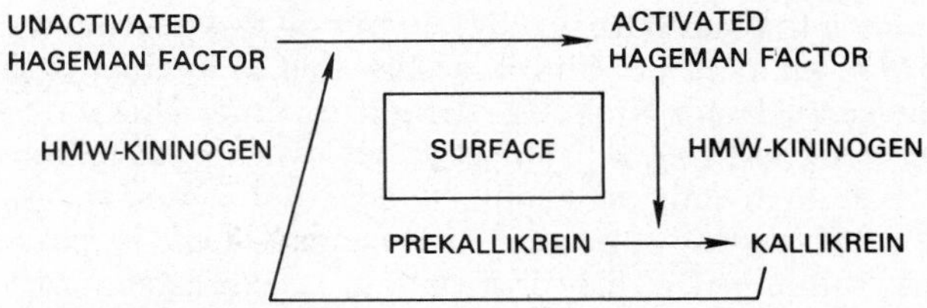


**Figure 8–4.** Schematic diagram of the reciprocal activation of surface-bound Hageman factor and prekallikrein that is catalyzed by HMW kininogen.

It should be emphasized that the surface and the active site of kallikrein were required for this activation of Hageman factor[99,101] to proceed. Thus kallikrein did not correct prekallikrein deficient plasma in the absence of a surface,[96,101] DFP-kallikrein did not correct prekallikrein deficient plasma in the presence of a surface,[99,101] and DFP-kallikrein would not activate purified surface-bound Hageman factor.[101] The surface has been estimated to augment the rate of cleavage of Hageman factor by kallikrein by as much as 50-fold.[102] Thus the surface appears to augment the rate of interaction of the reactants, and, in particular, render the Hageman factor a better substrate for plasma kallikrein. The ability of HMW kininogen to augment the function of activated Hageman factor has been estimated to be 3- to 4-fold, while its effect upon the activation of Hageman factor yields a 40-fold enhancement.[101] When combined with the surface, the rate is augmented 6000-fold. It is likely that changes observed upon binding of Hageman factor to surfaces or ellagic acid[103] may relate to the increased rate of cleavage of Hageman factor rather than the generation of a new active site in the Hageman factor.

More recent studies have attempted to further delineate the molecular mechanism by which HMW kininogen affects both the activation of Hageman factor as well as the effect of HFa upon its substrates. Wiggins and colleagues[104] determined that the quantity of prekallikrein and factor XI bound to the surface in HMW kininogen deficient plasma is diminished and that the rate of cleavage by surface bound Hageman factor was abnormal. These data appear consistent with Figure 8–3, in which HMW kininogen is the "bridge" by which prekallikrein and factor XI are attached to surfaces. However, using purified proteins in aqueous solution and a kaolin surface, Silverberg and colleagues[105] have shown that prekallikrein and factor XI bind to kaolin equally well in the presence or absence of HMW kininogen but that activation is markedly diminished when HMW kininogen is absent. These results indicate that with a surface such as kaolin, HMW kininogen binding of prekallikrein and factor XI allow them to attach to the surface in a conformation that facilitates cleavage by HFa. The fact that the quantity of prekallikrein and factor XI bound in plasma is indeed less than normal in the absence of HMW kininogen was reproduced but appears less important than the way in which binding occurs. Other data have further delineated the role of HMW kininogen upon the activation of Hageman factor by kallikrein. Once prekallikrein is converted to kallikrein, a fraction of the kallikrein can dissociate from the HMW kininogen,[106] and it is then able to interact with Hageman factor molecules bound to other sites or to adjacent particles.[105,107] Interestingly, when prekallikrein is bound directly to kaolin, it does not dissociate. In this fashion, the activation of Hageman factor is markedly amplified. This dissociation is consistent with observations that the binding constant of the prekallikrein–HMW kininogen complex is such that at plasma concentration, about 10 percent of prekallikrein should be free,[106] and other studies have demonstrated this small fraction of unbound prekallikrein.[108] In the presence of a surface with an equilibrium between bound and unbound prekallikrein, some of the kallikrein formed would be expected to dissociate. Thus the effect of HMW kininogen upon Hageman factor activation is indirect, since it does not augment the intrinsic activity of kallikrein, nor does it directly affect the rate at which Hageman factor is cleaved. It appears to maximize the effective ratio of kallikrein to Hageman factor, thereby facilitating the enzymatic reaction. This is accomplished by its cofactor function for conversion of prekallikrein to kallikrein and then allowing dissociation of kallikrein to sites of bound Hageman factor.[105]

**Activation of Hageman Factor: Autoactivation upon Negatively Charged Surfaces.** One of the enigmas faced when considering the initiation of contact activation is the fact that all of the enzymes involved exist in the circulation in a precursor form. Thus, it is unclear how the first active site is created to initiate the cascade. Studies pertaining to this issue generally focus upon Hageman factor as the starting point of the cascade, as depicted in Figure 8–1. Earlier studies presented evidence to suggest that when Hageman factor is bound to a surface, it undergoes a conformational change[103,109] and exposes an active site. Other studies failed to demonstrate active site formation in the absence of proteolysis.[97,99,101,102,110] On the other hand, some publications have presented data to suggest that rabbit, bovine,[111–113] and human[114] Hageman factor possess significant intrinsic enzymatic activity when surface bound in the absence of any cleavage and proposed the possibility of a substrate-induced conformational change in Hageman factor that facilitates the process.[112] In fact, data using bovine Hageman factor indicated that HFa is only 3- to 4-fold better than native, uncleaved HF in activating prekallikrein and factor XI.[111,112] Our own studies of human Hageman factor indicate that a different mechanism of initiation is involved. This was first suggested by observations made in rabbit[110] and human[115] Hageman factor in which purified Hageman factor slowly appeared to autoactivate upon binding to surfaces. For example, with time and in the absence of any identifiable contaminants, the Hageman factor was digested to yield both HFa and HFf, and incorporation of $^3$DFP into these activated forms was demonstrated.[115] Then in an attempt to prove that an autoactivation mechanism is operative, it was shown that the kinetics of the reaction indicate an accelerating reaction, i.e., a continuously increasing velocity as the concentration of activated enzyme increases[82] and that HFa can digest native HF to form more HFa[82] and then HFf.[116] When a careful estimate was made to quantitate the activity present in native, uncleaved Hageman factor it was found to be not greater than 1/4000 the activity of HFa.[117] Thus, if native HF possesses any intrinsic activity it is exceedingly small, and we suspect that putative intrinsic activity reported by others when the HF was not treated with potent HFa inactivators was due to traces of HFa present. Results similar to ours have been recently reported in preliminary form.[118]

The initial cleavage of human Hageman factor has been reported to occur within a disulfide bridge in such a way that the product is the same size as the starting material.[119,120] This is shown in Figure 8–5 as cleavage at site 1. A second cleavage occurs at site 2 and then at site 3 to yield the 28,500 and 30,000 molecular weight forms of HFf.[116,121] Although cleavage at sites 2 and 3 occur in sequence, i.e., 2 precedes 3, we usually obtain a mixture of these two forms in which a 28,000-dalton heavy chain (the same as the light chain of HFa) is disulfide linked to light chains of either 2000 or 500. Since the rate of autoactivation is much slower than the rate of Hageman factor activation by kallikrein,[116] most HFa and HFf formed are dependent upon the reciprocal activation by kallikrein. But we envision the autoactivation mechanism as the initiating reaction, and both are depicted in Figure 8–6. When the products of autoactivation are examined in the absence of any prekallikrein, an additional active enzyme of molecular weight 40,000 is seen[116,121] in quantities about equal to that of HFf. This represents one of the intermediate-sized active moieties originally described.[81] However, it is either not formed by kallikrein digestion of Hageman factor, or it is further degraded to HFf so rapidly that it is not seen when normal plasma is examined. Theoretically, it should be one of the products evident when prekallikrein deficient plasma is activated; it is thought that the gradual autocorrection of the partial thromboplastin time seen in this plasma is a reflection of Hageman factor autoactivation.

**Identification of Permeability Factor of Dilution**

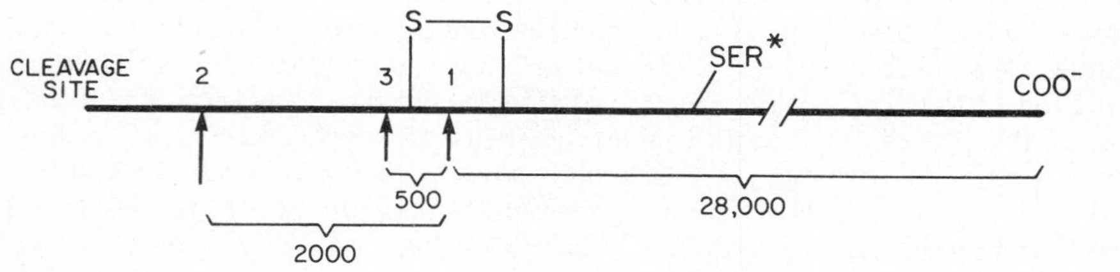


**Figure 8–5.** Cleavage sites in Hageman factor required for activation. HFa is formed by cleavage at site 1 within the disulfide bridge, while the two molecular forms of HFf are formed by cleavage at sites 2 and 3.

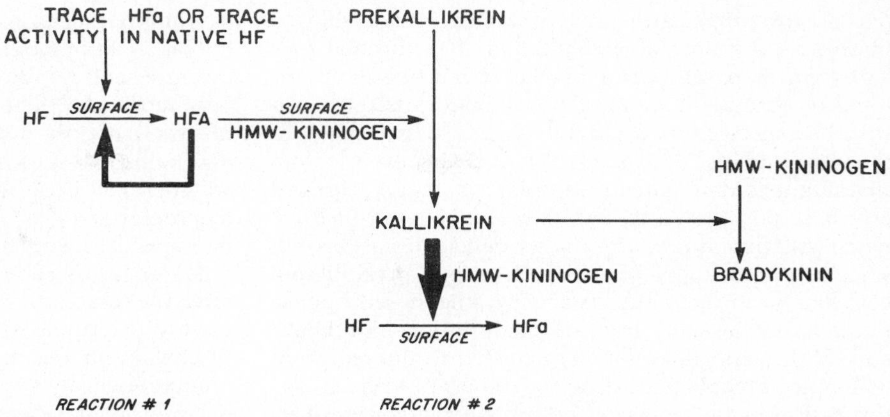


**Figure 8–6.** Diagram of the Hageman factor–dependent pathways, indicating the two-step process for HF activation. An autoactivation step is followed by reciprocal interaction with prekallikrein (kallikrein) for which HMW-kininogen acts as a cofactor. Digestion of HMW kininogen then generates bradykinin.

**(PF/dil) as Activated Hageman Factor.** Dilution of normal plasma obtained from several animal species in a glass vessel led to the formation of a permeability factor that was detected when the diluted plasma was injected into guinea pig skin.[13,14,122–125] The factor was found in a globulin-containing fraction of plasma; therefore the increase in vascular permeability was not attributable to the direct injection of bradykinin into the skin. Generation of PF/dil was shown to require the presence of Hageman factor;[14,126,127] thus neither dilution of normal plasma in a plastic vessel nor dilution of Hageman factor deficient plasma in a glass vessel generated permeability enhancing activity. Furthermore antiserum to human Hageman factor appeared to inhibit the formation of PF/dil when added prior to dilution, but did not inhibit PF/dil activity once it had formed.[128] Thus Hageman factor was required for the formation of PF/dil but did not appear to be identical to PF/dil. It was proposed that a precursor molecule (pro-PF/dil) exists that is activated by Hageman factor to PF/dil and that PF/dil could in turn convert prekallikrein to kallikrein.[14,15,126–130] When attempts to isolate PF/dil were initially made, a $\beta$ globulin fraction of human plasma was identified which could increase vascular permeability when injected into guinea pig skin. It could also generate bradykinin upon incubation with fresh plasma but not heat-inactivated plasma (plasma that is heated to 61° C for 2 hours destroys prekallikrein but not HMW kininogen).[131,132] PF/dil was therefore thought to be a prekallikrein activator. Subsequently, Kaplan and Austen attempted to purify PF/dil[133] and thereby isolated the Hageman factor fragments.[80] It therefore appeared that activated Hageman factor could directly convert prekallikrein to kallikrein and that PF/dil was, in fact, a form of activated Hageman factor.[80] Subsequently an anti-Hageman factor immunoadsorbent was used to remove PF/dil activity from diluted human plasma.[134] However, neither of these studies identified the particular molecular form of HFa present in diluted plasma, and it was suggested that a mixture of active fragments was present.[70,80] A later study by Oh-Ishi and Webster[135] confirmed the association of PF/dil activity with multiple molecular forms of activated Hageman factor.

It is likely that Hageman factor is activated in diluted plasma in the fluid phase as well as at the surface, and that dilution minimizes inhibition of the various Hageman factor fragments formed. Consistent with the conclusion that PF/dil is a form of activated HF are observations that both prekallikrein in HMW kininogen deficient plasmas possess an abnormality in the surface-dependent generation of PF/dil.[19,20,22,27,31] Each of these plasmas has also been shown to possess a diminished rate of liberation of Hageman factor fragments from the surface.[119] When PF/dil is injected into the skin of an animal, the generation of bradykinin locally might account for the enhanced vascular permeability. However, PF/dil activity has been shown to be expressed normally upon injection into the skin of a prekallikrein deficient patient, suggesting that plasma prekallikrein is not required at this stage of the assay and that bradykinin may not be the mediator of the enhanced permeability.[136,137] Identification of other permeability factors that may be generated and an examination of the direct effect of activated HF upon blood vessels may lead to new concepts relating the activation of the intrinsic coagulation pathway to the inflammatory response.

## PREKALLIKREIN

**Properties of Human Prekallikrein.** The molecular weights reported for human prekallikrein as assessed by gel filtration have ranged from 100,000 to 127,000. However, when purified prekallikrein was examined by SDS gel electrophoresis, two molecular variants were identified at 88,000 and 85,000 daltons and have been designated prekallikrein I and II, respectively. Upon immunoelectrophoresis, in 1 percent agar at pH 8.3, prekallikrein migrated as a fast $\gamma$ globulin, and its isoelectric point was determined to be between 8.5 and 9.0 (peak value at 8.7), utilizing ampholytes that ranged from pH 7 to 10.

**Assays of Prekallikrein and Kallikrein.** The correction of the abnormal partial thromboplastin time of prekallikrein deficient plasma can provide a very sensitive assay for prekallikrein, since reconstitution to a level of only 5 percent of normal plasma prekallikrein fully corrects the coagulation defect.[19,20] The prekallikrein concentration can be expressed as a percent of normal plasma concentration by comparison with the partial thromboplastin time obtained, using diluted plasma as a source of prekallikrein. If a purified prekallikrein preparation is available, it can be serially diluted to generate a standard curve, and unknowns can then be expressed on a weight basis. The limitations of this assay are as follows: (1) active coagulation factors that might contaminate the sample (e.g., factor XIa) will give false positives, although they can be controlled for by coagulation assays using other deficient plasmas; (2) since a level of only 5 percent of normal prekallikrein completely corrects the deficiency, the dose-response range is narrow and accurate quantitation is difficult; and (3) the assay does not distinguish prekallikrein from kallikrein. Prekallikrein deficiency appears to be an autosomal recessive trait, and both homozygotes and heterozygotes can be detected using a coagulation assay if celite or kaolin (rather than ellagic acid) is used as the surface.[138] The cold dependent activation of factor VII can also be used as an assay for prekallikrein[139] if one has ruled out Hageman factor deficiency. The requirement for HMW kininogen in the performance of this last test, however, has not been defined.

Synthetic substrates that are specific for kallikrein are available and can be utilized to assay for either kallikrein or prekallikrein. For example, $\alpha$-benzoyl-L-prolyl-L-phenylalanyl-L-arginyl-*p*-nitroanilide can be used in a simple and rapid colorimetric assay.[85] Quantitative assessment of kallikrein activity with this assay appears to correlate with proteolytic activity. The potential contribution by contaminating enzymes is small, since the substrate is highly specific for kallikrein. However, when assaying plasma samples, the kallikrein-$\alpha_2$ macroglobulin complex retains significant activity for low molecular weight substrates;[140,141] thus a falsely elevated estimate may result.

Using H-D-pro-phe-arg-*p*-nitroanilide and dextran sulfate as the plasma activator, assays that measure prekallikrein by its conversion to kallikrein have been reported using varying conditions of time and temperature.[142,143] More recently an assay for prekallikrein was devised utilizing kaolin activation of chloroform-treated plasma, and 78 percent of the absolute amount of prekallikrein in plasma was actually measured,[143] which compared favorably with other assays utilizing synthetic substrates and was more accurate than coagulation assays.

The synthetic substrate tosyl-arginine methyl ester (TAME)[145] has been used to quantitate preparations of partially purified kallikrein or to assess kallikrein generated upon kaolin activation of human plasma.[146–148] Kallikrein accounted for virtually all the TAME-esterase activity generated during the first few minutes of incubation of plasma with kaolin, and the kinetics of bradykinin generation, as assessed by radioimmunoassay,[149] paralleled the rate of ester hydrolysis.[150] Nevertheless, this substrate is not specific for kallikrein, and it is less sensitive than the assay utilizing synthetic *p*-nitroanilides. $^3$H-TAME has been utilized to improve the sensitivity as well as the ease of performance of the assay;[151] the $^3$H-methanol liberated is extracted with scintillation fluid and directly counted.

Kallikrein or prekallikrein antigen can be determined by radial immunodiffusion using a monospecific antiserum,[152] and a radioimmunoassay for prekallikrein has been reported.[153] The latter assay is sensitive and specific; however, it does not distinguish between prekallikrein and kallikrein. Further studies are needed to determine whether kallikrein bound to either $C\bar{1}$ INH[154] or $\alpha_2$ macroglobulin[155] is detected before such an assay could be applied to activated plasma.

Nevertheless such an assay can be utilized to determine the total antigen content of plasma[156] and has been used to determine that some patients with Fletcher trait (prekallikrein deficiency) contain a nonfunctional but immunologically reactive form of prekallikrein.[157] Similar molecular heterogeneity of patients with Hageman factor deficiency has been shown using anti-Hageman factor antibody,[158] and the protein in one patient has been shown to be noncleavable using the usual enzymes.[159] Another potential complication with regard to both immunochemical and functional determination of prekallikrein/kallikrein is that binding to HMW kininogen affects the prekallikrein determination;[108] thus determination of prekallikrein in plasma deficient in HMW kininogen requires reconstitution with HMW kininogen. Similar results were obtained using Laurell rocket electroimmunodiffusion,[160] although there is lack of agreement regarding the quantitation of prekallikrein in HMW kininogen deficient plasma.[108,160,161]

Kallikrein can also be determined by its ability to liberate bradykinin from kininogen. Kallikrein or Hageman factor fragment-activated prekallikrein is incubated for 5 minutes either with heat-inactivated plasma prepared at 61° C for 2 hours[162] or with a source of purified HMW kininogen. The bradykinin generated can then be assayed by its ability to contract a smooth muscle such as a guinea pig ileum.[163] If the kininogen source is incubated with kallikrein ranging from 0.1 to 5 percent by weight, a proportionate increase in the bradykinin liberated results. This assay is sensitive (can detect as little as 2 ng bradykinin), is not affected by most buffer constituents, and is highly specific for kallikrein. However, it is only semiquantitative. Use of a radioimmunoassay for bradykinin[149] can improve the reproducibility of the method. This approach is quite useful for following kallikrein (or prekallikrein) activity during isolation procedures but cannot be utilized as an assay for plasma kallikrein or prekallikrein.

**The Mechanism of Activation of Human Prekallikrein.** Activation of human prekallikrein by HFa proceeds by limited proteolytic digestion. Each of the molecular forms of prekallikrein seen at 88,000 and 85,000 daltons is cleaved, and upon reduction a two-chain disulfide-linked enzyme results. A heavy chain of 52,000 daltons is linked to a light chain of either 36,000 or 33,000 daltons corresponding to the two forms of the starting material.[164] When activation was carried out in the presence of $^3$H-DFP, all the $^3$H was seen in the light chains, indicating that this portion of the molecule contains the active site of kallikrein.[145] The evidence that both molecular weight forms represent prekallikrein include the following: (1) both were cleaved by Hageman factor fragments and yielded similar activation patterns, (2) they were not interconvertible upon activation by Hageman factor or incubation or prekallikrein with kallikrein, (3) they contained the same antigenic determinants, (4) DFP was incorporated into the light chains of each molecular form of the active enzymes, and (5) neither band was seen when prekallikrein deficient plasma was fractionated.[164] Similar results have been reported by other workers,[165] and kinetic studies of the activation of purified prekallikrein by HFf[166] have been reported. The heavy and light chains of reduced and alkylated kallikrein have been recently purified; the heavy chain was shown to possess the binding site for HMW kininogen, while the light chain retained enzymatic activity characteristic of kallikrein.[167]

Prekallikrein has been purified in other species, and its mechanism of activation has been examined. Bovine prekallikrein[168–170] was shown to be a single chain proenzyme that was digested by bovine Hageman factor to yield a two-chain disulfide-linked enzyme in a fashion analogous to that seen in man. Guinea pig prekallikrein is activated similarly.[171] Rabbit prekallikrein was found to be a $\beta$ globulin with a molecular weight of 90,000 daltons and an isoelectric point of 5.9.[172] Upon conversion to kallikrein, not only was a kinin-generating enzyme formed but the kallikrein was found to shorten the PTT of rabbit plasma and human kallikrein behaved similarly.[173] Thus the function of kallikrein as a coagulation factor can be detected in rabbit plasma. Addition of kallikrein to human plasma or to congenitally deficient plasmas (other than Fletcher trait) has no effect. When the mechanism of conversion of rabbit prekallikrein to kallikrein was examined, activation was associated with the loss of an 8000-dalton peptide.[172] However, when the mechanism was examined in greater detail, activation in the presence of trasylol yielded conversion to a two-chain disulfide-linked enzyme without any change in molecular weight.[174] Since trasylol inactivates kallikrein but not Hageman factor,[93] it appeared that the peptide released was secondary to digestion of prekallikrein (or kallikrein) by the kallikrein produced. This phenomenon has also been observed for human prekallikrein. Digestion of $^{125}$I prekallikrein with 5 percent nonradiolabeled kallikrein followed by SDS gel electrophoresis and autoradiography resulted in the formation of a prekallikrein that was diminished in size by approximately 10,000 daltons.[164] The molecule remained as a single chain, and no conversion to kallikrein was detected.

The enzyme kallikrein has at least three substrates in plasma that are relevant to coagulation, fibrinolysis, and kinin formation, as shown in Figure 8–7. The interaction with Hageman factor has been discussed above, and the interaction of kallikrein with HMW kininogen and plasminogen will be described presently.

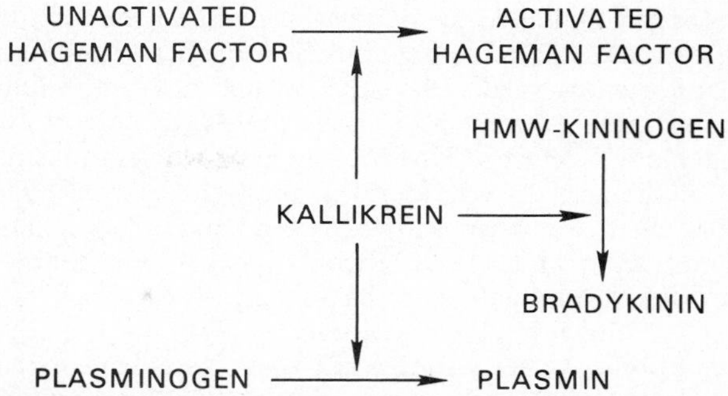


**Figure 8–7.** Diagram of the interaction of kallikrein with three of its substrates—Hageman factor, HMW kininogen, and plasminogen.

## HMW KININOGEN

**Plasma Kininogens.** The number of kininogens circulating in plasma had been a controversial issue; it was resolved largely as a consequence of the discovery of plasmas deficient in HMW kininogen. In 1966, two highly purified human kininogens (I and II) were isolated which had a molecular weight of approximately 50,000 as estimated by gel filtration and sucrose density ultracentrifugation.[175] Kininogen I appeared to have the bradykinin moiety at the C-terminus because its kinin-forming capacity was inactivated by carboxypeptidase B. However, kininogen II was not inactivated by exopeptidases and appeared to have the bradykinin located within the molecule. Given our present information, both these kininogens would be considered low molecular weight kininogen, and kininogen I might represent a partially degraded form. Soon thereafter, Jacobsen demonstrated the presence of two different kininogens in various mammalian plasmas.[176–178] These consisted of a high molecular weight form of about 200,000 daltons that was rapidly cleaved by plasma kallikrein, and a low molecular weight kininogen of 60,000 daltons that was slowly cleaved by plasma kallikrein. Tissue kallikreins appeared to digest both forms of kininogen at the same rate. Several investigators subsequently reported finding only the low molecular weight form in human plasma,[90,179–181] while others have found both high and low molecular weight forms in human[182–186] and bovine plasmas.[187,188] The discovery of plasmas that are deficient in kininogen (particularly HMW kininogen) has demonstrated that the two molecular weight forms do indeed exist in plasma, and confirmed earlier observations that HMW kininogen represents approximately 15 to 20 percent of the total plasma kininogen.[189] Furthermore, careful analysis of the kinetics of cleavage of high and low molecular weight kininogens demonstrated that high molecular weight kininogen is clearly the preferred substrate for plasma kallikrein.[189] The Km and k/cat for the cleavage of HMW kininogen by plasma kallikrein were 115 to 2.7, respectively, while the Km and k/cat for the cleavage of low molecular weight kininogen were 3.7 and 3.2, respectively.[189]

**Properties of Human HMW Kininogen.** Purified HMW kininogen[189a] had a molecular weight of 210,000 upon Sephadex G-200 gel filtration, an isoelectric point of 4.3, and a molecular weight of 120,000 when assessed by SDS gel electrophoresis. Over 90 percent of the material remained at 120,000 daltons after reduction, indicating that the HMW kininogen isolated was a single chain. When a time course of digestion of human HMW-kininogen by kallikrein was performed and the mixture reduced and alkylated, separation into a heavy and light chain was observed. When the isolated heavy and light chains were examined for their ability to correct the coagulation defect in HMW kininogen deficient plasma, all of the activity was found in the light chain.[189a] The light chain was then shown to bind prekallikrein and factor XI[106] and attach them to negatively charged surfaces.[105] Similar results have been observed by others;[192-196] however, the molecular weight of the light chain obtained has varied while there is agreement that the heavy chain is approximately 62,000 to 66,000. Schiffman and colleagues[196] presented evidence that following the initial cleavage, both heavy and light chains are of equal size at 65,000. Then the light chain is further digested to yield a 54,000 light chain. Other workers have not observed a light chain equal in size to a heavy chain but have reported a light chain of 56,000 that is then further degraded to 45,000,[193] while some have found the light chain to be yet smaller, between 37,000 and 44,000.[189a,194] All forms of the light chain isolated possess the same functional capability, and it is clear that once HMW kininogen is initially cleaved to liberate bradykinin, further digestion of the light chain occurs to yield products of differing molecular weight. These observations are consistent with earlier work demonstrating that kallikrein cleavage of human HMW kininogen does not diminish its coagulant activity.[33,37] However, excessive in vitro digestion of the light chain by kallikrein can destroy such activity.[184]

Studies of bovine HMW kininogen have conclusively demonstrated that bradykinin is located at the center of the molecule; thus two cleavages by plasma kallikrein are necessary in order to liberate bradykinin.[198,199] An illustration of the cleavages in HMW kininogen observed upon digestion by kallikrein are shown in Figure 8–8. Early studies of bovine HMW kininogen have suggested that a partially cleaved form of HMW kininogen in which only one of the two bond cleavages needed to liberate bradykinin has occurred may be a superior cofactor to that of the native molecule or the isolated light chain.[200,201] The degree to which this is important in man is unclear, but some evidence to suggest that cleavage of HMW kininogen augments its activity has been presented.[202] Further, the ability of HMW kininogen to displace fibrinogen from the surface may relate to such activity.[203]

Antibody to HMW kininogen has been prepared and used to determine the distinguishing features of HMW kininogen and LMW kininogen. A sheep was immunized with kininogen and the sheep plasma adsorbed with Williams trait plasma to yield an antibody that reacts with both high and low molecular weight kininogens. When the sheep antiserum was adsorbed with Fitzgerald trait plasma (which has significant quantities of LMW kininogen), an antiserum that was monospecific for HMW kininogen resulted. When each of these antisera was reacted with normal plasma, the pattern shown in Figure 8–9 was seen. Two arcs that fuse at one end are seen with the antikininogen serum, indicating a reaction

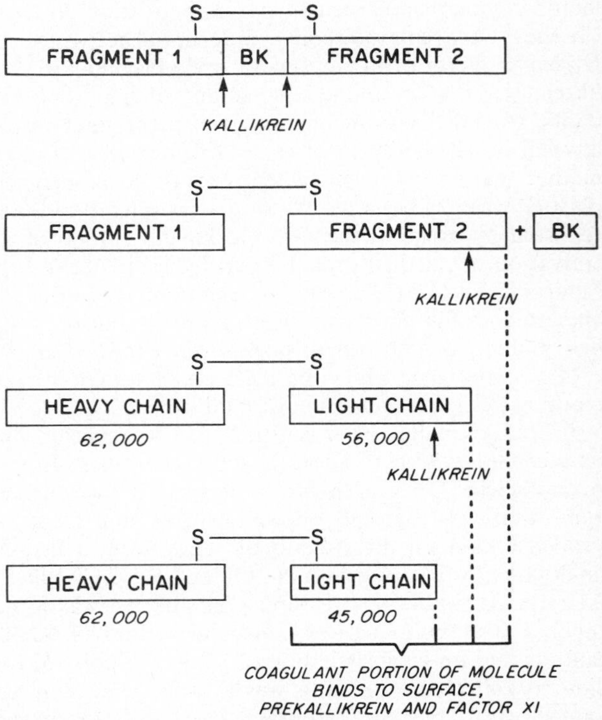


**Figure 8–8.** Steps by which HMW kininogen is cleaved by plasma kallikrein. Digestion at two sites within a disulfide bridge is required for release of kinin, and two chains of approximately equal size are left disulfide linked. Rapid further cleavage of one chain yields the 56,000 light chain (the major product) followed by a second slower cleavage to a 45,000 final product. The function of this light "chain" is as indicated.

of partial antigenic identity (upper trough). When normal plasma was reacted against the anti-HMW kininogen serum placed in the lower trough, only the inner arc was seen. When this latter antiserum was then reacted with the isolated HMW kininogen heavy and light chains, a precipitin was obtained only with the light chain. Thus the light chain appeared to possess the major antigenic determinants that distinguish HMW kininogen from LMW kininogen.[189a,195] Furthermore, the data demonstrated that the antigens they share were associated with the heavy chain, as has been reported when the chains of bovine kininogens were compared.[204-206]

**Assay of HMW Kininogens.** The presence of HMW kininogen can be assessed by cleavage with plasma kallikrein, urinary kallikrein,[207,208] or trypsin. The enzyme is inactivated by boiling[209] or by further incubation with soybean trypsin inhibitor. In each instance, the bradykinin generated is determined by either bioassay or radioimmunoassay. This method, however, does not distinguish HMW kininogen from LMW kininogen, and the known difference in their rate of cleavage by plasma kallikrein cannot be readily used to construct a simple assay. Clearly the ability of HMW kininogen to correct the prolonged partial thromboplastin time of HMW kininogen deficient plasma provides a specific and readily performed assay. Since reconstitution of this plasma with 10 to 12 percent of normal HMW kininogen completely

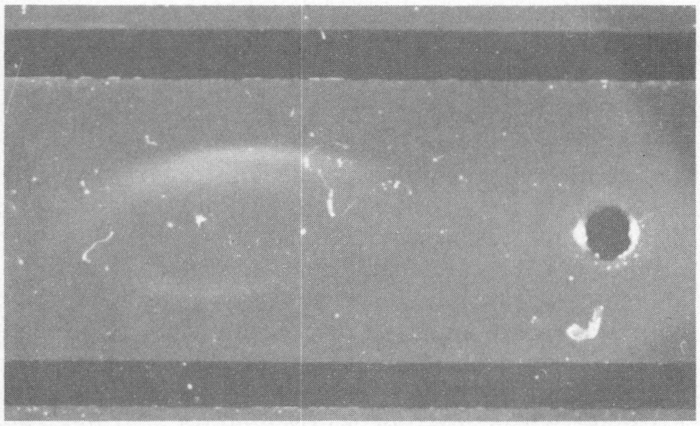

**Figure 8–9.** Immunoelectrophoresis of normal plasma reacted against antibody to human kininogens (upper trough) and against antibody rendered specific for HMW kininogen (lower trough). A line of partial identity is seen.

corrects the functional abnormality, significant dilution of normal plasma must be made in order to obtain a dose response between 0 and 12 percent of normal so that a standard curve can be constructed. Unknowns can be diluted and compared with the standards and expressed as a percent of normal HMW kininogen or in units per milliliter if the quantity of HMW kininogen present in plasma is set at 1.0 unit. If purified HMW kininogen is available, the HMW kininogen content of normal plasma can be expressed in $\mu$g per milliliter based upon either functional or antigenic analysis. We have found close agreement between the functional and antigenic determinations of plasma HMW kininogen and estimate the normal plasma level to be between 70 and 90 $\mu$g per milliliter. Since HMW kininogen is relatively plentiful in plasma and monospecific antisera can be prepared, HMW kininogen antigen could be measured by radial immunodiffusion, counterimmunoelectrophoresis, or radioimmunoassay.[160,210] Recently, an assay for HMW kininogen antigen using hemagglutination inhibition has been reported,[161] which is both sensitive and specific.

## FACTOR XI

**Properties of Purified Factor XI.** Factor XI[211] is a $\gamma$ globulin of molecular weight 158,000[19,96] as assessed by SDS gel electrophoresis and has an isoelectric point of 9.1.[212]

**Assays for Factor XI.** The standard assay of factor XI is a coagulation assay in which the partial thromboplastin time of factor XI deficient plasma is corrected. It is performed essentially as described above for either Hageman factor or HMW kininogen. Factor XIa appears to have weak esterolytic activity;[19] however, there is no known synthetic substrate that is specifically digested by factor XIa. The concentration of factor XI in plasma is only about 4 to 7 ng per milliliter,[19,96] which limits the ability to see precipitin lines when whole plasma is reacted with monospecific antisera to factor XI. Thus radial immunodiffusion or electroimmunodiffusion assays may not be feasible. A radioimmunoassay for factor XI has been described,[213] which represents the most sensitive way of determining factor XI; it does not, however, distinguish factor XI from factor XIa, and it is therefore not useful as a measure of activation. Nevertheless antisera to human factor XI have been prepared[96,214,215] and used to distinguish the homozygous from the heterozygous deficiency by functional inhibition of coagulant activity.[215]

**Activation of Human Factor XI.** Purified preparations of human factor XI have a molecular weight of 155,000 to 160,000 upon SDS gel electrophoresis; however, upon reduction, the molecular weight is 80,000 to 82,000,[19,215,216] and only a single band is seen. Thus it appears that factor XI is a two-chain molecule and the two constituent chains are virtually the same size. A similar observation was made when highly purified bovine factor XI was examined,[217] and thus far incorporation of high concentrations of benzamidine and DFP into the isolation procedure has not resulted in the formation of a single-chain form of factor XI.

Cleavage of human factor XI by trypsin,[19,218,219] Hageman factor fragments,[96,98,212] or surface-bound activated Hageman factor[220,221] resulted in cleavage of the 80,000 dalton chains within a disulfide bridge. Thus in the absence of reduction, the molecular weights of factor XI and factor XIa were essentially the same.[70,214,218,222] However, upon reduction, the two 80,000 chains of the starting material appeared to be cleaved to chains of 50,000 and 30,000. Factor XIa has been shown to be a serine protease[223] that can be inhibited by DFP. When factor XI was activated by Hageman factor, inactivated by $^3$H-DFP, and reduced, $^3$H-DFP was incorporated into the 30,000-dalton light chain.[220] When binding of antithrombin III-heparin by factor XIa was quantitated, two moles of antithrombin III appeared to be found by each mole of factor XIa, suggesting that there are two active sites in factor XIa, one for each light chain present.[221]

Factor XI circulates as a complex with HMW kininogen,[43] the rate of conversion of factor XI to factor XIa is augmented by HMW kininogen,[37,97–101] and the rate of formation of activated Hageman factor (and factor XIa) is dependent upon prekallikrein.[20–22,97–99,101] Yet prekallikrein circulates complexed to different HMW kininogen molecules from those of factor XI;[43] thus a mechanism must exist in which Hageman factor that is activated by kallikrein can interact with the factor XI–HMW kininogen complex. Binding of factor XI to surfaces is augmented by HMW kininogen in a plasma milieu,[104,105] and, as is the case for prekallikrein,[105] the HMW kininogen appears to counteract competing plasma proteins that inhibit factor XI binding.[224] Factor XIa attachment to the HMW kininogen appears to reside in the heavy chain.[225] A case of acquired factor XI deficiency has been reported in which an IgG antifactor XI was shown to inhibit its interaction with HMW kininogen and its ability to be activated and cleaved by HFa.[226]

The ability of factor XIa to completely correct the

coagulation defect of Hageman factor, prekallikrein, or HMW kininogen deficient plasmas, and the normal rate of generation of plasmin and bradykinin upon activation of factor XI deficient plasma, indicate that in a practical sense activation of factor XIa represents the second step in the intrinsic coagulation pathway. It may, however, play an alternative role in the initial step when prekallikrein is absent.[227]

## THE ROLE OF THE EARLY STEPS OF THE INTRINSIC COAGULATION PATHWAY IN FIBRINOLYSIS

Hageman factor dependent conversion of plasminogen to plasmin is readily demonstrable in whole plasma.[10,11,228] Since prekallikrein and HMW kininogen are required for optimal activation and function of Hageman factor, they are also required for activation of the Hageman factor dependent fibrinolytic pathway. However, identification of the molecule or molecules that directly convert plasminogen to plasmin has been the subject of numerous investigations, and the results have not been clear. Colman[229] first reported that incubation of kallikrein with plasminogen leads to the generation of plasmin, and the kinetics of the reaction appeared to be stoichiometric. Ogston and colleagues[230] demonstrated a cofactor required for Hageman factor dependent fibrinolysis that appeared to be distinguishable from kallikrein and factor XIa. However, it was clearly present in plasma fractions containing these factors. The assay for this protein was dependent upon reconstitution of glass-adsorbed plasma from which the fibrinolytic factor had been depleted. This "Hageman factor cofactor" had a molecular weight of 160,000, and it migrated with the $\gamma$ globulins. Kaplan and Austen subsequently demonstrated a Hageman factor–activatable plasma factor called plasminogen proactivator, which, upon activation, was able to directly convert plasminogen to plasmin.[231] These authors proposed that the plasminogen activator derived was responsible for the plasminogen-converting activity in kallikrein preparations. The demonstration of plasminogen proactivator activity in the $\gamma$ globulin fraction of prekallikrein deficient plasma appeared to confirm their interpretation.[231] This postulate was challenged by Laake and Vennerod based upon their inability to separate prekallikrein from plasminogen proactivator, and they concluded that kallikrein and plasminogen-activating activities are functions of the same molecule.[232] When these authors examined the $\gamma$ globulin effluent obtained from prekallikrein deficient plasma, no plasminogen activator or proactivator activity was observed.[233]

The successful purification of human prekallikrein has shed further light upon this question. First, when human prekallikrein was isolated in the presence of proteolytic inhibitors, the prekallikrein and plasminogen proactivator activities coincided and the two-banded pattern was shown to represent prekallikrein heterogeneity rather than two separate Hageman factor substrates.[164] Second, kallikrein was shown to cleave prekallikrein and decrease its molecular weight by 10,000 daltons; this difference in size corresponded to the previously reported difference in size between prekallikrein and plasminogen proactivator.[234] Finally, fractionation of prekallikrein deficient plasma demonstrated that the plasminogen proactivator activity seen associated with prekallikrein was absent.[164] Hence the conclusion was reached that prekallikrein is a plasminogen proactivator and that the previous reported activity was a property of prekallikrein and/or the prekallikrein degradation product. However, plasminogen-activating activity was again found in the $\gamma$ globulin fraction of normal plasma[235] which was not attributable to prekallikrein, and this same activity was found in prekallikrein deficient plasma. Further fractionation of this material demonstrated that the activity was superimposed upon factor XI.[164] Isolation of the plasminogen proactivator activity present in prekallikrein plasma was then identified as factor XI, and factor XIa was shown to directly convert plasminogen to plasmin.[236]

The observation that plasminogen-activating activity does indeed reside in the $\gamma$ globulin effluent of prekallikrein deficient plasma has been confirmed;[237] however, these authors did not demonstrate that the activity was Hageman factor activatable and considered prekallikrein to be the only plasminogen proactivator. Clearly, the gradual conversion of plasminogen to plasmin observed in prekallikrein deficient plasma is secondary to a Hageman factor dependent enzyme that is not kallikrein. When the fibrinolytic activity of factor XI deficient plasma was examined, its rate of activation was normal, but it failed to generate a normal amount of plasmin. Reconstitution with purified factor XI corrected this abnormality.[238] A single report has presented evidence that activated Hageman factor itself can function as a weak plasminogen activator;[239] however, when experiments are performed in which the fibrinolytic capacity of prekallikrein is assessed (i.e., Hageman factor fragments plus plasminogen), the contribution of HFf is less than 5 percent of the activity seen with kallikrein.[236] Thus larger quantities of activated Hageman factor may be required for this effect to reach significant levels. It appears clear that prekallikrein is a plasminogen proactivator, factor XI may function as a second proactivator, and HFa or HFf may directly contribute to plasminogen activation.

The identity of the Hageman factor cofactor is not clear; however, the function these authors observed does not appear to be distinguishable from that of the known Hageman factor substrates. Glass adsorbed plasma, used in the assay for the Hageman factor cofactor, has been shown to be depleted of prekallikrein;[240] thus the kallikrein present in Hageman factor cofactor preparations may contribute to the fibrinolysis observed by its effect upon Hageman factor activation. Yet the molecular weight reported for this factor was quite different from kallikrein, and the factor appeared to be separable from the bulk of kallikrein but not from factor XI.[230,241] The active factor was also inhibited by $\alpha_1$ antitrypsin, a property it shares with factor XIa.[242] The molecular properties of this cofactor most closely resemble the activity we have observed with our factor XI preparation; thus it is possible that the activity being measured was a function of more than one protein.

Further studies in whole plasma are needed to distinguish the effect of kallikrein upon fibrinolysis via its ability to activate Hageman factor from its ability to convert plasminogen to plasmin. It is of interest that one estimate of the direct contribution of kallikrein to the conversion of plasminogen to plasmin was approximately 50 percent[241] of the total Hageman factor dependent fibrinolytic activity present in plasma.

A summary of the known interactions leading to coagulation, fibrinolysis, and kinin formation is shown in Figure 8–10.

## CONTROL MECHANISMS

The binding of Hageman factor to surfaces is markedly inhibited by the presence of plasma, and the effect is attributable to many plasma fractions and does not, therefore, appear to be specific.[243] Nevertheless, such inhibition would serve to limit in vivo activation at the very first step. In vitro studies of Hageman factor activation have demonstrated that excess HMW kininogen also appears to be inhibitory.[102, 103] There is approximately twice the plasma concentration of HMW kininogen needed to bind all the prekallikrein and factor XI.[42,43,106] Since HMW kininogen is normally present in excess, activation in plasma may be suboptimal. This possibility has not, however, been examined. Once activation proceeds beyond the initial cleavage of Hageman factor, fragmentation of the Hageman factor occurs and the prealbumin fragment is liberated from the surface[119] and can continue to function as a prekallikrein activator in the fluid phase. The consequence of this step would be to divert the pathway from coagulation to fibrinolysis and kinin generation, as originally proposed by Kaplan and Austen.[81] The major inhibitor of activated Hageman factor[244] and Hageman factor fragments[245] is the inhibitor of the activated first component of complement ($C\bar{1}$ INH). The $C\bar{1}$ INH has been shown to bind[95] and irreversibly inactivate the Hageman factor fragments. Antithrombin III has also been shown to bind and inactivate HFa and HFf as well as an unfragmented form of Hageman factor in which the active site was available; however, the inactivation observed was slower than that obtained with comparable concentrations of $C\bar{1}$ INH.[246] Heparin markedly accelerated the binding and inactivation of Hageman factor by antithrombin III such that the reaction was virtually complete within 30 seconds. There was no inhibition of activated Hageman factor by $\alpha_2$ macroglobulin, $\alpha_1$ antitrypsin, $\alpha_1$ antichymotrypsin, and inter $\alpha$ trypsin inhibitor.

The major inhibitor of plasma kallikrein also appears to be $C\bar{1}$ INH, which has been shown to bind to the active site of the enzyme such that all esterase and proteolytic activities were inhibited[154,247] and a 1:1 stoichiometric complex was formed.[248] $\alpha_2$ Macroglobulin functions as a second kallikrein inhibitor,[155] although complete inactivation does not result; most of the esterase activity and a small fraction of residual proteolytic activity remain.[140] It is likely that $\alpha_2$ macroglobulin inhibits by sterically interfering with the function of the active site without actually binding to it. Of particular

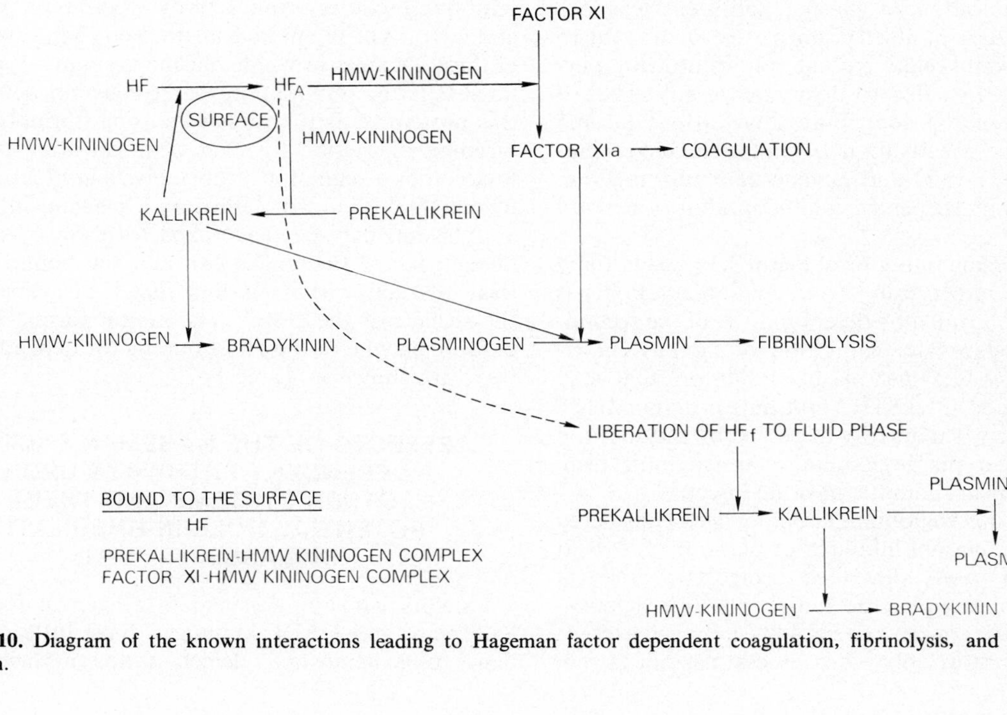


**Figure 8–10.** Diagram of the known interactions leading to Hageman factor dependent coagulation, fibrinolysis, and the generation of bradykinin.

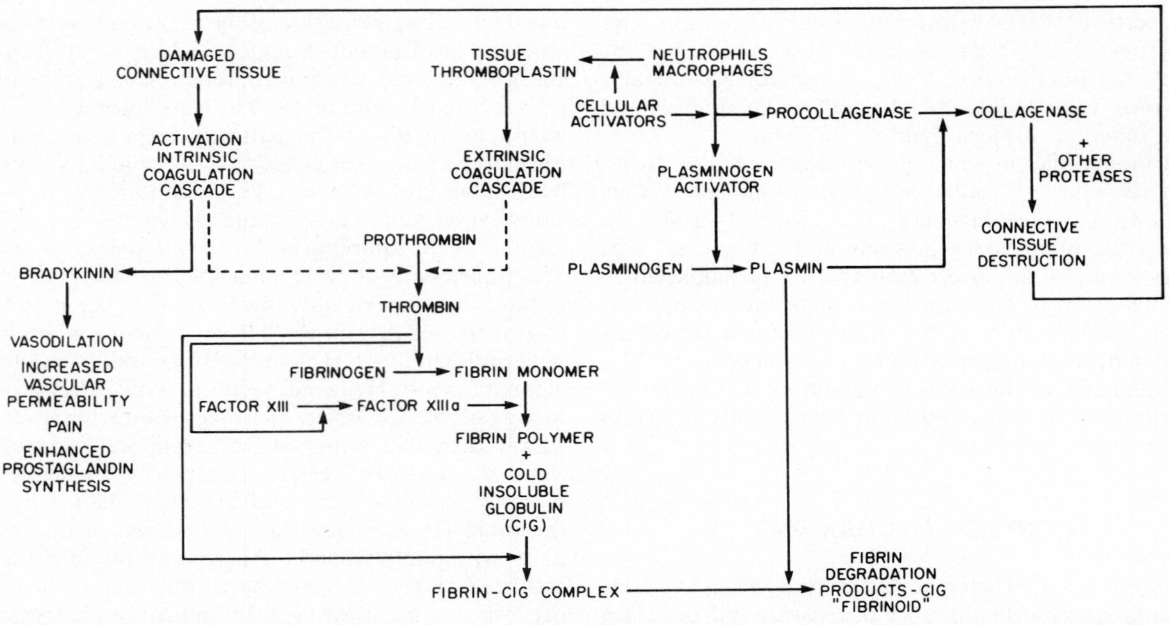


**Figure 8–11.** Diagram depicting the roles of the coagulation cascades in inflammation. The extrinsic pathway appears to be recruited by release of tissue factor from activated cells and interaction of coagulation, and fibrinolytic proteases yield deposition of "fibrinoid." Damaged connective tissue can serve as a surface upon which initiation of the intrinsic coagulation pathway can occur with formation of bradykinin.

interest is that the residual activity of the kallikrein–$\alpha_2$ macroglobulin complex resists further inactivation by C$\bar{1}$ INH; thus if there is continual activation of this pathway under normal conditions, this is one form in which a trace quantity of active enzyme could persist in plasma. Antithrombin III can also function as an inhibitor of plasma kallikrein,[249] although there is not agreement regarding the magnitude of augmentation in the presence of heparin.[250,251] Under conditions in which antithrombin III–heparin rapidly inactivated Hageman factor, little inhibition of plasma kallikrein was obtained.[246] Although $\alpha_1$ antitrypsin had been thought to inhibit plasma kallikrein,[247] recent studies utilizing purified $\alpha_1$ antitrypsin failed to demonstrate any effect.[212] Recent studies of the contribution of various plasma inhibitors to the inactivation of kallikrein have demonstrated that C$\bar{1}$ INH and $\alpha_2$ macroglobulin together account for about 90 percent of the inhibitory activity of plasma.[252, 253]

The major plasma inhibitor of factor XIa was initially shown to be $\alpha_1$ antitrypsin,[212] and this observation has been recently confirmed by determination of the second-order rate constants for inhibition of factor XIa by plasma proteases.[254] Other plasma inhibitors that may contribute include C$\bar{1}$ INH[244] and antithrombin III.[255] The latter activity is markedly increased by the addition of heparin while $\alpha_2$ macroglobulin, $\alpha_1$ antichymotrypsin, and inter-$\alpha$ trypsin inhibitor have no effect.[212]

Although $\alpha_2$ macroglobulin had long been considered to be the major plasma inhibitor of plasmin,[141, 256, 257] it is clear that a newly described proteolytic inhibitor called $\alpha_2$ antiplasmin is the major plasmin inactivator.[258-260] Since the concentration of plasminogen exceeds that of the inhibitor, only when excess plasmin is generated does significant binding to $\alpha_2$ macroglobulin result.[261,262] Other inhibitors of plasmin demonstrable in vitro include $\alpha_1$ antitrypsin[257] and C$\bar{1}$ INH;[263,264] however, it is clear that these contribute little in whole plasma. Antithrombin III can also function as a plasmin inhibitor; however, its effect is not significant unless it is assayed in the presence of heparin.[265] An extensive review of the inhibitory effect of $\alpha_2$ macroglobulin and antithrombin III upon activated coagulation factors has been published.[266] The inhibitory spectrum of $\alpha_2$ plasmin inhibitor includes weak activity upon HFf, kallikrein, and factor XIa,[267] but its contribution to the inactivation of these enzymes in whole plasma is small. Of particular interest is the observation that congenital deficiency of this protein leads to excessive plasma fibrinolysis and a bleeding diathesis,[268-271] thus demonstrating its critical function as a regulator of fibrinolysis in blood. In order to manifest its in vivo effect as a plasmin inhibitor $\alpha_2$ antiplasmin may be crosslinked to fibrin by fibrin-stabilizing factor (factor XIIIa), and the bound inhibitor then interacts within plasmin that is also bound along the surface of the clot.[272] The major plasma inhibitors of each enzyme of the Hageman factor dependent pathways are shown in Table 8–1.

## EFFECTS OF THE HAGEMAN FACTOR DEPENDENT PATHWAYS UPON OTHER SYSTEMS AND THEIR POTENTIAL ROLE IN RHEUMATIC DISEASES (Fig. 8–11)

Patients who are deficient in Hageman factor, prekallikrein, and HMW kininogen have little or no evidence of a hemostatic defect, although their plasmas

**Table 8–1.** Inhibitors of Enzymes of the Hageman Factor Dependent Pathways

| Enzyme | Inhibitors |
|---|---|
| HFa, HFf | $C\bar{1}$ INH |
| Kallikrein | $C\bar{1}$ INH |
| | $\alpha_2$ Macroglobulin |
| Factor XIa | $C\bar{1}$ INH |
| | $\alpha_1$ Antitrypsin |
| Plasmin | $\alpha_2$ Antiplasmin |
| | $\alpha_2$ Macroglobulin |

possess profound in vitro abnormalities. Since these are the only deficiencies in which there is simultaneous impairment of coagulation, fibrinolysis, and kinin generation, it is possible that the latter defects are somehow protective and diminish the incidence of bleeding. It is also possible that the normal function of this pathway is not to produce a blood clot but to regulate blood flow via the vasodilator activity of bradykinin and/or to contribute to the body's ability to respond to injury and generate an inflammatory response. Bradykinin not only acts as a vasodilator but also increases vascular permeability, causes a burning sensation upon contact with sensory nerve endings, and in high concentrations can cause hypotension.[273] Kallikrein has been shown to aggregate neutrophils[274] and to possess chemotactic activity for human neutrophils and monocytes[275,276] and could thereby act to recruit these cells into sites of tissue injury. Consistent with this possibility is the observation that the chemotactic activity seen in serum was diminished when prekallikrein deficient plasma was examined.[21] Surprisingly, skin windows placed in HMW kininogen deficient plasma revealed a markedly augmented infiltration with neutrophils,[277] suggesting that HMW kininogen or a fragment derived from HMW kininogen functions to inhibit cellular infiltration. The Hageman factor dependent pathways may also play a role in the complement pathways. Thus Hageman factor deficient plasma had an abnormal rate of activation of the alternative complement pathway.[278] In addition, patients with hereditary angioedema who lack $C\bar{1}$ INH have "spontaneous" activation of Cl, which appears to be dependent upon Hageman factor.[279] Studies by Ghebrehiwet and colleagues[280,281] have demonstrated that HFf can directly activate Cl by cleavage of the $C\bar{1}r$ subcomponent. Thus in the absence of $C\bar{1}$ INH, not only is Cl more likely to autoactivate[282,283] but further enzymatic digestion by HFf (and perhaps other enzymes) may lead to the profound consumption of C4 and C2 seen during attacks of swelling. Other possible interactions between these cascades, whose importance is less clear, include the ability of kallikrein to activate factor B[284] and the ability of plasmin to activate C1s[285] and cleave C3.[286] Numerical evidence regarding the pathogenesis of hereditary angioedema is of particular note; induced skin blisters in such patients have been shown to possess elevated levels of kallikrein[287] and spontaneous generation of bradykinin has been observed upon incubating such plasma in nonactivating surfaces[288] while massive activation of only the complement cascade failed to generate a contractile or vasoactive factor.[288]

The role of the Hageman factor dependent pathways in rheumatic diseases has not been systematically explored, and much work in this area is required. It is not likely that it is the primary mediator pathway activated in such disorders, since immune complexes do not directly initiate the cascade, and at least one patient with Hageman factor deficiency has been reported with rheumatoid arthritis.[289] Although uric acid and pyrophosphate crystals can initiate Hageman factor activation in vitro,[50] this potential contribution to the joint inflammation seen in gout and pseudogout has not been quantitated relative to the other effects of such crystals upon the complement cascade[290,291] and phagocytosis. Recently the activation of Hageman factor by sodium urate crystals has been examined in plasma and joint fluid. Hageman factor cleavage was shown to be dependent upon the presence of prekallikrein and HMW kininogen, and both HFa and HFf were generated.[292]

The observation that exposure to connective tissue elements can initiate the Hageman factor dependent pathways requires confirmation, and the specific connective tissue element responsible for such activity needs to be identified. Certainly, if damaged connective tissue secondary to inflammation initiated by immune complexes and complement or by cellular immune reactions can then lead to recruitment of these pathways, perpetuation of the inflammatory process might result. Thus the ability of bradykinin to increase vascular permeability would increase swelling and augment the local deposition of immune complexes and complement. Bradykinin would also increase the pain perceived by interaction with pain receptors. Plasmin has been identified as an enzyme that can convert a synovial procollagenase to a collagenase;[293] thus the fibrinolytic pathway may thereby augment connective tissue destruction. It is possible that activated Hageman factor or kallikrein might have additional effects upon the enzymes present in connective tissue or perhaps direct effects upon connective tissue itself. Kallikrein might also contribute to the influx of neutrophils and monocytes seen. In addition, local coagulation and fibrinolysis undoubtedly are responsible for the presence of fibrin degradation products or "fibrinoid" that is routinely seen in the lesions of virtually all the connective tissue disorders. Yet the relative contributions of the intrinsic and extrinsic coagulation pathways to the deposition of "fibrinoid" is unknown.

The critical components of the Hageman factor dependent pathways have been identified, their major interactions have been elucidated, and we actually possess sensitive functional assays for each component but also possess monospecific antisera that can be utilized to quantitate each component as a protein. In addition, further studies can be performed by radiolabeling purified preparations of each factor. Thus the reagents and techniques are now available with which to evaluate the possible contribution of these pathways to virtually any disorder, and future studies should be specifically focused upon the rheumatic diseases.

## Acknowledgment

The excellent typing and editing of this manuscript by Ms. Madeline Lee, Ms. Mavis Bolotsky, and Ms. Barbara Sykes are gratefully acknowledged.

## References

1. Bordet, J., and Genou, O.: Recherches sur la coagulation du sang et les serums anticoagulants. Ann. Inst. Pasteur 15:129, 1901.
2. Shafrir, E., and de Vries, A.: Studies on the clot-promoting activity of glass. J. Clin. Invest. 35:1183, 1956.
3. Margolis, J.: Glass surface and blood coagulation. Nature 178:805, 1956.
4. Hubbard, D., and Lucas, G.L.: Ionic charges of glass surfaces and other materials and their possible role in the coagulation of blood. J. Appl. Physiol. 15:265, 1960.
5. Ratnoff, O.D., and Colopy, J.E.: A familial hemorrhagic trait associated with a deficiency of clot-promoting fraction of plasma. J. Clin. Invest. 34:602, 1955.
6. Ratnoff, O.D., and Rosenblum, J.M.: Role of Hageman factor in the initiation of clotting by glass: Evidence that glass frees Hageman factor inhibition. Am. J. Med. 25:160, 1958.
7. Ratnoff, O.D., and Davie, E.W.: The purification of activated Hageman factor (activated XII). Biochemistry 1:967, 1962.
8. Speer, R.J., Ridgway, H., and Hill, J.M.: Activation of human Hageman factor (XII). Thromb. Diath. Haemorrhag. 14:1, 1965.
9. Donaldson, V.H., and Ratnoff, O.D.: Hageman factor: Alterations in physical properties during activation. Science 150:754, 1965.
10. Niewiarowski, S., and Prow-Wartelle, O.: Role du facteur contact (Facteur Hageman) dans la fibrinolyse. Thromb. Diath. Haemorrhag. 3:593, 1959.
11. Iatridis, S.G., and Ferguson, J.H.: Active Hageman factor. A plasma lysokinase of the human fibrinolytic system. J. Clin. Invest. 41:1277, 1962.
12. Margolis, J.: Plasma pain-producing substance and blood clotting. Nature 180:1464, 1957.
13. Margolis, J.: Activation of a permeability factor in plasma by contact with glass. Nature 180:635, 1958.
14. Margolis, J.: Activation of plasma by contact with glass. Evidence for a common reaction which releases plasma kinin and initiates coagulation. J. Physiol. 144:1, 1959.
15. Margolis, J.: The interrelationship of coagulation of plasma and release of peptides. Ann. N.Y. Acad. Sci. 104:133, 1963.
16. Hathaway, W.E., Belhausen, L.P., and Hathaway, H.S.: Evidence of a new plasma coagulation factor. I. Case report, coagulation studies and physiochemical properties. Blood 26:521, 1965.
17. Hattersley, P.G., and Hayse, D.: Fletcher factor deficiency. A report of three unrelated cases. Br. J. Haematol. 18:411, 1970.
18. Hathaway, W.E., and Alsever, J.: The relation of "Fletcher factor" to factors XI and XII. Br. J. Haematol. 18:161, 1970.
19. Wuepper, K.D.: Biochemistry and biology of components of the plasma kinin-forming system. *In* Lepow, I.H., and Ward, A. (eds.): Inflammation: Mechanisms and Control. New York, Academic Press, 1972, pp. 93–117.
20. Wuepper, K.D.: Prekallikrein deficiency in man. J. Exp. Med. 138:1345, 1973.
21. Weiss, A.S., Gallin, J.I., and Kaplan, A.P.: Fletcher factor deficiency. Abnormalities of coagulation, fibrinolysis, chemotactic activity, and kinin generation attributable to absence of prekallikrein. J. Clin. Invest. 53:622, 1974.
22. Saito, H., Ratnoff, O.D., and Donaldson, V.H.: Defective activation of clotting, fibrinolytic, and permeability enhancing systems in human Fletcher trait plasma. Circ. Res. 34:641, 1974.
23. Webster, M.E.: Human plasma kallikrein, its activation and pathologic role. Fed. Proc. 27:84, 1968.
24. Webster, M.E., and Pierce, J.V.: Activators of Hageman factor (factor XII): Identification and relationship to kallikrein-kinin system. Fed. Proc. 32:845, 1973.
25. Schiffman, S., and Lee, P.: Preparation, characterization, activation of a highly purified factor XI. Evidence that a hitherto unrecognized plasma activity participates in the interaction of factors XI and XII. Br. J. Haematol. 27:101, 1974.
26. Colman, R.W., Bagdasarian, A., Talamo, R.C., and Kaplan, A.P.: Williams trait: A new deficiency with abnormal levels of prekallikrein, plasminogen proactivator, and kininogen. *In* Pisano, J.J., and Austen, K.F. (eds.): The Chemistry and Biology of the Kallikrein-Kinin System in Health and Disease. Fogarty International Proceedings No. 27. Washington, D.C., U.S. Government Printing Office, 1974, pp. 65–72.
27. Saito, H., and Ratnoff, O.D.: Fitzgerald trait: An asymptomatic disorder with impaired blood coagulation, fibrinolysis, kinin generation, and generation of permeability factor of dilution. *In* Pisano, J.J., and Austen, K.F. (eds.): The Chemistry and Biology of the Kallikrein-Kinin System in Health and Disease. Fogarty International Proceedings No. 27. Washington, D.C., U.S. Government Printing Office, 1974, pp. 73–74.
28. LaCombe, M.J.: Déficit constitutionnel en un nouveau facteur de la coagulation intervenant au niveau de contact: Le facteur "Flaujeac." C. R. Acad. Sci. (D) 280:1039, 1975.
29. Waldman, R., and Abraham, J.: Fitzgerald factor: A heretofore unrecognized coagulation factor. Blood 46:761, 1975.
30. Saito, H., Ratnoff, O.D., Waldmann, R., and Abraham, J.P.: Fitzgerald trait. Deficiency of a hitherto unrecognized agent, Fitzgerald factor, participating in surface-mediated reactions of clotting, fibrinolysis, generation of kinins, and the property of diluted plasma enhancing vascular permeability (PF-dil). J. Clin. Invest. 55:1082, 1975.
31. Wuepper, K.D., Miller, D.R., and LaCombe, M.J.: Flaujeac trait: Deficiency of kininogen in man. Fed. Proc. 34:859, 1975.
32. Wuepper, K.D., Miller, D.R., and LaCombe, M.J.: Flaujeac trait. Deficiency of human plasma kininogen. J. Clin. Invest. 56:1663, 1975.
33. Colman, R.W., Bagdasarian, A., Talamo, R.C., Seavey, M., Scott, C.F., and Kaplan, A.P.: Williams trait: Combined deficiency of plasma plasminogen proactivator, kininogen, and a new procoagulant factor. Fed. Proc. 34:859, 1975.
34. Colman, R.W., Bagdasarian, A., Talamo, R.C., Scott, C.F., Seavey, M., Guimaraes, J.A., Pierce, J.V., and Kaplan, A.P.: Williams trait. Human kininogen deficiency with diminished levels of plasminogen proactivator and prekallikrein associated with abnormalities of the Hageman factor-dependent pathways. J. Clin. Invest. 56:1650, 1975.
35. Donaldson, V.H., Glueck, H.I., Miller, M.A., Movat, H.Z., and Habal, F.: Kininogen deficiency in Fitzgerald trait: Role of high molecular weight kininogen in clotting and fibrinolysis. J. Lab. Clin. Med. 87:327, 1976.
36. Schiffman, S., Lee, P., and Waldmann, R.: Identity of contact activation cofactor and Fitzgerald factor. Thromb. Res. 6:451, 1975.
37. Schiffman, S., and Lee, P.: Partial purification and characterization of contact activation cofactor. J. Clin. Invest. 56:1082, 1975.
38. Schiffman, S., Lee, P., Feinstein, D.I., and Pecci, R.: Relationship of contact activation cofactor (CAC) procoagulant activity to kininogen. Blood 49:935, 1977.
39. Ratnoff, O.D., Davie, E.W., and Mallet, D.L.: Studies on the action of Hageman factor: Evidence that activated Hageman factor in turn activates plasma thromboplastin antecedent. J. Clin. Invest. 40:803, 1961.
40. Wendel, U., Vogt, W., and Seidel, G.: Purification and some properties of a kininogenase from human plasma activated by surface contact. Hoppe Seylers Z. Physiol. Chem. 353:1591, 1972.
41. Nagasawa, S., and Nakayasu, T.: Human plasma prekallikrein as a protein complex. J. Biochem. 74:401, 1973.
42. Mandle, R., Jr., Colman, R.W., and Kaplan, A.P.: Identification of prekallikrein and HMW-kininogen as a circulating complex in human plasma. Proc. Natl. Acad. Sci. USA 73:4179, 1976.
43. Thompson, R.E., Mandle, R., Jr., and Kaplan, A.P.: Association of factor XI and high molecular weight kininogen in human plasma. J. Clin. Invest. 60:1376, 1977.
44. Ratnoff, O.D.: The biology and pathology of the initial stages of blood coagulation. Prog. Hematol. 5:204, 1966.
45. Margolis, J.: The effect of colloidal silica on blood coagulation. Aust. J. Exp. Biol. Med. Sci. 39:249, 1961.
46. Ratnoff, O.D., and Crum, J.D.: Activation of Hageman factor by solutions of ellagic acid. J. Lab. Clin. Med. 63:359, 1964.
47. Schwartz, H.J., and Kellermeyer, R.W.: Carrageenan and delayed hypersensitivity. II. Activation of Hageman factor by carrageenan and its possible significance. Proc. Soc. Exp. Biol. Med. 132:1021, 1969.
48. Kellermeyer, W.F., Jr., and Kellermeyer, R.W.: Hageman factor activation and kinin formation in human plasma induced by cellulose sulfate solutions. Proc. Soc. Exp. Biol. Med. 130:1310, 1969.
49. Kluft, C.: Assay for prekallikrein levels and prekallikrein activation in human plasma using dextran sulphate as a soluble activator. Thromb. Haemostasis 38:220, 1977.
50. Kellermeyer, R.W., and Breckenridge, R.T.: The inflammatory process in acute gouty arthritis. I. Activation of Hageman factor by sodium urate crystals. J. Lab. Clin. Med. 65:307, 1965.
51. Ratnoff, O.D.: Activation of Hageman factor by L-homocysteine. Science 29:1007, 1968.
52. Moskowitz, R.W., Schwartz, H.J., Michel, B., Ratnoff, O.D., and Astrup, T.: Generation of kinin-like agents by chondroitin sulfate, heparin, chitin sulfate, and human articular cartilage: Possible pathophysiologic implications. J. Lab. Clin. Med. 76:790, 1970.

53. Nossel, H.L.: Activation of factors XII (Hageman) and XI (PTA) by skin contact. Proc. Soc. Exp. Biol. Med. 122:16, 1966.
54. Margolis, J.: Activation of Hageman factor saturated fatty acids. Aust. J. Exp. Biol. Med. Sci. 40:505, 1962.
55. Botti, R.E., and Ratnoff, O.D.: The clot-promoting effect of soaps of long chain saturated fatty acids. J. Clin. Invest. 42:1569, 1963.
56. Didisheim, P., and Mibashan, R.S.: Activation of Hageman factor (factor XII) by long chain saturated fatty acids. Thromb. Diath. Haemorrh. 9:346, 1963.
57. Morrison, D.C., and Cochrane, C.G.: Direct evidence for Hageman factor (factor XII) activation by bacterial lipopolysaccharides (endotoxins). J. Exp. Med. 140:787, 1974.
58. McKay, D.G., Muller-Berghaus, G., and Gruse, V.: Activation of Hageman factor by ellagic acid and the generalized Shwartzman reaction. Am. J. Pathol. 54:393, 1969.
59. Pettinger, W.A., and Young, R.: Endotoxin-induced kinin (bradykinin) formation: Activation of Hageman factor and plasma kallikrein in human plasma. Life Sci. 9:313, 1970.
60. Kimball, H.R., Melmon, K.L., and Wolff, S.M.: Endotoxin-induced kinin production in man. Proc. Soc. Exp. Biol. Med. 139:1078, 1972.
61. Mason, J.W., Kleeberg, U., Dolan, P., and Colman, R.W.: Plasma kallikrein and Hageman factor in gram-negative bacteremia. Ann. Intern. Med. 73:545, 1970.
62. Rodriguez-Erdmann, F.: Studies on the pathogenesis of the generalized Schwartzman reaction. III. Trigger mechanism for the activation of the prothrombin molecule, Thromb. Diath. Haemorrh. 12:471, 1964.
63. Ulevitch, R.J., Cochrane, C.G., Henson, P.M., Morrison, D.C., and Doe, W.I.: Mediation systems in bacterial lipopolysaccharide-induced hypotension and disseminated intravascular coagulation. I. The role of complement. J. Exp. Med. 142:1570, 1975.
64. Eisen, V., and Smith, H.G.: Plasma kinin formation by complexes of aggregated $\gamma$-globulins and serum proteins. Br. J. Exp. Pathol. 51:328, 1970.
65. Movat, H.Z., and DiLorenzo, N.L.: Activation of the plasma kinin system by antigen-antibody aggregates. I. Generation of permeability factor in guinea pig serum. Lab. Invest. 19:187, 1968.
66. Movat, H.Z., DiLorenzo, N.L., and Treloar, M.P.: Activation of the plasma kinin system by antigen-antibody aggregates. II. Isolation of permeability enhancing and kinin releasing fractions from activated guinea pig serum. Lab. Invest. 19:201, 1968.
67. Movat, H.Z., Treloar, M.P., and Takeuchi, Y.: A small molecular weight permeability factor in guinea pig serum: Adsorption to antigen-antibody aggregates. J. Immunol. 103:875, 1969.
68. Epstein, W.V., Tan, M., and Melman, K.L.: Rheumatoid factor and kinin generation. Ann. N.Y. Acad. Sci. 168:173, 1969.
69. Cochrane, C.G., and Wuepper, K.D.: The kinin-forming system: Delineation and activation. *In* Miescher, P. (ed.): Immunopathology. Basel, Schwabe and Company, 1972, pp. 220–235.
70. Kaplan, A.P., Spragg, J., and Austen, K.F.: The bradykinin-forming system in man. *In* Austen, K.F., and Becker, E.L. (eds.): Biochemistry of the Acute Allergic Reaction. Oxford, Blackwell Scientific Publications Ltd., 1971, pp. 279–298.
71. Cochrane, C.G., Wuepper, K.D., Aiken, B.S., Revak, S.D., and Spiegelberg, H.L.: The interaction of Hageman factor and immune complexes. J. Clin. Invest. 51:2736, 1972.
72. Niewiarowski, S., Bankowski, E., and Rogowicka, J.: Studies on the adsorption and activation of Hageman factor (factor XII) by collagen and elastin. Thromb. Diath. Hemorrhag. 14:387, 1965.
73. Wilner, G.D., Nossel, H.L., and LeRoy, E.C.: Activation of Hageman factor by collagen. J. Clin. Invest. 47:2608, 1968.
74. Cochrane, C.G., Revak, S.D., Aiken, B.S., and Wuepper, K.D.: The structural characteristics and activation of Hageman factor. *In* Lepow, I.H., and Ward, P.A.: Inflammation: Mechanisms and Control. New York, Academic Press, 1972, pp. 119–138.
75. Harpel, P.C.: Studies on the interaction between collagen and a plasma kallikrein-like activity. Evidence for a surface-active enzyme system. J. Clin. Invest. 51:1813, 1972.
76. Griffin, J.H., Harper, A., and Cochrane, C.G.: Studies on the activation of human blood coagulation factor XII (Hageman factor) by soluble collagen. Fed. Proc. 34:860, 1975.
77. Meier, H.L., and Kaplan, A.P.: Evaluation of potential initiators of the Hageman factor (HF) dependent pathways. Fed. Proc. 37:12, 1978.
78. Revak, S.D., Cochrane, C.G., Johnston, A., and Hugli, T.: Structural changes accompanying enzymatic activation of Hageman factor. J. Clin. Invest. 54:619, 1974.
79. Proctor, R.R., and Rapaport, S.I.: The partial thromboplastin time with kaolin: A simple screening test for first stage plasma clotting deficiencies. Am. J. Clin. Pathol. 35:212, 1961.
80. Kaplan, A.P., and Austen, K.E.: A prealbumin activator of prekallikrein. J. Immunol. 105:802, 1970.
81. Kaplan, A.P., and Austen, K.F.: A prealbumin activator of prekallikrein. II. Derivation of activators of prekallikrein from active Hageman factor by digestion with plasmin. J. Exp. Med. 133:672–712, 1971.
82. Silverberg, M., Dunn, J.T., Garen, L., and Kaplan, A.P.: Autoactivation of human Hageman factor: Demonstration utilizing a synthetic substrate. J. Biol. Chem. 255:7281, 1980.
82a. Kaplan A.P., and Harpel, P.C.: Activation of the intrinsic coagulation-kinin system: Quantitation of activated Hageman factor-$C\bar{1}$ INH complexes by an enzyme-linked immununosorbent assay. Clin. Res. 31:483a, 1983.
83. Lewin, M.F., Kaplan, A.P. and Harpel P.C.: Studies of $C\bar{1}$ inactivator–plasma kallikrein complexes in purified systems and in plasma. Quantification by an enzyme-linked differential antibody immunosorbant assay. J. Biol. Chem. 258:6415, 1983.
84. Harpel, P.C.: $\alpha$2 Plasmin inhibitor and $\alpha$2 macroglobulin-plasmin complexes in plasma. Quantitation by an enzyme-linked differential antibody immunosorbent assay. J. Clin. Invest. 68:46, 1981.
85. Amandsen, E., Svendsen, L., Vennerod, A.M., and Laake, K.: Determination of plasma kallikrein with a new chromogenic tripeptide derivative. *In* Pisano, J.J., and Austen, K.F.: Chemistry and Biology of the Kallikrein-Kinin System in Health and Disease. Fogarty International Proceedings No. 27. Washington, D.C., U.S. Government Printing Office, 1974, pp. 215–220.
86. Saito, H., Ratnoff, O.D., and Pensky, J.: Radioimmunoassay of human Hageman factor (factor XII). J. Lab. Clin. Med. 88:506, 1976.
87. Wuepper, K.D., Tucker, E.S., III, and Cochrane, C.G.: Plasma kinin system: Proenzyme components. J. Immunol. 105:1307, 1970.
88. Treloar, M.P., and Movat, H.Z.: Isolation of two small molecular activators of the plasma kinin system in the guinea pig. Fed. Proc. 59:576, 1970.
89. Movat, H.Z., Poon, M.C., and Tukeuchi, Y.: The kinin system of human plasma. I. Isolation of a low molecular weight activator of prekallikrein. Int. Arch. Allergy Appl. Immunol. 40:89, 1971.
90. Wuepper, K.D., and Cochrane, C.G.: Isolation and mechanism of activation of components of the plasma kinin-forming system. *In* Austen, K.F., and Becker, E.L. (eds.): The Biochemistry of the Acute Allergic Reactions—Second International Symposium. Oxford, Blackwell Scientific Publications Ltd., 1971, pp. 299–320.
91. Cochrane, C.G., and Wuepper, K.D.: The first component of the kinin-forming system in human and rabbit plasma. Its relationship to clotting factor XII (Hageman factor). J. Exp. Med. 134:986, 1971.
92. Soltay, M.J., Movat, H.Z., and Ozge-Anwar, A.H.: The kinin system of human plasma. V. The probable derivative of prekallikrein activator from activated Hageman factor. Proc. Soc. Exp. Biol. Med. 138:952, 1972.
93. Burrowes, C.E., Movat, H.Z., and Soltay, M.J.: The kinin system of human plasma. VI. The action of plasmin. Proc. Soc. Exp. Biol. Med. 135:959, 1975.
94. Cochrane, C.G., Revak, S.D., and Wuepper, K.D.: Activation of Hageman factor in solid and fluid phases. J. Exp. Med. 138:1564, 1973.
95. Revak, S.D., and Cochrane, C.G.: The relationship of structure and function in human Hageman factor. The association of enzymatic and binding activities with separate regions of the molecule. J. Clin. Invest. 57:852, 1976.
96. Kaplan, A.P., Meier, H.L., Yecies, L.D., and Heck, L.W.: Hageman factor and its substrates: The role of factor XI (PTA), prekallikrein, and plasminogen proactivator in coagulation, fibrinolysis, and kinin-generation. *In* Pisano, J.J., and Austen, K.F. (eds.): Chemistry and Biology of the Kallikrein-Kinin System in Health and Disease. Fogarty International Center Proceedings No. 27. Washington, D.C., U.S. Government Printing Office, 1974, pp. 237–254.
97. Griffin, J.H., and Cochrane, C.G.: Mechanism for the involvement of high molecular weight kininogen in surface-dependent reactions of Hageman factor. Proc. Natl. Acad. Sci. USA 73:2559, 1976.
98. Kaplan, A.P., Meier, H.L., and Mandle, R., Jr.: The Hageman factor dependent pathways of coagulation, fibrinolysis, and kinin-generation. Semin. Thromb. Haemostasis 3:1, 1976.
99. Meier, H.L., Scott, C.F., Mandle, R., Jr., Webster, M.E., Pierce, J.V., Colman, R.W., and Kaplan, A.P.: Requirements for contact activation of human Hageman factor. Ann. N.Y. Acad. Sci. 283:93, 1977.
100. Liu, C.Y., Scott, C.F., Bagdasarian, A., Pierce, J.V., Kaplan, A.P., and Colman, R.W.: Potentiation of the function of Hageman factor fragments by high molecular weight kininogen. J. Clin. Invest. 60:7, 1977.
101. Meier, H.L., Pierce, J.V., Colman, R.W., and Kaplan, A.P.: Activation and function of human Hageman factor. The role of high molecular weight kininogen and prekallikrein. J. Clin. Invest. 60:18, 1977.
102. Griffin, J.H.: Role of surface in surface-dependent activation of Hageman factor (blood coagulation factor XII). Proc. Natl. Acad. Sci. 75:1998, 1978.
103. McMillin, C.R., Saito, H., Ratnoff, O.D., and Walton, A.G.: The secondary structure of human Hageman factor (Factor XII) and its alteration by activating agents. J. Clin. Invest. 54:1312, 1974.
104. Wiggins, R.C., Bouma, B.N., Cochrane, C.G., and Griffin, J.H.: Role of

high molecular weight kininogen in surface-binding and activation of coagulation factor XI and prekallikrein. Proc. Natl. Acad. Sci. 77:4636, 1977.

105. Silverberg, M., Nicoll, J.E., and Kaplan, A.P.: The mechanism by which the light chain of cleaved HMW-kininogen augments the activation of prekallikrein, factor XI, and Hageman factor. Thromb. Res. 20:173, 1980.
106. Thompson, R.E., Mandle, R., Jr., and Kaplan, A.P.: Studies of the binding of prekallikrein and factor XI to high molecular weight kininogen and its light chain. Proc. Natl. Acad. Sci. 76:4862, 1979.
107. Cochrane, C.G., and Revak, S.D.: Dissemination of contact activation in plasma by plasma kallikrein. J. Exp. Med. 152:608, 1980.
108. Scott, C.F., and Colman, R.W.: Function and immunochemistry of prekallikrein-high molecular weight kininogen complex in plasma. J. Clin. Invest. 65:413, 1980.
109. Fair, B.D., Saito, H., Ratnoff, O.D., and Rippon, W.B.: Detection by fluorescence of structural changes accompanying the activation of Hageman factor (factor XII). Proc. Soc. Exp. Biol. Med. 55:199, 1977.
110. Wiggins, R.C., and Cochrane, C.G.: The autoactivation of rabbit Hageman factor. J. Exp. Med. 150:1122, 1979.
111. Kurachi, K., Fujikawa, K., and Davie, E.W.: Mechanism of activation of bovine factor XI by factor XII and factor XIIa. Biochemistry 19:1330, 1980.
112. Heimark, R.L., Kurachi, K., Fujikawa, K., and Davie, E.W.: Surface activation of blood coagulation, fibrinolysis, and kinin formation. Nature 456, 1980.
113. Sugo, T., Hamaguchi, A., Shimada, J., Kato, H., and Iwanaga, S.: Mechanism of surface-mediated activation of bovine factor XII and plasma prekallikrein. J. Biochem. 92:689, 1982.
114. Ratnoff, O.D., and Saito, H.: Amidolytic properties of single-chain activated Hageman factor. Proc. Natl. Acad. Sci. 76:1461, 1979.
115. Miller, G., Silverberg, M., and Kaplan, A.P.: Autoactivatability of human Hageman factor (factor XII). Biochem. Biophys. Res. Commun. 92:803, 1980.
116. Dunn, J.T., Silverberg, M., and Kaplan, A.P.: The cleavage and formation of activated human Hageman factor by autodigestion and by kallikrein. J. Biol. Chem. 275:1779, 1982.
117. Silverberg, M., and Kaplan, A.P.: Enzymatic activities of activated and zymogen forms of human Hageman factor (factor XII). Blood 60:64, 1982.
118. Tankersley, D.L., and Finlayson, J.S.: Kinetics of activation and autoactivation of factor XII (Hageman factor). Circ. Supp. II. 66:296, 1982.
119. Revak, S.D., Cochrane, C.G., and Griffin, J.H.: The binding and cleavage characteristics of human Hageman factor during contact activation. A comparison of normal plasma with plasmas deficient in factor XI, prekallikrein, or high molecular weight kininogen. J. Clin. Invest. 59:1167, 1977.
120. Revak, S.D., Cochrane, C.G., Bouma, B.N., and Griffin, J.H.: Surface and fluid phase activities of two forms of activated Hageman factor produced during contact activation of plasma. J. Exp. Med. 147:719, 1978.
121. Dunn, J.T., and Kaplan, A.P.: Formation and structure of human Hageman factor fragments. J. Clin. Invest. 70:627, 1982.
122. Mackay, M.E., Miles, A.A., Schacter, C.B., and Wilhelm, D.L.: Susceptibility of the guinea pig to pharmacological factors from its own serum. Nature 172:714, 1953.
123. Stewart, P.B., and Bliss, J.Q.: The permeability increasing factor in diluted human plasma. Br. J. Exp. Path. 38:462, 1957.
124. Mill, P.J., Elder, J.M., Miles, A.A., and Wilhelm, D.L.: Enzyme-like globulins from serum reproducing the vascular phenomena of inflammation. VI. Isolation and properties of permeability factor and its inhibition in human plasma. Br. J. Exp. Path. 39:343, 1958.
125. Elder, J.M., and Wilhelm, D.L.: Enzyme-like globulins from serum producing the vascular phenomena of inflammation. V. Active permeability factor in human serum. Br. J. Exp. Path. 39:23, 1958.
126. Ratnoff, O.D., and Miles, A.A.: Activation of a vascular permeability increasing factor in human plasma incubated with purified activated Hageman factor. J. Lab. Clin. Med. 60:1009, 1962.
127. Ratnoff, O.D., and Miles, A.A.: The induction of permeability increasing activity in human plasma by activated Hageman factor. Br. J. Exp. Path. 45:328, 1964.
128. Kellermeyer, R.W., and Ratnoff, O.D.: Abolition of the permeability-enhancing properties of Hageman factor by specific antiserum. J. Lab. Clin. Med. 70:356, 1967.
129. Webster, M.E., and Ratnoff, O.D.: Role of Hageman factor in the activation of vasodilator activity in human plasma. Nature 192:180, 1961.
130. Webster, M.E., and Pierce, J.V.: Studies on the enzymes involved in the activation of human plasma kallikrein. *In* Rocha e Silva, M., and Rothschild, H.A. (eds.): International Symposium on Vasoactive Polypeptides: Bradykinin and Related Kinins. New York, Plenum Publishing Company, 1967, pp. 155–160.
131. Kagen, L.J., Leddy, J.P., and Becker, E.L.: Isolation of two permeability globulins from human plasma. Nature 197:693, 1963.
132. Kagen, L.J., Leddy, J.P., and Becker, E.L.: The presence of two permeability globulins in human serum. J. Clin. Invest. 42:1353, 1963.
133. Kaplan, A.P., Spragg, J., Gigli, I., and Austen, K.F.: Purification of kallikrein and PF/dil and their interaction with kininogen and with $C\bar{1}$ Inhibitor ($C\bar{1}$ INH). Fed. Proc. 29:491, 1970.
134. Johnston, A.R., Cochrane, C.G., and Revak, S.D.: The relationship between PF/dil and activated Hageman factor. J. Immunol. 113:103, 1974.
135. Oh-Ishi, S., and Webster, M.E.: Vascular permeability factors PF/nat and PF/dil: Their relationship to Hageman factor and the kallikrein-kinin system. Biochem. Pharm. 24:591, 1975.
136. Wuepper, K.D.: Plasma prekallikrein: Its characterization, mechanism of activation, and inherited deficiency in man. *In* Pisano, J.J., and Austen, K.F. (eds.): Chemistry and Biology and the Kallikrein-Kinin System in Health and Disease. Fogarty International Center Proceedings No. 27, Washington, D.C., U.S. Government Printing Office, 1974, pp. 37–51.
137. Hathaway, W.E., Wuepper, K.D., Weston, W.L., Hambert, J.R., Rivers, R.P.A., Genton, E., August, C.S., Montgomery, R.R., and Moss, M.F.: Clinical and physiologic studies of two siblings with prekallikren (Fletcher factor) deficiency. Am. J. Med. 60:654, 1976.
138. Abildgaard, C.F., and Harrison, J.: Fletcher factor deficiency: Family study and detection. Blood 43:641, 1974.
139. Stormorken, H., and Abildgaard, C.F.: The Fletcher factor—prekallikrein deficiency: A diagnostic test which identifies heterozygotes. Thromb. Res. 5:375, 1974.
140. Harpel, P.C.: Studies on human plasma $\alpha_2$ macroglobulin enzyme interactions. Evidence for proteolytic modification of the subunit chain structures. J. Exp. Med. 138:508, 1973.
141. Harpel, P.C., and Mosesson, M.W.: Degradation of human fibrinogen by plasma $\alpha_1$-macroglobulin-enzyme complexes. J. Clin. Invest. 52:2175, 1973.
142. Kluft, C.: Determination of prekallikrein in plasma: Optional condition for activation of prekallikrein. J. Lab. Clin. Med. 91:83, 1978.
143. Friberger, P., Eriksson, E., Constavsson, S., and Cleson, G.: Determination of prekallikrein in plasma by means of a chromogenic tripeptide substrate for plasma kallikrein. *In* Fugii, S., Moriya, H., and Suzuki, T. (eds.): Kinins II—Biochemistry, Pathophysiology, and Clinical Aspects. New York, Plenum Press, 1979, pp. 67–82.
144. Fisher, C.A., Schmaier, A.H., Addonizio, P., and Colman, R.W.: Assay of prekallikrein in human plasma: Comparison of amidolytic, esterolytic, coagulation, and immunochemical assays. Blood 59:963, 1982.
145. Webster, M.E., and Pierce, J.V.: Action of kallikreins on synthetic ester substrates. Proc. Soc. Exp. Biol. Med. 107:186, 1961.
146. Colman, R.W., Mason, J.W., and Sherry, S.: The kallikreinogen-kallikrein enzyme system of human plasma: Assay of components and observations in disease states. Ann. Intern. Med. 71:763, 1969.
147. Colman, R.W., Mattler, L., and Sherry, S.: Studies on the prekallikrein (kallikreinogen)-kallikrein enzyme system of human plasma. I. Isolation and purification of plasma kallikreins. J. Clin. Invest. 48:11, 1969.
148. Colman, R.W., Mattler, L., and Sherry, S.: Studies on the prekallikrein (kallikreinogen)-kallikrein enzyme system of human plasma. II. Evidence relating the kaolin-activated arginine esterase to plasma kallikrein. J. Clin. Invest. 48:23, 1969.
149. Talamo, R.C., Haber, E., and Austen, K.F.: A radioimmuno-assay for bradykinin in plasma and synovial fluid. J. Lab. Clin. Med. 74:816, 1969.
150. Gireg, G.J.D., Talamo, R.C., and Colman, R.W.: The kinetics of the release of bradykinin by kallikrein in normal human plasma. J. Lab. Clin. Med. 80:496, 1972.
151. Imanari, T., Kaizu, T., Yoshida, H., Yates, K., Pierce, J.V., and Pisano, J.J.: Radiochemical assay for human urinary, salivary, and plasma kallikreins. *In* Pisano, J.J., and Austen, K.F. (eds.): Chemistry and Biology of the Kallikrein-Kinin System in Health and Diseases. Fogarty International Center Proceedings No. 27. Washington, D.C., U.S. Government Printing Office, 1974, pp. 205–213.
152. Bagdasarian, A., Lahiri, B., Talamo, R.C., Wong, P., and Colman, R.W.: Immunochemical studies of plasma kallikrein. J. Clin. Invest. 54:1444, 1974.
153. Saito, H., and Poon, M.C.: Radioimmunoassay for a human plasma prekallikrein (Fletcher factor). Fed. Proc. 36:329, 1977.
154. Gigli, I., Mason, J.W., Colman, R.W., and Austen, K.F.: Interaction of plasma kallikrein with $C\bar{1}$ Inhibitor. J. Immunol. 104:574, 1970.
155. Harpel, P.C.: Human plasma $\alpha_2$ macroglobulin. An inhibitor of plasma kallikrein. J. Exp. Med. 132:329, 1970.
156. Saito, M., Poon, M.C., Vivic, W., Goldsmith, G.H., Jr., and Menitove, J.E.: Human plasma prekallikrein (Fletcher factor) clotting activity and antigen in health and disease. J. Lab. Clin. Med. 92:84, 1978.
157. Saito, H., Goodnough, L.T., Soria, J., Soria, C., Aznar, J., and Espana, F.: Heterogeneity of human prekallikrein deficiency (Fletcher trait).

Evidence that five of 18 cases are positive for cross-reacting material. N. Engl. J. Med. 305:910, 1981.
158. Saito, H., Ratnoff, O. D., and Pensky, J.: Radioimmunoassay of human Hageman factor (factor XII) J. Lab. Clin. Med. 88:506, 1976.
159. Saito, H., and Scialla S.J.: Isolation and properties of an abnormal Hageman factor (factor XII) molecule in a cross-reacting material-positive Hageman trait plasma. J. Clin. Invest. 68:1028, 1981.
160. Bouma, B.N., Kerbiriou, D.M., Vlooswijk, R.A.A., and Griffin, J.H.: Immunochemical studies of prekallikrein, kallikrein, and high-molecular weight kininogen in normal and deficient plasmas and in normal plasmas after cold-dependent activation. J. Lab. Clin. Med. 96:693, 1980.
161. Donaldson, V.M., Kleniewski, J., Saito, H., and Sayed, J.K.: Prekallikrein deficiency in a kindred with kininogen deficiency and Fitzgerald trait clotting defect. Evidence that high molecular weight kininogen and prekallikrein exist as a complex in normal human plasma. J. Clin. Invest. 60:571, 1977.
162. Jonasson, O., and Becker, E.L.: Release of kallikrein from guinea pig lung during anaphylaxis. J. Exp. Med. 123:509, 1966.
163. Rocha e Silva, M., Beraldo, W.T., and Rosenfeld, G.: Bradykinin, hypotensive and smooth muscle stimulating factor released from plasma globulin by snake venom and trypsin. Am. J. Physiol. 156:261, 1949.
164. Mandle, R., Jr., and Kaplan, A.P.: Hageman factor substrates. Human plasma prekallikrein. Mechanism of activation by Hageman factor and participation in Hageman factor-dependent fibrinolysis. J. Biol. Chem. 252:6097, 1977.
165. Bouma, B.N., Miles, L.A., Baretta, G., and Griffin, J.H. Human plasma prekallikrein. Studies of its activation by activated factor XII and of its inactivation by diisopropyl phosphofluoridate. Biochemistry 19:1151, 1980.
166. Tankersley, D.I., Fournel, M.A., and Schroeder, D.D. Kinetics of activation of prekallikrein by prekallikrein activator. Biochemistry 19:3121, 1980.
167. Van der Graff, F., Tans, G., Bouma, B.N., and Griffin, J.H.: Isolation and functional properties of the heavy and light chains of human plasma kallikrein. J. Biol. Chem. 257:14300, 1982.
168. Nagasawa, S., Takahashi, H., Koida, M., and Suzuki, T.: Partial purification of bovine plasma kallikreinogen, its activation by the Hageman factor. Biochem. Biophys. Res. Commun. 32:644, 1968.
169. Takahashi, H., Nagasawa, S., and Suzuki, T.: Studies on prekallikrein of bovine plasma. I. Purification and properties. J. Biochem. 71:471, 1972.
170. Takahashi, H., Nagasawa, S., and Suzuki, T.: Studies on prekallikrein of bovine plasma II. Activation of prekallikrein with proteinases and properties of kallikrein activated by bovine Hageman factor. J. Biochem. 87:23, 1980.
171. Yamamoto, T., Kozono, K., Okamoto, T., Kato, H., and Kamabara, T.: Purification of guinea-pig plasma prekallikrein. Activation by prekallikrein activator derived from guinea pig skin. Biochem. et Biophys. Acta 614:511, 1980.
172. Wuepper, K.D., and Cochrane, C.G.: Plasma prekallikrein: Isolation, characterization and mechanism of activation. J. Exp. Med. 135:1, 1972.
173. Wuepper, K.D., and Cochrane, C.G.: Effect of plasma kallikrein on coagulation in vitro. Proc. Soc. Exp. Biol. Med. 141:271, 1972.
174. Johnson, A.R., Ulevitch, R.J., and Ryan, K.: Biochemical and biological properties of rabbit prekallikrein. Fed. Proc. 35:693, 1976.
175. Pierce, J.V., and Webster, M.E.: The purification and some properties of two different kallidinogens. *In* Erdos, E.G., Back, N., and Sicuteri, F. (eds.): Hypotensive Peptides. New York, Springer-Verlag, 1966, pp. 130–138.
176. Jacobsen, S.: Substrates from plasma kinin-forming enzymes in human, dog, and rabbit plasmas. Br. J. Pharmacol. 26:403, 1966.
177. Jacobsen, S.: Substrates for plasma kinin-forming enzymes in rat and guinea pig plasma. Br. J. Pharmacol. 28:64, 1966.
178. Jacobsen, S., and Kriz, M.: Some data on two purified kininogens from human plasma. Br. J. Pharmacol. 29:25, 1967.
179. Spragg, J., Haber, E., and Austen, K.F.: The preparation of human kininogen and the elicitation of antibody for use in a radial immunodiffusion assay. J. Immunol. 104:1348, 1970.
180. Spragg, J., and Austen, K.F.: The preparation of human kininogen. II. Further characterization of purified human kininogen. J. Immunol. 107:1512, 1971.
181. Spragg, J., and Austen, K.F.: Preparation of human kininogen. III. Enzymatic digestion and modification. Biochem. Pharmacol. 23:781, 1974.
182. Pierce, J.V.: Purification of mammalian kallikreins, kininogens and kinins. *In* Erdos, E.G. (ed.): Handbook of Experimental Pharmacology. New York, Springer-Verlag, 1970, Vol. 25, pp. 21–51.
183. Habal, F.M., and Movat, H.Z.: Kininogens of human plasma. Res. Commun. Chem. Path. Pharmacol. 4:477, 1972.
184. Habal, F.M., Movat, H.Z., and Burrowes, C.E.: Isolation of two functionally different kininogens from human plasma—separation from proteinase inhibitors and interaction with plasma kallikrein. Biochem. Pharmacol. 23:2291, 1974.
185. Habal, F.M., and Movat, H.Z.: Some physicochemical and functional differences between low and high molecular weight kininogens of human plasma. *In* Pisano, J.J., and Austen, K.F. (eds.): The Chemistry and Biology of the Kallikrein-Kinin System in Health and Disease. Fogarty International Center Proceedings No. 27. Washington, D.C., U.S. Government Printing Office, 1974, pp. 129–131.
186. Habal, F.M., Underdown, B.J., and Movat, H.Z.: Further characterization of human plasma kininogens. Biochem. Pharmacol. 24:1241, 1975.
187. Suzuki, T., Mizushima, Y., Sato, T., and Iwanaga, S.: Purification of bovine bradykininogen. J. Biochem. 57:14, 1965.
188. Yano, M., Nagasawa, S., Hairuchi, K., and Suzuki, T.: Separation of a new substrate, kininogen I, for plasma kallikrein in bovine plasma. J. Biochem. 62:504, 1967.
189. Pierce, J.V., and Guimaraes, J.A.: Further characterization of highly purified human plasma kininogens. *In* Pisano, J.J., and Austen, K.F. (eds.): Chemistry and Biology of the Kallikrein-Kinin System in Health and Disease. Fogarty International Center Proceedings No. 27. Washington, D.C., U.S. Government Printing Office, 1974, pp. 121–127.
189a. Thompson, R.E., Mandle R.J., and Kaplan, A.P.: Characterization of human high molecular weight kininogen: Procoagulant activity associated with the light chain of kinin-free high molecular weight kininogen, J. Exp. Med. 147:488, 1978.
190. Saito, H.: Purification of high molecular weight kininogen and the role of this agent in blood coagulation. J. Clin. Invest. 60:584, 1977.
191. Nakayasa, T., and Nagasawa, S.: Studies on human kininogens I. Isolation characterization, and cleavage by plasma kallikrein of high molecular weight (HMW) kininogen. J. Biochem. 85:249, 1979.
192. Mori, K., and Nagasawa, S.: Studies on human high molecular weight (HMW) kininogen II. Structural change of HMW-kininogen by the action of human plasma kallikrein. J. Biochem. 89:1465, 1981.
193. Mori, K., Sakamoto, W., and Nagasawa, S.: Studies on human high molecular weight (HMW) kininogen III. Cleavage of HMW kininogen by the action of human salivary kallikrein. J. Biochem. 90:503, 1981.
194. Kerbiriou, D.M., and Griffin, J.H.: Human high molecular weight kininogen. Studies of structure-function relationships and of proteolysis of the molecule occurring during contact activation of plasma. J. Biol. Chem. 254:12020, 1979.
195. Kerbiriou, D.M., Bouma, B.N., and Griffin, J.H.: Immunochemical studies of human high molecular weight kininogen and of its complexes with plasma prekallikrein or kallikrein. J. Biol. Chem. 255:3952, 1980.
196. Schiffman, S., Mannhalter, C., and Tynerk, D.: Human high molecular weight kininogen. Effects of cleavage by kallikrein on protein structure and procoagulant activity. J. Biol. Chem. 255:6433, 1980.
197. Chan, J.Y.C., Habal, F.M., Burrowes, C.C., and Movat, H.Z.: Interaction between factor XII (Hageman factor), high molecular weight kininogen and prekallikrein. Thromb. Res. 9:423, 1976.
198. Han, Y.N., Kato, H., Iwanaga, S., and Suzuki, T.: Primary structure of bovine high molecular weight kininogen. The amino acid sequence of a glycopeptide (fragment) following the C-terminus of the bradykinin moiety. J. Biochem. 79:1201, 1976.
199. Han, Y.N., Kato, M., Iwanaga, S., and Suzaki, T.: Bovine plasma high molecular weight kininogen; the amino acid sequence of fragment 1 (glycopeptide) released by the action of plasma kallikrein and its location in the precursor molecule. FEBS Lett 67:197, 1976.
200. Scicli, A.G., Waldmann, R., Guimaraes, J.A., Scicli, G., Carretero, O.A., Kato, H., Han, Y.N., and Iwanaga, S.: Relationship between structure and correcting activity of bovine high molecular weight kininogen upon the clotting time of Fitzgerald-trait plasma. J. Exp. Med. 145:847, 1979.
201. Sugo, T., Kato, H., Iwanaga, S., and Fujii, S.: The accelerating effect of bovine plasma HMW kininogen on the surface-mediated activation of factor XII: Generation of a derivative form (active kininogen) with maximal cofactor activity by limited proteolysis. Thromb. Res. 24:329, 1981.
202. Sugo, T., Kato H., Iwanaga, S., and Fujii, S.: The accelerating effect of bovine plasma HMW kininogen on the surface-mediated activation of factor XII: Generation of a derivative form (active kininogen) with maximal cofactor activity by limited proteolysis. Thromb. Res. 24:329, 1981.
203. Vroman, L., Adams A.L., Fischer, G.C., and Munoz, P.C.: Interaction of high molecular weight kininogen, factor XII, and fibrinogen in plasma at interfaces. Blood 55:156, 1980.
204. Kato, H., Han, Y.N., Iwanaga, S., Suzuki, T., and Komiya, M.: Bovine plasma HMW and HMW kininogens. Structural differences between heavy and light chains derived from the kinin-free proteins. J. Biochem. 80:1299, 1966.
205. Komiya, M., Kato, H., and Suzuki, T.: Homology between bovine high molecular weight and low molecular weight kininogens. Biochem. Biophys. Res. Commun. 49:1438, 1972.
206. Komiya, M., Kato, H., and Suzuki, T.: Bovine plasma kininogens III. Structural comparison of high molecular weight and low molecular weight kininogens. J. Biochem. 76:833, 1974.

207. Prado, E.S., Prado, J.L., and Brandi, C.M.W.: Further purification and some properties of horse urinary kallikrein. Arch. Int. Pharmacodyn. 137:358, 1962.
208. Webster, M.E., and Prado, E.S.: Glandular kallikreins from horse and human urine and from hog pancreas. Methods Enzymol. 19:681, 1970.
209. Diniz, C.R., and Carvalho, I.F.: A micromethod for determination of bradykininogen under several conditions. Ann. N.Y. Acad. Sci. 104:77, 1963.
210. Proud, D., Pierce, J.V., and Pisano, J.J.: Radioimmunoassay of human high molecular weight kininogen in normal and deficient plasmas. J. Lab. Clin. Med. 95:563, 1980.
211. Rosenthal, R.L., Dreskin, O.H., and Rosenthal, N.: New hemophilia-like disease caused by deficiency of a third plasma thromboplastin factor. Proc. Soc. Exp. Biol. Med. 82:171, 1953.
212. Heck, L.W., and Kaplan, A.P.: Substrates of human Hageman factor. I. Isolation and characterization of PTA (Factor XI) and its inhibition by $\alpha_1$ antitrypsin. J. Exp. Med. 140:1615, 1630, 1974.
213. Saito, H., and Goldsmith, G.H., Jr.: Plasma thromboplastin antecedent (PTA, factor XI): A specific and sensitive radioimmunoassay. Blood 50:377, 1977.
214. Forbes, C.D., and Ratnoff, O.D.: Studies on plasma thromboplastin antecedent (factor XI), PTA deficiency, and inhibition of PTA by plasma, pharmacologic inhibitors, and specific antiserum. J. Lab. Clin. Med. 79:113, 1972.
215. Rimon, A., Schiffman, S., Feinstein, D.I., and Rapaport, S.I.: Factor XI activity and factor XI antigen in homozygous and heterozygous factor XI deficiency. Blood 48:165, 1976.
216. Chan, J.Y.C., and Movat, H.Z.: Purification of factor XII (Hageman factor) from human plasma. Thromb. Res. 8:337, 1976.
217. Kaode, T., Hermodson, M.A., and Davie, E.W.: Active site of bovine Hageman factor XI (plasma thromboplastin antecedent). Nature 266:729, 1977.
218. Saito, H., Ratnoff, O.D., Marshall, J.S., and Pensky, J.: Partial purification of plasma thromboplastin antecedent (factor XI) and its activation by trypsin. J. Clin. Invest. 52:850, 1973.
219. Mannhalter, C., Schiffman, S., and Jacobs, A.: Trypsin activation of human factor XI. J. Biol. Chem. 255:2667, 1980.
220. Bouma, B.N., and Griffin, J.H.: Human blood coagulation factor XI: Purification, properties and mechanism of activated Factor XII. J. Biol. Chem. 252:6432, 1977.
221. Kurachi, K., and Davie, E.W.: Activation of human factor XI (plasma thromboplastin antecedent) by factor XIIa (activated Hageman factor). Biochemistry 16:5831, 1977.
222. Ratnoff, O.D.: Studies on the product of the reaction between activated Hageman factor (factor XII) and plasma thromboplastin antecedent. J. Lab. Clin. Med. 80:704, 1972.
223. Kingdon, H.S., Davie, E.W., and Ratnoff, O.D.: The reaction between activated plasma thromboplastin antecedent and diisopropyl-phosphofluoridate. Biochemistry 3:166, 1964.
224. Schiffman, S., and Margalit, R.: Factor XI adsorption to surface: Interaction of high molecular weight kininogen (HMWK) and a plasma adsorption inhibitor. Blood 56:168, 1980.
225. Schiffman, S., and Mannhalter, C.: Surface adsorption of factor XI. Association of adsorption sites with the heavy chain of activated factor XI.
226. Stern, D.M., Nossel, H.L., and Owen, J.: Acquired antibody to factor XI in a patient with congenital factor XI deficiency. J. Clin. Invest. 69:1270, 1982.
227. Meier, M.L., Thompson, R.E., and Kaplan, A.P.: Ativation of Hageman factor by factor XIa–HMW–kininogen. Thromb. Haemostasis 38:14, 1977.
228. McDonagh, K.S., and Ferguson, J.H.: Studies on the participation of Hageman factor in fibrinolysis. Thromb. Diath. Haemorrh. 24:1, 1970.
229. Colman, R.W.: Activation of plasminogen by human plasma kallikrein. Biochem. Biophys. Res. Commun. 351:273, 1969.
230. Ogston, D., Ogston, C.M., Ratnoff, O.D., and Forbes, C.O.: Studies on a complex mechanism for the activation of plasminogen by kaolin and by chloroform: The participation of Hageman factor and additional cofactors. J. Clin. Invest. 48:1786, 1969.
231. Kaplan, A.P., Goetzl, E.J., and Austen, K.F.: The fibrinolytic pathway of human plasma. II. Generation of chemotactic activity by activation of plasminogen proactivator. J. Clin. Invest. 52:2591, 1973.
232. Laake, K., and Vennerod, A.M.: Factor XII-induced fibrinolysis. Studies on the separation of prekallikrein, plasminogen proactivator, and factor XI in human plasma. Thromb. Res. 4:285, 1974.
233. Vennerod, A.M., and Laake, K.: Prekallikrein and plasminogen proactivator: Absence of plasminogen proactivator in Fletcher factor deficient plasma. Thromb. Res. 8:519, 1976.
234. Kaplan, A.P., and Austen, K.F.: The fibrinolytic pathway of human plasma. Isolation and characterization of the plasminogen proactivator. J. Exp. Med. 136:1378, 1972.
235. Mandle, R., Jr., and Kaplan, A.P.: Plasminogen proactivators of human plasma: Relationship to prekallikrein and factor XI. Fed. Proc. 36:329, 1977.
236. Mandle, R., Jr., and Kaplan, A.P.: Hageman factor-dependent fibrinolysis: Generation of fibrinolytic activity by the interaction of human activated factor XI and plasminogen. Blood 54:850, 1979.
237. Bouma, B.N., and Griffin, J.H.: Human prekallikrein (plasminogen proactivator): Purification, characterization and activation by activated factor XII. Thromb. Haemostasis 38:136, 1977.
238. Saito, H.: The participation of plasma thromboplastin antecedent (Factor XI) in contact-activated fibrinolysis. Proc. Soc. Exp. Biol. Med. 164:153, 1980.
239. Goldsmith, G.H., Saito, H., and Ratnoff, O.D.: The activation of plasminogen by Hageman factor (factor XII) and Hageman factor fragments. J. Clin. Invest. 62:54, 1978.
240. Wuepper, K.D.: Prekallikrein–Hageman factor cofactor–Fletcher factor: Are they identical? Clin. Res. 21:484, 1973.
241. Kluft, C.: An inventory of plasminogen activators in human plasma. Thromb. Haemostasis 38:134, 1977.
242. Robyn, J.C., Ogston, D., and Douglas, A.T.: Further purification and properties of Hageman factor cofactor. Biochim. Biophys. Acta 271:371, 1972.
243. Saito, H., Ratnoff, O.D., Donaldson, V.H., Haney, G., and Pensky, J.: Inhibition of the adsorption of Hageman factor (factor XII) to glass by normal plasma. J. Lab. Clin. Med. 84:62, 1974.
244. Forbes, C.O., Pensky, J., and Ratnoff, O.D.: Inhibition of activated Hageman factor and activated plasma thromboplastin antecedent by purified $C\bar{1}$ inactivator. J. Lab. Clin. Med. 76:809, 1970.
245. Schreiber, A.D., Kaplan, A.P., and Austen, K.F.: Inhibition by $C\bar{1}$ INH of Hageman factor fragment activation of coagulation, fibrinolysis, and kinin-generation. J. Clin. Invest. 52:1402, 1973.
246. Stead, N.W., Kaplan, A.P., and Rosenberg, R.D.: The inhibition of human activated Hageman factor (HF) by human antithrombin-heparin cofactor (AT). J. Biol. Chem. 251:6481, 1976.
247. McConnell, D.J.: Inhibitors of kallikrein in human plasma. J. Clin. Invest. 51:1611, 1972.
248. Harpel, P.C.: Circulating inhibitors of human plasma kallikrein. *In* Pisano, J.J., and Austen, K.F. (eds.): Chemistry and Biology of the Kallikrein-Kinin System in Health and Disease. Fogarty International Center Proceedings No. 27. Washington, D.C., U.S. Government Printing Office, 1974, pp. 169–177.
249. Lahiri, B., Rosenberg, R., Mitchell, R.C., Bagdasarian, A., and Colman, R.W.: Antithrombin III. An inhibitor of plasma kallikrein. Fed. Proc. 33:642, 1974.
250. Burrowes, C.E., Habal, F.M., and Movat, H.Z.: The inhibition of human plasma kallikrein by antithrombin III. Thromb. Res. 7:175, 1975.
251. Vennerod, A.M., Laake, K., Solberg, A.K., and Stromland, S.: Inactivation and binding of human plasma kallikrein by antithrombin III. Thromb. Res. 9:457, 1976.
252. Schapira, M., Scott, C.F., and Colman, R.W.: Contribution of plasma protease inhibitor to the inactivation of kallikrein in plasma. J. Clin. Invest. 65:462, 1982.
253. Van der Graaf, F., Koedam, J.A., and Bouma, B.N.: Inactivation of kallikrein in human plasma. J. Clin. Invest. 71:149, 1983.
254. Scott, C.F., Schapira, M., James, H.L., Cohen, A.B., and Colman, R.W.: Inactivation of factor XIa by plasma protease inhibitor. Predominant role of $\alpha_1$ proteinase inhibitor and protective effect of high molecular weight kininogen. J. Clin. Invest. 69:844, 1982.
255. Damus, P.S., Hicks, M., and Rosenberg, R.D.: Anticoagulant action of heparin. Nature 246:355, 1973.
256. Ganrot, P.O.: Inhibition of plasmin activity by $\alpha_2$ macroglobulin. Clin. Chim. Acta 16:328, 1967.
257. Schreiber, A.D., Kaplan, A.P., and Austen, K.F.: Plasma inhibitors of the components of the fibrinolytic pathway in man. J. Clin. Invest. 52:1394, 1973.
258. Collen, D.: Identification and some properties of a new fast-reacting plasmin inhibitor in human plasma. Eur. J. Biochem. 69:209, 1976.
259. Moroi, M., and Aoki, N.: Isolation and characterization of $\alpha_2$ plasmin inhibitor from human plasma. J. Biol. Chem. 251:5956, 1976.
260. Mullertz, S., and Clemmensen, I.: The primary inhibitor of plasmin in human plasma. Biochem. J. 159:545, 1976.
261. Harpel, P.C.: Plasmin inhibitor interactions. The effectiveness of $\alpha_2$ plasmin inhibitor in the presence of $\alpha_2$ macroglobulin. J. Exp. Med. 146:1033, 1977.
262. Aoki, N., Moroi, M., Matsuda, M., and Tachiya, K.: The behavior of $\alpha_2$ plasmin inhibitor in fibrinolytic states. J. Clin. Invest. 60:361, 1977.
263. Harpel, P.C.: $C\bar{1}$ inactivator inhibition by plasmin. J. Clin. Invest. 49:569, 1970.
264. Harpel, P.C., and Cooper, N.R.: Studies on human plasma $C\bar{1}$ inactivator-enzyme interactions. I. Mechanisms of interaction with $C\bar{1}s$, plasmin, and trypsin. J. Clin. Invest. 55:593, 1975.
265. Highsmith, R.F., and Rosenberg, R.D.: The inhibition of human plasmin by human antithrombin-heparin cofactor. J. Biol. Chem. 249:4335, 1974.

266. Harpel, P.C., and Rosenberg, R.D.: $\alpha_2$-Macroglobulin and antithrombin-heparin cofactor. *In* Spaet, T.H. (ed.): Modulators of Hemostatic and Inflammatory Reactions. New York, Grune & Stratton, 1976, pp. 145–191.
267. Saito, H., Goldsmith, G.H., Moroi, M., and Aoki, N.: Inhibitory spectrum of $\alpha_2$ plasmin inhibitor. Proc. Natl. Acad. Sci. 76:2013, 1979.
268. Koie, K., Ogata, K., Kamiya, T., and Takamatsu, J.: $\alpha_2$-Plasmin-inhibitor deficiency. Lancet 2:1334, 1978.
269. Aoki, N., Saito, H., Kamiya, T., Koie, K., Sakata, Y., and Kobakura, M.: Congenital deficiency of $\alpha_2$ plasmin inhibitor associated with severe hemorrhagic tendency. J. Clin. Invest. 63:877, 1979.
270. Kluft, C., Vellenga, E., Brommer, E.J.P., and Wijngaards, G.: A familial hemorrhagic diathesis in a Dutch family: An inherited deficiency of $\alpha_2$ antiplasmin. Blood 59:1169, 1982.
271. Miles, L.A., Plow, E.F., Donnelly, K.J., Hougie, C., and Griffin, J.H.: A bleeding disorder due to deficiency of $\alpha_2$-antiplasmin. Blood 59:1246, 1982.
272. Sakata, Y., and Aoki, N.: Significance of cross-linking of $\alpha_2$ plasmin inhibitor to fibrin in inhibition of fibrinolysis and in hemostasis. J. Clin. Invest. 69:536, 1982.
273. Rocha e Silva, M.: The kinin trail: Possible significance of bradykinin and related kinins to autopharmacology. *In* Maxwell, R.A., and Acheson, G. (eds.): Pharmacology and the Future of Man. Vol. 5. Basel, S. Karger, 1972, pp. 250–266.
274. Schapira, M., Despland, E., Scott, C.F., Boxer, L.A., and Colman, R.W.: Purified human kallikrein aggregates human blood neutrophils. J. Clin. Invest. 69:1199, 1982.
275. Kaplan, A.P., Kay, A.B., and Austin, K.F.: A prealbumin activator of prekallikrein III. Appearance of chemotactic activity in human neutrophils by the conversion of human prekallikrein to kallikrein. J. Exp. Med. 135:81, 1972.
276. Gallin, J.I., and Kaplan, A.P.: Mononuclear cell chemotactic activity of kallikrein and plasminogen activator and its inhibition by $C\bar{1}$ INH and $\alpha_2$ macroglobulin. J. Immunol. 113:1928, 1974.
277. Waldmann, R., Rebuck, J.W., Saito, H., Abraham, J.P., Caldwell, J., and Ratnoff, O.D.: Fitzgerald factor: A hitherto unrecognized coagulation factor. Lancet 1:949, 1975.
278. Gigli, I., Koethe, S., and Austen, K.F.: Participation of an early component of complement and Hageman factor in C3 destruction by zymosan. Clin. Immunol. Immunopathol. 4:189, 1975.
279. Donaldson, V.H.: Mechanism of activation of C'1 esterase in hereditary angioneurotic edema in vitro. The role of Hageman factor, a clot-promoting agent. J. Exp. Med. 127:411, 1967.
280. Ghebrehiwet, B., Silverberg, M., and Kaplan, A.P.: Activation of the classical pathway of complement by Hageman factor fragment. J. Exp. Med. 153:665, 1981.
281. Ghebrehiwet, B., Randazzo, B.P., Dunn, J.T., Silverberg, M., and Kaplan, A.P.: Mechanisms of activation of the classical pathway of complement by Hageman factor fragment. J. Clin. Invest. 71:1450, 1983.
282. Ziccardi, R.J.: Spontaneous activation of the first component of human complement ($C\bar{1}$) by an intramolecular autocatalytic mechanism. J. Immunol. 128:2500, 1982.
283. Ziccardi, R.J.: A new role for $C\bar{1}$-inhibitor in homeostasis: Control of activation of the first component of human complement. J. Immunol. 128:2505, 1982.
284. DiScipis, R.G.: The activation of the alternative pathway C3 convertase by human plasma kallikrein. Immunology 45:587, 1982.
285. Ratnoff, O.D., and Naff, G.B.: The conversion of $C\bar{1}s$ and C'1 esterase by plasmin and trypsin. J. Exp. Med. 125:337, 1961.
286. Ward, P.A.: A plasmin-split fragment of C3 as a new chemotactic factor. J. Exp. Med. 126:189, 1967.
287. Curd, J.G., Prograis, L.J., Jr., and Cochrane, C.G.: Detection of active kallikrein in induced blister fluids of hereditary angioedema patients. J. Exp. Med. 152:742, 1980.
288. Fields, T., Ghebrehiwet, B., and Kaplan, A.P.: Kinin formation in hereditary angioedema plasma: Evidence against kinin derivation from C2 and in support of "spontaneous" formation of bradykinin. J. Allergy Clin. Immunol. 72:54, 1983.
289. Donaldson, V.H., Glueck, H.I., and Fleming, T.: Rheumatoid arthritis in a patient with Hageman trait. N. Engl. J. Med. 286:529, 1972.
290. Giclas, P.C., Ginsberg, M.H., and Cooper, N.R.: Immunoglobulin G independent activation of the classical complement pathway by monosodium urate crystals. J. Clin. Invest. 63:759, 1979.
291. Fields, T.R., Abramson, S.P., Weissman, G., Kaplan, A.P., and Ghebrehiwet, B.: Activation of the alternative pathway of complement by monosodium urate crystals. Clin. Immunol. Immunopathol 26:249, 1983.
292. Ginsberg, M., Jaques, B., Cochrane, C.G., and Griffin, J.H.: Urate crystal-dependent cleavage of Hageman factor in human plasma and synovial fluid. J. Lab. Clin. Med. 95:497, 1980.
293. Ward, Z., Mainardi, C.L., Vater, C.A., and Harris, E.D., Jr.: Endogenous activation of collagenase by rheumatoid synovial cells: Evidence for the role of plasminogen activator. N. Engl. J. Med. 296:1017, 1977.

# Chapter 9

# Cellular Components of Inflammation: Granulocytes

*Edward J. Goetzl and Ira M. Goldstein*

## INTRODUCTION

The influx and participation of granulocytes are constant features of acute, subacute, and some forms of chronic inflammation. Granulocytes play a central role in host defense, but if they accumulate in excessive numbers, persist, and are activated in an uncontrolled manner, the result may be deleterious to host tissues. Neutrophils can ingest and destroy bacteria, but they also mediate some types of necrotizing vasculitis. Similarly, eosinophils appear to contain parasitic invasion but may contribute to the endocardial fibrosis associated with sustained hypereosinophilia. The capacity of basophil mediators to increase the local delivery of antibodies and complement by increasing vascular permeability is still hypothetical in most instances, and the basophil continues to be identified principally with allergic reactions and some delayed cutaneous hypersensitivity states. This chapter will delineate the cellular characteristics and unique biochemical capabilities of the different subclasses of granulocytes, which account for both general and specialized functions. Deficiencies in function that may underlie increased susceptibility of some patients to infections will be discussed. The possible involvement of granulocytes in some rheumatic diseases will be explored by considering their roles in tissue damage.

## THE ORIGIN, DISTRIBUTION, AND FATE OF GRANULOCYTES

Granulocytes are derived in adults from pluripotential cells of the bone marrow, which are termed stem cells. Stem cells have the potential for both self-renewal and differentiation into the progenitors of granulocytes. The initial phases of differentiation in the bone marrow commit the cells to development into one type of granulocyte and lead to specific sensitivity to principles that regulate the production and terminal differentiation of that line of granulocytes. The results of studies of the capacity of bone marrow cells to form hematopoietic colonies in the spleens of lethally irradiated mice[1] and of human bone marrow cells to form clonal colonies of hematopoietic cells in agarose and other gelled media in vitro[2] have elucidated some characteristics of the progenitor cells of colony-forming units (CFUs). For example, each type of granulocyte is derived from a different subclass of progenitor cells, which are stimulated to proliferate and differentiate by structurally and functionally distinct glycoprotein colony-stimulating activities from several cellular sources.[1,3]

The terminal stages of proliferation and development of granulocytes in the bone marrow consist of a series of cell divisions that lead to the appearance of class-specific nuclear morphology and unique cytoplasmic granules, which distinguish the mature nonmitotic members of each subclass of granulocytes. All granulocyte precursors during the late blast and promyelocyte stages synthesize enzymes, other proteins, and smaller factors that are stored in the cytoplasmic secretory granules. Other cellular properties critical to the effector functions of granulocytes also develop during the later stages of maturation. Receptors appear for the Fc portion of immunoglobulin molecules, for complement components, and for lectins, and Ia antigens disappear during neutrophil differentiation.[4,5] Neutrophils and eosinophils acquire or increase their ability to phagocytize and respond to specific chemotactic factors.[6]

The apparent morphologic and constitutive differences among subclasses of granulocytes are accompanied by a striking divergence of cellular kinetics, tissue distribution, and function. While the knowledge of human granulocytes is incomplete, several studies have revealed a marrow storage compartment, intravascular circulating and marginated pools, and tissue representation for both neutrophils and eosinophils. Mature neutrophils and eosinophils remain in the marrow compartment for approximately 5 and 3 to 4 days, respectively, and circulate for about 10 and 12 hours, respectively, before entering the tissues.[7,8] A high percentage of the mature eosinophils and a smaller number of the basophils are located normally in tissues, while neutrophils are found in tissues only in relation to foci of irritation or infection. The tissue eosinophils are distributed in lymphoid organs and below the epithelial surfaces of the skin, lungs, intestines, and genitourinary tract.[8,9] Despite the differences in normal tissue representation, any significant influx of neutrophils, eosinophils, or basophils requires recruitment from the circulating pools. While some data suggest that eosinophils and basophils persist in tissue for much longer periods than neutrophils, the mechanism of the elimination of granulocytes is still unknown. However, recirculation of tissue granulocytes appears to be an uncommon and quantitatively insignificant phenomenon.

## CELLULAR FUNCTIONS OF GRANULOCYTES

**Regulation of Granulocyte Migration.** Granulocyte chemotaxis is initiated by the presentation to the cells of a concentration gradient of a specific stimulus and leads to the accumulation of granulocytes at tissue sites of inflammation.[10] Chemokinesis is the enhancement of random migration of granulocytes that is evoked as a function of stimulus concentration irrespective of a gradient. Both the development of in vitro methods for the quantitation of granulocyte migration and the availability of purified and synthetic principals have fostered intensive investigations of the stimulation of migration, have permitted the distinction between chemokinesis and chemotaxis, and have led to the understanding of several types of inhibitory mechanisms. In those assays that are modifications of Boyden's technique,[11] one or more micropore filters are employed to separate the granulocytes from the stimulus. Following routine fixation, a variety of granulocyte stains can be used, and the response is quantified by microscopically enumerating the cells within the filter. For the techniques that utilize radiolabeled granulocytes and a pair of micropore filters, quantification is based on counting the cell-associated radioactivity in the filter farther from the source of granulocytes. With the former approach, the use of selective stains precludes the necessity for prior purification of the target granulocytes,[12] and the cells can be counted at multiple levels within the micropore filter to establish the distance traveled by the "leading front."[13] The modifications using cells prelabeled with $^{51}Cr$ or other isotopes are highly objective and especially well suited to clinical studies of cellular migration defects as the granulocytes must migrate through the first filter to be counted in the second filter, a distance greater than that of conventional assays.[14] However, the radioassays require essentially total purification of cells in order to allow the radioactivity to be equated with a given population of granulocytes.[15] The newly developed agarose well assays[16] are also dependent on the use of purified cells, unless the agarose is removed to permit the staining and identification of the granulocytes that have migrated out of the wells. The need for only a relatively small number of granulocytes per assay and the ease of macroscopic assessment of maximal migratory responses are the primary advantages of the agarose well techniques.

The initial event in the stimulation of granulocyte chemotaxis involves the activation of the pathways for generation of specific chemotactic factors. Alterations of basement membrane or collagen structure activate Hageman factor,[17] which subsequently converts prekallikrein to kallikrein, a kinin-generating enzyme with chemotactic activity.[18] Activation by immune complexes of the classic complement pathway and by microbial polysaccharides of the alternative complement pathway elaborates chemotactic fragments, most notably the minor fragment of the fifth component, C5a,[19] or complexes such as $\overline{C567}$,[20] while the alternative pathway alone contributes the chemotactic factor C3bBb[21]. IgE-dependent activation of human mast cell–rich tissues releases both the eosinophil chemotactic factor of anaphylaxis (ECF-A),[22,23] which is composed in part of two acidic tetrapeptides,[24] and neutrophil chemotactic activities, consisting of high molecular weight proteins. The IgE-directed stimulation of mast cells also results in the elaboration of lipid chemotactic and chemokinetic factors, the most potent of which are lipoxygenase products of arachidonic acid.[25-27] Chemotactic factors for granulocytes and other leukocytes can be classified according to their structural properties (Table 9–1). While many of the protein complexes or fragments with chemotactic activity are derived from the complement pathways, large peptides and proteins liberated as a result of the proteolysis of fibrin and collagen also attract granulocytes in vitro.[28,29] The expression of chemotactic activity by the enzymatic factors is dependent on the integrity of their active site, as exemplified by the chemotactic inactivity of prekallikrein, which does not possess the capacity to generate bradykinin, and by the comparable degree of inhibition of both the chemotactic and kinin-generating activities of kallikrein by increasing concentrations of diisopropylfluorophosphate.[30] The peptides of ECF-A and other low molecular weight peptides and amines are cellular products released upon specific activation of the host cells or, in the case of bacterial factors,[31] during phases of rapid bacterial growth. Numerous chemotactic lymphokines have been described, which are proteins that vary in heat stability, size, and charge.[32] The lipid chemotactic factors that have been defined are either components of bacterial cell walls[33]

**Table 9–1.** The Structural Diversity and Specificity of Natural Factors Chemotactic for Human Granulocytes and Monocytes

| Class | Factor | Source | Molecular Weight | Structural Characteristics | Cellular Preference | Other Functions |
|---|---|---|---|---|---|---|
| I. Protein fragments or complexes | C5a | Complement pathways C5 proteolysis | 17,000 | Basic protein | N,E,B,M | Chemotactic deactivation; Mast cell degranulation; Smooth muscle contraction |
| | $\overline{C567}$ | Complement pathways | 435,000 | Protein complex | N,E | Lysis of bacteria |
| | Fibrin fragments | Fibrinolysis | 30,000-50,000 | Proteins | N,E,M | Chemotactic deactivation |
| | Collagen fragments | Collagenolysis | 300-1000 | Peptides | M,N | Fibroblast attraction |
| II. Enzymes | Plasma kallikrein | Kinin-generating sequence | 108,000 | γ-globulin | N | Bradykinin generation; Chemotactic deactivation |
| | C3bBb | Alternative complement pathway | 234,000 | Protein complex | N | Chemotactic deactivation |
| III. Cellular peptides or amines | ECF-A peptides | Mast cells | 360-390 | Acidic peptides | E>N | Chemotactic deactivation; Increase in eosinophil C3b receptors |
| | Histamine | Mast cells | 111 | Amine | E>N | Chemotactic facilitation and deactivation; Increase in eosinophil C3b receptors |
| | Bacterial soluble factors | Bacteria | 300-1000 | Peptides | N | — |
| IV. Lymphokines | | Lymphocytes | 20,000-60,000 | Protein | E,N | — |
| | | Lymphocytes | 12,500 | Protein | M | — |
| | | Lymphocytes | 12,500 | ? | B | |
| V. Lipids | $LTB_4$ | Arachidonate lipoxygenase | 340 | | E>N | Chemokinetic stimulation; Chemotactic deactivation |
| | HHT | Arachidonate cyclooxygenase | 280 | — | E>N | Chemokinetic stimulation; Chemotactic deactivation |
| | Bacterial lipids | Bacteria | — | Lipoproteins and lipids | N,M | — |

N = Neutrophil. E = Eosinophil. B = Basophil. M = Mononuclear leukocyte. LT = Leukotriene. HHT = 12-L-OH-5,8,10-heptadecatrienoic acid.

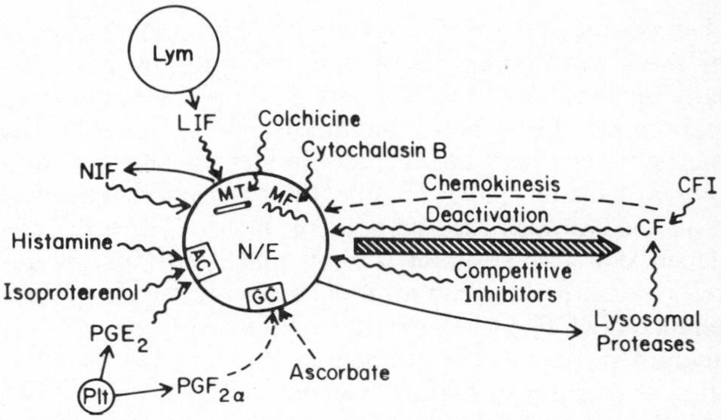


**Figure 9–1.** Regulation of granulocyte chemotaxis. N = Neutrophil. E = Eosinophil. Lym = Lymphocyte. Plt = Platelet. NIF = Neutrophil immobilizing factor. LIF = Leukocyte inhibition factor. ⇝ = Inhibitory effect. CF = Chemotactic factor. CFI = Chemotactic factor inactivator. AC = Adenylate cyclase. GC = Guanylate cyclase. MT = Microtubule. MF = Actin microfilament. ▨➔ = Chemotaxis. ⟶ = Release or generation. - - -> = Enhancing effect.

or lipoxygenase metabolites of arachidonic acid or related fatty acids.[34-36] The latter pathways are of special significance as the generation of the potent chemotactic fatty acid designated 5(S),12(R)-dihydroxy-eicosa-6,14 cis-8,10 trans-tetraenoic acid (leukotriene $B_4$)[26,27] by 5-lipoxygenases is not inhibited by the currently available nonsteroidal anti-inflammatory drugs.

The second aspect of the modulation of chemotaxis is the potency and leukocyte specificity of each stimulus. While for many chemotactic factors the potential range of responder leukocytes has not been explored, the cellular preference of some principals has been delineated. C5a attracts eosinophils, neutrophils, basophils, and monocytes with comparable activity.[37,38] In contrast, kallikrein preferentially attracts neutrophils and monocytes,[30] leukotriene $B_4$ is more active for neutrophils and eosinophils than monocytes, and ECF-A is most chemotactic for eosinophils, although it has some activity for neutrophils.[24,39] This aspect of regulation of chemotaxis and some of the other effects of chemotactic factors on granulocytes are functions of the properties of specific subsets of receptors, each of which is committed to one chemotactic factor.[10] A third regulatory dimension encompasses inactivators and inhibitors of chemotactic factors (Fig. 9-1). The anaphylatoxin inactivator acts to diminish the chemotactic potential of C5a[19,40] and leads to a dependence on a serum protein, termed the C5a des Arg "cochemotaxin," for the expression of maximal chemotactic activity.[19] The chemotactic factor inactivator, which is composed of at least two aminopeptidases, irreversibly destroys a variety of chemotactic factors.[41,42] Lysosomal proteases of granulocytes themselves inactivate C5a and possibly other protein chemotactic factors.[43] The inhibitor of the activated first component of complement, C$\bar{1}$INH, and $\alpha_2$-macroglobulin reversibly suppress the chemotactic activity of kallikrein.[30] The fourth level of regulation is granulocyte-directed and includes noncytotoxic factors which specifically influence the responsiveness of the stimulated population of cells irrespective of the nature of the chemotactic factor (Fig. 9-1). The chemotactic principals themselves reduce responsiveness through a process which has been designated chemotactic deactivation.[31,44,45] Chemotactic deactivation by any factor has a leukocyte specificity comparable to its chemotactic specificity,[39] but the biochemical mechanisms have not been elucidated. Concentrations of several chemotactic stimuli that are equal to or greater than maximally chemotactic levels induce a state of relative chemotactic unresponsiveness, which is not restricted to the initial stimulus and is mediated by an increase in granulocyte adherence.

A wide range of nonchemotactic agents specifically influence the chemotactic responses of granulocytes with or without affecting other functions (Fig. 9-1). At noncytotoxic concentrations, colchicine and cytochalasin B inhibit both chemotaxis and phagocytosis by actions on the microtubules and actin filaments, respectively.[46-49] In contrast, the release of lysosomal enzymes from granulocytes that are engaged in phagocytosis or are stimulated by the introduction of some chemotactic factors is inhibited by colchicine and markedly enhanced by cytochalasin B.[48-50] Amphotericin inhibits granulocyte chemotaxis, presumably by disorganizing the structure of plasma membrane sterols, but only inhibits phagocytosis at much higher concentrations than would be attainable in vivo during antifungal therapy.[51] Exogenous 3',5'-adenosine monophosphate (cyclic AMP) and agonists that elevate intracellular levels of cyclic AMP in granulocytes, including $\beta$-adrenergic agents, prostaglandins of the E series, and histamine acting through an $H_2$ receptor, inhibit chemotaxis with far less effect on phagocytosis.[52,53] Although ascorbic acid, serotonin, and prostaglandin $F_{2\alpha}$ ($PGF_{2\alpha}$) enhance both the random and chemotactic migration of granulocytes at concentrations known to raise the intracellular levels of 3',5'-guanosine monophosphate (cyclic GMP) in mononuclear leukocytes, comparable elevations of cyclic GMP levels have not been demonstrable in granulocytes.[53,55] Of the few principles which have been recognized to directly facilitate migration in vitro, ascorbic acid is of special interest. Levels of ascorbic acid ranging from 10- to 50-fold the normal plasma concentration induce a several-fold enhancement of random and directed migration of granulocytes and mononuclear leukocytes and a concomitant stimulation of hexose monophosphate shunt activity, without affecting phagocytosis.[54] Ascorbic acid has reversed the chemotactic and other functional deficiencies in granulocytes of patients with the Chédiak-Higashi syndrome[56] and the Quie-Hill syndrome[57] both in vitro and in vivo. Several naturally occurring peptides and proteins modulate granulocyte migration with both cellular and functional specificity, but the mechanisms of their effects are unknown. The neutrophil immobilizing factor (NIF) is composed of two basic lysosomal peptides of approximately 4000 daltons that are derived from human neutrophils or mononuclear leukocytes.[58] NIF lacks chemotactic activity, but suppresses the random and directed migration of neutrophils and eosinophils without influencing their metabolism, phagocytic capacity, or adherence to surfaces, and is without any action on monocytes.[59,60] Plasma proteins with other recognized humoral functions, such as $\alpha_1$-antitrypsin and $\alpha_2$-macroglobulin, can directly influence neutrophil random migration and chemotactic responsiveness, but do not alter phagocytosis.[61]

The interest in granulocyte migration has been heightened by observations of the modulatory effects of numerous other relevant cell types and by the evolving evidence for activities of chemotactic factors which bear on granulocyte functions other than migration. Proteases released upon stimulation of human platelets degrade C5 in a manner which releases chemotactic fragments.[62] Platelet aggregation, which activates the arachidonate oxygenases and provides a supply of substrate,[63] leads not only to the release of the chemotactic principal, 12-L-hydroxy-eicosatetraenoic acid (12-HETE), but also to the elaboration of $PGF_{2\alpha}$ and $PGE_2$ which are positively and negatively chemokinetic for granulocytes, respectively.[10] The interaction of human lymphocytes with mitogens or specific antigen generates and releases a 23,000 molecular weight esterase, termed the leukocyte inhibitory factor (LIF), which suppresses neutrophil but not mononuclear leukocyte migration from capillary tubes[64,65] and inhibits the random and chemotactic migration of neutrophils in modified Boyden micropore filter chambers.[66] Incubation of neutrophils with LIF releases additional inhibitory activity (Fig. 9–1), which resembles NIF by virtue of its molecular weight, susceptibility to inactivation by trypsin, and noncytotoxic preferential inhibition of granulocyte migration, as compared to that of mononuclear leukocytes.[66] Thus a spectrum of lymphokines may stimulate leukocyte chemotaxis, directly inhibit leukocyte responses to chemotactic factors, and induce the release of chemotactic inhibitors from the target granulocytes. Chemotactic factors not only are capable of evoking chemotactic and chemokinetic responses and of inducing chemotactic deactivation, but also stimulate neutrophil adherence, aggregation[67] and release of lysosomal enzymes,[68] and modulate the expression of plasma membrane C3b receptors on human eosinophils.[69] Treatment of eosinophils with chemotactic concentrations of the tetrapeptides of ECF-A led to a significant increase in the number of C3b receptors per cosinophil, an effect that was also observed upon the addition of histamine but was not reproduced by other mediators.[69]

## CHARACTERISTICS OF GRANULOCYTE INTERACTIONS WITH PARTICULATE STIMULI

### Recognition—Neutrophil Receptors for Immunoglobulins and Complement

Wright and Douglas,[70] in 1903, observed that fresh serum greatly enhanced ingestion and killing of bacteria by peripheral blood neutrophils. Numerous investigators subsequently established that there are two major constituents of serum (i.e., opsonins) that act upon certain bacteria, fungi, and other particles to increase their palatability. One is heat stable (56° C for 30 minutes) and present primarily in immune serum. The other is heat labile and present in fresh normal serum. The heat-stable constituent is recognized now as immunoglobulin (i.e., antibody) of the IgG class. The Fc regions of IgG immunoglobulins that have been altered as a consequence of either aggregation or binding to antigen attach to specific receptors ("Fc receptors" or "IgG recptors") on the plasma membrane of neutrophils (Table 9–2). Thus, neutrophils "recognize" particles sensitized with IgG antibody.

Heat-labile opsonic activity is attributable primarily to a fragment of the third component of complement. When complement is activated by either the classical or the alternative pathways, C3 is cleaved into two fragments, C3a and C3b. The larger of these fragments, C3b, is capable of becoming attached to the surfaces of cells and other particles (including bacteria and fungi).[71] C3b renders the particles to which it is attached recognizable by neutrophils and mediates firm particle–neutrophil adherence through interactions with "C3b receptors" (Table 9–2). The nature of the neutrophil receptors for IgG and C3b, as well as the consequences of receptor-ligand binding, are discussed in sections that follow.

**IgG Receptors.** After it was established that antigen-antibody complexes and antibody-coated particles are recognized by mononuclear phagocytes,[72] evidence appeared of receptors for immunoglobulins on the surface of neutrophils.[73,75] Henson,[73] for example, demonstrated that sheep erythrocytes sensitized with IgG antibody adhere to human, rabbit, and guinea pig neutrophils. Minimal adherence was noted when IgM antibody was used. Messner and Jelinek[76] extended these findings and provided evidence that receptors for the Fc regions of human IgG antibodies exist on both human neutrophils

**Table 9–2.** Properties of Human Neutrophil Immunoglobulin and Complement Receptors

| Immunoglobulin Receptor | Complement Receptor |
|---|---|
| Recognizes Fc regions of IgG (and some IgA immunoglobulins) | Recognizes C3b fragment of native C3 |
| Present on 75 to 90 percent of neutrophils in peripheral blood | Present on greater than 90 percent of neutrophils in peripheral blood |
| Not affected by trypsin | Trypsin-sensitive |
| Receptor-mediated functions unaffected by reduced temperatures, EDTA, $H_2O_2$, and hydrocortisone | Receptor-mediated functions inhibited by reduced temperatures, EDTA, $H_2O_2$, hydrocortisone, and trypan blue |
| Mobile in plane of neutrophil surface membrane | Distributed uniformly in clusters on the neutrophil surface |
| "Macromolecule(s)" with a molecular weight of 52,000 to 64,000 | Glycoprotein with a molecular weight of 205,000 |

and monocytes. They demonstrated that adherence of sensitized human erythrocytes to monolayers of neutrophils could be inhibited by native IgG, myeloma globulins of the $IgG_1$ and $IgG_3$ subclasses, and isolated Fc (but not Fab) fragments. Subsequent studies have established that 75 to 90 percent of human peripheral blood neutrophils bear receptors on their surface for IgG-coated particles.[77,78] Attachment of IgG-coated particles to human neutrophils does not require divalent cations,[73,74] nor is it influenced by reduced temperatures (e.g., 4° C) or prior treatment of cells with trypsin.[77]

The specificity of the immunoglobulin receptor on neutrophils has been confirmed in several studies. Sajnani and colleagues,[79,80] for example, demonstrated by fluorescence microscopy that human neutrophils bind isolated Fc fragments as well as intact IgG. Attempts to demonstrate binding of IgM to human neutrophils generally have not been successful.[73,74,76] Similarly, neutrophils appear to lack receptors for IgE and IgD.[73,81] Evidence has been provided recently that some phagocytic cells possess different receptors for monomeric immunoglobulins and for aggregated (or complexed) immunoglobulins.[82] This could explain the finding that whereas neutrophils bind unaggregated immunoglobulins only of the $IgG_1$ and $IgG_3$ subclasses[81] aggregated IgG of all four subclasses can bind to and stimulate these cells.[83]

As indicated above, binding to neutrophils of antigen-antibody complexes, immunoglobulin-coated particles, and aggregated immunoglobulins depends upon the integrity of the Fc regions of the immunoglobulin molecules. Binding to neutrophils of either aggregated or antigen-complexed immunoglobulins exceeds that of the corresponding monomeric immunoglobulin molecules. At least two hypotheses have been formulated to account for these observations. One hypothesis assumes that although monomeric immunoglobulins have an exposed binding site on their Fc regions available for attachment to neutrophils, univalent binding is unstable. More stable, and therefore detectable, binding results only from the formation of complexes with mulitple sites. Thus, stable binding of polyvalent antigen-antibody complexes or of immunoglobulin aggregates would result from cooperative binding to Fc receptors of several molecules (which exponentially increases binding of the whole complex).[75] The alternative hypothesis suggests that either aggregation of immunoglobulins or interactions between antibodies and antigens produce changes in the conformation of immunoglobulin molecules.[84] Such conformational changes would expose sites capable of interacting with the neutrophil surface. Thus, the tertiary structure of intact immunoglobulins may influence binding to neutrophils.

Fc receptors on human neutrophils have been visualized indirectly by fluorescence microscopy as well as by electron microscopy and shown to be mobile in the plane of the neutrophil plasma membrane.[79,80,85] Interestingly, a very close correlation was observed between Fc receptor redistribution and immune complex–induced neutrophil responses, suggesting a relationship between activation of neutrophils and surface receptor mobility.

Macromolecules with Fc receptor activity have been isolated from leukocytes of several species.[86,87] Kulczycki and colleagues,[87] for example, subjected solubilized, radiolabeled surface proteins of human neutrophils and mononuclear cells to repetitive affinity chromatography and succeeded in purifying material capable of binding specifically to Fc fragments of IgG. Neither Fab fragments nor IgM bound to the isolated receptorlike macromolecules. Analysis of the purified Fc-binding material by sodium dodecylsulfate polyacrylamide gel electrophoresis revealed a single, broad, 52,000 to 64,000 molecular weight band.

**Complement Receptors.** Although it was appreciated for many years that complement components on the surfaces of antibody-sensitized particles facilitated phagocytosis by neutrophils,[88,89] it was not until 1968 that evidence was reported of a complement receptor on the neutrophil surface membrane. Lay and Nussenzweig[74] observed that sheep erythrocytes sensitized with rabbit IgM antibodies did not adhere to isolate mouse peripheral blood neutrophils unless they were first incubated with fresh mouse serum for 30 minutes at 37° C. Adherence to neutrophils of sheep erythrocytes sensitized with IgG antibody also was enhanced after incubation with fresh mouse serum. Subsequent studies in the mouse, rabbit, guinea pig, and man have established that neutrophils possess receptors on their surface for fragments of the third component of complement (primarily C3b).[73,77,90–94] In man, such receptors can be demonstrated on greater than 90 percent of neutrophils in peripheral blood.[94] Binding to human neutrophils of particles coated with fragments of C3 is inhibited by treating cells with trypsin[73,74] and by reduced temperatures (4° C).[74,77] Binding can also be modulated by divalent cations (particularly $Mg^{2+}$).[95,96]

The function of C3 receptors on human neutrophils can be influenced by other agents. Boxer and colleagues,[77] for example, were able to inhibit attachment of complement-coated particles to human neutrophils by exposing these cells to the sulfhydryl-blocking agent *N*-ethylmaleimide as well as to hydrogen peroxide and hydrocortisone. Results similar to these were obtained by Guckian and associates[97] when human neutrophils were exposed to the vital dye trypan blue. The precise mechanisms whereby these compounds interfere with the function of neutrophil complement receptors are unknown.

Structurally specific receptors for C3b have been identified on the surface of neutrophils and have been isolated from these cells.[98–100] The human neutrophil C3b receptor is a glycoprotein with an apparent molecular weight of 205,000.[98] It appears to be similar to, or identical with, C3b receptors on human erythrocytes, B lymphocytes, and monocytes.[98] When examined at 0° C by indirect immunofluorescence, C3b receptors on human neutrophils appeared to be distributed in a random fashion in small clusters on the plasma membrane.[99] Interestingly, rapid receptor-mediated endocytosis of soluble ligands was observed when neutrophils were warmed to 37° C. It is not known yet whether aggregation of C3b receptors is a prerequisite for C3-dependent cytoadherence. More work is required to elucidate the mechanisms whereby receptor–ligand interactions promote specific neutrophil functions, such as adherence to particles or surfaces, phagocytosis, alterations in oxidative metabolism, and degranulation (see below).

It should not be concluded from the foregoing discussion that neutrophils only recognize particles or surfaces coated with fragments of C3 and/or IgG. It also should not be concluded that recognition is mediated only by structurally specific surface membrane receptors. Indeed, the term "receptor" need only imply an ability of neutrophils to recognize a given molecule and to be activated by it. Whereas molecular entities within (or on) the neutrophil surface membrane are presumed to mediate these functions, the presence of some of these only can be inferred. Receptors for some ligands have neither been identified nor isolated. Consequently, it is best to consider neutrophil surface membrane receptors as "recognition units," which may or may not be represented by specific single molecules or even by complex intramembranous structures. Recognition units, by necessity, would be linked to "effector units" (of similarly vague composition), which trigger or initiate specific cellular functions.

## Phagocytosis

When contact is established between a neutrophil and a suitable particle, the particle is ingested by the cell, a process termed phagocytosis. Direct observations of phagocytosis by light microscopy and by electron microscopy have revealed that attachment of a neutrophil to a suitable small particle results in the formation, at the site of attachment, of pseudopodia, which surround the particle and ultimately fuse at its distal pole.[101] The process of particle engulfment by neutrophils requires energy (supplied by anaerobic glycolysis) as well as complex interactions between cytoplasmic contractile proteins (i.e., actin and myosin) and the plasma membrane.[102,103]

Whereas neutrophils appear capable of ingesting seemingly "inert" particles (e.g., polystyrene latex beads), particularly under conditions in which particle-cell contact is maximized, opsonins such as C3b or IgG clearly increase the rate and extent of particle uptake. Stossel,[95] for example, found that particle-bound C3 fragments markedly accelerated maximal rates of ingestion by human neutrophils of albumin-coated paraffin oil particles. Interestingly, whereas opsonically active C3 and IgG increased the $V_{max}$ of the ingestion rate, only IgG altered the apparent $K_m$ of the reaction (markedly decreasing it). It was concluded that while both C3 and IgG increase the rate of ingestion, only IgG increases the affinity of the particle for some "catalytic site" that activates internalization. In a subsequent study, Stossel and colleagues[104] demonstrated that human peripheral blood neutrophils ingest lipopolysaccharide-coated paraffin oil droplets only if fragments of C3 are attached to the surfaces of these particles. Binding of radiolabeled C3 to these particles correlated precisely with their ingestibility.

**Table 9–3.** Roles Played by Neutrophil Immunoglobulin and Complement Receptors in Adherence and Phagocytosis*

| | Adherence | Phagocytosis |
|---|---|---|
| EA (IgM) | — | — |
| EA (IgG) | + | + |
| EA (IgM-C3b) | +++ | — |
| EA (IgG-C3b) | +++ | +++ |

*Adapted from Ehlenberger and Nussenzweig.[24] Sheep erythrocytes (E) sensitized with IgM or IgG antibodies (A) with or without complement (C3b).

More recent work has shed additional light on the roles played by C3 fragments and IgG in promoting particle recognition and phagocytosis by neutrophils. By using erythrocytes coated with IgG and/or C3b, several investigators have demonstrated that the neutrophil C3b receptor is involved primarily in recognition and attachment and only inefficiently promotes ingestion of bound or adherent particles. In contrast, particle binding to the neutrophil IgG receptor, while less efficient, appears necessary for the induction of optimal phagocytosis.[90,92,93] Thus, C3b and IgG have separate but synergistic roles in phagocytosis (Table 9–3). Depending upon the experimental conditions, the presence of particle-bound C3b is able to reduce by 100-fold the amount of IgG required to promote engulfment of particles. Under certain conditions, C3b receptors may serve to overcome electrostatic repulsion and permit contact between the neutrophil surface and moieties on particles that promote engulfment. The role of C3b in opsonization is mainly one of establishing contact between particles and phagocytes.

Neutrophils are capable of ingesting certain particles in the complete absence of complement or immunoglobulins. It is likely that such particles have chemical moieties on their surfaces that not only permit attachment by neutrophils but also behave as "surrogate immunoglobulins" and promote ingestion. Indeed, it has been demonstrated that particles requiring only C3b on their surfaces for optimal ingestion by neutrophils are ingestible in the native state if particle–cell contact is enhanced.[95]

How does IgG promote ingestion of particles? Although it has been suggested that phagocytosis occurs as a consequence of perturbation of the neutrophil cell membrane,[105] there is no direct evidence relating the ability of "altered" IgG to perturb artificial lipid bilayers with the ability to promote ingestion of particles.[106] Indeed, there is evidence to suggest that membrane perturbation may not be sufficient to induce phagocytosis. Stendahl and associates,[107] for example, demonstrated that whereas opsonized *Salmonella typhimurium* 395 MS and nonopsonized *S. typhimurium* 395 MR 10 are ingested by neutrophils to the same extent, only the opsonized bacteria perturb liposomal membranes. An alternative explanation for the role that IgG plays in promoting phagocytosis has been proposed by Griffin and co-workers.[108] These investigators suggested that phagocytosis results only from a sequential interaction of ligands and receptors around the surface of a particle (the "zipper" theory). They would suggest that the distribution of C3b moieties on the surface of a sensitized erythrocyte and C3b receptors on the surface of a neutrophil would not permit sufficient interactions of ligands and receptors around the entire particle. Cooperation with Fc receptors, however, would permit optimal ligand–receptor interactions and engulfment of the particle. A great deal more must be learned of the mechanisms whereby attachment of particles to the neutrophil surface membrane ultimately leads to phagocytosis.

## Lysosomes and Neutrophil Degranulation

Lysosomes are a class of subcellular organelles that contain various hydrolytic enzymes, predominantly with acid pH optima, bound in latent form within a relatively impermeable membrane.[109] Lysosomal granules of phagocytic cells constitute their vacuolar system, or internal digestive system. Human neutrophils contain two major types of lysosomal granules, distinguishable by their morphology, staining characteristics, and enzyme content. Azurophil granules, which contain peroxidase and other lysosomal hydrolases, appear in the cytoplasm of neutrophils during the promyelocyte stage of development and arise from the concave surface of the Golgi complex. Specific granules, on the other hand, are formed from the convex face of the Golgi complex during the myelocyte stage of development and contain predominantly lysozyme and the iron-binding protein lactoferrin.[110,111] Alkaline phosphatase is not a granule associated enzyme in human neutrophils but is associated only with the plasma membrane.[112,113] In rabbit neutrophils, however, 90 percent of total cellular alkaline phosphatase sediments with specific granules.[114]

Zonal sedimentation, velocity sedimentation, and isopycnic equilibration techniques have enabled investigators to localize more precisely most of the granule-associated enzymes of human neutrophils. It has been established, for example, that azurophil granules contain all of the myeloperoxidase and β-glucuronidase found in these cells.[112,113] Azurophil granules also contain all of the elastase and cathepsin G,[115] the bulk of other acid glycosidases, and approximately 50 percent of the lysozyme in human neutrophils.[112,113] Specific granules, on the other hand, contain all of the lactoferrin in these cells and the remainder of their lysozyme.[112,116] Specific granules also contain latent collagenase[117] and vitamin $B_{12}$-binding protein.[118] Less well-defined human neutrophil granules contain *N*-acetyl-β-glucosaminidase and a latent, neutral gelatinase.[113] Human neutrophils, therefore, contain granule-associated enzymes capable of hydrolysing a wide variety of both natural and synthetic substrates, including simple and complex polysaccharides, oligopeptides, and phosphate esters (Table 9–4). The roles played by these enzymes in maintaining normal host defenses and in mediating inflammation have been the subject of several reviews[119-123] and are discussed elsewhere in this volume (Chapter 12).

**Degranulation.** As indicated in previous sections, phagocytosis by neutrophils entails recognition of the particle to be ingested, binding of the particle to the cell surface, and finally, engulfment of the particle within a vacuole and closure of the plasma membrane. Shortly after, or coincident with these events, lysosomal granules fuse with those portions of the plasma membrane that constitute the phagocytic vacuole (or "phagosome").[124] Membrane fusion leads to the discharge of lysosomal enzymes and other granule constituents into the newly formed, or forming, phagosome (the process of "degranulation")[125] (Fig. 9–2). The resultant structure has been termed a phagolysosome.[124] Phagolysosomes, therefore, contain not only acid hydrolases but also substrate. In phagocytic cells, formation of phagolysosomes is crucial for normal host defenses.[126] It is within phagolysosomes, for example, that killing and digestion of microorganisms take place.[125] Stossel and colleagues[127] isolated phagolysosomes from human and guinea pig neutrophils and confirmed biochemically that degranulation occurs coincidentally with ingestion. Based on the kinetics of particle uptake and translocation of granule constituents into phagolysosomes, these investigators concluded that the "triggering" mechanisms for both phagocytosis and degranulation may be similar or identical.

Degranulation of neutrophils is not a uniform process. Azurophil and specific granules discharge their contents at different rates during phagocytosis.[127-129] Bainton[129]

**Table 9–4.** Some Lysosomal Constituents of Human Neutrophils

| Azurophil Granules | Specific Granules | Others |
|---|---|---|
| Myeloperoxidase | Lactoferrin | Latent gelatinase |
| β-Glucuronidase (other glycosidases) | Vitamin $B_{12}$-binding protein | *N*-acetyl-β-glucosaminidase |
| Lysozyme (50 percent) | Lysozyme (50 percent) | |
| Phospholipase | Latent collagenase | |
| Ribonuclease | | |
| Elastase | | |
| Cathepsin G | | |

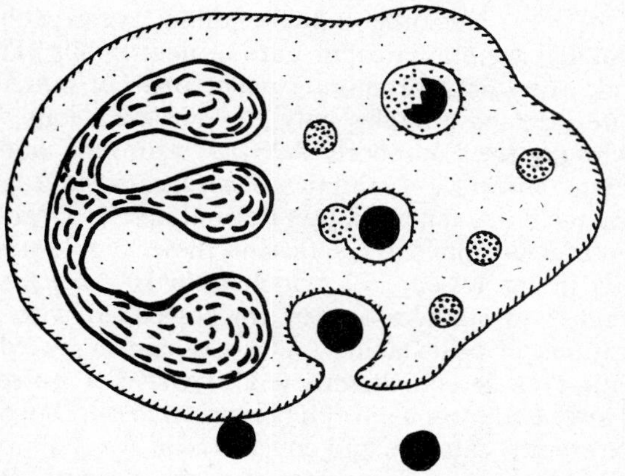

**Figure 9–2.** Neutrophil degranulation. Following phagocytosis, membrane fusion leads to the discharge of lysosomal constituents into newly formed, or forming, phagosomes.

found that specific granules of rabbit neutrophils fuse with phagosomes and discharge their contents more rapidly than azurophil granules. In addition, although azurophil and specific granules discharge their contents during phagocytosis, specific granule constituents appear to be more accessible for extracellular release.[128,130,131] Finally, based on the responses of neutrophils to mechanical and other nonphagocytic stimuli, it has been suggested that specific granules actually may be secretory granules and that their contents function extracellularly rather than intracellularly.[130,132,133] The precise mechanism whereby specific granules fuse so readily with portions of the neutrophil plasma membrane has not been elucidated. It has been found, however, that azurophil and specific granules differ with respect to their content of cholesterol, phospholipid, and protein.[134]

**Extracellular Release of Neutrophil Lysosomal Constituents.** Whereas the contents of neutrophil granules most often are discharged intracellularly into phagosomes, under certain circumstances they can be released extracellularly. One mechanism whereby granule constituents are extruded from neutrophils is simply "cell death" (Fig. 9–3*A*). When neutrophils are exposed to a variety of toxins, injury to the plasma membrane is an early consequence, and ultimately, all intracellular materials are released from the injured cells, including those ordinarily sequestered within azurophil and specific granules. Biologic detergents, for example, act in this manner to cause primary lysis of cell membranes and, only subsequently, disruption of cytoplasmic granules.[135] Under these circumstances, cytoplasmic enzymes and other cellular constituents, in addition to lysosomal hydrolases, are released into the medium surrounding dead and dying neutrophils.

Another mechanism by which lysosomal constituents can be released from neutrophils conforms to the "suicide sac" hypothesis of de Duve and Wattiaux.[136] Under some circumstances, materials gain access to the interior of the cells' vacuolar system wherein they cause membranes of lysosomes to rupture (Fig. 9–3*B*). Such damage of lysosomal membranes subsequently leads to release from neutrophils of cytoplasmic enzymes and other intracellular constituents as the cells die as a consequence of "perforation from within" of their vacuolar system.[137,138] Crystalline substances, such as monosodium urate and silica, act on neutrophils (and other phagocytic cells) in this fashion.[137–141]

Yet another mechanism of enzyme release from neutrophils involves the discharge of lysosomal constituents into the medium surrounding intact cells engaging in phagocytosis. Such release is not accompanied by leakage of cytoplasmic enzymes and appears to be due to the extrusion of lysosomal granule contents from incompletely sealed phagosomes, open at their external borders to the extracellular space but already joined at their internal borders by lysosomal granules actively discharging their contents (Fig. 9–3*C*). The cell engaging in phagocytosis remains viable, but its released lysosomal enzymes are free to act extracellularly. This probably is a common mechanism whereby neutrophils provoke tissue injury in a variety of disease states.[120,123]

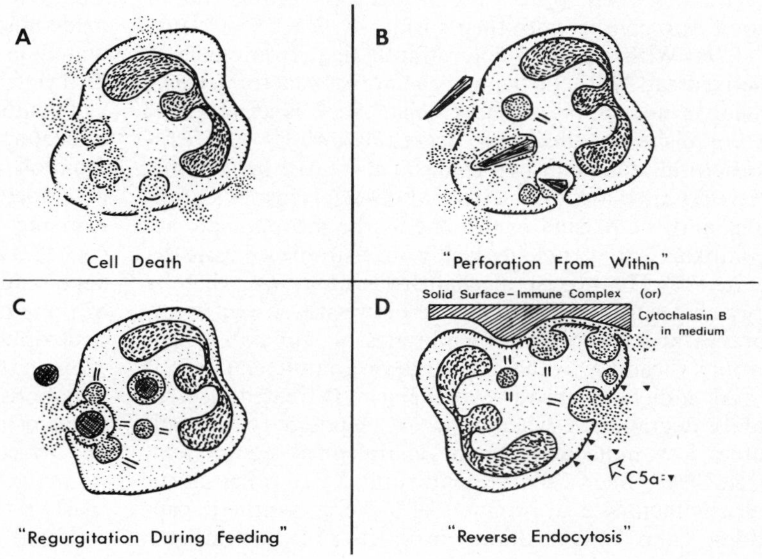


**Figure 9–3.** Extracellular release of neutrophil lysosomal constituents. *A*, Cell death. *B*, Perforation from within. *C*, Regurgitation during feeding. *D*, Reverse endocytosis.

Biochemical and morphologic evidence for this mechanism, which has been termed "regurgitation during feeding,"[137,138] has been presented for several experimental systems involving particle ingestion by neutrophils.[83,137,138,142–148]

Phagocytosis per se is not an absolute prerequisite for degranulation by neutrophils. In fact, there is a substantial amount of evidence indicating that degranulation of neutrophils can be provoked not only by appropriate ligand–surface membrane receptor interactions but also by "nonspecific" membrane perturbation. For example, when neutrophils encounter either immune complexes or aggregated immunoglobulins deposited on solid surfaces (e.g., micropore filters, collagen membranes), the cells adhere to these surfaces and selectively release a portion of their granule contents[138,142–145,148–150] (Fig. 9–3*D*). A similar phenomenon occurs when adherent cells encounter some soluble stimuli, such as the complement component, C5a.[50] Lysosomal enzyme release under these conditions occurs by a process of "reverse endocytosis"[138] or "frustrated phagocytosis,"[150] during which merger of granules with the plasma membrane results in discharge of granule constituents directly to the outside of cells as though into phagosomes. Phagocytosis per se does not occur, and the viability of adherent cells is not altered. This mechanism of granule constituent release from neutrophils very likely is relevant to the pathogenesis of tissue injury in a variety of diseases in which immune complexes are deposited on cell surfaces or extracellular structures, such as vascular basement membranes and articular cartilage.[120,123,149]

Lysosomal enzyme release from neutrophils by the mechanism of "reverse endocytosis" is facilitated greatly when cells are treated with the fungal metabolite cytochalasin B. Cytochalasin B interferes with the function of cytoplasmic microfilaments and inhibits membrane transport of sugars and nucleosides in cultured cells.[151–154] Cytochalasin B-treated neutrophils are unable to ingest particles, but nevertheless, release, or secrete, lysosomal but not cytoplasmic constituents (i.e., degranulate) when appropriate particles or soluble stimuli come into contact with their surfaces[48–50,68,148,154–157] (Fig. 9–3*D*). With some soluble stimuli (e.g., complement-derived and synthetic peptide chemotactic factors), treatment of neutrophils with cytochalasin B is an absolute prerequisite for maximal degranulation.[68,155,156] Ultrastructural studies of cytochalasin B-treated neutrophils have revealed membrane fusion between lysosomal granules and the plasma membrane as the morphologic accompaniment of biochemically measurable enzyme release.[49,156] The precise mechanism is unknown whereby cytochalasin B facilitates fusion between lysosomal membranes and the plasma membranes of stimulated neutrophils leading to the discharge of granule contents.

As indicated above, cytochalasin B-treated neutrophils degranulate when they are exposed to the soluble, low molecular weight complement component, C5a.[50,146,156] Such cells respond similarly to other chemotactic factors, e.g., products of bacteria, synthetic peptides, and oxygenation products of arachidonic acid.[50,155,158,159] Yet other soluble stimuli are capable of provoking degranulation of normal neutrophils. These include the tumor-promoting agent phorbol myristate acetate (specific granules only),[160,161] calcium ions with or without the ionophore, A23187 (azurophil and/or specific granules),[162,163] and the cell surface-reactive lectin concanavalin A (specific granules only).[164,165] Degranulation of neutrophils in response to these soluble stimuli occurs in the absence of cytochalasin B, particles, or adherence to surfaces and is not associated with any alterations of cell viability. The mechanism by which specific granule constituents (e.g., lysozyme) are selectively released from neutrophils exposed to phorbol myristate acetate, calcium, and concanavalin A is unknown. Some data, however, suggest that the limiting membranes of specific granules have unique physical and/or chemical properties that facilitate fusion with the neutrophil plasma membrane.[134]

## OXIDATIVE METABOLISM

### Cellular and Biochemical Aspects

Encounters between phagocytic leukocytes and appropriate particulate stimuli lead to increased consumption by the leukocytes of molecular oxygen.[102,121] The bulk of oxygen that is consumed is reduced to water through the formation of several highly reactive intermediates. Oxygen, in its ground state, contains two unpaired electrons with parallel spins. Since these present a "barrier" to the insertion of additional pairs of electrons, ground state oxygen "prefers" to be reduced by univalent, or single electron steps. When oxygen accepts a single electron, it is converted to the superoxide anion radical. In human neutrophils, a pyridine nucleotide-dependent oxidase, localized to either an intracellular granule fraction or the plasma membrane,[165-167] appears to catalyze this reaction. It has been demonstrated conclusively that the bulk of oxygen that is consumed by stimulated neutrophils is converted directly to superoxide anion radicals.[168] In addition to superoxide, stimulated neutrophils generate hydrogen peroxide,[169] hydroxyl radicals,[170] and, perhaps, singlet oxygen.[171] Concomitantly, there is stimulation of the hexose monophosphate shunt pathway of glucose oxidation and iodination of protein (mediated by the granule enzyme myeloperoxidase).[172,173] The increased ability of phagocytosing neutrophils to reduce nitroblue tetrazolium (NBT) dye is a reflection of the enhanced generation of superoxide anion radicals[174] (Fig. 9–4). The importance of these metabolic events to the microbicidal activity of neutrophils has been reviewed extensively.[102,121,175]

As is the case with degranulation, enhanced oxidative metabolism by neutrophils can be stimulated in the absence of phagocytosis. For example, neutrophils adherent to certain nonphagocytizable surfaces have been observed to increase their oxidative metabolism, particularly if the surfaces are coated with immune complexes, aggregated IgG, or the opsonic fragment of the third

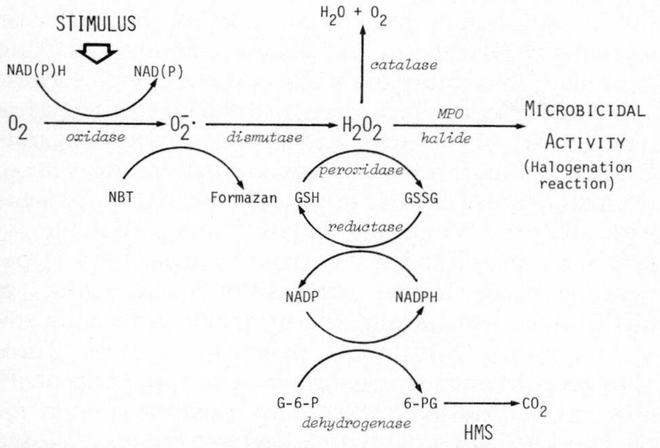


**Figure 9–4.** Changes in oxidative metabolism following stimulation of neutrophils. *NBT* = Nitroblue tetrazolium. *MPO* = Myeloperoxidase. *GSH* = Reduced glutathione. *G-6-P* = Glucose-6-phosphate. *HMS* = Hexose monophosphate shunt.

component of complement (C3b).[145,149] Similarly, neutrophils exposed to certain soluble stimuli have been demonstrated to increase their oxygen uptake, production of superoxide anion, hexose monophosphate shunt activity, and nitroblue tetrazolium dye reduction. These soluble stimuli include immune complexes, aggregates of IgG, and chemotactic factors (e.g., C5a) as well as a variety of surface-reactive compounds, such as phospholipase *c*, phorbol myristate acetate, concanavalin A, and digitonin.[145,146,165,176-180] The metabolic responses of neutrophils to these soluble stimuli require intact, viable cells and resemble closely those observed during phagocytosis.

It appears that cell surface stimulation of neutrophils is sufficient, in the absence of phagocytosis, to provoke the degranulation and the burst of oxidative metabolism that ordinarily accompany ingestion of particles. What is the relation between these two responses of neutrophils to stimulation? Whereas it is true that when normal neutrophils are allowed to ingest particles, the two responses appear to be inseparable, studies with nonphagocytic stimuli indicate that they can occur independently. For example, it has been demonstrated that there is no significant correlation between the ability of various stimuli to provoke lysosomal enzyme release from neutrophils (i.e., degranulation) and their ability to enhance generation of superoxide anion.[146]

Measurements of extracellular superoxide anion, as performed in most studies of stimulated neutrophils, presumably reflect not only the production of this radical but also the activity of endogenous superoxide dismutase and, possibly, the rate of release of superoxide from the cytoplasm to the extracellular fluid. The demonstration that neutrophils contain superoxide dismutase in their cytosol satisfied the requirement for a protective mechanism against the potentially injurious effects of superoxide anion radicals and led to the suggestion that production of superoxide takes place on the outer surface of the cell membrane as well as in phagocytic vacuoles that are formed by invaginations of this membrane[165,181] (Fig. 9–5). The hypothesis that the neutrophil superoxide-generating system is localized to the plasma membrane is attractive. Surface generation of superoxide would allow for its concentration within phagocytic vacuoles and provides a convenient explanation for the extracellular recovery of this highly reactive free radical. By conversion to freely diffusible hydrogen peroxide, extracellular or intraphagosomal superoxide anion radicals can mediate all of the biochemical events that ordinarily accompany particle contact, phagocytosis, and microbial killing.

## Oxygen-Derived Free Radicals as Mediators of Inflammation

Some recent observations have led to the suggestion that oxygen-derived free radicals are important mediators of inflammation and tissue injury. First, oxygen-derived free radicals injure tissues (e.g., damage lipid membranes) and irreversibly alter macromolecules (Table 9-5). Second, superoxide dismutase and other scavengers of oxygen-derived free radicals prevent tissue injury in vitro and possess anti-inflammatory activity in vivo. Further, some commonly used anti-inflammatory drugs either scavenge oxygen-derived free radicals directly (i.e., exhibit superoxide dismutase-like activity) or inhibit production of oxygen-derived free radicals by phagocytic cells.

**Oxygen-Derived Free Radicals Injure Tissues and Irreversibly Alter Macromolecules.** A role for oxygen-derived free radicals in the injury of biomembranes has been demonstrated in several experimental systems. Target cells have included human erythrocytes,[182] human neutrophils,[183] and cultured human endothelial cells.[184] The precise nature of the reactive molecules that mediate injury to biomembranes is unknown. Results of most studies, however, indicate roles for both superoxide anion radicals and hydrogen peroxide or, more specifically, for products of their interaction such as hydroxyl radicals and singlet oxygen. These reactive species can produce lipid peroxides, and it is likely that lipid peroxidation is responsible for altering membrane integrity.

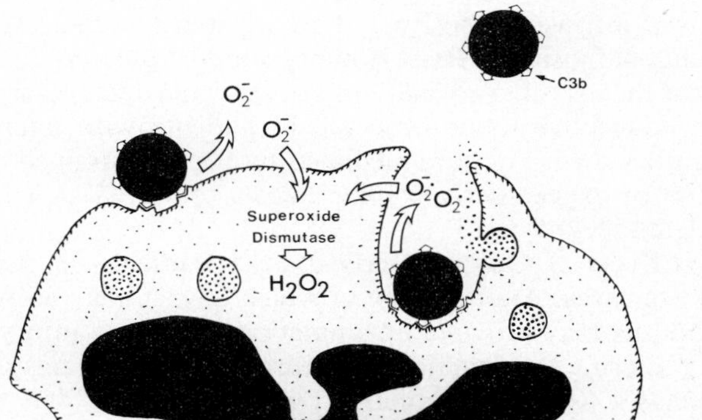


**Figure 9–5.** Generation of superoxide at the surface of a human neutrophil: response to particulate stimuli (from Goldstein, I.M.: Curr. Topics Hematol. 2:145, 1979.)

**Table 9–5.** Macromolecules Altered by Oxygen-Derived Free Radicals

| |
|---|
| Hyaluronic acid |
| Collagen and tropocollagen |
| $\alpha$-1-Proteinase inhibitor |
| Arachidonic acid |
| DNA |

In addition to damaging cells and tissues directly, oxygen-derived free radicals may provoke inflammation and tissue injury indirectly by irreversibly altering macromolecules. Several observations are particularly relevant to the possible roles played by oxygen-derived free radicals in provoking tissue injury in patients with arthritis. A number of investigators,[185-189] for example, have demonstrated that oxygen-derived free radicals, generated by the aerobic action of xanthine oxidase on either xanthine or hypoxanthine,[190] "degrade" bovine synovial fluid as well as purified hyaluronic acid. "Degradation" was manifested by a marked reduction in relative viscosity and by the inability of the treated synovial fluid to form a mucin clot. Depolymerization of hyaluronic acid also was demonstrated.[188] Addition of either catalase or superoxide dismutase provided protection against the "degradation," indicating that both hydrogen peroxide and superoxide were participants in the reaction. Normal synovial fluid was found to contain barely detectable levels of catalase and approximately 1 nanogram per milliliter of superoxide dismutase.[185] Interestingly, superoxide dismutase activity could not be detected at all in synovial fluids from patients with rheumatoid arthritis.[191] Furthermore, Rister and colleagues[192] reported that neutrophils from children with rheumatoid arthritis contain less superoxide dismutase activity than neutrophils from normal controls.

Another macromolecule that can be altered by oxygen-derived free radicals is collagen. Collagen solutions fail to gel normally and exhibit a slightly lower intrinsic viscosity after exposure to a superoxide-generating system (i.e., xanthine oxidase and hypoxanthine).[193] Soluble tropocollagen also does not gel properly (when heated) after exposure to chemically generated singlet oxygen.[194] After exposure to singlet oxygen, tropocollagen has a lower intrinsic viscosity and an apparently altered subunit composition. These findings support the hypothesis that the loss of synovial fluid viscosity and some changes in connective tissue observed in patients with inflammatory arthritides are mediated by the unrestrained action of oxygen-derived free radicals produced by stimulated leukocytes.[185]

**Effects of Oxygen-Derived Free Radicals on Antiproteinases.** Another way in which oxygen-derived free radicals may provoke inflammation and tissue injury is by altering the function of naturally occurring antiproteinases. Carp and Janoff[195] reported recently that superoxide anion radicals and hydrogen peroxide, produced by stimulated human neutrophils, were capable of inactivating $\alpha_1$-proteinase inhibitor. Inactivation was attributed to oxidation of methionine thioether residues (to sulfoxides) in or near the active site of the proteinase inhibitor.[196] Oxidized $\alpha_1$-proteinase inhibitor was found to be incapable of forming stable complexes with elastase and, consequently, incapable of influencing the elastolytic activity of the enzyme.[196] A recent report suggests that altered antiproteinase function may be relevant to the pathogenesis of tissue injury observed in patients with arthritis. Wong and Travis[197] found that the $\alpha_1$-proteinase inhibitor isolated from synovial fluid of patients with rheumatoid arthritis contained residues of methionine sulfoxide and was incapable of forming stable complexes with porcine pancreatic elastase. These findings confirmed that naturally occurring antiproteinases can be oxidized in vivo, and provided support for the hypothesis that oxygen-derived free radicals released from phagocytic leukocytes may mediate inflammation and tissue injury by altering the balance between proteinases (also released from these cells) and naturally occurring antiproteinases. Such an imbalance could render adjacent tissues and/or other macromolecules more susceptible to proteolytic attack.

**Effects of Oxygen-Derived Free Radicals on Lipids—Generation of Chemoattractants.** As indicated above, it appears that oxygen-derived free radicals alter the integrity of biomembranes by provoking lipid peroxidation. Hydroxyl radicals, for example, are capable of abstracting hydrogen atoms from allylic positions of unsaturated lipids to yield hydroperoxides.[198] Hydroperoxides also may be formed by the direct action of singlet oxygen on polyunsaturated fatty acids.[199] Peroxidation of unsaturated fatty acids after their exposure to simple superoxide-generating systems also has been demonstrated.[200]

As discussed elsewhere in this volume (Chapter 6), oxidized fatty acids have attracted a great deal of attention recently because of the roles they may play in provoking inflammation. It is possible, for example, that hydroxy and dihydroxy derivatives of arachidonic acid with chemotactic activity are responsible, in part, for provoking the accumulation of neutrophils in inflamed joints.[201] Since conversion of arachidonic acid to chemotactically active hydroxy derivatives proceeds through the formation of hydroperoxides, it is not surprising that similar derivatives can be generated nonenzymatically by free radical-mediated reactions. Turner and colleagues,[34,202] for example, found that exposure of arachidonic acid either to air for 24 hours or to ultraviolet irradiation resulted in the generation of oxidized lipids that were chemotactic for human neutrophils.

Recently, Perez and colleagues[203] described another mechanism whereby arachidonic acid could be converted nonenzymatically to biologically active products. These investigators found that chemotactic activity for human neutrophils was generated upon exposure of arachidonic acid to a superoxide-generating system consisting of xanthine oxidase and acetaldehyde. Generation of chemotactic activity in this experimental system was time dependent and could be inhibited significantly by scavengers of singlet oxygen, as well as by scavengers of superoxide, hydrogen peroxide, and hydroxyl radicals.

Silica gel thin-layer radiochromatography demonstrated a product with chemotactic activity that was distinct from that of unaltered arachidonic acid and 12-hydroxyeicosatetraenoic acid (12-HETE). The isolated product was chemotactic for human neutrophils at a concentration (approximate) of 3.0 ng per ml and chemokinetic at concentrations of 0.75 to 1.5 ng per ml.

Another chemoattractant formed by the action of oxygen-derived free radicals was described recently by Petrone and colleagues.[204] These investigators found that potent chemotactic activity for human neutrophils could be generated in vitro by exposing normal human plasma to a source of superoxide anion radicals (i.e., xanthine oxidase and xanthine). Generation of chemotactic activity in this system was inhibited by superoxide dismutase but not by catalase. When plasma that had been exposed to superoxide anion radicals was injected intradermally into rats, large numbers of neutrophils accumulated at the injection sites. A similar response was observed when rats were injected intradermally with xanthine oxidase and xanthine. No leukocyte infiltration was observed, however, if superoxide dismutase was injected simultaneously with the enzyme and substrate.

The chemotactic activity that was formed by exposing plasma to superoxide was heat labile (56° C for 30 minutes), nondialyzable, and stable to lyophilization. The bulk of the activity was recovered after gel filtration and ion exchange chromatography of superoxide-treated plasma in fractions containing albumin. Albumin itself, however, was not chemotactic. Rather, the chemotactic factor appeared to consist of a chloroform-extractable component (i.e., lipid) that was bound to albumin. Since the nature of the lipid was not determined, it is intriguing to speculate that it may be a hydroperoxy or hydroxy derivative of arachidonic acid.

**Superoxide Dismutase and Other Scavengers of Oxygen-Derived Free Radicals Possess Anti-Inflammatory Activity.** For organisms to survive in an aerobic environment, they must be protected from the potentially toxic effects of oxygen-derived free radicals and singlet oxygen. Protection of cells from the potentially injurious superoxide anion radical is provided primarily by superoxide dismutases, intracellular enzymes that catalyze dismutation of superoxide to hydrogen peroxide and oxygen. Eukaryotic organisms contain two distinct types of superoxide dismutases: a manganese-containing mitochondrial enzyme and a copper- and zinc-containing cytoplasmic enzyme.[205] By scavenging superoxide and thereby preventing either spontaneous dismutation or reactions between superoxide and hydrogen peroxide, superoxide dismutase also prevents the formation of toxic hydroxyl radicals and singlet oxygen.

In 1968, Huber and colleagues[206] reported the isolation and purification from bovine liver of an anti-inflammatory, copper-containing protein. This protein, termed orgotein, exhibited potent anti-inflammatory activity in several animal models of acute and chronic inflammation.[207] When administered subcutaneously to either rats or mice, orgotein effectively suppressed carrageenan-induced paw edema, abscess formation, and pleurisy. In guinea pigs, orgotein inhibited the vascular damage and neutrophil infiltration of skin observed as a consequence of reversed passive Arthus reactions. Orgotein also inhibited adjuvant-induced paw edema and arthritis in rats. Finally, orgotein suppressed anti-DNA antibody formation, as well as autoimmune glomerulonephritis, in NZB $\times$ NZW $F_1$ hybrid mice. It is appreciated now that orgotein is identical with bovine liver superoxide dismutase.[190,207]

Other studies in experimental animals have confirmed some of the seemingly remarkable anti-inflammatory effects of superoxide dismutase. Oyanagui,[208] for example, found that native superoxide dismutase from bovine liver, when administered intravenously to rats, completely suppressed carrageenan-induced paw edema. McCormick and colleagues[209] found that superoxide dismutase blocked immune complex–induced dermal vascular injury (i.e., Arthus reactions) in rats, as well as the early phases of immune complex–induced lung injury (i.e., edema, hemorrhage, and neutrophil accumulation). Neither heat-inactivated superoxide dismutase nor catalase affected the Arthus reactions in skin and lung, suggesting that the enzymatic activity of native superoxide dismutase was required for its anti-inflammatory effects.

Since superoxide dismutase (i.e., orgotein) was reported to be effective in the treatment of periostitis and arthritis in horses and dogs,[210,211] attention naturally was directed at the possibility that it might also be effective in the treatment of arthritis in man. Lund-Oleson and Menander[212] reported that treatment with multiple intra-articular injections of orgotein produced beneficial effects (e.g., decreased pain and swelling, increased range of motion and overall functional status) in 16 of 22 patients with osteoarthritis. It is noteworthy that Rosner and colleagues[213] found that intra-articular injections of orgotein did not ameliorate experimentally induced osteoarthritis in rabbits. In a very recent study, Goebel and colleagues[214] found that intra-articular injections of orgotein (4 mg per week for 6 weeks) in patients with classical rheumatoid arthritis resulted in significant improvement of several clinical parameters, including pain, morning stiffness, and range of motion. Orgotein also depressed significantly the levels in synovial fluid of rheumatoid factors, prostaglandin $E_2$, and lactate dehydrogenase. It should be emphasized that in all of the studies that have been reported to date of the effects of superoxide dismutase therapy in man, insufficient data preclude critical analysis of the results. Consequently, results of more rigorously controlled prospective clinical trials are required before any conclusions can be reached concerning the efficacy in man of treatment with superoxide dismutase.

One mechanism whereby superoxide dismutase may inhibit inflammatory reactions is through effects on other anti-inflammatory substances (e.g., protection of naturally occurring antiproteinases from oxidant-induced inactivation).[195] Another mechanism involves free radical-mediated generation of chemotactic activity for neutrophils. By preventing formation of chemotactic products by the action of oxygen-derived free radicals on either arachidonic acid[203] or substrates in plasma,[204] superoxide dismutase could prevent accumulation of neutrophils at foci of inflammation. Such an effect would serve to limit amplification of inflammatory reactions.

**Effects of Anti-Inflammatory Drugs on Oxygen-Derived Free Radicals.** Some commonly used potent anti-inflammatory drugs can influence oxygen-derived free radicals in two general ways (which may account for at least some of their anti-inflammatory effects). First, several drugs have been found capable of inhibiting production of oxygen-derived free radicals by appropriately stimulated phagocytic cells. Goldstein and colleagues,[215] for example, demonstrated that anti-inflammatory adrenal corticosteriods inhibit production of superoxide anion radicals by human neutrophils exposed to aggregated human IgG, opsonized zymosan particles, and the complement component C5a. Lehmeyer and Johnston[216] found that adrenal corticosteroids also were capable of inhibiting generation of superoxide anion radicals by human neutrophils and monocytes exposed to nonphagocytizable surfaces coated with aggregated IgG (an in vitro model of immunologically induced inflammation).

Another way in which commonly used anti-inflammatory drugs may influence oxygen-derived free radicals is by directly scavenging these reactive molecules. A number of drugs, for example, have been found capable of preventing the loss of relative viscosity that occurs when synovial fluid is exposed to xanthine oxidase and hypoxanthine.[189,217] Copper (II) chelates of salicylates, for example, have been demonstrated to possess superoxide dismutase-like activity,[218] as have low molecular weight cupric peptides.[219] In the absence of copper, these compounds do not exhibit superoxide-scavenging activity. It is of some interest that copper chelates of some commonly used drugs appear to have greater anti-inflammatory potency in vivo than the native compounds.[220] Whether this is due to their superoxide dismutase-like activity has not been determined.

## GRANULOCYTES AS SOURCES OF PEPTIDE AND LIPID MEDIATORS OF INFLAMMATION

The full range of functional capabilities of each class of granulocytes is developed fully by the generation of an array of fatty acid and phospholipid mediators, and by the liberation of peptide mediators from plasma protein precursors by granulocyte proteinases. The activity of many of the neutrophil proteinases is regulated by $\alpha$-globulin inhibitors. Although $\alpha_1$-proteinase inhibitor plays a relatively restricted role in the control of the plasma enzymes of coagulation, kinin generation, and fibrinolysis,[30] in comparison to the other $\alpha$-globulin inhibitors, it is a critical inhibitor of a wide spectrum of neutrophil-derived proteases. The $\alpha_1$-proteinase-inhibitable enzymes of neutrophils that are granule associated include the neutral proteases,[221] elastase,[221,222] and a family of cationic proteins with chymotrypsinlike, bactericidal, and phagocytosis-enhancing activities.[223] Inhibition of neutrophil elastase by $\alpha$-globulins is associated with the formation of complexes that exhibit an enzyme to inhibitor ratio of 1:1 for $\alpha_1$-proteinase inhibitor and 2:1 for $\alpha_2$ macroglobulin.[224] However, the quantitative predominance of $\alpha_1$-proteinase inhibitor over $\alpha_2$ macroglobulin in normal serum suggests that it is the dominant inhibitor. The overall significance of this regulatory role of $\alpha_1$-proteinase inhibitor is emphasized by the observation that one half of the elastase-inhibiting capacity of serum from individuals with homozygous deficiency of $\alpha_1$-proteinase inhibitor (PiZZ), containing less than 15 percent of the normal levels of $\alpha_1$-proteinase inhibitor, was nonetheless attributable to the residual $\alpha_1$-proteinase inhibitor.[224]

In addition to the lysosomal proteinases with broad activity, neutrophils possess proteinases that express specific activity for the liberation of potent peptide mediators from plasma proteins. Angiotensin II, assessed by both radioimmunoassay and smooth muscle contractile activity, is generated directly from plasma angiotensinogen by neutrophil cathepsin G, without the appearance of angiotensin I or the participation of angiotensin-converting enzyme.[225,226] Neutrophils also possess enzymatic pathways for the production of bradykinin and other kinins, which may be important fluid-phase mediators in some types of inflammation.[227,228] The generation of angiotensin II and kinins by neutrophils is controlled by two normally occurring classes of plasma proteins: $\alpha_1$-proteinase inhibitor and other $\alpha$-globulins, which block the activity of cathepsin G and kininogenases, and plasma inactivators that enzymatically degrade the peptide mediators.[225-227] Highly purified cathepsin G and the native cathepsin G in neutrophils are exquisitely sensitive to the inhibitory effect of $\alpha_1$-proteinase inhibitor. Less than 1 percent of the $\alpha_1$-proteinase inhibitor in 1 ml of normal human blood totally inhibits the expression of the cathepsin G of the 3 to 5 $\times 10^6$ neutrophils that would be present in the 1 ml portion of blood. The plasma inactivator of angiotensin II resembles kininase I and the anaphylatoxin inactivator in that it has a molecular weight of 300,000 to 350,000 and its activity is heat labile and calcium dependent.[227] As $\alpha_1$-proteinase inhibitor regulates both general and specific proteases of neutrophils, it is of considerable interest that a deficiency in serum $\alpha_1$-proteinase inhibitor is associated with the premature development of severe pulmonary emphysema and hepatic cirrhosis.[229,230] The increased incidence of the diseases noted suggests that a depression in the local tissue concentrations of $\alpha_1$-proteinase inhibitor accompanied the serum deficiency and resulted in a relative excess of free protease activities in some tissues, which led to proteolytic tissue damage and the secondary development of fibrosis. Evidence has emerged that extends the relevance of these findings to the rheumatic diseases, as a higher incidence of rheumatoid arthritis and juvenile rheumatoid arthritis was found in some groups of subjects who are severely deficient in $\alpha_1$-proteinase inhibitor.[231]

The recognition of the roles played by oxygenation products of arachidonic acid in inflammation led to the definition of the structures of several such products of granulocytes. The principal products and the quantities of each vary significantly for the different types of granulocytes. Prostaglandin $E_2$ ($PGE_2$) is the major cyclooxygenase metabolite of neutrophils and eosinophils, while $PGD_2$ predominates for basophils.[232] The 5-lipoxygenase pathway is the most active in neutrophils and basophils, but the distribution of leukotrienes (LTs) differs substantially. Neutrophils generate $LTB_4$, which is a potent stimulus of PMN leukocyte function and may endogenously amplify neutrophil chemotaxis and protein secretion elicited by other agonists.[26,27] $LTB_4$ is also an immunosuppressive factor, which stimulates suppressor T-lymphocyte function.[27,233] Basophils secrete large quantities of $LTB_4$ and the C-6 peptide leukotriene $LTD_4$, which is a potent mediator of smooth muscle contraction and increased vascular permeability, which appear to be important in allergic reactions and asthma.[234] In contrast, the 15-lipoxygenase predominates in eosinophils, with the generation of a series of 14,15-di-HETEs, 8,15-di-HETEs, and 5,15-di-HETEs,[235] which demonstrate effects on PMN leukocytes similar to those of $LTB_4$ but are far less potent.[236] Basophils and neutrophils are, in addition, capable of synthesizing and secreting 1-O-hexadecyl-2-acetyl-sn-glyceryl-3-phosphorylcholine, which is a platelet-activating factor (PAF) that induces platelet aggregation and the release of granule constituents from human and rabbit platelets in vitro[237] and rabbit platelets in vivo.[238] Thus granulocytes have the capacity to contribute to inflammation not only by cellular activities but also by the elaboration of a wide range of peptide and lipid mediators.

## GENERATION AND RELEASE OF CHEMICAL MEDIATORS OF THE BASOPHIL

The bridging of basophil membrane–bound IgE by specific antigen or anti-IgE, or the exposure of basophils to fluid phase immunological principals such as C5a or platelet factor 4 leads to the intracellular generation of unstored mediators and their release along with the preformed chemical mediators of the basophil.[239-241] Basophils differ from mast cells with respect to origin, tissue distribution, some cellular constituents, and their patterns of involvement in hypersensitivity reactions. Both cell types, however, may serve a central role in immediate-type hypersensitivity reactions by virtue of the brief interval required for mobilization of their full capacity to secrete a wide array of chemical mediators. Less is known for basophils than for mast cells of the biochemical events of activation, the structures of some of the mediators, and the mechanisms of cellular regulation of immediate hypersensitivity reactions.[242] The release of histamine from human basophils by IgE-dependent mechanisms and by C5a differs with respect to temperature optimum, time course, and the desensitizing activity of each stimulus, but both pathways of activation share with mast cell mechanisms a dependence on extracellular calcium.[240] Further, the immunological release of basophil mediators is inhibited by agents that elevate the intracellular levels of cyclic AMP in a manner comparable to cyclic AMP inhibition of mast cell activation.[243,244] Morphologic studies of human basophils that were challenged in various reactions revealed two patterns of degranulation.[245] One pattern, which is characteristic of anaphylactic reactions, exhibited prominent fusion of the membranes of adjacent granules and of granule membranes with the plasma membrane. The other pattern, typically seen in human allergic contact dermatitis, consisted of multiple cytoplasmic membrane–bound vesicles that were presumably derived from the granules and in many instances were in communication with the plasma membrane, suggesting "piecemeal" release of mediators without granule movement or loss of integrity. The primary mediators of the basophil, like those of the mast cell, may be viewed as belonging to two classes, namely those that are present totally preformed prior to challenge and those that are unstored and must be generated from inactive precursors subsequent to immunological activation (Table 9–6). Histamine, heparin,[246] and several leukocyte chemotactic factors[247] are in the former category, while $LTD_4$, $LTB_4$, phospholipid platelet-activating factor (PAF),[248] and other leukocyte chemotactic factors[249] cannot be detected in unchallenged basophils. The histamine content and the fraction of total proteoglycans accounted for by heparin both appear to be lower in the basophil than in the mast cell. Esterases of varying specificities have been identified in the granules of guinea pig basophils.[250] Both high and low molecular weight preformed leukocyte chemotactic factors have been extracted from human leukemic basophils,[247] but neither has been characterized structurally or functionally beyond its chemotactic preference for neutrophils and eosinophils, respectively. The SRS-A activity generated by basophils is attributable to $LTD_4$, as contrasted with $LTC_4$ or a mixture of $LTC_4$ and $LTD_4$ for different types of mast cells.[251] PAF from rabbit or human basophils results in platelet aggregation, stimulates the platelet release reaction, and appears to be the low molecular weight phospholipid 1-O-hexadecyl-2-acetyl-sn-glyceryl-3-phosphorylcholine, which is susceptible to inactivation by several phospholipases,[248,252] as is the case for some PAFs of mast cell origin.[253] A chemotactic factor which preferentially attracts eosinophils is generated from human basophils by immunological challenge, as well as from other human leukocytes during phagocytosis or exposure to the calcium ionophore A23187.[249,254] The major lipid chemotactic agent secreted by basophils is $LTB_4$.

Delayed hypersensitivity responses are recognized to be heterogeneous reactions that involve predominantly lymphocytes and macrophages, but basophils are substantial components in some instances.[255] Infiltrates of basophils that appear with a delayed time course are especially prominent in cutaneous contact reactions, Jones-Mote reactions to proteins, some instances of al-

**Table 9–6.** Chemical Mediators of the Basophilic Granulocyte

| Type | Mediator | Structural Characteristics | Assay(s) | Other Functions | Inactivation |
|---|---|---|---|---|---|
| Preformed | Histamine | β-Imidazolyl-ethylamine, molecular weight 111 | Contraction of guinea pig ileum<br>Radiolabeling by histamine *N*-methyltransferase | Increased vascular permeability<br>Enhancement of eosinophil migration | Histaminase<br>Histamine *N*-methyltransferase |
| | Leukotactic activities | Molecular weight > 150,000 | Chemotactic attraction of granulocytes (N > E)* | Chemotactic deactivation of granulocytes | – |
| | | Molecular weight ≃ 300–1000 | Chemotactic attraction of granulocytes (E > N) | Chemotactic deactivation of granulocytes | – |
| | Heparin | Acidic proteoglycan, molecular weight ≃ 1 million | Antithrombin III activation | Anticoagulation | – |
| | Chymase | – | Hydrolysis of synthetic esters | – | – |
| | Tryptase | – | Hydrolysis of synthetic esters | – | – |
| Unstored | Slow reacting substance of anaphylaxis (SRS-A) | $LTD_4$ | Contraction of antihistamine-treated guinea pig ileum | Contraction of human bronchiole | Peroxidase |
| | Leukotactic activity | $LTB_4$ | Chemotactic attraction of granulocytes (E > N) | Increased vascular permeability | |
| | Platelet activating factor (PAF9) | 1-O-hexadecyl-2-acetyl-sn-glyceryl-3-phosphoryl-choline | Release of $^{14}C$-5-OH-tryptamine from platelets | Platelet aggregation | Phospholipases |

*Abbreviations used are the same as in Table 9–1.

lograft rejection, and many tissue responses to tumors as well as viral and parasitic infections.[256] That basophil mediators may modulate mononuclear leukocyte function in such reactions has been suggested by a relative deficiency of macrophages in basophil-rich infiltrates and, in some cases, by lower concentrations of lymphokines than are found associated with classic delayed hypersensitivity reactions.[257] Both mast cells and basophils are common in subsynovial connective tissues, but any role in synovial inflammation remains speculative. The predominant possibilities are based on the observations that the chemical mediators that alter microvascular permeability enhance the local deposition of immune complexes,[258] and that mast cells and basophils release factors that are chemotactic for lymphocytes as well as granulocytes.

## ABNORMALITIES OF NEUTROPHIL FUNCTION IN HUMAN DISEASE

Neutrophils of some subjects predisposed to an increased incidence of bacterial infections may exhibit severe isolated defects in phagocytosis, in the absence of other functional abnormalities. Such defects may be considered in terms of the stages of the phagocytic process, and accordingly classified as predominantly ineffective opsonization, disordered ingestion, or deficient degranulation and/or metabolic activation.[259] These phagocytic abnormalities are largely congenital disorders or transient states, and none is associated with excessive spontaneous inflammation or rheumatic disease-like syndromes. In contrast, abnormalities in neutrophil chemotaxis with or without defects in random migration, phagocytosis, or other functions are linked both to defects in host defense against infections and to the development of a variety of inflammatory diseases. As such in vitro abnormalities have been reviewed recently,[260,261] this chapter will cover only illustrative examples and conditions relevant to the rheumatic diseases (Tables 9–7 and 9–8). Defects in chemotaxis resulting from intrinsic cellular disorders are subdivided into the permanent types, which are largely congenital, and the transient types, which include states of bone marrow development, viral and overwhelming bacterial infections, and some of the rheumatic diseases (Table 9–7). The neutrophils in the permanent states exhibit numerous functional abnormalities, and the patients are universally more susceptible to pyogenic infections. Neutropenia may occur as well, which presumably reflects in part abnormal migration and efflux from the bone marrow. It is of special interest that neutrophil migration in some cases of both the Chédiak-Higashi and the Quie-Hill syndromes may respond in vitro and in vivo to ascorbic acid.[56,57] The mechanism of enhancement of migration by ascorbic acid is unknown in the latter condition, but in the Chédiak-Higashi leukocytes ascorbic acid depresses the abnormally high intracellular level of cyclic AMP and concomitantly restores microtubule function to normal.[262] In the category of transient defects, the neutrophil abnormalities generally only respond to successful management of the basic disease. One notable exception is in viral infections, in which mononuclear leukocyte and, in some cases, neutrophil defects in migration are strikingly reversed by levamisole.[263]

Discrepancies exist among the results of several studies of neutrophil migration and other functions in the rheumatic diseases. Differences in in vitro methodology may be the basis for some of the discrepant results, as a double filter radiomigration assay, which requires that the neutrophils migrate farther than in single filter assays, has proved to be more sensitive than the conven-

**Table 9–7.** Defects In Neutrophil In Vitro Chemotaxis in Human Diseases

| Level of Defect | Disorder | Other Leukocyte-Related Abnormalities | Clinical Features |
|---|---|---|---|
| *Cellular* | | | |
| Permanent | Lazy leukocyte syndrome | Neutropenia, decreased neutrophil mobilization from bone marrow, depressed random migration of neutrophils | Recurrent upper respiratory infections, gingivitis, stomatitis |
| | Chédiak-Higashi syndrome | Neutropenia, defective bactericidal activity and decreased deformability of neutrophils, defective monocyte chemotaxis | Recurrent pyogenic infections, lymphoma-like phase |
| | Quie-Hill syndrome | Depressed random migration of neutrophils, defective monocyte random and chemotactic migration | Respiratory, cutaneous and ocular staphylococcal and *Candida* infections; eczema, peripheral eosinophilia, elevated serum IgE level |
| | Defective actin polymerization | Depressed neutrophil random migration and phagocytosis, but enhanced degranulation | Recurrent infections |
| Transient or episodic | Viral infections | — | Measles, influenza |
| | Septicemia | Depressed random migration and phagocytosis, morphologic abnormalities | Overwhelming bacterial infection |
| | Bone marrow transplantation | — | Subjects exhibiting graft-vs.-host reactions and treated with anti-thymocyte sera |
| | Neonatal period | Decreased neutrophil deformability, defective monocyte chemotaxis | — |
| | Rheumatoid arthritis | Depressed phagocytosis, serum inhibitors of chemotaxis in some patients | |
| | Felty's syndrome | Neutropenia, immunoglobulin inclusions | — |
| | Systemic lupus erythematosus | Neutropenia, anti-leukocyte antibodies, serum may not generate a normal level of chemotactic activity | — |
| *Fluid phase* | | | |
| Inadequate generation of chemotactic activity | Clr deficiency | Delayed generation of serum chemotactic activity | Systemic lupus erythematosus and dermatomyositis-like states, necrotizing angiitis |
| | C4 deficiency | Delayed generation of serum chemotactic activity | Systemic lupus erythematosus and dermatomyositis-like states, necrotizing angiitis |
| | C2 deficiency | Delayed generation of serum chemotactic activity | Systemic lupus erythematosus and dermatomyositis-like states, necrotizing angiitis |
| | C3 deficiency | Serum also lacks opsonic and bactericidal activity | Recurrent gram-positive and gram-negative infections |
| | C5 deficiency | May be co-existent inhibitors of chemotaxis | Systemic lupus erythematosus–like state and recurrent infections |
| | C7 deficiency | — | Scleroderma-like syndrome |
| | Mucocutaneous candidiasis, Wiskott-Aldrich syndrome | Decreased generation of lymphocyte-derived chemotactic activity: inhibitors of monocyte migration; deficient delayed hypersensitivity | Frequent infections |
| Excessive chemotactic factor inactivation or inhibition | Hodgkin's disease | High serum levels of normally occurring α-globulin aminopeptidases | Recurrent infections |
| | Lepromatous leprosy | High serum levels of normally occurring α-globulin aminopeptidases | Recurrent infections |
| | Sarcoidosis | High serum levels of normally occurring α-globulin aminopeptidases | Recurrent infections |
| | Hypogammaglobulinemia | High serum levels of normally occurring α-globulin aminopeptidases | Recurrent infections |
| | Cirrhosis in alcoholics | High serum levels of normally occurring α-globulin aminopeptidases | Recurrent infections |
| | Hypocomplementemic nephritis | Serum inhibitor of complement-derived factors | — |
| Leukocyte-directed inhibition | Elevated levels of IgA polymers | Leukocytosis, absent cutaneous delayed hypersensitivity | Recurrent respiratory and cutaneous infections |
| | Recurrent infections in childhood | Reversible inhibitor of chemotaxis | Respiratory and cutaneous infections |

tional Boyden assays in detecting the intrinsic abnormalities of neutrophils in rheumatic diseases.[14,264] The relationship of the neutrophil defects in rheumatic diseases to circulating antileukocyte antibodies or other inhibitors or to the prior in vivo phagocytosis of immune complexes by the neutrophils is not fully understood.[265] However, it appears that such qualitative abnormalities rather than coexisting neutropenia are the major determinant of the increased rate of infections in such patients.[266]

## ABNORMAL NEUTROPHIL FUNCTIONS ASSOCIATED WITH RHEUMATIC DISEASES

**Systemic Lupus Erythematosus.** Among patients with rheumatic diseases, those with systemic lupus erythematous (SLE) suffer most frequently from severe bacterial infections.[267] Although therapy with adrenal corticosteroids (and other immunosuppressive and/or cytotoxic drugs) very likely is a contributory factor,[268] there is

**Table 9–8.** Excessive Neutrophil In Vitro Chemotaxis in Human Diseases

| Level of Defect | Disorder | Other Leukocyte-Related Abnormalities | Special Clinical Features |
|---|---|---|---|
| *Cellular* | | | |
| Permanent | – | | |
| Transient or episodic | Acute bacterial infections | Leukocytosis | Moderately severe infections with host compensation |
| | Behçet's disease | | |
| | Reactive arthritis (HLA-B27 positive) | | |
| *Fluid phase* | | | |
| Increased generation of chemotactic activity | Cold urticaria | Mast cell–derived chemotactic factors, in vivo chemotactic deactivation of neutrophils | Chemotactic activity observed only in blood from cold-challenged area |
| | Bullous pemphigoid | In vivo chemotactic deactivation of eosinophils, lymphocyte migration–enhancing factors in bullous fluid | – |
| | Psoriasis | Arachidonic acid and complement-derived chemotactic factors | – |
| | Gout | Chemotactic glycoprotein of 8400 molecular weight derived from neutrophils phagocytosing crystals | – |
| | Rheumatoid arthritis | C5-derived chemotactic factor and $LTB_4$ in synovial fluid | – |
| Deficient chemotactic factor inactivation | Alpha$_1$-antitrypsin deficiency | Decreased serum levels of chemotactic factor–inactivating $\alpha$-globulin aminopeptidase | Pulmonary and hepatic tissue damage and fibrosis |
| Leukocyte-directed enhancement | Pyoderma gangrenosum | Plasma protein migration–enhancing factor of 160,000 molecular weight | Joint and cutaneous necrotizing inflammation |
| | Corticosteroid therapy | Neutrophil migration–enhancing factor derived from mononuclear leukocytes | – |

ample evidence that the disease itself is associated with altered host defenses against infection. Several functions of neutrophils have been found to be abnormal in patients with SLE. Goetzl,[264] for example, found neutrophils from four untreated patients with SLE less responsive to a standard chemotactic stimulus than cells from either normal controls or patients with other rheumatic diseases (i.e., rheumatoid arthritis, Felty's syndrome). A similar abnormality of neutrophil migration was reported by Landry[269] in six of 14 untreated patients with SLE. In yet another study, Clark and colleagues[266] found reduced amounts of complement-derived chemotactic activity (25 to 58 percent of controls) in endotoxin-activated serum from 10 of 24 patients with SLE. Neutrophils from all but one patient, however, migrated normally toward a standard, complement-derived chemotactic stimulus. Patients with the apparent abnormality in chemotactic factor generation were generally younger, had an earlier age of onset of SLE, and had a history of serious pyogenic infections. The precise nature of the abnormality observed in sera from these patients was not determined. It is likely, however, that these sera contained the inhibitor of complement (C5)-derived chemotactic activity described subsequently by Perez and colleagues.[270] This inhibitor does not act directly on neutrophils and does not affect the chemotactic activity exhibited by either synthetic peptides or filtrates prepared from cultures of *Escherichia coli* (bacterial chemotactic factors). Rather, it acts specifically and reversibly to inhibit the chemotactic activity exhibited by "complexes" of C5a des Arg and a naturally occurring serum protein, termed the cochemotaxin.[271,272] The inhibitor was isolated and purified from SLE serum and was found to be a heat stable (56° C for 30 minutes) cationic protein with a molecular weight of approximately 69,000.[271] Interestingly, patients with SLE whose serum contains the inhibitor have more active disease clinically and appear to have more frequent bacterial infections than patients whose serum does not contain the inhibitor.[273] It is possible, therefore, that this inhibitor of C5-derived chemotactic activity contributes, in part, to the increased susceptibility of patients with SLE to severe bacterial infections.

Neutrophils from some patients with SLE also exhibit abnormalities involving recognition and phagocytosis. Landry,[269] for example, found subnormal rates of particle ingestion by neutrophils from six of 25 untreated patients with SLE. In another report, Brandt and Hedberg[274] found that neutrophils from seven patients with SLE (receiving steroid therapy) had reduced phagocytic activity when compared with neutrophils from 12 normal controls and seven patients with rheumatoid arthritis. Phagocytosis was not reduced when normal cells were suspended in SLE plasma. In contrast to these findings, Zurier[275] reported that serum from 22 of 30 patients with SLE interfered significantly with particle uptake by normal neutrophils. Inhibitory activity in serum did not correlate with disease activity, levels of complement ($CH_{50}$ and C3), or corticosteroid therapy and was not influenced by mixing with normal serum. The nature of this "inhibitor" was not determined. It is of interest that Temple and Loewi[276] found that sera from SLE patients significantly inhibited the uptake by human blood monocytes of sheep erythrocytes coated with antibody. This effect was attributed to immune complexes in the sera that presumably were capable of binding preemptively to Fc receptors on the normal cells.

Support for the possibility that phagocytic cells in patients with SLE have impaired surface receptor function has been provided by the studies of Frank and colleagues.[277] These investigators measured the in vivo clearance of isologous erythrocytes coated with either C3b or IgG in patients with SLE. Four of eight patients were found to have a major defect in clearance mediated by Fc receptors. These four had the highest levels of circulating immune complexes as assessed by Clq-serum binding activity. Several patients also had defects in clearance mediated by C3b receptors. It should be noted that these experiments did not establish whether the defects were a cause or a consequence of circulating immune complexes (e.g., pre-emptive binding of ligands to receptors). Three groups of investigators reported recently that erythrocytes from patients with SLE possess decreased numbers of surface receptors for C3b.[278-280] Whereas one group concluded that this abnormality was acquired (as a consequence of disease activity),[278] the other two presented evidence that it was inherited.[279,280] It was suggested that the occurrence of SLE in individuals having reduced numbers of erythrocyte C3b receptors results from an impairment in complement-dependent clearance of potentially pathogenetic immune complexes.

Whereas detailed studies of the oxidative metabolism of neutrophils from patients with SLE have not been reported, abnormal nitroblue tetrazolium dye reduction by these cells has been observed.[281] Insofar as this may be an indicator of abnormal superoxide anion generation,[174] this finding suggests that the oxidative metabolism of neutrophils from some patients with SLE may be impaired. Degranulation of neutrophils from patients with SLE also has not been studied in detail. Zurier,[275] however, did find that SLE sera that inhibited particle ingestion by normal neutrophils also suppressed extracellular release of lysosomal enzymes.

**Rheumatoid Arthritis.** Patients with rheumatoid arthritis (RA) also exhibit an unusual susceptibility to bacterial infections,[282] as well as abnormalities of neutrophil function. Several investigators[283-285] have reported that neutrophils from the peripheral blood of some patients with RA have an impaired ability to respond to chemotactic stimuli and to ingest suitably opsonized particles in vitro. Mowat and Baum,[283] for example, found that the mean chemotactic index measured with neutrophils from 24 patients with definite RA was significantly less than that measured with cells from an equal number of normal controls matched for age and sex. As an explanation for this abnormality, it has been observed that incubation of normal neutrophils with serum from some patients with RA impairs their capacity to migrate randomly and/or in a directed fashion.[283,285,286] Identical results have been obtained when normal neutrophils were exposed to preformed immune complexes, particularly complexes containing rheumatoid factor.[283] Exposure of normal neutrophils to either RA serum or immune complexes also impairs phagocytosis and killing of bacteria.[287-289] Turner and colleagues[289] observed that phagocytosis of yeast particles by normal peripheral blood neutrophils was decreased if the cells were preincubated with complexes prepared with aggregated human IgG and sera from patients with high-titer rheumatoid factor. In fact, there was a significant correlation between the log of the reciprocal of the rheumatoid factor titer in sera used to prepare complexes and the phagocytic capacity exhibited by test neutrophils. Thus, it appears that the functional abnormalities exhibited by neutrophils from patients with RA occur largely as a consequence of encounters with immune complexes either in vivo or in vitro. Since such encounters are most likely to occur in the inflamed rheumatoid joint, it is not surprising that synovial fluid neutrophils from patients with RA exhibit the most severe abnormalities of chemotaxis and phagocytosis.[289-291] RA synovial fluid also interferes with ingestion of opsonized particles by normal leukocytes.[276,289] These findings may be relevant to the fact that septic arthritis is a particularly common complication of RA.[292]

The abnormalities of neutrophil functions observed in patients with Felty's syndrome also appear to be attributable to encounters with circulating immune complexes. Neutrophils from patients with Felty's syndrome exhibit abnormal chemotaxis in vitro[293] as well as abnormal phagocytosis and bacterial killing.[294] Immunoglobulin-containing inclusions have been seen in these cells by immunofluorescence and electron microscopy.[294] Normal neutrophils develop similar inclusions when they are incubated with serum from patients with Felty's syndrome.[265] It has been suggested that phagocytosis of circulating immune complexes by neutrophils may not only interfere with the function of these cells in combating infection, but also may render them susceptible to removal from the circulation.[265] It is noteworthy that bacterial infections in patients with Felty's syndrome are not always associated with decreased numbers of circulating neutrophils.[295]

Not all of the abnormalities of neutrophil function observed in patients with RA are attributable to encounters in vivo with immune complexes.[296,297] Hanlon and colleagues,[297] for example, described deficient generation of chemotactic activity in RA serum after incubation with *E. coli* lipopolysaccharide. This abnormality was associated with the presence of a heat stable (56° C for 30 minutes) inhibitor of chemotaxis, the potency of which was inversely related to the level of chemotactic activity generated in the rheumatoid sera.

It should be mentioned that some investigators have failed to detect abnormalities of neutrophil function in patients with RA.[274,281] Notably, van de Stadt and colleagues[298] found that if precautions were taken to prevent phagocytosis of immune complexes during the isolation of neutrophils from either peripheral blood or synovial fluid of patients with RA, the cells functioned in vitro quite normally. Oxygen uptake, extracellular release of lysosomal enzymes, and the granule enzyme content of RA neutrophils were comparable to that of peripheral blood neutrophils from healthy volunteer blood donors.

## OTHER RHEUMATIC SYNDROMES AND INFLAMMATORY STATES ASSOCIATED WITH ABNORMALITIES OF NEUTROPHIL FUNCTION

With the exception of a single report describing impaired directed migration of neutrophils from patients with juvenile rheumatoid arthritis,[283] most investigators have failed to detect defective neutrophil functions in patients with rheumatic diseases other than SLE and RA.[299-302] In fact, the chemotactic responsiveness of neutrophils has been found to be enhanced in some children with chronic arthritis,[299] patients with Behçet's disease,[300] and some patients with reactive arthritis following yersinia infections.[302] Interestingly, enhanced neutrophil migration (both chemokinesis and chemotaxis) was observed only with cells from patients with reactive arthritis who were HLA-B27 positive. Furthermore, enhanced chemokinetic and chemotactic responses to zymosan-activated serum were observed with neutrophils from HLA-B27 positive individuals irrespective of whether they suffered from either yersinia infections or arthritis. Finally, when activated with zymosan, sera from HLA-B27 positive patients and controls were significantly more chemokinetic than zymosan-activated sera from HLA-B27 negative individuals. These results suggest that the responsiveness of neutrophils to complement-derived chemotactic stimuli is regulated in some fashion by genes associated with the major histocompatibility complex. The increased chemokinetic activity of activated serum from HLA-B27 positive individuals, as well as the enhanced ability of neutrophils from these individuals to migrate in a directed fashion, may con tribute to the pathogenesis of "B27-associated" inflammatory arthritides.

An inadequate capacity to generate chemotactic activity in serum, with no demonstrable intrinsic neutrophil defect, is frequently associated with a rheumatic disease-like syndrome, most notably in the cases attributable to a deficiency of a complement component (Table 9–7). Patients lacking an early component of the classic pathway, namely Clr, C4, or C2, are subject to an increased incidence of an SLE-like illness or, more rarely, a dermatomyositis-like syndrome or necrotizing angiitis.[303,304] Patients lacking one of the terminal components, C5, C6, or C7, occasionally present with either an SLE-like disease or, in one instance, Raynaud's syndrome with scleroderma-like features.[305,306] C6-deficient serum develops normal chemotactic activity, however, in contrast to the abnormality in C5- or C7-deficient serum. As the defect in chemotactic activity in C7-deficient serum was originally presumed to reflect the decreased formation of the $\overline{C567}$ chemotactic factor, the normal chemotactic activity of C6-deficient sera, which would also fail to generate $\overline{C567}$, lends substantial credence to those reports of the generation of normal chemotactic activity in C7-deficient serum. Patients deficient in C3, a component critical to both the classic and alternative pathways, have a more pronounced serum abnormality relative to neutrophil function than individuals deficient in other complement components. C3-deficient patients are predisposed to recurrent severe infections, but do not develop rheumatic syndromes at an increased frequency.[307] Children with Wiskott-Aldrich syndrome and mucocutaneous candidiasis exhibit a variety of lymphocyte abnormalities, including decreased generation of chemotactic lymphokines, a defect that may possibly be related to their frequent incidence of infections.[308] A diverse group of diseases, previously related only by a common predisposition to frequent infections, characteristically leads to elevated serum levels of one or more aminopeptidases normally present in serum and known to degradatively inactive numerous chemotactic factors.[309,310] In several other conditions associated with recurrent infections or the occurrence of spontaneous inflammatory disease, serum factors have been detected which either inhibit the activity of chemotactic stimuli or suppress the chemotactic responsiveness of the neutrophils. A serum principal in hypocomplementemic nephritis appears to be a relatively selective inhibitor of complement-derived chemotactic activity.[311] Neutrophil-directed inhibitors have been found in rare children with multiple episodes of pulmonary and cutaneous infections, and the effect of these inhibitors was reversible upon washing the neutrophils.[312] Polymeric IgA is a neutrophil-directed inhibitor of chemotaxis[313] and has been related to in vivo defects in the neutrophil chemotactic responses of a group of patients with elevated serum levels of polymeric IgA in association with neutrophilic leukocytosis and absent cutaneous delayed hypersensitivity.

In comparison with the human diseases that are characteristically associated with defects in neutrophil chemotaxis, those conditions related to excessive neutrophil chemotactic activity in vitro are largely inflammatory disorders without deficiencies of host resistance (Table 9–8). The only subjects documented to have intrinsically hyperactive neutrophils have been those mounting an appropriate response to acute bacterial infections,[314] and some patients with Behçet's disease[300] or reactive arthritis in association with HLA-B27 antigen.[302] For other patients with chemotactically hyperactive neutrophils, the abnormalities have been predominantly in the fluid phase. The local generation of mast cell–derived chemotactic factors in quantities exceeding an apparent physiological need has been observed in acute cold urticaria and in bullous pemphigoid.[315,316] In both instances, eosinophil and neutrophil chemotactic activities were detected in association with the lesions, and the granulocytes exposed to the elevated local concentrations of the stimuli were chemotactically hyporesponsive in vitro, suggesting that in vivo chemotactic deactivation had occurred. High local concentrations of specific granulocyte chemotactic factors also have been found in samples of skin or synovial tissues of patients with psoriasis, gout, and rheumatoid arthritis, and the characteristics of these principals will be presented below. Defects in the in vitro modulation of chemotaxis have been recorded in $\alpha_1$-proteinase inhibitor deficiency, in which a concomitant deficiency exists in the $\alpha$-globulin chemotactic factor inactivator,[317] but the clinical significance of this finding is uncertain. Neutrophils in mixed leukocyte suspensions are chemotactically hyperactive following corticosteroid therapy as a result of the elaboration of a mononuclear leukocyte–derived factor that enhances the chemotactic responsiveness of neutrophils.[318] A naturally occurring leukocyte migration–enhancing principal has been found in sera of rare patients with pyoderma gangrenosum, characterized by episodes of sterile pyarthrosis and cutaneous inflammation.[319] This migration-enhancing factor was recovered from serum by Sephadex G-200 gel filtration and found to have a molecular weight of approximately 160,000. The partially purified principal enhanced the random migration of purified normal human neutrophils and mononuclear leukocytes by up to 200 percent without specifically influencing chemotaxis. Trauma or other stimuli which alter microvascular permeability may lead to an accumulation of this serum factor in tissues of such patients, with resultant excessive influx of leukocytes and heightened local activity of neutrophils and mononuclear leukocytes in the inflammatory exudate.

## SPECIFIC CHEMOTACTIC FACTORS IN RHEUMATIC DISORDERS

The possibility that one pathway for the generation of chemotactic activity may predominate in a given disease has been explored using relevant biological fluids or cell extracts for the absorption of known chemotactic principals with specific antisera and for the purification of the existing chemotactic activities. Initial efforts indicated that the major chemotactic factors for neutrophils in rheumatoid synovial fluid and in extracts of cutaneous lesions in a rat model for vasculitis were fragments of C5 of approximately 17,000 molecular weight that were analogous to C5a, while fragments of C3 appeared to account for the bulk of the neutrophil chemotactic activity in synovial fluid of some nonrheumatoid arthritides and in pericardial fluid following limited myocardial infarctions in rats.[320] Analyses of fluid phase and tissue enzymes capable of cleaving C5 and C3 suggested that the major protease that generated chemotactic fragments from C5 in rheumatoid synovial fluid was derived from the neutrophils themselves,[321] while in nonrheumatoid effusions the C3-directed protease was from the synovial tissue.[322] In other analyses, $LTB_4$ and C5a were the principal chemotactic factors of synovial fluid from patients with rheumatoid arthritis, while $LTB_4$ predominated in the spondyloarthritis.[201] Despite the demonstration of additional specific chemotactic factors and inhibitors in synovial fluid and tissue from patients with rheumatoid arthritis, in vitro studies have not provided an adequate explanation for the preferential accumulation of neutrophils in the synovial fluid and of mononuclear leukocytes in synovial tissue. The task of explaining the basis for the neutrophil infiltration in psoriatic skin has led to the discovery of at least two classes of factors which may stimulate neutrophil chemotaxis into the cutaneous lesions. Lipid analyses of extracts of psoriatic plaques have revealed increased levels of arachidonic acid and its lipoxygenase metabolites, especially the chemotactic factors 12-HETE and $LTB_4$, as compared to uninvolved skin of psoriasis patients and to normal skin.[323] Further, the levels of lipoxygenase metabolites and other arachidonate derivatives were suppressed by topical therapy with corticosteroids. A second neutrophil chemotactic factor identified in psoriatic scales was a protein of molecular weight 12,500 by Sephadex G-75 filtration.[324] The expression of the chemotactic activity of this principal was dependent on the presence of C3 or C5, which suggested it was a protease capable of generating chemotactic fragments from the complement components. This factor may be a portion of the 28,000 molecular weight neutral protease of human skin since the intact protease is present at higher concentrations in psoriatic skin than in normal skin, and has the capacity to generate C5-dependent chemotactic activity by a reaction that is blocked by some esterase inhibitors such as diisopropyl fluorophosphate, soybean trypsin inhibitor, and $\alpha_2$-macroglobulin.[325]

The chemotactic activity that appears rapidly in synovial fluid during acute gouty attacks is derived largely from the neutrophils phagocytizing monosodium urate crystals. Both human and rabbit granulocytes exposed to monosodium urate or calcium pyrophosphate crystals release an 8400 molecular weight glycoprotein that is chemotactic for neutrophils and mononuclear leukocytes.[326] The factor is not preformed, but appears in the lysosomal granular fraction during phagocytosis. The production and release of the factor require endocytosis of the crystals and are blocked by actinomycin D, colchicine, cytochalasin B, indomethacin, phenylbutazone, and some protease-esterase inhibitors including trasylol and epsilon-aminocaproic acid.[327] This neutrophil-derived factor, like other chemotactic principals, induces chemotactic deactivation and augments the release of lysosomal enzymes from neutrophils in the presence of cytochalasin B. Injection of the purified factor into rabbit joints led to the influx of neutrophils into the synovial tissues, without a significant increase in vascular permeability, as assessed by the rate of transport of circulating $^{125}I$-albumin into the joint space. The leukocyte infiltration of the joints injected with the purified chemotactic factor that had been generated in vitro was comparable in magnitude to that seen in joints injected with monosodium urate crystals, but the peak response was achieved at 90 minutes in contrast to over 300 minutes with the crystals.

## SPECIAL FUNCTIONS OF THE EOSINOPHIL AND THE SPECTRUM OF HYPEREOSINOPHILIC DISEASES

The eosinophil is a characteristic constituent of the tissue response evoked by immunological reactions of various types. Eosinophils are especially prominent in both the early and late cellular infiltrates of immediate-type hypersensitivity reactions,[328,329] which presumably reflects the release of numerous mast cell–derived eosinophilotactic factors. Eosinophils possess many of the general functional capabilities of neutrophils, which are often expressed at reduced levels relative to those of neutrophils.

Eosinophil granules contain a wide array of enzymes generally comparable to those found in lysosomes of neutrophilic leukocytes, although the human eosinophil lacks lysozyme.[8,9] A number of constituents of the eosinophil, however, are not present in the neutrophil. Eosinophil peroxidase, found in the large granule of the cell, differs physiochemically and functionally from neutrophil myeloperoxidase.[330] The enzyme lysophospholipase, prominent in the eosinophil and associated with eosinophil membranes, is the sole constituent of the distinctive dipyramidal Charcot-Leyden crystals, found in human tissues and fluids, such as sputum and feces, in a number of eosinophilic disease processes.[331,332] Lysophospholipase, which is found in eosinophils and basophils, is absent from neutrophils. In addition, several unique cationic proteins are present in the large granule of the eosinophil, including the major basic protein in the crystalloid core of the granule, eosinophil cationic protein, and another basic protein with neurotoxic properties.[333,334]

Membrane receptors for immunoglobulins and complement components are expressed on the surface of the eosinophil. Receptors for immunoglobulins G and E and for the components of complement C3b and C3d are demonstrable on the plasma membrane of eosinophils.[8,9] In addition, tissue eosinophils also fulfill at least two unique roles in defending the sensitized host. The eosinophil is specially endowed with high concentrations of a range of specific enzymes capable of degrading mediators released by immunologically activated mast cells and basophils. Eosinophil histaminase, like that of the neutrophil, is a diamine oxidase that oxidatively deaminates histamine with a pH optimum of 6.0 to 8.0.[335] Phospholipase D, which is preferentially contained in eosinophils as compared to neutrophils and mononuclear leukocytes degrades some forms of phospholipid PAF with the same pH optimum of 4.5 to 6.0 at which it most efficiently cleaves synthetic phospholipids.[253] Eosinophil-derived peroxidase inactivates $LTC_4$ by conversion to $LTC_4$-sulfone and to two 6-trans isomers of $LTB_4$, in the presence of $H_2O_2$ and chloride ion.[336] The peroxidatic inactivation of $LTC_4$ by intact eosinophils is dependent on the stimulation of maximum oxidative activity and is suppressed by sodium azide or catalase. The rate of degradation of $LTC_4$ by intact eosinophils is far greater than that for the isolated peroxidase, suggesting that intracellular peroxidation may account for the conversion of $LTC_4$ in vivo. In contrast, the actions of histaminase and phospholipase D on mediators are believed to be dependent on prior degranulation of the eosinophils.

As a further mechanism for the containment of immediate-type hypersensitivity reactions, eosinophils apparently preferentially phagocytose extruded mast cell granules,[337] which avidly retain both macromolecular heparin and a cationic chymotrypsin-like protease that is active while still in the granule.[338] A recently recognized additional capacity of the eosinophil, which bridges its activities in the traditional immune response[339] and its direct functions in host defense, is the IgG antibody–dependent destruction of schistosomulae[340] and schistosoma eggs[341] in vitro that is appreciated as enhanced helminthicidal activity in vivo.[342] The special ability of eosinophils to damage nonphagocytosable parasites may be related to their substantial concentrations of various phospholipases, some of which are associated with the plasma membrane, and to the sustained production and release of high levels of superoxide anion.[343] Other special functions have been proposed for the eosinophil, including preferential phagocytosis of *Mycoplasma* and soluble immune complexes, predominantly those containing IgE, binding and inactivation of estrogens, and participation in fibrinolytic reactions.[344]

Marked peripheral blood and tissue eosinophilia commonly accompanies allergic and parasitic diseases.[345-348] Eosinophilia in the absence of these precipitating factors, however, is less well defined and has been classified either according to the affected organ system or in terms of the overall clinical presentation. The term hypereosinophilic syndrome[349,350] has been applied to the range of entities within this spectrum which present with involvement of critical organs (Table 9–9). The pulmonary eosinophilias are the most common form and vary from the transient pulmonary infiltrates of Löffler's syndrome to the more chronic lesions associated with endomyocardial fibrosis and cardiac failure.[351,352] In general, Löffler's syndrome, bronchopulmonary aspergillosis, and tropical eosinophilia are responsive to therapy, whereas chronic eosinophilic pneumonitides with substantial abnormalities in pulmonary function, pulmonary eosinophilias with endomyocardial fibrosis, and polyarteritis with pulmonary involvement are more resistant to drug treatment.[350-353]

The extraction of tumor tissues obtained from three subjects with anaplastic squamous cell carcinoma of the lung, associated with peripheral blood hypereosinophilia and eosinophil infiltration of the tumors and surrounding normal lung tissue, led to the recognition of a low molecular weight eosinophil chemotactic peptide which is apparently unique to the tumors.[354] The approximate content of low molecular weight eosinophil chemotactic activity per milligram of tumor tissue was 2 to 35 times the level of activity in normal human lung tissue and far exceeded that in tumors not associated with eosinophilia. Further purification of the tumor-related eosinophil chemotactic factor, obtained from tissue extracts and cell culture supernatants, showed it to be comparable in size to the ECF-A tetrapeptides, but less acidic. Eosinophils from one of the patients were chemotactically unresponsive in vitro during the entire course, while those from a second patient exhibited normal chemotaxis initially but became hyporesponsive to C5 fragments and the tumor-derived factor at a time when the peripheral blood eosinophilia achieved a maximal level and the tumor eosinophil chemotactic factor first was detected in the urine. As the migration of eosinophils from both patients was enhanced by ascorbate, the selective chemotactic unresponsiveness was attributed to in vivo deactivation. In the disseminated hypereosinophilic syndromes and the rare cases of eosinophilic leukemia, the eosinophils exhibit profound morphological abnormal-

**Table 9–9.** Hypereosinophilic Syndromes

| Category | Organ Involvement | Pathological and Clinical Features | Morphological Characteristics of Eosinophils | Therapy |
|---|---|---|---|---|
| Löffler's syndrome | Transient pulmonary infiltrates | No vascular involvement, bronchospasm in some patients | Normal | Corticosteroids |
| Chronic eosinophilic pneumonitis | Pulmonary eosinophilic infiltrates | Altered pulmonary mechanics, impaired gas exchange | Normal | Corticosteroids |
| Tropical eosinophilia | Pulmonary eosinophilic infiltrates | Nocturnal bronchospasm, may be altered pulmonary mechanics | May be vacuolization | Diethylcarbamazine |
| Pulmonary eosinophilic angiitis | Pulmonary and usually systemic angiitis | Necrotizing granulomatous angiitis with vascular and parenchymal fibrosis; bronchospasm common | Normal | Generally resistant to anti-inflammatory therapy |
| Löffler's endomyocardial fibrosis | Cardiac and pulmonary eosinophilic infiltrates | Subendocardial eosinophilic infiltration and fibrosis, myocardial failure with early dyskinesis | May be vacuolization and hypogranulation | No specific treatment, related to level and duration of eosinophilic states |
| Other localized eosinophilias | Diffuse fasciitis with eosinophilia | Fibrosis and chronic inflammation of deep fascia of legs, arms, and trunk, large joint contractures, peripheral blood and variable tissue eosinophilia | Normal | Corticosteroids |
| Eosinophilia with large cell bronchogenic carcinoma | Tumor, normal pulmonary and cardiac tissue | Local tumor extension, pulmonary and endomyocardial fibrosis | May be vacuolization and hypogranulation | No specific treatment |
| Disseminated hypereosinophilic syndrome | Cutaneous, lymph node, liver, spleen, cranial and peripheral nerves, pulmonary and cardiac infiltrates | Predominantly adult males, neurological disease and endomyocardial fibrosis frequently fatal | Generally abnormal mature eosinophils | Hydroxyurea |
| Eosinophilic leukemia | Similar to disseminated hypereosinophilic syndrome | Thrombocytopenia | Increased bone marrow and circulating blasts, eosinophil chromosomal abnormalities | Insufficient experience with any drug |

ities and the prognosis for survival of such patients is poor.[350,351] Some of the eosinophil degranulation and vacuolization that have been observed may be secondary to therapy,[355] but studies of eosinophil function have not been performed systematically. Recent evidence supports the use of hydroxyurea as the drug of choice in aggressive hypereosinophilic syndromes.[356]

In the rheumatic diseases, substantial eosinophilia has been found in rheumatoid arthritis, in association with an increased incidence of extra-articular manifestations of disease,[357] polyarteritis with pulmonary involvement,[353] and occasional other states in an acute or accelerated phase. Eosinophilic fasciitis[358] is a localized infiltration of the connective tissues of the upper and lower extremities which may lead to fibrosis and significant functional losses. Thus, while eosinophils predominantly fulfill a protective role, they apparently are capable of injuring host tissues in some inflammatory reactions. As eosinophils, unlike neutrophils, are largely located in tissue spaces below the body surfaces both normally and in allergic and other transient reactive states, their capacity to damage autologous tissues and lead to fibrosis must be dependent not on redistribution, but on special conditions or pathways of activation which are not fully understood.

## References


1. Price, G.B., and McCulloch, E.A.: Cell surfaces and the regulation of hemopoiesis. Semin. Hematol. 15:283, 1978.
2. Bradley, T.R., and Metcalf, D.: The growth of mouse bone marrow cells in vitro. Aust. J. Exp. Biol. Med. Sci. 44:287, 1966.
3. Metcalf, D.: Studies on colony formation in vitro by mouse bone marrow cells. I. Continuous cluster formation and relation of clusters to colonies. J. Cell Physiol. 74:323, 1969.
4. Ross, G.D., Jarowski, C.I., Rabellino, E.M., and Winchester, R.J.: The sequential appearance of Ia-like antigens and two different complement receptors during the maturation of human neutrophils. J. Exp. Med. 147:730, 1978.
5. Bainton, D.F.: Differentiation of human neutrophilic granulocytes: Normal and abnormal. *In* Greenwalt, T.J., and Jamieson, G.A. (eds.): Progress in Clinical and Biological Research. Vol. 13. New York, Alan R. Liss, Inc., 1977.
6. Lichtman, M.A.: Cellular deformability during maturation of the myeloblast. Possible role in marrow egress. N. Engl. J. Med. 283:943, 1970.
7. Cronkite, E.P., and Vincent, P.: Granulocytopoiesis. Ser. Haem. II:3, 1969.
8. Weller, P.F., and Goetzl, E.J.: The regulatory and effector roles of eosinophils. Adv. Immunol. 27:339, 1979.
9. Weller, P.F., and Goetzl, E.J.: The human eosinophil: Roles in host defense and tissue injury. Am. J. Pathol. 100:791, 1980.
10. Snyderman, R., and Goetzl, E.J.: Molecular and cellular mechanisms of leukocyte chemotaxis. Science 213:830, 1981.
11. Boyden, S.: The chemotactic effect of mixtures of antibody and antigen on the polymorphonuclear leukocytes. J. Exp. Med. 115:453, 1962.
12. Wilkinson, P.C., and Allan, R.B.: Assay systems for measuring leukocyte locomotion: An overview. *In* Gallin, J.I., and Quie, P.G. (eds.): Leukocyte Chemotaxis: Methods, Physiology, and Clinical Implications. New York, Raven Press, 1978.
13. Zigmond, S.H., and Hirsch, J.G.: Leukocyte locomotion and chemotaxis: New methods for evaluation and demonstration of a cell-derived chemotactic factor. J. Exp. Med. 137:387, 1973.
14. Gallin, J.I., Clark, R.A., and Goetzl, E.J.: Radioassay of leukocyte locomotion: A sensitive technique for clinical studies. *In* Gallin, J.I., and Quie, P.G. (eds.): Leukocyte Chemotaxis: Methods, Physiology, and Clinical Implications. New York, Raven Press, 1978.
15. Goetzl, E.J., and Austen, K.F.: A method for assessing the in vitro chemotactic response of neutrophils utilizing $^{51}$Cr-labeled human leukocytes. Immunol. Commun. 1:142, 1972.
16. Nelson, R.D., Quie, P.G., and Simmons, R.L.: Chemotaxis under agarose: A new and simple method for measuring chemotaxis and spontaneous migration of human polymorphonuclear leukocytes and monocytes. J. Immunol. 115:1650, 1975.
17. Revak, S.D., and Cochrane, C.G.: The relationship of structure and

function in human Hageman factor. The association of enzymatic and binding activities with separate regions of the molecule. J. Clin. Invest. 57:852, 1976.
18. Kaplan, A.P., Kay, A.B., and Austen, K.F.: A prealbumin activator of prekallikrein, III. Appearance of chemotactic activity for human neutrophils by the conversion of human prekallikrein to kallikrein. J. Exp. Med. 135:81, 1972.
19. Fernandez, H.N., Henson, P.M., Otani, A., and Hugli, T.E.: Chemotactic response to human C3a and C5a anaphylatoxins. I. Evaluation of C3a and C5a leukotaxin in vitro and under simulated in vivo conditions. J. Immunol. 120:109, 1978.
20. Lachmann, P.J., Kay, A.B., and Thompson, R.A.: The chemotactic activity for neutrophil and eosinophil leukocytes of the trimolecular complex of the fifth, sixth, and seventh components of human complement ($\overline{C567}$) prepared in free solution by the "reactive lysis" procedure. Immunology 19:985, 1970.
21. Ruddy, S., Austen, K.F., and Goetzl, E.J.: Chemotactic activity derived from interaction of factors $\overline{D}$ and B of the properdin pathway with cobra venom factor or C3b. J. Clin. Invest. 55:587, 1975.
22. Kay, A.B., Stechschulte, D.J., and Austen, K.F.: An eosinophil leukocyte chemotactic factor of anaphylaxis. J. Exp. Med. 133:602, 1971.
23. Kay, A.B., and Austen, K.F.: The IgE-mediated release of an eosinophil leukocyte chemotactic factor from human lung. J. Immunol. 107:899, 1971.
24. Goetzl, E.J., and Austen, K.F.: Purification and synthesis of eosinophilotactic tetrapeptides of human lung tissue: Identification as eosinophil chemotactic factor of anaphylaxis. Proc. Natl. Acad. Sci. USA 72:4123, 1975.
25. Valone, F.H., and Goetzl, E.J.: Immunological release in the rat peritoneal cavity of lipid chemotactic and chemokinetic factors for polymorphonuclear leukocytes. J. Immunol. 120:102, 1978.
26. Goetzl, E.J.: Oxygenation products of arachidonic acid as mediators of hypersensitivity and inflammation. Med. Clin. North Am. 65:809, 1981.
27. Goetzl, E.J.: Leukocyte recognition and metabolism of leukotrienes. Fed. Proc., 42:3128, 1983.
28. Richardson, D.L., Pepper, D.S., and Kay, A.B.: Chemotaxis for human monocytes by fibrinogen-derived peptides. Br. J. Haematol. 32:507, 1976.
29. Postlethwaite, A.E., and Kang, A.H.: Collagen- and collagen peptide–induced chemotaxis of human blood monocytes. J. Exp. Med. 143:1299, 1976.
30. Goetzl, E.J., Schreiber, A.D., and Austen, K.F.: Chemotactic activity of components of the kallikrein-kinin and fibrinolytic sequences. *In* Pisano, J. (ed.): Chemistry and Biology of the Kallikrein-Kinin System in Health and Disease, Bethesda, Md., National Institute of Health, 1977.
31. Becker, E.L.: The relationship of the chemotactic behavior of the complement-derived factor C3a, C5a, and $\overline{C567}$ and a bacterial factor to their ability to activate the proesterase 1 of rabbit polymorphonuclear leukocytes. J. Exp. Med. 135:376, 1972.
32. Altman, L.C.: Chemotactic lymphokines: A review. *In* Gallin, J.I., and Quie, P.G. (eds.): Leukocyte Chemotaxis: Methods, Physiology, and Clinical Implications. New York, Raven Press, 1978.
33. Tainer, J.A., Turner, S.R., and Lynn, W.S.: New aspects of chemotaxis: Specific target cell attraction by lipid and lipoprotein fractions of *Escherichia coli* chemotactic factor. Am. J. Pathol. 81:401, 1975.
34. Turner, S.R., Tainer, J.A., and Lynn, W.S.: Biogenesis of chemotactic molecules by the arachidonic lipoxygenase system of platelets. Nature 257:680, 1975.
35. Goetzl, E.J., Woods, J.M., and Gorman, R.R.: Stimulation of human eosinophil and neutrophil polymorphonuclear leukocyte chemotaxis and random migration by 12-L-hydroxy-5,8,10,14-eicosatetraenoic acid (HETE). J. Clin. Invest. 59:179, 1977.
36. Goetzl, E.J., and Gorman, R.R.: Chemotactic and chemokinetic stimulation of human eosinophils and neutrophil polymorphonuclear leukocytes by 12-L-hydroxy-5,8,10-heptadecatrienoic acid (HHT). J. Immunol. 120:526, 1978.
37. Goetzl, E.J.: Modulation of human eosinophil polymorphonuclear leukocyte migration and function. Am. J. Pathol. 95:419, 1976.
38. Kay, A.B., and Austen, K.F.: Chemotaxis of human basophil leukocytes. Clin. Exp. Immunol. 11:557, 1972.
39. Goetzl, E.J., Wasserman, S.I., and Austen, K.F.: Modulation of the eosinophil chemotactic response in immediate hypersensitivity. *In* Brent, L., and Holborow, J. (eds.): Progress in Immunology II. Vol. 4. Amsterdam, North-Holland Publishing Company, 1974.
40. Valotta, E.H., and Müller-Eberhard, H.J.: Formation of C3a and C5a anaphylatoxins in whole serum after inhibition of the anaphylatoxin inactivator. J. Exp. Med. 137:1109, 1973.
41. Berenberg, J.L., and Ward, P.A.: The chemotactic factor inactivator in normal human serum. J. Clin. Invest. 52:1200, 1973.
42. Till, G., and Ward, P.A.: Two distinct chemotactic factor inactivators in normal human serum. J. Immunol. 114:843, 1975.
43. Wright, D.G., and Gallin, J.I.: Modulation of the inflammatory response by products released from human polymorphonuclear leukocytes during phagocytosis: Generation and inactivation of the chemotactic factor C5a. Inflammation 1:23, 1975.
44. Ward, P.A., and Becker, E.L.: The deactivation of rabbit neutrophils by chemotactic factor and the nature of the activatable esterase. J. Exp. Med. 127:693, 1968.
45. Ward, P.A., and Becker, E.L.: Biochemical demonstration of the activatable esterase of the rabbit neutrophil involved in the chemotactic response. J. Immunol. 105:1057, 1970.
46. Caner, J.E.Z.: Colchicine inhibition of chemotaxis. Arthritis Rheum. 8:757, 1965.
47. Becker, E.L., Davis, A.T., Estensen, R.D., and Quie, P.G.: Cytochalasin B: IV, Inhibition and stimulation of chemotaxis of rabbit and human polymorphonuclear leukocytes. J. Immunol. 108:396, 1972.
48. Zurier, R.B., Weissman, G., Hoffstein, S., Kammerman, S., and Tai, H.H.: Mechanism of lysosomal enzyme release from human leukocytes. II. Effects of cyclic AMP and cyclic GMP, autonomic agents, and agents which affect microtubule function. J. Clin. Invest. 53:297, 1974.
49. Zurier, R.B., Hoffstein, S., and Weissman, G.: Cytochalasin B: Effect on lysosomal enzyme release from human leukocytes. Proc. Natl. Acad. Sci. USA 70:844, 1973.
50. Becker, E.L., Showell, H.J., Henson, P.M., and Hsu, L.S.: The ability of chemotactic factors to induce lysosomal enzyme release: I. The characteristics of the release, the importance of surfaces and the relation of the enzyme release to chemotactic responsiveness. J. Immunol. 112:2047, 1974.
51. Björksten, B., Ray, C., and Quie, P.G.: Inhibition of human neutrophil chemotaxis and chemiluminescence by amphotericin B. Infect. Immun. 14:315, 1976.
52. Hatch, G.E., Nichols, W.K., and Hill, H.R.: Cyclic nucleotide changes in human neutrophils induced by chemoattractants and chemotactic modulators. J. Immunol. 119:450, 1976.
53. Hill, H.R., Estensen, R.D., Quie, P.G., Hogan, N.A., and Goldberg, N.D.: Modulation of human neutrophil chemotactic responses by cyclic 3′,5′ guanosine monophosphate and cyclic 3′,5′ adenosine monophosphate. Metabolism 24:447, 1975.
54. Goetzl, E.J., Wasserman, S.I., Gigli, I., and Austen, K.F.: Enhancement of random migration and chemotactic response of human leukocytes by ascorbic acid. J. Clin. Invest. 53:813, 1974.
55. Sandler, J.A., Gallin, J.I., and Vaughan, M.: Effects of serotonin, carbamylcholine, and ascorbic acid on leukocyte cyclic GMP and chemotaxis. J. Cell Biol. 67:480, 1975.
56. Boxer, L.A., Watanage, A.M., Rister, M., Besch, H.R., Jr., Allen, J., and Baehner, R.L.: Correction of leukocyte function in Chédjak-Higashi syndrome by ascorbate. N. Engl. J. Med. 295:1041, 1976.
57. Foster, C.S., and Goetzl, E.J.: Impaired neutrophil and monocyte chemotaxis in a patient with atopy, hyperimmunoglobulinemia E and recurrent infection: Effects of ascorbate therapy. Arch. Ophthalmol. 96:2069, 1978.
58. Watt, K.W.K., Brightman, I.L., and Goetzl, E.J.: Isolation of two polypeptides comprising the neutrophil-immobilizing factor of human leukocytes. Immunology 48:79, 1983.
59. Goetzl, E.J., and Austen, K.F.: A neutrophil immobilizing factor derived from human leukocytes. I. Generation and partial characterization. J. Exp. Med. 136:1564, 1972.
60. Goetzl, E.J., Gigli, I., Wasserman, S.I., and Austen, K.F.: A neutrophil immobilizing factor derived from human leukocytes. II. Specificity of action on polymorphonuclear leukocyte mobility. J. Immunol. 111:938, 1973.
61. Goetzl, E.J.: Modulation of human neutrophil polymorphonuclear leukocyte migration of human plasma alpha-globulin inhibitors and synthetic esterase inhibitors. Immunology 29:1419, 1973.
62. Weksler, B.B., and Coupal, C.E.: Platelet-dependent generation of chemotactic activity in serum. J. Exp. Med. 137:1419, 1973.
63. Samuelsson, B., Hamberg, M., Malmsten, C., and Svensson, J.: The role of prostaglandin endoperoxides and thromboxanes in platelet aggregation. *In* Samuelsson, B., and Paoletti, R. (eds.): Advances in Prostaglandin and Thromboxane Research, Vol. 2. New York, Raven Press, 1976.
64. Rocklin, R.E.: Products of activated lymphocytes: Leukocyte inhibitory factor (LIF) distinct from migration inhibitory factor (MIF). J. Immunol. 112:1461, 1974.
65. Rocklin, R.E.: Partial characterization of leukocyte inhibitory factor by concanavalin A–stimulated human lymphocytes (LIF con A). J. Immunol. 114:1161, 1975.
66. Goetzl, E.J., and Rocklin, R.E.: Amplification of the activity of human leukocyte inhibitory factor (LIF) by the generation of a low molecular weight inhibitor of PMN leukocyte chemotaxis, J. Immunol. 121:891, 1978.
67. Craddock, P.R., White, J.G., and Jacob, H.S.: Potentiation of complement

(C5a)-induced granulocyte aggregation by cytochalasin B. J. Lab. Clin. Med. 91:490, 1978.

68. Showell, H.J., Freer, R.J., Zigmond, S.H., Shiffman, E., Aswanikumar, S., Corcoran, B., and Becker, E.L.: The structure-activity relations of synthetic peptides as chemotactic factors and inducers of lysosomal enzyme secretion of neutrophils. J. Exp. Med. 143:1154, 1976.
69. Anwar, A.R.E., and Kay, A.B.: The ECF-A tetrapeptides and histamine selectivity enhance human eosinophil complement receptors. Nature 269:522, 1977.
70. Wright, A.E., and Douglas, S.R.: An experimental investigation of the role of blood fluids in connection with phagocytosis. Proc. R. Soc. Lond. Biol. 72:357, 1903.
71. Bokisch, V.A., Dierich, M.P., and Müller-Eberhard, H.J.: Third component of complement (C3): Structural properties in relation to functions. Proc. Natl. Acad. Sci. USA 72:1989, 1975.
72. Cline, M.J., and Lehrer, R.I.: Phagocytosis by human monocytes. Blood 32:423, 1968.
73. Henson, P.M.: The adherence of leukocytes and platelets induced by fixed IgG antibody or complement. Immunology 16:107, 1969.
74. Lay, W.H., and Nussenzweig, V.: Receptors for complement on leukocytes. J. Exp. Med. 128:991, 1968.
75. Phillips-Quagliata, J.M., Levine, B.B., and Uhr, J.W.: Studies on the mechanism of binding of immune complexes to phagocytes. Nature (Lond.) 222:1290, 1969.
76. Messner, R.P., and Jelinek, J.: Receptors for human $\gamma$G globulin on human neutrophils. J. Clin. Invest. 49:2165, 1970.
77. Boxer, L.A., Richardson, S.B., and Baehner, R.L.: Effects of surface-active agents on neutrophil receptors. Infect. Immun. 21:28, 1978.
78. Klempner, M.S., and Gallin, J.I.: Separation and functional characterization of human neutrophil subpopulations. Blood 51:659, 1978.
79. Sajnani, A.N., Ranadive, N.S., and Movat, H.Z.: The visualization of receptors for the Fc portion of the IgG molecule on human neutrophil leukocytes. Life Sci. 14:2427, 1974.
80. Sajnani, A.N., Ranadive, N.S., and Movat, H.Z.: Redistribution of immunoglobulin receptors on human neutrophils and its relationship to the release of lysosomal enzymes. Lab. Invest. 35:143, 1976.
81. Lawrence, D.A., Weigle, W.O., and Spiegelberg, H.L.: Immunoglobulins cytophilic for human lymphocytes, monocytes, and neutrophils. J. Clin. Invest. 55:368, 1975.
82. Walker, W.S.: Separate Fc receptors for immunoglobulin IgG2a and IgG2b on an established cell line of mouse macrophages. J. Immunol. 116:911, 1976.
83. Henson, P.M., Johnson, H.B., and Spiegelberg, H.L.: The release of granule enzymes from human neutrophils stimulated by aggregated immunoglobulins of different classes and subclasses. J. Immunol. 109:1182, 1972.
84. Schlessinger, J., Steinberg, I.Z., Givol, D., Hochman, J., and Pecht, I.: Antigen-induced conformational changes in antibodies and their Fab fragments studies by circular polarization of fluorescence. Proc. Natl. Acad. Sci. USA 72:2775, 1975.
85. An, T.: Fc receptors on human neutrophils: electron microscopic study of natural surface distribution. Immunology 40:1, 1980.
86. Loube, S.R., McNabb, T.C., and Dorrington, K.J.: Isolation of an Fc $\gamma$-binding protein from the cell membrane of a macrophage-like cell line (P388$D_1$) after detergent solubilization. J. Immunol. 120:709, 1978.
87. Kulczycki, A. Jr., Solanki, L., and Cohen, L.: Isolation and partial characterization of Fc $\gamma$-binding proteins of human leukocytes. J. Clin. Invest. 68:1558, 1981.
88. Ward, H.K., and Enders, J.F.: An analysis of the opsonic and tropic action of normal and immune sera based on experiments with the pneumococcus. J. Exp. Med. 57:527, 1933.
89. Nelson, D.S.: Immune adherence. *In* Wolstenholme, G.E.W., and Knight, J. (eds.): Ciba Foundation Symposium: Complement. Boston. Little, Brown and Co., 1965.
90. Mantovani, B.: Different roles of IgG and complement receptors in phagocytosis by polymorphonuclear leukocytes. J. Immunol. 115:15, 1975.
91. Gigli, I., and Nelson, R.A.: Complement dependent immune phagocytosis. I. Requirements for C'1, C'4, C'2, C'3. Exp. Cell Res. 51:45,1968.
92. Scribner, D.J., and Fahrney, D.: Neutrophil receptors for IgG and complement: Their roles in the attachment and ingestion phases of phagocytosis. J. Immunol. 116:892, 1976.
93. Ehlenberger, A.G., and Nussenzweig, V.: The role of membrane receptors for C3b and C3d in phagocytosis. J. Exp. Med. 145:357, 1977.
94. Pross, S.H., Hallock, J.A., Armstrong, R., and Fishel, C.W.: Complement and Fc receptors on cord blood and adult neutrophils. Pediatr. Res. 11:135, 1977.
95. Stossel, T.P.: Quantitative studies of phagocytosis. Kinetic effects of cations and heat-labile opsonin. J. Cell Biol. 58:346, 1973.
96. Stossel, T.P., Alper, C.A., and Rosen, F.S.: Serum-dependent phagocytosis of paraffin oil emulsified with bacterial lipopolysaccharide. J. Exp. Med. 137:690, 1973.
97. Guckian, J.C., Christensen, W.D., and Fine, D.P.: Trypan blue inhibits complement-mediated phagocytosis by human polymorphonuclear leukocytes. J. Immunol. 120:1580, 1978.
98. Fearon, D.T.: Identification of the membrane glycoprotein that is the C3b receptor of the human erythrocyte, polymorphonuclear leukocyte, B lymphocyte and monocyte. J. Exp. Med. 152:20, 1980.
99. Fearon, D.T., Kaneko, I., and Thomson, G.G.: Membrane distribution and adsorptive endocytosis by C3b receptors on human polymorphonuclear leukocytes. J. Exp. Med. 153:1615, 1981.
100. Ross, G.D., and Lambris, J.D.: Identification of a C3bi specific membrane complement receptor that is expressed on lymphocytes, monocytes, neutrophils, and erythrocytes. J. Exp. Med. 155:96, 1982.
101. Moore, P.L., Bank, H.L., Brissie, N.T., and Spicer, S.S.: Phagocytosis of bacteria by polymorphonuclear leukocytes. A freeze-fracture, scanning electron microscope, and thin-section investigation of membrane structure. J. Cell Biol. 76:158, 1978.
102. Karnovsky, M.L.: The metabolism of leukocytes. Semin. Hematol. 5:156, 1968.
103. Boxer, L.A., and Stossel, T.P.: Interactions of actin, myosin and an actin-binding protein of chronic myelogenous leukemia granulocytes. J. Clin. Invest. 56:964, 1976.
104. Stossel, T.P., Field, R.J., Gitlin, J.D., Alper, C.A., and Rosen, F.S.: The opsonic fragment of the third component of human complement (C3). J. Exp. Med 141:1329, 1975.
105. Patriarca, P., Cramer, R., Moncalvo, S., Rossi, F., and Romeo, D.: Enzymatic basis of metabolic stimulation in leukocytes during phagocytosis: the role of activated NADPH oxidase. Arch. Biochem. Biophys. 145:255, 1971.
106. Tagesson, C., Magnusson, K.-E., and Stendahl, O.: Physicochemical consequences of opsonization: perturbation of liposomal membranes by *Salmonella typhimurium* 395 MS opsonized with IgG antibodies. J. Immunol. 119:609, 1977.
107. Stendahl, O., Hed, J., Kihlstrom, E., Magnusson, K.-E., and Tagesson, C.: Phagocytic internalization and the requirement for membrane perturbation. FEBS Lett. 81:118, 1977.
108. Griffin, F.M. Jr., Griffin, J.A., Leider, J.E., and Silverstein, S.C.: Studies on the mechanism of phagocytosis. I. Requirements for circumferential attachment of particle-bound ligands to specific receptors on the macrophage plasma membrane. J. Exp. Med. 142:1263, 1975.
109. de Duve, C., Pressman, B.C., Gianetto, R., Wattiaux, R., and Appelmans, F.: Tissue fractionation studies. 6. Intracellular distribution patterns of enzymes in rat liver tissue. Biochem. J. 60:604, 1955.
110. Bainton, D.F., Ullyot, J.L., and Farquhar, M.G.: The development of neutrophilic polymorphonuclear leukocytes in human bone marrow. Origin and content of azurophil and specific granules. J. Exp. Med. 134:907, 1971.
111. Spitznagel, J.K., Dalldorf, M.G., Leffell, M.S., Folds, J.D., Welsh, I.R.H., Conney, M.H., and Martin, L.E.: Character of azurophil and specific granules purified from human polymorphonuclear leukocytes. Lab. Invest. 30:774, 1974.
112. West, B.C., Rosenthal, A.S., Gelb, N.A., and Kimball, H.R.: Separation and characterization of human neutrophil granules. Am. J. Pathol. 77:41, 1974.
113. Dewald, B., Bretz, U., and Baggiolini, M.: Release of gelatinase from a novel secretory compartment of human neutrophils. J. Clin. Invest. 70:518, 1982.
114. Zeya, H.I., and Spitznagel, J.K.: Characterization of cationic protein-bearing granules of polymorphonuclear leukocytes. Lab. Invest. 24:229, 1971.
115. Folds, J.D., Welsh, I.R.H., and Spitznagel, J.K.: Neutral proteases confined to one class of lysosomes of human polymorphonuclear leukocytes. Proc. Soc. Exp. Biol. Med. 139:461, 1972.
116. Leffell, M.S., and Spitznagel, J.K.: Association of lactoferrin with lysozyme in granules of human polymorphonuclear leukocytes. Infect. Immun. 6:761, 1972.
117. Murphy, G., Bretz, U., Baggiolini, M., and Reynolds, J.J.: The latent collagenase and gelatinase of human polymorphonuclear neutrophil leukocytes. Biochem. J. 192:517, 1980.
118. Kane, S.P., and Peters, T.J.: Analytical subcellular fractionation of human granulocytes with reference to the localization of vitamin $B_{12}$-binding proteins. Clin. Sci. Mol. Med. 49:171, 1975.
119. Goldstein, I.M.: Lysosomal hydrolases and inflammatory materials. In Weissmann, G.(ed.): Mediators of Inflammation. New York, Plenum Press, 1973.
120. Goldstein, I.M.: Polymorphonuclear leukocyte lysosomes and immune tissue injury. Prog. Allergy 20:301, 1976.
121. Babior, B.M.: Oxygen-dependent microbial killing by phagocytes. N. Engl. J. Med. 298:659, 1978.
122. Weissmann, G., Smolen, J.E., and Korchak, H.M.: Release of inflammatory mediators from stimulated neutrophils. N. Engl. J. Med. 303:27, 1980.
123. Weissmann, G.: Activation of neutrophils and the lesions of rheumatoid arthritis. J. Lab. Clin. Med. 100:322, 1982.

124. Straus, W.: Occurrence of phagosomes and phagolysosomes in different segments of the nephron in relation to the reabsorption, transport, digestion, and extrusion of intravenously injected horseradish peroxidase. J. Cell Biol. 21:295, 1964.
125. Hirsch, J.G., and Cohn, Z.A.: Degranulation of polymorphonuclear leukocytes following phagocytosis of microorganisms. J. Exp. Med. 112:1005, 1960.
126. Densen, P., and Mandell, G.L.: Gonococcal interactions with polymorphonuclear neutrophils. Importance of the phagosome for bactericidal activity. J. Clin. Invest. 62:1161, 1978.
127. Stossel, T.P., Pollard, T.D., Mason, R.J., and Vaughan, M.: Isolation and properties of phagocytic vesicles from polymorphonuclear leukocytes. J. Clin. Invest. 50:1745, 1971.
128. Leffell, M.S., and Spitznagel, J.K.: Intracellular and extracellular degranulation of human polymorphonuclear azurophil and specific granules induced by immune complexes. Infect. Immun. 10:1241, 1974.
129. Bainton, D.F.: Sequential degranulation of the two types of polymorphonuclear leukocyte granules during phagocytosis of microorganisms. J. Cell Biol. 58:249, 1973.
130. Leffell, M.S., and Spitznagel, J.K.: Fate of human lactoferrin and myeloperoxidase in phagocytizing human neutrophils: effects of immunoglobulin G subclasses and immune complexes on latex beads. Infect. Immun. 12:813, 1975.
131. Bentwood, B.J., and Henson, P.M.: The sequential release of granule constituents from human neutrophils. J. Immunol. 124:855, 1980.
132. Wright, D.G., Bralove, D.A., and Gallin, J.I.: The differential mobilization of human neutrophil granules. Effects of phorbol myristate acetate and ionophore A23187. Am. J. Pathol. 87:273, 1977.
133. Wright, D.G., and Gallin, J.I.: Secretory responses of human neutrophils: exocytosis of specific (secondary) granules by human neutrophils during adherence in vitro and during exudation in vivo. J. Immunol. 123:285, 1979.
134. Nachman, R., Hirsch, J.G., and Baggiolini, M.: Studies on isolated membranes of azurophil and specific granules from rabbit polymorphonuclear leukocytes. J. Cell Biol. 54:133, 1972.
135. Weissmann, G., Hirschhorn, R., and Krakauer, K.: Effect of mellitin upon cellular and lysosomal membranes. Biochem. Pharmacol. 18:1771, 1969.
136. de Duve, C., and Wattiaux, R.: Functions of lysosomes. Annu. Rev. Physiol. 28:435, 1966.
137. Weissmann, G., Zurier, R.B., Spieler, P.J., and Goldstein, I.M.: Mechanisms of lysosomal enzyme release from leukocytes exposed to immune complexes and other particles. J. Exp. Med. 134:149s, 1971.
138. Weissmann, G., Zurier, R.B., and Hoffstein, S.: Leukocytic proteases and the immunologic release of lysosomal enzymes. Am. J. Pathol. 68:539, 1972.
139. Weissmann, G., and Rita, G.A.: Molecular basis of gouty inflammation: interaction of monosodium urate crystals with lysosomes and liposomes. Nature New Biol. 240:167, 1972.
140. Schumacher, H.R., and Phelps, P.: Sequential changes in human polymorphonuclear leukocytes after urate crystal phagocytosis. An electron microscopic study. Arthritis Rheum. 14:513, 1971.
141. Allison, A.C., Harrington, J.S., and Birbeck, M.: An examination of the cytotoxic effects of silica on macrophages. J. Exp. Med. 124:141, 1968.
142. Hawkins, D.: Neutrophilic leukocytes in immunological reactions. Evidence for the selective release of lysosomal constituents. J. Immunol. 108:310, 1972.
143. Henson, P.M.: Interaction of cells with immune complexes. Adherence, release of constituents, and tissue injury. J. Exp. Med. 134:114s, 1971.
144. Henson, P.M.: Pathologic mechanisms in neutrophil-mediated injury. Am. J. Pathol. 68:593, 1972.
145. Henson, P.M., and Oades, Z.G.: Stimulation of human neutrophils by soluble and insoluble immunoglobulin aggregates. Secretion of granule constituents and increased oxidation of glucose. J. Clin. Invest. 56:1053, 1975.
146. Goldstein, I.M., Roos, D., Weissmann, G., and Kaplan, H.: Complement and immunoglobulins stimulate superoxide production by human leukocytes independently of phagocytosis. J. Clin. Invest. 56:1155, 1975.
147. Wright, D.G., and Malawista, S.E.: The mobilization and extracellular release of granular enzymes from human leukocytes during phagocytosis. J. Cell Biol. 53:788, 1972.
148. Zurier, R.B., Hoffstein, S., and Weissmann, G.: Mechanisms of lysosomal enzyme release from leukocytes. I. Effect of cyclic nucleotides and colchicine. J. Cell Biol. 58:27, 1973.
149. Johnston, R.B. Jr., and Lehmeyer, J.E.: Elaboration of toxic oxygen byproducts by neutrophils in a model of immune complex disease. J. Clin. Invest. 57:836, 1976.
150. Henson, P.M.: The immunologic release of constituents from neutrophil leukocytes. I. The role of antibody and complement on nonphagocytosable surfaces or phagocytosable particles. J. Immunol. 107:1535, 1971.
151. Carter, S.B.: Effects of cytochalasin on mammalian cells. Nature (Lond.) 213:261, 1967.
152. Hartwig, J.H., and Stossel, T.P.: Interactions of actin, myosin, and an actin-binding protein of rabbit pulmonary macrophages. III. Effects of cytochalasin B. J. Cell Biol. 71:295, 1976.
153. Plagemann, P.G.W., and Estensen, R.D.: Cytochalasin B. VI. Competitive inhibition of nucleotide transport by cultured Novikoff rat hepatoma cells. J. Cell Biol. 55:179, 1972.
154. Zigmond, S.H., and Hirsch, J.G.: Effects of cytochalasin B on polymorphonuclear leukocyte locomotion, phagocytosis, and glycolysis. Exp. Cell Res. 73:383, 1972.
155. Becker, E.L.: Some interrelationships of neutrophil chemotaxis, lysosomal enzyme secretion, and phagocytosis as revealed by synthetic peptides. Am. J. Pathol. 85:385, 1976.
156. Goldstein, I., Hoffstein, S., Gallin J., and Weissmann, G.: Mechanisms of lysosomal enzyme release from human leukocytes: microtubule assembly and membrane fusion induced by a component of complement. Proc. Natl. Acad. Sci. USA 70:2916, 1973.
157. Hawkins, D.: Neutrophilic leukocytes in immunologic reactions in vitro. Effect of cytochalasin B. J. Immunol. 110:294, 1973.
158. Stenson, W.F., and Parker, C.W.: Monohydroxyeicosatetraenoic acids (HETEs) induce degranulation of human neutrophils. J. Immunol. 124:2100, 1980.
159. O'Flaherty, J.T., Wykle, R.L., Lees, C.J., Shewmake, T., McCall, C.E., and Thomas, M.J.: Neutrophil degranulating action of 5,12-dihydroxy-6,8,10,14-eicosatetraenoic acid and 1-O-alkyl-2-O-acetyl-sn-glycero-3-phosphocholine. Am. J. Pathol. 105:264, 1981.
160. Estensen, R.D., White, J.G., and Holmes, B.: Specific degranulation of human polymorphonuclear leukocytes. Nature (Lond.) 248:347, 1974.
161. Goldstein, I.M., Hoffstein, S.T., and Weissmann, G.: Mechanisms of lysosomal enzyme release from human polymorphonuclear leukocytes. Effects of phorbol myristate acetate. J. Cell Biol. 66:647, 1975.
162. Goldstein, I.M., Horn, J.K., Kaplan, H.B., and Weissmann, G.: Calcium-induced lysozyme secretion from human polymorphonuclear leukocytes. Biochem. Biophys. Res. Commun. 60:807, 1974.
163. Goldstein, I.M., Hoffstein, S.T., and Weissmann, G.: Influence of divalent cations upon complement-mediated enzyme release from human polymorphonuclear leukocytes. J. Immunol. 115:665, 1975.
164. Hoffstein, S., Soberman, R., Goldstein, I., and Weissmann, G.: Concanavalin A induces microtubule assembly and specific granule discharge in human polymorphonuclear leukocytes. J. Cell Biol. 68:781, 1976.
165. Goldstein, I.M., Cerqueira, M., Lind, S., and Kaplan, H.B.: Evidence that the superoxide generating system of human leukocytes is associated with the cell surface. J. Clin. Invest. 59:249, 1977.
166. Iverson, D., DeChatelet, L.R., Spitznagel, J.K., and Wang, P.: Comparison of NADH and NADPH oxidase activities in granules isolated from human polymorphonuclear leukocytes with a fluorometric assay. J. Clin. Invest. 59:282, 1977.
167. Tauber, A.I., and Goetzl, E.J.: Structural and catalytic properties of the solubilized superoxide-generating activity of human polymorphonuclear leukocytes. I. Solubilization, stabilization in solution, and partial characterization. Biochemistry 18:5576, 1979.
168. Root, R.K., and Metcalf, J.A.: $H_2O_2$ release from human granulocytes during phagocytosis. Relationship to superoxide anion formation and cellular catabolism of $H_2O_2$: studies with normal and cytochalasin B-treated cells. J. Clin. Invest. 60:1266, 1977.
169. Root, R.K., Metcalf, J., Oshino, N., and Chance, B.: $H_2O_2$ release from human granulocytes during phagocytosis. I. Documentation, quantitation, and some regulating factors. J. Clin. Invest. 55:945, 1975.
170. Tauber, A.I., and Babior, B.M.: Evidence for hydroxyl radical production by human neutrophils. J. Clin. Invest. 60:374, 1977.
171. Krinsky, N.I.: Singlet excited oxygen as a mediator of the antibacterial action of leukocytes. Science 186:363, 1974.
172. Root, R.K., and Stossel, T.P.: Myeloperoxidase-mediated iodination by granulocytes. Intracellular site of operation and some regulating factors. J. Clin. Invest. 53:1207, 1974.
173. Klebanoff, S.J.: Iodination of bacteria: a bactericidal mechanism. J. Exp. Med. 126:1063, 1967.
174. Baehner, R.L., Boxer, L.A., and Davis, J.: The biochemical basis of nitroblue tetrazolium reduction in normal human and chronic granulomatous disease polymorphonuclear leukocytes. Blood 48:309, 1976.
175. DeChatelet, L.R.: Oxidative bactericidal mechanisms of polymorphonuclear leukocytes. J. Infect. Dis. 131:295, 1975.
176. Goetzl, E.J., and Austen, K.F.: Stimulation of human neutrophil leukocyte aerobic glucose metabolism by purified chemotactic factors. J. Clin. Invest. 53:591, 1974.
Goldstein, I.M., Kaplan, H.B., Radin, A., and Frosch, M.: Independent effects of IgG and complement upon human polymorphonuclear leukocyte function. J. Immunol. 117:1282, 1976.
178. Kaplan, S.S., Finch, S.C., and Basford, R.E.: Polymorphonuclear leukocyte activation: effects of phospholipase *c*. Proc. Soc. Exp. Biol. Med. 140:540, 1972.

179. DeChatelet, L.R., Shirley, P.S., and Johnston, R.B., Jr.: Effect of phorbol myristate acetate on the oxidative metabolism of human polymorphonuclear leukocytes. Blood. 47:545, 1976.
180. Cohen, H.J., and Chovaniec, M.E.: Superoxide generation by digitonin-stimulated guinea pig granulocytes. A basis for a continuous assay for monitoring superoxide production for the study of the activation of the generating system. J. Clin. Invest. 61:1081, 1978.
181. Salin, M.C., and McCord, J.M.: Superoxide dismutases in polymorphonuclear leukocytes. J. Clin. Invest. 54:1005, 1974.
182. Lynch, R.E., and Fridovich, I.: Effects of superoxide on the erythrocyte membrane. J. Biol. Chem. 253:1838, 1978.
183. Salin, M.C., and McCord, J.M.: Free radicals and inflammation. Protection of phagocytosing leukocytes by superoxide dismutase. J. Clin. Invest. 56:1319, 1975.
184. Sacks, T., Moldow, C.F., Craddock, P.R., Bowers, T.K., and Jacob, H.S.: Oxygen radicals mediate endothelial cell damage by complement-stimulated granulocytes: An in vitro model of immune vascular damage. J. Clin. Invest. 62:1161, 1978.
185. McCord, J.M.: Free radicals and inflammation: protection of synovial fluid by superoxide dismutase. Science 185:529, 1974.
186. Moore, J.S., Phillips, G.O., Davies, J.V., and Dodgson, K.S.: Reactions of connective tissue and related polyanions with hydrated electrons and hydroxyl radicals. Carbohyd. Res. 12:253, 1970.
187. Halliwell, B.: Superoxide-dependent formation of hydroxyl radicals in the presence of iron salts. Its role in degradation of hyaluronic acid by a superoxide-generating system. FEBS Lett. 96:238, 1978.
188. Greenwald, R.A., and Moy, W.W.: Effect of oxygen-derived free radicals on hyaluronic acid. Arthritis Rheum. 23:455, 1980.
189. Puig-Parellada, P., and Planas, J.M.: Synovial fluid degradation induced by free radicals: in vitro action of several free radical scavengers and anti-inflammatory drugs. Biochem. Pharmacol. 27:535, 1978.
190. McCord, J.M., and Fridovich, I.: Superoxide dismutase. An enzymic function for erythrocuprein (hemocuprein). J. Biol. Chem. 244:6049, 1969.
191. Blake, D.R., Hall, N.D., Treby, D.A., Halliwell, B., and Gutteridge, J.M.C.: Protection against superoxide and hydrogen peroxide in synovial fluid from rheumatoid patients. Clin. Sci. 61:483, 1981.
192. Rister, M., and Bauermeister, K.: Superoxide-dismutase and superoxide-radical-release in rheumatoid arthritis. Klin. Wochenschr. 60:561, 1982.
193. Greenwald, R.A., and Moy, W.W.: Inhibition of collagen gelation by action of the superoxide radical. Arthritis Rheum. 22:251, 1979.
194. Venkatasubramanian, K., and Joseph, K.T.: Action of singlet oxygen on collagen. Ind. J. Biochem. Biophys. 14:217, 1977.
195. Carp, H., and Janoff, A.: Potential mediator of inflammation. Phagocyte-derived oxidants suppress the elastase-inhibitory capacity of $\alpha_1$-proteinase inhibitor in vitro. J. Clin. Invest. 66:987, 1980.
196. Johnson, D., and Travis, J.: The oxidative inactivation of human $\alpha$-1-proteinase inhibitor: further evidence for methionine at the reactive center. J. Biol. Chem. 254:4022, 1979.
197. Wong, P.S., and Travis, J.: Isolation and properties of oxidized $\alpha$-1-proteinase inhibitor from human rheumatoid synovial fluid. Biochem. Biophys. Res. Commun. 96:1449, 1980.
198. Tien, M., Svingen, B.A., and Aust, S.D.: An investigation into the role of hydroxyl radical in xanthine oxidase–dependent lipid peroxidation. Arch. Biochem. Biophys. 216:142, 1982.
199. Rawls, H.R., and van Santen, P.J.: A possible role for singlet oxygen in the initiation of fatty acid autooxidation. J. Am. Oil Chem. Soc. 47:121, 1969.
200. Kellogg, E.W. III, and Fridovich, I.: Superoxide, hydrogen peroxide, and singlet oxygen in lipid peroxidation by a xanthine oxidase system. J. Biol. Chem. 250:8812, 1975.
201. Klickstein, L.B., Shapleigh, C., and Goetzl, E.J.: Lipoxygenation of arachidonic acid as a source of polymorphonuclear leukocyte chemotactic factors in synovial fluid and tissue in rheumatoid arthritis and spondyloarthritis. J. Clin. Invest. 66:1166, 1980.
202. Turner, S.R., Campbell, J.A., and Lynn, W.S.: Polymorphonuclear leukocyte chemotaxis toward oxidized lipid components of cell membranes. J. Exp. Med. 141:437, 1975.
203. Perez, H.D., Weksler, B.B., and Goldstein, I.M.: Generation of a chemotactic lipid from arachidonic acid by exposure to a superoxide-generating system. Inflammation 4:313, 1980.
204. Petrone, W.F., English, D.K., Wong, K., and McCord, J.M.: Free radicals and inflammation: superoxide-dependent activation of a neutrophil chemotactic factor in plasma. Proc. Natl. Acad. Sci. USA 77:1159, 1980.
205. Fridovich, I.: Superoxide dismutases. Annu. Rev. Biochem. 44:147, 1975.
206. Huber, W., Schulte, T.L., Carson, S., Goldhamer, R.E., and Vogin, E.E.: Some chemical and pharmacological properties of a novel antiinflammatory protein. Toxicol. Appl. Pharmacol. 12:308, 1968.
207. Huber, W., and Saifer, M.G.P.: Orgotein, the drug version of bovine Cu-Zn superoxide dismutase: I. A summary account of safety and pharmacology in laboratory animals. *In* Michelson, A.M., McCord, J.M., and Fridovich, I. (eds.): Superoxide and Superoxide Dismutases. London, Academic Press, 1977.
208. Oyanagui, Y.: Participation of superoxide anions at the prostaglandin phase of carrageenan foot-oedema. Biochem. Pharmacol. 25:1465, 1976.
209. McCormick, J.R., Harkin, M.M., Johnson, K.J., and Ward, P.A.: Suppression by superoxide dismutase of immune-complex-induced pulmonary alveolitis and dermal inflammation. Am. J. Pathol. 102:55, 1981.
210. Cushing, L.S., Decker, W.E., Santos, F.K., Schutle, T.L., and Huber, W.: Orgotein therapy for inflammation in horses. Mod. Vet. Pact. 54:17, 1973.
211. Breshears, D.E., Brown, C.D., Riffel, D.M., Cobble, R.J., and Cheesman, S.F.: Evaluation of orgotein in treatment of locomotor dysfunction in dogs. Mod. Vet. Pract. 55:85, 1974.
212. Lund-Oleson, K., and Menander, K.B.: Orgotein: a new anti-inflammatory metalloprotein drug: preliminary evaluation of clinical efficacy and safety in degenerative joint disease. Curr. Therap. Res. 16:706, 1974.
213. Rosner, I.A., Goldberg, V.M., Getzy, L., and Moskowitz, R.W.: A trial of intraarticular orgotein, a superoxide dismutase, in experimentally-induced osteoarthritis. J. Rheumatol. 7:24, 1980.
214. Goebel, K.M., Storck, U., and Neurath, F.: Intrasynovial orgotein therapy in rheumatoid arthritis. Lancet 1:1015, 1981.
215. Goldstein, I.M., Roos, D., Weissmann, G., and Kaplan, H.B.: Influence of corticosteroids on human polymorphonuclear leukocyte function in vitro. Reduction of lysosomal enzyme release and superoxide production. Inflammation 1:305, 1976.
216. Lehmeyer, J.E., and Johnston, R.B. Jr.: Effect of anti-inflammatory drugs and agents that elevate intracellular cyclic AMP on the release of toxic oxygen metabolites by phagocytes. Clin. Immunol. Immunopathol. 9:482, 1978.
217. Greenwald, R.A.: Effects of oxygen-derived free radicals on connective tissue macromolecules: inhibition by copper-penicillamine complex. J. Rheumatol. 8:9, 1981.
218. Younes, M., Lengfelder, E., Zienau, S., and Weser, U.: Pulse radiolytically generated superoxide and Cu (II)-salicylates. Biochem. Biophys. Res. Commun. 81:576, 1978.
219. Weinstein, J., and Bielski, B.H.J.: Reaction of superoxide radicals with copper (II)-histidine complexes. J. Am. Chem. Soc. 102:4916, 1980.
220. Sorenson, J.R.J.: Some copper coordination compounds and their anti-inflammatory and antiulcer activities. Inflammation 1:317, 1976.
221. Ohlsson, K.: Neutral leucocyte proteases and elastase inhibited by plasma $\alpha_1$-antitrypsin. Scand. J. Lab. Invest. 28:251, 1971.
222. Janoff, A.: Neutrophil proteases in inflammation. Ann. Rev. Med. 23:177, 1972.
223. Venge, P., Olsson, I., and Odeberg, H.: Cationic proteins of human granulocytes. V. Interaction with plasma protein inhibitors. Scand. J. Lab. Invest. 35:737, 1975.
224. Ohlsson, K., and Olsson, I.: Neutral proteases of human granulocytes. III. Interaction between human granulocyte elastase and plasma protease inhibitors. Scand. J. Clin. Lab. Invest. 34:349, 1974.
225. Wintroub, B.U., Goetzl, E.J., and Austen, K.F.: A neutrophil-dependent pathway for the generation of a neutral peptide mediator: Partial characterization of components and control by $\alpha_1$-antitrypsin. J. Exp. Med. 140:812, 1974.
226. Wintroub, B.U., Klickstein, L.B., and Watt, K.W.K.: A human neutrophil-dependent pathway for generation of angiotensin II. Purification of the product and identification as angiotensin II. J. Clin. Invest. 68:484, 1981.
227. Wintroub, B.U., and Austen, K.F.: Interaction of neutrophil-bound enzymes with plasma protein substrates. *In* Miescher, P.A. (ed.): Immunopathology. Vol. VII. Basel, Schwabe & Company, 1977.
228. Greenbaum, L.M.: Leukocyte kininogenases and leukokinins from normal and malignant cells. Am. J. Pathol. 68:613, 1972.
229. Eriksson, S.: Studies in $\alpha_1$-antitrypsin deficiency. Acta Med. Scand. (Suppl.)432:1, 1965.
230. Eriksson, S., and Larson, C.: Purification and partial characterization of PAS-positive inclusion bodies from the liver in alpha$_1$-antitrypsin deficiency. N. Engl. J. Med. 292:176, 1975.
231. Sjöblom, K.G., and Wolheim, F.A.: $\alpha_1$-Antitrypsin phenotypes and rheumatic diseases. Lancet 2:41, 1977.
232. Jakschik, B.A., Lee, L.N., Shuffer, G., Parker, C.W.: Arachidonic acid metabolism in rat basophilic leukemia (RBL-1) cells. Prostaglandins 16:733, 1978.
233. Payan, D.G., and Goetzl, E.J.: Specific suppression of human T-lymphocyte function by leukotriene $B_4$. J. Immunol. 131:551, 1983.
234. Lewis, R.A., and Austen, K.F.: Mediation of local homeostasis and inflammation by leukotrienes and other mast cell-dependent compounds. Nature 293:103, 1982.
235. Turk, J., Maas, R.L., Brash, A.R., Roberts, L.J., and Oates, J.A.: Arachidonic acid 15-lipoxygenase products from human eosinophils. J. Biol. Chem. 257:7068, 1982.

236. Shak, S., Perez, H.D., Goldyne, M., Gold, W., and Goldstein, I.M.: A novel dioxygenation product of arachidonic acid possesses potent chemotactic activity for human polymorphonuclear leukocytes. Clin. Res. 31:47A, 1983.
237. Hanahan, D.J., Demopoulos, C.A., Liehr, J., and Pinckard, R.N.: Identification of platelet activating factor isolated from rabbit basophils as acetyl glyceryl ether phosphorylcholine. J. Biol. Chem. 255:5514, 1980.
238. McManus, L.M., Morley, C.A., Levine, S.P., and Pinckard, R.N.: Platelet activating factor (PAF) induced release of platelet factor 4 (PF4) in vitro and during IgE anaphylaxis in the rabbit. J. Immunol. 123:2835, 1979.
239. Osler, A.G., Lichtenstein, L.M., and Levy, D.A.: In vitro studies of human reaginic allergy. Adv. Immunol. 8:183, 1968.
240. Siraganian, R.P., and Hook, W.A.: Complement-induced histamine release from human basophils. II. Mechanisms of the histamine release reaction. J. Immunol. 116:639, 1976.
241. Brindley, L.L., Sweet, J.M., and Goetzl, E.J.: Stimulation of histamine release from human basophils by human platelet factor 4. J. Clin. Invest. 72:1218, 1983.
242. Goetzl, E.J.: Mast cell-mediated reactions of host defense and tissue injury: The regulatory role of epsinophil polymorphonuclear leukocytes. Inflammation 2:239, 1977.
243. Lichtenstein, L.M., and Gillespie, E.: Inhibition of histamine release by histamine is controlled by an $H_2$ receptor. Nature 244:287, 1973.
244. Lichtenstein, L.M., and Margolis, S.: Histamine release in vitro: Inhibition by catecholamines and methylxanthines. Science 161:902, 1968.
245. Dvorak, A.M., Mihm, M.C., Jr., and Dvorak, H.F.: Degranulation of basophilic leukocytes in allergic contact dermatitis reactions in man. J. Immunol. 116:687, 1976.
246. Olsson, I., Berg, B., Fransson, L.A., and Norden, A.: The identity of the metachromatic substance of basophilic leukocytes. Scand. J. Haematol. 7:440, 1970.
247. Lewis, R.A., Goetzl, E.J., Wasserman, S.I., Valone, F.H., Rubin, R.H., and Austen, K.F.: The release of four mediators of immediate hypersensitivity from human leukemic basophils. J. Immunol. 114:87, 1975.
248. Benveniste, J., Henson, P.H., and Cochrane, C.G.: Leukocyte-dependent histamine release from rabbit platelets. J. Exp. Med. 136:1365, 1972.
249. Czarnetski, B.M., König, W., and Lichtenstein, L.M.: Antigen-induced eosinophil chemotactic factor (ECF) release by human leukocytes. Inflammation 1:201, 1976.
250. Orenstein, N.S., Hammand, M.E., Dvorak, H.F., and Feder, J.: Esterase and protease activity of purified guinea pig basophil granules. Biochem. Biophys. Res. Commun. 72:230, 1976.
251. Payan, D.G., Goldman, D.W. and Goetzl, E.J.: Biochemical and cellular characteristics of the regulation of human leukocyte function by lipoxygenase products of arachidonic acid. *In* Chakrin, L.W., and Bailey, D.M., (eds.): Biochemical and Cellular Characteristics of the Regulation of Human Leukocyte Function by Lipoxygenase Products of Arachidonic Acid. New York, Academic Press, Inc., in press.
252. Benveniste, J.: Platelet activating factor, a new mediator of anaphylaxis and immune complex deposition from human and rabbit basophils. Nature 249:581, 1974.
253. Kater, L.A., Goetzl, E.J., and Austen, K.F.: Isolation of human eosinophil phospholipase D. J. Clin. Invest. 57:1173, 1976.
254. Czarnetski, B., König, W., and Lichtenstein, L.M.: Eosinophil chemotactic factor (ECF). I. Release from polymorphonuclear leukocytes by the calcium inophore A23187. J. Immunol. 117:229, 1976.
255. Richerson, H.A., Dvorak, H.F., and Leskowitz, S.: Cutaneous basophil hypersensitivity. I. A new look at the Jones-Mote reaction, general characteristics. J. Exp. Med. 132:546, 1970.
256. Dvorak, H.F., and Dvorak, A.M.: Cutaneous basophil hypersensitivity. *In* Brent, L., and Holborow, J. (eds.): Progress in Immunology II, Vol. 3. Amsterdam, North-Holland Publishing Company, 1974.
257. Bast, R.C., Jr., Simpson, B.A., and Dvorak, H.F.: Heterogeneity of the cellular immune response. II. The role of adjuvant. Lymphocyte stimulation in cutaneous basophil hypersensitivity. J. Exp. Med. 133:202, 1971.
258. Cochrane, C.G., and Koffler, D.: Immune complex disease in experimental animals. Adv. Immunol. 16:185, 1973.
259. Stossel, T.P.: Phagocytosis. N. Engl. J. Med. 290:717, 774, 833, 1974.
260. Quie, P.G., and Cates, K.L.: Chemical conditions associated with defective polymorphonuclear leukocyte chemotaxis. Am. J. Pathol. 88:711, 1977.
261. Clark, R.A.: Disorders of granulocyte chemotaxis. *In* Gallin, J.I., and Quie, P.G. (eds.): Leukocyte Chemotaxis: Methods, Physiology, and Clinical Implications. New York, Raven Press, 1978.
262. Oliver, J.M., and Zurier, R.B.: Correction of characteristic abnormalities of microtubule function and granule morphology in Chédiak-Higashi syndrome with cholinergic agonists. J. Clin. Invest. 57:1239, 1976.
263. Pike, M.C., Daniels, C.A., and Snyderman, R.: Influenza induced depression of monocyte chemotaxis: Reversal by levamisole. Cell. Immunol. 32:234, 1977.
264. Goetzl, E.J.: Defective responsiveness to ascorbic acid of neutrophil random and chemotactic migration in Felty's syndrome and systemic lupus erythematosus. Ann. Rheum. Dis. 35:510, 1976.
265. Hurd, E.R., Andreis, and Ziff, M.: Phagocytosis of immune complexes by polymorphonuclear leukocytes in patients with Felty's syndrome. Clin. Exp. Immunol. 28:413, 1977.
266. Clark, R.A., Kimball, H.R., and Decker, J.L.: Neutrophil chemotaxis in systemic lupus erythematosus. Ann. Rheum. Dis. 33:167, 1974.
267. Perez, H.D., and Goldstein, I.M.: Infection and host defenses in systemic lupus erythematosus. In Franklin, E.C. (ed.): Clinical Immunology Update. New York, Elsevier, 1979.
268. Staples, P.J., Gerding, D.N., Decker, J.L., and Gordon, R.S.: Incidence of infection in systemic lupus erythematosus. Arthritis Rheum. 17:1, 1974.
269. Landry, M.: Phagocyte function and cell-mediated immunity in systemic lupus erythematosus. Arch. Dermatol. 113:147, 1977.
270. Perez, H.D., Lipton, M., and Goldstein, I.M.: A specific inhibitor of complement (C5)-derived chemotactic activity in serum from patients with systemic lupus erythematosus. J. Clin. Invest. 62:29, 1978.
271. Perez, H.D., Goldstein, I.M., Chernoff, D., Webster, R.O., and Henson, P.M.: Chemotactic activity of C5a des Arg: evidence of a requirement for an anionic peptide "helper factor" and inhibition by a cationic protein in serum from patients with systemic lupus erythematosus. Mole. Immunol. 17:163, 1980.
272. Perez, H.D., Goldstein, I.M., Webster, R.O., and Henson, P.M.: Enhancement of the chemotactic activity of human C5a des Arg by an anionic polypeptide ("cochemotaxin") in normal human serum and plasma. J. Immunol. 126:800, 1981.
273. Perez, H.D., Andron, R.I., and Goldstein, I.M.: Infection in patients with systemic lupus erythematosus. Association with a serum inhibitor of complement-derived chemotactic activity. Arthritis Rheum. 22:1326, 1979.
274. Brandt, L., and Hedberg, H.: Impaired phagocytosis by peripheral blood granulocytes in systemic lupus erythematosus. Scand. J. Haematol. 6:348, 1969.
275. Zurier, R.B.: Reduction of phagocytosis and lysosomal enzyme release from human leukocytes by serum from patients with systemic lupus erythematosus. Arthritis Rheum. 19:73, 1976.
276. Temple, A., and Loewi, G.: The effect of sera from patients with connective tissue diseases on red cell binding and phagocytosis by monocytes. Immunology 33:109, 1977.
277. Frank, M.M., Hamburger, M.I., Lawley, T.J., Kimberly, R.P., and Plotz, P.H.: Defective reticuloendothelial system Fc-receptor function in systemic lupus erythematosus. N. Engl. J. Med. 300:518, 1979.
278. Iida, K., Mornaghi, R., and Nussenzweig, V.: Complement receptor ($CR_1$) deficiency in erythrocytes from patients with systemic lupus erythematosus. J. Exp. Med. 155:1427, 1982.
279. Miyakawa, Y., Yamada, A., Kosaka, K., Tsuda, F., Kosugi, E., and Mayumi, M.: Defective immune-adherence (C3b) receptor on erythrocytes from patients with systemic lupus erythematosus. Lancet 2:493, 1981.
280. Wilson, J.G., Wong, W.W., Schur, P.H., and Fearon, D.T.: Mode of inheritance of decreased C3b receptors on erythrocytes of patients with systemic lupus erythematosus. N. Engl. J. Med. 307:981, 1982.
281. Wenger, M.E., and Bole, G.G.: Nitroblue tetrazolium dye reduction by peripheral blood leukocytes from rheumatoid arthritis and systemic lupus erythematosus patients measured by a histochemical and spectrophotometric method. J. Lab. Clin. Med. 82:513, 1973.
282. Baum, J.: Infection in rheumatoid arthritis. Arthritis Rheum. 14:135, 1971.
283. Mowat, A.G., and Baum, J.: Chemotaxis of polymorphonuclear leukocytes from patients with rheumatoid arthritis. J. Clin. Invest. 50:2541, 1971.
284. Hallgren, R., Hakansson, L., and Venge, P.: Kinetic studies of phagocytosis. I. The serum independent particle uptake by PMN from patients with rheumatoid arthritis and systemic lupus erythematosus. Arthritis Rheum. 21:107, 1978.
285. Attia, W.M., Clark, H.W., Brown, T.M., Ali, M.K.H., and Bellanti, J.A.: Inhibition of polymorphonuclear leukocyte migration by sera of patients with rheumatoid arthritis. Ann. Allergy 48:21, 1982.
286. Kemp, A.S., Roberts-Thomson, P., Neoh, S.H., and Brown, S.: Inhibition of neutrophil migration by sera from patients with rheumatoid arthritis. Clin. Exp. Immunol. 36:423, 1979.
287. Attia, W.M., Shams, A.H., Ali, M.K.H., Clark, H.W., Brown, T.M., and Bellanti, J.A.: Studies of phagocytic cell function in rheumatoid arthritis. I. Phagocytic and metabolic abnormalities of neutrophils. Ann. Allergy 48:279, 1982.
288. Attia, W.M., Shams, A.H., Ali, M.K.H., Jang, L.W., Clark, H.W., Brown, T.M., and Bellanti, J.A.: Studies of phagocytic cell functions in rheumatoid arthritis. II. Effects of serum factors on phagocytic and metabolic activities of neutrophils. Ann. Allergy 48:283, 1982.
289. Turner, R.A., Schumacher, H.R., and Myers, A.R.: Phagocytic function

of polymorphonuclear leukocytes in rheumatic diseases. J. Clin. Invest. 52:1632, 1973.

290. Bodel, P.T., and Hollingsworth, J.W.: Comparative morphology, respiration and phagocytic function of leucocytes from blood and joint fluid in rheumatoid arthritis. J. Clin. Invest. 45:580, 1966.
291. Kemp, A.S., Brown, S., Brooks, P.M., and Neoh, S.H.: Migration of blood and synovial fluid neutrophils obtained from patients with rheumatoid arthritis. Clin. Exp. Immunol. 39:240, 1980.
292. Karten, I.:Septic arthritis complicating rheumatoid arthritis. Ann. Intern. Med. 70:1147, 1969.
293. Zivkovic, M., and Baum, J.: Chemotaxis of polymorphonuclear leukocytes from patients with systemic lupus erythematosus and Felty's syndrome. Immunol. Commun. 1:39, 1972.
294. Gupta, R.C., Laforce, F.M., and Mills, D.M.: Polymorphonuclear leukocyte inclusions and impaired bacterial killing in patients with Felty's syndrome. J. Lab. Clin. Med. 88:183, 1976.
295. Ruderman, M., Miller, L.M., and Pinals, R.S.: Clinical and serologic observations on 27 patients with Felty's syndrome. Arthritis Rheum. 11:37, 1968.
296. Walker, J.R., Smith, M.J.H., and James D.W.: A comparison of two *in vitro* methods for studying a defect in leucocyte movement in rheumatoid arthritis. Int. Arch. Allergy Appl. Immunol. 59:343, 1979.
297. Hanlon, S.M., Panayi, G.S., and Laurent, R.: Defective polymorphonuclear leucocyte chemotaxis in rheumatoid arthritis associated with a serum inhibitor. Ann. Rheum. Dis. 39:68, 1980.
298. van de Stadt, R.J., van de Voorde-Vissers, E., and Feltkamp-Vroom, T.M.: Metabolic and secretory properties of peripheral and synovial granulocytes in rheumatoid arthritis. Arthritis Rheum. 23:17, 1980.
299. Trung, P.H., Prieur, A.M., and Griscelli, C.: Neutrophil chemotaxis in juvenile chronic arthritis. Ann. Rheum. Dis. 39:481, 1980.
300. Djawari, D., Hornstein, O.P., and Schotz, J.: Enhancement of granulocyte chemotaxis in Behçet's disease. Arch. Dermatol. Res. 270:81, 1981.
301. Mowat, A.G.: Neutrophil chemotaxis in ankylosing spondylitis, Reiter's disease, and polymyalgia rheumatica. Ann. Rheum. Dis. 37:9, 1978.
302. Leirisalo, M., Repo, H., Tiilikainen, A., Kosunen, T.U., and Laitinen, O.: Chemotaxis in yersinia arthritis. HLA-B27 positive neutrophils show high stimulated motility in vitro. Arthritis Rheum. 23:1036, 1980.
303. Day, N.K., Gieger, H., Stroud, R., DeBracco, M., Manacado, B., Windhorst, D., and Good, R.A.: Cr deficiency: An inborn error associated with cutaneous and renal disease. J. Clin. Invest. 51:1102, 1972.
304. Glass, D., Raum, D., Stillman, J.S., and Schur, P.H.: Inherited deficiency of the second component of complement. Rheumatic disease associations. J. Clin. Invest. 58:853, 1976.
305. Rosenfeld, S.I., Kelly, M.D., and Leddy, J.P.: Hereditary deficiency of the fifth component of complement in man. I. Clinical, immunochemical and family studies. J. Clin. Invest. 57:1626, 1976.
306. Wellek, B., and Opferkuch, W.: A case of deficiency of the seventh component of complement in man. Clin. Exp. Immunol. 19:223, 1975.
307. Ballow, M., Shira, J.E., Harden, Yang, S.Y., and Day, N.K.: Complete absence of the third component of complement in man. J. Clin. Invest. 56:703, 1975.
308. Altman, L.C., Snyderman, R., and Blaese, R.M.: Abnormalities of chemotactic lymphokine synthesis and mononuclear leukocyte chemotaxis in Wiskott-Aldrich syndrome. J. Clin. Invest. 54:486, 1974.
309. Maderazo, E.G., Ward, P.A., Woronick, C.L., Kubik, J., and DeGraff, A.C.: Leukotactic dysfunction in sarcoidosis. Ann. Intern. Med. 84:414, 1976.
310. Ward, P.A., Goralnick, S., and Bullock, W.E.: Defective leukotaxis in patients with lepromatous leprosy. J. Lab. Clin. Med. 87:1025, 1976.
311. Gewurz, H., Page, A.R., Pickering, R.J., and Good, R.A.: Complement activity and inflammatory neutrophil exudation in man. Int. Arch. Allergy Appl. Immunol. 32:64, 1967.
312. Ward, P.A., and Schlegel, R.A.: Impaired leucotactic responsiveness in a child with recurrent infections. Lancet 2:344, 1969.
313. Van Epps, D.E., and Williams, R.C., Jr.: Suppression of leukocyte chemotaxis by human IgA myeloma components. J. Exp. Med. 144:1227, 1976.
314. Hill, H.R., Gerrard, J.M., Hogan, N.A., and Quie, P.G.: Hyperactivity of neutrophil leukotactic responses during active bacterial infection. J. Clin. Invest. 53:996, 1974.
315. Soter, N.A., Wasserman, S.I., and Austen, K.F.: Cold urticaria: Release into the circulation of histamine and eosinophil chemotactic factor of anaphylaxis during cold challenge. N. Engl. J. Med. 294:687, 1976.
316. Wintroub, B.U., Mihm, M.C., Jr., Goetzl, E.J., Soter, N.A., and Austen, K.F.: Morphologic and functional evidence for the release of mast cell products in bullous pemphigoid. N. Engl. J. Med. 298:417, 1978.
317. Ward, P.A., and Talamo, R.C.: Deficiency of the chemotactic factor inactivator in human sera with $\alpha_1$-antitrypsin deficiency. J. Clin. Invest. 52:516, 1973.
318. Stevenson, R.D.: Effect of steroid therapy on in vitro polymorph migration. Clin. Exp. Immunol. 23:285, 1976.
319. Jacobs, J.C., and Goetzl, E.J.: "Streaking leukocyte factor," arthritis, and pyoderma gangrenosum. Pediatrics 56:570, 1975.
320. Ward, P.A.: Leukotactic factors in health and disease. Am. J. Pathol. 64:521, 1971.
321. Ward, P.A., and Hill, J.H.: C5 chemotactic fragments produced by an enzyme in lysosomal granules of neutrophils J. Immunol. 104:535, 1970.
322. Hill, J.H., and Ward, P.A.: C3 leukotactic factors produced by a tissue protease. J. Exp. Med. 103:505, 1969.
323. Hammarstrom, S., Hamberg, M., Samuelsson, B., Duell, E.A., Stawiski, M., and Voorhees, J.J.: Increased concentration of nonesterified arachidonic acid. 12L-hydroxy-5,8,10,14-eicosatetraenoic acid, prostaglandin $E_2$ and prostaglandin $F_{2\alpha}$ in epidermis of psoriasis. Proc. Natl. Acad. Sci. USA 72:5130, 1975.
324. Jagani, H., and Ofugi, S.: Characterization of a leukotactic factor derived from psoriatic scale. Br. J. Dermatol. 97:509, 1977.
325. Lazarus, G.S., Yost, F.J., Jr., and Thomas, C.A.: Polymorphonuclear leukocytes: Possible mechanism of accumulation in psoriasis. Science 198:1162, 1977.
326. Spilberg, I., Gallacher, A., Mehta, J.M., and Mandell, B.: Urate crystal induced chemotactic factor: Isolation and partial characterization. J. Clin. Invest. 58:815, 1976.
327 Spilberg, I., Gallacher, A., Mandell, B., and Rosenberg, D.: A mechanism of action for non-steroidal anti-inflammatory agents in calcium pyrophosphate dihydrate (CPPD) crystal induced arthritis. Agents Actions 7:153, 1977.
328. Dolovich, J., Hargreave, F.E., Chalmers, R., Shier, K.J., Gauldie, J., and Bienenstock, J.: Late cutaneous allergic responses in isolated IgE-dependent reactions. J. Allergy Clin. Immunol. 49:43, 1972.
329. Hargreave, F.E., and Pepys, J.: Allergic respiratory reactions in bird fanciers provoked by allergen inhalation provocation test. Relation to clinical features and allergic mechanism. J. Allergy Clin. Immunol. 50:157, 1973.
330. Klebanoff, S.J., Jong, E.C., and Henderson, Jr., W.R.: The eosinophil peroxidase: Purification and biologic properties. *In* Mahmoud, A.F., and Austen, K.F. (eds.): The Eosinophil in Health and Disease, New York, Grune & Stratton, 1980.
331. Weller, P.F., Goetzl, E.J., and Austen, K.F.: Identification of human eosinophil lysophospholipase as the constituent of Charcot-Leyden crystals. Proc. Natl. Acad. Sci. 77:7440, 1980.
332. Gleich, G.J., Loegering, D.A., Mann, K.G., and Maldonado, J.E.: Comparative properties of the Charcot-Leyden crystal protein and the major basic protein from human eosinophils. J. Clin. Invest. 57:633, 1976.
333. Olsson, I., Venge, P., Spitznagel, J.K., and Lehrer, R.I.: Arginine-rich cationic proteins of human eosinophil granules. Comparison of the constituents of eosinophilic and neutrophilic leukocytes. Lab. Invest. 36:493, 1977.
334. Venge, P., Dahl, R., Fredens, K., Hällgren, R., and Peterson, C.: Eosinophil cationic proteins (ECP and EPX) in health and disease. *In* Yoshida, T., and Torisu, M., (eds.): Immunobiology of the Eosinophil, New York, Elsevier Science Publishing Co., Inc., 1983.
335. Zeiger, R.S., Yurdin, D.L., and Colten, H.R.: Histamine metabolism. II. Cellular and subcellular localization of the catabolic enzymes, histaminase and histamine methyl transferase in human leukocytes. J. Allergy Clin. Immunol. 58:172, 1976.
336. Goetzl, E.J.: The conversion of leukotriene $C_4$ to isomers of leukotriene $B_4$ by human eosinophil peroxidase. Biochem. Biophys. Res. Commun. 106:270, 1982.
337. Welsh, R.A., and Geer, J.C.: Phagocytosis of mast cell granules by the eosinophilic leukocyte in the rat. Am. J. Pathol. 35:103, 1959.
338. Yurt, R.W., and Austen, K.F.: Cascade events in mast cell activation and function. *In* Lepow, I. (ed.): Proteolysis, Demineralization and Other Degradative Processes. New York, Academic Press, 1978.
339. Litt, M.: Studies in experimental eosinophilia. VII. Eosinophils in lymph nodes during the first 24 hours following primary antigenic stimulation. J. Immunol. 93:807, 1964.
340. Butterworth, A.E., David, J.R., Franks, D., Mahmoud, A.A.F., David, R.H., Sturrack, R.F., and Houba, V.: Antibody-dependent eosinophil-mediated damage to $^{51}Cr$ labeled schistosomula of *Schistosoma mansoni*: Damage by purified eosinophils. J. Exp. Med. 145:136, 1977.
341. James, S.L., and Colley, D.G.: Eosinophil-mediated destruction of *Schistosoma mansoni* eggs. J. Reticuloendothel. Soc. 20:359, 1976.
342. Mahmoud, A.A.F., Warren, K.S., and Peters, P.A.: A role for the eosinophil in acquired resistance to *Schistosoma mansoni* infection as determined by anti-eosinophil serum. J. Exp. Med. 142:805, 1975.
343. Tauber, A.I., Goetzl, E.J., and Babior, B.M.: Unique characteristics of superoxide production by human eosinophils in eosinophilic states. Inflammation 3:261, 1979.
344. Goetzl, E.J., Wasserman, S.I., and Austen, K.F.: Eosinophil polymorphonuclear leukocyte function in immediate hypersensitivity. Arch. Pathol. 99:1, 1975.
345. Ansari, A., and Williams, J.F.: The eosinophilic response of the rat to infection with *Taenia taeniaeformis*. J. Parasitol. 62:728, 1976.

346. Gelfand, M., and Bernberg, H.: Tropical eosinophilic syndrome: A clinical description of the disorder as seen in S. Rhodesia. Cent. Afr. J. Med. 5:405, 1959.
347. Lowell, F.C.: Clinical aspects of eosinophilia in atopic disease. JAMA 202:875, 1967.
348. Zolov, D.M., and Levine, B.B.: Correlation of blood eosinophilia with antibody classes. Int. Arch. Allergy 35:179, 1969.
349. Hardy, W.R., and Anderson, R.E.: The hypereosinophilic syndromes. Ann. Intern. Med. 68:1220, 1968.
350. Chusid, M.J., Dale, D.C., West, B.C., and Wolff, S.M.: The hypereosinophilic syndrome: Analysis of fourteen cases with review of the literature. Medicine 54:1, 1975.
351. Zucker-Franklin, D.: Eosinophil function and disorders. Adv. Intern. Med. 19:1, 1974.
352. Brockington, T.F., and Olsen, E.G.J.: Löffler's endocarditis and Davies' endomyocardial fibrosis. Am. Heart J. 85:308, 1973.
353. Crofton, J.W., and Douglas, A.C.: Pulmonary eosinophilia, polyarteritis nodosa, and Wegener's granulomatosis. *In* Crofton, J.W., and Douglas, A.C. (eds.): Respiratory Diseases. Oxford, Blackwell Scientific Publications, 1969.
354. Goetzl, E.J., Tashjian, A.H., Jr., Rubin, R.H., and Austen, K.F.: Production of a low molecular weight eosinophil polymorphonuclear leukocyte chemotactic factor by anaplastic squamous cell carcinomas of human lung. J. Clin. Invest. 61:770, 1978.
355. Kelenyi, G., Nemeth, A., Istvan, L., and Mohay, A.: Effect of corticosteroids on eosinophil leukocytes in hypereosinophilic syndromes. Acta Haematol. 49:235, 1973.
356. Parrillo, J.E., Fauci, A.S., and Wolff, S.M.: The hypereosinophilic syndrome: Dramatic response to therapeutic intervention. Trans. Am. Assoc. Physicians 90:135, 1977.
357. Panush, R.S., Franco, A.E., and Schur, P.H.: Rheumatoid arthritis associated with eosinophilia. Ann. Intern. Med. 75:199, 1971.
358. Shulman, L.E.: Diffuse fasciitis with eosinophilia: A new syndrome. Trans. Am. Assoc. Physicians 88:80, 1975.

# Chapter 10

# Cellular Components of Inflammation: Monocytes and Macrophages

*Carl F. Nathan and Zanvil A. Cohn*

## INTRODUCTION

Metchnikoff discovered phagocytosis in 1880, and soon thereafter designated one type of large phagocyte the macrophage.[1] A century later, phagocytosis remains central to our understanding of the physiology of this cell. Indeed, phagocytosis by macrophages is crucial to survival of the organism, for such diverse functions as remodeling tissue during normal growth and wound healing, clearance of senescent erythrocytes and neutrophils, and destruction of invading microbes.

Nonetheless, after 80 years in which phagocytosis received most of the attention in investigations on macrophages, the last 20 years have introduced entirely new concepts of macrophage function. First, it has become clear that the ability of macrophages to secrete soluble factors is as important as their ability to ingest particulates. Macrophage secretory products are more numerous and diverse in composition and function than those known for any other cell of the immune system. They endow the macrophage with the capacity to exert potent effects of both pro- and anti-inflammatory nature and to regulate the function of other cells. Prominent among these secretory factors are hydrolytic enzymes, products of oxidative metabolism (the reactive oxygen intermediates and the oxygenated derivatives of arachidonic acid), and the protein interleukin-1, which affects lymphocytes, hepatocytes, fibroblasts, synoviocytes, and cells in the hypothalamus.

Second, the classical notion that macrophages are involved in delayed-type hypersensitivity remains valid but too restrictive; macrophages have the capacity to participate in immediate hypersensitivity reactions as well. Third, the distribution of macrophages in pathologic sites is broader than earlier believed. It is now appreciated that macrophages are prominent not only in granulomas but also in the lesions of atherosclerosis and glomerulonephritis. Macrophages line not only the hepatic and splenic sinusoids but also the renal tubules and the surfaces of bone.

Other recent advances include the identification of molecules secreted by lymphocytes that regulate macrophage function, and the definition of mechanisms by which macrophages kill other cells, both microbial and mammalian. Sharper tools, especially monoclonal antibodies, have allowed us to dissect away from macrophages some of the functions to which they once laid exclusive claim, such as initiating T lymphocyte activation, a role now known to belong primarily to dendritic cells. Monoclonal antibodies and related techniques are throwing the macrophage surface into a relief of ligand-binding receptors and differentiation antigens. The function of purified receptors is under analysis at the biophysical level. Finally, for the first time since Metchnikoff observed phagocytosis in the starfish, studies of the macrophages of man now rival reports on cells from laboratory animals.

What follows is a brief summary of macrophage ontogeny, structure, and function. Many facts and citations in an enormous literature have been omitted. The reader seeking these will have to turn both to older books[2-7] and to the most recent volumes of journals of immunology, cell biology, biochemistry, pathology, and medicine.

## THE LIFE CYCLE OF MONONUCLEAR PHAGOCYTES

When colloidal dyes are injected intravenously, they are taken up by histiocytes, fibrocytes, and endothelial cells. Beginning with Aschoff in the 1920s, histologists grouped such cells together as the reticuloendothelial system (RES). In 1970, however, appreciation that the RES comprises cells of different lineages led to a more restricted definition of the mononuclear phagocyte system, based on appropriate morphology, an avid phagocytic capacity for antibody-coated particles, and a common origin in the bone marrow.[8] The cells that make up the mononuclear phagocyte system are listed in Table 10–1. In the 1980s, there has been a return to staining patterns in tissues as an aid in identifying mononuclear phagocytes. This time, however, the stains are not colloidal dyes, but reagents that detect monoclonal antibodies binding specifically to macrophages in tissue sections. Such techniques are continuing to yield new information about the distribution of macrophages in normal and inflamed organs.[9,10]

**The Marrow Progenitors.** Monocytes arise from precursors in the bone marrow.[11,12] It is not yet certain whether there is a separate or shared stem cell for monocytes and granulocytes. Murine monoblasts grown in liquid culture appear as round cells, 10 to 12 microns in diameter, with a small rim of basophilic cytoplasm containing few granules. Like their progeny, monoblasts ruffle their membranes, adhere to glass, phagocytize, display Fc receptors, and stain positively for nonspecific esterase and peroxidase. Murine monoblasts divide once, giving rise to two promonocytes, with a cycle time of about 12 hours.[13,14]

Compared to the monoblast, the murine promonocyte is larger (14 to 20 microns), with an indented nucleus and more vigorous phagocytic activity. Its pool size ($5 \times 10^5$) is only twice that of the monoblast, representing 0.25 percent of nucleated marrow cells. Its cycle time is about 16 hours.[13,15,16] In man, promonocytes represent some 2.9 percent of nucleated marrow cells, with a pool size of $6 \times 10^8$ per kg.[17-21]

**The Circulating Monocyte.** In contrast to neutrophils, the marrow reserve of preformed monocytes is small. Just 2 hours (in the mouse)[22] or 19 to 60 hours (in man)[18,19] after they are formed, monocytes are released in G1 phase[18] into the blood, where they circulate with a half-life of 22 hours in the mouse[16] and from 8 to 71 hours in man.[18,20] Monocytes leave the circulating pool at random[16] by marginating in capillaries, the marginating pool being some 3.5 times the size of the circulating pool.[21] Monocytes emigrate[23] into an extravascular pool, which is vast compared to that in the blood[24] and from which re-entry into the blood is rare.[19]

During inflammation, monocyte production is increased by several adaptations. The promonocyte pool expands, the proportion of promonocytes in cycle increases, the promonocyte cycle time decreases, and monocytes are released into the circulation more promptly after their formation. In this manner, the monocyte birth rate may increase 2- to 4-fold within 12 to 15 hours of an inflammatory stimulus.[16,25]

Thus, compared to granulocytes, monocytes have a much smaller marrow reserve, a more limited capacity to augment production under stress, a longer intravascular half-life, and a relatively larger extravascular compartment. During experimentally induced inflammation, up to 70 percent of the marrow production of monocytes may emigrate to the inflamed site, so that there may be insufficient reserve to supply subsequent inflammatory foci.

In culture, monocytes increase in size, display more mitochondria and lysosomes, and develop enhanced receptor-mediated phagocytic activity and diminished production of reactive oxygen intermediates, thereby coming to resemble tissue macrophages.[26-31]

**The Tissue Macrophage.** Tissue macrophages arise in two ways: by emigration from the blood and by proliferation of precursors in local sites. The relative predominance of these two sources in the steady state is difficult to establish, since the cells that proliferate locally themselves arise in the marrow. Most studies favor a primarily hematopoietic origin not only for peritoneal macrophages[23,32,33] but also for those of skin,[34] lung,[35] liver,[36,37] and brain.[38] In the mouse in the normal steady state, 56 percent of blood monocytes settle in the liver as Kupffer cells, 15 percent exit to the pulmonary alveoli, 8 percent emigrate into the peritoneal cavity, and 21 percent distribute to other tissues.[39]

With local inflammation, both the influx of blood monocytes and the local proliferation of tissue precursors may increase dramatically.[12,40-43] In chronic inflammatory foci, granulomas arise with both local replication and hematogenous replenishment of their constituent cells,[44,45] sometimes with a high turnover, as in tuberculous lesions. During long-term culture, monocyte-derived macrophages take on the appearance of "epithelioid cells," with a decreased vacuolar apparatus (suggesting less endocytic activity) and increased rough endoplasmic reticulum (suggesting increased secretory activity).[26,44,46] During prolonged culture, monocyte-derived macrophages also fuse to form multinucleated giant cells.[26,46,47] Giant cell formation is augmented by mediators from antigen- or mitogen-stimulated lymphocytes.[47] Epithelioid cells and multinucleated giant cells arising from monocytes in vitro closely resemble the mononuclear phagocytes of granulomas.[48]

In the tissues, in response to lymphocyte mediators and complement components, macrophages may become "activated," a process leading to dramatic structural and functional changes, of which over 50 have been enumerated. Macrophage activation is discussed more fully at the end of this chapter.

In rodents in the steady state, the turnover time of

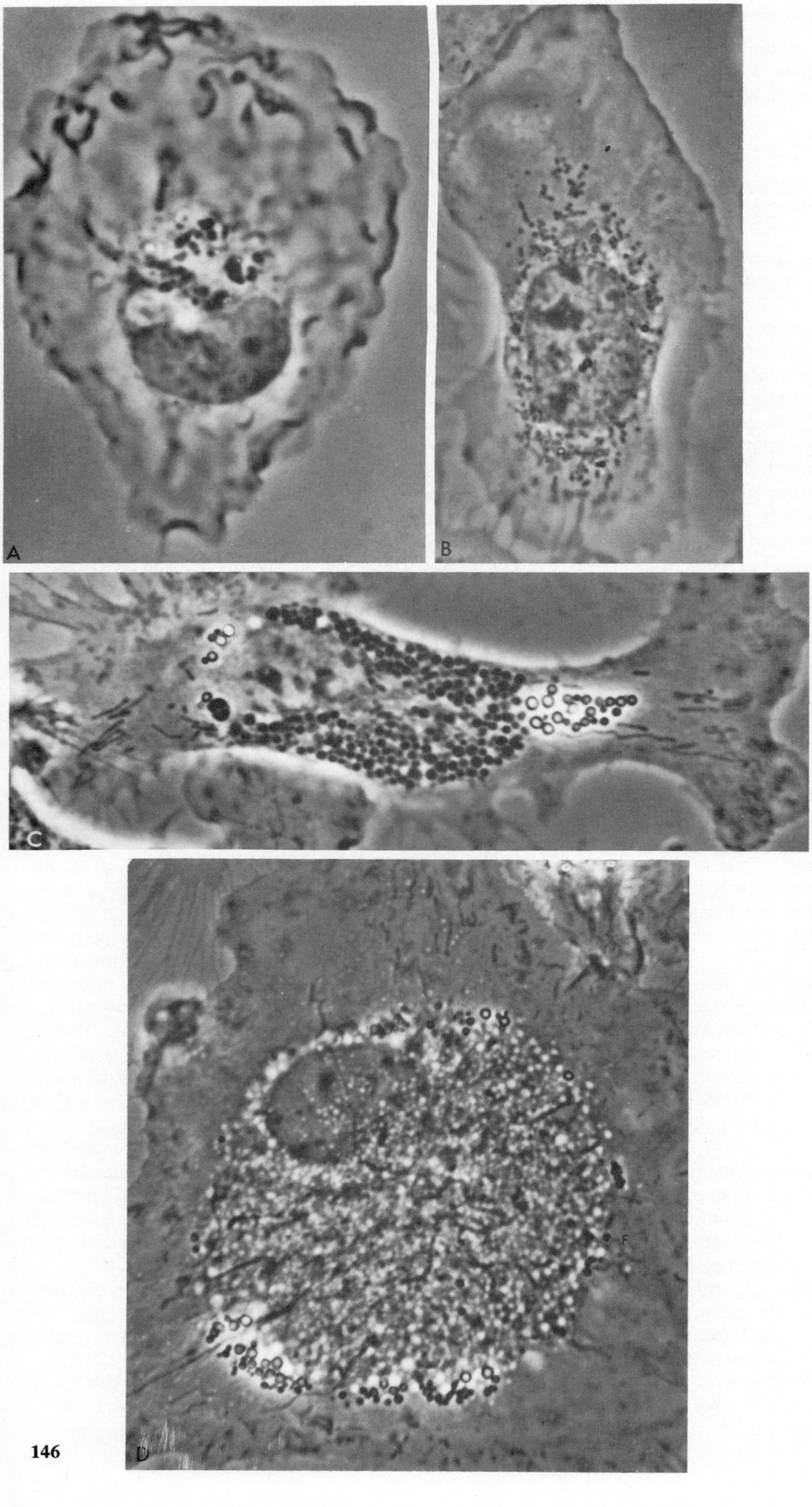


**Figure 10–1.** The morphologic heterogeneity of mononuclear phagocyte populations. Phase contrast × 2000. *A*, Human blood monocyte shortly after isolation and attachment to glass substrate. The reniform nucleus, small numbers of phase dense lysosomes in the nuclear "hof," and ruffled peripheral membrane are all typical of this class of cell. *B*, Resident macrophage obtained from the unstimulated peritoneal cavity of the mouse. The cell has spread on its substrate and in many ways is similar to the blood monocyte. The short, dense organelles surrounding the nucleus are largely mitochondria. *C*, A serous cavity macrophage which has accumulated large numbers of phase dense lysosomes. These are relatively uniform in size as a consequence of their pinocytic origin. Macrophages which interiorize large particles, such as the alveolar cell, exhibit a much more heterogeneous array. *D*, A macrophage obtained from an inflamed peritoneum some days after the acute insult. This cell is larger in size, and exhibits an extensive perinuclear vacuolar apparatus filled with endocytic vesicles and phagolysosomes.

**Table 10–1.** Mononuclear Phagocytes: Pools and Populations*

| Bone Marrow | Blood | Tissue (Resident Populations) |
|---|---|---|
| Multipotential stem cell | Monocyte | Bone (osteoclasts)? |
| Committed stem cell | | Bone marrow |
| Monoblast } | | CNS (CSF, microglia?) |
| Promonocyte } ~ $10^6$ | | Liver (Kupffer cell) |
| Monocyte } | | Lung (Alveolar macrophage, Interstitial macrophage) |
| | | Lymph node |
| | | Perivascular connective tissue |
| | | Serous cavities—peritoneum |
| | | pleura |
| | | synovium |
| | | Spleen |
| | | Skin connective tissue |
| | | Synovial membrane (type A cell) |
| Production rate: $1–2 \times 10^6$/day | $1–2 \times 10^6$ T½ 24–30 hours in circulation | Tissue pool $> 10^8$ Survival time 15– > 60 days |

*Murine

tissue macrophages ranges from 20 to 60 days.[23] The fate of senescent macrophages is not clear. The lung and gut may represent important routes of their loss.

**Control Mechanisms.** Products of antigen-stimulated lymphocytes, injected in vivo, increase the number of peritoneal macrophages synthesizing DNA.[49] Injection of irritants into nonsensitized animals results in the appearance in the serum of a protein of 18,000 to 24,000 daltons molecular mass, which elicits a brisk and selective monocytopoiesis when injected into normal hosts.[50] In vitro, glycoproteins from stimulated lymphocytes and fibroblasts trigger the replication of cells that give rise to colonies of macrophages or of macrophages and granulocytes (colony-stimulating factors).[51-53] Factors such as these may regulate the kinetics of mononuclear phagocytes. However, more work is needed to establish their physiologic role.

## DYNAMIC ASPECTS OF MACROPHAGE STRUCTURE

**The Plasma Membrane.** The capacity of the macrophage to recognize foreign or damaged autologous materials upon contact, the dramatic responses triggered by such recognition, and the large flux of membrane during endocytosis have directed the interest of many biologists to the macrophage plasma membrane. Fruitful approaches have included study of membrane proteins and lipids, transport systems, ectoenzymes, antigens, and receptors.

Exogenous proteins found on the surface of peritoneal macrophages include immunoglobulin[54] and fibrinogen-fibrin.[55] Procoagulant activity appears on the surface of mononuclear phagocytes after exposure to endotoxin, antigen-antibody complexes, and C3b or after phagocytosis.[56]

The intrinsic membrane proteins of macrophage membranes turn over rapidly even in the absence of phagocytosis, with a half-life of about 7 hours.[57] During phagocytosis, ectoenzymes are internalized and inactivated even faster.[58] For example, the half-life for 5′-nucleotidase falls to about 2 hours.[59] Macrophages taken from inflammatory sites have lower levels of 5′-nucleotidase[60] and alkaline phosphodiesterase[61] than those from uninflamed sites, probably reflecting their greater pinocytic activity,[62] with faster turnover of these ectoenzymes. During phagocytosis and pinocytosis, individual proteins are represented in the endocytic vacuoles with little alteration from their distribution on the plasma membrane itself. With immunologic activation of macrophages, major protease-sensitive surface glycoproteins of 160,000 daltons (gp160 in the guinea pig and probably F4/80 in the mouse) are dramatically decreased.[63,64]

The membrane lipids are in a state of dynamic equilibrium, which is well illustrated by cholesterol. The mouse macrophage does not synthesize cholesterol, but takes it up from serum lipoproteins into a rapidly exchanging plasma membrane compartment, and a smaller, slowly exchanging lysosomal membrane compartment.[65] While there is little increased turnover of phospholipids during phagocytosis, and no net increase, membrane cholesterol and phospholipids do begin to increase 4 to 8 hours later, to an extent proportionate to the phagocytic load.[65,66] The fatty acid composition of the macrophage plasma membrane influences its viscosity, as reflected in the activation energy for phagocytosis. Thus, a high level of saturated fatty acids in the culture medium leads to corresponding changes in the membrane, which then behaves as if it were stiffer.[67] A major membrane component is arachidonate, which in the mouse represents up to 25 percent of total macrophage fatty acid in phospholipid and serves as an important reservoir for the formation of cyclo-oxygenase and lipoxygenase products, both by the macrophage itself and perhaps also by neighboring granulocytes, as discussed later in this chapter.

A large number of antigens have recently been characterized on the macrophage surface with the aid of monoclonal antibodies. Many of these are shared with other cells, such as class I products of the major histocompatibility complex (e.g., HLA-A, B, and C antigens),[68] class II products (Ia and HLA-DR antigens),[69,70] and various antigens common to macrophages and certain other cells such as granulocytes and natural killer cells,[71] neurons,[72] or T lymphocytes.[73] Another group of antigens, partially overlapping with those just mentioned, are displayed by the plasma membrane receptors described below.[74] Of special interest, however, are the apparently macrophage-specific antigens, such as F4/80 in the mouse[75] and 3C10 in man,[10] as well as the differentiation antigens that mark subsets of macrophages, such as those that have undergone immunologic activation.[76] The antibodies of the last two categories represent powerful tools that are likely to provide considerable new information in the next few years.

**Plasma Membrane Receptors.** The macrophage continually samples and senses its environment through specific receptors. In turn, engagement of the receptors can trigger the secretion of numerous products, described below, through which the macrophage influences its environment. While some macrophage receptors are intracellular, like those for steroids, most are located on the plasma membrane. Macrophage receptors are listed in Table 10–2.

Receptors for the Fc portion of immunoglobulin permit the macrophage to ingest antibody-coated particles[77-80] and to secrete reactive oxygen intermediates,[81,82] oxidation products of arachidonic acid,[83] and lysosomal hydrolases.[84] In the mouse, macrophages display three different receptors for IgG.[80] In other species, Fc receptors for IgE have also been described on mononuclear phagocytes.[85-87] The trypsin-sensitive Fc receptor on mouse macrophages binds IgG2a monomers as cytophilic antibody, that is, antibody that binds to the cell without first reacting with antigen. Normal mouse peritoneal macrophages have about $1 \times 10^5$ such receptors. The number of receptors quadruples after injection of mice with certain inflammatory agents.[80] In vivo, ambient IgG could rapidly displace any given molecule of monomer from this Fc receptor, suggesting that it may not efficiently mediate phagocytosis so much as help localize antigen to the surface. Firm attachment and subsequent ingestion are probably mediated by the trypsin-resistant Fc receptor, which binds antigen-antibody complexes as well as IgG1 and IgG2b monomers. Mouse macrophages display about 5 to $8 \times 10^5$ such sites per cell,[80] although the number falls with macrophage activation.[82] In man, the monocyte displays an Fc receptor with the same specificity as that on the neutrophil. As the cell matures into a macrophage, a receptor analogous to the trypsin-resistant mouse macrophage receptor appears.[88] The latter receptor can be induced on both myeloid cells and on monocytes by gamma-interferon.[89]

The trypsin-resistant mouse macrophage Fc receptor has been purified through the use of a monoclonal antibody.[90] The purified receptor, a glycoprotein with a molecular mass of about 55,000 daltons, orients in lipid bilayers in such a manner that it specifically binds immune complexes added to the same side of the artificial membrane. Upon binding ligand, the lipid-moored receptor behaves as a ligand-dependent cation channel. That is, it permits a brief flux of cations (especially $Na^+$) to cross the membrane.[91] It remains to be demonstrated whether this cation flux is in fact responsible for triggering ingestion and secretion in macrophages.

There are at least three types of complement receptors

**Table 10–2.** Ligands for Macrophage Receptors

| | |
|---|---|
| *Immunoglobulin and Complement* | *Lipoproteins* |
| IgG1, IgG2b (murine) | LDL (apo-E) |
| IgG2a (murine) | Modified LDL |
| IgG3 (murine) | β-VLDL |
| IgG1, IgG3 monomers (human) | *Peptides* |
| IgG complexes (human) | Neuropeptides (enkephalins, endorphins) |
| IgE | Arginine vasopressin |
| C3b, C4b | *N*-formylated peptides from bacteria, mitochondria |
| C3bi | *Polysaccharides* |
| C3d | Lipopolysaccharide endotoxin |
| C5a | Carbohydrates on certain cells |
| *Other Proteins* | *Other* |
| Mannosyl-, fucosyl-, *N*-acetylglucosaminyl-terminal glycoproteins | Adrenergic agents |
| α2-macroglobulin–protease complexes | Cholinergic agents |
| Fibronectin | Phorbol diesters |
| Fibrin | Histamine |
| Lactoferrin | |
| Colony-stimulating factors | |
| Migration inhibitory and macrophage activation factors | |
| Insulin | |
| Factors VII, VIIa | |
| Interferons | |

on mononuclear phagocytes.[74,79,92-96] They are under complex regulation. For example, complement-coated particles bind to resident mouse peritoneal macrophages without triggering ingestion.[94] In this setting, their function may be to enhance the capacity of limiting amounts of antibody to mediate ingestion through the Fc receptor. However, as macrophages phagocytize, they release a factor that stimulates T lymphocytes to release another factor. Within seconds, the latter factor capacitates the macrophage complement receptor to mediate not only attachment but ingestion as well.[97] Macrophages taken from inflammatory sites already have this capacity. Macrophages derived from culture of human monocytes, like resident mouse peritoneal macrophages, bind but do not efficiently ingest complement-coated particles. However, exposure to a fibronectin-coated surface or to certain amyloid-related proteins quickly capacitates their complement receptors for ingestion.[98,99]

Binding of C5a anaphylatoxin to its receptor on macrophages triggers the release of interleukin-1,[96] which in turn enhances T-lymphocyte proliferation and the development of antibody-forming cells. Numerous other effects of interleukin-1, including pyrogenicity, are described later.

While galactose-terminal asialoglycoproteins are cleared from the circulation by hepatocytes, glycoproteins terminating in mannose, fucose, or *N*-acetylglucosamine are cleared by Kupffer cells and other macrophages through specific receptors.[100] Complexes of proteases with $\alpha_2$-macroglobulin are rapidly taken up by macrophages, even though proteases alone and the inhibitor alone are not.[101] Such a mechanism could be important for in vivo clearance of thrombin, plasmin, kallikrein, and active complement components.

Macrophages have receptors for the lymphokines that affect their behavior, such as migration inhibitory factor (MIF),[102] colony-stimulating factor,[103] and interferons. The MIF receptor appears to be a glycolipid[102] with a terminal fucose[104] important for its function.

Macrophage receptors for lipoproteins are of great interest in view of the monocyte or macrophage origin of many lipid-laden foam cells found in atheromatous plaques. Macrophages ingest low density lipoproteins (LDL) poorly,[105] but avidly ingest modified LDL.[106,107] This was first demonstrated with acetylated, maleylated, or malondialdehyde-treated LDL. It is doubtful that such LDL are physiologic. However, endothelial cells modify LDL in such a way that they are taken up by macrophages through the modified LDL receptor.[108] Foam cells can be generated in vitro by presenting macrophages either with modified LDL[106-108] or with $\beta$-migrating very low density lipoproteins from hyperlipidemic subjects.[109-111] It is of interest that maleylated bovine serum albumin, which may interact with the modified LDL receptor on macrophages, triggers the secretion of proteases, including plasminogen activator.[112] The pathophysiologic consequences of receptor-mediated macrophage interaction with lipoproteins remain to be fully explored.

Macrophage receptors for cholinergic agents[113] and for histamine[114] have been demonstrated only by pharmacologic criteria and are not yet characterized physicochemically. Nonetheless, they illustrate the responsiveness of the cell to the rapidly shifting environment of inflammatory sites.

**The Vacuolar Apparatus.** Through its vacuolar system, the macrophage both samples and modifies its environment at a prodigious rate. Combined morphometric and functional studies indicate that an unstimulated mouse peritoneal macrophage cultured in 20 percent fetal bovine serum forms at least 125 pinocytic vacuoles per minute, representing 0.43 percent of the cell volume of 395 cubic microns and 3.1 percent of the surface area of 825 square micons. Thus, even in the absence of a phagocytic load, the macrophage interiorizes the equivalent of its entire surface area every 33 minutes.[115] During phagocytosis, the cell can wrap in membrane each of some 150 to 200 latex beads with a diameter of 1 micron, thus interiorizing nearly its entire initial surface area in the form of phagosomes.[116]

Pinosomes flow through the cell, apparently guided by microtubules radiating from the centrioles, toward the perinuclear region. Here, lysosomes (see Chapter 9) have been formed by budding off the Golgi saccules, after being filled with acid hydrolases synthesized in the

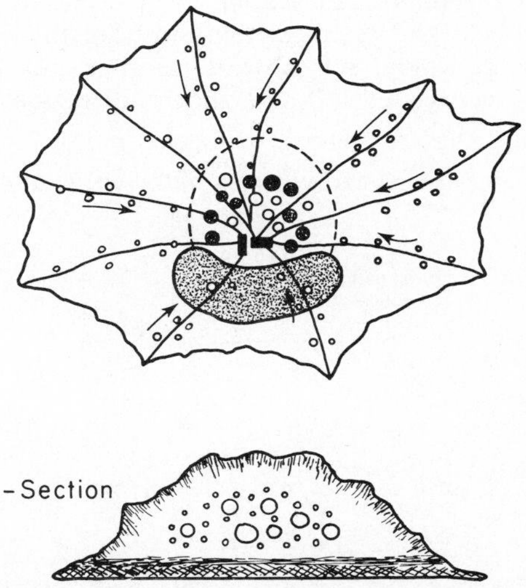


**Figure 10–2.** Organization and polarization of the macrophage cytoplasm. *Upper,* Schematic representation of a mononuclear phagocyte. Microtubules radiate from the two centrioles, spreading into the peripheral cytoplasm like spokes on a wheel and ending in proximity to the plasma membrane. These structures form a matrix along which endocytic vesicles, generated from the plasma membrane, flow centripetally (arrow) and congregate in the centrosphere area (outlined by the dotted line). Here, in the perinuclear region, fusion between endocytic vesicles and primary and secondary lysosomes takes place. This fusion of organelle membranes mixes exogenous substrates and acid hydrolases, leading to the intracellular digestion of most naturally occurring macromoles. *Lower,* A cross section through a spread macrophage pseudopod to illustrate the organization of contractile elements. On the superior surface, amorphous actin filaments decorate the inner surface of the plasma membrane and adjacent cytoplasm. In the central region microtubule bundles and the larger endocytic vesicles are mixed. Cells which attach to a substrate often demonstrate bundles of microfilament parallel to the cell membrane.

rough endoplasmic reticulum. These primary lysosomes fuse with incoming endosomes, the pH of which has already become acidic,[117] to form secondary lysosomes.[118-120] Both primary and secondary lysosomes may fuse with phagosomes. During pinocytosis, the size of the secondary lysosome compartment remains constant at about 2.5 percent of the cell's volume; yet, each hour, the secondary lysosome compartment accommodates a flux of incoming vesicles 10 times its own volume.[115] This implies that there is a recycling mechanism by which most of the pinocytosed fluid is expelled from the cell and the vesicles are reincorporated into the plasma membrane. Recycling of membrane proteins from phagolysosomes to plasma membrane has indeed been demonstrated, and is extremely rapid.[121]

In 1963, phase contrast cinemicrographs dramatically demonstrated the fusion of macrophage lysosomes with incoming vacuoles containing bacteria, and the discharge of lysosomal contents into the space around the microbes.[122] Lysosomes have been shown to contain over 40 hydrolytic enzymes. It became clear that this was the manner in which macrophages degrade endocytosed foreign matter. Tracer studies revealed that within about 2 hours, bacterial macromolecules were degraded to acid-soluble fragments.[123] Proteins, for example, were broken down into amino acids and dipeptides, which then escaped into the cytoplasm.[124]

**The Cytoskeletal Apparatus.** The muscles of the macrophage lie in the hyaline ectoplasm beneath the plasma membrane, where a meshwork of filaments excludes most other organelles[125] and undergoes regional sol-gel transitions and contractions. These appear to be responsible for membrane ruffling, pseudopod formation, and locomotion.[126] The main constituent of the microfilaments is actin, the most abundant protein of macrophages, accounting for 12 percent of cellular protein.[127] The globular form (G-actin) is a 42-kilodalton monomer that tends to polymerize into the F (filament) form until restrained by two factors; acumentin, a 65-kilodalton globular protein that caps the pointed end of the nascent chain in a calcium-insensitive manner;[128] and gelsolin, a 91-kilodalton globular protein that caps the barbed end of the filament only after binding $Ca^{++}$ in the micromolar range. When the concentration of $Ca^{++}$ falls, gelsolin releases F-actin and polymerization can proceed.[129] Actin filaments alone produce a weak meshwork. A rigid gel ensues when the filaments are crosslinked by actin-binding protein, which constitutes about 1 percent of macrophage protein. The 270-kilodalton monomers of the actin-binding protein dimer are joined to each other head-to-head, leaving two tails, each of which is free to bind an actin filament with high affinity,[130] resulting in branching and crosslinking. Contraction of actin filaments is the function of macrophage myosin, a $Mg^{++}$-ATPase hexamer of two 200-kilodalton heavy chains and two pairs of light chains of 20 kilodaltons and 15 kilodaltons, representing about 0.7 to 1.5 percent of macrophage protein.[127] Thus, local transients in $Ca^{++}$ concentration appear to control the length, branching, and rigidity of the filaments that form the skeleton upon which myosin contracts.

The role of microtubules in macrophages is less clear. When the microtubules are disrupted by colchicine, pinocytic vacuoles move about the cell in a disorderly manner, but phagocytosis can proceed.[131] Likewise, colchicine-treated cells lose directionality of migration in a chemotactic gradient but retain motility. Thus, microtubules may serve in part to provide polarity to the cell.

Selected Properties and Dynamics of the Vacuolar Apparatus of Macrophages

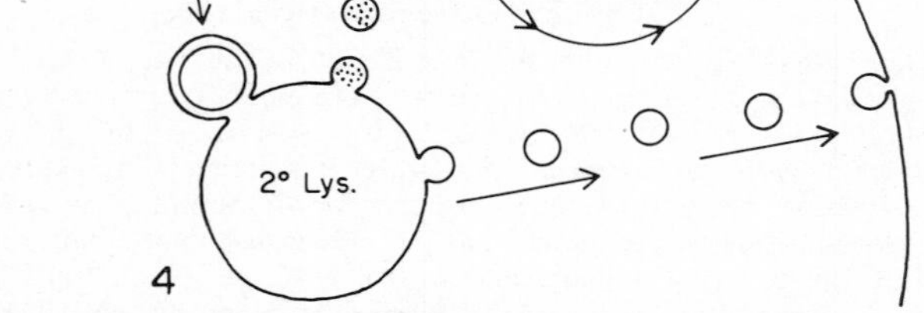

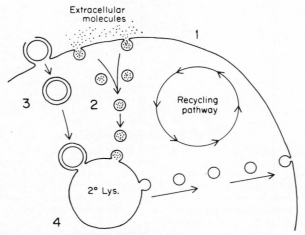


**Figure 10–3.** Exogenous solutes and particulates, which are either recognized and bound by plasma membrane receptors (adsorption) or free in the medium (fluid phase), are internalized via plasma-membrane-derived vesicles and vacuoles. The major portion of these organelles traverses the cytoplasm and fuses with secondary lysosomes. Selected contents remain within the lysosome. The membrane pinches off and the resulting vesicle returns to the cell surface. In such a manner membrane is reutilized for multiple bouts of endocytosis and maintains the volume and surface of the cell without the need for extensive membrane synthesis.

## THE CONGREGATION OF MACROPHAGES IN INFLAMMATORY SITES

**Model in Man: The Skin Window.** For macrophages to accumulate in an inflammatory focus, circulating monocytes must adhere to nearby endothelium, penetrate between cells and through the basement membrane, emigrate into the perivascular space, migrate to the tissue site, and remain there, where they are likely to become activated, and where a proportion of them may proliferate. The technique most often applied in man to assess the adequacy of macrophage mobilization in inflammatory sites is the skin window popularized by Rebuck and Crowley.[132] Sterile glass coverslips, applied sequentially to an area of abraded skin, with or without soluble antigen, permit direct visualization of the accumulation of monocytes and their maturation into macrophages, from about the sixth through the fortieth hour. However, to study separately each phase of the congregation of macrophages in inflammatory sites, it has been necessary to resort to in vitro models.

**Sticking and Spreading.** Macrophages both stick and spread rapidly on surfaces coated with antigen-antibody complexes, polyanions, or certain lectins. On uncoated glass or plastic and on collagen, sticking is rapid, but spreading occurs more slowly, requiring up to 24 hours for normal mouse peritoneal macrophages. Spreading can be enhanced by adding a variety of agents to the medium, including ATP and certain proteases.[133]

Unlike normal mouse peritoneal macrophages, macrophages from inflammatory exudates spread almost immediately on glass or plastic. This is probably related to the fact that activation of either the coagulation or the complement cascades generates activities in plasma or serum that promote rapid and dramatic spreading when added to normal macrophages.[136] Purified plasmin and complement component fragment Bb both cause macrophages to spread on glass.[135] The mechanism of this reaction is not understood.

Macrophage receptors for fibronectin[136] mediate the adherence of the cells to fibronectin-coated surfaces. Blood vessels produce fibronectin in response to injury.[137] In vivo, receptor-mediated adherence of monocytes to fibronectin or fibrin[138] may play a role in adherence within the vessels in inflamed tissue.

**Migration Through Tissues.** How mononuclear phagocytes make or find a path through connective tissue is not certain. This remarkable ability to wander, which macrophages share with malignant cells, is probably mediated by neutral proteases. Plasminogen activator is secreted by both macrophages[139] and malignant cells and is required for their ability to migrate in vitro. Macrophage elastase[140] and collagenases[141,142] are also active at extracellular pH. Unlike granulocyte elastase, macrophage elastase is resistant to inhibition by $\alpha_1$-protease inhibitor, and in fact, cleaves the inhibitor.[143] Macrophage elastase also degrades fibronectin, laminin, proteoglycans, and denatured collagen.[144] One macrophage collagenase is active against collagen types I, II, and III; another degrades type V collagen. In vitro, macrophages digest the extracellular matrix around them to lucent zones.[145,146] Similar events probably accompany the migration of the cells through tissue in vivo.

**Chemotaxis.** No less remarkable than the ability of macrophages to penetrate tissue is the directionality and speed that can be imparted to their movement. Numerous substances generated during the inflammatory response have the capacity both to enhance the speed of macrophage movement (chemokinesis) and to orient movement in the direction of increasing concentration of the agent (chemotaxis). Such factors are derived from plasma, from connective tissue, and from other cells (Table 10–3).

Among factors derived from plasma, the foremost chemotaxin for macrophages is C5a.[147] Macrophages have specific receptors for this anaphylatoxin,[148] which may be released as a consequence of complement activation by antigen-antibody complexes, by bacterial lipopolysaccharides, or by thrombin-coated platelets,[149] as well as by the direct action of cell-derived proteases on C5.[147] Such proteases may be released from damaged cells, from granulocytes,[150] or from macrophages themselves.[147] Other plasma-derived chemotactic factors for macrophages include thrombin,[151] a factor arising during the conversion of prekallikrein to kallikrein,[152] and denatured albumin.[153]

**Table 10–3.** Factors Chemotactic for Macrophages

| |
|---|
| *From Plasma* |
| C5a |
| Thrombin* |
| Kallikrein |
| Denatured albumin |
| *From Connective Tissue* |
| Fibronectin fragments* |
| Elastin fragments* |
| Collagen and collagen fragments* |
| Desmosine |
| Fluids from resorbing bone* |
| *From Host Cells* |
| Lymphocytes: chemotactic factor* |
| Phagocytes: lipoxygenase products |
| Platelets: platelet factor 4 |
| Fibroblasts: fibroblast-derived factor |
| Erythrocytes: denatured hemoglobin |
| Tumor cells: chemotactic polypeptides* |
| Many cells: formylated mitochondrial peptides† |
| *From Bacteria* |
| *N*-formylmethionyl peptides |
| Phospholipids* |
| Others |

*Relatively selective for macrophages rather than neutrophils.
†Chemotactic activity demonstrated only for neutrophils but expected for macrophages as well.

Proteolytic fragments of fibronectin are chemotactic for monocytes, whereas intact fibronectin is not.[154] Proteases that can cleave fibronectin include thrombin, macrophage elastase, and plasmin. Macrophages, of course, can promote the generation of plasmin by secreting plasminogen activator. Fibronectin fragments are also chemotactic for fibroblasts.[158] Other components of connective tissue with chemotactic activity for macrophages include fragments derived from the action of neutrophil elastase on vascular and tendinous elastin,[156,157] desmosine,[157] and collagen and its collagenase fragments.[158] In addition, culture fluids from resorbing bone are chemotactic for monocytes.[159]

Lymphocytes, neutrophils, platelets, erythrocytes, fibroblasts, tumor cells, and other cells can each release chemotaxins for macrophages. For example, lymphocytes release a chemotactic protein when encountering an antigen to which the host has been sensitized,[160] or when B lymphocytes are stimulated by bacterial lipopolysaccharide, antigen-antibody complexes, or aggregated immunoglobulin.[161] Lymphocyte-derived chemotactic factor appears to be the major chemotaxin produced in vivo when antigen is injected into the peritoneal cavity of immunized guinea pigs.[162] Neutrophil granules appear to be important. Thus, a patient with an apparently isolated deficiency of the specific granules of neutrophils failed to accumulate monocytes normally in skin windows, although the monocytes themselves responded even better than normally to standard test agents in vitro.[163] Platelet factor 4 is a monocyte chemotaxin.[164] The chemotactic activity of denatured hemoglobin has been related to the hydrophobicity of the unfolded chains.[153] The ability of tumor cells to secrete chemotaxins in vitro correlates with the content of macrophages in the tumors in vivo.[165]

Bacteria produce a variety of chemotaxins for macrophages. *Corynebacterium* and *Listeria* are of special interest, because they are intracellular pathogens of macrophages.[153] Formylation of terminal methionyl residues on peptides appears to be restricted to microbes and mitochondria. Macrophages have receptors for formylated peptides and respond to them chemotactically.[166] This may provide a detection system both for bacterial invasion and for tissue destruction that has resulted in spillage of mitochondrial contents.[167].

At least eight of the known chemotaxins attract macrophages much more efficiently than neutrophils. These are thrombin, collagen, fibronectin fragments, elastin fragments, fluids from resorbing bone, the lymphocyte-derived factor, tumor factors,[168] and a phospholipid from *C. parvum.* The specificity exhibited by these factors raises but does not adequately answer the important question of what controls the orderly succession of cell types in an inflammatory focus.

Factors influencing macrophage responsiveness to chemotactic stimuli are beginning to be recognized. Peritoneal macrophages from mice injected with BCG are more chemotactically responsive in vitro than resident peritoneal macrophages or blood monocytes.[169] Not only do tumor cells make chemotaxins, but they also release factors that decrease the chemotactic responsiveness of macrophages to other stimuli in vivo and in vitro.[170-172] Some such factors are immunologically related to envelope proteins of retroviruses, even when derived from human[173] or murine[174] tumors not shedding virus. Finally, tumor cells sometimes inactivate other chemotaxins directly.[175]

**Retention of Macrophages.** Antigen- or mitogen-stimulated lymphocytes release not only a chemotactic factor for macrophages but also physicochemically distinct substances[176] that inhibit macrophage migration (MIFs).[177,178] It has been suggested that MIF might serve to retain macrophages at the site of delayed hypersensitivity reactions. In addition, activation of complement produces factors, such as Bb, which inhibit migration of macrophages in vitro in a manner like that of MIF.[179] Finally, macrophages in delayed hypersensitivity lesions are invested in a basket of fibrin strands, which may also favor their retention at the site.[180]

Thus, proteases, complement and coagulation components, lymphocyte-derived factors, bacterial products, and substances released by tumor cells all have the direct or indirect potential both to enhance and to retard macrophage migration. It remains enigmatic how these are regulated to yield the reproducible, coordinated accumulation of cells seen in the skin window. Equally obscure are the messages, if any, that retract these commands to congregate.

## INTAKE: ENDOCYTOSIS

**Recognition and Attachment.** One of the most fascinating aspects of phagocytosis is the cell's ability to discriminate between normal self components on the one hand and damaged self or foreign particles on the other.[181,182] The recognition process is subserved in part by receptors. As discussed earlier, there are at least three classes of receptors for opsonized particles, that is, receptors for immunoglobulin, complement, or fibronectin. In addition, there are receptors that bind ligands without the mediation of opsonins, such as the receptor for mannose-terminal glycoproteins and the receptors for lipoprotein particles. Beyond this, there are particles that are avidly ingested, for which neither an opsonin nor a receptor is known. Examples are polystyrene latex beads and aldehyde-treated erythrocytes.[183] No single physicochemical feature of such particles seems adequate to explain their recognition. Some bacteria are phagocytized without opsonins, while others have antiphagocytic proteins that must be neutralized by opsonins before ingestion will occur. Other particles, such as mycoplasma, will attach to macrophages without triggering ingestion. When antimycoplasma antibody is added, the microbes are promptly engulfed.[184] Some ligand-receptor systems may interact synergistically in promoting ingestion. Illustrations involving antibody and complement, as well as fibronectin and complement, were discussed above. Thus, many mechanisms have evolved for the recognition of particles for phagocytosis, not all of which are yet understood.

**Triggering of Ingestion.** The macrophage surface response to a phagocytic stimulus is segmental, not global. This has been demonstrated by adding both C3b-coated and IgG-coated particles to resident mouse peritoneal macrophages in the cold. The C3 receptors on such cells mediate attachment but not ingestion. When the cells were warmed, they engulfed only the IgG-coated particles, while excluding the others.[185] When particles were coated with IgG on only one hemisphere, phagocytic vacuoles enclosed such particles only as far as the margin of opsonization. When the naked hemisphere was then opsonized, the macrophages completed enclosure.[186,187] Thus, ingestion is not triggered by point attachment, but requires continuous approximation, or "zippering," of receptors to opsonized sites over the entire surface of the particle. When the number of ligands per unit area of the opsonized surface is high, the apposition of the macrophage to the particle is so close that soluble proteins of molecular mass about 60 kilodaltons are excluded.[188] Thus, in the case of particles whose uptake is dependent on Fc receptors, tight surface-to-surface apposition proceeds under finely regulated local control until the macrophage membrane fuses over the top of the particle. It is unknown how these events are regulated, what restricts the diffusible signals, if any, to such a short range of action during ligand-receptor interaction, and whether the same sequence operates in the case of other ligand-receptor combinations that lead to ingestion.

**Metabolism During Phagocytosis.** Particle ingestion

by macrophages is usually accompanied by a respiratory burst similar to that in neutrophils and eosinophils (Fig. 10–4).[189] That is, there is a dramatic increase in oxygen consumption, during which a reduced nicotinamide adenine dinucleotide phosphate-dependent, flavoprotein-dependent oxidase, probably with a cytochrome b cofactor and a ubiquinone, reduces molecular oxygen to superoxide in or near the plasma membrane. Superoxide anion dismutates, in large part, to hydrogen peroxide. A portion of the peroxide diffuses from the cell, but some of it is catabolized either by catalase or by glutathione peroxidase. Glutathione is regenerated in reduced form by glutathione reductase in concert with NADPH. The NADPH for this last step, as well as that responsible for the initial reduction of oxygen, derives from the hexose monophosphate shunt, whose cycling of glucose to $CO_2$ spins faster to accommodate the increased reduction of oxygen. Meanwhile, superoxide and hydrogen peroxide can interact to give rise to hydroxyl radical. In monocytes, which contain myeloperoxidase, hypohalous ions are also formed.

A second, much smaller respiratory burst is initiated with similar kinetics by many of the same stimuli. It is immediately preceded by activation of phospholipases, which release arachidonic acid from cellular phospholipids. The free arachidonate is then oxygenated by either of two enzymes, cyclo-oxygenase or lipoxygenase, whose products are then further metabolized to produce a shower of pharmacologically active products.

Historically, the respiratory burst has been intimately linked to phagocytosis. However, the two processes are now known to be dissociable. Thus, there are many soluble agents that trigger the respiratory burst without phagocytosis, although they may lead to vacuole formation. These include antigen-antibody complexes, C5a, lectins, fatty acids, ionophores, and tumor promoters.[190] The respiratory burst can also be triggered by opsonized particles, when phagocytosis is blocked with microfilament-disrupting cytochalasins. Moreover, phagocytosis can proceed without the respiratory burst. This is seen with certain particles, like some preparations of latex, or with certain phagocytes, like those from patients with chronic granulomatous disease, which often lack the cytochrome cofactor of the oxidase.[191] Thus, the respiratory burst is a normal but by no means essential accompaniment of phagocytosis. It is more important for the microbicidal or inflammatory consequences of ingestion than for translocation of the particle into the cell.

If the extra respiration of phagocytosis is thus not devoted to recovery of utilizable chemical energy, what does fuel the musclelike movements that phagocytosis entails? It now appears that glycolysis generates ATP, which in turn maintains a large pool of creatine phosphate. The high energy bond in creatine phosphate is probably the proximate energy source for phagocytosis in macrophages.[192]

## OUTPUT: THE SECRETIONS OF MACROPHAGES

The inflammatory response is subject to influence at nearly every point by one or another macrophage secretory product, acting over a range as short as a few microns, or in the case of endogenous pyrogen, at a distance as great as two meters.

The enormous secretory repertoire is under complex regulation. Some products are secreted constitutively, others almost instantaneously following ligand-receptor

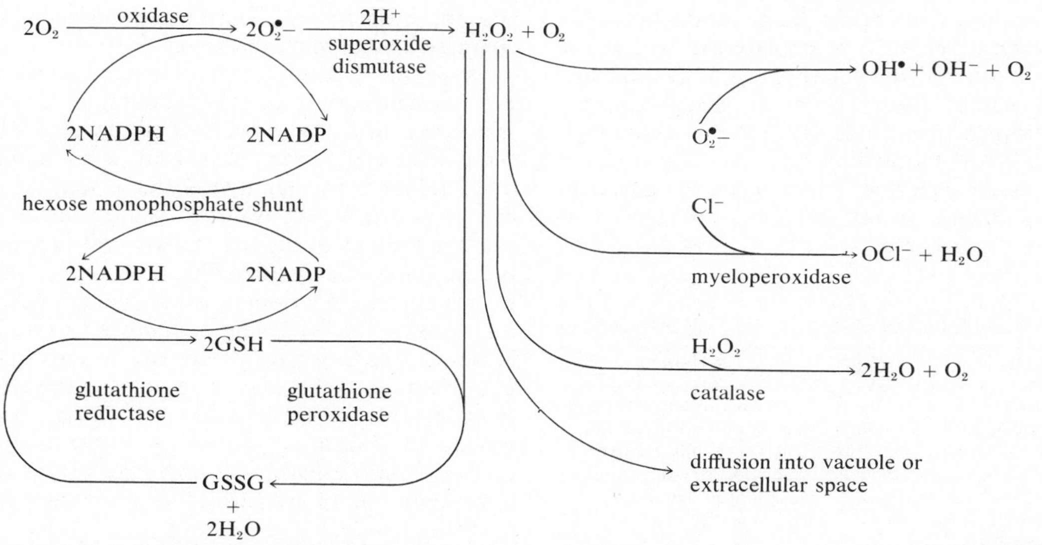


**Figure 10–4.** Metabolic pathways in the respiratory burst. These pathways appear to be the same in mononuclear phagocytes as in neutrophils, except that the activities of the various enzymes vary greatly in mononuclear phagocytes, depending on their source, manner of elicitation, maturity, and level of activation. Singlet oxygen could theoretically be produced at many points, such as by the reaction of hypochlorous ion with hydrogen peroxide; superoxide with hydrogen peroxide; hydrogen peroxide with hydrogen peroxide; or hydroxyl radical with superoxide. The overall effect is the consumption of glucose and oxygen and the production of carbon dioxide and water, with the generation of reactive metabolites of oxygen as intermediates.

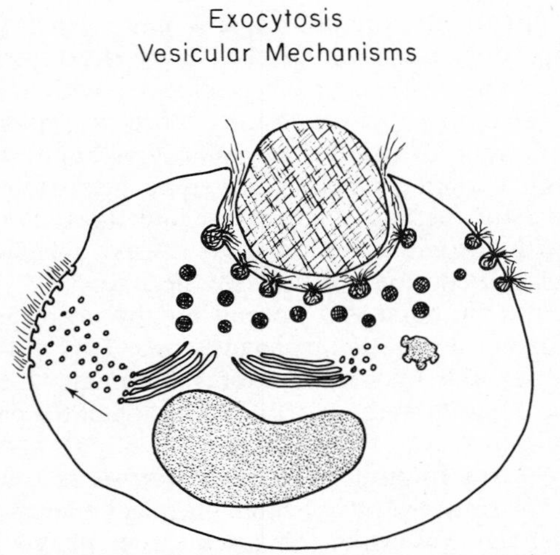


**Figure 10–5.** Possible mechanisms for the release and secretion of macromolecular products. *Left,* Small secretory vesicles derived from the endoplasmic reticulum-Golgi network fuse with the plasma membrane, liberating their contents to the extracellular space. This is analogous to secretion in the hepatocyte. *Superior,* Preformed secondary lysosomes or digestive bodies fuse with an unclosed phagocytic vacuole, thereby liberating their acid hydrolases. This may occur when the cell attaches to an irregular surface or following the phagocytosis of large, unusually shaped particles. *Right,* Secondary lysosomes fuse directly with the plasma membrane. This event occurs rarely under normal circumstances but is enhanced by agents which interfere with the distribution of contractile elements and allow these organelles closer access to the membrane.

interaction, still others only days after a stimulus. These patterns are illustrated in Table 10–4. In addition, the state of macrophage activation profoundly affects secretory capacity, but differently for different products. The macrophage itself is subject to influence by many of its own secretions, which can interact with macrophage receptors or which can generate other substances that do so. Finally, some macrophage products can interact with each other, or can regulate the function of cells, which in turn affect macrophage activation and secretion. A partial listing of macrophage secretory products is furnished in Table 10–5. Some of the individual products are highlighted below.

**Complement.** Complement components can affect the locomotive, endocytic, metabolic, and secretory behavior of the macrophage. Yet, the macrophage itself secretes many of the factors of the classical and alternative pathways and their regulators, omitting only the terminal components.[193-198] Perhaps through the action of other proteases on macrophage-derived complement components, macrophage culture supernatants may also contain cleavage products such as Bb, C3b, and C3a.[193] As noted earlier, Bb inhibits macrophage migration. C3b stimulates monocyte release of prostaglandins.[199] Prostaglandins, in turn, inhibit the secretion of C2 by monocytes.[200] In contrast, antigen-stimulated lymphocytes release a factor that enhances monocyte secretion of C2.[201] This is of considerable interest, because the low level of C2 in serum and the instability of the C42 complex may make C2 rate-limiting for classical pathway activation in extravascular sites. Finally, the C3a anaphylatoxin stimulates thromboxane release from guinea pig macrophages.[202] C3a also suppresses the ability of human helper T lymphocytes to release certain lymphocyte mediators.[203] It is not yet known whether the mediators whose release is suppressed include the one that enhances monocyte C2 synthesis.

**Table 10–4.** Regulation of Secretion from Macrophages

| Stimuli | Lag* | Products |
|---|---|---|
| None (constitutive) | — | Lysozyme, lipoprotein lipase |
| Phorbol myristate acetate | Seconds | Reactive $O_2$ intermediates |
| Immune complexes | Seconds | Reactive $O_2$ intermediates |
| | Minutes | Arachidonate metabolites |
| Endocytosis | Hours | Plasminogen activator |
| Redox agents, endocytosis, C′-activators without added complement | Days | Lysosomal hydrolases |
| Lymphocyte mediators | Days | Lysosomal hydrolases |

*Influenced by assay sensitivity.

**Coagulation Factors.** Several coagulation factors are secreted by macrophages,[204,205] as is an enzyme that promotes thrombolysis (plasminogen activator)[139] and inhibitors of thrombolytic enzymes (plasmin inhibitors).[206,207] Perhaps of equal importance, however, are surface activities involved in coagulation which are not secreted. These include inducible tissue factor activity (binding and activation of factor VII)[208] and a prothrombinase activity.[209] The prothrombinase is rapidly induced 10,000-fold when antigen-antibody complexes or bacterial lipopolysaccharides interact with lymphocytes that share Ia-like antigens with the monocytes.[209] The procoagulant activities of stimulated monocytes may account for the deposition of fibrin in delayed hypersensitivity sites.[210] It is the fibrin that appears to account in large part for the induration and swelling characteristic of such reactions.[180]

**Lysozyme.** Quantitatively, lysozyme is one of the major macrophage secretory products.[211] Its synthesis, which is constitutive, accounts for up to 2.5 percent of cellular protein per day. Lysozyme is a cationic protein of 14 kilodaltons that hydrolyzes a specific glucosidic link in bacterial cell walls. It is not known what advantage accrues to the host by committing such a large portion of the biosynthetic capacity of the macrophage to this enzyme in a noninducible manner, other than its well-known role in lysing a number of Gram-positive bacteria. These organisms are not usually regarded as pathogenic, but this may be thanks to the efficiency of lysozyme. Markedly elevated levels of the enzyme in the blood and urine are characteristic of the monocytic and myelomonocytic leukemias and may play a role in the hyperkaliuretic tubulopathy that sometimes accompanies them.

**Plasminogen Activator.** The secretion of plasminogen activator[139] is of special interest because of the numerous effects of the enzyme itself (it may, for example, act as a mitogen for lymphocytes) and of plasmin, whose for-

**Table 10–5.** Secretory Products of Mononuclear Phagocytes

| | | |
|---|---|---|
| *Complement Components* | *Binding Proteins* | *Factors Regulating Synthesis of Substances by Other Cells* |
| C1 | Transferrin | Hepatocytes |
| C4 | Transcobalamin II | Serum amyloid A |
| C2 | Fibronectin | Serum amyloid P |
| C3 | 95K Gelatin-binding protein | Haptoglobin |
| C5 | Apolipoprotein E | Synovial lining cells |
| Factor B | *Oligopeptides* | Collagenase |
| Factor D | Glutathione | Plasminogen activator |
| Properdin | *Bioactive Lipids* | Prostaglandins |
| C3b inactivator | Arachidonate metabolites | Chondrocytes |
| $\beta$1H | Prostaglandin $E_2$ | Prostaglandins |
| *Coagulation Factors* | Prostaglandin $F_{2\alpha}$ | Adipocytes |
| X | 6-keto-Prostaglandin $F_{1\alpha}$ (from prostacyclin) | Lipoprotein lipase |
| IX | Thromboxane $B_2$ (from $A_2$) | Acetyl Co-A carboxylase |
| VII | Leukotrienes B, C, D, E | Fatty acid synthetase |
| V | Monohydroxyeicosatetraenoic acids (5-; 12-; 15-) | *Factors Promoting Replication of:* |
| Thromboplastin | Dihydroxyeicosatetraenoic acids | Lymphocytes (including interleukin-1) |
| Prothrombin | Platelet-activating factors (including 1-O-alkyl-2-acetyl-*sn*-glyceryl-3-phosphorylcholine) | Myeloid precursors (including colony-stimulating factors; factor inducing monocytopoiesis) |
| *Other Enzymes* | *Nucleosides and Metabolites* | Erythroid precursors (including erythropoietin) |
| Lysozyme | Thymidine | Fibroblasts |
| Neutral proteases | Uracil | Smooth muscle cells |
| Plasminogen activator | Uric acid | Microvasculature |
| Collagenase | *Reactive Metabolites of Oxygen* | *Factors Inhibiting Replication of:* |
| Elastase | Superoxide | Lymphocytes |
| Angiotensin-convertase | Hydrogen peroxide | Myeloid precursors |
| Acid hydrolases | Hydroxyl radical | Mesangial cells |
| Proteases | Hypohalous acids | Tumor cells |
| Lipases | *Chemotactic Factors* | Viruses (interferon) |
| (deoxy) Ribonucleases | For neutrophils | *Listeria monocytogenes* |
| Phosphatases | For eosinophils | *Other Hormonelike Factors* |
| Glycosidases | For fibroblasts | Endogenous pyrogens |
| Sulfatases | | Insulin-like activity |
| Arginase | | Thymosin B4 |
| Lipoprotein lipase | | |
| Phospholipase $A_2$ | | |
| *Enzyme Inhibitors* | | |
| Plasmin inhibitors | | |
| $\alpha_2$-Macroglobulin | | |
| $\alpha_1$-Antiprotease | | |
| Phospholipase $A_2$ inhibitor (steroid-induced) | | |

mation it catalyzes. Plasmin not only lyses fibrin but activates C1 and C3 and cleaves activated Hageman factor to subunits that promote the conversion of prekallikrein to kallikrein. Plasmin degrades glycoprotein in extracellular matrix and accelerates degradation by elastase.[144-146] Macrophages secrete plasminogen activator continuously after exposure to mediators from antigen-stimulated T lymphocytes.[212,213] Activated macrophages secrete even more plasminogen activator during phagocytosis;[214] secretion subsides as the phagocytic particles are degraded. However, nonphagocytizable immune complexes fixed to a surface shut off plasminogen activator release from human monocytes.[215]

**Collagenase and Elastase.** Macrophages secrete another group of proteases, which like plasminogen activator are active at neutral pH and which are likely to play a role in degradation of connective tissue. This group includes collagenases,[141,142,216] elastase,[140,217-219] gelatinase,[218] azocaseinase,[218] and others. The various enzymes are secreted following phagocytosis,[142] exposure to endotoxin,[220] interaction with immune complexes,[215] or incubation in lymphocyte mediators. Macrophage elastase, a metalloenzyme distinct from the neutrophil serine enzyme, degrades not only elastin but also $\alpha_1$-protease inhibitor,[143] immunoglobulin,[221] plasminogen, fibrinogen, fibrin, fibronectin, laminin, and proteoglycans.[144-146] Destruction of $\alpha_1$-protease inhibitor by macrophage elastase would favor the action of neutrophil elastase in the same site.

**Acid Hydrolases.** A large number of hydrolases, active at acid pH, are present in macrophage lysosomes,[118] and increase in amount with activation of the cells.[119,217] The type-specific polysaccharide and peptidoglycans of streptococcal cell walls, which induce chronic inflammatory lesions in vivo, lead both to augmentation of lysosomal enzyme levels in cultured macrophages and to the discharge of such enzymes into the culture medium.[222] A large number of other microbial materials or polysaccharides have a similar effect, including endotoxin, BCG, *C. parvum,* yeast cell walls, dental plaque, carrageenan, and dextran sulfates. Such substances are also capable of activating complement by the alternative pathway, and with a similar rank order of potency.[223] Lysosomal enzyme release is also triggered by engagement of Fc[84] and complement[223] receptors and by incubation in lymphocyte mediators.[216]

Thus, lysosomal acid hydrolases may contribute to tissue breakdown when there is a sufficiently low pH extracellularly, or when portions of the matrix are ingested by macrophages[146] into phagolysosomes, which have an acid milieu.[224] Among the substances susceptible to degradation by macrophage acid hydrolases are collagen, cartilage, basement membrane, proteoglycans, immunoglobulin, kininogen, and complement components.[225]

**Protease Inhibitors.** Plasminogen activator, plasmin, collagenase, elastase, thrombin, kallikrein, and a variety of other proteases are all inhibited by $\alpha_2$-macroglobulin.[226] Alpha$_2$-macroglobulin also enhances the ability of lymphocyte-derived migration inhibitory factor to retard macrophage motility.[227] Human monocytes synthesize and secrete substantial amounts of this protein in culture (about 50 ng per $10^6$ cells per day),[228] as do human alveolar macrophages.[229] Recently, macrophages have also been found to synthesize and secrete $\alpha_1$-protease inhibitor.[230-232] It may seem paradoxical that macrophages secrete not only elastase[140,217-219] but also two protease inhibitors, one of which is a substrate for elastase[143] and one of which is an inhibitor of it.[226]

**Bioactive Lipids.** Engagement of Fc receptors, ingestion of particles, or exposure to other membrane-active agents trigger the rapid release from macrophages of a variety of oxygenation products of arachidonic acid that are likely to be of critical importance in the inflammatory response.[233-249]

This assertion rests on the following points. First, the proportion of phospholipid fatty acid that is arachidonate is much higher in macrophages (about 26 percent in the mouse) than in most other cell types. The mouse macrophage is capable of putting 45 percent of this fatty acid at the disposal of cyclo-oxygenase and lipoxygenase within minutes of a membrane stimulus without suffering a loss of viability.[236,238,242] As a consequence, the quantities of arachidonate oxygenation products secreted by mouse macrophages (e.g., 33 nmol per mg cell protein) are enormous in comparison with other cells, such as guinea pig neutrophils (e.g., 0.044 nmol per mg cell protein in one comparable study; see Table 10–6). Second, the spectrum of arachidonate metabolites secreted by macrophages is wide and includes such important mediators as leukotriene C,[237,239,242,244] one of the slow-reacting substances of anaphylaxis, in quantity, as well as leukotriene B,[243] a potent chemotactic factor. Third, this secretory spectrum is profoundly influenced by the state of immunologic activation of the macrophage,[249] which suggests possible mechanisms of control during the evolution of an inflammatory response. Finally, macrophages are distributed in submucosal and perivascular sites, in the pulmonary alveoli and interstitium,[242] in the renal interstitium and juxtaglomerular apparatus,[9] and in other control points under normal steady-state conditions. Thus, it is plausible that macrophages could play a role as sentinels in the earliest stages of inflammation, releasing products that regulate vasodilation, constriction, and permeability, bronchial smooth muscle contractility, neutrophil and monocyte motility, lymphocyte function,[246,247] myeloid stem cell proliferation,[248] hepatic release of acute phase reactants,[249] and nociception. The fact that complexes of antigen with IgE are potent triggers of macrophage leukotriene release[239] supports the idea that macrophages may play a role in immediate hypersensitivity reactions.

**Table 10–6.** Metabolism of 20:4* from Endogenous Phospholipids of Mouse Tissue Macrophages in Response to a Triggering Agent (Zymosan)†

| Feature | Peritoneal Macrophages | | Pulmonary Macrophages | | Guinea pig PMN with A23187‡ |
|---|---|---|---|---|---|
| | *Resident* | *Activated* | *Tissue* | *Alveolar* | |
| Fatty acid | | | | | |
| Percentage of phospholipid | 26 | 25 | 23 | ND | |
| Percentage 20:4 released | 45 | 17 | 14 | 5.5 | |
| Percentage of released 20:4 oxygenated | 95 | 30 | 80 | 75 | |
| Pmol products/$\mu$g protein | 33 | 6 | 15 | 6 | 0.004 |
| *Cyclooxygenase products* | | | | | |
| $PGE_2$ | 18 (54)§ | 4 (65) | 2 (12) | 0.8 (13) | 0.002 |
| $PGI_2$ | 6 (20) | 0.02 (0.3) | 0.9 (6) | 0 | 0.001 |
| $TXA_2$ | 0 | 0.7 (17) | 1.2 (8) | 0.6 (10) | 0.010 |
| $PGF_2$ | 0 | 0 | 0 | 0 | 0.001 |
| *Lipoxygenase products* | | | | | |
| HETES | 3 (10) | 1 (15) | 5 (32) | 2 (39) | 0.030 |
| LTC | 5 (16) | 0.13 (2) | 3 (23) | 1 (13) | |

*20:4 = arachidonic acid.
†Compiled from Scott and colleagues, refs. 236, 238, and 242.
‡From ref. 245.
§Numbers in parentheses are percentage of released 20:4.

Table 10–6 presents quantitative data for arachidonate metabolites produced by tissue macrophages in the mouse. These data reflect only one of two major pathways utilized by these cells, that is, the endogenous pathway in which the substrate is derived from the phospholipid pool of the producing cell in response to a membrane-perturbing agent.[236] However, free arachidonate, such as might be released from damaged cells by phospholipases, is also rapidly oxygenated by macrophages in the absence of a stimulus.[240,241] This pathway is not demonstrably saturable when macrophages are repeatedly provided with free arachidonic acid at nontoxic concentrations in vitro. Thus, it could be quantitatively important. The distribution of products formed by the exogenous pathway is given in Table 10–7. In addition, the free arachidonate released by macrophages may markedly augment the production of leukotriene B by neutrophils in the same site.

The influence of immunologic activation on the secretion of arachidonate metabolites by murine macrophages is summarized in Table 10–8. Of note is the marked decrease in $PGE_2$, $PGI_2$, hydroxyeicosatetraenoic acids, and leukotriene C and the appearance of significant amounts of thromboxane. In the guinea pig, macrophage activation increases rather than decreases $PGE_2$ release.[250] It is of interest that activation also has opposite effects on the secretion of complement components by macrophages in these two species. The reasons for these differences are not understood.

In man, leukotriene $B_4$ is a prominent product of the stimulated alveolar macrophage[243] and probably represents one of the major sources of alveolar macrophage chemotactic activity for neutrophils.[251] Study of the human blood monocyte has been complicated by the rosetting of platelets to monocytes during most isolation procedures. Recent techniques have overcome this problem and have permitted the demonstration that the human blood monocyte is a potent source of thromboxane, fully equivalent to the platelet on a protein basis, and much higher than the neutrophil.[244] Depending on the stimulus, human blood monocytes also release substantial amounts of lipoxygenase products, including leukotrienes B and C.[244] Studies with other populations of human mononuclear phagocytes should soon be forthcoming.

**Table 10–7.** Metabolism of 20:4 by Mouse Peritoneal Macrophages Utilizing Exogenous Free Fatty Acid Without a Triggering Stimulus*

| Feature | Resident Macrophages | Activated Macrophages |
|---|---|---|
| Percentage 20:4 incorporated into cell phospholipid† | 34 | 70 |
| Percentage 20:4 oxygenated† | 65 | 17 |
| Metabolites (as percentage of 20:4 oxygenated)† | | |
| *Cyclooxygenase products* | | |
| $PGE_2$ | 8 | 6 |
| $PGI_2$ | 26 | 1 |
| $TXA_2$ | 0 | 2 |
| $PGF_{2\alpha}$ | 0 | 4 |
| *Lipoxygenase products* | | |
| HETES | 42‡ | 4 |
| LTC | 3 | 0 |

*Compiled from ref. 241.

†Within 5 minutes of supplying cells with up to 1 μM 20:4 in serum-free medium.

‡Within 60 minutes 50 percent of released or exogenously supplied mono-hydroxyeicosatetraenoic acids (mono-HETES) are metabolized to di-HETES.[240]

**Reactive Oxygen Intermediates.** As already noted, macrophages respond to immune complexes, phagocytic particles, and other membrane-active agents by secreting superoxide anion, hydrogen peroxide, hydroxyl radical, and in the case of monocytes, hypohalous acid, into phagosomes and into the extracellular space.[190] Immunologic activation markedly increases the ability of macrophages to secrete these products, both in laboratory animals[190,252-254] and in man.[225,256] In the mouse, many malignant cells and some nonmalignant cells secrete a product that selectively down-regulates the capacity of macrophages to secrete reactive oxygen intermediates.[257]

These products can inactivate thiol groups in enzymes, rearrange and break bonds in proteins, lipids, and nucleic acids, and initiate radical chain reactions capable of inflicting further damage of the same kind.[258] The primary evolutionary role of the leukocyte-derived reactive oxygen intermediates is probably microbicidal. However, their other pro- and anti-inflammatory effects are legion, as summarized in Table 10–9. In addition to cytotoxicity toward malignant and normal cells,[190] reactive oxygen intermediates can regulate the function of neutrophils, platelets, and lymphocytes in a noncytotoxic manner, which is not yet fully understood. Oxidation of critical methionyl residues can inactivate a number of humoral mediators or regulators of inflammation, including leukotriene C and $\alpha_1$-protease inhibitor.

It has already been noted that macrophages undergo two respiratory bursts simultaneously in response to many of the same stimuli: incomplete reduction of molecular oxygen to produce reactive intermediates, and oxygenation of arachidonic acid. In an immunologically activated mouse peritoneal macrophage, about 100 times more oxygen is consumed in the former path than in the latter. The two respiratory bursts may interact at the levels of initiation, radical formation and utilization, and glutathione oxidation and consumption, in ways not yet fully analyzed. It is of interest that the activities of these two respiratory bursts are often under reciprocal control during immunologic activation in the mouse.[238,252]

**Regulatory Factors for Other Cells.** One of the most rapidly growing areas in the study of macrophage secretory function concerns factors that regulate synthesis by or growth of other types of cells. Many of these factors have been identified only as bioactivities and may be chemically similar to each other or to macrophage products whose composition is already known. An example is the remarkable protein interleukin-1,[259] whose purification has been achieved.[260] Interleukin-1 appears

**Table 10–8.** Possible Shifts in Mouse Macrophage 20:4* Metabolites During an Inflammatory Response

| Metabolites | Early Inflammation: Resident Cells | | Late Inflammation: Activated Cells | |
|---|---|---|---|---|
| | *From Endogenous Phospholipid 20:4 With Trigger* | *From Exogenous Free Fatty Acid 20:4 Without Trigger*† | *From Endogenous Phospholipid 20:4 With Trigger* | *From Exogenous Free Fatty Acid 20:4 Without Trigger*† |
| $PGE_2$ | 18‡ | 0.6 | 4 | 0.03 |
| $PGI_2$ | 6 | 1.6 | 0.02 | 0.01 |
| $TXA_2$ | 0 | 0 | 0.7 | 0.01 |
| $PGF_2$ | 0 | 0 | 0 | 0.02 |
| HETES | 3 | 4.4 | 1 | 0.08 |
| LTC | 5 | 0.02 | 0.13 | 0 |

*20:4 = arachidonic acid.
†Assuming 1 μM exogenous 20:4 in serum-free conditions.
‡pmol per μg cell protein.

to be a major macrophage product involved in stimulation of thymocyte proliferation (lymphocyte-activating factor);[261] B lymphocyte proliferation;[262] hyperthermia (endogenous pyrogen);[263] synovial cell synthesis of prostaglandins, collagenase, and plasminogen activator;[264] fibroblast growth[265] and collagenase production;[266] and perhaps hepatocyte synthesis of acute phase reactants.[267,268] However, there are clearly different factors made by macrophages that promote the growth of myeloid cells and of erythrocytes,[269] including erythropoietin.[270] The nature of other macrophage growth factors for fibroblasts, smooth muscle cells, and endothelial cells[271,272] remains to be defined.

Macrophages release both an insulinlike activity[273] and a factor that inhibits the action of insulin on adipocytes, suppressing their activity of lipoprotein lipase,[274] acetyl Co-A carboxylase, and fatty acid synthetase.[275] The latter factor is secreted by macrophages challenged with endotoxin and may contribute to the hypertriglyceridemia of acute phase responses and the insulin resistance of chronic infection. Even though this macrophage product inhibits lipoprotein lipase in adipocytes, macrophages themselves spontaneously secrete lipoprotein lipase into the medium.[276,277]

Factors from macrophages that suppress the replication of other cells include tumor necrosis factor,[278] interferon,[279] arginase (which depletes arginine from the medium),[280] reactive oxygen intermediates,[281] prostaglandins,[247] and thymidine.[282] The interferon secreted by macrophages is probably usually of the alpha type, but secretion of gamma interferon has also been reported.[283,284] The question has not yet been settled whether the latter is in fact acid-labile alpha-interferon. The issue is of interest, because gamma-interferon is a potent macrophage-activating factor.[256]

**Table 10–9.** Effects of Reactive Oxygen Intermediates

| On Cells | On Extracellular Factors |
|---|---|
| Killing of viruses, bacteria, fungi, protozoa, nematodes, trematodes | Depolymerization of ground substance |
| Mutagenesis of bacteria | Aggregation of immunoglobulin |
| Killing of tumor cells | Inactivation of chemotactic peptides |
| Killing of erythrocytes, endothelial cells, fibroblasts, lung parenchyma, spermatazoa, platelets, leukocytes | Inactivation of leukotrienes and prostaglandins |
| Inhibition of leukocyte lysosomal enzyme release | Activation of chemotactic lipids |
| Noncytolytic triggering of platelet and mast cell secretion | Inactivation of met-enkephalin |
| Suppression of lymphocyte responses, directly or through oxidation of soluble immune response suppressor from T cells | Inactivation of $\alpha_1$-antiprotease |
| Suppression of natural killer cells | Inactivation of leukocyte lysosomal hydrolases |
| | Inactivation of bacterial toxins |

## ANTIMICROBIAL FUNCTIONS

**Spectrum.** Presumably, one of the functions of macrophages providing the greatest evolutionary pressure for their representation throughout the phyla is that of inactivating invading microbes. In general, the antimicrobial spectrum of macrophages exceeds that of neutrophils, although neutrophils kill many organisms more rapidly than macrophages. However, the chief distinction between the antimicrobial ability of macrophages and neutrophils consists in the inducibility of this function in macrophages. Thus, normal macrophages will often support or succumb to viruses, *Chlamydia, Rickettsia, Listeria, Legionella, Corynebacterium, Salmonella, Brucella, Pasteurella, Nocardia, Mycobacteria, Leishmania, Toxoplasma, Trypanosoma, Cryptococcus, or Aspergillus.* With "activation," however, macrophages can inhibit or destroy many of the same organisms.[285] In addition, macrophages can damage multicellular parasites such as schistosomula[286] and microfilariae[287] through attachment that does not lead to phagocytosis.

If macrophages are not sufficiently microbicidal, however, they may provide certain microbes with a sanctuary within which to replicate. *Legionella pneumophila* is such a pathogen.[288] In fact, some parasites exist in the tissues almost exclusively within macrophages. *Leishmania* is an important example.

**Mechanisms.** One of the major antimicrobial mechanisms of macrophages is the production of reactive oxygen intermediates (ROI).[190,289] This is true both for monocytes, which are richly endowed with myeloperoxidase, and for tissue macrophages, which are not. For *Toxoplasma, Leishmania, Trypanosoma, Candida,* and *Mycobacterium,* there is a close correlation between the antimicrobial activity of a given macrophage population and its capacity to secrete ROI. Similarly, there is a correlation between the ability of a pathogen to trigger the secretion of ROI during its ingestion and its susceptibility to killing by macrophages. The susceptibility of a microbe to killing by ROI often correlates with the susceptibility of the same organisms to killing by macrophages, and this in turn can be inversely related to the levels of antioxidant defense pathways in the parasites. Finally, experimental interventions that decrease the level of ROI within macrophages also decrease killing, and interventions that augment the level or the cytotoxic efficiency of ROI enhance killing. Thus there is abundant evidence (reviewed in ref. 289) to support the importance of oxygen-dependent antimicrobial mechanisms.

However, oxygen-independent antimicrobial mechanisms also function within macrophages.[289] This seems assured from the fact that the monocytes of patients with chronic granulomatous disease, which produce very little ROI during ingestion of parasites, have reduced but definite antimicrobial activity.[290] Chronic granulomatous disease macrophages can be activated by lymphocyte products to display enhanced antimicrobial activity, and this is not accompanied by increased secretion of ROI, nor is it impeded by interventions designed to lower the intracellular concentration of ROI.[291] Indeed, fibroblasts and endothelial cells can kill some of the same pathogens as macrophages without evidence for secretion of ROI.[291]

The nature of the oxygen-independent antimicrobial mechanisms of macrophages is not yet firmly established.[289,293] Contributory factors may include acidification of the phagosome, the action of cationic peptides and lysosomal hydrolases, the production of complement components and interferon, depletion of arginine by secretion of arginase, and sequestration of iron by iron-binding proteins. Finally, the possibility has been raised that withholding of a trophic factor, rather than provision of a toxic one, may contribute to the ability of activated macrophages to inhibit the replication of certain organisms that depend on parasitization of macrophages for their survival in the mammalian host.[289]

The importance of individual antimicrobial mechanisms can be inferred from the evasions employed by parasites during successful infection of macrophages. For example, *Toxoplasma gondii* enters nonactivated macrophages without triggering the usual production of ROI, although the macrophages are fully capable of being triggered by other agents. When the macrophages are activated, or when the parasite is coated with antibody, then its ingestion elicits a normal respiratory burst, and survival of the parasite is impaired.[290] *Brucella abortus* secretes an unusual adenylate cyclase, which is taken up by macrophages, acutely raises their cyclic adenosine monophosphate levels, and suppresses their ability to secrete ROI in response to any stimulus, including the ingestion of the bacterium.[294] *Mycobacterium tuberculosis* frustrates the ability of the macrophage to empty its lysosomes into the phagosome, apparently by means of sulfolipids, which prevent fusion of the membranes of these organelles.[295] *M. lepraemurium,* however, permits fusion of phagosomes and lysosomes to occur and survives nonetheless.[296] *Trypanosoma cruzi* breaks out of its phagolysosome to replicate within the cytoplasm.[297] The complexity of the behavior of parasites during and after their ingestion by macrophages testifies to the variability of antimicrobial mechanisms that may be paramount in individual macrophage–parasite combinations.

## ANTITUMOR FUNCTION

One of the most dramatic performances of the macrophage on the stage of the microscope is the destruction of malignant cells. Through a reaction resembling a receptor-ligand interaction, activated macrophages form a firm attachment with tumor cells and secrete a cytolytic factor whose action includes a proteolytic step.[298] Nonmalignant cells and nonactivated macrophages appear unable to participate in this form of binding and lysis.[6] Small amounts of hydrogen peroxide released from activated macrophages may interact synergistically with the cytolytic factor.[299] The actual basis of cytotoxicity is not yet clear but appears to involve damage to tumor cell mitochondria at specific sites in the respiratory chain in a pattern typical of peroxidative damage.[300]

Compared with the spontaneous cytolysis described above, even more rapid and extensive lysis of tumor cells can result from triggering the respiratory burst of the activated macrophage.[281] Antibody-coated tumor cells interacting with Fc receptors on the macrophage sometimes elicit their own destruction in this manner.[301] Oxidative injury also appears to account for the rapid lysis of tumor cells coated with eosinophil peroxidase and exposed to activated macrophages in the absence of any known stimulus of the macrophage respiratory burst.[302]

There are numerous lines of evidence to indicate that macrophages can kill tumor cells in vivo.[303] Recent attention has focused on the role of macrophages in the therapeutic effects of monoclonal antitumor antibodies[304] and of adjuvant-laden liposomes.[305]

Just as many microbes have found ways to evade destruction by macrophages, so do tumor cells suppress macrophage-mediated cytotoxicity. For example, tumor cell products have been found both in the mouse and in man that inhibit the ability of macrophages to accumulate in tumors.[173,174] A product of malignant cells selectively suppresses the ability of macrophages to secrete hydrogen peroxide[257] and to kill intracellular protozoa.[306] Finally, tumor cells catabolize macrophage cytotoxic factors and repair their lesions. Pharmacologic agents that interfere with these processes enhance macrophage-mediated cytotoxicity.[307,308]

## IMMUNOREGULATORY FUNCTIONS

**Helper Effects.** T and B lymphocytes are highly dependent on adherent mononuclear cells for many of their functions. Initial reports attributed this accessory cell activity solely to macrophages, a view that now requires revision. Most macrophage-rich populations, including those from human blood, contain small numbers of dendritic cells, which are also mononuclear, adherent, bone marrow-derived, and rich in Ia antigens in the mouse or in the homologous antigens in other species.[309] It has been clearly shown, however, that dendritic cells are distinct from macrophages. Indeed, these two populations are segregated from each other anatomically in lymph nodes, spleen, and dermis, although they circulate together in blood.[10] Almost all procedures used to deplete macrophages (including anti-Ia antibodies) also deplete dendritic cells and do not clarify which cell may be required. However, selective elimination of dendritic cells with specific monoclonal antibody plus complement removes nearly all accessory activity for mixed leukocyte reactions, generation of cytotoxic T lymphocytes, proliferation of T lymphocytes in response to periodate-treated cells or antigen, and development of antibody-secreting B lymphocytes.[310] Highly enriched populations of dendritic cells reconstitute the same responses. The numbers of dendritic cells needed to do so are consistent with their number in the unseparated lymphoid cell populations. In contrast, using monoclonal antibodies which spare dendritic cells, specific depletion of monocytes has little or no effect on the same immune responses.[311]

Nonetheless, macrophages or their secretory products clearly can promote lymphocyte viability and proliferation. Reconstitution of macrophage-depleted cultures with 2-mercaptoethanol and/or interleukin-1 often reestablishes much of the response. 2-Mercaptoethanol may substitute for glutathione, a macrophage secretory product;[312] interleukin-1 is also a macrophage product and has been discussed above.

One somewhat speculative way of viewing accessory cell function is as follows. Resting T lymphocytes require contact with both antigen and dendritic cells in order to initiate secretion of interleukin-2. After the onset of interleukin-2 secretion, dendritic cells are no longer required.[313] The magnitude of the ensuing response will be much greater in the presence of trophic factors derived from macrophages, especially interleukin-1, which augments interleukin-2 secretion by T lymphocytes.[314] In the presence of the antigen alone (without need for dendritic cells), antigen-responsive T lymphocytes express interleukin-2 receptors. Binding of interleukin-2 to these receptors drives proliferation. If some T lymphocytes are already activated at the time the experiment begins (that is, they are secreting interleukin-2), a dendritic cell requirement may not be evident, and the only accessory cell still augmenting the response may be the macrophage (or another cell that produces interleukin-1).

Another area of controversy concerns the presentation and processing of antigen by macrophages. In several experimental systems, optimal immunologic responses have occurred with 3 to 4 logs less antigen when the antigen was added in association with macrophage-rich populations than when added alone.[315] In part, this may represent the contribution of the trophic macrophage products discussed above, but additional factors are likely to be involved and are not yet fully understood. The ability to partially degrade antigens and select determinants under immune response gene control was also attributed to macrophages. That is, it was thought that macrophages from a nonresponder animal failed to present the appropriate determinant to T cells. Recently, further data obtained in the original experimental system have supported alternative interpretations.[316] Thus, portions of antigen indeed seem to be associated with macrophages, but it is doubtful that IR genes act by determining how macrophages catabolize a given antigen.

**Suppressor Effects.** Many of the same immunologic functions that are impaired by depleting adherent cells are also suboptimal when the number of adherent cells is higher than normal or when the macrophages among them are activated.[317] Depressed immunologic responses in vitro using lymphocytes from patients with myeloma, Hodgkin's disease, other malignancies, or fungal infections appear to be due to adherent suppressor cells, which in many cases are probably monocytes or macrophages.[318] The mechanism of suppression often seems to involve prostaglandin secretion by the adherent cells.[247,318] In some cases, inhibitory effects can be attributed to the secretion of hydrogen peroxide[318] or arginase.[280]

## SELECTIVE REMOVAL OF AUTOLOGOUS CELLS

Removal of senescent, damaged, and perhaps aberrant cells is one of the chief functions of macrophages. The process has been best studied with erythrocytes, which are subject to at least three kinds of changes that lead to their selective removal. These mechanisms, while imperfectly understood, can serve as models for the means by which macrophages may be signaled to remove other kinds of autologous cells.

**Senescent Cells.** Aged red cells are opsonized by an immunoglobulin present in normal human serum and are ingested by autologous macrophages.[319] This may be the mechanism by which macrophages, mostly in the spleen, daily remove some $3 \times 10^{11}$ red cells from the circulation, a meal of 2.7 kg of hemoglobin per year.[81] The antigen recognized on senescent red cells appears to be related to the transmembrane protein, band 3. It is not known how senescence leads to autoantigenicity of a tiny portion of band 3 sites per cell.[319] Macrophages also ingest senescent neutrophils.[320] The basis of recognition in this case is unknown. There are natural antibodies in man to desialyated cells[321] as well as antibody-independent receptors on monocytes for some desialylated erythrocytes.[322] Thus, loss of sialic acid may also provide a signal.[323]

**Cells Targeted by Autoimmune Reactions.** In immune hemolytic anemias, red cells are opsonized, pulled from the circulation by macrophages, and ingested or destroyed extracellulary. Spherocytes, the morphologic hallmark of such anemias, are red cells from which opsonized pieces of membrane have been plucked, reducing the surface-to-volume ratio. In a similar manner, ingestion of opsonized platelets by macrophages underlies autoimmune thrombocytopenia.[324]

**Metabolically Defective Cells.** Red cells that are abnormally susceptible to oxidant stress are removed by splenic and hepatic macrophages. For example, during infection, leukocytes engaged in phagocytosis release hydrogen peroxide, which depletes the glutathione of glucose-6-phosphate dehydrogenase–deficient red cells and leads to their destruction in the liver and spleen.[325]

**Wound Healing.** The rate of removal of fibrin, neutrophils, erythrocytes, and other debris from wounds and the local ingrowth of fibroblasts and vascular buds are markedly impaired when monocytopenia is induced.[326]

## EFFECTS OF ANTI-INFLAMMATORY DRUGS ON MACROPHAGES

**Glucocorticoids.** In man, intravenous hydrocortisone induces a profound monocytopenia, with a nadir at 4 to 7 hours and restoration of normal counts in 24 hours.[327] This time course suggests that redistribution of cells may be partly responsible for the changes. Prednisone depresses both the blood monocyte count and the accumulation of monocytes in skin windows. Both features normalize with alternate-day administration of the drug.[328] Epicutaneous application of glucocorticoids retards accumulation of monocytes in skin windows at the same site.[329] In the mouse, hydrocortisone causes a 35 percent drop in the number of marrow promonocytes. Mitotic activity is unaffected, and the monocyte production rate falls only 20 percent. However, the release of newly formed monocytes from the marrow is sharply curtailed, and peripheral monocytopenia is marked.[330]

Monocytes from prednisone-treated volunteers are subnormal in killing of *Staphylococcus* and *Candida* despite normal phagocytosis.[331] Macrophages from hydrocortisone-treated mice are 1000-fold more susceptible to murine hepatitis virus in vitro than those from untreated animals.[332]

In vitro, glucocorticoids retard the increases in size and lysosomal enzyme content that normally accompany the differentiation of monocytes into macrophages.[333] If the monocytes are exposed continuously to hydrocortisone for 4 days, their ability to release hydrogen peroxide is suppressed by over 90 percent. The 50 percent inhibitory concentration of hydrocortisone is only about 0.2 micromolar. However, if continuous exposure is limited to 2 days, there is no suppressive effect even from 10 micromolar hydrocortisone.[334] Thus, diurnal peaks of endogenous glucocorticoids, or alternate-day administration of the drugs, would not be expected to have the same effect as continuous maintenance of high blood levels. In vitro treatment of human monocytes with cortisone also suppressed their ability to bind erythrocytes opsonized with immunoglobulin or complement.[335]

In the mouse, treatment of macrophages in vitro with glucocorticoids suppresses glucose utilization and overall protein synthesis.[336] Thus it is not surprising that there is depressed expression or secretion of Ia antigens,[337] interleukin-1,[337] plasminogen activator, collagenase, elastase, and other neutral proteases.[338] In contrast, low-dose treatment of rat peritoneal macrophages with cortisol reportedly enhances their protein synthesis and their ability to resorb bone in vitro.[339] Glucocorticoids also inhibit macrophage spreading on glass[274] and response to migration inhibitory factor from lymphocytes.[341]

While not anti-inflammatory, the estrogenic steroids also affect macrophages. Phagocytic activity of the fixed macrophages, as measured by clearance studies, is increased by estrogenic but not androgenic hormones.[342] Changes in phagocytic activity attend the fluctuations in estrogenic levels during the menstrual cycle and pregnancy. Ovariectomy reduces the capacity of mice to resist virulent infections.[342]

**Gold Salts.** Gold salts accumulate in macrophage lysosomes, where they inhibit a number of enzymes.[343] The chemotactic response of human monocytes to formylated peptides is also inhibited by these agents.[344] Of considerable interest is the ability of therapeutically attained concentrations of gold salts to block the ability of lymphocyte mediators to enhance monocyte production of complement component C2 in the absence of demonstrable toxicity to the monocytes. Monocytes that are already activated by lymphokine are unaffected.[345] This raises the possibility that the delayed therapeutic benefits of gold salts in vivo could have to do, in part, with the time it takes activated macrophages in the joint to be replaced by new cells that have yet to be activated. In murine models, treatment with gold salts impairs the virucidal[346] and tumoricidal activity of macrophages.[347]

**D-Penicillamine.** The enhanced mitogen responses of lymphocytes from arthritic animals treated with D-penicillamine have been attributed in part to diminished suppressor activity of their macrophages.[348] The drug also seems to stimulate the uptake of aggregated immunoglobulin by macrophages.[349] In addition, this agent seems to protect $\alpha_1$-antiprotease from oxidative inactivation.[350] The mechanisms of these effects and their possible relevance to the anti-inflammatory action of D-penicillamine remain to be worked out.

**Cytotoxic Agents.** Azathioprine blocks mouse promonocytes in late S or G2 phase, resulting in a severe drop in monocyte production and failure of monocytes to accumulate in inflammatory exudates.[351] Cyclophosphamide also reduces marrow colony-forming cells, circulating monocyte levels, and accumulation of macrophages in inflammatory exudates.[352,353]

**Other Nonsteroidal Anti-Inflammatory Agents.** Many of these agents have the expected effect on macrophage synthesis of arachidonic acid metabolites, which may account in part for some of their beneficial effects in vivo.[354]

## AN OVERVIEW: MACROPHAGE ACTIVATION

Almost every structural or functional feature of macrophages has been reported to change when the hosts or the cells are treated in some way. This accounts for much of the fascination these cells hold for many investigators, and also for some of the difficulty the investigators have in communicating with each other. For example, any gradual augmentation may be called "activation," or the term may be used to refer to the effect of any stimulus, however prompt. However, there is a more restricted usage of the term, which forms a central thread in the study of macrophages from the time of Metchnikoff to the present day. It is fitting to conclude a description of macrophage physiology by retracing this thread.[289]

Metchnikoff observed that macrophages in infected hosts often responded more vigorously to the introduction of phagocytic particles. In 1939, Lurie clearly demonstrated that the macrophages from tuberculous animals were larger and more phagocytic than those from controls. In the 1960s, Mackaness and his colleagues revealed both the immunologic basis and the protective function of macrophage activation. They demonstrated that in the later stages of infection or after the host recovers, its lymphocytes, when encountering the antigens of the original infecting organism, confer upon macrophages an enhanced capacity to inhibit the intracellular replication of the same or unrelated pathogens. That is, induction of macrophage activation is immunologically specific, while its expression is nonspecific and consists, in its essence, of enhanced antimicrobial capacity.

At the same time that macrophages acquire enhanced antimicrobial capacity, they undergo innumerable other changes, such as increased spreading on glass and alterations in phagocytic activity, surface receptor function, and the content of organelles and enzymes. These changes, for a time, were also referred to as macrophage activation. In the mid and late 1970s, however, it became apparent that such changes could be induced by a variety of means in macrophages that did not express enhanced antimicrobial activity, that not all the changes appear concordantly, that macrophages with enhanced antimicrobial activity often exhibit decreases rather than increases in other functions, or that these other functions may change in different ways under different experimental conditions, without relation to antimicrobial activity. By the end of the decade, the only biochemical feature that could be firmly correlated with antimicrobial capacity was the ability to secrete hydrogen peroxide. This surely reflects the prominent role of reactive oxygen intermediates in the killing of intracellular pathogens by macrophages. However, it has become increasingly apparent that oxygen-independent antimicrobial mechanisms are important under certain conditions, and in these cases, peroxide-secretory capacity and antimicrobial activity can be dissociated.

Just as some workers use macrophage "activation" in the sense introduced by Mackaness, and others use it to refer to enhanced antitumor activity, or to enhanced peroxide-secretory capacity, or to any altered function, so there is divergence in usage of the term "macrophage activating factor." Recent evidence indicates that in the case of oxidative metabolism, killing of intracellular protozoal pathogens, and killing of extracellular tumor cells, the primary T-lymphocyte product that activates macrophages is gamma-interferon.[256] However, other macrophage-activating factors may remain to be defined in the same or other assays. What about activation of macrophages by non-T lymphocytes, by nonlymphoid cells, by humoral agents like complement, or by bacterial products like lipopolysaccharide and muramyl dipeptide? It is conceivable that these involve secretion of alpha- or beta-interferon, or act through the induction of interferon secretion by the macrophages themselves.[355] In this view, there would be a final common pathway for macrophage activation. Alternatively, there may be many ways to activate a macrophage. The consequences of activation are so dramatic for numerous functions of this ubiquitous cell that this question remains an area of intense research 100 years after it was raised.

### References


1. Metchnikoff, E.: Immunity in Infective Diseases. F.G. Binnie, trans. London, Cambridge University Press, 1905.
2. van Furth, R. (ed.): Mononuclear Phagocytes. Oxford, Blackwell Scientific Publications, 1970.
3. van Furth, R. (ed.): Mononuclear Phagocytes in Immunity, Infection and Pathology. Oxford, Blackwell Scientific Publications, 1975.
4. van Furth, R. (ed.): Mononuclear Phagocytes: Functional Aspects. The Hague, Martinus Nijhoff, 1980.
5. Nelson, D.W. (ed.): Immunobiology of the Macrophage. New York, Academic Press, 1976.
6. Fink, M.A. (ed.): The Macrophage in Neoplasia. New York, Academic Press, 1976.
7. Zweifach, B.W., Grant, L., and McCluskey, R.T. (eds.): The Inflammatory Process. 2nd ed. New York, Academic Press, 1973.
8. Langevoort, H.C., Cohn, Z.A., Hirsch, J.G., Humphrey, J.H., Spector, W.G., and van Furth, R.: The nomenclature of mononuclear phagocytes: Proposal for a new classification. *In* van Furth, R. (ed.): Mononuclear Phagocytes. Oxford, Blackwell Scientific Publications, 1970, p. 1.
9. Hume, D.A., and Gordon, S.: The mononuclear phagocyte system of the mouse defined by immunohistochemical localisation of antigen F4/80. Identification of resident macropahges in renal medullary and cortical interstitium and the juxtaglomerular complex. J. Exp. Med. 157:1704, 1983.
10. van Voorhis, W.C., Steinman, R.M., Hair, L.S., Luban, J., Witmer, M.D., Koide, S., and Cohn, Z.A.: Specific antimononuclear phagocyte monoclonal antibodies. Application to the purification of dendritic cells and the tissue localization of macrophages. J. Exp. Med. 158:126, 1983.
11. Volkman, A., and Gowans, J.L.: The origin of macrophages from bone marrow in the rat. Br. J. Exp. Pathol. 46:62, 1965.
12. van Furth, R., and Cohn, Z.A.: The origin and kinetics of mononuclear phagocytes. J. Exp. Med. 128:415, 1968.

13. Goud, T.J.L.M., Schotte, C., and van Furth, R.: Identification and characterization of the monoblast in mononuclear phagocyte colonies grown in vitro. J. Exp. Med. 142:1180, 1975.
14. Goud, T.J.L.M., and van Furth, R.: Proliferative characteristics of monoblasts grown in vitro. J. Exp. Med. 142:1200, 1975.
15. van Furth, R., Hirsch, J.G., and Fedorko, M.E.: Morphology and peroxidase cytochemistry of mouse promonocytes, monocytes, and macrophages. J. Exp. Med. 132:794, 1970.
16. van Furth, R.: Origin and kinetics of mononuclear phagocytes. Ann. N.Y. Acad. Sci. 278:161, 1976.
17. Meuret, G., Batara, E., and Furste, H.O. Monocytopoiesis in normal man: Pool size, proliferation activity and DNA synthesis time of promonocytes. Acta Haematol. 54:261, 1975.
18. Meuret, G., Bammert, J., and Hoffman, G.: Kinetics of human monocytopoiesis. Blood 44:801, 1974.
19. Whitelaw, D.M., and Batho, H.F.: Kinetics of monocytes. *In* van Furth, R. (ed.): Mononuclear Phagocytes in Immunity, Infection and Pathology. Oxford, Blackwell Scientific Publications, 1975, p. 175.
20. Whitelaw, D.M.: Observations on human monocyte kinetics after pulse labelling. Cell Tissue Kinet. 5:311, 1972.
21. Meuret, G., and Hoffmann, G.: Monocyte kinetic studies in normal and disease states. Br. J. Haematol. 24:275, 1973.
22. van Furth, R., and Diesselfhoff-den Dulk, M.C.: The kinetics of promonocytes and monocytes in the bone marrow. J. Exp. Med. 132:813, 1970.
23. Ebert, R.H., and Florey, H.W.: The extravascular development of the monocyte observed in vivo. Br. J. Exp. Pathol. 20:342, 1939.
24. van Furth, R.: Origin and kinetics of monocytes and macrophages. Semin. Hematol. 7:125, 1970.
25. Meuret, G., Detel, U., Kilz, H.P., Senn, H.J., and van Lessen, H.: Human monocytopoiesis in acute and chronic inflammation. Acta Haematol. 54:328, 1975.
26. Lewis, M.R.: The formation of macrophages, epithelioid cells and giant cells from leukocytes in incubated blood. Am. J. Pathol. 1:91, 1925.
27. Bennett, W.E., and Cohn, Z.A.: The isolation and selected properties of blood monocytes. J. Exp. Med. 123:145, 1966.
28. Johnson, W.D., Jr., Mei, B., and Cohn, Z.A.: The separation, long-term cultivation, and maturation of the human monocyte. J. Exp. Med. 146:1613, 1977.
29. Musson, R.A., Shafran, H., and Henson, P.M.: Intracellular levels and stimulated release of lysosomal enzymes from human peripheral blood monocytes and monocyte-derived macrophages. J. Reticuloendothel. Soc. 28:249, 1980.
30. Newman, S.L., Musson, R.A., and Henson, P.M.: Development of functional complement receptors during in vitro maturation of human monocytes into macrophages. J. Immunol. 125:2236, 1980.
31. Nakagawara, A., Nathan, C.F., and Cohn, Z.A.: Hydrogen peroxide metabolism in human monocytes during differentiation in vitro. J. Clin. Invest. 68:1243, 1981.
32. Volkman, A.: Disparity in origin of mononuclear phagocyte populations. J. Reticuloendothel. Soc. 19:249, 1976.
33. Shands, J.W., and Axelrod, B.J.: Mouse peritoneal macrophages: Tritiated thymidine labelling and cell kinetics. J. Reticuloendothel. Soc. 21:69, 1977.
34. Volkman, A.: Monocyte kinetics and their changes in infection. *In* Nelson, D.S. (ed.): Immunobiology of the Macrophage. New York, Academic Press, 1976, p. 294.
35. Pinkett, M.O., Cordrey, C.R., and Nowell, P.C.: Mixed hematopoietic and pulmonary origin of 'alveolar macrophages' as demonstrated by chromosome markers. Am. J. Pathol. 48:859, 1966.
36. Crofton, R.W., Martina, M.C., Diesselhoff-den Dulk, M.M.C., and van Furth, R.: The origin, kinetics, and characteristics of the Kupffer cells in the normal steady state. J. Exp. Med. 148:1, 1978.
37. Gale, R.P., Sparkes, R.S., and Golde, D.W.: Bone marrow origin of hepatic macrophages (Kupffer cells) in humans. Science 201:937, 1978.
38. Oehmichen, M.: Monocytic orign of microglia cells. *In* van Furth, R. (ed.): Mononuclear Phagocytes in Immunity, Infection and Pathology. Oxford, Blackwell Scientific Publications 1975, p. 223.
39. Blussé van Oud Ablas, A., and van Furth, R.: Origin, kinetics, and characteristics of pulmonary macrophages in the normal steady state. J. Exp. Med. 149:1504, 1979.
40. Evans, J.J., Cabral, L.J., Stephens R.J., and Freeman, G.: Cell division of alveolar macrophages in rat lung following exposure to $NO_2$. Am. J. Pathol. 70:199, 1973.
41. Steward, C.C., Lin, H.S., and Adles, C.: Proliferation and colony-forming ability of peritoneal exudate cells in liquid culture. J. Exp. Med. 141:1114, 1975.
42. Volkman, A., and Gowans, J.L.: The production of macrophages in the rat. Br. J. Exp. Pathol. 46:50, 1965.
43. North, R.J.: The mitotic potential of fixed phagocytes in the liver as revealed during the development of cellular immunity. J. Exp. Med. 130:315, 1969.
44. Spector, W.G., and Mariano, M.: Macrophage behaviour in experimental granulomas. *In* van Furth, R. (ed.): Mononuclear Phagocytes in Immunity, Infection and Pathology. Oxford, Blackwell Scientific Publications, 1975, p. 927.
45. Dannenberg, A.M., Ando, M., Shima, K., and Tsuda, T.: Macrophage turnover and activation in tuberculous granulomata. *In* van Furth, R. (ed.): Mononuclear Phagocytes in Immunity, Infection and Pathology. Oxford, Blackwell Scientific Publications, 1975, p. 959.
46. Sutton, J.S.: Ultrastructural aspects of in vitro development of monocytes into macrophages, epithelioid cells, and multinucleated giant cells. Natl. Cancer Inst. Monograph 26:71, 1967.
47. Postlethwaite, A.E., Jackson, B.K., Beachey, E.H., and Kang, A.H.: Formation of multinucleated giant cells from human monocyte precursors. Mediation by a soluble protein from antigen- and mitogen-stimulated lymphocytes. J. Exp. Med. 155:168, 1982.
48. Lewis, W.H.: The formation of giant cells in tissue cultures and their similarity to those in tuberculous lesions. Am. Rev. Tuberculosis 15:616, 1927.
49. Izumi, S., Penrose, J.M., More, D.G., and Nelson, D.S.: Further observation on the immunological induction of DNA synthesis in mouse peritoneal macrophages. Int. Arch. Allergy App. Immunol. 49:573, 1975.
50. van Waarde, D., Hulsing-Hesselink, E., and van Furth, R.: Properties of a factor increasing monocytopoiesis (FIM) occurring in serum during the early phase of an inflammatory reaction. Blood 50:727, 1977.
51. Chervenick, P., and Lobuglio, A.F.: Human blood monocytes: Stimulators of granulocyte and mononuclear colony formation in vitro. Science 78:164, 1972.
52. Parker, J.W., and Metcalf, D.: Production of colony-stimulating factor in mitogen-stimulated lymphocyte cultures. J. Immunol. 112:502, 1974.
53. Stanley, E.R., and Guilbert, L.J.: Regulation of macrophage production by a colony stimulating factor. *In* van Furth, R. (ed.): Mononuclear Phagocytes: Functional Aspects. The Hague, Martinus Nijhoff, 1980, p. 417.
54. Loor, kF., and Roelants, G.E.: The dynamic state of the macrophage plasma membrane. Attachment and fate of immunoglobulin, antigen, and lectins. Eur. J. Immunol. 4:649, 1974.
55. Colvin, R.B., and Dvorak, H.F.: Fibrinogen/fibrin on the surface of macrophages: Detection, distribution, binding requirements, and possible role in macrophage adherence phenomena. J. Exp. Med. 142:1337, 1975.
56. van Ginkel, C.J.W., and van Akan, W.G.: Generation of tissue thromboplastin by human monocytes. *In* van Furth, R. (ed.): Mononuclear Phagocytes: Functional Aspects. The Hague, Martinus Nijhoff, 1980, p. 1351.
57. Nachman, R.L., Ferris, B., and Hirsch, J.G.: Macrophage plasma membrane. II. Studies on synthesis and turnover of protein constituents. J. Exp. Med. 133:807, 1971.
58. Werb, Z., and Cohn, Z.A.: Plasma membrane synthesis in the macrophage following phagocytosis of polystyrene latex particles. J. Biol. Chem. 247:2439, 1972.
59. Edelson, P.J., and Cohn, Z.A.: 5′-Nucleotidase activity of mouse peritoneal macrophages. II. Cellular distribution and effects of endocytosis. J. Exp. Med. 144:1596, 1976.
60. Edelson, P.J., and Cohn, Z.A.: 5′-Nucleotidase activity of mouse peritoneal macrophages. I. Synthesis and degradation in resident and inflammatory populations. J. Exp. Med. 144:1581, 1976.
61. Edelson, P.J., and Erbs, C.: Plasma membrane localization and metabolism of alkaline phosphodiesterase I in mouse peritoneal macrophages. J. Exp. Med. 147:77, 1978.
62. Edelson, P.J., Zweibel, R., and Cohn, Z.A.: The pinocytic rate of activated macrophages. J. Exp. Med. 142:1150, 1975.
63. Ezekowitz, R.A.B., Austyn, J., Stahl, P.D., and Gordon, S.: Surface properties of bacillus Calmette-Guerin-activated mouse macrophages. Reduced expression of mannose-specific endocytosis, Fc receptors, and antigen F4‖80 accompanies induction of Ia. J. Exp. Med. 154:60, 1981.
64. Remold-O'Donnell, E., and Lewandrowski, K.: Decrease of the major surface glycoprotein gp160 in activated macrophages. Cell. Immunol. 70:85, 982.
65. Werb, Z., and Cohn, Z.A.: Cholesterol metabolism in the macrophages. I. The regulation of cholesterol exchange. J. Exp. Med. 134:1545, 1971.
66. Werb, Z.: Macrophage membrane synthesis. *In* van Furth, R. (ed.): Mononuclear Phagocytes in Immunity, Infection and Pathology. Oxford, Blackwell Scientific Publications, 1975, p. 331.
67. Mahoney, E.M., Hamill, A.L., Scott, W.A., and Cohn, Z.A.: Response of endocytosis to altered fatty acyl composition of macrophage phospholipids. Proc. Natl. Acad. Sci. USA 74:4895, 1977.
68. Shreffler, D.C., and David, C.S.: The H-2 major histocompatibility complex and the I immune response gene region: Genetic variation, function and organization. Adv. Immunol. 20:125, 1975.
69. Steeg, P.S., Moore, R.N., and Oppenheim, J.J.: Regulation of macrophage

Ia-antigen expression by products of activated spleen cells. J. Exp. Med. 152:1734, 1980.
70. Steinman, R.M., Nogueira, N., Witmer, M.D., Tydings, J.D., and Mellman, I.S.: Lymphokine enhances the expression and synthesis of Ia antigens on cultured mouse peritoneal macrophages. J. Exp. Med. 152:1248, 1980.
71. Todd, R.F., III, and Schlossman, S.F.: Analysis of antigenic determinants of human monocytes and macrophages. Blood 59:775, 1982.
72. Hogg, N., Slusarenko, M., Cohen, J., and Reiser, J.: Monoclonal antibody with specificity for monocytes and neurons. Cell 24:875, 1981.
73. LeBien, T.W., Kersey, J.H.,: A monoclonal antibody (TA-1) reactive with human T lymphocytes and monocytes. J. Immunol. 125:2208, 1980.
74. Beller, D.P., Springer, T.A., and Schreiber, R.D.: Anti-Mac-1 selectively inhibits the mouse and human type three complement receptor. J. Exp. Med. 156:1000, 1982.
75. Austyn, J.M., and Gordon S.: F4||80, a monoclonal antibody directed specifically against the mouse macrophage. Eur. J. Immunol. 11:805, 1981.
76. Taniyama, T., and Watanabe, T.: Establishment of hybridoma secreting a monoclonal antibody specific for activated tumoricidal macrophages. J. Exp. Med. 156:1286, 1982.
77. Berken, A., and Benacerraf, B.: Properties of antibodies cytophilic for macrophages. J. Exp. Med. 123:119, 1966.
78. Lobuglio, A.F., Cotran, R.S., and Jandl, J.H.: Red cells coated with immunoglobulin G: Binding and sphering by mononuclear cells in man. Science 158:1582, 1967.
79. Huber, H., Polley, M.J., Linscott, W.D., Fudenberg, H.H., and Muller-Eberhard, H.J.: Human monocytes: Distinct receptor sites for the third component of complement and for immunoglobulin G. Science 162:1281, 1968.
80. Unkeless, J.C., Fleit, H., and Mellman, I.S.: Structural aspects and heterogeneity of immunoglobulin Fc receptors. Adv. Immunol. 31:247, 1981.
81. Johnston, R.B., Jr., Lehmeyer, J., and Guthrie, L.: Generation of superoxide anion and chemiluminescence by human monocytes during phagocytosis and by contact with surface-bound immunoglobulin G. J. Exp. Med. 143:1551, 1978.
82. Ezekowitz, R.A.B., Bampton, M., and Gordon, S.: Macrophage activation selectively enhances expression of Fc receptors for IgG2a. J. Exp. Med. 157:807, 983.
83. Bonney, R.J., Naruns, P., Davies, P., and Humes, J.L.: Antigen-antibody complexes stimulate the synthesis and release of prostaglandins by mouse peritoneal macrophages. Prostaglandins 18:605, 1979.
84. Cardella, C.J., Davies, P., and Allison, A.C.: Immune complexes induce selective release of lysosomal hydrolases from macrophages. Nature 247:46, 1974.
85. Melewicz, F.M., and Spiegelberg, H.L.: Fc receptors for IgE on a subpopulation of human peripheral blood monocytes. J. Immunol. 125:1026, 1980.
86. Finbloom, D.S., and Metzger, H.: Binding of immunoglobulin E to the receptor on rat peritoneal macrophages. J. Immunol. 129:2004, 1982.
87. Joseph, M., Tonnel, A.-B., Torpier, G., and Capron, A.: Involvement of immunoglobulin E in the secretory processes of alveolar macrophages from asthmatic patients. J. Clin. Invest. 71:221, 1983.
88. Fleit, H.B., Wright, S.D., and Unkeless, J.C.: Human neutrophil Fc receptor distribution and structure. Proc. Natl. Acad. Sci. USA 79:3275, 1982.
89. Perussia, B., Dayton, E.T., Lazarus, R., Fanning, V., and Trinchieri, G.: Immune interferon induces the receptor for monomeric IgG1 on human monocytic and myeloid cells. J. Exp. Med., 158:1092, 1983.
90. Mellman, I.S., and Unkeless, J.C.: Purification of a functional mouse Fc receptor through the use of a monoclonal antibody. J. Exp. Med. 152:1048, 1980.
91. Young, J.D., Unkeless, J.C., Kaback, H.R., and Cohn, Z.A.: Mouse macrophage Fc receptor for IgG 2bγ1 in artificial and plasma membrane vesicles functions as a ligand-dependent ionophore. Proc. Natl. Acad. Sci. USA 80:1636, 1983.
92. Griffin, F.M., Jr., Bianco, C., and Silverstein, S.C.: Characterization of the macrophage receptor for complement and demonstration of its functional independence from the receptor for the Fc portion of immunoglobulin G. J. Exp. Med. 141:1269, 1975.
93. Ehlenberger, A.G., and Nussenzweig, V.: The role of membrane receptors for C3b and C3d in phagocytosis. J. Exp. Med. 145:357, 1977.
94. Bianco, C., Griffin, F.M., Jr., and Silverstein, S.C.: Studies of the macrophage complement receptor. Alteration of receptor function upon macrophage activation. J. Exp. Med. 141:1278, 1975.
95. Rabellino, E.M., Ross, G.D., and Polley, M.J.: Membrane receptors of mouse leukocytes. I. Two types of complement receptors for different regions of C3. J. Immunol. 120:879, 1978.
96. Goodman, M.G., Chenoweth, D.E., and Weigle, W.O.: Induction of interleukin 1 secretion and enhancement of humoral immunity by binding of human C5a to macrophage surface C5a receptors. J. Exp. Med. 156:912, 1982.
97. Griffin, J.A., and Griffin, F.M.: Augmentation of macrophage complement receptor function in vitro. I. Characterization of the cellular interactions required for the generation of a T-lymphocyte product that enhances macrophage complement receptor function. J. Exp. Med. 150:653, 1979.
98. Pemmier, C.G., Inada, S., Fries, L.F., Takahashi, T., Frank, M.M., and Brown, E.J.: Plasma fibronectin enhances the phagocytosis of opsonized particles by human peripheral blood monocytes. J. Exp. Med. 157:1844, 1983.
99. Wright, S.D., Craigmyle, L., and Silverstein, S.C.: Fibronectin and serum amyloid P-component stimulate C3b- and C3bi-mediated phagocytosis in cultured human monocytes. J. Exp. Med., 158:1338, 1983.
100. Stahl, P.D., Rodman, J.S., Miller, M.J., and Schlesinger, P.H.: Evidence for receptor-mediated binding of glycoproteins, glycoconjugates and lysosomal glycosidases by alveolar macrophages. Proc. Natl. Acad. Sci. USA 75:1399, 1978.
101. Debanne, M.T., Bell, R., and Dolovich, J.: Uptake of proteinase-macroglobulin complexes by macrophages. Biochim. Biophys. Acta 411: 295, 1975.
102. Liu, D.Y., Petschek, K.D., Remold, H.G., and David, J.R.: Isolation of a guinea pig macrophage glycolipid with the properties of the putative migration inhibitory factor receptor. J. Biol. Chem. 257:159, 1982.
103. Guilbert, L.J., and Stanley, E.R.: Specific interaction of murine colony-stimulating factor with mononuclear phagocytic cells. J. Cell Biol. 85:153, 1980.
104. Remold, H.G.: Requirement for α-L-fucose on the macrophage membrane receptor for MIF. J. Exp. Med. 138:1065, 1973.
105. Traber, M.G., and Kayden, H.J.: Low density lipoprotein receptor activity in human monocyte-derived macrophages and its relation to atheromatous lesions. Proc. Natl. Acad. Sci. USA 77:5466, 1980.
106. Goldstein, J.L., Ho, Y.K., Basu, S.K., and Brown, M.S.: Binding site on macrophages that mediates uptake and degradation of acetylated low density lipoprotein, producing massive cholesterol deposition. Proc. Natl. Acad. Sci. USA 76:33, 1979.
107. Fogelman, A.M., Shechter, I., Seager, J., Hokom, M., Child, J.S., and Edwards, P.A.: Malondialdehyde alteration of low density lipoproteins leads to cholesteryl ester accumulation in human monocyte-macrophages. Proc. Natl. Acad. Sci. 77:2214, 1980.
108. Henriksen, T., Mahoney, E.M., and Steinberg, D.: Enhanced macrophage degradation of low density lipoprotein previously incubated with cultured endothelial cells: recognition by receptors for acetylated low density lipoproteins. Proc. Natl. Acad. Sci. USA 78:6499, 1981.
109. Goldstein, J.L., Ho, Y.K., Brown, M.S., Innerarity, T.L., and Mahley, R.W.: Cholesteryl-ester accumulation in macrophages resulting from receptor-mediated uptake and degradation of hypercholesterolemic canine β-very low density lipoproteins. J. Biol. Chem. 255:1839, 1980.
110. Gianturco, S.H., Bradley, W.A., Gotto, A.M., Jr., Morrisett, J.D., and Peavy, D.L.: Hypertriglyceridemic very low density lipoproteins induce tryglyceride synthesis and accumulation in mouse peritoneal macrophages. J. Clin. Invest. 70:168, 1982.
111. van Lenten, B.J., Fogelman, A.M., Hokom, M.M., Benson, L., Haberland, M.E., and Edwards, P.A.: Regulation of the uptake and degradation of β-very low density lipoprotein in human monocyte macrophages. J. Biol. Chem. 258:5151, 1983.
112. Johnson, W.J., Pizzo, S.V., Imber, M.J., and Adams, D.O.: Receptors for maleylated proteins regulate secretion of neutral proteases by murine macrophages. Science 218:574, 1982.
113. Whaley, K., Lappin, D., and Barkas, T.: C2 synthesis by human monocytes is modulated by a nicotinic cholinergic receptor. Nature 293:580, 1981.
114. Diaz, P., Jones, D.G., and Kay, A.B.: Histamine receptors on guinea-pig alveolar macrophages: chemical specificity and the effects of H1- and H2-receptor agonists and antagonists. Clin. Exp. Immunol. 35:462, 1979.
115. Steinman, R.M., Brodie, S.E., and Cohn, Z.A.: Membrane flow during pinocytosis: A stereologic analysis. J. Cell Biol. 68:665, 1976.
116. Steinman, R.M., and Cohn, Z.A.: Endocytosis and the vacuolar apparatus. *In* Cook, J.A. (ed.): Biogenesis and Turnover of Membrane Macromolecules. New York, Raven Press, 1976, p. 1.
117. Galloway, C.J., Dean, G.E., Marsh, M., Rudnick, G., and Mellman, I.: Acidification of macrophage and fibroblast endocytic vesicles in vitro. Proc. Natl. Acad. Sci. USA 80:3334, 1983.
118. Cohn, Z.A., and Wiener, E.: The particulate hydrolases of macrophages. I. Comparative enzymology, isolation and properties. J. Exp. Med. 118:991, 1963.
119. Cohn, Z.A., and Wiener, E.: The particulate hydrolases of macrophages. II. Biochemical and morphological response to particle ingestion. J. Exp. Med. 118:1009, 1963.
120. Cohn, Z.A., Fedorko, M.E., and Hirsch, J.G.: The in vitro differentiation of mononuclear phagocytes. V. The formation of macrophage lysosomes. J. Exp. Med. 123:757, 1966.
121. Steinman, R.M., Mellman, I.S., Muller, W.A., and Cohn, Z.A.: Endo-

cytosis and the recycling of the plasma membrane. J. Cell Biol. 96:1, 1983.
122. Cohn, Z.A., Hirsch, J.G., and Wiener, E.: The cytoplasmic granules of phagocytic cells and the degradation of bacteria. *In* de Reuck, A.V.S., and Cameron, M.P. (eds.): Ciba Foundation Symposium on Lysosomes. London, J. and A. Churchill, 1963, p. 126.
123. Cohn, Z.A.: The fate of bacteria within phagocytic cells. I. The degradation of isotopically labelled bacteria by polymorphonuclear leukcoytes and macrophages. J. Exp. Med. 117:27, 1963.
124. Ehrenreich, B.A., and Cohn, Z.A.: The fate of peptides pinocytosed by macrophages in vitro. J. Exp. Med. 129:227, 1969.
125. Reaven, E.P., and Axline, S.G.: Subplasmalemmal microfilaments and microtubules in resting and phagocytizing cultivated macrophages. J. Cell Biol. 59:12, 1973.
126. Hartwig, J.H., and Stossel, T.P.: Macrophages: their use in elucidation of the cytoskeletal roles of actin. Meth. Cell Biol. 25:201, 1982.
127. Hartwig, J.H., and Stossel, T.P.: Isolation and properties of actin, myosin, and a new actin-binding protein in rabbit alveolar macrophages. J. Biol. Chem. 250:5696, 1975.
128. Southwick, F.S., and Hartwig, J.H.: Acumentin, a protein in macrophages which caps the 'pointed' end of actin filaments. Nature 297:303, 1982.
129. Yin, H.L., Hartwig, J.H., Maruyama, K., and Stossel, T.P.: $Ca^{2+}$ control of actin filament length. Effects of macrophage gelsolin on actin polymerization. J. Biol. Chem. 256:9693, 1981.
130. Brotschi, E.A., Hartwig, J.H., and Stossel, T.P.: The gelation of actin by actin-binding protein. J. Biol. Chem. 253:8988, 1978.
131. Bhisey, A.N., and Freed, J.J.: Altered movement of endosomes in colchicine-treated cultured macrophages. Exp. Cell Res. 64:430, 1971.
132. Rebuck, J.W., and Crowley, J.H.: A method of studying leukocytic functions in vivo. Ann. N.Y. Acad. Sci. 59:757, 1955.
133. Rabinovitch, M.: Macrophage spreading in vitro. *In* van Furth, R. (ed.): Mononuclear Phagocytes in Immunity, Infection and Pathology. London, Blackwell Scientific Publications, 1975, p. 369.
134. Bianco, C., Eden, A., and Cohn, Z.A.: The induction of macrophage spreading: Role of coagulation factors and the complement system. J. Exp. Med. 144:1531, 1976.
135. Götze, O., Bianco, C., Sundsmo, J.S., and Cohn, Z.A.: The stimulation of mononuclear phagocytes by components of the classical and the alternative pathways of complement activation. *In* van Furth, R. (ed.): Mononuclear Phagocytes: Functional Aspects. The Hague, Martinus Nijhoff, 1980, p. 1421.
136. Bevilacqua, M.P., Amrani, D., Mosesson, M.W., and Bianco, C.: Receptors for cold-insoluble globulin (plasma fibronectin) on human monocytes. J. Exp. Med. 153:42, 1981.
137. Clark, R.A.F., Quinn, J.H., Winn, H.J., Lanigan, J.M., Dellepella, P., and Colvin, R.B.: Fibronectin is produced by blood vessels in response to injury. J. Exp. Med. 156:646, 1982.
138. Sherman, L.A., and Lee, J.: Specific binding of soluble fibrin to macrophages. J. Exp. Med. 145:76, 1977.
139. Unkeless, J.C., Gordon, S.C., and Reich, E.: Secretiòn of plasminogen activator by stimulated macrophages. J. Exp. Med. 139:834, 1974.
140. Werb, Z., and Gordon, S.: Elastase secretion by stimulated macrophages. J. Exp. Med. 142:345, 1975.
141. Wahl, L.M., Wahl, S.M., Mergenhagen, S.E., and Martin, G.R.: Collagenase production by lymphokine-activated macrophages. Science 187:261, 1975.
142. Werb, Z., and Gordon, S.: Secretion of a specific collagenase by stimulated macrophages. J. Exp. Med. 142:345, 1975.
143. Banda, M.J., Clark, E.J., and Werb, Z.: Limited proteolysis by macrophage elastase inactivates human $\alpha_1$-protease inhibitor. J. Exp. Med. 152:1563, 1980.
144. Werb, Z., Banda, M.J., and Jones, P.A.: Degradation of connective tissue matrices by macrophages. I. Proteolysis of elastin, glycoproteins, and collagen by proteinases isolated from macrophages. J. Exp. Med. 152:1340, 1980.
145. Jones, P.A., and Werb, Z.: Degradation of connective tissue matrices by macrophages. II. Influence of the matrix composition on proteolysis of glycoproteins, elastin, and collagen by macrophages in culture. J. Exp. Med. 152:1527, 1980.
146. Werb, Z., Bainton, D.F., and Jones, P.A.: Degradation of connective tissue matrices by macrophages. III. Morphological and biochemical studies on extracellular, pericellular, and intracellular events in matrix proteolysis by macrophages in culture. J. Exp. Med. 152:1537, 1980.
147. Snyderman, R., and Mergenhagen, S.E.: Chemotaxis of macrophages. *In* Nelson, D.S. (ed.): Immunobiology of the Macrophage. New York, Academic Press, 1976, p. 323.
148. Chenoweth, D.E., Goodman, M.G., and Weigle, W.O.: Demonstration of a specific receptor for human C5a anaphylatoxin on murine macrophages. J. Exp. Med. 156:68, 1982.
149. Polley, M.J., and Nachman, R.: The human complement system in thrombin-mediated platelet function. J. Exp. Med. 147:1713, 1978.
150. Ward, P.A.: Chemotaxis of mononuclear cells. J. Exp. Med. 128:1201, 1968.
151. Bar-Shavit, R., Kahn, A., Fenton, J.W., II, and Wilner, G.D.: Chemotactic response of monocytes to thrombin. J. Cell Biol. 96:282, 1983.
152. Gallin, J.I., and Kaplan, A.P.: Mononuclear cell chemotactic activity of kallikrein and plasminogen activator and its inhibition by C*1* inhibitor and $\alpha_2$-macroglobulin. J. Immunol. 113:1928, 1974.
153. Wilkinson, P.C.: Cellular and molecular aspects of chemotaxis of macrophages and monocytes. *In* Nelson, D.S. (ed.): Immunobiology of the Macrophage. New York, Academic Press, 1976. p. 350.
154. Norris, D.A., Clark, R.A.F., Swigart, L.M., Huff, J.C., Weston, W.L., and Howell, S.E.: Fibronectin fragment(s) are chemotactic for human peripheral blood monocytes. J. Immunol. 129:1612, 1982.
155. Postlethwaite, A.E., Keski-Oja, J., Balian, G., and Kang, A.H.: Induction of fibroblast chemotaxis by fibronectin. Localization of the chemotactic region to a 140,000-molecular weight non-gelatin-binding fragment. J. Exp. Med. 153:494, 1981.
156. Hunninghake, G.W., Davidson, J.M., Rennard, S., Szapeil, S., Gadek, J. E., and Crystal, R.G.: Elastin fragments attract macrophage precursors to diseased sited in pulmonary emphysema. Science 212:925, 1981.
157. Senior, R.M., Griffin, G.L., and Mecham, R.P.: Chemotactic activity of elastin-derived peptides. J. Clin. Invest. 66:859, 1980.
158. Postlethwaite, A.E., and Kang, A.H.: Collagen- and collagen peptide-induced chemotaxis of human blood monocytes. J. Exp. Med. 143:1299, 1976.
159. Mundy, G.R., Varani J., Orr, W., Gondek, M.D., and Ward, P.A.: Resorbing bone is chemotactic for monocytes. Nature 275:132, 1978.
160. Ward, P.A., Remold, H.G., and David, J.R.: Leukotactic factor produced by sensitized lymphocytes. Science 163:1079, 1969.
161. Wahl, S.M., Iverson, G.M., and Oppenheim, J.J.: Induction of guinea pig B-cell lymphokine synthesis by mitogenic and nonmitogenic signals to Fc, Ig and C3 receptors. J. Exp. Med. 140:1631, 1974.
162. Postlethwaite, A.E., Arnold, E., and Snyderman, R.: Characterization of chemotactic activity produced in vivo by a cell-mediated immune reaction in the guinea pig. J. Immunol. 114:274, 1975.
163. Gallin, J.I., Fletcher, M.P. Seligmann, B.E., Hoffstein, S., Cehrs, K., and Mounessa, N.: Human neutrophil-specific granule deficiency: A model to assess the role of neutrophil-specific granules in the evolution of the inflammatory response. Blood 59:1317, 1982.
164. Deuel, T.F., Senior, R.M., Chang, D., Griffin, G.L., Heinrikson, R.L., and Kaiser, E.T.: Platelet factor 4 is chemotactic for neutrophils and monocytes. Proc. Natl. Acad. Sci. USA 78:4584, 1981.
165. Bottazzi, B., Polentaratti, N., Balsari, A., Boraschi, D., Ghezzi, P. Salmona, M., and Mantovani, A.: Chemotactic activity for mononuclear phagocytes of culture supernatants from murine and human tumor cells: Evidence for a role in the regulation of the macrophage content of neoplastic tissues. Int. J. Cancer 31:55, 1983.
166. Schiffman, E., Corcoran, B.A., and Wahl, S.M.: N-formylmethionyl peptides as chemoattractants for leukocytes. Proc. Natl. Acad. Sci. USA 72:1059, 1975.
167. Carp, H.: Mitochondrial N-formylmethionyl proteins as chemoattractants for neutrophils. J. Exp. Med. 155:264, 1982.
168. Meltzer, M.S., Stevenson, M.M., and Leonard E.J.: Characterization of macrophage chemotaxins in tumor cell cultures and comparison with lymphocyte-derived chemotactic factors. Cancer Res. 37:721, 1977.
169. Meltzer, M.S., Jones, E.E., and Boetcher, D.A.: Increased chemotactic response of macrophages from BCG-infected mice. Cell. Immunol. 17:268, 1975.
170. Boetcher, D.A., and Leonard, E.J.: Abnormal monocyte chemotactic response in cancer patients. J. Natl. Cancer Inst. 52:1091, 1974.
171. Snyderman, R., Pike, M.C., Blaylock, B.L., and Weinstein, P.: Effects of neoplasms on inflammation: Depression of macrophage accumulation after tumor implantation. J. Immunol. 116:585, 1976.
172. Stevenson, M.M., and Meltzer, M.S.: Depressed chemotactic responses in vitro of peritoneal macropahges from tumor-bearing mice. J. Natl. Cancer Inst. 57:847, 1976.
173. Cianciolo, G., Hunter, J., Silva, J., Haskill, J.S., and Snyderman, R.: Inhibitors of monocyte responses to chemotaxins are present in human cancerous effusions and react with protein of retroviruses. J. Clin. Invest. 68:831, 1981.
174. Cianciolo, G., Lostrom, M., Tam, M., and Snyderman, R.: Murine malignant cells synthesize a 19,000-dalton protein that is physicochemically and antigenically related to the immunosuppressive retroviral protein, P15E. J. Exp. Med. 158:885, 1983.
175. Brozna, J.P., and Ward, P.A.: Antileukotactic properties of tumor cells. J. Clin. Invest. 56:616, 1975.
176. Remold, H.G., McCarthy, P.L., Jr., and Mednis, A.D.: Purification of guinea pig pH 3 migration inhibitory factor. Proc. Natl. Acad. Sci. USA 78:4088, 1981.
177. David, J.R.: Delayed hypersensitivity in vitro: Its mediation by cell-free substances formed by lymphoid cell-antigen interaction. Proc. Natl. Acad. Sci. USA 56:72, 1966.
178. Bloom, B.R., and Bennet, B.: Mechanism of a reaction in vitro associated with delayed-type hypersensitivity. Science 153:80, 1966.
179. Bianco, C., Gotze, O., and Cohn, Z.A.: Complement, coagulation, and

mononuclear phagocytes. *In* van Furth, R. (ed.): Mononuclear Phagocytes: Functional Aspects. The Hague, Martinus Nijhoff, 1980, p. 1443.
180. Hopper, K.E., Geczy, C.L., and Davies, W.A.: A mechanism of migration inhibition in delayed-type hypersensitivity reactions. I. Fibrin deposition on the surface of elicited peritoneal macropahges in vivo. J. Immunol. 126:1052, 1981.
181. Silverstein, S.C., Steinman, R.M., and Cohn, Z.A.: Endocytosis. Ann. Rev. Biochem. 46:669, 1977.
182. Stossel, T.P.: Phagocytosis. N. Engl. J. Med. 209:717, 774, 833, 1974.
183. Rabinovitch, M.: Phagocytic recognition. *In* van Furth, R. (ed.): Mononuclear Phagocytes. Oxford, Blackwell Scientific Publications, 1970, p. 299.
184. Jones, T.C., and Hirsch, J.G.: The interaction in vitro of Mycoplasma pulmonis with mouse peritoneal macrophages and L-cells. J. Exp. Med. 133:231, 1971.
185. Griffin, F.M., Jr., and Silverstein, S.C.: Segmental response of the macrophage plasma membrane to a phagocytic stimulus. J. Exp. Med. 139:323, 1974.
186. Griffin, F.M., Jr., Griffin, J.A., Leider, J.E., and Silverstein, S.C.: Studies on the mechanism of phagocytosis. I. Requirements for circumferential attachment of particle-bound ligands to specific receptors on the macrophage plasma membrane. J. Exp. Med. 142:1263, 1975.
187. Griffin, F.M., Jr., Griffin, J.A., and Silverstein, S.C.: Studies on the mechanism of phagocytosis. II. The interaction of macrophages with anti-immunoglobulin IgG-coated bone marrow-derived lymphocytes. J. Exp. Med. 144:788, 1976.
188. Wright, S.D., and Silverstein, S.C.: Phagocytosing macrophages exclude soluble macromolecules from the zone of contact with ligand-coated targets. J. Cell Biol. 95:443a, 1982.
189. Babior, B.M.: Oxygen-dependent microbial killng by phagocytes. N. Engl. J. Med. 298:659, 1978.
190. Nathan, C.F.: Secretion of oxygen intermediates: role in effector functions of activated macrophages. Fed. Proc. 41:2206, 1982.
191. Segal, A.W., Cross, A.R., Garcia, R.C., Borregaard, N., Valerius, N. H., Soothill, J.F., and Jones, O.T.G.: Absence of cytochrome $b_{245}$ in chronic granulomatous disease: A multicenter European evaluation of its incidence and relevance. N. Engl. J. Med. 308:245, 1983.
192. Loike, J.D., Kozler, V.F., and Silverstein, S.C.: Increased ATP and creatine phosphate turnover in phagocytosing mouse peritoneal macrophages. J. Biol. Chem. 254:958, 1979.
193. Brade, V., and Bentley, C.: Synthesis and release of complement components by macrophages. *In* van Furth, R. (ed.): Mononuclear Phagocytes: Functional Aspects. The Hague, Martinus Nijhoff, 1980, p.1385.
194. Bentley, C., Fries, W., Brade, V.: Synthesis of factors D, B, and P of the alternative pathway of complement activation, as well as of C3, by guinea pig peritoneal macrophages in vitro. Immunology. 35:971, 1978.
195. Whaley, K.: Biosynthesis of the complement components and the regulatory proteins of the alternative pathway by human peripheral blood monocytes. J. Exp. Med. 151:501, 1980.
196. Zimmer, B, Hartung, H.-P., Scharfenberger, G., Bitter-Suermann, D., and Hadding, U.: Quantitative studies of the secretion of complement component C3 by resident, elicited and activated macrophages. Comparison with C2, C4 and lysosomal enzyme release. Eur. J. Immunol. 12:426, 1982.
197. Einstein, L.P., Hansen, P.J., Ballow, M., Davis, A.E., III, Davis, J.S., IV, Alper, C.A., Rosen, F.S., and Colten, H.R.: Biosynthesis of the third component of complement (C3) in vitro by monocytes from both normal and homozygous C3-deficient humans. J. Clin. Invest. 60:963, 1977.
198. Einstein, L.P., Schneeberger, E.E., and Colten, H.R.: Synthesis of the second component of complement by long-term primary cultures of human monocytes. J. Exp. Med. 143:114, 1976.
199. Rutherford, B., and Schenkein, H.A.: C3 cleavage products stimulate release of prostaglandins by human mononuclear phagocytes in vitro. J. Immunol. 130:874, 1983.
200. Lappin, D.F., and Whaley, K.: Prostaglandins and prostaglandin synthetase inhibitors regulate the synthesis of complement components by human monocytes. Clin. Exp. Immunol. 49:623, 1982.
201. Littman, B.H., and Ruddy, S.: Production of the second component of complement by human monocytes: Stimulation by antigen-activated lymphocytes or lymphokines. J. Exp. Med. 145:1344, 977.
202. Hartung, H.-P., Bitter-Suermann, D., and Hadding, U.: Induction of thromboxane release from macrophages by anaphylatoxic peptide C3a of complement and synthetic hexapeptide C3a 72-77. J. Immunol. 130:1345, 1983.
203. Payan, D.G., Trentham, D.E., and Goetzl, E.J.: Modulation of human lymphocyte function by C3a and C3a (70-77). J. Exp. Med. 156:756, 1982.
204. Osterud, B., Lindahl, U., and Seljelid, R.: Macrophages produce blood coagulation factors. FEBS Lett. 120:41, 1980.
205. Osterud, B., Bogwald, J., Lindahl, U., and Seljelid, R.: Production of blood coagulation factor V and tissue thromboplastin by macrophages in vitro. FEBS Lett. 127:154, 1981.
206. Klimetzek, V., and Sorg, C.: The production of fibrinolysis inhibitors as a parameter of the activation state in murine macrophages. Eur. J. Immunol. 9:618, 1979.
207. Chapman, H.A., Jr., Vavrin, Z., and Hibbs, J.B., Jr.: Macrophage fibrinolytic activity: Identification of two pathways of plasmin formation by intact cells and of a plasminogen activator inhibitor. Cell 28:653, 1982.
208. Broze, G.J., Jr.: Binding of human factor VII and VIIa to monocytes. J. Clin. Invest. 70:526, 1982.
209. Schwartz, B.S., Levy, G.A., Fair, D.S., and Edgington, T.S.: Murine lymphoid procoagulant activity induced by bacterial lipopolysaccharide and immune complexes is a monocyte prothrombinase. J. Exp. Med. 155:1464, 1982.
210. Hogg, N.: Human monocytes are associated with the formation of fibrin. J. Exp. Med. 157:473, 1983.
211. Gordon, S., Todd, J., and Cohn, Z.A.: In vitro synthesis and secretion of lysozyme by mononuclear phagocytes. J. Exp. Med. 139:1228, 1974.
212. Klimetzek, V., and Sorg, C.: Lymphokine-induced secretion of plasminogen activator by murine macrophages. Eur. J. Immunol. 7:185, 1977.
213. Vassalli, J.-D., and Reich, E.: Macrophage plasminogen activator: Induction by products of activated lymphoid cells. J. Exp. Med. 145:429, 1977.
214. Gordon, S., Unkeless, J.C., and Cohn, Z.A.: Induction of macrophage plasminogen activator by endotoxin stimulation and phagocytosis. J. Exp. Med. 140:995, 1975.
215. Ragsdale, C.G., and Arend, W.P.: Neutral protease secretion by human monocytes. Effect of surface-bound immune complexes. J. Exp. Med. 149:954, 1979.
216. Pantalone, R., and Page, R.C.: Enzyme production and secretion by lymphokine-activated macrophages. J. Reticuloendothel. Soc. 21:343, 1977.
217. Schnyder, J., and Baggiolini, M.: Secretion of lysosomal hydrolases by stimulated and nonstimulated macrophages. J. Exp. Med. 148:435, 1978.
218. Gordon, S., and Werb, Z.: Secretion of macrophage neutral proteinases is enhanced by colchicine. Proc. Natl. Acad. Sci. USA 73:872, 1976.
219. Levine, E.A., Senior, R.M., and Butler, J.V.: The elastase activity of alveolar macrophages: Measurements using synthetic substrates and elastin. Amer. Rev. Respir. Dis. 113:25, 1976.
220. Wahl. L.M., Wahl, S., Mergenhagen, S.E., and Martin, G.E.: Collagenase production by endotoxin-activated macrophages. Proc. Natl. Acad. Sci. USA 71:3598, 1974.
221. Banda, M.J., Clark, E.J., and Werb, Z.: Selective proteolysis of immunoglobulins by mouse macrophage elastase. J. Exp. Med. 157:1184, 1983.
222. Davies, P., Page, R.C., and Allison, A.C.: Changes in cellular enzyme levels and extracellular release of lysosomal acid hydrolases in macrophages exposed to group A streptococcal cell wall substance. J. Exp. Med. 139:1262, 1974.
223. Schorlemmer, H.V., Bitter-Suermann, D., and Allison, A.C.: Complement activation by the alternative pathway and macrophage enzyme secretion in the pathogenesis of chronic inflammation. Immunology 32:929, 1977.
224. Ohkuma, S., and Poole, B.: Fluorescence probe measurement of the intralysosomal pH in living cells and the perturbation of pH by various agents. Proc. Natl. Acad. Sci. 75:3327, 1978.
225. Davies, P., and Allison, A.C.: Secretion of macrophage enzymes in relation to the pathogenesis of chronic inflammation. *In* Nelson, D.S. (ed.): Immunobiology of the Macrophage. New York, Academic Press, 1976, p. 428.
226. Barrett, A.J., and Starkey, P.M.: The interaction of $\alpha_2$-macroglobulin with proteinases. Characteristics and specificity of the reaction, and a hypothesis concerning its molecular mechanism. Biochem. J. 133:709, 1973.
227. Remold, H., and Rosenberg, R.D.: Enhancement of migration inhibitory factor activity by plasma esterase inhibitors. J. Biol. Chem. 250:6608, 1975.
228. Hovi, T., Mosher, D., and Vaheri, A.: Cultured human monocytes synthesize and secrete $\alpha_2$-macroglobulin. J. Exp. Med. 145:1580, 1977.
229. White, R., Janoff, A., and Godfrey, H.P.: Secretion of $\alpha_2$-macroglobulin by human alveolar macrophages. Lung 158:9, 1980.
230. Wilson, G.B., Walker, J.H., Watkins, J.H., Jr., and Wolgroch, D.: Determination of subpopulations of leukocytes involved in the synthesis of $\alpha_1$-antitrypsin in vitro. Proc. Soc. Exp. Biol. Med. 164:105, 1980.
231. White, R., Lee, D., Habicht, G.S., and Janoff, A.: Secretion of $\alpha_1$-proteinase inhibitor by cultured rat alveolar macrophages. Am Rev. Resp. Dis. 123:447, 1981.
232. Boldt, D.H., Chan, S.K., and Keaton, K.: Cell surface $\alpha_1$-protease inhibitor on human peripheral mononuclear cells in culture. J. Immunol. 129:1830, 1982.
233. Humes, J.L., Bonney, R.J., Pelus, L., Dahlgren, M.E., Sadowski, S.J.,

Kuehl, F.A., Jr., and Davies, P.: Macrophages synthesize and release prostaglandins in response to inflammatory stimuli. Nature 269:149, 1977.
234. Kurland, J.I., and Bockman, R.: Prostaglandin E production by human blood monocytes and mouse peritoneal macrophages. J. Exp. Med. 147:952, 1978.
235. Bonney, R.J., Wightman, P.D., Davies, P., Sadowski, S.J., Kuehl, F.A., Jr., and Humes, J.L.: Regulation of prostaglandin synthesis and of the selective release of lysosomal hydrolases by mouse peritoneal macrophages. Bioch. J. 176:433, 1978.
236. Scott, W.A., Zrike, J.M., Hamill, A.L., Kempe, J., and Cohn, Z.A.: Regulation of arachidonic acid metabolites in macrophages. J. Exp. Med. 152:324, 1980.
237. Rouzer, C.A., Scott, W.A., Hamill, A.L., and Cohn, Z.A.: Dynamics of leukotriene C production by macrophages. J. Exp. Med. 152:1236, 1980.
238. Scott, W.A., Pawlowski, N.A., Murray, H.W., Andreach, M., Zrike, J., and Cohn, Z.A.: Regulation of arachidonic acid metabolism by macrophage activation. J. Exp. Med. 155:1148, 1982.
239. Rouzer, C.A., Scott, W.A., Hamill, A.L., Liu, F.-T., Katz, D.H., and Cohn, Z.A.: Secretion of leukotriene C and other arachidonic acid metabolites by macrophages challenged with immunoglobulin E immune complexes. J. Exp. Med. 156:1077, 1982.
240. Pawlowski, N.A., Scott, W.A., Andreach, M., and Cohn, Z.A.: Uptake and metabolism of monohydroxyeicosatetraenoic acids by macrophages. J. Exp. Med. 155:1653, 1982.
241. Scott, W.A., Pawlowski, N.A., Andreach, M., and Cohn, Z.A.: Resting macrophages produce distinct metabolites from exogenous arachidonic acid. J. Exp. Med. 155:535, 1982.
242. Rouzer, C.A., Scott, W.A., Hamill, A.L., and Cohn, Z.A.: Synthesis of leukotriene C and other arachidonic acid metabolites by mouse pulmonary macrophages. J. Exp. Med. 155:720, 1982.
243. Fels, A.O.S., Pawlowski, N.A., Cramer, E.B., King, T.K.C., Cohn, Z.A., and Scott, W.A.: Human alveolar macrophages produce leukotriene B4. Proc. Natl. Acad. Sci. USA 79:7866, 1982.
244. Pawlowski, N.A., Kaplan, G.A., Hamill, A.L., Cohn, Z.A., and Scott, W.A.: Arachidonic acid metabolism by human monocytes. Studies with platelet-depleted cultures. J. Exp. Med., 158:393, 1983.
245. Bokoch, G.M., and Reed, P.W.: Stimulation of arachidonic acid metabolism in the polymorphonuclear leukocyte by an *N*-formylated peptide. J. Biol. Chem. 255:10223, 1980.
246. Kurland, J.I., Kincade, P.W., and Moore, M.A.S.: Regulation of B-lymphocyte clonal proliferation by stimulatory and inhibitory macrophage-derived factors. J. Exp. Med. 146:1420, 1977.
247. Goodwin, J.S., Bankhurst, A.D., and Messner, R.P.: Suppression of human T-cell mitogenesis by prostaglandin. Existence of a prostaglandin-producing suppressor cell. J. Exp. Med. 146:1719, 1977.
248. Kurland, J.I., Broxmeyer, H.E., Pelus, L.M., Bockman, R.S., and Moore, M.A.S.: Role of monocyte-macrophage-derived colony-stimulating factor and prostaglandin E in the positive and negative feedback control of myeloid stem cell proliferation. Blood 52:388, 1978.
249. Voelkel, E.F., Levine, L., Alper, C.A., and Tashjian, A.H., Jr.: Acute phase reactants ceruloplasmin and haptoglobin and their relationship to plasma prostaglandins in rabbits bearing the $VX_2$ carcinoma. J. Exp. Med. 147:1078, 1978.
250. Friedman, S.A., Remold-O'Donnell, E., and Piessens, W.F.: Enhanced PGE production by MAF-treated peritoneal exudate macrophages. Cell. Immunol. 42:213, 1979.
251. Hunninghake, G.W., Gadek, J.E., Fales, H.M., and Crystal, R.G.: Human alveolar macrophage-derived chemotactic factor for neutrophils. Stimuli and partial characterization. J. Clin. Invest. 66:473, 1980.
252. Nathan, C.F., and Root, R.K.: Hydrogen peroxide release from mouse peritoneal macrophages. Dependence on sequential activation and triggering. J. Exp. Med. 146:1648, 1977.
253. Johnson, R.B., Jr., Godzik, C.A., and Cohn, Z.A.: Increased superoxide anion production by immunologically activated and chemically elicited macrophages. J. Exp. Med. 148:115, 1978.
254. Nathan, C., Nogueira, N., Juangbhanich, C., Ellis, J., and Cohn, Z.: Activation of macrophages in vivo and in vitro: Correlation between hydrogen peroxide release and killing of Trypanosoma cruzi. J. Exp. Med. 149:1056, 1979.
255. Nakagawara, A., DeSantis, N.M., Nogueira, N., and Nathan, C.F.: Lymphokines enhance the capacity of human monocytes to secrete reactive oxygen intermediates. J. Clin. Invest. 70:1042, 1982.
256. Nathan, C.F., Murray, H.W., Wiebe, M.E., and Rubin, B.Y.: Identification of interferon-$\gamma$ as the lymphokine which activates human macrophage oxidative metabolism and antimicrobial activity. J. Exp. Med. 158:670, 1983.
257. Szuro-Sudol, A., and Nathan, C.F.: Suppression of macrophage oxidative metabolism by products of malignant and nonmalignant cells. J. Exp. Med. 156:945, 1982.
258. Slater, T.F.: Free Radical Mechanisms in Tissue Injury. London, Pion Ltd, 1972.
259. Oppenheim, J.J., and Gery, I.: Interleukin 1 is more than an interleukin. Immunol. Today 3:113, 1982.
260. Mizel, S.B., and Mizel, D.: Purification to apparent homogeneity of murine interleukin 1. J. Immunol. 126:834, 1981.
261. Gery, I., Gershon, R.K., and Waksman, B.H.: Potentiation of the T lymphocyte response to mitogens. I. The responding cell. J. Exp. Med. 136:128, 1972.
262. Howard, M., Mizel, S.B., Lachman, L., Ansel, J., Johnson, B., and Paul, W.E.: Role of interleukin-1 in anti-immunoglobulin-induced B cell proliferation. J. Exp. Med. 157:1529, 1983.
263. Murphy, P.A., Simon, P.L., and Willoughby, W.F.: Endogenous pyrogens made by rabbit peritoneal exudate cells are identical with lymphocyte-activating factors made by rabbit alveolar macrophages. J. Immunol. 124:2498, 1980.
264. Mizel, S.B., Dayer, J.-M., Krane, S.M., and Mergenhagen, S.E.: Stimulation of rheumatoid synovial cell collagenase and prostaglandin production by partially purified lymphocyte-activating factor (interleukin 1). Proc. Natl. Acad. Sci. USA 78:2474, 1981.
265. Schmidt, J.A., Mizel, S.B., Cohen, D., and Green, I.: Interleukin 1, a potential regulator of fibroblast proliferation. J. Immunol. 128:2177, 1982.
266. Postlethwaite, A.E., Lachman, L.B., Mainardi, C.L., and Kang, A.H.: Interleukin 1 stimulation of collagenase production by cultured fibroblasts. J. Exp. Med. 157:801, 1983.
267. Sipe, J.D., Vogel, S.N., Ryan, J.L., McAdam, K.P.W.J., and Rosenstreich, D.L.: Detection of a mediator derived from endotoxin-stimulated macrophages that induces the acute phase serum amyloid A response in mice. J. Exp. Med. 150:597, 1979.
268. Le, P.T., Muller, T., and Mortensen, R.F.: Acute phase reactants of mice. I. Isolation of serum amyloid P-component (SAP) and its induction by a monokine. J. Immunol. 129:665, 1982.
269. Kurland, J.I., Meyers, P.A., and Moore, M.A.S.: Synthesis and release of erythroid colony- and burst-potentiating activities by purified populations of murine peritoneal macrophages. J. Exp. Med. 151:838, 1980.
270. Rich, I.N., Heit, W., and Kubanck, B.: Extrarenal erythropoietin production by macrophages. Blood 60:1007, 1982.
271. Leibovich, S.J., and Ross, R.: A macrophage-dependent factor that stimulates the proliferation of fibroblasts in vitro. Am. J. Pathol. 84:501, 1976.
272. Polverini, P.J., Cotran, R.S., Gimbrone, M.A., Jr., and Unanue, E.R.: Activated macrophages induce vascular proliferation. Nature 269:804, 1977.
273. Filkins, J.P.: Endotoxin-enhanced secretion of macrophage insulin-like activity. J. Reticuloendothel. Soc. 27:507, 1980.
274. Kawakami, M., and Cerami, A.: Studies of endotoxin-induced decrease in lipoprotein lipase activity. J. Exp. Med. 154:631, 1981.
275. Pekala, P.H., Kawakami, M., Angus, C.W., Lane, M., and Cerami, A.: A selective inhibition of the synthesis of the enzymes for de novo fatty acid biosynthesis by an endotoxin-induced mediator from exudate cells. Proc. Natl. Acad. Sci. USA 80:2743, 1983.
276. Mahoney, E.M., Khoo, J.C., and Steinberg, D.: Lipoprotein lipase secretion by human monocytes and rabbit alveolar macrophages in culture. Proc. Natl. Acad. Sci. USA 79:1639, 1982.
277. Chait, A., Iverius, P.-H., and Brunzell, J.D.: Lipoprotein lipase secretion by human monocyte-derived macropahges. J. Clin. Invest. 69:490, 1982.
278. Kull, F.C., Jr., and Cuatrecasas, P.: Preliminary characterization of the tumor cell cytotoxin in tumor necrosis serum. J. Immunol. 126:1279, 1981.
279. Smith, T.J., and Wagner, R.R.: Rabbit macrophage interferons. I. Conditions for biosynthesis by virus-infected and uninfected cells. J. Exp. Med. 125:559, 1967.
280. Kung, J.T., Brooks, S.B., Jakway, J.P., Leonard, L.L., and Talmage, D.W.: Suppression of in vitro cytotoxic response by macrophages due to induced arginase. J. Exp. Med. 146:665, 1977.
281. Nathan, C.F., Silverstein, S.C., Brukner, L.H., and Cohn, Z.A.: Extracellular cytolysis by activated macrophages and granulocytes. II. Hydrogen peroxide as a mediator of cytotoxicity. J. Exp. Med. 149:100, 1979.
282. Stadecker, M.J., Calderon, J., Karnovsky, M.L., and Unanue, E.R.: Synthesis and release of thymidine by macrophages. J. Immunol. 119:1738, 1977.
283. Neumann, C., and Sorg, C.: Immune interferon. I. Production by lymphokine-activated murine macrophages. Eur. J. Immunol. 7:719, 1977.
284. Olstad, R., Degre, M., and Seljelid, R.: Production of immune interferon (Type II) in cocultures of mouse peritoneal macrophages and syngeneic tumor cells. Scand. J. Immunol. 13:605, 1981.
285. Krahenbuhl, J.L., Remington, J.S., and McLeod, R.: Cytotoxic and microbicidal properties of macrophages. *In* van Furth, R. (ed.): Mononuclear Phagocytes: Functional Aspects. The Hague, Martinus Nijhoff, 1980, p. 1631.

286. Mahmoud, A., Peters, P.A.S., Civil, R.H., and Remington, J.S.: In vitro killing of schistosomula of Schistosoma mansoni by BCG and C. parvum-activated macrophages. J. Immunol. 122:1655, 1979.
287. Haque, A., Ouaissi, A., Joseph, M., Capron, M., and Capron, A.: IgE antibody in eosinophil- and macrophage-mediated in vitro killing of Dipetalonema viteae microfilariae. J. Immunol. 127:716, 1981.
288. Horwitz, M.A., and Silverstein, S.C.: Legionnaires' disease bacterium (*Legionella pneumophila*) multiplies intracellularly in human monocytes. J. Clin. Invest. 66:445, 1980.
289. Nathan, C.F.: Mechanisms of macrophage antimicrobial activity. Trans. Roy. Soc. Trop. Med. Hyg., 77:620, 1983.
290. Wilson, C.B., Tsai, V., and Remington, J.S.: Failure to trigger the oxidative metabolic burst by normal macrophages: Possible mechanism for survival of intracellular pathogens. J. Exp. Med. 151:328, 1980.
291. Murray, H.W., Byrne, G.I., Rothermel, C.D., and Cartelli, D.M.: Lymphokine enhances oxygen-independent activity against intracellular pathogens. J. Exp. Med. 158:234, 1983.
292. Wisseman, C.L., Jr., and Waddell, A.: Interferonlike factors from antigen- and mitogen-stimulated human leukocytes with antirickettsial and cytolytic actions of Rickettsia prowazekii. Infected human endothelial cells, fibroblasts, and macrophages. J. Exp. Med. 157:1780, 1983.
293. Klebanoff, S.J., and Hamon, C.B.: Antimicrobial systems of mononuclear phagocytes. *In* van Furth (ed.): Mononuclear Phagocytes in Immunity, Infection, and Pathology. Oxford, Blackwell Scientific Publications, 1975, p. 507.
294. Confer, D.L., and Eaton, J.W.: Phagocyte impotence caused by an invasive bacterial adenylate cyclase. Science 217:948, 1982.
295. Draper, P, and D'Arcy Hart, P.: Phagosomes, lysosomes, and mycobacteria: cellular and microbial aspects. *In* van Furth, R. (ed.): Mononuclear Phagocytes in Immunity, Infection, and Pathology. Oxford, Blackwell Scientific Publications, 1975, p. 575.
296. Goren, M.B.: Phagocyte lysosomes: Interactions with infectious agents, phagosomes and experimental perturbations in function. Ann. Rev. Microbiol. 31:507, 1977.
297. Nogueira, N., and Cohn, Z.A.: *Trypansosoma cruzi*: In vitro induction of macropahge microbicidal activity. J. Exp. Med. 148:288, 1978.
298. Adams, D.O., Johnson, W., and Marino, P.: Mechanisms of target recognition and destruction in macrophage-mediated tumor cytotoxicity. Fed. Proc. 41:2212, 1982.
299. Adams, D.O., Johnson, W.J., Fiorito, E., and Nathan, C.F.: Hydrogen peroxide and cytolytic factor can interact in effecting cytolysis of neoplastic targets. J. Immunol. 127:1973, 1981.
300. Granger, D.L., and Lehninger, A.L.: Sites of inhibition of mitochondrial electron transport in macrophage-injured neoplastic cells. J. Cell Biol. 95:527, 1982.
301. Nathan, C., and Cohn, Z.: Role of oxygen-dependent mechanisms in antibody-induced lysis of tumor cells by activated macrophages. J. Exp. Med. 152:198, 1980.
302. Nathan, C.F., and Klebanoff, S.J.: Augmentation of spontaneous macrophage-mediated cytolysis by eosinophil peroxidase. J. Exp. Med. 155:1291, 1982.
303. Nathan, C.F., Murray, H.W., and Cohn, Z.A.: Current concepts: the macrophage as an effector cell. N. Engl. J. Med. 303:622, 1980.
304. Herlyn, D., and Koprowski, H.: IgG2a monoclonal antibodies inhibit human tumor growth through interaction with effector cells. Proc. Natl. Acad. Sci. USA 79:4761, 1982.
305. Kleinerman, E.S., Erickson, K.L., Schroit, A.J., Fogler, W.E., and Fidler, I.J.: Activation of tumoricidal properties in human blood monocytes by liposomes containing lipophilic muramyl tripeptides. Cancer Res. 43:2010, 1983.
306. Szuro-Sudol, A., Murray, H.W., and Nathan, C.F.: Suppression of macrophage antimicrobial activity by a tumor cell product. J. Immunol. 131:384, 1983.
307. Nathan, C.F., Arrick, B.A., Murray, H.W., DeSantis, N.M., and Cohn, Z.A.: Tumor cell antioxidant defenses: Inhibition of the glutathione redox cycle enhances macrophage-mediated cytolysis. J. Exp. Med. 153:766, 1981.
308. Arrick, B.A., Nathan, C.F., Griffith, O.W., and Cohn, Z.A.: Glutathione depletion sensitizes tumor cells to oxidative cytolysis. J. Biol. Chem. 257:1231, 1982.
309. Steinman, R.M., and Nussenzweig, M.C.: Dendritic cells: features and functions. Immunol. Rev. 53:127, 1980.
310. Steinman, R.M., Gutchinov, B., Witmer, M.D., and Nussenzweig, M.C.: Dendritic cells are the principal stimulators of the primary mixed leukocyte reaction in mice. J. Exp. Med. 157:613, 1983.
311. van Voorhis, W.C., Valinsky, J., Hoffman, E., Luban, J., Hair, L.S., and Steinman, R.M.: Relative efficacy of human monocytes and dendritic cells as accessory cells for T cell replication. J. Exp. Med. 158:174, 1983.
312. Rouzer, C.A., Scott, W.A., Griffith, O.W., Hamill, A.L., and Cohn, Z.A.: Glutathione metabolism in resting and phagocytizing peritoneal macrophages. J. Biol. Chem. 257:2002, 1982.
313. Austyn, J.M., Steinman, R.M., Weinstein, D.E., Granelli-Piperno, A., and Palladino, M.: Dendritic cells initiate a two-stage mechanism for T lymphocyte proliferation. J. Exp. Med. 157:1101, 1983.
314. Smith, K.A., Lachman, L.B., Oppenheim, J.J., and Favata, M.F.: The functional relationship of the interleukins. J. Exp. Med. 151:1551, 1980.
315. Unanue, E.R.: The regulatory role of macrophages in antigenic stimulation. Adv. Immunol. 15:95, 1972.
316. Dos Reis, G.A., and Shevach, E.M.: Antigen-presenting cells from non-responder strain 2 guinea pigs are fully competent to present bovine insulin chain B to responder strain 13 T cells. Evidence against a determinant selection model and in favor of clonal deletion. J. Exp. Med. 157:1287, 1983.
317. Kirchner, H., Holden, H.T., and Herberman, R.B.: Splenic suppressor macrophages induced in mice by injection of *Corynebacterium parvum.* J. Immunol. 115:1212, 1975.
318. Fisher, R.I., and Bostick-Bruton, F.: Depressed T cell proliferation responses in Hodgkin's disease: role of monocyte-mediated suppression via prostaglandins and hydrogen peroxide. J. Immunol. 129:1770, 1982.
319. Kay, M.M.B., Goodman, S.R., Sorensen, K., Whitfield, C.F., Wong, P., Zaki, L., and Rudloff, V.: Senescent cell antigen is immunologically related to band 3. Proc. Natl. Acad. Sci. USA 80:1631, 1983.
320. Newman, S.L., Henson, J.E., and Henson, P.M.: Phagocytosis of senescent neutrophils by human monocyte-derived macrophages and rabbit inflammatory macrophages. J. Exp. Med. 154:430, 1982.
321. Rosenberg, S.A., and Rogentine, N.: Natural human antibodies to "hidden" membrane components. Nature New Biol. 239:203, 1972.
322. Czop, J.K., Fearon, D.T., and Austen, K.F.: Membrane sialic acid on target particles modulate their phagocytosis by a trypsin-sensitive mechanism on human monocytes. Proc. Natl. Acad. Sci. USA 75:3831, 1978.
323. Aminoff, D., Bruegge, W.F.V., Bell, W.C., Sarpolis, K., and Williams, R.: Role of sialic acid in survival of erythrocytes in the circulation: interaction of neuraminidase-treated and untreated erythrocytes with spleen and liver at the cellular level. Proc. Natl. Acad. Sci. USA 74:1521, 1977.
324. Ahn, Y.S., Byrnes, J.J., Harrington, W.J., Cayer, M.L., Smith, D.S., Bruskill, D.E., and Pall, L.M.: The treatment of idiopathic thrombocytopenia with vinblastine-loaded platelets. N. Engl. J. Med. 298:1101, 1978.
325. Baehner, R.L., Nathan, D.G., and Castle, W.B.: Oxidant injury of Caucasian glucose-6-phosphate dehydrogenase-deficient red blood cells by phagocytosing leukocytes during infection. J. Clin. Invest. 50:2466, 1971.
326. Leibovich, S.J., and Ross, R.: The role of the macrophage in wound repair. A study with hydrocortisone and anti-macrophage serum. Am. J. Path. 78:71, 1975.
327. Fauci, A.S., and Dale, D.C.: The effect of in vivo hydrocortisone on subpopulations of human lymphocytes. J. Clin. Invest. 53:240, 1974.
328. Dale, D.C., Fauci, A.S., and Wolff, S.M.: Alternate-day prednisone. Leukocyte kinetics and susceptibility to infections. N. Engl. J. Med. 291:1154, 1974.
329. Norris, D.A., Capin, L., Weston, W.L.: The effect of epicutaneous glucocorticoids on human monocyte and neutrophil migration in vivo. J. Invest. Dermatol. 78:386, 1982.
330. Thompson, J., and van Furth, R.: The effect of glucocorticoids on the proliferation and kinetics of promonocytes and monocytes of the bone marrow. J. Exp. Med. 137:10, 1973.
331. Rinehart, J.J., Sagone, A.L., Balcerzak, S.P., Ackerman, G.A., and Lobuglio, A.F.: Effects of corticosteroid therapy on human monocyte function. N. Engl. J. Med. 292:236, 1975.
332. Taylor, C.E., Weiser, W.Y., and Bang, F.B.: In vitro macrophage manifestation of cortisone-induced decrease in resistance to mouse hepatitis virus. J. Exp. Med. 153:732, 1981.
333. Rinehart, J.J., Wuest, D., and Ackerman, G.A.: Corticosteroid alterations of human monocyte to macrophage differentiation. J. Immunol. 129:1436, 1982.
334. Nakagawara, A., DeSantis, N.M., Nogueira, N., and Nathan, C.F.: Lymphokines enhance the capacity of human monocytes to secrete reactive oxygen intermediates. J. Clin. Invest. 70:1042, 1982.
335. Schreiber, A.D., Parsons, J. McDermott, P., and Cooper, R.A.: Effect of corticosteroids on the human monocyte IgG and complement receptors. J. Clin. Invest. 56:1189, 1975.
336. Norton, J.M., and Munck, A.: In vitro actions of glucocorticoids on murine macrophages: effects on glucose transport and metabolism, growth in culture, and protein synthesis. J. Immunol. 125:259, 1980.
337. Snyder, D.S., and Unanue, E.R.: Corticosteroids inhibit murine macrophage Ia expression and interleukin 1 production. J. Immunol. 129:1803, 1982.
338. Werb, Z.: Biochemical actions of glucocorticoids on macrophages in culture. Specific inhibition of elastase, collagenase, and plasminogen activator secretion and effects on other metabolic functions. J. Exp. Med. 147:1695, 1978.

339. Teitelbaum, S.L., Malone, J.D., and Kahn, A.J.: Glucocorticoid enhancement of bone resorption by rat peritoneal macrophages in vitro. Endocrinology 108:795, 1981.
340. Fauve, R.M., and Pierce-Chase, C.H.: Comparative effects of corticosteroids on host resistance to infection in relation to chemical structure. J. Exp. Med. 125:807, 1967.
341. Balow, J.E., and Rosenthal, A.S.: Glucocorticoid suppression of macrophage migration inhibitory factor. J. Exp. Med. 137:1031, 1973.
342. Vernon-Roberts, B.: The effect of steroid hormones on macrophage activity. Int. Rev. Cytol. 25:131, 1969.
343. Persellin, R.H., and Ziff, M.: The effect of gold salts on lysosomal enzymes of the peritoneal macrophage. Arthr. Rheum. 9:56, 1966.
344. Ho, P.P.K., Young, A.L., and Southard, G.L.: Chemotactic responses of human blood monocytes to the methyl ester of *N*-formylmethionylleucylphenylalanine and its inhibition by gold compounds. J. Cell Biol. 75:95a, 1977.
345. Littman, B.H., and Schwartz, P.: Gold inhibition of the production of the second complement component by lymphokine-stimulated human monocytes. Arthr. Rheum. 25:288, 1982.
346. Oaten, S.W., Jagelman, S., and Webb, H.E.: Further studies of macrophages in relationship to avirulent semliki forest virus infections. Br. J. Exp. Path. 61:150, 1980.
347. Ghaffar, A., McBride, W.H., and Cullen, R.T.: Interaction of tumor cells and activated macrophages in vitro: Modulation by Corynebacterium and gold salts. J. Reticuloendothel. Soc. 20:283, 1976.
348. Binderup, L., Bramm, E., and Arrigoni-Martelli, E.: Immunological effects of D-penicillamine during experimentally induced inflammation in rats. Scand. J. Immunol. 12:239, 1980.
349. Binderup, L., Bramm, E., and Arrigoni-Martelli, E.: Effect of D-penicillamine in vitro and in vivo on macrophage phagocytosis. Biochem. Pharmacol. 29:2273, 1980.
350. Skosey, J.L., Chow, D.C., Lichon, F., and Hinckley, C.C.: Drug interference with inactivation of serum alpha-1-proteinase inhibitor by oxygen radicals. *In* Greenwald, R.A., and Cohen, G. (eds.): Oxygen Radicals and Their Scavenger Systems. Vol. II. Cellular and Medical Aspects. New York, Elsevier, 1983, p. 264.
351. van Furth, R., Gassmann, E., and Diesselhoff-den Dulk, M.M.C.: The effect of azathioprine (Imuran) on the cell cycle of promonocytes and the production of monocytes in the bone marrow. J. Exp. Med. 141:531, 1975.
352. Buhles, W.C., Jr, and Shifrine, M.: Effects of cyclophosphamide on macrophage numbers, fucntions and progenitor cells. J. Reticuloendothel. Soc. 21:285, 1977.
353. Mantovani, A.: The interaction of cancer chemotherapy agents with mononuclear phagocytes. Adv. Pharmacol. Chemother. 19:35, 1982.
354. Schnyder, J., Dewald, B., and Baggiolini, M.: Effects of cyclooxygenase inhibitors and prostaglandin $E_2$ on macrophage activation in vitro. Prostaglandins 22:411, 1981.
355. Schultz, R.M., and Chirigos, M.A.: Selective neutralization by antiinterferon globulin of macrophage activation by L-cell interferon, *Brucella abortus* ether extract, *Salmonella typhimurium* lipopolysaccharide, and polyanions. Cell. Immunol. 48:52, 1979.

# Chapter 11
# Cellular Components of Inflammation: Platelets

*Peter M. Henson and John L. Gordon*

## INTRODUCTION

Because of their size, platelets, which are the smallest circulating element in mammalian blood, were discovered much later than the other blood cells. They were first described in the mid-nineteenth century, but even in the early years of the twentieth century their existence was not universally recognized.[1,2] During the first half of this century, most of the research on platelets was connected with their role in the clotting process, but in the past 20 years or so there has been an enormous upsurge of interest in platelet biology. This is partly because they are easily obtainable as a virtually homogeneous population and exhibit a wide variety of cellular reactions, e.g., adhesion, aggregation, active transport, degranulation, and prostaglandin synthesis. They are thus valuable cellular models for studying such processes. Equally important, however, is their participation in many biologic events apart from coagulation. Their paramount role in the cellular aspects of hemostasis and thrombosis is now well recognized, and they have been implicated in the maintenance of capillary integrity, in wound healing, in atherosclerosis, in transplant rejection, in the clearance of particles from the blood, and in inflammation.[3] It is their role in inflammation with which this chapter is concerned.

Because studies on platelets have developed so rapidly, it will not be possible to provide a comprehensive review of all the literature in this area. Accordingly we will use more general reviews or representative papers to illustrate a number of points in this discussion. For a more detailed analysis see reference 3. In addition it is important to emphasize at the outset that although platelets seem to participate in many aspects of inflammation, and certainly possess many properties that are consistent with a potential role in these processes, nevertheless proof of a requirement for these cells in inflammation and in rheumatic diseases is not yet available. Therefore, while platelets should certainly be considered as likely contributors to the pathogenesis of inflammation, they do not appear to be sufficient by themselves to induce an inflammatory response, nor are they necessary for one to occur. Futhermore, there is no evidence that platelets can penetrate intact vascular walls. Therefore one must presume that their activation is confined to the intravascular compartment. This is not to exclude the possibility that platelet-derived mediators might act extravascularly but suggests that the parent cell remains within the blood vessel.

**Platelet Constituents and Structural Organization.** Platelets are anucleate, discoid fragments of megakaryocyte cytoplasm, about 2 μm in diameter, formed by megakaryocyte pseudopodia extruding in the bone marrow and budding off platelets from the periphery. In healthy subjects 250,000 to 400,000 platelets per cubic millimeter circulate in peripheral blood, and platelet production is about 35,000 per cubic millimeter per day, although these values can vary greatly in disease states, including arthritis. The life span of platelets is around 10 days in man, circulating cells being removed either by the reticuloendothelial system when effete or by incorporation into hemostatic plugs or intravascular aggregates when exposed to stimuli. Specific glycoprotein receptors on the platelet membrane form the recognition sites for many such stimuli, and changes in other membrane glycoproteins regulate the removal of "spent" platelets. The composition of the platelet membrane changes with age,[4] and removal of up to 10 percent of the sialic acid in the membrane results in the immediate clearance of the cells from the circulation, although their response to stimuli is virtually unaffected.[5]

Beneath the platelet membrane is a peripheral bundle of microtubules, running in the equatorial plane (Fig. 11–1), which apparently acts as a cytoskeleton and helps to maintain the characteristic shape of platelets (microtubules are disorganized in stimulated platelets that have lost their discoid form). The contractile proteins actin and myosin are abundant in platelets and seem to play a vital role in responses to stimuli[6] (see below). Most of the major platelet organelles are shown in Figure 11–1. Dense granules (dg) contain vasoactive amines (chiefly serotonin), adenine nucleotides (chiefly ATP), and bivalent cations ($Ca^{2+}$, $Mg^{2+}$). Alpha granules ($\alpha$g) are less osmiophilic than dense granules, are numerous, and contain fibrinogen, heparin-binding proteins such as $\beta$-thromboglobulin and platelet factor 4, fibronectin, and platelet-derived growth factor (PDGF).[7,8] True lysosomes are present in small numbers and contain a conventional array of acid hydrolases. Glycogen granules (gg) are abundant, but mitochondira (m) are sparse, with few cristae, which is consistent with the platelet's energy being derived mainly from glycolysis rather than oxidative phosphorylation. Finally, the apparently empty vesicles (v) frequently seen in platelets are usually not enclosed vacuoles but parts of a complex, surface-connected canalicular system that is apparently involved in uptake and secretory processes (see below). Intimately involved with this canalicular system (but not evident in Fig. 11–1) is a network of dense tubules that are apparently the site of prostaglandin synthesis. A more detailed description of platelet ultrastructure and cytochemistry is given by White.[3,9]

The energy required to support the platelet's response to stimuli is supplied by a metabolic pool of ATP in the cytoplasm, which is in very slow equilibrium with the storage pool of ATP in the dense granules. The review by Holmsen[10] provides a detailed account of platelet metabolism.

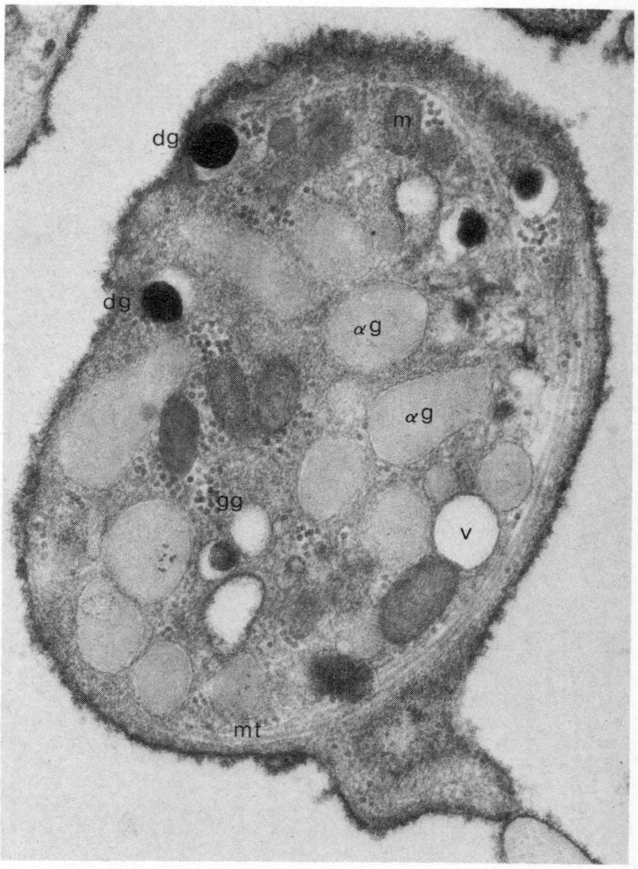


**Figure 11–1.** Platelet isolated from rabbit citrated platelet-rich plasma. $\times$ 45,000. $\alpha g$ = Alpha granules; $dg$ = dense granules; $gg$ = glycogen granules; $m$ = mitochondria; $mt$ = microtubules; $v$ = vesicles. (From MacIntyre, D.E., et al.: J. Cell Sci. 28:211, 1977.)

## PLATELET BIOLOGY

**Shape Change.** The first detectable response of platelets to most stimulants is extrusion of pseudopodia, with consequent loss of discoid shape (Fig. 11–2). This change in shape is extremely rapid and is not associated with any significant change in platelet volume. The intracellular events that accompany the shape change may represent a triggering mechanism, which leads in turn to the more profound cellular changes that regulate the processes of aggregation and secretion.[11] The mechanism of the shape change is unknown, but it is of interest that granulocytes also undergo profound alteration in shape as a very early step in stimulus-response coupling processes.[12]

**Adhesion.** Platelets adhere to many artificial surfaces, and, indeed, the production of surfaces that are "passive" to platelets is of considerable importance in the development of vascular prostheses and other appliances that must come in contact with blood. Of greater importance, particularly with regard to the inflammatory process, is the adhesion of platelets to biologic macromolecules. Most biopolymers (e.g., fibrin, proteoglycans, gelatin, elastin) are not good substrates for platelet adhesion, but platelets readily adhere to polymeric collagen[13] and other connective tissue elements, and this adhesion stimulates platelet secretion and aggregation. Platelet–collagen interaction may be biologically significant because the subendothelial region of the vascular wall contains these proteins; hence, when endothelial cells are

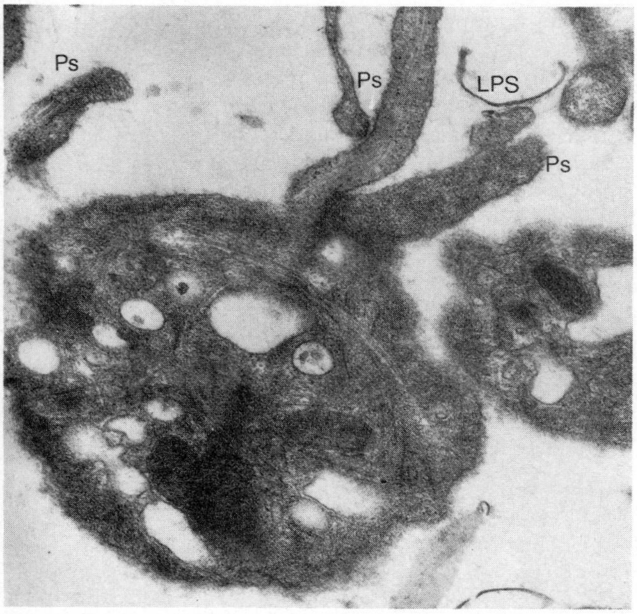


**Figure 11–2.** Rabbit platelets showing change in shape after exposure to bacterial endotoxin lipopolysaccharide. × 40,000. *LPS* = Lipopolysaccharide; *Ps* = pseudopodia. (From MacIntyre, D.E., et al.: J. Cell Sci. 28:211, 1977.)

damaged (or separated by vasodilation or by endothelial contraction), platelets can adhere to the exposed subendothelium (Fig. 11–3). This phenomenon of platelet accumulation at sites of vascular damage is fundamental to the physiologic and pathologic role of platelets and was recognized over a century ago[14] in studies with frog thrombocytes (the amphibian equivalent of the mammalian platelet). However, there has been some controversy as to which subendothelial constituent the platelets actually adhere to. Part of this confusion comes from the fact that adhesion and aggregation (stimulation) are separate events. Thus, aggregation of platelets in a test tube by collagen types I and III but not by type IV (basement membrane collagen) requires that there first be adhesion to the polymeric collagen and then secretion of aggregating constituents (ADP and/or thromboxane) (see below). More recently the importance of von Willebrand's factor in the interaction of platelet surface glycoprotein Ib and subendothelial constituents has been recognized.[15] Fibronectin, which is expressed on platelet surfaces following activation,[16] could also play a role in this process,[17] although others have questioned such a mechanism[18] and have implicated a separate collagen receptor on the platelet surface.

**Aggregation.** Several soluble biologic stimuli (e.g., ADP, serotonin, some prostaglandins, catecholamines, thrombin) can induce platelet aggregation. This is usually preceded by the extrusion of pseudopodia, and the aggregation response to the stimulant can be followed (if the stimulant concentration is high enough) by a secondary aggregation response caused by constituents (such as ADP or thromboxane $A_2$) secreted from the platelets initially stimulated. Aggregation requires extracellular $Ca^{2+}$ and fibrinogen, and the secretory response that results in secondary aggregation may be mediated by an increase in ionized calcium concentration in the platelet cytoplasm (see below). Consequently, aggregation and secretion can be induced by calcium ion-

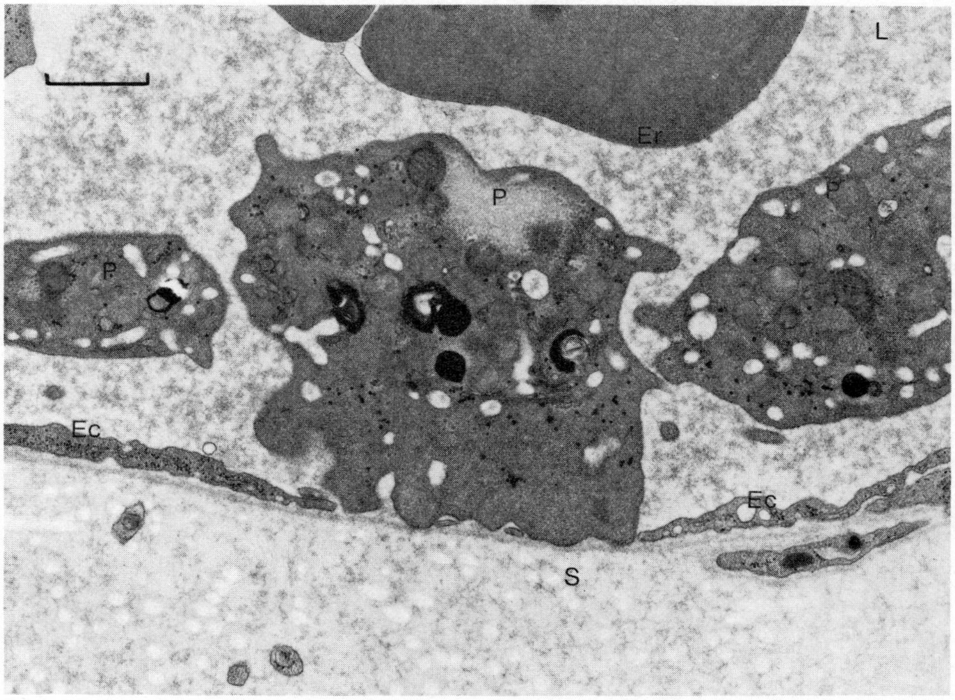


**Figure 11–3.** Platelet adhering to subendothelial basement membrane exposed between two endothelial cells. Bar indicates 1 μm. *Ec* = Endothelial cell; Er = erythrocyte; *L* = lumen of blood vessel; *P* = platelet; *S* = suendothelial basement membrane. (From Tranzer, J.P., and Baumgartner, H.R.: Nature 216:1126, 1967.)

ophores.[19] Particulate stimuli such as collagen and bacterial endotoxin also induce aggregation (Fig. 11–4), but the aggregation reaction follows initial adhesion between the platelets and the stimulant and depends on the secretion of aggregatory constituents from the platelets.

Platelet aggregation is the process mainly responsible for the early development of a hemostatic plug or thrombus, and because of its association with secretion it is also important in regulating the local concentrations in plasma or tissue of platelet constituents, some of which are powerful inflammatory agents (see Platelet Products with Potential Inflammatory Actions, below).

Recent work on the process of aggregation has begun to define its mechanism. Activated platelets develop binding sites for fibrinogen, which appear to involve in part the major surface glycoprotein Gp IIb-IIIa complex.[20,21] Additional work has suggested the involvement of an alpha granule–derived lectin termed thrombospondin, which may crosslink the fibrinogen molecules.[22]

**Secretion.** When stimulated, platelets can selectively release the contents of their dense granules and alpha granules and under some conditions, particularly with higher concentrations of stimulus, their lysosomal constituents. The adenine nucleotides and serotonin stored in the dense bodies can be released by stimulants such as ADP without significant secretion of alpha granule contents.[23] Stimulatory prostanoids evoke a similar pattern of secretion,[24] whereas "stronger" stimuli such as thrombin and collagen induce secretion of lysosomal hydrolases as well.[25-27] Blockade of platelet thromboxane

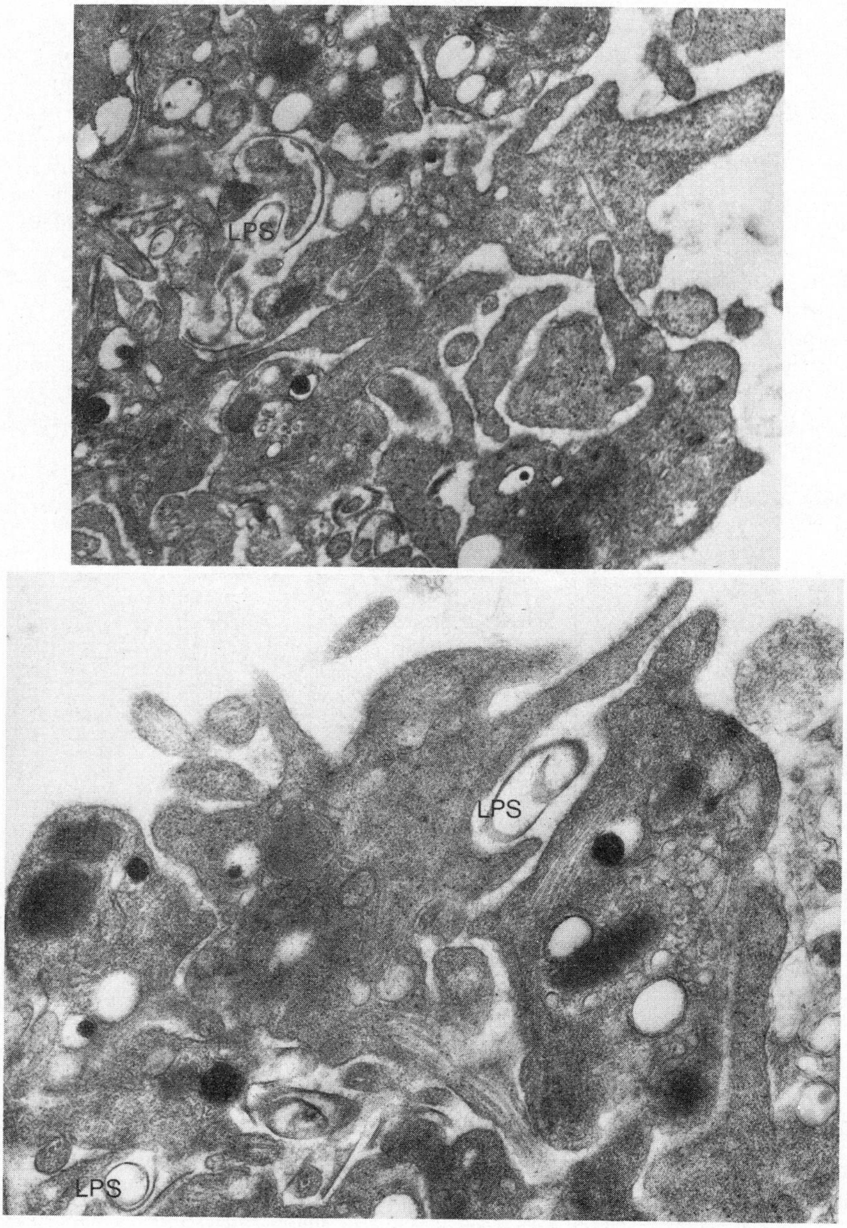


**Figure 11–4.** Platelet aggregation induced by bacterial endotoxin lipopolysaccharide (*LPS*). *A*, × 30,000. *B*, × 40,000. Note whorls of LPS between platelets and closely approximated platelet plasma membranes that retain their integrity. Granules and disrupted microtubles are visible within platelets. (From MacIntyre, D.E., et al.: J. Cell Sci. 28:211, 1977.)

synthesis by drugs such as aspirin can inhibit the secretion of platelet constituents by collagen, implying that here thromboxane synthesis is necessary for the secretory response.[27]

The cellular mechanisms regulating platelet secretion are not yet fully known, but the events seem to be very similar to those seen in other cells.[28] The process is initiated by a stimulant that binds to specific receptors on the platelet surface. This probably induces ionic alterations and depolarization[29] accompanied by an increase in cytoplasmic calcium ion concentration.[30] The platelet's contractile proteins (actin and myosin) are likely involved as well as a process of fusion of the granule membranes with the platelet plasma membrane (or some derivative of this) that results in extrusion of the granule contents. The exact morphologic mechanism for the discharge of dense bodies has not yet been clarified. Alpha granules on the other hand are thought to fuse first with each other to form a compound granule and then with the plasma membrane or the open canalicular system.[31] At least one intrinsic inhibitory pathway also exists: degranulation is readily inhibited if the level of cyclic AMP in platelets is raised,[32] either by stimulating the adenylate cyclase that forms cAMP or by inhibiting the phosphodiesterase that degrades it.

**Arachidonate Metabolism.** When platelets are exposed to a stimulus sufficiently powerful to induce degranulation, the arachidonic acid biosynthetic pathways are activated. Some of the products of this pathway have inflammatory activity (see below) and/or promote platelet aggregation and secretion. The main features of the pathway are outlined in Figure 11–5. General synthetic pathways and biologic activities of arachidonate derivatives are reviewed in Chapter 6. Briefly, activation of a phospholipase(s) associated with the platelet membrane liberates arachidonic acid from membrane phospholipids. This 20-carbon fatty acid is converted by a membrane-bound cyclo-oxygenase into labile intermediate compounds, the endoperoxides $PGG_2$ and $PGH_2$. These compounds, which can themselves induce platelet aggregation and secretion, are converted mainly to thromboxane (Tx)$A_2$, which is highly labile (half-life about 30 seconds) but is an extremely potent platelet stimulant[33] and vasoconstrictor. The metabolic product of $TxA_2$, known as $TxB_2$, is stable and readily measurable by radioimmunoassay but inactive on platelets. Small amounts of $PGD_2$, $PGE_2$, and $PGF_{2\alpha}$ are also formed from the endoperoxides. Although all are vasoactive, the only one with a powerful effect on platelets is $PGD_2$, which can inhibit platelet responses by stimulating adenylate cyclase,[34] thus elevating cyclic AMP. Through the lipo-oxygenase pathway, 12-hydroxytetraenoic acid (12-HETE) is produced in platelets. Interestingly, it has been suggested that platelets (12-lipo-oxygenase) and neutrophils (5-lipo-oxygenase) can cooperate to produce the important phlogistic agent $LTB_4$ (5,12-DiHETE) from arachidonic acid.[35] As we shall see later, cooperative interactions such as this between leukocytes and platelets may contribute significantly to inflammation. Finally, 12-hydroxy-5-*cis*,8,10-*trans*-heptadecatrienoic acid (HHT), together with the three-carbon fragment malondialdehyde (MDA), is produced from the endoperoxides. Although HHT and MDA are without effect on platelets, MDA can easily be measured either colorimetrically or fluorimetrically after combination with thiobarbituric acid, thus serving as a simple indicator of PG synthesis by platelets.

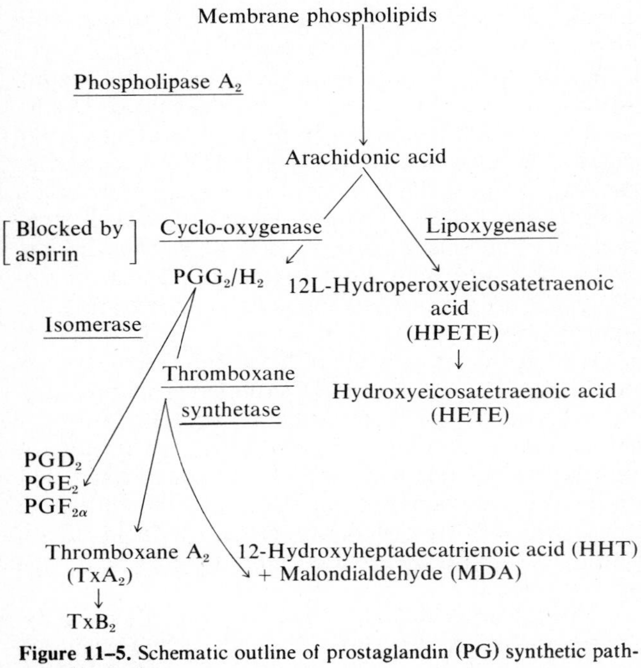


**Figure 11–5.** Schematic outline of prostaglandin (PG) synthetic pathways in platelets.

Nonsteroidal anti-inflammatory drugs such as aspirin and indomethacin block the cyclo-oxygenase and thus inhibit the platelet responses mediated by $TxA_2$ and the endoperoxides. The production of HHT, MDA, and the stable prostaglandins $D_2$, $E_2$ and $F_{2\alpha}$ is also prevented by these drugs, but they do not interfere with the formation of 12-HETE.

**Phospholipid Metabolism.** Stimulation of platelets by ligand–receptor interactions produces profound alteration in phospholipid metabolism, and it has been suggested that this participates in the stimulus-response coupling mechanism. Liberation of arachidonate has already been mentioned, and this appears to be derived from both phosphatidyl inositol and phosphatidyl choline, probably as as result of action of phospholipases C and $A_2$, respectively.[36,37] The so-called phosphoinositol (PI) cycle is activated, and both diacylglycerol (DAG) and phosphatidic acid (PA) are formed very early in the activation sequence. PA has been suggested to act as an ionophore, i.e., a molecule that promotes redistribution of calcium,[38] but this has been challenged.[37] DAG, on the other hand, acts as a cofactor for a unique protein kinase (protein kinase C), which is now felt to be important in cell activation.[36] By contrast, the arachidonate for thromboxane generation may well be derived via an as yet unidentified phospholipase $A_2$ ($PLA_2$) from other phospholipids, probably phosphatidyl choline. Interestingly, some of this substrate may have an ether-linked alkyl chain in the sn-1 position. The removal of arachidonate from this alkyl-acyl-glycero-phosphoryl choline would yield the precursor for the synthesis of platelet-activating factor (PAF) (see below). It should be emphasized, however, that platelet activation can proceed (following the appropriate stimuli) without participation of endogenous arachidonate derivatives and probably without the generation of PAF. However, these two lipid derivatives may significantly contribute to the amplification of the overall platelet response and thus lead to an explosive reaction, which can generate a significant thrombus, for example, before inhibitory processes take over.

**Uptake by Active Transport.** Platelets accumulate by active transport several vasoactive amines, which are then stored in the dense granules. The most striking example is serotonin, whose uptake by platelets has been studied for many years.[39] The transport process is highly efficient (see Fig. 11–6), and under normal circumstances all the serotonin in blood is carried in the platelet dense granules, which effectively isolates it from the vascular cells. The same system is used to transport dopamine, though with much lower affinity,[40] and norepinephrine is also transported into the platelet by the serotonin carrier, with even lower affinity (Olverman and Gordon, unpublished work).

Platelets also actively transport other vasoactive substances such as amino acids and adenosine, which provide fuel for the platelet's energy requirements. Adenosine is incorporated into the metabolic pool of adenine nucleotides, as is adenine.[41] The platelet's capacity to remove vasoactive agents such as adenosine from the plasma, though possibly important in inflammation, is subordinate to that of the vascular endothelial cells.[42]

**Uptake by Endocytosis.** Individual platelets, and platelet aggregates, can take up particulate materials of many kinds, such as lipid droplets, carbon particles, latex beads, and micro-organisms.[43] Whether this uptake represents genuine pinocytosis and phagocytosis, trapping of particles within the canalicular system, or in some cases merely incorporation of material within a platelet aggregate, is open to question. It is clear, however, that this is not just an in vitro phenomenon of academic interest; platelets can and do play an important role in removing some kinds of particulate material from the bloodstream.[44] This therefore merits further investigation, particularly with respect to the interaction of platelets and micro-organisms, a potentially important event in inflammation.

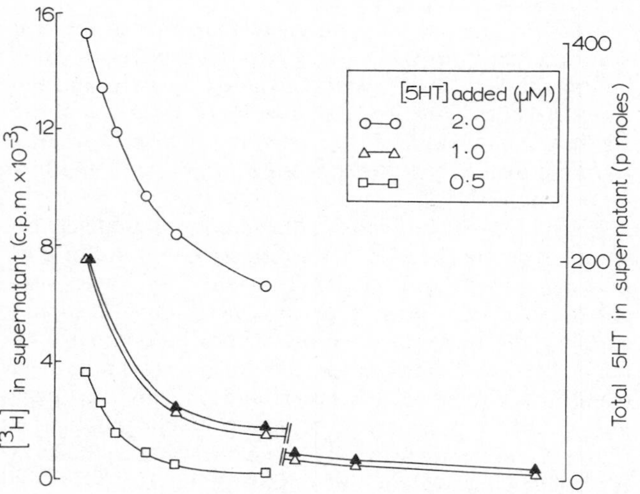


**Figure 11–6.** Uptake of [$^3$H]-5-hydroxytryptamine (serotonin; 5HT) by rat platelets in plasma. Samples of supernatant plasma were taken at the times shown for assay of total 5HT (closed symbols) and measurement of radioactivity (open symbols). Initial [$^3$H]-5HT concentrations added were (◯) 2 $\mu$m. (△) 1$\mu$M. (□) 0.5 $\mu$M. (From Drummond, A.H., and Gordon, J.L.: Br. J. Pharmacol. 56:417, 1976.)

## PLATELET PRODUCTS WITH POTENTIAL INFLAMMATORY ACTIONS

**Amines.** The amine content of human platelets is virtually all serotonin, although rabbit platelets are apparently unique in having a substantial content of histamine also.[45] These amines (as well as the small amounts of catecholamines also present in platelets) are stored in the dense granules, which possess an uptake mechanism capable of concentrating the amines transported from the extracellular medium into the platelet cytoplasm by the carrier on the plasma membrane. The amine content of platelets varies widely in different species, from about 3 to 60 nmole per mg cell protein, with values in man near the lower end of the range.[46]

Because the contents of dense granules are readily secreted by platelets, exposure of platelets to stimuli results in a high local concentration of serotonin in the plasma, which can have profound effects on vascular tone and permeability (Chapter 8). In addition, serotonin is a fibrogenic agent[47] and may therefore affect the connective tissue composition at sites of chronic inflammation. It is instructive to calculate the plasma concentration of serotonin that might be achieved around a human platelet aggregate; assuming $1 \times 10^9$ platelets form an aggregate at a site of local endothelial damage and release 50 percent of their serotonin (about 0.2 $\mu$g), then the serotonin concentration in the plasma (say, 0.1 ml in volume) around the aggregate is over 10 $\mu$M. In making this calculation it should be remembered that $10^9$ platelets are derived from about 3 ml blood, that an aggregate of $10^9$ platelets occupies only about 10 $\mu$l, and that platelets often release more than 50 percent of their serotonin.

**Arachidonate Products.** These have already been discussed above (see Arachidonate Synthesis). Thromboxane $A_2$ is a potent vasoconstrictor. Its role in inflammatory processes is not clear. Nevertheless (as outlined below) hemodynamic alterations are so important in inflammation that one cannot disregard the potential contribution of $TxA_2$. On the other hand, prostaglandins are secreted in such small amounts by platelets that although these molecules participate in inflammatory processes, the platelet does not seem to be an important source.

As indicated above, 12-HETE may have some chemotactic potential of its own but can be converted to $LTB_4$ by neutrophils. $LTB_4$ is an extremely potent chemoattractant and neutrophil stimulus and thus must be considered as a candidate for a platelet contribution to inflammation.

These mediators are all discussed in more detail in Chapter 6.

**Enzymes.** It has been known for some years that platelets contain acid hydrolases, such as $\beta$-glucuronidase, in lysosomal granules (see above). In addition to lysosomal glycosidases and acid phosphatase, platelets contain acid proteinases. Cathepsins A, C, D, and E have been described.[48] Cathepsin D is apparently the most prominent proteinase in human platelets, but, as with other platelet constituents, there are substantial interspecies variations. Neutral proteinases in platelets have been less well characterized; elastase, collagenase, and other neutral proteinases have been described, but the amounts of elastase and collagenase present per milligram of cell protein are very small compared with those in other cells such as neutrophils or those produced by macrophages. Indeed, some of these enzyme activities measured in "platelet" preparations may have been due to contaminating neutrophils,[48] although in the case of elastase there is apparently a small amount of activity in the platelets themselves.[49] This enzyme is not, however, readily detectable with substrates (including [$^3$H]-elastin) conventionally used to characterize the elastase in other cells, such as neutrophils.

The roles of the hydrolytic enzymes released by platelets remain to be determined. Most (if not all) of them are released when platelets are exposed to powerful stimuli such as thrombin and collagen. The ability of the acid hydrolases to attack components of connective tissue is presumably severely limited by the buffering action of the plasma surrounding platelets, which keeps the milieu around the platelets at a pH too alkaline for significant activity of acid hydrolases. Likewise, the platelet neutral proteinases would be affected by inhibitors such as $\alpha_1$-antitrypsin and $\alpha_2$-macroglobulin in the surrounding plasma. Therefore, it seems that such enzymes could only be effective in the immediate pericellular environment, where the access of plasma constituents might be restricted.

However, platelet neutral proteinases may play a role in generating phlogistic factors. For example, biologically active fragments of C5 are generated when platelets are activated in plasma.[50] This was shown to result from liberation of a platelet neutral proteinase. Such C5 fragments can themselves initiate a complete inflammatory reaction with both cellular infiltration and increased permeability.[51] Local production of such factors at the site of platelet–vessel wall interaction should therefore be considered as a candidate for initiation of some types of inflammatory reactions.

**Platelet-Derived Growth Factor.** Ross[52,53] described a low molecular weight protein from platelet granules that promoted proliferation of vascular smooth muscle cells. This molecule, platelet-derived growth factor (PDGF) has since been studied extensively. It has been purified, cloned, and sequenced and shows a fascinating homology in primary structure with an oncogene product.[54] Its receptors and growth-promoting effect on mesenchymal cells have also been well described,[55] and it may represent an important contribution to the repair processes following inflammation.

## INTERACTION OF PLATELETS WITH COMPONENTS OF THE INFLAMMATORY SYSTEM

**Purines.** There are three main aspects to the interactions between platelets and purines. First, ADP induces platelet aggregation (and a modest secretory response in human platelets) by combining with a specific receptor.[56] Second, adenosine inhibits platelet responses by interacting with another receptor[56] that is coupled to adenylate cyclase and thus elevates cyclic AMP in platelets. Finally, the ATP and ADP secreted during platelet degranulation are powerful vasoactive agents, largely because of their capacity to induce endothelium-dependent vasodilation,[57,58] a phenomenon in which endothelial cells are stimulated to release a mediator that relaxes the subjacent vascular smooth muscle. It should be emphasized that although ATP stimulates the release of $PGI_2$ from endothelial cells, $PGI_2$ is not the mediator of endothelium-dependent vasodilation.[60] Nucleotides can be released from cells other than platelets in response to a damaging stimulus—e.g., from erythrocytes and vascular endothelium[61]—and these extracellular nucleotides affect platelet function and vascular tone (see above); however, their effects are localized and transient, because nucleotides released into the plasma are rapidly metabolized, mainly by ectoenzymes located on the luminal surface of endothelial cells.[62] Adenosine, one of the products of such metabolism, induces vasodilation through a direct action on vascular smooth muscle, as well as by inhibiting platelet responsiveness.[56]

It may seen unusual to classify purines as components of the inflammatory system, but their powerful effects on vasoregulation suggest that their role in the inflammatory process may have been underrated (see also Chapter 21).

**Amines.** Amines are an important class of inflammatory mediators, chief among which are histamine and serotonin; catecholamines are also important because of their effects on blood flow. Platelets are unaffected by histamine but can be stimulated to aggregate and secrete by serotonin, epinephrine, norepinephrine, and (weakly) dopamine. Catecholamines induce aggregation with little or no shape change in human platelets. Serotonin is regarded as a weak platelet stimulant but is very sensitive to calcium ion concentration, and therefore anticoagulation with citrate can give a false picture.[63] Also aggregation is greatly potentiated when serotonin and a catecholamine are present together (Fig. 11–7). This is important because the circulating levels of catecholamines (in the nanomolar range) are too low to induce aggregation directly but can potentiate platelet responses to other stimuli. For example, platelet responsiveness is increased in subjects under stress,[64] and this may be correlated with increases in circulating catecholamines.

**Arachidonate Derivatives.** The arachidonate product that is the most powerful platelet stimulant is $TxA_2$, and the most potent inhibitory product is $PGI_2$ (prostacyclin). Both of these were discovered using platelets.[33,65] $TxA_2$ has already been discussed. $PGI_2$ and, to a lesser extent, $PGE_2$ inhibit platelet responses by activating adenylate cyclase and increasing the intracellular levels of cyclic AMP. $PGI_2$ has been suggested to contribute to the nonthrombogenic surface of the vascular endothelium, although other factors may also play a role in this important endothelial function.[66,67] Interestingly, as with platelets and neutrophils combining to synthesize $LTB_4$, platelet endoperoxides have been suggested to be "used" by endothelial cells to synthesize $PGI_2$.[68] Thus, cooperation between cells in the modulation of vascular responses is implied. Prostaglandins such as $PGI_2$ and $PGE_2$ are vasodilators in some vascular beds and thus may enhance vascular permeability and neutrophil migration in inflammation.

**Platelet-Activating Factor (PAF).** This phospholipid was first described as a platelet activator but is now known to have much broader biologic activities. The breadth is well illustrated in the recently published proceedings of the first international symposium on this molecule.[69] The structure of the PAF that is derived

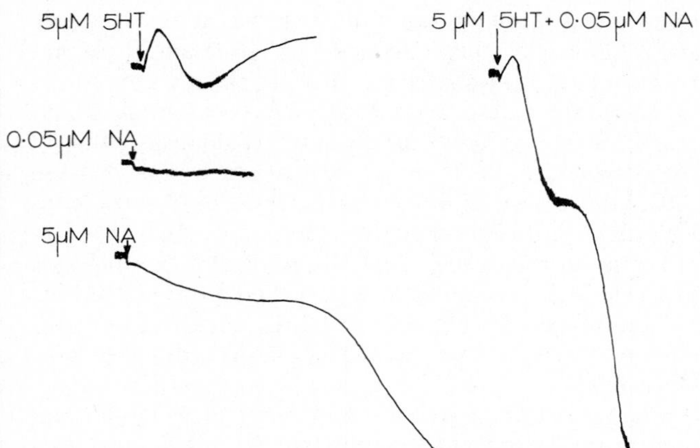


**Figure 11–7.** Platelet aggregation induced by 5-hydroxytryptamine (5HT) and by norepinephrine (noradrenaline [NA]), alone and in combination.

from rabbit basophils is 1-0-alkyl-2-acetyl-*sn*-glycero-3-phosphorylcholine. Molecule(s) derived from neutrophils, mononuclear phagocytes, endothelial cells, and the renal medulla are very similar, but their exact structure has not yet been determined.[69,70] As well as acting as a potent platelet stimulus, PAF (or acetyl-glyceryl-ether-phosphorylcholine [AGEPC] or [PAF acether][72]) contracts smooth muscle in a slow and prolonged fashion, activates neutrophils, and causes increased vascular permeability. Its actions in vivo also include induction of pulmonary hypertension and systemic hypotension.[70] Some of these effects are apparently mediated via its action on platelets; some, by other means. PAF is derived from ubiquitous membrane ether lipids. It is an extremely potent molecule (a few micrograms are lethal), and mammalian tissues and plasma contain a highly specific acetylhydrolase that inactivates the molecule.[72] These observations suggest that we may have to pay considerable attention to this group of compounds as inflammatory mediators in the future.

**Thrombin.** Thrombin is one of the most important physiologic activators of platelets and also plays a role in the inflammatory response around fibrin-cell clots. Lower concentrations of thrombin are needed to induce platelet secretion and aggregation than to clot fibrinogen, but despite many studies on the effect of thrombin on platelets no fully accepted explanation of its mechanism of action has yet emerged. The proteolytic action of thrombin is probably important for platelet stimulation, but the molecule also binds to receptors on the platelet surface.[71] The protein with which thrombin interacts to stimulate platelets is not fibrinogen; thrombin induces platelet secretion when fibrinogen is absent or blocked by antibodies,[72,73] although fibrinogen is a necessary cofactor for platelet aggregation.

**Other Coagulation Factors.** Platelets exhibit an intricate and intimate relationship with the process of coagulation. Additionally, the coagulation process is probably involved in inflammation; for example, fibrin deposition is a common occurrence. Nevertheless, the exact contribution of these elements to inflammation is as yet unclear, and, since coagulation is discussed in more detail in Chapter 8, it is only mentioned herein for completeness.

**Immune Stimuli and Complement Components.** For a recent review of immunologic reactions of platelets see reference 7. Platelets can be stimulated or damaged by several immunologic reactions (some complement mediated) in which the stimulus is not directed at the platelet in an immunologically specific sense. These immunologic reactions, in which the platelet is a "bystander," can be separated into two main classes, depending on whether the platelets are able to bind the third complement component C3b (i.e., are immune adherence positive) (see Chapter 7). Immune adherence is species dependent; platelets from many nonprimate species (e.g., rabbit, rat, mouse, guinea pig) are immune adherence positive and are consequently attracted to particles and surfaces that have fixed C3b.[74]

Immune adherence negative platelets (e.g., human)

react with aggregated gamma globulin, with IgG-coated surfaces, or with immune complexes containing IgG. This induces platelet secretion and, under appropriate conditions, aggregation, but not lysis. Complement activation is apparently not essential; indeed, the reactions proceed in platelet suspensions free of serum or plasma.[75] IgG stimulates platelets by interacting with a typical Fc receptor on the platelet membrane that is not one of the major glycoproteins.[76] This process can be markedly enhanced by the presence of lipopolysaccharide (endotoxin).[7] Activated zymosan (i.e., with C3b attached via the alternative pathway) also induces aggregation and secretion (but not lysis) in human platelets, whereas endotoxin alone does not,[77] but because zymosan readily accumulates IgG as well as C3b, and the attached C3b progressively decays to C3d (which is inactive), there is still some doubt about the mechanisms responsible for zymosan-induced stimulation of human platelets.

An interesting observation in relation to the interaction of platelets with complement components is that part of the Clq molecule is structurally similar to part of the collagen molecule, and Clq can inhibit platelet stimulation by collagen.[78,80] It has been suggested that complement activation is involved in platelet stimulation by collagen,[79] although this hypothesis now seems unlikely.

Polly and associates have studied another way in which platelets may interact with the complement system.[81] Assembly of components on the surface of the thrombin-activated platelet was suggested to represent a unique and perhaps important activating pathway for complement. Certainly various investigators have detected complement components on the surface of washed platelets (see reference 74), although whether this represented molecules trapped in the canalicular system is not clear.

Platelets participate in several immunologic reactions that result in inflammatory lesions (e.g., the Arthus and local Shwartzman reactions), and although their presence is apparently not always essential, there is no doubt that they often contribute to the biologic consequences.[82]

**Vascular Cells.** Changes in the vasculature (especially in the microcirculation) are central to the inflammatory process, as emphasized by Cohnheim almost a century ago. Since the participation of platelets in the body's response to a stimulus (whether "inflammatory" or otherwise) is necessarily an intravascular event, the interaction of platelets with vascular cells is of primary importance. The vascular cells involved are those of the endothelium and the underlying smooth muscle layer.

Under normal circumstances, platelets do not adhere to endothelial cells. This is partly because endothelium apparently does not present a surface "attractive" to platelets, and partly because endothelial cells synthesize and secrete prostacyclin ($PGI_2$) which, like $PGD_2$ and $PGE_1$, is a powerful adenylate cyclase stimulant and thus inhibits platelet secretion, aggregation, and adhesion.[66,67,83] In contrast to endothelium, vascular smooth muscle cells or fibroblasts readily induce platelet aggregation and secretion in vitro, possibly because of the connective tissue elements on their surface.[84] These in vitro findings are consistent with observations made in vivo; namely, that as long as the endothelial lining is maintained intact, platelets do not adhere in large numbers, but when endothelial damage occurs and the underlying connective tissue is exposed, then platelets adhere and form aggregates at these sites.

It is important to note that the preferential adhesion of platelets to vascular smooth muscle rather than endothelium is not a phenomenon observed with other cells such as leukocytes; granulocytes readily adhere to endothelial cells in vitro but have a lesser affinity for smooth muscle cells.[85]

**Mononuclear Phagocytes.** It has been established that platelet aggregates in vivo are eventually invaded by monocytes, and resolution of the thrombus is achieved by the monocytes phagocytizing platelet debris.[86] The signal for this phagocytosis has not yet been determined but may be similar to the mechanism by which senescent platelets are recognized as being ready for removal from the circulation; this recognition apparently involves a small reduction in platelet membrane sialic acid.[4,5] Interestingly, platelets appear to have some affinity for blood monocytes and may contribute to their adhesion to surfaces.[87]

The biochemical aspects of platelet-monocyte interactions have also been neglected. For example, although it seems likely that platelet constituents could affect the migration and endocytic activity of mononuclear phagocytes, this possibility has apparently not been investigated.

**Neutrophils.** Platelet aggregates that form in vivo or in vitro in a system with white cells present are frequently surrounded by PMN leukocytes in the form of "halos"[88] or "rosettes"[89] (Fig. 11–8). Similarly, the adhesion of platelets to blood vessels stripped of endothelial cells in vivo is followed by the attachment of leukocytes, and the leukocyte adhesion is a consequence of the presence of activated platelets rather than the loss of endothelium per se.[90] The leukocytes are apparently attracted by factors derived from the platelets, and the most likely candidates are C5a (formed in the plasma by the platelet proteinases)[50] or prostanoid products such as HETE and HHT or $LTB_4$.

The possible cooperation of platelets and neutrophils in synthesizing $LTB_4$ has already been mentioned. $LTB_4$ is an important neutrophil stimulant. In the other direction, neutrophils synthesize and secrete PAF, which can activate the platelets. This reciprocal activation may play an important role in the explosive early stages of inflammation. In addition, a recent report implicates platelet products in the enhancement of neutrophil-endothelial interactions,[91] i.e., the putative first step in leukocyte emigration.

It is clear that platelets may also interact with other circulating leukocytes. However, detailed mechanisms need further investigations.

**Fibroblasts.** Platelet-derived growth factor has already been mentioned and could contribute to fibroblast proliferation in the reparative phases of inflammation.

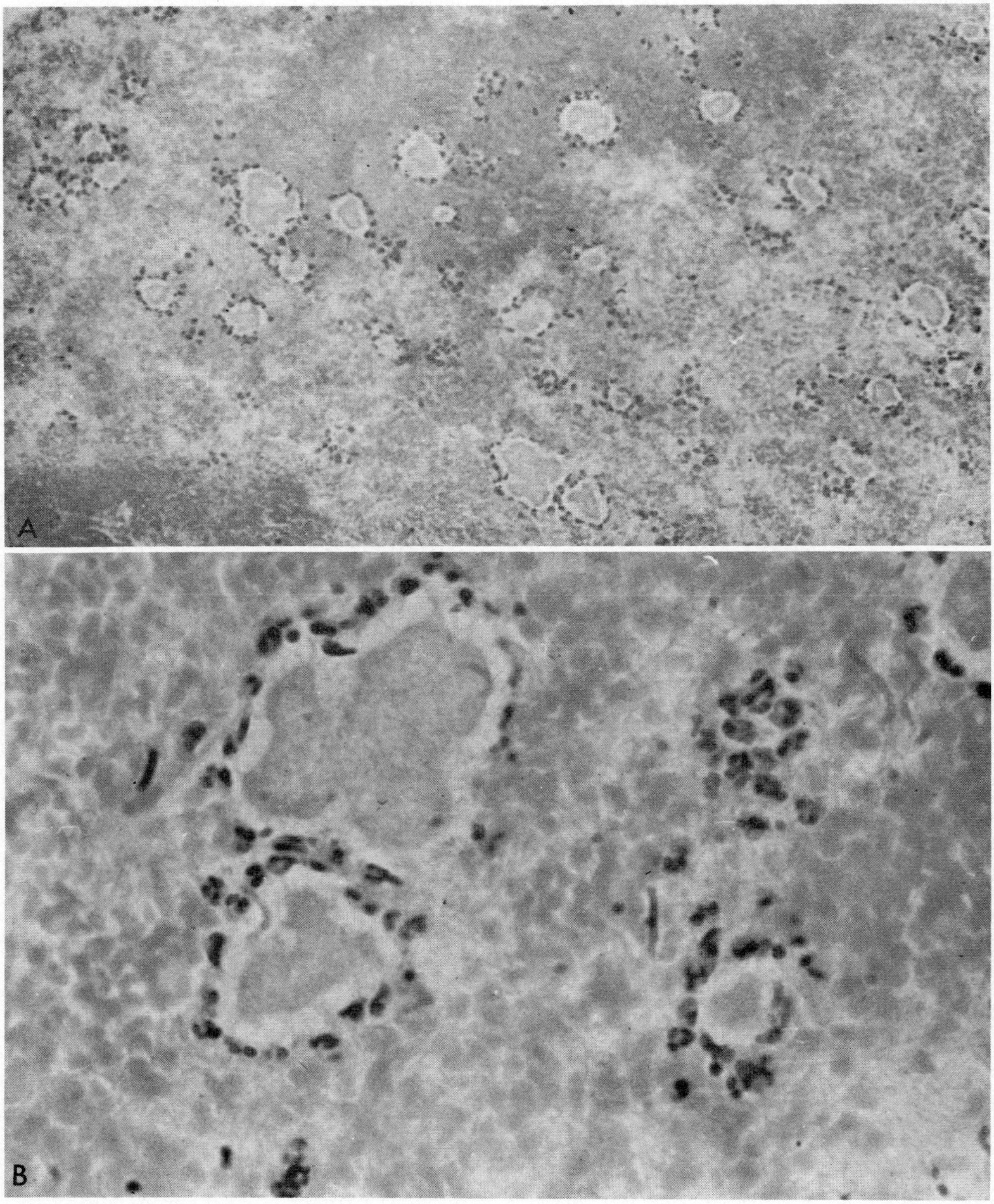


**Figure 11–8.** Platelet aggregates formed in vitro by rotating samples of recalcified citrated blood in plastic tubes. Aggregates are surrounded by "halos" of polymorphonuclear leukocytes. *A,* × 100. *B.* × 250.

However, like many aspects of platelet function, the in vivo involvement remains to be clarified.

## THE INFLAMMATORY PROCESS–A ROLE FOR PLATELETS?

Inflammation could be defined as a beneficial, nonspecific response of tissues to injury, which generally leads to resolution of the injury. As such, chronic inflammatory diseases might represent examples of continued or repetitive stimuli and/or abnormalities of the resolution process. In this context, chronic disease resulting from inflammatory processes might include persistent inflammation, permanent tissue destruction, or fibrosis. The last could be seen as a resolution that is inappropriate for the tissue, a last-ditch effect to repair the site of injury but one that does not allow restitution of normal tissue function. The inflammatory process can therefore be considered in three phases: initiation; resolution of the inflammation; and, lastly, resolution of the injury.

Initiation of inflammation involves alterations in blood vessel functions, emigration of leukocytes, and increased vascular permeability. Despite all the investigative efforts over the last 100 years, we still know surprisingly little about the details of these three processes. The contribution of hemodynamic alterations to inflammation has been known since the nineteenth century but has received a resurgence of interest following the recent suggestion that vasodilator prostaglandins ($PGE_2$, $PGI_2$) can enhance vascular permeability and increase neutrophil emigration.[92,93] Whether these effects are solely hemodynamic or whether they are the direct effects of the prostaglandins on the vessel wall and/or the leukocytes is not yet clear. The data do, however, suggest one area in which nonsteroidal anti-inflammatory cyclo-oxygenase inhibitors might be effective.

The emigration of leukocytes is also an area fraught with surprising mystery. Initial adhesion of leukocytes to the vascular endothelium is followed by migration between these cells and then across the barrier of the basement membrane (or basal lamina). The major site of emigration appears to be the postcapillary venules, but neutrophils can migrate through the walls of large arteries, veins, and capillaries.[94,95] Chemotactic factors apparently induce the expression of adhesive properties on the leukocytes, which induce the initial interaction with the endothelium. Subsequent events can be described only superficially, however. We[96] and Liotta's[97] group have suggested that cells migrate across basal laminae by digesting components of the connective tissue following release of proteases, but this hypothesis has not yet been proved in vivo. Additionally, the true nature and function of the putative chemotactic factors in these systems remain to be elucidated.

Increased permeability is also an integral component of inflammation. It has often been associated with the leukocytic phases of the inflammation,[92,95] but experiments have also suggested that leukocyte emigration and increased permeability are separable events.[96] While the suggested mechanisms for the permeability changes are beyond the scope of this chapter, it is noteworthy that leukocytes may "open" tight junctions between cells by release of neutral proteases or oxygen radicals (Parsons, Cott, Mason, and Henson, unpublished). This is an area of intense investigation in many centers, and evidence for specific mechanisms should be forthcoming in the near future.

Since most of the aforementioned processes occur in the blood vessels, platelets are potential candidates for contributing to these events. As indicated throughout this chapter, there is great *potential* for such platelet involvement but very little evidence that it actually occurs. Platelet depletion studies did not seem to alter significantly the induction of an Arthus reaction in the rabbit (Henson and Cochrane, 1969, unpublished). However, we know so much more about the systems involved now that it would seem appropriate to repeat this type of study with more detailed quantitative analysis of the effects of the depletion on the inflammatory process. Certainly platelets accumulate at sites of inflammation,[98,99] though whether as participants or as a consequence of the process is unclear.

With regard to termination of the inflammation itself (the shut-off mechanisms) we know even less, and the mechanisms involved in resolution and repair also require much more investigation. In these two areas, the role of platelets is largely unknown. Hints of a contribution come from the secretion and known effects of PDGF, but it may be that this molecule exerts its influence in vivo primarily on the blood vessel wall.

Future studies of the contribution of platelets to specific inflammatory processes should include the following:

1. Quantitative evidence of platelet accumulation
2. Morphologic evidence of platelet presence and secretion
3. The presence of platelet products
4. Prevention of effects by specific platelet inhibition or depletion
5. Prevention of effects by inhibition of the action of platelet products
6. Reproduction of the given effect by administration of platelets or the platelet product to the platelet-depleted system
7. Studies in animals or man with genetically malfunctioning platelets.

Clearly such investigations are easier in acute reactions, but even then they suffer from problems of specificity. Inflammation is a highly redundant process with many "collateral" mechanisms. Elimination of one component of the system often has little effect on the overall process because other cells and systems can take over, hence, the difficulty and fascination of research in this area.

## SUMMARY

The potential contributions of platelets to the inflammatory process are considerable, but their actual participation has not been established. Intravascular accumulation of platelets at sites of tissue injury has been clearly demonstrated,[99] and there have also been claims that platelets were present in inflammatory exudates,[100] but further investigations in the same laboratory revealed that these claims were incorrect.[101] It therefore appears that intact platelets are not found extravascularly at inflammatory sites. Indeed this might be expected, since the rapidity with which they adhere to vascular collagen would preclude their migration out of blood vessels. Nevertheless platelet constituents released intravascularly at an injury site may diffuse across the vessel wall[102] and could affect tissues in this manner.

It therefore appears that platelets may influence extravascular events in the inflammatory process to a limited extent through the actions of their secreted constituents, but their role in this respect would normally be subordinate to that of leukocytes. In intravascular events, however, platelets may play an important role, as the evidence summarized in this chapter demonstrates. This should be borne in mind when considering the vascular aspects of inflammation, as platelets can interact with many components of the inflammatory response. But as well as revealing potential biologic consequences, the study of such interactions can increase our understanding of the processes involved; as emphasized earlier in this chapter, platelets have been and will continue to be valuable cellular models for the biologist interested in adhesion, degranulation, and prostaglandin synthesis, and in the receptors and mediators that regulate these events.

## REFERENCES


1. Buckmaster, G.A.: The blood platelets. Sci. Prog. 1:73, 1906.
2. Robb-Smith, A.H.T.: Why the platelets were discovered. Br. J. Haematol. 13:618, 1967.
3. Gordon, J.L. (ed.): Platelets in Biology and Pathology 2. Amsterdam, Elsevier-North Holland-Biomedical Press, 1981.
4. George, J.N., and Lewis, P.C.: Studies on platelet plasma membranes. J. Lab. Clin. Med. 91:301, 1978.
5. Greenberg, J., Packham, M.A., Cazenave, J.P., Reimers, H.J., and Mustard, J.F.: Effects on platelet function of removal of platelet sialic acid by neuraminidase. Lab. Invest. 32:476, 1975.
6. Lind, S.E., and Stossel, T.P.: The microfilament network of the platelet. Prog Hemost. Thromb. 6:63, 1982.
7. Henson, P.M., and Ginsberg, M.H.: Immunological reactions of platelets. *In* Gordon, J.L. (ed): Platelets in Biology and Pathology 2. Amsterdam, Elsevier-North Holland-Biomedical Press, 1981.
8. Packham, M.A., and Mustard, J.F.: In vitro methods and the study of platelet mechanisms. Vox Sang. 40(Suppl. 1):22, 1981.
9. White, J.G.: Platelet morphology. *In* Johnson, S.A. (ed): The Circulating Platelet. New York, Academic Press. 1971.
10. Holmsen, H.: Energy metabolism in platelets. Vox Sang. 40(Suppl. 1):1, 1981.
11. Frojmovic, M.M., and Milton, J.G.: Human platelet size, shape and related functions in health and disease. Physiol. Rev. 62:185, 1982 .
12. Smith, C.W. and Hollens, J.C.: Motility and adhesiveness in human neutrophils: Redistribution of chemotactic factor induced adhesion sites. J. Clin. Invest. 65:804, 1980.
13. Gordon, J.L., and Dingle, J.T.: Binding of radiolabelled collagen to blood platelets. J. Cell Sci. 16:157, 1976.
14. Wharton-Jones, W.T.: On the state of the blood and blood vessels in inflammation. Guy's Hospital. Rep. Ser. 2 7:1, 1851.
15. Coller, B.S., Peerschke, E.I., Scudder, L.E., and Sullivan, C.A.: Studies with a murine monoclonal antibody that abolishes ristocetin-induced binding of von Willebrand factor to platelets: Additional evidence in support of GPIb as a platelet receptor for von Willebrand factor. Blood 61:99, 1983.
16. Ginsberg, M.H., Forsyth, J., Lightsey, A., Chediak, J., and Plow, E.F.: Reduced surface expression and binding of fibronectin by thrombin-stimulated thrombasthenic platelets. J. Clin. Invest. 71:619, 1983.
17. Bensusan, H.B., Koh, T.L., Henry, K.G., Murray, B.A., and Culp L.A.: Evidence that fibronectin is the collagen receptor on platelet membranes. Proc. Natl. Acad. Sci. 75:5864, 1978.
18. Chiang, T.M. and Kang, A.H.: Isolation and purification of collagen α 1(I) receptor from human platelet membrane. J. Biol. Chem. 257:7581, 1982.
19. Feinman, R.D., and Detwiler, T.C.: Platelet secretion induced by divalent calcium ionophores. Nature 249:172, 1974.
20. Di Minno, G., Thiagarajan, P., Perussia, B., Martinez, J., Shapiro, S., Trinchieri, G., and Murphy, S.: Exposure of platelet fibrinogen-binding sites by collagen, arachidonic acid, and ADP: Inhibition by a monoclonal antibody to the glycoprotein IIb-IIIa Complex. Blood 61:140, 1983.
21. Bennett, J.S., Hoxie, J.A., Leitman, S.F., Vilaire, G., and Cines, D.B.: Inhibition of fibrinogen binding to stimulated human platelets by a monoclonal antibody. Proc. Natl. Acad. Sci. 80:2417, 1983.
22. Jaffe, E.A., Leung, L.L.K., Nachman, R.L., Levin, R.I. and Mosher, D.F.: Thrombospondin is the endogenous lectin of human platelets. Nature 295:246, 1982.
23. Mills, D.C.B., Robb, I.A., and Roberts, G.C.K.: The release of nucleotides, 5-hydroxytryptamine and enzymes from human blood platelets during aggregation. J. Physiol. 195:715, 1968.
24. MacIntyre, D.E., Salzman, E.W., and Gordon, J.L.: Prostaglandin receptors on human platelets. Structure-activity relationships of stimulatory prostaglandins. Biochem. J. 174:921, 1978.
25. Holmsen, H., and Day, H.J.: The selectivity of the thrombin-induced platelet release reaction: Subcellular localization of released and retained constituents. J. Lab. Clin. Med. 75:840, 1970.
26. Gordon, J.L.: Blood platelet lysosomes and their contribution to the pathophysiological role of platelets. *In* Dingle, J.T., and Dean, R.T. (eds.): Lysosomes in Biology and Pathology, Vol. 4. Amsterdam, North-Holland, 1975.
27. MacIntyre, D.E., McMillan, R.M., and Gordon, J.L.: Secretion of lysosomal enzymes by platelets. Biochem. Soc. Trans. 5:1181, 1977.
28. Henson, P.M., Ginsberg, M.H. and Morrison, D.C.: Mechanisms of mediator release by inflammatory cells. *In* Poste, G. and Nicolson, G.L. (eds.): Membrane Fusion. Amsterdam, Elsevier-North Holland-Biomedical Press, 1978.
29. Friedhoff, L.T., and Sonenberg, M.: The membrane potential of human platelets. Blood 61:180, 1983.
30. Feinstein, M.B.: The role of calmodulin in hemostasis. Prog. Hemost. Thromb. 6:25, 1982.
31. Ginsberg, M.H., Taylor, L. and Painter R.G.: The mechanism of thrombin-induced platelet factor 4 release. Blood 55:661, 1980.
32. Haslam, R.J.: Roles of cyclic nucleotides in platelet function. *In* Biochemistry and Pharmacology of Platelets. Amsterdam, Elsevier, 1975.
33. Hamberg, M., Svensson, J., and Samuelsson, B.: Thromboxanes: A new group of biologically active compounds derived from prostaglandin endoperoxides. Proc. Natl. Acad. Sci. USA 72:2994, 1975.
34. Smith, J.B., Ingerman, C.M., and Silver, M.J.: Formation of prostaglandin D2 during endoperoxide-induced platelet aggregation. Thromb. Res. 9:413, 976.
35. Marcus, A.J., Brockman, M.J., Safier, G., Ullman, H.C., Islam, N., Sherman, C.N., Rutherford, L.E., Korchak, H.M., Weissmann, G.: Formation of leukotrienes and other hydroxy acids during platelet-neutrophil interactions in vitro. Biochem. Biophys. Res. Comm. 109:130, 1982.
36. Rittenhouse, S.E.: Inositol lipid metabolism in the responses of stimulated platelets. Cell Calcium 3:311, 1982.
37. Majerus, P.W., Prescott, S.M., Hoffman, S.C., Neufeld, E.J. and Wilson, D.B.: Uptake and release of arachidonate by platelets. Adv. Prostaglandin Thromboxane Leukotriene Res. 11:45, 1983.
38. Serhan, C., Anderson, P., Goodman, E., Dunham, P., and Weissmann, G.: Phosphatidate and oxidized fatty acids are calcium ionophores. J. Biol. Chem. 256:2736, 1981.
39. Sneddon, J.M.: Blood platelets as a model for mono-amine containing neurons. *In* Kerkut, G.A., and Phillis, J.W. (eds.): Progress in Neurobiology, Vol. 1. Oxford, Pergamon Press, 1973.
40. Gordon, J.L., and Olverman, H.J.: 5-Hydroxytryptamine and dopamine transport by rat and human platelets. Br. J. Pharmacol. 62:219, 1978.
41. Holmsen, H.: Platelet adenine nucleotide metabolism and platelet malfunction. *In* Caen, J. (ed): Platelet Aggregation. Paris, Masson, 1971.
42. Pearson, J.D., Carleton, J.S., Hutchings, A., and Gordon, J.L.: Uptake and metabolism of adenosine by pig aortic endothelial and smooth muscle cells in culture. Biochem. J. 170:265, 1978.
43. Mustard, J.F., and Packham, M.A.: Platelet phagocytosis. Ser. Haematol. 1:168, 1968.
44. Donald, K.J., and Tennent, R.J.: The relative roles of platelets and macrophages in clearing particles from the blood: the value of carbon

clearance as a measure of reticuloendothelial phagocytosis. J. Pathol. 117:235, 1975.
45. Humphrey, J.H., and Jacques, R.: The histamine and serotonin content of the platelets and polymorphonuclear leukocytes in various species. J. Physiol. 124:305, 1954.
46. DaPrada, M., Richards, J.R., and Kettler, R.: Amine storage organelles in platelets. *In* Gordon, J.L. (ed.): Platelets in Biology and Pathology 2. Amsterdam, Elsevier-North Holland Biomedical Press, 1981.
47. Aalto, M., and Kulonen, E.: Effects of serotonin, indomethacin and other antirheumatic drugs on the synthesis of collagen and other proteins in granulation tissue slices. Biochem. Pharmacol. 21:2835, 1972.
48. Ehrlich, H.P., and Gordon, J.L.: Proteinases and platelets. *In* Gordon, J.L. (ed.): Platelets in Biology and Pathology. Amsterdam, Elsevier-North Holland-Biomedical Press, 1976.
49. Homebeck, W., Starkey, P.M., Gordon, J.L., Legrand, Y., Pignaud, G., Robert, L., Caen, J.P., Ehrlich, H.P., and Barrett, A.J.: The elastase-like enzyme of platelets. Thrombos. Haemostas. 42:1681, 1980.
50. Weksler, B.B., and Coupal, C.E.: Platelet-dependent generation of chemotactic activity in serum. J. Exp. Med. 137:1419, 1973.
51. Larsen, G.L. and Henson, P.M.: Mediators in Inflammation. *In* Brass, A. (ed.): Annual Review of Immunology. Vol. 1. Palo Alto, Annual Reviews, Inc., 1983.
52. Ross, R., Glomset, J., Kariya, B., and Harker, L.: A platelet-dependent serum factor that stimulates the proliferation of arterial smooth muscle cells in vitro. Proc. Natl. Acad. Sci. USA 71:1207, 1974.
53. Ross, R., and Vogel, A.: The platelet-derived growth factor. Cell 14:203, 1978.
54. Doolittle, R.F., Hunkapiller, M.W., Hood, L.E., Devare, S.G., Robbins, K.E., Aaronson, S.A., and Antoniades, H.N.: Simian sarcoma virus *onc* gene, v-*sis*, is derived from the gene (or genes) encoding a platelet-derived growth factor. Science 221:275, 1983.
55. Stiles, C.D.: The molecular biology of platelet-derived growth factor. Cell 33:653, 1983.
56. Mills, D.C.B., Macfarlane, D.E., Lemmex, B.W.G., and Haslam, R.J.: Receptors for nucleosides and nucleotides on blood platelets. *In* Berne, R.M., Rall, T.W., and Rubio, R. (eds.): Regulatory Function of Adenosine. Boston, Marinus Nishoff, 1981.
57. Furchgott, R.F., and Zawadski, J.V.: The obligatory role of endothelial cells in the relaxation of arterial smooth muscle by acetylcholine. Nature 288:373, 1980.
58. DeMey, J.D., and Vanhoutte, P.M.: Role of the intima in cholinergic and purinergic relaxation of isolated canine femoral arteries. J. Physiol. 316:347, 1981.
59. Pearson, J.D., Slakey, L.L., and Gordon, J.L.; Stimulation of prostaglandin production through purinaceptors on cultured porcine endothelial cells. Biochem. J. 214:273, 1983.
60. Gordon, J.L., and Martin, W.: Stimulation of endothelial prostacyclin production plays no role in endothelium-dependent relaxation of the pig aorta. Br. J. Pharmacol. 80:179, 1983.
61. Pearson, J.D., and Gordon, J.L.: Vascular endothelial and smooth muscle cells in culture selectively release adenine nucleotides. Nature 281:384, 1979.
62. Gordon, J.L.: Vessel wall metabolism and vasoactive agents. *In* Woolf, N. (ed.): Biology and Pathology of the Vessel Wall. Eastbourne, Praeger, 1983.
63. Gordon, J.L., and Drummond, A.H.: Irreversible aggregation of pig platelets and release of intracellular constituents induced by 5-hydroxytryptamine. Biochem. Pharmacol. 24:33, 1975.
64. Gordon, J.L., Bowyer, D.E., Evans, D.W., and Mitchinson, M.J.: Human platelet reactivity during stressful diagnostic procedures. J. Clin. Pathol. 26:958, 1973.
65. Moncada, S., Gryglewski, R., Bunting, S., and Vane, J.R.: An enzyme isolated from arteries transforms prostaglandin endoperoxides to an unstable substance that inhibits platelet aggregation. Nature 263:663, 1976.
66. Gimbrone, M.A., and Buchanan, M.R.: Interactions of platelets and leukocytes with vascular endothelium: In vitro studies. Ann. N.Y. Acad. Sci. 401:171, 1982.
67. Weksler, B.B.: Prostacyclin Prog. Hemost. Thromb. 6:13, 1982.
68. Marcus, A.J., Weksler, B.B., Jaffe, E.A., and Brockman, M.J.: Synthesis of prostacyclin from platelet-derived endoperoxides by cultured human endothelial cells. J. Clin. Invest. 66:979, 1980.
69. First International Symposium on Platelet Activation Factor. J. Benveniste, editor. In press.
70. Lynch, J.M., Worthen, G.S., and Henson, P.H.: Mediators and the mechanism of their release: PAF. *In* Buckle, D.R., and Smith, H. (eds.): The Development of Antiasthma Drugs. In press.
71. Gordon, J.L. (ed.): Platelets in Biology and Pathology 2. *In* Dingle, J.T., and Gordon, J.L. (eds.): Research Monographs in Cell and Tissue Physiology. Vol. 5. Amsterdam. Elsevier/North-Holland, 1981.
72. Keenen, J.P., and Solum, N.O.: Quantitative studies on the release of platelet fibrinogen by thrombin. Br. J. Haematol. 23:461, 1972.
73. Tollefsen, D.M., and Majerus, P.W.: Inhibition of human platelet aggregation by monovalent antifibrinogen antibody fragments. J. Clin. Invest. 55:1259, 1975.
74. Henson, P.M.: The adherence of leukocytes and platelets induced by fixed IgG antibody or complement. Immunology 16:107, 969.
75. Pfueller, S.L., and Luscher, E.F.: The effects of aggregated immunoglobulins on human blood platelets in relation to their complement-fixing abilities. J. Immunol. 109:517, 526, 1972.
76. Pfueller, S.L., Jenkins, C.S.P., and Luscher, E.F.: A comparative study of the effect of modification of the surface of human platelets on the receptors for aggregated immunoglobulins and for ristocetin-von Willebrand factor. Biochim. Biophys. Acta 465:614, 1977.
77. Pfueller, S.L., and Luscher, E.F.: Studies of the mechanisms of the human platelet release reaction induced by immunologic stimuli. II. The effects of zymosan. J. Immunol. 112:1211, 1974.
78. Csako, G., and Suba, E.A.: A physiologic regulator of collagen-induced platelet aggregation: Inhibition by Clq. Thromb. Haemost. 45:110, 1981.
79. Chater, B.V.: The role of membrane-bound complement in the aggregation of mammalian platelets by collagen. Br. J. Haematol. 32:515, 1976.
80. Wautier, J.L., Legrand, Y.J., Fauvel, F. and Caen, J.P.: Inhibition of platelet collagen interactions by the Cls subcomponent of the first component of complement. Thromb. Res. 21:2, 1981.
81. Chater, B.V. The role of membrane-bound complement in the aggregation of mammalian platelets by collagen. Br. J. Haematol. 32:515, 1976.
82. Clark, W.F., Friesen, M., Linton, A.L., and Lindsay, R.M.: The platelet as a mediator of tissue damage in immune complex glomerulonephritis. Clin. Nephrol. 6:287, 1976.
83. Best, L.C., Martin, T.J., Russell, R.G.G., and Preston, F.E.: Prostacyclin increases cyclic AMP levels and adenylate cyclase activity in platelets. Nature 267:850, 1978.
84. MacIntyre, D.E., Pearson, J.D., and Gordon, J.L.: Localization and stimulation of prostacyclin production by vascular cells. Nature 271:549, 1978.
85. Beesley, J.E., Pearsons, J.D. Carleton, J.S., Hutchings, A., and Gordon, J.L.: Interaction of leukocytes with vernacular cells in culture. J. Cell Sci. 33:85, 1978.
86. Jorgensen, L., Rowsell, H.C., Hovig, T., and Mustard, J.F.: Resolution and organization of platelet-rich mural thrombi in carotid arteries of swine. Am. J. Pathol. 51:681, 1967.
87. Musson, R.A. and Henson, P.M.: Humoral and formed elements of blood modulate and response of peripheral blood monocytes. I. Plasma and serum inhibit and platelets enhance monocyte adherence. J. Immunol. 122:2026, 1979.
88. Sharp, A.A.: Platelet structure and function in relation to blood coagulation and haemostasis. *In* Chalmers, D.G., and Gresham, G.A. (eds.): Biological Aspects of Occlusive Vascular Disease. Cambridge, Cambridge University Press, 1964.
89. Giordano, N.D., Radivoyevitch, M., and Goodsitt, E.: Thrombus formation time in hemophilia: An in vitro study. Thromb. Diathes. Haemorrh. 20:596, 1968.
90. Baumgartner, H.R., and Muggli, R.: Adhesion and aggregation: Morphological demonstration and quantitation in vivo and in vitro. *In* Gordon, J.L. (ed.): Platelets in Biology and Pathology. Amsterdam, Elsevier-North Holland-Biomedical Press, 1976.
91. Boogaerts, M.A., Yamado, O., Jacob, H.S., Moldow, C.F.: Enhancement of granulocyte-endothelial cell adherence and granulocyte-induced cytotoxicity by platelet release products. PNAS 79:7019, 1982.
92. Williams, T.J. Jose, P.J., Wedmore, C.V., Peck, M.J., and Forrest, M.J.: Mechanisms underlying inflammatory edema. Adv. Prostaglandin Thromboxane Leukotriene Res. 11:33, 1983.
93. Larsen, G.L., and Henson, P.M.: Mediators of inflammation. *In* Brass, A. (ed.): Annual Review of Immunology. Volume 1. Palo Alto, Annual Reviews, Inc., 1983.
94. Issekutz A.C.: Effect of vasoactive agents on polymorphonuclear leukocyte emigration in vivo. Lab. Invest. 45:234, 1981.
95. Lipscomb, M.F., Onofrio, J.M., Nash, E.J., Pierce, A.K., and Toews, G.B.: A morphological study of the role of phagocytes in the clearance of Staphylococcus aureus from the lung. J. Reticuloendothel. Soc. 33:429, 1983.
96. Tonnesen, M., Smedly, L., Goins, A., and Henson, P.M.: Interaction between neutrophils and vascular endothelial cells. *In* Parnham, M.J., and Winkelmann, J. (eds.): Agents and Actions Supplements. Volume 11. 1st Cologne Atherosclerosis Conference. Basel, Birkhauser Verlag, 1982.
97. Russo, R.G., Liotta, L.A., Thorgeirsson, U., Brundage, R., and Schiffmann, E.: Polymorphonuclear leukocyte migration through human amnion membrane. J. Cell Biol. 91:459, 1981.
98. Henson, P.M., Larsen, G.L., Henson, J.E., Newman, S.L., Musson, R.A., and Leslie, C.C.: Resolution of pulmonary inflammation. In press.
99. Kravis, T.C., and Henson, P.M.: Accumulation of platelets at sites of

antigen-antibody-mediated injury: A possible role for IgE antibody and mast cells. J. Immunol. 118:1569, 1977.
100. Cotran, R.S.: The delayed and prolonged vascular leakage in inflammation. II. An electron microscopic study of the vascular response after thermal injury. Am. J. Pathol. 46:589, 1965.
101. Smith, M.J.H., Walker, J.R., Ford-Hutchinson, A.W., and Penington, D.G.: Platelets, prostaglandins and inflammation. Agents Actions 6:701, 1976.
102. Bolam, J.P., and Smith, M.J.H.: Platelets in inflammatory exudates. J Pharm. Pharmacol. 29:674, 1977.

### Acknowledgments

Supported in part by NIH Grants HL21565, HL28520, and GM24834.

# Chapter 12
# Proteinases in Joint Disease

*Alan J. Barrett and Jeremy Saklatvala*

## INTRODUCTION

Proteinases may be involved in several aspects of joint disease. For example, the formation of antibodies to immunoglobulins and collagen in rheumatoid arthritis may depend upon the formation of products of limited degradation of these proteins by extracellular proteinases.[1,2] Proteinases in the joints may also activate precursors of the complement and kinin systems to liberate polypeptide mediators of inflammation responsible for leukocyte chemotaxis, increased vascular permeability, and pain.[3,4] The formation of fibrin in the synovial fluid that is commonly seen in rheumatoid arthritis may arise from the action of proteinases other than thrombin on fibrinogen, or from the activation of prothrombin by an unusual mechanism. There is no doubt, however, that the aspect of joint pathology in which proteolytic enzymes are most strongly implicated by evidence currently available is that of the tissue damage that so often accompanies joint disease, and this will form the main topic of the present chapter.

## THE PROTEINASES OF THE JOINT

The proteases that are most important in the pathologic degradation of the extracellular structural proteins of connective tissues are those that cleave peptide bonds in the body of the protein chains, rather than simply releasing terminal residues; these are the *proteinases* or *endopeptidases.*[6,7] The enzymologist classifies the proteinases on the basis of the chemical groups responsible for catalytic activity. Four classes of proteinase are distinguished in this way: the *aspartic* (previously "acid" or "carboxyl"), *cysteine* (previously "thiol"), *serine,* and *metallo*-proteinases[5] (Table 12–1). Newly discovered proteinases can usually be assigned to one of these groups according to their response to appropriate active-site–directed inhibitors. Inhibitors also provide the most direct approach to identifying the proteinases active in biologic systems.

**Aspartic Proteinases—Cathepsin D.** It was recognized long ago that the stomach contains a proteinase, pepsin, capable of digesting proteins under the very acidic conditions of the stomach contents. Subsequently, it was discovered that many protozoa use intracellular "stomachs," or digestive vacuoles, to break down food particles, also under acidic conditions, and much more recently it has become clear that many mammalian cells carry out intracellular digestive processes at low pH. The most conspicuous of the acid-acting proteinases in cells is cathepsin D, an enzyme with many similarities to pepsin and evolved from the same primitive precursor. The vacuolar digestive system of mammalian cells is, of course, the lysosomal system, and several lines of evidence implicate this system in the pathology of inflammation. All nucleated cells seem to contain lysosomes, and all mammalian cells examined have been found to contain an enzyme with the properties of cathepsin D. Cathepsin D is the only aspartic proteinase likely to occur in the rheumatoid joint.

Cathepsin D[8-10] is an enzyme of molecular weight about 42,000 that is most active in the degradation of hemoglobin (a convenient test substrate) at about pH 3.5. Degradation of cartilage proteoglycan is most rapid at pH 5, but the enzyme shows little action on this or any other substrate above pH 6, and none at or above pH 7.

The mechanism of catalysis of the aspartic proteinases remains somewhat mysterious, but it is clear that there are at least two active groups, both being $\beta$-carboxyl groups of aspartic acid residues. The most useful reagent in the attribution of acid proteinase activity to aspartic proteinases is pepstatin.[11-13] This pentapeptide is produced by various species of *Streptomyces* and is a powerful and highly specific inhibitor of the aspartic proteinases. It has low toxicity and is suitable for inhibition of extracellular aspartic proteinase activity in biologic systems. Still more specific inhibition of cathepsin D can be produced with antibodies, however.[14]

The specificity of peptide bond cleavage by cathepsin D is relatively broad but shows a distinct preference for

**Table 12–1.** Classes of Proteinase (Endopeptidase) and Some of Their Characteristics

| | Aspartic | Cysteine | Serine | Metallo- |
|---|---|---|---|---|
| *Examples* | Pepsin<br>Cathepsin D<br>Renin | Cathepsin B<br>Cathepsin L | Trypsin<br>Chymotrypsin<br>Plasmin<br>Kallikrein<br>Elastases<br>Cathepsin G | Collagenase<br>Macrophage elastase<br>Gelatinase |
| *pH range for activity* | 3–6 | 3–7 | 6–10 | 6–9 |
| *Test inhibitors* | Pepstatin | E-64, leupeptin, thiol-blocking reagents | Dip-F,<br>Pms-F | 1,10-phenanthroline |
| *Major plasma inhibitors* | | $\alpha_2M$<br>$\alpha CPI$ | $\alpha_1$-$PI$<br>$\alpha_2M$<br>$\alpha_2M$ | $\alpha_2M$ |

Abbreviations: $\alpha_2$M: $\alpha_2$-macroglobulin; $\alpha_1$-PI: $\alpha_1$-proteinase inhibitor; Dip-F: diisopropyl fluorophosphate; Pms-F: phenylmethylsulfonylfluoride.

bonds flanked by hydrophobic amino acid residues. A sequence of at least five residues is generally required in a substrate, and no test substrate of really low molecular weight is available for routine use in the laboratory.

The degradation of cartilage proteoglycan by human cathepsin D has been characterized at the molecular level.[5-17] The enzyme cleaves the hyaluronic acid-binding region from the molecule and splits the polysaccharide-attachment region into rather large fragments (Fig. 12–1).

The structural integrity of collagen type II fibers is not detectably affected by cathepsin D, although some other types of collagen may have a few susceptible peptide bonds.[18-20]

In the body, any extracellular activity of cathepsin D is likely to be severely restricted by pH conditions, although it is possible that production of carbon dioxide and lactic acid by a cell creates pericellular regions of sufficiently low pH to allow the action of acid proteinases.[21] $\alpha_2$-Macroglobulin is capable of binding cathepsin D,[22] but little other inhibitory activity exists in mammalian tissues.

**Cysteine Proteinases—Cathepsins B and L.** Part of the acid proteinase activity of mammalian cells is expressed only in the presence of low molecular weight thiol compounds (e.g., glutathione, cysteine) and is destroyed by reagents that react with thiol groups (e.g., iodoacetate). This activity is attributable to the cysteine proteinases, the best known of which is lysosomal cathepsin B.

Human cathepsin B has been isolated and characterized.[3-5] It is a protein of about 25,000 molecular weight, with less activity against hemoglobin than cathepsin D but much more against collagen and gelatin. The optimum pH for the action of cathepsin B on its synthetic substrates is 6, but maximal activity against proteins may occur at a pH as low as 3, probably because the acidity sensitizes the substrate. Cathepsin B loses activity irreversibly above pH 7.

Cathepsin B is evolutionarily homologous with papain[26] and undoubtedly has a catalytic site in which the side chains of cysteine and histidine are active. The enzyme is best assayed fluorimetrically with the synthetic substrate benzyloxycarbonyl-arginyl-arginylmethylcoumarylamide.[25]

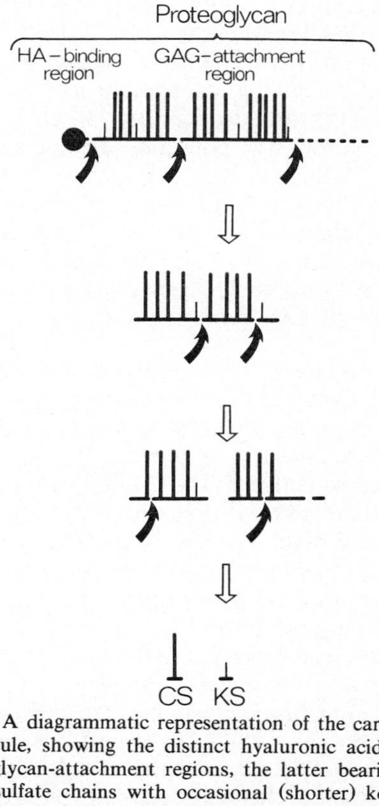


**Figure 12–1.** A diagrammatic representation of the cartilage proteoglycan molecule, showing the distinct hyaluronic acid-binding and glycosaminoglycan-attachment regions, the latter bearing groups of chondroitin sulfate chains with occasional (shorter) keratan sulfate chains. The arrows indicate points of proteolytic attack in the progressive degradation of the molecule. The sequence of events is the same for most proteinases, but some are able to take the process much further than others. Very early on, the hyaluronic acid-binding region is split off. Then large groups of polysaccharide chains are liberated, and these are further fragmented, but with no liberation of single polysaccharide chains until very late (and then only with the few proteinases of broadest specificity). (Redrawn from Roughley, P.J.: Biochem. J. 167:639, 1977).

In human tissues, the cysteine proteinase with greatest activity against collagen and proteoglycan is cathepsin L. Like cathepsin B, cathepsin L is a lysosomal enzyme, is active at acid pH, and is irreversibly denatured at neutral pH. At present, no convenient specific assay for cathepsin L has been discovered, but benzyloxycarbonyl-phenylalanyl-arginyl-methycoumarylamide is a sensitive substrate, and results can be corrected for the contribution from cathepin B.[25] Molar concentrations of active cathepsin B and cathepsin L can be determined by active site titration.[25] Cathepsins B and L both cleave the N-terminal peptides of collagen that contain the covalent crosslinks within and between molecules (see Chapter 12 and Fig. 12–2), but cathepsin L is very much the more active of the two.[27,28]

Cathepsin B cleaves the hyaluronic acid-binding region from cartilage proteoglycan and degrades the glycosaminoglycan-attachment region to rather small fragments.[15-17] Action on this substrate is rapid at pH 5 to 6.

Cathepsins B and L are inactivated by thiol-blocking reagents in general, but more selective inhibitors usable in biologic systems are leupeptin, E-64, and certain chloromethanes. Leupeptin is propionyl-leucyl-leucyl-L-argininaldehyde; it is a tight-binding reversible inhibitor of cathepsin B[29,30] (and cathepsin L). E-64, which is L-*trans*-epoxysuccinyl-leucylamido(4-guanidino) butane, is a very rapidly reacting irreversible inhibitor of these enzymes.[31] The synthetic peptidyl chloromethanes are notable for offering the potential of some selectivity of inhibition of cathepsin B or cathepsin L,[32] but the sensitivity of cathepsin B to benzyloxycarbonyl-phenylalanyl-phenylalanyl-chloromethane varies greatly between species, the human and rat enzymes being little affected. The lysosomal cysteine proteinases are also inhibited by protein inhibitors of the cystatin family.[32a,32b]

**Serine Proteinases.** The family of endopeptidases with a catalytically essential serine residue at their active site is by far the largest class of mammalian proteinases, and this may relate to the fact that these enzymes are ideally suited to acting in the conditions most common within cells and tissues: they are most active at about neutral pH and require no special co-factors. Their physiologic importance seems also to be reflected in the fact that 10 percent of the plasma protein is represented by serine proteinase inhibitors!

The serine proteinases include many of the proteins of the "cascades" of coagulation, fibrinolysis, complement, and kinins in the plasma, such as thrombin, plasmin, Cls, Clr, and kallikrein, as well as trypsin, chymotrypsin, and elastase from the exocrine pancreas. Of particular note to rheumatology are plasmin and the plasminogen activators, plasma kallikrein and the serine proteinases of the polymorphonuclear leukocytes, the lysosomal elastase and cathepsin G, both of which are major components of the azurophile granules of these cells (see Chapter 9).

***Plasmin.*** The inactive precursor of plasmin, plasminogen, occurs in the plasma at a concentration of about 20 mg per deciliter. Activation of the precursor can be brought about by a plasminogen activator system in the plasma, by bacterial components such as streptokinase, or by activators (which are themselves serine proteinases) produced by stimulation of various cells, including macrophages, synovial cells, and neutrophil leukocytes.[33-35] Activation by any of these agents is inhibited by 6-aminohexanoic acid and related antifibrinolytic compounds.[36]

Plasmin preferentially cleaves lysyl bonds. The enzyme seems to have evolved for the function of breaking down fibrin clots; not only is plasmin itself very active in degrading fibrin, but plasminogen has a high affinity for fibrin, so that a clot forms with a built-in mechanism for its own dissolution. (This may represent a common pattern for proteinases acting on insoluble proteins: elastase and collagenase also bind to their respective substrates.) Plasmin certainly has the capacity to degrade cartilage proteoglycan,[37] but it has little action on collagen, although it activates latent collagenase (see below).The major plasma inhibitors of plasmin are the $\alpha_2$-plasmin inhibitor and $\alpha_2$-macroglobulin.[38]

***Plasma Kallikrein.*** There are two distinct enzymes called kallikrein: tissue kallikrein and plasma kallikrein.[7] Plasma kallikrein is generated from the inactive precursor prokallikrein, by the action of coagulation factor XII (Hageman factor), or kallikrein itself.[39] Plasma kallikrein acts on high molecular weight kininogen to yield bradykinin, and the consequences of this are considered fully in Chapter 8.

Kallikrein also has the capacity to activate latent collagenase, and although active kallikrein is normally present in rheumatoid synovial fluid only at very low concentrations, it may be a significant activator.[40]

***Leukocyte Elastase.*** Elastin, the crosslinked structural protein important for the elastic strength of the arterial walls, the joint capsule, and skin, is highly resistant to proteolytic degradation, but it is attacked by the elastases of the pancreas and polymorphonuclear leukocytes. Unlike the collagenases, the elastases are by no means specific for the substrate after which they are named but have very broad proteolytic activity.

The polymorphonuclear leukocyte (lysosomal) elastase has not yet been positively detected in any other cells. It is a protein of about 28,000 molecular weight[41] that acts on cartilage proteoglycan to remove the hyaluronic acid–binding region, and then to fragment the glycosaminoglycan attachment region.[16,17,42]

The route by which leukocyte elastase degrades collagen fibers is illustrated diagrammatically in Figure 12–2.[43,44] The N-terminal peptides are degraded, with the elimination of the crosslinks that play a crucial part in the stabilization of collagen fibers. The individual molecules then separate and, if solubilized, denature in a few hours at 37° C, and are degraded to small peptides and amino acids by further proteolytic activity. Interestingly, the leukocyte elastase is several times more active against cartilage collagen (type II) than against type I collagen, whereas the reverse is true of the specific collagenases. The enzyme also degrades the type IV

is powerfully inhibited by chelating agents such as 1,10-phenanthroline, but these are too toxic for use in biologic systems. Some thiol compounds (e.g., thiorphan[65a] are effective inhibitors, and these might be applicable to biologic test systems. In rheumatology, it may be of interest that penicillamine (another thiol compound) is somewhat inhibitory.[66]

About 95 percent of the inhibitory capacity of plasma for collagenase is due to $\alpha_2$-macroglobulin, which reacts more slowly with the leukocyte collagenase than with that from other cells.[67] The lower molecular weight $\beta_1$-anticollagenase[68] and the closely related TIMP (tissue inhibitor of metalloproteinases) probably can enter cartilage matrix (unlike $\alpha_2$-macroglobulin) and might therefore be of significance in the control of collagenolysis.

Collagenase (like most of the other mammalian metalloproteinases) is commonly encountered in culture media and tissue preparations in an inactive or "latent" form. Typically, the latent collagenase can be activated by treatment with trypsin (or various other proteinases) or a mercurial compound such as aminophenylmercuric acetate. Probably, the latent collagenases are proenzymes requiring proteolytic activation. Evidence supporting this view comes from the synthesis of a single-chain latent collagenase in a cell free system with mRNA from synovial cells.[73] The mechanism of activation by the mercurial compounds remains to be explained, but the view that latent collagenase is an enzyme-inhibitor complex dissociable by the various activators is no longer widely held.

*Macrophage Elastase.* Stimulated macrophages secrete a metalloproteinase that degrades elastin, proteoglycan, and also protein inhibitors of other proteinases, including $\alpha_1$-proteinase inhibitor.[74-76a] If this enzyme is produced by the macrophage-like cells of the synovial lining, it certainly has the potential to contribute to tissue damage, but it is inhibited by $\alpha_2$-macroglobulin.

*Other Metalloproteinases.* In culture many types of cell have been shown to produce metalloproteinases in latent forms similar to those of collagenase. The enzymes are of two main types, a "gelatinase" active on denatured collagens and native collagen of types IV and V, and a general proteinase or "proteoglycanase" that readily hydrolyzes proteoglycan.[77] Neutrophil leukocytes contain a gelatinase in their "C particles" in addition to the collagenase of the specific granules.[72,78]

## ENDOGENOUS PROTEINASE INHIBITORS

Any assessment of the activities of proteinases in vivo must obviously take into account the naturally occurring inhibitors of the enzymes. In the context of the destruction of extracellular matrix components, the important inhibitors are those that derive from the plasma and those that are secreted by tissue cells.

**$\alpha_2$-Macroglobulin.** In general, the protein inhibitors of proteinases are easily classified as inhibitors of aspartic, cysteine, or serine proteinases or metalloproteinases, but $\alpha_2$-macroglobulin ($\alpha_2$M) is exceptional in inhibiting enzymes from all four groups, and the mechanism by which it does so is a unique form of protein–protein interaction. Each of the four identical subunits of $\alpha_2$M has near the center of its polypeptide chain a short sequence of amino acids that is highly sensitive to attack by the great majority of proteinases. When a proteinase cleaves this "bait region," it triggers a change in the shape of the $\alpha_2$M molecule, such that the proteinase molecule is physically trapped within it. The complexed enzyme molecule remains reactive with low molecular weight substrates and inhibitors that are able to diffuse to the interior of the trap but has little or no reactivity with large molecules, whether they be protein substrates, inhibitors, or antibodies. Since the original proposal of this remarkable mechanism of action by Barrett and Starkey,[22] a great deal more has been learned about the protein.[79,81,82] Particularly interesting has been the discovery that $\alpha_2$M contains a thiol ester group (formed between side-chains of neighboring cysteine and glutamic acid residues) that becomes chemically highly reactive in response to cleavage of the bait region and forms covalent links to the trapped proteinase molecule or other molecules that may be in the vicinity. This is a very similar reaction to that by which complement components C3 and C4 become linked to cell surfaces and immune complexes after their proteolytic activation, and indeed, they also contain thiol esters in sequences homologous with that of $\alpha_2$M. The covalent linking reaction of $\alpha_2$M does not contribute to its inhibition of proteinases, however, and the biologic significance of that reaction is not known.

In the course of its reaction with a proteinase, the $\alpha_2$M molecule acquires recognition sites for high affinity receptors on macrophages and some other cells. These cause the proteinase–$\alpha_2$M complexes to be removed from the plasma extremely rapidly.[83] $\alpha_2$M occurs in plasma at a concentration of about 250 mg per deciliter, but its molecular weight of 725,000 prevents it from escaping into the synovial fluid of a normal joint. In inflammation, however, it does escape, and rheumatoid synovial fluid holds about the same concentration as plasma. A difference is that $\alpha_2$M-proteinase complexes have a greater tendency to accumulate in synovial fluid than in plasma.

**Cysteine Proteinase Inhibitors.** The major extracellular inhibitor of the cysteine proteinases is $\alpha_2$M, but in addition these enzymes are specifically inhibited by a more minor plasma protein, $\alpha$-cysteine proteinase inhibitor ($\alpha$CPI).[84] $\alpha$CPI occurs in several forms of molecular weight 60,000 and greater; presumably it diffuses into the joint space from the circulation about as readily as albumin. $\alpha$CPI would probably enter cartilage matrix, whereas the $\alpha_2$M molecule is much too large to do so.

In human cells, there are two cytoplasmic inhibitors of cysteine proteinases, both of molecular weight about 13,000.[32b] Inhibitory activity corresponding to these was extracted from human articular cartilage,[86] but it was not shown whether it originated from the chondrocytes or the matrix.

**Serine Proteinase Inhibitors.** The inhibitors of serine proteinases in the joint are primarily those brought in in the plasma, which have been the subject of a recent review.[87] $\alpha_2$M is an important inhibitor of plasmin, kallikrein, leukocyte elastase, and cathepsin G, but plasmin is also powerfully inhibited by $\alpha_2$-antiplasmin, and kallikrein by $C\bar{1}$ inhibitor.

The leukocyte enzymes are inhibited by $\alpha_1$-proteinase inhibitor and for cathepsin G, $\alpha_1$-antichymotrypsin. These plasma proteins also enter the synovial fluid and penetrate cartilage to some extent.

**Metalloproteinase Inhibitors.** By far the major inhibitor of the collagenases and the other metalloproteinases in plasma and rheumatoid synovial fluid is $\alpha_2$M. A lower molecular weight inhibitor of collagenase ("$\beta_1$-anticollagenase") is present at very low concentrations in plasma.[68,88]

Various connective tissue cells produce a 30,000 molecular weight inhibitor of collagenase and other metalloproteinases (TIMP).[89]

## ARTICULAR TISSUE DAMAGE: THE MOLECULAR PROCESSES

As was mentioned above, the role of proteinases in causing damage to the articular cartilage and its underlying bone, with the likelihood of permanent impairment of joint function, is by far the most studied aspect of proteinases in rheumatology. Cartilage, bone, and tendon have each evolved to serve their physiologic functions by the development of extracellular matrices that comprise a large proportion of the mass of the tissue, but the matrices are chemically quite different and are subject to different forms of enzymic attack. None of these tissues has the capacity to repair itself with the full restoration of the original tissue structure.

**Cartilage.** In the remarkable extracellular matrix of cartilage, multimolecular assemblies of proteoglycan and collagen molecules interact to produce a rigid gel with very special physical properties, on which normal joint function depends.[90,91] Degradation of the molecules of either proteoglycan or collagen destroys this system, and the way in which this occurs is now understood in some detail.

***Proteoglycan.*** Since the cartilage proteoglycan is approximately 90 percent polysaccharide (see Chapter 15) it would be perfectly possible, in principle, for the degradation of the molecule to be mediated by polysaccharidases, but in fact, examination of the degradation products has tended to show the size of the polysaccharide chains to be unaltered, whereas the protein backbone is fragmented by the proteolytic attack. The backbone or "core protein" includes two regions, the glycosaminoglycan-attachment region, bearing clusters of covalently linked chondroitin sulfate and keratan sulfate chains, and the hyaluronic acid–binding region, which binds noncovalently to hyaluronic acid to assemble the multimolecular aggregates (Fig. 12–1). The binding to hyaluronic acid is stabilized by the participation of one or two "link proteins." The retention of proteoglycan in the matrix depends on the proteoglycan being assembled into these aggregate molecules, which are trapped within the three-dimensional meshwork of collagen fibers.[92]

The assay of enzymes active against proteoglycan is not an easy matter, since the physicochemical properties of the early products are not very different from those of the substrate. Model systems can be constructed, however, by trapping proteoglycan in polyacrylamide gels, which to some extent mimic the natural matrix.[93] Sensitive assays with reasonable quantitation can then be made with beads of this "synthetic matrix," in which the proteoglycan substrate is radiolabeled. The products are small enough to diffuse out of the gel and appear as radioactivity free in solution after removal of the beads.[94] Alternatively, release of nonradioactive proteoglycan from beads.[95] or from cartilage in culture is conveniently quantified by use of the metachromatic reaction of dimethylmethylene blue.[96]

The hyaluronic acid–binding region of the cartilage proteoglycan molecule is very susceptible to proteolysis, so that molecules in which there has been minimal degradation of the polysaccharide-attachment region often lack the capacity to bind to form aggregates. It is probable that loss of the hyaluronic acid–binding region is sufficient degradation to allow a proteoglycan molecule to diffuse out of the cartilage matrix, and thus make no further contribution to functional integrity of the tissue, and certainly very little degradation of the glycosaminoglycan-attachment region is required to allow this. Degradation of the polysaccharide-attachment region proceeds to different degrees with different proteinases; for example, cathepsin D liberates only rather large fragments bearing several polysaccharide chains, whereas cathepsin B takes the degradation further.[15-17] It is unclear as yet whether proteolysis of the link proteins occurs and, if so, what effect it has on the strength of the matrix.

The contribution made to the strength of cartilage matrix by the proteoglycan element is demonstrated by the effect of cathepsin D, which acts selectively on the proteoglycan. The enzyme causes a decrease in the resistance of the tissue to compression but not in the tensile stiffness at high stress. These changes in mechanical properties are explicable in terms of the model for the structure of cartilage matrix in which proteoglycan provides the resilient resistance to compression, whereas collagen is responsible for the tensile stiffness.[91]

***Collagen.*** The destruction of collagen is a process of especial interest in pathologic tissue damage for two reasons. First, it has seemed that the degradation of collagen is such a specific function of highly specialized enzymes that it may well be a rate-limiting process in tissue destruction. Second, there are strong indications that the capacity of a tissue to replace damaged collagenous elements with retention of the proper organization and structure may be so limited that the destruction of collagen is virtually irreparable. In particular, articular cartilage is irreversibly destroyed when the collagen component (type II) is degraded.

Collagen is largely polypeptide in nature, with some short carbohydrate side-chains. There is evidence for at least three distinct routes of proteolytic degradation (summarized in Fig. 12–5). Among the factors that will determine the relative importance of the various routes is the type of collagen involved; thus type II collagen (predominant in cartilage) is more resistant to the collagenases than is type I (present in tendon and bone) but more sensitive to the leukocyte elastase. Degradation of mature collagen must begin extracellularly, but it is thought to be completed intracellularly, and the uptake into the cells may occur at an early or late stage.

Mature collagen of adult cartilage exists as a network of fibers, each a bundle of collagen fibrils in which the molecules are aligned in the "quarter-stagger" array and covalently crosslinked (see Chapter 14). The intermolecular crosslinks of collagen are of great significance to its properties, conferring increased physical strength, raising the temperature for denaturation from 37° to above 50° C, and decreasing sensitivity to attack by collagenase 10-fold to 100-fold.[61,62]

Woolley and co-workers[60] have reported one of the few direct demonstrations that collagenase from rheumatoid synovium will degrade fibrous cartilage collagen, although more slowly than tendon collagen. If collagenase were to initiate the degradation of mature collagen fibers in vivo, it would be by cleavage of the helical regions of crosslinked molecules. Although the resulting A and B fragments would first be attached to other molecules, they would soon denature and become susceptible to nonspecific proteinases, including elastase, plasmin, and gelatinase.

An alternative form of attack on the collagen fibers may be mediated by the leukocyte elastase, or possibly by other nonspecific proteinases acting similarly.[43,44] The terminal, nonhelical peptides are cleaved by the elastase in such a way that the crosslinks are eliminated. The modified tropocollagen molecules then represent a highly susceptible substrate for the specific collagenase. Uncrosslinked molecules are more easily solubilized than crosslinked ones, and once solubilized, they denature quite rapidly at 37° C to give gelatin, which is rapidly degraded by almost any proteinase. Biomechanical measurements have shown that treatment of articular cartilage with leukocyte elastase markedly reduces its tensile stiffness and tensile strength.[97]

It is clear that there exists the third possibility of fragments of collagen fibers being taken up by cells and digested within the lysosomal system. The process has been studied in detail with the electron microscope for the fibroblasts of mouse periodontal ligament[98] and other cells and has been observed in a case of rheumatoid arthritis.[99] The lysosomal degradation of collagen would occur at the characteristic acid pH of these organelles and would be mediated by cysteine proteinases, cathepsin B, and cathepsin L, followed by exopeptidases, completing the degradation to very small peptides and amino acids. Even for the pathways of degradation initiated extracellularly by collagenase or elastase-like enzymes it is probable that the fragments are eventually taken into cells, either in the connective tissue itself or elsewhere in the body, for the final stages of breakdown.

**Bone.** The strength of bone is largely due to its mineral component, but the organic matrix of collagen, glycoprotein, and proteoglycan is formed first as the tissue develops, and is generally destroyed last as the tissue is broken down, since the mineral protects the organic component from enzymic attack.[100] Thus it seems that dissolution of the inorganic components of bone may be rate controlling in its resorption, and yet very little is known of the molecular mechanism by which this is brought about. Although bone cells or bone fragments in culture produce specific collagenase, some studies suggest that bone resorption in vitro is related more to activity of cysteine proteinases (e.g., cathepsin B or L) than to the classic metalloproteinases.

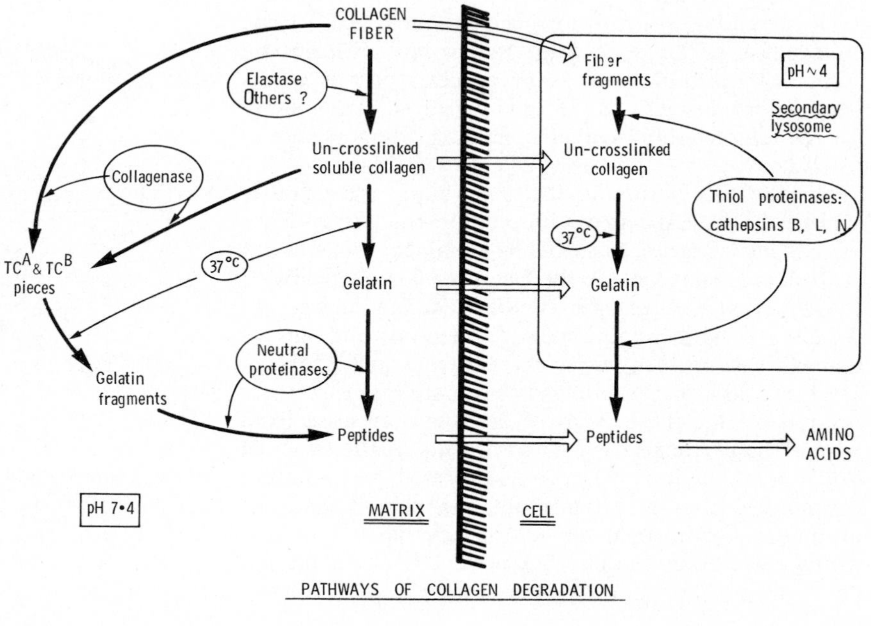

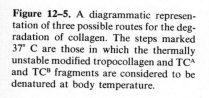

**Figure 12–5.** A diagrammatic representation of three possible routes for the degradation of collagen. The steps marked 37° C are those in which the thermally unstable modified tropocollagen and $TC^A$ and $TC^B$ fragments are considered to be denatured at body temperature.

**Tendon.** In rheumatoid arthritis, degradation of tendons can be a serious problem. The tendon is very largely composed of type I collagen in fiber bundles aligned parallel to the tensile stress; breakdown of the collagen leads to virtually complete destruction of the tissue and loss of its function.

## DEGRADATIVE PROTEINASES IN JOINT DISEASE: THEIR CELLULAR ORIGINS AND CONTROL PROCESSES

Since the various types of cells forming the articular tissues differ in the range of proteinases that they can produce, the questions of the identity of the proteinases responsible for tissue damage and their anatomic origin are closely linked. Two main lines of evidence may be considered in attempting to answer these questions: the anatomic locations of damage in the joint, and the capacity of the cells of each tissue within the joint to produce effective enzymes and to get them to the target tissues in an active state.

**The Anatomy of Joint Damage.** Much is written elsewhere in the present volume about the anatomy of joint damage, but certain points are of particular relevance to the questions of the identity and source of the degradation proteinases. In rheumatoid arthritis, the inflammatory changes affect the joint generally, and it is possible to argue in favor of the degradative enzymes originating from almost any of the cells that are present (Fig. 12–6). The apparent erosion of cartilage and bone at the margins of the articulating surface has suggested to many that the destructive enzymes arise from the adjacent soft tissue in a genuinely invasive process. That is to say that the enzymes are *extrinsic,* arising outside the target tissues, rather than *intrinsic.* This view seems to be supported by the demonstration of cathepsin D and collagenase at the pannus–cartilage junction.[101-103] Alternatively, it can be argued that the pannus is a form of granulation tissue produced in an attempt to heal areas of cartilage lysed by intrinsic enzymes. In this view, collagenase might arise from the pannus cells in the course of the (abortive) repair process, just as it has been reported that collagenase is produced, presumably for the remodeling of collagen, in the healing of dermal wounds.[104]

Besides the destruction at the margin of the articular surface that is associated with pannus, there is evidence of damage to other parts of the cartilage. Generalized loss of proteoglycan can be observed histologically.[105] Large areas of ulceration of the cartilage surface are commonly found remote from the pannus, and surface damage can be seen under the electron microscope in areas that are macroscropically normal.[106] The enzymes responsible for these types of damage may arise from within the cartilage itself or from cells in the synovial fluid in which it is bathed. Both cartilage and fluid contain enzymes and inhibitors (see below), and the arguments for intrinsic and extrinsic origins of the enzymes seem about equally balanced. Of course, a combination of the two is perfectly possible. The arguments relating to cartilage seem equally applicable to bone and tendon.

In osteoarthrosis, the lack of cellular infiltration of the synovium or synovial fluid makes an intrinsic mechanism of breakdown by enzymes from the chondrocytes themselves seem much more likely than an extrinsic attack by enzymes from outside the tissue. Normal cartilage matrix is known to show a slow but definite rate of turnover,[107] and it seems reasonable that the organized growth of cartilage would require the tissue cells to have the capacity to break down as well as to form the matrix in which they are embedded. It may well be that in osteoarthrosis one sees enhanced activity of the normal breakdown process.

**Proteinases and Their Inhibitors in Articular Cells and Tissues.** *Cartilage.* The major proteinases extractable from cartilage are the lysosomal acid proteinases cathepsin D and cathepsin B, both of which are highly effective in the degradation of cartilage proteoglycan in the range of pH 5 to 6.[108,109] Osteoarthrotic and osteophytic cartilage contains abnormally large amounts of both cathepsin D and cathepsin B.[109,110] Cathepsin D and other lysosomal enzymes are synthesized and secreted in greatly increased amounts by cartilage organ cultures stimulated to resorb with slight excess of retinol.[111] Attempts to block the breakdown of living cartilage in culture by inhibition of cathepsin D with pepstatin or antibodies have so far been unsuccessful, however, and this despite clear evidence that the pepstatin was present in the matrix at high concentration.[112]

Traces of a neutral proteinase have been detected in cartilage, and the enzyme has been characterized.[113] Extracts of cartilage contain inhibitors of cysteine, serine and metalloproteinases.[86] Articular cartilage explanted in organ culture produces collagenase[114] and other neutral metalloproteinases.[115] Chondrocytes in culture produce a spectrum of proteinases: collagenase, other

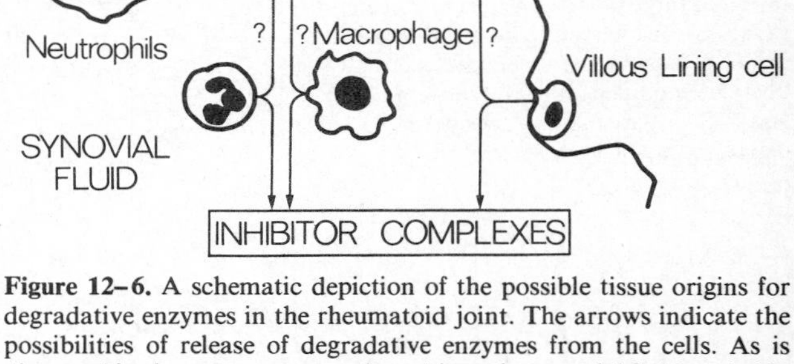

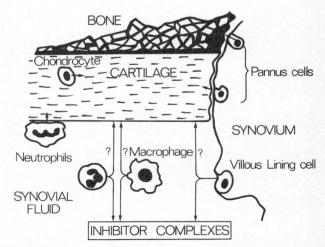


**Figure 12–6.** A schematic depiction of the possible tissue origins for degradative enzymes in the rheumatoid joint. The arrows indicate the possibilities of release of degradative enzymes from the cells. As is discussed in the text, enzymes released into the synovial fluid probably mainly form inhibitor complexes.

metalloproteinases[116,117] and plasminogen activator.[118] Cultured cartilage and chondrocytes also produce an inhibitor of metalloproteinases (TIMP).[119]

***Synovium.*** Rheumatoid synovium ex vivo contains a variety of proteinases that reflect its cellular heterogeneity; these include cathepsin D,[101,120,121] cathepsin G, elastase, unidentified serine proteinases,[122] and small amounts of collagenase.[123] Collagenase is secreted into the medium in quantity by rheumatoid synovium in culture, and this led to the first observation of a mammalian collagenase.[124] Subsequently, culture experiments have shown the production of collagenase by synovium from other arthritides, and from normal joints.[54,55]

The rheumatoid synovium collagenase has been purified,[60] and immunohistochemical studies have shown it to be present at some areas of the synovium–cartilage junction in some rheumatoid joints.[103] It is not known which cell type produces the collagenase at the junction, but collagenase can be secreted by both fibroblastic cells and macrophages (see above). Cultures of adherent cells obtained by enzymic disaggregation of rheumatoid synovium produce collagenase,[125] and immunofluorescent localization of the enzyme shows large amounts of it associated with small cells with long dendritic processes. These dendritic cells are morphologically different from any cells observed in the tissue.[126]

Relatively little attention has been paid to the occurrence of neutral proteinases other than collagenase in rheumatoid synovium, although they could well be important in cartilage breakdown. Removal of proteoglycan by such proteinases would render the collagen accessible to collagenase, and there is good reason to believe that proteoglycan is lost from the cartilage before the collagen. A gelatinase has been described in the culture medium of rheumatoid synovial tissue,[127] and two types of metalloproteinase have been detected from rabbit synovial fibroblasts[69] and from macrophages.[128] Synovial fibroblasts also make plasminogen activator.[129-131] Besides making proteinases, organ cultures of synovium also make the ubiquitious metalloproteinase inhibitor.[119]

***Synovial Fluid.*** In rheumatoid arthritis and other inflammatory joint diseases, large numbers of leukocytes may enter the synovial fluid. The human polymorphonuclear leukocyte is unusual among cells in having lysosomes containing neutral proteinases with only traces of acid proteinases. (Most cell types have acid proteinases in their lysosomes, and some species, e.g., rabbits, have predominantly acid proteinases in their polymorphonuclear cell granules.)[132] In human neutrophils, the azurophilic granules contain the serine enzymes, leukocyte elastase and cathepsin G,[133] and the specific granules contain two neutral metalloproteinases, a collagenase and a gelatinase, both being found in latent form.[59,78,134]

The leukocyte proteinases are released from the cells during phagocytosis. Elastase and collagenase are released on uptake of aggregated IgG,[135] and neutral proteinases are released when the cells are incubated with pieces of articular cartilage coated with IgG.[136] In the rheumatoid joint, release could accompany phagocytosis of immune complexes or tissue debris, or contact with a cartilage surface bearing immune complexes.

Proteinases of lymphocytes, monocytes, and macrophages have been little studied in man or animals. Human lymphocytes are known to contain a small amount of acid proteinase, probably cathepsin D,[137] and cathepsin D is present in rabbit macrophages.[138] Mouse macrophages have been shown to secrete collagenase, metalloproteinase and plasminogen activator in tissue culture,[33,71,74,76] and rabbit macrophages secrete a neutral metalloproteinase and collagenase.[75] Human platelets contain acid proteinases but not significant amounts of elastase or collagenase.[139-141]

Almost certainly there is release of proteinases into the synovial fluid in rheumatoid arthritis. Complexes of leukocyte elastase with $\alpha_1$-proteinase inhibitor have been found by crossed immunoelectrophoresis, and collagenase–$\alpha_2$M complexes have also been demonstrated.[142,143] The enhanced vascular permeability of the rheumatoid synovium allows even the high molecular weight plasma proteins such as $\alpha_2$M to equilibrate into the synovial fluid, so the fluid has essentially the same proteinase inhibitors as plasma. It has been calculated that the large numbers of neutrophils entering the synovial fluid (where they die and disintegrate within hours) could bring in large amounts of leukocyte proteinase,[44] but direct tests for active proteinases in rheumatoid synovial fluids have revealed only a small percentage (those with leukocyte counts exceeding 50,000 per cubic millimeter) with some collagenase activity.[144] Since it must be recognized that some findings of either free collagenase or proteinase-inhibitor complexes in synovial fluid could be due to breakage of cells during withdrawal of the fluid from the patient or subsequent storage, we feel that there is room for doubt as to whether proteinases are in excess over their inhibitors frequently enough to be of any real significance to the disease process. It is therefore uncertain whether any proteinases from cells of the synovial fluid or the synovial lining can traverse the fluid and damage the cartilage. It is conceivable, however, that membrane-bound or latent forms of the enzymes might escape synovial fluid inhibitors and then adhere to the cartilage surface and be activated locally. A proteinase-like metal-dependent enzyme associated with lipid, probably membrane fragments, is regularly found in rheumatoid synovial fluid.[145]

Another way in which the enzymes may evade the inhibitors is by direct release onto the cartilage surface by cells adherent to it. Such a process of "frustrated phagocytosis" might well be promoted by the presence of immune complexes at the cartilage surface,[146,147] and the effectiveness of this mechanism of circumventing proteinase inhibitors has been demonstrated directly in a model system.[148] Direct microscopic observations pointing strongly to a role for neutrophil leukocytes adherent to the cartilage surface in the erosion of the tissue have been reported.[149,150]

So far we have discussed enzymes originating from the cellular phase of the synovial fluid, but there are proenzymes of plasma proteinases in the bulk phase also. Plasminogen could be converted to plasmin by activators from synovial cells, and in septic arthritis activation might be by streptokinase or analogous bacterial products. Plasmin is a potent proteinase that will hydrolyze proteoglycan, and the possibility that it might play a role in cartilage degradation has been discussed.[37,129,151,152] Two considerations cast some doubt on the possibility of plasmin acting in the joint. (1) The synovial fluid contains very potent inhibitors derived from the plasma (notably the $\alpha_2$-plasmin inhibitor). (2) It is difficult to see why fibrin, the substrate for which plasmin has such high affinity, is abundant in rheumatoid joints if they contain the active enzyme.

There is some evidence for a proteinase activator in rheumatoid synovial fluid. As was mentioned earlier, the specific granules of the neutrophil contain latent forms of a collagenase and a gelatinase. A protein of about 35,000 molecular weight that will activate the latent forms of both collagenase and gelatinase has been isolated from rheumatoid synovial fluid.[153] Rheumatoid synovial cultures apparently produce an activator of the leukocyte gelatinase and collagenase that has similar properties to that in synovial fluid.[154] In other hands it has been shown that plasma kallikrein has the capacity to activate latent collagenase, and that the major activator in some samples of rheumatoid synovial fluid is identifiable as plasma kallikrein.[155]

## CONTROL PROCESSES

The current, widely held view is that resorption of connective tissues is brought about by the release of collagenase and other proteinases from cells. Various agents have been found to stimulate or inhibit release of collagenase. Anti-inflammatory steroids such as dexamethasone inhibit its production by synovial fibroblasts,[125] as do retinoids.[156] Agents stimulating collagenase production by synovial fibroblasts are phorbol myristate acetate,[157] cytochalasin B, vinblastine, aminophylline[158] and collagen.[159] Colchicine ($10^{-7}$ M) has a stimulatory effect on synovial organ cultures.[160]

Ingestion of nondigestible particles (mimicked experimentally with polystyrene latex) increases collagenase production by rabbit synovial fibroblasts and mouse peritoneal macrophages.[69,71]

To obtain collagenase from macrophages in culture it has been found necessary to stimulate them in some way. Thioglycolate has been used for mouse peritoneal macrophages; and the lipid A component of bacterial endotoxin, for cells from guinea pig peritoneum.[69-71] Whether or not these agents have similar effects in vivo is unknown.

Macrophages,[161] synovial fibroblasts,[162] and chondrocytes[116] are stimulated in vitro to produce collagenase by products of mononuclear leukocytes. The synovial cells and chondrocytes also make increased amounts of prostaglandin $E_2$[163-165] and plasminogen activator.[131] The "lymphokines" or "monokines" responsible for this stimulation have not been purified, but the activity is associated with a small protein (or proteins) of about 14,000 molecular weight called mononuclear cell factor.[163,166] Production of this mononuclear cell factor is stimulated in vitro by aggregated IgG, the Fc portion of IgG, concanavalin A,[167] native human collagens,[168] and products of activated lymphocytes.[169,170] There is now strong evidence that the activity of mononuclear cell factor is at least partly attributable to the monocyte-macrophage product interleukin I.[171,172] Interleukin I is a protein that enhances blastic stimulation of lymphocytes and was formerly called lymphocyte activating factor (LAF).[173] Another protein that may well be similar to interleukin I is catabolin, which is defined by its ability to induce resorption of cartilage matrix proteoglycans in vitro. It is made by synovium in organ culture,[174] by synovial fibroblasts[175] (especially if stimulated by phorbol myristate acetate), and by lectin-stimulated mononuclear leukocytes.[176] Pig catabolin is of 20,000 molecular weight and has a pI of 4.8[176a]; human catabolin is of similar size but has a pI of 5.2.[177] Leukocyte and fibroblast catabolins seem to be the same protein. The human catabolin is a more acid protein than human interleukin I, which has an isoelectric point of pH 6.8.[178] Purification of these proteins will enable their relationships and possible role in tissue resorption to be established.

Besides the secreted enzymes such as collagenase, the other group of proteinases that have been considered to be important in degradation are the lysosomal proteinases. Unlike the secreted proteinases, lysosomal hydrolases are stored in the cells and are normally discharged into intracellular digestive organelles, phagosomes. However, the neutral proteinases of polymorphonucear leukocytes may be released extracellularly during phagocytosis and by interaction of the cell with complement cleavage products (C5a).[179] Similarily the lysosomal enzymes of macrophages are released during phagocytosis and by C3a.[180]

The rheumatoid synovial cells in culture produce mainly latent enzymes, and the latent collagenase tends to bind to collagen.[181] Presumably the enzymes are initially latent in vivo, too, so their activation is obviously a potential control process. A variety of proteinases will activate latent collagenase, and plasmin has been proposed to play a significant role in rheumatoid arthritis, since the synovial fluid may contain large amounts of plasminogen, and rheumatoid synovial cells can produce plasminogen activators.[129-131] Plasma kallikrein may act in a similar way.[40] The latent collagenase does not interact with $\alpha_2$M but does bind to collagen (though less strongly than active enzyme). Latent collagenase could therefore evade $\alpha_2$M, bind to its substrate, and then be activated locally by plasmin.[129]

## CONCLUSIONS

Although we are not yet able to reach any definite conclusions as to the identity of proteinases important in joint diseases, there is reason for confidence that the foundation of knowledge at the molecular level that has been established during the past decade will form the basis for progress in the future.

One can speculate about the areas of current research that may prove particularly productive. The elucidation of the complex chemistry of the important structural molecules of connective tissues and the isolation of the major cellular proteinases are already allowing a clearer understanding of the precise way in which the proteinases could contribute to joint disease. The detailed characterization of degradation products formed in vivo may lead to the positive identification of some of the important enzymes.

Purification of the cellular proteinases has permitted the raising of specific antisera against them. The resulting immunochemical methods clearly have much to offer. Already antisera are being used to show which cells release particular enzymes; they are potentially useful also for specific immunoinhibition, ultrasensitive immunoassays, and study of synthesis and turnover of the enzymes. Further use of these techniques may follow from refinement of methods for raising specific antisera with very small amounts of pure immunogen, or with only partially purified immunogen. Such advances should allow more work with enzymes from diseased human tissues, for the small amounts of human articular tissues available usually preclude the complete purification of enzymes from this source, although cultivation of the tissue in vitro has been helpful.

The discovery of better substrates and inhibitors has a crucial role to play in the study of the physiologic functions of proteinases. The specificity and sensitivity of assays with synthetic substrates are becoming greater, and the extent to which these can be used in place of less convenient assays with complex substrates is becoming clearer. A powerful armory of proteinase inhibitors of microbial and synthetic origin has now become available and awaits full exploitation in appropriately designed biologic test systems.

A major area for future work is that of the natural regulation of the catabolic enzymes, including controls of synthesis and translocation. The question of the nature of latent collagenase will presumably be answered following the complete purification of greater amounts of material, but the larger question of the reactivity or otherwise of masked forms of the cellular proteinases with inhibitors may remain for some time. There are interesting indications of ways in which proteinases in the extracellular fluid can escape binding by the proteinase inhibitors and subsequently show activity perhaps after adsorption to collagen or proteoglycan.

Another topic of major interest is the possibility that regions of low pH around cells are sufficiently acid to allow extracellular activity of the lysosomal acid proteinases. Conversely, further evidence as to the part played by endocytosis and intracellular digestion in catabolism of connective tissue matrices will be welcome.

These, then, seem to be some of the important directions for future research into the role of cellular proteinases in joint disease.

## References


1. Fehr, K., Velvart, M., Böni, A., Watanabe, H., Spycher, M.A., and Rüttner, J.R.: Experimental arthritis of rabbits caused by intra-articular injection of autologous Fab2 produced by digestion of IgG with cathepsin D. 1. Microscopical and immunohistochemical findings in short-term experiments. Ann. Rheum. Dis. 35:85, 1976.
2. Trentham, D.E., Townes, A.S., and Kang, A.H.: Autoimmunity to type II collagen: An experimental model of arthritis. J. Exp. Med. 146:857, 1977.
3. Ward, P.A.: Complement-dependent phlogistic factors in rheumatoid synovial fluids. Ann. N.Y. Acad. Sci. 256:169, 1975.
4. Hayashi, H.: The intracellular neutral SH-dependent protease associated with inflammatory reactions. Int. Rev. Cytol. 40:101, 1975.
5. Barrett, A.J.: Introduction: the classification of proteinases. In Evered, D., and Whelan, J. (eds.): Protein Degradation in Health and Disease (Ciba Foundation Symposium 75). Amsterdam, Excerpta Medica, 1980, pp. 1–13.
6. Barrett, A.J. (ed.): Proteinases in Mammalian Cells and Tissues. Amsterdam, North-Holland Publishing Co., 1977.
7. Barrett, A.J., and McDonald, J.K.: Mammalian Proteases. A Glossary and Bibliography. London, Academic Press, 1980.
8. Barrett, A.J.: Cathepsin D and other carboxyl proteinases. In Barrett A.J. (ed.): Proteinases of Mammalian Cells and Tissues. Amsterdam, North-Holland Publishing Company, 1977, pp. 209–248.
9. Barrett, A.J.: Cathepsin D. Purification of isoenzymes from human and chicken liver. Biochem. J. 117:601, 1970.
10. Takahashi, T., and Tang, J.: Cathepsin D from porcine and bovine spleen. Methods Enzymol. 80:565, 1981.
11. Barrett, A.J., and Dingle, J.T.: The inhibition of tissue acid proteinases by pepstatin. Biochem. J. 127:439, 1972.
12. Dingle, J.T., Barrett, A.J., Poole, A.R., and Stovin, P.: Inhibition by pepstatin of human cartilage degradation. Biochem. J. 127:443, 1972.
13. Knight, C.G., and Barrett, A.J.: Interaction of human cathepsin D with the inhibitor pepstatin. Biochem. J. 115:117, 1975.
14. Dingle, J.T., Barrett, A.J., and Weston, P.D.: Cathepsin D. Characteristics of immunoinhibition and the confirmation of a role in cartilage breakdown. Biochem. J. 123:1, 1971.
15. Morrison, R.I.G., Barrett, A.J., Dingle, J.T., and Prior, D.: Cathepsins B1 and D. Action on human cartilage proteoglycans. Biochim. Biophys. Acta 302:411, 1973.
16. Roughley, P.J., and Barrett, A.J.: The degradation of cartilage proteoglycans by tissue proteinases. Proteoglycan structure and its susceptibility to proteolysis. Biochem. J. 167:629, 1977.
17. Roughley, P.J.: The degradation of cartilage proteoglycans by tissue proteinases. Proteoglycan heterogeneity and the pathway of proteolytic degradation. Biochem. J. 167:639, 1977.
18. Harris, E.D., Jr., Lock, S., and Lin, T.-Y.: Limited degradation of gelatin substrate by cathepsin D. Conn. Tiss. Res. 1:103, 1972.
19. Burleigh, M.C., Barrett, A.J., and Lazarus, G.S.: Cathepsin B1. A lysosomal enzyme that degrades native collagen. Biochem. J. 137:387, 1974.
20. Scott, P.G., and Pearson, C.H.: Cathepsin D—cleavage of soluble collagen and cross-linked peptides. FEBS Lett. 88:41, 1978.
21. Dingle, J.T.: The secretion of enzymes into the pericellular environment. Phil. Trans. R. Soc. Lond. B 271:315, 1975.
22. Barrett, A.J., and Starkey, P.M.: The interaction of $\alpha_2$-macroglobulin with proteinases. Characteristics and specificity of the reaction and a hypothesis concerning its molecular mechanism. Biochem. J. 133:709, 1973.
23. Barrett, A.J.: Human cathepsin B1. Purification and some properties of the enzyme. Biochem. J. 131:809, 1973.
24. Barrett, A.J.: Cathepsin B and other thiol proteinases. In Barrett, A.J. (ed.): Proteinases of Mammalian Cells and Tissues. North-Holland Publishing Company, Amsterdam, 1977, pp. 181–208.
25. Barrett, A.J., and Kirschke, H.: Cathepsin B, cathepsin H and cathepsin L. Methods Enzymol. 80:535, 1981.
26. Pohl, J., Baudys, M., Tomasek, V., and Kostka, V.: Identification of the active site cysteine and of the disulphide bonds in the N-terminal part of bovine spleen cathepsin B. FEBS Lett. 142:23, 1982.
27. Burleigh, M.C., Barrett, A.J., and Lazarus, G.S.: Cathepsin B1. A lysosomal enzyme that degrades native collagen. Biochem. J. 137:387, 1974.
28. Kirschke, H., Kembhavi, A.A., Bohley, P., and Barrett, A.J.: Action of rat liver cathepsin L on collagen and other substrates. Biochem. J. 201:367, 1982.
29. Knight, C.G.: Human cathepsin B. Application of the substrate *N*-benzyloxycarbonyl-L-arginyl-L-arginine 2-naphthylamide to a study of the inhibition by leupeptin. Biochem. J. 189:447, 1980.
30. Baici, A., and Gyger-Marazzi, M.: The slow, tight-binding inhibition of cathepsin B by leupeptin. A hysteretic effect. Eur. J. Biochem. 129:33, 1982.
31. Barrett, A.J., Kembhayi, A.A., Brown, M.A., Kirschke, J., Knight, C.G., Tamai, M., and Hanada, K.: L-*Trans*-epoxysuccinyl-leucyl-amino(4-

guanidino)butane (E-64) and its analogues as inhibitors of cysteine proteinases including cathepsins B, H and L. Biochem. J. 201:189, 1982.
32. Shaw, E., and Green, G.D.J.: Inactivation of thiol proteases with peptidyl diazomethyl ketones. Methods Enzymol. 80:820, 1981.
32a. Anastasi, A., Brown, M.A., Kembhavi, A.A., Nicklin, M.J.H., Sayers, C.A., Sunter, D.C., and Barrett, A.J.: Cystatin, a protein inhibitor of cysteine proteinases. Improved purification from egg white, characterization, and detection in chicken serum. Biochem. J. 211:129, 1983.
32b. Green, G.D.J., Kembhavi, A.A., Davies, M.E., and Barrett, A.J.: Biochem. J. in press, 1984.
33. Unkeless, J.C., Gordon, S., and Reich, E.: Secretion of plasminogen activator by stimulated macrophages. J. Exp. Med. 139:834, 1974.
34. Granelli-Piperno, A., Vassalli, J.-D., and Reich, E.: Secretion of plasminogen activator by human polymorphonuclear leukocytes. Modulation by glucocortoids and other effectors. J. Exp. Med. 146:1693, 1978.
35. Werb, Z., and Aggeler, J.: Proteases induce secretion of collagenase and plasminogen activator by fibroblasts. Proc. Natl. Acad. Sci. USA 75:1839, 1978.
36. Okamoto, S., Oshiba, S., Mihara, H., and Okamoto, U.: Synthetic inhibitors of fibrinolysis: In vitro and in vivo mode of action. Ann. N.Y. Acad. Sci. 146:414, 1968.
37. Lack, C.H., and Rogers, H.J.: Action of plasmin on cartilage. Nature 182:948, 1958.
38. Harpel, P.C.: Plasmin inhibitor reactions. The effectiveness of $\alpha_2$-plasmin inhibitor in the presence of $\alpha_2$-macroglobulin. J. Exp. Med. 146:1033, 1977.
39. Heimark, R.L. and Davie, E.W.: Bovine and human plasma prekallikrein. Methods Enzymol. 80:157, 1981.
40. Nagase, H., Cawston, T.E., DeSilva, M. and Barrett, A.J.: Identification of plasma kallikrein as an activator of latent collagenase in rheumatoid synovial fluid. Biochim. Biophys. Acta 702:133, 1982.
41. Barrett, A.J.: Leukocyte elastase. Methods Enzymol. 80:581, 1981.
42. Keiser, H., Greenwald, R.A., Feinstein, G., and Janoff, A.: Degradation of cartilage proteoglycan by human leukocyte neutral proteases—a model of joint injury. II. Degradation of isolated bovine nasal cartilage proteoglycan. J. Clin. Invest. 57:625, 1976.
43. Starkey, P.M., Barrett, A.J., and Burleigh M.C.: The degradation of articular collagen by neutrophil proteinases. Biochim. Biophys. Acta 483:386, 1977.
44. Barrett, A.J.: The possible role of neutrophil proteinases in damage to articular cartilage. Agents Actions 8:11, 1978.
45. Davies, M., Barrett, A.J., Travis, J., Sanders, E., and Coles, G.A.: The degradation of human glomerular basement membrane with purified lysosomal proteinases: Evidence for the pathogenic role of the polymorphonuclear leucocyte in glomerulonephritis. Clin. Sci. Mol. Med. 54:233, 1978.
46. Mainardi, C.L., Dixit, S.N., and Kang, A.H.: Degradation of type IV (basement membrane) collagen by a proteinase isolated from human polymorphonuclear leukocyte granules. J. Biol. Chem. 255:5435, 1980.
47. Powers, J.C., Gupton, B.F., Harley, A.D., Nishono, N., and Whitely, R.J.: Specificity of porcine pancreatic elastase, human leucocyte elastase and cathepsin G. Inhibition with peptide chloromethyl ketones. Biochim. Biophys. Acta 485:156, 1977.
48. Baici, A., Salgam, P., Fehr, K., and Böni, A.: Inhibition of human elastase from polymorphonuclear leucocytes by gold sodium thiomalate and pentosan polysulfate (SP-54®). Biochem. Pharmacol. 30:703, 1981.
49. Ohlsson, K., and Ohlsson, L.: Neutral proteases of human granulocytes. III. Interaction between granulocyte elastase and plasma protease inhibitors. Scand. J. Clin. Lab. Invest. 34:349, 1974.
50. Barrett, A.J.: Cathepsin G. Methods Enzymol. 80:561, 1981.
51. Woodbury, R.G., Everitt, M.T., and Neurath, H.: Mast cell proteases. Methods Enzymol. 80:588, 1981.
52. Venge, P.: PMN proteases and their effects on complement components and neutrophil function. In Havermann, K. (ed.): Neutral Proteases of Human Polymorphonuclear Leukocytes. Baltimore, Urban & Schwartzenberg, 1978.
53. Venge, P., Ohlsson, I., and Odeberg, H.: Cationic proteins of human granulocytes. V. Interaction with plasma protease inhibitors. Scand. J. Clin. Lab. Invest. 35:737, 1975.
54. Harris, E.D. Jr., and Krane, S.M.: Collagenases. N. Engl. J. Med. 291:557, 605, 652, 1974.
55. Woolley, D.E., and Evanson, J.M. (eds.): Collagenase in Normal and Pathological Connective Tissues. New York, John Wiley and Sons, 1980.
56. Miller, E.J., Harris, E.D. Jr., Finch, J.E. Jr., Chung, E., McCroskery, P.A., and Butler, W.T.: Cleavage of type II and III collagens with mammalian collagenase: Site of cleavage and primary structure at the $NH_2$-terminal portion of the smaller fragment released from both collagens. Biochemistry 15:787, 1976.
57. Gross, J., Highberger, J.H., Johnson-Wint, B., and Biswas, C.: Mode of action and regulation of tissue collagenases. In Woolley, D.E., and Evanson, J.M. (eds.): Collagenase in Normal and Pathological Connective Tissues. New York, John Wiley & Sons, 1980, p. 11.
58. Welgus, H.G., Jeffrey, J.J., Stricklin, G.P., and Eisen, A.Z.: The gelatinolytic activity of human skin fibroblast collagenase. J. Biol. Chem. 257:11534, 1982.
59. Christner, P., Damato, D., Reinhart, M., and Abrams, W.: Purification of human neutrophil collagenase and production of a monospecific antiserum. Biochemistry 21:6005, 1982.
60. Woolley, D.E., Lindberg, K.A., Glanville, R.W., and Evanson, J.M.: Action of rheumatoid synovial collagenase on cartilage collagen. Different susceptibilities of cartilage and tendon collagen to collagenase attack. Eur. J. Biochem. 50:437, 1975.
61. Harris, E.D. Jr., and Farrell, M.E.: Resistance to collagenase. A characteristic of collagen fibrils crosslinked by formaldehyde. Biochim. Biophys. Acta 278:133, 1972.
62. Vater, C.A., Harris, E.D. Jr., and Siegel, R.C.: Native cross-links in collagen fibrils induce resistance to human synovial collagenase. Biochem. J. 181:639, 1979.
63. Cawston, T.E., and Barrett, A.J.: A rapid and reproducible assay for collagenase using [1-$^{14}$C]acetylated collagen. Anal. Biochem. 99:340, 1979.
64. Cawston, T.E., and Murphy, G.: Mammalian collagenases. Methods Enzymol. 80:711, 1981.
65. Cawston, T.E., and Tyler, J.A.: Purification of pig synovial collagenase to high specific activity. Biochem. J. 183:647, 1979.
65a. Dr G. Murphy, personal communication, 1983.
66. François, J., Cambie, E., and Fehr, J.: Collagenase inhibition by penicillamine. Ophthalmologica 166:222, 1973.
67. Werb, Z., Burleigh, M.C., Barrett, A.J., and Starkey, P.M.: The interaction of $\alpha_2$-macroglobulin with proteinases. Binding and inhibition of mammalian collagenase and other metal proteinases. Biochem. J. 139:359, 1974.
68. Wooley, D.E., Roberts, D.R., and Evanson, J.M.: Small molecular weight $\beta_1$ serum protein which specifically inhibits human collagenase. Nature 261:325, 1976.
69. Werb, Z., and Reynolds, J.J.: Purification and properties of a specific collagenase from rabbit synovial fibroblasts. Biochem. J. 151:645, 1975.
70. Wahl, L.M., Wahl, S.M., Mergenhagen, S.E., and Martin, G.R.: Collagenase production by endotoxin-activated macrophages. Proc. Natl. Acad. Sci. USA 71:3598, 1974.
71. Werb, Z., and Gordon, S.: Secretion of a specific collagenase by stimulated macrophages. J. Exp. Med. 1420:346, 1975.
72. Murphy, G., Reynolds, J.J., Bretz, U., and Baggiolini, M.: Collagenase is a component of the specific granules of human neutrophil leucocytes. Biochem. J. 162:195, 1977.
73. Nagase, H., Jackson, R.C., Brinckerhoff, C.E., Vater, C.A., and Harris, E.D. Jr.: A precursor form of latent collagenase produced in a cell-free system with mRNA from rabbit synovial cells. J. Biol. Chem. 256:11951, 1981.
74. Werb, Z., and Gordon, S.: Elastase secretion by stimulated macrophages. Characterization and regulation. J. Exp. Med. 142:361, 1975.
75. Hauser, P., and Vaes, G.: Degradation of cartilage proteoglycans by neutral proteinase secreted by rabbit bone-marrow macrophages in culture. Biochem. J. 172:275, 1978.
76. Banda, M.J., and Werb, Z.: Mouse macrophage elastase. Purification and characterization as a metalloproteinase. Biochem. J. 193:589, 1981.
76a. Banda, M.J., and Werb, Z.: Limited proteolysis by macrophage elastase inactivates human $\alpha_1$-proteinase inhibitor. J. Exp. Med. 152:1563, 1980.
77. Galloway, W.A., Murphy, G., Sandy, J.D., Gavrilovic, J., Cawston, T.E., and Reynolds, J.J.: Purification and characterization of a rabbit bone metalloproteinase that degrades proteoglycan and other connective tissue components. Biochem. J. 209:741, 1983.
78. Sopata, I.: Further purification and some properties of a gelatin-specific proteinase of human leucocytes. Biochim. Biophys. Acta 717:26, 1982.
79. Starkey, P.M., and Barrett, A. J.: $\alpha_2$-Macroglobulin: inhibitor of endopeptidase: In Barrett, A.J. (ed.): Proteinases in Mammalian Cells and Tissues. Amsterdam, North-Holland Publishing Company, 1977, pp. 663–696.
81. Starkey, P.M., and Barrett, A.J.: $\alpha_2$-Macroglobulin. A Remarkable Proteinase Inhibitor. London, Academic Press, in press, 1984.
82. Feinman, R. (ed.): $\alpha_2$-Macroglobulin. Ann. N.Y. Acad. Sci., in press, 1983.
83. Imber, M.J., and Pizzo, S.V.: Clearance and binding of two electrophoretically "fast" forms of human $\alpha_2$-macroglobulin. J. Biol. Chem. 256:8134, 1981.
84. Sasaki, M., Taniguchi, K., and Minakata, K.: Multimolecular forms of thiol proteinase inhibitor in human plasma. J. Biochem. 89:169, 1981.
85. Green, G.D.J., Kembhavi, A.A., Davies, M.E, and Barrett, A.J.: Biochem. J. in press, 1984.
86. Killackey, J.J., Roughley, P.J., and Mort, J.S.: Proteinase inhibitors of human articular cartilage. Collagen Ref. Res. 3:419, 1983.

87. Travis, J., and Salvesen, G.S.: Plasma proteinase inhibitors. Ann. Rev. Biochem., 52:655, 1983.
88. Macartney, H.W., and Tschesche, H.: Interaction of $\beta_1$-anticollagenase from human plasma with collagenase from various tissues and competition with $\alpha_2$-macroglobulin. Eur. J. Biochem. 130:93, 1983.
89. Cawston, T.E., Galloway, W.A., Mercer, E., Murphy, G., and Reynolds, J.J.: Purification of rabbit bone inhibitor of collagenase. Biochem. J. 195:159, 1981.
90. Harris, E.D. Jr., Parker, H.G., Radin, E.L., and Krane, S.M.: Effects of proteolytic enzymes on structural and mechanical properties of cartilage. Arthritis Rheum. 15:497, 1972.
91. Kempson, G.E., Tuke, M.A., Dingle, J.T., Barrett, A.J., and Horsefield, P.H.: The effects of proteolytic enzymes on the mechanical properties of adult human articular cartilage. Biochim. Biophys. Acta 428:741, 1976.
92. Pottenger, L.A., Lyon, N.B., Hecht, J.D., Neustadt, P.M., and Robinson, R.A.: Influence of cartilage particle size and proteoglycan aggregation on immobilization of proteoglycans. J. Biol. Chem. 257:11479, 1982.
93. Barrett, A.J.: Chondromucoprotein-degrading enzymes. Nature (London) 211:1188, 1966.
94. Dingle, J.T., Blow, A.M.J., Barrett, A.J., and Martin, P.E.N.: Proteoglycan-degrading enzymes. A radiochemical assay method and the detection of a new enzyme, cathepsin F. Biochem. J. 167:775, 1977.
95. Nagase, H., and Woessner, J.F.: An improved assay for proteases and polysaccharidases employing a cartilage proteolglycan substrate entrapped in polyacrylamide beads. Anal. Biochem. 107:385, 1980.
96. Farndale, R.W., Sayers, C.A., and Barrett, A.J.: A direct spectrophotometric microassay for sulphated glycosaminoglycans. Conect. Tissue Res. 9:247, 1982.
97. Bader, D.L., Kempson, G.E., Barrett, A.J., and Webb, W.: The effect of leucocyte elastase on the mechanical properties of adult articular cartilage in tension. Biochim. Biophys. Acta 677:103, 1981.
98. Garant, P.R.: Collagen resorption by fibroblasts—a theory of fibroblastic maintenance of the periodontal ligament. J. Periodont. 47:380, 1976.
99. Harris, E.D. Jr., Glauert, A.M., and Murley, A.H.G.: Intracellular collagen fibres at the pannus-cartilage junction in rheumatoid arthritis. Arthritis Rheum. 20:657, 1977.
100. Stern, B., Golub, L., and Goldhaber, P.: Effects of demineralization and parathyroid hormone on the availability of bone collagen to degradation by collagenase. J. Periodont. Res. 5:116, 1970.
101. Poole, A.R.: Immunocytochemical studies of the secretion of a proteolytic enzyme, cathepsin D, in relation to cartilage breakdown. *In* Burleigh, P.M.C., and Poole, A.R. (eds.): Dynamics of Connective Tissue Macromolecules. Amsterdam, North-Holland Publishing Company, 1975, pp. 357–383.
102. Poole, A.R., Hembry, R.M., and Dingle, J.T.: Cathepsin D in cartilage: The immunohistochemical demonstration of extracellular enzyme in normal and pathological conditions. J. Cell Sci. 14:139, 1974.
103. Woolley, D.E., Crossley, M.J., and Evanson, J.M.: Collagenase at sites of cartilage erosion in the rheumatoid joint. Arthritis Rheum. 20:1231, 1977.
104. Donoff, R.B., McLennan, J.E., and Grillo, H.C.: Preparation and properties of collagenase from epithelium and mesenchyme of healing mammalian wounds. Biochim. Biophys. Acta 277:639, 1971.
105. Hamerman, D.: Cartilage change in the rheumatoid joint. Clin. Orthopaed. 64:91, 1969.
106. Kimura, H., Tateishi, H., and Ziff, M.: Surface ultrastructure of rheumatoid articular cartilage. Arthritis Rheum. 20:1085, 1977.
107. Maroudas, A.: Glycosaminoglycan turnover in articular cartilage. Proc. Roy. Soc. B. 271:293, 1975.
108. Sapolsky, A.I., Howell, D.S., and Woessner, J.F. Jr.: Neutral proteases and cathepsin D in human articular cartilage. J. Clin. Invest. 53:1044, 1974.
109. Bayliss, M.T., and Ali, S.Y.: Studies on cathepsin B in human articular cartilage. Biochem. J. 171:149, 1978.
110. Sapolsky, A.I., Altman, R.D., Woessner, J.F. Jr., and Howell, D.: The action of cathepsin D in human articular cartilage on proteoglycans. J. Clin. Invest. 52:624, 1973.
111. Fell, H.B., and Dingle, J.T.: Studies on the mode of action of excess of vitamin A. Lysosomal protease and the degradation of cartilage matrix. Biochem. J. 87:403, 1963.
112. Hembry, R.M., Knight, C.G., Dingle, J.T. and Barrett, A.J.: Evidence that cathepsin D is not responsible for the resorption of cartilage matrix in culture. Biochim. Biophys. Acta 714:307, 1982.
113. Sapolsky, A.I., and Howell, D.S.: Further characterization of a neutral metalloproteinase isolated from human articular cartilage. Arthritis Rheum. 25:981, 1982.
114. Ehrlich, M.G., Mankin, J.H.J., Jones, H., Wright, R., Crispen, C., and Vigliani, G.: Collagenase and collagenase inhibitors in osteoarthritis and normal human cartilage. J. Clin. Invest. 59:226, 1977.
115. Murphy, C., McGuire, M.B., Russell, R.G.G., and Reynolds, J.J.: Characterization of collagenase, other metallo-proteinases and an inhibitor (TIMP) produced by human synovium and cartilage in culture. Clin. Sci. 61:711, 1981.
116. Deshmukh-Phadke, K., Nanda, S., and Lee, K.: Macrophage factor that induces neutral protease secretion by normal rabbit chondrocytes. Eur. J. Biochem. 104:175, 1980.
117. Morales, T.I., and Kuettner, K.E.: The properties of the neutral proteinase released by primary chondrocyte cultures and its action on proteoglycan aggregate. Biochim. Biophys. Acta 705:92, 1982.
118. Meats, J.E., McGuire, M.B., and Russell, R.G.G.: Human synovium releases a factor which stimulates chondrocyte production of $PGE_2$ and plasminogen activator. Nature 286:891, 1980.
119. Murphy, G., Cambray, G.J., Virani, N., Page-Thomas, D.P., and Reynolds, J.J.: The production in culture of metalloproteinases and an inhibitor by joint tissues from normal rabbits and from rabbits with a model arthritis. I. Synovium. Rheumatol. Int. 1:11, 1981.
120. Luscombe, M.: Acid phosphatase and catheptic activity in rheumatoid synovial tissue. Nature 197:1010, 1963.
121. Barrett, A.J.: The enzymic degradation of cartilage matrix. *In* Burleigh, P.M.C., and Poole, A.R. (eds.): Dynamics of Connective Tissue Macromolecules. Amsterdam, North-Holland Publishing Company, 1975, pp. 189–226.
122. Saklatvala, J., and Barrett, A.J.: Identification of proteinases in rheumatoid synovium. Detection of leukocyte elastase, cathepsin G and another serine proteinase. Biochim. Biophys. Acta 615:167–177, 1980.
123. Nagai, Y., and Hori, H.: Vertebrate collagenase: Direct extraction from animal skin and human synovial membrane. J. Biochem. 72:1147, 1972.
124. Evanson, J.M., Jeffrey, J.J., and Krane, S.M.: Studies on collagenase from rheumatoid synovium in tissue culture. J. Clin. Invest. 47:2639, 1968.
125. Dayer, J.-M., Krane, S.M., Russell, R.G.G., and Robinson, D.R.: Production of collagenase and prostaglandins by isolated adherent rheumatoid synovial cells. Proc. Natl. Acad. Sci. USA 73:945, 1976.
126. Woolley, D.E., Harris, E.D. Jr., Mainardi, C.L., and Brinckerhoff, C.E.: Collagenase immunolocalization in cultures of rheumatoid synovial cells. Science 200:773, 1978.
127. Harris, E.D. Jr., and Krane, S.M.: An endopeptidase from rheumatoid synovial tissue culture. Biochim. Biophys. Acta 258:566, 1972.
128. Hauser, P., and Vaes., G.: Degradation of cartilage proteoglycans by a neutral proteinase secreted by rabbit bone-marrow macrophages in culture. Biochem. J. 172:275, 1978.
129. Werb, Z., Mainardi, C.L., Vater, C.A., and Harris, E.D. Jr.: Endogeneous activation of latent collagenase by rheumatoid synovial cells. N. Engl. J. Med. 296:1017, 1977.
130. Berger, H.: Secretion of plasminogen activator by rheumatoid and nonrheumatoid synovial cells in culture. Arthritis Rheum. 20:1198, 1977.
131. Hamilton, J.A., and Slywka, J.: Stimulation of human synovial fibroblast plasminogen activator production by mononuclear cell supernatants. J. Immunol. 126:851, 1981.
132. Folds, J.D., Welsh, I.R.H., and Spitznagel, J.K.: Neutral proteases confined to one class of lysosomes of human polymorphonuclear leukocytes. Proc. Soc. Exp. Biol. Med. 139:461, 1972.
133. Dewald, B., Rindler-Ludwig, R., Bretz, U., and Baggiolini, M.: Subcellular localisation and heterogeneity of neutral proteases in neutrophilic polymorphonuclear leucocytes. J. Exp. Med. 141:709, 1975.
134. Tschesche, H., and Macartney, H.W.: A new principle of enzyme regulation of enzymic activity. Activation and regulation of human polymorphonuclear leukocyte collagenase via disulfide-thiol exchange as catalysed by the glutathione cycle in a peroxidase-coupled reaction to glucose metabolism. Eur. J. Biochem. 120:183, 1981.
135. Oronsky, A.L., Perper, R.J., and Schroder, H.C.: Phagocytic release and activation of human leukocyte procollagenase. Nature 246:417, 1973.
136. Oronsky, A., Ignarro, L., and Perper, R.: Release of cartilage mucopolysaccharide-degrading neutral protease from human leucocytes. J. Exp. Med. 138:461, 1973.
137. Stiles, M.A., and Fraenkel-Conrat, J.: Subcellular distribution of human leukocytic cathepsins. Blood 32:119, 1968.
138. Rojas-Espinosa, O., Dannenberg, A.M., Murphy, P.A., Straat, P.A., Huang, P.C., and James, S.P.: Purification and properties of the cathepsin D type proteinase from beef and rabbit lung and its identification in macrophages. Infect. Immun. 8:100, 1973.
139. Ehrlich, H.P., and Gordon, J.L.: Proteinases in platelets. In Gordon, J. (ed.): Platelets in Biology and Pathology. Amsterdam, North-Holland Publishing Company, 1976, pp. 353–372.
140. Starkey, P.M., Gordon, J., Ehrlich, H.P., and Barrett, A.J.: Do platelets contain elastase? Haemostasis 39:542, 1978.
141. Hornebeck, W., Starkey, P.M., Gordon, J.L., Legrand, Y., Pignaud, G., Robert, L., Caen, J.P., Ehrlich, H.P., and Barrett, A.J.: The elastase-like enzyme of platelets. Thromb. Haemostas. 42:1681, 1981.
142. Ohlsson, K.: $\alpha_1$-Antitrypsin and $\alpha_2$-macroglobulin. Interactions with human neutrophil collagenase and elastase. Ann. N.Y. Acad. Sci. 256:409, 1975.
143. Abe, S., and Nagai, Y.: Evidence for the presence of a complex of collagenase with $\alpha_2$-macroglobulin in human rheumatoid synovial fluid:

A possible regulatory mechanism of collagenase activity in vivo. J. Biochem. 73:897, 1973.
144. Harris, E.D. Jr., DiBona, D.R., and Krane, S.M.: Collagenasas in human synovial fluid. J. Clin. Invest. 48:2104, 1969.
145. Saklatvala, J.: Hydrolysis of elastase substrate succinyltrialanine nitroanalide by a metal-dependent enzyme in rheumatoid synovial fluid. J. Clin. Invest. 59:794, 1977.
146. Henson, P.M.: Mechanisms of release of granulocyte enzymes from human neutrophils phagocytosing aggregated immunoglobulin. An electron microscopic study. Arthritis Rheum. 16:208, 1973.
147. Cochrane, C.G.: Role of granulocytes in immune complex-induced tissue injuries. Inflammation 2:319, 1977.
148. Campbell, E.J., Senior, R.M., McDonald, J.A., and Cox, D.L.: Proteolysis by neutrophils. Relative importance of cell-substrate contact and oxidative inactivation of proteinase inhibitors in vitro. J. Clin. Invest. 70:845, 1982.
149. Mohr, W., and Menninger, H.: Polymorphonuclear granulocytes at the pannus-cartilage junction in rheumatoid arthritis. Arthritis Rheum. 23:1413, 1980.
150. Mohr, W., Wessinghage, D., and Kohley, G.: The role of neutrophil granulocytes in the rheumatoid tissue destruction. I. Light microscopic demonstration of neutrophil polymorphonuclear cells in rheumatoid nodules. Z. Rheumatol. 39:322, 1980.
151. Lack, C.H.: Chondrolysis in arthritis. J. Bone Joint. Surg. 41:384, 1959.
152. Christman, O.D., Southwick, W.O., and Fessel, J.M.: Plasmin and articular cartilage. Yale J. Bio. Med. 34:524, 1962.
153. Wize, J., Sopata, I., Wojtecka-Lukasik, E., Ksiezny, S., and Dancewicz, A.M.: Isolation, purification and properties of a factor from rheumatoid synovial fluid activating the latent forms of collagenolytic enzymes. Acta Biochim. Polon. 22:239, 1975.
154. Wize, J., Abgarowicz, T., Wojtecka-Lukasik, E., Ksiezny, S., and Dancewicz, A.M.: Activation of human leucocyte procollagenase by rheumatoid synovial tissue culture medium. Ann. Rheum. Dis. 34:520, 1975.
155. Nagase, H., Cawston, T.E., DeSilva, M., and Barrett, A.J.: Identification of plasma kallikrein as an activator of latent collagenase in rheumatoid synovial fluid. Biochim. Biophys. Acta 702:133, 1982.
156. Brinckerhoff, C.E., and Harris, E.D. Jr.: Modulation by retinoic acid and corticosteroids of collagenase production by rabbit synovial fibroblasts treated with phorbol myristate acetate or polyethylene glycol. Biochim. Biophys. Acta. 677:424, 1981.
157. Brinckerhoff, C.E., McMillan, R.M., Fahey, J.V., and Harris, E.D. Jr.: Collagenase production by synovial fibroblasts treated with phorbol myristate acetate. Arthritis Rheum. 22:1109, 1979.
158. Harris, E.D. Jr., Reynolds, J.J., and Werb, Z.: Cytochalasin B increases collagenase production by cells in vitro. Nature 257:243, 1975.
159. Biswas, C., and Dayer, J.-H.: Stimulation of collagenase production by collagen in mammalian cell cultures. Cell 18:1035, 1979.
160. Harris, E.D. Jr., and Krane, S.M.: Effects of colchicine on collagenase in cultures of rheumatoid synovium. Arthritis Rheum. 14:669, 1971.
161. Wahl, L.M., Wahl, S.M., Mergenhagen, S.E., and Martin, G.R.: Collagenase production by lymphokine-activated macrophages. Science 187:261, 1975.
162. Dayer, J.-M., Russell, R.G.G., and Krane, S.M.: Collagenase production by rheumatoid synovial cells. Stimulation by a human lymphocyte factor. Science 195:181, 1977.
163. Dayer, J.-M., Breard, J., Chess, L., and Krane, S.M.: Participation of monocyte-macrophages and lymphocytes in the production of a factor which stimulates collagenase release by rheumatoid synovial cells. J. Clin. Invest. 64:1386, 1979.
164. Dayer, J.-M., Robinson, D.R., and Krane, S.M.: Prostaglandin production by rheumatoid synovial cells. Stimulation by a factor from human mononuclear cells. J. Exp. Med. 145:1399, 1977.
165. Meats, J.E., McGuire, M.B., and Russell R.G.G.: Human synovium releases a factor which stimulates chondrocyte production of PGE and plasminogen activator. Nature 286:891, 1980.
166. Dayer, J.-M., Stephenson, M.L., Schmidt, E., Karge, W., and Krane, S.M.: Purification of a factor from blood monocyte-macrophages which stimulates the production of collagenase and prostaglandin $E_2$ by cells cultured from rheumatoid synovial tissues. FEBS Lett. 124:253, 1981.
167. Dayer, J.-M., Paswell, J.H., Schneeberger, E.E., and Krane, S.M.: Interactions among rheumatoid synovial cells and monocyte-macrophages: production of collagenase stimulating factor by human monocytes exposed to Con A or immunoglobulin Fc fragments. J. Immunol. 124:1712, 1980.
168. Dayer, J.-M., Trentham, D.E., and Krane, S.M.: Collagens act as ligands to stimulate human monocytes to produce mononuclear cell factor (MCF) and prostaglandins ($PGE_2$). Collagen Rel. Res. 2:523, 1982.
169. Amento, E.P., Kurnick, J.T., Epstein, A., and Krane, S.M.: Modulation of synovial cell products by a factor from a human cell line: T lymphocyte induction of a mononuclear cell factor. Proc. Natl. Acad. Sci. USA 79:5307, 1982.
170. Huybrechts-Godin, G., Hauser, P., and Vaes, G.: Macrophage-fibroblast interactions in collagenase production and cartilage degradation. Biochem. J. 184:643, 1979.
171. Mizel, S.B., Dayer, J.-M., Krane, S.M., and Mergenhagen, S.E.: Stimulation of rheumatoid synovial cell collagenase and prostaglandin production by partially purified lymphocyte activating factor (interleukin 1). Proc. Natl. Acad. Sci. USA 78:2474, 1981.
172. Postlethwaite, A.E., Lachman, L.B., Mainardi, C.L., and Kang, A.H.: Interleukin 1 stimulation of collagenase production by cultured fibroblasts. J. Exp. Med. 157:801, 1983.
173. Mizel, S.B., and Mizel, D.: Purification to apparent homogeneity of murine interleukin 1. J. Immunol. 126:834, 1981.
174. Saklatvala, J.: Characterization of catabolin, the major product of pig synovial tissue that induces resorption of cartilage proteoglycan in vitro. Biochem. J. 199:705, 1981.
175. Pilsworth, L.M., and Saklatvala, J.: The cartilage resorbing protein catabolin is made by synovial fibroblasts and its production is enhanced by phorbol myristate acetate. Biochem. J. 216:481, 1983.
176. Saklatvala, J., and Sarsfield, S.J.: Lymphocytes induce resorption of cartilage by producing catabolin. Biochem. J. 202:275, 1982.
176a. Saklatvala, J. Curry, V.A., and Sarsfield, S.J.: Purification to homogeneity of pig leucocyte catabolin, a protein that causes cartilage resorption in vitro. Biochem. J. 215:385, 1983.
177. Saklatvala, J., Sarsfield, S.J., and Pilsworth, L.M.C.: Characterization of proteins from human synovium and mononuclear leucocytes that induce resorption of cartilage proteoglycan in vitro. Biochem. J. 209:337, 1983.
178. Lachman, L.B., Hacker, M.P., and Handschumacher, R.E.: Partial purification of human lymphocyte activating factor (LAF) by ultrafiltration and electrophoretic techniques. J. Immunol. 119:2019, 1977.
179. Goldstein, I.M., Hoffstein, S., Gallin, J., and Weissmann, G.: Mechanisms of lysosomal enzyme release from human leukocytes. Microtubule assembly and membrane fusion induced by a component of complement. Proc. Natl. Acad. Sci. USA. 70:2916, 1973.
180. Schorlemmer, H.-U., Davies, P., and Allison, A.C.: Ability of activated complement components to induce lysosomal enzyme release from macrophages. Nature 261:48, 1976.
181. Vater, C.A., Mainardi, C.L., and Harris, E.D. Jr.: Binding of latent rheumatoid synovial collagenase to collagen fibrils, Biochim. Biophys. Acta 539:238, 1978.

# Chapter 13
# Connective Tissue: Small Blood Vessels and Capillaries

*Judah Folkman, Dianna Ausprunk, and Robert Langer*

## INTRODUCTION

Proliferation and regression of vascular endothelium play important roles in a variety of biologic processes. These include wound healing, inflammatory granulation tissue, some immunologic reactions, organization of thrombi, and growth of tumors. Vascular proliferation may determine the rate of progression of certain diseases, e.g., diabetic retinopathy, rheumatoid arthritis, and neoplasia.

Vascular endothelium throughout the body is generally of at least two types: (1) large vessel endothelium such as in the aorta and vena cava, and (2) capillary endothelium. Only recently has it been appreciated that there are some functional differences between these two kinds of endothelium. For example, in cell culture, there are differences in growth rate and response to specific growth factors, and morphologic differences. Here we will be concerned primarily with capillary endothelium.

## EMBRYOLOGY

It is not appropriate in this chapter to examine in detail the developmental biology of the vascular system. However, one general theme seems to have some bearing on capillary proliferation and arthritis. In the embryo, many organs do not originally contain or develop their own vessels. Instead, the anlage of such an organ is "invaded" by capillaries that later establish arterial and venous patterns unique to that organ. The vessels and their vascular endothelium, however, arise as a completely separate tissue[1] from primitive cells in the yolk sac that quickly differentiate into hematopoietic cells and vascular endothelial cells. Capillary tubes form. The capillaries grow, migrate, and invade the various organs. For example, the kidney of the mouse embryo is an avascular island of mesenchyme until day 11, when it is invaded by new capillary blood vessels. This has been elegantly confirmed by Ekblom's experiments in which mouse renal primordium was transplanted to the chorioallantoic membrane of the chick embryo.[2]

The liver anlage also begins as an avascular field of mesenchyme that is invaded by capillary sprouts. The same pattern is seen with the limb bud and bone.[3] Vessels enter the limb bud at a time when it is a small clump of cartilage cells. Chondrolysis occurs in the path of the advancing capillary tips. Bone formation follows. Vessel advance is finally halted at the end of the limb at the future joint cartilage. In certain cartilages, such as the human mandibular condyle, vascular canals and their contained vessels do not regress until the neonatal period.[4]

The development of mammalian joints is described in detail by O'Rahilly and Gardner[5] (see also Chapter 16). By the time the limb bud center contains mostly chondrocytes that have developed from mesenchyme, the synovial mesenchyme develops and is itself soon vascularized. Cavitation then takes place beneath the synovial membrane. Under normal conditions, once the joint cavity is formed, the vessels in the synovial membrane never contact the joint cartilage. However, in progressive stages of arthritis, these vessels generate the new capillaries that eventually contact and invade cartilage.

## MAINTENANCE OF NORMAL VASCULAR ENDOTHELIUM DURING ADULT LIFE

In the adult, vascular endothelium occupies an estimated 2 kg of the body weight. It is a ubiquitous tissue and represents a population of cells that undergo a very slow renewal. Mitoses are rarely encountered in adult endothelium, and autoradiographic studies with $^{3}$H-labeled thymidine have confirmed the rarity of cell division. However, there is considerable variability in the normal rate of endothelial labeling among different tissues. For example, the labeling index with $^{3}$H-thymidine was 0.13 percent in myocardial capillaries, while it was only 0.01 percent in the retina.[6] In fact, retinal vessels may be the most resistant to an angiogenic stimulus of any vascular bed. Most published $^{3}$H-thymidine labeling indices of capillary endothelium have been less than 1 percent, being most often in the vicinity of 0.1 percent.

Against this background of sluggish turnover, the capillary endothelium in some organs undergoes slow waves of proliferation in response to physiological stimuli. For example, endothelial proliferation occurs in the endometrium during the menstrual cycle and has been induced experimentally by diethylstilbestrol.[7] Also, capillaries around hair follicles undergo cyclic changes during the hair growth cycle.[8] It is not known what factors are responsible for the normal level of maintenance that keeps the whole vascular network coated with a monolayer of endothelium. Nor is it clear if certain diseases like scleroderma, in which capillaries appear to be disintegrating, result from diminution of some "maintenance" factor or appearance of a factor harmful to endothelial cells (see Chapter 76).

## NEOVASCULARIZATION

The term neovascularization is used for convenience to categorize those conditions in which capillary proliferation occurs beyond the normal requirements for maintenance. Examples are the capillary proliferation that takes place in the healing of large wounds; granulation tissue that follows necrotizing inflammation; delayed hypersensitivity reaction; diabetic retinopathy; retrolental fibroplasia; rheumatoid arthritis; and neoplasia.

Angiogenesis is the term generally used to describe the phenomenon that eventually generates new capillary blood vessels. The proliferation of capillaries has been studied extensively in such systems as the rabbit ear chamber, the hamster cheek pouch, and the cremaster muscle. The light and electron microscopic sequence of events in the formation of new capillary blood vessels has been well described.[9] In all these systems, wounds were used as the vascularization stimulus.

The study of tumor angiogenesis and the mechanisms of angiogenesis in general required the development of new techniques that could be quantitated. Also, methods were needed that would permit the study of biochemical compounds that would stimulate angiogenesis or inhibit it. Four methods, developed over the past decade, are now used by most investigators who study angiogenesis.

### New Methods of Studying Angiogenesis

**The Corneal Micropocket.** This technique permits the linear measurement of individual growing capillaries. Tumor implants (1 mm$^3$) are inserted into a pocket made in the cornea of a rabbit at a distance of 1 to 2 mm from the edge of the cornea and the normal vascular bed[10] (Fig. 13–1). New capillaries grow at right angles from the edge of the cornea and elongate toward the tumor at approximately 0.2 mm per day (Fig. 13–2). They are measured with a slit-lamp stereoscope. Tissues or biochemical compounds can be interposed between the tumor and its vascular bed. For example, the angiogenesis inhibitory property of protamine was demonstrated in this way.[11] The rabbit cornea has some unique anatomic features: It is avascular; new vessels grow into it in a two-dimensional plane; accurate measurements of vessel growth can be made; and, finally, the anatomic separation of the angiogenic stimulus from the responding vascular bed ensures easy identification of new vessels because they arise at right angles to the preexisting limbal vasculature. A disadvantage is that heterologous tumors, once vascularized, may excite an immune response. Subsequent immunologic neovascularization superimposed on tumor neovascularization may be confusing. This problem can be avoided by the implantation of mouse tumor into the cornea of inbred mice.[12] Nonspecific inflammation is another problem of this assay. Inflammatory agents can often be defined by their ability to attract leukocytes (mainly polymorphonuclear neutrophils, lymphocytes, or macrophages).[13] These cells then migrate rapidly into the cornea and may themselves elicit or enhance neovas cularization. For example, solutions that are hyperosmotic or of abnormally low or high pH are inflammatory. Whenever a new substance is tested for angiogenic activity, histologic sections are essential to determine if the angiogenesis has been induced directly or indirectly.

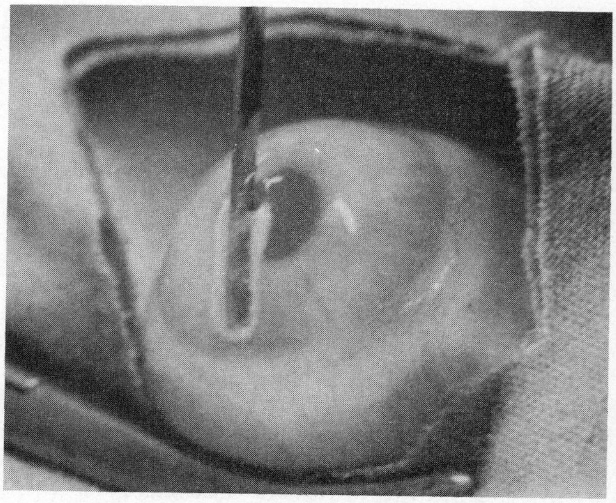

**Figure 13–1.** Method of implanting a sustained-release polymer pellet in the cornea. Through a small incision in the cornea, an intracorneal pocket is made with a spatula. The rabbit has been anesthetized. A slow-release polymer pellet is then implanted into the cornea.

**Sustained-Release Polymer Implants.** After the corneal micropocket technique was developed, the testing

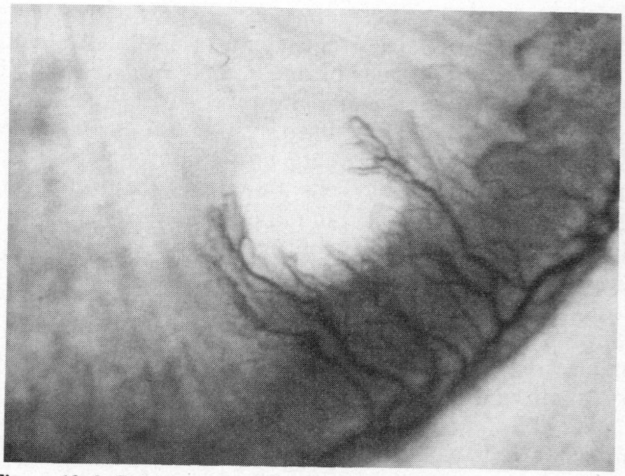

**Figure 13–2.** Rabbit cornea viewed through a slit-lamp stereoscope. A sustained-release pellet of ethylene vinyl acetate copolymer containing tumor-derived angiogenic activity has been implanted approximately 2 mm from the periphery of the cornea (limbus). New capillaries have grown toward the implant at a mean rate of approximately 0.2 mm/per day.

of fractions for angiogenesis activity required that they be released over a sustained period of time so that a concentration gradient could be established within the cornea. Two polymeric systems were developed that could release proteins and other macromolecules at approximately zero-order kinetics for periods of weeks to months.[14-16] These polymers are poly-hydroxyethyl methacrylate and ethylene-vinyl acetate co-polymer. They are not inflammatory when implanted as small pellets (1 mm$^3$) in the cornea.

**Chick Embryo–Chorioallantoic Membrane.** As biochemists attempted to purify angiogenic fractions from tumor and normal tissues, a need arose for a rapid screening assay for large numbers of test fractions that would be less expensive than rabbits and would avoid the problem of immunologic reactions. A method of dropping the chorioallantoic membrane and opening the eggshell to reveal a large expanse of chorioallantoic vascular membrane was previously described by Leighton.[17] We learned that the vessels of the chorioallantoic membrane grow rapidly until day 11, after which endothelial proliferation rapidly decreases.[18] Tumors or tumor fractions implanted on day 9 gave the most reproducible angiogenic response within 48 to 72 hours. This response could be recognized under a 6× stereoscope as new capillary loops converging on the implant.[18,19]

**Cloned Capillary Endothelial Cells.** Recently it has been possible to isolate cloned capillary endothelial cells and passage them in vitro for long periods of time.[20] This method is being used to test for endothelial cell mitogens. It has also confirmed in vivo observations implying that capillary growth is a multistep phenomenon that unfolds as an orderly sequence of events.

## Sequential Steps of Capillary Growth

By studying angiogenesis with these techniques, it has become clear that capillary growth takes place by a series of steps that are much the same regardless of the type of angiogenic stimulus. These steps can be summarized as follows: (i) New capillaries originate from small venules. Larger vessels with layers of smooth muscle do not usually give rise to capillary sprouts. (ii) Local degradation of the basement membrane on the side of the venule closest to the angiogenic stimulus[21] is one of the earliest events. Capillary endothelial cells stimulated in vitro by angiogenic substances secrete high concentrations of collagenase and plasminogen activator.[22,23] Also, fetal aortic endothelial cells degrade types IV and V collagen as they migrate when the stimulus for migration is an angiogenic factor.[24] These findings suggest that the local degradation of basement membrane in vivo is carried out directly by endothelial cells once they receive an angiogenic stimulus. (iii) Through this opening in the basement membrane, leader endothelial cells begin to migrate toward the angiogenic stimulus.[21] (iv) Endothelial cells that follow the leaders align in a bipolar fashion as the first sprout begins to form. (v) Lumen formation begins. In most examples of postembryonic angiogenesis, a lumen appears to be produced by a curvature that develops in the capillary endothelial cell, as if the cytoskeleton itself were responsible. This phenomenon has been observed in vivo in the cornea[21] and also in vitro.[25,26] However, during early embryonic angiogenesis lumen formation may take place by vacuole formation. This has also been observed in vivo[27] and in vitro.[25] (vi) Endothelial cells in the mid-section of the sprout begin to undergo mitosis. The leading capillary endothelial cells at the very tip of the sprout continue to migrate, but usually do not divide. (vii) Loop formation occurs next as individual sprouts join or anastomose with each other. These loops then elongate and may be the origin of additional sprouts. The loops continue to converge upon the angiogenic target. (viii) Flow begins sluggishly after loops have formed. (ix) Pericytes emerge along the length of the capillary sprouts. (x) Synthesis of new basement membrane follows.

When cloned capillary endothelial cells are cultured, i.e. "angiogenesis in vitro," most of these same events occur. Tubes form, branches appear, and whole capillary networks develop.[25] Maciag has shown that these in vitro "tubes" can also form from umbilical vein endothelial cells and that they are hollow and will carry fluid.[26] Fetal aortic endothelial cells can also generate tubes in culture.[28] Pericytes are absent in vitro. When these in vitro findings are taken together with in vivo observations, they suggest that all of the information necessary to form tubular structures and build an entire capillary network can be expressed by vascular endothelial cells. The program that is expressed seems to be similar for each type of angiogenic stimulus, whether the source of the stimulus is inflammatory, immunologic, or neoplastic.

## Modulation of the Rate of Capillary Growth

While the instructions for generating a capillary network originate from the vascular endothelial cell (once it is stimulated), the *rate* at which this endothelial cell program is revealed is modulated by several nonendothelial components. Two of these that have recently been studied in some detail are matrix components and mast cells.

**Matrix Components Modulate Endothelial Proliferation and Differentiation.** ***Collagen.*** When rat capillary endothelial cells are cultured on interstitial collagens (i.e., types I, III), they proliferate rapidly until a confluent monolayer is formed.[29] They form tubes only after very long periods of culture (i.e., 2 to 4 weeks). By contrast, when these cells are grown on basement membrane collagens (types IV and V), the cells do not proliferate but aggregate and form tubes early, i.e., after 4 days. Also, cells grown on basement membrane collagen produced more basement membrane constituents than did endothelial cells grown on interstitial collagen. In a confirmatory experiment, capillary endothelial cells were grown on either side of an amniotic membrane which was itself acellular. On the basement membrane surface these cells formed early tubelike structures and did not

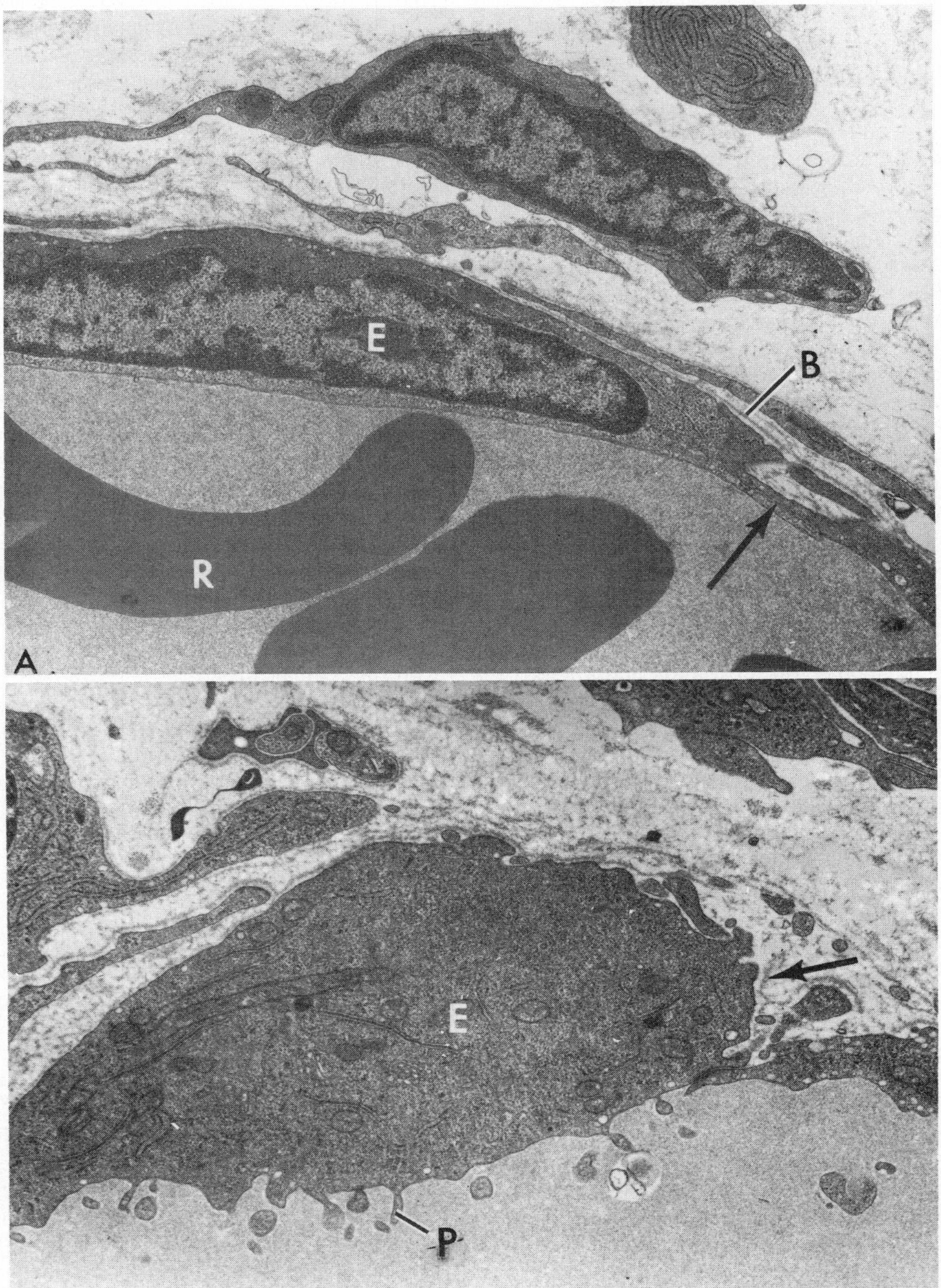


**Figure 13–3.** *A*, Electron micrograph of an endothelial cell (*E*) in a nonstimulated quiescent venule at the edge of the cornea, 2 days after implanting heat-killed tumor in a corneal pocket. The flattened cell has smooth contours, makes junctional contact with a neighboring cell (arrow), and is covered by a continuous basal lamina. (*B*). The vessel lumen contains erythrocytes (*R*). × 12,000. *B*, Endothelial cell (*E*) in a blood vessel at edge of cornea, 1 day after implanting live tumor in the cornea. The cell exhibits increased thickness, luminal projections (*P*), an increase in cytoplasmic organelles, and fragmentation of the basal lamina (arrow). × 13,500. (From Ausprunk, D.H., and Folkman, J.: Microvasc. Res. 14:53, 1977. With permission of the publisher.)

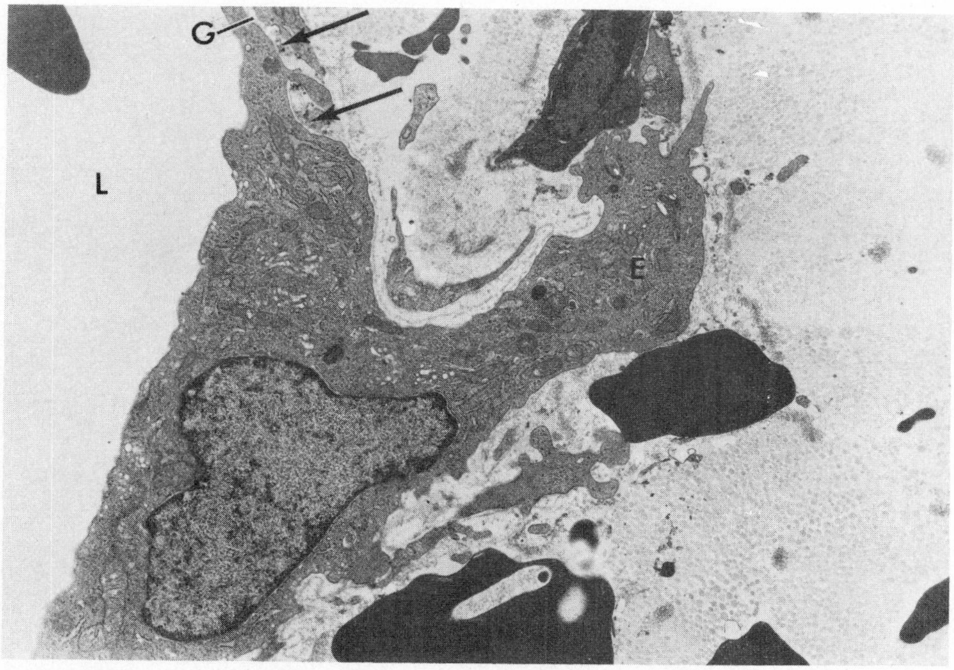


**Figure 13–4.** Limbal endothelial cell 2 days after tumor implant in cornea. A larger cytoplasmic extension (*E*) protudes into the perivascular connective tissue in the direction of the tumor implant. This pseudopod is mostly devoid of basal lamina. Carbon particles (arrows) have escaped from the vessel lumen (*L*) through a large intercellular gap (*G*). × 7700. (From Ausprunk, D.H., and Folkman, J.: J. Microvasc. Res. 14:53, 1977. With permission of the publisher.)

migrate through the basement membrane. In contrast, on the stromal surface (i.e., interstitial collagen) the endothelial cells proliferated and migrated into the stromal surface of the amnion. Tubelike structures occurred only occasionally and formed much later (21 days) and not until high cell densities were present. Taken together, these studies show that different collagenous components of extracellular matrix direct endothelial cells either toward proliferation and migration or toward tube formation. These collagenous components may have a similar role in vivo. Their relevance to neovascularization of the joint (as, for example, in rheumatoid arthritis) may be as follows: While vascular endothelium within the joint could be activated by angiogenic activity from macrophages or immune lymphocytes, whether or not they "invade" joint tissues may depend upon the state of collagen in the extravascular matrix.

*Glycosaminoglycans.* In mature resting (nonproliferating) capillaries, the basement membrane is rich in glycosaminoglycans, of which heparan sulfate is the most prominent. Highly sulfated glycosaminoglycans produced by vascular endothelial cells and incorporated in their matrix appear to help maintain the nonproliferative state of capillary endothelium. In contrast, proliferating capillaries have little or no basement membrane. Endothelial cells synthesize primarily nonsulfated glycosaminoglycans, mainly hyaluronate, which remain associated with the cells and are not secreted into the matrix. This GAG pattern has been observed during embryonic angiogenesis[30] and also in inflammatory and tumor angiogenesis.[31,32]

Whether the extent of GAG sulfation and collagen type act independently on capillary growth and maturation, or together, is unknown.

**Mast Cells Promote Angiogenesis But Cannot Initiate It.** Mast cells have been observed to accumulate around many types of solid tumors.[33] These cells are especially conspicuous in the neighborhood of in situ tumors prior to vascularization. In experimental studies with the chick embryo, mast cells accumulated at the site of the tumor extract within 24 hours after implantation and increased to 40-fold above normal mast cell density. Furthermore, mast cells preceded the new vessel sprouts that were converging upon the tumor site. However, mast cells added to the chorioallantoic membrane could not initiate angiogenesis.[34]

These findings suggested that mast cells might play an amplifying or a promoting role in the growth of new capillaries.

It has recently been reported that mast cells are significantly increased in the synovial membranes of patients with rheumatoid arthritis, and that mast cell counts were directly related to the intensity of clinical synovitis in the affected joint.[85]

**Heparin Is the Mediator by Which Mast Cells Amplify Capillary Growth.** After it became possible to grow capillary endothelial cells in long-term culture,[20] an assay was developed to measure their migration in vitro (chemokinesis).[35] This method was based upon phagokinetic

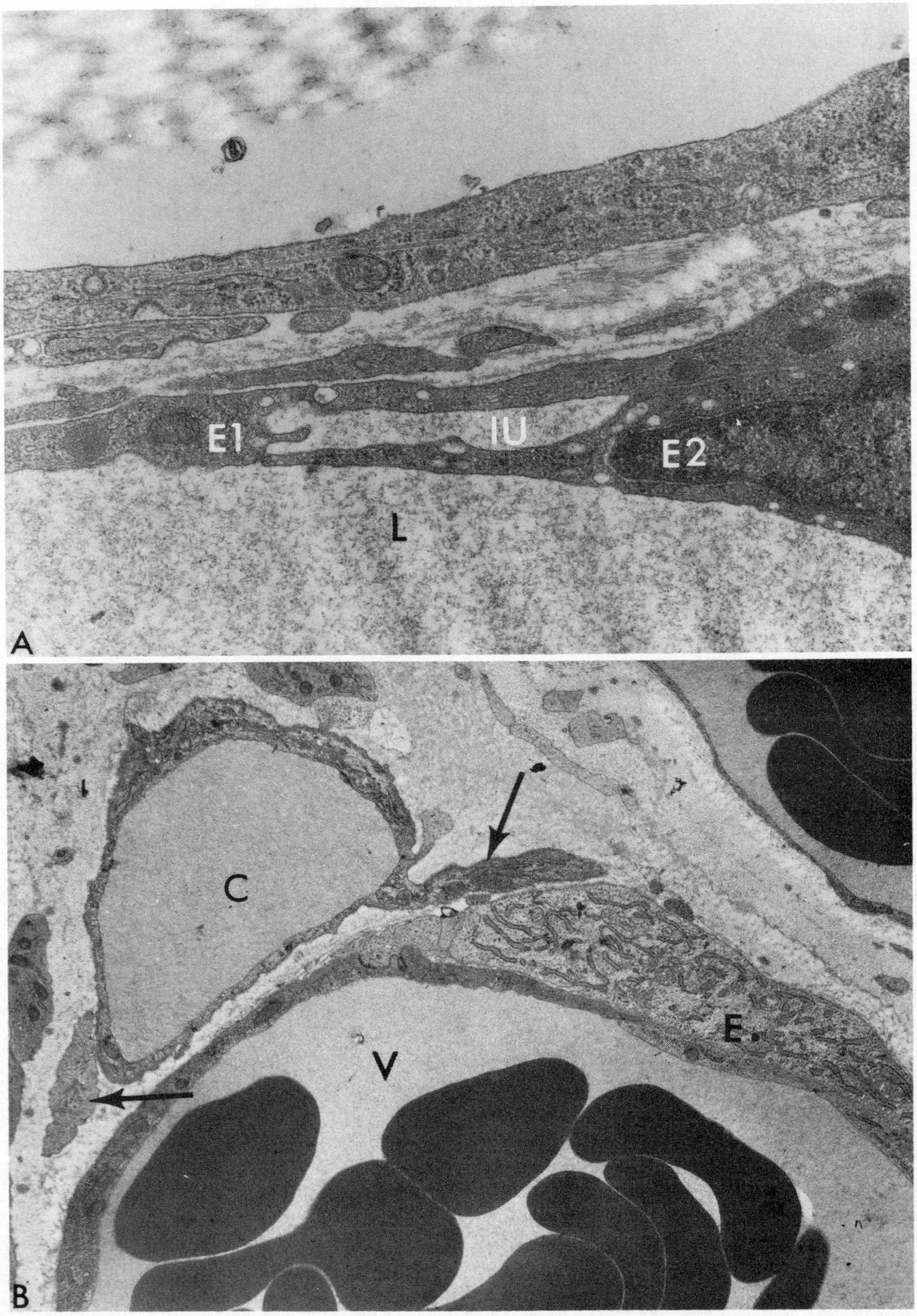


**Figure 13–5.** *A* A new lumen (*IU*) formed within the wall of an existing venule. It is the origin of a new capillary sprout, and is surrounded by two endothelial cells (*EI, E2*) that retain contact with the lumen (*L*) of the parent vessel. Two days after tumor implant. × 31,000. (From Ausprunk, D.H., and Folkman J.: Microvasc. Res. 14:53, 1977. With permission of the publisher.) *B*, A capillary sprout (*C*) adjacent to a preformed limbal venule (*V*) four days after tumor implant. The pseudopods (arrows) extending from the endothelial cells of the capillary suggest that the section is near the tip of this sprout. The double layer of active-appearing endothelial cells (*E*) in the venule indicates that the new capillary has probably budded from this vessel. × 6000.

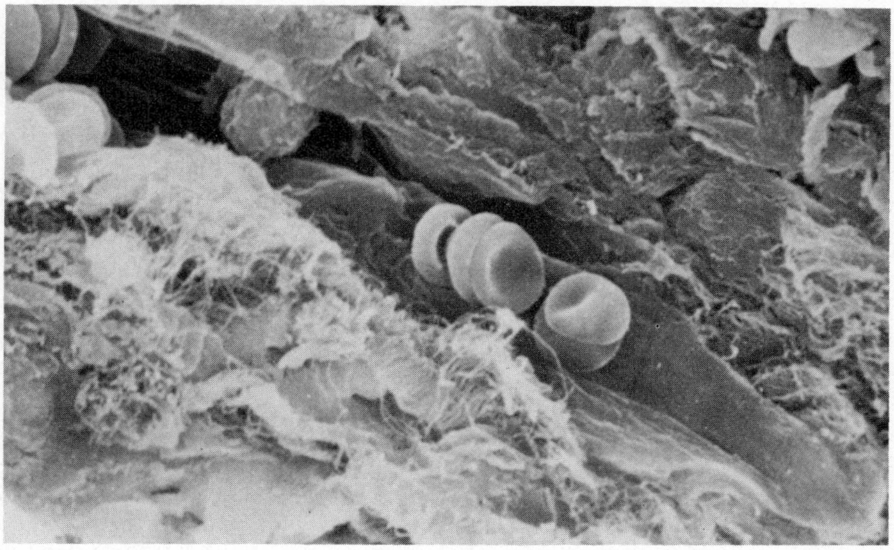

**Figure 13–6.** A later step in capillary formation. Endothelial cells align with each other, end to end, to form a sprout. The leading tip of such a sprout extends through collagen of the rabbit cornea. A lumen is beginning to form in the mid-section of this sprout. (Scanning electron micrograph × 2300.)

tracks, which cells make as they travel over colloidal gold and ingest it.[36] Culture medium conditioned by rat mast cells stimulated *migration* of capillary endothelial cells in vitro in a dose-dependent manner, but it did not stimulate proliferation[37] (Fig. 13–8).

These results suggest that mast cells may enhance angiogenesis by increasing the rate of directional migration of capillary endothelial cells toward an angiogenic stimulus such as tumor. When many mast cell products were tested, only heparin was found to significantly stimulate capillary endothelial cell migration.[37] Heparin could completely substitute for mast-cell-conditioned medium. Heparin antagonists such as protamine and heparinase blocked the stimulatory effect of heparin on capillary endothelial cell migration. When heparin was applied to the chorioallantoic membrane of the chick embryo at the time of implantation of tumor or tumor extract, angiogenesis was enhanced.[11] There was intense neovascularization at the site of tumor extracts within 1 day instead of 3 days as previously. Also, lower concentrations of tumor angiogenesis activity were detectable. Nonanticoagulant heparin lacking antithrombin III activity (supplied by Dr. Robert Rosenberg) also enhanced angiogenesis. Furthermore, neither heparin nor its nonanticoagulant subcomponents could initiate angiogenesis over a wide range of concentrations up to 500 times the enhancing dose.

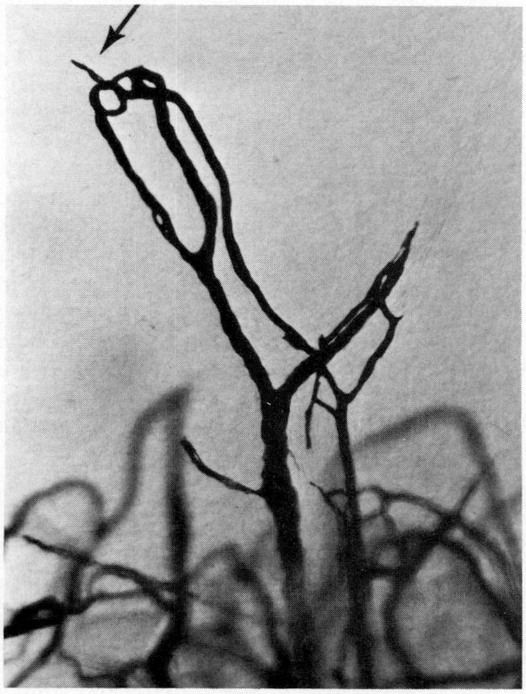

**Figure 13–7.** New capillary loop in cornea, showing beginning of another capillary sprout (arrow). × 160. India ink injection after implant of TAF pellet in cornea.

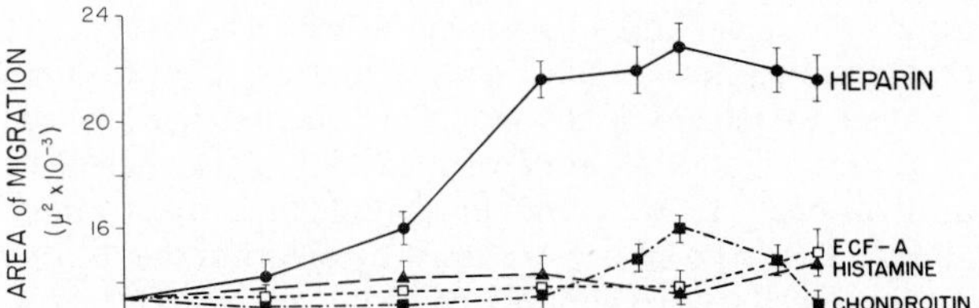

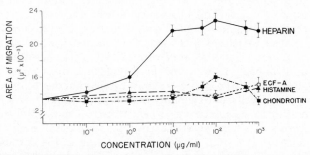

**Figure 13–8.** The effect of mast cell products on migration of bovine capillary endothelial cells. The mast cell products were dissolved in DMEM 10% calf serum and tested at log dose intervals from 10 ng to 1 mg/per ml. Heparin (solid circle); chondroitin sulfate A,B,C, (solid square); eosinophilic chemotactic factor-A (open square); and histamine phosphate (solid triangle). Each point represents the mean area of 100 phagokinetic tracks ± SEM. (Reprinted from *The Journal of Experimental Medicine* 152:931–944, 1980, with permission of the publisher.)

## Angiogenesis Factors from Non-neoplastic Cells

There are some recently discovered inducers of vascularization that may have an important role in mediating the neovascularization of the synovium in rheumatoid arthritis. Under certain conditions, lymphocytes and also macrophages have been found to liberate such substances.

**Lymphocytes.** Certain immune reactions are followed by neovascularization. The present experimental evidence suggests that white cells precede capillary invasion into the target tissue and then send back a diffusible signal that stimulates capillary proliferation. The best evidence so far comes from the studies of Sidky and Auerbach.[38] Originally Auerbach found that a rabbit's own lymph node implanted into its own cornea elicited neither neovascularization nor any other reaction. However, a lymph node implant from another outbred rabbit caused a weak vascular response after some delay. In contrast, a lymph node from a mouse produced a strong neovascular response. However, a lymph node from a nude mouse (thymic deficient) was unable to stimulate neovascularization in the rabbit eye.

Therefore, more extensive studies were undertaken using inbred mouse spleen cells. Those cells were injected intradermally into recipient normal animals that had been irradiated a few hours previously with 800 roentgens. After 2 to 3 days the animals were sacrificed, and the injection sites exposed by dissection. The number of new vessels was counted in the vascular response. No vascular response was seen in syngeneic combinations, i.e., donor spleen cells from the same animal strain. In contrast, allogeneic spleen cells inoculated into an irradiated normal recipient gave a typical vascular response.[39] Recent studies support these findings.[40] In other studies, an increase in capillary density[41] and extensive proliferation of postcapillary venular endothelium[42] were found in lymph nodes that were undergoing strong immunologic reactions.

**Macrophages.** Macrophages also appear capable of stimulating capillary endothelium under certain conditions. The first hint of this came from the observation that significant vascular endothelial proliferation and delayed hypersensitivity reactions occurred in the skin of guinea pigs at the time of maximal mononuclear cell infiltration.[43] It was further found that macrophages activated in vivo or in vitro and the medium conditioned by these cells were capable of inducing vascular proliferation in the guinea pig cornea.[44] Macrophages obtained from guinea pigs previously injected with paraffin oil or thioglycolate induced neovascularization in the cornea. Furthermore, macrophage-conditioned medium that had been dialyzed, concentrated, and impregnated into the cornea induced vessel growth. The microvascular responses were not associated with an acute inflammatory response. Also, the neovascularization could not be attributed solely to an immunologic reaction, because it was produced in a completely syngeneic cell system. In these and other studies, only activated macrophages (achieved either in vivo or in vitro) had the capacity to induce formation of new vessels, findings that parallel studies of enzymes and stimulatory factors released by macrophages (see Chapter 10).

Macrophages may play a key role as stimulators of blood vessel growth during wound healing.[45-47] Macrophages obtained from wounds have been shown to release angiogenic activity.[48] An angiogenic factor from wound fluid has been partially purified and found to be chemotactic for endothelial cells in vitro. It is a polypeptide with a molecular weight of approximately 10,000.[49] Furthermore, release of angiogenesis activity by wound macrophages was increased as local oxygen tension fell.

The increasing understanding about the angiogenic capacity of immune lymphocytes and activated macrophages may have important implications for arthritis. Synovial fluid from joints with rheumatoid arthritis contains angiogenic activity[50] and often has decreased oxygen tension. However, the cellular source of angiogenic activity in rheumatoid arthritis joint fluid has not been determined.

A factor has been discovered in the supernatant of proliferating fat cells (adipocytes) that stimulates capillary proliferation in vitro and angiogenesis in the chorioallantoic membrane. The adipocytes originated from 3T3 fibroblasts[51] that had differentiated in culture. Angiogenic activity was not found in the precursor cells.

At least six normal tissues have been reported to elicit angiogenesis during brief periods of their adult life. These are corpus luteum,[52,53] retina,[54,55] testicle,[56] skin,[57,58] salivary gland,[59] and kidney.[60] However, for each tissue, the cell or cells responsible for expressing angiogenic activity are unknown.

## Regression of Capillaries

Newly formed capillaries are not static but undergo remodeling. Some differentiate to form arterioles and venules, whereas others regress and disappear completely.[61] For example, certain vascular networks in the embryo seem to be intrinsically programmed for regression.[62] By contrast, tumor-induced vessels seem to depend for their maintenance upon the continuous presence of angiogenic activity at appropriate concentrations. By taking advantage of this short "half-life" of tumor-induced vessels, it has become possible to initiate capillary regression at will in the vascularized rabbit cornea. In this way, the topographic, histologic, and ultrastructural changes that occur in regressing capillaries can be precisely timed and sequenced.[63]

Pellets of ethylene-vinyl acetate co-polymer[63] were impregnated with partially purified tumor extracts that were angiogenic and implanted in corneal pockets 1.5 mm from the limbal vascular plexus. The polymer pellets were set to release up to 1 $\mu$g of this angiogenic protein per day for as long as 3 months. Four or 5 days after the implant, small capillaries penetrated the corneas and grew toward the polymer pellets at a rate of approximately 0.2 mm per day. They surrounded the polymers

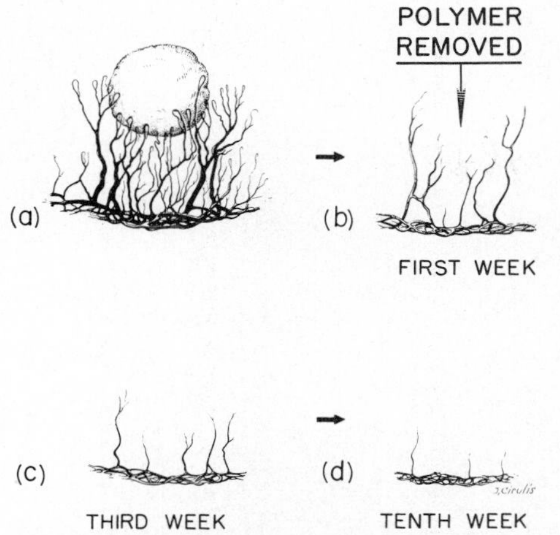


**Figure 13–9.** Diagram of the slit-lamp appearance of blood vessels in the cornea during regression. *a,* Before removing the TAF containing polymer, which had been implanted 10 to 12 days earlier. *b,* One week after polymer removal; only the largest vessels remain. *c,* These are thinner by the third week. *d,* Only two or three bloodless vessels persist to 10 weeks. (From Ausprunk, D.H., et al.: Lab. Invest. 38: 284, 1978. With permission of the publisher.)

by 10 to 12 days. Vessels then stopped growing but persisted in the cornea for at least 2 months if the polymer implants remained in place. However, if the pellets were removed 2 to 3 weeks after implantation, capillaries began to regress. The gross appearance in the slit-lamp stereoscope is shown schematically in Figure 13–9.

During regression, capillaries gradually narrow; by the end of the first week, the small distal branches disappear. Intravenously injected fluorescein appears rapidly in corneal vessels until 3 weeks after the onset of regression. Thereafter, vessels are not perfusable, as fluorescein cannot be detected by slit-lamp microscopy. At the microscopic level, the following sequence of morphologic changes occurs in the regressing vessels, regardless of vessel diameter or location within the vascular tree:

1. Endothelial cell changes and platelet sticking. One to 2 days after the removal of the stimulus, endothelial cells lining the distal corneal vessels contain swollen mitochondria and irregular cytoplasmic projections along their luminal surfaces (Fig. 13–10). Some cells become very thin or exhibit fenestrations. Fenestrated endothelium has never been observed in nonregressing corneal capillaries. Simultaneously, platelets adhere to the vessel wall (Fig. 13–11).

2. Stasis. Distal capillary branches become plugged with erythrocytes 1 to 2 days after removal of tumor angiogenesis pellets. However, larger, more proximal vessels are still perfused.

3. Endothelial cell degeneration. After stasis occurs, endothelial cells began to degenerate and lyse.

4. Removal of vessel debris. Dying endothelial cells are removed by macrophages. These mononuclear clear cells accumulate in the perivascular tissue of the cornea during the first week of regression (Fig. 13–12). They surround the degenerating capillaries and ingest the cell debris. By 6 to 10 weeks, only lipid-filled macrophages and some fibroblasts remain in most corneas.

Throughout the blood vessel regression, only an occasional polymorphonuclear neutrophil or mast cell is seen. The same sequence is observed when vessels regress after removal of different kinds of angiogenic stimuli, such as a sodium hydroxide pellet (e.g., vessels induced by an inflammatory stimulus instead of by tumor).

This corneal study has particular implications for cartilage, because both are avascular tissues that can be invaded by proliferating capillaries during certain pathologic states. The similar regressive behavior of blood vessels in these studies, whether induced by a neoplastic stimulus or an inflammatory stimulus, suggests that the fate of proliferating vessels is determined by a balance between the local environment and the continued presence of the vascularization stimulus. In normally vascularized tissue, such as a healed wound, regenerated blood vessels do not all regress.[64] Many are remodeled to restore the microvascular bed of the healed tissue. By contrast, the disappearance of *all* corneal vessels suggests that, whatever the stimulus for initiating vascularization, it must be continuously present to maintain the newly formed vessels and that it may be acting to overcome an inhibitor of angiogenesis in the cornea. The mechanism of regression is still unclear. That endothelial cells degenerate so soon after removal of the angiogenic stimulus implies that a humoral signal (in this case angiogenic activity from tumors) acts as a critically essen-

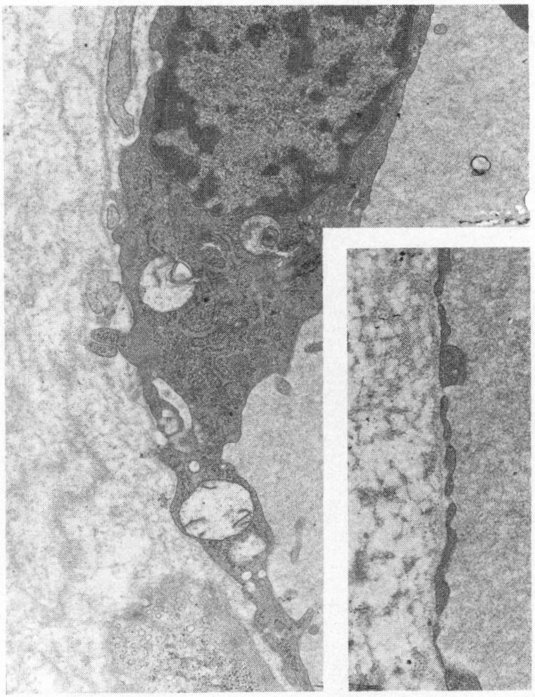

**Figure 13–10.** Sick endothelial cell in corneal capillary sprout, 1 day after removal of TAF polymer. Mitochondria are swollen, and the plasma membrane exhibits surface projection. × 19,500. *Inset:* Cell cytoplasm is attenuated and displays fenestrations. × 29,000. (From Ausprunk, D.H., et al.: Lab. Invest 38:284, 1978. With permission of the publisher.)

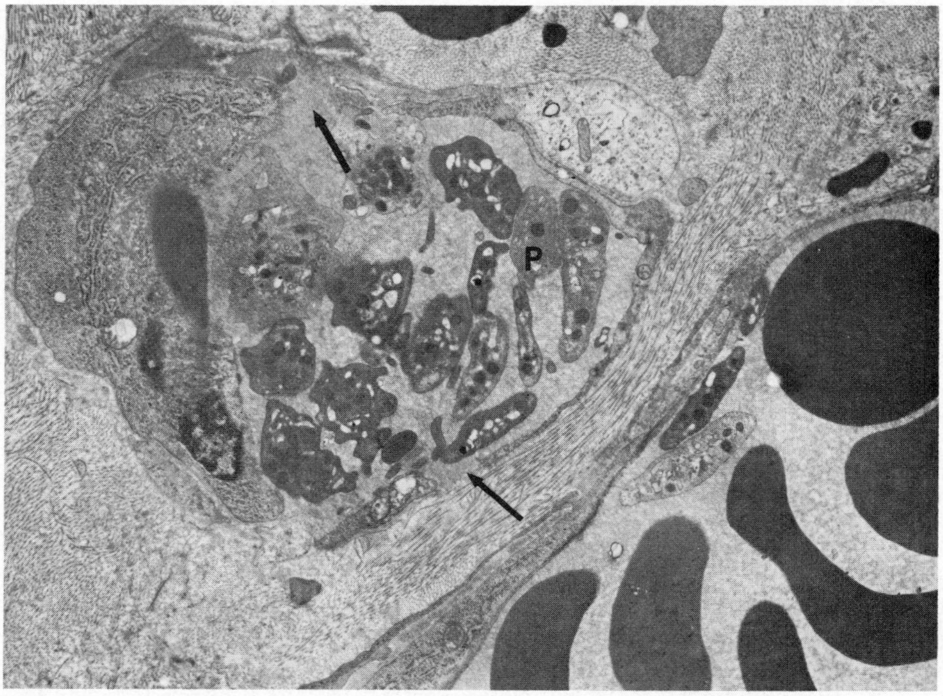


**Figure 13–11.** Platelets (*P*) accumulating in a small corneal blood vessel 2 days after removing a TAF polymer. Gaps (arrows) have formed between endothelial cells, permitting extravasation of vessel contents. The larger vessel is more normal in appearance except for a few platelets which adhere to the endothelium closest to the small vessel. × 9000. (From Ausprunk, D.H., et al.: Lab. Invest. 38:284, 1978. With permission of the publisher.)

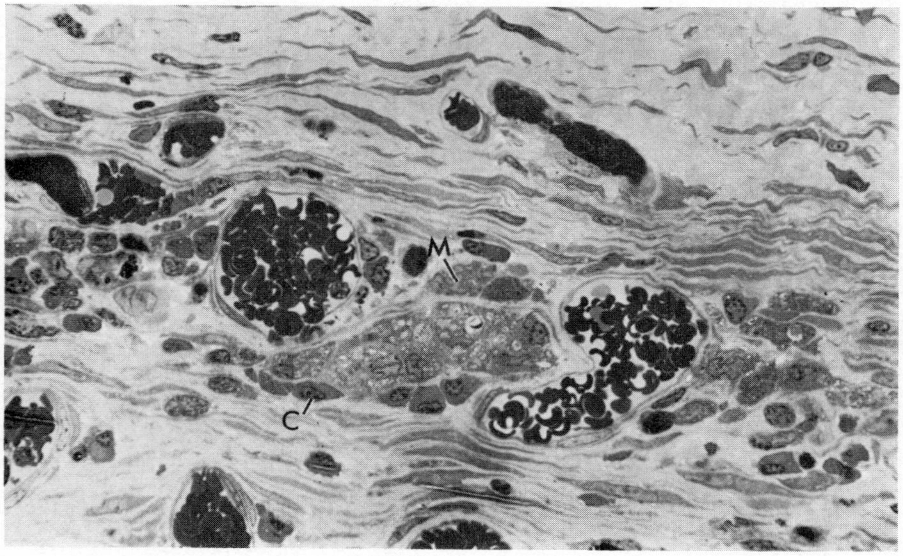


**Figure 13–12.** Regressing corneal vessels three days after removal of the TAF polymer. Monocytic cells (*C*) have infiltrated the perivascular stroma and are differentiating into macrophages (*M*). The smallest capillaries are plugged with erythrocytes × 900. (From Ausprunk, D.H., et al.: Lab. Invest. 38:284, 1978. With permission of the publisher.)

tial growth factor with a short half-life. Once there is blood stasis and macrophages have moved in, the process of regression appears to be irreversible.

## Angiogenesis Inhibitors

The term "antiangiogenesis" was proposed in 1972 to describe a potential therapy based on compounds that might specifically inhibit capillary proliferation.[65]

At that time, no such "angiogenesis inhibitor" existed. Clinical clues suggested that cartilage might contain such an inhibitor. For example, in mice, carcinomas induced in the ear by chemical carcinogens rarely infiltrate the cartilage but grow instead only in the surrounding tissues.[66] Furthermore, in certain human tumors, the field of neovascularization around the tumor stops at a cartilage interface. An example is squamous cell carcinoma of the trachea in which the tumor is unable to induce vascularization from the zone around the cartilage ring. Another example is osteogenic sarcoma, in which the tumor rarely enters the epiphyseal plate or the joint cartilage. Also, developmental studies on limb formation in the embryo have shown that vessels invade the field of chondrocytes that occupy the future central portion of a long bone. This is followed by chondrolysis and bone formation. However, zones of articular cartilage emerge in the neonatal period in an avascular state.[67]

The first experimental evidence for this inhibitor came from implants of cartilage in the chick embryo. It was reported that pieces of cartilage placed on the chorioallantoic membrane of the chick embryo did not become vascularized.[68] The general idea was proposed that cartilage may be resistant to "invasion" by a variety of tissues such as inflammatory cells, new vessels, and tumor cells, because cartilage contains certain protease inhibitors. In subsequent papers,[69,70] Kuettner and colleagues reported isolation of a trypsin inhibitor and a collagenase inhibitor from cartilage. Quantitation of the angiogenesis inhibiting capacity of cartilage was obtained by implanting 1-$mm^3$ pieces of fresh neonatal rabbit or calf cartilage into the cornea of the rabbit eye.[71,72]

The cartilage was positioned between the normal vascular bed of the limbus and a tumor implant in the cornea. In this experiment, vessels induced by the tumor had to pass through the zone of the cartilage before reaching the tumor. Fresh cartilage was capable of inhibiting new vessel growth for up to 3 months. In contrast, boiled cartilage or pieces of bone or other "control" tissues had no inhibitory effects; neovascularization continued unabated. Large vascularized tumors formed, and the rabbits had to be sacrificed by 3 weeks.

A partially purified angiogenesis inhibitor has been isolated from cartilage.[73] The active fraction contained several different proteins; the major one had a molecular weight of 16,000. It strongly inhibited proteinase activity. When impregnated into a sustained-release polymer pellet of ethylene-vinyl acetate co-polymer and implanted into the cornea, this fraction produced no detectable reaction by itself. However, when tumor was implanted behind the slow-release pellet, vessels induced by the tumor stopped growing as they approached the polymer implant containing the cartilage inhibitor.[73] In contrast, various controls and heat-degraded inhibitor had no effect. The active inhibitor fraction has been further purified. Infusion of this cartilage-derived inhibitor into the carotid artery of rabbits at concentrations of 1 mg per day inhibited tumor-induced vessels in the eye, with no detectable toxicity.[74]

The most potent inhibitor of neovascularization prepared by this method inhibits both trypsin and collagenase (type I) and shows two proteins with pKs of approximately 4.6 and 6.5 by isoelectric focusing. A second fraction with inhibitory activity toward trypsin can be isolated from cartilage by affinity chromatography and preparative gel electrophoresis or high pressure liquid chromatography.[75] However, this fraction does not have antiangiogenesis activity. The collagenase inhibitor has been purified several thousand–fold by ion exchange chromatography, molecular sieve chromatography, heparin-sepharose chromatography, and concanavalin A chromatography. While not enough of this material has been isolated to test its antiangiogenic activity, preliminary results show that it effectively inhibits cell migration in tissue culture in response to tumor-conditioned media or other growth factors.[76] It is possible that a mechanism of vessel inhibition involves the neutralization of proteolytic or collagenolytic activity found in blood vessels.

A recent study has shown that sharks, whose entire endoskeleton is cartilage and does not undergo ossification, have up to 100,000 times more angiogenesis inhibitor on a per organism basis than calf cartilage.[77] It is interesting to note that elasmobranchs such as sharks, in contrast to mammals, bony fishes, reptiles, and amphibians, rarely exhibit neoplasms.[78,79]

Another demonstration that normal cartilage can resist invasion by vascular endothelial cells has been made by Pauli and colleagues.[80] Small discs of bovine articular cartilage are used as a substratum for culturing vascular endothelial cells. The cartilage is extracted with guanidine hydrochloride to deplete the tissue of the soluble proteoglycan pool as well as the factor that inhibits neovascularization. Endothelial cells adhere to this devitalized cartilage and form a monolayer.[81] After 6 days of incubation, a basement-membrane-like matrix forms between the endothelial cells and the cartilage. The few microvilli on the basal surface of the endothelial cells do not reach the cartilage matrix. However, addition of heparin or tumor extract (Walker 256 carcinoma cells) to the medium stimulates the endothelial cells to penetrate the cartilage matrix with numerous microvilli.[82] The observation that salt-extracted, devitalized cartilage can be penetrated by stimulated endothelial cells yet remain impermeable to fibroblastic ingrowth further supports the hypothesis of Kuettner and colleagues that hyaline cartilage contains extractable components that specifically inhibit the invasive apparatus of potentially invasive cells.[81]

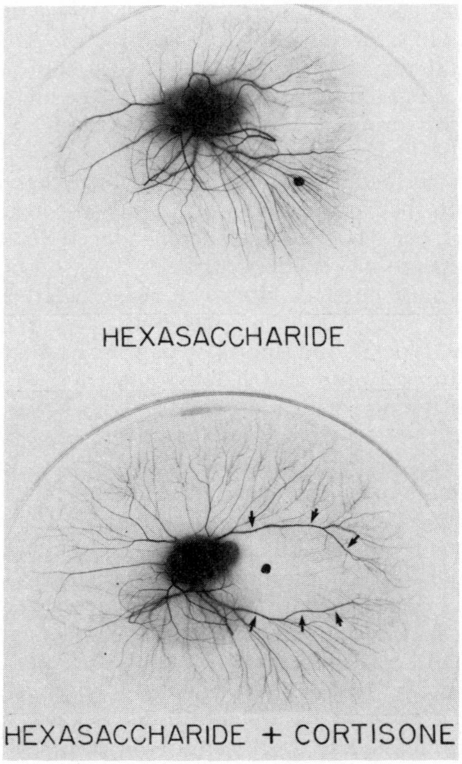


**Figure 13–13.** A method of using the chick embryo for detecting angiogenesis inhibitors. Embryonated embryos are grown in petri dishes. A 10 μl pellet of 0.5 percent methylcellulose is placed on the yolk sac vascular membrane at day 4, and an avascular zone appears at day 6 if the pellet contains an angiogenic inhibitor (in this case 100 μg cortisone acetate and 12 μcg hexasaccharide fragment of heparin). Another method is to use 50 μg of hydrocortisone, implant the methylcellulose pellet on the 6 day chorioallantoic membrane, and look for an avascular zone 48 hours later.

No one has yet completely purified the cartilage-derived angiogenesis inhibitor. Nonetheless, the presence of angiogenesis-inhibiting activity in cartilage provided a clue that angiogenesis inhibitors might also be found in other tissues or natural products.

Subsequently, protamine was found to be a potent angiogenesis inhibitor.[11] This discovery was made during experiments carried out to demonstrate that heparin could enhance or promote tumor angiogenesis. Protamine is a known antagonist of heparin, and it blocked the ability of mast cells or heparin to stimulate migration of capillary endothelial cells in vitro.[37] Protamine is an arginine-rich basic protein, with a relative molecular weight of 4300, found only in sperm. Protamine also reversed the heparin enhancement of tumor angiogenesis when it was mixed in a 2:1 ratio (wt/wt) with the heparin. When protamine concentrations were increased further, all angiogenesis in the chick embryo was inhibited, even in the absence of exogenous heparin. Further studies showed that protamine could inhibit angiogenesis regardless of whether the angiogenic source was embryologic, inflammatory, immunogenic, or neoplastic. When protamine was administered systemically, it inhibited angiogenesis in lung metastases, restricting these lesions to the avascular phase and markedly limiting their size. However, the toxic side effects of protamine, unrelated to its antiangiogenic activity (hypocalcemia and anaphylaxis), did not permit the use of sufficiently high doses to treat large primary tumors.

Recently, a more potent method of angiogenesis inhibition has been discovered (Fig. 13–13). During an experiment in which heparin was added to the chorioallantoic membrane to enhance tumor-induced angiogenesis, cortisone was also added. The rationale was that tumor angiogenesis, enhanced by heparin, might be made more conspicuous in the chick embryo bioassay if cortisone were added to suppress background inflammation on the membrane (usually due to eggshell dust). The result was unexpected. While heparin alone enhanced tumor angiogenesis and cortisone alone had little or no effect, angiogenesis was inhibited by the combination of heparin and cortisone.[83] Further experiments showed that heparin and cortisone, when administered together, abolished angiogenesis regardless of the type of angiogenic stimulus. Inflammatory, immunologic, embryologic, and neoplastic forms of angiogenesis were strongly inhibited. Furthermore, a nonanticoagulant fragment of heparin could substitute for whole heparin in this synergism. This fragment is a hexasaccharide with a molecular weight of about 1600. It has been further found that heparin administered orally is degraded into nonanticoagulant fragments that have similar antiangiogenic effects in the presence of cortisone. When mice bearing large tumor masses of B16 melanoma, Lewis lung carcinoma, or reticulum cell sarcoma were allowed to drink heparin and cortisone, the tumors regressed and in the majority of animals were completely eradicated. Metastases were so markedly reduced that the majority of animals remained tumor free after the angiogenesis inhibition was discontinued. Several further experiments showed that the tumor regression was specifically the result of angiogenesis inhibition and not the effect of cytotoxicity. In fact, cortisone alone increased the number of metastases while heparin had little effect. And, the combination of cortisone and heparin in tissue culture increased the proliferation rate of all these tumor lines.

The mechanism of angiogenesis inhibition by this heparin fragment in the presence of cortisone is unknown. Nevertheless, the potent angiogenesis inhibition that can be obtained when these two compounds are administered either locally or systemically raises the possibility of their use against the destructive neovascularization in the joints of certain patients with rheumatoid arthritis.

## Unanswered Questions

If an angiogenesis inhibitor as potent as the combination of hexa-saccharide and cortisone were available, could cartilage destruction be prevented? This and many other fundamental questions must be addressed before we can learn the full role of angiogenesis in diseases

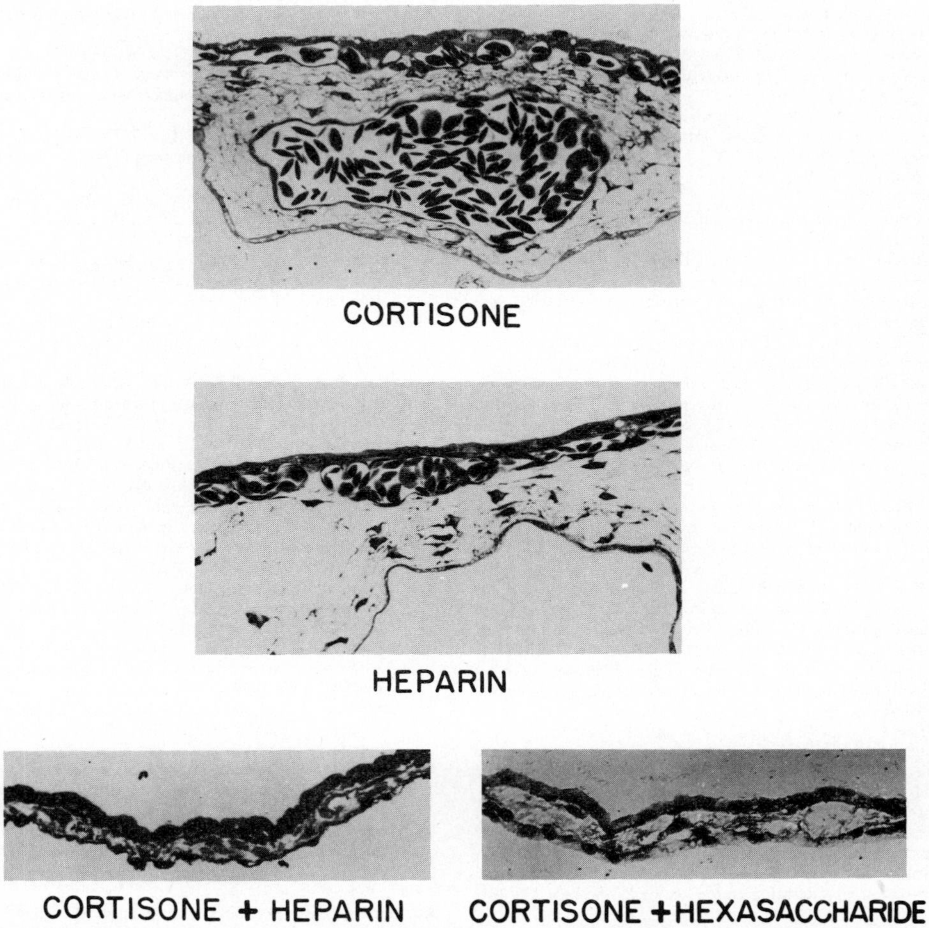


**Figure 13–14.** Inhibition of angiogenesis in the chorioallantoic membrane (CAM) of the chick embryo. Histologic cross-sections of 8 days CAMs. Test substances were implanted in a methylcellulose disc (10 $\mu$l) on day 6 and the histologic sections were made through this area on day 8. *A*, Cortisone alone: Ectoderm, vascular mesoderm and endoderm are normally developed. *B*, Heparin alone: All three layers are normally developed. *C*, Heparin plus cortisone: New vessel proliferation is inhibited in the mesoderm, leaving an avascular zone. *D* Hexasaccharide fragment of heparin plus cortisone: Similar avascular zone as produced in *C* and as viewed from above as seen in Figure 13–13. (From Folkman, et al.: Science 221:719, 1983, with permission of the publisher.)

such as rheumatoid arthritis. Some of these questions form the basis of investigations in other fields, such as tumor biology and diabetes research. For example: What are the requirements for the maintenance of endothelium in the normal microvasculature? How does a capillary, thinner than a hair, invade a tissue as tough as the cornea? What accounts for the directional growth of capillaries toward an angiogenic stimulus? Is there some undiscovered "chemotactic" mechanism for capillary endothelial cells that guides their migration? What is the role of fibrin? Could fibrin strands exuding from these capillary tips also help guide the migration of endothelium? Are angiogenesis inhibitors distributed in other normal tissues that parallel the angiogenesis inhibitor of cartilage? Finally, what are the signals that initiate capillary proliferation in the synovium, even before the formation of the pannus? Are these being secreted from activated macrophages or from sensitized lymphocytes? Once the angiogenesis stimulators from these cells have been identified, will they be detectable in the joint fluid in early phases of arthritis? Is there a vascular permeability factor in inflammatory fluid similar to the one reported from certain tumor cells?[84] Regardless of which field of investigation leads to explanations of these questions, at least one basic mechanism that is common to several chronic diseases may be revealed.

## References

1. Harr, J.A., and Ackerman, G.A.: A phase and electron microscopic study of vasculogenesis and erythropoiesis in the yolk sac of the mouse. Anat. Rec. 170:199, 1971.
2. Ekblom, P., Sariola, H., Karkinen, M., and Saxen, L.: The origin of the glomerular endothelium. Cell Differ. 11:35, 1982.
3. Smith, P.E., and Copenhaver, W.M.: Bailey's Textbook of Histology. Baltimore, Williams & Wilkins Company, 1953, p. 125.
4. Blackwood, H.J.J.: Vascularization of the condylar cartilage of the human mandible. J. Anat. 99:551, 1965.
5. O'Rahilly, R., and Gardner, E.: The embryology of movable joints. *In* Sokoloff, L. (ed.): The Joints and Synovial Fluid. Vol. I. New York, Academic Press, 1978.
6. Engerman, R.L., Pfaffenbach, D., and David, M.D.: Cell turnover of capillaries. Lab. Invest. 17:738, 1967.
7. Widman, J., and Cotran, R.S.: Personal communication.

8. Durward, A., and Randall, K.M.: Vascularity and patterns of growth of hair follicles. *In* Montagna, W. and Ellis, R.A. (eds.): The Biology of Hair Growth. New York, Academic Press, 1968.
9. Schoefl, G.I.: Growing capillaries: Their structure and permeability. Arch. Path. Anat. Physiol. 337:97, 1963.
10. Gimbrone, M.A., Jr., Cotran, R.S., Leapman, S.B., and Folkman, J.: Tumor growth and neovascularization: An experimental model using the rabbit cornea. JNCI 52:413, 1974.
11. Taylor, S., and Folkman, J.: Protamine is an inhibitor of angiogenesis. Nature 297:307, 982.
12. Muthukkaruppan, V., and Auerbach, R.: Angiogenesis in the mouse cornea. Science 205:1416, 1980.
13. Fromer, C.H., and Klinworth, G.K.: An evaluation of the role of leukocytes in the pathogenesis of experimentally induced corneal neovascularization. II. Studies on the effect of leukocytic elimination on corneal neovascularization. Am. J. Pathol. 81:531, 1975.
14. Langer, R.S., and Folkman, J.: Polymers for the sustained release of proteins and other macromolecules. Nature 263:797, 1976.
15. Rhine, W.D., Hseih, D.S., and Langer, R.S.: Polymers for sustained release of macromolecules. Procedure to fabricate reproducible delivery systems and control release kinetics. J. Pharm. Sci. 69:265, 1980.
16. Murray, J.B., Brown, L., Langer, R.S., and Klagsbrun, M.: A micro sustained release system for epidermal growth factor. In Vitro 19:743, 1983.
17. Leighton, J.: The Spread of Cancer. New York, Academic Press.
18. Knighton, D.R., Ausprunk, D., Tapper, D., and Folkman, J.: Avascular and vascular phases of tumour growth in the chick embryo. Br. J. Cancer 35:347, 1977.
19. Klagsbrun, M., Knighton, D., and Folkman, J.: Tumor angiogenesis activity in cells grown in tissue culture. Cancer Res. 36:110, 1976.
20. Folkman, J., Haudenschild, C.C., and Zetter, B.: Long-term culture of capillary endothelial cells. Proc. Natl. Acad. Sci. USA 76:5217, 1979.
21. Ausprunk, D.H., and Folkman, J.: Migration and proliferation of endothelial cells in preformed and newly formed blood vessels during tumor angiogenesis. Microvasc. Res. 14:53, 1977.
22. Rifkin, D.B., Gross, J.L., Moscatelli, D., and Jaffee, E.: Proteases and angiogenesis: Production of plasminogen activator and collagenese by endothelial cells. *In* Nosel, H., and Vogel, H.J. (eds.): Pathobiology of the Endothelial Cell. New York, Academic Press, 1982, p. 191.
23. Gross, J.L., Moscatelli, D., Jaffe, E.A., and Rifkin, D.B.: Plasminogen activator and collagenase production by cultured capillary endothelial cells. J. Cell Biol. 95:974, 1982.
24. Kalebio, T., Garbisa, S., Glaser, B., and Liotta, L.: Basement membrane collagen: Degradation by migrating endothelial cells. Science 221:281, 1983.
25. Folkman, J., and Haudenschild, C.: Angiogenesis in vitro. Nature 288:551, 1980.
26. Maciag, T., Hoover, G.A., van der Spek, J., Stemerman, M.B., and Weinster, R.: Growth and differentation of human umbilical-vein endothelial cells in culture. In Sato, G.H., Pardee, A.B., and Sirbasku, D.A. (eds.): Growth of Cells in Hormonally Defined Media. Book A (Cold Spring Harbor Conferences on Cell Proliferation). New York, Cold Spring Harbor Laboratories, 1982, p. 525.
27. Bar, T., and Wolff, J.R.: The formation of capillary basement membranes during internal vascularization of the rat's cerebral cortex. Z. Zellforsch. 133:231, 1972.
28. Feder, J., Marasa, J.C., and Olander, J.: The formation of capillary-like tubes by fetal calf aortic endothelial cells grown in vitro. In Vitro 18:303, 1982.
29. Madri, J.A., Williams, S.K., Wyatt, T., and Mezzio, C.: Capillary endothelial cell cultures: Pheontypic modulation by matrix components. J. Cell Biol. 97:153, 1983.
30. Ausprunk, D.H.: Synthesis of glycoproteins by endothelial cells in embryonic blood vessels. Dev. Biol. 90:79, 1982.
31. Ausprunk, D.H., and Boudreau, C.: Proteoglycans in the microvasculature. I. Histochemical localization in microscopic vessels of rabbit eyes. Am. J. Pathol. 103:353, 1981.
32. Ausprunk, D.H., and Boudreau, C.: Proteoglycans in the microvasculature. II. Proliferating capillaries of the rabbit cornea. Am. J. Pathol. 103:367, 1981.
33. Selye, H.: The Mast Cells. Washington, Butterworth Inc., 1965.
34. Kessler, D.A., Langer, R.S., Pless, N.A., and Folkman, J.: Mast cells and tumor angiogenesis. Int. J. Cancer 18:703, 1976.
35. Zetter, B.R.: Migration of capillary endothelial cells is stimulated by tumour-derived factors. Nature 285:41, 1980.
36. Albrecht-Buehler, G.: The phagokinetic tracks of 3T3 cells. Cell 11:395, 1977.
37. Azizkhan, R.G., Azizkhan, J.C., Zetter, B.R., and Folkman, J.: Mast cell heparin stimulates migration of capillary endothelial cells in vitro. J. Exp. Med. 152:931, 1980.
38. Sidky, Y., and Auerbach, R.: Lymphocyte-induced angiogenesis: A quantitative and sensitive assay of the graft-vs.-host reaction. J. Exp. Med. 141:1084, 1975.
39. Auerbach, R.: Angiogenesis-inducing factors: A review. Lymphokines 4:69, 1981.
40. Kaminski, M., Kaminski, G., and Majewski, S.: Local graft-versus-host reaction in mice evoked by Peyer's patch and other lymphoid tissue cells tested in a lymphocyte-induced angiogenesis assay. Folia Biol. 24:104, 1978.
41. Herman, P.G., Yamamoto, I., and Mellins, H.Z.: Blood microcirculation in the lymph node during the primary immune response. J. Exp. Med. 136:697, 1972.
42. Anderson, N.D., Anderson, A.O., and Wyllie, R.G.: Microvascular changes in lymph nodes during skin allografts. Am. J. Pathol. 81:131, 1975.
43. Polverini, P.J., Cotran, R.S., and Sholley, M.M.: Endothelial proliferation in the delayed hypersensitivity reaction: An autoradiographic study. J. Immunol. 118:529, 1977.
44. Polverini, P.J., Cotran, R.S., Gimbrone, M.A., Jr., and Unanue, E.R.: Activated macrophages induce vascular proliferation. Nature 269:804, 1977.
45. Clark, R.A., Stone, R.D., Leung, D.Y., Silver, I., Hohn, D.C., and Hunt, T.K.: Role of macrophages in wound healing. Surg. Forum 27:16, 1976.
46. Greenberg, G.B., and Hunt, T.K.: The proliferation response in vitro of vascular endothelial and smooth muscle cells exposed to wound fluids and macrophages. J. Cell Physiol. 97:353, 1978.
47. Thakral, K.K., Goodson, W.H., III, and Hunt, T.K.: Stimulation of wound blood vessel growth by wound macrophages. J. Surg. Res. 26:430, 1979.
48. Knighton, D.R., Silver, I.A., and Hunt, T.K.: Regulation of wound-healing angiogenesis—effect of oxygen gradients and inspired oxygen concentration. Surgery 90:262, 981.
49. Banda, M., Knighton, D.R., Hunt, T.K., and Werb, Z.: Isolation of a nonmitogenic angiogenesis factor from wound fluid. Proc. Natl. Acad. Sci. USA 79:7773, 1982.
50. Brown, R.A., Weiss, J.B., Tomlinson, I.W., Phillips, P., and Kumar, S.: Angiogenic factor from synovial fluid resembling that from tumours. Lancet 1:682, 1980.
51. Castellot, J.J., Jr., Karnovsky, M.J., and Spiegelman, B.M.: Potent stimulation of vascular endothelial cell growth by differentiated 3T3 adipocytes. Proc. Natl. Acad. Sci. USA 77:6007, 1980.
52. Jakob, W., Jentzsch, K.D., Mauersberger, B., and Oehme, P.: Demonstration of angiogenesis-activity in the corpus luteum of cattle. Exp. Pathol. (Jena) 13:321, 1977.
53. Gospodarowicz, D., and Thakral, K.K.: Production of a corpus luteum angiogenic factor responsible for proliferation of capillaries and neovascularization of the corpus luteum. Proc. Natl. Acad. Sci. USA 75:847, 1978.
54. Glaser, B.M., D'Amore, P., Michels, R., Patz, A., and Fenselau, A.: Demonstration of vasoproliferation activity from mammalian retina. J. Cell Biol. 84:298, 1980.
55. D'Amore, P., Glaser, B.M., Brunson, S.K., and Fenselau, A.H.: Angiogenic activity from bovine retina: Partial purification and characterization. Proc. Natl. Acad. Sci. USA 78:3068, 1981.
56. Huseby, R.A., Currie, C., Lagerborg, V.A., and Garb, S.: Angiogenesis about and within grafts of normal testicular tissue: A comparison with transplanted neoplastic tissue. Microvas. Res. 10:396, 1975.
57. Nishioka, K., and Ryan, T.J.: The influence of the epidermis and other tissues on blood vessel growth in the hamster cheek pouch. J. Invest. Dermatol. 58:33, 1972.
58. Wolf, J.E., and Harrison, R.G.: Demonstration and characterization of an epidermal angiogenic factor. J. Invest. Dermatol. 61:130, 1973.
59. Hoffman, H., McAuslan, B., Robertson, D., and Burnett, E.: An endothelial growth-stimulating factor from salivary glands. Exp. Cell Res. 102:269, 1976.
60. Warren, B.A., Greenblatt, M., and Kommineni, V.R.C.: Tumour angiogenesis: Ultrastructure of endothelial cells in mitosis. Br. J. Exp. Pathol. 53:215, 1972.
61. Jack, R.L.: Regression of the hyaloid vascular system. Am. J. Ophthalmol. 74:261, 1972.
62. Clark, E.R., and Clark, E.L.: Microscopic observations on the growth of blood capillaries in the living mammal. Am. J. Anat. 64:251, 939.
63. Ausprunk, D.H., Falterman, K., and Folkman, J.: The sequence of events in the regression of corneal capillaries. Lab. Invest. 38:284, 1978.
64. Jennings, M.A., and Florey, H.W.: Healing. *In* Florey, H.W. (ed.): General Pathology. Philadelphia, W. B. Saunders Company, 1970.
65. Folkman, J.: Anti-angiogenesis: New concept for therapy of solid tumors. Ann. of Surg. 175:409, 1972.
66. Dontenwill, W., Chevalier, H.J., and Reckzeh, G.: Growth of carcinomas in the region of the cartilage. JNCI 50:291, 1973.
67. Haraldson, S.: The vascular pattern of a growing and full-grown human epiphysis. Acta Anat. 48:156, 1962.
68. Eisenstein, R., Sorgente, N., Soble, L.W., Miller, A., and Kuettner, K.E.: The resistance of certain tissues to invasion. Am. J. Pathol. 73:675, 1973.
69. Kuettner, K.E., Croxen, R.L., Eisenstein, K., and Sorgente, N.: Proteinase inhibitor activity in connective tissues. Experientia 30:595, 1974.
70. Kuettner, K.E., Hiti, J., Eisenstein, R., and Harper, E.: Collagenase in-

hibition by cationic proteins derived from cartilage and aorta. Biochem. Biophys. Res. Commun. 72:40, 1976.
71. Brem, H., Arensman, R., and Folkman, J.: Inhibition of tumor angiogenesis by a diffusible factor from cartilage. *In* Slavkin, H.C., and Greulich, R.C. (eds.): Extracellular Matrix Influences on Gene Expression. New York, Academic Press, 1975.
72. Brem, H., and Folkman, J.: Inhibition of tumor angiogenesis mediated by cartilage. J. Exp. Med. 141:427, 1975.
73. Langer, R., Brem, H., Falterman, K., Klein, M., and Folkman, J.: Isolation of a cartilage factor that inhibits tumor neovascularization. Science 193:70, 1976.
74. Langer, R., Conn, H., Vacanti, J., Haudenschild, J., and Folkman, J.: Control of tumor growth in animals by infusion of an angiogenesis inhibitor. Proc. Natl. Acad. Sci. USA 77:4331, 1980.
75. Langer, R., and Murray, J.: Angiogenesis inhibitors and their delivery systems. Appl. Biochem. Biotech. 8:9, 1983.
76. Murray, J., Krochin, N., Hill, C., Zetter, B., and Langer, R.: Partial purification of a cartilage-derived collagenase inhibitor. Fed. Proc. 42:1889, 1983.
77. Lee, A., and Langer, R.: Shark cartilage contains inhibitors of tumor angiogenesis. Science, 221:1185, 1983.
78. Harshbarger, J.C.: Activities Report of Registry of Tumors in Lower Animals 1965–1973, Washington, D.C., Smithsonian Institute, 1974.
79. Prier, D.J., Fenstermacher, J.K., and Guarino, A.M.: A choroid plexus papilloma in an elasmobranch (*Squalus carcanthias*). JNCI 56:1207, 1976.
80. Pauli, B.U., Memoli, V.A., and Kuettner, K.E.: Regulation of invasion by cartilage-derived anti-invasion factor. JNCI 67:65, 1981.
81. Pauli, B.U., and Kuettner, K.E.: Vascularity of cartilage. *In* Hall, B.K. (ed.): Cartilage, Vol. 1. New York, Academic Press, 1983.
82. Kuettner, K.E., Memoli, V.A., Croxen, R.L., Madesen, L., and Pauli, B.U.: Anti-invasion factor mediates avascularity of hyaline. Semin. Arthritis Rheum. 11:67, 1981.
83. Folkman, J., Langer, R., Linhardt, R.J., Haudenschild, C., and Taylor, S.: Angiogenesis inhibition and tumor regression caused by a heparin or a heparin fragment in the presence of cortisone. Science, 221:719, 1983.
84. Senger, D.R., Galli, S.J., Dvorak, A.M., Perraszi, C.A., Harvey, V.S., and Dvorak, H.F.: Vascular permeability factor: A protein secreted by tumors that can cause ascites fluid accumulation. Fed. Proc. 41:4058, 1982.
85. Crisp, A.J., Chapman, C.M., Kirkham, S.E., Schiller, A.L., and Krane, S.M: Articular mastocytosis in rheumatoid arthritis. Arthritis Rheum., 1984, in press.

# Chapter 14

# Structural Proteins: Collagen, Elastin, and Fibronectin

*Jerome M. Seyer and Andrew H. Kang*

## INTRODUCTION

The connective tissues are those tissues that support and bind together the specialized elements of the body into functional, anatomic units. Thus, connective tissue is present in all internal organs, dermis, and blood vessels, and, in addition, forms the structural lattice of the bony skeleton and its attachments such as cartilage, ligaments, tendons, and fasciae. The most readily appreciated function of the tissue is to provide mechanical support and maintain structural integrity. However, it may also serve many other functions. For example, it plays an important role in regenerative and healing processes and is involved in inflammation. In the cornea, it must maintain transparency in addition to its supportive, structural role. In the kidney, the basement membrane of the renal glomerulus may function as a filtration barrier.

The connective tissues consist of cells and extracellular protein fibers, with an amorphous ground substance occupying the intercellular, interfibrillar space. Three kinds of fibers have been described: collagen, elastin, and reticulin, although the last may be closely related or identical chemically to collagen. The amorphous ground substance consists of acidic proteoglycans, glycoproteins such as fibronectin, laminin, chondronectin, and so on, and other less well characterized matrix components. Metabolism of these fibrous components as well as ground substance is governed by connective tissue cells, such as fibroblasts, chondroblasts, osteoblasts, and other cells extrinsic to the tissue.

## COLLAGEN

Collagen is the most ubiquitous and abundant protein in the animal kingdom. In most vertebrates, including humans, it comprises aproximately one third of total body proteins. It is also unique among proteins in that it undergoes a series of modifications in both primary and tertiary structure after the molecule is synthesized and excreted into the extracellular space. These changes have profound influence on the properties of the protein and, therefore, the extracellular tissues. Implicit in this is that these post-translational steps in collagen metabolism might be one of the sites of biologic control of the properties of connective tissue as well as the potential sites of pathologic processes.

### Structure of Collagen

The collagen molecule, which is the basic building unit of collagen fibers, has a highly asymmetric, rigid, rodlike structure. It is 1.5 nm in width and 300 nm in length and has a molecular weight of 285,000.[1-3] Amino acid composition of collagen from tissues of many different animals, including humans, has been well documented.[4-8] The composition of collagen from some of

**Table 14–1.** Compositional Characteristics of Different Collagens*

| | Major Interstitial Collagens | | | | Basement Membrane Collagen | | Pericellular Collagen | | |
|---|---|---|---|---|---|---|---|---|---|
| **Amino acid** | *α1(I)* | *α2(I)* | *α1(II)* | *α1(III)* | *α1(IV)* | *α2(IV)* | *α1(V)* | *α2(V)* | *α3(V)* |
| 3 OH-proline | 1.1 | 1.2 | 1.1 | 0 | 1 | 1 | 2.9 | 2.5 | 2.2 |
| 4 OH-proline | 114 | 105 | 96 | 126 | 122 | 107 | 109 | 109 | 92 |
| Aspartic acid | 46 | 45 | 36 | 42 | 45 | 50 | 50 | 51 | 42 |
| Threonine | 18 | 18 | 22 | 13 | 19 | 28 | 19 | 26 | 19 |
| Serine | 35 | 30 | 27 | 38 | 38 | 30 | 36 | 31 | 34 |
| Glutamic acid | 77 | 70 | 95 | 71 | 78 | 64 | 91 | 84 | 98 |
| Proline | 118 | 114 | 106 | 107 | 85 | 73 | 118 | 97 | 99 |
| Glycine | 330 | 331 | 334 | 352 | 334 | 328 | 344 | 341 | 332 |
| Alanine | 119 | 105 | 108 | 95 | 30 | 47 | 46 | 52 | 49 |
| Cystine/2 | 0 | 0 | 0 | 2 | 0 | 3 | 0 | 0 | 1 |
| Valine | 19 | 35 | 19 | 15 | 33 | 25 | 25 | 24 | 29 |
| Methionine | 7 | 8 | 11 | 8 | 15 | 14 | 8 | 11 | 8 |
| Isoleucine | 8 | 16 | 11 | 13 | 32 | 19 | 19 | 16 | 20 |
| Leucine | 20 | 33 | 27 | 23 | 52 | 56 | 39 | 35 | 56 |
| Tyrosine | 2 | 3 | 1 | 3 | 5 | 6 | 2 | 2 | 2 |
| Phenylalanine | 13 | 11 | 13 | 8 | 27 | 36 | 12 | 14 | 9 |
| Hydroxylysine | 10 | 12 | 18 | 6 | 50 | 39 | 35 | 24 | 43 |
| Lysine | 27 | 20 | 20 | 29 | 6 | 3 | 20 | 18 | 15 |
| Histidine | 4 | 10 | 2 | 6 | 6 | 5 | 8 | 11 | 14 |
| Arginine | 49 | 51 | 52 | 48 | 22 | 42 | 45 | 50 | 42 |
| Glucose | 1 | 1 | 5 | 1 | 44 | 29 | 18 | 10 | 17 |
| Galactose | 1 | 2 | 10 | 2 | 46 | 31 | 30 | 14 | 24 |

*Residues per 1000 total residues.

the representative tissues is presented in Table 14–1. Most striking is the constancy of the content of glycine (approximately one third of total residues) and imino acids (proline plus 3- and 4-hydroxyproline comprise approximately 20 percent). The amino acids 4-hydroxyproline and hydroxylysine occur exclusively in collagen, the Clq component of serum complement[9] and acetylcholinesterase.[10] A small amount of 4-hydroxyproline is also present in elastin (see Table 14–3). However, over 99 percent of total hydroxyproline in the body is found in collagen. Thus, studies on the turnover of the imino acids have been a convenient and useful tool in providing information on the metabolism of the protein.

The complete amino acid sequence of two genetically distinct collagen polypeptide chains, α1(I)[11] and α1(III),[12] have now been determined, and sufficient information is available on the remaining chains to indicate that collagen polypeptide chains consist of repeating triplet sequences of (Gly-X-Y)n (Fig. 14–1) where X and Y can be any amino acid but frequently are proline and 4-hydroxyproline, respectively. Short regions at each end of the molecule are nonhelical and differ markedly in amino acid content from the rest of the molecule. The significance of these regions will be discussed later in connection with crosslinking.

Chemical, physicochemical, and x-ray diffraction studies have established that the whole collagen molecule consists of three polypeptide chains, each of molecular weight 95,000 and each composed of approximately 1050 amino acid residues.[13-16] At least five different types of collagen have been identified in vertebrates (Table 14–2). Type I collagen is the principal form of collagen present in interstitial tissues, dermis, tendon, and bone.[1,4,6] It is composed of two identical polypeptide chains, designated α1(I), and one α2(I) chain, which differ from each other in amino acid composition and chromatographic behavior. Type I collagen, then, has the chain composition $[\alpha1(I)]_2\alpha2(I)$ In most of these tissues, an additional species of collagen, type III, is also found, though the proportion of type I and type III varies, depending on the tissue and the age of the animal.[6] The type III molecule is composed of three identical α chains, $[\alpha1(III)]_3$, which differ in amino acid composition from the chains of type I collagen. Collagen present in hyaline cartilage and vitreous of the eye (type II) is composed of three identical but distinct α chains $[\alpha1(II)]_3$.[5] The collagen present in basement membranes is referred to as type IV, which is composed of two nonidentical polypeptide chains α1(IV) and α2(IV) (for review see refs. 17 and 18). Both polypeptide chains have predominantly a Gly-X-Y sequence similar in length to the interstitial collagens with occasional interruptions. In addition, type IV molecules contain additional collagenous and noncollagenous segments at the amino and carboxyl ends in a manner similar to a procollagen molecule (see below). The molecular structure is still controversial at this time, but a heteropolymer $[\alpha1(IV)]_2\alpha2(IV)$ is favored. The large noncollagenous

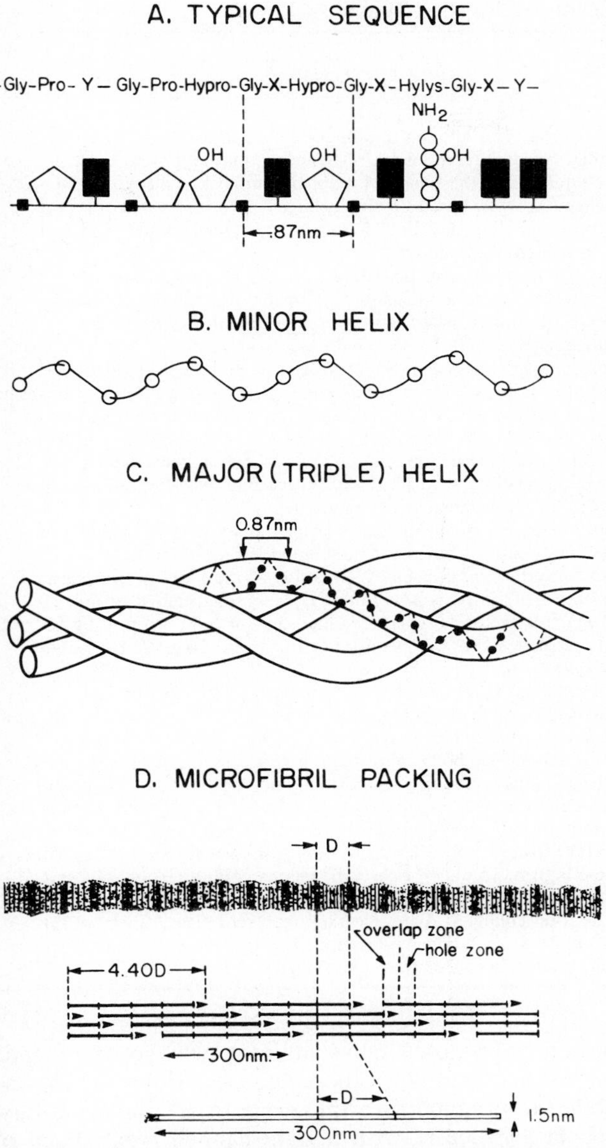


**Figure 14–1.** Diagrammatic representation of collagen structure. *A* shows that glycine occurs in every third position, and there are large amounts of proline and hydroxyproline in the other two positions. X and Y represent any amino acid. *B* shows an individual α chain in helix. *C* shows the triple helix. The individual α chains are left-handed helixes with approximately three residues per turn. *D* shows a stained microfibril of collagen exhibiting characteristic cross-striations with a regular repeat period (*D*) of approximately 68 nm, and a two-dimensional representation of the packing arrangement of collagen molecules in the microfibril. As discussed in the text, each collagen molecule has large numbers of darkly staining bands, and five of these separated by a regular distance of 68 nm account for the repeat period in the microfibril. (Adapted from similar presentations by Grant, M.E., and Prockop, D.J.: N. Engl. J. Med. 286:194, 1972, and Nimni, M.E.: Semin. Arthritis Rheum. 4:95, 1974, with permission of the authors and the publishers).

protein portion contains a heteropolysaccharide and many disulfide intrachain crosslinks.[19]

Type V collagen has recently been identified as a minor component of most tissues, including skin, liver, lung, placenta, and blood vessels, and has been referred to as possibly the exocytoskeleton of connective tissue cells.[20-22] It represents the major collagen product of certain smooth muscle cells in culture, but its biologic function remains uncertain. The type V collagen molecule consists of three polypeptide chains, α1(V), α2(V), and α3(V), and has a molecular structure of $[\alpha1(V)]_2$ α2(V) as the major form plus either $[\alpha3(V)]_3$ or [α1(V) α2(V) α3(V)] as a minor form. The major tissue source from which type V collagen has been obtained is the amnion/chorionic membrane, which contains only the α1(V) and α2(V) polypeptide chains. The placenta, in contrast, contains all three polypeptide chains. Hyaline cartilage, which, as stated previously, has type II collagen as its major interstitial collagen component, also contains minor amounts of a type-V-like collagen species, referred to as 1α, 2α, and 3α collagen polypeptide chains. While these polypeptide chains are similar to the α1(V), α2(V), and α3(V) collagen chains, some differences exist in amino acid composition and therefore in their amino acid sequence. It appears, therefore, that three clearly different collagen families may exist in vertebrate tissues. These may be classified as interstitial collagens (type I, II, and III), the basement membrane collagen (type IV), and the minor cytoskeleton collagens (type V and 1α, 2α, 3α). Type V collagen represents less than 6 percent of the total collagen in most tissues.

The search for additional, unidentified collagenous components in connective tissue continues, and many other less abundant collagen-like species will most likely be found. The complement component Clq, for example, contains a 72 amino acid, triple-helical segment of [Gly-X-Y] structure with 4-hydroxyproline occasionally in the Y position.[9] Acetylcholinesterase also has a short, less defined triple helical collagenous segment in the molecule.[10] More relevant to connective tissues, however, is the discovery of small quantities of high molecular weight collagenous complexes (HMC), which, with reduction of their disulfide bonds, yield three collagenous polypeptide chains of 45,000 to 55,000 molecular weight.[23] These short collagen polypeptide chains are genetically distinct from all of the above collagen types. Yet, it is clear that HMC exists as an intrinsic collagenous component of many tissues, including skin, liver, lung and placenta. A similar, but different, high molecular weight complex occurs in hyaline cartilage.[24] The tissue localization and functional significance of these unusual collagens remain uncertain, but it has been proposed that they may function as connecting or link proteins with collagens and other macromolecules.

As mentioned previously, the collagen chains contain a high content of the imino acids proline and hydroxyproline. The stereochemical configuration of the imino acid forces each of the α chains to assume a left-handed helical conformation (minor helix), with a residue repeat distance of 0.291 nm and a relative twist of 110 degrees, making the number of residues per turn of the helix 3.27 and the distance between each third glycine 0.87 nm (Fig. 14–1).[15] Thus, the minor helix of the collagen chains

**Table 14–2.** Distribution of Different Collagen Types

| Type | Molecular Structure | Location |
|---|---|---|
| I | $[\alpha 1(I)]_2\alpha 2(I)$ | This is the most abundant collagen found in the body. It is the major protein component of bone, tendon, and skin, but it is also ubiquitous in the body. Most of the initial knowledge of collagen chemistry was based on this collagen. A minor variant, type I trimer, $[\alpha 1(I)]_3$, has been found in embryonic tissue and some experimental systems. |
| II | $[\alpha 1(II)]_3$ | This is a cartilage-specific collagen, found also in certain eye structures and the vitreous. It is in the sole collagen of hyaline cartilage but is mixed with type I in certain fibrocartilage structures. |
| III | $[\alpha 1(III)]_3$ | This collagen was formerly considered to be reticulum, although this relationship remains circumstantial. It is generally found whenever type I is present but in increasing amounts in flexible tissues such as blood vessels, lung, and liver. It is also elevated in proliferating tissues, such as in fetal development, bone marrow, and early wound healing. A disulfide intramolecular crosslink is present in the COOH-terminal triple-helical region. |
| IV | $[\alpha 1(IV)]_2\alpha 2(IV)$ | This is a basement membrane–specific collagen. It is located in the lamina densa of basement membrane with high concentrations in the anterior lens capsule, glomerulus of the kidney, and placenta. Other structures such as $[\alpha 1(IV)]_3$ have not been ruled out. Segments of the polypeptide chain do not have a repeating [Gly-X-Y] sequence and are therefore subject to nonspecific proteolytic cleavage. |
| V | $[\alpha 1(V)]_2\alpha 2(V)$ and $\alpha 1(V)$, $\alpha 2(V)$, $\alpha 3(V)$ or $[\alpha 3(V)]_3$ | This collagen is thought to be a cell surface collagen or to be associated with the plasma membrane cells. It has been localized as the exocytoskeleton of connective tissue cells and is found throughout the body, with high concentrations in smooth muscle tissues such as amnionic/chorionic membranes and in capillary vasculature. The major structure is $[\alpha 1(V)]_2\alpha 2(V)$; but varying amounts of $[\alpha 3(V)]_3$ are also present. The presence of a different $\alpha 1(V)$, $\alpha 2(V)$, or $\alpha 3(V)$ molecule has been suggested in cartilage. |
| Unusual collagens | Disulfide-bonded high molecular weight aggregates of 45,000 to 55,000 daltons collagen chains | These high molecular weight collagenous complexes are widespread in connective tissue but generally represent less than 1 percent of the total collagen. Although they represent clearly distinct entities apart from the above collagen chains, their functional significance and molecular structure remain unsure. |

is nearly fully stretched, unlike the α helix found in most other proteins, which characteristically has an axial residue distance of 0.15 nm. The collagen chain minor helix also differs in that there are no hydrogen bonds between amino acids in the same chain due to the relatively large separation of the residues. Instead, the minor helix formed by each chain is stabilized by hydrogen bonds between it and the other two chains in the same collagen molecule.

The presence of glycine (which has no bulky side chain attached to its α carbon atom) at every third residue then allows three of the α chains to wind around a common axis, forming a right-handed super helix (Fig. 14–1). A cross-sectional visualization of the triple-helical structure would reveal only glycine in the central core, with the X and Y amino acid side-chains radiating away from the core. The three strands are stabilized by regularly occurring interchain hydrogen bonds. Hydroxyproline is known to exert a major stabilizing force in the triple helix presumably through hydrogen bond formation with its hydroxyl group. The exact number of hydrogen bonds used to maintain the triple helical structure is not known for certain. Two molecular models have been proposed, one containing two hydrogen bonds per triplet, and the other, one per triplet. Thus, the collagen monomer is a thin, long, rigid, three-stranded ropelike structure with a right-handed twist. Each of the strands itself is a left-handed helix.[15]

Sufficient information is built into the primary structure so that, under physiologic conditions of ionic strength, pH, and temperature, collagen molecules spontaneously aggregate into fibrils of the native type seen in tissues.[1,3] Examined with an electron microscope, each fibril can be seen to bear a characteristic repeating pattern of cross-striations of about 68 nm periodicity (Fig. 14–2). The periodicity of the cross-striations is explained by the fact that each collagen molecule (300 nm in length) has five charged regions 68 nm apart, which, using appropriate stains, appear as bands on electron microscopy, and by the highly ordered and regular way in which the collagen molecules are aligned within fibrils. As schematically depicted in Figure 14-1*D*, each neighboring row of collagen molecules is displaced along the long axis by a distance of 68 nm (a value of *D* in Fig. 14-1*D*). In addition, within the same row, there is a gap or "hole" of about 41 nm between the end of one mol-

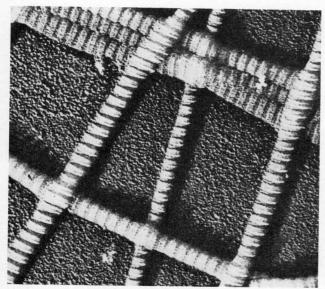

**Figure 14–2.** Native collagen fibril. Shadow-cast with platinum. The bar represents 0.2 μ × 70,000. (Courtesy of Dr. Jerome Gross.)

ecule and the beginning of the next (Fig. 14-1*D*). The "hole" created by this longitudinal displacement of the ends has attracted attention, because it may serve as a nidus for the deposition of hyroxyapatite crystals of bone.[25]

## Biosynthesis of Collagen

**Ribosomal Synthesis of Pro-α Chains on Polyribosomes.** As with all other known proteins, the peptide bonds linking the amino acids in the polypeptide chains of collagen are synthesized on ribosomal complexes containing mRNA (Fig.14–3).[26] Studies on the ribosomal clusters operating in collagen synthesis in fibroblasts indicate that associations of 23 to 60 ribosomes are involved and function with a monocistronic mRNA coding for single polypeptide chains larger than the α chains.[25,26] Recent evidence also has shown that the polypeptide chains of collagen synthesized by cells are indeed larger than the α chains with an estimated molecular weight of approximately 160,000.[26,27] This would require a 6 kilobase mRNA molecule. Each of the polypeptide

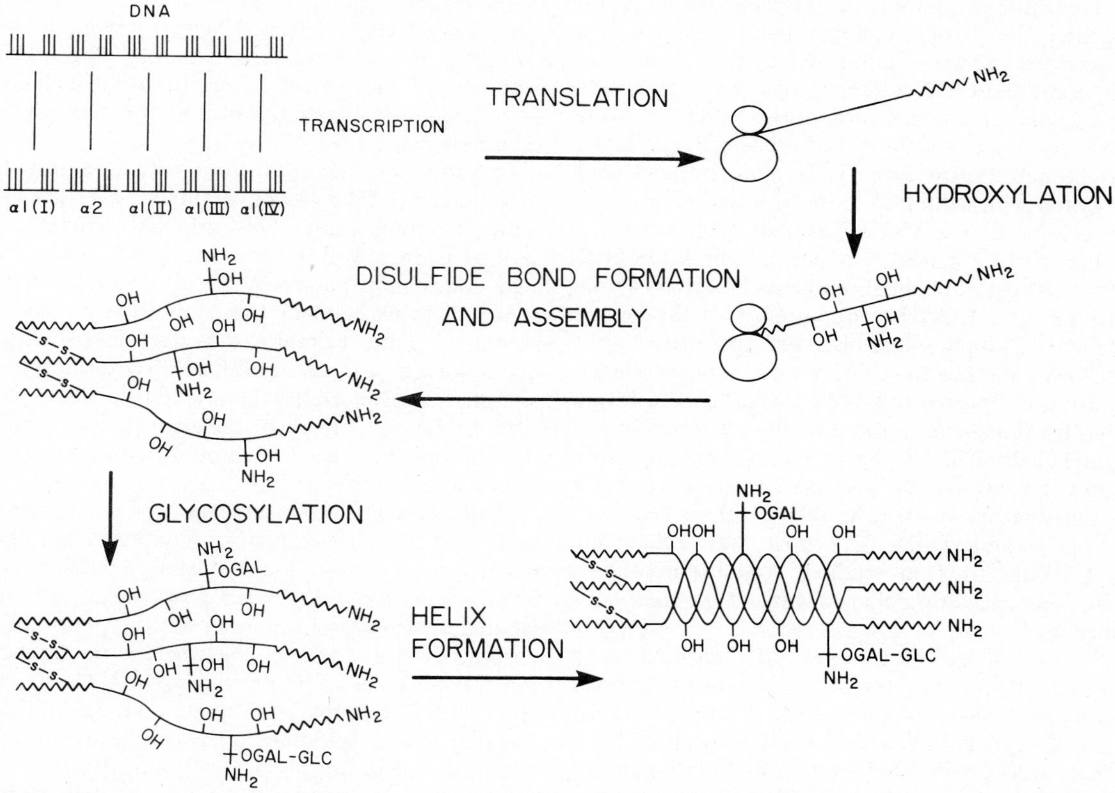


**Figure 14–3.** Biosynthesis of collagen. Each pro α chain is a distinct gene product. Messenger RNA is translated on membrane-bound ribosomes. As the pro α chains are being assembled and fed into the cisternae of the rough endoplasmic reticulum, certain prolyl and lysyl residues become hydroxylated by the action of prolyl and lysyl hydroxylases, and some of the susceptible hydroxylysyl residues are glycosylated by the action of glycosyl transferases. Following completion of the chain synthesis, chains align and disulfide bonds form at the COOH-terminal extension peptides. Helix formation then follows, and the assembled procollagen molecules are secreted to the extracellular space.

chains contains extensions of "noncollagenous" peptides at the $NH_2$- and COOH-termini.[28,29] These biosynthetic precursors of the collagen $\alpha$ chains have been designated pro-$\alpha$ chains. The role of the noncollagenous extension peptides is not known with certainty. Since the pro-$\alpha$ chains contain several residues of cystine in the extension peptides, it has been suggested that they facilitate the association of the three chains into a triple-helical structure (procollagen) by providing interchain disulfide bonds.[26,30] Since the $NH_2$-terminal end of a polypeptide chain is synthesized first,[31] association of these extensions on three separate pro-$\alpha$ chains might initiate the formation of a triple helix while the growing chains are still attached to ribosomes. Another role suggested for the extension peptides is that they render the procollagen molecule more soluble under physiologic conditions of pH, ionic strength, and temperature and keep the molecules from polymerizing into fibrils until transported into the extracellular space.[32] The $NH_2$-terminus of the procollagen polypeptide chain contains, in addition, a pre-pro segment (signal sequence), as do other newly synthesized proteins. This hydrophobic segment binds the molecule to the ribosome and is rapidly cleaved as the polypeptide chain passes through the membrane of the endoplasmic reticulum into the cisternae.[33]

**The Collagen Genes.** The five different collagen types thus far identified in mammalian systems are made up of nine genetically distinct collagen polypeptide chains, which therefore require a minimum of nine structural genes. Recombinant DNA technology has now made possible a partial characterization of the $\alpha 1$(I) and $\alpha 2$(I) genes (for review see refs. 34 and 35). The $\alpha 2$(I) collagen gene has been the most extensively characterized, and this discussion will be limited to its structure. The entire $\alpha 2$(I) gene consists of a 38-kilobase pair (kbp) segment, which codes for the helical region containing 338 Gly-X-Y triplets, short nonhelical telopeptide regions at the $NH_2$-terminal and COOH-terminal ends of the helical molecule, the 125-amino-acid $NH_2$-terminal procollagen $\alpha 2$(I) end-piece and the 264 COOH-terminal procollagen $\alpha 2$(I) end-piece representing 1442 amino acid residues, not including the signal peptide of the pre-procollagen polypeptide chain. The 38-kbp DNA has approximately eight times the number of base pairs required to code for the protein (Fig. 14–4). The RNA transcribed from this 38-kbp genomic DNA, like most other eukaryotic transcript RNAs thus far studied, contains numerous noncoding sequences (introns) that interrupt their coding sequences (exons).

The intron-exon structure was first identified using electron microscopic pictures of mRNA-DNA hybrids (Fig. 14–4) and was confirmed with the partial DNA sequence analysis. Utilizing the established amino acid sequence of $\alpha 2$(I), the DNA coding only the exon regions could be determined as well as the exact intron-exon junctions. Each exon is a multiple of the 9 bp, the required number of a single collagen triplet (Gly-X-Y), and begins by coding for Gly. An estimated 41 or 42 exons code for the complete triple-helical region; an additional 4 exons, for the COOH-terminal procollagen end-piece; and 2 or 3 exons, for the $NH_2$-terminal procollagen end-piece (Fig. 14–5). This suggests there must be at least 50 coding exons and an equal number of intervening introns. The DNA sequence of the introns segmenting the triple-helical coding exons has no repeating Gly-X-Y sequence; in fact little homology is found between intron and exon DNA sequences. The introns range in size from 86 bp to 2000 bp, and the length of the exons varies from 45 to 108 bp. Seven of the 14 exons thus far identified contain 54 bp each, and two contain 108 bp (multiple of 54), indicating a certain degree of repetition $(Gly\text{-}X\text{-}Y)_6$. The latter structure may represent a primordial gene which grew through duplication and recombination. Recombination between two exons at nonidentical positions within the 9 bp coding for the Gly-X-Y repeat is not possible, since it would result in disruption of the helical structure of collagen and thus be fatal. Therefore, the exon size must always be a multiple of 9 bp, and it is most frequently a 54-bp segment.

There are no definite exon-intron junctions separating either the triple-helical region, the telopeptides, or the initial segments of the procollagen end-piece. For example, the exon at the $NH_2$-terminal helical end codes for a COOH-terminal segment of the procollagen end-piece, all of the telopeptide, and the first three residues of the helical region. A somewhat similar situation occurs at the COOH-terminal helical region. These inclusive regions within one exon structure suggest that these segments of the nonhelical region are also highly conserved regions, especially around the procollagen peptidase cleavage sites.

In summary, the total amino acid sequence of the procollagen $\alpha 2$(I) molecule requires a 6-kb mRNA molecule for translation. This mRNA molecule is transcribed from a 38-kbp genomic DNA segment, which also codes approximately 50 interrupting intron segments. The excision of these multiple noncoding segments from the primary transcript RNA with subsequent splicing to form a 6-kb mRNA molecule requires complex nuclear multistep assembly process with possibly a nuclear control mechanism prior to the cytosol translation and post-translational control mechanisms of collagen synthesis.

**Protocollagen Hydroxylases.** As mentioned previously, the two characteristic amino acids of collagen are hydroxyproline and hydroxylysine. Neither of them, however, is genetically coded. Exogenously administered labeled hydroxyproline and hydroxylysine are not incorporated into collagen, and there is no clear evidence for the existence of hydroxyprolyl-tRNA or hydroxylysyl-tRNA. Isotopic experiments have established that the two amino acids are biosynthetically formed from precursor residues of proline and lysine in peptide chains, respectively, by the action of two specific oxygenases, *protocollagen proline hydroxylase* and *protocollagen lysine hydroxylase.*[26,36,37]

Protocollagen hydroxylases have now been isolated from various connective tissues in a highly purified state, and their requirements for the cofactors and the se-

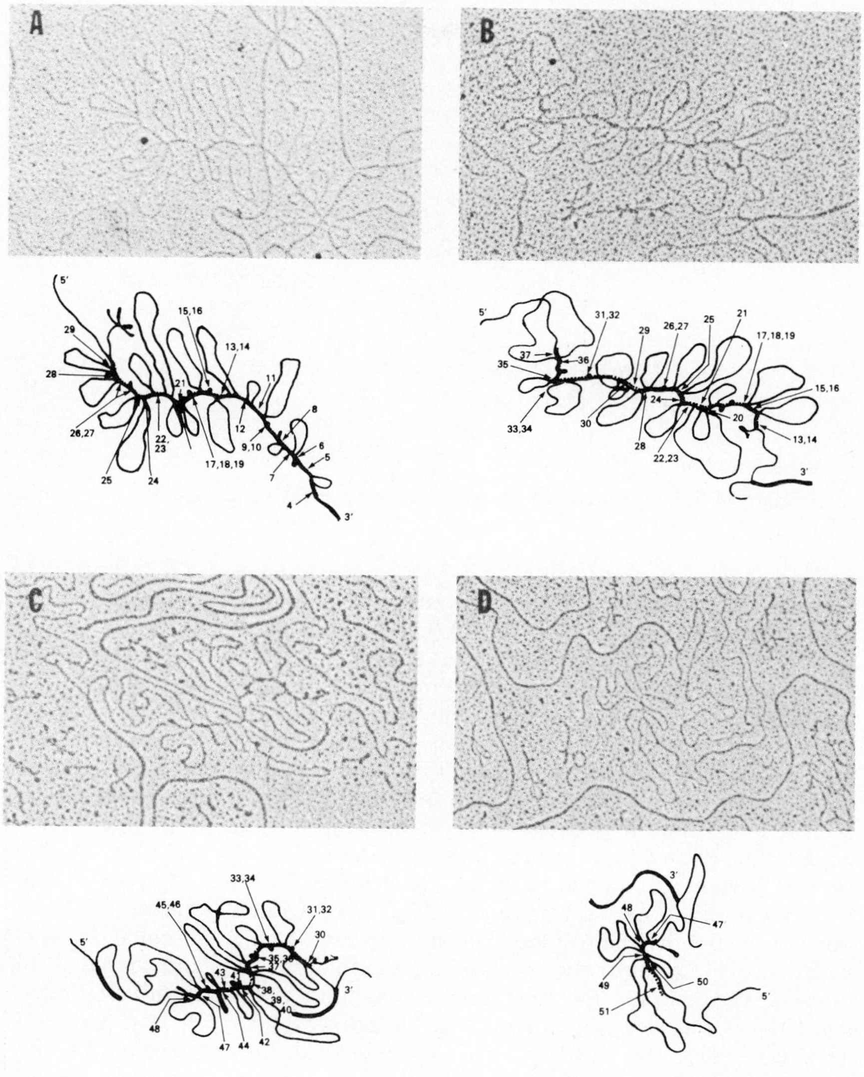


**Figure 14–4.** Electron microscopic pictures and diagrams of the hybrids between the DNAs of four representative overlapping clones and the chicken $\alpha 2$ mRNA. The coding sequences (exons) are numbered from the 3′ end of the gene. The loops and nodes represent intervening sequences (introns) of varying sizes. Measurements of these lengths provide evidence that the recombinant clones are truly overlapping. (From Ohkubo H., et al.: Proc. Natl. Acad. Sci. USA 77:7061, 1980, with permission of authors and publisher.)

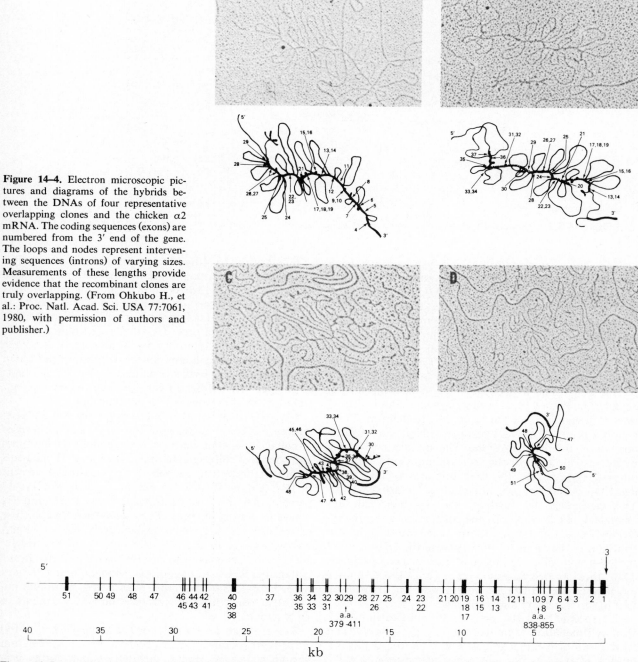

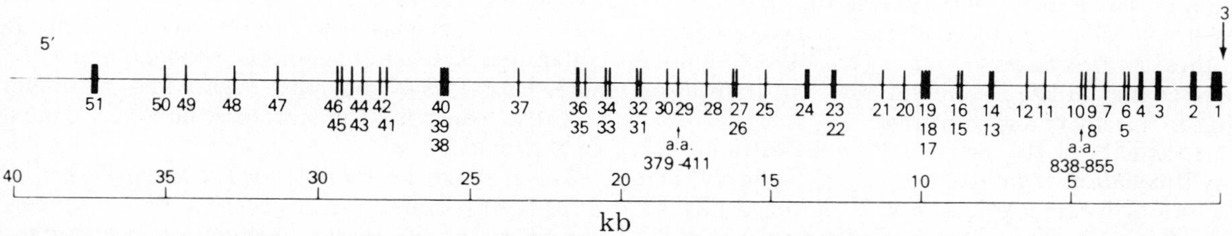


**Figure 14–5.** Graphic representation of measurements of coding and intervening sequences of the chicken $\alpha 2$ gene. The measurements were based on electromicroscopic pictures of DNA-mRNA hybrids (Fig. 14–4). Each vertical band represents the coding sequence or exon, and the lines between the bars correspond to intervening sequences or introns. Note that the coding information of the $\alpha 2$ collagen chain is divided into approximately 50 coding segments, which are separated by intervening sequences of various lengths. The length of the noncoding sequences varies but in general is much greater than the coding sequences. (From Ohkubo H., et al.: Proc. Natl. Acad. Sci. USA 77:7061, 1980, with permission of authors and publisher.)

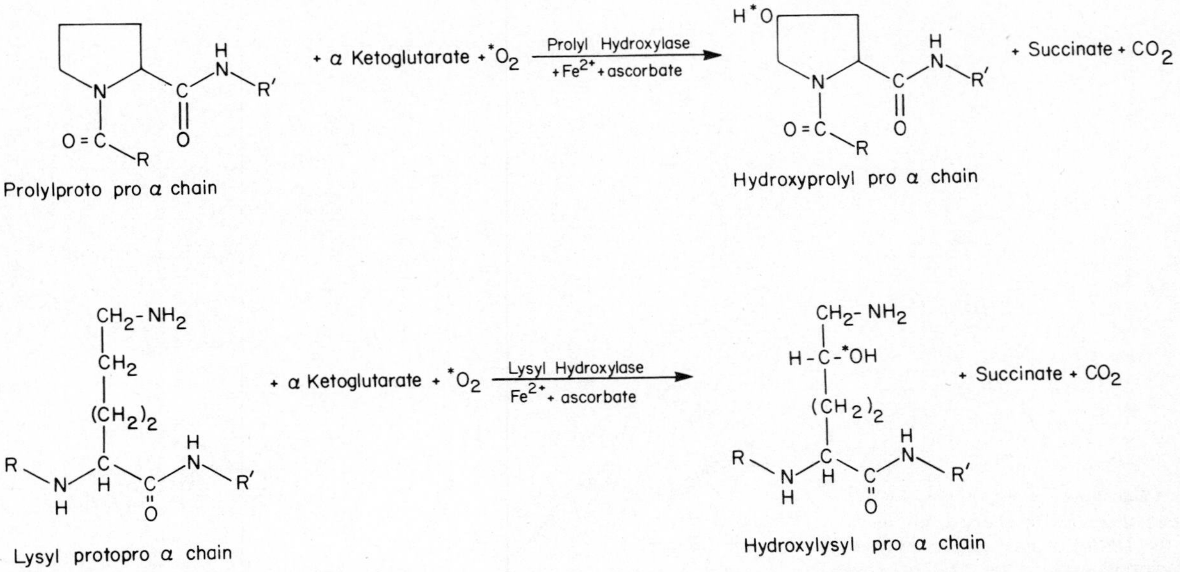


**Figure 14–6.** Biosynthesis of hydroxyproline and hydroxylysine. Unhydroxylated pro α chain is referred to as protopro α chain.

quence of the substrate prolyl and lysyl peptides have been characterized.[26,33] The enzyme systems require molecular oxygen (Km = $1 \times 10^{-5}$ M), $Fe^{2+}$ ions (Km = $1 \times 10^{-6}$ M) and α-ketoglutarate (Km = $5 \times 10^{-6}$ M) for their activity. The requirements for these substances are absolute and specific. The systems also require the presence of a reducing agent, but this agent is not specific and may be ascorbic acid or other reducing compounds. The mechanism of action of protocollagen proline and lysine hydroxylases has been proposed as depicted in Figure 14–6; protocollagen lysine hydroxylase is thought to act via a similar mechanism. Polypeptidyl proline forms a hydroperoxide at the 4 (trans) position of the proline residue. The anionic form of the hydroperoxide attacks the α-ketoglutarate to form an intermediate complex; this then is decarboxylated, yielding $CO_2$, succinate, and polypeptidyl hydroxyproline. This mechanism is consistent with the observed stoichiometry of the reactants, the concomitant decarboxylation of α-ketoglutarate to form succinate, and the distribution of the atoms of $^{18}O_2$ between the OH-group of the hydroxyproline residue and the formed succinate. Thus, these hydroxylases are among the class of unique oxygenases that utilize α-ketoglutarate and transfer an O atom to succinate and substrate.

The specificity of the enzymes for substrates is such that hydroxylation is limited to only those prolyl and lysyl residues located at position Y of the triplet sequence of (Gly-X-Y)n and never at position X.[14,26,36] Substrates of (Gly-X-Y)n in smaller than 50 triplets are poorly hydroxylated or not hydroxylated at all. Further, hydroxylation is possible only if the substrates are denatured and the triple-helical structure abolished. Although the precise intracellular site at which hydroxylation takes place is controversial, the major site of hydroxylation is probably the nascent chains, concurrent with translation on ribosomes.[26,36]

In addition to 4-hydroxyproline, there are smaller amounts of 3-hydroxyproline in various collagens (see Table 14–1). Very little is known about its biosynthesis or function. In the only case in which the residue is located in the type I collagen sequence, 3-hydroxyproline follows glycine and precedes 4-hydroxyproline.[12] No 3-hydroxyproline is found in type III collagen, but bovine type IV collagen contains up to 10 residues per chain in certain tissues. Evidence indicates that its synthesis is catalyzed by a different enzyme than the one responsible for the synthesis of 4-hydroxyproline.

**Glycosylation.** Another interesting feature of collagen structure is the occurrence of covalently bound hexoses in collagen. The amounts vary, depending on the types and source of collagens. In most type I and III collagens from vertebrates, the carbohydrate content is 1 percent or less; in type II, it is 5.5 percent; and in type IV, 12 percent. All the carbohydrates in type I, II, and III collagens consist of either the monosaccharide galactose or the disaccharide glucosylgalactose bound via O-glycosidic linkage to the δ-hydroxy group of hydroxylysine.[1,2] The same is true for the basement membrane collagen except that, in addition, small amounts of mannose, hexosamine, and other sugars may be bound covalently;[19] their linkage structure, however, remains to be elucidated.

The enzymes responsible for the glycosylation of hydroxylysyl residues of collagen have been isolated from various connective tissues, including kidney cortex, cartilage, and uterus.[26,39,40] Both *glucosyl-* and *galactosyltransferases* have been prepared. The UDP-galactose:hydroxylysine-collagen galactosyl transferase can transfer a galactose unit to a hydroxylysine residue of collagen. It cannot transfer galactose to free hydroxylysine or to small peptides containing hydroxylysine. The UDP–glucose:galactosyl–hydroxylysine–collagen glucosyl–transferase can transfer a glucose unit to hydroxylysine-linked galactose in either high or low molecular weight compounds. Both enzymes require a divalent cation, particularly $Mn^{2+}$, and they act in sequence so that galactose is added to hydroxylysine, and then glucose. It is not clear where these glycosyl transferases are located, and seemingly conflicting evidence locates these enzymes in either the cytoplasm or plasma membrane of cells.

**Secretion by the Cells.** Finally, the completed triple-stranded procollagen molecule is secreted by cells into the extracellular space, where the $NH_2$- and COOH-terminal extension peptides are proteolytically removed by the action of specific procollagen peptidases, yielding the triple helical collagen molecule (Fig. 14–7). Separate amino and carboxyl procollagen endopeptidases cleave pro $\alpha 1(I)$ and pro $\alpha 2(I)$ chains at specific sites.[41] The same excision of procollagen end-pieces occurs with type II, type III, and type V collagen, although different propeptidases are required. With type IV collagen, there is no evidence that any such processing of the procollagen molecule occurs, and it appears that the intact procollagen molecule may in fact be deposited in the tissue. The above procollagen peptidases are inhibited by EDTA but not by serine protease inhibitors.[42]

In summary, the biosynthesis of collagen has many similarities with that of other proteins, but it is distinguished by at least three prominent features: (1) the genomic structure is extremely large, i.e., eight times larger than necessary to code for the mRNA, (2) the protein is first synthesized in a precursor form known as procollagen, and (3) the biosynthesis involves several unusual post-translational modifications after assembly of amino acids into polypeptide chains. These include hydroxylation of certain prolyl and lysyl residues, glycosylation of certain hydroxylysyl residues, and the formation of disulfide linkages in the peptide extensions of procollagen. These post-translational changes are necessary for some of the biologic functions of collagen. In particular, the hydroxylation of peptidyl proline is essential for folding of the three polypeptide chains into the "correct" triple-helical structure. Hydroxylation of lysyl residues and glycosylation of the hydroxylysyl residues may influence the subsequent formation of interchain crosslinks (discussed below). The importance of these post-translational reactions has been further emphasized by the demonstration that if one or more of the reactions is interfered with, the secretion of procollagen by cells is markedly altered so that either it is not secreted or it is secreted at a reduced rate.

**Collagen Fibrillogenesis.** The mechanism for the formation of fibrils from the triple-helical molecules (Fig. 14–1) still remains unclear. At present, the process appears to involve formation of smaller aggregates from simple monomeric units (triple-helical molecules) with subsequent growth to intermediate size aggregates (for review see ref. 43). The collagen fibril formation then involves a stepwise formation from intermediate aggregates rather than from monomeric molecules. These monomeric procollagen molecules begin to aggregate in the secretory vacuoles of the cells. It is probably during this initial compartmentalization that other macromolecules such as proteoglycans exert influence on the aggregation state and ultimately fibrillogenesis. In this manner of using the same secretory vacuoles, the cell may regulate the stoichiometry of mixing of various connective tissue components and ultimately effect dif-

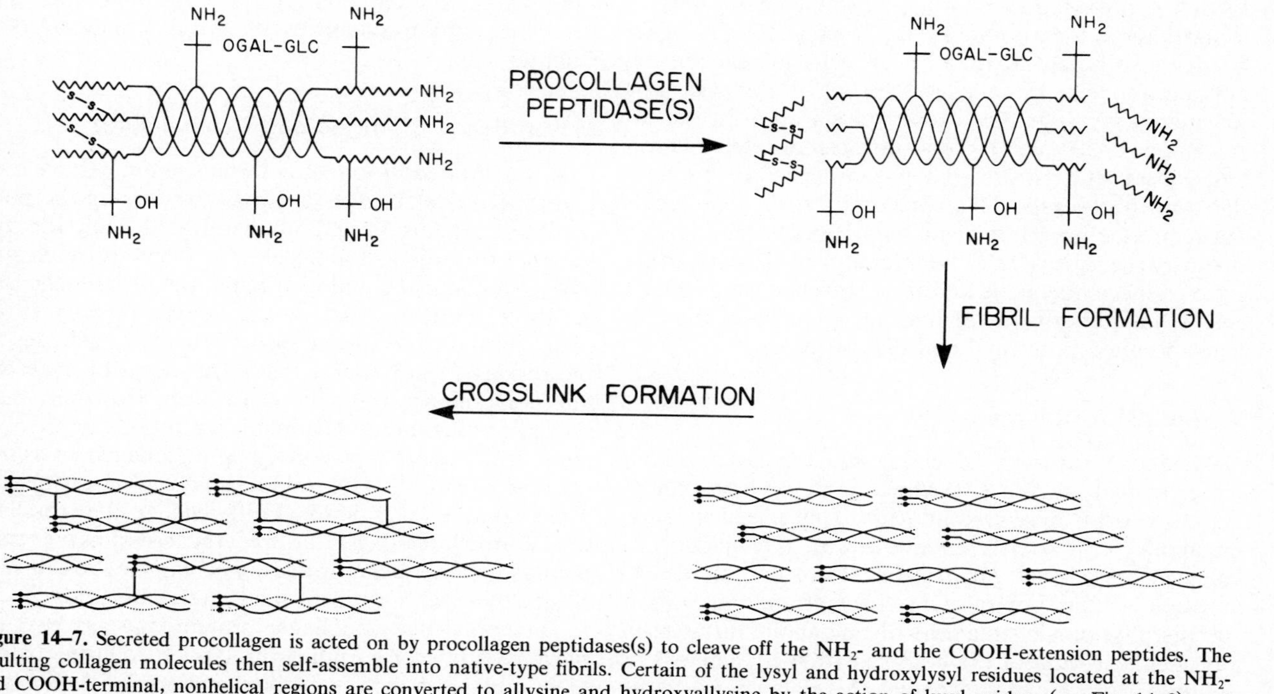


**Figure 14–7.** Secreted procollagen is acted on by procollagen peptidases(s) to cleave off the $NH_2$- and the COOH-extension peptides. The resulting collagen molecules then self-assemble into native-type fibrils. Certain of the lysyl and hydroxylysyl residues located at the $NH_2$- and COOH-terminal, nonhelical regions are converted to allysine and hydroxyallysine by the action of lysyl oxidase (see Fig. 14–8), and crosslinks form (see Fig. 14–9).

ferent morphologies of collagen fibrils. The formation of the small aggregates is most likely initiated through amino terminal–carboxyl terminal attachment of monomeric units by charge-charge interactions, since this process is dependent on the pH and ionic strength. This process sets up the 4D staggered dimers and trimers (Fig. 14–1). Lateral aggregation occurs subsequently by means of both hydrophobic and electrostatic interactions, with the basic unit being a stabilized 5-membered lateral fibril packing assembly. The aggregates then grow in length by the addition of other intermediate aggregates at the end of the subfibril and in width by lateral wrapping of subfibrils. The effects of other collagens and connective tissue macromolecules such as glycoproteins and proteoglycans continue to influence the process of these subassemblies. Ultrastructural data suggest that the latter assembly and fibril growth occur near the cell surface within its indentations. The process of fibrillogenesis therefore remains under continued cellular regulation and influence, since these recesses may act as a microenvironment of the cell surface.

**Intracellular Degradation.** Current evidence suggests that connective tissue cells may be highly inefficient in producing collagen molecules. Variable amounts (10 to 60 percent) of the newly synthesized collagen may be degraded intracellularly prior to secretion (for review, see ref. 44). The appearance of intracellular small peptide fragments of hydroxyproline and hydroxylysine provides unique markers for this process, since hydroxylation of these amino acidly occurs only after polypeptide chain synthesis. One source of this degraded collagen understandably comes from removal of abnormal collagen molecules or errors during synthesis. This is shown when cells are grown without ascorbic acid, which is needed for full hydroxylation, or when a proline analogue such as azetidine is incorporated into the polypeptide chains. It may also be an attempt by the cells to regulate the amount and type of collagen secreted by the cells. For instance, any agent that causes an elevation in the intracellular cAMP can increase intracellular degradation and consequently decrease collagen deposition by lung and skin fibroblasts. This appears to affect type I collagen production more than type III collagen. In this manner, the intracellular degradation of newly synthesized collagen may be an additional mechanism by which cells regulate both the quality and quantity of the collagen secreted in normal and disease states.

## Turnover of Collagen

Metabolic turnover of collagen, as measured in a whole animal or even in a whole tissue such as skin, is very low; $t^1/_2$ is measured in years. This extremely slow metabolic turnover is compatible with the function of collagen as a structural protein. However, this generalization should not obscure the fact that in several specific physiologic situations the metabolic turnover in a particular region of the body is extremely active. For example, during metamorphosis the collagenous tissue present in the tails of tadpoles is rapidly removed and that of back skin swiftly remodeled. Likewise, there must be an active turnover of the collagenous matrix during remodeling of bone. In patients with Paget's disease, in which there is markedly enhanced synthesis and resorption of bone, a marked increase in the urinary secretion of hydroxyproline, hydroxylysine, and its glycosides has been observed.[45-48] Since most hydroxyproline, hydroxylysine, and its glycosides in the blood are of collagenous origin, the urinary excretion of these compounds has been used as an index of collagen metabolism. Various metabolic studies have demonstrated that in states in which there is an increased breakdown of collagen, such as metastatic diseases of bone, hyperparathyroidism, and hyperthyroidism, the urinary excretion of the imino acid in the form of both free imino acid and oligopeptides and hydroxylysine glycosides is markedly increased; but that in states in which there is an increased synthesis of collagen, such as during growth, the urinary excretion of hydroxyproline in polypeptide form is increased.[46] Thus, an increase in the ratio of nondialyzable to low molecular weight hydroxyproline is found in states in which synthesis of collagen exceeds breakdown.

The mechanism of the resorption of collagen has been the subject of considerable interest, since collagen in the native state is resistant to attack by most proteolytic enzymes at physiologic pH and temperature, although it is degraded by a wide variety of proteolytic enzymes once the molecule is denatured (or the helical structures disrupted). It has recently been shown that physiologic breakdown of collagen is accomplished by the action of specific collagenases produced in extremely small amounts in situ where needed. Such specific collagenase activity has been demonstrated in many physiologic and pathologic situations, and the enzyme has been purified from several different sources.[49-51] Their molecular characteristics and mechanisms of action are detailed in Chapter 13.

## Maturational Changes and Crosslinking

After the deposition of collagen in the extracellular matrix, covalent bridges or crosslinks among the polypeptide $\alpha$ chains form both within the molecule and between the adjacent molecules.[52,53] There is much similarity in the crosslinking mechanism of collagen and elastin in that the crosslinks are derived from lysyl residues through the formation of reactive aldehydes by the action of *lysyl oxidase,*[54] and that some of the crosslink compounds are common to both. However, there are major differences. The first is the prominent involvement of the hydroxylysyl residues in collagen crosslinking rather than the lysyl residues solely as seen in elastin. The second is the functional difference in the crosslinkages formed. Collagen utilizes the crosslinking compounds for interchain bridges, whereas the crosslinks in elastin serve as both intra- and interchain bridges.

The knowledge of collagen crosslinking has been derived mostly from studies on type I collagen, which predominates in dermis, tendon, and bone. Specific lysyl and hydroxylysyl residues located in the nonhelical $NH_2$-

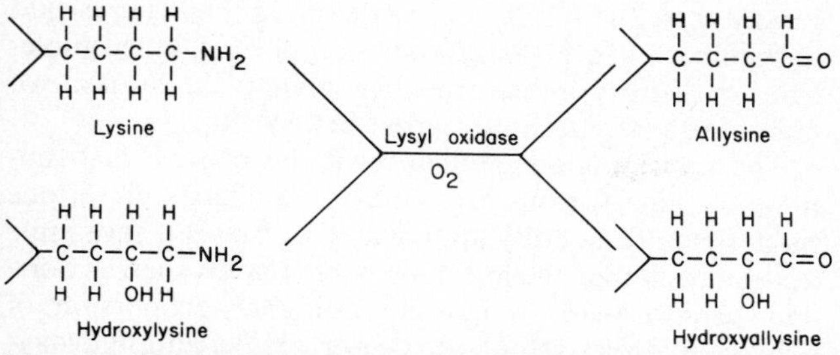


**Figure 14–8.** Oxidative deamination of peptide bound lysine and hydroxylysine by the action of lysyl. Allysine is formed both in collagen and elastin. Hydroxyallysine is found only in collagen.

and COOH-terminal regions of the α chains are converted to aldehydes, α-amino adipic-δ-semialdehyde (allysine, Fig. 14–8) and δ-hydroxy-α-amino adipic-δ-semialdehyde, respectively (hydroxyallysine, Fig. 14–8). These are catalyzed by the action of lysyl oxidase,[54] which is pyridoxal dependent and requires $Cu^{2+}$ for action. Apparently only the residues in the nonhelical portions of the collagen molecule are oxidatively deaminated, and the similar residues in the more rigid triple-helical region are not affected. Whether this is a result of enzyme specificity for a certain amino acid sequence present only in the $NH_2$- and COOH-termini, or a result of steric inaccessibility of the triple-helical region to the enzymes, is not known.

Once the aldehydes are formed, they undergo two basic types of reactions.[52,53] The first is the formation of aldamine bonds (Schiff bases) with ε-amino groups of lysine or hydroxylysine from an adjacent polypeptide chain, thus forming $\Delta^{6,7}$ dehydrolysinonorleucine, $\Delta^{6,7}$ dehydrohydroxylysinonorleucine, or $\Delta^{6,7}$ dehydrohydroxylysinohydroxynorleucine (Fig. 14–9). These compounds are unstable during acid hydrolysis and have been isolated from tissues in their reduced forms following chemical reduction with borohydride. The relative proportions of these aldamine crosslinks vary according to the source of tissues. Thus, hydroxylysinonorleucine predominates in dermal collagen, whereas hydroxylysinohydroxynorleucine represents the major aldamine crosslink in the more insoluble collagen present in bone and tendon. Lysinonorleucine is usually a minor component in normal collagenous tissues. Tissue differences in these aldamine crosslinks appear, therefore, to be controlled by the degree of post-translational lysyl hydroxylation.

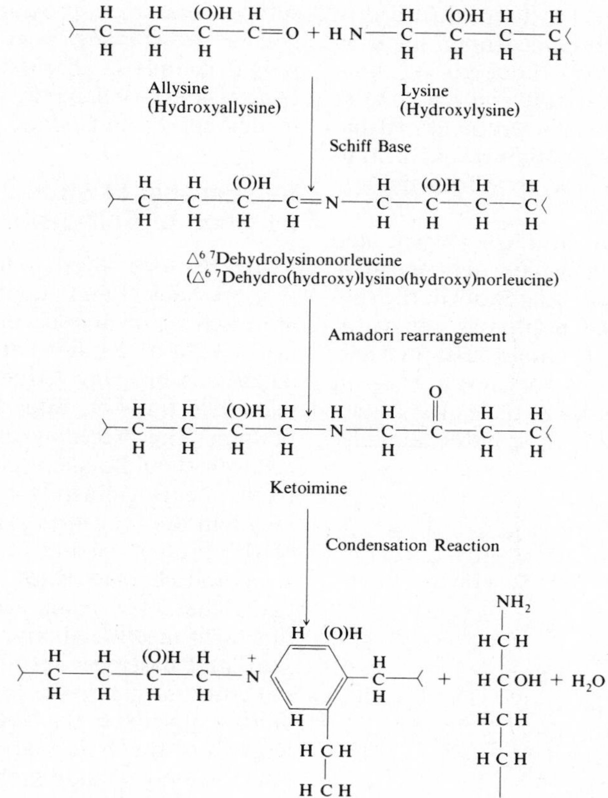


**Figure 14–9.** Aldamine crosslinks of collagen. Natural reduction of the double bond between N and C of the dehydro compounds apparently does not occur in collagen. In elastin, both dehydrolysinonorleucine and its reduced form lysinonorleucine are found. Hydroxylysine-containing crosslinks in collagen become stabilized by the formation of ketoimine structures by Amadori rearrangement. The proposed condensation of two ketoimine structures yields a hydroxypyridinium residue and free hydroxylysine.

These aldamine compounds apparently undergo Amadori rearrangement reactions to form keto-imine structures (Fig. 14–9), which are much more stable than the Schiff base forms and probably help explain the stability of the tissues to heat and dilute acid. A more stable trifunctional crosslink has recently been isolated from tendon, bone, and cartilage.[55] This crosslink, named hydroxypyridinoline (Fig. 14–9), appears to originate by the condensation of three amino acid side-chains (one hydroxylysine and two hydroxyallysine) to form a cyclic 3-hydroxypyridinoline. This crosslink compound, which links three collagen chains, increases in amount with age of the tissue and does not require prior borohydride reduction for its isolation. Its specific position within the collagen polypeptide chains remains undetermined.[55] The hexose-linked hydroxylysyl residues also participate as the amino donors to the aldamine bonds, especially in tissues of older animals. The compounds glucosylgalactosyl dehydrohydroxylysinohydroxynorleucine and galactosyl dehydrohydroxylysinohydroxynorleucine have been identified in mature dermis. What effects the sugar moiety imparts to the individual crosslinks are unknown.

The second basic type of crosslink compounds found in collagen originates from an aldol condensation reaction of two allysine residues with the formation of the corresponding dehydrated aldol (Fig. 14–10). This type of lysine-derived aldol crosslink has been identified in soft tissue collagens of dermis and tendon (and in elastin). The aldol condensate can undergo a further series of reactions with hydroxylysine and histidine to give rise to tri- and tetra-functional crosslinks, dehydrohydroxymerodesmosine, aldolhistidine, and histidinohydroxymerodesmosine.[2,56] These crosslinks link together three or four $\alpha$ chains.

It should be mentioned that although allysine and hydroxyallysine formation is enzymatically mediated, once these functional groups have been formed, the subsequent aldamine and aldol condensation as well as the histidine addition can proceed spontaneously in vitro. Whether this is also true in vivo is not known. It seems unnecessary, however, to hypothesize the existence of a separate enzyme system mediating these latter reactions.

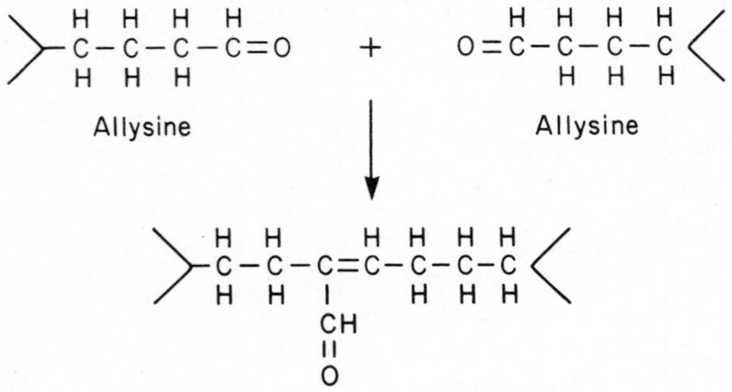


**Figure 14–10.** Aldol condensation product between two residues of allysine. This crosslink is found in both collagen and elastin.

In any case, the result of crosslinking of collagen is that it becomes then an enormous complex of macromolecules covalently linked together, giving rise to tissue of high tensile strength and great insolubility.

The physiologic significance of the relative distributions of these various crosslinks in collagens of various tissues cannot be fully appreciated at present. Available data suggest that the more insoluble tissues such as bone and tendon tend to contain a higher proportion of dehydrohydroxylysinohydroxynorleucine, and hydroxypyridinoline, whereas the tissues such as dermis, the collagen of which is slightly more soluble, contain a higher content of relatively less stable dehydrohydroxylysinonorleucine. Likewise, scar tissue of skin tends to contain a higher content of the more stable dehydrohydroxylysinohydroxynorleucine as compared with the normal skin.

The nature of crosslinks in type II, III, IV, and V collagens has not been investigated to the same extent as that of type I collagen. Presumably similar crosslinks will be found but with tissue-specific and age-specific variations. For instance, cartilage contains predominantly the more stable hydroxyallysine- and hydroxylysine-derived crosslinks. Type III collagen contains two cysteine residues at the COOH-terminus of the triple helix, and these participate in intramolecular crosslinks. Type IV contains numerous inter- and intrachain disulfide crosslinks, providing this collagen with even greater crosslinking capabilities. The high molecular weight complexes discussed earlier contain many cysteine residues, which may bind noncollagenous proteins to this poorly understood collagenous complex.[23,24]

## Relationship of Structure and Biologic Function of Collagen

In order for collagen to function as a structural protein in a mechanical and supportive role, several properties are essential or at least desirable; it must be insoluble in the kind of solutions encountered under physiologic conditions in living tissue; it must have a low overall metabolic turnover rate; and its tensile strength must be high. The preceding discussion on the structure of collagen should make it clear that collagen meets these requirements eminently well. Throughout the animal kingdom the rigid preservation of the general structure of the protein further attests to the suitability of its structural characteristics.

On the other hand, since collagen serves different functions in different tissues such as in bone, tendon, skin, and basement membrane, many variations in its structure must also be possible. Knowledge of the relationship between the biologic properties and the salient features of the molecular structure is of utmost importance in understanding structural bases for functional abnormalities found in pathologic states. In connective tissue it has been particularly difficult to obtain this type of information, largely because of the enormous complexity of the constituent macromolecules. Nevertheless, data are beginning to accumulate which have bearing on our understanding, and an attempt is made here to discuss the general principles of what is known about this important subject.

**Tissue-Specific Differences in Collagen Primary Structures.** The properties of the collagen molecule and the higher order of structures that collagen forms are dictated largely by the primary structure and the post-synthetic alterations discussed above, hydroxylation of prolyl and lysyl residues, glycosylation, proteolytic conversion of procollagen to collagen, and crosslinking. In some instances, tissue-specific differences in one or more aspects of the primary structure of collagen have been found. In addition, there are tissue-specific differences in the relative distribution of various types of collagens (Table 14–2).

*Soft Tissue Collagens.* Most soft tissues such as skin, tendon, and loose interstitial connective tissues of internal organs, including lung, liver, spleen, intestine, and uterus, contain two types of the protein present in the various tissues; however, these differ considerably. Although the data are not complete, they indicate that the loose connective tissues of the parenchymal organs contain 30 to 40 percent type III, the remainder being type I.[57] Tendon, on the other hand, consists predominantly of type I collagen, with only 5 to 10 percent type III. Skin is intermediate in this respect, with approximately 20 to 30 percent type III.[58] It would appear from this kind of survey that the tissues that require a high tensile strength are relatively richer in type I collagen than the loose connective tissues requiring a lesser degree of mechanical integrity. The findings that the relative content of type I collagen increases in the human dermis during late fetal development and early childhood[59] and that the relative content of type I collagen in scar tissues is increased during wound healing[59] provide support for this interpretation.

Nothing is known about the manner in which the two types of collagen molecules are organized within the tissues. The primary amino acid sequence of type I collagens in various tissues appears to be identical, and the same probably is true for type III collagens. The only differences known so far have been the microheterogeneity in the degree of hydroxylation of prolyl and lysyl residues and, therefore, the degree of glycosylation.[13] Although the data are not available, one can infer that there will be some differences in crosslinking arising from the variations in hydroxylysine and hydroxylysine glycosides.

The content of type IV and type V collagen in all tissues including skin is exceedingly small. Since type IV collagen represents the basement-membrane-specific collagen, its presence in any organ containing lamina densa must be expected.[60] In many cases, however, quantitation is impossible except by the immunofluorescent staining of such structures in connective tissues. Organs such as lung and liver understandably contain more basement membrane and type IV collagen than skin, bone, and tendon. The ubiquitous nature of type V collagen has also become more apparent. The fact that smooth muscle cells in culture produce greater amounts of type V collagen and tissues containing larger quantities of smooth muscle, i.e., placenta, lung, liver, and amnionic/chorionic membranes, contain up to 6 percent of their total collagen as type V led to the proposal that this was a smooth muscle collagen. The immunofluorescent studies, however, indicate that this collagen is associated primarily with the cell plasma membrane and not the interstitial mileu; hence its classification as an exocytoskeleton has developed. This may be important in cell–interstitial matrix interactions.[22]

*Bone Collagen.* Studies on the mineralization of bone and dentin indicate that this orderly process is governed by the ultrastructural organization of the collagen fibrils in these tissues, allowing specific compartmentalization of tissue spaces where mineralization can proceed.[25] Knowledge of the structure and properties of bone collagen is essential in understanding physiologic and pathologic bone formation.

Bone contains only type I collagen, and its $\alpha$ chain constitution and amino acid composition are indistinguishable from type I collagen of skin.[59] However, it has been shown, in bone, that the precursor lysyl residue for crosslinking located near the $NH_2$-termini of the $\alpha$ chains is partially hydroxylated, with the result that the predominant crosslink formed is dehydrohydroxylysinohydroxynorleucine. In addition, the content of polyfunctional crosslinks is lower than that found in skin. What effect these differences in crosslink structure have on fibril properties is difficult to assess. It seems likely that the intermolecular forces that stabilize the fibrillar organization may be influenced in some way so as to favor mineralization. The importance of the hole zone in the fibril packing in relation to mineralization was mentioned previously.

*Cartilage Collagen.* Hyaline cartilage, such as that from xiphoid and articular cartilage, contains largely type II collagen.[59] Fibrocartilages are composed of type II as well as type I collagen.[59] Type II collagen contains 5.5 percent carbohydrate by weight, as compared to the type I chains, which contain less than 1 percent.

Since the osseous tissues develop from cartilaginous structures, the implication of the finding is that there must exist a mechanism that controls the systematic replacement of one type of collagen molecule with another during osteogenesis. Theoretically, it is possible that a derangement in the control mechanism of the collagen turnover at this site could be the origin of some of the diseases of bone.

Cartilage also contains a type V–like collagen ($1\alpha$, $2\alpha$, and $3\alpha$ collagen chains). These appear to be different from their soft tissue type V collagen counterparts, although their function may be the same. Immunofluorescent studies of cartilaginous tissues have demonstrated their presence only around the chondrocytes as opposed to the bulk of the interstitial cartilage matrix.[22] These chains do, however, appear to be unique for cartilage in the same manner as type II collagen.

*Basement Membrane Collagen.* Recent studies have indicated that the major structural component of lamina densa is type IV collagen (Fig. 14–11). Tissues rich in

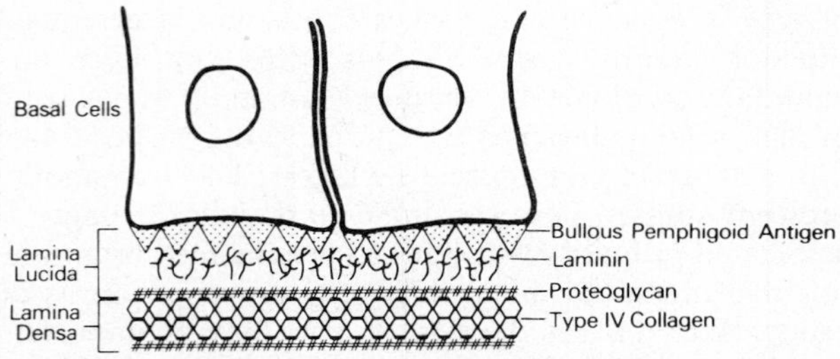


**Figure 14–11.** Schematic diagram of the epidermal basement membrane zone. Bullous pemphigoid antigen is localized to the lamina lucida by immunoelectron microscopy and is also closely associated with the basal cell plasma membrane. Laminin is localized to the lamina lucida as well and consists of three short chains as a long chain (molecular weights, 200,000 and 400,000). The basement membrane proteoglycan appears to be localized to both edges of the lamina densa. Type IV collagen is probably in a reticular pattern in the electron dense zone, the lamina densa. (From Stanley, J.R., et al.: J. Invest. Dermatol. 79:685, 1982, with permission of authors and publisher.)

basement membrane structures such as renal glomeruli and anterior lens capsule have been the major source of information on type IV collagen.[60-63] Two procollagen chains are synthesized by partial yolk sac cells, i.e., $\alpha 1(IV)$ and $\alpha 2(IV)$. Their molecular weights are 180,000 and 165,000, which are consistent with those of other procollagens. All of the post-translational modifications described above are necessary, except possibly for procollagen peptidase cleavage.

Evidence now suggests that the entire procollagen molecule is deposited into a loosely woven matrix unlike that observed with the interstitial collagens (Fig. 14–12). Both intermolecular disulfide and lysine-derived

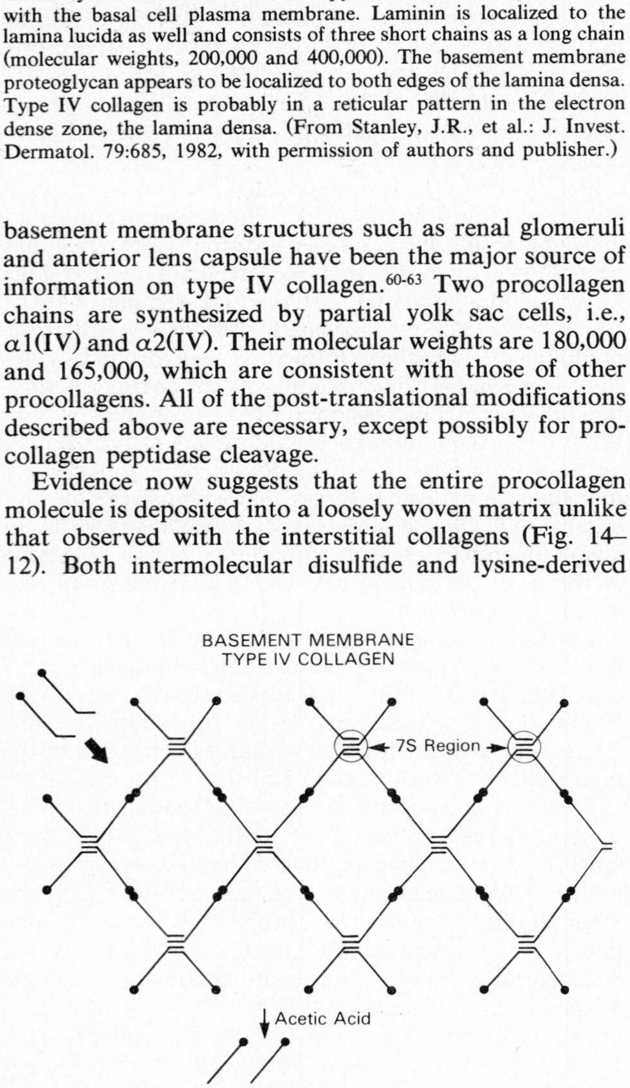


**Figure 14–12.** The model proposed for the arrangement of type IV collagen molecules in basement membrane. Type IV collagen molecules are incorporated into a netlike structure with the like ends of the molecule in apposition and presumably crosslinked. The 7S region refers to the part of the net where the $NH_2$-terminus of four triple-helical molecules align and form a very stable structure with both lysine-derived and disulfide inter- and intramolecular crosslinks. The COOH-terminal ends of the type IV molecules are "ball" shaped and presumably globular structures with uncertain crosslinks. (From Stanley, J.R., et al: J. Invest. Dermatol. 79:70s, 1982, with permission of authors and publisher.)

crosslinks contribute to its extreme insolubility. Most of the information on the structure of type IV collagen has been derived from limited pepsin digestion to produce $\alpha$ chain size molecules, $\alpha 1(IV)$ and $\alpha 2(IV)$, with amino acid compositions shown in Table 14–1. This pepsin-derived basement membrane collagen contains nearly one third glycine and has secondary and tertiary structures similar to other collagens.[61] The content of hydroxylysine is elevated, as is that of carbohydrate. Higher amounts of 3-hydroxyproline are present in bovine but not human placenta type IV collagen. One unusual characteristic is that in some cases, glycine does not appear at every third residue. Therefore, a less compact helix is present and nonspecific protease digestion can occur, such as with pepsin, to yield a heterogeneous mixture of collagenous components varying from $>220{,}000$ to 25,000 molecular weight. Amino acid sequence analyses have confirmed these "flaws" in the triplet sequence in type IV collagen chains, especially the $\alpha 2(IV)$ polypeptide chain. At present, it is uncertain whether the molecular structure consists of $[\alpha 1(IV)]_2$-$\alpha 2(IV)$ or two molecular forms having identical subunits. Quantitation is difficult because of the extreme susceptibility of the $\alpha 2(IV)$ polypeptide chain to nonspecific proteolysis even in its native state.

As stated previously, the type IV collagen appears to be deposited in the tissue as a large procollagen-like molecule. Immunofluorescent staining has pinpointed the location of this collagen in the lamina densa of the basement membrane. With milder extraction procedures and the use of a mouse tumor, several salient features have been demonstrated. The $NH_2$-terminal propeptide portion of the procollagen molecule contains collagenous regions rich in cysteine in addition to noncollagenous segments. Multiple disulfide and lysine-derived crosslinks are present in this domain, from which a highly crosslinked aggregate (referred to as 7S based on its sedimentation coefficient) can be obtained. In this complex, a minimum of 4 triple-helical molecules are densely crosslinked (see Fig. 14–12). The carboxyl-terminal region of the type IV procollagen molecule contains "ball-like" structures when visualized by rotary shadowing techniques. This, therefore, must contain a globular, non-triple-helical region as seen with the procollagen end-pieces of interstitial collagens.

In summary, several features of type IV collagn distinguish it from the interstitial collagens. Whether or not the entire procollagen molecule is indeed deposited in the tissue or an even larger polypeptide chain is synthesized remains a controversy. Regardless, previous dogma concerning strict structural characteristics of interstitial collagen does not hold true for type IV. The departure from or substitution of glycine at every third residue in limited areas of the triple-helical region of the polypeptide chain renders the native molecule susceptible to nonspecific protease cleavage by enzymes such as mast cell protease and elastase and enzymes from tumor cells, the latter being perhaps important in tumor invasion through basement membrane structures.[17,63]

***Reticulin.*** Reticulin is primarily a histologic phenomenon describing particular kinds of fibers that are abundantly seen in embryonic connective tissues and in some tissues of adults. In contrast to collagen fibers, which are in nonbranching coarse bundles, reticular fibers form a delicate network of freely branching fibers that stain black by a silver impregnation technique. It has long been assumed that during development these fine argyrophilic fibers are somehow transformed into the coarse strands of collagen fibers and lose argyrophilia, although in some tissues such as spleen, lymph nodes, liver, and bone marrow they persist throughout life.

The chemical and structural relationship between reticulin and collagen has long been controversial. A major problem has been to obtain reticulin in quantities sufficient for purification and analysis in a rigorous manner. Biochemical analysis[64,65] on the material obtained by microdissection showed that it has amino acid composition not dissimilar to that of collagen. In addition, a relatively large amount of carbohydrate was detected. It is, however, difficult to interpret the analytic data obtained from impure preparations. Ultrastructural studies with the electron microscope have demonstrated that reticulin possesses the same fine structure as collagen, with typical 64 nm periodicity. Since the cross-striation pattern as seen with the electron microscope is a reflection of the charged group distribution of the constituent amino acid side-chains, this suggests that reticulin has a primary structure very similar to or identical with collagen. Although the biologic function of reticulin is unknown, it seems reasonable to consider the possibility that reticulin may represent an embryonic form of collagen analogous to hemoglobin F. Reticulin is the first fibrous element to appear in embryonic connective tissue, which, in most tissues but not all, gives way to adult collagen during subsequent development. Although it is tempting to speculate on the possibility that reticulin may represent type III collagen, proof of the relationship has not been established.

**Immunochemistry of Collagens and Procollagen.** The complex structure of collagen is reflected by the different types of antigenic determinants that have been identified on the molecule. These can be defined as follows.[66,67]

1. *Helical determinants* depend on conformational factors inherent in the quaternary structure of the triple helix.

2. *Terminal determinants* are nonhelical and are different on both the $NH_2$-terminus and COOH-terminus of the molecule. Procollagen, with additional peptides on both ends of the molecule, produces different antibodies to the nonhelical portions from those of collagen itself.

3. *Central determinants* are unmasked after disruption of the helical structure and are a function of the primary sequence of the molecules. There is much interspecies cross-reaction of antibodies to these determinants but not of antibodies to the helical or terminal determinants.

Current data indicate that in mice the immune response to calf skin collagen is controlled by at least two genes.[68] One is the H-2 gene and represents a T-lymphocyte-dependent response. Another locus appears to be T-lymphocyte independent and responsible, in association with H-2, for high responsiveness to collagen.

Radioimmunoassay has been adapted to antibodies directed to the procollagen end-pieces of type I and type III collagen. After labeling the end-pieces with $^{125}$iodine, nanogram quantites of procollagen end-pieces were detected in serum.[69,70] Up to 200 ng of the procollagen end-pieces from type I collagen were detected, presumably being derived from normal bone remodeling. Five to 7 ng of type III procollagen end-pieces were detected, and this level was elevated in certain diseases with elevated collagen synthesis, namely alcoholic liver disease.[71]

The remainder of the collagen-like material in plasma represents the first component of complement, Clq.[9] Initial studies using this method have indicated that increased amounts of immunoreactive collagen can be found circulating (and in other body fluids) in patients with a number of other different disorders involving increased turnover of collagen.[72]

Studies of cell-mediated immunity to collagen and the role of this response in pathogenesis of inflammatory diseases of joints are described below.

**Biological Considerations.** Detailed clinical descriptions and some of the known defects of the collagen biosynthesis[73,74] and structure found in heritable disorders of connective tissues in humans are given in Chapter 105. In the present chapter, discussion will be confined to some of the animal disorders involving collagen that have been useful in our understanding of the human diseases, and to selected facets of collagen metabolism and structure in acquired disorders of humans.

*Animal Disorders. Lathyrism.* Lathyrism is an experimental disease state in animals caused by administering $\beta$-aminopropionitrile, $H_2N\text{-}CH_2\text{-}CH_2\text{-}C{\equiv}N$, a constituent of the sweet pea, *Lathyrus odoratus.* Administration of this agent to a wide variety of mammals and birds results in gross skeletal deformities as well as widely scattered abnormalities in the structure of connective tissue and an apparent failure in tensile strength. These include weakness of blood vessel walls with aneurysm formation or even rupture, slipped epiphyseal plates, avulsed tendons and ligaments, and weakness of fascial planes with subsequent hernia formation. The mechanism of action by $\beta$-aminopropionitrile in producing this remarkable disease state is now understood in detail.[75,76] It results from interference with aldehyde formation from the specific lysyl and hydroxylysyl residues by competitive inhibition of lysyl oxidase. Thus, there is an acquired failure of crosslinking of collagen in these animals resulting in marked diminution in tensile strength of the collagenous tissues, explaining the clinical abnormalities noted above. This conclusion is further supported by the observation that the state of lathyrism can be mimicked by agents such as D-penicillamine (Fig. 14–13), which also interfere with crosslinking but at a later step in the process.[77] The latter agent binds to the aldehydes already formed, preventing them from undergoing Schiff base formation or aldol condensation (Fig. 14–13). Thus, the importance of crosslinking to the proper functioning of collagen is established through

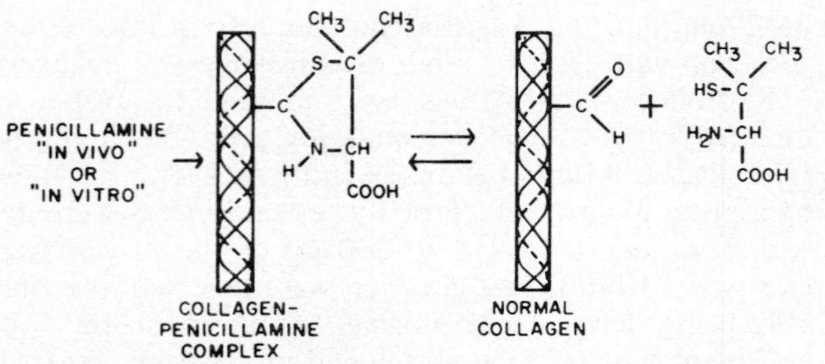


**Figure 14–13.** Schematic drawing of the mode of action of D-penicillamine. This compound interacts with aldehydes of collagen and prevents their subsequent aldamine or aldol condensation reactions. (From Nimni, M.E.: Semin. Arthritis Rheum. 4:95, 1974, with permission of author and publisher.)

our understanding of the biochemical pathogenesis of this disease state. The possible clinical importance of this is suggested by reports of side effects on connective tissues associated with the use of D-penicillamine in various situations. The side effects include poor wound healing,[78] hyperelastic skin, premature aging of skin, and other skin abnormalities.[79] An infant with widely scattered connective tissue malformation was born to a mother receiving penicillamine therapy for cystinuria during her pregnancy.[80] In homocystinuria (see Chapter 104), there is also an apparently acquired defect in collagen.[81] The mechanism of this defect may be similar to that produced by D-penicillamine, since both are structurally similar with adjacent aminothiol groups.

*Dermatosparaxis.* Dermatosparaxis, an inherited disease observed in cattle and sheep, is characterized by extreme fragility of skin and connective tissues. Morphologic studies have shown that there is a gross disorganization in the collagenous fibrils in connective-tissues with pseudofiber formation. Biochemically, collagen molecules extracted from the tissues of the affected animals contain a bulk of nonhelical $NH_2$-terminal extension peptides which have not been cleaved off from procollagen molecules. Called pN-collagen, these molecules have a molecular weight intermediate between that of procollagen and collagen, and cannot form native-type fibrils in vitro under conditions that favor polymerization of normal collagen. The defect has been shown to be the deficient activity of procollagen peptidase(s).[83] A similar enzymatic defect has been demonstrated in some patients with Ehlers-Danlos syndrome.[84]

*Acquired Disorders.* In many acquired human diseases, the pathologic processes seem to involve predominantly connective tissue, and the resultant destruction or alteration of the tissue plays a significant role in the genesis of morbid states. These include wound healing and its abnormal forms, including keloids, scurvy, several inflammatory diseases such as scleroderma and rheumatoid arthritis, corneal ulceration secondary to trauma or infection, and degenerative diseases of joints and several other unrelated diseases.

*Wound Healing.* Wound healing,[95] although not "pathologic," deserves a special consideration here because of the importance the metabolism of collagen plays in the process. If a wound is a break in the continuity of tissue, healing is the restoration of continuity of tissue. The process of wound healing may be divided into three phases: initial or lag phase, the phase of fibroplasia, and the phase of contraction of scar.

Following an injury, the hemostatic mechanism immediately comes into play, leading to the formation of clot. A firmly retracted clot not only stops bleeding but also provides support for the wound's edges, allowing proliferation and migration of capillary endothelial cells, fibroblasts, and epithelial cells. During this period of initial phase, there is active removal of cellular and other tissue debris, both within and outside the phagocytic cells. Of particular interest is the secretion of active collagenase by the epithelial cells and fibroblasts at the wound edge.[49]

The fibroblastic proliferation, which begins during the initial phase, reaches a maximum during the second phase (2 to 10 days after injury) and the cells begin to synthesize and secrete collagen. It is the collagen deposition that provides strength to the wound. After an adequate amount of collagen is deposited (10 to 14 days after injury), the fibroblasts begin to disappear from the scar, with gradual diminution and cessation of further collagen synthesis. Meanwhile, progressive crosslinking of the newly deposited collagen proceeds. This last phase is associated with increasing tensile strength of the wound, which reaches a maximum some 3 weeks following the initiation of healing.

The process of wound healing described above requires adequate general nutrition, blood supply, and control of infection. The precise factors that control the process are, however, not well understood. What is the message that attracts the fibroblast to the injured site? What messages do fibroblasts recognize to initiate and terminate the synthesis of collagen and collagenase? What is the biochemical event that transpires to bring about the contraction of the scar and the increase of tensile strength? The answers to these important questions must await further studies.

Evidence, however, is compelling for the crucial role of collagen metabolism in normal healing. Administration of $\beta$-aminopropionitrile (see Lathyrism, above) leads to marked weakness in tensile strength of wounds.[75] Presumably, this effect is mediated by its interference with crosslinking of collagen, discussed previously. This effect of the compound has been utilized for the treatment of conditions in which excessive contraction of scars in itself may be harmful, such as esophageal strictures following chemical or physical injuries and adhesions of tendons to tendon sheaths following repair of tendon disruption.

Likewise, scurvy, a state induced by a deficiency of ascorbic acid, is associated with poor wound healing as well as marked vascular fragility. As indicated previously, ascorbic acid probably serves as as cofactor in hydroxylation of proline and lysine during in vivo collagen biosynthesis. In vitro studies indicate that there is a marked diminution in collagen synthesis and secretion, and that extensively underhydroxylated collagen accumulates within cells in the absence of ascorbic acid.[96,97]

Lastly, an abnormality in collagen biosynthesis and/or degradation leads to defective wound healing such as keloid and hypertrophic scar. The precise defect or defects in these conditions, however, remain to be elucidated.

*Inflammation.* Recent studies have also implicated collagen and its degradative products in the process of inflammation. Evidence suggests that collagen and its breakdown products are directly chemotactic for blood monocytes and fibroblasts.[98,99] Since collagen is ubiquitous in all tissues, its chemotactic property may play a significant role in calling for monocytes and fibroblasts to clean up the tissue debris at the injury site during the early phase of inflammation, and begin to effect the synthesis of the extracellular matrix for healing.

In addition, data have been presented indicating that immunity against collagen or its fragments may play a role in the pathogenesis of chronic inflammation seen in scleroderma and rheumatoid arthritis,[93,94,100,101] in which there is a widespread inflammatory process taking place in various connective tissues with lymphocytic and monocytic infiltration. The histiologic features observed in these diseases are quite compatible with cellular immune-mediated inflammation. Thus, the discovery that the patients with these diseases possess evidence of cell-mediated immunity against collagen is of extreme interest in our understanding of the pathogenesis of these vexing conditions. There is also evidence that humoral immunity to collagen or its degradative products may be associated with the pathogenesis of rheumatoid arthritis.[93,94] In this connection, recent studies demonstrating induction of polyarthritis in rodents by immunization with purified type II collagen are of particular interest, and therefore the experimental model will be briefly described.

*Collagen-Induced Arthritis.* Chronic polyarthritis can be induced by immunization with heterologous or homologous type II collagen in susceptible animals.[85-88] This property appears to be unique for type II as opposed to type I, III, IV, or V collagen. Its triple-helical structure is also required, since denatured collagens are ineffective. Antibodies to type II collagen are normally not present in the animal but appear after immunization, and arthritis occurs when antibody levels are high. The major clinical manifestation of collagen-induced arthritis in rats and mice is an erosive, inflammatory polyarthritis affecting the peripheral joints.[89] Additionally, auricular chondritis[90] and sensory hearing loss[91] with vestibular dysfunction occur occasionally. The arthritic joints show proliferative synovitis with erosion of cartilage and bone resembling that seen in humans with chronic inflammatory arthritis.

A strong correlation exists between immunity to type II collagen and arthritis (for review, see ref. 92). Arthritis is associated with high levels of circulating IgG anti-collagen antibodies. Purified IgG antibodies from arthritic donors, when injected into a naive rat, can passively transfer the disease. In addition to the humoral immunity, the rats demonstrated an increased T-lymphocyte proliferative response suggesting a possible role for cell-mediated immunity in the disease. Subcutaneous injection of spleen cells containing covalently linked type II collagen induces cell-mediated immunity in the donor animal without antibody production or arthritis.[88] Immune tolerance to collagen-induced arthritis can also be developed using a single large intravenous injection of type II collagen either before or immediately after the primary immunization. The role of autoimmunity to collagen as a potential cause of inflammatory arthritis in man is less well understood. Many patients with rheumatoid arthritis have circulating antibodies to collagen in their serum.[93,94] It is unclear whether these autoantibodies are involved in the pathogenesis of arthritis or are the result of arthritis. Regardless, autoantibodies produced after the onset of arthritis may attack cartilage type II collagen, thus contributing to the inflammation and joint destruction.

More recently, several clones of monoclonal antibodies to type II collagen have been developed. At least one of the monoclonal antibodies can passively transfer arthritis in naive recipients, while others can protect the recipients from arthritis induction by active immunization. Taken together, these observations indicate that immune response directed to type II collagen can induce and perpetuate chronic polyarthritis in experimental animals.(see Chapter 58),

In addition, in patients with rheumatoid arthritis, an inflammatory disease that often results in severe destruction and deformities of joints, it has been found that the synovial tissue produces active collagenase capable of degrading native collagen (see Chapter 12). Although the primary cause of the disease is not known, it might be expected that inhibition of the collagenolytic enzyme may prevent or retard the destruction of the articular tissues. As yet, no attempt has been made to treat this condition with agents that inhibit the enzyme, such as EDTA, cysteine, macroglobulins, or other tissue-derived inhibitors.

In vitamin D–deficient rickets, it has been reported that the osteoid collagen is abnormally overglycosylated.[102] Whether this is a direct result of the deficiency of vitamin D per se or an indirect effect of the associated hypocalcemia is not known. Nonetheless, the common assumption that the defective bone formation in rickets is attributable to inadequate availability of mineral must be modified to include a defect in collagen structure as a factor.

Other biochemical alterations of connective tissue have been reported such as increased glycosylation of the renal basement membrane collagen in patients with diabetic nephropathy.[103] and alterations in the specific types of collagen deposited in liver cirrhosis and pulmonary fibrosis.[104,105] Although it is still premature to evaluate these findings, they do suggest a widespread involvement of the connective tissues in many pathologic states.

## ELASTIN

### Distribution and Mechanical Properties of Elastin

Elastin is the other major fibrous protein component of the extracellular connective tissue matrix. The yellow elastic ligaments such as the ligamenta flava of man or the ligamentum nuchae of grazing animals are largely composed of elastic fibers in close association with collagen and amorphous ground substance. Elastin also predominates in the media of large blood vessels. In contrast, the elastin content of other connective tissues such as dermis, tendon, and bone is low.

Elastin fiber exhibits some of the properties of an elastomer in that it has a high extensibility (i.e., the degree of elongation without irreversible changes per unit force applied to unit cross-sectional area is high). However, the tensile strength of elastin fibers is considerably less than that of collagen fibers. This is similar to the mechanical properties of rubber and is consistent with the function of elastin in relation to its distribution in arterial walls and ligaments. From consideration of its mechanical properties together with the ultrastructural and wide-angle x-ray diffraction studies showing no evidence of any repeating fine structure, it has been suggested that elastin is a three-dimensional network of randomly coiled polypetides joined together by covalent crosslinks.[2]

### Structure

Elastin is a highly insoluble protein and has been loosely defined as that protein material which remains after all other connective tissue components are removed. Virtually all the isolation methods for elastin for biochemical analyses have utilized the aforementioned principles.[2] The methods used to remove the non-elastin components have been variable but most commonly involve extracting the tissue with boiling water and/or hot alkali (0.1N NaOH at 95°) until no further protein components are solubilized. In an attempt to avoid these rather harsh treatments, other methods have also been tried in which the other connective tissue components are removed by the use of enzymes (trypsin, collagenase, and α-amylase) that do not attack elastin, in conjunction with various extracting solvents such as salt solutions, organic acids, or guanidine hydrochloride solutions.

Regardless of the method of preparation, the final products have an amino acid composition that is reasonably reproducible and constant (Table 14–3). The composition is unusual in several respects. As in collagen, glycine is one third of the total residues. The proline content is also similar. In contrast to collagen,

**Table 14–3.** Amino Acid Composition of Elastin, Tropoelastin, and Fibronectin*

| | Porcine Aortic Elastin† | Porcine Tropoelastin† | Fibronectin‡ |
|---|---|---|---|
| 4-Hydroxyproline | 15 | 11 | 0 |
| Aspartic acid | 9 | 3 | 94 |
| Threonine | 7 | 14 | 100 |
| Serine | 8 | 9 | 74 |
| Glutamic acid | 21 | 18 | 118 |
| Proline | 94 | 109 | 77 |
| Glycine | 329 | 334 | 106 |
| Alanine | 233 | 218 | 47 |
| Valine | 125 | 121 | 66 |
| Methionine | 2 | — | 13 |
| Isoleucine | 20 | 19 | 38 |
| Leucine | 57 | 46 | 55 |
| Tyrosine | 17 | 16 | 37 |
| Phenylalanine | 32 | 28 | 19 |
| 1/4 Isodesmosine | 8 | 0 | — |
| 1/4 Desmosine | 8 | 0 | — |
| Tryptophan | 0 | 0 | 36 |
| Lysine | 8 | 48 | 34 |
| Histidine | 1 | 0 | 16 |
| Arginine | 7 | 7 | 53 |

*Residues per 1000 total residues.
†From Sandberg, L.B., et al.: Biochemistry 8:2940, 1969.
‡From Yamata, K.M., et al.: Biochemistry 16:5532, 1977.

there is very little hydroxyproline and no hydroxylysine and a preponderance of the nonpolar amino acids, alanine, valine, isoleucine, and leucine. The polar amino acids, aspartic and glutamic acids, lysine, and arginine, are present in very small amounts, as are the hydroxyl amino acids.

Since elastin is insoluble, physicochemical studies to probe the molecular structure have been impossible to perform. Solubilization has been achieved only through limited disruption of the peptide bonds either by the use of weak acids or by the action of specific enzymes such as pancreatic elastase. Limited hydrolysis of elastin from bovine ligamentum nuchae by hot, dilute oxalic acid yields two fractions of solubilized polypeptides. On the basis of $NH_2$-terminal residue analyses and molecular weight determinations of these two fractions, it has been suggested that a considerable number of interchain crosslinks must be present in elastin.[2] This is not surprising, since it is well known among the polymer chemists that a rubber-like elastomer must contain a reasonable number of crosslinks in its structure. These crosslinks impose a mechanical restriction on the elastomer, so that while stretching under stress one chain does not slip completely past another, preserving the ability of the elastomer to return to its original size when the stress is removed.

### Crosslinks

There is a great deal of similarity between crosslinks of collagen and elastin. The basic difference is that no

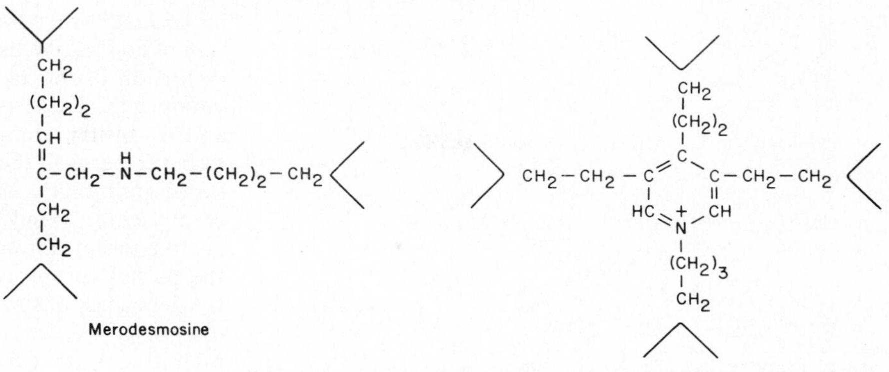


**Figure 14–14.** Structure of elastin crosslinks, merodesmosine and desmosine. An isomer of desmosine, isodesmosine, and their reduced and oxidized forms are also found in elastin.

hydroxylysine is present in elastin, so that all crosslinks in elastin are lysine derived. A second major difference is that in elastin, reduction of several of the crosslinks occurs spontaneously by unknown mechanisms. A final difference is the quantity of the crosslinks: collagen, for example, contains one to two lysine- or hydroxylysine-derived crosslinks per 1000 residues of amino acids, whereas elastin may have as many as 40 lysine-derived crosslinks per 1000 residues.[2]

Four basic types of compounds have been identified in elastin.[2] These are dehydrolysinonorleucine and its reduced form, lysinonorleucine (Fig. 14–9); the aldol condensation product of two residues of allysine (Fig. 14–10); dehydromerodesmosine and its reduced form, merodesmosine (Fig. 14–14); and desmosine (Fig. 14–14). Biosynthetically, all these compounds are derived from lysyl residues through allysine. The mechanism of formation of the aldol condensate and dehydrolysinonorleucine in elastin is identical with that described for collagen. Unlike collagen, in elastin some of the dehydro compound is reduced in vivo to lysinonorleucine. Presumably, this is catalyzed in vivo by an enzyme system, but such a system has not been characterized.

The biosynthetic origin of dehydromerodesmosine appears to be through aldamine bond formation between a residue each of the aldol condensate and lysine. The precise biosynthetic pathway for desmosine is less certain and has not been characterized.

The maturation of elastin, therefore, represents another case in which post-translational modifications of the protein are involved in determining the ultimate properties of the tissues. In comparison to collagen, elastin utilizes a much larger number of crosslinkages, both within and between the polypeptide chains.

## Tropoelastin

Unlike collagen, no soluble precursors of elastin can be found in extracts of normal tissues. This presumably is because of the low rate of synthesis and the rapidity with which the precursor forms are converted to mature, highly crosslinked elastin fibers via the enzyme lysyl oxidase. However, a soluble protein regarded by most investigators as the elastin precursor has been isolated from the aorta of piglets with copper deficiency,[106] a state in which there is a generalized inhibition of crosslinking in elastin. Since lysyl oxidase is a copper metalloenzyme, presumably copper deficiency leads to deficient biosynthesis of allysine so that normal crosslinking of elastin is prevented. Tropoelastin has also been isolated from animals treated with $\beta$-aminopropionitrile.[107]

The soluble protein, termed tropoelastin, has been purified and partially characterized.[2,106,107] It has a molecular weight of 67,000 daltons. Its amino acid composition is presented in Table 14–3, together with that of insoluble elastin prepared from normal animals. The composition is similar, except that tropoelastin lacks the normal crosslinks described previously, but instead has a much higher content of lysine. This is consistent with the fact that the crosslink compounds of mature elastin are derived from lysyl residues. The observed lysyl residue content of 47 in tropoelastin is compatible with the observed values (approximately 40 per 1000 residues) of various lysyl-derived crosslinks in mature elastin.

Much of the structural information of elastin has been derived from analyses of this tropoelastin molecule (for review, see ref. 108). The approximately 800 amino acid polypetide precursor contains large segments of hydrophobic amino acid residues which are interrupted with shorter segments of polyalanine sequence and clusters of lysine residues. The shorter segments are in alpha helix, but the larger hydrophobic regions possess a beta spiral structure with elastomeric properties. Within the hydrophobic regions a repeating pentapeptide (Pro-Gly-Val-Gly-Val) has been identified, which presumably imparts some unusual folding properties to the molecule. From this, it is evident that a collagen-like sequence [Gly-Val-Pro-Gly] occurs rather frequently. This would explain certain collagen-like properties of tropoelastin, such as its limited susceptibility to bacterial collagenase (Pro-Gly-X-Y) and also the observation of small amounts of hydroxyproline in tropoelastin. The sequence (Gly-X-Pro-Gly) is recognized by the enzyme prolyl hydroxylase. Only a small percentage of the proline residues, however, become hydroxylated.

The other unusual segments are the polyalanine regions. Each begins with tyrosine and exists as repeats

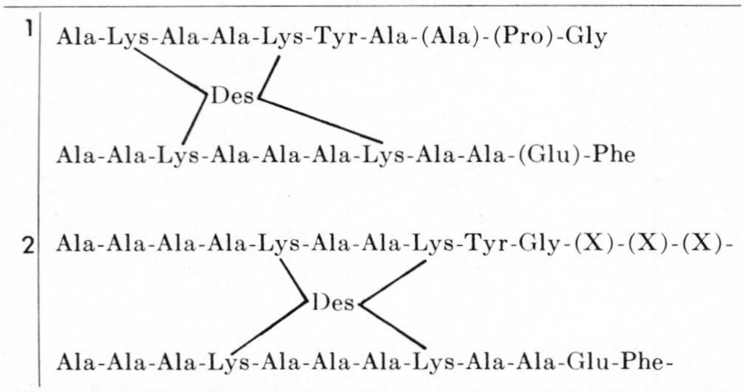


**Figure 14–15.** Amino acid sequence of two enzymatic fragments derived from mature elastin. (From Foster, J.A., et al.: J. Biol. Chem. 249:6191, 1974, with permission of authors and publisher.)

of two sequences, Ala-Ala-Lys and Ala-Ala-Ala-Lys.[109] This is of particular interest in view of the data describing the sequence of two crosslink peptides obtained from mature elastin from enzymatic digestion. Their sequence is shown in Figure 14–15. The clustering of alanyl residues adjacent to desmosine is noteworthy. The use of space-filling atomic models indicates that lysines separated by two or three alanyl residues in $\alpha$ helical conformation protrude on the same side of the helix. Hence, the sequence Lys-Ala-Ala-Lys allows the formation of dehydrolysinonorleucine, whereas the sequence Lys-Ala-Ala-Ala-Lys accommodates either aldol condensate or dehydrolysinonorleucine. Condensation of the two intrachain crosslinks could result in the formation of the interchain desmosine crosslinkages.

**Metabolism.** Ultrastructural studies indicate that the fibroblasts are the cell type producing elastin in most tissues. However, in the case of the arterial wall, the smooth muscle cells seem to be responsible for biogenesis of elastin. Elastin is synthesized on polysomes with a short leader sequence of about 25 residues[108] which is removed before tropoelastin is secreted. Regulation of elastin synthesis appears to be controlled at the pretranslational level, since the amount of elastin mRNA available is proportional to the level of elastin synthesis.[110] Utilizing a cDNA clone, a 3.5-kb mRNA was isolated and quantitated from chick aorta. The relative amount of elastin mRNA compared favorably with the functional elastin mRNA measured by elastin cell-free translation. Age-dependent changes in elastin synthesis also correlated with elastin mRNA content of the aorta.[111]

Very little is known about turnover of elastin. Even the existence of a physiologic elastolytic enzyme in connective tissue is not proved. The mammalian enzymes known to degrade elastin include polymorphonuclear leukocyte and pancreatic elastase (see Chapter 12).

Although little is known about the control in vivo of elastin turnover, there is a possible relationship between the absence of circulating elastase inhibitors and the development of destructive pulmonary disease seen in hereditary $\alpha_1$-proteinase inhibitor (formerly called $\alpha_1$-antitrypsin) deficiency.[112] In this disorder, the affected individuals suffer from gradual but progressive destruction of connective tissue of the lung, leading to a marked distortion in the architecture of the lung at a relatively young age. These patients are deficient in antielastase and $\alpha_1$-antitrypsin activity. The administration of elastase via aerosol therapy in mammals produces disordered pulmonary architecture similar to that seen in emphysema.[11] Since elastin is a major functional connective tissue component of the lung, it is possible that the pathologic process may be in some way related to the deficiency of the antienzyme activites. No large vessel disease is seen in this syndrome. Patients with rheumatoid arthritis carry normal amounts of this inhibitor in serum.

### Biologic Considerations, Copper Deficiency, and Lathyrism

Chick and swine fed a diet deficient in copper develop a clinical syndrome in which the main manifestation is vascular fragility with subcutaneous and internal hemorrhage.[114] Histologically, there is fragmentation of the elastic elements of the arterial wall and minute breaks in the internal elastic membrane of the arteries. Dissecting aneurysm of the aorta is usually observed. Elastin isolated from the diseased animals has been shown to be deficient in the content of the crosslink compounds but high in lysyl content as compared with the control.[107] In addition, there is evidence that collagen in these animals may be deficient in the content of collagen crosslinks.[115] It is now known that the defect in these animals is a failure of conversion of the lysyl residues to allysyl residues, thus blocking the crosslinking of elastin and collagen. The enzyme system involved in this deamination requires copper for action.

## FIBRONECTIN

Fibronectin is a high molecular weight glycoprotein that has rapidly gained prominence due to its cell surface interaction with extracellular matrix proteins. Its potential role in the control of cellular functions such as replication, motility, and differentiation has stimulated extensive studies from a variety of scientific disciplines (for review, see refs. 116 to 118). The name fibronectin (*fibra* [Lat.] = fiber; *nectene* [Lat.] = connect, link) is now accepted and replaces many others, such as cold insoluble globulin (plasma fibronectin), LETS protein, SF antigen, CSP, galactoprotein, and cell attachment factor. As early as 1940 it was identified as a cryoprecipitate of plasma; hence the early name was cold insoluble globulin. In connective tissue, its prominence became apparent as a cell attachment factor from serum which, in tissue culture, promoted binding of fibroblasts to collagen-coated surfaces.[119] It was later found to be a biosynthetic product of many different cell types in vitro. The multifaceted binding properties of this protein has led to identification of specific binding domains within its polypeptide structure. The rapid explosion of information on fibronectin has revealed its function in cell adhesion, connective tissue matrix formation, opsonization, blood coagulation and malignant transformation.

## Chemical Properties

Fibronectin exists as a 450,000-dalton, disulfide-linked dimer in plasma and tissue. With reduction, two equal- or nearly equal-sized polypeptide chains are released, with apparent molecular weights of 220,000 daltons each. Pyroglutamic acid was identified as the single $NH_2$-terminal amino acid of the intact dimer, and peptide maps of each of the individual polypeptide chains from plasma fibronectin monomers were identical, leading to the conclusion that it is a dimer of two identical polypeptides.[120] The amino acid composition of the intact fibronectin is presented in Table 14–3.

The precise relationship between plasma fibronectin, fibronectins on various cell surfaces, and tissue fibronectin remains unclear. All fibronectins examined thus far are immunochemically indistinguishable, even though the gel electrophoretic mobility may vary with species and source; and the extensive crossreactivity of antisera to fibronectin of widely diverse species further indicates its primary structure has been highly conserved during evolution.[121]

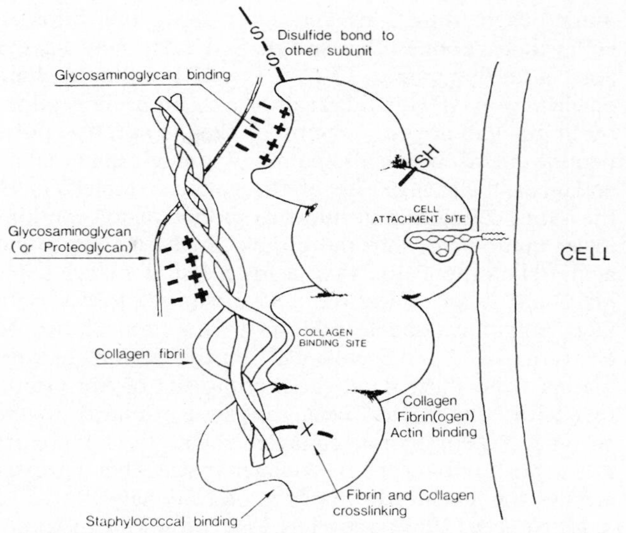


**Figure 14–16.** A model for the structure and interactions of fibronectin. Only a single subunit of fibronectin is shown, although identical sites are present with the other subunit. The specific molecules that interact are tabulated in Table 14–4. The free SH may be involved in certain interactions, and the X represents the site of covalent crosslinking via transglutaminase (Factor XIII of complement), which also crosslinks fibrin. The additional interaction of glycosaminoglycans to both fibronectin and collagen serve to stabilize this multimolecular complex. (From Rouslahti E., et al.: Coll. Res. 1:104, 1981, with permission of authors and publisher.)

## Interactions of Fibronectin

Most of the proposed biologic functions of fibronectin deal with its ability to adhere to cells and/or the extracellular matrix proteins, hence its role as an anchor protein in the extracellular matrix. This protein has been shown to interact with collagens, glycosaminoglycans, fibrinogen, actin, and certain gram-positive bacteria (Table 14–4). As more information is obtained, the list will presumably grow considerably, but, even now, the magnitude of the fibronectin involvement as a biologically active molecule in extracellular matrices must be appreciated. The adhesion is rapid, requires divalent cations, and is temperature-dependent, and cell adhesion is inhibited by cytochalasin B. The specific binding regions of the polypeptide structure have been classified as domains of the polypeptide chain (Fig. 14–16).

**Table 14–4.** Molecular Interactions of Fibronectin*

| Binding Site | Ligand | Comment |
|---|---|---|
| 1 | Collagen<br>Fibrin(ogen)<br>Actin | The same or adjacent binding sites in fibronectin |
| 2 | Heparin<br>Heparin sulfate<br>DNA<br>Dextran sulfate | A shared binding site |
| 3 | Hyaluronic acid | A binding site separate from the heparin binding site? |
| 4 | Staphylococci | A separate binding site in the N-terminal end of the fibronectin molecule |
| 5 | Cell surfaces | A separate binding site. Interacts with oligosaccharide portion of cell surface gangliosides? |

*From Rouslahti, E., et al.: Coll. Res. 1:98, 1981, with permission of authors and publisher.

**Collagen.** The binding properties of fibronectin with collagen have been studied in the greatest detail.[114] It was initially identified as a factor responsible for the attachment of cells in culture to collagen-coated surfaces. This cell adhesion was greatly enhanced by addition of serum or culture media now known to contain fibronectin. With time, cells can produce sufficient fibronectin to promote their own attachment.

All genetic types of collagen have been shown to bind fibronectin.[122] In fact, Clq of complement, which also contains a Gly-X-Y repeating structure, has affinity for fibronectin.[123] Several important observations have emerged from these collagen binding studies. Denatured collagens have a much greater affinity for fibronectin compared with their native counterparts. While this gelatin binding has been very exciting to cell attachment studies, its significance in connective tissue in vivo is uncertain, since gelatin is not a normal component of the extracellular matrix. The fact remains, however, that native collagens do bind fibronectin, and other macromolecules, such as hyaluronic acid and heparin sulfate, stabilize this attachment. From studies with denatured collagen and fragments from their chains, it appears that numerous binding sites may exist along the unfolded collagen backbone. One site in particular may have a great affinity, namely, CB-7 of the $\alpha 1(I)$ collagen chain or CB-5 of $\alpha 1(III)$.[117] These cyanogen bromide peptides occur in homologous regions of their respective polypeptide chains, which also contain the single mammalian collagenase cleavage site of the collagen molecule. In the native collagen molecule, this specific region contains fewer imino acids and more bulky hydrophobic amino acids. Hypothetically, this yields a less compact triple helix and is more accessible to disruptive forces.[124] In fact, polymorphonuclear elastase has been shown to cleave native type III collagen[125] in this region. Extrapolating from these data, the binding site of fibronectin to native collagen has been relegated primarily to the cleavage region of the collagen chain. It is therefore notsurprising that type III collagen (native) has a greater affinity for fibronectin than the other collagens.

**Fibrinogen.** Fibrinogen has long been known to coprecipitate with fibronectin (cold insoluble globulin) in the cold. It also becomes incorporated into a blood clot and becomes covalently crosslinked to fibrin via transglutaminase, the enzyme that crosslinks fibrin.[126] On the basis of these facts and the known cell attachment property of fibronectin, it has been proposed that fibronectin bound to a fibrin clot could provide an adhesive temporary matrix for cells to grow in. This would provide a scaffold then for early wound healing. This binding is inhibited by gelatin; hence the fibrinogen binding domain must be at or near the collagen binding domain. Although fibrinogen binding is very weak, the covalent linking of fibrin to fibronectin via the transglutaminase enzyme (Factor XIII) would provide a stable bond.[127]

**Glycosaminoglycans.** A number of polyanionic macromolecules bind to fibronectin. Heparin, heparin sulfate, dextran sulfate, and DNA compete with each other for binding to the fibronectin molecule, suggesting they all share the same binding site.[116] Hyaluronic acid also interacts but at a different domain of the fibronectin molecule.[129] Other polyanionic macromolecules such as chondroitin sulfates and dermatan sulfate do not bind, thereby demonstrating a certain degree of specificity.

Polyanionic binding can be augmented by gelatin-coated beads. In the presence of *both* fibronectin and glycosaminoglycan, the gelatin-coated beads agglutinated. Addition of heparin sulfate or hyaluronic acid to fibronectin-coated gelatin-Sepharose columns enhanced the stability of fibronectin-gelatin binding. This combined interaction of the three major components of extracellular matrix, fibronectin, glycosaminoglycan, and collagen, may serve as a model for the formation of extracellular matrix as an insoluble complex. In the presence of heparin, fibronectin will also precipitate native type I and type III collagen. Alone, neither fibronectin or heparin is effective. Therefore, this cooperative effect utilizing two distinct binding domains on the fibronectin molecule with enhancement of the binding affinity of native collagen to fibronectin makes this precipitation possible.

A similar situation occurs with fibrinogen. The addition of heparin to a solution of fibrinogen and fibronectin causes precipitation at low temperatures. Since fibrinogen occupies a site on the fibronectin molecule similar to that of collagen, a similar mechanism presumably exists. Therefore, the trimolecular complex may be a more physiologic situation to examine when studying the biologic significance of fibronectin in tissue matrix (Fig. 14–16).

**Cell Surfaces.** It is well-established that cell suspensions preferentially attach to surfaces in the presence of fibronectin. Furthermore, fibronectin provides a divalent cation-dependent linkage between collagen-coated surfaces and specific cells (Fig. 14–17). The presence of a specific cell attachment domain on the fibronectin molecule therefore comes as no surprise, and this domain is located at a distant site from the collagen, fibrinogen, and polyanionic macromolecular domain. The specific component of the cell membrane that is recognized by fibronectin has not been fully established. The current evidence based on binding inhibition studies with various gangliosides suggests that certain widely distributed cell surface oligosaccharides serve as these receptor sites.[129]

**Actin.** Fibronectin has been shown to bind directly to actin, and this binding can be inhibited by collagen, suggesting that the actin binding site is located in close proximity to the collagen and fibrin binding domain. Since actin is an intracellular protein, the significance of this specific binding remains unclear. The interaction of fibronectin with actin, an insoluble intracellular protein, may perhaps play a role in elimination of remnants of dead cells by utilizing the nonimmune opsonization ability of fibronectin. Alternatively, since both actin and fibronectin play a role in cell spreading, a possible communication between these two molecules through the cell membrane has been postulated (Fig. 14–17).

**Bacteria.** Another binding site on the fibronectin molecule has an affinity for specific gram-positive bacteria. Thus far, *Staphylococcus aureus*,[131] *Streptococcus pyogenes*,[132] and *Streptococcus pneumoniae*,[133] bind to a similar receptor on fibronectin at regions distinct from the collagen binding domain. The mucosal cell surface fibronectin serves as a receptor for the lipoteichoic acid–

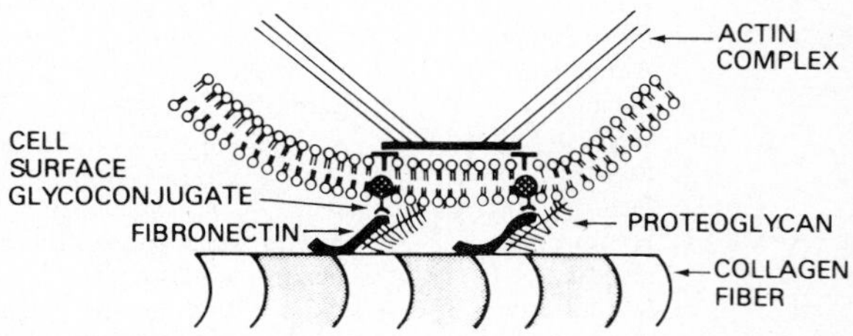


**Figure 14–17.** Schematic model of cell adhesion to fibronectin and collagen. Fibronectin contains a specific binding site for collagen and another for the cell surface. Collagen contains a specific binding region for fibronectin and a glycoconjugate, possibly a glycolipid in the cell membrane is recognized by fibronectin. Proteoglycans are also present and stabilize the interaction. The interaction, if any, between actin (intracellular) and fibronectin remains uncertain. (From Kleinman, H.K., et al.: J. Cell. Biol. 88:479, 1981, with permission of authors and publisher.)

mediated binding of Group A streptococci. This affinity is through the lipid region of the lipoteichoic acid to a fatty acid binding site on fibronectin. The binding of bacteria to fibronectin has been shown to enhance opsonization by circulating phagocytic cells. Gram-negative bacteria do not bind to fibronectin, but interestingly, *E. coli* does bind to laminin, the fibronectin counterpart in basement membrane tissue.[134]

The amount of information on fibronectin binding to proteins and cells has grown enormously in recent years, but with the complex nature of biologic systems, this information is probably far from complete. Already, fibronectin appears to be the "molecular fly paper" for many complex molecular structures. This ability to link molecules and cells via separate domains of the molecule alters the physical characteristics of these complexes and hence biologic properties of these unrelated components.

## Binding Sites on the Fibronectin Molecule

The designation of specific binding domains on fibronectin has been derived primarily by competitive inhibition of the various molecules in solution or on Sepharose affinity columns (for review, see ref. 118). Recent procedures have utilized large proteolytic fragments of fibronectin to pinpoint these areas. A 30,000 to 40,000 molecular weight $NH_2$-terminal fragment, which contains the collagen-binding region, has been isolated by gelatin-Sepharose affinity chromatography.[136] This was confirmed by the Dintzis procedure of short-term pulse labeling cells during polypeptide chain elongation.[137]

A tentative model for the fibronectin molecule has been presented in Figure 14–18. In this molecule, two similar 220,000 dalton subunits are linked via a disulfide bond near the COOH-terminus. The binding site for staphylococci occurs in the 27,000-dalton $NH_2$-terminal domain of fibronectin and may be obtained with mild tryptic digestion. This fragment was identified as the $NH_2$-terminal fragment by pulse labeling and by the fact that it contains a blocked $NH_2$-terminal (pyroglutamic acid). This fragment also contains the glutamic residue which becomes crosslinked to fibrin via the transglutaminase enzyme (Factor XIII) that crosslinks fibrin. The next binding domain is the collagen binding site. This was confirmed by isolation of a 72,000 MW fragment with a blocked $NH_2$-terminal which contains the gelatin-binding site. This fragment was further cleaved into two peptides, a 29,000 MW component (block $NH_2$-terminal) and a 43,000 MW fragment, which binds gelatin. The smallest fragment known to contain both the gelatin-binding domain and the cell attachment region was 130,000 MW. From this, it is assumed that these latter two domains must be considerably distant from each other. The smallest fragment known to contain the heparin-binding site, the cell attachment site, and the gelatin-binding domain is 200,000 MW, thereby placing the heparin-binding region near the COOH-terminus of the polypeptide chain. At least one and possibly two free SH groups are available. The free SH group at a position of about 170,000 MW from the $NH_2$-terminus of the polypeptide chain seems to participate in disulfide bond formation with the insoluble matrix at the cell surface. The location of the carbohydrate on the fibronectin molecule has been identified on a 40,000 MW gelatin-binding fragment in the hamster fibroblast fibronectin. However, as stated above, the degree of glycosylation is variable among species, and other carbohydrate regions may be found.

## Cell Origin and Tissue Distribution

Fibronectin, as stated previously, occurs as a circulating plasma fibronectin (soluble) and as that which is present in extracellular spaces (insoluble) (for review,

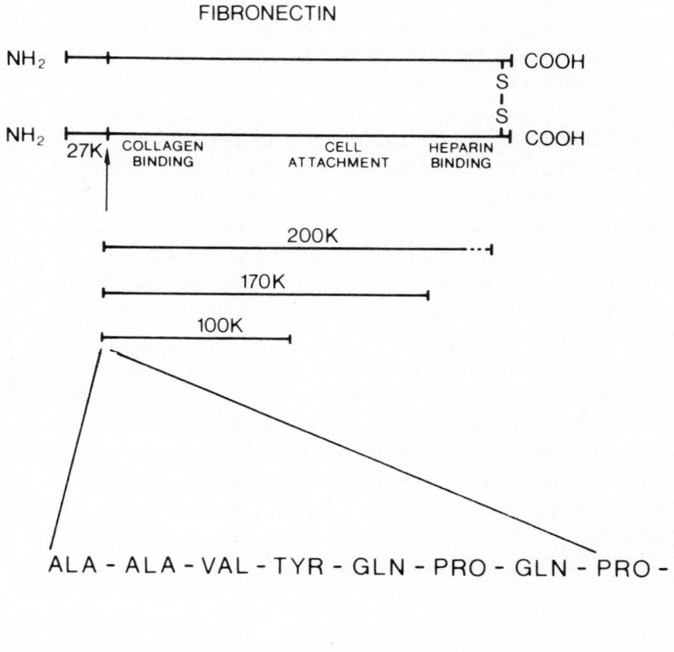


**Figure 14–18.** Schematic representation of plasmin-derived fragments from fibronectin and their localization in the fibronectin polypeptide. (From Ruoslahti E., et al.: J. Invest. Dermatol. 76:65s, 1982, with permission of authors and publisher.)

see ref. 116). Fibronectin levels in the plasma are quite high (300 μg per ml). Tissue fibronectin was first identified in fibroblast culture medium (up to 50 μg per ml at confluency). The cells of liver, kidney, gut, breast, and amnionic membranes produce fibronectin as do Schwann cells, macrophages, melanoma cells, endothelial cells, and undifferentiated chondrocytes. Endothelial cells and liver cells appear to be the source of plasma fibronectin. With cell cultures, fibronectin is found in the medium, at the cell surface, and in the extracellular matrix. An important fraction of the cell surface fibronectin is located at sites where the cells make contact with the substratum (Fig. 14–17). The cells may be detached by chelating agents and leave behind material that contains fibronectin and proteoglycans involved in cell attachment. Little is known about the physiologic significance of the culture medium fibronectin or the insoluble matrix fibronectin. These two latter fibronectin compartments appear to be in equilibrium with each other. In the same manner, when radiolabeled plasma fibronectin is injected into the same species, it becomes incorporated into the tissue matrix, indicating equilibration between body fluid and extracellular matrix fibronectin. The fibronectin in the tissue appears throughout loose connective tissues, with higher amounts at the interface between basement membrane and the cells. It is not, however, a component of basement membranes.

## Biologic Function and Significance of Fibronectin

The functional characteristics of fibronectin are derived primarily from its interaction properties (Table 14–4). It promotes cell attachment and spreading in vitro and presumably in vivo. The attachment of cells to an insoluble matrix is required for cell spreading and replication.

The circulating plasma fibronectin has been assigned a variety of roles in the cascade of wound healing events. It promotes adhesion and spreading of platelets on exposed collagen surfaces, binding of circulating cells to the fibrin clot and exposed collagen, binding to cell debris, thereby promoting nonimmune opsinization by phagocytic cells, and promoting fibroblast migration, via chemotaxis, to the damaged area for repair.[117]

The amount of fibronectin on the surface of malignantly transformed cells is greatly reduced. This is especially evident in experimental systems in which a shift of conditions to a transformation also results in a reduction in surface fibronectin.[116] When the conditions are reversed, the cells regain their normal morphology and cell surface fibronectin. The reduced amount of cell adhesion by malignant cells is thought to lead to increased invasive properties and metastases of these cells.

Fibronectin may play a role in directing differentiation and morphogenesis of certain cells. Myoblasts, for example, lose their ability to produce fibronectin prior to fusion into myotubules.[116] Chondrocytes also fail to produce this protein, but addition of exogenous fibronectin to the culture medium will cause the cells to dedifferentiate, assume a fibroblastic phenotype with lowered production of proteoglycans and cartilage-specific type II collagen, and induce the synthesis of endogenous fibronectin.[117]

There has been little conclusive information on abnormalities of fibronectin in diseased connective tissues. Skin lesions of scleroderma contain increased amounts of fibronectin as judged by immunofluorescent staining. Changes in fibronectin distribution are seen in various diseases affecting the skin. One must assume more alterations in matrix fibronectin will be identified as methodologies in this area improve.[116] Fibronectin has long been known to cause an enhancement of phagocytosis (opsonization) of gelatin-coated particles. More information is needed to determine the extent of this opsonization.

As alluded to earlier, some cells do not require fibronectin for attachment to native collagen. For example, baby hamster kidney (BHK) and BALB 3T3 cells attach more efficiently when fibronectin is added, but this requirement of fibronectin is not absolute. A controversy remains over whether these cells utilize exogenously added fibronectin or rapidly produce their own fibronectin or whether a different mechanism of cell attachment is possible for direct binding to native collagen or other surfaces. Additional unidentified glycoproteins may also mediate some cell attachment. These may be cell-specific and matrix-specific such as in cartilage.

Chondrocytes use another glycoprotein, chondronectin, to promote adherence. This protein has a molecular weight of 180,000 daltons, contains disulfide-linked chains, is present in serum, and is produced by cultured chondrocytes.[113] Although only a limited amount of information is available to date, it is presumed to be analogous in function to fibronectin.

Epithelial cells attach preferentially to type IV collagen in basement membrane. This adhesion is slow and not stimulated by fibronectin. In this case, laminin, another glycoprotein is apparently the attachment factor for these cells. Laminin is an 800,000-dalton glycoprotein found in basement membranes, and like fibronectin, apparently binds to the substrate (type IV collagen), and then the cells bind to the laminin–type IV collagen complex (Fig. 14–11). Some cells, such as regenerating rat liver hepatocytes, produce both laminin and fibronectin and may perhaps use both mechanisms for cell adhesions.[116] With metastatic cells, the target organ of a specific cell invasion and tumorigenicity may be dependent on the genetically programmed specific attachment protein of the metastatic cell. Clearly, the role of fibronectin and other adherence-promoting glycoproteins in biologic systems is exceedingly complex due to its multivalent capabilities and their widely diverse biologic activities.

## REFERENCES

1. Traub, W., and Piez, K.A.: The chemistry and structure of collagen. Adv. Prot. Chem. 25:243, 1971.
2. Gallop, P.M., Blumenfeld, O.O., and Seifter, S.: Structure and metabolism of connective tissue proteins. Ann. Rev. Biochem. 41:617, 1972.

3. Gross, J., Highberger, J.H., and Schmitt, F.O.: Collagen structures considered as states of aggregation of a kinetic unit. The tropocollagen particle. Proc. Natl. Acad. Sci. USA 40:679, 1954.
4. Epstein, E.H., Scott, R.D., Miller, E.J., and Piez, K.A.: Isolation and characterization of the peptides derived from soluble human and baboon skin collagen after CNBr cleavage. J. Biol. Chem. 246:1718, 1971.
5. Miller, E.J., and Lunde, L.G.: Isolation and characterization of the CNBr peptides from the $\alpha1$(II) chain of bovine and human cartilage collagen. Biochemistry 12:3153, 1973.
6. Chung, E., Keele, E.M., and Miller, E.J.: Isolation and characterization of CNBr peptides from $\alpha1$(II) chain of human collagen. Biochemistry 13:3463, 1974.
7. Kefalides, N.A.: Isolation of a collagen from basement membranes containing three identical $\alpha$ chains. Biochem. Biophys. Res. Commun. 45:226, 1971.
8. Bornstein, P., and Traub, W.: The chemistry and biology of collagen. *In* Neurath. H. (ed.): The Proteins. Vol. 4. 3rd ed. New York, Academic Press, 1979.
9. Reid, K.: A collagen-like amino acid sequence in a polypeptide chain of human Clq (a subcomponent of the first component of complement). Biochem. J. 141:189, 1974.
10. Rosenberry, T., and Richardson, J.: Structure of 18S and 14S acetylcholinesterase. Biochemistry 16:3550, 1977.
11. Seyer, J.M., and Kang, A.H.: Covalent structure of collagen: Amino acid sequence of $\alpha1$(III)-CB9 from type III collagen of human liver. Biochemistry 20:2621, 1981.
12. Highberger, J.H., Corbett, C., Dixit, S.N., Yu, W., Seyer, J.M., Kang, A.H., and Gross, J.: The amino acid sequence of chick skin collagen $\alpha1$(I)-CB8 and the complete primary structure of the helical portion of the chick skin collagen $\alpha1$(I) chain. Biochemistry 21:2048, 1982.
13. Piez, K.A.: Primary structure (of collagen). *In* Ramachandran, G.N., and Reddi, A.H. (eds.): Biochemistry of Collagen. New York and London, Plenum Press, 1976.
14. Hulmes, D.J.S., and Miller, A., Parry, D.A.D., Piez, K.A., and Woodhead-Galloway, J.: Analysis of the primary structure of collagen for the origins of molecular packing. J. Mol. Biol. 79:137, 1973.
15. Ramachandran, G.N., and Ramakrishnan, C.: Molecular structure (of collagen). *In* Ramachandran, G.N., and Reddi, A.H. (eds.): Biochemistry of Collagen. New York and London, Plenum Press, 1976.
16. Piez, K.A., Eigner, E.A., and Lewis, M.S.: The chromatographic separation and amino acid composition of the subunits of several collagens. Biochemistry 2:58, 1963.
17. Bornstein, P., and Sage, H.: Structurally distinct collagen types. Ann. Rev. Biochem. 49:957, 1980.
18. Burgeson, R.E.: Genetic heterogeneity of collagens. J. Invest. Dermatol. 79:25, 1982.
19. Kefalides, N.A.: Structure and biosynthesis of basement membranes. Int. Rev. Conn. Tissue Res. 6:63, 1973.
20. Chung, E., Rhodes, R.K., and Miller, E.J.: Isolation of three collagenous components of probable basement membrane origin from several tissues. Biochem. Biophys. Res. Commun. 71:1167, 1976.
21. Burgeson, R.E., El Adli, F.A., Kaitila, I.I., and Hollister, D.W.: Fetal membrane collagens: Identification of two new collagen $\alpha$ chains. Proc. Natl. Acad. Sci. USA 73:2579, 1976.
22. Gay, S., Rhodes, R.K., Gay, R.E., and Miller, E.J.: Collagen molecules composed of $\alpha1$(V) chains (B-chains): An apparent localization in the excytoskeleton. Coll Res. 1:53, 1981.
23. Furato, D.K., and Miller, E.J.: Isolation of a unique collagenous fraction from limited pepsin digests of human placental tissue. J. Biol. Chem. 255:290, 1980.
24. Reese, C.A., and Mayne, R.: Minor collagens of chick hyaline cartilage. Biochemistry 20:918, 1981.
25. Glimcher, M.J., and Krane, S.M.: The organization and structure of bone and the mechanism of calcification. *In* Gould, B.S., and Ramachandran, G.N. (eds.): A Treatise on Collagen, Vol. II. London and New York, Academic Press, 1968.
26. Prockop, D.J., Berg, R.A., and Kivirrikko, K.: Intracellular steps in the biosynthesis of collagen. *In* Ramachandran, G.N., and Reddi, A.H. (eds.): Biochemistry of Collagen. New York and London, Plenum Press, 1976.
27. Bornstein, P.: The biosynthesis of collagen. Ann. Rev. Biochem. 43:567, 1974.
28. Monson, J.M., Click, E.M., and Bornstein, P.: Further characterization of procollagen. Purification and analysis of the pro $\alpha1$ chain of chick bone procollagen. Biochemistry 14:4088, 1975.
29. Morris, N.P., Fessler, L.I., Weinstock, A., and Fessler, J.H.: Procollagen assembly and secretion in embryonic chick bone. J. Biol. Chem. 250:5719, 1975.
30. Uitto, J., and Prockop, D.J.: Rate of helix formation by intracellular procollagen and protocollagen. Evidence for a role for disulfide bonds. Biochem. Biophys. Res. Commun. 55:904, 1973.
31. Vuust, J., and Piez, K.A.: A kinetic study of collagen biosynthesis. J. Biol. Chem. 247:856, 1972.
32. Layman, D.L., McGoodwin, E.B., and Martin, G.R.: The nature of collagen synthesized by cultured human fibroblasts. Proc. Natl. Acad. Sci., USA 68:454, 1971.
33. Graves, P.N., Olsen, B.R., Fietzek, P.P., Prockop, D.J., and Monson, J.M.: Comparison of the $NH_2$-terminal sequence of chick type I preprocollagen chains synthesized in an mRNA-dependent reticulocyte lysate. Eur. J. Biochem. 118:363, 1981.
34. Wozney, J., Hanahaw, D., Tate, V., Boedtker, H., and Doty, P.: Structure of the pro $\alpha2$(I) collagen gene. Nature 294:129, 1981.
35. Tolstoshev, P., and Crystal, R.G.: The collagen alpha-2 chain gene. J. Invest. Dermatol. 79:60, 1982.
36. Grant, M.E., and Prockop, D.J.: The biosynthesis of collagen. N. Engl. J. Med. 286:194, 242, 291, 1972.
37. Cardinale, G.J., and Udenfriend, S.: Prolyl hydroxylase. Adv. Enzymol. 41:245, 1974.
38. Kuutti, E.R., Tuderman, L., and Kivvirikko, K.I.: Human prolyl hydroxylase. Purification, characterization, and preparation of antiserum to the enzyme. Eur. J. Biochem. 57:181, 1975.
39. Myllylä, R., Risteli, L., and Kivvirikko, K.I.: Assay of collagen galactosyltransferase and collagen glucosyltransferase activities and characterization of enzyme reactions with transferases from chick embryo cartilage. Eur. J. Biochem. 52:401, 1975.
40. Myllylä, R., Risteli, L., and Kivvirrikko, K.I.: Collagen glucosyltransferase. Partial purification and characterization of the enzyme from whole chick embryos and chick-embryo cartilage. Eur. J. Biochem. 61:59, 1976.
41. Tuderman, L., Kivvirikko, K., and Prockop, D.J.: Partial purification and characterization of neutral protease which cleaves the N-terminal propeptides from procollagen. Biochemistry 17:2948, 1978.
42. Leung, M.K.K., Fessler, L.I., Greenberg, D.B., and Fesler, J.H.: Separate amino acid carboxyl procollagen peptidases in chick embryo tendon. J. Biol. Chem. 254:224, 1979.
43. Trelstad, R.L., Birk, D.E., and Silver, F.H.: Collagen fibrillogenesis in tissues, in solution, and from modeling: A synthesis. J. Invest. Dermatol. 79:109, 1982.
44. Rennard, S.E., Steir, L.E., and Crystal, R.G.: Intracellular degradation of newly synthesized collagen. J. Invest. Dermatol. 79:77, 1982.
45. Kivvirikko, K.I.: Urinary excretion of hydroxyproline in health and disease. Int. Rev. Conn. Tissue Res. 5:93, 1970.
46. Krane, S.M., Munoz, A.J., and Harris, E.D., Jr.: Urinary polypeptides related to collagen synthesis. J. Clin. Invest. 49:716, 1970.
47. Askenasi, R.: Urinary hydroxylysine and hydroxylysyl glycoside excretions in normal and pathologic states. J. Lab. Clin. Med. 83:673, 1974.
48. Krane, S.M., Kantrowitz, F.G., Byrne, M., Pinnell, S.R., and Singer, F.R.: Urinary excretion of hydroxylysine and its glycosides as an index of collagen degradation. J. Clin. Invest. 59:819, 1977.
49. Gross, J.: Aspects of the animal collagenase. *In* Ramachandran, G.N., and Reddi, A.H. (eds.): Biochemistry of Collagen. New York and London, Plenum Press, 1976.
50. Harris, E.D., and Krane, S.M.: Collagenases. N. Engl. J. Med. 291:557, 605, 652, 1974.
51. Evanson, J.M., Jeffrey, J.J., and Krane, S.M.: Studies on collagenase from rheumatoid synovium in tissue culture. J. Clin. Invest. 47:2639, 1968.
52. Tanzer, M.L.: Cross-linking (of collagen). *In* Ramachandran, G.N., Reddi, A.H. (eds.): Biochemistry of Collagen. New York and London, Plenum Press, 1976.
53. Gallop, P.M., and Paz, M.A.: Posttranslational protein modifications with special attention to collagen and elastin. Physiol. Rev. 55:418, 1975.
54. Siegel, R.C.: Collagen crosslinking; Purification and substrate specificity of lysyl oxidase. J. Biol. Chem. 251:5779, 1976.
55. Fujimoto, D., Moriguchi, T., Ishida, T., and Hayashi, H.: The structure of pyridinoline: a collagen crosslink. Biochem. Biophys. Res. Commun. 84:52, 1978.
56. Bornstein, P.H., and Mechanic, G.L.: A natural histidine-based imminium crosslink in collagen and its location. J. Biol. Chem. 255:10414, 1980.
57. Epstein, E.H., and Munderloh, N.H.: Isolation and characterization of CNBr peptides of human $[\alpha1(IV)]_3$ collagen and tissue distribution of $[\alpha1(I)]_2\alpha2$ and $[\alpha1(III)]_3$ collagens J. Biol. Chem. 250:9304, 1975.
58. Bailey, A.J., Bazin, S., Sims, T.J., Lelous, M., Nicoletis, C., and Dalauncy, A.: Characterization of the collagen of human hypertrophic and normal scars. Biochim. Biophys. Acta 405:412, 1975.
59. Miller, E.J.: A review of biochemical studies on the genetically distinct collagens of the skeletal system. Clin. Orthop. Relat. Res. 92:260, 1973.
60. Foidant, J.M., and Yaar, M.: Type IV collagen, laminin, and fibronectin at the dermal-epidermal junction. Front Matrix Biol. Vol. 8. Basel, S. Karger, 1981, pp. 175–188.
61. Kresina, T.F., and Miller, E.J.: Isolation and characterization of basement membrane collagen from human placental tissue: Evidence of the pres-

ence of two genetically distinct collagen chains. Biochemistry 18:3089, 1979.
62. Timpl, R., Wiedemann, H., von Delden, V., Furthmayr, H., and Kühn, K.: A network model for the organization of type IV collagen molecules in basement membranes. Eur. J. Biochem. 120:203, 1981.
63. Sage, H.: Collagen of basement membranes. J. Invest. Dermatol. 79:51, 1982.
64. Valdrighi, L., and Vidol, B.C.: Silver impregnation: Collagenic and reticular fibers and the ground substance. Ann. Histochim. 16:29, 1971.
65. Windrum, G.M., Kent, P.W., and Eastoe, J.E.: Constitution of human renal reticulin. Br. J. Exp. Path. 36:49, 1955.
66. Furthmayer, H., and Timpl, R.: Immunochemistry of collagens and procollagens. *In* Hall, D.A., and Jackson, D.S. (eds.): International Review of Connective Tissue Research, Volume 7. New York, Academic Press, 1976, pp.61–99.
67. Beil, W., Timpl, R., and Furthmayer, H.: Conformation dependence of antigenic determinants on the collagen molecule. Immunology 24:13, 1973.
68. Nowack, H., Hahn, E., David, C.S., Timpl, R., and Götze, D.: Immune response to calf collagen Type I in mice: A combined control of Ir-1A and H-2 linked genes. Immunogenetics 2:331, 1975.
69. Taubman, M.B., Goldberg, B., and Sherr, C.J.: Radioimmunoassay for human procollagen. Science 186:1115, 1974.
70. Keiser, H., LeRoy, E.C., Udenfriend, S., and Sjoerdsma, A.: Collagen-like protein in human plasma. Science 142:1678, 1963.
71. Rohde, H., Vargas, L., Hahn, E., Kalbfleisch, H., Brugeura, M., and Timpl, R.: Radioimmunoassay for type III procollagen peptide and its application to human liver disease. Eur. J. Clin. Invest. 9:451, 1979.
72. Taubman, M.B., Kammerman, S., and Goldberg, B.: Radioimmunoassay of procollagen in serum of patients with Paget's disease of bone. Proc. Soc. Exp. Biol. Med. 152:284, 1976.
73. McKusick, V.A.: Heritable Disorders of Connective Tissue. 4th ed. St. Louis, C.V. Mosby Company, p. 192.
74. Pinnell, S.R.: Disorders of collagen. *In* Stanbury, J.B., Wyngaarden, J.B., and Fredrickson, D.S. (eds.): The Metabolic Basis of Inherited Disease. 4th ed. New York, McGraw-Hill Book Company, 1978.
75. Gross, J.: Collagen biology: Structure, degradation and disease. Harvey Lect. 68:351, 1974.
76. Narayanan, A.S., Siegel, R.C., and Martin, G.R.: On the inhibition of lysyl oxidase by $\beta$-aminopropionitrile. Biochem. Biophys. Res. Commun. 46:745, 1972.
77. Nimni, M.E., and Deshmukh, G.N.: Collagen defect induced by penicillamine. Nature 240:220, 1972.
78. Burry, H.C.: Penicillamine and wound healing: A potential hazard? Postgrad. Med. J. (Suppl.) 50:75, 1974.
79. Scheinberg, I.H.: Uses and usefulness of penicillamine. N. Engl. J. Med. 292:1080, 1975.
80. Mjolerod, I.K., Rasmussen, K., Dommerud, S.A., and Gjeruldsen, S.T.: Congenital connective tissue defect probably due to D-penicillamine treatment in pregnancy. Lancet 1:673, 1971.
81. Kang, A.H., and Trelstad, R.L.: A collagen defect in homocystinuria. J. Clin. Invest. 52:2571, 1973.
82. Helbe, O., and Ness, N.N.: A hereditary skin defect in sheep. Acta Vet. Scand. 13:443, 1972.
83. Lenaers, A., Ansay, M., Nusgens, B.V., and Lapiere, C.M.: Collagen made of extended $\alpha$ chains: Procollagen in genetically defective dermatosparaxic calves. Eur. J. Biochem. 23:533, 1971.
84. Lichtenstein, J.R., Kohn, L.D., Martin, G.R., Byers, P., and McKusick, V.A.: Procollagen peptidase deficiency in a form of the Ehlers-Danlos syndrome. Trans. Assoc. Am. Physicians 86:333, 1973.
85. Trentham, D.E., Townes, A.S., and Kang, A.H.: Autoimmunity to type II collagen: An experimental model of arthritis. J. Exp. Med. 146:857, 1977.
86. Trentham, D.E., Townes, A.S., Kang, A.H., and David, J.R.: Humoral and cellular sensitivity to collagen in type II collagen-induced arthritis in rats. J. Clin. Invest. 61:89, 1978.
87. Stuart, J.M., Cremer, M.A., Townes, A.S., and Kang, A.H.: Collagen-induced arthritis in rats: Evaluation of early immunologic events. Arthritis Rheum. 12:1344, 1979.
88. Trentham, D.E., Dynesius, R.A., and David, J.R.: Passive transfer by cells of type II collagen-induced arthritis in rats. J. Clin. Invest. 62:359, 1978.
89. Cremer, M.A., Pitcock, J.A., Stuart, J.M., Kang, A.H., and Townes, A.S.: Auricular chondritis in rats: An experimental model of relapsing polychondritis induced with type II collagen. J. Exp. Med. 154:535, 1981.
90. Yoo, T.J., Stuart, J.M., Kang, A.H., Townes, A.S., and Tomoda, K.: Type II collagen autoimmunity in otosclerosis and Meniere's disease. Science 217:1153, 1982.
91. Yoo, T.J., Tomoda, K., Stuart, J.M., Cremer, M.A., Kang, A.H., and Townes, A.S.: Type II collagen induced autoimmune sensorineural hearing loss and vestibular dysfunction in rats. Ann. Otol. Rhinol. Larynol., in press, 1983.
92. Stuart, J.M., Townes, A.S., and Kang, A.H.: The role of collagen autoimmunity in animal models and human diseases. J. Invest. Dermatol. 79:121, 1982.
93. Postlethwaite, A.E., and Kang, A.H.: Collagen and collagen peptide-induced chemotaxis of human blood monocytes. J. Exp. Med. 143:1299, 1976.
94. Postlethwaite, A.E., Seyer, J.M., and Kang, A.H.: Induction of fibroblast chemotaxis by type I, II, and III collagens and collagen degradation peptides. Proc. Natl. Acad. Sci. USA 75:871, 1978.
95. Peacock, E., and Van Winkle, W.V.: Wound Repair. 2nd ed. Philadelphia, W.B. Saunders Company, 1976.
96. Fernandez-Madrid, F.: Collagen biosynthesis. Clin. Orthop. 68:163, 1970.
97. Blanck, T.J., and Peterkofsky, B.: Stimulation of collagen secretion by ascorbic acid in fibroblasts. Arch. Biochem. Biophys. 17:259, 1975.
98. Stuart, J.M., Postlethwaite, A.E., and Kang, A.H.: Evidence for cell-mediated immunity to collagen in progressive systemic sclerosis. J. Lab. Clin. Med. 88:601, 1976.
99. Trentham, D.E., Dynesius, R.A., Rocklin, R.E., and David, J.R.: Cellular sensitivity to collagen in rheumatoid arthritis. N. Engl. J. Med. 299:327, 1978.
100. Andriopoules, N.A., Mestecky, J., Miller, E.J., and Bradley, E.L.: Antibodies to native and denatured collagens in sera of patients with rheumatoid arthritis. Arthritis Rheum. 19:613, 1976.
101. Cracchiolo, A., Michaeli, D., Goldberg, L.S., and Fudenberg, H.H.: The occurrence of antibodies to collagen in synovial fluids. Clin. Immunol. Immunopathol. 3:567, 1975.
102. Toole, B.P., Kang, A.H., Trelstad, R.L., and Gross, J.: Collagen heterogeneity within different growth regions of long bones of rachitic and nonrachitic chicks. Biochem. J. 127:715, 1972.
103. Beisswenger, P.J., and Spiro, R.G.: Studies on the human glomerular basement membrane: Composition, nature of carbohydrate units and chemical changes in diabetes mellitus. Diabetes 22:180, 1973.
104. Seyer, J.M., Hutcheson, E.T., and Kang, A.H.: Collagen polymorphism in idiopathic pulmonary fibrosis. J. Clin. Invest. 57:1498, 1976.
105. Seyer, J.M., Hutcheson, E.T., and Kang, A.H.: Collagen polymorphism in normal and cirrhotic human liver. J. Clin. Invest. 59:241, 1977.
106. Sandberg, L.B., Weissman, N., and Smith, D.W.: The purification and partial characterization of a soluble elastin-like protein from copper-deficient porcine aorta. Biochemistry 8:2940, 1969.
107. Foster, J.A., Shapiro, R., Voynow, P., Crombie, G., Faris, B., and Franzblau, C.: Isolation of soluble elastin from lathyritic chicks: Comparison of tropoelastin from copper deficient pigs. Biochemistry 14:5343, 1975.
108. Sandberg, L.B., Soskel, N.J., and Wolt, M.S.: Structure of the elastic fiber: An overview. J. Invest. Dermatol. 79:128, 1982.
109. Foster, J.A., Bruenger, E., Gray, W.R., and Sandberg, L.: Isolation and amino acid sequences of tropoelastin peptides. J. Biol. Chem. 248:2876, 1973.
110. Burnett, W., Yoon, K., Finnigan-Bunick, A., and Rosenbloom, J.: Control of elastin synthesis. J. Invest. Dermatol. 79:138, 1982.
111. Burnett, W., Yoon, K., and Rosenbloom, J.: Construction, identification and characterization of a chick elastin cDNA clone. Biochem. Biophys. Res. Commun. 99:364, 1981.
112. Stevens, P.M., Hrilica, V.S., Johnson, P.C., and Bell, R.L.: Pathophysiology of hereditary emphysema. Ann. Intern. Med. 74:672, 1971.
113. Kühn, C., Yu, S., Chraplyvy, M., Lander, H.E., and Senior, R.M.: The induction of emphysema with elastase. II. Changes in connective tissue. Lab. Invest. 34:372, 1976.
114. Carnes, W.H.: Role of copper in connective tissue metabolism. Fed. Proc. 30:995, 1971.
115. Chou, W.S., Savage, J.E., and O'Dell, B.L.: Role of copper in biosynthesis of intramolecular crosslinks in chick tendon collagen. J. Biol. Chem. 244:5785, 1969.
116. Ruoslahti, E., Engvall, E., and Jayman, E.G.: Fibronectin: Current concepts of its structure and function. Coll. Res. 1:95, 1981.
117. Kleinman, H.K., Klebe, R.J., and Martin, G.R.: Role of collagenous matrices in the adhesion and growth of cells. J. Cell Biol. 88:473, 1981.
118. Ruoslahti, E., Pierschbacher, M., Engvall, E., Oldberg, A., and Hayman, E.G.: Molecular and biological interactions of fibronectin. J. Invest. Dermatol. 79:65, 1982.
119. Klebe, R.J.: Isolation of a collagen-dependent cell attachment factor. Nature 250:248, 1974.
120. Mosesson, M.W., Chen, A.B., and Huseby, R.M.: The cold-insoluble globulin of human plasma: Studies of its essential structural features. Biochim. Biophys. Acta 386:509, 1975.
121. Ruoslahti, E., and Engvall, E.: Immunochemical and collagen-binding properties of fibronectin. Ann. N.Y. Acad. Sci. 312:198, 1978.
122. Engvall, E., and Ruoslahti, E., and Miller, E.J.: Affinity of fibronectin to collagen of different genetic types and to fibronectin. J. Exp. Med. 147:1584, 1978.
123. Porter, R.R., and Reid, K.B.M.: The biochemistry of complement. Nature 285:699, 1978.
124. Highberger, J.H., Corbett, C., and Gross, J.: Isolation and characterization of a peptide containing the site of cleavage of the chick skin

collagen αl(I) chain by animal collagenases. Biochem. Biophys. Res. Commun. 89:202, 1979.
125. Mainardi, C.L., Hasty, D.L., Seyer, J.M., and Kang, A.H.: Specific cleavage of human type III collagen by human polymorphonuclear leukocyte elastase. J. Biol. Chem. 255:12006, 1980.
126. Mosher, D.F.: Crosslinking of cold insoluble globulin by fibrin stabilizing factor. J. Biol. Chem. 250:6614, 1975.
127. Grinnell, F., Feld, M., and Minter, D.: Fibroblast adhesion to fibronectin and fibrin substrate: Requirement for cold-insoluble globulin (plasma fibronectin). Cell 19:517, 1980.
128. Yamata, K.M., Kennedy, D.W., Kimato, K., and Pratt: Characterization of fibronectin interaction with glycosaminoglycans and identification of active proteolytic fragments. J. Biol. Chem. 255:6055, 1980.
129. Kleinman, H.K., Martin G.R., and Fishman, P.H.: Ganglioside inhibition of the fibronectin-mediated cell adhesion to collagen. Proc. Natl. Acad. Sci. USA 76:3367, 1979.
130. Keski-Oja, J., Sen, A., and Todara, G.J.: Direct association of fibronectin and actin molecules in vitro. J. Cell Biol. 85:527, 1980.
131. Kuersela, P.: Fibronectin binds to *Staphylococcus aureus.* Nature 276:718, 1978.
132. Simpson, W.A., Hasty, D.L., Mason, J.M., and Beachey, E.H.: Fibronectin mediates the binding of streptocococci to human polymorphonuclear leukocytes. Infect. Immun. 37:805, 1982.
133. Simpson, W.A., and Beachey, E.H.: Adherence of group A streptococci to fibronectin on oral epithelial cells. Infect. Immun. 39:275, 1983.
134. Speziale, P., Höök, M., Wadström, T., Timpl, R.: Binding of the basement membrane protein laminin to *Escherichia coli.* FEBS Lett. 146:55, 1982.
135. Balian, G., Click, E.M., Crouch, E., Davidson, J.M., and Bornstein, P.: Isolation of a collagen-binding fragment from fibronectin and cold-insoluble globulin. J. Biol. Chem. 254:1429, 1979.
136. Wagner, D.D., and Haynes, R.O.: Topological arrangement of the major structural features of fibronectin. J. Biol. Chem. 255:4304, 1980.
137. Hewitt, A.T., Varner, H.H., and Martin, G.H.: Isolation of chondronectin. *In* Furthmayr, H. (ed.): Immunochemistry of Collagen. Vol. I: Methods. Boca Raton, Florida, CRS Press, 1982.
138. Terranova, V.P., Rohrback, D.H., and Martin, G.R.: Role of laminin in the attachment of PAM 212 (epithelial) cell to basement membrane collagen. Cell, 22:719, 1980.

# Chapter 15
# Glycosaminoglycans

*Kenneth D. Brandt, M.D.*

## NOMENCLATURE

"Glycosaminoglycan" (GAG) is the term currently used to designate members of the class of compounds formerly called "acid mucopolysaccharides." It represents a shortening of "glycosaminoglucuronoglycan," the designation proposed by Jeanloz[1] for these long-chain, unbranched carbohydrate polymers (-glycans) composed of repeating disaccharide units, one constituent of which is an aminosugar (glycosamino-) and the other a hexuronic acid (glucurono-). Since keratan sulfate contains galactose instead of hexuronic acid, it is not a glycosamino*glucurono*glycan and hence is an exception to this rule of generic structure. Glycosaminoglycan, therefore, is both a simpler and more accurate designation for this class of compounds.

## GAG COMPOSITION AND STRUCTURE

Several clear, concise reviews of GAG structure have been published.[2-4] The relevant features will be summarized here. Seven GAGs have been characterized: (1) hyaluronic acid, (2) chondroitin 4-sulfate, (3) chondroitin 6-sulfate, (4) dermatan sulfate, (5) heparan sulfate, (6) heparin, and (7) keratan sulfate. The current nomenclature, which has evolved as the molecular structures of these GAGs have become known, and their old synonyms, are shown in Table 15–1. Each GAG is distinguished by the composition of its disaccharide repeating units, the location and number of its sulfate groups, and the position and configuration of its glycosidic linkages (Table 15–2; Fig. 15–1). Hyaluronic acid and the chondroitin sulfates are homogeneous chains, showing unvarying repetition of their basic disaccharide units, whereas other GAGs, for example, heparin, heparan sulfate, and dermatan sulfate, contain variations in their repeating units, either in block structures or in a less well-ordered fashion.

GAGs are very widely distributed in animal tissues. They do not normally occur in vivo as free polymers, however, but as protein-carbohydrate complexes (proteoglycans:protein-polysaccharides), i.e., complex molecules in which many GAG chains are linked covalently to protein via an intercalated specific linkage region involving the terminal reducing sugar of the chain. Proteoglycans differ structurally from glycoproteins; in the latter the carbohydrate exists as heteropolysaccharides rather than as homogeneous disaccharide repeating units.

GAGs are synthesized and secreted by connective tissue cells (e.g., fibroblasts and chondrocytes) and play an essential role in maintaining the structural integrity

**Table 15–1.** Current and Old Nomenclature of Glycosaminoglycans

| New Term | Old Term |
|---|---|
| Hyaluronic acid | Hyaluronic acid |
| Chondroitin 4-sulfate | Chondroitin sulfate A |
| Chondroitin 6-sulfate | Chondroitin sulfate C |
| Dermatan sulfate | Chondroitin sulfate B |
| Heparan sulfate | Heparitin sulfate; heparin monosulfate |
| Heparin | Heparin |
| Keratan sulfate | Keratosulfate |
| Glycosaminoglycan | Acid mucopolysaccharide |
| Proteoglycan | Chondromucoprotein; protein-polysaccharide complex |

**Table 15–2.** Composition, Structure and Occurrence of Glycosaminoglycans

| Compound | Monosaccharides in Disaccharide Repeating Unit | Molecular Weight (X 10⁻³) | *N*-Acetyl Groups | *O*-Sulfate Groups | *N*-Sulfate Groups | Sulfate (Moles per Disaccharide Unit) | Examples of Sites of Occurrence |
|---|---|---|---|---|---|---|---|
| Hyaluronic acid | D-glucosamine + D-glucuronic acid | 4–8 | + | — | — | 0 | Synovial fluid, umbilical cord, vitreous humor, skin cartilage |
| Chondroitin 4-sulfate | D-galactosamine + D-glucuronic acid | 5–50 | + | + | — | 0.1–1.3 | Cartilage, cornea, skin, bone |
| Chondroitin 6-sulfate | D-galactosamine + D-glucuronic acid | 5–50 | + | + | — | 0.1–1.3 | Arterial wall, leukocytes, platelets |
| Dermatan sulfate | D-galactosamine + L-iduronic acid or D-glucuronic acid | 15–40 | + | + | — | 1.0–3.0 | Skin, heart valve, arterial wall, tendon |
| Heparan sulfate | D-glucosamine + L-iduronic acid or D-glucuronic acid | 50 | + | + | + | 0.4–2.0 | Lung, arterial wall |
| Heparin | D-glucosamine + L-iduronic acid or D-glucuronic acid | 4–25 | + | + | ++ | 1.6–3.0 | Mast cells (lung, liver, skin, intestinal mucosa) |
| Keratan sulfate | D-glucosamine + galactose | 4–19 | + | + | — | 0.9–1.8 | Cartilage, cornea, intervertebral disc |

of connective tissue. In addition, some GAGs are synthesized and stored within specialized cells in the circulation, e.g., platelets and leukocytes,[5] where they may have an intracellular structural role. Heparan sulfate, which is present on the cell surface, mediates fibroblast adhesion,[6] and the heparan sulfate proteoglycan on the surface of endothelial cells functions as an anticoagulant[7] and, by binding lipoprotein lipase, may help regulate removal of triacylglycerol fatty acids from the circulation.[8] Heparin is synthesized and stored in tissue mast cells and hence is not a component of connective tissue. It is, however, secreted into the connective tissue where it is an anticoagulant and perhaps has other functions, but no structural role.

**Hyaluronic Acid.** Hyaluronic acid preparations vary greatly in chain length and, therefore, in molecular weight, depending on the tissue of origin (Table 15–2).[9] Their disaccharide repeating units contain one molecule of *N*-acetyl-D-glucosamine and one of D-glucuronic acid in 1→3 glycosidic linkage (Fig. 15–1). The repeating unit undergoes no further modification. Hyaluronic acid is the predominant GAG in synovial fluid, vitreous humor, and umbilical cord, and occurs in lesser proportions in most tissues of the body, and in all cartilage, where it serves as an integral part of proteoglycan aggregates (see below).

**Chondroitin 4- and Chondroitin 6-Sulfate.** The repeating disaccharides of the chondroitin sulfate 4- and 6- isomers are identical except for the position of their substituent sulfate moieties. The chondroitin sulfates are the most abundant of the GAGs in the body and occur in both skeletal and soft connective tissues; they are the predominant GAGs of articular cartilage. The 4-sulfate isomer is characteristic of embryonic and immature cartilage, while the tissue content of chondroitin 6-sulfate increases with maturation. Chondroitin 4-sulfate has also been identified in leukocytes and platelets.[5]

Chondroitin sulfate chains are shorter than those of hyaluronic acid, and consist of some 20 to 100 repeating units, which account for average molecular weights of about 5000 to 50,000 (Table 15–2). Each repeating unit consists of *N*-acetyl-D-galactosamine and D-glucuronic acid in 1→3 glyosidic linkage. The sulfate groups are situated on the galactosamine (Fig. 15–1). In some cases chondroitin sulfate chains may be hybrids, with some galactosamine residues bearing sulfate in the 4- position and others in the 6- position.[10] Occasionally, the glucuronic acid moiety also may contain ester sulfate.

**Dermatan Sulfate.** Dermatan sulfate differs from chondroitin sulfate in that it contains predominantly L-iduronic acid rather than D-glucuronic acid. (Iduronic acid is the carbon-5 epimer of glucuronic acid). The uronosyl linkage is 1→3, as in hyaluronic acid and the chondroitin sulfates. Since the purified GAG chain invariably contains some D-glucuronic acid residues,[11] which are in disaccharide units identical to those of chondroitin sulfate, dermatan sulfate can be regarded as a hybrid molecule, or a co-polymer of chondroitin sulfate. Dermatan sulfate is found chiefly in skin, heart valves, tendon, and arterial wall. In the skin, dermatan sulfate is copolymerized with chondroitin 4-sulfate, whereas the dermatan sulfate in umbilical cord is copolymerized with chondroitin 6-sulfate.[11] In some cases dermatan sulfate may contain more than one sulfate group per disaccharide unit.[12]

In vitro, dermatan sulfate proteoglycans exhibit a strong ability to precipitate tropocollagen from solution at physiologic pH and ionic strength, which is not seen with chondroitin sulfate proteoglycans.[13] It has been suggested that the main function of dermatan sulfate may be related to the formation of collagen fibers.[14] In vivo, dermatan sulfate is very closely associated with collagen.[15]

**Heparan Sulfate.** Heparan sulfate is found in significant quantities in lung and in blood vessel walls, where it probably plays a structural role, and is associated with amyloid fibrils in the connective tissue.[16] Heparan sulfate occurs predominantly in the microenvironment of the cell. It is present at the external surface of a number of cell types grown in vitro,[17] and in the extracellular matrix synthesized by fibroblast-like cells in culture.[18] It is also a constituent of the glomerular basement membrane,[19,20] but it is not a constituent of skeletal tissue.

Heparan sulfate contains some disaccharide repeating units comprised of D-glucosamine and D-glucuronic acid, and others composed of D-glucosamine and L-iduronic acid. It differs from all of the GAGs mentioned previously with respect to its glycosidic linkage, since its uronosyl linkages are 1→4, rather than 1→3. Heparan sulfate and heparin uniquely contain *N*-sulfate groups in addition to *O*-sulfate groups on the glucosamine residues (Table 15–2).

**Heparin.** Heparin bears close structural similarity to heparan sulfate, and it has been considered that these two GAGs make up a family of related molecules. There is evidence to suggest that heparan sulfate may be a normal precursor in the biosynthesis of heparin.[21,22] Thus, heparin consists of disaccharide repeating units containing D-glucosamine and either D-glucuronic or L-iduronic acid. The uronosyl linkage is 1→4, with an α-configuration, which distinguishes it from the chondroitin sulfates and keratan sulfate, which contain β 1→3 uronosyl linkages. In contrast to heparan sulfate, nearly all of the glucosamine residues of heparin are *N*-sulfated and many of the uronic acid moieties also bear sulfate groups.[23] Furthermore, while heparan sulfate exists in

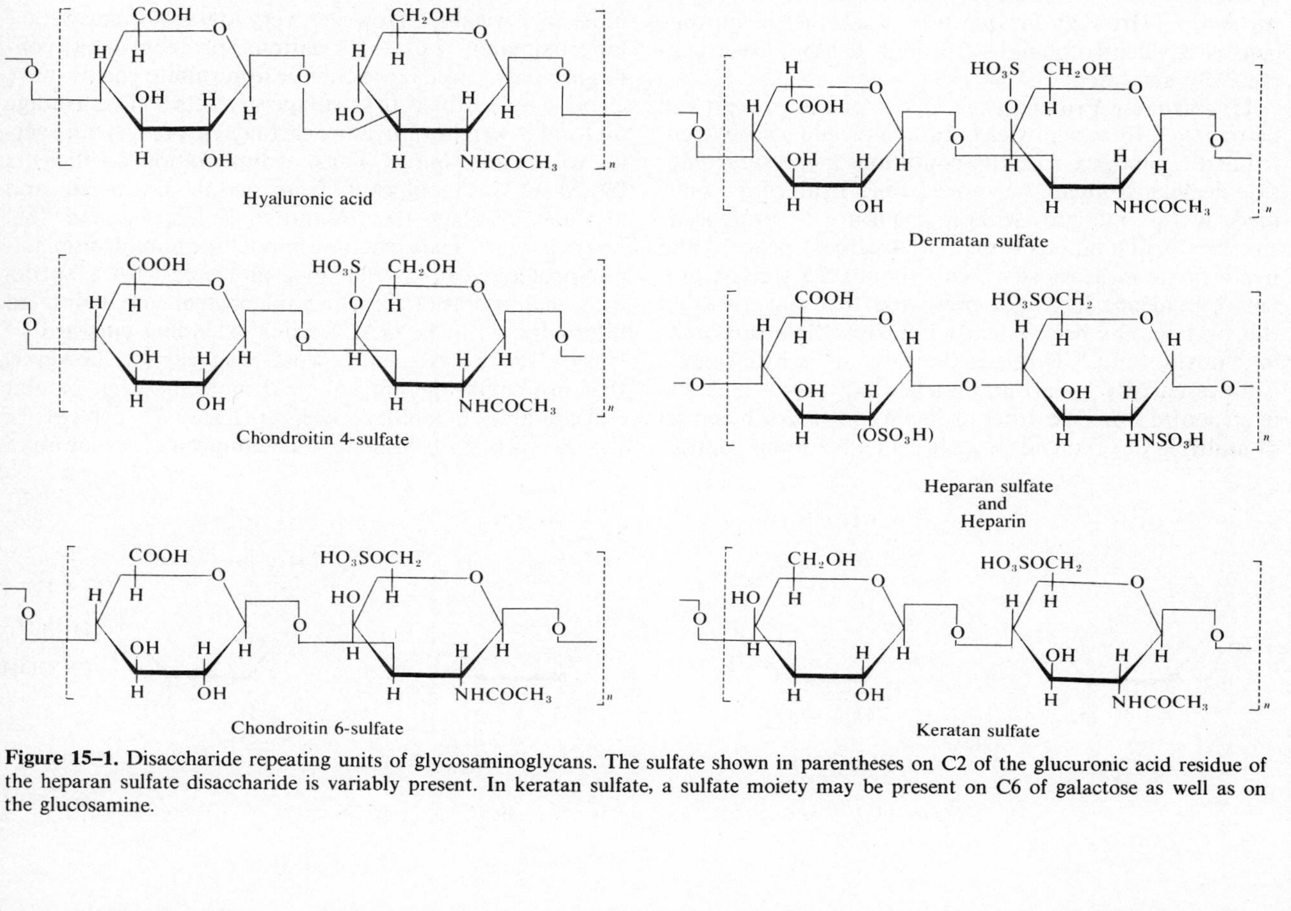


**Figure 15–1.** Disaccharide repeating units of glycosaminoglycans. The sulfate shown in parentheses on C2 of the glucuronic acid residue of the heparan sulfate disaccharide is variably present. In keratan sulfate, a sulfate moiety may be present on C6 of galactose as well as on the glucosamine.

extracellular locations, heparin is stored in the specific granules of the tissue mast cell.

**Keratan Sulfate.** Keratan sulfate contains a repeating disaccharide unit made up of galactose linked in a $\beta$-configuration $1 \rightarrow 3$ to *N*-acetylglucosamine. Sulfate may be present at C-6 of the glucosamine and also on the galactose residues. Keratan sulfate has been reported to show a good amount of compositional heterogeneity, and to contain small amounts of mannose, fucose, sialic acid, xylose, and *N*-acetyl galactosamine.[24,25] More recent data, however, indicate that these sugars are not components of the GAG chain itself but constituents of oligosaccharides situated in the keratan sulfate–rich region of the proteoglycan[26] (see below).

Two types of keratan sulfate have been characterized: Type I occurs in cornea, and Type II in cartilage and nucleus pulposus.[27,28] In cartilage proteoglycans, keratan sulfate and chondroitin sulfate are covalently linked to the same protein core. The linkage to protein of Type I and Type II keratan sulfate, however, is not the same. In cornea the link appears to be *N*-glycosidic, involving *N*-acetyl glucosamine and asparagine.[29] In cartilage, however, the linkage is *O*-glycosidic and involves the hydroxyaminoacids, threonine or serine,[30] and *N*-acetyl galactosamine.[31]

## LINKAGE OF GAGs TO PROTEIN

There is now clear evidence that most of the GAGs in cartilage exist as proteoglycans, covalently linked to protein,[32,33] although the question of whether hyaluronic acid is covalently bound to protein has not been conclusively answered.

**Hyaluronate-Proteoglycan.** Most of the protein can be removed from synovial fluid hyaluronic acid by centrifugation under associative conditions in a cesium chloride density gradient.[34] Synovial fluid hyaluronate purified by this method, without exposure to proteolytic enzymes, still contains some 2 to 4 percent protein, and hyaluronate from rooster comb about 0.35 percent protein.[35] Evidence has been presented that suggests that this protein may be covalently linked to the hyaluronate in synovial fluid.[36] If this is the case, since hyaluronate is an essentially linear, unbranched polymer,[37] it differs in structure from the other proteoglycans, which consist of multiple GAG chains attached to a common peptide. On the other hand, when cultures of Swarm rat chondrosarcoma were labeled with $^3$H-lysine, no $^3$H-labeled molecules, and therefore no core protein, was found to be associated with the hyaluronate.[38]

**Chondroitin Sulfate–Keratan Sulfate Proteoglycans.** The most extensively studied proteoglycan is the chondroitin 4-sulfate–keratan sulfate protein of cartilage. The demonstration of a covalent linkage between the GAG and protein was provided by Muir,[39] who noted that after exhaustive treatment with proteolytic enzymes, purified chondroitin sulfate preparations retained an abundance of serine. The structure of the chondroitin 4-sulfate linkage region was subsequently worked out[40,41] and was shown to consist of serine, xylose, galactose, and glucuronic acid, in molar ratios of 1:1:2:1. The chondroitin sulfate is covalently attached via an *O*-glycosidic bond between xylose and the hydroxyl group of serine on the protein core of the proteoglycan (Fig. 15–2). About 50 percent of the total serine of the proteoglycan is occupied in linkage of chondroitin sulfate chains.[42] A linkage structure identical to that described above for 4-sulfate proteoglycans has been described for proteoglycans of chondroitin 6-sulfate, dermatan sulfate, heparan sulfate, and heparin.[43,44]

The protein core of a typical cartilage proteoglycan has a molecular weight of approximately 200,000 daltons. It constitutes about 5 to 10 percent of the total weight of the molecule, and contains approximately 100 chondroitin sulfate chains and 60 keratan sulfate chains covalently bound to the protein. The complete proteoglycan molecule thus averages 1 to 4 $\times$ $10^6$ daltons in molecular weight.[33] However, very low molecular weight (approximately 7.6 $\times$ $10^4$ daltons) proteoglycans, containing only 1 to 2 large chondroitin sulfate chains, have also been identified in cartilage extracts.[45] The average molecular weight of hyaline cartilage proteoglycans varies with their source. Thus, sedimentation coefficients ($S^o_{20}$,S) of proteoglycans from nasal, traceheal, and articular cartilage were found to be 25, 20, and 16S, respectively.[46] The structural model for chondroitin sulfate-proteoglycans is that of a molecule with a bottle-brush configuration, in which the protein core is situated internally, with the GAG chains extending outward[47,48] (Fig. 15–3). Recent work suggests, however, that proteoglycans are not rigid molecules, but exhibit considerable flexibility over at least 80 percent of the core protein backbone.[49] The molecular structure of

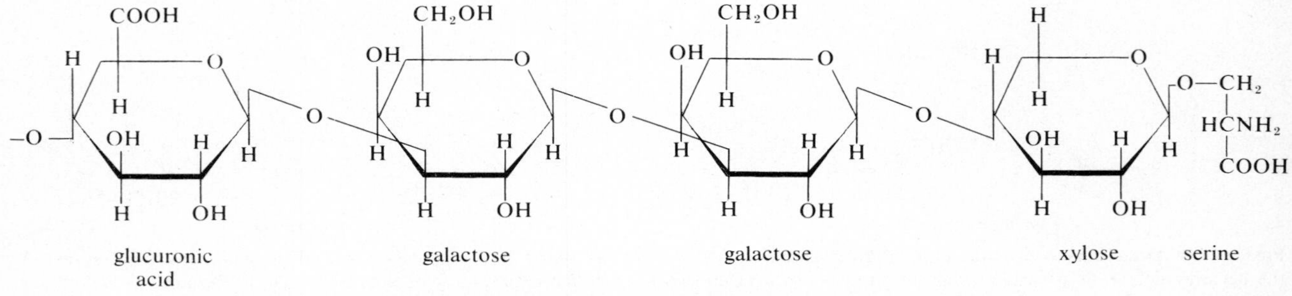


**Figure 15–2.** Structure of the common linkage region of proteoglycans.

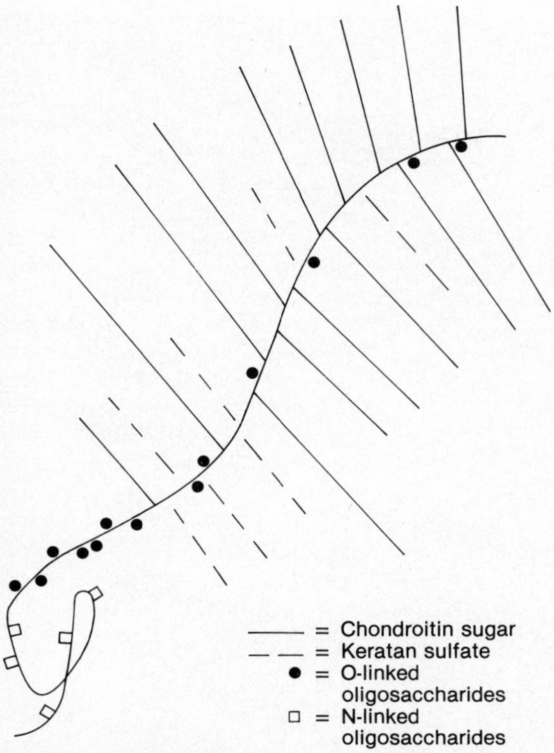


**Figure 15–3.** Proteoglycan molecule, depicting bottle-brush configuration and heterogeneity of the core protein with respect to attachment sites for chondroitin sulfate and keratan sulfate, and hyaluronate-binding region.

the proteoglycan renders it especially vulnerable to degradation by proteolytic enzymes, so that cleavage of only one or two peptide bonds on the protein core will destroy the molecule.[39]

The GAGs are not homogeneously distributed along the protein core of the proteoglycan, but most of the chondroitin sulfate chains are attached near the C-terminal end, while the N-terminal portion is devoid of polysaccharide and constitutes a hyaluronate-binding region whose integrity is crucial for aggregation[50,51] (Fig. 15–1). Most of the keratan sulfate is attached to the protein near the hyaluronate-binding region, in a region proximal to the attachment sites of most of the chondroitin sulfate chains.

The hyaluronate-binding region appears to have the same structure whenever present, and it is found on most proteoglycans. However, some nonaggregating proteoglycans with a high molecular weight appear to lack the hyaluronate-binding region and the adjacent keratan-sulfate–rich segment.[52] The very low molecular weight ($7.6 \times 10^4$ daltons) proteoglycan mentioned above also does not interact with hyaluronate.[45] Its protein core (apparent molecular weight $= 1.5 \times 10^4$ daltons) has an amino acid composition that is different from that of other cartilage proteoglycans, but similar to that found in low molecular weight proteoglycans from sclera, tendon, aorta, and cornea.

The polysaccharide attachment region of the aggregating proteoglycans varies in length; proteoglycans from young cartilage appear to have a longer chondroitin sulfate attachment region than those from older cartilage.[53]

Recently, small oligosaccharide chains containing sialic acid have been shown to be integral constituents of cartilage proteoglycans.[26] Two classes of oligosaccharides have been described: the first, which is of larger size, contains mannose, galactose, glucosamine, and sialic acid and is linked to an asparagine molecule on the core protein via an *N*-glycosidic bond. The second class of oligosaccharide contains galactosamine, galactose, and glucosamine, in addition to sialic acid, and is linked to serine or threonine on the core protein via an *O*-glycosidic bond involving *N*-acetylgalactosamine.

The structure of the *O*-linked oligosaccharides markedly resembles that of the keratan sulfate linkage region, and it is likely, therefore, that they represent a biosynthetic precursor of keratan sulfate. Consistent with this possibility is the observation that an inverse relationship exists between the number of *O*-linked oligosaccharides and the number of keratan sulfate chains at various ages and in various cartilages.[26,54] Furthermore, in view of the evidence that the uptake of glycoproteins, including lysosomal enzymes, by cells is mediated by receptors that recognize specific monosaccharide markers carried on the oligosaccharide chains of the glycoproteins,[55-58] it is possible that the oligosaccharides on proteoglycans serve similarly as markers to facilitate their uptake by cells.

Indeed, studies indicate that sulfated proteoglycans are internalized by skin fibroblasts by endocytosis, following their association with binding sites on the cell surface.[59] GAGs and other anionic macromolecules inhibit the endocytosis of sulfated proteoglycans noncompetitively, and do not interact with the cell surface receptors for the sulfated proteoglycans, suggesting that the core protein is required for binding to the cell surface. The data suggest also that a recycling of the receptors occurs between the endocytotic vesicles and/or lysosomes and the cell surface.[59]

The molecular structure of the proteoglycans accounts for some of the unique biological properties of articular cartilage. Due to their high carboxylate and sulfate content GAGs are polyanions, possessing a high negative charge density. Adjacent GAG chains on the proteoglycan, therefore, strongly repel each other. Because of this charge repulsion, the protein core and the GAG chains tend to be fully extended in the cartilage so that each proteoglycan, in attempting to occupy the largest possible molecular domain, encompasses a very large volume of water. The hydroxyl groups on the GAGs, furthermore, are highly hydrophilic. These factors thus account for the very high water content of articular cartilage (some 70 to 80 percent of the total weight), and its elastic resistance to compression.

Articular cartilage proteoglycans inhibit fibroblast spreading and adhesion to collagenous substrates.[60] On the basis of this data it has been hypothesized that loss of proteoglycans from the cartilage in rheumatoid arthritis may be necessary for invasion of the surface by the cells in the pannus.

In normal articular cartilage about 75 percent of the proteoglycans exist in aggregates, in which many individual molecules are noncovalently associated with a long, chainlike molecule of hyaluronic acid[61,62] (Fig. 15–4). Link proteins, which constitute about 3 percent of the weight of the complex, stabilize the proteoglycan-hyaluronate interaction.[50] Two link proteins, with molecular weights of approximately 44,000 and 48,000 daltons, respectively, have been identified. The larger contains 9.5 percent carbohydrate while the smaller, whose amino acid composition is similar, contains only 3 percent carbohydrate and is presumed to be a degradation product of the larger.[63,64] These molecular interactions account for sedimentation coefficients ($S_{20^\circ w}$) of 60 to 70 S and molecular weights of $1 \times 10^8$ daltons exhibited by the aggregates. Recent evidence suggests that the interaction of link with hyaluronate may induce a structural change in the latter, leading to a larger aggregate than that seen with equimolar concentrations of proteoglycans and of hyaluronate in the absence of link.[65]

The proteoglycan-hyaluronate interaction has been examined in detail[66] by viscometry and molecular sieve chromatography. From these studies, on the basis of average molecular weights of proteoglycans and hyaluronate (approximately $0.5 \times 10^6$ daltons), a model for the aggregate was derived.[67] The dimensions of the model closely approximate those calculated from electron photomicrographs of aggregates.[68] Figure 15–5 shows the ultrastructure of a PG aggregate, published by Rosenberg and associates.[68] Weaving through the structure is the backbone of the aggregate, the chain of hyaluronic acid. The "side chains" represent individual proteoglycan molecules (monomers) noncovalently linked to the hyaluronate backbone. The cartilage hyaluronate molecules range from about 4000 to 40,000 Å in length, and the number of proteoglycan subunits per aggregate is roughly proportional to the length of the hyaluronate. Some 30 to 60 repeating disaccharide units of hyaluronic acid are present between adjacent proteoglycans. The binding region for each proteoglycan occupies some 5 to 10 disaccharide units of the hyaluronate.[68,69] Decasaccharides of hyaluronic acid compete strongly with high molecular weight hyaluronic acid and effectively inhibit the interaction, whereas smaller oligosaccharides have little effect on aggregation.[69,70]

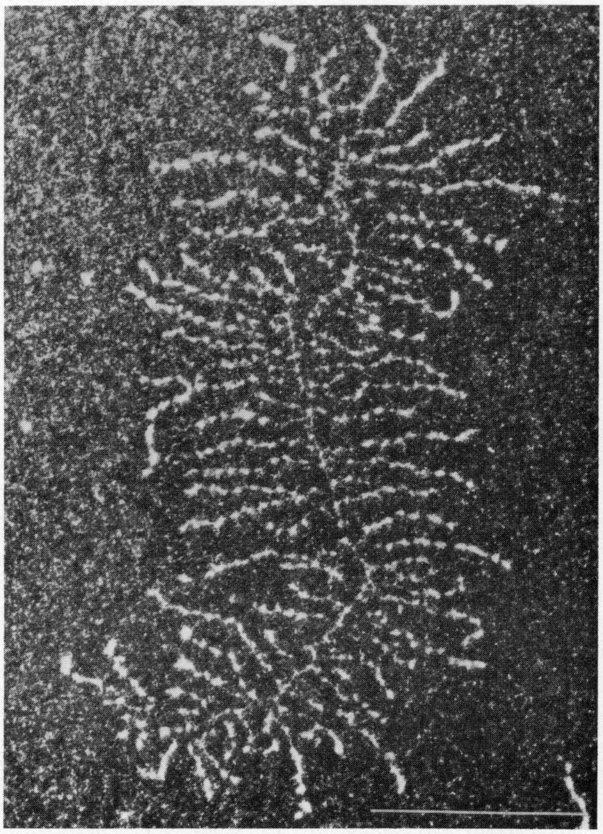

**Figure 15–5.** Dark-field electron photomicrograph of a proteoglycan aggregate. The central core is comprised of a molecule of hyaluronic acid. The appended "side chains" represent individual proteoglycans. The length of the white bar in the lower right hand corner represents 0.5 m (magnification = 120,000). (From Rosenberg, L., Hellmann, W., Kleinschmidt, A.K.: J. Biol. Chem. 250:1877, 1975.)

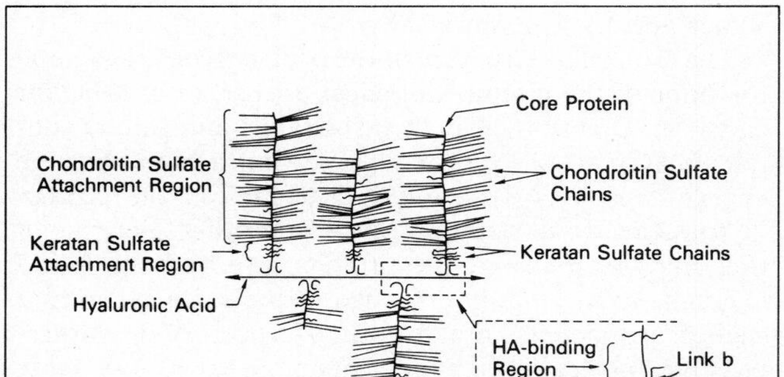

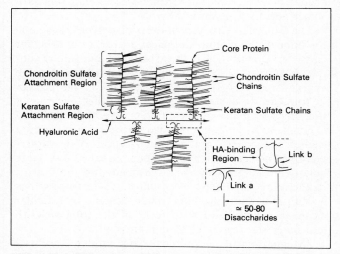

**Figure 15–4.** Schematic model for structure of cartilage proteoglycans and for a portion of a proteoglycan aggregate. (From Hascall, V.C.: J. Supramolecular Struct. 7:101, 1977.)

The aggregation phenomenon is phenotypic of cartilage and is highly specific. Cartilage proteoglycans will interact only with hyaluronate and not with other GAGs.[71] Aggregation presumably helps constrain individual proteoglycans (which themselves may have molecular weights greater than $1 \times 10^6$ daltons) in the collagen meshwork. Although proteoglycan monomers interact more extensively among themselves than aggregates, interactions among aggregates are much stronger than those among monomers. Furthermore, the stiffening of an interacting network of monomers produced by shear forces relaxes much more quickly than the shear stiffening of a network of interacting aggregates.[72] In addition, aggregation may help protect proteoglycans from proteolytic degradation.[50]

Aggregation may also modulate cartilage metabolism, since hyaluronic acid, if free and not combined with proteoglycans, inhibits proteoglycan synthesis in chondrocyte cultures.[71,73] There is also evidence that proteoglycan aggregates inhibit calcification of cartilage,[74] presumably by shielding minute crystal particles and preventing their further growth.[75] Proteoglycan aggregates may prevent urate, as well as calcium, from precipitating in cartilage, since they retard precipitation of monosodium urate from supersaturated solutions, whereas equimolar concentrations of nonaggregated proteoglycans do not.[76]

Recently, a chondroitin-sulfate proteoglycan that inhibits Clq, the first component of complement, has been identified in serum.[77] This molecule contains less than 1 percent glucosamine and presumably lacks keratan sulfate. Since it does not form a complex with hyaluronic acid or contain any chondroitin 6-sulfate, its origin is presumably noncartilaginous. Interaction between the inhibitor and Clq was evident in 0.15M NaCl, suggesting that it may have some importance under physiologic conditions.

**Heparin-Proteoglycan.** Studies of heparin-proteoglycans have yielded seemingly contradictory results. Heparin is synthesized by mast cells, which store it in specific cytoplasmic granules. In some tissues, e.g., bovine liver capsule, heparin occurs as free GAG chains, with a molecular weight less than $1 \times 10^4$ daltons,[78] a value comparable to that of the commercial heparin used as an anticoagulant. Heparin isolated from rat peritoneal mast cells, in contrast, has a molecular weight of about $7.5 \times 10^5$ daltons and appears to consist of multiple GAG chains joined to a protein core.[79] This complex is notably resistant to proteolysis. It is possible that single-chain forms of heparin represent reaction products resulting from cleavage of peptide-bound chains by specific endoglycosidases.[80]

## GAG BIOSYNTHESIS

Present information suggests that the protein core is synthesized in a conventional manner on a ribosomal template, and the carbohydrate chains are assembled post-translationally,[81,82] one sugar at a time, starting with the attachment of xylose to serine in a structurally specific linkage region. Sulfation takes place after the appropriate monosaccharide has been linked into the growing chain. The sugars and the sulfate residues each are derived from "activated" precursors, i.e., uridine sugar nucleotides and phosphoadenosine-5′-phosphosulfate, respectively. Elongation of the GAG chain, and its sulfation, occur in the endoplasmic reticulum and Golgi complex as the core protein progresses from the polyribosomes to the exterior of the cell.

The requisite sugar nucleotides that serve as monosaccharide precursors of the growing chain of repeating disaccharides are synthesized from D-glucose, as shown in Figure 15–6. Details of the enzymatic steps involved have been reviewed.[2,3] The UDP-sugars are then transferred sequentially to the growing GAG chain (or its linkage region).

Intracellular levels of UDP derivatives are controlled to some extent by feedback inhibition. For example, increasing levels of UDP-xylose inhibit UDP-glucose dehydrogenase, which converts UDP-glucose to UDP-glucuronic acid, the immediate precursor of UDP-xylose.[3] Similarly, excessive levels of UDP-*N*-acetylglucosamine inhibit formation of glucosamine 6-phosphate from fructose 6-phosphate and glutamine[3] (Fig. 15–6). Since xylose is the initial sugar to be added to protein in GAG chain synthesis, a deficiency of acceptor protein will lead to accumulation of UDP-xylose which, by the negative feedback mechanism described above, can suppress formation of UDP-glucuronic acid, inhibiting further GAG chain synthesis.

For the biosynthesis of a chondroitin sulfate chain several transferase steps are required, involving a variety of glycosyltransferases and one sulfotransferase (Fig. 15–7). The first reaction involves xylosyltransferase, which

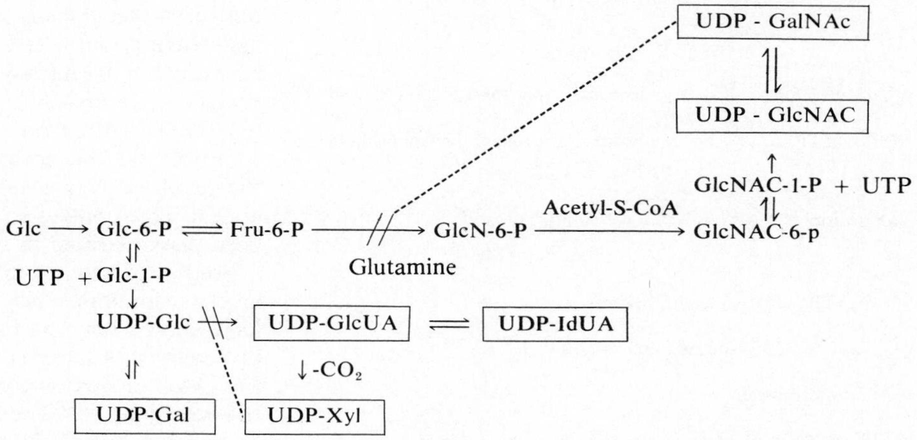


**Figure 15–6.** Nucleotide sugars involved in biosynthesis of GAGs and relevant sugar interconversions. Dotted lines indicate sites of feedback inhibition.

- Serine (on core protein) -

① Xylosyl transferase

② Galactosyl transferase

③ Galactosyl transferase

④ Glucuronic acid transferase

⑤ N-acetylgalactosamine transferase

⑥ Sequential action of No. 4 and No. 5 for lengthening of chain

⑦ Sulfotransferase

**Figure 15–7.** Enzymes involved in biosynthesis of a chrondroitin sulfate chain and its specific linkage region on a proteoglycan. The glycosyl transferases act on UDP-sugars and the sulfotransferase on PAPS.

effects the transfer of xylose from UDP-xylose to serine on the protein core.[83] The next two reactions involve galactosyltransferase, which transfers two moles of galactose from UDP-galactose.[84] This is followed by the addition of the first *N*-acetylglucuronic acid residue, which is covalently bound to the second galactose residue by the action of *O*-glucuronic acid transferase on UDP-*N*-acetylglucuronic acid. Growth of the chondroitin sulfate chain then occurs by alternating transfer of *N*-acetylgalactosamine and D-glucuronic acid residues from their respective UDP-derivatives, mediated by their specific transferases (Fig. 15–7).

Sulfation of the GAG, which occurs during or after growth of the chain, requires 3-phosphoadenosyl-5-phosphosulfate (PAPS) as an intermediate.[85] Sulfate is then transferred from PAPS to the GAG chain in a reaction catalyzed by sulfotransferase (Fig. 15–8). There is no evidence that sulfated polymers can be synthesized from sulfated monosaccharide nucleotide precursors. Thus, UDP-*N*-acetylgalactosamine sulfate was not incorporated into chondroitin sulfate in epiphyseal cartilage.[86] The *N*-sulfate groups of heparan sulfate and of heparin are synthesized by displacement of pre-existing *N*-acetyl groups.[87] The chondroitin sulfate chains within a single proteoglycan molecule are heterogeneous with respect to chain length, degree of sulfation, and the location of the sulfate groups (position 4 or 6 of the galactosamine), but the factors that account for these differences are not entirely clear. It has been suggested that differences in molecular size of GAGs may be due to partial degradation of the chains.[88]

Whether the sulfotransferases lack specificity or whether different enzymes are involved in sulfation of the 4- and 6- positions of the galactosamine in chondroitin sulfate remains uncertain. The conformation of the acceptor monosaccharides and the adjacent sugar residues may influence the position of sulfation. For example, dermatan sulfate from umbilical cord contains 6-sulfate on galactosamine groups situated next to glucuronic acid residues, and chiefly 4-sulfate on those near iduronic residues.[89] Other evidence suggests the presence of specific sulfatases in embryonic chick cartilage that catalyze sulfation of specific hydroxyl groups of hexosamine residues. Robinson and Dorfman[90] found that the proportions of chondroitin 4-sulfate and 6-sulfate varied with the stage of development of the embryo, and that the proportion of the isomeric chondroitin sulfates synthesized in vitro was similar to that found in ovo at the same stage of development. A cell-free system synthesized both isomers in the presence of PAPS, but the proportion of chondroitin 4-sulfate was affected by pH and length of incubation, suggesting the presence of two sulfotransferases.[91]

sulfate + ATP —①→ adenosine-5′ phosphosulfate (APS) + PPi

APS + ATP —②→ 3′ phosphoadenosine-5′ phosphosulfate (PAPS) + ADP

chondroitin + PAPS —③→ chondroitin sulfate + phospho AMP

① = ATP: sulfate adenyltransferase

② = ATP: adenylsulfate-3′ phosphotransferase

③ = sulfotransferase

**Figure 15–8.** Enzymatic reactions in sulfation of chondroitin.

## GAG DEGRADATION

Degradation of the PG involves breakdown of the GAG chain, desulfation of the sugars, and proteolysis. The loss of cartilage matrix that results from intravenous injection of the proteolytic enzyme papain[92] illustrates the importance of the protein core to the structural integrity of the proteoglycan. Rupture of only one or two peptide bonds will cause the molecule to fall apart.[39] Cartilage contains lysosomal acid proteases, which degrade proteoglycans (e.g., cathepsin D),[93] but which have an acid pH optimum and are not active at pH 7, i.e., the pH of the extracellular ground substance. It is likely, therefore, that these acid proteases play a role in digestion of proteoglycans intracellulary, and in the immediate vicinity of the cell, but not in the expanse of matrix between the chondrocytes. On the other hand, neutral proteases are present in cartilage and will degrade proteoglycans at neutral pH 7,[94] and are presumably responsible for the normal turnover of proteoglycans in the territory between the cells. The neutral proteases appear to be controlled by potent inhibitors, which have been demonstrated in normal cartilage.[95,96]

Studies of newly synthesized cartilage proteoglycans, labeled simultaneously with $^{14}$C-lysine and $^{35}$S-sulfate, have shown that the protein and GAG moieties of the proteoglycan turn over concomitantly.[97] Degradation of the GAG chains of proteoglycans occurs principally in the lysosomes.[98,99] The most well-defined GAG lyase is the hyaluronidase from testes, which degrades hyaluronic acid to a family of even-numbered oligosaccharides, with tetrasaccharides predominating.[100] The enzyme is an endo-$\beta$-*N*-acetylhexosaminidase, and thus degrades chondroitin, chondroitin 4-sulfate, and chondroitin 6-sulfate, yielding oligosaccharide products similar in size to those that result from its action on hyaluronic acid.[101,102] Since dermatan sulfate is a chondroitin sulfate copolymer, it will also be partially degraded by these enzymes.

Endoglycosidases that degrade the iduronic acid–containing portions of dermatan sulfate or heparan sulfate, or that break down keratan sulfate, have not yet been identified in mammalian tissues. Heparin and heparan sulfate, however, are degraded by an enzyme produced by adapted strains of *Flavobacterium heparinum.*[102] This enzyme specificity may explain why chondroitin sulfate, even when injected in large amounts, is extensively degraded, whereas other mucopolysaccharides can be largely recovered in an unaltered state from the tissues and urine.[103] On the other hand, normal urine contains small quantities of GAGs, about two thirds of which are derived from chondroitin sulfate, and the remainder from chondroitin, heparan sulfate, dermatan sulfate, hyaluronic acid, and keratan sulfate.[104] The chondroitin sulfate in urine has a lower molecular weight and less sulfate than that in tissue, and is bound to a smaller protein fragment, indicative of its degraded state.

Hyaluronidase has been demonstrated in a variety of mammalian tissues in addition to testis, including liver, skin, and synovium,[105] although earlier studies failed to find evidence of hyaluronidase in articular cartilage.[105] Recently, by use of a viscometric technique more sensitive than the previously employed colorimetric methods, hyaluronidase activity was demonstrated in normal articular cartilage.[106] The activity, which had a pH optimum around 3, appeared to be specific (it could not be demonstrated when chondroitin was employed as substrate) and was related to the concentration of cyclic adenosine monophosphate in the tissue.

Other glycosidases, i.e., exoglycosidases, are required to complete the breakdown to monosaccharides of the oligosaccharides resulting from the action of hyaluronidase on GAGs. Glucuronidase and *N*-acetylhexosaminidases are lysosomal exo-enzymes, capable of cleaving terminal nonreducing glucuronic acid or hexosamine residues, respectively, from oligo- or polysaccharides. Lysosomes also contain $\beta$-xylosidase, $\beta$-galactosidase, and $\alpha$-iduronidase.[107] As indicated above, xylose and galactose occur in minor and major amounts, respectively, in keratan sulfate and also in the GAG-protein linkage region common to these proteoglycans; $\alpha$-L-iduronic acid is a constituent of dermatan sulfate, heparan sulfate, and heparin.

Lysosomal sulfatases are responsible for the desulfation of GAGs. Activity of sulfatases against intact GAG chains has not been demonstrated, but they may act on the terminal nonreducing end of sulfated oligosaccharides, or monosaccharides. A deficiency of sulfoiduronate sulfatase is the basic defect in Hurler's syndrome and deficiency of a sulfamidase specific for terminal hexosaminyl residues has been identified in another mucopolysaccharidosis, Sanfilippo A disease.

## GAGs IN THE GENETIC MUCOPOLYSACCHARIDOSES

While the excessive breakdown of GAGs in articular cartilage is important in the pathogenesis of various joint diseases (e.g., osteoarthritis, rheumatoid arthritis), incomplete degradation of GAGs is the essence of another group of disorders—the genetic mucopolysaccharidoses. A detailed description of the clinical features of these diseases is beyond the scope of this chapter but may be found elsewhere.[108] This section will review the specific biochemical abnormalities in the mucopolysaccharidoses and emphasize the relationship of these disorders to normal GAG catabolism.

The mucopolysaccharidoses are storage disorders in which the lysosomal breakdown of GAGs is incomplete, so that partially degraded GAGs are retained in lysosomes[109] within the tissues and excreted in elevated amounts in the urine. Since the demonstration by Danes and Bearn that fibroblasts cultured from the skin of patients with Hurler's syndrome show metachromasia and accumulate GAGs,[110] tissue culture has been widely applied to the study of the mucopolysaccharidoses. It was subsequently shown, on the basis of kinetics of $^{35}SO_4$ accumulation in cultured fibroblasts from patients with Hurler's and Hunter's syndromes, that the GAG accumulation was due to defective degradation[111] rather than to abnormalities in GAG synthesis or secretion. Furthermore, it was found that cocultivation of Hurler and Hunter cells resulted in mutual correction of the excessive GAG accumulation.[112] Correction of the metabolic defect in the fibroblasts could also be achieved by use of culture medium, tissue extracts, or urine from patients with any genotype except that of the patient from whom the fibroblasts were derived;[113] thus, material from patients with various mucopolysaccharidoses cross-corrected each other's defects. This led to the recognition that the various mucopolysaccharidoses were each associated with deficiencies in specific lysosomal hydrolases involved in normal GAG catabolism.

Except for the Morquio syndrome, which involves a defect in breakdown of keratan sulfate, all the other presently classified mucopolysaccharidoses involve a disturbance in the breakdown of dermatan sulfate and/or heparan sulfate by lysosomal exoenzymes, i.e., glycosides and sulfatases. These exoenzymes cleave the chains from their nonreducing termini and sequentially remove sulfate groups and sugar residues as they become exposed. For complete degradation of a GAG chain, multiple enzymes are thus required. If any are missing, the degradative sequence is blocked. Some further degradation may occur through the action of lysosomal endoglycosidases (e.g., hyaluronidase), but in the absence of the exoenzyme complete degradation cannot occur. Thus, in patients with a mucopolysaccharidosis, elevated levels of degradation fragments of the GAGs are found in urine and within lysosomes. Figure 15–9 schematically depicts portions of GAG chains and indicates the specific defects in lysosomal degradative enzymes that have been identified in the mucopolysaccharidoses.

The "corrective factors" described above have proved to be the lysosomal hydrolases missing from the fibroblasts.[114,115] Uptake of the missing enzyme by the cell does not occur simply by endocytosis, but the enzyme is taken up selectively by the cells, which appear to have a specific receptor on their surface that recognizes a specific marker associated with the carbohydrate portion of lysosomal enzymes.

In I-cell (inclusion cell) disease (mucolipidosis II) and pseudo-Hurler dystrophy (mucolipidosis III)[116] glycosidases, sulfatases, and cathepsins required for GAG degradation, as well as a number of enzymes associated with sphingolipid metabolism, are not packaged into lysosomes, but are secreted extracellularly. The clinical features of I-cell disease resemble those of Hurler's syndrome (i.e., retarded psychomotor development, progressive organomegaly, skeletal abnormalities, restricted joint mobility). Most patients die by age 6. Pseudo-Hurler polydystrophy resembles the Maroteaux-Lamy syndrome (mucopolysacchidosis VI), in which the lysosomal enzyme *N*-acetylgalactosamine 4-sulfatase is deficient.[108] In contrast to the mucopolysaccharidoses, however, in which the primary abnormality is a genetic defect in the synthesis of a specific lysosomal enzyme, in I-cell and the pseudo-Hurler disorder the enzymes are synthesized normally. Many of them are present in strikingly large amounts in plasma and other body fluids in vivo, and in the tissue culture medium when fibroblasts from afflicted individuals are cultured in vitro.

The basic defect in these disorders lies in the post-

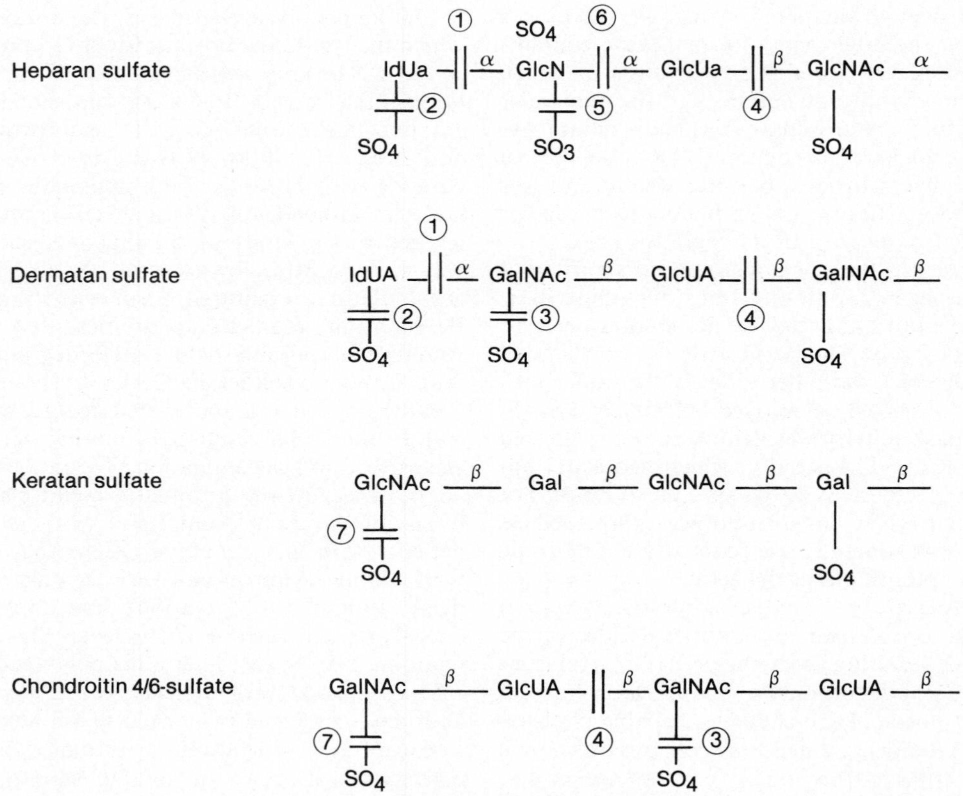


**Figure 15–9.** Enzyme defects in mucopolysaccaridoses.

| *Enzyme* | *Substrate* | *Deficiency Disease* |
|---|---|---|
| ① α-L-iduronidase | heparan sulfate; dermatan sulfate | Hurler's and Scheie's syndromes |
| ② iduronate sulfatase | heparan sulfate; dermatan sulfate | Hunter's syndrome |
| ③ N-acetylgalactosamine 4-sulfatase | dermatan sulfate; chondroitin sulfate | Maroteaux-Lamy syndrome |
| ④ β-glucuronidase | chondroitin sulfate; heparan sulfate; dermatan sulfate | Glucuronidase deficiency |
| ⑤ heparan N-sulfatase (sulfamidase) | heparan sulfate | Sanfilippo's A syndrome |
| ⑥ α-*N*-acetylglucosaminidase | heparan sulfate | Sanfilippo's B syndrome |
| ⑦ *N*-acetylhexosamine 6-sulfatase | keratan sulfate; chonroitin 6-sulfate | Morquio's syndrome |

translational modification of the acid hydrolases, and is marked by a deficiency of the mannose-6-phosphate receptor, which is present on normal hydrolases and is essential for mediating the uptake of the hydrolase by lysosomes.[55] The biochemical defect resides in the enzymatic pathway that phosphorylates mannose residues on the oligosaccharide chains of the newly synthesized hydrolases. In normal fibroblasts, this is accomplished by initial transfer of phosphate together with *N*-acetylglucosamine from UDP-*N*-acetylglucosamine, resulting in formation of a mannose-P-*N*-acetylglucosamine diester,[117] which is subsequently cleaved, leaving the mannose phosphate.[118] Patients with I-cell disease lack the specific UDP-*N*-acetylglucosamine phosphotransferase involved in this process,[119,120] while in fibroblasts from patients with pseudo-Hurler dystrophy the reaction proceeds at a very low rate.[120]

## PHYSICAL PROPERTIES OF GAGs IN RELATION TO THEIR STRUCTURE

How do GAGs subserve a structural role in connective tissue? There is considerable evidence that GAGs in certain tissues, such as cartilage and umbilical cord, exist not as solutions but as gels.[121] In hyaline cartilage and intervertebral disc, for example, GAGs may account for as much as 10 percent of the wet weight of the tissue. Because of their enormous hydrodynamic volumes (Fig. 15–10) (which, for hyaluronate and cartilage proteoglycan are 1000 and 100 times, respectively, larger than the volumes occupied by the dehydrated molecules) their solute domains are very large. For this reason, at concentrations of approximately 1 mg per $cm^3$ and 10 mg per $cm^3$, respectively, which are achieved in vivo, hyaluronate and cartilage proteoglycan molecules will begin to entangle with themselves; at higher concentrations a continuous overlapping molecular network will exist. The entanglement will tend to immobilize the proteoglycans in the tissues, achieving physical stability. The specific association of cartilage proteoglycans with hyaluronic acid, leading to formation of aggregates stabilized by link glycoproteins,[50,61] also may provide mechanical stability to cartilage. The entangled and/or aggregated proteoglycans are further constrained physically by the fibrous network of connective tissue (collagen, elastin). The proteoglycan gels prevent the gross flow of water through the tissues, although individual water molecules and small solutes diffuse readily through the gel. Large molecules, however, such as proteins, are excluded from the domain of the proteoglycan.[121,122] The diffusion of larger molecules through cartilage is limited by size and steric configuration, as well as by charge.[123] Larger molecules, therefore, such as albumin, are effectively excluded from the tissue, as reflected by studies of Maroudas showing that the partition coefficients for albumin, transferrin, and IgG were only about 0.01, in comparison with a value of 1 for proline.[123]

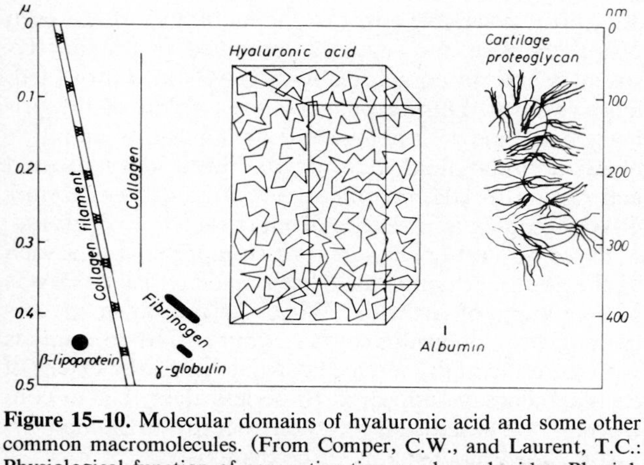


**Figure 15–10.** Molecular domains of hyaluronic acid and some other common macromolecules. (From Comper, C.W., and Laurent, T.C.: Physiological function of connective tissue polysaccharides. Physiol. Rev. 58:255, 1978.)

Because of their polyanionicity and the localization of sulfate and carboxyl groups within the molecule, the negative charge concentration within the domain of a proteoglycan is very high. The proteoglycan thus is able to participate extensively in intermolecular electrostatic interactions with adjacent molecules, such as collagen. In addition, transport of ions through connective tissue, osmotic pressure effects, and the distribution of other ions (Donnan effect) are affected considerably by the composition and concentration of the proteoglycans in tissue, and their macromolecular organization. Detailed discussion of these aspects of connective tissue physiology may be found in reference 121.

## ROLE OF HYALURONATE IN SKELETAL MORPHOGENESIS

GAGs appear to play an essential role in embryologic differentiation. For example, during morphogenesis of the limb bud at a stage characterized by extensive cell migration, hyaluronic acid accumulates in the tissues. For cell differentiation to occur the hyaluronate must be removed. Hyaluronidase can be detected, in association with a fall in GAG content of the tissue, at the onset of differentiation, as marked by the appearance of metachromasia and increase in synthesis of chondroitin sulfate.[124,125]

Hyaluronic acid, when added at an appropriate stage, can inhibit the normal formation of cartilage nodules in cultures of cells from chick embryo somites,[126] although chondroitin sulfates, heparin, or other biologic polyanions (e.g., nucleic acids) do not have this effect. A hyaluronate surface coat may regulate cell-cell interactions. Thus, in vitro, hyaluronidase digestion of endogenous surface-bound hyaluronate inhibits receptor-mediated aggregation of simian virus 40–transformed 3T3 cells.[127] The same effect was observed upon addition of a large excess of exogenous hyaluronate, which presumably caused all receptor sites to be occupied, thereby preventing crossbridging and inhibiting cell aggregation.[127] It has been considered possible that a similar phenomenon might affect embryonic cells in vivo. Thus, the hyaluronate concentrations present in the pathways of migration of embryonic cells may prevent cells from adhering to one another, thereby facilitating movement by preventing interactions that would immobilize the cells.[128] In addition, since cell movement requires sequential attachments and detachments of localized areas of the cell surface, hyaluronate interposed between the cell and the substratum may facilitate detachment, and hence cell migration. Hyaluronate has been shown to be a component of cell "foot pads"[129] and to interact specifically with fibronectin, another component of these structures.[130]

Hyaluronate is an extremely potent inhibitor of proteoglycan synthesis[131] by chondrocytes; as little as 0.005 $\mu$g per ml decreases $^{35}SO_4$ incorporation into chondroitin sulfate, whereas other polyanions have no effect even at much higher concentrations.[132] Furthermore, this inhibitory effect of hyaluronic acid on GAG synthesis is specific for chondrocytes, since synthesis of sulfated GAGs by fibroblasts is unaffected by concentrations of hyaluronic acid as high as 10 $\mu$g per ml.

$^{14}$C-labeled hyaluronic acid is taken up by cells, and this uptake can be diminished by unlabeled hyaluronate. Since the label and the inhibition of GAG synthesis can be removed by mild trypsinization, it appears to be associated with the surface of the chondrocyte.[133] The inhibitory effect of hyaluronate can be abolished by benzyl-$\beta$-D-xyloside (an exogenous initiator of GAG chain polymerization), suggesting that hyaluronate acts by interfering with initiation of the GAG chain (and thus the proteoglycan) by specifically inhibiting formation of the core protein or, perhaps, of the xylosyl transferase that initiates synthesis of chondroitin sulfate chains on the protein. In contrast to hyaluronic acid, sulfated GAGs stimulate GAG synthesis by chondrocytes, although relatively high concentrations are required and no evidence for a receptor-mediated mechanism has been noted.[134] Thus, the GAG composition and concentration in the extracellular matrix appear to influence cell differentiation in the skeleton, and the metabolism of mature cells in connective tissue.

## GAGs AS REGULATORS OF CARTILAGE MINERALIZATION

Chains of chondroitin sulfate have been shown to bind $Ca^{+2}$, but $Ca^{+2}$ binding is much greater when the chondroitin sulfate is present in cartilage proteoglycan,[135,136] suggesting that individual calcium ions were each bound by two sulfate groups, located on adjacent GAG chains of the proteoglycan. Endochondral calcification is accompanied by a sharp decrease in the chondroitin sulfate content of the tissue.[137] It has been proposed that the binding of calcium by proteoglycans raises the local calcium concentration in the cartilage, increasing the local pH and thereby causing an influx of phosphate and hydroxyl ions, leading to precipitation of calcium salts.[138] On the other hand, proteoglycans, especially when present as very large aggregates, may inhibit the sedimentation of precipitating calcium phosphate.[139] The inhibitory effect of aggregates, as opposed to nonaggregated proteoglycans, on calcification is not due to differential calcium binding affinity. It has been suggested that the aggregate provides a physical shield to prevent growth of minute calcium crystals.[140] Evidence indicates that in vivo the onset of calcification in cartilage is associated with disaggregation of proteoglycans. It is unlikely that disaggregation in these circumstances is effected by proteolytic enzymes, since there is no indication that individual proteoglycans are degraded, and it seems unlikely that a protease in calcifying cartilage would selectively attack proteoglycans in aggregates. Lysozyme, a low molecular weight cationic protein that is present in cartilage in large amounts,[141] has been shown to cause disaggregation of proteoglycans in vitro. The mechanisms of calcification in fracture callus may be similar to those of endochondral calcification in skeletal growth. Thus, in healing of rat tibial fractures a rise in lysozyme was associated with a decrease in proteoglycan aggregation prior to mineralization of the callus.[142]

## BINDING OF GAGs TO LYSOSOMAL ENZYMES

Because of the pre-eminent role of lysosomal enzymes as mediators of tissue damage in rheumatic disease, it is relevant that GAGs have been identified as components of primary lysosomes and have been shown to affect the activity of lysosomal enzymes. When chondroitin sulfate, dermatan sulfate, and heparin were added to lysosomal hydrolases the activity of the latter was augmented or decreased. The increase in acid hydrolase activity was proposed to be due to protection of the enzyme from degradation by lysosomal proteases.[143] Lysosomal enzymes in polymorphonuclear leukocytes have been shown to interact with GAGs in pH-dependent reversible electrostatic binding.[144] It has been postulated that the enzymes contained in primary lysosomes exist in complexes with GAGs in a protected, inactive form. During phagocytosis, fusion of the primary lysosome with phagosome would lead to an influx of extracellular fluid, diluting the intralysosomal fluid and raising its pH, causing dissociation of the enzyme-GAG complex and release of intact active hydrolases.

Based on a rationale stemming from observations such as the above, attempts have been made to utilize GAGs in treatment of arthritis. When Arteparon, a glycosaminoglycan polysulfate, was administered to animals with experimentally induced osteoarthritis, the extent of cartilage damage appeared to be less than that in controls.[145,146] The efficacy of such therapy in human arthritis, however, remains to be demonstrated.[147]

## FUNCTION OF GAGs IN THE CLOTTING OF BLOOD

**Anticoagulant Function of Heparin.** Heparin is synthesized and stored within mast cells in the connective tissue, in the vicinity of blood vessels. Despite the ability of exogenous heparin to inhibit clotting of blood, whether it is present in the plasma under physiological conditions is not resolved.[148] Thus, the function of endogenous heparin in anticoagulation is not entirely clear. Notably, native heparin possessed only about 10 percent of the anticoagulant activity of commercial heparin.[149]

The molecular mechanisms underlying heparin's activity as an anticoagulant have recently been reviewed in detail.[150] The action of heparin as an anticoagulant appears to be indirect. It binds to a plasma protease inhibitor, antithrombin (antithrombin III), and markedly accelerates the rate at which the latter forms stable, equimolar complexes with serine proteases of the hemostatic cascade, neutralizing their activity.[151] Antithrombin, which is an $\alpha$-globulin (molecular weight = about $5.5 \times 10^4$ daltons), inactivates thrombin stoichiometrically.[150] The interaction involves an attack by thrombin of a specific Arg-Ser bond on the inhibitor. In the presence of heparin, formation of the antithrombin-thrombin complex is accelerated up to 2000-fold, preventing formation of fibrin. Other serine proteases in the coagulation system (Factors $IX_a$, $X_a$, $XI_a$, $XII_a$) are similarly inactivated by antithrombin, by reactions that are also greatly increased by the presence of heparin.

Heparin catalyzes the antithrombin-protease reaction. Since it is not consumed during the reaction, upon release from the antithrombin-protease complex it is available again for binding to another molecule of antithrombin.[150] Plasmin, a component of the fibrinolytic system, appears to be inactivated in the same way. Evidence indicates that heparin binds to lysine residues in antithrombin, inducing a conformational change in the inhibitor, which makes its reactive site more accessible to the active center of thrombin and the other serine proteases.[151]

Heparin preparations vary considerably with respect to molecular size, glucuronic acid:iduronic acid molar ratios, degrees of *N*-acetylation, and amounts of ester and *N*-sulfation. However, changes in none of these molecular parameters have shown a high degree of correlation with the anticoagulation activity of the molecule, suggesting that a highly defined, specific molecular structure may not be required for anticoagulant activity.[152] Recently, however, highly purified commercial heparin was shown to contain two distinct forms, separable by sucrose density gradient centrifugation: about one third of the molecules bound to antithrombin and had potent anticoagulant activity; the remaining two thirds could not form a stable complex with antithrombin and had minimal anticoagulant activity.[152] Similar results have been obtained with heparin from a murine mastocytoma.[153] The antithrombin-binding region in heparin contains a pentasaccharide with a unique glucosamine-3-0-sulfate group, which is not present in other regions of the molecule, or in heparin with low affinity for antithrombin.[151] Also, the biological function of the majority of the heparin molecules (which are poor anticoagulants), and whether the heparin that binds to antithrombin has other (nonanticoagulant) function in vivo, remain to be determined.[154]

**Procoagulant Function of Platelet Factor 4-Proteoglycan Complex.** Platelets contain a chondroitin 4-sulfate proteoglycan[5] in their cytoplasmic granules, where it exists in a complex with platelet factor 4 (PF4).[155] The latter has the ability to neutralize the anticoagulant effect of heparin in plasma after release from the platelets and, therefore, may be of clinical significance in relation to heparin therapy. Its physiologic role, however, is not clear.

The proteoglycan-PF4 complex is dissociable at high ionic strength into the proteoglycan carrier (MW = 59,000 daltons) and PF4 (MW = 29,000 daltons). The proteoglycan contains four chains of chondroitin 4-sulfate (MW = 12,000 daltons each), covalently linked to a single polypeptide. When fully saturated with PF4, the molecular weight of the complex is about 350,000 daltons, indicating that it occurs as a dimer, with each monomer comprised of 4 molecules of PF4 and one molecule of proteoglycan.[149]

Other GAGs are able to displace PF4 from the proteoglycan carrier. Heparin has the highest, and hyaluronic acid the lowest, affinity from the protein; in general, binding appears to be promoted by high charge density and by L-iduronic acid residues. Thus, heparan sulfate and dermatan sulfate, which are present in blood vessel walls, could, by displacing PF4 from its proteoglycan carrier, serve to control its deposition locally on the vessel wall.

**Anticoagulant Function of Heparan Sulfate.** While the above interaction between heparan sulfate and the PF4-proteoglycan complex would imply a potential coagulation-promoting role for this GAG, heparan sulfate proteoglycans on the surface of vascular endothelial cells have been shown also to interact with one of the enzymes of the thromboplastin pathway, thereby inhibiting conversion of prothrombin to thrombin.[7] This action could have some importance in vivo in maintaining the fluidity of the blood within the vascular tree.

The heparan sulfate proteoglycan on the surface of endothelial cells of aorta has been shown also to bind lipoprotein lipase, the extrahepatic enzyme that is responsible for hydrolysis of plasma triacylglycerol.[8] A recent study showed that at saturation $1.24 \times 10^{11}$ molecules of lipoprotein lipase were bound per cm of intact porcine aortic endothelium.[8] Binding was reduced by prior trypsinization, which would have degraded the heparan-sulfate proteoglycan, and was reversed by exogenous heparin. (It is well known that heparin administration releases the lipase into the circulation in vivo.) The porcine endothelium was shown to have available at its surface approximately $5.4 \times 10^{11}$ chains of heparan sulfate per $cm^2$, suggesting that lipoprotein lipase may interact with approximately 25 percent of the available GAG chains.[8]

Studies of the heparan sulfate proteoglycan–cell interaction indicate that binding of the proteoglycan to the surface of hepatocytes requires intact GAG chains.[17] Since exogenous heparin displaces about two thirds of the endogenous heparan sulfate proteoglycans from the cell, the polysaccharide receptor is involved also in their association with the cell surface. Furthermore, the ability of heparin to displace endogenous heparan sulfate was proportional to the molecular weight.

## POSSIBLE ROLE OF HEPARIN IN INFLAMMATION

The mast cell is an important effector of inflammation via release of the biologically active substances (histamine, serotonin, eosinophilic chemotactic factor of anaphylaxis, and so on) contained in its cytoplasmic granules. Since these granules also contain its heparin, it is relevant to examine the possible functions of this GAG that may be unrelated to its effects on clotting. Several lines of evidence point to the likelihood that heparin has such functions.

Commercial heparin has been shown to be anticomplementary, and it inhibits both the classical and alternative pathways.[156,157] Heparin enhances the activity of the inhibitor of the first component of the complement ($C\bar{1}$ INH) on activated $C\bar{1}$.[157] Commercial heparin also inhibits the binding of C1q to immune complexes,[156] the interaction of C1s with C4 and C2,[158] the binding of C2 to the C4b receptor,[159] and formation, or binding, of the trimolecular complex C567.[160]

In addition, native heparin has been shown to mask the active site of chymase,[161] a chymotrypsin-like enzyme contained in the mast cell granules, which is released upon degranulation of the cell induced by immunologic or nonimmunologic stimuli. Additional evidence indicates that heparin suppresses the in vitro assay for macrophage-inhibitor factor (MIF).[162]

Recently, it has been shown that macrophages, which occur in association with mast cells in the tissues, produce and secrete coagulation enzymes.[163] Mouse peritoneal macrophages produce the proteinase precursors needed for formation of fibrin via the extrinsic pathway (factor VII, factor X, prothrombin) and also tissue thromboplastin and factor V, which are required for activation of the enzymes.[150] Thromboplastin production, which triggers the extrinsic pathway, results from interaction of macrophages with activated T lymphocytes.[164,165] Thus, the coagulation mechanism of the macrophage may be activated in the course of a cellular immune response, and may explain synovial fibrin deposition in joint diseases such as rheumatoid arthritis. This fibrin-generating system is susceptible to inhibition by heparin.[150]

From the foregoing it is apparent that heparin may possess a potential for modulating immediate hypersensitivity reactions, complement-mediated immunologic reactions (involving both classical and alternative pathways), and delayed hypersensitivity.

## HEPARIN-INDUCED OSTEOPOROSIS

In 1965, Griffith and associates reported spontaneous vertebral and/or rib fractures in 6 of 10 patients treated with 15,000 to 30,000 units of heparin for 6 months or longer.[166] Marked osteopenia was noted radiologically, and serum concentrations of calcium, phosphorus, and alkaline phosphatase, and renal tubular resorption of phosphate, were normal. The complication appeared to be dose related, since no symptoms of osteoporosis were noted in 107 patients who received 10,000 units of heparin or less daily for up to 15 years. Several subsequent reports have confirmed that osteoporosis and fractures may occur as a result of high-dose heparin therapy.[167-171] The true frequency of heparin-induced osteopenia is unknown, but x-ray changes and clinical evidence of fracture appear to be much less common than the 60 percent prevalence reported initially.[166]

The mechanism(s) underlying the effect of heparin on bone are unclear; data suggest that heparin may interfere with osteoblastic activity, or with bone crystal nucleation and enchondral ossification.[172] Other data suggest that heparin may act as a cofactor for the action of parathyroid hormone on bone.[173] The calcium-mobilizing effect of heparin on bone may also be direct, and may occur even in the absence of parathyroid hormone.[174] Mast cells are associated with the multinucleated cells (osteoclasts) that resorb bone, and heparin may be an *endogenous* cofactor in bone resorption in normal individuals. Consistent with this possibility, protamine was recently shown to decrease the resorption of devitalized bone particles implanted subcutaneously in normal rats.[175]

### References

1. Jeanloz, R.W.: The nomenclature of acid mucopolysaccharides. Arthritis Rheum. 3:323, 1960.
2. Lamberg, S.I., and Stoolmiller, A.C.: Glycosaminoglycans. A biochemical and clinical review. J. Invest. Derm. 63:433, 1974.
3. Silbert J.E.: Structure and metabolism of proteoglycans and glycosaminoglycans. J. Invest. Derm. 79:31s, 1982.
4. Lindahl, U., and Hook, M.: Glycosaminoglycans and their binding to biological macromolecules. Ann. Rev. Biochem. 47:385, 1978.
5. Olsson, I., and Gardell, S.: The isolation and characterization of glycosaminoglycans from human leukocytes and platelets. Biochim. Biophys. Acta 141:348, 1967.
6. Laterra, J., Silbert, J.E., and Culp, L.A.: Cell surface heparan sulfate mediates some adhesive responses to glycosaminoglycan-binding matrices, including fibronectin. J. Cell Biol. 96:112, 1983.
7. Buonassisi, V., and Colburn, P.: Biological significance of heparan sulfate proteoglycans. Ann. N.Y. Acad. Sci. 401:76, 1982.
8. Williams, M.P., Streeter, H.B., Wusteman, F.S., and Cryer, A.: Heparan sulphate and the binding of lipoprotein lipase to porcine thoracic aorta endothelium. Biochim. Biophys. Acta 756:83, 1983.
9. Mathews, M.B.: Macromolecular evolution of connective tissue. Biol. Rev. 42:499, 1967.
10. Antonopoulos, C.A., Engfeldt, B., Gardell, S., Hjertquist, S., and Solheim, K.: Isolation and identification of the glycosaminoglycans from fracture callus. Biochim. Biophys. Acta 101:150, 1965.
11. Fransson, L.A., and Roden, L.: Structure of dermatan sulfate. II. Characterization of products obtained by hyaluronidase digestion of dermatan sulfate. J. Biol. Chem. 242:4170, 1967.
12. Suzuki, S., Saito, H., Yamagata, I., Anno, K., Seno, N., Kawai, Y., and

Furuhashi, T.: Formation of three types of disulfated disaccharides from chondroitin sulfates by chondroitinase digestion. J. Biol. Chem. 243:1543, 1968.

13. Toole, B.P., and Lowther, D.: Dermatan sulphate protein: Isolation from and interaction with collagen. Arch Biochem. 128:567, 1968.
14. Mathews, M.B., and Decker, L.: The effect of acid mucopolysaccharide proteins on fibril formation from collagen solutions. Biochem. J. 109:517, 1968.
15. Toole, B.P., and Lowther, D.: The isolation of dermatan sulphate protein complex from bovine heart valves. Biochim. Biophys. Acta 101:364, 1965.
16. Brandt, K.D., Skinner, M., and Cohen, A.S.: Characterization of the mucopolysaccharides associated with fractions of guanidine-denatured amyloid fibrils. Clin. Chim. Acta 55:295, 1974.
17. Kjellen, L., Oldberg, A., and Hook, M.: Cell-surface heparan sulfate. Mechanisms of proteoglycan-cell association. J. Biol. Chem. 255:10407, 1980.
18. Rollins, B.J., and Culp, L.A.: Glycosaminoglycans in the substrate adhesion sites of normal and virus-transformed murine cells. Biochemistry 18:141, 1979.
19. Kanwar, Y.S., and Farquhar, M.G.: Presence of heparan sulfate in the glomerular basement membranes. Proc. Natl. Acad. Sci. U.S.A. 76:1303, 1979.
20. Kanwar, Y.S., and Farquhar, M.G.: Isolation of glycosaminoglycans (heparan sulfate) from glomerular basement membranes. Proc. Natl. Acad. Sci. U.S.A. 76, 4493, 1979.
21. Lindahl, U., and Backstrom, G.: Biosynthesis of L-iduronic acid in heparin: Epimerization of D-glucuronic acid on the polymer level. Biochem. Biophys. Res. Commun. 46:985, 1972.
22. Helting, T., and Lindahl, U.: Occurrence and biosynthesis of $\beta$-glucuronidic linkages in heparin. J. Biol. Chem. 246:5442, 1971.
23. Foster, A.B., Hanison, R., Inch, T.D., Stacey, M., and Webber, J.M.: Amino sugars and related compounds. IX. Periodate oxidation of heparin and some related substances. J. Chem. Soc. pp. 2279–2287, 1963.
24. Hirano, S., Hoffman, P., and Meyer, K.: The structure of keratosulfate of bovine cornea. J. Org. Chem. 26:5064, 1961.
25. Baldini, G., Brovelli, A., and Castellani, A.A.: Gas chromatography identification of neutral sugars in keratan sulfates from different sources. Ital. Biochem. J. 17:257, 1968.
26. Lohmander, L.S., DeLuca, S., Nilsson, B., Hascall, V.C., Caputo, C.B., Kimura, J.H., and Heinegard, D.K.: Oligosaccharides on proteoglycans from the Swarm rat chondrosarcoma. J. Biol. Chem. 255:6084, 1980.
27. Bhavanadan, V.P., and Meyer, K.: Studies on keratosulfates: Methylation, desulfation and acid hydrolysis studies in old human cartilage keratosulfate. J. Biol. Chem. 243:1052, 1968.
28. Bhavanadan, V.P., and Meyer, K.: Studies on keratosulfates: Methylation and partial acid hydrolysis of bovine corneal keratosulfate. J. Biol. Chem. 242:4352, 1967.
29. Nilsson, B., Nakazawa, K., Hassell, J.R., Newsome, D.A., and Hascall, V.G.: Structure of oligosaccharides and the linkage region between keratan sulfate and the core protein on proteoglycans from monkey cornea. J. Biol. Chem. 258:6056, 1983.
30. Seno, N., Meyer, K., Anderson, B., and Hoffman, P.: Variations in keratosulfates. J. Biol. Chem. 240:1005, 1965.
31. Bray, B., Lieberman, R., and Meyer, K.: Structure of human skeletal keratosulfate. The linkage region. J. Biol. Chem. 242:3373, 1967.
32. Muir, H., and Hardingham, T.E.: Structure of proteoglycans. *In* Whelan, W.J. (ed.): Biochemistry of Carbohydrates. MTP International Review of Science. Vol. 5. London, Butterworths, 1975, pp. 153–222.
33. Mathews, M.B.: Connective Tissue. Macromolecular Structure and Evolution. New York, Springer, 1975, p. 318.
34. Silpanata, P., Dunstone, J.R., and Ogston, A.G.: Fractionation of a hyaluronic acid preparation in a density gradient. Biochem. J. 109:43, 1968.
35. Swann, D.A.: Studies of hyaluronic acid. I. The preparation and properties of rooster comb hyaluronic acid. Biochim. Biophys. Acta 156:17, 1968.
36. Scher, I., and Hamerman, D.: Isolation of human synovial fluid hyaluronate by density-gradient ultracentrifugation and evaluation of its protein content. Biochem. J. 126:1073, 1972.
37. Fessler, J.H., and Fessler, L.I.: Electron microscopic visualization of the polysaccharide hyaluronic acid. Proc. Natl. Acad. Sci. USA 56:141, 1966.
38. Mason, R.M., d'Arville, C., Kimura, J.H., and Hascell, V.C.: Absence of covalently linked core protein from newly synthesized hyaluronate. Biochem. J. 207:445, 1982.
39. Muir, H.: The nature of the link between protein and carbohydrate of a chondroitin sulphate complex from hyaline cartilage. Biochem. J. 69:195, 1958.
40. Lindahl, U., and Roden, L.: The chondroitin 4-sulfate-protein linkage. J. Biol. Chem. 241:2113, 1966.
41. Roden, L., and Smith, R.: Structure of the neutral trisaccharide region of the chondroitin 4-sulfate protein linkage region. J. Biol. Chem. 241:5949, 1966.
42. Baker, J.R., Roden, L., and Stoolmiller, A.C.: Biosynthesis of chondroitin sulfate proteoglycan: Xylosyl transfer to Smith-degraded cartilage proteoglycan and other exogenous acceptors. J. Biol. Chem. 247:3838, 1972.
43. Roden, L.: Linkage of acid mucopolysaccharides to protein. *In* Rossi, E. and Stahl, E. (eds.): Biochemistry of Glycoproteins and Related Substances. Basel, Karger, 1968, pp. 185–202.
44. Lindahl, U.: The structures of xyloserine and galactosyl-xyloserine from heparin. Biochim. Biophys. Acta 130:361, 1966.
45. Heinegard, D., Paulsson, M., Inerot, S., and Carlstrom, C.: A novel low-molecular-weight chondroitin sulphate proteoglycan isolated from cartilage. Biochem. J. 197:355, 1981.
46. Rosenberg, L.: Structure of cartilage proteoglycans. *In* Burleigh, P.M.C., and Poole, A.R. (eds.): Dynamics of Connective Tissue Macromolecules. Amsterdam, North Holland Publishers, 1975, p. 105.
47. Mathews, M.B., and Lozaityte, I.: Sodium chrondroitin sulfate-protein complexes of cartilage. I. Molecular weight and shape. Arch. Biochem. Biophys. 74:158, 1958.
48. Partridge, S.M., Davis, H.F., and Adair, G.S.: The chemistry of connective tissue and the constitution of the chondroitin sulphate protein complex in cartilage. Biochem. J. 79:15, 1961.
49. Torchia, D.A., Hason, M.A., and Hascall, V.C.: $^{13}C$ Nuclear magnetic resonance suggests a flexible proteoglycan core protein. J. Biol. Chem. 256:7129, 1981.
50. Heinegard, D., and Hascall, V.S.: Aggregation of cartilage proteoglycans. III. Characteristics of the proteins isolated from trypsin digests of aggregates. J. Biol. Chem. 249:4250, 1974.
51. Brandt, K.D., Palmoski, M., and Perricone, E.: Aggregation of cartilage proteoglycans. II. Evidence for the presence of a hyaluronate-binding region on proteoglycans from osteoarthritic cartilage. Arthritis Rheum. 19:1308. 1976.
52. Heinegard, D., and Hascall, V.: Characteristics of the nonaggregating proteoglycans isolated from bovine nasal cartilage. J. Biol. Chem. 254:927, 1979.
53. Heinegard, D., Paulsson, M., and Sonmarin, Y.: Proteoglycans and matrix proteins in cartilage. Prog. Clin. Biol. Res. 110B:35, 1983.
54. Sweet, M.B.E., Thonar, E.J.-M.A., and Marsh, J.: Age-related changes in proteoglycan structure. Arch. Biochem. Biophys. 198:439, 1979.
55. Willingham, M.C., Pastan, I.H., Sahagian, G.G., Jourdian, G.W., and Neufeld, E.F.: Morphologic study of the internalization of a lysosomal enzyme by the mannose 6-phosphate receptor in cultured Chinese hamster ovary cells. Proc. Natl. Acad. Sci. 78:6967, 1981.
56. Ashwell, G., and Morell, A.G.: The role of surface carbohydrates in the hepatic recognition and transport of circulating glycoproteins. Adv. Enzymol. 41:99, 1974.
57. Hudgin, R.L., Pricer, W.E., Jr., Ashwell, G., Stockert, R.J., and Morell, A.G.: The isolation of properties of a rabbit liver binding protein specific for asialoglycoproteins. J. Biol. Chem. 249:5536, 1974.
58. Lunney, J., and Ashwell, G.: A hepatic receptor of avian origin capable of binding specifically modified glycoproteins. Proc. Natl. Acad. Sci. U.S.A. 73:341, 1976.
59. Prinz, R., Schwermann, J., Buddecke, E., and von Figura, K.: Endocytosis of sulphated proteoglycans by cultured skin fibroblasts. Biochem. J. 176:671, 1978.
60. Rich, A.M., Pearlstein, E., Weissmann, G., and Hoffstein, S.: Cartilage proteoglycans inhibit fibronectin-mediated adhesion. Nature 293:224, 1981.
61. Hascall, V.C., and Heinegard, D.: Aggregation of cartilage proteoglycans. I. The role of hyaluronic acid. J. Biol. Chem. 249:4232, 1974.
62. Hardingham, T.E., and Muir, H.: Hyaluronic acid in cartilage and proteoglycan aggregation. Biochem. J. 139:565, 1974.
63. Baker, J., and Caterson, B.: The isolation and characterization of the link proteins from proteoglycan aggregates of bovine nasal cartilage. J. Biol. Chem. 254:2387, 1979.
64. Baker, J. and Caterson, B.: The link proteins. Glycoconjugate Res. 1:329, 1979.
65. Pita, J.C., Howell, D.S., Goldberg, V.M., and Moskowitz, R.W.: Proteoglycan aggregation in normal and experimental osteoarthritic articular cartilage. Trans. Orthop. Res. Soc. 8:171, 1983.
66. Hardingham, T.E., and Muir, H.: The specific interaction of hyaluronic acid with cartilage proteoglycans. Biochim. Biophys. Acta 279:401, 1972.
67. Hardingham, T.E., and Muir, H.: The function of hyaluronic acid in proteoglycan aggregation. *In* Ali, S.Y., Elves, M.W., and Leaback, D.H. (eds.): Normal and Osteoarthrotic Articular Cartilage. London, Institute of Orthopaedics, 1974, pp. 51–63.
68. Rosenberg, L., Hellmann, W., and Kleinschmidt, A.K.: Electron microscopic studies of proteoglycan aggregates from bovine articular cartilage. J. Biol. Chem. 250:1877, 1975.

69. Hardingham, T.E., and Muir, H.: Binding of oligosaccharides of hyaluronic acid to proteoglycans. Biochem. J. 135:905, 1973.
70. Hascall, V.C., and Heinegard, D.: Aggregation of cartilage proteoglycans. II. Oligosaccharide competitors of the proteoglycan-hyaluronic acid interaction. J. Biol. Chem. 249:4242, 1974.
71. Wiebkin, O.W., Hardingham, T.E., and Muir, H.: The interaction of proteoglycans and hyaluronic acid and the effect of hyaluronic acid on proteoglycan synthesis by chondrocytes of adult cartilage. *In* Burleigh, P.M.C., and Poole, A.R. (eds.): Dynamics of Connective Tissue Macromolecules. Amsterdam, North-Holland, 1975, pp. 81–104.
72. Mak, A.F., Mow, V.C., and Lai, W.M.: Predictions of the number and strength of the proteoglycan-proteoglycan interactions from viscometric data. Trans. Orthop. Res. Soc. 10:3, 1983.
73. Toole, B.P.: Hyaluronate and hyaluronidase in morphogenesis and differentiation. Am. Zool. 13:1061, 1973.
74. Howell, D.S., Pita, J.C., Marquez, J.F., et al.: Demonstration of macromolecular inhibitor(s) of calcification and nucleaton factor(s) in fluid from calcifying sites in cartilage. J. Clin. Invest. 48:630, 1969.
75. Cuervo, L.A., Pita, J.C., and Howell, D.S.: Inhibition of calcium phosphate mineral growth by proteoglycan aggregate fractions in a synthetic lymph. Calcif. Tiss. Res. 13:1, 1973.
76. Perricone, E., and Brandt, K.: Enhancement of urate solubility by connective tissue. I. Effect of proteoglycan aggregates and buffer cation. Arthritis Rheum. 21:453, 1978.
77. Silvestri, L., Baker, J.R., Roden, L., and Stroud, R.M.: The Clq inhibitor in serum is a chondroitin 4-sulfate proteoglycan. J. Biol. Chem. 256:7383, 1981.
78. Jansson, L., Ogren, S., and Lindahl, U.: Macromolecular properties and end-group analysis of heparin isolated from bovine liver capsule. Biochem. J. 145:53, 1975.
79. Yurt, R.W., Leid, R.W., Austen, K.F., and Silbert, J.E.: Native heparin from rat peritoneal mast cells. J. Biol. Chem. 252:518, 1977.
80. Robinson, H.C., Horner, A.A., Höök, M., Ögren, S., and Lindahl, U.: A proteoglycan form of heparin and its degeneration to single chain molecules. J. Biol. Chem. 253:6687, 1978.
81. Telser, A., Robinson, H.C., and Dorfman, A.: The biosynthesis of chondroitin-sulfate protein complex. Proc. Natl. Acad. Sci. USA 54:912, 1965.
82. Cole, N.N., and Lowther, D.A.: The inhibition of chondroitin sulfate protein synthesis by cycloheximide. FEBS Lett. 2:351, 1969.
83. Stoolmiller, A.C., Horwitz, A.L., and Dorfman, A.: Biosynthesis of the chondroitin sulfate proteoglycan. Purification and properties of xylosyltransferase. J. Biol. Chem. 247:3525, 1972.
84. Helting, T., and Rodin, L.: Biosynthesis of chondroitin sulfate. I. Galactosyl transfer in the formation of the carbohydrate-protein linkage region. J. Biol. Chem. 244:2790, 1968.
85. Robbins, P.W., and Lippmann, F.: Isolation and identification of active sulfate. J. Biol. Chem. 229:837, 1957.
86. Picard, J., Gardais, A., and Dubernand, L.: Presence of sulphated nucleotides in the epiphyseal growth cartilage of the rat. Nature 202:1213, 1964.
87. Silbert, J.E.: Biosynthesis of heparin. IV. N-Deacetylation of a precursor glycosaminoglycan. J. Biol. Chem. 242:5153, 1967.
88. Olssen, I.: The intracellular transport of glycosaminoglycans (mucopolysaccharides) in human leukocytes. Exp. Cell. Res. 54:318, 1969.
89. Fransson, L-A.: Structure of dermatan sulfate. III. The hybrid structure of dermatan sulfate from umbilical cord. J. Biol. Chem. 243:1504, 1968.
90. Robinson, H.C., and Dorfman, A.: The sulfation of chondroitin sulfate in embryonic chick cartilage epiphyses. J. Biol. Chem. 244:348, 1969.
91. Robinson, H.C.: The sulphation of chondroitin sulphate in embryonic chicken cartilage. Biochem. J. 113:543, 1969.
92. Thomas, L.: The effect of papain, vitamin A and cortisone on cartilage matrix in vivo. Biophys. J. 4(Suppl.):207, 1964.
93. Sapolsky, A.I., Altman, R.D., and Howell, D.S.: Cathepsin D activity in normal and osteoarthritic human cartilage. Fed. Proc. 32:1489, 1973.
94. Sapolsky, A.I., Howell, D.S., and Woessner, J.F., Jr.: Neutral proteases and cathepsin D in human articular cartilage. J. Clin. Invest. 53:1044, 1974.
95. Kuettner, K.E., Harper, E., and Eisenstein, R.: Protease inhibitors in cartilage. Arthritis Rheum. 20(Suppl.):S124, 1977.
96. Knight, J.A., Stephens, R.W., Bushell, G.R., Ghosh, P., and Taylor, T.K.F.: Neutral protease inhibitors from human intervertebral disc and femoral head articular cartilage. Biochim. Biophys. Acta 584:304, 1979.
97. Gross, J.I., Mathews, M.B., and Dorfman, A.: Sodium chondroitin sulfate-protein complexes of cartilage. J. Biol. Chem. 235:2889, 1960.
98. Hutterer, F.: Degradation of mucopolysaccharides by hepatic lysosomes. Biochim. Biophys. Acta 115:312, 1966.
99. Aronson, N.N., and Davidson, E.A.: Lysosomal hyaluronidase from rat liver. I. Preparation. J. Biol. Chem. 242:437, 1967.
100. Weissmann, B., Meyer, K., Sampson, P., and Linker, A.: Isolation of oligosaccharides enzymatically produced from hyaluronic acid. J. Biol. Chem. 208:417, 1954.
101. Hoffman, P., Meyer, K., and Linker, A.: Transglycosylation during the mixed digestion of hyaluronic acid and chondroitin sulfate by testicular hyaluronidase. J. Biol. Chem. 219:653, 1956.
102. Linker, A., and Hovingh, P.: The enzymic degradation of heparin and heparitin sulfate. I. The fractionation of crude heparinase from flavobacteria. J. Biol. Chem. 240:3724, 1965.
103. Kaplan, D., and Meyer, K.: The fate of injected mucopolysaccharides. J. Clin. Invest. 41:743, 1962.
104. Varadi, D.P., Cifonelli, J.A., and Dorfman, A.: The acid mucopolysaccharides in normal urine. Biochim. Biophys. Acta 141:103, 1967.
105. Bollet, A.J., Bonner, W.M., and Nance, J.L.: The presence of hyaluronidase in various mammalian tissues. J. Biol. Chem. 238:3522, 1963.
106. Stack, M.T., and Brandt, K.D.: Identification and characterization of articular cartilage hyaluronidase. Arthritis Rheum. 25:S100, 1982.
107. van Hoof, F., and Hers, H.G.: The abnormalities of lysosomal enzymes in mucopolysaccharidoses. Eur. J. Biochem. 7:34, 1968.
108. McKusick, V.A. and Neufeld, E.F.: The mucopolysaccharide storage diseases. *In* Stanbury, J.B., Wyngaarden, J.B., Fredrickson, D.S., Goldstein, J.L., and Brown, M.S. (eds.): The Metabolic Basis of Inherited Disease. 5th ed. New York, McGraw-Hill Book Company, 1983, p. 751.
109. van Hoof, F., and Hers, H.G.: L'ultrastructure des cellules hepatiques dans la maladie de Hurler. Compt. Rend. Acad. Sci. 259:1281, 1964.
110. Danes, B.S., and Bearn, A.G.: Hurler's syndrome: Demonstration of an inherited disorder of connective tissue in cell culture. Science 149:987, 1965.
111. Fratantoni, J.C., Hall, C.W., and Heufeld, E.F.: The defect in Hurler's and Hunter's syndromes: Faulty degradation of mucopolysaccharides. Proc. Natl. Acad. Sci. USA 60:699, 1968.
112. Fratantoni, J.C., Hall, C.W., and Neufeld, E.F.: Hurler and Hunter syndromes: Mutual correction of the defect in cultured fibroblasts. Science 162:570, 1968.
113. Neufeld, E.F., and Cantz, M.J.: Corrective factors for inborn errors of mucopolysaccharide metabolism. Ann. N.Y. Acad. Sci. 179:580, 1970.
114. Neufeld, E.F.: The biochemical basis for mucopolysaccharidoses and mucolipidoses. Prog. Med. Genet. 10:81, 1974.
115. Neufeld, E.F.: The enzymology of inherited mucopolysaccharide storage disorders. Trends Biochem. Sci. 2:25, 1977.
116. Neufeld, E.F., and McKusick, V.A.: Disorders of lysosomal enzyme synthesis and localization: I-cell disease and pseudo-Hurler polydystrophy. *In* Stanbury, J.B. Wyngaarden, J.B., Fredrickson, D.S., Goldstein, J.L., and Brown, M.S. (eds.): The Metabolic Basis of Inherited Disease. 5th ed. New York, McGraw-Hill Book Company, 1983, p. 778.
117. Hasilik, A., Klein, U., Waheed, A., Strecker, G., and von Figura, K.: Phosphorylated oligosaccharides in lysosomal enzymes: Identification of α-N-acetylglucosamine (1) phospho (6) mannose diester groups. Proc. Natl. Acad. Sci. USA 77:7074, 1980.
118. Varki, A., and Kornfeld, S.: Identification of a rate liver α-N-acetylglucosaminyl phosphodiesterase capable of removing "blocking" α-N-acetylglucosamine residues from phosphorylated high mannase oligosaccharides of lysosomal enzymes. J. Biol. Chem. 255:8398, 1980.
119. Hasilik, A., Waheed, A., and von Figura, K.: Enzymatic phosphorylation of lysosomal enzymes in the presence of UDP-N-acetylglucosamine. Absence of the activity in I-cell fibroblasts. Biochem. Biophys. Res. Commun. 98:761, 1981.
120. Reitman, A.L., Varki, A., and Kornfeld, S.: Fibroblasts from patients with I-cell disease and pseudo-Hurler polydystrophy are deficient in uridine 5′-diphosphate-N-acetylglucosamine: Glycoprotein N-acetylglucosaminylphosphotransferase activity. J. Clin. Invest. 67:1574, 1981.
121. Comper, C.W., and Laurent, T.C.: Physiological function of connective tissue polysaccharides. Physiol. Rev. 58:255, 1978.
122. Ogston, A.G., and Phelps, C.F.: The partition of solutes between buffer solutions containing hyaluronic acid. Biochem. J. 78:827, 1961.
123. Maroudas, A.: Physical chemistry of articular cartilage and the intervertebral disc. *In* Sokoloff, L. (ed.): The Joints and Synovial Fluid. Vol. II. New York, Academic Press, 1980, p. 239.
124. Toole, B.P.: Hyaluronate turnover during chondrogenesis in the developing chick limb and axial skeleton. Dev. Biol. 29:321, 1972.
125. Toole, B.P., and Linsenmayer, T.F.: Newer knowledge of skeletogenesis. Clin. Orthop. 129:258, 1977.
126. Toole, B.P., Jackson, G., and Gross, J.: Hyaluronate in morphogenesis: Inhibition of chondrogenesis in vitro. Proc. Natl. Acad. Sci. USA 69:1384, 1972.
127. Underhill, C.B., and Dorfman, A.: The role of hyaluronic acid in intercellular adhesion of cultured mouse cells. Exp. Cell Res. 117:155, 1978.
128. Toole, B.P.: Developmental role of hyaluronate. Conn. Tiss. Res. 10:93, 1982.
129. Culp, L.A.: Molecular composition and origin of substrate-attached material from normal and virus-transformed cells. J. Supramol. Struct. 5:239, 1976.

130. Yamada, K., Kennedy, D.W., Kimata, K., and Pratt, R.M.: Characterization of fibronectin interactions with glycosaminoglycans and identification of active proteolytic fragments. J. Biol. Chem. 255:6055, 1980.
131. Solursh, M., Vaerewyck, S.A., and Reiter, R.S.: Depression by hyaluronic acid of glycosaminoglycan synthesis by chick cultured embryo chondrocytes. Dev. Biol. 41:233, 1974.
132. Wiebkin, O.W., Hardingham, T.E., and Muir, H.: The interaction of proteoglycans and hyaluronic acid and the effect of hyaluronic acid on proteoglycan synthesis by chondrocytes of adult cartilage. *In* Burleigh, P.M.C., and Poole, A.R. (eds.): Dynamics of Connective Tissue Macromolecules. Amsterdam, North-Holland, 1975, p. 81.
133. Wiebkin, O.W., Hardingham, T.E., and Muir, H.: Hyaluronic acid-proteoglycan interaction and the influence of hyaluronic acid on proteoglycan synthesis by chondrocytes from adult cartilage. *In* Slavkin, H., and Greulich, R.C. (eds.): Extracellular Matrix Influences on Gene Expression. New York, Academic Press, 1975, pp. 209–223.
134. Nevo, Z., and Dorfman, A.: Stimulation of chondromucoprotein synthesis in chondrocytes by extracellular chondromucoprotein. Proc. Natl. Acad. Sci. USA 69:2069, 1972.
135. Farber, S.J., and Schubert, M.: The binding of cations by chondroitin sulfate. J. Clin. Invest. 36:1715, 1957.
136. Woodward, C., and Davidson, E.A.: Structure-function relationships of protein polysaccharide complexes: Specific ion-binding properties. Proc. Natl. Acad. Sci. USA 60:201, 1968.
137. DeBarnard, B., Stagni, N., Colautti, I., et al.: Glycosaminoglycans and endochondral calcification. Clin. Orthop. 126:285, 1977.
138. Waddell, W.J.: A molecular mechanism for biological calcification. Biochem. Biophys. Res. Commun. 49:127, 1972.
139. Howell, D.S., Pita, J.C., Marquez, J.F., et al.: Demonstration of macromolecular inhibitor(s) of calcification and nucleation factor(s) in fluid from calcifying sites in cartilage. J. Clin. Invest. 48:630, 1969.
140. Cuervo, L.A., Pita, J.C., and Howell, D.S.: Inhibition of calcium phosphate mineral growth by proteoglycan aggregate fractions in a synthetic lymph. Calcif. Tiss. Res. 13:1, 1973.
141. Pita, J.C., Muller, F., and Howell, D.S.: Disaggregation of proteoglycan aggregate during endochondral calcification. Physiological role of cartilage lysozyme. *In* Burleigh, P.M.C., and Poole, A.R. (eds.): Dynamics of Connective Tissue Macromolecules. Cambridge, North-Holland, 1974, p. 247.
142. Greenwald, R.A., and Lane, J.M.: Proteoglycan and lysozyme content of healing fracture callus. Trans. Orthop. Res. Soc. 3:33, 1978.
143. Kint, J.A., Dacremont, G., Carton, D., Orye, E., and Hooft, C.: Mucopolysaccharidosis: Secondarily induced abnormal distribution of lysosomal isoenzymes. Science 181:352, 1973.
144. Avila, J.L., and Convit, J.: Inhibition of leukocytic lysosomal enzymes by glycosaminoglycans in vitro. Biochem. J. 152:57, 1975.
145. Ueno, R.: Ergebnisse der behandlung mit einem mucopolysaccharid-polyschwefelsaureester bei der experimentellen arthrose des kniegelenks. Z. Orthop. 111:886, 1973.
146. Dustmann, H.O., Puhl, W., and Martin, K.: Der Einfluss intraartikularer arteparoninjektionen bei arthrose. Z. Orthop. 112:1188, 1974.
147. Fife, R.S., and Brandt, K.D.: Experimental modes of therapy in osteoarthritis. *In* Moskowitz, R.W., Howell, D.S., Goldberg, V.M., and Mankin, H.J. (eds.): Osteoarthritis Diagnosis and Management. In Press.
148. Horner, A.A.: Demonstration of endogenous heparin in rat blood. Adv. Exp. Med. Biol. 52:85, 1975.
149. Lindahl, U., and Hook, M.: Glycosaminoglycans and their binding to biological macromolecules. Ann. Rev. Biochem. 47:385, 1978.
150. Bjork, I., and Lindahl, U.: Mechanism of the anticoagulant action of heparin. Molecular and Cellular Biochemistry 48:161, 1982.
151. Rosenberg, R.D., and Damus, P.S.: The purification and mechanism of action of human antithrombin-heparin cofactor. J. Biol. Chem. 248:6490, 1973.
152. Lam, L.H., Silbert, J.E., and Rosenberg, R.D.: The separation of active and inactive forms of heparin. Biochem. Biophys. Res. Commun. 69:570, 1976.
153. Lewis, R.G., Spencer, A.F., and Silbert, J.E.: Biosynthesis of glycosaminoglycans by cultured mastocytoma cells. Biochem. J. 134:455, 1973.
154. Jacques, L.B.: Heparin: An old drug with a new paradigm. Science 206:528, 1979.
155. Barber, A.J., Kaser-Glanzmann, R., Jakabova, M., and Luscher, E.F.: Characterization of a chondroitin 4-sulfate proteoglycan carrier for heparin neutralizing activity (platelet factor 4) released from human blood platelets. Biochim. Biophys. Acta 286:312, 1972.
156. Raepple, E., Hill, H., and Loos, M.: Mode of interaction of different polyanions with the first (Cl,$\bar{\text{Cl}}$), the second (C2) and the fourth (C4) component of complement. I. Immunochemistry 13:251, 1976.
157. Rent, R., Myhrman, R., Fiedel, B.A., and Gewurz, H.: Potentiation of Cl-esterase inhibitor activity by heparin. Clin. Exp. Immunol. 23:264, 1976.
158. Loos, M., Volanakis, J.E., and Stroud, R.M.: Mode of interaction of different polyanions with the first (Cl,$\bar{\text{Cl}}$), the second (C2) and the fourth (C4) component of complement. III. Immunochemistry 13:789, 1976.
159. Loos, M., Volanakis, J.E., and Stroud, R.M.: Mode of interaction of different polyanions with the first (Cl,$\bar{\text{Cl}}$), the second (C2) and the fourth (C4) component of complement. II. Immunochemistry 13:257, 1976.
160. Baker, P.J., Liat, T.F., McLeod, B.C., Behrends, C.L., and Bewurz, H.: Studies on the inhibition of C56-induced lysis (reactive lysis). VI. Modulation of C56-induced lysis by polyanions and polycations. J. Immunol. 114:554, 1975.
161. Yurt, R.W., and Austen, K.F.: Preparative purification of the rat mast cell chymase. Characterization and interaction with granule components. J. Exp. Med. 146:1405, 1977.
162. Makinen, I., Totterman, T.H., Gordin, A., and Weber, T.H.: Migration inhibition factor and the blood clotting system: Effects of defibrination, heparin and thrombin. Clin. Exp. Immunol. 29:181, 1977.
163. Oslerud, B., Bogwald, J., Lindahl, U., and Seljelid, R.: Production of blood coagulation factor V and tissue thromboplastin by macrophages in vitro. FEBS Lett. 127:154, 1981.
164. Levy, G.A., and Edgington, T.S.: Lymphocyte cooperation is required for amplification of macrophage procoagulant activity. J. Exp. Med. 151:1232, 1980.
165. Greczy, C.L., and Hopper, K.E.: A mechanism of migration inhibition in delayed-type hypersensitivity reactions. J. Immunol. 126:1059, 1981.
166. Griffith, G.C., Nichols, G., Jr., Asher, J., and Flanegan, B.: Heparin osteoporosis. JAMA 193:91, 1965.
167. Miller, W.E., and deWolfe, V.G.: Osteoporosis resulting from heparin therapy. Cleveland Clin. Quart. 33:31, 1966.
168. Sackler, J.P., and Liu, L.: Heparin-induced osteoporosis. Br. J. Radiol. 46:548, 1973.
169. Squires, J.W., and Pinch, L.W.: Heparin-induced spinal fractures. JAMA 241:2417, 1979.
170. Wise, P.H., and Hall, A.J.: Heparin-induced osteopenia in pregnancy. Br. Med. J. 11:110, 1980.
171. Rupp, W.M., McCarthy, H.B., Rohde, T.D., Blackshear, P.J., Goldenberg, F.J., and Buchwald, H.: Risk of osteoporosis in patients treated with long-term intravenous heparin therapy. Curr. Surg. 39:419, 1982.
172. Avioli, L.: Heparin-induced osteopenia: an appraisal. Adv. Exp. Med. Biol. 52:375, 1975.
173. Goldhaber, P.: Heparin enhancement of factors stimulating bone resorption in tissue culture. Science 147:407, 1965.
174. Jowsey, J., Adams, P., and Schlein, A.P.: Calcium metabolism in response to heparin administration. Calc. Tiss. Res. 6:249, 1970.
175. Glowacki, J.: Heparin's role in bone resorption. Calcif. Tiss. Int. 35:641, 1983.

# Chapter 16
# Biology of the Joint

*Edward D. Harris, Jr.*

## INTRODUCTION

Joints hold the end or the periphery of bone in apposition to an adjacent bone. Joints that have essentially no motion (e.g., the fibrous joints in the skull vault) are of no concern to rheumatologists. An increase in the potential for motion of joints is accompanied by an increased potential for trauma; motion also accentuates inflammation when it occurs in the joint, hastening deterioration. Thus, for the rheumatologist and orthopedic surgeon, the study of joints must link biology to motion.

## CLASSIFICATION OF JOINTS

The function of each joint is closely linked to its structure. Some joints have a wide range of motion but little intrinsic stability (e.g., the knee, shoulder). Others have minimal movement and need little if any stabilization from overlying muscle groups (e.g., the sacroiliac joints). It is useful for students of joint disease to recognize two basic types of articulation: (1) *synovial or diarthrodial joints* (Fig. 16–1), which are articulations with free movement, with synovial membrane lining a joint cavity, and (2) *synarthroses*, which have very little movement. There are four subclassifications of synarthroses: (a) *Symphyses*: a fibrocartilaginous disc separates bone ends that are joined by firm ligaments (e.g., symphysis pubis and intervertebral joints). (b) *Synchondroses*: bone ends are covered with articular cartilage, but there is no synovium or significant joint cavity (e.g., sternomanubrial joint). (c) *Syndesmoses*: bones are joined directly by fibrous ligaments without a cartilagenous interface (e.g., the distal tibiofibular articulation, the only joint of this type outside the cranial vault). (d) *Synostoses*: bone bridges between bones, producing ankylosis.

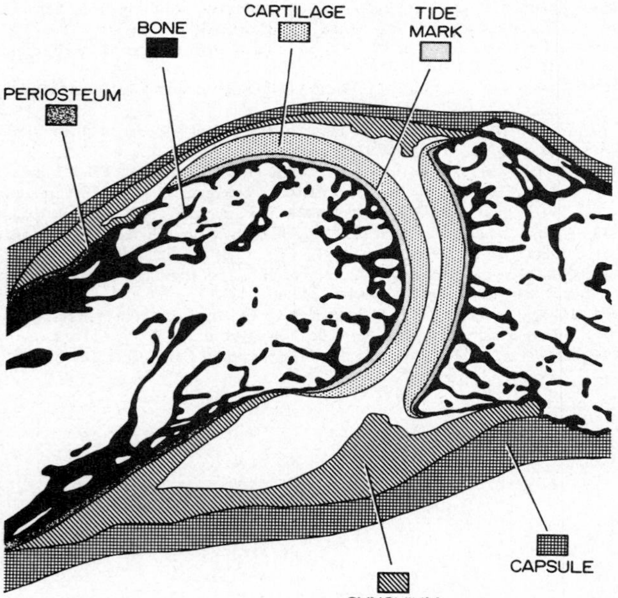


**Figure 16–1.** A diagram of a normal human interphalangeal joint in sagittal section, as an example of a synovial or diarthrodial joint. The "tidemark" represents the calcified cartilage which bonds articular cartilage to the subchondral bony plate. (From Sokoloff, L., and Bland, J.H.: The Musculoskeletal System. Baltimore, Williams & Wilkins Company, 1975).

Among synovial joints there are great differences in structure, and therefore function. For instance, the humeroulnar joint is a true hinge joint limited to motion in one plane, whereas the spherical hip joint, a ball (the femoral head) and socket (the acetabulum) joint, has motion in all directions and rotations. Accompanying the relative restrictions upon planes of motion of the elbow there is an intrinsic stability; the hinge construction needs little surrounding muscle to stablize it. Conversely, the freedom of motion inherent in the structure of a ball-and-socket joint such as the hip or shoulder demands that a very powerful musculature be developed to provide stability and to prevent frequent subluxation.

Details of structure and range of motion of individual joints are discussed in detail in Chapter 24.

## DEVELOPMENTAL BIOLOGY OF THE DIARTHRODIAL JOINT

Extensive histochemical studies of embryonic human specimens have provided much data about the sequence of joint development in the fetus[1] (Fig. 16–2). Experimental work to supplement these descriptive studies has been done in other vertebrate species, especially the chick.

Genetic information controlling the development of joints is expressed by cells in the *apical ectodermal* ridge of the embryo.[2] Excision of this ridge prevents normal joint development by removing competence of the distal mesenchyme to form organized limb components.[3]

The normal sequences following induction of limb bud formation are described very well by O'Rahilly and Gardner.[1] A summary follows.

*1. Condensation.* Condensation of mesenchyme by cellular aggregation forms a blastema. This occurs shortly after limb buds appear[4] and is believed to occur before a cartilaginous matrix is formed (i.e., chondrification).

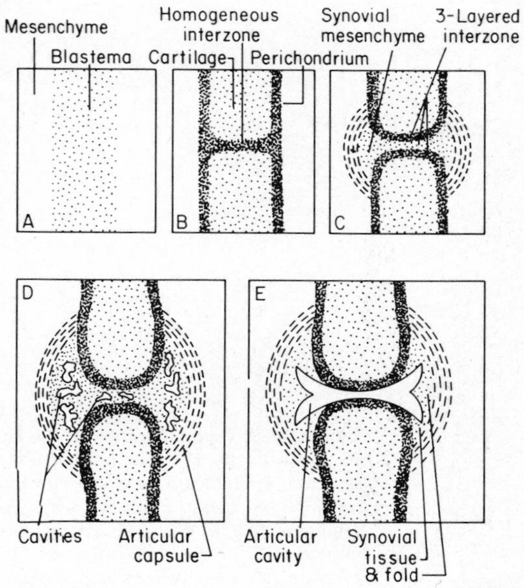


**Figure 16–2.** Diagram of the development of a synovial joint. Joints develop from the blastema, not the surrounding mesenchyme. Chondrification has occurred in *B.* The *interzone* remains avascular and highly cellular. The *synovial mesenchyme* develops from the periphery of the interzone (*C*) and becomes vascularized. Following shortly after differentiation of synovial membrane is *cavitation,* which may begin centrally in the interzone or peripherally (*D*) and merge to form the joint cavity. (From O'Rahilly, R., and Gardner, E.,: In Sokoloff, L. [ed.]: The Joints and Synovial Fluid, Vol. 1, New York, Academic Press, 1978.)

*2. Chondrification* (Fig. 16–3). This begins in the regions of future bones and effectively divides the blastema. Intercellular sulfated material accumulates, and this can be demonstrated by radioautography.[6] In the human, chondrification can be detected when the emryo is as small as 11.7 mm (stage 17 of embryologic development).[5]

*3. Interzones, the Future Joints.* The space between segments undergoing chondrification remains as avascular, homogeneous, densely cellular areas that secrete material staining intensely for polysaccharides (probably chondroitin sulfate).[7] This extracellular material appears almost to force the interzone cells apart. The border of each interzone is continuous at the periphery of this evolving joint with perichondrium and serves as an appositional growth zone for the preskeletal segments.

*4. Formation of Synovial Mesenchyme.* The synovium differentiates from the periphery of the interzone. It probably orginates from the blastema and not from the surrounding general mesenchyme.[7,8] In addition to the synovial lining, joint capsule, intracapsular ligaments, menisci, and tendons all develop from the synovial mesenchyme. Unlike the central interzone or its chondrogenous borders, the synovial mesenchyme becomes vascularized. A dense capillary network develops in the subsynovial tissue. The tough joint capsule evolves as a structural continuum from the more cellular and vascular subsynovial tissue.[9]

This vascularization is the critical point of development of synovial tissue. Among other phenomena it permits delivery of extrablastemal cells to the developing synovium. These extrablastemal cells include *mast cells* (appearing when the embryo is approximately 80 mm in crown-rump length) and *macrophages* that become histiocytes.[9] The macrophages have been identified by the presence of cytoplasmic granules that stain for acid phosphatase or esterases and by their signs of motility. Although not proved, it is presumed that these macrophages arise from primitive endothelial cells, are released into the lumen of primitive vessels, and move to the surrounding tissue.[10]

*5. Formation of the Joint Cavity.* Cavitation occurs at about the time the synovial mesenchyme differentiates into a membrane (Fig. 16–4). The precise mechanisms causing cavitation have not been completely defined. Extracellular matrix destruction by enzymes is probably the final pathway, and the interzone cells are probably programmed to release the enzymes that degrade the extracellular material. In chick embryos it has been shown that movement of the limb is essential for normal cavitation,[11,12] but similar experiments in developing human embryonic joints have yielded conflicting views.[13,14]

The cavity begins in the central interzone, which is, in effect, absorbed into each adjacent chondrogenous zone, which evolves into the underlying articular cartilage surface. Thus, when the joint cavity has formed, the joint is lined at all surfaces either by hyaline cartilage or by synovial membrane. These two very different tissues merge at the periphery of the joint, where the cartilage melds into bone. A potential space in the body has developed without any basement membrane below the lining cell surface. This absence of any epithelial tissue is a major determinant of joint physiology.

Direct experimental evidence is lacking as to when sodium hyaluronate (characteristic of joint fluid) first appears in the newly formed cavity. Synovial fibroblasts synthesize and release hyaluronate which is admixed with a protein-rich filtrate of blood to form synovial fluid. It is assured, therefore, that true synovial fluid cannot form until the synovial mesenchyme has vascularized and cellular differentiation in lining cells has progressed sufficiently to result in hyaluronate synthesis.

The entire development from a cellular but undifferentiated blastema to structures resembling an adult joint occurs in the human from about 4½ to 7 weeks after fertilization.[1] By this time all large synovial joints have recognizable cavities and are, functionally, true joints. Formation of joints occurs prior to many other crucial phases of musculoskeletal development, including vascularization of epiphyseal cartilage (8 to 12 weeks), appearance of villous folds in synovium (10 to 12 weeks), evolution of bursae (after 3 or 4 months), and appearance of fat pads (4 to 5 months).

In contrast to other joints, the temporomandibular joint develops slowly, with cavitation at a crown-rump length of 57 to 75 mm (i.e., well into the fetal stage).[15,16] This retardation may be related to the fact that this joint

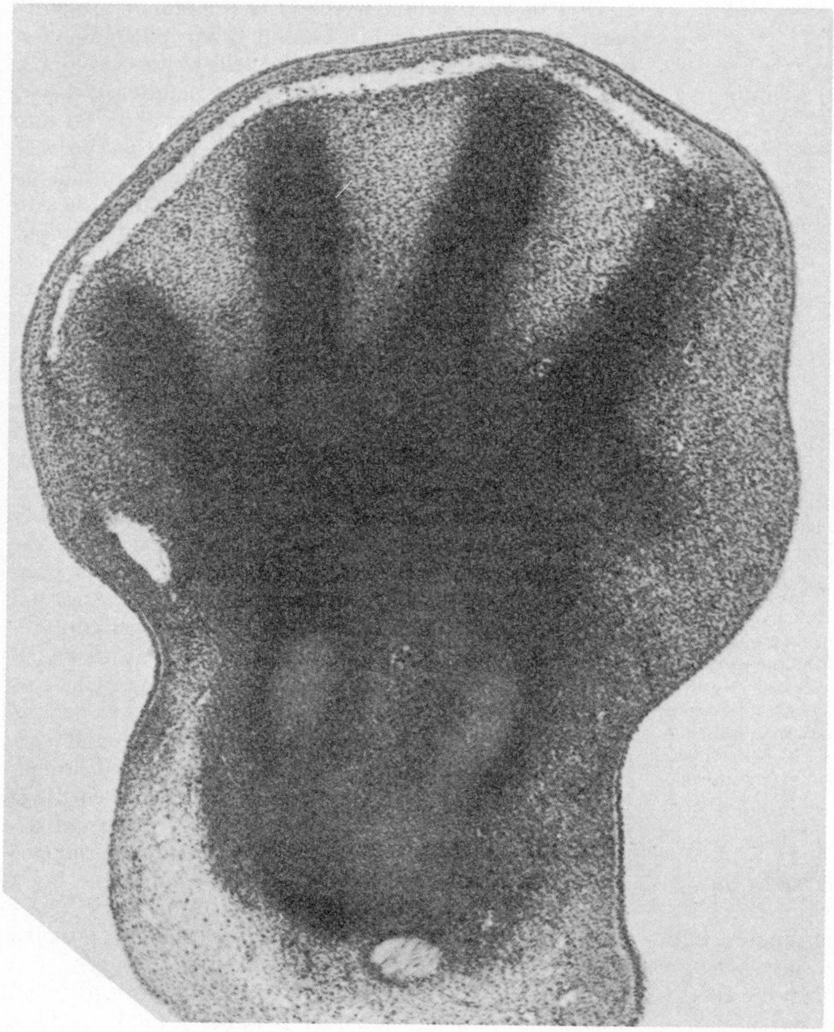

**Figure 16–3.** Coronal section of the hand at 11.7 mm (stage 17). The blastema with its increased cellularity serves to outline the form of the hand. Faint lightening in the region of the third and fourth metacarpals indicates very early chondrification. The radius and ulna are further along in chondrification. (From O'Rahilly, R.: Irish J. Med. Sci. 6:456, 1957).

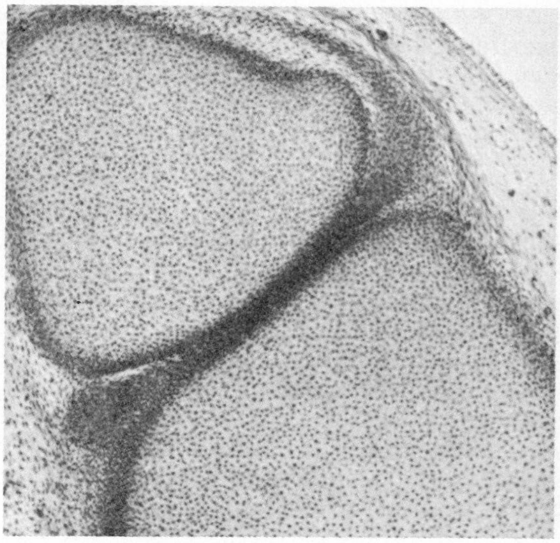

**Figure 16–4.** The embryonic joint developing between the femur and tibia at 31 mm (stage 23). The lateral meniscus is outlined by cavitation on the femoral side. Cavitation will subsequently spread in a medial direction as well as developing spontaneously at other foci. (From Gardner, E., and O'Rahilly, R.: J. Anat. 102:289, 1968)

develops in the absence of a continuous blastema and that its completion is related to insertion of a fibrocartilaginous disc between bone ends[15,17] derived from muscular and mesenchymal derivatives of the first pharyngeal arch.[16]

Synostoses (cartilaginous and fibrous joints) are presumed to evolve similarly, with the important exceptions that synovial mesenchyme is not formed and cavitation does not occur. Indeed, the "fused" peripheral joints induced in chicken embryos by paralyzing their limbs[18] resemble symphyses, with fibrocartilaginous plates developing between hyaline cartilage at the ends of bones. It may be that these joints develop as they do because there is relatively little motion during their development.

Human vertebrae and intervertebral discs probably develop as units from material arising from somites that form a homogeneous blastema.[19] The embryonic intervertebral discs serve as chondrogenous zones (both rostral and caudal) for the evolving vertebral bodies. The embryonic "disc" is replaced after it ceases chondrifying by the annulus fibrosus[20,21] (Fig. 16–5). It seems possible that since the nucleus pulposus contains proteoglycans as well as type II (cartilaginous) collagen,[22-24] it may represent segmented inclusions of the original embryonic disc still active in chondrification.

## ORGANIZATION OF THE MATURE JOINT

The mature joint is a complex structure. Understanding it demands consideration of biomechanics (see Chapter 20) and analysis of the different function of each joint, which is determined in turn by the anatomy peculiar to each joint.

In the following section, components of the "typical" synovial joint will be described.

**Muscles, Tendons, and Ligaments.** The physiology of muscle is described in detail in Chapter 18. It is sufficient here to emphasize only the direct correlation between muscle mass around a joint relative to its normal motion in different planes, such as the hip and shoulder. The shoulder, for example, is surrounded by bulky musculature with multiple components. This is essential to allow control of its many arcs of motions: forward flexion, 160 degrees; backward extension, 50 degrees; abduction, 170 degrees; adduction, 50 degrees; rotation (internal, 70 degrees; external, 70 to 90 degrees). In contrast, peripheral joints are not stablized by contracting muscle mass but rather by their anatomy, which restricts planes of normal motion, and by dense ligaments, which are structurally a part of the joint capsule.

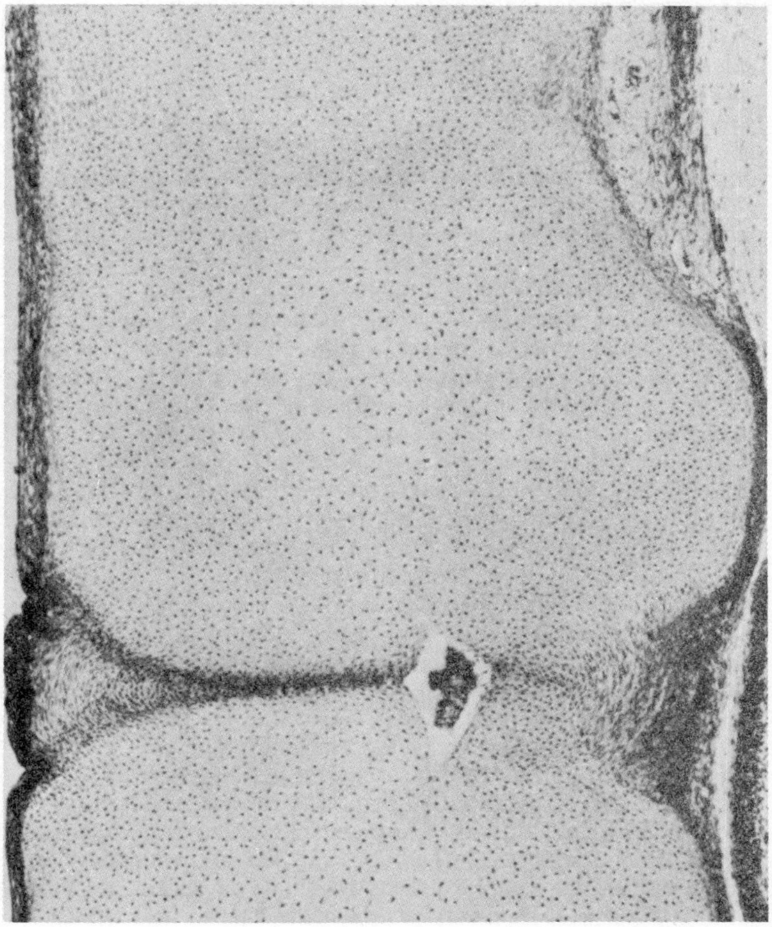

**Figure 16–5.** At 50 mm human fetal development, the body of the second and third cervical vertebrae has completed chondrification. The anulus fibrosus is beginning to differentiate at the periphery of the interzone (which in this section contains a nub of persisting notochord). (From O'Rahilly, R., and Gardner, E.: In Sokoloff, L. [ed.]: The Joint and Synovial Fluid, New York, Academic Press, 1978.)

The ankle, for example, moves in one plane through limited arcs: flexion, 50 degrees, and extension, 20 degrees. Muscle mass is directly proportional to stability of certain joints such as the knee. Joint effusions produce reflex inhibition of muscle contraction,[25] and muscle atrophy around a painful (and therefore hypomobile) joint occurs within days. It is unusual for the muscle/tendon apparatus to fail, but when it does, it is secondary to enormous, quickly generated forces across a joint. The site of failure is usually at the tendinous insertion into bone.

Individual variability in passive joint motion has a broad range, from the muscled athlete often at risk for muscle "pulls and strains" to the "loosed-jointed" asthenic person who suffers frequent joint sprains, who may have a predisposition to develop osteoarthritis,[26] and who may resemble those with Ehlers-Danlos type III syndromes (see Chapter 105).

Tendons act as functional and anatomic bridges between muscle and bone. As described by Canoso,[27] in addition to focusing the force of a large mass of muscle into a localized area on bone, tendons can, by splitting to form numerous insertions on different bones, transmit the force of a single muscle to different bones (e.g., the multiple distal insertions of the tibialis posterior). In development, muscle is not necessary for early differentiation of tendons, but without muscle (and muscle contraction?) sustained development of tendons fails.[28] Tendons are formed of logitudinally arranged type I collagen bundles interlaced by a delicate reticular network of type III collagen blood vessels, lymphatics, and possibly thin cellular processes of fibroblasts which can provide cell to cell contact.[29] The principal cell product for export from tendon fibroblasts is type I collagen, although they also synthesize proteoglycans (always a part of the connective tissue matrix) and other proteins (e.g., inhibitor[s] of metalloproteinases and collagenases, which have potential for degrading tendon components).

Most tendon attachments to bone are a highly specialized complex of tiers through which collagen fibers blend into fibrocartilage; then mineralized fibrocartilage merges into bone.[30] "Sharpey's perforating fibers," the tendon fibrils that have been seen to run through the periosteum and become continuous with outer bone lamellae (i.e., a functional staple), may be important at tendon insertions where there are no intervening tiers of fibrocartilage. An example of this type is the insertion of the pectoralis major tendon into the humerus.[31]

Many tendons, particularly those with a large range of motion, run through vascularized, discontinuous sheaths of collagen lined with mesenchymal cells resembling synovium. Tendon sheaths provide gliding function, which probably is enhanced by hyaluronic acid produced by the lining cells.[32] Loss of gliding function by formation of fibrous adhesions between tendons and their sheaths occurs when inflammation or surgical scar is followed by long periods of immobilization.

Pain of tendinous origin, tendinous calcification, and tendon rupture are complex pathophysiologic processes that have not been thoroughly evaluated. Factors involved at different times to a greater or lesser degree are (1) ageing processes, including loss of extracellular water and an increase in intermolecular crosslinks of collagen; (2) traumatically induced ischemic areas in tendon; (3) iatrogenic factors, including intratendon injection of glucocorticoids; (4) deposition of calcium hydroxyapatite crystals (perhaps enhanced by presence of the calcium-binding amino acid $\gamma$-carboxyglutamic acid [Gla]).[33]

There are few anatomic and structural differences between ligaments and tendons. The obvious one is that one set of the end of tendon collagen fibrils are intertwined and braided among the fibrillar endomysium that surrounds each individual muscle fiber, whereas both ends of ligaments insert into bone on either side of a joint. Often the latter are recognized only as hypertrophied components of the fibrous joint capsule. Some ligaments have a much higher ratio of elastin to collagen (1:4) than do tendons (1:50).[27] The ligamentum flavum, which holds adjacent vertebral laminae in place, is an example of these. The ligament that sustains the greatest stress during normal function is the plantar ligament of the foot, which has a large functional role in keeping the longitudinal arch of the foot raised. Ligaments and tendons synthesize substances that regulate connective tissue metabolism locally. In addition to collagen, for instance, tendon cells produce collagenase in latent form as well as inhibitors of collagenolytic enzymes.

The stabilization of joints is in part a function of ligaments, capsule, and menisci of joints. In the knee (the most studied of all joints), the medial collateral ligaments and anterior cruciate ligaments form a resistant couple for stability when there is little or no load upon the joint. During load-bearing conditions there is an increasing contribution to stability from the joint surfaces themselves as compressive load increases. The components that provide surface stability are friction (minimal) between the joint surfaces, deformation of the cartilage, and geometrical conformity of the condyles.

**Bursae.** The many bursae in the human body serve to facilitate gliding function much as a tendon sheath facilitates movement of the tendon within, enabling low friction motion of one tissue over another. Bursae are closed sacs, lined sparsely with mesenchymal cells similar to synovial cells. Although most bursae differentiate concurrently with synovial joints during embryogenesis, during life new bursae may develop in response to stress and previously existing ones may become hypertrophied.[34] During life, again in response to stress (i.e., inflammation or trauma), deep bursae often develop communications with joints.[27] Examples of this include (1) iliopsoas bursa—hip joint; (2) subacromial bursae—glenohumeral joint; these develop secondary to degenerative or inflammatory involvement of the rotator cuff tendons; and (3) gastrocnemius or semimembranous bursae—knee joint. It is unusual for subcutaneous bursae (e.g., the prepatellar bursa or olecranon bursa) to develop communication with the underlying joint. Bursal fluid, even when the bursa is infected or host to an attack of gout, rarely generates an inflammatory response (measured by numbers of PMN leukocytes) that a similar process does within a joint.[35] This may be related to a lesser degree of vascularization of bursae.

**Vascular and Nerve Supply to the Joint.** Arterial and venous networks of the joint are complex and are characterized by arteriovenous anastomoses that communicate freely with the vascular supply to periosteum and to periarticular bone.[36] As large synovial arteries enter the deep layers of the synovium near the capsule, they give off branches, which branch again to form "microvascular units" in the subsynovial layers. As in other tissues, precapillary arterioles probably play a major role in controlling circulation to the lining layer. The surface area of the synovial capillary bed is very large and, as it runs only a few cell layers deep to the surface, it has a role in trans-synovial exchange of molecules that may explain the propensity of diarthrodial joints to develop effusions and hemarthroses.

Heat (up to an intra-articular temperature of 40° C) increases blood flow through synovial capillaries.[37] Exercise, although resulting in an increase in periarticular muscle blood flow, may actually result in a decrease in the clearance rate of small molecules.[38] Immobilization, in experimental animals, actually decreases the number of capillary plexi as well as blood flow in joints.[37] Pressure also has an effect on blood flow. Effusions can act to tamponade blood supply, and it is possible that large effusions could virtually shut off blood flow to superficial lining layers.

Synovial capillaries are fenestrated; they contain small pores covered by a thin membrane[38,39] (Fig. 16–6). These fenestrations may facilitate rapid exchange of small molecules (e.g., glucose, lactate, and so on) with the synovial fluid.

Dissection studies have shown that each joint has a dual nerve supply: (1) specific articular nerves that penetrate the capsule as independent branches of adjacent peripheral nerves and (2) articular branches that arise from related muscle nerves.[39] The definition of joint position and the detection of joint motion are monitored separately and by a combination of multiple inputs from different receptors in varied systems. Dee has summarized data indicating that nerve endings in muscle as well as in the joint capsule are involved in articular kinesthetic sensation.[40] Patients who have had capsulectomy along with total hip replacement[41] or surgical removal of proximal interphalangeal or metacarpophalangeal joints of the hand[42] still retain good joint position sensation.

**The Subchondral Bone.** The microstructure of bone in the plate beneath the calcified base of articular cartilage may have many effects upon the cartilage above it. The subchondral bone of the knee is formed from a meshwork of fine trabeculae of less than 0.2 mm diameter and in a density of fewer than 2 per mm of bone. The stiffness of subchondral bone, and thus the impact transmitted to cartilage during weight bearing or effort, may be a factor in the health of normal articular cartilage.[43]

**Articular Cartilage—the Unique Functional Struc-**

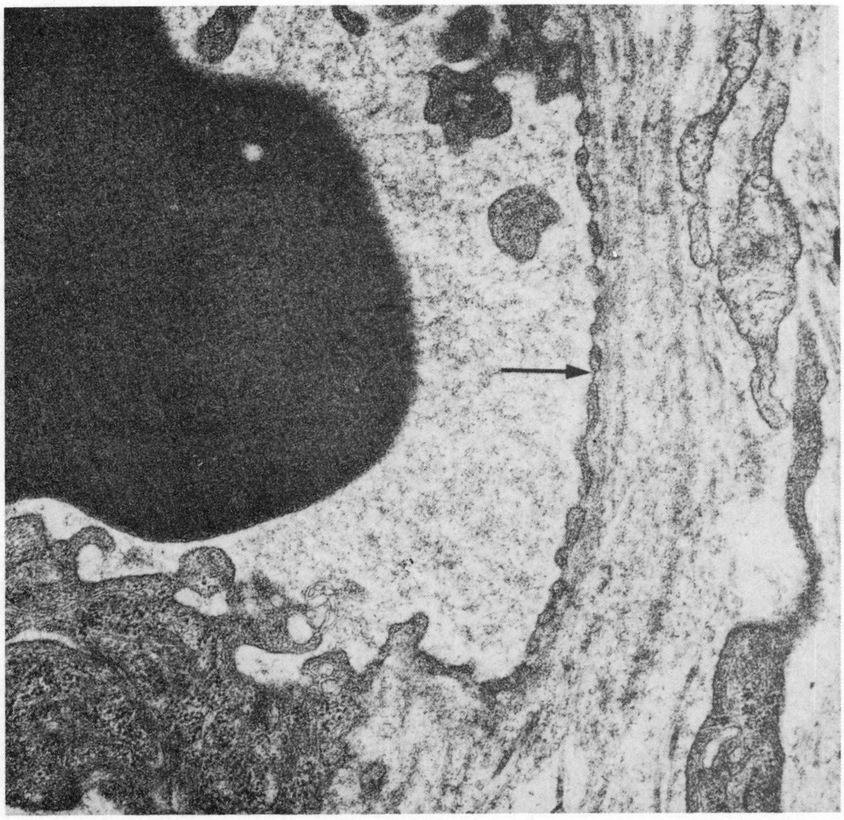

**Figure 16–6.** Fenestrated blood capillary in human synovium. This capillary is situated just beneath the lining layer. Pores in endothelium are indicated by the arrow. A red blood cell lies in the lumen of the capillary. × 11,000. (From Bassleer, R., et al.: Histological structure and functions of synovium. In Franchimont, P. [ed.]: Articular Synovium: Anatomy, Physiology, Pathology, Pharmacology, and Therapy. Basel, Karger, 1982, pp. 1–26.)

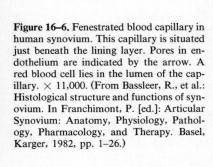

**ture of Joints.** Articular cartilage is highly differentiated and has physical properties that no other tissue or synthetic product of bioengineering laboratories can equal. Articular cartilage must provide a smooth, resilient surface for joint motion under conditions of either intense pressure or high velocity, or both. At the same time the cartilage must retain capacity for maintenance without morphologic change and in the absence of any blood vessels to carry in nutrients and remove products of chondrocyte metabolism and matrix turnover. While endowed with a capacity for maintenance, articular cartilage cannot effectively regenerate itself, and this imposes a limitation on the organism—a need to protect articular cartilage from destruction.

Articular cartilage is composed principally of collagen and proteoglycans. The structure and biology of these components are discussed in detail in Chapters 14 and 15.

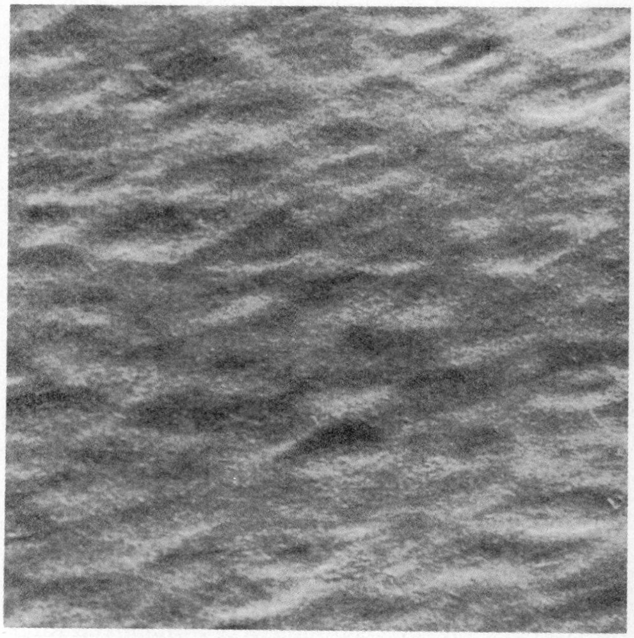

**Figure 16–8.** Scanning electron microscopic view of the "pits" found on the surface of articular cartilage. This view is of adult rabbit cartilage at ~500 magnification. It is not known whether the depressions are present in vivo or whether they represent artifacts produced by desiccation and shrinkage during preparation for microscopy. Prominent ridgings of the surface of articular cartilage reported by earlier investigators are probably true cutting artifacts. Surface irregularity of some magnitude is essential for the full development of hypothesis of squeeze-film lubrication in which, during weight-bearing, interstitial fluid from cartilage matrix would be trapped in surface depressions (or between ridges) and prevent direct cartilage-cartilage contact. (From Ghadially, F. N., et al.: J. Anat. 121:119, 1976).

## ORGANIZATION OF ARTICULAR CARTILAGE

Intensive study of the articular cartilage from the metacarpophalangeal joints of young steers has provided the most recent and precise data on the organization of this tissue.[44,45] Figure 16–7 is a diagrammatic representation of the various zones and regions of cartilage.

The *superficial zone* (5 to 10 percent of total thickness) has a reduced metachromatic staining for glycosaminoglycans and a rich content of immunoreactive proteoglycan core protein and link protein. Called the lamina splendens, this is probably composed of hyaluronic acid and/or absorbed glycoproteins.[46] The superficial zone is covered at the cartilage surface by a layer of thin fibrils (4 to 10 μm in diameter), which are arranged in a random fashion up to several microns in depth. Early studies using scanning electron microscopy showed ridges and undulations in the cartilage surface.[47,48] Other investigators believe that these undulations are artifacts of cutting and fixation.[49,50] Instead, there is evidence[51-53] that there are shallow pits or round undulations in the surface contour (10 to 40 μm in diameter and 1 to 6 μm deep), which may represent underlying lacunae of chondrocytes (Fig. 16–8). It is not known whether these depressions exist in vivo, although those who study joint lubrication have often used the existence of undulations as evidence of crucial "trapped" reservoirs for squeeze-film lubrication.

Collagen fibril diameters in this and the other zones are listed in Table 16–1. In pericellular areas collagen fibril diameters are much less than in territorial and interterritorial areas. Type II collagen represents approximately 85 to 90 percent of the total tissue collagen in articular cartilage. Type V collagen also is found in cartilage, primarily in a pericellular location near chondrocytes.[54] Thus, the narrow diameter pericellular fibrils probably represent type V collagen.

Proteoglycan and link proteins are organized in territorial and pericellular regions of the deep zone in a manner similar to that of comparable regions in the superficial and middle zones.[44,45] Immunoelectron mi-

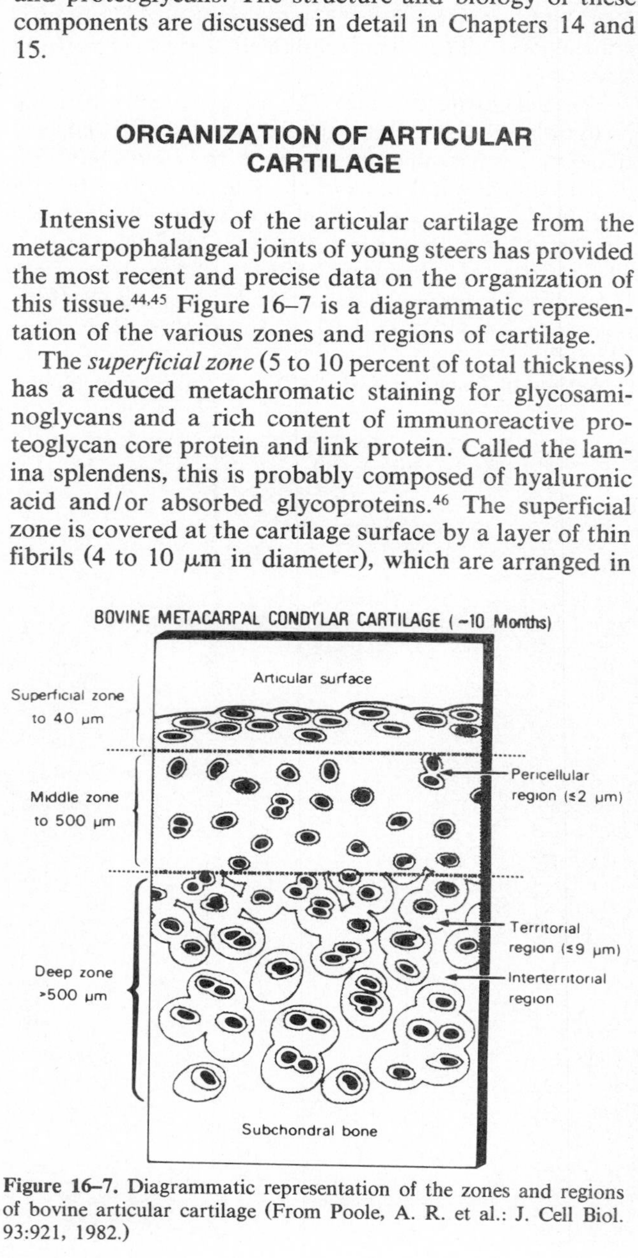


**Figure 16–7.** Diagrammatic representation of the zones and regions of bovine articular cartilage (From Poole, A. R. et al.: J. Cell Biol. 93:921, 1982.)

**Table 16–1.** Collagen Fibril Diameters*

| Zone/Region | Diameter (nm) |
|---|---|
| | *mean* ± *SD (n)* |
| Superficial zone | |
| 1. Pericellular | 15.4 ± 8.3 (18) |
| 2. Territorial | 29.2 ± 5.4 (22) |
| Middle zone | |
| 3. Pericellular | 21.5 ± 12.7 (18) |
| 4. Territorial | 31.8 ± 5.0 (23) |
| Deep zone | |
| 5. Pericellular | 19.0 ± 4.4 (23) |
| 6. Territorial | 48.5 ± 7.0 (23) |
| 7. Interterritorial | 57.5 ± 7.6 (25) |

*From Poole, A.R. et al.: J. Cell Biol. 93:921, 1982.

All measurements were made from one experiment (BC14). Student's $t$ test analyses revealed that the following were significantly different from each other ($P < 0.001$): *1* and *2*, *3* and *4*, *5* and *6*, *6* and *7*, *4* and *6*, *4* and *7*.

croscopic studies have revealed that the interterritorial regions of the deep zone differ markedly in organization from the territorial regions of the deep zone. The territorial regions revealed minimal evidence for link protein, whereas only the interterritorial regions of the deep zone revealed staining patterns consistent with structural organization of hyaluronate, link protein, proteoglycan core protein, and glycosaminoglycans as large aggregates.

These large aggregates and the large amount of $H_2O$ bound to them form a massive polyanionic complex that has a large domain and the capacity to resist compressive force; compression shrinks the domain of each aggregate, increasing the electronegative repellent force. In addition, the charge effects cause a resistance to bound water flow. The effect, in biomechanical terms, is to make the cartilage elastic, so that after compression is released, the aggregated proteoglycans return to their fully extended state from forces generated by mutual repulsion of negatively charged groups.

It has been suggested that since the interterritorial regions have widely spaced, thick collagen fibrils and large amounts of link-stabilized proteoglycans, it is this area of cartilage that has the greatest compressibility.[44,45] The nature of the association of proteoglycans and hyaluronic acid with collagen is complex.[55] Certain fractions of proteoglycans may affect the formation of fibrils,[56] while others may inhibit calcification in articular cartilage.[57] Significantly, fractions of proteoglycans capable of inhibiting mineral crystal formation are absent from calcifying cartilage.[58]

**Cartilage Glycoproteins.** Glycoproteins are present in collagen in a concentration inverse to that of collagen.[59] Lysozyme and other cationic glycoproteins of low molecular weight are present in cartilage, probably synthesized by chondrocytes. Some of these cationic proteins have the capacity to inhibit proteolytic enzymes[60-62] and tumor neovascularization[63] and retard the development of osteoclasts.[64] These factors are of particular interest because avascular cartilage is generally resistant to invasion by tumors. The proteinase (trypsin) inhibitors in cartilage appear to be identical to the well-known bovine pancreatic trypsin inhibitor described by Kunitz.[62] The collagenase inhibitor found in cartilage is a molecular species separate from the serine or thiol proteinase inhibitors.[65]

**Cartilage Water and Small Solutes.** Amidst collagen fibers is a heterogeneous collection of water and ground substance. Water content is about 70 to 75 percent of the wet weight,[66] and in many cases this rises to over 80 percent near the surface.

Micropuncture studies of articular cartilage have revealed an electrolyte concentration in this extracellular fluid similar to that in plasma except for a pH of 7.1 to 7.2.[67] Interestingly, at the growth area of articular cartilage around hypertrophic cells the pH is higher, a factor that may facilitate the mechanism of calcification near the tidemark.

As reviewed by Mankin[68] most of the water of articular cartilage is bound loosely within the matrix and exchanges readily with water in synovial fluid. The cartilage glycosaminoglycan do not appear to be essential for water binding; in osteoarthritis, when proteoglycans content is decreased, water content in cartilage can be increased by as much as 8 percent[69] due to loss of restraint of GAG and to collagen network defects.

It is of interest that movement of uncharged small solutes, such as glucose, is not impaired by diffusion through matrices containing large amounts of glycosaminoglycans, and Hadler has reviewed studies indicating that diffusivity of small molecules through hyaluronate is actually enhanced.[70] If applicable to articular cartilage in vivo, this phenomenon would facilitate nutrient exchange during compressive force on cartilage.

**Chondrocytes.** Chondrocytes exist in relative isolation, living singly or in pairs or with a few other cells in clusters. In addition, they are highly specialized and express the capacity to synthesize matrix components (e.g., collagen, proteoglycans, noncollagenous acidic glycoproteins, chondronectin, small cationic polypeptides, and other glycoproteins) as well as enzymes (e.g., collagenase, neutral proteinases, and cathepsins) capable of breaking down matrix components. Chondrocytes lie in a zone of finely textured matrix containing abundant ground substance but only a few collagen fibers.[71] Taking into consideration mean cell size and density, Stockwell and Meachim[72] have estimated that the volume of cartilage occupied by cells is between 0.4 and 2.0 percent of total cartilage volume. The "lacunae" seen around chondrocytes prepared for light microscopy are probably shrinkage artifacts.[73] Preparations of articular cartilage prepared for transmission electron microscopy show cells with rounded or oval nuclei that sometimes contain fibrous laminae (up to 95 nm thick, particularly in chondrocytes involved, apparently, in repair of tissue defects).[74] Rough endoplasmic reticulum and the Golgi complex are most developed in chondrocytes of zones II and III. Short cell processes are seen on all chondrocytes but are better developed in cells of deeper zones[75] and may play a role in transport of cellular enzymes to the extracellular space and/or in pinocytotic

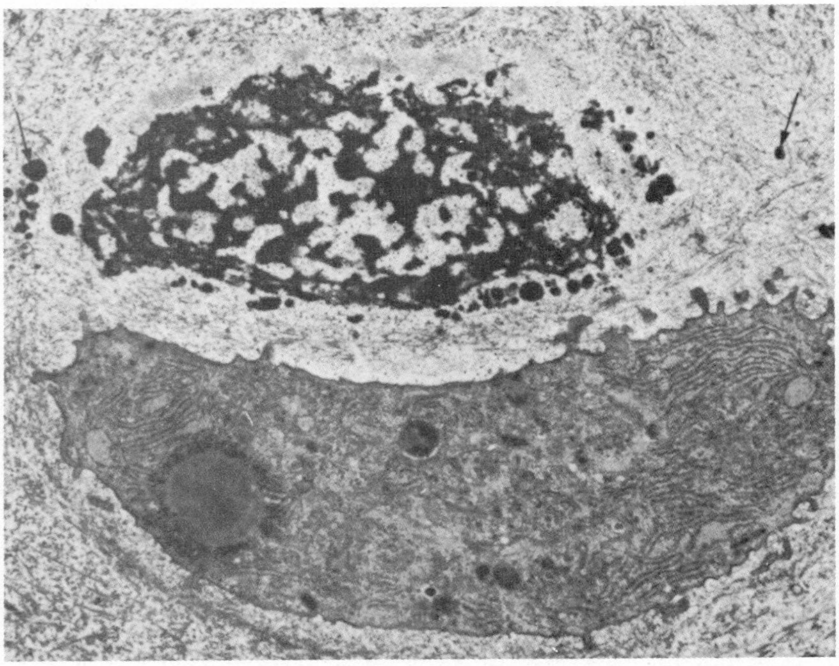

**Figure 16–9.** In situ necrosis and disintegration of one of two chondrocytes in articular cartilage. Such finds indicate that chondrocytes do replicate in normal cartilage, because despite the findings of dead or effete chondrocytes in cartilage sections it is recognized that the cell concentration in human articular cartilage does not change during aging. (From Ghadially, F. N.: In Sokoloff, L. [ed.]: The Joints and Synovial Fluid, Vol. 1, New York, Acadamic Press, 1978.)

function. Chondrocytes certainly have a phagocytic function and can be shown to take up red blood cell products in chronic hemarthrosis[76] (see Chapter 100). Cartilage cells die in situ from time to time. Necrotic remnants of cells are found adjacent to healthy cells(Fig. 16–9). Since data by Stockwell[77] have shown that the cell density of the full thickness of human adult femoral condylar cartilage is $14.5 \pm 3.0 \times 10^3$ cells per cubic millimeter from age 20 through 80 years, it follows that new chondrocytes arise by mitosis to replace dead ones. Despite this logical extrapolation of data, mitoses are not observed in normal adult articular cartilage.[78]

Since William Hunter's observations in 1743 that adult articular cartilage contains no blood vessels,[79] there has been debate about how chondrocytes receive nutrients, although numerous studies have confirmed an early study by Bywaters[80] that articular cartilage principally utilizes anaerobic glycolysis for energy production.

In the growing child, active enchondral ossification occurs at the base of articular cartilage just as it does at the growth plate (primary epiphysis). Here, in the hypertrophic zone of cartilage, blood vessels penetrate between columns of chondrocytes. The cartilage is calcified and subsequently is replaced by true bone. It is likely that diffusion from these tiny end capillaries through matrix to chondrocytes occurs. This mechanism is unlikely in the adult, although there is an argument over whether the "tidemark" (the dense calcified plate of articular cartilage) is or is not bridged by capillaries. Some studies[81,82] have described partial defects in the osteocartilaginous barrier. Collins[83] has suggested that the existence of this calcified barrier characterizes a "stable" contact, which, whether in a joint, rib, or intervertebral disc, prevents passage of anything across the barrier.

In contrast, morphologic, physiologic, and pathologic studies have confirmed that solutes pass easily from the synovial fluid into cartilage and that cartilage does not survive without contact with synovial fluid in vivo. Strangeways provided early support for the concept of nutrition by diffusion by noting that loose bodies of cartilage in joints actually grow in size.[84] In experimental systems it has been shown that sufficient agitation of synovial fluid results in nourishment of even the deepest layers of articular cartilage.[85]

There are three potential mechanisms for nutrient transfer within cartilage matrix: diffusion, active transport by chondrocytes, and pumping by intermittent compression of cartilage matrix. Maroudas and coworkers[86] have demonstrated that molecules the size of hemoglobin ($Mr$ 65,000) are the largest that can diffuse through normal articular cartilage. Fortunately, the molecular weight of solutes needed for cellular metabolism is small enough to permit adequately diffusion within the cartilage of mobilized, healthy joints.

Intermittent compression serving as a pump mechanism for solute exchange in cartilage is a concept that has arisen from observations that joint immobilization[87] or dislocation[88] or other events that interfere with normal movement of one articular surface upon its counterpart lead to degenerative changes in cartilage. Exercise, in contrast, increases solute penetration into cartilage in experimental systems.[85] Pressing filter paper against cartilage squeezes out liquid that has the ionic composition of extracellular fluid.[89] McCutchen[90] suggested that during weight bearing, fluid escapes from the load-bearing region by flow to other cartilage sites and into grooves in the slightly irregular cartilage surface. When the load was removed, cartilage would re-expand and draw back fluid. Nutrients could be exchanged with waste materials during such a process. Whether diffusion, even boosted by pressure, could occur fast enough for this weeping lubrication to facilitate solute exchange and penetration is hotly debated but is supported by studies showing free exchange of water between cartilage and synovial fluid and the enchanced diffusivity of solutes in a matrix of hyaluronate.

*Characteristics of Chondrocytes in Vitro.* The specialized nature of chondrocytes is emphasized when these cells are separated from their matrix environment and grown in cell culture. The expression of the chondrogenic phenotype in vitro has been shown to be susceptible to many environmental factors.

In general, chondrocytes placed in monolayer culture shift from synthesis of type II to type I collagen[91] and produce a different amount and type of glycosaminoglycans[92] than they do in vivo or in organ culture. If placed into suspension (spinner) cultures from monolayer cultures, rabbit chondrocytes begin to express once again the capability of synthesizing type II collagen[93] as well as cartilage-specific proteoglycans.[94] If cultured in soft agar in low density,[95] chondrocytes thrive and continue to express their capability to produce type II collagen and large amounts of glycosaminoglycans, which appear as a "lake" around the chondrocytes (Fig. 16–10). Addition to the agar cultures of growth factors (e.g., epidermal growth factor) results in a proliferation of chondrocytes, which aggregate as balls of cells, although the surrounding lake of glycosaminoglycans becomes much smaller when expressed as area per cell.[95] Thus, the growth and the extracellular matrix production of these cells in culture can be dissociated by the addition of exogenous agents.

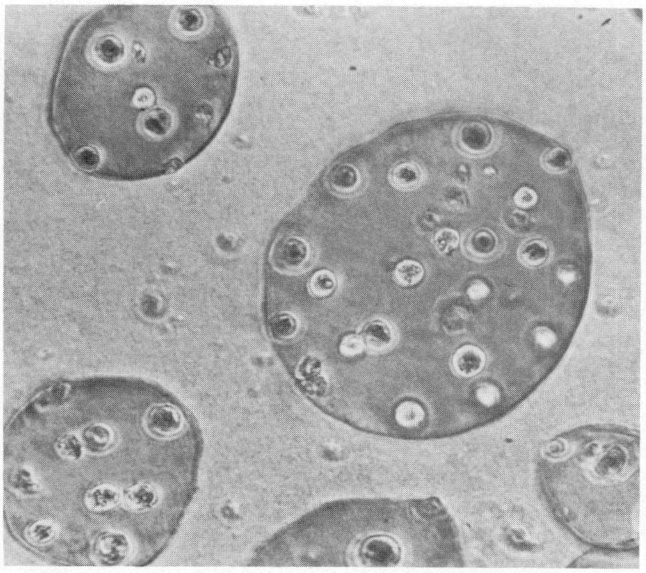

**Figure 16–10.** Chondrocytes in organ culture. This represents a 21 day culture pf rabbit articular condrocytes that had been dissociated into a single cell suspension and cultured in 0.25% agar and F-12 medium with 10 percent fetal calf serum as described by Benya and Straffer (Cell 30:215, 1982). Note the "islands" of chondrocytes surrounded by "lakes" of glycosaminoglycans (proteoglycans) that have been stained by alcian blue dye. × 100. (From Skantze, K. A. et al. in press.)

**Joint Lubrication.** This complicated subject has been reviewed effectively for physicians by Wright and Dowson[96] and in more detail by McCutchen[97] and Swanson.[98]

Although there have been at least 12 distinct mechanisms put forth to explain part or all of joint lubrication, most fall into two basic categories: (1) *fluid-film lubrication,* in which cartilage surfaces are separated by a fluid film, and (2) *boundary lubrication,* in which surface-to-surface contact exists, with protection and a decreased coefficient of friction offered by special molecules attached to cartilage surfaces. Variants of these may evolve as follows: (a) squeeze film lubrication, in which, as discussed above, a film of fluid is trapped between opposing cartilage surfaces and, because the fluid film is noncompressible, prevents the surfaces from touching.[99] This is very similar, of course, to weeping lubrication;[100] (b) boosted lubrication,[101,102] in which pools of synovial fluid are compressed, as in weeping lubrication, but at high load the low molecular weight solute is driven back into cartilage or to non-weight-bearing fluid, leaving hyaluronate ("mucin") concentrates to bear weight; and (c) elastohydrodynamic lubrication,[103] in which the viscosity and shear rate (hence, the coefficient of friction) is reduced because cartilage surfaces are deformable by a combination of tangential stretching and compression of the opposing surfaces.

In reality, several of these mechanisms and mixtures of them are involved in lubrication at both high and low loads and velocity imposed by daily activities. While walking, the load on weight-bearing joints (hip and knee) rises to three or four times body weight, yet is reduced to a fraction of body weight moments later. Thus, during the walking cycle,[96] three distinct modes may lubricate the knee: (1) As the heel hits the walking surface, impact is high and load maximal. Squeeze-film lubrication could protect the surfaces from direct contact and attenutate the force of impact. (2) As the point of contact shifts from heel to toe, a combination of many mechanisms may apply. Cartilage may be deformed by sheer forces which minimize surface-surface motion (elastohydrodynamic lubrication). Boundary lubrication is always available if cartilage surfaces approximate each other sufficiently, although the evidence suggests that boundary mechanisms fail during high load (see below). (3) After toe-off, the knee is in a minimal load situation, and the simplest of hydrodynamic lubrication mechanisms may be useful.

In Figure 16–11 a mechanism is portrayed for both enhanced perfusion and lubrication of cartilage-cartilage surfaces during weight bearing; this is "squeeze-film" lubrication.

Hyaluronate, the extremely large and viscous molecule found in abundance in synovial fluid, is probably not involved in cartilage-cartilage lubrication. Hyalu-

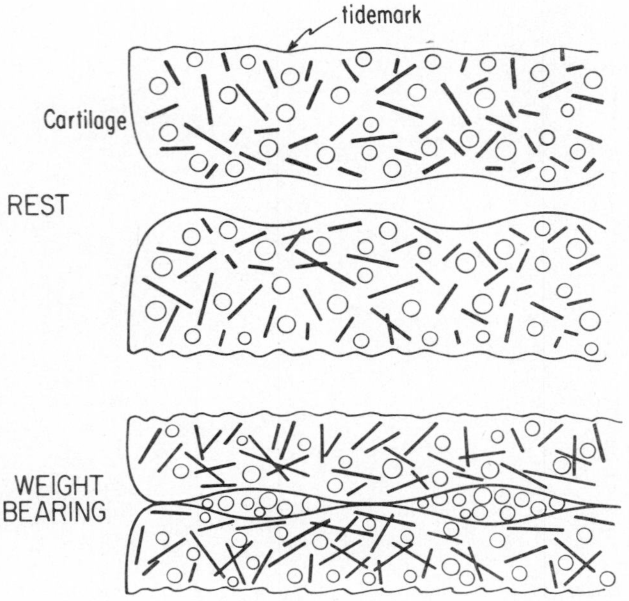


**Figure 16–11.** A scheme of a possible mechanism for both cartilage lubrication and provision of nutrition to chondrocytes. Two opposing articular surfaces are shown at rest and during weight bearing. The lines indicate collagen fibrils within cartilage. The circles represent solute, the interstitial fluid. Proteoglycans are not included for sake of clarity. During weight bearing the cartilage is compressed. Fluid is driven out of the cartilage into the intercondylar space. When weight bearing is released, solute (presumably having exchanged cellular metabolites for nutrients) is resorbed as cartilage re-expands.[90]

ronidase treatment did not inhibit lubrication capability of synovial fluid at low load, while trypsin (with the capability of digesting glycoproteins) in synovial fluid did eliminate lubricating ability.[104] The compound responsible for cartilage-cartilage lubrication has been purified. It is glycoprotein of molecular weight of 225,000 daltons and has been named *lubricin.* This molecule, synthesized by synovial cells, is 200 nm in length and 1 to 2 nm in diameter. The exact structure-function relationships of this molecule remain unknown,[105] but it appears to be the primary boundary lubricant in mammalian joints. Another boundary lubricant may be fat. Lipid is reported to comprise 1 to 2 percent of dry weight of cartilage,[106] and experimental treatment of cartilage surfaces with fat solvents has impaired lubrication qualities of the tissue.[107]

It is also important to realize that articular surfaces are protected by other mechanisms not involving lubrication. During impact loading, muscles and bone absorb the great majority of force and energy, leaving only a small amount to be absorbed by cartilage itself.[108] Finely tuned neuromuscular reflexes are essential for this system to work effectively. It is possible that small failures in these reflex arcs may lead to insufficient attenuation of impact loading resulting in degenerative changes in joints and subchondral bone (i.e., Charcot's arthropathy).

**Mechanical Properties of Cartilage During Load.** The most important function of cartilage—its ability to be compressed by a load and recover from this deformity—has been an object of research since Bar's studies in 1926[109] (Fig. 16–12). When a load is applied to cartilage, there is a rapid ("instantaneous") indentation, followed by a time-dependent creep phase during which indentation increases while load remains constant. On removal of the load there is an initial immediate recovery, followed by a long, sustained recovery to normal volume. The initial rapid deformation results from a bulk movement of water and compression of collagen fibers. In the second, time-dependent compression (called "creep"), water flows through the matrix.

From studies of the bone-bone contact in the absence of cartilage, it has become apparent that a function of cartilage, in addition to providing low-friction movement at high speeds, may be to absorb some of the energy of impact loading by deforming and effectively spreading a load over a broad area. Freeman and Kempson[110] have put forth the argument that in normal cartilage both collagen and proteoglycans contribute to load carriage. Tensile strength of the collagen resists deformation and maintains the basic structural framework to allow proteoglycans to remain in place. The proteoglycans, through strong charge interactions with water, control solute flow and therefore the absolute and time-dependent deformation by weight bearing.

Studies of matrix-depleted cartilage have helped clarify the relative roles of collagen and proteoglycans in the function of cartilage. Using canine articular cartilage slices, it was demonstrated that cartilage incubated with collagenase became filmy, flimsy, and transparent (Fig. 16–13); it was devoid of tensile strength.[111] Similar slices incubated with trypsin sufficient to deplete matrix proteoglycans did not change in gross appearance; however, the physical qualities changed. Control slices were relatively rigid, while trypsin-treated slices were easily bent

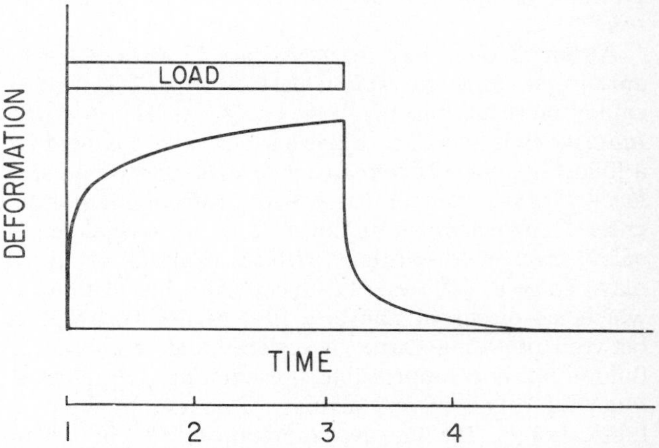


**Figure 16–12.** A typical curve of deformation of articular cartilage by a load as a function of time. The four phases expressed as a function of time are as follows: 1 = instantaneous deformation coincident with application of the load; 2 = slow deformation which gradually slows in rate of deformation; 3 = instantaneous recovery; 4 = time - dependent recovery to normal cartilage thickness. (After Bär[83] and Kempson.[88])

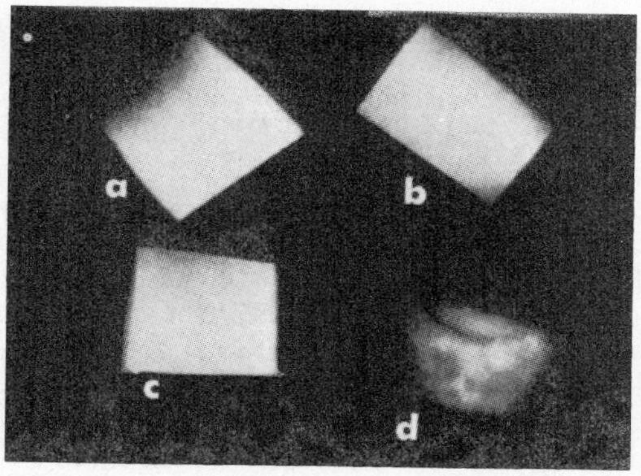


**Figure 16–13.** Effect of collagenase and trypsin on canine patellar cartilage slices. Each piece was incubated separately; buffer was 0.1 M Tris-HCl, 0.005 M in $CaCl_2$, pH 7.6 *a*, Buffer only; *b*, trypsin, 15 μg in buffer; *c*, trypsin, 10 μg in buffer; *d*, synovial coll agenase (partially purified) in buffer. Approximately 35 percent of the collagen was removed from the collagenase-treated sample, < 5 percent from the trypsin-treated samples, and none from the control sample. (From Harris, E.D., Jr., et al.: Excerpta Medica International Congress Series No. 229 , Immunopathology of Inflammation, 1970.)

in half. More detailed studies to measure deformation revealed that proteoglycan-depleted cartilage had lost its ability to rebound from a deforming load; it had lost compressive stiffness.[112,113] In similar experiments, using cathepsin D, British investigators[114] freed 50 percent of tissue uronic acid without releasing any hydroxyproline (a collagen marker). This produced a 50 percent reduction in compressive stiffness.

**Repair of Cartilage.** Healing of cartilage defects that do not penetrate the subchondral bone plate is dependent entirely on surviving chondrocytes near the margins of injury. In man, essentially no repair is generated by these cells.[115] Occasionally, the chondrocytes proliferate to form clones in "brood capsules," but the clefts in cartilage do not heal. Defects will remain without progression so long as the subchondral bony plate remains intact.

In deeper injury through the subchondral plate there is extensive fibroblastic proliferation in the defect, but seldom is true hyaline cartilage produced. More often a fibrocartilaginous scar results from this extrinsic repair effort.[115,116] Thus, repair of articular cartilage is not programmed well in human biologic systems; the emphasis is on protection from damage. In the early stages of osteoarthritis, however, there is considerable increase in new matrix synthesis, which may retard progression of destructive disease (see Chapter 88).

**Aging of Articular Cartilage.** The thickness of articular cartilage in mammalian limbs has been found to be related to body weight, to hip-to-shoulder length, and to the area of the tibial plateau.[117] Cartilage thickness is asymmetrical over the surface of weight-bearing joints.[118] On the surface of the human femoral head, cartilage is thickest on the anterosuperior surface of the femoral head and increases with age. The increased thickness has not been related to fibrillation of the cartilage[119] and cannot be interpreted as a change associated with early osteoarthrosis.

The overall cellularity of cartilage does not change with age nor does the fluid content or total amounts of collagen and glycosaminoglycan.[120] Changes in color appear; adult cartilage develops a yellow tinge, but there is no evidence that this pigment has any functional significance. As mentioned above, cartilage collagen fibers in aged articular cartilage are thicker than those in cartilage of younger people.

In contrast to the lack of change in normal cartilage with age, it must be recognized that cartilage fibrillation is an age-related process.[121] Fibrillation, however, cannot be considered as necessarily leading to osteoarthritis, and may best be considered a "regressive change." It often occurs first at the periphery of joint surfaces.[119,122] Fibrillation is initially confined to the superficial layers of cartilage. The cartilage shows foci of mild splitting and fraying. Surface "pits" develop, and grossly the surface develops a "matte" appearance instead of a "gloss" appearance. It has been suggested that clefts develop at the base of small splits in the surface.

Chemical analysis of fibrillated areas of cartilage has shown a depletion of glycosaminoglycans with normal collagen concentration.[123,124] Comparative stiffness of the cartilage is decreased. If fibrillation progresses into deeper layers of cartilage, an abnormal multicellular cluster of chondrocytes that stain intensely for glycosaminoglycans is found at the base of clefts.[125] The fibrillated areas by this time are noticeably softer or malacic. Freeman and Meachim[120] have presented a reasonable argument for the hypothesis that fibrillation begins with fatigue fracture of superficial collagen bundles. This results in superficial clefts, which deepen if the process continues. See Chapter 88 for a detailed discussion of the A's in osteoarthritis.

## SYNOVIUM

The synovial membrane covers all intra-articular structures except for articular cartilage and the central portions of fibrocartilaginous menisci,[83] and for localized "bare areas" where bone is exposed. As mentioned in the discussion of embryologic development of joints, the synovium has at least two unusual features. (1) It develops from the blastema from which the skeleton evolves and not from the general mesenchyme. (2) Although it lines a closed space in the body, there is no epithelial tissue in the synovium and therefore no basement membrane or structural barrier between synovial fluid and synovial blood vessels.

**Organization of the Synovium.** The absence of a basement membrane assures a continuation of morphology as well as of function. Although the outer layers of the joint capsule are relatively acellular and formed of thick interwining bands of collagen fibers that do not resemble the highly cellular synovial lining, the change from one to the other is not abrupt. The cells below the lining layers resemble lining cells, but there is more connective tissue. Continuing centrifugally, the cells appear more as fibroblasts. Fat cells increase in number, larger blood

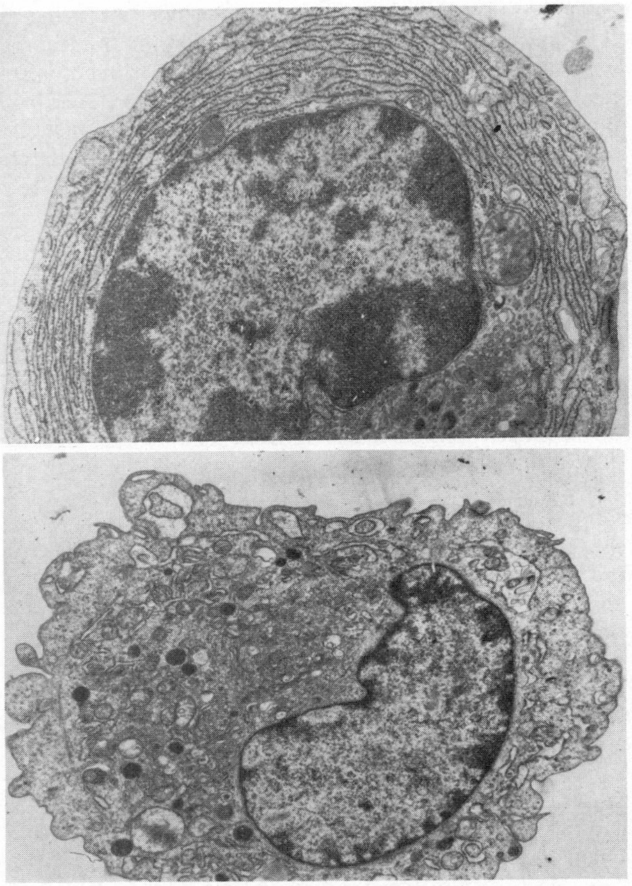

A

B

**Figure 16–14.** *A,* Type A human synovial cell with many undulations in the cell membrane, vacuoles, and inclusions. This cell presumably has phagocytic capabilities and is thought of as a macrophage × 11,200. (Courtesy of Donald Gates.) *B,* Type B human synovial cell with a very well-developed endoplasmic reticulum. This cell presumably has capabilities for snythesis of protein × 17,500. (Courtesy of Donald Gates.) It must be emphasized that there are many synovial cells with organelles developed for both synthetic and phagocytic function. In addition, it is possible that individuals cells may be modulated from cel ls with synthetic to ones with phagocytic function.

vessels are seen, and dense bands of collagen appear. The ligaments that span joints and confer stability on them are continuous with the outer layers of capsule in many joints. With this concept of a structural continuum established, however, it is convenient to divide the lining into (1) the intima or synovial lining, (2) subsynovial tissue, and (3) the joint capsule.

The synovial lining layer is discontinuous. In some areas where the synovium is subjected to pressure and over ligaments and tendons, the cells are widely separated; at these loci, the extracellular connective tissue, not synovial cells, constitutes the lining layer.[126] Intra-articular fat pads are usually covered by a single layer of synovial cells. In other areas not subject to trauma, the synovial cells often accumulate in layers three to four cells deep (Fig. 16–14). Viewed under a tangential light source, a faint pebbling can be seen, which represents microvilli.

**Synovial Lining Cells.** Barland and colleagues defined two principal types of synovial lining cells[127] (Fig.16–14), and their existence has been confirmed by others.[128] *Type A cells* (macrophage-like) contain a prominent Golgi complex and many microvesicles, various and heterogeneous inclusions (residual bodies), and lysosomes. The nucleus contains dense chromatin. Microfilaments are abundant, lying in the long axis of the cell. Frequent thin cell processes stretching into the adjacent matrix are seen. *Type B cells* (fibroblast-like) have a prominent, rough endoplasmic reticulum with few cell processes and vacuoles. Nuclear chromatin is less dense, and nucleoli are more developed. Cytoplasmic vacuoles and vesicles are rare.

It has been natural to ascribe phagocytic and, therefore, macrophage-like function to type A cells and synthetic or fibroblast-like function to type B cells.[129,130] This, however, may be a naive assumption. It ignores the facts that one cell may have more than one function and that, in response to different stimuli, cells can modulate their internal structure as their function changes. A number of observations support this. (1) Type C cells or intermediate synovial cells have been described which have endoplasmic reticulum and Golgi complexes and vacuoles.[130] (2) Using stains for RNA on ribosomes (an acceptable index of synthetic function in cells), only a few cells stain positively in normal synovium. Staining increases in intensity and appears in increased numbers of cells if a joint has been traumatized;[131] in severe inflammatory states no cells without a developed endoplasmic reticulum are observed. Synovial cells that appear morphologically to be fibroblasts nevertheless demonstrate macrophage-like function in response to certain stimuli. Rabbit synovial "fibroblasts," for example, actively phagocytose latex particles[132] (Fig. 16–15). Gold salts injected into the synovial cavity are rapidly taken up in pinocytotic vesicles,[133] and iron pigment is readily engulfed after intra-articular hemorrhage in hemophilia[134] (also see Chapter 100). Evidence is mounting that type A cells may synthesize and secrete

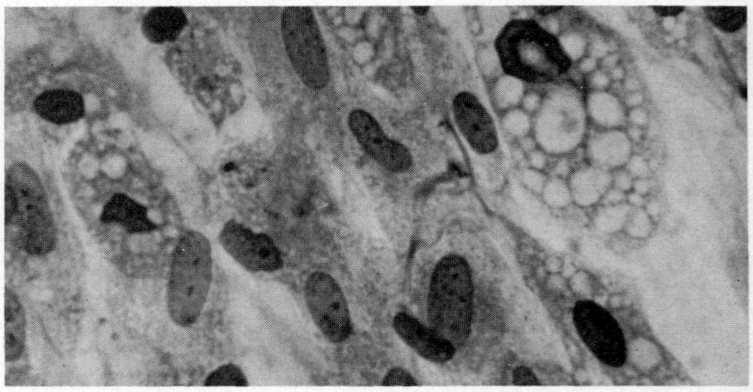

**Figure 16–15.** Rabbit synovial fibroblasts in cell culture have the capacity to phagocytose latex particles (these are 0.05 to 0.15 μm in diameter). The patchy uptake is apparent in this photograph (×400); some cells have phagocytosed particles, while other have not. Yet, all appeared the same on microscopic examination prior to being exposed to latex. These cell populations, having been exposed to latex, or other inert but phagocytosable substance, produce and release large amounts of collagenase.[105]

hyaluronic acid. The firmest data are the demonstrations by ultrastructural studies that hyaluronic acid is found both in the Golgi complex and in large secretory vacuoles of these "phagocytic cells."[135]

It may be reasonable to consider the synovial lining cell as one with multiple phenotypic possibilities and to resist categorizing it by its morphologic resemblance at certain stages to other, better characterized cells. As noted by Ghadially, "[Type A and B may be cells] whose difference in morphology reflects the function they are performing at a given moment."[136]

Fibronectin[137] and probably laminin[138] are secreted by synovial cells. These glycoproteins may aid in attachment of cells to underlying matrix.[138-141] In cell culture, synovial cells synthesize collagen (types I and III), latent collagenase, latent proteinases, an activator of collagenase, inhibitors of neutral metalloproteinases, hyaluronic acid, proteoglycans, and many other minor and nonidentified matrix constituents. Normal synovium in culture can be induced to produce a substance named "catabolin," which appears to stimulate chondrocytes to release enzymes that degrade the proteoglycans matrix in cartilage.[142,143] A similar messenger molecule(s) is found in human rheumatoid synovium.

**Synovial Fluid.** Fluid in normal joints is present in small quantities sufficient to coat multiple folds of synovial membrane. Small pools collect in recesses in the joint, but in the normal state there is never sufficient volume to distend the joint or to separate redundant surfaces of synovium one from the other.

As in other systems, more is known about abnormal synovial fluid than normal because there is an excess of the former. Truly normal synovial fluid is rarely analyzed. The largest accumulation of data was by Ropes and Bauer,[144] and their treatise is still a valuable reference. Synovial fluid is a filtrate of plasma that passes through the fenestrations of subsynovial capillary endothelium into the extracellular space, where it joins with hyaluronic acid that is secreted by synovial cells and achieves an equilibrium with free fluid in the joint space. Rates of transfer from capillaries to the interstitial fluid and of diffusion through this tissue are affected by many factors. Each component of synovial fluid must be considered separately. (The procedure for aspiration and analysis of synovial fluid is outlined in Chapters 37 and 38.)

***Components of Synovial Fluid Originating in Plasma.*** *Small Molecules.* Most of small molecules pass through synovial interstitium by a process of free diffusion.[145] The concentration of electrolytes is the same as in plasma. Cations that bind significantly to protein are present in concentrations consistent with the lower concentrations of serum proteins present in synovial fluid (see below). The concentration of glucose in synovial fluid is close to that of plasma.[146] However, in the nonsteady state glucose enters the joint space at a rate faster than expected from its molecular size,[145] indicating facilitated diffusion or active transport of this molecule into (but not out of) joints. It seems likely, therefore, that to explain low levels of glucose in sepsis or severe inflammation one must invoke both impaired delivery and increased utilization by synovial components.

*Large Molecules.* Proteins are present in synovial fluid in concentration inversely proportional to molecular size.[147] The cause of this selective retardation of large molecule flux into synovial fluid is due in part to regulation by the extracellular matrix of synovium; when plasma is filtered through hyaluronic acid, an ultrafiltrate is produced with a composition similar to that found in normal synovial fluid.[148] Hyaluronic acid in interstitial tissues probably acts as a molecular filter; by its large domain it excludes large solute molecules from passing through into synovial fluid. Because of their large size, molecules such as $\alpha_2$-macroglobulin (the principle proteinase inhibitor of plasma), fibrinogen, and IgM are present in only small quantities in noninflammatory synovial fluid. In inflammatory synovial fluids this selective exclusion is altered,[147] perhaps because of increased size of endothelial cell fenestrations or because interstitial hyaluronate-protein complexes are fragmented by enzymes associated with the inflammatory process. Thus, larger proteins enter synovial fluid, enabling it to form fibrin clots and to have higher concentrations of proteinase inhibitors. Details of the structure of hyaluronic acid are found in Chapter 15.

***Removal of Material from Synovial Fluid.*** The synovial lining cells phagocytize debris presented at the fluid-cell interface. In addition, the lymphatic system can enhance removal of synovial fluid macromolecules. All large molecules appear to leave the joint at equivalent rates, unlike the rate (inversely proportional to molecular weight) at which they enter the joint space.[149] There is indirect evidence to suggest that this clearing mechanism is inadequate to the task presented in severe inflammation of joints. For instance, the synovial fluid appears to act as a "sink" for complement components in rheumatoid arthritis.[150] In severe inflammation, proteinases released by leukocytes drawn by chemotactic factors accumulate within the joint fluid and soon saturate the inhibitors present there.[151,152]

***Other Aspects of Synovial Physiology.*** *Intra-Articular Temperature.* The vascular system of the extremities acts as a countercurrent distribution system for temperature of tissues. Although core body temperature in most human beings varies little from the mean of 37° C, it is likely that temperatures reflect more the temperature of overlying soft tissues. For example, the metacarpophalangeal joint, one with very little overlying insulation of fat or muscle, has intra-articular temperatures that parallel those of skin closely between the resting temperatures and 39 to 40° C created by insertion of the hand into an electric mitten[153] (Fig. 16–16). The knee joint temperature is not so simple a function. Although intra-articular temperatures are always below 36° C (at ambient temperatures of around 20° C), there are wide variations noted between joint and skin temperature.[154] In addition, cold or hot packs reflexly change knee joint temperatures in the opposite direction.[155] Similarly, painful stimuli (e.g., apprehension, alarm, or smoking) lower the skin temperature and elevate the joint temperature.

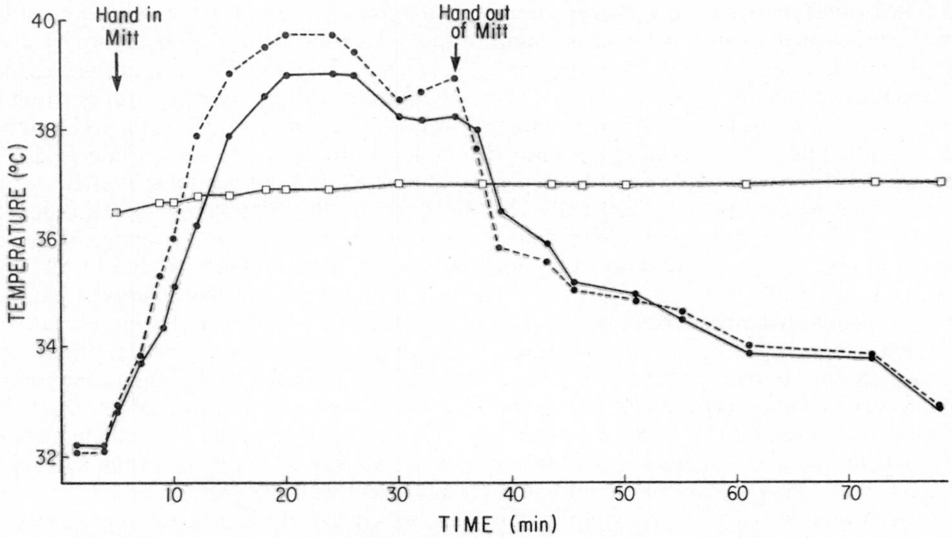


**Figure 16–16.** A sterile needle temperature probe was inserted into the left second metacarpophalangeal joint of a physician (E. D. Harris, Jr.) without joint disease. Skin and intra-articular temperatures were monitored by a Thermalert (Bailey Instruments, Saddle Brook, N.J.). An electric mitten was put on at the time indicated and removed 30 minutes later. □-□ Body core temperature: •——• = intra-articular temperature; •——• = skin temperature over the same joint. (See ref. 157.)

Non-weight-bearing active movements increase intra-articular temperature as much as 1° C, a phenomenon probably best explained by an increased subsynovial tissue blood flow.

The reason for interest in these data is that rates of enzyme action are a direct function of temperature. Connective tissue metabolism is generally studied in vitro at 37° C, yet tissues in joints do not reach this temperature except during inflamed states. Biochemical reactions that proceed vigorously at 37° C may at 32° be altered sufficiently so that the net effect would be movement of a metabolic pathway in the opposite direction, or retardation of rates of reaction. For instance, the rate of destruction of articular cartilage collagen fibers by synovial collagenase is significant at 37° C; at 32° it is imperceptible.[156] In addition, large increases in the rate of hyaluronic acid synthesis occur over an 8° C temperature change (30 to 38° C) in both normal and rheumatoid cell lines in culture, whereas glucose utilization and lactate production increase only slightly.[157]

**Intra-articular Pressure.** The joint cavity is a potential space. The small amount of synovial fluid present lines synovial surfaces but does not separate them. Indeed, the pressure within normal joints may be a negative one compared with ambient atmospheric pressure.[158] Negative pressure must be very large within finger joints during the "knuckle-cracking" process, which is a nervous (and/or aggravating) habit of some persons. During this procedure of pulling rapidly on a relaxed phalanx, a gas bubble is created within the joint, which cavitates with a cracking sound, liberating energy in the form of heat and sound.[159] This cavitation is the same process that destroys propellers of steamships; presumably, if repeated frequently enough, it could destroy a joint. The normal negative pressure in the joint plays a role in stabilizing articular surfaces against one another.

The presence of a synovial effusion changes all this. Intra-articular pressure becomes positive, and roentgenograms may show a widening of the apparent joint space as the articulating surfaces are forced apart. Pressure within a joint is perceived by humans as an uncomfortable sensation; a patient with a knee effusion rests it in a position of slight flexion, the position at which pressure is minimal[160] (see Chapter 29). Full flexion or extension increases pressures within joints containing effusions and may be sufficient to rupture a joint capsule.[161] High intra-articular pressure may compromise synovial blood flow. Inflammed, chronic proliferative synovitis generates a thickened joint capsule, which gradually, perhaps secondary to increased joint pressure, becomes redundant and stretched and demonstrates decreased compliance.[162] Pressure in these joints may be minimal until a critical volume at which the noncompliant capsule stretches no more and intra-articular pressure soars to produce rupture or even penetration through weakened bone to form subchondral cysts.[163,164] It is likely that increased intra-articular pressure in the presence of effusions affects synovial blood flow.[165]

## References

1. O'Rahilly, R., and Gardner, E.: The embryology of movable joints. *In* Sokoloff, L. (ed.): The Joints and Synovial Fluid. Vol I. New York, Academic Press, 1978, pp. 49–97.
2. Saunders, J.W.: Developmental control of three-dimensional polarity in the avian limb. Ann. N.Y. Acad. Sci. 193:29, 1972.
3. Stocum, D.L.: Outgrowth and pattern formation during limb ontogeny and regeneration. Differentiation 3:167, 1975.
4. O'Rahilly, R.: The development of joints. Irish J. Med. Sci. 6:456, 1957.
5. Thorogood, P.V., and Hinchcliffe, J.R.: An analysis of the condensation process during chondrogenesis in the embryonic chick hind limb. J. Embryol. Exp. Morphol. 33:581, 1975.
6. Friberg, V., and Ringertz, N.R.: An autoradiographic study on the uptake of radiosulfate in the rat embryo. J. Embryol. Exp. Morphol. 4:313, 1956.
7. Anderson, H., and Bro-Rasmussen, F.: Histochemical studies on the

histogenesis of the joints in human fetuses with special reference to the development of the joint cavities in the hand and foot. Am. J. Anat. 108:111, 1961.
8. Warsilev, W.: Elektronenmikroskopische und histochemische Untersuchungen zur Entwicklung des Kniegelenkes der Ratte. Z. Anat. Entwicklungsgesh. 137:221, 1972.
9. Anderson, H.: Development morphology and histochemistry of the early synovial tissue in human foetuses. Acta Anat. 58:90, 1964.
10. Bloom, W., and Fawcett, D.W.: A Textbook of Histology. 8th ed. Philadelphia, W.B. Saunders Company, 1972.
11. Drachman, D.B., and Sokoloff, L.: The role of movement in embryonic joint development. Dev. Biol. 14:401, 1966.
12. Murray, P.D.F., and Drachman, D.B.: The role of movement in the development of joints and related structures: The head and neck in the chick embryo. J. Embryol. Exp. Morphol. 22:349, 1969.
13. Yasuda, Y.: Differentiation of human limb buds in vitro. Anat. Rec. 175:561, 1973.
14. Rajan, K.T., and Merker, H.J.: Joint formation in culture. Ann. Rheum. Dis. 34:200, 1975.
15. Symons, N.B.B.: The development of the human mandibular joint. J. Anat. 86:326, 1952.
16. Moffett, B.C.: The prenatal development of the human temporomandibular joint. Contrib. Embryol. Carnegie Inst. 36:19, 1957.
17. Levy, B.M.: Embryological development of the temporomandibular joint. *In* Sarnat, B.G. (ed.): The Temporomandibular Joint. 2nd ed. Springfield, Ill., Charles C Thomas, 1964, pp. 59–70.
18. Bradley, S.J.: An analysis of self-differentiation of chick limb buds in chorio-allantoic grafts. J. Anat. 107:479, 1970.
19. Bauer, R.: Zur Problem der Neugliederung der Wurbelsaule. Acta Anat. 72:321, 1969.
20. Peacock, A.: Observations on the pre-natal development of the intervertebral disc in man. J. Anat. 85:260, 1951.
21. Walmsley, R.: The development and growth of the intervertebral disc. Endinburgh Med. J. 60:341, 1953.
22. Eyre, D.R., and Muri, H.: Collagen polymorphism: Two molecular species in pig intervertebral discs. FEBS Lett. 42:192, 1974.
23. Linsenmeyer, T.F., Trelstad, R.L., and Gross, J.: The collagen of chick embryonic notochord. Biochem. Biophys. Res. Commun. 53:39, 1973.
24. Herbert, C.M., Lindberg, K.A., Jayson, M.I.V., and Bailey, A.J.: Changes in the collagen of human intervertebral discs during aging and degenerative joint disease. J. Mol. Med. 1:79, 1975.
25. Jayson, M.I.V.: Inter-articular pressure. Clin. Rheum. Dis. 7:149, 1981.
26. Bird, H.A., Tribe, C.R., and Bacon, P.A.: Joint hypermobility leading to osteoarthritis and chondrocalcinosis. Ann. Rheum. Dis. 37:203, 1978.
27. Canoso, J.J.: Bursae, tendons and ligaments. Clin. Rheum. Dis. 7:189, 1981.
28. Kieny, M. and Chevallier, A.: Autonomy of tendon development in the embryonic duck wing. J. Embryol. Exp. Morphol. 49:153, 1979.
29. Gay, S., and Miller, E.J.: Collagen in the Physiology and Pathology of Connective Tissue. Stuttgart and New York, Gustav Fisher, 1978.
30. Cooper, R.R., and Misol, S.: Tendon and ligament insertion. A light and electron microscopic study. J. Bone Joint Surg. 52A:1, 1970.
31. Dorfl, J.: Vessels in the region of tendinous insertions. Chondroapophyseal insertion. Folia Morphol. 17:74, 1969.
32. Swann, D.A.: Macromolecules of synovial fluid. *In* Sokoloff, L. (ed): The Joints and Synovial Fluid. New York, Academic Press, 1978, pp. 407–435.
33. Glimcher, M.J., Brickley-Parsons, D., and Kossiva, D.: Phosphopeptides and γ-carboxyglutamic acid-containing peptides in calcified turkey tendon: Their absence in uncalcified tendon. Calcif. Tissue Int. 27:281, 1979.
34. Kuhns, J.G.: Adventitious bursa. Arch. Surg. 46:687, 1943.
35. Canoso, J.J., and Yood, R.A.: Reaction of superficial bursae to specific disease stimuli. Arthritis Rheum. 22:1361, 1979.
36. Liew, M., and Dick, C.: The anatomy and physiology of blood flow in a diarthrodial joint. Clin. Rheum. Dis. 7:131, 1981.
37. Lindstrom, J.: Microvascular anatomy of synovial tissue. Acta Rheum. Scand. (Suppl.) 7:1, 963.
38. Suter, J., and Majno, G.: Ultrastructure of the joint capsule in the rat: Presence of two kinds of capillaries. Nature 202:920, 1964.
39. Schumacher, H.R.: The microvasculature of the synovial membrane of the monkey: Ultrastructural studies. Arthritis Rheum. 112:387, 1969.
40. Dee, R.: Structure and function of hip joint innervation. Ann. R. Coll. Surg. Engl. 45:357, 1969.
41. Griff, P., Finerman, G.A., and Riley, L.H.R.: Joint position sense after total hip replacement. J. Bone Joint Surg. 55A:1016, 1973.
42. Cross, M.J., and McCloskey, D.I.: Position sense following surgical removal of joints in man. Brain Res. 55:443, 1973.
43. Pugh, J.W., Radin, E.L., and Rose, R.M.: Quantitative studies of human subchondral cancellous bone. J. Bone Joint Surg. 56A:313, 1974.
44. Poole, A.R., Pidoux, I., Reiner, A., Tang, L.-H., Choi, H., and Rosenberg, L.: Localization of proteoglycan monomer and link protein in the matrix of bovine articular cartilage: An immunohistochemical study. J. Histochem. Cytochem. 28:621, 1980.
45. Poole, A.R., Pidoux, I., Reiner, A., and Rosenberg, L.: An immunoelectron microscope study of the organization of proteoglycan monomer, link protein, and collagen in the matrix of articular cartilage. J. Cell. Biol. 93:921, 1982.
46. Balacz, E.A., Bloom, G.D., and Swann, D.A.: Fine structure and glycosaminoglycan content of the surface layer of articular cartilage. Fed. Proc. 25:1813, 966.
47. Redler, I., and Zimmy, M.L.: Scanning electron microscopy and abnormal articular cartilage and synovium. J. Bone Joint Surg. 52A:1395, 1970.
48. Gardner, D.L.: The influence of microscopic technology on knowledge of cartilage surface structure. Ann. Rheum. Dis. 31:235, 1972.
49. Clarke, I.C.: Human articular surface contours and related surface depression frequency studies. Ann. Rheum. Dis. 30:15, 1971.
50. Clarke, I.C.: Surface characteristics of human articular cartilage—a scanning electron microscope study. J. Anat. 108:23, 1971.
51. Gardner, D.L., and McGilliwray, D.C.: Living articular cartilage is not smooth. Ann. Rheum. Dis. 30:3, 1971.
52. Clarke, I.C.: Human articular surface contours and related surface depression frequency studies. Ann. Rheum. Dis. 30:15, 1971.
53. Ghadially, F.N., Ghadially, J.A., Oryschak, A.F., and Yong, N.K.: Experimental production of ridges on rabbit articular cartilage: A scanning electron microscopic study. J. Anat. 121:119, 1976.
54. Burgeson, R.E., Hebda, P.A., Morris, N.P., and Hollister, D.W.: Human cartilage collagens. Comparison of cartilage collagens with human type V collagen. J. Biol. Chem. 257:7852, 1982.
55. Hardingham, T.E., and Muir, H.: The specific interaction of hyaluronic acid with cartilage proteoglycans. Biochim. Biophys. Acta 279:401, 1972.
56. Poole, B.P., and Lowther, D.A.: The effect of chondroitin sulfate protein on the formation of collagen fibrils in vitro. Biochem. J. 109:857, 1968.
57. DiSalvo, J., and Schubert, M.: Specific interaction of some cartilage protein polysaccharides with freshly precipitating calcium phosphate. J. Biol. Chem. 242:705, 1967.
58. Howell, D.S., Pita, J.C., Marquez, J.F., and Galtes, R.A.: Demonstration of macromolecular inhibitors of calcification and nucleation factor(s) in fluid from calcifying sites in cartilage. J. Clin. Invest. 48:630, 1969.
59. Muir, H., Bullough, P., and Maroudas, A.: The distribution of collagen in human articular cartilage with some of its physiological implications. J. Bone Joint Surg. 52B:554, 1970.
60. Kuettner, K.F., Hiti, J., Eisenstein, R., and Harper, E.: Collagenase inhibition by cationic proteins derived from cartilage and aorta. Biochem. Biophys. Res. Commun. 72:40, 1976.
61. Keuttner, K.E., Soble, L., Croxen, R.L., Marczynska, B., Hiti, J., and Harper, E.: Tumor cell collagenase and its inhibitions by a cartilage-derived protease inhibitor. Science 196:653, 1977.
62. Rifkin, D.B., and Crowe, R.M.: Isolation of a protease inhibitor from tissues resistant to tumor invasion. Hoppe Seyler's Z. Physiol. Chem. 358:1525, 1977.
63. Langer, R., Brem, H., Flaterman, K., Klein, M., and Folkman, J.: Isolation of a cartilage factor that inhibits tumor neovascularization. Science 193:70, 1976.
64. Horton, J.E., Wezeman, F.H., and Kuettner, K.E.: Inhibition of bone resorption in vitro by a cartilage-derived anticollagenase factor. Science 199:1342, 1978.
65. Roughley, P.J., Murphy, G., and Barrett, A.J.: Proteinase inhibitors of bovine nasal cartilage. Biochem. J. 169:721, 1978.
66. Linn, F.C., and Sokoloff, L.: Movement and composition of interstitial fluid of cartilage. Arthritis Rheum. 8:481, 1965.
67. Pita, J.C., and Howell, D.S.: Micro-biochemical studies of cartilage. *In* Sokoloff, L. (ed.): The Joints and Synovial Fluid. Vol. 1. New York, Academic Press, 1978, pp. 273–330.
68. Mankin, H.J.: The water of articular cartilage. *In* Simon, W.H. (ed.): The Human Joint in Health and Disease. Philadelphia, University of Pennsylvania Press, 1978, pp. 37–42.
69. Bollet, A.J., and Nance, J.L.: Biochemical findings in normal and osteoarthritic articular cartilage. II. Chondroitin sulfate concentration and chain length, water and ash content. J. Clin. Invest. 45:1170, 1966.
70. Hadler, N.M.: The biology of the extracellular space. Clin. Rheum. Dis. 7:71, 1981.
71. Ghadially, F.N.: Fine structure of joints. *In* Sokoloff, L. (ed.): The Joints and Synovial Fluid. Vol. I. New York, Academic Press, 1978, pp. 105–176.
72. Stockwell, R.A., and Meachim, G.: The chondrocytes. *In* Freeman, M.A.R. (ed.): Adult Articular Cartilage. London, Pitman Medical, 1979, pp. 69–145.
73. Davies, D.V., Barnett, C.H., Cochrane, W., and Palfrey, A.J.: Electron microscopy of articular cartilage in the young adult rabbit. Ann. Rheum. Dis. 21:11, 1962.
74. Ghadially, F.N.: Waxing and waning of nuclear fibrous lamina. Arch. Pathol. 94:303, 1972.
75. Ghadially, F.N., Meachim, G., and Collins, D.H.: Extracellular lipid in

the matrix of human articular cartilage. Ann. Rheum. Dis. 24:136, 1965.
76. Ghadially, F.N., Oryshak, A.F., Ailsby, R.L., and Mehta, P.N.: Electron-probe X-ray analysis of siderosomes in haemarthrotic articular cartilage. Virchows Arch. B. 16:43, 1974.
77. Stockwell, R.A.: The cell density of human articular and costal cartilage. J. Anat. 101:753, 1967.
78. Stockwell, R.A., and Meachim, G.: The chondrocytes. *In* Freeman, M.A.R. (ed.): Adult Articular Cartilage. New York, Grune & Stratton, 1974, pp. 51–99.
79. Hunter, W.: On the structure and diseases of articulating cartilage. Philos. Trans. 42:514, 1743.
80. Bywaters, E.G.L.: The metabolism of joint tissues. J. Pathol. Bact. 44:247, 1937.
81. Woods, G.C., Greenwald, A.J., and Haynes, D.W.: Subchondral vascularity in the human femoral head. Ann. Rheum. Dis. 29:138, 1970.
82. Mitul, M.A., and Millington, P.F.: Osseous pathway of nutrition to articular cartilage of the human femoral head. Lancet 1:842, 1970.
83. Collins, D.H.: The Pathology of Articular and Spinal Diseases. London, Arnold, 1949.
84. Strangeways, T.S.P.: The nutrition of articular cartilage. Br. Med. J. 1:661, 1920.
85. Maroudas, A., Bullough, P., Swanson, S.A.V., and Freeman, M.A.R.: The permeability of articular cartilage. J. Bone Joint Surg. 50B:166, 1968.
86. Maroudas, A.: Physico-chemical properties of articular cartilage. *In* Freeman, M.A.R. (ed.): Adult Articular Cartilage. New York, Grune & Stratton, 1974, pp. 131–170.
87. Sood, S.C.: A study of the effects of experimental immobilization on rabbit articular cartilage. J. Anat. 108:497, 1971.
88. Bennett, G., and Baner, W.: Joint changes resulting from patellar displacement and their relation to degenerative hip disease. J. Bone Joint Surg. 19A:667, 1937.
89. Lewis, P.R., and McCutchen, C.W.: Experimental evidence for weeping lubrication in mammalian joints. Nature 184:1285, 1959.
90. McCutchen, C.W.: An approximate equation for weeping lubrication, solved with an electrical analogue. Ann. Rheum. Dis. 34 (Suppl. 2):85, 1975.
91. Layman, D.L., Sokoloff, L., and Miller, E.J.: Collagen synthesis by articular chondrocytes in monolayer culture. Exp. Cell. Res. 73:107, 1972.
92. Srivastava, V.M.L., Malemud, C.J., and Sokoloff, L.: Chondroid expression by lapine articular chondrocytes in spinner culture following monolayer growth. Connect. Tissue Res. 2:127, 1974.
93. Norby, D.P., Malemud, C.J., and Sokoloff, L.: Differences in the collagen types synthesized by lapine articular chondrocytes in spinner and monolayer cultures. Arthritis Rheum. 20:709, 1977.
94. Wiebkin, O.W., and Muir, H.: Synthesis of cartilage-specific proteoglycan by suspension cultures of adult chondrocytes. Biochem. J. 164:269, 1977.
95. Skantze, K.A., Brinckerhoff, C.E., Collier, J.P., and Harris, E.D., Jr.: Modulation of chrondrocyte function in agar culture. Abstr. Arthritis Rheum. 26:41, 1983.
96. Wright, V., and Dowson, D.: Lubrication and cartilage. J. Anat. 121:107, 1976.
97. McCutchen, C.W.: Lubrication of joints. In Sokoloff, L. (ed.): The Joints and Synovial Fluid. Vol I. New York, Academic Press, 1978, pp. 437–477.
98. Swanson, S.A.V.: Lubrication. *In* Freeman, M.A.R. (ed.): Adult Articular Cartilage. New York, Grune & Stratton, 1977, pp. 247–277.
99. Fein, R.S.: Are synovial joints squeeze-film lubricated? Proc. Inst. Mech. Eng. London 181:125, 1967.
100. McCutchen, C.W.: Animal joints and weeping lubrication. New Scientist 15:412, 1962.
101. Dowson, D., Unsworth, A., and Wright, V.: Analysis of boosted lubrication in human joints. J. Mech. Eng. Sci. 12:364, 1970.
102. Walker, P.S., Dowson, D., Longfield, M.D., and Wright, V.: "Boosted lubrication" in synovial joints by fluid entrapment and enrichment. Ann. Rheum. Dis. 27:512, 1968.
103. Dintenfass, L.: Lubrication in synovial joints. Nature 197:496, 1963.
104. Radin, E.L., Swann, D.A., and Weisser, P.A.: Separation of hyaluronate-free lubricating fraction from synovial fluid. Nature 288:377, 1970.
105. Swamm, D.A.: Structure and function of lubricin, the glycoprotein responsible for the boundary lubrication of articular cartilage. *In* Franchimont, P. (ed.): Articular Synovium. Basel, Karger, 1982, pp. 45–58.
106. Stockwell, R.A.: Lipid content of human costal and articular cartilage. Ann. Rheum. Dis. 26:481, 1967.
107. Little, T., Freeman, M.A.R., and Swanson, S.A.V.: Experiments on friction in the human hip joint. *In* Wright, V. (ed.): Lubrication and Wear Joints. London, Sector, 1969, p. 110.
108. Radin, E.L., and Paul, I.L.: A consolidated concept of joint lubrication. J. Bone Joint Surg. 54A:607, 1972.
109. Bar, E.: Elasticitätsprüfungen der Gelenkknorpel. Arch. J. Entwicklungsmech. Organ. 108:739, 1926.
110. Freeman, M.A.R., and Kempson, G.E.: Load carriage. *In* Freeman, M.A.R. (ed.): Adult Articular Cartilage. New York, Grune & Stratton, 1974, pp. 228–246.
111. Harris, E.D., Jr., DiBona, D.R., and Krane, S.M.: A mechanism for cartilage destruction in rheumatoid arthritis. Trans. Assoc. Am. Physicians. 83:267, 1970.
112. Harris, E.D., Jr., Parker, H.G., Radin, E.L., and Krane, S.M.: Effects of proteolytic enzymes on structural and mechanical properties of cartilage. Arthritis Rheum. 15:497, 1972.
113. Kempson, G.E., Muir, H., Swanson, S.A.V., and Freeman, M.A.R.: Correlations between stiffness and the chemical constituents of cartilage on the human femoral head. Biochim. Biophys. Acta 215:70, 1970.
114. Kempson, G.E.: Mechanical properties of articular cartilage. *In* Freeman, M.A.R. (ed.): Adult Articular Cartilage. New York, Grune & Stratton, 1974, p. 196.
115. Landelles, J.W.: The reactions of injured human articular cartilage. J. Bone Joint Surg. 39B:548, 1957.
116. Meachim, G., and Osborne, G.V.: Repair at the femoral articular cartilage surface in osteoarthritis of the hip. J. Pathol. 102:1, 1970.
117. Simon, W.H.: Scale effects in animal joints. I. Articular cartilage thickness and compressive stress. Arthritis Rheum. 13:244, 1970.
118. Armstron, C.G., and Gardner, D.L.: Thickness and distribution of human femoral head articular cartilage. Changes with age. Ann. Rheum. Dis. 36:407, 1977.
119. Byers, P.D., Contepomi, C.A., and Farker, T.A.: A postmortem study of the hip joint. Ann. Rheum. Dis. 29:15, 1970.
120. Freeman, M.A.R., and Meachim, G.: Aging, degeneration and remodeling of articular cartilage. *In* Freeman, M.A.R. (ed.): Adult Articular Cartilage. New York, Grune & Stratton, 1973, pp. 287–330.
121. Collins, D.H., and Meachim, G.: Sulphate ($^{35}SO_4$) fixation by human articular cartilage compared in the knee and shoulder joints. Ann. Rheum. Dis. 20:117, 1961.
122. Meachim, G.: Light microscopy of Indian ink preparations of fibrillated cartilage. Ann. Rheum. Dis. 31:457, 1972.
123. Bollet, A.J., and Nance, J.L.: Biochemical findings in normal and osteoarthritic articular cartilage. II. Chondroitin sulfate concentration and chain length, water, and ash content. J. Clin. Invest. 45:1170, 1966.
124. Mankin, H.J., and Lippiello, L.: Biochemical and metabolic abnormalities in articular cartilage from osteoarthritic human hips. J. Bone Joint Surg. 52A:424, 1970.
125. Collins, D.H., and McElligott, T.F.: Sulfate ($^{35}SO_4$) uptake by chondrocytes in relation to histological changes in osteoarthritic human articular cartilage. Ann. Rheum. Dis. 19:318, 1960.
126. Bassleer R, Lhoest-Ganthier, M.-P., Renard, A-M., Heinen, E., and Goessins, G.: Histological structure and functions of synovium. *In* Franchimont, P. (ed.): Articular Synovium, Basel, Karger, 1982, pp. 1–26.
127. Barland, P., Novikoff, A.B., and Hamerman, D.: Electron microscopy of the human synovial membrane. J. Cell. Biol. 14:207, 1962.
128. Ghadially, F.N., and Roy, S.: Ultrastructure of synovial joints, in health and disease. London, Butterworth, 1969.
129. Hirobata, H., and Kobayaski, I.: Fine structure of the synovial tissue in rheumatoid arthritis. Kobe J. Med. Sci. 10:195, 1964.
130. Krey, P.R., Cohen, A.S., Smith, C.B., and Finland, M.: The human fetal synovium. Histology, fine structure and changes in organ culture. Arthritis Rheum. 14:319, 1971.
131. Roy, S., Ghadially, F.N., and Crane, W.A.J.: Synovial membrane in traumatic effusion. Ultrastructure and autoradiography with tritiated leucine. Ann. Rheum. Dis. 25:259, 1966.
132. Werb, Z., and Reynolds, J.J.: Stimulation by endocytosis of the secretion of collagenase and neutral proteinases from rabbit synovial fibroblasts. J. Exp. Med. 140:1482, 1976.
133. Norton, W.L., Lewis, D.C., and Ziff, M.: Electron-dense deposits following injection of gold sodium thiomalate and thiomalic acid. Arthritis Rheum. 11:436, 1968.
134. Ghadially, F.N., Ailsby, R.L., and Yong, N.K.: Ultrastructure of the hemophilic synovial membrane and electron-probe X-ray analysis of haemosiderin. J. Pathol. 120:201, 1976.
135. Roy, S., and Ghadially, F.N.: Synthesis of hyaluronic acid by synovial cells. J. Pathol. Bacteriol. 93:555, 1967.
136. Ghadially, F.N.: Fine structure of joints. *In* Sokoloff, L. (ed.): The Joints and Synovial Fluid. New York, Academic Press, 1978, p. 140.
137. Hynes, R.O.: Cell surface proteins and malignant transformation. Biochim. Biophys. Acta 458:73, 1976.
138. Clemmensen, I., Holund, B., and Andersen, R.B.: Fibrin and fibronectin in rheumatoid synovial membrane and rheumatoid synovial fluid. Arthritis Rheum. 26:497, 1983.
139. Ali, I.V., Mautner, V., Lanza, R., and Hynes, R.O.: Restoration of normal morphology, adhesion and cytoskeleton sensitive surface protein. Cell 11:115, 1977.

140. Yamada, K.M., and Weston, J.A.: Isolation of a major cell surface glycoprotein from fibroblasts. Proc. Natl. Acad. Sci. USA 71:3492, 1974.
141. Hynes, R.O.: Alteration of cell-surface proteins by viral transformation and proteolysis. Proc. Natl. Acad. Sci. USA 70:3170, 1973.
142. Fell, H.B., and Jubb, R.W.: The effect of synovial tissue on the breakdown of articlar cartilage in organ culture. Arthritis Rheum. 20:1359, 1977.
143. Dingle, J.T., Saklatvata, J., Hembry, R., Tyler, J.: A cartilage catabolic factor from synovium. Biochem. J. 184:177, 1979.
144. Ropes, M.W., and Bauer, W.: Synovial Fluid Changes in Joint Diseases. Cambridge, Harvard University Press, 1953.
145. Simkin, P.A., and Pizzoro, J.E.: Transynovial exchange of small molecules in normal human subjects. J. Appl. Physiol. 36:581, 1974.
146. Ropes, M.W., Muller, A.F., and Bauer, W.: The entrance of glucose and other sugars into joints. Arthritis Rheum. 3:496, 1960.
147. Kushner, I., and Somerville, J.A.: Permeability of human synovial membrane to plasma proteins. Arthritis Rheum. 14:560, 1971.
148. Nettelbladt, E., Sundblad, L., and Jonsson, E.: Permeability of the synovial membrane to proteins. Acta. Rheum. Scand. 9:28, 1963.
149. Brown, D.L., Cooper, A.G., and Bluestone, R.: Exchange of IgM and albumin between plasma and synovial fluid in rheumatoid arthritis. Ann. Rheum. Dis. 29:644, 1969.
150. Ruddy, S.: Synovial fluid: Mirror of the inflammatory lesion in rheumatoid arthritis. *In* Harris, E.D., Jr. (ed.): Rheumatoid Arthritis. New York, Medcom Press, 1974, pp. 58–71.
151. Harris, E.D., Jr., Faulkner, C.S., II, and Brown, F.E.: Collagenolytic systems in rheumatoid arthritis. Clin. Orthop. 110:303, 1975.
152. Abe, S., and Nagai, Y.: Evidence for the presence of a complex of collagenase with $\alpha_2$-macroglobulin in human rheumatoid synovial fluid: A possible regulatory mechanism of collagenase activity in vivo. J. Biochem. 73:897, 1973.
153. Mainardi, C.L., Walter, J.M., Spiegel, P.K., Goldkamp, O.G., and Harris, E.D., Jr.: The lack of effect of daily heat therapy on the progression of rheumatoid arthritis. Arch. Phys. Med. Rehab. 60:390, 1979.
154. Horvath, S.M., and Hollander, J.L.: Intra-articular temperature as a measure of joint reaction. J. Clin. Invest. 28:469, 1949.
155. Hollander, J.L., and Horvath, S.M.: The influence of physical therapy procedures on the intra-articular temperature of normal and arthritic subjects. Am. J. Med. Sci. 218:543, 1949.
156. Harris, E.D., Jr., and McCroskery, P.A.: The influence of temperature and fibril stability on degradation of cartilage collagen by rheumatoid synovial collagenase. N. Engl. J. Med. 290:1, 1974.
157. Castor, C.W., and Yaron, M.: Connective tissue activation. VIII. The effects of temperature studied in vitro. Arch. Phys. Med. Rehab. 57:5, 1976.
158. Mueller, W.: Über den negativen Luftdruck im Gelenkram. Dtsch. Z. Chirurgie 218:395, 1929.
159. Unsworth, A., Dowson, D., and Wright, V.: "Cracking Joints." A bioengineering study of cavitation in the metacarpophalangeal joint. Ann. Rheum. Dis. 30:348, 1971.
160. Jayson, M.I.V., and Dixon, A.St.J.: Intra-articular pressure in rheumatoid arthritis of the knee. III. Pressure changes during joint use. Ann. Rheum. Dis. 29:401, 1970.
161. Jayson, M.I.V., and Dixon, A.St.J.: Valvular mechanisms in juxta-articular cyts. Ann. Rheum. Dis. 29:415, 1970.
162. Myers, D.B., and Palmer, D.G.: Capsular compliance and pressure-volume relationships in normal and arthritic knees. J. Bone Joint Surg. 54B:710, 1972.
163. Jayson, M.I.V., Rubenstein, D., and Dixon, A.St.J.: Intra-articular pressure and rheumatoid geodes (bone 'cysts'). Ann. Rheum. Dis. 29:496, 1970.
164. Magyer, E., Talerman, A., Feher, M., and Wonters, H.W.: The pathogenesis of the subchondral pseudocysts in rheumatoid arthritis. Clin. Orthop. 100:341, 1974.
165. Jayson, M.I.V., and Dixon, A.St.J.: Intra-articular pressure in rheumatoid arthritis of the knee. II. Effect of intra-articular pressure on blood circulation to the synovium. Ann. Rheum. Dis. 29:266, 1970.

# Chapter 17
# Formation and Resorption of Bone

*Clement B. Sledge*

## INTRODUCTION

The skeleton serves both a mechanical and a metabolic role. As an internal, articulated strut it provides the framework of the body, protects vital organs, and facilitates locomotion. Although these functions are important, especially in relation to arthritis, they are clearly secondary to the homeostatic role of the skeleton. As an ion-reservoir, the skeleton contains 99 percent of the total body calcium, 85 percent of the phosphorus, and 66 percent of the magnesium.[1] The maintenance of serum calcium ion concentration is vital to survival; it is therefore the role of the skeleton as a source of reserve calcium that occupies primary importance. Diseases that produce excessive loss of calcium (e.g., hyperparathyroidism, renal disease) may weaken the skeleton to the point of mechanical failure while serum calcium levels are maintained within a close range. A skeletal system that is mechanically inadequate (osteogenesis imperfecta, severe osteoporosis, multiple fractures) will continue its metabolic role and maintain a normal serum ($Ca^{++}$).

Paradoxical features of bone are its hardness and its ability to heal without a scar. Hardness suggests an inert character, which belies the constant turnover and internal remodeling that eventually result in the obliteration of the scars left by fractures, infections, and loss of blood supply.

The word bone is used to describe both the tissue and the organ. In the former sense it denotes a special mineralized connective tissue; in the latter it includes cartilage and hematopoietic and adipose tissues. Bones, as organs, are the structural elements of the body and as such are dealt with in standard textbooks of orthopedics. This chapter is devoted to a brief review of mechanisms of bone *tissue* formation and resorption, to provide a background for the discussion of metabolic bone disease and the alterations in bone structure that accompany rheumatoid arthritis.

## BONE AS A TISSUE

**Bone Cells.** Osteogenic cells (osteoblasts, osteoclasts, and osteocytes) cover all bone surfaces except those of

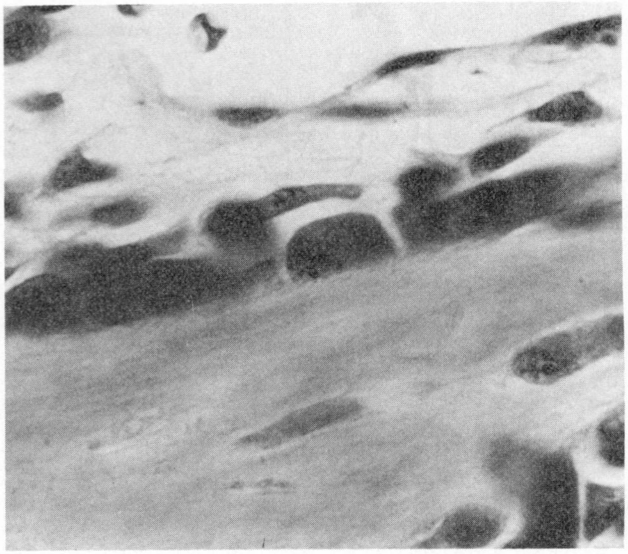

**Figure 17–1.** Polyhedral osteoblasts lying on the surface of newly formed bone matrix. (From Jowsey, J.: Metabolic Diseases of Bone. Philadelphia, W.B. Saunders Company, 1977. Courtesy of Dr. B. Boothroyd.)

the sinuses of the adult skull.[2] Thus, all interactions of the skeleton with the body in general are mediated by these cells, which constitute a functional continuum resembling a membrane.[3] Young[4] stated that "each problem in bone physiology may be considered in the light of the relative distribution of bone cells among their various functional roles, for this system of cells acts as the 'final common path' through which the great variety of stimuli affecting bone must pass."

All the osteogenic cells are felt to arise from a common stem cell, a mononuclear blood cell, which, when identified by its spatial relation to bone, is termed an "osteoprogenitor cell."[5] Reacting to mechanical, chemical, or hormonal stimuli, these pleuripotent cells "modulate" to a functional-blast or -clast. The term modulation indicates that this change in functional state is only temporary, as opposed to permanent change or "differentiation." Numerous studies have shown conversion from one functional type to another within the osteogenic series.[6-9] The naming of these cells therefore depends upon location and presumed function or upon demonstration of specific cytoplasmic elements.

***Osteoblasts.*** These are plump cuboidal cells usually seen as a layer, one cell thick, applied to the surface of bone (Fig. 17–1). These features help distinguish the osteoblasts from osteo-progenitor cells, which are not polygonal but flattened and are not found in sheets or applied to bone surfaces.[10] The osteoblasts are linked to one another by tight junctions, so that the environment of bone surface can be altered from that of the general extracellular fluid space.[11] This ability of the osteoblast to produce a localized change in environment may be important in the formation of new bone and/or its mineralization. Electron microscopy reveals an extremely abundant rough endoplasmic reticulum with cisternae and a well developed Golgi body as well as abundant free ribosomes.[12] The Golgi body may be visible by light microscopy, and the ribosomes produce the basophilia seen in hematoxylin and eosin section.

The major function of the osteoblast is to produce osteoid,[13] composed chiefly of collagen and proteoglycans. The former is classified as a type I collagen and appears to be similar to that found in skin and tendon.[14,15] The formation and secretion of this collagen appears identical to collagen formation in other cells, with formation on the rough endoplasmic reticulum of a procollagen which is secreted from the dilated cisternae into the extracellular space on the bone side of the osteoblast.[16] Extracellular modification, with removal of terminal regions and the formation of inter- and intramolecular cross-links, results in fibril deposition. The collagen fibrils are deposited as sheets about 3 to 10 μm in thickness, with the individual fibrils oriented in parallel array within each sheet.[17] These sheets, or lamellae, tend to lie parallel to the long axis of the bone, with adjacent lamellae alternating about 30 degrees from this axis.[18,19] The collagen bundles thus alternate by about

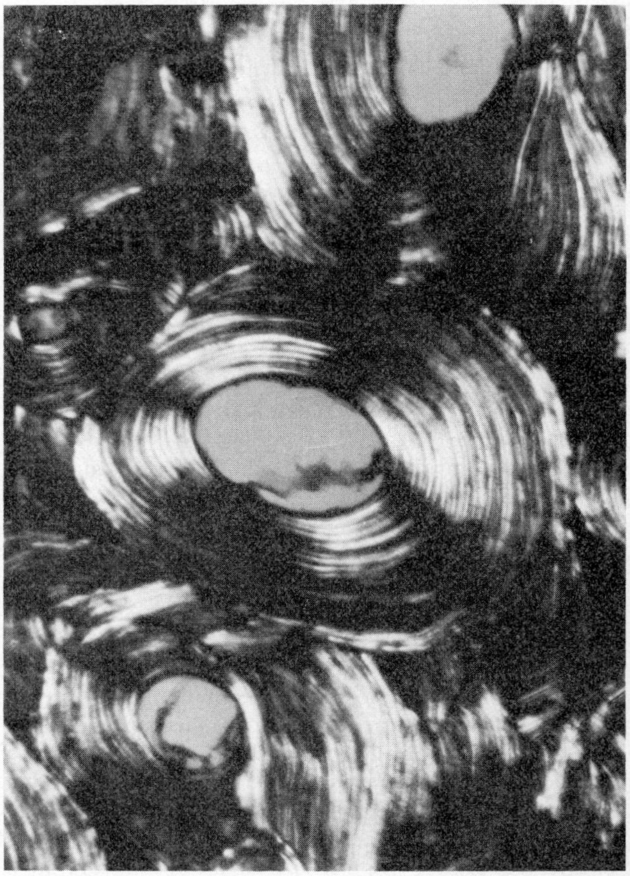

**Figure 17–2.** Ground section of bone photographed with polarized light showing the concentric lamellar structure of the basic unit of mature bone, the osteon. The central vascular canal (empty in this preparation) is surrounded by multiple lamellae of bone. The adjacent lamellae are composed of collagen bundles with differing orientations, giving rise to alternating light and dark bands in polarized light.

60 degrees from lamella to lamella, providing tensile strength and a characteristic appearance under polarized light microscopy (Fig. 17–2).

The "functional life" of the osteoblast in man is unknown. Estimates vary from 3 days in young rabbits[7,20] to 54 days in aged mice.[21] Jowsey[22] estimates that each osteoblast produces a seam of osteoid about 15 μm thick, at a rate of 1 μm per day. The functional life in man would thus be 15 days. During this span, each osteoblast has produced 1500 cubic μm of new bone matrix.

*Osteocytes.* As new osteoid is laid down, osteoblasts become encased within the lacunae of the new bone, becoming osteocytes. At one time these cells were considered effete and unresponsive. It is now known that under stress conditions (e.g., PTH stimulation, calcium deprivation) the osteocyte participates in resorption of the surrounding bone.[23-25] This process, termed osteocytic osteolysis, is probably responsible for the moment-to-moment maintenance of serum calcium, since it can be evoked rapidly, rather than depending upon the induction of new multinucleated osteoclasts. When the period of stress is over, the osteocyte replaces the lost bone around its lacuna and returns to a resting state. The osteocyte, therefore, rather than being effete, is capable of both bone resorption and formation, but quantitative data are lacking.[26]

Each osteocyte in its lacuna is connected to adjacent osteocytes by way of cytoplasmic extensions extending through tunnels (canaliculi) radiating outward from the central vascular canal (Fig. 17–3). These provide a pathway of nutrition through the dense bone matrix and connect each osteocyte via gap junctions.[27] The volume of bone occupied by this system has been estimated at 4 to 6 percent for canaliculi and 1 to 2 percent for lacunae.[28] The surface area of the lacunar and canalicular system has been estimated to be at least 250 sq meters per liter of calcified bone matrix and communicates with a submicroscopic, interfibrillar space representing 35,000 sq mm per cubic millimeter. Exchange of mineral across this enormous surface is very rapid and is under the control of the osteocyte.[29]

*Osteoclasts.* Where bone is being removed or internally remodeled, large multinucleate cells are seen lying in irregular resorption cavities known as Howship's lacunae (Fig. 17–4). These cells vary in size from 200 to 200,000 sq μm, with from 2 to 100 or more nuclei.[30] The cell surface applied to bone is characterized by a brush or ruffled border where active bone resorption occurs.[31] The cytoplasm is often foamy, owing to the large number of digestive vacuoles and vesicles. There are numerous lysosomal bodies, which contain histochemically demonstrable acid hydrolases.[32,33] In remodeling bone, there are normally many more osteoblasts than osteoclasts (22 to 1 in the growing rabbit),[34] suggesting much greater efficiency on the part of the osteoclast. Figures for humans are lacking, but Jowsey[35] suggests that it is reasonable to multiply osteoclast nuclei by 6 to estimate the activity equivalent of the osteoblast. These ratios are of interest, since they allow an estimate of metabolic activity in histologic sections of bone. Because of osteocytic osteolysis and variable resorption rates by individual osteoclasts,[36] however, the method is only semiquantitative.

Osteoclasts are seen in increased numbers during rapid remodeling, as in the metaphysis of growing bone, and in response to parathyroid hormone. Even when bone resorption is produced by other factors, such as hyperoxia or vitamin A, osteoclasts are seen, suggesting that they participate in bone resorption even though the process may be initiated by mononuclear cells.[37]

The origin, functional span, and fate of the osteoclast have been debated for years. Three theories of origin suggest that osteoclasts arise from specific "pre-osteo-

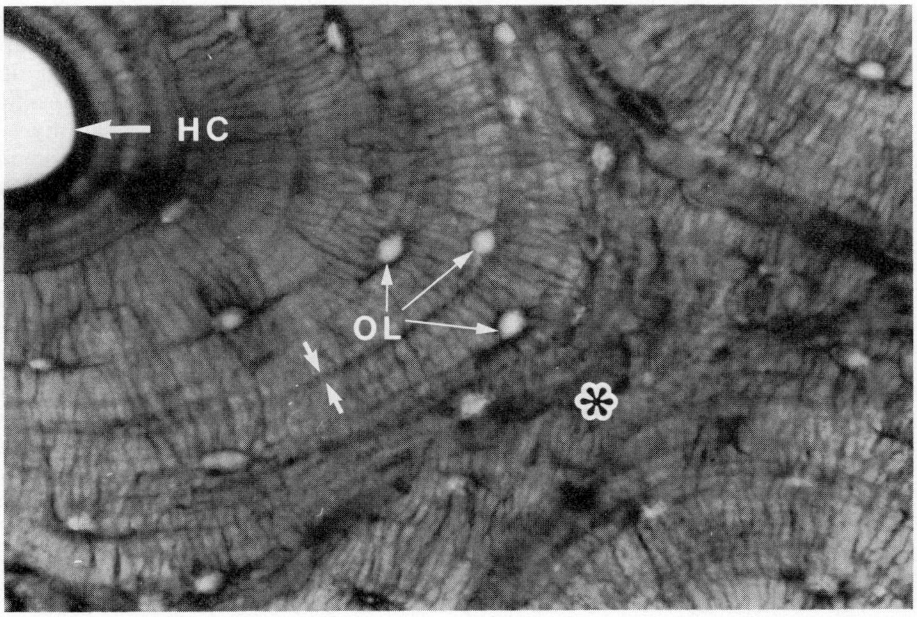


**Figure 17–3.** Ground section of bone photographed in normal light showing empty osteocyte lacunae (OL) connected by fine darkly stained canaliculi. The central haversian canal (HC) is seen in the upper left hand corner; the reversal line (*) marking the junction between two adjacent osteons and the cement line (→ ←) separating adjacent lamellae are seen.

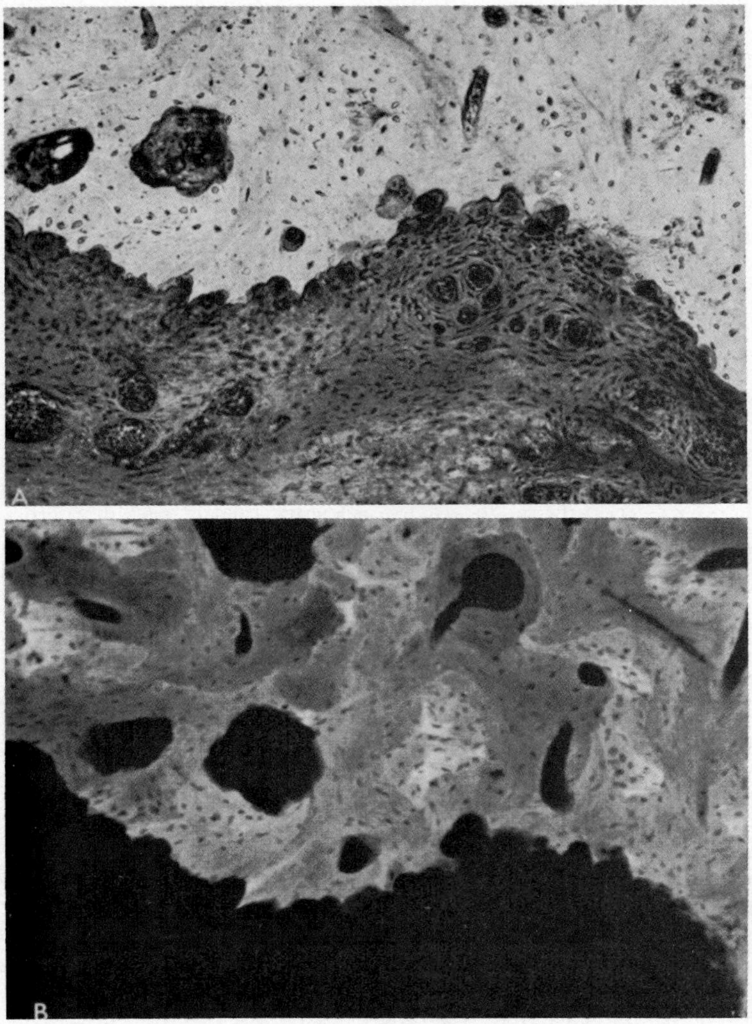

**Figure 17–4.** *A,* Paragon-stained mineralized section with large multinucleate osteoclasts lying along the pale staining bone surface. *B,* Microradiograph of the same area showing Howship's lacunae in the areas of osteoclastic resorption. (From Jowsey, J., and Gordan, G.: *In* Bourne, G.H. [ed.]: The Biochemistry and Physiology of Bone. Vol. III. 2nd ed. New York, Academic Press, 1972, pp. 201–238.)

clasts" found on bone surfaces as resting mononuclear cells;[34,38] arise from the same pool of undifferentiated "osteo-progenitor cells" that gives origin to osteoblasts;[8] or arise from wandering phagocytes.[39,40] A recent convincing review of available information gives strong support to the concept that osteoclasts arise from mononuclear lymphoid cells of the monocyte-macrophage series.[41] Whatever their origin, increased numbers of osteoclasts can be seen within 17 to 24 hours after injection of parathyroid hormone into experimental animals.[42]

The life span and ultimate fate of the osteoclast are also obscure. Tissue culture experiments suggest a life span of from 48 to 72 hours[43] to 3 days.[5] No convincing evidence has been found to suggest that osteoclasts can give rise to mononuclear cells. They thus appear to arise from mononuclear cells in response to various stimuli, carry out bone resorption, and then shed nuclei and finally disappear when stimuli to resorption (PTH, OAF, etc.) are removed or when there is no bone matrix left to be resorbed.[41]

Mast cells are seen in increased numbers in direct contact with resorbing bone surfaces in a number of conditions (lathyrism, PTH excess, mast cell disease), leading to the suggestion that they too can produce bone resorption.[44-46] Since heparin can enhance the resorptive response to parathyroid hormone[47] and produce osteoporosis after chronic administration,[48-50] it is interesting to speculate on the role, if any, of the mast cell content of this polysaccharide in bone resorption.

Myeloma cells also appear to resorb bone directly, as do some other malignant cells.[51] In addition, leukocytes produce a factor called osteoclast-activating factor (OAF) that stimulates osteoclastic activity and bone resorption.[52]

Thyroxin stimulates both bone formation and resorption, especially the latter.[53,54] Glucocorticoids have complex effects on bone formation and resorption, depending on the model used[55] and method of stimulation, whether PTH[56] or vitamin D metabolites[57] or prostaglandins.[58]

In clinical situations such as corticosteroid treatment of asthma[56] or rheumatoid arthritis,[56,57] bone loss may be severe, owing to a primary decrease in bone formation accompanied by hypercalciuria that leads to secondary hyperparathyroidism with increased bone resorption.[59]

Prostaglandins probably do not play a role in normal bone turnover,[60] but may be influential in pathological bone resorption by tumors[61] and inflammatory processes such as rheumatoid arthritis.[62,63] For a more detailed discussion of the role of hormones and other factors affecting bone growth and remodeling see Chapter 106 and reference 64.

**Organization of Bone.** Bone can be classified in a number of ways: (1) by its gross appearance (cortical or cancellous); (2) by its microscopic appearance (lamellar, woven, or haversian); or (3) on the basis of its origin (endochondral or intramembranous).[17]

Classification based on gross appearance has only limited usefulness, and that based on developmental origin suggests differences which do not exist since both endochondral and intramembranous bone are usually intermixed and indistinguishable. For our purposes, therefore, a system of classification based on microscopic appearance will be used.[65]

- Bone
  - Lamellar
    - Circumferential
    - Concentric
    - Interstitial
  - Nonlamellar (woven)

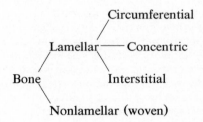

Nonlamellar or woven bone is the result of rapid bone formation. It is characteristic of embryonic and fetal development, but when seen in the adult is always pathological (i.e., tumor bone or fracture healing).

Lamellar bone can be packed tightly to form the cortex of a bone or loosely, as in cancellous bone[66,67] (Fig. 17–5).

After formation of the periosteal cuff surrounding the primary center of ossification, bone grows in diameter by one of two methods. During rapid growth, spicules of new bone are formed perpendicular to the surface, allowing maximal radial expansion with minimal material. Later, the gaps between the spicules are filled in by lamellar bone surrounding individual periosteal blood vessels which parallel the long axis of the bone (Fig. 17–6). These systems of lamellar bone surrounding a blood vessel are known as haversian systems or osteons.[68] An osteon that is formed de novo is referred to as a primary osteon, while one that is formed to replace a pre-existing bone structure is known as a secondary osteon.

When slow diametric growth occurs, seams of new bone are laid on the existing surface (Fig. 17–7*A*). These *circumferential* lamellae resemble the layers of an onion and provide a strong laminated structure like plywood. Indeed, the collagen bundles in adjacent lamellae alternate in direction from layer to layer, maximizing strength in all planes.[69] Later, for maximal strength, the circumferential lamellae are replaced by individual concentric lamellar systems; when these replace pre-existing bone (lamellar, woven, or earlier osteonal bone), they are

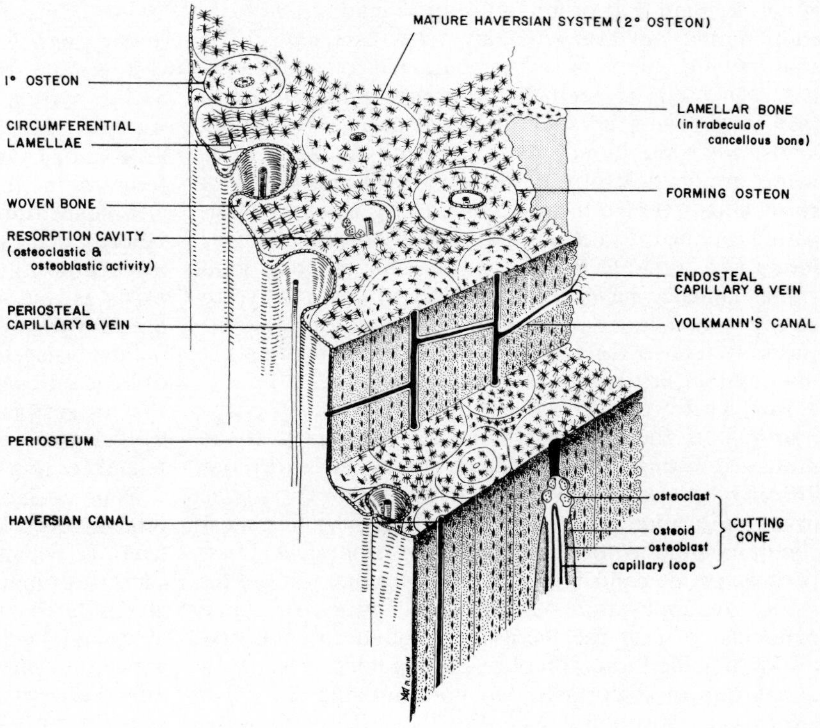


**Figure 17–5.** Diagrammatic representation of the structure of human cortical bone.

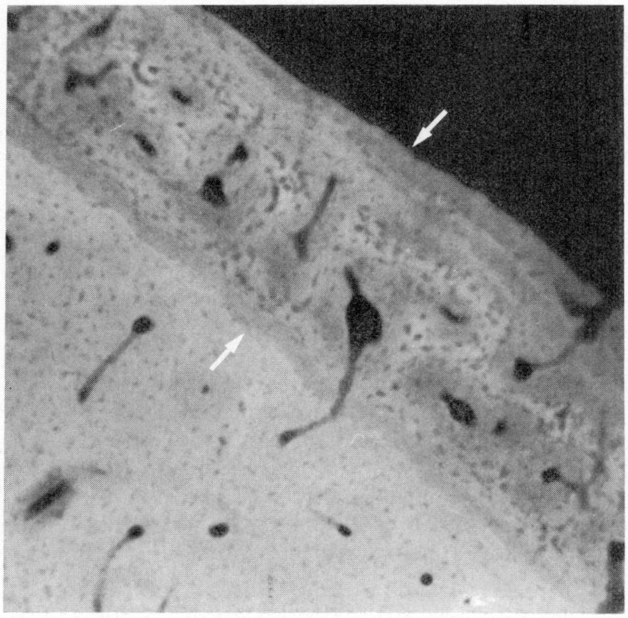

**Figure 17–6.** Outer cortex of bone showing the results of rapid periosteal bone formation producing woven bone, followed by the slower formation of primary osteons surrounding blood vessels.

termed secondary osteons and constitute the bulk of adult bone[70] (Fig. 17–7*B*). Remnants of pre-existing osteons and circumferential lamellae persist between newer, complete osteons. These fragments are called interstitial lamellae (Fig. 17–8).

The mechanical strength of fully mature osteonal bone is greater than that of immature bone composed of circumferential lamellae with only a few osteons.[71,72] The analogy of a bundle of straws compared to a solid stick has been used; as bending forces are applied to each, they bend. The solid stick breaks at fairly low bending loads, while the bundle of straws with the same mass will continue to deform rather than break. Each twig of straw slips, relative to adjacent bundles, thereby dissipating applied forces and avoiding excessive tensile forces and ultimate failure. In the same manner, individual lamellae have been observed to slip relative to adjacent lamellae, dissipating energy and allowing the entire system to react in a more elastic manner rather than sustain brittle failure or fracture.[18,71]

In order to replace pre-existing bone, it must first be resorbed. If the structural function of bone is to be preserved during this remodeling, it must be carried out little by little with the simultaneous removal of bone from one location and its deposition elsewhere. The most common stimulus for this remodeling is physical stress. If excessive demand is placed upon a bone (or the direction of application of force is changed), the bone remodels to meet the increased demand.[73,74] The first response is the formation of a "cutting cone" composed of a group of osteoclasts that bore into the old bone, creating a resorption cavity (Fig. 17–7*B*). In the wake of this resorptive process, a capillary grows in, surrounded by osteoblasts constructing a new haversian system.[75,76] In the absence of unusual physical demands, the process of conversion and remodeling of immature bone is quite orderly and predictable. Indeed, Kerley[70] has quantified the percentage of the cross section of the tibia that has been converted into mature osteonal bone and has related this percent conversion to the age of the individual. The resulting graph of percent osteonal bone versus age has been useful in forensic medicine and archeology in determining the age at death of skeletal remains.

When bone is being resorbed, osteoclasts are seen lying in irregular Howship's lacunae, the irregular margins of which allow one to recognize resorption even if the osteoclasts themselves are not seen (microradiographs, ground sections). When resorption is completed, these irregularities are smoothed out before new bone formation begins. This process leaves a boundary, which is visible in histologic sections as a "reversal line." If the resorbed bone is to be replaced by new bone, the reversal line clearly demarcates the junction between old and new bone. A similar line, called a "cement line," is seen between the adjacent lamellae of bone (Fig. 17–3).

During growth in diameter new bone is added peripherally (appositional growth) and old bone is resorbed on the inner or parallel surface (endosteal resorption). Some of the old cortical bone is spared during the process of removal on the endosteal surface and becomes a component of the cancellous structure. The appearance of these trabeculae of cancellous bone reflects this origin, and fragments of osteons as well as new lamellae and abundant cement lines are seen (Fig. 17–9). In places, trabeculae are covered with osteoblasts making new bone, while in other places osteoclasts are seen eroding the surface. By this process of resorption and formation, orientation of the trabeculae is changed to meet the altered forces produced by longitudinal growth or change in alignment secondary to disease or fracture.[74]

**Composition of Bone.** Newly synthesized bone matrix, before calcification, is called osteoid. The precise chemical composition is unknown, since the material normally exists as thin seams scattered throughout the skeleton, mixed with mineralized bone, cells, and marrow elements. Separation has been attempted by fragmentation of bone followed by density separation based on the fact that osteoid is less dense than mineralized bone (1.46 vs. 2.2 grams per milliliter).[77] Analysis of material obtained by this technique is shown in Table 17–1.

Bone collagen is classified as type I[78] and resembles other type I collagens found in skin and tendon. It differs from the collagen of cartilage (type II) in several salient aspects, primarily in that the latter contains much more glycosylated hydroxylysine. Cartilage collagen is also more resistant to degradation by collagenase than is bone collagen. More subtle, but important, differences exist between bone collagen and other type I collagens,[79,80] and these are discussed below.

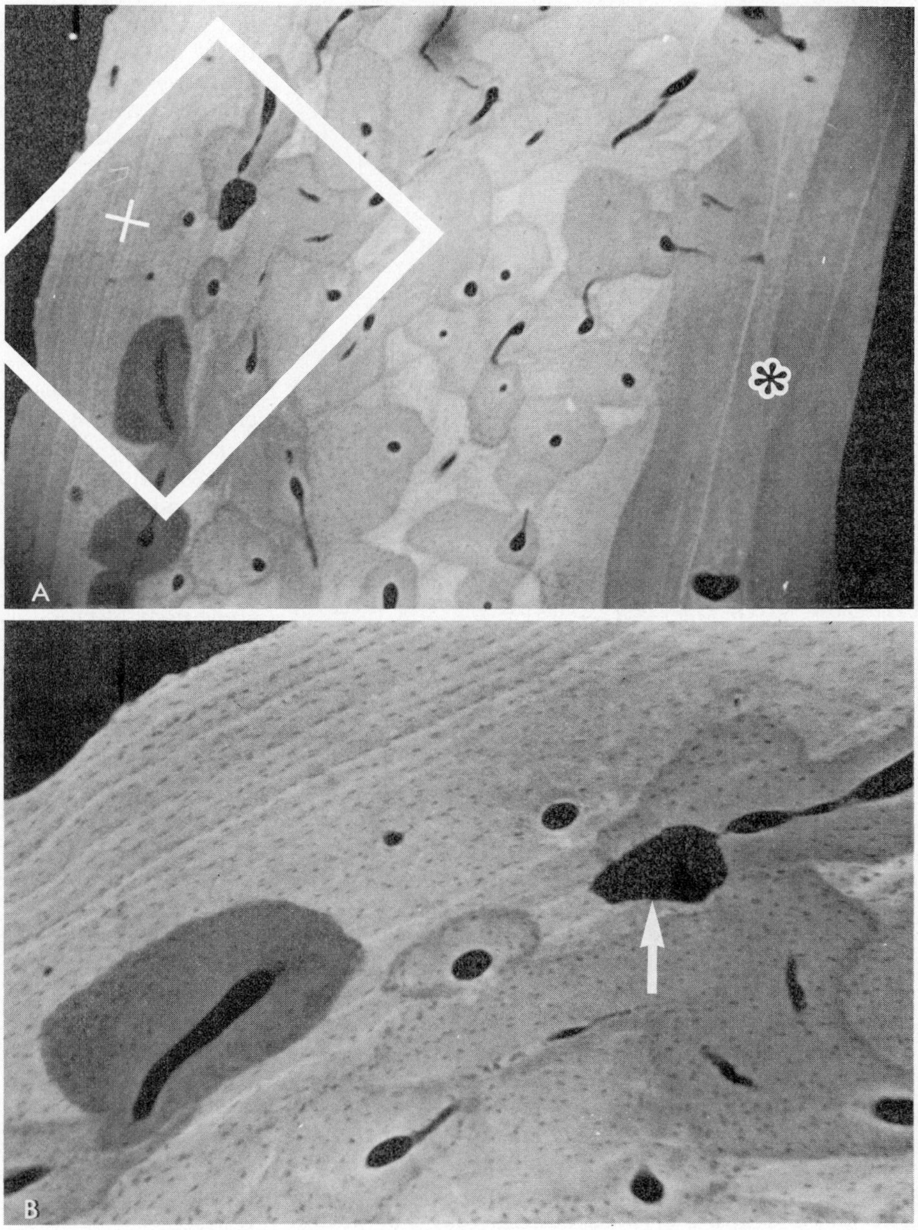


**Figure 17–7.** *A*, Microradiograph of the full thickness of cortical bone showing outer (+) and inner (*) circumferential lamellae with concentric (osteonal) bone in the center. *B*, Enlarged section of a portion of *A*, Showing a resorption cavity (→) with irregular margins, "burrowing" into the older circumferential lamellar bone.

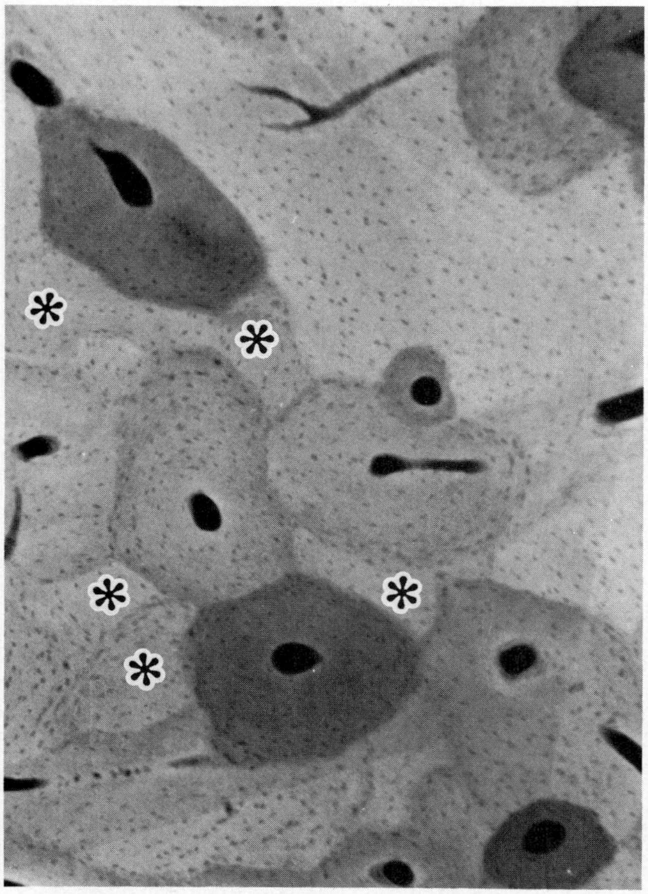

**Figure 17–8.** Microradiograph of cortical bone showing osteons in varying degrees of mineralization with numerous interstitial fragments (*).

The polysaccharides of bone have been difficult to analyze.[81,82] Chondroitin sulfate linked to protein and resembling the proteoglycan of cartilage has been identified by Herring,[83] who has also isolated a glycoprotein that represents the majority of the noncollagenous portion of bone matrix. A fraction rich in sialic acid, sialoprotein, has been characterized and is thought to be unique to bone. Lipids and phospholipids have also been identified but poorly characterized.[83,84]

Bone mineral is referred to as hydroxyapatite [$Ca_{10}(PO_4)_6 \bullet (OH)_2$] but is quite different from naturally occuring apatite, containing a number of impurities, including sodium, fluorine, strontium, lead, and radium. The initial deposits of bone mineral may not be hydroxyapatite but amorphous calcium phosphate (ACP)[85] or octacalcium phosphate (OCP),[86] which are gradually transformed to more crystalline hydroxyapatite. The enormous surface area of ACP, with its hydration shell, provides an immense surface for exchange. This is reflected in the greater avidity of new bone for "bone-seeking" isotopes (technetium, fluorine, strontium) and the greater rate of calcium exchange in young as opposed to old subjects. Vaughan estimates that 100 percent of bone surfaces are available for exchange at the age of 1 year compared with 1 to 2 percent in adults.[87]

**Mineralization.** The process by which unmineralized bone matrix is converted to calcified bone remains incompletely understood. There are two leading theories. The first suggests a central role for collagen as a "nucleator," with proteoglycans and other minor constituents serving as inhibitors, protecting noncalcifying tissues.[88,89] The second theory suggests that mineral-rich lipid vesicles are produced by calcifying tissues (cartilage and bone) and that these vesicles serve as the initial foci of mineralization, which then spreads to permeate the entire structure.[90,91] Current evidence points to a role for these vesicles in the calcification of growth cartilage,[92] but supports the principal role of collagen in bone mineralization.[93]

Body fluids are supersaturated with respect to hydroxyapatite. If type I collagen is capable of nucleating crystals of hydroxyapatite from such solutions, why do not ligaments, skin, and tendon normally calcify? Convincing evidence has been accumulated that the proteoglycans found in these noncalcifying collagenous structures prevent mineral deposition (see reference 93 for review). Enzymatic removal of these blocking substances would allow mineral deposition. An abrupt loss of sulfated proteoglycan at the calcification front has been shown,[89] confirming earlier, in vitro demonstrations that collagen "contaminated" with proteoglycan did not include mineralization as effectively as did purified type I collagen.

There is general agreement that early in the mineralization process crystals of hydroxyapatite are seen within collagen fibrils, reproducing the 640 Å periodicity and apparently lying in "holes" in the collagen fibril.[94] The initial localization of mineral to these "hole" regions is presumably due to both spatial and chemical factors. The water that is displaced during mineralization (Table 17–1) presumably is concentrated in the holes, and the organic phosphate groups, which institute crystal nucleation, are concentrated nearby.[95] As crystal growth occurs, mineralization spreads beyond the hole region but remains largely or wholly within the fibrils, which are held together by strong interfibrillar and interfiber

**Table 17-1.** Composition of Bone*

| | Osteoid | "New" Bone | "Old" Bone |
|---|---|---|---|
| Density | 1.460 | 2.005 | 2.211 |
| Collagen | 31.99% | 25.85% | 23.63% |
| Other protein | 12.87 | 11.31 | 1.56 |
| Mucopolysaccharides | 1.64 | 0.83 | 0.75 |
| Mineral | 11.07 | 39.25 | 54.59 |
| Water | 20.15 | 15.15 | 17.45 |
| Total | 77.7% | 92.4% | 98% |

*Composition given as percent dry weight. After Herring, G.M.: *In* Bourne, G.H. (ed.): The Biochemistry and Physiology of Bone, Vol. I. 2nd ed. New York, Academic Press, 1972, p. 127. Data from Pugliarello, M.C., et al.: Calc. Tissue Res. 5:108, 1970.

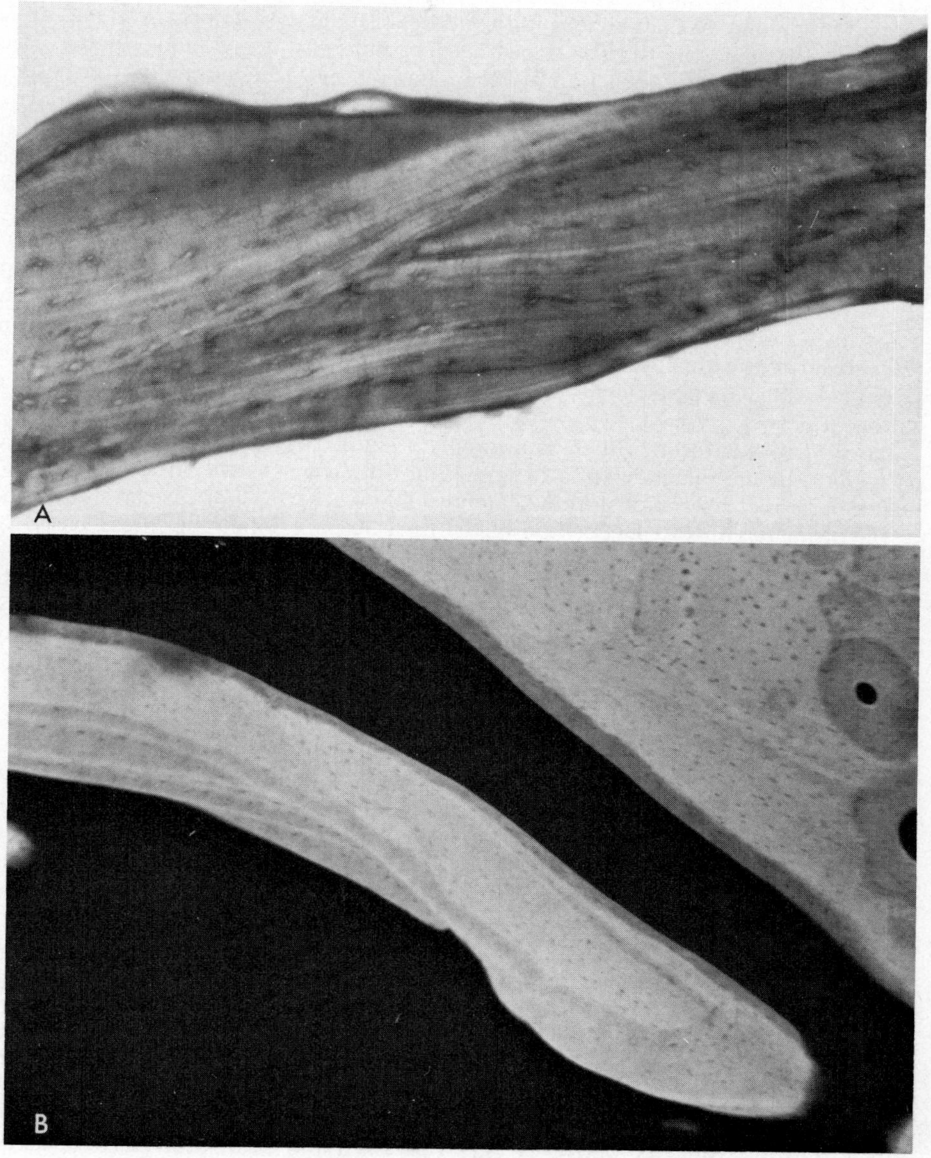


**Figure 17–9.** *A*, Ground section of cancellous bone showing a single trabecula composed of multiple lamellae of bone and numerous osteocytes. *B*, Microradiograph of a trabecula adjacent to the inner cortex of bone. Growth of the trabecula by the addition of new seams of lamellar bone is clearly seen.

bonds. The total amount of mineral that can be accommodated by this theory—two thirds of the weight of the tissue—is the amount measured in mature, fully calcified bone. In tissues that do not normally calcify, the "holes" are smaller, but the lack of strong inter- and intramolecular bonds allows more mineral to be deposited outside of the fibrils. Thus, these structures may contain more mineral than bone, and the mineral is both within and outside the fibril.[93] It has been postulated that in calcific "bursitis" or tendinitis, the inflammatory process produces enzymatic loss of the protective proteoglycan, allowing the exposed collagen fibrils to nucleate hydroxyapatite from the supersaturated interstitial fluid.

A vitamin K–dependent calcium-building amino acid residue, γ-carboxyglutamic acid, has been identified in bone, calcifying cartilage, and various pathologic calcifications.[96,97] The parent protein, named osteocalcin, constitutes only 0.5 to 1 percent of total bone protein (20 percent of the noncollagenous protein) but may represent a critical regulatory mechanism in the mineralization of tissues.[98]

After osteoid is formed, there is normally a lag of 10 to 15 days before mineralization begins. Following this lag, mineral increases almost immediately to 70 percent of the ultimate content. Deposition of the final 30 percent may take several months.[99] In undemineralized ground sections, microradiography demonstrates differences in the calcium content of various osteons, thus allowing separation into "old" or "new" osteons based on mineral content (Fig. 17–7). In addition, very young osteons, in the process of formation, have large central vascular canals which narrow with maturity. Remodeling rates can thus be inferred from morphological characteristics.[99]

## BONES AS ORGANS

**General Considerations.** Bones are remarkably well suited for their structural role. As hollow tubes, they combine maximal strength with minimal weight. This strength-to-weight ratio is further enhanced by the microscopic arrangement of the collagen within the bone and the two-phase composition of collagen and mineral. The tensile strength of the bone approximates that of cast iron; its bending strength is between that of oak and cast iron, while its weight is only one third the weight of the latter.

Because of its strength, the shaft of a bone can be quite narrow for its length. In order to distribute forces on the articular cartilage, thereby minimizing wear and the deleterious effects of excessive force on the articular chondrocyte, the end of the bone flares to a larger diameter. The type and distribution of material also change to minimize weight and protect the articular cartilage (see discussion in Chapter 18) (Fig. 17–10). Additionally, bone responds to the physical demands placed upon it, not only by changes in size but by changes in shape and internal structure. The skeleton also reconstitutes itself after fracture in such a way that its form-function relationship is maintained. In order to meet these demands, bone is constantly being internally remodeled by a complex and interrelated sequence of resorption and formation which is never entirely quiescent and is capable of responding to metabolic demands without loss of structural integrity.

As organs, bones are composed of marrow, cartilage, nerves and blood vessels, and the periosteal covering. Functionally, the origins and insertions of muscles should also be included.

In childhood and early adult life, marrow is hematopoietic in most of the bones. With advancing age, this red marrow retreats from the appendicular skeleton and occupies the flat bones, vertebral bodies, and epiphyseal ends of the larger tubular bones such as the humerus and femur. As hematopoietic red marrow is lost, it is replaced by fatty yellow marrow. This process begins at about the sixth year and is complete by the eighteenth. Since the red marrow is much more vascular than the fatty marrow, the ends of the long bones, the vertebra, and the flat bones are metabolically more responsive, and it is here that the changes of systemic disease are usually first apparent.

For ease of discussion, the long bones are divided into anatomic areas based on the zones of growing bones: the juxta-articular or epiphyseal area (on the articular side of the growth plate), the metaphysis (the tapered portion from the epiphysis to the straight tubular midsection), and the diaphysis (the shaft). Although these regions are imprecise and are used somewhat differently by anatomists and radiologists, they are useful for descriptive purposes.

Most of the bones of the skeleton are first formed in the embryo as cartilaginous models, which are later resorbed and replaced by bone tissue. The cartilage model (anlage) is formed by the condensation of mesenchymal cells in the developing limb bud. The shape of the anlage resembles that of the adult bone and is genetically determined. The bone that replaces it, however, is greatly influenced by physical factors (e.g., weight bearing, muscle pull), and remodels constantly as these forces change (Wolff's law).[73]

At the stage of the cartilage anlage, bone as an organ is composed entirely of cartilage.[1] The anlage expands and elongates by interstitial growth in which chondrocytes divide, enlarge, and surround themselves with a new matrix.[100] As growth continues, the limits of diffusion are reached and materials can no longer diffuse into the avascular cartilage model. The oldest and most centrally placed cells become hypertrophic, and the matrix surrounding them becomes encrusted with mineral deposits (the "primary center of ossification"). At about the same time, cells in the connective tissues surrounding the anlage (perichondrium) begin to lay down bone tissue and form a collar of bone around the center of the cartilage model. At about the time it is formed, it is pierced by a capillary, which invades the calcified cartilage matrix and begins to hollow out the center of the anlage, replacing the excavated cartilage with bone and

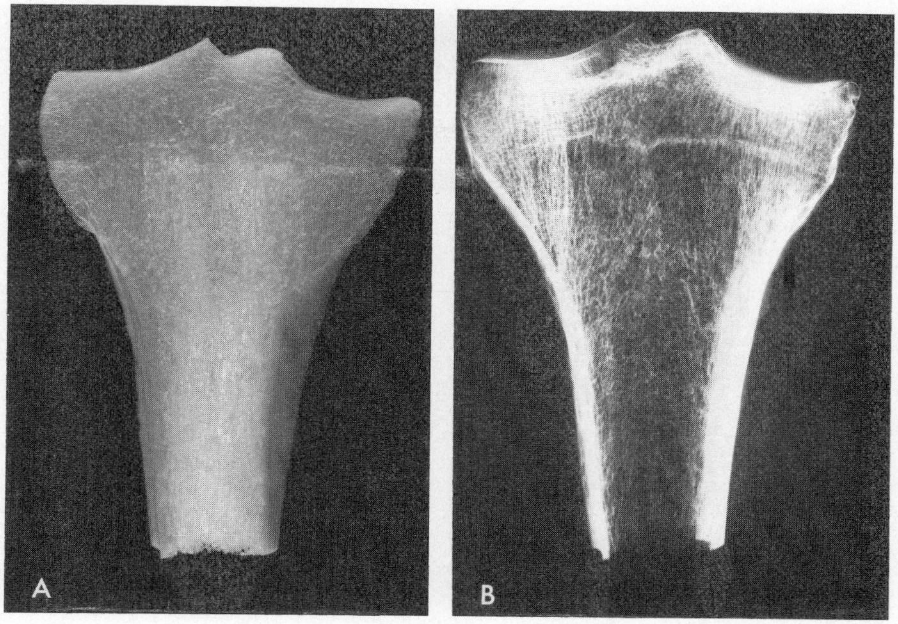


**Figure 17–10.** *A,* Macerated preparation of the human knee showing the trabecular structure which supports the flared articular surface. *B,* Radiograph of the specimen shown in *A.*

creating the primitive marrow space. This process of vascular invasion of the cartilage model, followed by bone deposition, is referred to as endochondral ossification. The process continues until the entire shaft of the anlage is replaced by marrow and bone, confining the growth process of chondrocyte multiplication to the epiphyseal ends of the bone. As these enlarge, the centrally placed chondrocytes again find themselves too far removed from a blood supply to exist by diffusion. The process of chondrocyte death followed by vascular invasion and bone formation is repeated, this time producing the "secondary center of ossification" in the epiphysis. The growth process continues between these two centers of ossification, confined to a relatively thin disc of cartilage called the physis, growth plate, or epiphyseal plate. A similar zone of proliferating cells exists under the articular cartilage as a "microepiphyseal plate." Both areas respond to growth hormone (via somatomedin) and provide longitudinal growth of the bone and enlargement of the articular end to maintain an appropriate size and shape for the weight-bearing surface (Fig. 17–11).

While growth in length occurs at the growth plate, growth in diameter occurs by the centrifugal deposition of bone by cells on the surface—so-called periosteal osteoblasts.[101]

This process of adding new bone to the exterior surface and resorbing bone from the inner surface continues throughout life. When "rate-linked," the mass and strength of the skeleton remain constant; however, aging and hormonal changes lead to alterations in shape and strength. "The outer, subperiosteal surface undergoes lifelong apposition, more in the male than in the female, with a classic 'adolescent spurt' and with a slower rate of gain thereafter, through to the end of life. The inner, endosteal bone surface undergoes resorption from childhood until adolescence, an appositional phase from middle adolescence through the end of the fourth decade, and then a second resorptive phase thereafter—demonstrably larger in the female and of greater consequence."[102]

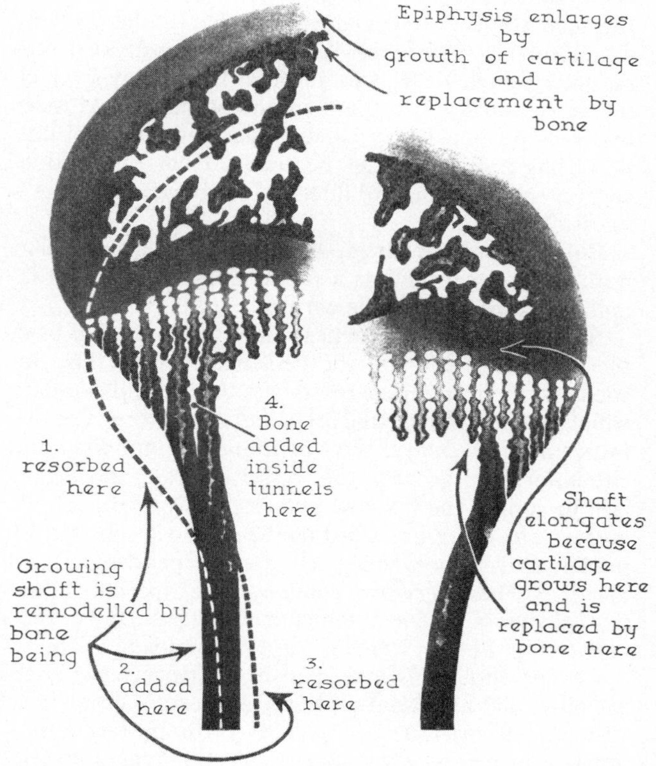


**Figure 17–11.** Diagram of the articular end of the bone showing the process of addition of new bone and removal of old bone which allows the articular end to increase in size while maintaining its shape during longitudinal growth. (From Ham, A.W.: J. Bone Joint Surg. 34A:701, 1952.)

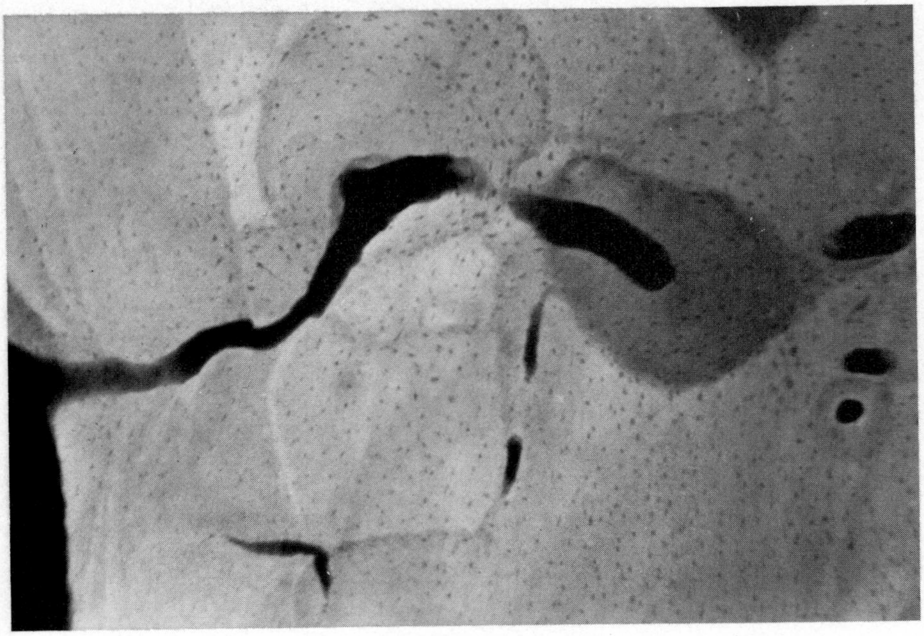

**Figure 17–12.** Endosteal capillary penetrating the inner cortex to communicate with two haversian canals, providing an anastomotic communication between the nutrient artery, periosteal arteries, and capillaries traveling longitudinally within the haversian canal.

**Periosteum.** When enlargement of the cartilaginous anlage first begins, a condensed layer of mesenchyme develops around it as a membrane of cells and collagen. While this tissue surrounds the cartilage model, it is called *perichondrium*. As cartilage is replaced by bone, the membrane is renamed *periosteum*. In the growing skeleton, this periosteum is rather clearly divided into an inner cellular layer and an outer fibrous layer which merges gradually into the surrounding muscle. Muscles take origin from the periosteum and tendons insert into it. Collagen bundles can be traced from the tendon, through periosteum, and directly into bone as Sharpey's fibers.[103]

**Blood Supply of Bone.** Bone is extremely vascular, both as an organ and as a tissue, and receives approximately 10 percent of the cardiac output.[104]

Blood supply to the cortical diaphysis is derived from the nutrient artery and the periosteal vessels. The nutrient artery (or arteries) represents the original capillary which pierced the cartilaginous anlage to form the primitive marrow cavity. With continued longitudinal and circumferential growth, this vessel enlarges and arborizes to supply the marrow and inner two thirds of the cortex. The outer one third of the cortex is supplied by numerous vessels which perforate the periosteum and cortex.[105] These *periosteal capillaries* are especially abundant at sites of tendon and ligament insertion and muscle origin (Fig. 17–12). In the metaphyseal ends of the bone, where metabolism is most active, the periosteal vessels are large and abundant and they are also referred to as *metaphyseal arteries*, although they are entirely analogous to the periosteal capillaries. The third set of vessels, the *epiphyseal arteries*, supply the subarticular ends of the bones and assume special importance because of the growth process in this area and the vulnerability of these vessels to injury (Fig. 17–13).

During infancy and adolescence, the epiphyseal (growth) plate serves as a barrier separating the epiphysis from the metaphysis. Although a few vessels crossing the plate have been described, it is widely accepted that there is no effective circulation across the plate. The epiphyses therefore exist with an isolated blood supply via the epiphyseal arteries. In most joints, there are abundant soft tissue attachments to the epiphyses (muscles, ligaments, capsule), so that numerous vessels supply the bone through these attachments (Fig. 17–14*A*). In a few locations, such as the proximal femur, the entire epiphysis may be intraarticular and therefore covered by articular cartilage. Since neither this cartilage nor the growth cartilage is penetrated by vessels, the few epiphyseal arteries must pass alongside the growth plate, covered by a thin layer of periosteum, to perforate the epiphysis[106] (Fig. 17–14*B*). The route of blood supply is extremely vulnerable to trauma (fractures through the growth plate), increased intra-articular pressure (joint infections or bleeding into the joint), or idiopathic interruption (Legg-Perthes disease in children, avascular necrosis in adults).

Epiphyseal vessels arborize within the bony nucleus to supply the marrow, cancellous bone, and the crucial dividing chondrocytes in the microepiphyseal plates in the depths of the articular cartilage and the growth plate itself (Fig. 17–14*C*). Because of this, interruption of the vessels leads to cessation of longitudinal growth and loss of further diametric growth of the epiphysis and joint surface.

In contrast to the critical role of epiphyseal vessels during growth, the metaphyseal vessels are responsible only for resorption of the growth plate prior to its replacement by bone. Interruption of these vessels therefore will lead only to temporary loss of this function with increased thickness of the growth plate owing to

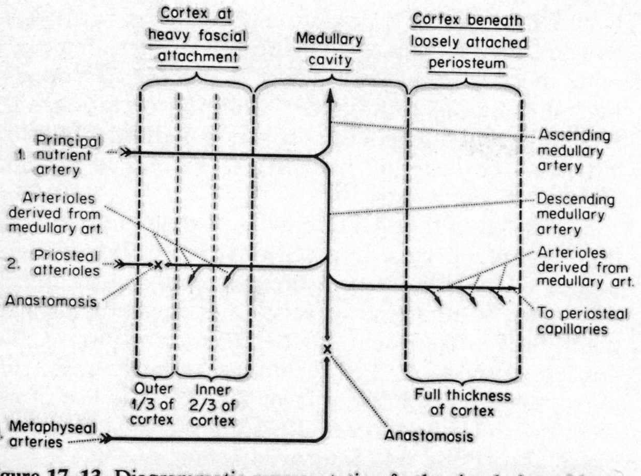


**Figure 17–13.** Diagrammatic representation fo the circulation of bone emphasizing the multiple communications seen at the site of heavy fascial attachment contrasted with the sparse communication in other areas. (From Rhinelander, F.W.: *In* Bourne, G.H. [ed.]: The Biochemistry and Physiology of Bone. Vol. II. 2nd ed. New York, Academic Press, 1972.)

accumulation of chondrocytes and matrix. Upon re-establishment of the metaphyseal blood supply, the thickened plate is resorbed to its normal thickness and growth is not affected.[107]

Even in growing bones there is an abundant system of anastomoses between metaphyseal, periosteal, and nutrient arteries. Interruption of a single system results in limited changes in bone. With termination of longitudinal growth and obliteration of the growth plate, anastomoses are established between the metaphyseal system and the epiphyseal system, thereby interconnecting the entire blood supply of the bone. For this reason, elevation of the periosteum (dissecting infection or surgical approaches) or obliteration of the nutrient artery (intra-articular fixation devices or infection) have only limited effects on the blood supply to the entire bone.[105]

Within the cortex of bone, capillaries travel primarily in the longitudinal direction within haversian canals. Occasional branching is seen, and lateral communications with the periosteal vessels through Volkmann's canals provide collateral circulation.[68] The usual haversian system is 100 $\mu$m or less in diameter; thus individual osteocytes are not more than 50 $\mu$m from their blood supply. The rich system of canaliculi radiating out from the central canal enhances microcirculation to the most distant osteocytes.

Although the periosteum and marrow have long been known to be innervated with sensory and autonomic fibers, nerves within the haversian canals have only recently been described.[19]

Neural, hormonal, and metabolic factors affecting the blood supply to bone have been discussed by Shim,[104] and the effects of loss of blood to cortical and cancellous bone are discussed in Chapter 107.

**Assessment of Bone Formation and Resorption.** Because of the close relationship between bone form and function, estimates of skeletal metabolic activity can be made by morphologic techniques that assess the amount of either bone or mineral. The simplest technique is a visual assessment of mineral quantity on routine clinical radiographs. The technique is insensitive (30 percent of vertebral mass must be removed before it is detected by this technique[108]) and inaccurate (varying technical factors such as kilovoltage and exposure change the radiographic appearance[109]). The use of a densitometer, multiple scans of the same bone, and inclusion of a reference aluminum step wedge increase the accuracy of the technique and have allowed useful estimates of bone loss caused by bed rest[110] and the weightlessness of space flight.[111]

Estimates of cortical thickness, either metacarpal or vertebral body, have been used to follow age-related and pathological loss of bone mass and the response to therapy in osteoporosis.[112,113] The most useful of these techniques involves the determination of the combined cortical thickness of a reference bone, usually a metacarpal, although the humerus, clavicle, and phalanges have been used.[114] The thickness of the two cortices is measured

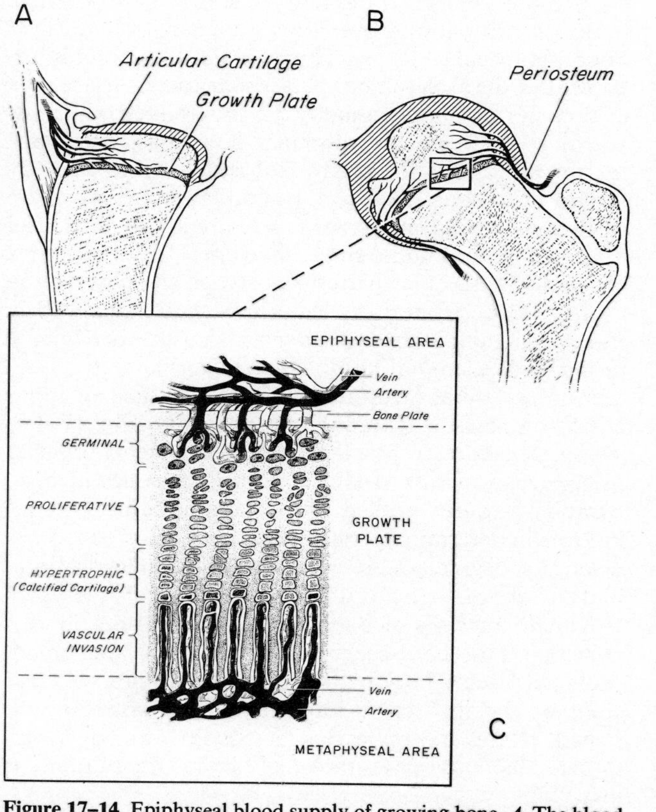


**Figure 17–14.** Epiphyseal blood supply of growing bone. *A*, The blood supply of most secondary centers of ossification is abundant by virtue of the numerous soft tissue attachments. *B*, Certain secondary centers, such as the proximal femur, are devoid of soft tissue attachments, and the blood supply therefore follows a tenuous route through the joint where it is liable to injury. *C*, Diagrammatic representation of the blood supply to the growth plate showing the contribution of the epiphyseal artery to the germinal portion of the growth plate. (From Sledge, C.B.: *In* Cave, E.F., et al. [eds.]: Trauma Management. Chicago, Year Book Medical Publishers, 1974.)

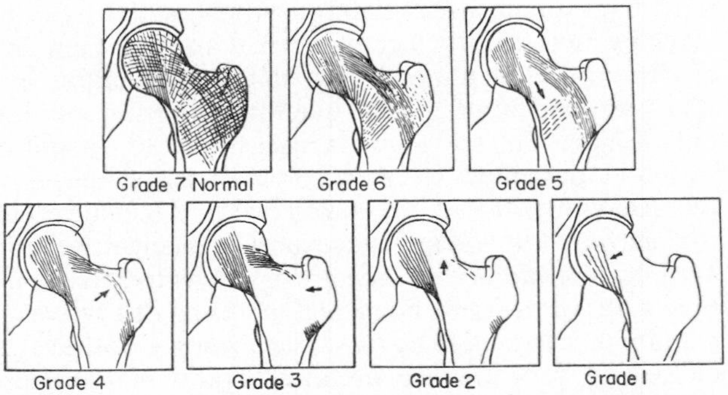


**Figure 17–15.** Singh index of trabecular patterns, illustrating the progressive stages of trabecular loss in osteoporosis. (From Jowsey, J.: Metabolic Diseases of Bone. Philadelphia, W.B. Saunders Company, 1977.)

and expressed as a ratio of that thickness to the diameter of the bone. Although having the advantage of simplicity, this technique is not as accurate as the quantitative radiographic technique discussed in the preceding paragraph.[109]

Because both bone formation and bone resorption are surface phenomena, trabecular bone is a more sensitive indicator of bone turnover than are changes in cortical bone. Trabeculae of cancellous bone occupy only 20 percent of the skeleton but present the same surface area as does cortical bone, roughly 5.5 square meters.[115] Furthermore, decreases in trabecular bone mass occur primarily by loss of the entire trabecula, rather than by thinning.[116] Thus, losses of trabecular bone are more easily detected in radiographs than are losses of cortical bone. Singh and colleagues[117] have developed an index of femoral trabecular patterns based on the observation that the trabeculae of the femoral neck are arranged in three predominant groups: a vertical compressive bundle in the medial femoral head, a curved vertial tensile bundle in the lateral head and neck region, and an interconnecting bundle lying more horizontally (Fig. 17–15). These groups of trabeculae are lost in reverse order in osteoporosis, giving rise to a sequential series of radiographic patterns graded 1 to 7. The usefulness of this index is in determining when bone loss, or osteoporosis, reaches a degree which endangers the mechanical stability of the skeleton and produces a risk of fracture.

Kinetic analyses of bone turnover, based on the disappearance of bone-seeking isotopes from the blood, provided useful information in early studies, but are complex and difficult to interpret. The information obtained relates to mineral metabolism and turnover, rather than to new rates of bone deposition or loss.[118-120]

Gamma-emitting bone-seeking isotopes that can be imaged with a gamma camera can provide visual and quantitative information on bone turnover. It is not clear to what degree bone formation and blood supply contribute to localization of the isotope; therefore these techniques are largely qualitative (see Chapter 40).

Total body bone mass can be determined by neutron activation analysis whereby stable body calcium ($^{48}Ca$) is converted to $^{49}Ca$, which emits gamma rays with a half-life of 8.8 minutes. Quantitative determination of bone mass with an accuracy of 1 percent has been reported using this technique.[121] Comparison between this technique and the photon absorption method (see below) suggests the latter is less precise in measuring small changes in bone mass.[122,123]

Variations in the characteristics of x-ray emissions and film processing gave imprecision to radiographic techniques of bone mass measurement and led to the development of mono-energetic sources of gamma rays and quantitative determinations of their absorption. Called photon absorption, the technique is fairly rapid and inexpensive but relatively insensitive.[124] The use of two different isotope sources allows subtraction of the soft tissue absorption and improved accuracy.[125]

New developments in computerized axial tomography have largely supplanted both total body neutron activation and photon absorption as methods of determining bone mineral content. Multiple "cuts" through one or more vertebral bodies can be averaged by the computer, obviating many of the sampling problems inherent in other methods, and giving calcium content with an accuracy of $\pm 3$ percent.[126,127]

The unique nature of bone collagen has given rise to other techniques of estimating skeletal turnover based on analysis of urinary hydroxyproline[128] and glycosylated hydroxylysines.[129] Because it is not entirely possible to distinguish between fragments of collagen resulting from bone breakdown and those resulting from increased but faulty synthesis, these techniques are only semiquantitative, but their simplicity and noninvasiveness are attractive.

**Bone Biopsy.** The techniques of determination of skeletal and/or mineral mass described above are useful and accurate to varying degrees but produce results that are largely "net effects." They do not clearly discern between decreased formation and increased resorption; nor do they separate changes in matrix metabolism from those of mineral balance. In osteomalacia, for example, bone mass and bone mineral changes may be masked by coexisting osteoporosis.[130] Bone biopsy, in addition to providing material for the usual histological evaluation of disease processes in the skeleton, has been developed into an extremely useful and accurate method of measuring bone metabolism.[131] The interested reader is referred to the excellent monograph by Jowsey,[10] the discussion by Byers,[132] and a monograph on noninvasive bone measurements edited by Dequeker and Johnston.[133]

## References

1. Krane, S.M., and Potts, J.T., Jr.: Skeletal remodeling and factors influencing bone and bone mineral metabolism. *In* Thorn, G.W., Adams, R.D., Braunwald, E., Isselbacher, K.J., and Petersdorf, R.G. (eds.): Harrison's Principles of Internal Medicine. New York, McGraw-Hill Book Company, 1972.
2. Vaughan, J.M.: Osteogenic cells. *In* The Physiology of Bone. Oxford, Oxford University Press, 1970, p. 23.
3. Neuman, W.F., and Ramp, W.K.: The concept of a bone membrane: Some implications. *In* Nichols, G., Jr., and Wasserman, R.H. (eds.): Cellular Mechanisms for Calcium Transfer and Homeostasis. New York, Academic Press, 1971, p. 197.

4. Young, R.W.: Nucleic acids, protein synthesis and bone. Clin. Orthop. 26:147, 1963.
5. Young, R.W.: Cell proliferation and specialization during endochondral osteogenesis in young rats. J. Cell Biol. 14:357, 1962.
6. Tonna, E.A., and Cronkite, E.P.: Histochemical and autoradiographic studies on the effects of aging on the mucopolysaccharides of the periosteum. J. Biophys. Biochem. Cytol. 6:171, 1959.
7. Owen, M.E.: Cell population kinetics of an osteogenic tissue. J. Cell Biol. 19:19, 1963.
8. Young, R.W.: Autoradiographic studies on postnatal growth of the skull in young rats injected with tritiated glycine. Anat. Rec. 143:1, 1962.
9. Young, R.W.: Specialization of bone cells. *In* Frost, H.M. (ed.): Bone Biodynamics. Boston, Little, Brown & Company, 1964.
10. Jowsey, J.: Metabolic Disease of Bone. Philadelphia, W.B. Saunders Company, 1977, p. 59.
11. Weinger, J.M., and Holtrop, M.E.: An ultrastructural study of bone cells: the occurrence of microtubules, microfilaments and tight junctions. Calcif. Tissue Res. 14:15, 1974.
12. Pritchard, J.J.: The osteoblast. *In* Bourne, G.H. (ed.): The Biochemistry and Physiology of Bone, Vol. I. 2nd ed. New York, Academic Press, 1972, p. 21.
13. Carneiro, J., and Leblond, C.P.: Role of osteoblasts and odontoblasts in secreting the collagen of bone and dentin, as shown by radioautography in mice given tritium-labelled glycine. Exp. Cell Res. 18:291, 1959.
14. Miller, E.J., Martin, G.R., Piez, K.A., and Powers, M.J.: Characterization of chick bone collagen and compositional changes associated with maturation. J. Biol. Chem. 242:5481, 1967.
15. Miller, E.J.: A review of biochemical studies on the genetically distinct collagens of the skeletal system. Clin. Orthop. 91:260, 1973.
16. Prockop, D.J., Kivirikko, K.I., Tuderman, L., and Guzman, N.A.: The biosynthesis of collagen and its disorders. N. Engl. J. Med. 301:13, 77, 1979.
17. Pritchard, J.J.: General histology of bone. *In* Bourne, G.H. (ed.): The Biochemistry and Physiology of Bone, Vol. I. 2nd ed. New York, Academic Press, 1972, p. 15.
18. Gebhardt, W.: Über funktionel wichtige Anordnungsweisen der feineren und grosseren Bauelemente des wirbeltier Knockens. 2. Spezieller Teil. Der Bau Der Haversischen Lamellen Systeme und seine functionelle Bedeutung. Arch. Entwicklungsmech. Organismen. 20:187, 1906.
19. Cooper, R.R., James, M.D., Milgram, J.W., and Robinson, R.A.: Morphology of the osteon. J. Bone Joint Surg. 48A:1239, 1966.
20. Owen, M.: Cellular dynamics of bone. *In* Bourne, G.H. (ed.): The Biochemistry and Physiology of Bone, Vol. III. 2nd ed. New York, Academic Press, 1972, p. 271.
21. Tonna, E.A.: A study of osteocyte formation and distribution in aging mice complemented with $^3$H-proline autoradiography. J. Gerontol. 21:124, 1966.
22. Jowsey, J.: Metabolic Diseases of Bone. Philadelphia, W.B. Saunders Company, 1977, p. 61.
23. Ruth, E.B.: Further observations on histological evidence of osseous tissue resorption (abstract). Anat. Rec. 118:347, 1954.
24. Bélanger, L.F.: Osteocytic resorption. *In* Bourne, G.H. (ed.): The Biochemistry and Physiology of Bone, Vol. III. 2nd ed. New York, Academic Press, 1972, p. 239.
25. Duriez, J.: Les modifications calciques péri-ostéocytaires; étude microradiographique à l'analyseur automatique d'images. Nouv. Presse Med. 3:2007, 1974.
26. Liu, C.C., Baylink, D.J., and Wergedahl, J.: Vitamin D—enhanced osteoclastic bone resorption at vascular canals. Endocrinology 95:1011, 1974.
27. Holtrop, M.E., and Weinger, J.M.: Ultrastructural evidence for a transport system in bone. *In* Talmage, R.V., and Munson, P.L. (eds.): Calcium, Parathyroid Hormone and the Calcitonins. Excerpta Medica International Congress Series No. 243. Amsterdam, Excerpta Medica Foundation, 1972, p. 365.
28. Robinson, R.A.: Observations regarding compartments for tracer calcium in the body. *In* Frost, H.M. (ed.): Bone Biodynamics. Boston, Little, Brown & Company, 1964.
29. Baud, C.A.: The fine structure of normal and parathormone-treated bone cells. *In* Galliard, P.J., Van Den Hoof, A., and Steendijk, R. (eds.): Fourth European Symposium on Calcified Tissues. Excerpta Medica International Congress Series No. 120. Amsterdam, Excerpta Medica Foundation, 1966, p. 4.
30. Hancox, N.M.: The Osteoclast. *In* Bourne, G.H. (ed.): The Biochemistry and Physiology of Bone, Vol. I. 2nd ed. New York, Academic Press, 1972, p. 45.
31. Holtrop, M.E., Raisz, L.G., and Simmons, H.: The effects of PTH, colchicine and calcitonin on the ultrastructure and activity of osteoclasts in organ culture. J. Cell Biol. 60:346, 1974.
32. Walker, D.G.: Enzymatic and electron microscopic analysis of isolated osteoclasts. Calcif. Tissue Res. 9:296, 1972.
33. Vaes, G.: Lysosomes and the cellular physiology of bone resorption. *In* Dingle, J.T., and Fell, H.B. (eds.): Lysosomes in Biology and Pathology, Vol. 1. Amsterdam, North-Holland Publishers, 1969, p. 217.
34. Owen, M.: The origin of bone cells. Int. Rev. Cytol. 28:213, 1970.
35. Jowsey, J.: Metabolic Diseases of Bone. Philadelphia, W.B. Saunders Co., 1977, p. 73.
36. Jaworski, Z.F.G., and Lok, E.: The rate of osteoclastic bone erosion in Haversian remodeling sites of adult dog's rib. Calcif. Tissue Res. 10:103, 1972.
37. Sledge, C.B.: Biochemical events in the epiphyseal plate and their physiological control. Clin. Orthop. Rel. Res. 61:37, 1968.
38. Scott, B.L.: The occurrence of specific cytoplasmic granules in the osteoclast. J. Ultrastruct. Res. 19:417, 1967.
39. Fischman, D.A., and Hay, E.D.: Origin of osteoclasts from mononuclear leukocytes in regenerating newt limbs. Anat. Rec. 143:329, 1962.
40. Jee, W.S.S., and Nolan, P.D.: Origin of osteoclasts from the fusion of phagocytes. Nature 200:225, 1963.
41. Bonucci, E.: New knowledge on the origin, function and fate of osteoclasts. Clin. Orthop. Rel. Res. 158:252, 1981.
42. Bingham, P.J., Brazell, I.A., and Owen, M.: The effect of parathyroid extract on cellular activity and plasma calcium levels in vivo. J. Endocrinol. 45:387, 1969.
43. Hancox, N.M.: The osteoclast. *In* Willmer, E.N. (ed.): Cells and Tissues in Culture, Vol. 2. New York, Academic Press, 1965, p. 261.
44. Frame, B., and Nixon, R.K.: Bone marrow mast cells in osteoporosis of aging. N. Engl. J. Med. 279:626, 1968.
45. Severson, A.R.: Mast cells in areas of experimental bone resorption and remodeling. Br. J. Exp. Pathol. 50:17, 1969.
46. Camus, J.P., Prier, A., Lièvre, J.A., Stephan, J.C., and Laveant, C.: L'ostéoporose mastocytaire. Rev. Rhumat. 46:29, 1979.
47. Goldhaber, P.: Heparin enhancement of factors stimulating bone resorption in tissue culture. Science 147:407, 1965.
48. Griffith, G.C., Nichols, G., Jr., Asher, J.D., and Flanagan, B.: Heparin osteoporosis. JAMA 193:91, 1965.
49. Squires, J.W., and Pinch, L.W.: Heparin-induced spinal fractures. JAMA 241:2417, 1979.
50. Henderson, R.G., Russell, R.G.G., Earnshaw, M.J., Ledingham, J.G.G., Oliver, D.O., and Woods, C.G.: Loss of metacarpal and iliac bone in chronic renal failure: Influence of haemodialysis, parathyroid activity, type of renal disease, physical activity and heparin consumption. Clin. Sci. 56:317, 1979.
51. Mundy, G.R., Raisz, L.G., Cooper, R.A., Schechter, G.P., and Salmon, S.E.: Evidence for the secretion of an osteoclast stimulating factor in myeloma. N. Engl. J. Med. 21:1041, 1974.
52. Raisz, L.G., Luben, R.A., Mundy, G.R., Dietrich, J.W., Horton, J.E., and Trummel, C.L.: Effect of osteoclast activating factor from human leukocytes on bone metabolism. J. Clin. Invest. 56:408, 1975.
53. Krane, S.M., Brownell, G.L., Stanbury, J.B., and Corrigan, H.: The effect of thyroid disease on calcium metabolism in man. J. Clin. Invest. 35:874, 1956.
54. Mundy, G.R., Shapiro, J.L., Bandelin, J.G., Canalis, E.M., and Raisz, L.G.: Direct stimulation of bone resorption by thyroid hormones. J. Clin. J. Invest. 58:529, 1976.
55. Adinoff, A.D., and Hollister, J.R.: Steroid-induced fractures and bone loss in patients with asthma. N. Engl. J. Med. 309:265, 1983.
56. Hahn, T.J.: Corticosteroid-induced osteopenia. Arch. Intern. Med. 138:882, 1978.
57. Gluck, O.S., Murphy, W.A., Hahn, T.J., and Hahn, B.: Bone loss in adults receiving alternate day glucocorticoid therapy: A comparison with daily therapy. Arthritis Rheum. 24:892, 1981.
58. Chyun, Y.S., and Raisz, L.G.: Opposing effects of prostaglandin $E_2$ and cortisol on bone growth factor in organ culture. Clin. Res. 30:387A, 1982.
59. Suzuki, Y., Ichikawa, Y., Saito, E., and Homma, M.: Importance of increased urinary calcium excretion in the development of secondary hyperparathyroidism of patients under glucocorticoid therapy. Metabolism 32:151, 1983.
60. Klein, D.C., and Raisz, L.G.: Prostaglandin: Stimulation of bone resorption in tissue culture. Endocrinology 86:1436, 1970.
61. Tashjian, A.H., Jr., Voelkel, E.F., Levine, L., and Goldhaber, P.: Evidence that the bone resorption-stimulating factor produced by mouse fibrosarcoma cells is prostaglandin $E_2$: A new model for the hypercalcemia of cancer. J. Exp. Med. 136:1329, 1972.
62. Raisz, L.G., Sandberg, A., Goodson, J.M., Simmons, H.A., and Mergenhagen, S.E.: Complement-dependent stimulation of prostaglandin synthesis and bone resorption. Science 185:789, 1974.
63. Robinson, D.R., McGuire, M.B., and Levine, L.: Prostaglandins in the rheumatic diseases. Ann. N.Y. Acad. Sci. 256:318, 1975.
64. Raisz, L.G., and Kream, B.E.: Regulation of bone formation: N. Engl. J. Med. 309:29 (Part I), 309:83 (Part II), 1983.
65. Weidenreich, F.: Das Knochengewebe. *In* von Möllendorff, W. (ed.): Handbuch der mikroskopischen Anatomie des Menschen, Vol. 2. Berlin and New York, Springer-Verlag, 1930, p. 408.

66. Boyde, A., and Hobdell, M.H.: Scanning electron microscopy of lamellar bone. Z. Zellforsch. 93:213, 1969.
67. Dyson, E.D., Jackson, C.K., and Whitehouse, W.J.: Scanning electron microscope studies of human trabecular bone. Nature 225:957, 1970.
68. Cohen, J., and Harris, W.H.: The three-dimensional anatomy of haversian systems. J. Bone Joint Surg. 40A:419, 1958.
69. Boyde, A.: Scanning electron microscopic studies of bone. *In* Bourne, G.H. (ed.): The Biochemistry and Physiology of Bone, Vol. I. 2nd ed. New York, Academic Press, 1972, p. 259.
70. Kerley, E.R.: The Microscopic Determination of Age in Human Bone. University of Michigan, Ph.D. Anthropology, 1962.
71. Tischendorf, F.: Die mechanische Reaktion der haversschen Systeme und ihrer Lamellen auf experimentelle Belastung (nebst Bemerkungen zur Histogenese des lamellaren Knochengwebes). Wilhelm Roux Arch. Entwicklungsmechanik 146:661, 1954.
72. Ascenzi, A., and Bell, G.H.: Bone as a mechanical engineering problem. *In* Bourne, G.H. (ed.): The Biochemistry and Physiology of Bone, Vol. I. 2nd ed. New York, Academic Press, 1972, p. 311.
73. Wolff, J.: Das Gesetz der Transformation der Knochen. Berlin, Hirschwald, 1892.
74. Koch, J.C.: The laws of bone architecture. Am. J. Anat. 21:177, 1917.
75. Lacroix, P.: The internal remodeling of bones. *In* Bourne, G.H. (ed.): The Biochemistry and Physiology of Bone, Vol. III. 2nd ed. New York, Academic Press, 1972, p. 119.
76. Johnson, L.C.: Morphologic analysis in pathology: The kinetics of disease and general biology of bone. *In* Frost, H.M. (ed.): Bone Biodynamics. Boston, Little, Brown & Company, 1964, p. 543.
77. Pugliarello, M.C., Vittur, F., de Bernard, B., Bonucci, E., and Ascenzi, A.: Chemical modifications in osteones during calcification. Calc. Tissue Res. 5:108, 1970.
78. Miller, E.J., and Matukas, V.J.: Chick cartilage collagen: A new type of alpha-1 chain not present in bone or skin of the species. Proc. Natl. Acad. Sci. 64:1264, 1969.
79. Glimcher, M.J.: Studies of the structure, organization and reactivity of bone collagen. *In* Gibson, T. (ed.): Proceedings of the International Symposium on Wound Healing. Montreaux Found. Intern. Coop. Med. Sci., 1975, p. 253.
80. Pinnell, S.R., Fox, R., and Krane, S.M.: Human collagens: Differences in glycosylated hydroxylysines in skin and bone. Biochim. Biophys. Acta. 229:119, 1971.
81. Herring, G.M.: The chemical structure of tendon cartilage, dentin and bone matrix. Clin. Orthop. 60:261, 1968.
82. Castellani, A.A.: Protein-polysaccharides from ossifying cartilage and cornea. *In* Fitton-Jackson, S., Harkness, R.D., Partridge, S.M., and Tristram, G.R. (eds.): Structure and Function of Connective and Skeletal Tissue. London, Butterworths, 1965, p. 131.
83. Herring, G.M.: The organic matrix of bone. *In* Bourne, G.H. (ed.): The Biochemistry and Physiology of Bone, Vol. I. 2nd ed. New York, Academic Press, 1972, p. 127.
84. Shapiro, I.M., Wuthier, R.E., and Irving, J.T.: A study of the phospholipids of bovine dental tissues. I. Arch. Oral Biol. 11:501, 1966.
85. Posner, A.S.: Crystal chemistry of bone mineral. Physiol. Rev. 49:760, 1969.
86. Brown, W.E.: Crystal growth of bone mineral. Clin. Orthop. 44:205, 1966.
87. Vaughan, J.M.: Osteogenic cells. *In* The Physiology of Bone. Oxford, Oxford University Press, 1970, p. 110.
88. Glimcher, M.J., and Krane, S.M.: The organization and structure of bone and the mechanism of calcification. *In* Ramachandran, G.N., and Gould, B.S. (eds.): Treatise on Collagen, Vol. IIB, Biology of Collagen. New York, Academic Press, 1968, p. 68.
89. Baylink, D., Wergedal, J., and Thompson, E.: Loss of protein polysaccharides at sites where bone mineralization is initiated. J. Histochem. Cytochem. 20:279, 1972.
90. Anderson, H.C.: Vesicles associated with calcification in the matrix of epiphyseal cartilage. J. Cell Biol. 41:59, 1969.
91. Bonucci, E.: The locus of initial calcification in cartilage and bone. Clin. Orthop. 78:108, 1971.
92. Ali, S.Y., Sajdera, S.W., and Anderson, H.C.: Isolation and characterization of calcifying matrix vesicles from epiphyseal cartilage. Proc. Natl. Acad. Sci. 67:1513, 1970.
93. Glimcher, M.J.: Composition, structure and organization of bone and other mineralized tissues and the mechanism of calcification. Handbook of Physiology: Endocrinology, VII. Baltimore, Williams & Wilkins Company, 1976, p. 25.
94. Hodge, A.J., and Petruska, J.A.: Recent studies with the electron microscope on ordered aggregates of the tropocollagen macromolecule. *In* Ramachandran, G.N. (ed.): Aspects of Protein Structure. New York, Academic Press, 1963, p. 289.
95. Krane, S.M., Stone, M.J., Francois, C.J., and Glimcher, M.J.: Collagens and gelatins as phosphoryl acceptors for protein phosphokinase. Biochim. Biophys. Acta III:562, 1965.
96. Gallop, P.M., Lian, J.B., and Hauschka, P.Z.: Carboxylated calcium-binding proteins and vitamin K. N. Engl. J. Med. 302:1460, 1980.
97. Lian, J.B., Pachman, L.M., Gundberg, C.M., Partridge, R.E., and Maryjowski, M.C.: Gamma-carboxyglutamate excretion and calcinosis in juvenile dermatomyositis. Arthritis Rheum. 25:1094, 1982.
98. Gundberg, C.M., Lian, J.B., and Gallop, P.M.: Measurements of gamma-carboxyglutamate and circulating osteocalcin in normal children and adults. Clin. Chem. Acta 128:1, 1983.
99. Jowsey, J.: Microradiography: A morphologic approach to quantitating bone turnover. Excerpta Medica International Congress Series No. 270. Amsterdam, Excerpta Medica Foundation, 1972, p. 114.
100. Gardner, E.: Osteogenesis in the human embryo and fetus. *In* Bourne, G.H. (ed.): The Biochemistry and Physiology of Bone, Vol. III, 2nd ed. New York, Academic Press, 1972.
101. Sissons, A.: The growth of bone. *In* Bourne, G.H. (ed.) :The Biochemistry and Physiology of Bone, Vol. III. 2nd ed. New York, Academic Press, 1972.
102. Garn, S.M.: The course of bone gain and the phases of bone loss. Orthop. Clin. North Am. 3:503, 1972.
103. Cooper, R.R., and Misol, S.: Tendon and ligament insertion: A light and electron microscopic study. J. Bone Joint Surg. 52A:1, 1970.
104. Shim, S.S.: Physiology of blood circulation of bone. J. Bone Joint Surg. 50A:812, 1968.
105. Rhinelander, F.W.: Circulation of bone. *In* Bourne, G.H. (ed.): The Biochemistry and Physiology of Bone, Vol. II. 2nd ed. New York, Academic Press, 1972.
106. Sledge, C.B.: Epiphyseal injuries. *In* Cave, E.F., Burke, J.F. and Boyd, R.J. (eds): Trauma Management. Chicago, Year Book Medical Publishers, 1974.
107. Trueta, J.: Studies of the Development and Decay of the Human Frame. Philadelphia, W.B. Saunders Company, 1968.
108. Reifenstein, E.C., Jr.: Definitions, terminology and classification of metabolic bone disorders. Clin. Orthop. 9:30, 1957.
109. Shimmins, J., Anderson, J.B., Smith, D.A., and Aitken, M.: The accuracy and reproducibility of bone mineral measurements "in vivo." Clin. Radiol. 23:42, 1972.
110. Donaldson, C.L., Hulley, S.B., Vogel, J.M., Hattner, R.S., Bayers, J.H., and McMillan, D.E.: Effect of prolonged bedrest on bone mineral. Metabolism 19:1071, 1970.
111. Mack, P.B., LaChance, P.A., Vose, G.P., and Vogt, F.B.: Bone demineralization of foot and hand of Gemini-Titan IV, V, and VII astronauts during orbital flight. Am. J. Roentgenol. Rad. Ther. Nucl. Med. 100:503, 1967.
112. Barnett, E., and Nordin, B.E.C.: The radiological diagnosis of osteoporosis: A new approach. Clin. Radiol. 11:166, 1960.
113. Meema, H.E.: Cortical bone atrophy and osteoporosis as a manifestation of aging. Am. J. Roentgenol. Rad. Ther. Nucl. Med. 89:1287, 1963.
114. Meema, H.E., and Meema, S.: Prevention of postmenopausal osteoporosis by hormone treatment of the menopause. Can. Med. Assoc. J. 99:248, 1968.
115. Jowsey, J.: Metabolic Diseases of Bone. Philadelphia, W.B. Saunders Company, 1977, p. 45.
116. Wakamatsu, E., and Sissons, H.A.: The cancellous bone of the iliac crest. Calcif. Tissue Res. 4:147, 1969.
117. Singh, M., Riggs, B.L., Beabout, J.W., and Jowsey, J.: Femoral trabecular pattern index for evaluation of spinal osteoporosis: A detailed methodologic description. Mayo Clin. Proc. 48:184, 1973.
118. Heaney, R.P., and Whedon, G.D.: Radiocalcium studies of bone formation rate in human metabolic bone disease. J. Clin. Endocrinol. Metabol. 18:1246, 1958.
119. Neer, R., Berman, M., Fisher, L., and Rosenberg, L.E.: Multicompartmental analysis of calcium kinetics in normal adult males. J. Clin. Invest. 46:1364, 1967.
120. Marshall, J.H.: Measurements and models of skeletal metabolism. *In* Comar, C.L., and Bronner, F. (eds.): Mineral Metabolism, Vol. III. New York, Academic Press, 1969.
121. Cohn, S.H., Shukla, K.K., Dombrowski, C.S., and Fairchild, R.G.: Design and calibration of a "broad-beam" $^{238}$Pu, Be neutron source for total body neutron activation analysis. J. Nucl. Med. 13:487, 1972.
122. Aloia, J.F., Ellis, K., Zanzi, I., and Cohn, S.H.: Photon absorptimetry and skeletal mass in the treatment of osteoporosis. J. Nucl. Med. 16:196, 1975.
123. Goldsmith, N.E., Johnston, J.O., Ury, H., Vose, G., and Colbert, C.: Bone mineral estimation in normal and osteoporotic women: A comparability trial of four methods and seven bone sites. J. Bone Joint Surg. 53A:83, 1971.
124. Cameron, J.R., and Sorenson, J.: Measurement of bone mineral in vivo: An improved method. Science 142:230, 1963.
125. Hansson, T.H., Ross, R.O., and Nachemson, A.: Development of osteopenia in the fourth lumbar vertebra during prolonged bed rest after operation for scoliosis. Acta Orthop. Scand. 46:621, 1975.

126. Genant, H.K., and Body, D.: Quantitative bone mineral analysis using dual energy computed tomography. Invest. Radiol. 12:545, 1977.
127. Genant, H.K., Turski, P.A., and Moss, A.A.: Advances in CT assessment of metabolic and endocrine disorders. Adv. Intern. Med. 28:409, 1983.
128. Krane, S.M., Munoz, A.J., and Harris, E.D., Jr.: Urinary polypeptides related to collagen synthesis. J. Clin. Invest. 49:716, 1970.
129. Nagant de Deuxchaisnes, C., and Krane, S.M.: The treatment of adult phosphate diabetes and Fanconi syndrome with neutral sodium phosphate. Am. J. Med. 43:508, 1967.
130. Chalmers, J., Conacher, W.D.H., Gardner, D.L., and Scott, P.: Osteomalacia—a common disease in elderly women. J. Bone Joint Surg. 49B:403, 1967.
131. Jowsey, J., Kelly, P.J., Riggs, B.L., Bianco, A.J., Scholz, D.A., and Gershon-Cohen, J.: Quantitative microradiographic studies of normal and osteoporotic bone. J. Bone Joint Surg. 47A:785, 1965.
132. Byers, P.D.: The diagnostic value of bone biopsies. *In* Avioli, L.V., and Krane, S.M. (eds.): Metabolic Bone Disease, Vol. I. New York, Academic Press, 1977.
133. Dequeker, J., and Johnston, C.C., Jr.: Non-invasive Bone Measurements: Methodological Problems, Oxford, Eng., Wash. D.C., IRL Press, 1982.

# Chapter 18

# Structure and Function of the Motor Unit

*Walter G. Bradley and Paul F. Good*

## INTRODUCTION

The function of the muscles is to produce force and movement. Their structure and biochemistry are intimately directed to this end, and the control of their activity is achieved through the motor nerves. This chapter provides a brief outline of current knowledge of neuromuscular function.

## ANATOMY

The motor unit is the functional unit of striated muscle activity. It consists of an alpha motoneuron in the anterior horn of the spinal cord or the motor nuclei of the brainstem, its peripheral axon, and the muscle fibers on which it synapses. The number of muscle fibers in a motor unit ranges from the tens in the extraocular muscles to the thousands in the large proximal limb muscles. The domain of one motor unit is intermingled with the domains of other units and covers an area of 5 to 10 mm in transverse section. Motor units are of three distinct functional and biochemical types: slow twitch (S, type 1), fast twitch, fatigue resistant (FR, type 2A), and fast twitch, easily fatigued (FF, type 2B). The slow twitch fibers rely predominantly on mitochondrial oxidative metabolism for energy production. They have slower rates of contraction and relaxation, and their motoneuron fires more tonically than in type 2 units. The FF (type 2B) fibers rely predominantly on glycolysis and intracellular stores of glycogen for energy supply, fire phasically in short bursts, and are rapidly fatigued. The type 2A fibers are fast-contracting fibers and have both high glycolytic and high mitochondrial activity; they are thus fatigue resistant. Though it is standard to teach that slow motor units are used for maintaining posture and that fast motor units are used for rapid movements, recent evidence indicates that in man this distinction is less than absolute.

The myosin ATPase, which is responsible for the transduction of biochemical energy to contractile force, is different in type 1 and type 2 fibers with regard to pH optima and stability. These differences form the basis of the myosin ATPase stains used for the histochemical typing of muscle fibers.

A single muscle *fiber* (Fig. 18–1) is the cellular unit of the muscle. Each fiber is a syncytium of postmitotic myoblasts. Each fiber has a basal lamina which surrounds it and is bound together with other fibers into bundles of *fascicles* by a thin layer of collagen, the *endomysium.* Thicker sheets of collagen, the *perimysium,* bind fascicles together and surround the entire muscle (*epimysium*). The muscle fibers can course the entire length of a muscle (up to 34 cm in the human sartorius muscle) or can insert laterally into tendons (pennate muscles) or, rarely, can make muscle-muscle attachments. Muscle fibers vary in diameter from 10 to 100 $\mu$m, with a mean diameter in normal muscle of about 50 $\mu$m. The collagen of the tendon (or other connective tissue) is physically attached to the basal lamina of the muscle fiber. Muscle is invested with a capillary bed, intramuscular nerves, and a specialized sensory organ, the *spindle,* composed of 4 to 12 *intrafusal* muscle fibers and associated with $\gamma$ motor and sensory nerve fibers.

The extrafusal muscle fibers contain up to thousands of postmitotic nuclei, which were the original nuclei of the mononucleated myoblasts. They are oriented longitudinally beneath the muscle fiber plasma membrane (the *sarcolemma*) and are called sarcolemmal nuclei.

## CONTRACTILE PROTEINS

The predominant constituents (about 75 percent) of the muscle fiber cytoplasm (*sarcoplasm*) are the myofibrils, which consist predominantly of the contractile proteins, actin and myosin.

*Actin* (Figure 18-2) is a globular single-chain protein

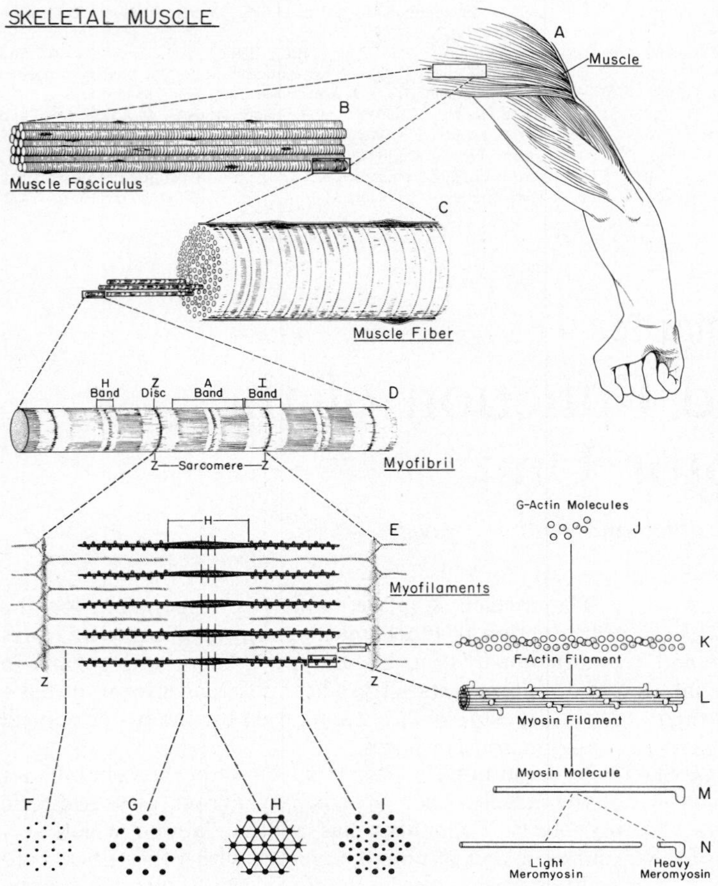


**Figure 18–1.** Diagram of the organization of skeletal muscle from the gross to the molecular level. *F, G, H,* and *I* are cross sections of the levels indicated. (From Bloom, W., and Fawcett, D.W.: A Textbook of Histology. 10th ed. Philadelphia, W. B. Saunders Co., 1975.)

(G-actin) with a molecular weight of about 42,000 daltons and a diameter of 5.5 nm. It will polymerize into a double-stranded helical filament (F-actin). This helix has a half pitch or repeating distance of 38.5 nm. Each molecule of G-actin can bind to the head of a myosin molecule. Associated with each strand of F-actin is one molecule of *tropomyosin* extending along seven molecules of G-actin and one molecule of *troponin* at the end of each tropomyosin molecule. These are regulatory proteins involved in the control of muscular contraction and relaxation.

*Myosin* (Fig. 18–3) is a large, elongated molecule of about 460,000 daltons. It is about 160 nm long with a globular head at one end. It is composed of two identical heavy chains that are predominantly $\alpha$ helical and are supercoiled around each other. At one end, the heavy chains are folded into globular structures, which, along with four light chains, form the head. The myosin mol-

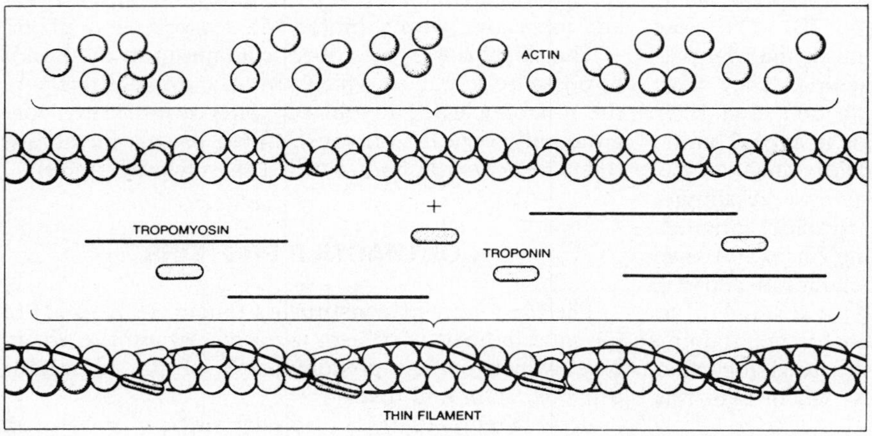


**Figure 18–2.** A thin filament contains actin, tropomyosin, and troponin molecules, assembled as shown schematically here. The spherical actin molecules are arranged like a double string of beads twisted to form a helix. A tropomyosin molecule extends along seven actin molecules, and there is one troponin molecule near the end of each tropomyosin. (From Murray, J.M., and Weber, A.: The cooperative action of muscle proteins. Copyright © 1974 by Scientific American, Inc. All rights reserved.)
batch 18 p. 288

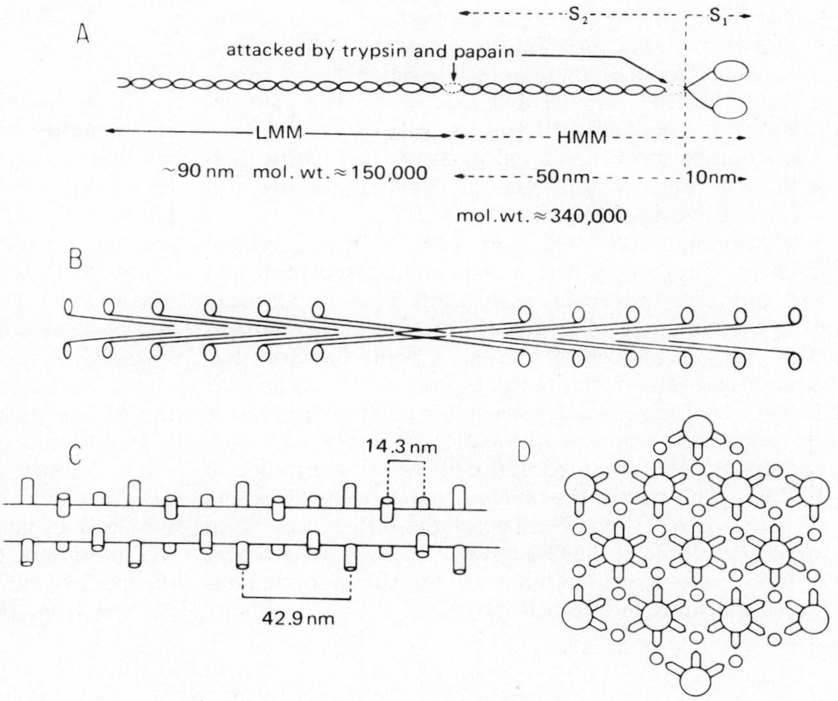


**Figure 18–3.** *A,* A diagram of the myosin molecule with its two identical sub-units. The enzyme trypsin preferentially cleaves the molecule in two between the parts labeled as heavy meromyosin (HMM) and light meromyosin (LMM) because of their relative molecular weights. Further enzymatic digestion of HMM produces subfragments $S_1$ and $S_2$. *B,* A diagram showing the arrangement of myosin molecules in a filament. The heads of the molecules are oriented towards the two ends, while the tails of the molecules are oriented towards the center. *C,* X-ray diffraction patterns indicate that the filament in part *B* is twisted into a helix with a spacing of about 43 nm. The heads of the myosin molecules, here indicated by pegs, would then be spaced just above 14 nm apart and rotated 120 degrees from each other. *D,* Cross-sectional diagram showing that over a distance of 43 nm crossbridges from each thick filament will project toward all six neighboring thin filaments in the hexagonal array. (From Stein, R.B.: Nerve and Muscle: Membranes, Cells, and Systems. New York, Plenum Press, 1980.)
p. 289

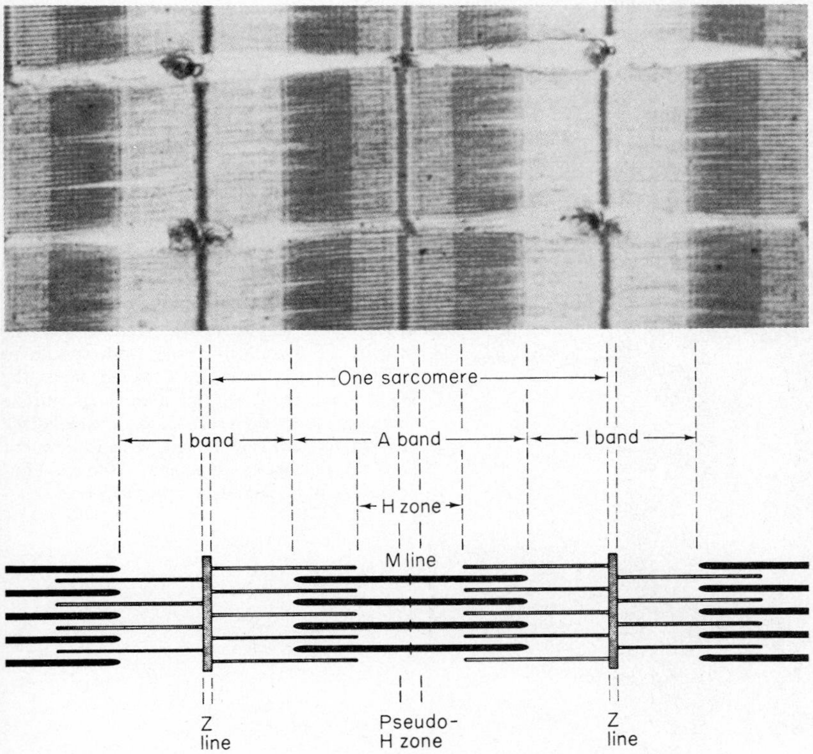


**Figure 18–4.** Longitudinal section of frog sartorius muscle (top) together with diagram showing the overlap of filaments that gives rise to the band pattern. The A band is most dense in its lateral zones, where the thick and thin filaments overlap. The central zone of the A band (the H zone) is less dense, since it contains thick filaments only. The I bands are less dense still because they contain only thin filaments. The sarcomere length here is about 2.5μm. (From Huxley, H.E.: Molecular basis of contraction in cross striated muscle. *In,* The Structure and Function of Muscle. Vol. 1. Bourne, G.H.: New York, Academic Press, 1972.)
p. 289

ecule can be split by trypsin into a part containing about 96 nm of the tail, called light meromyosin (LMM), and the remainder, including the head, called heavy meromyosin (HMM). The HMM can be further split by papain into the head ($S_1$) and the rest of the tail ($S_2$). The subunits form functional parts of the myosin molecule. The myosin head has the enzymatic activity of ATPase (myosin ATPase).

Myosin molecules will aggregate to form a myosin filament. They begin with a tail-to-tail association and add additional molecules with heads all pointing away from the initiation point, toward the end of the filament (Fig. 18–3). This central initiation point therefore has no myosin heads (forming the M line, described below). The myosin filament is constructed so that myosin heads are paired on opposite sides of a filament and each additional pair is rotated 120 degrees, at a distance of 14.3 nm. This causes the repeat distance to be three sets of pairs, or 42.9 nm. Neither of these distances is an integral multiple of the G-actin size or the F-actin repeat distance, which has significance for the smooth contraction of muscle (see below).

## ULTRASTRUCTURE OF THE MUSCLE FIBER

The contractile filaments are bound together in parallel bundles to form a *myofibril.* The actin filaments are bound together at the *Z line* and interdigitate in a hexagonal pattern with the myosin filaments, which are bound together at their central zone (the *M line*). The area from one Z line to the next, a *sarcomere* (Figs. 18–1 and 18–4), is composed of the region of actin filaments alone (the *I* [*isotropic*] *band,* which is about 1 μm at rest), the region of myosin filaments with or without interdigitating actin (the *A* [anisotropic] *band,* which is about 1.6 μm at rest), and the region on either side of the M line with no actin (*the H zone*).

In addition to the contractile proteins there are two sets of tubules running among the myofibrils (Fig. 18–5). There is a transverse system (the *T tubules*). Each T tubule is an invagination of sarcolemma, which runs to the interior of the fiber at the A-I band junction. The other set of tubules, the *sarcoplasmic reticulum* (SR), is derived from the cellular endoplasmic reticulum. The

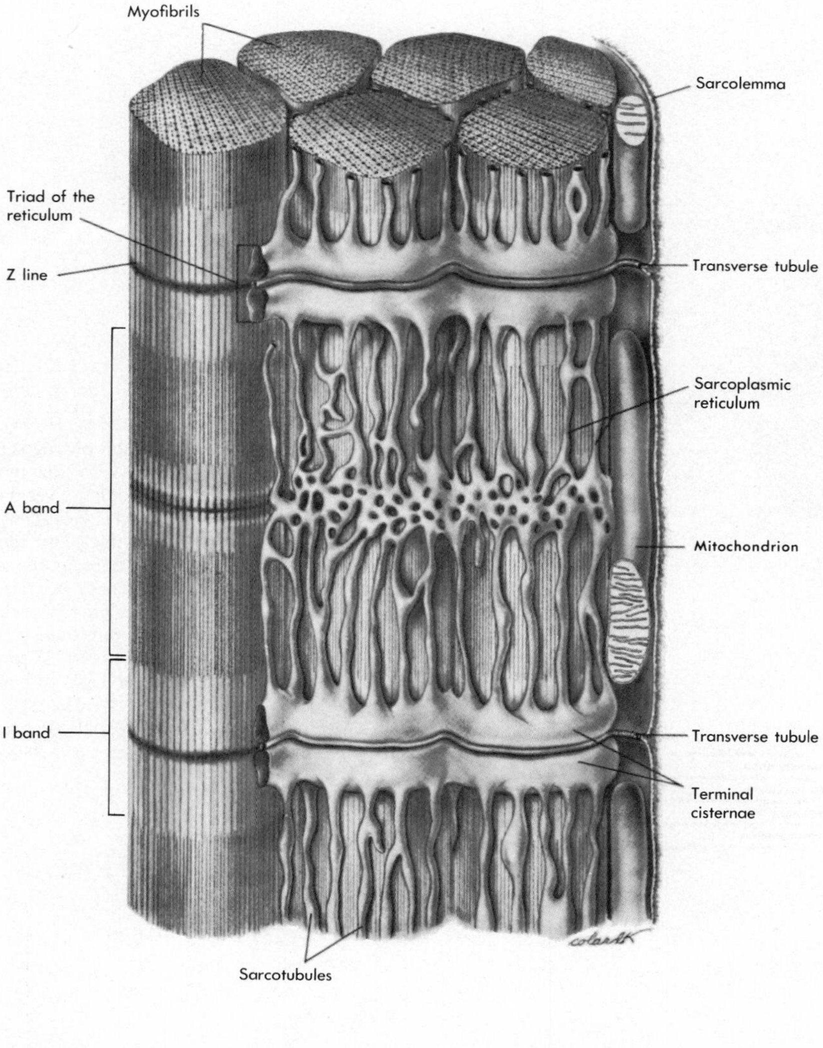


**Figure 18–5.** Schematic representation of the distribution of the sarcoplasmic reticulum around the myofibrils of skeletal muscle. The longitudinal sarcotubules are confluent with transverse elements called the terminal cisternae. A slender transverse tubule (T tubule) extending inward from the sarcolemma is flanked by two terminal cisternae to form the so-called triads of the reticulum. The location of these with respect to the cross banded pattern of the myofibrils varies from species to species. In frog muscle, depicted here, the triads are at the Z line. In mammalian muscle there are two to each sarcomere, located at the A-I junctions. (From Bloom, W., and Fawcett, D.W., A Textbook of Histology. 10th ed., Philadelphia, W.B. Saunders Co., 1975.)

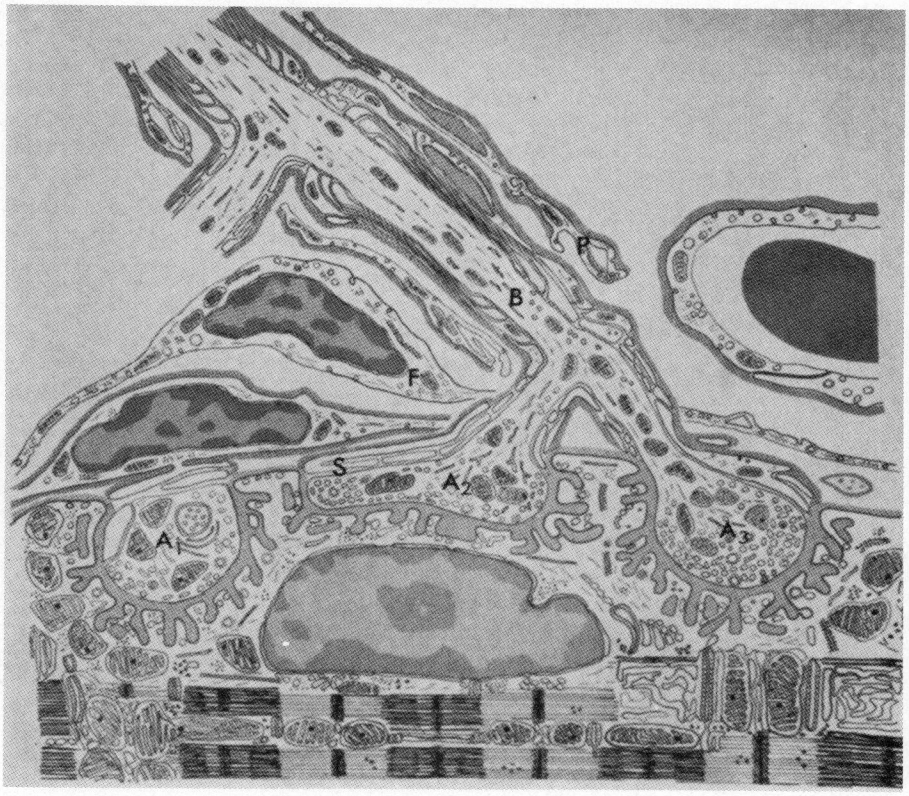


**Figure 18–6.** Vertebrate neuromuscular junction showing relationship of axon (*B*) and axon terminals ($A_1$, $A_2$, $A_3$) with Schwann cells (*S*) and perineural cells (*P*). Fibrocyte (*F*) lies adjacent to a Schwann cell. Basement lamina covering the muscle fiber and within the subneurial clefts is indicated by dots and Schwann cell basement lamina by crosshatching. Note presence of mitochondria, coated vesicles, and synaptic vesicles in all terminals. (From Hubbard, J.I.: Microphysiology of vertebrate neuromuscular transmission. Physiol. Rev. 53:674, 1973.)

SR runs essentially longitudinally, surrounds the myofibrils, and abuts the T tubules in a specialized structure, the *triad.* Also among the myofibrils are mitochondria, glycogen granules, lipid droplets, etc.

## THE NEUROMUSCULAR JUNCTION

The sarcolemma has a specialization at the location of the motoneuron axon terminal, the *motor endplate* (Fig. 18–6). This is a complex folding of the sarcolemma into the *primary synaptic cleft,* which conforms to the axon surface and from which project the *secondary synaptic clefts.* On the apex of each fold between the secondary synaptic clefts lie the *acetylcholine receptors (AChR),* which are proteins embedded in the plasma membrane. These AChR bind acetylcholine (ACh), the neurotransmitter of the neuromuscular junction.

Approximately 1 to 1.5 μm from the neuromuscular junction the nerve fiber loses its perineurial sheath, and the myelin is lost from the Schwann cell as well. A thin layer of Schwann cell cytoplasm continues until it meets the sarcolemma, where its basal lamina fuses with that of the muscle fiber. This fused basal lamina continues between the axon terminal and the sarcolemma. There is a 40- to 60-nm gap between the axon and the muscle fiber, the *synaptic gap.* Bound to the basal lamina of the synaptic gap is the enzyme *acetylcholinesterase (AChE),* which hydrolyzes the transmitter ACh.

The axon terminal contains unit membrane–bound *synaptic vesicles,* 40 to 50 nm in diameter, containing ACh, large coated vesicles about 100 nm in diameter, mitochondria, neurotubules, and neurofilaments.

## PHYSIOLOGY OF THE MOTOR UNIT

The internal and external environments of nerve and muscle cells are quite different. Internally the concentration of potassium is high, and there is an electrical potential or voltage difference (polarization) of 70 to 90 mV negative with respect to the outside. Externally there is a high concentration of sodium, chloride, and calcium with respect to the inside. The resting potential (−70 mV) corresponds to the potassium equilibrium potential, since the cell membrane is freely permeable to potassium ion. The positive external potential resists the tendency for the potassium ion to flow outward toward its chemical equilibrium point. The resting membrane potential is created and maintained by the presence internally of large impermeable negative ions and the sodium pump, which extrudes sodium from the cell.

The sarcolemma contains voltage-dependent sodium channels, which run from the outside of the sarcolemma to the inside. At rest these are mainly closed (i.e., there is only a small resting permeability to sodium). A small depolarization opens some channels, increasing the sodium permeability, and thus tending to increase the depolarization. Below a threshold (about 20 to 30 mV) of depolarization this influx will be balanced by the efflux of the much more highly permeable potassium ion. At the *critical membrane depolarization potential* (that potential required to generate an action potential), the inward sodium current becomes regenerative, opening all the sodium channels, leading to depolarization of the sarcolemma to the sodium equilibrium potential of 20 mV positive internally. The sodium channels have an active closure mechanism, which terminates the influx of sodium. Repolarization is achieved by the opening of separate potassium channels, which allow the potassium ions to flow outward, restoring the resting membrane potential. The sodium is extruded by the sodium pump.

In the motoneuron the action potential is initiated in the cell body and propagated down the axon to the axon terminal. There the action potential opens specific calcium channels, which allow the entry into the axon terminal of calcium ions. The increase in intraterminal calcium concentration initiates release of the synaptic vesicles containing ACh. ACh is synthesized by the acetylation of choline by acetylcoenzyme A catalyzed by choline acetyltransferase (ChAT). There are about $10^4$ molecules of ACh in each synaptic vesicle. Random events will allow the occasional discharge of one synaptic vesicle of ACh (*one quantum*). The ACh diffuses across the synaptic gap and binds to the AChR on the motor endplate membrane. This binding changes the physical conformation of the receptor and opens an ion channel permeable to sodium and other ions. Subsequently, the ACh is released from the receptor and hydrolyzed by AChE in the synaptic gap into choline and acetate. The choline is then taken up by the axonal terminal and synthesized to acetylcholine.

The depolarization of the motor endplate produced by one quantum of ACh (*miniature endplate potential*) is about 0.5 mV. The action potential reaching the axon terminal causes the release of 100 to 300 synaptic vesicles into the synaptic gap. This will depolarize the postsynaptic muscle membrane by about 50 mV, which is greater than the critical depolarization potential of the muscle membrane.

## EXCITATION-CONTRACTION COUPLING

Activation of the muscle contractile mechanism is achieved by the propagation of an action potential along the muscle fiber and into the T-tubule system. The depolarization of the T-tubules induces the release of calcium ion from the SR into the sarcoplasm. The mechanism is not completely understood, but the coupling between the T-tubules and SR is mediated either by depolarization of the SR or, more likely, by influx of calcium from the extracellular to the intracellular space at the T-tubules, which induces further release of calcium from the SR (calcium-mediated calcium release).

The increased sarcoplasmic calcium binds to the troponin molecule on the actin filament, exposing the binding site on the G-actin monomer for the head of the myosin molecule. This process, from T-tubule depolarization to contraction, is termed *excitation-contraction coupling*.

## THE BIOCHEMISTRY OF CONTRACTION

In the resting state (Fig. 18–7) the myosin head has a molecule of ATP bound to it. The entry of calcium into the sarcoplasm from the longitudinal sarcoplasm reticulum produces a calcium-troponin complex, the formation of which exposes the actin binding site and pro-

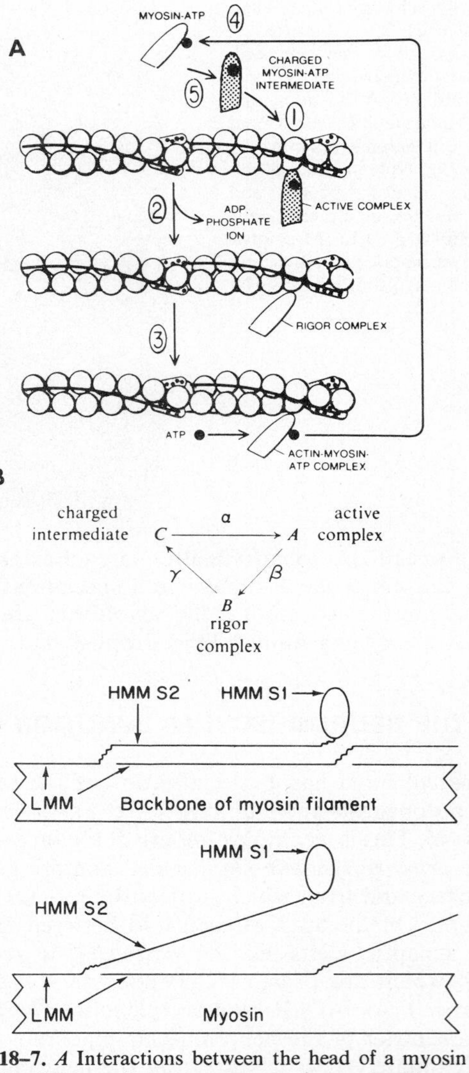


**Figure 18–7.** *A* Interactions between the head of a myosin molecule and a thin filament during one contraction cycle. The parts of the cycle are numbered and described in more detail in the text. *B*, For analysis of the overall kinetics of the cycle, it can be simplified, perhaps to as few as three rate-limiting steps. (From Stien, R. B. Nerve and Muscle: Membranes, Cells and Systems. New York, Plenum Press, 1980.), *C* Suggested behavior of myosin molecules in the thick filaments. The light meromyosin (LMM) of the molecule is bonded into the backbone of the filament, while the linear portion of the heavy meromyosin (HMM) component can tilt further out from the filament (by bending at the HMM–LMM junction), allowing the globular part of HMM (that is, the SI fragment) to attach to actin over a range of different side spacings while maintaining the same orientation. (From Huxley, H.E.: Molecular basis of contraction in cross striated muscle. *In* Bourne, G.H. (ed.): The Structure and Function of Muscle. Vol. 1. New York, Academic Press, 1972.)

duces an activated actin-myosin-ATP complex. The myosin molecule is bent away from the myosin filament at the HMM-LMM junction to reach the actin filament and achieve this binding. The myosin ATPase of the myosin head cleaves the ATP, yielding energy that rotates the myosin head about the $S_1$-$S_2$ junction. This moves the actin and myosin relative to one another (*sliding filaments*), producing muscle contraction. Dissociation from the myosin head of ADP and inorganic phosphate produces the low energy *rigor complex* (also found in rigor mortis). The binding of a molecule of ATP allows the dissociation of actin and myosin and the spontaneous return of the myosin head to its resting position. If calcium ions remain in high concentration in the sarcoplasm from repeated muscle action potentials, the actin and myosin filaments continue to slide past each other, producing further muscle contraction. The previously discussed lack of matching between the repeat distances of the action and myosin monomers allows a continuous application of force rather than a saltatory effect, which would result from the cross-bridges all lining up and rotating together.

The nerve and muscle action potentials can arrive at a higher frequency than the contraction cycling of actin-myosin, allowing a continuous contraction of the muscle fibers.

ATP-dependent reabsorption of sarcoplasmic calcium ions into the longitudinal SR occurs when the muscle action potentials cease. This allows regenerated ATP to remain bound to the myosin heads and removes the trigger for activation of actin and myosin. The tension produced by sliding of the filaments is removed, and the filaments return to their preactivated position. Thus, relaxation as well as contraction is an energy-dependent process.

## MUSCLE ENERGY METABOLISM

The high energy compound ATP is replenished by the transfer of high-energy phosphate to ADP from *creatine phosphate*. This transfer is catalyzed by the enzyme *creatine kinase (CK)*. Rapid muscle contraction, as in sprinting, depends on the *glycolytic pathway* for the anaerobic production of ATP by conversion of glycogen to lactate (see Fig. 18–8). More sustained exertion depends on the oxidative metabolism initially of pyruvate produced by glycolysis (see Fig. 18–8), and later of *free fatty acids* derived from lipid droplets in the muscle fibers and fat depots of the body (see Fig. 18–9). Long-chain fatty acids cannot enter mitochondria. They must first be activated to fatty acylcoenzyme A, which is then converted to fatty acylcarnitine by carnitine palmityl transferase. The fatty acylcarnitine then enters the mitochondria and is reconverted to fatty acylcoenzyme A. It is then subject to beta oxidation for the production of ATP via the Krebs cycle and the mitochondrial electron transport chain.

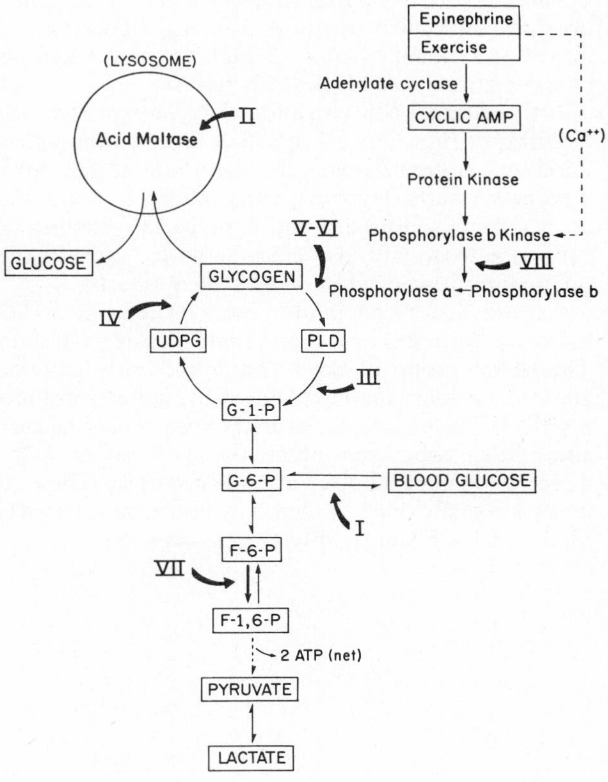


**Figure 18–8.** Scheme of glycogen metabolism and glycolysis. Roman numerals refer to glycogen storage diseases and indicate the sites of metabolic block due to deficiency of the following enzymes: I, glucose-6-phosphatase; II, acid maltase; III, debrancher; IV, brancher; V, muscle phosphorylase; VI, liver phosphorylase; VII, muscle phosphofructokinase; VIII, liver dephosphophosphorylase kinase (G-1-P—glucose-1-phosphate; G-6P—glucose-6-phosphate; F-6-P—fructose-6-phosphate; F-1, 6-P—fructose-1, 6-diphosphate; UDPG—uridine diphosphate-glucose; PLD—phosphorylase limit dextrin). (From DiMauro, S.D., Metabolic myopathies. *In* Vinken, P.J., and Bruyn, G.W. (eds.): Handbook of Clinical Neurology. Vol. 41. North-Holland Publishing Co., Amsterdam, 1979.)

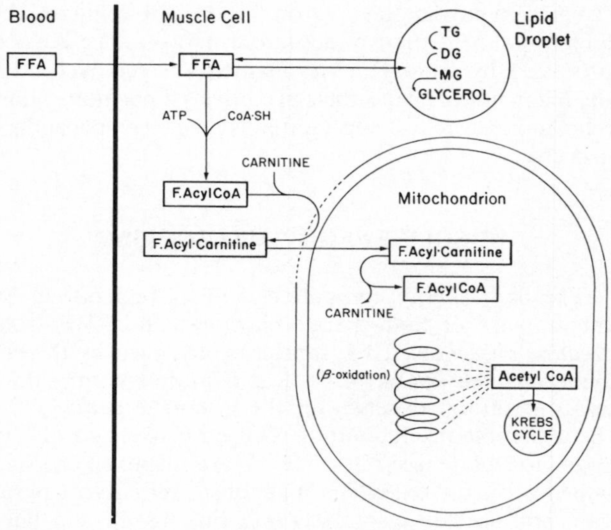


**Figure 18–9.** Scheme of intracellular long-chain fatty acid metabolism (FAA—free fatty acids; TG—triglyceride; DG—diglyceride; MG—monoglyceride). (From DiMauro, S.D.: Metabolic Myopathies. *In* Vinke, P.J., and Bruyn, G.W. (eds.); Handbook of Clinical Neurology. Vol. 41. North-Holland Publishing Co., Amsterdam, 1979.)

## THE PHARMACOLOGY OF THE MOTOR UNIT

The nerve and muscle membranes are extremely sensitive to external ionic concentrations. As mentioned previously, ACh release requires external calcium as does excitation-contraction coupling. Therefore, removal of external calcium or high external magnesium concentrations will block ACh release.

If the external concentration of potassium falls below 2.5 mEq or rises above 7 mEq per liter, action potential initiation and conduction are compromised and muscle weakness results. Hypercalcemia (above 12 mg per ml), as in vitamin D intoxication, hyperparathyroidism, and carcinomatosis, will also cause lethargy and weakness, due mainly to central nervous system effects.

Certain drugs can inhibit the synthesis of ACh by blocking the uptake of choline into the nerve terminal. The major group of these compounds are quaternary ammonium ions, the best known being hemicholinium-3 (HC-3). They compete with choline for choline carrier sites. Other drugs can inhibit the synthesis of ACh by directly blocking choline acetyltransferase. These generally are analogs of choline or acetylcoenzymes, which bind to ChAT and modify the enzyme.

There are many animal venoms and toxins that have their effect on the nerve terminal as well as on the postsynaptic membrane (see below). The release of ACh is blocked by botulinum toxin, probably by reduction of the sensitivity of the ACh release mechanism to intracellular calcium. Beta-bungarotoxin has an effect similar to botulinum toxin. The venom of the black widow spider produces paralysis by causing the uncontrolled release of all the synaptic vesicles into the synaptic gap. Puffer fish toxin (tetrodotoxin) and paralytic shellfish poison (saxitoxin) selectively block sodium channels in nerve and muscle membranes, abolishing excitability. Local anesthetic drugs such as procaine and lidocaine block both sodium and potassium channels.

Other drugs act on the postsynaptic muscle membrane. Compounds such as decamethonium and succinylcholine depolarize the membrane by binding to the AChR, opening the ion channel, but are not hydrolyzed by AChE. Curarelike drugs and the α-bungarotoxin (cf. above) fraction of the venom of the Taiwan multibanded krait (*Bungarus multicinctus*) bind to the AChR without depolarization, thus preventing acetylcholine from binding and initiating an endplate potential.

In myasthenia gravis the body has produced immune antibodies against the acetylcholine receptor, which attack it and vastly reduce the number of receptors available for binding ACh. This large loss of ion channels diminishes the muscle's ability to produce an endplate potential, leading to rapid fatigability and weakness. *Anticholinesterases* such as neostigmine (Prostigmin), pyridostigmine (Mestinon), edrophonium (Tensilon), physostigmine (Eserine), as well as some "nerve gases" and organophosphorus insecticides, allow the accumulation of acetylcholine and therefore the increased function of the remaining AChR, partially reversing the effects of the lost AChR. In the healthy individual these lead to paralysis by continuous depolarization of the muscle membrane by nonhydrolysis of acetylcholine.

### References

1. Katz, B.: Nerve, Muscle and Synapse. New York, McGraw Hill, 1966.
2. Bourne, G.H. (ed.): The Structure and Function of Muscle. New York, Academic Press, 1972.
3. Stein, R.B.: Nerve and Muscle: Membranes, Cells and Systems. New York, Plenum Press, 1980.
4. Hubbard, J.I.: Microphysiology of vertebrate neuromuscular transmission. Physiol. Rev. 53:674, 1973.
5. Pepe, R.A., Sanger, J.W., and Nachmias, V.T. (eds.): Motility in Cell Function. New York, Academic Press, 1979.
6. Squire, J.: The Structural Basis of Muscular Contraction. New York, Plenum Press, 1981.
7. Bowman, W.C.: Pharmacology of Neuromuscular Function. Baltimore, University Park Press, 1980.

# Chapter 19

# Peripheral Nerve: Structure, Function, and Dysfunction

*John E. Castaldo and José Ochoa*

## INTRODUCTION

Disorders of the nerve fiber may affect the peripheral motor, sensory, or autonomic units in various combinations to produce muscle weakness, atrophy, skin numbness, paresthesias, pain, or dysautonomia. The specific constellation of symptoms and signs, and the tempo of evolution of neural dysfunction, judiciously interpreted in the light of nerve pathophysiology, provide useful preliminary evidence on the kind of pathology and the types of nerve fibers affected. Clinical electrophysiology sharpens detection of subclinical damage while clarifying the kind of primary nerve fiber pathology and its extent, if diffuse, as well as its precise location, if focal. Finally, neuromuscular biopsy endorses the indirect clinical and neurophysiological criteria for the type of fiber affected and the kind of nerve fiber pathology while potentially disclosing an etiology. What follows is an attempt to correlate normal and abnormal structure and function of peripheral nerve in order to optimize the clinical evaluation, diagnosis, and early treatment of peripheral neuropathy.

## GENERAL ORGANIZATION OF THE PERIPHERAL NERVOUS SYSTEM

The peripheral nervous system is functionally organized into sensory, motor, and autonomic components. *Motor* nerve fibers emerge from anterior horn cell bodies in the spinal cord and from analogous brainstem nuclei. They exit via specific cranial nerves and anterior roots in the spinal cord to innervate extrafusal and intrafusal striated muscle fibers. The cell bodies of bipolar primary *sensory* neurons reside in dorsal root or cranial nerve ganglia. Sensory neurons give rise to fibers that innervate sensory receptors in skin, muscle, and deep tissues. Preganglionic sympathetic *autonomic* nerve cell bodies reside in the intermediolateral gray columns of the thoracic and first and second lumbar segments of the spinal cord. Preganglionic fibers emerge with ventral roots and enter the sympathetic chain as white rami to synapse with multipolar sympathetic ganglion cells. These neurons then give rise to postganglionic unmyelinated axons, which emerge from the ganglia as gray rami and innervate sweat glands and smooth muscle of blood vessels, hair, and other effector organs. Preganglionic neurons of the parasympathetic system reside in the brainstem, integrating functions of cranial nerves III, VII, IX, and X and in the S2 through S4 segments of the spinal cord. Axons from these cell bodies synapse in ganglia in close proximity to the smooth muscle, heart muscle, and glandular tissue they innervate.

## GROSS STRUCTURE OF NERVE TRUNKS

Nerve trunks are composed of groups of macroscopic nerve fascicles bound together in a connective epineurial sheath. Within a laminated cellular perineurium, fascicles contain microscopic myelinated and unmyelinated fibers suspended amid collagen, at pressures of 0.4 to 2.9 mm Hg[1,2] (Fig. 19–1). Polygonal perineurial cells, linked by tight junctions and layered in concentric sleeves, constitute the major diffusion barrier within nerve.[3-5] This structure is instrumental in protecting the endoneurial fascicular contents from microorganisms and macromolecular substances, in particular, toxins and antigens.[6] While perineurial permeability may be altered in mechanical crush injuries to nerve, it is remarkably resistant to ischemia[7] and to mediators of the inflammatory response. Perineurium is also an effective barrier to pus cells, even when it is contiguous to tissue abscesses.[8]

Peripheral nerves are abundantly vascularized throughout their length by a widely anastomotic network of longitudinal and segmental arteries.[9,10] Nutrient arteries penetrate perineurium and form an endoneurial plexus composed largely of capillaries, which supply longitudinal segments of nerves. Small vessel occlusive disease with resultant damage to peripheral nerve most commonly occurs at the level of the epineurial arterioles and may occur in conjunction with a number of systemic diseases, including diabetes, polyarteritis, rheumatoid arthritis (RA), and systemic lupus erythematosus (SLE) as well as the cryoglobulinemic states. Intrafascicular capillaries are the site of the blood-nerve barrier (Fig. 19–2). Nutrients and metabolites that ultimately reach endoneurium must meet permeability requirements of the capillary endothelium.[11] Integrity of the endoneurium is fundamental for efficient nerve fiber regeneration of axons subsequent to wallerian degeneration. In particular, continuity of the basal lamina tubes of damaged nerve fibers allows regenerating nerve fibers to elongate through their original Schwann cell columns to be paired eventually with their target muscle fibers or sensory end organs.

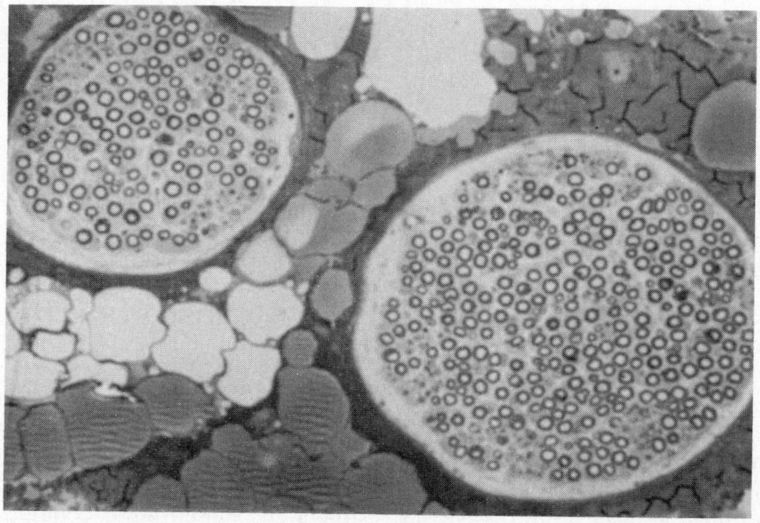

**Figure 19–1.** Light micrograph of part of a normal human nerve in cross section. Abundant myelinated fibers are seen within two nerve fascicles, which are defined by thin perineurial sheaths. Connective tissue and fat globules intervene (glutaraldehyde-Epon-toluidine blue).

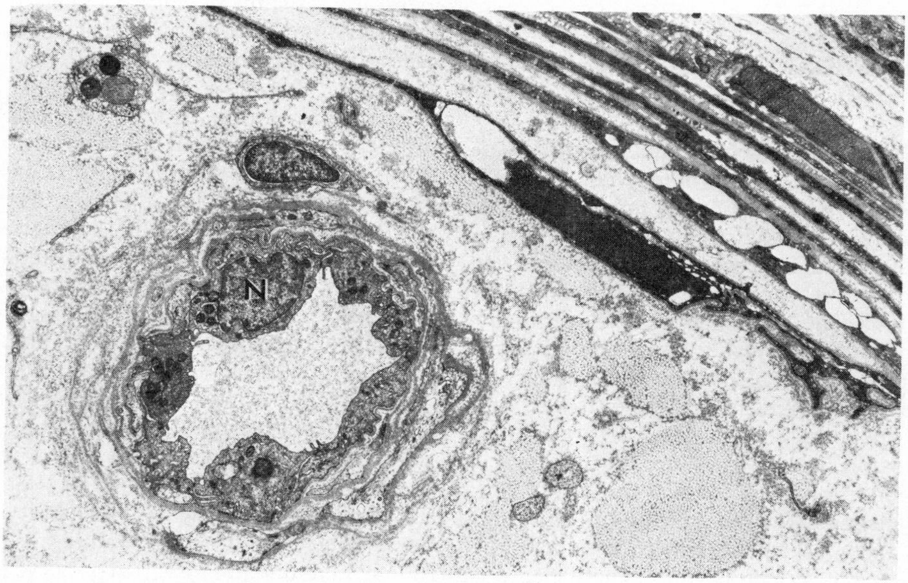


**Figure 19–2.** Electron-micrograph of cross section at the periphery of a normal human nerve fascicle. Slender perineurial cell processes course diagonally at top right. A capillary shows section across endothelial cell nucleus its lumen is filled with amorphous (plasma) material. The capillary as well as the perineurial cell surface are dressed by basal lamina. (glutaraldehyde-Epon-toluidine blue).

## NERVE FIBER POPULATIONS AND SOME OF THEIR SELECTIVE DISORDERS

Most peripheral nerves contain mixtures of myelinated and unmyelinated fibers. Nothing in the fiber structure distinguishes sensory myelinated fibers from motor myelinated fibers or sensory unmyelinated fibers from autonomic unmyelinated fibers. In nerves to human skin, unmyelinated fibers are three to four times more numerous than myelinated fibers. In terms of fiber diameters, most nerves contain two populations of myelinated fibers and a single one of unmyelinated fibers (Fig. 19–3*A*). The fact that nerve conduction velocity is a function of axonal diameter (and degree of myelination) is reflected in the compound nerve action potential (NAP). When a nerve trunk is supramaximally stimulated at one point, the compound nature of the propagated wave can be displayed oscillographically by recording at a suitable conduction distance. The different elevations reflect more or less synchronous conduction along nerve fibers of the different populations.[12]

The modern classification of the components in the sensory NAP includes A-alpha (30 to 72 meters per second), A-delta (4 to 30 meters per second), and C (0.4 to 2 meters per second).[13] In human nerves, the fastest component of the sensory NAP can be comfortably recorded through the skin with surface electrodes.[14] All three components can be recorded in vitro following nerve biopsy[15] (Fig. 19–3*B*).

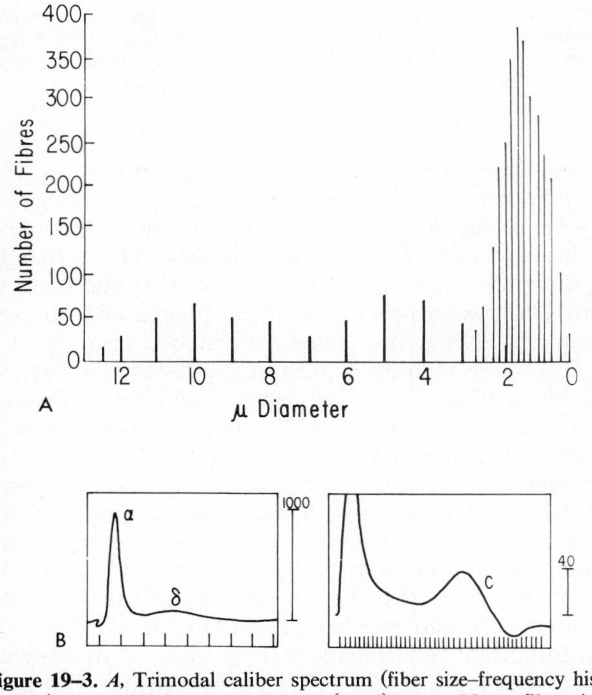


**Figure 19–3.** *A*, Trimodal caliber spectrum (fiber size–frequency histogram) of normal human cutaneous (sural) nerve. Nerve fibers increase in number as they decrease in diameter. (Modified from Ochoa, J. and Mair, W.G.P. Acta Neuropathol. 13:197, 1969.) *B*, Diagrammatic representation of compound action potential of normal human sural nerve recorded in vitro, showing Aα, Aβ and C fiber potentials. (Modified from Dyck, P.J. et al.: Arch. Neurol. 20:490, 1969.)

In nerves to skin, the large diameter myelinated fibers connect with low threshold mechanoreceptor units (RA, SA-I,SA-II) while A-delta fibers connect with cold units and with nociceptive units for sharp, "first" pain. Within the unmyelinated population and together with efferent sympathetic fibers are represented two categories of afferent cutaneous units: the high threshold nociceptive units for dull, "second" (C-type) pain and units for warmth.[16]

In nerves to muscle, the largest diameter myelinated fibers are proprioceptive spindle afferents, whereas the smallest are the fusimotor fibers destined for the end plates of intrafusal muscle. Unmyelinated fibers connected to muscle are sympathetic efferent or sensory afferent; the latter are probably concerned mostly with pain rather than with thermal sensation.

Diseases causing selective loss of unmyelinated fibers abolish C-type pain and itch and warmth sensations and also cause dysautonomia.[17] These diseases erase the C elevation in the compound NAP recorded in vitro, without affecting maximal motor conduction velocity or the fast component of the sensory nerve action potentials. On the other hand, selective block of myelinated fiber activity (for example, through the ischemic block induced by placing a pneumatic cuff around a limb at suprasystolic pressure for about 30 minutes) causes paralysis and sensory loss, except for warmth and C-type pain.[18,19] Acute local nerve lesions caused by mechanical trauma tend to affect all nerve fiber types. "Neurapraxia" from acute local nerve compression is an exception in that it causes a specific pathologic lesion with conduction block of large diameter myelinated fibers only.[20]

## AXONS AND AXOPLASM

Ultrastructurally, *axoplasm* contains smooth endoplasmic reticulum, mitochondria, and numerous microtubules and neurofilaments. Microtubules are well categorized as 240-Å (24-nm) diameter helical chains of dimer proteins with a central core of about 14 nm. These cytoskeletal structures probably play key roles as conduits for subcellular particle movements.[21] That particle movements occur in axons has been accepted for years. Weiss and Hiscoe[22] showed that placing a ligature around an axon or regenerating nerve resulted in focal distention of the axon proximal to the constricting band. They concluded that a continuous cellulofugal flow of axonal contents arises from neuronal perikaryon and is essential for maturation, maintenance, and regeneration of distal nerve fibers. Proteins and nutrients stored within the neuronal cell body must be conveyed along the nerve fiber; this is accomplished by *fast* and *slow axoplasmic transport mechanisms.* In addition to the anterograde trophic influences of the cell bodies on nerve fibers, Schwann cells, and effector organs, axoplasmic transport is also channeled in a *retrograde* manner, allowing the periphery to feed back to the soma. Nerve growth factor is one example of a substance carried by retrograde transport; it is believed that feedback suppression due to axonal injury might trigger the necessary cellular reactions for nerve regeneration (chromatolysis).[23] Other substances carried by retrograde transport include tetanospasmin (tetanus toxin), herpes virus, and the useful cytologic marker, horseradish peroxidase.

Definitive measurements of axoplasmic flow were obtained in the 1960s from studies using isotope labeled tracers. Calculated flow rates of 1 to 3 mm per day were in keeping with the known rates of elongation of regenerating axons and with the simple early idea of "perpetual" bulk translocation of axoplasm. This slow transport system, however, did not account for why wallerian degeneration occurred so rapidly within a nerve only a few days after its transection. Interruption of a "fast" axoplasmic transport system was soon postulated and, in the late 1960s, transport systems attaining flow rates of 50 to 2000 mm per day were documented in different animal models.[24-26]

The mechanism underlying *fast axoplasmic transport* is incompletely understood. It is not dependent on propulsive force exerted in the neuronal cell body, but is dependent on local supplies of energy. The "transport filament" theory of Ochs proposes that the ATP activates crossbridges between bits of filaments that carry the transported material on axonal microtubules[27] (Fig. 19–4). The "sliding vesicle" theory also implicates microtubules as the guiding framework for fast transport.[24] These theories are supported by observations that colchicine and vinca alkaloid agents, which arrest mitosis by binding to microtubular subunits, also block fast transport in low doses. However, higher doses of these agents block *slow axonal transport* and electron microscopic studies of nerve after treatment with these agents have shown microtubules to be intact.[28] This evidence, along with critical studies of fast axoplasm recovery time after rewarming from cold injury, suggests that colchicine and vinblastine may exert their effects in some way other than through disaggregation of microtubular systems.[29] Other subcellular organelles may be crucial to the system of particle transport. Droz and colleagues have emphasized the importance of the longitudinal smooth endoplasmic reticulum in *fast axoplasmic transport* and demonstrated the passage of substances from axon to myelin by direct diffusion and by distribution via Schmidt-Lanterman clefts.[30]

As to the *slow axoplasmic displacement*, its physical mechanism also remains unknown; peristaltic waves have not been demonstrated in vivo in undisturbed nerve fibers. While a portion of the substances transported are "absorbed" as they pass down the axon or are used for renewal of material at the axon terminals, a portion are "*turned around*" and channeled in retrograde manner.

Defects in neuronal synthesis or axonal transport of materials cause various grades of atrophy or frank disintegration of the motor, sensory, and autonomic nerve fibers and target organs. The worst example is *wallerian*

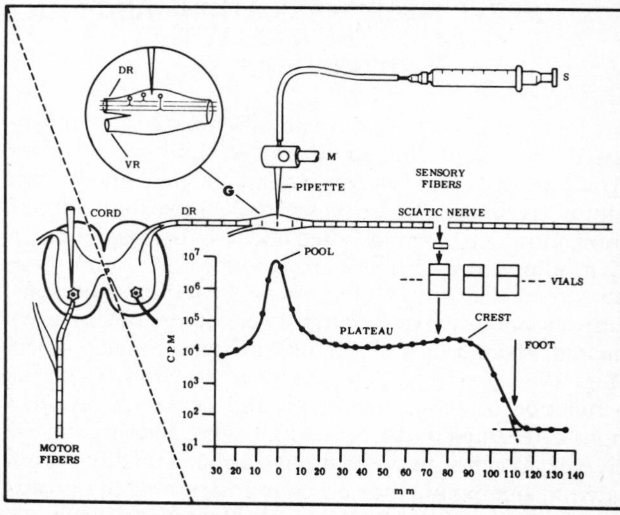


**Figure 19–4.** Injection and sampling technique showing transport. The L7 ganglion shown in the insert contains T-shaped neurons with one branch ascending in the dorsal root, the other descending in the sciatic nerve. A pipette containing $^3H$-leucine is passed into the ganglion; after its injection and the incorporation of precursor, the downflow of labeled components in the fibers is sampled at various times by sacrificing the animal and sectioning the nerve. Each segment is placed in a vial and solubilized; scintillation fluid is added; and the activity is counted. The outflow pattern is displayed on the ordinate log scale; the abscissa is in millimeters, taking the distance from the center of the ganglion as zero. A high level of activity is seen remaining in the ganglion region; more distally, a plateau rises to a crest before abruptly falling at the front of the crest to baseline levels. For motoneurons the left-hand side of the cord undergoes an injection of the precursor into the L7 cell body region followed by removal of ventral root and sciatic nerve at a later time for a similar treatment and display of outflow. (Reproduced by permission from Ochs, S. and Worth, R.M.: In Waxman, S.G.: Physiology and Pathobiology of Axons. New York, Raven Press, 1978, pp. 251–264.)

*degeneration*, by which anatomic interruption of the axon leads to fragmentation and resorption of axons and myelin in the distal stump and "denervation atrophy" of target organs. Empty Schwann cell columns (bands of Büngner), well characterized by electron microscopy, testify to past degeneration of myelinated and unmyelinated fibers, a useful pathologic criterion (Fig. 19–5).[31]

In a large number of neurologic diseases, a "dying-back" pattern of structural decay is observed, affecting first the most distal parts of the longest nerve fibers and spreading centripetally.[32] It is attributable to defective synthesis or flow of "trophic" material. Such a pattern explains distal emphasis of weakness, wasting, sensory loss, and reflex change. More recently, the expression *central-peripheral distal axonopathy* has been used to emphasize that often there is simultaneous involvement of the central and peripheral nervous systems[33] (Fig. 19–6). Important refinements in the concept of dying-back have been made as the result of experiments with neurotoxic agents that interfere with neuronal cell processing and axoplasmic transport.[34-42]

**Axonal Regeneration.** Even during the administration of toxic substances that cause axonal damage and degeneration, axonal *regeneration* may occur. In general,

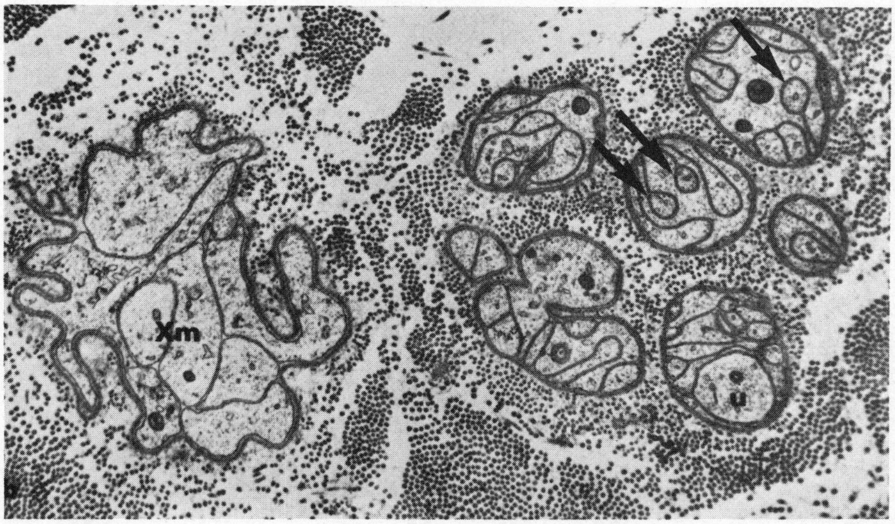


**Figure 19–5.** Electron micrograph of cross-section through "denervated" or "empty" Schwann cell bands from human sural nerve. Large isolated, irregular band on the left (*Xm*) is typically ex-myelinated. On the right, smaller, grouped, more regularly shaped bands, one of which still contains a surviving unmyelinated axon (*u*), two of which contain probably axonal sprouts (arrows), while the remaining three are "denervated." (× 11,600) (Reproduced by permission from Ochoa, J.: Proceedings of the VIth International Congress of Neuropathology, p. 589, Masson et Cie, Paris, 1970.)

regeneration of an axon involves a number of steps, including (a) synthesis of new structural material; (b) its transport down the axon; (c) elongation of the new sprouts (at about 1 mm per day) consequent to locomotion of the growth cone and insertion of new material at the tip; (d) guidance of the sprouts to a peripheral target to re-establish a functional connection; and (e) myelination and maturation in diameter.

Predictably, in the dying-back axonopathies, the process of regeneration is upset,[43] and interference of growth cone dynamics may arrest elongation of new axons, at least as seen in tissue culture experimentation.[44] Regenerating axons that fail to establish functional connections with a peripheral target remain immature, and excess numbers of them are produced. Immature axon sprouts may behave abnormally as impulse generators.[45,46] In cross sections of nerves, regenerating myelinated axons are often grouped in characteristic "clusters" (Fig. 19–7), whereas regenerating unmyelinating axons distort the unimodal size-frequency histogram of axon diameters. These are further pathologic criteria substantiating past axonal degeneration.[47]

**Schwann Cells and Myelin.** There is a single kind of Schwann cell. Nevertheless, axons may be myelinated or unmyelinated. This is dependent upon the message given by the axon to its satellite cell. Groups of unmyelinated axons are packaged communally within Schwann cell chains, each axon separated from the others by enveloping Schwann cell cytoplasm whose cell tongues interdigitate to define the *mesaxon* (Fig. 19–8).

Individualization of a single axon in an exclusive Schwann cell is a prerequisite for myelination. During development, axons destined to become large in diameter myelinate first and more abundantly. Such early, short myelin segments are more exposed to developmental stretch, especially in the limbs. As a result, in the adult, large diameter axons have thicker and longer myelin segments than small axons. New myelin segments laid on axons that regenerate in nerves of adults remain short. This constitutes yet another useful pathologic criterion[48,49] (Fig. 19–9).

Schwann cell cytoplasm is found internal to (adaxonal) and external to myelin sheaths. The adaxonal cytoplasm is traversed by the inner mesaxon and communicates with Schwann cell cytoplasm external to myelin through the Schmidt-Lanterman clefts. The *internode* (or segment) is that section of a nerve fiber subserved by a single Schwann cell bounded at its extremities by nodes of Ranvier. The node is enveloped by contiguous Schwann cells which interdigitate multiple fingerlike projections from cytoplasm external to myelin. External to Schwann cell plasma membrane lies a continuous *basement membrane (basal lamina) sleeve* to which collagen is intimately attached.

Within spinal roots, a short distance from the spinal cord, Schwann cells are abruptly replaced by oligodendroglia at nodes of Ranvier.[50,51] At this level, epineurium becomes dura mater, but endoneurium persists as far as the junction of roots with central nervous tissue. Inner layers of perineurium merge with the root sheath, which is in continuity with the subarachnoid space.

The myelin sheath is a compound unit membrane appendage and arises after cytoplasmic resorption of a Schwann cell process that has wrapped about an axon.[52,53] The concentric lamellae of the myelin spiral have a periodicity of 150 to 180 Å between *major dense lines.* These are separated by a less electron dense *intraperiod line* (Fig. 19–10). The darker staining, major dense line is formed by a fusion of the internal cytoplasmic faces of Schwann cell membrane, while the fain-

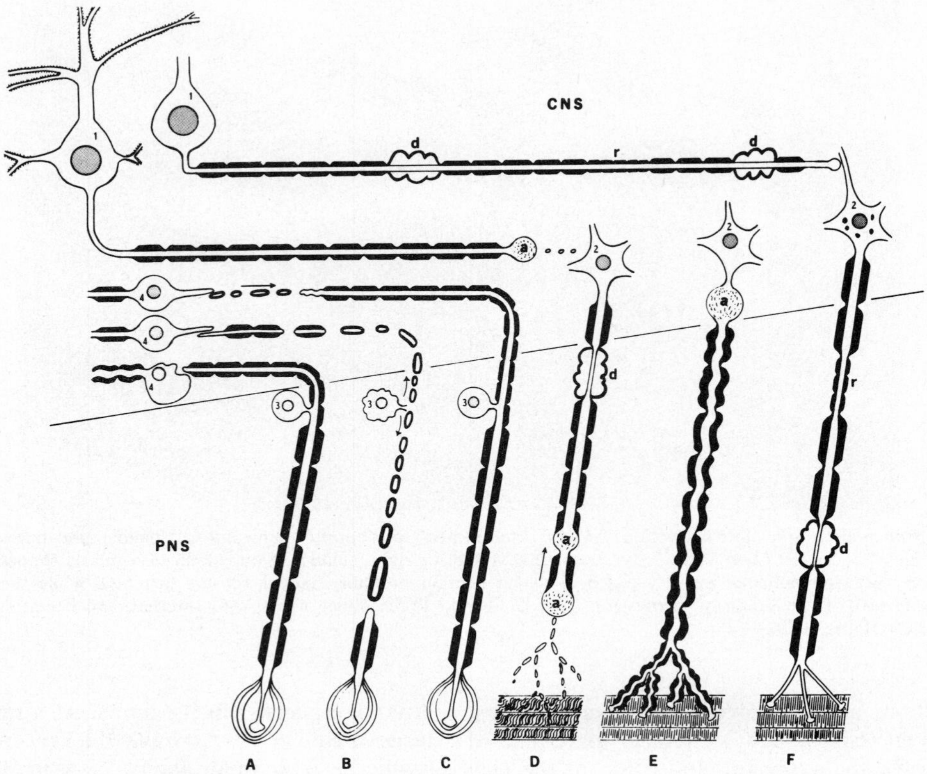


**Figure 19–6.** Cellular target sites of some neurotoxic chemicals illustrated by upper (*1*) and lower (*2*) motor neurons, dorsal root ganglion cells (*3*), and second order sensory neurons (*4*) in the gracile nucleus of the medulla oblongata. The central nervous system (CNS) is represented above the sloping horizontal line; the peripheral nervous system (MNS), below. The peripheral receptors on fibers *A–C* are Pacinian corpuscles. Fibers *D–F* innervate extrafusal muscle fibers. *A,* Neuronopathy: The excitotoxin alanosine acts as a false transmitter at neuron 4, causing maintained depolarization leading to cellular damage. *B,* Neuronopathy: Doxorubicin irreversibly damages neuron *3*, resulting in a rapid anterograde (arrows) pattern of total axonal breakdown and myelin loss. *C,* Central distal axonopathy: Clioquinol induces retrograde degeneration of the central axonal process of the dorsal root ganglion cell (*3*) but leaves the cell and peripheral process intact. *D,* Central-peripheral distal axonopathy: 2,5-hexanedione causes retrograde axonal degeneration (*a*) to develop slowly in long and large central and peripheral axons. Muscle atrophy will occur unless axons regenerate and sprouts reinnervate the muscle. The anterior horn cell (*2*) is left intact, and eventually (after months to years) a secondary demyelination in the ventral root ensues (*d*). *E,* IDPN causes a giant axonal swelling (*a*) to develop in the intraspinal portion of the axon; the distal axon at the distal axon attenuates but does not degenerate. *F,* Myelinopathy: AETT causes myelin bubbling (*d*) focally along the axon of large diameter central (*1*) and peripheral (*2*) axons. Axonal denudation is followed by remyelination: this is occurring in the ventral roots (*r*) and medulla oblongata when demyelination (*d*) is in progress in the peripheral nerve and elsewhere. A similar process would occur in a primary disease of the myelinating cell except that remyelination might not occur during intoxication. (Reproduced by permission from Spencer, P., and Schaumburg, H., (ed.): Experimental and Clinical Neurotoxicology. Baltimore, Williams & Wilkins, 1980, pp. 92–99.)

ter staining, intraperiod line represents its paired apposed external surfaces.

Peripheral myelin is composed of water (40 percent net weight), lipids (75 percent dry weight), and protein (25 percent).[54] It is structurally quite different from central myelin, containing less glycolipid and more sphingomyelin in polyunsaturated fatty acid than its central counterpart. Myelin proteins and lipids are interesting in that they are immunogenic and may play a role in experimental "allergic neuritis" in animals and in idiopathic inflammatory demyelinating neuropathy in man.[55]

**Axolemma.** Like the surface membranes of other electrically excitable cells, the unit membrane enveloping the axon is specialized to generate all-or-nothing action potentials in response to adequate excitation. A difference of $-15$ to $-100$ mV electrochemical potential exists between the inside of any cell and the extracellular fluid of warm-blooded animals. This is generated largely by selective permeability features of the resting membrane and by the fact that various species of ions (chiefly sodium, potassium, chloride, and large protein anions) are unequally distributed across the plasma membrane. Intracellular potassium and large impermeable protein anions exceed extracellular concentrations of these ions by a ratio of 50:1. At rest, the axolemma is selectively permeable to potassium ions, which tend to diffuse outward along their chemical concentration gradient. Net potassium efflux leads to the progressive development of a transmembrane voltage that apposes further outward potassium movement. Such is the *potassium equilibrium potential* ($E_k$); it largely determines the value of

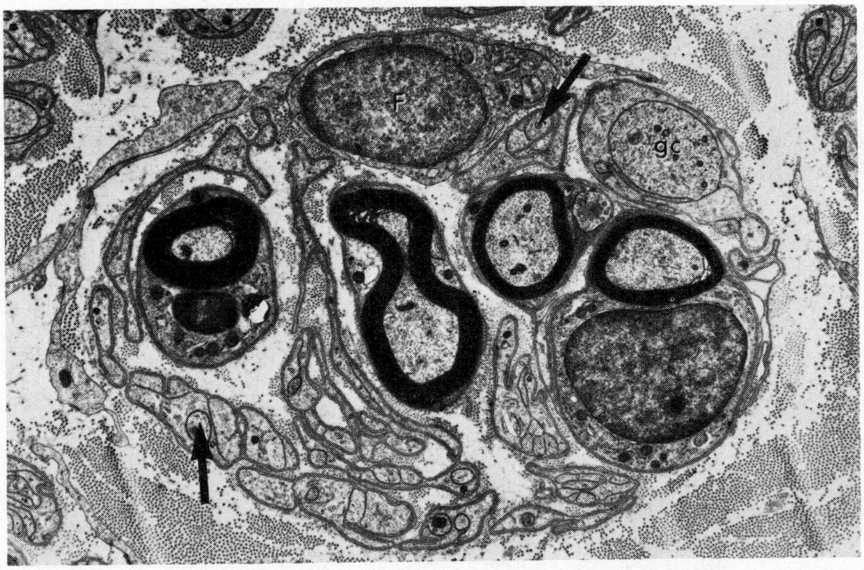


**Figure 19–7.** Cross section of a cluster of regenerated fibers from the sural nerve of a patient with isoniazid neuropathy. Within the unit there are small myelinated fibers and axons devoid of myelin (arrows) suspended in their Schwann cells. A "growth cone" (*gc*) also occurs. The various subunits and the fibroblast (*F*) fit to complement an oval pattern. (Osmium tetroxide immersion fixation, × 7200.) (Reproduced by permission from Ochoa, J.: In Dyck, P.J., et al. (eds.): Peripheral Neuropathy. Philadelphia, W.B. Saunders Co., 1975, pp. 131–150.)

the membrane potential at rest. The resting membrane is to some extent also permeable to sodium ions. Since the concentration of sodium is higher outside the cell than inside the cell, sodium passively "leaks" into the cell, propelled there by electrochemical forces. This inward flow of positive charges tends to balance the ionic disequilibrium and to decrease the resting membrane potential established by the potassium leak outward. Maintenance of the steady concentration gradient across the membrane is secured by active transport of sodium ions outward and potassium ions inward against their concentration gradients at the expense of ATP.

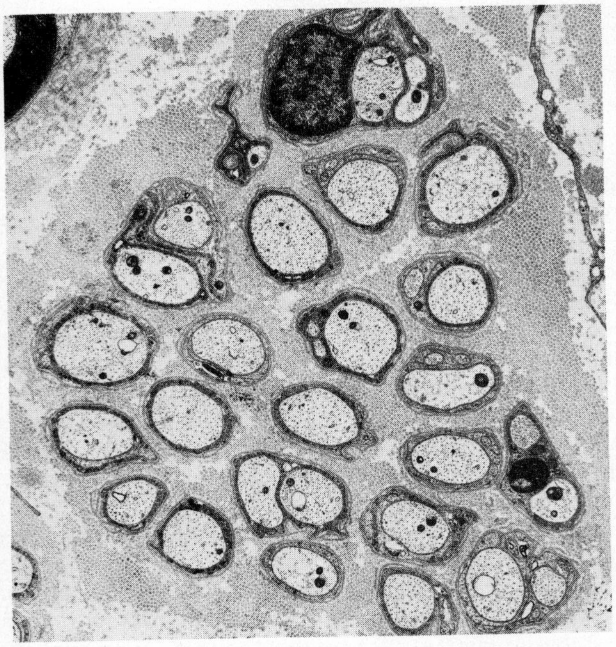

**Figure 19–8.** Electron micrograph across normal human unmyelinated fibers. Multiple axons devoid of myelin congregate in space, wrapped individually or in subgroups by Schwann cell processes which separate the axons from the collagen-rich endoneurial spaces.

The above description concerns the axolemma at rest. But this electrically excitable membrane contains ion-specific, voltage-dependent channels through which ions can move to generate action potentials. These channels may be opened or closed depending on the electrical potential across the membrane. At resting membrane potential (polarized negatively inside to about −80 mV), the channels are closed but available for activation. Depolarization of the membrane may occur by application of cathode current to the nerve membrane, by mechanical deformation of axolemma, or naturally by the arrival of positive charges to the inside of the axon during propagation of action potentials. At an intracellular potential difference of about −50 mV, threshold is reached for opening (activation; m) of voltage-dependent sodium channels in the axolemma. This permits the sudden influx of sodium along its concentration and electrochemical gradients in a positive feedback fashion. Indeed, the rapid influx of sodium further depolarizes the membrane, which activates more voltage-dependent sodium channels, thus accelerating the course of the all-or-none depolarizing shift, which eventually overshoots zero potential. After a few milliseconds, sodium influx is interrupted by voltage-dependent closure (h) of sodium channels. During this same period, there is opening of voltage-regulated potassium channels. This allows for rapid efflux of positive charges, which repolarize the membrane potential down toward its original potassium (resting) equilibrium potential. The system remains *refractory* (unexcitable) for 2 to 4 msec, since sodium

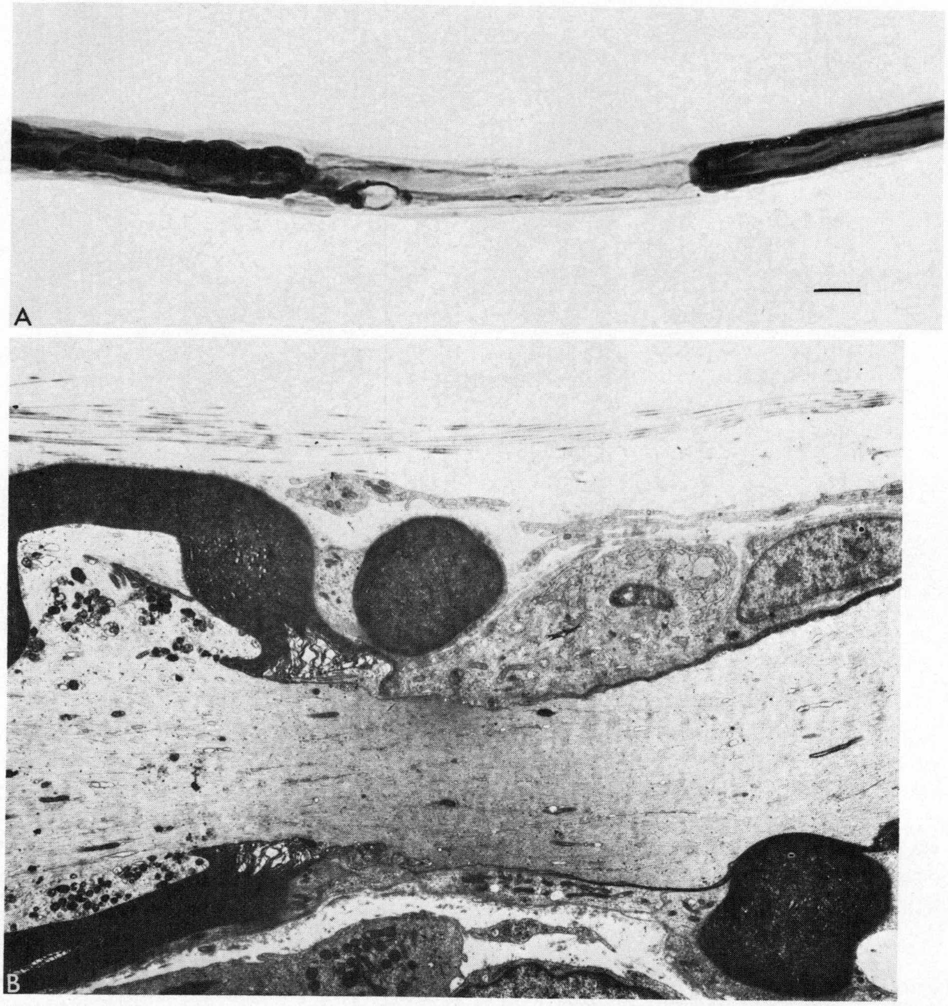

**Figure 19–9.** *A,* Thinly remyelinated segment intercalated in fiber microdissected from baboon sciatic nerve during repair of paranodal invagination and demyelination (bar = 10 μm). *B,* Low-power electron micrograph after ultrathin sectioning of the fiber above. It shows detail of the node on the left. (× 5500) (Reproduced by permission from Ochoa, J.: J. Neurol. Sci. 17:103, 1972.)

inactivation gates will remain shut until the membrane fully repolarizes. This absolute refractory period sets the limit for the maximum firing rates that can be triggered in nerve fibers (Fig. 19–11). It is more prolonged in unmyelinated than in myelinated fibers. Prolonged inactivation of the sodium conductance may occur if the membrane does not repolarize, a recognized cause being the chronic extracellular accumulation of potassium ions.[56]

The density of sodium and potassium channels can in principle be estimated through the use of labeled neurotoxins that bind specifically to either.[57-59] Unmyelinated axons have relatively few scattered sodium channels and relatively abundant potassium channels. Myelinated axons have abundant sodium channels concentrated at the nodes of Ranvier and at the initial segment of the axon. This is probably the basis for special cytochemical reactivity of the axolemma at those sites.[60] The potassium channels in myelinated axons are hidden under the myelin. Such channel formulae may explain why myelinated axons (particularly sensory axons) *accommodate* little and are easily induced into spontaneous impulse generation.[46,59]

Decreased membrane excitability may result from deviations in the resting membrane potential related to abnormal ionic concentration. It may also result from blocking activation of sodium channels, for example, by certain specific neurotoxins or by local anesthetic drugs. As mentioned earlier, the membrane may remain unexcitable if the inactivation gates are not reopened after an action potential.

Spontaneous impulse generation from nerve fibers may produce a variety of abnormal sensory phenomena, inclusive of paresthesias and perhaps neuralgic pains. Ectopic impulse generation is thought to result from membrane insults, such as the abolition of sodium inactivation caused by certain neurotoxins or drugs, or the blocking of potassium channels by similar means,

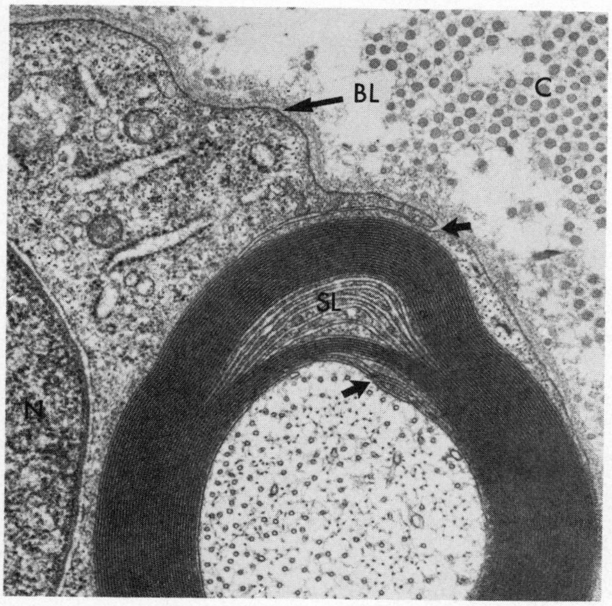


Figure 19–10. Electron micrograph across normal human myelinated fiber. Sector of nucleus (*N*) is seen to the left of sector of myelinated axon. Regular myelin periodicity is disturbed by a partial Schmidt-Lanterman cleft (*SL*). Note external and internal mesaxons (arrowed) and tubular and filamentous contents of axoplasm. A basal lamina (*BL*) separates the Schwann cell membrane from endoneurial collagen fibrils (*C*).

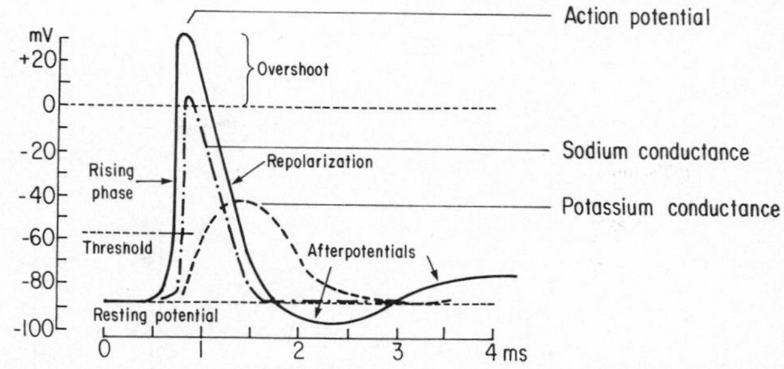


**Figure 19–11.** Time course of the action potential and of the associated changes in sodium and potassium permeabilities. (Modified from Dudel, J.: *In* Schmidt, R. F.: Fundamentals of Neurophysiology. New York, Springer, 1978.)

or deviations in the time or voltage dependence of subpopulations of sodium channels, allowing the extemporaneous channel opening (m-h overlap).[46] One form of spontaneous impulse generation, postischemic paresthesia, is less readily elicited in patients with certain neuropathies. One explanation for this observation is that potassium channels become exposed through paranodal myelin defects, thus increasing accommodation.

Propagation of the action potential occurs along the membrane owing to the fact that influx of ions moves longitudinally within the axon. If axons acted as though they were inert cables, the propagated longitudinal current would fall off exponentially with distance, owing to outward current leakage. However, the potential change propagates along the whole length of unmyelinated axons without decreasing in amplitude. This is because the positively charged longitudinal current brings to threshold neighboring points in the excitable membrane. Indeed, upon turning outward through the membrane, the internal longitudinal current initiates voltage-dependent excitation of ion channels in every point visited. This in turn supplies fresh inward current for further depolarization for neighboring regions of the membrane. The velocity of propagation of the action potential is dependent upon several factors:

a. It increases together with the magnitude of the sodium (sodium channel density), since a greater internal longitudinal current will accelerate the excitation of adjacent membrane.

b. It increases markedly with increased membrane resistance (for example, myelin), since the longitudinal current will hardly weaken with distance. Thus, conduction time along the internodal portions of the myelinated axons is negligible but is delayed at the naked nodal portions. Here the progressive depolarization comparatively slowly builds up to the threshold for channel opening. The term "saltatory" conduction expresses such excitation jumping from node to node (Fig 19–12*A*).

c. It increases with the diameter of the axon, since the resistance to the flow of internal longitudinal current is inversely proportional to the square of the axon diameter.

Pathologically, conduction of the action potential is slowed along thin regenerated axons. Nerve conduction is also slowed in partially demyelinated axons and in nerves with presumably abnormal membrane composition. Slowing of conduction in demyelinated axons may either reflect abnormally delayed "saltation" or the development of internodal voltage-dependent channels and continuous conduction, as occurs normally in unmyelinated fibers[62-64] (Fig. 19–12*B*). Slowing of conduction may also occur in severe axonopathies such as acute intermittent porphyria, uremia, and certain heavy metal poisonings. This is not necessarily due to drop out of fast conducting axons; it may be due to secondary demyelination in these disorders. Conduction of the action potential may be completely blocked in severe demyelination. A few layers of remyelination may transform conduction block into slowed conduction and hence restore strength to a nerve-muscle preparation (see Fig. 19–9). Patchy demyelination affecting many nerve fibers slows their conduction to different extents. Functions requiring synchronous conduction of nerve volleys, as in tendon reflexes and vibration sense, are selectively upset. Equally, compound nerve action potentials recorded locally become dispersed and are ultimately unobtainable from desynchronization of impulses.

## THE CLINICAL SYNDROME OF PERIPHERAL NEUROPATHY

Peripheral nerve disorders may be broadly categorized into two groups based on their clinical pattern of extent.

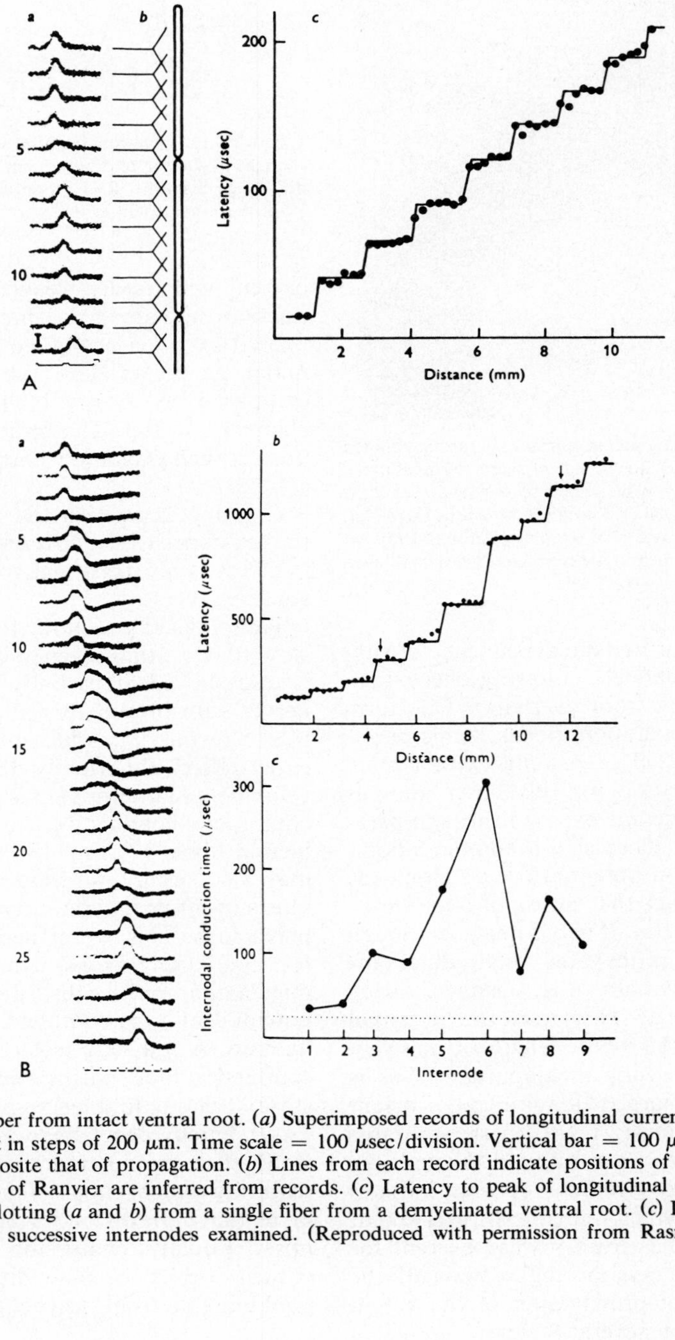


**Figure 19–12.** *A*, Normal single fiber from intact ventral root. (*a*) Superimposed records of longitudinal current from a single fiber as electrode pair was moved along ventral root in steps of 200 μm. Time scale = 100 μsec/division. Vertical bar = 100 μV. Upward deflection represents current flowing in a direction opposite that of propagation. (*b*) Lines from each record indicate positions of the electrode with respect to the diagrammatic fiber. Sites of nodes of Ranvier are inferred from records. (*c*) Latency to peak of longitudinal current as a function of distance along the fiber. *B*, Records and plotting (*a* and *b*) from a single fiber from a demyelinated ventral root. (*c*) Data of *b* replotted as internodal conduction time for each of nine successive internodes examined. (Reproduced with permission from Rasminsky, M., and Sears, T.A.: J. Physiol. 227:323, 1972.)

They are either more or less symmetrical polyneuropathies or a focal injury of a single nerve trunk, designated mononeuropathy. Polyneuropathies are diffuse disorders of peripheral nerves presenting as muscle weakness, with or without wasting, areflexia, and sensory and autonomic disturbance, in a distal-greater-than-proximal distribution, usually in the feet and legs before the hands and arms. The term polyradiculoneuropathy is used to emphasize symmetrical involvement of spinal roots as well as nerve trunks. Polyneuropathies may be genetically inherited or acquired from a host of metabolic, toxic, infectious, or nutritional insults. As shown in Table 19–1, it is possible to subclassify polyneuropathies as primarily due to axonal degeneration or as primarily due to demyelination of nerve fibers. Useful and usually accurate insights into the kind of pathology affecting nerve fibers can be derived from measurements of nerve conduction velocity.[65] Even morphologically, however, this distinction is not pure in many disease states. Chronic axonal degenerations may be preceded by axonal atrophy accompanied by secondary demyelination. Similarly, primary demyelinating diseases, especially if chronic, may be associated with some degree of secondary axonal degeneration.

Mononeuropathies may occur from chronic entrapment or acute mechanical compression, from ischemia, from neoplastic infiltration, or from granulomatous disease. At times, multiple mononeuropathies (often termed mononeuritis multiplex) may become so widespread and confluent in an individual as to resemble polyneuropathy. In these cases thorough electrophysiologic study may differentiate the two and may precisely localize the sites of the lesions, thus calling for appropriate tissue biopsy and medical or surgical intervention when indicated.

Neuropathies may present as acute (less than one week), subacute (less than one month), or chronic (greater than one month) disorders and they may be predominantly motor, sensory, autonomic, or mixed, depending on the type of function involved at presentation. Weakness with minor sensory complaint is often seen in idiopathic inflammatory demyelinating polyneuropathy (Guillain-Barré syndrome), lead intoxication, porphyria, diphtheritic neuropathy, and in some forms of hereditary peroneal muscular atrophy.[66,67] Minor sensory symptoms are often neglected and may be elicited only by careful questioning. A genuinely pure motor neuron syndrome of a subacute or chronic nature is rarely due to polyneuropathy and, after appropriate screening tests, most often proves to be a form of anterior horn cell disease.

Predominant sensory involvement is a common feature of many polyneuropathies, including leprosy, diabetes, amyloid neuropathy, uremia, vitamin $B_6$ and $B_{12}$

**Table 19–1.** Common Causes of Polyneuropathy in Man

| Marked Axonal Degeneration | Marked Demyelination |
|---|---|
| *Acquired* | |
| *Metabolic* | *Metabolic* |
| Vitamin deficiency ($B_1$, $B_6$, $B_{12}$, folic acid, nicotinic acid) | Carcinoma (remote effect) |
| Diabetes | Lymphoma, myeloma, dysproteinemias |
| Uremia | Diabetes |
| | Hypothyroidism |
| | Liver failure |
| *Toxic* | *Toxic* |
| Heavy metals (lead, arsenic, mercury, thallium, gold, etc.) | Diphtheria |
| Inorganic compounds (nitrous oxide, etc.) | Buckthorn toxin |
| Organic compounds (alcohol, organomercury, organophosphorus (TOCP), hexacarbons (*n*-hexane, MnBK, kepone, etc.), acrylamide, carbon disulfide, hexachlorophene, dietary cyanides) | *Inflammatory* |
| Drugs (vincristine, vinblastine, isoniazid (B6), nitrogen mustards, cliquinol, thalidomide, nitrofurantoin, phenytoin, dapsone, disulfiram, perhexiline) | Guillain-Barré syndrome (autoimmune and variants) |
| *Collagen vascular disease and sarcoidosis* | |
| *Leprosy* | *Leprosy* |
| *Genetic* | |
| *Degenerative* | *Degenerative* |
| Porphyria | Hypertrophic Charcot-Marie-Tooth disease |
| Neuronal-type Charcot-Marie-Tooth disease | H.N. of Dejerine-Sottas type |
| Friedreich's ataxia | Refsum's disease |
| Ataxia telangiectasia | Metachromatic leukodystrophy |
| Bassen-Kornzweig syndrome (abetalipoproteinemia) | Adrenomyeloneuropathy |
| Primary amyloidosis | Krabbe's disease |
| Hereditary sensory neuropathies | Liability to pressure palsies |
| Tangier disease (alphalipoproteinemia) | |
| Fabry's disease | |
| Leigh's disease | |
| Familial dysautonomia | |
| Giant axonal neuropathy (?) | |
| | *Dysgenetic (?)* |
| | Arrested myelinogenesis |

deficiencies, arteritis, alcoholic neuropathy, hereditary sensory neuropathy, and a form of carcinomatous neuropathy.

**Symptoms and Signs of Neuropathy.** Paresthesias of "burning," "pins and needles," and "tingling" qualities, pain (aching, brief stabbing, etc.), and numbness in a stocking-glove distribution are common symptoms of polyneuropathy. The sensation of a bandlike constriction about a limb or a feeling of swelling in the limb is sometimes volunteered. "Restless legs," a nondescript discomfort in the calves, which usually occurs while sitting or during sleep and is relieved with movement of the legs, may herald early polyneuropathy. Atypically, sensory manifestations may occur in a proximal distribution. This has been described in acute intermittent porphyria,[68,69] Tangier disease,[70] and leprosy. In lepromatous leprosy, the pattern of sensory loss can be related to the fact that bacilli proliferate in nerves of cooler tissues, thus sparing midline, palms, axillae, and the warm regions of the face.[71]

On examination, weakness is greater in a distal rather than proximal distribution in most forms of polyneuropathy and is usually seen in feet before hands. There are several notable exceptions to this rule, however. In lead neuropathy, wrist drop from radial nerve dysfunction classically is reputed to precede onset of weakness in the lower limbs. Proximal weakness greater than distal is commonly encountered in cases of inflammatory demyelinating polyneuropathy and in acute intermittent porphyria. The explanation for this is unclear. Thomas suggests this may be due to the fact that proximal portions of limbs are supplied by nerve fibers of greater diameter than those supplying distal extremities. Hence, the myelin of these fibers may be more susceptible to certain metabolic or immunogenic injury.[72]

Cranial nerve involvement in polyneuropathy is uncommon on the whole. Ophthalmoplegia, in particular when in combination with global areflexia and ataxia, should be considered to be the Miller-Fisher variant of inflammatory polyneuropathy until proven otherwise.[73] Patchy involvement of mixed motor and sensory cranial nerves, as well as the nerves in the extremities, may be seen in diabetes, sarcoidosis, carcinomatosis, Tangier's disease, leprosy, and in various forms of arteritis.

Muscle wasting is not to be expected in pure demyelinating neuropathy or in axonal neuropathies of recent onset. The deformities associated with chronic muscle wasting may be characteristically revealing. For example, pes cavus, usually signifying inherited axonal neuropathy and, of course, the various clawhands point to lesions of particular isolated nerves. Fasciculations from involuntary contraction of individual motor units are commonly found in motor neuropathies by careful scrutiny of skin overlying muscle groups. These may be identified as spontaneous, fine, irregular twitches of muscle that occur at rest and are usually not strong enough to displace a joint. It is now generally agreed that the origin of fasciculations may be the ectopic generation of nerve impulses propagated from anywhere along the motor neuron.[74,75] The abnormal mechanisms responsible for development of ectopic impulse generation in nerve fibers have been analyzed by Diamond and colleagues.[46]

Intact tendon (stretch) reflexes require the normal functioning of spindle afferent nerve fibers and alpha motor neuron fibers to extrafusal muscle. In addition, these reflexes require gamma motor neuron output for appropriate tuning of the intrafusal spindle apparatus. In polyneuropathy, reflexes are most often lost or diminished following the axonal dying-back pattern of sensorimotor dysfunction or as a result of demyelination with desynchronization of the nerve volleys required for the compound muscle response. Similarly, in mononeuropathies, reflexes are diminished in a focal pattern that often clarifies the exact root or nerve involved. Brisk reflexes in the setting of a polyneuropathy should suggest concurrent damage of spinal cord and peripheral nerves, as may be seen in vitamin $B_{12}$ deficiency,[76,77] porphyric neuropathy,[69,78] adrenomyeloneuropathy,[79] and in some neuropathies caused by toxic agents, for example, triorthocresyl phosphate[80] and nitrous oxide.[81] It should be remembered that *joint deformity* might be a consequence of peripheral neuropathy. Indeed, Charcot joints, thought to result from loss of joint nociception, can be a dramatic manifestation of chronic sensory neuropathies, inclusive of diabetic neuropathy and Charcot-Marie-Tooth disease.

## NEUROPATHIES OF SPECIAL INTEREST TO RHEUMATOLOGISTS

**Neuropathies Associated with the Arteritides.** *Rheumatoid Arthritis.* Peripheral neuropathy may be a particularly vexing complication to patients already weakened and disabled from rheumatoid arthritis (RA). While its precise incidence in the rheumatoid population is unknown, peripheral neuropathy, excluding entrapment syndromes, has been reported in 1.2 to 9.8 percent of cases.[82,83] Electrophysiologic examination of muscle and nerve shows abnormalities in 85 percent of patients with RA who have no specific neurologic complaints.[84]

The neuropathy usually presents insidiously as a symmetrical, predominantly sensory abnormality with numbness, tingling, or burning of distal extremities. Subtle motor deficits are difficult to quantitate in patients with joint pain or deformity, but a degree of muscle wasting and weakness is usually present.[82,85] The clinical picture is characterized by a distal loss of vibration sense and proprioception, although all modalities are affected to some degree.[86-88] Less commonly, abrupt painful asymmetric mononeuropathy or a fairly symmetric chronic sensorimotor neuropathy may arise as a complication of systemic arteritis in RA. The distal sensorimotor polyneuropathy resembling infectious polyneuritis may present abruptly or with stuttering progression over several months.[82,85] Most commonly this type of neuropathy is seen in patients with severe, long-standing disease who are on steroids or experiencing rapid change in steroid doses. Commonly, these patients demonstrate severe joint deformities, rheumatoid nodules, high titers of rheumatoid factor, diminished serum complement, high ESR, anemia, anorexia, and fever.[85,87,89,90]

There is now considerable evidence indicating that these deficits are a result of axonal degeneration of nerve fibers due to occlusion of vasa nervorum and resultant ischemia of nerve trunks. Perivascular mononuclear infiltrates, fibrinoid necrosis of media with polymorphonuclear infiltrates, arteriolar intimal proliferation, perivascular hemorrhages, fibrosis, and small vessel occlusions are documented evidence of diffuse necrotizing angiopathy of peripheral nerve in these patients.[91,92] Ischemia occurs most commonly in the middle of the upper arm and thigh, with a striking central fascicular pattern of maximal nerve fiber damage. Between axilla and elbow and between hip and thigh, portions of nerve receive relatively few nutrient arteries; hence, there are diminished systems of collateral circulation.[9] Under conditions of widespread inflammation and occlusion of vasa nervorum, these regions of nerve may represent watershed zones of selective ischemic vulnerability.[91,93] Electrophysiologic and histologic studies have documented axonal degeneration with some segmental demyelination.[86] Myelinated fibers sustain most of the damage with relatively less involvement of smaller unmyelinated fibers.[94] This may reflect a greater vulnerability of myelinated fibers to ischemia.[95-98]

The etiology of rheumatoid vasculitis is unknown, although its correlation with high titers of rheumatoid factor, low serum complement, and the presence of 7S IgM suggests it may be immune mediated. The definitive diagnosis may be aided by skin, rectal, muscle, or nerve biopsy.[90,94,99] The overall mortality of patients with rheumatoid neuropathy due to vasculitis approaches 30 to 50 percent, and aggressive management with steroids, cyclophosphamide, penicillamine, and/or plasmapheresis has been advocated.[88,92,99]

*Polyarteritis Nodosa.* This disorder is a systemic vasculitis of small and medium-sized arteries, occurring throughout the body. Peripheral neuropathy is common in this disorder and has been reported in up to 52 percent of cases.[100] While mononeuritis multiplex (with the onset of weakness, pain, numbness, and paresthesia radiating down an arm or a leg) is often described as the classic form of neuropathy in this disorder,[101] polyneuropathy may indeed be more common.[90] Mononeuritis multiplex may, however, become so extensive and confluent as to resemble a symmetrical "pseudo"-polyneuropathy. Electrophysiologic testing will identify subclinical polyneuropathy in a substantial number of neurologically asymptomatic patients with systemic vasculitis and thus aid in the early recognition and treatment of this disorder.

The clinical features of neuropathy due to polyarteritis nodosa are largely similar to those secondary to the arteritis of RA, though differences have been described. Polyarteritis neuropathy has been cited as more commonly asymmetrical, primarily motor, and rarely pure sensory, while rheumatoid neuropathy is commonly a symmetrical, distal, predominantly sensory polyneuropathy.[89] These characteristics are unreliable in differentiating the two diseases, however, and nerve biopsy of either may give similar pathologic appearances. Nevertheless, peripheral neuropathy as a presenting complaint is uncommon in RA but common in polyarteritis nodosa, and should initiate a careful search for other signs of systemic vasculitis.

Peripheral neuropathy due to vasculitis may be seen in a variety of other connective tissue diseases including Churg-Strauss' arteritis, systemic lupus erythematosus, Sjögren's syndrome, cranial arteritis, and Wegener's granulomatosis.[82] The clinical features commonly take the form of mononeuritis multiplex or symmetrical sensory polyneuropathy. The frequency of peripheral neuropathy in Sjögren's syndrome may approach 60 percent of cases,[102] and has recently been shown to correlate with high titers of anti-Ro (SSA) antibodies in these patients.[103] Electrophysiologic studies and neuropathology document ischemic centrofascicular nerve lesions with axonal degeneration likely due to vasculitic changes in vasa nervorum.[94]

*Peripheral Neuropathy and Dysimmunoglobulinemia.* Neuropathy may develop in association with dysimmunoglobulinemia in a number of systemic disorders, including myeloma, cryoglobulinemic states, Waldenström's macroglobulinemia, solitary plasmacytoma, amyloidosis, and "benign" monoclonal gammopathies, unaccompanied by cancer or systemic illness. The pathophysiology of neuropathy in these illnesses is disputed. Theories have incriminated subperineurial immunoglobulin deposition, serum hyperviscosity due to paraproteins, direct infiltration of nerve by tumor cells, and metabolic or immunologic injury of nerve.[104]

Peripheral neuropathy may be seen in association with systemic *amyloidosis* in approximately 15 percent of cases.[105] Typically, it presents as a moderate to severe sensorimotor-autonomic neuropathy which comes on in the late decades of life and is associated with systemic cardiac, renal, hematologic, or gastrointestinal involvement in approximately one half of cases.[106] The polyneuropathy usually begins with positive sensory symptoms in lower limbs described as a stabbing, prickling, piercing, burning, or "painful" numbness. The dysesthesias predominate over sensory loss and, in some cases, may be incapacitating enough to prohibit weight bearing and may require narcotics. Pain, cold, and warm sensations are disproportionately affected early in the disease, beginning in the distal extremities and progressing proximally.[107] Disturbances of proprioception and light touch may follow in similar fashion and are accompanied by symmetrical distal weakness, usually beginning in extensor muscles of the feet and progressing to complete disability in some cases.[108]

Autonomic dysfunction typified by postural hypotension, diarrhea, impotence, and bladder incontinence in men is common. Serum protein electrophoresis may be abnormal in 50 percent of cases, and monoclonal proteins may be found in 90 percent when urine and serum are examined simultaneously. The diagnosis is often made by rectal biopsy, but when neuropathy is present, amyloid may be identified by sural nerve biopsy in virtually all cases.[106]

Electromyographic studies usually confirm primary distal axonal degeneration, though the mechanism of neural injury is uncertain.[106,108] Amyloid deposits within epineural arteries may lead to small vessel occlusion and nerve ischemia.[109] This by itself would not explain the selective small fiber dropout witnessed early in the course of the disease.

***Macroglobulinemia.*** The term macroglobulinemia was first coined by Waldenström and categorizes a group of patients with hepatosplenomegaly, anemia, weight loss, malaise, bleeding diathesis, and an elevated level of 19S IgM found on immunoelectrophoresis of plasma[110] (see Chapter 84). Commonly, these patients have an elevated ESR and lymphoid proliferation of bone marrow, lymph nodes, spleen, and other tissues. Peripheral neuropathy occurs in up to 25 percent of cases of macroglobulinemia[111,112] and may be associated with chronic lymphocytic leukemia, lymphosarcoma, carcinoma, cirrhosis of the liver, and a variety of connective tissue disorders.[113]

A heterogenous pattern of peripheral nerve dysfunction may occur, including mononeuropathy, mononeuritis multiplex, and pure sensory, sensorimotor, and predominantly motor (resembling Guillain-Barré) and cranial neuropathies.[112,114,115] Most commonly, however, patients suffer a symmetrical distal sensory syndrome, involving spontaneous pain, paresthesias, and numbness, which usually precedes the onset of weakness and muscle cramps and occasionally antedates other protean manifestations of the disease.[116,117]

Histopathologic examination of involved nerves shows partial demyelination of nerve fibers. Often scattered lymphocytic infiltrates are seen around small and medium-sized vessels. Ultrastructural examination of nerve may reveal occasional plasma cells within endoneurium.[118] Amyloid deposits within nerve fascicles may be identified on Congo red stain in a small percentage of patients with macroglobulinemia and neuropathy.

The pathogenesis of peripheral neuropathy is uncertain, but to date much evidence has been collected implying that IgM paraproteins may be directed against peripheral myelin. Iwashita and colleagues[104] identified IgM paraprotein deposits in perineurium and vasa nervorum in a patient with Waldenström's macroglobulinemia. Others have demonstrated large deposits of macroglobulin in the myelin sheath of nerve fibers associated with a marked distortion of myelin lamellae and swelling of the mesaxon.[118-120] More recently, Latov and colleagues[120] demonstrated abnormal activity of IgM immunoglobulin against peripheral nerve myelin using complement fixation and immunoglobulin techniques in a patient with IgM monoclonal gammopathy and demyelinating peripheral neuropathy. In this case, marked clinical improvement was obtained through reduction of serum paraprotein by means of plasmapheresis, prednisone, and chlorambucil, suggesting that IgM-mediated demyelination is the primary pathophysiology in this disorder. Using the immunoperoxidase technique, Abrams and colleagues[121] later demonstrated immunohistochemical binding of IgM paraproteins in 10 patients with peripheral neuropathy and plasma cell dyscrasia. Binding of IgM paraprotein to peripheral myelin and to axons was seen in seven cases. Subsequently, myelin-associated glycoprotein was demonstrated as the likely antigen in patients with antimyelin IgM antibodies.[122]

***Multiple Myeloma.*** This is a disease characterized by malignant proliferation of plasma cell lines that infiltrate bone marrow and other tissues and commonly produce abnormal quantities of immunoglobulins in serum and urine. Evidence of peripheral neuropathy is reported in 5 to 13 percent of cases[123,124] and may be found histologically or electrophysiologically in 40 to 60 percent of cases when neurologically asymptomatic patients are included in studies.[124,125] The neuropathy may occur in the disorder with or without amyloidosis and, in both forms, has been associated with axonal degeneration and segmental demyelination.[126,127] However, amyloid deposition in nerve is rarely found and is thought to play no role in the development of neuropathy.[114,128]

The neuropathy of myeloma without amyloidosis is not stereotyped and may present as a pure sensory, mild sensorimotor, or subacute relapsing polyneuropathy. Neuropathy in myeloma may also be associated with systemic amyloidosis and has the same features of amyloid neuropathy described earlier. Long-term survival of patients is uncommon in this disease but most often is seen in patients with a good response to chemotherapy.[129] The use of alkylating agents and other forms of chemotherapy in this disease, however, does not seem to alter the continuous progression of neuropathy in patients who suffer from it.

***Osteosclerotic Myeloma.*** A rare form of myeloma seen in younger, healthier individuals, osteosclerotic myeloma is associated with peripheral neuropathy in 50 percent of cases.[126,130,131] In these patients, polyneuropathy is characterized by a predominantly symmetrical distal motor weakness, which overshadows sensory loss and may mimic the presentation of chronic inflammatory demyelinating neuropathy.[130] The abnormal monoclonal "spike" may be missed on routine serum protein electrophoresis; for this reason, skeletal survey and serum immunoelectrophoresis are recommended for definitive diagnosis in selected patients. Surgical extirpation of a solitary plasmacytoma may be curative.[131] Tumoricidal radiation therapy and chemotherapy are associated with improvement of polyneuropathy in some patients.[132,133] The exact role that monoclonal antibody plays in the pathogenesis of polyneuropathy in this disorder is unknown.

***Cryoglobulinemia.*** Cryoglobulins are immunoglobulins that precipitate at 4°C and redissolve upon rewarming (see Chapter 84). They may be characterized as either monoclonal IgM or IgG in patients with plasma cell dyscrasia, or as mixed polyclonal comprised of two or more immunoglobulins, usually IgM and IgG; this latter group is associated with infection, liver disease, and collagen vascular diseases such as rheumatoid arthritis, systemic lupus erythematosus, and polyarteritis nodosa.[134]

Peripheral neuropathy has been reported to occur in up to 15 percent of cases of cryoglobulinema and is usually characterized by symmetrical, subacute motor-sensory polyneuropathy or mononeuritis multiplex.[112,135] Electrophysiology of muscle and nerve may show evidence for axonal degeneration. On nerve biopsy, vasculitis of medium and small size epineurial arteries and perivascular infiltration of lymphocytes in plasma cells may be seen.[136] Abnormal immunoglobulin deposits in perineurial capillaries and throughout subperineurial and endoneurial subspaces have been demonstrated.[135,137,138]

While the pathogenesis of axonal degeneration in cryoglobulinemic states is uncertain, the evidence for an ischemic factor is attractive and plasmapheresis may be beneficial in some patients.[137]

**Sarcoid Neuropathy.** Sarcoidosis is a systemic granulomatous disease of unknown etiology that most commonly involves lung, lymph nodes, parotid glands, spleen, skin, and eyes (see Chapter 93). A wide variety of central and peripheral nervous system disturbances are reported in about 5 percent of cases.[139-141] Of these, the most remarkable feature of neurologic sarcoid is the occurrence of multiple relapsing and remitting cranial nerve palsies, involvement of the VII cranial nerve being the single most common.[141-144] Polyneuropathy is a rare development but may present as a subacute or chronic symmetrical sensorimotor disturbance or as an acute mononeuritis or Guillain-Barré syndrome.[145-148]

The pathogenesis of sarcoid neuropathy is not well categorized, and there have been few histopathologic studies.[142,146,147] Electrophysiologic data has shown evidence for axonal degeneration with[146,149] or without[141,147] segmental demyelination. Panarteritis in sarcoid neuropathy has been documented by others and has been cited as a possible underlying etiology to the neuropathy.[147] Frank infiltration of nerve by granuloma, however, has also been documented on nerve biopsy in this disorder and may play a role in subsequent nerve injury.[142,146,147,149]

The natural history of sarcoid neuropathy is difficult to establish. Most patients with peripheral neurologic symptoms and sarcoidosis are treated with high-dose glucocorticoids, and the general prognosis is favorable in most cases. Whether a good prognosis is due to the self-limiting nature of the disease or the use of corticosteroids is currently unknown.[140,142,143]

**Leprosy of the Peripheral Nervous System.** Leprosy is a chronic, disabling disease of superficial body parts caused by the acid-fast bacillus *Mycobacterium leprae.* The disease is of relatively low contagiousness and is common to tropical and subtropical areas of the world, with endemic foci in India, Spain, Portugal, Mexico, and portions of the southern United States.[150] In part as a result of the increasing influx of Hispanic and Southeast Asian immigrants, the incidence of leprosy has risen sharply in the United States, particularly in the cities of New York, San Francisco, and Los Angeles.[151] Since the disease is not readily recognized by many physicians, it may go undiagnosed for many years, mimicking a variety of neurologic, rheumatologic, and dermatologic syndromes.[152]

A wide clinical pathologic spectrum of the disease is seen, ranging from the well circumscribed, slowly progressive tuberculoid form to the rapidly proliferating, widely disseminating lepromatous type. The form of leprosy that develops depends, to a large extent, on host response factors. Patients with lepromatous leprosy display abnormalities of cellular immunity characterized by delayed hypersensitivity reactions and impaired lymphocyte transformation while retaining normal humoral response mechanisms.[153-156] Inability to contain the infection results in unchecked proliferation of bacilli and extensive hematogenous spread to skin, mucous membranes, eyes, upper respiratory tract, and peripheral nerves.

In all forms of leprosy, sensory loss is the hallmark of neurologic involvement and is commonly the first manifestation of the disease.[157-160] In lepromatous leprosy, the pattern of neurologic deficit can be shown to occur in tissues of cooler body temperature where bacilli tend to reproduce most readily.[158] The pinnae of the ears, dorsal surfaces of the hands and feet, dorsomedial surfaces of the forearm, and anterolateral aspects of the legs are the areas most commonly involved. The precise sequence of sensory modality loss is disputed.[157] Commonly, however, patients retain the ability to differentiate sharp from blunt sensation while demonstrating a remarkable insensitivity to pain. The skin is marked by numerous deep lacerations, abrasions, contusions, and burns in various stages of healing, suffered, without comment or notice, while performing the routine chores of life. Modalities of light touch, proprioception, and vibration sense may be variably lost as the disease progresses. Motor strength and deep tendon reflexes are typically preserved well into advanced stages of the illness.

Hypertrophic nerves are common in leprosy and predispose the patient to a variety of compression neuropathy syndromes. Motor and sensory nerve conduction studies may reveal mononeuropathy multiplex with focal slowing in several nerves at common sites of nerve entrapment and enlargement. Electromyography may show evidence of chronic denervation of involved muscle groups.[157,161,162]

Peripheral neuropathy in leprosy results from direct invasion of nerve by the bacillus, an unusual but consistent characteristic of infection with *Mycobacterium leprae.* The histopathology of nerve lesions is usually diagnostic. Typically there is marked proliferation of perineurium and intraneural fibrous tissue, with an increased number of endoneurial collagen fibrils seen. There is hypertrophy of Schwann cells with the formation of multiple cytoplasmic protrusions. *Mycobacterium leprae* may be seen singly or in aggregates within

Schwann cells as well as within scattered foamy macrophages and other inflammatory cells throughout an involved nerve. Foamy degeneration of Schwann cells associated with myelinated and unmyelinated axons may be seen, with little or no involvement of axoplasm and myelin.[163] In lepromatous leprosy, acid-fast stains may reveal large numbers of bacilli invading epineurium, perineurium, and occasionally endoneurial blood vessels, even in asymptomatic patients with the disease.[157,159,163] It has been speculated that these bacilli may gain access to peripheral nerves by primary invasion of Schwann cell cytoplasm. Sporadic Schwann cell degeneration from bacterial infestation could ultimately lead to focal demyelination and secondary axonal degeneration, thus explaining focal slowing of nerve conduction in these patients.[161,163,164] When erythema nodosum is associated with lepromatous leprosy, the histopathology of nerve lesions shows foci of an acute angiitis, largely of small arteries and arterioles within perineurium. Inflammatory infiltrates, vascular occlusions, and subsequent intraneural edema may result in segmental infarction of neural elements or multiple microabscesses of neural trunks.[165]

Treatment of leprosy with adequate doses of diaminodiphenylsulfone, rifampin, or both is the mainstay of therapy. When antibacterial therapy is provided early in the course of the disease, it will halt the progression of the destructive process and promote natural recovery of the neuropathy.[151,157] Surgical intervention for cosmesis, stabilization of joints, transposition, and drainage of entrapped or infected nerves is often beneficial.[166]

## MECHANICAL INJURIES OF NERVE

Mechanical injuries of nerve are a common complication of rheumatologic illness. The degree, character, and duration of neuropathy in these patients depend on the type of nerve fiber damage and the efficiency of repair processes, when they occur. Nerve injury may be broadly classified as acute or chronic, with the type of structural damage differing dramatically in each. The histopathologic features of acute and chronic compressive neuropathies, as studied in animal models, provide insight into their nature and mechanism and thus a scientific approach to their management.

**Acute Nerve Compression.** Acute compressive nerve injury may result in sensorimotor deficit or paresthesias, which may be completely and rapidly reversible or virtually permanent. Early clinical manifestations of nerve dysfunction (numbness, paralysis, paresthesia, and pain) may provide little clue as to the nature of the underlying pathology or the possibility of recovery. Short-lasting compression of peripheral nerve above systolic pressure results in a *rapidly reversed physiologic block* of nerve conduction. Lewis, Pickering, and Rothschild, in pneumatic tourniquet experiments conducted on themselves, elegantly demonstrated that this is a result of nerve ischemia rather than the direct effect of high pressure on nerve.[18] In addition, they established the sequence of sensory modality loss during progressive nerve ischemia and described in detail the quality of paresthesia perceived during recovery from the ischemic insult.

Typically, if a pneumatic cuff is placed proximally on an arm at suprasystolic pressures, numbness is detected in the fingertips within 13 to 15 minutes. Loss of light touch and pressure modalities spreads centripetally toward the tourniquet at about 3 to 4 cm per minute. Pain, cold, and warm modalities are later lost in a similar fashion within 30 to 40 minutes. Weakness starts distally and spreads centrally soon after anesthesia, with complete paralysis occurring by 30 to 40 minutes of limb ischemia. If the tourniquet is removed at this point, recovery is normally always accompanied by tingling paresthesias, which may become uncomfortably intense and last for some four to six minutes. Sensory deficits are usually fully restored within 30 seconds and full muscle power some time after 10 minutes.

That this sequence of sensorimotor nerve disturbance is due to ischemia and not direct pressure on nerve was established by placing a second pneumatic cuff on the extremity, proximal to the first, just before the time of distal cuff release. Release of the distal cuff and hence release of local nerve compression without restoration of blood supply, failed to result in recovery of neural deficits. The stereotyped sequence of sensory modality loss suggested to Lewis and colleagues that the excitable membrane function of myelinated nerve fibers may be more vulnerable to ischemia; this has recently been corroborated by others.[95,167-169]

Regarding the pathophysiology of postischemic paresthesia, there is much evidence favoring nerve fibers as their site of origin.[170-172] Torebjörk and colleagues[172] and Ochoa and colleagues,[173] using intraneural microelectrode recording from sensory fascicles, concluded that the paroxysmal discharges recorded from single sensory units during postischemic paresthesias are generated ectopically along nerve fibers and not primarily from skin receptors.

As early as 1876, Erb described a type of nerve dysfunction that is more prolonged than the typical reversible physiologic block yet less severe than that resulting from nerve section.[174] Seddon called this *neurapraxia* (Saturday night paralysis) and noted the absence of muscle atrophy and the usually rapid recovery.[175] Denny-Brown and Brenner[176] demonstrated that neurapraxia could be produced in experimental animals with the use of a pneumatic cuff, and the end result was segmental demyelination of nerve. They erroneously concluded, however, that this lesion was ischemic in nature—a complication of the ischemic paralysis described earlier by Lewis, Pickering, and Rothschild.[18] Gilliatt and associates showed later that the demyelinating lesions occurred only in portions of nerve corresponding to the edges of the cuff, where pressure gradients are greatest. The mechanical nature of the neurapraxic lesion nerve was elucidated by Ochoa and colleagues[177] and is depicted in Figure 19–13*A* through *D*. Axoplasm and myelin are displaced outwardly from sites of compression, corresponding to cuff edges. Nodes

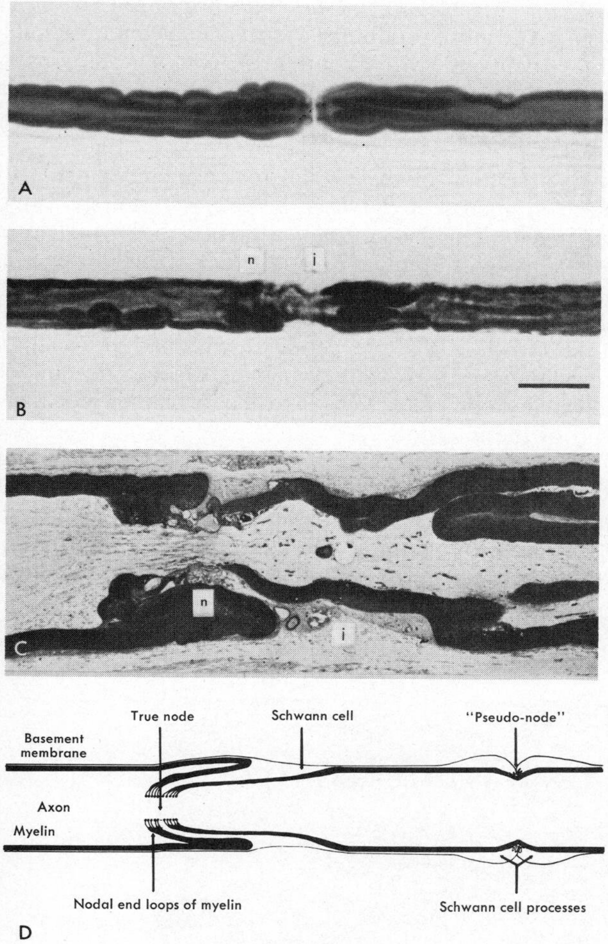


**Figure 19–13.** *A*, Normal myelinated fiber microdissected from baboon tibial nerve after fixation in buffered glutaraldehyde and postfixation in osmium tetroxide. Note myelin gap at node of Ranvier. *B*, Occlusion of nodal gap with invagination (intussusception) of adjacent myelin segments. Myelin has stretched beyond original site of node marked by indentation *j* to reach *n*. Fiber was microdissected from baboon tibial nerve soon after acute compression with pneumatic cuff, leading to neurapraxia. Bar = 20 $\mu$m. *C*, Low-power electron micrograph of abnormal myelinated fiber from baboon ulnar nerve soon after compression, leading to neurapraxia. Original site of node is marked by indentation at site of Schwann cell junction *j*. Note new position of node covered by infolded myelin, *n*. *D*, Diagram describing primary lesion of myelinated fibers underlying neurapraxia. Myelin segment on right has partially invaginated segment on left. (*B* and *C* from Rudge, P., Ochoa, J., and Gilliatt, R.W.: J. Neurol. Sci. 23:403, 1974; *D* from Ochoa, J., Fowler, T.J., and Gilliatt, R.W.: In Desmedt, J.E. (ed.): New Developments in Electromyography and Clinical Neurophysiology. Vol. 2. Karger, Basel, 1973).

of Ranvier prolapse into paranodal regions a considerable distance from their normal anatomic sites.

More severe forms of nerve injury may result in significant disruption of endoneurial elements. The term *axonotmesis* is used to indicate that the distal portion of the axon is physically separated from the neuronal cell body. Unlike neurapraxic lesions, in axonotmesis, disruption of axonal transport at the site of the lesion results in wallerian degeneration, chromatolysis of parent cell body, some degree of retrograde axonal degeneration, and target tissue atrophy. After three to five days, electrodiagnostic tests will distinguish this lesion from neurapraxia in that wallerian degeneration leads to total inexcitability of distal nerve segments.

Nerve regeneration is preceded by Schwann cell proliferation to form cellular columns, known as bands of Büngner, within the basal lamina tubes. Nerve sprouts from the tips of proximal stump axons slowly advance through these columns to regenerate the distal axons at a rate of approximately 1 mm per day.[178] Myelination proceeds centrifugally down nerve fibers soon after Schwann cells reorganize, to establish one satellite cell per internode segment.[179,180]

Prognosis for functional recovery is favorable in axonotmesis with preservation of original basal lamina tubes because guidance of regenerating axons to their original peripheral targets is accurate. If a mechanical injury is sufficient to disrupt the normal architecture of nerve fibers, with destruction of the anatomic integrity of endoneurium, the term *neurotmesis* is used. In contrast to axonotmesis, regeneration of axons to their original targets is unlikely and the functional outcome is poor. In addition, regenerating fibers may be unable to proceed beyond the site of injury and, instead, ball-up and entwine to form a painful neuroma.[181-183]

**Chronic Nerve Compression.** If a nerve fiber is chronically constricted or entrapped, there may be slowing or a block of nerve impulse conduction through the area of compression and histologic evidence for demyelination. Single nerve fiber histopathology of this type of nerve injury, however, demonstrates a physical distortion of fiber architecture quite unlike that of acute injuries. Dr. Nakano discusses the various nerve entrapment syndromes in Chapter 110. In this section we will describe the fine structural pathology in these lesions which, to a large degree, explains the pathophysiology of nerve dysfunction.

A naturally occurring animal model for chronic compressive nerve lesions was identified in elderly guinea pigs in the 1960s by Fullerton and Gilliatt.[184,185] They found that these animals had a high incidence of carpal tunnel syndrome at the wrist and that the severity of the entrapment could be predicted from the results of nerve conduction studies. Conduction delay and, eventually, conduction block were associated with progressively severe focal demyelinating nerve lesions extending a few millimeters in length under the flexor retinaculum. In severe cases, there was gross narrowing of the nerve trunk with evidence of wallerian degeneration of myelinated fibers at the level of compression.

Ochoa and Marotte[186] studied these animals at very early stages of nerve entrapment when nerve conduction studies were still normal. They found that along stretches of several millimeters proximal and distal to the entrapment, myelin internodes were distorted into tapered "tadpole"-appearing segments with bulbous ends always polarized away from the site of compression. A schematic illustration of how chronic compression appears at different stages in its development is shown

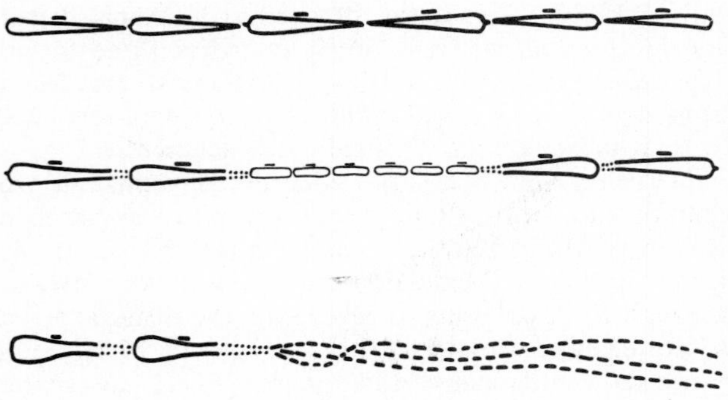

**Figure 19–14.** *A*, Diagram showing distorted myelin segments from median nerve of young guinea pig. Note reversal of polarity at the wrist. *B*, Further distortion and exposure of the axon proximal and distal to the site of entrapment. The median nerve under the carpal tunnel has lost its original myelin segments. Multiple, short remyelinated internodes repair the lesion. *C*, Advanced lesion with massive bulbs and axonal wallerian degeneration and regeneration. (Reproduced by permission from Ochoa, J.: In Omer, G.E., and Spinner, M. (eds.): Management of Peripheral Nerve Problems. Philadelphia, W.B. Saunders Co., 1980, pp. 487–501.)

in Figure 19–14*A* to *C*. The more prolonged the nerve injury, the more pronounced is the demyelination under the carpal band, with abnormal segments heading away from the entrapment site. In severe lesions, wallerian degeneration and regeneration are identified (Figure 19–14*C*).

Examination of these abnormal myelin segments by electron microscopy reveals the pathophysiology. Internal myelin lamellae normally attached to the axolemma at the node of Ranvier are retracted along the fiber at tapered ends of the "tadpole" segment, resulting in buckling of redundant myelin at the bulbous ends (Fig. 19–15). The likely sequence of demyelination, then, is through progressive retraction of unattached myelin, followed by complete demyelination of the axon at one end of the internode.

Ultrastructural examination of entrapment neuropathies in man corroborate the histopathology obtained in animal models.[187] Ochoa has suggested that detachment of terminal loops and subsequent myelin deformation may be due to repeated longitudinal stretching or fric-

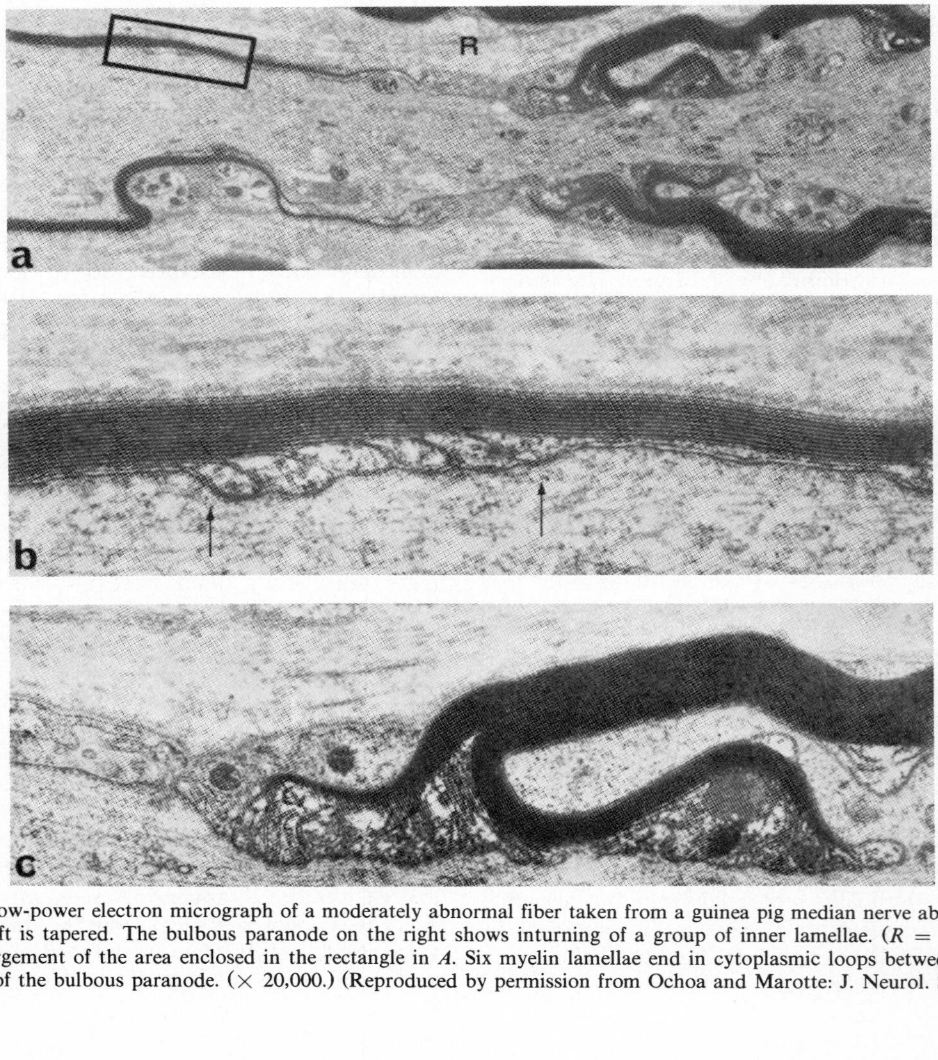


**Figure 19–15.** *A*, Low-power electron micrograph of a moderately abnormal fiber taken from a guinea pig median nerve above the wrist. The paranode on the left is tapered. The bulbous paranode on the right shows inturning of a group of inner lamellae. (*R* = node of Ranvier.) (× 7000.) *B*, Enlargement of the area enclosed in the rectangle in *A*. Six myelin lamellae end in cytoplasmic loops between the arrows. (× 48,000.) *C*, Detail of the bulbous paranode. (× 20,000.) (Reproduced by permission from Ochoa and Marotte: J. Neurol. Sci. 19:491, 1973.)

tion against flexor tendons, producing pressure waves that propagate away from the entrapment.[61]

## AGING OF THE PERIPHERAL NERVOUS SYSTEM

A variety of age-related changes in the peripheral nervous system are commonly seen in uncomplicated senesence.[188-190] Beginning at 50 years of age, there is diminished appreciation of vibratory sense (128 cps tuning fork) in the lower extremities, particularly at the great toe, with no appreciable loss in upper extremities.[191-194] Less dramatic changes in perception of light touch, proprioception, pain, and thermal sense may be expected with increasing age.[193-195,196] Muscle wasting, particularly of thigh, calf, and dorsal interossei, not associated with much weakness, fasciculation, or fibrillation, is common in the elderly and not necessarily related to disuse.[197,198] Reduction or loss of ankle jerks with normal or diminished knee and upper extremity reflexes in aging individuals is a common finding.[193,199,200]

The histopathologic changes associated with these clinical findings are multivariable.[189] The causes of the age-related changes in the peripheral nervous system are largely unknown and await futher study.

## LABORATORY INVESTIGATIONS

Complete neurologic and electrodiagnostic evaluation should precede indiscriminate laboratory investigation of peripheral neuropathy. The history, neurologic examination, and neurophysiology should help broadly categorize the neuropathy as acquired versus inherited, axonal versus demyelinating, mononeuropathy multiplex versus polyneuropathy. In acquired neuropathies, those clues should guide the physician toward an appropriate laboratory search for uremia, diabetes, vitamin $B_{12}$ deficiency, heavy metal poisoning, collagen vascular disease, dysproteinemia, sarcoidosis, or other likely entities. Following inconclusive neurologic and electrodiagnostic studies and a negative routine laboratory screen, further investigation may include the following in selected patients: (a.) special assays for serum vitamin, enzyme, or metabolite levels (e.g., phytanic acid deficiency in Refsum's disease); (b.) detection of porphyrin metabolites; (c.) serum and cerebrospinal fluid examination with focus on protein electrophoresis and immunoelectrophoresis when indicated; (d.) bone marrow microscopy; (e.) urine screen for metachromatic material and serum lysosomal analysis for inborn errors of metabolism; (f.) organ function tests (liver, thyroid, adrenal, pituitary); and (g.) appropriate screens for occult malignancy.

The search for toxic etiologies to peripheral neuropathy should rely more heavily on epidemiologic data than on laboratory investigation. Heavy metal screening in blood and urine should be complemented by assays of nail and hair for toxic exposure.

Finally, nerve biopsy can firmly establish the diagnosis in a number of neuropathies. These include leprosy, primary amyloidosis, metachromatic leukodystrophy, Fabry's disease, familial liability to pressure palsies, and the vasculitides.

## References


1. Low, P.A., Marchand F., and Dyck, P.J.: Measurement of endoneurial fluid pressure with polyethylene matrix capsules. Brain Res. 122:373, 1977.
2. Low, P.A., Dyck P.J., and Schmelzer, J.D.: Mammalian peripheral nerve sheath has unique responses to chronic elevations of endoneurial fluid pressure. Exp. Neurol. 70:300, 1980.
3. Thomas, P.K.: The connective tissue of peripheral nerve: An electron microscope study. J. Anat. 97:35, 1963.
4. Olsson, Y., Kristensson K., and Klatzo, J.: Permeability of blood vessels and connective tissue sheath in the peripheral nervous system to exogenous protein. Acta Neuro. Pathol. (Supplement) 5:61, 1971.
5. Olsson, Y., and Reese, T.S.: Permeability of vasa nervorum and perineurium in mouse sciatic nerve studied by fluorescence and electron microscopy. J. Neuropathol. Exp. Neurol. 30:105, 1971.
6. Waggener, J.P., Bunn, S.M., and Beggs, J.: The diffusion of ferritin within the peripheral nerve sheath: An electron microscopy study. J. Neuropathol. Exp. Neurol. 24:430, 1965.
7. Lundborg, G., Nordborg, C., Rydevik, B., and Olsson, Y.: The effect of ischemia on the permeability of the perineurium to protein tracers in rabbit tibial nerve. Acta Neurol. Scand. 49:287, 1973.
8. Denny-Brown, P.: Importance of neural fibroblasts in the regeneration of nerve. Arch. Neurol. Psychiatry 55:171, 1946.
9. Adams, W.E.: The blood supply of nerves. 1. Historical review. J. Anat. 76:323, 1942.
10. Sunderland, S.: Nerve and Nerve Injuries. Edinburgh, London, and New York, Churchill Livingstone, 1978.
11. Olsson, Y.: Vascular permeability in the peripheral nervous system. *In* Dyck, P.J., Thomas, P.K., and Lambert, E.H. (eds.): Peripheral Neuropathy. Philadelphia, W.B. Saunders Company, 1975, pp. 190–200.
12. Erlanger, J., and Gasser, H.S.: The compound nature of the action current of nerve as disclosed by the cathode ray oscillograph. Am. J. Physiol. 70:624, 1924.
13. Burgess, P.R., and Perl, E.R.: Cutaneous mechanoreceptors and nocireceptors. *In* Iggo, A. (ed.): Handbook of Sensory Physiology. Vol. 2. Berlin, Springer Verlag, 1973, pp. 29–78.
14. Dawson, G.D.: The relative excitability and conduction velocity of sensory and motor nerve fibers in man. J. Physiol. 131:436, 1956.
15. Lambert, E.H., and Dyck, P.J.: Compound action potentials of sural nerve in vitro in peripheral neuropathy. *In* Dyck, P.J., Thomas, P.K., and Lambert, E.H. (eds.): Peripheral Neuropathy. Philadelphia, W.B. Saunders Company, 1975, pp. 427–441.
16. Vallbo, A.B., Hagbarth, K.-E., Torebjörk, H.E., and Wallin, B.G.: Somatosensory, proprioceptive, and sympathetic activity in human peripheral nerves. Physiol. Rev. 59:920, 1979.
17. Dyck, J.P., and Lambert, E.H.: Dissociated sensation in amyloidosis. Arch. Neurol. 20:490, 1969.
18. Lewis, T., Pickering, G.W., and Rothschild, P.: Centripetal paralysis arising out of arrested blood flow to the limb, including notes on a form of tingling. Heart 16:1, 1931.
19. Kugelberg, E.: Accommodation in human nerves. Acta Physiol. Scand. 8(Suppl. 24):105, 1944.
20. Ochoa, J., Fowler, T.J., and Gilliatt, R.W.: Anatomical changes in peripheral nerves compressed by pneumatic tourniquet. J. Anat. 113:433, 1972.
21. Tsukita, S., and Ishikawa, H.: The cytoskeleton in myelinated axons: Serial section study. Biomed. Res. 2:424, 1981.
22. Weiss, P., and Hiscoe, H.B.: Experiments on the mechanism of nerve growth. J. Exp. Zool. 107:315, 1948.
23. Levi-Montalcini, R., and Angeletti, P.U.: Essential role of the nerve growth factor in the survival and maintenance of dissociated sensory and sympathetic embryonic nerve cells in vitro. Dev. Biol. 7:653, 1963.
24. Schmitt, F.O.: Fibrous proteins—neuronal organelles. Proc. Natl. Acad. Sci. USA 60:1092, 1968.
25. Dahlström, A.: Axoplasmic transport (with particular respect to adrenergic neurons). Philos. Trans. R. Soc. Lond. (Biol.) 261:1325, 1971.
26. Schmitt, F.O., and Samson, F.E.: Neuronal fibrous proteins. Neurosci. Res. Program Bull. 6:113, 1968.
27. Ochs, S.: Fast axoplasmic transport-energy metabolism and mechanism. *In* Hubbard, J.I. (ed.): The Vertebrate Peripheral Nervous System. New York, Plenum Press, 1974.
28. Samson, F.E.: Mechanism of axoplasmic transport. J. Neurobiol. 2:347, 1971.

29. Ochs, S.: Axoplasmic transport—a basis for neural pathology. *In* Dyck, P.J., Thomas, P.K., and Lambert, E.H. (eds.): Peripheral Neuropathy. Philadelphia, W.B. Saunders Company, 1975, pp. 213–230.
30. Droz, B., and Barondes, S.H.: Nerve endings: Rapid appearance of labeled protein shown by electron microscopic radioautography. Science 165:1131, 1969.
31. Ochoa, J., and Mair, W.G.P.: The normal sural nerve in man. II. Changes in axons and Schwann cells due to age. Acta Neuropathol. 13:217, 1969.
32. Cavanagh, J.B.: The significance of the "dying-back" process in experimental and human neurological disease. Int. Rev. Exp. Pathol. 3:219, 1964.
33. Spencer, P.S., and Schaumburg, H.H.: Ultrastructural studies of the dying-back process. IV. Differential vulnerability of PNS and CNS fibers in experimental central-peripheral distal axonopathies. J. Neuropathol. Exp. Neurol. 36:300, 1977.
34. Mendell, J.R., and Sahenk, Z.: Interference of neuronal processing and axoplasmic transport by toxic chemicals. *In* Spencer, P.S., and Schaumburg, H.H. (eds.): Experimental and Clinical Neurotoxicology. Baltimore, Williams and Wilkins Co., 1980.
35. Cho, E.-S., Schaumburg, H.H., and Spencer, P.S.: Adriamycin produces ganglioradiculopathy in rats. J. Neuropathol. Exp. Neurol. 36:597, 1977.
36. Cavanagh, J.B., and Chen, F.C.K.: The effect of methyl-mercury-decyandiamide on the peripheral nerves and spinal cord of rats. Acta Neuropathol. 19:208, 1971.
37. Chou, S.-M., and Hartmann, H.A.: Electron microscopy of focal neuroaxonal lesions produced by B, B-iminodipropionitrite (IDPN) in rats. Acta Neuropathol. 4:590, 1965.
38. Prineas, J.W.: The pathogenesis of dying-back polyneuropathies. Part II. An ultrastructural study of experimental acrylamide intoxication in the cat. J. Neuropathol. Exp. Neurol. 28:598, 1969.
39. Schaumburg, H.H., and Spencer, P.S.: Degeneration in central and peripheral nervous systems produced by pure n-hexane: An experimental study. Brain 99:183, 1976.
40. Clark, A., Griffin, J.W., Price, D.L., Carroll, P., and Hoffman, P.: Pathogenesis of neurofilamentary swellings in B, B-iminodipropionitrite (IDPN): Role of slow axonal transport. Neurology 28a:357, 1978.
41. Sahenk, Z., and Mendell, J.R.: Abnormal retrograde axoplasmic transport in the pathogenesis of the experimental dying-back neuropathy of BOTZ. Neurology 28a:357, 1978.
42. Thomas, P.K.: The selective vulnerability of the centripetal axons of primary sensory neurons. Lecture: Physiologic approaches to neuromuscular disease. Presented at the Mayo Clinic, Department of Neurology, Rochester, Minnesota, April 25, 1982.
43. Morgan-Hughes, J.A., Sinclair, S., and Durston, J.H.: The pattern of peripheral nerve regeneration induced by crush in rats with severe acrylamide neuropathy. Brain 97:235, 1974.
44. Yamada, K.M., Spooner, B.S., and Wessells, N.K.: Axon growth: Roles of microfilaments and microtubules. Proc. Natl. Acad. Sci. USA 66:1206, 1970.
45. Wall, P.D., and Gutnick, M.: Properties of afferent nerve impulses originating from a neuroma. Nature 248:740, 1974.
46. Diamond, J., Ochoa, J., and Culp, W.J.: An introduction to abnormal nerves and muscles as impulse generators. *In* Culp, W.J., and Ochoa, J. (eds.): Abnormal Nerves and Muscles As Impulse Generators. New York, Oxford University Press, 1982.
47. Ochoa, J.: Isoniazid neuropathy in man: Quantitative electron microscope study. Brain 93:831, 1970.
48. Fullerton, P., Gilliatt, R., Lascelles, R., and Morgan-Hughes, J.: The relationship between fiber diameter and internodal length in chronic neuropathy. J. Physiol. 178:26P, 1965.
49. Vizoso, A.D., and Young, J.Z.: Internodal length and fiber diameter in developing and regenerating nerves. J. Anat. 82:110, 1948.
50. Steer, J.M.: Some observations on the fine structure of rat dorsal spinal nerve roots. J. Anat. 109:467, 1971.
51. Maxwell, D.S., Kruger, L., and Pineda, A.: The trigeminal nerve root with special reference to the central peripheral transition zone: An electron microscope study in macaques. Anat. Rec. 164:113, 1969.
52. Geren, B.B.: The formation from the Schwann cell surface of myelin in the peripheral nerves of chick embryos. Exp. Cell Res. 7:558, 1954.
53. Robertson, J.D.: The ultrastructure of adult vertebrate peripheral myelinated nerve fibers in relation to myelinogenesis. J. Biophys. Biochem. Cytol. 1:271, 1955.
54. Bradley, W.G.: Disorders of Peripheral Nerves. Oxford, Blackwell Scientific Publications, 1974.
55. Waksman, B.H., and Adams, R.D.: Allergic neuritis: An experimental disease of rabbits induced by the injection of peripheral nervous tissue and adjuvant. J. Exp. Med. 102:213, 1955.
56. Rogart, R.B., and Stampfli, R.: Voltage clamp studies of mammalian myelinated nerve. *In* Culp, W.J., and Ochoa, J. (eds.): Abnormal Nerves and Muscles as Impulse Generators. New York, Oxford University Press, 1982, pp. 193–210.
57. Ritchie, J.M., and Rogart, R.B.: The density of sodium channels in mammalian myelinated nerve fibers and the nature of the axonal membrane under the myelin sheath. Proc. Natl. Acad. Sci. USA 74:211, 1977.
58. Barchi, R.L., Weigele, J.B., and Cohen, S.A.: Biochemical approaches to the sodium channel: Saxitoxin binding component from mammalian excitable membrane. *In* Culp, W.J., and Ochoa, J., (eds.): Abnormal Nerves and Muscles as Impulse Generators. New York, Oxford University Press, 1982, pp. 130–151.
59. Culp, W.J.: Scorpion neurotoxins as affinity reagents for voltage-dependent sodium channel components. *In* Culp, W.J., and Ochoa, J., (eds.): Abnormal Nerves and Muscles as Impulse Generators. New York, Oxford University Press, 1982, pp. 151–162.
60. Waxman, S.G.: Variations in axonal morphology and their functional significance. *In* Waxman, S.G. (ed.): Physiology and Pathobiology of Axons. New York, Raven Press, 1978.
61. Ochoa, J.: Nerve fiber pathology in acute and chronic compression. *In* Omer, G.E., and Spinner, M. (eds.): Management of Peripheral Nerve Problems. Philadelphia, W.B. Saunders Company, 1980, p. 47.
62. Rasminsky, M.: Physiology of conduction in demyelinated axons. *In* Waxman, S.G. (ed.): Physiology and Pathobiology of Axons. New York, Raven Press, 1978, p. 361.
63. Bostok, H., and Sears, T.A.: The internodal axon membrane: Electrical excitability and continuous conduction in segmental demyelination. J. Physiol. 280:273, 1978.
64. Bostok, H.: Conduction changes in mammalian axons following experimental demyelination. *In* Culp, W.J., and Ochoa, J. (eds.): Abnormal Nerves and Muscles as Impulse Generators. New York, Oxford University Press, 1982, pp. 236–252.
65. Gilliatt, R.W.: Nerve conduction in human and experimental neuropathies. Proc. R. Soc. Med. 59:989, 1966.
66. Dyck, P.J., and Lambert, E.H.: Lower motor and primary sensory neuron diseases with peroneal muscular atrophy. I. Neurologic, genetic and electrophysiologic findings in hereditary polyneuropathies. Arch. Neurol. 18:603, 1968.
67. Dyck, P.J., and Lambert, E.H.: Lower motor and primary sensory neuron diseases with peroneal muscular atrophy. II. Neurologic, genetic and electrophysiological findings in various neuronal degenerations. Arch. Neurol. 18:619, 1968.
68. Ridley, A.: The neuropathy of acute intermittent porphyria. Q. J. Med. 38:307, 1969.
69. Cavanagh, J.B., and Mellick, R.S.: On the nature of the peripheral nerve lesions associated with acute intermittent porphyria. J. Neurol. Neurosurg. Psychiatry 28:320, 1965.
70. Kocen, R.S., Thomas, P.K., Kink, R.H.M., and Haas, L.F.: Nerve biopsy findings in two cases of Tangier disease. Acta Neuropathol. 26:317, 1973.
71. Sabin, T.D.: Temperature-linked sensory loss: A unique pattern in leprosy. Arch. Neurol. 20:257, 1969.
72. Thomas, P.K.: Symptomatology and differential diagnosis of peripheral neuropathy. Clinical features and differential diagnosis. *In* Dyck, P.J., Thomas, P.K., and Lambert, E.H. (eds.): Peripheral Neuropathy. Philadelphia, W.B. Saunders Company, 1975, pp. 495–512.
73. Fisher, M.: An unusual variant of acute idiopathic polyneuritis (syndrome of ophthalmoplegia, ataxia and areflexia). N. Engl. J. Med. 255:57, 1956.
74. Wertstein, A.: The origin of fasciculations in motor neuron disease. Ann. Neurol., 5:295, 1979.
75. Roth, G.: The origin of fasciculations. Ann. Neurol. 12:542, 1982.
76. Woltmann, H.W.: The nervous symptoms in pernicious anemia: An analysis of 150 cases. Am. J. Med. Sci. 173:400, 1919.
77. Victor, M.: Polyneuropathy due to nutritional deficiency and alcoholism. *In* Dyck, P.J., Thomas, P.K., and Lambert, E.H. (eds.): Peripheral Neuropathy. Philadelphia, W.B. Saunders Company, 1975, pp. 1030–1066.
78. Ridley, A.: Porphyric neuropathy. *In* Dyck, P.J., Thomas, P.K., and Lambert, E.H. (eds.): Peripheral Neuropathy. Philadelphia, W.B. Saunders Company, 1975, pp. 942–955.
79. Griffin, J.W., Goren, E., Schaumburg, H., Engel, W.K., and Loriaux, L.: Adrenomyeloneuropathy: A probable variant of adrenoleukodystrophy. I. Clinical and endocrinologic aspects. Neurology 27:1107, 1977.
80. Cavanagh, J.B.: Peripheral nerve changes in orthocresyl phosphate poisoning of the cat. J. Pathol. Bacteriol. 87:365, 1964.
81. Layzer, R.B.: Myeloneuropathy after prolonged exposure to nitrous oxide. Lancet 2:1227, 1978.
82. Conn, D.L., and Dyck, P.J.: Angiopathic neuropathy in connective tissue diseases. In Dyck, P.J., Thomas, P.K., and Lambert, E.H. (eds.): Peripheral Neuropathy. Philadelphia, W.B. Saunders Company, 1975, pp. 1149–1165.
83. Johnson, R.L., Smyth, C.J., Holt, G.W., Lubckenco, A., and Valentine, E.: Steroid therapy and vascular lesions in rheumatoid arthritis. Arthritis Rheum. 2:224, 1959.

84. Good, A.F., Christopher, R.P., Koepke, G.H., Bender, L.F., and Tarter, M.: Peripheral neuropathy associated with rheumatoid arthritis: A clinical and electrodiagnostic study of 70 consecutive rheumatoid arthritis patients. Ann. Intern. Med. 63:87, 1965.
85. Pallis, C.A., and Scott, J.T.: Peripheral neuropathy in rheumatoid arthritis. Br. Med. J. I:1141, 1965.
86. Weller, R.O., Bruckner, F.E., and Chamberlain, M.A.: Rheumatoid neuropathy: A histological and electrophysiological study. J. Neurol. Neurosurg. Psychiatry 33:592, 1970.
87. Irby, R., Adams, R.A., and Toone, E.C.: Peripheral neuritis associated with rheumatoid arthritis. Arthritis Rheum. 1:44, 1958.
88. Ferguson, R.H., and Slocumb, C.H.: Peripheral neuropathy in rheumatoid arthritis. Bull. Rheum. Dis. II:251, 1961.
89. Hart, F.D., and Golding, J.R.: Rheumatoid neuropathy. Br. Med. J. 1:1594, 1960.
90. Wees, S.J., Sun Woo, I.N., and Joong Oh, S.: Sural nerve biopsy in systemic necrotizing vasculitis. Am. J. Med. 71:525, 1981.
91. Dyck, P.J., Conn, D.L., and Okazaki, H.: Necrotizing angiopathic neuropathy: Three-dimensional morphology of fiber degeneration related to sites of occluded vessels. Mayo Clin. Proc. 47:461, 1972.
92. Conn, D.L., McDuffee, F.C., and Dyck, P.J.: Immunopathologic study of sural nerves in rheumatoid arthritis. Arthritis Rheum. 15:135, 1972.
93. Moore, P.M., and Fauce, A.S.: Neurologic manifestations of systemic vasculitis. A retrospective and prospective study of the clinicopathologic features and responses to therapy in 25 patients. Am. J. Med. 71:517, 1981.
94. Peyronnard, J.M., Charron, L., Beaudet F., and Couture, F.: Vasculitic neuropathy in rheumatoid disease and Sjögren's syndrome. Neurology 32:839, 1982.
95. Fox, J.D., and Kenmore, P.I.: The effect of ischemia on nerve conduction. Exp. Neurol. 17:403, 1967.
96. Garven, H.S.D., Gairns, F.W., and Smith, G.: The nerve fiber populations of the nerves of the leg in chronic occlusive arterial disease in man. Scott. Med. J. 7:250, 1962.
97. Hess, K., Eames, R.A., Darveniza, P., and Gilliatt, R.W.: Acute ischemic neuropathy in the rabbit. J. Neurol. Sci. 44:19, 1979.
98. Korthals, J.K., and Wisnuwski, H.M.: Peripheral nerve ischemia. I. Experimental model. J. Neurol. Sci. 24:65, 1975.
99. Scott, D.G., Bacon, P.A., and Tribe, C.R.: Systemic rheumatoid vasculitis: A clinical and laboratory study of 50 cases. Medicine 60:288, 1981.
100. Frohnert, P.P., and Sheps, S.G.: Long-term follow-up study of periarteritis nodosa. Am. J. Med. 43:8, 1967.
101. Lovelace, R.E.: Mononeuritis multiplex in polyarteritis nodosa. Neurology 14:434, 1964.
102. Alexander, E.L., Provost, T., Stevens, M.B., and Alexander, G.: Neurologic complications of primary Sjögren's syndrome. Medicine 61:247, 1982.
103. Alexander, G.E., Provost, T.T., Stevens, M.B., and Alexander, E.L.: Sjögren's syndrome: Central nervous system manifestations. Neurology 31:1391, 1981.
104. Iwashita, H., Argyrakis, A., Lowetzseh, K., and Spaar, F.-W.: Polyneuropathy in Waldenström's macroglobulinemia. J. Neurol. Sci. 21:341, 1974.
105. Kyle, R.A., and Bayrd, E.D.: Amyloidosis: A review of 236 cases. Medicine (Baltimore) 54:271, 1975.
106. Kelly, J., Kyle, R., and O'Brien, P.: The natural history of peripheral neuropathy in primary systemic amyloidosis. Ann. Neurol. 6:1, 1979.
107. Dyck, P.J., and Lambert, E.H.: Dissociated sensation in amyloidosis. Arch. Neurol. 20:490, 1969.
108. Blom, S., Steen, L., and Zetterlund, B.: Familial amyloidosis with polyneuropathy-Type I: A neurophysiological study of peripheral nerve function. Acta Neurol. Scand. 63:99, 1981.
109. Cohen, A.S., and Benson, M.: Amyloid neuropathy. *In* Dyck, P.J., Thomas, P.K., and Lambert, E.H. (eds.): Peripheral Neuropathy. Philadelphia, W.B. Saunders Company, 1975, pp. 1012–1029.
110. Waldenström, J.: Incipient myelomatosis or "essential" hyperglobulinemia with fibrinogopenia-A new syndrome? Acta Med. Scand. 117:216, 1944.
111. Fahey, J.L., Barth, W.F., and Solomon, A.: Serum hyperviscosity syndrome. JAMA 192:464, 1965.
112. Logothetis, J.P., Silverstein, P., and Coe, J.: Neurologic aspects of Waldenström's macroglobulinemia. Arch. Neurol. 5:564, 1960.
113. Waldenström, J.: Studies on "abnormal" serum globulins (M-components) in myeloma macroglobulinasemia and related disease: Clinical diagnosis and biochemical finding in material of 296 sera with M type marrow Y globulins. Acta Med. Scand. 170(Suppl. 367):110, 1961.
114. McLeod, J.G., and Walsh, J.C.: Neuropathies associated with paraproteinemias and dysproteinemias. *In* Dyck, P.J., Thomas, P.K., and Lambert, E.H. (eds.): Peripheral Neuropathy. Philadelphia, W.B. Saunders Company, 1975, pp. 1012–1029.
115. Kreindler, A., and Macover-Patrichi, M.: Recurrent cranial nerve palsies of dysglobulinaemic origin. J. Neurol. Sci. 6:117, 1968.
116. Darnley, J.D.: Polyneuropathy in Waldenström's macroglobulinemia. Neurology 12:617, 1962.
117. Aarseth, S., Ofstad, E., and Torvek, A.: Macroglobulinaemia Waldenström: A case with haemolytic syndrome and involvement of the nervous system. Acta Med. Scand. 169:691, 1961.
118. Vital, C., Valeat, J., Deminiere, C., et al.: Peripheral nerve damage during multiple myeloma and Waldenström's macroglobulinemia. An ultrastructural and immunopathologic study. Cancer 50:1491, 1982.
119. Propp, R.P., Means, E., Derbel, R., et al.: Waldenström's macroglobulinemia and neuropathy. Deposition of M component in myelin sheaths. Neurology 25:980, 1975.
120. Latov, N., Sherman, W., Nemni, R., Galassi, G., Shyong, J., Penn, A., Chess, L. Olarte, M., Rowland, L., and Osserman, E.: Plasma-cell dyscrasia and peripheral neuropathy with monoclonal antibody to peripheral nerve myelin. N. Engl. J. Med. 303:618, 1980.
121. Abrams, G., Latov, N., Hays, A., Shermann, W., and Zimmerman, E.: Immunocytochemical studies of human peripheral nerve with serum from patients with polyneuropathy and paraproteinemia. Neurology 32:821, 1982.
122. Braun, P.E., Latov, N., and Freil, M.D.: MAG is the antigen for a monoclonal antibody in patients with a demyelinating neuropathy. Trans. Am. Soc. Neurochem. 13:230, 1982.
123. Silverstein, A., and Doniger, D.E.: Neurologic complications of myelomatosis. Arch. Neurol. 9:534, 1963.
124. Walsh, J.C.: The neuropathy of multiple myeloma: An electrophysiological histological study. Arch. Neurol. 25:404, 1971.
125. Hesselvik, M.: Neuropathological studies on myelomatosis. Acta Neurol. Scand. 45:95, 1969.
126. Kelly, J.J., Kyle, R.A., Miles, J.M., O'Brien, P.C., and Dyck, P.J.: The spectrum of peripheral neuropathy in myeloma. Neurology 31:24, 1981.
127. Victor, M., Banker, B.Q., and Adams, R.D.: The neuropathy of multiple myeloma. J. Neurol. Neurosurg. Psychiatry 21:73, 1958.
128. Campbell, A.M., and Halford, M.: Syndrome of diarrhoea and peripheral nerve changes due to generalized vascular disease. Br. Med. J. 2:1509, 1964.
129. Kyle, R.: Long-term survival in multiple myeloma. N. Engl. J. Med. 308:314, 1983.
130. Kelly, J.J., Kyle, R.A., Miles, J.M., and Dyck, P.J.: Osteosclerotic myeloma and peripheral neuropathy. Neurology 33:202, 1983.
131. Waldenström, J.G., Adner, A., Gydell, K., and Zettervall, O.: Osteosclerotic " plasmacytoma" with polyneuropathy, hypertrichosis, and diabetes. Acta Med. Scand. 203:297, 1978.
132. Morley, J.B., and Schwieger, A.C.: The relation between chronic polyneuropathy and osteosclerotic myeloma. J. Neurol. Neurosurg. Psychiatry 30:432, 1967.
133. Read, D., and Warlow, C.: Peripheral neuropathy and solitary plasmacytoma. J. Neurol. Neurosurg. Psychiatry 41:177, 1978.
134. Brouet, J.C., Clauvel, J.P., Danon, F., Klein, M., and Seligman, M.: Biologic and clinical significances of cryoglobulins: A report of 86 cases. Am. J. Med. 57:775, 1974.
135. Konesi, T., Saida, K., Ohnishi, A., and Nishitani, H.: Perineuritis in mononeuritis multiplex with cryoglobulinemia. Muscle Nerve 5:173, 1982.
136. Cream, J.J., Hern, J.E.C., Hughes, R., and MacKenzie, I.: Mixed or immune complex cryoglobulinaemia and neuropathy. J. Neurol. Neurosurg. Psychiatry 37:82, 1974.
137. Chad, D., Parisher, K., Bradley, W., et al.: The pathogenesis of cryoglobulinemic neuropathy. Neurology 32:725, 1982.
138. Vallat, J.M., Desproges-Gotteron, R., Leboutet, M., Loubet, A., Gaulde, N., and Treves, R.: Cryoglobulinemic neuropathy: A pathological study. Ann. Neurol. 8:179, 1980.
139. Maycock, R.L., Bertrand, P., Morrison, C.E., and Scott, J.: Manifestations of sarcoidosis. Am. J. Med. 35:67, 1963.
140. Delaney, P.: Neurologic manifestations in sarcoidosis. Review of the literature, with a report of 23 cases. Ann. Intern. Med. 87:336, 1977.
141. Silverstein, A., Feur, M.M., and Seltzbach, L.E.: Neurologic sarcoidosis. Arch. Neurol. 12:1, 1965.
142. Matthews, W.B.: Sarcoid neuropathy. *In* Dyke, P.J., Thomas, P.K., and Lambert, E.H. (eds.): Peripheral Neuropathy. Philadelphia, W.B. Saunders Company, 1975, pp. 1199–1226.
143. Jefferson, M.: Sarcoidosis of the nervous system. Brain 80:540, 1957.
144. Tharp, B.R., and Pfeiffer, J.B.: Sarcoidosis and the acoustic nerve. Arch. Otolaryngol. 90:360, 1969.
145. Strickland, G.T., and Moser, K.M.: Sarcoidosis with a Landry-Guillain-Barré syndrome and clinical response to corticosteroids. Am. J. Med. 43:131, 1967.
146. Nemni, R., Galassi, G., Cohen, M., Hays, A., Gould, R., Singh, N., Bressman, S., and Gamboa, E.: Symmetric sarcoid polyneuropathy: Analysis of a sural nerve biopsy. Neurology 31:1217, 1981.
147. Oh, S.J.: Sarcoid polyneuropathy: A histologically proven case. Ann. Neurol. 7:178, 1980.

148. Colover, J.: Sarcoidosis with involvement of the nervous system. Brain 71:451, 1948.
149. Wells, C.E.C.: The natural history of neurosarcoidosis. Proc. R. Soc. Med. 60:1172, 1967.
150. Bechelli, L.M., and Martinez, D.V.: The leprosy problem in the world. Bull. WHO 34:811, 1966.
151. Levis, W.R., and Hedrick, J.L.: Rising incidence of leprosy in the United States. N. Engl. J. Med. 304:363, 1981.
152. Sabin, T.B.: Neurologic features of lepromatous leprosy. Am. Fam. Physician 4:84, 1971.
153. Sheagren, J.N., Block, J.B., Trautman, J.R., and Wolff, S.M.: Immunologic reactivity in patients with leprosy. Ann. Intern. Med. 70:295, 1969.
154. Nath, I., and Singh, R.: The suppressive effect of M. leprae. Clin. Exp. Immunol. 41:406, 1980.
155. Bullock, W.E.: Studies of immune mechanisms in leprosy. I. Depression of delayed allergic response to skin test antigens. N. Engl. J. Med. 278:298, 1968.
156. Turk, J.L., and Waters, M.E.R.: Cell-mediated immunity in patients with leprosy. Lancet 2:243, 1969.
157. Sabin, T.D., and Swift, T.R.: Leprosy. *In* Dyck, P.J., Thomas, P.K., and Lambert, E.H. (eds.): Peripheral Neuropathy. Philadelphia, W.B. Saunders Company, 1975, pp. 1166–1199.
158. Sabin, T.D., and Ebner, J.D.: Patterns of sensory loss in lepromatous leprosy. Int. J. Lepr. 37:239, 1969.
159. Pedley, J.C., Harman, D.J., Waudy, H., and McDougall, A.C.: Leprosy in peripheral nerves: Histopathological findings in 119 untreated patients in Nepal. J. Neurol. Neurosurg. Psychiatry 43(3):198, 1980.
160. Dastur, D.K.: Cutaneous nerve in leprosy: The relationship between histopathology and cutaneous sensitivity. Brain 78:615, 1955.
161. Rosenberg, R.N., and Lovelace, R.E.: Mononeuritis multiplex in lepromatous leprosy. Arch. Neurol. 19:310, 1968.
162. Kopell, H.P., and Thompson, W.A.C.: Peripheral Entrapment Neuropathies. Baltimore, Williams and Wilkins, 1965.
163. Job, C.K.: *Mycobacterium leprae* in nerve lesions in lepromatous leprosy. An electron microscopic study. Arch. Pathol. 89:195, 1970.
164. Dastur, D.K.: Lepromatous leprosy as a model of Schwann cell pathology and lysosomal activity. Clin. Exp. Neurol. 16:277, 1979.
165. Enna, C.D., and Brand, P.W.: Peripheral nerve abscess in leprosy. Lepr. Rev. 41:175, 1970.
166. Brand, P.W.: Treatment of leprosy: The role of surgery. N. Engl. J. Med. 254:64, 1956.
167. Behse, F., and Buckthal, F.: Slowing in maximum nerve conduction velocity during acute hypoxia due to block of large fibers or to slowing along all fibers. 21st Scandinavian Congress of Neurology, Stockholm, June 1975.
168. Caruso, G., Labianca, O., and Ferrannini, E.: Effects of ischemia on sensory protential of normal subjects of different ages. J. Neurol. Neurosurg. Psychiatry 36:455, 1973.
169. Caruso, G., Santoro, L., Perretti, A., and Amantin, B.: Recovery of sensory potentials after ischemic block by pneumatic compression of varying duration. Proceedings of the International Symposium on Peripheral Neuropathies, Milan, June 1978.
170. Kugelberg, E., and Cobb, W.: Repetitive discharges in human motor nerve fibers during the postischemic state. J. Neurol. Neurosurg. Psychiatry 14:88, 1951.
171. Merrington, W.R., and Nathan, P.W.: A study of postischemic paresthesiae. J. Neurol. Neurosurg. Psychiatry 12:1, 1949.
172. Torebjörk, H.E., Ochoa, J.L., and McCann, F.V.: Paresthesiae: Abnormal impulse generation in sensory nerve fibers in man. Acta Physiologica Scand. 105:518, 1979.
173. Ochoa, J.L., and Torebjörk, H.E.: Paresthesiae from ectopic impulse generation in human sensory nerves. Brain 103:835, 1980.
174. Erb, W.: Diseases of the peripheral cerebrospinal nerves. *In* Ziemssen, H. Von (ed.): Cyclopedia of the Practice of Medicine. Vol. XI. London, Samson, Low, Marston, Searle and Rivington, 1876.
175. Seddon, H.J.: Three types of nerve injury. Brain 66:237, 1943.
176. Denny-Brown, D., and Brenner, C.: Paralysis of nerve induced by direct pressure and by tourniquet. Arch. Neurol. Psychiatry 51:1, 1944.
177. Ochoa, J., Danta, G., Fowler, T.J., and Gilliatt, R.W.: Nature of the nerve lesion caused by pneumatic tourniquet. Nature 233:265, 1971.
178. Lubinska, L.: Axoplasmic streaming in regenerating and in normal nerve fibers. *In* Singer, M., and Schade, J.P. (eds.): Progress in Brain Research. Vol. 13, Mechanisms of Neural Regeneration. Amsterdam, Elsevier Publishing Co., 1964, pp. 1–77.
179. Hiscoe, H.B.: Distribution of nodes and incisurae in normal and regenerated nerve fibers. Anat. Rec. 99:447, 1947.
180. Lubinska, L.: Demyelination and remyelination in the proximal parts of regenerated nerve fiber. J. Comp. Neurol. 117:275, 1961.
181. Seddon, H.J.: Peripheral nerve injuries in Great Britain during World War II: A review. Arch. Neurol. Psychiatry 63:171, 1950.
182. Seltzer, C.A., and Sevor, M.: Ephaptic transmission in chronically damaged peripheral nerves. Neurology 29:1061, 1979.
183. Ochoa, J.: Pain in local nerve lesions. *In* Culp, W., and Ochoa, J. (eds.): Abnormal Nerves and Muscles as Impulse Generators. New York, Oxford University Press, 1982.
184. Fullerton, P.M.: The effect of ischemia on nerve conduction in carpal tunnel syndrome. J. Neurol. Neurosurg. Psychiatry 26:385, 1963.
185. Fullerton, P.M., and Gilliatt, R.W.: Median and ulnar neuropathy in the guinea pig. J. Neurol. Neurosurg. Psychiatry 30:393, 1967.
186. Ochoa, J., and Marotte L.: Nature of the nerve lesion underlying chronic entrapment. J. Neurol. Sci. 19:49, 1973.
187. Neary, D., Ochoa, J., and Gilliatt, R.W.: Subclinical entrapment neuropathy in man. J. Neurol. Sci. 24:283, 1975.
188. Schaumburg, H.H., Spencer, P.S., and Ochoa, J.: The aging human peripheral nervous system. *In* Katzman, R., and Terry, R.D. (eds.): The Neurology of Aging, Philadelphia, F.A. Davis Co., 1983.
189. Spencer, P.S., and Ochoa, J.: The mammalian peripheral nervous system in old age. *In* Johnson, J.E., Jr. (ed.): Aging and Cell Structure. Vol. I. New York, Plenum Press, 1981.
190. Jenkyn, L.R., and Reeves, A.G.: Neurologic signs in uncomplicated aging (senescence). Semin. Neurol. 1:21, 1981.
191. Steiness, I.: Vibration perception in normal subjects. Acta Med. Scand. 158:315, 1957.
192. Pearson, G.H.: Effect of age on vibratory sensibility. Arch. Neurol. Psychiatry 20:482, 1928.
193. Critchley, M.: The neurology of old age. Lancet 1:1221, 1931.
194. Goldberg, J.M., and Lindblom, U.: Standardized method of determining vibratory perception thresholds for diagnosis and screening in neurological investigation. J. Neurol. Neurosurg. Psychiatry 42:793, 1979.
195. Potvin, A.R., Syndulko, K., Tourtellotte, W.W., Lemman, J.A., and Potvin, J.H.: Human neurologic function and the aging process. J. Am. Geriatr. Soc. 28:1, 1980.
196. Dyck, P.J., Curtis, D.J., Bushek, W., and Offord, K.: Description of "Minnesota thermal discs" and normal values of cutaneous thermal discrimination in man. Neurology 24:325, 1974.
197. Prakash, C., and Stern, G.: Neurological signs in the elderly. Age Ageing 2:24, 1973.
198. Carter, A.B.: The neurologic aspects of aging. *In* Rossman, I. (ed.): Clinical Geriatrics. Second edition. Philadelphia, J.B. Lippincott, 1979.
199. Jenkyn, L.R., Walsh, D.B., Walsh, B.T., Culver, C.M., and Reeves, A.G.: The nuchocephalic reflex. J. Neurol. Neurosurg. Psychiatry 38:561, 1975.
200. Klawans, H.L., Tupo, H.M., Ostfeld, A.M., Shekelli, R.B., and Killridge, J.A.: Neurologic examination in an elderly population. Dis. Nerv. Syst. 32:374, 1971.

# Chapter 20
# Biomechanics of Joints

*Sheldon R. Simon*

## INTRODUCTION

Webster's Third New International Dictionary defines that specialized organ system of the body called a joint as the "point of contact between elements of an animal skeleton . . . with the parts . . . that surround and support it." It continues to describe a joint in more general terms as "an area at which two ends, surfaces, or edges are *attached*," "the junction of two or more members of a *framed structure*," "a fracture or crack in rock *not accompanied by dislocation*," and "a part or *space* included between two articulations" (emphasis added). Mechanics is defined as that "branch of physical science that deals with energy and forces" and their effect on bodies, and the "practical application of mechanics to the design, construction, or operation of machines," and "of the nature of or resembling a machine especially in routine or automatic performance." In describing the biomechanics of joints how many of these definitions apply? The answer is simpler than the explanation: all of them and more.

All joints in the body exist as the point, place, crack, or junction where at least two skeletal members attach, and all joints essentially consist of the same elements of the space between the members and the parts that surround, support, and stabilize it. However, the location of each joint in its proximal or distal, upper or lower position sufficiently alters the mechanics to make it uniquely distinct (e.g., hip joint, knee joint, elbow joints, or finger joints).[1-7]

Animal joints are classified into groups according to the biologic nature of the materials and the amount of relative motion between the articular ends of the bones. In general three types of joints exist:[8] (1) fibrous joints or synarthroses: joints with no relative motion; (2) cartilaginous joints or amphiarthroses: joints with little or no relative motion; and (3) diarthrodial or synovial joints: joints with large degrees of motion.[9-15] Whether mechanical conditions have created distinct individual joint constructs or biological design has designated their uniquely specified mechanics is not known; but as we shall see, when joint destruction is present and treatment is attempted, the outcome of the situation is heavily dependent upon the mechanics.

## BIOMECHANICS OF NORMAL JOINTS

**Joint Stability.** All joints have the potential to move. True joint movement is the relative change in position of one skeletal member in relation to its adjacent one. When we pick up a glass and bring it to our mouth, our wrist moves from a position on the table to one adjacent to our face. This type of movement may be considered extremity movement and total joint displacement, rather than true joint movement. There are six possible types of motion about three perpendicular axes: three rotational and three translational (Fig. 20–1). In general most joint motion is only minimally translational and is primarily rotational.[9-17] If the motion were solely rotational, at any instant, the center of the radius of the arc of motion would repeatedly be at the same point. However, there exists a small component of translational movement, and the deviation from absolute rotatory motion may be noted by the changes in the path of the joint's "instantaneous centers of rotation" (Fig. 20–2). These centers have been measured for the shoulder, elbow, wrist, knee, and ankle and found to vary only slightly from true arcs of rotation.[18-28] However, this minimal translation or deviation from it may be detrimental to the joints.

The inability of the structures making up a joint to limit translational motions and to restrict some rotational arcs of motion is considered subluxation or dislocation of the joint. To stabilize joints and maintain them moving principally in rotational arcs, three anatomical structures are utilized: bones, ligaments, and muscles. These three structures contribute to different extents at different joints.

The first structure to be considered is bone. The contours of the ends of each bone are unique for each joint and each side of a joint. No two are alike. Although in general one side of a joint may be considered concave in shape and the other side convex, at each joint significant deviations exist in each of the three rotational planes in the radius of curvature, and in the amount of the arc of curvature that is present. Since bone is the most rigid anatomical structure, in any rotational plane the greater the arc of motion enclosed by bone, the greater the amount of inherent stability that exists. For example, at the hip the spherical head of the femur is almost enclosed by a hemispherical arc of bony acetabulum, whereas the shoulder, with a similar shape but a much flatter radius of curvature and a less enclosed humeral head is markedly different in the ease with which it can be subluxed or dislocated (Fig. 20–3).[19,30]

If stability is desired and the contour of the bone is inadequate to achieve it, a second structure is available—ligaments. The ability of ligaments to restrict displacement absolutely is not as good as that of bone but is perfectly adequate under most circumstances and situations. The intrinsic properties of ligaments are different from those of bone in several aspects. Unlike bone, ligament cannot provide stability against translational mo-

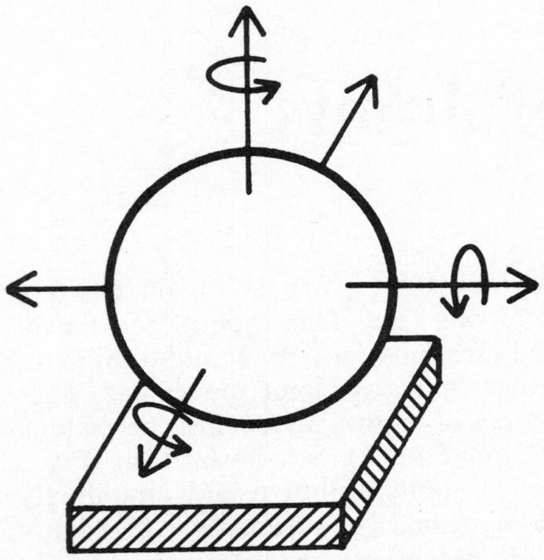

Figure 20–1. All motions of two adjacent bodies relative to each other consist of translational motions along three mutually perpendicular axes and three rotational motions about these same three axes.

tions in any direction which is across or perpendicular to its major axis—it is not "solid enough." The medial collateral ligament of the knee, for example, will not prevent anterior-posterior (AP) or medial-lateral translational motions by itself (Fig. 20–4). Ligaments resist motions that are situated in the plane in which the ligament lies. Furthermore, when ligaments are called upon to resist displacement in such a direction, they are not only weaker than bone in being able to do so, but also will yield or stretch.[31-37] In certain circumstances this feature seems to be a desirable one, as ligaments are commonly used throughout the body as structural joint stabilizers.[38-54] Most often they complement the effect of bony contouring by limiting the degree of *allowable* rotatory motion rather than by preventing translation. The control of translational motions, which can lead to subluxation or dislocation, is left in most cases for bone.[38-41,48,49] At the ankle, the deltoid and lateral ligaments limit varus-valgus rotation in the same plane as the tibial-fibular ankle mortise limits medial-lateral translation (Fig. 20–5). In other circumstances bone and ligaments function in different planes. For example, at the elbow, bony contouring in the AP plane limits AP translation, while ligaments in the medial-lateral plane limit varus-valgus rotation.

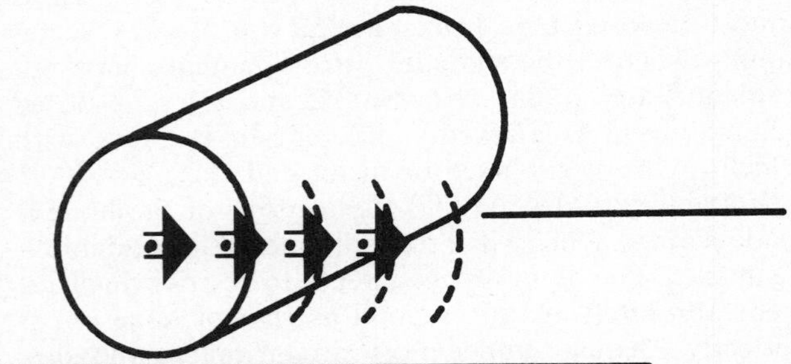

Figure 20–2. If a body rotates in place, the center of its rotation does not move. If the body translates as it rotates, movement of the center of rotation reflects this motion.

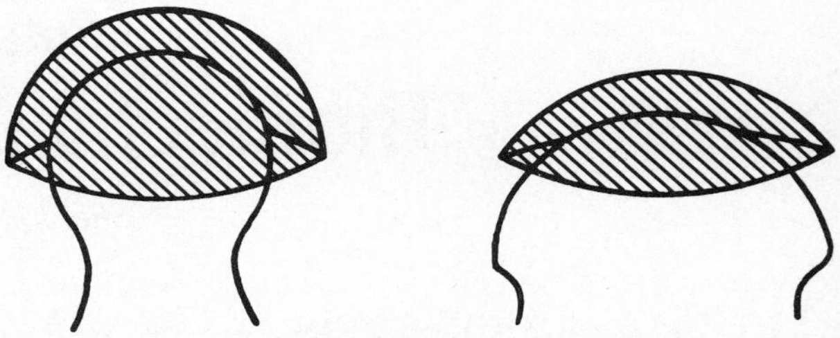

Figure 20–3. Both the hip and shoulder joints have no rotational restrictions and have similar ball-in-socket shapes. The glenoid socket does not stabilize the humeral head as well as the acetabulum stabilizes the femoral head.

At certain joints the forces in a given rotational plane are minimal and a single ligament may act alone. If the forces are high, several ligaments, or a markedly thickened or structurally modified and strengthened ligament, or even the complementary action of a third structural member, muscle, may be present.[58-69] For example, to control varus-valgus and internal-external rotation in the medial-lateral plane of the knee, bone and ligaments are complemented by multiple muscles such as the hamstrings (Fig. 20–6).[42-69] Another example is the spine, where the posterior ligamentous elements are multiple, with each one having a different basic structure and anatomic size, and they work in combination with the extensor paraspinal muscle group to prevent excessive flexion.

The muscle-tendon complex, similar to ligaments in the manner in which it stabilizes a joint, is unlike either bone or ligament in its capability to respond, as it first must be activated. Of all three structural "stabilizers," muscle is the only one which can be controlled during the immediate action. It can thus act as a stabilizer and resist rotatory motions created by external forces or can itself create unstable rotatory motions.[58-69]

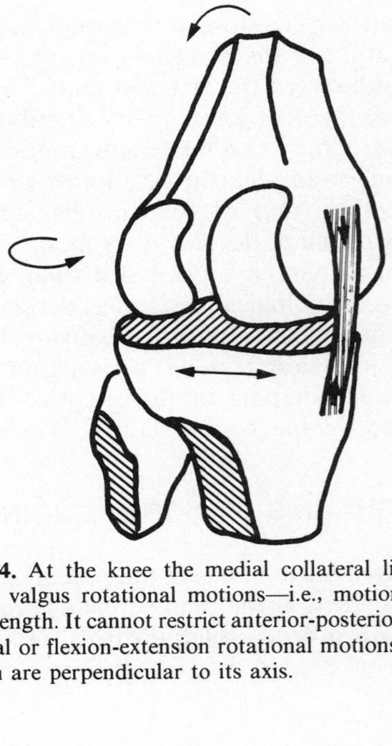

Figure 20–4. At the knee the medial collateral ligament can only restrict the valgus rotational motions—i.e., motions parallel to the ligament's length. It cannot restrict anterior-posterior or medial-lateral translational or flexion-extension rotational motions of the joint, motions which are perpendicular to its axis.

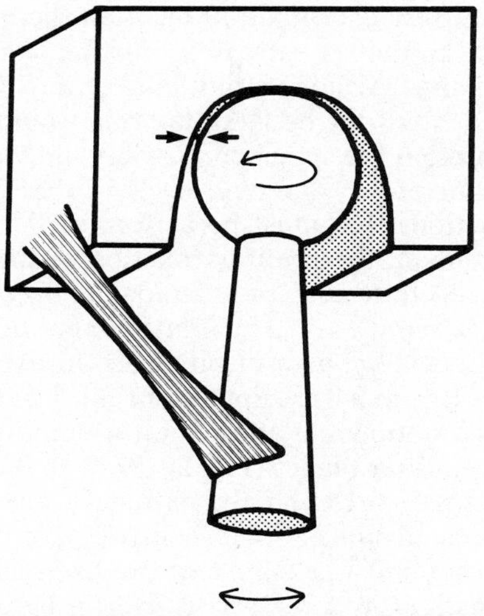

**Figure 20–5.** Ankle stability in the medial-lateral plane is maintained by a combination of bony contouring limiting translational movements and ligaments limiting rotational movements.

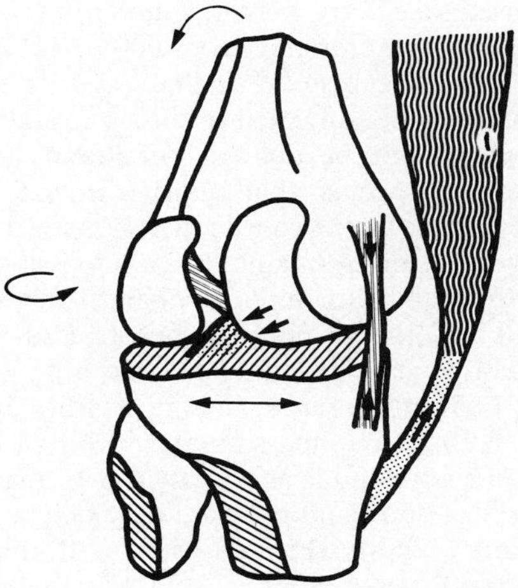

**Figure 20–6.** At the knee, bony contouring (tibial spine) only stabilizes medial-lateral translational motion. To control all the other motions that this joint undergoes, multiple ligaments of different sizes and shapes as well as muscles in many planes are needed.

The intricate balance among the three structural stabilizers, bone, ligament, and muscle, is best illustrated by the spine. To protect the spinal cord while still allowing rotatory motions of the trunk to occur, a sophisticated mechanical stabilizing arrangement has evolved. Each intervertebral segment has unique modification of all three structures to satisfy differing mechanical conditions yet maintain balance. The intervertebral unit is composed of two joints (one disc, an amphiarthritic joint, and two diarthrodial facet joints), multiple ligaments (anterior and posterior longitudinal ligaments, ligamentum flavum, and interspinous ligaments), and paraspinal muscles. The disc, unlike other amphiarthritic joints, is a very important joint, being the major supporting unit between the vertebral bony units and maintaining the vertical rigidity of the entire system.[70,71] This biological structure with its central nucleus pulposus and surrounding ligamentous anulus fibrosus may be compared to a hydrostatic balloon set in a coffee can; the nucleus is resistant to being vertically deformed because no significant sideways displacement is permitted by the anulus fibrosus (Fig. 20–7*A*). Although the disc will stabilize vertical loads and prevent vertical translation, it does not stabilize horizontal translation.[72] When a person sits, stands, or bends forward, whether to tie a shoelace or pick up a weight, the body's weight is located anterior to the spine. This configuration would not only compress the disc but would also topple the spine by creating forces tending to tilt and slide one vertebral unit over the one below it. To prevent the sliding, "slipping" motions, each vertebral body must overhang the one below it. This arrangement is provided by the facet joints, located posteriorly and laterally. They provide little vertical support for body weight but prevent AP and medial-lateral translational motions (Fig. 20–7*B*). However, movements in rotational arcs whose axes cross at the posterior central portion of the disc are still allowed. Depending on the degree to which the translational sliding motions in any direction need be restricted, the joints are oriented differently in the atlantoaxial region, cervical spine region, and thoracic and lumbar spine regions. Within the planes and motions so allowed, the ligaments and muscles then limit the *extent* and control the degree and speed with which such motions occur, acting as the major source of stability to rotation (Fig. 20–7*C*).[72-89] However, a price is paid for the use of muscle effort. To control forward trunk flexion the erector spinae muscles must exert large forces

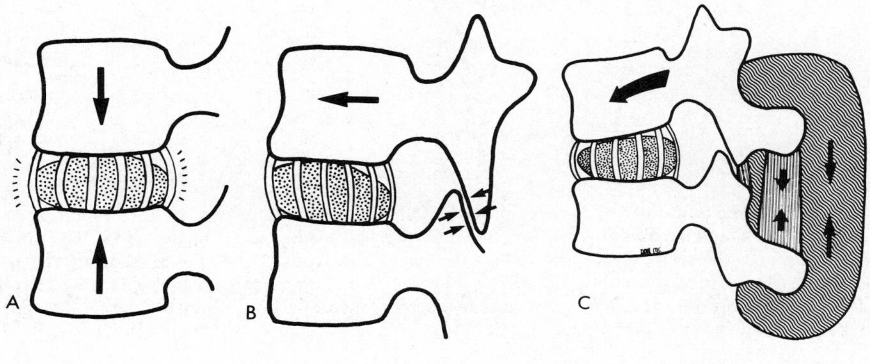


**Figure 20–7.** The intervertebral unit of the spine has multiple structures contributing to its stability. The disc (*A*) prevents vertical translational motions, like a balloon placed in a coffee can. The facet joints (*B*) prevent forward translation, permitting the more proximal vertebrae only to rotate about the more distal one in a prescribed arc. Multiple ligaments and paraspinal muscles control the speed and extent within this arc of movement through their "clamping" effect on the posterior elements (*C*).

to counterbalance body weight. These forces cause large compression forces, ranging from 600 to 1500 lbs, to be exerted across the disc.[86,90,91] The intervertebral discs cannot routinely be subjected to these extreme pressures, as they would not be able to withstand them. Thus investigators suspected that another structure besides the spine might play a role in trunk stability. At first sight it seems unreasonable to assume any pressure transfers through the trunk other than through the spine, because all the other structures are soft. However, a soft material can be arranged in such a way that use is made of its tensile strength, rather than its rigidity, to transmit pressures.[92] In a manner similar to the way the disc controls and withstands the vertical pressures imposed upon it, intra-abdominal pressure may play a significant role in trunk stability (Fig. 20–8).[86-94] Although the abdominal muscle is potentially a source to reduce the load across the disc regardless of its strength, in certain situations it may not be utilized, and its effect in reducing disc loads has therefore been disputed.[89,93,94]

**Joint Motions.** As a consequence of bone, ligaments, and muscles contributing to joint stability to various degrees and in various planes, each joint in the body is distinct with regard to both the types of motions that exist and the degree to which each is allowed.[95-98] While some joints have grossly similar movements, for example, hip and shoulder, knee and elbow, ankle and wrist, the combinations of the three structural units comprising them are different and appear related to the external force demands and functional requirements imposed upon them.

The spine, while providing support for the body above it and protecting the spinal cord within it, must have some degree of flexibility to allow proper sensing of the head and proper coordination between the head, upper extremities, and lower extremities for the vital functions of daily living. Although motions at any given joint cannot and need not be large (as this would place too great a strain on the spinal cord at any individual level), they are different at different levels of the spine owing to the functions that must be performed.[75,99-102]

In the human, the primary function of the upper extremities is to transport and manipulate objects; that of the lower extremities is to facilitate locomotion. To provide for the wide sphere of influence an extremity can encompass, the most proximal joint must have the widest range of motion and allow rotatory motions of large degrees in all three planes (Fig. 20–9).[103,104] Because most of the external forces on the extremity are exerted at some distance from the joint, controlling muscle forces about the joint must be high. One can liken this situation to that existing on a seesaw. If even a light weight is placed far out on one side of the fulcrum, it must be balanced by another, much larger weight close in on the other side of the fulcrum. Further, the fulcrum must be sufficiently stable that the plank does not slide from side to side.

In vertebrate animals, the joint established at the shoulder to suit these demands is a ball-and-socket joint—large enclosing stable bony contours with large muscle masses that obviate the need for intricate ligamentous systems. In the human the hip maintains the same functional characteristics as in other animals, namely that of balancing a large mass (body weight) at very frequent intervals, and also maintains the same

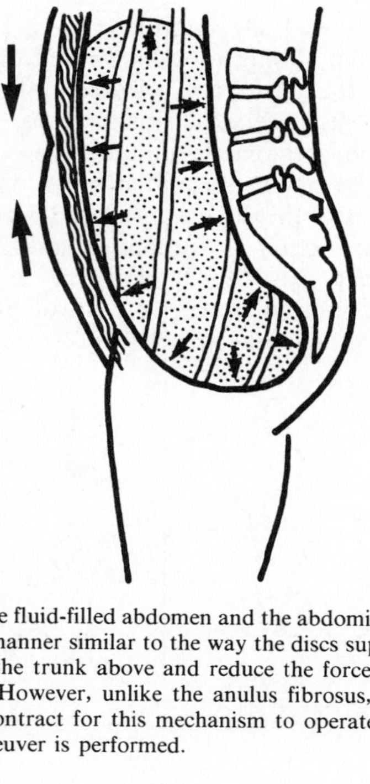

**Figure 20–8.** The fluid-filled abdomen and the abdominal musculature around it, in a manner similar to the way the discs support loads, can act to support the trunk above and reduce the forces and loads the disc must feel. However, unlike the anulus fibrosus, the abdominal muscles must contract for this mechanism to operate, such as when a Valsalva maneuver is performed.

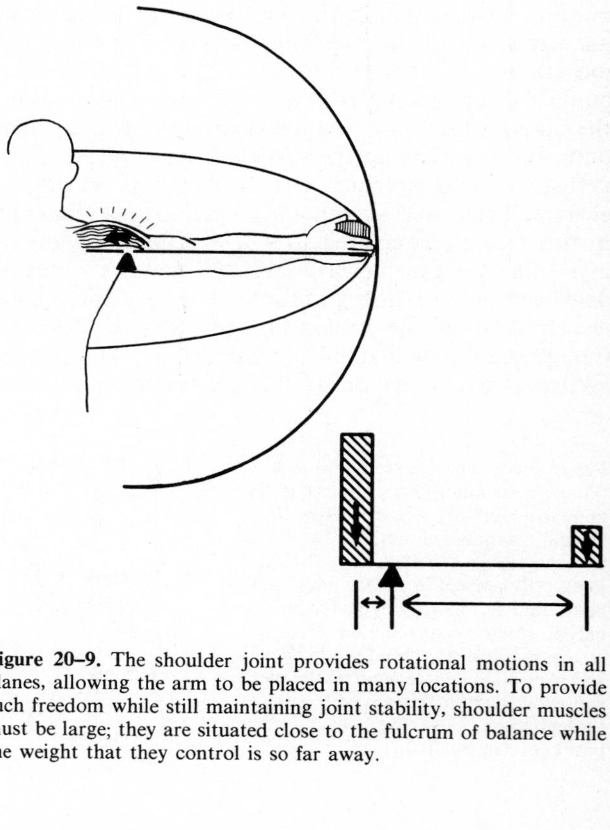

**Figure 20–9.** The shoulder joint provides rotational motions in all planes, allowing the arm to be placed in many locations. To provide such freedom while still maintaining joint stability, shoulder muscles must be large; they are situated close to the fulcrum of balance while the weight that they control is so far away.

bone and muscle characteristics. The shoulder, however, reduced in its demand of weight and repetitive use, relies less on bony stability but retains its muscle mass.[104-106]

In order for an extremity to cover all areas within the range allowed, a means must be provided to alter its length. It would not be advisable to have the bones of the upper and lower arm or leg extend and shorten in piston-like manner, as a number of repetitions in combination with high imposed loads would place too great a strain on the bony structures.[107,108] The rotational motion of the elbow or knee joint allows overall limb length changes only if both adjacent limb segments move (Fig. 20–10). This movement can occur only if motion at another, more proximal joint occurs simultaneously and coordination and synchronization between the two joints are maintained. In some circumstances the existing mechanism for this process is a passive one. During the initiation of the swing phase of walking or while climbing stairs, hip flexors flex the hip, while the knee flexes passively; the inertia of the shank lagging behind that of the actively mobile femur creates knee flexion and a relative shortening of the limb's length to provide floor or step clearance. In other circumstances muscles must be utilized.[107-110] Although neurologic control could coordinate separate muscles about each joint to perform the task, it is often more efficient to provide control with a single muscle which spans two joints. Such muscles are used when a repetitious act of limb shortening or lengthening occurs in which one joint does not move or is moving in a direction to stretch the muscle and the other rotates in an opposite direction to take advantage of the active contraction of the muscle. The two-joint muscles act to move one joint while the other remains in a stable position or is controlled by other forces.[110,111]

**Joint Forces.** Control of movement by muscles has several distinguishing features that are important to joint mechanics. Because all muscle-tendon systems cross a joint, their contraction creates a force at the joint regardless of whether their effort is for the purpose of causing active rotation or for inhibiting the movement that might be created by body inertia. No muscle goes through a joint; rather, all known biological muscle systems span the periphery of the joint. A major advantage is thereby obtained in controlling rotational motion. The torque or force causing rotational motion is not merely the contractile force produced by the muscle but is the product of this force multiplied by the distance between the joint's center of rotation and the tendon (Figs. 20–9 and 20–11). The tendon placed at the periphery of the joint gives the muscle a mechanical advantage in creating the greatest torque with the least effort.[1-7,112-125]

In addition to the torque that rotates the joint, muscle contraction produces additional types of forces at the joint. One is compression, which tends to squeeze the joint together (Fig. 20–12). This force is considerable, and in most of the weight-bearing joints of the lower extremities it can be up to three to four times body weight.[113-122] As will be discussed below (joint lubrication), the joint takes advantage of this situation for the purposes of its own lubrication. This force also maintains stability against forces that might pivot a joint open (Figs. 20–6, 20–7*C*, 20–9, 20–11, and 20–13). However, in so doing it creates relatively high forces that the joint

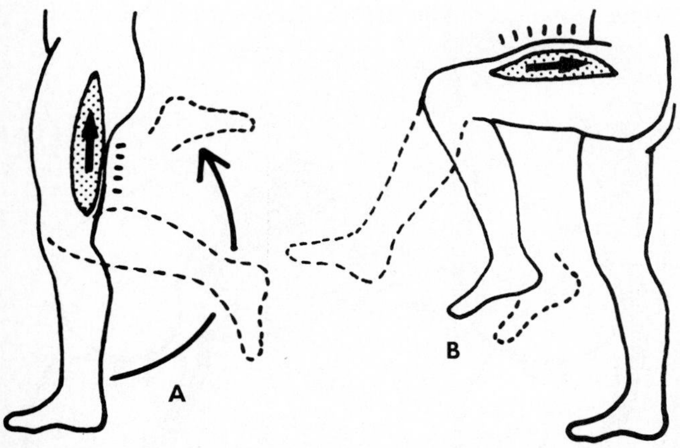


**Figure 20–10.** If the femur is stationary (*A*), knee motions alone are not an effective means of producing limb shortening. Under such circumstances the foot can move only in a single prescribed 180 degrees arc behind the knee. However, if at the same time the thigh is allowed to move by rotatory motions produced about the hip (*B*), the limb can be shortened or placed within a wide spherical volume.

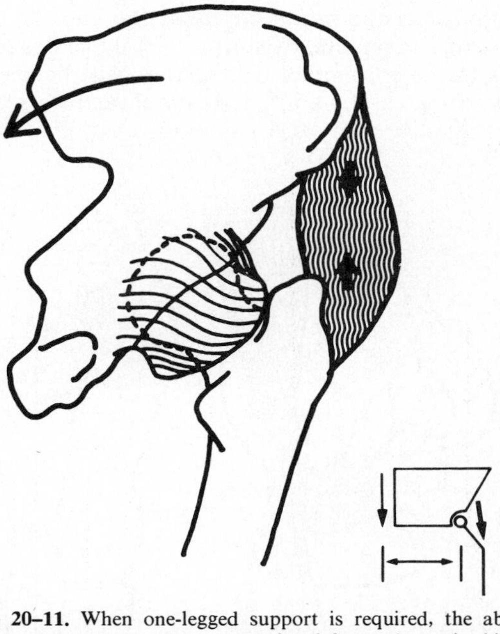

**Figure 20–11.** When one-legged support is required, the abductor muscles contract to produce a rotational force about the hip joint opposite to that produced by body weight. The farther away the muscle-tendon complex is from the center of the joint, the lower the muscle force needs to be to create the same rotational force. In most cases the muscle-tendon complex's distance from the center of the joint is less than that of the weight it is trying to counteract. This produces a larger force in the muscles than the weight it balances. As a consequence during the functional activities of daily living the major muscles about the hip typically produce forces two to four times body weight.

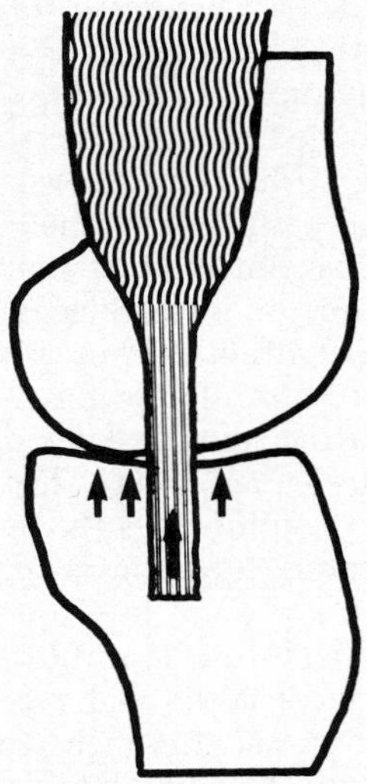

**Figure 20–12.** The force that a muscle produces tends to squeeze or compress the joint it spans.

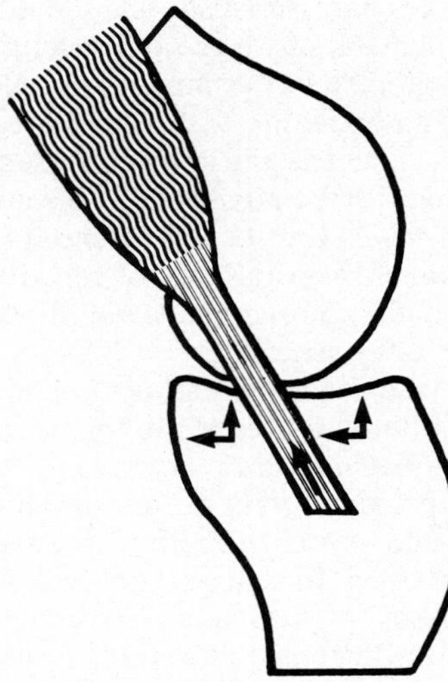

**Figure 20–14.** In many areas, the muscles placed on the concave, medial, or lateral sides of the joint become more parallel to the surface of the joint as the joint is flexed. Joint compressive forces are reduced but shear forces arise.

surface must withstand. Further, in certain movements as the joint is rotated to positions of greater flexion, the muscles become more parallel to the joint surface (Fig. 20–14). In many cases the shear force or rotational torque parallel to the joint line is helpful in stabilizing the joint against inertial or weight-bearing forces that tend to translate the two sides of the joint apart.[118-125] Rotational torque produced about the knee of a skier traversing a mountain, twisting outward over his planted ski, is but one example. However, as will be discussed below, in cases of joint instability shear forces can be detrimental.[126-133] In other cases, such as the flexor tendons of the fingers, pulleys are provided to maintain a constant direction of pull across the joint (Fig. 20–15).

**Joint Control.** If muscles were to act continuously with the same degree of forceful contraction, the nature of stresses placed upon the joint would merely depend upon the angular position of the joint relative to the direction of muscle pull. But such is not the case. Joint motions allow multiple functional body activities. The neurologic control system and muscle physiology that could dictate such continuous constant force situations would not be efficient, either in performing the activity or in preserving energy. Rather, the total magnitude of the forces as well as the time that the joint feels them in compression or shear fluctuates and depends on what the specific functional activity is, how the activity is performed, how fast it is completed, and when in the time sequence of the act the forces are observed.[134-150]

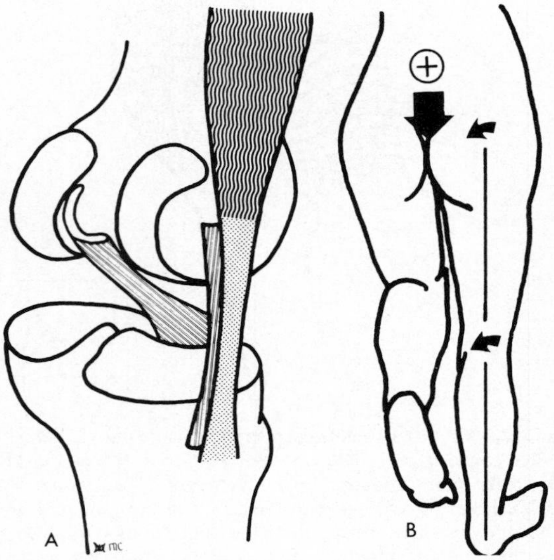


**Figure 20–13.** Being eccentrically placed, a muscle will produce compressive force that will prevent a joint from pivoting open. At the knee the vastus lateralis assists knee ligaments (*A*), preventing body weight medially placed from opening up the lateral side of the joint during one-legged support (*B*).

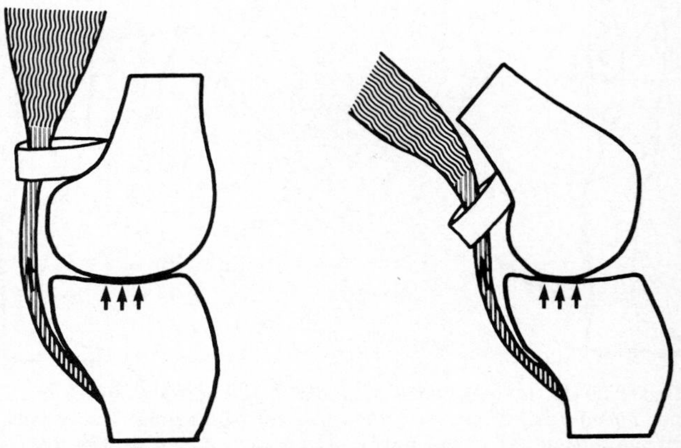

**Figure 20–15.** At certain joints pulleys located proximal to the joint maintain flexor tendons at fixed distances and orientation to the joint's surface.

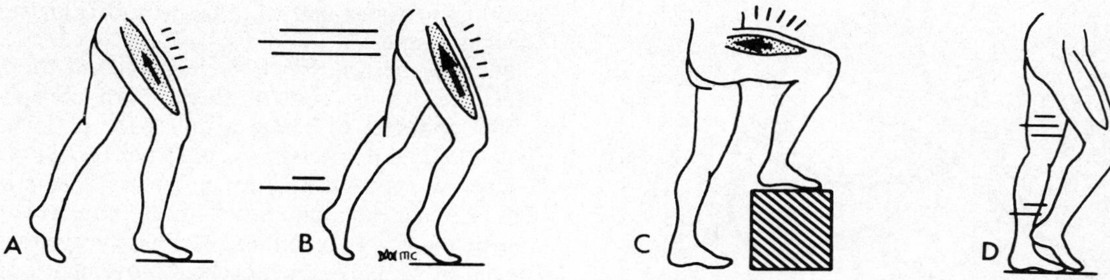


**Figure 20–16.** The muscle activity of the quadriceps will depend upon the type of activity that is being performed—i.e., the early stance phase of walking (*A*), running (*B*), going up stairs (*C*), and the early wing phase of walking or running (*D*).

At the knee joint, while walking, 15 to 20 degrees of knee flexion occurs in the early stance phase. The quadriceps muscle attempts to prevent collapse of the leg under the body's weight as the leg is decelerating. Most of the force exerted at this joint is compressive in nature. If the individual walks faster, greater muscle activity is needed for deceleration with the knee in a relatively similar position, thereby creating higher compressive loads across the joint (Fig. 20–16).[141-145] Quadriceps activity increases even further during the act of running, where again it is needed for decelerative purposes. It also increases in rising from a chair or climbing stairs to lift the body to a greater height rather than to control deceleration.[146,147] In the latter case, the knee is in greater flexion and, in addition to compression forces, higher shear forces arise. In contrast, during the swing phase of walking an equal and even greater degree of flexion occurs, but no significant muscle activity is present about the knee and joint forces are thus minimal. The activity of the quadriceps and the consequent forces at the knee joint during such highly repetitive activities are relatively the same from person to person, appearing to be dictated by single, fixed, preprogrammed neurological responses. Other joints engaged in repetitive activities in which overall efficiency and energy are prime considerations function in a manner similar to the knee.

In activities involving less repetitive motions, the consistency in the manner in which such activities are performed varies from person to person and from time to time in the same person. As an example, activities involving joints of the spine, such as bending or lifting, are dictated by factors in addition to a single, fixed, preprogrammed, neurologic response. These factors seem to be related to the fact that activities that require the involvement of the low back region can also require the participation of one or more joints of the upper or lower extremities.

One factor relates to an individual's *potential* to perform a task in a chosen manner. This ability depends on the strength of various muscle groups in different parts of the body. For example, a person wishing to bend over and pick something up may accomplish this task by keeping the legs straight and bending from the back and hips (Fig. 20–17*A*). The person may pick up the object in this manner because of habit, but he or she must also have the appropriate strength in the back muscles to withstand the brunt of the lifting that will be required of these tissues. Alternatively, the person may desire to bend at the hips, knees, and ankles, keeping the back straight, and therefore lift the object by utilizing the leg muscles (Fig. 20–17*B*). If this method is chosen, there must exist sufficient strength in the leg muscles.[149,150] A person may also chose to utilize a combination of these two methods, employing both back and lower extremity muscles (Fig. 20–17*C*).

Another factor relates to the "psychological bent" of the person. Because of overall temperament and manner, each individual can perform the same task in a unique way (Figs. 20–17 to 20–19).[101,110] If a specific function (bending) is performed utilizing lower extremity segment motions and upper extremity segment motions in combination with the back "correctly," less stress may be placed on the lower lumbar region. One might liken this to "good or bad form" observed on the part of someone playing an individual sport. Proper form not only utilizes other joints but relates to the speed and frequency with which a movement at any particular joint occurs (Figs. 20–18 and 20–19). Alterations in the speed the limbs move during any given interval time in which a given function occurs will place certain stresses on the muscular tissues and/or the joints at various intervals owing to the fact that large acceleration and deceleration forces will occur. One could liken this situation to viewing someone swinging a golf club or tennis racket. One might note that the person may not be using his or her body to the extent required for proper form. The person might be swinging rapidly at the onset of stroke prior to hitting the ball, and minimizing the follow-up after the ball is

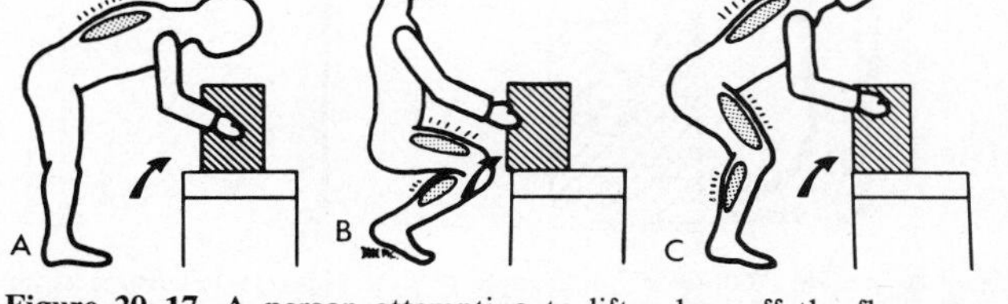


**Figure 20–17.** A person attempting to lift a box off the floor may utilize hip, trunk, and arm motions (*A*), hip, knee, and ankle motions (*B*), or a combination of all of these (*C*). Muscles needed, and the magnitude of the force from each that is required, will be dependent upon which method the individual chooses.

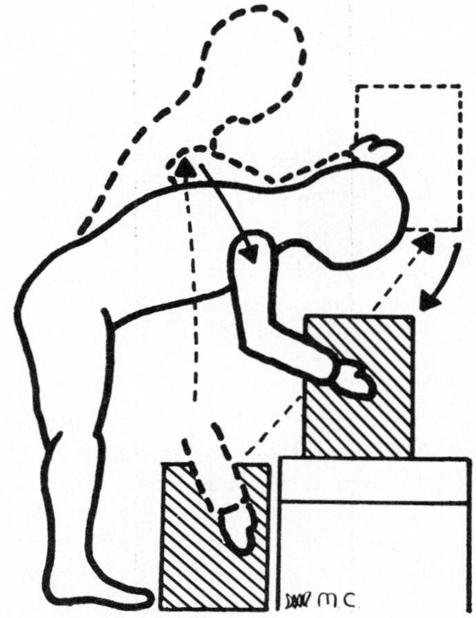

**Figure 20–18.** Whatever muscles a person chooses to utilize when lifting a box off the floor, nonpurposeful movement may be employed, such as overshooting the table and then setting the box back down. Muscles needed for such unnecessary movements create additional forces and stresses across respective joints.

hit. This type of movement would cause increased stresses in certain muscles and at certain arcs of joint motion in the initial part of the stroke, while reducing those which would occur normally in the latter part of the stroke. Thus, the same function utilizing relatively the same neurologic controlling programs can produce different forces in different joints in the same individual at different times and in different individuals acting at the same time.

**Joint Structure.** Body movements and the muscular effort needed to control them, both constrained by joints, combine to create a multitude of joint stresses that mandate a specialized construct for the joint itself to prevent its failure.[151] As an example, it is estimated that in 1 year each joint in the lower extremity undergoes approximately two million oscillatory cycles solely in the act of walking. Each cyclical movement occurs over a period of approximately 1 second or less, and the loads imposed upon the joint are not only three to four times body weight but are of very brief duration (three tenths of a second), making these loads impulsive and of more potential damage than a constant steady load alone. Such conditions of heavy loads and pressures (up to 5 times body weight and 5 MN per square meter), low speeds (sliding speeds of less than 65 mm per second), and intermittent oscillatory motion (about 1 to 2 cycles per second) are extremely severe for weight-bearing joints; yet animal joints last longer than any man-made joint thus far devised (wear rate about 2 $\mu$g per hour). The way in which these joints function mechanically seems to have dictated a specific structure, anatomic form, and mechanism to ensure their survival. Over the past 50 years considerable investigation has led to the understanding that all aspects of a joint structure are related and that each serves a specific need for the mechanical survival of the joint—be it synovial fluid and articular cartilage surfaces to withstand the interfacial frictional forces created, the biochemical composition and geometrical distribution of water and organic matrix within the articular cartilage to provide "micromovement" and conformational load bearing, or the highly specialized subchondral trabecular bone arrangement to absorb some of the shock of impulsive loading. Each aspect of the joint structure appears to be optimized to allow joint movement to occur, reduce the mechanical forces that it must withstand, and provide some way to nourish and protect the cells needed for self-repair.

***Minimization of Frictional Forces.*** The rotational movements of a joint, constrained by bony contours and ligamentous tissues, create a sliding motion of one articular surface on another. Such a motion should create shearing or frictional forces between the two surfaces which would be expected to cause joint breakdown, yet joints do not wear down by rubbing.

Frictional force is defined as the resistance one surface exerts on the other to impede its progress.[152] Such resistance depends upon the compressional load that is imposed across the two surfaces, the nature of the material and smoothness of the surfaces themselves, and the presence and characteristics of any material interposed between the two surfaces (a lubricant) which prevents the two sides from coming in contact with each other (Fig. 20–20). Under a standard load and a standard force to move one surface over another, the resistance to movement may be quantitated by a unitless number called the "coefficient of friction." The lower this number is, the more slippery is the movement of

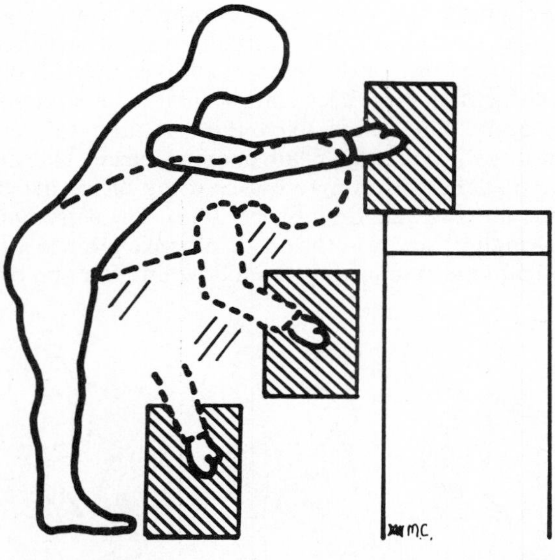

**Figure 20–19.** Whatever method a person chooses to utilize when lifting a box off the floor, different speeds may be employed during different intervals of the act. Changes in speed require muscles to control body weight and inertial acceleration and decelerations, creating additional, often unnecessary forces and stresses across the joints if "improper form" is used.

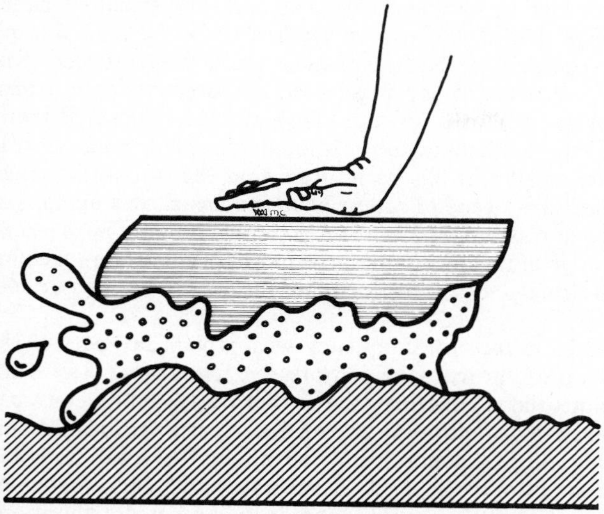

**Figure 20–20.** The ease with which one surface may be slid over another is dependent upon the compressive load, the characteristics of the two opposing materials and their surfaces, and the nature of the material interposed between the two surfaces.

the two surfaces, and the lower the shear forces created between them. Good man-made joints, such as steel-on-steel lubricated by oil, operate at coefficients of friction between 0.1 and 0.5, whereas an ice skate moving on ice with a film of water between the two is about 0.01. Biological joints operate at coefficients of friction between 0.02 and 0.002, nearly one tenth to one hundredth that of what humans can at present design![153-155] Thus, if a 70-kilogram man walks and creates a 200-kilogram compressive force across the joint, the shear or frictional force felt at the joint would only be 0.2 kilogram.

The low frictional forces minimizing surface wear appear to be related to a number of biological constructs of the joint which are present at the surface, above the surface in the intervening fluid, and below the surface.

The porous deformable collagen surface is arranged with its fibers parallel to the surface of the joint. This layer has the highest concentration of collagen fibers in the joint,[156] and this factor plus its orientation may be considered ideal for preserving surface integrity.[156-160] Any shear forces generated may disrupt the surface by pulling the material apart (tensile stretch). Collagen is strongest in the direction parallel to its fiber length and more resistant to breaking when it is pulled apart rather than squeezed together along this axis. However, this structural feature resists only the shear forces that might be imposed.[161,162] It does little to reduce the overall magnitude of the shear forces the joint must bear.

Articular cartilage, with an intact surface layer but without any fluid imbibed within it, has a coefficient of friction of 0.3. If saline is added, the cartilage imbibes this fluid like a sponge; when the surfaces are now slid against each other, the coefficient of friction is reduced to 0.1 to 0.02.[163,164] If a glycoprotein fraction[165] molecule in the concentrations found in synovial fluid is added to the saline, the coefficient of friction is further reduced to 0.02 to 0.002.[164-167] (It appears that the exact coefficient of friction at any given time depends on the loading configuration, joint position, and magnitude and speed of the joint's motion.) The porosity of the cartilage soaked with fluid and an active lubricant in the synovial fluid are both major features that *reduce* the shear forces that the articular surface feels. How they interact to produce this low level of frictional resistance is still a matter of controversy, and many theories have been proposed.[167-179] Common to all theories is the movement of fluid in and out of the porous cartilage. McCutchen[164] postulated that as the cartilage is compressed, the fluid from within seeps out and forms a layer separating the two surfaces, thereby lubricating the joint. This theory is called weeping lubrication. In contrast, Walker and co-workers[167] postulated that when compression exists across the joint, it causes the fluid at the surface where compression is occurring to move into the articular cartilage; the fluid inside then moves sideways to areas that are not compressed; and the central cartilage, which is compressed, deforms. Because of their size, the "slippery" synovial fluid macromolecules[180-184] are trapped and concentrated in pools on the surface, thereby lowering the coefficient of friction.[170,172-175] This mechanism is called boosted lubrication. The accumulating evidence seems to indicate that under different loading conditions and movement speeds, one of the two fluid flow mechanisms dominates and that in most circumstances a combination of these two mechanisms may exist. While no one denies the existence of either mechanism, the two theories are somewhat contradictory as to how the fluid moves in the area of compression. Recent theoretical evidence and in vitro tests from Mow and co-workers[177-179] suggest that, in general, in the trailing area of compression, fluid is imbibed into articular surface, while at the same time at the leading edge where compression is developing, fluid is expressed (Fig. 20–21).

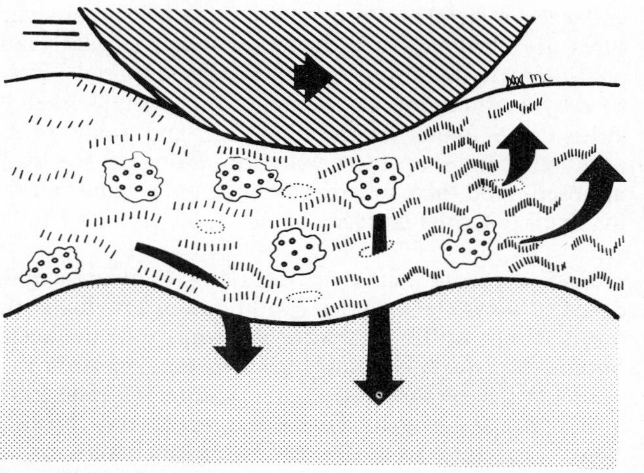

**Figure 20–21.** To minimize the resistance of moving one cartilage surface over another, the porous cartilaginous surface is layered with viscous macromolecules, but primarily weeps synovial fluid dialysate at the leading edge, absorbs this fluid in the trailing area, and deforms in the "area of contact," allowing the two cartilaginous surfaces to be kept apart.

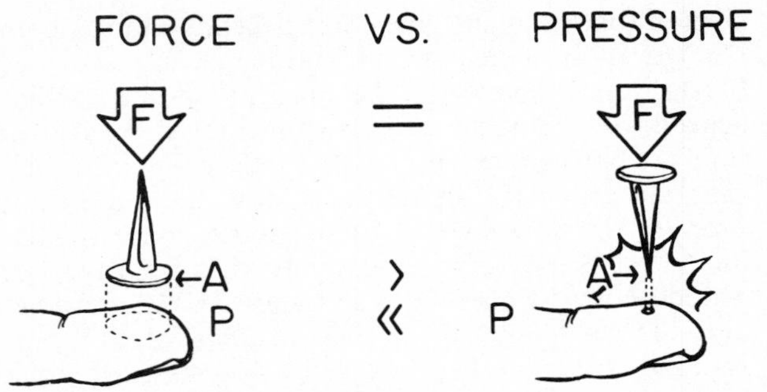


**Figure 20–22.** An individual's response to a tack pressed into a finger is dependent upon the pressure of stress that tack exerts at the skin. The force may be the same whether the point of the tack or the head of the tack is pressed against the skin, but the skin will feel worse when the same force is exerted over a smaller area (point).

Regardless of how this controversy is resolved, it is clear that each component of the joint surface appears to be important in determining the final reduction in shear forces. The mechanism is so efficient that in normal joints such forces do not appear to be the major cause of surface breakdown.

***Maximization of Contact Area.*** As with shear forces, the joint handles the compressive forces it receives by having a structure which both minimizes and withstands these loads. One important feature is contact area. The breakdown of any structure depends not only upon the total force it receives but also upon the size of the area that receives it. For example, if a tack is pressed into a person's finger, there is a big difference in the individual's reaction to it, depending upon whether the needle point of the tack or the flat part of the tack comes in contact with the skin (Fig. 20–22). In the former case, a given force is distributed over a very small area and the stress created (force per unit area) is much greater than in the latter case when the force is distributed over a larger area. Despite the wide variation in the shapes and sizes of distal and proximal joints, their gross structures are designed to provide a contact surface commensurate with the magnitude of the imposed forces, thereby maintaining approximately the same level of stress at all joints. At the hip, knee, and ankle joints, although joint shapes are markedly different, the loads imposed upon them are approximately the same and the maximal potential surface contact areas are of a similar size.

Each of these joints provides this contact area in different ways.[185-187] Under conditions of low loads the hip does not utilize the entire hemisphere of the acetabulum to provide contact; rather, a small portion in a peripheral horseshoe shape is utilized.[188-190] The knee, although appearing to have a large potential cartilaginous contacting area, actually has a small one, owing to the convex nature of the surfaces of both the femoral and tibial articulations. Recent evidence, however, has shown that the load-bearing contact area is greater owing to the fact that the meniscus plays an important function in transmitting loads.[191-194] At the ankle the contact area of the tibial-talar joint is potentially smaller than that of the hip but is increased by the load-sharing properties of the fibular-talar joint.[195] This latter joint can bear up to one sixth of the compressive forces transmitted from the joint to the shank.[196] In the small joints of the hands and feet, although the joint contact areas are smaller, it has been found that the forces they must bear are less, and recent evidence has shown again that compressive stresses of the joint are roughly in the same range of magnitude as those found in the larger "weight-bearing joints," approximately 5.0 MN per square meter.[197]

To reduce the frequency with which any part of the joint might feel such compressive loads, at any joint the potential contacting area is not always completely utilized. The deforming properties of cartilage and the surrounding subchondral bone allow the total potential contacting surfaces to exist only under high loads. At lower loads less surface area is in contact. Furthermore, the location of the contact area changes, dependent upon the angular position of the joint. Studies have shown that a changing contact area allows for continued circulation of fluid along the surface interface and the entrance and exit of synovial fluid into cartilage, thereby permitting all aspects of the articular cartilage to be nourished.[198,199] The changing areas of contact along the surface also provide a mechanism to entrap fluid under high loads when it is most needed for lubrication purposes. Lest one believe that this design is perfect, it is to be emphasized that at best the stress levels achieved appear to be relatively the same in all joints only within a certain range. Different joints do appear to have different ratios of maximal force to contacting area, and this fact may explain why certain joints are more susceptible to degenerative arthritis.[197]

**Resistance to Compressive Stresses.** Alterations in the contact area tend to reduce the stresses in articular cartilage, and cartilage is constructed in an ideal way to withstand the final compressive stress level.[201] It has two components: a liquid and a solid. The liquid is a dialysate of synovial fluid and possesses the mechanical property of incompressibility.[202,203] However, for this property to be effective and withstand the compressive loads that joints sustain, like the nucleus pulposus of the disc, this liquid must be contained. The cartilage matrix, as previously described, grossly resembles a sponge with multiple pores. The small diameter (60 Å) of these pores and their arrangement in random circuitous "tunnels" prevent large molecules from entering the cartilage, and offer considerable resistance to the direct flow in and out of the cartilage and from side to side within the cartilage (Fig. 20–23).[204-210] These characteristics provide the mechanism for the fluid to support the load.

At any instant, only a part of the whole joint is load bearing or compressed. If one part is in compression, an adjacent area is being stretched and pulled apart. This situation places high stresses of both compression and tension on the organic matrix of cartilage. The organic matrix of cartilage is a fiber-reinforced composite consisting primarily of collagen and proteoglycans and is designed to resist compression and tension. Collagen is distributed throughout the tissue with definite ultrastructure, while the proteoglycans are dispersed and immobilized in the interfibular space. Many of the proteoglycan subunits (PGS) are found in aggregates (PGA) associated with hyaluronic acid, which immobilize and anchor the subunits. Although the nature of the interaction between collagen and PGA is not known, recent evidence indicates that these interactions are responsible for the structural integrity of the tissues and the ability of cartilage to function as a bearing material. The matrix component of articular cartilage has greater mechanical resistance to being stretched apart[209,210] in a direction parallel to the oscillating direction of movement and perpendicular to the orientation of surface collagen bundles. Although many recent scanning electron microscope studies have shown that the distribution of collagen fibers in the middle and deep zones is random when the joint is unloaded,[211,212] in vitro studies have clearly indicated that their mechanical properties and the fluid flow through them are not uniform in all directions and at all levels.[213] Further, the collagen fibers of the midzone, although randomly distributed when the joint is unloaded, alter their alignment under compression to provide maximal resistance against load.[214] Such changes not only allow the matrix itself to accommodate the imposed loads better but also decrease the pore size and increase resistance to fluid flow through the cartilage. Recent studies have shown that the permeability of the tissue (ease of fluid flow) decreases exponentially[207] and the mechanical strength of cartilage increases as greater loads are imposed.[215] Such findings are dependent on age and on the depth of the cartilage layer examined, for the greater the depth the larger these factors become.[216,217]

The electrical properties of the proteoglycans and their interaction with the surrounding substances also contribute to the mechanical strength of cartilage. The carboxyl and sulfate groups of the glycosaminoglycan are endowed with highly polyanionic charge characteristics.[218-221] This charge correlates with the negative fixed charge density found in articular cartilage, which increases with the depth from the articular surface. At the surface the content of hexosamine is 3 to 8.5 percent of the dry weight of cartilage; with increasing depth it increases to 35 percent, and then gradually decreases to approximately 5.5 percent at the tidemark.[222] The large proteoglycan molecules are fixed and highly charged and hold a large volume of water. Under compressive loads these molecules "open up," exposing a greater charge to the surrounding fluid and offering increasing electrical resistance to the flow of such fluid away from it, thereby increasing the mechanical strength of the cartilage. Further, the synovial fluid dialysate itself consists of charged particles, and their movement is impeded by the repelling electrical barriers they encounter (known as streaming potential).[223-236]

Both the fluid and the organic matrix of cartilage are uniquely designed to complement each other in maintaining the integrity of the structure in the face of repeated compressive stresses. Yet ultimately, as a consequence of various arthritis diseases, cartilage in most cases weakens and tears apart.[237-241]

***Additional Resistance to Compressive Loads.*** It has long been recognized that subchondral bone has a lattice arrangement with a specific orientation at each joint with respect to the surface. Subchondral bone in certain areas shows a high concentration of trabeculae, while in others the trabeculae may occupy a broader total cross-sectional area with its outer cortical margins "flaring" out. Over the past decade Radin and others investigating the mechanical properties of the subchondral bone appear to have confirmed the ideas of earlier clinical workers that this specialization provides a means for absorbing some of the compressible impulses the

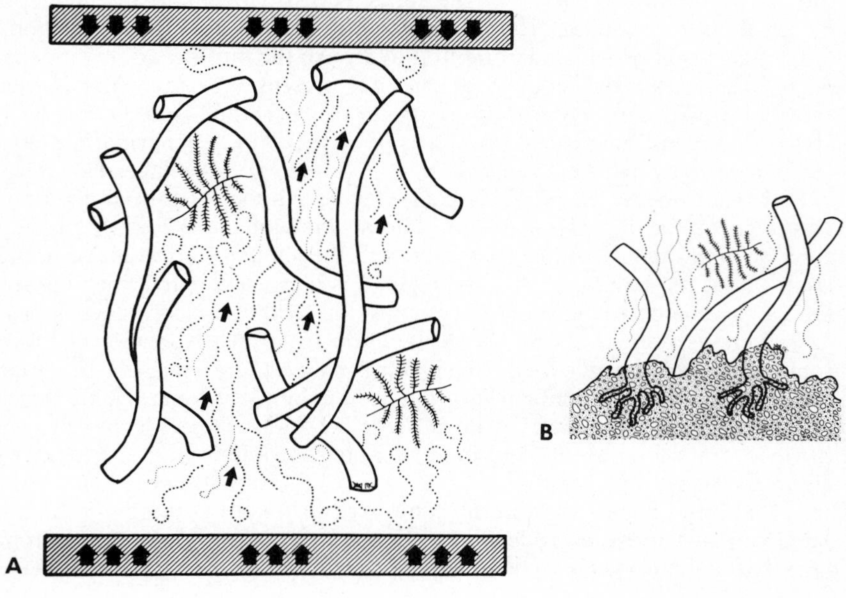


**Figure 20–23.** Cartilage is composed of a liquid and a multi-component solid, consisting of collagen and hydrophilic proteoglycan molecules. In the middle layer (*A*) the mechanical and electrical properties and architectural design of the solid "contain" the fluid, preventing it from being compressed, while still allowing fluid flow providing nourishment for cartilage cells. In the deepest zone (*B*), though the content of proteoglycans decreases, the collagen is secured tightly to subchondral bone similar to liquid-solid properties.

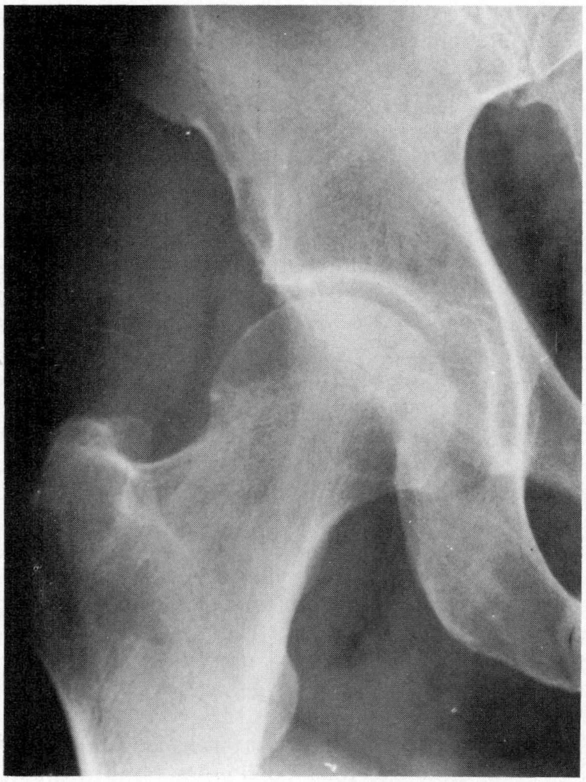

**Figure 20–24.** At the hip, trabecular bone in the femoral head is concentrated along an axis 160 degrees to the vertical where the greatest concentration of forces occurs. In contrast, the trabecular bone on the acetabular side flares out to occupy a greater area than the joint's contacting surface, distributing the same forces over a wide area, thereby reducing the stresses and allowing some of the stresses to be absorbed by bone deformation.

joint receives.[242-253] This mechanism can be viewed in the following way. If a hardball hits one's hand, the shock of impact can be reduced if the hand moves away from the ball; some of the energy of the shock is dissipated by the motion produced. The trabeculae arranged in a lattice-like array provide micromotion to absorb the impact. The greater the amount of material present (in areas of trabecular concentration) or the greater the ability of any one area to deform (areas of bone flaring), the more energy can be absorbed.

Perhaps no better example of this system exists than that seen at the hip (Fig. 20–24). The acetabulum is concave, and under low loads contact with the femur is made about its periphery; thus as the load is increased, the surface tends to flare out. This plus the fact that more bone is present allows the acetabulum to absorb some of the compressive load. The femur is convex, and thus in its peripheral contact with the acetabulum it is "clamped" and "squeezed" from all sides. To absorb the load, trabeculae are present in greater concentration along the lines of greatest force.

The ability of the subchondral bone to absorb compressive loads provides added protection for the cartilage. Although cartilage is very compliant, it is thin and is limited in its ability to absorb impulsive loads; one would not like to fall 10 feet onto a mattress 1 inch thick laid on a concrete floor, no matter how soft the mattress is!

## BIOMECHANICS OF JOINT DEGENERATION

Under normal conditions joints last. The fact that an individual can get at least 40 to 50 years of good service from almost all the joints is ample tribute to nature's grand design and marvelous mechanical structural architecture. Yet under certain conditions these structures do "wear out," and their loss is markedly disabling. To provide for their proper restoration requires therapeutic modalities which take into account how the entire mechanical system has broken down.

Normal function of any joint requires that all structures (cartilage, bone, ligaments, and muscles) act in combination to allow smooth steady motion while still maintaining stability. However, since this system is so delicately balanced and since relatively low safety factors exist within any given structure, alteration of any individual component alters the balance and often leads to mechanical breakdown of the entire joint system. Although many different factors may initiate joint destruction, it is the mechanical factors which lead to chronic joint dysfunction, and it is the total system that must be repaired. Knowledge of how this mechanical breakdown occurs and how the body can compensate for it leads to a better understanding of why function at some joints is more readily restored than at others and what must or can be done to any aspect of the system to prevent total joint destruction. An examination of different types of "joint disease" and their effects on various joints illustrate this concept.

**Hip Degeneration—Chemical Breakdown of the Organic Matrix of Cartilage.** Over one million persons over the age of 60 have impaired locomotion because of hip dysfunction. Symptoms may be present for many years before the dysfunction becomes disabling. When the cause is rheumatoid arthritis, the initial symptoms may be due to a synovitis or the earliest onset of direct enzymatic destruction of the organic matrix of the cartilage. The chemical effect clearly is aggravated even by normal external mechanical stresses that the body imposes upon the weakened bearing surface. Often when the disease is "burned out" or, as in juvenile rheumatoid arthritis, quiescent for many years, cartilage destruction continues to progress because of the alteration in balance between the forces sustained and the structure which is present to withstand them. Pain while walking or moving the hip implies that this imbalance is too great. Since little biochemical "repair" is possible, the body must use compensatory mechanisms to reduce the forces across the hip joint and to overcome lost hip motion.[253,254] As most of the forces across the joint or any joint arise from muscle action, such action must be reduced in magnitude, duration, and frequency. At the hip the greatest muscle forces in walking arise during the stance phase and are needed to counteract the body's weight and the body's inertial forces as the trunk moves over and around the involved hip. The body weight is medial to the hip joint on a long fulcrum (Fig. 20–11).[139] To balance this weight with minimal abductor effort, the trunk may shift so that the weight is brought closer to the center of the fulcrum over the hip joint itself.[258,259] To balance the inertial forces which occur in slowing down and speeding up the leg during the various aspects of the gait cycle, and to minimize the muscular effort about the hip, an individual may reduce the walking speed. But this reduction will increase the duration of the muscle's action in any given cycle, unless the stance phase on that side is shortened; thus, an asymmetric gait is produced. These factors—trunk shift, pelvic drop, slower walking speed, and a shortened stance phase on the involved side—are the characteristics of a Trendelenburg antalgic gait. The greater the number of these factors that are present and the more severe they are, the greater need to lower the forces across the joint and the more severe the state of joint degeneration. If forces are to be reduced further, the entire body weight cannot be transmitted through the leg; a substitute "peg leg" must be utilized, i.e., transmission to the ground via the arm by use of a cane or crutch.[259]

Although such mechanisms can reduce the forces, motions, and, therefore, pain, significant consequences result. With decreased stimulation muscles atrophy, and subchondral bone resorption and joint contractures (secondary to decreased motion) will progress even when the disease itself is quiescent. If pain is dramatically eliminated (disease remission or successful use of medications or surgical replacement of the joint), limitations to normal functional ability are eliminated without rapid concomitant restoration of bone structure, muscle strength, or loss of contractures.[260] Improvement in function occurs, with increased walking speed and greater joint forces.[261] This situation, over time, may be detrimental in that subchondral bone collapse may occur and the protective influence that this bone has upon the cartilage is lost. The problem is further compounded by the fact that weak muscles and/or joint contractures in the face of subchondral weakness may alter the locus, direction, and distribution of the forces across the joint, concentrating the stresses in some areas and possibly increasing the stresses in other areas not designed to cope with them. This situation may lead to further cartilage breakdown and to preferential breakdown in particular locations leading to lateral or medial femoral displacement (femoral subluxation or protrusion) (Fig. 20–25). Although localized areas of breakdown are often seen at the hip, they do not lead to a significant loss of stability and dislocation. Nevertheless, progressive joint destruction can be viewed as a vicious spiral. Each cycle is initiated by cartilage breakdown, causing compensa-

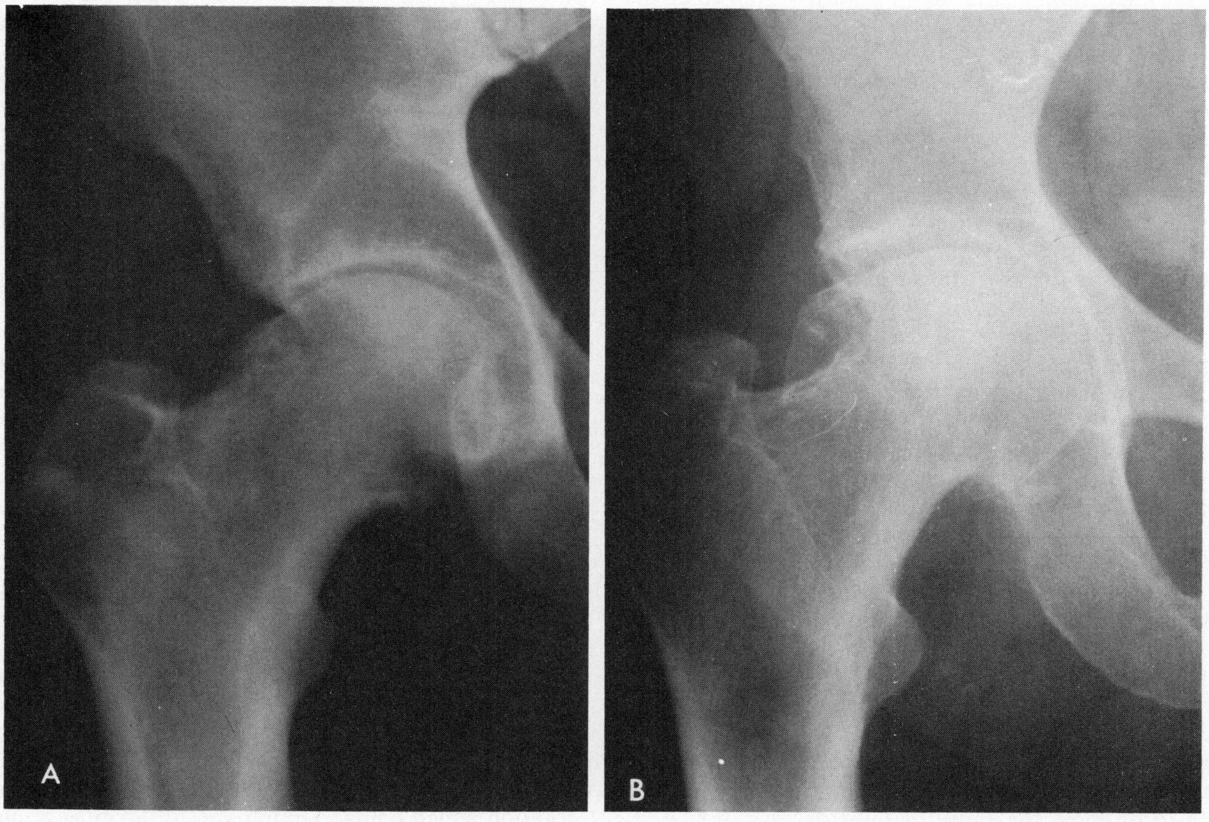


**Figure 20–25.** Two radiographic examples of moderate arthritis at the hip joint. Loss of cartilage can preferentially occur on the lateral side of the joint (*A*) or on the medial side (*B*).

tory body reactions; total joint changes occur which eventually stop because of medical intervention or disease quiescence; function consequently improves with a relative increase in "abnormal" forces over unprotected weakened surfaces, leading to further mechanical joint destruction.

Although the example cited above illustrates the situation if rheumatoid arthritis is the initiating factor, the consequent mechanical-biological steps in the cycle leading to joint destruction occur in a variety of other diseases leading to hip arthritis. In degenerative arthritis, whose cause is still unknown but is currently viewed as an initial weakening of the mechanical structure of cartilage or bone (owing to congenital microstructural abnormalities, normal aging, or impulsive, repetitive overstressing), the delicate balance of imposed stresses and structural resistance is altered and the cycle is initiated (see Chapter 88). From the onset of symptoms to final complete hip dysfunction can take many years. Thus, the cycle may not be rapid, and the individual and his or her practitioner can keep the imbalance small enough to prevent rapid acceleration of the process. How severe and chronic the initiating cause is, how effectively medical treatments produce disease remission, whether available compensatory mechanisms are adequate, whether an individual can sufficiently invoke such mechanisms or is limited by physical, psychological, or social factors, and how well the practitioner can understand and relate to the patient what is necessary to slow down the process are all important in the rapidity with which joint disability progresses.

The practitioner can control only some of these factors but must be aware of all of them and understand their interaction. In a patient who already has arthritic changes, the achievement of relief of pain or reduction in inflammatory reaction with medications does not imply that the patient can return to a full, active life. The need for caution and an awareness of the detrimental effects that activities such as sports can have must be understood by the practitioner and conveyed to the patient. Individuals who are in active jobs—e.g., are on their feet all day—may still need some reduction in their normal functional activities; they may require continued use of a cane or a reduction in the total number of "poundings" the joint will feel in a given day, month, or year. The physician must ensure that a proper range of motion is present and that muscle strength is maintained at the involved joints and about all other joints for proper compensations to occur.

**Knee Arthritis—Instability and Ligamentous Injury.** Arthritis of the knee constitutes almost as great an incidence of locomotion disability as does that of the hip.[262] A comparison of the biomechanics of these two joints illustrates (1) how different joints have different safety factors in the balance between the stresses imposed on them and the structural resistance to the stresses and (2) how damage to structures in the joint system other than cartilage can cause joint degeneration.

In most cases the cause of joint degeneration is the same in the knee as it is in the hip—idiopathic degenerative joint disease or rheumatoid arthritis. Unlike the hip, cartilage destruction in its initial stages often is not uniform over the entire cartilage surface of the knee. In degenerative joint disease the medial compartment is usually more involved; in rheumatoid arthritis it is the lateral compartment. This fact has three consequences: (1) As cartilage breakdown occurs, a varus-valgus angle forms which concentrates the force in the area of cartilage degeneration and further enhances the tendency toward mechanical breakdown. (2) Differential compartment destruction may be associated, with the joint surfaces losing their parallelism with the horizontal plane when the body is upright. Vertical body loads will then begin to have a greater tendency to create high shear or translational forces, which themselves are potentially highly damaging to the cartilage. (3) Such changes, by their effect on the surrounding ligaments, may indirectly affect the cartilage by stretching and weakening the ligaments. Since the knee is so dependent on ligaments for stability, ligamentous laxity eventually can allow even greater abnormally directed shear motions and forces.

As with degeneration at the hip, an individual's attempt to compensate for knee joint damage is aimed primarily at reducing joint load. During walking an individual can reduce the joint load by decreasing walking speed to decrease quadriceps activity.[263,264] Joint stability (maintenance of knee extension) may still be retained by leaning the trunk forward over the knee in the stance phase. However, in so doing the posterior capsule is abnormally stretched and the muscle, relatively little used, becomes weakened. The deficiency of bony contouring in the sagittal plane to stabilize the knee can eventually lead to increased AP translational motion with consequent abnormal shear forces that further aggravate cartilage damage. In the coronal plane the major compensatory action would be a shift of the trunk in a direction away from the compartment most involved. Because of the trunk's position this shift can only be made to a very limited degree. Ligamentous contractures can further nullify this compensating attempt.

On the concave side of a varus-valgus angulation (medial collateral ligament when the joint goes into varus, lateral collateral ligament when it goes into valgus) a contracture may result. Such contractures will even further limit the individual's compensatory attempt to redistribute the forces more appropriately.[265,266] If sufficiently severe, this lack of compensatory mechanisms, added to the aforementioned factors, may be accompanied by rapid, unremitting joint destruction, created not by the basic underlying disease but by the consequent superimposed mechanical conditions.

Thus, in contrast to the stabilizing effect of bony contours at the hip, the use of ligamentous constraints in normal knees to stabilize and limit certain motions, and the use of muscles to stabilize the joint in other directions, places the joint in an extremely precarious situation which tends to amplify even the most minimal joint damage.

These conditions also make the knee more susceptible to arthritis from those traumatic incidents which, by their nature, damage only ligaments and other soft tissues.[50-52,267-270] Increasingly, ligamentous injuries are becoming a larger cause of knee joint dysfunction. Often, after an injury to the knee that affects only the ligaments, laxity may remain despite proper medical management. Because the fibers have stretched or scarred, weaker ligaments result and their stabilizing effect is diminished. If the medial collateral ligament is damaged, varus-valgus rotational motions can occur, allowing the joint to open and close and thereby creating more severe impact on the cartilage bed. If the posterior or anterior cruciate ligaments or posterior medial or lateral capsular ligaments are damaged, AP or internal-external rotational translational motions can now occur with a magnitude which the femoral-tibial cartilage was not designed to withstand. Meniscal injuries will increase the stresses the joint surface feels by concentrating the load transmitted through the joint to a smaller area. Commonly, when such injuries exist (ligaments and menisci) even without direct cartilage damage, the eventual outcome is the same—cartilage destruction and arthritis.[271]

**Low Back Pain—Total System Destruction.** If knee arthritis illustrates how the various components of the joint system are affected when any single element is damaged, and how difficult it therefore is to compensate mechanically, low back problems epitomize this situation. When one considers how each component of this joint system—disc, facet joints, ligaments, and muscles—is so specifically designed to control a given aspect of joint stability and motion, it is not hard to see why back problems are so difficult for the patient and the clinician to manage. Many different diseases cause low back problems; one of these, "disc degeneration," will be used as an illustration. (See also Chapter 30.)

Disc degeneration constitutes the leading cause of morbidity in middle age.[272-280] The initial symptom is back pain.[281-286] Such pain must be compensated for by reducing the forces across the disc and reducing the movements of the joint. Again, as in the hip or knee joint, as the major load is not body weight but muscle activity, use of paraspinal muscles must be decreased in frequency and/or lessened in magnitude. However, to reduce motion while an individual is upright, the muscles must function as an internal brace. So long as the patient attempts to function, a vicious cycle is established: the upright position leads to back pain, back pain leads to muscle spasm, muscle spasm leads to increased disc pressure, and disc pressure leads to more back pain. Unlike the hip or knee, as long as a vertical position is maintained, muscle activity will be present as long as the body's center of gravity is in front of the disc and pressure will exist across the disc.

The patient's ability to compensate for back pain is extremely limited because, in the upright position, loads must remain across the disc. Medications, besides being directed toward the original source of pain, must be given to break ths cycle. Since the trunk does not have another side to help compensate for its disability, if medication proves ineffective, two additional measures can be tried: bed rest, which eliminates all vertical loading on the back; or bracing, which allows the abdomen to work like a disc to support the spine or restrict motion. Each of these measures has the detrimental effect of causing muscle atrophy, and prolonged use can have a markedly adverse effect on the long-term prognosis. If atrophy is present, support is lost; and although the total force across the disc may be decreased, the stability of the intervertebral joint is also decreased. This loss must be taken up by high strains on the disc, facet joints, or ligaments.

Since low back disorders are such a common disability, many attempts have been made to reduce their rate of occurrence in industrial settings. Since the middle 1930s, it has generally been recommended that all lifting activities be carried out with the back near vertical and the knees and hips bent.[287] The advocates of this method have been so enthusiastic and persistent in regard to training programs that nearly every major industry has adopted this method to the exclusion of any other method regardless of the size, shape, or weight of the object to be lifted, the person's ability to lift, or the desire to do it in the proper fashion.[288] In view of the popularization of the theory of correct lifting methods, it was expected that the incidence of low back injury would be significantly reduced. However, studies conducted in Britain and Canada offer clear evidence that there is no such reduction in the number of back injuries due to lifting and handling activities.[89]

A skepticism regarding the proper way to lift emerged from these and similar studies, and some investigators sought the reasons for the apparent failure of the instructional programs that had been designed to promote correct lifting. A photographic study of the actual lifting techniques of industrial workers showed that a wide variety of lifting methods were employed, and that the prescribed manner of lifting with a straight back and bent knees was seldom used.[89] Results indicated either that the indoctrination was insufficient or that the workers preferred to use another method even though they understood the "proper" lifting technique. In any case, the proper lifting method was not used consistently, so it could not be expected to contribute to a reduction in the incidence of low back injuries even if it were a truly superior technique.

A study that attempted to calculate the forces in the lower trunk during various acts of lifting was reported by Park and Chaffin.[287] This study indicated that the proper lifting method increased the compressive load on the lumbosacral disc by over 50 percent of that incurred by the "improper" method under certain specific conditions. Generally the straight-back, bent-knees method induced larger compressive forces whenever the object to be lifted was sufficiently heavy, and was too large to be lifted "between the knees," thus preventing the efficiency of a near vertical positioning of the upper extremities.

Brown[288] found that the greatest energy cost occurs with the straight-back, bent-knees method; this result is not unexpected, since the proper method requires an additional mass, i.e., the thighs and lower trunk, to be moved against gravity. Thus, if a person must continually perform this manner of lift throughout the working day, a great deal of unnecessary fatigue would develop, and therefore this method is not appropriate for prolonged repetitive tasks.

Since the training of individuals to lift "properly" has not been effective in reducing the incidence of low back problems,[288,289] studies were carried out to determine the maximal load acceptable to industrial workers during various lifting tasks.[290,291] The amount of weight to be lifted was adjusted according to the subject's assessment after the individual was informed of the duration, frequency, and conditions of the task at hand. With such facts, it was found that an ergonomic approach by "designing the job to fit the worker"[292] can reduce the incidence of low back disorders. Further, a study of preemployment static strength testing showed that a correlation exists between the type of job that a person has to do, the incidence of low back pain, and the static strength that a person has.[293-300]

If such techniques are not utilized or are ineffective, since joint destruction has begun, and although both the clinician and the patient are aware of it, little compensation is invoked and the delicate balance between stresses imposed and joint resistance to them has been tipped in the wrong direction. With time, even when nerve root irritation does not intervene, there frequently occurs a gradual loss of disc height, which further upsets the balance among disc, facet, ligaments, and muscle function. With disc narrowing, facet joint subluxation can result, causing higher stresses in the area of the joint still in contact and eventually leading to facet arthritis. With loss of disc height, normal ligament length is also reduced. The ligaments either can maintain a lax position, in which case they offer less protection to the disc, or can contract and be put on stretch, thereby becoming a source of pain themselves. Similarly, muscles may become slightly lax or operate at the lower end of their length-tension curve and be unable to control movement properly. Such lack of control creates abnormally high accelerative or decelerative forces in the disc, facet joints, or ligaments, thereby adding to the forces imposed upon these structures. Although such disc height loss, facet joint subluxation, ligamentous laxity, or muscle laxity may seem small in absolute magnitude, one must realize that in comparison to the total normal length of these structures, such changes may constitute a 25 to 50 percent difference.

## References


1. Morris, J.M.: Biomechanics of the spine. Arch. Surg. 107:418, 1973.
2. Lucas, D.B.: Biomechanics of the shoulder joint. Arch. Surg. 107:425, 1973.
3. Morris, J.M.: Biomechanical aspects of the hip joint. Orthop. Clin. North Am. 2:33, 1971.
4. Radin, E.L.: Biomechanics of the knee joint. Its implication in the design of replacements. Orthop. Clin. North Am. 4:539, 1973.
5. Frankel, V.H.: Biomechanics of the knee. Orthop. Clin. North Am. 2:175, 1971.
6. Kaufer, J.: Mechanical function of the patella. J. Bone Joint Surg. 53A:155, 1971.
7. Frankel, V.H.: Biomechanics of the musculoskeletal system. Introduction. Arch. Surg. 107:405, 1973.
8. Goss, C.M.: Gray's Anatomy of the Human Body. Philadelphia, Lea & Febiger, 1973, Chapter 4.
9. Walmsley, T.: On the form of the surface of diarthroses. Proc. Anat. Soc., Great Britain and Ireland, 1918.
10. Walmsley, T.: The articular mechanism of the diarthroses. J. Bone Joint Surg. 10:40, 1928.
11. MacConaill, M.A.: The movements of bones and joints. J. Bone Joint Surg. 31B:100, 1949.
12. Barnett, C.H., Davies, D.V., and MacConaill, M.A.: Synovial Joints—Their Structure and Mechanics. London, Longmans, 1961.
13. Steindler, A.: Kinesiology of the Human Body. Springfield, Ill., Charles C Thomas, 1955.
14. Langa, G.S.: The morphology and function of the human joint. Acta Anat. 55:16, 1963.
15. Landsmeer, J.M.F.: Power grip and precision handling. Ann. Rheum. Dis. 21:164, 1962.
16. Goodfellow, J., and O'Connor, J.: The mechanics of the knee and problems in reconstructive surgery. J. Bone Joint Surg. 60:358, 1978.
17. Frigerio, N.A., Stowe, R.S., and Howe, J.W.: Movement of the sacroiliac joint. Clin. Orthop. 100:379, 1974.
18. Poppen, N.K., and Walker, P.S.: Normal and abnormal motion of the shoulder. J. Bone Joint Surg. 58A:195, 1976.
19. Morrey, B.F., and Chao, E.Y.S.: Passive motion of the elbow joint. J. Bone Joint Surg. 58A:501, 1976.
20. Chao, E.Y.S., and Morrey, B.F.: Three-dimensional rotation of the elbow. J. Biomechanics 11:57, 1978.
21. Youm, Y., Dryer, R.F., Thambyrajah, K., et al.: Biomechanical analysis of forearm pronation-supination and elbow flexion-extension. J. Biomechanics 12:245, 1979.
22. McMurty, R.Y., Youm, Y., and Flatt, A.E., et al: Kinematics of the wrist. II. Clinical applications. J. Bone Joint Surg. 60A:955, 1978.
23. Youm, Y., McMurty, R.Y., Flatt, A.E., et al.: Kinematics of the wrist. I. An experimental study of radial ulnar deviation and flexion-extension. J. Bone Joint Surg. 60A:423, 1978.
24. Youm, Y., Gillespie, T.E., Flatt, A.E., et al.: Kinematic investigation of normal MCP joint. J. Biomechanics 11:109, 1978.
25. Frankel, V.H., Burstein, A.H., and Brooks, D.B.: Biomechanics of internal derangement of the knee. Pathomechanics as determined by analysis of the instant centers of motion. J. Bone Joint Surg. 53A:945, 1971.
26. Walker, P.S., Shoji, J., and Erkman, M.J.: The rotational axis of the knee and its significance to prosthesis design. Clin. Orthop. 89:160, 1972.
27. Soudan, K., Auderkercke, and Martens, M.: Methods, difficulties and inaccuracies in the study of human joint kinematics and pathokinematics by the instant axis concept. Example: The knee joint. J. Biomechanics 12:27, 1979.
28. Laurin, C., and Mathiev, J.: Sagittal mobility of the normal ankle. Clin. Orthop. 108:99, 1975.
29. Rothman, R.H., Marvel, J.P., Jr., and Heppenstall, R.B.: Anatomic considerations in glenohumeral joint. Orthop. Clin. North Am. 6:341, 1975.
30. Clark, I.C., and Amstutz, H.C.: Human hip geometry and hemiarthroplasty selection. Proceedings of the Hip Society, 1975. *In* The Hip. St. Louis, C. V. Mosby Company, 1975.
31. Benedict, J.V., Walker, L.B., and Harris, E.H.: Stress-strain characteristics and tensile strength of unembalmed human tendon. J. Biomechanics 1:53, 1968.
32. Blanton, P.L., and Biggs, N.L.: Ultimate tensile strength of fetal and adult human tendons. J. Biomechanics 3:181, 1970.
33. Crisp, J.D.C.: Properties of tendon and skin. *In* Fung, Y.C., Perrone, N., and Anliker, M. (eds.): Biomechanics, Its Foundations and Objectives. Englewood Cliffs, N.J., Prentice-Hall, 1972.
34. Noyes, F.R., DeLucas, J.L., and Torvik, P.J.: Biomechanics of anterior cruciate ligament failure: An analysis of strain rate sensitivity and mechanisms of failure in primates. J. Bone Joint Surg. 56A:236, 1974.
35. Kennedy, J.C., Hawkins, R.J., Willis, R.B., et al.: Tension studies of human knee ligaments. J. Bone Joint Surg. 58A:350, 1977.
36. Noyes, F.R., Torvik, P.J., Hyde, M.S., et al.: Biomechanics of ligament failure. J. Bone Joint Surg. 56A:1406, 1974.
37. Noyes, F.R., and Groud, E.S.: The strength of the anterior cruciate ligament in humans and Rhesus monkeys. J. Bone Joint Surg. 58A:1074, 1976.
38. Rosenorn, M., and Pederson, E.B.: The significance of the coracoclavicular ligament in experimental dislocation of the acromoclavicular joint. Acta Orthop. Scand. 45:346, 1974.
39. Ogden, J.A.: The anatomy and function of the proximal tibiofibular joint. Clin. Orthop. 101:186, 1974.
40. Ogden, J.A.: Subluxation and dislocation of the proximal tibiofibular joint. J. Bone Joint Surg. 56A:145, 1974.

41. Moseley, H.F., and Overgaard, B.: The anterior capsule mechanism in recurrent anterior dislocation of the shoulder. J. Bone Joint Surg. 44B:913, 1962.
42. Brantigan, O.C., and Voshell, A.F.: The mechanics of the ligaments and menisci of the knee joint. J. Bone Joint Surg. 23:44, 1941.
43. Trent, P.S., Walker, P.S., and Wolf, B.: Ligament length patterns, strengths and rotational axes of the knee joint. Clin. Orthop. 117:263, 1976.
44. Hsieh, H-H., and Walker, P.S.: Stabilizing mechanisms of the loaded and unloaded knee joint. J. Bone Joint Surg. 58A:87, 1976.
45. Fowler, P.J.: Medial and anterior instability of the knee. An anatomical and clinical study using stress machines. J. Bone Joint Surg. 53A:1257, 1971.
46. Kennedy, J.C., Weinberg, H.W., and Wilson, A.S.: The anatomy and function of the anterior cruciate ligament. As determined by clinical and morphological studies. J. Bone Joint Surg. 56A:223, 1974.
47. Shaw, J.A., and Murray, D.G.: The longitudinal axis of the knee and the role of the cruciate ligaments in controlling transverse rotation. J. Bone Joint Surg. 56A:1603, 1974.
48. Girgis, F.G., Marshall, J.L., and Monajem, A.R.S.: The cruciate ligaments of the knee joint. Anatomical, functional and experimental analysis. Clin. Orthop. 106:216, 1975.
49. Furman, W., Marshall, J.L., and Girgis, F.G.: The anterior cruciate ligament. J. Bone Joint Surg. 58A:179, 1976.
50. Hughston, J.C., Cross, M.J., and Andrews, J.R.: Classification of lateral ligament instability of the knee. J. Bone Joint Surg. 56A:1539, 1974.
51. Hughston, J.C., Andrews, J.R., Cross, M.J., et al.: Classification of knee ligament instabilities. Part I: The medial compartment and cruciate ligaments. J. Bone Joint Surg. 58A:159, 1976.
52. Hughston, J.C., Andrews, J.R., Cross, M.J., et al.: Classification of knee ligament instabilities. Part II: The lateral compartment. J. Bone Joint Surg. 58A:173, 1976.
53. Wang, C.J., and Walker, P.S.: Rotatory laxity of the human knee joint. J. Bone Joint Surg. 56A:161, 1974.
54. Warren, L.A., Marshall, J.L., and Griggs, F.: The prime static stabilizer of the medial side of the knee. J. Bone Joint Surg. 56A:665, 1974.
55. Noyes, F.R., Grood, E.S., Butler, D.L., and Malek, M.: Clinical laxity tests and functional stability of the knee: Biomechanical concepts. Clin. Orthop. 146:84, 1980.
56. Grood, E.S., Noyes, F.R., Butler, D.L., and Suntay, W.S.: Ligamentous and capsular restraints preventing straight medial and lateral laxity in intact human cadaver knees. J. Bone Joint Surg. 63A:1257, 1981.
57. Noyes, F.R., Grood, E.S., Butler, D.L., and Paulos, L.E.: Clinical biomechanics of the knee-ligament restraints and functional stability. *In* The American Academy of Orthopaedic Surgeons: Symposium on the Athlete's Knee: Surgical Repair and Reconstruction. St. Louis, C. V. Mosby, 1980.
58. White, A.A., III, and Raphael, I.G.: The effect of quadriceps loads and knee position on strain measurements of the tibial collateral ligament. An experimental study on human amputation specimens. Acta Orthop. Scand. 43:176. 1972.
59. Bose, K., and Chong, K.C.: The clinical manifestations and pathomechanics of contracture of the extensor mechanism of the knee. J. Bone Joint Surg. 58B:478, 1976.
60. Sylvia, L.E.: A more exact measurement of the sagittal stability of the knee joint. Acta Orthop. Scand. 46:1008, 1975.
61. Basmajian, J.V., and Bazant, F.J.: Factors preventing downward dislocation of the adducted shoulder—an electromyographic and morphological study. J. Bone Joint Surg. 41A:1182, 1959.
62. Linscheid, R.L., Dobyns, J.H., Beabout, J.W., et al.: Traumatic instability of the wrist. Diagnosis, classification, and pathomechanics. J. Bone Joint Surg. 54A:1612, 1972.
63. Smith, R.J.: Post-traumatic instability of the metacarpophalangeal joint of the thumb. J. Bone Joint Surg. 59A:14, 1977.
64. Coventry, M.B., and Tapper, E.M.: Pelvic instability: A consequence of removing iliac bone for grafting. J. Bone Joint Surg. 54A:83, 1972.
65. Marshall, J.L., Girgis, F.G., and Zelko, R.R.: The biceps femoris tendon and its functional significance. J. Bone Joint Surg. 54A:1444, 1972.
66. Noyes, F.R., and Sonstegard, D.G.: Biomechanical function of the pes anserinus at the knee and the effect of its transplantation. J. Bone Joint Surg. 55A:1225, 1973.
67. Poe, M.H., Johnson, R.J., and Brown, D.W.: The role of the musculature in injuries to the medial collateral ligament. J. Bone Joint Surg. 61A:398, 1979.
68. Symeonides, P.P.: The significance of the subscapularis muscle in the pathogenesis of recurrent anterior dislocation of the shoulder. J. Bone Joint Surg. 54B:476, 1972.
69. Weisman, H.J., Simon, S.R., Ewald, F.C., et al.: Total hip replacement with and without osteotomy of the greater trochanter: Clinical and biomechanical comparisons in the same patients. J. Bone Joint Surg. 60A:203, 1978.
70. Parke, W.W., and Schiff, D.C.M.: The applied anatomy of the intervertebral disc. Orthop. Clin. North Am. 2:309, 1971.
71. Markolf, K.L., and Morris, J.M.: The structural components of the intervertebral disc. A study of their contributions to the ability of the disc to withstand compressive forces. J. Bone Joint Surg. 56A:675, 1974.
72. MacNab, I.: The traction spur. An indicator of segmental instability. J. Bone Joint Surg. 53A:663, 1971.
73. Palacios, E., Brackett, C.E., and Leary, D.J.: Ossification of the posterior longitudinal ligament associated with a herniated intervertebral disk. Radiology 100:313, 1971.
74. Markolf, K.L.: Deformation of the thoracolumbar intervertebral joints in response to external loads: A biomechanical study using autopsy material. J. Bone Joint Surg. 54A:511, 1972.
75. White, A.A., III, and Panjabi, J.M.: Clinical Biomechanics of the Spine. Philadelphia, J. B. Lippincott Company, 1978.
76. Radin, E.L., Simon, S.R., and Rose, R.M.: Practical Biomechanics for the Orthopedic Surgeon. New York, John Wiley & Sons, 1978.
77. Fielding, J.W., Gehran, G., Van, B., et al.: Tears of the transverse ligament of the atlas. A clinical and biomechanical study. J. Bone Joint Surg. 56A:1683, 1974.
78. Callahan, R.A., Johnson, R.M., Margolis, R.N., et al.: Cervical facet fusion for control of instability following laminectomy. J. Bone Joint Surg. 59A:991, 1977.
79. Bauze, R.J., and Ardran, G.M.: Proceedings: The mechanism of forward dislocation in the human cervical spine. J. Bone Joint Surg. 57B:253, 1975.
80. White, A.A., III, and Hirsch, C.: The significance of the vertebral posterior elements in the mechanics of the thoracic spine. Clin. Orthop. 81:2, 1971.
81. Panjabi, M.M., Brand, R.A., Jr., and White, A.A., III: Mechanical properties of the human thoracic spine as shown by three-dimensional load-displacement curves. J. Bone Joint Surg. 58A:642, 1976.
82. Lin, H.S., Liu, Y.K., and Atems, K.H.: Mechanical response of the lumbar intervertebral joint under physiological loading (complex). J. Bone Joint Surg. 60A:41, 1978.
83. Howes, R.G., and Isdale, I.C.: The loose back: An unrecognized syndrome. Rheumatol. Phys. Med. 11:72, 1971.
84. Liu, Y.K., Ray, G., and Hirsch, C.: The resistance of the lumbar spine to direct shear. Orthop. Clin. North Am. 1:33, 1975.
85. Floyd, W.F., and Silver, P.H.: The function of the erectors spinae muscles in certain movements and postures in man. J. Physiol. 129:184, 1955.
86. Morris, J.M., Lucas, D.B., and Bresler, B.: Role of the trunk in stability of the spine. J. Bone Joint Surg. 43A:327, 1961.
87. Morris, J.M., Benner, G., and Lucas, D.G.: An electromyographic study of the intrinsic muscles of the back in man. J. Anat. 96:509, 1962.
88. Asmussen, E.: The functions of the back muscles in standing and while holding weights. Prog. Phys. Ther. 1:87, 1979.
89. Asmussen, E., Dahlerup, J.V., and Fredsted, A.: Quantitative Evaluation of the Activity of the Back Muscles in Lifting. Communications from the Danish National Association for Infantile Paralysis, p. 21, 1965.
90. Nachemson, A., and Morris, J.M.: In vivo measurements of intradiscal pressure. J. Bone Joint Surg. 45A:1077, 1964.
91. Nachemson, A.: The effect of forward leaning on lumbar intradiscal pressure. Acta Orthop. Scand. 35:314, 1965.
92. Bartelink, D.L.: Role of abdominal pressure in relieving the pressure on the lumbar intervertebral discs. J. Bone Joint Surg. 39B:718, 1957.
93. Eie, N., and When, P.: Measurements of the intra-abdominal pressure in relation to weight bearing of the lumbosacral spine. J. Oslo City Hosp. 12:205, 1962.
94. Asmussen, E., and Poulsen, E.: On the Role of Intraabdominal Pressure in Relieving the Back Muscles While Holding Weights in a Forward Inclined Position. Communications from the Danish National Association for Infantile Paralysis, p. 28, 1968.
95. American Academy of Orthopaedic Surgeons: Joint Motion: Method of Measuring and Recording. Chicago, American Academy of Orthopaedic Surgeons, 1965.
96. Kapandji, I.A.: The Physiology of Joints. 2nd ed. Edinburgh, E.R.S. Livingstone, 1970.
97. Boone, D.C., and Azen, S.P.: Normal range of motion of joints in male subjects. J. Bone Joint Surg. 61A:756, 1979.
98. Plagenhoff, S.: Patterns of Human Motion. Englewood Cliffs, N.J., Prentice-Hall, 1971.
99. Panjabi, M.M.: Experimental determination of spinal motion in segment behavior. Orthop. Clin. North Am. 8:169, 1977.
100. Pennal, G.F., Conn, G.S., McDonald, G., et al.: Motion studies of the lumbar spine: A preliminary report. J. Bone Joint Surg. 54B:442, 1972.
101. Davis, P.R., Troup, J.D., and Barnard, J.H.: Movements of the thoracic and lumbar spine when lifting: A chronocyclophotographic study. J. Anat. 99:13, 1965.
102. Kulak, R.F., Schultz, A.B., Belytschko, T., et al.: Biomechanical characteristics of vertebral motion segments and intervertebral discs. Orthop. Clin. North Am. 6:121, 1975.
103. Cleland, J.: The shoulder-girdle and its movements. Lancet, Feb. 19, 1881, p. 283.

104. Saha, A.K.: Theory of Shoulder Mechanism. Springfield, Ill., Charles C Thomas, 1961.
105. Saha, A.K.: Dynamic stability of the glenohumeral joint. Acta Orthop. Scand. 42:491, 1971.
106. Saha, A.K.: Mechanics of elevation of glenohumeral joint. Its application in rehabilitation of flail shoulder in upper brachial plexus injuries and poliomyelitis and in replacement of the upper humerus by prosthesis. Acta Orthop. Scand. 44:668, 1973.
107. Blacharski, P.A., Somerset, JH., and Murray, D.G.: A three-dimensional study of the kinematics of the human knee. J. Biomechanics 8:375, 1975.
108. Hallen, L.G., and Lindahl, O.: The "screw-home" movement in the knee joint. Acta Orthop. Scand. 37:97, 1966.
109. Murray, M.P.: Gait as a total pattern of movement—including a bibliography on gait. Am. J. Phys. Med. 46:290, 1967.
110. Eberhart, H.D., Inman, V.T., et al.: Fundamental Studies of Human Locomotion and Other Information Relating to Design of Artificial Limbs. Report to the Committee on Artificial Limbs, National Research Council. Washington, D.C., 1945–47.
111. Waters, R.L., Perry, J., McDaniels, J.M., et al.: The relative strength of the hamstrings during hip extension. J. Bone Joint Surg. 56A:1592, 1974.
112. Brand, P.W.: Biomechanics of tendon transfer. Orthop. Clin. North Am. 5:205, 1974.
113. Denham, R.A.: Hip mechanics. J. Bone Joint Surg. 41B:550, 1959.
114. McLeish, R.D., and Charnley, J.: Abduction forces in the one-legged stance. J. Biomechanics 3:191, 1970.
115. Johnston, R.C.: Mechanical considerations of the hip joint. Arch. Surg. 107:411, 1973.
116. Rydell, N.: Forces in the hip joint. II. Intravital studies. *In* Kenedi, R.M. (ed.): Biomechanics and Related Bioengineering Topics. London, Pergamon Press, 1965.
117. Rydell, N.: Biomechanics of the hip-joint. Clin. Orthop. 92:6, 1973.
118. Morrison, J.B.: Function of the knee joint in various activities. Med. Biol. Eng. 4:573, 1969.
119. Morrison, J.B.: The mechanics of the knee joint in relation to normal walking. J. Biomechanics 3:51, 1970.
120. Paul, J.P.: Force actions transmitted in the knee of normal subjects and by prosthetic joint replacements. Institute of Mechanical Engineering Conference on Total Knee Replacement, London, September, 1974.
121. Sammarco, G.J., Burstein, A.H., and Frankel, V.H.: Biomechanics of the ankle: A kinematic study. Orthop. Clin. North Am. 4:75, 1973.
122. Brewster, R.C., Chao, E.Y., and Stauffer, R.N.: Force analysis of the ankle joint during the stance phase of gait. 27th Proceedings of the Annual Conference on Engineering in Medicine and Biology, Philadelphia, 1974, p. 368.
123. DeLuca, C.J., and Forrest, W.F.: Force analysis of individual muscles acting simultaneously on the shoulder joint during isometric abduction. J. Biomechanics 6:385, 1973.
124. Dvir, Z., and Berme, N.: The shoulder complex in elevation of the arm: A mechanism approach. J. Biomechanics 11:219, 1978.
125. Cooney, W.P., III, and Chao, E.Y.S.: Biomechanical analysis of static forces in the thumb during hand function. J. Bone Joint Surg. 59A:27, 1977.
126. Swanson, A.B., and Swanson, G.D.: Pathogenesis and pathomechanics of rheumatoid deformities in the hand and wrist. Orthop. Clin. North Am. 4:1039, 1973.
127. Hakstian, R.W., and Tubiana, R.: Ulnar deviation of the fingers. J. Bone Joint Surg. 49A:299, 1967.
128. Flatt, A.E.: The pathomechanics of ulnar drift. Social and Rehabilitation Services Final Report. Grant No. RD, 226M, 1971.
129. Wise, K.S.: The anatomy of the metacarpo-phalangeal joints, with observations of the aetiology of ulnar drift. J. Bone Joint Surg. 57B:485, 1975.
130. Smith, R.J.: Balance and kinetics of the fingers under normal and pathological conditions. Clin. Orthop. 104:92, 1974.
131. Hueston, J.T., and Wilson, W.F.: The role of the intrinsic muscles in the production of metacarpophalangeal subluxation in the rheumatoid hand. Plast. Reconstr. Surg. 52:342, 1973.
132. Pieron, A.P.: The mechanism of the first carpometacarpal (CMC) joint. An anatomical and mechanical analysis. Acta Orthop. Scand. (Suppl.) 48:1, 1973.
133. Hirsch, D., Page, D., Miller, D., Dumbleton, J.G., and Miller, E.H.: A biomechanical analysis of the metacarpophalangeal joint of the thumb. J. Biomechanics 7:343, 1974.
134. Johns, R.J., and Draper, I.T.: The control of movement in normal subjects. Bull. Johns Hopkins Hosp. 115:447, 1964.
135. Haffajee, D., Moritz, U., and Svantesson, G.: Isometric knee extension strength as a function of joint angle, muscle length and motor unit activity. Acta Orthop. Scand. 43:138, 1972.
136. Basmajian, J.V., and Latif, A.: Integrated actions and functions of the chief flexors of the elbow. J. Bone Joint Surg. 39A:1106, 1957.
137. Landsmeer, J.M.F.: The coordination of finger-joint motions. J. Bone Joint Surg. 45:1654, 1963.
138. Basmajian, J.V., and Travill, A.: Electromyography of the pronator muscles in the forearm. Anat. Rec. 139:45, 1961.
139. Barnett, C.H., and Harding, D.: The activity of antagonist muscles during voluntary movement. Ann. Phys. Med. 2:290, 1955.
140. Basmajian, J.V.: Muscles Alive—Their Functions Revealed by Electromyography. Baltimore, Williams & Wilkins Company, 1974.
141. Basmajian, J.V., and Bentzon, J.W.: An electromyographic study of certain muscles of the leg and foot in the standing position. Surg. Gynecol. Obstet. 98:662, 1954.
142. Elftman, H.: Biomechanics of muscle with particular application to studies of gait. J. Bone Joint Surg. 48A:363, 1966.
143. Mann, R.A., Hagy, J.L., and Simon, S.R.: Biomechanics of Gait. A Critical Visual Analysis. Instructional Course Lectures, The American Academy of Orthopaedic Surgeons, March 1975.
144. Bigland, B., and Lippold, O.J.C.: The relation between force, velocity and integrated activity in human muscles. J. Physiol. 123:214, 1954.
145. Stern, J.T.: Investigations concerning the theory of spurt and shunt muscles. J. Biomechanics 4:437, 1971.
146. Joseph, J., and Watson, R.: Telemetering electromyography of muscles used in walking up and down stairs. J. Bone Joint Surg. 49B:774, 1967.
147. Andriacchi, T.P., Andersson, G.B.J., Fermier, R.W., et al.: A study of lower limb mechanics during stair climbing. J. Bone Joint Surg. (in press).
148. Andersson, B.J., Ortengren, R., Nachemson, A.L., Elfstrom, G., and Broman, H.: The sitting posture: An electromyographic and discometric study. Orthop. Clin. North Am. 6:105, 1975.
149. Farfan, H.F.: Muscular mechanism of the lumbar spine and the position of power and efficiency. Orthop. Clin. North Am. 6:135, 1975.
150. Davis, P.R.: Posture of the trunk during the lifting of weights. Br. Med. J. 5114:87, 1959.
151. Mow, V.C., and Lai, W.M.: Selected unresolved problems in synovial joint biomechanics. ASME, 1979 Biomechanics Symposium, AMD-32, p. 19.
152. Naylor, H.: Bearings and lubrication. Chart. Mech. Eng. 12:642, 1965.
153. Archard, J.F., and Hirst, W.: The wear of metals under unlubricated conditions. Proc. R. Soc. London, 236A:397, 1956.
154. Unsworth, A., Dowson, D., and Wright, V.: The frictional behavior of human synovial joints. Part I. Natural joints. J. Lubrication Tech. 97F:369, 1975.
155. Simon, S.R., Paul, I.L., Rose, R.M., and Radin, E.L.: "Stiction-friction" of total hip prostheses and its relationship to loosening. J. Bone Joint Surg. 57A:226, 1975.
156. Muir, H., Bullough, P., and Maroudas, A.: The distribution of collagen in human articular cartilage with some of its physiological implications. J. Bone Joint Surg. 52B:554, 1970.
157. Sayles, R.S., Thomas, T.R., Anderson, J., Haslock, I., and Unsworth, A.: Measurement of the surface microgeometry of articular cartilage. J. Biomechanics. 12:257, 1979.
158. Gardner, D.L., and McGillivray, D.C.: Living articular cartilage is not smooth. Ann. Rheum. Dis. 30:3, 1971.
159. Gardner, D.L., and McGillivray, D.C.: Surface structures of articular cartilage. Ann. Rheum. Dis. 30:10, 1971.
160. Clarke, I.C.: Human articular surface contours and related surface depression frequency studies. Ann. Rheum. Dis. 30:15, 1971.
161. Archard, J.F.: Surface topography and tribology. Tribology 7:213, 1974.
162. Archard, J.F., and Kirk, M.T.: Influence of elastic modulus on the lubrication of point contacts. Lubrication and Wear Convention. Proc. Inst. Mech. Engrs., London 117:181, 1963.
163. Jones, E.S.: Joint lubrication. Lancet 226:1426, 1934.
164. McCutchen, C.W.: The frictional properties of animal joints. Wear 5:1, 1962.
165. Linn, F.C.: Lubrication of animal joints. J. Bone Joint Surg. 49A:1079, 1967.
166. Linn, F.C., and Radin, E.L.: Lubrication of animal joints. Arthritis Rheum. 2:674, 1968.
167. Walker, P.S., Dowson, D., Longfield, M.D., et al.: Boosted lubrication in synovial joints by fluid entrapment and enrichment. Ann. Rheum. Dis. 27:512, 1968.
168. MacConaill, M.A.: The movements of bones and joints. II. The synovial fluid and its assistants. J. Bone Joint Surg. 32B:244, 1950.
169. McCutchen, C.W., and Lewis, P.R.: Mechanism of animal joints. Nature 184:1284, 1959.
170. Dintenfass, L.: Rheology of synovial fluid and its role in joint lubrication. *In* Copley, A.L. (ed.): Proceedings of the International Congress on Rheology, Part IV. New York, Wiley Interscience, 1963, pp. 489–503.
171. McCutchen, C.W.: Boundary lubrication by synovial fluids: Demonstration and possible osmotic explanation. Fed. Proc. 25:1061, 1966.
172. Dowson, D.: Modes of lubrication in human joints. Symposium on Lubrication and Wear in Living and Artificial Human Joints. Proc. Inst. Mech. Engrs., London 181:45, 1967.

173. Linn, F.C.: Lubrication of animal joints. II. The mechanism. J. Biomechanics 1:193, 1968.
174. Longfield, M.D., Dowson, D., Walker, P.S., et al.: Boosted lubrication of human joints by fluid enrichment and entrapment. Bio-Med. Engr. 4:517, 1969.
175. Walker, P.S., Unsworth, A., Dowson, D., et al.: Modes of aggregation of hyaluronic acid protein complex on the surface of articular cartilage. Ann. Rheum. Dis. 29:591, 1970.
176. Radin, E.L., and Paul, I.L.: A consolidated concept of joint lubrication. J. Bone Joint Surg. 54A:607, 1972.
177. Ling, F.F.: A new model of articular cartilage in human joints. J. Lubrication Tech. 96:449, 1974.
178. Torzilli, P.A., and Mow, V.C.: On the fundamental fluid transport mechanisms through normal and pathological articular cartilage during function. II. The analysis, solution and conclusions. J. Biomechanics 9:587, 1976.
179. Mansour, J.M., and Mow, V.C.: On the natural lubrication of synovial joints: Normal and degenerate. J. Lubrication Tech. 99:163, 1977.
180. Ogston, A.G., and Stanier, J.E.: The physiological function of hyaluronic acid in synovial fluid; viscous elastic and lubricant properties. J. Physiol. 119:244, 1953.
181. Laurent, T.C.: Physico-chemical Studies on Hyaluronic Acid. Uppsala, Sweden, Almquist & Wiksell, 1957, pp. 1–28.
182. Balazs, E.A., Watson, D., Duff, I.F., et al.: Hyaluronic acid in synovial fluid. I. Molecular parameters of hyaluronic acid in normal and arthritic human fluids. Arthritis Rheum. 10:357, 1967.
183. Davis, D.V., and Palfrey, A.F.: Some of the physical properties of normal and pathological synovial fluids. J. Biomechanics 1:79, 1968.
184. Maroudas, A.: Studies on the formation of hyaluronic acid films. *In* Wright, V. (ed.): Lubrication and Wear in Joints. Philadelphia, J.B. Lippincott Company, 1969.
185. Bullough, P.G., Goodfellow, J.B., Greenwald, A.S., et al.: Incongruent surfaces in the human joint. Nature 217:1290, 1968.
186. Oberlander, W.: On biomechanics of joints. The influence of functional cartilage swelling on the congruity of regular curved joints. J. Biomechanics 11:151, 1978.
187. Simon, W.H., Friedenberg, S., and Richardson, S.: Joint congruence. A correlation of joint congruence and thickness of articular cartilage in dogs. J. Bone Joint Surg. 55A:1614, 1973.
188. Greenwald, A.S., and Haynes, D.W.: Weight-bearing areas in the human hip joint. J. Bone Joint Surg. 54B:157, 1972.
189. Day, W.H., Swanson, S.A.V., and Freeman, M.A.R.: Contact pressures in the loaded human cadaver hip. J. Bone Joint Surg. 57B:302, 1975.
190. Armstrong, C.G., Bahrani, A.S., and Gardner, D.L.: In vitro measurement of articular cartilage deformation in the intact human hip joint under load. J. Bone Joint Surg. 61A:744–755, 1979.
191. Walker, P.S., and Hajek, J.V.: The load-bearing areas in the knee joint. J. Biomechanics 5:581, 1972.
192. Kettlkamp, D.B., and Jacobs, A.W.: Tibiofemoral contact area—determination and implications. J. Bone Joint Surg. 54A:349, 1972.
193. Maquet, P.G., Van de Berg, A.J., and Simoret, J.C.: Femorotibial weight-bearing areas. Experimental determination. J. Bone Joint Surg. 57A:766, 1975.
194. Walker, P.S., and Erkman, J.J.: The role of the menisci in force transmission across the knee. Clin. Orthop. 109:184, 1975.
195. Greenwald, A.S., and Matejczyk, M-B.: A contact area study of the human ankle joint. Orthop. Rev. 6:85, August 1967.
196. Lambert, K.L.: The weight-bearing function of the fibula. A strain gauge study. J. Bone Joint Surg. 53A:507, 1971.
197. Walker, P.S.: Human Joints and Their Artificial Replacements. Springfield, Ill., Charles C Thomas, 1977.
198. Salter, R.B., and Field, P.: The effects of continuous compression on living articular cartilage. J. Bone Joint Surg. 42A:31, 1960.
199. Mankin, H., and Thrasher, A.Z.: Water content and binding in normal and osteoarthritic human cartilage. J. Bone Joint Surg. 57A:76, 1975.
200. Radin, E., Paul, I., and Rose, R.: Role of mechanical factors in the pathogenesis of primary osteoarthritis. Lancet 1:519, 1972.
201. Freeman, M.A.R.: Articular Cartilage. New York, Grune & Stratton, 1974.
202. MacConaill, M.A.: The movement of bones and joints. IV. The mechanical structure of articulating cartilage. J. Bone Joint Surg. 33B:251, 1951.
203. Linn, F.C., and Sokoloff, L.: Movement and composition of interstitial fluid of cartilage. Arthritis Rheum. 8:481, 1965.
204. Eisenfeld, J., Mow, V.C., and Lipshitz, H.: The mathematical analysis of stress relaxation in articular cartilage during compression. Math. Biosci. 39:97, 1978.
205. Mow, V.C.: Biphasic rheological properties of cartilage. Bull. Hosp. Joint Dis. 38:121, 1977.
206. Hayes, W.C., and Mockros, L.F.: Viscoelastic properties of human articular cartilage. J. Appl. Physiol. 31:562, 1971.
207. Mansour, J.M., and Mow, V.C.: The permeability of articular cartilage under compressive strain and at high pressures. J. Bone Joint Surg. 58A:509, 1976.
208. Camosso, M.E., and Marotti, G.: The mechanical behavior of articular cartilage under compressive stress. J. Bone Joint Surg. 44A:699, 1962.
209. Kempson, G.E.: Mechanical properties of articular cartilage. *In* Freeman, M.A.R. (ed.): Adult Articular Cartilage. New York, Grune & Stratton, 1979, p. 197.
210. Woo, S.L-Y., Akeson, W.H., and Jemmott, C.F.: Measurement of non-homogeneous, directional mechanical properties of articular cartilage in tension. J. Biomechanics 9:785, 1976.
211. Redler, I.: A scanning electron microscopic study of human normal and osteoarthritis articular cartilage. Clin. Orthop. 103:262, 1974.
212. Redler, I., and Zimmy, M.: Scanning electron microscopy of normal and abnormal articular cartilage and synovium. J. Bone Joint Surg. 52A:1395, 1970.
213. Lane, J.M., and Weiss, C.: Review of articular cartilage collagen research. Arthritis Rheum. 18:553, 1975.
214. Roth, V., and Mow, V.C.: Finite element analysis of contact problems for indentation of articular cartilage. *In* Grood, E.S., and Smith, C.R. (eds.): Advances in Bioengineering. New York, American Society of Mechanical Engineers, 1977, pp. 47–48.
215. Maroudas, A.: Physico-chemical properties of articular cartilage. *In* Freeman, M.A.R. (ed.): Adult Articular Cartilage. New York, Grune & Stratton, 1974.
216. Bullough, P.G., and Goodfellow, J.: The significance of the fine structure of articular cartilage. J. Bone Joint Surg. 50B:852, 1968.
217. Roth, V., Wirth, C., Mow, V.C., et al.: Variation of tensile properties of articular cartilage with age. Transactions, 24th Annual Meeting of the Orthopedic Research Society, Dallas, Texas, 3:9, 1978.
218. Mathews, M.B., and Lozaityte, I.: Sodium chondroitin sulfate-protein complexes of cartilage. I. Molecular weight and shape. Arch. Biochem. Biophys. 74:158, 1978.
219. Muir, H.: The nature of the link between protein and carbohydrate of a chondroitin sulphate complex from hyaline cartilage. Biochem. J. 69:195, 1958.
220. Partridge, S.M., Davis, H.F., and Adair, F.S.: The chemistry of connective tissues. 6. The constitution of the chondroitin sulphate-protein complex in cartilage. Biochem. J. 79:15, 1961.
221. Rosenberg, L.: Cartilage proteoglycans. Fed. Proc. 32:1467, 1973.
222. Lipshitz, H., Etheridge, R., and Glimcher, M.J.: Changes in the hexosamine content and swelling ratio of articular cartilage as a function of depth from the surface. J. Bone Joint Surg. 58A:1149, 1976.
223. Lipshitz, H., Etheridge, R., and Glimcher, M.J.: In vitro wear of articular cartilage. J. Bone Joint Surg. 57A:527, 1975.
224. Maroudas, A., Muir, H., and Wingham, J.: The correlation of fixed negative charge with glycosaminoglycan content of human articular cartilage. Biochim. Biophys. Acta 177:492, 1969.
225. Maroudas, A.: Physiochemical properties of cartilage in the light of ion-exchange theory. Biophys. J. 8:575, 1968.
226. Maroudas, A.: Biophysical chemistry of cartilaginous tissues with special reference to solute and fluid transport. Biorheology 12:233, 1975.
227. Gordon, S.S., Mow, V.C., Lee, R., et al.: Permeability and transport properties of articular cartilage. Proceedings, 3rd International Congress of Biorheology, La Jolla, California, 1978, p. 175.
228. Sokoloff, L.: Elasticity of articular cartilage: Effect of ions and viscous solutions. Science 141:1055, 1963.
229. Picheny, M.A., and Grodzinsky, A.J.: Method for measurement of charge in collagen and polyelectrolyte composite materials. Biopolymers 15:1845, 1976.
230. Nussbaum, J.H., and Grodzinsky, A.J.: $H^+$ binding and diffusion-reaction rates in collagen electromechanics. *In* Ostrander, L.E. (ed.): Proceedings, 7th New England (Northeast) Bioengineering Congress, 1979, pp. 61–64.
231. Grodzinsky, A.J., and Shoenfeld, N.A.: Tensile forces induced in collagen by means of electromechanochemical transductive coupling. Polymer 18:421, 1977.
232. Grodzinsky, A.J., Lipschitz, H., and Glimcher, M.J.: Electromechanical properties of articular cartilage during compression and stress relaxation. Nature 275:448, 1978.
233. Grodzinsky, A.J., Roth, V., Fox, P., et al.: The influence of electrochemical transduction on matrix interactions in articular cartilage. Transactions, 25th Annual Meeting, Orthopedic Research Society, San Francisco, 4:141, 1979.
234. Grodzinsky, A.J., and Eisenberg, S.R.: Double layer mediated energy conversion with a protein membrane using an imposed frequency and wavelength. J. Electrostatics 5:33, 1978.
235. Grodzinsky, A.J., and Melcher, J.R.: Electromechanical transduction with charged polyelectrolyte membranes. IEEE Trans. Biomed. Eng. 23:421, 1976.
236. Lotke, P.A., Black, J., and Richardson, S.: Electromechanical properties in human articular cartilage. J. Bone Joint Surg. 56A:1040, 1974.
237. Meachim, G., Ghadially, F., and Collins, D.M.: Regressive changes in

the superficial layer of human articular cartilage. Ann. Rheum. Dis. 24:23, 1965.
238. Goodfellow, J.W., and Bullough, P.G.: The pattern of aging of the articular cartilage of the elbow joint. J. Bone Joint Surg. 49B:175, 1967.
239. Mankin, H.J.: The reaction of articular cartilage to injury and osteoarthritis (first of two parts). N. Engl. J. Med. 291:1285, 1974.
240. Krane, S.M.: Joint erosion in rheumatoid arthritis. Arthritis Rheum. 17:206, 1974.
241. Muir, H.: Molecular approach to understanding of osteoarthrosis. Ann. Rheum. Dis. 36:199, 1977.
242. Radin, E.L., Paul, I.L., and Lowy, M.: A comparison of the dynamic force-transmitting properties of subchondral bone and articular cartilage. J. Bone Joint Surg. 52A:444, 1970.
243. Radin, E.L., and Paul, L.: Importance of bone in sparing articular cartilage from impact. Clin. Orthop. 78:342, 1971.
244. Chamay, A., and Tschantz, P.: Mechanical influences in bone remodeling. Experimental research on Wolff's law. J. Biomechanics 5:173, 1972.
245. Dickson, R.A.: The assessment of hand function. II. Forces and bone density, a relationship in the hand. Hand 5:15, 1973.
246. Pugh, J.W., Rose, R.M., and Radin, E.L.: Elastic and viscoelastic properties of trabecular bone: Dependence on structure. J. Biomechanics 6:475, 1973.
247. Pugh, J.W., Rose, R.M., and Radin, E.L.: A possible mechanism of Wolff's law: Trabecular microfractures. Arch. Intern. Physiol. Biochim. 81:27, 1973.
248. Behrens, J.C., Walker, P.S., and Shoji, H.: Variations in strength and structure of cancellous bone at the knee. J. Biomechanics 7:201, 1974.
249. Pugh, J.W., Radin, E.L., and Rose, R.M.: Quantitative studies of human subchondral cancellous bone. Its relationship to the state of its overlying cartilage. J. Bone Joint Surg. 56A:313, 1974.
250. Leriem, P., et al.: Hardness of the subchondral bone of the tibial condyles in the normal state and in osteoarthritis and rheumatoid arthritis. Acta Orthop. Scand. 45:614, 1974.
251. Raux, P., Townsend, P.R., Meigel, R., et al.: Trabecular architecture of the human patella. J. Biomechanics 8:1, 1975.
252. Bullough, P., Goodfellow, J., and O'Connor, J.: The relationship between degenerative changes and load-bearing in the human hip. J. Bone Joint Surg. 55B:746, 1973.
253. F. Pauwel's Der Schenkelhalsbruch: Ein mechanisches Problem: Grundlagen Heilungsvorganges. Prognose und kausale Therapie: Zeitchrift für orthopadische Chirurgie, Vol. 63. Stuttgart, Enke, 1935.
254. Murray, M.P., Gore, D.R., and Clarkson, B.H.: Walking patterns of patients with unilateral hip pain due to osteoarthritis and avascular necrosis. J. Bone Joint Surg. 53A:259, 1971.
255. Murray, M.P., Brewer, B., and Zuege, R.C.: Kinesiologic measurements of functional performance before and after McKee-Farrar total hip replacement. A study of thirty patients with rheumatoid arthritis, osteoarthritis, or avascular necrosis of the femoral head. J. Bone Joint Surg. 54A:237, 1972.
256. Gord, D.R., Murray, M.P., and Sepic, S.B.: Walking patterns of men with unilateral surgical hip fusion. J. Bone Joint Surg. 57A:759, 1975.
257. Hauge, M.F.: The knee in patients with hip joint ankylosis. Clinical survey and bio-mechanical aspects. Acta Orthop. Scand. 44:485, 1973.
258. Johnston, R.C., Brand, R.A., and Crowinshield, R.D.: Reconstruction of the hip. A mathematical approach to determine optimum geometric relationships. J. Bone Joint Surg. 61A:639, 1979.
259. Blount, W.: Don't throw away the cane. J. Bone Joint Surg. 38A:695, 1956.
260. Gore, D.R., Murray, M.P., Gardner, G.M., et al.: Roentgenographic measurements after Muller total hip replacement. J. Bone Joint Surg. 59A:948, 1977.
261. Stauffer, R.N., Smidt, G.L., and Wadsworth, J.B.: Clinical and biomechanical analysis of gait following Charnley total hip replacement. Clin. Orthop. 99:70, 1974.
262. Cracchiolo, A. (ed.): Statistics of total knee replacement. Clin. Orthop. Rel. Res. 120:2085, 1976.
263. Reilly, D.T., and Martens, M.: Experimental analysis of the quadriceps muscle force and patello-femoral joint reaction force for various activities. Acta Orthop. Scand. 43:126, 1972.
264. Zdravkovic, D., and Damholt, V.: Knee and quadriceps function after fracture of the femur. Acta Orthop. Scand. 42:460, 1971.
265. Kostuik, J.P., Schmidt, O., Harris, W.R., and Wooldridge, C.: A study of weight transmission through the knee joint with applied varus and valgus loads. Clin. Orthop. 108:95, 1975.
266. Kellelkamp, D.B.: Clinical implications of knee biomechanics. Arch. Surg. 107:406, 1973.
267. Hughston, J.C., and Eilers, A.F.: The role of the posterior oblique ligament in repairs of acute medial (collateral) ligament tears of the knee. J. Bone Joint Surg. 55:923, 1973.
268. Harrington, K.: Degenerative arthritis of the ankle secondary to long-standing lateral ligament instability. J. Bone Joint Surg. 61A:347, 1979.
269. Lew, W.D., and Lewis, J.L.: An anthropometric scaling method with application to the knee joint. J. Biomechanics 10:171, 1977.
270. Lewis, J.L., and Lew, W.D.: A method for locating an optimal "fixed" axis of rotation for the human knee joint. J. Biomech. Eng. 100:187, 1978.
271. Krause, W.R., Pope, M.H., Johnson, R., et al.: Mechanical changes in the knee after menisectomy. J. Bone Joint Surg. 58A:599, 1976.
272. Snook, S.H., and Ciriello, V.M.: Low back pain in industry. ASSE J. 17:17, 1972.
273. Bond, M.B.: Low back injuries in industry. Indust. Med. Surg. 39:204, 1970.
274. National Center for Health Statistics: Prevalence of chronic skin and musculo-skeletal conditions, United States 1969. Series 10, No. 92, 1974.
275. Rowe, M.L.: Low back pain in industry. J. Occup. Med. 11:161, 1969.
276. National Center for Health Statistics: Limitation of Activity Due to Chronic Conditions, United States, 1969 and 1970. Series, 10, No. 80, 1973.
277. National Center for Health Statistics: Types of Injuries. Incidence and Associated Disability, United States, July 1965–1967. Series 10, No. 57, 1969.
278. Rowe, M.L.: Low back disability in industry: Updated position. J. Occup. Med. 13:476, 1971.
279. Horal, J.: The clinical appearance of low back disorders in the city of Gothenburg, Sweden. Acta Orthop. Scand. Suppl. No. 118, 1969.
280. Kosiak, M., Aurelius, J.R., and Hatfield, W.F.: Backache in industry. J. Occup. Med. 8:51, 1966.
281. Hirsch, C.: Etiology and pathogenesis of low back pain. Israel J. Med. Sci. 2:362, 1966.
282. Farfan, H.F., Huberdeau, R.M., and Dubow, H.I.: Lumbar intervertebral disc degeneration: The influence of geometrical features on the pattern of disc degeneration—a post mortem study. J. Bone Joint Surg. 54A:492, 1972.
283. Fahrni, W.H.: Conservative treatment of lumbar disc degeneration: Our primary responsibility. Orthop. Clin. North Am. 6:93, 1975.
284. Nachemson, A.: Towards a better understanding of low-back pain: A review of the mechanics of the lumbar disc. Rheumatol. Rehabil. 14:129, 1975.
285. Cailliet, R.: Lowback Pain Syndrome. Philadelphia, F. A. Davis, 1962.
286. Magora, A.: Investigation of the relationship between low back pain and occupation. Indust. Med. Surg. 39:504, 1970.
287. Park, K.S., and Chaffin, D.B.: Methods of manual load lifting: A biomechanical evaluation of an old problem. Technical report, University of Michigan, Department of Industrial and Operations Engineering, Ann Arbor, Michigan, 1973.
288. Brown, J.R.: Manual Lifting and Related Fields: An Annotated Bibliography. Labour Safety Council of Ontario. Ontario, Ministry of Labour, 1972.
289. Snook, S.H.: The design of manual handling tasks. Ergonomics 21:963, 1978.
290. Snook, S.H., and Ciriello, V.M.: Maximum weights and work loads acceptable to female workers. J. Occup. Med. 16:527, 1974.
291. Snook, S.H., and Irvine, C.H.: Maximum acceptable weight of lift. Am. Indust. Hyg. Assoc. J. 28:322, 1967.
292. Snook, S.H., Campanelli, R.A., and Hart, J.W.: A study of three preventive approaches to low back injury. J. Occup. Med. 20:478, 1978.
293. Chaffin, D.B., Herrin, C.D., Keyerling, W.M., et al.: Preemployment strength testing in selecting workers for materials handling jobs. NIOSH Contract No. CDC-99-74-62, May 1977.
294. Chaffin, D.B.: Human strength capability and low-back pain. J. Occup. Med. 16:248, 1974.
295. Chaffin, D.B.: Biomechanics of manual materials handling and lowback pain. *In* Zenz, C. (ed.): Occupational Medicine: Principles and Practical Applications. Chicago, Year Book Medical Publishers, 1975, Chapter 19.
296. Chaffin, D.B., and Park, K.S.: A longitudinal study of lowback pain as associated with occupational weight lifting factors. Am. Indust. Assoc. J. 34:513, 1973.
297. Chaffin, D.B., Herrin, C.D., Keyserling, W.M., et al.: Preemployment Strength Testing in Selecting Workers for Manual Handling Jobs. Washington, D.C., U.S. Department of Health, Education and Welfare, CDC-99-74-72, 1976.
298. Pedersen, O.F., Petersen, R., and Staffeldt, E.S.: Back pain and isometric back muscle strength of workers in a Danish factory. Scand. J. Rehabil. Med. 7:125, 1975.
299. Poulsen, E.: Prediction of maximum loads in lifting from measurements of muscular strength. Communications from the Danish National Association for Infantile Paralysis, 1970, 31.
300. Chaffin, D.B., Herrin, G.D., and Keyserling, W.M.: Preemployment strength testing, an updated position. J. Occup. Med. 20:No. 6, 403, 78.

# Chapter 21

# Purine and Deoxypurine Metabolism

*Thomas D. Palella and William N. Kelley*

Recognition of the role of purines in human disease began with the observation that uric acid, a purine base, was a component of some renal calculi,[1] and in its ionized form, monosodium urate, was (1) a major constituent of tophi,[2] (2) elevated in the serum of gouty patients,[3] and (3) present, in its crystalline form, in synovial fluid during the acute attack of gouty arthritis.[4] In more recent years the role in human disease of other purines such as xanthine, hypoxanthine, adenine, and 2,8-dihydroxyadenine, as well as the potential role of the deoxypurines, deoxyguanosine and deoxyadenosine, has become increasingly apparent. In this chapter we will trace (1) the reactions by which purine compounds are synthesized, interconverted, salvaged, degraded, and eventually oxidized to uric acid; (2) the mechanisms by which these pathways are controlled in man; (3) the mechanisms by which the final degradative product of the pathway, uric acid, is excreted and/or degraded; and (4) the physical properties of uric acid.

## BIOCHEMISTRY OF PURINE COMPOUNDS

The parent compound, the purine base, is composed of a six-membered pyrimidine ring fused to the five-membered imidazole ring. The origins of individual atoms of the purine ring are as follows: carbon atoms 4 and 5 and nitrogen atom 7 come from glycine;[5-7] carbon atoms 2 and 8 come from formate;[7,8] carbon atom 6 comes from $CO_2$;[6,9] nitrogen atoms 3 and 9 come from the amide nitrogen of glutamine;[10-12] and nitrogen atom 1 comes from aspartic acid.[11] These precursor-product relationships are shown in Figure 21-1.

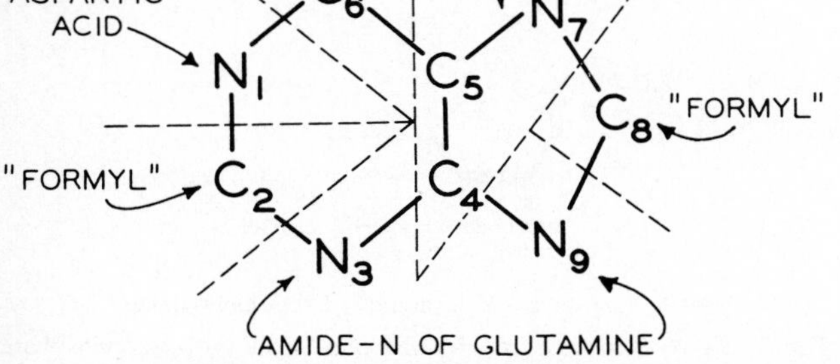


**Figure 21–1.** Origins of atoms of the purine ring.

The most important purine bases are adenine, guanine, hypoxanthine, xanthine, and uric acid (Fig. 21-2). The purines all show lactam-lactim isomerism and may be written in either form, as shown for uric acid in Figure 21-2*B*.

Purine nucleosides are composed of a purine base plus a pentose joined to the base by a $\beta$-*N*-glycosyl bond between carbon atom 1 of the pentose and nitrogen atom 9 of the purine base. There are two series of nucleosides: the ribonucleosides, which contain D-ribose as the sugar component, and the deoxyribonucleosides, which contain 2-deoxy-D-ribose (Fig. 21-3).

Purine nucleotides and deoxynucleotides consist of a nucleoside or deoxynucleoside with a phosphate group in ester linkage with carbon 5 of the pentose (Fig. 21-

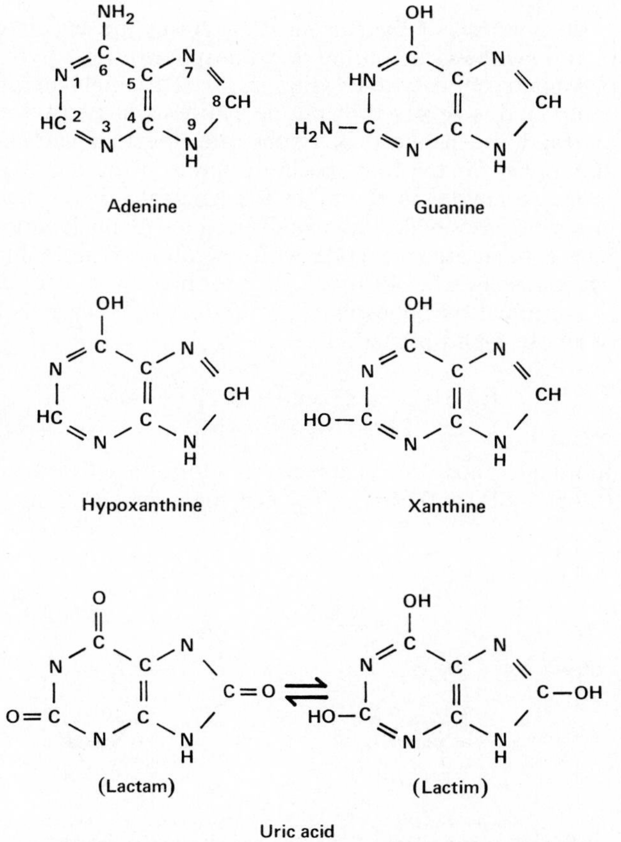


**Figure 21–2.** Structures of the purine bases, adenine, guanine, hypoxanthine, xanthine, and uric acid. All purine bases may exist in the lactam form in a reversible manner as shown for uric acid.

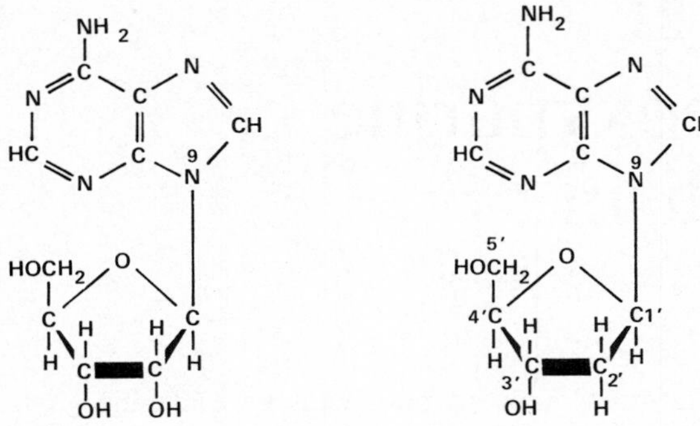


Adenosine          2' – Deoxyadenosine

**Figure 21–3.** Structures of adenosine and 2'-deoxyadenosine as examples of nucleosides and 2'-deoxynucleosides, respectively.

4). The nucleosides and deoxynucleosides may exist as 5'-monophosphates, 5'-diphosphates, and 5'-triphosphates (Fig. 21-5). The phosphoric acid residues of these compounds are designated by the symbols α, β, and γ. These compounds serve (1) as building blocks for RNA and DNA; (2) as precursors of the cyclic nucleotides, adenosine 3',5'-cyclic phosphate, and guanosine 3',5'-cyclic phosphate; (3) as a source of chemical energy; and (4) as precursors of various purine cofactors and coenzymes such as nicotinamide adenine dinucleotide (NAD).

**Biosynthesis of the Purine Ring.** A key intermediate in the synthesis of purine is 5-phosphoribosyl-1-pyrophosphate (PP-ribose-P) (Fig. 21-6). This high-energy compound is involved in purine synthesis in two types of reactions: in one it is a substrate, together with L-glutamine, for the first specific reaction of purine synthesis de novo;[13] in the other it participates in salvage of purine bases which are reconverted to ribonucleotides by a condensation reaction with liberation of inorganic pyrophosphate.[14,15] PP-ribose-P is formed by transfer of the terminal pyrophosphate group of ATP to carbon 1 of ribose 5-phosphate:[16,17]

$$\text{Ribose-5-phosphate} + \text{ATP} \xrightarrow{Mg^{2+}} \text{PP-ribose-P} + \text{AMP} \qquad (1)$$

Inorganic phosphate is a required allosteric activator of PP-ribose-P synthetase.[18] The enzyme is subject to met-

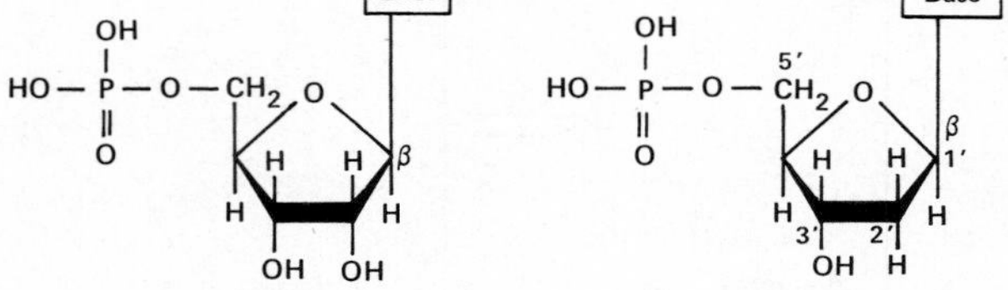


Ribonucleoside 5' – monophosphates          2' – Deoxyribonucleoside 5' – monophosphates

**Figure 21–4.** General structures of nucleoside and deoxynucleoside 5'-monophosphates.

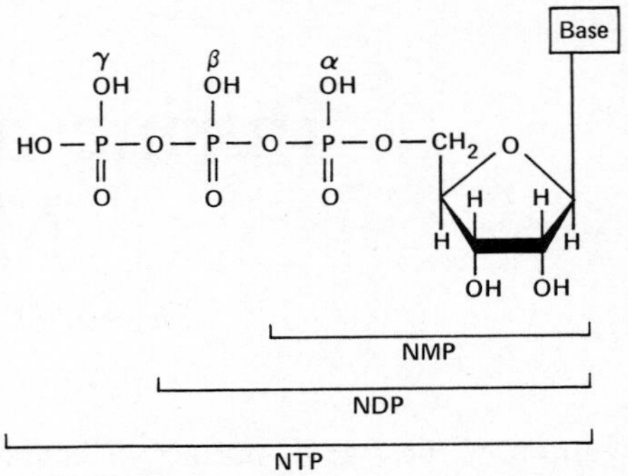


**Figure 21–5.** Comparison of the structures of nucleoside, mono-, di-, and triphosphates.

abolic regulation by purine and pyrimidine ribonucleotides and certain other compounds.[19]

The first specific step of purine synthesis de novo is that in which the highly labile amino sugar, 5-β-phospho-D-ribosyl-1-amine, is generated. There are three known reactions for synthesis of phosphoribosylamine. In the best studied of the three,[12,13,20] the amide group of glutamine is transferred to PP-ribose-P and inorganic pyrophosphate is displaced. There is simultaneously an inversion of substituents at carbon 1 with formation of the β linkage characteristic of the glycosidic bond of all naturally occurring ribonucleotides (Fig. 21-7).[13]

$$\alpha\text{-PP-ribose-P} + \text{glutamine} + H_2O \xrightarrow{Mg^{2+}} \beta\text{-phosphoribosylamine} + \text{glutamic acid} + PP_i \qquad (2)$$

This reaction which is catalyzed by anidophasphoribosyltransferase, is irreversible, and an important site of feedback control of purine synthesis. Other potential pathways for the synthesis of phosphoribosylamine include the direct reaction of PP-ribose-P with ammonia and a direct reaction of ribose-5-phosphate with ammonia. The contribution of this latter reaction in mammalian cells is probably insignificant. Cultured mammalian cell lines deficient in the first two synthetic reactions for phosphoribosylamine are auxotrophic for purines, despite the presence of the direct condensation of ammonia and ribose-5-phosphate.[21,22,23] The aminotransferase reaction, whereby ammonia and PP-ribose-P condense enzymatically, has been shown to contribute to de novo purine synthesis in human lymphocytes. In these same studies, the inhibitory effects of purine nucleotides were independent of the origin of the amine nitrogen.[24]

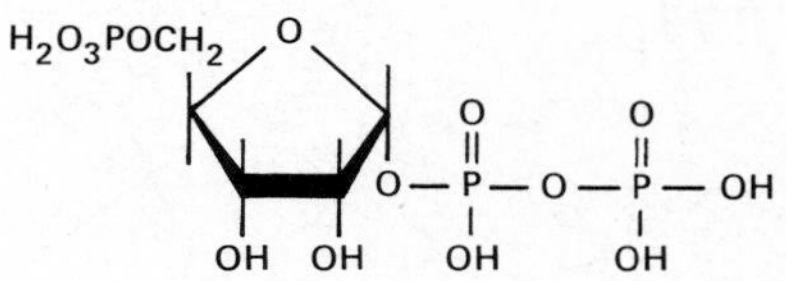


α – 5 – phospho – D – ribosyl – 1 – pyrophosphate

**Figure 21–6.** Structure of α-5-phospho-D-ribosyl-l-pyrophosphate (PP-ribose-l').

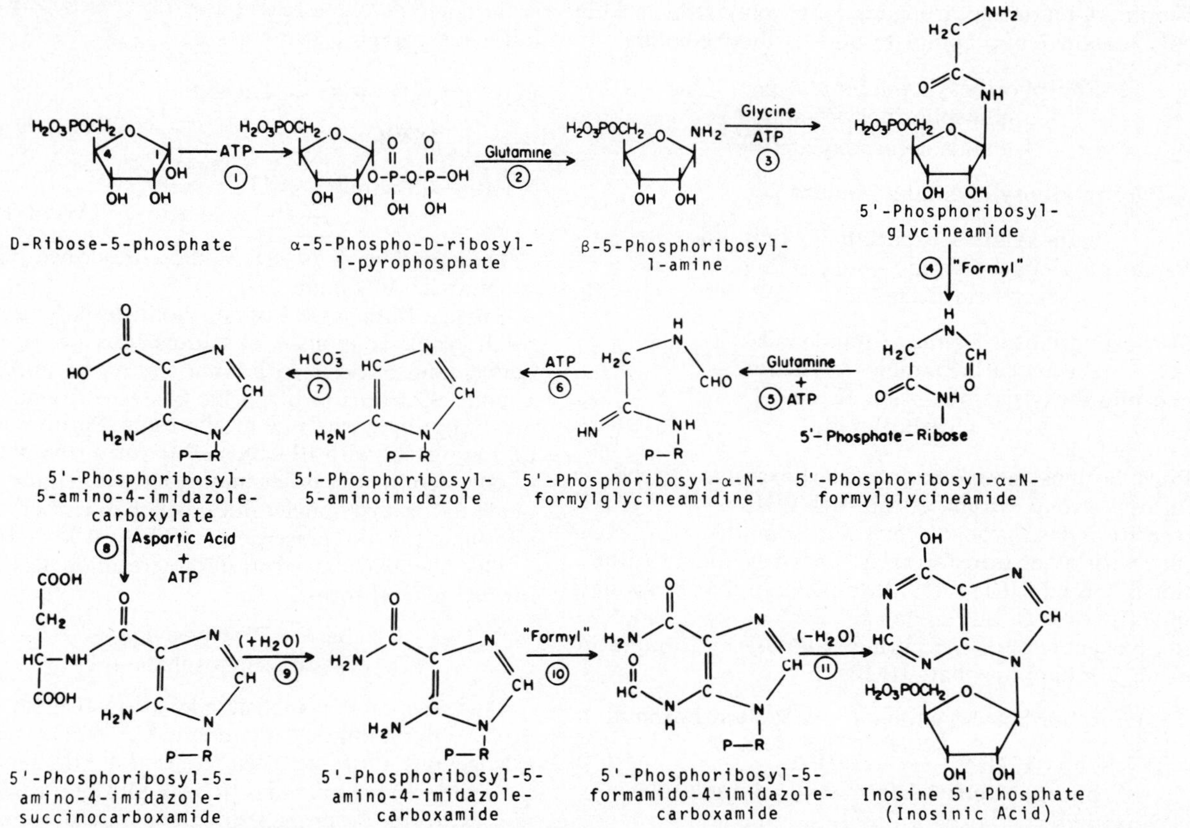


**Figure 21–7.** Biosynthesis of the purine ring. The encircled numbers in this figure refer to numbered reactions in the text. (From Wyngaarden, J.B., and Kelley, W.N.: Gout and Hyperuricemia. New York, Grune and Stratton, 1976.)

The stepwise synthesis of the purine ring is shown in Figure 21-7. Phosphoribosylamine is conjugated with glycine to yield 5′-phosphoribosylglycineamide, the first intermediate in which one finds the fundamental components of a nucleotide—namely, the combination of base, sugar, and phosphoric acid. ATP is involved in this reaction as an energy source.[12,25,26] Nucleotides of adenine and guanine show no inhibitory effects upon the enzyme catalyzing this reaction.[27]

$$\text{Phosphoribosylamine} + \text{glycine} + \text{ATP} \xrightarrow{Mg^{2+}} \text{5}'\text{-phosphoribosylglycineamide (PRG)} + \text{ADP} + P_i \quad (3)$$

Phosphoribosylglycineamide receives a one-carbon "formyl" unit from $N^5,N^{10}$-methenyltetrahydrofolic acid ($N^5,N^{10}$-methenyl-THFA).[28,29] The transformylase activity has been shown to proceed through a direct displacement mechanism involving only formyl donor (10-CHO-$H_4$ folate) and formyl acceptor.[30]

$$\text{Phosphoribosylglycineamide} + N^5,N^{10}\text{-methenyl-THFA} + H_2O \rightarrow \text{phosphoribosyl-}\alpha\text{-}N\text{-formylglycineamide} + \text{THFA} + H^+ \quad (4)$$

Next, the amide group of glutamine is transferred to phosphoribosylglycineamide to form the corresponding amidine compound,[31-33] following which ring closure generates the five-membered imidazole ring.[34] Each of these reactions requires ATP as an energy source and magnesium. The ring-closure reaction requires potassium as well.

$$\text{5}'\text{-Phosphoribosyl-}\alpha\text{-}N\text{-formylglycineamide} + \text{glutamine} + \text{ATP} + H_2O \xrightarrow{Mg^{2+}} \text{5}'\text{-phosphoribosyl-}\alpha\text{-}N\text{-formylglycineamidine} + \text{glutamic acid} + \text{ADP} + P_i \quad (5)$$

$$\text{5}'\text{-phosphoribosyl-}\alpha\text{-}N\text{-formylglycineamidine} + \text{ATP} \xrightarrow{Mg^{2+}, K^+} \text{5}'\text{-phosphoribosyl-5-aminoimidazole} + \text{ADP} + P_i \quad (6)$$

5′-Phosphoribosyl-5-aminoimidazole now receives a carboxyl group at carbon 4 by a reversible $CO_2$ fixation reaction that requires a high concentration of bicarbonate.[35] The carboxyl serves as a point for condensation of this intermediate with aspartic acid through an amide linkage involving another ATP as source of energy.[35] Hydrolysis of the intermediate yields 5′-phosphoribosyl-

5-amino-4-imidazolecarboxamide, a compound lacking only carbon 2 of a complete purine ribonucleotide.

$$\text{5}'\text{-Phosphoribosylaminoimidazole} + CO_2 \longrightarrow \text{5}'\text{-phosphoribosyl-5-amino-4-imidazolecarboxylate} \quad (7)$$

$$\text{5}'\text{-Phosphoribosyl-5-amino-4-imidazole-carboxylate} + \text{aspartate} + \text{ATP} \xrightarrow{Mg^{2+}} \text{5}'\text{-phosphoribosyl-5-amino-4-imidazole-succinocarboxamide} + \text{ADP} + P_i \quad (8)$$

$$\text{5}'\text{-Phosphoribosyl-5-amino-4-imidazole-succinocarboxamide} \longrightarrow \text{fumarate} + \text{5}'\text{-phosphoribosyl-5-amino-4-imidazole-carboxamide} \quad (9)$$

Phosphoribosylaminoimidazolecarboxamide receives a formyl group from $N^{10}$-formyl-THFA.[36,37] AICAR transformylase probably exists in a multienzyme complex with other transformylase enzymes and a "trifunctional" protein. The actual carbon donor may be formate directly through this complex.[38] Ring closure completes the biosynthesis of the purine structure by forming inosine 5′-monophosphate (IMP):[37]

$$\text{5}'\text{-Phosphoribosyl-5-amino-4-imidazolecarboxamide} + N^{10}\text{-formyl-THFA} \xrightarrow{K^+} + \text{THFA} \quad (10)$$

5′-phosphoribosyl-5-formamido-4-inudazole-carboxamide

$$\text{5}'\text{-Phosphoribosyl-5-formamido-4-imidazolecarboxamide} \longrightarrow \text{IMP} + H_2O \quad (11)$$

**Biosynthesis of Other Nucleotides.** Inosinic acid may be considered the parent purine compound. It is an intermediate in the formation of adenylic acid (adenosine 5′-monophosphate, AMP) and guanylic acid (guanosine 5′-monophosphate, GMP), the major purine nucleotide components of nucleic acids. Conversion of inosinic acid to adenylic acid occurs in two steps. There is an initial condensation of inosinic acid with aspartic acid to form adenylosuccinic acid (AMP-S).[39,40] Energy for this reaction is derived from guanosine triphosphate.[41-44] Cleavage of adenylosuccinic acid yields adenylic acid and fumaric acid. This reaction is freely reversible;[41] it is analogous to cleavage of phosphoribosylaminoimidazole-succinocarboxamide (reaction 9) and is probably catalyzed by the same enzyme, adenylosuccinate lyase.

$$\text{IMP} + \text{L-asparate} + \text{GTP} \xrightarrow{Mg^{2+}} \text{AMP-S} + \text{GDP} + P_i \quad (12)$$

$$\text{AMP-S} \longrightarrow \text{AMP} + \text{fumarate} \quad (13)$$

Conversion of inosinic acid to guanylic acid also occurs in two steps. There is first an irreversible oxidation of inosinic acid to xanthosine 5′-monophosphate (XMP), with nicotinamide adenine dinucleotide (NAD) as hydrogen acceptor.[45-47] The second reaction involves amination of XMP at the 2 position, and the specific donor is the amide group of glutamine.[48,49] The second step requires ATP. These reactions proceed according to the following overall schemes:

$$\text{IMP} + \text{NAD}^+ H_2O \xrightarrow{K^+} \text{XMP} + \text{NADH} + H^+ \quad (14)$$

$$\text{XMP} + \text{glutamine} + \text{ATP} \xrightarrow{Mg^{2+}} \text{GMP} + \text{glutamic acid} + \text{AMP} + P_i \quad (15)$$

These pathways as well as those described below are summarized in Figure 21-8.

**Salvage Pathways.** Purine ribonucleosides and bases result from catabolism of endogenous or ingested ribonucleotides, or from administration of purine compounds. Conversion of purine bases to ribonucleotides may occur by one of two mechanisms. Purine bases may be conjugated with PP-ribose-P to form ribonucleotides in one step, or the bases may react with ribose 1-phosphate to form ribonucleosides, which may then be phosphorylated in the presence of ATP to ribonucleotides.

The phosphoribosyltransferase reaction has the following general form:

$$\text{Base} + \text{PP-ribose-P} \longrightarrow \text{base-ribosephosphate} + P_i \quad (16)$$

This reaction is responsible for the conversion of purines,[14,15] pyrimidines,[50] nicotinamide,[51] and certain other nitrogenous bases to their respective ribonucleotides. Two different mammalian purine phosphoribosyltransferases (formerly termed ribonucleotide pyrophosphorylases) have been identified: one, ademine phosphoribosyltransferase (APRT), acting on AIC and adenine (Reaction 4, Fig. 21-8),[14,52] the other, hypoxanthine-guanine phosphoribosyltransferese (HPRT), acting on hypoxanthine and guanine (Reaction 2, Fig. 21-8).[15,53] APRT will also accept adenine analogues such as 2,6-diaminopurine and 8-azadenine. HPRT will catalyze the

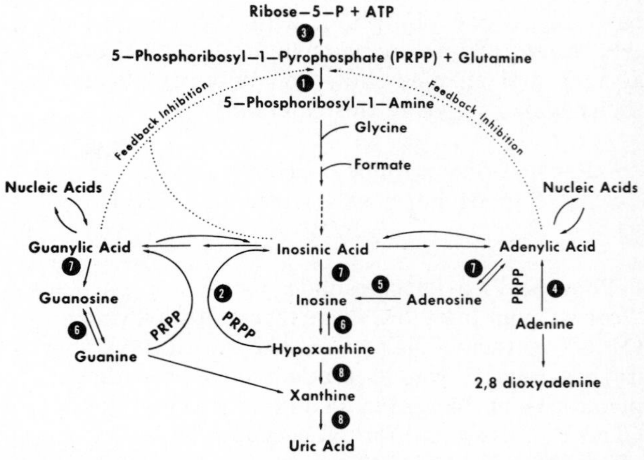


**Figure 21–8.** Outline of purine metabolism. (1) Amidophosphoribosyltransferase; (2) hypoxanthine-guanine phosphoribosyltransferase; (3) PRPP synthetase; (4) adenine phosphoribosyltransferase; (5) adenosine deaminase; (6) purine nucleoside phosphorylase; (7) 5′-nucleotidase; (8) xanthine oxidase. (From Seegmiller, J.E. et al.: Science 155:1682, 1967.)

conversion of xanthine to XMP, but at only about 0.3 percent of the rate of the reaction with hypoxanthine or guanine.[54] HPRT will also catalyze the conversion of 6-thiopurine,[15] 6-thioguanine, 8-azaguanine, allopurinol,[55] and oxipurinol[56] to their respective ribonucleotides. In man, HPRT activity is widely distributed and is especially rich in brain, where activity is greatest in basal ganglia.[57] Activity is low in muscle and bone marrow.[57] The $K_{eq}$ of both phosphoribosyltransferases is far toward the ribonucleotide; a value of 290 has been estimated for APRT.[52] Both phosphoribosyltransferases are inhibited by purine ribonucleoside monophosphates. Adenine phosphoribosyltransferase is inhibited by adenylic acid.[52] Hypoxanthine- guanine phosphoribosyltransferase is inhibited by inosinic acid and guanylic acid whether the substrate is hypoxanthine or guanine.[53] The inhibitions are formally competitive against PP-ribose-P, but appear to involve mutually exclusive binding rather than product inhibition at the substrate site.[58]

The two-step pathway has the following general form:

$$\text{Base} + \text{(deoxy)ribose 1-phosphate} \longrightarrow \text{base-(deoxy)ribose} + P_i \quad (17)$$

$$\text{Base} - \text{(deoxy)ribose} + \text{ATP} \longrightarrow \text{base-(deoxy)ribosephosphate} + \text{ADP} \quad (18)$$

Reaction 17 is catalyzed by purine nucleoside phosphorylase, an enzyme widely distributed in mammalian tissue and active with guanine, with hypoxanthine, and, to a lesser extent, with xanthine (Reaction 6, Fig. 21-8). Deoxyribose 1-phosphate may substitute for ribose 1-phosphate. The erythrocyte enzyme does not accept adenine,[59,60] but adenosine appears to be cleaved by the purine nucleoside phosphorylase of liver.[61] In the case of hypoxanthine, the equilibrium point is far toward the ribonucleoside. The phosphorylase has been extensively studied in human erythrocytes.[60,62]

Reaction 18 is catalyzed by a nucleoside or deoxynucleoside kinase. Kinases capable of catalyzing the phosphorylation of inosine or guanosine have been described in animal tissues,[63] and labeled inosine is incorporated into adenine and guanine nucleotides in liver of both normal and HPRT-deficient subjects.[64] These kinases appear to be absent in human fibroblasts.[65] In contrast, deoxyguanosine and deoxyinosine are readily converted to their respective monophosphates in a reaction that appears to be catalyzed by deoxycytidine kinase.[66] Adenosine kinase is an active enzyme, widely distributed in mammalian tissues, that is capable of catalyzing the phosphorylation of both adenosine and deoxyadenosine.[67,68] Adenosine kinase is inhibited by AMP and ADP, both of which are products of the reaction. Inhibition constants are of the order of the physiologic concentrations of each and may thus indicate a regulatory role for the adenine nucleotides.[69] The phosphorylation of deoxyadenosine may also be catalyzed by kinases other than adenosine kinase.[70-74]

Studies in subjects who lack activity of HPRT, and of their cells in culture, indicate that HPRT is normally responsible for a much more extensive recycling of purine bases into nucleotide pools than was initially appreciated. By contrast, recycling of hypoxanthine and guanine via the nucleoside phosphorylase-nucleoside kinase route is not very active. While this two-step pathway does not appear to be important in the normal salvage of purine nucleosides or bases, salvage of deoxynucleosides by the appropriate kinase appears to occur in patients lacking adenosine deaminase[75,76] or purine nucleoside phosphorylase.[77]

**Nucleic Acid Catabolism.** Enzymatic hydrolysis of polynucleotide chains of nucleic acid occurs through the action of various nucleases.[78] The major products released by ribonuclease a and b and by deoxyribonuclease I and II are oligonucleotides. The oligonucleotides are further cleaved by phosphodiesterases to yield 5′- and 3′-mononucleotides.

The mononucleotides are split by group-specific 5′-nucleotidases,[79] as well as by nonspecific phosphatases,[80] to yield the corresponding purine or pyrimidine nucleoside and orthophosphate. At least one form of 5′-nucleotidase is localized in the external surface of the plasma membrane (ecto-5′-nucleotidase). This enzyme is selectively present on the surface of B lymphocytes. In diseases associated with low levels of B lymphocytes (e.g., hypogammaglobulenemia) it appears to be deficient when mixed lymphocyte populations are studied.[81,82] Ecto-5′-nucleotidase appears to have little role in the regulation of intracellular nucleotide metabolism.[83] The purine nucleoside or deoxynucleoside is then split by purine nucleoside phosphorylase to yield a free purine base and ribose 1-phosphate or deoxyribose 1-phosphate as described above.

$$\text{Purine(deoxy)mononucleotide} \longrightarrow \text{purine(deoxy)nucleoside} + P_i \quad (19)$$

$$\text{Purine(deoxy)nucleoside} + P_i \longrightarrow \text{purine base} + \text{(deoxy)ribose 1-phosphate} \quad (20)$$

In addition to these general reactions, adenylic acid and adenosine are acted upon by specific deaminating enzymes. Adenylic acid is converted to inosinic acid by adenylic acid deaminase (Fig. 21-8)[84] and adenosine or deoxyadenosine to inosine or deoxyinosine by adenosine deaminase (Reaction 5, Fig. 21-8).[85] Guanylic acid may be deaminated to inosinic acid in bacteria. These various reactions and their controls may serve to provide the cell with the proper balance of adenyl and guanyl ribonucleotides, and also allow for replenishment of one from the other when necessary.

**Formation of Uric Acid.** The free purine bases that result from nucleoside cleavage are adenine, guanine, hypoxanthine, and xanthine. Since purine nucleoside phosphorylase acts most readily on inosine and guanosine,[59] the major bases generated are very likely hypoxanthine and guanine. Guanine is deaminated to xanthine by guanase (Fig. 21-8). Hypoxanthine is oxidized to xanthine by xanthine oxidase and then further oxidized to uric acid by the same enzyme (Reaction 8, Fig. 21-8).[86] Thus, whereas adenine, hypoxanthine, and guanine arise exclusively by cleavage of the corresponding nucleoside, xanthine potentially has three direct precursors—namely, xanthosine (or deoxyxanthosine), hypoxanthine, and guanine.

In man, xanthine oxidase is found in high activity only in liver and small intestinal mucosa.[87,88] Because of this restricted distribution of xanthine oxidase, uric acid synthesis appears largely to be a hepatic process in man. Presumably purine degradation products of other tissues are transported to the liver for further oxidation. Plasma contains small quantities of xanthine and hypoxanthine, together amounting to about 0.1 to 0.3 mg per 100 ml,[89,90] but no other uric acid precursors have been detected in normal plasma in significant quantity, with the possible exception of IMP following anoxic muscle injury.[91]

## REGULATION OF PURINE METABOLISM

**Nucleotide Synthesis de Novo.** Data obtained in bacterial,[92] avian,[93,94] and mammalian[95-98] systems indicate that adenylic acid (AMP) and guanylic acid (GMP) inhibit amidophosphoribosyltransferase (Reaction 1, Fig. 21-8), the initial and rate-limiting step of de novo purine biosynthesis, by interacting at separate sites on the enzyme termed the 6-amino and 6-hydroxy sites, respectively. Inhibition of the human enzyme by purine nucleotides is competitive with respect to PP-ribose-P, and the kinetics of the reaction shift from a hyperbolic to a sigmoidal function when PP-ribose-P is the variable substrate. Adenylic acid and guanylic acid are also inhibitors of formylglycinamide ribonucleotide (FGAR) amidotransferase, although the importance of this feedback site to the control of the rate of purine synthesis de novo is not established.[99]

A regulatory role of PP-ribose-P was suggested by several observations in human cell culture as well as in man in vivo.[100-103] Under normal conditions depletion of PP-ribose-P in vitro and in vivo decreases the rate of purine biosynthesis de novo.[100-103] Elevation of PP-ribose-P by several different mechanisms is associated with an increased rate of purine biosynthesis de novo.[101,104,105] In addition, when PP-ribose-P concentrations are initially elevated and then reduced to levels that are still supranormal, there is no inhibitory effect on purine biosynthesis de novo.[100] Finally, the normal intracellular concentration of PP-ribose-P is considerably less than the Michaelis constant established for amidophosphoribosyltransferase in lower organisms[92,106-108] or in mammalian cells.

The mechanism by which PP-ribose-P and purine ribonucleotides interact to regulate the activity of amidophosphoribosyltransferase was provided by direct study of the enzyme from a human source, and, in subsequent studies, from Chinese hamster fibroblasts and mouse liver.[109,110] Two forms of human amidophosphoribosyltransferase are apparent following gel filtration; the small form has a molecular weight of about 133,000, and the large form has a molecular weight of about 270,000.[98] The larger species appears to be catalytically inactive, while the smaller species appears to be catalytically active. Purine ribonucleotides shift the active smaller species to the inactive larger molecular species: PP-ribose-P converts the large inactive species back to the small active species (Fig. 21-9). Direct in vivo conformation of this model has now been obtained in mouse liver.[110]

**Regulation of Purine Ribonucleotide Interconversions.** The first branch point in the pathway leading to the synthesis de novo of adenylic acid and guanylic acid occurs with the synthesis of inosinic acid (Fig. 21-8). In bacterial systems each nucleotide appears to regulate its own de novo formation by inhibiting the appropriate nucleotide interconversion; guanylic acid inhibits inosinic acid dehydrogenase that catalyzes the formation of xanthylic acid (XMP) from inosinic acid,[47,111] adenylic acid inhibits the formation of adenylosuccinic acid (AMP-S) from inosinic acid that is catalyzed by adenylosuccinic acid synthetase.[42] An analysis, however, of the regulation of adenylosuccinic acid synthetase[44] and inosinic acid dehydrogenase[112] from a human source suggests that the utilization of inosinic acid by each of the alternative pathways may be governed by the intracellular concentration of GTP. GTP is a substrate of adenylosuccinate synthetase with a $K_m$ ranging from 31 to $72 \mu M$[44] and an inhibitor of inosinic acid dehydrogenase.[112] While those observations cannot be applied directly to the setting in vivo, they suggest that as inosinic acid is formed, it is utilized for the synthesis of XMP, guanylic acid (GMP), GDP, and GTP. As GTP reaches a critical concentration in the cell, probably in the micromolar range, it may then increase the activity of AMP-S synthetase, allowing inosinic acid to be effectively utilized in the synthesis of adenylic acid. As GTP reaches an even higher level, not only can it promote the flux of inosinic acid in the direction of adenylic acid, but it can then function as a direct inhibitor of the conversion of inosinic acid to XMP and thus guanylic acid. Indirect evidence in support of this mode of regulation derives from studies with cultured murine lymphoma cells partially deficient in adenylosuccinic acid synthetase. AMP synthesis is maintained at the expense of elevated GTP and IMP.[113]

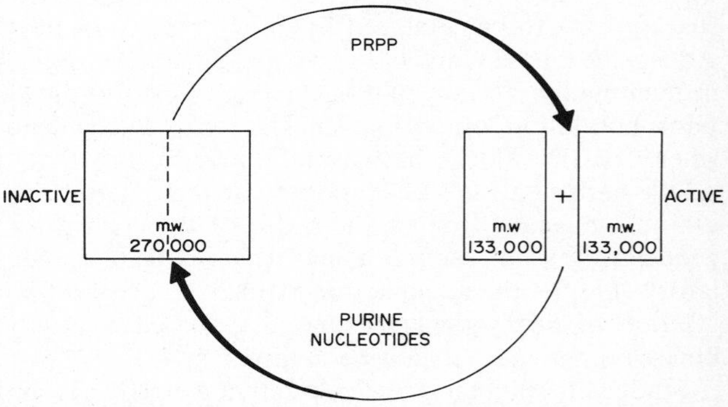


**Figure 21–9** Model of interconversion of small (active) and large (inactive) forms of amidophosphoribosyltransferase. (From Kelley, W.N., et al.: Arthritis Rheum. 18:673, 1975.)

**Ribonucleotide Cleavage.** In circumstances in which accelerated purine biosynthesis de novo results in production of a surfeit of inosinic acid, there is a rapid conversion of the excess ribonucleotide to uric acid. The controls that lead to this result rather than to continual expansion of pools of adenyl and guanyl nucleotides, are not well characterized, but may depend on tight regulation of nucleotide biosynthetic pathways plus improved competition of 5′-nucleotidase for inosinic acid as its concentration is raised.

A comparison of the $K_m$ values of cytoplasmic 5′-nucleotidases with reactions of inosinic acid leading to synthesis of adenylic acid or guanylic acid suggest that increasing concentrations of inosinic acid will saturate adenylosuccinic acid synthetase and inosinic acid dehydrogenase first and then activate the 5′-nucleotidase reaction. The latter will lead to hydrolysis of inosinic acid to inosine, which can then be cleaved by phosphorolysis to form hypoxanthine, followed by oxidation to xanthine and uric acid. Adenylic acid and guanylic acid may be relatively protected from this fate by their higher $K_m$ values and slower rates of hydrolysis in the 5′-nucleotidase reaction and by their conversions to triphosphates, which are poor 5′-nucleotidase substrates.[114,115,116]

**Purine Salvage.** As described earlier, the purine phosphoribosyltransferases are inhibited by the nucleoside monophosphate products of each reaction. Whether such product inhibition is of any physiologic significance in the control of these pathways remains uncertain.

## ORIGIN OF URIC ACID IN MAN

**The Exogenous Contribution.** Unless an individual is in a total fast or ingesting a highly artificial purine-free diet, there is a significant exogenous contribution to the body load and urinary excretion of uric acid. The magnitude of this contribution depends on both the amount and type of purine in the diet, but it is often considerable. For example, when Griebsch and Zollner[117] placed healthy young males on an isocaloric purine-free formula diet, serum urate values declined in 10 days from about 4.9 mg per 100 ml to 3.1 ± 0.4 mg per 100 ml, and urinary excretion of uric acid declined from 500 to 600 mg per day to 336 ± 39 mg per day. Roughly 50 percent of the RNA purines and 25 percent of DNA purines are absorbed and excreted in the urine as uric acid.[118] The difference between amounts of purine administered and excreted may be due to partial hydrolysis, incomplete absorption, enteric decomposition, suppression of purine synthesis de novo, or a combination of some or all of these factors.[117]

**Endogenous Formation of Uric Acid.** Urinary uric acid excretion declines to constant low values after 5 to 7 days of dietary purine elimination or severe restriction. Mean values then range from 336 ± 39 to 426 ± 81 mg per 24 hours. These values reflect the continued synthesis and turnover of endogenous purines. However, the urinary uric acid excretion accounts for only a part of the daily disposition of uric acid. Another part is disposed of by extrarenal routes. Thus, the true rate of endogenous purine turnover cannot be accurately determined by measurement of urinary uric acid excretion but requires the use of isotope dilution techniques in subjects in whom the exogenous contribution has been reduced to a minimum by severe dietary purine restriction.

## EXTRARENAL DISPOSITION OF URIC ACID

**Recovery Studies.** Urinary recoveries of intravenously administered uric acid are incomplete in normal subjects. Over 50 years ago Folin and colleagues[119] and Koehler[120] reported urinary recoveries of unlabeled uric acid that ranged from 28 to 91 percent, and averaged about 50 percent. More recently recoveries of infused $^{15}N$-uric acid or 2-$^{14}C$-uric acid ranging from 55 to 95 percent have been reported.[121-124] The average of 14 studies with $^{15}N$-uric acid was 75.6 percent. These studies suggested extrarenal disposal of 25 to 50 percent of infused uric acid.

Studies of the turnover of uric acid in normal man have uniformly shown that the quantity of uric acid turning over each day exceeds the quantity appearing in urine. Surplus amounts have ranged from 100 to 365 mg per day.[125-127] Thus, these studies also indicate that a significant quantity of uric acid is disposed of by routes other than the kidney. In fact, in comparative studies the fraction of the turnover appearing in urine is essentially the same as the fraction of injected isotopic uric acid recovered in urine.[57,128,129]

Sorensen[126] estimated that 100 mg or more of uric acid enters the alimentary tract in saliva, gastric juice, and bile. An equal quantity may enter in pancreatic and intestinal juices. These quantities of uric acid are larger than once thought[130,131] and are sufficient to account for the degradation of one third of the uric acid normally turned over each day.

The total amount of uricolysis that can be attributed to human tissues is unknown but has been estimated to be less than 2 percent of the turnover of the uric acid pool.[132] Thus, for all practical purposes, extrarenal disposal of uric acid is synonymous with intestinal uricolysis.

## RENAL HANDLING OF URIC ACID IN NORMAL MAN

Initially it was thought that renal excretion of uric acid in man occurred by glomerular filtration followed by extensive, though incomplete, tubular reabsorption.[133] Next, a three-component system was proposed on the basis of evidence for tubular secretion of uric acid in animals and man.[134] More recently several investigators have proposed a four-component model: of glomerular filtration, early proximal tubular reabsorption, tubular secretion, and finally postsecretory tubular reabsorption.

Within the vertebrate phylum there is an impressive

variety of patterns for the renal disposition of uric acid. In some animals net secretion of urate is the rule—e.g., birds,[135] reptiles,[136,137] guinea pigs,[138] Dalmatian coach hounds,[139] and certain species of monkeys.[140] In others net reabsorption is the rule—e.g., rats,[141,142] non-Dalmatian dogs,[139] cats,[138] several species of New World monkeys,[140] the great apes,[140] and man.[133] In many of these species there is evidence for bidirectional transport. In some species in which net secretion occurs, clearance ratios (i.e., $C_{urate}/C_{inulin}$) fall below 1.0 in the presence of inhibitors of urate secretion.[138,143,144] In almost all animals exhibiting net reabsorption, there is evidence that secretion of urate also occurs but is normally masked by extensive reabsorption.[144-152]

The species most nearly comparable to man in the renal handling of urate is the chimpanzee, and next the *Cebus* monkey. The ratio, $C_{urate}/GFR$, is about 0.07 to 0.11 in these species,[145,146,153] as in man. Both species respond appropriately to substances that are uricosuric in man.[153-156] The discussion to follow will emphasize studies performed in man or in these lower primates.

**Glomerular Filtration of Uric Acid.** Glomerular ultrafiltration of uric acid was first conclusively demonstrated by micropuncture studies of Bowman's space in the snake and frog in which urate concentrations in the glomerular fluid were the same as in plasma.[157] Although comparable studies have not been performed with a mammalian glomerulus, micropuncture of the earliest portion of the proximal tubule of the rat also discloses urate concentrations of tubular fluid equal to those of plasma.[147] It is reasonable to assume that ultrafiltration of uric acid also occurs in man.

Whether all urate in plasma is freely filterable at the glomerulus is uncertain. While some urate may be bound to plasma protein, this fraction is currently thought to be small, perhaps less than 5 percent. If the fraction is larger, as some studies suggest, binding could result in the incomplete filtration of urate at the glomerulus.

**Reabsorption of Uric Acid.** Comparisons of renal clearance of uric acid with those of inulin or creatinine disclose a mean ratio of about 0.07 to 0.10 in normal human subjects. If complete glomerular ultrafiltration of plasma urate is assumed, such clearance ratios indicate tubular reabsorption of at least 90 to 93 percent of filtered urate.

Almost all studies of uric acid reabsorption indicate that the process takes place in the proximal tubule. Most localizations have been made with the stop-flow technique in lower animals. Results of free-flow micropuncture studies in *Cebus albifrons* are essentially in accord with results of stopflow experiments in specifying that most urate reabsorption occurs in the proximal tubule.[158] However, distal tubular fluid contains a greater fraction of filtered urate than does final urine. This finding, confirmed in additional animals,[159] may signify reabsorption of a small fraction of filtered or secreted urate in collecting ducts. Thus, although net urate reabsorption occurs largely in proximal tubules in all animals in which the process has been localized (with the exception of the rat, in which it may take place in the loop of Henle), the possibility exists of reabsorption in more distal segments, at least in certain animals.

Available evidence suggests that urate reabsorption occurs by a mechanism of *active transport.* In lower animals ouabain and metabolic poisons inhibit urate reabsorption.[152,160] In rats, the net urate reabsorption in the proximal tubule is an active transport process, although passive movement of urate into and out of the proximal tubule has been demonstrated.[161] This active transport mechanism has been shown to have saturable kinetics, indicating that urate reabsorption in the rat proximal tubule is probably carrier mediated.[162] By way of contrast, urate reabsorption in the rabbit proximal tubule has been shown to consist of both passive and facilitated mechanisms. In these studies, it appeared that the net absorptive flux in the rabbit proximal tubule was passive.[163] In nonhuman primates and in man the concentration of uric acid in urine may approach one tenth the concentration in plasma during diuresis and inhibition of urate secretion with pyrazinoate.[164] In free-flowing micropuncture samples in the chimpanzee and monkey, the concentrations of urate average 0.6 of the concentrations in plasma, and in individual samples may be as low as 0.2. Thus, urate reabsorption may occur against a concentration gradient. According to Weiner and Fanelli[159] the transepithelial potential difference in the proximal tubule is too small to account for this phenomenon by passive forces.

There is a close link between reabsorption of sodium and reabsorption of a number of other components of the glomerular filtrate such as glucose,[165] phosphate,[166] calcium,[167] and bicarbonate,[168] and also uric acid.[167,169,170] In conditions associated with an increase in proximal reabsorption of sodium the clearance of uric acid is reduced (Table 21-1); in conditions leading to decreased proximal reabsorption of sodium the clearance of uric acid is increased (Table 21-2). In addition, sodium reabsorption per nephron is decreased[171] and uric acid excretion per nephron is increased[172] in chronic renal failure in man.

The responses of proximal sodium reabsorption to changes in extracellular fluid volume or filtration fraction have been attributed to changes of hydrostatic and effective oncotic pressure ("physical factors") in the peritubular capillaries.[173] Tubular reabsorption of many solutes in addition to sodium is affected.[167] Uric acid is among the solutes that respond to changes in "physical factors."[170]

The pH of the fluid in the proximal tubule is approximately the same as that of plasma.[174] Since the $pK_{a1}$ of uric acid is 5.75, over 98 percent of this compound will be in the form of the monovalent urate ion in the proximal tubule. Excretion of uric acid is largely independent of changes of pH of urine,[175] but acidification is a distal tubular function, and would not be expected to affect proximal processes. In highly acidified distal tubular fluid, uric acid will be minimally ionized. One might anticipate that uric acid would then undergo reabsorption by nonionic diffusion. If so, the contribution to urate reabsorption is too small to be readily

**Table 21–1.** Conditions Associated with Hyperuricemia or Reduced Renal Uric Acid Clearance*

| Condition | $\Delta$ Serum Urate | $\Delta$ Uric Acid Clearance | $\Delta$ Extracellular Fluid Volume | $\Delta$ Filtration Fraction | Predicted $\Delta$ Proximal Tubular Sodium Reabsorption† |
|---|---|---|---|---|---|
| Salt restriction | ↑ | ↓ | ↓ | — | ↑ |
| Diuretic therapy without salt replacement | ↑ | ↓ | ↓ | — | ↑ |
| Diabetes insipidus | ↑ | ↓ | ↓ | ↑ | ↑ |
| Hypertension | ↑ | ↓ | — | ↑ | ↑ |
| Angiotensin infusion (without increased lactate or ketones) | — | ↓ | — | ↑ | ↑ |
| Norepinephrine (without increased lactate or ketones) | — | ↓ | — | ↑ | ↑ |

*From Holmes, E. W., et al.: Kidney Int. 2:115, 1972. Reproduced with permission.
†Proximal tubular sodium reabsorption was not evaluated directly in the reported studies; the changes listed represent a prediction from the observed changes in extracellular fluid volume and filtration fraction.

detected, for unlike other weak organic acids, the overall process of uric acid reabsorption does not follow principles of nonionic diffusion.[159]

**Secretion of Uric Acid.** The first evidence for uric acid secretion in man was published in 1950, when Praetorius and Kirk[176] reported the case of a young man with a plasma urate concentration of less than 0.6 mg per 100 ml, and a urate/inulin clearance ratio of 1.46. Subsequently, Gutman and coworkers[148] achieved urate/inulin clearance ratios as high as 1.23 in normal subjects following urate loading, mannitol diuresis, and large doses of probenecid. Each of these studies indicated net tubular secretion of urate in man under these special conditions. The biphasic effects of salicylate upon uric acid excretion were interpreted as representing inhibition of urate secretion with urate retention at low salicylate doses plus inhibition of urate reabsorption with urate diuresis at higher salicylate doses.[177] More recently Diamond and colleagues[178] have suggested that this apparent paradoxical effect of salicylate on uric acid excretion is due to inhibition of reabsorption by salicylate itself with inhibition of secretion due to a metabolite, salicylurate. Irrespective of the mechanism, bidirectional transport of uric acid is apparent.

The site within the nephron of man where uric acid secretion occurs is not definitely established. In the only study of this process in man, the proximal nephron transported uric acid from plasma to tubular fluid but the distal nephron was unable to do so.[179]

In animals in which net secretion occurs, urate moves into the proximal lumen against an electrical potential difference. Thus, the process qualifies as an active transport mechanism. In animals in which net movement of urate is reabsorptive, secretory flux of urate normally proceeds in the direction of a favorable concentration gradient. However, the process can be inhibited by certain chemicals[151,152,180,181] and possesses specificity; it cannot therefore represent simple diffusion. Weiner and Fanelli[159] have evidence that the mechanism is capable of transport against a gradient and is therefore active. In the chimpanzee,[182] the mercurial diuretic mersalyl is sufficiently uricosuric to unmask net secretion of urate. These results suggest a model involving two oppositely oriented active transport systems in the proximal tubule.

Although a number of authors have expressed the view that urate is secreted by the same mechanism responsible for the secretion of other organic anions, e.g., p-aminohippurate (PAH),[151,183] there is reason to consider an alternative hypothesis—namely, that urate and PAH are secreted by different transport systems. Two types of observation support this concept. In the reptile, transport of PAH and urate is not strictly coextensive along the nephron. In the chimpanzee[164,165] and man,[184] pyrazinoate reduces urate excretion to very low levels at concentrations that do not influence clearance or $T_m$ of PAH.

A number of organic acids will inhibit uric acid excretion in animals and man. These include lactate,[185,186]

**Table 21–2.** Conditions Associated with Reduction in Serum Urate Levels*

| Condition | $\Delta$ Serum Urate | $\Delta$ Uric Acid Clearance | $\Delta$ Extracellular Fluid Volume | $\Delta$ Filtration Fraction | Predicted $\Delta$ Proximal Tubular Sodium Reabsorption |
|---|---|---|---|---|---|
| Salt | ↓ | ↑ | ↑ | — | ↓ |
| Diuretic therapy with salt replacement | ↓ | ↑ | ↑ | — | ↓ |
| Inappropriate secretion of ADH | ↓ | ↑ | ↑ | — | ↓ |
| Pregnancy (early) | ↓ | ↑ | ↑ | — | ↓ |

*From Holmes, E. W., et al.: Kidney Int. 2:115, 1972. Reproduced with permission.

β-hydroxybutyrate,[187] acetoacetate,[187] and branched-chain keto acids.[188] These effects have been interpreted as representing inhibition of tubular secretion of urate,[177,189] for which there is evidence in micropuncture studies.[190]

**Postsecretory Reabsorption.** A number of observations have proved difficult to accommodate within the model of filtration, early proximal reabsorption, and later proximal secretion. In patients with Wilson's disease[191] or Hodgkin's disease,[192] and hypouricemia associated with raised renal urate clearance values, pyrazinamide suppresses the hyperuricosuria. In both chimpanzee[146] and man[134,193] the uricosuric response to probenecid is virtually abolished by pretreatment with pyrazinamide or pyrazinoate. Finally, the uricosuric responses to intravenous chlorothiazide[134] or volume expansion with hypertonic sodium chloride[194] are substantially diminished by pretreatment with pyrazinamide. If these effects were to be interpreted within the three-component model, one would need to conclude that the renal tubular dysfunctions of Wilson's and Hodgkin's diseases, and the administration of probenecid, chlorothiazide, and saline, resulted in enhanced tubular secretion of urate which was suppressible by pyrazinamide.

In 1973, Steele and Boner,[193] Steele,[195] and Diamond and Paolino[196] proposed a more tenable model to account for these observations, in which extensive postsecretory reabsorption of urate was postulated. In this model the effects of pyrazinamide are explained in terms of reduced secretory delivery to the late reabsorptive sites. The location of the postsecretory reabsorptive process could be coextensive with the secretory mechanism, or separate and distal to it, or both. Fanelli and Weiner have attempted to demonstrate that the observations upon which this model is based are consistent with coextensive secretion and reabsorption.[197] The latter possibilities are supported in some animals by evidence for urate reabsorption beyond the proximal tubule, as cited above. A patient with renal urate wasting, presumably on the basis of a defect in postsecretory reabsorption, has now been described.[198] Additionally, in two kindreds with familial hyperuricemia due to diminished renal clearance of urate it was proposed that the defect was due to increased postsecretory reabsorption.[199] Thus postsecretory reabsorption may be more important than previously recognized.

**Quantitative Estimates of Reabsorption and Secretion.** The existence of bidirectional uric acid transport in man is certain from the evidence cited above. However, the relative contributions of tubular reabsorption and tubular secretion have been difficult to ascertain. In man mean urate/inulin (or creatinine) ratios of 1.23 to 1.46 have been observed in unusual situations[148,176] In the chimpanzee a ratio of 1.78 was observed following administration of mersalyl.[159] These figures provide minimal estimates of unidirectional urate secretion, for there is no evidence in any of these studies that urate reabsorption was reduced to zero or that secretion was unimpaired by the drugs or procedures employed. The data suggest that secretion may be of the same order of magnitude as filtration, and therefore, that reabsorption may be very much greater than might be deduced from control clearance periods.

**Additional Factors Controlling Renal Clearance of Uric Acid in Normal Subjects. Urine Flow.** In 1940, Brochner-Mortensen[200] observed that uric acid excretion and clearance were increased at high rates of urine flow in man. He reported an augmentation limit of 2 ml per minute, above which further increases of rates of urine flow did not affect uric acid clearance. Others have reported that uric acid excretion in dogs is also dependent on the rate of urine flow.[144,150]

More recently, Diamond and colleagues[201] found that uric acid excretion increased from 290 to 410 μg per minute as urine flow increased from 2.7 to 6.4 ml per minute in response to oral and intravenous fluid loading in man. The effects of flow may be difficult to distinguish from those of osmotic diuresis.[202] Nevertheless, both the basal uric acid excretion and the increment accompanying diuresis were greatly reduced by pyrazinamide. Diamond and Meisel[203] suggest that the uricosuria of water diuresis can be attributed to diminished postsecretory reabsorption of urate, perhaps in the collecting duct.

*Estrogens.* The serum urate concentration is relatively low in children; increases in males and to a lesser extent also in females at puberty; and in females increases again at the menopause. Changes in renal urate clearance are at least partly responsible. Wolfson and colleagues[204] and Scott and Pollard[205] observed that the mean clearance of uric acid was 2.3 and 1.2 ml per minute higher in females than in males. Nicholls and associates[206] found that exogenous estrogens produced a significant increase in mean $C^{urate}$ values from 6.3 to 9.1 ml per minute in 22 transsexual males.

*Surgery.* Snaith and Scott[207] observed an increase in the excretion of uric acid, and in the urinary uric acid-to-creatinine ratio, in 10 patients undergoing abdominal surgery. Little or no change in serum urate concentration occurred. Factors such as anesthetics, increased endogenous steroids, intravenous fluids, intestinal manipulation, and vagotomy were suggested as possibly affecting urate clearance. The only patient not exhibiting a postoperative increase in uric acid excretion was one of two who did not have a vagotomy.

*Autonomic Nervous System.* In 1937, Grabfield[208] noted that the uricosuric effect of cincophen depended on an intact renal nerve supply in the dog. Denervation increased the renal clearance of uric acid to values attained with cincophen in the intact dog. Cincophen had no additional uricosuric effect in the denervated dog. The effects of cincophen were blocked by ergotamine but not by atropine. Excretion of allantoin, which is cleared by glomerular filtration without subsequent tubular reabsorption, was unchanged by denervation.

Postlethwaite and colleagues[209] noted that several anticholinergic agents increased renal clearance of uric acid in some subjects. One interpretation is that the parasympathetic nervous system plays a role in controlling the renal excretion of uric acid, perhaps through an effect on peritubular blood flow.

## Physical Properties of Uric Acid

**Ionization and Salt Formation.** The weakly acidic nature of uric acid is due to ionization of hydrogen atoms at position 9 ($pK_a = 5.75$) and position 3 ($pK_a = 10.3$).[210] The hydrogen atoms at positions 1 and 7 do not ionize significantly. The ionized forms of uric acid readily form salts such as mono- and disodium or potassium urates. In extracellular fluids in which sodium is the principal cation, about 98 percent of uric acid is in the form of the monosodium salt at pH 7.4. When the solubility limits of body fluids are exceeded, the crystals that occur in the synovial fluid or the tophi of gouty patients are composed of monosodium urate monohydrate.

**Solubility in Water.** Monosodium urate is soluble in water to the extent of 120 mg per 100 ml, compared with the much more limited solubility of uric acid in water of only 6.5 mg per 100 ml.[210] The solubility product of monosodium urate is $4.9 \times 10^{-5}$. Based on this value, aqueous solutions having the sodium content of serum, 0.13 M, are saturated with urate at 6.4 mg per 100 ml at 37° C.[210] Allen and colleagues[211] and Loeb[212] have found that urate solubility in solutions of 140 mEq per liter sodium content is markedly temperature dependent, with a two-fold drop in solubility between 37 and 25° C (Table 21-3). Wilcox and colleagues[213] have carefully reinvestigated the solubility of uric acid and monosodium urate, and have found that both are dependent on pH; with increasing pH uric acid is more soluble, whereas monosodium urate is less. The solubility of monosodium urate is dependent on sodium concentration and ionic strength as well. No stoichiometric relationship between urate and sodium (or potassium) exists. Binding of monovalent cations is a complex function of crystal shape, ion concentration, time, pH, and ion competition.[214]

**Solubility in Plasma.** The solubility of urate in plasma is somewhat greater than the saturation value in aqueous solutions of 0.13 M sodium. Actual determinations of solubility of monosodium urate in human plasma (or serum) indicate that saturation occurs at concentrations of about 7 mg per 100 ml.[215,216] Considerably higher concentrations of monosodium urate in plasma can be achieved in supersaturated solutions. Concentrations approaching 400 mg per 100 ml can be obtained by dissolving free uric acid in serum at 38° C.[215] These solutions are unstable, and monosodium urate readily precipitates out. At somewhat lower concentrations of 100 to 200 mg per 100 ml the solution may remain in a stable supersaturated state for longer periods of time, and no crystallization may occur for 24 hours or more, or until a seed crystal of monosodium urate is added. Stable supersaturated solutions of monosodium urate ranging up to 40 to 90 mg per 100 ml have been observed in patients with leukemia or lymphoma following aggressive therapy with cytotoxic drugs in the absence of allopurinol therapy.[217,218] The factors responsible for enhanced urate solubility in such patients are not clear, and may include both the natural tendency for urate to form stable supersaturated solutions and an increase in plasma of substances capable of solubilizing urate.[219] However, even at these remarkable plasma concentrations, all urate is digestible by uricase.[217]

The physicochemical state of urate in plasma has been a controversial subject for decades. Some early investigators claimed substantial binding of urate to nondiffusible elements of plasma,[220] whereas others concluded that all urate was in true solution because it was readily ultrafilterable[221] and dialyzable.[222] Even studies of urate localization following filter paper electrophoresis of serum yielded conflicting data in different laboratories.[223] In one laboratory a careful study of urate binding[225] disclosed no more than 4 to 5 percent of urate bound to plasma protein, a figure agreeing with results of earlier studies in vitro using equilibrium dialysis,[222] as well as with more recent studies in vivo.[226] These studies confirm that the binding of uric acid to plasma proteins at 37° C is small and probably of little physiological significance.

**Solubility in Urine.** As the urine is acidified along the renal tubule a portion of urinary urate is converted to uric acid. The solubility of uric acid in aqueous solutions is substantially less than that of urate. At pH 5 urine is saturated with uric acid at 15 mg per 100 ml, whereas at pH 7 urine will accommodate 158 to 200 mg per 100 ml in solution.[210,216] The limited solubility of uric acid in urine of pH 5 is of particular significance in patients with gout, many of whom display a tendency toward excretion of unusually acidic urine.

At any pH value human urine will dissolve more urate than can be carried in water. The solubilizing effects of urine have been attributed to urea,[227] proteins, and a mucopolysaccharide that resembles the Tamm-Horsfall mucopolysaccharide.[228,229] It was initially anticipated

**Table 21-3.** Solubility of Urate Ion ($U^-$) as a Function of Temperature in the Presence of 140 mM $Na^+$*

| Temperature (°C) | Maximal Equilibrium Concentration of $U^-$ in the Presence of 140 mM $Na^+$ (mg/100 ml) |
|---|---|
| 37 | 6.8 |
| 35 | 6.0 |
| 30 | 4.5 |
| 25 | 3.3 |
| 20 | 2.5 |
| 15 | 1.8 |
| 10 | 1.2 |

*From Loeb, J. N.: Arthritis Rheum. 8:1123, 1965. Reproduced by permission.

that habitual uric acid stone formers would show deficits of this mucopolysaccharide, but this could not be demonstrated.[229]

**Crystalline Forms.** Monosodium urate occurs as a monohydrate and forms crystals that are needle- or bar-shaped in a monoclinic or triclinic system. When rapidly crystallized from pure solutions, the crystals are very fine and appear amorphous.

Free uric acid crystallizes from pure solutions in an orthorhombic system, forming rhombic plates. Crystals formed in urine incorporate pigments and exist in a variety of crystalline forms. Tissue deposits are composed of monosodium urate monohydrate, and urinary stones largely of uric acid.[230,231] Both urate and uric acid crystals show strong negative birefringence when viewed under polarized light. With the use of a red compensator, urate cyrstals are yellow when oriented in parallel with the axis of polarization, and blue when perpendicular (see Chapter 38). These features permit ready identification of urate cyrstals in synovial fluid, leukocytes, or tissue deposits, and thus constitute an important diagnostic aid.[232,233]

The clinical features of gout and related disorders are reviewed in Chapter 86.

## References


1. Scheele, K.W.: Examen chemicum calculi urinarii. Opuscula 2:73, 1776.
2. Wollaston, W.H.: On gouty and urinary concretions. Philos. Trans. R. Soc. Lond. 87:386, 1797.
3. Garrod, A.B.: Observations on certain pathological conditions of the blood and urine in gout, rheumatism and Bright's disease. Trans. M-Chir. Soc. Edinburgh 31:83, 1848.
4. Freudweiler, M.: Experimentelle Untersuchungen über das Wesen der Gichtknoten. Deutsch. Arch. Klin. Med. 63:266, 1899.
5. Shemin, D., and Rittenberg, D.: On the utilization of glycine for uric acid synthesis in man. J. Biol. Chem. 167:875, 1947.
6. Buchanan, J.M., Sonne, J.C., and Delluva, A.M.: Biologic precursors of uric acid. II. The role of lactate, glycine, and carbon dioxide as precursors of the carbon chain and nitrogen atom 7 of uric acid. J. Biol. Chem. 173:81, 1948.
7. Karlson, J.L., and Barker, H.A.: Biosynthesis of uric acid labeled with radioactive carbon. J. Biol. Chem. 177:597, 1949.
8. Sonne, J.C., Buchanan, J.M., and Delluva, A.M.: Biological precursors of uric acid. I. The role of lactate, acetate and formate in synthesis of the ureido groups of uric acid. J. Biol. Chem. 173:69, 1948.
9. Heinrich, M.R., and Wilson, D.W.: Biosynthesis of nucleic acid components studied with $C^{14}$. I. Purines and pyrimidines in the rat. J. Biol. Chem. 186:447, 1950.
10. Sonn, J.C., Lin, I., and Buchanan, J.M.: Biosynthesis of the purines. IX. Precursors of the nitrogen atoms of the purine ring. J. Biol. Chem. 220:369, 1956.
11. Levenberg, B., Hartman, S.C., and Buchanan, J.M.: Biosynthesis of the purines. X. Further studies in vitro on the metabolic origin of nitrogen atoms 1 and 3 of the purine ring. J. Biol. Chem. 220:379, 1956.
12. Goldthwait, D.A., Peabody, R.A., and Greenberg, G.R.: On the mechanism of synthesis of glycinamide ribotide and its formyl derivative. J. Biol. Chem. 221:569, 1956.
13. Hartman, S.C., and Buchanan, J.M.: Biosynthesis of the purines. XXI. 5-phosphoribosylpyrophosphate-amidotransferase. J. Biol. Chem. 233: 451, 1958.
14. Flaks, J.G., Erwin, M.J., and Buchanan, J.M.: Biosynthesis of the purines. XVI. The synthesis of adenosine 5'-phosphate and 5'-amino-4-imidazolecarboxamide ribotide by a nucleotide pyrophosphorylase. J. Biol. Chem. 228:201, 1957.
15. Lukens, L.N., and Herrington, K.A.: Enzymic synthesis and properties of 6-mercaptopurine ribotide. Biochim. Biophys. Acta 24:432, 1957.
16. Kornberg, A., Lieberman, I., and Simms, E.S.: Enzymatic synthesis and properties of 5-phosphoribosylpyrophosphate. J. Biol. Chem. 215:389, 1955.
17. Remy, C.N., Remy, W.T., and Buchanan, J.M.: Biosynthesis of the purines. VIII. Enzymatic synthesis and utilization of 5-phosphoribosylprophosphate. J. Biol. Chem. 217:855, 1955.
18. Switzer, R.L.: Regulation and mechanism of phosphoribosylpyrophosphate synthetase. I. Purification and properties of the enzyme from *Salmonella typhimurium.* J. Biol. Chem. 244:2854, 1959.
19. Fox, I.H., and Kelley, W.N.: Human phosphoribosylpyrophosphate synthetase: Kinetic mechanism and endproduct inhibition. J. Biol. Chem. 247:2126, 1972.
20. Goldthwait, D.A.: 5-Phosphoribosylamine, a precursor of glycinamide ribotide. J. Biol. Chem. 222:1051, 1956.
21. Feldman, R.I., and Taylor, M.W.: Purine mutants of mammalian cell lines. II. Identification of a phosphoribosylpyrophosphate amidotransferase deficient mutant of Chinese hamster lung cells. Biochem. Genet. 13:227, 1975.
22. Holmes, E.W., King, G.L., Leyva, A., and Singer, S.C.: A purine auxotroph deficient in phosphoribosylpyrophosphate amidotransferase and phosphoribosylpyrophosphate amidotransferase activities with normal activity of ribose-5-phosphate aminotransferase, Proc. Natl. Acad. Sci. (Wash.) 73:2458, 1976.
23. Oates, D.C., and Patterson, D.: Biochemical genetics of Chinese hamster cell mutants with deviant pruine metabolism: Characterization of Chinese hamster call mutants defective in phosphoribosylpyrophosphate amidotransferase and phosphoribosylglycinamide sythetase and an examination of alternatives to the first step of purine biosynthesis. Somatic Cell Genet. 3:561, 1977.
24. McCarvus, E., Fahey, D., Sauer, D., and Rowe, P.B.: De novo purine synthesis in human lymphocytes: Partial co-purification of the enzymes and some properties of the pathway. J. Biol. Chem. 258:1851, 1983.
25. Harman, S.C., Levenberg, B., and Buchanan, J.M.: Biosynthesis of the purines. XI. Structure, enzymatic synthesis, and metabolism of glycinamide ribotide and (α-N-formyl) glycinamide ribotide. J. Biol. Chem. 221:1057. 1956.
26. Hartman, S.C., and Buchanan, J.M.: Biosynthesis of the purines. XXII. 2-Amino-N-ribosylacetamide-5'-phosphate kinosynthetase. J. Biol. Chem. 223:456, 1958.
27. Nierlich, D.P., and Magasanik, B.: Phosphoribosylglycinamide synthetase of *Aerobacter aerogenes.* J. Biol. Chem. 240:366, 1965.
28. Warren, L., and Buchanan, J.M.: Biosynthesis of the purines. XIX. 2-Amino-N-ribosylacetamide-5'-phosphate (glycinamide ribotide) transformylase. J. Biol. Chem. 229:613, 1957.
29. Warren, L., Flaks, J.G., and Buchanan, J.M.: Biosynthesis of the purines. XX. Integration of enzymatic transformylation reactions. J. Biol. Chem. 229:627, 1957.
30. Smith, G.K., Mueller, W.T., Slieker, L.J., et al.: Direct transfer of one-carbon units in the transformylations of de novo purine biosynthesis. Biochemistry 21:2870, 1982.
31. Mizobuchi, K., and Buchanan, J.M.: Biosynthesis of the purines: Purification and properties of formylglycinamide ribonucleotide amidotransferase from chicken liver. J. Biol. Chem. 243:4842, 1968.
32. Mizobuchi, K., and Buchanan, J.M.: Biosynthesis of the purines: Isolation and characterization of formylglycinamide ribonucleotide amidotransferase-glutamyl complex. J. Biol. Chem. 243:4853, 1968.
33. Mizobuchi, K., Kenyon, G.L., and Buchanan, J.M.: Binding of formylglylcinamide ribonucleotide and adenosine triphosphate to formylglycinamide ribonucleotide amidotransferase. J. Biol. Chem. 243:4863, 1968.
34. Levenberg, B., and Buchanan, J.M.: Biosynthesis of the purines. XII. Structure enzymatic, synthesis, and metabolism of 5-aminoimidazole ribotide. J. Biol. Chem. 224:1005, 1957.
35. Lukens, L.N., and Buchanan, J.B.: Further intermediates in the biosynthesis of inosinic acid de novo. J. Am. Chem. Soc. 79:1511, 1957.
36. Flaks, J.G., Warren, L., and Buchanan, J.M.: Biosynthesis of the purines. XVII. Further studies of the inosinic acid transformylase system. J. Biol. Chem. 228:215, 1957.
37. Flaks, J.G., Erwin, M.J., and Buchanan, J.M.: Biosynthesis of the purines. XVII. 5-Amino-1-ribosyl-4-imidazole-carboxamide 5'-phosphate transformylase and inosinicase. J. Biol. Chem. 229:603, 1957.
38. Smith, G.K., Mueller, W.T., Wasserman, G.F., et al.: Characterization of the enzyme complex involving the folate-requiring enzymes of de novo purine biosynthesis. Biochemistry 19:4313, 1980.
39. Carter, C.E., and Cohen, C.H.: The preparation and properties of adenylosuccinase and adenylosuccinic acid. J. Biol. Chem. 222:17, 1956.
40. Joklik, W.K.: Adenine succinic acid and adenylosuccinic acid from mammalian liver: Isolation and identification. Biochem. J. 66:333, 1957.
41. Lieberman, I.: Enzymatic synthesis of adenosine 5'-phosphate from inosine 5'-phosphate. J. Biol. Chem. 223:327, 1956.
42. Wyngaarden, J.B., and Greenland, R.A.: The inhibition of succinoadenylate kinosynthetase of *Escherichia coli* by adenosine and guanosine 5'-monophosphates. J. Biol. Chem. 238:1054, 1963.
43. Murihead, K.M., and Bishop, S.H.: Purification of adenylosuccinate synthetase from rabbit skeletal muscle. J. Biol. Chem. 249:459, 1974.
44. Van Der Weyden, M., and Kelley, W.N.: Human adenylosuccinate synthetase. Partial purification kinetic and regulatory properties of the enzyme. J. Biol. Chem. 249:7282, 1974.
45. Magasanik, B., Moyed, H.S., and Gehring, L.B.: Enzymes essential for

the biosynthesis of nucleic acid guanine: Iinosine-5′-phosphate dehydrogenase of *Aerobacter aerogenes.* J. Biol. Chem. 226:339, 1957.
46. Lagerkvist, U.: Biosynthesis of guanosine 5′-phosphate. I. Xanthosine 5′-phosphate as an intermediate. J. Biol. Chem. 223:138, 1958.
47. Mager, J., and Magasanik, B.: Guanosine 5′-phosphate reductase and its role in the interconversion of purine nucleotides. J. Biol. Chem. 235:1474, 1960.
48. Lagerkvist, U.: Biosynthesis of guanosine 5′-phosphate. II. Amination of xanthosine 5′-phosphate by purified enzymes from pigeon liver. J. Biol. Chem. 223:143, 1958.
49. Abrams, R., and Bentley, M.: Biosynthesis of nucleic acid purines. III. Guanosine 5′-phosphate formation from xanthosine 5′-phosphate and L -glutamine. Arch. Biochem. 79:91, 1959.
50. Lieberman, I., Kornberg, A., and Simms, E.S.: Enzymatic synthesis of pyrimidine nucleotides: Orotidine-5′-phosphate and uridine-5′phosphate J. Biol. Chem. 215:403, 1955.
51. Preiss, J., and Handler, P.: Enzymatic synthesis of nicotinamide mononucleotide. J. Biol. Chem. 255:759, 1957.
52. Hori, M., and Henderson, J.F.: Kinetic studies of adenine phosphoribosyltransferase. J. Biol. Chem. 241:3304, 1966.
53. Henderson, J.F., Brox, L.W., Kelley, W.N., et al.: Kinetic studies of hypoxanthine-guanine phosphoribosyltransferase. J. Biol. Chem. 243:2514, 1968.
54. Kelley, W.N., Rosenbloom, F.M., Henderson, J.F., et al.: Xanthine phosphoribosyltransferase in man. Relationship of hypoxanthine-guanine phosphoribosyltransferase. Biochem. Biophys. Res. Commun. 28:340, 1967.
55. McCollister, R.J., Gilbert, W.R., Jr., Ashton, D.M. et al.: Pseudofeedback inhibition of purine synthesis by 6-mercaptopurine ribonucleotide and other purine analogues. J. Biol. Chem. 239:1560, 1964.
56. Krenitsky, T.A., Papaioannou, R., and Elion, G.B.: Human hypoxanthine phosphoribosyltransferase. J. Biol. Chem. 244:1263, 1969.
57. Kelley, W.N., Greene, M.L., Rosenbloom, F.M., et al.: Hypoxanthine-guanine phosphoribosyltransferase deficiency in gout. Ann. Intern. Med. 70:155, 1969.
58. Henderson, J.K.: Kinetic properties of hypoxanthine-guanine and adenine phosphoribosyltransferases. Fed. Proc. 27:1053, 1968.
59. Friedkin, N., and Kalckar, H.: Nucleoside phosphorylases. *In* Boyer, P.D., Lardy, H., and Myrback, K. (eds.): The Enzymes, Vol. 5. New York, Academic Press, 1961, p. 237.
60. Krenitsky, T.A., Elion, G.B., Henderson, A.M., et al.: Inhibition of human purine nucleoside phosphorylase: Studies with intact erythrocytes and the purified enzyme. J. Biol. Chem. 243:2876, 1968.
61. Zimmerman, T.P., Gersten, N., and Miech, R.P.: Adenine and adenosine metabolism in liver. Proc. Am. Assoc. Cancer Res. 11:87, 1970.
62. Sandberg, A.A., Lee, G.R., Cartwright, G.E., et al.: Purine nucleoside phosphorylase activity of blood. I. Erythrocytes. J. Clin. Invest. 34:1823, 1955.
63. Pierre, K.J., and LePage, G.A.: Formation of inosine-5′-monophosphate by a kinase in cell-free extracts of Ehrlich ascites cells in vitro. Proc. Soc. Exp. Biol. Med. 127:342, 1968.
64. Wada, Y., Arakawa, T., and Koizumi, K.: Lesch-Nyhan syndrome: Autopsy findings and in vitro study of incorporation of $^{14}C$-8-inosine into uric acid, guanosine-monophosphate and adenosine-monophosphate in the liver. Tohoku J. Exp. Med. 95:253, 1968.
65. Friedman, T., Seegmiller, J.E., and Subak-Sharpe, J.H.: Evidence against the existence of guanosine and inosine kinases in human fibroblasts in tissue culture. Exp. Cell Res. 56:425, 1969.
66. Gudas, L.J., Allman, B., Cohen, A., and Martin, D.W.: Deoxyguanosine toxicity in a mouse T lymphoma: Relationship to purine nucleoside phosphorylase-associated immune dysfunction. Cell 14:531, 1978.
67. Capputo, R.: The enzymatic synthesis of adenylic acid. Adenosine kinase. J. Biol. Chem. 189:801, 1951.
68. Kornberg, A., and Pricer, W.E., Jr.: Enzymatic phosphorylation of adenosine and 2,6-diaminopurine riboside, J. Biol. Chem. 193:481, 1951.
69. Palella, T.D., Andres, C.M., and Fox, I.H.: Human placental adenosine kinase: Kinetic mechanism and inhibition. J. Biol. Chem. 255:5264, 1980.
70. Streeter, D.G., Simon, L.N., Robins, R.K., and Miller, J.P.: The phosphorylation of ribavirin by deoxyadenosine kinase from rat liver. Differentiation between adenosine and deoxyadenosine kinase. Biochemistry 13:4543, 1974.
71. Krygier, V., and Momparler, L.: Mammalian deoxynucleoside kinase. II. Deoxyadenosine kinase: Purification and properties. J. Biol. Chem. 246:2745, 1971.
72. Krygier, V., and Momparler, L.: Mammalian deoxynucleoside kinase. III. Deoxyadenosine kinase. Inhibition by nucleotides and kinetic studies. J. Biol. Chem. 246:2752, 1971.
73. Carson, D.A., Kaye, J., and Seegmiller, J.E.: Lymphospecific toxicity in adenosine deaminase deficiency and purine nucleoside phosphorylase deficiency: Possible role of nucleoside kinase(s). Proc. Natl. Acad. Sci. USA 74:5677, 1977.
74. Fox, I.H., and Kelley, W.N.: The role of adenosine and 2′-deoxyadenosine in mammalian cells. Ann. Rev. Biochem. 47:566, 1978.
75. Coleman, M.A., Donofrio, J., Hutton, J.J., and Hahn, L.: Identification and quantitation of adenine deoxynucleotides in erythrocytes of a patient with adenosine deaminase deficiency and severe combined immunodeficiency. J. Biol. Chem. 253:1619, 1978.
76. Cohen, A., Hirschhorn, R., Horowitz, S.D., Rubinstein, A., Polmar, S.H., Hong, R., and Martin, D.W.: Deoxyadenosine triphosphate as a potentially toxic metabolite in adenosine deaminase deficiency. Proc. Natl. Acad. Sci. USA 75:472, 1978.
77. Martin, W.D., Gudas, L.J., Cohen A., and Ammann, A.J.: The common molecular mechanism of immune dysfunction in the inherited deficiencies of adenosine deaminase and purine nucleoside phosphorylase. Clin. Res. 26:501A, 1978.
78. Heppel, L.A., and Rabinowitz, J.C.: Enzymology of nucleic acids, purines, and pyrimidines. Ann. Rev. Biochem. 27:613, 1958.
79. Heppel, L.A., and Hilmoe, R.J.: Purification and properties of 5′-nucleotidase. J. Biol. Chem. 188:665, 1951.
80. Schmidt, G.: Nucleases and enzymes attacking nucleic acid components. *In* Chargaff, E., and Davidson J.N. (eds.): The Nucleic Acids, Vol. 1. New York, Academic Press, 1955, p. 555.
81. Johnson, S.M., Asherson, G.L., Watts, R.W.E., et al.: Lymphocyte purine 5′-nucleotidase deficiency in primary hypogammaglobulinemia. Lancet 1:168, 1977.
82. Edwards, N.L., Magilavy, D.B., Cassidy, J.T., and Fox, I.H.: Lymphocyte ecto-5′-nucleotidase deficiency in agammaglobulinemia. Science 201:628, 1978.
83. Edwards, N.L., Recker, D., Montredi, J., et al.: Regulation of purine metabolism by plasma membrane and cytoplasmic 5′-nucleotidoses. Am. J. Physiol. 243:C270, 1982.
84. Nikiforuk, G., and Colowick, S.P.: The purification and properties of 5-adenylic acid deaminase from muscle. J. Biol. Chem. 219:119, 1956.
85. Kalckar, H.M.: Differential spectrophotometry of purine compounds by means of specific enzymes. III. Studies of the enzymes of purine metabolism. J. Biol. Chem. 167:461, 1947.
86. Bergmann, F., and Dikstein, S.: Studies on uric acid and related compounds. III. Observations on the specificity of mammalian xanthine oxidase. J. Biol. Chem. 223:765, 1956.
87. Engleman, K., Watts, R.W.E., Klinenberg, J.R., et al.: Clinical physiological and biochemical studies of a patient with xanthinuria and pheochromocytoma. Am. J. Med. 37:839, 1964.
88. Watts, R.W.E., Watts, J.E.M., and Seegmiller, J.E.: Xanthine oxidase activity in human tissues and its inhibition by allopurinol (4-hydropyrazolo(3,4-d)pyrimidine). J. Lab. Clin. Med. 66:688, 1965.
89. Segal, S., and Wyngaarden, J.B.: Plasma glutamine and oxypurine content in patients with gout. Proc. Soc. Exp. Biol. Med. 88:342, 1955.
90. Jorgensen, S., and Poulsen, H.E.: Enzymatic determination of hypoxanthine and xanthine in human plasma and urine. Acta Pharmacol. 11:223, 1955.
91. Hoffman, G.T., Rottino, A., and Albaum, H.G.: Levels of nucleotide in the blood during shock. Science 114:188, 1951.
92. Nierlich, D.P., and Magasanik, B.: Regulation of purine ribonucleotide synthesis by end product inhibition: The effect of adenine and guanine ribonucleotides on the 5′-phos-phoribosylpyrophosphate amidotransferase of *Aerobacter aerogenes.* J. Biol. Chem. 240:358, 1965.
93. Wyngaarden, J.B., and Ashton, D.M.: The regulation of activity of phosphoribosylpyrophosphate amidotransferase by purine ribonucleotides: A potential feedback control of purine biosynthesis. J. Biol. Chem. 234:1492, 1959.
94. Caskey, C.T., Ashton, D.M., and Wyngaarden, J.B.: The enzymology of feedback inhibition of glutamine phosphoribosylpyrophosphate amidotransferase by purine ribonucleotides. J. Biol. Chem. 239:2570, 1964.
95. Henderson, J.F.: Feedback inhibition of purine biosynthesis in ascites tumor cells. J. Biol. Chem. 237:2631, 1962.
96. Holmes, E.W., McDonald, J.A., McCord, M.M., Wyngaarden, J.B., and Kelley, W.N.: Human glutamine phosphoribosylpyrophosphate amidotransferase: Kinetic and regulatory properties. J. Biol. Chem. 248:144, 1973.
97. Wood, A.W., and Seegmiller, J.E.: Properties of 5-phosphoribosyl-1-pyrophosphate amidotransferase from human lymphoblasts. J. Biol. Chem. 248:138, 1973.
98. Holmes, E.W., Wyngaarden, J.B., and Kelley, W.N.: Human glutamine phosphoribosylpyrophosphate amidotransferase: Two molecular forms interconvertible by purine ribonucleotide and phosphoribosylpyrophosphate. J. Biol. Chem. 248:6035, 1973.
99. Howard, W.J., and Appel, S.I.: Control of purine biosynthesis: FGAR amidotransferase (abstr.) Clin. Res. 16:344, 1968.
100. Kelley, W.N., Fox, I.H., and Wyngaarden, J.B.: Regulation of purine biosynthesis in cultured human cells. I. Effects of orotic acid. Biochim. Biophys. Acta 215:512, 1970.
101. Kelley, W.N., Fox, I.H., and Wyngaarden, J.B.: Essential role of phos-

phoribosylpyrophosphate (PRPP) in regulation of purine biosynthesis in cultured human fibroblasts. Clin. Res. 18:457, 1970.
102. Fox, I.H., and Kelley, W.N.: Phosphoribosylpyrophosphate in man: Biochemical and clinical significance. Ann. Intern. Med. 74:424, 1971.
103. Kelley, W.N., Greene, M.L., Fox, I.H., Rosenbloom, F.M., Levy, R.H., and Seegmiller, J.E.: Effects of orotic acid on purine and lipoprotein metabolism in man. Metabolism 19:1025, 1970.
104. Henderson, J.F., and Khoo, M.K.Y.: Synthesis of 5-phosphoribosyl-1-pyrophosphate from glucose in Ehrlich ascites tumor cells in vitro. J. Biol. Chem. 240:2349, 1965.
105. Lindsay, R.H., Cash, A.G., and Hill, J.B.: TSH stimulation of orotic acid conversion of pyrimidine nucleotides and RNA in bovine thyroid. Endocrinology 84:534, 1969.
106. Rottman, F., and Guarino, A.J.: The inhibition of phosphoribosylpyrophosphate amidotransferase activity by cordecepin monophosphate. Biochim. Biophys. Acta 89:465, 1964.
107. Nagy, M.: Regulation of biosynthesis of purine nucleotides in *Schizosaccharomyces pombe.* I. Properties of the phosphoribosylpyrophosphate glutamine amidotransferase of the wild strain and of a mutant desensitized towards feedback modifiers. Biochim. Biophys. Acta 198:471, 1970.
108. Rowe, P.B., Coleman, M.D., and Wyngaarden, J.B.: Glutamine phosphoribosylpyrophosphate amidotransferase: Catalytic and conformational heterogeneity of the pigeon liver enzyme. Biochemistry 9:1498, 1970.
109. King G., Meade, J.C., Borinous, C.G. and Holmes, E.W.: Demonstration of ammonia utilization for purine biosynthesis by the intact cell and characterization of the enzymatic activity catalyzing this reaction. Metabolism 28:348, 1979.
110. Itakura, M., Sabina, R., Heald, P. and Holmes, E.W.: Basis for the control of purine biosynthesis by purine ribonucleotides. J. Clin. Invest, 67:994, 1981.
111. Magasanik, B., and Karibian, D.: Purine nucleotide cycles and their metabolic role. J. Biol. Chem. 235:2672, 1960.
112. Holmes, E.W., Pehlke, D.M., and Kelley, W.N.: The role of human inosinic acid dehydrogenase in the control of purine biosynthesis de novo. Biochim. Biophys. Acta 364:209, 1974.
113. Ullman, B., Wormstead, M.A., Cohen, M.B., and Martin, D.W.: Purine oversecretion in cultured murine lymphoma cells deficient in adenylosuccinate synthetase: Genetic model for hyperuricemia and gout. Proc. Natl. Acad. Sci. (USA) 79:2673, 1982.
114. Wyngaarden, J.B., and Kelley, W.N.: Gout and Hyperuricemia. New York, Grune & Stratton, 1976.
115. Fox, I.H.: Metabolic basis for disorders of purine nucleotide degradation. Metabolism 30:616, 1981.
116. Bagnora, A.S., and Hershfield, M.S.: Mechanism of deoxyadenosine-induced catabolism of adenine ribonucleotides in adenosine deaminase-inhibited human T lymphoblastoid cells.: Proc. Natl. Acad. Sci. (USA) 79:2673, 1982.
117. Griebsch, A., and Zollner, N.: Effect of ribonucleotides given orally on uric acid production in man. *In* Sperling, O., de Vries, A., and Wygaarden, J.B. (eds.): Purine Metabolism in Man, Vol. 41B. New York, Plenum Press, 1974, p. 443.
118. Zollner, N.: Influence of various purines on uric acid metabolism. Bibl. "Nutr. Diet." No. 19. Basel, Karger, 1973, pp.34–43.
119. Folin, O., Berglund, H., and Derick, C.: The uric acid problem: An experimental study on animals and man, including gouty subjects. J. Biol. Chem. 60:361, 1924.
120. Koehler, A.E.: Uric acid excretion. J. Biol. Chem. 60:721, 1924.
121. Buzard, J., Bishop, C., and Talbott, J.H.: Recovery in humans of intravenously injected isotopic uric acid. J. Biol. Chem. 196:179, 1952.
122. Wyngaarden, J.B.: The effect of phenylbutazone on uric acid metabolism in two normal subjects. J. Clin. Invest. 34:256, 1955.
123. Sorensen, L.B.: The elimination of uric acid in man studies by means of $C^{14}$-labeled uric acid. Scand. J. Clin. Lab. Invest. 12(Suppl. 54):1, 1960.
124. Spilman, E.L.: Uric acid synthesis in the nongouty and gouty human (abstr.) Fed. Proc. 13:302, 1954.
125. Benedict, J.D., Forsham, P.H., and Stetten, DeW., Jr.: The metabolism of uric acid in the normal and gouty human studied with the aid of isotopic uric acid. J. Biol. Chem. 18:183, 1949.
126. Sorensen, L.B.: Degradation of uric acid in man. Metabolism 8:687, 1959.
127. Scott, J.T., Holloway, V.P., Glass, H.I., et al.: Studies of uric acid pool size and turnover rate. Ann. Rheum. Dis. 28:366, 1969.
128. Seegmiller, J.D., Grayzel, A.I., Laster, L., et al.: Uric acid production in gout. J. Clin. Invest. 40:1304, 1961.
129. Kelley, W.N., Rosenbloom, F.M., Seegmiller, J.E., et al.: Excessive production of uric acid in type I glycogen storage disease. J. Pediat. 72:488, 1968.
130. Lucke, H.: Das Harnsaureproblem and seine klinische Bedeutung. Ergeb. Inn. Med. Kinderheilk. 44:499, 1932.
131. Kurti, L.: Untersuchungen uber den Harnsaurestoffwechsel bei Nierenkranken. Z. Klin. Med. 122:585, 1932.
132. Wyngaarden, J.B.: Gout. *In* Stanbury, J.B., Wyngaarden, J.B., and Fredrickson, D.S., (eds.): The Metabolic Basis of Inherited Disease. New York, McGraw-Hill Book Company, 1960, p. 728.
133. Berliner, R.W., Hilton, J.G., Yu, T-F., et al.: The renal mechanism for urate excretion in man. J. Clin. Invest. 29:296, 1950.
134. Gutman, W.B., and Yu, T-F.: A three-component system for regulation of renal excretion of urate in man. Trans. Assoc. Am. Physicians 74:353, 1961.
135. Shannon, J.A.: The excretion of uric acid by the chicken. J. Cell. Comp. Physiol. 11:135, 1938.
136. Dantzler, W.H.: Comparison of renal tubular transport of urate and PAH in water snakes. Evidence for differences in mechanisms and sites of transport. Comp. Biochem. Physiol. 34:609, 1970.
137. Dantzler, W.H.: Characteristics of urate transport by isolated perfused snake proximal renal tubules. Am. J. Physiol. 224:445, 1973.
138. Mudge, G.H., McAlary, B., and Berndt, W.O.: Renal transport of uric acid in the guinea pig. Am. J. Physiol. 214:875, 1969.
139. Kessler, R.H., Hierholzer, K., and Gurd, R.S.: Localization of urate transport in the nephron of mongrel and Dalmatian dog kidney. Am. J. Physiol. 197:601, 1959.
140. Fanelli, G.M., Bohn, D., and Russo, H.F.: Renal clearance of uric acid in non-human primates. Comp. Biochem. Physiol. 33:459, 1970.
141. Boudry, J.F.: Mécanismes de l'excretion d'acide urique chez le rat. Pfluegers Arch. Ges. Physiol. 328:265, 1971.
142. Boudry, J.F.: Effet d'inhibiteurs des transports transtubulaires sur l'execretion renale d'acide urique chez le rat. Pfluegers Arch. Ges. Physiol. 328:279, 1971.
143. Berger, L., Yu, T-F., and Gutman, A.B.: Effects of drugs that alter uric acid excretion in man on uric acid clearance in the chicken. Am. J. Physiol. 198:575, 1960.
144. Yu, T-F., Berger, L., Kupfer, S., et al.: Tubular secretion of urate in the dog. Am. J. Physiol. 199:1199, 1960.
145. Fanelli, G.M., Jr., Bohn, D., and Stafford, S.: Functional characteristics of renal urate transport in the *Cebus* monkey. Am. J. Physiol. 218:627, 1970.
146. Fanelli, G.M., Jr., Bohn, D.L., and Reilly, S.S.: Renal urate transport in the chimpanzee. Am. J. Physiol. 220:613, 1971.
147. Greger, R., Lang, F., and Deetjen, P.: Handling of uric acid by the rat kidney. I. Microanalysis of uric acid in proximal tubular fluid. Eur. J. Physiol. 324:279, 1971.
148. Gutman, A.B., Yu, T-F., and Berger, L.: Tubular secretion of urate in man. J. Clin. Invest. 39:1778, 1959.
149. Lathem, W., Davis, B.B., and Rodnan, G.P.: Renal tubular secretion of uric acid in the mongrel dog. Am. J. Physiol. 199:9, 1960.
150. Mudge, G.H., Cucchi, J., Platts, M., et al.: Renal excretion of uric acid in the dog. Am. J. Physiol. 215:404, 1968.
151. Nolan, R.P., and Foulkes, E.C.: Studies on renal urate secretion in the dog. J. Pharmacol. Exp. Ther. 179:429, 1971.
152. Zins, G.R., and Weiner, I.M.: Bidirectional urate transport limited to the proximal tubule in dogs. Am. J. Physiol. 215:411, 1968.
153. Blanchard, K.C., Maroske, D., May, D.G., et al.: Uricosuric potency of 2-substituted analogs of probenecid. J. Pharmacol. Exp. Ther. 180:397, 1972.
154. Fannelli, G.M., Jr., Bohn., D.L., and Reilly, S.S.: Renal effects of uricosuric agents in the *Cebus* monkey. J. Pharmacol. Exp. Ther. 175:259, 1970.
155. Fanelli, G.M., Jr., Bohn, D.L., and Reilly, S.S.: Renal effects of uricosuric agents in the chimpanzee. J. Pharmacol. Exp. Ther. 177:591, 1971.
156. Fanelli, G.M., Jr., Bohn, D.L., Reilly, S.S., et al.: Renal excretion and uricosuric properties of halofenate, a hypolipidemic uricosuric agent, in the chimpanzee. J. Pharmacol. Exp. Ther. 180:377, 1972.
157. Bordley, J., III, and Richards, A.N.: Quantitative studies of the composition of glomerular urine. VIII. The concentration of uric acid in glomerular urine of snakes and frogs, determined by an ultramicro adaption of Folin's method. J. Biol. Chem. 101:193, 1933.
158. Roch-Ramel, F., and Weiner, I.M.: Excretion of urate by the kidneys of *Cebus* monkeys: A micropuncture study. Am. J. Physiol. 224:1369, 1973.
159. Weiner, I.M., and Fanelli, G.M., Jr.: Renal urate excretion in animal models. Nephron 14:33, 1975.
160. Berndt, W.O., and Beechwood, E.C.: Influence of inorganic electrolytes and ouabain on uric acid transport. Am. J. Physiol. 208:642, 1965.
161. Weinman, E.J., Senekjian, H.O., Sansom, S.C. et al.: Evidence for active and passive urate transport in the rate proximal tubule. Am. J. Physiol. 240:F90, 1981.
162. Sansom, S.C., Senekjian, H.O., Knight, T.F. et al.: Determination of the apparent transport constants for urate absorption in the rate proximal tubule. Am. J. Physiol. 240:F406, 1981.
163. Senekjian, H.O., Knight, T.F., and Weinman, E.J.: Urate transport by the isolated perfused $S_2$ segment of the rabbit. Am. J. Physiol. 240:F530, 1981.
164. Fanelli, G.M., Jr., and Weiner, I.M.: Pyrazinoate excretion in the chim-

panzee. Relation to urate disposition and the actions of uricosuric drugs. J. Clin. Invest. 52:1946, 1973.
165. Robson, A.M., Srivastave, P.L., and Bricker, N.S.: The influence of saline loading on renal glucose reabsorption in the rat. J. Clin. Invest. 47:329, 1968.
166. Bricker, N.S.: On the pathogenesis of the uremic state: The "trade-off hypothesis." N. Engl. J. Med. 286:1093, 1972.
167. Cannon, P.J., Svahn, D.S., and DeMartini, F.E.: The influence of hypertonic saline infusion upon the fractional reabsorption of urate and other ions in normal and hypertensive man. Circulation 41:97, 1970.
168. Kurtzman, N.A.: Regulation of renal bicarbonate reabsorption by extracellular volume. J. Clin. Invest. 49:586, 1970.
169. Holmes, E.W., Kelley W.N., and Wyngaarden, J.B.: The kidney and uric acid excretion in man. Kidney Int. 2:115, 1972.
170. Weinman, E.J., Eknoyan, G., and Suki, W.N.: The influence of the extracellular fluid volume on the tubular reabsorption of uric acid. J. Clin. Invest. 55:283, 1975.
171. Kahn, T., Mohammed, G., and Stein R.M.: Alterations in renal tubular sodium and water reabsorption in chronic renal disease in man. Kidney Int. 2:164, 1972.
172. Steele, T.H., and Rieselbach, R.E.: The contributions of residual nephrons within the chronically diseased kidney to urate homeostasis in man. Am. J. Med. 43:876, 1967.
173. Martino J.A., and Earley, L.E.: Demonstration of a role of physical factors as determinants of the nutriuretic response to volume expansion. J. Clin. Invest. 56:1963, 1967.
174. Malnic, G., Aires, M.M., and Giebisch, G.: Micropuncture study of renal tubular hydrogen ion transport in the rat. Am. J. Physiol. 222:147, 1972.
175. Weiner, I.M., and Mudge, F.H.: Renal tubular mechanisms for excretion of organic acids and bases. Am. J. Med. 36:743, 1964.
176. Praetorius, D., and Kirk, J.E.: Hypouricemia: With evidence for tubular elimination of uric acid. J. Lab. Clin. Med. 35:865, 1950.
177. Yu, T-F., and Gutman, A.B.: Study of the paradoxical effects of salicylate in low, intermediate and high dosage on the renal mechanisms for excretion of urate in man. J. Clin. Invest. 38:1298, 1959.
178. Diamond, H.S., Sterba, G., Jayadeven, K., and Meisel, A.D.: On the mechanism of the paradoxical effect of salicylate on urate excretion. *In* Ropado, A. Watts, R.W.E., and DeBruyn, C.H.M. (eds.): Third International Symposium on Purine Metabolism in Man. New York, Plenum Publishing Co., 1980, pp. 221–225.
179. Podevin, R., Ardaillou, R., Paillar, F., et al.: Étude chez l'homme de la cinétique d'apparition dans l'urine de l'acide urique-2$^{14}$C. Nephron 5:134, 1968.
180. Nechay, B.R., and Nechay, L.: Effects of probenecid, sodium lactate, 2, 4-dinitrophenol, and pyrazinamide on renal secretion of uric acid in chickens. J. Pharmacol. Exp. Ther. 126:291, 1959.
181. Moller, J.V.: The tubular site of urate transport in the rabbit kidney and the effect of probenecid on urate secretion. Acta Pharmacol. Toxicol. 23:329, 1965.
182. Fanelli, G.M., Jr., Bohn, D.L., Reilly, S.S., et al.: Effects of mercurial diuretics on renal transport of urate in the chimpanzee. Am. J. Physiol. 224:985, 1973.
183. Moller, J.V.: The relation between secretion of urate and p-aminohippurate in the rabbit kidney. J. Physiol. 192:505, 1967.
184. Boner, G., Steele, T.H.: Relationship of urate and p-aminohippurate secretion in man. Am. J. Physiol. 225:100, 1973.
185. Yu, T-F., Sirota, J.H., Berger, L., et al.: Effect of sodium lactate infusion on urate clearance in man. Proc. Soc. Exp. Biol. Med. 96:809, 1957.
186. Reem, G.H., and Vanamee, P.: Effect of sodium lactate on urate clearance in the Dalmatian and mongrel dog. Am. J. Physiol. 207:113, 1964.
187. Goldfinger, S., Klinenberg, J.R., and Seegmiller, J.E.: Renal retention of uric acid induced by infusion of betahydroxybutyrate and acetoacetate. N. Engl. J. Med. 272:351, 1965.
188. Schulman, J.F., Lustberg, T.J., Kennedy, J.L., et al.: A new variant of maple syrup urine disease (branched chain ketoaciduria). Clinical and biochemical evaluation. Am. J. Med. 49:118, 1970.
189. Gutman, A.B., and Yu, T-F.: Renal mechanisms for regulation of uric acid excretion, with special reference to normal and gouty man. Semin. Arthritis Rheum. 2:1, 1972.
190. Greger, R., Lang, R., and Deetjen, P.: Handling of uric acid by the rat kidney. II. Microperfusion studies on bidirectional transport of uric acid in the proximal tubule. Eur. J. Physiol. 335:257, 1972.
191. Wilson, D.M., and Goldstein, N.P.: Renal urate excretion in patients with Wilson's disease. Kidney Int. 4:331, 1973.
192. Bennet, J.S., Bond, J., Singer, I., et al.: Hypouricemia in Hodgkin's disease. Ann. Intern. Med. 76:751, 1972.
193. Steele, T.H., and Boner G.: Origins of the uricosuric response, J. Clin. Invest. 52:1368, 1973.
194. Manuel, M.A., and Steele, T.H.: Pyrazinamide suppression of the uricosuric response to sodium chloride infusion. J. Lab. Clin. Med. 83:417, 1974.
195. Steele, T.H.: Urate secretion in man: The pyrazinamide suppression test. Ann. Intern. Med. 79:734, 1973.
196. Diamond, H.S., and Paolino, J.S.: Evidence for a postsecretory reabsorptive site for uric acid in man. J. Clin. Invest. 52:1491, 1973.
197. Fanelli, G.M. Jr., and Werner, I.M.: Urate excretion: Drug interactions. J. Pharmacol. Exp. Therap. 210:186, 1979.
198. Tofuku, Y., Mitsuhiko, K. and Takeda, R.: Hypouricemia due to renal urate wasting. Nephron 30:39, 1982.
199. Stapleton, F.B., Nyhan, W.L., et al.: Renal pathogenesis of familial hyperuricemia: Studies in two kindreds. Pediatr. Res. 15:1447, 1981.
200. Brochner-Mortensen, K.: The uric acid content in blood and urine in health and disease. Medicine 19:161, 1940.
201. Diamond, H.S., Lazarus, R., Kaplan, E., et al.: Effect of urine flow rate on uric acid excretion in man. Arthritis Rheum. 15:338, 1972.
202. Skeith, M.D., Healy, L.A., and Cutler, R.E.: Urate excretion during mannitol and glucose diuresis. J. Lab. Clin. Med. 70:213, 1967.
203. Diamond, H.S., and Meisel, A.D.: Collecting duct urate reabsorption in man. Program abstracts, 39th Annual Meeting of American Rheumatism Association, Section of Arthritis Foundation, New Orleans, June 4–6, 1977.
204. Wolfson, W.Q., Hunt, H.D., Levine, R., et al.: The transport and excretion or uric acid in man; sex difference and urate metabolism with note on clinical and laboratory findings in gouty women. J. Clin. Endocrinol. Metab. 9:749, 1949.
205. Scott, J.T., and Pollard, A.D.: Uric acid excretion in the relatives of patients with gout. Ann. Rheum. Dis. 29:397, 1970.
206. Nicholls, A., Snaith, M.L., and Scott, J.T.: Effect of oestrogen therapy on plasma and urinary levels of uric acid. Br. Med. J. 1:449, 1973.
207. Snaith, M.L., and Scott, J.T.: Uric acid excretion and surgery. Ann. Rheum. Dis. 31:162, 1972.
208. Grabfield, B.P.: A pharmacologic study of the mechanism of gout. Ann. Intern. Med. 11:651, 1937.
209. Postlethwaite, A.E., Ramsdell, C.M., and Kelley, W.N.: Uricosuric effect of an anticholinergic agent in hyperuricemic subjects. Arch. Intern. Med. 134:270, 1974.
210. Peters, J.P., and Van Slyke, K.K.: Quantitative Clinical Chemistry, Vol. 1. 2nd ed. Baltimore, Williams & Wilkins Company, 1946, p. 937.
211. Allen, D.J., Milosovich, G., and Mattocks, A.M.: Inhibition of monosodium urate crystal growth. Arthritis Rheum. 8:1123, 1965.
212. Loeb, J.N.: The influence of temperature on the solubility of monosodium urate. Arthritis Rheum. 15:189, 1972.
213. Wilcox, W.R., Khalaf, A., Weinberger, A., et al.: The solubility of uric acid and monosodium urate. Med. Biol. Eng. 10:522, 1972.
214. McNabb, R.A., and McNabb, F.M.A.: Physiological chemistry of uric acid: solubility, colloid and ion-binding properties. Comp. Biochem. Physiol. 67A:27, 1980.
215. Seegmiller, J.E.: The acute attack of gouty arthritis. Arthritis Rheum. 8:714, 1965.
216. Klinenberg, J.R., Goldfinger, S.E., and Seegmiller, J.E.: The effectiveness of a xanthine oxidase inhibitor on the treatment of gout. Ann. Intern. Med. 62:639, 1965.
217. Gold, G.L., and Fritz, R.D.: Hyperuricemia associated with the treatment of acute leukemia. Ann. Intern. Med. 47:428, 1957.
218. Kjellstrand, C.M., Campbell, D.C., III, von Hartizseh, B., et al.: Hyperuricemic acute renal failure. Arch. Intern. Med. 133:349, 1974.
219. Alvsaker, J.O.: Uric acid in human plasma. V. Isolation and identification of plasma proteins interacting with urate. Scand. J. Clin. Lab. Invest. 18:228, 1966.
220. Adlersberg, D., Grishman, E., and Sobotka, H.: Uric acid partition in gout and hepatic disease. Arch. Intern. Med. 70:101, 1942.
221. Yu, T-F., and Gutman, A.B.: Ultrafilterability of plasma urate in man. Proc. Soc. Exp. Biol. Med. 84:21, 1953.
222. Wyngaarden, J.B.: Uric acid. *In* Piersol, G.M. (ed.): The Cyclopedia of Medicine, Surgery. Specialties. Philadelphia, F.A. Davis Company, 1955, p. 341.
223. Morris, J.E.: The transport of uric acid in serum. Am. J. Med. Sci. 235:43, 1958.
224. Villa, L., Robecchi, A., and Ballabio, C.B.: Physiopathology clinical manifestations, and treatment of gout. Part I. Physiopathology and pathogenesis. Ann. Rheum. Dis. 17:9, 1958.
225. Kovarsky, J., Holmes, E., and Kelley, W.N.: Absence of significant urate binding to human serum proteins. J. Lab. Clin. Med. 93:85, 1979.
226. Postlethwaite, A.E., Gutman, R.A., and Kelley, W.N.: Salicylate-mediated increase in urate removal during hemodialysis: Evidence of urate binding to protein in vivo. Metabolism 23:771, 1974.
227. Medes, G.: Solubility of calcium oxalate and uric acid in solutions of urea. Proc. Soc. Exp. Biol. Med. 30:281, 1932.
228. Atsmon, A., De Vries, A., and Frank, M.: Uric Acid Lithiasis. Amsterdam, Elsevier, 1963, p. 63.
229. Sperling, O., De Vries, A., and Kedem, O.: Studies on the etiology of uric acid lithiasis. IV. Urinary non-dialyzable substances in idiopathic uric acid lithiasis. J. Urol. 94:286, 1965.

230. Prien, E.L., and Prien, E.L., Jr.: Composition and structure of urinary stone. Am. J. Med. 45:654, 1968.
231. Howell, R.R., Eanes, E.D., and Seegmiller, J.E.: X-ray diffraction studies on the tophaceous deposits in gout. Arthritis Rheum. 6:97, 1963.
232. McCarty, D.J., Jr., and Hollander, J.L.: Identification of urate crystals in gouty synovial fluid. Ann. Intern. Med. 54:452, 1961.
233. Zwaifler, N.J., and Pekin, T.J.: Significance of urate crystals in synovial fluids. Arch Intern. Med. 111:99, 1963.
234. Seegmiller, J.E., Rosenbloom, F.M., and Kelley, W.N.: An enzyme defect associated with a sex-linked human neurological disorder and excessive purine synthesis. Science 155:1682, 1967.
235. Kelley, W.N., Holmes, E.W., and van der Weyden, M.B.: Current concepts on the regulation of purine biosynthesis de novo in man. Arthritis Rheum. 18:673, 1975.

# Chapter 22
# Nutrition and Rheumatic Diseases

*Edward A. Mascioli and George L. Blackburn*

## INTRODUCTION

Nutrition is an important science interacting with rheumatic diseases. A major focus of nutrition deals with nutrient intake to preserve and sustain immune competence and the host's defenses to inflammatory insults. In turn, a primary role of the body's response to inflammation involves the breakdown of various body tissues to effect a redistribution of nutrients, which, if unrecognized and untreated, can lead to nutritional deficiencies and malnutrition and subsequent morbidity and mortality.

Given the recent development of techniques for measuring the metabolic response to inflammation, the development of biometric parameters to assess nutritional deficiencies, and the development of new nutritional support techniques, it is possible to utilize the science of nutrition in the treatment of rheumatic diseases. Nutritional intervention in the area of rheumatology need not be restricted to correcting deficiencies that result from anorexia and catabolism associated with rheumatologic conditions; very promising work is being done in treating and palliating the inflammatory response to rheumatologic disease by altering the inflammatory response, particularly by way of dietary manipulation to alter ptostaglandin production and by the administration of vitamin A derivatives.

The main focus of this chapter will be the indications and requirements for nutritional support of the rheumatology patient. Included is a discussion of various metabolic changes that occur with inflammation. Changes in specific nutrients will also be addressed as well as the therapeutic trials designed to restore the normal concentrations of nutrients following inflammation and arthritis. Direct potential therapeutic interventions involving nutritional therapies will be addressed, followed by the role of overnutrition (obesity) and its impact on rheumatologic diseases.

## NUTRITION ASSESSMENT AND BODY COMPOSITION

The various tissues of the body are not equivalent with regard to their water, fat, protein and mineral composition. More importantly, in starvation, with and without added inflammation, there are significant differences as to what tissues account for the observed weight losses. After adaptation to simple starvation, adipose tissue accounts for most (90 percent) of the loss. However, an inflammatory disease process coupled with anorexia will lead to proportionately much greater losses of lean tissues (50 percent), those metabolically functioning tissues containing most of the body's protein, such as skeletal muscle (Fig. 22–1). Before making a diagnosis of malnutrition, a nutritional assessment is performed with normal body composition in mind (Table 22–1).

The patient's weight for height is a traditional approach. Standardized tables have been assembled (Table 22–2) to help gauge the adequacy of the patient's weight. A more discerning parameter is the recent involuntary loss of weight. As a rule, loss of 5 percent of the patient's normal weight over a 1-month interval or loss of 10

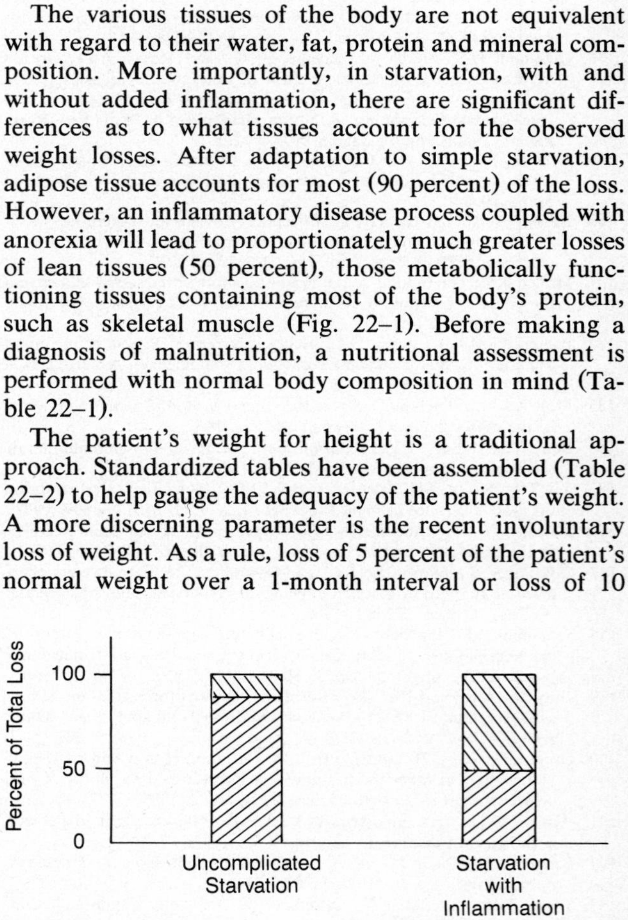


**Figure 22–1.** Differential tissue losses from uncomplicated starvation and starvation associated with inflammation. ▨ denotes fat loss; ▧ denotes lean tissue loss.

**Table 22–1.** The Major Parameters for the Assessment of Nutritional Status, With Corresponding Components of Body Composition*

| Body Composition | Percent Body Weight | Protein (kg) (Total = 13 kg) | Nutritional Assessment |
|---|---|---|---|
| Fat (160,000 calories) | 20 | | Triceps skin fold (mm) |
| Skin; Skeleton | 9 | 6.3 | |
| Extracellular Fluid | 20 | 0.7 | |
| Viscera | 11 | 1.5 | Albumin, total lymphocyte count, delayed hypersensitivity |
| Skeletal muscle | 40 | 4.5 | Arm muscle circumference (cm) |

*Adapted from Moore, F.D., and Brannan, M.F.: Manual of Surgical Nutrition. American College of Surgeons. Philadelphia, W. B. Saunders Co., 1975.

percent over a 6-month interval should be considered significant weight loss. As discussed later, this weight loss puts the patient at increased risk.

Other parameters that are conveniently available in the clinical setting and have utility in a nutritional assessment include serum albumin, the total lymphocyte count, and cutaneous delayed hypersensitivity to common antigens. The serum albumin level, although affected by several factors, is a very good indicator of the adequacy of the patient's protein intake over the prior 2 to 3 weeks. In addition, it serves as an indicator of the degree of catabolic stress the patient is undergoing. The total lymphocyte count, obtained as the product of the total white blood cell count and the percentage of lymphocytes, often mirrors albumin as an indicator of malnutrition. Measuring the patient's ability to mount appropriate type 4 immunologic reactions to intradermally placed skin test antigens is a third approach to assessing the impact malnutrition has had on the functioning tissues of the body. These parameters are needed to diagnose the type of malnutrition and are powerful predictors of subsequent morbidity and mortality.

Protein-calorie malnutrition (PCM) has two major subcategories. Marasmus is defined by the patient's weight being less than 80 percent of the standard for his height. Marasmus is usually the result of starvation or semistarvation without added catabolic stresses such as infections, surgery, or inflammatory processes. Since most of this weight loss has been at the expense of adipose tissue, albumin, total lymphocyte count, and skin test reactivity are usually at normally expected values. Hypoalbuminemic malnutrition or adult kwashiorkor gives a reverse picture. Body weight for height is often at or above the standard. However, significant deficits in serum albumin, total lymphocyte count, and skin test reactivity are found. The albumin level is below 3 g/dl, the total lymphocyte count is less than 1200 per mm$^3$, and the patient fails to react to intradermally placed antigens such as *Candida,* mumps, or tetanus. Hypoalbuminemic malnutrition carries a higher mortality than does marasmus. The difference in pathogenesis of this form of malnutrition is the concomitant presence of a catabolic stress such as inflammation or infection.

There are other parameters that are utilized in the more complete nutritional assessment.[1] However, Seltzer[2-4] has popularized an abbreviated assessment consisting of serum albumin, total lymphocyte count, and involuntary weight loss of 10 pounds or more in the prior 6 months. This assessment was performed in surgical patients on admission to the hospital, and a 19-fold increase in mortality was found among the malnourished patients. How nutritional assessment can help to have an impact on the patient's course will become more evident after a discussion of protein-calorie malnutrition.

**Table 22–2.** Ideal Weight for Height

**Males**

| *Height (cm)* | *Weight (kg)* | *Height (cm)* | *Weight (kg)* | *Height (cm)* | *Weight (kg)* |
|---|---|---|---|---|---|
| 145 | 51.9 | 159 | 59.9 | 173 | 68.7 |
| 146 | 52.4 | 160 | 60.5 | 174 | 69.4 |
| 147 | 52.9 | 161 | 61.1 | 175 | 70.1 |
| 148 | 53.5 | 162 | 61.7 | 176 | 70.8 |
| 149 | 54.0 | 163 | 62.3 | 177 | 71.6 |
| 150 | 54.5 | 164 | 62.9 | 178 | 72.4 |
| 151 | 55.0 | 165 | 63.5 | 179 | 73.3 |
| 152 | 55.6 | 166 | 64.0 | 180 | 74.2 |
| 153 | 56.1 | 167 | 64.6 | 181 | 75.0 |
| 154 | 56.6 | 168 | 65.2 | 182 | 75.8 |
| 155 | 57.2 | 169 | 65.9 | 183 | 76.5 |
| 156 | 57.9 | 170 | 66.6 | 184 | 77.3 |
| 157 | 58.6 | 171 | 67.3 | 185 | 78.1 |
| 158 | 59.3 | 172 | 68.0 | 186 | 78.9 |

**Females**

| *Height (cm)* | *Weight (kg)* | *Height (cm)* | *Weight (kg)* | *Height (cm)* | *Weight (kg)* |
|---|---|---|---|---|---|
| 140 | 44.9 | 150 | 50.4 | 160 | 56.2 |
| 141 | 45.4 | 151 | 51.0 | 161 | 56.9 |
| 142 | 45.9 | 152 | 51.5 | 162 | 57.6 |
| 143 | 46.4 | 153 | 52.0 | 163 | 58.3 |
| 144 | 47.0 | 154 | 52.5 | 164 | 58.9 |
| 145 | 47.5 | 155 | 53.1 | 165 | 59.5 |
| 146 | 48.0 | 156 | 53.7 | 166 | 60.1 |
| 147 | 48.6 | 157 | 54.3 | 167 | 60.7 |
| 148 | 49.2 | 158 | 54.9 | 168 | 61.4 |
| 149 | 49.8 | 159 | 55.5 | 169 | 62.1 |

This table corrects the 1959 Metropolitan Standards to nude weight without shoe heels. Adapted from Jelliffe, D.B.: The Assessment of the Nutritional Status of the Community. Geneva, W.H.O., 1966.

## METABOLIC RESPONSE TO INFLAMMATION

With any systemic metabolic insult to the body, whether it be infection, trauma, surgery, or inflammatory process, there is a remarkably consistent and universal metabolic and hormonal response. Any stimulus leading to a sufficient amount of inflammatory activity involving white blood cells serves as the initiator of this process. Stimulated mononuclear phagocytes release a polypeptide, variously called leukocyte pyrogen (LP), interleukin 1(IL 1), or leukocyte endogenous mediator (LEM).[5] This polypeptide then acts on many tissues, causing fever, modulation of the immune response, and a redirection of tissue proteins (to name just a few). We shall concern ourselves with the metabolic and nutritional consequences of inflammation. The reader is referred to the earlier chapters of this text for more detail on the other processes present with inflammation.

Inflammatory arthritides, although not eliciting the same magnitude of a metabolic response as trauma or a burn, for example, can be nutritionally as detrimental because of their chronicity. Increased energy expenditure occurs early, in part to support a fever, and is supported by catecholamine-mediated lipolysis and glycogenolysis. Hyperglycemia, hypoinsulinemia, and high free fatty acid levels due to release from adipose tissue serve to increase the energy substrate availability for increased energy expenditure. This is termed the acute phase response to injury.[6] After the acute phase, lasting from 1 to 3 days, comes the adaptive phase. Since the inflammatory insult has persisted, other hormonal inputs occur. This phase is dominated by increased endogenous glucocorticosteroid secretion. This leads to hyperglycemia, hyperinsulinemia, and increased protein catabolism (especially in skeletal muscle), leading to protein breakdown. The increased amino acids exiting from skeletal muscle as well as connective tissue serve as precursors for new hepatic synthesis of the so-called acute phase reactants. Among these are fibrinogen, ceruloplasmin, $\alpha_1$-antitrypsin, and other plasma globulins.

The redistributed amino acids also serve as carbon skeletons in gluconeogenesis, which is augmented owing to the glucocorticoid effect. The consequently increased ureagenesis accounts for the excessive nitrogen loss seen in periods of catabolic stress. Exogenously supplied protein, either from the diet or given intravenously, is used much less efficiently for protein synthesis because of the enhanced gluconeogenesis. Therefore the patient's protein requirement, for the maintenance of a net protein balance, is increased. Convalescence can only begin after the inflammatory stimulus lessens sufficiently to allow glucocorticoid secretion to approach the normal diurnal pattern, thereby restoring protein utilization efficiency. The obvious inciting event is IL 1–mediated inflammation, but an understanding of the ensuing metabolic response can lead to more rational nutritional therapy until the inflammation is eliminated. An unfortunate accompaniment to this response is anorexia, serving to thwart the physician's attempts at nutritional management. Pragmatic approaches to solutions of this problem are discussed later in this chapter.

Several nutrients have been specifically investigated because of observed changes related directly or inversely to the activity of the underlying rheumatologic disease. Most of the work has been done in patients with rheumatoid arthritis, and most therapeutic interventions have been equivocal at best. This is perhaps explained by the changes being a consequence of the metabolic response to inflammation, rather than being etiologic in nature.

**Histidine.** Many studies have shown a decreased histidine concentration in the blood of patients with rheumatoid arthritis. Gerber[7] reviews these reports and documents statistically significant correlations with more conventional clinical parameters used to monitor disease activity. Direct correlations were found between hypohistidinemia and hematocrit and grip strength, whereas inverse correlations were found with erythrocyte sedimentation rate, duration of morning stiffness, walking time, rheumatoid factor, and the duration of arthritis. Other patients, defined only as a group without rheumatoid arthritis, had normal histidine levels. A subsequent report demonstrated that patients with rheumatoid arthritis normalized their serum histidine concentrations within 1 hour of an oral dose of histidine.[8] This implies that the defect is not due to a malabsorption disorder. Comparing relatives of patients with rheumatoid arthritis, Kirkham and co-workers showed that hypohistidinemia was an acquired feature of the disease and not predictive of risk. Histidine levels were followed in patients receiving drug therapy.[10,11] In spite of clinical improvement there were no changes in histidine levels after treatment with gold, prednisone, or hydroxychloroquine. However, coincident with clinical improvement, normalization of hypohistidinemia was seen following D-penicillamine therapy. This discrepancy further calls into question any role histidine could play in the pathogenesis of rheumatoid arthritis or as a form of therapy in this disorder. Gerber has proposed a mechanism for hypohistidinemia in the pathogenesis of rheumatoid arthritis,[12] but clinical evaluation is lacking.

**Iron.** It is well-known that a hypoferremic anemia (also known as the anemia of chronic disease) often accompanies active rheumatoid arthritis.[13] The anemia is also characterized by occasional hypochromia, a decrease in the total iron-binding capacity, a reduced ratio of iron to total iron-binding capacity, decreased marrow sideroblasts, and an increase in marrow reticuloendothelial iron. The anemia has been shown to have normal or even slightly increased erythropoiesis, increased ineffective erythropoiesis and a decreased mean red cell life span.[14] The shortened life span is due to some as yet unexplained hemolysis. The anemia is also due to some degree of failure of the marrow to respond sufficiently to the hemolysis. This may be related to inadequate release of iron from the reticuloendothelial cells.

It is very important to differentiate the anemia of chronic disease from that of iron deficiency. This is because the anemia of iron deficiency, unlike that of chronic disease, is responsive to iron administration. Establishing a firm diagnosis of iron deficiency anemia in the rheumatoid arthritis patient can be difficult. Because of the coexisting anemia of chronic disease, serum iron, total iron-binding capacity, the ratio of iron to total iron-binding capacity, and red blood cell indices are not specific. The serum ferritin level, normally low in iron deficiency (reflecting minimal or absent iron stores), rises with concomitant inflammation.[15] The lower end of the normal range is 12 $\mu$g per liter, but in patients with rheumatoid arthritis and no iron stores demonstrable on bone marrow biopsy, the mean value is 38 $\mu$g per liter.[16] This highlights the lack of sensitivity but enhanced specificity of a low serum ferritin in patients with rheumatoid arthritis. If the serum ferritin is normal or elevated, iron deficiency is not ruled out, since the ferritin may be spuriously elevated owing to inflammation. In this case, a bone marrow biopsy and Prussian blue staining for iron should be performed to directly assess iron stores.

**Zinc.** Serum zinc levels have been shown to be low in patients with rheumatoid arthritis.[17] They have also been shown to correlate inversely with osteoporosis associated with rheumatoid arthritis.[18] Balogh and colleagues found zinc levels to correlate directly with serum albumin and inversely with the erythrocyte sedimentation rate and serum globulins but not to correlate with joint tenderness.[19] Simkin argued that the changes in zinc levels were more than changes merely associated with the inflammation of rheumatoid arthritis.[20] He felt that oral supplementation with zinc, given its anti-inflammatory properties, would favorably affect the course of patients with rheumatoid arthritis. In a double-blind trial of 24 patients, positive results were seen in the treatment group for some clinical parameters but not in the erythrocyte sedimentation ratio or hematocrit. Kennedy, Bessent, and Reynolds divided 14 rheumatoid arthritis patients into two equal groups depending on their respective whole-body zinc amounts.[21] The half with the lowest zinc amounts were treated with zinc, while the other half received penicillamine. Neither group showed any statistically significant changes in clinical or laboratory parameters nor in whole-body zinc over the course of the 8-week trial. Despite large differences in whole-body zinc amounts between the two groups before the trial, there were no differences in severity of disease. Further negative evidence of a beneficial effect from zinc supplementation in rheumatoid arthritis came from Job and colleagues[22] and Mettingly and Mowat.[23] The trials lasted 4 and 6 months, respectively, and no statistically significant differences were detected in clinical or laboratory parameters between the treatment and placebo groups. In sum, the published reports to date relate changes in plasma zinc levels to the inflammation of rheumatoid arthritis and attribute no convincing etiologic nor therapeutic role to zinc.

**Copper.** It has been discovered that serum copper levels rise in patients with rheumatoid arthritis.[24] Since 90 percent of the serum copper is complexed to ceruloplasmin, an acute phase reactant protein, these levels rise as well in rheumatoid arthritis patients.[25] Direct correlations with disease activity, articular index, erythrocyte sedimentation rate, and antioxidant activity of the serum were found with serum copper and ceruloplasmin, whereas inverse correlations were found with serum iron and serum zinc.[26-28] In patients with severe disease, values twice normal can be found, a range similar to that seen with estrogen administration. Antirheumatic drugs that are associated with a lowering of copper levels include glucocorticosteroids, gold, and penicillamine. Because of ceruloplasmin's role as an antioxidant, it has been hypothesized to act as a free-radical scavenger in rheumatoid synovial effusions.[29] Other workers, however, have not found enhanced levels of ceruloplasmin in synovial fluid.[30] It must again be concluded that the changes observed in this nutrient, copper, are secondary to systemic inflammation and not nutritional aberrations.

## SURVEYS OF MALNUTRITION

For the practitioner unfamiliar with currently accepted nutritional standards, the prevalence of malnutrition among hospitalized patients will seem astounding. Many different surveys have been done by various groups, all with similar results. Bistrian and colleagues surveyed the entire surgical patient population of an urban municipal hospital on one day.[31] Using the anthropometric measures of triceps skin fold and arm muscle circumference and serum albumin levels, the prevalence rate for protein-calorie malnutrition was 50 percent. In a similar survey conducted among medical patients in the same hospital, a rate of protein-calorie malnutrition comparable to that found in the surgical patients was found.[32] Differences were more depletion on a calorie basis (less weight/height and smaller triceps skin folds) and less depletion on a protein basis (greater arm muscle circumference and greater serum albumin levels) among medical patients as compared with surgical patients. In surveys done on orthopedic patients specifically, similar results were obtained. Dreblow and colleagues found a prevalence of 48 percent among 82 consecutively admitted orthopedic patients.[33] McFarlane studied 65 consecutively admitted fractured hip patients to a community hospital.[34] Although the prevalence of protein-calorie malnutrition was not as great as in the studies cited above, it was still noteworthy. Over one third of the group was anergic to skin test antigens on admission and 20 percent of those initially positive became negative over 1 week after surgery. The only statistically significant difference between those patients who developed anergy and those who remained immunocompetent was age; most of the patients in the former group were older than 85 years. One third of the total series had measurements less than 85 percent of the standard for arm muscle circumference, whereas 10 percent were less than a comparable value for weight for height. This discrepancy probably reflects the age-associated decline in muscle mass with its replacement by adipose tissue.

Lom-Orta and colleagues reported on five patients

with systemic lupus erythematosus as well as concomitant, severe protein-calorie malnutrition.[35] They speculated that the origin of the observed hypocomplementemia in these patients may have been due to poor production rather than increased utilization. In work done with young women suffering from anorexia nervosa, multiple complement proteins of the alternate pathway were observed to rise from deficient to normal levels coincident with feeding.[36] This highlights the need to consider two possible causes for hypocomplementemia in the rheumatologic patient—decreased synthesis secondary to malnutrition as well as increased utilization due to an inflammatory process. In 24 patients with classic rheumatoid arthritis or rheumatoid spondylitis, Pettersson and colleagues showed either malnutrition or malabsorption or both in over one half of the cases.[37] Folic acid deficiency, abnormal D-xylose absorption tests, and intestinal amyloidosis demonstrated by biopsy were among their criteria. In 1963, Eising summarized much earlier literature concerning arthritis and nutrition and remarked on the equivocal nature of the studies taken as a whole.[38] The weights and dietary intakes of patients with rheumatoid arthritis and degenerative arthritis were also analyzed. The only statistically significant differences were in body weight and acidic residues of the respective diets. The rheumatoid arthritis patients were shown to average 10 pounds below their recommended weights, whereas the patients with degenerative arthritis averaged 15 pounds above their recommended weights. The above studies all support a finding of malnutrition among the rheumatologic patient to varying degrees. It is reasonable to ask ourselves what impact malnutrition has on the subsequent course of the patient.

**Malnutrition and Prognosis.** In studies done on general surgical patients, mortality during the hospital stay was directly related to the presence of protein-calorie malnutrition. Meakins and colleagues found a mortality rate of 74 percent among anergic patients, whereas for immunocompetent patients, mortality was only 5 percent.[39] In a similar study, albumin levels, transferrin levels, and immunocompetence were found to be the only statistically significant predictors of complications among 16 factors studied.[40]

Other nutritional and anthropometric measures as well as in vivo and in vitro immunologic tests did not reliably predict outcome. In a study of orthopedic patients, the patients with three abnormal nutritional markers had longer hospital stays than those without.[33] These reports all point to an etiologic role for malnutrition and complications. The primary complications are an increased incidence of infection or sepsis and poor wound healing.

**Nutritional Intervention.** Given the malnourished patient's increased risk for complications, work has been done to evaluate preoperative nutritional support in decreasing predicted risk. Three studies have recently shown quite striking benefits of total parenteral nutrition among malnourished patients facing surgery, chemotherapy, or radiation therapy.[41-43] Nutritional therapy was shown to effect a three- to sixfold reduction in morbidity and mortality.[41] Although no comparable trials have yet been published on rheumatologic patients not undergoing surgery, given our understanding of the metabolic response to a catabolic insult, we would expect a similar benefit of nutritional support in the rheumatologic patient, though perhaps not of the same magnitude because the insult is less. A potential mechanism through which this effect may occur is enhanced production of leukocyte endogenous mediator (LEM). As shown by Hoffman-Goetz and colleagues, production of LEM was impaired in leukocytes from malnourished patients but was restored after a period of nutritional support.[44] Conceivably the normalized production of LEM could be the route through which enhanced survival has been seen with nutritional support, by allowing the patient to optimally mobilize energy and protein stores to meet the catabolic, inflammatory insult. Whatever the mechanism, it is clear that full nutritional support is indicated wherever and whenever the physician encounters a malnourished patient.

## NUTRITIONAL REQUIREMENTS

Nearly 40 individual substances are required by adults for a healthy nutritional intake. We will discuss some of the requirements, but the reader is referred to other sources for more detailed discussions of the various nutrients required for an adequate diet.[45]

**Energy.** Many factors affect the energy requirement of the individual. Age, sex, physical activity, weight, and degree of systemic inflammation all interact to help determine energy needs. Some factors change, often on a daily basis. Nevertheless, estimates can and should be made so that proper amounts of calories can be given. The basal energy expenditure (BEE) is the amount of energy the patient would burn at rest, free of illness, in 24 hours. A reasonable estimate of the BEE for an individual patient can be made from the Harris-Benedict equation.[46] For men the kilocaloric requirement is estimated by the following:

$$\text{BEE} = 655 + 13.8 \times \text{Weight} + 5.0 \times \text{Height} - 6.8 \times \text{Age}$$

For women it is as follows:

$$\text{BEE} = 655 + 9.6 \times \text{Weight} + 1.8 \times \text{Height} - 4.7 \times \text{Age}$$

Weight is in kilograms, height is in centimeters, and age is in years.

For a patient for whom enteral intake is feasible, approximately 125 percent of their calculated BEE should be given if weight maintenance is the goal of nutritional therapy. If weight gain is needed, then 150 percent of the BEE should be ingested by the patient. Since energy sources delivered parenterally are utilized less efficiently, 175 percent of the BEE is needed for anabolism to occur by this route.[46] A quicker, less accurate method, but one which is certainly justifiable in the clinical situation, is to estimate the patient's caloric requirement using 25 to 30 kilocalories per kilogram of body weight. Since the figures are approximate, this approach gives an adequate estimate.

**Protein.** The Food and Nutrition Board set, as a safe estimate of protein requirements, a value of 0.8 gram protein per kilogram of body weight per day.[45] Owing to the enhanced gluconeogenesis occurring in the metabolic response to injury, greater amounts of protein than normal are oxidized. Therefore more protein should be ingested to keep the patient in a state of no net protein loss. Consequently the protein requirement should be based on a factor of 1.0 to 1.5 grams of dietary protein per kilogram of body weight per day. Given adequate energy intakes, this is sufficient to keep all but the most catabolic patients in nitrogen balance. For a reference 70-kg man, this is approximately 90 grams of protein per day, which is the amount in the typical American diet.

Additional nutrients, such as vitamins, minerals, and trace elements, are vitally important in a complete nutritional intake. Other than specific reference to a few nutrients in regard to rheumatologic diseases, no further mention of these nutrients will be made in this chapter. The interested reader is referred to other sources for further discussion.[45]

## NUTRITIONAL THERAPY APPROACHES

The start of any nutritional therapy depends on an accurate assessment of the nutritional status of the patient as well as the establishment of nutritional goals. If the patient is not depleted nutritionally or has normal levels of serum albumin and is immunocompetent, then maintenance of the nutritional state is indicated. However, if the patient has suffered recent weight loss, is anergic or has a low serum albumin level, and is facing an additional catabolic insult such as surgery, then full nutritional repletion is warranted. Elective surgery should be delayed, if possible, until immunocompetence is restored. This usually necessitates a week of nutritional intervention.

**Choice of Feeding Approach.** Significant advances have been made in methods of feeding patients. No longer is it justified to allow a patient to starve if voluntary oral intake is insufficient. Many products and techniques have become available, allowing the physician many means for the successful treatment of malnutrition.

Once the patient's nutritional status is assessed, therapeutic goals outlined, and nutritional requirements estimated, daily counts of the caloric and protein contents of the food ingested are made by a dietitian. If consistently below requirements, nutritional intervention is in order (Fig. 22–2). Oral supplements are first used in an attempt to reach calculated requirements. These are available in innumerable flavors and formulations and are "complete" nutritionally; that is, they contain protein, carbohydrate, fat, and micronutrients.[47] Other more specialized formulas exist and are used depending on the inadequacy of the patient's gastrointestinal tract or the presence of renal, hepatic, or cardiac failure. The invaluable aid of a dietitian is essential in situations such as these.

If the patient is unable or unwilling to eat sufficient

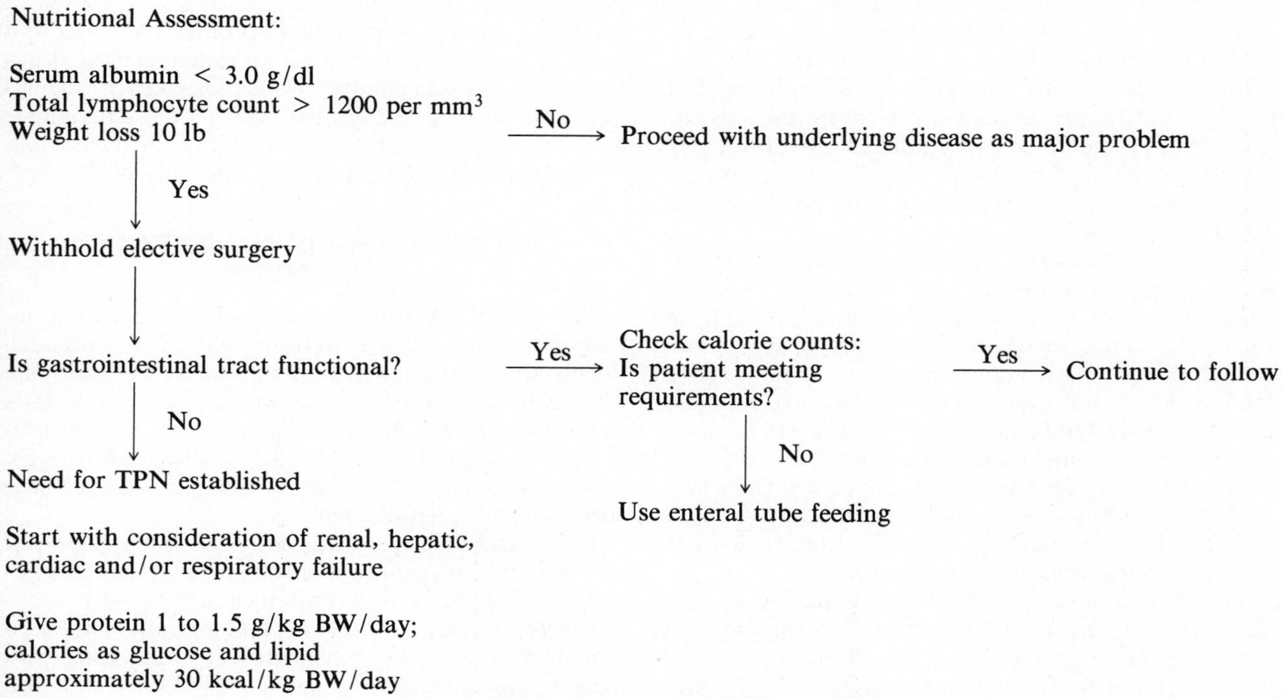
Nutritional Assessment:
Serum albumin < 3.0 g/dl
Total lymphocyte count > 1200 per mm³
Weight loss 10 lb
No
Proceed with underlying disease as major problem
Yes
Withhold elective surgery
Is gastrointestinal tract functional?
Yes
Check calorie counts:
Is patient meeting requirements?
Yes
Continue to follow
No
Use enteral tube feeding
No
Need for TPN established
Start with consideration of renal, hepatic, cardiac and/or respiratory failure
Give protein 1 to 1.5 g/kg BW/day; calories as glucose and lipid approximately 30 kcal/kg BW/day

**Figure 22–2.** Algorithm for nutritional management.

amounts and has a functioning gastrointestinal tract, then a nasoenteral feeding tube should be passed. There are many available, but common features include a small diameter and pliability for optimal patient comfort. These are easily and rapidly passed with little or no trauma, which is quite in contrast to the experience with a larger, stiff tube for nasogastric aspiration. The use of nasoenteral tubes has been reviewed recently.[48] This simple technique should be utilized for many patients at risk for malnutrition.

For those patients whose gastrointestinal tract is unable to accommodate their nutritional requirements, a parenteral route must be used. Fortunately the delivery of total parenteral nutrition (TPN) has developed into a readily available technique whereby patients can be maintained in near optimal health for years in spite of no oral intake. TPN supplies the patient with all nutritional requirements, including water, calories, protein, fat, vitamins, minerals, and salts. Since the final solution is hypertonic, it must be infused through a large, high-flow central vein. Given the mechanical, metabolic, and infectious complications that can arise with TPN, it is strongly advised that only those physicians familiar with the procedure administer it.[49]

## FURTHER NUTRITIONAL CONSIDERATIONS

**Ascorbic Acid.** Severe deficiency of dietary ascorbic acid, vitamin C, results in the clinical syndrome known as scurvy. One biochemical role ascorbic acid has is as a coenzyme in collagen biosynthesis. The clinical manifestations of scurvy are thought to be due to a defect in collagen synthesis. Signs and symptoms include recurrent hemarthroses, bleeding gums, perifollicular hemorrhages, and purpura and ecchymoses.[50] Today in the United States scurvy is usually seen in the elderly who subsist on processed foods or in alcoholics.

Since patients with scurvy are often suffering from multiple nutritional deficiencies, hemarthroses secondary to scurvy should be easily differentiated from other non-nutritional arthritides. If the diagnostic work-up leads to joint aspiration, the diagnostic possibilities are certainly narrowed.

**Selenium.** Selenium, a trace mineral, has recently been shown to be an essential nutrient for humans.[51,52] Among clinical the symptoms of selenium deficiency are arthritis, myalgias, and a congestive cardiomyopathy mostly seen in children. An individual patient maintained on total parenteral nutrition was reported to have developed debilitating myalgias and muscle tenderness in her lower extremities.[53] Examination of her nervous system and upper extremities revealed no abnormalities. Coincident with this syndrome was a very low blood level of selenium. The symptoms resolved after one week of intravenous selenium supplementation.

The amount of selenium in the diet is dependent upon the amount found in the soil on which the food was grown. Large geographic areas with deficient soil selenium include New Zealand and a large area of China. Keshan disease, originally thought to be caused by food toxins, is now believed due to selenium deficiency.[54] Keshan disease, endemic in the area of China with low soil selenium, is characterized by a congestive cardiomyopathy in children and an episodic, recurring arthritis over the years involving the spine and peripheral joints, leading to a disabling premature osteoarthritis. In a large-scale trial involving dietary supplementation of selenium in Chinese children, the incidence of cardiomyopathy was drastically reduced; but to date, there has been no published report of changes in the incidence of the arthritis.[55,56]

**Pyridoxine.** Vitamin $B_6$ (pyridoxine) levels have been found to be low in patients suffering from rheumatoid arthritis.[57-60] The question of whether this is, through some unknown mechanism, an etiology of rheumatoid arthritis has been investigated by the use of therapeutic trials. Ellis and Presley did find some improvement with arthritis of the hands and in carpal tunnel syndrome.[61] However, other trials have not shown this effect. Bruckner and co-workers failed to see any improvement in neuropathies due to rheumatoid disease.[62] In a double-blind trial of 21 patients, no change in clinical parameters or in erythrocyte sedimentation rate was seen in vitamin $B_6$ deficient patients, in spite of tripling of pre-treatment plasma pyridoxine levels.[60] The conclusion that we can draw from these studies is that in spite of the high prevalence of nutritional deficiencies in arthritis patients, correction of the deficits is indicated from a nutritional viewpoint and not from a rheumatologic one.

**Retinoic Acid.** Retinoic acid is the acid form of retinol, or vitamin A. It has been shown recently that the all-*trans* as well as the 13-*cis* isomers of retinoic acid can inhibit collagenase and prostaglandin $E_2$ production from cultures of rheumatoid synovial cells.[63] A mechanism thought responsible for the beneficial effect of corticosteroids in rheumatoid arthritis is the inhibition of collagenase and prostaglandin $E_2$ production by synovial cells; in contrast nonsteroidal anti-inflammatory drugs block only prostaglandin production. Given the remarkable success and relative safety of 13-*cis* retinoic acid in severe acne, the use of this drug in rheumatoid arthritis patients may prove to be clinically justifiable.[64]

## PROSTAGLANDINS AND DIETARY FATTY ACIDS

The central role prostaglandins play in mediating inflammation (see Chapter 6) has recently led to research in this area on the possible development of nutritional interventions to modify inflammatory processes. It is important to keep in mind the many different prostaglandins, each with its own specific effects on specific tissues, including those that enhance as well as those that suppress inflammation.

Zurier and colleagues demonstrated prolongation of survival and prevention of anemia and glomerulonephritis in NZB/NZW $F_1$ hybrid mice (a strain that spontaneously develops a disease pathologically similar to human systemic lupus erythematosus) when treated with daily subcutaneous prostaglandin $E_1$ ($PGE_1$).[65,66] Oral administration of a stable analog of $PGE_1$,15-(S)-15-

methyl prostaglandin $E_1$, has been shown to ameliorate the damage from immune complex–induced vasculitis as well as adjuvant-induced polyarthritis.[67,68] This experimental rat model has led to further experiments with dietary manipulations of essential fatty acid content, because essential fatty acids serve as the precursors of prostaglandins.

Humoral immunity in mice was found to be significantly impaired when the animals were made deficient in essential fatty acids.[69] In the murine lupus model, Hurd and co-workers found a striking increase in survival and prevention of glomerulonephritis among essential-fatty-acid-deficient mice.[70,71] The treated mice were shown to develop antibodies to double-stranded DNA, but at a later age than the control animals. Mice treated with $PGE_1$ fared better than controls but not as well as the essential-fatty-acid-deficient animals. In a different approach, Prickett and colleagues treated NZB/NZW mice with diets enriched with eicosopentaenoic acid.[72] This fatty acid is a precursor of prostaglandin $E_3$ and is thought to interfere with the metabolism of arachidonic acid, an essential fatty acid, to other prostaglandins and thromboxanes. The treated animals did have lower levels of arachidonic acid but were not deficient in essential fatty acids. Probably the effect of eicosapentaenoic acid is exerted through prostaglandin metabolism but other than through depletion of arachidonic acid, as occurs in essential fatty acid deficiency. Dihomo-gamma-linolenic acid is a fatty acid that serves as a precursor of prostaglandin $E_1$. A rich source of this fatty acid is the oil of the evening primrose plant. Kunkel and associates have shown a beneficial effect from dietary supplementation of this oil, using an adjuvant-induced polyarthritis model in rats.[73] The mechanism thought to be operative in this situation is enhanced endogenous production of $PGE_1$ due to increased precursor concentration, leading to a less enhanced inflammatory response to the injected adjuvant.

No in vivo work in this area for humans has been published as yet; but in vitro data do exist, and they show that the synovium of patients with rheumatoid arthritis produces significant amounts of prostaglandins.[74] It has been recently shown that the dietary mix of fatty acids can significantly alter the fatty acid profile seen in plasma phospholipids, triglycerides, sterol esters, and platelet lipids.[75,76] These studies show that adults fed diets enriched with fish oils, abundant sources of eicosapentaenoic acid, demonstrated changes in lipid profiles within four weeks of the new diet. These studies and the work to date in animal models set the stage for therapeutic dietary trials in patients with arthritis.

## OBESITY

**Gout.** Gout and obesity are directly associated. In the Framingham Heart Study, over 5000 patients were followed longitudinally. The study revealed that patients with gout or hyperuricemia were on the average 10 percent heavier than nongouty or nonhyperuricemic subjects.[78] The relationship was linear; that is, the greater the degree of obesity, the greater the chance of gout. With weight loss, uric acid levels tend to decrease.[79] However, in diets sufficiently restrictive in calories as to allow starvation ketosis to occur, transient hyperuricemia may result from renal tubular excretion competition between urate and ketone bodies.[80] When starvation ketosis is abolished, urate levels return to baseline values. (See Chapters 21 and 86 for further discussion.)

**Degenerative Joint Disease.** A direct correlation exists between obesity and osteoarthritis of weight-bearing joints.[38] There is also an increased prevalence of osteoarthritis in non-weight-bearing joints of obese patients.[81] The prevalence of osteoarthritis among the obese is approximately twice that for the normal-weighted individual, for both weight-bearing as well as non-weight-bearing joints. The mechanism for this increase is thought to be mechanical in origin, but this certainly cannot be the process in non-weight-bearing joints.

## References


1. Blackburn, G.L., Bistrian, B.R., Maini, B.S., Schlamm, H.T., and Smith, M.F.: Nutritional and metabolic assessment of the hospitalized patient. JPEN 1:11, 1977.
2. Seltzer, M.H., Bastidas, J.A., Cooper, D., Engler, P., Slocum, B., and Fletcher, H.S.: Instant nutritional assessment. JPEN 3:157, 1979.
3. Seltzer, M.H., Fletcher, H.S., Slocum, B.A., and Engler, P.E.: Instant nutritional assessment in the intensive care unit. JPEN 5:70, 1981.
4. Seltzer, M.H., Slocum, B.A., Cataldi-Betcher, E.L., Fileti, C., and Gerson, N.: Instant nutritional assessment: absolute weight loss and surgical mortality. JPEN 6:218, 1982.
5. Dinarello, C.A., and Wolff, S.M.: Molecular basis of fever in humans. Am. J. Med. 72:799, 1982.
6. Blackburn, G.L., and Bistrian, B.R.: Nutritional care of the injured and/or septic patient. Surg. Clin. North Am. 56:1195, 1976.
7. Gerber, D.A.: Low free serum histidine concentration in rheumatoid arthritis. J. Clin. Invest. 55:1164, 1975.
8. Gerber, D.A., Tanenbaum, L., and Ahrens, M.: Free serum histidine levels in patients with rheumatoid arthritis and control subjects following an oral load of free L-histidine. Metabolism. 25:655, 1976.
9. Kirkham, J., Lowe, J., Bird, H.A., and Wright, V.: Serum histidine in rheumatoid arthritis: a family study. Ann. Rheum. Dis. 40:501, 1981.
10. Pickup, M.E., Dixon, J.S., Lowe, J.R., and Wright, V.: Serum histidine in rheumatoid arthritis: changes induced by antirheumatic drug therapy. J. Rheumatol. 7:71, 1980.
11. Gerber, D.A.: Antirheumatic drugs, the ESR and the hypohistidinemia of rheumatoid arthritis. J. Rheumatol. 4:40, 1977.
12. Gerber, D.A.: Inhibition of denaturation of human gamma globulin by a mixture of L-histidine, L-cystine, and copper and its clinical implications in rheumatoid arthritis. Arthritis Rheum. 19:593, 1976.
13. Cartwright, G.E.: The anemia of chronic disorders. Semin. Hematol. 3:351, 1966.
14. Dinant, H.J., and DeMaat, C.E.M.: Erythropoiesis and mean red-cell lifespan in normal subjects and in patients with the anemia of active rheumatoid arthritis. Br. J. Hematol. 39:437, 1978.
15. Blake, D.R., and Bacon, P.A.: Serum ferritin and rheumatoid disease. Br. Med. J. 282:1273, 1981.
16. Bentley, D.P. and Williams, P.: Serum ferritin concentration as an index of storage iron in rheumatoid arthritis. J. Clin. Pathol. 27:786, 1974.
17. Niedermeier, W., Prillaman, W.W., and Griggs, J.H.: The effect of chrysotherapy on trace metals in patients with rheumatoid arthritis. Arthritis Rheum. 14:533, 1971.
18. Kennedy, A.C., Fell, G.S., Rooney, P.J., Stevens, W.H., Dick, W.C., and Buchanan, W.W.: Zinc: its relationship to osteoporosis in rheumatoid arthritis. Scand. J. Rheumatol. 4:243, 1975.
19. Balogh, Z., El-Ghobarey, A.F., Fell, G.S., Brown, D.H., Dunlop, J., and Dick, W.C.: Plasma zinc and its relationship to clinical symptoms and drug treatment in rheumatoid arthritis. Ann. Rheum. Dis. 39:329, 1980.
20. Simkin, P.A.: Oral zinc sulfate in rheumatoid arthritis. Lancet 2:539, 1976.
21. Kennedy, A.C., Bessent, R.G., and Reynolds, P.M.G.: Effect of oral zinc sulfate and penicillamine on zinc metabolism in patients with rheumatoid arthritis. J. Rheumatol. 7:639, 1980.
22. Job, C., Menkes, C.J., and Delbarre, F.: Zinc sulfate in the treatment of rheumatoid arthritis. Arthritis Rheum. 23:1408, 1980.
23. Mattingly, P.C., and Mowat, A.G.: Zinc sulfate in rheumatoid arthritis. Ann. Rheum. Dis. 41:456, 1982.
24. Scudder, P.R., Al-Timimi, D., McMurray, W:, White, A.G., Zoob, B.C.,

and Dormandy, T.L.: Serum copper and related variables in rheumatoid arthritis. Ann. Rheum. Dis. 37:67, 1978.
25. Scudder, P.R., McMurray, W., White, A.G., and Dormandy, T.L.: Synovial fluid copper and related variables in rheumatoid and degenerative arthritis. Ann. Rheum. Dis. 37:71, 1978.
26. Pryzanski, W., Russell, M.L., Gordon, D.A., and Ogryzlo, M.A.: Serum and synovial fluid proteins in rheumatoid arthritis and degenerative joint diseases. Am. J. Med. Sci. 265:483, 1973.
27. Brown, D.H., Buchanan, W.W., El-Ghobarey, A.F., Smith, W.E., and Teape, J.: Serum copper and its relationship to clinical symptoms in rheumatoid arthritis. Ann. Rheum. Dis. 38:174, 1979.
28. Banford, J.C., Brown, D.H., Hazelton, R.A., McNeil, C.J., Sturrock, R.D., and Smith, W.E.: Serum copper and erythrocyte superoxide dismutase in rheumatoid arthritis. Ann. Rheum. Dis. 41:458, 1982.
29. Lunec, J., Halloran, S.P., White, A.G., and Dormandy, T.L.: Free-radical oxidation (peroxidation) products in serum and synovial fluid in rheumatoid arthritis. J. Rheumatol. 8:233, 1981.
30. Blake, D.R., Hall, N.D., Treby, D.A., Halliwell, B., and Gutteridge, J.M.C.: Protection against superoxide and hydrogen peroxide in synovial fluid from rheumatoid patients. Clin. Sci. 61:483, 1981.
31. Bistrian, B.R., Blackburn, G.L., Hallowell, E., and Heddle, R.: Protein status of general surgical patients. JAMA 230:858, 1974.
32. Bistrian, B.R., Blackburn, G.L., Vitale, J., Cochran, D., and Naylor J.: Prevalence of malnutrition in general medical patients. JAMA 235:1567, 1976.
33. Dreblow, D.M., Anderson, C.F., and Moxness, K.: Nutritional assessment of orthopedic patients. Mayo Clin. Proc. 56:51, 1981.
34. McFarlane, D.S.: The role of nutrition in the metabolic response to trauma and in the production of endogenous pyrogen. Master's Thesis, University of Edinburgh, Scotland, 1982.
35. Lom-Orta, H., Diaz-Jouanen, E., and Alarcon-Segovia, D.: Protein calorie malnutrition and systemic lupus erythematosus. J. Rheumatol. 7:178, 1980.
36. Wyatt, R.J., Farrell, M., Berry, P.L., Forristal, J., Maloney, M.J., and West, C.D.: Reduced alternative complement pathway control protein levels in anorexia nervosa: response to parenteral alimentation. Am. J. Clin. Nutr. 35:973, 1982.
37. Pettersson, T., Wegelius, O., and Skrifvars, B.: Gastro-intestinal disturbances in patients with severe rheumatoid arthritis. Acta. Med. Scand. 188:139, 1970.
38. Eising, L.: Dietary intake in patients with arthritis and other chronic diseases. J. Bone Joint Surg. 45:69, 1963.
39. Meakins, J.L., Pietsch, J.B., Bubenick, O., Kelly, R., Rode, H., Gordon, J., and MacLean, L.D.: Delayed hypersensitivity: indicator of acquired failure of host defenses in sepsis and trauma. Ann. Surg. 186:241, 1977.
40. Mullen, J.L., Gertner, M.H., Buzby, G.P., Goodhart, G.L., and Rosato, E.F.: Implications of malnutrition in the surgical patient. Arch. Surg. 114:121, 1979.
41. Mullen, J.L., Buzby, G.P., Matthews, D.C., Smale, B.F., and Rosato, E.F.: Reduction of operative morbidity and mortality by combined preoperative and postoperative nutritional support. Ann. Surg. 192:604, 1980.
42. Daly, J.M., Dudrick, S.J., and Copeland, E.M.: Intravenous hyperalimentation: effect on delayed cutaneous hypersensitivity in cancer patients. Ann. Surg. 192:587, 1980.
43. Smale, B.F., Mullen, J.L., Buzby, G.P., and Rosato, E.F.: The efficacy of nutritional assessment and support in cancer surgery. Cancer 47:2375, 1981.
44. Hoffman-Goetz, L., McFarlane, D., Bistrian, B.R., and Blackburn, G.L.: Febrile and plasma iron responses of rabbits injected with endogenous pyrogen from malnourished patients. Am. J. Clin. Nutr. 34:1109, 1981.
45. Food and Nutrition Board, National Research Council: Recommended Dietary Allowances, 9th ed. Washington, D.C., National Academy of Science, 1980.
46. Rutten, P., Blackburn, G.L., Flatt, J.P., Hallowell, E., and Cochran, D.: Determination of optimal hyperalimentation infusion rate. J. Surg. Res. 18:477, 1975.
47. Bothe, A., Wade, J.E., and Blackburn, G.L.: Enteral nutrition—an overview. *In* Hill, G.L. (ed.): Nutrition and the Surgical Patient. London, Churchill Livingstone, 1981.
48. Orr, G., Wade, J., Bothe, A., and Blackburn, G.L.: Alternatives to total parenteral nutrition in the critically ill patient. Crit. Care Med. 8:29, 1980.
49. Blackburn, G.L., Maini, B.S., and Pierce, E.C.: Nutrition in the critically ill patient. Anesthesiology 47:181, 1977.
50. Hodges, R.E., Hood, J., Canham, J.E., Sauberlich, H.E., and Baker, E.M.: Clinical manifestations of ascorbic acid deficiency in man. Am. J. Clin. Nutr. 24:432, 1971.
51. Young, V.R.: Selenium: a case for its essentiality in man. N. Engl. J. Med. 304:1228, 1981.
52. Johnson, R.A., Baker, S.S., Fallon, J.T., Maynard, E.P., Ruskin, J.N., Wen, Z., Ge, K., and Cohen, H.J.: An occidental case of cardiomyopathy and selenum deficiency. N. Engl. J. Med. 304:1210, 1981.
53. VanRij, A.M., Thomson, C.D., McKenzie, J.M., and Robinson, M.F.: Selenium deficiency in total parenteral nutrition. Am. J. Clin. Nutr. 32:2076, 1979.
54. Keshan Disease Research Group of the Chinese Academy of Medical Sciences, Beijing: Epidemiologic studies on the etiologic relationship of selenium and Keshan Disease. Chinese Med. J. (Engl.) 92:477, 1979.
55. Keshan Disease Research Group of the Chinese Academy of Medical Sciences, Beijing: Observations on effect of sodium selenite in prevention of Keshan disease. Chinese Med. J. (Engl.) 92:471, 1979.
56. Anonymous. Prevention of Keshan cardiomyopathy by sodium selenite. Nutr. Rev. 38:278, 1980.
57. Houpt, J.B., Ogryzlo, M.A., and Hunt, M.: Tryptophan metabolism in man (with special reference to rheumatoid arthritis and scleroderma). Semin. Arthritis Rheum. 2:333, 1973.
58. Jaffe, I.A., and Altman, K.: The effect of pyridoxine on the abnormal tryptophan metabolism in rheumatoid arthritis. Arthritis Rheum. 7:319, 1964.
59. Anderson, B.B., Peart, M.D., and Fulford Jones, C.E.: The measurement of serum pyridoxal by a microbiological assay using *Lactobacillus casei.* J. Clin. Pathol. 23:232, 1970.
60. Schumacher, H.R., Bernhart, F.W., and György, P.: Vitamin $B_6$ levels in rheumatoid arthritis: effect of treatment. Am. J. Clin. Nutr. 28:1200, 1975.
61. Ellis, J.M., and Presley, J.: Vitamin $B_6$: The Doctor's Report. New York, Harper & Row, 1973, p. 39.
62. Bruckner, F.E., Smith, H.G., Lakatos, C., and Chamberlain, M.H.: Tryptophan metabolism in rheumatoid neuropathies. Ann. Rheum. Dis. 31:311, 1972.
63. Brinckerhoff, C.E., McMillan, R.M., Dayer, J.M., and Harris, E.D.: Inhibition by retinoic acid of collagenase production in rheumatoid synovial cells. N. Engl. J. Med. 303:432, 1980.
64. Peck, G.L., Olsen, T.G., Yoder, F.W., Strauss, J.S., Downing, D.T., Pandya, M., Butkus, D., and Arnaud-Battandien, J.: Prolonged remissions of cystic and conglobate acne with 13-*cis*-retinoic acid. N. Engl. J. Med. 300:329, 1979.
65. Zurier, R.B., Sayadoff, D.M., Torrey, S.B., and Rothfield, N.F.: Prostaglandin $E_1$ treatment of NZB/NZW mice. Prolonged survival of female mice. Arthritis Rheum. 20:723, 1977.
66. Zurier, R.B., Damjanov, I., Sayadoff, D.M., and Rothfield, N.F.: Prostaglandin $E_1$ treatment of NZB/NZW $F_1$ hybrid mice. Prevention of glomerulonephritis. Arthritis Rheum. 20:1449, 1977.
67. Kunkel, S.L., Thrall, R.S., Kunkel, R.G., McCormick, J.R., Ward, P.A., and Zurier, R.B.: Suppression of immune complex vasculitis in rats by prostaglandin. J. Clin. Invest. 64:1525, 1979.
68. Kunkel, S.L., Ogawa, H., Conran, P.B., Ward, P.A., and Zurier, R.B.: Suppression of acute and chronic inflammation by orally administered prostaglandins. Arthritis Rheum. 24:1151, 1981.
69. De Wille, J.W., Fraker, P.J., and Romsos, D.R.: Effects of essential fatty acid deficiency, and various levels of dietary polyunsaturated fatty acids, on humoral immunity in mice. J. Nutr. 109:1018, 1979.
70. Hurd, E.R., Johnston, J.M., Okita, J.R., McDonald, P.C., Ziff, M., and Gilliam, J.N.: Prevention of glomerulonephritis and prolonged survival in New Zealand Black/New Zealand White $F_1$ hybrid mice fed an essential fatty acid deficient diet. J. Clin. Invest. 67:476, 1981.
71. Hurd, E.R., and Gilliam, J.N.: Beneficial effect of an essential fatty acid deficient diet in NZB/NZW $F_1$ mice. J. Invest. Dermatol. 77:381, 1981.
72. Prickett, J.D., Robinson, D.R., and Steinberg, A.D.: Dietary enrichment with the polyunsaturated fatty acid eicosapentaenoic acid prevents proteinuria and prolongs survival in NZB $\times$ NZW $F_1$ mice. J. Clin. Invest. 68:556, 1981.
73. Kunkel, S.L., Ogawa, H., Ward, P.A., and Zurier, R.B.: Suppression of chronic inflammation by evening primrose oil. Prog. Lipid Res. 20:885, 981.
74. Sturge, R.A., Yates, D.B., Gordon, D., Franco, M., Paul, W., Bray, A., and Morley, J.: Prostaglandin production in arthritis. Ann. Rheum. Dis. 37:315, 1978.
75. Bronsgeest-Schoute, H.C., Van Gent, C.M., Luten, J.B., and Ruiter, A.: The effect of various intakes of $\omega 3$ fatty acids on the blood lipid composition in healthy human subjects. Am. J. Clin. Nutr. 34:1752, 1981.
76. Goodnight, S.H., Harris, W.S., and Connor, W.E.: The effects of dietary $\omega 3$ fatty acids on platelet composition and function in man: a prospective, controlled study. Blood 58:880, 1981.
77. Acheson, R.M., and O'Brien, W.M.: Dependence of serum uric acid on hemoglobin and other factors in the general population. Lancet 2:777, 1966.
78. Hall, A.P., Barry, P.E., Dawber, T.R., and McNamara, P.M.: Epidemiology of gout and hyperuricemia. A long-term population study. Am. J. Med. 42:27, 1967.
79. Nicholls, A., and Scott, J.T.: Effect of weight-loss on plasma and urinary levels of uric acid. Lancet 2:1223, 1972.
80. Lecoq, F.R., and McPhaul, J.J.: The effects of starvation, high fat diets and ketone infusions on uric acid balance. Metabolism 14:186, 1965.
81. Kellgren, J.H.: Osteoarthrosis in patients and populations. Br. Med. J. 2:1, 1961.

# Section II
# General Approach to the Patient

## Chapter 23
## General Approach to the Rheumatic Disease Patient

*James F. Fries*

### INTRODUCTION

The intrinsic nature of the rheumatic diseases poses an ultimate challenge to the skill and humanity of the managing physician. The chronicity of disease processes, their variability, their tendency to exacerbate and remit, their biochemical and immunologic complexity, their unknown pathogenesis, their variable response to specific treatment, and the myriad ways in which the diseases affect the patient's life style, family relationships, self-image, and employability combine to complicate the therapeutic equation. Complex therapeutic decisions must be made for the most part without adequate experimental justification and evaluated against a poorly understood natural history.

Within the complicated mixture of fact and opinion which constitutes the literature of rheumatic disease lies a strategy which forms the basis for contemporary management of the rheumatic disease patient. Essentially, this strategy requires quite simply that the rheumatic disease patient be treated as an individual and that therapeutic decisions be based upon individual circumstances.[1,2] Further, decisions are modified in a continuing feedback between application of treatment and observed response. Decisions evolve and change with time as appropriate to the trends, tempo, and previous response of the disease in the particular patient. The broad principles underlying this strategy are set forth in this chapter. Despite the generalizations required by this topic, it is hoped that the reader will find a structure which will aid in understanding the specific chapters to follow.

In the old view, arthritis was a single disease, about which "nothing much could be done" and for which aspirin was the best, perhaps the only, medication. The inadequacy of this perception should be too obvious to merit mention, but even today it is shared by large segments of the lay community, a surprising number of physicians in practice, and many members of policy-making political bodies. Its lingering effects are found in hospitals whose laboratories offer an "arthritis profile" and in management approaches based upon monolithic "pyramids." The following paragraphs develop an approach to selective individualized management based upon six major management questions.

### WHAT IS WRONG WITH THIS PATIENT?

Diagnosis in the rheumatic diseases has been overemphasized. On the one hand, current classifications frequently contain patients with features of several diagnostic entities, often termed "overlap" patients, with no absolute diagnosis possible. On the other hand, patients with the same diagnosis often should be managed very differently. Modern management individualizes therapy within diagnostic categories, based upon subgroups of patients with differing prognoses and therapeutic requirements.

Management in the rheumatic diseases is more closely linked to the underlying pathophysiologic process than to the specific disease entity. Simple decision aphorisms, such as, "Do not use an anti-inflammatory agent if there is no evidence of inflammation," can be obscured by excessive reliance upon a link between diagnostic category and treatment. Even such a basic concept as "inflammation" has different therapeutic implications, depending upon the underlying pathophysiology. The inflamed synovial membrane typical of rheumatoid arthritis responds to a different spectrum of anti-inflammatory agents than does the inflammation of ligamentous insertions typical of ankylosing spondylitis, or the inflammation within the joint space induced by crystals.

Eight specific types of musculoskeletal pathology are distinguished by history and physical examination in most patients[3] and provide a framework for pathophysiologic categorization. These categories are not entirely mutually exclusive, but correct categorization of the predominant pathophysiology in a given patient is usually straightforward. The eight categories are discussed below and are listed in Table 23–1, together with the prototype disease of the category, examples of the most useful laboratory tests for that category, and typical treatments required. The management implications for each category are surprisingly distinct, and provide guidelines for the ordering of laboratory investigations and the selection of initial treatment.

**Synovitis.** Inflammation of the synovial membrane with eventual damage to surrounding joint structures is most strikingly manifested in the disease rheumatoid arthritis. The synovium is tender, thickened, and palpable, and often may demonstrate heat and, less often, redness. Joint destruction is presumed to be caused by the enzymatic products of inflammation and may occur slowly over many years. Management is based upon reducing the inflammation and thereby reducing the rate of damage to joint structures. In the laboratory, the sedimentation rate is consistently elevated with significant synovitis, and the latex fixation or other tests for rheumatoid arthritis are often useful for further categorization. A wide range of pharmacologic and other treatments may be required, and many patients require sequential trial with a variety of agents. Some useful drugs, such as gold, penicillamine, and hydroxychloroquine, appear to be therapeutically ineffective in any other disease category, and others, such as aspirin, find their greatest use here.

**Enthesopathy.** Inflammation here is most marked at the enthesis, that transition region where ligament attaches to bone.[4] Such inflammation is the hallmark of a family of rheumatic diseases of which the most common is ankylosing spondylitis. The distribution of musculoskeletal involvement follows the location of regions of enthesis throughout the body. The marked predilection for the sacroiliac joints, heels, and spine illustrates involvement of areas characterized by ligament and tendon attachment rather than synovium. This pathophysiology has been recognized only in the last several years and provides a unifying observation upon which to base the observed clinical features of the diseases and their typical response to specific therapy. Nonsteroidal anti-inflammatory agents, in particular indomethacin, phenylbutazone, and naproxen, are therapeutically effective and are well tolerated over the long term. The spectrum of effective anti-inflammatory drugs is different from that used for synovitis.

**Cartilage Degeneration.** Degenerative and other processes can cause fraying and destruction of the articular cartilage, with injury to the underlying subchondral bone. This occurrence is usually termed osteoarthritis or osteoarthrosis, and a group of specific syndromes is recognized within this category. Narrowing of the apparent joint space and development of spurs make radiography the most useful investigation; other laboratory aids are predictably negative. Few patients have significant inflammation, and it is not surprising that anti-inflammatory treatment is not frequently useful. The analgesic effects of aspirin or nonsteroidal anti-inflammatory agents may be helpful; doses required for optimal effect are often considerably less than doses required for anti-inflammatory effects with the same compound. Treatment is symptomatic and seldom dramatically effective.

**Crystal-Induced Synovitis.** Microcrystalline arthritis occurs when crystals forming in the synovial fluid (or injected therein) induce an inflammatory reaction in the joint fluid and the surrounding synovium. Gout is the prototypic disease, with inflammation induced by crystals of sodium urate. Similar syndromes may occur with crystals of several other types. The rapid, acute inflammatory response creates a rather sudden onset, increasing to very intense inflammation within a period of hours, with slow resolution without treatment over a period of a few days to a few weeks. The physical factors underlying crystal formation ensure that only one or at most a few joints are involved at a time. The crucial laboratory observation is inspection of aspirated joint fluid for crystals under polarized light. Drugs inhibiting the mobilization of polymorphonuclear leukocytes are particularly effective, as exemplified by colchicine, a drug with little effect in any other rheumatic disease category.

**Joint Infection.** The synovium encloses a body space that can be the site of direct infection by microorganisms. Critical to investigation of the patient with suspected joint infection are aspiration and culture of the joint fluid and, in many instances, culture of other body fluids as well. Treatment, obviously, consists of a specific antibiotic.

**Myositis.** Inflammation of muscle occurs in two closely related diseases, dermatomyositis and polymyositis, and in a distant relative, polymyalgia rheumatica. Determination of muscle enzymes and histologic examination of involved muscle are the critical labora-

**Table 23–1.** Categories of Rheumatic Disease

| Pathology | Prototype | Most Useful Tests | Typical Treatment |
|---|---|---|---|
| Synovitis | Rheumatoid arthritis | Latex, erythrocyte sedimentation rate | Acetylsalicylic acid, gold |
| Enthesopathy | Ankylosing spondylitis | Sacroiliac radiographs, B27 | Indomethacin |
| Cartilage degeneration | Osteoarthritis | Radiographs of affected areas | Analgesic |
| Crystal-induced synovitis | Gout | Joint fluid crystal examination | Colchicine |
| Joint infection | Staphylococcal | Joint fluid culture | Antibiotics |
| Myositis | Dermatomyositis | Muscle enzymes, muscle biopsy | Corticosteroids |
| Focal conditions | Tennis elbow | None, radiographs of affected area | Localized |
| Generalized conditions | Fibrositis | Erythrocyte sedimentation rate | Conservative |

tory observations. In polymyalgia, the sedimentation rate separates this disease from the final category below. Corticosteroids are almost always required and, in contrast to every other rheumatic disease category, are usually required at the outset.

**Focal Conditions.** A wide variety of conditions affecting the musculoskeletal system do not truly warrant the term "disease." Tendinitis, bursitis, low back strain, calcific tendinitis, and a variety of others can affect almost any area of the body and are among the most common medical problems of the population. Laboratory aids are few, although radiography may be occasionally useful in locating calcium deposits or spurs. The therapeutic approach, unfortunately often neglected, is to apply localized treatment measures. Treatment of the entire organism when the problem exists only in one small area is seldom rewarding. Splints, slings, heat, or local injection constitutes the most reasonable initial approach.

**Generalized Conditions.** A variety of poorly defined entities fall into this poorly defined category. Terms such as "fibrositis" or the "chronic muscle contraction syndrome" are sometimes used to indicate the likelihood of organic disease. The terms "psychogenic rheumatism" or "nonarticular rheumatism" or "depressive equivalent" are frequently used to suggest an emotional component to such complaints. These patients are rich in symptoms but poor in objective pathology. The conditions may be extremely troublesome for the individual but are not progressive and do not result in physical crippling. Laboratory aids, such as the sedimentation rate, are normal and are employed only to rule out other categories. Treatment is best termed "conservative." The therapeutic approaches listed for other categories are unlikely to help, and the physician who attempts major pharmacologic intervention rather than reassurance, life style counseling, and support often ends up with a drug-dependent patient who gets no better.

These eight categories and the brief descriptions above are supported by generalizations that will find some exceptions. However, Table 23–1 suggests quite specific directions in which laboratory investigation and the therapeutic approach may begin. The experienced physician will soon move far beyond this table, but it has provided for us an extraordinarily useful framework upon which to build the clinical knowledge of the young physician.

## WHAT INVESTIGATIONS, IF ANY, ARE REQUIRED?

One in six visits by a patient to a health professional is for a musculoskeletal complaint.[3] The great majority of such physician visits occur for the category of "focal conditions" and do not pose a major hazard to the health of the patient. The overwhelming majority of such complaints are easily identified as self-limited. Optimal management includes the ruling out of significant illness, advice about activity or rest, reassurance, occasionally symptomatic medication, and transmission of the expectation that the natural healing process will resolve the difficulty. The usual healing period for minor musculoskeletal problems requires 2 to 6 weeks, depending on the magnitude of the often inapparent injury, with the healing process beginning again from the start if there is reinjury during this period. Healing cannot be pharmacologically accelerated. Thus, optimal treatment requires "masterly inactivity," with confident reliance upon the natural healing process. Inappropriate management can lead to investigative mishaps, therapeutic side reactions, and an intensity of focus upon the problem entirely inappropriate to its magnitude.

Ulysses, it is said, went off to fight the Trojan War. Battle completed, he attempted to return home but found it necessary to pass through a series of dramatic crises and often unpleasant adventures in order finally, after 20 years, to arrive once again at his starting point. The "Ulysses syndrome" in medicine consists of a series of adverse events stemming from a procedure or a therapy that should never have been undertaken, and sometimes requiring heroic measures just to get back to the starting point. The careful rheumatic disease clinician uses *time* to establish the trends and tempo of the condition in the individual, and to remove the self-limited condition from the hazard of inappropriate response.

A critical clinical decision, therefore, is whether the problem requires immediate investigation and action, or whether the decision to investigate or treat can be postponed with profit until the course of the disease and the magnitude of the appropriate response may be better estimated.[5]

The algorithm of Figure 23–1 displays the major con-

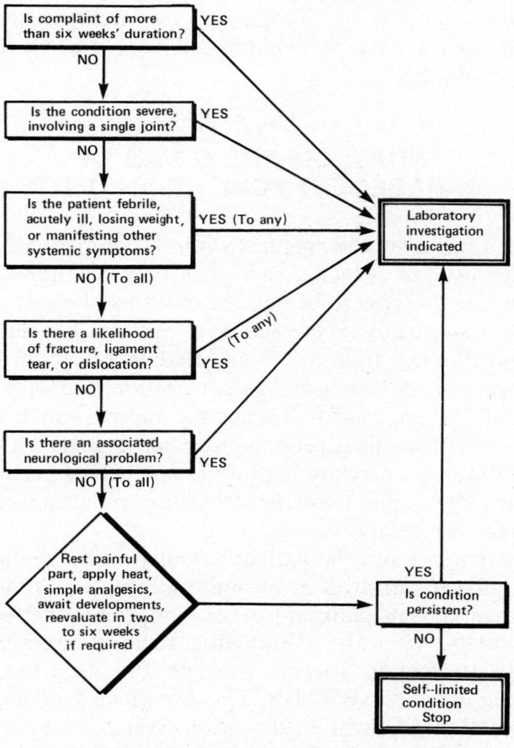


**Figure 23–1.** The initial approach to the patient.

siderations that determine the need for immediate investigation. Chronicity is the most frequent indication for more elaborate investigation and management. For most complaints, an observation period of approximately 6 weeks is appropriate. Four major exceptions obtain. First, a condition that is severe and involves a single joint or at most a few joints is much more likely, paradoxically, to require immediate attention than is a widespread arthritis. Acute gouty arthritis and infections of the joint space each require immediate attention. In contrast, in rheumatoid arthritis a period of 6 weeks is required before the criteria for diagnosis can even be met, and management in the first days of disease is most appropriately conservative. Many "possible rheumatoid arthritis" patients or patients with a "rheumatoid arthritis-like" illness will have minor problems that disappear as the viral or minor hypersensitivity reaction subsides.

Second, a patient who is febrile, systemically ill, and otherwise showing signs of major disease of multiple organs deserves immediate attention. Endocarditis, neoplasm, tuberculosis, and other major illnesses are frequently identified at this stage through musculoskeletal clues, and a connective tissue disease with systemic manifestations deserves immediate attention. Third, if the problem is associated with significant trauma, the possible need for immediate orthopedic management should be considered. And fourth, an associated neurologic problem such as carpal tunnel syndrome, sciatic nerve pain radiation, or cervical nerve root compression syndromes is benefited by immediate attention. These indications are relatively unusual in practice. When this algorithm is applied, the large majority of patients with initial complaints of "joint pain" or "arthritis" will be found not to have serious conditions requiring immediate evaluation.

## WHAT ARE THE GOALS OF MANAGEMENT FOR THIS PATIENT?

With increasing sophistication in laboratory aids and biochemical knowledge, there has been a tendency for management goals to be defined in terms of easily measured, numerically expressed test results. The level of autoantibodies, titer of rheumatoid factor, number of radiographic erosions, and sedimentation rate have often become the criteria for therapeutic success. Such measurements of medical process have value only to the extent that they correlate with illness perceived eventually by the patient, and unfortunately the correlations in each instance are poor.

The patient and the patient's family are more directly interested in survival, in normal mobility and function, in absence from pain and other symptoms, in freedom of toxicity from the therapeutic regimen, and in the ability to remain solvent through the duration of a chronic disease. ARAMIS (The American Rheumatism Association Medical Information System) and several multipurpose arthritis centers have recently employed the five "D's" (death, disability, discomfort, drug toxicity, and dollar cost) as dimensions for describing patient outcome (Fig. 23–2). The disability dimension is meant to include psychological disability as well as physical, and the discomfort dimension to include functional symptoms as well as physical ones.[6] Carefully validated instruments, usually self-administered patient questionnaires, now allow accurate and reproducible measurement of the "quality of life" dimensions.[7] New patient record formats allow serial notation of these values over time. Figure 23–3*A* and *B* reproduces the disability and pain sections of the Health Assessment Questionnaire (HAQ) of the Stanford Arthritis Center together with scoring conventions.[7]

Patients have very individual preferences for the values which they place upon one outcome dimension relative to others. Thus, a treatment strategy expected to minimize disability but with a small potential hazard of iatrogenic death will be embraced enthusiastically by some patients and shunned by others. In some disease areas, such as oncology, the single outcome dimension of death suffices to dominate most clinical decisions. In the rheumatic diseases, value trade-offs between outcome dimensions must be predicated upon the values of the patient after informed explanation, with the expectation that these values will not always perfectly match the physician's view.[8]

The setting of goals logically must precede development of the individual management strategy.[9] In some instances a limited goal, such as regaining the ability to walk, may be dramatically useful to the patient and far more valuable than a modest reduction in the general severity of the disease. Some very worthy goals may not be achievable in the particular instance, and their pursuit will only increase the dimension of therapeutic toxicity. The question "What is desirable?" is subordinate to "What is achievable?" for the individual patient.

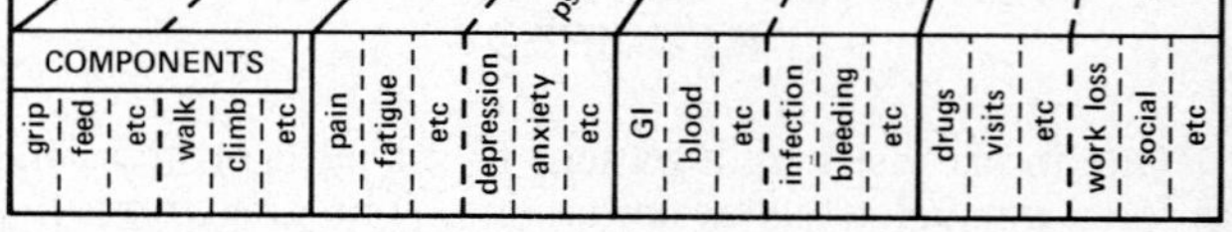

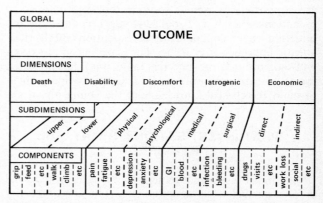


**Figure 23–2.** Conceptualization of "outcome" as a hierarchy of dimensions, subdimensions, and components which collectively include all patient concerns allows particular observations to be placed in the context of other relevant events, provides perspective on the role of a specific assessment, and permits the investigator to select appropriate measures for each study while maintaining some comparability with the results of others.

## OVER WHAT TIME PERIOD SHOULD THE GOALS BE ACHIEVED?

A chronic disease can be psychologically as well as physically devastating, and the difficulties of adjustment are difficult to overstate. In general, management strategies are designed to provide the most favorable outcomes across each outcome dimension, and also along the time dimension representing the duration of the illness. Frequently, agents dramatically effective over the short term are available. Corticosteroids, narcotic analgesics, and intra-articular injections often have this characteristic. Unfortunately, the agent that provides the best initial response may not provide the best long-term outcome.

The experienced clinician spends a great deal of time discussing with the patient the time period for response as well as the expected magnitude of response. In general, simple and nontoxic measures are used first and hazardous medications withheld unless the simpler approaches fail. But the individual patient frequently poses special considerations requiring modification of such rational progressions. Thus, the tempo of disease may be such that serious joint destruction appears likely over a short period of months and the therapeutic progression thus requires acceleration. A major therapeutic attempt with an agent such as gold, penicillamine, or an immunosuppressant may require many months until the expected date of response; meanwhile, the patient may have exhausted sick leave, leading to a forced retirement because of disability. Additional use of a more immediately effective agent, such as prednisone, might well be indicated under such circumstances. In a patient of advanced age, concern about eventual hazard of malignancy secondary to a drug might well be smaller. In a vigorous and active male patient, concern about corticosteroid osteopenia over long administration of such a drug might be less. In a young patient, the expectation for patient outcome might be integrated over 20 to 30 years. In the older patient, both the risks and the benefits of treatment might be reduced, but not by the same amount. Again, the necessity for the individual program is seen.

The inexperienced clinician is often trapped by taking the short view of a chronic illness. The quack practitioner more intentionally follows the strategy of attempting to maximize immediate benefits at the expense of future problems. A chronic disease cannot be managed by tactics; it requires a long-term strategy, shared and negotiated with the patient.

This strategy requires tactical modification at nearly every physician-patient encounter. At each visit, new information is always present, even if it is only the information about what has transpired in response to the last set of decisions. Decision is thus followed by observation, then by further decision, and then by another period of observation. The decision strategy is flexible and, in the final analysis, frequently empiric.

## WHAT THERAPEUTIC STRATEGY IS MOST LIKELY TO ACHIEVE THE GOALS?

Treatment is frequently discussed only in terms of available pharmacologic agents. This myopic view neglects the dominant contributions often afforded by reconstructive surgical procedures, by the use of appliances and devices to allow handicapped individuals to function more normally, or by personal interaction designed to increase the motivation and self-image of the patient.

A drug-based strategy tends to find its greatest use in early, systemic, inflammatory disease processes. Orthopedic approaches tend to have greatest utility if the number of joints or regions involved is small, if major problems are concentrated in a single anatomic region, or if the inflammatory process has "burned out." Improvement after occupational therapy intervention is often seen in individuals with moderate to major disability who require adaptive devices to render the environment somewhat more friendly. The will of the patient to live normally sometimes can be more important to outcome than any specific therapy. Indeed, medical therapy that interferes with mental or emotional adaptation frequently appears to make things worse.

The novice at managing rheumatic diseases employs only a limited therapeutic repertoire. Typically, the patient requires a diverse program individualized to specific needs and frequently making use of a variety of individuals and skills in the community as well as within the medical establishment. Development of rational strategies requires intimate knowledge of the strengths and weaknesses of all available therapeutic modalities. The physician cannot manage rheumatic disease patients effectively without having either direct knowledge of community resources and the techniques of adjacent disciplines or a good working relationship and individuals who possess these skills.

## DOES THE PATIENT UNDERSTAND ENOUGH TO ACHIEVE THE GOALS?

The partnership between physician and patient, often eulogized but seldom practiced, is of particular importance in management of a difficult chronic disease. The informed patient brings tremendous strength to the therapeutic encounter. Transmission of knowledge about the disease process to the patient, appropriately individualized to the particular situation, is a therapeutic imperative.[10]

Consider some of the outside factors that operate if the partnership is not well established and the patient is told to take aspirin. Frequent reports in the lay media describe the hazards of aspirin, advertisements suggest that you don't need a doctor for aspirin, colloquialisms associate aspirin with neglect on the part of the physi-

## HEALTH ASSESSMENT QUESTIONNAIRE

OFFICE USE ONLY

Name ______________________

Date ______________________

TOR NO: ________

In this section we are interested in learning how your illness affects your ability to function in daily life. Please feel free to add any comments on the back of this page.

- **Please check the one response which best describes your usual abilities OVER THE PAST WEEK:**

| | Without ANY Difficulty | With SOME Difficulty | With MUCH Difficulty | UNABLE To Do | |
|---|---|---|---|---|---|
| **DRESSING & GROOMING** | | | | | (246) ______ |
| Are you able to: | | | | | |
| –Dress yourself, including tying shoelaces and doing buttons? | ______ | ______ | ______ | ______ | |
| –Shampoo your hair? | ______ | ______ | ______ | ______ | |
| **ARISING** | | | | | (217) ______ |
| Are you able to: | | | | | |
| –Stand up from an armless straight chair? | ______ | ______ | ______ | ______ | |
| –Get in and out of bed? | ______ | ______ | ______ | ______ | |
| **EATING** | | | | | (235) ______ |
| Are you able to: | | | | | |
| –Cut your meat? | ______ | ______ | ______ | ______ | |
| –Lift a full cup or glass to your mouth? | ______ | ______ | ______ | ______ | |
| –Open a new milk carton? | ______ | ______ | ______ | ______ | |
| **WALKING** | | | | | (220) ______ |
| Are you able to: | | | | | |
| –Walk outdoors on flat ground? | ______ | ______ | ______ | ______ | |
| –Climb up five steps? | ______ | ______ | ______ | ______ | |

- **Please check any AIDS OR DEVICES that you usually use for any of these activities:**

____ Cane

____ Devices Used for Dressing (button hook, zipper pull, long-handled shoe horn, etc.)

____ Walker

____ Built Up or Special Utensils

____ Crutches

____ Special or Built Up Chair

____ Wheelchair

____ Other (Specify: ______________________)

- **Please check any categories for which you usually need HELP FROM ANOTHER PERSON:**

____ Dressing and Grooming

____ Eating

____ Arising

____ Walking

—1— Stanford Arthritis Center Disability and Discomfort Scales, 1981

**Figure 23–3.** *A,* Page 1, The Health Assessment Questionnaire (HAO), Disability Dimension. *B,* Page 2, Disability and Pain Dimensions. Columns are scored 0, 1, 2, 3, and are parallel in structure to ARA Functional Class scores of I, II, III, and IV. The highest score for each component is used. A notation of use of aids, devices, or help from another requires a minimal score of 2 for the corresponding component. Component scores are added, then divided by 8 in order to calculate the Disability Index.

OFFICE USE ONLY

• **Please check the one response which best describes your usual abilities OVER THE PAST WEEK:**

| | Without ANY Difficulty | With SOME Difficulty | With MUCH Difficulty | UNABLE To Do | |
|---|---|---|---|---|---|
| **HYGIENE** | | | | | (251) ______ |
| Are you able to: | | | | | |
| —Wash and dry your entire body? | ______ | ______ | ______ | ______ | |
| —Take a tub bath? | ______ | ______ | ______ | ______ | |
| —Get on and off the toilet? | ______ | ______ | ______ | ______ | |
| **REACH** | | | | | (210) ______ |
| Are you able to: | | | | | |
| —Reach and get down a 5 pound object (such as a bag of sugar) from just above your head? | ______ | ______ | ______ | ______ | |
| —Bend down to pick up clothing from the floor? | ______ | ______ | ______ | ______ | |
| **GRIP** | | | | | (216) ______ |
| Are you able to: | | | | | |
| —Open car doors? | ______ | ______ | ______ | ______ | |
| —Open jars which have been previously opened? | ______ | ______ | ______ | ______ | |
| —Turn faucets on and off? | ______ | ______ | ______ | ______ | |
| **ACTIVITIES** | | | | | (368) ______ |
| Are you able to: | | | | | |
| —Run errands and shop? | ______ | ______ | ______ | ______ | |
| —Get in and out of a car? | ______ | ______ | ______ | ______ | |
| —Do chores such as vacuuming or yardwork? | ______ | ______ | ______ | ______ | |

• **Please check any AIDS OR DEVICES that you usually use for any of these activities:**

______ Raised Toilet Seat

______ Bathtub Seat

______ Jar Opener (for jars previously opened)

______ Bathtub Bar

______ Long-Handled Appliances for Reach

______ Long-Handled Appliances in Bathroom

Other (Specify ______________________________)

• **Please check any categories for which you usually need HELP FROM ANOTHER PERSON:**

______ Hygiene

______ Reach

______ Gripping and Opening Things

______ Errands and Chores

We are also interested in learning whether or not you are affected by pain because of your illness.

• **How much pain have you had because of your illness IN THE PAST WEEK?** (700) ______

*PLACE A MARK ON THE LINE TO INDICATE THE SEVERITY OF THE PAIN*

NO PAIN ———————————————————— VERY SEVERE PAIN

0 ———————————————————— 100

—2— Stanford Arthritis Center Disability and Discomfort Scales, 1981 cian, and the lack of requirement for prescription suggests a minor and ineffective remedy. For anti-inflammatory treatment with aspirin the physician may aim for a rather narrow therapeutic range just below toxicity and far above the doses to which the public is accustomed. During the establishment of dosage the patient is almost certain to run into one or another side effect even though the drug later may be well tolerated over the long term. The informed patient must know that anti-inflammatory and analgesic activities of aspirin are different, that a particular therapeutic range is desired, that the drug will be active against the inflammatory process itself, that many weeks may be required to see the full effects of the drug, and so forth. In the absence of such information, it is extremely unusual for a patient to do well on acetylsalicylic acid; patient education becomes a prerequisite for therapeutic success.

The patient with arthritis is under intense psychologic pressures. Self-image is threatened by diseases that may cripple or prevent remunerative employment. The possibility of dependence upon others in the future is often present. The patient's expectations for the future are frequently drawn from the most unfortunate individuals whom the patient has encountered. Recognition that every patient with arthritis has significant fears is essential to good management. Direct discussion of expectation is essential. For the most part, positive expectations are the most realistic. Only 15 per cent of patients with rheumatoid arthritis, for example, actually experience severe "crippling," and many of these instances are probably preventable. A patient should almost never be told to expect to become housebound, wheelchair bound, or bedridden. The expectation for gradually increasing disease activity is likewise unfortunate, since the disease activity will usually subside, even after many years. Most clinicians believe that the patient with positive expectations comes to a better outcome. While direct inference of causality is not warranted from this association, it is reasonable to assume as an operational principle that restoration of hope and a positive self-image are beneficial therapeutic adjuncts.

The informed patient is more likely to comply with a particular therapeutic regimen and will report more reliably the effects, good or bad, of that regimen. The physician making a series of clinical decisions with the patient over a long period is heavily influenced by the patient's report of success or failure with a previous regimen. This report must be as accurate as possible, and the accuracy depends upon the directness of the patient-physician communication.

Advice for living is frequently requested of the physician. While it is well known that splinting, hospitalization, bed rest, and other techniques of resting inflamed joints decrease inflammation temporarily, it is not clear that these effects persist beyond the period of rest. Costs incurred by such treatment in terms of muscle wasting, osteopenia, and loss of social image detract from the temporary gain. As a general rule, we find employment preferred to disability retirement by our patients, and attempt in the therapeutic relationship to guide the patient into activities consistent with a normal or nearly normal life.

Unrealistic expectations and inadequate patient education are probably the major causes of a burgeoning business in quack treatment of arthritis. The charlatan promises a quick and easy response to a difficult and chronic disease. The patient must be armed to recognize the intrinsic falsity of such superficially attractive claims and the losses in courage, independence, and money that may result. The obscenity of the quack who makes a living by defrauding patients with arthritis focuses the attention of most physicians upon the outrage. At a more basic level, however, the patient susceptible to the claims of the quack does not have a confident and informed relationship with his personal physician.

We do not like to think of patients with arthritis as "victims." Illness of some type at some point is a universal human occurrence. The various forms of arthritis may be worse than some illnesses and less bad than others. The repressed hostility emanating from "Why did this have to happen to me?" is not constructive to an optimal life adjustment. Most persons with arthritis are independent and healthy despite the arthritis. This independence is the final goal of the individualized management strategy.

## References

1. Urowitz, M.B.: SLE subsets—divide and conquer. J. Rheumatol. 4:332, 1977.
2. Fries, J.F., and Holman, H.R.: Systemic Lupus Erythematosus: A Clinical Analysis. Philadelphia, W.B. Saunders Company, 1975.
3. Fries, J.F., and Mitchell, D.M.: Joint pain or arthritis. JAMA 235:199, 1976.
4. Calin, A.C., and Fries, J.F.: Ankylosing Spondylitis; Discussions in Patient Management. Garden City, N.Y., Medical Examination Publishing Company, 1978.
5. Vickery, D.F., and Fries, J.F.: Take Care of Yourself: A Consumer's Guide to Medical Care. Reading, Massachusetts, Addison-Wesley Publishing Company, 1976.
6. Fries, J.F.: Education for outcome. J. Rheumatol. 5:1, 1978.
7. Fries, J.F.: Toward an understanding of patient outcome measurement. Arthritis Rheum. 26:697–704, 1983.
8. Murphy, E.A.: The Logic of Medicine. Baltimore, Johns Hopkins University Press, 1976.
9. Feinstein, A.R.: Clinical Judgment. Baltimore, Waverly Press, 1967.
10. Tumulty, P.A.: The Effective Clinician. Philadelphia, W.B. Saunders Company, 1973.

# Chapter 24
# Examination of the Joints

*Clement J. Michet and Gene G. Hunder*

## HISTORY IN THE PATIENT WITH MUSCULOSKELETAL DISEASE

A detailed description of symptoms related to the musculoskeletal system will provide much of the information necessary to making a diagnosis. The goal of the interview is to understand precisely what the patient means by what is said about symptoms. In obtaining a history of the patient's illness the physician must probe for details of the sequence and severity of symptoms and patterns of progression, exacerbation, or remission. The effects of the previous therapy, associated diseases, and stress must be elucidated. The impact of the disease on the patient must be defined.

The effects of current or previous therapy on the course of the illness are important. Frequently, these are not volunteered by the patient. Assessment of compliance is extremely important; even an ideal therapeutic regimen will fail if the patient does not comply with the outlined program.

The patient's behavior usually provides clues to the nature of the illness and the patient's response to it. It is important to determine whether the patient is reacting appropriately to an illness or is overly concerned or has ignored the joint symptoms. The patient's understanding of his illness will affect his response to it.

**Pain.** Pain is the complaint that most commonly brings the patient with musculoskeletal disease to the physician. Pain is a complex subjective sensation that is often difficult to define, explain, or measure. It has different meanings to different people and even to the same person at different times. Response to pain is affected by the patient's current emotional status as well as previous experiences, including observations of others in pain.

Pain must be localized anatomically. If the pain is in a joint, an articular disorder is likely to be present. Pain between joints may suggest bone or muscle disease or referred pain. Pain in bursal areas, fascial planes, or along tendons, ligaments, or nerve distributions suggests disease in these structures. Pain arising from deeper structures is often less focal than pain originating from superficial tissues. Pain in small joints of the hand or feet tends to be more accurately localized than pain in larger more proximal joints such as the shoulder, hip, or spine. Pain from the hip joint, for example, may be felt in the groin, buttock, or over the greater trochanter or referred to the anterior portion of the thigh or knee. When pain is diffuse, variable, poorly described, or unrelated to anatomic structures, a functional problem or fibromyalgia may be suspected.

Although variable from one patient to another, the character of the pain often helps in understanding the patient's illness. For example, "aching" in a joint area suggests an arthritic disorder, whereas "burning" or "prickling" in an extremity may indicate a neuropathy. An "intolerable" or "excruciating" pain in a patient who otherwise is able to carry out normal activities suggests that emotional factors may be amplifying symptoms.

The presence or absence of pain at rest usually helps the evaluation. Joint pain present both at rest and with movement is more suggestive of an inflammatory process, whereas pain mainly or only during motion often indicates a mechanical disorder such as degenerative arthritis or traumatic arthritis. However, many patients with more advanced degenerative joint disease of the hip or spine also have pain at night.

**Swelling.** An important finding in rheumatic diseases is swelling. Patients vary in their perception of swelling and ability to describe it. The interviewer needs to determine where and when the swelling occurs; it is helpful to learn whether the swelling is visible to others. Description of the exact location of the swelling helps in understanding whether the swelling conforms to an anatomically discrete area such as a particular joint, bursa, or other specific extra-articular area. An obese person may interpret normal collections of adipose tissue over the medial aspects of the elbow or knee and lateral aspect of the ankle as swellings.

Information about the onset, persistence, and influencing factors help define the nature of the swelling. Discomfort with use of the swollen part may indicate synovitis or bursitis because of tension on these tissues during motion of a joint. However, when inflamed tissues are not put under stress during joint movement, pain is minimal; for example, movement of the knee is generally painless in cases of prepatellar bursitis. Swelling in a confined area such as a synovial sac or bursa is most painful when it has developed acutely. In such instances, even light palpation may be intolerable. In chronic swelling when the synovial sac has stretched or when the distention has developed gradually, pain is generally less severe.

**Limitation of Motion.** Patients with rheumatic disorders frequently complain of limitation of motion. Determination of the extent of disability resulting from lack of motion is important. The length of time restrictions of motion have been present can be helpful in predicting reversibility of the disability. It is helpful also to know whether the limitation of motion began abruptly, as with a tendon rupture or onset of psychogenic episode, or gradually as in slowly progressive inflammatory disease.

**Stiffness.** Stiffness is a word that has different meanings to different patients. Some equate it with pain or fatigue; others equate it with soreness, weakness or restrictions of movement; and still others use the term without being able to tell clearly what they feel. Most rheumatologists define stiffness as discomfort perceived by the patient attempting to move joints after a period of inactivity. When it occurs, stiffness or "gelling" usually develops after inactivity of one or more hours. Mild stiffness may resolve within a few minutes. When severe, as in rheumatoid arthritis or polymyalgia rheumatica, the stiffness may improve only over one to several hours.

Morning stiffness can be a prodromal symptom of arthritis, and it is a criterion of the American Rheumatism Association for the diagnosis of rheumatoid arthritis. (See Chapter 60.) It should be differentiated from the discomfort associated with movement of a mechanically damaged joint. Morning stiffness associated with noninflammatory joint diseases is almost always of short duration, usually less than one-half hour, and of less severity than stiffness of inflammatory joint disease. In addition, in mechanical, degenerative, or other destructive joint disease, the degree of stiffness is related to the extent of overuse of the damaged joint and responds usually within a few days to adequate limitation of the use of the affected joint. In degenerative joint disease stiffness may be more noticeable during the day after resting an hour or more than it is in the morning.

The absence of stiffness does not exclude the possibility of the presence of systemic inflammatory rheumatic diseases such as rheumatoid arthritis, but its absence is uncommon. Stiffness from neurologic disorders of the Parkinsonism type, without a recognized inflammatory basis, also occurs and sometimes is conspicuous, although the "limbering up" component is lacking.

**Weakness.** When present, a loss of motor power or muscular strength is nearly always objectively demonstrable during the examination, at least in relation to what a patient was formerly able to do. True weakness can be noted only when muscles are actively being used. In musculoskeletal disorders weakness is usually persistent rather than intermittent. Muscle weakness as a result of inflammatory myopathies occurs typically in proximal portions of the extremities, whereas weakness caused by most neuropathies is found in a distal or peripheral parts.

**Fatigue.** A common and important complaint of many patients with musculoskeletal disease, fatigue is nonetheless an imprecise term. It can be defined as an inclination to rest even though pain and weakness are not limiting factors. It implies exhaustion and depletion of energy. Fatigue is a normal phenomenon after variable degrees of activity but resolves after rest. In rheumatic diseases fatigue may be prominent even when the patient has not been active physically. If the arthritis improves, fatigue tends to lessen. In the absence of organic disease, anxiety and muscular tension or related emotional states are prominent factors in producing chronic fatigue. Patients with an inflammatory arthritis may complain of weakness when they are experiencing stiffness. The differentiation from stiffness and weakness may be facilitated by remembering that stiffness is a discomfort during movement and weakness is an inability to move normally against resistance. Fatigue may be sensed when the patient is resting and is an aversion to activity.

## CLASSIFICATION OF THE JOINTS

Joints are of three main types: synarthroses (immobile articulations), such as suture joints between the bones of the skull; amphiarthroses (slightly movable joints), such as those between the vertebral bodies and the inferior tibial-fibular articulation; and diarthroses (freely movable articulations), such as the knee.

Diarthrodial joints are the most common joints of the body and damage to them by disease causes most disability. The articulating ends of the bones forming a diarthrodial joint are covered by cartilage and are enclosed in a capsule of fibrous tissue (Fig. 24–1). The structure and physiology of diarthrodial joints are discussed in detail in Chapter 16.

Diarthrodial joints have been classified further according to the shapes of the surfaces that articulate. The shape of the articulating surface along with the supporting ligaments determines the type and the extent of motion in the joint. *Plane joints* allow only gliding movements. Articular surfaces of this type of joint are planar or flat or slightly curved. Carpal and tarsal joints are of this type. *Spheroidal joints*, also called ball and socket joints, are formed by the articulation of a rounded convex surface with a cuplike cavity. The distal bone is thus capable of a wide variety of movements, including rotation and circumduction. The shoulder and hip joint are examples of spheroidal joints. *Cotylic joints* are sim-

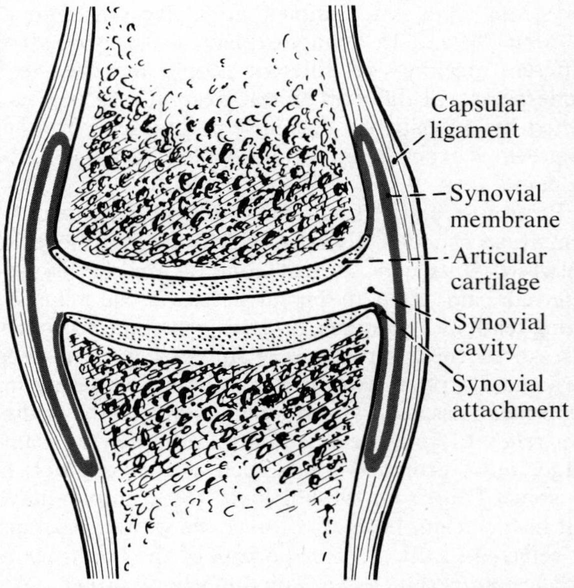


**Figure 24–1.** Schematic diagram of a diathrodial joint. (From Polley, H.F., and Hunder, G.G.: Rheumatologic Interviewing and Physical Examination of the Joints. Philadelphia, W.B. Saunders Company, 1978.)

ilar to spheroidal joints, but the articular surfaces resemble an ellipse rather than a circle. Movement is less free than in spheroidal joints, since rotation is not permitted. The metacarpophalangeal joints of the hand and radiocarpal joint are examples of cotylic joints. *Hinge joints* permit motion in only one plane, namely flexion and extension. Examples are interphalangeal joints of the hand and the humeral-ulnar joint. *Condylar joints* articulate by two distinct articular surfaces whose movements are not dissociable. Each of the surfaces is referred to as a condyle. The knee is an example and has two femoral condyles and two tibial condyles. *Trochoid* or *pivot joints* move in rotation only. The proximal radioulnar and atlanto-odontal (medial atlantoaxial) joints are examples. *Sellar joints* have saddle-shaped articular surfaces. All motions are permitted except axial rotation. The carpometacarpal joint of the thumb is an example.

## SYSTEMIC METHOD OF EXAMINATION

As with the general physical examination, a systematic method of examining joints is the quickest and easiest way of obtaining a thorough assessment of the status of the joints. Many rheumatologists begin with the joints of the upper extremities and proceed to the joints of the trunk and lower extremity, but each examiner should establish his or her own routine. Gentle handling of tender and painful joints will enhance cooperation by the patient and allow an accurate evaluation of the joints.

**Important Physical Signs of Arthritis.** The general aim of the examination of the joints is to detect abnormalities in structure and function of joints. Some of the more common signs of articular disease are swelling, tenderness, limitation of motion, and instability.

***Swelling.*** Swelling about a joint may be caused by intra-articular effusion; synovial thickening; periarticular soft tissue inflammation, such as bursitis or tendinitis; bony enlargement; or extra-articular fat pads. All need to be differentiated from each other. Familiarity with the anatomic configuration of the synovial membrane in various joints aids in differentiating soft tissue swelling due to synovitis (articular effusion or synovial thickening) from swelling of periarticular tissues. The presence of an effusion of a joint is often visible or palpable as bulging of the joint capsule. The presence of palpable fluid in a joint in the absence of immediately preceding trauma usually indicates synovitis. The normal synovial membrane is too thin to palpate, whereas the thickened synovial membrane in rheumatoid arthritis may have a "doughy" or "boggy" consistency. In some joints the extent of the synovial cavity can be delineated on physical examination by compressing the fluid into one of the extreme limits of synovial reflection. The edge of the resulting bulge may thus be palpated more easily. If this palpable edge is within the anatomic confines of the synovial membrane and disappears on release of the compression, the distention may be regarded as representing synovial effusion; if it persists, it is an indication of a thickened synovial membrane. Reliable differentiation between synovial membrane thickening and effusion is not always possible by physical examination. Occasional intrasynovial loose bodies or fibrin clots may be palpated.

Localization of tenderness by palpation should help determine whether the reaction is intra-articular or in a periarticular structure such as a fat pad, tendon attachments, ligaments, bursae, muscles, or skin.

***Limitation of Motion.*** Since *limitation of motion* is a common manifestation of articular disease, it is important to know the normal type and range of motion of each joint in order to detect restriction resulting from abnormalities of the joint or adjacent structures. In patients with joint disease, passive range of motion is often greater than active motion, providing the patient is relaxed during the examination. This may be due to pain, weakness, or the state of the articular or periarticular structures.

***Crepitation.*** A palpable or audible grating or crunching sensation produced by motion, crepitation may or may not be accompanied by discomfort. Crepitation occurs when roughened articular or extra-articular surfaces are rubbed together, either by active motion or by manual compression. Fine crepitation is often palpable over joints involved by chronic inflammatory arthritis and usually indicates roughening of the opposing cartilage surfaces as a result of erosion or the presence of granulation tissue. Coarse crepitation is also due to irregularity of the cartilage surfaces caused by either inflammatory or noninflammatory arthritis. Bone-on-bone crepitus produces a higher frequency palpable and audible "squeak." Crepitation from within the joints should be differentiated from cracking sounds caused by the slipping of ligaments or tendons over bony surfaces during motion. The latter are usually less significant to the diagnosis of joint disease and may be heard over many normal joints. In scleroderma a peculiar coarse, creaking, leathery crepitation may be palpable or audible about various joints and tendon sheaths.

***Deformity.*** A deformity is a malalignment of the joint and may occur as a bony enlargement, articular subluxation, contracture, or ankylosis in abnormal positions. Deformed joints do not function normally, usually restrict activities, and may be associated with pain when put under stressful use.

***Instability.*** Joint instability is present when the joint has greater than normal movement in any plane. Subluxation is defined as a partial displacement of the articular surfaces with some persistent joint surface-to-surface contact, whereas a dislocated joint has lost all cartilage surface contact. Instability is best determined by supporting the joint between the examiner's two hands and stressing the adjacent bones in directions in which the normal joint does not move.

Muscle testing is covered in Chapters 18 and 27.

**Recording the Joint Examination.** A permanent record of examination of the joints is of importance in determining the status and following the progress of arthritic diseases. A variety of methods have been described. To avoid a cumbersome chart, suitable abbreviations for joints can be used such as TM for temporomandibular or SC for sternoclavicular. In recording the degree of swelling (S), tenderness (T), and limitation of motion (L) of a joint, a quantitative estimate of gradation based on a system of grades from 0 (normal) to 4 (highly abnormal) is convenient. The abbreviation S refers to synovial effusion, thickening, or a combination of these. Tenderness of structures other than joints should be specifically described. In the case of limitation of motion, L, grade 1 may be used to indicate about 25 percent loss of motion; grade 2, about 50 percent loss; grade 3, about 75 percent loss; and grade 4, 100 percent loss or ankylosis. In most instances, when more accuracy is desired, it is preferable to record degrees of motion in one or more joints using a goniometer. A table can be constructed with a column for each S, T, and L and the findings recorded for each joint.

A still more abbreviated, narrative form of recording the joint examination may be used, especially when a limited number of joints are involved. An example is as follows: Lt Sh $S_0$, $T_2$, $L_1$; Rt Wr $S_2$, $T_2$, $L_1$; Lt-$MCP_{1\ and\ 2}$ $S_1$, $T_0$, $L_1$; Rt knee $S_1$ (bulge), $T_0$, $L_1$ (lacks 10° of extension).

Alternative methods include the following: the use of a schematic skeleton with marked articulations that may be used to record the status of individual joints (Fig. 24–2); determination of the total number of tender and/or swollen joints and the use of this number as a joint count or joint index; measurement of the size of joints by use of a tape measure or jeweler's ring; determination of the degree of warmth by use of thermography; and measurement of the amount of tenderness by use of a dolorimeter. Grip strength can be measured by asking a patient to squeeze a partially inflated (20 mm Hg) sphygmomanometer cuff. The use of joints can be assessed by determining the speed and the ability to perform other specified coordinated functions.

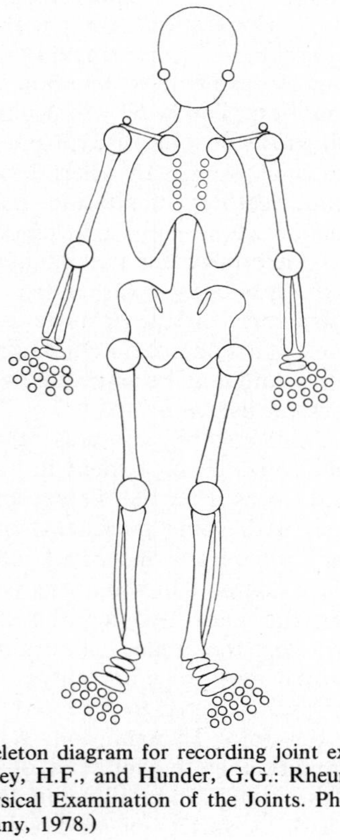

**Figure 24–2.** Skeleton diagram for recording joint examination findings. (From Polley, H.F., and Hunder, G.G.: Rheumatologic Interviewing and Physical Examination of the Joints. Philadelphia, W.B. Saunders Company, 1978.)

## EXAMINATION OF SPECIFIC JOINTS

**Temporomandibular Joint.** The temporomandibular joint is formed by the condyle of the mandible and the fossa of the temporal bone just anterior to the external auditory canal. It is uncommon for this joint to be visibly swollen. The joint is palpated by placing a finger just anterior to the external auditory canal and asking the patient to open and close the mouth and to move the mandible from side to side. Because of normal differences in soft tissue thickness, the presence of synovial thickness or swelling of minimal or moderate degree can be detected most easily if the synovitis is unilateral or asymmetrical. Vertical movement of the temporomandibular joint can be measured by determining the space between the upper and lower incisor teeth with the patient's mouth open maximally. This distance is normally 3 to 6 cm. Lateral movement can be determined by using incisor teeth as landmarks.

Many forms of arthritis affect the temporomandibular joints. Juvenile rheumatoid arthritis commonly affects these joints and may produce arrest of bone growth of the mandible with resultant micrognathia. Audible or palpable crepitus or clicking occur frequently in those without evidence of severe arthritis.

**Cricoarytenoid Joint.** The paired cricoarytenoid joints are formed by the articulation of the base of the small pyramidal arytenoid cartilage and the upper posterolateral border of the cricoid cartilage. The vocal ligaments (cords) are attached to the arytenoid cartilages. The cricoarytenoid joints are normally very mobile diarthrodial joints that move both medially and laterally and rotate during opening and closing of the vocal cords.

Examination of these joints is performed by direct or indirect laryngoscopy. Erythema, swelling, and lack of mobility during phonation may result from inflammation of the joints.

The cricoarytenoid joints may be affected in rheumatoid arthritis, trauma, and infection. Involvement in rheumatoid arthritis is more common than clinically apparent. Early symptoms include a sense of fullness or discomfort in the throat that is worse upon speaking or swallowing. Hoarseness may occur, and significant airway obstruction has been reported.

**Sternoclavicular, Manubriosternal, and Sternocostal Joints.** The medial ends of the clavicles articulate on each side of the sternum at its upper end to form the sternoclavicular joints. The articulations of the first ribs and the sternum (sternocostal joints) are immediately caudad. The articulation of the manubrium and body of the sternum is at the level of the attachment of the second costal cartilage to the sternum. The third through seventh sternocostal joints articulate distally along the lateral borders of the sternum. The sternoclavicular joints are the only articulations in this group that are always diarthrodial in form. The others may be amphiarthroses or synchondroses. The sternoclavicular joints are the only true points of articulation of the shoulder girdle with the trunk. These joints lie beneath the skin, and thus any synovitis is visible and easily palpated. Movement of these joints is slight and cannot be measured accurately.

Involvement of the sternoclavicular joints is common in ankylosing spondylitis, rheumatoid arthritis, and degenerative arthritis but is frequently overlooked. The sternoclavicular joint also may be the site of septic arthritis, especially in drug abusers. Tenderness of the manubriosternal or costosternal joints is much more frequent than actual swelling. Many older patients with no systemic rheumatic disorder may be found to have tender sternocostal joints or costal cartilages (costochondritis). Actual swelling of the upper costal cartilages or areas of the costochondral junctions (Tietze's syndrome) is uncommon.

**Acromioclavicular Joint.** The acromioclavicular joint is formed by the lateral end of the clavicle and medial margin of the acromion process of the scapula. Bony enlargement of this joint is often seen in middle-aged or older persons, but soft tissue swelling is not usually visible or palpable. Local tenderness, or pain with adduction of the arm across the front of the chest, helps pinpoint the involvement to this joint. Arthritis of the acromioclavicular joint is usually secondary to trauma lending to degenerative disease. It is not usually severely affected in rheumatoid arthritis. Movement occurs at this joint during shoulder motion, but actual measurements need not be made in the routine joint examination.

**Shoulder.** The glenohumeral joint is formed by the articulation of the head of the humerus and the shallow glenoid cavity of the scapula (glenoid fossa). Details of shoulder anatomy are presented in Chapter 29. Two outpouchings of synovium perforate the shoulder capsule; one contains the long head of the biceps along the bicipital groove of the humerus, and the other is located under the subscapularis tendon.

The rotator cuff of the shoulder is the term used for the broad, flat, conjoined tendons of the supraspinatus, infraspinatus, teres minor, and subscapularis muscles. Tendons of the first three muscles insert into the superior and posterolateral surface of the greater tubercle (tuberosity) of the humerus as a group. When the shoulder is passively extended, a portion of the rotator cuff moves out from under the anterolateral border of the acromion where this portion of the rotator cuff may be palpated. Alternatively, the posterior portion of the rotator cuff can be palpated inferior to the posterolateral border of the acromion when the patient adducts the arm across the chest.

The subacromial bursa lies under the acromion process and extends anterolaterally beyond the edge of the acromion under the deltoid muscle. It overlies the rotator cuff. The bursa facilitates movement of the greater tuberosity of the humerus beneath the acromion during abduction of the arm.

The shoulders should be inspected for evidence of swelling, muscular atrophy, and muscle fasciculations. Alteration of normal bony landmarks should be noted. If the shoulder is dislocated anteriorly, as is most common, the rounded lateral aspect of the shoulder is lost and it appears flattened. To cause visible distention of the articular capsule, a moderate to large effusion must be present. In such cases, distention usually occurs over the anterior aspect of the joint. Lesser effusions may be palpated by alternate ballottement of the anterior and lateral aspects of the shoulder. Large effusions of the subacromial bursa may produce a localized swelling under the deltoid that may be confused with swelling of the shoulder joint.

A systematic examination of the shoulder includes palpation of the acromioclavicular joint, rotator cuff, region of the subacromial bursa, the bicipital (intertubercular) groove, and the anterior, lateral and posterior aspects of the glenohumeral joint and articular capsule. Details of this examination in specific disease states are given in Chapter 29.

Normally motion of the shoulder and arm is a combination of shoulder girdle and shoulder joint movement. The ball and socket glenohumeral joint is capable of movement in any direction, as is the shoulder girdle on the chest wall. The overall motion of the shoulder can be assessed by moving the shoulder through a full range of motion actively or passively. Shoulder motion can be considered normal if the patient can make a full circle of the arms from the sides of the body anteriorly up over the head at 180 degrees and back down to the original position. To test glenohumeral motion, the examiner fixes the scapula with one hand or prevents the shoulder girdle from moving upward by placing one hand over the top of the acromion while the shoulder again is put through an active and passive range of motion. Normally the glenohumeral joint can be abducted to 90 degrees and rotated internally and externally 90 degrees. Many conditions of the shoulder or periarticular structures may cause restriction of shoulder motion (Fig. 24–3).

In most cases, the muscles of the shoulders can be tested adequately with the patient sitting. Muscle function can be assessed by testing flexion, extension, abduction, adduction, and rotation. Prime movers of flexion are the anterior portion of the deltoid muscles (C5 and 6) and the coracobrachialis muscles (C5 and 6). The latissimus dorsi (C5 and 6), teres major (C5 and 6), and deltoid (C5 and 6) muscles are the prime movers of shoulder extension. Abduction is carried out by the middle fibers of the deltoid (C5 and 6) and supraspinatus (C5) muscles. Prime movers of adduction are the pectoralis major (C5-8, T1) and latissimus dorsi (C5, 6) and teres minor (C5, 6) muscles. The prime movers of medial rotation are the subscapularis, pectoralis major, and teres major muscles.

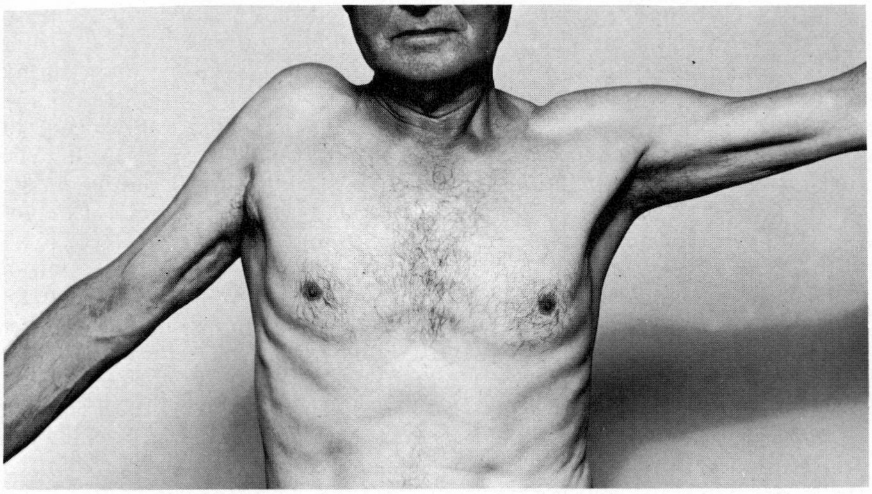

**Figure 24–3.** Attempted abduction of the right arm in a patient with a rotator cuff tear. (From Polley, H.F., and Hunder, G.G.: Rheumatologic Interviewing and Physical Examination of the Joints. Philadelphia, W.B. Saunders Company, 1978.)

Many diseases cause referred pain to the shoulder area and thereby mimic shoulder joint disease. Heart disease, pleural involvement, and hiatal hernia may produce pain referred to the shoulder. Subphrenic inflammation may affect the diaphragm and, through this, cause referred pain to the shoulder or neck. Conditions of the cervical portion of the spinal column, nerve roots, or peripheral nerves in the upper extremity may be frequent sources of shoulder pain and disability. When pain in the shoulder is not related to use of the shoulder and when the examination indicates a completely normal shoulder, referred pain should be considered as a possible cause of the symptoms.

**Elbow.** The elbow joint (see also Chapter 115) is composed of three bony articulations. The principal one is the humeroulnar joint, which is a hinge joint. The radiohumeral and proximal radioulnar articulations allow rotation of the forearm.

To examine the elbow joint, the examiner's thumb is placed between the lateral epicondyle and the olecranon process in the lateral para-olecranon groove and one or two fingers are placed in the corresponding groove medial to the olecranon (Fig. 24–4). The elbow should be relaxed and moved passively through flexion, extension, and rotation. Limitation of motion and crepitus may thus be noted. Synovial swelling is most easily palpated as it bulges under the examiner's thumb when the elbow is passively extended fully. At times synovial membrane can be palpated over the posterior aspect of the joint between the olecranon process and distal humerus. Synovitis is commonly associated with limitation of extension of the joint.

The olecranon bursa overlies the olecranon process of the ulna. Olecranon bursitis is common after repeated or chronic local trauma or occurs in rheumatic diseases such as rheumatoid arthritis and tophaceous gout.

The medial and lateral epicondyles of the humerus and tendinous attachments are common sites of tenderness (tennis elbow, lateral or medial epicondylitis).

Muscle function of the elbow can be assessed by testing flexion and extension. The prime movers of flexion are the biceps brachii (C5, 6), brachialis (C5, 6) and brachioradialis (C5, 6) muscles. The prime mover of extension is the triceps brachii muscle (C7, 8).

**Wrist and Carpal Joints.** The wrist is a complex joint (see also Chapter 114). The true wrist or radiocarpal articulation is formed proximally by the distal end of the radius and the articular disc and distally by a row of three of the carpal bones, the scaphoid, the lunate, and the triangular. The distal radioulnar joint is usually separated from the wrist joint. The mid-carpal joints are formed by the junction of the proximal and distal rows of the carpal bones, which are, from radial to the ulnar side, the trapezium, trapezoid, capitate, and ha-

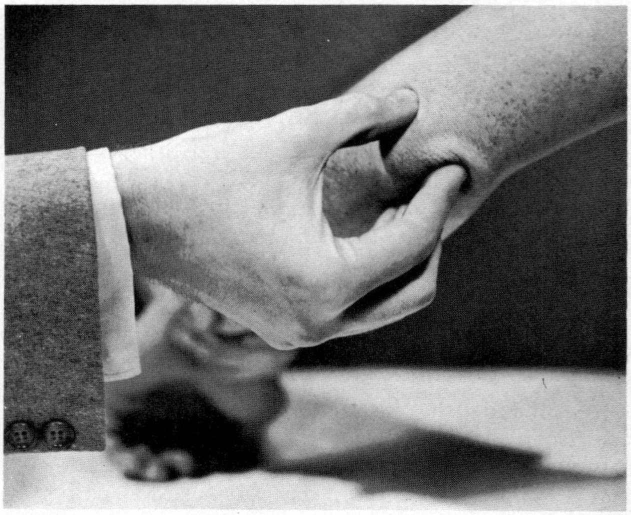

**Figure 24–4.** Palpation of the paraolecranon grooves of the elbow joint. (From Polley, H.F., and Hunder, G.G.: Rheumatologic Interviewing and Physical Examination of the Joints. Philadelphia, W.B. Saunders Company, 1978.)

mate. The mid-carpal and carpometacarpal articular cavities often communicate.

The long flexor tendons of the muscles of the forearm cross the front of the wrist and are enclosed in a flexor tendon sheath under the flexor retinaculum (transverse carpal ligament). The flexor retinaculum and the underlying carpal bones form the carpal tunnel. The median nerve also runs through the carpal tunnel superficial to the flexor tendons. The extensor tendons of the forearm pass under the extensor retinaculum (dorsal carpal ligament) enclosed in a synovial sheath.

The palmar aponeurosis (fascia) spreads out into the palm from the flexor retinaculum. In *Dupuytren's contracture* the palmar aponeurosis becomes thickened and contracted drawing one or more fingers into flexion at the metacarpophalangeal joint. The fourth finger is usually affected earliest, then the fifth and the third. The first two digits are rarely involved. The skin frequently feels adherent to the palmar fascia.

A *ganglion* is a cystic enlargement arising from a joint capsule; it characteristically occurs on the dorsum of the wrist between the tendons of the common extensors of the digits and the radial extensors at the base of the second metacarpal bone.

Subluxation of the ulna occurs secondary to chronic inflammatory arthritis. The subluxed ulna appears as a prominence on the dorsolateral wrist and presses against the extensor digitorum communis tendons, especially those of the fourth and fifth digits. Attrition may result in rupture of these tendons. The long extensor tendon of the thumb is also particularly vulnerable to wear and fraying as a result of its course over bony prominences.

Swelling of the wrist may be due to involvement of the sheaths of the tendons crossing the wrist and/or the wrist joint itself. When swelling is due to tenosynovitis, the outpouching tends to be more localized and is altered by flexing and extending the fingers (Fig. 24–5). Articular swelling is more diffuse and protrudes anteriorly and posteriorly from under the tendons.

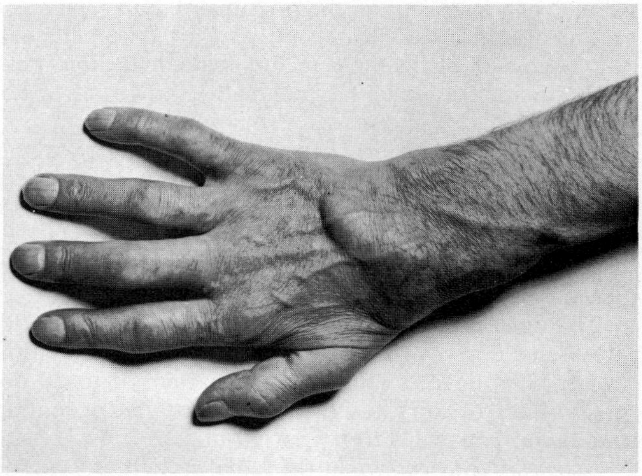

**Figure 24–5.** Localized swelling of the dorsal wrist tenosynovium in a patient with rheumatoid arthritis. (From Polley, H.F., and Hunder, G.G.: Rheumatologic Interviewing and Physical Examination of the Joints. Philadelphia, W.B. Saunders Company, 1978.)

Synovitis of the wrist joint is detected most reliably by palpating over the dorsal surface (Fig. 24–6). Because of structures overlying both the dorsal and palmar aspects of the wrist, accurate localization of the margins of the synovial membrane may be difficult. To examine the wrist the physician should palpate or pinch this joint gently between the thumbs and fingers to detect abnormalities of bony and soft tissue structures. Swelling in hypertrophic osteoarthropathy, if present, extends proximal to the wrist and does not have the typical consistency of either synovial fluid swelling or pitting edema. In addition, clubbing may be present.

*Tenosynovitis* and *trigger finger* can be detected by palpating crepitus or nodules along the tendons in the palm while the patient slowly flexes and extends the fingers. Tendon nodules causing triggering usually occur at the level of the metacarpal heads, where a thickening

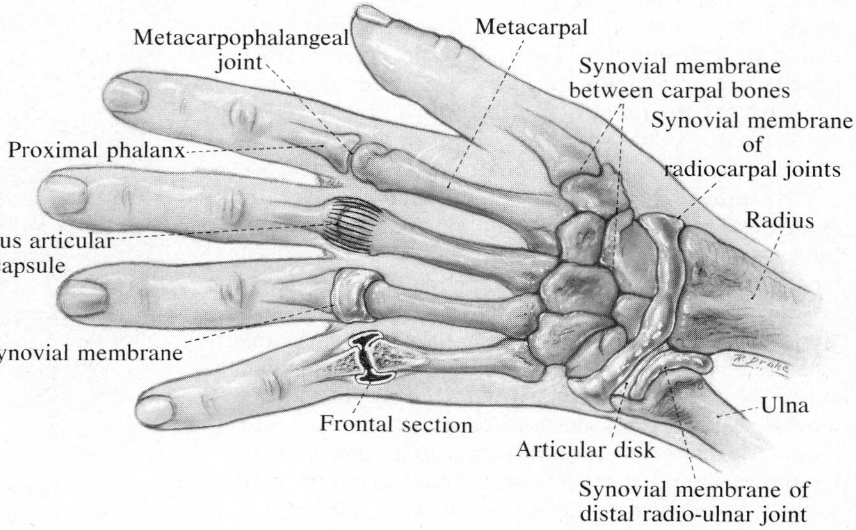


**Figure 24–6.** Illustration of the relationship of the synovial membranes of the wrist and carpal and metacarpal joints to the surrounding bony structures. (From Polley, H.F., and Hunder, G.G.: Rheumatologic Interviewing and Physical Examination of the Joints. Philadelphia, W.B. Saunders Company, 1978.)

of the deep fascia forms the proximal annular ligament in the sheath of the flexor tendons (proximal pulley).

Movements of the wrist include palmar flexion (flexion), dorsiflexion (extension), radial deviation, ulnar deviation, and circumduction. Pronation and supination of the hand and forearm occur primarily at the proximal and distal radioulnar joints. The only carpometacarpal joint that moves to any degree is the carpometacarpal joint of the thumb, which possesses the movements of a sellar joint. Crepitus at this joint is commmon in degenerative arthritis.

The wrist can normally be extended to about 70 degrees and flexed to 80 or 90 degrees. Ulnar deviation averages 50 degrees and radial deviation 20 to 30 degrees. Loss of dorsiflexion is the most incapacitating functional impairment of wrist motion.

*Stenosing tenosynovitis* at the radial styloid process (de Quervain's tenosynovitis) characteristically involves the long abductor and short extensor tendons of the thumb. Tenderness near the radial styloid process can be localized to these tendons by having the patient make a fist with the thumb in the palm of his hand. The examiner then moves the patient's wrist into ulnar deviation. The development of severe pain over the radial styloid is a positive Finkelstein's test and is caused by stretching the thumb tendons in the stenosed sheath.

*Carpal tunnel syndrome* results from pressure on the median nerve in the carpal tunnel and is discussed in detail in Chapter 110.

Muscle function of the wrist can be measured by testing flexion and extension, and supination and pronation of the forearm. Prime movers in wrist flexion are the flexor carpi radialis (C6, 7) and flexor carpi ulnaris (C8, T1) muscles. Each of these two muscles can be tested separately. This can be accomplished if the examiner provides resistance to flexion at the base of the second metacarpal bone in the direction of extension and ulnar deviation in the case of the flexor carpi radialis and resistance at the base of the fifth metacarpal in the direction of extension and radial deviation in the case of the flexor carpi ulnaris. The prime extensions of the wrist are the extensor carpi radialis longus (C6, 7), extensor carpi radialis brevis (C6, 7), and extensor carpi ulnaris (C7, 8) muscles. The radial and ulnar extensor muscles can also be tested separately. Prime movers in supination of the forearm are the biceps brachii (C5, 6) and supinator (C6). Prime movers in pronation are the pronator teres (C6, 7) and pronator quadratus (C8, T1).

**Metacarpophalangeal, Proximal, and Distal Interphalangeal Joints.** The metacarpophalangeal joints are hinge joints. Lateral collateral ligaments that are loose in extension tighten in flexion, thereby preventing lateral movement of the digits. The extensor tendons that cross the dorsum of each joint strengthen the articular capsule. When the extensor tendon of the digit reaches the distal end of the metacarpal head, it is joined by fibers of the interossei and lumbricales and expands over the entire dorsum of the metacarpophalangeal joint and on to the dorsum of the adjacent phalanx. This expansion of the extensor mechanism is known as the extensor hood.

The proximal and distal interphalangeal joints are also hinge joints. The ligaments of the interphalangeal joints resemble those of the metacarpophalangeal joints. When the fingers are flexed, the bases of the proximal phalanges slide toward the palmar side of the heads of the metacarpal bones. The metacarpal heads form the rounded prominences of the knuckles with the metacarpal joint spaces lying about 1 cm distal to the apices of the prominences.

The skin on the palmar surface of the hand is relatively thick and covers a fat pad between it and the metacarpophalangeal joint. This makes palpation of the palmar surface of the joint more difficult than the dorsal surfaces.

Swelling of the fingers may result from articular or periarticular causes. Synovial swelling produces symmetrical enlargement of a joint itself, whereas extra-articular swelling may be diffuse, extending beyond the joints, or asymmetrical, involving only one side of the digit or joint (Fig. 24–7). Chronic swelling and distention of the metacarpophalangeal joints tends to produce stretching and laxity of the articular capsule and ligaments. This laxity, combined with muscle imbalance and other forces, results in the extensor tendons of the digits slipping off the metacarpal heads to the ulnar sides of the joints. The abnormal pull of the displaced tendons is one of the factors that causes ulnar deviation of the fingers in chronic inflammatory arthritis.

"*Swan-neck*" deformity describes the appearance of a finger in which there is a flexion contracture of the metacarpophalangeal joint, hyperextension of the proximal interphalangeal joint, and flexion of the distal interphalangeal joint. These changes are produced by contraction of the interossei and other muscles that flex the metacarpophalangeal joints and extend the proximal interphalangeal joints. This deformity is characteristic of

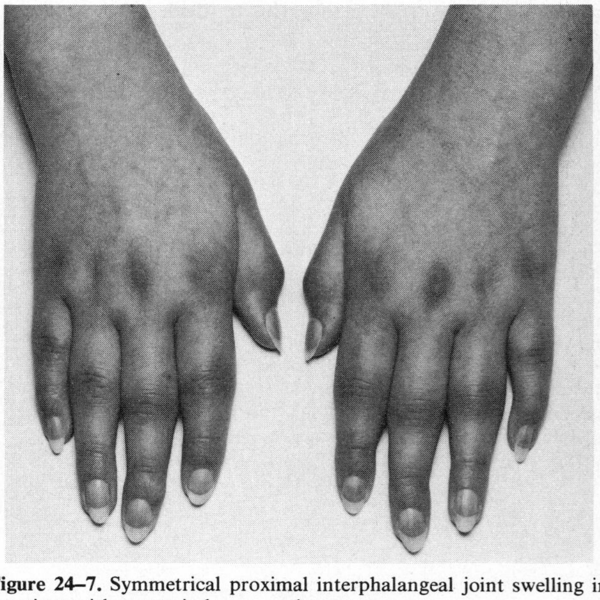

**Figure 24–7.** Symmetrical proximal interphalangeal joint swelling in a patient with systemic lupus erythematosus.

rheumatoid arthritis but may be seen in other chronic arthritides such as lupus erythematosus (Fig. 24–8).

The term "*boutonnière*" deformity is used to describe a finger with a flexion contracture of the proximal interphalangeal joint associated with hyperextension of the distal interphalangeal joint. The deformity is relatively common in rheumatoid arthritis and results when the central slip of the extensor tendon of the proximal interphalangeal joint becomes detached from the base of the middle phalanx, allowing palmar dislocation of the lateral bands. The dislocated bands cross the fulcrum of the joint and then act as flexors instead of extensors of the joint.

Another abnormality is "telescoping" or shortening of the digits produced by resorption of the ends of the phalanges secondary to destructive arthropathy. Shortening of the fingers is associated with wrinkling of the skin over involved joints and also is called "opera-glass hand" or "la main en lorgnette." Bony hypertrophic or osteophytic articular nodules on the distal interphalangeal joints are called *Heberden's nodes,* and when they are located on the proximal interphalangeal joints are called *Bouchard's nodes.*

The metacarpophalangeal joints are palpated on the dorsal aspect of the metacarpal heads on each side of the extensor tendons (Fig. 24–9) with the proximal phalanges flexed 20 to 30 degrees. Small amounts of swelling in one or more joints can best be detected by comparing the joints in question with others. Synovitis of metacarpophalangeal joints is often associated with lateral compression tenderness, which can be elicited by gently squeezing the patient's hand at the level of the joints.

The proximal and distal interphalangeal joints are best examined by palpating gently over the lateral and medial aspects of the joint where the flexor and extensor tendons do not interfere with assessment of the synovial membrane. Alternatively, the joint can be compressed anteroposteriorly by the thumb and index finger of one of the examiner's hands while the other thumb and index finger palpate for synovial distention medially and laterally (Fig. 24–10).

The presence of clubbing of the fingernails can be detected by repeated gentle palpation of the distal nail edge with one hand while using the other hand to palpate the proximal edge of the nail for elevation from the nail bed. Alternatively, the examiner can palpate the proximal edge of the patient's nail with the tip of one or more fingers or thumbs pointing distally (same direction as the patient's fingers). When clubbing is present, the proximal edge of the nail "floats" in its bed.

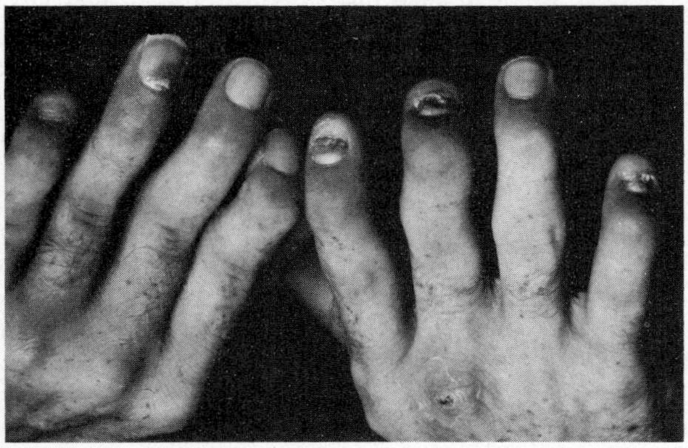

**Figure 24–8.** Swan neck deformities in a patient with chronic Reiter's syndrome.

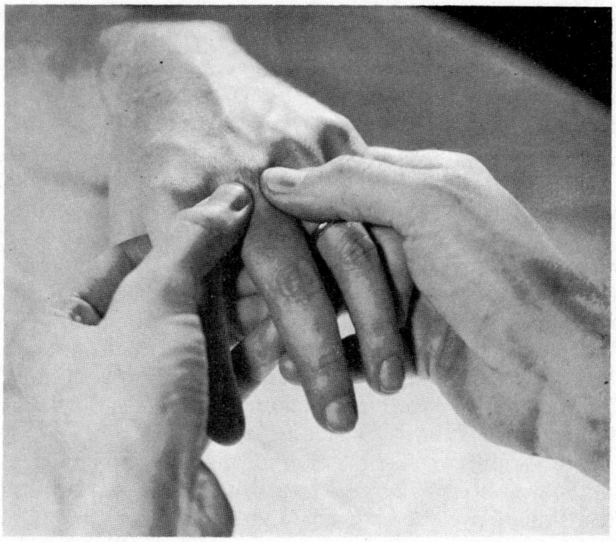

**Figure 24–9.** Palpation of the metacarpophalangeal joints. The examiner's thumbs palpate the dorsal aspect of the joint while the index fingers palpate the volar aspect of the metacarpal head. (From Polley, H.F., and Hunder, G.G.: Rheumatologic Interviewing and Physical Examination of the Joints. Philadelphia, W.B. Saunders Company, 1978.)

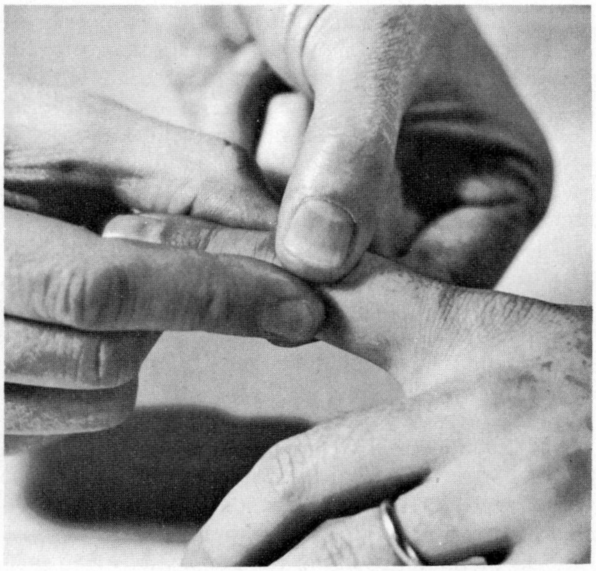

**Figure 24–10.** Palpation of the proximal interphalangeal joint. Anteroposterior compression of the joint by the examiner's thumb and index finger while the other thumb and index finger palpate for medial and lateral synovial distention. (From Polley, H.F., and Hunder, G.G.: Rheumatologic Interviewing and Physical Examination of the Joints. Philadelphia, W.B. Saunders Company, 1978.)

A general assessment of the strength of the hands can be made when the patient makes a tight fist by gripping two or more of the examiner's fingers. A more accurate measure, which can be used in comparative studies, is obtained having the patient squeeze a partially inflated sphygmomanometer (at 20 mm Hg).

It is often helpful to test strength of the fingers separately. The prime movers of flexion of the second through fifth metacarpophalangeal joints are the dorsal and palmar interosseus muscles (C8, T1). The lumbrical muscles (C6, 7, 8) flex the metacarpophalangeal joints when the proximal phalangeal joints are extended. The flexors of the proximal interphalangeal joints are the flexor digitorum superficialis muscles (C7, 8, T1) and the flexor of the distal interphalangeal joints is the flexor digitorum profundus muscle (C7, 8, T1).

The prime extensors of the metacarpophalangeal joints and interphalangeal joints of the second through fifth fingers are the extensor digitorum communis (C6, 7, 8), the extensor indicis proprius (C6, 7, 8), and the extensor digiti minimi (C7) muscles. The interossei and lumbrical muscles simultaneously flex the metacarpophalangeal joints and extend the interphalangeal joints. The dorsal interosseus muscles (C8, T1) and abductor digiti minimi (C8) abduct the fingers, whereas the palmar interosseus muscles adduct the fingers.

The thumb is moved by a number of muscles. Prime flexor of the first metacarpophalangeal joint is the flexor pollicus brevis muscle (C6, 7, 8, T1). The prime flexor of the first interphalangeal joint is the flexor pollicus longus muscle (C8, T1). The metacarpophalangeal joint of the thumb is extended by the extensor pollicus brevis muscle, and the prime extensor of the interphalangeal joint is the extensor pollicus longus muscle (C6-8).

The prime abductors of the thumb are the abductor pollicis longus (C6, 7) and the abductor pollicis brevis (C6, 7) muscles. Motion takes place primarily at the carpometacarpal joint. The prime mover in thumb adduction is the adductor pollicis muscle (C8, T1). Motion takes place primarily at the carpometacarpal joint. The prime movers in opposition of the thumb and fifth fingers are the opponens pollicis muscles (C6, 7) and opponens digiti minimi muscle (C8, T1).

**Spine and Sacroiliac Joints.** In conjunction with muscles and ligaments, the bony structure of the spinal column allows for upright posture and provides for flexion of the trunk and rotation of the head. The spine has four normal curves, including the two anterior convexities in the cervical and lumbar region and the two posterior convexities in the thoracic and sacrococcygeal regions. Each vertebra consists of two segments, the anterior portion, including the vertebral body and disc, and the posterior portion or vertebral arch. Details of spinal anatomy are found in Chapters 28 and 30.

The sacroiliac joints are of particular interest to rheumatologists. At the caudal end of the spine the triangular-shaped sacral segment of the vertebral column articulates with the bony pelvis via the sacroiliac joints. The sacroiliac joints function to transmit the upper body weight to the pelvis and legs. The upper two thirds of the joint is in an oblique plane and the tuberosities of the posterior iliac crests project medially beyond the joints and overlie them. The lower one third of the joint articulates in the anteroposterior plane with the ilium. Because of the bony shape of the joint and the strong ligaments there is essentially no motion across the sacroiliac joint in adults.

Additional stability of the vertebral column is provided for by ligaments. The strong anterior longitudinal ligament supplies reinforcement to the anterior annulus fibrosus and also limits spine extension. The posterior longitudinal ligament provides less support. Limitation of spinal flexion and lateral bending are provided by the interspinous ligaments. Between the laminae are the elastic ligamenta flava, which help return the vertebral column to its initial position after movement.

Motion of the spine is dependent upon multiple muscle groups. The intrinsic back muscles, including the long sacrospinalis, act as spine extensors. The abdominal wall muscles, including the internal and external obliques and the rectus abdominous, are the major flexors of the spine. They are assisted by muscles anterior to the spine, including the quadratus lumborum and the psoas muscles. Lateral bending and rotation occur with unilateral contraction of the abdominal and intrinsic back muscles with contralateral simultaneous relaxation.

The landmark surface anatomy of the back is important in order to localize the site of pathologic involvement. It is best appreciated with the patient standing with the entire back, posterior shoulder, and legs exposed to the examiner. The subject should stand in a relaxed manner with the feet slightly separated and the hips and knees fully extended. Arms should be at the sides. In the midline, the seventh cervical and first thoracic spinous processes are prominent at the base of the neck. Because of the caudal sloping projection of the thoracic spinous processes, the tips of the spinous processes overlie the adjacent inferior thoracic vertebral body. In the lumbar region, the spinous processes overlie the corresponding vertebral body. With the arms relaxed and held at the sides, the inferior angles of the scapulae lie in the horizontal line that intersects the spine of the seventh thoracic vertebra. The horizontal line between the highest point of each iliac crest intersects the fourth lumbar vertebra. The sacral dimples overlie the posterior superior iliac spines and mark the level of the second sacral vertebra. Medial to the posterior superior iliac spine is the mid portion of the sacroiliac joint.

Inspection of the spine from behind includes notation of scars, asymmetry of shoulder elevation, scapular prominence, height of iliac crests, and gluteal creases. The examiner should draw an imaginary vertical line from the first thoracic process to the sacrum. If the line does not fall on the sacral midline, a lateral list of spinal tilt is present. A compensatory scoliosis may obscure a lateral tilt.

If a scoliosis is present, it is described by the direction of the convexity. A functional versus structural scoliosis should be differentiated by examining the patient in a forward bending position. While a functional scoliosis will disappear, a structural scoliosis will not, and may actually be accentuated. A rotational thoracic scoliosis will create a prominent hump on the side of the convexity. At times, a very mild curvature may not be appreciated unless the thorax is observed with the examiner seated in front of the patient who bends forward with the arms extended in front of the body. Similarly, while a lumbar scoliosis may cause prominence of the sacrospinalis muscle on the side of the convexity, a mild curve may be appreciated only by careful palpation of the spinous processes.

Pelvic tilt may accompany a scoliosis. This is identified by noting one superior iliac crest higher than the other. The scoliotic convexity will be toward the lower side. If the pelvic tilt and scoliosis are related to an anatomic leg length discrepancy, they should be abolished by leveling the pelvis with support under the short leg. With the pelvis leveled, a persistent scoliosis is related to spinal column disease.

Additional spinal deformities are noted by observing the patient from the side. Thoracic kyphosis may be either structural or postural. In young persons, elimination of postural kyphosis may be observed with the patient lying in the prone position of hyperextending the spine or with the patient standing with the shoulders back. In older adults with postural kyphosis correction may not be possible. In addition, a postural kyphosis tends to cause a smooth symmetrical forward curve of the spine with forward bending, while a structural kyphosis may appear to originate at a specific segmental level. Hyperlordosis, loss of lordosis, forward pelvic tilt, and head protrusion are also best observed from the side.

Muscle spasm may be recognized by prominent paravertebral musculature, usually asymmetrical. While palpation can be performed with the patient erect, fixed spasm is best appreciated with the patient prone with a pillow under the abdomen. Palpation should begin at a site distant to the location of pain and discomfort, as indicated by the patient. This will allow assessment of general muscle tone and the overall level of the patient's reactivity and pain tolerance. To localize areas of tenderness, it is important to use a systematic approach to palpation, beginning with the spinous processes. Localized levels of bony tenderness should be noted, as well as levels of step-off as observed in spondylolisthesis. Bony palpation is then followed by palpation of the paravertebral musculature. Additional sites of tenderness, such as fatty nodules or ligaments, should be noted. The buttock is palpated for areas of gluteus muscle attachment tenderness, trochanteric bursitis, ischial tuberosity bursitis, and sciatic notch tenderness. Percussion of tender areas may help localize the painful structures. Tenderness elicited by reflex hammer or fingertip percussion over a vertebral body suggests disease in that specific spinal segment.

Observation of lumbar spine range of motion is performed with the examiner standing to the side of and behind the patient. With the knees kept straight, the patient is instructed to bend forward to attempt to touch the floor. Normally, a flattening of the lumbar lordosis will occur; persistence of lordosis suggests paravertebral muscle spasm or intrinsic spine deformity. Although the recording of the finger-to-floor distance is often cited as a method of estimating lumbar spine flexion, it is inaccurate, since the majority of motion measured is due to hip flexion. The contribution made by hip flexion may be eliminated by grasping the patient around the hips to stabilize the pelvis. Lumbar flexion is normally up to 45 degrees.

The *Schober test,* as used by Moll and Wright, is another method for reproducibly measuring lumbar flexion.[3] It is commonly employed to evaluate spondylitis. A skin mark is placed in the midline at the level of the sacral dimples. Two additional marks are placed 10 cm above and 5 cm below the first mark. The patient is then instructed to bend forward as far as possible. The distance between the upper and lower marks is measured and the difference between the resting 15 cm and flexion measurement is calculated. Normal distraction of the marks is 5 cm. Movement of the marks less than 5 cm indicates abnormally decreased lumbar spine flexion secondary to enthesopathy or to hyperostosis or severe muscle spasm.

With forward flexion, the ease with which the patient moves should be observed. "Corkscrewing," with rotation to one side during flexion, suggests muscle spasm. A break in the normal rhythm of motion should be noted, such as a catch with resuming the upright position, in which the patient completes the motion of standing upright by bending the hips and knees to move the pelvis under the spine, rather than to further extend a painful spine. Corkscrew motion and catching are most often seen in lumbar disc disease. Lateral bending is observed with the examiner standing behind the patient. The patient should stand with feet apart and bend by sliding the hand down the lateral thigh. Lateral bending is estimated by observing the degrees of distraction from vertical of an imaginary line from the lumbosacral level to the occiput. Motion may be estimated in degrees, with normal to 30 degrees or more.

Extension is performed with the physician stabilizing the pelvis with one hand firmly over the sacrum and the other over the upper anterior thigh. With extension, the normal lordosis should increase. Motion is estimated in degrees, and the normal is up to 30 to 40 degrees from the vertical.

Thoracolumbar spine motion may be estimated by the degree of spine rotation. With the physician stabilizing the pelvis, motion is recorded in degrees; normal rotation is 30 degrees or more. With the exception of rotation, the use of goniometer usually does not provide any improvement in estimation of degrees of spinal motion.[4]

Costovertebral motion, often reduced in ankylosing spondylitis, is estimated by the change in chest circumference with inspiration and expiration. The usual site for measuring chest motion is at the nipple line in males and just above the line in females. The extent of chest expansion from full expiration to full inspiration is measured with a tape measure. Normally, there is at least a 5 to 6 cm difference in healthy young adults.

The sacroiliac joint is first evaluated by identifying the joint with palpation. The joint is under the sacral dimple or is found by palpating medially to the posterior iliac spine. The *Gaenslen test* is performed as the patient lies at the edge of the table. In this test the leg and thigh closest to the edge are hyperextended over the side of the table by lowering toward the floor. The other leg is held in a knee chest position by the patient in order to fix the pelvis. If the sacroiliac joint is the origin of the patient's back pain, the maneuver will elicit pain in the joint on the hyperextended side. The maneuver is repeated by hyperextending the other leg over the other side of the table. The sacroiliac joint can also be stressed by applying pelvic compression. The patient is instructed to lie on his side. The examiner places downward compression against the lateral iliac crest. Caution should be exercised in the interpretation of these maneuvers to examine the sacroiliac joints. A recent prospective study has shown that they lack specificity and are not capable of distinguishing sacroiliac pathology from other causes of low back pain.[5]

Examination of the patient with back pain should always include a neurologic examination, including reflexes, straight leg raising, muscle strength, and sensory testing. In performing the tests for straight leg raising, the examiner should not interpret the occurrence of all lumbosacral pain as a positive test, since pelvic rotation with leg raising will cause pain in a diseased lumbrosacral segment. In addition, pain in the posterior thigh caused by tight hamstrings should not be confused with a positive test. Pain aggravated by ankle dorsiflexion and relieved by knee flexion supports a positive straight leg test. The bowstring test is good supporting evidence for root tension: With the knee flexed and the pain relieved, firm pressure applied by the thumbs into the popliteal space may reproduce the pain. The crossed straight leg test, in which the elevation of the uninvolved leg causes pain in the opposite affected leg, is a reliable sign of nerve root tension.

Because low back pain is often a social problem involving medical-legal or work disability issues, the examiner should be aware of signs during the examination that suggest a nonorganic basis to the patient's complaints. A group of five standardized nonorganic signs has been suggested in which the presence of three or more is thought to be significant.[6] First, tenderness over a wide area of skin to light pinching, as well as extensive deep tenderness over more than one anatomic structure, suggests nonorganic tenderness. Second, simulation of movements that created pain during the examination should be performed in a manner by which the actual structure does not move. These include painful axial loading of the lumbar spine by placing downward pressure on the patient's skull, and the provocation of back pain by rotating both the shoulders and pelvis in the same plane. Third, the examiner should use distraction testing, in which a painful part of the examination is repeated in another painless manner. Fourth, regional weakness and sensory changes in a nonanatomic distribution are important to note, as well as cogwheel giving way on muscle testing. Fifth, overreaction to minimal stimuli should be noted.

No examination of the patient with low back pain is complete without an abdominal examination for masses and aortic aneurysms and a pelvic-rectal examination. The supine lithotomy position is best for providing an adequate rectal examination of the coccyx, sacrum, and surrounding tissues. Tenderness of the piriformis muscle, as seen in pelvic floor myalgias or the piriformis syndrome, should be noted.[7] The coccyx may be palpated for tenderness and mobility with the index finger in the rectum and the thumb outside.

Cervical spine motion is measured by observing flexion and extension (nodding), supplied primarily by the atlantooccipital joint; rotation, primarily the atlantoaxial joint; and lateral bending motion from the C2-7. Flexion of the chin towards the chest is normally about 45 degrees; rotation of the chin towards the shoulder is about 60 to 90 degrees and extension is about 50 to 60 degrees. Lateral bending with the head towards the shoulder should be performed without elevation of the ipsilateral shoulder girdle. Pain occurring on the ipsilateral side of the neck with lateral bending suggest apophyseal joint disease, while the presence of contralateral pain suggests a muscular or ligamentous origin.

The cervical spinous processes can be palpated from C2 to C7. C1 is not palpable. The surrounding soft tissue should be palpated for tenderness and spasm. Palpation should extend to include the trapezius muscles, interscapular musculature, and sternocleidomastoid muscles. It is important to palpate for greater occipital nerve tenderness at the base of the occiput in patients with occipital headaches or pain.

In evaluating patients with possible cervical radicular symptoms, the *foramen compression test*, or *Spurling maneuver*, is used. This examination should only be done after radiographic examination of the cervical spine has been performed and fractures or lytic lesions of the vertebrae or odontoid are known to be absent. The patient's head is placed in hyperextension or tilted toward the side of the radicular symptoms. Pressure is placed on the top of the patient's skull for 10 seconds. The test is positive if the symptoms are reproduced or aggravated by the maneuver.

Atlantoaxial subluxation may be observed at times by noticing a change in the smooth rhythm of flexion and extension. The patient may be aware of a clicking or jerking sensation. The jerking motion may be observed or palpated in the upper cervical spine. The subluxation may be palpated using a finger to examine the patient's posterior pharyngeal wall while the neck moves in flexion and extension. Radiographic analysis of the cervical spine in flexion and extension remains the most accurate means of assessing subluxation.

The occiput-to-wall measurement as well as overall

height of the patient is a useful test for following upper spine involvement in ankylosing spondylitis. The patient is instructed to stand with the back against the wall and heels as close to the wall as possible. With the chin level, the neck is extended to bring the occiput to the wall. The distance remaining between the head and the wall is measured in centimeters.

**Hip.** The hip joint is a spheroidal or ball and socket joint consisting of the rounded head of the femur and the cup-shaped acetabulum (see also Chapter 120). Stability of the joint is ensured by the fibrocartilaginous rim of the glenoid labrum and the dense articular capsule and surrounding ligaments, including the iliofemoral, pubofemoral, and ischiocapsular ligaments that reinforce the capsule. The hip joint is also surrounded by powerful muscle groups. The primary hip flexor is the iliopsoas muscle assisted by the sartorius and the rectus femoris muscles. Hip adduction is accomplished by the three adductors, the longus, brevis, and magnus plus the gracilis and pectineus muscles. The gluteus medius is the major hip abductor, while the gluteus maximus and hamstrings extend the hip. There are several clinically important bursae about the hip joint. Anteriorly, the iliopsoas bursa lies between the psoas muscle and the joint surface. The trochanteric bursa lies between the gluteus maximus muscle and the posterolateral greater trochanter, and the ischiogluteal bursa overlies the ischial tuberosity.

Examination of the hip begins by observing the patient's stance and gait. The patient should stand in front of the examiner so that the anterior iliac spines are visible. If pelvic tilt or obliquity is present, it may be related to a structural scoliosis, anatomic leg length discrepancy, or hip disease. Hip contractures may result in abduction or adduction deformities. To compensate for an adduction contracture, the pelvis is tilted upward on the side of the contracture. This allows the legs to be parallel during walking and weight bearing. With a fixed abduction deformity, the pelvis becomes elevated on the normal side during standing or walking. This causes an apparent shortening of the normal leg and forces the patient to stand or walk on the toes of the normal side or to flex the knee on the abnormal leg.

Viewed from the rear, with the legs parallel, the patient with hip disease and an adducted hip contracture may have asymmetrical gluteal folds due to pelvic tilt with the diseased side elevated. In this situation, the patient is unable to stand with the foot of the involved leg flat on the floor. In abduction contracture, the findings are reversed; with both legs extended and parallel the uninvolved side is elevated.

A hip flexion deformity commonly occurs in diseases of the hip but is often overlooked. Unilateral flexion of the hip in the standing position reduces weight bearing on the involved side, and relaxes the joint capsule, causing less pain. This posture may be noted when observing the patient from the side. There is a hyperlordotic curve of the lumbar spine to compensate for lack of full hip extension.

The patient with possible hip disease should be observed walking. With a normal gait, the abductors of the weight-bearing leg contract to hold the pelvis level or elevate the non-weight-bearing side slightly. Two abnormalities of gait may be observed in hip disease. With a painful hip, the most common abnormality is the antalgic gait. In this gait, the person leans over the diseased hip during the phase of weight bearing on that hip, placing the body weight directly over the joint to avoid painful contraction of the hip abductors. Alternatively, a Trendelenburg gait may develop. Here, with weight bearing on the affected side, the pelvis drops and the trunk shifts to the normal side. While the antalgic gait is said to be seen with painful hips and the Trendelenburg gait in conditions with weak hip abductors, neither gait is specific and either accompanies a painful hip.

The *Trendelenburg test* is a measure of the gluteus medius hip abductor weakness. The patient is asked to stand bearing weight only on the involved side. Normally, the abductors will hold the pelvis level or the nonsupported side slightly elevated. If the non-weight-bearing side drops, the test is positive for weakness of the weight-bearing gluteus medius. This test is nonspecific and may be observed in primary neurologic or muscle disorders or in a variety of hip diseases, leading to weakness of the abductors, including coxa vara, congenital dislocation, slipped capital femoral epiphysis, or femoral neck fracture. A mild Trendelenburg gait is seen commonly in normal persons.

The patient is next examined in the supine position. The presence of a hip flexion contracture is suggested by persistence of lumbar lordosis and pelvic tilt, masking the contracture by allowing the involved leg to remain in contact with the examination table. The *Thomas test* will demonstrate the flexion contracture. In this test the opposite hip is fully flexed, to flatten the lumbar lordosis and fix the pelvis. The involved leg should then be extended towards the table as far as possible. The diseased hip's flexion contracture will become more obvious and can be estimated in degrees from full extension. While the patient is supine, measurement for leg length discrepancy is performed with the legs fully extended. To detect true leg length discrepancy, each leg is measured from the anterior superior iliac spine to the medial malleolus. A difference of 1 cm or less is unlikely to cause any abnormality of gait. An apparent leg length discrepancy may result from pelvic tilt or abduction or adduction contractures of the hip.

The hip joint range of motion includes flexion, extension, abduction, adduction, and internal and external rotation and circumduction. The degree of flexion permitted varies with the manner in which it is assessed. When the knee is held flexed 90 degrees, the hip normally flexes to an angle of 120 degrees between the thigh and long axis of the body. If the knee is held in extension, the hamstrings limit the hip flexion to about 90 degrees. Abduction is measured with the patient still supine with the leg in an extended position perpendicular to the pelvis. Pelvic stabilization is achieved by placing one arm across the pelvis with the hand on the opposite anterior iliac spine. With the other hand, the examiner grasps the patient's ankle and abducts the leg until the pelvis is noted to begin moving. Normally, abduction is to approximately 45 degrees. The maneuver is repeated on the other side. The examiner may also stand at the foot of the table, grasp both ankles and simultaneously abduct the legs. Differences between the two hips can be appreciated, and the intermalleolar distance is measured. Abduction is commonly limited in hip joint disease. Adduction is tested by grasping the ankle and raising the leg off the examination table by flexing the hip enough to allow the tested leg to cross over the opposite leg. Normal adduction is to about 20 to 30 degrees. Hip rotation may be tested with both hip and knee flexed to 90 degrees or with the leg extended. In the flexed position, external rotation is performed by moving the foot medially and internal rotation is performed by moving the foot laterally.

Normal hip external rotation is to 45 degrees, and internal rotation is to 40 degrees. These figures vary somewhat in normals. There is also a difference in rotation between the flexed and extended hip. Owing to the increased stabilization of the joint by the surrounding ligaments in the extended position, rotation decreases with extension. To test hip rotation, the extended leg is grasped above the ankle and rotated externally and internally from the neutral position. Limitation of internal rotation of the hip is a very sensitive indicator of hip joint disease.

Extension is tested with the patient in the prone position. Estimating actual hip joint extension can be difficult, since some of the apparent motion arises from hyperextension of the lumbar spine, pelvis rotation, motion of the buttock soft tissue, and flexion of the opposite hip. The pelvis and lumbar spine are partially immobilized by placing one arm across the posterior iliac crest and lower lumbar spine. The examiner places the other hand under the thigh with the knee flexed and hyperextends the thigh. Normal extension ranges up to 10 to 20 degrees. Limitation of extension is most often secondary to a hip flexion contracture.

The iliotibial band is a part of the fascia lata extending from the iliac crest, sacrum, and ischium over the greater trochanter to the lateral femoral condyle, tibial condyle, and fibular head and along the lateral intermuscular system, separating the hamstrings from the vastus lateralis. The tensor fascia lata may cause an audible snap as it slips over the greater trochanter if the weight-bearing leg moves from hip flexion and adduction to a neutral position, as in climbing stairs. Most commonly observed in young women, the "snapping" hip usually does not cause any significant degree of pain.

In patients complaining of lateral hip pain, the soft tissues over the greater trochanter should be palpated for tenderness. The lateral surface of the trochanter is tender in cases of trochanteric bursitis. Swelling occasionally may be palpable and helps to differentiate actual bursitis from gluteus tendinitis or attachment tenderness in which there is posterolateral trochanteric tenderness without swelling. If lateral tenderness without swelling is present, differentiation between the two conditions can be difficult. The pain of trochanteric bursitis is aggravated by actively resisted abduction of the hip.

Patients complaining of anterior hip or groin pain should be examined for iliopsoas bursitis. Swelling and tenderness may be noted in the middle one third of the inguinal ligament lateral to the femoral pulse. The pain is aggravated by hip extension and reduced by flexion. The bursitis may be a localized problem or represent extension of hip synovitis to the bursa, since there is communication between the two structures in approximately 15 percent of cases. In the latter instance, the bursitis actually represents a synovial cyst. It is impossible to differentiate a bursitis from a cyst on examination. If the patient is tender in the region of the iliopsoas bursa but no swelling is palpable, it is not possible to differentiate this condition from an overlying tendonitis of the iliopsoas muscle. The inguinal region should be carefully palpated for other abnormalities such as hernias, femoral aneurysms, adenopathy, tumor, and psoas abscess masses.

Muscle strength testing should include the hip flexors, extensors, abductors, and adductors. The primary hip flexor is the iliopsoas muscle (L2, L3). Flexion may be tested with the patient sitting at the end of the table. The pelvis is stabilized by placing one hand on the ipsilateral iliac crest while the patient actively flexes the hip. The examiner uses the other hand to exert downward pressure against the thigh proximal to the knee. A second approach is to have the patient assume the supine position and hold the leg to be tested in 90 degrees of flexion at the hip while the examiner attempts to straighten the hip. Hip extension is tested with the patient lying prone. The primary hip extensor is the gluteus maximus muscle (L5, S1). With the knee flexed to remove hamstring action, the patient is instructed to extend the hip and thigh off the surface of the table as the examiner places one forearm across the posterior iliac crest to stabilize the pelvis while the other hand presses down against the thigh. The major hip abductor is the gluteus medius (L4, L5). Hip abductor strength is tested with the patient lying on his side. The upper abducting leg should be slightly extended to eliminate contribution from the hip flexors and tensor fascia lata. The examiner must stabilize the pelvis by placing one hand downward against the iliac crest to prevent the lateral trunk muscles from elevating the pelvis and leg off the table. The patient is instructed to abduct the thigh and leg while the examiner places downward pressure with his other hand against the distal lateral thigh. The leg nearest the table is then tested for hip adduction. The primary adductor is the adductor longus (L3, L4). The examiner holds the upper leg in slight abduction while the patient adducts the lower leg off the table against the resistance of the examiner's other hand proximal to the knee.

An alternative method for testing abduction and adduction enables the examiner to compare the two legs simultaneously. The patient lies supine with the legs fully extended and the hips moderately abducted. To test abduction, the patient actively pushes out against the examiners resistance against the lateral malleoli. Adduction is tested by movement against resistance at the medial malleoli.

**Knee.** The knee is a compound condylar joint with three articulations, the patellofemoral and the lateral and medial tibial femoral condyles with their fibrocartilaginous menisci. The joint is stabilized by the articular capsule, the ligamentum patellae, the medial and lateral collateral and anterior and posterior cruciate ligaments. The collateral ligaments provide medial and lateral stability, while the cruciates provide anteroposterior support and rotatory stability. Normal knee motion is a combination of flexion or extension and rotation. With flexion the tibia internally rotates, and with extension it externally rotates on the femur. The surrounding synovial membrane is the largest of any of the body's joints; it extends up to 6 cm proximal to the joint as the suprapatellar pouch beneath the quadriceps femoris muscle. There are several clinically significant bursae about the knee, including the superficial prepatellar bursa, the superficial and deep infrapatellar bursae, the anserine bursa distal to the medial tibial plateau, and the posterior medial semimembranous and posterolateral gastrocnemius bursae (Fig. 24–11). Knee extension is provided for primarily by the quadriceps femoris muscle and flexion by the hamstrings. The biceps femoris externally rotates the lower leg on the femur, while the popliteus and semitendinous muscles supply internal rotation.

Examination of the knees should always include observation of the standing patient. Weight bearing will place deforming stress on the knees. *Genu varum* or lateral deviation of the knee joint (with medial deviation of the lower leg), *genu valgum* or medial deviation of the knee (and lateral deviation of the lower leg), and genu recurvatum or posterior bowing are often more easily appreciated in the standing patient. Limp, flexion contracture, locking, or giving away should be noted. Locking is the sudden loss of ability to extend the knee; it is painful and may be associated with an audible noise such as a click, pop, or snap.

Asymmetry from swelling or muscle atrophy may be noted on initial inspection. Patellar malalignment should be noted, including high-riding or laterally displaced patellas. The examiner should inspect the knee from the rear to identify popliteal swelling due to a popliteal or Baker's cyst, which is most commonly a medial semimembranous bursal swelling. If the calves appear asymmetric, measurement of calf circumference should be performed when the patient is lying on the examination table. Popliteal cysts may dissect down into the calf muscles, producing enlargement and palpable fullness. Edema may be present if the cyst causes secondary venous or lymphatic obstruction. Acute dissection or rupture of a popliteal cyst can mimic thrombophlebitis, the so-called pseudothrombophlebitis syndrome, with local pain, heat, redness, and swelling.

The patient is next examined in the supine position. Inability to fully extend the knee may be related to a flexion contracture or a large synovial effusion. Suprapatellar swelling with fullness of the distal anterior thigh that obliterates the normal depressed contours along the side of the patella usually indicates a knee joint effusion or synovitis. Localized swelling over the surface of the patella is generally secondary to prepatellar bursitis, while localized anterolateral or medial swelling along the joint line may represent cystic swelling of menisci.

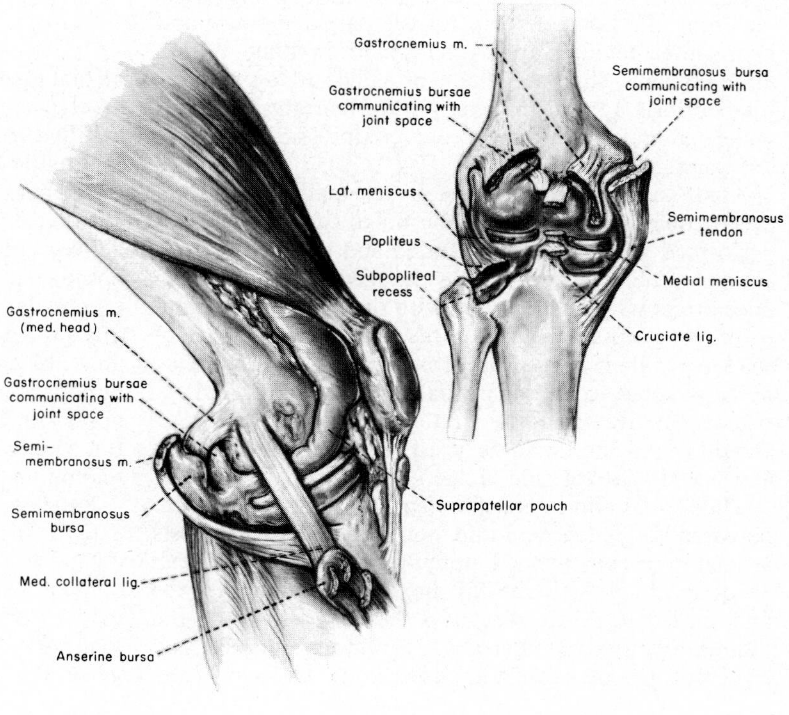


**Figure 24–11.** Medial and posterior aspects of the knee with important muscle attachments and bursae illustrated. (From Polley, H.F., and Hunder, G.G.: Rheumatologic Interviewing and Physical Examination of the Joints. Philadelphia, W.B. Saunders Company, 1978.)

Quadriceps femoris muscle atrophy usually develops in chronic arthritis of the knee. Atrophy of the vastus medalis is the earliest change and may be appreciated by comparing the two thighs for medial asymmetry and circumference. Usually measurement of the thigh circumference is performed at approximately 15 cm above the joint to avoid spurious results due to suprapatellar effusions.

To adequately palpate the knee, the joint must be relaxed. This is usually best accomplished with the patient supine, and the knees fully extended as possible and not touching. Palpation should begin over the anterior thigh approximately 10 cm above the patella. In order to identify the superior margin of the suprapatellar pouch, which is an extension of the knee joint cavity, the examiner should palpate the tissues moving distally towards the knee. Swelling, warmth, thickness, nodules, loose bodies, tenderness, should be noted. A thickened synovial membrane has a "boggy," doughy consistency different from the surrounding soft tissue and muscle. It is usually palpated earlier over the medial aspect of the suprapatellar pouch and medial tibiofemoral joint. To enhance detection of knee fluid, any fluid in the suprapatellar pouch is compressed with the palm of one hand placed just proximal to the patella. The synovial fluid forced into the inferior distal articular cavity is then palpated with the opposite thumb and index finger laterally and medially to the patella. If the examiner alternates compression and release of the suprapatellar pouch, the synovial thickening can be differentiated from a synovial effusion, since the effusion will intermittently distend the joint capsule under the thumb and index finger of the opposite hand, while the synovial thickening will not. The examiner should be cautious not to compress the suprapatellar pouch too firmly or push the tissues distally because the patella or normal soft tissue, including the fat pads, will fill the palpated space and be misinterpreted as synovitis or joint swelling. With a large effusion, the patella can be ballotted by pushing it posteriorly against the femur with the right forefinger while maintaining suprapatellar compression with the left hand.

At the other extreme, effusions as small as 4 to 8 ml can be detected by eliciting the bulge sign. This test is performed with the knee extended and relaxed. The examiner strokes or compresses the medial aspect of the knee proximally and laterally with the palm of one hand to move the fluid from the area. The lateral aspect of the knee is then tapped or stroked, and a fluid wave or bulge is noted to appear medially (Fig. 24–12*A* and *B*). If not positive with the first attempt, the maneuver should be repeated with the pressure applied to the other areas of the lateral side of the knee.

The medial and lateral tibiofemoral joint margins are palpated for tenderness and bony lipping or exostosis as seen in osteoarthritis. Palpating the joint margins can be done easily with the hip flexed to 45 degrees, the knee flexed to 90 degrees, and the foot resting on the examining table. Tenderness over joint margins may represent articular cartilage disease, involvement of the medial meniscus or anterior cruciate ligament, or lateral involvement of the collateral ligament, iliotibial band, or fibial head.

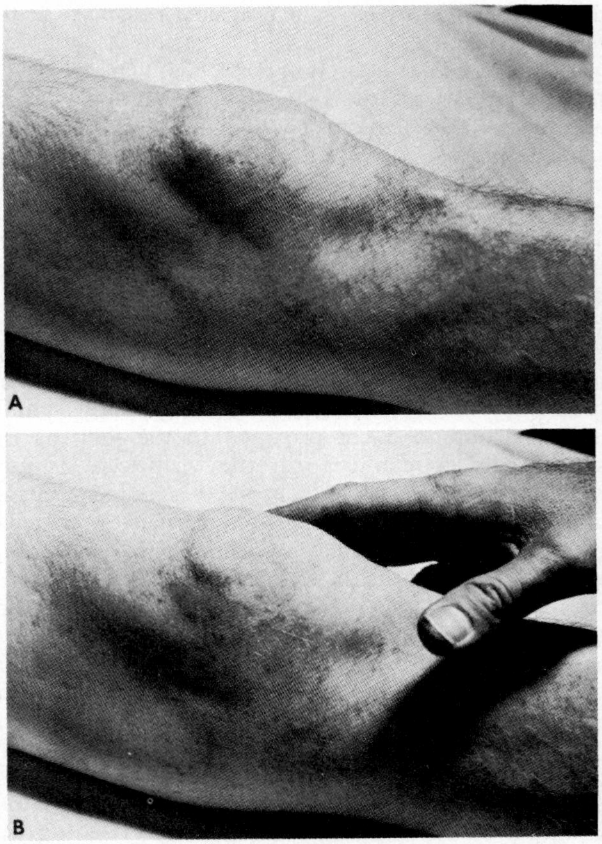

A

B

**Figure 24–12.** Demonstration of the bulge sign for a small synovial knee effusion. The medial aspect of the knee has been shaded to move the synovial fluid from this area (shaded depressed area in *A*). *B* shows bulge in previously shaded area after lateral aspect of the knee has been happed. (From Polley, H.F., and Hunder, G.G.: Rheumatologic Interviewing and Physical Examination of the Joints. Philadelphia, W.B. Saunders Company, 1978.)

Bursitis can be differentiated from articular synovitis by palpation of localized tenderness and swelling. The anserine bursa is located at the medial tibial plateau between the medial collateral ligament and the tendons of the sartorius, gracilis, and semitendinous muscles. The prepatellar bursa, if quite swollen, can be mistakenly interpreted as knee joint synovitis unless the bursal margins are carefully outlined by palpation. Infrapatellar bursitis is palpated either overlying the infrapatellar tendon at the level of the tibia (superficial) or lying beneath the tendon (deep). The infrapatellar fat pad beneath the tendon at the level of the joint line may also be tender.

Patellar palpation is best performed with the knee extended and relaxed. The patella is compressed and moved so that its entire articular surface will come into contact with the underlying femur. Slight crepitation may be observed in many normally functioning knees. Pain with crepitation may suggest patellofemoral degenerative arthritis or chondromalacia patellae. Retropatellar pain occurring with active knee flexion and extension and secondary to patellofemoral disease may be differentiated from tibiofemoral articular pain. To test this the examiner should attempt to lift the patella away from the knee while passively moving it through range of motion. Painless motion during this maneuver indicates that the patellofemoral joint is the source of the difficulty. In addition, the *patellar inhibition test* will also help to clarify the presence of patellofemoral arthritis. In this test the examiner compresses the patella distally away from the femoral condyles while instructing the patient to isometrically contract the quadriceps. Sudden patellar pain and quadriceps relaxation are interpreted as a positive test for chondromalacia, but frequency of false positives is very high.

The patella should be checked for stability in patients suspected of having recurrent patellar dislocation. The patella is pushed laterally with the patient supine and the knee extended and relaxed. A distressed reaction from the patient is considered a positive *apprehension test.* Subluxation of the patella can also be appreciated while moving the knee through range of motion from 0 to 90 degrees flexion or back to full extension.

Another cause of joint snapping and symptoms suggesting an internal derangement is the *plica syndrome* caused by bands of synovial tissue.[8] In cases of mediopatellar plica syndrome, a tender bandlike structure may be palpated parallel to the medial border of the patella. During flexion and extension, a palpable or audible snap is appreciated. Patellar crepitance may also be noted.

Ligamentous instability is tested by applying valgus and varus stress to the knee and by using the drawer test. The knee should be extended and relaxed. The *abduction* or *valgus test* is performed by stabilizing the lower femur while placing a valgus stress on the knee by abducting the lower leg with the other hand placed proximal to the ankle. A medial joint line separation with the knee fully extended indicates a tear of the medial compartment ligaments plus the posterior cruciate ligament. The test is then performed with the knee in 30 degrees of flexion. If the test is negative at 0 degrees but positive at 30 degrees, the instability represents a tear of the medial compartment ligaments with the posterior cruciate ligament remaining intact. The adduction or varus test is then performed at 0 degrees. Separation of the lateral joint line indicates a lateral compartment ligament tear with an associated tear of the posterior cruciate ligament. Rotatory instability of the knee may also exist. The *jerk test* measures anterolateral instability.[9] With the hip flexed to 45 degrees and the knee to 90 degrees, the tibia is internally rotated while valgus stress is applied to the knee. The leg is extended and at approximately 30 degrees of flexion subluxation of the lateral femorotibial articulation is appreciated. With further extension, the articulation relocates. The change in acceleration rate of the two joint surfaces (during the maneuver) is felt as a sudden jerk.

The degree of ligamentous laxity observed during testing should be graded on a scale of 1 to 3.[9] A mild grade 1 instability indicates that the joint surfaces separate 5 mm or less; moderate grade 2 represents a separation of 5 to 10 mm. A severe instability, grade 3, is a separation greater than 10 mm. In cases of trauma, opening of the joint space indicates ligamentous instability secondary to rupture or stretching of the ligaments. However, in cases of chronic arthritis of the tibiofemoral compartment, there may be apparent medial or lateral separation due to the "pseudolaxity" created by loss of cartilage and bone. If the ligaments are intact, the resulting degree of valgus or varus displacement with stressing will not be any greater than in the normal knee.

The *drawer test* is performed with the hip flexed to 45 degrees and the knee to 90 degrees. To stabilize the knee, the examiner either sits on the foot while grasping the posterior calf with both hands or supports the lower leg between his lateral chest wall and forearm. The anterior drawer test is performed by pulling the tibia forward. This maneuver has been said to test whether the anterior cruciate ligament is intact. However, anterior subluxation may actually represent more complex instability.[9] With the tibia in neutral, a positive anterior drawer test in which the lateral tibial plateau subluxes forward while the medial stays in normal position represent anterolateral rotatory instability. If both plateaus sublux, tears of the middle one third of the medial and lateral capsular ligaments are present. If the subluxation is not present with the tibia internally rotated, the posterior cruciate ligament is intact. A positive anterior drawer test with the leg in external rotation represents a tear of the medial capsular ligament. A posterior drawer test in a chronically unstable knee suggests that damage has occurred to the posterior cruciate ligament.

Meniscal injury should also be tested for during the survey for joint instability. Symptoms that suggest a meniscal tear include locking during extension, joint clicking or popping during motion, and localized line tenderness along the joint. To examine the medial meniscus, the medial tibiofemoral joint line should be palpated with the lower leg internally rotated and the knee flexed to 90 degrees. Localized tenderness suggests involvement of the medial meniscus. With the knee flexed to 90 degrees, the lateral joint line is palpated for localized tenderness that would indicate lateral meniscal injury. The *McMurray test* is performed to elicit evidence of a posterior meniscal tear. In this, the patient's knee is placed in full extension and the examiner places one hand over the knee with the fingers along the side of the knee along one joint line and the thumb along the other side. The other hand holds the leg at the ankle and is used to flex, extend, and rotate the lower leg. With the knee flexed and the lower leg externally rotated 15 degrees, a palpable or audible snap occurring when the knee is extended from full to 90 degrees of flexion is a positive test and suggests a tear of the medial meniscus. A lateral snap or click occurring with the knee internally rotated 30 degrees and moved into extension suggests a lateral meniscal tear. In addition, a positive lateral test may represent a tear of the popliteus tendon, which can accompany a lateral meniscal tear. The *Apley maneuver* also tests for a torn meniscus. With the patient lying prone and the knee flexed to 90 degrees, the examiner places downward compression on the foot while rotating the tibia on the femur. Pain elicited during this maneuver suggests a meniscal tear. The *distraction test* is then performed by the examiner placing his knee on the patient's posterior thigh to stabilize the leg while applying an upward distractive force on the foot. Pain from rotating the tibia suggests ligament damage.

Range of motion of the knee in flexion and extension should be from full extension (zero degrees), to full flexion of 120 to 150 degrees. Some normal persons may be able to hyperextend to up to 15 degrees. Loss of full extension due to a flexion contracture is a common finding that accompanies chronic arthritis of the knee. In advanced arthritis, such as seen in some cases of rheumatoid arthritis, a posterior subluxation of the tibia on the femur may be observed.

Muscle strength testing includes testing flexion supplied by the hamstrings, i.e., the biceps femoris, semitendinosus, and semimembranosus (L5-S3) and extension supplied by the quadriceps femoris (L2-4). The hamstrings are tested best with the patient prone and attempting to flex the knee from 90 degrees to beyond. The ankle should be kept in neutral position or dorsiflexed to remove gastrocnemius action. With the leg externally rotated, the biceps femoris, which inserts on the fibula and lateral tibia, is primarily tested, while flexion with internal rotation tests the semitendinosus and semimembranosus muscles, which insert on the medial side of the tibia. Extension is tested with the patient sitting upright with the knee fully extended. The examiner stabilizes the thigh with downward pressure just proximal to the knee and places downward pressure at the ankle to test the knee extensors.

**Ankle and Foot.** The ankle is a hinged joint, and movement is limited to plantar flexion and dorsiflexion. It is formed by the distal ends of the tibia and fibula and proximal aspect of the body of the talus. The tibia forms the weight-bearing portion of the ankle joint; the fibula articulates on the side of the tibia. The malleoli of the tibia and fibula extend downward beyond the weight-bearing part of the joint and articulate with the sides of the talus. Malleoli provide lateral stability by enveloping the talus in a mortise-like fashion.

The articular capsule of the ankle is lax on the anterior and posterior aspects of the joint, allowing extension and flexion, but is tightly bound bilaterally by ligaments. The synovial membrane of the ankle on the inside of the capsule usually does not communicate with any other joints, bursae, or tendon sheaths in the region of the ankle or foot.

Strong medial and lateral ligaments of the ankle contribute to the lateral stability of the joint. The medial or deltoid ligament, the only ligament on the medial side of the ankle, is a triangle-shaped fibrous band that tends to resist eversion of the foot. It may be torn in eversion sprains of the ankles. The lateral ligaments of the foot consist of three distinct bands forming the posterior talofibular, the calcaneofibular, and the anterior talofibular ligaments. These ligaments may be torn in inversion sprains of the ankle. All tendons crossing the ankle joint lie superficial to the articular capsule and are enclosed in synovial sheaths (~ 8 cm in length) for part of their course across the ankle. On the anterior aspect of the ankle the tendons and synovial tendon sheaths of the tibialis anterior, extensor digitorum longus, peroneus tertius, and extensor hallucis longus overlie the articular capsule and synovial membrane. On the medial side of the ankle posteriorly and inferiorly to the medial malleolus lie the flexor tendons and tendon sheaths of the tibialis posterior, flexor digitorum longus, and flexor hallucis longus (Fig. 24–13). All three of these muscles plantar flex and supinate the foot. The tendon of the flexor hallucis longus is located more posteriorly than the other flexor tendons and lies beneath the Achilles' tendon for part of its course. The tendo calcaneus (Achilles' tendon) is a common tendon of the gastrocnemius and soleus muscles and inserts into the posterior surface of the calcaneus, where it is subject to external trauma, various inflammatory reactions, and irritations from bony spurs beneath it. On the lateral aspect of the ankle, posteriorly and inferiorly to the lateral malleolus, a synovial sheath encloses the tendons of the peroneus longus and peroneus brevis. These muscles extend the ankle (plantar flex) and evert (pronate) the foot. Each of the tendons adjacent to the ankle may be involved separately in traumatic or disease processes.

There are three sets of fibrous bands or retinacula that hold down the tendons that cross the ankle in their passage to the foot. The extensor retinaculum consists of a superior part (transverse crural ligament) in the anterior and inferior portions of the leg and an inferior part in the proximal portion of the dorsum of the foot. The flexor retinaculum is a thickened fibrous band on the medial side of the ankle. On the lateral side of the ankle the peroneal retinaculum forms a superior and an inferior fibrous band. These bands bind down tendons of the peroneus longus and peroneus brevis as they cross the lateral aspect of the ankle.

The intertarsal joints provide additional mobility to the foot. The intertarsal joints allow the foot to be everted and abducted (pronated) or inverted and adducted (supinated) to maintain the arch of the foot during weight bearing. Intertarsal ligaments on the undersurface of the foot are particularly strong. The arch is supported also by the plantar aponeurosis, the short muscles of the foot, and the long tendons that cross the ankle in their course into the sole of the foot. The subtalar (talocalcaneal) joint permits inversion and eversion of the foot. No muscles insert on the talus.

The plantar aponeurosis or fascia is a fibrous structure of great strength that extends from the calcaneus forward as a single band, which then divides at about the middle of the foot into portions for each of the five toes. The plantar aponeurosis becomes thinner as it extends distally in a fashion similar to that of the palmar aponeurosis in the hands and fingers. The area of the plantar aponeurosis near the attachment to the calcaneus is particularly subject to the effects of trauma and inflam-

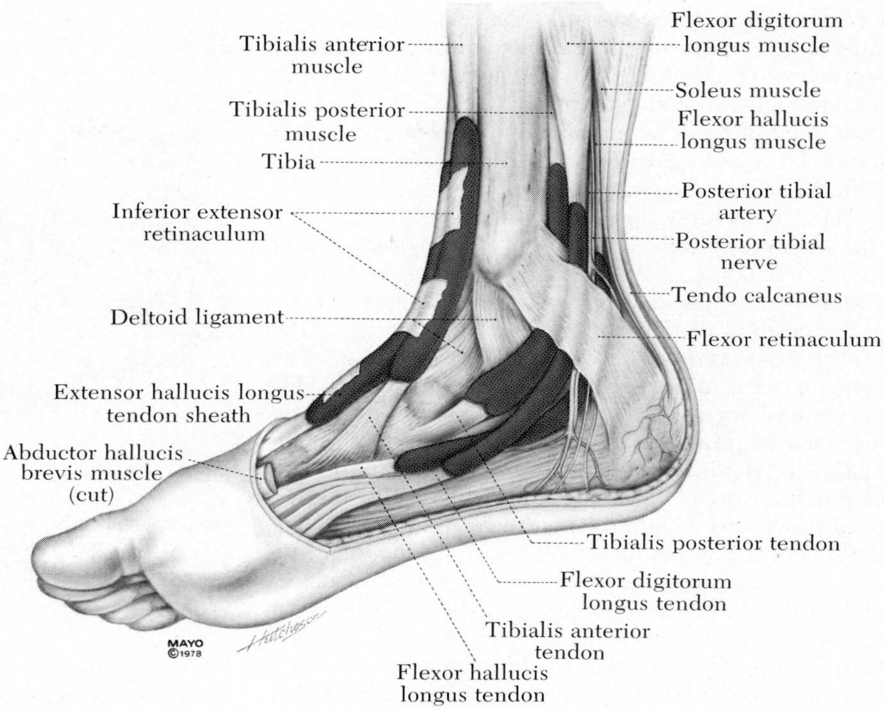


**Figure 24–13.** Medial aspect of the ankle demonstrating the relationships between the tendons, ligaments, and posterior tibial artery and nerve. (From Polley, H.F., and Hunder, G.G.: Rheumatologic Interviewing and Physical Examination of the Joints. Philadelphia, W.B. Saunders Company, 1978.)

matory reactions. Bony spurs are likely to form at this area.

Each of the metatarsophalangeal and interphalangeal joints has an articular capsule lined with synovial membrane. The extensor tendon completes the capsule dorsally, and the collateral ligaments strengthen the capsule on its sides and the plantar ligaments support the plantar portion of the capsule. The metatarsophalangeal joints normally undergo less flexion than the metacarpophalangeal joints.

Bursae in the foot are commonly located on the sides of the first and fifth metatarsophalangeal joints and about the heel, especially between the skin and Achilles' tendon, between the Achilles' tendon and calcaneus, and between the skin on the sole and plantar surface of both the calcaneous and metatarsal heads. Subcutaneous bursae are likely to develop in areas that are subject to abnormal weight bearing or friction. Thus, a bursal reaction may form between the thickened skin (callus) and the underlying bony prominence of the first metatarsal head in a hallux valgus deformity of the great toe.

The foot and ankle should be inspected while the patient is standing, walking, and in a non-weight-bearing position. The feet can be compared with each other for evidence of localized or diffuse swelling or atrophy, the position of nodules, cutaneous changes, and appearance of the nails (Fig. 24–14). The location of calluses and subcutaneous bursae should be noted because they indicate areas of pressure or friction due to alterations in foot structure.

Synovial swelling of the ankle joint is most likely to cause fullness over the anterior or anterolateral aspect of the joint, since the capsule is more lax in this area. Mild swelling of the joint may not be apparent on inspection because of the many structures that cross the joint superficially to the synovial membrane. Efforts should be made to differentiate between superficial linear swelling localized to the distribution of the tendon sheaths from more diffuse fullness and swelling due to involvement of the ankle joint. Similarly, it is difficult to observe synovitis of the intertarsal joints. Intertarsal joint synovitis may produce an erythematous puffiness or fullness over the dorsum of the foot. Chronic inflammation of structures around the ligaments that hold the

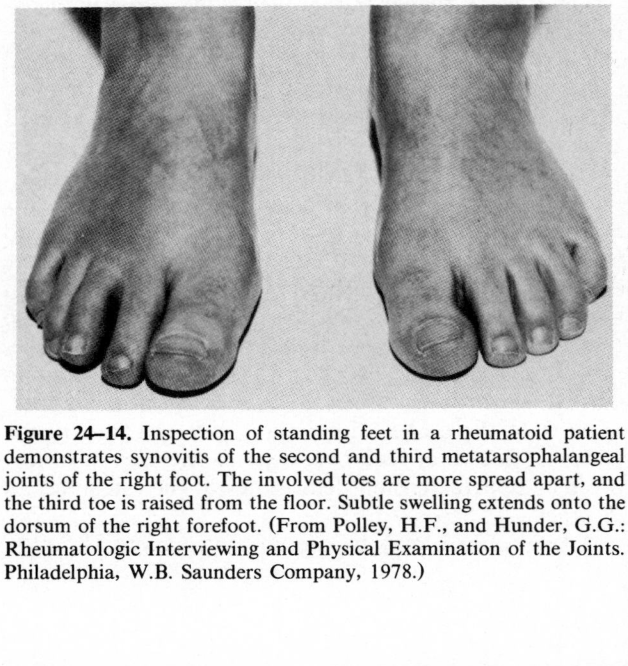

**Figure 24–14.** Inspection of standing feet in a rheumatoid patient demonstrates synovitis of the second and third metatarsophalangeal joints of the right foot. The involved toes are more spread apart, and the third toe is raised from the floor. Subtle swelling extends onto the dorsum of the right forefoot. (From Polley, H.F., and Hunder, G.G.: Rheumatologic Interviewing and Physical Examination of the Joints. Philadelphia, W.B. Saunders Company, 1978.)

forefoot together may result in weakening of these ligaments and spreading of the metatarsals, resulting in separation of the toes and widening of the forefoot. Swelling of the metatarsophalangeal joints produces thickening of the forefoot, which may keep some of the toes from touching the floor when the patient is sitting with the feet in a resting position.

There are several abnormal positions of the foot that should be recognized. Lowering of the longitudinal arch (pes valgoplanus or flat foot) or elevation of the longitudinal arch (pes cavus) may be seen. Talipes equinus is the position of the foot in plantar flexion and often results from contracture of the Achilles' tendon. This tends to occur in patients who are confined to bed. The presence of varus or valgus positions of the heel is determined by noting the deviation of the foot either medially or laterally, respectively. Inversion of the foot (supination) exists when the sole of the foot is turned inward, and eversion of the foot (pronation) exists when the sole of the foot is turned outward. Adduction of the foot is present when the forepart of the foot is displaced inward in relation to the midline of the leg. Abduction of the foot occurs when the forepart of the foot is displaced outward in relation to the midline of the limb. The various abnormal positions are often combined in deformities of the foot or may be associated with abnormalities of the knees.

The most common deformity of the great toe is *hallux valgus.* This is a lateral or outward deviation of the great toe resulting in an abnormal angulation and rotation of the first metatarsophalangeal joint. The first metatarsal bone deviates medially, which increases the width of the forefoot and produces a prominence of the first metatarsal head. The big toe may overlap, or underlie the second toe. A callus and bursal reaction are commonly found over the prominence of the medial aspect of the head of the first metatarsal bone. *Hallux rigidus* is the term used when motion at the first metatarsophalangeal joint is markedly reduced.

The typical "hammer toe" deformity consists of hyperextension at the metatarsophalangeal joint and flexion at the proximal interphalangeal joint. The distal interphalangeal joint may be straight or hyperextended. When the distal interphalangeal joint remains straight and the tip of the toe touches the floor, the deformity also is referred to as "mallet toe." A "cock-up toe" refers to a dorsal subluxation of the proximal phalanx on the metatarsal head (Fig. 24–15). The metatarsal head becomes depressed towards the sole of the foot, where it can be palpated readily. The tip of the toe is elevated above the surface on which the foot is resting. Cock-up toes occur in patients with arthritis at the metatarsophalangeal joint, whereas hammer toes may occur in patients with or without joint disease. Various combinations of these alterations may be found in arthritic patients. Severe articular damage of the toes also may produce hyperextension deformities of the phalanges of the toes.

A painful heel may be caused by a variety of conditions such as osseus spurs, Achilles' tendinitis, calcaneal bursitis, fractures, periostitis, osteomyelitis, or tumors. Careful localization of swelling and tenderness by palpation may help reveal the cause of the symptoms. The Achilles' tendon is subjected to local trauma because of its prominent location and also because of the magnitude of stress applied to it during walking and other activities. Palpable swelling and tenderness at the attachment of the Achilles' tendon to the calcaneus suggest Achilles' tendinitis. Attempts should be made to distinguish by palpation more superficial swelling about the tendon due to local irritation from a deep bursal reaction, since the latter often signifies inflammation due to a systemic disease such as rheumatoid arthritis or ankylosing spondylitis. Xanthomas, tophi, rheumatoid nodules, or fibrous calluses may be palpable in the Achilles' tendon.

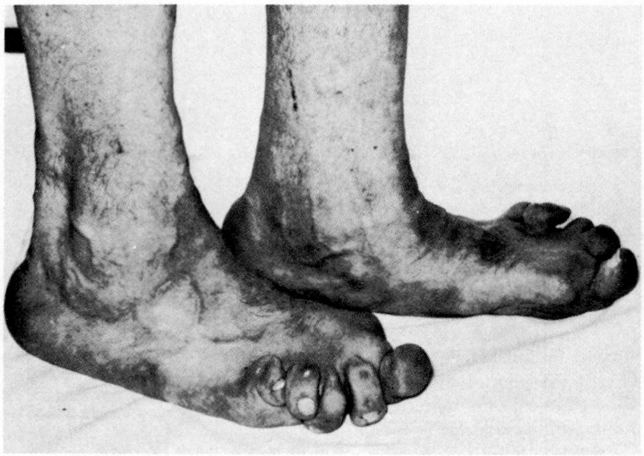

**Figure 24–15.** Rheumatoid foot demonstrating cock-up toe deformities of the fourth and fifth toes as well as loss of the longitudinal arch and pronation of the left foot due to subtalar joint involvement. (From Polley, H.F., and Hunder, G.G.: Rheumatologic Interviewing and Physical Examination of the Joints. Philadelphia, W.B. Saunders Company, 1978.)

Complete or partial rupture of the Achilles' tendon is usually a sudden event and generally occurs during a burst of unaccustomed physical activity. Pain, swelling, ecchymosis, and tenderness are present at the site of the tear, but the swelling may become more diffuse and include the region of the ankle joint. Tenderness over the Achilles' tendon and a visible or palpable depression in the tendon at the site of the separation help in recognition of this condition.

When the Achilles' tendon has been ruptured, a defect in the tendon may be palpable. Pain in the Achilles' tendon region with flexion of the foot against resistance is present in partial tears. When the tear is complete, squeezing the calf while the patient is lying prone with the feet over the edge of the examining table will fail to cause plantar flexion of the foot. Rupture of the Achilles' tendon may be confused with thrombophlebitis or with rupture of fibers of the gastrocnemius muscle or plantaris tendon.

Periostitis associated with pain and tenderness diffusely over the calcaneus or over a localized area may be seen in Reiter's disease or ankylosing spondylitis.

Pain and tenderness in the heel with weight bearing may be seen occasionally in adolescence. The syndrome is self-limited and has been attributed to calcaneal epiphysitis or tenosynovitis of the Achilles' tendon at the level of its insertion into the os calcis. There is no swelling, but the posterior superior portion of the os calcis is tender when palpated.

Plantar fasciitis is a condition in which the patient has pain under the calcaneus on weight bearing and tenderness under the anterior portion of the heel. It is commonly attributed to excessive standing or walking, especially when the patient has been unaccustomed to such activity. But often such a history cannot be elicited. Radiographs may or may not show a bony spur at the attachment of the plantar fascia to the calcaneus.

The metatarsophalangeal joints should be palpated between the examiner's thumb and forefinger. On the plantar surface the soft tissues consist of thick skin, superficial fascia, and adipose tissue. On the dorsal surface the normal soft tissues are not as thick, and the outline of the metatarsophalangeal joint can be determined more precisely. Changes from normal depend on the amount of atrophy of fat pads and other subcutaneous tissue that may be associated with metatarsalgia. Synovitis causes thickness of the soft tissues in the area of these joints, which is most readily detected by palpating the joint margins on their dorsal surfaces. Tenderness on lateral compression of the metatarsophalangeal joints may be noted with mild synovitis of these joints. Dorsal subluxation of the metatarsophalangeal joints may result from chronic synovitis in which the capsule is stretched and soft tissue forces elevate the base of the proximal phalanges on the metatarsal head. A step upward of the base of the proximal phalanx can be palpated in most instances and may be associated with a cock-up deformity. Chronic synovitis also may result in separation of the toes and widening of the forefoot.

The proximal and distal interphalangeal joints of the toes are palpated between the thumb and index finger in a manner similar to palpation of the corresponding joints in the fingers. Synovitis usually is detected best on the medial and lateral aspects of these joints while varying degrees of pressure are applied by the palpating fingers to determine the presence of swelling, tenderness, or warmth. Synovitis of the interphalangeal joints may cause diffuse swelling of the entire toe, a finding sometimes referred to as "*sausage toe.*"

From the normal position of rest in which there is a right angle between the leg and foot, labeled 0 degrees, the ankle normally allows about 20 degrees of dorsiflexion and about 45 degrees of plantar flexion. Inversion and eversion of the foot occur mainly at the subtalar and other intertarsal joints. From the normal position of the foot the subtalar joint normally permits about 20 degrees of eversion and 30 degrees of inversion. To test the subtalar joint the examiner grasps the calcaneus with one hand and attempts to invert and evert it, holding the ankle motionless. To move the mid-tarsal joints the examiner holds the calcaneus in one hand and the forefoot in the other and rotates the mid-foot in both directions in relation to the calcaneus. Both feet should be compared. The metatarsophalangeal joint of the great toe extends to about 80 degrees and flexes to about 35 degrees. The second through fifth toes move only about 45 degrees in either direction. Flexion of the interphalangeal joints varies among individuals, but generally the interphalangeal joints flex to 40 or 50 degrees.

A general assessment of muscular strength of the ankle can be obtained by asking the patient to lift the weight of the body on the toes and heels. If the patient can walk on toes and heels, the muscle strength of the flexors and extensors of the ankle can be considered normal. In many instances, however, joint pains may prevent the patient from walking, or it is desired to test muscles individually.

Prime movers in plantar flexion of the ankle are the gastrocnemius (S1,2) and the soleus (S1,2) muscles. The prime mover in dorsiflexion and inversion of the foot is the tibialis anterior muscle (L4,5, S1). The examiner applies graded resistance on the medial and dorsal aspect of the foot when testing the tibialis anterior muscle. The prime mover in inversion is the tibialis posterior muscle (L5, S1). To test the tibialis posterior muscle the foot should be in plantar flexion. The examiner applies graded resistance on the medial border of the forefoot while the patient attempts to invert the foot. The prime movers in eversion of the foot are the peroneus longus (L4, 5, S1) and peroneus brevis (L4, 5, S1) muscles.

The prime mover in flexion of the first metatarsophalangeal joint is the flexor hallucis brevis muscle (L4, 5, S1). The prime mover in flexion of the interphalangeal joint of this toe is the flexor hallucis longus muscle (L5, S1, 2). The prime mover in extension of the first metatarsophalangeal joint is the extensor digitorum brevis (L5, S1), and the prime mover in extension of the interphalangeal joint is the extensor hallucis longus (L4, 5, S1). Prime movers in flexion of the second through fifth metatarsophalangeal joints are the lumbrical muscles (L4, 5). The interosseus muscles and flexor digitiquinti muscles also function in flexion.

The prime mover in flexion of the proximal interphalangeal joints of the toes is the flexor digitorum brevis (L4, 5), and the prime mover in flexion of the distal interphalangeal joints of these toes is the flexor digitorum longus (L5, S1).

The prime movers in extension of the second through fifth metatarsophalangeal joints and interphalangeal joints are the extensor digitorum longus (L4, 5, S1) and extensor digitorum brevis (L5, S1) muscles. Because of the shortness of the toes and underdeveloped state of their muscles, it is often difficult to distinguish between function at the proximal and distal interphalangeal joints.

When the synovial tendon sheaths become inflamed

(tenosynovitis) as they cross the ankle, the superficial linear swelling and fullness of tenosynovitis should be differentiated from the more generalized swelling and tenderness found in synovitis of the ankle joint. At times the swelling of the tendon sheath is obscured by a more diffuse overlying edema, but when the edema is reduced by rest in bed and elevation of the extremity, careful palpation may show that the swelling and tenderness follow the line of a tendon. Tenosynovitis frequently causes pain on movement of the involved tendon. Thus, inversion or eversion of the foot against resistance may cause pain when there is a synovial reaction on the respective medial or lateral aspect of the foot or ankle. However, failure to produce pain with these maneuvers does not exclude a tenosynovial reaction.

Metatarsalgia, or pain and tenderness of the plantar surface of the heads of the metatarsal bones or metatarsophalangeal joints, is a common complaint, which occurs alone or in association with many local and systemic conditions. In youth, trauma and osteochondritis of the second metatarsal head are common causes. In the adult, any disturbance that can affect the feet can manifest itself in the metatarsophalangeal joint region of one or both feet. Patients with metatarsalgia may have atrophy of fat pads under these joints.

Interdigital neuroma, or *Morton's toe,* is a fusiform enlargement of an interdigital nerve. It must be differentiated from metatarsalgia. Interdigital neuroma is most commonly located between or distal to the heads of the third and fourth metatarsal bones. It is often bilateral and more common in women. Pain associated with interdigital neuroma is sharp or burning in quality and occurs initially with activity and later also at rest. Sharply localized tenderness is characteristic and is present in the soft fleshy tissues either between or distal to the heads of the third and fourth metatarsals, less often between the second and third toes. The location of tenderness helps differentiate it from metatarsophalangeal joint disease. Altered sensation or decreased 2-point discrimination may be found over the skin between the third and fourth toes. Occasionally large interdigital neuromas may be palpable and movable between the heads of the metatarsals.

"*March foot*" is caused by severe or prolonged use of the foot, such as during strenuous walking and usually is caused by a transverse fracture of the metatarsal shaft. The second metatarsal is affected most frequently and the third metatarsal next most frequently. However, any of the metatarsals can be involved. Localized pain develops over the dorsum of the forefoot, causing the patient to limp. The most common and significant findings on physical examination are palpable tenderness and swelling over the fracture. The diagnosis is confirmed by roentgenograms or bone scans of the foot. March fracture may also occur in the calcaneus or the lower part of the tibia or fibula.

Reflex sympathetic dystrophy is an incompletely understood syndrome that involves the entire foot and ankle and easily can be mistaken for an atypical polyarthritis. It can be a sequel to, or complication of, trauma or synovitis, but frequently it has no obvious or detectable organic cause. Typically the foot is cyanotic or mottled, edematous, tender, cool, moist, and shiny. Hyperalgesia, although present, often does not conform to any definite nerve distribution.

When transient or regional osteoporosis involves the foot, it is similar to reflex dystrophy in some ways. Tenderness of the tarsal and metatarsal bones is present, and weight bearing is painful. In transient osteoporosis, however, the color of the skin is likely to be more normal, but occasionally some evidence of inflammation is present. In addition, in transient osteoporosis recurrences may be seen, and the knee and hip may also be involved. In this syndrome, the findings generally resolve in 4 to 8 months.

Tarsal tunnel syndrome is discussed in detail in Chapter 110. Excess accumulation of fat, tenosynovitis, fibrosis, or trauma may produce symptoms of the tarsal tunnel syndrome. Characteristic symptoms include burning pain, tingling, or numbness in the toes, forefoot, or heel in the distribution of the particular branch or branches entrapped.

*Tinel's sign* may be elicited by tapping over the posterior tibial nerve at the site of compression. Decreased sensation to pinprick or to 2-point discrimination is found earlier and more commonly than weakness or atrophy of the foot muscles. Electromyograms may show an increase in the nerve conduction time of the entrapped nerve.

## References

1. Polley, H.F., and Hunder, G.G.: Rheumatological Interviewing and Physical Examination of the Joints. 2nd ed. Philadelphia, W.B. Saunders Company, 1978.
2. Hoppenfeld, S.: Physical Examination of the Spine and Extremities. Englewood Cliffs, New Jersey, Appleton-Century-Crofts, 1976.
3. Moll, J.M.H., and Wright, V.: Normal range of spinal mobility. An objective clinical study. Ann. Rheum. Dis. 30:381, 1971.
4. Nelson, M.A., Allen, P., Clamp, S.E., and DeDombal, F.T.: Reliability and reproducibility in low back pain. Spine 4:97, 1979.
5. Russell, A.S., Maksymowych, W., and LeClercq, S.: Clinical examination of the sacroiliac joints: A prospective study. Arthritis Rheum. 24:1575, 1981.
6. Waddell, G., McCulloch, J.A., Kummel, E., and Venner, R.M.: Nonorganic physical signs in low back pain. Spine 5:117, 1980.
7. Pace, J.B., and Nogle, D.: Piriform syndrome. West. J. Med. 124:435, 1976.
8. Hardaker, W.T., Whipple, T.L., and Bassett, F.H.: Diagnosis and treatment of the plica syndrome of the knee. J. Bone Joint Surg. 62A:221, 1980.
9. Hughston, J.C., Andrews, J.R., Cross, M.J., and Moschi, A.: Classification of knee ligament instabilities. Part I. The medial compartment and cruciate ligaments. J. Bone Joint Surg. 58A:159, 1976.

# Chapter 25

# Approach to Monarticular Arthritis

*Frank R. Schmid*

## GENERAL CONSIDERATIONS

No other presentation for a rheumatic disease tests the physician's knowledge and skill as does monarticular arthritis. Often the onset is acute and the threat of infection real, so that urgency is required in decision making; sometimes the involved joint is the only apparent abnormality, so that every clue must be gleaned from the history, systemic and local examination, and the laboratory to make a diagnosis. While the challenge is demanding and, perhaps for that reason, exciting, solution of the problem can often be the most rewarding experience in rheumatology.

**Definition of Monarticular Arthritis.** Diarthrodial joints throughout the body have the same basic composition: synovium, capsule, articular cartilage, and bone. Periarticular structures such as tendons and bursae, although lacking bone and cartilage, have a similar synovial lining. Thus, they undergo many of the same pathologic processes as joints. Since they are anatomically adjacent to joints, their involvement may be mistakenly attributed to the joint itself unless a careful examination is performed. For these reasons, the approach to their management is included along with that of the joints under the overall chapter heading, monarticular arthritis.

By definition, monarticular means one joint or joint-related structure. In practice, involvement of as many as two or three separate joints still qualifies as a monarticular problem because of the frequency with which the classic monarticular syndromes are actually oligoarticular (Table 25–1). Involvement of more than this number of joint structures, however, even if the development is migratory and noncumulative, tends to suggest an entirely different set of causes.

Obviously every patient who ultimately has polyarthritis must at some point during the onset have a monarticular syndrome, if only for a short while. Therefore, awareness of subsequent polyarticular spread and the diagnostic possibilities that this raises must be kept in mind when the patient is first seen. Appropriate studies to test for their presence must be carried out. However, further discussion of such polyarthritic diseases as rheumatoid arthritis, rheumatic fever, and generalized osteoarthritis is not included in this chapter unless the duration of the monarticular phase is prolonged (Table 25-2). A related point to remember is that some patients present with a false monarticular history. Lesser degrees of involvement in other joints are ignored because attention becomes focused upon the major process in one or two joints. The true polyarthritic nature of the disease will be uncovered only by a careful and complete examination.

**Broad Spectrum of Possible Diagnoses.** Monarticular arthritis can be caused by many factors: genetic and biochemical abnormalities, as seen in the structural defects of the inherited connective tissue diseases as hy-

**Table 25–1.** Monarticular Diseases

| |
|---|
| Septic arthritis[1-4] |
| Gout[5] |
| Pseudogout[6] |
| Traumatic arthritis |
| Neuropathic arthropathy[7] |
| Mechanical derangement of joint |
| Localized syndromes (tendinitis, bursitis) |
| Arthritis with bleeding–clotting disorders (hemophilia, von Willebrand's disease, anticoagulant use)[8,9,10] |
| Familial Mediterranean fever[11] |
| Gaucher's disease[12] |
| Hyperlipoproteinemia (type II)[13] |
| Congenital dysplasia of hip |
| Juvenile osteochondroses |
| Avascular necrosis of bone[14] |
| Osteochondritis dissecans[15] |
| Loose joint body |
| Foreign body |
| Pigmented villonodular synovitis[16] |
| Synovioma[17] |
| Juxta-articular bone tumors[18-20] |
| Osteochondromatosis[21] |
| Fat necrosis in pancreatic disease[22] |

**Table 25–2.** Polyarticular Diseases with Frequent Monarticular Component

| |
|---|
| Reiter's syndrome[23] |
| Juvenile rheumatoid arthritis (including ankylosing spondylitis)[24] |
| Psoriatic arthritis[25,26] |
| Colitic arthritis, Whipple's arthritis[27-29] |
| Sarcoid arthritis[30] |
| Pseudogout[6] |
| Arthritis with bleeding–clotting disorders (hemophilia, scurvy, von Willebrand's disease)[8,9,10] |
| Hemochromatosis[31] |
| Septic arthritis (especially due to *N. gonorrhoeae* and *meningitidis*)*[4] |
| Osteoarthritis (selected sites, as hip)[32] |
| Amyloid arthritis[33] |
| Relapsing polychondritis[34] |
| Hyperlipoproteinemia (Types II, IV)[35,36] |

*Onset is frequently polyarticular before monarticular localization. Other syndromes usually have monarticular presentation initially.

permobility and in gout; trauma; infection; neoplasia; hormonal changes, as in parathyroid disease and pseudogout; immunologic mechanisms, as in amyloidosis; and finally, for the majority of patients, a nonspecific inflammatory process. The diagnostic net must be cast widely at the outset to ensure that the unusual cause for monarthritis is not overlooked.

Systemic diseases often include joint involvement in their spectrum of symptoms, in part because the connective tissue of joints is duplicated throughout the supporting structures of various parenchymal organs and also in part because a disorder in the mechanical function of joints is so readily perceived by the patient even if only minor. Therefore, a thorough general history and examination are mandatory. Focus upon the painful or swollen joint alone will not allow the correct diagnosis to be made in many cases. However, because so much of the severity of the illness falls upon one or just a few joint structures rather than multiple joint structures, the role of local factors in the causation of monarticular arthritis is usually more evident than in polyarticular arthritis. In fact, it may be helpful to analyze the patient's problem from the standpoint of the reason why one particular joint became involved and not another. For example, even though the bacteremia that precedes most cases of septic arthritis could potentially allow any joint in the body to become infected, only one or two, perhaps because of prior trauma, actually do become involved. Another example is the unusual instance in which a foreign body such as a plant thorn might have been introduced into the joint. This event may not be recalled by the patient unless all circumstances connected with the prior history of the involved part are reviewed.

The lesson in monarticular arthritis is that while no less a general history and examination are required than for any general medical problem, a more meticulous inspection of the local site adds insight into the pathogenesis and sometimes the specific cause.

**Urgency for Diagnosis and Treatment.** Among the prominent causes for monarthritis is infectious arthritis. Suspicion for this diagnosis must be raised upon initial examination even if the severity of joint pain and swelling is only minimal. Sometimes, as in the elderly or debilitated, systemic findings of sepsis may be absent. Since cure of this disease is possible and full restoration of joint function expected, confirmation or exclusion of this entity assumes major importance in the first few hours and days. In addition, other possible causes for monarticular arthritis, such as gout and pseudogout, are painful and disabling. Diagnosis of these diseases can be verified easily and quickly by examination of joint fluid, so that undue delay in making the diagnosis is not warranted. For these reasons, every patient with an undiagnosed monarticular arthritis should be considered a medical emergency.

**Planning Ahead.** Along with dispatch in handling the multiple aspects of examination and laboratory procedures, the physician must make both immediate and long-range decisions within the larger framework of a comprehensive approach to the problem. Less obvious diagnostic possibilities must be pursued as more likely ones are being investigated. Furthermore, no treatment carried out early should alter important clinical findings. Thus, use of anti-inflammatory drugs such as corticosteroids or even aspirin at the outset may mask some of the indicators of disease, e.g., fever and inflammation, that must be observed if one is monitoring the response of an infectious process to treatment. Drugs such as codeine should be given instead for pain relief.

In this chapter, the approach to diagnosis and management will be covered in a chronologic fashion in much the same manner as is seen in practice. Emphasis will be placed upon the use of a predetermined plan that can be followed for patients with monarthritis (Table 25–3).

## INITIAL HISTORY AND EXAMINATION

**The Involved Joint.** Initial attention is directed to the patient's presenting complaint, the involved joint. Diagnostic clues can be obtained by analysis of events that may have precipitated the problem, by the type of onset, and by the nature of the findings both within and around the joint.

***Precipitating Factors.*** When recognized, trauma to a limb may readily be shown to account for a painful or swollen joint. Occasionally, instances of trauma are more elusive, as for example when the patient is unable to provide an accurate history because of stupor from alcoholism, drug addiction, or an illness such as diabetic coma. In these cases, monarthritis may be the direct result of an unappreciated injury, although septic arthritis too is a well known complication of each of these situations. In other cases joint or bone disease caused by trauma may not show external evidence of soft tissue injury such as bruising or laceration, thus obscuring the diagnosis. A march fracture of a metatarsal may not be suspected on physical appearance or may not even be visible on the roentgenogram until callus appears weeks later. Meanwhile attention may be directed toward a presumed arthritis of an adjacent metatarsophalangeal or intertarsal joint as the cause of the problem. As noted earlier, a history of a penetrating injury that occurred days or weeks earlier may not be forthcoming unless a specific inquiry is made. Only then may it be obvious that a foreign body could have entered the joint. Trauma can also cause disease in more insidious ways. Forces applied for long periods of time to the arm of a cellist or violinist, to the forefoot of a ballet dancer, or to the shoulders of a gymnast can at one moment of time induce musculoskeletal symptoms in a joint or tendon. The patient who is hypermobile experiences long continued stress that can also produce an overt synovitis at some point, as in the metacarpophalangeal joint of the hand of a laboratory technician who had done extensive pipetting.

Other precipitating events for monarticular arthritis include the classic story of surgery or myocardial infarction 5 to 7 days before the abrupt onset of gout; the role of drugs such as corticosteroids in the development of aseptic necrosis; and the triggering effect of infection due to certain gram-negative bacilli such as *Salmonella* in causing the appearance of one or two swollen joints in Reiter's syndrome.

Further examples of precipitating factors for monarticular arthritis could be given, but these should suffice to underline the critical importance of their recognition in defining the cause of the disease. Caution is in order, however, in accepting each triggering event at face value. The arthritis presumed to have been induced by an identifiable precipitating factor must still be confirmed by more direct evidence, as discussed below. In some cases, the suspected precipitating factor may be largely irrelevant to the subsequent arthritis.

*Type of Onset.* Most patients with monarticular arthritis have an acute onset, with the peak intensity of symptoms reached in a few days' time. As such, a fairly exact time of onset can be given. In a few cases, the acuteness can be as dramatic as in gout. The patient may retire for the night perfectly well and be awakened before morning by exquisite pain in the joint. Less often, the onset is insidious, as might occur in some patients with psoriatic arthritis or sarcoidosis or with a more chronic presentation of chondrocalcinosis.

*Age and Sex.* Generally these characteristics afford some help in approaching the diagnosis. Male patients account for the largest fraction of cases of gouty arthritis, Reiter's syndrome, Whipple's disease, and the peripheral arthritis of juvenile ankylosing spondylitis. Female patients more often are candidates for a polyarthritic syndrome but are at greater risk for monarticular arthritis related to the gonococcus or hypermobility. Youngsters tend to be the victims of inherited and congenital disorders such as acetabular dysplasia of the hip or juvenile osteochondritis, and, with regard to septic arthritis, to be infected with *Hemophilus* species. Some diseases, such as chondrocalcinosis, are much more common in aged people. Gout when it occurs in women almost always appears postmenopausally.

*Anatomic Localization of Joint Disease.* Certain joints have the undeserved reputation of being so closely associated with certain types of arthritis that their involvement is tantamount to the diagnosis. Inflammation of the first metatarsal-phalangeal joint of the foot or podagra, although characteristic of gout, in fact can be found in other forms of arthritis. Similarly, heel pain, particularly at the weight-bearing portion of the calcaneus, is often found in Reiter's syndrome and in other spondyloarthropathies but again is not diagnostic. Distal interphalangeal joint involvement occurs in many diseases but is a more characteristic feature of osteoarthritis (Heberden's nodes), psoriatic arthritis, and, rarely, lupus erythematosus. The first carpometacarpal joint at the base of the thumb is often tender in patients with osteoarthritis who have Heberden's nodes. Thus, the specific site of the arthritis, while helpful, can only be suggestive in arriving at a diagnosis.

Inflammation of a single joint with rapid extension to an adjacent joint along with considerable overlying soft tissue swelling is a characteristic feature in gout, the so-called satellite phenomenon. Migratory polyarthritis of short duration followed by localization of the infection to but one of two joints is often seen in some forms of infectious arthritis such as gonococcal arthritis. However, by its very nature, monarticular or oligoarticular disease will be confined to but a few joints so that various anatomic or temporal patterns of involvement that could aid the diagnosis will not usually be seen.

*Articular vs. Periarticular Involvement.* A detailed history and examination will indicate whether the symptomatic musculoskeletal structure is actually within the joint and, if so, in which portion of the joint, or whether it is periarticular, involving the associated ligaments, tendons, or other supporting structures (Table 25-4). The physician, on examination, should gently pinpoint the exact source of pain with slight pressure over different parts of the joint. With confidence gained from the patient in this manner, motion of the part can be attempted. A primary intra-articular problem can be shown to encompass the entire circumference of a joint or to be localized within a portion of the joint, as, for example, a meniscal cartilage tear in the knee. Periarticular disease, in contrast, is confined to the unique region that conforms to the outline of the involved structures, as, for instance, the linear pattern of pain and swelling overlying the thumb extensor tendons near the wrist in de Quervain's disease.

Disease in other tissues of the extremity can mimic musculoskeletal symptoms. Neurologic pain has a burning or tingling quality and may follow the distribution of a dermatome or a peripheral nerve. As such it can occur as part of an unrelated disease or at times as a symptom resulting from a primary arthritic disease, as, for instance, compression of the median nerve in the carpal tunnel. Ischemic vascular disease is expressed as pallor or cyanosis, sometimes with but often without changes in the major pulses if vessels of small caliber are involved. Occasionally, the circulatory disturbance is the direct cause of both the musculoskeletal and vascular symptoms, as in polyarteritis nodosa. In gout and in the rarer disease of familial Mediterranean fever, a diffuse subcutaneous swelling and erythema can appear in an extremity and be confused with an infectious cellulitis. Therefore, in the approach to the patient who presents with symptoms in an extremity or the trunk, precision in interpretation of the clinical findings by a detailed history and a systemic examination of the affected part is required to define the problem accurately.

*Symptoms of Joint Disease.* Pain, whether severe or mild, is a cardinal feature of joint disease and can be felt directly at the site of involvement or referred to tissues at a distance from the joint. A well known example of referred pain is the pattern of pain felt in the anterior thigh or knee region caused by hip joint disease. Glenohumeral pain may be referred to the deltoid, and knee pain may be felt in the gastrocnemius muscle. In each case, careful examination will fail to reveal objective

**Table 25–3.** Algorithm for the Diagnosis of Monarticular Arthritis

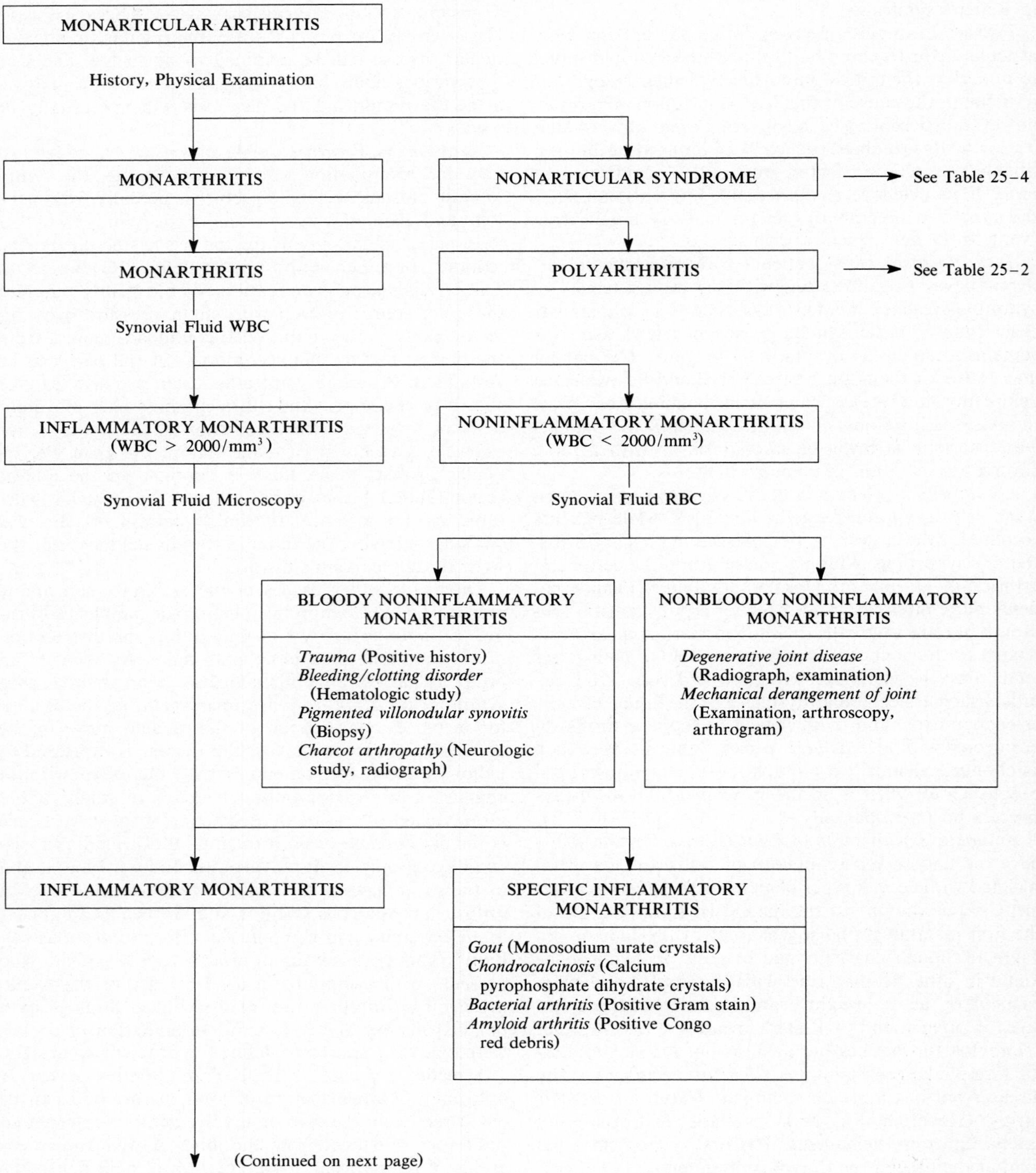


(Continued on next page)

(Continued from previous page)

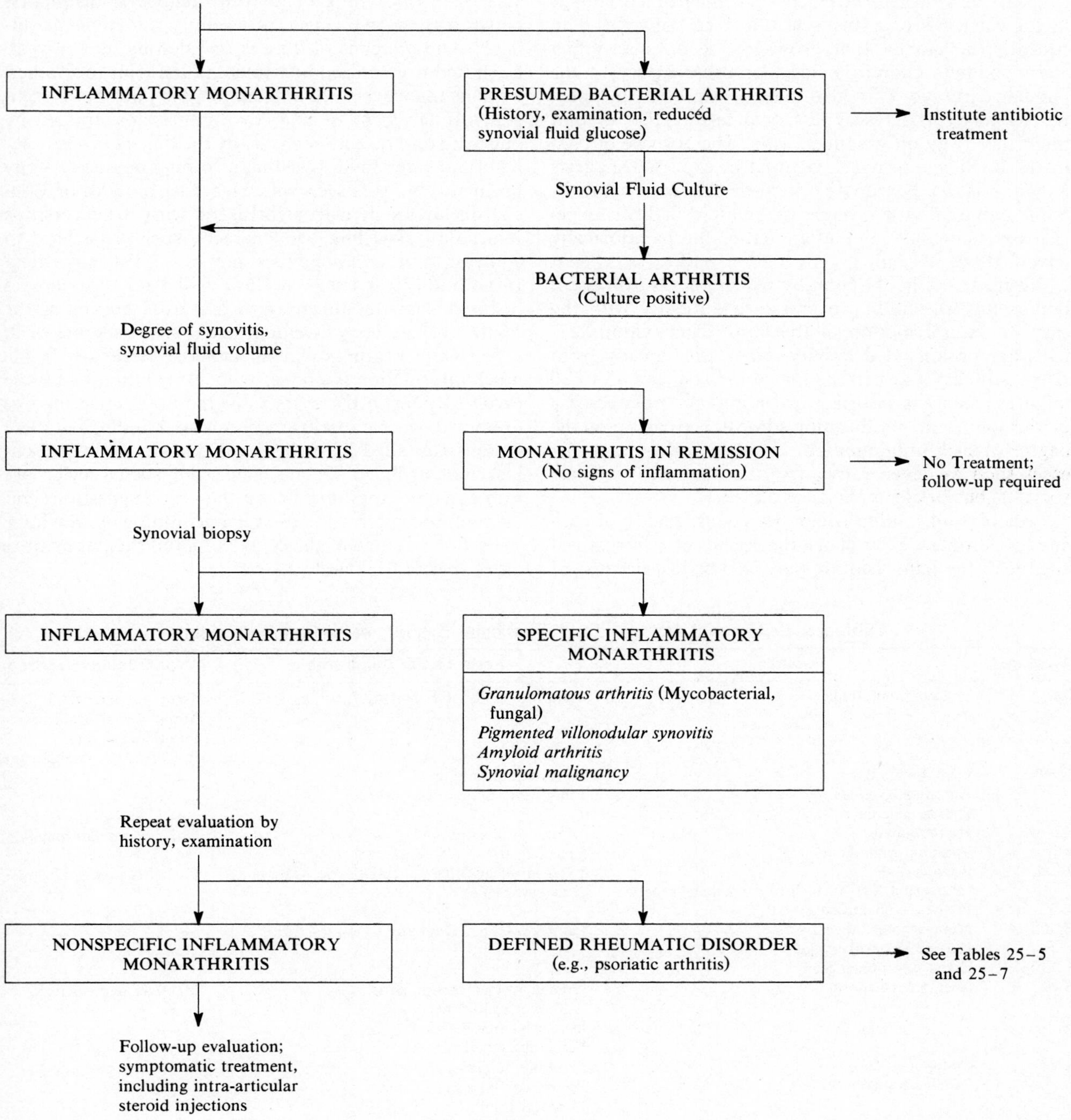


This algorithm may be used in the analysis of the problem presented by a patient with monarticular arthritis. The time frame development of these steps is several weeks. At each step the scope of diagnostic possibilities is named within the box; directions for further evaluation follow if the diagnosis has not been ascertained within the flow chart itself or by reference to tables in this chapter.

findings at the site of the referred pain, but pain, swelling, or limitation of motion can be detected in the involved joint. The relationship of pain to other factors can be a clue to the diagnosis. Pain at rest suggests inflammation of the joint structure; pain on use tends to speak for a mechanical defect such as cartilage damage in osteoarthritis or a meniscal injury to the knee. Pain beneath the patella that grows worse on descending stairs suggests chondromalacia or other injury to the patellar cartilage. Pain also may be expressed in unexpected ways, as in weakness or a feeling that a joint might give way on weight-bearing. The absence of pain in circumstances in which it might be expected suggests a diagnosis of a neuropathic joint or Charcot's arthritis. Some children with juvenile rheumatoid arthritis experience considerable joint inflammation but paradoxically have little or no pain.

Stiffness may be the term by which pain is expressed, but usually the finding expresses a difficulty with the easy or natural motion of the joint. This symptom is felt after prolonged inactivity, often after arising from sleep. Stiffness that persists for periods beyond 15 to 30 minutes usually is associated with inflammatory disease of the joint, and its duration affords a measure of the degree of such inflammation. However, other joint diseases such as degenerative arthritis may also have associated but briefer periods of stiffness.

Loss of joint motion occurs as a consequence of pain and/or stiffness as well as the result of a structural change in the joint. Motion may also be lost because of rupture of a tendon or a muscle attachment. Detection of this latter possibility requires meticulous examination of the joint structure for absence of tendon tightening on attempts at motion.

Swelling may be due to effusion within the joint capsule or to thickening of joint structures. A distinction between these two causes of swelling sometimes is difficult. The presence of fluid is revealed by its ability to be shifted from one compartment of the joint to another. Various maneuvers are applied for this purpose. In general, displacement of fluid by compression applied by one hand and detection of this by the fingers of the other hand indicates fluid. Swelling also may be due to bony proliferation, as is seen with Heberden's nodes or Bouchard's nodes in osteoarthritis or with a neuropathic joint. Bony swelling will characteristically be hard in contrast to the soft boggy reaction of soft tissue swelling. In addition, soft tissue swelling will tend to assume a fusiform shape conforming to the gross outline of the joint, whereas bony swelling tends to be asymmetrical.

**Systemic Features of Monarticular Arthritis.** While much information is gained by focusing attention on the involved joint, other systems of the body must also be examined, since either overt or minimal findings in these regions can shed light on the diagnosis of the musculoskeletal problem. Details concerning such a review are presented in other portions of this text; suggestions concerning the application of systemic findings to the interpretation of some of the causes of monarticular arthritis are presented in Table 25–5.

**Table 25–4.** Regional Articular and Periarticular Syndromes of Peripheral Joints

| Region | Joint | Periarticular Syndrome | Nonarticular Syndrome |
|---|---|---|---|
| Jaw | Temporomandibular | Temporomandibular joint dysfunction | Temporal arteritis<br>Molar dental problems<br>Parotid swelling<br>Preauricular lymphadenitis |
| Shoulder | Glenohumeral<br>Acromioclavicular<br>Sternoclavicular | Subacromial bursitis<br>Long head bicipital tendinitis | |
| Elbow | Humeroulnar<br>Proximal radioulnar | Olecranon bursitis<br>Epicondylitis | Ulnar nerve entrapment |
| Wrist | Radiocarpal<br>Intercarpal, second to fifth carpometacarpal<br>First carpometacarpal | Extensor tendinitis (including de Quervain's tenosynovitis) | Carpal tunnel syndrome |
| Hand | Metacarpophalangeal<br>Proximal interphalangeal<br>Distal interphalangeal | Palmar fasciitis (Dupuytren's contracture) | |
| Hip | Acetabular-femoral | Greater trochanteric bursitis<br>Adductor syndrome<br>Ischial bursitis<br>Fascia lata syndrome | Meralgia paresthetica |
| Knee | Condylar-tibial<br>Patellar-condylar | Anserine bursitis<br>Prepatellar bursitis<br>Meniscal injury<br>Ligamentous tear–laxity | |
| Ankle | Tibiotalar<br>Subtalar (talonavicular, calcaneocuboid, talocalcaneal) | Peroneal tendinitis<br>Subachilles bursitis<br>Calcaneal fasciitis | Tarsal tunnel syndrome |
| Foot | Intertalar<br>Metatarsophalangeal<br>Interphalangeal | First metatarsophalangeal bursitis (bunion) | Morton's neuroma |

**Table 25–5.** Systemic Features of Monarticular Arthritis

| System | Mono- or Oligoarticular Arthritis |
|---|---|
| Skin | Juvenile chronic arthritis (Still's variety) |
| | Psoriatic arthritis |
| | Reiter's syndrome |
| | Colitic arthritis |
| | Sarcoid arthritis |
| | Familial Mediterranean fever |
| | Septic arthritis (esp. *N. gonorrhoeae* and *meningitidis*) |
| | Hyperlipoproteinemia |
| | Hemochromatosis |
| | Hemophilia, scurvy |
| | Fat necrosis due to pancreatic disease |
| | Amyloidosis |
| Nasopharynx and ear | Reiter's syndrome |
| | Gout |
| | Relapsing polychondritis |
| Eye | Juvenile rheumatoid arthritis |
| | Reiter's syndrome |
| | Relapsing polychondritis |
| | Sarcoid arthritis |
| Gastrointestinal tract | Colitic arthritis |
| | Whipple's disease |
| | Hemochromatosis |
| | Fat necrosis due to pancreatic disease |
| Heart and circulation | Amyloidosis |
| | Reiter's syndrome |
| | Relapsing polychondritis |
| Respiratory tract | Sarcoidosis |
| | Relapsing polychondritis |
| Nervous system | Neuropathic arthropathy |
| Renal system | Amyloidosis |
| | Gout |
| Hematologic system | Hemophilia |
| | Gaucher's disease |
| | Hemochromatosis |

## IMMEDIATE LABORATORY STUDIES

**Joint Fluid Examination.** Patients with monarticular arthritis may demonstrate a joint effusion, and its possible presence should be carefully sought. Even a trace amount of excess joint fluid can be aspirated and used for microscopic examination or for culture. The selection of which tests should be run when only a small volume of sample is available must take into account the most likely diagnoses being considered, but as a general rule should include a wet-mount preparation for a semiquantitative assessment of the number and type of cells and the demonstration of monosodium urate or calcium pyrophosphate dihydrate crystals; a gram-stained smear for rapid identification of the common bacterial invaders of the joint; and finally a standard culture preparation. All these critical procedures can be performed with as little as 2 or 3 drops of fluid. Given a larger amount of fluid, a more extended analysis can be performed (Table 25–6).

**Urine, Blood, and Other Body Fluid Examinations.** Conventional laboratory procedures may provide valuable information that can direct the physician's attention toward the appropriate diagnosis (Table 25–7).

**Roentgenograms and Radioisotopic Scans.** Most often the roentgenogram of the involved site will reveal normal bone density and structure and a preserved cartilage space. Nevertheless, films should always be obtained at the outset, both of the affected and of the contralateral joint. Comparison of the films of paired joints is especially valuable in monarticular arthritis, since the normal joint acts as a control for the diseased joint and permits greater confidence in the interpretation of borderline abnormalities. Sometimes, as in chondrocalcinosis, the stippled line of calcific density on the articular surface can be seen in both the inflamed and the quiescent joint, thereby adding to the confidence of the diagnosis. Even totally normal films have value. They offer a baseline against which the efficacy of treatment can be measured. Findings that can be noted on roentgenograms are listed in Table 25–7.

In contrast, radioisotopic scans are often positive even in the early stages of disease and regardless of the type of process affecting the joint (Table 25–7). For this purpose, radioactive technetium is usually coupled to a polyphosphonate compound that has a preferential affinity for sites of active bone metabolism. Superficial joints can be more accurately appraised by clinical examination, but in deep-seated joints such as the hip or the shoulder as well as the spine, the scan can indicate that the site of pathology is confined within the joint or the bone rather than spread out into the surrounding soft tissues. Distinction between cellulitis and synovitis is possible by this method. The scan also can help identify areas of aseptic necrosis. Patients in whom uncertainty exists about the anatomic localization of disease should be checked by the radioisotopic scan; in others, this procedure may not be required.

## IMMEDIATE MANAGEMENT

Apart from the urgency to begin treatment at once for a potential joint infection even before the diagnosis is confirmed or for a crystal-induced arthritis, the natural course of the disease can well be observed during the first few days. Drugs that might modify the inflammatory response, such as corticosteroids, and even nonsteroidal anti-inflammatory drugs, such as aspirin, should be withheld. Comfort for the patient can be achieved by the use of splints or other supportive devices and an analgesic medication such as codeine or propoxyphene. Intra-articular injection of corticosteroids should be avoided, not only because of its dramatic effect on the reduction of inflammation but also because it can facilitate extension of an infectious process.

In monarticular arthritis, three common situations present during the first few days that require special mention. Foremost is consideration of septic arthritis. All patients with monarticular arthritis must be consid-

**Table 25–6.** Diagnostic Findings from Joint Fluid Examination in Monarticular Arthritis (After Harris)

| Test | Finding | Possible Diagnosis |
|---|---|---|
| Appearance | Bloody | Traumatic arthritis |
| | | Bleeding/clotting disorder |
| | | Neuropathic arthropathy |
| | | Pigmented villonodular synovitis |
| | Turbid | Septic arthritis |
| | | Other inflammatory arthritides |
| | Clear | Degenerative joint disease |
| | | Mechanical derangement of joint |
| White blood cell count | $< 2000/mm^3$ | Osteoarthritis |
| | | Amyloidosis |
| | | Osteochondromatosis |
| | | Osteochondritis dissecans |
| | | Gaucher's disease |
| | | Hemochromatosis |
| | | Arthritis with pancreatic disease |
| | $2000–50{,}000/mm^3$ | Juvenile chronic arthritis |
| | | Psoriatic arthritis |
| | | Reiter's syndrome |
| | | Colitic arthritis |
| | | Familial Mediterranean fever |
| | | Gout |
| | | Pseudogout |
| | | Septic arthritis |
| | $> 50{,}000/mm^3$ | Septic arthritis |
| | | Gout |
| | | Pseudogout |
| | | Reiter's syndrome |
| Microscopy, wet mount | Sodium monourate crystals | Gout[37] |
| | Calcium pyrophosphate dihydrate crystals | Pseudogout[6] |
| | Lipid droplets | Traumatic arthritis, arthritis with pancreatic disease[22,38] |
| Glucose (simultaneous blood glucose normal) | $< 20$ mg% | Septic arthritis |
| | $> 20$ mg% | Septic arthritis |
| | | Nonseptic inflammatory arthritides |
| Wright's stained smear | Mononuclear phagocytic cells | Reiter's disease (nonspecific)[39] |
| Gram-stained smear/culture | Gram-positive and gram-negative microorganisms | Septic arthritis[2] |
| Miscellaneous stained smear | Acid-fast microorganisms | Tuberculous, lepromatous arthritis[40] |
| | PAS-positive fungal bodies | Fungal arthritis[1,3] |
| | Congo red positive debris | Amyloid arthritis[41] |
| | PAS-positive intracellular inclusions | Whipple's disease[42] |

ered candidates for this disease until it has been definitely excluded. Next is the approach that can be taken when a crystal-induced arthritis such as gout or pseudogout is thought to exist. Lastly, the most common situation is represented by those patients with an inflammatory disease not caused by either of these specific conditions. Further details concerning the diagnosis and management of each of these diseases, as well as the host of others that might present as a monarticular arthritis, are given elsewhere in this text.

**Possible Septic Arthritis.** Clues that an infection is a probable diagnosis may be found in the history and examination as well as in the joint fluid. Demonstration of microorganisms on smear of joint fluid is absolute evidence of infection; indirect evidence might be a markedly decreased synovial fluid glucose concentration in a turbid fluid containing large numbers of polymorphonuclear leukocytes. However, infection may still have to be considered in the absence of these findings. In gonococcal arthritis, the smear and indeed the culture may be negative and the synovial fluid glucose only moderately decreased. Whenever the clinical findings suggest the possibility of infection, the proper course of action is to initiate antibiotic treatment, preferably intravenously or intramuscularly, and to monitor the response of the patient during the next several days. In gonococcal disease, the decrease in joint swelling and the return of the synovial fluid abnormalities toward normal usually occur in this time. Disease caused by other microorganisms may respond more slowly, but even if the response to antibiotic therapy directed at the presumed infectious agent is not completely convincing, results of the culture will be returned during this period. Based upon whether the culture is positive or negative, a more rational therapeutic decision can then be made.

**Possible Crystal-Induced Arthritis.** In almost every instance, the diagnosis of gout or pseudogout can be made with absolute certainty within the first several hours by careful examination of joint fluid for the appropriate crystal: a strongly negative needle-shaped

**Table 25–7.** Diagnostic Findings from Laboratory Tests and Procedure in Monarticular Arthritis*

| Test | Finding | Possible Diagnosis |
|---|---|---|
| Urinalysis | Protein | Amyloidosis |
| | WBC/RBC | Gout |
| | Stones | Gout |
| Hematology | Leukocytosis | Septic arthritis |
| | | Gout (mild elevation) |
| | Bleeding/clotting abnormality | Hemophilia, scurvy |
| Sedimentation rate | Elevated | Inflammatory arthritides |
| C-reactive protein | | |
| Chemistry | | |
| Urea nitrogen, creatinine | Elevated | Amyloidosis, gout |
| SGOT, LDH | Elevated | Hemochromatosis |
| Uric acid | Elevated | Gout |
| Globulin | Elevated | Sarcoidosis, amyloidosis |
| Calcium | Elevated | Pseudogout, sarcoidosis |
| Amylase | Elevated | Fat necrosis in pancreatic disease |
| Cholesterol | Elevated | Hyperlipoproteinemia |
| Radiology | Normal bone film | Inflammatory arthritides (early or mild) |
| | Bone erosion/cartilage loss | Neuropathic arthropathy |
| | | Gout (tophi) |
| | | Juvenile chronic arthritis (late) |
| | | Septic arthritis |
| | | Avascular necrosis |
| | Lytic lesions/cysts | Juxta-articular bone tumors |
| | | Osteoarthritis |
| | | Osteochondritis dissecans |
| | Calcification (articular and/or synovial) | Pseudogout |
| | | Osteochondromatosis |
| Radioisotopic scan | Polyphosphonate localization | Most arthropathies |

*Excluding synovial fluid analysis.

monosodium urate crystal or a weakly positive needle- or rhomboid-shaped calcium pyrophosphate dihydrate crystal. Once the diagnosis is made, specific therapy can be started. In most patients with gout, colchicine can be used, either orally or by intravenous injection. The latter technique reduces the likelihood of such gastrointestinal side effects as nausea, vomiting, and diarrhea. Colchicine remains one of the relatively few drugs that are effective in one or only a few diseases. The dramatic improvement in pain and the slower reduction of swelling within the first 24 hours of its use are strong evidence for a diagnosis of gout. Another situation in which it may be effective is familial Mediterranean fever, but this disease can be distinguished from gout on clinical grounds and by the absence of crystals in joint fluid. Alternative drugs would be the nonsteroidal anti-inflammatory compounds, but, as opposed to the selectivity of colchicine for gout, these drugs are wholly nonspecific in their ability to control inflammation. They are more reasonable for treatment of pseudogout, in which the action of colchicine is usually far less effective.

**Nonspecific Inflammatory Monarthritis.** The dilemma faced most often is the management of the patient with but one or two inflamed joints in whom no data that could establish a diagnosis are available within the first 24 to 72 hours. In some of these patients, infection may still be a consideration. Whenever this possibility cannot be definitely excluded, one might choose a course of antibiotics or perhaps just observation. Pain relief should be attempted by drugs or physical measures that will not modify the inflammatory process. Antipyretic drugs such as aspirin or acetaminophen and the nonsteroidal anti-inflammatory drugs should not be used. Fever and the possibility of extension of arthritis to other joints are helpful indicators of the nature of the underlying disease. Once sufficient evidence is at hand that infection is no longer a likely problem, then analgesic or anti-inflammatory treatment may be employed.

In the past, the striking effect of aspirin in rheumatic fever led to the notion that it could be used in a therapeutic trial in this disease. If an arthritic process rapidly abates, perhaps in 2 to 3 days, during the use of aspirin, rheumatic fever might well be considered; but, unfortunately from the standpoint of the selectivity of aspirin, other unrelated inflammatory arthritides do also. Thus, as indicated above, aspirin and other nonsteroidal anti-inflammatory drugs should only be prescribed in the initial phases of management, particularly in monarticular arthritis, after careful consideration has been given to the need to monitor the natural course of the illness, especially to response of more truly specific drugs as colchicine or an antibiotic drug.

Generally, early in the evaluation of the patient with monarticular arthritis, the physician will choose between colchicine, an antibiotic, aspirin, or observation for the reasons described above.

## REASSESSMENT

**Diagnosis Confirmed.** During the first week, a diagnosis will have been established for most patients with an arthritis whose cause or pathogenesis is well understood. Some solutions will be direct, as is often the case with, among others, gout, pseudogout, septic arthritis, and traumatic arthritis. Other solutions will be reached upon completion of special diagnostic studies or after the appearance of additional clinical findings, as with the recognition of the bowel lesion of regional enteritis in a puzzling case of oligoarthritis or the detection of a *Salmonella* species in the stool culture of a HLA-B27 positive young adult with a similar arthritis.

**Diagnosis Unconfirmed.** Other patients, perhaps even a majority, with monarticular arthritis remain an enigma. With mixed emotions, the physician will observe that a large number undergo a spontaneous remission, leaving unanswered, at least for the moment, why the disease occurred and whether it will return. For most of these patients, optimism is in order. The frequency of unexplained types of monarthritis is much higher than is generally realized, with only a small portion likely to recur. In part this is due to the one-time nature of the illness: a viral disease or a traumatic event. Even for conditions that are thought to be progressive and persistent, such as rheumatoid arthritis, it is reasonable to assume that mild forms of disease occur that undergo a spontaneous cure.

In some patients, arthritis may persist, still lacking a definite diagnosis. In these, the dictum postulated above, that one should observe their natural history without modification by treatment, may now pay off. Some will slowly develop additional features of their illness. Although most patients with psoriatic arthritis show skin lesions before arthritis, a few develop psoriatic plaques later, thus providing an explanation for the previously unknown type of oligoarthritis. The rare syndrome of systemic fat necrosis seen with chronic pancreatitis or pancreatic carcinoma becomes obvious upon the radiologic demonstration of calcific deposits in the pancreas, a high serum amylase, or the necrotic lesion in a biopsy of the subcutaneous adipose tissue. In others, concern for a possible infection may remain, so that additional diagnostic tests will be required.

Among such procedures are those that provide more information about the diseased joint. A tomogram can reveal details of a juxta-articular bone tumor, osteomyelitis, osteochondromatosis, avascular necrosis, juvenile osteochondrosis, or osteochondritis dissecans. A dye and/or air-contrast arthrogram can define a meniscal tear or the filling defect of nonradiopaque osteochondromatosis. Computerized tomograms can define abnormalities of an internal structure with increasingly distinct precision, particularly if the structure has a density that contrasts with that of surrounding tissues. Metal, bone, or calcified tissues stand out, as does adipose tissue, against connective tissues and muscle, tendons, and capsule. This method can help identify foreign bodies such as plant thorns or tumors within the joint. Synovial biopsy can provide direct information about the pathology of the disease.[43] In pigmented villonodular synovitis, the brownish, hemosiderin-laden tissue can be diagnostic. The electron-dense bodies of Whipple's disease have been found in synovium as well as in the small bowel mucosa. The granulomatous lesions of sarcoid and tuberculosis can be seen, with the further opportunity provided by the biopsy to inoculate tissue samples into appropriate culture media. In mycobacterial infections, including leprosy and atypical tuberculosis in addition to infection with *M. tuberculosis,* in fungal infections, and in infections caused by some common pyogenic invaders such as staphylococci and gonococci, culture of synovial tissue has proved to be positive when culture of joint fluid remained negative.

Direct inspection of the synovium can be accomplished by use of open biopsy rather than closed needle biopsy. Instances when this may be helpful are, for example, the diagnosis of a foreign body in synovium or the opportunity to exclude a mechanical defect such as a torn cartilage in a chronically inflamed joint. Some of these problems can now be more conveniently explored by arthroscopy.[44] This procedure allows inspection of the interior of large joints, especially the knee, and biopsy under direct vision of selected areas of synovium or cartilage.

## THE UNDIAGNOSED MONARTICULAR ARTHRITIS

For those patients in whom a diagnosis of a persistent arthritis cannot be made despite all tests, therapy with intra-articular steroid may be useful. Negative cultures and tissue examination will have excluded all reasonable possibility of sepsis. Control of synovitis is sometimes dramatic by this approach, particularly when combined with a period of several weeks of either immobilization or absence of weight bearing. Injections can be repeated at intervals of at least 2 to 3 months; if after several injections, such maneuvers fail to control the disease, synovectomy should be considered, in the hope that this surgical approach will permit eradication of the process, or at least give information about the cause of the arthritis. Close cooperation among the various physicians involved in the care of the patient—the primary physician, the rheumatologist, the orthopedic surgeon, and others, including the team from rehabilitation medicine—is the best way to manage these difficult cases. Not only must all efforts to eliminate the disease be carried out before a state of chronic disability is accepted; appropriate planning for future activities at home or at work is also necessary.

Although most cases of monarticular arthritis yield a satisfactory answer, the temptation to apply a specific diagnostic label to the truly undiagnosed case should be scrupulously avoided even if it offends the physician's pride. Some problems are idiopathic. The main reason for use of a term as "nonspecific inflammatory monarthritis" is to encourage future studies to help clarify the diagnosis. Periodic reviews at appointed intervals offer both the patient and the physician the opportunity to observe new developments. The uncomfortable presence of these patients with a nonspecific arthritis has been a strong challenge to clinical investigators. Their efforts have led to renewed interest in synovial histopathology, to the acceptance of diagnostic arthroscopy, and to a detailed analysis of all circumstances surrounding the earliest stages of such cases. In the future, these approaches along with others will reduce still further the numbers of patients for whom no exact diagnosis can be made.

## References


1. Schumacher, H.R.: Joint pathology in infectious arthritis. Clin. Rheum. Dis. 4:33, 1978.
2. Goldenberg, D.L., and Cohen, A.S.: Acute infectious arthritis. A review of patients with nongonococcal joint infections (with emphasis on therapy and prognosis). Am. J. Med. 60:369, 1976.
3. Goldenberg, D.L., and Cohen, A.S.: Arthritis due to tuberculous and fungal microorganisms. Clin. Rheum. Dis. 4:211, 1978.
4. Brogadir, S.P., Schimmer, B.M., and Myers, A.R.: Spectrum of the gonococcal arthritis-dermatitis syndrome. Semin. Arthritis Rheum. 8:177, 1979.
5. Grahame, R., and Scott, J.T.: Clinical survey of 354 patients with gout. Ann. Rheum. Dis. 29:461, 1970.
6. McCarty, D.J.: Calcium pyrophosphate dihydrate deposition disease—1975. Arthritis Rheum. 19:275, 1976.
7. Katz, I., Rainowitz, J.G., and Dziadiw, R.: Early changes in Charcot's joints. Am. J. Roentgenol. 86:965, 1961.
8. Hilgartner, M.W.: Hemophilic arthropathy. Adv. Pediatr. 21:139, 1975.
9. Ahlberg, A., and Silwer, J.: Arthropathy in von Willebrand's disease. Acta Orthop. Scand. 41:539, 1970.
10. Wild, J.H., and Zvaifler, N.J.: Hemarthrosis associated with sodium warfarin therapy. Arthritis Rheum. 19:98, 1976.
11. Heller, H., Gafni, J., Michaeli, D., Shahin, N., Sohar, E., Ehrlich, G., Karten, I., and Sokoloff, L.: Arthritis of familial Mediterranean fever (FMF). Arthritis Rheum. 9:1, 1966.
12. Silverstein, M.N., and Kelly, P.J.: Osteoarticular manifestations of Gaucher's disease. Am. J. Med. Sc. 253:569, 1967.
13. Glueck, C.J., Levy, R.I., and Fredrickson, D.S.: Acute tendinitis and arthritis. A presenting symptom of familial Type II hyperlipoproteinemia. JAMA 206:2895, 1968.
14. Martel, W., and Sitterly, B.H.: Roentgenologic manifestations of osteonecrosis. Am. J. Roentgenol. 106:509, 1969.
15. Bauer, G.C.H.: Osteonecrosis of the knee. Clin. Orthop. 130:210, 1978.
16. Byers, P.D., Cotton, R.E., Deacon, R.W., Lowy, M., Newman, P.H., Sissons, H.A., and Thomas, A.D.: The diagnosis and treatment of pigmented villonodular synovitis. J. Bone Joint Surg. 50B:290, 1968.
17. Cadman, N.L., Soule, E.H., and Kelly, P.J.: Synovial sarcoma: An analysis of 134 tumors. Cancer 18:613, 1965.
18. Calabro, J.J.: Cancer and arthritis. Arthritis Rheum. 10:553, 1967.
19. Goldenberg, D.L., Kelley, W., and Gibbons, R.B.: Metastatic adenocarcinoma of synovium presenting as an acute arthritis. Arthritis Rheum. 18:107, 1975.
20. Lagier, R.: Synovial reaction caused by adjacent malignant tumors: Anatomico-pathological study of three cases. J. Rheumatol. 4:65, 1977.
21. Milgram, J.W.: Synovial osteochondromatosis: A histologic study of 30 cases. J. Bone Joint Surg. 59A:792, 1977.
22. Gibson, T., Schumacher, H.R., Pascual, E., and Brighton, C.: Arthropathy, skin and bone lesions in pancreatic disease. J. Rheum. 2:7, 1975.
23. Calin, A.: Reiter's syndrome. Med. Clin. North Am. 61:365, 1977.
24. Cassidy, J.T., Brody, G.L., and Martel, W.: Monarticular juvenile rheumatoid arthritis. J. Pediatr. 70:867, 1967.
25. Sherman, M.: Psoriatic arthritis: Observations on the clinical, roentgenographic and pathological changes. J. Bone Joint Surg. 34A:831, 1952.
26. Wright, V.: Psoriasis and arthritis. Ann. Rheum. Dis. 15:348, 1956.
27. Haslock, I., and Wright, V.: The musculo-skeletal complications of Crohn's disease. Medicine 52:217, 1973.
28. Wright, V., and Watkinson, G.: The arthritis of ulcerative colitis. Br. Med. J. 2:670, 1965.
29. Kelly, J.J. III, and Weisiger, B.B.: The arthritis of Whipple's disease. Arthritis Rheum. 6:615, 1963.
30. Spilberg, I., Siltzbach, L.E., and McEwen, C.E.: The arthritis of sarcoidosis. Arthritis Rheum. 12:126, 1969.
31. Dymock, I.W., Hamilton, E.B.D., Laws, J.W., and Williams, R.: Arthropathy of haemochromatosis. Clinical and radiologic analysis of 63 patients with iron overload. Ann. Rheum. Dis. 29:469, 1970.
32. Solomon, L.: Patterns of osteoarthritis of the hip. J. Bone Joint Surg. 58B:176, 1976.
33. Cohen, A.S., and Canoso, J.J.: Rheumatological aspects of amyloid disease. Clin. Rheum. Dis. 1:149, 1975.
34. O'Hanlan, M., McAdam, L.P., Bluestone, R., and Pearson, C.M.: The arthropathy of relapsing polychondritis. Arthritis Rheum. 19:191, 1976.
35. Khachadurian, A.K.: Migratory polyarthritis in familial hypercholesterolemia (Type II hyperlipoproteinemia). Arthritis Rheum. 11:385, 1968.
36. Goldman, J.A., Abrams, N.R., Glueck, C.J., Steiner, P., and Herman, J.H.: Musculoskeletal disorders associated with Type IV hyperlipoproteinemia. Lancet 2:449, 1972.
37. McCarty, D.J., and Hollander, J.L.: Identification of urate crystals in gouty synovial fluid. Ann. Intern. Med. 54:452, 1961.
38. Graham, J., and Goldman, J.A.: Fat droplets and synovial fluid leukocytes in traumatic arthritis. Arthritis Rheum. 21:76, 1978.
39. Pekin, T.J. Jr., Malinin, T.I., Zvaifler, N.J.: Unusual synovial fluid findings in Reiter's syndrome. Ann. Intern. Med. 66:677, 1967.
40. Wallace, R., and Cohen, A.S.: Tuberculous arthritis. A report of two cases with a review of biopsy and synovial fluid findings. Am. J. Med. 61:277, 1976.
41. Gordon, D.A., Pruzanski, W., and Ogryzlo, M.A.: Synovial fluid examination for the diagnosis of amyloidosis. Ann. Rheum. Dis. 32:428, 1973.
42. Hawkins, C.F., Farr, M., Morris, C.J., Hoare, A.M., and Williamson, N.: Detection by electron microscope of rod-shaped organisms in synovial membrane from a patient with the arthritis of Whipple's disease. Ann. Rheum. Dis. 35:502, 1976.
43. Goldenberg, D.L., and Cohen, A.S.: Synovial membrane histopathology in the differential diagnosis of rheumatoid arthritis, gout, pseudogout, systemic lupus erythematosus, infectious arthritis and degenerative joint disease. Medicine 57:239, 1978.
44. Johnson, L.L.: Comprehensive Arthroscopic Examination of the Knee. St. Louis, C.V. Mosby Co., 1977.

# Chapter 26
# Polyarticular Arthritis

*Ronald J. Anderson*

## THE DIFFERENTIAL DIAGNOSIS OF POLYARTICULAR SYMPTOMS

In evaluating a patient with polyarticular joint complaints the initial decision is to determine whether one is dealing with (1) polyarticular synovitis, (2) multiple structural lesions, or (3) diffuse myalgias. There are several features of the latter two conditions that permit one to make such a diagnosis based primarily on history and physical examination alone (Table 26–1).

## MULTIPLE STRUCTURAL LESIONS

Although degenerative joint disease is most frequently a monarticular process, it may occur in either a symmetrical or a polyarticular fashion. The occurrence of premature polyarticular degenerative joint disease should alert one to the possibility of a primary defect in cartilage metabolism such as is seen in either hemachromatosis or ochronosis.

### Features of Structural Lesions

**Historical Features.** *Progressive Increase in Symptoms.* Because of the irreversibility of cartilage loss, the symptoms tend to become progressively more severe. However, because of the gradual process of cartilage wear, the time course necessary for the development of these symptoms is prolonged and usually entails several years.

*Absence of Symptoms at Rest.* As the genesis of pain in structural lesions would appear to be due to the opposition of two imperfect surfaces against each other, the predominant early symptoms of structural lesions occur only with use. It is only late in the course of the degenerative process that pain at rest occurs.

*Absence of Reversible "Flares."* As the process is a gradual degenerative one, "flares" of increased symptoms are rare and should be attributed to some other cause (e.g., bursitis, pseudogout) rather than to an increase in cartilage degeneration itself.

*Lack of Response to Anti-inflammatory Therapy.* Because synovitis or other inflammatory conditions play little or no role in causing symptoms, the clinical response to the use of these agents is minimal. A frequent exception, however, is a beneficial symptomatic response to indomethacin seen in osteoarthritis of the hip.

*Absence of Systemic Symptoms.* Since the disease process is local and primarily degenerative, there is an absence of systemic malaise or other generalized symptoms.

*Absence of Prolonged Morning Stiffness.* Morning stiffness in structural lesions is a "gelling" phenomenon, with maximal relief occurring in 5 to 10 minutes. This is in contradistinction to the chronic rheumatic diseases, which have prolonged morning stiffness.

**Objective Data.** 1. Localization to weight-bearing joints. It is unusual for degenerative changes to occur in such non-weight-bearing joints as the shoulder, elbow, wrist, or metacarpal-phalangeal joints.

2. Radiographic evidence of cartilage loss in the involved joints.

3. Radiographic evidence of hypertrophic new bone formation. This feature is absent in the synovitic conditions because the erosive inflammatory process precludes new bone formation. Because significant synovitis is not seen in osteoarthritis, the reparative process is allowed to occur and hypertrophic spurs are frequently seen.

4. Noninflammatory characteristics of synovial fluid.

### Diffuse Myalgia

This entity encompasses a large group of conditions, the primary features of which are benignity, nonprogressiveness, and generally an absence of physical findings. The symptoms seem to arise out of the muscles

**Table 26–1.** Cardinal Distinctions Between Structural and Synovial Lesions

| Structural Lesions | Synovial Lesions |
|---|---|
| *Subjective Features* | |
| Symptoms only with use | Symptoms at rest |
| "Gelling" phenomenon | Morning stiffness common |
| Progressive worsening course | Variable course |
| Flares not seen | Flares common |
| Minimal response to medical treatment | Patient often benefits from medical treatment |
| Patient systematically well | Patient often systemically ill |
| *Objective Features* | |
| Crepitus and bony hypertrophy on physical examination | Soft tissue swelling on physical examination |
| Noninflammatory joint fluid | Inflammatory joint fluid |
| X-ray: | X-ray: |
| Usually positive | Negative early in course |
| Local cartilage loss | Diffuse cartilage loss |
| Often new bone growth | No new bone growth |
| Weight-bearing joints involved | Any joint involved (e.g., elbow) |
| *Therapy* | |
| Surgical | Medical |

and periarticular structures. Patients with these complaints range from a group of patients best described as "achey" to another group who appear to use their symptoms for secondary gain. The "genuinely achey" group would seem to be analogous to patients with a spastic colon in that they are anatomically normal and do not develop any specific lesion. Laboratory examinations in the rheumatic diseases are relatively nonspecific. In the area of "false-positives" approximately 30 percent of "normals" will be latex positive, ANA positive, or hyperuricemic. It may also be stated, parenthetically, that no one over age 40 has a normal spinal radiograph. In regard to "false-negatives," skeletal radiographs are invariably normal in early synovitis, and the latex, ANA, and serum uric acid are frequently normal in those patients afflicted with the corresponding conditions. Therefore, as in most of rheumatology, it may be said regarding benign myalgias that if the physician does not know whether a patient is sick or not prior to laboratory evaluation, the laboratory and radiologic data will not answer this basic question.

## FEATURES OF BENIGN MYALGIAS

**Intermittent Pattern of Symptoms with Asymptomatic Intervals.** This pattern is frequently abrupt in onset, with symptoms lasting only several minutes to hours, a distinguishing point from synovitis, in which the inflammatory process can seldom arise and subside in less than 3 days. The major value of this historical feature is in the differentiation from the generally irreversible structural lesions, which, with the exception of a deranged knee meniscus, are never intermittent. A corollary of this feature is that radiographic abnormalities of an intermittently asymptomatic joint are meaningless, as the radiograph shows irreversible changes that can never improve.

**Lack of Functional Loss.** There is no functional loss, or what functional loss exists is "illogical." Any condition with the ability to alter or destroy the anatomy of a joint will be associated with a dysfunction or loss of function of that particular joint. For example, patients with diseases affecting the hands will become unable to open jars or turn faucets. Hip or knee disease is associated with an inability to arise from a bathtub or a low chair. These specific dysfunctions are virtually universally found in disorders of these joints, and their absence implies that a significant disorder of these joints does not exist. Patients with benign myalgias, on the other hand, do not lose function over time, or whatever function they do lose is illogical (e.g., the patient no longer is employed but he still goes bowling). The usual history obtained is: "I've slowed down," but one cannot elicit a specific function that the patient cannot do.

**Negative or Static Physical Examination.** The physical examination is negative or static over an extended period of time. Occasionally a patient will be examined on a "good day" when he is asymptomatic and the physical examination is negative. If this is the situation and the patient states, "You should have seen me 10 days ago when I was bad," the logical diagnostic approach is to have him return on a day when he is symptomatic and examine him at that time to determine if a change has occurred. If, on the other hand, the examination is negative in a patient with persistent symptoms, a logical approach is to record functions quantitatively (e.g., grip strengths, range of motion, timed walk of 50 feet) and then re-examine the patient several months later. If the measurements are unchanged, one can infer that no active destructive process, despite persistent symptoms, has occurred during the interim.

## THE DIAGNOSIS OF SYNOVITIS

The ultimate requirement for the diagnosis of synovitis is the demonstration of inflammatory changes in a joint. The techniques used to perform this are as follows.

**Evaluation of Historical Features.** The author's experience has lead him to believe that patients are frequently unreliable in describing swelling within their own joints. More credence may be lent to a description by family members of the appearance of the joint, particularly when it is unilateral. The description by the patient of swelling in joints in which synovitis is never physically apparent (i.e., spine or hips) leads the physician to doubt the patient's reliability as an examiner of himself. However, several historical features are valuable.

*The Significance of Morning Stiffness.* Any musculoskeletal disorder, even a sprained ankle, has accentuated symptoms following prolonged immobility. However, in benign myalgias, most of the acute inflammatory disorders such as gout, and osteoarthritis, in general the stiffness tends to be short lived, and maximal alleviation of the symptoms is noted after 5 to 10 minutes of activity. In contrast, in the chronic inflammatory disorders (rheumatoid arthritis, spondylitis, psoriatic arthritis, and systemic lupus erythematosus), the morning stiffness tends to be prolonged for several hours' duration. This is not only a subjective phenomenon. Objective signs of synovitis may be detected on early-morning examinations but disappear as the day progresses. Measurements of joint function (i.e., grip strengths) also tend to improve in the same pattern.

It is advisable to quantitate the duration of morning stiffness in a standardized fashion. A phrase such as: "How long does it take, once you get up in the morning, until you're as good as you'll ever be?" usually will result in a reproducibly quantitative answer. The duration is a valuable bit of data for two reasons:

1. Significant (greater than one hour) morning stiffness tends to differentiate the chronic inflammatory processes from other disorders.

2. The duration of morning stiffness tends to parallel the severity of the synovitis. This is of particular value in assessing the effectiveness of anti-inflammatory therapy in patients whose symptoms represent a combina-

tion of potentially reversible synovitis and irreversible structural lesions. In such patients, a remission may be associated with a complete disappearance of morning stiffness but only minor or no improvement in the functional status. As medical therapy has the ability only to alter the reversible inflammatory aspects of these conditions, it becomes apparent that the duration of morning stiffness serves as a useful parameter in evaluating the effectiveness of such therapy.

*Gradual Variability of Course.* The inflammatory process of synovitis is potentially reversible, and periods of remission when the patient may be asymptomatic are seen in several conditions of this type. The minimal time required for a joint to become inflamed and then totally remit would seem to be in the range of 36 to 48 hours. Symptomatic flares in benign myalgias tend to be brief periods of symptoms lasting less than 24 hours.

It is more common for the synovitis to follow a course of gradual variability, with a rate of change measured in weeks and months. Specific dysfunctions occur during periods of synovitic activity, a distinguishing point in comparison with benign myalgias.

In contradistinction, the symptoms of structural lesions, with the exception of a deranged meniscus of the knee, are persistent and progressive in severity.

*Symptoms at Rest.* The presence of pain at rest is a feature of synovitis, neuropathies, and periarticular lesions (tendinitis, bursitis). Rest pain is seen in structural lesions only in the most far-advanced conditions in which a several-year history of increasing pain with activity is obtained.

*Rapidity of Onset of Symptoms and Flares of Accentuated Activity.* The degeneration of articular cartilage is a gradual process. Flares are rarely seen, and rapid improvement from accentuated symptoms is never seen. On the other hand, flares are common with synovitis.

**Physical Examination.** The appearance of an obviously inflamed, swollen joint makes the diagnosis easy. On the other hand, the hip and the spine will never appear swollen on physical examination, and one is forced to rely upon range of motion to elicit an objective abnormality. In addition, palpable effusions are rarely seen in the shoulder joint and are frequently subtle in the metacarpophalangeal and tarsal joints. In these latter two regions, one may employ examination techniques aimed at demonstrating spasm and shortening of muscles adjacent to inflamed joints. These techniques are as follows:

*Bunnel's Sign.* The intrinsic muscles of the hand, which consist of the lumbricales and the interossei, arise from the metacarpals, pass across the metacarpophalangeal joint, and serve to flex the metacarpophalangeal joint and extend the proximal interphalangeal joint. In the inflammation of the metacarpophalangeal joint, these muscles become tight and produce a situation in which proximal interphalangeal flexion is limited when the metacarpophalangeals are extended but normal when the metacarpophalangeals are flexed. Because the metacarpophalangeals are exclusively involved in synovitic processes and are not affected by osteoarthritis or Bouchard's nodes, this sign is pathognomonic of synovitis of the metacarpophalangeal joint. In addition, in a patient with obvious synovitis it will distinguish between proximal interphalangeal and metacarpophalangeal disease as the cause of proximal interphalangeal dysfunction.

The principle of Bunnel's sign is also useful as a screening technique in evaluating generalized hand stiffness. A patient who can fully extend his fingers and also touch his fingertips to his palms with his metacarpophalangeals extended has normal metacarpophalangeals, proximal interphalangeals, and distal interphalangeals (Fig. 26-1; see Plate I, p. xxxv).

*Peroneal Spasm.* The peroneal muscles arise from the lateral calf, run across the tarsal bones, and serve to evert the foot. In tarsal inflammation, particularly of the talonavicular joint (the tarsal joint most commonly involved in rheumatoid arthritis), the peroneal musculature tightens up and everts the foot, and pain localized to the peroneal area is felt on forced inversion of the ankle. The associated tenderness localized to the talonavicular joint adds specificity to this maneuver (Fig. 26–2).

**Laboratory Examination.** The only direct technique of establishing the presence of synovitis in an inflamed joint is the determination of the white blood cell (WBC) count within the synovial fluids (Table 26–2).

The major diagnostic distinction that may be made based upon the synovial fluid WBC count is between an inflammatory condition and normal or osteoarthritic joint fluid. Although patients with septic arthritis may present with pus, they may also have a WBC count in the range found with sterile inflammatory conditions.

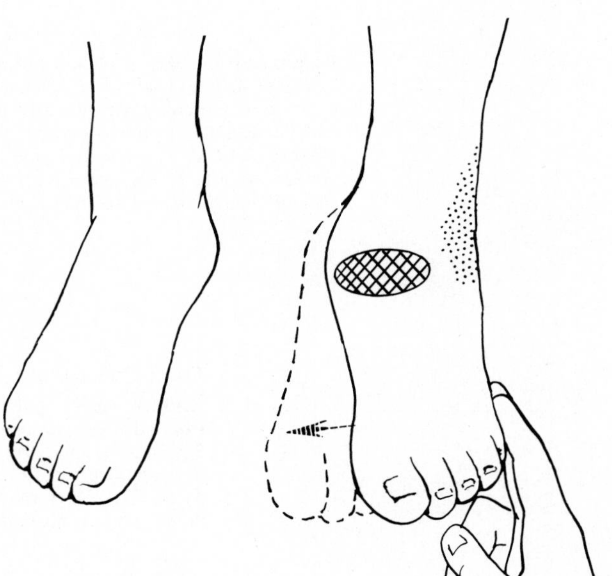

**Figure 26–2.** Peroneal spasm. Tenderness to palpation over the talonavicular-joint (cross-hatched area) in conjunction with painful spasm within the peroneal musculature (dotted area) upon passive inversion of the foot is indicative of talonavicular synovitis.

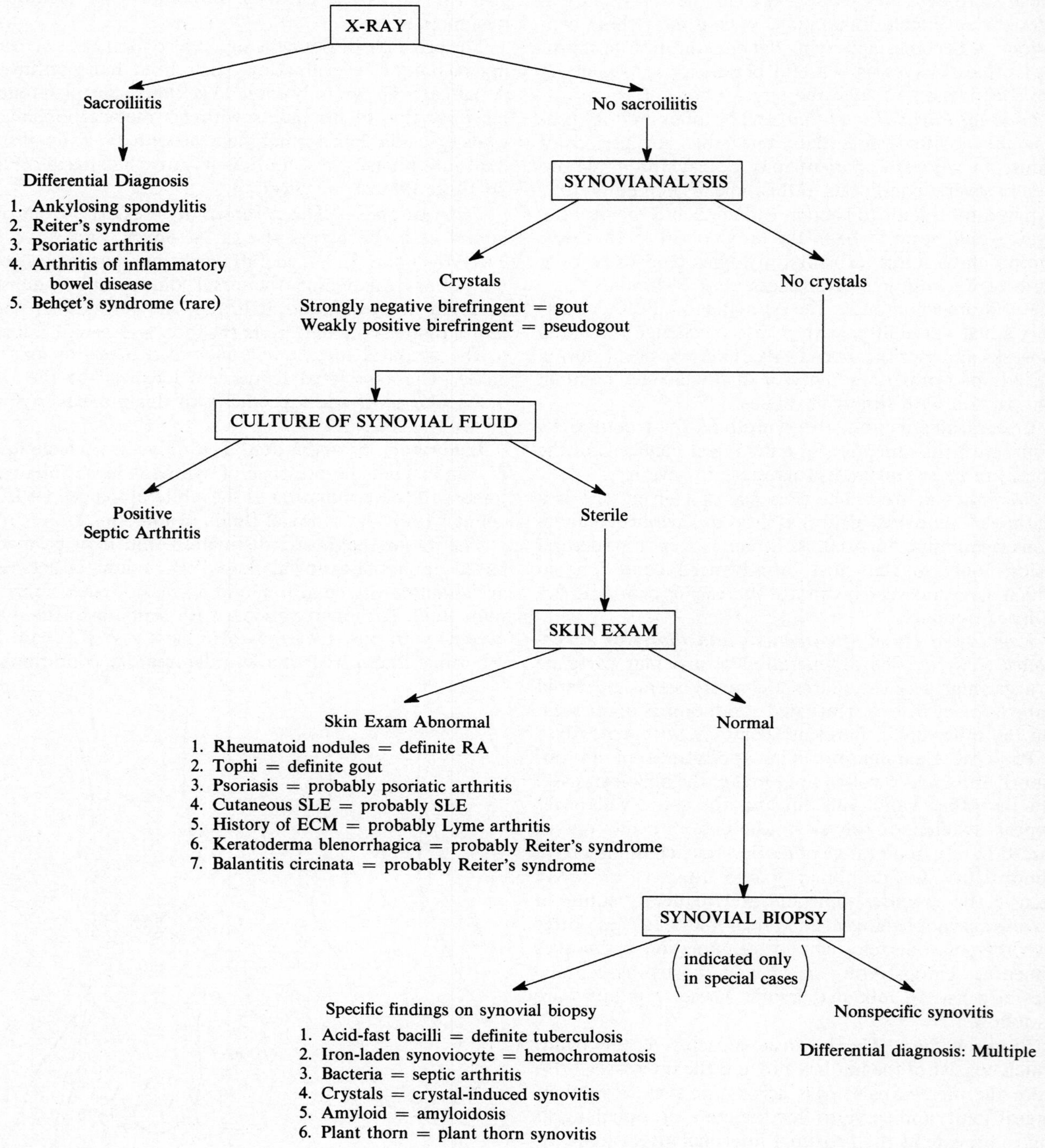
X-RAY
Sacroiliitis
No sacroiliitis
Differential Diagnosis
1. Ankylosing spondylitis
2. Reiter's syndrome
3. Psoriatic arthritis
4. Arthritis of inflammatory bowel disease
5. Behçet's syndrome (rare)
SYNOVIANALYSIS
Crystals
Strongly negative birefringent = gout
Weakly positive birefringent = pseudogout
No crystals
CULTURE OF SYNOVIAL FLUID
Positive
Septic Arthritis
Sterile
SKIN EXAM
Skin Exam Abnormal
1. Rheumatoid nodules = definite RA
2. Tophi = definite gout
3. Psoriasis = probably psoriatic arthritis
4. Cutaneous SLE = probably SLE
5. History of ECM = probably Lyme arthritis
6. Keratoderma blenorrhagica = probably Reiter's syndrome
7. Balantitis circinata = probably Reiter's syndrome
Normal
SYNOVIAL BIOPSY
(indicated only in special cases)
Specific findings on synovial biopsy
1. Acid-fast bacilli = definite tuberculosis
2. Iron-laden synoviocyte = hemochromatosis
3. Bacteria = septic arthritis
4. Crystals = crystal-induced synovitis
5. Amyloid = amyloidosis
6. Plant thorn = plant thorn synovitis
Nonspecific synovitis
Differential diagnosis: Multiple

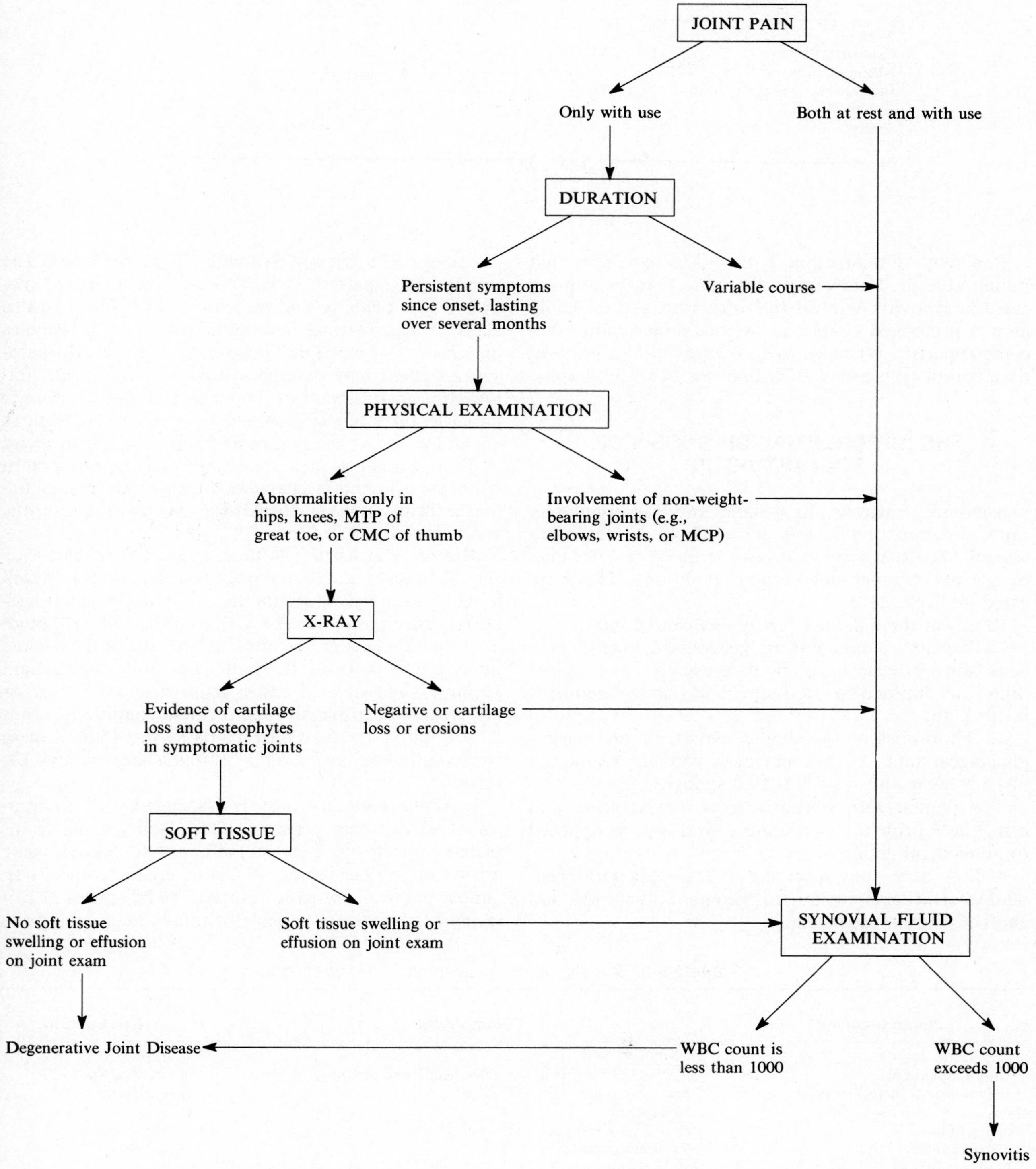
JOINT PAIN
Only with use
Both at rest and with use
DURATION
Persistent symptoms since onset, lasting over several months
Variable course
PHYSICAL EXAMINATION
Abnormalities only in hips, knees, MTP of great toe, or CMC of thumb
Involvement of non-weight-bearing joints (e.g., elbows, wrists, or MCP)
X-RAY
Evidence of cartilage loss and osteophytes in symptomatic joints
Negative or cartilage loss or erosions
SOFT TISSUE
No soft tissue swelling or effusion on joint exam
Soft tissue swelling or effusion on joint exam
SYNOVIAL FLUID EXAMINATION
Degenerative Joint Disease
WBC count is less than 1000
WBC count exceeds 1000
Synovitis

**Table 26–2.** White Blood Cell Count ($\times 10^3$)

| Condition | 0 | 1 | 2 | 4 | 8 | 16 | 32 | 64 | 128 | Pus |
|---|---|---|---|---|---|---|---|---|---|---|
| Normal | — | | | | | | | | | |
| Osteoarthritis | — | — | | | | | | | | |
| Rheumatoid arthritis | | — | — | — | — | — | — | — | | |
| Juvenile rheumatoid arthritis | | — | — | — | — | — | — | — | | |
| Gout | | | | | — | — | — | — | | |
| Sepsis | | | | | | | — | — | — | — |

**Radiologic Examination.** It is well to remember that radiographs predominantly show bone, that the primary event in synovitis involves the soft tissue, and that only after a prolonged course do osseous abnormalities become apparent. When synovitis is equivocal on physical examination, it is even less distinct on roentgenography.

## THE DIFFERENTIAL DIAGNOSIS OF POLYARTHRITIS

**Anatomic Patterns.** In general any condition may cause inflammation in any joint. However, there are several joints that seem to have a specificity, in a negative or positive manner, for certain conditions. These are listed in Table 26–3.

Based on these data, a few points can be made:

1. Patients complaining of generalized musculoskeletal pain who also have jaw pain usually have "something," as opposed to "nothing," and that "something" is not gout.
2. Deformities of the elbows, wrists, or metacarpophalangeal joints, even in an elderly patient, are due not just to "wear and tear" but to a synovitic process.
3. A patient with urethritis, fever, polyarthritis, and a *stiff neck* probably has Reiter's syndrome as opposed to gonococcal arthritis.
4. Low back pain occurring in a patient with rheumatoid arthritis is not due to rheumatoid arthritis, and another cause must be sought.

**Temporal Patterns of Synovitis.** *Additive Pattern.* The term additive pattern is used to describe a clinical syndrome that tends to add on features as it flares and to subtract these features in a similar manner as it becomes quiescent. For example, in systemic lupus erythematosus, a patient may develop synovitis of the wrists, followed by involvement of the knees and elbows. All the initial features of the disease persist while new features are added on. As the syndrome remits, the features tend to disappear in a sequential manner. This type of pattern is nonspecific and is characteristically seen in rheumatoid arthritis, lupus erythematosus, postrubella arthritis, and spondylitis.

*Migratory Pattern.* The term migratory polyarthritis should be restricted to describe those situations in which initially inflamed joints totally remit while, simultaneously, other joints become actively inflamed. Although occasionally seen in rheumatoid arthritis and systemic lupus erythematosus, the pattern is quite unique and strongly suggestive of either acute rheumatic fever or gonococcal arthritis. In each of these conditions, a migratory polyarthritis is characteristic. In addition, these two conditions have several distinguishing clinical features.

1. Acute rheumatic fever is associated with a migratory synovitis that peaks in 12 to 24 hours and completely subsides in a given joint in 2 to 5 days while arising in another region. A characteristic feature is an almost uniform dramatic response to full doses of salicylates, which seem capable of totally suppressing the

**Table 26–3.** Specific Joint Involvement in Polyarthritis

| Joints Involved | Common With | Not Seen In |
|---|---|---|
| Temporomandibular | Rheumatoid arthritis, juvenile rheumatoid arthritis, psoriasis | Gout, myalgias |
| Elbows, wrists, metacarpophalangeals | Any synovitis | Osteoarthritis |
| Hips | Nonspecific | Gout |
| Ankles (only) | Erythema nodosum | |
| Cricoarytenoid | Rheumatoid arthritis | All other |
| Talonavicular | Rheumatoid arthritis | |
| Cervical spine | Rheumatoid arthritis, juvenile rheumatoid arthritis, psoriasis, osteoarthritis, spondylitis, myalgias | Gout, gonococcal arthritis |
| Thoracolumbar spine | Spondylitis: Ankylosing spondylitis; Psoriasis; Reiter's syndrome; Inflammatory bowel disease | Gout, rheumatoid arthritis |

synovitis within 2 to 4 days after the initiation of therapy. If the salicylates are abruptly discontinued, the synovitis tends to reappear in a few days' time.

2. Gonococcal arthritis has two major patterns of joint involvement.[1,2] One pattern involves a migratory polyarthritis and tenosynovitis, predominantly of the small joints; bacteremia; petechial skin lesions, which progress to pustules; and sterile synovial fluid. Because of the difficulty of aspirating fluid from either the small joints or the inflamed tenosynovium, samples of synovial fluid are seldom obtainable for culture. The second pattern, which may be the initial presentation or may occur following an initial migratory polyarthritis, is the "septic joint" syndrome in which the presentation is of an acute septic, usually monarticular, arthritis. In these patients the blood cultures are often sterile and the synovial fluid cultures are often positive. Skin lesions are rarely reported in this presentation.

In 1974 Brandt and colleagues,[3] on the other hand, had surveyed 31 patients with acute arthritis and proved gonococcal infection. Although the presence of positive blood and synovial fluid cultures was mutually exclusive, they found no correlation between the source of the positive culture and the clinical picture. In addition, the clinical features were variable, and two distinct patterns were not seen.

Despite these conflicting reports, several points seem to be in agreement and of definite clinical value:

1. Positive cultures of either the synovial fluid or the blood seem to be mutually exclusive, and either may occur in any presentation. Therefore appropriate diagnosis requires bacteriologic examination from both sources.

2. Migratory polyarthritis should alert the physician to the possibility of gonococcal arthritis. This is particularly important also in evaluating a patient with acute, apparently septic monarticular arthritis. There is essentially no other condition except gonococcal arthritis in which an antecedent history of migratory polyarthritis will be obtained prior to the onset of acute monarticular arthritis. Therefore, one should always search for this history when evaluating a patient with a hot, inflamed joint.

Meningococcemia may have a presentation identical with that of gonococcal arthritis. With regard to patient screening, all patients with a migratory pattern of synovitis warrant immediate and complete evaluation, as the two predominant conditions associated with this pattern are both significantly treatable and ominous.

***Palindromic or Intermittent Patterns.*** The term palindromic polyarthritis is used to describe those conditions associated with repetitive attacks of polyarticular synovitis that completely remit without sequelae or spread to other joints. Migratory conditions have already been discussed elsewhere. In evaluating patients with these complaints, two useful points should come to mind:

1. The definition of a palindromic state requires a period of observation to establish that the condition will spontaneously remit. Despite this, a prior history of palindromic flares makes it more likely that the current process will follow the same pattern.

2. At the time of initial examination the patient may be completely asymptomatic with a negative physical examination. Rather than obtaining laboratory data blindly and randomly, it is best to request that the patient return during a symptomatic interval when the true nature of the lesion may better be evaluated.

There is some value in separating palindromic conditions according to temporal patterns based upon the duration of inflammation. Short courses (2 to 3 days) are almost exclusively seen in rheumatoid arthritis, although they may also occur in sarcoidosis, familial Mediterranean fever, and sickle cell anemia.[4] Longer courses (7 to 100 days) occur in the peripheral synovitis of spondylitis, the arthropathy of inflammatory bowel disease,[5] Whipple's disease,[6] the polyarthritis associated with intestinal bypass,[7] Behçet's syndrome,[8] familial Mediterranean fever, and sickle cell anemia.[4] Acute polyarthritis has also been described in gout as an initial presentation. In 1974 Hadler and colleagues[9] reviewed the records of 1830 patients discharged from the Massachusetts General Hospital with the diagnosis of gout, gouty arthritis, or hyperuricemia. Of these patients 34 presented with acute polyarticular gout confirmed by the identification of sodium urate crystals in the synovial fluid. Twelve patients within this subgroup of 34 had polyarthritis as the initial manifestation of gout. The unique features of the presentation were asymmetry and preponderant involvement of the foot, ankle, and knee.

While polyarticular gout, particularly as an initial manifestation of the disease, would appear to be decidedly rare, "cluster attacks" of polyarthritis are not rare in pseudogout.[10]

**Fever and Polyarticular Arthritis.** The presence of fever may serve as an important clue in the diagnosis of polyarthritis. Septic arthritis is discussed elsewhere, and only the sterile processes will be discussed here. Any synovitic process may be associated with a fever, which tends to reflect the activity of the apparent synovitis. Gout would be a classic example of this situation, and temperatures in the 100 to 102° F range are not uncommon.[9] The examiner is usually able to examine the joint, assay the degree of inflammation, and make a relatively accurate guess as to what level of fever will be found.

On the other hand, there are several sterile processes that may present as polyarthritis in which the fever would appear to be in excess of the degree of inflammation observable in the joints. In this situation the cause of the excessive fever would seem to be an inflammatory process not readily apparent on physical examination. Conditions in which this is the case are as follows:

1. Rheumatoid arthritis. The excessive fever is often due to one of three situations: (a) vasculitis; (b) serositis affecting the pleura or pericardium; or (c) a recent abrupt decrease in the steroid dose in a patient maintained on chronic steroids (this may occur even though an adequate physiologic dose of steroids is administered).

2. Systemic lupus erythematosus.
3. Erythema nodosum. Fever can occur even in the absence of skin or joint lesions.
4. Familial Mediterranean fever.
5. Henoch-Schönlein purpura.
6. Behçet's syndrome.
7. Acute rheumatic fever.
8. Whipple's disease.
9. Lyme arthritis.
10. Sarcoidosis with or without erythema nodosum.
11. Juvenile rheumatoid arthritis. In the Still's disease variant of this disorder, fever without synovitis, or fever tremendously in excess of that expected from the apparent synovitis, is the rule. The characteristic truncal, evanescent skin rash is often the only observable lesion, and the true cause of the fever is not known. When the presentation occurs in adulthood, the diagnosis may be particularly obscure.[11]
12. Inflammatory bowel disease. The bowel lesion may be either inapparent or quiescent. Clubbing of the fingers is a distinctive and almost diagnostic feature of this condition if it is present and if subacute bacterial endocarditis has been excluded in a patient with febrile polyarthritis.
13. Reiter's syndrome and ankylosing spondylitis. The articulations of the spine are sufficiently "buried" so that inflammation is not apparent to palpation. This is a possible explanation for the fever's being often in excess of the apparent joint inflammation.

## PATTERNS OF THERAPEUTIC RESPONSE

Therapeutic response to specific pharmacologic agents is highly variable in the rheumatic diseases, and few firm conclusions can be drawn. Even the classic specificity of colchicine for gout suffers from the sizable proportion of gouty attacks that do not respond, and the ability of colchicine to abort attacks of familial Mediterranean fever and occasionally erythema nodosum. Diagnostic decisions based on this type of evidence are usually not sound. However, a few points may be of diagnostic value:

1. The dramatic response of acute rheumatic fever to salicylates seems highly specific. Usually the findings and symptoms may be completely suppressed when therapeutic levels of the drug are obtained.
2. Indomethacin and phenylbutazone are usually equipotent to the other nonsteroidal anti-inflammatory agents in most polyarticular inflammatory diseases. However, in gout and the spondyloarthropathies they are usually dramatically more effective.
3. The institution of steroids in a prednisone dose of about 20 mg per day usually will initially almost completely suppress the synovitic features of rheumatoid arthritis and systemic lupus erythematosus but often will have little effect upon the synovitis of the spondyloarthropathies.

## SYSTEMIC ASSOCIATIONS WITH POLYARTICULAR ARTHRITIS

Under this heading, associations will be recorded between polyarthritis and lesions or specific diseases of other organ systems. As pulmonary diseases are not covered separately in this text, they will be discussed here in somewhat greater depth.

**Pulmonary Manifestations of Rheumatic Diseases.** *Tracheolaryngeal Lesions.* Inflammation of the cricoarytenoid joint is a common manifestation of rheumatoid arthritis and is seen in virtually no other form of polyarthritis. Symptoms are chronic laryngeal pain and dysphonia, often accentuated with morning stiffness. A dysphagia of the globus hystericus type may also be seen. Tracheal pain is a common feature of relapsing polychondritis, and tracheal collapse is a fatal complication of this rare condition. The chronic mucous membrane dryness of Sjögren's syndrome may also provoke laryngeal symptoms.

*Bronchial Lesions.* An undocumented clinical suspicion exists that chronic bronchitis is more common in rheumatoid arthritis. The only documented lesion is atrophy of the glands of the respiratory tract in Sjögren's syndrome.

*Pulmonary Fibrosis.* Symptoms of dyspnea usually present only in the later stages of fibrosis owing to the tendency of patients to decrease their activity in accordance with their reduced pulmonary function. This is particularly significant in evaluating patients with crippling disorders who, because their primary musculoskeletal disease limits their exercise capacity, are seldom stressed to the limits of their pulmonary capacity. The exact incidence of parenchymal pulmonary dysfunction in the rheumatic diseases is unknown and varies with the sensitivity of the assay employed.

Pulmonary fibrosis is seen frequently in rheumatoid arthritis, systemic lupus erythematosus, polymyositis or dermatomyositis, and scleroderma. It appears to be much less common in the spondyloarthropathies. The current understanding implies that the disorder encompasses a spectrum that probably progresses from alveolitis to interstitial fibrosis. One cannot distinguish between the different arthropathies based on the pulmonary features; nor can the pulmonary lesion be distinguished from idiopathic pulmonary fibrosis.[12,13]

*Pulmonary Infiltrates.* Pulmonary infiltrates are relatively common as a transient event in systermic lupus erythematosus and may occur in any vasculitis, particularly in Wegener's granulomatosis, and rarely in Sjögren's syndrome.

*Pulmonary Nodules.* Among the rheumatic diseases, nodules occur almost exclusively in rheumatoid arthritis. They are usually multiple, do not calcify, and range from 0.5 to 5 cm in diameter. Rheumatoid pulmonary nodule formation is associated with peripheral nodules, a higher titer of rheumatoid factor, the male gender, and pneumoconiotic exposure. Their natural tendency to involute and their multiplicity tend to differentiate them from malignant nodules.

*Lesions of the Pulmonary Vasculature.* Pulmonary hypertension may develop secondary to the chronic hypoxia associated with pulmonary fibrosis or may arise de novo and not correlate with either arterial hypoxia or pulmonary fibrosis. In the latter situation Raynaud's phenomenon is usually present and the condition is seen in scleroderma, other rheumatic disorders with Raynaud's phenomenon, or Raynaud's syndrome alone.

*Pleural Disorders.* Inflammatory pleuritis is a common manifestation of rheumatoid arthritis, systemic lupus erythematosus, and the other vasculitides. It is not seen in noninflammatory rheumatic disorders and has not been described in psoriatic arthritis, Reiter's syndrome, or the spondyloarthropathies. The fluid characteristically will have a leukocytosis, elevation of the lactic dehydrogenase, and a protein content consistent with an exudate. In rheumatoid arthritis a low glucose content, usually less than 10 mg per 100 ml, is almost pathognomonic of the disease but is not universally seen in rheumatoid pleural effusions.

**Dermatological Manifestations of Polyarticular Arthritis.** This topic is covered in Chapter 36, and will be discussed here only briefly.

*Nodules.* These lesions are almost exclusively seen in rheumatoid arthritis and gout. There is a predilection in both conditions for them to form on the olecranon surfaces. Although the biopsy of each is distinctive, the appearance on physical examination may be identical. Several features tend to distinguish the two:

1. Rheumatoid nodules may occur simultaneously, soon after, or even prior to the onset of rheumatoid arthritis. Tophi occur later and are seldom evident within the first 2 years of the disease. Therefore, a patient with polyarthritis of less than 2 years' duration and olecranon nodules probably has rheumatoid arthritis.
2. Aspiration of tophi will reveal urate crystals.
3. Rheumatoid nodules usually arise abruptly, with a definite inflammatory reaction, and tend to regress in size with time. Tophi increase in size in a gradual manner and an inflammatory reaction is seldom seen, particularly early in their course.

*Erythema.* In Still's disease a transient, primarily truncal rash with the Koebner phenomenon is characteristic. It is usually seen in the late afternoon.

*Squamous Eruptions.* These are characteristic of Reiter's syndrome and psoriasis and are indistinguishable from each other by both physical and histological examination. Subungual hyperkeratoses are also seen in both diseases. Pitting of the nails seems to be limited to psoriasis.

*Pustules.* These are found in neisserial bacteremia and usually occur distally, progressing from papules to vesicles to pustules.

*Urticaria.* This may be seen in any vasculitis but is found most characteristically in the arthritis seen in the preicteric phase of infectious hepatitis.

*Scarring.* Any deep vasculitis may result in scarring. Paradoxically the relatively benign condition discoid lupus erythematosus tends to produce a scarring alopecia, which is rare in the more malignant condition, systemic lupus erythematosus. Behçet's syndrome produces scarring and has two associated unique features: the oral mucosal ulcerations usually heal to form a "pursed-lipped" appearance; and scars and phlebitis often occur at phlebotomy sites, a finding not seen in other conditions causing polyarticular disease.

**Renal and Urological Manifestations of Polyarticular Disease.** Nephritis is seen commonly in systemic lupus erythematosus, Wegener's granulomatosis, and the other vasculitides. It is virtually absent in rheumatoid arthritis. The resulting hematuria could also be associated with the nephrolithiasis seen in gout or hyperparathyroidism and its associated chondrocalcinosis. Phenacetin and cyclophosphamide are two commonly used drugs in arthritis which may also be associated with hematuria.

Proteinuria may be a feature of any nephritis or amyloidosis, or may be due to the toxicity of either gold or penicillamine.

Urethritis is essentially exclusively seen with gonococcal arthritis and Reiter's syndrome. Painless penile skin lesions often accompany Reiter's syndrome. Painful penile lesions are seen in Behçet's syndrome.

**Cardiac Manifestations of Polyarticular Disease.** Pericarditis is commonly seen in rheumatoid arthritis and systemic lupus erythematosus. It is also seen in scleroderma and may serve as an indicator of precipitant renal failure.[14]

Cardiomyopathies may be a clinical problem most commonly in amyloidosis, hemochromatosis, and scleroderma. Valvular heart disease is seen in subacute bacterial endocarditis and acute rheumatic fever. It has also been a rare clinical problem in rheumatoid arthritis, systemic lupus erythematosus, and ankylosing spondylitis—usually in the later stages of these diseases.

**Hepatic Manifestations of Polyarticular Disease.** Despite their tendency to involve almost all organs within the body, the systemic rheumatic diseases in general create little in the way of hepatic dysfunction, and most postmortem studies in these conditions describe only minimal abnormalities. Elevations of the hepatocellular enzymes (e.g., SGOT, SGPT) are found primarily in two situations: (1) in hepatitis-associated arthritis, and (2) in patients with either juvenile rheumatoid arthritis or systemic lupus erythematosus receiving salicylates.[15,16] The abnormally elevated enzymes will revert with the cessation of salicylates. Hepatomegaly or cirrhosis should alert the clinician to the possibility of amyloidosis, Wilson's disease, or hemochromatosis.

**Gastrointestinal Manifestations of Polyarticular Disease.** The vast majority of the anti-inflammatory medications are ulcerogenic, so it is difficult to define the specific effect of the drug or the disease upon this condition. Esophageal dysfunction is a common lesion in scleroderma, in any condition associated with Raynaud's phenomenon, or in Raynaud's phenomenon alone.

Diarrhea or the presence of malabsorption should alert one to the possibility of inflammatory bowel disease, scleroderma with small bowel atony, or Whipple's disease. Diarrhea may also frequently precede the onset of typical Reiter's syndrome, which may occur after *Salmonella, Shigella,* or *Yersinia* infections.

**Neurologic Manifestations of Polyarticular Disease.** Peripheral neuropathies may be found in all forms of vasculitis, usually as a result of an infarction of the *vasa nervorum* or secondary to entrapments as is discussed in Chapter 3. Vertebral instability can lead to the development of a myelopathy. This is most commonly seen in association with the later stages of rheumatoid arthritis. The *cauda equina* syndrome has been described in far-advanced ankylosing spondylitis.[17] Neither of these syndromes is seen early in the course of the disease, however, so they are not distinguishing features in the differential diagnosis of polyarthritis of recent onset. Seizures or diffuse abnormalities of cerebral functions are features usually associated with systemic lupus. However, Lyme arthritis, Behçet's syndrome, and the use of ibuprofen in patients with systemic lupus[18] may be associated with a picture of aseptic meningitis.

## References

1. Holmes, K.K., Counts, G.W., and Beaty, H.N.: Disseminated gonococcal infection. Ann. Intern. Med. 74:979, 1971.
2. Keiser, H., Ruben, E.L., Wolinsky, E., and Kushner, I.: Clinical forms of gonococcal arthritis. N. Engl. J. Med. 279:234, 1968.
3. Brandt, K.D., Cathcart, E.S., and Cohen, A.S.: Gonococcal arthritis. Clinical features correlated with blood, synovial fluid, and genitourinary cultures. Arthritis Rheum. 17:503, 1974.
4. Schumacher, H.R., Andrews, R., and McLaughlin, G.: Arthropathy in sickle cell disease. Ann. Intern. Med. 78:203, 1973.
5. Haslock, I., and Wright, V.: The musculoskeletal complications of Crohn's disease. Medicine 52:217, 1973.
6. Caughey, D.E., and Bywaters, E.G.L.: The arthritis of Whipple's syndrome. Ann. Rheum. Dis. 22:327, 1963.
7. Shagrin, J.W., Frame, B., and Duncan, H.: Polyarthritis in obese patients with intestinal bypass. Ann. Intern. Med. 75:377, 1971.
8. O'Duffy, J.D., Carney, J.A., and Deodhar, S.: Behçet's disease: Report of 10 cases, 3 new manifestations. Ann. Intern. Med. 75:561, 1971.
9. Hadler, N.M., Franck, W.A., Bress, N.M., and Robinson, D.R.: Acute polyarticular gout. Am. J. Med. 56:715, 1974.
10. McCarty, D.J.: Diagnostic mimicry in arthritis—patterns of joint involvement associated with calcium pyrophosphate dihydrate crystal deposits. Bull. Rheum. Dis. 25:803, 1975.
11. Bujak, J.S., Aptekar, R.G., Decker, J.L., et al.: Juvenile rheumatoid arthritis presenting in the adult as fever of unknown origin. Medicine 52:431, 1973.
12. Crystal, R.G., Fulmer, J.D., Roberts, W.C., Moss, M.L., Line, B.R., and Reynolds, H.Y.: Idiopathic pulmonary fibrosis, Ann. Intern. Med. 85:769, 1976.
13. Walker, W.C., and Wright, V.: Pulmonary lesions and rheumatoid arthritis. Medicine 47:501, 1968.
14. McWhorter, J.E., IV, and LeRoy, E.C.: Pericardial disease in scleroderma (systemic sclerosis). Am. J. Med. 56:566, 1974.
15. Rich, R.R., and Johnson, J.S.: Salicylate hepatotoxicity in patients with JRA. Arthritis Rheum. 16:1, 1973.
16. Seaman, W.E., Ishak, K.G., and Plotz, P.H.: Aspirin-induced hepatotoxicity in patients with systemic lupus erythematosus. Ann. Intern. Med. 80:1, 1974.
17. Gordon, A.L., and Yudell, A.: Cauda equina lesion associated with ankylosing spondylitis. Ann. Intern. Med. 78:555, 1973.
18. Widener, H.L., and Littman, B.H.: Ibuprofen-induced meningitis in systemic lupus erythematosus. JAMA 239:1062, 1978.

# Chapter 27
# Muscle Weakness

*Walter G. Bradley*

## INTRODUCTION

The techniques of history-taking and examination of patients are part of the basic tools of the trade of medicine. Nevertheless, it is always instructive to watch an expert in any specialty handling the interview and examination of a patient with a disease within his area. Speed, accuracy, and completeness come from years of experience.

The doctor who is asked to give a diagnostic opinion should approach the patient like a detective, albeit a sympathetic one, with every faculty attuned to the task. One of the key attributes of the great detective in fact or fiction is intuition—that is, the feeling that all is not as it should be. This is no sixth sense, but rather the ability to collect every piece of data, to make judgments on the reliability of the data, to match them against a vast experience of similar situations, and to see where the fault lies and where further investigation is required.

This is the era of science in medicine. No sooner is a symptom recorded than a list of investigations flashes into mind. It is important to reiterate the old teaching that the way to come to a diagnosis is through the history, examination, and formulation of a differential diagnosis, before it is possible to plan the investigations. The finding of a raised creatine kinase (CK) does not necessarily prove the presence of a diffuse muscle disease. Intramuscular injections, excessive exercise, focal muscle injury, and ischemic heart disease may all produce a raised serum CK. The findings in a muscle biopsy of necrosis and regeneration of muscle fibers may be due to a muscular dystrophy or polymyositis, and the diagnosis may depend on the clinical picture rather than the muscle pathology.

This chapter is aimed at providing a framework for searching out all relevant clues from patients complaining of muscle weakness. The various conditions that may cause muscle weakness are briefly considered in Chapter 79. The diagnostic tests of value in defining and separating conditions considered in the differential diagnosis are outlined in Chapter 47.

## HISTORY OF THE PRESENT ILLNESS

It is curious how infrequently patients complain of the loss of a motor function when suffering from muscle weakness. They usually use terms like "tiredness" or "fatigue," rather than complaining of difficulty with performing a certain action, such as climbing stairs or doing their hair. This may be because the universal experience of muscle fatigue or tiredness on prolonged exercise, which is built into our linguistic framework, is equated with the symptoms of excessive exertion required to perform a standard task by a person with muscle weakness.

Sometimes the term "numbness" or "deadness" is used to indicate muscle weakness, though further questioning indicates the absence of true sensory loss. The patient is using the term to draw an analogy with the paralysis of an arm following sleeping on it at night, and of the loss of function following a dental anesthetic. It is thus important that the physician-detective try to find out exactly what the patient is experiencing. It is classic teaching that the patient should be allowed to tell his own story in his own words, but this should not be construed as preventing the questioning of the patient to clarify his words. Such *positive history-taking* should be directed to allow the physician to understand the symptoms just as well as if he had experienced them himself.

It is extremely difficult to quantify symptoms of weakness or fatigability. The only way in which this can be achieved is to relate it to functional capacity. If the patient complains of leg weakness, how far can he walk on the flat? Can he climb stairs with or without the bannisters? Can he get up out of a chair or off the floor? Is the weakness proximal or distal? For instance, is the main difficulty in getting up from a chair, or does the patient trip easily? If the complaints are of weakness of the arms, is it distal or proximal? Is there difficulty in opening bottles and holding tools, or is lifting objects above the head or doing the hair difficult?

The time-scale of the development of the symptoms is important. Was it sudden, gradual, or episodic? This is of diagnostic importance, since every disease has a different time course. If the weakness is variable, what are the modifying factors, such as diet, exercise, or environmental temperature?

## SYSTEMATIC INQUIRY

As can be seen from the paragraphs above, the physician-detective is more than a passive recorder of the patient's words when taking the history of the illness. The physician will already have asked many questions by the time the patient has completed the story to his own satisfaction. At that time there will still be many other points of systematic inquiry which need to be checked.

Patients may not complain of extraocular, facial, bulbar, or neck weakness, particularly if these are mild. Has anyone commented on a change in the facial appearance? Has there been any diplopia or difficulty in keeping the eyelids opened, as in myasthenia gravis? Are the muscles of mastication weak on chewing steak? Is there difficulty in swallowing (a symptom which is present in about a quarter of the patients with polymyositis, and about which patients rarely complain)? Do liquids go up the nose or into the larynx on swallowing, indicating bulbar involvement? Is there any difficulty in lifting the head off the pillow, suggesting weakness of neck flexion, or difficulty in holding up the head while working at the desk, suggesting weakness of neck extensors? Has there been any change in the posture, or wasting of muscles? Have the shoulders changed, or is there an alteration in the gait? Has there been any pain? If so, is it spontaneous pain, tenderness to palpation, or cramps after exercise or at rest? Pain and tenderness of the muscles after exercise are frequently present in normal individuals. If the patient is weak, increased exertion is required to perform the same tasks, with consequently greater postexertional pain. It is thus important to assess complaints of pain or tenderness carefully. Is it a prominent feature, or is it simply compatible with the degree of weakness? Pain and weakness are often symptoms of a local arthropathy, and separation of muscle pains from joint pains is often difficult despite detailed questioning.

Cramps are common in the general population, and some individuals are particularly susceptible. Cramps are particularly prominent in patients with upper motor neuron diseases, including multiple sclerosis and amyotrophic lateral sclerosis (ALS), but may also occur in the muscular dystrophies and polymyositis. This is the time to seek for clues about whether muscle weakness may be due to upper motor neuron conditions by inquiring about flexion spasms and sphincter control. Inquiries about sensory symptoms will help indicate the presence of a peripheral neuropathy or central nervous disease. Muscle fasciculations are an important symptom of lower motor neuron degeneration, as in ALS. Has the patient been aware of flickering of the muscles, and if so, in what distributions? Has there been any change in the urine suggestive of myoglobinuria? Myoglobinuria occurs if there is massive muscle breakdown in acute polymyositis, acute rhabdomyolysis, carnitine palmityl-transferase deficiency, and a number of other conditions.

A search for symptoms of systemic disease—endocrine, metabolic, dietary, respiratory, intestinal, immunologic, or inflammatory—is of major importance. Muscle weakness may be due to metabolic aberrations related to many primary diseases of other systems of the body. Weakness may also be due to peripheral nerve or skeletal muscle damage from toxic exposures in the patient's occupation or hobbies, or pharmaceutical or self-abusive drugs.

## PAST HISTORY

Patients will often forget many past illnesses, even hospitalizations and surgical procedures. These illnesses may be of considerable significance, and it is important to spend time delving into the past. A previous cancer operation may be relevant in a man of 60 with dermatomyositis. A blind loop syndrome from gastric resection might be a cause of a painful proximal myopathy from malabsorption of vitamin D. There are great satisfactions for the physician-detective in the past history.

## FAMILY HISTORY

Many of the neuromuscular diseases run in families. Some, such as facioscapulohumeral (FSH) muscular dystrophy, dystrophia myotonica, and peroneal muscular atrophy, are dominantly inherited, and the condition is passed on by an affected parent. Some, such as Duchenne muscular dystrophy, are X-linked recessive conditions, affecting only males but transmitted by females, so that a search of the maternal line for affected male relatives is needed. Some, for example, limb-girdle muscular dystrophy and infantile spinal muscular atrophy (Werdnig-Hoffmann disease), are inherited as recessive traits, and a history of consanguinity or affected sibs may be present.

In an overt disease such as peroneal muscular atrophy, patients often recognize their own condition and know which individuals in the family are also affected. However, formes frustes of the condition are frequent in such diseases. Knowledge of this allows search among relatives for the presence of such features as high arches, difficulty in obtaining shoes, and the development of calluses, which may indicate that the individual bears the gene for the disease. A vague history of a child who died with paralysis or a diagnosis of "polio" may be of relevance. Further information and search of medical records may be helpful when there are any pointers toward inherited disease.

Sometimes a patient will deny a family history in a disease that is frequently dominantly inherited. There are many possibilities: Inheritance may be through an individual who has a forme fruste of the disease. There may have been a spontaneous mutation or a rare autosomal recessive form of inheritance. The social parents may not be the biological parents. There may be poor family contact so that a child does not know about his parents. Sometimes patients will accept a feature as a family characteristic and not think it relates to a disease. The typical "fruity" transverse or pouting smile and drooped shoulders of FSH muscular dystrophy are examples in point. Sometimes there is a positive attempt to cover up a disease; this is particularly true in dystrophia myotonica, in which patients often refuse permission for contact to be made with relatives, and relatives may refuse to have anything to do with the inquiring physician.

Family photographs are useful for recognizing ocular myopathy, FSH dystrophy, and dystrophia myotonica. A careful search of the family history is important, since it may aid and confirm the diagnosis in the patient. Diagnosing the familial condition may avoid complex investigations. It may also lead to important genetic counseling for the patient and relatives.

## EXAMINATION

The specialist in rheumatology, neurology, neuromuscular disease, or any other field must be a good general physician. The complete physical examination is an obligatory part of the examination of any patient complaining of muscle weakness. For instance, detection of an endocrine disturbance or carcinoma may reveal the cause of the muscle disease.

In examining the neuromuscular apparatus, as in any other part of the body, a systematic approach is essential. The neuromuscular examination includes inspection, palpation, assessment of contractures, assessment of muscle strength, and elicitation of tendon reflexes.

**Inspection.** *General.* The patient should be undressed to the underclothes or completely, and observed standing and walking. If standing or walking is impossible, that must be recorded. When standing is there any unusual postural change, such as hyperlordosis, kyphoscoliosis, or fixed flexion of a joint? Is there any wasting of muscles such as the "champagne bottle" or more severe "hock bottle" wasting of the distal legs seen in peroneal muscular atrophy? Are the shoulders forwardly ptosed as in limb-girdle dystrophy, or horizontally drooped as in FSH dystrophy? In the latter, outward rotation of the shoulder blades may cause the angle of the scapula to rise and bulge into the line of the shoulders, producing a spurious appearance of muscularity. Hypertrophy of calf and other muscles may be seen in X-linked and some other muscular dystrophies.

*Regional.* Is the face normal at rest, or is there abnormal posture of the eyes, eyelids, or lips? Is there any abnormal asymmetry, ptosis, or strabismus? The lips are abnormally pouting in FSH dystrophy, and may droop in the other facial myopathies. This is the stage at which to examine the facial muscles, as well as the cranial nerves, skull, and cranial vasculature. Is there eyelid ptosis from weakness of the levator palpebrae superioris? Is there difficulty on burying the eyelashes, indicating weakness of the orbicularis oculi? A horizontal smile is due to weakness of the levator anguli oris, and difficulty in puffing out the cheeks may be due to weakness of the orbicularis oris, preventing the air from being held anteriorly, or, less commonly, to palatal weakness, preventing the air from being held posteriorly. The bulk of the temporalis and masseter muscles should be checked. Is the tongue normal in size and movements, or is it wasted and fasciculating? Most normal individuals find it difficult to keep the tongue still, so that it is generally advisable to diagnose fasciculation from denervation only when wasting is present.

Is the neck normal in position? The head may be thrust forward due to neck extensor weakness, perhaps caused by polymyositis or some other proximal myopathy. Wasting of the sternomastoid muscles occurs in dystrophia myotonica. Are the shoulder or arm muscles wasted? For instance, wasting of the deltoid muscle, causing the shoulder to be sharply right-angled, is not common in a muscular dystrophy but may occur in polymyositis. Is there any wasting of the muscles of the arms or legs, and any abnormal posture such as the claw hand of an ulnar palsy or pes cavus? Keep watch for fasciculations, small spontaneous twitches of groups of muscle fibers causing dimpling of the skin. Tapping the muscle may sometimes bring these out, but they must be distinguished from the normal twitches seen in poorly relaxed muscles and after heavy exertion.

Inspection should always include examination of the gait. Is it waddling (Trendelenburg gait), indicating weakness of hip abduction? Or is the abdomen thrust forward (the aldermanic gait) as a result of weakness of hip extensors? Are the arms and hips used excessively in walking, indicating weakness of hip flexors? Is there a footdrop, indicated by high-stepping? Excessive wearing of the toes of the shoes may prove the presence of the footdrop. There are many techniques for recording gaits, including force plates, cinematographic means, and computerized facilities, but these are still in the realm of research into their clinical usefulness and will not be discussed here.

**Palpation.** Palpation is best done during the examination of each muscle when the object is to assess (1) *bulk*—the grade of atrophy in percentage of expected bulk for the sex, age, and body habitus; (2) *consistency*—normal, fibrotic, or abnormally soft; or (3) *strength,* which is detailed below. During examination of the consistency of the muscle, tenderness to pressure should also be assessed.

**Determination of Contractures.** In clinical terms, contracture indicates restriction of the normal range of movement of a joint. There are several causes of this, including alteration of the joint surfaces, excessive thickening of the joint capsule or ligaments, and alterations of the muscles and tendons. Contraction caused by the muscles and tendons may be recognized by variation in the range of restriction in relation to differing positions of intervening joints. Thus clawed fingers may be due to alterations of the ligaments and joints, or to contracture of the long flexor muscles of the fingers. In the latter case, the fingers may be straightened when the wrist is hyperflexed.

The exact basis of this type of contracture of skeletal muscle is not certain. It is seen in conditions in which muscle damage produces fibrosis, such as the muscular dystrophies and polymyositis, and may also be seen in muscles chronically denervated, for instance by poliomyelitis or by chronic spinal muscular atrophy. Probably the amount of collagen deposited around the muscle fibers in these conditions reduces the normal degree of stretch of each muscle fiber.

It is important to assess the degree of contracture prior to attempting to assess voluntary strength of a muscle. Strength can only be assessed over the range of free movement of the joint and muscle. The examiner tests the strength by pulling against a contracting muscle; if he is pulling against a fibrotic contracture, he may get a false impression of muscle strength. The degree of contracture of the muscle can be measured with a simple protractor.

**Muscle Strength Testing.** There are many different ways to assess the strength of a muscle: the maximum force on voluntary contraction of that muscle; that maximum force expressed as a percentage of the expected normal for the age, sex, and body habitus; the duration for which it is possible to maintain a given percentage of the maximum voluntary contraction; whether a certain action is possible, such as, for the deltoid muscle, lifting the extended arm to 90 degrees away from the body; or the time taken to perform a certain action, such as the biceps lifting 10 kg ten times at maximum speed. Consideration of the more important of these parameters is given below.

It is important that the examiner have a good knowledge of myology and neurology, particularly with regard to the action and range of each muscle. The body functions in terms of whole movements, often produced by several muscles. To isolate and test only one muscle is difficult. Patients with weakness of one muscle learn trick maneuvers involving various agonists. It is essential to have knowledge of such trick movements, and of the correct position for examining each muscle in as pure isolation as possible.

Several other factors must also be taken into account in assessing muscle strength. The degree of extension of a muscle governs its power output; it is weakest at the extremes of contraction or relaxation, and strongest in the mid-range of movement. The apparent contradiction to this rule provided by the quadriceps femoris muscle, which appears strongest in full extension, is due to the mechanical locking of the knee joint in that position. Thus the quadriceps muscle strength must be tested in midposition.The effect of gravity must not be forgotten; when tested with the patient supine, the hip flexors appear weaker than with the body vertical owing to the necessity of lifting the additional weight of the leg in the supine position.

It is also important to recognize that the maximum voluntary strength of a muscle is proportional to the amount of effort expended by the subject. In experimental terms the maximum strength of an animal muscle produced by nerve stimulation is several times that exerted by the animal in maximum voluntary contraction. Thus, because of central nervous phenomena, the maximum *voluntary* contraction is less than the *absolute* maximum. Similarly "fatigue," i.e., the loss of ability to sustain a maximum effort, is a central rather than a peripheral phenomenon. If the subject *does not want* to exert full effort, either consciously or unconsciously, then the muscle will appear weak. The examiner must be on the continuous lookout for such central phenomena related to muscle strength. Thus conscious malingering may produce inability to contract the quadriceps against gravity, although the patient gets up from a chair readily. Wavering or variability of effort with a sudden "give" may be due either to psychogenic causes or to local pain.

*Clinical Assessment.* The strength of each muscle group can be assessed by simply finding how much effort the examiner has to impose to overcome maximum contraction. Details of the techniques for estimation of the strength of each muscle are outside the scope of this chapter, and readers should consult Walton and Gardner-Medwin (1981),[1] the Medical Research Council War Memorandum (1943),[2] and the Mayo Clinic "Clinical Examinations in Neurology."[3]

*Medical Research Council (MRC) Grading of Strength (1943).* Muscle strength can be quantitated in a crude but reproducible fashion on the following grades: 5—normal power; 4—muscle contraction possible against gravity and resistance combined; 3—muscle contraction possible only against gravity; 2—movement of a joint possible with gravity eliminated but not possible against gravity; 1—flicker of contraction; 0—no contraction.

The grades are relatively absolute, and different observers are generally concordant in their observations. However, MRC grade 4 encompasses the vast majority of clinically weak muscles, and any attempt to subdivide this category into 4 minus, 4, and 4 plus returns subjectivity to the field.

*Muscle Dynamometry.* Numerous systems of measuring muscle strength have been devised. Among the simplest are the various pulley and weight or spring balance devices. Optimally the limb is placed in a frame so that the joint is in its midposition of movement, and only the muscle under test can move the joint. Consideration must be given to whether the contraction is to be isometric, i.e., in which no movement shall result from the contraction, or whether it is to be isotonic, in which case the range of movement must be defined. During repeated tests the power usually increases for a few times owing to a learning effect; it then reaches a plateau and eventually fades owing to fatigue. It is thus important to take measurements in a standardized fashion, frequently as the maximum of the first three contractions. Vigorous reinforcement and urging by the examiner are necessary to obtain the *maximum* voluntary contraction.

The apparatus required for such measurements as those outlined above is cumbersome, and a useful compromise between dynamometry and clinical examination is a hand-held dynamometer. Various models are available. The strictures already described above in relation to the clinical examination without additional apparatus apply equally to dynamometry, and the need for a rigorously standardized technique must be emphasized.

*Functional Tests.* Tests of the all-or-none ability to perform an action or of the time taken to perform such an action are of major help in muscle assessment, particularly in serial studies of a patient. The ability or inability to rise from the floor is one such test. Aberrations of the method of rising from the floor, including the Gower's maneuver, offer refinements of characterization.[4] The time that a patient takes to get from sitting on the floor to the vertical may be used for monitor of muscle power when weakness of hip and knee extensors becomes significant. Similar tests include the time to get out of a chair, to walk a measured distance on the flat, to climb a standard flight of stairs, to hold the legs horizontally without support, or to hold the extended arms horizontally.

**Tendon Reflexes.** Elicitation of the tendon reflexes is a standard part of medical training and will not be described in detail here. The patient should be completely relaxed and the muscle in midposition. The tendon should be carefully struck a sharp blow. Reflexes should be categorized as 0 absent; $\pm$ present only with reinforcement maneuvers such as jaw or hand clenching; 1+ present but depressed; 2+ normal; 3+ exaggerated; 4+ sustained clonus.

It is important to know the changes in reflex patterns with age, including the loss of the ankle jerks in many patients over the age of 60. The pattern of reflex change is important in the diagnosis of the cause of muscle weakness. Thus upper motor neuron disease causes exaggeration of reflexes with spread of the reflex beyond the nerve and myotomal supply of the muscle which is struck. In addition, there are pathological reflexes indicative of upper motor neuron damage, such as extensor plantar responses. Lower motor neuron disease generally causes depressed or lost reflexes, particularly if this is due to a peripheral neuropathy affecting both the sensory and the motor fibers, and particularly in demyelinating rather than axonal diseases. Neuronal degenerations of either the anterior horn cell or the dorsal root ganglion tend to cause the reflexes to be lost rather later than in peripheral neuropathies. In amyotrophic lateral sclerosis, coexistent upper motor neuron motor disease causes increased reflexes in muscles that are atrophied owing to lower motor neuron damage, thus producing a characteristic clinical picture. Loss of tendon reflexes in primary muscle disease is probably due to involvement of muscle spindles, and possibly due to secondary involvement of intramuscular nerves. Only late in the disease is extrafusal muscle fiber damage sufficiently severe as to abolish reflexes. Thus, in primary muscle disease, the reflexes may be relatively spared compared with peripheral nerve disease until there is a greater degree of muscle weakness and wasting. In polymyositis, surprisingly, the tendon reflexes may occasionally be somewhat exaggerated. The explanation for this is not clear but may be related to membrane damage in muscle spindles causing hyperexcitability.

The distribution of reflex change may be characteristic. In muscular dystrophy such as that of Duchenne, the ankle jerks may be preserved though the knee and biceps reflexes are lost. In a distal polyneuropathy the peripheral reflexes such as the ankle jerk may be lost, while proximal reflexes such as those of the knee and elbow may remain.

**The Examination of the Peripheral Nervous System.** The recognition of whether weakness is due to skeletal muscle or nervous system damage relates to the distribution of the muscle weakness and the presence or absence of associated features. Distal muscle weakness is usually of peripheral nerve origin, while proximal muscle weakness is more likely to be due to a primary muscle problem. A specific distribution of muscle weakness may be diagnostic, as in the patterns seen in muscular dystrophy, in an upper motor neuron lesion, or in a peripheral nerve or root lesion. Thus in a muscular dystrophy such as that of Duchenne or Becker, the muscles earliest and most severely affected are the quadriceps, hip flexors, hip extensors, anterior tibialis, biceps, and brachioradialis, while others such as the gastrocnemius, triceps, deltoids, wrist flexors, and extensors are spared until later. This specific distribution cannot be explained on the basis of any root or peripheral nerve distribution.

In a chronic spinal muscular atrophy, the distribution of muscle involvement may be very variable. Commonly all muscles are very atrophic, but certain muscles or muscle groups are particularly weak. The distribution of muscle involvement, whatever its specific pattern, again cannot be explained on the basis of any nerve or root involvement. It may, in fact, imitate the distribution of a muscular dystrophy, when the term "pseudomyopathic spinal muscular atrophy" is applied. Further investigations are then required to separate the muscular dystrophy and spinal muscular atrophy.

In an upper motor neuron disease, the characteristic distribution of muscle weakness is concentrated in the extensors of the upper limbs, the deltoid, triceps, and wrist and finger extensors, and in the flexors of the lower limbs, the hip flexors, hamstrings, and anterior tibialis muscles. Here, the presence of the associated features of increased tendon jerks and pathologic reflexes confirms the anatomic diagnosis. In a lesion of one or more peripheral nerves or roots, the pattern of nerve and superficial sensory involvement is such that it can be explained solely and entirely from the known distribution of the nerve(s) or root(s). A knowledge of the myotonal and dermatomal map[5] is essential.

The presence of definite sensory loss proves that the nervous system is involved. Detailed individual examination of all modalities of sensation over the whole of the body is required.

As an aid to anatomic diagnosis it is best to tabulate the distribution of muscle weakness and sensory impairment, first listing the clearcut abnormalities and then listing more dubious abnormalities. It is important to develop a mental image of the dermatomes, myotomes, and peripheral nerve distribution in the body, having tables and figures[5] readily available for repeated comparison.

## SUMMARY AND CONCLUSIONS

The diagnostic interview is a major part of the investigation of every patient, and this is particularly so in those with muscle weakness. It provides a guide to further investigation by laboratory and other procedures. These investigations are considered elsewhere; those dealing with the investigations of a patient with neuromuscular symptoms and signs are dealt with in Chapter 47. By the end of the interview and examination, the physician-detective should have a clear idea of the differential diagnosis, and thus the investigations required. Such investigations should always be directed; the shotgun approach is both expensive and sometimes misleading.

A final word is necessary concerning the diagnosis of neuromuscular involvement in the presence of rheumatologic conditions, for this is often difficult. Local joint pain makes it impossible for patients to exert their maximum voluntary effort, with resultant *apparent* weakness. Disuse of a limb from pain causes muscle atrophy, predominantly of type 2 muscle fibers. It is thus important to assess as well as possible the degree of joint involvement and consequent joint pain. At times it is clear that the degree of weakness and atrophy may simply be ascribable to the joint problems. At other times it is difficult to exclude some degree of neuromuscular involvement, and the investigations outlined in Chapter 47 are then required. The importance of recognizing the superimposition of a neuromuscular involvement upon the underlying rheumatologic condition is that the prognosis may be altered by such involvement, and the treatment may have to be altered to take account of this involvement. For instance, the development of polymyositis during the course of progressive systemic sclerosis may necessitate the addition of glucocorticoids or immunomodulation drugs to the treatment regimen; the development of a multiple mononeuropathy in rheumatoid arthritis may indicate the appearance of a diffuse vasculitis.

### References

1. Gardner-Medwin, D.: The clinical examination of the neuromuscular system. *In* Walton, Sir John (ed.): Disorders of Voluntary Muscle. 4th ed. Edinburgh, Churchill Livingstone, 1981. p. 448.
2. Medical Research Council War Memorandum, No. 7. Revised 2nd ed. London, HMSO, 1943.
3. Mayo Clinic Staff: Clinical Examinations in Neurology. 4th ed. Philadelphia, W.B. Saunders Company, 1977.
4. Brooke, M.H.: A Clinician's View of Neuromuscular Diseases. Baltimore, Williams & Wilkins Company, 1977.
5. Bradley, W.G.: Disorders of Peripheral Nerves. Oxford, Blackwell Scientific Publications, 1974.

# Chapter 28
# Neck Pain

*Kenneth K. Nakano*

## INTRODUCTION

When localized by a patient to the neck, pain can often produce a confusing diagnostic problem. Pain can originate from the involved tissues or may be so perceived but due to referral from another site (Table 28–1). Musculoskeletal conditions involve neurologic tissues, and the converse appears equally true.

Neck pain in clinical practice occurs slightly less frequently than low back pain; a major difference is that neck pain becomes far less disabling, seldom compromising work capacity. Neck stiffness exists as a common disorder; for the age group 25 to 29 years of age in our working population there is a 25 to 30 percent frequency of one or more attacks of stiff neck.[1] For the work population over 45 years of age this figure rises to 50 percent. Episodes of "simple" stiff neck last 1 to 4 days and seldom require medical care. Brachial neuralgia (pain radiating to the shoulder and arm) occurs later in life than stiff neck, with a frequency of 5 to 10 percent in the 25 to 29 year age group and subsequently rising to 25 to 40 percent after age 45. Overall, 45 percent of working men experience at least one attack of stiff neck, 23 percent report at least one attack of brachial neuralgia, and 51 percent suffer both these symptoms. The frequency of brachial neuralgia is approximately three times higher in those who complain of stiff neck, suggesting common factors in their pathogensis.

Pain in the neck exists in all occupational groups. Stiff neck appears first, followed by headache and shoulder-arm pain.[1] The pain-sensitive structures of the neck include the ligaments, the nerve roots, the articular facets and capsules, the muscles, and the dura. Pain in the neck region can originate from many tissue sites and result from a number of mechanisms (Table 28–2).

**Table 28–1.** Structures Causing Neck Pain

| |
|---|
| Acromioclavicular joint |
| Heart and coronary artery disease |
| Apex of lung, Pancoast's tumor, bronchogenic cancer (C3, C4, C5 nerve roots in common) |
| Diaphragm muscle (C3, C4, C5 innervation) |
| Gallbladder |
| Spinal cord tumor |
| Temporomandibular joint |
| Fibrositis and fibromyositis syndromes (upper thoracic spine, proximal arm and shoulder) |
| Aorta |
| Pancreas |
| Disorders of any somatic or visceral structure (produces cervical nerve root irritation) |
| Peripheral nerves |
| Central nervous system (posterior fossa lesions) |
| Hiatus hernia (C3, C4, C5) |
| Gastric ulcer |

**Table 28–2.** Cervical Spine Syndromes

| |
|---|
| **Localized Neck Disorders** |
| Osteoarthritis (apophyseal joints, C1-C2-C3 levels most often) |
| Rheumatoid arthritis (atlantoaxial) |
| Juvenile rheumatoid arthritis |
| Sternocleidomastoid tendinitis |
| Acute posterior cervical strain |
| Pharyngeal infections |
| Cervical lymphadenitis |
| Osteomyelitis (staphylococcal, tuberculosis) |
| Meningitis |
| Ankylosing spondylitis |
| Paget's disease |
| Torticollis (congenital, spasmodic, drug-involved, hysterical) |
| Neoplasms (primary or metastatic) |
| Occipital neuralgia (greater and lesser occipital nerves) |
| Diffuse idiopathic skeletal hyperostosis |
| Rheumatic fever (infrequently) |
| Gout (infrequently) |
| **Lesions Producing Neck and Shoulder Pain** |
| Postural disorders |
| Rheumatoid arthritis |
| Fibrositis syndromes |
| Musculoligamentous injuries to neck and shoulder |
| Osteoarthritis (apophyseal and Luschka) |
| Cervical spondylosis |
| Intervertebral osteoarthritis |
| Thoracic outlet syndromes |
| Nerve injuries (serratus anterior, C3-C4 nerve root, long thoracic nerve) |
| **Lesions Producing Predominantly Shoulder Pain** |
| Rotator cuff tears and tendinitis |
| Calcareous tendinitis |
| Subacromial bursitis |
| Bicipital tendinitis |
| Adhesive capsulitis |
| Reflex sympathetic dystrophy |
| Frozen shoulder syndromes |
| Acromioclavicular secondary osteoarthritis |
| Glenohumeral arthritis |
| Septic arthritis |
| Tumors of the shoulder |
| **Lesions Producing Neck and Head Pain with Radiation** |
| Cervical spondylosis |
| Rheumatoid arthritis |
| Intervertebral disc protrusion |
| Osteoarthritis (apophyseal and Luschka joints; intervertebral disc; osteoarthritis) |
| Spinal cord tumors |
| Cervical Neurovascular syndromes |
| Cervical rib |
| Scalene muscle |
| Hyperabduction syndrome |
| Rib-clavicle compression |

Normal function of the cervical spine requires physiologic movements of the joints, bones, spinal cord, nerve roots through the intervertebral foramina, muscles, ligaments, tendons, fascia, sympathetic nervous system, and the vascular supply of all these structures. Since most structures in the neck potentially become pain sensitive, a knowledge of the dermatome pattern of pain distribution is necessary in clinical diagnosis.

## ANATOMY AND BIOMECHANICS

The most mobile segment of the spine is the neck. Through a cylinder connecting the head to the thorax pass structures requiring the greatest protection and possessing the least: the carotid and vertebral arteries, the spinal cord, and the spinal nerve roots. The head, weighing 6 to 8 pounds, balances on the seven cervical vertebrae in a flexible chain held together by 14 apophyseal joints, 5 intervertebral discs, 12 joints of Luschka, and a system of ligaments (anterior longitudinal, posterior longitudinal, ligmentum flavum, interspinous and ligamentum nuchae) and muscles (14 paired anterior, lateral and posterior) (Figs. 28–1 and 28–2).

The shape and mode of articulation of the joints influence the axes and ranges of movement of the neck. Plates of avascular hyaline cartilage cover, and the intervertebral discs unite, the articular surfaces of the vertebral bodies. The intervertebral discs increase in area from below the axis (C2) downwards, and the cervical lordosis results from their wedge shape (Figs. 28–1 and 28–2). The thickness of the discs vary; the two deepest lie below the sixth and fifth vertebra, respectively. Each intervertebral disc consists of fibrocartilage and contains a nucleus pulposus, which, in turn, changes in shape but cannot be compressed.

Anterior and posterior longitudinal ligaments extend up to the occipital bone and down into the sacrum, joining the vertebral bodies. The anterior longitudinal ligament attaches to the bodies and becomes tightly fixed at the discs (Fig. 28–2); a sudden extending force may rupture it and lead to severe hyperextension associated with damage to the spinal cord. The posterior ligament attaches to the discs and adjacent bones but not to the center.

The specialized atlanto-occipital and atlantoaxial joints are controlled by intersegmental muscles. The head and atlas move together around the odontoid peg and the upper articular facets of the axis (Fig. 28–1*B*), the long transverse processes of the atlas providing the levers used in rotation. The anterior surface of the odontoid process articulates with the posterior surface of the anterior arch of the atlas. The total excursion of the head can be measured in flexion, extension, rotation, and lateral flexion (Table 28–3). The overall range of movement in the sagittal plane (flexion and extension) approximates 90 degrees, about three quarters being due to extension.[2] Approximately 10 degrees of flexion and 25 degrees of extension occur at the atlanto-occipital joints.[3] In this range of movement, the ligaments help protect the spinal cord from damage by the normal,

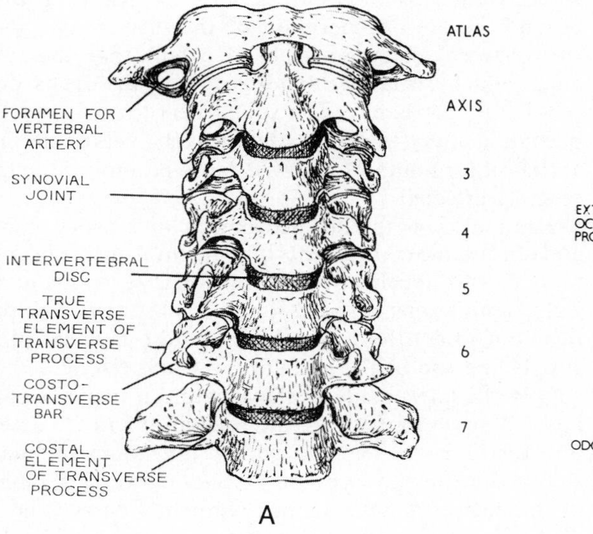


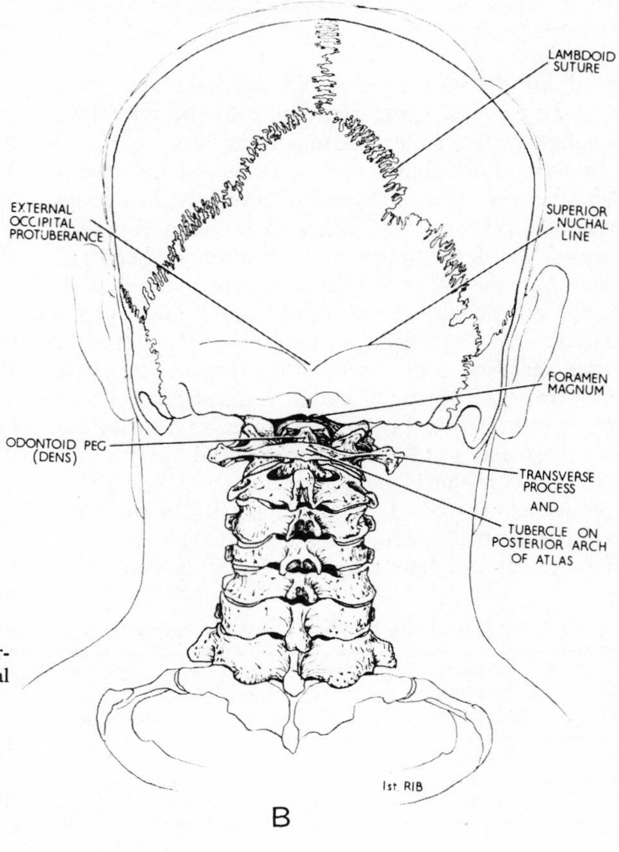


**Figure 28–1.** *A,* Cervical spine: anterior view of articulated cervical vertebrae. *B,* Posterior view of the skull, seven cervical vertebrae and first thoracic vertebra.

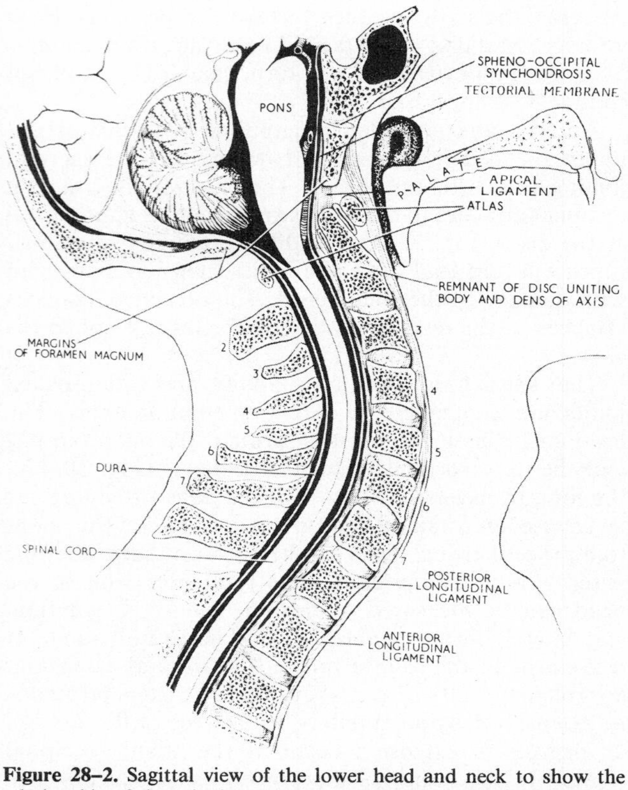


**Figure 28–2.** Sagittal view of the lower head and neck to show the relationship of the spinal cord and brainstem to the bones, ligaments, and joints between the bodies of the cervical vertebrae. The cervical lordosis can be seen as can the relationship of the anterior and posterior longitudinal ligaments to intervertebral discs and the ligaments at the craniovertebral junction.

fractured, or dislocated odontoid process. The lower parts of the cervical spine contribute to the remainder of full range in this plane. The maximum range of movement between individual vertebrae occurs at the level of the joints between the fourth and fifth vertebrae in young children and between the fifth and sixth in teenagers and adults. The total range of rotation of the head and neck encompasses 80 to 90 degrees. Approximately 35 to 45 degrees occurs at the atlantoaxial joint and is associated with a screwing movement of the upper on the lower vertebra, a movement that reduces the cross-sectional area of the spinal canal. Lateral flexion does not occur in isolation but accompanies some rotation. Usually there exists about 30 degrees of lateral mobility on both sides in the lower cervical spine.[3] The spinal canal shortens on the side of the concavity of the spine and lengthens on the side of the convexity.

With age, the nucleus pulposus becomes vulnerable to acute and chronic trauma.[4] With loss of disc substance the annulus fibrosus may bulge into the spinal canal, and on account of its eccentric position, the nucleus tends to prolapse backward if any tear develops in the annulus. The commonest sites for both types of herniation are the most mobile regions (viz., at C5-C6 and C6-C7). With degenerative changes, the disc space narrows and the spinal column shortens. The intervertebral foramina become narrowed, movements become restricted, and unusual mechanical strains on the synovial joints result. These changes may be confined to a localized area or may become widespread in generalized degenerative disease. The formation of osteophytes leads to encroachment on the spinal canal and intervertebral foramina. The canal may also be further narrowed by bulging of the ligamenta flava. Changes in the caliber of the vertebral arteries can result because of degenerative changes in the joints of the cervical spine. Arterial branches supplying joints and nervous tissue can be constricted at rest and further obstructed with movement. Occasionally, with severe vertebral artery stenosis, syncope results from rotation of the head.

**Table 28–3.** Age and the Normal Cervical Spine Motion

| Age in Years | Flexion Extension (degrees) | Lateral Rotation (degrees) | Lateral Flexion (degrees) |
|---|---|---|---|
| < 30 | 90 | 90 | 45 |
| 31–50 | 70 | 90 | 45 |
| > 50 | 60 | 90 | 30 |

Mere bony changes do not necessarily correspond to the segmental level of neurologic damage. Two reasons exist for this. The first relates to the disproportionate growth of the spinal cord and column. The first thoracic segment of the spinal cord lies opposite the seventh cervical vertebra (Fig. 28–2), and the upper rootlets of the lower cervical and first thoracic nerves cross over two intervertebral discs, while normally the lower rootlets of these two nerves cross only one disc (Fig. 28–3). Second, severe degeneration of the discs may shorten the vertebral canal to such an extent that the spinal cord, which remains unaltered in length, drops down relative to the bones. The spinal nerve roots may then become acutely folded as they travel toward the intervertebral foramina, the lowest roots becoming the most severely affected.

Familiarity with the distribution of sensory, motor, and autonomic components in segmental nerves becomes necessary for localization of neurologic segments in clinical examinations (Fig. 28–4 and Table 28–4). For practical purposes, the lower fibers of the cervical plexus supply the top of the shoulder; C5 and C6 nerve roots supply the lateral side of the arm and forearm; C6, C7, and C8 nerve roots innervate the hand; and C8 extends into the forearm. The T1 segment innervates the medial side of the arm and forearm. Visceral pain can be referred in some cases to well-defined segmental areas (Fig. 28–5); for example, pain of the point of the shoulder (C3-C4) may be associated with acute cholecystitis. The segmental supplies of individual muscles are listed in Table 28–4.

**Nerve Root Compression.** Normally a radicular nerve occupies 20 to 25 percent of the intervertebral foramen. There may be considerable variation in the anatomy of the lower cervical nerves and their root pouches, and as age advances, they become relatively fixed and vulnerable to damage.[5] Two types of disc lesions cause pressure on the radicular nerves or nerve roots: first, a dorsolat-

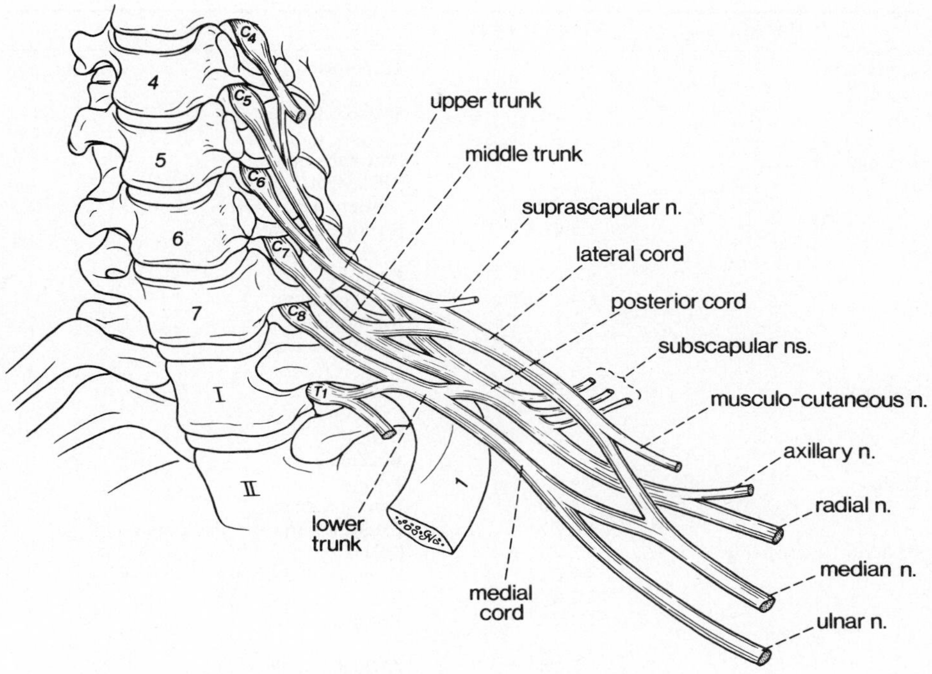


**Figure 28–3.** Brachial plexus and lower cervical spine. Note nerve roots, trunk, cords, and the peripheral nerves. The brachial plexus goes under the clavicle and over the first rib, accompanied by the subclavian artery and vein.

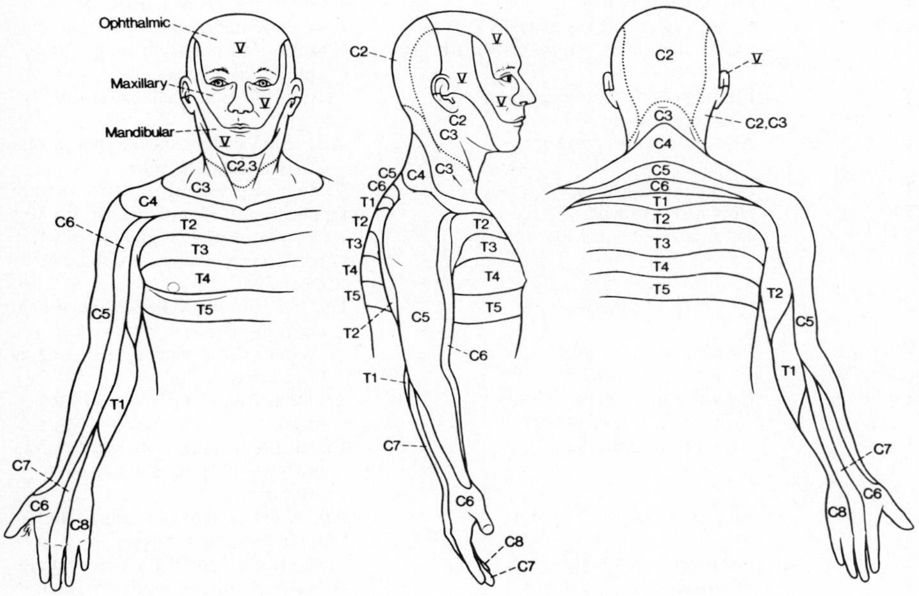

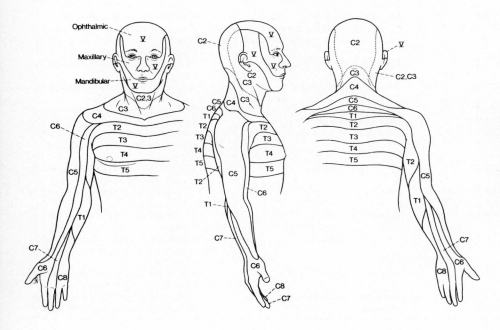


**Figure 28–4.** Dermatome distribution of nerve fibers from C1 through T5 carrying senses of pain, heat, cold, vibration, and touch to the head, neck, arm, hand, and thoracic area. The sclerotomes and myotomes will be similar but with some overlap. Pain arising from structures deep to the deep fascia (myotome and sclerotome) do not precisely follow the dermatome distribution.

**Table 28–4.** Nerves and Tests of Principal Muscles

| Nerve | Nerve R oots | Muscle | Test |
|---|---|---|---|
| Accessory | Spinal | Trapezius | Elevation of shoulders<br>Abduction of scapula |
| | Spinal | Sternocleidomastoid | Tilting of head to same side with rotation to opposite side |
| Brachial Plexus | | Pectoralis major | |
| | C5,C6 | Clavicular part | Adduction of arm |
| | C7,C8,T1 | Sternocostal part | Adduction, forward depression of arm |
| | C5,C6,C7 | Serratus anterior | Fixation of scapula during forward thrusting of the arm |
| | C4,C5 | Rhomboid | Elevation and fixation of scapula |
| | C4,C5,C6 | Supraspinatus | Initiate abduction arm |
| | (C4),C5,C6 | Infraspinatus | External rotation arm |
| | C6,C7,C8 | Latissimus dorsi | Adduction of horizontal, externally rotated arm, coughing |
| Axillary | C5,C6 | Deltoid | Lateral and forward elevation of arm to horizontal |
| Musculocutaneous | C5,C6 | Biceps<br>Brachialis | Flexion of supinated forearm |
| Radial | C6,C7,C8 | Triceps | Extension of forearm |
| | C5,C6 | Brachioradialis | Flexion of semiprone forearm |
| | C6,C7 | Extensor carpi radialis longus | Extension of wrist to radial side |
| Posterior Interosseous | C5,C6 | Supinator | Supination of extended forearm |
| | C7,C8 | Extensor digitorum | Extension of proximal phalanges |
| | C7,C8 | Extensor carpi ulnaris | Extension of wrist to ulnar side |
| | C7,C8 | Extensor indicis | Extension of proximal phalanx of index finger |
| | C7,C8 | Abductor pollicis longus | Abduction of first metacarpal in plane at right angle to palm |
| | C7,C8 | Extensor pollicis longus | Extension of first interphalangeal joint |
| | C7,C8 | Extensor pollicis brevis | Extension at first metacarpophalangeal joint |
| Median | C6,C7 | Pronator teres | Pronation of extended forearm |
| | C6,C7 | Flexor carpi radialis | Flexion of wrist to radial side |
| | C7,C8,T1 | Flexor digitorum superficialis | Flexion of middle phalanges |
| | C8,T1 | Flexor digitorum profundus (lateral part) | Flexion of terminal phalanges, index and middle fingers |
| | C8,T1 | Flexor pollicis longus (anterior interosseous nerve) | Flexion of distal phalanx, thumb |
| | C8,T1 | Abductor pollicis brevis | Abduction of first metacarpal in plane at right angle to palm |
| | C8,T1 | Flexor pollicis brevis | Flexion of proximal phalanx, thumb |
| | C8,T1 | Opponens pollicis | Opposition of thumb against 5th finger |
| | C8,T1 | 1st and 2nd lumbricals | Extension of middle phalanges while proximal phalanges are fixed in extension |
| Ulnar | C7,C8 | Flexor carpi ulnaris | Observe tendons while testing abductor digiti minimi |
| | C8,T1 | Flexor digitorum profundus (medial part) | Flexion of distal phalanges of ring and little fingers |
| | C8,T1 | Hypothenar muscles | Abduction and opposition of little finger |
| | C8,T1 | 3rd and 4th lumbricals | Extension of middle phalanges while proximal-phalanges are fixed in extension |
| | C8,T1 | Adductor pollicis | Adduction of thumb against palmar surface of index finger |
| | C8,T1 | Flexor pollicis brevis | Flexion of proximal phalanx, thumb |
| | C8,T1 | Interossei | Abduction and adduction of fingers |

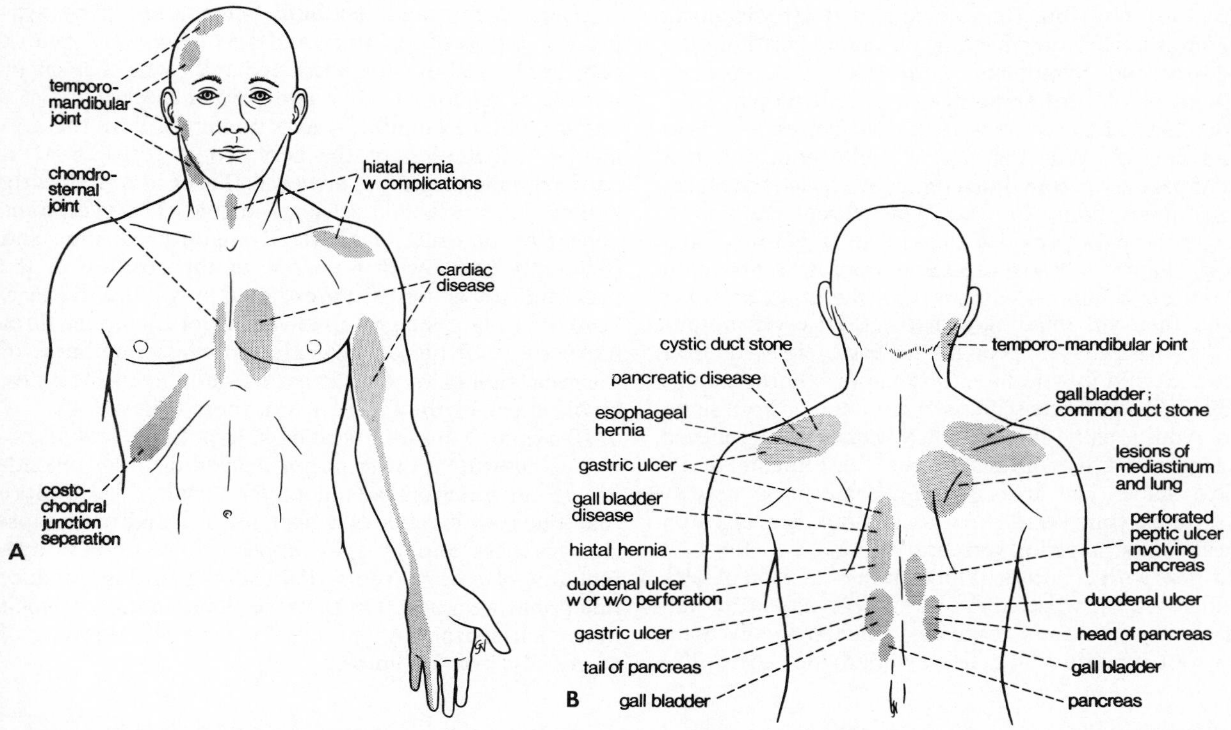


**Figure 28–5.** Patterns of reflexly referred pain from visceral and somatic structures. Anterior distribution (*A*); posterior distribution (*B*).

eral protrusion that does not invade the intervertebral foramen but compresses the intrameningeal nerve roots against the vertebral laminae; and second, an intraforaminal protrusion from the uncinate part of the disc that compresses the radicular nerve against the articular process. The extent of root compression depends on the angulation of the radicular nerve and its location in the foramen as well as on the size and position of the protrusion. Marginal lipping of the vertebrae and narrowing of the discs lead to secondary osteophyte formation of the articular processes and consequent posterolateral narrowing of the foramen.

**Blood Supply.** Variations in the pattern of blood vessels in the cervical spinal cord exist, but the main blood supply comes through a few major articular arteries.[6] The anterior and posterior spinal arteries act more as connecting links than as main channels of blood. The blood supply to the spinal cord can be impaired in patients with cervical spondylosis when one or more radicular arteries become compressed. The resultant ischemia may be either continuous or intermittent, and sometimes the maximum impairment occurs only when the head is in a certain position (usually extension).

The vertebral arteries vary in size, and one (usually the left) may be larger than the other. The vertebral arteries lie within the vertebral canal, on their medial aspect closely related to the neurocentral joint, and pass immediately anterior to the emerging cervical nerve roots. Each nerve root receives a small arterial branch. Spondylotic changes of the cervical vertebrae may displace the artery laterally and, in severe cases, posteriorly as well. The degree of displacement depends on the size and position of the body prominence that arises as a result of spondylosis. Atheroma of the vertebral artery also may be important in the production of symptoms. Cerebellar infarction may result from a critical reduction of blood flow to the vertebral artery in the neck. When the block occurs in the cervical part of the vertebral artery, the cerebellar infarcts tend to be bilateral, approximately symmetrical, and in the territory of the superior cerebellar artery. Most often the obstruction will be incomplete, and blood flow may be reduced only when the patient turns or extends his head. Rotation and extension of the head to one side can obstruct the contralateral vertebral artery; and in patients with atherosclerosis, rotation and extension of the head can produce posterior circulation abnormalities such as nystagmus, vertigo, weakness, dysarthria, drop attacks, and a Babinski response. An anterior spinal-artery–spinal-cord syndrome results either from compromise of the anterior spinal artery or from compression of one of the main radicular arteries by osteophytes or adhesions associated with nerve root-sleeve fibrosis. In diseases involving the major blood vessels (e.g., arteriosclerosis, diabetes, syphilis) the blood supply of the spinal cord may be impaired, especially if the condition is associated with spondylosis.

## CLINICAL EVALUATION

The essential means in the diagnosis and management of cervical pain include elicitation of the history and the physical examination. Radiologic and electrodiagnostic procedures assist in confirming the clinical formulation.

**History and Symptoms.** ***Pain.*** The most common symptom of cervical spine disorders will be pain (Fig. 28–6). Cervical nerve root irritation causes a well-localized area of pain (Fig. 28–4), while poorly defined areas of pain arise from deep connective tissue structures, muscle, joint, bone, or disc. The patient's ability to describe the pain provides the examiner with essential clues to diagnosis. Retro-orbital, temporal, and occipital pain reflects a referral pattern from the atlas, axis, and C3 and their surrounding structures. In cervical spine disorders pain may appear in the back, sides, or front of the neck and may radiate to the upper thoracic spine, shoulders, or scapular regions or into one or both upper limbs. Additionally, this pain may be produced, relieved, or exaggerated by various normal movements of the cervical spine. The areas of pain designation may be tender (e.g., transverse process, spinous process, apophyseal joints, anterior vertebral bodies).

Stiffness with consequent limitation of motion of neck, shoulder, elbow, wrist, and even fingers may occur subsequent to prior injury response, articular involvement, nerve root irritation, or reflex sympathetic dystrophy.

Tenosynovitis and tendinitis often accompany syndromes of the cervical spine and may involve the rotator cuff; tendons about the wrist or hand, with stenosis or fibrosis of tendon sheaths; and palmar fascia.

***Paresthesias.*** Numbness and tingling follow the segmental distribution of the nerve roots (Fig. 28–4) in cervical spine disorders; however, this occurs frequently without demonstrable sensory change. The symptoms appear on one side or bilaterally upon awakening and frequently abate with a change in the position of the neck and upper limbs. Paresthesias involving the face, head, or tongue suggest involvement of the upper three nerve roots of the cervical plexus, while numbness of the neck, shoulders, arm, forearms, and fingers indicates, involvement of the C5-T1 nerve roots (Fig. 28–4).

***Weakness.*** Muscular weakness, hypotonia, and fasciculation indicate a lower motor neuron disorder secondary to an anterior radiculopathy (Table 28–4). More than one root innervates a given muscle, and when muscle weakness and atrophy appear, they suggest dysfunction of several roots. Pain and guarding produce functional weakness. On the other hand, a motor deficit may elicit sensory symptoms, for example, a feeling of "heaviness" of the limbs.

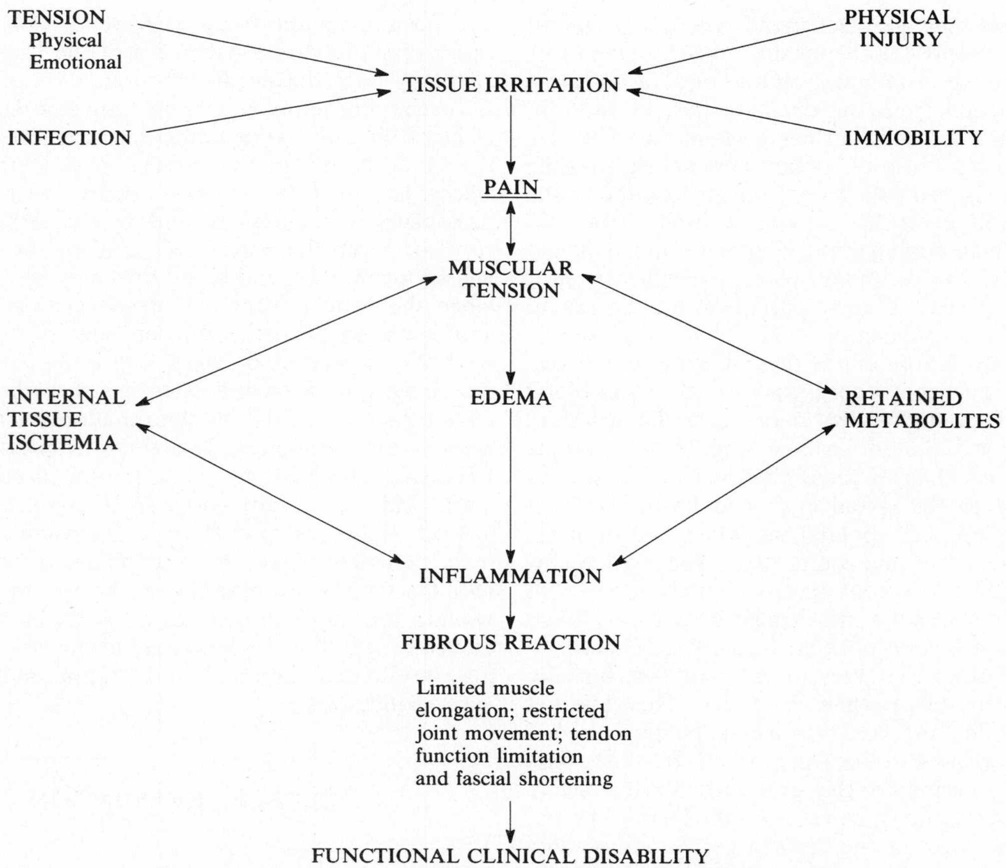


**Figure 28–6.** Mechanisms producing neck pain and disability.

*Headache and Occipital Neuralgia.* Head pain appears commonly and is characteristic of cervical spine disorders and results from nerve root compression, vertebral artery pressure, compression of sympathetic nerves, autonomic dysfunction, and posterior occipital muscle spasm as well as from osteoarthritic changes of the apophyseal joints of the upper three cervical vertebrae.[7] Occipital headache occurs commonly in the age group in which spondylosis appears, and becomes associated with pain in the neck and upper limbs. The pain may, in turn, spread to the eye region and may become dull rather than pulsating. It will be aggravated by strain, sneeze, and cough as well as by movements of the head and neck. Furthermore, the headache begins upon arising and worsens as the day progresses.

*Pseudoangina Pectoris.* A lesion at C6 and C7 may produce neurologic or myalgic pain with tenderness in the precordium or scapular region, raising confusion with angina pectoris. Pain from C6 and C7 may become compressive or may be increased with exercise, referred down the arm, aggravated by neck movement, or associated with torticollis or muscle spasm in the neck. Differentiation between heart disease and a radiculopathy can be made in the presence of other neurologic signs of C6-C7 dysfunction (e.g., muscle weakness, fasciculation, sensory changes). However, difficulty will arise in clinical situations in which true angina and pseudoangina coexist.

*Eye Symptoms.* "Blurring" of vision relieved by changing neck position, increased tearing, pain in one or both eyes, retro-orbital pain, and descriptions of the eyes being "pulled backward or pushed forward" may be reported by the patient with a cervical spine disorder. These symptoms result from irritation of the cervical sympathetic nerve supply to eye structures via the plexuses surrounding the vertebral and internal carotid arteries and their branches.

*Ear Symptoms.* Changes in equilibrium develop with irritation of sympathetic plexuses surrounding the vertebral arteries or with vascular insufficiency of these same arteries. Associated gait disturbances with or without tinnitus and altered auditory acuity result from vascular insufficiency secondary to vasospasm or compression of the vertebral arteries by cervical structures.

*Throat Symptoms.* Dysphagia results from muscle spasm, anterior osteophyte compression of the pharynx and esophagus, or abnormalities of cervical cranial nerve and sympathetic communications.

*Miscellaneous Symptoms.* Occasionally, bizarre symptoms appear in patients with cervical spine disorders. Dyspnea ("can't get a deep breath . . . or enough air") results from a C3-C4-C5 deficit (innervation of the respiratory muscles). Cardiac palpitations and tachycardia associated with unusual positions or hyperextension of the neck appear with irritation of the C4 nerve root, which innervates the diaphragm and pericardium, or with irritation of the cardiac sympathetic nerve supply. Nausea and emesis, ill-defined pain, and paresthesias may accompany spinal cord compression. Drop attacks, with abrupt loss of proprioception, and collapse without loss of consciousness may suggest posterior circulation insufficiency.

A complex variety of symptoms and signs result from cervical nerve root dysfunction, sympathetic nervous system involvement, cervical spinal cord compression, and posterior circulation insufficiency as well as diseases and injury of cervical bone, muscles, and joints. The clinician must consider all of these factors in evaluating patients with neck pain before diagnosing the symptoms as "functional" or psychoneurotic.

**Clinical Examination.** Systematic examination of patients with cervical spine syndromes includes head, neck, upper thoracic spine, shoulders, arms, forearms, wrists, and hands with the patient fully undressed. The clinician observes the patient's posture, movements, facial expression, gait, and various positions (e.g., sitting, standing, supine). As the patient walks into the office, the clinician observes the patient's head position and how naturally and rhythmically the head and neck move with body movement.

The neck should be inspected for normal anatomic position of the hyoid bone, thyroid cartilage, and thyroid gland and for normal cervical lordosis as well as scars or pigmentation. Palpation of bony structures in the neck should be performed with the patient supine in order to relax the overlying muscles. In palpating the anterior neck, the examiner stands at the patient's side and supports the neck from behind with one hand, palpating with the other, relaxing the spine as much as possible. The horseshoe-shaped hyoid bone lies above the thyroid cartilage and is at the level of the C3 vertebra. With the index finger and thumb (pincerlike) the examiner feels the stem of the horseshoe, and as the patient swallows, the hyoid bone moves up and then down. The thyroid cartilage possesses a superior notch and a flaring upper portion (sits at the C4 vertebra level); the lower border lies at the C5 level. Below the lower border of the thyroid cartilage the examiner palpates the first cricoid ring (opposite the C6 vertebra), and this will be the upper border of the trachea and just superior to the site of emergency tracheostomy. The cricoid ring moves with swallowing. About 2 to 3 cm lateral to the first cricoid ring, the carotid tubercle, the anterior tubercle of the transverse process of C6, can be felt. The carotid arteries lie adjacent to the tubercle, and their pulsation can be appreciated. Palpation of both carotid tubercles simultaneously results in restriction of carotid arterial flow, causing a carotid reflex. The carotid tubercle proves useful as a landmark in stellate sympathetic ganglion injections. The transverse process of C1 lies between the angle of the jaw and the styloid process of the skull. Since it will be the broadest transverse process of the cervical spine, palpation will be facilitated. Normal anatomic movements of the atlanto-occipital and atlantoaxial joints and bony structures can be appreciated by a lateral sliding movement, holding the atlas between the thumb and index finger by the transverse processes.

The posterior landmarks of the cervical spine include the occiput, inion, superior nuchal line, mastoid process, spinous processes of each vertebra, and apophyseal joints. Initially, the examiner palpates the occiput, then the inion, marking the center point of the superior nuchal line (the line will feel like a transverse ridge extending out on both sides of the inion). The round mastoid process sits at the lateral edge of the superior nuchal line (Fig. 28–1*B*). The spinous process of the axis (C2) can be palpated below the indented area immediately under the occiput. As each spinous process from C2 to T1 is palpated, the examiner notes the cervical lordosis. Occasionally the bifid spinous processes of C3 to C6 can be appreciated. The C7 (vertebra prominens) and T1 spinous processes will be larger than the others. Alignment of the spinous processes should be noted. The apophyseal joints can be felt as small rounded domes deep to the trapezius muscles about 1 inch lateral to the spinous processes. In order to palpate these joints the patient must be relaxed, as spasm and tension preclude access on examination. The joint involved can be determined by alignment with the hyoid bone at C3, the thyroid cartilage at C4 and C5, and the first cricoid ring at C6. These joints often become tender with osteoarthritis, especially in the upper cervical spine, whereas the C5-C6, C6-C7 level will be most often involved in cervical spondylosis.

Examination of soft tissues in the neck should be divided into two anatomic areas, anterior and posterior, the anterior being bordered laterally by the two sternocleidomastoid muscles, superiorly by the mandible, and inferiorly by the suprasternal notch (an upside-down triangle); the posterior aspect includes the whole area posterior to the lateral border of the sternocleidomastoid muscle. The supine position appears optimal in the examination. Anteriorly the sternocleidomastoid muscle can be examined by asking the patient to turn the head to the opposite side; the muscle then stands out and can be palpated from origin to insertion. The opposite muscle can be compared for any discrepancies in size, bulges, or strength. Hyperextension injuries overstretch the muscle, with resultant hemorrhage into the tissue. Localized swelling may be due to hematomas. In torticollis the sternocleidomastoid muscles will be involved. The lymph node chain resides along the medial border of the sternocleidomastoid muscle and in the normal situation cannot be palpated. Small tender lymph nodes can be palpated if they are enlarged secondary to infections (throat, ear), metastases, or primary tumor. Enlarged lymph nodes may, in turn, produce torticollis. The thyroid gland overlies the thyroid cartilage in an H pattern, the bar being the isthmus between the two laterally situated lobes. Normally, the thyroid gland will be smooth and palpable without enlargement. Diffuse enlargement of the thyroid gland, cysts, nodules, or tenderness from thyroiditis should be noted. The carotid arteries, best felt near the carotid tubercle on C6, should be examined separately, owing to the carotid reflex secondary to simultaneous palpation. Normally carotid pulsation should be symmetric.

The parotid gland overlies part of the sharp angle of the mandible, which is usually indistinct to palpation; but when the parotid gland is enlarged, the usually sharp and bony angle of the mandible feels soft and boggy owing to overlying glandular tissue (e.g., mumps, Sjögren's syndrome, and endocrine disorders). The supraclavicular fossa above the clavicle should be examined for lymph nodes, unusual excursion with respiration, swelling, fat accumulation, and asymmetry with the opposite side. The platysma muscle crosses the supraclavicular fossa but will be too thin to alter the contour of the fossa. Observation during voluntary platysma contracture may reveal lumps or asymmetry. The apex and dome of the lung extend up into the supraclavicular fossa. At times cervical ribs can be palpated.

Posteriorly, with the patient sitting, the clinician examines the trapezius muscle, lymph nodes, the greater occipital nerves, and the superior nuchal ligament. The trapezius muscle origin extends from the inion to the spinous process of T12 and inserts laterally in a continuous arc into the clavicle, the acromion, and the spine of the scapula. The trapezius should be felt from origin to insertion, beginning high up on the neck. Flexion injuries may traumatize the trapezius, and hematomas in the muscle occur frequently. Furthermore, the trapezius will be the site of focal points of pain and tenderness in fibrositis syndromes. Two trapezius muscles should be palpated bilaterally and simultaneously, while looking for tenderness, lumps and swelling, and asymmetry of the two muscles. Embryologically the trapezius and sternocleidomastoid muscles begin as one muscle and later split, but they retain a common attachment along the base of the skull to the mastoid process and their nerve supply remains the same, the spinal accessory nerve (ninth cranial nerve). The lymph node chain lies at the anterolateral border of the trapezius and normally cannot be palpated. The greater occipital nerves sit laterally to the inion, extending up in the scalp, and can be easily palpated when tender and inflamed. Commonly a flexion-extension injury of the spine produces traumatic inflammation and swelling of the occipital nerves with resultant painful occipital neuralgia, a frequent cause of headache. The superior nuchal ligament arises from the anion and extends to C7 and T1 spinous processes. It will be under the examining finger when the physician is feeling the spinous processes. It may become tender, irregular, and lumpy if overstretched or injured.

***Range of Motion.*** There exists a large range of motion of the cervical spine (Table 28–3), which, in turn, provides a wide scope of vision and is essential to the sense of balance. The basic movements of the neck include flexion, extension, lateral flexion to the right and left, and rotation to the right and left. About half of the total flexion and extension of the neck occurs at the occiput-C1 level, the other half being equally distributed among the other six cervical vertebra, with a slight increase at the C5-C6 level. Approximately half of rotation occurs at the atlantoaxial joint (odontoid); the other half distributes equally among the other five vertebrae. All vertebrae share in lateral flexion. A decrease in specific motion may occur with blocking at a joint, pain, fibrous contractures, bony ankylosis, muscle spasm, mechanical alteration in joint and skeletal structures, or a tense and uncooperative patient. Other causes of muscle spasm include injury to muscles, involuntary splinting over painful joints or skeletal structures, and irritation or compression of cervical nerve roots of the spinal cord.

All range of cervical spine motion should be performed as follows: (1) actively and to the extreme of motion (to assess muscle function and strength), as observed by the examiner; (2) passively (to assess nonmobile structures, ligaments, capsules, and fascia), by which the examiner moves the relaxed cervical spine through all its motions; and (3) against resistance (to study origin and insertions of tendon and ligaments and assess motor strength), with each motion maximally attempted against force of the examiner's hand.

*Flexion and Extension.* The patient nods his head forward and touches chin to sternum. If one of the examiner's fingers can be placed between the patient's chin and sternum, there exists 10 degrees' limitation of flexion while 30 degrees of limitation exists if three fingers can be inserted within the above area. Observation of the curve of the cervical spine should be done as the examiner instructs the patient to look from floor to ceiling. The arc of neck motion normally remains smooth and not halting or irregular. In full hyperextension the base of the occiput normally touches the spinous process of T1.

*Lateral Flexion.* The patient attempts to touch his ear to his shoulder without rotation or shoulder shrugging. Normal people can laterally flex 45 degrees in either direction.

*Rotation.* The patient rotates the head maximally, usually being able to bring his chin into alignment with his shoulder. Normally, the motion remains smooth, while torticollis restricts motion.

*Passive Range of Motion.* The examiner asks for complete relaxation and takes the patient's head firmly in his hands, putting the spine through maximal flexion, extension, lateral flexion, and rotation. Passive motion may be more extensive than active motion if muscles remain stiff, painful, or possess involuntary spasm. In cases of head or cervical spine injury, passive range of motion should not be done because of the risk of neurologic trauma to an unstable spine.

*Motion Against Resistance.* All ranges of neck motion can be performed with the examiner offering firm resistance to each movement. The anchorage of muscle, tendon insertion and origin, muscle strength, and muscular function should be assessed. This phase of the examination should be performed with the patient seated. The primary (sternocleidomastoids) and secondary (three scalenes and small prevertebral muscles) flexors of the neck can be assessed by the examiner placing his left hand flat on the patient's upper sternum and his right (resisting) hand, with the palm cupped, on the patient's forehead; the patient then flexes his neck, slowly increasing the power to maximal pressure. The primary (paravertebral extensor mass, splenius and semispinalis capitis, and trapezius muscles) and secondary extensor muscles (small intrinsic neck muscles) should be assessed by the examiner placing his left hand over the patient's upper posterior chest and scapular area, with his right palm cupped over the patient's occiput; the patient then gradually increases neck extension to his maximum. Lateral flexor muscles (three scalenes and the small intrinsic neck muscles) can be examined by placing the examiner's left hand on the patient's shoulder (for stability) and his right palm (fingers extended) against the side of the patient's head; the patient then laterally flexes against the examiner's resistance. The rotators of the neck (sternocleidomastoid and intrinsic neck muscles) can be tested to right lateral rotation by placing the stabilizing left hand of the examiner on the patient's left shoulder and his right hand along the right side of the patient's mandible while the patient rotates against resistance. Left rotation is tested in the reverse fashion. Either sternocleidomastoid muscle functioning alone provides the main pull to the side being tested.

**Special Clinical Tests of the Cervical Spine.** ***Head Compression Test (Fig. 28–7).*** With narrowing of the intervertebral foramina, pressure and shearing forces on the apophyseal joint surfaces, intervertebral disc compression, or pressure on stiff ligamentous and muscle structures there will be pain on compression of the head onto the cervical spine. If radicular pain or paresthesias with referral to the upper limb occur with the head compression test, it strongly suggests nerve root irritation. On the other hand, if the pain remains in the neck, soft connective tissues or joints appear as the pain-sensitive structures involved. The test should be performed with the patient sitting; the examiner places one hand across the other on the top of the patient's head with gradually increased downward pressure; the patient then reports any pain or paresthesias and its distribution. Application of pressure may also be down with the head tilted to either side, backward, or forward.

***Head Distraction Test (Fig. 28–7).*** This test should be done with the patient seated; the open palm of the examiner's hand should be placed under the patient's chin.

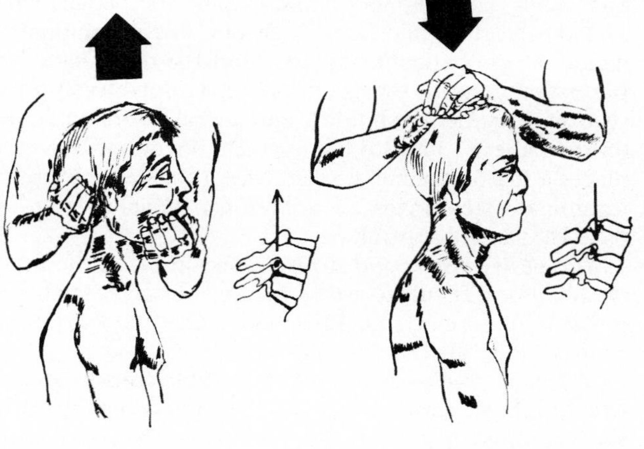


**Figure 28–7.** Neck compression and distraction tests in the examination of patients with cervical spine syndromes.

while the examiner's other hand goes under the patient's occiput; gradually the force of lifting the patient's head increases, removing the weight of the skull and distracting the foramina, discs, and joints. Nerve root compression may be relieved, with disappearance of symptoms with opening of the intervertebral foramina or extension of the disc spaces. Additionally, pressure on joint capsules of apophyseal joints diminishes with head distraction.

***Valsalva Maneuver.*** Holding one's breath against a closed glottis raises intrathecal pressure. If an intraspinal tumor or a herniated disc exists in a person, then this test will produce pain, which radiates in a dermatome distribution. Vigorous cough or sneeze, likewise, will elicit pain in the above situations.

***Dysphagia Test.*** Soft tissue swelling, hematoma, vertebral subluxation, or cervical osteophytic projections produce pain or restriction to swallowing.

***Ophthalmologic Tests.*** Pupillary signs may differ from one side to the other or vary from one time to another in certain patients with cervical spine disorders, thereby indicating irritability of sympathetic nerve supply in the neck controlling the pupillary muscles. This should not be confused with Horner's syndrome, which follows complete interruption or paralysis of the sympathetic fibers, resulting in miosis, vasomotor and sweating changes, and ptosis on the affected side.

***Adson Test.*** The Adson test examines the subclavian artery when it may be compressed by a cervical rib, the scalene muscles, or other thoracic outlet abnormalities. The examiner palpates the patient's radial pulse in abduction, extension, and external rotation of the arm. The patient then takes a deep inspiration while rotating his head maximally toward the side being tested. With subclavian artery compression there results a marked decrease in volume or absence of the radial pulse on the affected side.

***Shoulder Depression Test.*** This test indirectly determines if there exists irritation on compression of nerve root, dural root sleeve fibrosis or adhesions, foraminal encroachment, or adjacent joint capsule thickening and adhesions. The examiner stands beside the patient who tilts the head to one side. With one of the examiner's hands on the patient's shoulder and the other hand on the patient's head, the examiner exerts downward pressure on the patient's shoulder and lateral flexion pressure on the patient's head in the opposite direction. This test places a tug on the nerve roots; with root sleeve fibrosis, foraminal osteophytes, or adhesions, radicular pain or paresthesias often result.

***Muscle Weakness and Atrophy.*** Weakness of the muscles may be difficult to assess, as innervation of shoulder girdle, arm, forearm and muscles occurs by two or more roots (Table 28–4).

Muscular weakness has many possible causes; to narrow the choice down to one or a few, one must ascertain the anatomic localization of the patient's complaints. Tables 28–5 and 28–6 provide guidelines and offer differential clinical features separating upper and lower motor neuron weakness. Atrophy may follow weakness owing to disuse or pain. Interossei hand muscle atrophy can appear with cervical spine disease (Fig. 28–8).

**Table 28–5.** Clinical Features Differentiating Upper and Lower Motor Neuron Weakness

| Clinical Feature | Upper Motor Neuron Weakness | Lower Motor Neuron Weakness |
|---|---|---|
| Weakness | Greater in extensors of upper limbs and in flexors of lower limbs (pyramidal distribution); usually involves one side of body but may also produce paraparesis, quadriparesis, or (rarely) monoparesis; usually does not produce weakness in one muscle group or bilateral cranial weakness | Nonpyramidal distribution; May be present in one muscle group; paraparesis, quadriparesis, and bilateral cranial nerve weakness also seen |
| Deep tendon reflexes | Usually increased, but acutely may be decreased; also may be decreased with parietal and cerebellar lesions | Decreased |
| Tone to passive motion | Increased; may be decreased with cerebellar and parietal lesions | Decreased |
| Pathologic reflexes | Babinski and others | Absent |
| associated | Defect of cortical association areas; frontal-release signs defect of sensation; cerebellar defects; cranial nerve defects | Cranial nerve signs; sensory sign |

***Reflexes.*** Reflexes indicate the state of the nervous system and its afferent pathways (Table 28–7). Certain abnormal reflexes appear only with spasticity and paralysis; these indicate injury to the corticospinal tract. The primary deep tendon reflexes (Table 28–8 and 28–9), abdominal reflexes, and plantar responses should be routinely examined; bulbocavernosus and anal reflexes should be tested in all suspected lower spinal cord (conus or cauda equina) lesions and in cases of sphincter disturbances.

In eliciting the deep-tendon reflexes, adequate relaxation of the patient and a mild degree of passive tension on the muscle becomes essential, especially in the radial (supinator) and ankle jerks. The examiner varies the tension on the muscle by manipulating the joint, and reinforcement procedures enable the patient to relax completely, as by pulling one of his hands with the other (Jendrassik maneuver). When the examiner elicits the triceps jerk, the small contraction of the triceps muscle should be disregarded, for most muscles will contract if directly percussed.

The tendon jerk normally occurs in only a part of each muscle, and in a myopathy, the reflex jerk may be

**Table 28–6.** Differentiating Symptoms of Lower Motor Neuron Weakness

| Signs and Symptoms | Neuropathy | Myopathy* | Motor Neuron or Anterior Horn Cell Dysfunction | Neuromuscular Junction Dysfunction |
|---|---|---|---|---|
| Weakness | Mainly distal or nerve distribution | Proximal | May be distal or proximal and involve midline muscles (neck flexor weak) | Mainly bulbar respiratory, and proximal |
| Deep tendon reflexes | Decreased | Decreased | Increased | Normal |
| Myotatic reflexes | Increased | Decreased | Increased | Normal |
| Sensory loss paresthesias | Usually present | Absent | Absent | Absent |
| Fasciculations | May be present | Absent | Present | Absent |
| Atrophy | May be present | May be present | Present | Absent |
| Fatigue | Mild | Mild | Mild | Severe |
| Tenderness | May have dysesthesias | May be present | Cramps | Absent |

*Myoglobinuria or myotonia may differentiate certain myopathies.

lost in the quadriceps through wasting in the vastus internus, though the power of contraction of the remainder persists to a fair degree. Some clinically normal people show reduced reflexes, and before the examiner decides, he should ascertain whether there exists other evidence of peripheral nerve (sensory loss, atrophy, etc.) or muscle disease.

***Examination of Related Area.*** Shoulder lesions may closely mimic cervical spine disease, and a complete shoulder examination becomes necessary in these situations. The shoulder syndromes usually demonstrate little or no neurologic involvement. Rotator cuff tendinitis, calcareous deposits in tendons, and capsulitis often coexist with cervical spine disease. Reflex sympathetic dystrophy may occur, with the initial triggering pain mechanism arising in the spine. Similar changes may occur at the elbow, wrist, and fingers. Finger motion may be limited because of swelling secondary to circulatory reflex ischemic changes from sympathetic nerve irritation. Fibrous nodules and contracture of palmar fascia occur following cervical spine disease or injury.

Infections of the temporomandibular joint, teeth, lower jaw, or scalp may refer pain to the temporomandibular joint area and to the neck. The jaw reflex (mediated by the fifth cranial nerve and involving the masseter and temporalis muscles) can be examined by placing the index finger on the mental area of the chin with the patient's mouth in the rest position (slightly open); a reflex hammer then taps the fingers and the jaw reflexly closes. An absent or decreased jaw jerk suggests abnormality in the course of the trigeminal nerve, while a brisk reflex suggests an upper motor neuron lesion. The jaw jerk proves useful in separating cervical spine disease from primary trigeminal nerve dysfunction.

**Radiographic Examination.** X-rays are essential in evaluation of the patient with a cervical spine disorder. The clinicians should assess both the clinical and the radiographic studies of his patient and not depend solely on the radiologist. Clinical correlation will be necessary, as gross radiologic signs and abnormalities may be associated with minimal or no clinical disturbance while the reverse situation (minimal radiographic change and neurolgic signs) may also occur.

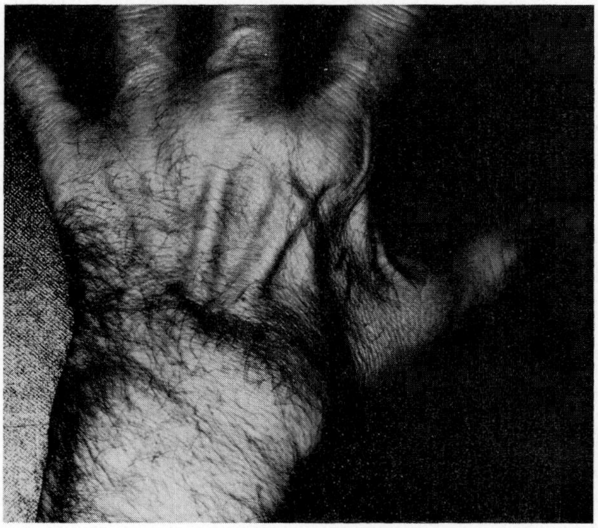

**Figure 28–8.** Interossei hand muscle weakness in a patient with severe cervical spondylosis.

**Table 28–7.** Relation of Reflexes to Peripheral Nerves and Spinal Cord Segments

| Reflex | Site and Mode of Elicitation | Response | Muscle(s) | Peripheral Nerve(s) | Cord Segment |
|---|---|---|---|---|---|
| Scapulohumeral reflex | Tap on lower end of medial border of scapula | Adduction and lateral rotation of dependent arm | Infraspinatus and teres minor | Suprascapular (axillary) | C4 to C6 |
| Biceps jerk | Tap on tendon of biceps brachii | Flexion at elbow | Biceps brachii | Musculocutaneous | C5 and C6 |
| Supinator jerk (also called radial reflex) | Tap on distal end of radius | Flexion at elbow | Brachioradialis (and biceps brachii and brachialis) | Radial (musculocutaneous) | C5 and C6 |
| Triceps jerk | Tap on tendon of triceps brachii above olecranon, with elbow flexed | Extension at elbow | Triceps brachii | Radial | C7 and C8 |
| Thumb reflex | Tap on tendon of flexor pollicis longus in distal third of forearm | Flexion of terminal phalanx of thumb | Flexor pollicis longus | Median | C6 to C8 |
| Extensor finger and hand jerk | Tap on posterior aspect of wrist just proximal to radiocarpal joint | Extension of hand and fingers (inconstant) | Extensors of hand and fingers | Radial | C6 to C8 |
| Flexor finger jerk | Tap on examiner's thumb placed on palm of hand; sharp tap on tips of flexed fingers (Tromner's sign) | Flexion of fingers | Flexor digitorum superficialis (and profundus) | Median | C7 and C8 (T1) |
| Epigastric reflex (exteroceptive) | Brisk stroking of skin downwards from nipple in mammillary line | Retraction of epigastrium | Transversus abdominis | Intercostal | T5 and T6 |
| Abdominal skin reflex (exteroceptive) | Brisk stroking of skin of abdominal wall in lateromedial direction | Shift of skin of abdomen and displacement of umbilicus | Muscles of abdominal wall | Intercostal, hypogastric, and ilioinguinal | T6 and T12 |
| Cremasteric reflex (exteroceptive) | Stroking skin on medial aspect of thigh (pinching adductor muscles) | Elevation of testis | Cremaster | Genital branch of genitofemoral | L2 and L3 (L1) |
| Adductor reflex | Tap on medial condyle of femur | Adduction of leg | Adductors of thigh | Obturator | L2, L3, and L4 |
| Knee jerk | Tap on tendon of quadriceps femoris below patella | Extension at knee | Quadriceps femoris | Femoral | (L2), L3, and L4 |
| Gluteal reflex (exteroceptive) | Stroking skin over gluteal region | Tightening of buttock (inconstant) | Gluteus medius and gluteus maximus | Superior and inferior gluteal | L4, L5, and S1 |
| Posterior tibial reflex | Tap on tendon of tibialis posterior behind medial malleolus | Supination of foot (inconstant) | Tibialis posterior | Tibial | L5 |
| Semimembranosus and semitendinosus reflex | Tap on medial hamstring tendons (patient prone and knee slightly flexed) | Contraction of semimembranosus and semitendinosus muscles | Semimembranosus and semitendinosus | Sciatic | S1 |
| Biceps femoris reflex | Tap on lateral hamstring tendon (patient prone and knee slightly flexed) | Contraction of biceps femoris | Biceps femoris | Sciatic | S1 and S2 |
| Ankle jerk | Tap on tendo calcaneus | Plantar flexion of foot | Triceps surae and other flexors of foot | Tibial | S1 and S2 |
| Bulbocavernosus reflex (exteroceptive) | Gentle squeezing of glans penis or pinching of skin of dorsum of penis | Contraction of bulbocavernosus muscle, palpable at root of penis | Bulbocavernosus | Pudendal | S3 and S4 |
| Anal reflex (exteroceptive) | Scratch or prick of perianal skin (patient lying on side) | Visible contraction of anus | Sphincter ani externus | Pudendal | S5 |

**Table 28–8.** The Six Primary Reflexes

| Reflex | Nerve Roots Necessary for Reflex | Muscle Carrying Out the Reflex |
|---|---|---|
| Ankle jerk | S1 | Gastrocnemius |
| Posterior tibial | L5 | Posterior tibial |
| Knee | L2-L4 | Quadriceps |
| Biceps | C5, C6 | Biceps |
| Radial | C5, C6 | Brachioradialis |
| Triceps | (C6), C7, C8 | Triceps |

Routine x-ray views include (1) anteroposterior views of the atlas and axis through the open mouth (Fig. 28–9); (2) anteroposterior views of the lower five vertebra; (3) lateral views in flexion, neutral, and extension (Fig. 28–10); and (4) both right and left oblique (Fig. 28–11) views.

Planograms and tomograms may be necessary in certain instances (e.g., trauma, tumors, infection). Nuclear bone scans can be used in patients suspected of having infection, tumor, certain metabolic diseases, and compression fractures. Computed tomography (CT) scan and myelography with iodinated contrast material will be necessary in cervical disc disease, tumors, and syringomyelia.

**Electrodiagnostic Studies: Electromyography (EMG), Nerve Conduction Velocities (NCV), Somatosensory Evoked Responses (SER).** Various EMG, NCV, and SER patterns help differentiate the normal from diffuse polyneuropathy, focal entrapment neuropathy, radiculopathy, myopathy, disorders of the neuromuscular junction (e.g., myasthenia gravis), and anterior horn cell disease (e.g., amyotrophic lateral sclerosis) (Table 28–10). No one feature of the EMG (except for true myotonia) gives a diagnosis; rather, it requires the summated information of needle EMG coupled with NCV and SER as well as the clinical examination as performed by a clinician.

Clinicians often face the problem of a patient with weakness. Weakness, in turn, may be secondary to disease within the muscle, nerve, neuromuscular junction, or upper motor neuron (spinal cord, brainstem, or cerebrum) (Tables 28–5 and 28–6). The specific need for definitive therapy, including surgery, can be established only when the physician becomes aware of the cause, extent, and prognosis of the weakness. Evaluation of the electrical activity of muscle tissue and of muscle response to nerve stimulation solves many of these problems.

**Other Laboratory Tests.** The clinical laboratory offers some help in diagnosis and management of neck pain in specific diseases (e.g., rheumatoid arthritis, hyperparathyroidism, multiple myeloma, ankylosing spondylitis, and metastatic malignant cancer). Cerebrospinal fluid (CSF) evaluation should be done in patients with neck pain suspected of having infection (meningitis, meningismus) or subarachnoid hemorrhage. In the latter conditions, the CSF will be diagnostic.

**Table 28–9.** Four Point Grading Scale for Reflexes

| Grade | State of Reflexes |
|---|---|
| 0 | Absent despite full relaxation and reinforcement maneuvers |
| 1 | Reduced but not absent |
| 2 | Normal physiologic reflexes |
| 3 | Increased response but no reduplication or excessive spread |
| 4 | Marked increase with reduplication, clonus, and spread |

## DIFFERENTIAL DIAGNOSIS

Many clinical conditions arising outside the cervical spine but perceived in or about the neck area (Fig. 28–5) mimic cervical nerve root irritation, muscle spasm, ligament strain, bone disease, and joint disorders. Although Table 28–1 lists multiple structures potentially causing neck pain, clinical evaluation usually differentiates between the entities.

Disorders of somatic or visceral structures having cervical nerve root innervation (same embryologic origin) cause pain felt in the neck. Since these areas constitute reflexly referred pain along the segmental distribution of the nerve roots, such areas of referral will not be tender on deep palpation. Areas of superficial peripheral tenderness develop owing to reflex or direct sympathetic irritation secondary to vasomotor changes. Referred painful areas do not have muscle spasm and often will be described as having a burning or cramping sensation. Nausea, emesis, and pallor may accompany this type of pain.

Peripheral neuropathy may produce pain both proximal as well as distal to the irritative site. However, muscle spasm will not be associated with peripheral neuropathy. Spinal cord tumor produces a poorly localized and ill-defined neck pain, hyper-reflexia, spasticity; immobilization will not relieve the pain, and deep tenderness and local muscle spasms will be absent. Furthermore, in spinal cord lesions there exists paralysis or weakness below the cord level (not dermatome) associated with sensory changes and Babinski signs. Cerebral or subarachnoid hemorrhage, meningitis, head and neck trauma, or a central tumor produces cervical spine pain, mimicking cervical spine syndromes producing nerve root irritation. In these instances the clinical examination, CT scan, CSF tests, and angiographic studies will differentiate between the various conditions.

An important point to remember in the differential diagnosis of neck pain is that compression or irritation of cervical nerve roots with radiation of pain is associated with deep tenderness at the site of pain. Segmental areas of deep tenderness that are not painful until palpated indicate nerve root involvement. A 1 percent injection of lidocaine in the painful area results in transient reproduction of the radicular pain followed by relief from pain for days or weeks in the patient with nerve root irritation. If local anesthetic injection fails to reproduce (and relieve) the pain, one then looks at potential visceral or somatic structures having the same segmental nerve supply.

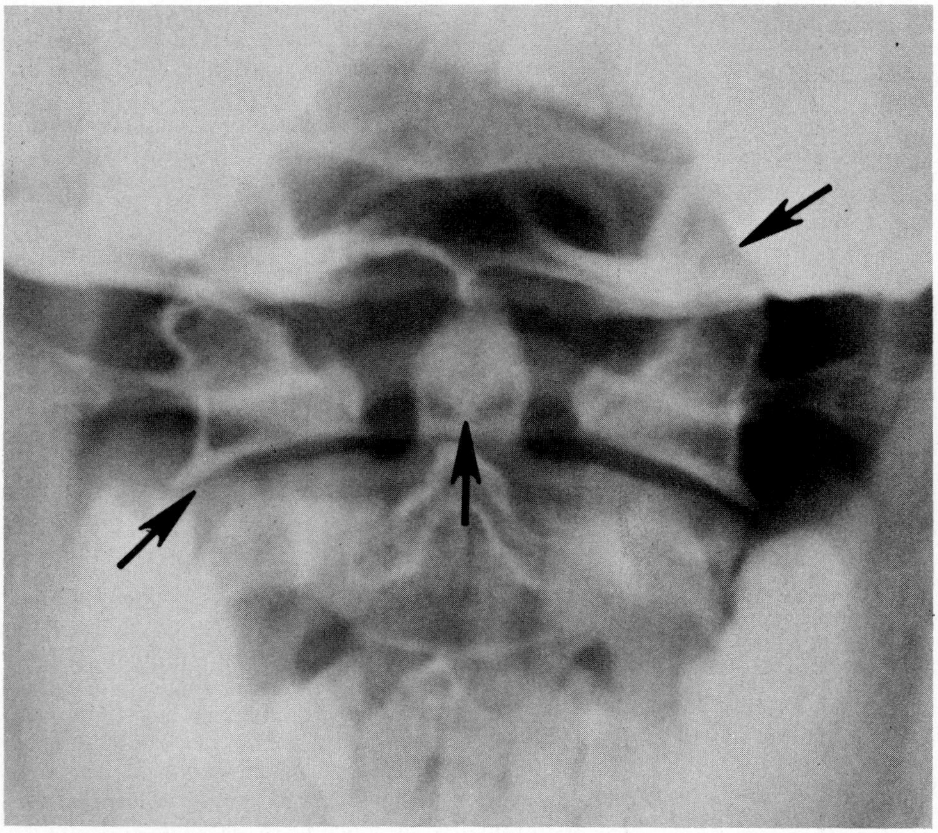

**Figure 28–9.** Open mouth cervical spine x-ray showing the atlanto-occipital relationship, symmetry, joint space, and the bony configuration. The atlas-axis relationship and odontoid can also be seen. The arrow to the left shows the atlanto-axial joint; the middle arrow, the odontoid process; and the arrow to the right, the atlanto-occipital joint.

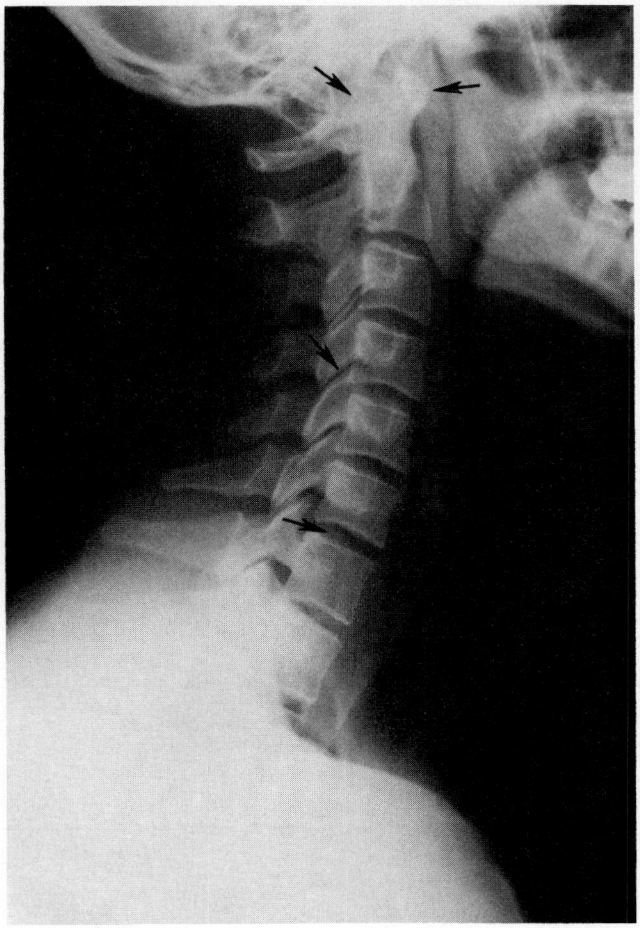

**Figure 28–10.** Lateral x-ray view showing the normal cervical lordosis with anterior convexity; spinous processes and the apophyseal joints are seen. The lower arrow marks the C6-C7 disc space. The upper right arrow shows the anterior arch of the atlas while the upper left arrow shows the posterior surface of the odontoid. In a C1-C2 subluxation, the space between the posterior surface of the arch of the atlas and the anterior surface of the odontoid opens up (normal will be up to 2.5 mm); this is seen best in flexion. The sagittal diameter may be measured from the middle of each vertebra to the point of union of the lamina; 10 mm or less will usually indicate pathologic narrowing and a myelopathy.

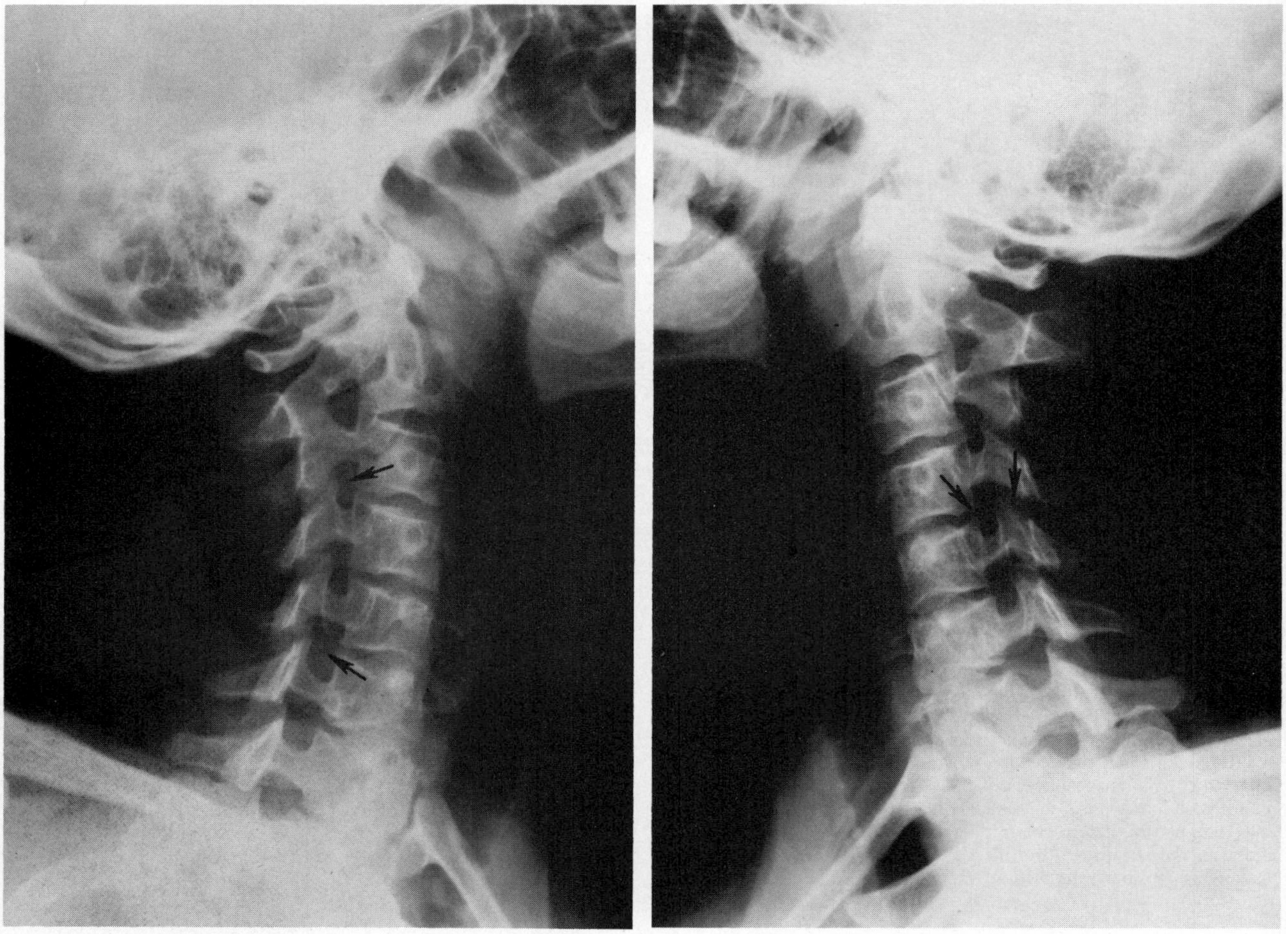

A B

**Figure 28–11.** Oblique cervical x-rays display the intervertebral foramina, normally 10 mm vertical height and 5 mm transverse. Osteophyte projection from the uncovertebral joints, the vertebrae themselves, and the apophyseal joints can be seen (arrows).

**Table 28–10.** Summary of EMG, NCV, and SER Findings by Location in Disease in the Motor Unit

| | **Location** | | | | | | |
|---|---|---|---|---|---|---|---|
| | *Spinal Cord* | | *Nerve Root* | | | | *Muscle* |
| **Study** | *Anterior Horn Cell* | *Anterior Motor* | *Dorsal Pre-* | *Ganglion Post-* | *Peripheral Nerve* | *Neuromuscular Junction* | |
| Motor NCV | N | N | N | N | + | N | N |
| Sensory NCV | N | N | N | ± | + | N | N |
| EMG | + | + | N | N | + | ± | + |
| Repetitive stimulation | ± | ± | N | N | ± | + | N |
| F wave | + | + | N | N | + | N | N |
| H reflex | + | + | + | + | + | N | N |
| SER | ± | ± | + | + | + | N | N |

N = Normal
+ = Abnormal
± = Occasional Abnormality
SER = Somatosensory Evoked Response

Neck pain occurs in malingerers, depressed individuals, patients seeking compensation, hysterical and psychoneurotic patients, and automobile accident victims. If these patients possess no concomitant nerve root irritation, then they will derive no relief from local anesthesia injected in the painful area(s). Absence of muscle spasm, an antalgic position, and feigning of limitation of motion should arouse the examiner's suspicion.

Skilled clinical elicitation of historical data and the physical examination constitute the principal and most reproducible means of making a differential diagnosis[6,8,9] (Fig. 28–12). In evaluating the patient with neck pain the examiner soon realizes that there may be a syndrome of neck pain alone, head and neck pain, neck and shoulder pain, shoulder pain alone, shoulder and arm pain, or just arm, forearm, hand, or finger pain. Symptoms of altered sensation and vascular insufficiency often accompany the complaint of neck pain. Symptoms or signs arising in the head and upper cervical spine arise only from structures at the C1 to C4 level; symptoms in the lower neck, shoulder, and arm arise from structures at the C4 to T1 levels. When the examiner observes muscle weakness in the patient with neck pain, he must differentiate among nerve root compromise, myelopathy, pe-

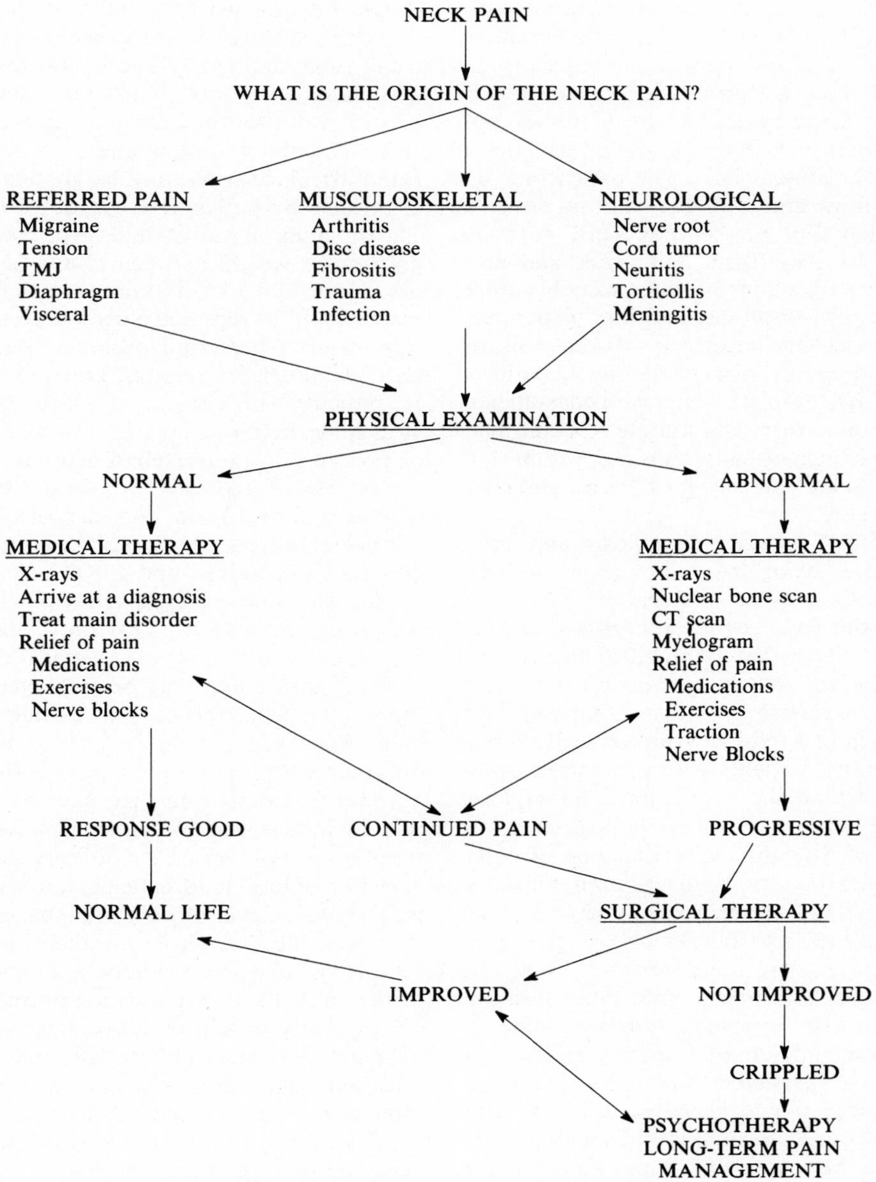


**Figure 28–12.** Algorithm for the clinical evaluation of patients with neck pain.

ripheral neuropathy, and a primary muscle disease (Table 6).

## TREATMENT

**Medical Regimen.** Opinions differ as to the best treatment of neck pain and the various cervical spine syndromes discussed in this chapter. Cautious clinical, electrodiagnostic, and x-ray assessment must precede the planning of treatment, and it becomes important to exclude other causes of pain in the neck and upper limbs before treatment commences. In any treatment regimen, the clinician must consider the following: (1) severity of the symptoms, (2) the presence or absence of neurologic findings, and (3) the severity of the condition as seen by electrodiagnostic evaluation and radiographic procedures (which may necessitate CT and myelography).

***Bed Rest.*** Medical therapy aims at the relief of pain and stiffness in the neck and arms. Bed rest should be reserved for severe acute cases, for chronic cases with an acute exacerbation of symptoms, or for patients in whom ambulatory treatment fails. The patient lies flat in bed with one pillow and with the head in the most comfortable position. For the relief of pain, adequate analgesics should be prescribed. Salicylates and anti-inflammatory and analgesic medications usually suffice; however, if severe pain develops, codeine, meperidine, or morphine may become necessary. Muscle relaxant medications, hypnotics, or diazepam may be utilized concomitantly. With complete bed rest and sufficient analgesic, anti-inflammatory, and muscle relaxant medications, acute neck pain usually subsides within 7 to 10 days. When the acute pain subsides, the patient commences active exercises.

***Cervical Collar.*** In cervical spondylosis and other musculoskeletal-type syndromes, limitation of neck movement benefits the patient, and cervical collars can be used to achieve this end. The several types of cervical collars range from those that immobilize the cervical spine to those intended merely to provide temporary support and limit excessive movement. Patients with nerve root pain often find relief of symptoms after wearing a collar. Generally, patients with generalized spondylosis do less well than those with focal spondylosis. Before prescribing a cervical collar, it is essential to assess the degree of disability, and the type of collar selected should depend on the degree of immobilization desired. Felt, foam, and rubber collars restrict gross movement, while plastic and plaster collars give more secure immobilization. Any collar must fit well and maintain the neck in the most comfortable position. Most people dislike wearing collars; however, some patients seem to become addicted to wearing collars, and it becomes difficult to persuade them to remove them. In general, the patient should leave his collar off after about 2 months to prevent weakness and wasting of the neck muscles. After the acute painful stage abates, active exercise in conjunction with collar use is encouraged.

***Traction.*** Traction, either continuous or intermittent, should be considered when bed rest fails. Continuous traction should be reserved for more severe cases with symptoms of nerve root compression. Many patients cannot tolerate traction, and a few will become worse with it. Analgesics and muscle relaxants can be used in doses sufficient to prevent restlessness. Sometimes it becomes necessary to set up a traction apparatus utilizing only 5 pounds of weight; this keeps the patient immobile in bed and avoids the unpleasant effects of heavier traction. There exists some difference in opinion as to the correct direction of pull in traction. Some authors feel that the most comfortable position should be found and traction exerted in this direction; others recommend that the head be in extension, while other authorities consider slight flexion as the best postion. A weight of 10 pounds should be attached to a pulley at the head of the bed, and the bed raised to increase the pull and prevent the trunk from sliding up. The weight may be increased to 20 pounds according to muscular development or may be varied during the day: some authorities recommend 10 to 12 pounds by day and 5 to 8 pounds at night.[10] Intermittent traction may be applied manually or mechanically by pulley and weight with the head halter. The direction of pull should be in the most comfortable position. A weight between 15 and 25 pounds and traction applied for 15 to 20 minutes generally suffice. Treatment should be repeated daily if necessary. Occasionally, side effects of traction occur, and rarely, hemianopic visual field defects develop. Traction appears unsuitable for patients with visible gross x-ray changes of the cervical spine, because of danger of spinal cord compression or pressure on the vertebral arteries.

***Exercises.*** Active exercises should be utilized in most regimens of treatment. The exercises can be grouped as follows: (1) anterior-neck-mobilizing exercises, (2) shoulder-raising exercises, and (3) muscle-strengthening exercises. Shoulder exercises, aimed at elevating the shoulder girdle and relieving drag on the nerve roots, can be combined with the use of a cervical collar.

Head positioning may be employed to relieve symptoms, as placing the head in certain positions relieves pain. The head should be carried at all times in its optimum position of slight flexion with the chin indrawn.

***Other Measures.*** Massage may be useful in patients with painful muscle spasms; however, in most cases massage is not prescribed in cervical spine disorders. Injection of local anesthetic or steroids into painful areas may provide relief of pain and spasm with subsequent improvement in cervical movement. Ice applied to painful areas in the acute situations often helps, while heat in the form of ultrasound or infrared radiations helps subsequently to relieve muscle spasm.

Sometimes catastrophes, with severe neurologic complications and even death, have occurred with neck manipulation as a treatment of neck pain.[11] These complications usually result from vascular disturbances of the vertebral arteries, which appear to be particularly vulnerable at the first cervical vertebra where they enter the skull. Rotation and hyperextension can become dangerous movements.

**Surgery.** Two main groups of patients appear appropriate for surgical consideration.[12] In the first group, symptoms relate principally to the nerve roots emerging from the cervical spine, and the condition presents itself with either neck or arm pain. In the second situation, a slowly progressive spinal cord syndrome involves the legs first and then the arms.

Careful clinical investigation supplemented by EMG, NCV, and SER to exclude peripheral nerve disease becomes essential in patients with radicular symptoms.

**Patient Education.** Finally, an important aspect in the treatment of patients with neck pain entails "patient education." The clinician should define the problem, instruct the patient in the rationale of the treatment, and teach the patient how to care for his neck in standing, sitting, driving, and other activities of daily living.

## SUMMARY

Many medical conditions produce neck pain both locally and in its referred aspect. Confirming the source of dysfunction in the neck, understanding the mechanism by which the symptoms occur, and recognizing the tissues capable of eliciting clinical signs assume importance. A careful, thorough history and complete physical examination usually reveal the problem clearly. When the clinician recognizes which symptoms can be reproduced and which movements and positions reproduce them, he will arrive at a diagnosis and direct effective therapy. Following the principals so established reaffirms the fact that a diagnosis need not be a diagnosis of exclusion.

## References

1. Holt, L.: Frequency of symptoms for different age groups and professions. *In* Hirsch, C., and Zotterman, Y. (eds.): Cervical Pain. New York, Pergamon Press, 1971, pp. 17–20.
2. Waltz, T.A.: Physical factors in the production of the myelopathy of cervical spondylosis. Brain 90:395, 1967.
3. Penning, L.: Functional Pathology of the Cervical Spine. Amsterdam, Excerpta Medica, 1968.
4. Schmorl, G., and Junghans, H.: The Human Spine in Health and Disease. New York, Grune and Stratton, 1959.
5. Brain, W.R.: Some unsolved problems in cervical spondylosis. Br. Med. J. 1:771, 1963.
6. Nakano, K.K.: Neurology of Musculoskeletal and Rheumatic Disorders. Boston, Houghton-Mifflin, 1979.
7. Bull, J.W.D., Nixon, W.L.B., and Pratt, R.T.C.: The radiological criteria and familial occurrence of primary basilar impression. Brain 78:229, 1956.
8. Hoppenfeld, S.: Orthopaedic Neurology. Philadelphia, J.B. Lippincott Company, 1977.
9. Cailliet, R.: Neck and Arm Pain. Philadelphia, F.A. Davis Company, 1964.
10. Cyriax, J.: Textbook of Orthopedic Medicine. Volume 2. London, Cassell, 1965.
11. Miller, R.G., and Burton, R.: Stroke following chiropractic manipulation of the spine. JAMA 229:189, 1974.
12. Dunsker, S.B.: Cervical Spondylosis. Seminars in Neurological Surgery. New York, Raven Press, 1981.

# Chapter 29
# The Painful Shoulder

*Thomas S. Thornhill*

## INTRODUCTION

Pain about the shoulder girdle is one of the more common patient problems seen in an outpatient setting. The clinician must differentiate between pain from a local musculoskeletal problem and that referred from another source. Owing to its role as the link between the thorax and the upper extremity and the close proximity of major neurovascular structures, shoulder pain is frequently an early manifestation of systemic disease. The purpose of this chapter is to provide the reader with practical guidelines for the diagnosis and treatment of painful shoulder disorders seen in a rheumatology practice. A detailed analysis of shoulder problems and the treatment of major trauma are beyond the scope of this chapter and have been covered by other authors.[1-5] The conditions to be discussed are divided, albeit artificially, into (1) disorders of the periarticular structures, (2) disorders of the glenohumeral joint, and (3) regional disorders (Table 29–1).

## DIAGNOSTIC AIDS

**Anatomy.** An understanding of the structural and functional anatomy is a requisite for the clinician treating shoulder pain. One must visualize the three dimensional relationships, the muscular function, the ligamentous and tendinous attachments, and the routing of neurovascular structures. Figure 29–1 shows the musculoskeletal and topographic localization of pain in association with common shoulder disorders. By understanding the relationship between the rotator cuff and the subacromial region bounded inferiorly by the humeral head and superiorly by the undersurface of the acromion, the clinician not only can visualize the problems of an im-

**Table 29–1.** Common Causes of Shoulder Pain

**I. Periarticular Disorders**
1. Rotator cuff tendinitis/impingement syndrome
2. Calcific tendinitis
3. Rotator cuff tear
4. Bicipital tendinitis
5. Acromioclavicular arthritis

**II. Glenohumeral Disorders**
1. Inflammatory arthritis
2. Osteoarthritis
3. Osteonecrosis
4. Cuff arthropathy
5. Septic arthritis
6. Glenoid labral tears
7. Adhesive capsulitis

**III. Regional Disorders**
1. Cervical radiculopathy
2. Brachial neuritis
3. Nerve entrapment syndromes
4. Sternoclavicular arthritis
5. Reflex sympathetic dystrophy
6. Fibrositis
7. Neoplasms
8. Miscellaneous
   - Gallbladder disease
   - Splenic trauma
   - Subphrenic abscess
   - Myocardial infarction
   - Thyroid disease
   - Diabetes mellitus
   - Renal osteodystrophy

pingement syndrome but can also accurately aspirate and inject this space. Knowledge of the route of the tendon of the long head of the biceps through the bicipital groove and onto the superior aspect of the glenoid helps in an understanding of bicipital tendinitis. Before attempting to diagnose and treat shoulder pain the reader should review in some detail one of the many sources describing the structural and functional relationships of the shoulder girdle.[2,3]

**History.** Most shoulder problems can be diagnosed by taking a detailed history. The association with trauma, the rapidity of onset, and the character and localization of the pain will frequently lead the clinician to the proper diagnosis. For instance, dislocations of the glenohumeral joint are usually associated with a force directed to the arm with the shoulder in an abducted and externally rotated position, while dislocations of the acromioclavicular joint are usually due to direct trauma to the shoulder. The gradual onset of pain in the subacromial region that is worse on forward elevation of the shoulder is characteristic of rotator cuff tendinitis with impingement. The presence of a snap or click on forward elevation frequently will indicate rotator cuff tear associated with impingement. The burning quality and characteristic radiation of pain are indicative of a neuropathic process.

**Physical Examination.** A detailed physical and neurologic examination with particular attention to the involved extremity is essential. Careful recording of range of motion should include both active and passive forward flexion, abduction, internal and external rotation in a neutral position and at 90 degrees of abduction, and forward elevation. Forward elevation is defined as the arc between forward flexion and abduction and represents the most important arc in terms of placing the hand into a functional position. Abduction should be divided into that which occurs at the glenohumeral joint and that which occurs at the scapulothoracic joint. Careful recording of these values on serial examination will aid in judging response to therapy.

The localization of tenderness can help differentiate common entities such as glenoid labral tears, rotator cuff tendinitis, and bicipital tendinitis. While all three are associated with tenderness in the anterior aspect of the shoulder, the tenderness of rotator cuff tendinitis is generally subacromial and that of bicipital tendinitis migrates laterally and superiorly as the shoulder is abducted and externally rotated. Tenderness in the quadrilateral space or suprascapular notch is frequently associated with nerve entrapment syndromes. Neurologic examination should include sensory testing of the upper extremity with particular reference to the area innervated by the axillary nerve. All muscle systems should be graded and recorded, and the presence of atrophy or fasciculations noted.

Examination of the ipsilateral elbow, wrist, and hand is important not only in planning therapy but also in determining functional expectations.

**Plain Radiographs.** For most nontraumatic painful shoulder syndromes the use of an anteroposterior or glenohumeral view of the involved shoulder in internal and external rotation will suffice. In cases of trauma, a "trauma series," involving an anteroposterior view, scapular Y view, and axillary view, has become standard protocol. In cases of suspected acromioclavicular joint injury, an AP view of the shoulder with a weight held in the ipsilateral hand will frequently demonstrate subluxation at the AC joint.

**Scintigraphy.** $^{99}$Technetium-MDP or gallium may be of diagnostic help in evaluating the painful shoulder. This benefit usually occurs when evaluating skeletal lesions about the shoulder joint. Bone scans are generally not helpful in the diagnosis of non-neoplastic or noninfectious shoulder disease.

**Arthrography.** Single-contrast arthrography, double-contrast arthrography, and double-contrast arthrotomography are valuable tools in evaluating problems of the rotator cuff, the glenoid labrum, the biceps tendon, and the shoulder capsule.[6-9] Figure 29–2 shows a normal double-contrast arthrogram of the shoulder. Rotator cuff tears can be demonstrated by both single- and double-contrast studies. The proponents of double-contrast arthrography feel that the extent of the tear, the preferred surgical approach, and the quality of the rotator cuff tissue are best determined by double-contrast studies.[7-9] Figure 29–3 demonstrates extravasation of contrast into the subacromial space from a rotator cuff tear. Arthrography can be misleading by underestimating the extent of a rotator cuff tear.

Tears of the glenoid labrum without shoulder dislocation are now being recognized as sources of anterior

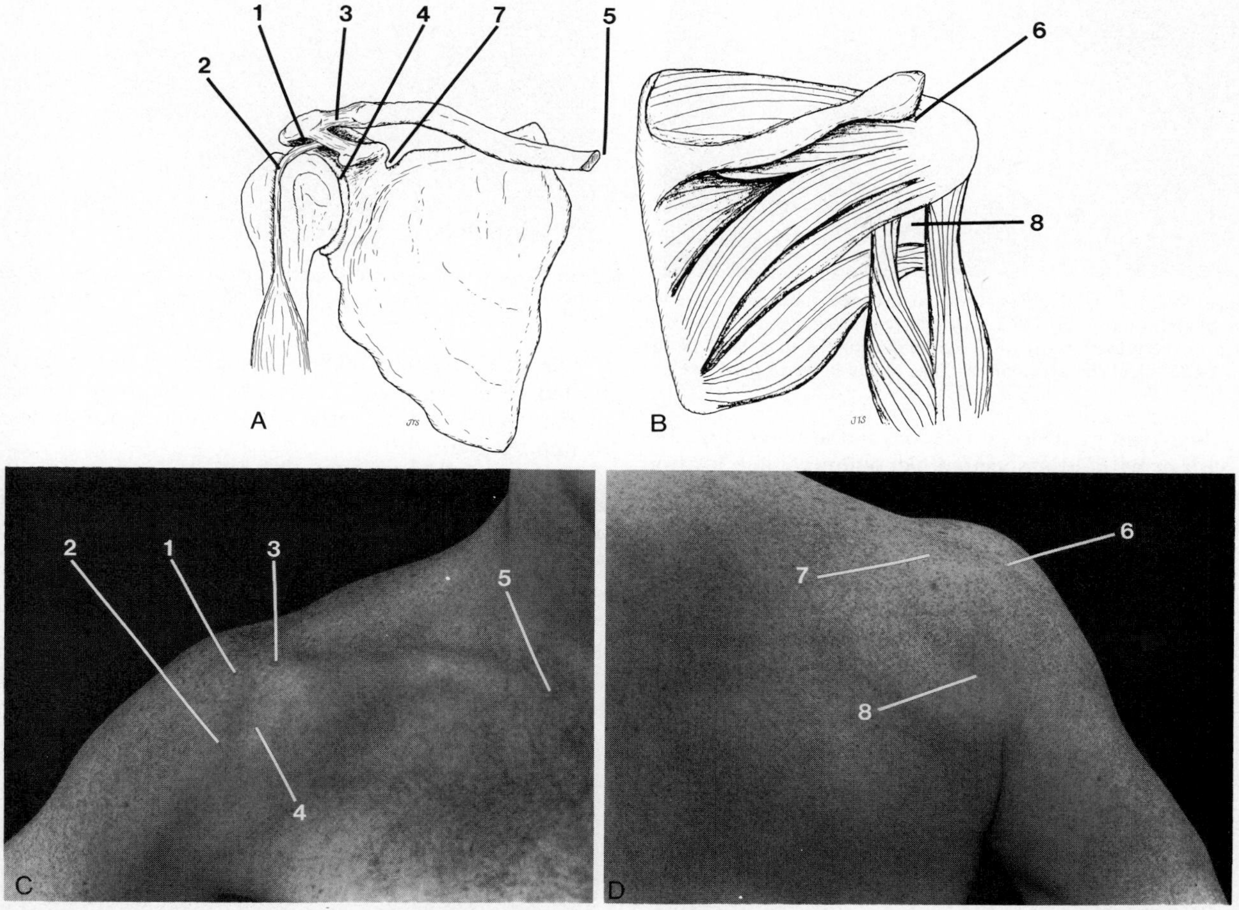


**Figure 29–1.** Musculoskeletal (*A* and *B*) and topographical (*C* and *D*) areas localizing pain and tenderness associated with specific shoulder problems. *1*, Subacromial space (rotator cuff tendinitis/impingement syndrome, calcific tendinitis, rotator cuff tear). *2*, Bicipital groove (bicipital tendinitis, biceps tendon subluxation and tear). *3*, Acromioclavicular joint. *4*, Anterior glenohumeral joint (glenohumeral arthritis, osteonecrosis, glenoid labral tears, adhesive capsulitis). *5*, Sternoclavicular joint. *6*, Posterior edge of acromion (rotator cuff tendinitis, calcific tendinitis, rotator cuff tear). *7*, Suprascapular notch (suprascapular nerve entrapment). *8*, Quadrilateral space (axillary nerve entrapment). These areas of pain and tenderness frequently overlap.

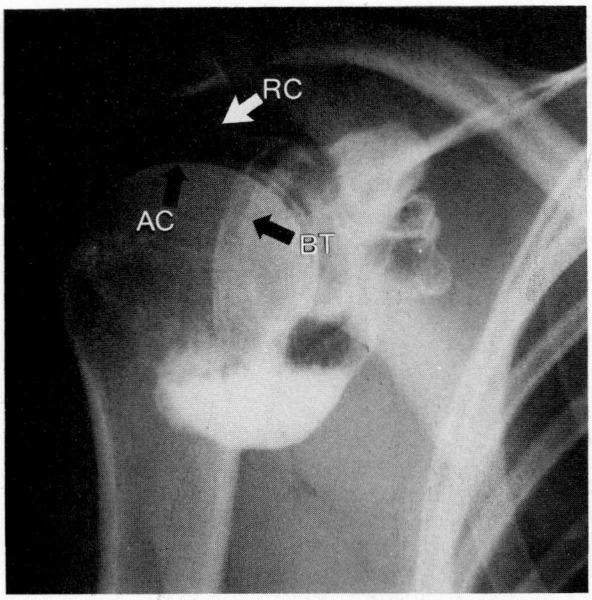


**Figure 29–2.** Normal double-contrast arthrogram showing the inferior edge of the rotator cuff (*RC*) as it courses through the subacromial space to the greater tuberosity; the tendon of the long head of the biceps (*BT*); and the articular cartilage of the humeral head (*AC*).

shoulder pain in athletes. Glenoid labral tears (Fig. 29–4) with or without associated glenohumeral subluxation can frequently be identified by double-contrast arthrotomography.[9] Shoulder arthrography can confirm a diagnosis of adhesive capsulitis by showing a contracted capsule with an obliterated axillary recess (Fig. 29–5).

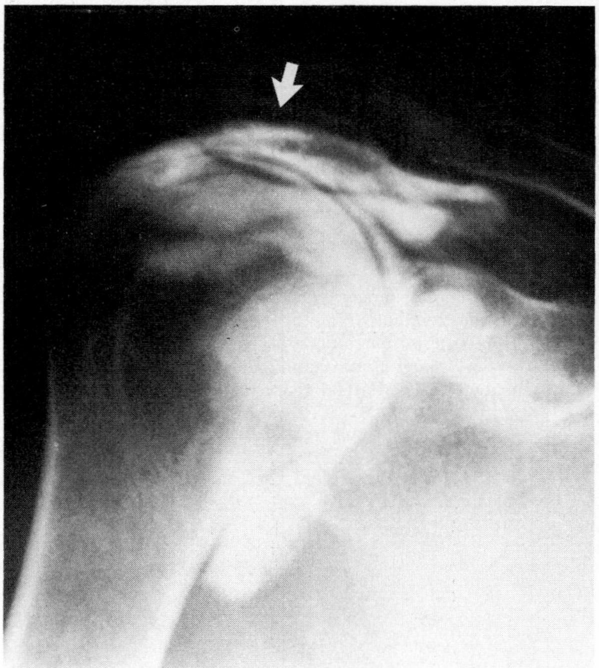

**Figure 29–3.** Single-contrast arthrogram demonstrating a massive rotator cuff tear with extravasation of contrast into the subacromial space (see arrow).

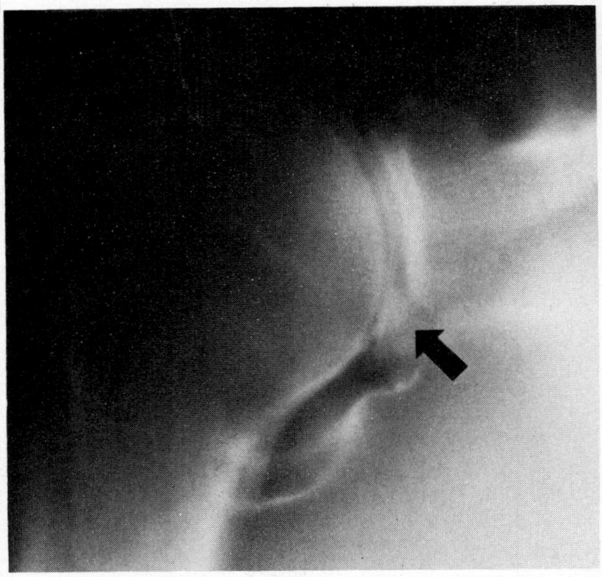

**Figure 29–4.** A double-contrast arthrotomogram demonstrating a tear of the anteroinferior portion of the glenoid labrum (see arrow).

The use of subacromial bursography has been reported to be beneficial in visualizing the outer surface of the rotator cuff and the subacromial space in cases of impingement.[10,11]

**Computed Tomography.** CT has been shown to be helpful in evaluating the musculoskeletal system, but its use around the shoulder has been limited (see Chapter 40).

**Electromyography and Nerve Conduction Velocity Studies.** EMG and NCV studies can be helpful in differentiating shoulder pain from pain of neurogenic origin (see Chapter 47). They may also be beneficial in deter-

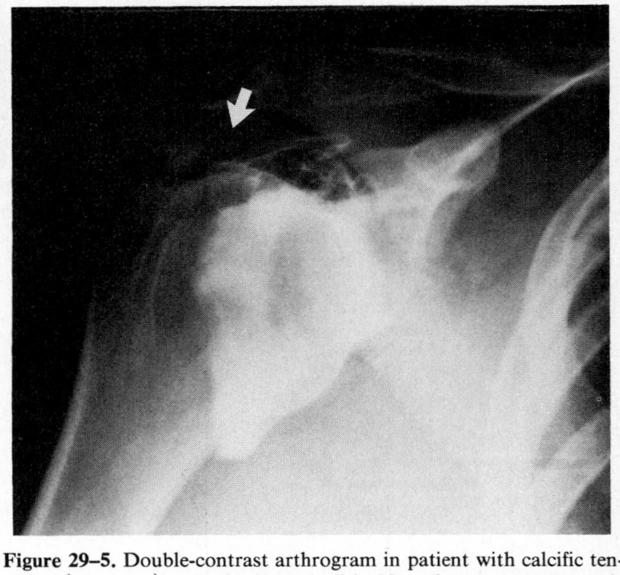

**Figure 29–5.** Double-contrast arthrogram in patient with calcific tendinitis (see arrow) and adhesive capsulitis. Note the contracted capsule with diminution of the synovial space and obliteration of the axillary recess.

mining the localization of neurogenic pain to a particular cervical root, the brachial plexus, or a peripheral nerve.[12,13]

**Arthroscopy.** Diagnostic arthroscopy and arthroscopic surgery have greatly aided in the diagnosis and treatment of knee injuries (see Chapter 41). Recent interest has focused on the use of arthroscopy for glenohumeral pain. It has been recommended for evaluating glenohumeral synovitis, articular cartilage damage, loose bodies and particularly for the diagnosis of labral tears. The added benefit of arthroscopy over arthrography remains to be shown. Arthroscopic surgery of the shoulder to date has been limited to removal of loose bodies and shaving of injuries of the glenoid labrum.

**Injection.** Injection of local anesthetics and corticosteroids is an extremely useful technique for both the diagnosis and treatment of shoulder pain (see Chapter 37). The physician must have a thorough knowledge of the anatomy of the shoulder girdle and a presumptive diagnosis in order to direct the injection properly. Injection of referred pain areas may be misleading. For example, in the patient with lateral arm pain due to deltoid bursal involvement from calcific tendinitis of the supraspinatus tendon, injection should be in the subacromial space and not the area of referred pain in the deltoid muscle.

It is often better to use a posterior subacromial approach when injecting a rotator cuff tendinitis in a patient with anterior impingement symptoms, as it is not only easier to enter the subacromial region posteriorly but also less traumatic to the contracted anterior structures.

The instillation of rapidly acting local anesthetics can be beneficial in determining the source of shoulder pain. Obliteration of pain, for instance, by injection of a local anesthetic along the bicipital groove can confirm a diagnosis of bicipital tendinitis. The use of local anesthetics is somewhat less helpful when injecting the subacromial space, owing to its extensive communications with the rest of the shoulder girdle, but relief of symptoms by such an injection can rule out pain from conditions such as cervical radiculopathy or an entrapment neuropathy.

## PERIARTICULAR DISORDERS

**Rotator Cuff Tendinitis/Impingement Syndrome.** The majority of painful nontraumatic conditions about the shoulder joint are caused by tendinitis of the rotator cuff. E.A. Codman published his classic text reviewing the nature of these lesions and pointed out their importance in work-related disabilities.[1] Degenerative tendinitis has been labeled pericapsulitis, subacromial bursitis, subdeltoid bursitis, supraspinatus tendinitis, rotator cuff tear, and impingement syndrome. The variation in clinical description, method of treatment, and response to treatment perhaps is due to descriptions of the same condition at various points in time. Neer has clarified this condition by pointing out the various stages in which this disorder presents.[14] Though stratified into three stages the process represents a continuum of inflammation, degeneration, and attrition of the rotator cuff by impingement on the anterior edge and undersurface of the anterior third of the acromion, the coracoacromial ligament, and occasionally the acromioclavicular joint.[15] The wear and attritional tears of the cuff occur in the supraspinatus tendon and may extend into the infraspinatus and the long head of the biceps.[16] The mechanical impingement of the rotator cuff may be influenced by variations in the shape and slope of the acromion.[16,17]

According to Neer,[14] the three stages of impingement are as follows: *Stage I, edema and hemorrhage,* usually occurs in active individuals younger than age 25 who engage in activities requiring excessive overhead arm usage. In stage I, treatment is conservative, and the patient generally responds to rest, nonsteroidal antiinflammatory agents, and occasional corticosteroid injection. *Stage II, fibrosis and tendinitis,* represents the biologic response of fibrosis and thickening due to repeated episodes of mechanical impingement. This stage is usually seen in active individuals between 25 and 40 years of age. They may respond to conservative treatment as in stage I but experience recurrent attacks. *Stage III, rotator cuff tears, biceps rupture, and bone changes,* rarely appears before the age of 40 years. Stage III represents the attritional wear of the supraspinatus tendon and occasionally the infraspinatus and long head of the biceps from repeated impingement. Patients with stage III disease present with varying weakness, crepitus, and supraspinatus atrophy, depending upon the extent of the tear and its chronicity.

The predominant feature of degenerative tendinitis is pain. The pain can be sudden and incapacitating or present as a dull ache. It can be focal and pinpointed as an area of tenderness along the anterior edge of the acromion (see Fig. 29–1). It also may present as a diffuse pain around the anterolateral or even posterior edge of the acromion or, at times, radiate to the subdeltoid bursa. This pain can be differentiated from other nontraumatic painful conditions about the shoulder by its position and response to treatment. For instance, the tenderness from bicipital tendinitis will follow the bicipital groove as the arm is externally rotated. Tenderness from a glenoid labral tear is generally beneath the coracoid and over the anterior edge of the glenoid. The impingement sign as elicited in Figure 29–6 is useful in the diagnosis of rotator cuff tendinitis. The patient with stage I and even stage II disease will frequently describe a catch as the arm is brought to an overhead position. They will frequently raise their arm by abduction and rotation to bypass the painful "spot." This observation underscores the Codman paradox, which states that the arm can be brought fully overhead from an anatomic position by either external rotation and abduction in the coronal plane or internal rotation and forward flexion in the sagittal plane.[1] In patients with focal tenderness of the supraspinatus the pain may disappear under the edge of the acromion as the arm is abducted (Dawbarn's sign).[3] Instillation of short-acting local anesthetics into

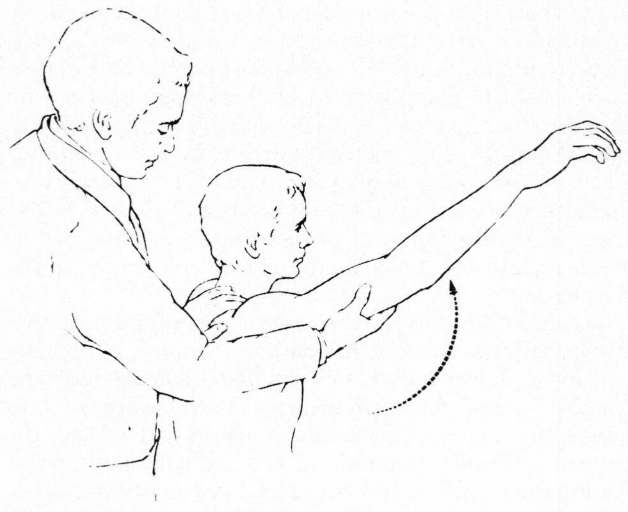

**Figure 29–6.** The "impingement sign" is elicited by forced forward elevation of the arm. Pain results as the greater tuberosity impinges on the acromion. The examiner's hand prevents scapular rotation. This maneuver may be positive in other periarticular disorders. (Reproduced with permission from Neer, C.S., II: Clin. Orthop. 173:70, 1983.)

the subacromial space can frequently obliterate the symptoms and confirm the diagnosis of degenerative tendinitis with impingement. It is important to remember that trigger point injection alone can be misleading and that injection of the subacromial space is necessary to assure validity of this diagnostic test.

Radiographs in the early stages of degenerative tendinitis with impingement are normal. As the disease progresses there may be some sclerosis, cyst formation, and eburnation of the anterior third of the acromion and the greater tuberosity. An anterior acromial traction spur may appear on the undersurface of the acromion lateral to the acromioclavicular joint and represent contracture of the coracoacromial ligament. The late radiographic findings include narrowing of the acromiohumeral gap, superior subluxation of the humeral head in relationship to the glenoid, and erosive changes of the anterior acromion.[18] Arthrography, as discussed earlier, can be helpful in diagnosing a full-thickness tear of the rotator cuff in association with stage III disease.

The choice of treatment, and frequently its result, is a function of the stage of the impingement. In stage I disease, in which there is little mechanical impingement, most patients will respond to rest. It is important not to immobilize the shoulder for any period of time, as contraction of the shoulder capsule and periarticular structures can produce an adhesive capsulitis. After a period of rest, a progressive program of stretching and strengthening exercises will generally restore the shoulder to normal function. Use of aspirin and other nonsteroidal antiinflammatory agents may shorten the symptomatic period. Modalities such as ultrasound, neuroprobe, and transcutaneous electrical nerve stimulation (TENS) are generally not necessary. Patients with stage I and stage II disease may have a dramatic response to local injection of corticosteroids. In stage II disease, in which there is fibrosis and thickening anteriorly, it is frequently better to inject through a posterior approach. The author prefers a combination of 3 ml of 1 percent xylocaine, 3 ml of 0.5 percent bupivacaine and 20 mg of triamcinolone. This combines a short-acting anesthetic for diagnostic purposes, a longer-acting anesthetic for analgesic purposes, and a steroid preparation in a depot form. Neer has suggested that the patient with refractory stage II disease may respond to division of the coracoacromial ligament and bursectomy of the subacromial bursa. Division of the coracoacromial ligament alone has been performed under a local anesthetic.

Treatment of stage III disease depends upon the chronicity of the symptoms and the presence or absence of a rotator cuff tear. Neer recommends arthrography in those patients over 40 years of age who fail to respond to conservative treatment or experience sudden weakness of abduction and external rotation suggesting extension of a tear.[14] The surgical treatment of choice is an anterior acromioplasty.[15] Lateral acromionectomies and complete acromionectomies unnecessarily weaken the deltoid muscle.[18] Indications for anterior acromioplasty include (1) failure to respond to one year of conservative therapy and (2) chronic impingement and a rotator cuff tear shown on arthrography. The surgical technique and rehabilitation measures are beyond the scope of this discussion.[14,15]

**Calcific Tendinitis.** While most rotator cuff tendinitis probably represents one of the stages of mechanical impingement, there appears to be a subset of patients predisposed to inflammation in this area. These patients frequently have bilateral disease and give a history of other periarticular conditions such as trochanteric bursitis of the hip or symptoms of fibrositis. One particular subset within this group is made up of those individuals with calcific tendinitis.

Calcific tendinitis is a painful condition about the rotator cuff in association with deposition of calcium salts, primarily hydroxyapatite.[19,21,22] It is most common in patients over 30 years of age and shows a predilection for females.[19,20] While more common in the right shoulder, there is at least a 6 percent incidence of bilaterality.[19] Codman pointed out the localization of the calcification within the tendon of the supraspinatus.[1] He provided a detailed description of the symptoms and natural history of this condition. In describing the phases of pain, spasm, limitation of motion and atrophy, he pointed out the lack of correlation between symptoms and the size of the calcific deposit. According to Codman the natural history includes degeneration of the supraspinatus tendon, calcification, and eventual rupture into the subacromial bursa. During this latter phase, pain and decreased motion can lead to adhesive capsulitis (Fig. 29–5).

The pathogenesis of calcific tendinitis of the supraspinatus is recognized as a degenerative process with secondary calcification within the tendon fibers.[1,19,21,22] The localization of the calcium within the supraspinatus is most likely due to one of two reasons. Many of these patients have an early stage of impingement, and it is the supraspinatus that is compressed by the anterior portion of the acromion.[14,15] This longstanding impingement may lead to local degeneration of the tendon fibers. In patients without impingement the localization of the calcium within the supraspinatus may be related to the blood supply of the rotator cuff, which normally comes from an anastomatic network of vessels from either the greater tuberosity or the bellies of the short rotator muscles.[21] The watershed of these sources is just medial to the tendinous attachment of the supraspinatus.[23] Rathburn and MacNab referred to this watershed as the "critical zone" and pointed out that during adduction this area was rendered ischemic.[24]

The stimulation for calcification in calcific tendinitis has been the focus of considerable study.[4,21,22,25] Steinbrocker postulated that the process begins with necrosis and fraying of the tendon fibers, with secondary formation of a fibrinoid mass surrounded by leukocytes. This mass then serves as a template for calcification.[25] Others have suggested that the process of degeneration of the tendon causes formation of small particles consisting primarily of calcium salts.[4] The hyperemia associated with the acute episode would cause coalescence of the calcium with formation of a liquified calcium mass. As the increased vascularity subsides, this calcified mass would return to its "dry state."

It is also possible that the hypervascularity may, in fact, "wash out" an inhibitor substance and allow calcification to occur on the denuded fibers of the frayed tendon. It would be attractive to consider proteoglycans in this inhibitory role, as they are ubiquitous in tendons and articular cartilage, both of which do not calcify in the normal state.

Uhthoff has proposed that the pathogenesis of this process is not associated inflammation or scarring but suggests that the primary stimulus is hypoxia, which results in transformation of portions of the tendon into fibrocartilage.[21] The chondrocytes then would mediate calcification in a way similar to that occurring in the calcifying zone of the epiphyseal plate. In a subsequent study it was pointed out that the ultrastructure of calcifying tendinitis failed to demonstrate the arrangement or cell types seen in the epiphyseal plate.[22] The calcification occurred in extracellular matrix vesicles located in areas that had undergone fibrocartilagenous transformation. The authors pointed out the similarity to extracellular vesicles noted in other normal and pathologic conditions.[22] After calcification, the foci became surrounded by mononuclear and multinucleated cells, with phagocytized material within the cytoplasm.[21] Vascular invasion occurred as part of the reparative process. By restoring normal perfusion and oxygen tension to the tissue, the calcium could then be resorbed and the tendon returned to its normal state.[21]

Treatment of calcific tendinitis depends upon the clinical presentation and the presence of associated impingement. These patients can present with an acute inflammatory reaction that may resemble gout. They seem to be the most acutely painful patients with rotator cuff tendinitis. The acute inflammation can be treated with local corticosteroid injection or the use of nonsteroidal agents or both. On occasion the use of ultrasound may be of some benefit. If there is associated impingement, treatment depends upon the stage of presentation, as discussed earlier. The radiographic appearance of the calcification can direct and perhaps predict the response to therapy. In the resorptive phase, the deposits appear floccular, suggesting that the process is in the phase of repair and that a conservative program is indicated. Those patients with discrete calcification and perhaps associated adhesive capsulitis (Fig. 29–5) may be at a stable phase at which the calcium produces a mechanical block and is unlikely to be resorbed. In patients who have failed to respond to conservative means, excision of the calcium salts and decompression of associated impingement is indicated.

**Rotator Cuff Tear.** Spontaneous tear of the rotator cuff in an otherwise normal individual is rare.[14] It can occur in patients with rheumatoid arthritis or lupus as part of the pathologic process with invasion from underlying pannus. Metabolic conditions such as renal osteodystrophy or agents such as corticosteroids are occasionally associated with spontaneous cuff tears.

Most patients will report a traumatic episode such as falling upon an outstretched arm of lifting a heavy object. The usual presenting symptoms are pain and weakness of abduction and external rotation. There may be associated crepitus and even a palpable defect. Longstanding tears are generally associated with atrophy of the supraspinatus and infraspinatus muscles.

It may be difficult to differentiate a partial thickness cuff tear from a painful tendinitis. Plain radiographs are helpful only during a later stage of the process when there may be narrowing of the acromiohumeral gap, proximal subluxation of the humeral head, and even erosion on the undersurface of the acromion.[27] Arthrography, as reported earlier, is helpful in diagnosing an acute tear but frequently underestimates its size.

Because of the overlap in diagnosis of complete tears and incomplete lesions, it is difficult to develop a rational form of treatment. DePalma reports that 90 percent of patients with rotator cuff tears respond to conservative measures such as rest, analgesics, anti-inflammatory agents, and physiotherapy.[28]

During the acute phase of pain the arm may be supported in a sling, but early restoration of motion is important to prevent adhesive capsulitis. Instillation of corticosteroids into the subacromial bursa may provide dramatic relief of symptoms.

Consideration of surgical treatment depends upon the patient's symptoms, the functional demand, and the etiology of the tear. Most acute tears represent extension of a tear associated with chronic impingement.[14] Patients in this group who fail to respond to conservative means should be treated by an anterior acromioplasty with rotator cuff repair.

In elderly patients whose pain and weakness do not create a functional problem, a conservative program is preferable. Wolfgang pointed out that surgical results were less satisfactory with advancing patient age.[29] Earnshaw reviewed 37 patients who had undergone rotator cuff repair and found an overall 65 percent with good results.[30] Patients in the fourth and fifth decades of life generally did well, while only 60 percent of patients in the sixth and seventh decades had a good result. In their study, the mechanism of injury, the extent of the tear, and the timing of repair had no influence on the outcome. The authors pointed out that most shoulders showed radiographic progression of proximal subluxation despite surgical repair. In this small series, good functional results were reported in two patients with irreparable tears and in some patients with postoperative arthrograms showing leakage of contrast. They concluded that relief of impingement and debridement of the edge of the tear were important determinants in the relief of symptoms.[30]

The surgical approach, technique of repair, and postoperative management are beyond the scope of this discussion and are well covered in other sources.[2,3,28,30,31]

**Bicipital Tendinitis and Rupture.** Bicipital tendinitis, subluxation of the biceps tendon within the bicipital groove, and rupture of the long head of the biceps are generally associated with anterior shoulder pain.

The long head of the biceps is an intracapsular and extrasynovial structure. It passes through the bicipital groove and over the head of the humerus and inserts on the superior rim of the glenoid (see Fig. 29–1*A*).[32] The biceps tendon aids in flexion of the forearm, supination of the pronated forearm if the elbow is flexed, and forward elevation of the shoulder.[3] As it crosses the humeral head, the biceps tendon is fixed within the bicipital groove. Meyer described a bony ridge on the lesser tuberosity and suggested this as a source of tendon wear and eventual rupture.[33] Shallowness of this groove has been reported as a cause of subluxation and dislocation of the bicipital tendon.[34]

Crenshaw and Kilgore reported that the early phases of bicipital tendinitis were associated with hypervascularity, edema of the tendon, and tenosynovitis.[35] Persistence of this process leads to adhesions between the tendon and its sheath, with impairment of the normal gliding mechanism in the groove. Stretching of these adhesions may be associated with chronic bicipital tendinitis.[34] The diagnosis of bicipital tendinitis is based upon the localization of tenderness (see Fig. 29–1). It is often confused with impingement symptoms and, in fact, is frequently seen in association with an impingement syndrome.[14] Isolated bicipital tendinitis can be differentiated by the fact that the tender area will migrate with the bicipital groove as the arm is abducted and externally rotated. There are many eponyms associated with tests to identify bicipital tendinitis.[3] Yergason's supination sign refers to pain in the bicipital groove when the examiner resists supination of the pronated forearm with the elbow at 90 degrees. Ludington's sign refers to pain in the bicipital groove when the patient interlocks his fingers on top of the head and actively abducts the arms.

Treatment is generally conservative and consists of rest, analgesics, nonsteroidal agents, and local injection of corticosteroids. The use of ultrasound and neuroprobe is more beneficial in this condition than in isolated rotator cuff tendinitis.

Patients with refractory bicipital tendinitis and recurrent symptoms of subluxation are treated by opening the bicipital groove and resecting the proximal portion of the tendon with either tenodesis of the distal portion into the groove or transfer to the coracoid process. The proponents of tenodesis believe that this prevents proximal migration of the humeral head, while those who advocate transfer to the coracoid feel that it maintains biceps power.

Rupture of the long head of the biceps is easily diagnosed by the appearance of the contracted belly of the biceps muscle ("Popeye sign"). The patient will frequently relate a snap and acute pain in association with lifting an object. In older patients, in whom rupture is due to attrition, presentation is frequently spontaneous and is associated with few or no symptoms. Acute ruptures in young active individuals are best treated surgically with either tenodesis of the distal stump into the bicipital groove or transfer to the coracoid. Patients with longstanding symptoms of impingement and acute biceps tendon rupture are treated with anterior acromioplasty and tenodesis of the distal stump into the bicipital groove. In older patients without symptoms of impingement, a conservative program is preferable, as these patients are generally asymptomatic and have sufficient strength and the contracted belly of the biceps muscle serves to impress their grandchildren.

**Acromioclavicular Arthritis.** The majority of painful conditions about the acromioclavicular joint are the result of trauma with resultant acromioclavicular joint instability, meniscal tears, and secondary degenerative change.[36] Most patients present with a history of direct trauma to the shoulder girdle. The pain may be generalized, but tenderness and, at times, crepitus can be palpated directly over the acromioclavicular joint. The pain is increased by abduction of the arm and particularly by adducting the arm across the chest and compressing the joint.[2]

Plain radiographs may be normal unless there is a true dislocation or degenerative change. It is important to differentiate the traction spur at the insertion of the coracoacromial ligament from an osteophyte associated with degenerative change of the joint. An anteroposterior radiograph with the patient holding a weight in the ipsilateral hand may demonstrate joint instability in acute cases.

Acute injuries are treated by rest, strapping, or surgical repair, depending upon the degree of instability and the functional demand of the patient. Acute injuries without subluxation (grade I) or partial subluxation (grade II) are best treated by conservative means. Complete dislocations (grade III) are treated by early mobilization, strapping to reduce the dislocation, or surgical repair according to the patient's functional demand and the surgeon's preference.[36-38]

Patients with degenerative change in the acromioclavicular joint and symptoms that cannot be controlled by conservative means are best treated by debridement of the joint and resection of the distal clavicle.[37,39] At no time should this joint be surgically fused.

## GLENOHUMERAL DISORDERS

The various arthritides that affect the shoulder joint are discussed in detail in other chapters. They are presented here in order to discuss aspects that are unique to the glenohumeral joint.

The usual presentation of intra-articular disorders is pain with motion. The pain is generalized throughout the shoulder girdle and at times referred to the neck, back, and upper arm. The usual response to pain is to decrease glenohumeral motion and to substitute for it with increased scapulothoracic mobility. Patients with adequate elbow and scapulothoracic motion require little glenohumeral motion for activities of daily living; in fact, patients with glenohumeral arthrodesis can achieve adequate function.[40,41] The secondary response to pain, therefore, is diminution of motion and secondary soft tissue contractures with muscle atrophy. With increasing weakness and involvement of adjacent joints, the pain, limitation of motion, and weakness cause a substantial functional deficit.

**Inflammatory Arthritis.** While the most common inflammatory arthritis involving the shoulder joint is rheumatoid arthritis, other systemic disorders such as systemic lupus erythematosus, psoriatic arthritis, ankylosing spondylitis, Reiter's syndrome, and scleroderma may cause glenohumeral arthritis. The pathogenesis of the joint involvement in these conditions is discussed in detail in other chapters.

All patients with significant involvement present with pain. The limitation of motion is either secondary to splinting of the joint with secondary soft tissue contractures or primary soft tissue involvement with scarring or rupture. Plain radiographs will confirm glenohumeral involvement (Fig. 29–7*A*). There is narrowing of the glenohumeral joint space, with erosion and cyst formation without significant sclerosis or osteophytes. As the disease progresses, superior and posterior erosion of the glenoid with proximal subluxation of the humeral head may occur. Eventually, there may be secondary degenerative changes and even osteonecrosis of the humeral head.

Treatment is initially conservative and directed towards control of pain, inducing a systemic remission (see Chapter 63) and maintaining joint motion by physical therapy. The use of intra-articular corticosteroids may be beneficial in controlling local synovitis. In rheumatoid arthritis, the involvement of periarticular structures with subacromial bursitis and rupture of the rotator cuff magnifies the functional deficit.

Once the synovial cartilage interactions produce significant symptoms and radiographic changes that cannot be controlled by conventional therapy, glenohumeral resurfacing should be considered. The treatment of choice is an unconstrained shoulder arthroplasty of the type reported in detail in Chapter 115.[42,43] Total shoulder arthroplasty is best performed in patients with rheumatoid arthritis before end-stage bony erosion and soft tissue contractions have occurred.[44]

Acute inflammatory arthritis of the glenohumeral joint may also occur in association with gout, pseudogout, hydroxyapatite deposition of renal osteodystrophy, and recurrent hemophilic hemarthrosis.

**Osteoarthritis.** Osteoarthritis of the glenohumeral joint is less common than in the hip, its counterpart in the lower extremity. This is a result of both the non-weight-bearing characteristics of the shoulder joint and the distribution of forces throughout the shoulder girdle.

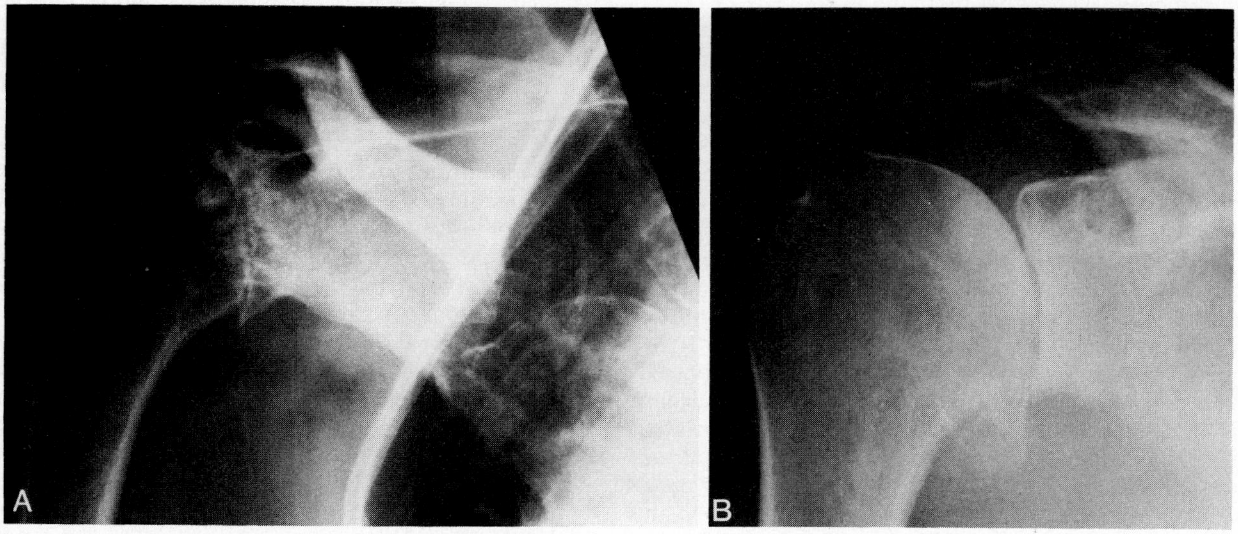


**Figure 29–7.** Plain radiographs demonstrating (*A*) rheumatoid arthritis with loss of joint space, cyst formation, glenohumeral erosion, and early proximal subluxation of the humerus indicating a rotator cuff tear. *B*, Osteoarthritis with narrowing of the glenohumeral joint space, sclerosis, and osteophyte formation. Note the preservation of the subacromial space, suggesting an intact rotator cuff.

Osteoarthritis is divided into those conditions associated with high unit loading of articular cartilage and those in which there is an intrinsic abnormality within the cartilage that causes abnormal wear at normal loads. Since the shoulder is normally a non-weight-bearing joint and less susceptible to repeated high loading, the presence of osteoarthritis of the glenohumeral joint should alert the physician to consider other associated factors. Has the patient engaged in unusual activities such as boxing, heavy construction, or chronic use of a pneumatic hammer? Is there some disorder such as epiphyseal dysplasia that has created joint incongruity with high unit loading of the articular cartilage? Is this a neuropathic process caused by diabetes, syringomyelia or leprosy? Is there associated hemachromatosis, hemophilia, or gout that may have altered the ability of articular cartilage to withstand normal loading? Is unrecognized chronic dislocation responsible?

Pain is the usual presentation, but it is generally not as acute or associated with the spasm seen in inflammatory conditions. Plain radiographs show narrowing of the glenohumeral joint, osteophyte formation, sclerosis, and some cyst formation (Fig. 29–7*B*). As the rotator cuff is generally intact there is less bony erosion of the glenoid and proximal subluxation of the humerus.

Patients with osteoarthritis of the glenohumeral joint frequently do well by functional adjustment and conservative therapy. Analgesics and nonsteroidal agents may provide symptomatic relief. The use of corticosteroid injections is less beneficial unless there is evidence of synovitis. Those patients with severe involvement who fail to respond are best treated by shoulder arthroplasty[42-44] (see Chapter 116).

**Osteonecrosis.** Osteonecrosis of the shoulder refers to necrosis of the humeral head seen in association with a variety of conditions. Symptoms are due to synovitis and joint incongruity secondary to resorption, repair, and remodeling. The pathogenesis and various etiologies are discussed in Chapter 107.

The most common cause of osteonecrosis of the shoulder is avascularity due to fractures through the anatomic neck of the humerus.[45] Fracture through this area disrupts the intramedullary and capsular blood supplies to the humeral head. Another common cause of osteonecrosis of the shoulder is steroid therapy in conjunction with organ transplantation, systemic lupus erythematosus, or asthma.

The mechanism by which steroids are associated with osteonecrosis is unknown. There appears to be a host susceptibility, which may be genetically predetermined. Patients will generally develop osteonecrosis shortly following steroid use, although symptoms may not present for a considerable period. At least in renal transplant patients, the association of osteonecrosis is independent of steroid dosage. The proposed pathogenesis of steroid-induced osteonecrosis includes increased free fatty acids with obliteration of intramedullary blood supply and steroid-induced vasculitis. This may elevate the intramedullary pressures within the humeral head and cause bone ischemia and death.[46] Other conditions associated with osteonecrosis of the humeral head include systemic lupus erythematosus, hemoglobinopathies, pancreatitis, and hyperbarism.

Early diagnosis is difficult, as there is frequently a considerable delay until symptoms are present. Bone scans may be helpful in early cases before radiographic changes are present. Plain radiographs demonstrate progressive phases of necrosis and repair and are discussed in detail in Chapter 107. In the early stages, the films may be normal or show either osteopenia or bony sclerosis. A crescent sign representing subchondral fracture or demarcation of the necrotic segment will appear during the reparative process. Patients who fail to remodel will show collapse of the humeral head with secondary degenerative changes.

There is often a considerable discrepancy between symptoms and radiographic involvement. Patients with extensive bony changes may be asymptomatic. Treatment should be directed by the patient's symptoms rather than the radiographs and is similar to that for osteoarthritis. Patients with severe symptoms that cannot be controlled by conservative means are best treated with an unconstrained shoulder arthroplasty or hemiarthroplasty.[42]

**Cuff Arthropathy.** Neer and colleagues have reported an unusual condition in which untreated massive tears of the rotator cuff with proximal migration of the humeral head are associated with erosion of the humeral surface.[17] The erosion of the humeral head is different from that seen in other arthritides and is presumed to be due to a combination of mechanical factors and nutritional factors. As the humeral head migrates superiorly, it is no longer contained and its cartilage cannot be nourished by the synovial fluid.

Patients with cuff tear arthropathies present a difficult therapeutic problem, as the bony erosion and disruption of the cuff jeopardizes the functional result from an unconstrained prosthesis.[44] In such patients a constrained total shoulder arthroplasty may be indicated.[47,48]

**Septic Arthritis.** Septic arthritis can masquerade as any of the conditions listed under periarticular or glenohumeral disorders. Sepsis must be included in any differential diagnosis of shoulder pain, as early recognition and prompt treatment are necessary to achieve a good functional result. The diagnosis is confirmed by joint aspiration with synovianalysis and culture. Cultures should include aerobic, anaerobic, mycobacterial, and fungal studies. Septic arthritis is extensively covered in Chapters 96, 97, and 98.

**Glenoid Labral Tears.** The increasing popularity of throwing sports and racket sports in 25- to 60-year-old individuals has led to the recognition of tears of the glenoid labrum as a cause of anterior shoulder pain (see Fig. 29–1).

This diagnosis is easily confused with rotator cuff tendinitis or bicipital tendinitis and can best be confirmed by double-contrast arthrotomography[9] or arthroscopy (see Fig. 29–4). Glenoid labral tears may be seen in association with anterior or even posterior instability. Surgical treatment is directed toward excision or repair of the torn labral portion and correction of any joint instability.

**Adhesive Capsulitis.** Adhesive capsulitis, or "frozen shoulder," is a condition characterized by limitation of motion of the shoulder joint with pain at the extremes of motion. It was first described by Putnam in 1882[49] and later by Codman.[1] The initial presentation is pain, which is generalized and referred to the upper arm, the back, and the neck. As the pain increases, loss of joint motion ensues. The process is generally self-limiting and in most cases resolves spontaneously within 10 months unless there is an underlying problem.

Adhesive capsulitis is slightly more common in females than in males.[50] There is usually an underlying condition producing pain and restricted motion of the glenohumeral joint. Adhesive capsulitis may be seen as an end result of rotator cuff tendinitis, calcific tendinitis (see Fig. 29–5), bicipital tendinitis, and glenohumeral arthritis.[51,52] It is also seen in a variety of conditions, including apical lung tumors, pulmonary tuberculosis, cervical radiculopathy, and postmyocardial infarction.[51-54]

DePalma reported that any condition that hindered scapulohumeral motion caused muscular inactivity and predisposed the patient to adhesive capsulitis.[52] Neviaser[55] found capsular adhesions to the underlying humeral head upon surgical exploration for adhesive capsulitis.

It is unclear whether the contracture of the shoulder capsule is a passive process related to lack of motion or an active process associated with capsular inflammation. Bulgen and colleagues reported an association between adhesive capsulitis and HLA-B27 antigen positivity.[56] He also reported decreased IgA levels in patients with the condition.[57] Lundberg and Neviaser failed to demonstrate synovitis or capsular inflammation when surgically exploring patients with adhesive capsulitis.[55,58]

Treatment of adhesive capsulitis is directed towards pain relief, restoration of function, and correction of the underlying cause. Many patients will have associated depression or emotional lability either as an underlying problem or secondary to their pain and functional limitation. The physician must direct a long-term therapy program and reassure the patient that this condition is usually self-limiting. As symptoms may last for a year, daily visits to the physical therapist become impractical and a home program should be outlined.

In patients with restriction of motion that prevents activities of daily living, a closed manipulation is indicated. This is best achieved at the time of arthrography (to confirm the diagnosis) and entails passive manipulation after the joint is inflated with a local anesthetic. The combination of inflating the joint and passive manipulation may free some adhesions and improve joint motion. On occasion, a general anesthetic is indicated for closed manipulation. Surgical intervention for adhesive capsulitis should be limited to treatment of an underlying problem such as calcific tendinitis or an impingement syndrome.

## REGIONAL DISORDERS

Because the shoulder girdle connects the thorax with the upper extremity and the major neurovascular structures pass in close proximity to the joint, shoulder pain is a hallmark of many nonarticular conditions.

**Cervical Radiculopathy.** Cervical neck pain, with or without radiculopathy, may be associated with shoulder pain. When cervical radiculopathy presents as shoulder pain, it is frequently due to involvement of the upper cervical roots. It can be differentiated from shoulder pain on the basis of history, physical examination, electromyographs, cervical radiographs, and myelography when indicated. Since conditions causing cervical neck pain and those causing shoulder pain, such as calcific tendinitis and cervical radiculopathy, may co-exist, it is often difficult to distinguish which lesion is causing the symptoms. These conditions can often be distinguished by injection of local anesthetics to block certain components of the pain.

As cervical neck pain is reviewed extensively in Chapter 28 its diagnosis and treatment will not be discussed here.

**Brachial Neuritis.** In the 1940s, Spillane,[59] and Parsonage and Turner[60,61] described a painful condition of the shoulder associated with limitation of motion. As the pain subsided and motion improved, muscle weakness and atrophy became apparent.[62] The deltoid, supraspinatus, infraspinatus, biceps, and triceps are the most frequently involved muscles,[62] although diaphragmatic paralysis has also been reported.[61] The etiology remains unclear, but the clustering of cases suggests a viral or postviral syndrome.[60,61] Occasionally an associated influenza-like syndrome or previous vaccination has been reported.[62]

The prognosis for recovery is excellent, although full recovery may take two to three years. Tsiaris reported 80 percent recovery within two years and more than 90 percent by the end of three years.[63]

**Nerve Entrapment Syndromes.** Entrapment of peripheral nerves as either a primary or a secondary process may present with pain about the shoulder girdle. The clinical picture and neurophysiology of nerve entrapment syndromes are covered in Chapter 110 and in other detailed sources.[64-67] Two entrapment neuropathies, namely, axillary nerve entrapment and suprascapular nerve entrapment, are frequently overlooked and bear further discussion.

The axillary nerve arises from the posterior cord of the brachial plexus and exits posteriorly through the quadrilateral space. This space is bordered superiorly by the teres major, inferiorly by the teres minor, medially by the long head of the triceps, and laterally by the humeral shaft and lateral triceps heads. After sending a sensory branch to the upper lateral cutaneous surface and a motor branch to the teres minor, the nerve courses anteriorly to innervate the deltoid.[32]

Entrapment of the axillary nerve as it exits through the quadrilateral space is an infrequent cause of pain, weakness, and atrophy about the shoulder girdle. It is most commonly seen in the dominant shoulder of young athletic individuals such as pitchers, tennis players, and swimmers who function with excessive overhead activity. The pain may occur throughout the shoulder girdle and radiate down the arm in a nondermatomal pattern. It may be elicited by abduction and external rotation or by palpation of the quadrilateral space (see Fig. 29–1).

This condition represents entrapment of the axillary nerve as it leaves the posterior cord, penetrates the quadrilateral space, and moves anteriorly to innervate the deltoid. On surgical exploration the nerve has been found to be tethered upon the aponeurosis of the hypertrophied muscle or by fibrous bands encroaching upon the quadrilateral space.[68]

The suprascapular nerve is a branch of the upper trunk of the brachial plexus formed by the 5th and 6th cervical nerves. It passes obliquely beneath the trapezius and crosses the scapula through the suprascapular notch.[32] The suprascapular nerve has no cutaneous sensory branches, but supplies motor branches to the supraspinatus and infraspinatus muscles.

The suprascapular nerve entrapment syndrome is the result of compression and tethering of the nerve as it passes through the suprascapular notch. Rengachary and colleagues described variations in the size and shape of the fossa and the suprascapular ligament, which forms its superior border. The authors demonstrated variations in the fossa from a complete bony foramen to a smooth depression on the upper border of the scapula.[69] Patients with a true bony foramen or a deep notch should be more susceptible to the development of entrapment in this area.

The primary symptom is pain, which generally is described as a deep ache felt over the upper border and body of the scapula. The pain is well localized and does not radiate down the arm. Any activity that brings the scapula forward, such as reaching across the chest, may aggravate the pain.[70] Palpation of the suprascapular notch may elicit local tenderness (see Fig. 29–1).

Since the suprascapular nerve has no cutaneous innervation, there is no associated numbness, tingling, or paresthesias. With time, the patients will develop atrophy and weakness of the supraspinatus and infraspinatus muscles. This syndrome must be differentiated from rotator cuff tendinitis, which also could be associated with a similar pattern of pain and muscle atrophy.[71] It also must be differentiated from brachial neuritis and a cervical radiculopathy involving the 5th and 6th roots.[72] Selective EMG determinations of the supraspinatus and infraspinatus may reveal motor atrophy. Instillation of local anesthetics into the supraspinous notch may relieve the symptoms.

As with axillary nerve entrapment, this syndrome is often associated with athletic young individuals with excessive overhead activity. It has also been reported in relationship to trauma.[73,74] Once confirmed, the treatment of choice is surgical decompression of the suprascapular notch. If the entrapment is in association with trauma, a substantial period of time should be given to rule out a neuropraxia, which is likely to resolve.

**Sternoclavicular Arthritis.** Occasionally, traumatic and nontraumatic conditions can cause pain about the sternoclavicular joint (see Fig. 29–1). The most common problem is ligamentous injury and painful subluxation or dislocation. This can be diagnosed by palpable instability and crepitus over the sternoclavicular joint. Sternoclavicular views may radiographically demonstrate dislocation.[37]

Inflammatory arthritis of the sternoclavicular joint has been seen in association with rheumatoid arthritis, ankylosing spondylitis, and septic arthritis. Two other conditions involving the sternoclavicular joint are Tietze's syndrome, a painful nonsuppurative swelling of the joint and adjacent sternochondral junctions, and Friedrich's disease, a painful osteonecrosis of the sternal end of the clavicle.[3]

**Reflex Sympathetic Dystrophy.** Since its original description by Weir Mitchell in 1864,[75] reflex sympathetic dystrophy (RSD) has remained a poorly understood and frequently overlooked condition. Its etiology is unknown but may be related to sympathetic overflow or short circuiting of impulses through the sympathetic system. Any clinician dealing with painful disorders must be familiar with the diagnosis and treatment of this condition. Bonica has provided an excellent review, which covers the clinical presentation, the various stages of the disease, and the importance of early intervention to ensure a successful outcome.[76]

Reflex sympathetic dystrophy has been confusingly called causalgia, shoulder-hand syndrome, and Sudeck's atrophy. It is generally associated with minor trauma and is to be differentiated from causalgia that involves trauma to major nerve trunks.[76] RSD is divided into three phases, which are important in the determination of the stage of involvement and the mode of treatment.[77] Phase one is characterized by sympathetic overflow with diffuse swelling, pain, increased vascularity, and radiographic evidence of demineralization. If left untreated for 3 to 6 months, this may progress to phase two, which is characterized by atrophy. The extremity may now be cold and shiny with atrophy of the skin and muscles. Phase three refers to progression of the trophic changes, with irreversible flexion contractures and a pale, cold, painful extremity. It has been speculated that phase one is related to a peripheral short circuiting of nerve impulses, phase two represents short circuiting through the internuncial pool in the spinal cord, and phase three is controlled by higher thalamic centers.[76,77]

Steinbocker reported that as long as there is evidence of vasomotor activity with swelling and hyperemia, there remains a chance for recovery.[78] Once the trophic phase two or three is established, the prognosis for recovery is poor. Prompt recognition of the syndrome is important, as early intervention to control pain is mandatory. Careful supervision and reassurance are critical, as many of these patients are emotionally labile, as a result of either their pain or an underlying problem. The syndrome may be remarkably reversed by a sympathetic block. Patients who receive transient relief from sympathetic blockade may be helped by surgical sympathectomy.

**Fibrositis.** Fibrositis and other diffuse musculoskeletal syndromes are characterized by multiple trigger points about the shoulder girdle. This subject is discussed in Chapter 32.

**Neoplasms.** Primary and metastatic neoplasms may cause shoulder pain by direct invasion of the musculoskeletal system or by compression with referred pain.[2,66] Primary tumors are more likely to occur in younger individuals. The more common lesions have a typical distribution, such as the predilection of a chondroblastoma for the proximal humeral epiphysis or of an osteogenic sarcoma for the metaphysis.[79] The differential diagnosis of spontaneous onset of shoulder pain in older individuals should include metastatic lesions and myeloma. Neoplasms are best identified by plain radiographs, $^{99}$Tc-MDP scintigraphy, and computed tomography.

The Pancoast or apical lung tumor may present as shoulder pain owing to invasion of the brachial plexus.[52,80] With invasion of the cervical sympathetic chain the patient may also develop Horner's syndrome.

**Miscellaneous.** A variety of other conditions may present as shoulder pain and should be mentioned in this discussion. Acute abdominal disorders such as gallbladder disease, splenic injuries, and subphrenic abscess can refer pain to the shoulder. The pain of acute angina and myocardial infarction may be referred to the left shoulder and down the inner aspect of the left arm. Metabolic disorders such as hypo- and hyperthyroidism,[81] diabetes mellitus,[82] and secondary hyperparathyroidism in association with renal osteodystrophy are infrequently associated with pain about the shoulder girdle.

## References


1. Codman, E.A.: The Shoulder-Rupture of the Supraspinatus Tendon and Other Lesions in or about the Subacromial Bursa. Boston, Thomas Todd Company, Printer, 1934.
2. Bateman, J.E.: The Shoulder and Neck. 2nd ed. Philadelphia, W. B. Saunders Company, 1978.
3. Post, M.: The Shoulder—Surgical and Nonsurgical Management. Philadelphia, Lea & Febiger, 1978.
4. Cailliet, R.: Shoulder Pain. 2nd ed. Philadelphia, F. A. Davis Company, 1981.
5. Greep, J.M., Lemmens, H.A.J., Roos, D.B., and Urschel, H.C.: Pain in Shoulder and Arm. An Integrated View. The Hague, Martinus Nijhoff, 1979.
6. Goldman, A.B.: Shoulder Arthrography. Boston, Little, Brown & Company, 1982.
7. Goldman, A.B., and Ghelman, B.: The double contrast shoulder arthrogram. A review of 158 studies. Radiology 127:655, 1978.
8. Mink, J., and Harris, E.: Double contrast shoulder arthrography: Its use in evaluation of rotator cuff tears. Ortho. Trans. 7:71, 1983.
9. Braunstein, E.M., and O'Connor, G.: Double-contrast arthrotomography of the shoulder. J. Bone Joint Surg. 64A:192, 1982.
10. Strizak, A.M., Danzig, L., Jackson, D.W., Greenway, D., Resnick, D., and Staple, T.: Subacromial bursography. J. Bone Joint Surg. 64A:196, 1982.
11. Lie, S.: Subacromial bursography. Radiology 144:626, 1982.
12. Nakano, K.K.: Neurology of Musculoskeletal and Rheumatic Disorders. Boston, Houghton Mifflin, 1979.
13. Leffert, R.D.: Brachial plexus injuries. N. Engl. J. Med. 291:1059, 1974.
14. Neer, C.S., II: Impingement lesions. Clin. Orthop. 173:70, 1983.
15. Neer, C.S., II: Anterior acromioplasty for the chronic impingement syndrome in the shoulder. A preliminary report. J. Bone Joint Surg. 54A:41, 1972.
16. Neer, C.S., II, Bigliani, L.U., and Hawkins, R.J.: Rupture of the long head of the biceps related to subacromial impingment. Ortho. Trans. 1:111, 1977.
17. Neer, C.S., II, Craig, E.V., Fukada, H., and Mendoza, F.X.: Cuff tear arthropathy. Exhibit at the annual meeting of the American Academy of Orthopedic Surgeons. Jan., 1982.
18. Neer, C.S., II, and Marberry, T.A.: On the disadvantages of radical acromionectomy. J. Bone Joint Surg. 63A:416, 1981.
19. McKendry, R.J.R., Uhthoff, H.K., Sarkar, K., and Hyslop, P.: Calcifying tendinitis of the shoulder: Prognostic value of clinical, histologic, and radiographic features in 57 surgically treated cases. J. Rheumatol. 9:75, 1982.
20. Vebostad, A.: Calcific tendinitis in the shoulder region. A review of 43 operated shoulders. Acta. Orthop. Scan. 46:205, 1975.
21. Uhthoff, H.K., Sarkar, K., and Maynard, J.A.: Calcifying tendinitis, a new concept of its pathogenesis. Clin. Orthop. 118:164, 1976.
22. Sarkar, K., and Uhthoff, H.K.: Ultrastructural localization of calcium in calcifying tendinitis. Arch. Pathol. Lab. Med. 102:266, 1978.
23. Moseley, H.F., and Goldie, I.: The arterial pattern of the rotator cuff of the shoulder. J. Bone Joint Surg. 45B:780, 1963.
24. Rathburn, J.B., and MacNab, I.: The microvascular pattern of the rotator cuff. J. Bone Joint Surg. 52B:540, 1970.
25. Steinbrocker, O.: The Painful Shoulder. *In* Hollander, J.E. (ed.): Arthritis and Allied Conditions. 8th ed. Philadelphia, Lea & Febiger, 1972.
26. Thompson, G.R., Ting, Y.M., Riggs, G.A., Fenn, M.E., and Denning, R.M.: Calcific tendinitis and soft tissue calcification resembling gout. JAMA 203:122, 1968.
27. Kotzen, L.M.: Roentgen diagnosis of rotator cuff tear. Am. J. Roentgenol. 112:507, 1971.
28. De Palma, A.F.: Surgery of the Shoulder, 2nd ed. Philadelphia, J. B. Lippincott Company, 1973.
29. Wolfgang, G.L.: Surgical repair of tears of the rotator cuff of the shoulder. Factors influencing the result. J. Bone Joint Surg. 56A:14, 1974.
30. Earnshaw, P., Desjardins, D., Sarkar, K., and Uhthoff, H.K.: Rotator cuff tears: The role of surgery. Can. J. Surg. 25:60, 1982.
31. Post, M., Silver, R., and Singh, M.: Rotator cuff tear, diagnosis and treatment. Clin. Orthop. 173:78, 1983.
32. Goss, C.M.: Gray's Anatomy of the Human Body. 28th ed. Philadelphia, Lea & Febiger, 1966.
33. Meyer, A.W.: Spontaneous dislocation and destruction of the tendon of the long head of the biceps brachii, fifty-nine instances. Arch. Surg. 17:493, 1928.
34. Hitchcock, H.H., and Bechtol, C.O.: Painful shoulder. Observations on the role of the tendon of the long head of the biceps brachii in its causation. J. Bone Joint Surg. 30A:263, 1948.
35. Crenshaw, A.H., and Kilgore, W.E.: Surgical treatment of bicipital tenosynovitis. J. Bone Joint Surg. 48A:1496, 1966.
36. Wright, P.E.: Dislocations. *In* Edmonson, A.S., and Crenshaw, A.H. (eds.): Campbell's Operative Orthopedics. St. Louis, C. V. Mosby Company, 1980.
37. Rockwood, C.A., Jr.: Fractures and dislocations of the shoulder. Part II. *In* Rockwood, C.A., Jr., and Green, D.P. (eds.) Fractures. Philadelphia, J. B. Lippincott Company, 1975.
38. Glick, J.: Acromioclavicular dislocations in athletes. Orthop. Rev. 1:31, 1972.
39. Taylor, G.M., and Tooke, M.: Degeneration of the acromioclavicular joint as a cause of shoulder pain. J. Bone Joint Surg. 59B:507, 1977.
40. Cofield, R.H., and Briggs, B.T.: Glenohumeral arthrodesis. J. Bone Joint Surg. 61A:668, 1979.
41. Rowe, C.R.: Arthrodesis of the shoulder used in treating painful conditions. Clin. Orthop. 173:92, 1983.
42. Neer, C.S., II, Watson, K.C., and Stanton, F.J.: Recent experience in total shoulder replacement. J. Bone Joint Surg. 64A:319, 1982.
43. Cofield, R.H.: Unconstrained total shoulder prosthesis. Clin. Orthop. 173:97, 1983.
44. Thornhill, T.S., Karr, M.J., Averill, R.M., Batte, N.J., Thomas, W.H., and Sledge, C.B.: Total shoulder arthroplasty, the Brigham Experience. 50th Annual Meeting of the American Academy of Orthopedic Surgeons, Anaheim, March, 1983.
45. Neer, C.S., II: Fracture and Dislocations of the Shoulder. Part I. *In* Rockwood, C.A., Jr., and Green, D.P. (eds.): Fractures. Philadelphia, J. B. Lippincott, Company, 1975.
46. Ficat, R.P., and Arlet, J.: Ischemia and Necrosis of the Bone. Baltimore, Williams & Wilkins Company, 1980.

47. Post, M., Haskell, S.S., and Jablon, M.: Total shoulder replacement with a constrained prosthesis. J. Bone Joint Surg. 62A:327, 1980.
48. Post, M., and Jablon, M.: Constrained total shoulder arthroplasty: Long-term follow-up observations. Clin. Orthop. 173:109, 1983.
49. Putnam, J.J.: The treatment of a form of painful periarthritis of the shoulder. Boston Med. Surg. J. 107:536, 1882.
50. Lippman, R.K.: Frozen shoulder; periarthritis; bicipital tenosynovitis. Arch. Surg. 47:283, 1943.
51. McLaughlin, H.L.: The "frozen shoulder." Clin. Orthop. 20:126, 1961.
52. DePalma, A.F.: Loss of scapulohumeral motion (frozen shoulder). Ann. Surg. 135:193, 1952.
53. Johnson, J.T.H.: Frozen shoulder syndrome in patients with pulmonary tuberculosis. J. Bone Joint Surg. 41A:877, 1959.
54. Dee, P.E., Smith, R.G., Gullickson, M.J., and Ballinger, C.S.: The orthopedist and apical lung carcinoma. J. Bone Joint Surg. 42A:605, 1960.
55. Neviaser, J.S.: Adhesive capsulitis of the shoulder. A study of the pathological findings in periarthritis of the shoulder. J. Bone Joint Surg. 27:211, 1945.
56. Bulgen, D.Y., Hazelman, B.L., and Voak, D.: HLA-B27 and frozen shoulder. Lancet 1:1042, 1976.
57. Bulgen, D.Y., Hazelman, B.L., Ward, M., and McCallum, M.: Immunological studies in frozen shoulder. Ann. Rheum. Dis. 37:135, 1978.
58. Lundberg, B.J.: The frozen shoulder. Acta Orthop. Scand. Suppl. 19, 1969.
59. Spillane, J.D.: Localized neuritis of the shoulder girdle. A report of 46 cases in the MEF. Lancet 2:532, 1943.
60. Parsonage, M.J., and Turner, J.W.A.: Neurologic amyotrophy. The shoulder-girdle syndrome. Lancet 1:973, 1948.
61. Turner, J.W.A., and Parsonage, M.J.: Neurologic amyotrophy (paralytic brachial neuritis). With special reference to prognosis. Lancet 2:209, 1957.
62. Bacevich, B.B.: Paralytic brachial neuritis. J. Bone Joint Surg. 58A:262, 1976.
63. Tsiaris, P., Dyck, P.J., and Mulder, D.W.: Natural history of brachial plexus neuropathy. Arch. Neurol. 27:109, 1972.
64. Omer, G.E., Jr., and Spinner, M.: Management of Peripheral Nerve Problems. Philadelphia, W. B. Saunders Company, 1980.
65. Kelly, T.R.: Thoracic outlet syndrome, current concepts and treatment. Ann. Surg. 190:657, 1979.
66. Brown, C.: Compressive invasive referred pain to the shoulder. Clin. Orthop. 173:55, 1983.
67. Bateman, J.E.: Neurologic painful conditions affecting the shoulder. Clin. Orthop. 173:44, 1983.
68. Cahill, B.R.: Quadrilateral space syndrome. *In* Omer, G.E., Jr., and Spinner, M.D. (eds.): Management of Peripheral Nerve Problems. Philadelphia, W. B. Saunders Company, 1980.
69. Rengachary, S.S., Neft, J.P., Singer, P.A., and Brackett, C.E.: Suprascapular entrapment neuropathy: A clinical, anatomical and comparative study. Neurosurgery 5:441, 1979.
70. Kopell, H.P., and Thompson, W.A.L.: Pain and the frozen shoulder. Surg. Gynecol. Obstet. 109:92, 1959.
71. Drez, D.: Suprascapular neuropathy in the differential diagnosis of rotator cuff injuries. Am. J. Sports Med. 4:43, 1976.
72. Khalili, A.A.: Neuromuscular electrodiagnostic studies in entrapment neuropathy of the suprascapular nerve. Orthop. Rev. 3:27, 1974.
73. Rask, M.R.: Suprascapular nerve entrapment. A report of two cases treated with suprascapular notch resection. Clin. Orthop. 123:73, 1977.
74. Solheim, L.F., and Roaas, A.: Compression of the suprascapular nerve after fracture of the scapula notch. Acta Orthop. Scand. 49:338, 1978.
75. Mitchell, S.W.: Phantom limbs. Lippincott's, Mag. 8:563, 1871.
76. Bonica, J.J.: Causalgia and other reflex dystrophies. *In* Bonica, J.J. (ed.): Management of Pain. Philadelphia, Lea & Febiger, 1979.
77. Evans, J.A.: Reflex sympathetic dystrophy. Surg. Gynecol. Obstet. 82:36, 1946.
78. Steinbocker, O.: The shoulder-hand syndrome: Present perspective. Arch. Phys. Med. 49:388, 1968.
79. Dahlin, D.C.: Bone Tumors. Springfield, Charles C Thomas, 1978.
80. Pancoast, H.K.: Importance of careful roentgen ray investigation of apical chest tumors. JAMA 83:1407, 1924.
81. Golding, D.N.: Hypothyroidism presenting with musculoskeletal syndromes. Ann. Rheum. Dis. 29:10, 1970.
82. Bridgman, J.F.: Periarthritis of the shoulder and diabetes mellitus. Ann. Rheum. Dis. 31:69, 1972.

# Chapter 30
# Low Back Pain

*Stephen J. Lipson*

## INCIDENCE AND DISABILITY

Low back pain is extremely common, is estimated to affect about 65 to 80 percent of populations sampled,[1-3] and accounts for one third of rheumatic complaints.[4] Particular groups, notably those doing heavy industrial labor, have a higher incidence.[5] Back pain has accounted for a 63 percent rate of sick leave among manual laborers,[6] about 500 work days lost per 1000 workers per year,[7] prolonged disability with pain of up to 3 months' duration in 87 percent of those afflicted,[8] and a 60 percent incidence of recurrent bouts of pain in the first year of an attack. Back pain accounts for 4.2 percent of all consultations in general practice in Great Britain[4,9] where 1.1 million persons see general practitioners for a total of 3.1 million consultations per year[10] and where it creates an annual cost of over 500 million dollars in medical care, disability benefits, and lost work. In the United States, a family practice study over a 3-year period showed that 11 percent of men and 9.5 percent of women reported low back pain.[11] Associated risk factors are considered to be occupation, anxiety, depression, pregnancy, and cigarette smoking.[11] Over 5 billion dollars are spent annually for diagnosis and treatment, while lost productivity, compensation payments, and litigation costs add up to more than 14 billion dollars per year.[12]

## OVERALL ADVANCES

The understanding of back disorders has tended to be overshadowed by the syndrome of the herniated nucleus pulposus as delineated by Mixter and Barr.[13] Disc herniations, however, account for only 5 percent of back disorders[14] and do not increase in incidence with a heavy lifting population,[15] as does low back pain. More recent progress in back pain has been directed away from this limited condition. Improvement in the understanding and management of low back pain has come from the recognition of the multiple factors involved in disability secondary to low back pain, methods to elucidate better the source of the pain and therefore attempt more specific therapy, definition of the syndromes, which encompass types of spinal disorders and their pathology, advances in radiologic imaging techniques, subsequent refinements of operative indications, and, finally, improved operative techniques. It is the goal of this chapter to review these advances, except for operative techniques, in terms of patient evaluation and disease states with consideration of any known underlying pathophysiology. An intended emphasis is placed on disc degeneration. Tumors, traumatic fractures, and metabolic bone disease are not discussed.

## BACK PAIN AND CLINICAL EVALUATION

**Relevant Anatomy and Pain Sources.** Adjacent vertebrae are connected by an articular triad composed of the intervertebral disc anteriorly and two zygoapophyseal facet joints lined with synovium posteriorly. The unit is further stabilized by the anterior longitudinal ligament on the ventral side of the intervertebral disc and the posterior longitudinal ligament on the dorsal side. The latter is thinner and consists of bands fanning out over the posterior surface of the disc and loosely attached to it. In the vertebral arches the ligamentum flavum acts as a ligament and blends into the medial superior aspect of the facet joint capsule; it may prevent the synovium from being pinched in the joint during motion and protect the spinal nerves from protrusion of the capsule into the spinal nerve foramen. The interspinous ligament runs between the posterior spinous processes and is a true ligament. The supraspinous ligament connects the spinous processes.

The muscles of the lumbar region are the sacrospinalis and multifidus muscles. The sacrospinalis attaches to the posterior surface of the sacrum and iliac crest, inserts at the lateral angulus of the ribs, and acts as the posterior longitudinal support. The multifidus covers the intervertebral facet joints while running from the mamillary and transverse processes to insert on the spinous process one or two vertebrae above. These act as rotator muscles of the spine. The abdominal muscles via the abdomen provide anterior support to the spine.

The innervation of the lumbar spine has been well reviewed.[16] It consists of the sinuvertebral nerve and the posterior primary ramus (Fig. 30–1). The sinuvertebral nerve, first described by Luschka,[17] arises from the anterior aspect of the spinal nerve just distal to the spinal ganglion. After turning medially it is joined by a sympathetic branch from the ramus communicans, and the composite nerve passes through the intervertebral foramen into the spinal canal where it branches. Adjacent to the posterior longitudinal ligament it divides into ascending, descending, and transverse branches anastomosing with branches from the contralateral side and adjacent levels above and below. The branches are felt

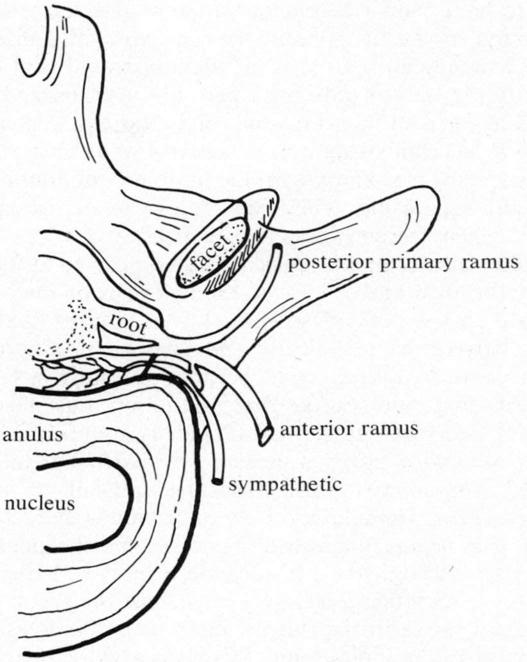


**Figure 30–1.** The innervation of the spine showing the relationships of the posterior primary ramus and the sinuvertebral nerve.

to innervate the vertebral body, laminae, intervertebral discs at the same level and one above and below, the posterior longitudinal ligament, the internal vertebral plexus, the epidural tissues, and the dura. The normal intervertebral disc is believed to be innervated only to the extent of the outer layers of the anulus fibrosus.

The posterior primary ramus arises from the spinal nerve just lateral to the intervertebral foramen in association with the major branch, the anterior ramus. It then divides into medial and lateral branches. The medial branch descends in a notch posterior to the transverse process and is covered by the medial part of the intertransverse ligament. It immediately gives off a small branch to the inferior part of the capsule of the facet joint. The medial branch then continues caudally, innervating the dorsal musculature, anastomosing with nerves from adjacent levels, and then innervating the superior part of the capsule of the facet joint below. The lateral branches of the upper three lumbar levels have cutaneous nerves reaching as far as the greater trochanter, and the two lower lumbar posterior primary rami have no skin supply.

There have been a number of clinical experimental studies to demonstrate pain sources in the low back. Smyth and Wright[18] used nylon thread loops to stimulate structures. The dura, ligamentum flavum, and interspinous ligaments were insensitive. The anulus gave back pain, and the nerve root caused sciatic pain when stimulated. Kellgren[19] injected hypertonic saline into spinal muscles and interspinous ligaments and produced back pain with sclerotomal referral. Hirsch[20] also injected hypertonic saline into the facet joint, which gave back pain with sclerotomal referral. Injection of the disc gave severe back pain resembling patients' attacks, whereas injection of the ligamentum flavum gave mild discomfort. Mooney and Robertson[21] demonstrated that facet irritation gave not only back pain but also marked patterns of referred pain into the thigh and leg, depending upon level. Hamstring muscle activity was enhanced, as evidenced by electromyographic findings and diminished straight leg raising. There was return of depressed reflexes when the facet was anesthetized.

Pain sources in the back, then, appear to originate from the disc and the facet joint. The root may contribute to the pain of sciatica, but it is clear that the pain pattern seen clinically can also be produced by facet joint irritation. It is because of the overlap of contributing pain sources that evaluation must be done carefully to sort out the pathologically significant anatomy; otherwise, surgical measures in particular may be aimed at noncontributing structures and fail.

**Presenting Complaints.** Low back pain is age related. Back pain begins in the second decade, and the incidence increases through the fifth decade of life[1] and then decreases.[3,22] Sciatica is rarely seen before the second decade and peaks in the third.[23] Back pain is increased in heavy lifting laborers,[5] and therefore a work history is necessary both for documentation and for purposes of certifying disability. Pain presents with a number of patterns, and the history will facilitate an accurate assessment of what is or is not its cause. Traditional analysis of low back pain demonstrates that the pain is usefully categorized as local, radicular, referred, or spasmodic.[24]

Local pain, presumably from a pathologic process stimulating sensory nerve endings, is usually steady, is occasionally intermittent, changes with position, is sharp or dull, and is felt in the affected part. It most often gives reflex paravertebral spasm.

Referred pain from pelvic and abdominal viscera is referred to dermatomal areas and takes on a deep and aching characteristic. Referred pain from spinal sources is noted in the sacroiliac area, buttocks, and posterior thigh and is noted as sclerotomal pain, since the referral area has the same embryonic origin as the mesodermal tissue involved.

Radicular pain relates to a spinal nerve root distribution, worsens with root stretching maneuvers such as bending, and usually improves with rest. If pain is worsened by rest, particularly at night, a spinal cord tumor may be suspected. The pain has neurologic characteristics of paresthesias and numbness, and there may be associated motor weakness. The characteristic of walking giving rise to the spinal claudication symptom of spinal stenosis should be noted, as well as the effect of sitting, which will improve spinal stenosis symptoms but worsen those of disc herniation. Bladder, bowel, and sexual function should be determined, since they are involved in central midline herniations of the disc, conus tumors, and occasionally spinal stenosis. Pain from muscular spasm will have cramping, achy characteristics, usually in the sacrospinalis and gluteus maximus. A summary of the characteristics of back pain of various origins is given in Table 30–1.

A useful analysis of back pain arises out of an evaluation of further mechanical relationships of the pain. These mechanical relationships reflect the pathophysiologic origins of the pain. Low back pain and the pain of disc herniation tend to worsen with postural positions of prolonged duration. Positions that increase intradiscal pressure exacerbate pain; those that decrease pressure improve the pain, as outlined by the intradiscal pressure measurements done by Nachemson.[71] However, it is not established that intradiscal pressure causes pain, only that this relationship exists. Another pattern of pain, commonly seen in degenerative spinal stenosis, is that of neurogenic claudication, pain produced in the back or leg by walking or by assuming an erect position. This pain tends to be more diffuse than the pain caused during root entrapment by a herniated lumbar disc. In neurogenic claudication, when the spine is in flexion, room in the lumbar canal enlarges and the pain lessens. A summary of mechanical relationships is given in Table 30–2.

A past medical history of medications, other medical conditions, and a family history, especially of arthritic diseases, is necessary. It is useful at the initial encounter to ascertain work status, compensation, litigation, disability at work and home, and the patient's own assessment of how well he is coping with his affliction, as these factors can markedly alter the assessment, management, and outcome of treatment.[25-28]

**Physical Examination.** Examination should be done

**Table 30–1.** Summary of the Characteristics of Low Back Pain of Various Origins

| Source of Pain | Distribution | Nature | Aggravating Factors | Neurologic Changes |
|---|---|---|---|---|
| Spinal pain | Sclerotomal<br>Local | Sharp<br>Dull | Motion | None |
| Discogenic pain | Sclerotomal | Deep, aching | Increased intradiscal pressure, e.g., bending, sitting, Valsalva maneuver | None |
| Nerve root pain | Radicular | Paresthesias<br>Numbness | Root stretching | Present |
| Multiple lumbar spinal stenosis pain | Radicular<br>Sclerotomal | Paresthesias<br>Spinal claudication pattern | Lumbar extension<br>Walking | Present |
| Referred visceral pain | Dermatomal | Deep, aching | Related to affected organ | None |

**Table 30–2.** Mechanical Relationships Noted in Discogenic Low Back Pain and Herniated Nucleus Pulposus as Compared with Spinal Stenosis

| | Herniated Nucleus Pulposus/Discogenic Low Back Pain | Spinal Stenosis |
|---|---|---|
| Standing/walking | ▼ | ▲ |
| Sitting | ▲ | ▼ |
| Valsalva maneuver | ▲ | — |
| Bending | ▲ | — |
| Lifting | ▲ | — |
| Bed rest | ▼ | ▼ |

with the patient undressed. The spine and stance are inspected while the patient is standing to note lumbar lordosis, thoracic kyphos, scoliosis, tilt from "sciatic scoliosis," flexed lower extremities to relieve root tension, muscle spasm, and skin nevi over the spine. Gait and motion are noted, including toe and heel gait, to determine muscular weakness and to observe any inconsistent or exaggerated posturing.

Forward bending is measured and can be crudely quantitated by an estimate of flexion or the distance of the fingers from the floor. Lateral bending may be asymmetric with unilateral root entrapment. Hyperextension will elicit pain from inflamed facet joints. The spine is palpated to determine local tenderness, the stepoff of spondylolisthesis, or the defect of spina bifida, and percussed to produce local pain or sciatica and in the costovertebral angle to elicit pain of renal origin. The iliac crests are palpated and may be tender, particularly over the posterior iliac spine where local injection may give symptomatic relief. The sciatic nerve is palpated in its notch and along its course to determine hyperesthesia and tenderness. Calf tenderness may be found, reflecting sciatic hyperesthesia.

A thorough neurologic examination is done for objective signs of lumbar root involvement. In disc herniations, L5-S1 and L4-5 are most common, followed by L3-4. Disc herniations at L5-S1 usually involve the S1 root, L4-5 the L5 root, and L3-4 the L4 root. L4-5 herniation may involve both the L5 and S1 roots, and there is a 10 percent incidence of two-level herniations.[29] The neurologic findings are summarized in Table 30–3. The findings according to level should be regarded as guidelines since, although these patterns are generally accurate as to level of entrapment, they can be misleading. The distribution of paresis in the lower extremity in herniated discs at the L4-5 and L5-S1 levels was studied by Weber,[30] who noted that although there is localization of paresis according to nerve root, in 30 to 40 percent of other muscle groups in the lower extremity are also affected. Impairment of the knee jerk has been shown to be affected more often by L4-5 herniations than by those at L3-4.[31] Neurologic assessment must be done carefully, since often only subtle motor weakness is present and must be elicited by repetitive testing. This is particularly true for the gastrosoleus, which is so powerful that manual testing may not demonstrate weakness. Repetitive toe lifts while standing on one foot are useful in this respect, as is examining a toe-toe and heel-heel gait. Reflexes can be enhanced by an isometric maneuver with the hands or, in the case of the ankle jerk, having the patient kneel on a chair. Sensory findings are often confusing and must be mapped carefully. It is of value to perform both pin and vibration tests to ascertain that all columns of the cord are intact.

The patient can then be placed supine and thigh and leg girths measured for atrophy. Leg lengths are measured, since leg length inequality may be associated with back pain that can be helped symptomatically with a shoe lift. Maneuvers are then done to stretch the sciatic nerve and elicit pain. Straight leg raising is done by lifting the leg by the heel with the knee extended until the patient expresses pain and the hamstrings tighten. The site of the pain is asked, since only radicular pain, not back pain, is indicative of a herniated disc. The test is of value only with distal roots and is therefore most accurate with lesions involving the L5 and S1 roots. Young patients have a marked tendency toward a positive straight leg raising test with disc herniations. Its absence fairly accurately excludes a disc herniation up to the age of 30, when it no longer excludes the diagnosis.[32] Variations of the straight leg raising test include dorsiflexion of the foot at the end point of straight leg raising to further stretch the sciatic nerve. Lasègue's test is done by having the hip and knee flexed and then

**Table 30–3.** Nerve Root Findings

| Nerve Root | Pain and Dysesthesia | Weakness and Atrophy | Decreased Reflexes |
|---|---|---|---|
| L4 | Posterolateral thigh across knee<br>Anteromedial leg | Quadriceps | Knee jerk |
| L5 | Posterior thigh<br>Anterolateral leg<br>Medial foot and hallux | Tibialis anterior<br>Extensor hallucis longus<br>Atrophied anterior compartment of the leg | None or decreased tibialis posterior |
| S1 | Posterior thigh<br>Posterior leg<br>Posterolateral foot<br>Lateral toes | Gastrosoleus | Ankle jerk |
| Sacral roots S2-4 | Buttocks and perineum<br>Posterior thigh<br>Posterior leg<br>Plantar foot | Gluteus maximus<br>Hamstrings<br>Gastrosoleus<br>Foot intrinsics and long flexors<br>Anal and bladder sphincters | Ankle jerk<br>Absent plantar toe responses |

slowly extending the knee. It can also be done with the patient seated over the side of the examining table. The crossed straight leg raising test is done by elevating the leg contralateral to the symptomatic side. Reproduction of radicular pain by this maneuver is considered the most indicative sign of disc herniation.[31]

To stretch the more proximal roots to the femoral nerve, the patient is turned prone and the Ely test for rectus femoris contracture done. The knee is flexed and the hip is hyperextended. This motion will be limited by irritation of the L3 and L4 roots. The Patrick or fabere test, to implicate the sacroiliac rather than the hip joint, is done by flexing, abducting, externally rotating, and extending the hip (giving rise to the mnemonic "fabere").[33] A painful response points to the sacroiliac joint as the source of the complaint.

If it is felt that the patient has too much emotional overlay, is too coached in examination by multiple previous consultations, or is guilty of outright malingering, there are some tests to help reveal this. In straight leg raising, the foot is both dorsiflexed and plantar flexed to ascertain the correct anatomical result. When the patient is sitting on the table, the knees are casually extended to note the presence of Lasègue's sign and to see if the patient sits back to relax sciatic tension. With the patient supine, he is asked to do an active straight leg raising maneuver while the examiner's hand is under the contralateral heel. A true effort will give a downward push on the opposite heel, while a feigned attempt will not produce it. A true list will persist while bending forward in a chair. These and other useful tests are reviewed elsewhere.[34,35]

An assessment of peripheral circulation should be performed as well as abdominal, rectal, and pelvic examination, since the source of some back pain may be found here. Chest expansion is measured with a tape measure as a screen for ankylosing spondylitis; it is highly significant when chest excursion is reduced to 1 inch.

**Laboratory Examination.** It is useful to perform a simple battery of tests as a screen for metabolic and specific diseases early on in the assessment and management of back pain. These, like the initial radiograph of the spine, provide a baseline for the exclusion of some diseases as the underlying cause of the pain. They can be tailored when appropriate. The tests include a complete blood count, sedimentation rate, rheumatoid factor, antinuclear antibodies, serum calcium, phosphorus, alkaline phosphatase, acid phosphatase when appropriate, uric acid, blood sugar, immunoelectrophoresis, protein electrophoresis, and urinalysis.

**Psychologic Evaluation.** For better or worse, back pain involves a significant number of emotional factors, and it is necessary to recognize them early in assessing pain. When personality factors are unfavorable, management will be unsuccessful no matter how skillfully performed.[27] Fortunately, emotional factors can be made more objective by psychological testing. The Minnesota Multiphasic Personality Inventory (MMPI) has become the most accurate guideline for detecting personality traits that will predict poor results.[28,36] The hysteria (Hy) and hypochondriasis (Hs) scales of the MMPI have been shown to be the best predictors of a symptomatic result of surgery and chemonucleolysis for disc disease. A simple pain diagram has been correlated with the MMPI.[37] This makes it possible to have a quick, simple office assessment of personality traits that may confuse pain assessment. These tests cannot be used in an absolute sense to rule in or out functional versus organic pain,[38] but help in deciding whether to pursue invasive therapy, to seek psychologic and psychiatric consultation, or, in the case of chronic pain, to enter into behavior modification by operant conditioning.[39,40]

Anatomically based aid is given by the Pentothal interview,[41] utilizing the straight leg raising test. The patient's straight leg raising endpoint is established, and he is then given intravenous Pentothal anesthesia until a noxious stimulus such as toe squeeze or heel cord pinching no longer produces a response. The anesthetic is allowed to wear off, and at intervals the noxious stimulus, given in the limb examined, is tested. Upon return of a response such as a grimace, deep sigh, or withdrawal, the straight leg raising is repeated. If there is organic disease and lumbar root irritation, an appropriate response to this noxious stimulus will be registered. In this manner, further information as to the severity and organic nature of the pain described is gained.

**Radiologic Evaluation.** ***Plain Radiographs and Common Anomalies of the Low Back.*** The lumbosacral spine film is a necessary part of early evaluation. A lateral lumbosacral radiograph delivers a 2 rem skin dose, which is 15 times the exposure delivered by a chest radiograph.[42] Although the yield of causes of low back pain by radiography is low and the radiation dose relatively high, it serves to rule out serious conditions such as tumor and infection. It should be obtained with some discretion. One study has shown that the risks and costs of obtaining a lumbar radiograph at the initial visit does not justify the small associated benefit.[43] The standard anteroposterior, lateral, coned-down lateral, and 45-degree oblique views comprise the standard series. Early signs of disc degeneration are decreased height of the anterior disc space and anteroposterior intervertebral shift on flexion-extension lateral views.[44] The so-called vacuum sign of intranuclear gas also reflects disc degeneration.[45] Later radiographic signs of disc degeneration are further collapse of the disc space, sclerosis, and osteophyte formation. Osteophytes also occur in Reiter's syndrome, ankylosing spondylitis, and psoriatic arthritis. The presence of disc degeneration radiographically does not imply that a disc is the cause of pain. Lawrence[46] surveyed lumbosacral spine films in persons 35 years of age and older. Sixty-five percent of the males and 52 percent of the females showed disc degeneration, but in only 13 percent were there symptoms of pain. Nerve root involvement occurred in only 10 percent of those with signs of moderate to severe degeneration. In a large series of disc herniations proved at operation, the plain radiograph predicted a correct diagnosis in only 34 percent of cases.[47] Epstein[48] found 46 percent narrowing at L5-S1 and only 25 percent narrowing at L4-5 in 300 proved herniations. Therefore a disc can often appear radiographically normal when it is symptomatic, and when a disc is symptomatic, radiography is not an accurate predictor of the symptomatic level.

Various structural anomalies, definable on plain radiographs and associated with back pain and disc degeneration, have been reviewed.[49] A defect in the pars interarticularis (spondylolysis) increases the likelihood of symptomatic back pain by about 25 percent. Disc herniation, however, is unusual. The incidence of disc degeneration defined by discogram is increased by bilateral pars defects, and the degeneration is felt to be more rapidly progressive. Wiltse[49] believes that unilateral pars defects increase the rate of disc degeneration. Tropism, or a rotational asymmetry of the lumbosacral facets from a sagittal to a coronal direction, produces accelerated disc degeneration. Farfan and Sullivan[50] found a 23 percent incidence of asymmetry in asymptomatic backs. In symptomatic backs they found a very high incidence of asymmetry and disc herniations on the side of the more coronal facet.

Scoliosis in the thoracolumbar region does not increase the incidence of low back pain up to the age of 56.[4,5,51] There is progressive disc degeneration at the apex of the curve in progressive scoliotic curves. Lumbar lordosis does not increase the incidence of back pain.[1,5] Lumbosacral tilt from a unilateral anomalous lumbosacral facet or unilateral hypoplasia of the sacrum and pelvis is not known to produce rapid disc degeneration, although it might be expected to.[49] Leg length discrepancy producing tilt is known not to produce symptoms with up to 1 to 2 cm of discrepancy.[1,5] With greater than 4.5 cm of discrepancy, the incidence of back pain increases.[49]

Spina bifida occulta does not produce back pain.[1,5] Transitional vertebrae are either a sacralized lumbar vertebra or a lumbarized sacral vertebra, and neither produces increased back pain.[1,5] Five percent of people have six lumbar vertebrae, 2.5 percent have four, and the rest have the usual five.[52] Wiltse[49] advances a guideline that the more sacralized a vertebra, the more vestigial its disc and the less likely it is to herniate. If there is disc herniation, it is usually at the level above the transitional vertebra.

***Bone Scan.*** Bone scanning with $^{99}$Tc diphosphonate can be of use in defining the origin of back pain in some situations. It can demonstrate bony infections or tumors, and is useful in detecting early evidence of ankylosing spondylitis with increased activity in the sacroiliac, facet, and costovertebral joints. A developing pars interarticularis defect, not visible on plain radiography, can be demonstrated by bone scan. Advanced degenerative disc and facet disease produces increased uptake, and bone scan yields little useful information.[53] Ga-citrate scanning offers the possibility of early diagnosis of infections.[54]

***Discography.*** Discography, the injection of radiologic water-soluble contrast material into the intervertebral disc, is felt to be a safe procedure and has been used since 1948.[55] Some large series have revealed no complications,[56,57] although there are reports of occasional infections, ranging from 1 in 622[58] to 1 in 2500.[59] The effect of puncture of the disc has been examined. Discography in dogs with followup at 6 to 12 months did not reveal significant radiologic or histologic changes.[60] Nuclear herniation with protruded disc has been caused with a 20-gauge needle in dogs,[61] and in clinical studies changes have varied from none at 1 to 3 months[58,62] to loss of disc height in about one fourth of patients 12 months after discography.[63]

Disc degeneration evidenced by discography increases with age and progression down the lumbar spine.[58] In cadavers, 90 percent of lumbar discs are normal in the age group 14 to 34 years, but only 5 percent are normal at 60 years.[64] Holt[65] found 34 percent degenerative changes in normal volunteers. Because of the marked prevalence of age-related disc degeneration, discography has been felt to be of little use in correctly diagnosing a herniated disc and was a reliable diagnostic method in only 30 percent of cases of surgically proved disc herniation.[47]

In normal discs it is difficult to inject more than 1 ml of contrast material into the nucleus. There is marked resistance to the injection but no pain. A degenerative disc is usually easy to inject, although firm resistance is reported in 15 percent of a large series.[59] The injection may be painful in up to two thirds of degenerative discs,[59] but pain may also be produced by injection of the anulus and by an irritant in the contrast medium. The radiologic appearance of degeneration is that of diffusion of contrast material through the disc and occasional extravasation through anular cracks into the epidural space. The appearance is variable and of no significance in diagnosing symptomatic herniation. Pain can be of diagnostic value, but only if it reproduces the symptomatic pain.[41] Discography produces back pain in 15 percent of normal males,[65] so that the simple production of pain is not diagnostic.

Discography in the lumbar spine, then, has certain indications.[41] It is useful in assessing the state of degeneration in a disc above the level of a proposed fusion, since that disc will be subject to progressive degeneration and will fail if unrecognized degeneration already exists. If myelography is negative but disc herniation is still suspected, discography can help define the disc degeneration. In patients in whom there is intractable low back pain without evidence of disc degeneration on the plain radiograph, discography can demonstrate the degeneration. The source of usual pain patterns may be confirmed by its reproduction on discography. Discography is routinely used in chemonucleolysis prior to the injection of chymopapain to ensure that a normal disc is not injected. Macnab[41] assesses a symptomatic pseudarthrosis, following fusion, by discography. Disc injection at the level of pseudarthrosis is painful, but it is painless if the fusion is solid. He feels that this technique is 80 percent reliable.

***Myelography.*** Myelography is used as a preoperative

investigation, not as a diagnostic technique.[29,41] It is recommended preoperatively for two reasons: (1) it will reveal a tumor presenting as a disc herniation which might be missed if it is not at the level examined at surgery; and (2) it more precisely localizes the site of disc herniation and root entrapment. Lateral bony root entrapments may present with a negative myelogram. Diffuse anular bulges will give a waisted, hourglass appearance. Multiple disc herniations occur with a 5 to 10 percent incidence.[42] Myelographic information will thus allow the surgeon to modify his approach so that excessive exposure will be avoided, minimizing postoperative perineural scarring. As has been previously noted, neurologic examination is not completely accurate in localizing the level of involvement. In disc herniations, neurologic symptoms associated with the last two lowest spaces point to the correct level only about 60 percent of the time.[31] Neurologic signs are more accurate, reaching 75 to 80 percent.[31] Myelography is accurate 80 to 90 percent of the time,[47,66,67] but it is not foolproof in that lateral disc herniations are detected in only 70 to 80 percent of myelograms[42] and 11 percent of cases of sciatica have a negative myelogram as well as a negative neurologic exam.[68] Over two thirds of disc herniations with false-negative myelography are in the L5-S1 space,[31] because the dural sac may be short or may lie away from the disc by 3 to 4 mm.

Traditional myelography has been done with Pantopaque (iodophenylundelic acid), which is an oil-soluble contrast medium. The complications are numerous and include fever, headache, nausea, meningismus, backache, urinary changes, paresthesias, ileus, and acute and chronic arachnoiditis. Complications related to technique include extradural injections, epidural hematomas, contrast retention, venous intravasation, pulmonary embolism, epidermoid cyst formation, chronic dural leaks, chemical arachnoiditis secondary to the mixing of blood with Pantopaque, and others that are well reviewed.[69,70] Complications are infrequent, but the most common are the acute, transient systemic reactions secondary to inflammation caused by the Pantopaque, the extradural or mixed injection, and retention of contrast caused by faulty technique.[69]

Water-soluble myelography has replaced oil-soluble myelography and has been used extensively in Europe. Oil-soluble contrasts are now banned in Scandinavia.[71] Meglumine[70] and more recently metrizamide[71] are the agents used. These water-soluble contrast media are found to fill the root sleeves more completely because of their solubility in cerebrospinal fluid and their low viscosity. Therefore lateral disc herniations are more readily detected. These agents are less inflammatory and they are resorbed, leaving no retained contrast. The major complications are those of meningeal irritation, increased radicular symptoms, transient hypotension, and seizures.[70] Metrizamide is the most improved of the contrasts, but is still regarded as epileptogenic. It is reported to have 95 percent accuracy in disc herniations.[71]

The abnormalities noted on myelography vary with the size and location of the lesion. Lateral disc herniations usually cause incomplete filling of the root sleeve, lateral dural sac indentation, and a double density of the sac (Fig. 30–2). Central midline herniations often give a complete block with ventral indentation. Sequestered free fragments may migrate and will be seen as circumscribed masses. Chronic degeneration with a diffuse anular bulge will give a waisted, hourglass appearance at the level of the disc space and osteophytes (Fig. 30–3). Artifacts encountered are from the needle, hematomas, and scarring from previous surgery.

***Lumbar Epidural Venography.*** Lumbar epidural venography is of particular use in demonstrating lumbar disc herniation and has achieved success by selective catheterization of the ascending lumbar veins.[72] The ascending lumbar veins off the external iliac veins and ascending sacral veins off the internal iliac veins are catheterized, and defects in filling of the anterior internal vertebral and radicular veins are noted (Fig. 30–4). In Macnab's series,[72] the diagnostic accuracy of venography was 98 percent, compared with 90 percent for myelography, in patients with lumbar disc herniation and no prior surgery. It cannot distinguish postoperative scarring from recurrent disc herniation. Epidural venography is indicated in patients who have not had a previous operation and in those patients in whom the myelogram is normal or equivocal but in whom there is a strong clinical suspicion of disc herniation.

***Computed Tomography.*** Computed tomography (CT) has replaced many of the alternative methods of radiologic imaging described above. With fourth-generation scanners, the need for myelography has decreased and therefore the morbidity of investigation has decreased. CT scanning has the disadvantage of not being useful as a screening procedure, as myelography is, and may not visualize intradural lesions unless contrast is present intrathecally. The reliability of CT scanning in detecting herniated disc appears to be well over 95 percent. Herniated disc can be easily visualized on thin-cut CT scan, as seen in Figure 30–5. Spinal stenosis can be visualized as in Figure 30–6, with bulging of the disc, thickening of the ligamentum flavum, osteophytic entrapment from the facets, and the obliteration of epidural fat.

These techniques should be reserved for cases in which there is clinical suspicion of an anatomic lesion. Imaging techniques should not be used to find a lesion and thereby provide a presumptive diagnosis of the cause of pain. If one uses this latter approach, false positives from asymptomatic degeneration will confuse the evaluation. Such degeneration in the cervical and lumbar region was found following myelography in 28 percent of patients who had no spinal symptoms and were being studied for other reasons.[73]

***Other Techniques.*** Epidurography is a technique of injecting epidural water-soluble contrast medium to outline the dural sac and root sleeves.[74] It is placed via the sacral hiatus, but in one series 7.5 percent of patients could not be injected successfully.[67] Subarachnoid injections carry a risk of seizure and death.

Nerve root infiltration is of value in localizing the

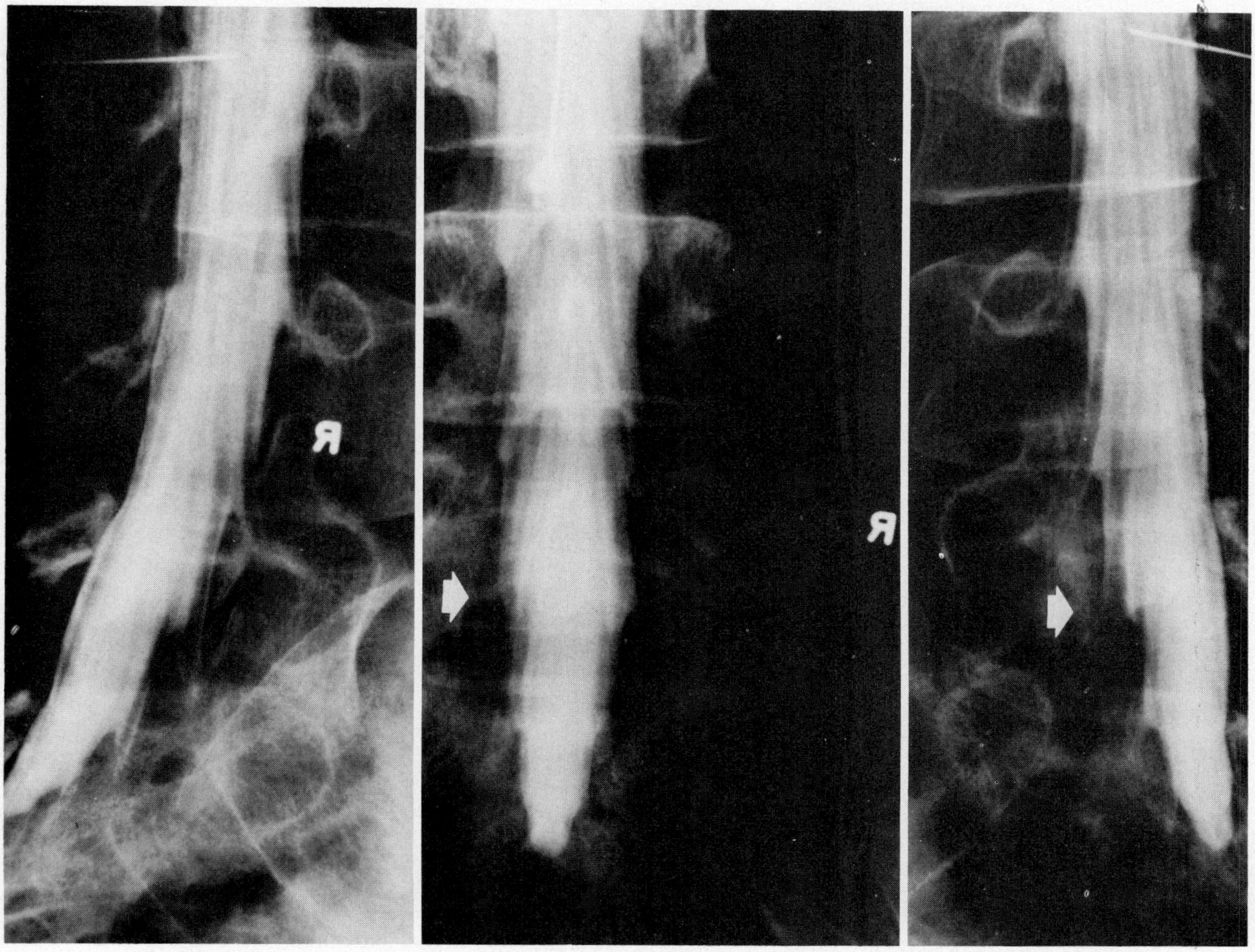

**Figure 30–2.** A metrizamide myelogram with L5-S1 herniated nucleus pulposus and root sleeve cutoff (arrows).

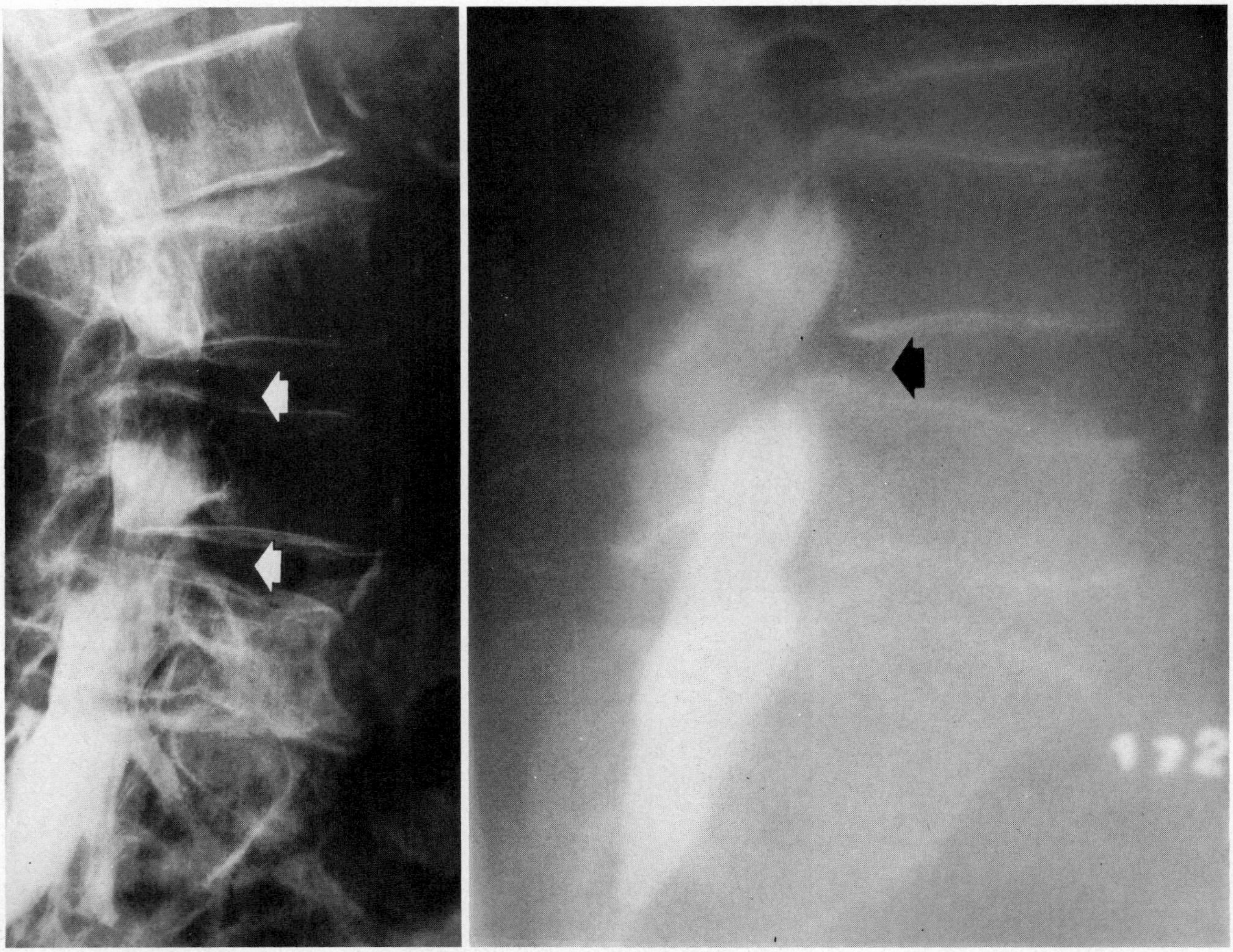

**Figure 30–3.** A metrizamide myelogram of a patient with degenerative spinal stenosis demonstrating central exclusion of the contrast with the hourglass configuration at the level of the discs (arrows). Tomography was used to enhance visualization.

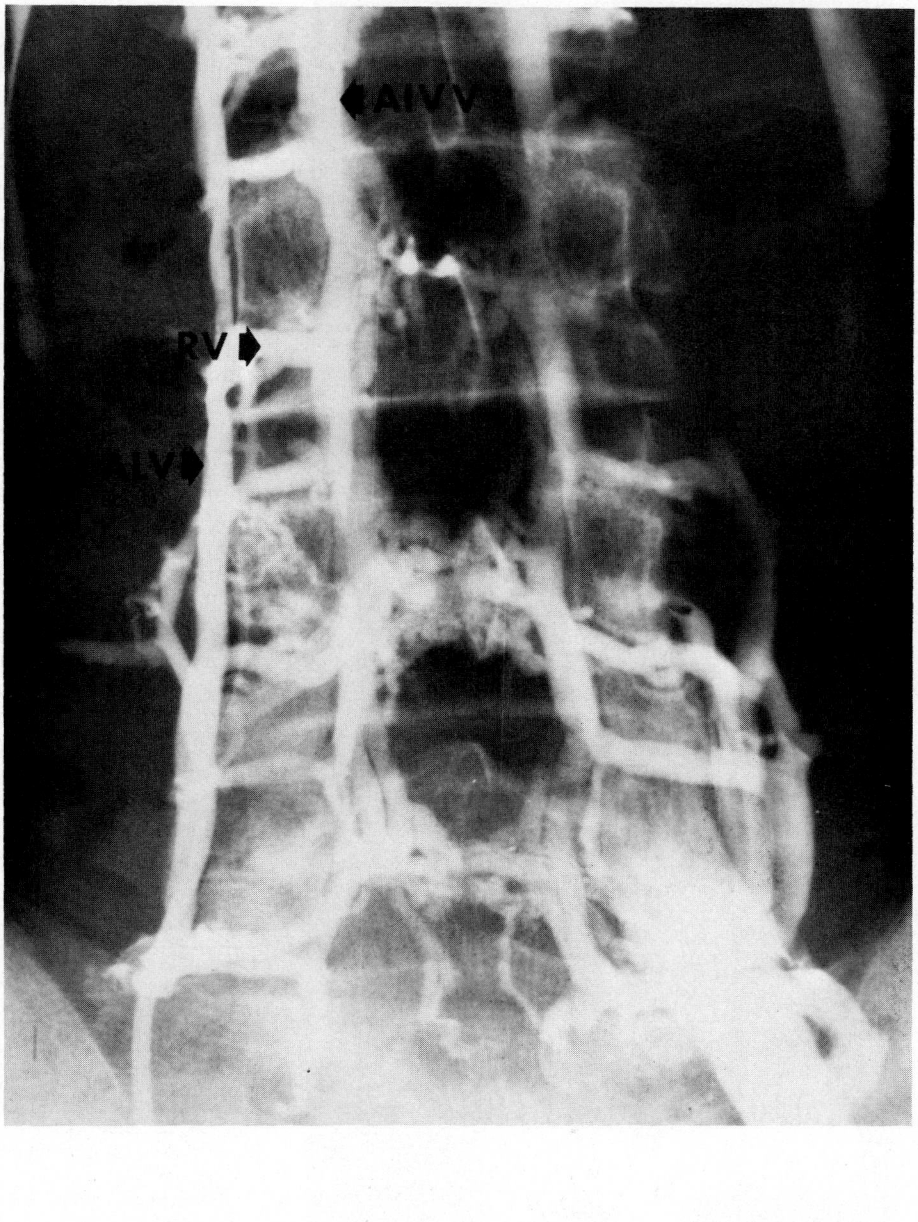


**Figure 30–4.** Normal lumbar epidural venogram demonstrating the radicular vein (*RV*), ascending lumbar vein (*ALV*), and anterior internal vertebral vein (*AIVV*).

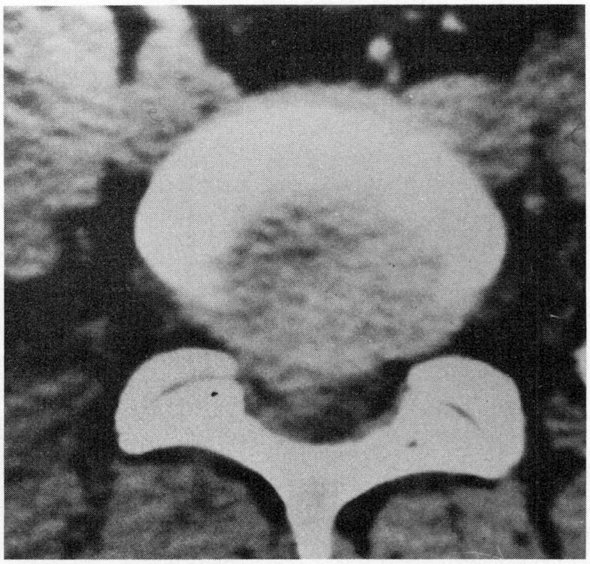

**Figure 30–5.** Computerized tomographic scan of a herniated intervertebral disc with unilateral obliteration of the root by disc material.

level of root involvement.[41] It is done under image intensification with oil-soluble contrast medium injected into the sleeve for definition and Xylocaine injected to determine if clinical relief of pain occurs.

Facet blocks offer both a diagnostic and therapeutic measure for relief of back pain.[21,53] Under image intensification a needle is placed into the facet joint. Water-soluble contrast can be used to outline the facet and a local anesthetic and/or a deposteroid injected for prolonged relief of symptoms. The relief of pain is the only endpoint of significance.

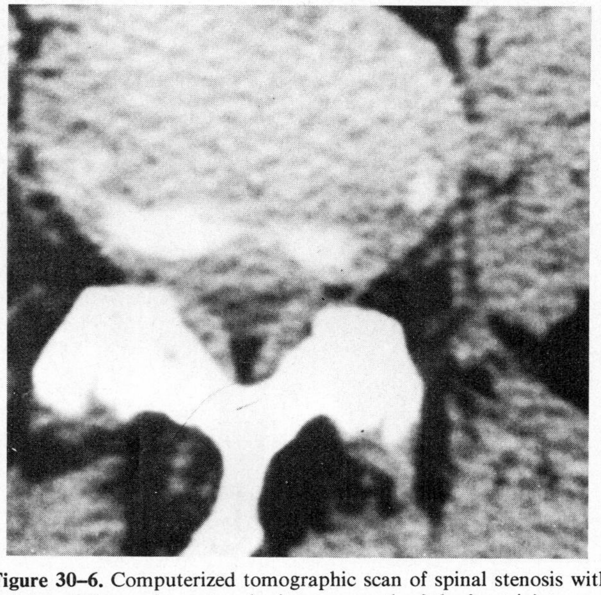

**Figure 30–6.** Computerized tomographic scan of spinal stenosis with bulging of the anulus, osteophytic overgrowth of the facet joints, and thickening of the ligamentum flavum.

## DISEASE STATES

**Degenerative Disc Disease.** ***Spinal Stenosis and Lumbar Root Entrapment.*** Intervertebral disc degeneration is the central factor in many of the conditions of age-related degenerative disease of the lumbar spine. As already noted under Radiologic Evaluation, disc degeneration progresses with age and as one progresses down the lumbar spine. Mixter and Barr[13] first emphasized the role of herniation of the nucleus pulposus in producing lumbar root entrapment. In more recent years, much work has focused on disc degeneration itself and lumbar root entrapment as a result of anatomical changes secondary to disc degeneration. Clinically, lumbar root entrapment is now encompassed in the broad classification of spinal stenosis,[75] which includes narrowing of the spinal canal, nerve root canals, and intervertebral foramina. The process may be local, segmental, or generalized. It may be secondary to soft tissue or bone and may involve the canal, dural sac, or both. This definition includes classical disc herniation and a variety of entrapment syndromes described by Macnab.[76] The classification of spinal stenosis is outlined in Table 30–4.[75]

Historically, spinal stenosis was originally used to describe root entrapment caused by a congenital narrowing of the spinal canal produced by thickening of the neural arches, interpedicular narrowing, and a trefoil configuration of the canal.[77,78] The term was subsequently extended[79,80] to include degenerative and other changes causing root entrapment (illustrated in Fig. 30–7). Prior to their inclusion in the definition of spinal stenosis, it was already known that degenerative changes caused root entrapment,[81] and it had been shown that in an already compromised canal, small changes causing further root entrapment can have marked neurologic consequences.[82] Iatrogenic spinal stenosis has been shown to produce symptomatic narrowing of the canal by thickening of the laminae after decortication—particularly after posterior fusion. Scar tissue from laminectomy may cause compression. Epidural fat involved

**Table 30–4.** Classification of Spinal Stenosis

| |
|---|
| Congenital |
| Idiopathic |
| Achondroplastic |
| Acquired stenosis |
| Degenerative |
| Central portion of the spinal canal |
| Lateral portion of the spinal canal |
| Degenerative spondylolisthesis |
| Combined—any combination of congenital, degenerative, and disc herniations |
| Spondylolytic, spondylolisthetic |
| Iatrogenic |
| Postlaminectomy |
| Postfusion |
| Postchemonucleolysis |
| Post-traumatic |
| Miscellaneous |
| Paget's disease |
| Fluorosis |

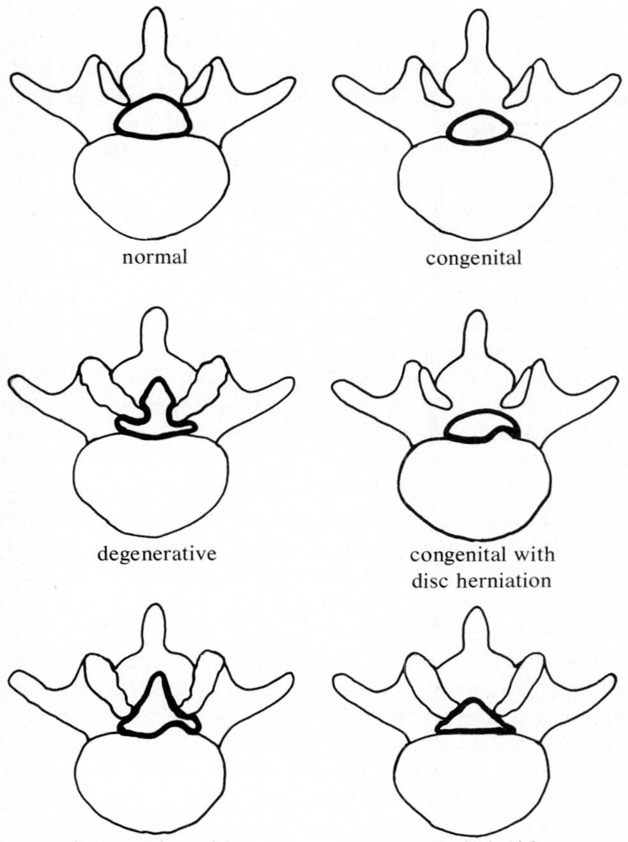


**Figure 30–7.** Outlines of the cross section of the spinal canal in different types of spinal stenosis.

in lipomatosis can cause spinal stenosis.[83] Degenerative stenosis is the most common kind of spinal stenosis encountered.[84]

In the following paragraphs we will review what is known about degenerative disc disease and then consider the clinical states of lumbar root entrapment which result from these changes.

***Pathologic Changes.*** The changes in the intervertebral disc with age have been well documented[85-87] and involve the central nucleus pulposus, the surrounding anulus fibrosus, and the cartilaginous endplates on the adjacent vertebral bodies. By the third decade the incidence of progressive degenerative change in the lumbar intervertebral disc shows a marked increase. In the cartilaginous endplate, early changes of fibrillation occur without evidence of repair. Some fissures and fibrous invasion occur, and breaks in the endplate with nuclear extrusion are seen. In the fourth and fifth decades the endplate is thinned and sometimes absent, and nuclear extrusion with Schmorl's node formation is more frequent. Calcium salts are deposited and progress from this stage on. The chondrocytes of the endplate show signs of senescence and frank necrosis. At older ages the changes are more progressive, with gradual loss of the endplate.

The anulus is well developed by 6 months of life, and in the first decade it fills with ground substance and attaches to the anterior and posterior longitudinal ligaments. The fibers are distinct, but by the end of the second decade the tissue is more hyalinized and less cellular. It then becomes coarse with fissuring, signs of cell death, deposition of pigment, and vascularization. In the fifth decade the anulus loses its lamellar distinction, the fibrils shorten and thicken, and there is hypocellularity. Degeneration is progressive with fissuring, nuclear herniation, and vascular invasion.

The nucleus pulposus starts as a cellular structure with a gelatinous matrix. In the first decade the notochordal cells disappear and fibroblasts distribute toward the periphery. Vacuoles are present in the nucleus pulposus. This arrangement is preserved into the second decade when it gradually loses its mucoid appearance and a fibrillar network appears. The nucleus-anulus border becomes less distinct in the third decade, and by the fourth decade it is obscured by a proliferation of fibrous tissue and cartilage cells. The fibrous change continues with pigment formation, desiccation, cleft formation, and calcium salt deposition. The pathology of symptomatic discs is the same, except that the changes appear more advanced than one might expect on an age basis.[87] Work over recent years has sought to delineate the causes of these changes and has focused on the biochemistry, immunology, nutrition, and biomechanics of the disc.

***Biochemical Changes.*** Investigations on the biochemical changes with age and degeneration have been reviewed,[88-90] and work has focused on the changes in the collagen and proteoglycans of the intervertebral disc. The collagen of the disc is known to exhibit polymorphism and to change with age. Eyre and Muir[91] demonstrated types I and II collagen in the anulus fibrosus of young pigs, but only type II in the nucleus. They later demonstrated a smooth transition of types I and II with respect to outer versus inner parts of the anulus.[92] Other workers[93,94] have found evidence of type I collagen in degenerated nuclei, implying new collagen synthesis, but of an inappropriate type. The collagen crosslinks in aging discs change,[95] and interactions with proteoglycans are altered.[96] Noncollagenous proteins change in disc degeneration with the appearance and progressive accumulation of $\beta$-proteins,[97] but the significance of these changes is unclear.[90]

The proteoglycans of the disc are known to change with age.[98] With age and progression down the lumbar spine the composition of the proteoglycans in the anulus and the nucleus changes in that in both regions the size of the proteoglycans decreases, the keratan sulfate content increases, and they become less extractable.[99] Hyaluronate content parallels the distribution of proteoglycans in the disc, increases with age, and is present in adequate amounts to permit complete aggregation of available proteoglycans.[100] Proteoglycan structure in the human disc is similar to proteoglycans from cartilage except for a shorter core protein region. Anular proteoglycans have higher aggregation properties than do nuclear proteoglycans.[101] The water content of the disc decreases with age but may be due not so much to simple changes in the osmotic properties of the proteoglycans as to alterations in matrix interactions.[102]

***Role of Immunity.*** Bobechko and Hirsch[103] postulated an autoimmune mechanism of disc degeneration after autologous nucleus pulposus implanted in rabbit ears caused lymph node stimulation. Humoral antibodies have not been found in patients with disc disease,[104,105] but leukocyte migration inhibition[105,106] and lymphocyte transformation[107,108] have been demonstrated in disc material. A proteoglycan fraction may be the antigenic stimulus.[108] Previous work on uncomplicated disc degeneration and nuclear herniation in the human[86,88,109] and experimental animal herniation[110] have not shown inflammatory infiltrates, although they have been observed in nerve roots involved in disc herniations.[111] The nucleus implants of Bobechko and Hirsch[103] also did not show cellular infiltrates. There is no evidence, therefore, that the target tissue is involved in a cell-mediated immune response, although it may contain something that exhibits lymphokine activity. Further work is needed to clarify the possible involvement of the immune mechanism in disc degeneration.

***Disc Nutrition.*** Intradiscal pH measurements show that the pH is low in degenerated discs.[112] This was found to be due to increased lactate levels.[113] Since lactate is a product of anaerobic metabolism and the disc in young adults is avascular, disc nutrition was investigated to determine a possible contributing factor. Solute diffusion occurs through the anulus and central portion of the endplate[114] where vascular contacts are made. These contacts are reduced in degeneration. The cellularity of the disc is greatest in the anulus,[115] and by calculating energy requirements it was found that the center of the disc was unable to support much cellular activity. Glucose and oxygen enter the disc via the endplate and anulus,[115] but sulfate, an anion, is partially excluded by the polyanionic glycosaminoglycans of the nucleus and enters primarily by the anulus.[115] It is postulated that changes in the endplate with a consequence of nutritional deprivation may have a role in disc degeneration.

***Biomechanical Factors.*** Mechanical factors are of importance in disc degeneration, and not just those due to an upright position, since dogs and other animals have disc degeneration.[117,118] The area of the spine subjected to the most mechanical stress appears to fail. Extensive intradiscal pressure studies have been performed and reviewed by Nachemson[71] and have shown that the nucleus acts as a liquid contained by the anular fibers. When the disc is loaded, intradiscal pressure exceeds the applied axial force with particularly high tensile stresses in the posterior anulus where herniations are most common. Axial loads per se produce failure first in the vertebral body with fracture of the subchondral endplate.[119] Schmorl's nodes can result, representing nuclear herniations through an endplate fracture.[120] Farfan[121] believes that rotational forces are the most important forces involved, producing early outer anular cracks with progression of the cracks until a radial fissure forms, allowing nuclear herniation. Progressive damage occurs with degenerative changes occurring in the posterior facet joints. A complete biomechanical description of the disc is not yet available, and there is a need to correlate the mechanical data with biologic status.[122]

Intradiscal pressure measurements by Nachemson[71] have given invaluable insight into measures used in the management of low back pain and its prevention. Postural and dynamic lifting measurements have shown the optimal positions to minimize intradiscal pressure. Lumbar supports are of benefit, and isometric exercises reduce the load delivered to the lumbar spine by traditional exercises. In this manner patients can be guided to better back hygiene and particularly stressful maneuvers can be avoided.

***Clinical States and Treatment.*** Degenerative disc disease can present with backache and no nerve root entrapment or with nerve root involvement with or without backache. As the disc degenerates, segmental instability is produced and abnormal degrees of motion are permitted. This produces excessive motion and subluxation in the facet joints which undergo small degrees of trauma and can fracture.[43] As the disc loses height, further subluxation of the facets occurs, and degenerative arthritis in these joints is the sequela. Disc degeneration may remain asymptomatic, may be symptomatic because of changes in the disc itself, or may be symptomatic because of trauma in the facet joints and ligaments. Root entrapment occurs when roots are involved in disc herniations or entrapment by settling structures or osteophytic processes, yielding pain with discogenic or neurogenic claudication mechanics. The differences are presumably on the basis of different pathophysiologic mechanisms involving nociception to a radicular irritation or inflammatory phenomenon versus radicular ischemia.

Backache without nerve involvement is managed conservatively. Pain can be prolonged, lasting up to 3 months in 87 percent of those affected,[8] and has a 60 percent incidence of recurrent bouts within the first year of an attack. It is managed with bedrest, analgesics, muscle relaxants, corsets, weight loss, and exercises that emphasize back stretching and abdominal strengthening. Bed rest can decrease discomfort and hasten recovery, but analgesics do not speed recovery and nonsteroidal anti-inflammatories are ineffective.[123] Outlines of treatment programs vary with the treating physician but usually follow these measures.[34,124] Spinal fusion may be warranted in cases of chronic backache, but thorough investigation of the patient, including a psychological assessment,[124,125] is required to give some preoperative estimate of the likelihood of success.

Lumbar nerve root entrapment in disc degeneration was classically ascribed to disc herniation.[13] With anular radial fissures, the nucleus, as long as it is mobile, can herniate. The nomenclature describing disc herniations has been confusing, but certain patterns are established (Fig. 30–8). If the nucleus is confined by a few outer

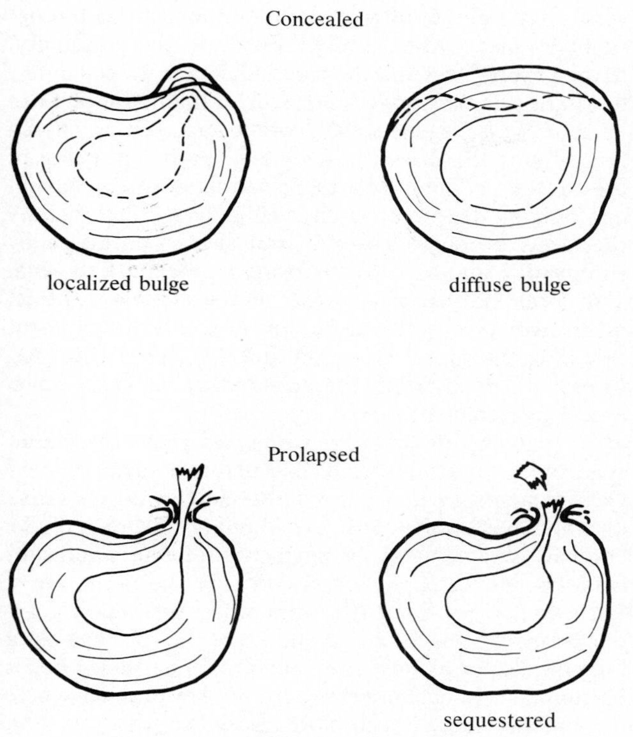


**Figure 30–8.** A classification of disc herniations.

anular fibers so that it does not enter the epidural space, it may present as a concealed disc with a localized or diffuse anular bulge. If the anular fibers are disrupted so that the nucleus leaves the confines of the anulus and enters the epidural space, it is prolapsed. If a piece of herniated material breaks off and is free in the epidural space, it is a sequestered disc or free fragment. The mechanism of root pain is not clear. Originally it was thought to be compression, but root compression is not necessarily found at surgery. All observers agree that involved roots exhibit stages of inflammation and that these inflamed roots will reproduce sciatic symptoms when stimulated. There is biopsy substantiation of intraneural inflammation.[111] Possible mechanisms of neural damage have been reviewed by Murphy.[126]

Symptoms of disc herniation may include backache, backache and sciatica, sciatica, and those of cauda equina compression. The onset is usually sudden and severe. Sciatic symptoms are radicular in nature and are exacerbated by activities such as Valsalva maneuvers and bending, which increase intradiscal pressure. Signs present are those reflecting root tension; these have been outlined previously. The phenomenon of sciatic scoliosis may suggest the relation of the herniation to the root. If the herniation is lateral to the root, the patient leans away from the symptomatic side. He leans toward the symptomatic side if the herniation is medial to the root. The clinical examination is directed toward establishing the diagnosis as accurately as possible. Neurologic symptoms give the correct level only 46 percent of the time,[47] whereas signs raise the accuracy to about 75 percent. Complete loss of a reflex is much more reliable as a diagnostic sign than simple depression.[31] A positive straight leg raising test is 75 to 80 percent diagnostically accurate, with crossed straight leg raising almost pathognomonic for disc herniation. Electromyography raises diagnostic accuracy to 80 percent.[127] Plain radiographs are essentially nondiagnostic. Water-soluble myelography raises accuracy to 90 to 95 percent.

Conservative therapy for disc herniation centers on bed rest, analgesics, muscle relaxants, and anti-inflammatory medications. Pelvic traction may be of benefit in some patients. The degree of bed rest is dependent on the severity of symptoms. Once they abate, a program of exercises and back protection is started. For severe symptoms more enforced bed rest over a 2-week period is used. Most disc herniations respond to conservative therapy, but in those that are unresponsive further measures may be needed.

Chemonucleolysis, the injection of chymopapain into the disc space, is now available in the United States. When previously in use it had about a 75 percent rate of good results, about the same as laminectomy and discectomy.[128] More recent studies indicate an 89 percent good result.[129] It is indicated in patients with a proven disc herniation who would otherwise be surgical candidates. Other techniques available for symptomatic relief are facet blocks[21] and radiofrequency facet denervation.[53] Intrathecal and epidural steroids have had some success in the symptomatic relief of discogenic pain,[130] although some authors find it no better than placebo.[131] Nerve root sleeve infiltrations with steroid may give relief.[124] Intradiscal steroids have been used.[132]

The one indisputable indication for surgery for removal of a disc is the cauda equina syndrome, in which a central midline herniation causes paralysis of the sacral roots, with bladder and bowel dysfunction and inability to walk (see Table 30–2). It occurs in about 2.4 percent of operative disc herniations.[133] The loss of bladder and bowel function is disastrous and return is limited, so that this entity is a true surgical emergency. Perineal anesthesia seldom recovers, and bladder paralysis may have a worse rate of recovery than somatic sensory deficits.[134]

Other indications for laminectomy are marked muscular weakness and progressive neurologic deficit in spite of bed rest.[124,125] There have been studies to dispute these indications as absolute. Andersson and Carlsson[135] found that the time since onset, duration of symptoms, and operative findings have no relationship to the return of motor activity in foot drop secondary to disc herniation. Estimates of motor return after loss from disc herniation are 50[23] to 80[136] percent and are not different in operative compared with nonoperative patients. After 1 year of followup the prognosis of motor return is no better after delayed surgery than with conservative therapy. Immediate surgical treatment is regarded as adequate therapy for the pain of disc herniation, but there is some doubt as to the use of paresis as an indication.[30]

Relative indications for laminectomy are intolerable

pain unrelieved by bed rest and recurrent episodes of incapacitating pain. Laminectomy for definite disc herniation remains a highly successful procedure.[2,68,133] Hirsch and Nachemson[68] reported that if disc herniation is a prolapse, 96 percent of operative patients have improvement. If concealed disc herniation is found with scarring and inflammation the predominant findings, 70 percent of patients have relief regardless of whether or not the disc is removed. Improvement in these patients is a matter of degree, and only 15 percent have complete and permanent relief. The remainder are improved but have recurrent symptoms. About one third will have persistent backache after discectomy.[133] The relationship between complete prolapse and a high degree of relief after surgery has been substantiated in other series.[133] Negative explorations prolong disability.[23] The overall long-term relief of sciatica has been shown to be the same in operative versus nonoperative patients, although the operative patients achieve their degree of relief more rapidly.[23] These studies imply that a relative indication for surgery offering optimal results is the emotionally stable patient with unequivocal disc herniation who for personal and socioeconomic reasons cannot sustain prolonged or repeated bouts of incapacitating pain. The most common cause for surgical failure is poor initial patient selection.[137]

Adhesive radiculitis is a condition in which the nerve root is found to be extensively involved in fibrous tissue in proximity to a disc space. It is presumably the result of chronic inflammation and clinically presents with persistent sciatic pain. Neurolysis is the only treatment, but the results are variable.

The remainder of the lumbar root entrapment syndromes fall into the broad definition of degenerative spinal stenosis. They are predominantly bony entrapments. As these are changes resulting from more advanced disc degeneration, they usually occur in patients over age 50. Prior to this, disc herniation is the common cause of radicular pain, but over age 50 bony entrapment predominates. The entrapment may be more lateral, giving only root symptoms, or more central, giving cauda equina symptoms. Unlike those with disc herniations, patients with these spinal stenosis syndromes have a long history of back pain and more recent sciatica. There is often a claudicating character to the pain, with pain in the back or in the legs with walking. The pain is not relieved by standing still but rather by flexing the back, as in sitting. Therefore these patients can walk up hills more easily than down and can bicycle, but cannot tolerate lumbar extension. These changes are usually progressive. There may be bowel and bladder symptoms, with the latter mimicking prostatic bladder outlet obstruction. These patients do not give marked root tension signs such as straight leg raising and may have multiple levels of root involvement. Radiographs reveal changes of degenerative disc disease with disc height narrowing, facet subluxation and degeneration, retrolisthesis, and pseudospondylolisthesis. The cross section of the spinal canal is difficult to visualize, but can be done with transverse axial tomography,[138] and computed axial tomography[139] has dramatically lessened the difficulty. Myelography[84] reveals the canal diameter. In the anteroposterior dimension it is normally a minimum of 14 to 15 mm.[140,141] Degenerative stenotic changes are noted centrally at the discs, producing hourglass waisting of the contrast column by a thickened ligamentum flavum and bulging degenerative discs (Fig. 30–3). Peripherally the facets produce "cut-off" root sleeves produced by subluxation and osteophyte formation, leading to canal and foraminal encroachment. Water-soluble contrast media will give better definition of lateral entrapment by filling the root sleeve more fully. CT scan (Fig. 30–6) easily demonstrates the entrapment via disc, bone, and ligamentum flavum.

Macnab has described a variety of root entrapment syndromes resulting from degenerative change.[41,76,124] Central stenosis can occur with the bulging degenerative disc and posteriorly with a "shingling" overlap of the laminae, thickening of the ligamentum flavum, and subluxation and osteophyte formation in the facet joints. Subarticular entrapment occurs when the superior articular facet enlarges and compresses the root against a bulging disc or against the dorsum of a vertebral body. Foraminal encroachment occurs in the foramen where the superior facet lies in close relationship to the root. With subluxation and osteophytic outgrowths from the facet and the vertebral body, the root may be entrapped. Pedicular kinking occurs when there is loss of disc height, particularly asymmetrically whereby the root is kinked by the descending pedicle and commonly is entrapped between a bulging disc and a pedicle about it. Extraforaminal entrapment occurs after the root has left the foramen where it may be involved in diffuse or discrete anular bulge and, in the case of L5, trapped by the corporotransverse ligament against the sacral ala.

The treatment of all these spinal stenosis syndromes with severe symptoms is surgical, with emphasis placed on adequate decompression of the entrapped roots.[76,142] Once the symptoms are severe, they tend not to improve. If symptoms are not severe, regimens of back protection, isometric exercises, back supports, and anti-inflammatory medications are used. Operation is withheld until symptoms are no longer tolerable. Neurologic changes are not usually severe enough to warrant surgery. The symptomatic relief offered by adequate surgical decompression is considered particularly good.[142]

**Systemic Inflammatory Disease of the Low Back.** Rheumatoid arthritis is known to involve the lumbar spine. An increased incidence of subluxation and disc narrowing, apophyseal destruction, and osteoporosis was found in rheumatoid patients.[143] Rheumatoid erosions in facet joints have been demonstrated by stereoscopic radiographic examination.[144]

The inflammatory spondyloarthropathies, of which ankylosing spondylitis is the prototype, produce back pain of a diffuse and often severe nature.[145-149] They are discussed in detail in Section VI.

Hyperostotic spondylosis, described by Forestier and

Rotes-Querol,[150] is a disease of new bone formation in the thoracic and thoracolumbar spine. The spine stiffens and spurs form at multiple levels, often forming a bony ankylosis more marked on the right side of the spine. The disc spaces remain intact.[151] There may be subperiosteal new bone formation in the pelvis.[152] The cause is unknown, but there is associated glucose intolerance, diabetes, and obesity.[153]

**Infections.** ***Pyogenic Vertebral Osteomyelitis.*** Hematogenous osteomyelitis has a predilection for the vertebral column,[154,155] and pyogenic vertebral osteomyelitis has a predilection for older adults.[156] This is felt to be secondary to the marked vascularity of adult vertebrae[154] with seeding of the capillary beds at the endplate while the disc has no vascular channels in the adult.[157] An associated causative factor is that the incidence of urinary tract infections rises in adults, and these organisms may be seeded to the vertebrae by Batson's plexus, the vertebral, ascending lumbar, and sacral veins, freely communicating with the external vertebral, internal vertebral, and intraosseous vertebral veins.[158,159] Pyogenic infection then starts in the vertebral body and frequently involves the next body by spread to the epidural space and formation of an abscess, with compression, fracture, and collapse of the involved vertebra and spinal cord vascular compromise. These complications, plus bacteremia, accounted for most of the deaths in the older literature. Mortality now is expected to be less than 10 percent.[160]

*Staphylococcus aureus* traditionally has been the responsible organism, but gram-negative bacilli, especially related to genitourinary manipulations, are increasingly common.[156,161-163]

Patients present with backache of slow onset with or without radicular symptoms, low-grade fever, night sweats, and weight loss.[164] Paravertebral and hamstring spasms are present. Diabetes is frequently associated and should be sought.[155,165] The sedimentation rate is elevated, but the white blood cell count may be normal. Early radiographic signs are an eroded subchondral endplate, followed by involvement of the adjacent vertebra and loss of disc height. There is progressive loss of disc height over 6 to 8 weeks, progressive bony destruction, and reactive bone formation. Serial radiographs help to confirm the diagnosis.[166] Bone scan is useful in early detection. Multiple blood cultures and urine cultures should be obtained to determine the responsible organism. A biopsy for culture, either by closed Craig needle biopsy or open biopsy, is strongly advised, especially if blood cultures are negative. Antibiotics are recommended for 6 weeks[156] with monitoring of blood levels of the appropriate antibiotic to achieve bactericidal levels. The sedimentation rate can be used to follow the disease.[165,167] Bed rest is used during the treatment period, and a plaster jacket is used for 3 months. Fusion occurs in half the patients within 1 year, and most patients obliterate the disc space over 2 years.

***Disc Space Infections.*** Disc space infections can result from any procedure inoculating the disc space. The most common is disc excision, the incidence of which is estimated to be 1 to 2.8 percent.[168,169] The hallmark of the disease is severe, excruciating pain, which may have an onset as late as 3 months postoperatively; in some cases, however, postoperative pain may not disappear but increase. There is marked muscle spasm. Laboratory evidence is not present or is obscured by the recent operation, although an elevated sedimentation rate after operation will normally fall over 3 months. Aspiration biopsy of the disc space is needed to determine the specific organism and its antibiotic sensitivity. Radiographic signs include dissolution of the subchondral bone but lag behind clinical signs by 2 to 3 weeks. There is a progression of loss of disc space height and sclerotic bony reaction.[170] Bone scan is of no diagnostic value because of postoperative changes. The disc space often goes on to fusion when infected.[171] Treatment is with antibiotics and cast immobilization.

Disc space infections in children are different from pyogenic vertebral osteomyelitis and offer a different prognosis.[172] They also differ from adult postoperative disc space infections. An irritable child will have progressive backache or limp, or refuse to walk. Night pain is common. There is paravertebral spasm. Early radiographic findings are absent. Later, progressive loss of disc space height with irregularity of the vertebral endplates is seen. The sedimentation rate is elevated. *Staphylococcus aureus* is the most common organism. Gallium bone scan may be useful for early detection.[54] Treatment is aimed toward 6 to 12 weeks of immobilization in a body jacket or spica cast. Antibiotics are not necessarily indicated and may not affect prognosis. They should be used when pain is not relieved by immobilization, when paravertebral spasm does not subside, or if the sedimentation rate remains elevated and the child is systemically ill. Aspiration biopsy is recommended if there are progressive and prolonged symptoms despite prolonged immobilization.

***Other Infections of the Spine.*** Nontubercular granulomatous infections of the spine are widely reported and have been reviewed by Pritchard.[173] Blastomycosis in the vertebrae infects the disc space, adjacent bodies, and frequently the adjacent ribs. Cryptococcosis of the spine is uncommon and is thought to be hematogenous in origin. It produces little periosteal reaction and has lucent lesions. Actinomycosis may involve the anterior and posterior elements and has a tendency toward paravertebral abscesses. The vertebral body produces a "soap bubble" radiographic appearance, and the disc is spared. Coccidioidomycosis usually causes multiple vertebral lesions with relative sparing of the disc space. Brucellosis has a spondylitic form with involvement of the disc and adjacent vertebra.

Tuberculosis of the spine is now found primarily in third world countries. The spine accounts for about half the cases of bone and joint tuberculosis. There is a predilection for L1 to be the most commonly involved vertebra, and this is thought to be due to invasion by bacteria transported from the urinary tract via Batson's plexus.[174] The vertebral body is invaded and the disc is spared. The symptoms are insidious backache, increasing over many months. Constitutional symptoms can usually be elicited and paravertebral spasm with an acute kyphosis is found on examination. The sedimentation rate is elevated. Radiographs initially reveal osteopenia, followed by erosion on each side of the disc. Collapse follows, producing a variety of radiographic signs described by Hodgson[174] as concertina collapse, aneurysmal syndrome, lateral deviation, bony bridging, reversal of height-width ratio of the body, and wedging of the intervertebral disc. Paraplegia is a relatively frequent complication. Management is with multiple drug therapy; there is debate about the role of surgery and immobilization.[173]

Syphilitic spondylitis is rare,[120] and occurs secondary to gummatous destruction with collapse and a great deal of reactive bone. The more common manifestation is that of destructive change with excessive bony reaction from a Charcot neuropathic arthropathy, usually at the thoracolumbar junction.

Hydatid disease of bone is known but rare. The midthoracic spine is usually involved and the vertebral body is permeated by cysts, which often progress into the spinal canal. Vertebral collapse is common because of pathologic fractures. The incidence of paraplegia is high, as is the mortality.[175]

**Spondylolysis and Spondylolisthesis.** Spondylolisthesis designates a slipping of one vertebra forward on the one below. Spondylolysis indicates a separation at the pars interarticularis, permitting the slipping or "olisthesis." A classification of spondylolysis and spondylolisthesis has been proposed (Table 30–5).[176] Spondylolysis and, more frequently, spondylolisthesis can be involved with back pain. As previously noted, a pars interarticularis defect increases the incidence of back pain.[49] A vertebra may slip forward on the one below as a whole, or it may separate at the isthmus and slip. The entire unit may slip with subluxated posterior facets in degenerative or pseudospondylolisthesis. The slippage is graded either as a percent subluxation or I to IV by quarterly increments of slipping.

In the dysplastic type there is congenital dysplasia of the upper sacrum or the neural arch of L5 and the lowest free lumbar vertebra slips forward, usually in adolescence. The pars may remain unchanged, and the slippage will not exceed 25 percent, preventing cauda equina paralysis. Usually the pars elongates or separates. Dysplastic changes of the upper sacrum with inadequate development of the L5 to S1 facets most commonly produce the instability.[177] The pars is often dysplastic, and the sacrum and L5 may have a wide spina bifida, giving rise to a high-grade slippage. It appears to be twice as common in girls as in boys.[176]

Isthmic spondylolisthesis involves a lesion in the pars interarticularis. The lytic lesion is a separation of the pars and is a fatigue fracture.[178] It is the most common type in patients less than 50 years old and is rarely seen in those less than 5 years old. The incidence in white children is 5 percent at 7 years and increases to 5.8 percent by 18 years old, mostly during the 11- to 15-year-old period.[176] There is a hereditary component,[179] the incidence increasing to 35 percent in families in which one member has spondylolysis or spondylolisthesis. Female gymnasts have been noted to have a fourfold increase in pars defects and spondylolisthesis,[180] and football interior linemen have an even higher incidence over the normal population.[181] Of the mechanical forces involved—flexion overload, unbalanced shear forces, and forced rotation—it is not yet known[182,183] which is primarily responsible for the slippage.

Elongation of the pars without separation is the same disease as the lytic lesion, but with repeated microfractures healing in an elongated position. The pars may taper out and then separate, in which case the defect is reclassified as lytic. Acute pars fractures are secondary to trauma and usually have only spondylolysis without slippage.

Degenerative spondylolisthesis is secondary to degenerative disc disease, with intersegmental instability[81,120] producing a local spinal stenosis. It is seldom seen before the age of 50, is ten times more frequent at L4 than at L5 or L3, is six times more frequent in women, and is three times more frequent in blacks. Sacralization is four times more frequent in degenerative spondylolisthesis as in the general population. It does not occur with spina bifida or isthmic spondylolisthesis, and the slippage is never more than 30 percent. Predisposing factors are a straight, stable lumbosacral joint putting more stress on the L4-5 facets. The disc and ligaments degenerate and allow hypermobility and facet degeneration, permitting forward slipping.[184]

Traumatic spondylolisthesis is secondary to a fracture in the posterior elements other than the pars such as a facet or pedicle.[176]

Pathological spondylolisthesis is due to a local or generalized bone disease in the pedicle, pars, or facets, where the forward forces are inadequately opposed and forward slippage results. It is known in osteopetrosis with pars fractures giving spondylolysis, arthrogryposis in Eskimos,[185] Paget's disease with pars elongation, syphilis secondary to gummas,[186] neurogenic arthropathies, tuberculous spondylitis, giant cell tumors of the posterior elements, and metastatic tumors.[177] Spondylolysis and spondylolisthesis aquisita are known to occur at the upper end of lumbar spine fusions[187-192] and are reported below a thoracolumbar scoliosis fusion.[193]

**Table 30–5.** Classification of Spondylolysis and Spondylolisthesis

| |
|---|
| Dysplastic—congenital abnormalities of the upper sacrum or the arch of L5 allow the olisthesis |
| Isthmic—a pars interarticularis lesion of one of three types: |
| Lytic—fatigue fracture of the pars |
| Elongated, but intact pars |
| Acute fracture |
| Degenerative—secondary to longstanding intervertebral instability |
| Traumatic—secondary to bony fractures in areas other than the pars |
| Pathological—secondary to generalized or local bone disease |

These are complications and are not seen with lateral fusions.[176]

Management of spondylolisthesis is age and lesion dependent. Wiltse and Jackson[194] have provided guidelines for the management of children with spondylolisthesis. A child, especially if less than 10 years old, who is found to have an isthmic spondylolisthesis is examined, and radiographs obtained, every 4 months for a year, then every 6 months up to the age of 15, then annually until growth is completed. This is especially important in girls, who have twice the incidence of high-grade olisthesis (slippage). In cases with up to 25 percent slippage and without symptoms, the child is followed and advised to avoid a career of heavy labor. In those with up to 50 percent slippage without symptoms, avoidance of traumatic sports is recommended. Those children with symptoms but recovery by conservative measures are followed. In a child with greater than 50 percent slippage, fusion is recommended regardless of symptoms. A child with persistent symptoms regardless of degree of slippage is advised to undergo fusion. A child less than 10 years old with a 50 percent slippage is often fused. Slippage will usually occur before 18 years of age if it is going to occur and rarely past 25 years of age. The most rapid slippage is between 9 and 15 years of age.[195] The onset of pain may be sudden and produce a "listhetic crisis" with the sudden onset of backache. On examination, a rigid lumbar spine, spastic scoliosis, flattened sacrum, and often hamstring spasm are found. There is usually no nerve root involvement; but if such involvement is present, laminectomy and possibly decompression will be required in addition to lumbosacral fusion.[124]

The presence of a pars defect does not mean that it is always the cause of back pain. Macnab[124] examined a large series of patients with backache and found a 7.6 percent incidence of pars defects, similar to the overall incidence in asymptomatic individuals. Dividing these patients by age, he showed that for those over 40 years of age the incidence is the same as in the general population. Under 26, however, about 19 percent of symptomatic individuals had a defect. Therefore if the patient is younger than 26, the defect is probably the cause of the back pain. Between ages 26 and 40 it is possibly the cause. Over age 40 it is rarely the cause.

Root irritation can occur with lytic spondylolisthesis by a variety of mechanisms. The neural arch of L5 may rotate forward on the sacrum and encroach on the foramen. Small ossicles and traction spurs make foraminal encroachment worse. Bony entrapment, described by Macnab,[124] occurs with forward and downward descent. The pedicles may kink the roots. Disc degeneration with bulging may cause entrapment lateral to the foramen. The corporotransverse ligament of L5 may compress the L5 root against the sacral ala with descent of L5. Disc herniation of L4-5 may involve the L5 root. Disc degeneration itself may be painful, and in patients over 35 lumbodorsal disc degeneration may be symptomatic.[124] Therefore clinical evaluation with myelography and root sleeve injection is necessary in the older patient with back pain and spondylolisthesis. Foramenotomy may be necessary with fusion if there is a long history of backache. In this case discography is used to determine the upper extent of the fusion. If there is L4-5 degeneration or the slip is greater than 50 percent, an L4-S1 fusion is indicated.

In adults older than 40 with painful spondylolisthesis, the Gill procedure of removal of the loose posterior elements has been successful.[196] In adults without evidence of root entrapment and minimal slip, Newman[197] recommends direct repair of the defect.

Degenerative spondylolisthesis is a form of local spinal stenosis and a result of disc degeneration. It produces root entrapment and cauda equina symptoms with back pain, sciatic symptoms, and occasionally spinal claudication symptoms. Ten percent of Rosenberg's series[184] came to decompression. The question of fusion is unresolved. Guidelines of management are essentially those for degenerative disc disease and spinal stenosis.

**Nonspinal Sources of Back Pain.** Back pain can occur from disorders of the abdominal, retroperitoneal, and pelvic viscera, but it is rarely the only symptom. Pain is referred in a dermatomal distribution from viscera and is not aggravated by activity or relieved by rest, as is most pain of spinal origin. Peptic ulcer disease, gastric, duodenal, and pancreatic tumors, retroperitoneal lymphoma, sarcoma, and colonic tumors can all give rise to back pain. Retroperitoneal bleeding in anticoagulated patients can give back pain. In the pelvis, endometriosis and uterine, cervical, and bladder invasive carcinoma may give back pain, and tumors invading the lumbosacral plexus give rise to radicular pain. Sacral menstrual pain occurs, and uterine malposition and prolapse can give rise to sacral pain with standing. Fibroids may cause back pain. Chronic prostatitis can give sacral pain. Renal pain is located in the costovertebral angle and frequently radiates to the groin and testis.

Abdominal aortic aneurysm may give rise to back pain, which is particularly acute during dissection. Intermittent claudication of peripheral vascular disease may mimic sciatic pain and can be confused with spinal stenosis, but can be differentiated by the relief of vascular claudication pain on standing still.

## References


1. Horal, J.: The clinical appearance of low back disorders in the city of Gothenburg, Sweden. Acta Orthop. Scand. Suppl. 118, 1969.
2. Hirsch, C.: Efficiency of surgery in low-back disorders. J. Bone Joint Surg. 47A:991, 1965.
3. Kelsey, J.L., and White, A.A.: Epidemiology and impact of low back pain. Spine 5:133, 1980.
4. Wood, P.H.N., and MacLeish, C.L.: Digest of data on the rheumatic diseases. 5. Morbidity in industry and rheumatism in general practice. Ann. Rheum. Dis. 33:93, 1974.
5. Hult, L.: The Munk Fors investigation. Acta Orthop. Scand. Suppl. 16, 1954.
6. Anderson, J.A.D.: Back pain in industry. *In* Jayson, M. (ed.): The Lumbar Spine and Back Pain. London, Sector Publishing, Ltd., 1976.
7. Glover, J.R.: Prevention of back pain. *In* Jayson, M. (ed.): The Lumbar Spine and Back Pain. London, Sector Publishing, Ltd., 1976.
8. Berquist-Ullman, M., and Larsson, U.: Acute low back pain in industry. Acta Orthop. Scand. Suppl. 170, 1977.
9. Wood, P.H.N.: Epidemiology of back pain. *In* Jayson, M. (ed.): The Lumbar Spine and Back Pain. London, Sector Publishing, Ltd., 1976.

10. Benn, R.T., and Wood, P.H.N.: Pain in the back: An attempt to estimate the size of the problem. Rheum. Rehab. 14:121, 1975.
11. Frymoyer, J.W., Pope, M.H., Cogtanza, M.C., Rosa, J.C., Goggin, J.E., and Wilder, D.G.: Epidemiologic studies of low back pain. Spine 5:419, 1980.
12. Akeson, W.H., and Murphy, R.W.: Low back pain. Clin. Orthop. 129:2, 1977.
13. Mixter, W.J., and Barr, J.S.: Rupture of the intervertebral disc with involvement of the spinal canal: N. Engl. J. Med. 211:210, 1934.
14. Hirsch, C.: Etiology and pathogenesis of low back pain. Israel J. Med. Sci. 2:362, 1966.
15. Kelsey, J.L.: An epidemiological study of acutely herniated lumbar intervertebral discs. Rheum. Rehab. 14:144, 1975.
16. Edgar, M.A., and Ghadially, J.A.: Innervation of the lumbar spine. Clin. Orthop. 115:35, 1976.
17. Luschka, H.: Die Nerven des menschlichen Wibelkanales. Verlag der H. Lappschen Buchhandelung P. V. 4850:8:1, 1850.
18. Smyth, M.J., and Wright, V.J.: Sciatica and the intervertebral disk. An experimental study. J. Bone Joint Surg. 40A:1401, 1958.
19. Kellgren, J.H.: Observations on referred pain arising from muscle. Clin. Sci. 3:175, 1938.
20. Hirsch, C., Ingelmark, B., and Miller, M.: The anatomical basis for low back pain. Acta Orthop. Scand. 33:1, 1963.
21. Mooney, V., and Robertson, J.: The facet syndrome. Clin. Orthop. 115:149, 1976.
22. Nachemson, A.L.: The natural course of low back pain. *In* White, A.A. and Gordon, S.L. (eds.): A.A.O.S. Symposium on Idiopathic Low Back Pain. St. Louis, C. V. Mosby Company, 1982, p. 46.
23. Hakelius, A.: Long term follow-up in sciatica. Acta Orthop. Scand. Suppl. 129, 1972.
24. Mankin, H.J., and Adams, R.D.: Pain in the back and neck. *In* Thorn, G.W., Adams, R.D., Braunwald, E., Isselbacher, K.J., and Petersdorf, R.G. (eds.): Harrison's Principles of Internal Medicine. 8th ed. New York, McGraw-Hill Book Company, 1977.
25. Macnab, I.: The "whiplash syndrome." Orthop. Clin. North Am. 2:389, 1971.
26. Wilfling, F.J., Klonoff, H., and Kokan, P.: Psychological, demographic and orthopaedic factors associated with prediction of outcome of spinal fusion. Clin. Orthop. 90:153, 1973.
27. White, A.W.M.: The compensation back. Applied Therap. 8:871, 1966.
28. Wiltse, L.L., and Rocchio, P.D.: Preoperative psychologic tests as predictors of success of chemonucleolysis in the treatment of low-back syndrome. J. Bone Joint Surg. 57A:478, 1975.
29. Rothman, R.H., and Simeone, F.A.: Lumbar disc disease. *In* Rothman, R.H., and Simeone, F.A. (eds.): The Spine. Philadelphia, W. B. Saunders Company, 1975.
30. Weber, H.: The effect of delayed disc surgery on muscular paresis. Acta Orthop. Scand. 46:631, 1975.
31. Hakelius, A., and Hindmarsh, J.: The significance of neurologic signs and myelographic findings in the diagnosis of lumbar root compression. Acta Orthop. Scand. 43:239, 1972.
32. Sprangfort, E.: Lasegue's sign in patients with lumbar disc herniation. Acta Orthop. Scand. 42:459, 1971.
33. Hoppenfeld, S.: Physical Examination of the Spine and Extremities. New York, Appleton-Century Crofts, 1976.
34. Finneson, B.E.: Low Back Pain. Philadelphia, J. B. Lippincott Company, 1973.
35. Wiltse, L.L.: Lumbosacral strain and instability. *In* American Academy of Orthopedic Surgeons: Symposium on the Spine. St. Louis, C. V. Mosby Company, 1969.
36. Caldwell, A.B., and Chase, C.: Diagnosis and treatment of personality factors in low back pain. Clin. Orthop. 129:141, 1977.
37. Ransford, A.O., Cairns, D., and Mooney, V.: The pain drawing as an aid to the psychologic evaluation of patients with low back pain. Spine 1:127, 1976.
38. Sternbach, R.A.: Psychologic aspects of chronic pain. Clin. Orthop. 129:150, 1977.
39. Fordyce, W.E., Fowler, R.S., Lehman, J.F., DeLateur, B.J., Sand, P.L., and Trieschmann, R.B.: Operant conditioning in the treatment of chronic pain. Arch. Phys. Med. Rehab. 54:399, 1973.
40. Anderson, T.P., Cole, T.M., Gullickson, G., Hudgens, A., and Roberts, A.H.: Behavior modification of chronic pain: A treatment program by a multidisciplinary team. Clin. Orthop. 129:97, 1977.
41. Macnab, I.: Surgical treatment of degenerative disc disease of the lumbar spine. *In* McKibbin, B. (ed.): Recent Advances in Orthopaedics. Edinburgh, Churchill Livingstone, 1975.
42. Park, W.: Radiological investigation of the intervertebral disc. *In* Jayson, M. (ed.): The Lumbar Spine and Back Pain. London, Sector Publishing, Ltd., 1976.
43. Liang, M., and Komaroff, A.L.: Roentgenograms in primary care patients with acute low back pain. A cost-effective analysis. Arch. Intern. Med. 142:1108, 1982.
44. Harris, R.I., and Macnab, I.: Structural changes in the lumbar intervertebral discs. Their relationship to low back pain and sciatica. J. Bone Joint Surg. 36B:304, 1954.
45. Edeiken, J., and Pitt, M.J.: The radiologic diagnosis of disc disease. Orthop. Clin. North Am. 2:405, 1971.
46. Lawrence, J.S.: Disc degeneration. Its frequency and relationship to symptoms. Ann. Rheum. Dis. 28:121, 1969.
47. Hakelius, A., and Hindmarsh, J.: The comparative reliability of preoperative diagnostic methods in lumbar disc surgery. Acta Orthop. Scand. 43:234, 1972.
48. Epstein, B.: The Spine. A Radiological Text and Atlas. 3rd ed. Philadelphia, Lea & Febiger, 1969.
49. Wiltse, L.L.: The effect of common anomalies of the lumbar spine upon disc degeneration and low back pain. Orthop. Clin. North Am. 2:569, 1971.
50. Farfan, H.F., and Sullivan, J.D.: The relation of facet orientation to intervertebral disc failure. Can. J. Surg. 10:179, 1967.
51. Collis, D.K., and Ponseti, I.V.: Long term followup of patients with idiopathic scoliosis not treated surgically. J. Bone Joint Surg. 51A:425, 1969.
52. Roche, M.B., and Rowe, G.G.: The incidence of separate neural arch and coincident bone variations. Anat. Rec. 109:233, 1951.
53. Shealy, C.N.: Facet denervation in the management of back and sciatic pain. Clin. Orthop. 115:157, 1976.
54. Norris, S.H., Ehrlich, M.G., McKusick, K., and Provine, H.: The radioisotope study of an experimental model of disc space infection. J. Bone Joint Surg. 60B:281, 1978.
55. Lindblom, K.: Diagnostic puncture of intervertebral discs in sciatica. Acta Orthop. Scand. 7:321, 1948.
56. Cloward, R.B., and Buzaid, L.L.: Discography technique—indications and evaluation of normal and abnormal intervertebral disc. Am. J. Roentgenol. 68:552, 1952.
57. Collis, J.S., and Gardner, W.J.: Lumbar discography—an analysis of 1000 cases. J. Neurosurg. 19:452, 1962.
58. Massie, W.K., and Stevens, D.B.: A critical evaluation of discography. J. Bone Joint Surg. 49A:1243, 1967.
59. Wiley, J.J., Macnab, I., and Wortzman, G.: Lumbar discography and its applications. Can. J. Surg. 11:280, 1968.
60. Garrick, J.G., and Sullivan, C.R.: Long-term effects of diskography in dogs. Minn. Med. 53:81, 1970.
61. Key, J.A., and Ford, L.T.: Experimental intervertebral disc lesions. J. Bone Joint Surg. 30A:621, 1948.
62. Goldie, I.: Intervertebral disc changes after discography. Acta Chir. Scand. 113:438, 1957.
63. DeSeze, S., and Levernieux, J.: Accidents in discography. Rev. Rheum. 19:1027, 1952.
64. Gresham, J.L., and Miller, R.: Evaluation of the lumbar spine by diskography and its use in selection of proper treatment of the herniated disk syndrome. Clin. Orthop. 67:29, 1969.
65. Holt, E.P.: The question of lumbar discography. J. Bone Joint Surg. 50A:720, 1968.
66. Friberg, S., and Hult, L.: Comparative study of Abrodil myelogram and operative findings in low back pain and sciatica. Acta Orthop. Scand. 20:303, 1951.
67. Luyendijk, W., and Van Voorthuisen, A.E.: Contrast examination of the spinal epidural space. Acta Radiol. Scand. 5:1051, 1966.
68. Hirsch, C., and Nachemson, A.: The reliability of lumbar disc surgery. Clin. Orthop. 29:189, 1963.
69. Post, M.J.D., Brown, M.D., and Gargano, F.P.: The technique and interpretation of lumbar myelograms. Spine 2:214, 1977.
70. McNeill, T.W., Huncke, B., Kornblatt, I., Stiehl, J., and Kahn, H.A.:A new advance in water-soluble myelography. Spine 1:72, 1976.
71. Nachemson, A.: The lumbar spine. An orthopaedic challenge. Spine 1:59, 1976.
72. Macnab, I., St. Louis, E.L., Grabias, S.L., and Jacob, R.: Selective ascending lumbosacral venography in the assessment of lumbar-disc herniation. J. Bone Joint Surg. 58A:1093, 1976.
73. Hitselberger, W.A., and Witten, R.M.: Abnormal myelograms in asymptomatic patients. J. Neurosurg. 32:132, 1970.
74. Mathews, J.A.: Epidurography—a technique for diagnosis and research. *In* Jayson, M. (ed.): The Lumbar Spine and Back Pain. London, Sector Publishing, Ltd., 1976.
75. Arnoldi, C.C., Brodsky, A.E., Cauchoix, J., Crock, H.V., Dommisse, G.F., Edgar, M.A., Gargano, F.P., Jacobson, R.E., Kirkaldy-Willis, W.H., Kurihara, A., Langerskjold, A., Macnab, I., McIvor, G.W.D., Newman, P.H., Paine, K.W.E., Russin, L.A., Sheldon, J., Tile, M., Urist, M.R., Wilson, W.E., and Wiltse, L.L.: Lumbar spinal stenosis and nerve root entrapment syndrome. Definition and classification. Clin. Orthop. 115:4, 1976.
76. Macnab, I.: Negative disc exploration. An analysis of causes of nerve-root involvement in sixty-eight patients. J. Bone Joint Surg. 53A:891, 1971.

77. Verbeist, H.: A radicular syndrome from developmental narrowing of the lumbar vertebral canal. J. Bone Joint Surg. 36B:230, 1954.
78. Verbeist, H.: Further experiences on the pathological influence on the developmental narrowness of the lumbar vertebral canal. J. Bone Joint Surg. 37B:576, 1955.
79. Kirkaldy-Willis, W.H., Paine, K.W.E., Cauchoix, J., and McIvor, G.W.D.: Lumbar spinal stenosis. Clin. Orthop. 99:30, 1974.
80. Schatzker, J., and Pennal, G.F.: Spinal stenosis. A cause of cauda equina compression. J. Bone Joint Surg. 50B:606, 1968.
81. Macnab, I.: Spondylolisthesis with an intact neural arch. The so-called pseudospondylolisthesis. J. Bone Joint Surg. 32B:325, 1950.
82. Schlesinger, E.B., and Taveres, J.M.: Factors in the production of "cauda equina" syndromes in lumbar discs. Trans. Am. Neurol. Assoc. 78:263, 1953.
83. Lipson, S.J., Naheedy, M.H., Kaplan, M.M., and Bienfang, D.C.: Spinal stenosis caused by epidural lipomatosis in Cushing's syndrome. N. Engl. J. Med. 302:36, 1980.
84. McIvor, G.W.D., and Kirkaldy-Willis, W.H.: Pathologic and myelographic changes in the major types of lumbar spinal stenosis. Clin. Orthop. 115:72, 1976.
85. Coventry, M.B., Ghormley, R.K., and Kernohan, J.W.: The intervertebral disc: Its microscopic anatomy and pathology. Part II. Changes in the intervertebral disc concomitant with age. J. Bone Joint Surg. 27A:233, 1945.
86. Coventry, M.B., Ghormley, R.I., and Kernohan, J.W.: The intervertebral disc: Its microscopic anatomy and pathology. Part III. Pathological changes in the intervertebral disc. J. Bone Joint Surg. 27A:460, 1945.
87. Eckert, C., and Decker, A.: Pathological studies of intervertebral discs. J. Bone Joint Surg. 29A:447, 1947.
88. Naylor, A.: Intervertebral disc prolapse and degeneration. The biochemical and biophysical approach. Spine 1:108, 1976.
89. Bushell, G.R., Ghosh, P., Taylor, T.K.F., and Akeson, W.H.: Proteoglycan chemistry of the intervertebral disks. Clin. Orthop. 129:115, 1977.
90. Ghosh, P., Bushell, G.R., Taylor, T.K.F., and Akeson, W.H.: Collagens, elastin and noncollagenous protein of the intervertebral disk. Clin. Orthop. 129:124, 1977.
91. Eyre, D.R., and Muir, H.: Collagen polymorphism: Two molecular species in pig intervertebral disc. FEBS Letters 42:192, 1974.
92. Eyre, D.R., and Muir, H.: Types I and II collagens in intervertebral disc. Interchanging radial distributions in annulus fibrosus. Biochem. J. 157:267, 1976.
93. Herbert, C.M., Lindberg, K.A., Jayson, M.I.V., and Bailey, A.J.: Intervertebral disc collagen in degenerative disc disease. Ann. Rheum. Dis. 34:467, 1975.
94. Naylor, A., Shentall, R.D., and Micklethwaite, B.: An electron microscopic study of segment long spacing collagen from the intervertebral disc. Orthop. Clin. North Am. 8:217, 1977.
95. Herbert, C.M., Lindberg, K.A., Jayson, M.I.V., and Bailey, A.J.: Changes in collagen of human intervertebral disks during aging and degenerative disk disease. J. Molec. Med. 1:79, 1975.
96. Pearson, C.H., Happey, F., Naylor, A., and Turner, R.L.: Collagens and associated glycoproteins in the human intervertebral disk. Variations in sugar and amino acid composition in relation to location and age. Ann. Rheum. Dis. 31:45, 1972.
97. Blakely, P.R., Happey, F., Naylor, A., and Turner, R.L.: Protein in the nucleus pulposus of the intervertebral disk. Nature 195:73, 1962.
98. Gower, W.E., and Pedrini, V.: Age-related variations in proteinpolysaccharides from human nucleus pulposus, annulus fibrosus and costal cartilage. J. Bone Joint Surg. 51A:1154, 1969.
99. Adams, P., and Muir, H.: Qualitative changes with age of proteoglycans of human lumbar discs. Ann. Rheum. Dis. 35:289, 1976.
100. Hardingham, T.E., and Adams, P.: A method for the determination of hyaluronate in the presence of other glycosaminoglycans and its application to human intervertebral disc. Biochem. J. 159:143, 1976.
101. Stevens, R.L., Ewins, R.J.F., and Muir, H.: Proteoglycans of the intervertebral disc: Homology of structure with laryngeal proteoglycans. Biochem. J. 179:561, 1979.
102. Comper, W.D., and Preston, B.N.: Model connective tissue systems. A study of polyion-mobile ion and of excluded volume interactions of proteoglycans. Biochem. J. 143:1, 1974.
103. Bobechko, W.P., and Hirsch, C.: Autoimmune response to nucleus pulposus in the rabbit. J. Bone Joint Surg. 47B:574, 1965.
104. Naylor, A., Happey, F., Turner, R.L., Shentall, R.D., West, D.C., and Richardson, C.: Enzymic and immunological activity in the intervertebral disc. Orthop. Clin. North Am. 6:51, 1975.
105. Gertzbein, S.D., Tile, M., Gross, A., and Falk, R.: Autoimmunity in degenerative disc disease of the lumbar spine. Orthop. Clin. North Am. 6:67, 1975.
106. Elves, M.W., Bucknill, T., and Sullivan, M.F.: In vitro inhibition of leucocyte migration in patients with intervertebral disc lesions. Orthop. Clin. North Am. 6:59, 1975.
107. Gertzbein, S.D., Tait, J.H., and Devlin, S.R.: The stimulation of lymphocytes by nucleus pulposus in patients with degenerative disc disease of the lumbar spine. Clin. Orthop. 123:149, 1977.
108. Bisla, R.S., Marchisello, P.J., Lockshin, M.D., Hart D.M., Marcus, R.E., and Granda, J.: Autoimmunological basis of disk degeneration. Clin. Orthop. 121:206, 1976.
109. Lindblom, K., and Hultqvist, G.: Absorption of protruded disc tissue. J. Bone Joint Surg. 32A:557, 1950.
110. Smith, J.W., and Walmsley, R.: Experimental incision of the intervertebral disc. J. Bone Joint Surg. 33B:612, 1951.
111. Lindahl, O., and Rexed, G.: Histologic changes in spinal nerve roots of operated cases of sciatica. Acta Orthop. Scand. 20:215, 1951.
112. Nachemson, A.: Intradiscal measurements of pH in patients with lumbar rhizopathies. Acta Orthop. Scand. 40:23, 1969.
113. Diamant, B., Karlsson, J., and Nachemson, A.: Correlation between lactate levels and pH in discs of patients with lumbar rhizopathies. Experientia 24:1195, 1968.
114. Nachemson, A., Lewin, T., Maroudas, A., and Freeman, M.A.R.: In vitro diffusion of dye through endplates in the annulus fibrosus of human lumbar intervertebral disks. Acta Orthop. Scand. 41:589, 1970.
115. Maroudas, A., Stockwell, R.A., Nachemson, A., and Urban, J.: Factors involved in the nutrition of human lumbar intervertebral disk: Cellularity and diffusion of glucose in vitro. J. Anat. 120:113, 1975.
116. Urban, J.P.G., Holm, S., Maroudas, A., and Nachemson, A.: Nutrition of the intervertebral disk. An in vivo study of solute transport. Clin. Orthop. 129:101, 1977.
117. Olsson, S.E.: On disc protrusion in dog. Acta Orthop. Scand. Suppl. 8, 1951.
118. Hansen, H.J.: Comparative views on the pathology of disk degeneration in animals. Lab. Invest. 8:1242, 1959.
119. Rolander, S.D., and Blair, W.E.: Deformation and fracture of the lumbar vertebral endplate. Orthop. Clin. North Am. 6:75, 1975.
120. Junghanns, H., and Schmorl, G.: The Human Spine in Health and Disease. New York, Grune & Stratton, 1959.
121. Farfan, H.E.: A reorientation in the surgical approach to degenerative lumbar intervertebral joint disease. Orthop. Clin. North Am. 8:9, 1977.
122. Akeson, W.H., Woo, S.L.Y., Taylor, T.K.F., Ghosh, P., and Bushell, G.R.: Biomechanics and biochemistry of the intervertebral disks: The need for correlation studies. Clin. Orthop. 129:133, 1977.
123. Wiesel, J.W., Cuckler, J.M., DeLuca, F., James, F., Zeide, M.S., and Rothman, R.H.: Acute low back pain. An objective analysis of conservative therapy. Spine 5:324, 1980.
124. Macnab, I.: Backache. Baltimore, Williams & Wilkins Company, 1977.
125. Wiltse, L.L.: Surgery for intervertebral disk disease of the lumbar spine. Clin. Orthop. 129:22, 1977.
126. Murphy, R.W.: Nerve roots and spinal nerves in degenerative disk disease. Clin. Orthop. 129:47, 1977.
127. Knuttson, B.: Comparative value of electromyographic, myelographic and clinical neurological examination in diagnosis of lumbar root compression syndrome. Acta Orthop. Scand. Suppl. 49, 1961.
128. Nordby, E.J., and Brown, M.D.: Present status of chymopapain and chemonucleolysis. Clin. Orthop. 129:79, 1977.
129. McCulloch, J.A.: Chemonucleolysis: Experience with 2000 cases. Clin. Orthop. 146:128, 1980.
130. Brown, F.W.: Management of diskogenic pain using epidural and intrathecal steroids. Clin. Orthop. 129:72, 1977.
131. Snoek, W., Weber, H., and Jorgensen, B.: Double blind evaluation of extradural methylprednisolone for herniated lumbar discs. Acta Orthop. Scand. 48:635, 1977.
132. Feffer, H.L.: Therapeutic intradiscal hydrocortisone. A long term study. Clin. Orthop. 67:100, 1969.
133. Spangfort, E.V.: The lumbar disc herniation. A computer aided analysis of 2,504 operations. Acta Orthop. Scand. Suppl. 142, 1972.
134. Scott, R.J.: Bladder paralysis in cauda equina lesions from disc prolapse. J. Bone Joint Surg. 47B:224, 1965.
135. Andersson, H., and Carlsson, C.A.: Prognosis of operatively treated lumbar disc herniation causing foot extensor paralysis. Acta Chir. Scand. 132:501, 1966.
136. Weber, H.: An evaluation of conservative and surgical treatment of lumbar disc protrusion. J. Oslo City Hosp. 20:81, 1970.
137. Spengler, D.M., Freeman, C., Westbrook, R., and Miller, J.W.: Low back pain following multiple spine procedures. Failure of initial selection? Spine 5:356, 1980.
138. Sheldon, J.J., Russin, L.A., and Gargano, F.P.: Lumbar spinal stenosis. Radiographic diagnosis with special reference to transverse axial tomography. Clin. Orthop. 115:53, 1976.
139. Hammerschlag, S.B., Wolpert, S.M., and Carter, B.L.: Computed tomography of the spinal canal. Radiology 121:361, 1976.
140. Eisenstein, S.: Measurements of the lumbar spinal canal in 2 racial groups. Clin. Orthop. 115:53, 1976.
141. Paine, K.W.E., and Huang, P.W.H.: Lumbar disc syndrome. J. Neurosurg. 37:75, 1972.

142. Wiltse, L.L., Kirkaldy-Willis, W.H., and McIvor, G.W.D.: The treatment of spinal stenosis. Clin. Orthop. 115:83, 1976.
143. Lawrence, J.S., Sharp, J., Ball, J., and Bier, F.: Rheumatoid arthritis of the lumbar spine. Ann. Rheum. Dis. 23:205, 1964.
144. Sims-Williams, H., Jayson, M.I.V., and Baddeley, H.: Rheumatoid involvement of the lumbar spine. Ann. Rheum. Dis. 36:524, 1977.
145. West, H.F.: The aetiology of ankylosing spondylitis. Ann. Rheum. Dis. 8:143, 1949.
146. Lawrence, J.S.: The prevalence of arthritis. Br. J. Clin. Pract. 17:699, 1963.
147. deBlecourt, J.J., and deBlecourt-Meindersma, T.: Hereditary factors in rheumatoid arthritis and ankylosing spondylitis. Ann. Rheum. Dis. 20:215, 1961.
148. Schlosstein, L., Terasaki, P.I., Bluestone, R., and Pearson, C.M.: High association of HL-A antigen W27 with ankylosing spondylitis. N. Engl. J. Med. 288:704, 1973.
149. Brewerton, D.A., Caffrey, M., Hart, F.D., James, D.C.O., Nicholls, A., and Sturrock, R.D.: Ankylosing spondylitis and HL-A-27. Lancet 1:904, 1973.
150. Forestier, J., and Rotes-Querol, J.: Senile ankylosing hyperostosis of the spine. Ann. Rheum. Dis. 9:321, 1950.
151. Vernon-Roberts, B., Pirie, C.J., and Trenwith, V.: Pathology of the dorsal spine in ankylosing hyperostosis. Ann. Rheum. Dis. 33:281, 1974.
152. Harris, J., Carter, A.R., Glick, R.N., and Storey, G.O.: Ankylosing hyperostosis: Clinical and radiological features. Ann. Rheum. Dis. 33:210, 1974.
153. Julkunen, H., Heinonen, O.P., and Pyorala, K.: Hyperostosis of the spine in an adult population. Its relation to hyperglycemia and obesity. Ann. Rheum. Dis. 30:605, 1971.
154. Wiley, A.M., and Trueta, J.: The vascular anatomy of the spine and its relation to pyogenic vertebral osteomyelitis. J. Bone Joint Surg. 41B:796, 1959.
155. Stone, D.B., and Bonfiglio, M.: Pyogenic vertebral osteomyelitis: A diagnostic pitfall for the internist. Arch. Intern. Med. 112:491, 1963.
156. Waldvogel, F.A., Medoff, G., and Swartz, M.N.: Osteomyelitis: A review of clinical features, therapeutic considerations and unusual aspects (third of three parts). N. Engl. J. Med. 282:316, 1970.
157. Crock, H.V., Yoshzava, H., and Kame, S.K.: Observations on the venous drainage of the human vertebral body. J. Bone Joint Surg. 55B:528, 1973.
158. Batson, O.V.: The function of the vertebral veins and their role in the spread of metastasis. Ann. Surg. 112:138, 1940.
159. Batson, O.V.: The vertebral vein system. Am. J. Roentgenol. 78:195, 1957.
160. Musher, D.M., Thorsteinsson, S.B., Minuth, J.N., and Luchi, R.J.: Vertebral osteomyelitis: Still a diagnostic pitfall. Arch. Intern. Med. 136:105, 1976.
161. Stauffer, R.N.: Pyogenic vertebral osteomyelitis. Orthop. Clin. North Am. 6:1015, 1975.
162. Wedge, J.H., Onyschak, A.F., Robertson, D.E., and Kirkaldy-Willis, W.H.: Atypical manifestations of spinal infections. Clin. Orthop. 123:155, 1977.
163. Ross, P.M., and Fleming J.L.: Vertebral body osteomyelitis: Spectrum and natural history. Clin. Orthop. 118:190, 1976.
164. Bonfiglio, M., Lange, T.A., and Kim, Y.M.: Pyogenic vertebral osteomyelitis. Clin. Orthop. 96:234, 1973.
165. Garcia, A., and Grantham, S.A.: Hematogenous pyogenic vertebral osteomyelitis. J. Bone Joint Surg. 42A:429, 1960.
166. Guri, J.P.: Pyogenic osteomyelitis of the spine. Differential diagnosis through clinical and roentgenographic observations. J. Bone Joint Surg. 28A:29, 1946.
167. Griffiths, H.E.D., and Jones, D.M.: Pyogenic infection of the spine. J. Bone Joint Surg. 53B:383, 1971.
168. Ford, L.T., and Key, J.A.: Postoperative infection of the intervertebral disc space. South. Med. J. 48:1295, 1955.
169. Pilgaard, S.: Discitis (closed space infection) following removal of lumbar intervertebral disc. J. Bone Joint Surg. 51A: 713, 1969.
170. Thibodeau, A.A.: Closed space infection following removal of lumbar intervertebral disc. J. Bone Joint Surg. 50A:400, 1968.
171. Sullivan, C.R., Bickel, W.H., and Svien, H.J.: Infections of vertebral interspaces after operations on the intervertebral disks. JAMA 166:1973, 1958.
172. Boston, H.C., Bianco, A.J., and Rhodes, K.H.: Disk space infections in children. Orthop. Clin. North Am. 6:953, 1975.
173. Pritchard, D.J.: Granulomatous infections of bones and joints. Orthop. Clin. North Am. 6:1029, 1975.
174. Hodgson, A.R.: Infectious disease of the spine. *In* Rothman, R H., and Simeone, F. A. (eds.): The Spine. Philadelphia, W. B. Saunders Company, 1975.
175. Alldred, A.J., and Nisket, N.W.: Hydatid disease of bone in Australasia. J. Bone Joint Surg. 46B:260, 1964.
176. Wiltse, L.L., Newman, P.H., and Macnab, I.: Classification of spondylolysis and spondylolisthesis. Clin. Orthop. 117:30, 1976.
177. Taillard, W.F.: Etiology of spondylolisthesis. Clin. Orthop. 117:30, 1976.
178. Wiltse, L.L., Widell, E.H., and Jackson, D.W.: Fatigue fracture: The basic lesion in isthmic spondylolisthesis. J. Bone Joint Surg. 57A:17, 1975.
179. Wiltse, L.L.: Etiology of spondylolisthesis. Clin. Orthop. 10:45, 1957.
180. Jackson, D.W., Wiltse, L.L., and Cirincione, R.J.: Spondylolysis in the female gymnast. Clin. Orthop. 117:68, 1976.
181. Ferguson, R.J.: Low-back pain in college football lineman. J. Bone Joint Surg. 56A:1300, 1974.
182. Farfan, H.F., Osteria, V., and Lamy, C.: The mechanical etiology of spondylolysis and spondylolisthesis. Clin. Orthop. 117:40, 1976.
183. Troup, J.D.G.: Mechanical factors in spondylolisthesis and spondylolysis. Clin. Orthop. 117:59, 1976.
184. Rosenberg, N.J.: Degenerative spondylolisthesis. J. Bone Joint Surg. 57A:4, 1975.
185. Petajan, J., Momberger, G., Aase, J., and Wright, D.G.: Arthrogryposis syndrome (Kusokwim disease) in the Eskimo. JAMA 209:1481, 1969.
186. Karaharjii, E., and Hummuksela, M.: Possible syphilitic spondylitis. Acta Orthop. Scand. 44:289, 1973.
187. Anderson, C.E.: Spondyloschisis following spine fusion. J. Bone Joint Surg. 38A:1142, 1956.
188. Harris, R.I., and Wiley, J.J.: Acquired spondylolisthesis as a sequel to spine fusion. J. Bone Joint Surg. 45A:1159, 1963.
189. Unander-Scharin, L.: A case of spondylolisthesis lumbalis aquisita. Acta Orthop. Scand. 19:536, 1950.
190. DePalma, A.F., and Marme, P.J.: Spondylolysis following spine fusion. Clin. Orthop. 15:208, 1959.
191. Harrington, P.R., and Tullos, H.S.: Spondylolisthesis in children. Clin. Orthop. 79:75, 1971.
192. Strayer, L.M., Risser, J.C., and Waugh, T.R.: Results of spine fusion for scoliosis twenty-five years or more after surgery. J. Bone Joint Surg. 51A:205, 1969.
193. Tietjen, R., and Morgenstern, J.M.: Spondylolisthesis following surgical fusion for scoliosis. Clin. Orthop. 117:176, 1976.
194. Wiltse, L.L., and Jackson, D.W.: Treatment of spondylolisthesis and spondylolysis in children. Clin. Orthop. 117:92, 1976.
195. Laurent, L.E., and Einola, S.: Spondylolischisis in children and adolescents. Acta Orthop. Scand. 82:45, 1961.
Osterman, K., Lindholm, T.S., and Laurent, L.E.: Late results of removal of the loose posterior element (Gill's operation) in the treatment of lytic lumbar spondylolisthesis. Clin. Orthop. 117:121, 1976.
197. Newman, P.H.: Surgical treatment for spondylolisthesis in the adult. Clin. Orthop. 117:106, 1976.

# Chapter 31
# The Painful Foot

*Bruce Wood*

## THE NORMAL FOOT

Normal feet should perhaps be defined as feet capable of providing pain-free function throughout a wide range of reasonable physical activities. More rigid definitions of normal structure and function become difficult as one encounters numerous structural variations which offer little or no impediment to function. Obversely, feet that could by other criteria be defined as "normal" may present severe functional limitations and challenge the most astute clinician.

The foot is an extremely adaptive organ, capable of functioning under extreme conditions imposed by both environmental and activity demands. Numerous small joints provide flexibility and adaptability; and yet when needed for walking or running propulsion, these same joints under the combined forces of gravity and muscle action transform the foot into an efficient rigid propulsive lever.[1]

The skin on the weight-bearing plantar surface is thick and, together with the dense fat pads under the calcaneus and metatarsal heads, provides protection against shear and impact stress.

The transition from normality to presentation of symptoms is often a gradual process clinically, except in the presence of acute traumatic, inflammatory, or infectious processes.

Symptoms presenting in the foot may be the first indication of numerous systemic disorders, such as diabetes mellitus, rheumatoid arthritis, gout, and occlusive vascular diseases. It is important when evaluating foot symptoms to consider the systemic ramifications that may be a factor in foot pain or dysfunction. The occurrence of swelling, sensory changes, skin changes, and deformity, while often found as local problems, may be associated with systemic disorders as well.

## OSTEOARTHRITIS—DEGENERATIVE JOINT DISEASE

A National Health survey conducted between 1960 and 1962 showed a prevalance of osteoarthritis in feet to be nearly 20 percent in a population between 18 and 79 years of age. As would be expected, the incidence rose sharply in the fifth and sixth decades. At ages 75 to 79 the incidence was 48.6 percent for males and 53.1 percent for females. In this same age group moderate to severe arthritis was three times more prevalent in women, with 14.6 percent of women and 4.8 percent of men being reported with foot involvement.[2]

From a biomechanical standpoint, any change in the functional mechanisms of the foot may produce pain and dysfunction. Continued use or overuse of biomechanically deficient feet, together with trauma, is probably the most common precipating factor in secondary degenerative joint disease in the foot. The first metatarsophalangeal joint is a frequent site for a variety of degenerative changes ranging from cartilage erosion and bursitis to joint rigidity secondary to osteophyte formation with or without the presence of bunions and hallux valgus.

**The Hallux and Lesser Toes.** Among the most common and easily identified deformities are bunions, hallux valgus, and hammer toes. Hallux valgus refers to an abnormal position of the great or first toe in which the toe is deviated laterally or in a fibular direction. In relation to the sagittal plane of the body, this change may be defined as a position of abduction. Occasionally the toe will also rotate or evert about its long axis. The deformity occurs principally at the first metatarsophalangeal joint, where positional changes ranging from slight deviation to frank dislocation are found. In addition to the deviation of the first toe, the first metatarsal usually deviates medially or to a position of adduction in relation to the sagittal plane. In the presence of this deformity, the head of the first metatarsal becomes prominent medially. This bony prominence, or bunion, may be normal in size or may be significantly enlarged. As static deformities, symptoms may be less severe than suggested by the deformity; but under the stress of function, particularly in a shoe incapable of accommodating the deformity, pain and secondary lesions occur frequently. In the absence of inflammatory or other connective tissue disorders, these deformities are probably related to inherited structural factors. Persons, particularly between the ages of 30 and 50, with such predisposing factors are likely to develop these deformities, especially in the presence of obesity, inappropriate shoes, and prolonged periods of overuse of their feet.[1,31] These deformities do not usually occur as single entities but rather are seen in combination. The lateral displacement of the hallux interferes with the lesser toes and may lead to contracture deformities and overlapping toes. The hammer toe is the most common lesser toe deformity and may occur singly or multiply. The deformity is characterized by hyperextension at the metatarsophalangeal joint and marked flexion at the proximal interphalangeal joint.

Dorsally contracted digits, particularly the second toe, may exert retrograde and plantar forces on the metatarsal heads, causing pain and perhaps skin lesions under the metatarsal heads. Frequently corns may develop secondary to shoe pressure over the prominent proximal interphalangeal joints. As these deformities develop, muscle imbalances occur, which encourage further progressions of the deformity.[4,5]

**Gout.** The classic picture of gout at the first metatarsophalangeal joint, podagra, is usually quite evident with a history of sudden onset and rather extreme pain to both touch and motion. The adjacent soft tissues and skin are moderately inflamed and swollen. The necessary differential diagnosis from infection in some cases is made by the absence of streaks and node hypertrophy as well as by the response to medication. Often the acute attack has subsided before the laboratory has confirmed the presence of synovial fluid crystals or determined serum uric acid levels. (See Chapter 86.) Tophaceous gout often leaves residual foot deformities requiring special shoe modifications to prevent excess weight bearing and subsequent tissue breakdown over prominent tophaceous lesions. Occasionally surgical reconstruction of deformities is necessary.

Osteophytes over the dorsal area of the first metatarsophalangeal joint may initially cause an extensor tendinitis resulting from the irritation of tendon and sheath as the tendon glides over or is pressed against the bony prominence. Further growth of osteophytes results in painful impingement (hallux limitus, Fig. 31–1), reducing the capability of dorsiflexion, a motion essential in each normal gait cycle. The end result is hallux rigidus when no motion is possible. Although interfering with gait and shoe fit, the rigid toe is much less painful than hallux limitus. Local inflammation of the tendon, synovium, or bursa may be treated with moist heat and steroid injections. An extended shank, sole stiffener, and rocker bar are shoe modifications that may decrease the need for full range of motion and therefore reduce pain. The eventual treatment often involves an arthroplasty to remove the osteophytes or, with cartilage damage, either a fusion or joint replacement procedure.

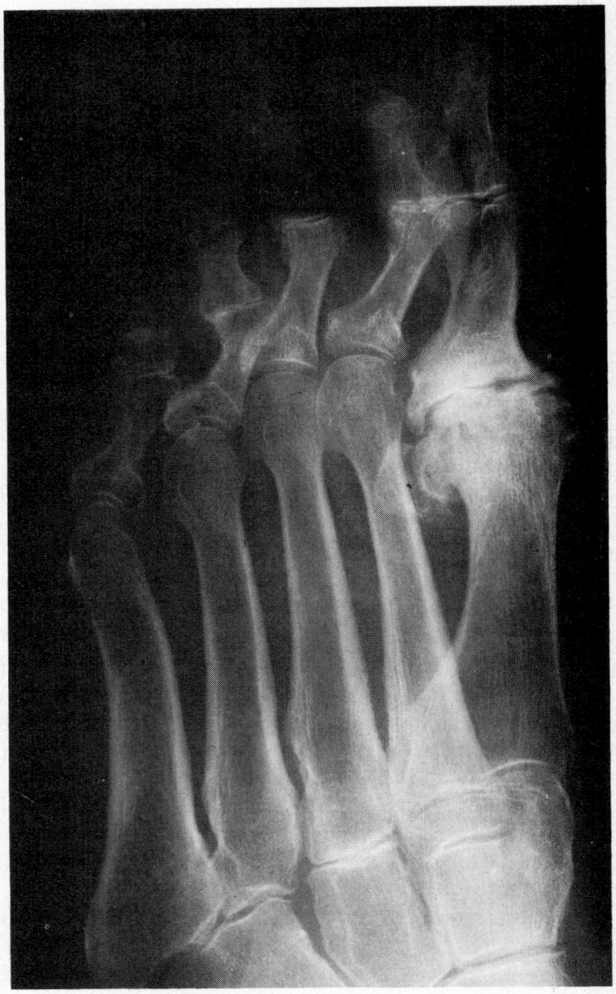

**Figure 31–1.** Hallux limitus showing degenerative joint changes with osteophytes.

The patient with chronic pronation, particularly when the foot is subjected to excessive occupational or athletic stress and obesity, exerts high stresses upon improperly aligned midtarsal joints, leading to the formation of osteophytes dorsally at the talonavicular, navicular-cuneiform, and cuneiform-metatarsal joints. Although conclusive studies are not available, the talonavicular joint may well be the most commonly involved foot joint in osteoarthritis.[6] As with the first metatarsophalangeal joint, the extensor tendons lying over these prominences frequently develop tendinitis, especially when shoe pressures are excessive. Arthritis in this area is initially treated with appropriately fitted shoes and an orthosis to control pronation. Occasionally arthroplasty or fusion is indicated.

On a theoretical if not practical basis, degenerative joint disease secondary to chronic excessive pronation could be prevented if proper control of pronation is initiated early and maintained on a continuous basis.

**Heel Pain.** Chronic pronation results in attempts to stretch the medial and plantar connective tissue structures, especially the plantar calcaneonavicular or Spring ligament, the capsule of the calcaneotalonavicular joint, and the plantar fascia, an extensive and complex band of fibers binding the joints of the foot together plantarly.[7] The fascia is subjected to considerable tension, particularly at the area of its medial and plantar attachments to the tuberosity of the calcaneus. Continued tension of this inelastic tissue may result in periostitis at the calcaneal attachment, with eventual proliferative changes producing a plantar calcaneal spur. As with the calcaneal valgus and pronation seen in rheumatoid arthritis, the first concern is the mechanical control of the deformity and its causes. This may be done initially with a supportive dressing of adhesive tape and felt, followed with an orthosis. Following initial mechanical support, heat, ultrasound, anti-inflammatory agents, and injection may be used.

The etiology of heel pain includes numerous other medical and orthopedic diseases, ranging from ischemia and nerve entrapment to bursitis and fat pad atrophy. Identifying and managing the underlying disease or deformity is the obvious direction to follow, while local treatment is often less obvious.

There are three principal bursae and six major medial, lateral, and posterior tendons subject to inflammation in the heel area.[8,9] The Achilles, peroneus longus, and posterior tibial tendons are most frequently involved with tendinitis. The anatomic bursae are located as follows: (1) retrocalcaneal, located between the Achilles tendon and the posterior surface of the calcaneus just above the Achilles insertion; (2) superficial, located between the tendon and the overlying fascia; and (3) plantar calcaneal, located between the plantar aponeurosis (fascia) and the calcaneus. Inflammation of the posterior bursae may be in conjunction with or confused with Achilles tendinitis and is frequently caused and certainly aggravated by a rigid shoe counter, particularly in high heeled shoes or pumps. Occasionally a bony prominence is present at the posterior lateral aspect of the calcaneus, which, when subjected to shoe irritation, may develop a periostitis or adventitious bursitis. Rest, heat, protective padding, and occasionally steroid injection may help.

Caution must be exercised when considering a steroid injection in the region of the Achilles insertion, as tendon rupture and soft tissue necrosis have been reported in this area following such injections. In some instances these "pump bumps" may require surgical removal. Achilles tendinitis will have pain, swelling, and possibly heat and crepitus along its course just proximal to its insertion, while bursitis is more localized to the anatomic location of the bursae. Plantar bursitis may not be distinguishable from fasciitis or periostitis. Each is appropriately treated with rest, heat, anti-inflammatory drugs, or injection. A heel lift may be a helpful adjunct inasmuch as it reduces stress slightly in the region of the Achilles insertion. Short-term use of a short leg cast is sometimes necessary for this and other inflammatory conditions of foot and ankle structures. Chronic inflammation in the area of the retrocalcaneal bursa may cause erosive changes of the posterior aspect of the calcaneus. The quality and quantity of the plantar calcaneal fat pad can be readily palpated. On weight bearing it will occasionally bulge both medially and laterally owing to weakness or herniation of its fascial covering. This can sometimes be helped with a plastic heel cup and/or a 1/2 inch thickness of Plastazote or similar cushioning substance. Rheumatoid nodules directly under the calcaneus, as in other weight-bearing areas, may be protected with a suitable cushion or aperture pad but may ultimately require excision. Sudden onset of pain in the heel area during activity of a strenuous nature may indicate rupture of the plantaris tendon, a small but lengthy tendon which inserts laterally either into the calcaneus or Achilles tendon.

## NEUROPATHIC ARTHROPATHY—CHARCOT'S JOINT

While most inflammatory and degenerative connective tissue diseases of the foot are pain producing and disabling, Charcot joint disease or neuropathic arthropathy is unique for developing only in the presence of neuropathy. The loss of pain and proprioceptive responses allows joints and their soft tissues to exceed normal ranges of motion and develop significant joint instability. Ultimately, dislocation and deformity occur. Associated with the destructive process are swelling and hyperemia. Trauma, often only normal weight bearing on insensitive joints, is always a factor in this process. Diabetes mellitus is the most commonly associated disease, but neuropathic arthropathy may occur in a variety of neurologic diseases which are accompanied by diminished sensation and position sense such as tertiary syphilis, leprosy, and syringomyelia.

Typically, on initial presentation, Charcot feet are warm, swollen, and relatively nonpainful in proportion to clinical appearances. A common deformity is a broadening of the midtarsal region and a rocker bottom foot caused by collapse and destruction of the midtarsal structures. In the diabetic a strong pulse may be present. Charcot's joint should be suspected in the presence of long-term diabetes mellitus, swelling, and pain-free joint destruction out of proportion to the patient's complaint. Neuropathic ulcers may also be present, particularly on the sole of the foot. These may lead to osteomyelitis of the underlying weight-bearing bone, producing a very confusing radiographic picture. Initial treatment of non-weight-bearing rest in a nondependent position should be continued until swelling and erythema subside. This is followed by non-weight-bearing cast immobilization until complete bone repair is demonstrated radiographically. Ultimately the patient will require shoes which accurately accommodate and support the foot and therefore prevent further trauma and destruction.[1,10]

## RHEUMATOID ARTHRITIS

The management and prevention of pain, deformity, and dysfunction in the rheumatoid arthritic foot have become increasingly important as total knee and hip joint replacement procedures provide significant and predictable improvement in lower extremity function. The goal of management, as with other joints, is to prevent or reduce deformity and pain and maintain or increase function.

It is important to differentiate between dysfunction resulting from an active inflammatory process and that resulting from structural or mechanical changes and certain pre-existing biomechanical defects. Within a large cross section of persons foot problems and minor disabilities are common, and when rheumatoid arthritis is superimposed, it is too easy to ascribe all foot pain to the rheumatoid arthritis.[11] This consideration is particularly important in the patient who has a preexisting peripheral vascular disease, neuropathy, diabetes mellitus, or structural abnormality.[12,13]

The foot presents no exception to the desirability of providing a team approach to management of rheumatoid arthritis, with rheumatologists, orthopedists, podiatrists, physical therapists, and orthotists working closely together. The treatment and management approach will vary, depending on the stage of the disease and the extent of functional loss, with prevention of pain and deformity being indicated in the early stages and surgical correction of deformity in the later stages.[14] In stages I and II early foot symptoms result from the inflammation, swelling, and thickening of synovial tissues and the accompanying inability to achieve free moving joint and muscle function both at rest and on weight bearing. In stages III and IV, following structural damage to the bones and joints, pain may be related to attempts to bear weight on mechanically altered structures, and frequently both inflammatory and structural changes will be responsible concurrently for pain.

**History.** Initial symptoms of rheumatoid arthritis are reported to appear in the feet in 17 to 20 percent of patients, while throughout the course of the disease foot involvement may reach 90 percent. Patients with early foot involvement will often report aching, pain, swelling, and change in their manner of walking. Less commonly encountered is pain of a sharp or shooting nature. The early symptoms are most frequent in the forefoot.[1,15,16] Initial swelling is often noted with the need, particularly by women, to change to a larger size shoe but without improvement of symptoms. Pain and dysfunction usually increase following periods of rest, particularly in early morning. Because of the diffuse nature of pain in the arthritic foot, patients are often unable to identify, locate, and quantify specific areas of pain; therefore close manual examination is needed. A careful foot history should determine any pre-existing congenital, familial, or acquired deformities as well as functional disabilities and limitations and the need for prior foot care.[17] Answers to this line of questioning will help differentiate present symptoms and may also be of assistance in treatment. As an example, calcaneal valgus and flat feet may occur with or without symptoms in the nonarthritic patient. Such a pre-existing situation could increase the severity of both deformity and pain if rheumatoid arthritis were to involve the rear foot[18-21] and should be treated early in the attempt to correct and prevent deformities. It is important to inquire about a person's prearthritic abilities. The patient with a pre-existing pronated foot or calcaneal valgus invariably reports, for example, poor ice skating ability because of "weak ankles," or in other sports a tendency to "sprain" or turn the ankles. Inquiry about relative pain and comfort associated with various shoe styles, materials, and walking surfaces can be helpful in selecting changes which will benefit the patient. The person whose forefoot pain is lessened while walking on a thick, well-padded carpet can be expected to do well with properly fitted compliant footwear or Plastazote* inner soles. Forefoot pain, particularly in patients with depressed metatarsal heads and displaced or absent fat pads, will often be likened to walking on marbles or a bed of coals.[3] A history of ankle pain or weakness often cannot be accepted as stated, for frequently the source of pain or instability is in the subtalar and talonavicular joints.[22] Associated with talonavicular disease, peroneal muscle spasm can be a frequent source of leg pain.

**Evaluation.** Early diagnostic and evaluative processes should include recording baseline data to include neurological, vascular, and integumentary systems as well as assessments of gait function, deformity, range of motion, and relative muscle strengths. This baseline information is an essential reference point for measuring both progress and future treatment requirements. Note that the posterior tibial pulse may often be obscured by swelling and thickening in the tarsal tunnel area and that occasionally the posterior tibial nerve may be compressed in this same area.[23,24]

It is helpful to observe walking gait both with and without shoes, but pain may limit this examination to stance only. Normal heel-to-toe gait is a complicated mechanical function in which the posterior-lateral aspect of the heel strikes the walking surface and weight is rapidly transmitted along the lateral margin of the foot and across the ball of the foot, where a compliant fat pad absorbs some of the shear and impact force. During the gait cycle, the foot briefly pronates and then supinates just before push-off.[25,26] Any mechanical or disease process interfering with this function may produce pain.

Such mechanical shortcomings are of particular importance when the foot attempts to accommodate to the surface incongruities or otherwise uneven and inclined terrain. Pain and functional limitations of the knee and hip joints will also affect gait and foot function and must be considered in evaluation.[27] The rheumatoid patient with forefoot involvement often fails to push off from the ball of the foot and toes but rather will slide, shuffle, or lift the foot and place it forward. With rearfoot deformity, the foot may remain pronated (flattened) throughout the gait cycle. Biomechanically, long-term weight bearing on a pronated foot may encourage the development of further forefoot deformity and pain, especially hallux valgus, splaying, and metatarsalgia. Excessive pronations may also increase the internal rotary motion of the entire lower extremity, with resulting torsional stresses having an effect at both the knee and hip joints.[25]

Observe the standing and walking foot from all angles. At normal stance, the foot presents an upright calcaneus and straight Achilles tendon when viewed from behind. The rheumatoid foot, particularly with subtalar or talonavicular joint involvement, often presents a valgus attitude of the calcaneus and a flattening of the medial longitudinal arch (Fig. 31–2). In addition, the navicular becomes prominent medially and small skin creases may appear lateral to the heel. Typical forefoot deformities are easily recognized and consist of dorsally contracted digits or the so-called cockup toe deformity with dorsiflexion at the metatarsophalangeal joint and flexion of one or both of the interphalangeal joints.[1] Occasionally the interphalangeal joints will resemble swan neck or boutonnière deformities as seen in fingers. Hallux valgus, or hallux abductus, in which the great toe deviates laterally, is frequently seen, as in the prominent medial bunion whose apparent size is often accentuated by a

*Smith and Nephew, Ltd., Hertfordshire, England.

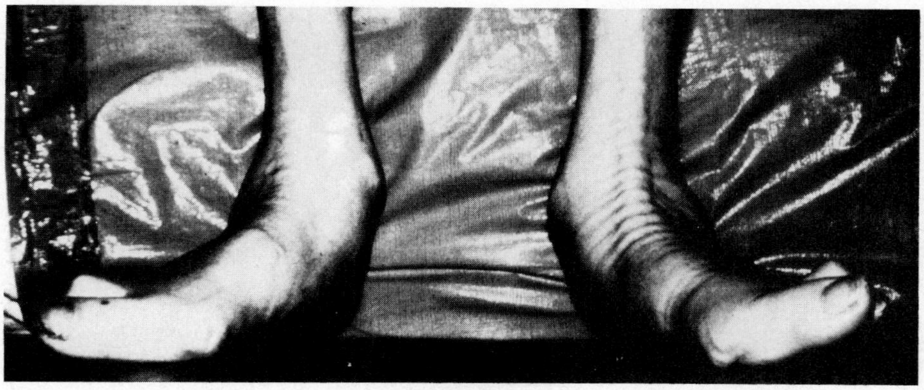

**Figure 31–2.** Rheumatoid foot showing calcaneal valgue, hallux abductus, bunions, and cockup toes.

splaying of the forefoot in the region of the metatarsal heads. The lesser toes, in addition to dorsal contraction, may also deviate laterally (fibular deviation) and often overlap one another or the great toe[28,29] (Fig. 31–3).

**Range of Motion.** Normal gait function requires an adequate joint excursion but with defined limits at each extreme, and it is necessary for all lower extremity joints to work in close harmony with each other. The range of motion may be decreased by fibrous ankylosis and bony impingement, soft tissue contractures, and pain, as well as by other extra-articular changes occurring in response to the disease. Similarly, joint excursions can be increased following destruction of the joint or its related supportive structures. Additionally, whether excursion is altered or not, the formal relation of one joint to another can be altered and thus affect function. An example of this is found with marked valgus deformity of the knee in the presence of normal ankle and foot joints. The valgus deformity at the knee is compensated for by a marked varus position in the subtalar joint.

The active and passive range of motion of the ankle, subtalar, midtarsal, and metatarsophalangeal joints should be recorded, and the strength of the muscles

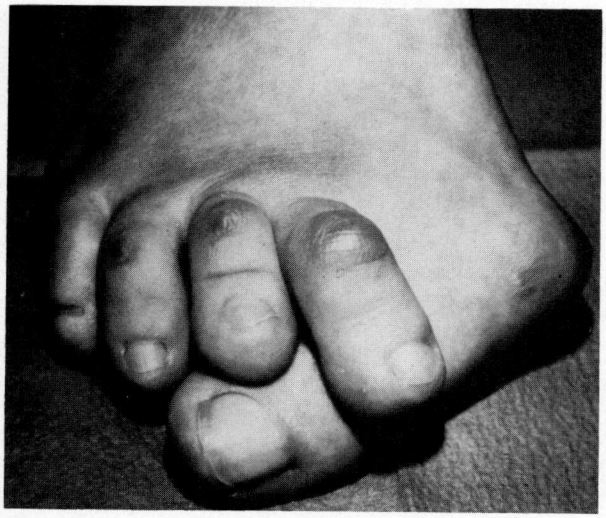

**Figure 31–3.** Hallux abductus, overlapping toes, splaying of forefoot, and bunion.

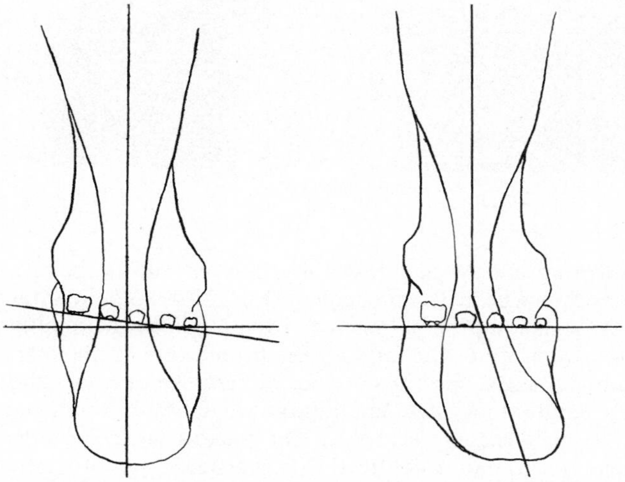

**Figure 31–4.** *Left,* Non–weight-bearing foot depicting forefoot varus. *Right,* Compensatory rearfoot valgus as foot bears weight.

controlling these joints should be evaluated. The relationship of the forefoot to the rearfoot and of the rearfoot to the leg both on weight bearing and at rest should be noted, as well as the sites of pain with both active and passive motion. One will frequently note that the forefoot is in a varus position relative to the rearfoot, that is, the forefoot is in an inverted position relative to the heel. This may represent a compensatory adaptation to a rearfoot valgus[25] (Fig. 31–4); however, it is also seen in the nonarthritic foot in a large population cross section and often precedes and causes the compensatory rearfoot valgus. Deformity at the metatarsophalangeal joint may advance to the point of subluxation or dislocation with the base of one or more proximal phalanges displaced over the metatarsal head. This may be appreciated by palpation and is readily seen on radiographs.

**Palpation.** On examination note the presence of thickening or swelling and heat, particularly in the region of the ankle, at the Achilles tendon, and both dorsally and plantarly at the metatarsophalangeal joints. Note the locations of tenderness of both articular and nonarticular structures. Associated with cockup toes, the anatomical plantar fat pad which protects the ball of the foot from

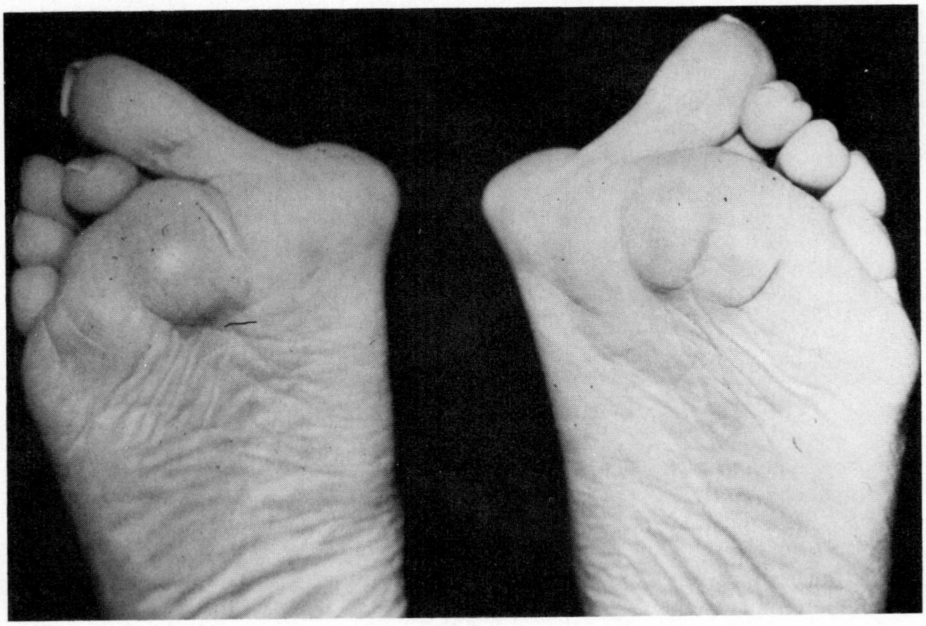

Figure 31–5. Prominent metatarsal heads and atrophic fat pads.

shearing and impact stress is displaced anteriorly to a position where it is ineffective (Fig. 31–5). The plantar surface should be palpated to evaluate both the quality and quantity of the fat pad, the prominence of the metatarsal heads, and the presence of keratoses, bursae, and rheumatoid nodules. In addition, the fat pads under the heel may become atrophic. The plantar surface of the heel is a common site for the occurrence of symptomatic rheumatoid nodules. A Harris Mat imprint may be used to provide a graphic representation of those areas, particularly in the forefoot, which are subject to the greatest amounts of weight-bearing stress. Its principal value is in documentation and confirmation of clinical findings noted on careful manual examination (Fig. 31–6).

Examination of shoe wear on both the sole and inner sole provides further evidence of weight-bearing stress areas, while the heel and shoe counter provide graphic evidence of rearfoot deformity.

**Tenderness.** Inflammation can cause pain, swelling, or thickening of the joints of the ankle or foot; pain that is not significantly changed by rest is most likely secondary to inflammation. Common sites include the Achilles tendon along its distal portion and at its insertion. Localized tenderness anterior to the tendon just proximal to its insertion may represent a bursitis as well as tendinitis of the Achilles and its sheath.[8,9] Compression of the heel and palpation of the plantar surface of the os calcis may elicit pain, especially with Reiter's syndrome and psoriatic arthritis. Palpation medially and laterally at the talocalcaneal joint yields confusing results. Thickening of the joint synovium may cause pain, but along the medial aspect other sources of pain could be tendinitis or nerve entrapment in the tarsal tunnel. The metatarsal compression test, performed by compressing the metatarsal bones together, elicits pain between metatarsal heads in the presence of synovitis (Fig. 31–7). When compressing or squeezing this area, it is important that the pressure be exerted on the shafts of the first and fifth metatarsals rather than over the metatarsophalangeal joint. Further confirmation is made by palpating in the intermetatarsal head space. A more selective procedure to localize inflammatory pain con-

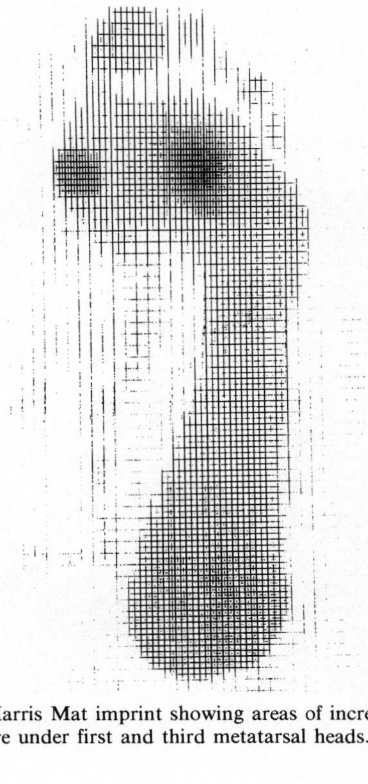

Figure 31–6. Harris Mat imprint showing areas of increased weight-bearing pressure under first and third metatarsal heads.

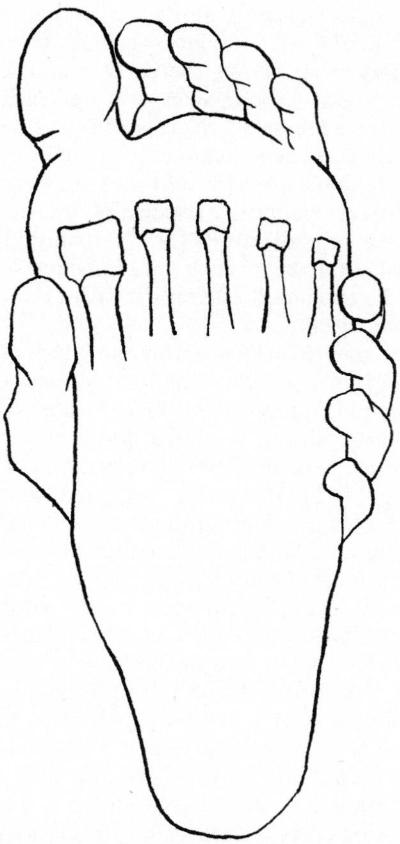

**Figure 31–7.** Metatarsal compression test exerts pressure on tissues in the intermetatarsal head spaces.

sists of dorsiflexing the toes, if not already in a cockup position, and applying direct digital pressure plantarly and distally at the point where the base of the toe joins the metatarsal head (Fig. 31–8*A*). This test can be used to distinguish between synovial joint pain and metatarsal head pain secondary to mechanical problems, which is noted by applying pressure directly on the plantar weight-bearing surface of the metatarsal head (Fig. 31–8*B*). Extensor tendinitis can be appreciated by applying gentle pressure over each extensor tendon while putting the digit through a full range of motion. Pain may be elicited, and additionally a fine crepitus may be felt. Plantar metatarsal head pain secondary to mechanical forces occurs most often under the second and third heads and somewhat less frequently under the fourth head. The fifth head and first, under which glide the sesamoid bones, are less frequently involved. The previously mentioned pronated foot with a varus forefoot exerts considerable stress on the second metatarsal and relatively less on the first, and it will be commonly noted in this circumstance that the second metatarsal head will be the most tender.[25] Radiography of the chronically pronated foot may demonstrate a relative hypertrophy of the second metatarsal shaft.

**Skin Changes.** The skin and its lesions are a good barometer of foot health and may indicate the extent of occlusive vascular disease, rheumatoid vasculitis, and the locations and effects of weight bearing and shoe pressure stresses.[30,31] Note especially the presence and locations of pressure-induced lesions such as corns and calluses, and particularly note if these lesions have ulcerated or become infected. It is not unusual to find a hematoma or extravasated blood under or within these keratotic lesions, particularly under the metatarsal heads and over the proximal interphalangeal joints of cockup toes. This is not only an indication of the degree of trauma inflicted upon the area, but more importantly represents a high risk area where continued trauma could be expected to produce an ulceration or abscess. Ulceration may be of a low grade, slowly evolving nature and is easily overlooked.

Careful debridement of plantar and digital lesions is essential both to aid in relief of pain and also to locate and treat ulcerations. Proprietary medications should never be used by patients to treat corns and calluses. Ulcerations are especially prevalent in those patients on long-term steroid therapy, as well as in patients with diabetes mellitus, large and small vessel disease, peripheral neuropathy, vasculitis, plantarly located nodules, and absent or atrophic plantar fat pads.[32] Ulcerative lesions and abscesses take on an even greater significance when joint replacement surgery of the hip and lower extremity has been performed or is contemplated, for these lesions may seed infection to the operated joint. Patients with vasculitis or on steroid therapy may develop small hemorrhagic lesions, and when located in the subungual or periungual areas these may become a focus for infection.

Verrucous lesions are not common in the adult population but when present are usually painful. These lesions can be distinguished from corns and calluses by

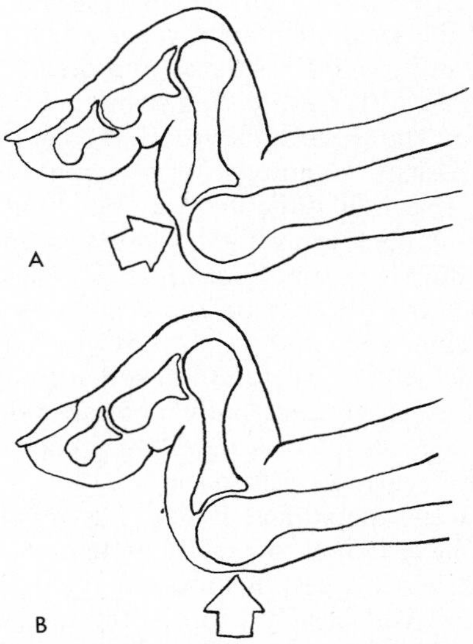


**Figure 31–8.** *A*, Pressure applied at the joint space and capsule may differentiate pain secondary to synovitis. *B*, Pain in response to pressure directly on the metatarsal head is more likely to be of mechanical origin.

the presence of multiple papillae with dark-colored blood clots of pinpoint size which bleed freely when the surface callus is removed. Rheumatoid nodules are frequently noted in the foot, appearing usually adjacent to bony prominences in both the forefoot and heel areas. They may be a source of pain from shoe and weight-bearing pressure, and may also occasionally ulcerate or become abscessed.

The arthritic patient often has difficulty caring for nails, and family members and nurses are often fearful or unwilling to perform this task. The periungual and subungual tissue offer a fertile medium for both bacterial and mycotic infection. Neglected nails, particularly in the presence of digital deformity, will frequently abrade or lacerate adjacent soft tissues, causing both pain and infection. Repetitive pressure of as little as 5 pounds per square inch, a quantity easily achieved with shoe pressure upon thickened nails, will cause development of subungual abscesses, especially in the diabetic, vascular diseased, neuropathic, or debilitated patient.[12] Such subungual abscesses may readily initiate an osteomyelitis of the distal phalanx. Appropriate attention to and care of the nails constitute a small but essential element in the management of the rheumatoid foot. Intertriginous areas of skin must be protected from maceration, abrasion, and infection.

The periodic care of even minor lesions could be essential to the health of the arthritic patient, particularly in the presence of lower extremity joint replacements.

**Radiography.** Radiography is essential to proper evaluation to assess both the extent of bone and joint destruction and the functional and mechanical alterations, as well as the approaches to be taken to deal with these problems. The standard views, anteroposterior, lateral, and lateral oblique, will be adequate in most instances; however, the medial oblique may occasionally be helpful. Less frequently required but of great value when taken properly are the Harris view, which displays the subtalar joints, and the axial metatarsal view, which profiles the weight-bearing condylar sufaces and sesamoids in the ball of the foot. When evaluating structural relationships and changes, the three standard views should be taken with the patient standing. With some radiographic equipment this is a difficult task, but relatively inexpensive equipment is available which is specially designed for weight-bearing foot films. The significance of a weight-bearing film can be appreciated by comparing weight-bearing and non-weight-bearing views of the same foot. It will be noted that most deformities become much more apparent or actually increase under the force of gravity and weight bearing. This is particularly true with valgus rearfoot deformities, hallux valgus, and splaying of the metatarsal heads. The location of the metatarsal head lesions is usually quite obvious in rheumatoid feet; when questions arise, a small lead marker on the lesion will clearly identify the metatarsal head associated with the lesion.

Less conventional radiological techniques may be of value in selected cases. Fine detail radiography with optical magnification has the capability of identifying erosive changes in small joints earlier and in a detail not appreciated with standard views.[33] This technique may also aid in clarifying the early presence of osteomyelitis, although a bone scan is more sensitive in this important determination. Xerography, as well as fine detail and magnification, can be of value in more clearly defining soft tissue changes and masses. Persistent pain and an elusive diagnosis, especially in the rear- and midfoot, may be indications for CT scanning. The talocaneal joints and the angular relationships of the tarsal joints can be evaluated effectively with this technique.[34] (See Chapter 39.)

**Rearfoot and Midfoot.** Patients will frequently attribute symptoms of pain, swelling, stiffness, and weakness to the ankle when in fact their disease is more likely to be in the subtalar or midtarsal joints.[20] In one clinical study, rearfoot pain interfered with walking in 16 percent of patients, while 42 percent reported some rearfoot disability.[20] Normal ankles move in one plane only, that being flexion and extension (dorsiflexion) in the sagittal plane. Motion of the foot from side to side (inversion and eversion) occurs primarily in the subtalar joint. Normal subtalar motion is about 30 degrees; when measured from a neutral position, inversion is greater than eversion in a 2:1 ratio. Reports of physical examination of these joints are often confusing, and clinicians should be encouraged to distinguish clearly between the motions of the true ankle joint and the subtalar joint. Occasionally following ankle sprains or fracture, a small amount of inversion or eversion will occur in the unstable ankle joint.

Calcaneal valgus is the most common rearfoot deformity, and it may involve any or all of the talocalcaneal (subtalar), talonavicular, and calcaneocuboid joints. These joints may be severely involved with joint loss, decreased motion, and severe pain and yet show no valgus deformity. At the other extreme the rearfoot valgus may be great enough to cause bone and soft tissue impingement of the calcaneus against the fibula.[20]

The talonavicular joint margins can be palpated medially and plantarly just behind the navicular tuberosity. The talonavicular joint with its associated soft tissue structures is a vitally essential component in the normal foot and is often the site of early symptoms and clinical findings in conditions ranging from functional overuse syndromes to the rheumatoid foot with rearfoot involvement. Tenderness at this location could be fascial, ligamentous, muscular, or synovial in origin. Often associated with advanced disease and deformity in this region is peroneal muscle spasm, which can be a source of significant lateral leg pain.[21] Confirmation of peroneal spasm can be determined by the following test. With the patient at rest, apply enough force to the lateral side of the fifth metatarsal head to push the forefoot into a position of adduction. Repeat this motion several times rapidly, and peroneal spasm and involuntary forefoot abduction will occur.

When ankle dorsiflexion is limited to 0 or less, pronation and forefoot abduction may occur to compensate for loss of this essential ankle motion.[22,25] The limitation of dorsiflexion may be caused by articular changes in the ankle or by a tight or shortened gastrocnemius-soleus group or Achilles tendon. When examining ankle joint motion, the ranges should be evaluated with the knee in full extension as well as in 90 degrees of flexion. If ankle dorsiflexion increases beyond neutral with the knee in flexion, the limiting factor is the gastrocnemius, which arises from the femoral condyles. Calcaneal varus deformity (inversion) occurs rarely in adult rheumatoid arthritis but is more frequently seen in juvenile rheumatoid arthritis.[20] When present in adults, it is more likely to be a deformity occurring in the ankle, where owing to bone and cartilage erosions the talus becomes inverted within the ankle mortise.

**Conservative Management.** *General Principles.* During stages I and II when secondary deformity is less likely to be a problem, pre-existing mechanically induced lesions and deformities should be dealt with, especially chronic pronation and calcaneovalgus, for in the presence of rheumatoid arthritis these deformities are likely to increase. While inflammatory processes are active, particularly if multiple foot joints are involved, local mechanical therapy is of limited value; however, this is an appropriate time to outline changes in both foot use and foot wear. A change to shoes designed for function and comfort is helpful, especially for female patients whose shoes are often uncomfortable for even a normal foot. Appropriate exercise and activity programs should be encouraged as tolerated. Inappropriate activity would include contact sports and activities involving high foot-to-ground impact and shearing forces such as tennis and racquet ball; more suitable activities include bicycling, either stationary or two- or three-wheeled, swimming, and certainly walking on a compliant yet smooth surface such as a golf course or well groomed park. Rough and uneven surfaces requiring compensatory inversion and eversion may be difficult, especially with later stages of disease. Static active, passive, and isometric exercise of all joints, but especially the ankle, subtalar, and metatarsophalangeal joints, is encouraged within reasonable limits for maintaining both muscle tone and strength and joint mobility. The use of moist heat applications may be helpful for temporary relief of pain and stiffness. Polypropylene ankle-foot orthoses may be used as a night or resting splint. Generally when used as a night splint, these devices do not require custom fabrication, although stock splints may require the addition or modification of Velcro strapping for both comfort of fit and maintenance of position.

*Footwear.* Comfort is the essential quality for footwear in rheumatoid arthritis. A comfortable shoe should be lightweight and flexible with room to accommodate forefoot deformity; it should have a low heel of 3/16 to ½ inch of height, and a sole thick enough to protect the foot from mechanical surface trauma and compliant to cushion impact. The upper leather should be soft and pliable with a minimum of stitching and decoration, and should have a laced closure. The ideal shoe would have a natural crepe sole ½ inch thick with a totally plain glove leather upper and a combination last to ensure adequate fit for both rear- and forefoot. The problem of closure in the presence of limited hand function is solved either with a Velcro strap or by using elastic shoelaces, which eliminate the task of tying. The traditional so-called "orthopedic shoe" is of limited value except in the presence of minimal deformity and discomfort. With more severe deformity this shoe is often uncomfortable until the supporting counter has broken down, at which point the initial supportive value of the shoe is lost. Custom-fabricated stabilizing or supportive devices can be added to the comfortable shoe when needed without compromising comfort and fit. Adding inserts or orthoses to deal with forefoot problems usually increases the difficulty of shoe fitting. The Extra Depth Shoe* has a removable innersole which when removed increases the depth of the shoe by ¼ inch, which is usually ample to accept both deformed toes and an effective plantar insert (Fig. 31–9). Molded or "space" shoes, although good conceptually, have definite limitations with rheumatoid feet as they are usually too stiff and noncompliant. Any increase of deformity or swelling results in an uncomfortably poor fit. Some manufacturers are now using removable molded Plastazote or Aliplast inserts, which are an improvement. This shoe is most suitable for the fixed rigid deformity or for some osteoarthritic feet. The Plastazote sandal introduced by Paul Brand, M.D., has been successfully adapted as either a shoe or sandal for many patients other than those with the neuropathic lesions of Hansen's disease for whom it was originally designed (Fig. 31–10). The experience at the Robert B. Brigham Hospital has demonstrated a 25 percent reduction in surgery on the rheumatoid foot since the introduction of this material. Some manufacturers have developed a nonmolded shoe and sandal utilizing Plastazote (Fig. 31–11).†

*The Forefoot.* Treatment of plantar forefoot pain involves two principles, the first being provision of a compliant stress absorbing surface for weight bearing, and the second, redistribution of weight-bearing forces. The placement of compliant accommodative weight dispersive devices within a shoe is subject to obvious space limitations, and for this reason the extra depth shoe is often used. Microcellular rubber, closed cell neoprene, and closed cell foamed polyethylenes are representative of compliant materials available. In addition to these, materials such as adhesive-backed felt, cork, rubber, or leather can be used to fabricate accommodative weight distributing padding. Plastazote and Aliplast may be heated and molded to the contour of the foot or may be inserted without heating as an inner sole. Molded orthoses from these materials are capable of not only providing stress and impact absorbing qualities under metatarsal heads but also allowing the entire plantar surface of the foot to bear weight, thereby shifting some weight bearing away from metatarsal heads. Using a combination of materials, including the more firm varieties of Plastazote and Aliplast, these devices can also

*P.W. Minor & Son, Inc., Batavia, New York 14020.
†AliMed, Inc., Boston, Massachusetts 02111.

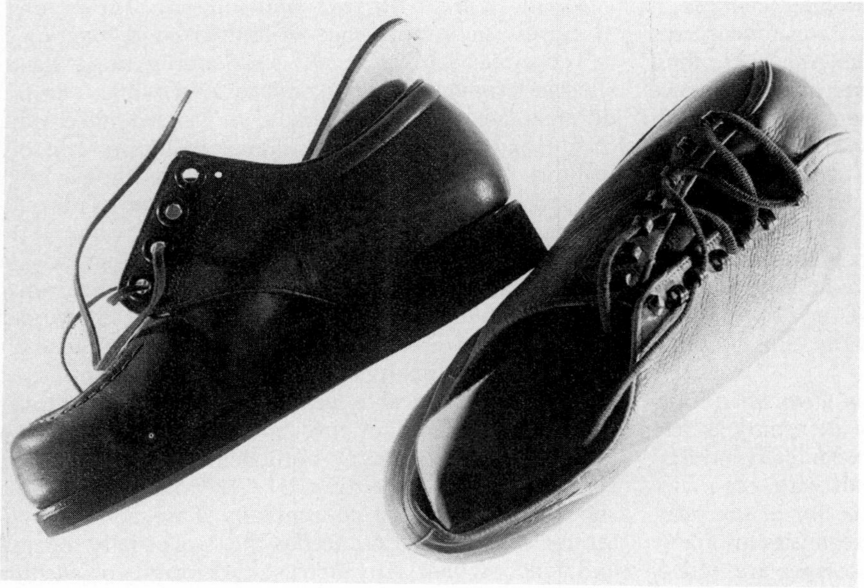

**Figure 31–9.** Extra Depth Shoes showing removable innersoles in variations of style and closure (manufactured by P.W. Minor & Son, Inc., Batavia, New York 14020).

be used for long arch support in the less severe cases of pronation of mid- and rearfoot disease. The same concept of distributing weight over the entire sole can be effective for both the treatment and prevention of plantar skin lesions, including ulcers, corns, and calluses. The addition of forefoot accommodative apertures either directly to the inside of the shoe itself or to the shoe insert is effective in unloading a specific head or heads. When multiple heads, usually more than two, are involved, a metatarsal bar can be added to the orthoses just behind the metatarsal head area. This has the effect of shifting the weight to an area proximal to the heads (Fig. 31–9).

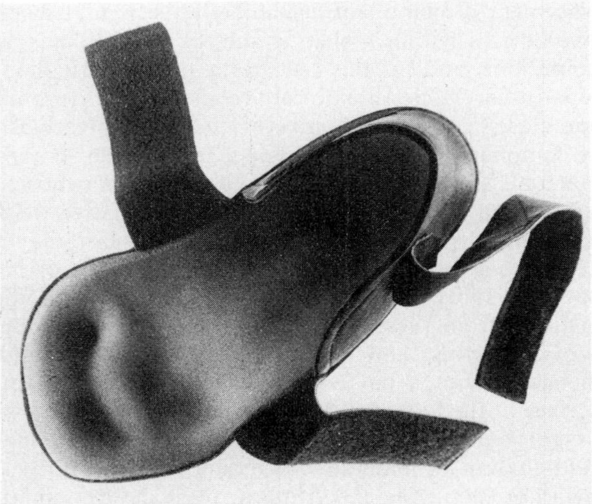

**Figure 31–10.** Plastazote sandal with polypropylene rearfoot stabilizer (by Barry Bent, Robert B. Brigham Division, Brigham and Women's Hospital).

*Orthoses.* Custom-made orthoses can also be ordered for accommodating or cushioning forefoot lesions. As with rearfoot devices, they are best made from plaster foot molds in preference to using paper tracings. Skilled technical help for the fabrication of these devices is often difficult to locate. Most large urban areas will have laboratories with some experience in this area. As an alternative there are numerous laboratories having nationwide service via mail. Generally these laboratories provide clear instructions for selecting and ordering their devices.

Splinting and exercise may be of value in retarding the development of deformity but are of limited value once significant joint destruction and deformity have occurred. Splinting and protective padding or shielding of the toes are helpful in reducing irritation of the soft tissues caused by pressure from shoes. An effective device for both splinting and protection can be molded from MPC.* Polyurethane foam impregnated with liquid latex rubber can also be fabricated as a protective shield or splint. MPC splints can also be used to maintain digital alignments during forefoot postoperative periods. The use of splints and wedges to correct hallux valgus deformity is of no value; because of the great forces acting on this deformity, a wedge between the great and second toes may increase the fibular displacement of the lesser toes. Occasionally hyperextension will occur at the interphalangeal joint of the great toe with or without hallux valgus or rigidus. This is a painful deformity, and the site is subject to chronic ulceration. Although surgical intervention is often required, an accommodative orthotic or MPC protective splint may be of value.

*Siebe Norton Inc., Cranston, Rhode Island 02920.

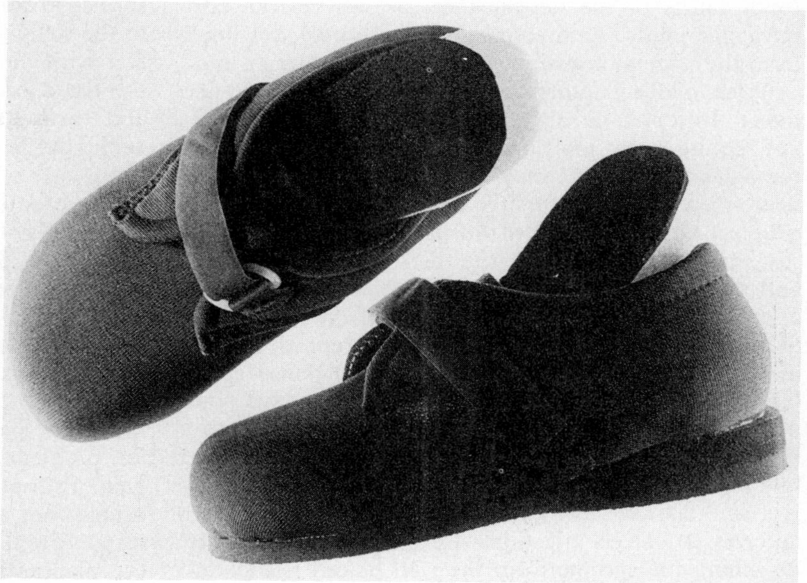

**Figure 31–11.** AliMed Plastazote Shoe showing removable innersole and Velcro closure (manufactured by AliMed, Inc., Boston, Massachusetts 02111).

*Shoe Modifications.* The same principles of redistribution of weight can be applied directly to the sole of the shoe. Plantation crepe soles can be added to almost any shoe to cushion impact. Metatarsal bars likewise provide a quick and simple modification. The major drawback to bars is that when improperly placed, an unfortunately frequent occurrence, they will increase pain. To be effective the front edge of the bar must be located proximal to the metatarsal heads. This location can be determined by noting the location of wear of both the inner and outer soles. Transferable marks placed on the metatarsal heads with ball-point pen, lipstick, or marker pens will be imprinted within the shoe after a few steps and will provide an accurate placement. Many orthopedic shoe repair shops and orthotics laboratories have shoe-stretching apparatus (such as a Eupedus device) which can selectively stretch a shoe to accommodate a digital deformity.

For patients able to play golf, the removal of cleats, particularly from the forefoot area, will reduce some of the shearing and torsional stresses induced by golf shoes; however, in general, the more flexible crepe sole shoe is probably more appropriate.

The molded Plastazote shoe provides the ultimate in forefoot protection. When the need to protect the forefoot maximally is combined with rearfoot deformity requiring stabilization, a shoe utilizing a polypropylene rearfoot stabilizer in addition to the Plastazote forefoot can be made. The use of thin-soled elevated heel shoes with narrow toes should be discouraged both from a comfort standpoint and from the fact that they will increase forefoot deformity. As a practical matter this rule can be broken for occasional social functions.

*Injections.* Polyarticular inflammatory foot pain is best managed with rest, heat, and systemic treatment; however, recalcitrant pain, particularly when located within a specific joint or joints, may be selectively treated with an injection of steroids, as can bursae and tendon sheaths.[8,9] The foot, particularly its plantar and interdigital spaces, is a potentially dirty area surgically, and careful skin preparation is essential. Sterile technique, including gloving, is advised. Steroid injections into deep areas, particularly the plantar heel area, are easier when preceded by injection of anesthetic. With the exception of the ankle and subtalar joints, the foot joints should be treated as small joints in terms of the quantity and strength of steroid to be injected. Reference to anatomic diagrams is helpful unless one is familiar with foot joints. Tuberculin syringes provide excellent control with both insertion and introduction of fluids when dealing with small joints and superficial bursae and tendon sheaths. Aspiration from bursae and the ankle joint for purposes of fluid examination and volume reduction can be readily accomplished; the smaller joints, except in the presence of significant effusion, can be most difficult to enter for either aspiration or injection. The metatarsophalangeal and talonavicular joints are most readily entered by attempting to follow the natural joint contours rather than through a vertical approach to the joint space. Care must be taken when injecting in the region of the Achilles tendon and its adjacent bursae, as rupture of the Achilles tendon has been reported following steroid injection.

The subtalar joint can be entered with a 1½-inch needle inserted at a point anterior to the fibula approximately 1 cm from its tip, directing the needle in a posterior, plantar, and medial direction. This provides entrance into the sinus tarsi. From this point, redirecting to a medial direction permits entrance into the extensive capsular complex, which includes the middle and anterior facets of the talocalcaneal as well as the talonavicular joints. Redirecting to a more posterior angle from the original insertion will locate the posterior joint.

Other midfoot joints are very difficult to locate and inject. Intermetatarsal head synovitis or bursitis does not require direct joint penetration, but a deposit along the sides of the joint may be helpful. Plantar heel injections, whether for bursitis, fasciitis, or heel spurs, are simplest when approached medially. Entrance is made just above the junction of the thick tough plantar skin and the much more delicate skin of the upper foot and at a point medial to the attachment of the plantar fascia. Skin in this area is much more readily prepped, and the injection is far less painful. In addition, since spurs, fasciitis, or bursae are rarely limited to the pencil point of bone spur seen on x-ray, medial injection allows a broader deposition of steroid in the region of pain and inflammation. When properly located, this injection site is a safe distance away from the posterior tibial nerve and vessels. Deep injections are often made easier by detaching the syringe from the well placed needle and reloading with steroid. This is likely to be less traumatic and probably is more accurate.

***Rearfoot.*** Moderate deformity occurring on weight bearing in a foot capable of resupinating before toe off can be treated with an orthosis designed to control or minimize pronation.[26] In the presence of more severe deformities with joint destruction but with the capability for passive motion, the aim of an orthosis is to restore normal structural and functional alignment, reduce pain, and prevent further deformity.

Following total knee replacement procedures in which a significant valgus or varus deformity has been reduced, the foot frequently requires modification of shoes or orthotic appliances. With an adequate supple subtalar range of motion, the foot may easily accommodate to the correct functional planes. With limited subtalar motion the stabilizing orthoses can be used in an attempt to make a gradual realignment. When this fails or in the presence of a rigid joint, shoes and orthoses must be constructed that will provide adequate distribution of weight-bearing forces without increasing stress to the midtarsal and subtalar joints. The use of orthoses to realign these rearfoot joints may be a long-term treatment requiring periodic modifications of the device or fabication of new devices as changes in structural relationship occur. If bony ankylosis occurs with the subtalar and midtarsal joints in an adequate functional position, the use of a stabilizing orthosis may be discontinued. This procedure is followed also in candidates for talonavicular fusion or triple arthrodesis and may also be used postoperatively following cast immobilization.

Stabilizing orthoses may be constructed from a variety of materials, including Fiberglas, Rohadur, nylon, polypropylene, Celastic, and Cutter Cast. Such devices are fabricated over a plaster model of the foot. The cast for the model or mold is made with the foot held in the position which the orthosis is intended to maintain. The surface in contact with the foot is contoured to conform to the weight-bearing surfaces, while the surface in contact with the shoe is flattened. Modifying the angle of the flattened surface allows adjustment of the valgus and varus attitude. In some instances in which both ankle and rearfoot joints are involved, a polypropylene drop foot orthosis can be fabricated to support and stabilize both joint complexes. When a stabilizing orthosis fails to achieve relief of pain, a plaster cast may be used for 3 to 4 weeks, to be followed again with an orthosis and physical therapy. These conservative measures deserve trial before resorting to rear foot surgery. (See Chapter 118.) In addition to rheumatoid arthritis, Reiter's disease and psoriasis may present painful inflammatory periosteal changes, particularly in the rearfoot area. Reiter's disease especially presents a frustrating problem as one attempts to resolve or reduce heel pain. Psoriatic and Reiter's periostitis of the heel are usually not mechanical in origin and therefore do not respond well to orthotics designed to reduce traction on the plantar fascia. The use of Plastazote inserts, heel cups, and cushion-soled shoes is helpful. Rest, application of moist heat, and occasionally the timely injection of steroids may be of benefit.

## JUVENILE RHEUMATOID ARTHRITIS

The juvenile rheumatoid arthritic presents difficult challenges from the standpoint of both preventing and correcting or accommodating foot deformities. Early detection of structural changes and institution of appropriate shoes, orthoses, splints, and physical therapy are necessary.[35,36] The physically active child should be watched for any tendency toward deformity, particularly in the rear- and midfoot, where, in contrast to the adult calcaneal valgus deformity, equinovarus deformity is more frequently encountered. Appropriate shoes and/or orthoses should be utilized to minimize or prevent this deformity. Night splints and foot boards may also be needed. The juvenile rheumatoid arthritic is often an unreliable historian and reporter, and treatment requirements and decisions must be based largely on clinical judgment. Correction of deformities before the occurrence of fibrous ankylosis is essential if proper functional alignments are to be achieved and maintained. Active and passive range of motion and muscle strengthening exercises should be encouraged at an early stage as pain tolerance permits. Once fibrous or bony ankylosis has occurred, correction is difficult at best and surgical revision may ultimately be required.

## SUMMARY

Early detection and treatment of deformity and pain with proper shoes, exercise, orthoses, and splints when needed may prevent, delay, or minimize disability. Soft, compliant, nonrestrictive footwear with low heels and crepe soles together with supportive, stabilizing, compliant, or accommodative orthoses and shoe modifications will often increase levels of function and comfort. For purposes other than splinting and rest, or treatment of pre-existing deformity, other local medical and surgical techniques are most useful following effective systemic management of the inflammatory disease. The management of the rheumatoid arthritic foot requires that patients be informed of the nature and course of treatment and that realistic goals and limitations be set. The criteria for lower extremity surgical intervention are such that major foot surgical procedures and joint replacements are often of low priority and in most instances are best performed late. The presence of deformity is not by itself justification for intervention, and indeed surgical intervention usually should follow failure of conservative measures.[4,5,37]

## References

1. Inman, V.T., and DuVries, H.: DuVries' Surgery of the Foot. 3rd ed. St. Louis, C. V. Mosby Company, 1973.
2. National Health Survey Vital and Health Statistics: Data. United States DHEW Publication, No. 1000, Series 11,20:9, 1966.
3. Stott, J.R.P., Hutton, W.C., and Stokes, I.A.F.: Forces under the foot. J. Bone Joint Surg. 55B:335, 1973.
4. Giannestras, N.: Foot Disorders, Medical and Surgical Management. 2nd ed. Philadelphia, Lea & Febiger, 1973.
5. Kelikian, H.: Hallux Valgus and Allied Deformities of the Forefoot. Philadelphia, W. B. Saunders Company, 1965.
6. Roth, D.R.: Talonavicular joint osteoarthritis (osteoarthrisis). JAPA 72:237, 1982.
7. Furey, J.G.F.: Plantar fasciitis, J. Bone Joint Surg. 57A:672, 1975.
8. Kech, S.W., and Kelly, P.J.: Bursitis of the posterior part of the heel. J. Bone Joint Surg. 47A:267, 1965.
9. Cozen, L.: Bursitis of the heel. Am. J. Orthop. 3:372, 1961.
10. Frykeberg, R.G., and Kozak, G.P.: Neuropathic arthropathy in the diabetic foot. Fam. Phys. 17:105, 1978.
11. Clark, M.: Trouble with Feet. London, G. Bell, 1969. p. 13.
12. Brand, P.W.: Repetitive Stress on Insensitive Feet—The Pathology and Management of Plantar Ulceration in Neurotrophic Feet. SRSG No. RC-75, MPO, U.S. Public Health Service, 1975.
13. Hall, O.C., and Brand, P.W.: The etiology of the neuropathic ulcer. JAPA 69:173, 1979.
14. Steinbrocker, O., Traeger, C.H., and Batterman, R.C.: Therapeutic criteria in rheumatoid arthritis. JAMA 140:659, 1949.
15. Vainio, S.: The rheumatoid foot: A clinical study with pathological roentgenological comments. Ann. Chir. Gynaec. Fenn. 45:Suppl. 1, 1956.
16. Black, J.R., Cahalin, C., and Germain, B.F.: Pedal morbidity in rheumatic diseases. JAPA 72:360, 1982.
17. Taylor, P.M.: A review of changes of the hands and feet in rheumatoid arthritis. JAPA 68:817, 1978.
18. D'Amico, J.C.: The pathomechanics of adult rheumatoid arthritis affecting the foot. JAPA 66:227, 1976.
19. Harris, R.L.: Rigid valgus foot. J. Bone Joint Surg. 37A:169, 1955.
20. King, J., Burke, D., and Freeman, M.A.R.: The incidence of pain in the rheumatoid hind foot and the significance of calcaneo-fibular impingement. Int. Orthop. 2:255, 1978.
21. Harris, R.I., and Beath, T.: Etiology of peroneal spastic flatfoot. J. Bone Joint Surg. 30B:624, 1948.
22. Inman, V.T.: The Joints of the Ankle. Baltimore, Williams & Wilkins Company, 1976.
23. Chater, E.H.: Tarsal tunnel syndrome in rheumatoid arthritis. Br. Med. J. 3:406, 1970.
24. Kopell, H.P., and Thompson, W.A.L.: Peripheral Entrapment Neuropathies. Baltimore, Williams & Wilkins Company, 1963.
25. Sgarlato, T.E.: A Compendium of Podiatric Biomechanics. San Francisco, California College of Podiatric Medicine, 1971.
26. Root, M., Orien, W., and Weed, J.: Abnormal Function of the foot. Los Angeles, Clinical Biomechanics Inc., 1978.
27. Close, J.R.: Functional Anatomy of the Extremities. Springfield, Ill., Charles C Thomas, 1973.
28. Benson, G.M., and Johnson, E.W.: Management of the foot in the rheumatoid arthritic. Orthop. Clin. North Am. 2:733, 1971.
29. Kuhns, J.G.: The foot in chronic arthritis. Clin. Orthop. 16:141, 1960.
30. Wilkinson, M., and Torrance, W.N.: Clinical background of rheumatoid vascular disease. Ann. Rheum. Dis. 26:475, 1967.
31. Soter, N.A., Austen, K.F., and Gigli, I.: Urticaria and arthralgias as manifestation of necrotizing angiitis (vasculitis). J. Invest. Dermatol. 63:485, 1974.
32. Scott, J.T.: Digital arteritis in rheumatoid disease. Ann. Rheum. Dis. 20:224, 1961.
33. Mall, J.C., Genant, H.K., Silcox, D.C., and McCarty, D.J.: The efficacy of fine-detailed radiography in the evaluation of patients with rheumatoid arthritis. Radiology 112:37, 1974.
34. Seltzer, S.: Unpublished data, Department of Radiology, Brigham and Womens Hospital, 1983.
35. Donovan, W.: Proceedings of the First ARA Conference on the Rheumatic Diseases of Childhood, March 1974.
36. Calabro, J.J., Katz, R.M., and Maltz, B.A.: A critical appraisal of juvenile rheumatoid arthritis. Clin. Orthop. 74:100, 1971.
37. Clayton, M.L.: Surgery of the forefoot in rheumatoid arthritis. Clin. Orthop.16:136, 1960.

# Chapter 32

# "Fibrositis" and Other Diffuse Musculoskeletal Syndromes

*Hugh Smythe*

## INTRODUCTION

Patients often describe trunk or limb pain unaccompanied by new findings on physical or radiologic examination. In these circumstances, approaches to diagnosis may reflect several levels of clinical skill. Most commonly and superficially, this symptom is attributed to "arthritis," "bursitis," "nerve compression," or "fibrositis," on the basis of evidence that is trivial or irrelevant. A more skilled examiner may recognize that the joints, bursae, and nervous system are essentially normal, leaving the patient and physician incompletely reassured and leaving also a natural suspicion that either the patient or the diagnostic effort is inadequate. With still more care, previously unsuspected points of tenderness may be found; but there has been so little definition and discussion of the significance of these tender points that confident and accurate diagnosis is by no means assured. To the beginner, problems in diagnosis emerge from the diffuse and vague localization of much pain of deep origin and the absence of obvious findings in the area of complaint. At the more advanced level, a wealth of physical findings exist, and the problem lies in assessment of the significance of newly discovered sites of deep tenderness.

Often deep tenderness indicates subtle local pathology—an enthesopathy, a bursitis, or a soft tissue injury. More often, however, there is no histologically definable local pathology. Recent controlled studies have confirmed and extended our knowledge of the clinical associations of these findings.[1-3] The concept of pain amplification syndromes (Table 32–1) has been introduced to group these conditions. The term amplification implies that the increase in pain or tenderness has resulted from altered physiological mechanisms, independent of psychological influences. The effect is selective, not diffuse. Some sites become tender, but background pain threshold is unaltered.[2]

**Referred Pain and Associated Phenomena.** ***Body Image.***[4] When a pin is stuck into a finger, the patient can accurately localize the site of the injury and identify the nature of the stimulus. With eyes closed, he can summon up an image of the finger—extended or flexed, accurately located in space—and draw a picture of the part and the site of injury. This kind of detailed knowledge of the position and environment of the hand is essential to function, and a considerable area of cerebral cortex is assigned to processing this information.

However, we have no comparable need for information about deeply lying structures, and no comparable cortical mechanism exists. We have no "body image" of these deeply lying structures, and pain arising in them cannot therefore be accurately located. The pain must be referred; it is misinterpreted as arising from other areas that are within the body image. This spread of pain is not dependent on nerve root compression, and the dysesthesia in the fourth and fifth fingers produced by trauma to the ulnar nerve is not a good general illustration of the nature of referred pain.

***Quality of Referred Pain.*** The quality of referred pain is determined more by the site to which it is referred than by the nature of the original pain stimulus. Anginal pain is of course not localized to the myocardium, as we have no body image of the heart muscle. It may be felt in the precordial region, where it is appreciated as a heaviness or a crushing pressure. It may be referred to the shoulder region, where it is felt as a deep ache, perhaps exacerbated by a draft. It may be referred to the forearm or hand, which may be described as dead, numb, woody, or swollen. The same pain, arising in the same area of heart muscle, and traveling by the same pathways to association areas in the cerebral cortex, may simultaneously give three very different kinds of sensory impression to the patient struggling to find words to accurately describe the nature of his distress. The qualities of deadness, numbness, and swelling associated with distal referral should be particularly noted, as they are common to many pains referred distally in the limbs, and commonly are misinterpreted as evidence of neural involvement.

***Referred Tenderness.*** The development of tenderness ("hyperalgesia") in areas to which pain is referred is part of all the classic descriptions of referred pain.[4-7] In these accounts, however, an inordinate emphasis has been placed on the development of exagerated skin tenderness, "cutaneous hyperalgesia." Deep referred tenderness is much more common than skin tenderness.

***Associated Features.*** Two separate kinds of phenomena are commonly associated with referred pain; together they can give rise to the bizarre association of pain and numbness. Tenderness, involuntary muscle spasm, inhibition of voluntary motion, and increased blood flow belong to the first category and can be thought of as protective in nature, though often mislocated. Referred muscle spasm, interfering with some function, may give rise to deep "clicks" or "clunks" in otherwise normal structures, such as the temporomandibular joints (from cervical spine), scapulae (from neck or shoulder), or greater trochanter (from low back).

A provisional diagnosis is made on the basis of the carefully gathered initial clinical evidence, and then alternative diagnoses are considered. This process raises reasonable doubts, which must be resolved by review of specific features in history or examination, by special investigations, by a therapeutic trial, or not at all. With nonarticular rheumatic disease, the special investigations are mostly not helpful. They are useful only in the diagnosis of degeneration, fracture, tumor, abscess, or systemic disease. Most nonarticular pain is not due to these

**Table 32–1.** Pain Amplification Syndromes

| |
|---|
| Group One: Tenderness at "Fibrositic" Sites |
| 1. Referred pain syndromes |
| 2. "Fibrositis" syndrome |
| 3. Experimental sleep deprivation |
| 4. Narcotic withdrawal |
| 5. Others |
| Group Two: Tenderness of Different Distribution |
| 1. Reflex dystrophies |
| 2. Tender shins of steroid therapy |

**Table 32–2.** Special Features of Referred Tenderness

| |
|---|
| 1. Usually distal to primary lesion |
| 2. Often not in region of maximum pain |
| 3. Deep more than cutaneous |
| 4. Often unknown to patient |
| 5. Most at predictable sites* |
| 6. Often relieved by local anesthesia or counterirritant therapy |

*See Table 32–4 and Figure 32–1.

**Table 32–3.** Local Causes of Soft Tissue Pain

1. Bursitis, tendinitis, tenosynovitis
2. Phlebitis, vasculitis, panniculitis
3. Bone-tendon junction syndromes, muscle-tendon junction syndromes, hematoma in muscle, postexercise myalgia
4. Referred pain syndromes
   - Reflex dystophies
   - Nerve entrapment syndromes
   - Pain with central nervous system disease
   - Traumatic neuromas
5. Writer's cramp, other habit spasms

conditions, and in most situations the correct diagnosis comes from a specifically directed review of the history and physical findings.

## THE POINT COUNT

In order to review the findings on physical examination while assessing alternative diagnoses, the clinician must have a systemic and effective approach to the examination of the peripheral joints, of the spine, and of the nonarticular regions. There must be a practiced familiarity with the sites in which tenderness is likely to occur and a technique that measures the quantity of tenderness, allowing for differences among individuals in general responses to pain stimulus. One approach is to do a "point count," analogous to the "joint count" inevitably used in assessing changes in the severity of peripheral joint inflammation. The basic idea is simple enough, and to the novice examiner there are only two methodologic problems: where to press and how hard to press.

A list of 14 sites at which tenderness may be found has been published,[13] and is reviewed in Table 32–4 and Figure 32–1. This list is not all-inclusive and certainly need not be carved in stone, but it remains a useful start. The firmness of pressure is determined by using as reference sites clinically "silent" areas—the lower ribs, the forearm or thigh muscles, and the fat pad lateral to the knee. For humanity as well as precision, one works at the threshold of tenderness, reducing the stimulus for generally tender individuals. Pressure over the target site

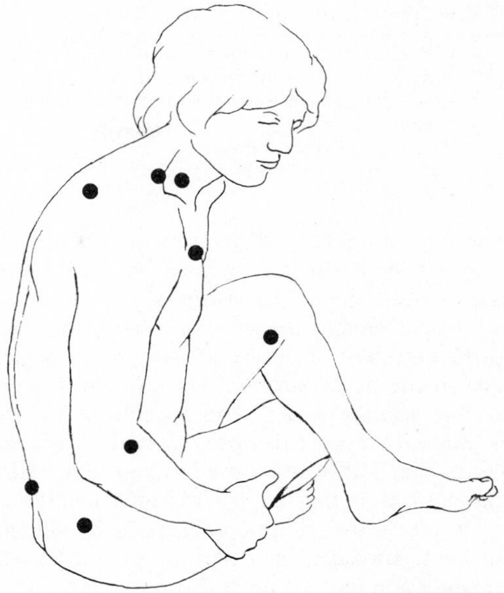

**Figure 32–1.** Characteristic sites of referred tenderness.

should be somewhat less firm, about 80 percent of the pressure over adjacent nontender areas, and the site scored positive only if very distinct tenderness is reported. This comparison of two sites, target and reference, may have to be done with some care, as the patient often assumes that the exquisite tenderness is due to unnecessary roughness and must be assured that the pressure on the "target" site is in fact less than on the "reference" area. The quantity of tenderness may then be scored in terms of the number of tender points and the distribution of these points examined for clues as to the underlying mechanisms. A small number of points, clustered in a single region, unassociated with diffuse aching stiffness and fatigue, suggests a referred pain syndrome. A large number of tender sites, spread widely and symmetrically, with systemic symptoms, suggests the "fibrositis" syndrome.

**Table 32–4.** The Point Count: 14 Tender Sites

| | | |
|---|---|---|
| **Trapezius,** midpoint of upper fold | R | 1 |
| | L | 2 |
| **Costochondral junctions,** second; maximum just lateral to junctions on upper surface | R<br>L | 3<br>4 |
| **Lateral epicondyles,** tennis elbow sites, 2 cm distal to epicondyles, within muscle that tenses when long finger is actually extended | R<br>L | 5<br>6 |
| **Supraspinatus,** at origins, above scapular spine near the medial border | R<br>L | 7<br>8 |
| **Low cervical,** anterior aspects of intertransverse C4-6 | | 9 |
| **Low lumbar,** interspinous ligaments L4-S1 | | 10 |
| **Gluteus medius,** upper outer quadrants of buttocks, in anterior fold of muscle | R<br>L | 11<br>12 |
| **Medial fat pad,** overlying medial collateral ligament of the knee, proximal to the joint line | R<br>L | 13<br>14 |

## THE "FIBROSITIS" SYNDROME

The "fibrositis" syndrome is a pain amplification syndrome, the essential clinical feature of which is the presence of a large number of specifically tender sites. While there are complex interactions between personality and pathogenesis in these patients, the evidence to be discussed below indicates that the magnification is not purely psychogenic, i.e., at the interpretive level, but physiogenic, predominantly a quantitative change in physiologically normal pain mechanisms. Four lines of evidence support this belief: the predictability of the tender sites, the reactive hyperemia, the strong association with a specific sleep disturbance, and the temporary reproduction of the syndrome in normal subjects.

**Clinical Picture.** The pain or aching is widespread, poorly circumscribed and deep, and is referred to mus-

**Table 32–5.** Cardinal Features of "Fibrositis"

1. Diffuse aching pain, stiffness, weakness
2. High point count, diffuse distribution
3. High sensitivity to internal and external stimuli
4. Nonrestorative sleep
5. Perfectionistic personality

cles or bony prominences. When central, it has an aching character; when peripheral, it may feel like a swelling, stiffness, or numbness. The stiffness is an increase of a sense of tissue tension or of muscular effort required toward the extremes of range. These symptoms are concentrated in the broad areas of reference of the cervical and lumbar segments and tend to shift with time, so that the patients recurrently present with "new" sites of complaints. The stiffness is noted at rest, is worse in the morning, and is increased by weather changes, cold, fatigue, or excess use. Simple analgesics are disappointing, but heat, massage, or a holiday may give relief.

The exhaustion may be most disabling and not clearly related to lack of rest. It is often marked in the morning and paralyzes as well as punishes initiative.

The patients emphasize their exhaustion but many minimize their sleep disturbance. They may have been light sleepers for years and relate their frequent and prolonged wakefulness to pain. Virtually all arise feeling unrefreshed (this is the key question to ask), more exhausted than at bedtime the night before. After stress, they may spend whole nights without sleep (see Table 32–6).

They are sensitive to cold, noise, and environmental irritants. Visceral sensations may be equally amplified. An example is urinary frequency, particularly nocturnal, due to a sense of bladder fullness despite small urinary volume. There is usually no pain on urination, and cultures are sterile, but recurrent cystitis is frequently misdiagnosed and inappropriately treated. The association of the irritable bowel syndrome with "fibrositis" has been well documented.[1]

These patients are apprehensive and relax poorly during examination, with spasmodic, inappropriate muscle contractions interrupting active and passive motion; a full range is achieved only after gentle persistence. Grip strength and other muscle power as measured by a modified blood pressure cuff is half normal or less and is

**Table 32–6.** Symptoms of Sleep Disturbance*

| Symptom | "Fibrositis" Group (n = 22) | Control Group (n = 22) |
|---|---|---|
| Waking with aching, stiffness | 100 percent | 23 percent |
| Tired during the day | 100 | 41 |
| Waking tired | 95 | 32 |
| Waking frequently | 68 | 59 |
| Difficulty falling asleep | 36 | 23 |
| Waking early | 36 | 36 |

*After Campbell, S.M., Clark, S., Findall, E.A., et al.: Clinical characteristics of fibrositis. Arthritis Rheum. 26:817, 983.

inconstant and poorly sustained. Yet the muscles show the conditioning effect of isometric exercise; they tend to be well preserved, in striking contrast to the weakness described and displayed. Tenderness is not simply reported; it may be demonstrated by sudden dramatic twisting leaps, the highly characteristic "jump sign." The interview is exhausting for the examiner as well as the patient, a significant sign given the professional experience of the physician, indicative of the stresses between the patient and the environment.

**The Tender Points.** Most of the multiple other points are unknown to the patient and are often not central to the areas of pain. They can be readily found because of their remarkably constant location. The published list (see Table 32–4 and Fig. 32–1) is by no means exclusive. Tenderness at the medial epicondyle, the lower pole of the coracoid process, the other costochondral junctions, and the margins of the greater trochanters and patellae is almost equally common. The cervical tenderness is most often missed or underestimated. The anterior aspects of the lower intertransverse spaces are strikingly more tender than lateral or posterior aspects of transverse processes or interspinous ligaments. The carefully controlled dolorimeter study of Campbell and associates[2] has shown the efficiency of specific point tenderness in differentiating between normal and "fibrositic" subjects (Fig. 32–2).

The tenderness involves a variety of tissues, including muscle, bone, fibrous tissue, and subcutaneous fat, and extensive histologic and electromyographic studies have not identified any concentration of neural structures or other consistent histologic bases.[14-16] They tend to be firmer than surrounding tissues.

Skinfold tenderness and reactive hyperemia are important witnesses to diagnosis and to underlying mechanisms. Both are most marked in the upper scapular region. Hyperesthesia to pinprick is much less marked. Both occur in the general regions of sites of deep tenderness and so are found at the tennis elbow and costochondral sites. The erythema is uncommon distally in the limbs or in the lower half of the body. Absence of laboratory evidence of inflammatory or muscle damage is a defined requirement for the diagnosis of "primary" fibrositis; but it must be re-emphasized that fibrositic mechanisms ("secondary fibrositis") commonly complicate the assessment and therapy of rheumatoid arthritis and other diseases.

**The "Fibrositic" Personality.**

> . . . In the morning she was asked how she slept. "Oh, terribly badly!" said the Princess. "I have scarcely shut my eyes the whole night. Heaven only knows what was in the bed, but I was lying on something hard, so that I am black and blue all over. . . ." Nobody but a real princess could be as sensitive as that. So the prince took her for his wife, for now he knew he had a real princess. (From "The Princess and the Pea," *Arthur Rackham Fairy Book.*)

These patients set high standards and are as demanding of themselves as of others. They are caring, honest, tidy, committed, moral, industrious—virtuous

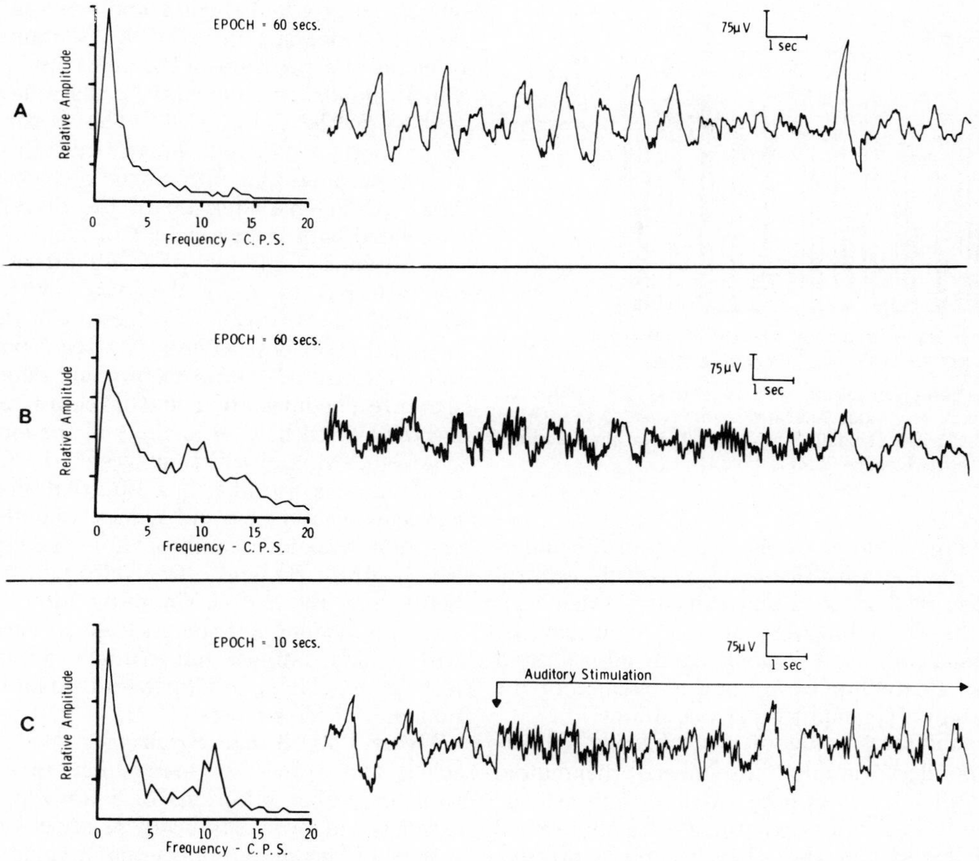


**Figure 32–2.** *A,* Frequency spectra and raw EEG from NREM (stage 4) sleep in a healthy 25-year-old subject. The spectrum shows that most amplitude is concentrated at 1 cps (delta). *B,* NREM sleep in a 42-year-old "fibrositis" patient. The spectrum shows amplitude at both 1 cps (delta) and 8–10 cps (alpha). *C,* NREM sleep of a healthy 21-year-old subject during stage 4 sleep deprivation. In the EEG there is a clear association between external arousal (auditory stimulation) and alpha onset. Again the frequency spectrum (obtained by 10-second analysis from stimulus onset) shows amplitude concentrated in the delta and alpha bands. (From Moldofsky, H., et al.: Psychosomat. Med. *37*:341, 1975.)

to a fault. Their perfectionism can be trying, but they are often very effective in their chosen field of activity and have unusual loyalty from employers and family. They are not abnormal, just characteristic. They deeply resent any suggestion that they are using their illness as a crutch, as they drive themselves harder than most, and dislike other crutches, such as alcohol and prescribed medication. They are not depressed,[17] and the concept of "masked depression" may have arisen because of the response of "fibrositic" symptoms to tricyclic medication.

**The Sleep Disturbance.** As yet unconfirmed key studies have provided evidence of a specific disturbance in sleep physiology. In the first study,[18] 10 "fibrositic" subjects showed a decrease in stages 3 and 4 slow-wave sleep, with intrusion of a rapid alpha rhythm, as determined by computer analysis of the energy frequency spectra (Fig. 32–3), and all showed an overnight increase in tenderness measured by dolorimeter. These observations have since been confirmed and extended in studies of a large number of other patients.[19,20] High-energy bursts of alpha waves intruding into slow-wave sleep was described by Hauri and Hawkins as alpha-delta sleep,[21] and its association with aching, fatigue, and stiffness described.[22] This more florid pattern can be read by eye, and was recognized in 8 of 26 "chronic pain" patients.[23] Other studies on this point have been done,[2] but they have not been published in detail.

In another study, experimental reproduction of aspects of the "fibrositis" syndrome was achieved in healthy university students.[24] After control nights, for three nights they were deprived of rapid eye movement (REM), or stage 4 non-REM, sleep, by a buzzer, supplemented when necessary by hand arousal. The buzzer caused a rapid alpha rhythm to appear in the EEG superimposed on the slow-wave pattern, to mimic the pattern seen in the "fibrositis" patients. No increase in tenderness was associated with REM deprivation, but disturbance of slow-wave non-REM sleep was associated with a marked overnight increase in tenderness scores and symptoms of anorexia, overwhelming physical tiredness, and heaviness (Fig. 32–3).

**"Fibrositic" Features and Other Rheumatic Diseases.** Therapy is often determined by the urgency of the pa-

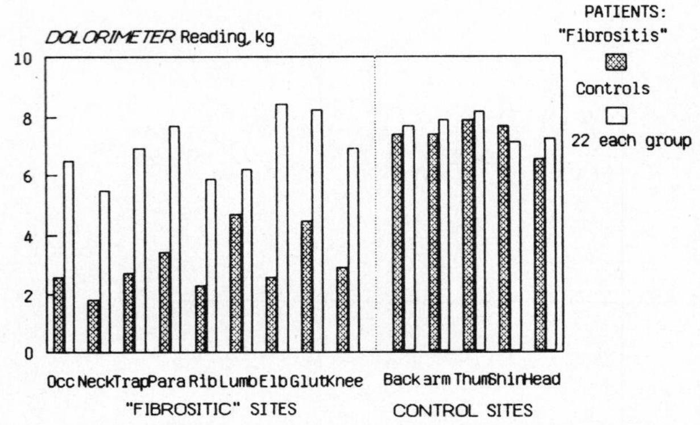


**Figure 32–3.** Tenderness at selected sites in patients with "fibrositis" and in controls. A low value indicates a more tender site. (After Campbell, S.M., Clark, S., Tindall, E. A., et al.: Clinical characteristics of fibrositis. Arthritis Rheum. 26:817, 1983.)

tient's complaints and not by the severity of the underlying disease. Patients with rheumatoid arthritis, cervical or lumbar disc disease, or a whole host of other conditions may have amplification of their symptoms by "fibrositic" mechanisms. The point count allows rapid recognition of this complication and avoidance of the excess of therapy that might otherwise follow.

Moldofsky and Chester identified a subgroup of "paradoxical responders" among hospitalized rheumatoid patients, identified by worsening mood with improving disease.[25] When first admitted, these patients seemed cheerful and cooperative; but they became depressed, complaining, and agitated as treatment progressed. They were more likely to receive prolonged hospitalization, extensive investigation, and hazardous medical and surgical therapies, with increased morbidity and even mortality. "The squeaky wheel gets the grease." Almost half the hospitalized rheumatoid patients showed this pattern, and on examination the "fibrositic" sites were characteristically more tender than their swollen joints.

**Prevalence, Criteria, and Nomenclature.** Figure 32–4 shows the number of tender points recorded in an

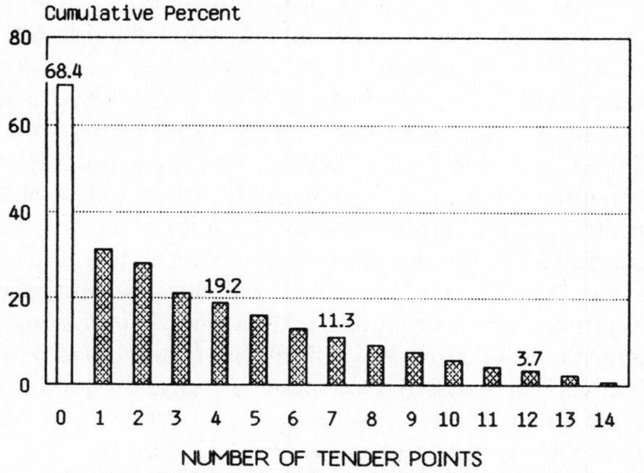


**Figure 32–4.** Prevalence of "fibrositic" tender points in 980 mixed rheumatic patients. (Data from Wolfe, F.: 1983.)

unselected group of rheumatic disease patients.[3] Clearly the prevalence of "fibrositis" in this population will be intolerably dependent on the point count criterion chosen. In published studies, the criteria have varied from 4 of 53 points[1] to 12 of 14.[16] The 20 percent with 4 or more points will include a majority with simple referred pain syndromes and without the other features listed in Table 32–2, characteristic of the disabling syndrome associated with large numbers of points. The pathogenesis, prognosis, and therapy are all different, and it seems inappropriate to apply the same name, be it "fibromyalgia"[1] or "fibrositis," to these very different groups. It would seem best to imbed "trigger points" and "localized fibrositis" within the primary diagnosis of which these are a manifestation, and develop a new name stressing the altered pain physiology of the more generalized syndrome. Moldofsky has suggested the "rheumatic pain modulation syndrome,"[26] a title that shares the disadvantages of other current names, that they are archaic and nonphysiologic, and therefore unsaleable to internists, neurologists, and other colleagues. The criteria are better than the names. Choosing subjects with a sufficient number of tender points leads to a group of patients with aching, fatigue, and irritable everything,[1] and selecting for aching and fatigue leads to patients with large numbers of tender points.[2]

**Other Polymyalgic Syndromes.** Widespread muscle aching and stiffness are seen acutely in association with viral and other infections or following unaccustomed exercise, and more chronically in association with a large variety of rheumatic, infectious, myopathic, endocrine, or malignant disorders. These manifestations have not been closely observed and warrant disciplined study. In acute illness the symptoms and tenderness are usually diffusely spread throughout the muscles, especially proximal muscles. About half the patients with the chronic syndromes show concentration of tenderness at "fibrositic" sites; but in others the tenderness is more diffuse, often with restriction of shoulder or other joint movement. In summary, almost any systemic disease, whether infectious, autoimmune, neoplastic, or metabolic in origin, may cause diffuse aching. In addition, the anxieties and frustrations of undiagnosed illness may unmask "fibrositic" elements in predisposed individuals.

## PSYCHOGENIC MUSCULOSKELETAL PAIN SYNDROMES

For psychological reasons, symptoms may be invented or magnified, willfully or unconsciously. These classic varieties of psychiatric illness are relatively easy to suspect and to understand because of the obvious inconsistencies, exaggerations, emotional manipulations, and secondary gains. There remain two very difficult questions that frequently arise: (1) Does this obviously disturbed patient have an underlying organic disease? (2) By what mechanisms do psychological storms produce physiological changes?

Neither of these questions has received the attention

it deserves. The individual patient will require close and often repeated study with objective clinical and laboratory techniques; with such study, the number of symptoms resulting from purely cortical invention becomes very small. Magnification and modification of symptoms are common, and the interaction of personality and physical disability is so strong that psychogenic enhancement of tissue change is a distinct possibility. These questions require restatement in terms of phenomena that can be studied quantitatively. Many of the instruments used in these studies are inappropriate for rheumatology patients, scoring symptoms of disease and normal reactions to them as attributes of psychogenic origin.

## PSYCHOGENIC REGIONAL PAIN OR HYSTERIA

Regional or generalized pain may be an important symptom in patients with hysteria of the classic type described by Charcot, Freud, and others, or it may be seen in patients with depression, schizophrenia, other neuroses, or even organic brain syndromes.[27]

The pain is regional rather than segmental and affects areas with large cortical or emotional representation, such as the face, anterior chest, or limbs. The boundary of the region affected is often sharply defined, at the root of a limb or the midline, but can be shifted dramatically by suggestion. There is often an extraordinary mixture of skin hyperesthesia plus numbness—marked distress when a hair is twitched but total inability to feel a pin. These features do not of course rule out the possibility of coexistent organic disease. Limitation of joint movement in these patients may stubbornly persist despite gently persistent persuasion, and re-examination after intravenous diazepam or Pentothal may be necessary. This examination should be carried out only with informed consent and detailed descriptive notes and in the presence of a qualified anesthetist and other witnesses.

## OTHER SOFT TISSUE PAIN SYNDROMES

**Diffuse Idiopathic Skeletal Hyperostosis (DISH, Ankylosing Hyperostosis, Forestier's Disease).** The criteria for diagnosis of this syndrome are radiologic and spinal. Extraspinal involvement was described by Forestier and colleagues[28,29] and emphasized by Resnick and colleagues[30,31] with ossification of ligamentous attachments to bone at multiple sites. The diagnosis cannot now be made in the absence of extensive ossification, obviously a late event. Many of these patients describe widespread trunk and limb aching for decades prior to diagnosis, with points of tenderness where fibrous tissues attach to bone—a distribution quite different from the "fibrositic" points. This condition develops in heavy-boned, thick-limbed individuals, and must be considered, along with trauma and the B27-associated anthropathies, in the differential diagnosis in patients presenting with pain under the heel or at other bone-tendon junction syndromes.

**Tender Shins with Steroid Therapy.** Slocumb[32] described "myalgias" associated with cortisone therapy, and later Rotstein and Good[33] described the occurrence of striking tenderness of the "muscles of the extremities" in five patients receiving high doses of oral steroids, coining the term "steroid pseudo-rheumatism." The tenderness is maximal in the lower legs, and affects bone, skin, tendon, and muscle but spares the feet. It is commonly associated with a waxlike shiny atrophy of the skin but not with edema, evidence of neuropathy, or tenderness at "fibrositic" sites. It is overwhelmingly associated with steroid therapy and may lessen if steroids are withdrawn but may also occasionally be seen in patients with maturity-onset diabetes. Its pathogenesis is unknown.

**Malignant Hyperthermia Syndrome.** Chronic widespread aching and stiffness have recently been emphasized as being characteristic and suggestive of the malignant hyperthermia syndrome,[34] a warning that general anesthesia may precipitate a catastrophe. The condition is fortunately rare, and the diagnosis is virtually impossible to confirm prior to the occurrence of a near-fatal event. Symptom analysis has therefore been retrospective in badly frightened patients and has not been sufficiently detailed to separate those caused by interaction of events and personality.

## PROBLEMS IN THERAPY

The explanations are the most important and a difficult part of the treatment program. Multiple factors often combine to produce symptoms in patients with nonarticular rheumatism, and the therapeutic discussion may involve one or all of the following topics: (1) referred pain, tenderness, and reflex responses; (2) mechanical stress in neck and lower back; (3) the sleep disturbance; (4) measures for pain relief; and (5) attitudes and expectations.

One cannot cover all the areas in one interview, and the most urgent should be selected for explanations in depth. There may be varying emphasis on mechanical or "fibrositic" amplifying factors, but the same patterns occur so commonly that a printed handout covering this ground briefly may be of more value in this than in any other field of rheumatology. All explanations begin with the reassurance that the pain is real, not imaginary or neurotic in origin, a reassurance needed because of the absence of anatomic changes in the areas of pain.

**Referred Pain, Tenderness, and Reflex Responses.** The patient is given a brief but specific account of referred pain. All pain of deep origin is necessarily referred. The mental equipment to permit us to visualize our pancreas, apophyseal joints, or acetabulum does not exist, and pain arising in these structures is necessarily misinterpreted as arising in other structures sharing the same nerve supply and familiar enough to be included in the body image. The areas to which pain is referred often develop secondary reflex changes, misguided but protective in intent, including deep tenderness, circulatory changes, and strange mixtures of increased muscle tone and inhibition of voluntary action, and of pain and subjective numbness.

**Mechanical Stresses in Neck and Low Back.** For very good mechanical reasons, two regions of the spine account for the vast majority of complaints. No treatment program is adequate that fails to identify and correct these underlying mechanical problems, which are very often overlooked or neglected.

The cervical spine is particularly subjected to stresses during sleep. The skull and thorax are supported, but the neck forms an unsupported bridge, subjected to the compressive forces that give stability to the arch in architecture. Furthermore, the thoracic vertebrae are lifted by the support of the ribs, and the cervical vertebrae sag, inducing shear stresses. Slight exaggeration of these forces during examination with the patient in the sleeping position will reproduce the pain, which can be relieved nicely by using the examiner's forearm to provide support under the arch of the neck. The cause and the cure have been demonstrated, and it remains necessary only to find a similarly pleasant and effective support. A pair of cervical ruffs may be made by enclosing two 8-inch by 24-inch dressing pads within tubes of 3-inch stockinette; these should be loosely tied in front and worn during sleep as a pillow, not a splint. Neck-support pillows may give cooler long-term comfort, or a regular pillow can be doubled over and used with the fold under the neck. A variety of physical therapies can also be useful if gently applied; but 15 minutes of therapy three times weekly will not solve the problem if 8 hours per night is spent making it worse.

The lower lumbar spine is at the extreme limit of hyperextension in virtually all patients with low back problems, and many have such weak abdominal muscles they can neither improve their posture nor develop a positive intra-abdominal pressure during lifting to spare their back. The investigation and therapy are similar, using sit-ups with neck, trunk, hips, and knees flexed (for safety) and feet held. The test or exercise progresses through levels of difficulty, beginning with arms outstretched; then hands to opposite shoulders; hands behind neck; and finally arms behind head, with fingers touching opposite ears. Five repetitions faithfully performed once daily will restore abdominal power to level 3 or 4 within weeks, even for the aged. Postural training is designed to avoid lumbar hyperextension. The ideal is that of the athlete, with knees bent and spine slightly flexed. To be avoided is the military posture: chest out, shoulders back, and swaybacked.

The sleep disturbance is little helped by barbiturates, which do not restore the normal sleep pattern. Chlorpromazine is effective[20] in restoring deep sleep and relieving pain but leaves such unpleasant morning lethargy that it is unsuitable for long-term use. The benzodiazepines, such as diazepam, 5 to 20 mg at night, are occasionally helpful symptomatically. They do not abolish alpha intrusion into slow-wave sleep and are often ineffective. Tricyclic antidepressants, such as amitriptyline or imipramine, can reduce alpha intrusion, and with an effect better sustained over prolonged periods.[22] In modest doses there is little effect for several hours after ingestion, but the quality of late morning sleep is improved. Some patients report frightening dreams, and others are sensitive to morning lethargy, so that appropriate evening dosage of amitriptyline may vary widely from 10 to 75 mg.

**Counterirritant Therapies.** A wide variety of popular or unusual therapies, including massage, heat, liniments, steroid injections, ethyl chloride spray, and acupuncture, are helpful in relieving pain. The "gate" theory of Melzack and Wall[8] has provided theoretical respectability, and recent studies have provided evidence for involvement of endorphins in the analgesic effect.[9] Factors influencing choice of counterirritant technique will include simplicity, safety, and availability and economy on one hand and maximal placebo effect on the other.

**Compliance and Noncompliance.** Among the most common reasons for failure to respond to conservative therapy is the failure to use it. The term noncompliance suggests that the fault lies with the patient. A better term might be faulty doctor-patient interaction, as noncompliant patients may have inadequate understanding of the program proposed and may have such apprehension of the doctor's anger that they will not reveal to the doctor their omissions and their reasons. Faced with failure, the patient and the doctor tend to try something new; this is ineffective strategy if the new remedy is similar to the old, and a dangerous decision if a hazardous course is taken unnecessarily. A certain decisiveness on the part of the therapist is obviously essential, but anger and ultimatums usually lead to evasions or countermanipulations. It is better to reduce the opportunities for personality conflicts, and to reinforce the continuing direction of therapy by sharing when possible clinical and laboratory evidence of improvement and compliance. The diary system can be very helpful, with the patient recording such variables as weight, abdominal muscle power, sedimentation rate, and salicylate level, with clearly defined target levels. Then the battle is between the patient and the chart, with the physician standing by as a helpful friend.

**Attitudes and Expectations.** Patients who are sensitive and perfectionistic set too high standards for themselves and may have to be specifically advised to take a holiday totally away from continuing responsibilities and cares. Such holidays should be consciously scheduled to take place once a year, once a month, once a week, and once a day. These patients are very sensitive to any implications that they are "quitters" or "fakers"—they are more characteristically unusually loyal and effective but at too high a cost.

Tension normally and necessarily accompanies major effort. It is normal for an athlete preparing for a major event to develop sweaty palms, a rapid heart rate, and the other physical responses to anticipated challenge. The body responds similarly to intellectual or emotional challenges, and this build-up of tension is essential to optimal performance. When the challenge is undramatic, is repeated daily, and arises from normal job and family duties, the relationship between tension and response to challenge may be inapparent or devalued. The defect does not lie in the exposure to tension but in the failure to get out from under self-imposed loads. Any variety of recreational release may be considered, but preference should be given to activities that give pleasure, are social, and involve physical activity. These patients are not helped by narrowing the scope of their life, and it is extremely important that their work patterns not be interrupted.

## References


1. Yunus, M., Masi, A.T., Calabro, J.J., Miller, K.A., and Feigenbaum, S.L.: Primary fibromyalgia (fibrositis): Clinical study of 50 patients with matched normal controls. Semin. Arthritis Rheum. 11:151, 1981.
2. Campbell, S.M., Clark, S., Tindall, E.A., Forehand, M.E., and Bennett, R.H.O.: Clinical characteristics of fibrositis. Arthritis Rheum. 26:817, 1983.
3. Wolfe, F., and Cathey, M.A.: Prevalence of primary and secondary fibrositis. J. Rheumatol. 10:965, 1983.
4. Kellgren, J.H.: Deep pain sensibility. Lancet 1:943, 1949.
5. Kellgren, J.H.: Observations on referred pain arising from muscle. Clin. Sci. 3:174, 1938.
6. Kellgren, J.H.: On distribution of pain arising from deep somatic structures with charts of segmental pain areas. Clin. Sci. 4:35, 1939.
7. Lewis, T., and Kellgren, J.H.: Observations relating to referred pain, visceromotor reflexes and other associated phenomena. Clin. Sci. 4:47, 1939.
8. Melzack, R., and Wall, P.D.: Pain mechanisms: A new theory. Science 150:971.
9. Pomeranz, B.: Do endorphins mediate acupuncture analgesia? *In* Costa, E., and Trabucchi, M. (eds.): The Endorphins. Advances in Biochemical Psychopharmacology. Vol. 18. New York, Raven Press, 1977, p. 351.
10. Hinoki, M., and Niki, H.: Role of the sympathetic nervous system in the formation of the traumatic vertigo of cervical origin. Acta. Otolaryngol. 330(Suppl.):185, 1975.
11. Toglia, J.V.: Acute flexion-extension injury of the neck. Electronystagmographic study of 309 cases. Neurology 25:808, 1976.
12. Moldofsky, H.: Occupational cramp. J. Psychosomat. Res. 15:439, 1971.
13. Smythe, H.A., and Moldofsky, H.: Two contributions to understanding of the "fibrositis" syndrome. Bull. Rheum. Dis. 28:298, 1977.
14. Simons, D.G.: Muscle pain syndromes. Part 1. Am. J. Phys. Med. 54:289, 1975.
15. Simons, D.G. Muscle pain syndromes. Part 2. Am. J. Phys. Med. 55:15, 1976.
16. Smythe, H.A.: Nonarticular rheumatism and the "fibrositis" syndrome. *In* Hollander, J.L., and McCarty, D.J., Jr. (eds.): Arthritis and Allied Conditions. 8th ed. Philadelphia, Lea & Febiger, 1972.
17. Payne, T.C., Leavitt, F., Garron, D.C., Katz, R.S., Golden, H.E., Glickman, P.B., and Vanderplate, C.: Fibrositis and psychogenic disturbance. Arthritis Rheum. 25:213–217, 1982.
18. Moldofsky, H., Scarisbrick, P., England, R., and Smythe, H.: Musculoskeletal symptoms and non-REM sleep disturbance in patients with "fibrositis syndrome" and healthy subjects. Psychosomat. Med. 37:341, 1975.
19. Moldofsky, H., and Scarisbrick, P.: Induction of neurasthenic musculoskeletal pain syndrome by selective sleep stage deprivation. Psychosomat. Med. 38:35, 1976.
20. Moldofsky, H., and Lue, F.: Alpha and delta EEG frequencies, pain and mood in "fibrositic" patients treated with chlorpromazine and L-tryptophan. EEG Clin. Neurophysiol. 50:71, 1980.
21. Hauri, P., and Hawkins, D.R.: Alpha-delta sleep. Electroencephalogr. Clin. Neurophysiol. 34:233, 1973.
22. Hauri, P.: The Sleep Disorders. Kalamazoo, The Upjohn Co., 1977, p. 51.
23. Wittig, R.M., Zorick, F.J., Blumer, D., Heilbronn, M., and Roth, T.: Disturbed sleep in patients complaining of chronic pain. J. Nerv. Ment. Dis. 170:429, 1982.
24. Moldofsky, H., and Scarisbrick, P.: Induction of neuresthenic musculoskeletal pain syndrome by selective stage sleep deprivation. Psychosomat. Med. 38:35, 1976.
25. Moldofsky, H., and Chester, W.J.: Pain and mood patterns in patients with rheumatoid arthritis. Psychosomat. Med. 32:309, 1970.
26. Moldofsky, H.: Rheumatic pain modulation syndrome: The interrelationships between sleep, central nervous system serotonin, and pain. *In* Critchley, M., Friedman, A.P., Sicuteri, F. (eds.): Advances in Neurology. Vol. 33. New York, Raven Press, 1982, p. 51.
27. Walters, A.: Psychogenic regional pain alias hysterical pain. Brain 84:1, 1961.
28. Forestier, J., and Rotes-Querol, J.: Senile ankylosing hyperostosis of the spine. Ann. Rheum. Dis. 9:321, 1950.
29. Forestier, J., and Lagier, R.: Vertebral ankylosing hyperostosis: Morphological basis, clinical manifestations, situation and diagnosis. *In* Hill, A. (ed.).: Modern Trends in Rheumatology. Vol. 2. London, Butterworths, 1971, p. 323.
30. Resnick, D., Shall, S.R., and Robins, J.M.: Diffuse idiopathic skeletal hyperostosis (DISH): Forestier's disease with extraspinal manifestations. Radiology 115:513, 1975.
31. Utsinger, P.D., Resnick, D., and Shapiro, R.: Diffuse skeletal abnormalities in Forestier's disease. Arch. Intern. Med. 136:763, 1976.
32. Slocumb, C.H.: Symposium on certain problems are arising from clinical use of cortisone. Mayo Clin. Proc. 28:655, 1973.
33. Rotstein, J., and Good, B.A.: Steroid pseudorheumatism. Arch. Intern. Med. 99:545, 1957.
34. Henschel, E.O. (ed.): Malignant Hyperthermia: Current Concepts. New York, Appleton-Century-Crofts, 1977.


# Chapter 33

# Approach to the Patient with Hyperuricemia

*William N. Kelley*

Evaluation of the patient with hyperuricemia is directed toward answering the following questions: (1) Does the patient really have hyperuricemia? (2) Has damage to tissues or organs occurred as a result? (3) Are associated findings present? (4) What is the cause? (5) What, if anything, should be done? From a practical standpoint these inquiries are pursued simultaneously, since decisions about the significance of hyperuricemia and about therapy depend on the answers to all of them.

## WHAT IS HYPERURICEMIA AND DOES THE PATIENT HAVE IT?

The serum urate value is elevated in an absolute sense when it exceeds the limit of solubility of monosodium urate in serum. At 37° C the saturation value of urate in plasma is about 7.0 mg per 100 ml; a value above this concentration represents supersaturation in a physicochemical sense. The serum urate concentration is elevated in a relative sense when it exceeds the upper limit of an arbitrary normal range, which is usually defined as the mean serum urate value plus two standard deviations in a sex- and age-matched healthy population. In most epidemiological studies, the upper limit has been rounded off at 7.0 mg per 100 ml in men and 6.0 mg per 100 ml in women. Finally, a serum urate value in excess of 7.0 mg per 100 ml begins to carry an increased risk of gouty arthritis or renal stones.

Many factors, including sex and age, have an important influence on the serum urate concentration. The serum urate concentration before puberty in both boys and girls averages approximately 3.6 mg per 100 ml. After the onset of puberty, the levels rise in males more than in females. Values in males reach a plateau in the early 20's and are essentially stable thereafter. Values in females are constant at a lower level than those found in males from age 20 through 40. With menopause the values in women rise and approach or equal those in men. Differences in the serum urate levels with sex and age are thought to be related to differences in the renal clearance of urate, perhaps determined, in turn, by the endogenous levels of estrogens and androgens. In addition to age and sex, other factors, including obesity, muscle mass, warm ambient temperature, higher social status, achievement, and intelligence, appear to correlate with a higher serum urate concentration.

Interpretation of the serum urate level must also take into account the laboratory method employed. Fluorimetric methods and most automated techniques will measure materials other than urate and may give higher values than the more specific uricase method. In addition, there may be substantial variation over a period of time in any single individual, an observation attributable to many causes, including some of the variables described above. Accordingly, a single serum urate value is of considerably less value than several determinations over time.

Hyperuricemia by one or more of the aforementioned definitions has been described in 2.3 to 17.6 percent of the populations studied. In one hospitalized population in the United States, 13.2 percent of all adult men exhibited a serum urate concentration in excess of 7.0 mg per 100 ml.[1]

## HAS TISSUE OR ORGAN DAMAGE OCCURRED OWING TO THE HYPERURICEMIA?

Assessment of tissue damage that might be attributed to hyperuricemia is of major importance in the patient with arthritis, subcutaneous nodules, erosions or other changes on radiographs, aseptic necrosis, nephrolithiasis, or renal insufficiency. Any other clinical signs and symptoms that might result from sustained hyperuricemia would be rare in the absence of at least one of the above.

**Arthritis.** In the hyperuricemic patient with active joint disease, the most useful diagnostic test is direct examination of the synovial fluid. According to current dogma, the demonstration of intracellular monosodium urate crystals establishes the diagnosis of gout; it does not, of course, exclude other diseases that may occur simultaneously, e.g., septic arthritis, pseudogout, osteoarthritis, fractures, or torn ligaments or tendons, and these possibilities may have to be excluded. Intracellular monosodium urate crystals can be demonstrated in virtually all patients with gout if synovial fluid from the appropriate joint is carefully examined using compensated polarized light microscopy within the first 24 to 48 hours after onset of the attack. Thus, failure to demonstrate intracellular urate crystals in synovial fluid obtained from an acutely inflamed joint makes the diagnosis of gout highly unlikely as the cause of an acute episode of synovitis. However, when patients are examined several days after the onset of acute synovitis, the likelihood of finding urate crystals declines and the urate crystals observed may not be located in polymorphonuclear leukocytes. Extracellular urate crystals can be found in synovial fluid of 70 percent of gouty patients even during the intercritical period when they are asymptomatic.[2] The finding of extracellular urate crystals in synovial fluid does not carry the same degree of specificity for diagnosing gout as does the demonstration of intracellular urate crystals. This conclusion is based on the following observations. Although the patient with uncomplicated asymptomatic hyperuricemia rarely ($<5$ percent) exhibits extracellular urate crystals in synovial fluid, as many as 20 percent of patients with hyperuricemia secondary to renal failure may have extracellular urate crystals in the absence of any history of arthritis.[2]

When synovial fluid cannot be obtained or active joint disease is not present at the time of examination, the relationship of hyperuricemia to the clinical symptoms may be more difficult to evaluate. If there is a history of classic podagra or of an acute monoarticular arthritis strongly suggestive of gouty arthritis and dramatically responsive to colchicine, a working assumption that the patient has gout is justified. The diagnosis should be documented with demonstration of urate crystals at the first opportunity.

**Nodules.** The finding of subcutaneous nodules in the hyperuricemic subject raises the possibility that these are tophaceous deposits. The history is important in this connection, since tophi rarely occur without preceding gouty arthritis. However, if a question exists as to the nature of the nodule or deposit, material should be obtained for microscopic examination. This may be done most easily by closed aspiration of the nodule under aseptic conditions, using a sterile 22-gauge needle. Injection of a small amount of sterile saline may enhance the recovery of urate crystals if no material is obtained with aspiration alone. Suspected tophi in the helix of the ear can be confirmed by gentle abrasion of the skin and blotting the denuded surface with a sterile slide. If urate crystals are demonstrated, the nodule represents a tophus. If crystals are not demonstrated with this procedure, open surgical biopsy of the lesion may be performed. The tissue obtained at that time should be fixed in absolute alcohol in order to avoid dissolution of crystals if present.

Serologic tests for rheumatoid factor are also helpful in evaluating the patient with subcutaneous nodules. If the lesion is a rheumatoid nodule, over 90 percent of patients will have a positive screening test for rheumatoid factor and the test will usually remain positive at serum dilutions of 1:80 or greater. Only 30 percent of patients with gout exhibit positive screening tests for rheumatoid factor, and these are usually of low titer.

**Radiographic Findings.** Bony erosions seen on roentgenograms in a patient with hyperuricemia can present a difficult diagnostic problem. From a practical standpoint, erosions resulting from gout represent tophi, and consequently, they are usually preceded by a history of gouty arthritis. Tophi are not always evident in subcutaneous tissues on physical examination, however, at the time bony erosions are noted on roentgenograms. The radiographic appearance of the erosions may be of some help in determining the etiology of this lesion. Should this history be inconsistent with gout and the radiologic features atypical for gout, one would ordinarily assume that the erosions were not due to deposition of monosodium urate crystals. Biopsy may be indicated, particularly if a neoplastic lesion or infection is possible.

Tophi in the subcutaneous tissues are usually radiolucent, but they can become radiopaque if calcium is deposited in these lesions. In the latter circumstances radiographic examination may reveal the presence of tophaceous deposits, but physical examination will usually detect tophi in subcutaneous tissues before they are evident on roentenograms.

A possible relationship between hyperuricemia and aseptic necrosis of the femoral heads is suggested by the observation that aseptic necrosis may occur with an increased incidence in patients without gout and by the finding of monosodium urate crystals in synovium obtained from the hip at the time of surgery, even in some patients who give no history of gouty arthritis. Even though this relationship is not firmly established, it may be reasonable to consider treating the hyperuricemia if the necrosis is unilateral, or in an early stage if bilateral.

**Nephrolithiasis.** A history or laboratory finding indicative of a renal calculus provides information important to the future management of the patient. In contrast to the situation observed with tophi, renal calculi may antedate the onset of gouty arthritis. The typical uric acid stone is radiolucent and therefore is not visible on routine radiologic examination of the abdomen. It will appear as a filling defect with the use of radiopaque contrast material. As such it may be confused with other radiolucent stones, such as those composed of xanthine and adenine (which are very rare), as well as with tumors or blood clots. If a stone is passed or retrieved at surgery, it is important that it be subjected to chemical analysis.

The importance of hyperuricemia in patients with radiopaque stones deserves emphasis. First, radiopaque stones occur more commonly in patients with gout than in a nongouty population. In addition, reduction of uric acid production (and hence concentration in the urine) with allopurinol is associated with a striking decrease in the frequency of radiopaque stones containing calcium in both hyperuricemic and nonhyperuricemic subjects (Chapter 86). It is possible that the initial nidus for opaque stones in this setting is crystals of urate or uric acid. Whether or not this hypothesis accounts for the observation, the therapeutic implications are clear. Hyperuricemic subjects with calcium stones, but not other radiopaque stones such as magnesium ammonium phosphate or cystine, may benefit from a trial with allopurinol. In nonhyperuricemic subjects with hyperuricosuria ($>$ 800 and $>$ 750 mg of uric acid excreted per 24 hrs for men and women, respectively) who repetitively form calcium-containing stones a trial of allopurinol may also be indicated.[3]

**Renal Insufficiency.** One of the most difficult problems facing the clinician lies in his attempt to determine the relationship of hyperuricemia and renal insufficiency in the patient presenting with both abnormalities. In assessing the relationship between hyperuricemia and renal insufficiency it is important to consider the mechanisms by which uric acid and/or urate may injure the kidney. Urate can precipitate in the interstitium of the kidney, leading to slowly progressive renal insufficiency referred to as *urate nephropathy*; uric acid can precipitate in the collecting tubules, leading to acute renal failure, which is referred to as *uric acid nephropathy*; or uric acid crystals can grow into *calculi*, which leads to obstruction and/or infection of the kidney. If the patient has a history of gout preceding renal insufficiency and there is no evidence to suggest another cause of renal disease, such as hypertension or lead exposure, one may assume that urate nephropathy is the etiology of the renal failure. Attempts to reduce uric acid production are justified in that setting, in order to prevent further progress of the putative urate nephropathy. The patient with hyperuricemia and renal disease without a previous history of gout presents a more difficult problem. Since an understanding of the relationship of asymptomatic hyperuricemia to chronic renal disease is an important element in directing management of the former, this issue is discussed extensively later in this chapter. In the patient with acute renal failure, uric acid nephropathy should be considered. This entity is more likely to be encountered in patients with malignancies undergoing chemotherapy or radiation treatment than in gouty patients, with the exception of those individuals with inherited enzyme abnormalities leading to marked purine overproduction. The uric acid:creatinine ratio in a random urine sample from such a patient may help in his evaluation. The finding of a ratio in excess of 1.0 in a patient with acute renal insufficiency is indicative of a substantial increase in uric acid production and raises the possibility that uric acid deposition in the nephron or collecting system may be contributing to the renal insufficiency.[4] In this situation vigorous therapy is indicated. The more common finding in acute renal failure is a ratio of less than 1.0. In this situation the hyperuricemia may be due entirely to the renal disease and associated factors such as acidosis and dehydration. A history of renal calculi, especially if the stone is demonstrated to contain uric acid and/or calcium, may be another indication for antihyperuricemic therapy in the patient with renal insufficiency.

A general approach to the hyperuricemic patient is summarized in Figure 33–1. Most hyperuricemic patients will have no evidence of end-organ damage and thus have asymptomatic hyperuricemia. Management of asymptomatic hyperuricemia will depend on the associated findings and the cause of the hyperuricemia, as discussed in the following paragraphs.

## ARE ASSOCIATED FINDINGS PRESENT?

Hyperuricemia and gout may be associated with obesity, ethanol consumption, and hypertension in a significant percentage of individuals. As a consequence it is not uncommon to also find glucose intolerance, hypertriglyceridemia, atherosclerosis, and renal, hepatic, and ischemic heart disease in hyperuricemic individuals. In evaluating hyperuricemic subjects it is important to keep these associated problems in mind. It may be justified to include a complete blood count, urinalysis, 2-hour postprandial blood sugar, fasting triglycerides, creatinine, liver panel, electrocardiogram, and chest x-ray in the evaluation of the hyperuricemic patient who is overweight or hypertensive or consumes significant amounts of ethanol. In the normotensive hyperuricemic patient who is not overweight and does not drink, a search for these associated findings would probably not be cost effective.

## WHAT IS THE CAUSE OF HYPERURICEMIA?

Hyperuricemia may be defined as primary, first in order of time or development, or secondary, second in order of time or development (see Chapter 86).[5] In the latter setting, the hyperuricemia develops in the course of another disease or as a consequence of its therapy. Hyperuricemia, whether primary or secondary, may be due to overproduction of purines, reduced renal clearance of uric acid, or a combination of the two processes.

In 70 percent of hyperuricemic patients an underlying cause of hyperuricemia can be readily defined by history and physical examination.[1] Hyperuricemia may be the initial clue to the presence of a previously unsuspected disorder. In addition, the nature of the underlying cause may be useful in predicting the potential consequence, if any, of the chemical abnormality. Thus the possibility of an underlying cause should be explored in every hyperuricemic patient.

A scheme for investigating the cause of hyperuricemia, including the secondary causes, is summarized in Figure 33–2. It would seem most reasonable that one be guided by the initial history and physical examination. If an acquired cause commonly associated with normal uric acid excretion is present in the patient with asymptomatic hyperuricemia, further evaluation is probably unnecessary. If the patient has an underlying disorder usually associated with an overproduction of uric acid, determination of 24-hour urinary uric acid may be useful. The higher the urinary uric acid in this group of patients, the higher the incidence of renal calculi[6] and acute uric acid nephropathy,[7] and thus the more likely that treatment will be indicated. If no findings suggestive of a secondary cause are forthcoming, then 24-hour urinary uric acid should be measured in those with a serum urate in excess of 11 mg per 100 ml. Further rationale underlying this approach is described later in this chapter under Management of Hyperuricemia.

## THE GENERAL WORKUP

At this point the general workup of the patient with hyperuricemia may be reviewed.

**History.** In beginning to sort out clues that will help in directing the physician toward a correct understanding of the problem, it is useful to formulate questions that will decide the following:

1. Is the hyperuricemia primary or secondary? (a) Is the patient obese? If so, for how long? (b) Does the patient consume alcohol regularly and liberally? (c) Has the patient consumed unbonded alcohol? (d) Is the patient taking thiazide diuretics, salicylates, or other drugs? (e) Is there evidence of volume depletion? (f) Is there a history suggestive of renal disease? (g) Is there a history suggestive of a myeloproliferative syndrome, chronic hemolytic anemia, or solid tumor malignancy?
2. Is there a history of acute arthritic attacks? If so, what was their character? Was there a response to colchicine? Has the patient noted any tophi?
3. Is there a history of kidney stones?
4. Has there been hypertension or any history of cardiovascular disease?
5. Is there a family history of hyperuricemia, gout, kidney stones, or renal disease?

**Physical Examination.** Special attention should be directed toward the following:

1. Habitus should be noted, and height and weight recorded.
2. Is there plethora or pallor? Is there lymphadenopathy, splenomegaly, or hepatomegaly?
3. What is the status of the vascular system? Is there evidence of present or previous hypertension?
4. Are there tophi present in the ears, tendons, joints, digits, or fingertips? Is joint disease present?

**Laboratory Data.** The need for laboratory studies will depend on the severity of the hyperuricemia and findings elicited from history and physical examination. In general, the laboratory studies will be those that would be

**Figure 33–1.** Treatment decision diagram for hyperuricemia.

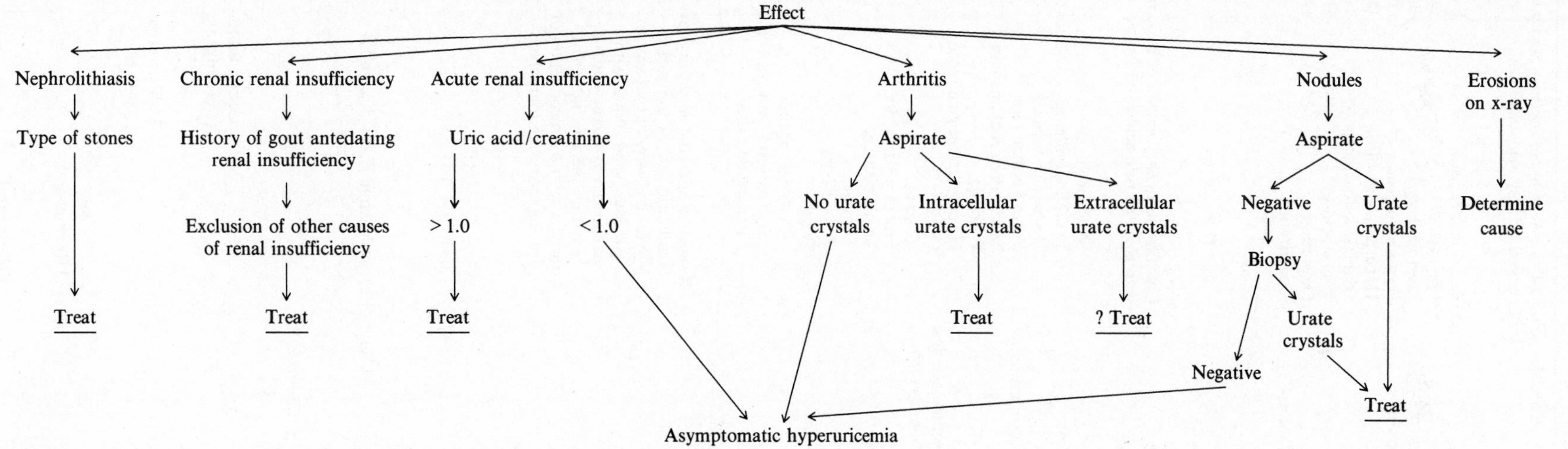

**Figure 33–2.** Evaluation of the patient with hyperuricemia.

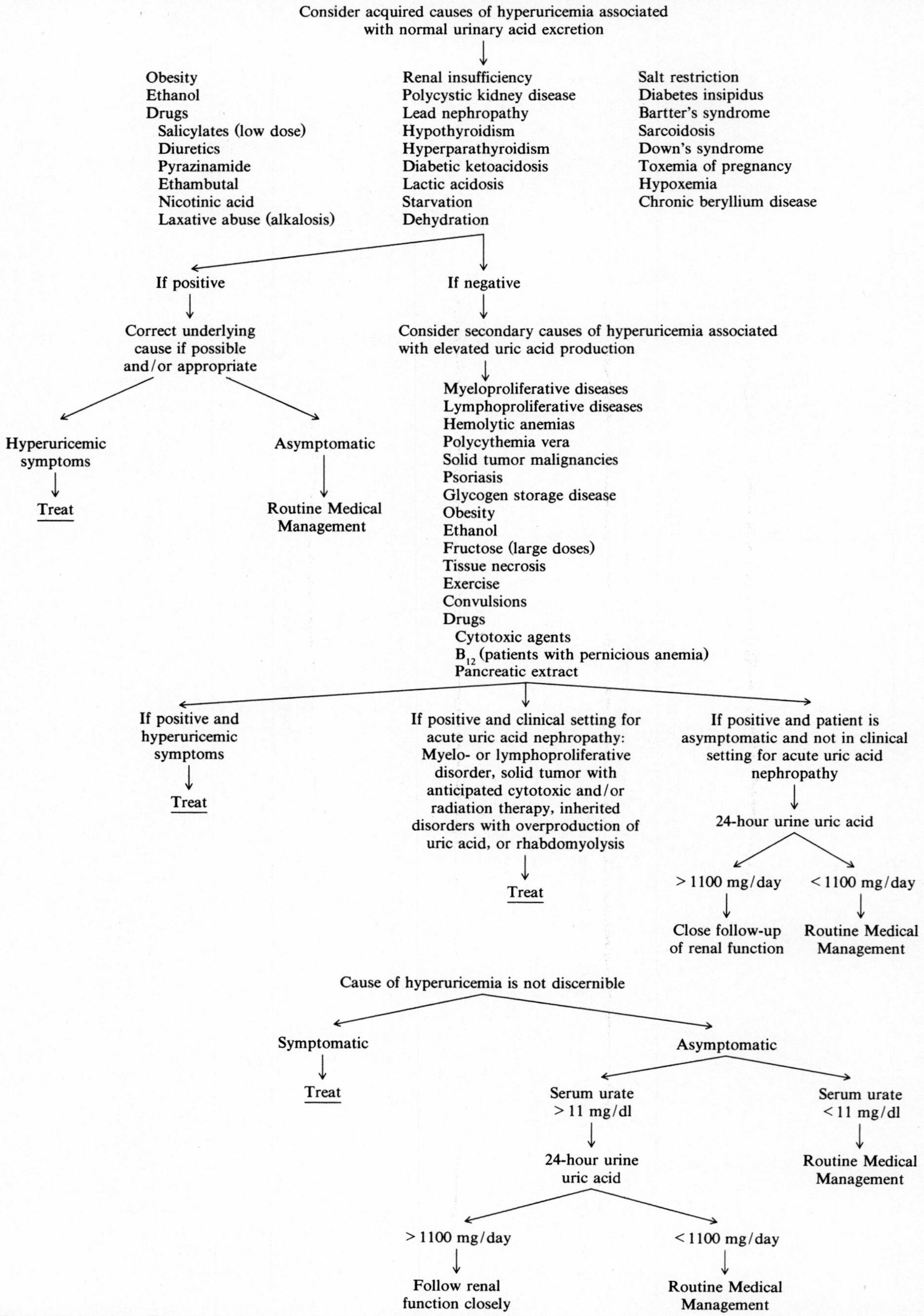

Consider acquired causes of hyperuricemia associated with normal urinary acid excretion
Obesity
Ethanol
Drugs
Salicylates (low dose)
Diuretics
Pyrazinamide
Ethambutal
Nicotinic acid
Laxative abuse (alkalosis)
Renal insufficiency
Polycystic kidney disease
Lead nephropathy
Hypothyroidism
Hyperparathyroidism
Diabetic ketoacidosis
Lactic acidosis
Starvation
Dehydration
Salt restriction
Diabetes insipidus
Bartter's syndrome
Sarcoidosis
Down's syndrome
Toxemia of pregnancy
Hypoxemia
Chronic beryllium disease
If positive
Correct underlying cause if possible and/or appropriate
Hyperuricemic symptoms
Treat
Asymptomatic
Routine Medical Management
If negative
Consider secondary causes of hyperuricemia associated with elevated uric acid production
Myeloproliferative diseases
Lymphoproliferative diseases
Hemolytic anemias
Polycythemia vera
Solid tumor malignancies
Psoriasis
Glycogen storage disease
Obesity
Ethanol
Fructose (large doses)
Tissue necrosis
Exercise
Convulsions
Drugs
Cytotoxic agents
$B_{12}$ (patients with pernicious anemia)
Pancreatic extract
If positive and hyperuricemic symptoms
Treat
If positive and clinical setting for acute uric acid nephropathy: Myelo- or lymphoproliferative disorder, solid tumor with anticipated cytotoxic and/or radiation therapy, inherited disorders with overproduction of uric acid, or rhabdomyolysis
Treat
If positive and patient is asymptomatic and not in clinical setting for acute uric acid nephropathy
24-hour urine uric acid
> 1100 mg/day
Close follow-up of renal function
< 1100 mg/day
Routine Medical Management
Cause of hyperuricemia is not discernible
Symptomatic
Treat
Asymptomatic
Serum urate > 11 mg/dl
24-hour urine uric acid
> 1100 mg/day
Follow renal function closely
< 1100 mg/day
Routine Medical Management
Serum urate < 11 mg/dl
Routine Medical Management

indicated because of the basic disease process whether or not the patient had hyperuricemia or gout. Some of these have been reviewed earlier in the chapter. Several special tests, however, are worthy of emphasis.

1. The most useful of special tests in determining whether the hyperuricemic patient has gout are those that may disclose urate crystals: (a) Synovial fluid analysis. Note should be made of gross appearance, total and differential cell count, bacteria if present, quality of the mucin clot, and crystals if present. The fluid should be examined with standard light, as well as with polarized light microscopy (see Chapter 38). (b) Needle aspiration or biopsy of suspected superficial or bony tophus with search for urate crystals.

2. If a renal stone is recovered, it should be analyzed for uric acid and other constituents by the most definitive methods available. If there is a history of renal colic, IVP may be required to visualize radiolucent stones.

3. If there is a suspicion of lead-induced hyperuricemia or gout, one should perform a calcium EDTA-infusion test with measurement of urinary lead, or analyze erythrocyte δ-aminolevulinic acid dehydratase activity.

## MANAGEMENT OF HYPERURICEMIA

The management of patients with symptoms related to hyperuricemia is discussed in detail in Chapter 86. In general, such patients should be treated with antihyperuricemic agents. The decision of whether or not to treat hyperuricemia uncomplicated by articular gout, urolithiasis, or nephropathy is an exercise in clinical judgment on which there is less than universal agreement among physicians. The lack of unanimity reflects the paucity of firm data on hyperuricemia as an independent risk factor for hypertension, atherosclerosis, and renal disease. The weight of evidence favors the view that hyperuricemia is directly important only as it may predispose to articular tophi, gout, urate nephropathy, uric acid stones, and acute uric acid nephropathy. Accordingly, the risks engendered by asymptomatic hyperuricemia can be reduced to the statistical risks of development of these manifestations and their consequences.

The magnitude of the risk of articular gout or tophi is related to the degree and duration of hyperuricemia and the sex and age of the patient. Gouty arthritis and tophi are treatable and reversible whenever they occur and by themselves are not life threatening. It would be reasonable to withhold antihyperuricemic therapy in patients with hyperuricemia if the only goal of such therapy was to prevent the development of gout. Clearly, such therapy could be instituted when these manifestations occurred.

Urate nephropathy is an entity that may not be reversible. This manifestation is difficult to document, is probably a very late event, and is very rarely reported to occur in the absence of previous episodes of gouty arthritis.

Several studies relevant to the relationship between hyperuricemia and urate nephropathy deserve comment in this regard. In one study, no examples of renal disease were found in 15 patients at the time of their initial gouty attack.[8] Another group of investigators has evaluated renal function in asymptomatic hyperuricemic subjects.[9] Studies performed included the examination of urinary sediment, urine culture, Pitressin concentration test, PSP excretion, intravenous pyelogram, glomerular filtration rate, 24-hour urinary protein, and an acid load test. Abnormality in one or more of these tests was found in 63 percent of the hyperuricemic individuals. The Pitressin concentration test, PSP excretion, and acid load tests were the studies most frequently found to be abnormal. From these data, however, one cannot tell (1) if these abnormalities were due to an adverse effect of an increased filtered load of urate, (2) if hyperuricemia is simply a very sensitive marker for intrinsic renal disease, or (3) if hyperuricemia is a reflection of a fundamental metabolic disturbance that also affects renal tubular function. In a subsequent study renal function was monitored prospectively with serum creatinine determination for 8 years in 113 asymptomatic hyperuricemic subjects and 193 normouricemic patients.[10] During this extended follow-up the development of azotemia, as reflected by an increase in serum creatinine concentration, was not different in the hyperuricemic and control subjects. To the extent that an increase in serum creatinine concentration can be used to detect urate nephropathy, we conclude from this study that this particular abnormality is not a major contributor to renal dysfunction in hyperuricemic subjects who do not have articular manifestations of gout.

Urate nephropathy may not be a very common cause of renal dysfunction even in the patient with gout. In one study of 524 gouty patients followed for up to 12 years, hyperuricemia alone appeared to have no deleterious effect on renal function.[11] Renal functional deterioration was mainly associated with aging, renal vascular disease, renal calculi, and pyelonephritis, and the correlation with hypertension and resultant nephrosclerosis was much stronger than with hyperuricemia. In another study of 168 gouty patients followed for 10 years, the development of azotemia appeared to be unrelated to control of the hyperuricemia and was mild when it occurred.[10] Thus, although an association appears to exist between gout and renal disease, a causal role of the hyperuricemia per se in the production of urate nephropathy has yet to be established.

The lack of proof of a direct causal role of hyperuricemia in the genesis of urate nephropathy serves to emphasize the importance of a study designed to determine if control of hyperuricemia has an effect on renal function; one such short-term study exists. A study of 116 patients followed for a mean of 2.5 years compared the effects of allopurinol and placebo therapy in nongouty patients matched for serum urate concentration, mean creatinine clearance, blood pressure, and body weight.[12] No statistically significant differences were consistently found between the placebo-treated and allopurinol-treated groups, and it was concluded that normalization of the plasma urate concentration did not significantly alter renal function.

At present, therefore, the available data, which are admittedly incomplete, suggest that (1) renal function is not necessarily affected in an adverse manner by an elevated serum urate concentration; (2) the renal disease that accompanies hyperuricemia may often be related to inadequately controlled hypertension; and (3) correction of hyperuricemia has no apparent effect on renal function. When these observations are coupled with the side effects of the antihyperuricemic drugs, our current recommendation is that asymptomatic hyperuricemia per se is not an indication for antihyperuricemic agents if the goal is to prevent urate nephropathy.

Uric acid nephrolithiasis and calcium oxalate nephrolithiasis occur more commonly in the patient with hyperuricemia or hyperuricaciduria. Fessel[10] found an incidence of one stone per 114 patients per year in gouty patients, one stone per 295 patients per year in subjects with asymptomatic hyperuricemia, and one stone per 852 patients per year in normouricemic control subjects. In a careful long-term follow-up of gouty patients by Yu and Gutman,[13] the risk of uric acid nephrolithiasis was related to the height of the serum urate level and, to a greater degree, to the magnitude of urinary uric acid excretion. For example, risk of stone formation was less than 20 percent if the serum urate level was 7.1 to 9.0 mg per 100 ml, and reached 50 percent if it was over 13 mg per 100 ml. In similar patients the risk of nephrolithiasis was less than 21 percent if urinary uric acid excretion was less than 700 mg per day and increased substantially with uric acid excretion over 700 mg per day, reaching 50 percent if the excretion was over 1100 mg per day.

The most common type of stone in patients with gout is a uric acid calculus, but gouty subjects also have an increased prevalence of calcium-containing stones. From 1 to 3 percent of the gouty population have a history of calcium stone formation as compared with an overall prevalence of calcium stones in the population of about 0.1 percent. In addition, patients selected because of calcium oxalate or calcium phosphate stones have a high prevalence of hyperuricemia. In one series the mean serum urate in 67 patients with calcium oxalate stones was 7.2 mg per 100 ml compared with the mean serum urate in 10 patients with uric acid stones of 7.8 mg per 100 ml.[14] Perhaps more importantly, Coe and Kavalach[15] noted that 46 of 105 male patients and 9 of 41 female patients with idiopathic recurrent calcium stone disease had a urinary uric acid value over 750 (females) or 800 (males) mg per day while on an unrestricted diet. Hyperuricemia occurred in only 26 of the 55 hyperuricosuric patients. These studies have clearly identified a relationship between hyperuricemia, hyperuricaciduria, and idiopathic calcium oxalate nephrolithiasis. The incidence of calcium oxalate stone disease in a group of patients with asymptomatic hyperuricemia, however, has not been determined.

While both uric acid and calcium nephrolithiasis are often responsive to appropriate therapeutic regimens, including allopurinol, several observations militate against routine antihyperuricemic prophylaxis in asymptomatic patients at putative risk for developing renal stone disease: (1) The actual prevalence of stone disease in the asymptomatic patient with hyperuricemia is only twice as high as it is in the normouricemic population. (2) When a stone is formed, it rarely produces a life-threatening or irreversible series of events. In fact, stone disease related to hyperuricemia and/or hyperuricaciduria is often reversible with appropriate therapy. At this point, in the author's opinion, antihyperuricemic therapy should not be instituted as prophylaxis against the development of stone disease but should be started promptly with discovery of a stone in the hyperuricemic or hyperuricaciduric patient. Identification of the patient with a substantial risk of developing a stone in the future may be valuable to the physician in counseling the patient and in recommending frequency of follow-up visits (see below).

Uric acid nephropathy is a severe form of acute renal failure that may occur in hyperuricemic subjects as a result of the precipitation of uric acid crystals in collecting ducts and ureters. This condition occurs most commonly (1) in patients with profound overproduction of uric acid, particularly those with leukemia or lymphoma subjected to aggressive chemotherapy, (2) in patients with gout and marked hyperuricaciduria, and possibly (3) in patients after severe exercise or convulsions. Postmortem studies in patients with acute uric acid nephropathy reveal intraluminal precipitates of uric acid with dilatation of proximal tubules. Therapy designed to decrease the formation of uric acid and to increase the fraction of uric acid present as the more soluble ionized form, monosodium urate, is highly effective in the prevention or reversal of this process. Indeed, it is in this small group of patients that prophylactic antihyperuricemic therapy may be useful.

Based on the considerations discussed above the author has developed an approach to the hyperuricemic patient, and it is summarized in Figure 33–2. Determine, if possible, whether the patient has one of the conditions listed in this figure which might account for the hyperuricemia. If the underlying cause cannot be corrected, a decision regarding therapy and future management is required. When a symptom such as articular gout, tophi, bone lesions, or renal calculi is documented, antihyperuricemic therapy is justified. In the absence of symptoms, the following guidelines are helpful: (1) If the hyperuricemia is associated with one of the conditions that leads to a decrease in renal clearance of urate, the patient can be observed, without instituting hypouricemic therapy, at intervals dictated by his other medical problems. (2) If the hyperuricemia is related to one of the conditions associated with increased uric acid production, these patients may be at greater risk of developing renal calculi or acute uric acid nephropathy. In clinical settings in which acute uric acid nephropathy is likely, prophylactic treatment is probably justified. In other situations, although immediate antihyperuricemic therapy may not be indicated, quantitation of 24-hour urine uric acid excretion may be helpful in directing future management of the hyperuricemic subject. Based on studies of gouty patients and subject with malignancies, we have selected 1100 mg of uric acid excreted per day as a cut-off for potentially identifying those patients at higher risk for developing renal calculi and acute uric acid nephropathy. In our opinion those individuals who excrete >1100 mg of uric acid per day warrant close follow-up of their renal function and immediate therapy at the first onset of symptoms or evidence of renal dysfunction. (3) If the probable cause of hyperuricemia cannot be determined to identify those patients with increased uric acid production and excretion, the serum urate concentration may be indicative of the amount of uric acid excreted in the urine. Studies in nongouty subjects with normal renal function have demonstrated that there is an abrupt increase in the rate of excretion of urinary uric acid when the serum urate concentration is increased to ≃11 mg per 100 ml, and the amount of uric acid excreted at these rates exceeds 1000 mg per day.[16] In our opinion those patients with serum urate concentrations of >11 mg per 100 ml in whom a secondary cause of hyperuricemia cannot be determined deserve further evaluation with quantitation of 24-hour urine uric acid excretion. This level of serum urate concentration should not lead to the unnecessary evaluation of large numbers of asymptomatic hyperuricemic subjects, but should identify those patients who need further evaluation and close follow-up of their renal function.

## References


1. Paulus, H.E., Coutts, A., Calabro, J.J., et al.: Clinical significance of hyperuricemia in routinely screened hospitalized men. JAMA 211:277, 1970.
2. Rouault, T., Caldwell, D.S., and Holmes, E.W.: Aspiration of the asymptomatic metatarsophalangeal joint in gouty patients and hyperuricemic controls. Arth. Rheum. 25:209, 1982.
3. Coe, F.L.: Hyperuricosuric calcium oxalate nephrolithiasis. Contemporary Issues in Nephrology 5:116, 1980.
4. Kelton, J., Kelley, W.N., and Holmes, E.W.: A rapid method for the diagnosis of acute uric acid nephropathy. Arch. Intern. Med. 138:612, 1978.
5. Wyngaarden, J.B., and Kelley, W.N.: Gout and Hyperuricemia. New York, Grune & Stratton, 1976.
6. Boyce, W.H., Garvey, F.K., and Strawcutter, H.E.: Incidence of urinary calculi among patients in general hospitals, 1948 to 1952. JAMA 161:1437, 1956.
7. Rieselbach, R.E., Bentzel, C.J., Cotlove, E., et al.: Uric acid excretion and renal function in the acute hyperuricemia of leukemia: Pathogenesis and therapy of uric acid nephropathy. Am. J. Med. 37:872, 1964.
8. Colton, R.S., Ward, L.E., Maher, F.I., et al.: Occult renal impairment in gouty and hyperuricemic individuals. Am. J. Med. Sci. 252:575, 1966.
9. Klinenberg, J.R., Dornfield, L.P., and Gonick, H.C.: Renal function in patients with asymptomatic hyperuricemia (abstr.). Arthritis Rheum. 12:307, 1969.
10. Fessel, W.J.: Renal outcomes of gout and hyperuricemia. Am. J. Med. 67:74, 1979.
11. Berger, L., and Yu, T-F.: Renal function in gout. IV. An analysis of 524 gouty subjects including long-term follow-up studies. Am. J. Med. 59:605, 1975.
12. Rosenfeld, J.B.: Effect of long-term allopurinol administration on serial GFR in normotensive and hypertensive hyperuricemic subjects. *In* Sperling, O., de Vries, A., and Wyngaarden, J.B. (eds.): Purine Metabolism in Man. New York, Plenum Press, 1974, p. 581.
13. Yu, T-F., and Gutman, A.B.: Uric acid nephrolithiasis in gout. Predisposing factors. Ann. Intern. Med. 67:1133, 1967.
14. Smith, M.J.V., Hunt, L.D., King, J.S., Jr., et al.: Uricemia and urolithiasis. J. Urol. 101:637, 1969.
15. Coe, F.L., and Kavalach, A.G.: Hypercalcemia and hyperuricosuria in patients with calcium nephrolithiasis. N. Engl. J. Med. 291:1344, 1974.
16. Wyngaarden, J.B.: Gout. Adv. Metab. Dis. 2:1, 1965.


# Chapter 34
# Psychological and Sexual Health in Rheumatic Diseases

*Barbara Figley Banwell and Beth Ziebell*

## INTRODUCTION

Patients with rheumatic diseases are among those who need comprehensive health care. The types of care that physiatrists, physical therapists, and occupational therapists can offer are described in Chapter 111, and the help that can be gained by close collaboration with orthopedists is discussed in Chapters 112 through 121.

It is not a paradox that the rheumatologist, a subspecialist within the specialty of internal medicine, must be concerned with providing comprehensive care to patients, since he or she is often the co-ordinator of treatment activities. Comprehensive care includes a commitment to understanding emotional responses to chronic disease and knowledge sufficient to treat normal, exaggerated, and pathologic psychological reactions to chronic diseases or to refer the patient to qualified mental health professionals. The most compelling reason for such an approach is that most patients and health care professionals would agree that comprehensive care with sensitive and knowledgeable appreciation of psychosocial-sexual issues has a positive effect on outcome and attitude. There is a growing body of information in the literature that describes psychosocial and biologic variables as they shape and are shaped by the pattern of chronic recurring illness. A number of studies can be cited that trace physiologic responses to emotional states and the behaviors that accompany or result from those states.[1-3] Knowledge of these psychological factors influences the success of management and treatment programs in rheumatic disease.[4-11]

This chapter will discuss the following points: (1) specific features of rheumatic disease that are likely to evoke a psychological response, (2) common emotional responses to rheumatic disease, (3) a framework, for management of psychosocial problems in rheumatology, including the behavioral aspects of pain, (4) a framework for recognition and management of sexual problems in rheumatic disease, (5) methods and data pertinent to psychobiosocial research in rheumatic diseases, and (6) the psychosocial factors in juvenile arthritis.

## FEATURES OF RHEUMATIC DISEASES THAT EVOKE PSYCHOLOGICAL RESPONSES

Psychological reaction to rheumatic disease is an interaction between the disease, its treatment, and the patients' perception of their illness. Some features of the disease are more likely than others to have psychological effects. However, one should not assume that all patients have similar reactions, since people perceive and experience symptoms differently.[12] Illness and disability represent catastrophic events to some people; to others they are an expected part of the human experience.[13]

The first psychological reactions are evoked by the symptoms or diagnosis of arthritis. The prior state of good health is disrupted. Some people consider good health a principal goal in life and pride themselves on its achievement and maintenance. Others have taken good health for granted. Good health is intimately related in some to self-respect, and even temporary change in health status may carry with it a sense of loss or vulnerability. The diagnosis of arthritis, so often associated with "wearing out" or old age, may carry a special negative meaning. Terms such as "chronic disease," "rheumatism," or "crippling" carry strong connotations in many subcultures of our society.

*Change in physical appearance* that results in disrupted body image can occur as a result of disease or treatment and is difficult to handle for the average patient. An attractive body image is particularly important for the patient whose self-esteem is already eroded by pain, loss of function, and decreased activity. An obvious disability can be a barrier to satisfactory social interaction.[14,15] The malar rash and alopecia of systematic lupus erythematosus, the swollen joints of rheumatoid arthritis, and the drawn appearance of those with scleroderma are sometimes the most disturbing symptoms of the disease. When drug treatment causes changes in physical appearance, the patient may be reluctant to take the medication and compliance with medication schedules may be threatened. For example, many patients fear rejection because of a changed physical appearance produced by corticosteroids. Each person considers his appearance a part of his identity and self-image; a change in this self-perception may have a greater or lesser impact than might be predicted. It is the physician's responsibility to be aware of how patients react to physical changes.

*Pain* exerts a powerful influence upon the personality and emotions. Whether intermittent or persistent, it dulls the environment and interrupts well-established patterns of behavior. Pain interferes with intellectual and emotional functioning.[16,17] The "chronic pain syndrome," in which pain becomes interwoven with a series of behavioral responses and patterns, is frequently seen in rheumatic diseases. Family interactions, particularly intimate ones involving broad and deep emotion, undergo stress when one member is in pain. In addition to the reaction to pain, many patients are affected by the anticipation of pain, a phenomenon that affects even the pain-free segments of their lives. This reaction to anticipated pain may change activity patterns more than pain itself. Pain is the most disconcerting problem encountered by the patient with a rheumatic disease. Chronic pain in the patient with arthritis will be discussed in a later section.

*Weakness, fatigue, and loss of energy* are discouraging concomitants of rheumatic disease. "If I just didn't get so tired" is a frequent complaint in almost every diagnostic category. Those who value accomplishment and achievement seem particularly dismayed by lack of energy. "Strength" is often defined culturally as a personality characteristic rather than a measure of the ability to do physical work. Thus, physical weakness may represent to the patient a character or personality flaw. This is complicated by the fact that persons with rheumatic diseases are often advised to rest and avoid hard physical tasks as a part of treatment. This contrasts with cultural advice to "fight the disease" or "conquer the symptoms."

*The loss of functional ability* is the result of pain, weakness, or other physiological impairment. The significance of the patient's functional loss is by no means correlated with the number of joints or muscles involved. The patient's perception of disability is subjective.[18] Those who do not easily adapt to change may experience prolonged depression or anger. Many adults are socially defined primarily by the name of their occupation—e.g., cooks, teachers, truck drivers, painters, or surgeons. Loss of the ability to carry out these tasks and function in these roles may cause loss of social identity and diminished self-esteem, even though function in another role would be quite possible.

When loss of function causes *dependence on others,* the effect may be even more devastating. Independence has great cultural significance, particularly for men. However, women forced to be dependent may be no less depressed than men. Dependence means seeking and requesting assistance, and asking for help is a difficult task. It involves timing (neither too soon nor too late), judgment (asking the right person), and humility. Each request presents the risk of rejection for the patient needing help. The helper is also at risk, and must be skilled in offering assistance without exerting control. Being helpful without being patronizing is a difficult skill. This tenuous interaction is repeated many times daily for those who are not independent. Independence is a quality achieved throughout life by accomplishing a series of tasks that began in childhood. For most people, losing independence symbolizes a return to previous states of immaturity. This reaches its ultimate expression in those patients who are unable to perform tasks of personal hygiene. Many patients express the view that the ongoing negotiation of assistance is one of the most difficult challenges of arthritis.

One last feature that has considerable psychological impact is the *financial cost of chronic illness.* Even with excellent comprehensive health insurance plans, many patients must still pay for drugs or laboratory tests. Common aspirin can become expensive when taken in large quantities over a period of years. In long-term illnesses, the costs of treatment, travel for medical care, special equipment, and child and home care can strain resources.

Although discussion to this point has centered upon the patient, the family and others who interact closely with the patient can also be expected to react to their perceptions of the disease. Their interactions with the patient will be tempered by their own experiences with illness. Medical personnel do not encounter all family members and are thus often unaware of their concerns. As the disease interferes with the patient's ability to fulfill his or her role within the family, conflicts and misunderstandings can develop. Family members are often confused about the fluctuating symptoms and function of the patient. When good communication does not exist between family members, problems and feelings often go unrecognized and unresolved. Resentment, anger, and depression have been described within many families. Patterns of reaction will be influenced by previous family patterns and structure. It is heartening to note in some families that adjustment has improved after participation in therapeutic programs.[19,20]

## PSYCHOLOGICAL RESPONSES COMMON TO RHEUMATIC DISEASES

As the individual notices symptoms of disease, the initial response is *anxiety.* Fear and uneasiness grow as symptoms persist. Anxiety can precipitate positive action: the patient may seek medical advice. In contrast, it may also engender *denial* as the patient ignores symptoms or insists they have no meaning. Another component of denial may involve rejection of assistance. A form of denial is manifest in those who wander from specialist to specialist in search of assurance that they will "get well." When pain becomes constant or when a diagnosis of arthritis is made, most patients begin to accept or reach equilibrium with their disease. Seeking medical evaluation, diagnosis, and treatment represents a reasonable attempt to deal with circumstances.

*Anger* is a frequent response to disease or disability. Anger may be generated about the injustice of illness,

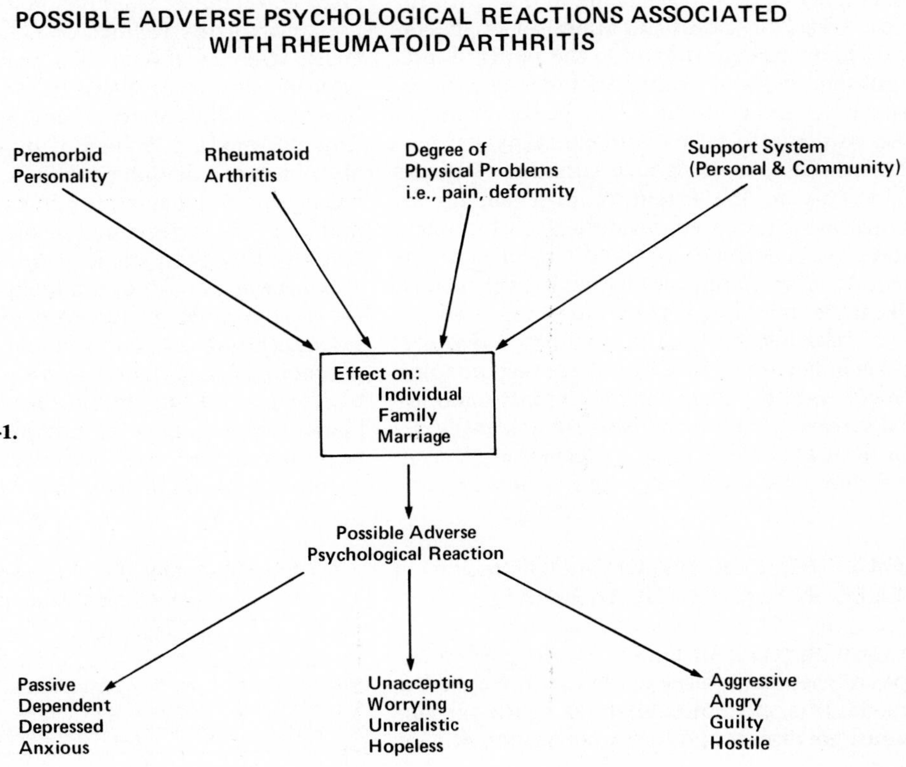


Figure 34–1.

dependency, pain, the interruption of life patterns, or the moratorium on opportunity induced by functional handicap. Anger may be poorly focused and expressed in the most convenient way at the time, frequently being directed inappropriately at family or friends. Patients who refuse medication or resist educational programs may be expressing anger in the only way available to them. Persons with physical disabilities may have lost access to the usual means by which anger is diffused. They cannot easily "get away from things," engage in vigorous physical activity, or risk expressing emotions spontaneously. Unexpressed or unrecognized anger often leads to adverse reactions, among them depression.

*Depression* is one of the most commonly noted emotions in people with arthritis. A study of 50 psychiatric consultations for hospitalized arthritis patients revealed depression to be the most common psychological diagnosis.[21] It is a natural reaction to actual or perceived loss, and may be a useful temporary defense, allowing one to rest and reorder life's priorities. However, prolonged depression results in loss of energy and motivation. In rheumatic diseases it appears to accentuate pain and to be counterproductive to the therapy designed to strengthen muscles and restore function.

The reactions described above can be experienced at varied times throughout the course of one chronic illness. Each new symptom, frustration, or exacerbation of disease activity stimulates responses, which usually are consistent in the same patient. It is important for patient, family, and health professionals to recognize that experiencing these emotions again and again is not regression.

Ideally, as the patient experiences emotional responses to a disease activity, a decision is made to deal with the circumstances based on a realistic appraisal of the situation. The coping resources include the patient's previously established ways of dealing with personal problems, external help, and the influence of the environment. The decision to come to terms is made many times in the course of disease, in each new situation. Patients differ considerably in the extent of their coping resources. Adjustment is sometimes influenced by others who facilitate its occurrence or create barriers to its development. It is an important psychological mechanism which enables individuals to continue a satisfactory life in spite of impaired health and diminished abilities. Adjustment is easier to achieve from the stage of anger and resentment resulting from the development and activity of the disease, and is progressively less easily attained from the stages of depression, decreased physical activity, and diminished self-image and/or invalidism.

## MANAGEMENT OF PSYCHOLOGICAL ISSUES IN RHEUMATIC DISEASES

There are two purposes for understanding psychological concepts in rheumatic disease: (1) to appreciate the role of personality and emotional states in the physiologic mechanism of disease and the response to treatment and (2) to facilitate successful psychologic adaptation to disease and its consequences. The physician should develop a conceptual framework that incorporates these concepts into a philosophy of treatment. A longitudinal approach, including assessment and appropriate intervention in psychosocial events, is ideal both as a treatment and as a research model.[20] A comprehensive model will include preventive, therapeutic, and rehabilitative components.

Discussion of health issues, including psychological components, occurs best in an atmosphere of trust and acceptance. Time must be provided for thorough assessment and understanding of the psychodynamics of specific situations. Time should be allotted for communication with other health professionals who contribute to the care of the patient.

Effective use of health professionals knowledgeable about arthritis is often the solution to providing comprehensive care with minimal cost of physician's time. During their longer treatment contacts therapists and nurses often make observations about a patient's emotional status that the physicians may miss.

Consideration of psychosocial issues and concerns must be based upon effective assessment of the patient's personal and social adjustment. This evaluation may be accomplished by psychometric testing,[22] interview, observation, or other clinical data collection methods. Each professional who participates in the treatment activities should develop a knowledge of the psychological status of the patient and the family. Included in the health interview must be a series of questions about psychological issues. Such questions might include the following: (1) How have your symptoms affected your life? (2) How have those around you been affected? (3) What are some of the feelings or emotions you have experienced lately? (4) What has been the biggest change in your life since your illness or symptoms began? (5) How have you adjusted to situations like this in the past? This information, enhanced by observations and available history, should provide a sense of the patient's recent emotional state, the effect of the disease upon the patient's life style, and the previous coping strategies employed by the patient (Table 34–1).

A network of resources, including lay support groups (often sponsored by such organizations as the Arthritis Foundation or the Lupus Foundation), social workers, psychologists, and others, is invaluable for complete patient care (Table 34–2). Group interaction is particularly useful because it provides the members an opportunity to test new patterns and behavior in an atmosphere of familiarity and trust. Groups can be

**Table 34–1.** Questions to Elicit Information About Psychological Issues in Arthritis

1. How have your symptoms affected your life?
2. How have those around you been affected?
3. What feelings have you experienced lately?
4. What is the biggest change in your life in the past year?
5. What has helped you cope with arthritis?

**Table 34–2.** Some Resources for Psychological Support

| |
|---|
| Arthritis health professionals |
| physicians |
| psychologists |
| social workers |
| nurses |
| therapists |
| Mutual support groups (e.g., Arthritis Foundation, Lupus Foundation) |
| Community mental health agencies |
| Clergy |
| Family and friends |
| Self-help literature |

structured to include opportunities for education about disease and treatment, mutual support, expression of concerns, and skill training for dealing with these concerns. The leaders of groups concerned with persons affected by rheumatic disease should have knowledge of the specific disease and its effects. In one of the few controlled studies of the effects of group counseling, Kaplan and Kozin note its value in improving knowledge and self-concept.[23]

When considering the best treatment for emotional problems, Achterberg-Lawlis[24] has found, "The traditional mental health models for therapy simply appear unacceptable for people who are brought together with a common diagnosis of arthritis." A stress management approach for dealing with psychosocial issues is often more acceptable for people who are hesitant to discuss feelings and emotions and for those who believe their problems are entirely physical. Some people even consider a suggestion for psychological help to be a strong criticism, whereas nearly everyone today accepts the logic of the importance of managing stress well.

A good stress management program includes better communication skills; assertiveness training; dealing with the negative emotions of anger, depression, worry, and guilt; relaxation techniques; pain management, and development of a less stressful lifestyle. All of these stress management concepts contribute to emotional health.

Following initial assessment, the physician should continue to both observe the patient's psychological health and be closely in touch with members of the patient care team who are directly involved with the patient's emotional health. Some indicators to be aware of include behavior changes, sleep patterns, sexual interest, personal appearance, work difficulties, and personal interactions with family and friends. Subsequent interviews should assess the patient's physical and emotional reactions to the treatment program. The patient and family should be given an opportunity to express opinions regarding the effect of medication and therapy. Faithfulness to treatment regimens should be monitored both for the sake of successful treatment and as an indicator of psychologic status.

In addition to the best possible medical and psychological management of the patient with arthritis, patients benefit from being involved in a "wellness" approach to their care. In such a wellness[25] approach, the patient will learn that everyone can be healthier than they are, in spite of having arthritis or any other chronic disease or disability. The patients discover that there are many aspects of their lives that only they can control, such as diet, exercise, personal growth and development, maintaining satisfying relationships, personal habits such as smoking, stress management, attitudes, lifestyle, and nonpharmaceutical pain management. The awareness of the many factors that contribute to a total health picture for each person can be taught in groups or on an individual basis by the physician or other health care providers. Psychological health can be improved when people give up a helpless, passive attitude and become more active in their own health care.

Until this point, the information presented has emphasized the patient and family as recipients of services and attention. It is also worthwhile to consider influencing the social and physical environment in which these persons live. Social and personal attitudes are in many instances the cause of depression, loss, and hopelessness among persons affected by chronic disease or disability.[26] Support is needed to provide barrier-free physical environments, accessible transportation, and nondiscriminatory employment for the handicapped. Equitable Social Security, medical care programs, and educational opportunities for the physically exceptional can provide wide-reaching impact on the consequences of disease.

In a study examining the relative contributions of selected disease, social, and work-related factors to disability status in a population of 180 people with rheumatoid arthritis, it was determined that social and work factors combined have a far larger effect on work disability than all disease factors.[27] The work factors of "control over the pace" and "activities of the job" had the greatest effect on continued employment, and "self-employment" was the favored work status. It was suggested that work disability is not strongly associated with the physical requirements of the job among persons with rheumatoid arthritis. These findings imply that the probability of work disability could be reduced by more flexible roles and pace in work settings. The responsibility of educating employers and other labor-management personnel lies with the physician or other health professional, and a climate of social responsibility makes the success of such efforts more likely.

The trauma of rheumatic disease might not be as overwhelming if the opportunity to fulfill roles and responsibilities within society were better protected.

## BEHAVIORAL ASPECTS OF PAIN

Pain is perhaps the most potent stimulus of adverse psychological reactions for people experiencing arthritis. Although recent developments in the scientific study of pain have produced a greater understanding of some of its mechanisms and characteristics,[28,29] many misconceptions prevail about the experience and management of pain. These misconceptions and misunderstandings contribute to inadequate pain management techniques by health professionals. Many physicians who encounter patients with primary pain problems are frustrated both by the patient and by the failure of traditionally prescribed treatments.[30] Because patients with primary pain problems are so difficult to treat, and the impact of their disability so significant, multidisciplinary pain management programs have been developed.[31] These programs attempt to treat the complex psychological components of the experience in addition to the physical symptoms. These units are established on the premise that every pain patient who truly wants to get better can be helped at least to some degree. This basic premise has yet to be refuted.

In all pain programs, an individual management program is developed for each patient. A broad range of available techniques could include biofeedback, group and individual psychotherapy, heat or cold modalities, electrotherapy, hypnosis, therapeutic massage, exercise, and relaxation techniques. Various drug therapies and nerve blocks might be included, but the emphasis is on patient participation and the utilization of the person's inner resources. Every effort is made to eliminate feelings of helplessness and hopelessness. Numerous studies have been done to assess the effectiveness of behavorial pain management programs. Gottlieb and colleagues[32] reported 50 of 72 patients to have attained a preset level of satisfactory functioning. A significant level of improvement was retained on a 1-month follow-up. Thirty-six chronic pain patients with histories of treatment failure in other modalities were enrolled in the behavioral program summarized by Fordyce and colleagues.[33] On follow-up 22 months post-treatment, the patients reported a stable and significant decrease in pain intensity as well as a significant decrease in the degree to which pain interfered with activities. Pain management programs continue to develop with emphasis on rehabilitation principles and careful evaluation.

There are several characteristics of arthritis pain that set this condition apart from other pain management problems. First, arthritis pain is not one pain, but many pains, ranging in nature from acute to chronic. People with arthritis must learn to live and function with chronic pain while still attending to the signals of acute pain. Patient education materials for people with arthritis emphasize the need to "respect pain"[34] and "alter activities which cause pain lasting more than 1–2 hours,"[35] thus clearly implying the control that pain is to have over the patient's life. While it is relatively easy to cope with acute pain of short duration, facing a lifetime with pain as a constant companion can be an overwhelming experience. Even when arthritis is well managed or in remission, serious pain often still exists because of remaining joint damage. Guidelines for dealing with this type of pain may be very different from those for dealing with acute inflammatory pain. Another factor that makes arthritis pain difficult to manage is the unpredictable course and nature of the disease. Unexpected pain and flare-ups make long-range planning virtually an impossibility for the patient and family. And finally, patients who experience pain from arthritis are frequently told by health professionals and other advisors that because there is no cure for arthritis, they must "learn to live with it," thus reinforcing their hopelessness and diminishing their belief in the ability to alleviate the distress.

Therefore, the first challenge in developing a pain management program for arthritis patients is to help them to become less passive and begin to accept some personal responsibility for their own comfort level. This initial phase is primarily educational, teaching the relationship between stress, muscle tension, and feelings of pain. This framework of personal responsibility and control over the physical experience is the basis for positive management of pain in arthritis.

Once a stress management program is underway, the specific problem of dealing with pain can be addressed. Patients with arthritis react quite differently both to pain and to pain management techniques, so a many faceted approach is generally best. Because pain is a personal and subjective experience, every person with an ongoing, chronic pain problem will benefit from developing his own personal "bag of tricks" containing tried and proven ideas and techniques that are effective in reducing the pain experience for that individual.

The three major categories of useful techniques for nonmedicinal management of pain are physical measures, distraction, and relaxation. These measures, used individually or in combination, are central in the long-term management of arthritis pain (Fig. 34–2).

Physical measures often originate in a medical environment even though the patient will then have the responsibility for carrying them out at home. The patient may receive information from the physician, physical therapist, or occupational therapist about such things as paraffin dips for hands, warm showers and baths, hot or cold packs, exercises, splinting, and so on. In this category also belongs appropriate shoes and clothing, self-help devices, and joint protection.

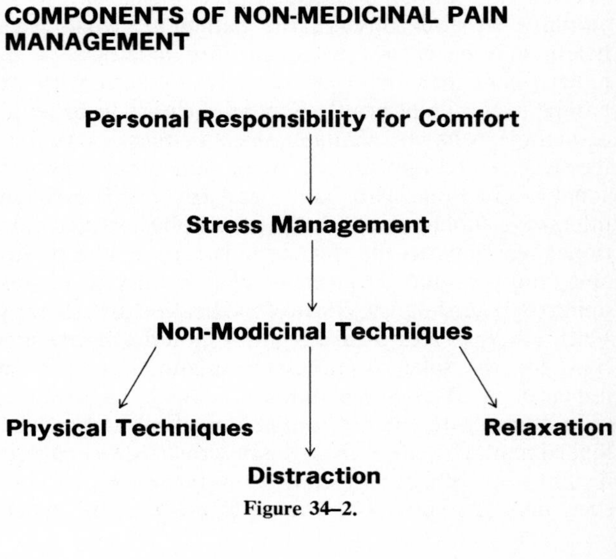


Figure 34–2.

A VARIETY OF AVAILABLE RELAXATION METHODS

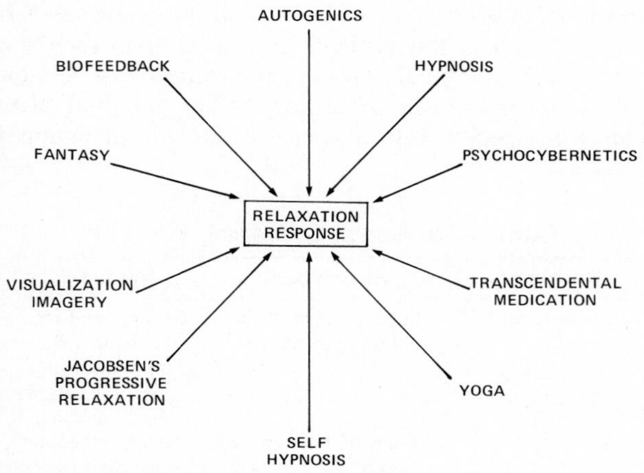


**Figure 34–3.**

Distraction techniques are useful because nearly everyone is capable of forgetting pain when their attention becomes focused on something else. What takes the person's mind off himself? Because of the personal nature of this activity, each person will need to find his own list of items that divert attention from the pain, at least for short periods of time. Chronic pain is easier to live with if one is able to achieve periods of relief. For one person, listening to music might be effective; for another, playing with a puppy or grandchild or both. The list of possibilities is endless and includes such diverse activities as working puzzles, singing, or doing crafts.

The third category of pain relief measures is relaxation. Tension always intensifies pain, so that decreased tension, both physical and emotional, provides comfort and relief. Being deeply relaxed in mind and body can profoundly diminish the experience of pain. There are many different kinds of relaxation methods, including Jacobson's Progressive Relaxation,[36] Yoga,[37] Autogenic Training,[38] and Transcendental Meditation[39] (Fig. 34–3). Benson simplifies the matter of choice by explaining that the outcome is more important than the specific technique used.[40]

One more adjunct to pain management is counseling or psychotherapy. If a patient's personal life is unsettled and unhappy, the resulting stress and tension cannot help but worsen existing pain problems. When emotions can be maintained on a relatively even level, people seem to be better able to manage the pain caused by arthritis.

As each person accumulates his own personal "bag of tricks," he can continue to add ideas as he learns and tries new things. Of course, gathering this collection of helpful pain management tools and skills is only the beginning, since they must be used and practiced in order to be effective. Patients can make a valuable contribution to their pain management when they are taught the necessary skills.

In summary, only the rare patient with arthritis will be in need of a formal comprehensive chronic pain management program. On the other hand, certain components of these programs such as stress management and relaxation are appropriate for almost any arthritis patient with pain. No health professional should ever advise a person with arthritis to simply "learn to live with pain." Patients have a right to learn about the rich repertoire of creative alternatives for dealing with pain rather than hearing a statement of helplessness.

## SEXUAL HEALTH AND RHEUMATIC DISEASE

Sexual health is vulnerable to the effects of rheumatic disease. Sexuality is a concept that should be viewed from several perspectives. In the broad sense, it embodies all those aspects of personality relating to masculinity and femininity, including factors such as gender identity and behavior, self-perception, societal and personal roles, and interpersonal skills. In contrast, the narrow definition focuses on genital behavior and expressions. To the individual, sexuality is a construct of life experiences framed by values and attitudes. It is probably impossible for one person to define sexuality for another; yet it is useful to strive for mutual understanding.

One's perception of self as a sexual person is likely to be influenced by the physical changes caused by chronic disease. In rheumatic disease, whether acute or chronic, the characteristics of pain, loss of function, and physical change may disrupt many components of the life pattern, including sexual health. A seldom recognized consideration is that some drugs used in the treatment of rheumatic disease affect sexuality. They may also alter physical appearance and thus affect sexual interest or energy. Cytotoxic agents may be toxic to sperm and öocytes and/or may induce fetal wastage or sterility.

Although sexuality is gaining wider acceptance as a legitimate concern for health care professionals, adequate resources of skill, knowledge, and attitudes within the medical community remain to be developed to provide needed and appropriate services. A significant body of information now exists regarding sexuality in neuromuscular disabilities such as quadriplegia or paraplegia.[41,42] Although some aspects of this knowledge are relevant to rheumatic disease, there are some differences. It must be recognized that achieving satisfactory adjustments regarding sexuality may be particularly complicated by the fluctuating nature of the physical and emotional states that occur in rheumatic diseases.

The health practitioner who seeks to develop an approach that considers the sexual health of patients must first possess three requisite qualities: (1) recognition of the sexual aspects of his or her own personality ("comfort" with sexuality), (2) a commitment to respect the personal attitudes and values of others, and (3) a commitment and adherence to ethical professional standards regarding sex education, counseling, and therapy. Knowledge of anatomy, sexual physiology, and the manner in which sexual functioning might be affected by disease or disability is essential.

Approaches to sexuality should be sensitive and nonsexist. Perhaps because of the predominance of rheumatic disease in females, an inordinate portion of existing literature about sexuality and arthritis deals with women's sexual concerns. The sexual role of women is often described as the more passive and their societal role as that of traditional feminine homemaker. Men are usually described by their professional or work roles. If family and societal roles are to be considered as an aspect of sexuality, then consideration should be given to the woman whose work or professional career is interrupted by arthritis, and to the man whose domestic interests and roles are rendered difficult to fulfill.

Lief[43] has described the following as the effective physician's tasks in dealing with the sexual problems of patients, but these are certainly applicable to all health practitioners: (1) Be comfortable with sexual topics. (2) Listen well and know how to take a sexual history. (3) Show concern for the patient's feelings. (4) Judge whether the sexual problems identified are within the practitioner's competence, and, if the patient is in agreement, set up a plan of treatment with the patient's full knowledge and consent. (5) For problems not within the practitioner's competence, refer the patient to another professional person who has the required knowledge and skills. The physician may choose also not to deal with dysfunction that predated the disease or disability. Appropriate referral may be effective in this situation. The goal of intervention is to provide the recipient with information and assistance so that ultimately he or she can make decisions about sexuality within his or her own value system.

Creating an atmosphere in which discussion of sexual issues can occur is the first and most important step in any program. It has often been observed that patients rarely initiate discussion of sexual concerns, and yet this does not indicate a lack of importance of such concerns. Gathering information as part of a total health assessment provides a comfortable avenue for discussion for both health professionals and patients with sexual concerns. A few carefully worded questions about sexual function can show that the subject is open for discussion and is viewed as a health concern. The initial interview need not be a detailed sex history but will serve to identify areas of change or difficulty. If concerns are expressed, the subsequent information obtained should detail (1) the duration of the problem, (2) how it affects the patient at this time, (3) what, if anything, helps, (4) what the patient believes is the cause, and (5) how the patient feels about dealing with the problem. With this information, professionals can make a decision about their competence to work with the patient and whether the patient desires assistance at this time. Asking all patients about sexual concerns provides an opportunity to learn from patients who have made satisfactory adjustment. Interviews at this level also provide the opportunity to introduce ideas and concepts which can reduce vulnerability to sexual dysfunction.

In one study a comprehensive plan to consider sexuality in rheumatic disease not only resulted in greater attention to patient concerns; it also provided an opportunity to document problems and interventions.[44] In this study, half the patients indicated that they had concerns about sexual function, and some identified multiple problems. Table 34–3 depicts ten potential problems, the specific information needed for assessment,

**Table 34–3.** Sexual Counseling Protocol*

| Problem | Assessment | Intervention |
|---|---|---|
| Pain or weakness | Specify cause, location, and nature | Recommend measures to relieve or minimize, i.e., position, warm bath, medication |
| Fatigue | Time of day, cause, nature | Pacing, scheduling, establishing priorities |
| Lack of interest | Determine influencing factors, i.e., medication, disease activity, depression | Educate to promote understanding of the effect of pain, fatigue, and disease activity on interest |
| Limited range of motion | Define functional limitations | Suggestions about positioning, alternative forms of expression |
| Lack of lubrication | Determine cause | Suggest psychological or physical measures as indicated |
| Erectile difficulties | Determine contributing factors, i.e., medical or psychological | Consider altering medications if possible; appropriate counseling measures |
| Fear of pregnancy, interfering medical problems (e.g., vaginal or penile ulcers, urinary tract infection) | Refer to physican or nurse to determine appropriate medical intervention; assess implications for individual and/or partner | Recommend appropriate medical measures; provide counseling regarding impact of decisions |
| Feelings of unattractiveness | Determine if perception is by self, partner, and/or others | Promote positive body image and acceptance of body, enhance feelings of self-worth |
| Problems with partner | Assess cause, e.g., fear of causing pain, partner's disinterest, responsibility for satisfaction, sexual roles, general relationship problems | Education and counseling as appropriate |
| Lack of partner | Evaluate possibilities for meeting other people, individual's own response | Discuss self-pleasuring, affirmation of self, encourage social contacts |

*From Ferguson, K., and Figley, B.: Sexuality Disability 2:130,1979.

and examples of interventions. It demonstrates that concerns range from physical to psychological and require a variety of strategies. In an interdisciplinary approach, the physical therapist may be the most appropriate person to work with problems of sexual functioning that are due to limited range of motion or weakness; the social worker may best address issues of emotions, personality, or interpersonal relationships; the occupational therapist may offer principles of pacing and energy conservation which enable the patient to deal with fatigue and function; education by the nurse about the disease and medications may prepare the patient and family to cope with aspects of the disease that have implications for sexual function. The physician will view concerns in the context of the total health picture. Issues of birth control, fertility, or contraindication to pregnancy can be best addressed by the physician. By expressing interest, the physician who acts as coordinator of services also sanctions sexuality as a health concern. It should be noted that none of these people require highly trained or developed skills in sex therapy in order to contribute to a positive approach to sexual health.

It is important to plan a system for documentation of sexual issues in the patient's medical record. The record must accurately convey information to other medical staff without violating sensitivities or confidentiality. Documentation will avoid duplication of professional efforts and improve communication.

One conceptual model of a structured approach to sexual health is known as the PLISSIT model.[45] It describes the need for varying levels and types of education or intervention regarding sexuality. The model demonstrates that by offering permission to talk about sexual issues, providing limited information to those with questions and specific suggestions for specific concerns, there will be only a few people who require intensive therapy.

## PSYCHOSOCIAL RESEARCH IN RHEUMATIC DISEASES; METHODOLOGY AND RESULTS

Many investigators have attempted to define psychologic concepts in rheumatic disease.[46] Their methods ranged from personal viewpoints based upon clinical observation[47,48] to intricate designs evaluating dependent and independent variables in controlled settings on multiple population samples.[2,11,20] Most populations studied have been patients with rheumatoid arthritis. Although early case studies were impressionistic and descriptive, they did generate interest and energy for future studies. More recent work has produced a wealth of descriptive data enticing to many. Nevertheless one must make careful assessment and interpretation of each study.

Studies of psychological factors in arthritis have been carried out by researchers in various disciplines and orientations, including rheumatology, psychiatry, sociology, and psychology. The scope and focus of a particular study may be influenced by the professional or philosophical orientation of the researcher; the social scientist may be unfamiliar with the subtleties of rheumatic disease, a rheumatologist not aware of the intricacies of psychological testing. These differences should be recognized and appreciated by the reader.

An assumption persists through much of the literature that persons of one diagnostic category represent a homogeneous group. However, clinical experience reveals that people with rheumatoid arthritis or lupus erythematosus, for instance, are heterogeneous. They are different in terms of severity and activity of disease, physical function or disability, sex, age, serology, and length of symptoms. These differences should be stated and defined as completely as possible. Experimental and control groups should be utilized with dependent and independent variables stated.

Several techniques have been used to observe or measure psychologic variables. Many early studies which produced "personality profiles" were based on case studies and interviews in therapy settings.[48,49] The case study approach represents a subjective and minimally controlled research strategy. Some later designs have included a combination of interview and testing in attempts to gain more objective information. Interpretive tests such as the Rorschach, Thematic Apperception Test (TAT), and Draw-a-Person (DAP) were at times utilized in attempts to construct personality descriptions unique to persons with arthritis.[50,51] It must be recognized that these tests and the validity of interpretation may be particularly affected by the method of administration, scoring, and circumstances of testing.

Self-report questionnaires are another method designed to obtain information without the intervening influence of the interviewer.[52] These seem to provide relevant information regarding perception and knowledge of disease or physical and functional status, but more extensive interpretation may lead to subjective decision on the part of the interpreter. Fries has confirmed the usefulness of one self-report scale.[53]

The Minnesota Multiphasic Personality Inventory is a long and complex psychometric instrument,[54] used in some of the studies which sought quantitative and objective descriptors.[55-57] The personality profiles have been standardized with nonclinical, psychiatric, and other criterion groups in the interest of extending usefulness. Moos and Solomon[56] point out that the demonstrated differences between arthritis and nonarthritis populations may be due to variables other than diagnosis such as physical disability or pain. Some test items have content only indirectly related to or influenced by arthritis. The implications of these on the validity of this instrument have been pointed out by Nalven and O'Brien.[58]

These issues in methodology are not presented in skepticism of earlier research, but rather to encourage caution in interpretation of biopsychosocial research and to provide guidelines for assessment. A systemized evaluation will include consideration of (1) orientation of the researcher, (2) description of experimental and control samples, (3) inclusion of control groups, (4) variables measured, (5) instruments of evaluation, and (6) whether the hypothesis was answered by the methods employed.

Much of the existing literature about psychologic concepts in rheumatoid arthritis addresses two questions: (1) Do common personality patterns and characteristics exist among those with rheumatoid disease—i.e., is there a rheumatoid personality? (2) What relationship exists between biological and psychosocial variables in rheumatoid arthritis?

A number of investigators have assessed patients with arthritis for common premorbid personality patterns.[46-48] They argue that some patterns predisposed a person to develop the disease. Most of the characteristics cited were described with negative words like "self-punitive," "rigid," "depressed," and "angry." It was suggested[50,58,59] that persons with rheumatoid arthritis repress hostility and direct rage against themselves. Other authors believe that patients with rheumatoid arthritis had often endured negative life experiences such as poor parental relationships, stressful marriage, or separation. However, the methodological problems inherent in these studies have been emphasized in recent reviews.[60-62] It is now concluded by these recent reviewers that many but not all patients with rheumatoid arthritis demonstrate certain common personality characteristics, but that these patterns are probably a result of the disease process rather than factors related to the development of rheumatoid arthritis.

There is a striking lack of research describing the presence or development of positive emotional states even though practitioners recognize that some people do manage to adjust to disease. Characteristics such as flexibility, confidence, and sense of humor are seldom measured or discussed. An urgent need exists for longitudinal studies tracing the course of adjustment and coping. As suggested by Crown and Crown,[12] such research would document the experiences of people with arthritis as they learn to live in spite of diminished resources of energy, mobility, skill, and strength. Studies with this perspective have great instructive and therapeutic value.

Another category of research has examined the relationship between psychological and physiological variables. It has been suggested that psychological and biological variables interact to influence the onset, pattern, and course of rheumatoid arthritis.[63] In a group of adult monozygotic twins, all of whom were discordant for rheumatoid arthritis, evidence was found for stress as the initiating factor in those who developed rheumatoid arthritis.[64] Solomon and colleagues reviewed the literature about the relationship of immunity, emotions, and stress.[65] They hypothesized a central mechanism which controls the immune system and links the physical and emotional affective systems with physiological responses, but the data to support this are tentative. Many more studies are in progress about these relationships; and this promises to be a major focus of research, particularly since it has preventive and therapeutic meaning.

There is growing interest in the relationship of psychosocial factors to other rheumatic diseases such as SLE, primary gout, and juvenile rheumatoid arthritis. In gout, Katz and Weiner[2] have developed a model demonstrating that some gouty attacks are precipitated by definite and predictable factors (see also Chapter 86). These precipitants include alcohol, dietary indiscretion, and/or noncompliance in taking medications. In some instances these factors lead to other, more direct precipitating causes. For example, stress in the job setting may lead to consumption of alcohol and noncompliance with medication, leading to an attack of gout. In systemic lupus erythematosus the neurologic involvement of the central nervous system complicates assessment. Psychological change may be due to disease pathology (organic) or emotional reaction to the symptoms (functional). Existing research in SLE has been reviewed by Gurland et al.[66] Compared with the psychological literature in rheumatoid arthritis, research in other rheumatic diseases is sparse.

Several important factors have emerged in recent years that contribute to a better understanding of psychological issues in rheumatic disease through expanded research. Among these factors are the following:

1. The overall increased interest and support for comprehensive multidisciplinary arthritis management programs such as the Multipurpose Arthritis Centers created by the National Institutes of Health in 1976. These Centers and others have provided a focus for the innovation, implementation, and evaluation of creative arthritis management strategies. The emphasis on program evaluation has served to foster more critical thinking among arthritis health professionals.

2. The growth of behavioral medicine, which seeks to link the biology and pathophysiology of disease and its treatment to associated psychological factors. Many new approaches to psychological assessment and intervention have thus taken into account the physical as well as the emotional or affective aspect of the individual patient, yielding a more unified and cohesive body of information. Behavioral medicine is experiencing particular growth in the field of rehabilitation, where function is usually more important than cure. Behavioral research in such areas as compliance with exercise[67,68] and control of Raynaud's phenomenon[69] is especially applicable to rheumatic disease. Achterberg has demonstrated the positive affect of relaxation training on functional indices in patients with rheumatoid arthritis.[70] While admittedly in early stages, such research does attempt to measure the outcomes of particular behavioral techniques in treatment.

3. The development of standardized, computer systems of patient classification and description such as ARAMIS (American Rheumatism Association Medical Information System). These systems facilitate the aggregation of large sample populations and information resources. In such systems, information about patients from all parts of the country and world can be assimilated and analyzed.

4. The creation of new multidimensional health status indices either appropriate for or specific to the rheumatic diseases. These instruments, such as the Arthritis Impact Measurement Scale,[71,72] the Sickness Impact Profile,[73] and the Stanford Health Assessment Questionnaire,[74]

measure discrete physical, emotional, and social factors and produce as well a summative score of the particular construct of items. These instruments are, as a rule, convenient and practical to administer, thus encouraging more widespread utilization. The instruments have provided a better method of defining the problems encountered by the person with arthritis and recognizing the inter-relationship of these problems. As validation of these instruments continues, more information will be obtained about their utility in detecting change along health status levels.

The expanding field of research in psychological issues in rheumatic disease seeks both to describe the current status of the individual with arthritis and to evaluate the effects of intervention. More emphasis now is placed on the therapeutic value of understanding these issues, rather than simply describing an existing personality construct.

## PSYCHOLOGICAL FACTORS IN JUVENILE ARTHRITIS

Children with arthritis have been studied extensively for psychological variables. However, these investigations have suffered from the same problems as the work that has been reported in adults. The investigations are made following the development of the disease process so that the psychological factors noted in the patients are colored by the disability itself.

Even though there is a variability in the types and activity of juvenile arthritis (JA)—changed from the former term of juvenile rheumatoid arthritis JRA to include all forms of childhood arthritis—data obtained from these children are usually pooled and reported for JA as a single disease entity. In one exception McAnarney and her colleagues did a detailed investigation of 42 children from a pediatric rheumatology clinic.[75] As would be expected, they found that children with arthritis had more psychological problems than the normal controls. Surprisingly, children who were in Functional Class 1 (without evidence of disability) had more psychosocial problems than children who had moderate to severe functional disability. During the childhood years the children with mono- or pauciarticular disease appeared to have more problems in coping with their illness than did those who had polyarthritis with obvious disability. The authors felt that the latter group were more recognizable as handicapped and thus had more allowances made for them by parents and teachers, whereas the children with minimal disease, such as an involved knee or ankle concealed by trousers, were not thought to be sick or disabled. However, such children still might have joint involvement and pain, take medication, and be seen at regular intervals by a physician, indicating at least, to the children themselves, that they have an active and chronic disease. The expectations by parents, teachers, and peers that these children should behave and perform normally is probably the unsettling feature in their lives.

In psychological studies of a number of children, a Paris group found that before the age of 7 the defense mechanisms in children with juvenile rheumatoid arthritis were poor.[76,77] Beyond age 8, boys appeared to show more rigidity and obsessional features, whereas the girls were able to show variety in their responses and more compensation for depression. It was also noted that these children did well intellectually but performed poorly in social settings.[77]

It has also been found that arthritic children are unusually expressive in physical and motor actions.[78] They also show significantly higher activity in tasks emphasizing motor skills compared to verbal tests. The investigators also looked at the responses of the parents to the disease; as might be expected, there were feelings of guilt in the mothers, who thought that they might have contributed to the appearance of the disease.

Recently studies have emphasized life stresses as precipitating factors in the onset of juvenile arthritis. In one, 50 patients with JA were studied in Finland.[79] The investigators found a depressive reaction in 17 of the children, and in 13 of this group depression occurred after the onset of JA. Disturbed father-child relationships were observed in 46 percent of the families. Problems in sibling interrelationships were uncommon. Evidence of an increased intensity of overprotection in the mother-child relationship was not found. The two most frequent family problems were divorce or marital separation (18.5 percent) and death or hospitalization of a parent because of serious illness (11 percent). The investigators could not find a typical personality profile in the children. The life stress factors were present during the year before the onset of the JA in 37 percent of the patients.

In the Pediatric Arthritis Clinic in Rochester, New York, 88 patients with JA and their families were surveyed.[80] There was a high frequency of broken homes (Table 34–4), as defined by a home in which there had been divorce, separation, or death of a parent.

Statistical analysis showed this population of JA to be consonant with a sample of about 3000 children in this region. In the large control group the frequency of single-parent homes was 10.6 percent. This was significantly different from the data obtained with JRA (28.4 percent). It is obvious that although divorce, separation, and death are discrete events, situations may persist over a period of time within the household which could be

**Table 34–4.** Frequency of Broken Homes Among Children With JA*

| Population | Parents (%) *Married* | Parents (%) *Unmarried*† | Single Parent(%) |
|---|---|---|---|
| JA | 69.3 | 28.4 | 2.3 |
| Control | 87.6 | 10.6 | 1.8 |
| Welfare | 21.0 | 35.8 | 43.2 |

*From Henoch, M., Batson, J., and Baum, J.: Psychosocial factors in juvenile rheumatoid arthritis. Arthritis Rheum. 21:229, 1978.

†Divorce, separation, death.

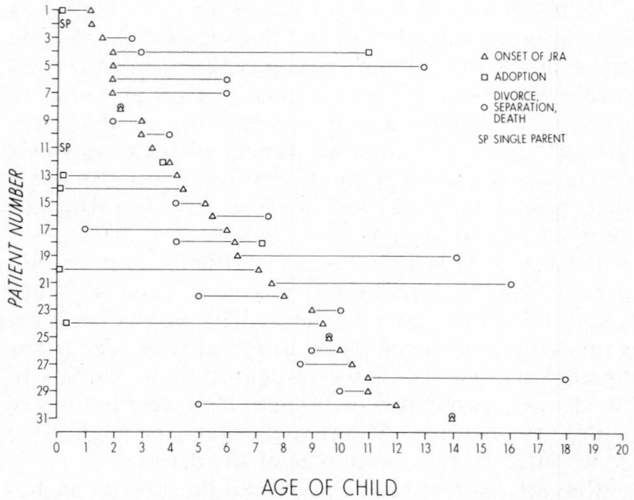


**Figure 34–4.** The time span of events in the lives of the children with JRA who have been adopted, or who come from broken or single parent homes, is presented. Each set of points connected by a line represents the time period between the event and the onset of disease for the individual patients. (From Henoch, M.J., Batson, J.W., and Baum, J.: Arthritis Rheum. 21:229, 1978.)

viewed as more traumatic than the actual separation or divorce. A more precise relationship is shown in Figure 34–4, which depicts the occurrence of the family trauma in relation to the onset of the arthritis in the child. Even with the noted variability, it was found that 48 percent of the events took place within the 2-year period preceding or following the development of arthritis in the child.

On the basis of these and Rimon's studies, a strong correlation has been found between stressful family life events and the development of juvenile rheumatoid arthritis.[79,80]

Others have noted that children with JA had problems achieving emotional separation from their mothers, a tendency to depression, and an impairment in their ability to show anger.[81] Again, these findings are consistent with the reactions of any patient with a chronic disease who is forced to become dependent. In some children it is particularly striking, because at the age when children are expected to show more independence from their parents, they often have the frustration of becoming more and more dependent.

Because of the potentially serious impact that childhood illness can have on personality development, intervention strategies have been developed that can help families as well as children with arthritis.

Parent support groups have been formed in many communities. These groups offer emotional support, understanding, and education to parents who have been previously quite isolated because of the relatively small number of children with arthritis. Parents are often given the advice that their child with arthritis should lead as normal a life as possible without clear information about how to incorporate this concept into everyday life.[82] In conjunction with studies of the child's perception of the disease and experience of pain in juvenile chronic arthritis, Beales and colleagues point out that the child may have inaccurate interpretations of joint sensations and changes. Formal education and counseling sessions for the child and family are recommended to improve understanding and prevent unnecessary fears and fantasies.[83]

Parents and teachers usually need help in understanding that too much overprotection and pity rob the child of the chance to be strong and feel good about himself. The experiences the young child has as a child strongly influence the personality traits he will have as an adult.

Teen groups or rap sessions can be of great value for helping young people in this age group understand and cope with the many personal problems of adjustment that are a part of having arthritis. Often previously isolated, these teens appreciate the support and problem-solving advice from other kids their age who also have arthritis. They often feel better understood by their peers than by family or medical care providers.

Now that Public Law 94-142 (The Education for All Handicapped Children Act) has been in place for some time, support services should be provided in schools for all children. However, in reality one cannot expect even necessary services to be provided automatically because of the budget problems within school districts. Often it is necessary for parents and sometimes physicians to fight hard to obtain essential programs for individual children.

With the present emphasis on "mainstreaming," some children with quite severe handicaps may find themselves in a regular classroom for the first time. If there are any significant adjustment problems, the child might need the support of a psychologist or social worker trained to deal with school problems.

Many school districts now have a program called "adapted physical education" that allows all youngsters to participate in physical education according to their abilities. Unfortunately, one cannot assume that the physical education teacher has any expertise in childhood arthritis. It is more and more apparent that even when services are mandated by public law, there is not a guarantee of appropriate or adequate treatment. Thus, all of these activities need to be closely monitored by the rheumatology team, extending their scope of interest from the medical setting into the community itself.

## A VIEW TO THE FUTURE

In looking to the future with regard to psychological issues in rheumatic disease, several intriguing questions can be considered. What is the impact of "holistic" philosophy on the care of arthritis? Who should be primarily responsible for the emotional and mental health care of the patient with arthritis? To what extent does this care belong in the medical as opposed to community mental health or lay volunteer organizations? How does one measure the outcome of attention to psychological health, and if such outcome measures do not indicate

← Death Sickness Average Wellness High Level Wellness →

← TRADITIONAL MEDICINE →

all resources directed toward
taking care of illness

MANPOWER TRAINING
RESEARCH
INSTITUTIONS
PATIENT CARE

← HOLISTIC HEALTH CARE →

includes resources of TRADITIONAL MEDICINE *plus*
emotional and spiritual aspects of life and personal responsibility for health

PREVENTION
SPIRITUAL AND EMOTIONAL RESOLUTION
EDUCATION ABOUT NUTRITION, EXERCISE
HABIT CONTROL (Smoking, Weight, Stress)

**Figure 34–5.** A model of holistic health care.

an improved physical condition, how much effort and therapy ought to be afforded them?

First, the question of "holistic" approaches to arthritis. Such approaches are based on the philosophy that the patient is a whole person, and that any disease affects all aspects of being, not simply the physical being. "Holistic" approaches include emphasis on health as well as illness and tend to be more positive in nature (Fig. 34–5) with significant attention to psychological issues. Yet they also include activities which, while not in the category of "quackery," are sometimes unproven or untested by traditional measures. The previously discussed "wellness" approaches may be considered in the category of "holistic" medicine. Holistic medicine has appeal for many people and should be at least understood by the more traditional medical community. Evaluation of the various approaches as they relate to arthritis care should be supported and vigorously pursued.

Who is primarily responsible for mental and emotional health of the patient with arthritis? In multidisciplinary settings where physicians, social workers, nurses, and therapists—and sometimes clerical staff and maintenance personnel—have been trained in listening skills and supportive counseling, the primary responsibility must be assigned by some method in order to avoid conflict of advice and wasted effort. When is referral to psychiatry indicated? Does every patient with significant depression warrant psychiatric evaluation, or can this become the function of a highly trained nurse or social worker? What is the place of the psychologist or psychometrician, and how are their skills best used?

To what extent does psychological care belong in the medical system, where costs are high and continuing to rise? Recently, more attention has been given to programs of Arthritis Self Management skills, including many strategies to cope with psychological concerns.[84] The question of how much medical supervision is needed for such lay or volunteer programs has not yet been answered. What is the role of the community health program, and how much information about the medical aspects of arthritis is necessary for effective psychotherapy?

Finally, how are the outcomes of attention to psychological needs measured, and if a positive effect is not documented, how is the value of such attention justified to the medical community? In previous times the focus was to ascertain and describe various psychological health issues associated with arthritis. Now that a body of knowledge about those issues has been accumulated, the focus shifts to dealing with the concerns raised by them.

## CONCLUSION

The symptoms and consequences of rheumatic disease can cause a variety of emotional reactions in patients and their families. These reactions are not specific to the diagnosis of the disease, but rather to the nature of the changes brought about by disease. Most people initially experience negative emotional reactions such as anxiety, fear, denial, and depression. These psychological states and altered sexual function need not and usually do not remain unchanged throughout the course of disease. It is possible for those affected by rheumatic disease to evolve psychologically to more positive states of adjustment. One strategy for helping people with arthritis achieve better psychological health is through stress and pain management techniques. Children with arthritis and their families require particular support and understanding so that the label of "sick child" does not preclude experiences for growth and development. Responsibility for psychological health and quality of life should be shared by health care professionals and the person with arthritis.

## References


1. Moos, R.H., and Solomon, G.F.: Personality correlates of the rapidity of progression of rheumatoid arthritis. Ann. Rheum. Dis. 23:145, 1964.
2. Katz, J.L., and Weiner, H.: Psychobiological variables in the onset and recurrence of gouty arthritis: A chronic disease model. J. Chron. Dis. 28:51, 1975.
3. Solomon, G.F., Amkraut, A.A., and Kasper, P.: Immunity, emotions, and stress. Ann. Clin. Res. 6:313, 1974.
4. Carpenter, J.O., and Davis, L.J.: Medical recommendations—followed or ignored? Factors influencing compliance in arthritis. Arch. Phys. Med. Rehabil. 57:241, 1976.
5. Ferguson, K., and Bole, G.G.: Family support, health beliefs, and therapeutic compliance in patients with rheumatoid arthritis. Pat. Counsel. Health Ed. 2:101, 1979.
6. Moldofsky, H., and Rothman, A.I.: Personality, disease parameters and medication in rheumatoid arthritis. J. Chron. Dis. 24:363, 1971.
7. Rosillo, R.H., and Vogel, M.L.: Correlation of psychological variables and progress in physical rehabilitation. I. Degree of disability and denial of illness. Arch. Phys. Med. 51:227, 1970.
8. Vogel, M.L., and Rosillo, R.H.: Correlation of psychological variables and progress in physical rehabilitation. II. Motivation, attitude and flexibility of goals. Dis. Nerv. Syst. 30:593, 1969.
9. Vogel, M.L., and Rosillo, R.H.: Correlation of psychological variables and progress in physical rehabilitation. III. Ego functions and defensive and adaptive mechanism. Arch. Phys. Med. 52:15, 1971.
10. Rosillo, R.H., and Vogel, M.L.: Correlation of psychological variables and progress in physical rehabilitation. IV. The relation of body image to success of physical rehabilitation. Arch. Phys. Med. 52:182, 1971.
11. Earle, J.R., et al.: Psycho-social adjustment of rheumatoid arthritis patients from two alternative treatment settings. J. Rheumatol. 6:80, 1979.
12. Crown, S., and Crown, J.M.: Personality in early rheumatoid arthritis. J. Psychosomat. Res. 17:189, 1973.
13. Edwards, M.H.: The relationship of the arthritis patient to the community. *In* Lamont-Havers, R.W., and Hislop, H.J. (eds.): Arthritis and Related Disorders. New York, American Physical Therapy Association, 1965.
14. Comer, R.J., and Piliavin, J.A.: The effects of physical deviation on face-to-face interaction. J. Pers. Soc. Psychol. 23:33, 1972.
15. Goffman, E.: Stigma: Notes on the Management of Spoiled Identity. Englewood Cliffs, N.J., Prentice-Hall, 1969.
16. Moldofsky, H., and Chester, W.J.: Pain and mood patterns in patients with rheumatoid arthritis. Psychosomat. Med. 32:309, 1970.
17. Petrie, A.: Individuality in Pain and Suffering. Chicago, University of Chicago Press, 1969.
18. Moos, R.H., and Solomon, G.F.: Personality correlates of the degree of functional incapacity of patients with physical disease. J. Chron. Dis. 18:1019, 1965.
19. Katz, S. Vignos, P.J., Moskowitz, R.W., Thompson, H.M., and Svec, K.H.: Comprehensive outpatient care in rheumatoid arthritis: A controlled study. JAMA 206:1244, 1968.
20. Vignos, P.J., Thompson, H.M., Katz, S., Moskowitz, R.W., Fink, S., and Svec, K.H.: Comprehensive care and psycho-social factors in rehabilitation in chronic rheumatoid arthritis: A controlled study. J. Chron. Dis. 25:388, 1972.
21. Rogers, M.P., Reich, P., Kelly, M.J., and Liang, M.H.: Psychiatric consultation among hospitalized arthritis patients. Gen. Hosp. Psychiatry 2:89, 1980.
22. Shontz, F.C., and Fink, S.L.: A method for evaluating psychosocial adjustment of the chronically ill. Am. J. Phys. Med. 40:63, 1962.
23. Kaplan, S., and Kozin, F.: A controlled study of group counseling in rheumatoid arthritis. J. Rheumatol. 8:91, 1981.
24. Achterberg-Lawlis, J.: The psychological dimensions of arthritis. J. Consult. Clin. Psychol. 50:984, 1982.
25. Zeibell, B.: Wellness: An Arthritis Reality. Dubuque, Kendall Hunt, 1981.
26. Comer, R.J., and Piliavin, J.A.: As others see us: Attitudes of physically handicapped and normals toward own and other groups. Rehabil. Lit. 36:206, 1975.
27. Yelin, E., Meenan, R., Nevitt, M., and Epstein, W.: Work disability in rheumatoid arthritis: effects of disease, social, and work factors. Ann. Intern. Med. 93:551, 1980.
28. Melzack, R., and Wall, P.N.: Pain mechanisms: A new theory. Science 150:971, 1975.
29. Lim, R.K.S.: Neuropharmacology of pain and analgesia. *In* Pharmacology of Pain. Elmsford, New York, Pergamon, 1968.
30. Reuler, J.B., Girard, D.E., Nardone, D.A.: The chronic pain syndrome: Misconceptions and management. Ann. Intern. Med. 93:588, 1980.
31. Bonica, J.J.: Organization and function of a pain clinic. Adv. Neurol. 4:563, 1974.
32. Gottlieb, H., Strite, L.C., Koller, R., Madorsky, A., Hockersmith, V., Kleeman, M., and Wagner, T.: Comprehensive rehabilitation of patients having chronic low back pain. Arch. Phys. Med. Rehabil. 58:101, 1977.
33. Fordyce, W.E., Fowler, R., Lehmann, J., DeLateur, R., Sand, P., and Trieschmann, R.: Operant conditioning in the treatment of chronic clinical pain. Arch. Phys. Med. Rehabil. 54:399, 1973.
34. Melvin, J.: Rheumatic Disease. Occupational Therapy and Rehabilitation. Philadelphia, F.A. Davis Company, 1982, p. 353.
35. Haviland, N., Kamil-Miller, L., and Sliwa, J.: A Workbook for Consumers with Arthritis. Rockville, Maryland, AOTA, 1978.
36. Jacobson, E.: You Must Relax. New York, McGraw-Hill, 1976.
37. Hrena, S.F.: Yoga and Medicine: The Merging of Yogic Concepts with Modern Medicine Knowledge. New York, Penguin, 1973.
38. Shealy, C.N.: 90 Days to Self-health. New York, Bantam Books, 1978.
39. Bloomfield, H.H., Cain, M.P., Jaffe, D.T., and Kory, R.B.: TM*: Discovering Inner Energy and Overcoming Stress. New York, Dell, 1975.
40. Benson, H.: The Relaxation Response. 1st ed. New York, Avon, 1975.
41. Griffith, E.B., et al.: Sexual functioning in spinal cord injured patients: A review. Arch. Phys. Med. Rehabil. 56:18, 1975.
42. Cole, T.M.: Sexuality and the Spinal Cord Injured. *In* Green, R. (ed.): Human Sexuality: A Health Practitioner's Text. Baltimore, Williams & Wilkins Company, 1975, Chapter 12.
43. Lief, H.: Sexual knowledge, attitudes and behavior of medical students; implications for medical practice. *In* Abse, D.W., Nash, E.M., and London, L.M. (eds.): Marital and Sexual Counseling in Medical Practice. Hagerstown, Md., Harper & Row, 1974.
44. Ferguson, K., and Figley, B.: Sexuality and rheumatic disease: A prospective study. Sexuality Disability 2:130, 1979.
45. Annon, J.: The Behavioral Treatment of Sexual Problems. Honolulu, Kapiolani Health Services, 1974.
46. Ludwig, A.: Rheumatoid arthritis. *In* Wittkower, E.D., and Cleghorn, R.A. (eds.): Recent Developments in Psychosomatic Medicine. Philadelphia, J.B. Lippincott Company, 1954, pp. 232–244.
47. Dunbar, H.F.: Psychosomatic Diagnosis. New York, Paul Hoeber, 1943.
48. Robinson, C.E.: Emotional factors and rheumatoid arthritis. Can. Med. Assoc. J. 77:344, 1957.
49. Alexander, F.: Psychosomatic Medicine. New York, W.W. Norton, 1950.
50. Cleveland, S.E., and Fisher, S.: Behavior and unconscious fantasies of patients with rheumatoid arthritis. Psychosomat. Med. 16:327, 1954.
51. Cormier, B.M., and Wittkower, E.D.: Psychological aspects of rheumatoid arthritis. Can. Med. Assoc. J. 77:533, 1957.
52. Edwards, M.H., et al.: Patient's attitudes and knowledge concerning arthritis. Arthritis Rheum. 7:425, 1964.
53. Fries, J.F., Spitz, P.W., and Kraine, R.G.: Measurement of patient outcome in arthritis. Arthritis Rheum. 23:137, 1980.
54. Dahlstrom, W.G., et al.: An MMPI Handbook. Revised ed. Minneapolis, University of Minnesota Press, 1972.
55. Nalven, F.B., and O'Brien, J.F.: Personality patterns of rheumatoid arthritis patients. Arthritis Rheum. 7:18, 1964.
56. Moos, R.H., and Solomon, G.F.: Minnesota Multiphasic Personality Inventory response patterns in patients with rheumatoid arthritis. J. Psychosomat. Res. 8:17, 1964.
57. Bourestom, N.C., and Howard, M.T.: Personality characteristics of three disability groups. Arch. Phys. Med. Rehabil. 46:626, 1965.
58. Cobb, S.: Contained hostility in rheumatoid arthritis. Arthritis Rheum. 2:419, 1959.
59. Geist, H.: The Psychological Aspects of Rheumatoid Arthritis. Springfield, Ill., Charles C Thomas, 1966.
60. Scotch, N.A., and Geiger, H.J.: The epidemiology of rheumatoid arthritis: A review with special attention to social factors. J. Chron. Dis. 15:1037, 1962.
61. Hoffman, A.: Psychological factors associated with rheumatoid arthritis. Nurs. Res. 23:218, 1974.

62. Wolff, B.B.: Current psychosocial concepts in rheumatoid arthritis. Bull. Rheum. Dis. 22:656a, 1971–72.
63. Robinson, H., Kirk, R., Frye, R., and Robertson, J.T.: A psychological study of patients with rheumatoid arthritis and other painful diseases. J. Psychosomat. Res. 16:53, 1972.
64. Meyerowitz, S., Jacox, R.F., and Hess, D.W.: Monozygotic twins discordant from rheumatoid arthritis. Arthritis Rheum. 11:1, 1968.
65. Solomon, G.F., Amkraut, A.A., and Kasper, P.: Immunity, emotions and stress. Ann. Clin. Res. 6:313, 1974.
66. Gurland, B.J., Ganz, V.H., Fleiss, J.L., and Zubin, J.: The study of the psychiatric symptoms of systemic lupus erythematosus: A critical review. Psychosomat. Med. 34:199, 1972.
67. Waggoner, C.D., and Le Lieuvre, R.B.: A method to increase compliance to exercise regimens in rheumatoid arthritis patients. J. Behav. Med. 4:191, 1981.
68. Martin, J.E., and Dubbert, P.M.: Exercise applications and promotion in behavioral medicine: Current status and future directions. J. Consult. Clin. Psychol. 50:1004, 1982.
69. Surwit, R.S.: Behavioral treatment of Raynaud's syndrome in peripheral vascular disease. J. Consult. Clin. Psychol. 50:922, 1982.
70. Achterberg, J., Mc Graw, P., and Lawlis, G.F.: Rheumatoid arthritis: A study of relaxation and temperature biofeedback training as adjunctive therapy. Biofeedback Self Regul. 6:207, 223, 1981.
71. Meenan, R.F., Gertman, P.M., and Mason, J.H.: Measuring health status in arthritis. The Arthritis Impact Measurement Scales. Arthritis Rheum. 23:145, 1980.
72. Meenan, R.F., Gertman, P.M., and Mason, J.H.: The Arthritis Impact Measurement Scales: Further investigation of a health status measure. Arthritis Rheum. 25:1048, 1982.
73. Fries, J.F., Spitz, P.W., and Young, D.Y.: The dimensions of health outcomes; The Health Assessment Questionnaire, Disability and Pain Scales. J. Rheum. 9:789, 1982.
74. Deyo, R.A.: Physical and psychosocial function in rheumatoid arthritis. Clinical use of a self-administered health status instrument. Arch. Intern. Med. 142, 879, 1982.
75. McAnarney, E.R., Pless, I.B., Satterwhite, B., and Friedman, S.B.: Psychological problems in children with chronic juvenile arthritis. Pediatrics 53:523, 1974.
76. Rapoport, D., Hatt, A., Weil-Halpern, F., Hayem, F., and Mozziconacci, P.: La polyarthrite chronique juvenile dans la structure hospitaliere. IV. Étude psychologique des enfants atteints. Ann. Pédiat. 23:437, 1976.
77. Tursz, A.: La polyarthrite chronique juvenile dans la structure hospitaliere. V. Scolarité, vie sociale et familiale. Ann. Pédiat. 23:442, 1976.
78. Cleveland, S.E., Reitman, E.E., and Brewer, E.J., Jr.: Psychological factors in juvenile rheumatoid arthritis. Arthritis Rheum. 8:1152, 1965.
79. Rimon, R., Belmaker, R.H., and Ebstein, R.: Psychosomatic aspects of juvenile rheumatoid arthritis. Scand. J. Rheumatol. 6:1, 1977.
80. Henoch, M.J., Batson, J.W., and Baum, J.: Psychosocial factors in juvenile rheumatoid arthritis. Arthritis Rheum. 21:229, 1978.
81. Blom, G.E., and Nicholls, G.: Emotional factors in children with rheumatoid arthritis. Am. J. Orthopsychiat. 24:588, 1954.
82. Ziebell, B.A.: As Normal as Possible. 1st ed. Tucson, Arizona, Arthritis Foundation, Southern Arizona Chapter, 1976.
83. Beales, J.C., Keen, J.H., and Holt, P.J.: The child's perception of the disease and the experience of pain in juvenile chronic arthritis. J. Rheumatol. 10:61, 1983.
84. Lorig, K., and Fries, J.F.: The Arthritis Helpbook. Reading, Massachusetts, Addison Wesley, 1982.

# Chapter 35
# Ocular Manifestations of Rheumatic Diseases

*Andrew P. Ferry*

## INTRODUCTION

Not many of the detailed clinical studies of rheumatic diseases reported in the literature include a detailed ocular examination by an ophthalmologist as an integral part of the study. Although most rheumatologists are aware of eye involvement in rheumatic disease, they are not necessarily well informed about how often the eyes are involved in patients with rheumatic diseases, which ocular abnormalities are most likely to be present in each of these conditions, and what the management should entail. Many of the associated ocular lesions are potentially blinding. In some instances (e.g., rheumatoid scleritis) the presence of an ocular abnormality may be obvious on casual examination, but in other cases the presence of an ocular abnormality may be overlooked on careful rheumatologic examination. For example, it is well known that the uveitis that leads to cataract formation in juvenile rheumatoid arthritis is usually asymptomatic. This *demands* ocular examination as part of the management protocol for children with this disease. Furthermore, even when ocular symptoms are present, the patient may not report them to the rheumatologist. Patients seldom relate their ocular symptoms to their nonocular disorders.

Detailed ophthalmic examination should be included in the protocol for future prospective studies of the rheumatic diseases. This will benefit the individual patients involved and will help fill some of the many gaps that remain in our understanding of the various types of ocular lesions that develop in patients afflicted with rheumatic disease.

In some of the diseases within the purview of the rheumatologist (e.g., the mucopolysaccharidoses, ochronosis, and Marfan's syndrome) ocular involvement is an integral part of the disorder. These ocular abnormalities are described in the chapters of this book devoted to these particular rheumatic diseases. Ocular involvement may also occur in certain other diseases (e.g., hemochromatosis) which I have not included in this chapter because of their rarity.

The entities discussed in this chapter are rheumatic fever, rheumatoid arthritis, juvenile rheumatoid arthritis, ankylosing spondylitis, systemic lupus erythematosus, connective tissue diseases other than rheumatoid arthritis and lupus erythematosus (scleroderma, periarteritis nodosa, and polymyositis), giant cell arteritis and polymyalgia rheumatica, Wegener's granulomatosis, relapsing polychondritis, enteropathic arthropathy, sarcoidosis, amyloidosis, and gout.

## RHEUMATIC FEVER

Ocular complications are very uncommon in rheum atic fever. In a retrospective study of 200 patients with rheumatic fever examined at the Johns Hopkins Hospital, Smith found ocular manifestations in 12.[1] Most of these ocular lesions were inconsequential, and some probably were nonspecific responses to fever. Duke-Elder lists the following as ocular complications of rheumatic fever: palpebral edema, characteristic arborizations of the conjunctival vessels, subconjunctival hemorrhages, episcleritis and scleritis, and, more rarely, uveitis or embolic phenomena.[2]

## RHEUMATOID ARTHRITIS

The eyes are affected considerably more often and more seriously in patients with rheumatoid arthritis than in patients with rheumatic fever. Keratoconjunctivitis sicca is the most common ocular complication of rheumatoid arthritis in adults.[3] But the most dramatic complications occur in the sclera, episclera, and corneal periphery. Anterior uveitis, band keratopathy, secondary cataract, palpebral edema, orbital myositis, and transitory palsies of the oculomotor nerves are all uncommon complications (although anterior uveitis and band keratopathy do occur with increased frequency in juvenile rheumatoid arthritis).

**Keratoconjunctivitis Sicca.** The normal precorneal tear film has a rather complex structure. It consists of three layers: (1) the outermost, oily layer derived from the palpebral sebaceous glands; (2) the innermost, mucoid layer derived from conjunctival goblet cell secretions; and (3) a watery, middle layer interposed between the oily and mucoid layers. The watery layer is formed by the secretions of the main and accessory lacrimal glands.

Keratoconjunctivitis sicca results from a decreased amount of tear elaboration by the main and accessory lacrimal glands. This failure of lacrimal secretion is caused by atrophic and cirrhotic changes in the lacrimal glands and leads to reduction of the middle layer of the precorneal tear film, the latter becoming attenuated and more viscous. Patients with keratoconjunctivitis sicca have tear lysozyme levels that are below normal.

Dryness of the mouth and oropharynx consequent to salivary gland atrophy is a frequent associated finding. This combination of xerostomia and keratoconjunctivitis sicca is commonly referred to as the *sicca syndrome.*[4] When associated with rheumatoid arthritis the resultant triad is known as *Sjögren's syndrome.* Components of the sicca syndrome have been found in up to one third of patients with rheumatoid arthritis, the incidence being particularly high in those patients with advanced joint disease. Sjögren's syndrome also has been described in patients with other connective tissue diseases, including systemic lupus erythematosus, polyarteritis nodosa, and scleroderma.

Keratoconjunctivitis sicca is usually of insidious onset and bilateral, occurs far more commonly in women than in men (about 90 percent of cases occur in women), and is extremely uncommon in those below age 40. Affected patients usually complain of itching or burning of the eyes. Photophobia is another common symptom. When first seen by the ophthalmologist, only a minority of these patients complain of ocular dryness. Because itching and burning of the eyes are such common symptoms among the general population, the presence of keratoconjunctivitis sicca often goes unsuspected by the ophthalmologist for months or years. Treatment of the supposed infection or allergy with various types of ointment only worsens the condition.

The eyes often appear slightly to moderately red and irritated (Fig. 35–1, Plate II, p. xxxvi). On slit-lamp biomicroscopic examination tiny, punctate gray opacities are seen that stain prominently with fluorescein solution. This epithelial keratopathy is usually most prominent in that portion of the cornea located in the interpalpebral fissure. Because this area is not covered by the lids during most of the waking hours it is particularly subject to drying. Rose bengal solution (1 percent) causes bright red staining of the abnormal corneal and conjunctival epithelium in the interpalpebral fissure. (Although much written about, rose bengal staining is used only infrequently by American ophthalmologists as a practical aid in diagnosis.)

In keratoconjunctivitis sicca the conjunctival goblet cells are stimulated to secrete an overabundance of mucus. A common finding is the presence of ropelike strands of mucus, often 1 cm or more long, arrayed over the eye or resting in the inferior fornix. Less often a so-called filamentary keratitis may develop. Plaques of diseased epithelium desquamate but remain attached to the adjacent epithelium at one end, forming epithelial filaments that may reach several millimeters in length and which simulate strands of mucus on clinical examination. A relatively rare complication of keratoconjunctivitis sicca is severe corneal opacification resulting from an infectious ulcer developing in the dry cornea.

When keratoconjunctivitis sicca is suspected, the Schirmer test of tear secretion often helps establish the diagnosis. This procedure can be carried out by the internist as well as by the ophthalmologist. A strip of filter paper that has been cut to size $5 \times 35$ mm is folded at one end, and the small, folded end is placed in the unanesthetized conjunctival sac (Fig. 35–2). At the end of 5 minutes the amount of wetting of the strip by tears is measured. Although there are many variables, such as the patient's age, 5 mm or less of wetting in 5 minutes is regarded as strongly indicating abnormally low tear secretion.

Patients with Sjögren's syndrome show a wide variety of organ-specific and non-organ-specific antibodies.[4] Rheumatoid factor tests are positive in 75 to 90 percent of the patients.

*Treatment* of keratoconjunctivitis sicca is unsatisfactory. Chronic replacement of tears by artificial substances is required. A variety of such agents are available. Some of the most popular ones at present are

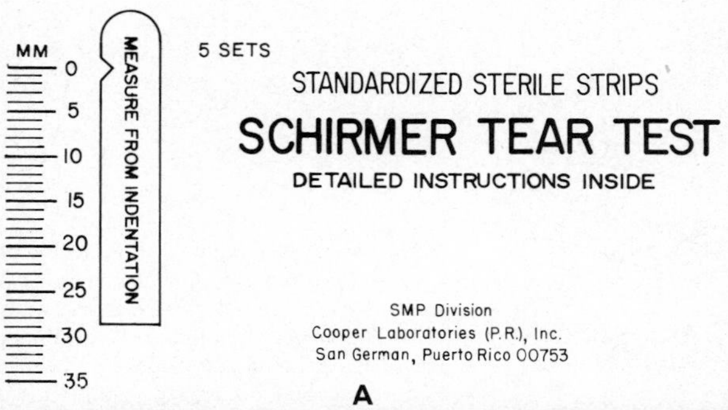


A

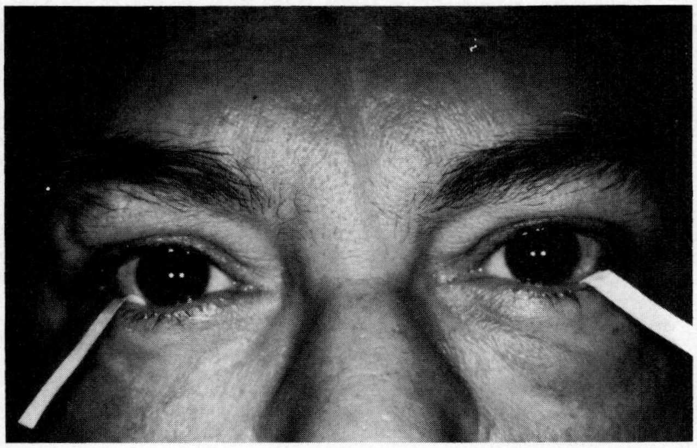

B

**Figure 35–2.** The Schirmer test. *A*, The paper strips are supplied in a packet bearing a scale in millimeters. *B*, Each test strip has been folded partially at its indented area, and the shorter end has been placed in the conjunctival sac. After remaining there for 5 minutes the strips will be removed and the extent of wetting will be measured against the millimeter scale.

Adsorbotear (Burton, Parsons), Tears Naturale (Alcon), and Liquifilm Tears (Allergan). These are helpful in mild to moderate cases and typically must be instilled at least four times daily. Slowly dissolving hydroxypropyl cellulose pellets (Lacriserts) that are placed in the lower conjunctival fornix once daily have recently become available and have allowed many patients to circumvent the need for frequent instillation of drops. Many patients with keratoconjunctivitis sicca go through periods in which their symptoms lessen markedly, or even disappear. During these asymptomatic periods the ophthalmologist may advise reducing the frequency with which the artificial tears are instilled. In unusually severe cases conservation of any tears available may be accomplished by occluding the lacrimal drainage apparatus. This is done by applying diathermy to the superior and inferior puncta and canaliculi. In extreme cases tarsorrhaphy is required to protect the cornea.

**Scleritis and Episcleritis.** ***Anatomy of Sclera and Episclera.*** The sclera is composed of three layers which, from without inward, are (1) the episcleral tissue, (2) the sclera proper, and (3) the lamina fusca (Fig. 35–3). The episclera is a loose structure of delicate fibrous and elastic tissue that is continuous superficially with the loose trabeculae of Tenon's space. (Tenon's capsule is covered, in turn, by the bulbar conjunctiva.) The loose structure of the episclera gradually gives way to a denser arrangement as the episclera merges with the sclera proper. The peculiar feature of the episclera is the large number of small vessels that it possesses in contradistinction to the sclera proper, which is almost avascular. The episcleral vessels are not seen easily in the uninflamed eye. But as soon as the eye becomes congested, three quite separate vascular plexuses become readily visible.[5]

The sclera proper is made up of a dense mass of fibrous tissue arranged in compact bundles. Each bundle consists of parallel collagenous fibers, interspersed among which are numerous elastic fibers. Between the bundles are the fixed cells of the scleral tissue (Fig. 35–3*B*). They are fibroblasts with small nuclei and long, branching processes.

***Incidence of Scleritis and Episcleritis in Rheumatoid Arthritis.*** It has been known for many years that the incidence of scleritis and episcleritis is higher in patients with rheumatoid arthritis than it is in the general population. In an attempt to determine the incidence of these inflammatory lesions in patients with rheumatoid arthritis, and to differentiate rheumatoid scleritis and episcleritis from nonrheumatoid scleritis and episcleritis, a cooperative study was undertaken by the Center for Rheumatic Diseases in Glasgow and the Tennent Institute of Ophthalmology in that city.[6]

Between 1965 and 1973, 4210 patients with rheumatoid arthritis were examined at the Center for Rheumatic Diseases. Twenty-eight (0.67 percent) had scleritis, and seven (0.17 percent) had episcleritis.[6] (One assumes that some patients in this cohort with rheumatoid arthritis who did not have episcleritis or scleritis at the time of initial examination will develop one of these lesions in the future, thereby increasing the overall incidence of scleritis and episcleritis in the group of 4210 patients.)

Correspondingly, in 1971 and 1972 a total of 27 patients with scleritis and 35 patients with episcleritis were seen at the Tennent Institute of Ophthalmology. Of the 27 patients with scleritis, nine (33 percent) had clinical and radiological evidence of rheumatoid arthritis. Of the 35 patients with episcleritis, two (6 percent) had rheumatoid arthritis.[6] Of the 159 patients with episcleritis reported from London by Watson and Hayreh, seven (4 percent) had rheumatoid arthritis, as did 21 (10 percent) of their 207 patients with scleritis.[5]

Combining their patients, investigators at the two cooperating institutions in Glasgow found that all nine of their patients with rheumatoid episcleritis, and 25 of their 37 patients with rheumatoid scleritis, were women.[6] Among nonrheumatoid patients with episcleritis, men and women were affected equally. But among nonrheumatoid patients with scleritis, women were affected about five times as often as were men.[6]

The mean age of all patients with rheumatoid scleritis, rheumatoid episcleritis, and nonrheumatoid scleritis was in the sixth decade. Patients with nonrheumatoid episcleritis were younger, having a mean age of 45 years.

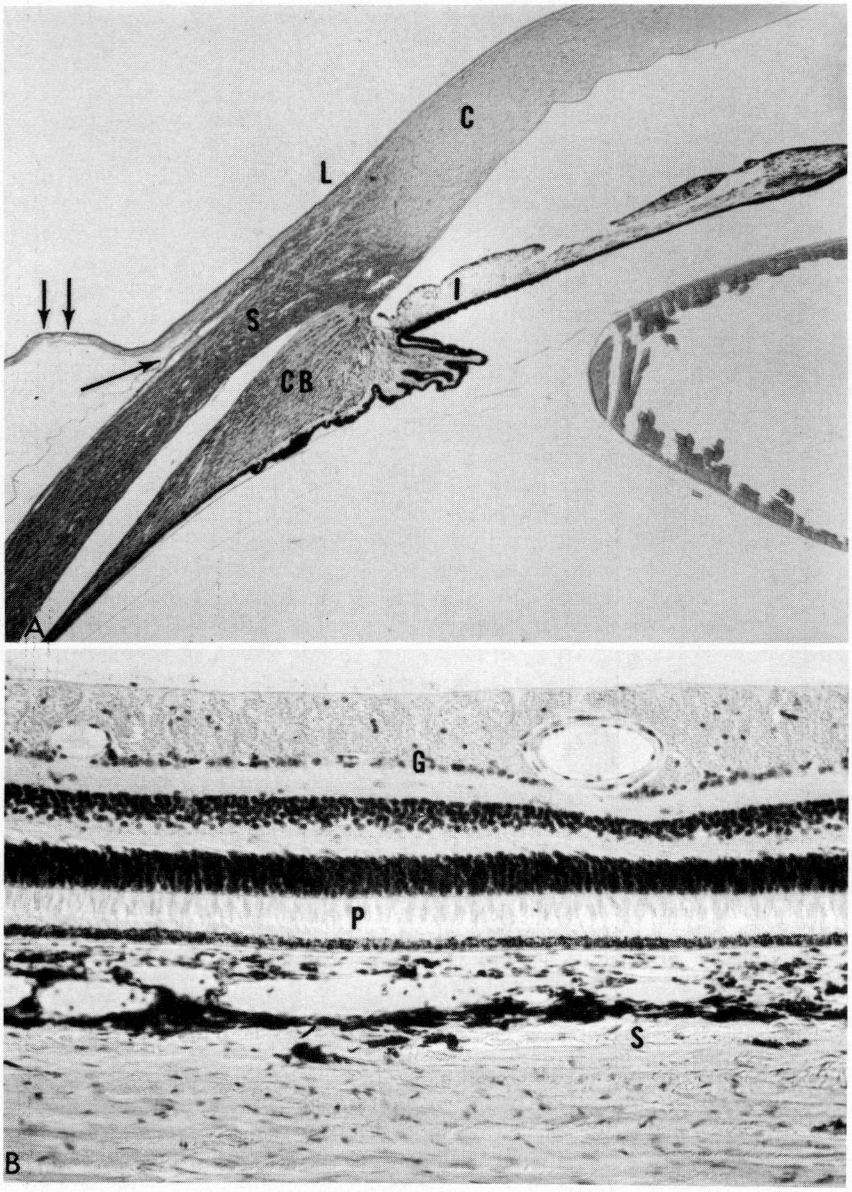


**Figure 35–3.** Normal eye. *A*, Anterior portion of a normal eye. The clear cornea (*C*) joins the opaque sclera (*S*) at the limbus (*L*). The bulbar conjunctiva (double arrows) is artifactitiously separated from the underlying Tenon's capsule (single arrow) and sclera at the left hand side of the field. Farther anteriorly the conjunctival epithelium merges with the corneal epithelium. The iris (*I*) merges posteriorly with the ciliary body (*CB*), the latter being separated artifactitiously from the overlying sclera. The periphery of the lens is visible behind the iris. Much of the lenticular substance has been lost in sectioning. Hematoxylin and eosin; magnification × 13. *B*, Wall of posterior portion of eye. The retina occupies the upper half of the field and the sclera fills the lower one fourth of the field. The choroid is interposed between the retina and sclera. The retinal layers are as follows: internal limiting membrane (top of the field), the nerve fiber layer (containing two prominent blood vessels), the ganglion cell layer (*G*), the inner plexiform layer, the inner nuclear layer, the outer plexiform layer, the outer nuclear layer, and the photoreceptors (rods and cones; *P*). The retinal pigment epithelium traverses the field below the photoreceptors. The choroid lines the outer surface of the retinal pigment epithelium and merges with the sclera at S. Only the inner half of the sclera is included in this field. Hematoxylin and eosin; magnification × 150.

With regard to bilaterality, among patients with rheumatoid scleritis both eyes were involved in 25 of 37 cases (68 percent). Among patients with rheumatoid episcleritis, both eyes were affected in about half the cases.[6]

Rheumatoid scleritis and rheumatoid episcleritis generally occur in patients whose arthritis is of longer duration than that of rheumatoid control patients. Also, patients with rheumatoid scleritis and episcleritis usually have more widespread systemic disease—particularly of the cardiovascular and respiratory systems—and have radiological evidence of more advanced joint disease than do rheumatoid control patients. Subcutaneous granulomatous nodules and atrophy of the skin are much more common in patients with rheumatoid scleritis and episcleritis than in rheumatoid control patients.[6]

The erythrocyte sedimentation rate is significantly higher in patients with rheumatoid scleritis and episcleritis than in rheumatoid control patients. Autoantibody studies in patients with rheumatoid scleritis and episcleritis show little variation from results expected in rheumatoid arthritis.[6]

***Signs and Symptoms of Scleritis and Episcleritis.*** Inflammatory lesions of the sclera and episclera have been subjected to a variety of classifications. For a traditional view the reader is referred to Duke-Elder's System of Ophthalmology.[7]

Scleritis and episcleritis are clinically distinct, with different symptoms, signs, and prognoses. They require different forms of management. From a series involving many years of experience in treating patients with scleral

**Table 35–1.** Classification of Episcleritis and Scleritis*

| | | | | |
|---|---|---|---|---|
| Episcleritis | | | | 217 eyes |
| Simple episcleritis | 170 | | | |
| Nodular episcleritis | 47 | | | |
| Scleritis | | | | 301 eyes |
| Anterior scleritis | 295 | | | |
| Diffuse scleritis | | 119 | | |
| Nodular scleritis | | 134 | | |
| Necrotizing scleritis | | 42 | | |
| With inflammation | | 29 | | |
| Without inflammation (scleromalacia perforans) | | 13 | | |
| Posterior scleritis | 6 | | | |

*From Watson, P. G., and Hayreh, S. S.: Br. J. Ophthalmol. *60*:163, 1976.

inflammatory disease, Watson and Hayreh have put forth a simplified classification which is useful clinically and which has gained wide acceptance[5] (Table 35–1).

*Visual Status.* Episcleritis rarely or never causes loss of vision. Scleritis may cause loss of vision by leading to one or more of a variety of complications such as uveitis, keratitis, or secondary cataract formation. In the series of Watson and Hayreh, 14 percent of patients with scleritis lost a significant amount of vision after the disease had been present for 1 year.[5]

*Pain.* Scleritis is one of the very few diseases that cause severe ocular pain. Some 60 percent of patients with scleritis have severe ocular pain. Although about half the patients with episcleritis will complain of ocular discomfort, severe pain is not a clinical feature of episcleritis.

*Redness.* In simple episcleritis the onset is often extremely rapid, the eye becoming flushed within several minutes of the beginning of symptoms. In nodular episcleritis and in scleritis the onset is much more gradual. In scleromalacia perforans there often is little or no redness of the eye at all.

It is of great importance to examine these patients in daylight, for this often is the only way to distinguish episcleritis from the much more serious scleral disease. In episcleritis the color is salmon-pink to bright red (Fig. 35–4, Plate II, p. xxxvi); in scleritis the redness has a deeper, purple hue (Fig. 35–5*B*, Plate II, p. xxxvi).

*Conjunctival Discharge.* This is not a feature of either scleritis or episcleritis. Indeed, if there is a discharge, and if it is anything but watery, the patient probably has neither of these disorders.

*Location of the Inflammatory Focus.* In episcleritis the areas in the interpalpebral fissures, both nasally and temporally, are most commonly affected (Fig. 35–4, Plate II, p. xxxvi). In scleritis there is no marked predilection for one meridian to be involved more often than the others, but scleritis does occur somewhat more often in the upper quadrants than in the lower quadrants of the sclera.

*Scleral Edema.* In scleritis there is scleral edema and involvement of the scleral vessels. With the slit-lamp biomicroscope scleral edema can be detected by observing the outward displacement of the deep vascular network of the episclera. Avascular zones of episclera may be identified overlying or adjacent to the site of severe necrotizing scleritis.

In episcleritis the sclera is not edematous. The episcleral vessels will be congested (Fig. 35–4, Plate II, p. xxxvi), and the episcleral tissues are infiltrated by inflammatory cells. (In scleritis, the overlying episclera will also be secondarily inflamed in many cases. But instillation of 1:1000 epinephrine or 2.5 percent phenylephrine in the conjunctival sac will constrict these secondarily affected superficial vessels, thereby revealing any underlying scleral disease.)

*Scleral Thinning.* In eyes that have been subjected to previous bouts of scleritis the sclera in the affected area often appears blue when viewed in daylight. (In daylight it is often possible to see areas of scleral thinning that are not recognizable with the slit-lamp biomicroscope or in rooms illuminated by tungsten or fluorescent lights.)

The blue color is imparted by the underlying ciliary body or choroid. In the past it had been assumed that the reason the uveal tract was more visible in these eyes was that the sclera had become thinned by the previous bout of inflammation. But more recently, it has become recognized that this increased visibility of the underlying uveal tract often is on the basis of increased scleral translucency, rather than scleral thinning. In the series of patients reported by Watson and Hayreh, scleral thinning occurred only in patients who had necrotizing scleritis.[5] Early in the pathogenesis of scleral thinning an avascular zone appears in the center of an area of scleritis. This avascular zone then breaks down to form a slough, the end result of which is an area of thinned sclera.

*Scleral Defects.* Scleral defects, as opposed to scleral thinning or increased scleral translucency, occur only in the severest forms of necrotizing disease.

Sir William Read, who was Royal Ophthalmologist in the reign of Queen Anne and who was unable to read or write, has been credited with the following description of the danger of perforation in deep scleritis: "For it is most certain that this horny membrane . . . by how much deeper the blister is hidden in the membrane . . . in danger to make an ulceration by breaking through the membrane, whereupon may ensue an utter loss and decay of all the humours."[6] But a different view of this worthy is provided by Garrison.[8] Sir William was a quack who started out as a tailor but set up as an oculist in London in 1694, having hired someone to write a book on ocular diseases in his name and having hired a poet to praise him in verse. His success attracted the attention of Queen Anne, whose bad eyesight made her an easy victim. After gaining her good graces Read was actually knighted and subsequently became oculist to George I.

In *necrotizing scleritis with adjacent inflammation* (see Table 35–1) the disease begins as a localized area of scleritis associated with severe congestion. About one fourth of these patients will also exhibit avascularity of a patch of episcleral tissue overlying or adjacent to the

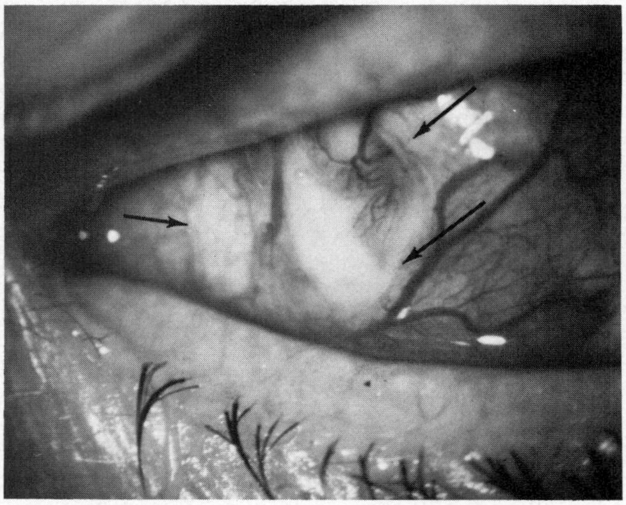

A

**Figure 35–5.** Necrotizing scleritis. *A,* The lesion is located in the temporal aspect of the right eye of a 77-year-old woman whose antinuclear antibody titer was markedly elevated. (The eye is adducted, the temporal periphery of the cornea and iris being just visible in the far right hand side of the field.) Arrows delineate the borders of the scleral ulceration. An oblong avascular patch of episclera extends across the center of the scleral defect, reaching the rim of the ulcer inferonasally. *B,* Same patient as shown in *A,* 2 weeks later (see Plate II, p. xxxvi).

area of scleral edema (Fig. 35–5*A*). The inflammation may remain localized or may spread in both directions around the globe. In those areas where necrosis has occurred there will be scleral thinning or even absence of the sclera, with exposure of the underlying uvea (Fig. 35–5*B*; Plate II, p. xxxvi).

In *necrotizing scleritis without adjacent inflammation* ("*scleromalacia perforans*"; see Table 35–1), the patient initially has no ocular symptoms in many cases. Either she or an acquaintance may notice a grayish or yellow scleral patch which already may have progressed to a complete loss of scleral tissue in a localized area. Any clinical evidence of inflammatory change is minimal. After a variable period the yellowish-gray area separates as a sequestrum together with the overlying episclera. The resulting defect is covered by a thin layer of conjunctiva. Although unsupported by sclera, the underlying uvea tends not to bulge through the defect unless the intraocular pressure becomes elevated (Fig. 35–6).

About half the patients with scleromalacia perforans have rheumatoid arthritis, usually of long standing. Virtually all these patients are women.

*Uveitis.* In episcleritis severe uveitis is rare. But careful examination of the anterior chamber with the slit-lamp biomicroscope will reveal evidence (cells and flare) of a mild anterior uveitis in a small minority of cases.

In scleritis, about one third of the patients will have an anterior uveitis (iridocyclitis) and a smaller number will have posterior uveitis (choroiditis). The uveitis is believed to be caused by inflamed sclera overlying the uveal tract. (But in patients with Wegener's granulomatosis and necrotizing scleritis I have found well-developed foci of granulomatous inflammation in the uveal tract, apparently unrelated to scleral disease, on histopathological examination of several eyes.) In adult rheumatoid arthritis, when scleritis is not present, the incidence of uveitis is believed to be no greater than it is in the nonrheumatoid population.

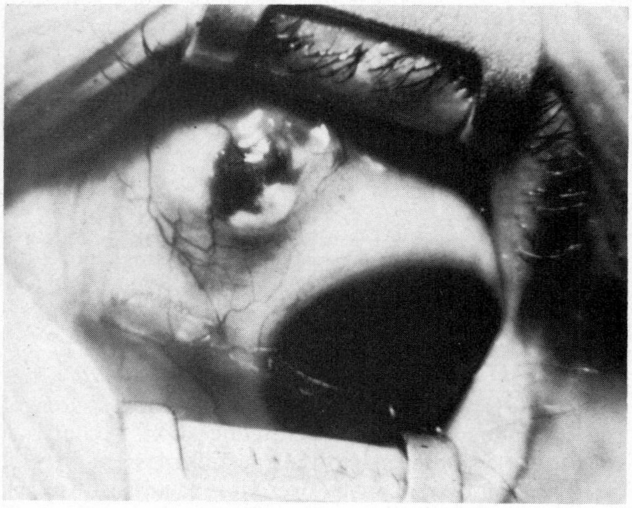

**Figure 35–6.** Scleromalacia perforans (necrotizing scleritis without adjacent inflammation) in a 54-year-old woman with severe rheumatoid arthritis. The left upper and lower eyelids are separated by a speculum and the eye is directed inferotemporally. The sclera has perforated supranasally, and the underlying uveal tissue bulges through the scleral defect. (Courtesy of Milton Boniuk, M.D.)

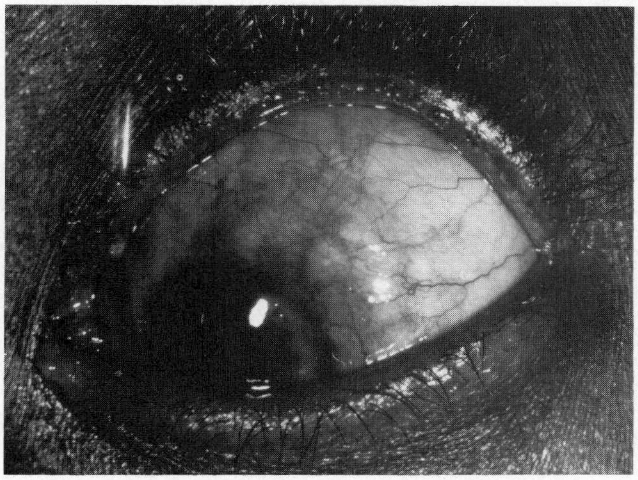

**Figure 35–7.** Nodular scleritis and sclerosing keratitis. Prominent scleral nodules are present just behind the limbus of the left eye superiorly and supratemporally. The nodules were immobile and were separate from the overlying, inflamed episcleral tissues. An area of sclerosing keratitis appears as the limbus-parallel grayish infiltrate in the corneal periphery, extending from the site of the reflex of the photographic flash to the point where the cornea is covered by the lower eyelid temporally. Slit-lamp biomicroscopic examination revealed that the corneal edema and vessels were located in the deepest layers of the corneal stroma.

*Keratitis.* Mild corneal changes occur in a small minority of patients with episcleritis, but these are never severe.

In patients with scleritis, corneal changes of a type characteristically seen in scleritis occur in about 30 percent of cases.[5] Two of the most important of these are sclerosing keratitis and marginal corneal ulcer ("ring ulcer"; "limbal guttering").

In sclerosing keratitis the cornea adjacent to the swollen sclera becomes edematous and blood vessels grow into this edematous zone. The patient shown in Figure 35–7 has both nodular scleritis (see Table 35–1) and sclerosing keratitis.

Marginal corneal ulcers (see Fig. 35–15, Plate II, p. xxxvi) are potentially devastating because of the risk of perforation. They occur in about 5 percent of all patients with scleritis. Marginal corneal ulcers are more common in patients whose scleritis is associated with rheumatoid arthritis and other connective tissue diseases than in nonrheumatoid patients with scleritis.

***Pathology of Scleritis and Episcleritis.*** The characteristic histologic picture in rheumatoid scleritis is a zonal type of granulomatous inflammatory reaction (Fig. 35–8). A central area of necrotic scleral collagen is surrounded by a palisade of epithelioid cells and giant cells. These epithelioid and giant cells are in turn surrounded by a mantle of chronic inflammatory cells, chiefly plasma cells and lymphocytes, which often involve the overlying episclera and the underlying uvea. In eyes with scleromalacia perforans the nongranulomatous component of the inflammatory reaction is often inconspicuous.

In simple episcleritis and in most cases of nodular episcleritis the usual histologic changes consist of hyperemia, edema, and infiltration by lymphocytes and plasma cells. But some rheumatoid episcleral nodules have exhibited all the features of subcutaneous rheumatoid nodules on pathologic examination (Fig. 35–9).[9]

***Treatment.*** Episcleritis is a benign, self-limiting disorder for which no treatment is necessary in most patients. There is a tendency for recurrence in many cases. Should it seem desirable to treat a particular patient, topical corticosteroids may be used.

Scleritis is a much more serious condition and requires skilled management. Topical corticosteroids alone are seldom effective in arresting the disease. Topical therapy with corticosteroids (e.g., prednisolone or dexamethasone) must be supplemented in most cases with systemic anti-inflammatory agents such as oxyphenbutazone, indomethacin, or prednisone. Complications of the scleritis (e.g., uveitis and secondary glaucoma) will require appropriate treatment by the ophthalmologist.

Some authorities believe that subconjunctival injection of corticosteroids, which is beneficial in various other types of ocular inflammation, is contraindicated in treating scleritis. In several cases patients have developed scleral thinning at the site of steroid injection. The relationship, if any, of the scleral thinning to the preceding subconjunctival injection of corticosteroids has not been established.

In extreme cases more heroic forms of medical and surgical treatment have been used. A variety of antimetabolites and alkylating compounds, including methotrexate, 5-fluorouracil, azathioprine, chlorambucil, nitrogen mustard, duazomycin, and cyclophosphamide, have been used with favorable results. Among these drugs, the one now believed to be most effective is cyclophosphamide (Cytoxan). Scleral grafting has been done to bridge over gaps that have developed at the site of necrotizing scleritis. Donor sclera, fascia lata, and periosteum are some of the substances that have been used for this purpose.

## JUVENILE RHEUMATOID ARTHRITIS (STILL'S DISEASE)

Juvenile rheumatoid arthritis differs from adult rheumatoid arthritis in many ways that are well known to the rheumatologist. These differences include both clin-

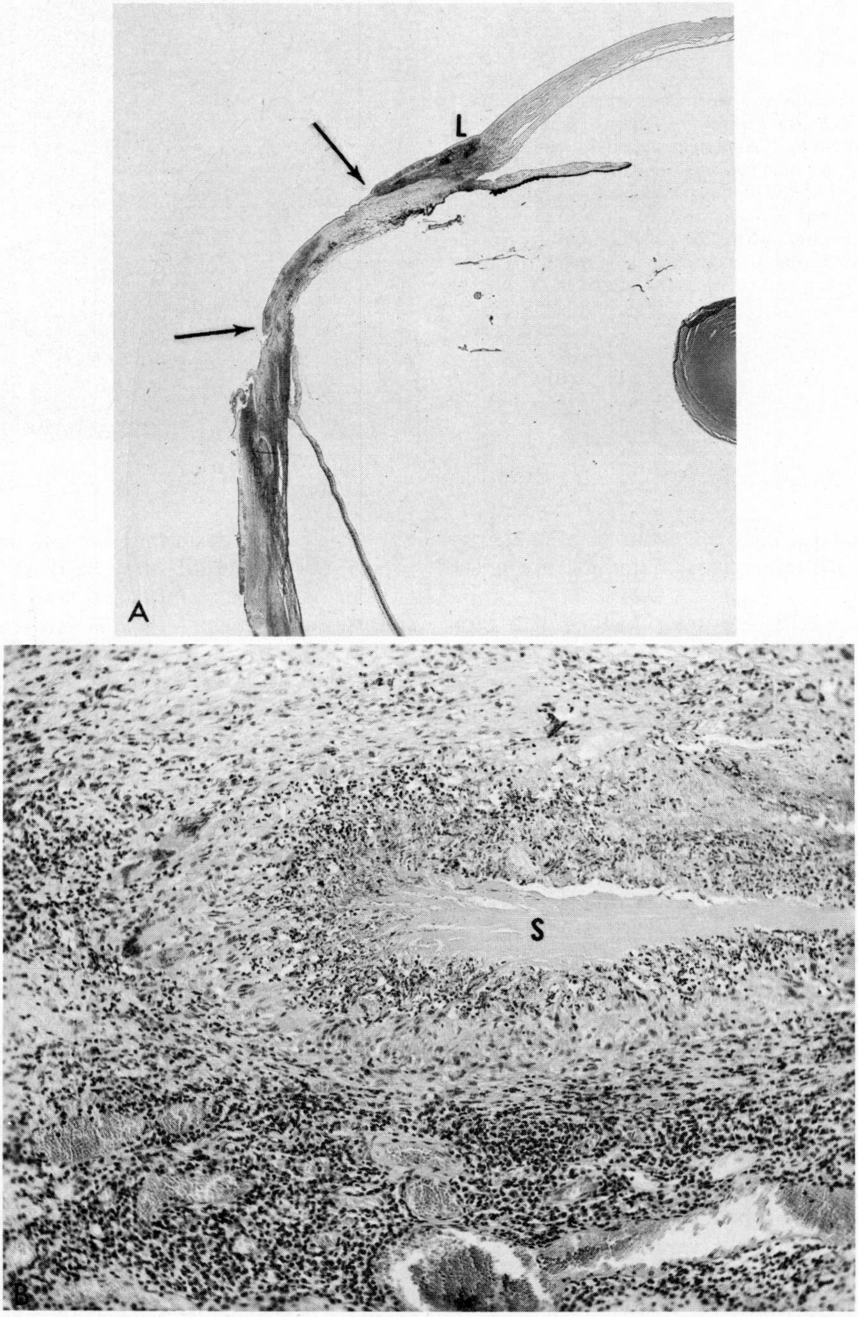


**Figure 35–8.** Granulomatous scleritis. A 64-year-old woman who had rheumatoid arthritis with crippling deformities for several years consulted an ophthalmologist because of gradual diminution of vision over a 6-month period. He observed a lesion that "... perforated and destroyed the sclera at about three o'clock." The ophthalmologist did not suspect the possibility of rheumatoid scleritis with perforation and exposure of the uvea. Rather, he made a diagnosis of malignant melanoma of the ciliary body with perforation of the overlying sclera, and enucleated the eye. *A,* The sclera has been destroyed by an inflammatory process from the limbus (*L*) to the equatorial region of the eye at the bottom of the field. It is completely absent in the zone between the arrows, thereby exposing the underlying ciliary body. Hematoxylin and eosin; magnification × 6; Armed Forces Institute of Pathology Negative Number 57-1167. (Courtesy of Lorenz E. Zimmerman, M.D.) *B,* In this field only a small island of necrotic sclera (*S*) remains. It is being attacked and surmounted by polymorphonuclear neutrophils and a mantle of epithelioid cells. Several well-developed giant cells are present at the left hand side of the field, directly opposite the scleral fragment. The granulomatous inflammatory reaction is surrounded, in turn, by an outpouring of inflammatory cells consisting chiefly of plasma cells and lymphocytes. These are seen best in the lower portion of the field. Hematoxylin and eosin; magnification × 115; Armed Forces Institute of Pathology Negative Number 57-1163. (Courtesy of Lorenz E. Zimmerman, M.D.)

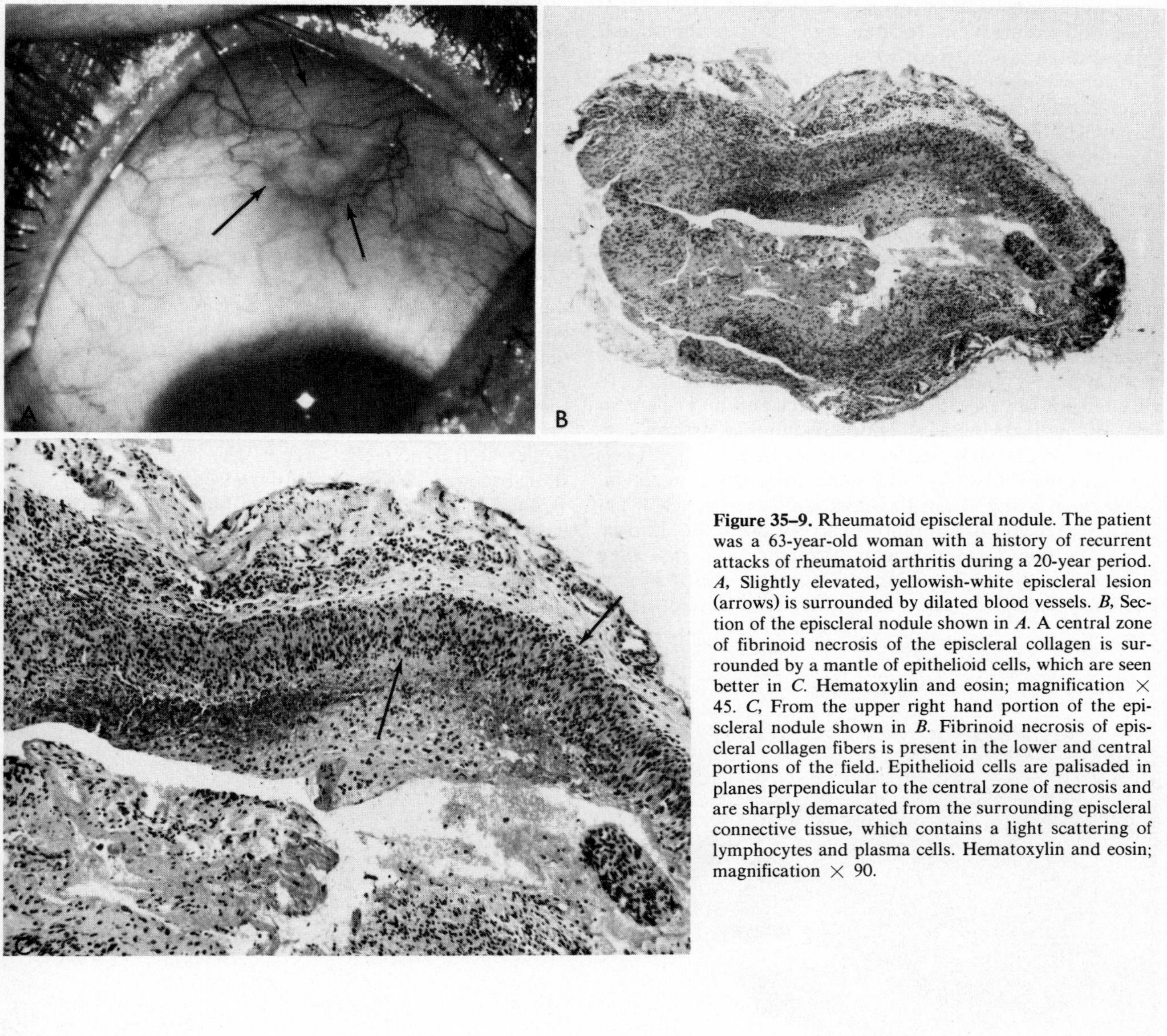

**Figure 35–9.** Rheumatoid episcleral nodule. The patient was a 63-year-old woman with a history of recurrent attacks of rheumatoid arthritis during a 20-year period. *A*, Slightly elevated, yellowish-white episcleral lesion (arrows) is surrounded by dilated blood vessels. *B*, Section of the episcleral nodule shown in *A*. A central zone of fibrinoid necrosis of the episcleral collagen is surrounded by a mantle of epithelioid cells, which are seen better in *C*. Hematoxylin and eosin; magnification × 45. *C*, From the upper right hand portion of the episcleral nodule shown in *B*. Fibrinoid necrosis of episcleral collagen fibers is present in the lower and central portions of the field. Epithelioid cells are palisaded in planes perpendicular to the central zone of necrosis and are sharply demarcated from the surrounding episcleral connective tissue, which contains a light scattering of lymphocytes and plasma cells. Hematoxylin and eosin; magnification × 90.

ical and laboratory features. For example, in juvenile rheumatoid arthritis no more than 10 percent of sera are positive in the commonly employed tests for rheumatoid factor. The frequency of antinuclear antibody is higher in children with rheumatoid arthritis than in adults with rheumatoid arthritis. These two disorders also differ in the nature of associated ocular involvement. In juvenile rheumatoid arthritis the classic triad of ocular lesions consists of anterior uveitis, band keratopathy, and secondary cataract. In adults with rheumatoid arthritis, uveitis (except as a complication of scleritis) probably occurs no more often than it does in the general population. And, except for individuals who have scleritis or who have drug-induced lenticular opacities, cataract is no more common in these adults than in normal controls. Nor is band keratopathy a feature of adult rheumatoid arthritis. Conversely, scleritis and keratitis, both of which are major problems in adult rheumatoid arthritis, are seldom seen in patients with juvenile rheumatoid arthritis. Keratitis sicca, which is so common in adults with rheumatoid arthritis, occurs only rarely in children with rheumatoid arthritis.

In virtually all cases the *uveitis* is an anterior uveitis (iridocyclitis). It is of nongranulomatous type (epithelioid cells and giant cells are not components of the inflammatory exudate) and is bilateral in about 50 to 70 percent of cases. Iridocyclitis occurred in 17 percent of 210 patients with juvenile rheumatoid arthritis reported by Chylack and co-workers in Boston.[10] Girls are affected more often than are boys, the ratio of involvement being 2:1 in the aforementioned series of patients.[10] Uveitis is far more likely to occur in children with the mono-pauciarticular form of the disease than in those with polyarticular involvement, and it is particularly likely to occur in children who develop rheumatoid arthritis before 4 years of age. Kanski studied 160 patients (102 girls and 58 boys) with anterior uveitis and seronegative juvenile arthritis.[11] *Chronic* uveitis occurred in 131 patients, 76 percent of whom were girls. (This is only slightly higher than would be expected from the proportion of girls in the study: 64 percent.) The remaining 29 patients with anterior uveitis had an *acute* form of uveitis, and 27 of them were boys. The acute form of iridocyclitis is bilateral in only about 15 percent of cases.

*Band keratopathy* occurs as a complication of iridocyclitis in many children whose uveitis is of a *chronic* nature. The incidence often has been put at about 50 percent. Band keratopathy occurred in 41 percent of the eyes that had a chronic anterior uveitis in Kanski's series. But Chylack and co-workers found band keratopathy in only 13 percent of the eyes with anterior uveitis in their study.[10]

Band keratopathy is not pathognomonic of juvenile rheumatoid arthritis. It occurs in a variety of other disorders and results from deposition of calcium in Bowman's layer (Fig. 35–10). Typically, the first areas of the cornea to be involved are located just inside the limbus nasally and temporally. Calcification of Bowman's layer then progresses across the cornea, eventually connecting the two original sites of involvement. The result is a band-like opacity located in the interpalpebral fissure. Although a slit-lamp biomicroscope is required to detect the incipient stage of the lesion, the opacity soon becomes visible to the naked eye.

The cause and pathogenesis of band keratopathy are unknown. Calcium and phosphorus metabolism are no different in the affected children than in those who do not develop band keratopathy. The fact that the calcification is usually confined to the zone of the interpal-

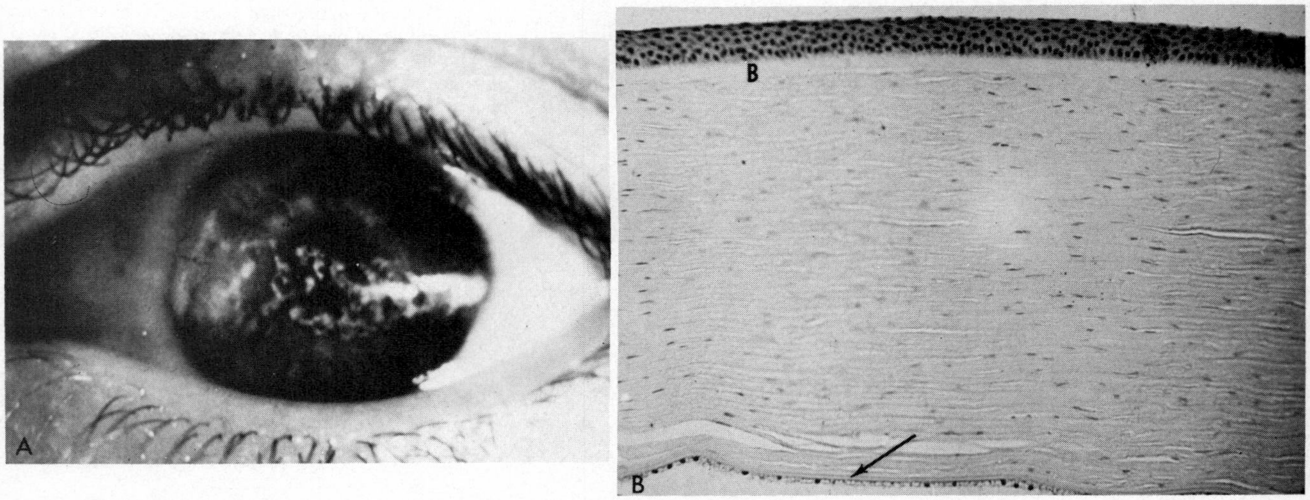


**Figure 35–10.** *A*, Band keratopathy in a 12-year-old girl with severe juvenile rheumatoid arthritis. (Courtesy of Torrence A. Makley, M.D.) *B*, Normal cornea. Bowman's layer (B, upper left), a modified portion of the stroma, is the clear zone traversing the cornea beneath the epithelium. In band keratopathy calcium is deposited in Bowman's layer. Beneath Bowman's layer lies the stroma proper, consisting of collagenous lamellae, keratocytes, and ground substance. Descemet's membrane (arrow) is elaborated by the single layered corneal endothelium, behind which lies the anterior chamber. Hematoxylin and eosin; magnification × 120.

pebral fissure suggests that drying of the cornea may play a role in deposition of calcium in this region.

*Cataract* is said to occur as a complication in about half of the children who have *chronic* uveitis,[12] and developed in 42 percent of the eyes with chronic iridocyclitis in Kanski's study.[11] But Chylack and co-workers found cataract in only 22 percent of eyes with uveitis.[10] The lower incidence of band keratopathy and secondary cataract in the patients reported by these investigators may reflect their diligent search for early, and often asymptomatic, uveitis, thereby enabling institution of appropriate therapy.

*Treatment* of eyes affected with the *acute* form of anterior uveitis is usually relatively simple, the inflammation responding well to topical medications. Because these eyes usually exhibit pain and redness that is obvious to the parents and to the rheumatologist, there seldom is any delay in beginning treatment. Serious ocular complications (e.g., cataract and band keratopathy) seldom occur.[11] In Kanski's study of 29 patients with the acute type of anterior uveitis, the mean age at onset of arthritis was 11.5 years. On followup, 21 of the 29 patients had developed typical ankylosing spondylitis, and five patients had sacroiliitis.

*Treatment* of the *chronic* form of uveitis is often difficult, but about 40 percent of cases can be brought under control in 3 months or less.[10] The mainstays of therapy are topical corticosteroids and atropine. Systemic corticosteroids may be required to treat those eyes that fail to respond to topical medications. Immunosuppressive drugs other than corticosteroids have seldom been used in treating iridocyclitis occurring in patients with juvenile rheumatoid arthritis.[11] This is attributable both to the lack of convincing evidence for their effectiveness and to the rheumatologist's reluctance to subject these young individuals to the major toxic effects of chemotherapy.

Chelation of the calcium in Bowman's layer with topically applied sodium versenate solution will result in clearing of band keratopathy and improvement of vision in many cases. In those children who eventually require ocular surgery (e.g., for a cataract dense enough to cause major visual loss or for glaucoma consequent to synechia formation) the results are often discouraging.

Many observers have commented on the lack of symptoms reported by children with the *chronic* form of uveitis when the ocular inflammation begins. Only a minority report symptoms of iridocyclitis or exhibit evidence of ocular inflammation that is apparent to their parents or to the rheumatologist. In view of this often asymptomatic onset of ocular inflammation, and because treatment of the uveitis at an early stage will often forestall development of complications such as band keratopathy and cataract, it is of great importance that children with rheumatoid arthritis be subjected to periodic examination by an ophthalmologist in a search for anterior uveitis. A 6-month interval between ophthalmic examinations would be appropriate in most cases. The children who are at greatest risk are those with the pauciarticular form of the disease, and they should be seen, at least initially, at even more frequent intervals.

## ANKYLOSING SPONDYLITIS

Because one third to one half of the patients with ankylosing spondylitis exhibit synovitis in peripheral joints, the disease was formerly viewed as a variant of rheumatoid arthritis. But ankylosing spondylitis differs from rheumatoid arthritis in several ways: (1) Preponderance of involvement in men (male:female ratio 8:1). (2) Evidence of genetic transmission in related kindreds. (The disease is 30 times more prevalent among the relatives of spondylitis patients than in relatives of controls. The striking association of ankylosing spondylitis with the histocompatibility antigen HLA-B27 provides further insight into the genetic aspect of this disorder.) (3) The absence of rheumatoid factor and rheumatoid nodules. (4) Prominent calcification of the longitudinal ligaments of the peripheral portions of the intervertebral discs. (5) A tendency to bony ankylosis. (An ophthalmologic aphorism is that a young man with anterior uveitis who has difficulty in placing his chin in the slit-lamp apparatus should be suspected of having ankylosing spondylitis.) (6) The association of certain extra-articular manifestations, such as iridocyclitis and aortitis. (7) Symptomatic benefit with medications that are only minimally effective in rheumatoid arthritis (e.g., phenylbutazone and indomethacin).[13]

In various series, from 4 to 50 percent of patients with ankylosing spondylitis have had an anterior uveitis, with 25 percent being, perhaps, the most commonly accepted figure. Recent studies suggest that among patients with ankylosing spondylitis, uveitis occurs far more commonly in those who are HLA-B27 positive than it does in those who are HLA-B27 negative. Although uveitis may be the presenting sign of the disease, characteristically the ocular inflammation develops in a patient already known to have spondylitis. Typically the inflammation is an acute, nongranulomatous anterior uveitis. The signs and symptoms include photophobia, some decrease in visual acuity, a variable degree of ocular pain, congestion of the episcleral vessels, fine cellular precipitates on the corneal endothelium, cells and flare in the anterior chamber, and miosis. A severe plastic iritis, with formation of dense synechiae, is decidedly uncommon.[14]

Treatment of the iridocyclitis consists of the usual topical corticosteroids, cycloplegics (e.g., atropine), and mydriatics. The iritis generally runs a favorable course and tends to clear in 3 to 6 weeks, with few sequelae. Relapses are typical of the disease and may occur repeatedly over the course of many years.[13]

## SYSTEMIC LUPUS ERYTHEMATOSUS

In the realm of the ophthalmologist the most common manifestation of this disease is the *butterfly eruption,*[15] which occurs in some 40 percent of cases and which is discussed in Chapter 36. Signs and symptoms of *central nervous system* involvement occur in some 30 percent of patients with systemic lupus erythematosus, and some of these individuals will be seen by the ophthalmologist because of ptosis, diplopia, or nystagmus.[16]

With regard to the *eye* itself, "cotton wool patches" in the retina often have been cited as being the most common lesion, followed in frequency by corneal and conjunctival involvement, with only a very occasional patient exhibiting uveitis or scleritis. But one encounters difficulty in attempting to determine the incidence of ocular involvement in systemic lupus erythematosus. For example, many observers have remarked that the retinal lesions occur much more often in acutely ill patients than they do in those who are in remission or who have only a relatively mild form of the disease. The investigation of Gold and co-workers, in which they reported the ocular findings in their 61 patients with systemic lupus erythematosus and reviewed ten similar series reported in the literature by other workers, is of interest in this regard.[17] They found retinal hemorrhages reported in from 5 to 28 percent of cases (not one of their 61 patients had a retinal hemorrhage) and cotton wool spots described in from 6 to 28 percent of cases (only 3 percent of their patients had cotton wool spots). Gold and associates remarked that all 61 of their patients had been referred to them for ocular examination from the systemic lupus erythematosus clinic at Bellevue Hospital. Most of these patients had been treated already with systemic antimalarials and/or corticosteroids, and were no longer acutely ill.

Another consideration in determining the incidence of ocular involvement in systemic lupus erythematosus is the fact that greater clinical awareness and better laboratory diagnostic aids in recent years have led to the detection of many mild cases of lupus. These patients are the very ones who are least likely to exhibit ocular complications.

**Retinopathy.** Retinal damage from antimalarials used in treating systemic lupus erythematosus is a greater cause of visual loss than is retinal involvement occurring in the natural course of the disease.

*Cotton wool spots* occur in lupus and in a variety of other disorders, most notably the "connective tissue" diseases, vascular hypertension, central retinal vein occlusion, diabetic retinopathy, papilledema, the dysproteinemias, leukemia, and severe anemia.[18] On ophthalmoscopic examination one or more (but usually less than ten) cotton wool spots are seen. They occur preferentially in the posterior part of the retina, rendering them detectable by casual examination. The optic nerve head is often involved. Each cotton wool spot appears as a grayish-white, soft, fluffy exudate, usually situated more closely to the arterioles than to the veins, lying in the inner layers of the retina and bulging slightly toward the vitreous body (Fig. 35–11). They are small, averaging about one third of a disc diameter in width. (The normal diameter of the optic nerve head is from 1.5 to 2.0 mm.) Cotton wool spots usually clear within 1 to 3 months of their appearance.

Pathologic examination of tissue from a cotton wool spot confirms the clinical impression that the lesion involves chiefly the inner retinal layers (Fig. 35–12). The ganglion cell nerve fiber layer is greatly thickened in a disciform, sharply circumscribed fashion. In this region some of the nerve fibers have been interrupted, and in many cases "*cytoid bodies*" are seen. The latter are globular bodies, 10 to 20 microns in diameter. Each bears a superficial resemblance to a cell because of a centrally located structure simulating a nucleus. (Thus, "cotton wool spot" is an ophthalmoscopic term, and "cytoid body" is a histologic feature of the cotton wool spot.)

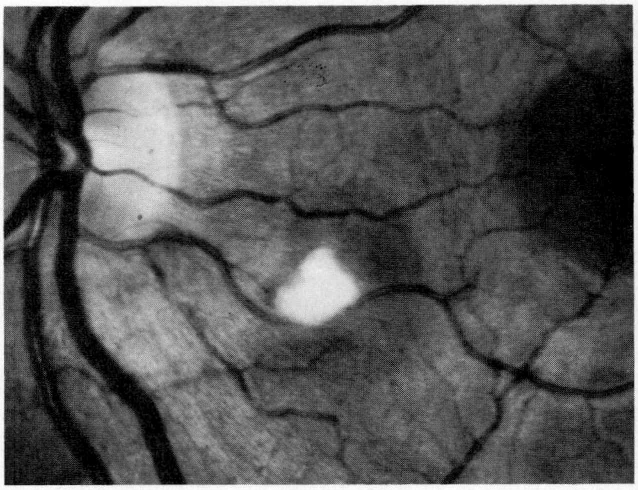

**Figure 35–11.** A typical cotton wool spot in a young woman with systemic lupus erythematosus. The lesion is situated along the upper border of a retinal arteriole, about midway between the optic nerve head and the macula.

The nature of cytoid bodies has been argued since their discovery in 1856. In recent years Wolter has shown conclusively that cytoid bodies arise from the axons of retinal ganglion cells. The axons of the retinal ganglion cells have their synapses in the lateral geniculate body. In a patient with a cotton wool spot these nerve fibers become interrupted as they course through the lesion which is located between the ganglion cell and the optic nerve head. Prominent terminal swelling of the axonal stump on the side remaining in contact with the retinal ganglion cell occurs. This bulbous terminal swelling of the interrupted nerve fiber, together with aggregation of the lipid debris of the degenerating axonal structures to form a pseudonucleus, constitutes a cytoid body.[18]

It is generally agreed that focal ischemia is the cause of cotton wool spots and the cotton wool spot is, therefore, a microinfarct of the retina. The precise nature of the vascular insufficiency is unsettled. Recent work suggests that the white material seen in a cotton wool spot may consist at least partially of accumulated axoplasmic debris at the site of an obstruction in the normal orthograde axoplasmic transportation system in axons of retinal ganglion cells.

*Hemorrhages* in the inner retinal layers are another feature of the retinopathy occurring in systemic lupus erythematosus. And, as is true of cotton wool spots,

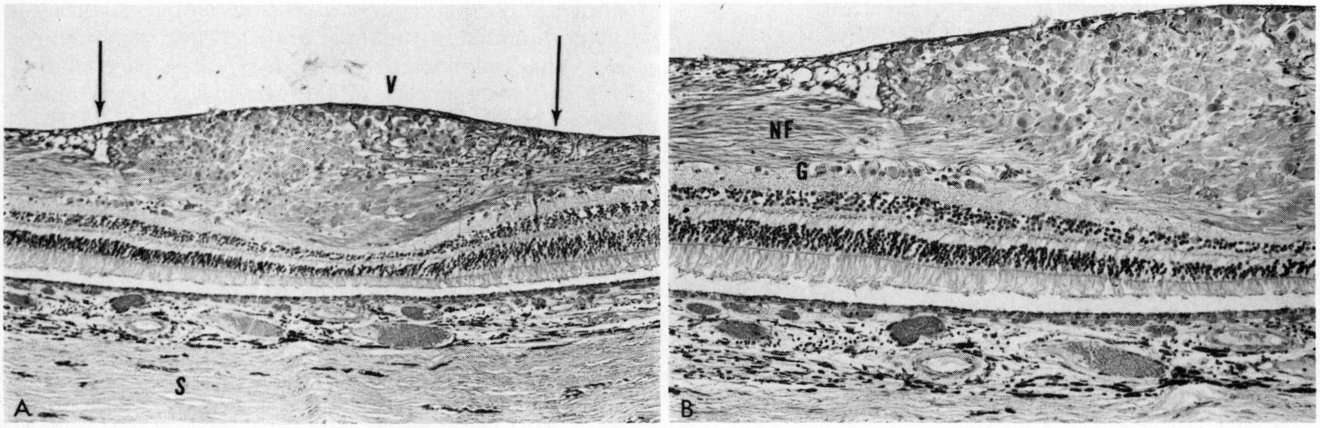


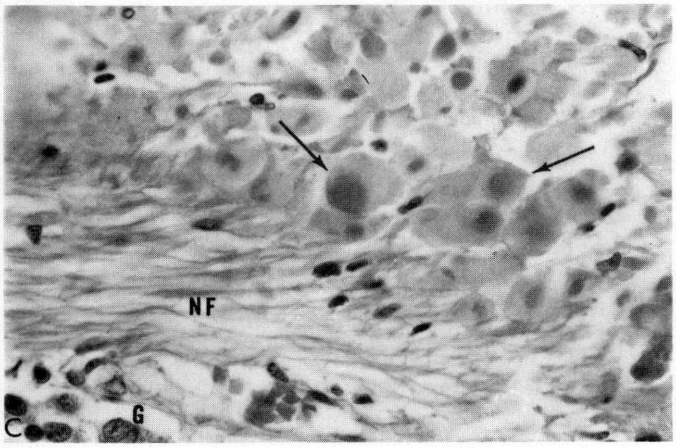


**Figure 35–12.** A cotton wool spot in the retina of a 26-year-old woman who died of systemic lupus erythematosus. *A* (compare with Fig. 35-3*B*). The ganglion cell nerve fiber layer is greatly thickened in a disciform, sharply circumscribed fashion (arrows). It bulges internally toward the vitreous body (V), and also externally, distorting the inner nuclear layer of the retina. The rods and cones are separated artifactitiously from the underlying layer of retinal pigment epithelium. *S* = Sclera. Hematoxylin and eosin; magnification × 75. *B*, Same lesion shown in *A*. Nerve fibers (*NF*) are interrupted as they enter the area of the cotton wool spot. Many "cytoid bodies" are visible in the lesion. *G* = Ganglion cell layer of retina. Hematoxylin and eosin; magnification × 120. *C*, From near the center of the field shown in *B*. Many "cytoid bodies" (arrows) are present. *NF* = Nerve fiber layer of retina. *G* = Retinal ganglion cell. Hematoxylin and eosin; magnification × 480.

they are not necessarily mere reflections of a concomitant vascular hypertension. They can result from an independent effect of the disease on the retinal tissues and they are found in the absence of hypertension.[17] Other retinal lesions that may occur with or without concomitant hypertension are retinal *microaneurysms, arteriovenous crossing changes,* and *arteriolar narrowing.*[17]

**Corneal and Conjunctival Lesions.** A variety of these have been described.[19] The most common are *conjunctivitis* (3 to 20 percent of cases) and mild *epithelial degeneration,* rendering the affected cells stainable with topical fluorescein.[17] *Sjögren's syndrome* has been documented in association with various connective tissue diseases, including systemic lupus erythematosus, and any of these may replace rheumatoid arthritis in the classic triad of Sjögren's syndrome.[4]

## CONNECTIVE TISSUE DISEASES OTHER THAN RHEUMATOID ARTHRITIS AND LUPUS ERYTHEMATOSUS

*Scleroderma* (systemic sclerosis) is a rare disease. Some three to five new cases per million population appear each year in the United States. In this disorder the ocular adnexa and the outer coats of the eye are affected relatively often, but involvement of the inner eye, particularly the retina, is unusual.[20] The most common finding is tightness of the eyelids. Keratoconjunctivitis sicca and Sjögren's syndrome occur less often.

Ocular involvement is uncommon in *periarteritis nodosa* (polyarteritis nodosa.) Reported abnormalities of the outer coats of the eye include chemosis (conjunctival edema), subconjunctival hemorrhages, conjunctivitis, keratitis, scleritis, marginal corneal ulceration, and Sjögren's syndrome. Choroidal angiitis has been found in many eyes examined post mortem, but clinical signs of choroidal involvement are seen only seldom. Retinal lesions are rarer than choroidal involvement, and the majority of these result from the effects of vascular hypertension upon the retinal vessels.[21]

Involvement of the eye is rare in *polymyositis* and in *dermatomyositis.* Conjunctivitis, episcleritis, iritis, and retinal cotton wool spots have been reported. The eyelids are involved more often. A peculiar bluish to violaceous ("heliotrope") erythematous suffusion develops in the eyelids in many cases and is often associated with closely set telangiectasias of the palpebral skin and with marked palpebral edema. The orbicularis oculi muscles and the extraocular muscles may participate in the widespread myositis, leading to pain, tenderness, oculomotor palsies, and nystagmus.[22]

## GIANT CELL ARTERITIS (TEMPORAL ARTERITIS, CRANIAL ARTERITIS) AND POLYMYALGIA RHEUMATICA

The association of giant cell arteritis with polymyalgia rheumatica is discussed in Chapter 73. Henkind and Gold have emphasized that the incidence of giant cell arteritis in patients with polymyalgia rheumatica is much higher than the often cited 20 percent.[23] For those patients with polymyalgia rheumatica who do *not* have clinical evidence of giant cell arteritis and whose symptoms are controllable with small amounts of corticosteroids (10 mg or less of prednisone daily), the risk of visual complications is far lower than it is for patients with polymyalgia rheumatica who have clinical evidence of giant cell arteritis. Spiera and Davison followed for a minimum of 4 years 56 patients with polymyalgia rheumatica who had no clinical evidence of giant cell arteritis. None became blind or developed any other visual disturbance.[24] The outlook is much grimmer for patients with giant cell arteritis. Ocular involvement formerly occurred in 40 to 50 percent of patients, with unilateral blindness developing in 10 to 15 percent, and both eyes becoming blind in 12 to 15 percent.[25] Blindness in these patients is particularly unfortunate because it is usually preventable if the disease is diagnosed promptly and corticosteroids are administered immediately. In a recently reported series of cases, 15 of 126 patients with giant cell arteritis (12 percent) suffered ocular complications.[26] Earlier diagnosis and awareness of the need for immediate treatment probably account for the decreased frequency with which visual catastrophes currently occur in patients with giant cell arteritis.

The systemic disorder known today as "giant cell arteritis" was described first by the British ophthalmologist Jonathan Hutchinson in 1890. Subsequently it was studied in detail by others and was given the name "temporal arteritis" because involvement of the temporal arteries is a dominating feature. But because many patients also have evidence of involvement of other arteries in the cranial region (e.g., the cerebral and lingual arteries), there has been a more recent tendency to supplant the term "temporal arteritis" with the designation "cranial arteritis." Other authors prefer the term "giant cell arteritis" because, although the brunt of the disease is borne by the carotid arteries and their branches, other vessels (e.g., the aorta, innominate, subclavian, and coronary arteries) have been involved in many cases. Furthermore, this designation emphasizes one of the salient histologic features of the lesion. HLA tissue typing for A, B, and C antigens has been unremarkable in patients with giant cell arteritis, as have serum levels of IgA, IgG, IgM, antinuclear antibodies, and complement components C3 and C4.

A frequent characteristic feature is the presence of a prominent, thickened, tortuous, tender temporal artery that often shows no pulsation. An affected artery exhibits patchy areas of necrosis in the tunica media with fragmentation of the internal elastic lamina. A prominent granulomatous inflammatory reaction, with many giant cells, is found in the necrotic areas, particularly along the outer aspect of the internal elastic lamina, while marked fibrosis occurs on the intimal side. This diffuse, chronic, granulomatous inflammatory reaction produces such a severe amount of intimal reaction that the vascular lumen may be occluded (Fig. 35–13).

Only the ocular symptoms and signs occurring in this systemic disease will be considered here. The ocular complications of giant cell arteritis appear within several weeks or months of the onset of systemic manifestations. Typically the visual loss is abrupt and progresses rapidly to blindness. Less often the blindness is preceded by episodes of unilateral visual loss (amaurosis fugax). Both eyes often are affected, the second eye becoming involved from 1 day to 3 weeks after the first. Visual loss may be complete or may be limited to a sector of the visual field. When only part of the visual field is lost, an inferior altitudinal defect is the most common finding.

The visual loss results from ischemic infarction of the optic nerve (ischemic optic neuropathy) caused by giant cell arteritis involving branches of the ophthalmic artery supplying the optic nerve. Much less often the central retinal artery is occluded. The site of predilection for optic nerve involvement is just behind the lamina cribrosa. Low-grade papilledema results and the swollen optic nerve head tends to be more pallid than is the disc in cases of inflammatory optic neuritis (Fig. 35–14).

The presence of giant cell arteritis should be suspected in any patient above age 50 years with abrupt visual loss and ischemic optic neuropathy. The erythrocyte sedimentation rate should be determined immediately. It usually is elevated markedly in giant cell arteritis; but if the patient has been taking corticosteroids, it may be only slightly increased or even normal. If the sedimentation rate is found to be elevated, or if the patient has other evidence of giant cell arteritis, systemic corticosteroids should be administered immediately in large doses (60 to 120 mg of prednisone or its equivalent daily), and the temporal artery should be biopsied. Institution of corticosteroid therapy should not await the biopsy report. A negative temporal artery biopsy does not rule out the presence of giant cell arteritis. Skip areas of involvement occur. As the erythrocyte sedimentation rate falls, the dose of corticosteroids may be decreased to the lowest level sufficient to maintain the sedimentation rate at a normal level for at least 4 to 6 months, after which the steroids may be cautiously discontinued. If the temporal artery biopsy was negative, but the trial of corticosteroids has lowered a high sedimentation rate to normal, continued treatment is probably warranted. A patient with a normal sedimentation rate and a negative temporal artery biopsy is unlikely to have the disease and should not be subjected to the hazards of long-term, high-dose corticosteroid therapy.

Corticosteroid therapy usually will prevent involvement of the second eye, but only seldom will it improve vision in the first eye to be affected in patients with giant cell arteritis.

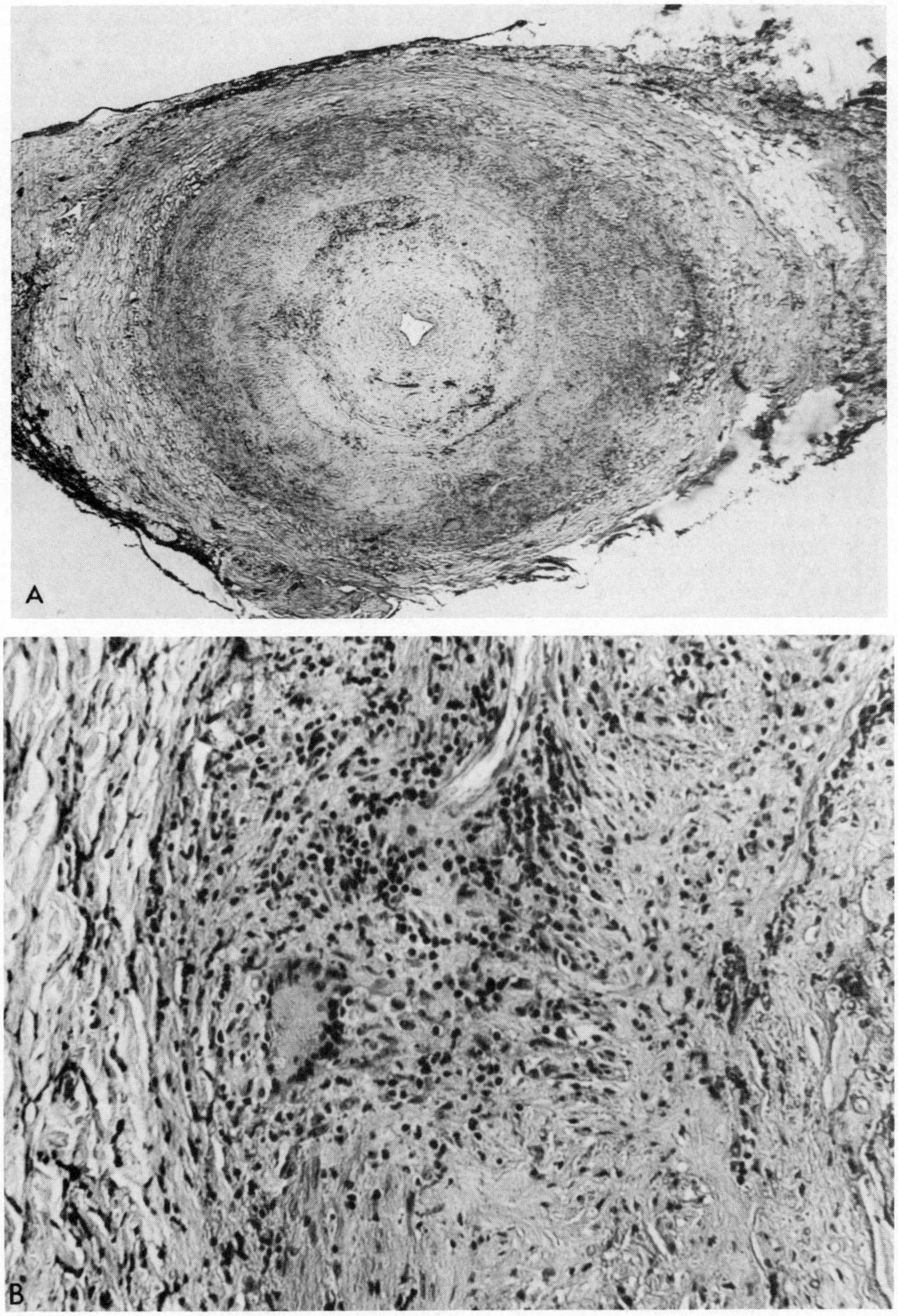


**Figure 35–13.** Giant cell arteritis. *A,* The temporal artery's lumen has been reduced profoundly in diameter by the inflammatory process in its wall and by subintimal proliferation. Hematoxylin and eosin; magnification × 30. *B,* In many areas epithelioid cells have fused to form giant cells. A prominent giant cell is located just to the left of the center of this field. Many lymphocytes and plasma cells also are present. Hematoxylin and eosin; magnification × 150.

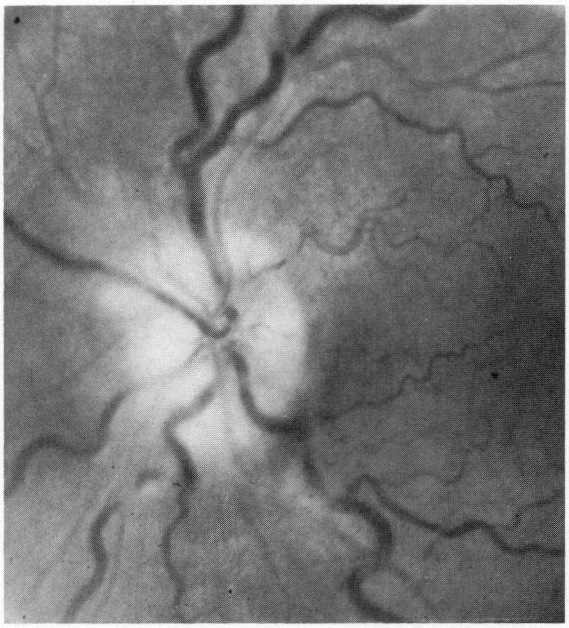

**Figure 35–14.** Giant cell arteritis. (Same patient whose temporal artery biopsy is shown in Fig 35–13.) The optic nerve head is edematous. Retinal arteriolar narrowing is present. The retinal veins are slightly dilated, and the venous blood column is darker than normal. (A nuclear cataract was present, rendering the fundus details slightly indistinct.)

## WEGENER'S GRANULOMATOSIS

The classic triad of Wegener's granulomatosis consists of granulomas of the upper or lower respiratory tract, focal necrotizing glomerulonephritis, and arteritis. But, as Wegener has emphasized, the condition should not be considered primarily an angiitis.[27] Angiitis is a prominent feature in the lungs in some patients, but it is not responsible for the extravascular granulomatous lesions. In some cases it is difficult or impossible to demonstrate angiitis.

Ocular involvement is common in Wegener's granulomatosis and may be the first sign of the disease.[28] Haynes and colleagues reported the ocular findings in 29 patients with Wegener's granulomatosis seen at the National Institutes of Health during a 15-year span and reviewed ocular involvement in cases reported in the English language literature since 1957.[29] Among the overall total of 342 patients, 39 percent had ocular disease. In 286 of the 342 patients the nature of the ocular involvement had been recorded. The most common abnormalities among these 286 patients were proptosis (18 percent); conjunctivitis, scleritis, episcleritis, or corneoscleral ulcer (16 percent); vasculitis of retina or optic nerve (8 percent); dacryocystitis (inflammation of the tear sac; 3 percent); and uveitis (2 percent).

I have seen several patients in whom ring ulcers of the corneal periphery were the initial sign of Wegener's granulomatosis.[28] The woman whose eye is shown in Figure 35–15, Plate II, p. xxxvi; had been treated initially for conjunctivitis. When I first examined her, 3 weeks after the onset of her ocular symptoms, she had a deep ring ulcer in the superotemporal periphery of her cornea. She also gave a history of recent weight loss and had several areas of cutaneous ulceration over her lower legs. Examination of her urine disclosed the presence of albuminuria and erythrocyte casts. Pulmonary cavities were demonstrated on roentgenography. The corneal lesion progressed and she soon developed a necrotizing scleritis of the type seen in rheumatoid arthritis. Death occurred from a cerebral hemorrhage 14 months after the onset of her symptoms. On pathological examination of the affected eye a granulomatous reaction to collagen fibers was found in the corneal ring ulcer and in the broad area of necrotizing scleritis (Fig. 35–16). There was no evidence of vasculitis in serial sections of the entire eye.

Although topical and systemic corticosteroids often are helpful in controlling some of the ocular lesions that occur in Wegener's granulomatosis, cyclophosphamide (Cytoxan) is regarded currently as the drug of choice in treating this disorder.[29]

## RELAPSING POLYCHONDRITIS

Relapsing polychondritis is a rare disorder characterized by inflammation and destruction of cartilage. The condition has some features of rheumatoid arthritis, Wegener's granulomatosis, and midline lethal granuloma. The cause and pathogenesis are unknown.

Although the human eye does not contain cartilage, ocular involvement in relapsing polychondritis is common, occurring in about 65 percent of cases. Hyaline cartilage, such as articular cartilage, contains exclusively type II collagen. Fibrocartilages are composed of type II as well as type I collagen. With regard to the eye, corneal collagen is type I. Type II collagen is found in the retina and the vitreous body, but neither of these two tissues is an ocular site of predilection for involvement in relapsing polychrondritis. The most common ocular abnormalities associated with this disorder are episcleritis, iritis, and conjunctivitis.[23,30]

## ENTEROPATHIC ARTHROPATHY

The disorders of main interest in this group are ulcerative colitis, Crohn's disease, and Whipple's disease.

The reported incidence of arthritis complicating *ulcerative colitis* and *Crohn's disease* is generally in the range of 10 percent, although Greenstein and associates reported involvement in 53 of 202 patients (26 percent) with ulcerative colitis and in 111 of 498 patients with Crohn's disease (22 percent).[31] The most common rheumatic pattern is an asymmetric polyarthritis involving a few joints. The reported incidence of spondylitis, which is indistinguishable from ankylosing spondylitis, in patients with ulcerative colitis and Crohn's disease varies from 2 to 6 percent. In contrast to Crohn's disease, the

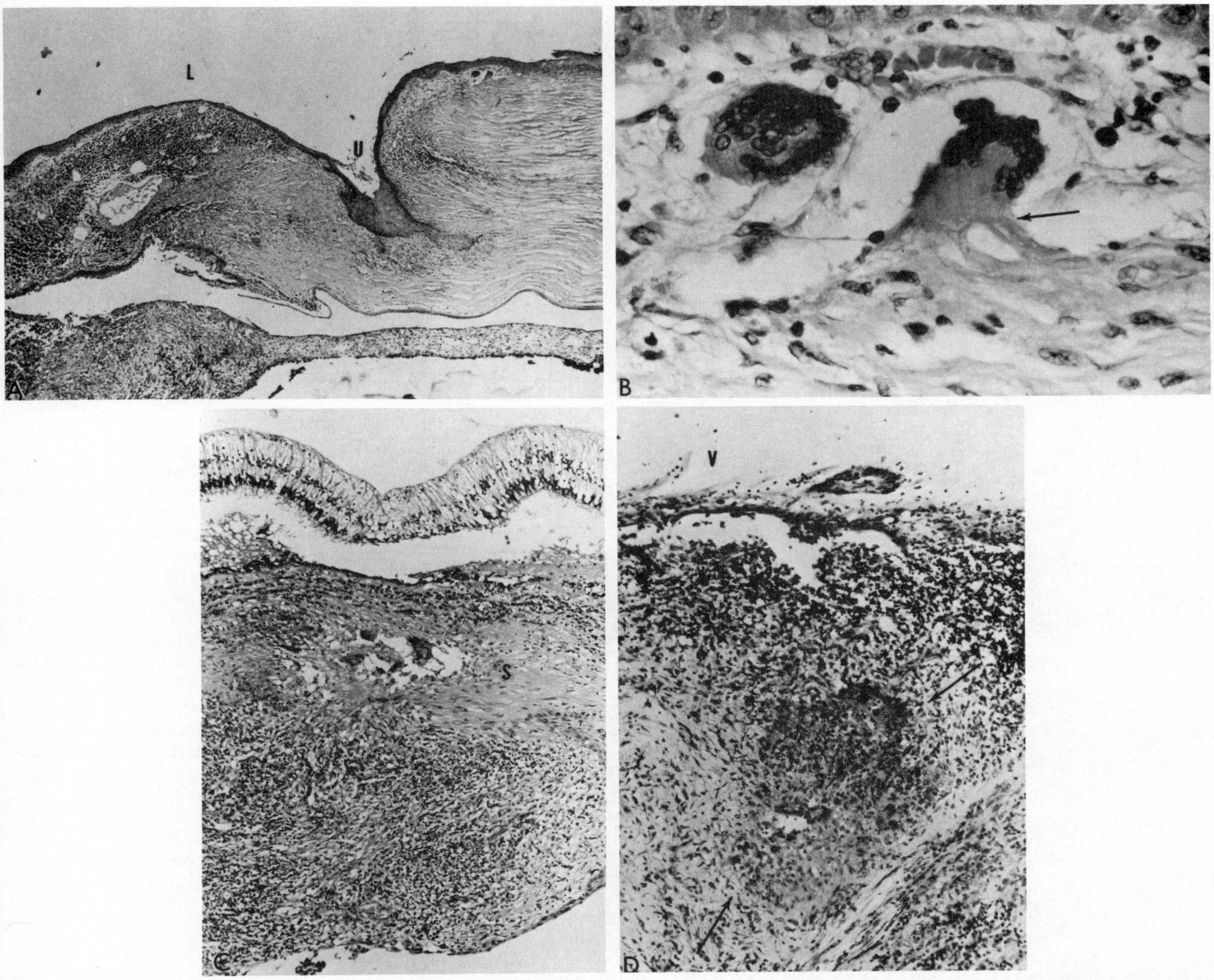


**Figure 35–16.** Wegener's granulomatosis. (From the same patient whose eye is shown in Fig. 35–15.) *A,* In this plane of section the corneal ring ulcer (U) has become re-epithelialized. Epithelioid cells and giant cells attack the interrupted corneal collagen fibers. The limbal tissues (*L*) and the anterior portion of the sclera (left hand side of field) are severely necrotic. Hematoxylin and eosin; magnification × 30. *B,* Higher magnification of superficial portion of corneal ulcer shown in *A.* Two large giant cells are present. One of them is apposed to the interrupted collagen fibers (arrow) in the wall of the ulcer. Corneal collagen is type 1. Hematoxylin and eosin; magnification × 480. *C,* Most of the sclera (*S*) has been destroyed. Giant cells (the most prominent ones are located near the center of the field) attack the remaining scleral collagen fibers. The undulating structure traversing the upper portion of the field is the retina. Hematoxylin and eosin; magnification × 75. *D,* Epithelioid cells and giant cells form a granulomatous lesion (arrows) in ciliary body. *V* = Vitreous body. Hematoxylin and eosin; magnification × 95.

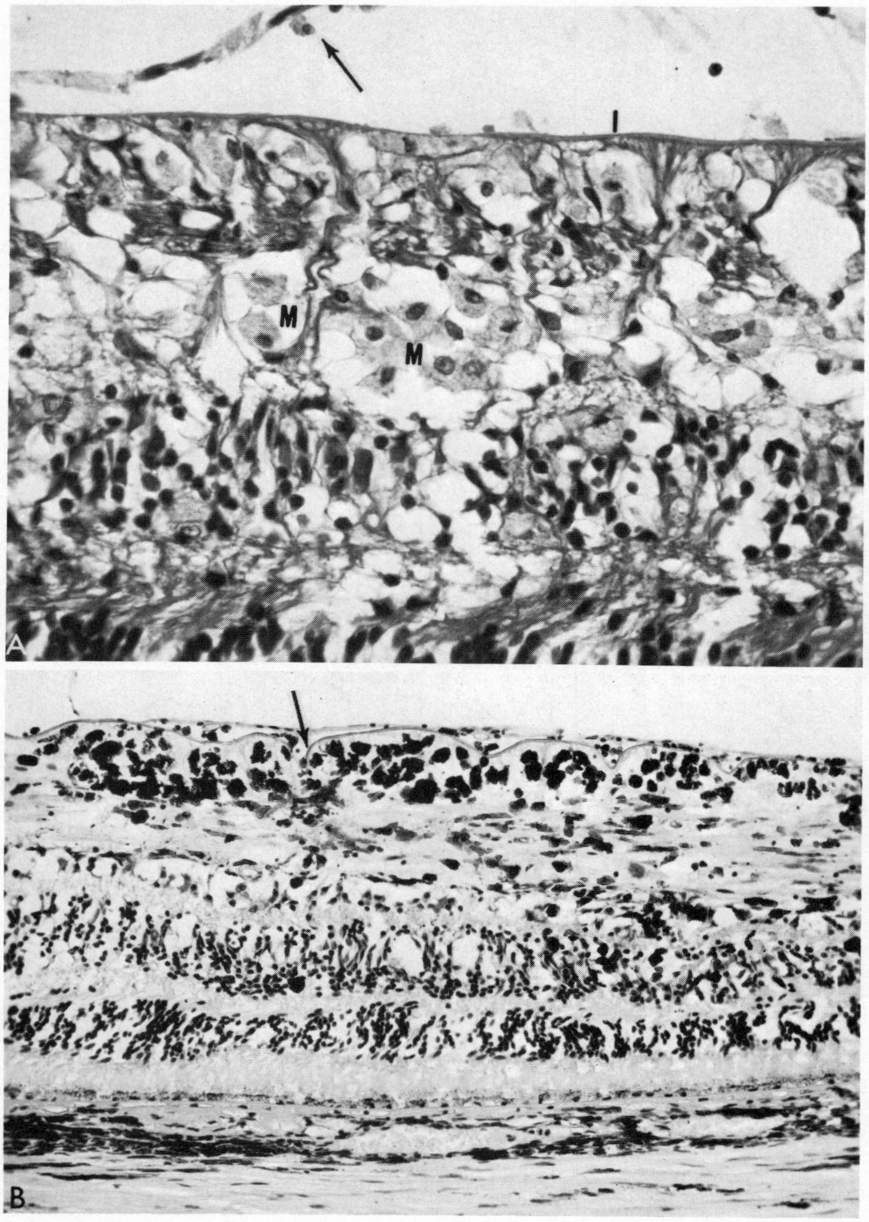


**Figure 35–17.** Whipple's disease. The patient was a 52-year-old man with vitreous body opacities thought to be on the basis of a uveitis. He had a 25-year history of intermittent polyarthritis and was regarded as having rheumatoid arthritis. The presence of Whipple's disease was diagnosed only on postmortem examination. *A*, The inner retinal layers are infiltrated by macrophages (*M*) with pale-blue cytoplasm and eccentric or paracentral small nuclei. Several macrophages (arrow) have migrated across the internal limiting membrane (*I*) into the vitreous body. Hematoxylin and eosin; magnification × 400. Armed Forces Institute of Pathology Negative Number 77-7146. (Courtesy of Ramon L. Font, M.D.) *B*, The retinal nerve fiber layer contains myriads of macrophages with intensely PAS-positive cytoplasm. Many macrophages have traversed the wrinkled internal limiting membrane (arrow) and are interposed between it and a fine preretinal membrane. The choroid and the inner layers of the sclera are present at the bottom of the field. (Compare with Fig. 35-3*B*.) PAS-hematoxylin; magnification × 170. Armed Forces Institute of Pathology Negative Number 77-7147. (Courtesy of Ramon L. Font, M.D.)

extraintestinal manifestations of ulcerative colitis (involvement of joints, eyes, and skin) seldom precede the intestinal symptoms.

There is an increased incidence of uveitis, particularly iritis, in patients with ulcerative colitis. Episcleritis and (rarely) marginal ring ulceration of the cornea are other types of ocular abnormalities that occur in these individuals. Patients with ulcerative colitis and spondylitis are much more likely to have iritis than are those without such joint involvement.[23] For example, Wright and colleagues found that 12 percent of 144 patients with ulcerative colitis had iritis and 17 percent had spondylitis.[32] There was a close association of uveitis with sacroiliac involvement. Of their 25 patients with spondylitis and ulcerative colitis, 13 (52 percent) had uveitis. But among the patients with colitis who did not have spondylitis, only 3 percent had uveitis.

Ocular involvement was found in 41 of 820 patients with Crohn's disease (5 percent).[31,33] (But because not all of the 820 individuals had undergone ophthalmologic examination, the prevalence of ocular involvement was undoubtedly higher than the reported 5 percent.) The most common ocular disorders were conjunctivitis, episcleritis, uveitis (especially iridocyclitis), and peripheral corneal ulceration.[31,33] Ocular lesions were much more common in those patients whose disease affected the colon than in those whose disease was in the small intestine.[31] (Similarly, joint involvement was also much more prevalent in patients whose Crohn's disease occurred in the colon than in those whose disease was limited to the small bowel.[31]) And there was a striking association of ocular involvement with joint involvement: Those patients with Crohn's disease who had joint lesions were far more likely to also have ocular lesions than were those patients with Crohn's disease whose joints were unaffected.[33]

In patients with *Whipple's disease* there is heavy infiltration of the intestinal wall and lymphatics by macrophages filled with glycoprotein. Steatorrhea and diarrhea are frequent signs. Nondeforming migratory arthritis is common and is often the initial complaint. Fever occurs in about one third of patients with Whipple's disease. Many of these individuals have been regarded erroneously as having rheumatoid arthritis.

Opacities in the vitreous body are the most common ocular abnormality in patients with Whipple's disease. They consist of macrophages that have migrated from the inner layers of the retina into the vitreous body. Thus, the basic abnormality is a retinitis (Fig. 35–17). The strong PAS-positivity of the macrophages' cytoplasm is attributed to the high content of polysaccharides present in bacterial wall remnants that are located within the cytoplasmic granules.[34] Electron microscopic examination of these macrophages in the retina and vitreous body has displayed intracytoplasmic, degenerating, rod-shaped bacteria and membranous structures identical with those seen in the intestine, brain, heart, and other tissues of patients with Whipple's disease.[34]

## SARCOIDOSIS

The eyes and ocular adnexa are involved in many patients with sarcoidosis. The precise incidence varies widely in different studies and depends upon several factors. Involvement of the eyes in about 25 percent of patients with sarcoidosis is a widely accepted approximation. Considerable suffering and visual loss often occur.

*Uveitis* is the most common type of ocular involvement.[35] It is granulomatous in nature, is usually bilateral, and characteristically affects the anterior uvea (iris and ciliary body) more often and more severely than it does the posterior uvea (choroid). The severe inflammation leads to cataract formation and, by adhesion of the iris to the corneal periphery (anterior synechia formation) or by adhesion of the iris to the lens (posterior synechia formation), may result in chronic secondary glaucoma (Fig. 35–18). Much less often inflammation of the posterior portion of the uveal tract (choroid) predominates. A relatively common event is the development of *retinal perivasculitis.* The inflammatory cells aggregated about the retinal vessels account for the ophthalmoscopic picture known as "candle wax drippings." *Optic neuritis* and central nervous system sarcoidosis occur more often in patients with retinal perivasculitis than in those who do not have retinal lesions. Corticosteroids, topically and systemically, and topical atropine are the mainstays in treating sarcoid uveitis.

Involvement of the *outer coats* of the eye occurs much less often than do uveitis and retinitis. Major scleral

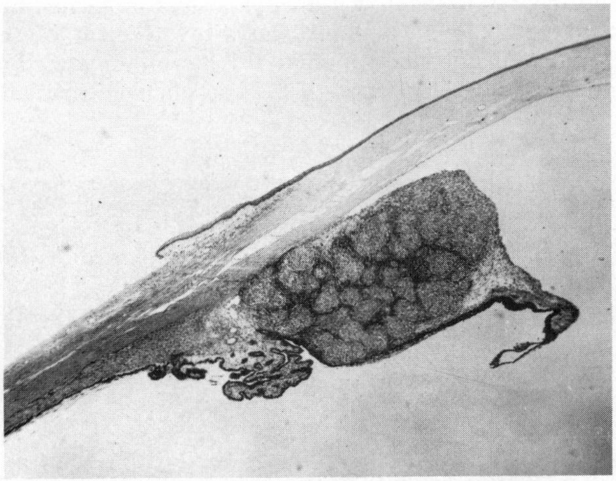

**Figure 35–18.** Iridocyclitis in sarcoidosis. The peripheral and midzones of the iris are massively infiltrated by discrete, noncaseating epithelioid cell tubercles. The pupillary zone of the iris is uninvolved and, in this plane of section, only the most anterior aspect of the ciliary body participates in the inflammatory reaction. Peripheral anterior synechia formation (adhesion of the iris to the anterior chamber angle structures and to the corneal periphery) has caused obstruction of the major outflow channels of the aqueous humor, resulting in intractable secondary glaucoma. Hematoxylin and eosin; magnification × 20. (Courtesy of Lorenz E. Zimmerman, M.D.)

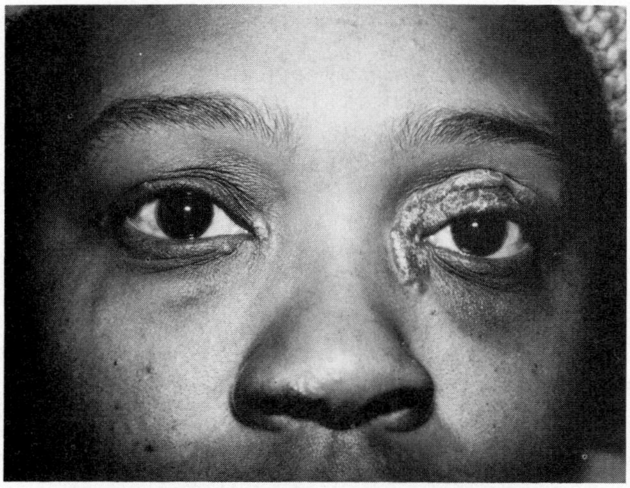

**Figure 35–19.** Sarcoidosis of eyelids. The inflammatory infiltrate has caused plaque-like thickening of the skin of the left upper lid and the left inner canthus. Smaller lesions are present in the right lower lid, the right inner canthus, and near the tip of the nose.

lesions are great rarities. But particularly in patients with erythema nodosum small granulomatous lesions may develop in the episclera or in the outer scleral layers. In patients with hypercalcemia calcium deposition in Bowman's layer may cause band keratopathy.

Involvement of the *ocular adnexa* is common. The eyelids often are affected (Fig. 35–19). The lacrimal glands and fornical conjunctiva also are involved frequently. Although sarcoidosis of the main and accessory lacrimal glands may lead to diminished tear formation and thereby to keratoconjunctivitis sicca in a small minority of patients, in most cases involvement of the lacrimal gland and conjunctiva is asymptomatic. But simple clinical inspection of the conjunctiva, especially the conjunctiva in the inferior fornix, and the lacrimal gland often will reveal abnormalities in the form of conjunctival nodules and lacrimal gland enlargement (Fig. 35–20).

The lacrimal gland and conjunctiva are located superficially and are readily available for *biopsy.* In an unpublished series of patients at The Mount Sinai Hospital in New York with "proved" systemic sarcoidosis, biopsy of the lacrimal gland exhibited noncaseating epithelioid cell tubercles in 25 percent of patients in whom the lacrimal glands were of normal size, and in 75 percent of those in whom the lacrimal glands were enlarged. At the University of Pennsylvania, biopsy of conjunctiva that appeared normal clinically was performed in 146 patients who were being evaluated for sarcoidosis. In 55 patients the diagnosis of systemic sarcoidosis was established by transbronchial biopsy, mediastinoscopy with biopsy, liver biopsy, or biopsy of another nonocular site. Thirty of these 55 patients (55 percent) with sarcoidosis documented by biopsy of a nonocular site also had positive conjunctival biopsies.[36]

Biopsy of the conjunctiva or lacrimal gland has many advantages over such invasive procedures as biopsy of a scalene lymph node, mediastinoscopy, or the recently introduced transbronchial biopsy of the lung. These latter procedures require hospitalization and, in the case of mediastinoscopy, subjection of the patient to general anesthesia. Because the cutaneous tuberculin test is positive in 20 to 40 percent of patients with sarcoidosis, the significance and specificity of granulomas found in mediastinal and scalene lymph nodes are open to question and require the most careful professional judgment. (But tuberculosis of the conjunctiva is rare—so rare that I have never seen a case. Thus, upon detecting a conjunctival granuloma with the histologic features of sarcoidosis the ophthalmic pathologist, unlike the general surgical pathologist examining a mediastinal or scalene

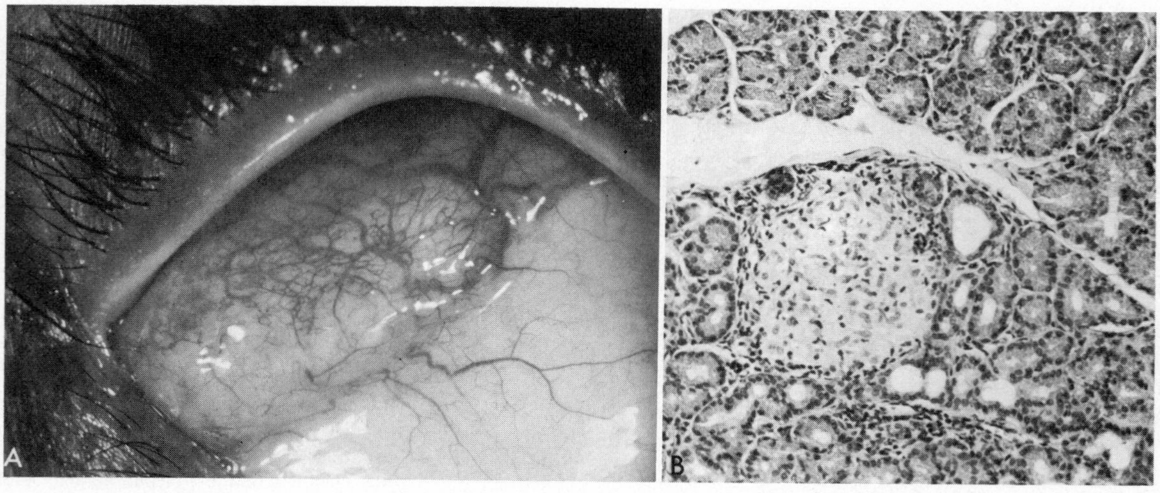


**Figure 35–20.** Sarcoidosis of lacrimal gland. *A,* The right upper lid is partially everted for photographic purposes, and the patient is directing her gaze inferonasally. The palpebral lobe of the lacrimal gland is moderately to markedly enlarged. *B,* Biopsy of the lacrimal gland revealed many discrete, noncaseating epithelioid cell tubercles of the type seen near the center of the field. Hematoxylin and eosin; magnification × 150.

lymph node, seldom is concerned about the possibility that the lesion might really be of tuberculous origin.)

The yield of positive biopsies is higher with the invasive procedures noted above, wherein positive results are obtained in 70 to 90 percent of cases, than it is in biopsies of the conjunctiva or lacrimal gland. But the yield of positive results in patients with proved sarcoidosis whose conjunctiva and lacrimal glands appear normal on clinical examination ranges from 25 to 55 percent.[36] And the yield is even higher in patients with obvious conjunctival nodules or with frank lacrimal gland enlargement. Biopsy of the conjunctiva or lacrimal gland is accomplished in a matter of a few minutes on an outpatient basis, using a local anesthetic. Conjunctival biopsy is well known to be a safe procedure, and none of the 115 patients who have undergone lacrimal gland biopsy on my service have developed any complication. Thus, when attempting to establish histologic confirmation in a patient suspected of having sarcoidosis, it seems prudent to offer her biopsy of the lacrimal gland or conjunctiva. Should these simple procedures prove negative (the results will be available within a day or two), the patient can then be subjected to the more formidable invasive procedures involving thoracic surgery.

Although the Kveim-Siltzbach test is a satisfactory and noninvasive way of establishing a tissue diagnosis, it entails a number of disadvantages: (1) the antigen is not widely available; (2) the clinician must wait a month to 6 weeks before obtaining the result; (3) biopsy of the skin is required eventually; and (4) the test is often negative in the later stages of sarcoidosis.

Thus, instead of merely referring the patient with suspected sarcoidosis to the ophthalmologist for ocular examination, I believe the internist should suggest that biopsy of the lacrimal gland and/or conjunctiva be done if a histologic diagnosis has not been established already.

Detection of altered levels of serum angiotensin converting enzyme (ACE) may also be helpful in establishing the diagnosis of sarcoidosis. In a series of patients with sarcoid uveitis studied at the Medical College of Virginia, both serum lysozyme and serum ACE were elevated in 90 percent. We have also been studying tear enzymes in patients with sarcoid uveitis. Dr. Robert S. Weinberg found a remarkably high correlation between levels of ACE in the serum and in the tears of patients with sarcoid uveitis. In the normal population, tear lysozyme levels usually are very high, but this does not appear to be the case with tear ACE levels. Thus, based on these preliminary observations, it appears that studying tear ACE levels in patients suspected of having sarcoid uveitis may be of great help in establishing the diagnosis.

## AMYLOIDOSIS

*Secondary systemic amyloidosis* (pattern II type, perireticulin type) is a well-known complication of chronic inflammatory diseases, including rheumatoid arthritis and other connective tissue disorders. In secondary amyloidosis small, clinically unimportant deposits of ocular amyloid have been described only rarely, and ophthalmic signs attributable to the presence of amyloid are virtually unknown.[37]

But in *primary systemic amyloidosis* (pattern I type, pericollagenous type) ocular involvement occurs often.[37,38] Amyloid depositions in the collagenous sheaths of the retinal vessels are visible ophthalmoscopically as "vascular sheathing." From this pericollagenous location the amyloid passes into the vitreous body, resulting in opacities of a peculiar type that often reduce vision severely (Fig. 35–21, Plate II, p. xxxvi). Involvement of the uvea, particularly the choroid, is common but usually causes no clinical symptoms. Amyloid deposition in the trabecular meshwork drainage apparatus of the anterior chamber is often a cause of intractable open angle glaucoma. Lattice dystrophy of the cornea results from amyloid deposition in the corneal stroma. (The amyloid is arranged in a network configuration; hence the descriptive clinical term "lattice dystrophy.")

In primary systemic amyloidosis conjunctival involvement is very rare, but the skin of the eyelids is a site of predilection, the palpebral skin being affected more often in this disease than is any other cutaneous site in the body. Amyloid deposition in the soft tissues of the orbit may cause proptosis, and involvement of the orbital nerves produces a variety of abnormalities such as ophthalmoplegia and pupillary disturbances.[37]

## GOUT

In the latter part of the nineteenth century and the first part of the twentieth century gout was accorded a major role in the causation of a broad variety of ocular disease. "Gouty iritis" was a frequently used term, and as many as 3.5 percent of all cases of iritis were attributed to gout. Today gout is seldom listed in tabulations of the causes of uveitis. Although gout is now less common than in the days when overindulgence in food and drink was the necessary attribute of a gentleman, it is obvious that the term "gouty iritis" was in many cases merely a convenient label assigned on most unconvincing evidence to many cases of ocular inflammation. Features of gouty iritis were as follows: (1) the onset was abrupt, and the iritis was preceded by inflammation of the outer coats of the eye (conjunctiva, episclera, and sclera); (2) the eye was intensely congested and very painful; (3) the attack preceded or accompanied an attack of acute gouty arthritis; (4) the attack was of short duration—a matter of only several days; and (5) relatively complete resolution, with few postinflammatory sequelae, was the rule.

A variety of other ocular abnormalities were also attributed to gout: (1) "the gouty hot eye" of Jonathan Hutchinson, wherein the eyes appeared chronically red and irritated, this persistent state being subject to periodic exacerbations; (2) gouty episcleritis and scleritis; and (3) tophi in the eyelids.

In the 1960s, when allopurinol was being evaluated

for its potential in treating patients with gout, I had the opportunity to perform complete eye examinations on 70 patients being cared for by Drs. Alexander Gutman and Tsai-Fan Yü. Most of these patients had severe gouty arthritis and had been selected for inclusion in this study because their disease was not controllable with conventional medications. Not one of these patients with severe gouty arthritis had uveitis, a history of uveitis, or residual evidence of past uveitis on ocular examination. But almost all of them exhibited congestion of the conjunctival and episcleral vessels, and in nearly half of the patients redness of the eyes was a source of cosmetic concern. There were no other noteworthy ocular findings in these 70 patients with severe gouty arthritis.

## Acknowledgment

Supported in part by a grant from the National Society Southern Dames of America.

## References

1. Smith, J.L.: Ocular complications of rheumatic fever and rheumatoid arthritis. Am. J. Ophthalmol. 43:575, 1957.
2. Duke-Elder, S., and Soley, R.E.: Summary of Systemic Ophthalmology. Vol. XV *in* System of Ophthalmology (Duke-Elder, S., ed.). St. Louis, C. V. Mosby Company, 1976, p. 139.
3. Ibid., p. 15.
4. Duke-Elder, S., and MacFaul, P.A.: The Ocular Adnexa. Vol. XIII *in* System of Ophthalmology (Duke-Elder, S., ed.). St. Louis, C. V. Mosby Company, 1974, pp. 625–635.
5. Watson, P.G., and Hayreh, S.S.: Scleritis and episcleritis. Br. J. Ophthalmol. 60:163, 1976.
6. McGavin, D.D., Williamson, J., Forrester, J.V., Foulds, W.S., Buchanan, W.W., Dick, W.C., Lee, P., Macsween, R.N., and Whaley, K.: Episcleritis and scleritis. A study of their clinical manifestations and association with rheumatoid arthritis. Br. J. Ophthalmol. 60:192, 1976.
7. Duke-Elder, S., and Leigh, A.G.: Diseases of the Outer Eye. Vol. VIII *in* System of Ophthalmology (Duke-Elder, S., ed.). St. Louis, C. V. Mosby Company, 1965, pp. 1003–1049.
8. Garrison, F.H.: An Introduction to the History of Medicine. 4th ed. Philadelphia, W. B. Saunders Company, 1929, p. 385.
9. Ferry, A.P.: The histopathology of rheumatoid episcleral nodules. An extra-articular manifestation of rheumatoid arthritis. Arch. Ophthalmol. 82:77, 1969.
10. Chylack, L.T., Bienfang, D.C., Bellows, A.R., and Stillman, J.S.: Ocular manifestations of juvenile rheumatoid arthritis. Am. J. Ophthalmol. 79:1026, 1975.
11. Kanski, J.J.: Anterior uveitis in juvenile rheumatoid arthritis. Arch. Ophthalmol. 95:1794–1797, 1977.
12. Duke-Elder, S., and Perkins, E.S.: Diseases of the Uveal Tract. Vol. IX *in* System of Ophthalmology (Duke-Elder, S., ed.). St. Louis, C. V. Mosby Company, 1966, pp. 533–553.
13. Christian, C.L.: Ankylosing spondylitis. *In* Wyngaarden, J.B., Smith, L.H. (eds.): Cecil Textbook of Medicine. 16th ed. Philadelphia, W. B. Saunders Company, 1982, pp. 878–1879.
14. Duke-Elder, S., and Perkins, E.S.: Diseases of the Uveal Tract. Vol. IX *in* System of Ophthalmology (Duke-Elder, S., ed.). St. Louis, C. V. Mosby Company, 1966, pp. 542–544.
15. Duke-Elder, S., and MacFaul, P.A.: The Ocular Adnexa. Vol. XIII *in* System of Ophthalmology (Duke-Elder, S., ed.). St. Louis, C. V. Mosby Company, 1974, pp. 321–327.
16. Lessell, S.: The neuro-ophthalmology of systemic lupus erythematosus. Doc. Ophthalmol. 47:13, 1979.
17. Gold, D.H., Morris, D.A., and Henkind, P.: Ocular findings in systemic lupus erythematosus. Br. J. Ophthalmol. 56:800, 1972.
18. Ferry, A.P.: Retinal cotton wool spots and cytoid bodies. Mt. Sinai J. Med. 39:604, 1972.
19. Duke-Elder, S., and Leigh, A.G.: Diseases of the Outer Eye. Vol. VIII *in* System of Ophthalmology (Duke-Elder, S., ed.). St. Louis, C. V. Mosby Company, 1965, pp. 1098–1100.
20. Duke-Elder, S., and Soley, R.E.: Summary of Systemic Ophthalmology. Vol. XV *in* System of Ophthalmology (Duke-Elder, S., ed.). St. Louis, C. V. Mosby Company, 1976, p. 145.
21. Ibid., p. 129.
22. Ibid, p. 43.
23. Henkind, P., and Gold, D.H.: Ocular manifestations of rheumatic disorders. Rheumatology 4:13, 1973.
24. Spiera, H., and Davison, S.: Long-term follow-up of polymyalgia rheumatica. Mt. Sinai J. Med. 45:225, 1978.
25. Duke-Elder, S., and Scott, G.I.: Neuro-Ophthalmology. Vol. XII *in* System of Ophthalmology (Duke-Elder, S., ed.). St. Louis, C. V. Mosby Company, 1971, pp. 116–122.
26. Bengtsson, B.-A., and Malmvall, B.-E.: The epidemiology of giant cell arteritis, including temporal arteritis and polymyalgia rheumatica. Incidences of different clinical presentations and eye complications. Arthritis Rheum. 24:899, 1981.
27. Wegener, F.: About the so-called Wegener's granulomatosis with special reference to the generalized vascular lesions. Morgagni 1:5, 1968.
28. Ferry, A.P., and Leopold, I.H.: Marginal (ring) corneal ulcer as presenting manifestation of Wegener's granuloma. A clinicopathologic study. Trans. Am. Acad. Ophthalmol. Otolaryngol. 74:1276, 1970.
29. Haynes, B.F., Fishman, M.L., Fauci, A.S., and Wolff, S.M.: The ocular manifestations of Wegener's granulomatosis. Fifteen years (*sic*) experience and review of the literature. Am. J. Med. 63:131, 1977.
30. Anderson, W.B.: Ocular lesions in relapsing polychondritis and other rheumatoid syndromes. Am. J. Ophthalmol. 64:35, 1967.
31. Greenstein, A.J., Janowitz, H.D., and Sachar, D.B.: The extra-intestinal complications of Crohn's disease and ulcerative colitis: A study of 700 patients. Medicine 55:401, 1976.
32. Wright, R., Lumsden, K., Luntz, M.H., Sevel, D., and Truelove, S.C.: Abnormalities of the sacro-iliac joints and uveitis in ulcerative colitis. Quart. J. Med. 34:229, 1965.
33. Hopkins, D.J., Horan, E., Burton, I.L., Clamp, S.E., de Dombal, F.T., and Goligher, J.C.: Ocular disorders in a series of 332 patients with Crohn's disease. Br. J. Ophthalmol. 58:732, 1974.
34. Font, R.L., Rao, N.A., Issarescu, S., and McEntee, W.J.: Ocular involvement in Whipple's disease. Light and electron microscopic observations. Arch. Ophthalmol. 96:1431, 1978.
35. Duke-Elder, S., and Soley, R.E.: Summary of Systemic Ophthalmology. Vol. XV *in* System of Ophthalmology (Duke-Elder, S., ed.). St. Louis, C. V. Mosby Company, 1976, p. 143.
36. Nichols, C.W., Eagle, R.C., Yanoff, M., and Menocal, N.G.: Conjunctival biopsy as an aid in the evaluation of the patient with suspected sarcoidosis. Ophthalmology 87:287, 1980.
37. Ferry, A.P., and Lieberman, T.W.: Bilateral amyloidosis of the vitreous body. Arch. Ophthalmol. 94:982, 1976.
38. Duke-Elder, S., and Soley, R.E.: Summary of Systemic Ophthalmology. Vol. XV *in* System of Ophthalmology (Duke-Elder, S., ed.). St. Louis, C. V. Mosby Company, 1976, p. 9.

# Chapter 36
# Cutaneous Manifestations of Rheumatic Disorders

*Nicholas A. Soter*

## INTRODUCTION

Dermatologic lesions may indicate associated disorders of organ systems other than the skin. The presence of skin lesions is especially noteworthy in patients with rheumatic diseases. Thus, the integument should be assessed with the same precision that is devoted to an examination of the joints and musculoskeletal system. In addition, it is important to ascertain whether topical medicaments have been applied to the skin inasmuch as these therapeutic agents can modify the gross and histopathologic features of the dermatologic lesions.

## INTERPRETATION OF ALTERATIONS IN THE SKIN

**Visual Examination of the Skin.** Skin lesions may be the presenting complaint of the patient, may occur in association with other symptoms and signs, such as fever or arthralgia, or may be incidental findings observed during the routine physical examination. When examining the skin, one should consider the specific type of lesion and its configuration or shape as well as distribution. Eruptions may be localized or generalized. When the eruption occurs in bilateral and symmetrical distribution, the pathologic stimulus is usually endogenous or is hematogenously disseminated.

**Aids in Examination of the Skin.** Certain signs are recognized more easily by magnification of the skin lesions. Sidelighting of the skin lesions, which is preferably done in a darkened room, is often required to detect slight degrees of elevation or depression. The technique known as diascopy is performed by firmly pressing a piece of glass, such as a microscope slide, over a skin lesion; in the examination of erythematous lesions, blanching reflects capillary dilatation and lack of blanching reflects extravasated blood. Diascopy thus permits the differentiation of purpura from the erythema of vasodilatation. Diascopy performed on dermal papules may show a yellow-brown appearance that is characteristic of granulomas, which occur in such disorders as sarcoid of the skin.

Wood's lamp, which emits long-wave ultraviolet light (360 nm), is useful in the assessment of variations in skin pigmentation. When hyperpigmentation occurs in the epidermis, the pigmented areas show an increased intensity under Wood's lamp, which is not seen when the pigmentation occurs in the dermis. Areas of depigmentation appear more prominent when the melanocyte has been destroyed; in contrast, the hypopigmentation of impaired melanogenesis with intact melanocytes is not enhanced with Wood's lamp examination.

All lesions consisting of crusts and purulent exudates should be examined with Gram's stain and bacterial cultures.

The application of 10 percent potassium hydroxide to a portion of scale, which is then gently heated and examined with a light microscope, is used to search for fungi.

The microscopic examination of cells obtained from the base of vesicles, known as the Tzanck test, may allow the detection of isolated epithelial cells that occur in the pemphigus group of disorders or the giant cells with multiple nuclei that are present in herpes simplex or varicella-zoster viruses. Material obtained from the base of a vesicle is applied to a glass slide and stained with Giemsa's or Wright's reagent for examination.

Microscopic examination of skin lesions is particularly useful, since biopsy specimens are easily obtained for diagnosis by the use of a skin trephine or punch. A tubular blade is rotated between the thumb and index finger to cut through the entire thickness of the abnormal skin; the resulting cylinder of skin is secured with forceps and is cut at its base with a scissors. This simple operation is performed after local anesthesia, preferably with a solution without epinephrine which could theoretically alter blood vessels. Specimens from nodular lesions are best obtained by incision with a scalpel.

**Classification of Skin Lesions.** A macule is a circumscribed area of alteration in normal skin color without elevation or depression of its surface relative to the surrounding skin. Macules may be of any size and are the result of pigmentary or vascular abnormalities of the skin.

A papule is a solid lesion, most of which is elevated above, rather than deep within, the plane of the surrounding skin. The elevation may be caused by localized hyperplasia of cellular elements in the dermis or epidermis, by metabolic deposits in the dermis, or by dermal edema.

A nodule is a solid, round, or ellipsoidal lesion usually located in the dermis or subcutaneous tissue; however, it may occur in the epidermis. The depth of involvement rather than the diameter primarily differentiates a nodule from a papule. Nodules result from infiltrates, neoplasms, or metabolic deposits in the dermis or subcutaneous tissue and often indicate systemic disease.

A plaque is an elevation above the skin surface that occupies a relatively large surface area in comparison with its height above the skin. Frequently, it is formed by the confluence of papules.

A wheal is an edematous, flat-topped, erythematous elevation of the skin that is evanescent. Wheals reflect edema in the superficial layer of the dermis; when the edema occurs in the deep dermis or subcutaneous tissue, the term angioedema is used.

Vesicles and bullae are circumscribed elevated lesions containing fluid. They arise either from separation within the epidermis (intraepidermal vesiculation) or from separation at the dermoepidermal junction (subepidermal vesiculation).

A pustule is a circumscribed elevation of the skin that contains a neutrophilic polymorphonuclear cell infiltrate that may be white, yellow, or greenish yellow. These lesions may be sterile, as in psoriasis, or may reflect a purulent exudate. All pustules should be examined with Gram's stain and culture.

Erosions are superficial lesions in which there is destruction of the epidermis; when there is extension into the dermis, the lesion becomes an ulcer.

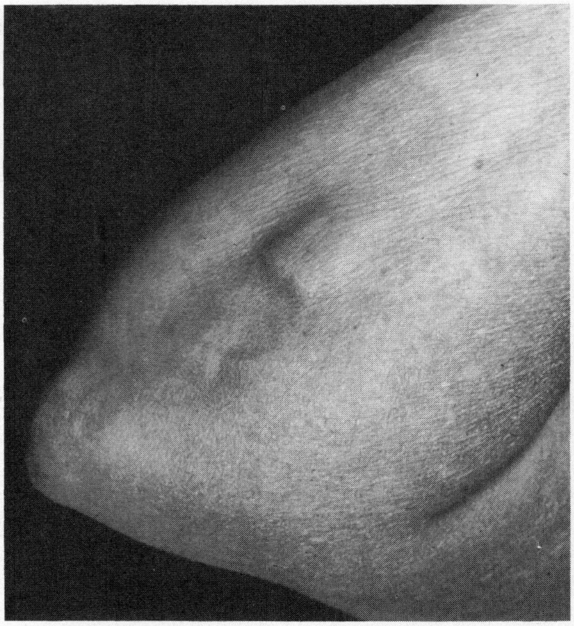

**Figure 36–1.** Rheumatoid nodule. Subcutaneous nodule over the ulnar aspect of the forearm in a patient with rheumatoid arthritis.

## CUTANEOUS MANIFESTATIONS OF CERTAIN RHEUMATOLOGIC DISORDERS

**Rheumatoid Arthritis.** A variety of skin alterations occur in patients with rheumatoid arthritis; the most frequently recognized lesion is the rheumatoid nodule (Fig. 36–1).[1,2] These lesions occur over areas subjected to trauma or pressure, especially the ulnar aspect of the forearm and the lumbosacral area. They vary in size up to several centimeters in diameter, are firm in consistency, and may ulcerate after trauma. These subcutaneous nodules occur in approximately 20 percent of patients with rheumatoid arthritis, especially in those individuals with severe forms of the disease and rheumatoid factor.

The skin is often pale, translucent, and atrophic, especially over the hands, fingers, and toes. The presence of swelling of the proximal interphalangeal joints in addition to the atrophic skin may mimic the appearance of sclerodactyly. Palmar erythema is a frequent feature; however, its presence does not imply underlying liver disease. A few patients manifest telangiectases of the nail folds. Raynaud's phenomenon may occur, as well as a bluish coloration over the distal portions of the toes. Although longitudinal ridges with beading of the nail plate are claimed to be present more frequently in patients with rheumatoid arthritis,[3] the fact that this change also occurs in a high proportion of normal people casts doubt on this association.[4] Pyoderma gangrenosum occasionally may occur in individuals with severe rheumatoid arthritis.[5]

Vasculitis in patients with rheumatoid arthritis appears as a variety of syndromes; the clinical and pathologic features reflect involvement of vessels of different sizes.[6] Rheumatoid vasculitis is frequently described as an arteritis that involves the small arteries, such as the vasa nervorum and the digital arteries (Fig. 36–2). The clinical features in these patients with severe rheumatoid arthritis include a peripheral neuropathy, digital gangrene, nailfold infarcts, cutaneous ulcers, and, in some instances, pericarditis as well as coronary or mesenteric arteritis.[7,8] Patients with nodular and erosive disease and high titers of rheumatoid factor are particularly prone to develop arteritis.[9]

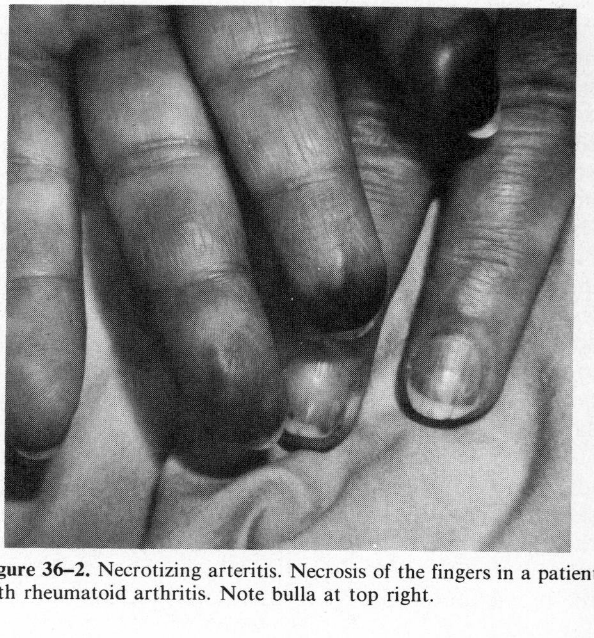

**Figure 36–2.** Necrotizing arteritis. Necrosis of the fingers in a patient with rheumatoid arthritis. Note bulla at top right.

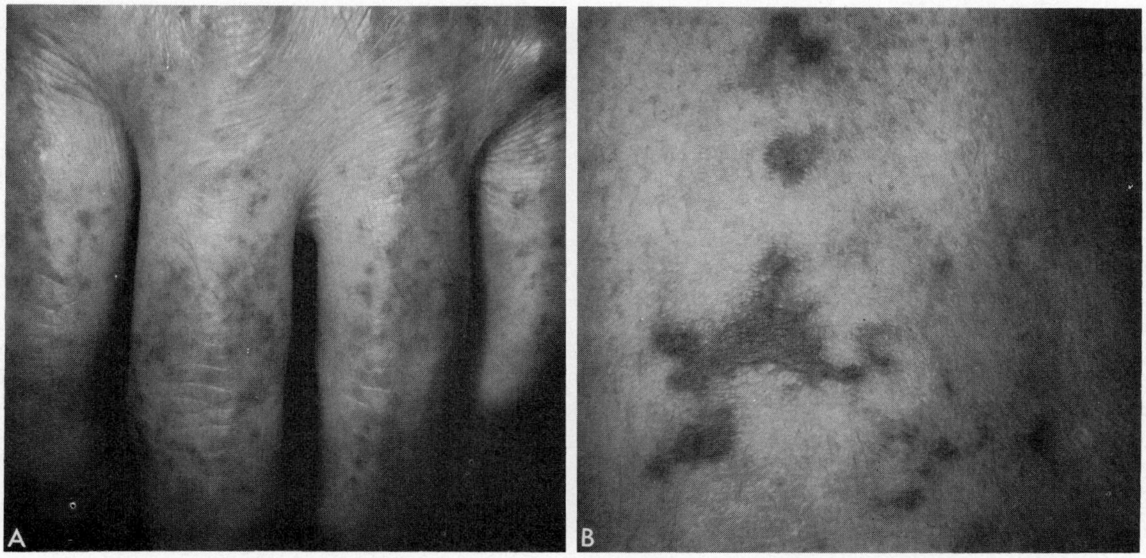


**Figure 36–3.** Necrotizing venulitis. *A*, Palpable purpura over the dorsum of the fingers in a patient with rheumatoid arthritis. *B*, Necrosis in a reticulate array over the thigh.
batch 36 p. 535

Occasional patients experience involvement of medium rather than small arteries. The segmental pathologic lesions in these instances resemble those of polyarteritis nodosa.[10] These individuals manifest a form of arteritis with clinical features similar to those of patients with vasculitis of small arteries.

A common form of necrotizing vasculitis in patients with rheumatoid arthritis involves the venules, especially of the skin. *Cutaneous necrotizing venulitis* is recognized as erythematous papules (palpable purpura), in which the erythema does not blanch when pressed (Fig. 36–3). These vascular lesions may occur over any portion of the body; however, they most often appear on the lower extremities or over dependent areas in recumbent patients. The venular lesions are not related to the duration of the arthritis but rather are associated with severe articular disease, which is generally but not invariably seropositive. The duration and evolution of the venulitis do seem to correlate with the levels of rheumatoid factor and involvement of the complement system.[11] In one study, when the palpable purpura was present less than 1 month, rheumatoid factor levels tended to be low or absent, and the complement system was normal. When the skin lesions were present longer than 1 month, the rheumatoid factor titer was high, and hypocomplementemia was present. Arteritic, arteriolar, and venular lesions may coexist in the same patient.[11]

**Sjögren's Syndrome.** The dermatologic manifestations in patients with Sjögren's syndrome usually reflect glandular dysfunction with desiccation of the skin and mucous membranes and less frequently are a manifestation of involvement of blood vessels. Approximately 50 percent of individuals manifest dry skin (xerosis); however, the ability to sweat is normal as assessed by pilocarpine iontophoresis, and the sweat contains normal amounts of sodium and chloride.[12] The mucous membranes of the eyes, oral cavity (including the tongue), and vagina are usually involved in the sicca complex. A burning sensation of the eyes may occur with erythema, pruritus, a decreased ability to form tears, and the accumulation of inspissated rope-like material at the inner canthus. The lack of tears is confirmed by decreased wetting of a measured distance of filter paper strips placed under the eyelids (Schirmer test); however, this test should be used only for screening patients inasmuch as false-positive tests may be obtained in elderly persons. The oral cavity and tongue may be red and dry with oral erosions and decreased amounts of saliva. Scaling of the lips and fissures at the angles of the mouth may be noted; the teeth readily decay. Desiccation of the vagina is manifested as burning, pruritus, and dyspareunia. Enlargement of parotid glands is frequently noted; Raynaud's phenomenon may occur.

Cutaneous necrotizing venulitis[11] occurs in patients with Sjögren's syndrome[13] with or without underlying cryoglobulinemia. The venular lesions are present predominantly over the lower extremities, appear after exercise, and are associated with hyperpigmentation and cutaneous ulcers. Autoantibodies to small-molecular-weight ribonucleoprotein Ro(SS-A) are noted in individuals with Sjögren's syndrome and systemic or cutaneous necrotizing vasculitis with hematologic and serologic abnormalities.[14] Sjögren's syndrome occurs in association with other disorders such as hypergammaglobulinemic purpura, systemic lupus erythematosus, scleroderma, biliary cirrhosis, and lymphoproliferative disorders;[15] certain dermatologic features may thus reflect the coexistent disorder.

**Spondyloarthropathies.** ***Reiter's Syndrome.*** Reiter's syndrome[16] is recognized as a clinical symptom complex which consists of conjunctivitis, urethritis, arthritis, and skin lesions and usually occurs in men. The conjunctivitis and urethritis tend to be transient in contrast to the arthritis and skin manifestations. Approximately 50 to 80 percent of patients experience mucocutaneous alterations[17] with involvement of the acral regions, especially soles, toes, and fingers. The most characteristic skin lesions, which are rare, begin as vesicles on erythematous bases, become sterile pustules, evolve to manifest keratotic scale, and are known as *keratoderma blennorrhagica* (Fig. 36–4). In addition, keratotic papules and plaques occur on the scalp and elsewhere on the skin. These psoriasiform plaques are reminiscent of psoriasis. Indeed, there have been patients reported with both Reiter's syndrome and psoriasis, yet the skin lesions in these two disorders are often difficult or impossible to distinguish clinically and histologically.[18] This relation between Reiter's syndrome and psoriasis takes on even greater importance, owing to the association of the histocompatibility antigen HLA-B27 with each disorder.[19,20] Sterile pustules develop beneath the nail plate; onychodystrophy frequently is noted.

Conjunctivitis, which occurs in 50 percent of patients,[21,22] is usually bilateral; a sterile purulent exudate frequently is noted. Balanitis occurs in 25 percent of individuals; it appears as papules and plaques with scale over the glans. Mouth erosions have been noted.

***Psoriatic Arthritis.*** Psoriasis occurs in a variety of patterns and may be associated with several forms of arthritis. Classic psoriasis appears as papules and plaques with layers of scales; the individual lesion (Fig. 36–5) is erythematous, covered with layers of silver-white scale, and rather sharply demarcated from adjacent uninvolved skin. Removing the scale results in punctate bleeding that reflects rupture of the superficial blood vessels in the tips of the dermal papillae (Auspitz sign). Individual lesions heal with transient hyperpigmentation or hypopigmentation.

Psoriasis may occur over any portion of the integument, especially the elbows, knees, lumbosacral area,

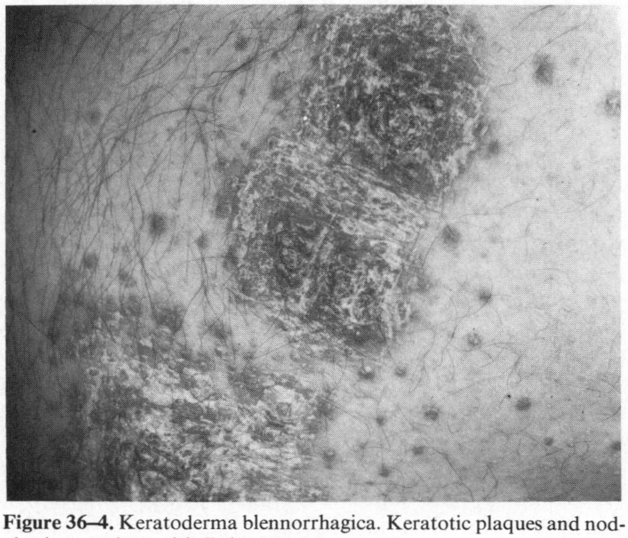

**Figure 36–4.** Keratoderma blennorrhagica. Keratotic plaques and nodules in a patient with Reiter's syndrome.

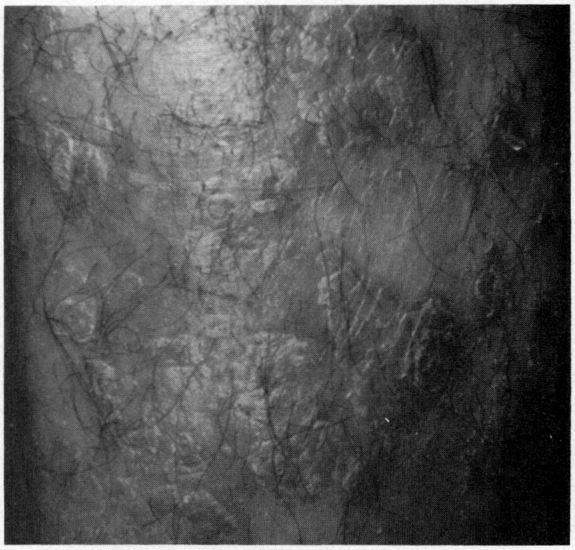

**Figure 36–5.** Psoriasis. Erythematous plaques with layers of scale.

scalp, gluteal cleft, and genitalia. The glans penis is frequently affected; the oral mucosa is infrequently involved, and the tongue is rarely affected.[23] The extent of involvement is quite variable and may range from minimal lesions of the elbows and knees to extensive numbers of lesions scattered over the skin. Uncommonly, there are considerable numbers of small, drop-like plaques designated as guttate psoriasis. Rarely fissures and scale of the distal portions of the fingers may be a predominant manifestation.[24] The skin lesions often appear at sites of trauma (Koebner reaction or isomorphic phenomenon).[25,26] Although the stimulus is usually mechanical, excess exposure to sunlight and the administration of drugs have been implicated.

The nails[27] are frequently affected; the extent of involvement varies in severity and may include one or several nails. The nail plate manifests a translucent quality with a yellow or brown coloration. There may be subungual accumulations of keratotic material, which frequently contains *Candida* species or *Pseudomonas* species; however, dermatophyte infections are rare.[28] The most widely recognized alteration of the nail plate is the presence of discrete pits (Fig. 36–6).

Generalized erythroderma or exfoliative dermatitis has been reported to occur in 20 percent of patients with psoriasis.[29-32] This reaction may develop spontaneously or occur after systemic illness, the administration of medications, or excessive exposure to the sun. Associated abnormalities include abnormal thermoregulation, increased transepidermal water loss, enhanced absorption of topically applied medicaments, loss of protein and iron,[33] and the possibility of high-output cardiac failure in persons with heart disorders.[34]

Pustular types of psoriasis are uncommon and occur in two forms: one is generalized[35,36] and the other is localized to the palms and soles.[37] Patients with generalized pustular psoriasis manifest an extensive sterile

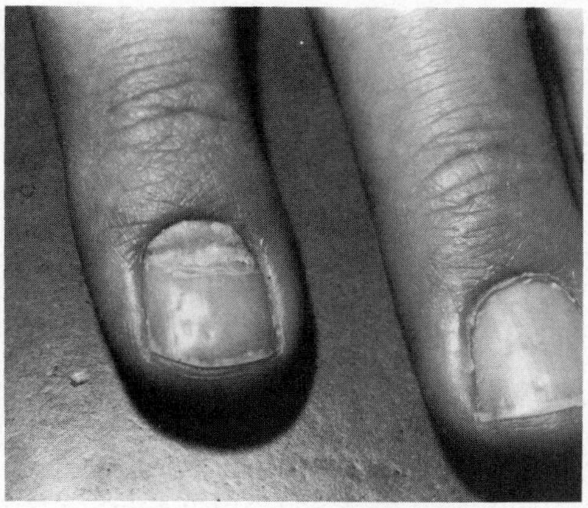

**Figure 36–6.** Psoriasis. Onychodystrophy of the proximal portion of the nail plate with pits.

pustular eruption that may involve the mucous membranes. The onset is sudden with pyrexia and other signs of systemic toxicity, such as myalgia and arthralgia. The skin lesions consist of superficial pustules that may evolve into large purulent areas; existing psoriatic plaques may also contain sterile pustules. The episodes of pustules may continue over intervals of days to weeks. It has been suggested that patients with psoriatic arthritis are more likely to develop generalized pustular psoriasis than are patients without arthritis.[38,39]

Localized pustular psoriasis of the palms and soles is bilateral and recalcitrant without systemic manifestations. Onychodystrophy is common, and the plaques of ordinary psoriasis may be found elsewhere.

There are increased numbers of *Staphylococcus aureus* on lesional skin of patients with psoriasis.[40] Shedding of scale has been suggested as a source of hospital infection.[41]

Psoriasis may occur in association with various forms of inflammatory arthritis[42,43] (see Chapters 58 to 67), which include asymmetric oligoarthritis, symmetric arthritis, spondyloarthritis, and arthritis mutilans. The presence of psoriasis in patients with rheumatoid arthritis is considered to be the coincidental association of two common disorders. Onychodystrophy in patients with symmetric psoriatic arthritis may help to differentiate them from patients with rheumatoid arthritis.

**Lupus Erythematosus.** Lupus erythematosus may occur as a systemic disease or as a disorder, in which the lesions are restricted to the skin. The term *discoid lupus erythematosus*[44,45] has been used to refer to disease restricted to the skin as well as to refer to the gross appearance of the atrophic skin lesions irrespective of whether there is systemic disease. The term *subacute cutaneous lupus erythematosus* defines a mild systemic form with symmetrical, nonscarring skin lesions.[46] When lupus erythematosus is restricted to the skin, available data suggest that fewer than 5 percent of individuals are at risk to develop systemic disease. These data, however, are influenced by definition, vary in studies from different centers, and need re-examination.

The skin is involved at some time during the course of disease in approximately 80 percent of patients with lupus erythematosus.[47] The most widely recognized manifestation is an erythematous eruption (butterfly rash) over the malar areas of the face (Fig. 36–7), which occurs in patients with acute exacerbations of systemic lupus erythematosus. Rarely, bullous skin lesions occur that contain aggregates of neutrophilic leukocytes in the superficial dermis.[48]

The discoid skin lesion in patients with lupus erythematosus is a circumscribed, slightly indurated, red-purple plaque which manifests scaling, follicular plugs, telangiectases, atrophy, and hyperpigmentation or hypopigmentation (Fig. 36–8). The pigmentary alterations are especially prominent in black patients, in whom the cosmetic alteration may be disfiguring. The cutaneous lesions may be single but are usually multiple and occur over any portion of the body, including the scalp. In some individuals there is a predilection for sun-exposed areas. The skin lesions are usually asymptomatic.

Skin lesions in subacute cutaneous lupus erythematosus are symmetrical and affect the neck, extensor surfaces of the arms, and the upper portions of the trunk. The early lesions are edematous and erythematous papules and plaques that evolve into lesions with scales, producing a psoriasiform picture, or into annular polycyclic or figurate configurations.[46,49] These individuals have a mild systemic illness with fever, arthralgia, and malaise and without central nervous system and pro-

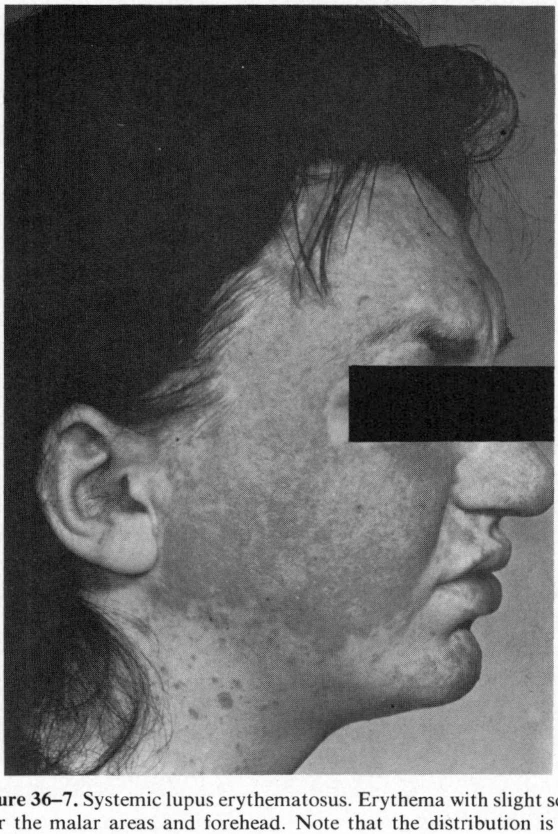

**Figure 36–7.** Systemic lupus erythematosus. Erythema with slight scale over the malar areas and forehead. Note that the distribution is determined by exposure to sunlight.

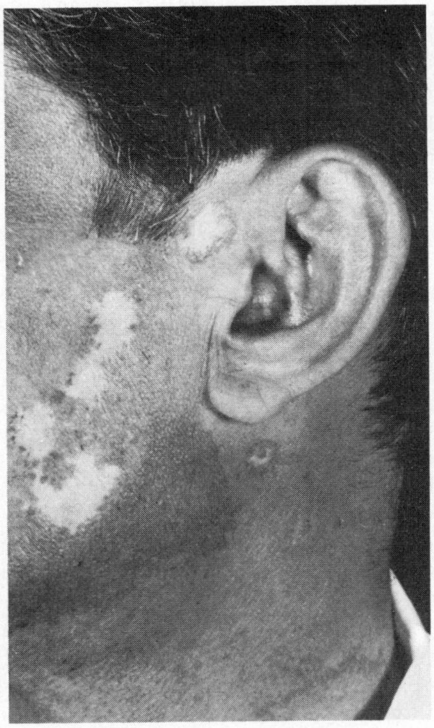

**Figure 36–8.** Cutaneous lupus erythematosus. Circumscribed atrophic patches with hypopigmentation and hyperpigmentation on the face.

gressive renal disease. There is an association with HLA-B8 and DR3 as well as anti-Ro and anti-La antibodies.[50,51]

Alopecia is common in patients with lupus erythematosus; it occurs in both scarring and nonscarring forms. Atrophic patches are present as solitary or multiple areas with the characteristic features of erythema, scale, follicular plugs, and pigmentary alterations. Diffuse hair loss without scarring may occur, especially in individuals with subacute cutaneous lupus erythematosus or with systemic lupus erythematosus.

Although many patients with subacute or systemic lupus erythematosus develop telangiectases over the nail folds, this sign also occurs in patients with rheumatoid arthritis, dermatomyositis, and scleroderma.[52]

A variety of other skin lesions occur in patients with lupus erythematosus. Raynaud's phenomenon is reported to occur in 10 to 30 percent, and episodes of urticaria or angioedema may be a manifestation.[53] The urticarial lesions in some instances have been shown to be a manifestation of underlying necrotizing venulitis.[54] Another manifestation of cutaneous necrotizing venulitis is palpable purpura, which appears to occur during exacerbations of the systemic disease.[11] Involvement of larger arterial blood vessels is present as peripheral gangrene.[55] In addition, flat purpura and petechiae may occur as manifestations of thrombocytopenia or the administration of corticosteroid preparations. Livedo reticularis may be present as a reticulate, erythematous mottling of the skin.

Photosensitivity[56,57] occurs in at least one third of patients with systemic lupus erythematosus and may be associated with flares of both the cutaneous and the systemic manifestations of the disease. The skin lesions have been experimentally induced by exposure to discrete wavelengths of light from an artificial light source.[58]

The oral and lingual lesions are more common in patients with systemic lupus erythematosus and consist of erythematous patches, dilated blood vessels, and erosions, which are frequently painful. Ulcers of the nasal septum may occur.

A rare skin manifestation is panniculitis (lupus profundus),[59] which appears as firm, deep nodules that have a predilection for the face, buttocks, and upper arms. The overlying skin may be erythematous, atrophic, or ulcerated. Healing results in a depressed scar.

Direct immunofluorescence techniques have been applied to the study of the skin of patients with lupus erythematosus as an aid in diagnosis and prognosis.[60-64] This procedure is known as the *lupus band test* (Fig. 36–9). In the skin lesions of both systemic and cutaneous lupus erythematosus, immunoglobulins and complement proteins are deposited in a granular pattern along the dermoepidermal junction in 90 to 95 percent of patients, whereas these immunoreactants are detected in uninvolved non-sun-exposed skin of approximately 50 percent of patients with systemic but not cutaneous lupus erythematosus—an important distinguishing feature. When uninvolved sun-exposed skin is examined, the lupus band test is usually negative in cutaneous lupus erythematosus and is positive in about 80 percent of individuals with systemic lupus erythematosus.[65]

The types of immunoglobulins detected in the deposited materials include mainly IgG and IgM. Complement factors from both the classic activating and amplification pathways are deposited at the same site,[66-68] notably Clq, C4, C3, properdin, and B as well as those

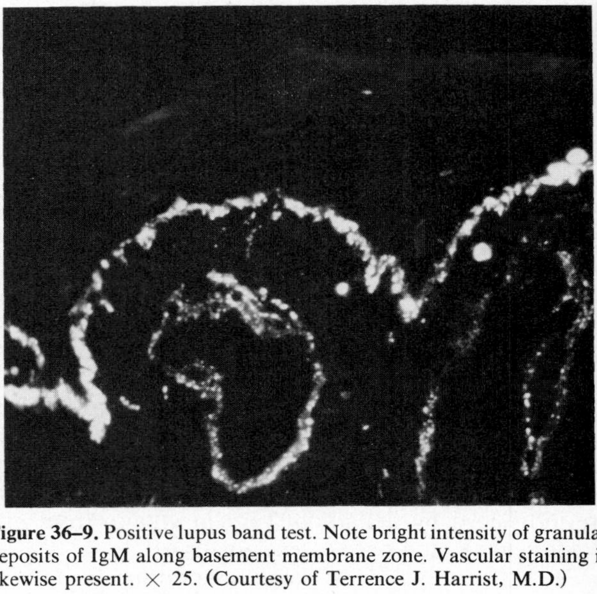

**Figure 36–9.** Positive lupus band test. Note bright intensity of granular deposits of IgM along basement membrane zone. Vascular staining is likewise present. × 25. (Courtesy of Terrence J. Harrist, M.D.)

of the terminal membrane attack complex, C5b, C6-C9.[69]

It has been suggested that the deposition of immunoreactants in uninvolved non-sun-exposed skin of patients with systemic lupus erythematosus can be correlated with renal disease.[70-72] This observation at present remains speculative inasmuch as there are reports unable to confirm it.[73,74] The suggestion has been offered that direct immunofluorescence techniques may have value as an indicator of the efficacy of therapy, especially with immunosuppressive agents;[75] however, long-term data in humans are unavailable.

**Mixed Connective Tissue Disease.** Mixed connective tissue disease is a disorder with clinical features of systemic lupus erythematosus, scleroderma, and/or polymyositis in association with circulating antibody to a saline-soluble nuclear antigen.[76] The dermatologic manifestations include a diffuse nonscarring alopecia, areas of hyperpigmentation and hypopigmentation, sclerodactyly, sclerosis reminiscent of the alterations observed in patients with scleroderma, and a variety of skin changes similar to those observed in patients with lupus erythematosus.[77] Raynaud's phenomenon is frequently present.

**Necrotizing Vasculitides.** *Necrotizing angiitis* or *vasculitis* is a term applied to disorders in which there is segmental inflammation with fibrinoid necrosis of the blood vessels. Clinical syndromes are based on criteria that include the gross and histologic appearance of the vascular lesions, the caliber of the affected blood vessels,[78-80] the frequency of involvement of specific organs, and the absence or presence of hematological and serological abnormalities. Although all sizes of blood vessels may be affected, necrotizing vasculitis of the skin in the majority of instances involves venules.[81-83] Cutaneous necrotizing venulitis may occur in association with coexistent chronic diseases, may be precipitated by infections or drugs, or may develop for unknown reasons.[84]

Although the manifestations of cutaneous necrotizing venulitis are polymorphous, the most characteristic lesion is an erythematous papule, in which the erythema does not blanch when the skin is pressed (*palpable purpura*) (Fig. 36–10; for color of part *B* see Plate III, p. xxxvii),[11,85] Transient areas of urticaria or angioedema are less frequent manifestations;[86-90] rarely, punctate petechiae are noted in the edematous lesions. Nodules, pustules,[91] vesicles, ulcers, necrosis, and a netlike mottling of the skin (livedo reticularis) may occur. Occasionally there is subcutaneous edema in the area of the vascular lesions.

The vascular eruption most often appears on the lower extremities and frequently over dependent portions of the body or areas under local pressure. The lesions may occur anywhere on the skin, but are uncommon on the face, palms, soles, and mucous membranes. The skin lesions occur in episodes that may recur for various periods of time ranging from weeks to years. Palpable purpuric lesions persist from 1 to 4 weeks and then resolve, leaving hyperpigmentation and/or atrophic scars. The urticarial lesions, which may last fewer than

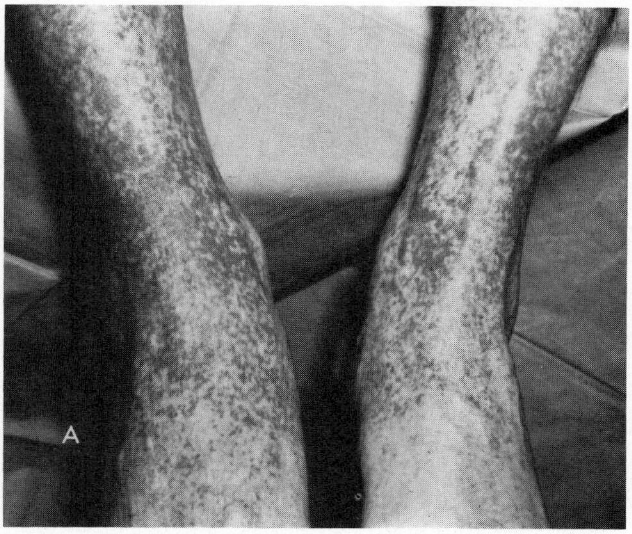


**Figure 36–10.** *A*, Necrotizing venulitis. Palpable purpura distributed over the lower extremities. *B*, Close-up view of the lesions (see Plate III, p. xxxvii).

24 hours and at times up to 72 hours, resolve without residua except for occasional hyperpigmentation. Lesional symptoms include pruritus or burning and, less commonly, pain. Rarely, there are no symptoms. An episode of cutaneous vascular lesions may be attended by pyrexia, malaise, arthralgias, or myalgias. When present, associated systemic involvement of the small blood vessels most commonly occurs in kidneys, muscles, peripheral nerves, gastrointestinal tract, and joints.

Involvement of large blood vessels occurs in periarteritis nodosa, which is recognized in the skin as nodular lesions over an artery,[92-94] and giant cell (temporal) arteritis, which is present as erythema overlying the affected vessel.[95] Both Wegener's granulomatosis[96] and granulomatous angiitis (Churg-Strauss)[97,98] affect large and small vessels; the skin lesions in both disorders are present as erythematous nodules with or without necrosis and a variety of less specific erythematous, edematous, purpuric, papular, and pustular lesions.

Cutaneous necrotizing venulitis has been associated with collagen-vascular diseases, notably rheumatoid arthritis, Sjögren's syndrome, and systemic lupus erythematosus, as previously mentioned.

Hypergammaglobulinemic purpura, defined by the presence of circulating intermediate-sized complexes of immunoglobulin with sedimentation rates between 9S and 17S,[99] occurs predominantly in older women and may be associated with Sjögren's syndrome, systemic lupus erythematosus, and chronic lymphocytic lymphoma.[100] The recurrent purpuric skin lesions are a manifestation of necrotizing venulitis.

Cutaneous necrotizing venulitis also has been reported in association with lymphoproliferative disorders, especially Hodgkin's disease and lymphosarcoma.[101]

Cryoglobulins may occur in patients with cutaneous necrotizing venulitis with and without concomitant collagen-vascular and lymphoproliferative disorders,[11,102] in patients with hepatitis B virus,[103,104] and idiopathically.[105]

Infections and drugs are known to precipitate cutaneous necrotizing venulitis. The most commonly recognized infectious agents are hepatitis B virus[103,104,106] Group A streptococci.[107] *Staphylococcus aureus,*[107] and *Mycobacterium leprae.*[107-109] In hepatitis B virus disease, transient urticaria may be present early in the course and represents immune complex–induced vasculitis.[104] Episodes of palpable purpura may occur in patients with chronic active hepatitis.[110]

The most commonly incriminated medications are sulfonamides, thiazides, penicillin, and serum. Inasmuch as this is an infrequent form of drug-induced reaction, the literature consists of case reports rather than prospective or retrospective studies.

Genetic C2 deficiency has been noted in patients with cutaneous necrotizing venulitis[111,112] that was labeled anaphylactoid purpura.

In perhaps 50 percent of instances the cause of cutaneous necrotizing venulitis remains unknown. The Henoch-Schönlein syndrome or anaphylactoid purpura is the most widely recognized subgroup. A history of upper respiratory tract symptoms and signs is occasionally obtained. The syndrome, which occurs predominantly in children[113] and less frequently in adults,[114] includes involvement of the skin, joints, gastrointestinal tract, and kidneys.

The urticarial form of cutaneous necrotizing venulitis[86-90] (Fig. 36–11, Plate III, p. xxxvii) affects mainly women and is associated with arthralgias that tend to be episodic and are related in time to the appearance of the skin lesions. Abdominal pain, lymphadenopathy, and diffuse glomerulonephritis[86,90,115,116] have also been reported. Additional skin manifestations include occasional macular erythema, angioedema, and foci of purpura. This array of cutaneous lesions may have led to the description of similar patients with hypocomplementemia and Clq precipitins under the terms systemic lupus erythematosus–like syndrome and erythema multiforme.[117-121]

Erythema elevatum diutinum[122,123] consists of erythematous papules, plaques, and nodules predominantly disposed over the buttocks and extensor surfaces and is often accompanied by arthralgias of the associated joint. Other systemic manifestations are lacking.

**Dermatomyositis-Polymyositis.** A variety of cutaneous lesions, which develop insidiously or abruptly, occur in patients with dermatomyositis-polymyositis. Inasmuch as the clinical features and histopathologic alterations in involved muscles are similar in the absence or presence of skin lesions, dermatomyositis and polymyositis are considered as manifestations of a single disease. Dermatomyositis occurs in approximately 25 percent of patients with polymyositis. The most characteristic skin changes are periorbital edema and a purple-red color of the eyelids, which is frequently described as heliotrope.[124] Erythematous macules with scale occur on the face, scalp, neck, and upper portion of the trunk. Especially characteristic are purple-red papules that evolve into atrophic plaques with telangiectases and pigmentary alterations (Fig. 36–12); these lesions, known as Gottron's sign, occur over the dorsal aspects of the interphalangeal joints. Ulcers of the oral mucous membranes may occur;[125] less frequently the conjunctivae and genitalia are affected. Various degrees of alopecia may be present; telangiectases are noted frequently over the nail folds.

Calcification has been noted in both muscle and subcutaneous tissues; this change is more frequent when the disease begins in childhood.[126] Calcification occurs especially over the shoulders, elbows, and buttocks, and is rare over the fingers in contrast to scleroderma.[128] Cutaneous ulcers and sinuses may develop after the extrusion of deposited calcium. Raynaud's phenomenon may be present in adults but is rare in children. Children often manifest facial erythema[127] and involvement of blood vessels of the gastrointestinal tract leading to intestinal perforation.[128]

The skin manifestations[129] in patients with dermatomyositis are at times reminiscent of those occurring in individuals with systemic lupus erythematosus and scleroderma. Occasionally a reticulated erythema known as poikiloderma is noted with telangiectases, atrophy, and pigmentary alterations.

Although the emergence of dermatomyositis in persons past middle age has been associated with the presence of internal malignant disorders, the reported frequency is undoubtedly too high.

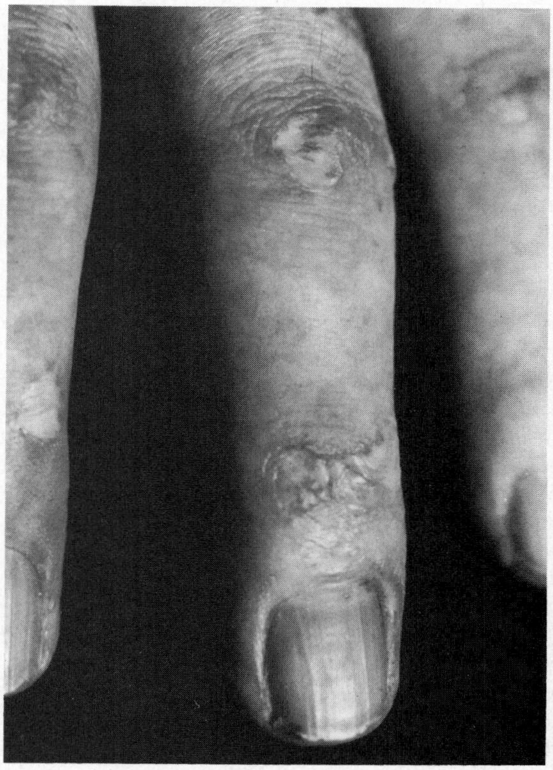

**Figure 36–12.** Dermatomyositis. Atrophic plaques with telangiectases and pigmentary alterations over the interphalangeal joints of the fingers. Note telangiectases of the nail folds.

**Scleroderma.** Scleroderma may occur as a systemic disorder or as various localized forms that primarily affect the skin (see Chapters 76 and 77). The most common type is *morphea,* in which the skin lesions are present as circumscribed areas of atrophy with an ivory color in the center and a violet hue at the periphery. The lesions of morphea commonly persist for years; however, they may disappear spontaneously, healing with or without residual pigmentary alterations. Rarely, morphea may progress to systemic scleroderma.[130,131]

Linear scleroderma appears in a bandlike distribution. The lower extremities are most frequently affected.[132] In addition to the skin, underlying muscles and bones may be involved with deformities. Linear scleroderma begins most frequently during the first two decades of life. It has been associated with abnormalities of the axial skeleton, especially occult spina bifida.[133] Other variants of scleroderma include frontal or frontoparietal involvement of the head known as *coup de sabre,* which is characterized by an atrophic furrow that extends below the plane of the skin, and progressive facial hemiatrophy (Parry-Romberg syndrome).

In systemic scleroderma[134] or progressive systemic sclerosis the cutaneous alterations especially affect the face and hands. Features include a masklike expressionless face with a fixed stare, inability to wrinkle the forehead, tightening of the skin over the nose with a beaklike appearance, and restriction of the mouth with radial folds and a loss of tissue such that the teeth are prominent. An early sign is indolent nonpitting edema over the dorsum of the fingers, hands, and forearms. Sclerodactyly is noted with tapered fingers over which the skin is atrophic; flexion contractures may be present. Raynaud's phenomenon is common; recurrent painful ulcers occur over the fingers and toes (Fig. 36–13). Cutaneous calcification may be present, especially about the fingers, elbows, and knees; when calcification occurs in association with Raynaud's phenomenon, sclerodactyly, and telangiectases, the clinical symptom complex is known as the CRST syndrome. Although this form of scleroderma is alleged to pursue a more benign course,[135] pulmonary hypertension[136] and esophageal abnormalities have been reported.

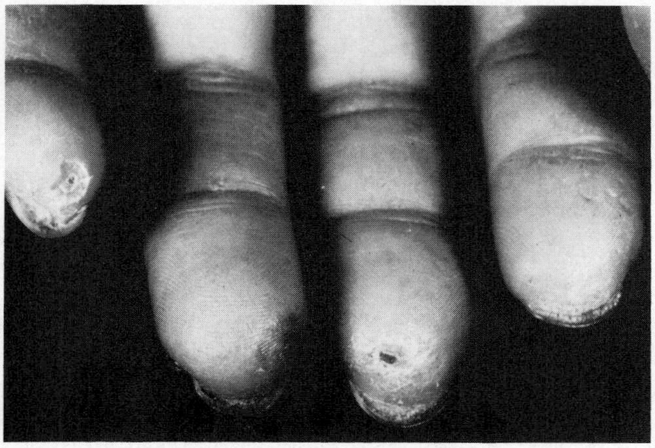

**Figure 36–13.** Scleroderma. Ulcers and scars of the tips of the digits in an individual with Raynaud's phenomenon.

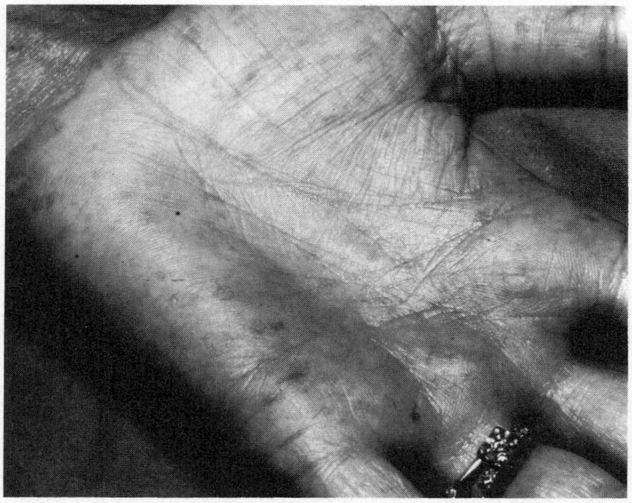

**Figure 36–14.** Scleroderma. Telangiectases and telangiectatic macules over the palms.

Telangiectases occur commonly, especially on the nail folds; telangiectatic macules, which are square, may involve the face, lips, tongue, and hands (Fig. 36–14). Other features may include generalized hyperpigmentation and alopecia.

Disorders with cutaneous sclerosis that should be considered in the differential diagnosis of scleroderma include eosinophilic fasciitis,[137] porphyria cutanea tarda, papular mucinosis (scleromyxedema),[138] lichen sclerosus et atrophicus, melorheostosis,[139,140] and the chronic form of graft-versus-host disease.[141]

**Juvenile Rheumatoid Arthritis.** The cutaneous eruptions that occur in association with juvenile rheumatoid arthritis are not adequately characterized. The most frequently recognized form is an evanescent, erythematous eruption that accompanies the late afternoon temperature rise in 25 to 40 percent of patients.[142,143] The skin lesions appear as small erythematous or salmon-colored macules and papules distributed over the face, trunk, and extremities. They are usually not pruritic and once formed do not move or enlarge. They occur when the disease is active, subside with remission, and heal without residua. Subcutaneous nodules may be noted and must be differentiated from the subcutaneous form of granuloma annulare.[144]

**Rheumatic Fever.** A variety of erythematous eruptions have been noted in patients with rheumatic fever.[145] The most specific eruption is *erythema marginatum.*[146,147] It appears as erythematous rings, usually with raised margins, that rapidly spread peripherally to form polycyclic or geographic outlines, leaving a pale or pigmented center. The essential feature is the rapid spread, which may be 2 to 10 mm in 12 hours.[148] The lesions occur on the trunk and extremities; they are rarely pruritic. The flat or macular form is known as *erythema circinatum.* Both erythema marginatum and circinatum are usually associated with carditis and are unaffected by treatment of the underlying disease. Small, multiple subcutaneous nodules may be noted over the hands, elbows, and occiput.[149]

A rare manifestation is *erythema papulatum,* which appears as indolent papules, especially over the elbows and knees.[150]

**Infiltrative Systemic Diseases.** ***Amyloid.*** Amyloid may be present as a primary cutaneous disease, may occur with genetic disorders, or may be associated in a secondary fashion with chronic inflammatory conditions.[151,152] Skin lesions occur in primary amyloid; secondary amyloid rarely has skin lesions. It is of note, however, that clinically uninvolved skin may contain amyloid deposits in both primary and secondary types, suggesting that a skin biopsy of such uninvolved skin can have a high diagnostic yield.[153]

The skin lesions appear as firm papules that are translucent and occur on the face (especially about the eyes), neck, intertriginous areas, and extremities. They vary in color from rose to yellow to brown; pruritus is absent. A conspicuous feature is hemorrhage; in fact the tendency to develop purpura is the basis for a diagnostic maneuver, in which purpura develops after a blunt instrument is used to traumatize the lesions.[154] Ecchymoses may occur in the absence of papules. Macroglossia is present in 25 to 40 percent of patients and appears with papules of the tongue; it is occasionally accompanied by ulcers and purpura.

Other clinical disorders associated with amyloid include familial Mediterranean fever, in which erythema and lesions resembling those of erysipelas occur; the syndrome of amyloid, urticaria, and deafness,[155,156] in which papules are present over the trunk; the Portuguese form, in which hyperkeratosis and ulcers of the feet occur;[157] and the carpal tunnel syndrome.

***Sarcoid.*** A variety of cutaneous manifestations have been noted in patients with sarcoid.[158] Skin lesions occur in 25 percent of patients, and erythema nodosum occurs in 30 percent.[159-161] The most characteristic lesions ob served in the United States are yellow-brown to violaceous papules and plaques with a predilection for the face, especially the alae nasi and the periocular areas (Fig. 36–15). Similar lesions may be widely distributed over the trunk and extremities. The papules may arise in a scar,[160] a valuable diagnostic sign. Especially in Europe, livid purple plaques have been described on the nose, cheeks, and lobes of the ear; these lesions are known as *lupus pernio.*[158] Other skin manifestations include an ichthyosiform dermatosis over the lower legs, subcutaneous calcification,[162] and areas of hypopigmentation.[163] The relation of the cutaneous lesions with specific internal manifestations and with prognosis is not adequately documented.

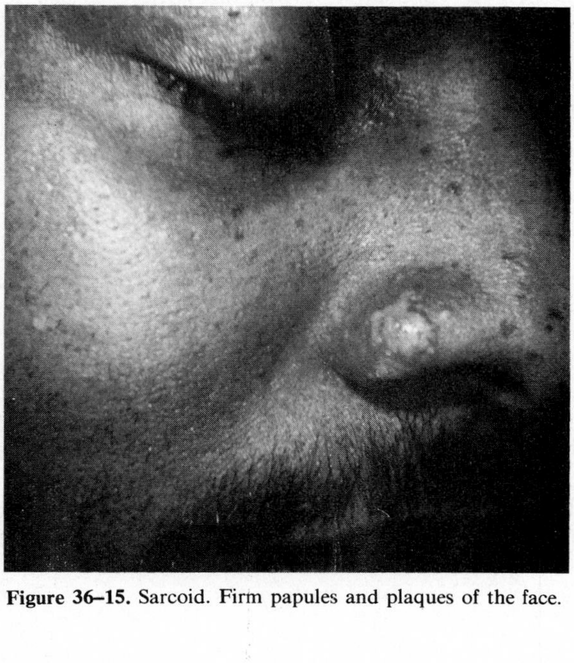

**Figure 36–15.** Sarcoid. Firm papules and plaques of the face.

## References


1. Collins, D.H.: The subcutaneous nodule of rheumatoid arthritis. J. Pathol. Bacteriol. 45:97, 1937.
2. Bennett, G.A., Zeller, J.W., and Bauer, W.: Subcutaneous nodules of rheumatoid arthritis and rheumatic fever: A pathologic study. Arch. Pathol. 30:70, 1940.
3. Hamilton, E.B.D.: Nail studies in rheumatoid arthritis. Ann. Rheum. Dis. 19:167, 1960.
4. Samman, P.D.: The Nails in Disease. London, Heinemann Medical Books, Ltd., 1965, p. 67.
5. Stolman, C.P., Rosenthal, D., Yaworsky, R., and Horan, F.: Pyoderma gangrenosum and rheumatoid arthritis. Arch. Dermatol. 111:1020, 1975.
6. Glass, D.N., Soter, N.A., and Schur, P.H.: Rheumatoid vasculitis. Arthritis Rheum. 19:950, 1976.
7. Sokoloff, L., Wilens, S.L., and Bunim, J.J.: Arteritis of striated muscle in rheumatoid arthritis. Am. J. Pathol. 27:157, 1951.
8. Schmid, F.R., Cooper, N.S., Ziff, M., and McEwen, C.: Arteritis in rheumatoid arthritis. Am. J. Med. 30:56, 1961.
9. Mongan, E.S., Cass, R.M., Jacox, R.F., and Vaughan, J.H.: A study of the relation of seronegative and seropositive rheumatoid arthritis to each other and to necrotizing vasculitis. Am. J. Med. 47:23, 1969.
10. Sokoloff, L., and Bunim, J.J.: Vascular lesions in rheumatoid arthritis. J. Chronic Dis. 5:668, 1957.
11. Soter, N.A., Austen, K.F., and Gigli, I.: The complement system in necrotizing angiitis of the skin. Analysis of complement component activities in serum of patients with concomitant collagen-vascular diseases. J. Invest. Dermatol. 63:219, 1974.
12. Bloch, K.J., Buchanan, W.W., Wohl, M.J., and Bunim, J.J.: Sjögren's syndrome: A clinical, pathological, and serological study of sixty-two cases. Medicine 44:187, 1965.
13. Shearn, M.A.: Sjögren's syndrome. Semin. Arthritis Rheum. 2:165, 1972.
14. Alexander, E.L., Arnett, F.C., Provost, T.T., and Stevens, M.B.: Sjögren's syndrome: association of anti-Ro (SS-A) antibodies with vasculitis, hematologic abnormalities, and serologic hyperreactivity. Ann. Intern. Med. 98:155, 1983.
15. Bloch, K.J., and Bunim, J.J.: Sjögren's syndrome and its relation to connective tissue diseases. J. Chronic Dis. 16:915, 1963.
16. Weinberger, H.W., Ropes, M.W., Kulka, J.P., and Bauer, W.: Reiter's syndrome, clinical and pathologic observations. A long term study of 16 cases. Medicine 41:35, 1962.
17. Montgomery, M.M., Poske, R.M., Barton, E.M., Foxworthy, D.T., and Baker, L.A.: The mucocutaneous lesions of Reiter's syndrome. Ann. Intern. Med. 51:99, 1959.
18. Wright, V., and Reed, W.B.: The link between Reiter's syndrome and psoriatic arthritis. Ann. Rheum. Dis. 23:12, 1964.
19. Brewerton, D.A., Caffrey, M., Nicholls, A., Walters, D., and James, D.C.O.: Acute anterior uveitis and HL-A 27. Lancet 2:994, 1973.
20. Lambert, J.R., Wright, V., Farjah, S.M., and Moll, J.M.H.: Histocompatibility antigens in psoriatic arthritis. Ann. Rheum. Dis. 35:526, 1976.
21. Csonka, G.W.: The course of Reiter's syndrome, Br. Med. J. 1:1088, 1958.
22. Hancock, J.: Surface manifestations of Reiter's disease in the male. Br. J. Vener. Dis. 36:36, 1960.
23. Schuppner, H.J.: Das klinische Bild der Schleimhautbeteiligung bei Psoriasis pustulosa. Arch. Klin. Exp. Dermatol. 209:600, 1960.
24. Baer, R.L., and Witten, V.H.: Psoriasis: A discussion of selected aspects.

*In* Baer, R.L., and Witten, V.H. (eds.): Yearbook of Dermatology, 1961–1962 Series. Chicago, Year Book Medical Publishers, 1962, p. 9.
25. Farber, E.M., Roth, R.J., Aschheim, E., Eddy, D.D., and Epinette, W.W.: Role of trauma in isomorphic response in psoriasis. Arch. Dermatol. 91:246, 1965.
26. Reinertson, R.P.: Vascular trauma and pathogenesis of the Koebner reaction in psoriasis. J. Invest. Dermatol. 30:283, 1958.
27. Zaias, N.: Psoriasis of the nail: A clinical-pathologic study. Arch. Dermatol. 99:567, 1969.
28. White, C.J., and Laipply, T.C.: Histopathology of nail diseases. J. Invest. Dermatol. 19:121, 1952.
29. Montgomery, H.: Exfoliative dermatitis and malignant erythroderma: The value and limitations of histopathologic studies. Arch. Dermatol. Syphilol. 27:253, 1933.
30. Wilson, H.T.H.: Exfoliative dermatitis: Its etiology and prognosis. Arch. Dermatol. Syphilol. 69:577, 1954.
31. Gentele, H., Lodin, A., and Skog, E.: Dermatitis exfoliativa. Acta Dermatol. Venereol. 38:296, 1958.
32. Abrahams, I., McCarthy, J.T., and Sanders, S.L.: 101 cases of exfoliative dermatitis. Arch. Dermatol. 87:96, 1963.
33. Marks, J., and Shuster, S.: Iron metabolism in skin disease. Arch. Dermatol. 98:469, 1968.
34. Fox, R.H., Shuster, S., Williams, R., Marks, J., Goldsmith, R., and Condon, R.E.: Cardiovascular, metabolic, and thermoregulatory disturbances with patients with erythrodermic skin diseases. Br. Med. J. 1:619, 1965.
35. von Zumbusch, L.R.: Psoriasis und pustulöses exanthem. Arch Dermatol. Syphilis 99:335, 1909–1910.
36. Tolman, M.M., and Moschella, S.L.: Pustular psoriasis (von Zumbusch). Arch. Dermatol. 81:400, 1960.
37. Barber, H.W.: Acrodermatitis continua vel perstans (dermatitis repens) and psoriasis pustulosa. Br. J. Dermatol. Syphilol. 42:500, 1930.
38. Ingram, J.T.: Pustular psoriasis. Arch. Dermatol. 77:314, 1958.
39. Champion, R.H.: Generalized pustular psoriasis. Br. J. Dermatol. 71:384, 1959.
40. Marples, R.R., Heaton, C.L., and Kligman, A.M.: *Staphylococcus aureus* in psoriasis. Arch. Dermatol. 107:568, 1973.
41. Payne, R.W.: Severe outbreak of surgical sepsis due to *Staphylococcus aureus* of unusual type and origin. Br. Med. J. 4:17, 1967.
42. Moll, J.M.H., and Wright, V.: Psoriatic arthritis. Semin. Arthritis Rheum. 3:55, 1963.
43. Kammer, G.M., Soter, N.A., Gibson, D.J., and Schur, P.H.: Psoriatic arthritis: a clinical, immunologic and HLA study of 100 patients. Semin. Arthritis Rheum. 9:75, 1979.
44. Rothfield, N.F., March, C.H., Miescher, P., and McEwen, C.: Chronic discoid lupus erythematosus: Study of 65 patients and 65 controls. N. Engl. J. Med. 269:1155, 1963.
45. Beck, J.S., and Rowell, N.R.: Discoid lupus erythematosus: A study of clinical features and biochemical and serological abnormalities in 120 patients with observation on relationship of this disease to systemic lupus erythematosus. Quart. J. Med. 35:119, 1966.
46. Sontheimer, R.D., Thomas, J.R., and Gilliam J.N.: Subacute cutaneous lupus erythematosus—a cutaneous marker for a distinct LE subset. Arch. Dermatol. 115:1409, 1979.
47. Tuffanelli, D.L., and Dubois, E.L.: Cutaneous manifestation of systemic lupus erythematosus. Arch. Dermatol. 90:377, 1964.
48. Hall, R.P., Lawley, T.J., Smith, H.R., and Katz, S.I.: Bullous eruption of systemic lupus erythematosus. Dramatic response to dapsone therapy. Ann. Intern. Med. 97:165, 1982.
49. Gilliam, J.N., and Sontheimer, R.D.: Distinctive cutaneous subsets in the spectrum of lupus erythematosus. J. Am. Acad. Dermatol. 4:471, 1981.
50. Sontheimer, R.D., Stastny, P., and Gilliam, J.N.: HLA associations in subacute cutaneous lupus erythematosus. J. Clin. Invest. 67:312, 1981.
51. Sontheimer, R.D., Stastny, P., Maddison, P., Reichlin, M., and Gilliam, J.N.: Anti-Ro and La antibodies and further HLA associations in subacute cutaneous lupus erythematosus (SCLE). Arthritis Rheum. 23:750, 1980.
52. Ross, J.P.: Nail fold capillaroscopy—a useful aid in the diagnosis of collagen vascular diseases. J. Invest. Dermatol. 47:282, 1966.
53. Harvey, A.M., Shulman, L.E., Tumulty, P.A., Conley, C.L., and Schoenrich, E.H.: Systemic lupus erythematosus: Review of the literature and clinical analysis of 138 cases. Medicine 33:291, 1954.
54. O'Loughlin, S., Schroeter, A.L., and Jordon, R.E.: Chronic urticaria-like lesions in systemic lupus erythematosus: A review of 12 cases. Arch. Dermatol. 114:879, 1978.
55. Dubois, E.L., and Arterberry, J.D.: Gangrene as a manifestation of systemic lupus erythematosus. JAMA 181:366, 1962.
56. Epstein, J.H., Tuffanelli, D.L., and Dubois, E.L.: Light sensitivity and lupus erythematosus. Arch. Dermatol. 91:483, 1965.
57. Baer, R.L. and Harber, L.C.: Photobiology of lupus erythematosus. Arch. Dermatol. 92:124, 1965.
58. Freeman, R.G., Knox, J.M., and Owens, D.W.: Cutaneous lesions of lupus erythematosus induced by monochromatic light. Arch. Dermatol. 100:677, 1969.
59. Tuffanelli, D.L.: Lupus erythematosus panniculitis (profundus): Clinical and immunologic studies. Arch. Dermatol. 103:231, 1971.
60. Burnham, T.K., Neblett, T.R., and Fine, G.: The application of the fluorescent antibody technique to the investigation of lupus erythematosus and various dermatoses. J. Invest. Dermatol. 41:451, 1963.
61. Cormane, R.H.: "Bound" globulin in the skin of patients with chronic discoid lupus erythematosus and systemic lupus erythematosus. Lancet 1:534, 1964.
62. Tan, E.M., and Kunkel, H.G.: An immunofluorescent study of the skin lesions in systemic lupus erythematosus. Arthritis Rheum. 9:37, 1966.
63. Tuffanelli, D.L., Kay, D., and Fukuyama, K.: Dermal-epidermal junction in lupus erythematosus. Arch. Dermatol. 99:652, 1969.
64. Harrist, T.J., and Mihm, M.C. Jr.: The specificity and clinical usefulness of the lupus band test. Arthritis Rheum. 23:479, 1980.
65. Provost, T.T., Andres, G., Maddison, P.J., and Reichlin, M.: Lupus band test in untreated SLE patients. Correlation of immunoglobulin deposition in the skin of the extensor forearm with clinical renal disease and serological abnormalities. J. Invest. Dermatol. 74:407, 1980.
66. Jordon, R.E., Schroeter, A.L., and Winkelmann, R.K.: Dermoepidermal deposition of complement components and properdin in systemic lupus erythematosus. Br. J. Dermatol. 92:263, 1975.
67. Schrager, M.A., and Rothfield, N.F.: Clinical significance of serum properdin levels and properdin deposition in the dermo-epidermal junction in systemic lupus erythematosus. J. Clin. Invest. 57:212, 1976.
68. Provost, T.T., and Tomasi, T.B.: Evidence for complement activation via the alternate pathway in skin diseases. I. Herpes gestationis, systemic lupus erythematosus, and bullous pemphigoid. J. Clin. Invest. 52:1779, 1973.
69. Biesecker, G., Lavin, L., Ziskind, M., and Koffler, D.: Cutaneous localization of the membrane attack complex in discoid and systemic lupus erythematosus. N. Engl. J. Med. 306:264, 1982.
70. Pohle, E.L., and Tuffanelli, D.L.: Study of cutaneous lupus by immunohistochemical methods. Arch. Dermatol. 97:520, 1968.
71. Gilliam, N.J., Cheatum, D.E., Hurd, E.R., Stastny, P., and Ziff, M.: Immunoglobulin in clinically uninvolved skin in systemic lupus erythematosus: Association with renal disease. J. Clin. Invest. 53:1434, 1974.
72. Dantzig, P.I., Mauro, J., Rayhanzadeh, S., and Rudofsky, U.H.: The significance of a positive cutaneous immunofluorescence test in systemic lupus erythematosus. Br. J. Dermatol. 93:531, 1975.
73. Caperton, E.M. Jr., Bean, S.F., and Dick, F.R.: Immunofluorescent skin test in systemic lupus erythematosus: Lack of relationship with renal disease. JAMA 222:935, 1972.
74. Grossman, J., Callerame, M.L., and Condemi, J.J.: Skin immunofluorescence studies on lupus erythematosus and other antinuclear-antibody-positive diseases. Ann. Intern. Med. 80:496, 1974.
75. Gilliam, J.N.: The significance of cutaneous immunoglobulin deposits in lupus erythematosus and NZB/NZW $F_1$ hybrid mice. J. Invest. Dermatol. 65:154, 1975.
76. Sharp, G.C., Irvin, W.S., LaRoque, R.L., Velez, C., Daly, V., Kaiser, A.D., and Holman, H.R.: Association of antibodies to different nuclear antigens with clinical patterns of rheumatic disease and responsiveness to therapy. J. Clin. Invest. 50:350, 1971.
77. Gilliam, J.N., and Prystowsky, S.D.: Mixed connective tissue disease syndrome: Cutaneous manifestations of patients with epidermal nuclear staining and high titer serum antibody to ribonuclease-sensitive extractable nuclear antigen. Arch. Dermatol. 113:583, 1977.
78. Zeek, P.M.: Periarteritis nodosa: A critical review. Am. J. Clin. Pathol. 22:777, 1952.
79. Zeek, P.M.: Periarteritis nodosa and other forms of necrotizing angitis. N. Engl. J. Med. 248:764, 1953.
80. Fauci, A.S., Haynes, B.F., and Katz, P.: The spectrum of vasculitis: Clinical, pathologic, immunologic, and therapeutic considerations. Ann. Intern. Med. 89:660, 1978.
81. Copeman, P.W.M., and Ryan, T.J.: The problem of classification of cutaneous angiitis with reference to histopathology and pathogenesis. Br. J. Dermatol. 82(Suppl. 5):2, 1970.
82. Soter, N.A., Mihm, M.C., Jr., Gigli, I., Dvorak, H.F., and Austen, K.F.: Two distinct cellular patterns in cutaneous necrotizing angiitis. J. Invest. Dermatol. 66:344, 1976.
83. Braverman, I.M., and Yen, A.: Demonstration of immune complexes in spontaneous and histamine-induced lesions and in normal skin of patients with leukocytoclastic angiitis. J. Invest. Dermatol. 64:105, 1975.
84. Soter, N.A., and Austen, K.F.: Cutaneous necrotizing angiitis. *In* Samter, M., et al. (eds.): Immunological Diseases. Boston, Little, Brown & Company, 1978, pp. 993–1001.
85. Braverman, I.M.: The angiitides, *In* Skin Signs of Systemic Disease. Philadelphia, W.B. Saunders Company, 1970, p. 199.
86. McDuffee, F.D., Sams, W.M., Jr., Maldonado, J.E., Andreini, P.H.,

Conn, D.L., and Samayoa, E.A.: Hypocomplementemia with cutaneous vasculitis and arthritis: Possible immune complex syndrome. Mayo Clin. Proc. 48:340, 1973.
87. Soter, N.A., Austen, K.F., and Gigli, I.: Urticaria and arthralgias as manifestations of necrotizing angiitis (vasculitis). J. Invest. Dermatol. 63:485, 1974.
88. Soter, N.A.: Chronic urticaria as a manifestation of necrotizing venulitis. N. Engl. J. Med. 296:1440, 1977.
89. Monroe, E.W.: Urticarial vasculitis: an updated review. J. Am. Acad. Dermatol. 5:88, 1981.
90. Sanchez, N.P., Winkelmann, R.K., Schroeter, A.L., and Dicken, C.H.: The clinical and histopathologic spectrums of urticarial vasculitis: Study of 40 cases. J. Am. Acad. Dermatol. 7:599,. 1982.
91. Diaz, L.A., Provost, T.T., and Tomasi, T.B., Jr.; Pustular necrotizing angiitis. Arch. Dermatol. 108:114, 1973.
92. Borrie, P.: Cutaneous polyarteritis nodosa. Br. J. Dermatol. 87:87, 1972.
93. Diaz-Perez, J.L., and Winkelmann, R.K.: Cutaneous periarteritis nodosa. Arch. Dermatol. 110:407, 1974.
94. Kussmaul, A., and Maier, R.: Über eine bisher nicht beschriebene eigenthumliche Arterienerkrankung (Periarteritis nodosa), die mit Morbus brightii und rapid fortschreitender allgemeiner Muskellahmung einhergeht. Dtsch. Arch. Klin. Med. 1:484, 1866.
95. Hamilton, C.R., Jr., Shelley, W.M., and Tumulty, P.A.: Giant cell arteritis: Including temporal arteritis and polymyalgia rheumatica. Medicine 50:1, 1971.
96. Fauci, A.S., and Wolff, S.M.: Wegener's granulomatosis: Studies in eighteen patients and a review of the literature. Medicine 52:535, 1973.
97. Churg, J., and Strauss, L.: Allergic granulomatosis, allergic angiitis and periarteritis nodosa. Am. J. Pathol. 27:277, 1951.
98. Chumbley, L.C., Harrison, E.G., and DeRemee, R.A.: Allergic granulomatosis and angiitis (Churg-Strauss Syndrome): Report and analysis of 30 cases. Mayo Clin. Proc. 52:447, 1977.
99. Capra, J.D., Winchester, R.J., and Kunkel, H.G.: Hypergammaglobuli nemic purpura: Studies on the unusual anti-$\gamma$-globulins characteristic of the sera of these patients. Medicine 50:125, 1971.
100. Kyle, R.A., Gleich, G.J., Bayrd, E.D., and Vaughan, J.H.: Benign hypergammaglobulinemic purpura of Waldenström. Medicine 50:113, 1971.
101. Sams, W.M., Jr., Harville, D.D., and Winkelmann, R.K.: Necrotising vasculitis associated with lethal reticuloendothelial diseases. Br. J. Dermatol. 80:555, 1968.
102. Brouet, J.-C., Claurel, J.-P., Danon, F., Klein, M., and Seligmann, M.: Biologic and clinical significance of cryoglobulins: A report of 86 cases. Am. J. Med. 57:775, 1974.
103. Levo, Y., Gorevic, P.D., Kassab, H., Zucker-Franklin, D., Gigli, I., and Franklin, E.C.: Mixed cryoglobulinemia—an immune complex disease often associated with hepatitis B virus infection. Trans. Assoc. Am. Physicians 90:167, 1977.
104. Dienstag, J.L., Rhodes, A.R., Bhan, A.K., Dvorak, A.M., Mihm, M.C. Jr., and Wands, J.R.: Urticaria associated with acute viral hepatitis type B. Ann. Intern. Med. 89:34, 1978.
105. Meltzer, M., and Franklin, E.C.: Cryoglobulinemia—a study of twenty-nine patients. I. IgG and IgM cryoglobulins and factors affecting cryoprecipitability. Am. J. Med. 40:828, 1966.
106. Gower, R.G., Sausker, W.F., Kohler, P.F., Thorne, G.E., and McIntosh, R.M.: Small vessel vasculitis caused by hepatitis B virus immune complexes. Small vessel vasculitis and HBsAg. J. Allergy Clin. Immunol. 62:222, 1978.
107. Parish, W.E.: Cutaneous vasculitis: The occurrence of complexes of bacterial antigens with antibody, and of abnormalities associated with chronic inflammation. *In* Beutner, E.H., Chorzelski, T.P., Bean, S.F., and Jordon, R.E.: Immunopathology of the Skin; Labelled Antibody Studies. Chicago, Year Book Medical Publishers, Inc., 1974, p. 153.
108. Moschella, S.L.: The lepra reaction with necrotizing skin lesions: A report of six cases. Arch. Dermatol. 95:565, 1967.
109. Quismorio, F.P., Jr., Rea, T., Chandor, S., Levan, N., and Friou, G.J.: Lucio's phenomenon: An immune complex deposition syndrome in lepromatous leprosy. Clin. Immunol. Immunopathol. 9:184, 1978.
110. Duffy, J., Lidsky, M.D., Sharp, J.T., Davis, J.S., Person, D.A., Hollinger, F.B., and Min, K.-W.: Polyarthritis, polyarteritis, and hepatitis B. Medicine 55:19, 1976.
111. Sussman, M., Jones, J.H., Almeida, J.D., and Lachmann, P.J.: Deficiency of the second component of complement associated with anaphylactoid purpura and presence of mycoplasma in the serum. Clin. Exp. Immunol. 14:531, 1973.
112. Gelfand, E.W., Clarkson, J.E., and Minta, J.O.: Selective deficiency of the second component of complement in a patient with anaphylactoid purpura. Clin. Immunol. Immunopathol. 4:269, 1975.
113. Gairdner, D.: The Schönlein-Henoch syndrome (anaphylactoid purpura). Quart. J. Med. 66:95, 1948.
114. Cream, J.J., Gumpel, J.H., and Peachey, R.D.G.: Schönlein-Henoch purpura in the adult: A study of 77 adults with anaphylactoid or Schönlein-Henoch purpura. Quart. J. Med. 34:461, 1970.
115. Sissons, J.G.P., Williams, D.G., Peters, D.K., Boulton-Jones, J.M., and Goldsmith, H.J.: Skin lesions, angio-oedema, and hypocomplementaemia. Lancet 2:1350, 1974.
116. Feig, P.U., Soter, N.A., Yager, H.M., Caplan, L., and Rosen, S.: Vasculitis with urticaria, hypocomplementemia, and multiple system involvement. JAMA 236:2065, 1976.
117. Agnello, V., Winchester, R.J., and Kunkel, H.G.: Precipitin reactions of the C1q component of complement with aggregated $\gamma$-globulin and immune complexes in gel diffusion. Immunology 19:909, 1970.
118. Agnello, V., Koffler, D., Eisenberg, J.W., Winchester, R.J., and Kunkel, H.G.: C1q precipitins in the sera of patients with systemic lupus erythematosus and other hypocomplementemic states: Characterization of high and low molecular weight types. J. Exp. Med. 134:228s, 1971.
119. Agnello, V., Ruddy, S., Winchester, R.J., Christian, C.L., and Kunkel, H.G.: Hereditary C2 deficiency in systemic lupus erythematosus and acquired complement abnormalities in an unusual SLE-related syndrome. Birth Defects 11:312, 1975.
120. Agnello, V.: Association of systemic lupus erythematosus and SLE-like syndromes with hereditary and acquired complement deficiency states. Arthritis Rheum. 21(Suppl.5):S146, 1978.
121. Marder, F.J., Burch F.X., Schmid, F.R., Zeiss, C.R., and Gewurz, H.: Low molecular weight C1q-precipitins in hypocomplementemic vasculitis-urticaria syndrome: Partial purification and characterization as immunoglobulin. J. Immunol. 121:613, 1978.
122. Mraz, J.P., and Newcomer, V.D.: Erythema elevatum diutinum: Presentation of a case and evaluation of laboratory and immunological status. Arch. Dermatol. 96:235, 1967.
123. Katz, S.I., Gallin, J.I., Hertz, K.C., Fauci, A.S., and Lawley, T.J.: Erythema elevatum diutinum: Skin and systemic manifestations, immunologic studies, and successful treatment with dapsone. Medicine 56:443, 1977.
124. Keil, H.: The manifestations in the skin and mucous membranes in dermatomyositis, with special reference to the differential diagnosis from systemic lupus erythematosus. Ann. Intern. Med. 16:828, 1942.
125. O'Leary, P.A., and Waisman, M.: Dermatomyositis: A study of 40 cases. Arch. Dermatol. Syphilol. 41:1001, 1940.
126. Muller, S.A., Winkelmann, R.K., and Brunsting, L.A.: Calcinosis in dermatomyositis: Observations on course of disease in children and adults. Arch. Dermatol. 79:669, 1959.
127. Everett, M.A., and Curtis, A.D.: Dermatomyositis: A review of nineteen cases in adolescents and children. Arch. Intern. Med. 100:70, 1957.
128. Banker, B.Q., and Victor, M.: Dermatomyositis (systemic angiopathy) of childhood. Medicine 45:261, 1966.
129. Christianson, H.B., Brunsting, L.A., and Perry, H.O.: Dermatomyositis: Unusual features, complications, and treatment. Arch. Dermatol. 74:581, 1956.
130. Curtis, A.C., and Jansen, T.G.: The prognosis of localized scleroderma. Arch. Dermatol. 78:749, 1958.
131. Jabłońska, S., Bubnow, B., and Szczepański, A.: Morphea: Is it a separate entity or a variety of scleroderma? Dermatologica 125:140, 1962.
132. Christianson, H.B., Dorsey, C.S., O'Leary, P.A., and Kierland, R.R.: Localized scleroderma: A clinical study of two hundred thirty-five cases. Arch. Dermatol. 74:629, 1956.
133. Rubin, L.: Linear scleroderma: Association with abnormalities of spine and nervous system. Arch. Dermatol. Syphilol. 58:1, 1948.
134. Tuffanelli, D.L., and Winkelmann, R.K.: Systemic scleroderma: Clinical study of 727 cases. Arch. Dermatol. 84:359, 1961.
135. Carr, R.D., Heisel, E.B., and Stevenson, T.D.: CRST syndrome: Benign variant of scleroderma. Arch. Dermatol. 92:519, 1965.
136. Salerni, R., Rodnan, G.P., Leon, D.F., and Shaver, J.A.: Pulmonary hypertension in the CREST syndrome variant of progressive systemic sclerosis (scleroderma). Ann. Intern. Med. 86:394, 1977.
137. Schumacher, H.R.: A scleroderma-like syndrome with fasciitis, myositis, and eosinophilia. Ann. Intern. Med. 84:49, 1976.
138. Rudner, E.J., Mehregan, A., and Pinkus, H.: Scleromyxedema: A variant of lichen myxedematosus. Arch. Dermatol. 93:3, 1966.
139. Morris, J.M., Samilson, R.L., and Corley, C.L.: Melorheostosis: Review of the literature and report of an interesting case with a nineteen-year follow-up. J. Bone Joint Surg. 45:1191, 1963.
140. Wagers, L.T., Young, A.W., Jr., and Ryan, S.F.: Linear melorheostotic scleroderma. Br. J. Derm. 86:297, 1972.
141. Hood, A.F., Soter, N.A., Rappeport, J., and Gigli I.: Graft-versus-host reaction: cutaneous manifestations following bone marrow transplantation. Arch. Dermatol. 113:1087, 1977.
142. Isdale, I.C., and Bywaters, E.G.L.: The rash of rheumatoid arthritis and Still's disease. Quart. J. Med. 25:377, 1956.
143. Calabro, J.J., and Marchesano, J.M.: Rash associated with juvenile rheumatoid arthritis. J. Pediatr. 72:611, 1968.
144. Taranta, A.: Occurrence of rheumatic-like subcutaneous nodules without

evidence of joint or heart disease: Report of a case. N. Engl. J. Med. 266:13, 1962.
145. Canizares, O.: Cutaneous lesions of rheumatic fever: A clinical study in young adults. Arch. Dermatol. 76:702, 1957.
146. Perry, C.B.: Erythema marginatum (rheumaticum). Arch. Dis. Child. 12:233, 1937.
147. Keil, H.: The rheumatic erythemas: A critical survey. Ann. Intern. Med. 11:2223, 1938.
148. Bywaters, E.G.L.: Skin manifestations of rheumatic diseases. In Fitzpatrick, T.B., et al. (eds.): Dermatology in General Medicine. New York, McGraw-Hill Book Company, 1971, p. 1534.
149. Bywaters, E.G.L., and Thomas, G.T.: Bed rest, salicylates and steroid in rheumatic fever. Br. Med. J. 1:1628, 1961.
150. Bass, M.H.: The cutaneous manifestations of acute rheumatic fever in childhood. Med. Clin. North Am. 2:201, 1918.
151. Goltz, R.W.: Systematized amyloidosis: A review of the skin and mucous membrane lesions and a report of two cases. Medicine 31:381, 1952.
152. Rukavina, J.G., Block, W.D., Jackson, C.E., Falls, H.F., Carey, J.H., and Curtis A.C.: Primary systemic amyloidosis: A review and an experimental, genetic, and clinical study of 29 cases with particular emphasis on the familial form. Medicine 35:239, 1956.
153. Rubinow, A., and Cohen, A.S.: Skin involvement in generalized amyloidosis: A study of clinically involved and uninvolved skin in 50 patients with primary and secondary amyloidosis. Ann. Intern. Med. 88:781, 1978.
154. Hurley, H.J., and Weinberg, R.: Induced intralesional hemorrhage in primary systemic amyloidosis. Arch. Dermatol. 89:678, 1964.
155. Muckle, T.J., and Wells, M.: Urticaria, deafness and amyloidosis: A new heredo-familial syndrome. Quart. J. Med. 31:235, 1962.
Black, J.T.: Amyloidosis, deafness, urticaria, and limb pains: A hereditary syndrome. Ann. Intern. Med. 70:989, 1969.
157. Andrade, C.: A peculiar form of peripheral neuropathy: Familiar atypical generalized amyloidosis with special involvement of peripheral nerves. Brain 75:408, 1952.
158. James, D.G.: Dermatological aspects of sarcoidosis. Quart. J. Med. 28:109, 1959.
159. James, D.G., Thomson, A.D., and Willcox, A.: Erythema nodosum as a manifestation of sarcoidosis. Lancet 2:218, 1956.
160. Löfgren, S.: Erythema nodosum: Studies on etiology and pathogenesis in 185 adult cases. Acta Med. Scand. Suppl. 174, 1946.
161. Wood, B.T., Behlen, C.H., and Weary, P.E.: The association of sarcoidosis, erythema nodosum, and arthritis. Arch. Dermatol. 94:406, 1966.
162. Kroll, J.J., Shapiro, L., Koplon, B.S., and Feldman, F.: Subcutaneous sarcoidosis with calcification. Arch. Dermatol. 106:894, 1972.
163. Cornelius, C.E., Stein, K.M., Hanshaw, W.J., and Spolt, D.A.: Hypopigmentation and sarcoidosis. Arch. Dermatol. 108:249, 1973.

# Section III
# Diagnostic Tests

## Chapter 37
## Aspiration and Injection of Joints and Soft Tissues

*Duncan S. Owen, Jr.*

### INTRODUCTION

Shortly after systemic cortisone and hydrocortisone were first used in the management of rheumatoid arthritis, Dr. George Thorn[1] injected 10 mg of hydrocortisone into the knee joint of a patient with rheumatoid arthritis. The knee improved locally, but the patient also improved generally; it was concluded that the improvement resulted from systemic absorption of the intra-articularly injected material. No further studies of intra-articular corticosteroid injections were carried out until 1951, when Dr. Joseph Hollander and his associates[2] reported a study from their clinic at the University of Pennsylvania. In an early study from the Mayo Clinic[3] short-lived improvement of 2 to 8 days was reported in patients with rheumatoid arthritis or osteoarthritis following intra-articular injections of hydrocortisone. Ten years later a series of over 100,000 injections of joints, bursae, and tendon sheaths in 4000 patients was reported by Hollander and colleagues.[4] They called attention to the usefulness of intra-articular corticosteroids as temporary, palliative, repeatable, local adjunct treatments of a variety of rheumatic conditions[5] and to the more prolonged benefits afforded by preparations less rapidly hydrolyzed than hydrocortisone.

### MECHANISM(S) OF ACTION OF INTRASYNOVIAL CORTICOSTEROIDS

The anti-inflammatory mechanisms of corticosteroids are still not fully understood.[6] Early clinical studies demonstrated a decrease in erythema, swelling, heat, and tenderness to palpation of the inflamed joints.[3] An increase in viscosity and hyaluronate concentration of the synovial fluid was observed.[7] Studies with liver lysosomes indicated stabilization of the lysosomal membrane and prevention of release of lysosomal enzymes, which can induce further inflammation.[8-10] Experiments using phagocytic leukocytes and bacterial systems failed to document stabilization by hydrocortisone of the lysosomes in these cells.[11-13] Measurement of the action of hydrocortisone, dexamethasone, and prednisone on intact lysosomes isolated from human peripheral blood polymorphonuclear leukocytes demonstrated protection of these organelle membranes from either detergent lysis or heat incubation as assessed by the release of the lysosomal marker $\beta$-glucuronidase. Polymorphonuclear leukocyte lysosomes isolated from human volunteers treated with prednisolone were no more stable than those from untreated normals, and the serum from these treated volunteers did not protect intact lysosomes from detergent lysis.[14] The investigators felt the anti-inflammatory activity of corticosteroids was best explained by inhibitory effects on cellular metabolism rather than by their direct interaction with lysosomal membranes.

There is evidence of an anti-inflammatory effect mediated by a peptide hormone that inhibits polymorphonuclear microtubular assembly.[15] Many peptide hormones are believed to act by increasing the action of adenosine monophosphate within target cells, and this mechanism could explain the inhibitory effect of corticosteroids on phagocytic cells.

Corticosteroids are potent inhibitors of prostaglandin synthesis by several types of cells and tissues, including rheumatoid synovial tissue.[16-20] One of the effects is a decreased release of arachidonic acid from phospholipids.[19-21] Since only unesterified fatty acids are used by cyclooxygenase, this decreased release of arachidonic acid depresses all cyclooxygenase-derived products.[22]

Corticosteroids decrease levels of serum immunoglobulins and complement.[23,24] One study of intra-articular corticosteroids demonstrated a transient decrease in synovial fluid complement.[25] In another study, 12 patients received intra-articular methylprednisolone. Six showed no alteration of synovial fluid total hemolytic complement, C4 protein level, or rheumatoid factor titer. The other 6 showed a 50 percent or greater change in only one of the synovial fluid values. Most had reductions in total leukocyte counts, polymorphonuclear leukocyte counts, and acid phosphatase levels.[26]

Dick and co-workers in 1970[27] reported the results of

studies using intra-articular radioactive xenon ($^{133}Xe$). They demonstrated a fall in the rate of disappearance of $^{133}Xe$ after an intra-articular injection of hydrocortisone hemisuccinate. They felt corticosteroids diminish synovial permeability. A 1979 study of patients with rheumatoid arthritis from this same laboratory,[28] using intra-articular $^{133}Xe$ and triamcinolone hexacetonide in one group of patients and $^{133}Xe$ and lidocaine in a second group, revealed no difference in the rate of clearance of $^{133}Xe$ after 40 minutes in the triamcinolone-treated group. Therefore, they felt triamcinolone had no immediate effect on synovial blood vessels. However, the lidocaine-treated group showed a decrease in the rate of $^{133}Xe$ clearance.

In 1982, Eymontt and colleagues[29] reported the effects of intra-articular triamcinolone hexacetonide, prednisolone tebutate, and saline administration on both synovial permeability and synovial fluid leukocyte counts in patients with symptomatic osteoarthritis. In their study, they employed a radioactive blood-pool tracer, $^{99m}Tc$ human serum albumin. Their results indicated that corticosteroids decrease synovial permeability but produce an increase in synovial fluid leukocytes.

## POTENTIAL SEQUELAE (TABLE 37–1)

In the late 1950s, there first appeared a few reports of Charcot-like arthropathy attributed to intra-articular corticosteroid therapy.[30,31] One study by Mankin and Conger, in 1966, reported that intra-articularly administered hydrocortisone acetate reduced the incorporation of glycine-$^3H$ into rabbit articular cartilage to approximately one-third of control values within 6 hours. They interpreted the decrease in utilization to a decrease in matrix protein synthesis caused by hydrocortisone.[32]

In 1969, Bentley and Goodfellow[33] advised strongly against recurrent intra-articular injections because of potential severe arthropathy.

In 1970, Moskowitz and associates showed that intra-articular triamcinolone acetonide produced nuclear degeneration of chondrocytes and prominent cyst formation.[34]

In 1972, Mankin, Zarins, and Jaffe reported that intramuscular cortisone reduced the incorporation of glycine-$^3H$, $^{35}SO_4$, and was associated with a progressive decline in the concentration of hexosamine.[35]

**Table 37–1.** Potential Sequelae from Intra-Articular and Soft Tissue Corticosteroid Injections

| |
|---|
| 1. Radiologic deterioration of joints—"steroid arthropathy"; Charcot-like arthropathy; osteonecrosis |
| 2. Iatrogenic infection—very low incidence |
| 3. Rupture of tendon |
| 4. Tissue atrophy and fat necrosis |
| 5. Nerve damage, e.g., inadvertent injection of median nerve in carpal tunnel syndrome |
| 6. "Postinjection flare" |
| 7. Uterine bleeding |
| 8. Pancreatitis |
| 9. Cushing's syndrome |

In 1975, Behrens and associates found an increased number of fissures in rabbit cartilage after intra-articular injections of hydrocortisone. Hexosamine incorporation decreased, as did synthesis of proteoglycans; collagen production was reduced to one-fifth. They hypothesized that the anti-anabolic effects of the corticosteroids cause a massive decrease in the synthesis of all major matrix components. The loss of proteoglycan content led to a decrease in cartilage stiffness such that the impact of cyclic loading with weight-bearing caused death of cells, cystic degeneration of matrix, and fissuring in the midzonal areas of weight-bearing surfaces.

Completely different data were reported in 1976 by Gibson and associates.[37] They repeatedly injected the knee joints of 10 *Macaca irus* monkeys with either methylprednisolone or a control solution. Minor degenerative changes of femoral condyles were shown by India ink staining and by a system of histochemical grading, but changes in the joints injected with corticosteroids were *not* significantly different from those seen in control joints.

In 1981, Tenenbaum and colleagues[38] reported on a continuing study of the long-term effects of intra-articular dexamethasone TBA on rabbit knee cartilage. There was an acceleration of the calcific degenerative arthropathy that occurs in mature New Zealand rabbits. Under these experimental conditions, the cartilage injury seems limited and did not progress with repeated injections.

In 1969, Sweetnam[39] cautioned against steroid injection of inflamed tendons in athletes because of the possibility of tendon rupture. Wrenn and associates[40] in 1954 demonstrated a 40 per cent reduction in tensile strength of a tendon after the use of corticosteroids. (We have rarely observed a rupture of the long head of the biceps tendon or Achilles tendon following the injection of the tendon sheath for tendinitis.) Other complications include soft-tissue atrophy, especially noted when the small joints such as finger proximal interphalangeal joints are injected. Periarticular calcifications and ecchymoses around the atrophied areas have been reported.[41]

The intra-articular injection of corticosteroids occassionally produces what has been called a "postinjection flare."[42] This increase in local inflammation may develop a few hours after injection and last up to 48 hours. The difficulty of distinguishing this reaction from an iatrogenic infection may be worrisome. The flare is noted more frequently with the needle-shaped corticosteroid crystals and may be a form of crystal-induced arthritis produced by synovial fluid leukocytes phagocytosing the crystals and subsequently releasing lysosomal enzymes.

Systemic absorption of intra-articular corticosteroid, or from other soft tissue injections, occurs in almost all patients. Usually, this is clinically manifested, for example, in a patient with rheumatoid arthritis, by subjective and objective improvement of inflamed joints other than the one(s) injected. There may be other effects, such as eosinopenia, lymphopenia, and, depending upon the corticosteroid injected, changes in serum and urine cortisol levels. There may be suppression of the hypothalamic-pituitary-adrenal axis.[43] Patients with diabetes mellitus may note a severalfold rise in their blood glucose levels.

Prominent erythema, warmth, and diaphoresis of the face and torso may occur within minutes to hours after an intra-articular corticosteroid injection.[44] This reaction is noted mainly with triamcinolone acetonide. Some feel it is an uncommon reaction, but we note it in greater than 10 percent of patients injected with this medication. Some of these patients note headache. In this regard, it resembles the nitratoid reaction occasionally observed with the injection of gold salts, especially gold sodium thiomalate. These corticosteroid reactions may last a few minutes to a few days. However, some patients are so frightened by these reactions they refuse further injections.

Abnormal uterine bleeding may occur from injection of corticosteroids, especially triamcinolone acetonide. The exact mechanisms are unknown, but ovulation may be inhibited.[45,46] Also, corticosteroids may produce uterine bleeding in a postmenopausal patient. This alarms both patient and physician.

Pancreatitis, apparently induced by injectable corticosteroids, is rarely noted.

## PRECAUTIONS

When performing arthrocenteses or soft-tissue injections, strict adherence to aseptic procedures is required. The physician should use the same precautions as for a lumbar spinal puncture. Iatrogenic infections may be disastrous but are rare if these precautions are taken. At the Medical College of Virginia we have observed one, or possibly two, infections in over 35,000 injections.

In theory, arthrocentesis may provide a focus for septic arthritis in a patient with bacteremia, such as staphylococcal endocarditis.[47] It is well known that a patient with damaged joints from, for example, rheumatoid arthritis, is more susceptible to developing spontaneous septic arthritis from blood-borne bacteria. Arthrocentesis in such instances has enabled rapid diagnosis and prevented the patient's joint from being destroyed. "Routine" therapeutic arthrocenteses should be avoided, however, if the patient is being treated for a condition associated with bacteremia.

Because of tissue atrophy with corticosteroids, one should use extreme caution when injecting near peripheral nerves. For example, carpal tunnel syndrome, either idiopathic or induced by rheumatoid arthritis, may be benefited by corticosteroid injection in the carpal tunnel. An injection directly into the median nerve could result in nerve necrosis or atrophy.

Gottlieb reported two cases of hypodermic needle separations during arthrocenteses.[48] It was recommended that the needles be inspected after arthrocentesis to ascertain that they are intact, and he advised keeping a hemostat within easy access to enable the operator to remove a separated needle from the soft tissues.

## EFFICACY OF INJECTIONS

**Intra-articular Injections.** Despite the fact thousands of intra-articular corticosteroid preparations have been injected in thousands of patients, there are few good studies of their efficacy.[49] The length of symptomatic improvement appears related to the particular preparation used. Most patients with rheumatoid arthritis will benefit from an injection, but the effect may last only days. Hydrocortisone acetate may give improvement for a few days to a week or more; and prednisolone tebutate, for two weeks or more. Triamcinolone hexacetonide, which is poorly water soluble and one of the longest-acting agents, has been shown to provide reversal of inflammation in some patients for longer periods.[41] As with oral nonsteroidal anti-inflammatory drugs, responses among different patients are extremely varied. If one or two injections prove ineffective or give only short-lived benefit, there is no logic in persistently injecting the same joint.

Results of injections in osteoarthritic joints conflict. The data range from no benefit to outstanding benefit.[1,50-52] The differences may relate in part to the joint injected. For example, degenerative arthritis of the first carpometacarpal joint is a fairly common and painful condition in which there is little synovial thickening or increase in synovial fluid. The injection of corticosteroid is often painful, probably because of the moderate to marked decrease in joint space, but dramatic symptomatic improvement usually occurs within 12 hours, and may last many months. This contrasts with injection for osteoarthritis of the hip, in which it is very difficult to know if the hip joint space has been entered, even with use of the fluoroscope as a guide. Improvement of hip symptoms within 12 to 24 hours after injection probably indicates the corticosteroid was injected intra-articularly, but benefit often lasts only 2 days to a week. The mechanical problem of bone rubbing against bone in a weight-bearing joint may be the reason for the short-lived benefit, and repeated injections may be expected to be of little value.

Osteoarthritis of the knee may be very painful and may be associated with large volumes of synovial fluid. Even though it is the usual practice to remove as much synovial fluid as possible, the efficacy of this procedure in osteoarthritis is questionable. Usually the corticosteroid injection is associated with dramatic symptomatic relief, which lasts days to weeks or more. If the injections give short-lived benefit, repeated injections are probably contraindicated because the primary problem is in the cartilage, and repeated injections could hasten cartilage deterioration for reasons previously outlined.

A weight-bearing joint probably should be rested as much as possible for 24 to 48 hours after injection. Additionally, some recommend resting all corticosteroid-injected joints for a prolonged period of time.[53] There is no consensus about this, however.

**Non-Articular Injections.** In contrast to intra-articular injections that are used adjunctively, certain soft-tissue inflammatory conditions may be more or less permanently eradicated by judicious injections of corticosteroids with or without local anesthetics.[54-57] The conditions having the longest benefits from injections are those precipitated by trauma, especially when the activity causing the inflammation is avoided. For example, a patient troubled by recurrent lateral epicondylitis who derives short-lived benefit from a corticosteroid injection into the inflamed area may improve more permanently by discontinuing golf or tennis.

Many cases of apparent tendinitis and bursitis may be secondary manifestations of rheumatoid arthritis, in which injections may give an outstanding initial benefit that, unfortunately, is temporary. In such patients appropriate treatment of the underlying disease should be instituted, and the injections must be considered as adjunctive management.

The poorly understood but apparently quite common "fibrositis syndrome"[58,59] is associated with various "trigger points" and is discussed in detail in Chapter 32. These exaggerated tender areas may respond dramatically to the injection of a local anesthetic directly into the most tender area, but the addition of a corticosteroid in the same syringe may give more lasting relief.

## TYPES OF PREPARATIONS

The original intra-articular corticosteroid, hydrocortisone acetate, is still available, is widely used, and is inexpensive. Other preparations of various potency and solubility are now available, and these are listed in Table 37–2. Few comparative studies of the efficacy or duration of action of the various agents have been reported. As previously mentioned, McCarty[41] has noted long-term benefits with triamcinolone hexacetonide, and thinks this is the least soluble and produces the most prolonged effect of the agents commercially available. Such "longer-acting and more potent" suspensions are much more expensive than hydrocortisone. Some investigators are of the opinion that the more potent preparations are also more efficacious,[49] but the evidence for this is not strong.

**Table 37–2.** Corticosteroids and Prednisone Equivalents*

| Intra-articular Preparations (generic name, strength, and trade names) | Prednisone Equivalents |
|---|---|
| Betamethasone sodium phosphate and acetate suspension<br>6 mg/ml (Celestone Soluspan) | 10 |
| Dexamethasone sodium phosphate<br>4 mg/ml (Decadron and Hexadrol) | 8 |
| Dexamethasone acetate<br>8 mg/ml (Decadron-LA) | 16 |
| Hydrocortisone acetate<br>25 mg/ml (Hydrocortone) | 1 |
| Methylprednisolone acetate<br>20, 40, and 80 mg/ml (Depo-Medrol) | 5, 10 and 20 |
| Prednisolone tebutate<br>20 mg/ml (Hydeltra-T.B.A.) | 4 |
| Triamcinolone acetonide<br>10 and 40 mg/ml (Kenalog-10 and Kenalog-40) | 2.5 and 10 |
| Triamcinolone hexacetonide<br>20 mg/ml (Aristospan) | 5 |

*One equivalent = 5 mg prednisone.

Many clinicians, over months or years of practice, have settled on a preparation that seems to have, in their opinion, good benefit and few side effects. Some prefer, for example, a preparation of a "short-acting" solution and a "long-acting" suspension of betamethasone (Celestone Soluspan). They feel the solution works rapidly and prevents the possibility of a postinjection flare. For the same reason, others prefer to inject a "short-acting" solution, such as dexamethasone sodium phosphate, together with a more long-acting suspension.

Mixing the corticosteroid suspension with a local anesthetic, particularly procaine or lidocaine, may be helpful when injecting small joints and tendons, thereby preventing the injection in a single area of a very concentrated suspension, which could produce soft-tissue atrophy. However, one must be concerned over the compatibility of the two preparations. In the Aristospan package brochure dated February, 1978, the following is written:

> Aristospan suspension may be mixed with 1% or 2% lidocaine hydrochloride, using the formulations which do not contain parabens. Similar local anesthetics may also be used. Diluents containing methylparaben, propylparaben, phenol, etc., should be avoided since these compounds may cause flocculation of the steroid.

A review of package inserts of intra-articular corticosteroids from the larger pharmaceutical companies revealed that most do not recommend the use of a mixture of corticosteroids and local anesthetics containing preservatives.

Local anesthetics usually contain preservatives. Ones without them are usually more expensive and are usually not available in the average arthrocentesis tray. Lidocaine for intravenous use does not contain preservatives. A brief survey of several rheumatologists and orthopedic surgeons throughout the country revealed that approximately one half used a corticosteroid and local anesthetic mixture, and only one was aware of the potential problem of flocculation. A few orthopedists, however, reported finding "steroid chalk" in joints, especially wrists, that had been injected with the "older steroids." There is no way of knowing if these joints had been injected with corticosteroid and local anesthetic combinations.

There is no consensus concerning the amount of material that should be injected into the various sized joints. Some clinicians tend to inject a smaller amount in volume of the "more potent" corticosteroids, but many, probably the majority, tend to inject 1 ml in the large joints and a lesser amount in the medium and small joints. Table 37–3 is a rough guide of the amount to be injected.

**Table 37–3.** Amount of Intra-Articular Corticosteroid for Injection

| Size of Joint | Examples | Range of Dosage |
|---|---|---|
| Large | Knees<br>Ankles<br>Shoulders | 1–2 ml |
| Medium | Elbows<br>Wrists | 0.5–1.0 ml |
| Small | Interphalangeal<br>Metacarpophalangeal | 0.1–0.5 ml |

## INDICATIONS

Intra-articular and soft-tissue corticosteroid injections are considered adjunctive therapy. Rarely are they considered primary therapy. Exceptions, as previously noted, include bursitis, tendinitis, or documented gout in a single joint. Table 37–4 lists the indications for intra-articular corticosteroid injections. This therapeutic list is not arranged in any particular order of preference or likelihood of response.

**Articular.** ***Rheumatoid Arthritis.*** Rheumatoid arthritis (with the possible exception of tendinitis and bursitis) is probably the one illness for which the most injections are given. The efficacy of injections in this illness is the most controversial, for reasons previously discussed. If systemic regimens were uniformly efficacious in patients with rheumatoid arthritis, there would be no need to inject corticosteroids in the joints. Since this is not the case, the judicious use of intra-articular corticosteroids may enable a patient to lead a more productive life and one of better quality. Injections may especially be indicated when the patient has failed to respond or when there are contraindications to nonsteroidal anti-inflammatory drugs, hydroxychloroquine, gold salts, or other systemic agents. Usually the injections will enable the patient to better participate in physical therapeutic procedures. The number of injections on a single day should be limited to two, but other joints may be injected on other days. There are no data as to how often the same joint may safely be re-injected. Not more than three times a year seems prudent.

***Gout.*** Acute gouty arthritis (monosodium urate monohydrate crystal deposition disease) on occasion is refractory to so-called conventional regimens, that is, colchicine, phenylbutazone, or other nonsteroidal anti-inflammatory drugs. If this is the case, and if phagocytized sodium urate crystals continue to be present in the synovial fluid, complete aspiration of the inflamed joint followed by corticosteroid injection may be helpful. One has to be very sure that an infectious process is not the reason for the persistent inflammation.

**Table 37–4.** Indications for Intra-articular Corticosteroid Injections

1. Rheumatoid arthritis
2. Gout
3. Pseudogout
4. Acute traumatic "arthritis"
5. Osteoarthritis
6. Synovitis of ipsilateral knee following total hip arthroplasty
7. Juvenile rheumatoid arthritis
8. Inflammatory bowel disease with peripheral joint involvement
9. Miscellaneous conditions with peripheral joint manifestations: ankylosing spondylitis, psoriatic arthritis, and Reiter's disease

***Pseudogout.*** The diagnosis of pseudogout (calcium pyrophosphate dihydrate crystal deposition disease) requires the identification of the calcium pyrosphosphate crystals in synovial fluid. Aspirating as much fluid as possible may alleviate not only pain but also inflammation. That is, aspiration may remove a sufficient number of crystals to reduce the inflammatory process. On occasion, however, the inflammatory response does not respond to this and/or the usual nonsteroidal anti-inflammatory drugs, and intra-articular corticosteroids prove efficacious.

***Acute Traumatic "Arthritis."*** Acute trauma to joints is usually treated with a conservative regimen of cold packs, rest, and, after an appropriate time, an increase in activity. Many feel that injuries to the soft tissues of the shoulder and ankle will cause serious sequelae if range of motion is not instituted after a short period of rest. Intra-articular corticosteroids may help in these situations by allowing early movement.

***Osteoarthritis.*** Osteoarthritic joints, as previously discussed, can be extremely painful. The efficacy of intra-articular corticosteroids is debated; however, on occasion injections give outstanding and prolonged benefit. This is especially true if inflammation is present and there is little cartilage loss. If one or two injections do not give benefit, there is no good reason to keep injecting the joint.

***Synovitis of Knee after Hip Arthroplasty.*** Synovitis of the ipsilateral knee after total hip arthroplasty is noted on occasion and may resolve spontaneously after a few days. It may persist, however, and injection of the knee with a corticosteroid usually is quite beneficial.

***Juvenile Rheumatoid Arthritis.*** In children with rheumatoid arthritis, the number of systemic drugs that can be administered is limited. The judicious use of intra-articular corticosteroids may prove quite helpful. This is especially true when only a few joints are involved; for example, in the pauci (oligo) articular type.

***Synovitis of Inflammatory Bowel Disease.*** Inflammatory gastrointestinal diseases may be associated with peripheral or axial arthritis. Sometimes, depending upon the type of intestinal disorder, an exacerbation of the intestinal problem is associated with an exacerbation of the joint symptoms. In certain situations, control of the intestinal disease also controls the joint disease. If, however, the arthropathy is not helped, injections of intra-articular corticosteroids may give rapid and prolonged relief.

***Miscellaneous.*** Peripheral joint manifestations of other inflammatory arthritides such as ankylosing spondylitis, psoriatic arthritis, and Reiter's disease may be benefited by intra-articular corticosteroids.

**Nonarticular.** Nonarticular inflammatory conditions may be greatly benefited by the injection of a corticosteroid with or without a local anesthetic. Table 37–5 lists various soft tissue conditions which may benefit from the injections.

***Shoulder.*** The main shoulder problems are bicipital tendinitis, subacromial bursitis, and supraspinatus tendinitis. As previously mentioned, these problems can be primary or part of a systemic problem, for example, rheumatoid arthritis. Injection of the specifically inflamed tendon or bursa usually gives relief within a few hours. However, when mixed with a local anesthetic, relief is usually immediate if the physician injected the correct area.

The possible sequelae of intratendinous injections have previously been mentioned. If the inflammatory problems involve the bicipital tendon or subacromial bursa, some physicians prefer to inject the shoulder joint directly. This seems especially true in patients with rheumatoid arthritis because arthrographic studies in these patients have frequently shown a communication between the subacromial bursa, the bicipital tendon sheath, and the shoulder joint. Thus, the drug can have a local effect in all these areas.

***Elbow.*** Inflammation of the elbow epicondylar areas is frequently noted in patients who are quite active in sports, especially tennis and golf. Lateral epicondylitis is frequently a sequela of these activities, and it can be very painful. Injecting the inflamed region can give good to excellent benefit. Mixing the corticosteroid with local anesthetic can give immediate benefit; however, when the effect of the local anesthetic subsides, there is frequently an exacerbation of pain, apparently as a result of a crystal-induced postinjection flare. Medial epicondylitis also can be very painful and usually responds well to an injection. However, one should be careful not to inject the nearby ulnar nerve.

**Table 37–5.** Indications for Non-articular Corticosteroid Injections

1. Shoulder
   a. Bicipital tendinitis
   b. Subacromial bursitis
   c. Supraspinatus tendinitis
2. Elbow
   a. Lateral epicondylitis—"tennis elbow"
   b. Medial epicondylitis—"golfer's elbow"
   c. Olecranon bursitis
   d. Cubital tunnel syndrome
3. Wrist and Hand
   a. Ganglion
   b. de Quervain's disease—stenosing tenosynovitis of extensor pollicis brevis and abductor pollicis longus
   c. Trigger (snapping) fingers
   d. Carpal tunnel syndrome
4. Hip
   a. Trochanteric bursitis
5. Knee
   a. Anserine bursitis
   b. Prepatella bursitis
6. Pelvis
   a. Ischial bursitis
   b. Iliopectineal bursitis
7. Back
   a. "Fibrositic" trigger points
8. Foot
   a. Achilles tendinitis
   b. Achilles bursitis
   c. Calcaneal bursitis
   d. Tarsal tunnel syndrome

Olecranon bursitis may be a primary condition, usually from trauma, but may be secondary to conditions such as gout, infection, and rheumatoid arthritis. Therefore, aspiration of the fluid and synovianalysis are essential before corticosteroids are injected.

Cubital tunnel syndrome, an entrapment of the ulnar nerve at the elbow, may be caused by tenosynovitis. The symptoms are usually more motor related than sensory. Injections can be administered by experienced operators; however, surgical decompression is usually necessary.[60]

***Wrist and Hand.*** A ganglion on the dorsal aspect of the wrist can be treated by aspiration and injection. Again, there may be considerable discomfort several hours after injection. Between two thirds and three fourths of patients have their ganglia "cured" by this conservative approach.[42,61]

Stenosing tenosynovitis of the extensor pollicis brevis and abductor pollicis longus (de Quervain's disease) may cause considerable discomfort over the distal aspect of the radius. Conservative management with corticosteroid and local anesthetic injection may be quite helpful.[57,62] If immediate benefit is noted, this usually indicates the injection was in the proper area. Recurrence is common, however.

Trigger and snapping fingers may be caused by a primary nonspecific hand flexor tenosynovitis or tenosynovitis of rheumatoid arthritis. The tendinous sheath injection of corticosteroid and local anesthetic has been shown to be efficacious in over 90 percent of the cases, and median length of relief has been two years.[55]

Carpal tunnel syndrome has multiple etiologies, but the rheumatoid and idiopathic types may be helped by corticosteroid injections. Extreme care is necessary to prevent median nerve damage.[62] One should receive personal instruction in this technique before attempting it.

***Hip.*** Trochanteric bursitis can give considerable discomfort and may be relieved by injections. There are one or more bursae about the femoral trochanter at the gluteal insertion. The tender region is easily palpated unless there is obesity.

***Knee.*** The anserine bursa is present on the medial aspect of the knee where the tendons of the sartorius, semitendinosus, and gracilus muscles insert on the tibia. When it is inflamed, there is pain, palpable swelling, and tenderness over the medial anterior aspect of the tibia just below the knee. There may be associated degenerative arthritis of the knee, obesity, or a history of physical activity such as jogging, frequent knee bending, or frequent going up and down stairs. Some authors do not consider the condition a true bursitis and classify it as Dercum's disease (painful adiposity) or place it in the "fibrositis syndrome" category.[58] Whatever one wishes to call it, most cases are greatly benefited by injection of corticosteroid and local anesthetic. If the material is injected in the proper place, immediate relief is usually experienced.

Prepatellar bursitis may be secondary to trauma, for example, "housemaid's knee," or could be secondary to systemic illnesses such as rheumatoid arthritis or gout. It may be asymptomatic or quite painful. Some patients request treatment for cosmetic reasons. If clinically indicated, the bursal fluid can be examined by techniques similar to those used for synovial fluid. Injections are usually effective.[63]

***Pelvis.*** Ischial or ischiogluteal bursitis may be more common than is generally thought and may be misdiagnosed as herniated nucleus pulposus, lumbosacral strain, or thrombophlebitis.[64] The ischiogluteal bursa overlies the sciatic nerve and the posterior femoral cutaneous nerve. Therefore, the pain may radiate and the wrong diagnosis may be made. Palpation over the ischial tuberosity should cause significant pain. Injections are helpful but are not recommended for the inexperienced operator.

Iliopectineal (iliopsoas) bursitis is an inflammation of the bursa that is located between the iliopsoas muscle and the iliopectineal eminence. It may communicate with the hip joint. There is tenderness over the anterior aspect of the hip in the region of the middle portion of the inguinal ligament. Hyperextension, adduction, or internal rotation of the hip elicits pain. Differential diagnoses include femoral hernia, psoas abscess, and septic arthritis of the hip. When these other diagnoses have been excluded, and if more conservative regimens have failed or are not practical, an injection of corticosteroid with or without local anesthetic can be tried.[65]

***Back.*** Painful subjective and objective areas of the back may be noted and may be difficult to explain anatomically. Tender areas to moderate deep palpation, the so-called "trigger points," may be noted especially around the upper medial border of the trapezius, various periscapular areas, inferior posterior cervical area, and presacral regions. The latter may represent herniated presacral fatpads. These painful areas may be part of the "fibrositis syndrome."[58] An injection of corticosteroid, local anesthetic, or a combination of the two, into the "trigger points" frequently gives relief.

***Foot.*** Achilles tendinitis may be secondary to trauma or to systemic illnesses such as rheumatoid arthritis or gout. The former may be associated with rheumatoid nodules in the tendon and the latter with tophi. Rest, analgesics, and anti-inflammatory medications are preferable to injections. If little benefit is obtained from these conservative measures, a small amount of a mixture of corticosteroid and local anesthetic may be injected.

Achilles bursitis may represent inflammation of the retrocalcaneal bursa between the calcaneus and Achilles tendon, or a subcutaneous bursitis between the skin and tendon. One should not forget the possibility of gout being the cause, and if the bursae are punctured, an attempt at aspiration is a good idea. The contents should then be examined. Conservative management of nonspecific bursitis is similar to that of Achilles tendinitis; but if this is ineffective, an injection may prove beneficial.

Calcaneal bursitis is an inflammation of the bursa at the attachment of the plantar fascia to the os calcis. Pain is present in the center of the plantar aspect of the heel. Conservative management such as a rubber doughnut may help. If not, an intrabursal injection of corticosteroid mixed with local anesthetic usually gives good relief, but the injection frequently causes considerable pain.

Tarsal tunnel syndrome is an entrapment neuropathy of all or part of the posterior tibial nerve as it passes under the flexor retinaculum of the ankle. Burning pain and paresthesias in the affected foot are the symptoms. Injections by an experienced operator may help, but relief is usually temporary.[66]

## CONTRAINDICATIONS TO INTRA-ARTICULAR CORTICOSTEROID INJECTIONS

The main contraindications to intra-articular corticosteroid injections are listed in Table 37–6. As previously stated, even though rare, iatrogenic infections occur. Therefore, it is essential to adhere to strict aseptic procedures, and certainly the physician must avoid inserting a needle through any area of cellulitis.

The previously mentioned bacteremia, as would be noted in certain cases of pneumonia, endocarditis, and pyelonephritis, is considered a contraindication by some. Therefore, if a patient is hospitalized for a condition that may be associated with bacteremia, and the patient concomitantly has active rheumatoid arthritis, it is probably wise not to institute therapeutic arthrocenteses and corticosteroid injections because of the possibility of an iatrogenic infection. (If one is concerned that bacteremia may have produced septic arthritis, arthrocentesis and special studies on the synovial fluid are mandatory.)

Instability of joints may be part of the Charcot-like arthropathy from intra-articular corticosteroids. Theoretically, further injections could make the instability worse. In general, joints of the spine are considered inaccessible, and injections are contraindicated because of potential sequelae. One should keep in mind that articular pain following trauma could represent an intra-articular fracture. Corticosteroid injection is contrain-

**Table 37–6.** Contraindications to Intra-Articular Corticosteroid Injections

1. Periarticular sepsis
2. Bacteremia
3. Unstable joints
4. Essentially inaccessible joints, e.g., spinal
5. Intra-articular fracture
6. Septic joint; do *not* forget possibility of tuberculosis
7. Possibly the nondiathrodial joints, e.g., symphysis pubis; however, sternomanubrial injections may prove very helpful on occasion
8. Marked juxta-articular osteoporosis
9. Failure to respond to prior injections
10. Blood clotting disorders
11. Probably total joint arthroplasty

dicated because of its potential for retarding the healing of a fracture.

Injection of a septic joint with a corticosteroid could greatly increase the morbidity of the infection. Purulent appearance of synovial fluid should alert the physician to this possibility, but tuberculous synovitis may produce a synovial fluid with minimal inflammatory findings, and the physician may thus be misled. The possibility should always be kept in mind and further studies of synovial fluid and even percutaneous synovial biopsy considered.

Nondiarthrodial joints, such as the symphysis pubis, are involved with certain arthritides, but these joints are difficult to inject. If they are accessible, injections are helpful on occasion, but several punctures may be necessary.

Juxta-articular osteoporosis of a marked degree may be worsened by intra-articular corticosteroid. This type of osteoporosis is more commonly seen in the patient with rheumatoid arthritis, and the arthritis itself plus lack of motion in the joint may be the main cause of the osteoporosis. Therefore, theoretically one or two corticosteroid injections may improve the problem. If one or two corticosteroid injections in the same joint provide no benefit, there is no sound reason to keep injecting it. Blood clotting disorders, such as factor VIII deficiency, may produce a destructive type of arthritis. Arthrocentesis could produce both intra-articular and external hemmorrhage. This problem should definitely be considered when undiagnosed synovitis is noted in a child.

There is an increased incidence of infections in the operated joints of patients who have total joint arthroplasties. These patients are seriously jeopardized by these injections. Even if these patients have an exacerbation of their primary disease—for example, rheumatoid arthritis—in their operated joints, it is probably unwise to inject these joints with corticosteroids.

## ANESTHESIA

As previously discussed, some physicians prefer mixing the corticosteroid with a local anesthetic, usually procaine or lidocaine, for two reasons. First, when injecting a bursa, tendon sheath, or periarticular region, this combination usually would give immediate subjective relief if the materials were injected in the proper space. This immediate benefit, of course, would be from the local anesthetic, not the corticosteroid, and the patients should be told they may experience further pain in an hour or two but should improve a few hours later, when the anti-inflammatory actions of the corticosteroids begin. Second, a mixture may be preferable because the corticosteroid would be diluted and there should be less soft tissue atrophy at the sites of injection.

A physician experienced in arthrocenteses may elect not to use any anesthesia when injecting large joints. If the patient is cooperative and relaxed, and if disposal needles are used, there should be very little pain associated with the arthrocenteses. If the physician is inexperienced or the patient is anxious and tense, a short burst of ethyl chloride spray on the skin over the joint to be injected is helpful.

The injection of a local anesthetic is the other option. First, a skin wheal should be made, followed by infiltration of the subcutaneous tissue and joint capsule. After a few minutes arthrocentesis can be performed and should be painless.

## TECHNIQUES

To perform an arthrocentesis, the specific area of the joint to be aspirated is palpated and is then marked with firm pressure with a ballpoint pen that has the writing portion retracted. This will leave an impression that will last 10 to 30 minutes. (The ballpoint pen technique can also be used with soft tissue injection.) Strict asepsis is important and deserves re-emphasis. The area to be aspirated or injected should be carefully cleansed with a good antiseptic, such as the iodinated compounds. Then the needle can be inserted through the ballpoint pen impression. This method does not require the use of rubber gloves.

A tray for arthrocentesis can be prepared and kept available for use. This includes the following items: alcohol sponges; iodine or merthiolate; pHisoHex; sterile gauze dressings (2 × 2); sterile disposable 2-, 10-, and 20-ml syringes; 18- and 20-gauge 1½ inch needles; 20-gauge spinal needles; 25-gauge ½ inch needles; plain test tubes; heparinized tubes; vial of normal saline solution; clean microscope slides and coverslips; heparin to add to heparinized tubes if a large amount of inflammatory fluid is to be placed in the tube; fingernail polish to seal wet preparation; chocolate agar plates or Thayer-Martin medium; tryptic soy broth for most bacteria; anaerobic transport medium (replace periodically to keep culture media from becoming outdated); tubes with fluoride for glucose; plastic adhesive bandages; ethyl chloride; hemostat; tourniquet for drawing of simultaneous blood samples; and 1 percent lidocaine.

**Articular.** *Knee.* The knee is the easiest joint to inject. If fluid is to be aspirated, the patient should be in a supine position with the knee fully extended. The puncture mark is made just posterior to the medial portion of the patella, and an 18 to 20 g, 1½ inch needle directed slightly posteriorly and slightly inferiorly. The joint space should be entered readily and synovial fluid easily aspirated. On occasion thickened synovium or villous projections may occlude the opening of the needle, and it may be necessary to rotate the needle to facilitate aspiration of fluid. An infrapatellar plica, a vestigial structure that is also called the ligamentum mucosum, may prevent adequate aspiration of the knee when using the medial approach.[67] However, the plica should not adversely affect aspiration from the lateral aspect. If corticosteroid is injected, one should not have any feeling of obstruction as it is being injected. The supine technique is illustrated in Figure 37–1. The patient

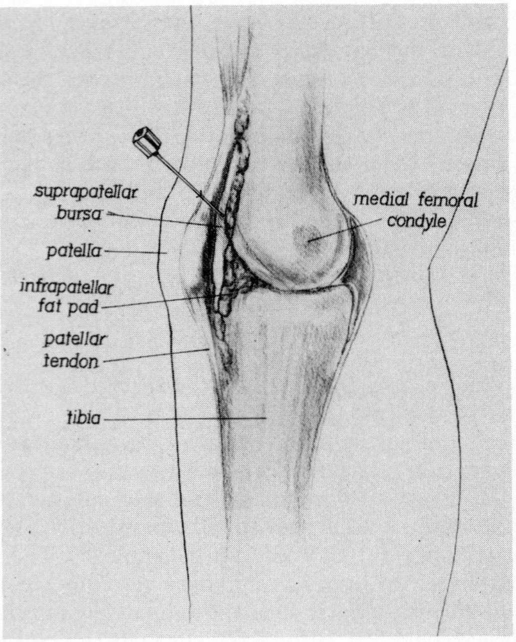


**Figure 37–1.** Diagram of knee arthrocentesis. The needle is inserted just posterior to the medial portion of the patella and is directed slightly posteriorly and slightly inferiorly.

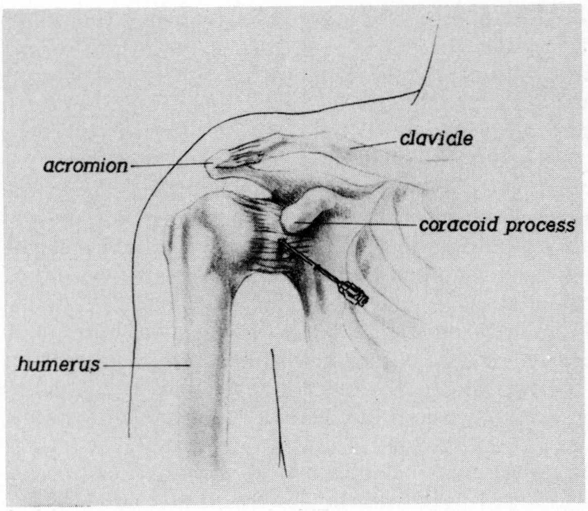


**Figure 37–2.** Diagram of shoulder arthrocentesis. With the shoulder externally rotated, the needle is inserted at a point just medial to the head of the humerus and slightly inferiorly and laterally to the coracoid process. The needle is then directed posteriorly and slightly superiorly and laterally.

should be relaxed if this technique is used. An anxious patient may tighten the patella to the point of making arthrocentesis very difficult. If this is the case or if fusion or osteophytes make the medial or lateral approaches to the knee joint very difficult, an easy technique, which usually avoids these problems, is to inject the knee with the patient sitting with the knee flexed. The mark is made at the medial aspect of the distal border of the patella, and the needle directed slightly superiorly towards the joint cavity. It is usually difficult to obtain fluid with this technique.

The suprapatellar "bursa" may be distended if a large amount of synovial fluid is present. In this instance, the "bursa" may be aspirated in a very easy and essential asymptomatic fashion.

***Shoulder.*** The shoulder arthrocentesis is most easily accomplished with the patient sitting and the shoulder externally rotated. A mark is made just medial to the head of the humerus and slightly inferiorly and laterally to the coracoid process. A 20 to 22 g, 1½ inch needle is directed posteriorly and slightly superiorly and laterally. One should be able to feel the needle enter the joint space. If bone is hit, the operator should pull back and redirect the needle at a slightly different angle. This technique is illustrated in Figure 37–2.

The acromioclavicular joint may be palpated as a groove at the lateral end of the clavicle just medial to the shoulder. A mark is made and a 22 to 26 g, ⅝ to 1 inch needle is carefully directed inferiorly. Rarely is synovial fluid obtained.

The sternoclavicular joint is most easily entered from a point directly anterior to the joint. Caution is necessary to avoid a pneumothorax. The space is fibrocartilaginous and rarely can fluid be aspirated.

***Ankle Joint.*** The patient should be supine and the leg-foot angle should be at 90 degrees. A mark is made just medial to the tibialis anterior tendon and lateral to the medial malleolus. A 20 to 22 g, 1½ inch needle is directed posteriorly and should enter the joint space easily without striking bone. Figure 37–3 illustrates injection of the ankle joint.

***Subtalar Ankle Joint.*** Again, the patient is supine and the leg-foot angle is at 90 degrees. A mark is made just

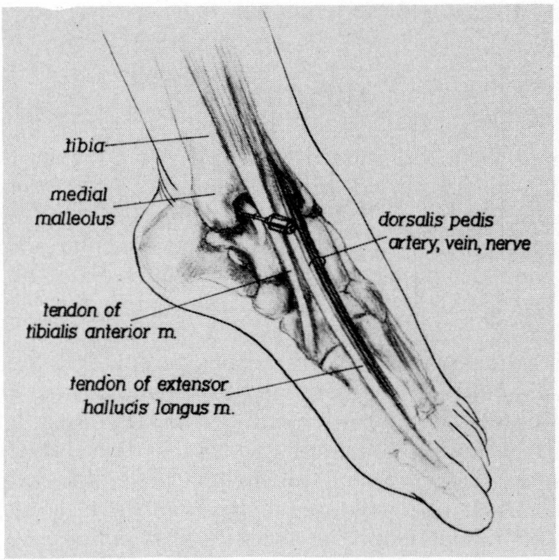


**Figure 37–3.** Diagram of ankle arthrocentesis. With the leg-foot angle at 90 degrees, the needle is inserted at a point just medial to the tibialis anterior tendon and just lateral to the medial malleolus. The needle is then directed posteriorly.

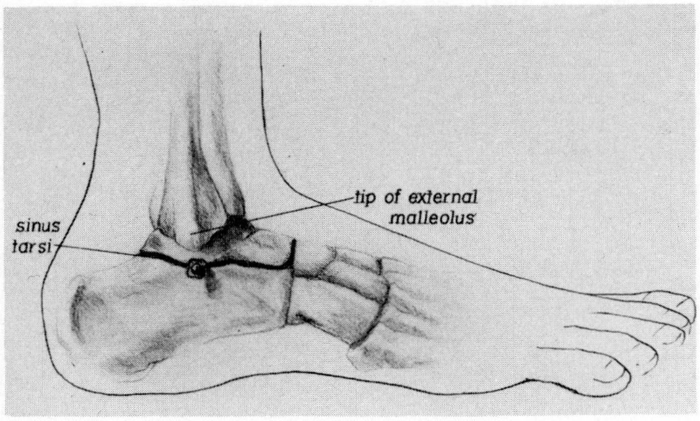


**Figure 37–4.** Diagram of ankle subtalar arthrocentesis. With the leg-foot angle at 90 degrees, the needle is inserted at a point just inferior to the tip of the lateral (external) malleolus and is directed perpendicularly.

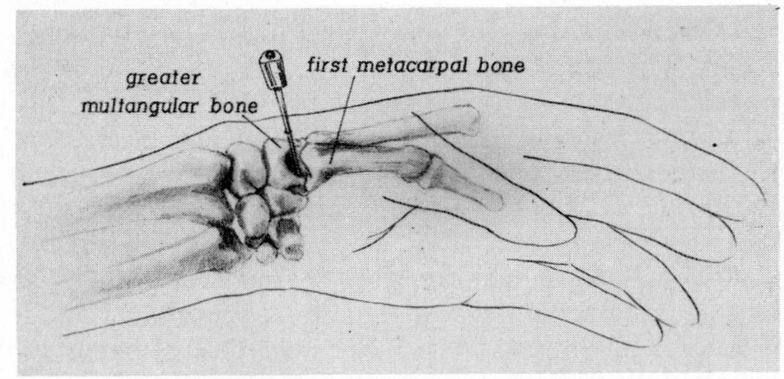


**Figure 37–6.** Diagram of first carpometacarpal arthrocentesis. The thumb is flexed across the palm toward the tip of the fifth finger. The needle is inserted at the base of the metacarpal bone away from the border of the snuffbox. It is then directed toward the proximal end of the fourth metacarpal.

inferior to the tip of the lateral malleolus. A 20 to 22 g, 1½ inch needle is directed perpendicular to the mark. With this joint, the needle may not enter the first time and another attempt or two may be necessary. Because of this and the associated pain, local anesthesia may be helpful. Figure 37–4 illustrates injection of this joint.

***Wrist.*** This is a complex joint, but fortunately most of the intercarpal spaces communicate. A mark is made just distal to the radius and just ulnar to the so-called anatomic snuff box. Usually a 24 to 26 g, ⅝ to 1 inch needle is adequate, and the injection is made perpendicular to the mark. If bone is hit, the needle should be pulled back and slightly redirected toward the thumb. This type of injection is illustrated in Figure 37–5.

***First Carpometacarpal Joint.*** Degenerative arthritis frequently involves this joint. Frequently the joint space is quite narrowed, and arthrocenteses may be difficult and painful. A few simple maneuvers may make the injection fairly easy. The thumb is flexed across the palm toward the tip of the fifth finger. A mark is made at the base of the first metacarpal bone away from the border of the snuff box. A 22 to 26 g, ⅝ to 1 inch needle is inserted at the mark and directed towards the proximal end of the fourth metacarpal. This approach avoids hitting the radial artery. Figure 37–6 illustrates injection of this joint.

***Metacarpophalangeal Joints and Finger Interphalangeal Joints.*** Synovitis in these joints usually causes the synovium to bulge dorsally, and a 24 to 26 g, ½ to ⅝ inch needle can be inserted on either side just under the extensor tendon mechanism. It is not necessary for the needle to be interposed between the articular surfaces. Some prefer having the fingers slightly flexed when injecting the metacarpophalangeal joints. It is unusual to obtain synovial fluid. When injecting corticosteroids, consider mixing them with a small amount of local anesthetic using the precautions previously discussed. This will distend the joint on all sides and possibly help prevent soft tissue atrophy. These injections are illustrated in Figure 37–7.

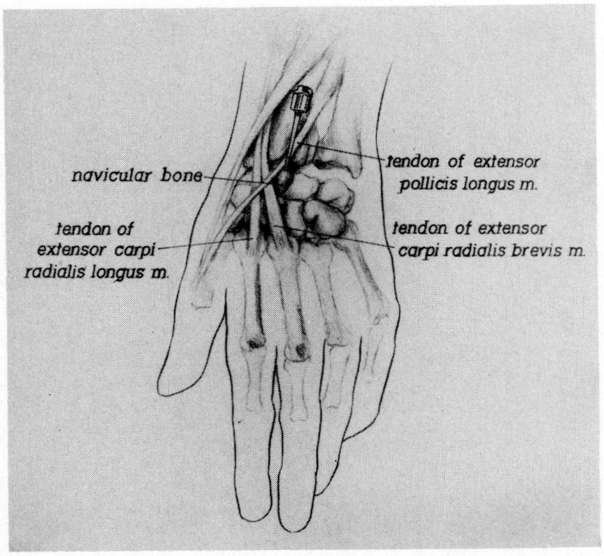


**Figure 37–5.** Diagram of wrist arthrocentesis. The needle is inserted at a point just distal to the radius and just ulnar to the anatomic snuffbox. It is then directed perpendicularly. If bone is hit, the needle should be pulled back and slightly redirected towards the thumb.

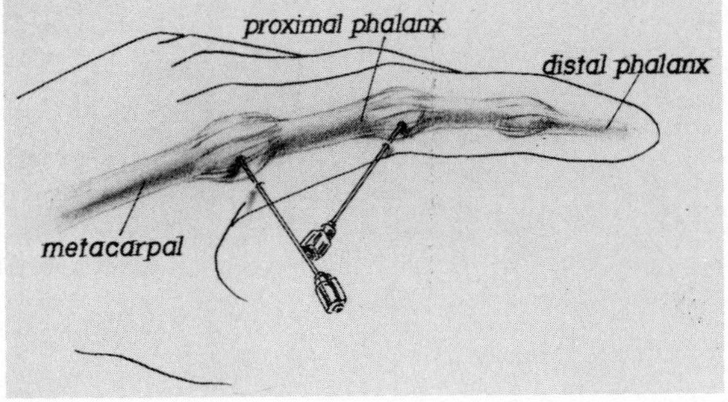


**Figure 37–7.** Diagram of metacarpophalangeal and interphalangeal arthrocenteses. With the digit straight or slightly flexed a small and short needle is inserted on either side just under the extensor tendon mechanism. It is not necessary for the needle to be interposed between the articular surfaces.

*Metatarsophalangeal Joints and Toe Interphalangeal Joints.* The techniques are quite similar to those of the metacarpophalangeal and finger interphalangeal joints, but many prefer to inject more dorsally and laterally to the extensor tendons. Marking the area(s) to be injected is helpful, as is gentle traction on the toe of each joint that is injected.

*Elbow.* A technique preferred by many is to have the elbow flexed at 90 degrees. The joint capsule will bulge if there is inflammation. A mark is made just below the lateral epicondyle of the humerus. A 22 g, 1 to 1½ inch needle is inserted at the mark and directed parallel to the shaft of the radius or can be directed perpendicular to the skin. Figure 37–8 illustrates these two approaches.

*Hip.* This is a very difficult joint to inject, even when using a fluoroscope as a guide. Rarely is the physician quite sure the joint has been entered; synovial fluid is rarely obtained. Two approaches can be used, anterior or lateral. A 20 g, 3½ inch spinal needle should be used for both approaches.

For the anterior approach, the patient is supine and the extremity fully extended and externally rotated. A mark should be made about 2 to 3 cms below the anterior superior iliac spine and 2 to 3 cms lateral to the femoral pulse. The needle is inserted at a 60-degree angle to the skin and directed posteriorly and medially until bone is hit. The needle is slightly withdrawn, and possibly a drop or two of synovial fluid can be obtained, indicating entry into the joint space.

Many prefer the lateral approach because the needle can "follow" the femoral neck into the joint. The patient is supine and the hips should be internally rotated—the knees apart and toes touching. A mark is made just anterior to the greater trochanter, and the needle is inserted and directed medially and slightly cephalad toward a point slightly below the middle of the inguinal ligament. One may feel the tip of the needle slide into the joint. Figure 37–9 illustrates the lateral approach to the hip joint.

*Temporomandibular Joint.* The temporomandibular joint is palpated as a depression just below the zygo-

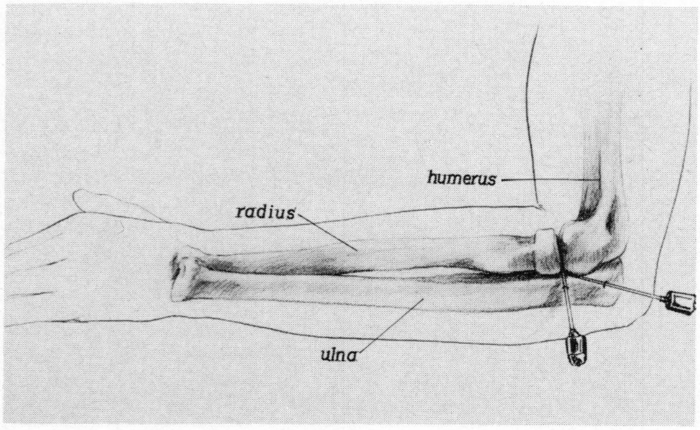


**Figure 37–8.** Diagram of elbow arthrocenteses illustrating parallel and perpendicular techniques. With the elbow flexed at 90 degrees, the needle is inserted just below the lateral epicondyle of the humerus and is directed parallel to the shaft of the radius, or it can be directed perpendicularly to the skin.

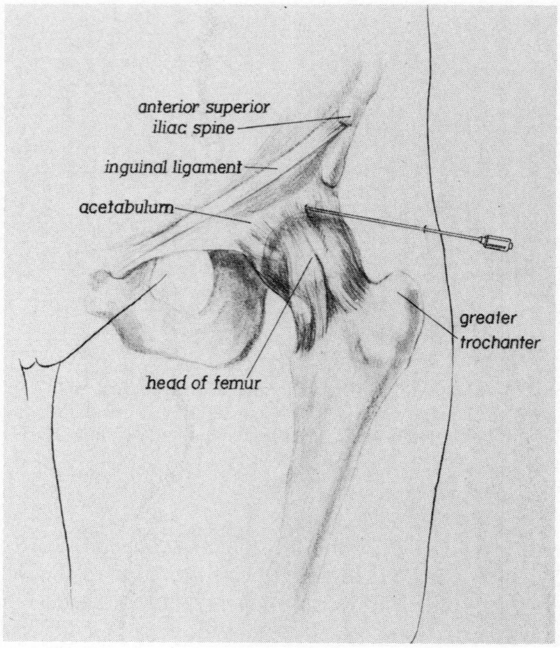


**Figure 37–9.** Diagram of hip arthrocentesis illustrating lateral technique. Using this technique, the patient is supine with the hips internally rotated—knees apart and toes touching. The needle is inserted just anterior to the greater trochanter and is directed medially and slightly cephalad toward a point slightly below the middle of the inguinal ligament. One may feel the needle slip into the joint. For the *anterior approach*, the patient is supine and the extremity fully extended and externally rotated. A mark is made 2 to 3 cm below the anterior superior iliac spine and 2 to 3 cm lateral to the femoral pulse. The needle is inserted at a 60-degree angle to the mark and directed posteriorly and medially until bone is hit.

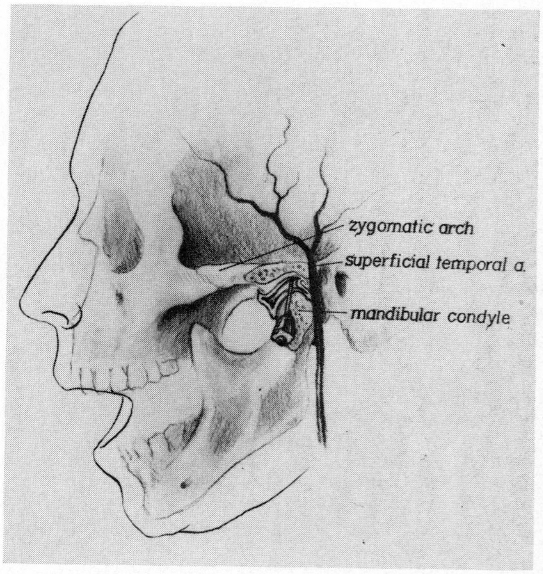


**Figure 37–10.** Diagram of temporomandibular arthrocentesis. With the mouth open, the joint space is palpated as a depression just below the zygomatic arch and 1 to 2 cm anterior to the tragus. The needle is inserted just perpendicular to the skin and directed slightly posteriorly and superiorly.

matic arch and 1 to 2 cms anterior to the tragus. The depression is more easily palpated by having the patient open and close the mouth. A mark is made and with the mouth open, a 22 g, ½ to 1 inch needle is inserted perpendicular to the skin and directed slightly posteriorly and superiorly. Figure 37–10 illustrates injection of the temporomandibular joint.

**Nonarticular.** ***Shoulder.*** Bicipital tendinitis can be treated by injecting the shoulder joint or by injecting the tendon sheath. The tendon is tender, is easily palpated in the bicipital groove of the humerus, and can be rolled from side to side. If it is elected to inject the sheath, the point of maximal tenderness is marked. A 22 g, 1½ inch needle is inserted in the sheath at the mark, and a portion of 0.5 ml of corticosteroid, with or without local anesthetic, is injected at this site. Then the needle is directed superiorly along the tendon, in the sheath, for about 2 to 3 cm, and more material is injected. The needle is then partially withdrawn and redirected inferiorly along the tendon for about 2 to 3 cm, and the remainder of the material injected. Figure 37–11 illustrates the bicipital tendon sheath injection.

Subacromial bursitis can be treated by injecting the shoulder joint or the bursa. The bursitis is frequently secondary to supraspinatus tendinitis. If only the subacromial bursa is to be injected, the most tender area is marked, and using a 20 to 22 g, 1 to 1½ inch needle, 0.5 ml corticosteroid with or without local anesthetic is injected. Calcification of the supraspinatus tendon may be present, and there may be an acute and severe pain. In this circumstance, one should consider aspirating and irrigating the bursa using a 16 to 18 g, 1½ inch needle. Then 0.5 to 1.0 ml of corticosteroid with or without local anesthetic can be injected. Figure 37–12 illustrates the injection of the subacromial bursa.

The supraspinatus tendon can be directly injected by palpating the groove between the acromium and the humerus on the lateral aspect of the shoulder and marking this spot. Then a 20 to 22 g, 1 to 1½ inch needle is directed medially on a horizontal plane for about 2.5 cm and 0.5 ml of corticosteroid and 2.5 to 4.0 ml of local anesthetic injected. The technique of injecting the supraspinatus tendon is also illustrated in Figure 37–12.

***Elbow.*** Lateral epicondylitis, or "tennis elbow," can be very painful, disabling, and chronic. With the elbow flexed and pronated, there is usually marked tenderness to palpation of a small area on the anterolateral surface of the external condyle of the humerus. This spot should be marked. A 20 to 22 g, 1 to 1½ inch needle is inserted about 2 cm distal to the mark, and 0.5 ml of corticosteroid mixed with 4 to 4.5 ml local anesthetic is injected in several small doses by injecting, withdrawing, redirecting the needle, and reinjecting the mixture. The injection of a "tennis elbow" is shown in Figure 37–13.

***"Nodule."*** A nodule—for example, in the olecranon region or on the proximal aspect of the extensor surface of the ulna—may be a diagnostic dilemma: is it a tophus or a rheumatoid nodule? A simple punch needle biopsy should answer the question. Figure 37–14 illustrates the technique. Prepare the nodule with an antiseptic solution. Then insert a disposable 18 to 20 g, 1 to 1½ inch needle at a 90-degree angle and rotate it. The needle is then retracted almost completely and is inserted at a

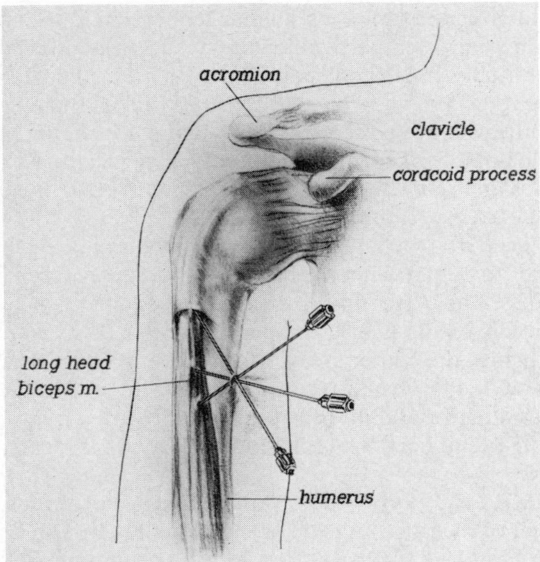


**Figure 37–11.** Diagram of bicipital tendon sheath injections. At the point of maximal tenderness, the needle is inserted just under the sheath, and corticosteroid, with or without local anesthetic, is injected. The needle can then be directed superiorly and then inferiorly, with further injections at each site.

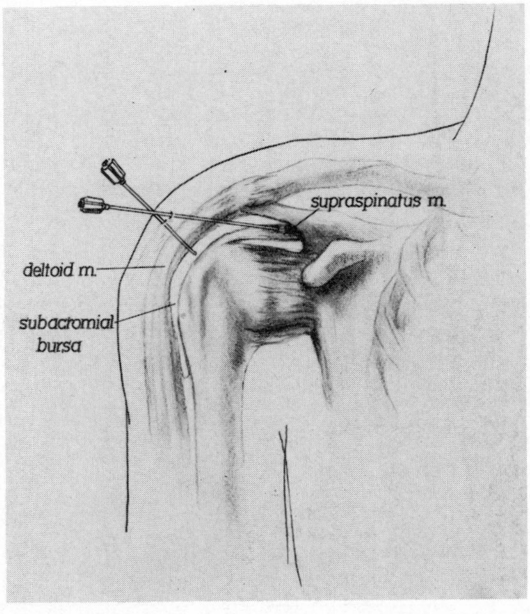


**Figure 37–12.** Diagram of subcromial bursa and supraspinatus tendon injections. For the subacromial bursa, the most tender area is palpated, and the needle is inserted directly into this area. To inject the supraspinatus tendon, the groove between the acromium and the humerus on the lateral aspect of the shoulder is palpated. The needle is inserted at this point and directed medially on a horizontal plane for 2.5 cm, and the materials are injected at this point.

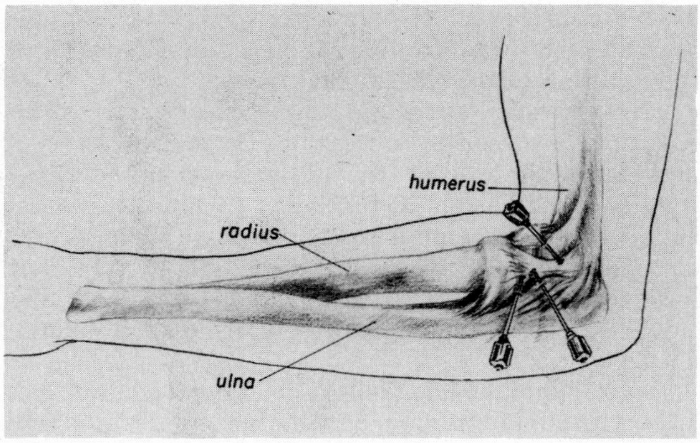


**Figure 37–13.** Diagram of "tennis elbow" injection(s). With the elbow flexed and pronated, the needle is inserted at the most tender area on the anterolateral aspect of the external condyle of the humerus. A combination of corticosteroid and local anesthetic is injected in several areas.

45-degree angle and again rotated (Fig. 37–14*A*). Repeat this in three other quadrants of the nodule. Remove the needle from the nodule and slightly loosen it. Pull back on the syringe plunger to the 2 to 3 ml level, tighten the needle, and expel the contents onto a microscopic slide. In addition, use a 25 g needle to pick out collected material from the biopsy needle (Fig. 37–14*B*). Examine the specimen under the microscope for sodium urate crystals, preferably using polarizing filters. With a little experience, you can virtually exclude the possibility of a tophus if no crystals are observed.

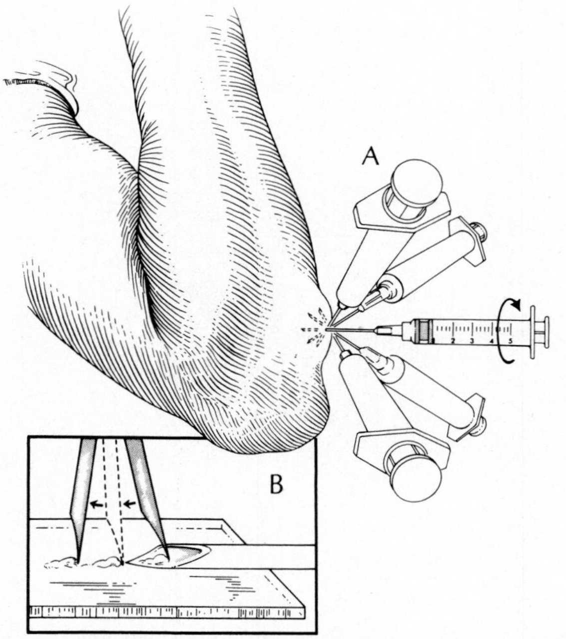


**Figure 37–14.** Diagram of punch needle biopsy of forearm nodule. The needle is inserted at a 90-degree angle and is rotated. The needle is then retraced almost completely, and is inserted at a 45-degree angle. Repeat this in three other quadrants (*A*). The contents of the needle are placed on a microscopic slide (*B*) and examined.

***Wrists and Hands.*** Aspiration of a ganglion on the dorsal aspect of the wrist is done by using an 18 g, 1½ inch needle. After as much material as possible is aspirated, 0.5 to 1.0 ml of an intra-articular corticosteroid is injected.

De Quervain's disease (stenosing tenosynovitis of the extensor pollicis brevis and abductor pollicis longus) may be helped by injection. The most tender area in the region of the radial styloid is located by performing a modified Finkelstein's test, clasping the fingers over the thumb and gradually flexing the wrist in ulnar deviation. The most tender point is marked. Then a 22 g, 1½ inch needle is inserted about 1 cm proximal to the most tender spot and directed almost parallel to the skin toward the styloid process. As the needle is being advanced in the tendon sheath, 0.5 ml of corticosteroid and 2.5 ml of local anesthetic can be injected.

Trigger fingers are usually associated with chronic stenosing tenosynovitis of the finger flexor tendons. The main pathology usually lies over the head of the metacarpal bones in the palm, and a localized swelling may be palpated in this area. A mark is made over the palmar aspect of the metacarpal head, a 22 g, 1½ inch needle is inserted at a 45-degree angle and then directed proximally, almost parallel to the skin, and a mixture of 0.5 ml of both corticosteroid and local anesthetic is injected. Lack of resistance during injection should indicate proper needle placement.

Carpal tunnel syndrome injections should not be performed by an inexperienced operator. Theoretically, an injection of a long-acting corticosteroid directly into the medial nerve will damage it. If one elects to perform the procedure, a mark is made over the carpal tunnel just on the ulnar side of the long palmar tendon. A 25 g, ⅝ inch needle is directed perpendicular to the mark and inserted its full length. If the needle meets obstruction, or if the patient experiences paresthesias, the needle should be withdrawn and redirected in a more ulnar fashion. An injection of 0.5 ml corticosteroid may give benefit. The carpal tunnel may be injected again, but if relief is short-lived, surgery should be considered.

***Hip.*** With trochanteric bursitis, there is an area that is tender to palpation in the region of the greater trochanter of the femur. After marking this area, a 20 to 22 g, 1½ to 3½ inch needle is inserted perpendicular to the skin directly into the tender area(s). Since several bursae may be inflamed, it is usually more effective to inject several areas superior and inferior to the mark with a mixture of 0.5 to 1.0 ml corticosteroid and 4.5 to 9.0 ml local anesthetic.

***Knee.*** Anserine bursitis produces pain on the medial aspect of the tibia. In this same region may be noted pain from a fat pad, from another bursa, or from medial collateral ligament strain. All may benefit from injection. The point of maximal tenderness is marked. A 20 to 22 g, 1½ inch needle is inserted perpendicular to the skin and continued until bone is hit. It is then withdrawn slightly and 0.25 to 0.50 ml corticosteroid and 2.5 to 4.5 ml local anesthetic injected.

The prepatellar bursa is easily aspirated. An 18 g, 1½ inch needle is recommended because sometimes the fluid is very gelatinous and difficult to obtain through a small-bore needle. After aspirating as much fluid as possible, 0.5 to 1.0 ml corticosteroid is injected. On occasion very little fluid is obtained during the initial aspiration, but reaspiration 24 hours after corticosteroid injection may yield a large amount of fluid.

***Pelvis.*** When inflamed, the ischial (ischiogluteal) bursa is usually easily palpated as a tender area when the patient is lying on his side with the knees flexed. Theoretically this position will cause the ischium to be more exposed and the gluteal muscles and sciatic nerve to be pulled away. The point of maximal tenderness is marked, and 0.5 to 1.0 ml corticosteroid and 2.5 to 4.0 ml of local anesthetic are mixed in a syringe with a 20 g, 3½ inch needle attached. It is helpful to "fix" the skin over the mark. Then the needle is inserted into the mark until bone is hit. The needle is withdrawn slightly and all the mixture injected; alternatively, the needle is redirected in one or two other directions and portions of the mixture injected.

Iliopectineal (iliopsoas) bursitis, as previously mentioned, must be differentiated from psoas abscess, femoral hernia, and septic arthritis of the hip. If one elects to inject the bursa, a 20 to 22 g, 3½ inch spinal needle is used. Many use the technique of hip arthrocentesis. A dose of 0.5 to 1.0 ml of corticosteroid is injected with or without 4 to 4.5 ml local anesthetic.

***Back.*** The "fibrositis syndrome" and the "trigger points" of the back have been briefly discussed. These "trigger points" can be marked and each injected with 0.25 ml corticosteroid or 1 ml or more of local anesthetic, or as many physicians prefer, a combination of the two. The shorter-acting corticosteroids, in contrast to the repository forms, have been recommended.[59] The physician must be careful to avoid injury to the underlying structures.

***Foot.*** Achilles tendinitis may respond to injection. If this is done, a 22 g, 1½ inch needle is inserted just under the tendon sheath and a mixture of 0.25 ml corticosteroid and 2.5 ml local anesthetic injected. Direct injection of the tendon should be avoided.

An inflammation of the subcutaneous Achilles bursa between the skin and tendon is usually readily palpable, can be marked, and should be easily aspirated with a 20 g, 1 inch needle. The retrocalcaneal bursa is located between the Achilles tendon and the posterior facet of the calcaneus. A lateral or medial approach is probably better. Careful injection of either location with 0.25 to 0.50 ml corticosteroid with or without local anesthetic is usually beneficial.

Calcaneal bursitis can be treated by inserting a 20 g, 1½ inch needle perpendicular to the plantar surface of the midcalcaneal region, pushing the needle in until bone is hit, withdrawing slightly, and injecting 0.5 ml corticosteroid and 3.5 ml local anesthetic.

## References

1. Hollander, J.L.: Arthrocentesis and intrasynovial therapy. *In* McCarty, D.J. (ed.): Arthritis and Allied Conditions. Philadelphia. Lea and Febiger, 1979.
2. Hollander, J.L.: The local effects of compound F(hydrocortisone) injected into joints. Bull. Rheum. Dis. 2:3, 1951.
3. Young, H.H., Ward, L.E., and Henderson, E.D.: The use of hydrocortisone acetate (compound F acetate) in the treatment of some common orthopaedic conditions. J. Bone Joint Surg. 36A:602, 1954.
4. Hollander, J.L., Jessar, R.A., and Brown, E.M., Jr.: Intrasynovial corticosteroid therapy: A decade of use. Bull. Rheum. Dis. 11:239, 1961.
5. Hollander, J.L.: Intrasynovial corticosteroid therapy in arthritis. Maryland State Med. J. 19:62, 1970.
6. Ragan, C., Howes, E.L., Plotz, C.M., Meyer, K., Blunt, J.W., and Lattes, R.: The effect of ACTH and cortisone on connective tissue. Bull. N.Y. Acad. Med. 26:251, 1950.
7. Jessar, R.A., Ganzell, M.A., and Ragan, C.: The action of hydrocortisone in synovial inflammation. J. Clin. Invest. 32:480, 1954.
8. de Duve, C., Wattiaux, R., and Wibo, M.: Effects of fat-soluble compounds on lysosomes in vitro. Biochem. Pharmacol. 9:97, 1962.
9. Weissman, G., and Thomas, L.: Studies on lysosomes: II. The effect of cortisone on the release of acid hydrolases from a large granule fraction of rabbit liver induced by an excess of vitamin A. J. Clin. Invest. 42:661, 1963.
10. Weissmann, G.: The role of lysosomes in inflammation and disease. Ann. Rev. Med. 18:97, 1967.
11. Wright, D.G., and Malawista, S.E.: Mobilization and extracellular release of granular enzymes from human leukocytes during phagocytosis: Inhibition by colchicine and cortisol but not by salicylate. Arthritis Rheum. 16:749, 1973.
12. Mandell, G.L., Rubin, W., and Hook, E.W.: The effect of an NADH oxidase inhibitor (hydrocortisone) on polymorphonuclear leukocyte bacterial activity. J. Clin. Invest. 49:1381, 1970.
13. Wiener, E., Marmary, Y., and Curelaru, Z.: The in vitro effect of hydrocortisone on the uptake and intracellular digestion of particulate matter by macrophages in culture. Lab. Invest. 26:220, 1972.
14. Persellin, R.H., and Ku, L.C.: Effects of steroid hormones on human polymorphonuclear leukocyte lysosomes. J. Clin. Invest. 54:919, 1974.
15. Stevenson, R.D.: Mechanism of anti-inflammatory action of glucocorticosteroids. Lancet. 1:225, 1977.
16. Lewis, G.P., and Piper, P.J.: Inhibition of release of prostaglandins as an explanation of some of the actions of anti-inflammatory corticosteroids. Nature 254:308, 1975.
17. Kantrowitz, F., Robinson, D.R., McGuire, M.B. and Levine, L.: Corticosteroids inhibit prostaglandin production by rheumatoid synovia. Nature 258:737, 1975.
18. Tashjian, A.H., Jr., Voelkel, E.F., McDonough, J., and Levine, L.: Hydrocortisone inhibits prostaglandin production by mouse fibrosarcoma cells. Nature 258:739, 1975.
19. Gryglewski, R.J.: Steroid hormones, anti-inflammatory steroids, and prostaglandins. Pharmacol. Res. Commun. 8:337, 1976.
20. Hong, S.-C.L., and Levine, L.: Inhibition of arachidonic acid release from cells as the biochemical action of anti-inflammatory corticosteroids. Proc. Natl. Acad. Sci. 73:1730, 1976.
21. Gryglewski, R.J., Panczenko, B., Korbut, R., Grodzinska, L., and Ocetkiewicz, A.: Corticosteroids inhibit prostaglandin release from perfused mesenteric blood vessels of rabbit and from perfused lungs of sensitized guinea pig. Prostaglandins 10:343, 1975.
22. Kuehl, F.A., Jr., and Egan, R.W.: Prostaglandins, arachidonic acid, and inflammation. Science 210:978, 1980.
23. Butler, W.T., and Rossen, R.D.: Effect of corticosteroids on immunity in man. I. Decreased serum IgG concentration caused by 3 or 5 days of high doses of methylprednisolone. J. Clin. Invest. 52:2629, 1973.
24. Atkinson, J.P., and Frank, M.M.: Effect of cortisone therapy on serum complement components. J. Immunol. 111:1061, 1973.
25. Hunder, G.G., and McDuffie, F.C.: Effect of intra-articular hydrocortisone on complement in synovial fluid. J. Lab. Clin. Med. 79:62, 1972.
26. Goetzl, E.J., Bianco, N.E., Alpert, J.S., Sledge, C.B., and Schur, P.H.: Effects of intra-articular corticosteroids in vivo on synovial fluid variables in rheumatoid synovitis. Ann. Rheum. Dis. 33:62, 1974.
27. Dick, W.C., Whaley, K., St. Onge, R.A., Downie, W.W., Doyle, J.A., Nuki, G., Gillespie, F.C., and Buchanan, W.W.: Clinical studies on inflammation in human knee joints: Xenon ($Xe^{133}$) clearances correlated with clinical assessment in various arthritides and studies on the effect of intra-articular administered hydrocortisone in rheumatoid arthritis. Clin. Sci. 38:123, 1970.
28. DeCeulaer, K., Balint, G., El-Ghobarey, A., and Dick, W.C.: Effects of corticosteroids and local anaesthetics applied directly to the synovial vascular bed. Ann. Rheum. Dis. 38:440, 1979.
29. Eymontt, M.J., Gordon, G.V., Schumacher, H.R., and Hansell, J.R.: The

effects on synovial permeability and synovial fluid leukocyte counts in symptomatic osteoarthritis after intra-articular corticosteroid administration. J. Rheumatol. 9:198, 1982.
30. Chandler, G.N., and Wright, V.: Deleterious effect of intra-articular hydrocortisone. Lancet 2:661, 1958.
31. Chandler, G.N., Wright, V., and Hartfall, S.J.: Intra-articular therapy in rheumatoid arthritis. Comparison of hydrocortisone tertiary butyl acetate and hydrocortisone acetate. Lancet 2:659, 1968.
32. Mankin, H.J., and Conger, K.A.: The acute effects of intra-articular hydrocortisone on articular cartilage in rabbits. J. Bone Joint Surg. 48A:1383, 1966.
33. Bentley, G., and Goodfellow, J.W.: Disorganization of the knees following intra-articular hydrocortisone injections. J. Bone Joint Surg. 51B:498, 1969.
34. Moskowitz, R.W., Davis, W., Sammarco, J., Mast, W., and Chase, S.W.: Experimentally induced corticosteroid arthropathy. Arthritis Rheum. 13:236, 1970.
35. Mankin, H.J., Zarins, A., and Jaffe, W.L.: The effect of systemic corticosteroids on rabbit articular cartilage. Arthritis Rheum. 15:593, 1972.
36. Behrens, F., Shepard, N., and Mitchell, N.: Alteration of rabbit articular cartilage by intra-articular injections of glucocorticosteroids. J. Bone Joint Surg. 57A:70, 1975.
37. Gibson, T., Barry, H.C., Poswillo, D., and Glass, J.: Effect of intra-articular corticosteroid injections on primate cartilage. Ann. Rheum. Dis. 36:74, 1976.
38. Tenenbaum, J., Pritzker, K.P.H., Gross, A.E., Cheng, P-T, Renlund, R.C., and Tenenbaum, H.: The effects of intraarticular corticosteroids on articular cartilage. Sem. Arthritis Rheum. 11:140, Suppl. 1, 1981.
39. Sweetnam, R.: Corticosteroid arthropathy and tendon rupture (editorial) J. Bone Joint Surg. 51B:397, 1969.
40. Wrenn, R.N., Goldner, J.L., and Markee, J.L.: An experimental study of the effect of cortisone on the healing process and tensile stength of tendons. J. Bone Joint Surg. 36A:588, 1954.
41. McCarty, D.J.: Treatment of rheumatoid joint inflammation with triamcinolone hexacetonide. Arthritis Rheum. 15:157, 1972.
42. McCarty, D.J., Jr., and Hogan, J.M.: Inflammatory reaction after intrasynovial injection of microcrystalline adrenocorticosteroid esters. Arthritis Rheum. 7:359, 1964.
43. Koehler, B.F., Urowitz, M.B., and Killinger, D.W.: The systemic effects of intra-articular corticosteroid. J. Rheum. 1:117, 1974.
44. Gottlieb, N.L., and Riskin, W.G.: Complications of local corticosteroid injections. JAMA 243:1547, 1980.
45. Carson, T.E., Daane, T.A., Lee, P.A., Tredway, D.R., and Wallin, J.D.: Effect of intramuscular triamcinolone acetonide on the human ovulatory cycle. Cutis 19:633, 1977.
46. Cunningham, G.R., Goldzieher, J.W., de la Pena, A., and Oliver, M.: The mechanism of ovulation inhibition by triamcinolone acetonide. J. Clin. Endocrinol. Metab. 46:8, 1978.
47. McCarty, D.J., Jr.. A basic guide to arthrocentesis. Hosp. Med. (Nov.) 4:77, 1968.
48. Gottlieb, N.L.: Hypodermic needle separation during arthrocentesis. Arthritis Rheum. 24:1593, 1981.
49. Fitzgerald, R.F., Jr.: Intrasynovial injection of steroids. Mayo Clin. Proc. 51:655, 1976.
50. Miller, J.H., White, J., and Norton, T.H.: The value of intra-articular injections in osteoarthritis of the knee. J. Bone Joint Surg. 40B:636, 1958.
51. Friedman, D.M., and Moore, M.F.: The efficacy of intra-articular corticosteroid for osteoarthritis of the knee. Arthritis Rheum. 21:556, 1978.
52. Utsinger, P.D., Resnick, D., Shapiro, R.F., and Wiesner, K.B.: Roentgenologic, immunologic, and therapeutic study of erosive (Inflammatory) osteoarthritis. Arch. Intern. Med. 138:693, 1978.
53. McCarty, D.J.: Intrasynovial therapy with adreno-corticosteroid esters. Wis. Med. J. 77:875, 1978.
54. Henderson, E.D., and Henderson, C.C.: The use of hydrocortisone acetate (compound F acetate) in the treatment of post-traumatic bursitis of the knee and elbow. Minn. Med. 36:142, 1953.
55. Gray, R.G., Kiem, I.M., and Gottlieb, N.L.: Intratendon sheath corticosteroid treatment of rheumatoid arthritis-associated and idiopathic hand flexor tenosynovitis. Arthritis Rheum. 21:92, 1978.
56. Steinbrocker, O.: Management of some non-articular rheumatic disorders. Mod. Treatment 1:1254, 1964.
57. Steinbrocker, O., and Neustadt, D.H.: Aspiration and injection therapy in arthritis and musculoskeletal disorders. Hagerstown, Md., Harper and Row, 1972.
58. Smythe, H.A., and Moldofsky, H.: Two contributions to understanding of the "fibrositis" syndrome. Bull. Rheum. Dis. 28:928, 1977.
59. Brown, B.B., Jr.: Diagnosis and therapy of common myofascial syndromes. JAMA 239:646, 1978.
60. Clark, C.B.: Cubital tunnel syndrome. JAMA 241:801, 1979.
61. Lapidus, P.W., and Guidotti, F.P.: Report on the treatment of one hundred and two ganglions. Bull. Hosp. Joint Dis. 28:50, 1967.
62. Phalen, G.S.: Soft tissue affection of the hand and wrist. Hosp. Med. 7:47, 1971.
63. Blau, S.P.: All those joint pains may not be arthritis. Drug Therapy (Nov.) 1976, p. 144.
64. Swartout, R., and Compere, E.L.: Ischiogluteal bursitis. JAMA 227:551, 1974.
65. Hucherson, D.C., and Freeman, G.E., Jr.: Iliopectineal bursitis: A cause of hip pain frequently unrecognized. Am. J. Orthop. 4:220, 1962.
66. Kaplan, P.E., and Kernahan, W.T.: Tarsal tunnel syndrome. J. Bone Joint Surg. 63A:96, 1981.
67. Hardaker, W.T., Whipple, T.L., and Bassett, F.H.: Diagnosis and treatment of the plica syndrome of the knee. J. Bone Joint Surg. 62A:221, 1980.

# Chapter 38
# Synovial Fluid Analysis

*H. Ralph Schumacher*

## INTRODUCTION

Joint fluid examination is to evaluation of joint disease as urinalysis is to renal disease. Analysis of joint fluid should be performed as part of the diagnostic evaluation in any patient with joint disease. Even small amounts of joint fluid can be aspirated and systematically examined. One to three drops of synovial fluid can be obtained from virtually any first MTP joint, for example.[1]

Some common diseases such as gout, pseudogout, septic arthritis, and systemic lupus erythematosus, as well as other less common diseases, can be quickly and definitively diagnosed by examination of joint fluid. Even if joint fluid examination is not diagnostic in other patients, it can be one of the most useful of a battery of clinical and laboratory tests used in differential diagnosis. Gross examination and leukocyte count as described later allow narrowing of diagnostic possibilities to the diseases causing "noninflammatory" effusions; "inflammatory" fluids, including septic effusions; and hemarthroses (Tables 38–1 to 38–3).

Even in patients in whom the diagnosis has been established, synovianalysis can show clues to new developments such as low-grade infection in a joint of a patient with lupus erythematosus or rheumatoid disease, superimposition of calcium pyrophosphate crystal deposition in osteoarthritis, or crystals of intra-articularly injected steroids causing a transient crystal-induced synovitis.

**TABLE 38–1.** "NONINFLAMMATORY" JOINT EFFUSIONS (LEUKOCYTE COUNT LESS THAN 2000 PER CUBIC MILLIMETER)

| |
|---|
| Osteoarthritis |
| Traumatic arthritis |
| Acromegaly |
| Gaucher's disease |
| Hemochromatosis |
| Hyperparathyroidism |
| Ochronosis |
| Paget's disease |
| Mechanical derangement |
| Erythema nodosum |
| Villonodular synovitis, tumors |
| Aseptic necrosis |
| Ehlers-Danlos syndrome |
| Sickle cell disease |
| Amyloidosis |
| Hypertrophic pulmonary osteoarthropathy |
| Pancreatitis |
| Osteochondritis dissecans |
| Charcot's joints |
| Wilson's disease |
| Epiphyseal dysplasias |

**TABLE 38–2.** INFLAMMATORY JOINT EFFUSIONS (LEUKOCYTE COUNT GREATER THAN 2000 PER CUBIC MILLIMETER)

| |
|---|
| Rheumatoid arthritis |
| Psoriatic arthritis |
| Reiter's syndrome |
| Ulcerative colitis |
| Regional enteritis |
| Postileal bypass arthritis |
| Ankylosing spondylitis |
| Juvenile rheumatoid arthritis |
| Rheumatic fever |
| Collagen-vascular disease |
| Systemic lupus erythematosus |
| Scleroderma |
| Polymyositis |
| Polychondritis |
| Polyarteritis |
| Polymyalgia rheumatica |
| Giant cell arteritis |
| Sjögren's syndrome |
| Wegener's granulomatosis |
| Goodpasture's syndrome |
| Henoch-Schönlein purpura |
| Familial Mediterranean fever |
| Whipple's disease |
| Behçet's syndrome |
| Erythema nodosum |
| Sarcoidosis |
| Multicentric reticulohistiocytosis |
| Erythema multiforme (Stevens-Johnson) |
| Postsalmonella, shigella, yersinia arthritis |
| Infectious arthritis |
| Parasitic |
| Viral (hepatitis, mumps, rubella, others) |
| Fungal |
| Mycoplasmal |
| Bacterial (staphylococcal, gonococcal, tuberculous, others) |
| Treponemal |
| Carcinoid |
| Subacute bacterial endocarditis |
| Crystal-induced arthritis |
| Gout |
| Pseudogout |
| Post-intra-articular steroid injection |
| Hydroxyapatite arthritis |
| Hyperlipoproteinemias |
| Serum sickness |
| Agammaglobulinemia |
| Leukemia |
| Hypersensitivity angiitis |
| Palindromic rheumatism |

**TABLE 38–3.** HEMARTHROSIS

| |
|---|
| Trauma with or without fractures |
| Pigmented villonodular synovitis |
| Synovioma, other tumors |
| Hemangioma |
| Charcot joint or other severe joint destruction |
| Hemophilia or other bleeding disorders |
| Von Willebrand's disease |
| Anticoagulant therapy |
| Myeloproliferative disease with thrombocytosis |
| Thrombocytopenia |
| Scurvy |
| Ruptured aneurysm |
| Arteriovenous fistula |
| Idiopathic |

Only by examining the joint fluid can one be best informed about what is occurring in that joint. Abnormal blood tests such as rheumatoid factor, antinuclear antibodies, and elevated uric acid can be misleading and do not establish the nature of disease in the joint.

Normal joint fluid is described in detail in Chapter 16. Briefly, normal synovial fluid is an ultrafiltrate of plasma, with only small amounts of larger molecular weight proteins such as fibrinogen, beta 1C globulin, and other globulins, to which has been added hyaluronate-protein produced in the synovial membrane. Normal fluid is compared with that seen in various diseases in Table 38–4.

## TECHNIQUE FOR ARTHROCENTESIS

The techniques used, appropriate precautions, and routes for arthrocentesis are described in Chapter 37.

If no fluid is identified in the syringe after attempted aspiration, try to express a drop of blood or tissue fluid from the needle. One can use such a single drop for examination for crystals, Gram stain, or culture. If no fluid is obtained and infection is suspected, irrigate the joint with a small amount of normal saline and culture this irrigating fluid. The patient should be fasting if synovial fluid and serum glucose are to be compared.

Consider the studies most likely to be helpful in each case before arthrocentesis and prepare a list of priorities for the fluid obtained. Not all tests by any means need be performed on each specimen.

## GROSS EXAMINATION

This can partly be done at the bedside to help plan which of the other studies are most pertinent and should be done on small volume effusions.

**Volume.** The amount of effusion can help serve as one measure of the severity of arthritis and can be used for comparison with previous arthrocenteses. Low volume does not mean absence of an important intra-articular process. Effusions may be difficult to aspirate because of thick fibrin, rice bodies, and other debris. Fluid may be loculated and not accessible by the route chosen.

**Viscosity.** This is estimated by watching the synovial fluid as it is slowly expressed from the syringe and by manipulating several drops of fluid between the thumb and index finger. Fluid of normal viscosity holds together and stretches to a string of 1 to 2 inches before separating. Low-viscosity fluid drips from a syringe like water. Recent studies show that viscosity is less reliable than previously thought in classification of effusions.[3] Very viscous fluid is seen in hypothyroid effusions and in ganglia. Viscosity is generally decreased in inflammation but also is low in edema fluid. Greater degrees of quantitation are generally not needed; but if they are desired, a simple technique using a white blood cell diluting pipette has been described.[3] Viscosity tends to parallel the concentration of hyaluronate, which is measured as uronic acid as a research tool.[2] In purulent effusions the massive numbers of leukocytes may make the fluid seem more viscous. The usual patterns of viscosity and many of the other examination findings are given in Table 38–4. Hyaluronidase can be used to de-

**Table 38–4.** Classification of Synovial Effusions*

| Gross Examination | Normal | "Noninflammatory" (Group I) | Inflammatory (Group II) | Septic (Group III) |
|---|---|---|---|---|
| Volume (ml) (knee) | <3.5 | Often >3.5 | Often >3.5 | Often >3.5 |
| Viscosity | High | High | Low | Variable |
| Color | Colorless to straw | Straw to yellow | Yellow | Variable |
| Clarity | Transparent | Transparent | Translucent | Opaque |
| Routine laboratory examination | | | | |
| WBC ($mm^3$) | <200 | 200 to 2000 | 2000 to 75,000 | Often >100,000† |
| PMN leukocytes (%) | <25 | <25 | >50 often | >75† |
| Culture | Negative | Negative | Negative | Often positive |
| Mucin clot | Firm | Firm | Friable | Friable |
| Glucose (AM fasting) | Nearly equal to blood | Nearly equal to blood | <50 mg% lower than blood | >50 mg% lower than blood |

*See Tables 38–1 and 38–2 for diseases in the noninflammatory and inflammatory groups.
†WBC and % PMN leukocytes will be less if organism is less virulent or partially treated.

crease synovial fluid viscosity before performing other tests, provided that the normal values using this enzyme have been standardized in the laboratory. Hyaluronidase use reportedly gives slightly higher synovial fluid leukocyte counts.[4]

**Color and Clarity (Fig. 38–1).** If print cannot be read easily through the fluid, the effusion is cloudy and this should suggest an inflammatory process. The plastic of some syringes makes fluids appear falsely cloudy, so fluids should be examined in glass. The value of gross examination in classifying effusions is summarized in Table 38–4. Generally, the more cloudy fluids have more cells, but not all very cloudy or opaque fluids are inflammatory. Microscopic examination is still needed to be certain that the opacity is not due to massive numbers of crystals, triglycerides, fibrin, amyloid, or cartilage fragments. Sometimes chronically inflamed joints have effusions containing rice bodies, which might also be confused grossly with pus. Rice bodies are end results of synovial proliferation and degeneration; they contain collagen, cell debris, and fibrin (Fig. 38–2, Plate IV, p. xxxviii).

Ochronotic fluid may be speckled with dark particles ("ground pepper" sign).[5] Black or gray debris from metal or plastic fragments after prosthetic arthroplasty can also discolor the fluid.[6]

Rheumatoid and other chronic effusions occasionally have a greenish hue; pigmented villonodular synovitis can be grossly bloody or may produce an orange-brown color. Gouty fluid tends to be unusually white when it contains massive amounts of crystals. Streaks of blood are the result of injury to a small vessel during the procedure. Causes of diffusely bloody fluid are listed in Table 38–3. Partially treated or low-grade infection can make the synovial fluid look like any other moderately inflammatory but not purulent fluid. Very slightly inflammatory or clear fluids are common in systemic lupus erythematosus, rheumatic fever, polymyositis, and scleroderma and can be seen in the interim between attacks of gout and pseudogout.

## LEUKOCYTE COUNT

Quantitation of the synovial fluid leukocyte count is a very important part of synovial fluid analysis, especially as it is the major basis for classification of an effusion as "septic," "inflammatory," or "noninflammatory" (Table 38–4). Note the many important systemic diseases such as hypertrophic pulmonary osteoarthropathy and sickle cell disease that can be associated with noninflammatory effusions. Synovial fluid leukocyte counts along with volumes can be used as a rough measure of the intensity of inflammation in sequential samples.

The standard white blood cell (WBC) counting chamber and techniques are used, except that ordinary WBC counting fluid should be replaced with normal or 0.3 percent saline. The 0.3 percent saline will lyse erythrocytes. The acid of ordinary WBC counting fluid clots synovial fluid and gives inaccurate leukocyte counts. The fluid should be placed in a heparinized tube and shaken to mix it thoroughly. The count must be done promptly, as there may be some spontaneous clotting and clumping of leukocytes. A small amount of methylene blue can be added for easier identification of leukocytes. Rheumatoid arthritis fluid usually has leukocyte counts from 2000 to 75,000. Counts over 60,000 should raise a suspicion of infection. However, it should be noted that partially treated infections or "low-grade" infections with gonococci, mycobacteria, and fungi often have lower leukocyte counts. Patients with rheumatoid disease, Reiter's syndrome, and crystal-induced arthritis may have counts over 100,000 WBC per cubic millimeter.

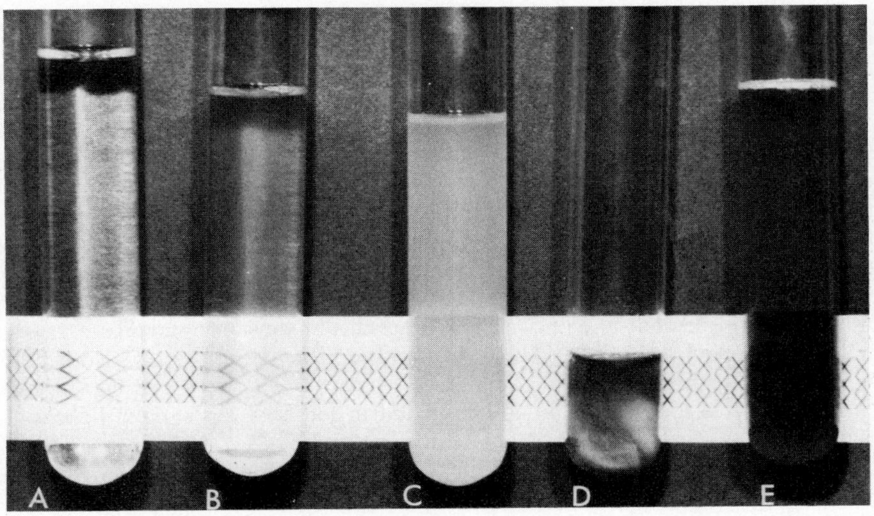


**Figure 38–1.** Synovial effusions. *A*, Normal or edema fluid is clear, pale yellow, or colorless. Print is easily read through the tube. *B*, Fluid from noninflammatory joint disease is yellow and clear. *C*, An inflammmatory effusion is cloudy and yellow. Print may be blurred or completely obliterated, depending on the number of leukocytes. The effusion is translucent. *D*, A purulent effusion from septic arthritis contains a dense clump that does not even allow light through the many leukocytes. *E*, Hemorrhagic fluid is red. The supernatant may be darker yellow-brown (xanthochromic). A traumatic tap is less uniform and often has blood streaks.

Leukocyte counts of 200 to 2000 per cubic millimeter have generally been termed noninflammatory. Actually, truly normal joint fluid usually has only up to 50 WBC per cubic millimeter, so that counts over 200 clearly represent at least a low-grade inflammatory response, which is seen, for example, in some patients with osteoarthritis. Patients who have predominantly degenerative arthritis, as in hemochromatosis, can have "inflammatory" effusions with high WBCs if associated chondrocalcinosis leads to crystal-induced arthritis. The significance of occasional erythrocytes has not been evaluated. Noncrenated red cells may have been introduced by the arthrocentesis.

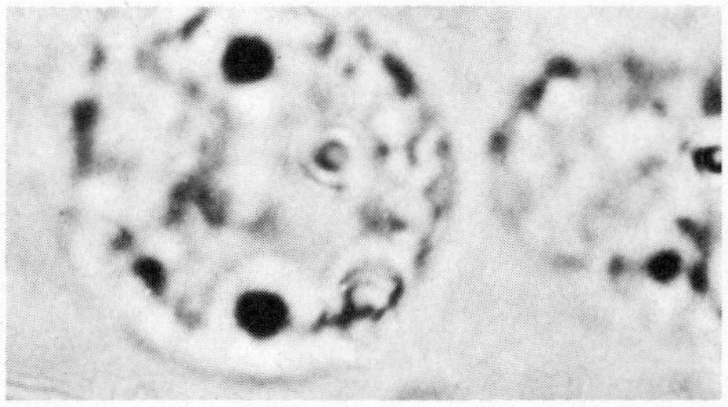

**Figure 38–3.** Synovial fluid leukocytes with cytoplasmic inclusions, "ragocytes," that have been felt to represent phagocytic vacuoles. Inclusions can appear pale or dark depending on focus.

## MICROSCOPIC STUDIES

**Wet Preparation.** Probably the single most important step in synovial fluid analysis is prompt microscopic examination of a fresh drop of synovial fluid as a wet preparation. Even if only a single drop of fluid is obtained with aspiration, this can be examined for crystals and other constituents as a wet preparation and then the same fluid allowed to dry for staining with Gram's stain if required. Express 1 to 3 drops of unadulterated synovial fluid from the syringe or transfer the fluid with a flamed loop onto a clean glass slide. We usually examine uncentrifuged fluids, but examination of a button after centrifugation can help concentrate rare crystals or cells in a clear-appearing fluid. Dirty slides can be washed in acetone and air dried. Lens paper used to clean slides can introduce birefringent paper fibrils.

Cover the drops of synovial fluid with a glass cover slip. If any delay is expected before examination, the cover slip margins may be sealed with nail polish. This allows several hours of delay, but slides may still dry out and produce birefringent drying artifacts if left overnight. Remember that the nail polish at the margins is birefringent with polarized light.

***Regular Light Microscopy.*** First examine each joint fluid with regular light microscopy. Red and white cells can be noted and their numbers estimated. Fragments of cartilage can be seen and, if numerous enough, concentrated by centrifugation and fixed for staining as a biopsy. Some leukocytes will be seen to contain cytoplasmic inclusions (Fig. 38–3) that have been felt to represent distended phagosomes and/or lipid droplets. Such cytoplasmic inclusion-containing cells[7] or "ragocytes" were first detected in rheumatoid arthritis but are also seen in other inflammatory arthropathies. Staining with fluorescein-conjugated antibodies to immunoglobulins and complement has shown these materials in vacuoles of some synovial fluid cells in rheumatoid arthritis and other diseases.

Erythrocytes may be noted to be sickled in patients with sickle cell disease or trait, but this does not establish that their current effusion is due to the sickle cell disease.

A variety of fibrillar materials can be seen in joint fluids. Some of these fibrils are fibrin, whereas others can be shown to be collagen from synovium or cartilage fragments.[8,9] Such fibrils (and crystals) can often be seen better by lowering the condenser or closing the diaphragm to produce a partial phase effect. Both collagen and fibrin are faintly birefringent. Ferrography has also been used to concentrate and analyze cartilage wear fragments.[10] Dark, irregularly shaped metal fragments can be seen in effusions of patients with implant arthroplasties.[6] Polymer fragments might also be seen.[11] The rare shards of ochronotic cartilage are yellow or ochre fragments with regular transmitted light microscopy[12] (Fig. 38–4, Plate IV, p. xxxviii).

Large numbers of lipid droplets may be noted in traumatic arthritis,[13,14] in inflammatory effusions of various types, including some otherwise unexplained effusions,[15] and in pancreatic fat necrosis,[16] or a few droplets can simply result from the arthrocentesis. Fat droplets should rise to the top of a spun specimen. Oil red O will stain lipid red. The origin and full significance of lipid droplets is not yet clear. In trauma some lipid presumably comes from marrow and synovium. Marrow spicules may be found if fracture into the joint has occurred. Such spicules tend to adhere to glass and must be sought carefully.[17]

Amorphous globular and irregular material, usually without birefringence, can be seen and can be due to amyloid masses[18] in patients with primary amyloid, multiple myeloma, and Waldenström's macroglobulinemia. Congo red will stain this pink or red on the wet preparation. Other globular or "coinlike" clumps can be seen from hydroxyapatite aggregates in joint and bursa fluids.[19] Apatite often appears to be phlogistic in bursae and joints.

Crystals can be noted with regular light microscopy and may be especially well seen with the illumination low or with the help of phase microscopy. Urate crystals are often acicular but may be blunt rods. Calcium pyrophosphate crystals can be rods or rhomboids. Other crystals also occasionally occur in joint fluids. All these crystals can be further differentiated with compensated polarized light.

***Compensated Polarized Light Microscopy.***[20,21] In a polarized light microscope, ordinary incandescent light is oriented in a single plane by a polarizer over the light source. When a second polarizer is added and rotated

90 degrees to the first, all light is blocked and the microscope field viewed through the ocular appears totally dark. If crystalline (birefringent) material is placed in the light path between the polarizers, light is deflected and split into fast and slow rays vibrating at different angles from the incident light. The vibration planes of these two new rays are mutually perpendicular, but neither is parallel to the original ray of plane polarized light. Some of these rays now pass through the second polarizer (also termed the analyzer) and are brightly visible on the dark field. This brightness is common to all birefringent material.

In clinical use different birefringent materials such as crystals can be distinguished in part by the altered behavior of light that passes through another birefringent structure (the compensator) placed between the first polarizer and the specimen. The compensator generally used is a "first order red plate," which eliminates green from the background and produces a rose-colored, instead of black, background field. The first order red compensator quality and thickness can be expressed numerically as 540 nm. If the slow ray of a birefringent crystal is parallel to the slow ray from the compensator, the additive effect of a urate or pyrophosphate crystal creates a value of about 700 nm and a blue color. If the same crystal is now rotated 90 degrees so that its fast ray is parallel to the compensator's slow ray, a color subtraction of the same number of nanometers will give a yellow color.

Monosodium urate crystals can be differentiated from calcium pyrophosphate dihydrate (CPPD) because with urate crystals the fast ray is in the long axis of the crystal, giving a yellow color when the crystal axis is parallel to the slow ray of the compensator. This is termed a negative optical sign or negative birefringence. CPPD crystals have their slow ray in the long axis of the crystal, and thus when parallel to the axis of slow vibration of the compensator they appear blue.

Monosodium urate crystals of gout tend to be 3 to 20$\mu$ long, rod or needle shaped, and very brightly negatively birefringent (Fig. 38–5, Plate IV, p. xxxviii). Crystals are generally identifiable within cells during active gouty arthritis. Crystals obtained from puncturing a tophus in a joint or elsewhere are often longer needles that are predominantly extracellular. Calcium pyrophosphate crystals have a weaker birefringence, are rarely as long as urates, are often rhomboid, and normally exhibit a blue color when the crystal axis is parallel to the slow ray of the compensator (i.e., positive optical sign or positive birefringence) (Fig. 38–6, Plate IV, p. xxxviii).

A variety of other birefringent materials will be seen on polarized light examinations of joint fluids. Depot corticosteroid preparations are crystalline[22] and can remain in joints or adjacent connective tissue for long periods after local injections. These crystals can be phagocytized and occasionally induce a transient inflammation several hours after intra-articular injections (Fig. 38–7), Plate V, p. xxxix). Corticosteroid crystals can appear as positively or negatively birefringent rods similar in size to urates or CPPD, as granules, or as irregular debris. Most other irregular birefringent material is artifact, such as dust from the slide or cover slip. Powder from rubber gloves is birefringent and generally shows a Maltese cross appearance.

Erroneous use of an oxalate[23] or lithium heparin[24] anticoagulant can introduce anticoagulant-derived crystals. Such crystals can be phagocytized by leukocytes in vitro and can thus be seen intracellulary. Oxalate and lithium heparin crystals are positively birefringent.

Cholesterol crystals can be seen in chronic joint effusions, especially in rheumatoid arthritis.[25] Crystals are usually platelike with a notch in one corner (Fig. 38–8, Plate V, p. xxxix) and larger than a cell, but crystals in cholesterol-laden effusions can occasionally also be negatively birefringent needles. Oxalate crystals recently described in joint effusions of patients with chronic renal failure may be pleomorphic but typically include some large bipyramidal forms.[26]

Calcium hydrogen phosphate dihydrate crystals are brightly positively birefringent and have been identified in joint fluids and tissues.[27,28] These crystals might be confused with CPPD and can only be definitely differentiated by x-ray diffraction. Apatite crystal clumps occasionally have some birefringence.

Commercial polarizing microscopes are readily available and should generally be used.[20] One can also obtain polarizing filters to be inserted in a regular light microscope. One filter is placed between the light source and condenser; another is placed above the objective or in the eyepiece. Filters are rotated until a black field is obtained. This produces the white birefringence that shows crystals more easily than ordinary light but cannot separate positive and negative birefringence. An effect similar to that obtained with a commercial compensated polarizing microscope can be achieved by applying two layers of cellophane tape to the top of a clean glass slide and placing this over the polarizing filter above the light source.[29,30] The long axis of the slide then is substituted for the axis of slow vibration of the first order red compensator. Some variation has been noted with different tapes; newer tapes that appear semiopaque before use do not appear to work. Before using such a set-up, findings should be clinically compared on several crystals with the findings using a commercial compensator.

Absolutely definitive diagnosis of crystals is made only by x-ray diffraction, but sufficient numbers of crystals are needed for this. Uricase digestion may be helpful in that urates but not other crystals will be digested with uricase.[31] Fortunately this is rarely required. Occasionally crystals of urate or CPPD are so few or so small that they are detected only by electron microscopy.(EM)[32,33] Urate crystals are dissolved out in usual electron microscopic preparations, but CPPD crystals are not. Individual apatite crystals can only be seen by EM. Electron diffraction or electron probe analysis can be done on such crystals, but techniques for this are less well standardized than those for x-ray diffraction.[19] Infrared spectroscopy using Fourier transformation or electron microscopy can identify small amounts of crystals mixed with other predominant crystals.

**Dried Smears for Staining.** Synovial smears are made using 1 to 2 drops of heparinized fluid on slides or coverslips in the same manner as with peripheral blood smears. If the leukocyte count is greater than approximately 5000, a good smear can generally be made from the whole fluid. Fluids with lower counts often produce better smears if the fluid is centrifuged and the button is resuspended in a few drops of the supernatant before smearing. It should be allowed to air dry.

***Wright's Stain.*** For this single most useful stain, cover the smear with Wright's stain and let it stand for 2 minutes. Add distilled water to the stain on the slide until a metallic sheen appears. Let this stand 4 to 5 minutes, wash with distilled water, air dry, and examine.

Smears should be examined briefly under low magnifications to look for such findings as LE cells. LE cells have so far been reported frequently in systemic lupus erythematosus and only very rarely in rheumatoid arthritis, but they need not be present in typical systemic lupus erythematosus. Round, homogeneous hematoxylin bodies might also suggest lupus erythematosus, although their specificity has not been evaluated in synovial fluids. Cartilage and synovial fragments may be seen and should be examined for any characteristic changes. Iron-laden chondrocytes have been seen in a cartilage fragment in hemochromatosis. Blue to brown pigmented debris or brown cytoplasmic granules can be seen in ochronosis. Bone marrow spicules with fat cells or other marrow elements may also be seen.

The smear is next examined carefully under oil immersion. Cells can be separated into polymorphonuclear leukocytes, monocytes, small lymphocytes, and large mononuclear cells. The latter probably include some transformed lymphocytes, monocytes, and synovial lining cells. Although classification of individual large mononuclear cells may be difficult, it may be worth attempting, since transformed lymphocytes are seen in rheumatoid arthritis and not in acute gout or pseudogout.[34] Other diseases have received insufficient study. Synovial lining cells (Fig. 38–9, Plate V, p. xxxix) typically are 20 to 40 $\mu$ in diameter, with an eccentric nucleus that occupies less than 50 percent of the cytoplasm. Some large monocyte-derived cells are similar in size, although they often have larger nuclei. These two large mononuclear cells can best distinguished with nonspecific esterase or Sudan black stains,[35] since these stains are positive in monocytes but not in most lining cells. Other large cells (15 to 25 $\mu$ in diameter) that have nuclei filling the majority of the cytoplasm and are Sudan negative are the transformed lymphocytes or lymphoblasts (Fig. 38–10, Plate V, p. xxxix). Both the lining cells and lymphoblasts often have prominent nucleoli. Mononuclear cells in joint fluid can now also be classified by monoclonal antibodies.[36] The percentage of polymorphonuclear cells (PMN) is helpful in distinguishing some diseases (see Table 38–4). Among the inflammatory effusions, lower polymorphonuclear cell counts have been seen in early rheumatoid arthritis, systemic lupus erythematosus, rheumatic fever, scleroderma, and chronic infections such as tuberculosis. Lining cells or large monocytes can be seen to have phagocytized polymorphonuclear leukocytes in a variety of diseases in which there are both exudation of neutrophils and lining cell proliferation. Such cells are common in Reiter's syndrome but are by no means diagnostic (Fig. 38–11). A variety of unidentified cells are also seen. These require further study, as they may be clues to presently unrecognized processes or mechanisms occurring in some patients. Dark purple inclusions in phagocytic cells can be from cell debris but also can be clumps of apatite crystals. Bacteria can occasionally be seen in cells even with Wright's stain. Urate or calcium pyrophosphate crystals can often be seen in Wright's stained specimens, although the urates are dissolved out of some smears.

Eosinophils are uncommon in differential counts, having been reported after arthrography with just air or contrast medium,[37,38] but also occasionally in a variety of other effusions.[37] Malignant cells can occasionally be identified in synovial fluid with Wright's or the Papanicolaou stain.[39]

***Gram's Stain.*** Smears for Gram's stain are made as for Wright's stain. Sometimes the addition of a single drop of serum to the slide prior to the drying stage allows better adherence of organisms. Flame the smear, specimen side down, three times through a blue flame. Let it cool and then flood the slide with crystal violet for 1 minute. Wash the slide with water, then flood with Gram's iodine and let it stand for 2 minutes. Pour off the iodine and wash the slide with 95 percent alcohol until it runs off clear. Flood the slide with Safranin for 30 seconds, wash it with water, and air dry. Bacteria can be quickly classified into broad groups, but mucin artifacts can be confusing. The absence of bacteria on Gram's stain is much too common in infection and does not rule out a septic joint.

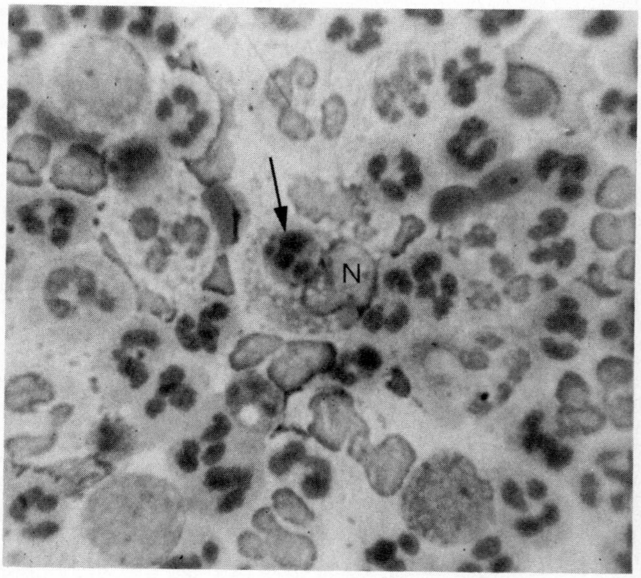


**Figure 38–11.** "Reiter's cell." This is a phagocytic mononuclear cell with its nucleus marked (N) that has phagocytized a polymorpho nuclear leukocyte (arrow) with a pyknotic nucleus.

*Other Stains.* Ziehl-Neelsen stain may be helpful in evaluation of possible tuberculosis, although cultures and synovial biopsy are often needed. Fat stains and alcian blue–PAS stains for proteoglycans (mucopolysaccharide) may show deposition of these materials in synovial macrophages. Other stains that may be useful include a Prussian blue stain that may show iron in synovial lining cells in pigmented villonodular synovitis or in hemochromatosis.

Amyloid deposits stained with Congo red show an apple-green birefringence on polarized light examination of wet smears of synovial fluid or of paraffin-embedded specimens.

The Von Kossa stain or Alizarin red S[40] will stain calcium- and phosphate-containing CPPD crystals or clumps of apatite crystals.

## SPECIAL TESTS

**Mucin Clot Test.**[41] Several drops of synovial fluid are added to about 20 ml of 5 percent acetic acid in a small beaker. Allow 1 minute for a "clot" to form and then shake the beaker. A good clot from normal or osteoarthritic fluid forms a firm mass that does not fragment on shaking. A poor clot, like those that result from many inflammatory effusions, fragments easily and forms flakes, shreds, and cloudiness in the surrounding fluid. Effusions from patients with systemic lupus erythematosus and rheumatic fever, although mildly inflammatory, often have good mucin clots.

Good mucin generally reflects the normal integrity of hyaluronate. Poor mucin indicates both dilution and destruction of hyaluronate protein (see Table 38–4). Unfortunately the mucin test and viscosity give only rough clues and are not as reliable as leukocyte counts in classification of effusions.

*Glucose.* Synovial fluid glucose can be measured by the standard Somogyi-Nelson true glucose method or the ortho-toluidine method and should be done simultaneously on fasting serum and synovial fluid for comparison[41] (see Table 38–4). Synovial fluid glucose concentration is normally very slightly less than that of blood glucose. Equilibration between blood and synovial fluid after a meal is slow and unpredictable, so that fasting levels are most reliable. Effusions for glucose should be placed in a fluoride tube to stop glucose metabolism in vitro by the synovial fluid leukocytes, which would further lower the glucose level. Glucose measurements should not have a high priority, but a very low level of glucose in the synovial fluid suggests joint infection. Most effusions in rheumatoid arthritis have a synovial fluid sugar level of less than half that of the blood, and some will be near zero.

*Complement.* Total hemolytic complement is determined by the technique of Kabat and Mayer.[42,43] Synovial fluid complement is predominantly of value when compared with serum levels and with serum and synovial fluid protein determinations. Fluid must be centrifuged promptly and the supernatant stored at −70° C. In rheumatoid arthritis the serum complement is usually normal, while the synovial fluid level is often less than 30 percent of this.

In systemic lupus erythematosus and hepatitis both serum and synovial fluid levels may be low. Synovial fluid complement levels in infectious arthritis, gout, and Reiter's syndrome may be high, but this is largely due to elevated serum levels. Beta$_1$ globulin can also be measured by immunodiffusion in addition to or instead of hemolytic complement. Prompt storage at −70° C is not as critical with this. It is useful to measure serum and synovial fluid protein[44] and globulin levels when evaluating complement, because synovial fluid complement may be very low in normal or noninflammatory fluids in which there is little escape of complement or other proteins into the joint space from the circulation.

**Cultures.** Prompt and careful culture of synovial fluid is very important if there is any suspicion of infection. Most bacteria will grow well in tryptic soy broth or sheep blood agar. Planting the cultures at the time of aspiration may be useful if prompt transport and handling in the laboratory cannot be assured. Try to obtain laboratory help in planning cultures needed. If certain organisms are a possibility, specific media are necessary. If anaerobic organisms are suspected, expel any air from the syringe and use anaerobic transport medium and/or take the fluid directly to the laboratory for planting on prereduced anaerobically sterile blood agar or a comparable culture medium.

Gonococci can be successfully cultured in only 25 to 30 percent of cases of apparent gonococcal arthritis. When this is suspected, plate the fluid immediately on chocolate agar or Thayer-Martin medium and have the culture continued in the laboratory under $CO_2$. There are $CO_2$ transport systems if delay is expected. If a mixed infection is possible, Thayer-Martin medium should retard the growth of organisms other than gonococci.

For suspected fungal infections the fluid should be transported in a sterile tube and processed in the laboratory for culture on Sabouraud's dextrose agar. Lowenstein-Jensen medium is used for mycobacterial infections.

**Other Tests.** Antinuclear factors, rheumatoid factor, immunoglobulins, and other substances involved in immune reactions can be measured in synovial fluid, but these assays have so far added little to the simple studies described here. Antinuclear factors, for example, are seen in synovial effusions in many conditions in which they are not identifiable in serum. Latex fixation tests for rheumatoid factor are occasionally positive in effusions when negative in the serum. However, the significance of such positive synovial fluids is not established. Several causes for false-positive tests for rheumatoid factor in synovial fluid have been described.[45] Immune complexes can be measured with a variety of techniques but are still largely investigational.

Other studies are not of much diagnostic value. The pH of normal fluid is 7.4, and this is slightly lower in inflammation.[46] Joint fluid $pO_2$ also falls in many inflammatory conditions. This tends to correlate with severity of leukocytosis and also with synovial fluid volume, which may lower $pO_2$ by affecting blood flow to the joint.[47] Total protein normally averages only 1.7 g per dl, but rises with inflammation. Uric acid, electrolytes, and urea nitrogen tend to reflect the serum values. Fibrinogen and its products are normally absent, so that normal fluid does not clot upon standing. Bence Jones kappa light chains have been demonstrated in amyloid arthropathy secondary to multiple myeloma. For research lymphokines, fibronectin, proteinases, and prostaglandins can be assayed in joint fluid.

Gas chromatography on synovial fluid has been suggested as an aid in identifying bacterial products in culture-negative infections.[48] Elevated synovial fluid lactic acid measurements have been found in untreated nongonococcal septic arthritis.[49] Succinic acid levels are also elevated in septic arthritis and tend to persist even after treatment.[50] Neither lactic nor succinic acid is specific for infection but may complement other tests for early diagnosis of infectious arthritis. Bacterial antigens can also be sought in synovial fluid by counter immunoelectrophoresis.

## References


1. Agudelo, C.A., Weinberger, A., Schumacher, H.R., Turner, R., and Molina, J.: Definitive diagnosis of gout by identification of urate crystals in asymptomatic metatarsophalangeal joints. Arthritis Rheum. 22:559, 1979.
2. Bitter, T., and Muir, H.M.: A modified uronic acid carbazole reaction. Anal. Biochem. 4:330, 1962.
3. Hasselbacher, P.: Measuring synovial fluid viscosity with a white blood cell diluting pipette. Arthritis Rheum. 19:1358, 1978.
4. Palmer, D.G.: Total leukocyte enumeration in pathologic synovial fluids. Am. J. Clin. Pathol. 49:812, 1968.
5. Hunter, T., Gordon, D.A., and Ogryzlo, M.A.: The ground pepper sign of synovial fluid; a new diagnostic feature of ochronosis. J. Rheum. 1:45, 1974.
6. Kitridou, R., Schumacher, H.R., Sbarbaro, J.L., and Hollander, J.L.: Recurrent hemarthrosis after prosthetic knee arthroplasty: Identification of metal particles in the synovial fluid. Arthritis Rheum. 12:520, 1969.
7. Hollander, J.L., McCarty, D.J., and Rawson, A.J.: The "RA cell," "ragocyte," or "inclusion body cell." Bull. Rheum. Dis. 16:382, 1965.
8. Kitridou, R., McCarty, D.J., Prockop, D.J., and Hummeler, K.: Identification of collagen in synovial fluid. Arthritis Rheum. 12:580, 1969.
9. Cheung, H.S., Ryan, L.M., Kozin, F., and McCarty, D.J.: Identification of collagen subtypes in synovial fluid sediments from arthritic patients. Am. J. Med. 68:73, 1980.
10. Evans, C.H., Mears, D.C., and Stanitski, C.L.: Ferrographic analysis of wear in human joints. J. Bone Joint Surg. 64B:572, 1982.
11. Crugnola, A., Schillar, A., and Radin, E.: Polymeric debris in synovium after total joint replacement: Histological identification. J. Bone Joint Surg. 59A:860, 1977.
12. Schumacher, H.R., and Holdsworth, D.E.: Ochronotic arthropathy. I. Clinicopathologic studies. Semin. Arthritis Rheum. 6:207, 1977.
13. Graham, J., and Goldman, J.A.: Fat droplets and synovial fluid leukocytes in traumatic arthritis. Arthritis Rheum. 21:76, 1978.
14. Weinberger, A., Schumacher, H.R.: Experimental joint trauma: Synovial response to blunt trauma and inflammatory response to intra-articular injection of fat. J. Rheum. 8:380–389, 1981.
15. Reginato, A.J., Schumacher, H.R., Allan, D., and Rabinowitz, J.L.: Acute monoarthritis with lipid liquid crystals. Arthritis Rheum. 25:S35, 1982 (Abst).
16. Gibson, T., Schumacher, H.R., Pascual, E., and Brighton, C.: Arthropathy, skin and bone lesions in pancreatic disease. J. Rheum. 2:7, 1975.
17. Lawrence, C., and Seife, B.: Bone marrow in joint fluid: A clue to fracture. Ann. Intern. Med. 74:740, 1971.
18. Gordon, O.A., Pruzanski, W., and Ogryzlo, M.A.: Synovial fluid examination from the diagnosis of amyloidosis. Ann. Rheum. Dis. 32:428, 1973.
19. Schumacher, H.R., Somlyo, A.P., Tse, R.L., and Maurer, K.: Apatite crystal associated arthritis. Ann. Intern. Med. 87:411, 1977.
20. Phelps, P., Steele, A.D., and McCarty, D.J.: Compensated polarized light microscopy. JAMA 203:508, 1968.
21. Gatter, R.A.: Use of the compensated polarizing microscope. Clin. Rheum. Dis. 3:91, 1977.
22. Kahn, C.B., Hollander, J.L., and Schumacher, H.R.: Corticosteroid crystals in synovial fluid. JAMA 211:807, 1970.
23. Schumacher, H.R.: Intracellular crystals in synovial fluid anticoagulated with oxalate. N. Engl. J. Med. 274:1372, 1966.
24. Tanphaichitr, K., Spilberg, I., and Hahn, B.: Lithium heparin crystals simulating calcium pyrophosphate dihydrate crystals in synovial fluid. Arthritis Rheum. 19:966, 1976 (letter).
25. Zuckner, J., Uddin, J., Gantner, G.E., and Dorner, R.W.: Cholesterol crystals in synovial fluid. Ann. Intern. Med. 60:436, 1964.
26. Hoffman, G., Schumacher, H.R., Paul, H., Cherian, V., Reed, R., Ramsay, A., and Franck, W.: Calcium oxalate microcrystalline associated arthritis in end stage renal disease. Ann. Int. Med. 97:36–42, 1982.
27. Moskowitz, R.W., Harris, B.K., Schwartz, A., and Marshall, G.: Chronic synovitis as a manifestation of calcium crystal deposition disease. Arthritis Rheum. 14:109, 1971.
28. Gaucher, A., Faure, G., Netter, P., Pourel, J., and Duheille, J.: Identification des cristaux observés dans les arthropathies destructrices de la chondrocalcinose. Rev. Rheum. 44:407, 1977.
29. Owen, D.S.: A cheap and useful compensated polarizing microscope. N. Engl. J. Med. 285:115, 1971.
30. Fagan, T.J., and Lidsky, M.D.: Compensated polarized light microscopy using cellophane adhesive tape. Arthritis Rheum. 17:256, 1974.
31. McCarty, D.J., and Hollander, J.L.: Identification of urate crystals in gouty synovial fluid. Ann. Intern. Med. 54:452, 1961.
32. Schumacher, H.R., Jimenez, S.A., Gibson, T., Pascual, E., Traycoff, R.B., Dorwart, B.B., and Reginato, A.J.: Acute gouty arthritis without urate crystals identified on initial examination of synovial fluid. Arthritis Rheum. 18:603, 1975.
33. Honig, S., Gorevic, P., Hoffstein, S., and Weissmann, G.: Crystal deposition disease, diagnosis by electron microscopy. Am. J. Med. 63:161, 1977.
34. Traycoff, R.B., Pascual, E., and Schumacher, H.R.: Mononuclear cells in human synovial fluid. Identification of lymphoblasts in rheumatoid arthritis. Arthritis Rheum. 19:743, 1976.
35. Shehan, H., and Storey, G.: An improved method of staining leukocyte granules with Sudan black. Br. J. Pathol. Bacteriol. 59:336, 1947.
36. Duclos, M., Zeidler, H., Liman, W., Pichler, W.J., Rieber, P., and Peter, H.H.: Characterization of blood and synovial fluid lymphocytes from patients with rheumatoid arthritis and other joint diseases by monoclonal antibodies (OKT Series) and acid $\alpha$-naphthyl esterase staining. Rheum. Internat. 2:75, 1982.
37. Hasselbacher, P., and Schumacher, H.R.: Synovial fluid eosinophilia following arthrography. J. Rheum. 5:173, 1978.
38. Murray, R.C., and Forrai, E.: Transitory eosinophilia localized in the knee joint after pneumarthrography. J. Bone Joint Surg. 32B:74, 1950.
39. Fam, A.G., Kolin, A., and Lewis, A.J.: Metastatic carcinomatous arthritis and carcinoma of the lung. J. Rheum. 7:98, 1980.
40. Paul, H., Reginato, A.J., and Schumacher, H.R.: Alizarin red S staining as a screening test to detect calcium compounds in synovial fluid. Arthritis Rheum. 26:191, 1983.
41. Ropes, M.M., and Bauer, W.: Synovial Fluid Changes in Joint Disease. Cambridge, Mass., Harvard University Press, 1953.
42. Pekin, I., and Zvaifler, N.J.: Hemolytic complement in synovial fluid. J. Clin. Invest. 43:1372, 1964.
43. Townes, A.S., and Sowa, J.M.: Complement in synovial fluid. Johns Hopkins Med. J. 125:23, 1970.
44. Bunch, T.W., Hunder, G.G., McDuffie, F.C., O'Brien, P.C., and Markowitz, H.: Synovial fluid complement determination as a diagnostic aid in inflammatory joint disease. Mayo Clin. Proc. 49:715, 1974.
45. Seward, C.W., and Osterland, C.K.: The pattern of anti-immunoglobulin activities in serum, pleural and synovial fluids. J. Lab. Clin. Med. 81:230, 1973.
46. Ward, T.T.: Acidosis of synovial fluid correlates with synovial fluid leukocytosis. Am. J. Med. 64:933, 1978.
47. Richman, A.I., Su, E.Y., and Ho, G.: Reciprocal relationship of synovial fluid volume and oxygen tension. Arthritis Rheum. 24:701, 1981.
48. Brooks, J.B., Kellogg, D.S., Alley, C.C., Short, H.B., Handsfield, H.H., and Huff, B.: Gas chromatography as a potential means of diagnosing arthritis. I. Differentiation between staphylococcal, streptococcal, gonococcal and traumatic arthritis. J. Infect. Dis. 129:660, 1974.
49. Brook, I.: Abnormalities in synovial fluid of patients with septic arthritis detected by gas-liquid chromatography. Ann. Rheum. Dis. 39:168, 1980.
50. Borenstein, D.G., Gibbs, C.A., and Jacobs, R.P.: Gas-liquid chromatographic analysis of synovial fluid. Arthritis Rheum. 25:947, 1982.

# Chapter 39
# Radiographic Evaluation of Articular Disorders

*Robert O. Cone, III, and Donald Resnick*

## INTRODUCTION

The radiographic examination is a keystone in the diagnosis and management of the patient with articular disease. In some patients the diagnosis may initially be suggested by radiographic techniques, while in other patients with a known clinical diagnosis, the extent and the severity of the disease process may be documented by such techniques. Furthermore, serial radiographic examinations provide evidence of the therapeutic response of the disease process.

In this chapter we will discuss radiographic techniques and modalities and cardinal roentgen signs of articular disease as well as the radiographic findings at specific "target" areas of the major articular disorders.

## RADIOGRAPHIC TECHNIQUES AND MODALITIES

**Plain Film Examination.** Appropriately selected plain films form the initial step in the radiologic evaluation of articular disease. The choice of radiographic projections for each anatomic area is a decision that deserves careful consideration. The need for a comprehensive examination to document the extent and configuration of the disease must be balanced with the consideration of expense, comfort, and radiation exposure to the patient, who may be expected to have numerous radiographic examinations over many years.

In most cases multiple radiographic projections of a number of joints are indicated. In Table 39–1, the suggested radiographic projections for the optimal evaluation of specific anatomic areas are listed. In the patient with monoarticular or pauciarticular disease, such a list may be closely followed. In the patient with polyarticular disease, however, obtaining the numerous radiographic views listed in Table 39–1 would be considered excessive in almost all cases. In these patients the initial radiographic examination should be individually tailored to as great an extent as is possible.

A "tailored" arthritis series is useful in those patients with polyarthritis who have either a known or a highly likely clinical diagnosis. In this setting, plain films are selected that most optimally visualize the major "target" areas of the disease as well as additional areas of clinical significance. For example, the patient with rheumatoid arthritis requires careful radiographic evaluation of the hands, wrists, feet, knees, shoulders, and cervical spine, whereas the patient with calcium pyrophosphate dihydrate (CPPD) crystal deposition disease usually requires analysis of only the hands, wrists, knees, and symphysis pubis.

The situation often arises in which a patient has polyarthritis without a specific clinical diagnosis. In this case, a "standard" arthritis series is useful. In this radiographic series, projections are selected to provide adequate visualization of a large number of major target areas with a minimum of radiation exposure. A suggested standard arthritis series, consisting of fifteen radiographs, is listed in Table 39–2.

The follow-up radiographic examination obtained during the course of treatment does not need to be as extensive as the initial survey. In many cases it can be limited to a few symptomatic areas or areas where unsuspected progression of disease may lead to catastrophic consequences, such as the cervical spine in patients with rheumatoid arthritis.

The intensifying screen in a radiographic film cassette combined with double emulsion radiographic film allows formation of a radiographic image with considerably less radiation exposure to the patient. A small decrease in radiographic resolution, however, is the price that is paid for this considerable diminution in radiation exposure. Occasionally, in evaluating diseases such as rheumatoid

**Table 39–1.** Radiographic Projections

| | |
|---|---|
| Hand | Posteroanterior, oblique |
| Wrist | Posteroanterior, oblique, lateral |
| Elbow | Anteroposterior, lateral |
| Shoulder | Anteroposterior with internal rotation of the humerus; anteroposterior with external rotation of the humerus |
| Foot | Anteroposterior, oblique, lateral (including calcaneus) |
| Ankle | Anteroposterior, lateral |
| Knee | Anteroposterior, lateral, "tunnel" (anteroposterior in semiflexion), axial patellar ("sunrise") |
| Hip | Anteroposterior of pelvis, anteroposterior of hip with internal rotation of leg, anteroposterior of hip with external rotation of leg ("frog leg") |
| Sacroiliac Joint | Anteroposterior, anteroposterior with 30 degrees cephalic angulation of central ray |
| Lumbar Spine | Anteroposterior, obliques, lateral, lateral coned-down to L5-S1 |
| Thoracic Spine | Anteroposterior, lateral |
| Cervical Spine | Anteroposterior, obliques, lateral with neck in flexion, lateral with neck in extension, "open-mouth" odontoid view |

**Table 39–2.** Arthritis Survey

| | |
|---|---|
| Hand and Wrist | Posteroanterior, obliques |
| Feet | Anteroposterior (2), obliques (2), lateral (2) |
| Knees | Anteroposterior (2), lateral (2) |
| Pelvis and Hips | Anteroposterior |
| Thorax and Shoulders | Anteroposterior |
| Cervical Spine | Lateral with neck in flexion |

arthritis, osteomyelitis, septic arthritis, or hyperparathyroidism, increased resolution may be important in establishing a diagnosis at an early stage.[1-3] In these instances, increased radiation exposure to a relatively radioresistant area of the body, such as the hand, the wrist, or the foot, may be acceptable in order to obtain important diagnostic information. With virtually any radiographic unit, use of single emulsion film and a nonscreen vacuum-packed cassette will allow high-resolution images to be obtained. Furthermore, optical or radiographic magnification can be extremely helpful. In the latter case, these images may be obtained using microfocal spot radiographic tubes, such as are present on many angiographic units, or specially designed magnification units. It should be emphasized that these are specialized techniques and should be used only in selected clinical situations.

Radiographs of an articulation obtained during weight-bearing or the application of stress or traction may provide valuable supplemental information to the plain film radiographic examination. Weight-bearing views of the knees are especially useful in the evaluation of patients with osteoarthritis[4] and may allow a more exact delineation of cartilaginous loss as well as abnormal varus or valgus angulation of the joint. Stress radiographs may be utilized to assess soft tissue and bony stability following injury to the knee, ankle, acromioclavicular joint, or first metacarpophalangeal joint.[5] Upright lateral radiographs of the lumbar spine obtained after prolonged standing may accentuate bony neural arch defects (spondylolysis) or intervertebral slippage (spondylolisthesis). Radiographs of the pelvis obtained with the patient standing on one leg at a time may demonstrate instability of the sacroiliac joint or symphysis pubis.[6]

Radiographs obtained during application of traction across a joint may prove useful in selected circumstances. Subtle transchondral fractures in osteonecrosis of the femoral head may be accentuated with this technique.[7] Such traction may also stimulate the release of gas, primarily nitrogen, into the joint cavity, an occurrence that usually excludes the presence of a joint effusion and allows visualization of a portion of the cartilaginous surface.

**Conventional Tomography.** Conventional tomography can aid in the identification of subtle abnormalities as well as in the more precise delineation of previously identified lesions. In some anatomic areas, such as the temporomandibular, sternoclavicular, and costovertebral articulations, plain radiographs are rarely adequate and tomography is often indicated.

**Arthrography and Bursography.** Injection of radiopaque contrast material or air, or both, into a joint or bursa may be essential in evaluating a number of articular disorders.[8] Contrast arthrography is most often utilized in the knee and shoulder to identify surgically repairable soft tissue injuries such as meniscal or rotator cuff tears. Aspiration-arthrography allows confirmation of suspected joint sepsis; fluoroscopically guided intra-articular needle placement is particularly useful in recovering fluid from deep articulations such as the glenohumeral joint or the hip. Subsequent instillation of a small amount of radiographic contrast agent verifies that the joint space was indeed entered and may also yield important information concerning the extent of periarticular soft tissue destruction. Evaluation of the patient with a painful total hip prosthesis is an important indication for aspiration-arthrography to conclusively differentiate between chronic infection and aseptic loosening of the prosthesis.[9] Air arthrography, usually combined with conventional tomography, is often of great value in the identification of transchondral fractures as well as intra-articular osteocartilaginous bodies. Arthrography may also provide a firm diagnosis in cases of pigmented villonodular synovitis[10] or idiopathic synovial osteochondromatosis.[11]

Bursography has its greatest value in evaluating lesions of the subacromial bursa in the shoulder.[12,13] In this location, bursitis, intrabursal osteocartilaginous bodies, partial rotator cuff tears, and causes of shoulder impingement may be identified. At the same time, instillation of local anesthetic agents or anti-inflammatory medications directly into the bursa serves as both a diagnostic and a therapeutic procedure.

**Computed Tomography.** Computed axial tomography has only recently been applied to the evaluation of diseases of the musculoskeletal system. These diseases include sacroiliitis[14] and a number of vertebral disorders, such as spinal stenosis, apophyseal joint osteoarthritis, ossification of the posterior intraspinal ligaments, and intervertebral disc herniation.[15] Analysis of bone mineral content in the axial skeleton with computed tomography is now performed in many medical centers.[16]

## RHEUMATOID ARTHRITIS

Rheumatoid arthritis is a common disease whose features are familiar to most physicians. For this reason it tends to be the clinical and radiographic standard against which other arthritides are evaluated. A thorough understanding of the roentgenographic features of this important disease provides a firm basis for evaluating articular disease in general.

**General Distribution.** Rheumatoid arthritis demonstrates a propensity toward symmetric involvement of synovial articulations. In the appendicular skeleton, the hands, wrists, feet, knees, hips, shoulders, and elbows are frequently affected. The small joints of the hands and feet are the earliest and most frequent sites of radiographic changes. In the axial skeleton, involvement of the cervical spine is common, while thoracolumbar and sacroiliac joint involvement is uncommon. Cartilaginous articulations, such as the symphysis pubis and manubriosternal joints, and entheses, where ligaments and tendons attach to bone, may be involved in rheumatoid arthritis, but such involvement is both less frequent and less severe than in the seronegative spondyloarthopathies.

**General Radiographic Features.** ***Symmetry.*** The symmetry of rheumatoid arthritis constitutes an important diagnostic criterion for this disease. Asymmetric involvement may be noted in male patients and in men and women with early disease or neurologic deficit.[17]

***Osteoporosis.*** Osteoporosis is a characteristic feature of rheumatoid arthritis. Early in the course of the disease, it tends to be localized to the juxta-articular region of the small peripheral joints. Later, generalized osteoporosis may be present in the axial and appendicular skeleton, often exacerbated by medications (i.e., salicylates, corticosteroids) and disuse or immobilization. In a few patients with rheumatoid arthritis, osteomalacia may be observed.[18]

***Soft Tissue Changes.*** Radiographic changes in the soft tissues can be of diagnostic importance in the patient with rheumatoid arthritis. Diffuse (fusiform) periarticular soft tissue swelling (Fig. 39–1) is an early finding about the small joints of the hands and feet. Intra-articular effusions are common radiographic findings in the knees, elbows, and ankles, producing characteristic displacements of adjacent fat planes. Occasionally, similar effusions in the small joints of the hand may lead to mild joint space widening. Bursal involvement can be identified as asymmetric soft tissue prominence, particularly in the knee (prepatellar bursa), elbow (olecranon bursa), heel (retrocalcaneal bursa), and shoulder (subacromial bursa). Tendinitis and tenosynovitis are most frequently identified in the wrist when involvement of the extensor carpi ulnaris tendon and its synovial sheath causes prominent soft tissue swelling adjacent to the ulnar styloid process. Rheumatoid nodules may occasionally be observed on radiographs as noncalcified, eccentric, lobular soft tissue masses, which may cause pressure erosion of adjacent bones.

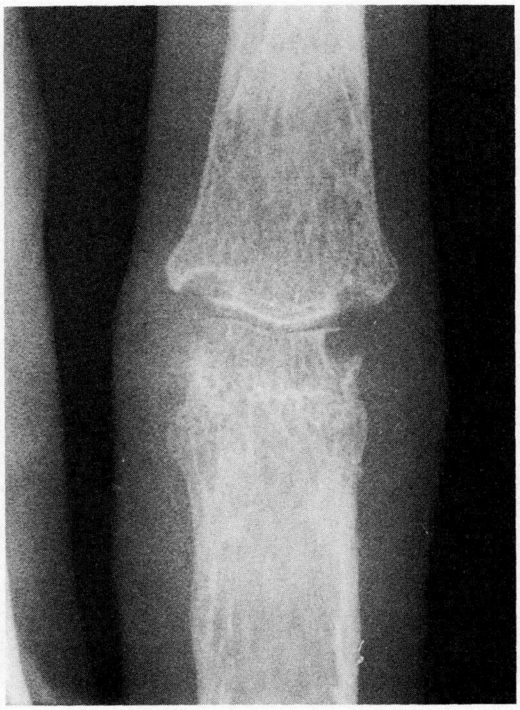

**Figure 39–1.** Rheumatoid arthritis. Marginal erosions are present on both sides of the interphalangeal joint. Joint space narrowing and fusiform soft tissue swelling are also evident.

***Joint Space Narrowing.*** Progressive joint space narrowing due to destruction of articular cartilage by pannus is another hallmark of rheumatoid arthritis, which may allow its differentiation from gout, a disease in which preservation of joint width is typical. In rheumatoid arthritis, the diffuse cartilaginous loss and the tendency toward pancompartmental involvement of complex joints, such as the knee and the wrist, limit additional diagnostic possibilities. Bony ankylosis is common only in the wrist and in the midfoot; it is distinctly unusual at other sites.

***Bony Erosions.*** Three types of bony erosions may be identified in rheumatoid arthritis. *Marginal erosions* occur at intra-articular sites that are not protected by overlying cartilage. Typically these "bare" areas are the initial points of attack by the proliferating synovial tissue (Fig. 39–1). *Compressive erosions* occur when collapse of osteoporotic subchondral bone leads to invagination of one bone into another. These changes occur at articulations exposed to strong muscular actions or significant weight-bearing forces. The most characteristic site of compressive erosion is the hip, where protrusio acetabuli may be identified (Fig. 39–2). Other important sites are at the metacarpophalangeal joints, where collapse of the base of a proximal phalanx by a metacarpal head produces a ball-in-socket-type articulation, and the radiocarpal joint of the wrist, where the scaphoid may appear to be "countersunk" into the distal radius. The third type of erosion seen in rheumatoid arthritis is *surface resorption,* usually related to inflammation of an adjacent tendon sheath (Fig. 39–3). This is an important finding in the wrist, where a characteristic erosion of the outer margin of the ulnar styloid process, due to externor carpi ulnaris tenosynovitis, provides an early radiographic sign of rheumatoid arthritis.

***Bony Cysts.*** Subchondral cystic lesions are frequent in rheumatoid arthritis and have been described as cysts, pseudocysts, geodes, and granulomas. Most commonly, multiple small, ill-defined subchondral radiolucencies are identified at any articulation involved in rheumatoid arthritis. The identification of larger cystic areas, especially in the hands and wrists of physically active men, has been termed rheumatoid arthritis of the robust reaction pattern.[19] Occasionally very large cystic lesions

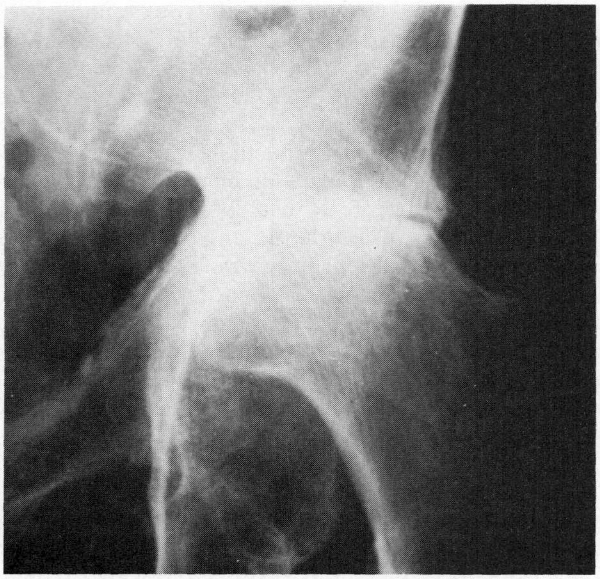

**Figure 39–2.** Rheumatoid arthritis. Symmetric destruction of the cartilaginous surface has resulted in axial migration of the femoral head. The femoral head has become small and flattened. Sclerosis is apparent.

may be encountered in the elbow (olecranon process of ulna, distal humerus), femoral neck, or knee (distal femur, proximal tibia, patella) and have been described as pseudocystic rheumatoid arthritis (Fig. 39–4).[20] These large lesions may subsequently fracture.

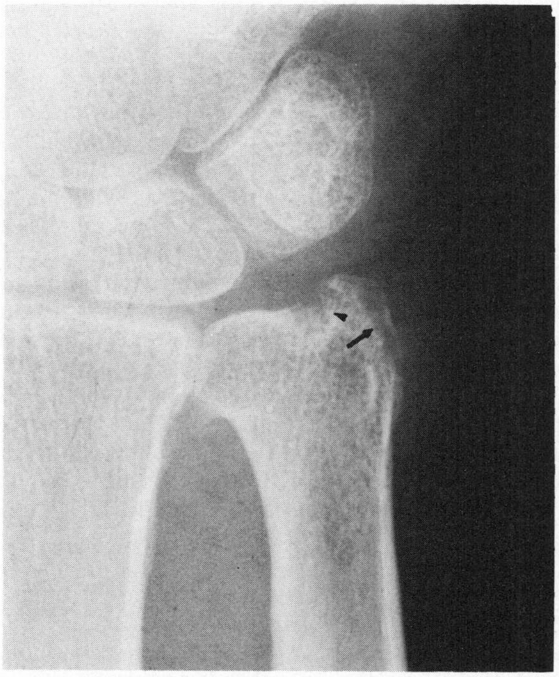

**Figure 39–3.** Rheumatoid arthritis. An osseous erosion is present in the lateral margin of the ulnar styloid (surface erosion) (arrow) due to synovitis of the extensor carpi ulnaris tendon sheath. A second erosion is present at the point of insertion of the triangular fibrocartilage on the ulnar head (arrowhead). (From Resnick, D., and Niwayama, G.: Diagnosis of Bone and Joint Disorders. Philadelphia, W.B. Saunders Co., 1981.)

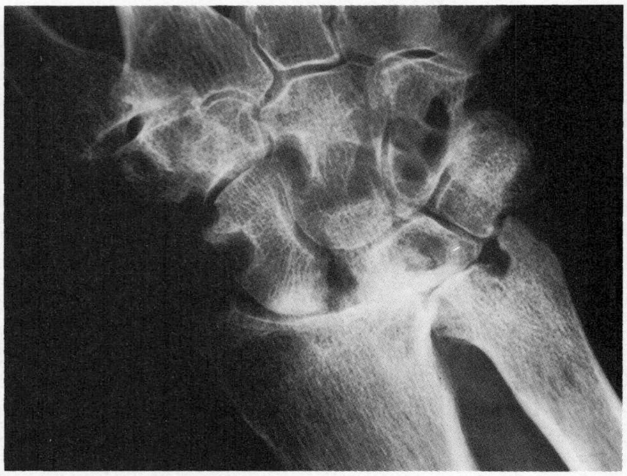

**Figure 39–4.** Pseudocystic rheumatoid arthritis. In this patient, large cystic erosions are present, giving the appearance of "hollow" carpal bones. Also note the narrowing of the radiocarpal joint with ulnar translocation of the carpus. (From Resnick, D., and Niwayama, G.: Diagnosis of Bone and Joint Disorders. Philadelphia, W.B. Saunders Co., 1981.)

***Deformities and Instabilities.*** Many types of articular deformity and instability are observed in rheumatoid arthritis (Fig. 39–5). Most of these relate to tendinous or ligamentous laxity or disruption, with alteration of the normal muscle pull across one or more articulations (e.g., boutonnière or swan-neck deformity of the fingers, ulnar deviation at the metacarpophalangeal joints, fibular deviation at the metatarsophalangeal joints, or at-

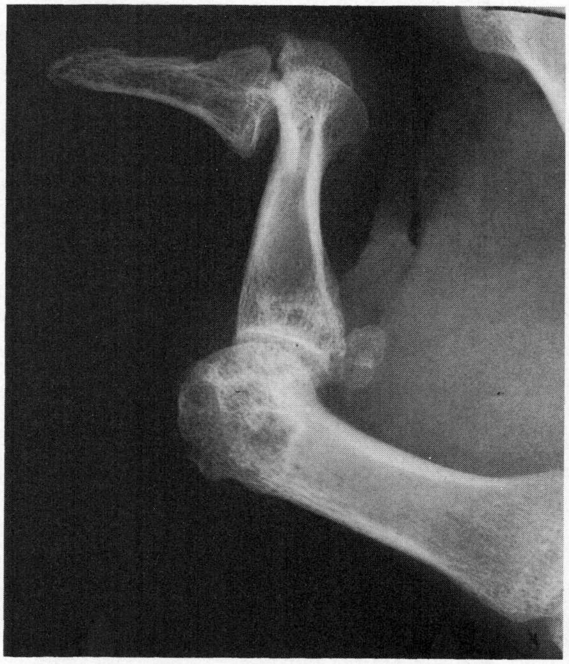

**Figure 39–5.** Rheumatoid arthritis. In this patient note the prominent thumb deformity with flexion at the metacarpophalangeal joint and extension of the interphalangeal joint. This constitutes the boutonnière deformity.

lanto-axial subluxation). In some cases, however, the abnormality may relate directly to bone or cartilage destruction (e.g., protrusio acetabuli). These characteristic deformities and instabilities are summarized in Table 39–3.

**Abnormalities at Specific Sites.** ***Hand.*** The target areas of rheumatoid arthritis in the hands are the metacarpophalangeal and proximal interphalangeal joints. The earliest changes consist of fusiform soft tissue swelling, juxta-articular osteoporosis, diffuse joint space loss, and marginal bony erosions (Fig. 39–1). A particularly characteristic finding is indistinctness and focal loss of continuity of the dorsoradial subchondral bone plate (dot-dash pattern) of the metacarpal head.[21] In general, these radiographic findings appear initially at the second and third metacarpophalangeal joints and third proximal interphalangeal joint. The marginal osseous erosions tend to be more prominent on the proximal bone of the articulation, which tends to have a larger bare area. With progression of the disease, large erosions, complete joint space obliteration, and finger deformities appear. The end stage is usually fibrous ankylosis of the articular cavity; bony ankylosis is rare in the hand but, when present, almost exclusively involves the proximal interphalangeal joints.[17]

**Wrist.** The wrist is a complex articulation that should properly be viewed as a series of distinct synovial compartments: (1) radiocarpal, (2) inferior radioulnar, (3) midcarpal, (4) pisotriquetral, (5) common carpometacarpal, and (6) first carpometacarpal. Rheumatoid arthritis demonstrates distinctive pancompartmental involvement of the wrist, which helps to differentiate it from other arthropathies.[22] The least commonly involved area is the first carpometacarpal compartment, which may be spared even in the presence of advanced disease elsewhere in the wrist.

The distal ulna, being bounded by three important sites of synovial proliferation, occupies a prominent role as a target area in rheumatoid arthritis[23] (Fig. 39–3). Erosions along the outer margin of the ulnar styloid are related to tenosynovitis of the extensor carpi ulnaris tendon; erosions of the styloid tip are related to involvement of the prestyloid recess of the radiocarpal compartment; and erosions of the base and juxta-articular area of the distal ulna indicate inferior radioulnar compartment involvement.

Early erosions may involve any bone in the wrist; in addition to the distal ulna, some of the more characteristic sites[24,25] include the radial styloid, lateral scaphoid waist, triquetrum, and pisiform. These changes may be manifested as distinct erosions or as cystic lesions which give the radiographic appearance of hollow carpal bones. With time, the characteristic pancompartmental involvement becomes evident with loss of articular spaces. Bony ankylosis of the carpus is a relatively common end result of advanced rheumatoid arthritis. In some cases diffuse carpal destruction may occur, culminating in complete disintegration of the wrist.

Numerous deformities related to soft tissue destruction and muscular imbalances may be seen. The most characteristic wrist deformities consist of ulnar translocation of the proximal carpal row, related to destruc-

**Table 39–3.** Instabilities and Deformities in Rheumatoid Arthritis

| Site | Name | Abnormality |
|---|---|---|
| Hand | | |
| D.I.P. joint | Mallet finger | Flexion D.I.P. |
| P.I.P. and D.I.P. joints | Boutonnière deformity | Flexion P.I.P., extension D.I.P. |
| | Swan-neck deformity | Extension P.I.P., flexion D.I.P. |
| M.C.P. joint | | Ulnar deviation |
| | | Volar subluxation |
| Wrist | | |
| Distal radioulnar joint | Caput ulna | Subluxation/dislocation D.R.U. joint |
| Radiocarpal joint | | Radial deviation |
| | | Ulnar translocation |
| Intercarpal joints | Scapholunate dissociation | Scapholunate space >2 mm |
| | Dorsal intercalary segment instability | Dorsiflexion lunate, volar flexion caphoid |
| | Volar intercalary segment instability | Volarflexion lunate, dorsiflexion scaphoid |
| | | Subluxation extensor carpi ulnaris tendon |
| Hip | Protrusio acetabuli | Acetabular wall medial to ilioischial line |
| | | >3 mm in male |
| | | >6 mm in female |
| Knee | Genu varus | Inward deviation of tibia |
| | Genu valgus | Outward deviation of tibia |
| Foot | | |
| First M.T.P. joint | Hallux valgus (bunion) | Lateral deviation first M.T.P. joint |
| M.T.P. (all) | | Fibular deviation M.T.P. joints (I–IV) |
| | | Plantar subluxation M.T.P. joints |
| | Cock-up toe | Hyperextension and dorsal subluxation M.T.P. |
| P.I.P. and D.I.P. | Hammer toe | Hyperflexion P.I.P. or D.I.P. |
| Cervical spine | | |
| Atlanto-axial joint | Atlanto-axial subluxation | Atlanto-odontoid space >3 mm |
| | Vertical atlanto-axial subluxation | Superior displacement odontoid |
| All levels | Stair-step deformity | Subluxation apophyseal joints |

tion of the triangular fibrocartilage-meniscus homologue complex, and radial deviation at the radiocarpal joint (Fig. 39–6).[26]

***Elbow.*** The elbow is a frequent site of abnormality, particularly in patients with advanced disease. In this area a common radiographic finding consists of a positive "fat pad" sign, representing displacement of the fat pads anterior and posterior to the distal humerus owing to intra-articular effusion or synovial hypertrophy.[27,28] Soft tissue swelling over the ulnar olecranon, related to olecranon bursitis, and about the proximal ulna, related to rheumatoid nodules, is another frequent finding. Eventually, extensive osteolysis of the humerus, radius, and ulna may resemble the findings in neuroarthropathy. Large medullary cystic lesions of the distal humerus and ulnar olecranon may be the sites of pathologic fracture.[29]

***Shoulder.*** Two main anatomic sites are frequently involved in rheumatoid arthritis of the shoulder, the glenohumeral and acromioclavicular joints. In the former location, changes of rheumatoid arthritis are prominent joint space narrowing, bony sclerosis, and cyst formation.[24] Osseous erosions are most prominent along the superolateral margin of the humerus, adjacent to the greater tuberosity, and may resemble the Hill-Sachs fracture associated with anterior shoulder dislocation. Erosions may be present at other sites on the proximal humerus and glenoid region of the scapula. Subacromial bursitis, bicipital tendinitis, and rotator cuff tears are frequent complications.

At the acromioclavicular joint, soft tissue swelling and erosions, which tend to be more prominent on the clavicular side of the joint, are early findings.[17] Later, destruction of a large portion of the distal clavicle may be seen.

***Foot.*** Sites of foot involvement in rheumatoid arthritis may be divided into the forefoot, the midfoot, and the heel. The forefoot is very commonly affected (80 to 90 percent) in rheumatoid arthritis, especially the metatarsophalangeal joints.[30-32] The earliest changes involve the metatarsal heads at the first and fifth metatarsophalangeal articulations (Fig. 39–7).[17] At the fifth metatarsophalangeal joint, an early and characteristic erosion occurs on the dorsolateral aspect of the metatarsal head and may be visualized only on oblique radiographs. At the first metatarsophalangeal joint, the earliest involvement is along the medial aspect of the metatarsal head, with later erosions involving the adjacent sesamoid bones. With progression, diffuse joint space loss and larger erosions may be seen. Forefoot deformities in rheumatoid arthritis include hallux valgus, hammer toes, and "cock-up" toes, as well as fibular deviation of the digits and plantar subluxation of the metatarsal heads.

In the midfoot, rheumatoid arthritis is characterized by diffuse joint space loss, bony sclerosis, and osteophytosis, with osseous erosions being uncommon.[17] Osseous fusion in longstanding disease is relatively common. Differentiation of this disease from degenerative, post-traumatic, or neuropathic disorders may be difficult in this region.

In the heel, abnormalities of rheumatoid arthritis are related to involvement of the retrocalcaneal bursa, Achilles tendon, and plantar fascia. With the utilization of soft tissue–enhancing radiographic techniques, swelling of the Achilles tendon (> 1 cm in diameter at the level of the posterosuperior margin of the calcaneus) or soft tissue masses adjacent to the posterosuperior margin

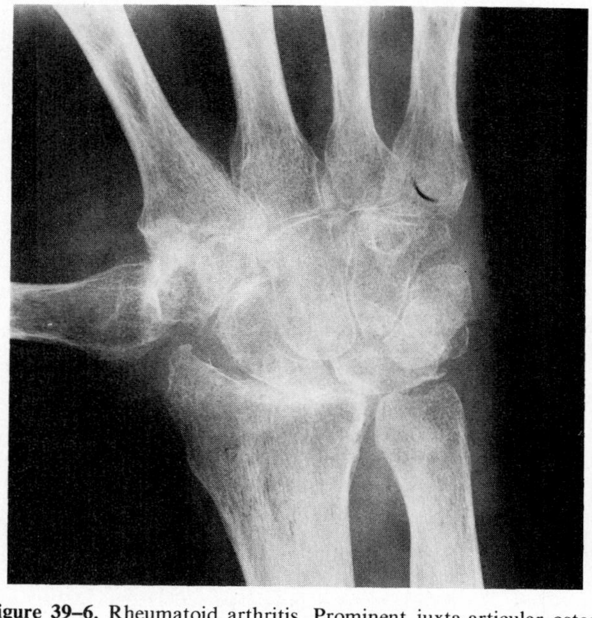

**Figure 39–6.** Rheumatoid arthritis. Prominent juxta-articular osteoporosis is present with radial deviation of the radiocarpal joint and ulnar translocation of the carpus. Extensive erosive changes of the radial and ulnar styloid processes and multiple carpal bones are also present. (From Resnick, D., and Niwayama, G.: Diagnosis of Bone and Joint Disorders. Philadelphia, W.B. Saunders Co., 1981.)

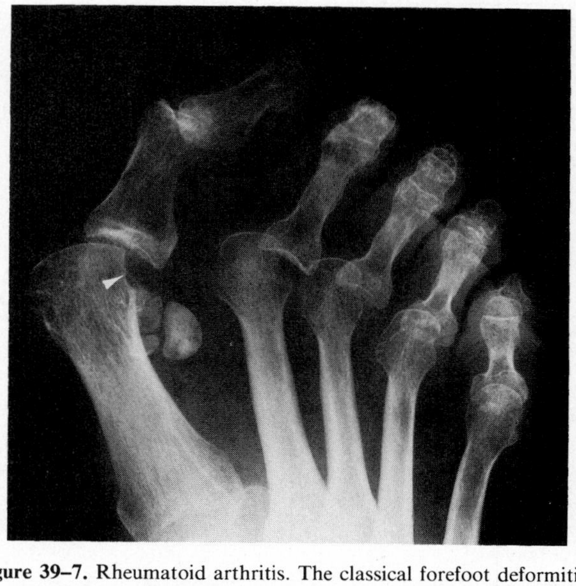

**Figure 39–7.** Rheumatoid arthritis. The classical forefoot deformities are well illustrated in this patient. Note the subluxation and fibular deviation at the MTP joints and the prominent marginal erosions of the first metatarsal head (arrowhead). (From Resnick, D., and Niwayama, G.: Diagnosis of Bone and Joint Disorders. Philadelphia, W.B. Saunders, Co., 1981.)

of the calcaneus as the result of an engorged retrocalcaneal bursa may be early findings.[17,33,34] Osseous erosions at the posterosuperior margin of the calcaneus (Fig. 39–8) are subsequently noted. Well-defined plantar calcaneal spurs, which are identical to those seen in "normal" individuals, can be distinguished from the fluffy, proliferative calcaneal excrescences seen in the seronegative spondyloarthropathies.

*Ankle.* Although the ankle may be the site of radiographically identifiable joint effusions in the patient with rheumatoid arthritis, bony changes at this site are relatively uncommon. In some cases diffuse osteoporosis and joint space narrowing as well as marginal and central bony erosions may be seen.[35] Rarely, with severe disease, loss of integrity of the ankle mortice may occur.

*Knee.* The knee is commonly affected in rheumatoid arthritis. Engorgement of the suprapatellar space of the knee joint by effusion or synovial hypertrophy is noted on the lateral radiographic projection. Small erosions along the medial and lateral margins of the tibia and femur are the earliest bony changes and are followed by joint space loss involving the medial femorotibial, lateral femorotibial, and patellofemoral compartments.[17] Subchondral cysts may be seen in the femoral condyles or proximal tibia, and subchondral sclerosis due to bony collapse may be prominent.[36] Varsus or valgus deformity of the knee joint or patellar instability may be present. Rupture of the quadriceps or patellar tendon may occur with corresponding abnormalities of the soft tissue shadows about the knee. The knee is also a common site of large synovial cysts, especially in the popliteal region.[37] These synovial cysts may extend along fascial planes for a considerable distance in a proximal or distal direction.

*Hip.* Hip involvement in rheumatoid arthritis is less common than knee involvement. A characteristic radiographic abnormality is diffuse concentric loss of articular space, with migration of the femoral head along the plane of the axis of the femoral neck.[38] Radiolucent zones at the bone cartilage junction of the femoral head are related to circumferential marginal erosions.[17] Central erosions of the femoral head and, less commonly, of the acetabulum may be seen. Occasionally large pseudocystic lesions of the femoral neck occur and are liable to pathologic fracture. Acetabular protrusion is present if the inner margin of the acetabulum is medial to the ilioischial line by 3 mm or more in men or 6 mm or more in women. Mild sclerosis and small osteophytes may be noted, related to secondary degenerative disease (osteoarthritis). Osteonecrosis of the femoral heads may be encountered in rheumatoid arthritis, usually in association with corticosteroid therapy.

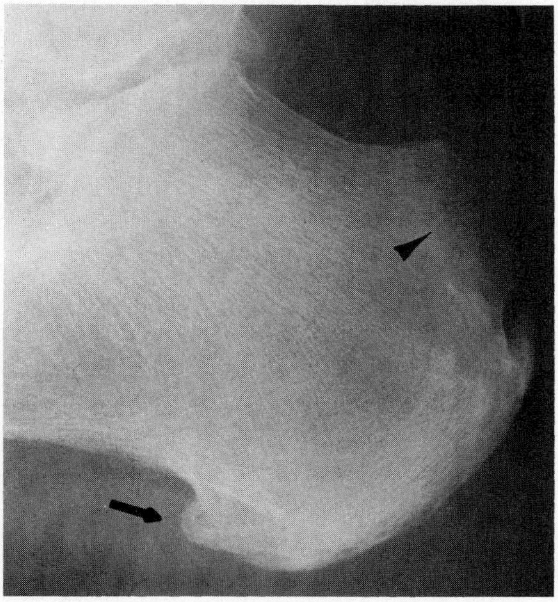

**Figure 39–8.** Rheumatoid arthritis. Erosions are present on the posterior (arrowhead) calcaneal surface. A plantar calcaneal spur is evident (arrow).

*Sacroiliac Joints.* Asymptomatic sacroiliac joint changes are common in rheumatoid arthritis of long duration.[40] In general the findings consist of bilateral but asymmetric bony erosions that primarily involve the iliac side of the synovial articulation.

*Spine.* The cervical spine is one of the more common and important areas of involvement in rheumatoid arthritis. The apophyseal joints of the cervical spine are diffusely affected with bony erosion, joint space narrowing and, eventually, subluxation that leads to a "stair-step" type of deformity (Fig. 39–9), with contiguous vertebral bodies being offset like the steps of a staircase.[42] Erosions and destruction involving the uncovertebral joints (Luschka) as well as the discovertebral junctions are also common. Between the spinous processes, the formation of adventitious bursae and their subsequent inflammation lead to characteristic erosions and a "sharpened" appearance of these processes on lateral radiographs of the cervical spine.

The most important site of cervical spine abnormality is the craniocervical junction. Erosions involving the anterior or posterior margins of the odontoid process as well as joint space narrowing and marginal osseous erosions involving the lateral occipito-atlanto-axial articulations are early findings.[42] Subsequently, laxity or destruction of the transverse atlanto-axial ligament can lead to horizontal (in the sagittal plane) atlanto-axial subluxation with encroachment of the odontoid process on the vertebral canal during flexion of the neck.[42,43] The diagnosis of this complication is based upon the identification of an abnormally wide space ($>5$ mm in the adult) between the posterior margin of the anterior arch of the atlas and the anterior surface of the odontoid process on lateral radiographs of the cervical spine exposed during flexion of the patient's neck. Large odontoid erosions may predispose to pathologic fracture. A second, less common but potentially fatal, pattern of cevical instability in rheumatoid arthritis is vertical atlanto-axial subluxation in which compression of the lateral masses of the atlas in association with disease of the lateral atlanto-axial and atlanto-occipital joints allows the odontoid process to be elevated vetically, becoming intimate with the brainstem.[44,45] Furthermore,

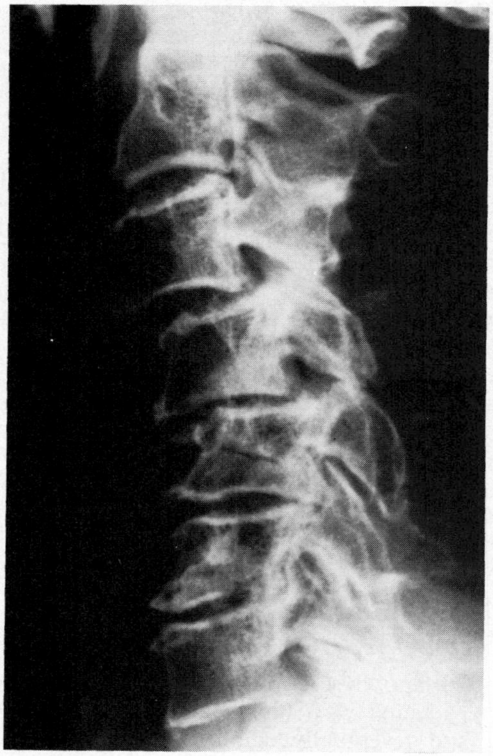

**Figure 39–9.** Rheumatoid arthritis. The "stair-step" deformity of the cervical spine is present with subluxation at multiple contiguous levels. Diffuse loss of intervertebral disc height and erosion of articular surfaces of the apophyseal joints are also present. (From Resnick, D., and Niwayama, G.: Diagnosis of Bone and Joint Disorders. Philadelphia, W.B. Saunders Co., 1981.)

occipito-atlanto-axial instability in the coronal plane can lead to lateral tilting of the head.

In contrast to the frequency of cervical spine involvement, changes in the thoracic and lumbar spine are uncommon in rheumatoid arthritis. However, erosive and destructive abnormalities about the lumbar apophyseal joints are well documented, as are irregularity, erosion, and loss of definition of the bony vertebral endplates.[17] Synovial cysts arising from the apophyseal joints are rare causes of neurologic symptoms and signs.[41]

***Other Locations.*** Other synovial joints that may be involved in rheumatoid arthritis include the temporomandibular and sternoclavicular joints. Not infrequently, cartilaginous articulations, such as the sternomanubrial joint and symphysis pubis, may show erosive change and narrowing.

## JUVENILE ARTHRITIS

**General Radiographic Features.** Juvenile arthritis (JA) is a generic term used to describe a group of childhood articular disorders that share, to a variable degree, certain clinical, laboratory, and radiologic features. Each specific subgroup of JA has its own distinctive radiographic appearance. However, many of the changes are nonspecific and related to effects of the disorder on growth and development of the immature skeleton. It is useful to first consider these general features of childhood arthritis prior to considering abnormalities in specific subgroups of disease.

***Growth Disturbances.***[46-48] Epiphyseal enlargement is a common feature of JA and is related to growth stimulation associated with epiphyseal hyperemia. The changes occur diffusely but often are most marked at the femoral condyles, humeral condyles, and radial head. Epiphyseal overgrowth is combined with subnormal growth of the diaphyseal portion of the bone, resulting in a constricted appearance to the diaphysis with "ballooning" of the epiphysis (Fig. 39–10). The time of appearance and the size of individual bones in the wrist and midfoot may be increased. In some cases, overall bone length may be diminished owing to premature closure of the physis or, in other cases, increased owing to hyperemia.

***Periostitis.***[48] Periostitis is a common and nonspecific component of virtually all forms of JA. This is in contrast to the specificity of periostitis in the differential diagnosis of adult arthropathies. In childhood the periosteum is relatively loosely attached to the underlying bone, a situation that allows it to be easily lifted and stimulated to produce new bone in response to inflammation. Periostitis is most common in the phalanges, metacarpals, and metatarsals but may occasionally be

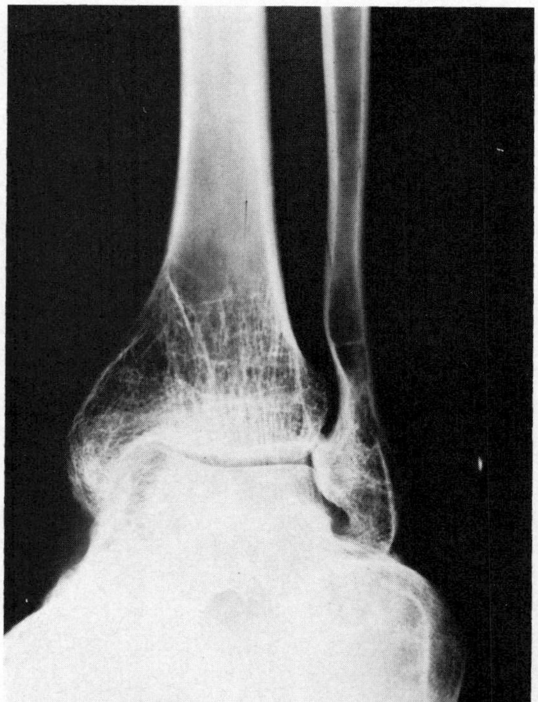

**Figure 39–10.** Juvenile chronic arthritis. Note the prominent juxta-articular osteoporosis with "ballooning" of the distal tibial and fibular epiphyses and a constricted appearance to the bone shafts.

seen in the metaphyses and diaphyses of long tubular bones. In the small bones of the hands and feet, exuberant periosteal new bone formation may result in a "squared" appearance.

***Epiphyseal Compression Fractures.***[48] Flattening and deformity of the epiphyseal centers in weight-bearing articulations are common in JA. Cupping of the epiphyseal centers of the proximal phalanges is also frequent. These changes are related to the abnormal stresses associated with joint contracture and subluxation acting on the osteoporotic epiphyses.

***Osteopenia.*** Osteopenia, representing increased skeletal radiolucency, is generally most striking in the metaphyseal region of a bone, resulting in the formation of horizontally oriented radiolucent metaphyseal bands.[48] These lucent bands are commonly noted in the femur, tibia, fibula, and radius and are identical to those seen in childhood leukemia, metastatic neuroblastoma, and congenital infections. With time, diffuse osteoporosis can develop. Growth recovery lines (Fig. 39–11) are thin, horizontally oriented radiodense bands visualized in the diametaphyseal region of tubular bones in children with chronic illness. Presumably they are manifestations of accelerated bone growth in the intervals following exacerbations of disease. Occasionally, widespread metaphyseal sclerosis is seen (Fig. 39–11).

**Juvenile-Onset Adult-Type (Seropositive) Rheumatoid Arthritis.** Soft tissue swelling, juxta-articular osteoporosis, and marginal erosions are present, as in the typical adult case.[46] However, two features help differentiate this disorder from adult-onset rheumatoid arthritis: the presence of periostitis, especially of the small bones of the hands and feet, and the frequent occurrence of prominent marginal erosions without associated joint space narrowing.[50,51]

**Seronegative Chronic Arthritis (Still's Disease).**[49] Classic systemic Still's disease is an acute systemic illness that rarely manifests radiographic articular changes.

Polyarticular disease may occur in the presence or absence of classic Still's disease. Symmetric involvement of the hands, wrists, knees, ankles, feet, and cervical spine is common. In the hands and feet, osteoporosis is associated with joint space narrowing, and the small bones assume a "squared" shape as a result of new bone formation. Osseous erosions are unusual in this disorder and, when present, are usually of small size. Intra-articular bony ankylosis (Fig. 39–12) is a common late complication in the small joints, in contrast to its rarity in adult-onset rheumatoid arthritis. In the larger articulations such as the knee and the hip, osteoporosis and epiphyseal overgrowth are the most typical manifestations, often occurring without joint space narrowing or bony erosions. The cervical spine is frequently the only spinal level involved in this disorder (Fig. 39–13); abnormalities predominate in the upper cervical region. The growth disturbance results in a constriction of vertebral body width and depth with relatively normal height, resulting in a slender, gracile appearance. Apophyseal joint space narrowing, bony ankylosis, and osseous erosions occur with hypoplasia of the intervertebral discs and bony ankylosis of vertebral bodies. As in adults, atlanto-axial subluxation is a frequent complication in children.

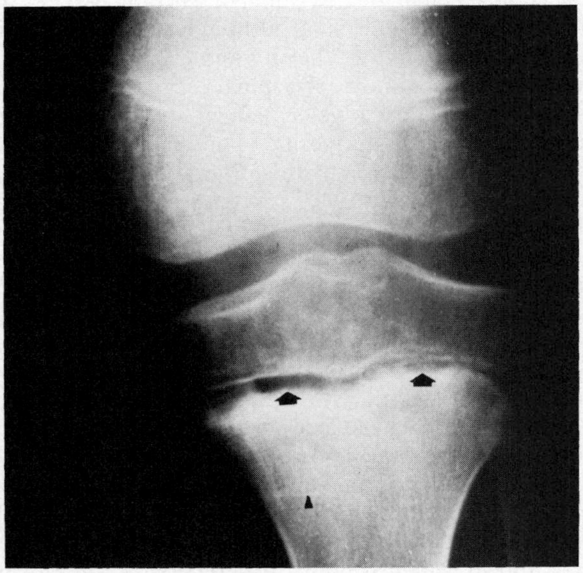

**Figure 39–11.** Juvenile chronic arthritis. There is overgrowth of the epiphyses about the knee. Juxta-articular osteoporosis is evident, with several horizontally oriented growth recovery lines (arrowhead). Metaphyseal sclerosis (arrows) can be visualized in the proximal tibia.

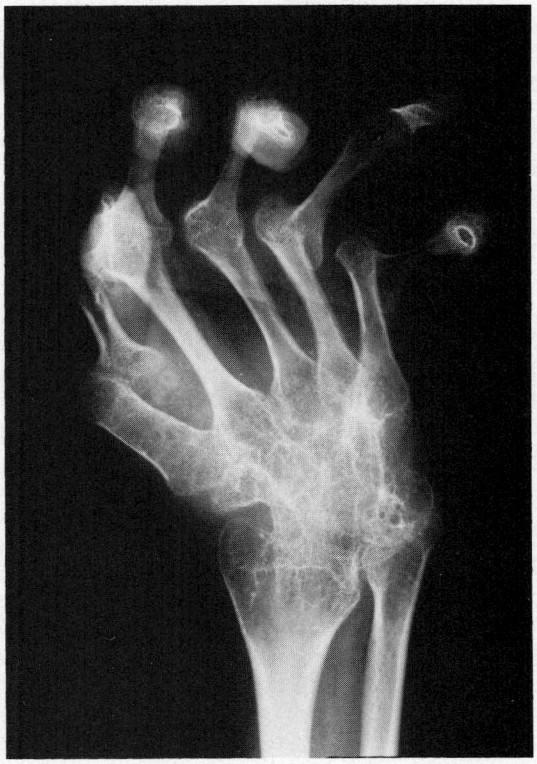

**Figure 39–12.** Juvenile chronic arthritis. There are prominent finger deformities, osteoporosis, and bony ankylosis, especially in the carpus. Note the elongated, slender appearance of the tubular bones, which is related to growth disturbance.

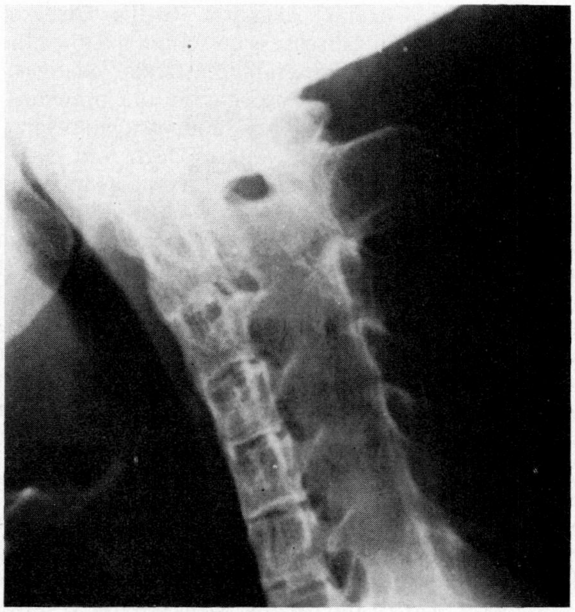

**Figure 39–13.** Juvenile chronic arthritis. Intervertebral and apophyseal joint bony ankylosis is present at multiple levels. The overall appearance of the cervical spine is gracile, owing to the relatively normal height of the vertebral bodies and the diminished anteroposterior vertebral diameter. (From Resnick, D., and Niwayama, G.: Diagnosis of Bone and Joint Disorders. Philadelphia, W.B. Saunders Co., 1981.)

Pauciarticular and monoarticular forms of seronegative chronic arthritis are occasionally seen.[51,52] Changes are generally confined to the larger articulations such as the knee, hip, ankle, elbow, and wrist; the small joints of the hands and feet are spared. Radiographic abnormalities are the same as those in the polyarticular pattern of disease.

**Juvenile-Onset Ankylosing Spondylitis.** Juvenile-onset ankylosing spondylitis is generally first manifest in the articulations of the lower extremity, particularly the hips, knees, ankles, and small joints of the feet.[46] The joints of the upper extremities are relatively spared. Sacroiliitis and spondylitis occur but are usually identified later in the course of the disease, in contrast to adult-onset ankylosing spondylitis. In the spine, thoracic and lumbar involvement is common with involvement of the cervical spine being distinctly unusual.

Radiographic changes in the peripheral skeleton consist of joint space narrowing, bony erosions and proliferation, and intra-articular osseous fusion.[53] Osteoporosis is frequently not prominent. In the sacroiliac articulations and the thoracolumbar spine, the radiographic changes are identical to those of adult-onset ankylosing spondylitis.[54] Useful features in differentiating this disorder from other types of JA include the absence of diffuse osteoporosis, relative sparing of the articulations of the upper extremity and cervical spine, and sacroiliitis and spondylitis.

**Juvenile-Onset Psoriatic Arthritis.** Juvenile-onset psoriatic arthritis is occasionally encountered. Radiographic changes simulate those in adults. Hand involvement is characterized by resorption of the terminal tufts of the distal phalanges and interphalangeal joint destruction.[49] Although sacroiliitis is common in this disorder, the normal indistinct appearance of the sacroiliac articulations in children and adolescents makes accurate radiographic diagnosis of sacroiliitis difficult.

**Adult-Onset Still's Disease.** Rarely, an adult patient may be encountered with a febrile illness identical to classic Still's disease.[55] When present, radiographic changes involve the wrists, knees, and fingers. Bony erosions are unusual. A peculiar tendency toward narrowing or ankylosis of the common carpometacarpal joint, especially that portion at the level of the second and third metacarpal bases, and the intercarpal joint in a pericapitate distribution has been reported.[97]

**Others.** Enteropathic arthropathy may be identified in childhood accompanying regional enteritis, ulcerative colitis, or bowel infections (*Salmonella, Shigella*). Its appearance is identical to that of juvenile-onset ankylosing spondylitis. Other rare causes of childhood arthropathy include systemic lupus erythematosus and familial Mediterranean fever.

## THE SERONEGATIVE SPONDYLOARTHROPATHIES

**Ankylosing Spondylitis.** Synovial and cartilaginous joints as well as sites of tendon and ligament insertion (entheses) may be involved in ankylosing spondylitis and the other seronegative spondyloarthropathies.[57,58] Axial skeletal involvement is characteristic, with a predilection for the sacroiliac, apophyseal, discovertebral, and costovertebral articulations. The initial sites of involvement are the sacroiliac joints and lumbosacral and thoracolumbar vertebral junctions. Subsequently, ascending and descending spinal disease may be encountered.[59,60] Peripheral joint involvement, although frequent (50 percent), is usually mild.[54] The hips and glenohumeral joints are the most common extraspinal locations of disease.

*Sacroiliac Joints.* Involvement of the sacroiliac joint is the hallmark of ankylosing spondylitis. It is difficult to verify the diagnosis of this disease in the absence of such involvement. Rarely, spinal disease occurs in the absence of significant sacroiliac joint abnormality. Sacroiliitis occurs early in the course of ankylosing spondylitis and is characteristically bilateral and symmetric in its distribution.[59-62] On rare occasions, initial unilateral or asymmetric sacroiliac joint changes are observed. Changes occur both in the synovial and the ligamentous portions of the joint, with the abnormalities being more prominent on the iliac side of the articulation.[58] Osteoporosis, subchondral bony resorption with loss of definition of the articular margins, and superficial osseous erosions are interspersed with focal areas of bony sclerosis. Radiographically, in this stage, the articulation may appear widened. With progression of the disease, a wide, ill-defined band of sclerosis is seen on the iliac side of the joint with larger subchondral erosions (Fig. 39–14). In the late proliferative stage, bony bridges trav-

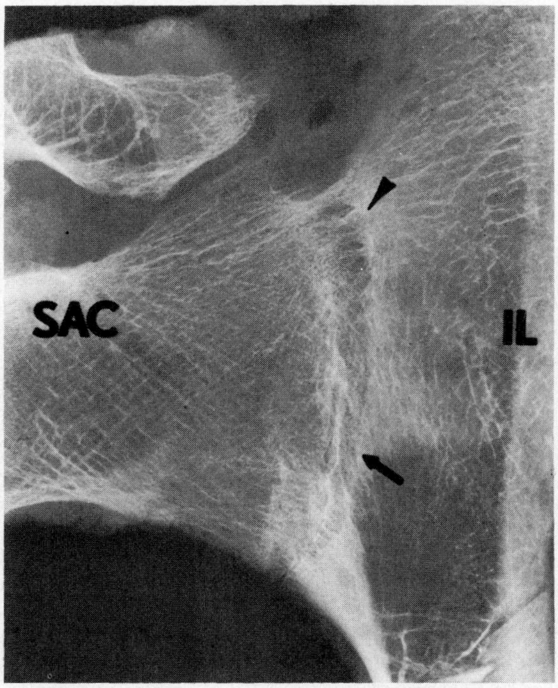


**Figure 39–15.** Ankylosing spondylitis. A specimen radiograph from a cadaver with the disease demonstrates complete intra-articular ankylosis of the ligamentous (arrowhead) and synovial (arrow) portions of the joint. (*SAC,* sacrum; *IL,* ilium).

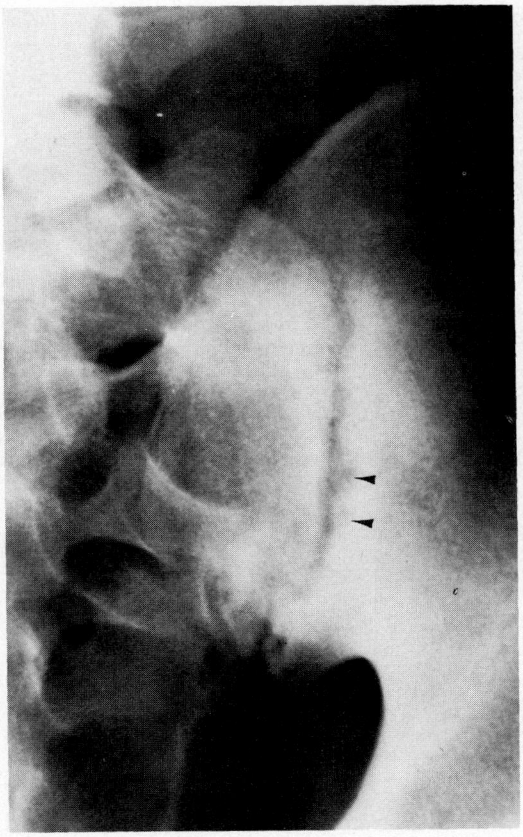

**Figure 39–14.** Ankylosing spondylitis. Note the ill-defined band of sclerosis and prominent erosions of the subchondral bone plate (arrowheads), which are most conspicuous on the iliac side of the articulation.

erse the joint space, initially isolating islands of intact cartilage. Such segmental ankylosis may be followed by complete intra-articular bony fusion (Fig. 39–15) and disappearance of the periarticular sclerosis. The ligamentous (syndesmotic) portions of the sacroiliac joint may also be affected, leading to bony erosions and proliferation. In general, involvement of the ligamentous portion of the articulation is less prominent in ankylosing spondylitis than in psoriatic arthritis and Reiter's syndrome.

***Spine.*** The initial sites of spinal involvement, especially in men, are the lumbosacral and thoracolumbar junctions. In women, the cervical spine may be affected at an early stage of disease. "Osteitis" is an initial finding, related to inflammation of the anterior portion of the discovertebral junction.[58] A focal erosive lesion at the anterosuperior and anteroinferior vertebral margins leads to loss of the normal concavity of the anterior aspect of the vertebral body, resulting in a "squared" configuration of the vertebral body in the lateral radiographic projection. This appearance is more easily identified in the lumbar spine as the thoracic vertebral bodies may normally have a squared appearance. In ankylosing spondylitis, bony sclerosis adjacent to the sites of erosion produces a "shiny corner" sign on radiographs.

Syndesmophytes are vertically oriented bony excrescences, which represent ossification of the outer fibers of the annulus fibrosus of the intervertebral disc.[63] They predominate on the anterior and lateral aspects of the spine and eventually bridge the intervertebral disc. (Fig. 39–16*A*). In the late stages of the disease, extensive syndesmophytic formation produces a smooth, undulating spinal contour, the "bamboo" spine.

It is of critical importance that the syndesmophytes that characterize ankylosing spondylitis (and enteropathic spondyloarthritis) be differentiated from other spinal and paraspinal bony excrescences (Figs. 39–16, 39–23, 39–38, and 39–39). Vertebral excrescences in spondylosis deformans arise several millimeters from the discovertebral junction, are triangular in shape, and demonstrate a horizontally oriented segment of variable length at their point of origin. In diffuse idiopathic skeletal hyperostosis (DISH), bone formation in the anterior longitudinal ligament results in a flowing pattern of ossification, thicker than that seen in ankylosing spondylitis. Such ossification is best demonstrated on lateral spine radiographs. Furthermore, in DISH, there is absence of erosion or bony ankylosis in the sacroiliac joints. The paravertebral ossifications that characterize psoriatic arthritis and Reiter's syndrome arise in an asymmetric fashion in the soft tissues adjacent to the outer layer of the annulus fibrosus. They are initially unattached to the vertebral body but, with time, they fuse with the margins of the vertebral body at a point several millimeters from the discovertebral junction.

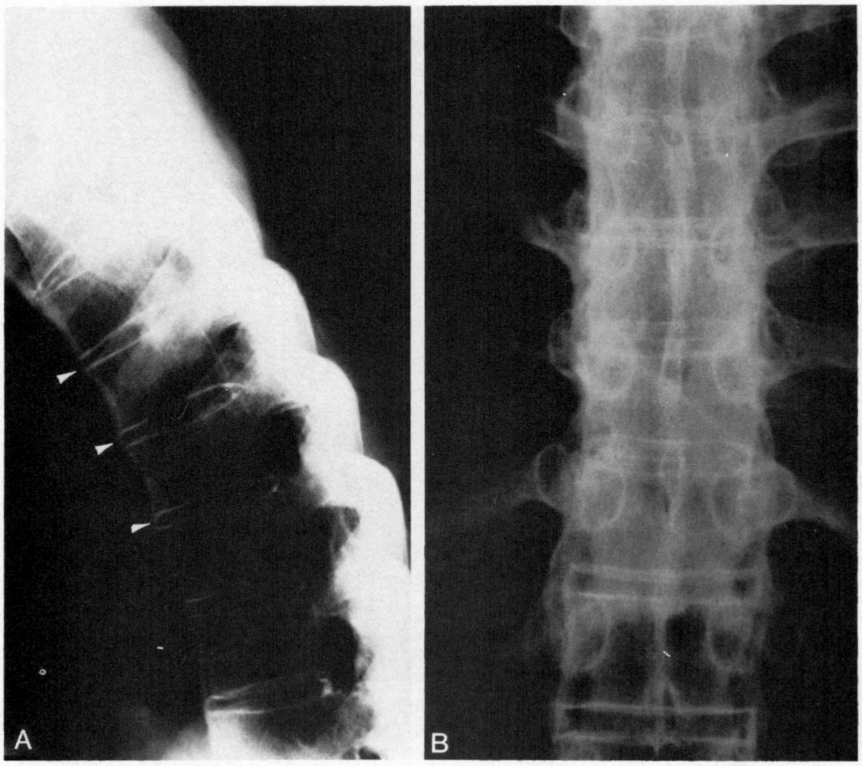


**Figure 39–16.** Ankylosing spondylitis. Lateral (*A*) and frontal (*B*) radiographs of the spine demonstrate complete intervertebral ankylosis, which produces the characteristic "bamboo spine" appearance. Note the thin, vertically oriented syndesmophytes (arrowheads) arising from the discovertebral junction, owing to ossification in the outermost layer of the annulus fibrosus.

Erosions at one or more discovertebral junctions can be prominent radiographic findings in ankylosing spondylitis. These may be classified as focal or diffuse.[64] Focal lesions may relate to intraosseous herniation of disc material (cartilaginous or Schmorl's node) or enthesitis. Diffuse destruction of the discovertebral junction may be related to a pseudarthrosis following fracture. Discal calcification is common and usually seen in association with apophyseal joint ankylosis at the same spinal level.

Early alterations in the apophyseal joints in the lumbar, thoracic, and cervical segments consist of ill-defined erosions accompanied by reactive sclerosis. Capsular ossification or intra-articular bony ankylosis may subsequently occur. On frontal radiographs of the spine, such ossification produces vertically oriented, parallel, radiodense bands, which, when combined with a central radiodense band related to ossification of the interspinous and supraspinous ligaments, lead to the "trolley-track" sign (Fig. 39–16*B*).[58]

Erosions of the odontoid process and atlanto-axial subluxation may be observed in ankylosing spondylitis, although with less frequency than in rheumatoid arthritis.[44,59] Ankylosis of the atlanto-axial articulation, either in its normal position or in a position of subluxation, may occasionally be noted. At other levels in the cervical spine, the changes, when present, are identical to those in the thoracolumbar spine.

***Extraspinal Locations.*** The hip is the most commonly involved peripheral articulation in ankylosing spondylitis, with the changes most frequently being bilateral and symmetrical in distribution.[65] Concentric joint space narrowing with axial migration of the femoral head and marginal osteophyte formation characterizes the hip disease of ankylosing spondylitis (Fig. 39–17). Osteophytes are first observed at the lateral margin of the femoral head-neck junction and, with progression, proliferate circumferentially to produce a characteristic "ring osteophyte."[65,66] Subchondral cysts and erosions as well as intra-articular bony ankylosis may be seen in some cases. Such hip disease can lead to significant clinical manifestations requiring surgical intervention. However, patients with ankylosing spondylitis who undergo hip surgery, including total joint replacement, are prone to develop exuberant deposits of juxta-articular heterotopic bone, which may severely restrict postoperative hip motion.[67]

The shoulder is the second most common peripheral site of involvement in ankylosing spondylitis.[54] Bilateral involvement is common; changes are osteoporosis, joint space narrowing, bony erosions, and rotator cuff disruption. A characteristic large destructive abnormality involving the superolateral aspect of the humeral head in this disease has been termed the "hatchet" sign[68] (Fig. 39–18).

Changes in other peripheral joints occur with variable frequency. In general, these changes, which are similar to but less extensive than those in the other seronegative spondyloarthropathies, include soft tissue swelling, mild osteoporosis, joint space narrowing, bony erosions, and osseous proliferation.[58] The erosions tend to be less prominent than in rheumatoid arthritis. The presence of bone proliferation (whiskering) and periostitis in an-

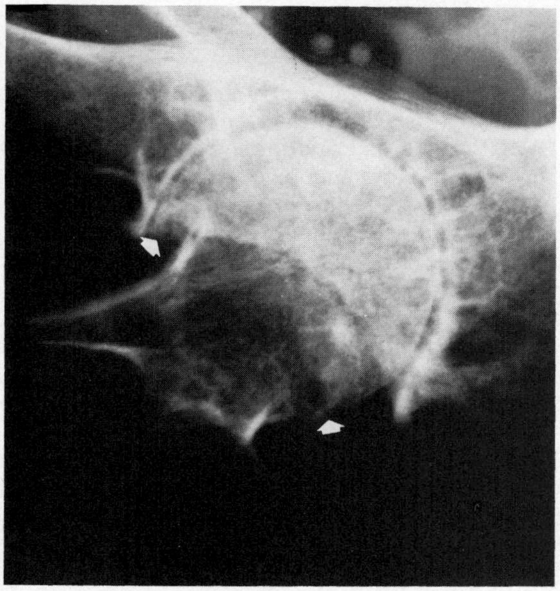

Figure 39–17. Ankylosing spondylitis. Concentric joint space narrowing with axial migration of the femoral head is present. Osteophytes (arrows) are present at the medial and lateral margins of the femoral head.

kylosing spondylitis (and the other seronegative spondyloarthropathies) is another helpful diagnostic feature.

Inflammation with bony proliferation at sites of tendon and ligament insertion (enthesopathy), especially those of the pelvis, patella, and calcaneus, is prominent in ankylosing spondylitis (as well as in the other seronegative spondyloarthropathies). Plantar and posterior calcaneal spurs are common and may be either well-defined or indistinct with feathery margins, representing the combination of erosive and proliferative change. Erosions of the posterior calcaneal margin due to inflammation in the retrocalcaneal bursa and thickening of the Achilles tendon may be present (Fig. 39–19).[34] The inflammatory enthesopathy of the seronegative spondyloarthropathies[58,69] differs from the degenerative enthesopathy seen in DISH (see Fig. 39–41). In the latter disease, bony outgrowths (enthesophytes) are sharply marginated and well-defined.

Other sites of involvement in ankylosing spondylitis[58] include the symphysis pubis and manubriosternal, temporomandibular, and sternoclavicular joints.

**Psoriatic Arthritis.** In general, psoriatic arthritis is asymmetric or unilateral with involvement of synovial and cartilaginous joints as well as entheses.[70] The most common sites of involvement are the interphalangeal joints of the hands and feet, metatarsophalangeal joints, metacarpophalangeal joints, sacroiliac joints, and spine. Changes in the knees, ankles, elbows, and wrists and manubriosternal, acromioclavicular, and sternoclavicular joints, as well as pelvic entheses, are not uncommon. Hip or glenohumeral joint involvement is rare.

The arthritis of psoriasis is associated with periarticular soft tissue swelling, which in some cases may be manifested by diffuse, sausage-like enlargement of an

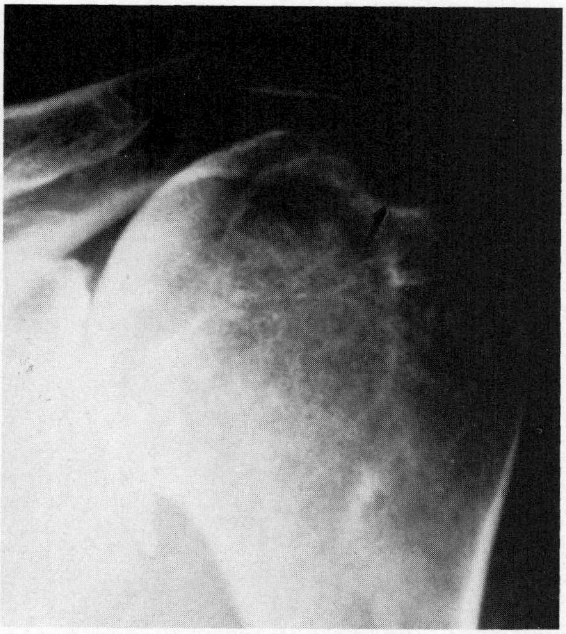

Figure 39–18. Ankylosing spondylitis. There is disruption of the musculotendinous rotator cuff with superior migration of the humeral head. The large erosion (arrow) of the superolateral aspect of the humeral head ("hatchet deformity") is a characteristic radiographic sign of the disease.

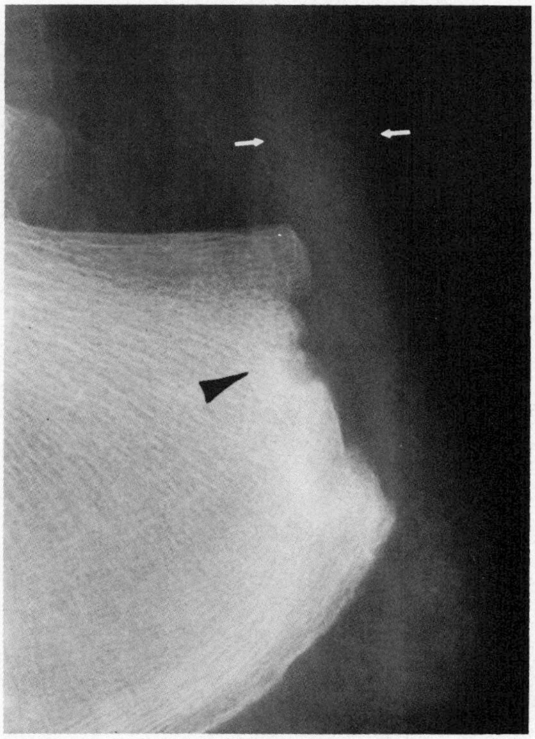

Figure 39–19. Ankylosing spondylitis. Erosive change of the posterior calcaneal margin is present (arrowhead) as well as thickening of the Achilles tendon (between arrows).

entire digit. The absence of osteoporosis is remarkable in many cases of psoriatic arthritis and is an important consideration in the differential diagnosis. However, osteoporosis may occasionally be evident; thus, its presence does not exclude the diagnosis of psoriatic arthritis. Joint space narrowing or widening may be encountered, the latter being more common in the small joints of the hands and feet. Erosions progress from marginal areas in a central direction, often resulting in a "whittled" or "pencil-in-cup" deformity of the involved articulation.[72] In cases in which this severe destructive change is predominant, in combination with marked joint deformity, the term *arthritis mutilans* is frequently used. Bony proliferation is a striking feature of psoriatic arthritis and the other seronegative spondyloarthropathies (Fig. 39–20).[73] Proliferation around erosions produces a "whiskered" appearance. Diaphyseal and metaphyseal periostitis is also common.[74] In fact, osseous proliferation involving the distal phalanges may produce diffuse increased radiodensity, termed the "ivory phalanx."[75] Intra-articular bony fusion, especially involving the proximal and distal interphalangeal joints of the hands and feet, is a common finding. An inflammatory enthesopathy consisting of fine, feathery, bony proliferation at sites of tendon and ligament insertion is also prominent in many cases.

***Hands.*** In the hands, involvement of the distal interphalangeal joints is frequent and may be unilateral or bilateral, symmetric or asymmetric in distribution (Fig. 39–20). Erosions occur at the joint margins and progress centrally, with irregular destructive changes. Protrusion of one joint surface into its articular counterpart produces the pencil-in-cup deformity. Resorption of the terminal tufts of the distal phalanges may be seen. Psoriatic arthritis can lead to intra-articular bony ankylosis, a finding that is rare in rheumatoid arthritis.

***Feet.*** Psoriatic arthritis involves two major areas in the foot: the forefoot and the calcaneus.[70] In the forefoot, changes are usually bilateral and asymmetric, predominating at the interphalangeal and metatarsophalangeal articulations. Marginal erosion, joint space narrowing (or widening), and bony proliferation are present, characteristically without significant osteoporosis. Severe destruction of the interphalangeal articulation of the great toe can be seen in psoriatic arthritis (and in Reiter's syndrome). Sesamoid involvement is also common in the foot as well as in the hand.

As in the other seronegative spondyloarthropathies, the combination of proliferative and erosive changes in the posterior and inferior surfaces of the calcaneus is an important radiographic finding of psoriatic arthritis. Erosions of the posterior surface of the calcaneus with surrounding proliferation adjacent to the retrocalcaneal bursa are common. Irregular and poorly defined spurs are typically present at the insertion of the plantar aponeurosis (Fig. 39–21), although in time, such spurs may become relatively well defined.

***Sacroiliac Joints.*** A bilateral and symmetric distribution constitutes the most common radiographic pattern of sacroiliac joint abnormalities in psoriatic arthritis, although asymmetric involvement is not rare (Fig. 39–22).[70,76] Initially subchondral bony erosions and ill-defined sclerosis with apparent joint space widening are noted, abnormalities identical to those in ankylosing spondylitis. However, the frequency of intra-articular

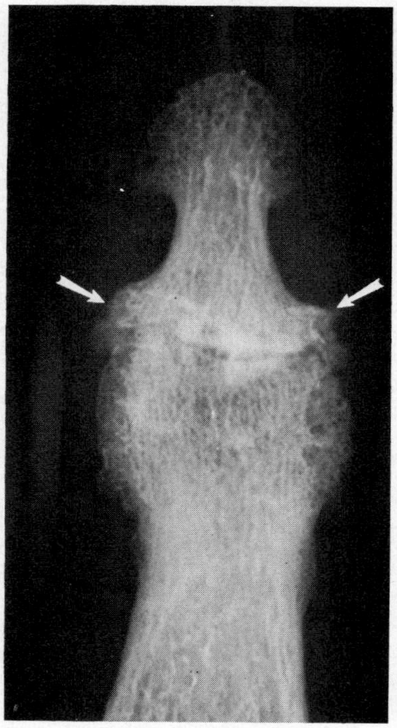

**Figure 39–20.** Psoriatic arthritis. The distal interphalangeal joint is narrowed, with proliferative bony erosions (arrows). Also note the prominent soft tissue swelling and the abnormality of the fingernail.

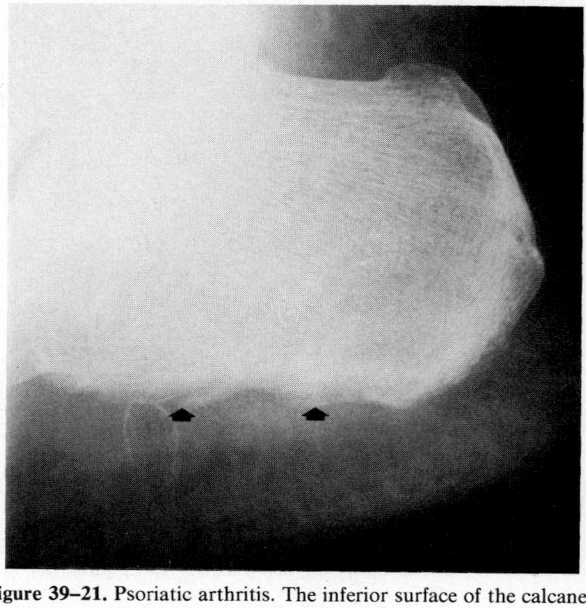

**Figure 39–21.** Psoriatic arthritis. The inferior surface of the calcaneus reveals the characteristic combination of erosive and proliferative changes (arrows) that form the hallmark of the seronegative spondyloarthropathies.

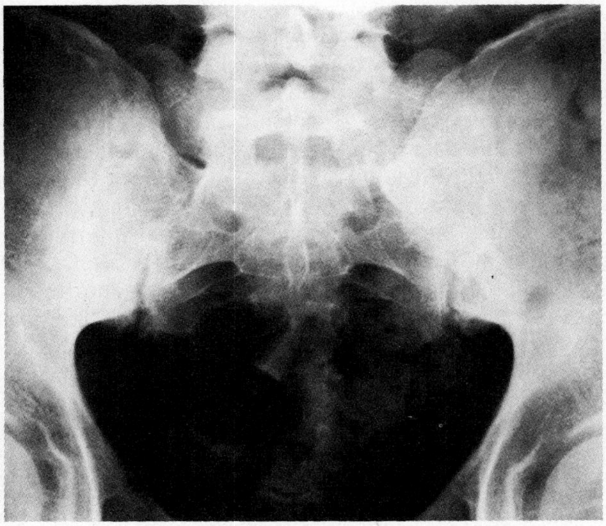

**Figure 39–22.** Psoriatic arthritis. Bilateral and asymmetric changes of the sacroiliac joints are present with erosions and sclerosis of the subchondral bone plate.

bony ankylosis in psoriatic arthritis is less than that in ankylosing spondylitis or the spondyloarthritis associated with inflammatory bowel diseases. Furthermore, in psoriatic arthritis (as in Reiter's syndrome), blurring and eburnation of apposing sacral and iliac surfaces within the ligamentous portion of the sacroiliac joint are more common than in ankylosing spondylitis.

***Spine.*** The characteristic spinal lesion of psoriatic arthritis (as well as Reiter's syndrome) is paravertebral ossification.[77] These ossifications initially appear as either thick and irregular or thin and curvilinear densities, asymmetrically distributed parallel to the lateral surface of the intervertebral disc and vertebral body (Fig. 39–23). At this stage, the outgrowths are not attached to the vertebral body, although in later stages, the ossific densities merge with the lateral margins of the vertebral body several millimeters distal to the discovertebral junction. Occasionally, syndesmophytes identical to those in ankylosing spondylitis do occur in psoriatic arthritis[70] and Reiter's syndrome; however, in the great majority of cases, they are interspersed with the more characteristic paravertebral ossifications. "Corner osteitis," vertebral body "squaring," and apophyseal joint ankylosis are less common than in ankylosing spondylitis.

Cervical spine changes in psoriatic arthritis may be dramatic, even in patients with minimal thoracolumbar spinal involvement.[76,78] Discovertebral joint irregularity with extensive bony proliferation about the anterior aspect of the vertebra and extensive apophyseal joint erosion and narrowing may be seen. Atlanto-axial subluxation is common.[76]

***Other Locations.*** In longstanding or severe disease, virtually any articulation may be involved. In most sites, the characteristic combination of erosive and proliferative change is present.

**Reiter's Syndrome.** Radiographic alterations occur in approximately 60 to 80 percent of patients with Reiter's syndrome.[79] These radiographic changes demonstrate morphologic characteristics that are virtually indistinguishable from those in the other seronegative spondyloarthropathies, especially psoriatic arthritis; differentiation is usually possible only by means of the distribution of abnormalities and the clinical history. Synovial joints, cartilaginous joints, and entheses may be affected. Characteristically these changes are bilateral and asymmetric, with a predilection for involvement of the lower extremity.[79]

The most common sites of involvement are the small joints of the foot and the posterior and inferior calcaneal surfaces, followed, in order of frequency, by the ankle and the knee. Involvement of the hip and upper extremity is considerably less common. In the axial skeleton the sacroiliac joints, spine, symphysis pubis, and manubriosternal joints are the most common sites of alteration.

The general radiographic features of Reiter's syndrome are soft tissue swelling, joint space narrowing, and bony erosion and proliferation. Osteoporosis is variable in frequency and extent but may be present during acute exacerbations of arthritis. Osseous proliferation at insertions of tendons and ligaments is a frequent finding, especially in the pelvis and the calcaneus.

***Feet and Ankles.*** Asymmetric abnormalities of the metatarsophalangeal and interphalangeal joints of the forefoot are the most common manifestations of Reiter's syndrome (Fig. 39–24).[80] Frequently, effusions in the

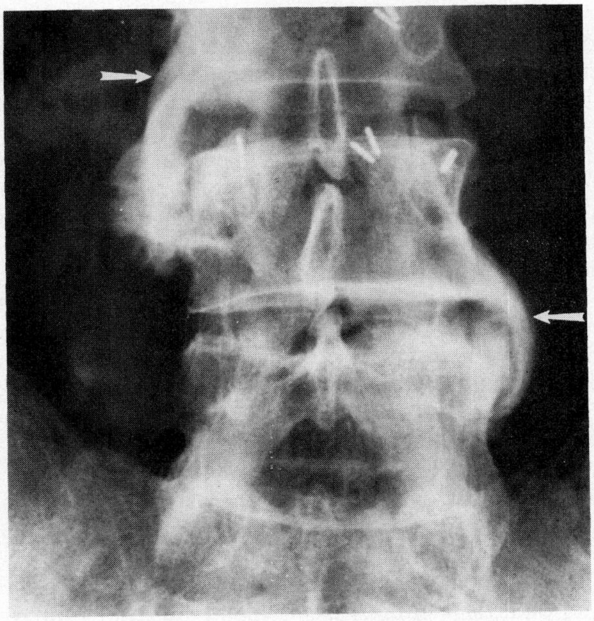

**Figure 39–23.** Psoriatic arthritis. Note the thick asymmetric paravertebral ossifications (arrows) arising from the vertebral margins in this patient with psoriatic spondylitis. These lesions, which are best visualized in the anteroposterior projection of the spine, are characteristic of psoriatic arthritis and Reiter's syndrome.

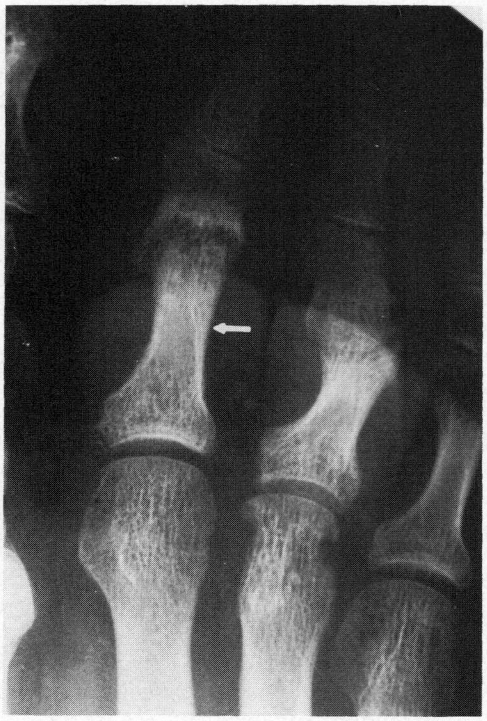

**Figure 39–24.** Reiter's syndrome. There is destructive change of the second and third proximal interphalangeal joints with subtle periosteal proliferative reaction along the phalangeal shafts (arrow). Marginal erosions of the metatarsal heads and proximal phalanges are also evident.

retrocalcaneal bursa may be identified as radiodense shadows obliterating the normal fat plane between the posterosuperior aspect of the calcaneus and the Achilles tendon.[34] Thickening of this tendon may also be evident. Ill-defined plantar calcaneal spurs are characteristic but, as in the other seronegative spondyloarthropathies, the spurs may be relatively well-defined in the later stages of the disease. Marginal erosions are somewhat uncommon about the ankle, but joint space narrowing, with adjacent soft tissue swelling, and fluffy periostitis of the distal tibia and fibula are seen.[79]

*Knee.* The most common abnormality in the knee in Reiter's syndrome is the presence of a joint effusion, which in some instances becomes massive. Osteoporosis, joint space narrowing, and periostitis of the patella and distal femoral shaft also occur. Bony erosions in the femur or tibia are rare.

*Sacroiliac Joints.* Sacroiliac joint abnormalities are common and may be bilateral and asymmetric or unilateral in distribution. These abnormalities are identical to those of psoriatic arthritis.

*Spine.* Spinal involvement is less frequent in Reiter's syndrome than in ankylosing spondylitis and psoriatic arthritis. Although in some instances the changes may be identical to those of ankylosing spondylitis, a more characteristic finding consists of asymmetrically distributed paravertebral ossifications involving the thoracolumbar spine.[81] Cervical spine involvement in unusual, and atlanto-axial subluxation is rare.

*Other Locations.* In the cartilaginous manubriosternal and pubic symphyseal articulations, the changes of Reiter's syndrome consist of erosions of the articular surfaces with adjacent bony proliferation and sclerosis.[79]

Severe and diffuse involvement of joints of the upper extremity is rare in Reiter's syndrome,[79] although scattered lesions, particularly in the proximal interphalangeal joints of the hands, may occasionally be seen. Distal interphalangeal or metacarpophalangeal joint alterations are less frequent. Fusiform or "sausage-like" soft tissue swelling, joint space narrowing, periarticular osteoporosis, and bony erosion and proliferation are observed.

**Enteropathic Arthropathies and Related Conditions.** The frequency of peripheral joint involvement in enteropathic arthritis is variable. Several types of involvement are seen:[82-86] a mild, inflammatory, self-limited peripheral arthritis in which the radiographic changes consist principally of soft tissue swelling and juxta-articular osteoporosis; a progressive, destructive peripheral arthropathy characterized by soft tissue swelling, variable osteoporosis, joint space narrowing, osseous erosions, bony proliferation; and sacroiliitis or spondylitis. In patients with spondyloarthritis the changes are identical to those in ankylosing spondylitis, although the male predominance of ankylosing spondylitis is less marked in this group of disorders and isolated sacroiliitis without spinal involvement is more common.

In primary biliary cirrhosis a severe destructive arthropathy of the hands has been described[87] characterized by the asymmetric distribution of well-defined marginal erosions primarily involving the proximal and distal interphalangeal joints with relative sparing of the metacarpophalangeal joints. Chondrocalcinosis may be present in some patients, and occasionally, severe involvement of the hips and shoulders resembling osteonecrosis has been noted.[88]

A number of pancreatic diseases, including carcinoma, inflammation, and pancreatic duct calculi, may be associated with a syndrome characterized by subcutaneous nodules, polyarthritis, and medullary fat necrosis.[89,90] The polyarthritis is radiographically nonspecific, with osteoporosis and soft tissue swelling being most commonly encountered. The radiographic appearance of medullary fat necrosis consists of diffuse osteolytic lesions with a "moth-eaten" appearance and periostitis. These changes closely resemble those of osteomyelitis and osteonecrosis.

## CONNECTIVE TISSUE DISEASES

A number of connective tissue disorders, including systemic lupus erythematosus, progressive systemic sclerosis, dermatomyositis, polymyositis, periarteritis nodosa, and mixed connective tissue disease, may be associated with musculoskeletal radiographic abnormalities.

**Systemic Lupus Erythematosus.** The roentgenographic changes of systemic lupus erythematosus (SLE) include symmetric polyarthritis, deforming nonerosive arthropathy, spontaneous tendon rupture, osteonecrosis, soft tissue calcification, infection, acrosclerosis, and tuftal resorption.[91-100] With the polyarthritis the radiographic changes are nonspecific and consist of soft tissue swelling and periarticular osteoporosis.[91,92]

Joint space narrowing and bony erosions are unusual. Deforming nonerosive arthropathy is seen in 5 to 40 percent of patients with SLE.[92] Symmetric involvement of the hands is typical. The specific type of deformity is variable.[91-93] Swan-neck or boutonnière deformity can be evident. Other deformities include hyperextension of the interphalangeal joint of the thumb, ulnar drift at the metacarpophalangeal joints, and subluxation of the first carpometacarpal joint (Fig. 39–25). It is the prominent thumb deformity that is especially characteristic of lupus arthropathy. Although bony and cartilaginous abnormalities are generally not present, joint space narrowing, "hook-like" erosions of the radial and volar aspects of the metacarpal heads, and subchondral cyst formation are occasionally encountered (Fig. 39–26).[95] The radiographic findings of osteonecrosis in patients with SLE include transchondral fractures, subchondral sclerosis with cyst formation, and osseous collapse. Secondary osteoarthritis may eventually be prominent.

Linear or nodular calcific deposits in the subcutaneous tissues, particularly in the lower extremities, may occasionally be seen in SLE.[97] Sclerosis (acrosclerosis) or resorption of the tufts of the terminal phalanges is occasionally evident in SLE.[100]

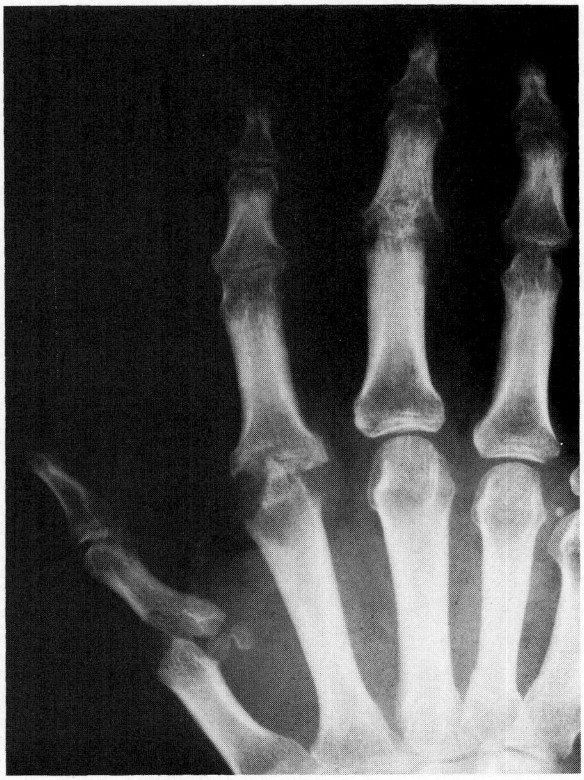

**Figure 39–26.** Systemic lupus erythematosus. An unusual pattern of involvement is seen. Severe erosive changes are present in the first and second metacarpophalangeal joints and third PIP joint. Juxta-articular osteoporosis is prominent.

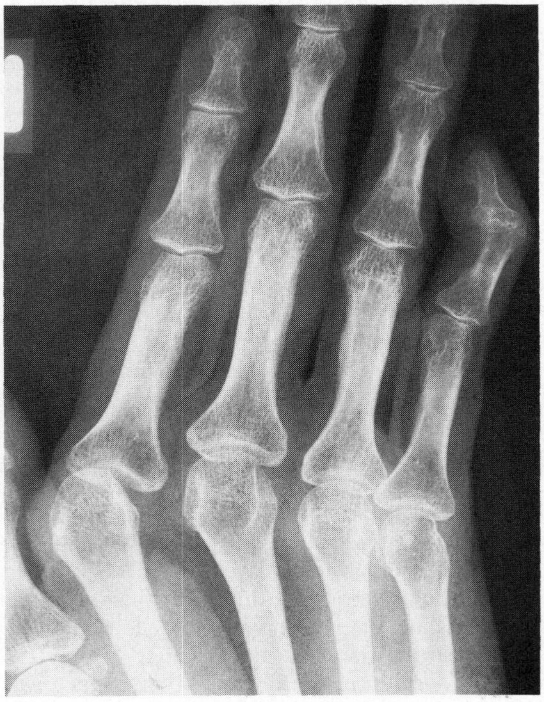

**Figure 39–25.** Systemic lupus erythematosus. This patient demonstrates juxta-articular osteoporosis with ulnar deviation at the metacarpophalangeal joints. No erosions are present.

**Progressive Systemic Sclerosis (PSS, Scleroderma).** Soft tissue or bony involvement in PSS is common. The radiographic abnormalities can be divided into four main categories:[100] (1) soft tissue resorption, (2) soft tissue calcification, (3) osteolysis, and (4) erosive articular disease.

Soft tissue resorption is most commonly noted in the fingertips in association with Raynaud's phenomenon (Fig. 39–27). Early changes can be identified by noting a reduction in the normal distance between the phalangeal tips and the skin (normal $\geq$ 20 percent of the transverse diameter of the base of the same distal phalanx).[131] In time the fingertip assumes a conical shape and soft tissue calcification is often present.

Soft tissue calcification is most common in the hand but may occur at virtually any site.[102,103] Calcification may be present in subcutaneous tissue, joint capsule, tendons, or ligaments (Fig. 39–28). The calcification typically is composed of hydroxyapatite crystals and has a soft cloudlike radiographic appearance. Occasionally large tumoral collections may be present adjacent to a joint. Intra-articular or intra-osseous calcification may also be noted (Fig. 39–29).

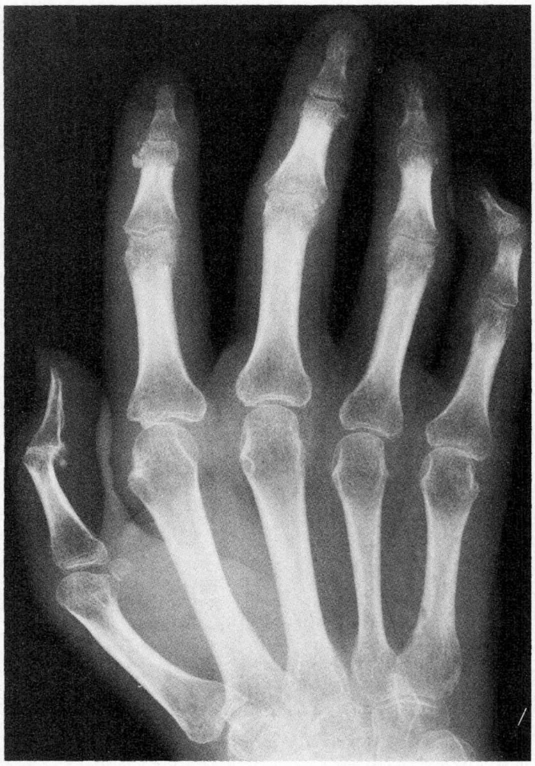

**Figure 39–27.** Scleroderma. Juxta-articular osteoporosis, soft tissue calcification, and resorption of the terminal tufts of the distal phalanges are present. Also note the tapered appearance of the soft tissues of the second finger and a hooklike erosion in the radial aspect of the third metacarpal head.

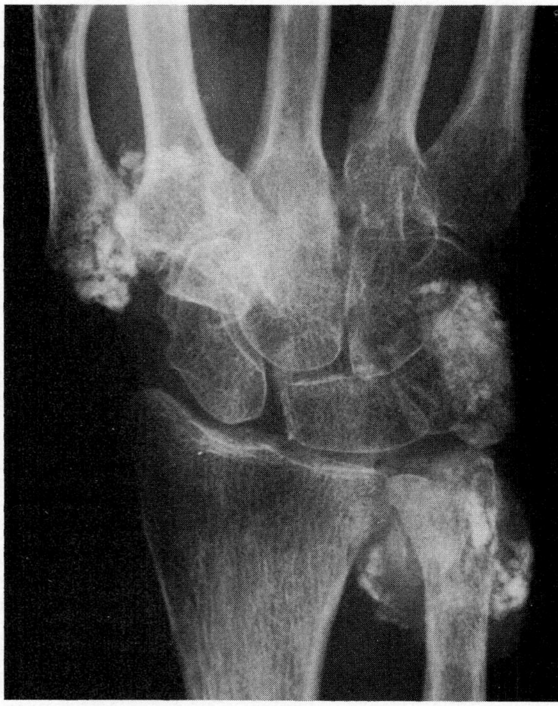

**Figure 39–29.** Scleroderma. Prominent soft tissue calcification and intra-articular calcification are present as well as severe erosive change of the first carpometacarpal joint. This is a characteristic "target" area of scleroderma. (From Resnick, D., and Niwayama, G.: Diagnosis of Bone and Joint Disorders. Philadelphia, W.B. Saunders, 1981.)

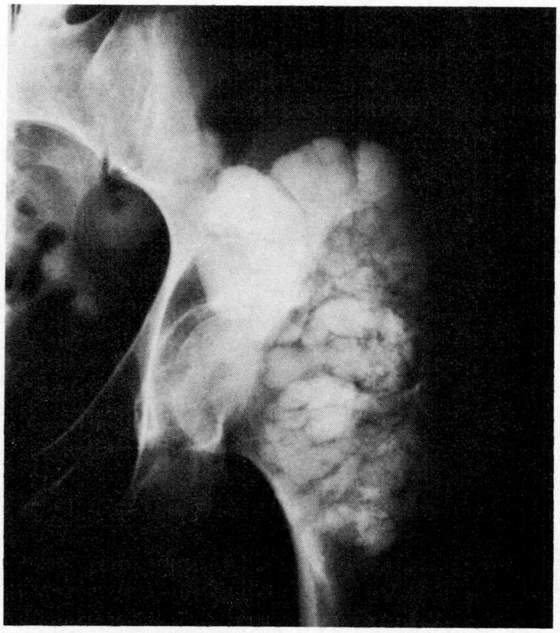

**Figure 39–28.** Scleroderma. A large tumoral calcific collection is present adjacent to the hip.

Extra-articular osteolysis is a frequent manifestation of PSS. The most common site is the tuft of the distal phalanx of the hand or occasionally the foot, usually in association with Raynaud's phenomenon and soft tissue calcification. The earliest change is in the volar aspect of the tuft with continuing resorption leading to a "sharpened" appearance of the phalanx (Fig. 39–30).[100] Elsewhere, thickening of the periodontal membrane about the roots of the teeth[104] or localized mandibular osteolysis may be seen, the latter predisposing to pathologic fracture.[105] Localized osteolysis involving the ribs, acromion, clavicle, radius, ulna, and cervical spine has also been reported.[106-109]

A severe articular disease consisting of joint space narrowing, marginal and central osseous erosions, and deformity may occur.[109] There is a distinctive tendency toward involvement of the first carpometacarpal joint (Fig. 39–29).[100] Indeed, bilateral destructive changes of the first carpometacarpal articulation with joint subluxation should arouse suspicion of PSS. Other relatively common sites of joint involvement in PSS include the distal interphalangeal, proximal interphalangeal, inferior radioulnar, and metatarsophalangeal joints.

**Dermatomyositis and Polymyositis.** Articular abnormalities in dermatomyositis and polymyositis are usually without radiographic manifestations, although periarticular soft tissue swelling and osteoporosis may occasionally be noted.[112] More dramatic roentgenographic

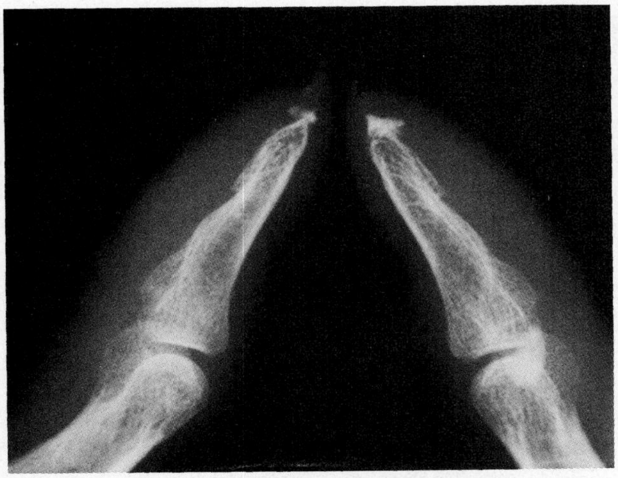

**Figure 39–30.** Scleroderma. There is osteolysis of the volar aspect of the distal phalanges of the thumbs with adjacent soft tissue calcification. Also note the tapered appearance of the adjacent soft tissues.

changes occur in the skeletal musculature, especially the large proximal muscle groups of the thorax, arm, forearm, thigh, and calf. Initial inflammation produces increased bulk and radiodensity of muscles with loss of the normal intermuscular fat planes.[113] In later stages, muscle atrophy or contractures may be prominent. The most characteristic soft tissue abnormality is calcification[114] in subcutaneous tissue, intermuscular fascia, tendons, or fat (Fig. 39–31). Subcutaneous calcific deposits simulate those of progressive systemic sclerosis, but the presence of marked linear calcific collections favors the diagnosis of polymyositis or dermatomyositis.

**Periarteritis Nodosa.** Plain film radiographic findings are unusual in this disorder, although joint effusions or periostitis of the tubular bones identical to that of hypertrophic osteoarthropathy may occasionally be seen.[115] Angiography is an important diagnostic modality in evaluating the extent of vascular damage in this disease.

**Mixed Connective Tissue Disease and "Overlap" Syndromes.** A broad spectrum of radiographic abnormalities may be present in mixed connective tissue disease (MCTD),[116,117] including soft tissue swelling and calcification, osteoporosis, joint space narrowing, bony erosions, and joint deformity. Useful radiographic clues include (1) a radiographic pattern suggestive of more than one collagen vascular disease, (2) an erosive arthropathy with an asymmetric distribution or with prominent involvement of the distal interphalangeal joints, and (3) sausage-like soft tissue swelling of a digit. However, none of these changes is specific for MCTD.

There is a group of patients with clinical and radiographic features of more than one collagen vascular disease in whom serologic testing fails to document the presence of MCTD. Such patients are considered to have an "overlap" syndrome. Roentgenographic alterations generally indicate findings of rheumatoid arthritis, SLE, PSS, and dermatomyositis in various combinations.

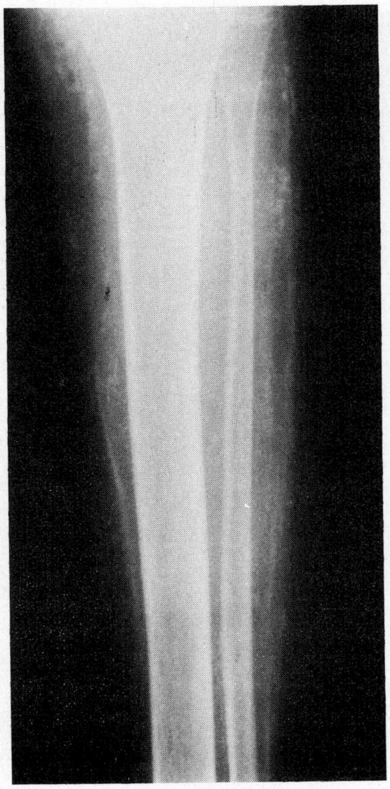

**Figure 39–31.** Dermatomyositis. There is prominent calcification of the subcutaneous tissue and the muscle in the leg.

## DEGENERATIVE JOINT DISEASE

The most characteristic sites of osteoarthritis (OA) include the proximal and distal interphalangeal joints of the hand, first carpometacarpal and trapezioscaphoid joints of the wrist, acromioclavicular and sacroiliac joints, hip, knee, and first metatarsophalangeal joint of the foot. Degenerative joint disease may also affect cartilaginous joints (such as the manubriosternal joint and symphysis pubis) and tendinous and ligamentous attachments to bone or entheses (such as in the pelvis, patella, and calcaneus). Degenerative disease of the spine is a separate subject and will be discussed later.

**Osteoarthritis.** In spite of a diversity of etiologies of OA, certain common radiographic characteristics allow a confident diagnosis in most cases. Joint space narrowing is a key diagnostic feature of the disease (Fig. 39–32).[118] In contrast to the inflammatory arthropathies, in which diffuse joint space narrowing of an involved articulation is expected, the joint space loss in OA tends to involve the portion of the joint exposed to the greatest stress (i.e., the lateral aspect of the hip, the medial compartment of the knee). Subchondral bone abnormalities are also characteristic of OA and include sclerosis (eburnation) and cyst formation, both of which predominate in the stressed area of the articulation. Subchondral

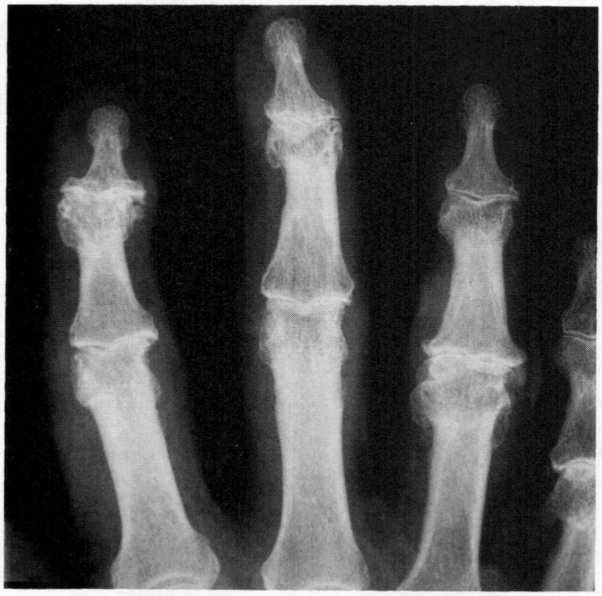

**Figure 39–32.** Osteoarthritis. There is narrowing of multiple interphalangeal joints with interdigitating osteophytes.

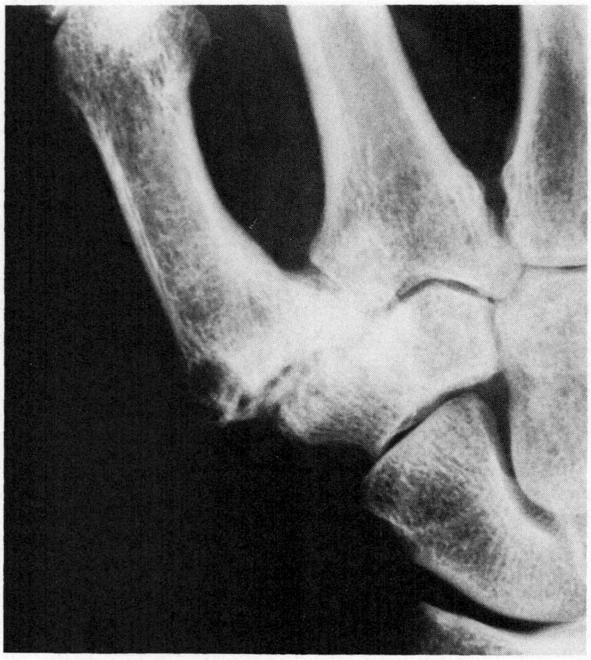

**Figure 39–33.** Osteoarthritis. Narrowing of the articular space and subchondral sclerosis about the first carpometacarpal joint are apparent.

eburnation results from cartilage denudation with subsequent bone-to-bone contact. The origin of subchondral cysts remains in debate.[119,120]

Osteophytes are the single most characteristic radiographic and pathologic abnormality in OA.[118] They tend to arise from endochondral ossification in areas of low stress where islands of cartilage are preserved, most commonly at joint margins. In some cases osteophytes may arise from the synovium or joint capsule.

***Hand and Wrist.*** The interphalangeal joints of the hand are frequent target areas of OA. (Fig. 39–32). The appearance of articular space narrowing with closely apposed interdigitating bony surfaces and marginal osteophytes is characteristic. Metacarpophalangeal joint involvement may also occur but not as an isolated event; rather, such involvement is associated with alterations at interphalangeal articulations. At the metacarpophalangeal joints, it is interosseous space narrowing that is the predominant abnormality. Osseous erosions are not apparent. The first carpometacarpal (trapeziometacarpal) joint is the characteristic site of degenerative abnormalities in the wrist (Fig. 39–33). Joint space narrowing with bony eburnation, subchondral cysts, and osteophyte formation is typical. Radial subluxation of the first metacarpal base is common. The trapezioscaphoid space is the only other common site of OA in the wrist; involvement at this site is generally combined with that at the first carpometacarpal joint. Trapezioscaphoid joint disease in the absence of first carpometacarpal joint involvement should suggest another diagnosis, especially calcium pyrophosphate crystal deposition disease. Similarly, a degenerative disease-like arthropathy elsewhere in the wrist, especially at the radiocarpal joint, in the absence of significant occupational or accidental trauma, is generally related to a disease other than OA.

***Sacroiliac Joint.*** OA of the sacroiliac joint is very common in the older age group. Joint space narrowing with a thin, well-defined band of subchondral sclerosis, especially in the ilium, is typically present. Osteophyte formation is most common at the superior and inferior margins of the synovium-lined portion of the joint. At the former location, these osteophytes may appear as localized radiodensities projected over the joint in the anteroposterior radiographic projection. Bony erosion and intra-articular osseous fusion are not features of OA of the sacroiliac joint.

***Hip.*** OA of the hip is exceedingly frequent and may lead to significant patient disability. In the typical case, cartilage loss is focal, involves the superolateral aspect of the joint, and leads to upward migration of the femoral head (Fig. 39–34). Osteophyte formation is most prominent at the lateral acetabular and medial femoral margins, often in combination with thickening (buttressing) of the cortex in the medial aspect of the femoral neck. Subchondral sclerosis and cyst formation on both sides of the joint space may be marked. Focal loss of cartilage on the medial aspect of the articulation occurs in approximately 20 percent of patients with OA. Diffuse loss of cartilage with axial migration of the femoral head (along the axis of the femoral neck) is rare in OA. This latter feature is important in the differentiation of OA from inflammatory arthropathies such as rheumatoid arthritis.

***Knee.*** The knee is a common site of OA. The most characteristic pattern of disease consists of involvement of the medial femorotibial compartment with joint space narrowing, osseous eburnation, subchondral cysts, and

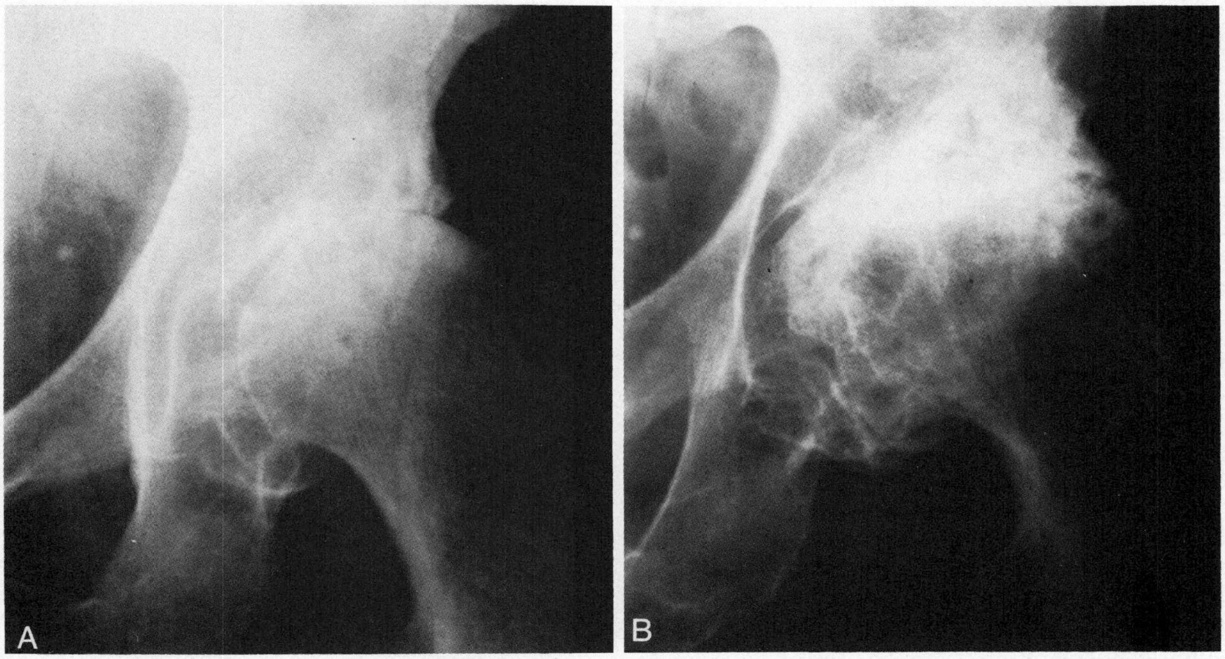


**Figure 39–34.** Osteoarthritis. Moderately advanced osteoarthritic changes are present in *A* with asymmetric joint space narrowing and superior migration of the femoral head. Eburnation and cystic changes are seen in the subchondral region. In *B* advanced changes have occurred, with collapse of the superior articular surface and the formation of large marginal osteophytes.

marginal osteophytes.[122] Sharpening of the tibial spines or the presence of osteophytes arising from the intercondylar notch of the femur may also be observed. A true assessment of cartilage destruction may not be possible on standard anteroposterior radiographs (obtained with the patient supine) but is better provided by radiographs obtained either in the "tunnel" projection (Fig. 39–35) or with the patient in a weight-bearing

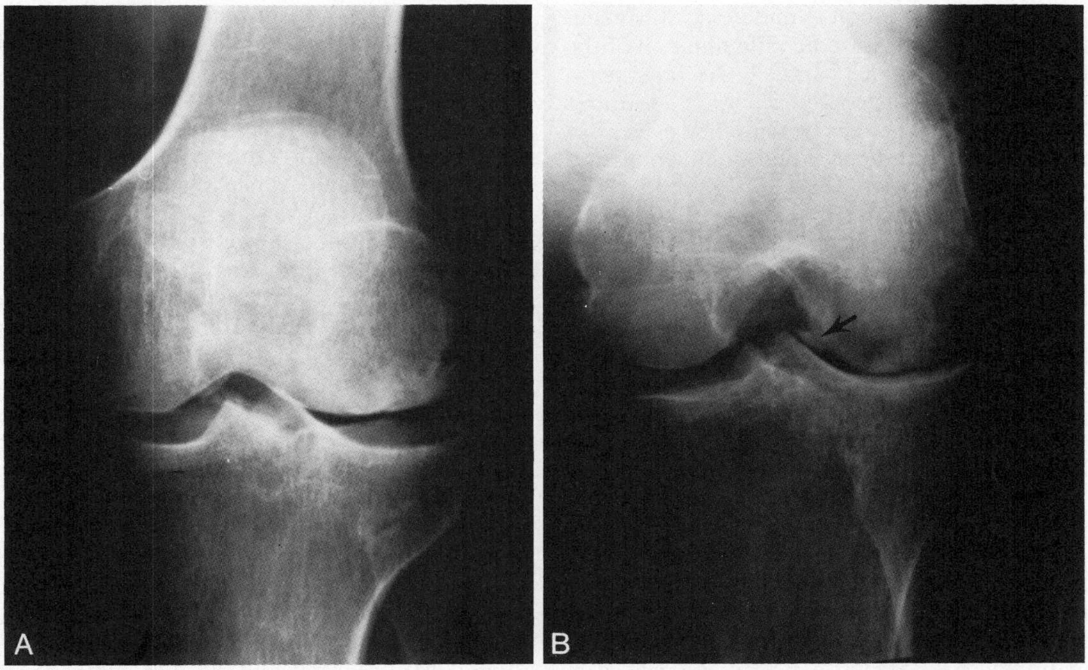


**Figure 39–35.** Osteoarthritis. Anteroposterior (*A*) and tunnel (*B*) projections reveal typical osteoarthritic changes of the knee. Note the asymmetric involvement with subchondral eburnation of the lateral articular surfaces. In this case the actual degree of joint space narrowing is much more apparent in the tunnel projection. An osteophyte arising from the intercondylar notch is identified (arrow).

position.[124] Varus angulation of the knee is the most common deformity in OA, reflecting the more severe involvement of the medial femorotibial compartment compared with the lateral one. Symmetric medial and lateral femorotibial compartment disease is unusual. Osteoarthritic changes in the patellofemoral compartment are also common, either in isolation or accompanying medial femorotibial compartment disease.

Osseous or cartilaginous debris may be present as intra-articular bodies ("joint mice") either free within the joint cavity or embedded in the synovial membrane. Degeneration of the fibrocartilaginous menisci is a typical feature of advanced OA.

*Foot.* OA in the foot typically affects the first metatarsophalangeal joint. Articular space narrowing, bony eburnation, osteophyte formation, and subchondral cysts are common. Hallux rigidus is a specific pattern of OA, which may be seen in adolescent or young adults; there is painful restriction of dorsiflexion at the first metatarsophalangeal joint.[124] Hallux valgus is another common pattern of OA about this joint, with lateral angulation of the first toe and prominent sclerosis, cyst formation, and osteophytosis on the medial aspect of the first metatarsal head.

*Other Locations.* Typical osteoarthritic changes in the elbows, acromioclavicular and glenohumeral joints, and ankles may be encountered, usually in patients with a history of trauma or pre-existing disease. In general, without such a history, a radiographic pattern consistent with OA[118] at an unusual site should suggest another disease process, including acromegaly, calcium pyrophosphate crystal deposition disease, ochronosis, and epiphyseal dysplasia.

**Inflammatory Osteoarthritis.** Inflammatory osteoarthritis is a disease most common in middle-aged women. It is characterized by acute episodic inflammation of the interphalangeal joints of the hand.[125] On roentgenograms, typical marginal osteophytes with or without bony erosions are seen. The erosions are first evident in the central portion of the subchondral bone, appearing as sharply marginated defects (Fig. 39–36).[118] Intra-articular ankylosis may subsequently result.[126] It must be emphasized that the clinical syndrome of inflammatory osteoarthritis can occur in the absence of radiographically demonstrable bony erosions; therefore, the term erosive osteoarthritis is not an ideal one for this disorder.

**Degenerative Enthesopathy.** Coarse bony proliferation at sites of ligamentous and tendinous attachment is a manifestation of a degenerative enthesopathy. This is most commonly observed in the pelvis, patella, ulnar olecranon, and calcaneus. The resulting bony excrescences are identical to those encountered in diffuse idiopathic skeletal hyperostosis. They are usually coarser and better defined than the outgrowths accompanying the inflammatory enthesopathy of the seronegative spondyloarthropathies.

**Degenerative Disease of the Spine.** The vertebral column is composed of a complex series of synovial, cartilaginous, and fibrous articulations. Degenerative diseases of the spine can involve any of these articulations

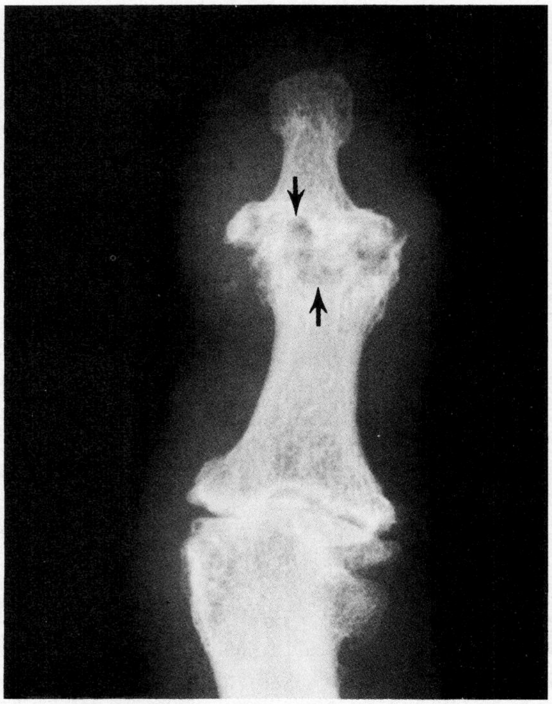

**Figure 39–36.** Inflammatory osteoarthritis. The combination of interphalangeal joint involvement, prominent marginal osteophytes, and central erosions of the articular surfaces (arrows) is characteristic of this disease. (From Resnick, D., and Niwayama, G.: Diagnosis of Bone and Joint Disorders. Philadelphia, W.B. Saunders Co., 1981.)

as well as ligamentous insertions (entheses).[128] Many distinct degenerative processes can be identified.

*Intervertebral (Osteo)chondrosis.* Primary degenerative disease of the nucleus pulposus of the intervertebral disc, termed intervertebral (osteo)chondrosis, is a common disorder, especially in the elderly, which may occur at any spinal level but is more commonly identified in the lumbar and cervical regions.[1]

The earliest radiographic change consists of linear or circular collections of gas ("vacuum phenomena") within the disc substance (Fig. 39–37).[129] These gas collections are more prominent on radiographs obtained with the spine in extension and may disappear in flexion. The presence of a vacuum phenomenon is a very useful observation, since it virtually excludes the possibility of infection.[130] Progressive narrowing of the intervertebral disc and sclerosis beneath the subchondral bone plate are additional manifestations of intervertebral (osteo)chondrosis. Herniation of portions of the intervertebral disc into the adjacent vertebral body (Schmorl's node, cartilaginous node) is a further radiographic sign. Small triangular osteophytes at the discovertebral junction are also seen (Fig. 39–37).

*Spondylosis Deformans.* Spondylosis deformans[127] refers to the formation of multiple large osteophytes predominantly along the anterior and lateral aspects of the vertebral bodies (Fig. 39–38).[131] These osteophytes may occur at any level; in the thoracic spine, they predom-

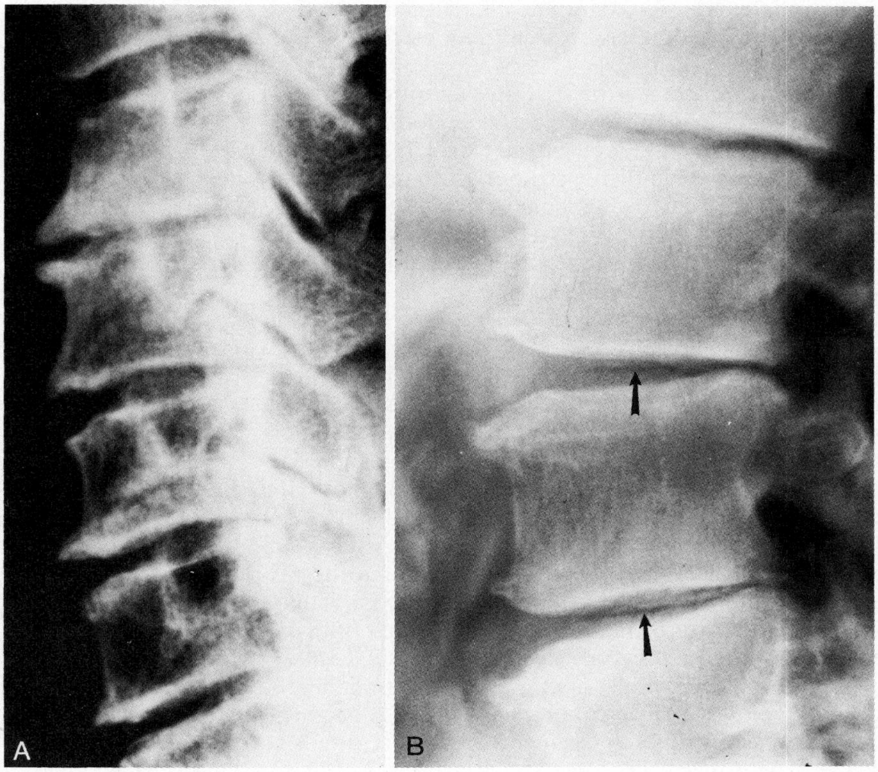


**Figure 39–37.** Intervertebral osteochondrosis. Lateral projections of the cervical spine (*A*) and lumbar spine (*B*) reveal typical abnormalities of intervertebral (osteo)chondrosis. Intervertebral disc space narrowing with sclerosis of the vertebral endplates and the formation of small triangular osteophytes from the anterior vertebral margins are evident. Prominent vacuum phenomena (arrows) are present in the lumbar spine. (From Resnick, D., and Niwayama, G.: Diagnosis of Bone and Joint Disorders. Philadelphia, W.B. Saunders Co., 1981.)

inate on the right side, presumably because their formation is inhibited on the left side by the constant pulsation of the descending thoracic aorta.[132] Narrowing of the intervertebral disc space, vacuum phenomena, and endplate bony sclerosis are not features of spondylosis deformans. The differentiation of the osteophytes of spondylosis deformans from the vertebral lesions of the seronegative spondyloarthropathies has been discussed previously.

*Apophyseal Joint Osteoarthritis.* The synovium-lined apophyseal joint is a frequent site of degenerative disease.[128] Changes are most common in the mid and lower cervical spine, the mid thoracic spine, and the lower lumbar spine. The radiographic changes are identical to those of OA in peripheral articulations,[133] with joint space narrowing, osseous eburnation, and marginal osteophyte formation. Capsular laxity may result in apophyseal joint malalignment. In this setting or with large osteophytes arising from the joint margins, impingement of a spinal nerve root within the neural foramen may occur.

*Uncovertebral Arthrosis.* Degenerative changes in the cervical uncovertebral articulations (Lushka) are often identified on the frontal radiograph of the cervical spine. The nature of this process is debated, since these articulations have been shown to represent intervertebral disc extensions in early life and to contain synovium-like

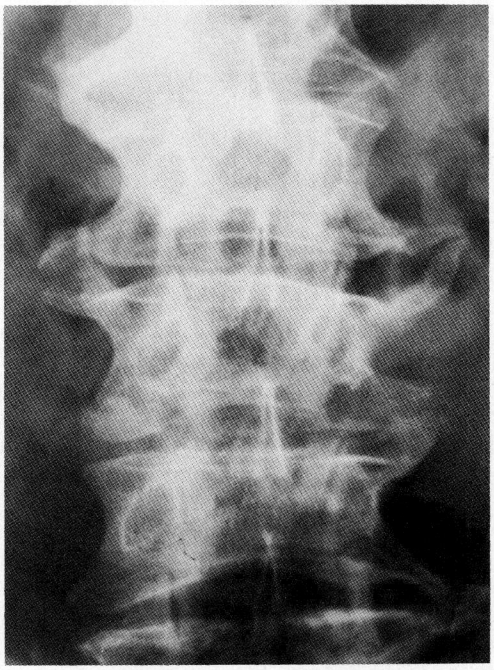

**Figure 39–38.** Spondylosis deformans. The frontal projection of the spine reveals multiple large interdigitating osteophytes arising from the lateral margins of the vertebral bodies. Note that the initial portion of the osteophytes has a horizontal orientation.

tissue in later life. Radiographic changes consist of osseous sclerosis, joint space loss, and osteophyte formation.

***Costovertebral Osteoarthritis.*** Osteoarthritic changes of the synovium-lined costovertebral joints are very common, especially at the level of the eleventh and twelfth ribs.[128] Radiographic demonstration of these abnormalities (joint space narrowing, bony sclerosis, osteophytes) is frequently difficult, owing to the superimposition of ribs and vertebral bodies over the articulations on conventional radiographic studies.

***Diffuse Idiopathic Skeletal Hyperostosis.*** Diffuse idiopathic skeletal hyperostosis (DISH) is a common degenerative enthesopathy and has been described under a variety of terms,[134-136] including Forestier's disease, spondylitis ossificans ligamentosa, spondylosis hyperostotica, and ankylosing hyperostosis of the spine. Although radiographic changes are evident in both the axial and the appendicular skeleton, the diagnosis of DISH is based on the presence of characteristic spinal alterations. In fact, the radiographic change in the vertebral column must fulfill three criteria before a diagnosis of DISH can be made: (1) the presence of flowing calcification or ossification along the anterolateral aspects of at least four contiguous vertebral levels, (2) relative preservation of intervertebral disc height in the involved vertebral segments without extensive changes of primary degenerative disc disease, and (3) the absence of apophyseal joint ankylosis or sacroiliac joint erosions, sclerosis, or intra-articular bony ankylosis.

The most characteristic radiographic abnormality of DISH is calcification and ossification of the anterior longitudinal ligament (ALL) of the spine.[137] This is most commonly identified in the mid thoracic spine but is also evident in the cervical and lumbar levels. Early in the disease, an undulating radiodense band forms along the anterolateral aspect of the spine separated from the anterior aspect of the vertebral body by a thin radiolucent line (Fig. 39–39); with progression of the disease, the lucency may disappear. These changes, which are best demonstrated in the lateral radiographic projection of the thoracic spine, may resemble the "bamboo spine" of ankylosing spondylitis but several important diagnostic features exist. Syndesmophytes arise from the anterosuperior and anteroinferior margins of the vertebral body, whereas the ossification in DISH attaches to the vertebral body several millimeters from these margins. In addition, syndesmophytes may be best seen in the frontal radiographic projection, in contrast to DISH, in which changes are most prominent on the lateral radiographic projection. The presence of sacroiliac joint erosions and intra-articular bony ankylosis of the sacroiliac or apophyseal joints in ankylosing spondylitis constitutes another important differential diagnostic point.

In the cervical spine, bony outgrowths characteristically appear at the anteroinferior margin of the vertebral body and extend inferiorly around the disc space. With progression, a thick, armorlike mass of bone bridges the intervertebral disc, leading to markedly diminished cervical motion and, in some cases, dysphagia (Fig. 39–40).[138] Linear or Y-shaped radiolucencies in the bony mass may be noted at the level of the intervertebral disc space owing to herniation of disc material into the ossific mass. Ossification adjacent to the inferior margin of the anterior arch of the atlas is common and may be confused with traumatic changes. Ossification of the posterior longitudinal ligament may be seen as a distinct entity but occurs with increased frequency in patients with DISH (Fig. 39–40).[139] DISH may also be associated with a rare syndrome, sternocostoclavicular hyperostosis (SCCH),[139,140] in which extensive ossification of the soft tissues between the anterior ribs, medial clavicle, and sternum is evident.

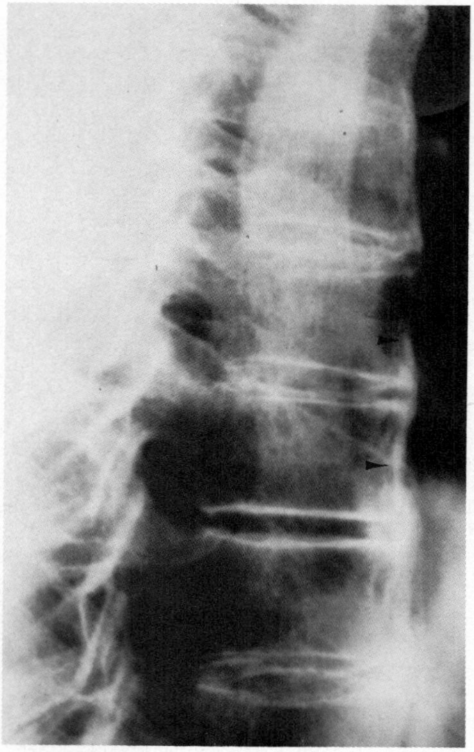

**Figure 39–39.** Diffuse idiopathic skeletal hyperostosis (DISH). The lateral view of the thoracic spine in this patient with DISH demonstrates ossification of the anterior longitudinal ligament (ALL). Note the characteristic lucencies between the ossified ALL and the anterior vertebral margin (arrowheads).

In the lumbar spine, changes of DISH resemble those in the cervical region; osteophytes are present.

Extraspinal manifestations of DISH[142] are especially common in the pelvis. Bony proliferation at sites of ligamentous and tendinous attachment (enthesopathy) results in the formation of coarse, well-marginated bony excrescences, in contrast to the fine, spiculated, ill-defined bony proliferative changes of the seronegative spondyloarthropathies (Fig. 39–41). Calcification of the iliolumbar and sacrotuberous ligaments is an additional characteristic feature (Fig. 39–42). Para-articular osteophytes are commonly noted about the hip and along the inferior aspect of the sacroiliac joints.

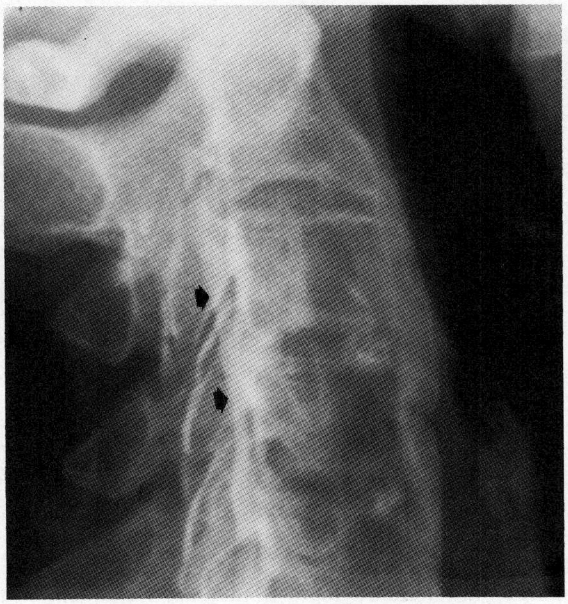

**Figure 39–40.** Diffuse idiopathic skeletal hyperostosis (DISH). The lateral view of the cervical spine in this patient demonstrates thick, flowing ossification along the anterior margins of the vertebral bodies. Ossification of the posterior longitudinal ligament (OPLL) is also present (arrows).

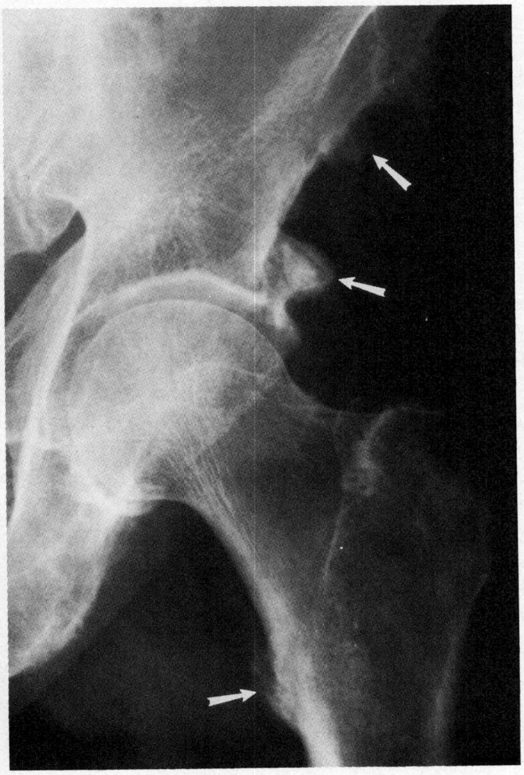

**Figure 39–41.** Diffuse idiopathic skeletal hyperostosis (DISH). The degenerative enthesopathy of DISH is well demonstrated with coarse bony excrescences arising from sites of ligament and tendon insertion along the lateral aspect of the ilium, superior acetabular margin, and lesser trochanter (arrows). This appearance differs from that of the finely spiculated inflammatory enthesopathy of the seronegative spondyloarthropathies.

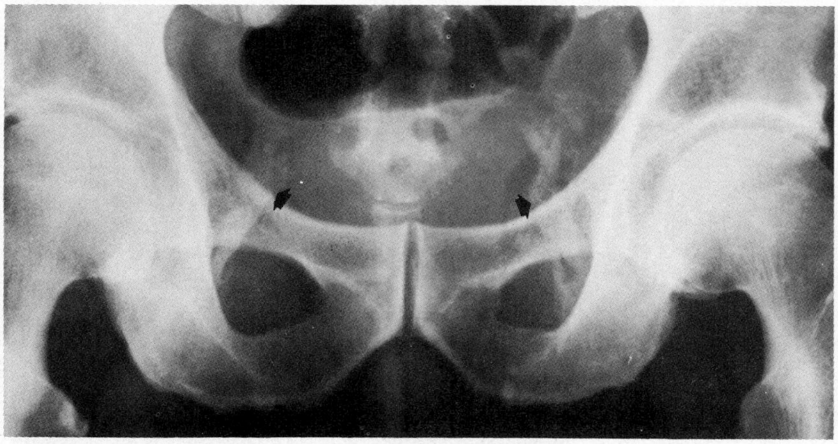

**Figure 39–42.** Diffuse idiopathic skeletal hyperostosis (DISH). Calcification of the sacrotuberous ligaments (arrows) has occurred.

Other extraspinal sites of prominent bony proliferation include the patellar poles, calcaneus, and olecranon process of the ulna. The "spurs" that form at these sites may be identical in appearance to localized degenerative changes in otherwise normal individuals, but they demonstrate a tendency toward increased size and multiplicity. In the hand, hyperostotic changes of the metacarpal and phalangeal heads, with proliferation in the terminal tufts, may be noted. Irregular excrescences may also be seen at the femoral trochanters, deltoid tuberosity of the humerus and anterior tibial tuberosity and about the interosseous membranes of the forearm and leg.

## NEUROARTHROPATHY

Neuroarthropathy (Charcot joint) refers to destructive and productive articular abnormalities occurring in association with loss of pain or proprioceptive sensation, or both. Although debate exists as to the precise pathogenesis of neuroarthropathy, it is believed that the cumulative effect of trauma and joint laxity due to relaxation of periarticular supporting structures is contributory.

One of the early radiographic changes of neuroarthropathy is the presence of a joint effusion, which may become large. Mild joint subluxation may then appear.[142] Subsequently, fragmentation of the articular surface occurs with eburnation of bony surfaces, leading, in time, to complete joint disorganization. These radiographic abnormalities have been subdivided into hypertrophic and atrophic types. The hypertrophic reaction is more common in central lesions, as in tabes dorsalis and syringomyelia. There is prominent periosteal new bone formation as well as metaplasia of the synovium with the formation of bone and cartilage within its deeper layers. Large osteocartilaginous bodies of synovial origin in combination with fragments originating from the articular surfaces result in a fragmented, disorganized articulation with a great deal of osseous debris (Fig. 39–43). The atrophic reaction occurs more commonly with diseases, such as diabetes mellitus, in which the abnormality involves the peripheral nerve (Fig. 39–44). Fragmentation occurs, but the osteocartilaginous debris is resorbed, resulting in disappearance of the articular surfaces. It should be emphasized that hypertrophic and atrophic patterns are not completely reliable in identifying the level of neurologic abnormality, since exceptions to these rules are common.

A great number of disorders lead to neuropathic changes. In general the morphologic aberrations produced by these disorders are similar; however, there are differences in articular distribution among these disorders, which provide clues to the specific diagnosis.

**Tabes Dorsalis.**[142-144] Five to 10 percent of patients with tabes dorsalis demonstrate neuroarthropathy. The articulations of the lower extremity are most commonly affected, with the knee and the hip being the most frequent target sites (Fig. 39–43*A* and *B*). Other sites include the ankle and the articulations in both the upper extremity and the spinal column. In peripheral joints, typic radiographic features are large effusions, bony eburnation, and fragmentation. Bilateral and symmetric changes are not uncommon. In the axial skeleton, intervertebral disc space narrowing, vertebral body sclerosis, and formation of large osteophytes may resemble the changes of unusually severe degenerative disease.

**Syringomyelia.**[145] Approximately 20 to 50 percent of patients with syringomyelia develop neuroarthropathy. There is a distinct predilection for upper extremity involvement, especially the glenohumeral joint, elbow, and wrist. Lower extremity or spinal alterations may occur in some cases. Bilateral and symmetric involvement is less frequent in syringomyelia than in tabes dorsalis.

**Diabetes Mellitus.**[146-148] Diabetes mellitus is probably the most common cause of neuroarthropathy, although less than 1 percent of patients with this disease develop such changes. The articulations of the foot are affected in the majority of cases, although the ankle, knee, spine, and joints of the upper extremity may occasionally be affected. Abnormalities predominate in the tarsal and tarsometatarsal articulations, consisting of bony ebur-

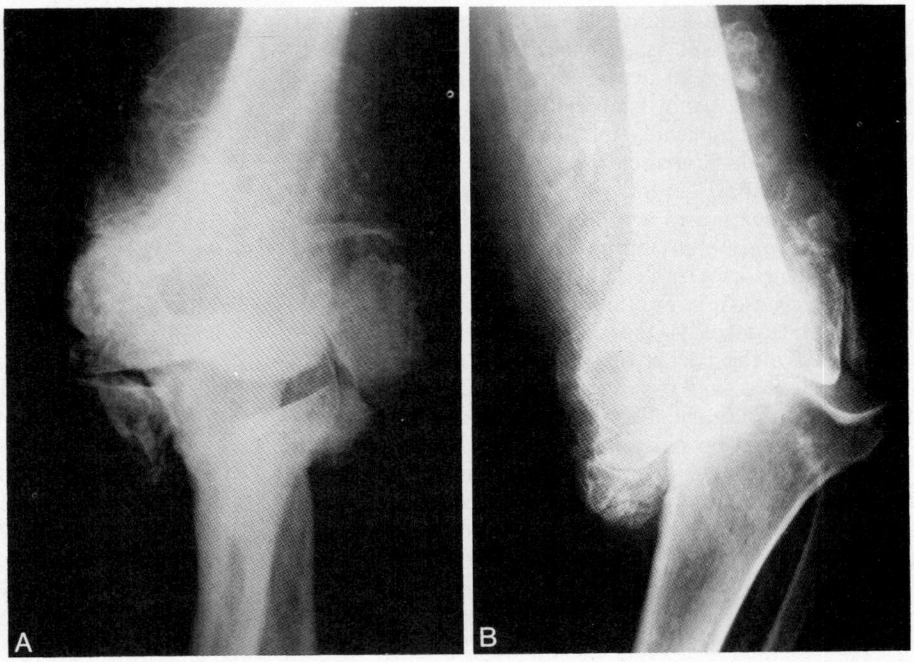


**Figure 39–43.** Tabes dorsalis with neuroarthropathy. Radiographs of the elbow (*A*) and knee (*B*) in patients with tabes dorsalis demonstrate changes of neuroarthropathy. Bony sclerosis, fragmentation, and instability of the joints are present with dramatic soft tissue swelling.

nation and fragmentation. Spontaneous fractures are common and a Lisfranc fracture-dislocation pattern may be seen (Fig. 39–44). In the forefoot a resorptive pattern is most typical, with tapering or "sharpening" of metatarsal and phalangeal shafts. Concurrent or superimposed infection is a common problem in the diabetic individual. There is great difficulty in differentiating the radiographic changes of neuroarthropathy from those of infection; however, the indistinctness of bony margins in infection compared with the sharp margins in neuroarthropathy aids in correct diagnosis.

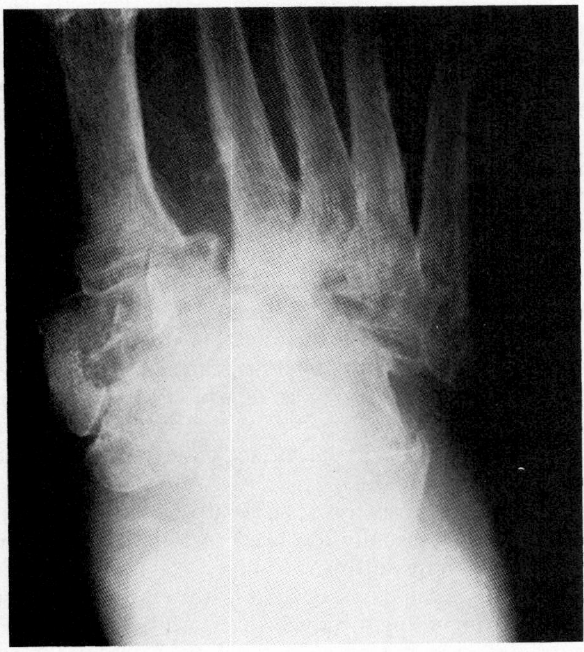

**Figure 39–44.** Diabetic neuroarthropathy. A Lisfranc's type of fracture-dislocation has occurred as a complication of neuroarthropathy in this diabetic patient. Note the lateral displacement of the second through fifth metatarsal bases with sclerosis and fragmentation of the adjacent tarsal bones.

**Other Disorders.** Although peripheral neuropathy is common in the alcoholic patient, neuroarthropathy is rare. It resembles that in diabetes mellitus with characteristic involvement of the articulations of the foot.[149] In amyloidosis, knee and ankle involvement is most typical.[150] Neuropathic changes in childhood should suggest the possibility of congenital indifference to pain or meningomyelocele.[142] In both of these disorders involvement of the ankle and tarsal articulations is seen, and changes may appear at the physis, or growth plate, with osseous irregularity, sclerosis, epiphyseal separation, and periostitis. An idiopathic form of neuroarthropathy of the elbow has been described, and neuroarthropathic changes have been observed following intra-articular administration of steroids.

## CRYSTAL-RELATED ARTHROPATHIES

Several types of articular disease are related to abnormal deposition or accumulation of crystalline material in and about articulations. These include gout, calcium pyrophosphate dihydrate (CPPD) crystal deposition disease, hemochromatosis, and hydroxyapatite crystal deposition disease (HADD).[151] Two other entities that may be included in this group are Wilson's disease and ochronosis (alkaptonuria).

**Gout.** The earliest radiographic change in gout consists of reversible soft tissue swelling about the involved articulation during an acute gouty attack. With chronicity of disease, tophi lead to nodular, lobulated soft tissue densities, especially in the feet, ankles, knees, elbows, and hands. Calcification within a tophus may be evident, particularly in individuals with gouty nephritis, whereas ossification of a tophus is rare.[151,152] Bony erosions are common in longstanding gout and may be intra-articular or extra-articular in location. Intra-articular erosions most commonly involve the joint margins and proceed centrally (Fig. 39–45). Extra-articular erosions involve the cortex of the bone, frequently in association with a soft tissue mass (tophus) (Fig. 39–46). These erosions are usually round or oval in shape, often with a sclerotic border and a "punched-out" appearance.[153] The presence of an "overhanging lip" of bone at the margin of an erosion is a characteristic feature of gout. Occasionally a more extensive proliferative bony reaction, presumably due to a reparative process, may be noted, typically at the first metatarsophalangeal joint, intertarsal joints, and knee.[155] The joint space is usually preserved in gouty arthritis until the late stages of the disease. In fact, the presence of prominent intra-articular osseous erosions with relative preservation of the joint space suggests the diagnosis of gout. Intra-articular bony ankylosis is occasionally seen, especially involving the interphalangeal joints of the hands and feet as well as the carpal region.[154] Although transient localized osteoporosis may be present during an acute gouty attack, extensive osteoporosis is not a feature of this disease.

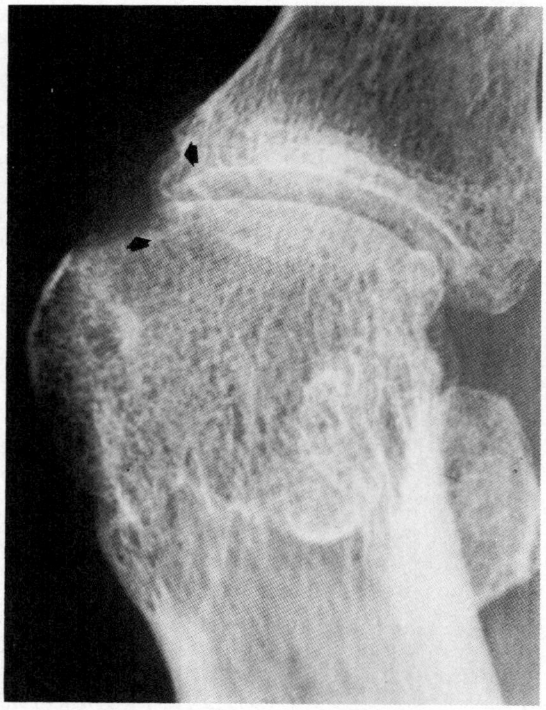

**Figure 39–45.** Gout. Typical erosions of the metatarsal head and proximal phalangeal base (arrows) are present in this patient with gouty arthritis of the first metatarsophalangeal joint.

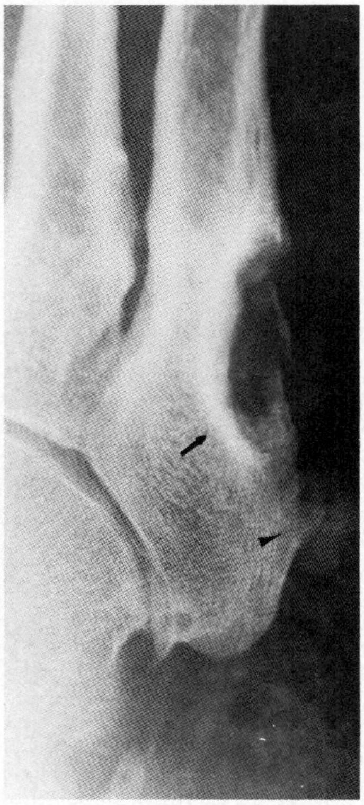

**Figure 39–46.** Gout. A large extra-articular erosion of the lateral aspect of the fifth metatarsal shaft is bordered by reactive bony sclerosis (arrow). A smaller erosion is present more proximally (arrowhead) with an adjacent calcified soft tissue tophus. (From Resnick, D., and Niwayama, G.: Diagnosis of Bone and Joint Disorders. Philadelphia, W.B. Saunders Co., 1981.)

The general radiographic features of gout are similar at all sites; however, involvement at several specific areas may be of diagnostic importance.[151] The first metatarsophalangeal joint is the most characteristic site of involvement (Fig. 39–45). Erosions are most frequent on the dorsal and medial aspects of the metatarsal head, usually in association with a hallux valgus deformity. They are best demonstrated in the oblique radiographic projection. In the hand, proximal and distal interphalangeal joint involvement is more common than metacarpophalangeal joint involvement. Wrist abnormality is frequently pancompartmental, but extensive involvement of the common carpometacarpal articulation is important, since this area is relatively spared in most other arthropathies. Erosions of the olecranon process of the elbow and the dorsal surface of the patella strongly suggest gouty bursitis.

Chondrocalcinosis is occasionally seen in patients with gout. It is usually localized to a few articulations and predominates in fibrocartilage.

Secondary gout is associated with a wide variety of situations, including glycogen storage disease (type I),[156] Lesch-Nyhan syndrome,[157] myeloproliferative disorders,[158] endocrine diseases,[159] and the administration of certain drugs.[160] In general, secondary gout resembles primary gout radiographically, although unusual sites may be affected.[156-160]

**Calcium Pyrophosphate Dihydrate (CPPD) Crystal Deposition Disease.** CPPD crystal deposition disease is characterized by the deposition of calcium pyrophosphate dihydrate crystals in hyaline cartilage and fibrocartilage as well as in synovium, capsule, tendons, and ligaments.[151] CPPD crystal deposition disease is a general term indicating the presence of CPPD crystal in or around joints. Chondrocalcinosis refers to calcification of hyaline cartilage or fibrocartilage, regardless of its etiology. Pyrophosphate arthropathy refers to a pattern of structural joint damage with or without radiographically demonstrable chondrocalcinosis. There are two main types of radiographic abnormalities in CPPD crystal deposition disease: (1) abnormal calcification and (2) destructive arthropathy. These changes may be present in combination or in isolation.

Abnormal calcification related to CPPD crystal deposition disease may be identified in articular or periarticular structures. The most comon intra-articular site of calcification is within cartilage, either hyaline cartilage or fibrocartilage (Fig. 39–47). Hyaline cartilage calcification may occur in any joint but is most common in the wrist, knee, elbow, and hip. It appears as thin curvilinear radiodensities parallel to, but distinct from, the subchondral bone plate.[151] Fibrocartilage calcification most commonly involves the menisci of the knee, triangular fibrocartilage of the wrist, symphysis pubis, annulus fibrosus of the intervertebral disc, or labra of the glenoid and acetabulum. (Fig. 39–48). It appears as thick, irregular radiodensities within the involved structure. Cloudlike or speckled radiodensities, representing calcific deposits within synovium, may be seen at many locations, including bursal cavities, but are most common about the wrist. Additional sites of calcification include joint capsule, tendons, bursae, and ligaments.[161] Calcification at these sites is less frequent than within cartilage.

Pyrophosphate arthropathy exhibits a degenerative disease–type pattern of structural joint disease. Its general radiographic features include a bilateral symmetric or asymmetric distribution and changes characterized by joint space narrowing, bony sclerosis, and prominent subchondral cysts.[161] The latter, representing an important diagnostic feature of the arthropathy, are frequently numerous and large and may simulate neoplasm. These cysts may progress rapidly in size, undermining the articular surface and resulting in collapse and deformity of the joint. At times, this progression may be so rapid as to resemble infection or neuroarthropathy (Fig. 39–49). In some patients, large osteophytes may be present about involved articulations.

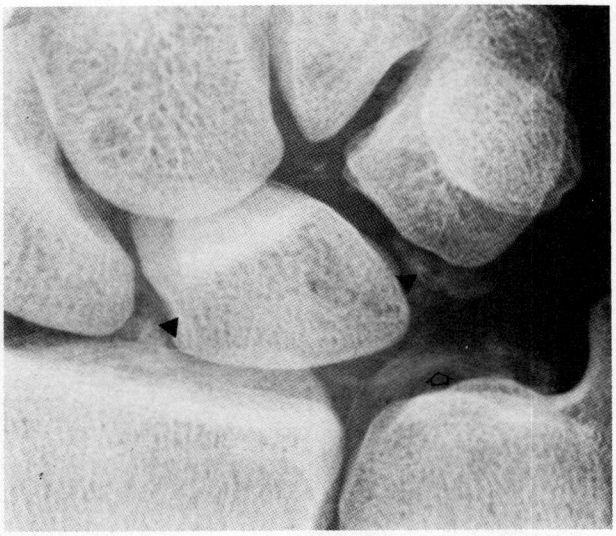

Figure 39–48. Calcium pyrophosphate crystal deposition disease. A frontal radiograph of the wrist demonstrates calcification of the triangular fibrocartilage (open arrow) and several intercarpal ligaments (arrowheads). (From Resnick, D., and Niwayama, G.: Diagnosis of Bone and Joint Disorders. Philadelphia, W.B. Saunders Co., 1981.)

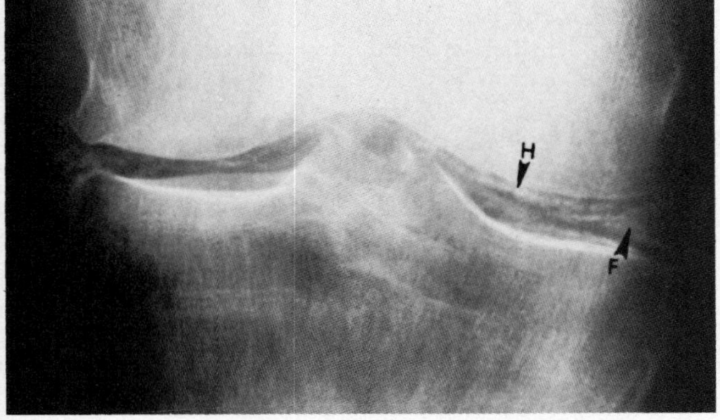


Figure 39–47. Calcium pyrophosphate crystal deposition disease. A frontal radiograph of the knee reveals calcification of hyaline articular cartilage (*H*) as well as fibrocartilaginous menisci (*F*). (From Resnick, D., and Niwayama, G.: Diagnosis of Bone and Joint Disorders. Philadelphia, W.B. Saunders Co., 1981.)

Pyrophosphate arthropathy is most commonly seen in the knee, wrist, and metacarpophalangeal joints, although any joint may be involved. The relatively common involvement of the wrist, elbow, and shoulder contrast with the situation in degenerative joint disease in which these areas are usually spared. In the hand there is a tendency toward selective involvement of the second and third metacarpophalangeal joints. In the wrist, the radioscaphoid space is frequently involved, with collapse of the proximal pole of the scaphoid into the distal radial articular surface (Fig. 39–50). Narrowing of the capitolunate space is also frequent, as is involvement of the trapezioscaphoid articulation with or without involvement of the first carpometacarpal joint. Associated calcification of the triangular fibrocartilage, intercarpal ligaments, or articular cartilage may be encountered. In the knee, the distribution of abnormalities may mimic that of osteoarthritis with involvement of the medial femorotibial and patellofemoral compartments. At times, there is isolated involvement of the patellofemoral space. In the hip, superior joint space narrowing, mimicking osteoarthritis, or axial migration of the femoral head, simulating rheumatoid arthritis, can be seen.

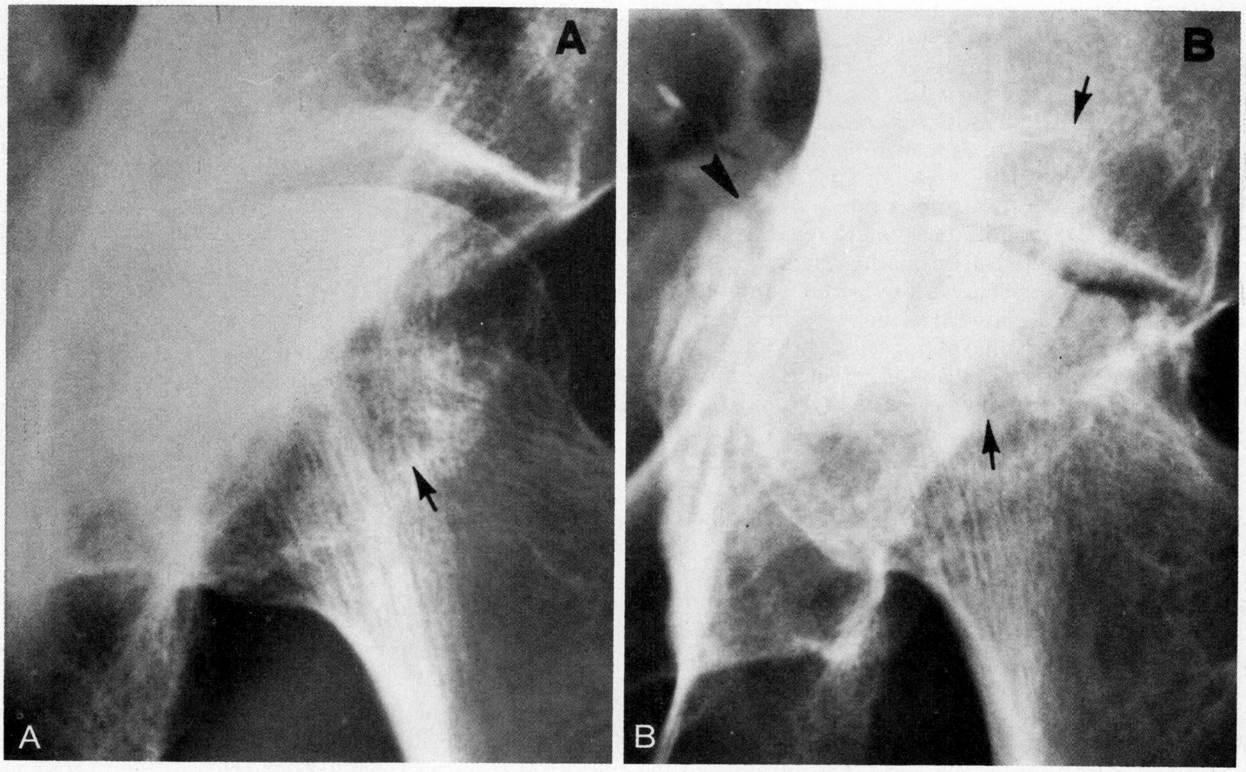


**Figure 39–49.** Calcium pyrophosphate crystal deposition disease. *A* and *B* are radiographs of the hip obtained 16 months apart. In *A*, there is preservation of the joint space with subtle cystic change within the femoral head (arrow). In *B*, there is collapse of the femoral head with large cystic lesions (arrows) and fragmentation of the acetabulum (arrowhead). This rapidly progressive arthropathy is characteristic of pyrophosphate arthropathy. (From Resnick, D., and Niwayama, G.: Diagnosis of Bone and Joint Disorders. Philadelphia, W.B. Saunders Co., 1981.)

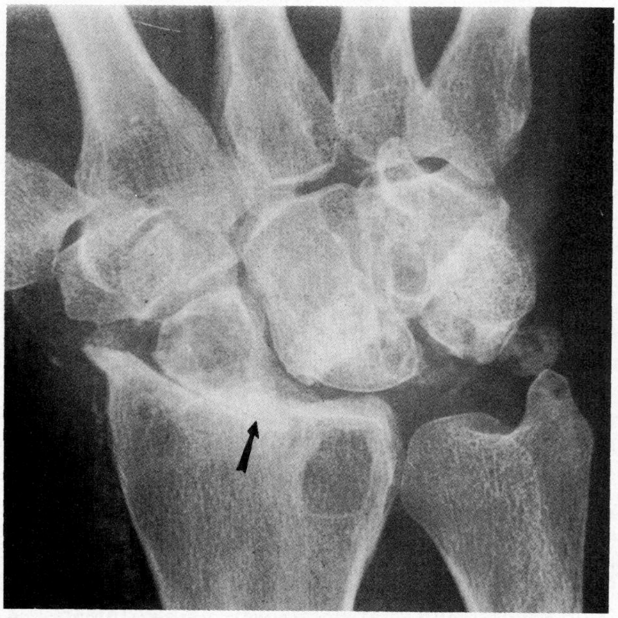

**Figure 39–50.** Calcium pyrophosphate crystal deposition disease. In this patient, the changes of pyrophosphate arthropathy include narrowing of the radiocarpal joint with collapse of the scaphoid into the radial articular surface (arrow) as well as the presence of numerous subchondral cystic lesions. Calcification of the triangular fibrocartilage can also be noted.

**Calcium Hydroxyapatite Crystal Deposition Disease (HADD).** HADD may be a primary idiopathic disorder or secondary to other diseases and is characterized by the deposition of calcium hydroxyapatite crystals in periarticular or, rarely, intra-articular structures. In idiopathic disease, calcification is most commonly seen about the shoulder, although involvement of the hand, wrist, hip, foot, and paraspinal tissues may be seen. Hydroxyapatite deposits appear on radiographs as soft, cloudlike densities within tendons, ligaments, joint capsules, bursae, and periarticular soft tissues. These deposits may vary in size from small collections, 1 to 2 mm in diameter, to large lobulated masses, many centimeters in diameter. On serial radiographs, deposits may enlarge, remain unchanged, or diminish in size. They can even disappear completely.

In the shoulder, HADD is most commonly identified in the supraspinatus tendon of the fibromuscular rotator cuff. Here, it is frequently referred to as calcific tendinitis, peritendinitis calcarea, or hydroxyapatite rheumatism (Fig. 39–51).[151] Other sites of calcification in the shoulder include the infraspinatus, teres minor, subscapularis, and bicipital tendons.[162] It should be emphasized that in most cases these deposits are not symptomatic; the majority of patients with shoulder discomfort and periarticular calcific deposits will have another cause of

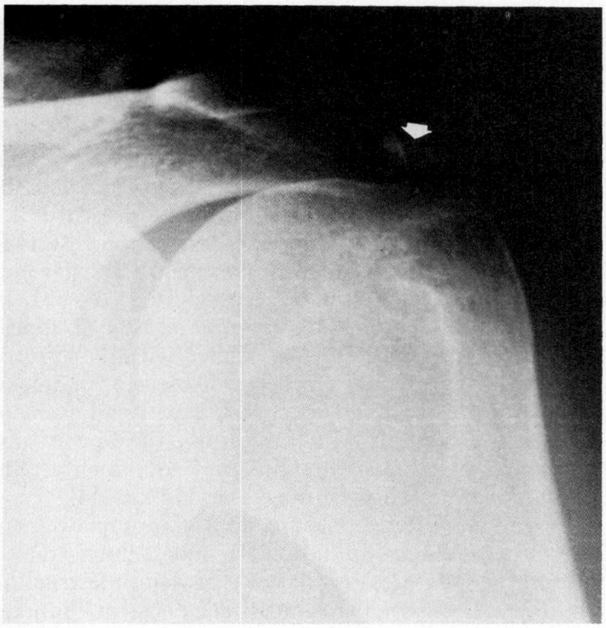

**Figure 39–51.** Hydroxyapatite crystal deposition disease. Calcification (arrow) of the supraspinatus tendon of the musculotendinous rotator cuff is present. This constitutes the single most common manifestation of this disorder. (From Resnick, D., and Niwayama, G.: Diagnosis of Bone and Joint Disease. Philadelphia, W.B. Saunders Co., 1981.)

pain, frequently subacromial bursitis or rotator cuff tendinitis.

Intra-articular HADD may be seen as an isolated event or in association with osteoarthritis or collagen vascular disease. Radiographically, cloudlike calcific collections within the joint are apparent. Rarely, severe articular destruction, especially in the glenohumeral joint, may be an associated feature.

Periarticular calcification, representing hydroxyapatite crystal deposition, is seen in a variety of disorders,[151] including hyperparathyroidism, renal osteodystrophy, collagen vascular diseases, hypoparathyroidism, milk-alkali syndrome, hypervitaminosis D, and sardoidosis.

**Hemochromatosis.** Radiographically the manifestations of hemochromatosis may be divided into three major categories: (1) osteoporosis, (2) articular calcification, and (3) structural joint damage.

Diffuse osteoporosis is an important feature of hemochromatosis,[163] in contrast to idiopathic CPPD crystal deposition disease, and may involve the axial and appendicular skeleton. In the spine, collapse of the vertebral endplates leads to biconcave deformities of the vertebral body ("fish" vertebra). Osteoporosis in the appendicular skeleton tends to be diffuse without a tendency toward a periarticular distribution.[165]

Articular calcification, related to CPPD crystal deposition (chondrocalcinosis), occurs in approximately 30 percent of patients with hemochromatosis.[151] In general this calcification is identical to that of idiopathic CPPD crystal deposition disease, but several characteristics may help to distinguish between these two disorders. In hemochromatosis, hyaline cartilage calcification tends to be more prominent and the fibrocartilage of the symphysis pubis is more commonly involved than in idiopathic CPPD crystal deposition disease.[151]

Structural articular alterations in hemochromatosis occur in slightly less than half of the cases.[166,167] In general, the arthropathy of hemochromatosis is similar to that of idiopathic CPPD crystal deposition disease with joint space narrowing and subchondral cyst formation being prominent features. Although the two disorders cannot be absolutely separated on a radiographic basis, several features may be useful in differential diagnosis.[151] "Hook" osteophytes are distinctive bony excrescences, most commonly identified at the radial margins of the metacarpal heads, in patients with hemochromatosis. These osteophytes tend to be small, triangular, and sharply defined (Fig. 39–52). They are not prominent in osteoarthritis or idiopathic CPPD crystal deposition disease. The distribution of abnormalities may also be a useful diagnostic feature. In both CPPD crystal deposition disease and hemochromatosis, the second and third metacarpophalangeal joints are the most commonly involved sites in the hands, but additional alterations of the fourth and fifth metacarpophalangeal joints are more frequent in hemochromatosis. In addition, the radiocarpal joint may be spared in hemochromatosis, whereas it is almost always involved in idiopathic CPPD crystal deposition disease. The arthropathy of hemochromatosis is usually slowly progressive in contrast to idiopathic pyrophosphate arthropathy, in which a rapidly progressive arthropathy may be seen.

**Wilson's Disease.** Wilson's disease is a rare inherited disorder characterized by abnormal accumulation of copper in body tissues. The age of onset is typically the first through fourth decades of life. The general radi-

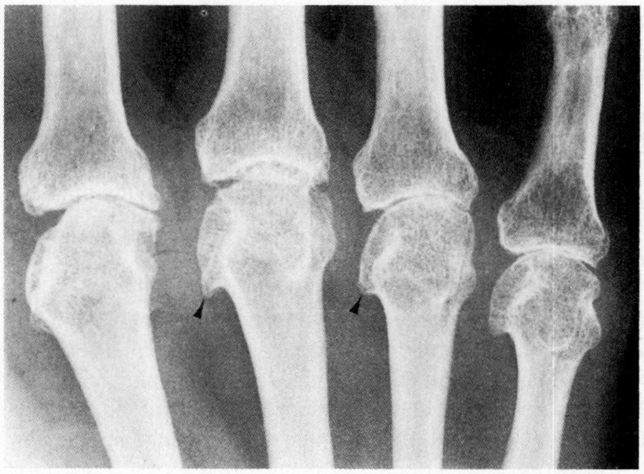

**Figure 39–52.** Hemochromatosis. There is joint space narrowing with erosive change about the second through fifth metacarpophalangeal joints. "Hook" osteophytes (arrowheads) occur at the radial margins of the metacarpal heads. (From Resnick, D., and Niwayama, G.: Diagnosis of Bone and Joint Disorders. Philadelphia, W.B. Saunders Co., 1981.)

ographic features consist of osteopenia and arthropathy.[151,168] Chondrocalcinosis has been considered an important feature of this disorder, but it appears to be very rare. Osteopenia, present in approximately 50 percent of patients, is most prominent in the hands, feet, and spine. It may relate to osteoporosis or osteomalacia, or both. Changes of rickets, with Looser's zones or "pseudofractures," are prominent in some cases.[169]

The arthropathy of Wilson's disease is most commonly identified in the wrist, hand, foot, hip, shoulder, elbow, and knee. Irregularity and indistinctness of the subchondral bone plate ("paintbrush" appearance) in combination with focal radiodense excrescences at the central and peripheral joint margins are characteristic. Subchondral cysts and focal areas of fragmentation of the articular surface may also be observed. An additional manifestation is the occurrence of small distinctly corticated ossicles about affected joints, especially prominent in the wrist. These structures resemble the accessory ossicles frequently seen in normal individuals but are more numerous and appear in unusual locations. Joint effusions are not prominent, but spiculated bony proliferative changes are frequently noted at entheses, resembling the inflammatory enthesopathy seen in the seronegative spondyloarthropathies.

**Ochronosis (Alkaptonuria).** The major radiographic features of ochronosis consist of osteoporosis, abnormal calcification and ossification, and arthropathy.[151] Osteoporosis, although generally diffuse in nature, is most prominent in the spine, where it may be associated with vertebral body collapse.[170]

Abnormal calcification and ossification are most prominent in the intervertebral discs, especially those in the lumbar spine. Additional sites of calcification and ossification include the symphysis pubis, costal cartilage, helix of the ear, and peripheral tendons and ligaments.[171] The crystals are composed of calcium hydroxyapatite and demonstrate a typical "cloudlike" appearance.

In the spine osteoporosis with waferlike calcification of the intervertebral disc is an early radiographic finding. Intervertebral disc narrowing with the formation of radiolucent discal collections (vacuum phenomena) are also common, often obscuring the calcification.[172] Progressive discal ossification and the formation of peripheral bony bridges in the outermost layer of the annulus fibrosus may lead to the appearance of a "bamboo spine," similar to that in ankylosing spondylitis. At some levels, osteophytes may also be prominent.

In the peripheral skeleton, the knees, hips, and shoulders are most commonly involved, with relative sparing of the small joints of the hands and feet.[172] In these locations, changes resemble those of degenerative joint disease; however, osteophytes and subchondral cysts are not prominent in ochronosis. In addition the location of abnormalities, such as the lateral femorotibial compartment of the knee, may help in differentiating ochronosis from OA. Occasionally, a rapidly progressing destructive peripheral arthropathy characterized by fragmentation of articular surfaces may be observed.

## SEPTIC ARTHRITIS

**Mechanisms.** In general the radiographic features of joint sepsis consist of periarticular soft tissue swelling, intra-articular effusions, cartilage destruction with joint space narrowing, and irregular erosions of the subchondral bone plate.[173-175] In the initial stage of disease, the joint may appear widened, owing to the presence of a large effusion, but rapid cartilage destruction results in articular space narrowing with confluent irregular erosions of the subchondral bone plate (Fig. 39–53). In children, epiphyseal centers may completely disappear as a result of the hyperemia associated with the infected joint. Diabetic patients are prone to develop indolent, slowly progressive joint infections, usually adjacent to soft tissue ulcerations. In this setting the loss of distinctiveness of articular margins may be the only radiographic manifestation of infection (Fig. 39–54).

In contrast to bacterial infection, granulomatous infection (tuberculosis and fungal) may demonstrate a more slowly progressive pattern of joint destruction (Fig. 39–55). Osseous erosions first appear at the joint margins ("bare" areas) where synovial inflammatory tissue is in direct contact with bone. In fact, prominent juxta-articular osteoporosis and marginal bone erosions, in the absence of significant joint space loss, are characteristics of granulomatous infection. The late complications of joint sepsis include intra-articular fibrous or bony ankylosis as well as joint instability. In the spine the latter complication may result in spinal cord or nerve root compromise.

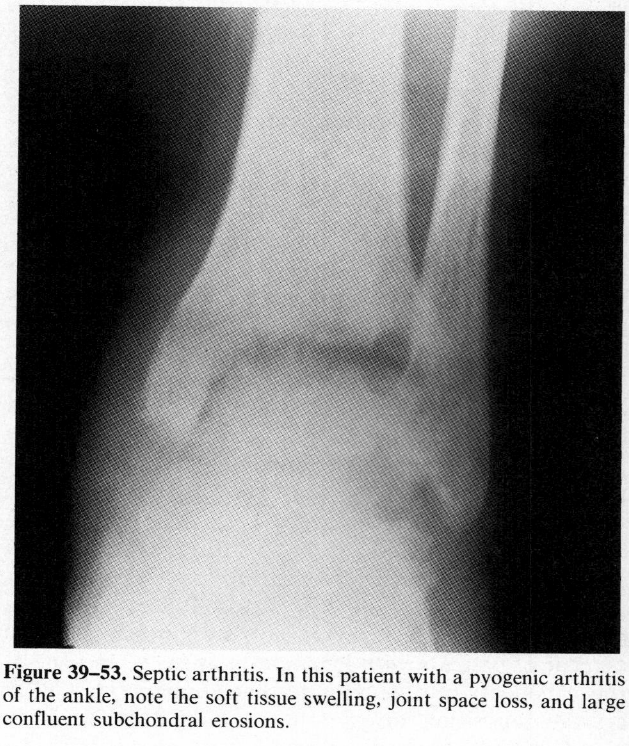

**Figure 39–53.** Septic arthritis. In this patient with a pyogenic arthritis of the ankle, note the soft tissue swelling, joint space loss, and large confluent subchondral erosions.

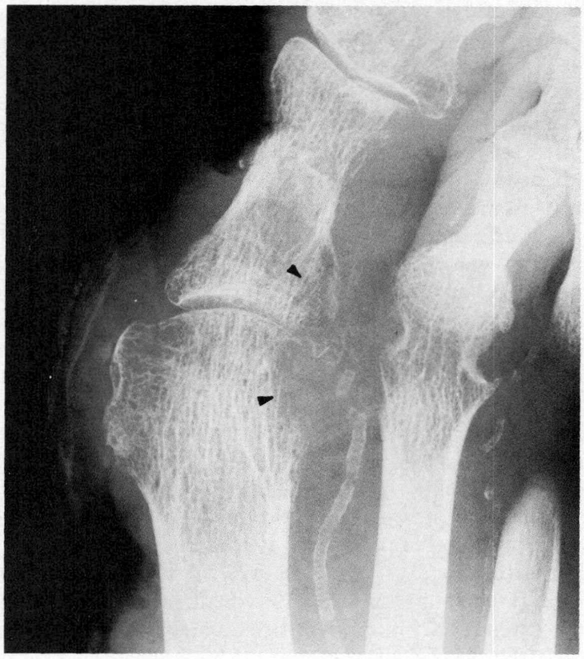

**Figure 39–54.** Septic arthritis. In this specimen radiograph of an infected foot in a diabetic patient, note the erosions of the lateral margins of the articular surfaces of the first metatarsal head and proximal phalanx (arrowheads).

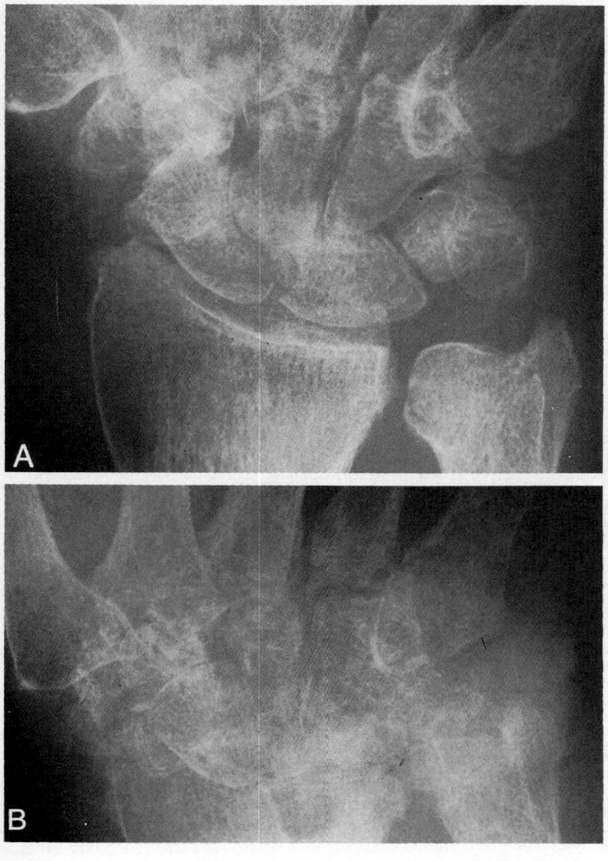


**Figure 39–55.** Tuberculosis. Note the gradual progression of destructive changes in radiographs obtained 18 months apart. In *A* there is prominent soft tissue swelling and osteoporosis with marginal osseous erosions at multiple sites. In *B* the process has progressed to virtually complete destruction of the carpus. A large erosion of the distal radius is also present.

The role of various imaging modalities in the diagnosis of joint sepsis should be emphasized. Early detection is important in order to avoid irreversible joint destruction, or in the child, significant growth disturbance. Radionuclide studies are useful in this regard, both in detecting infection early in the course of the disease and in documenting the extent of involvement. However, adjacent soft tissue or bone infections, recent surgery, or posttraumatic changes may render this important tool useless in some cases. Recognition of articular effusions and periarticular soft tissue swelling on roentgenograms is of critical importance in the early diagnosis of joint infection. Magnification radiography may provide additional diagnostic information, especially in the diabetic patient with a foot infection. Fluoroscopically guided aspiration may play an important role in the evaluation of joint sepsis, especially in deep joints such as the hip or the shoulder or in sites such as the spine where surgical exploration may be required. Although the principal aim of this procedure is to procure a specimen for laboratory analysis, instillation of a small amount of radiopaque contrast agent may be helpful in ascertaining the extent of articular destruction and in detecting extra-articular spread of contaminated material.

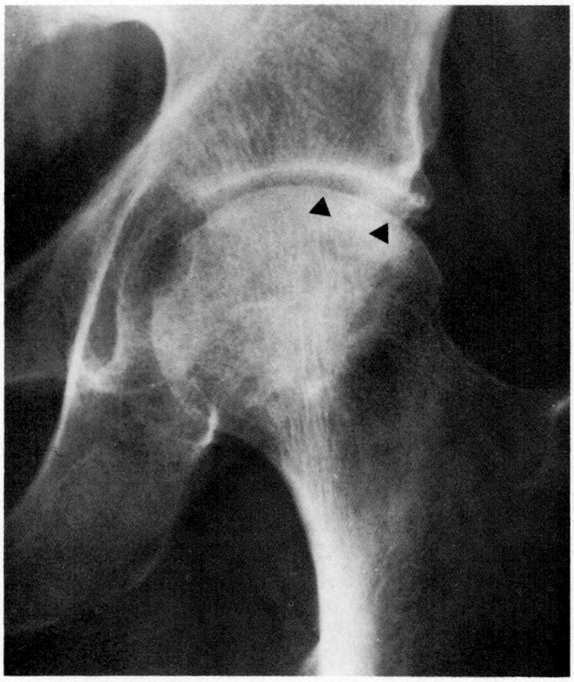

**Figure 39–56.** Osteonecrosis. An early radiographic change of osteonecrosis is an arclike radiolucent band (arrowheads) parallel to the articular surface.

## MISCELLANEOUS ARTHROPATHIES

**Osteonecrosis.** Early in the course of epiphyseal osteonecrosis, radiographic changes are not evident. Subsequently a characteristic progression of radiographic changes will be seen. The earliest findings are a subtle, arclike radiolucent subchondral band (crescent sign) and the formation of patchy subchondral lucent and sclerotic foci (Fig. 39–56). Fragmentation and collapse of the articular surface follow. The joint space is usually preserved until late in the course of the disease when secondary osteoarthritis may supervene.

A peculiar form of spontaneous osteonecrosis is seen in the knee, most commonly involving the medial femoral condyle. It is manifested by the sudden appearance of pain and the radiographic changes of sclerosis, flattening, and irregularity of the femoral surface (Fig. 39–57).

**Paget's Disease.** Articular disease is a recognized complication of Paget's disease. Gout,[176] CPPD crystal deposition disease,[177] and rheumatoid arthritis[176] have each been observed in patients with Paget's disease. More importantly, individuals with this disease demonstrate an increased incidence of osteoarthritis in association with juxta-articular pagetic bony involvement.[121] This is most common in the hip and knee. Although radiographic features resemble those in idiopathic osteoarthritis (Fig. 39–58), more specific changes, such as acetabular protrusion, may be seen.

**Acromegaly.** Acromegalic arthropathy most closely resembles degenerative joint disease. Some features that aid in its recognition are (1) increased soft tissue thickness (e.g., heel pad > 21 mm) (Fig. 39–59), (2) promi-

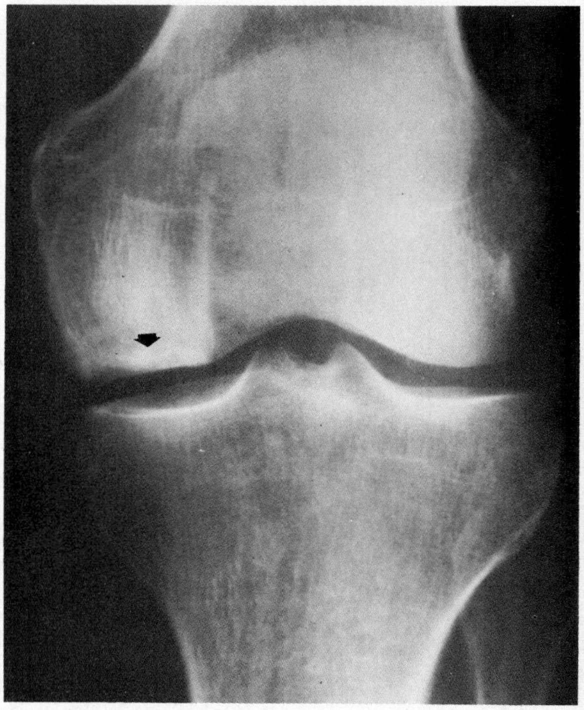

**Figure 39–57.** Spontaneous osteonecrosis. In this adult with the sudden onset of knee pain, the frontal radiograph demonstrates a defect in the articular surface of the medial femoral condyle (arrow). This is the characteristic location of this lesion. (From Resnick, D., and Niwayama, G.: Diagnosis of Bone and Joint Disorders. Philadelphia, W.B. Saunders Co., 1981.)

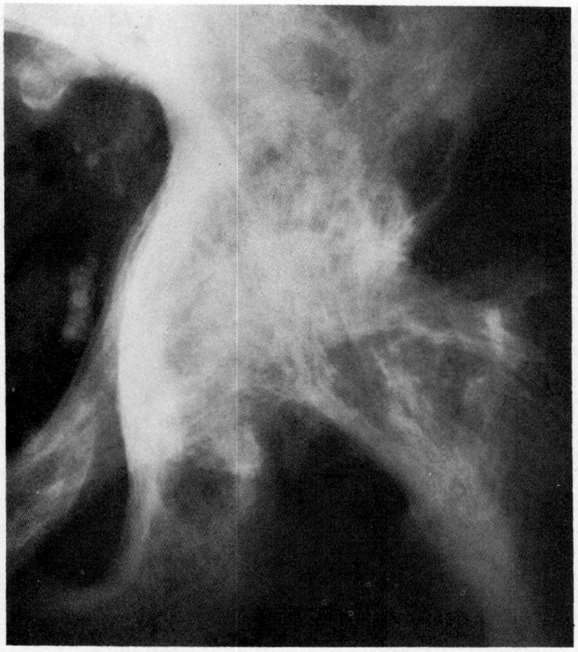

**Figure 39–58.** Paget's disease. Observe the prominent osteoarthritislike changes of the hip with asymmetric joint space loss and large marginal osteophytes. The juxta-articular bone is coarsened and enlarged.

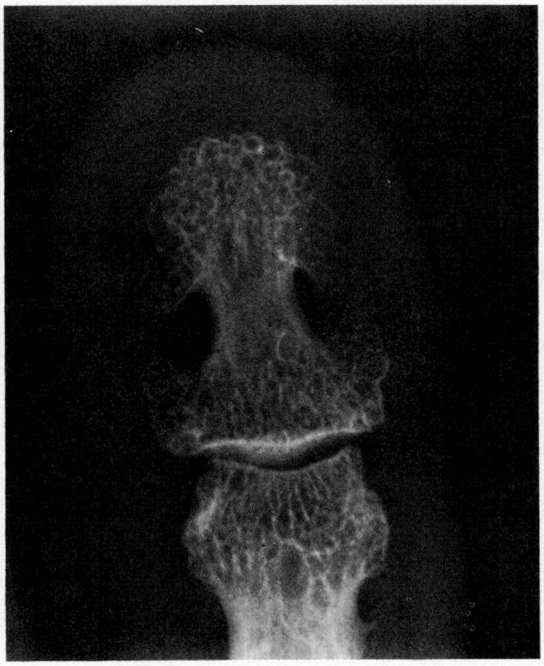

**Figure 39–60.** Acromegaly. There is proliferation of the margins of the base and terminal tuft of the distal phalanx resulting in the classic "arrowhead" appearance.

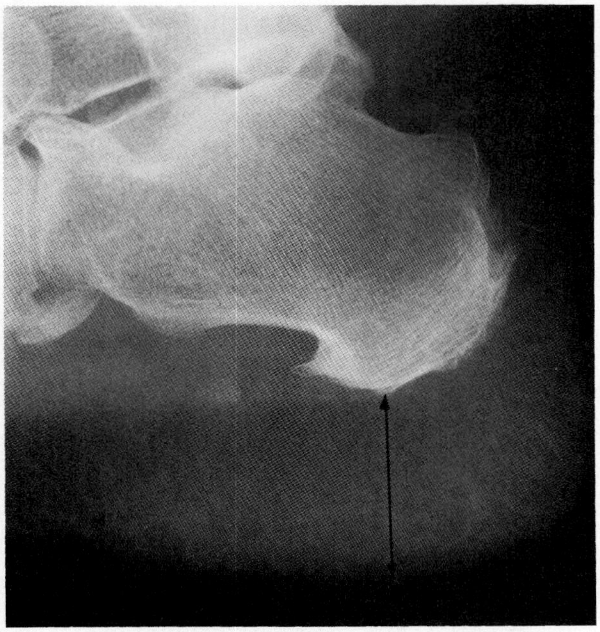

**Figure 39–59.** Acromegaly. Note the soft tissue prominence of the heel pad with the formation of multiple osteophytes from the plantar and posterior surfaces of the calcaneus. (From Resnick, D., and Niwayama, G.: Diagnosis of Bone and Joint Disorders. Philadelphia, W.B. Saunders Co., 1981.)

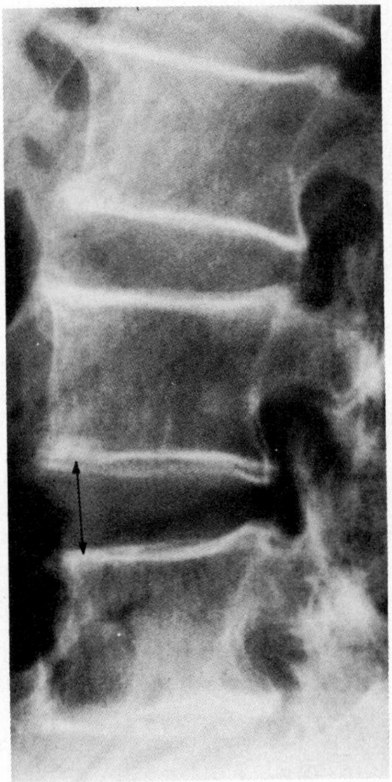

**Figure 39–61.** Acromegaly. In this case, the most striking finding is the abnormally increased height of the intervertebral disc spaces (between arrowheads). Note posterior concavity of the vertebral bodies and degenerative changes.

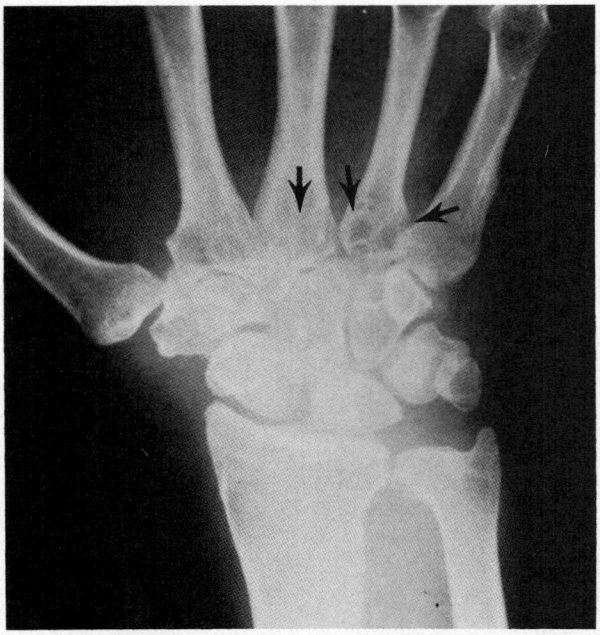

**Figure 39–62.** Amyloidosis. Observe the diffuse soft tissue swelling and the presence of destructive lesions in the third and fourth metacarpal bases (arrows), radius, and ulna.

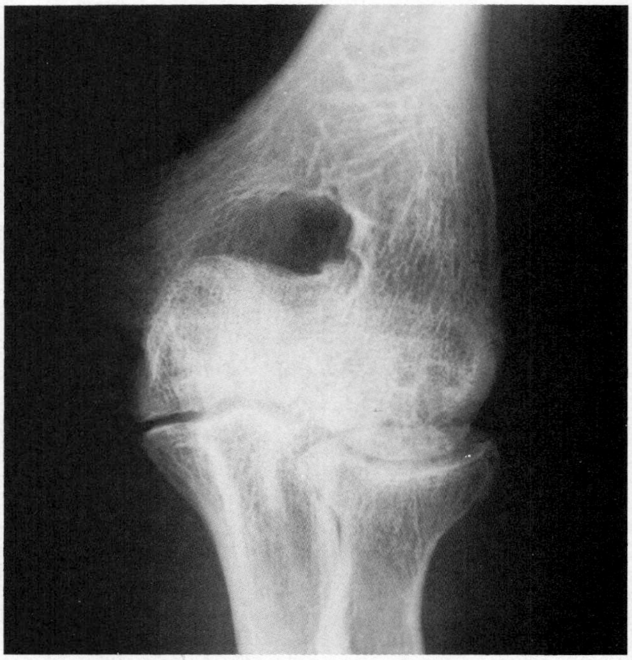

**Figure 39–63.** Hemophilia. There is overgrowth of the epiphyses, especially the radial head. Joint space narrowing and subchondral cysts are seen.

nent phalangeal tufts and bases ("arrowhead" phalanges) (Fig. 39–60), (3) "hooklike" osteophytes in the metacarpal heads, (4) joint space widening, (5) exuberant spinal osteophytosis with widened intervertebral discs (Fig. 39–61), and (6) prominent thoracic kyphosis.[178,179] In the later stages of the disease, loss of joint space becomes apparent. Acromegaly should be considered if a degenerative process occurs in an unusual articulation, such as the glenohumeral joint.

**Hemoglobinopathies.** Hemoglobinopathies may affect articular structures. The major changes in sickle cell anemia relate to vascular occlusion with osteonecrosis, which may involve epiphysis, metaphysis, or diaphysis of a tubular bone as well as flat bones. In sickle cell dactylitis (hand-foot syndrome), the changes of bone infarction are accompanied by prominent soft tissue swelling and exuberant periosteal reaction.[180] Osteomyelitis and, less commonly, septic arthritis can be seen in sickle cell anemia. Salmonella is frequently implicated.

**Amyloidosis.** Radiographically the diagnosis is suggested by the occurrence of a bilateral symmetric erosive arthropathy similar to rheumatoid arthritis but without joint space narrowing.[181,182] Large soft tissue masses and osteolytic defects in the diaphyses of tubular bones are other prominent findings in this disorder (Fig. 39–62).

**Hemophilia.** The arthropathy of hemophilia is related to destructive changes associated with repeated episodes of intra-articular hemorrhage (hemarthrosis).[183] Any joint may be involved, but changes in the knee, ankle, and elbow are most frequently identified. The earliest finding consists of juxta-articular soft tissue swelling with large intra-articular effusions. This is followed by prominent osteoporosis and, in the immature skeleton, by epiphyseal overgrowth (Fig. 39–63). Subchondral cysts and bony erosions appear, initially with preservation of the cartilaginous coat, and subsequently with cartilage destruction and joint space narrowing. Late abnormalities include complete joint disorganization

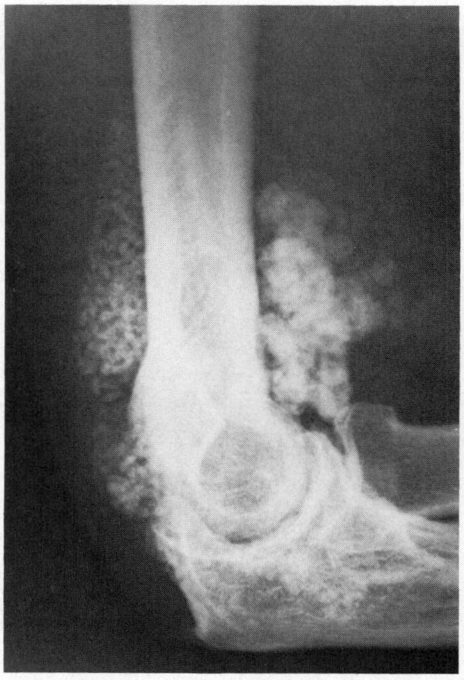

**Figure 39–64.** Idiopathic synovial (osteo)chondromatosis. A radiograph of the elbow reveals multiple calcified bodies of varying sizes within the confines of an enlarged joint capsule.

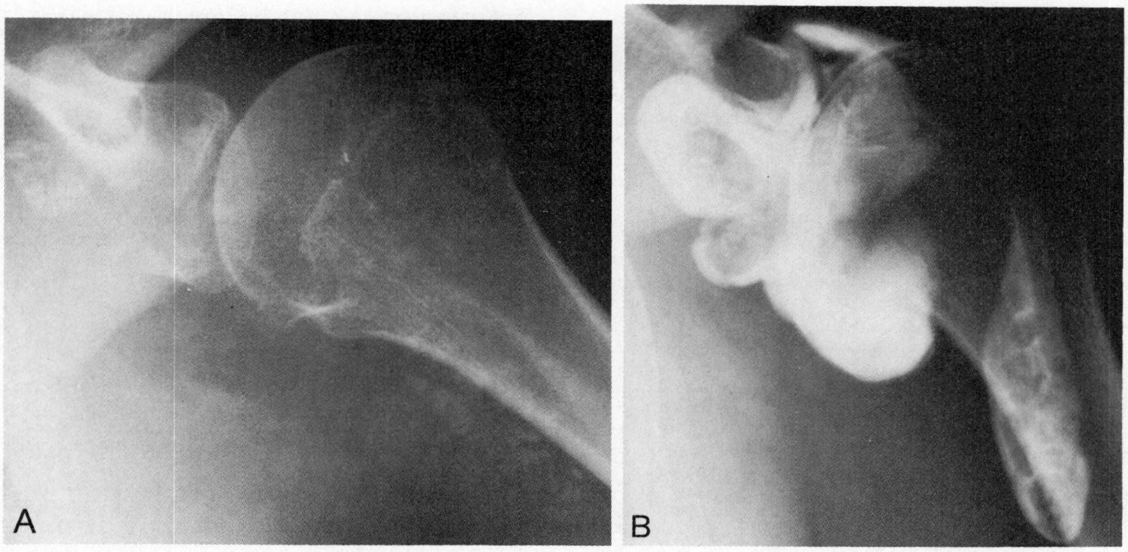


**Figure 39–65.** Idiopathic synovial (osteo)chondromatosis. A plain film (*A*) and arthrogram (*B*) reveal typical changes. In *A*, observe intra-articular calcified bodies along the synovial sheath of the bicipital tendons. The arthrogram defines multiple radiolucent filling defects.

with obliteration of the articular space, large bony erosions, and joint instability. In the knee, radiographic features of hemophilia include widening of the intercondylar notch of the distal femur and squaring of the inferior patellar pole. The radiographic features of hemophilia may be difficult to differentiate from those of juvenile chronic arthritis.

**Synovial (Osteo)chondromatosis and Pigmented Villonodular Synovitis.** The typical radiographic picture of synovial (osteo)chondromatosis is that of numerous calcific densities confined to the articular cavity (Fig. 39–64). Pressure erosions of adjacent bony surfaces may be seen. Osteoporosis and joint space narrowing are generally not prominent. In cases where the bodies are not calcified, arthrography may confirm the diagnosis (Fig. 39–65).

Multiple erosions and cysts on both sides of the joint are seen in pigmented villonodular synovitis. Osteoporosis and joint space narrowing are usually not prominent.[184,186] During arthrography, nodular soft tissue masses may be demonstrated and aspiration of joint fluid will yield a characteristic "rusty" fluid.

**Synovial Sarcoma.** The typical roentgenographic finding of a synovial sarcoma is a soft tissue mass, which contains calcification in approximately 30 percent of cases. Erosion of neighboring bone is seen in 25 to 35 percent of lesions.

## References


1. Mall, J.C., Genant, H.K., Silcox, D.C., and McCarty, D.J.: The efficacy of fine-detail radiography in the evaluation of patients with rheumatoid arthritis. Radiology 112:37, 1974.
2. Genant, H.K.: Magnification radiography. *In* Resnick, D., and Niwayama, G. (eds.) Diagnosis of Bone and Joint Disorders. Philadelphia, W. B. Saunders Company, 1981, p. 335.
3. Genant, H.K., Vardez Horst, J., Lanzl, L.H., Mall, J.C., and Doi, K.: Skeletal demineralization in primary hyperparathyroidism. *In* Mazesi, R.B. (ed.): Proceedings of the International Conference on Bone Mineral Measurement. Washington D.C., National Institute of Arthritis, Metabolism and Digestive Diseases, 1973, p. 177.
4. Leach, R.E., Grett, T., and Ferris, J.S.: Weight-bearing radiography in osteoarthritis of the knee. Radiology 97:265, 1970.
5. Resnick, D., and Danzig, L.: Arthrographic evaluation of injuries of the first metacarpophalangeal joint: Gamekeeper's Thumb. Am. J. Roentgenol. 126:1046, 1976.
6. Chamberlain, W.E.: The symphysis pubis in the roentgen examination of the sacroiliac joint. Am. J. Roentgenol. 24:621, 1930.
7. Martel, W., and Poznanski, A.K.: The value of traction during roentgenography of the hip. Radiology 94:497, 1970.
8. Resnick, D.: Arthrography, tenography and bursography. *In* Resnick, D., and Niwayama, G. (ed.): Diagnosis of Bone and Joint Disorders., Philadelphia, W. B. Saunders Company, 1981, p. 510.
9. Gelman, M., Coleman, R.E., Stevens, P.M., and Davey, B.W.: Radiography, radionuclide imaging, and arthrography in evaluation of painful total hip and knee replacements. Radiology 128:677, 1978.
10. Wolfe, R.D., and Giuliano, V.J.: Double-contrast arthrography in the diagnosis of pigmented villonudular synovitis of the knee. Am. J. Roentgenol. 110:793, 1970.
11. Prager, R.J., and Mall, J.C.: Arthrographic diagnosis of synovial chondromatosis. Am. J. Roentgenol. 127:344, 1976.
12. Strizak, A.M., Danzig, L.A., Jackson, D.W., Greenway, G., Resnick, D., and Staple, T.: Subacromial bursography: an anatomic and clinical study. J. Bone and Joint Surg. 64A:196, 1982.
13. Cone, R., Danzig, L., and Resnick, D.: The shoulder impingement syndrome. Radiology 150:29, 3, 10, 1984.
14. Carrera, G.F., Foley, W.D., Kozin, F., et al.: CT of sacroiliitis. Am. J. Roentgenol. 136:41, 1981.
15. Sheldon, J.J., Sersland, T., and Leboranc, J.: Computed tomography of the lower lumbar vertebral column. Radiology 124:183, 1977.
16. Genant, H.K.: Quantitative bone mineral analysis. *In* Resnick, D., and Niwayama, G. (eds.): Diagnosis of Bone and Joint Disorders. Philadelphia, W. B. Saunders Company, 1981, p. 686.
17. Resnick, D., and Niwayama, G.: Rheumatoid arthritis. *In* Resnick, D., and Niwayama, G. (eds.): Diagnosis of Bone and Joint Disorders. Philadelphia, W. B. Saunders Company, 1981, p. 906.
18. O'Driscoll, S., and O'Driscoll, M.: Osteomalacia in rheumatoid arthritis. Ann. Rheum. Dis. 39:1, 1980.
19. DeHaas, W.H.D., DeBoer, W., Griffin, F., and Oosten-Elst, P.: Rheumatoid arthritis of the robust reaction type. Ann. Rheum. Dis. 33:81, 1974.
20. Renneic, C., Mainzer, F., Multz, C.V., and Genant, H.K.: Subchondral pseudocysts in rheumatoid arthritis. Am. J. Roentgenol. 129:1069, 1977.
21. Norgaard, F.: Tidligste rontgenoligiske forandringer ved polyarthritis. Ugeskr. Laeger 125:1312, 1963.
22. Resnick, D.: Rheumatoid arthritis of the wrist. The compartmental approach. Med. Radiog. Photog. 52:50, 1976.
23. Resnick, D.: Rheumatoid arthritis of the wrist: Why the ulnar styloid? Radiolgy 112:29, 1974.

24. Berens, D.L., and Lin, R.K.: Roentgen Diagnosis of Rheumatoid Arthritis. Springfield, Ill., Charles C Thomas, 1969.
25. Resnick, D.: Early abnormalities of the pisiform and triquetrum in rheumatoid arthritis. Ann. Rheum. Dis. 35:46, 1976.
26. Linscheid, R.L.: The mechanical factors affecting deformity at the wrist in rheumatoid arthritis. *In* Proceedings of the twenty-fourth annual meeting of the American Society for Surgery of the Hand. New York, Jan. 17–18, 1969. J. Bone Joint Surg. 51A:790, 1969.
27. Jackman, R.J., and Pugh, D.G.: The positive elbow fat pad sign in rheumatoid arthritis. Am. J. Roentgenol. 108:812, 1970.
28. Weston, W.J.: The synovial changes at the elbow in rheumatoid arthritis. Australas. Radiog. 15:170, 1971.
29. Rappaport, A.S., Sosman, J.L., and Weissman, B.N.: Spontaneous fractures of the olecranon process in rheumatoid arthritis. Radiology 119:83, 1976.
30. Short, C.L. Bauer, W., and Reynolds, W.E.: Rheumatoid Arthritis. Cambridge, Massachusetts, Harvard University Press, 1957.
31. Thould, A.K., and Simon, G.: Assessment of the radiological changes in the hands and feet in rheumatoid arthritis. Ann. Rheum. Dis. 25:220, 1966.
32. Calabro, J.J.: The feet as an aid in the differential diagnosis of arthritis (abstr.). Arthritis Rheum. 3:435, 1960.
33. Bywaters, E.G.L.: Heel lesions in rheumatoid arthritis. Ann. Rheum. Dis. 13:42, 1954.
34. Resnick, D., Feingold, M.L., Curd, J., Niwayama, G., and Goergen, T.G.: Calcaneal abnormalities in articular disorders. Rheumatoid arthritis, ankylosing spondylitis, psoriatic arthritis, and Reiter's Syndrome. Radiology 125:355, 1977.
35. Kirkup, J.R.: Ankle and tarsal joints in rheumatoid arthritis. Scand. J. Rheumatol. 3:50, 1974.
36. Magayar, E., Talerman, A., Feher, M., and Wouters, H.W.: Giant bone cysts in rheumatoid arthritis. J. Bone Joint Surg. 56B:121, 1974.
37. Genovese, G.R., Jayson, M.I.J., and Dixon, A.S.: Protective value of synovial cysts in rheumatoid knees. Ann. Rheum. Dis. 31:179, 1972.
38. Resnick, D.: Patterns of migration of the femoral head in ostoearthritis of the hip: roentgenographic-pathologic correlation and comparison with rheumatoid arthritis. Am. J. Roentgenol. 124:62, 1975.
39. Armbuster, T., Guerra, J., Resnick, D., Georgen, J.G., Feingold, M.L., Niwayama, G., and Danzig, L.: The adult hip: An anatomic study. Part I. The bony landmarks. Radiology 128:1, 1978.
40. Sievers, K., and Caine, V.: The sacroiliac joint in rheumatoid arthritis in adult females. Acta Rheum. Scand. 9:222, 1963.
41. Linquist, P.R., and McDonnell, D.E.: Rheumatoid cyst causing extradural compression. J. Bone Joint Surg. 52A:1235, 1970.
42. Martel, W.: The occipito-atlanto-axial joints in rheumatoid arthritis. *In* Carter, M.E. (ed.): Radiological Aspects of Rheumatoid Disease. Proceedings of an international symposium, Amsterdam, 1963. Amsterdam, Excerpta Medica, 1964, p. 189.
43. Mathews, J.A.: Atlanto-axial subluxation in rheumatoid arthritis. A 5-year follow-up study. Ann. Rheum. Dis. 33:526, 1974.
44. Martel, W.: The occipito-atlanto-axial joints in rheumatoid arthritis and ankylosing spondylitis. Am. J. Roentgenol. 86:223, 1961.
45. Rana, N.A., Hancock, D.O., Taylor, A.R., and Hill, A.G.S.: Upward translocation of the dens in rheumatoid arthritis. J. Bone Joint Surg. 55B:471, 1973.
46. Ansell, B.M., and Kent, P.A.: Radiological changes in juvenile chronic polyarthritis. Skel. Radiol. 1:129, 1977.
47. Ansell, B.M., and Bywaters, E.G.L.: Growth in Still's Disease. Ann. Rheum. Dis. 15:295, 1956.
48. Martel, W., Holt, J.F., and Cassidy, J.T.: Roentgenologic manifestations of juvenile rheumatoid arthritis. Am. J. Roentgenol. 88:400, 1962.
49. Resnick, D., and Niwayama, G.: Juvenile chronic arthritis. *In* Resnick, D., and Niwayama, G. (ed.): Diagnosis of Bone and Joint Disease. Philadelphia, W. B. Saunders Company, 1981, p. 1008.
50. Ansell, B.M.: Chronic arthritis in childhood. Ann. Rheum. Dis. 37:107, 1978.
51. Schaller, J., and Wedgewood, R.J.: Juvenile rheumatoid arthritis: A review. Pediatrics 50:940, 1972.
52. Cassidy, J.T., Brody, G.L., and Martel, W.: Monoarticular juvenile rheumatoid arthritis. J. Pediatr. 70:867, 1967.
53. Kleinman, P., Rivelas, M., Schneider, R., and Kaye, J.J.: Juvenile ankylosing spondylitis. Radiology 125:775, 1977.
54. Resnick, D.: Patterns of peripheral joint disease in ankylosing spondylitis. Radiology 110:523, 1977.
55. Bywaters, E.G.L.: Still's disease in the adult. Ann. Rheum. Dis. 30:121, 1971.
56. Medsger, T.A. Jr., and Christy, W.C.: Carpal arthritis with ankylosis in late onset Still's disease. Arthritis Rheum. 19:232, 1976.
57. Bluestone, R.: Histocompatibility antigens and rheumatic disease. *In* Current Concepts. Kalamazoo, Michigan, Upjohn Company, 1978, p. 17.
58. Resnick, D., and Niwayama, G.: Ankylosing spondylitis. *In* Resnick, D., and Niwayama, G. (eds.): Diagnosis of Bone and Joint Disorders. Philadelphia, W. B. Saunders Company, 1981, p. 1040.
59. Wilkinson, M., and Bywaters, E.G.L.: Clinical features and course of ankylosing spondylitis as seen in a follow-up of 222 hospital referred cases. Ann. Rheum. Dis. 17:209, 1958.
60. Rosen, P.S., and Graham, D.C.: Ankylosing (Strumpell-Marie) Spondylitis (A clinical review of 128 cases). AIR 5:158, 1962.
61. Berens, D.L.: Roentgen features of ankylosing spondylitis. Clin. Orthop. Rel. Res. 74:20, 1971.
62. Resnick, D., Niwayama, G., and Goergen, T.G.: Comparison of radiographic abnormalities of the sacro-iliac joint in degenerative joint disease and ankylosing spondylitis. Am. J. Roentgenol. 128:189, 1977.
63. Forestier, J., Jacqueline, F., and Rotes-Querol, J.: Ankylosing Spondylitis. Springfield, Ill., Charles C Thomas, 1956.
64. Cawley, M.I.D., Chalmers, T.M., Kellgren, J.H., and Ball, J.: Destructive lesions of vertebral bodies in ankylosing spondylitis. Ann. Rheum. Dis. 31:345, 1972.
65. Dwosh, I.L., Resnick, D., and Becker, M.P.: Hip involvement in ankylosing spondylitis. Arthritis Rheum. 19:683, 1976.
66. Glick, E.N.: A radiological comparison of the hip joint in rheumatoid arthritis and ankylosing spondylitis. Proc. Roy. Soc. Med. 59:1229, 1976.
67. Resnick, D., Dwosh, I.L., Goergen, T.G., Shapiro, R.F., and D'Ambrosia, R.: Clinical and radiographic "reankylosis" following hip surgery in ankylosing spondylitis. Am. J. Roentgenol. 216:1181, 1976.
68. Rosen, P.S.: A unique shoulder lesion in ankylosing spondylitis. Clinical Comment. J. Rheum. 7:109, 1980.
69. Ball, J.: Enthesopathy of rheumatoid and ankylosing spondylitis. Ann. Rheum. Dis. 30:213, 1971.
70. Resnick, D., and Niwayama, G.: Psoriatic arthritis. *In* Resnick, D., and Niwayama, G. (eds.): Diagnosis of Bone and Joint Disorders. Philadelphia, W. B. Saunders Company, 1981, p. 1103.
71. Wright, V.: Psoriatic arthritis. *In* Scott, J.T. (ed.): Copeman's Textbook of the Rheumatic Diseases. 5th ed. Edinburgh, Churchill Livingstone, 1978, p. 537.
72. Zaias, N.: Psoriasis of the nail: A clinico-pathological study. Arch. Dermatol. 99:567, 1967.
73. Resnick, D., and Niwayama, G.: On the nature and significance of bony proliferation in "rheumatoid variant" disorders. Am. J. Roentgenol. 129:275, 1977.
74. Forrester, D.M., and Kirkpatrick, R.W.: Periostitis and pseudoperiostitis. Radiology 118:597, 1976.
75. Resnick, D., and Broderick, R.W.: Bony proliferation of terminal phalanges in psoriasis. The "Ivory" phalanx. J. Can. Assoc. Radiol. 28:187, 1977.
76. Killebrew, K., Gold, R.H., and Sholkoff, S.D.: Psoriatic spondylitis. Radiology 108:9, 1973.
77. Sundaram, M., and Patton, J.T.: Paravertebral ossification in psoriasis and Reiter's disease. Br. J. Radiol. 48:628, 1975.
78. Kaplan, D., Plotz, C.M., Nathanson, L., and Frank, L.: Cervical spine in psoriasis and psoriatic arthritis. Ann. Rheum. Dis. 23:50, 1964.
79. Resnick, D., and Niwayama, G.: Reiter's syndrome. *In* Resnick, D., and Niwayama, G. (eds.): Diagnosis of Bone and Joint Disorders, Philadelphia, W. B. Saunders Company, 1981, p. 1130.
80. Sholkoff, S.D., Glickman, M.G., and Steinback, H.L.: Roentgenology of Reiter's syndrome. Radiology 97:497, 1970.
81. Cliff, J.M.: Spinal bony bridging and carditis in Reiter's disease. Ann. Rheum. Dis. 30:171, 1971.
82. Resnick, D., and Niwayama, G.: Enteropathic arthropathies. *In* Resnick, D., and Niwayama, G. (eds.): Diagnosis of Bone and Joint Disorders. Philadelphia, W. B. Saunders Company, 1981, p. 1149.
83. Jayson, M.I.V., Salmon, P.R., and Harrison, W.J.: Inflammatory bowel disease in ankylosing spondylitis. Gut 11:506, 1970.
84. McEwen, C., Ditata, D., Lingg, C., Porini, A., Good, A., and Rankin, T.: Ankylosing spondylitis and spondylitis accompanying ulcerative colitis, regional enteritis, psoriasis, and Reiter's disease. Arthritis Rheum. 14:291, 1971.
85. Haslock, I.: Enteropathic arthritis. *In* Scott, J.T. (ed.): Copeman's Textbook of the Rheumatic Diseases. 5th ed. Edinburgh, Churchill Livingstone, 1978, p. 567.
86. Ferguson, R.H.: Enteropathic arthritis. *In* Hollander, J.L., and McCarty, D.J. (eds.): Arthritis and Allied Conditions. 8th ed. Philadelphia, Lea & Febiger, 1972, p. 846.
87. O'Connell, D.J., and Marx, W.J.: Hand changes in primary biliary cirrhosis. Radiology 129:31, 1978.
88. Clarke, A.K., Galbraith, R.M., Hamilton, E.B.D., and Williams, R.: Rheumatic disorders in primary biliary cirrhosis. Ann. Rheum. Dis. 37:42, 1978.
89. Lucas, P.F., and Owen, T.K.: Subcutaneous fat necrosis, "polyarthritis", and pancreatic disease. Gut 3:146, 1962.

90. Gibson, T.J., Schumacher, H.R., Pascual, E., Brighton, E., and Brighton, C.: Arthropathy, skin and bone lesions in pancreatic disease. J. Rheumatol. 2:7, 1975.
91. Labowitz, R., and Schumacher, H.R. Jr.: Articular manifestations of systemic lupus erythematosus. Ann. Int. Med. 74:911, 1971.
92. Weissman, B.N., Rappoport, A.S., Sosman, J.L., and Schur, P.H.: Radiographic findings in the hands in patients with systemic lupus erythematosus. Radiology 126:313, 1978.
93. Bleifield, C.J., and Inglis, A.E.: The hand in systemic lupus erythematosus. J. Bone Joint Surg. 56A:1207, 1974.
94. Bywaters, E.G.L.: Jaccoud's syndrome. A sequel to the joint involvement in systemic lupus erythematosus. Clin. Rheum. Dis. 1:125, 1975.
95. Twinning, R.H., Marcus, W.Y., and Garey, J.L.: Tendon rupture in systemic lupus erythematosus. JAMA 189:377, 1964.
96. Klippel, J.H., Gerber, L.H., Pollack, L., and Decker, J.L.: Avascular necroses in systemic lupus erythematosus. Silent symmetric osteonecrosis. Am. J. Med. 67:83, 1979.
97. Budin, J.A., and Feldman, F.: Soft tissue calcifications in systemic lupus erythematosus. Am. J. Roentgenol. 124:358, 1975.
98. Staples, P.J., Gerding, D.N., Decker, J.L., and Gordon, R.S. Jr.: Incidence of infection in systemic lupus erythematosus. Arthritis Rheum. 17:1, 1971.
99. Goodman, N.: The significance of terminal phalangeal osteosclerosis. Radiology 89:709, 1967.
100. Resnick, D.: Scleroderma (progressive systemic sclerosis). *In* Resnick, D., and Niwayama, G. (eds.): Diagnosis of Bone and Joint Disorders. Philadelphia, W. B. Saunders Company, 1981, p. 1204.
101. Poznanski, A.K.: The Hand in Radiologic Diagnosis. Philadelphia, W. B. Saunders Company, 1974, p. 531.
102. Thibierge, G., and Weissenbach, R.J.: Concretions calcare sous-cutanees et sclerodermie. Ann. Dermatol. Syphiligr. 2:129, 1911.
103. Muller, S.A., Brunsting, L.A., and Winkelmann, R.K.: Calcinosis cutis: Its relationship to scleroderma. Arch Dermatol. 80:15, 1959.
104. Rowell, N.R., and Hopper, F.E.: The periodontal membrane in systemic lupus erythematosus. Br. J. Dermatol. 93(Suppl.):23, 1975.
105. Seifert, M.H., Steigerwald, J.C., and Cliff, M.M.: Bone resorption of the mandible in progressive systemic sclerosis. Arthritis Rheum. 18:507, 1977.
106. Keats, T.E.: Rib erosions in scleroderma. Am. J. Roentgenol. 100:530, 1967.
107. Mezarsos, W.T.: The regional manifestations of scleroderma. Radiology 70:313, 1958.
108. Kemp Harper, R.A., and Jackson, D.C.: Progressive systemic sclerosis. Br. J. Radiol. 38:825, 1965.
109. Haverbush, T.J., Wilde, A.H., Hawk, W.A. Jr., and Scherbel, A.L.: Osteolysis of the ribs and cervical spine in progressive systemic sclerosis (scleroderma): A case report. J. Bone Joint Surg. 56A:637, 1974.
110. Lovell, C.R., and Jayson, M.I.V.: Joint involvement in systemic sclerosis. Scand. J. Rheumatol. 8:154, 1979.
111. Resnick, D.: Dermatomyositis and polymyositis. *In* Resnick, D., and Niwayama, G. (eds.): Diagnosis of Bone and Joint Disorders. Philadelphia, W. B. Saunders Company, 1981, p. 1230.
112. Schumacher, H.R., Schimmer, B., Gordon, G.V., Bookspan, M.A., Brogadir, S., and Dorwart, B.B.: Articular manifestations of polymyositis and dermatomyositis. Arthritis Rheum. 23:491, 1980.
113. Ozonoff, M.B., and Flynn, F.J. Jr.: Roentgenologic features of dermatomyositis of childhood. Am. J. Roentgenol. 118:206, 1973.
114. Sewell, J.R., Liyanage, B., and Ansell, B.M.: Calcinosis in juvenile dermatomyositis. Skel. Radiol. 3:137, 1978.
115. Resnick, D.: Polyarteritis nodosa and other vasculitides. *In* Resnick, D., and Niwayama, G. (eds.): Diagnosis of Bone and Joint Disorders. Philadelphia, W. B. Saunders Company, 1981, p. 1242.
116. Bennet, R.M., and O'Connell, D.J.: The arthritis of mixed conective tissue disease. Ann. Rheum. Dis. 37:397, 1978.
117. Ramos-Niembro, F., Alarcon-Segovia, D., and Hernandez-Ortiz, J.: Articular manifestations of mixed connective tissue disease. Arthritis Rheum. 22:43, 1979.
118. Resnick, D., and Niwayama, G.: Degenerative disease of extraspinal locations. *In* Resnick, D., and Niwayama, G. (eds.): Diagnosis of Bone and Joint Disorders. Philadelphia, W. B. Saunders Company, 1981, p. 1270.
119. Landells, J.W.: The bone cysts of osteoarthritis. J. Bone Joint Surg. 35B:643, 1953.
120. Ferguson, A.B.: The pathologic changes in degenerative arthritis of the hip and treatment by rotational osteotomy. J. Bone Joint Surg. 46A:1337, 1964.
121. Resnick, D.: Patterns of migration of the femoral head in osteoarthritis of the hip. Roentgenographic-pathologic correlation and comparison with rheumatoid arthritis. Am. J. Roentgenol. 124:62, 1975.
122. Thomas, R.H., Resnick, D., Alazraki, N.P., Daniel, D., and Greenfield, R.: Compartmental evaluation of osteoarthritis of the knee. A comparative study of available diagnostic modalities. Radiology 116:585, 1975.
123. Leach, R.E., Gregg, T., and Siber, F.J.: Weight-bearing radiography in osteoarthritis of the knee. Radiology 97:265, 1970.
124. Mann, R.A., Coughlin, M.J., and DuVries, H.L.: Hallux rigidus: A review of the literature and a method of treatment. Clin. Orthop. Rel. Res. 142:57, 1979.
125. Crain, D.C.: Interphalangeal osteoarthritis characterized by painful inflammatory episodes resulting in deformity of the proximal and distal articulations. JAMA 175:1049, 1961.
126. McEwen, C.: Osteoarthritis of the fingers with ankylosis. Arthritis Rheum. 11:734, 1968.
127. Resnick, D., and Niwayama, G.: Degenerative disease of the spine. *In* Resnick, D., and Niwayama, G. (eds.): Diagnosis of Bone and Joint Disorders. Philadelphia, W. B. Saunders Company, 1981, p. 1368.
128. Schmorl, G., and Junghanns, H.: The Human Spine in Health and Disease. 2nd ed. Translated by E.F. Besemann. New York, Grune & Stratton, 1971, p. 138.
129. Knutsson, F.: The vacuum phenomenon in the intervertebral discs. Acta Radiol. 23:173, 1942.
130. Kroker, P.: Sichtbare Rissbildungen in den Bandscheiben der Wirbelsaule. Fortschr. Geb. Roentgenstr. Nuklearmed. 72:1, 1949.
131. Bick, E.M.: Vertebral osteophytosis. Pathologic basis of its roentgenology. Am. J. Roentgenol. 73:979, 1955.
132. Goldberg, R.P., and Carter, B.L.: Absence of thoracic osteophytosis in the area adjacent to the aorta: Computed tomography demonstration. J. Comput. Assist. Tomogr. 2:173, 1978.
133. Hadley, L.A.: Anatomico-roentgenographic studies of the posterior spinal articulations. Am. J. Roentgenol. 86:270, 1961.
134. Resnick, D., and Niwayama, G.: Diffuse idiopathic skeletal hyperostosis (DISH): Ankylosing hyperostosis of Forestier and Rotes-Querol. *In* Resnick, D., and Niwayama, G. (eds.): Diagnosis of Bone and Joint Disorders. Philadelphia, W. B. Saunders Company, 1981, p. 1416.
135. Forestier, J., and Rotes-Querol, J.: Senile ankylosing hyperostosis of the spine. Ann. Rheum. Dis. 9:321, 1950.
136. Oppenheimer, A.: Calcification and ossification of vertebral ligaments (spondylosis ossificans ligamentosa): Roentgen study of pathogenesis and clinical significance. Radiology 38:160, 1940.
137. Resnick, D., and Niwayama, G.: Radiographic and pathologic features of spinal involvement in diffuse idiopathic skeletal hyperostosis (DISH). Radiology 119:559, 1976.
138. Bauer, F.: Dysphagia due to cervical spondylosis. J. Laryngol. Otol. 67:615, 1953.
139. Resnick, D., Guerra, J., Jr., Robinson, C.A., and Vint, V.C.: Association of diffuse idiopathic skeletal hyperostosis (DISH) and calcification and ossification of the posterior longitudinal ligament. Am. J. Roentgenol. 131:1049, 1978.
140. Kohler, H., Uehlinger, E., Kutzner, J., and West, T.B.: Sternocostoclavicular hyperostosis: Painful swelling of the sternum, clavicles, and upper ribs. Ann. Intern. Med. 87,192, 1977.
141. Resnick, D., Shaul, S.R., and Robins, J.M.: Diffuse idiopathic skeletal hyperostosis (DISH): Forestier's disease with extraspinal manifestations. Radiology 115:513, 1975.
142. Resnick, D.: Neuroarthropathy. *In* Resnick, D., and Niwayama, G. (eds.): Diagnosis of Bone and Joint Disorders. Philadelphia, W. B. Saunders Company, 1981, p. 2422.
143. Key, J.A.: Clinical observations on tabetic arthropathies (Charcot joints). Am. J. Syph. 14:429, 1932.
144. Pomeranz, M.M., and Rothberg, A.S.: A review of 58 cases of tabetic arthropathy. Am. J. Syph. 25:103, 1941.
145. Jaffe, H.L.: Metabolic, Degenerative and Inflammatory Diseases of Bones and Joints. Philadelphia, Lea & Febiger, 1972, p. 847.
146. Clouse, M.E., Gramm, H.F., Legg, M., and Flood, T.: Diabetic osteoarthropathy: clinical and roentgenographic observations in 90 cases. Am. J. Roentgenol. 121:22, 1974.
147. Gray, R.G., and Gottlieb, N.L.: Rheumatic disorders associated with diabetes mellitus: Literature review. Semin. Arthritis Rheum. 6:19, 1976.
148. Giesecke, S.B., Dalinka, M.K., and Kyle, G.C.: Lisfranc's fracture-dislocation: A manifestation of peripheral neuropathy. Am. J. Roentgenol. 131:139, 1978.
149. Thornhill, H.L., Richter, R.W., Shelton, M.L., and Johnson, C.A.: Neuropathic arthropathy (Charcot forefeet) in alcoholics. Orthop. Clin. N. Am. 4:7, 1973.
150. Peitzman, S.J., Miller, J.L., Ortega, L., Schumacher, H.R., and Fernandez, P.C.: Charcot arthropathy secondary to amyloid neuropathy. JAMA 235:1345, 1976.
151. Resnick, D., and Niwayama, G.: Crystal-induced and related diseases. *In* Resnick, D., and Niwayama, G. (eds.): Diagnosis of Bone and Joint Disorders. Philadelphia, W. B. Saunders Company, 1981, p. 1463.
152. Talbott, J.H.: Gout. 3rd ed. New York, Grune & Stratton, 1967.

153. Vyhanek, L., Lavicka, J., and Blahos, J.: Roentgenological findings in gout. Radiol. Clin. 28:256, 1960.
154. Good, A.E., and Rapp, R.: Bony ankylosis: A rare manifestation of gout. J. Rheumatol. 5:335, 1978.
155. Kawenoki-Minc, E., Eyman, E., Leo, W., and Werynska-Przybylska, J.: Zwyrodnienie stawow i kregoslupa u chorych na dne. Analiza 262 przypadkowdny. Reumatoligia 12:267, 1974.
156. von Hoyningen-Huene, C.B.J.: Gout and glycogen storage disease in preadolescent brothers. Arch. Intern. Med. 118:471, 1966.
157. Riley, J.D.: Gout and cerebral palsy in a three-year-old boy. Arch. Dis. Child. 35:293, 1960.
158. Gutman, A.B.: Primary and secondary gout. Ann. Intern. Med. 39:1062, 1953.
159. Grahme, R., Sutor, D.J., and Mitchener, M.B.: Crystal deposition in hyperparathyroidism. Ann. Rheum. Dis. 30:597, 1971.
160. Dmartini, F.E.: Hyperuricemia induced by drugs. Arthritis Rheum. 8:823, 1965.
161. Resnick, D., Niwayama, G., Goergen, T.G., Utsinger, P.D., Shapiro, R.F., Hasselwood, D.H., and Wiesner, K.B.: Clinical, radiographic and pathologic abnormalities in calcium pyrophosphate dihydrate deposition disease (CPPD): Pseudogout. Radiology 122:1, 1977.
162. Vigario, D.G., and Keats, T.E.: Localization of calcific deposits in the shoulder. Am. J. Roentgenol. 108:806, 1970.
163. Schumacher, H.R. Jr.: Hemochromatosis and arthritis. Arthritis Rheum. 7:41, 1964.
164. Hamilton, E., Williams, R., Barlow, K.A., and Smith, P.M.: The arthropathy of hemochromatosis. Q. J. Med. 37:171, 1968.
165. Atkins, C.J., McIvor, J., Smith, P.M., Hamilton, E., and Williams, R.: Chondrocalcinosis and arthropathy: Studies in haemochromatosis and in idiopathic chondrocalcinosis. Q. J. Med. 39:71, 1970.
166. Seze, S. de, Solnica, J., Mitrovic, D., Miravet, L., and Dorfmann, H.: Joint and bone disorders and hypoparathyroidism in hemochromatosis. Semin. Arthritis Rheum. 2:71, 1972.
167. Hirsch, J.H., Killien, C., and Troupin, R.H.: The arthropathy of hemochromatosis. Radiology 118:591, 1976.
168. Feller, E.R., and Schumacher, H.R.: Osteoarticular changes in Wilson's disease. Arthritis Rheum. 15:259, 1972.
169. Finby, N., and Bearn, A.G.: Roentgenographic abnormalities of the skeletal system in Wilson's disease (hepatolenticular degeneration). Am. J. Roentgenol. 79:603, 1958.
170. Cervenansky, J., Sitaj, S., and Urbanek, T.: Alkaptonuria and ochronosis. J. Bone Joint Surg. 41A:1169, 1959.
171. Mueller, M.N., Sorenson, L.B., Strandjord, N., and Kappas, A.: Alkaptonuria and ochronotic arthropathy. Med. Clin. North Am. 49:101, 1965.
172. Martin, W.J., Underahl, L.O., Mathieson, D.R., and Pugh, D.G.: Alkaptonuria: Report of 12 cases. Ann. Intern. Med. 42:1052, 1955.
173. Resnick, D., and Niwayama, G.: Osteomyelitis, septic arthritis, and soft tissue infection: the mechanisms and situations. *In* Resnick, D., and Niwayama, G. (eds.): Diagnosis of Bone and Joint Disorders. Philadelphia, W. B. Saunders Company, 1981, p. 2042.
174. Chuinard, R.G., and D'Ambrosia, R.: Human bite infections of the hand. J. Bone Joint Surg. 59A:416, 1977.
175. Patterson, F.P., and Brown, C.S.: Complications of total hip replacement arthroplasty. Orthop. Clin. North Am. 4:503, 1973.
176. Franck, W.A., Bress, N.M., Singer, F.R., and Krane, S.M.: Rheumatic manifestation of Paget's disease of bone. Am. J. Med. 56:592, 1974.
177. McCarty, D.J. Jr.: Pseudogout: articular chondrocalcinsis. *In* Hollander, J.L., and McCarty, D.J., Jr. (eds.): Arthritis and Related Disorders. 8th ed. Philadelphia, Lea & Febiger, 1972, p. 410.
178. Steinbach, H.L., and Russell, W.: Measurements of the heel pad as an aid to diagnosis of acromegaly. Radiology 82:418, 1964.
179. Lang, E.K., and Bessler, W.T.: The roentgenologic features of acromegaly. Am. J. Roentgenol. 86:321, 1961.
180. Watson, R.J., Burko, H., Megas, H., and Robinson, M.: Hand-foot syndrome in sickle cell disease in young children. Pediatrics 31:975, 1963.
181. Grossman, R.E., and Hensley, G.T.: Bone lesions in primary amyloidosis. Am. J. Roentgenol. 101:872, 1967.
182. Weinfield, A., Stern, M.H., and Marx, L.H.: Amyloid lesions of bone. Am. J. Roentgenol. 108:799, 1970.
183. Pettersson, H., Ahlberg, A., and Nilsson, I.M.: A radiologic classification of hemophilic arthropathy. Clin. Orthop. Rel. Res. 149:153, 1980.
184. Resnick, D.: Tumors and tumor-like lesions in or about joints. *In* Resnick, D., and Niwayama, G. (eds.): Diagnosis of Bone and Joint Disorders. Philadelphia, W. B. Saunders Company, 1981, p. 2638.
185. Prager, R.J., and Mall, J.C.: Arthrographic diagnosis of synovial chondromatosis. Am. J. Roentgenol. 127:344, 1976.
186. Breimer, C.W., and Freiberger, R.H.: Bone lesions associated with villonodular synovitis. Am. J. Roentgenol. 79:618, 1958.

# Chapter 40

# Nuclear Medicine, and Special Radiologic Imaging and Technique in the Diagnosis of Rheumatic Diseases

*Thomas C. Namey*

## INTRODUCTION

Prior to the advent of modern serologic studies, radiology was the physician's major ally in the diagnosis of rheumatic diseases. In recent years, electronic microcircuitry and information processing have re-expanded the radiologist's imaging armamentarium. Studies once available only at university centers are now commonplace in the community hospital: nuclear medicine, ultrasound, and computed tomography. Refinements and defined applications of existing studies in thermography, arthrography, and xeroradiography have increased their specific utilities. Cost effectiveness as well as outcome is a major concern and accentuates the need for a discussion of strategies in utilization of special imaging studies.

This chapter deals with this expanded technologic base, covering the uses of nuclear medicine, thermography, ultrasound, xeroradiography, arthrography, and computed tomography in the diagnosis of rheumatic diseases.

## NUCLEAR IMAGING

The uses of the early bone-seeking radionuclides, strontium-85 ($^{85}Sr$), strontium-87m ($^{87m}Sr$), and fluorine-18($^{18}F$), were generally restricted to the detection of metastatic or primary bone malignancies.[1-3] This was because of high cost or limited availability, excessive radiation per study ($^{85}Sr$), or a too short half-life ($^{87m}Sr$). In 1971, technetium-99m-phosphates were introduced. They had an optimal half-life (6 hours), low radiation dose to the patient, and low cost.[4,5] Early clinical trials verified the superior bone-imaging properties of the $^{99m}Tc$ phosphates, which were readily applicable to the evaluation of nonmalignant bone disease.[3,6] Gallium-67 ($^{67}Ga$), a radiolanthanide introduced in the search for alternative bone-seeking agents, was found to localize in lymphomas and other malignancies, but also in active pyogenic inflammatory sites to a greater degree than in bone.[7-8] $^{67}Ga$ scintiscanning has now proved to be a useful adjunct to $^{99m}Tc$-phosphate imaging of bone and joints.[9-11] The important properties and utilities of the radiopharmaceuticals used in rheumatic imaging, $^{99m}Tc$-pertechnetate, phosphate and sulfur colloid, and $^{67}Ga$, are discussed in the following sections and are summarized in Table 40–1.

**Radiotechnetium ($^{99m}$)Tc-Pertechnetate.** $^{99m}Tc$-pertechnetate binds primarily to serum albumin, and the free $TcO_4^-$ in equilibrium with albumin-bound $TcO_4^-$ is taken up rapidly by organs that "trap" iodide, including the thyroid, gastric mucosa, salivary glands, choroid plexus, and kidneys. Organ uptake may be competitively inhibited by administration of pharmacologic amounts of perchlorate ($C10_4^-$). Irrespective of $C10_4^-$ administration, sufficient pertechnetate is bound to albumin to serve as a "blood-pool" imaging agent if scintigraphy is performed within 5 to 15 minutes after administration.

Synovial inflammation increases articular blood flow and juxta-articular venous capacitance, the principal determinants of "blood-pool" size.[12-14] The inflamed synovium binds no more pertechnetate than normal tissue on a weight basis.[15] Radiopertechnetate joint scintigraphy is analogous to "nuclear thermography." Many studies have confirmed that *quantitative* $^{99m}Tc$-pertechnetate synovial scintigraphy provides a reliable, measurable, and reproducible index of acute articular inflammation.[14,16-19] Unfortunately the sensitivity for *qualitative* diagnostic imaging is too low relative to $^{99m}$technetium-phosphate bone and joint studies, and the primary utility for joint study is quantitative, where it retains practical superiority.

Salivary gland imaging remains the most important clinical utility of radiopertechnetate. Both qualitative salivary gland imaging and quantitative computer studies can be performed, supplying complementary data for diagnostic purposes in Sjögren's syndrome, sarcoidosis, and salivary duct obstruction.[20-22] Functional uptake occurs because the iodide-trapping mechanism of the salivary acini cannot distinguish iodide from pertechnetate. Abnormalities are defined by abnormally low rates of accumulation, assymmetric accumulation, overaccumulation (as in the case of duct calculi), and impaired excretion after standard stimuli to salivation (e.g., lemon juice or 500 mg. of ascorbic acid).[21,23-25]

**Technetium-99$^m$-Phosphates.** The initial mechanism considered responsible for osseous uptake of the $^{99m}Tc$-phosphates was ionic "adsorption" to the surface of microcrystalline hydroxyapatite by a phosphate–calcium ionic interaction.[26] Factors that would modify uptake by this mechanism include blood flow in tissues[27,28] and

**Table 40–1.** Commonly Used Radionuclide Imaging Agents

| Radiopharmaceutical | Half-Life (hours) | Photon(s) | Clinical Study |
|---|---|---|---|
| $^{99}Tc^m$ Pertechnetate | 6.1 | 140 | Quantitative synovial blood-pool imaging<br>Salivary gland imaging |
| $^{99}Tc^m$ Phosphates | 6.1 | 140 | Standard bone and joint scintigraphy<br>Quantitative bone and joint studies (i.e., sacroiliac joints)<br>Immediate blood-pool imaging |
| $^{99}Tc^m$ Sulfur colloids | 6.1 | 140 | Liver-spleen imaging<br>Bone marrow imaging—useful in avascular necrosis, bone infarcts |
| $^{67}$Gallium (citrate) | 78 | 93(40%)<br>184(24%)<br>296(22%)<br>388(7%) | Infection<br>Granulomatous disease, e.g., sarcoidosis<br>Lymphoreticular diseases (lymphoma, Hodgkin's disease)<br>Occult carcinoma |

the rate of bone turnover or remodeling, factors that alter the available surface area of hydroxyapatite.[29,30] However, the original premise of ionic binding has been challenged by observation in vivo, in which uptake occurs in tissue with little or no histochemical evidence for salts of calcium.[26]

An alternative mechanism is that uptake of $^{99m}$Tc-phosphates depends on binding to collagen, in the presence of normal blood flow.[31,32] There is a correlation between 5-hour bone–soft tissue uptake and urinary hydroxyproline excretion in renal osteodystrophy, Paget's disease, and hyperparathyroidism.[33] Hydroxyproline is found almost exclusively in collagen, the primary structural protein in bone. Because reutilization does not occur in vivo, urinary hydroxyproline reflects bone matrix degradation. In most circumstances, bone formation parallels bone destruction. Thus, an agent localized in areas of bone matrix synthesis will be paralleled by evidence for matrix breakdown. In three patient groups, including controls, patients with Paget's disease, and those with renal osteodystrophy, there was no difference in the early rate of accumulation in bone of $^{99m}$Tc-pyrophosphate, despite the increased osseous blood flow in Paget's disease. After 5 hours, the highest bone–soft tissue ratios occurred in the patients with Paget's disease and renal osteodystrophy. Patients with hyperparathyroidism maintained their increased 5-hour bone–soft tissue ratios for several weeks after parathyroidectomy during the phase of reparative bone formation, despite a marked decrease in bone turnover.[33,34]

In vitro incubation studies on the rat tibia with $^{99m}$Tc-pyrophosphate demonstrated a higher uptake in unmineralized osteoid than in bone (Fig. 40–1).[32] Using agents that inhibited crosslinking of collagen, data have been presented that indicate that immature, recently synthesized, incompletely crosslinked collagen is the substrate for $^{99m}$Tc-phosphate uptake. Garcia and coworkers showed that after intramuscular implants of bone-forming demineralized matrix and "bone-resorbing" dead bone, only the bone-forming system accumulated $^{99m}$Tc-pyrophosphate, whereas the lytic, bone-resorbing system accumulated less radiopharmaceutical than normal bone.[35] The "bone-seeking" technetium phosphates have a greater affinity for cartilage than for bone, and direct proof has been provided for nonmineral binding of technetium phosphates.[36]

In summary, factors associated with mineralization of bone appear to be responsible for the increased uptake of $^{99m}$Tc-phosphates in vivo. Increased uptake may be expected to occur in areas of hyperemia (probably secondary to an increase in absolute metabolic activity of the cells as well as in delivery of the carrier) and in areas of osteogenesis irrespective of the net accumulation or loss of bone. Decreased activity is seen in areas of mature, quiescent bone and in areas where the vascular supply is deficient or absent.

**Technetium Sulfur Colloid.** Technetium-99m sulfur colloid is an established imaging agent for liver and spleen. The reticuloendothelial cells of these organs phagocytize the radiolabeled sulfur colloid, providing an estimation of size and macrophage phagocytic capacity. Uptake also occurs in bone marrow but to a lesser extent with the sulfur colloid preparations used in liver–spleen scintigraphy. However, this uptake is enhanced in states in which marrow activity is increased, such as megaloblastic anemias, hemolytic anemias, and hemoglobinopathies and when reticuloendothelial tissue of the liver and spleen is bypassed or replaced, as in portal hypertension or metastatic carcinoma. The preferential uptake by the phagocytic cells of the liver and spleen of the sulfur colloid versus the marrow cells is a function of the size distribution of the sulfur colloid in standard preparations (a mean of 100 microns). The reticuloendothelial cells in the marrow optimally phagocytize particles in the range of 10 microns.[37] However, adequate imaging of bone marrow tissues can be accomplished when the vascular clearance of the larger particles has occurred, which is after 15 to 20 minutes in normal individuals.[38] Alternatively, preparations of sulfur colloid particles with a smaller size distribution or other colloid aggregates of $^{99m}$technetium, such as antimony colloid, will provide more efficient and selective marrow reticuloendothelial studies.[37] The clinical indications for bone-marrow imaging are avascular necrosis, bone infarction, viability of bone after fracture, and determination of erythropoietic marrow mass in disease states in which it is increased or decreased.

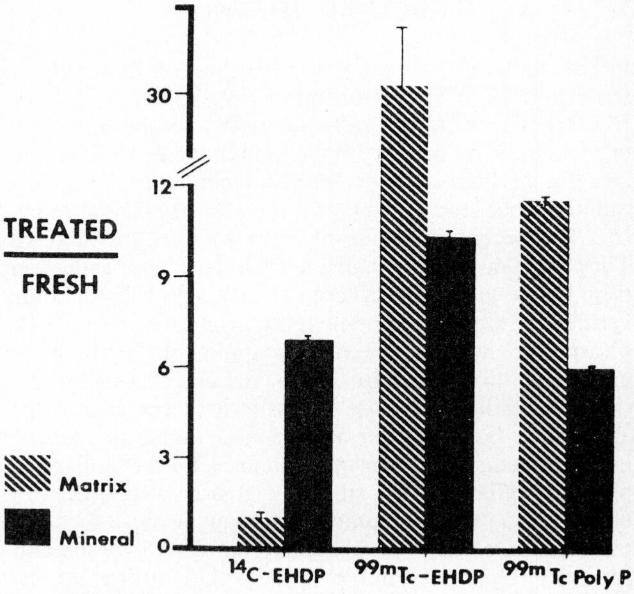

**Figure 40–1.** In vivo uptake ratios of treated bone to normal untreated bone with various radiopharmaceuticals. While $^{14}$C-EHDP exhibits preferential binding for bone mineral, the technetium-99m-phosphates bind to demineralized bone (matrix) to a greater extent than to the mineral. (From Rosenthall, L., and Kaye, M.: Semin. Nucl. Med. 6:59, 1976. Reprinted by permission.)

**$^{67}$Gallium.** While bone binds some ionic gallium, much greater uptake occurs by microsomes in nonosseous cells, particularly polymorphonuclear (PMN) leukocytes and monocytes.[39-44] Gallium binds to serum and cellular transferrin and lactoferrin, suggesting that molecular substrates for ferric ion are the principal determinants for tissue distribution of $^{67}$gallium in vivo (Fig. 40–2).[45-49] Cellular uptake is mediated by a transferrin-specific ferric ion receptor, although this may not be the mechanism for uptake in tumor tissue.[50,51] PMN leukocytes bind greater amounts of gallium than do lymphocytes, probably because of the high concentration of lactoferrin in PMN leukocytes, and this rapid uptake establishes the means by which $^{67}$Ga localizes at sites of infection and pus.[52] However, certain tumors take up gallium independent of leukocytes, enabling $^{67}$Ga imaging to aid in the diagnosis of occult tumors as well as infection.[8,50] Deferoxamine mesylate, a potent iron-chelating agent, has been shown to effectively displace bound $^{67}$Ga from tissues but increase target–nontarget tissue activity ratio.[53]

Because of different mechanisms for localization, $^{67}$Ga imaging complements $^{99m}$Tc-phosphate bone imaging in the detection of osteomyelitis and septic arthritis.[10,11,52] Imaging with $^{67}$Ga should always *follow* rather than *precede* the studies using radiotechnetium, because of its long half-life (70 hours). Imaging should be performed at 8 to 24 hours and again at 72 hours using $^{67}$Ga. Gallium is normally excreted in the terminal ileum, and normally some activity in the bowel may be seen. The multiple energies of emitted photons limit the resolution of radiogallium imaging and contribute to the substantially higher radiation dose used compared with radiotechnetium. The radiation exposure, while not excessive, should cause concern over the casual use of $^{67}$Ga imaging, particularly in children or women of child-bearing age.

## IMAGING METHODS AND DEVICES

The radioisotopes $^{99m}$Tc and $^{67}$Ga may be imaged with conventional rectilinear scanning devices or the Anger-type gamma scintillation camera, using several different collimators. Dual-probe scanners have shortened the time necessary to perform a skeletal or whole-body survey with any of the $^{99m}$Tc or $^{67}$Ga complexes. Nonetheless, the images obtained, although often sufficient for diagnostic purposes, do not contain the information density, resolution, or projections needed for complete studies.[3,11] The use of the Anger-type gamma camera is recommended for optimal visualization of abnormalities, since resolution is independent of the "focusing" effect seen in dual-crystal rectilinear scanning devices, and proximity of the lesion to the collimator surface leads to improved resolution.[1,11] For further definition, particularly of internal articulations that cannot closely approximate the collimator surface (e.g., hips and the axial skeleton), a pinhole collimator affords greater detail and magnification. This collimator is of particular value in pediatric imaging, since active epiphyseal growth plates often obscure early osseous inflammatory lesions.[11,54]

Survey scintigraphy with a rectilinear camera or gamma camera, followed by special views with a gamma camera employing a high-resolution parallel-hole or pinhole collimator, is the best approach in inflammatory bone or joint disease. Any abnormal or suspicious areas seen on the survey images and areas clinically suspect for osseous or articular involvement should be subjected to special study.[11] Finally, it is important to image the contralateral side for comparison, which increases accurate recognition of inflammatory lesions. Blood-pool imaging with immediate scanning after $^{99}$Tc$^{m}$-phosphate injection should be done if cellulitis or a soft tissue abscess is present and could obscure the diagnosis of an underlying bone lesion. Specialized or quantitative studies should be discussed in advance of imaging with the nuclear medicine specialist. Standard bone imaging is not optimal for assessment of inflammatory articular disease. Technicians and referring physicians acquaint themselves with the views constituting a "joint" scan.[55]

## PERIPHERAL JOINT SCINTIGRAPHY IN INFLAMMATORY ARTHRITIS

The first agents used to assess joint inflammation were blood-pool markers, labled albumin, and $^{99}TcO_4^-$.[56]

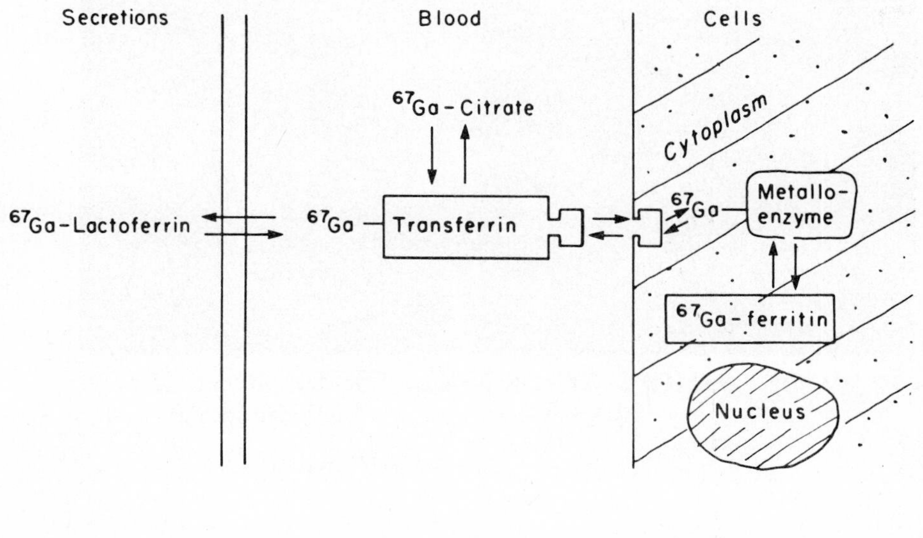


**Figure 40–2.** Proposed mechanism for cellular uptake of $^{67}$Ga-citrate by tumor cells and leukocytes. (From Larson, S.M.: Semin. Nucl. Med. 8:200, 1978. Reprinted by permission.)

While the low sensitivity of pertechnetates precluded broader diagnostic use, use of this isotope presented a new and relatively simple approach to quantifying inflammation and was particularly applicable to research. Superiority of the newer $^{99m}$Tc-phosphate bone-seeking radiotracers over blood-pool imaging with pertechnetate for diagnostic was demonstrated in 1975.[57] In some instances, articular "positivity" on $^{99m}$Tc-PYP scanning predated the patient's awareness of joint inflammation, which was confirmed by the development of clinical synovitis weeks to months after the joint scan.[57] Numerous studies have since appeared and confirmed the efficacy of joint scanning with the bone-seeking radiotracers in documenting preradiographic articular involvement in rheumatoid arthritis, psoriatic arthritis, ankylosing spondylitis, gout, and other arthropathies.[58-69] Arguments for the use of joint imaging include the following:

1. Extreme sensitivity. The presence of articular or juxta-articular inflammation is virtually excluded by the presence of a normal joint scan. This was suggested by the long-term follow-up of 22 patients with "polyarthralgias" who had negative or noninflammatory scintigrams. None demonstrated inflammatory joint disease, although one had SLE and two had polymyalgia rheumatica (now considered as having an inflammatory articular component by author)[70].

2. Reduced radiation. Judicious use of joint and bone scanning can reduce the radiation exposure in diagnosing inflammatory rheumatic diseases, since multiple joints are frequently radiographed before disease becomes radiographically manifest.[71-74] For conventional imaging, radiographic exposure is "additive." This is not true for scintimaging. Only one radiation dose is accrued per study no matter how many images are made during the radioisotopic procedure. This concern varies for the age and sex of the patient and for the joint in question. It is most critical in lumbosacral studies in women of childbearing age, since gonads cannot be shielded. Since sacroiliac disease develops more slowly in women than men, this point cannot be overemphasized.[75-77] Gonadal exposure approximates 390 mREM in women during conventional lumbosacral radiography versus 140 mREM for $^{99}$Tc$^{m}$- phosphate scintigraphy using 15 mCi of $^{99}$Tc$^{m}$-EHDP.[78,79]

3. Cost. This is often inapparent to many clinicians. While the cost of bone and joint imaging is higher than one or two conventional radiographs, once survey studies are considered or the number of joints radiographed increases, economic considerations favor the radioisotopic study. Technetium phosphate bone and joint studies remain substantially less costly than computed tomography.

4. Early diagnosis. Documentation of the pattern of articular disease is the most important consideration in establishing a specific diagnosis. In rheumatoid arthritis, considered to be a symmetric polyarticular disease, patients may initially present with asymmetric oligo- or monoarticular synovitis. Alternatively, disease activity in one joint may obscure pain at another joint. In early disease, when standard radiographs are normal, joint imaging has the greatest value in documenting clinical and subclinical synovitis and establishing the pattern of articular activity crucial to diagnosis[80-82] (Figs. 40–3 and 40–4).

In summary, joint imaging offers the most sensitive documentation of the extent and pattern of early arthritis.[57,59,60,63,64,66-69,83] Normal studies are useful in ruling

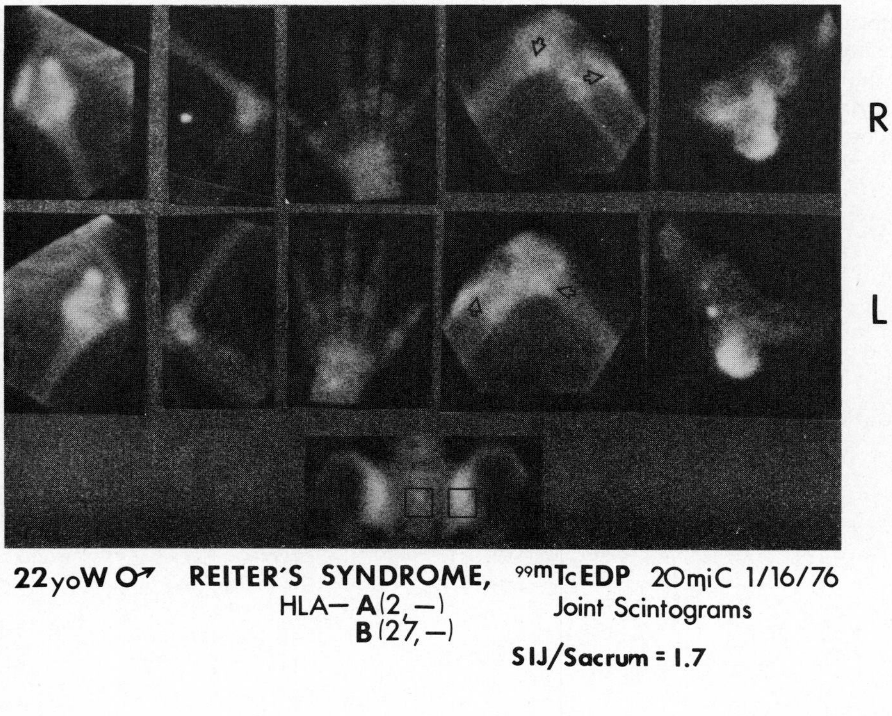


**Figure 40–3.** Reiter's syndrome. This joint scan is virtually diagnostic for Reiter's syndrome. Readily apparent is the periostitis of the os calcanei, or "lover's heels." In addition the patient has plantar fasciitis on the right, synovitis of the right ankle, sacroiliitis, and abnormally increased uptake at the knees and shoulders. The patient's initial complaint was right ankle pain following an episode of "presumed" gonococcal urethritis. Within two weeks, both heels and sacroiliac joints were symptomatic.

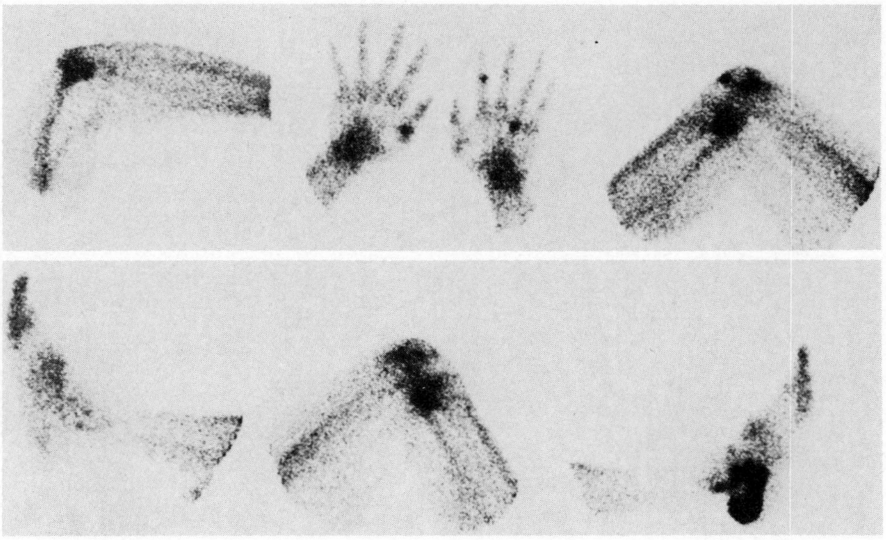

**Figure 40–4.** Technetium joint scan of a young male with acute reactive arthritis. Note the presence of tibial-fibular disease, which is occasionally seen in "enthesopathic" arthritis. This site of his knee pain was clinically "missed" by three different rheumatologists who examined the patient prior to imaging. Intense unilateral plantar fasciitis and asymmetric interphalangeal disease of the hands is also seen. QSS demonstrated unilateral (left) sacroiliitis (not shown).

out inflammatory arthropathy, as in the case of fibromyositis. The patient avoids multiple and expensive radiographs in preradiographic "early disease."

It is mandatory that joint imaging, when used, follow a specific protocol.[55] While it is true that no diagnosis is established by imaging one joint, the specificity for diagnosis comes from the composite pattern established by imaging multiple joints. Contralateral joints should be imaged for equal durations rather than by counts accumulated or activity. For some articulations, the subjective appreciation of inflammation is enhanced by a quantitative study, as is the case for the sacroiliac joints.[57,63,64,67]

**Rheumatoid Arthritis and Seronegative Spondyloarthropathies.** Scintimaging has been found to be a more sensitive indicator of disease activity compared with standard radiography, and the symmetric pattern of articular inflammation (particularly in the hands), which characterizes rheumatoid arthritis, can be distinguished from the rheumatoid variants, which tend toward asymmetry and greater axial involvement[68] (Fig. 40–5*A*, *B*, and *C*). Scintigraphic changes are, however, less specific than the radiographs in distinguishing between rheumatoid and seronegative diseases. Documentation of articular disease by scintimaging often antedates both clinical and radiographic abnormalities. Late abnormalities demonstrated by standard radiographic studies are more specific than are radioisotopic studies; early disease is more sensitively investigated by radionuclide joint imaging. This conclusion was confirmed in a comparison of $^{99m}$Tc-EHDP imaging with both $^{99}TcO_4^-$ imaging and fine-detail radiographs in hand studies in patients with rheumatoid arthritis.[58] It was concluded that the pattern of normal hand activity was maximal activity in the wrist, relative diminution in activity from the first to fifth MCPs, and a progressive decrease of activity from the proximal to more distal joints in each digit[58] (Fig. 40–5).

Lateral bone images of the ankle and heel are particularly important when imaging the feet in patients suspected of having Reiter's syndrome or psoriatic arthritis. Periostitis of the os calcis, plantar fasciitis, and Achilles tendonitis can and should be readily distinguished, since they are not typical in rheumatoid arthritis[67,68,84,85] (Figs. 40–3, 40–4, and 40–6). Asymmetric uptake in the metatarsal and interphalangeal joints of the feet or isolated distal interphalangeal uptake is also more characteristic of the rheumatoid variants.[67,68,84,85] Of unknown significance is the finding that patients with severe psoriasis demonstrate diffuse juxta-articular increased activity with $^{99m}$Tc-phosphate imaging.[85-87] This finding has focused interest on abnormal juxta-articular connective tissue metabolism in psoriasis. Other peripheral features of the spondyloarthropathies suggest manifestations of "enthesitis" and include insertional tendonitis, patellar involvement, and asymmetric oligoarthritis.[61,67,68,84]

In spondyloarthropathies, increased uptake may be seen in the sacroiliac joints, the lumbar, thoracic, and cervical spine, and the sternoclavicular and costoclavicular joints.[61,63,64,67-69,88] Focal disciitis can be noted, if present.[61,64,69,88] Intense sacroiliitis can often be identified, particularly if asymmetric or unilateral, without resorting to quantitative studies.[61,67-69,89] However, even though sacroiliac joint involvement may be noted visually, there is a great deal of observer error, since normal sacroiliac joints demonstrate a higher physiologic uptake than either adjacent iliac or sacral bone. Technical factors in imaging that affect contrast further impair visual estimation (Fig. 40–7), leading to attempts to quantify the uptake in the sacroiliac joints to aid in the documentation of inflammatory sacroiliitis.

***Quantitative Sacroiliac Joint Imaging.*** Techniques have been developed that interface a computer with the gamma camera to both document and quantify the presence of inflammatory sacroiliitis. The uptake of bone-seeking radiotracer at the sacroiliac joints is compared

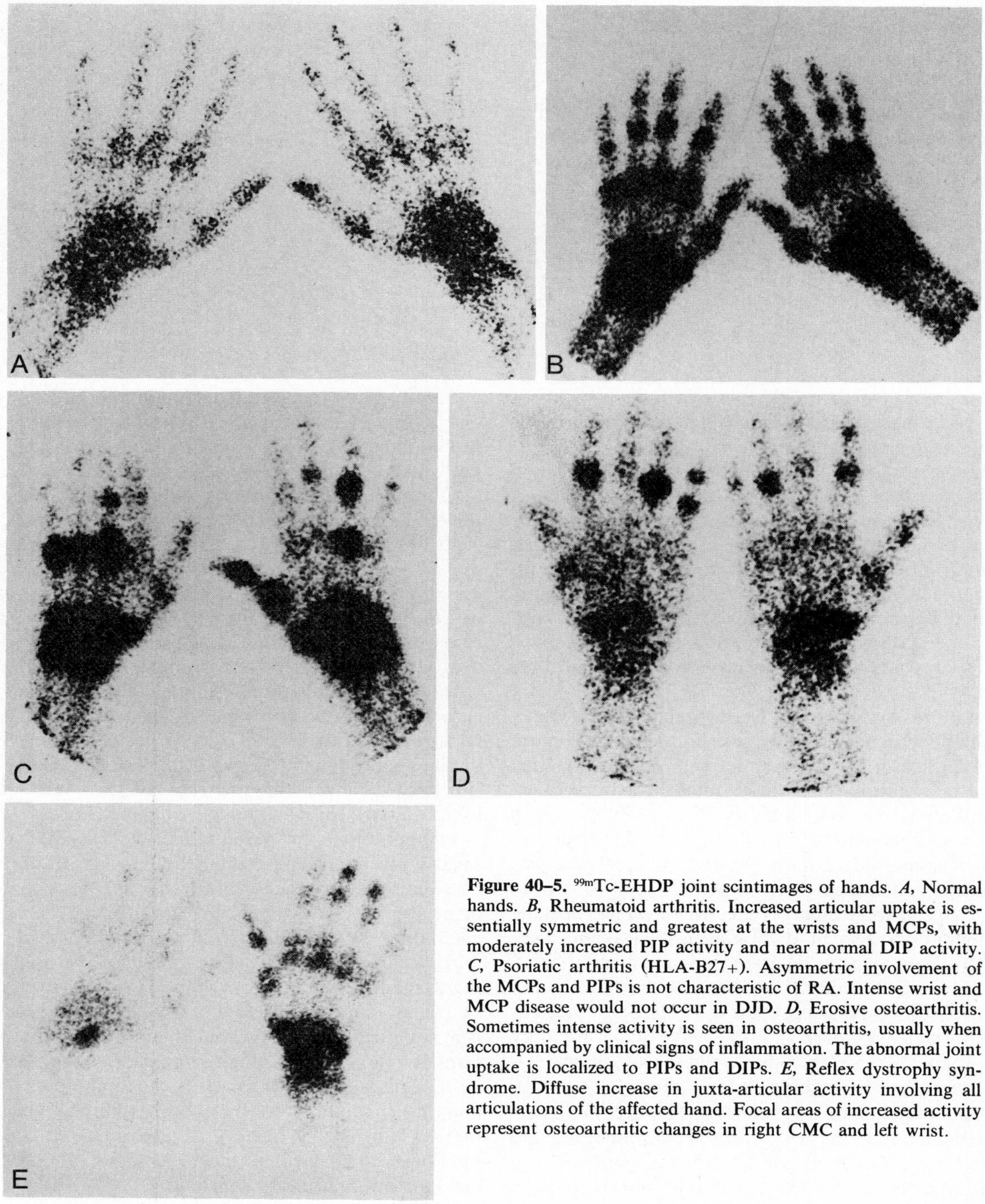


**Figure 40–5.** $^{99m}Tc$-EHDP joint scintimages of hands. *A*, Normal hands. *B*, Rheumatoid arthritis. Increased articular uptake is essentially symmetric and greatest at the wrists and MCPs, with moderately increased PIP activity and near normal DIP activity. *C*, Psoriatic arthritis (HLA-B27+). Asymmetric involvement of the MCPs and PIPs is not characteristic of RA. Intense wrist and MCP disease would not occur in DJD. *D*, Erosive osteoarthritis. Sometimes intense activity is seen in osteoarthritis, usually when accompanied by clinical signs of inflammation. The abnormal joint uptake is localized to PIPs and DIPs. *E*, Reflex dystrophy syndrome. Diffuse increase in juxta-articular activity involving all articulations of the affected hand. Focal areas of increased activity represent osteoarthritic changes in right CMC and left wrist.

Figure 40–6. Acute right Achilles tendinitis (black arrowhead). Some uptake is also seen in the tendon itself (white arrow). Radiographs were normal.

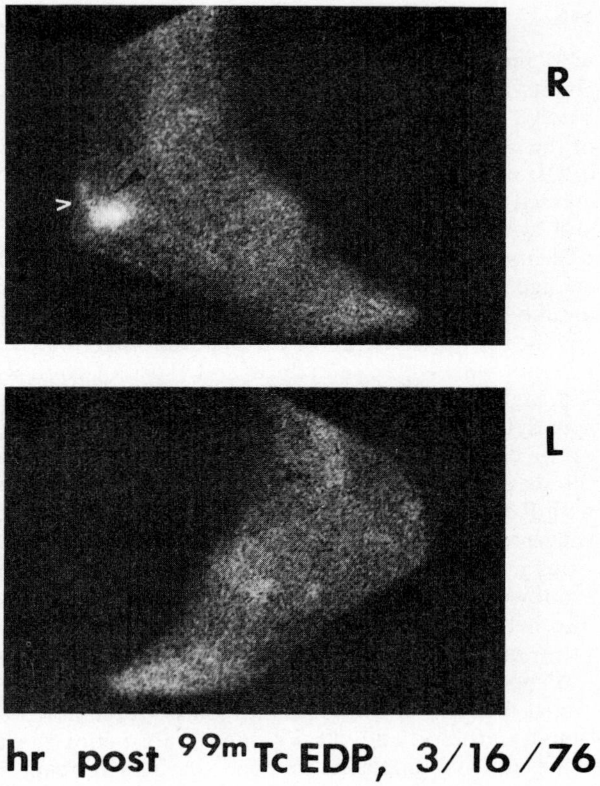


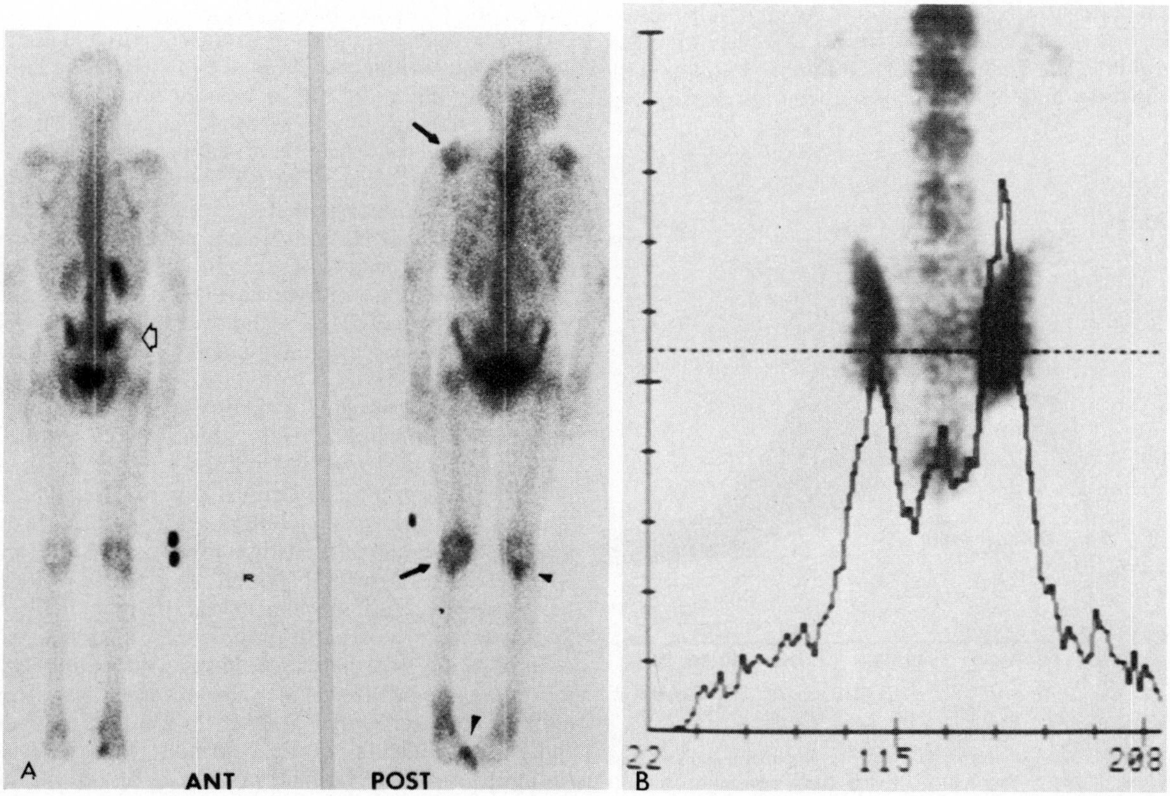


**Figure 40–7.** *A,* This 23-year-old male complained of right-sided low back pain, which he developed while working on an oil rig at sea. Because of "atypical" sciatica, a bone scan was performed and interpreted as normal. Closer inspection revealed relatively greater activity in the right sacroiliac joint, which was partially obscured by bladder activity (a technical mistake in bone imaging). Increased activity was also seen in the knees and right 1st MTP and DP of the foot. The patient underwent a myelogram, which was normal, but still had "exploratory" back surgery. *B,* Two months later, quantitative sacroiliac joint scintigraphy revealed definite, active, right-sided sacroiliitis. Patient was HLA-B27 positive.

with uptake at "normal" adjacent bone. The ratio of counts is expressed as an index. This procedure, quantitative sacroiliac scintigraphy (QSS), has become one of the more controversial areas of radioisotopic imaging in the diagnosis of rheumatic diseases. Historically, increased uptake of bone-seeking radiotracers, fluorine-18 and strontium-67, was seen in the sacroiliac joint of patients with sacroiliitis, often preceding radiographic change.[90-92] Early attempts to quantify sacroiliac joint uptake using the newer $^{99m}$Tc-phosphates demonstrated significant differences between the sacroiliac indices of patients with active sacroiliitis and those of controls.[93] The highest values appeared in patients with ankylosing spondylitis with early sacroiliitis (radiographic grade 1 or 2) compared with patients with advanced disease (grade 3 or 4)[93,94] (Fig. 40–8). In one study of patients with Reiter's syndrome, 24 of 33 had sacroiliitis by QSS, suggesting that sacroiliitis is more common than previously thought in acute Reiter's and is possibly overshadowed by peripheral disease in some and transient in others, since fewer would have been expected to develop radiographic disease.[89]

Proposed technical modifications for QSS are fractional analysis of the sacroiliac joints (three horizontal activity profiles) and "background" subtraction to eliminate activity unrelated to bone due to overlying soft tissue and incomplete vascular clearance[63] (Fig. 40–9).

In another study, employing background subtraction to calculate a single sacroiliac index, QSS was found to be of value in the diagnosis of sacroiliitis.[95] Patients with active disease had significantly higher indices than patients with a similar grade of radiographic sacroiliitis but with clinically inactive disease. Overlap between patients with back pain of a "mechanical" etiology and those with sacroiliitis was found, however.[95] A more recent study concluded that QSS was useful in the diagnosis of early sacroiliitis and suggested that multilevel analysis, background subtraction, and drug washout techniques improved reliability of the study.[96] Using similar techniques for QSS, a good discrimination between patients with early sacroiliitis and controls has been observed.[97]

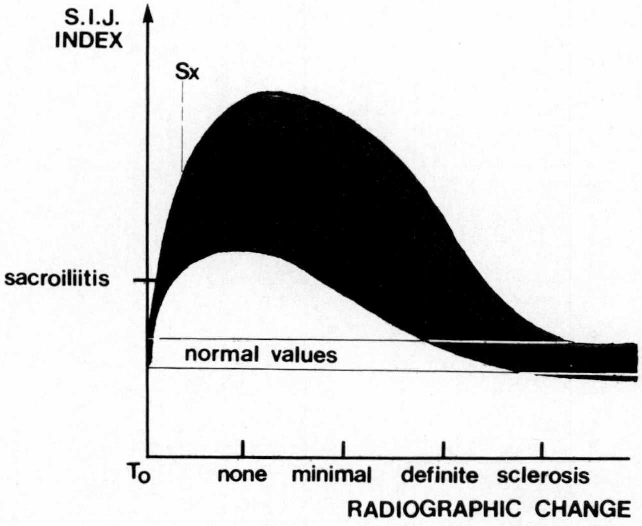


**Figure 40–8.** The relationships between sacroiliac joint indices by quantitative sacroiliac scintigraphy for *untreated* patients with various radiographic stages of sacroiliitis. In early *active* sacroiliitis, quantitative sacroiliac joint scintigraphy is more helpful than conventional x-rays. Once radiographic disease develops, the sacroiliac indices fall and become normal with complete sclerosis. Normal indices may be seen for any stage of disease, if inactive or successfully treated. (From Namey, T. et al.: Arthritis Rheum. 20:1058, 1977. Reprinted with permission.)

Other investigators, however, have reported results to the contrary.[98-103] Similar lack of correlation between increased sacroiliac joint uptake and the presence of radiographic disease or clinical disease has been reported.[98,99] Other investigators have reported some correlation of the sacroiliac index with QSS and the presence or absence of radiographic or clinical sacroiliitis, but they have noted poor specificity or too great an overlap with the broad range of normal values obtained for the quantitative sacroiliac study to be clinically useful.[100-102] Recently, a comparative study of the various techniques used for quantitative sacroiliac imaging was performed, with the conclusion that quantitative sacroiliac scintigraphy was useful as an objective tool for determination of sacroiliac joint inflammation, and that technical differences between the studies reported were the major reason for disparate results.[103]

Two long-term follow-up studies of patients identified as having sacroiliitis determined by QSS who had normal sacroiliac joint radiographs have been performed, concluding that QSS will identify patients with preradiographic sacroiliitis.[104,105] It is apparent, however, that not all patients with scintigraphic disease develop radiographic changes, and it is argued that clinical circumstances must be considered; an elevated sacroiliac index, while suggestive of sacroiliitis, is not specific.[104,105] Elevated sacroiliac indices have been demonstrated in sacroiliac ligament strain and metabolic bone disease and in those occasional patients with degenerative changes.[101,102]

Radiographic changes suggestive of "sacroiliitis" are not specific for inflammatory disease.[106] Likewise, inflammatory sacroiliitis is also known to occur in a number of inflammatory conditions not previously considered in the family of spondyloarthropathies; namely, gout, pseudogout, polymyalgia rheumatica, and familial Mediterranean fever.[106,107] Since "sacroiliitis" will eventually appear radiographically in many patients with paraplegia or hyperparathyroidism,[106] it seems reasonable to apply standards of specificity to quantitative sacroiliac scintigraphy when the accepted basis for diagnosis of "sacroiliitis" is itself fallible. It is probable that sacroiliitis is more common than previously thought, and this possibility is raised by the finding of "transient" sacroiliitis, present clinically and scintigraphically, in patients with Whipple's disease and acute sarcoid arthritis.[108,109] Both scintigraphic and radiographic sacroiliitis have recently been shown to be sequelae of both acute and chronic pelvic inflammatory

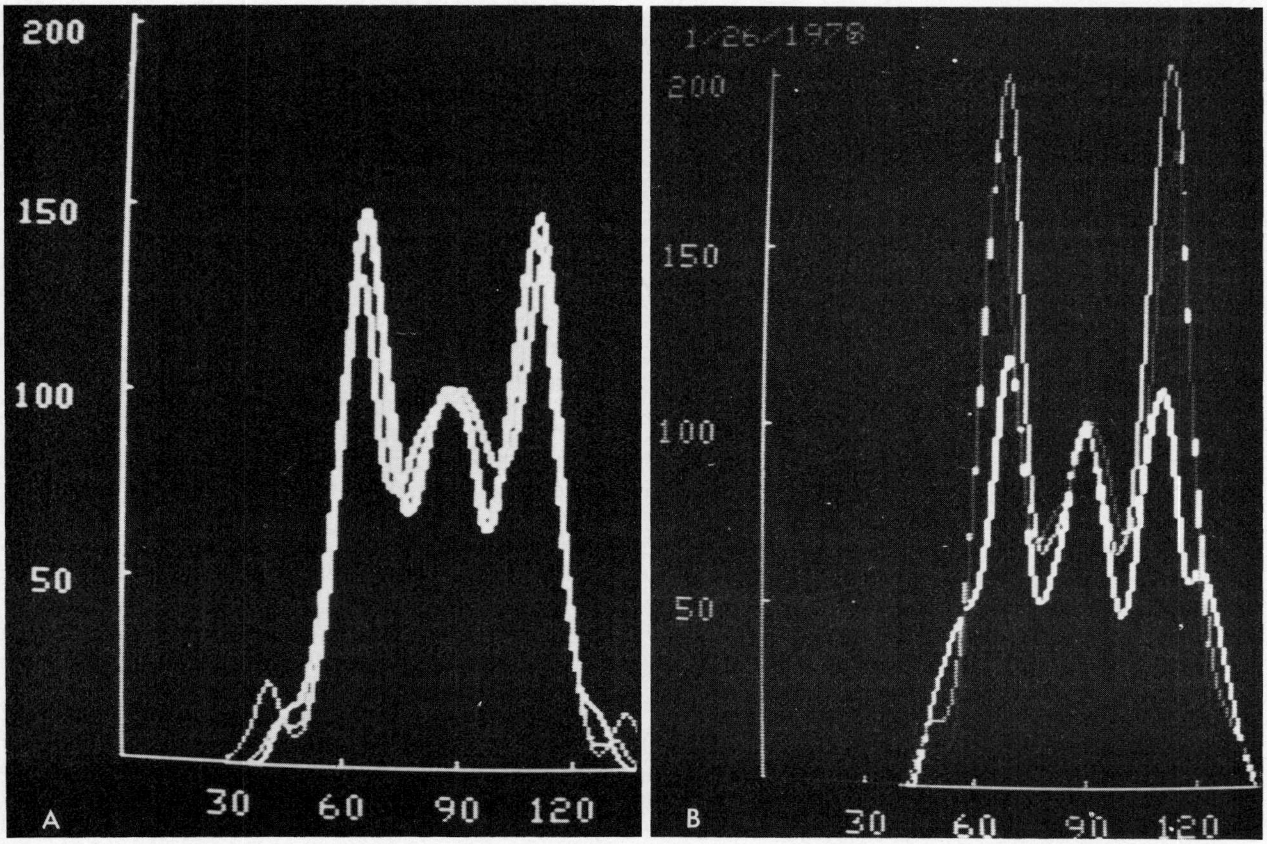


**Figure 40–9.** Composite profiles of three regions (upper, middle and lower thirds) of each sacroiliac joint generated by a computer macrofunction performing quantitative sacroiliac joint scintigraphy. The central sacral region for each profile is assigned a value of 100 for ease of visual interpretation of the sacroiliac peak to sacral peak ratio. By looking at the curves, the sacroiliac indices and asymmetry of activity can be assessed. *A* is a normal study. *B* represents the profile of a patient with ankylosing spondylitis of two years' duration. Activity is symmetric and greatest in the upper third of each sacroiliac joint.

disease.[110-112] Differences in the laterality of unilateral sacroiliitis demonstrated by QSS has been offered as support for the etiologic role of Batson's vertebral venous plexus in triggering inflammatory sacroiliitis.[112]

In summary, QSS appears to be an independently useful marker for sacroiliitis that is clinically active, if the procedure is methodologically sound. It is not specific for "inflammatory" sacroiliac disease and must be clinically evaluated with other findings in the overall assessment of the patient. QSS is most logically employed during the performance of peripheral joint scintigraphic studies rather than as an isolated procedure.

**Septic Arthritis.** The diagnosis of septic arthritis, in contrast to osteomyelitis, is usually made without resort to radionuclide imaging. This statement specifically excludes pyarthrosis of the hip, sacroiliac joint, and intervertebral discs, where the problems of clinical assessment and difficulty with arthrocentesis increase the importance of radioisotopic studies.[11] A number of recent clinical reports have suggested that $^{99m}$Tc-phosphate bone scintigraphy is an important indirect study in diagnosing septic sacroiliitis.[113-118] Also, several clinical situations generate a need to consider $^{99m}$Tc-phosphate or $^{67}$Ga scintigraphy: (1) the evaluation of arthritis in the patient with known osteomyelitis or endocarditis; (2) the patient with underlying rheumatic disease; (3) acute arthritis and coexistant hemoglobinopathy; (4) persistent joint pain and fever following joint prosthesis insertion[11,119-121]; and (5) cellulitis overlying the questionably inflamed joint.[122,123]

Both negative and positive studies are clinically relevant. Because most inflammatory arthropathies involve more than one articulation, the presence of monoarticular disease on the bone or joint scan should always include septic arthritis in the differential diagnosis.[11] The bone scan becomes positive between 24 and 48 hours after pyarthrosis develops.[11,120,121] It remains positive for weeks to months after therapy, depending on when therapy was initiated. Septic arthritis always increases activity on both sides of the joint(s) affected, particularly in juxtasynovial bone within the joint capsule, and this is a general rule for synovitis.[1,125] Bone scan positivity represents attempted osteogenesis of repair. The negative joint scan presents a strong argument against the diagnosis of pyarthroses, especially when there is no known underlying arthropathy.[11,124] Radiographic changes take 10 to 14 days to become manifest in septic arthritis, in contrast to the changes seen within 2 days on the bone or joint scan. They, too, may be ambiguous if coexistent arthropathy is present.[120-122]

Cellulitis without pyarthrosis will generate a positive "blood-pool" study with the bone-seeking tracer, while delayed "osseous" imaging reveals only normal or slightly increased bone activity.[11,117-121] Several groups have recommended inclusion of an immediate postinjection radionuclide angiogram with the "blood-pool" and osseous phases of bone imaging (the "three-phase" study), but rarely is this essential in ruling out pyarthrosis.[11] The blood-pool study is necessary, particularly when superficial edema or erythema suggestive of cellulitis is present. One important observation has been made regarding the significance of focal photon-lucency, or photopenia, on blood-pool imaging. The presence of joint effusion, particularly in the hip, may cause an area of nonactivity, a possible result of capsular pressure diminishing the venous blood-pool or the mass of the nonvascular effusion itself.[127,128] When identified, especially in the presence of increased periarticular uptake, it most likely signals the presence of effusion. The blood-pool study should be routinely requested when ordering a $^{99}$Tc$^{m}$-phosphate bone and joint scan for possible joint infection.

Sequential imaging with $^{67}$Ga should be considered when the $^{99m}$Tc-phosphate scan is difficult to interpret, as in the case of children, whose active epiphyseal growth centers normally demonstrate greater uptake than adjacent bone, or in patients with underlying inflammatory disease.[11,119-121,124] The benefit of dual studies with $^{99m}$Tc-phosphate/$^{67}$Ga in patients with rheumatoid arthritis and possible septic arthritis has been contested, however.[129] In the setting of a possible infected prosthesis, specifically in the hip, combined bone-gallium scanning does appear to enhance diagnostic accuracy.[130] $^{67}$Ga scintigraphy should always follow $^{99m}$Tc-phosphate imaging.[11,121,124] Early gallium scan positivity (increased activity seen on images obtained in the first 8 to 24 hours after administration of the $^{67}$Ga) is a feature of acute pyogenic inflammation. Late positivity with minimally increased joint uptake seen at 8 to 12 hours is more typical of chronic infection, such as fungal or tuberculous arthritis. The gallium scan may also demonstrate nonosseous involvement, which is not demonstrable by the bone scan or radiograph (Fig. 40–10).

**Osteomyelitis.** The results of most clinical reports establish the bone scan as a primary diagnostic tool in evaluating osteomyelitis in children and adults.[131-136] An abnormal bone scan is usually seen within 1 or 2 days after the initial spread of infection to bone (not including fungal or tuberculous disease), which is days to weeks before radiographic changes occur.[1,3,11,54,120,121] In one series of patients with osteomyelitis, 20 of 33 cases had radiographic abnormalities prior to bone imaging.[132] This underscores the fact that many patients present to the physician "late" in the disease course or elude diagnosis on first contact, a fact that reinforces the need to recognize the earliest radiographic changes. The sensitivity and specificity of radionuclide bone studies in diagnosing osteomyelitis approach or exceed 90 percent

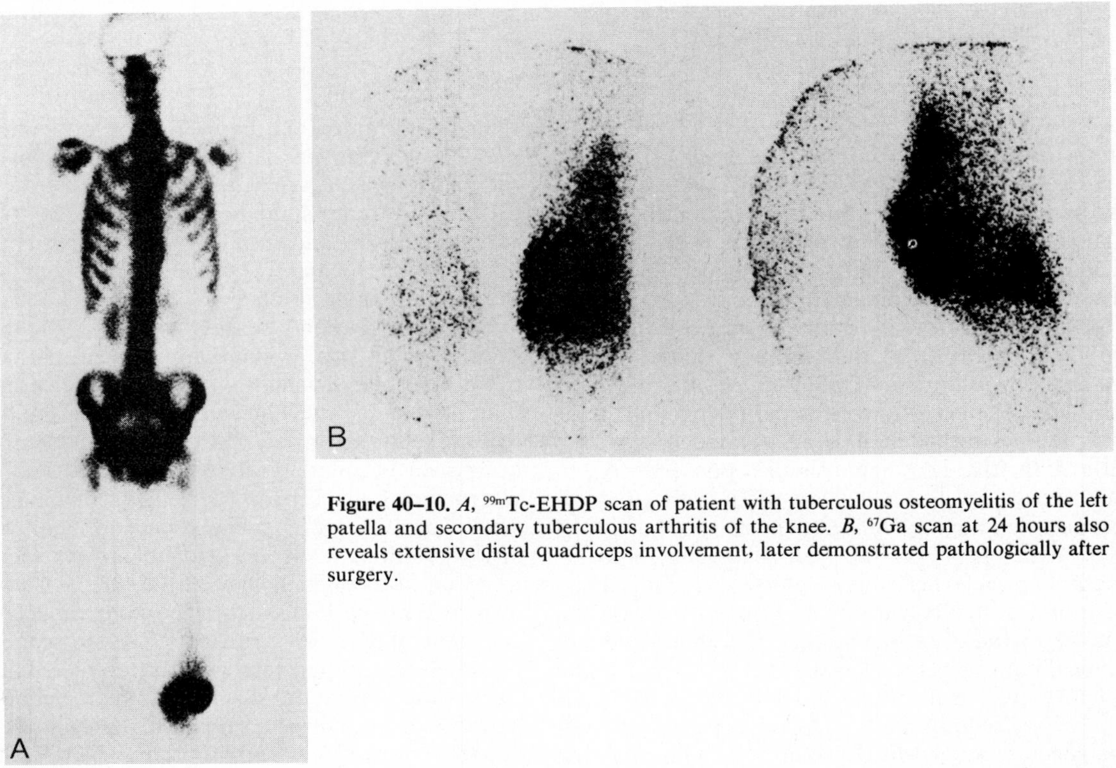

**Figure 40–10.** *A,* $^{99m}$Tc-EHDP scan of patient with tuberculous osteomyelitis of the left patella and secondary tuberculous arthritis of the knee. *B,* $^{67}$Ga scan at 24 hours also reveals extensive distal quadriceps involvement, later demonstrated pathologically after surgery.

in most series, if patients with sickle cell disease are excluded.[11,126,131,136] This is not true of neonates, in whom a much higher "false negativity" has been noted in "proven" osteomyelitis.[137-139]

The bone scan demonstrates an area of increased concentration of $^{99m}$Tc-phosphate at the site of osteomyelitis, with a diffuse, less intense perimeter of activity occurring in adjacent uninvolved bone secondary to hyperemia and increased metabolic activity (Fig. 40–11). This pattern may be absent acutely if septic embolization, medullary vessel thrombosis, or compression of the osseous microcirculation by subperiosteal or interosseous pus has occurred.[127,140-143] In these cases a transient central area of photon-lucency, or nonuptake, surrounded by an area of increased activity, may be seen. Exclusion of bone infarction is impossible at this stage.

In acute osteomyelitis, hyperemia increases distal bone and periarticular activity, which develop as a consequence of the central focus of acute osteomyelitis acting as a low resistance "shunt" augmenting distal blood flow.[11] This is a valuable clue in discriminating most acute forms of osteomyelitis from the subacute variant (Brodie's abscess) or chronic and/or granulomatous osteomyelitis (Fig. 40–12). Blood-pool imaging and immediate radionuclide angiography, in conjunction with the delayed osseous phase of bone imaging in suspected cases of osteomyelitis, do not increase the sensitivity of the scan in diagnosing osteomyelitis, but markedly decrease the rate of false-positive diagnosis and increase diagnostic accuracy.[126,144] Hence, specificity of diagnosis is augmented by radionuclide angiography and blood-pool studies in cases of suspect osteomyelitis, particularly in children with normally "hot" epiphyseal growth centers. Combination blood-pool studies are also particularly valuable in a patient with superficial ulcers or cellulitis and should precede static bone imaging.[144] Both radionuclide angiography and blood-pool imaging are important parts of the "complete" bone scan when osteomyelitis is considered as a possible diagnosis.

Sequential imaging with $^{67}$Ga citrate is helpful, particularly in children with possible hematogenous osteomyelitis, because of the proximity of metaphysis (the usual initial nidus of infection) to the epiphysis.[123,124] Gallium scanning may also better indicate disease activity if there is a question of recrudescence, since technetium bone scan positivity will lag behind relative clinical response, now reflecting osseous repair.[11,120,124] $^{67}$Ga scintigraphy has been shown to be valuable in detecting osteomyelitis following total joint replacement, when increased activity around the prosthesis on bone scan, normally present, may be impossible to differentiate from an infected prosthesis.[130]

**Bone Infarction and Avascular Necrosis.** Avascular necrosis of bone is a common complication of sickle cell anemia, fractures of the femoral neck, steroid therapy, pancreatitis, and numerous systemic entities (see Chapter 107). Radiography cannot detect the acute phase of avascular necrosis because of the equivalent densities of acutely devitalized and normal bone.[37,38,145,146] Hence, the changes that become radiographically manifest with time are those of subsequent repair, sclerosis, and damage to the articulating surfaces, if localized to subchondral bone.

Early attempts to detect avascular necrosis by scin-

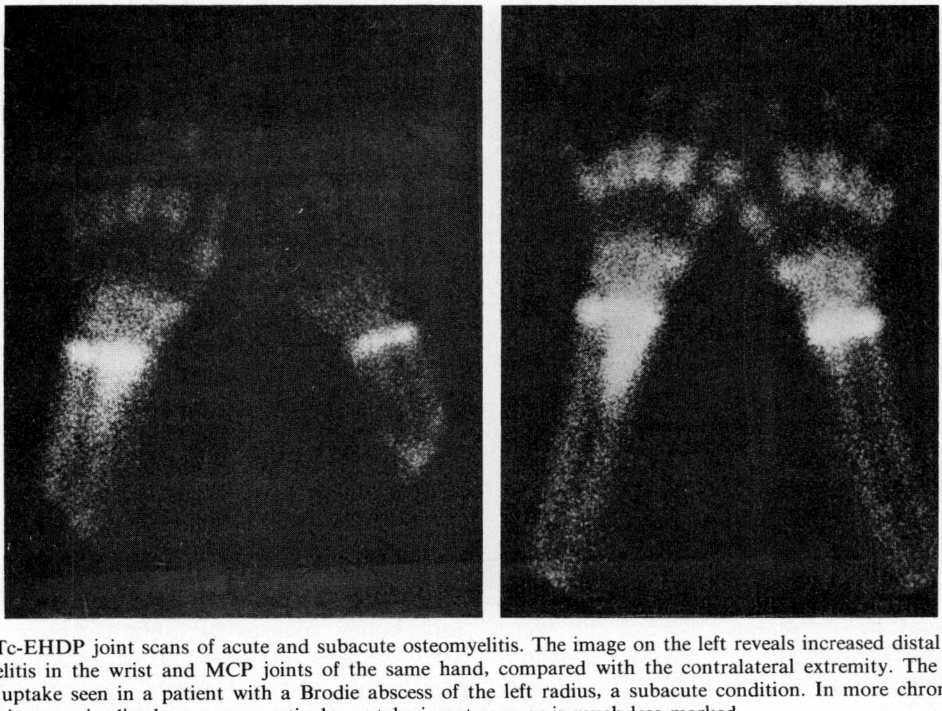

**Figure 40–11.** $^{99m}$Tc-EHDP joint scans of acute and subacute osteomyelitis. The image on the left reveals increased distal uptake beyond the focus of osteomyelitis in the wrist and MCP joints of the same hand, compared with the contralateral extremity. The study on the right demonstrates the uptake seen in a patient with a Brodie abscess of the left radius, a subacute condition. In more chronic osteomyelitis or joint infection, an increase in distal osseous or articular uptake is not seen or is much less marked.

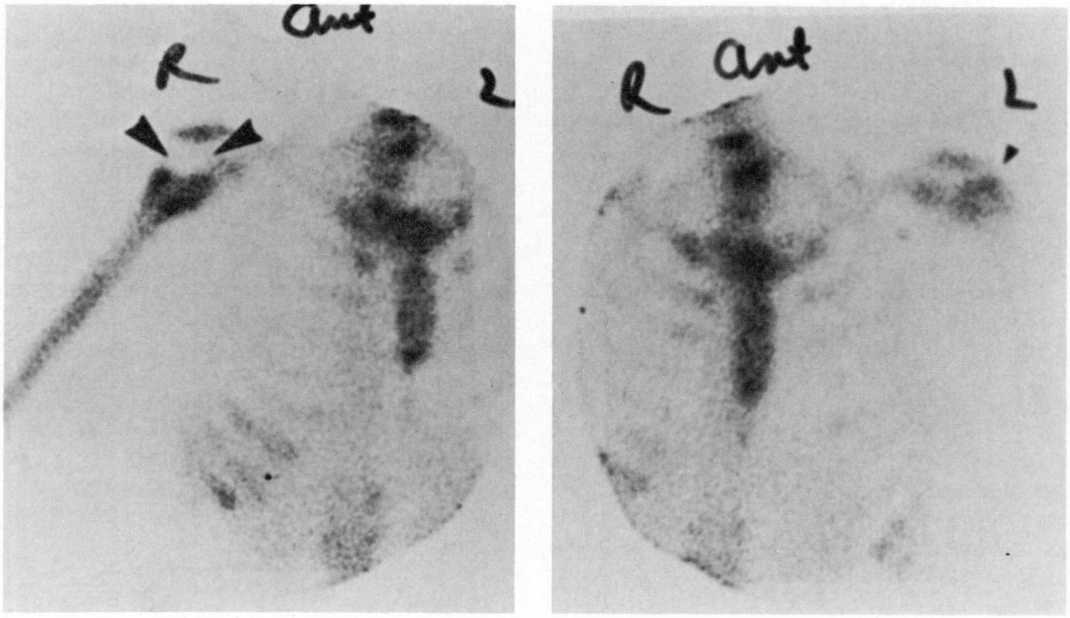


**Figure 40–12.** Acute ischemic necrosis of the right proximal humeral head seen in the bone scan of a 23-year-old female with acute sickle cell crisis. The entire area of infarction is seen as a region of nonuptake (large arrows) surrounded by an area of reactive, increased activity. The left shoulder is normal.

tigraphy were limited by the physical properties of the early bone-seeking tracers, $^{85}Sr$ and $^{18}F$. Both were ineffective in delineating the acute necrosis phase, and late uptake was nonspecific, requiring radiographic, arthrographic, or surgical confirmation of diagnosis.[145,147,148]

Once available, the clear superiority of the newer $^{99m}$Tc-phosphates in the diagnosis of avascular necrosis was readily demonstrated.[149-152] For the first time, the acute phase of injury, a region of nonuptake surrounded by an area of increased activity, could be routinely visualized, provided imaging was performed soon after the initial insult (Fig. 40–12). Once the reparative phase began, uptake nonspecifically increased without evidence for the once present avascular area, and differentiation of ischemic necrosis from inflammatory or severe degenerative arthritis would be impossible.

One recent study compared the $^{99m}$Tc-phosphate bone scan with radiograph sensitivity in detecting steroid-induced avascular necrosis of bone in 36 patients. The sensitivity of the scan was 89 versus 41 percent for radiography when compared with interosseous pressure measurements.[153] While the bone scan specificity was only 50 percent, the predictive value of the scan was 92 percent. In children, epiphyseal growth center activity often obscures bone scan evidence for avascular necrosis, unless high-resolution studies with a pinhole collimator are obtained.[152]

To effectively diagnose avascular necrosis in bone, marrow imaging with $^{99m}$Tc-sulfur colloid (SC) or antimony colloid may be necessary. $^{99m}$Tc-SC, the agent used for conventional liver/spleen imaging, is phagocytized by the reticuloendothelial cells of both liver-spleen (85 percent) and the bone marrow (15 percent). Because the large joints are anatomically far enough from the liver, imaging of bone is possible with the colloids, since some colloid is phagocytized by reticuloendothelial cells in bone marrow. Since both vascularity, necessary for delivery, and vital marrow, necessary for uptake, must be intact, $^{99m}$Tc-SC imaging demonstrates avascular necrosis with greater specificity, both in the acute phase (vascular flow interrupted) and the late phase (vital marrow has been replaced by fibrous marrow)[11,37,38,150] (Fig. 40–13).

Ischemic necroses of bone and marrow are frequent complications of many hemoglobinopathies and storage diseases, but they are by far most common in sickle cell disease. The differential diagnosis between infarction and infection is exceedingly difficult, and both may be present simultaneously. Roentgenographic evaluation is invariably negative in the early stages of both. Most episodes of infarction during sickle crisis are polycentric, which often aids in distinguishing between infarction and osteomyelitis. Scintigraphic bone imaging frequently reveals periostitis in the long bones, a known and common feature of bone infarction. Bone scan abnormalities also frequently suggest skull and vertebral involvement. In a study of 30 patients with sickle cell anemia by bone marrow imaging using $^{99}$Tc$^{m}$-SC, one half had evidence for previous bone infarction, i.e., photopenic areas representing regions of marrow fibrosis.[150] Because there is normally extreme marrow expansion in patients with sickle disease, previous infarction even in more distal long bones, such as the tibia or fibula, can usually be seen[150,152] (Fig. 40–14). This contrasts with the absence of active marrow at these sites in normals but emphasizes the reason for the inherent clinical advantage of $^{99m}$Tc-

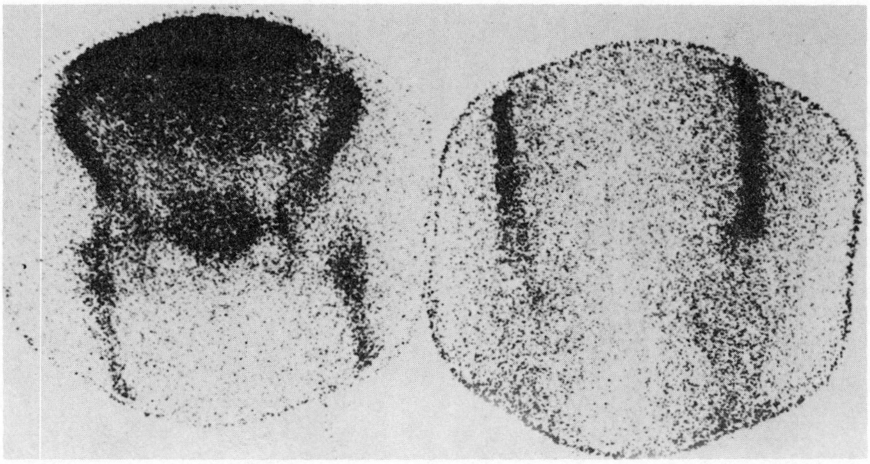

**Figure 40–13.** Avascular necrosis of the right femoral head documented by $^{99m}$Tc-SC scan. Note diminished uptake in the right femoral head compared with the left. Also note that in the normal individual, active marrow rarely extends below the knee. Compare with sickle cell patient in Figure 40–14.

SC imaging in sickle cell crisis. The bone scan will demonstrate a "mottled" pattern at these distal sites.[150]

Radiocolloid imaging for diagnosis of avascular necrosis is important in assessing viability of the femoral head after femoral neck fracture.[37,38] Colloid imaging has a 95 percent correlation with surgical findings in several reports.[37,38] The utility of sulfur colloid imaging is greatest in cases of unilateral avascular necrosis of the hip. This is because partial nonuptake in the femoral head is a normal finding in up to 40 percent of adults, but it is bilateral when present.[155,156] Unilateral nonuptake of $^{99m}$Tc-SC is generally significant and much more specific for the scintigraphic diagnosis of avascular necrosis.[155,156]

**Paget's Disease of Bone.** Radionuclide bone imaging with the $^{99m}$Tc-phosphates is the diagnostic procedure of choice in evaluating suspected or symptomatic Paget's disease.[157-167] The bone scan's sensitivity in detection and assessment of disease is superior to conventional radiography.[157-164,166,167] Scintigraphic changes will improve, but rarely revert to normal during or after treatment with mithramycin, calcitonin, or etidronate.[158,159,161,163,164,166-167] Bone scanning is more sensitive in detecting Paget's disease than measurement of serum alkaline phosphatase, which is frequently normal in mild or inactive disease.[158,160,165]

Paget's disease is most commonly polyostotic; multiple lesions are seen in 75 percent of patients[158-160] (Fig. 40–15). Diagnosis is rarely a problem in polyostotic disease, and differentiation between Paget's disease and osteomyelitis, tumor, or fracture is easily made. The difficulty lies in choosing between monostotic Paget's disease, when present, and metastatic disease in bone. Recent studies suggest that $^{67}$Ga scanning may be even more sensitive than bone scanning agents in diagnosing

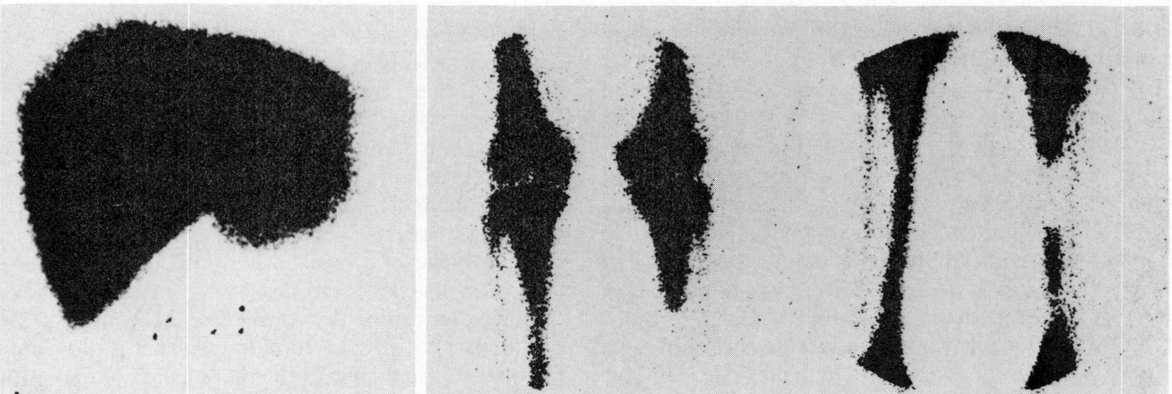


**Figure 40–14.** $^{99m}$Technetium sulfur colloid liver/spleen scan and bone marrow scan in acute sickle cell crisis. *A*, Liver is slightly enlarged, but spleen is not visualized due to acute "functional asplenia," often noted in sickle crisis. *B*, The marrow scan is typical of the patient with active compensatory erythropoiesis, with extreme proximal marrow extension through both tibias. The patient had severe left tibial pain, shown to represent acute bone infarction of the left tibia. Note central absence of marrow uptake of the $^{99m}$Tc-SC.

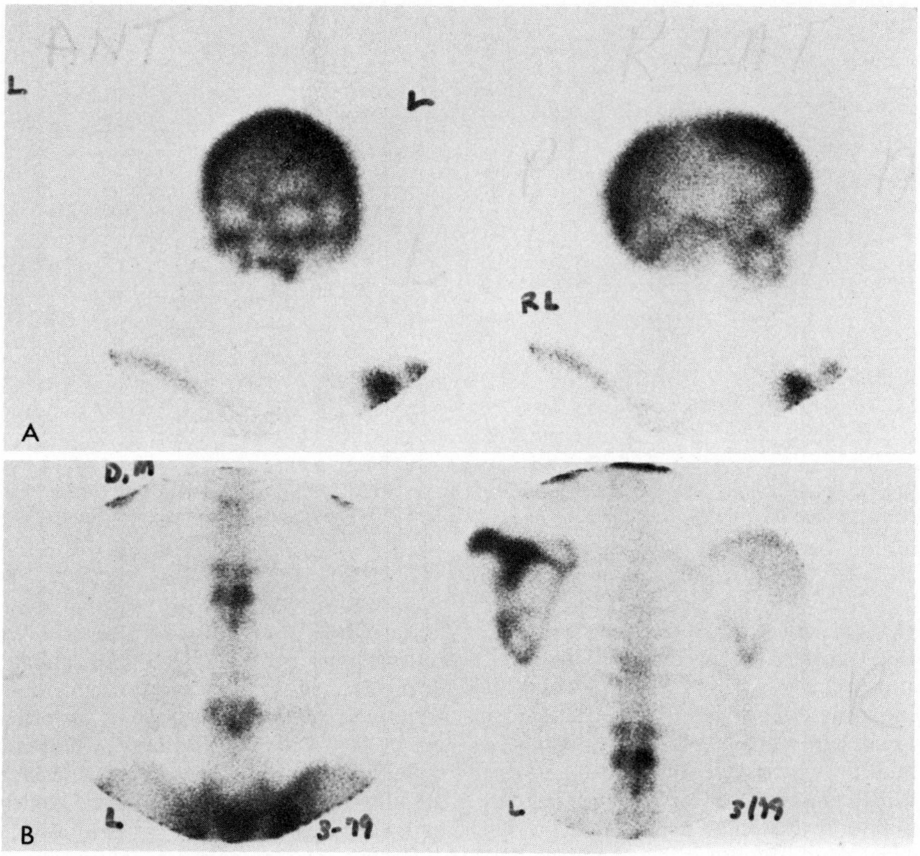


**Figure 40–15.** Paget's disease of bone. *A*, $^{99m}$Tc-EHDP scintimages of cranial involvement typical of some patients with Paget's disease; few other entities will demonstrate such widespread cranial increased activity. *B* illustrates the polycentric nature of Paget's disease. Left scapular, "skip" vertebral, sacral, and left scapular disease are present by the abnormal uptake. Such patterns are virtually diagnostic of Paget's disease.

Paget's disease and evaluating therapy, but considerations of increased cost, patient inconvenience, and radiation dosimetry make routine use as yet impractical.[168]

**Hypertrophic Osteoarthropathy and Periostitis.** Hypertrophic osteoarthropathy is a osseous disease frequently associated with pulmonary, cardiac, or hepatic disorders, characterized by periosteal inflammation and reaction primarily of long bones, although all bones may be affected (Fig. 40–16) (see Chapter 103). The patient may be symptomatic with diffuse periosteal pain for months before radiologic periosteal thickening or elevation is seen.[169-173] In the early symptomatic phase, radionuclide bone scanning may suggest the diagnosis.[171,172] Findings include increased periosteal activity, which generates the "double stripe" sign at the ends of long bones (femur or humerus). Scintigraphic periostitis may also be found at the radius, ulna, tibia, and fibula. A patchy "skip" pattern to the periostitis is not uncommon. Increased patellar uptake is frequent. The terminal phalanges rarely demonstrate a significant increase in activity, even with marked "clubbing." Or importance to the scintigraphic diagnosis is the presence of "articular sparing," despite the reported infrequent synovitis. Resolution of scintigraphic abnormalities will accompany resection of an etiologic pulmonary tumor or surgical correction of a cardiac left-to-right shunt, despite the persistence of radiographic findings.[172] "Spot" periostitis is sometimes seen following bone trauma and, when seen in children, should raise the possibility of the battered child syndrome and support such a diagnosis.[152]

**Reflex Sympathetic Dystrophy.** Reflex sympathetic dystrophy (RSD) is often post-traumatic and is considered to be an abnormal, excessive sympathetic nervous system response affecting distal extremities. Pain, swelling, and vasomotor disturbances are present with an initial increase in vascular flow and subsequent trophic dermal changes, radiographic osteoporosis, and juxta-articular erosions.[174,175] Unfortunately, early disease is frequently misdiagnosed when visible changes are minimal or absent, or is confused with local articular disease or nerve entrapment syndromes. Although 80 percent of patients with RSD develop eventual radiographic abnormalities that suggest the diagnosis, bone scintigraphy combined with early vascular studies presents a method of early diagnosis with objective findings that mirror abnormal physiology at a time when radiographs are normal.[174-181]

Scan findings include increased distal osseous uptake

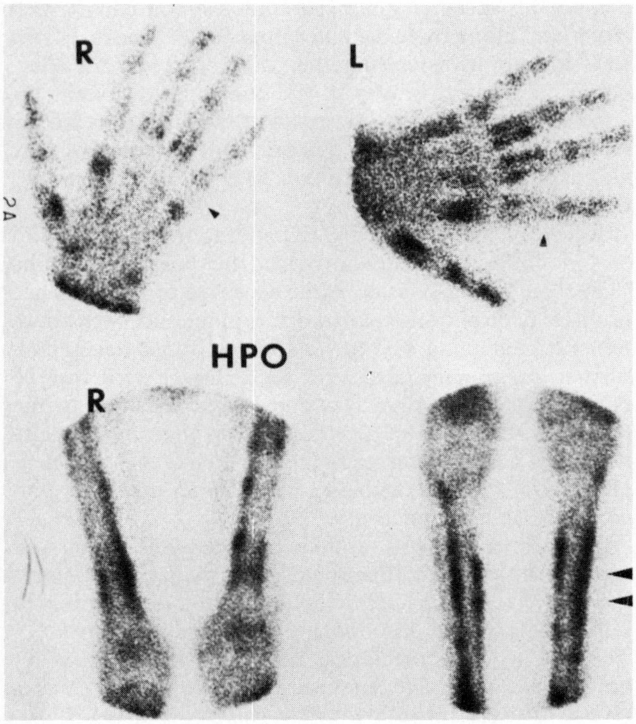


**Figure 40–16.** Increased periosteal activity on bone scan characteristic of hypertrophic osteoarthropathy. Activity is greatest in the long bones (large arrows) with occasional "skipping." Note that activity is *decreased* over articulations (small arrows). The periosteum of small bones is also involved. These scintigraphic findings will precede radiographic changes.

in the affected extremity with mild juxta-articular accentuation[126,175,178-180] (Fig. 40–5*E*). Bone activity is usually increased from the forearm or calf, extending distally, although increased activity may extend to the elbow or knee. When unilateral, these findings are relatively specific, although they have also been described in hemiplegia, following immobilization, or with diffuse cellulitis of the hand or foot.[181] The vascular flow studies demonstrate excessive arterial flow and the blood pool marked hyperemia on the affected side.[126,175,178-180] While RSD is clinically bilateral in one fourth of patients, scintigraphic studies have suggested a much higher frequency of bilaterality in clinically unilateral RSD. A few patients will develop changes of contralateral disease after bilaterality had been noted on the scan.[174,179,180] Carlson has verified the value of scanning for RSD of the lower limbs in patients whose disease followed a herniated lumbar disc.[177] It has also been seen in the lower extremities following sacroiliitis.[182] Abnormal scintigraphic changes revert with successful therapy and precede radiographic return to normalcy.[174,179,180]

**Orthopedic and Sports Medicine Applications.** Bone and joint scintigraphic examinations have been used by orthopedic surgeons to evaluate compartmental knee disease in planning arthrotomy and in interpreting pain after total hip or knee replacement.[183-185] In one study scintigraphy was compared with arthrography in confirming medial or lateral compartment degeneration and found to be as sensitive[183] (Fig. 40–17). The problem of possible loose prostheses is a major diagnostic dilemma in which $^{99m}$Tc-phosphate bone imaging appears clinically useful. When compared with standard radiographs in 20 patients with total hip replacement, scintigraphy and arthrography were of equal, but complementary value in identifying prosthetic loosening.[184] In another study evaluating 94 total hip prostheses, the bone scan was found to best differentiate loosening from infection.[186] Bone scintigraphy for loosening was used to study 35 patients with 39 total knee prostheses. The authors concluded that there were highly correlated findings on the bone scans that suggested loosening, and that while the scan could not serve as the sole method of evaluation, it was a useful adjunct to clinical criteria and conventional radiography.[187]

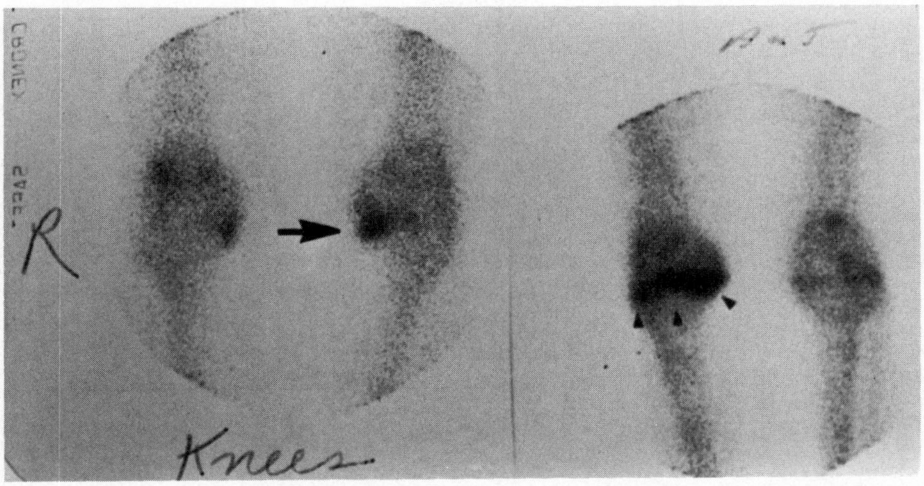


**Figure 40–17.** Medial compartment osteoarthritis of the left knee demonstrated by scintimaging with $^{99m}$Tc-EHDP in the left panel. The right panel reveals increased subchondral uptake increased across the entire tibial plateau, suggestive of severe osteoarthritis involving both medial and lateral compartments, much worse in the right knee.

Recently, nuclear arthrography using $^{99m}Tc$-sulfur colloid has been used to study prosthetic loosening.[188-190] Its theoretical advantages include the fact that any radioactivity at the bone–prosthesis interface will *always* be abnormal and indicates communication with the joint space.

Because of the extreme sensitivity of bone and joint scintigraphy, these studies have been used, with a great deal of clinical success, to evaluate the athlete with unexplained pain and normal radiographs. The conditions diagnosed or suggested by bone scan include "shin splints,"[191,192] stress fractures, including those of the sesamoids of the feet, femur and femoral neck, tarsal, and wrist;[193-198] traumatic periostitis of the heel and plantar fasciitis;[191,199] insertional tendinitis;[191] damage to the pars interarticularis;[200] severe trauma following car, cycle, or other collisions that result in possibly severe musculoskeletal injury.[201]

**$^{67}Ga$ and $^{99m}Tc$-pertechnetate Imaging in Sarcoidosis and Sjögren's Syndrome.** One of the first reports evaluating $^{67}Ga$ scanning included two patients with sarcoidosis, both of whom had positive scans.[9] One patient had marked perihilar uptake, and this has been subsequently demonstrated to be a significant finding in patients with sarcoidosis studied by $^{67}Ga$ imaging.[9,201,202] (Fig. 40–18). In another study, 9 of 27 patients had bilateral parotid uptake, a feature of sarcoid not typical for most other granulomatous or lymphomatous diseases.[203,204] Salivary uptake with $^{67}Ga$ is occasionally seen in Sjögren's syndrome but without coexistent hilar uptake.[205] Coupling the $^{67}Ga$ scan with the assay for angiontensin-converting enzyme (ACE) activity, Nosal and associates found that the combined studies increased the diagnostic specificity for sarcoidosis compared with either test alone by 98 versus 83 percent.[206] Because both tests are noninvasive, together they represent an alternative to surgical biopsy in the confirmation of the diagnosis of sarcoidosis. Increased uptake is also typically seen in the orbits, nasal mucosa, and smaller salivary glands, all of which are known sites of sarcoid activity (Fig. 40–18).

Recently, in one study of 12 patients with sarcoid and chronic hilar lymphadenopathy, the positivity of the $^{67}Ga$ scan or ACE-assay, while sensitive to the presence of disease, did not appear to discriminate between those patients remaining asymptomatic and those developing further pulmonary disease.[208] In a larger series of 54 patients, the $^{67}Ga$ scan was considered sensitive to the presence of disease (97 percent), but it did not correlate well with activity assessed clinically. However, the negative $^{67}Ga$ scan was considered to be an excellent predictor of clinical inactivity.[209]

The salivary gland uptake usually seen in sarcoid rarely progresses to functional abnormality demonstrable by $^{99m}Tc$-pertechnetate imaging but is common in both primary and secondary Sjögren's syndrome.[20-23,25] There is a good correlation between labial biopsy abnormalities and pertechnetate scanning, which is therefore held useful in following disease progression.[21-25]

## ARTHROGRAPHY

**Technical and Clinical Considerations.** Arthrography is the technique of radiographic visualization of intra-articular anatomy after arthrocentesis and instillation of

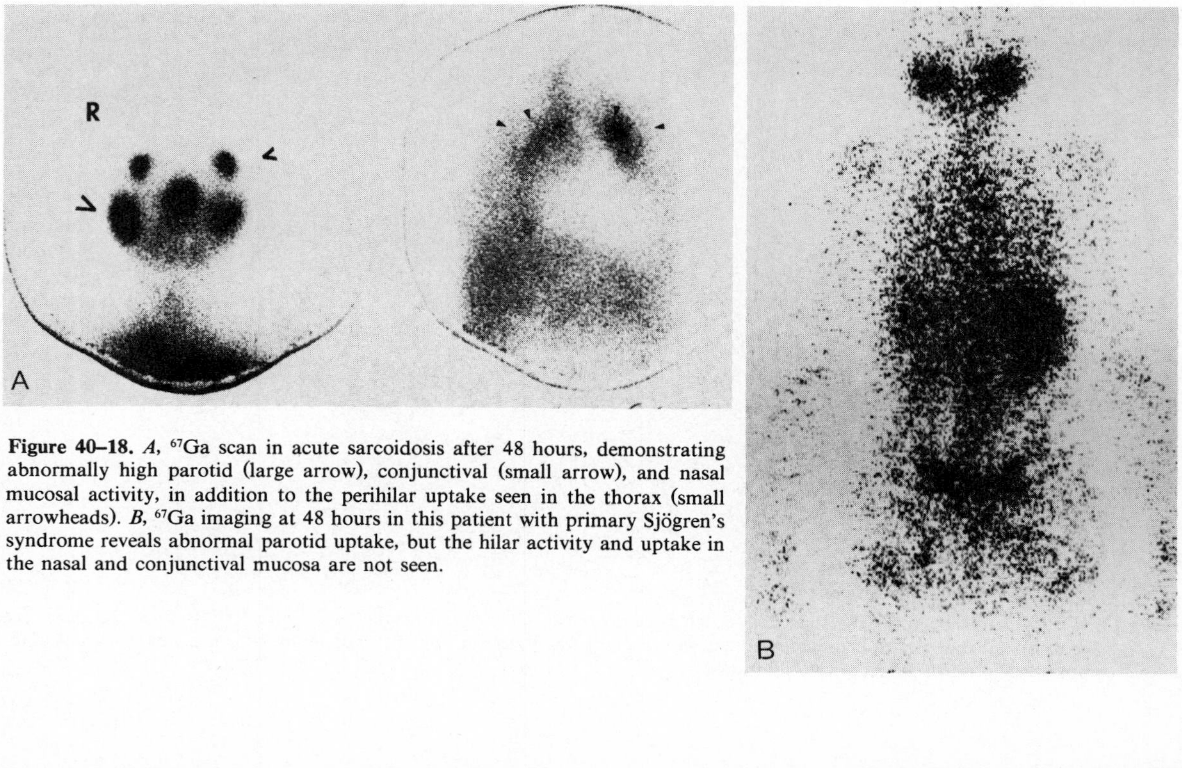


**Figure 40–18.** *A,* $^{67}Ga$ scan in acute sarcoidosis after 48 hours, demonstrating abnormally high parotid (large arrow), conjunctival (small arrow), and nasal mucosal activity, in addition to the perihilar uptake seen in the thorax (small arrowheads). *B,* $^{67}Ga$ imaging at 48 hours in this patient with primary Sjögren's syndrome reveals abnormal parotid uptake, but the hilar activity and uptake in the nasal and conjunctival mucosa are not seen.

a contrast agent, one of several radiopaque, iodinated, water-soluble compounds. The contrast medium may be used alone (single or positive contrast) or with injected air or $CO_2$ in a 1 to 5–10 ratio (double contrast). The amount injected is enough to mildly distend the joint capsule.[210-213] If joint effusion is present, the physician should send fluid for analysis prior to injection of contrast medium; if present in large amounts enough should be removed to prevent dilution of the contrast agent, particularly in double-contrast studies. Occasionally, air, $CO_2$, or other gas may be used above as a "contrast" agent if the patient is allergic to the iodinated contrast medium (negative contrast). The first arthrographic studies performed in Germany in 1905 used air for negative contrast.[214] Since then, extensive refinements have enhanced arthrographic studies: fluoroscopic guidance of the procedure and positioning; improved radiopaque media; stress devices for optimal opening of the joint space; spot filming of specific intra-articular structures; and finally the use of tomography or computed tomography in conjunction with standard imaging.[212,213,215-217]

Double-contrast studies are usually preferred because of superior detail and are most always indicated except for arthrography of the smaller joints, i.e., interphalangeal, or bursography, when the differences between the two methods are less significant. Although usually performed by a radiologist, simple studies may be performed by the rheumatologist or orthopedic surgeon in the outpatient setting if x-ray equipment is available and fluoroscopic guidance is unnecessary.[218]

Arthrography in adults (with the exception of certain hip arthrograms) does not require general anesthesia, although mild sedation may be of value, particularly in young children or infants. This contrasts with arthroscopy in which general or regional anesthesia is almost always required. The most common complication is increased articular pain in the first 24 hours after the completion of the study, which occurs in 25 percent of patients following knee arthrography and in up to 75 percent of patients undergoing shoulder study.[219,220] Mild synovitis secondary to the contrast agent is the most likely explanation rather than distention of the joint capsule.[212,213,218-222] The appearance of postprocedural pain is unrelated to sex, age of the patient, or arthrographic findings.[220] Double-contrast studies are usually better tolerated than positive-contrast arthrograms, but reaspiration of contrast agent (and air) after imaging does not lessen the likelihood of discomfort.[219] Reaspiration should be performed, nonetheless, in painful cases, in larger weight-bearing joints for psychic benefit, and to lessen mechanical discomfort. True allergic reactions to the contrast are uncommon. Pyogenic arthritis is rare, and the appearance of postprocedure pain is usually transient and benign and should not alarm either patient or clinician in the first 24 hours.[212,213,218-221]

Internal anatomic derangements are the single most common indication for arthrography. Usually the internal derangement is post-traumatic, but many arthrographically defined lesions develop as sequelae to underlying arthropathy, particularly in the shoulder and knee.[212,213,222] While virtually all articulations may be evaluated arthrographically, commonly studied joints include knee, shoulder, hip, ankle, wrist, elbow, and interphalangeal joints. Arthrographic technique is also frequently applied to juxta-articular structures, including bursa (bursography) and tendon sheaths.

**Arthrography of the Knee.** The most frequent indication for knee arthrography is confirmation of the presence or absence of clinically suspect meniscal injury[210-213] (Fig. 40–19). Medial meniscal tears predominate, since the medial meniscus is larger than the lateral meniscus and more vulnerable to trauma because of its firmer capsular attachment. Accuracy of arthrography in diagnosing medial meniscal lesions approaches 95 percent, when compared with findings at arthroscopy or surgery.[212,213] Lateral meniscal tears develop more frequently when knee stability is reduced by previous medial meniscal injury, ligamentous or capsular tears, adhesions, or osteoarthritis. Certain meniscal tears are common to specific settings. Vertical tears often follow acute trauma or athletic injury. Horizontal tears generally are seen in older individuals whose knees sustain continual stress, often occupational, without specific history of trauma. Osteonecrosis of the medial femoral condyle (most commonly developing in the sixth or seventh decade) was associated with medial meniscal tears in one report (21 of 27 patients), suggesting a causal relationship.[223]

Other indications for knee arthrography include the suspicion of loose bodies, abnormalities of articular cartilage, and ligamentous injury. Intra-articular loose bodies tend to migrate to synovial recesses or the intercondylar notch and are, hence, less accurately identified than meniscal lesions.[212,213] Cruciate ligamentous tears may be diagnosed, although the indications for arthrography in this instance are in question. Pathology of the posterior cruciate ligament poses more difficulty in delineation relative to the anterior.[224,225] Arthrography, although accurate in identifying anterior cruciate tear,

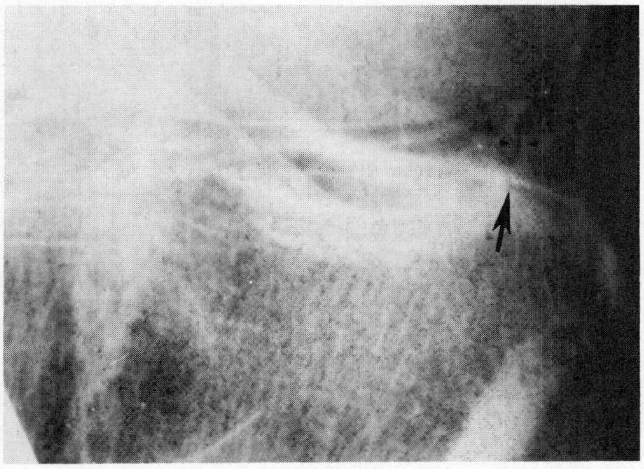

**Figure 40–19.** Medial meniscus "bucket handle" tear demonstrated by double-contrast arthrography. The tear is filled with air (arrows).

offers no diagnostic advantages over the simple "drawer" test.[226] Arthrographically demonstrable lesions of articular cartilage include osteochondritis dissecans, osteochondral fractures, and chondral fractures (which must be distinguished from each other), and chondromalacia patellae.[211-213,227,228]

Arthrography can usefully evaluate communicating cysts or bursae of the knee, particularly in patients with underlying inflammatory disease.[212,213,218,229,230] Fifty percent of all individuals have a posteromedial, synovia-lined bursa called the gastrocnemius-semimembranosus (G-S) bursa which communicates with the knee and is frequently bilateral. The G-S bursa may enlarge, causing pain with increased intra-articular pressure and chronic effusion (Fig. 40–20). The clinical term for the cyst in this clinical situation is Baker's cyst. While definition is possible with ultrasound or radioisotopic scanning, ultrasound cannot accurately delineate the ruptured cyst, nor identify internal derangement when it is etiologic. Arthrography is therefore preferred in the context of a Baker's cyst occurring with possible meniscal lesion, or if the possibility of rupture is a diagnostic consideration, or when surgical removal of a Baker's cyst is contemplated.[212,218,231]

Arthrography is useful in the preoperative evaluation of juxta- or intra-articular masses of the knee, particularly when combined with tomography. In cases of malignant or locally aggressive lesions for which amputation is *not* planned, preoperative arthrography can determine if synovial or capsular invasion is present.[228] In selected benign osseous and synovial lesions, including both intra- and extra-articular chondromatosis and pigmented villonodular synovitis, arthrography can be helpful in deciding whether an arthrotomy is needed, and if so, how extensive the surgical exploration should be.[228,232-234] Certain lesions, such as synovial plicae, are

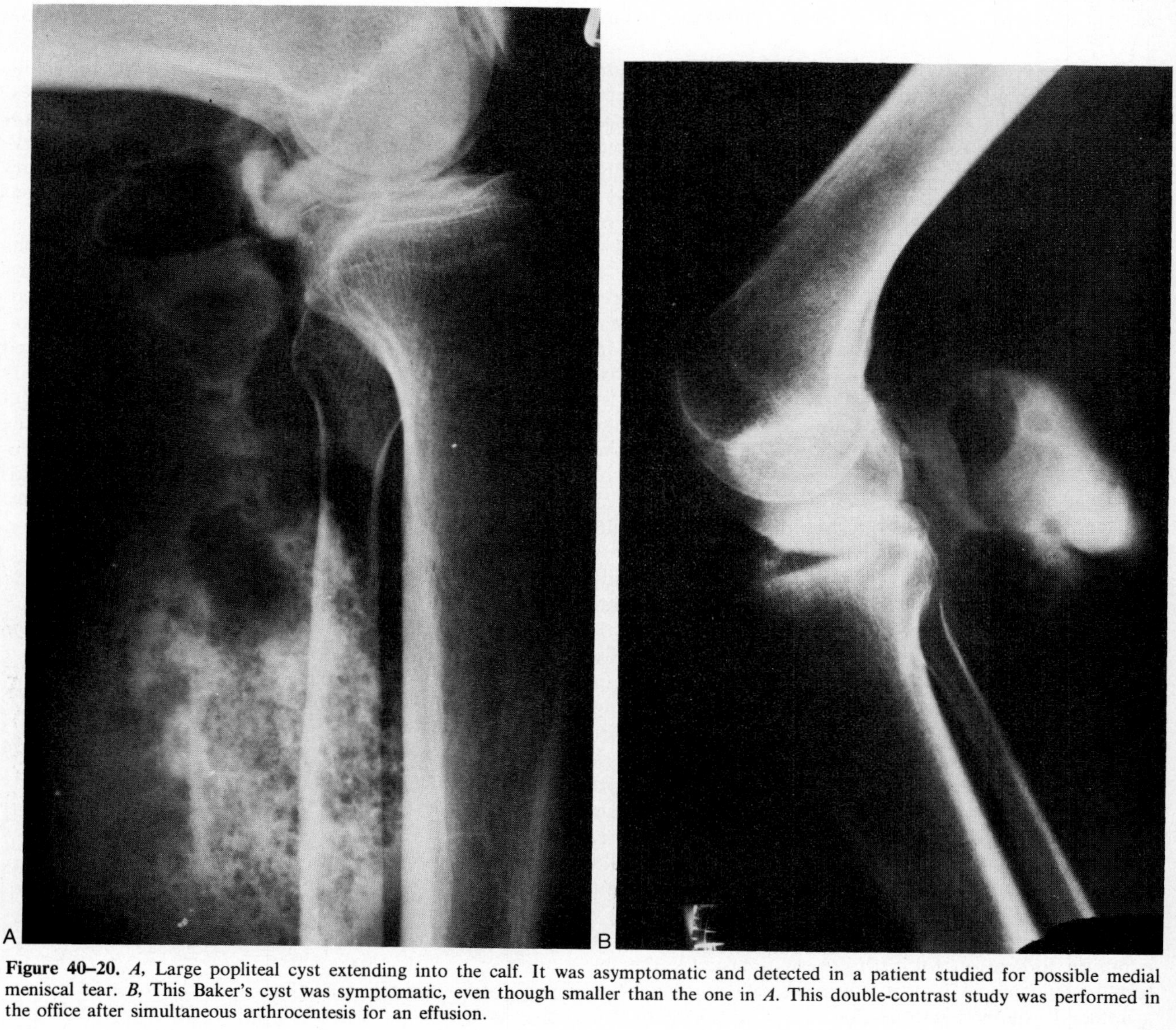


**Figure 40–20.** *A,* Large popliteal cyst extending into the calf. It was asymptomatic and detected in a patient studied for possible medial meniscal tear. *B,* This Baker's cyst was symptomatic, even though smaller than the one in *A.* This double-contrast study was performed in the office after simultaneous arthrocentesis for an effusion.

better dealt with by arthroscopy, since they are both diagnosed and treated with one procedure.[235]

**Arthrography of the Shoulder.** Arthrography to evaluate acute or chronic shoulder pain can demonstrate adhesive capsulitis, tears of the rotator cuff or joint capsule, lesions of the bicipital tendon, loose bodies, pigmented villonodular synovitis, and many other conditions.[212,222,236-238] It is also helpful in managing acute, recurrent, and chronic shoulder dislocation.[212,239,240] As with the knee, double-contrast studies are preferred for inherently greater anatomic detail (Fig. 40–21).

The rotator cuff is a musculotendinous aponeurosis of four muscles: the supraspinatus, infraspinatus, teres minor, and subscapularis. Damage occurs with acute or chronic dislocations or with chronic inflammation, as in patients with rheumatoid arthritis, calcific tendonitis, or pseudogout.[212,222,236,237] The usual presentation of rotator cuff tears is decreased range of motion with associated pain. The most common tear involves the supraspinatus tendon and separates the subacromial-subdeltoid bursa from the joint capsule. Diagnosis is made when contrast medium enters the subdeltoid bursa covering the greater tuberosity after instillation of the medium into the glenohumeral space[212,222,236,237] (Fig. 40–22). Tomography combined with double-contrast studies of the shoulder in rotator cuff tears has the ability to accurately demonstrate the size of the cuff tear and the thickness of remaining cuff tissue.[238] This information provides the surgeon with a better preoperative estimate of the difficulty of repair and prognosis for functional recovery.

Adhesive capsulitis (pericapsulitis), both a presentation or late complication of spondyloarthropathies, may also be post-traumatic or idiopathic. Exquisite pain, followed by progressively limited glenohumeral motion, with a concomitant decrease in external and internal rotation, is the characteristic clinical picture. During arthrography, much greater force than usual is required to instill both contrast medium and/or air, and the principal findings include a small capsular volume with (Fig. 40–23). Periarticular lymphatics are sometimes visualized because of the force required for injection.[218,222,236] Occasionally, the capsulitis appears treated as well as definitively diagnosed by the procedure, since large volumes of air and contrast medium can free capsular adhesions.[212,239] Since occult trauma to the rotator cuff is not uncommon, in instances of long-standing adhesive capsulitis arthrography may aid in the diagnosis of a coexistant rotator cuff tear.

The unstable, subluxing, or dislocating shoulder is probably better studied by arthrotomography, and in some instances by computed arthrotomography. Ten patients with unstable shoulders in which 3 had occult Hill-Sachs lesions were not successfully diagnosed by conventional studies.[240] Double-contrast arthrotomograms were also shown to be of value in lesions of the shoulder accompanied by known history of dislocation, since assessment of the integrity of the glenoid labrum has implications in the operative management of patients with shoulder trauma.[241] Subacromial bursography has been shown to be of value in differentiating "impinge-

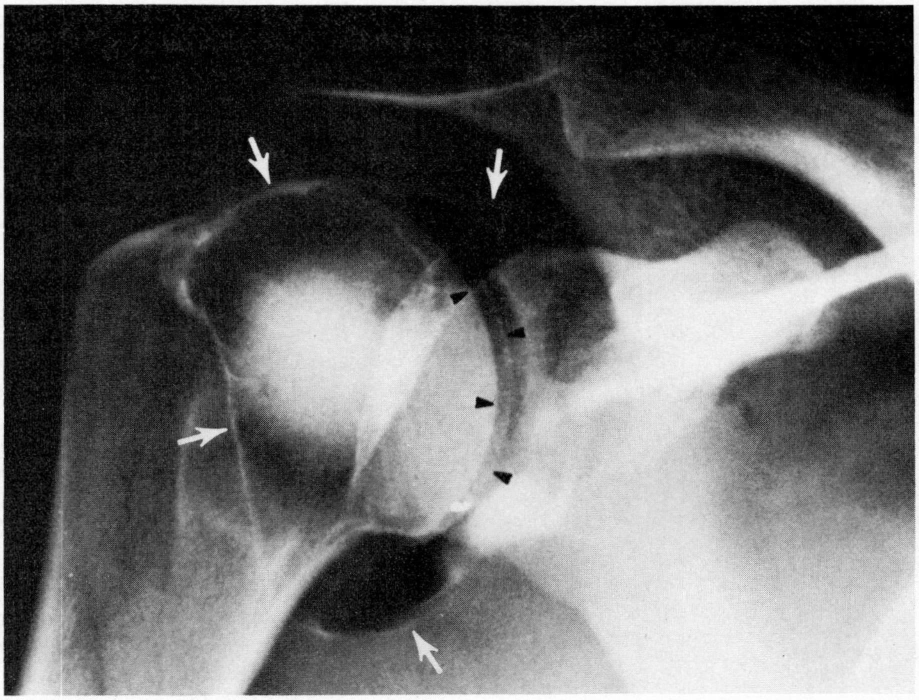

**Figure 40–21.** Normal double-contrast arthrogram of the shoulder. Positive contrast and air outline the joint capsule (white arrows) and humeral articular cartilage (black arrowheads). Note that *no* air is found adjacent to either acromion or the greater tuberosity. (Courtesy of William A. Murphy, M.D.)

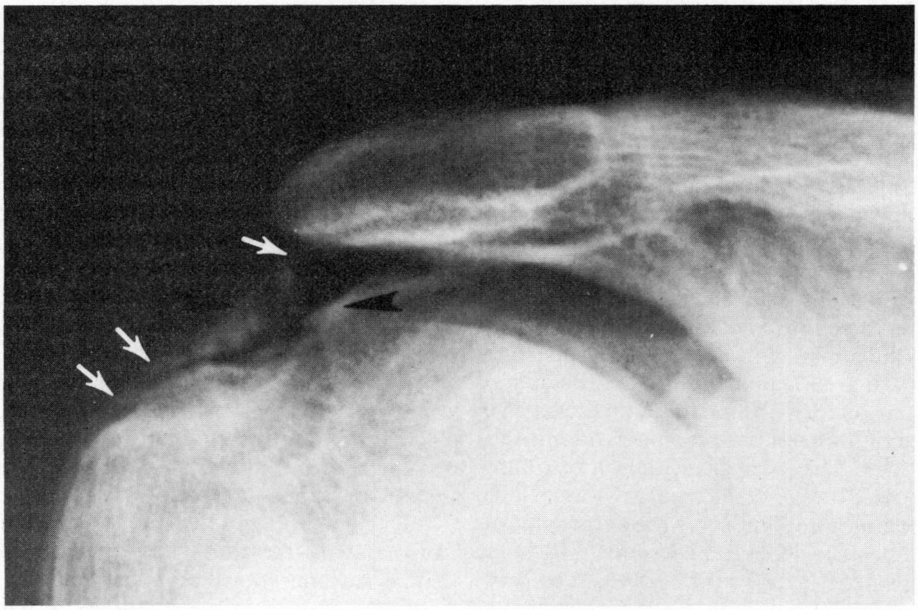

**Figure 40–22.** Rotator cuff tear. A double-contrast arthrogram demonstrates air in the subacromial and subdeltoid bursae (white arrows), which connects to the shoulder joint through the rotator cuff tear (black arrowheads). (Courtesy of William A. Murphy, M.D.)

ment syndrome" from subtle instability of the glenohumeral joint and/or rotator cuff disease. Strizak and associates suggested in their recent series that a normal bursogram literally rules out the diagnosis of chronic impingement syndrome.[243]

**Arthrography of the Hip.** Arthrography of the hip is technically much easier to perform than arthroscopy. Unexplained hip pain after total hip replacement with a differential diagnosis of loose hip prosthesis from hip infection and adhesive capsulitis represents a major indication in the adult.[212,221,243-245] Subtraction radiography is frequently necessary to differentiate contrast media surrounding the prosthesis, which has a similar radiopaque density. There is approximately a 20 to 50 percent error rate for arthrographic findings, compared with subsequent operative findings.[245,246] Errors are more likely to be false-positive for the acetabular component and false-negative for the femoral component in the diagnosis of loose prosthesis made on the basis of arthrography, although arthrography is more accurate than conventional radiography alone.[245] In one recent study, concomitant measuring of intracapsular pressure during arthrography was said to enhance the accuracy of the procedure.[246] A series has been reported of ten patients in whom intracapsular pressure recordings were made during arthrographic evaluation of loose hip prosthesis. A surprising finding was the evidence for postoperative adhesive capsulitis in five of the ten patients.[247] Hip arthrography has been used in infants to diagnose infection, congenital hip dislocation, and Legg-Calvé-Perthes disease.[212,221]

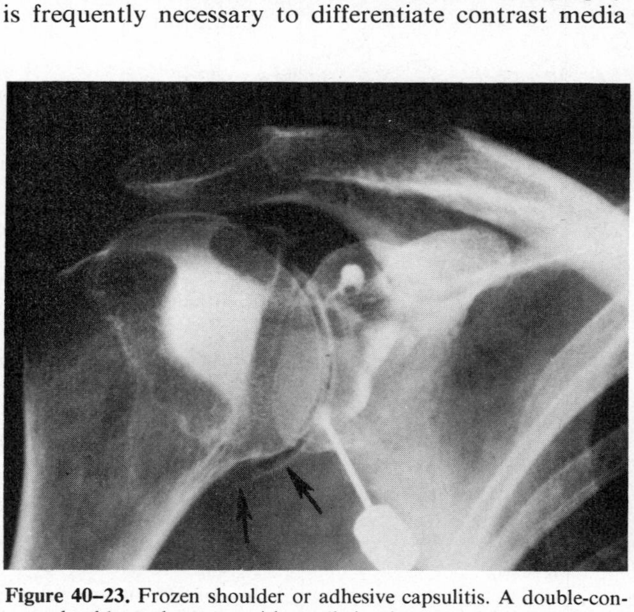

**Figure 40–23.** Frozen shoulder or adhesive capsulitis. A double-contrast shoulder arthrogram with needle in place reveals the small joint volume and obliteration of axial pouch recess.

**Arthrography of Other Articulations.** The ankle may be safely studied for diagnosis of ligament and capsular tears.[212,218,248-251] Since treatment modalities for various types of ankle sprains differ greatly, it is held by several authors that ankle arthrography is grossly underutilized by clinicians.[248-252] Elbow studies provide aid in diagnosis and management of ligamentous tears, loose bodies, chondromatosis, villonodular synovitis, and osteochondritis.[212,216] Arthrographic examination of the wrist is useful in planning the extent of surgical synovectomy or in evaluating the site of median nerve compression prior to surgical release or for patients with chronic posttraumatic pain.[212,218,253-256] Finger arthrography combined with magnification radiography was of use in defining the pathology of chronic finger pain in a series of fifteen patients. Both single and double-contrast studies were used.[257] Rheumatologists should also be aware of the use of arthrography in the diagnosis and management of patients with temporomandibular joint pain and dysfunction, which are characteristic of many inflammatory arthropathies.[258,259]

## ULTRASOUND

Ultrasonography, diagnostic imaging with high-frequency (1 to 5 megahertz) sound waves, represents a safe, noninvasive imaging technique for virtually all abdominal and pelvic organs, the heart (cardiac chambers, valves, and pericardium), and orbit of the eye. Applications have multiplied with the development of B-mode compound scanning and gray-scale imaging, which provide a two-dimensional echographic map based on the echoes arising from the boundaries of tissues with differential acoustic impedance, the product of the density of a substance multiplied by the speed of sound in the substance. The greater the difference in acoustic impedance, the larger the portion of sound reflected from the acoustic interface.[260,261] Bone presents a boundary with high reflectance (greater than 70 percent at the tissue–bone interface) too great for satisfactory echo imaging.[260,262] This has been the major drawback in musculoskeletal imaging. Collagen is responsible for the majority of internal echoes on gray-scale ultrasonography[262,263] and ultrasound has been described as a distribution and density map of the collagenous macrostructural support elements of human tissues.[264]

The general applications of ultrasound, mass delineation and determination of consistency, have proved valuable in delineating soft tissue lesions, such as tumors arising from the spine and bony pelvis.[260,265] The most specific musculoskeletal application has been the evaluation of the popliteal fossa and the noninvasive diagnosis of Baker's cyst.[266-271] Other uses particularly relevant to the rheumatologist include the echocardiographic diagnosis of pericardial disease and effusions in rheumatoid arthritis,[272-276] systemic lupus erythematosus,[277] scleroderma,[278] and other collagen vascular diseases;[279] the accurate detection of dilated bile ducts in the differentiation of medical versus surgical jaundice; and the diagnostic and therapeutic percutaneous biopsy or aspiration of viscera, masses, and cysts. The percutaneous localization of biopsy site by ultrasonography has been reported to be more accurate than corresponding radiographic or radioisotopic methods.[260] A preliminary report has suggested the sonographic diagnosis of preradiographic myositis ossificans.[280] No doubt many other uses will be proposed, but their specific role in disease management will be unclear until large prospective studies are completed.

**Ultrasonography of Baker's Cyst.** Although the presence of a popliteal mass should suggest the diagnosis of a Baker's cyst in a patient with rheumatoid arthritis or in an individual with a history of knee effusion, clinical definition is usually uncertain and it is difficult to distinguish such a cyst from hematoma, popliteal artery aneurysm, or lipoma[212,218,266-271,281] (Fig. 40–24). Problems arise when posterior calf pain, often accompanied by distal edema and dilated veins, makes the clinical distinction between acute thrombophlebitis impossible (i.e., the so-called pseudothrombophlebitis syndrome or PTS). Only 25 percent of patients in one series of 34 patients with the clinical entity of PTS had rupture or rupture concurrent with acute dissection.[282] While most patients with PTS could be sorted out by ultrasound and spared more invasive diagnostic procedures, two pitfalls become apparent. First, patients may have both thrombophlebitis *and* Baker's cyst.[283,284] Thus, caution must be entertained, even when a Baker's cyst is documented. Second, ultrasound studies will frequently miss cyst rupture.[212,218,266,269,282] If cyst rupture is considered, then arthrography may be indicated, particularly if surgery is entertained.

Reports on ultrasound studies of articulations other than the knee are lacking. While able to diagnose effusion, ultrasound is more expensive than needle aspi-

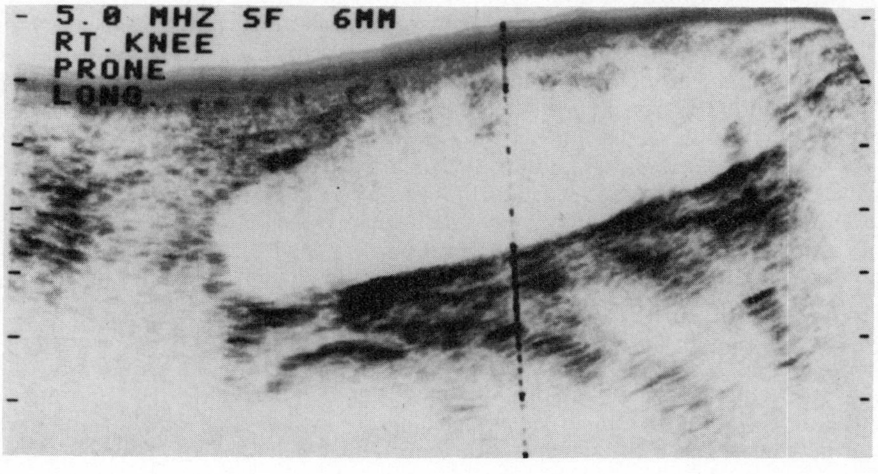


**Figure 40–24.** Ultrasound of Baker's cyst of the right knee.

ration and does not provide synovial fluid, which may be diagnostic. Although the latter procedure is *invasive*, in the hands of a skilled rheumatologist or orthopedic surgeon the procedure is rapid, simple, safe, and relatively painless. One study did combine ultrasound with arthrography successfully in evaluation of elbow, hip, and shoulder joints,[285] but it is unclear what was gained by the two procedures other than cost.

## THERMOGRAPHY

The development of modern thermography represents an interesting study in the application of technology. The existence of infrared emissions from the sun and other warm bodies was the observation of the royal astronomer to King George III of England, Sir William Herschel, in 1800. His son, John, took an interest in these studies and created the first primitive thermograph.[286] In 1880, Langley invented the bolometer, which was sensitive enough to detect a cow at 400 meters.[287] Hardy verified that human skin radiates infrared energy like the perfect "black body."[288] Interest in clinical applications waned until the use of thermography to detect night movements in World War II provided a technology for precise human measurements.

In 1949, Horvath and Hollander demonstrated the correlation between intra-articular temperature and clinical activity of the joint in patients with rheumatoid arthritis.[289] Skin temperature, lower than the tissue beneath it, is determined by the blood flow, the metabolic activity, and external temperature. This difference at the knee was shown by Hanson to be between 4 and 5 degrees Centigrade.[290] These facts form the basis for clinical assessment of inflammation by thermography.

Modern emission thermography utilizes equipment capable of 0.1°C temperature discrimination. This precision is available using modern electronic telethermography, which must be performed in a temperature-controlled room, whose technical features add to the cost of true quantitative thermography. Collins and associates have described a complicated "thermographic index" for normal joints, a basis for comparative thermographic assessment of inflammatory activity in joint disease,[291] but noted that there is a diurnal variation in the thermographic index. It has been used successfully in measuring the articular response to steroid injections, oral nonsteroidal drugs, penicillamine, and cytotoxic drugs.[292,293]

A second, less precise method of thermography more widely utilized employs a device for liquid crystal thermography (LCT). The "liquid" crystals are derivatives of cholesterol esters and polarize light in narrow wavebands. Phase transition with temperature is characterized by specific color-temperature response, allowing color thermography applications with color-temperature gradients of 0.2 to 0.4 degrees Centigrade in the most sensitive response zone.[294,295] Recently, these liquid crystals have been embedded in elastomeric sheets, which can be contoured to the torso, allowing for convenient application of thermographic studies at lower cost.[296] The area of study is restricted to the area covered by the liquid crystal sheeting and similar controlled temperature environs must be maintained for accuracy.

**Diagnosis of Low Back Pain.** One of the first clinical uses for thermography was in the evaluation of lumbar disc disease by Albert and associates in 1964,[297] and by several other groups who demonstrated abnormal infrared emission patterns in lumbar spine disease.[298-304] Because of a high frequency of thermographic abnormalities in lumbar disc disease, it has been argued that lumbar thermography might rationally precede myelography for evaluating patients with possible disc herniation.[299-301] The procedure has not gained widespread acceptance because of a high rate of false negatives,[301] although a claim has been entered for both higher accuracy (91 versus 86 percent) and fewer false negatives (1 versus 6 of 42 patients) for LCT compared with myelography in patients who had undergone subsequent surgery.[302,303] However, the precise surgical diagnosis was not given, nor was it correlated with clinical information or electromyographic findings in this study. In another report, thermography compared favorably with myelography in the diagnosis of disc herniation but was ineffective in diagnosis of spinal stenosis.[301] There is also a high false positive rate in diagnosing herniated disc in patients with spondylitis, many of whom present with symptoms of sciatica suggestive of disc disease.[305]

Unfortunately, the litigious nature of low back pain and the need for more accurate diagnosis has led to the publication of articles emphasizing the specificity of thermographic diagnosis in legal journals.[306] Diagnostic thermography has much potential in neurologic disease of the spine, and more critical studies are needed. Raskin has suggested that lumbar thermography also be used to screen for muscular and ligamentous injuries, since lumbar and paraspinal spasm is probably responsible for the abnormal heat pattern in noninflammatory lumbar disease, to add to the clinical impression with a perfectly noninvasive procedure.[301] Lumbar thermography has been applied to the diagnosis of metastatic spine disease and spondylitis.[307,308] Thermographic assessment of sacroiliitis in a study by Scott and associates suggested value only in serial follow-up of the individual patient rather than in comparison between patients.[309]

**Peripheral Disease.** Thermography has not been used for the diagnosis of peripheral arthritis, possibly because of the greater ease in clinically documenting peripheral synovitis versus axial inflammation. Nonetheless a consistent series of observations has verified the value of thermographic measurement of inflammation of peripheral joints.[291-293] Thermography has also been of value in quantifying the inflammation of adjuvant or carrageenan-induced arthritis in the rat, thereby providing a tool for drug study.[292] While skin temperature differs from the articular temperature by a near constant for each joint, early studies with radiometers suggested that skin temperature varies with blood flow measured by xenon clearance or plethysmography. Recent studies employing peripheral thermography suggest that this skin

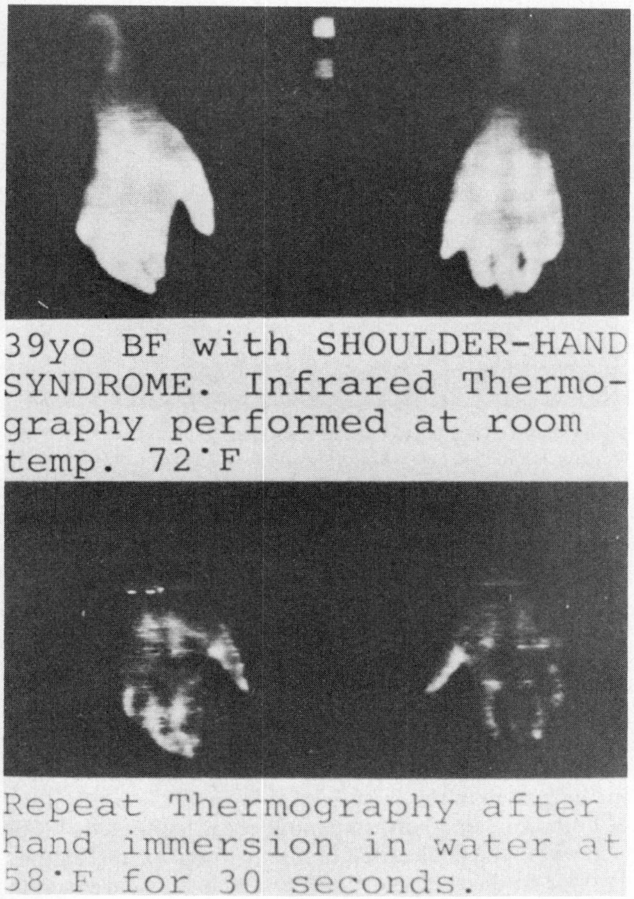
39yo BF with SHOULDER-HAND
SYNDROME. Infrared Thermography performed at room
temp. 72°F
Repeat Thermography after
hand immersion in water at
58°F for 30 seconds.

**Figure 40–25.** Abnormal distal hyperemia in reflex dystrophy contributing to the positive telethermogram. Diminished relative vasoconstriction was seen after immersion in cold water, indicating aberrant sympathetic outflow.

temperature variation renders the thermographic assessment of the small peripheral joints of the phalanges unsatisfactory, but the effect is inconsequential for quantifying inflammation of the knee, ankle, elbow, and wrists.[310] Thermography has been found useful in the evaluation of the reflex dystrophy syndrome (Fig. 40–25).

## COMPUTED TOMOGRAPHY

*Donald Resnick, M.D.*

In a little more than a decade since its introduction, computed tomography (CT) has already had a dramatic impact on the diagnosis of disease processes that affect virtually any organ system or tissue. In this brief time period, generations of CT scanners have appeared, each succeeding one striving for an increase in image resolution and a decrease in the time necessary for the examination.[311–314] Initially, CT scanners were found predominantly at a few large patient referral centers; subsequently, their numbers have increased at an incredible rate, and currently, they are found in even small and isolated hospitals as well as private medical offices.

The potential advantages of CT relative to conventional radiography are many, but foremost is an ability to display cross-sectional anatomy utilizing a series of images; these images, typically 2 to 13 mm in thickness, can be spaced at variable intervals, generally 2 to 10 mm apart. Specific x-ray attenuation values can be calculated for tissues within the slices and are expressed as CT numbers, usually on a scale of −1000 for air, 0 for water, and +1000 for dense bone.[311] The ability to differentiate among tissues with only subtle differences in radiodensity is, therefore, possible with CT and represents another significant advantage of this modality compared with routine radiography.

With regard to image format, a two-dimensional matrix of picture elements called pixels is displayed in a video monitor using, most commonly, shades of gray corresponding to the CT numbers. The range of such numbers can be adjusted by changing the window width and level in the monitor. Although cross-sectional image display is the classic format that is used, reconstruction of the image in a coronal or sagittal plane, or in any other plane, is possible.

The spatial resolution, a measure of image sharpness, is about 1.5 mm, slightly less than that for conventional radiography; the density resolution, a measure of the ability to differentiate subtle soft tissue densities, is about 0.5 percent greater than that for conventional radiography; and the radiation exposure for a series of images is in the acceptable range of 1 to 3 rads for the entire examination.[35]

In the last decade, the application of CT to the diagnosis of musculoskeletal disorders has been emphasized in hundreds of scientific articles. In general, CT is most valuable when utilized to evaluate regions such as the spine, pelvis, and hips, where anatomy is complex, and is less useful in the examination of the peripheral parts of the body. The following comments will serve as an overview of the more important clinical applications of this modality.

**Low Back Pain.** CT is quickly replacing myelography as the procedure of choice for the diagnosis of herniated intervertebral discs.[316,317] Methods of evaluation by CT vary with respect to slice interval and thickness as well as the utilization of either parallel cross-sectional images ("stacked coins") or images obtained along the axes of the intervertebral discs using angulation of the gantry. Furthermore, debate exists regarding the advantages of plain CT or that obtained following the introduction of intraspinal metrizamide,[318] and regarding the ability of reconstructed images in the sagittal or coronal plane to further increase the accuracy of CT in the diagnosis of discal herniation.[319] Although central herniation of the intervertebral disc is well evaluated with both myelography and CT, the latter modality is superior in the recognition of lateral lumbar disc herniation.[320]

With CT, a herniated disc appears as a soft tissue density located posterior to the normal intervertebral disc or vertebral body or both (Fig. 40–26). This density

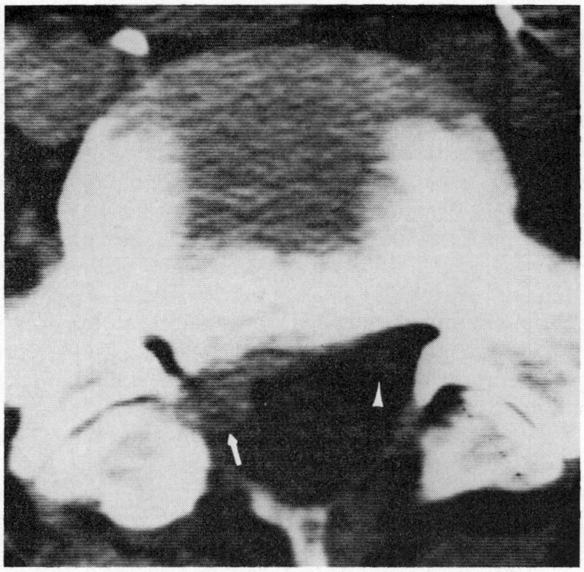

**Figure 40–26.** Herniation of an intervertebral disc. On this cross-sectional image at the level of the intervertebral disc, observe a soft tissue density protruding into the spinal canal (arrow), obliterating the adjacent nerve root. The root on the opposite site (arrowhead) is visible.

is generally easy to recognize, although differentiation from a bulging anulus fibrosus[319,321] and conjoined nerve roots[322] can present diagnostic difficulty.

The evaluation of spinal stenosis related to congenital or acquired disorders is well accomplished with CT.[323] The cross-sectional display of CT provides information regarding the anteroposterior and transverse diameters of the spinal canal, and measurements of the diameter can be compared with available normal values.[324] In this fashion, stenosis of the central canal, the lateral recesses, and the neural foramina can be detected.[325,326] Alterations of the apophyseal joints are also well shown.

High-resolution CT can be indispensable in the evaluation of patients with persistent or recurrent symptoms and signs following lumbar spine surgery.[327] In these individuals, routine radiography generally provides little diagnostic information. With CT, extradural fibrosis or hematoma, postlaminectomy pseudomeningocele, recurrent discal herniation, and postoperative bony stenosis can be accurately defined, although in some cases administration of intraspinal or intravenous contrast material may be required.[328]

**Sacroiliitis.** The precise role of CT in the diagnosis of sacroiliitis is not clear. Although some reports have indicated an increased sensitivity of this modality compared with conventional radiography in the detection of early or minor abnormalities of the sacroiliac articulation,[329,330] others disagree with this assessment.[331] Carefully performed investigations comparing CT and conventional tomography[332] in detecting sacroiliitis have not yet been provided. However, CT can be useful in delineating the extent of disease in patients with infective sacroiliitis (Fig. 40–27) and in evaluating those with ankylosing spondylitis who have the cauda equina syn-

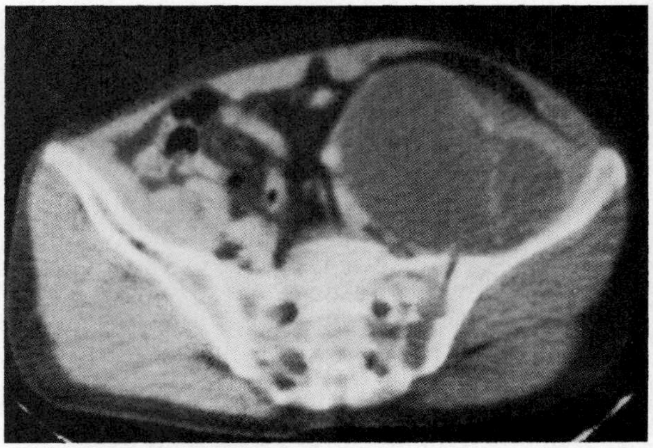

**Figure 40–27.** Tuberculosis of the sacroiliac joints. Observe the destruction of the left sacroiliac joint and a large cystic mass anterior to the articulation, representing soft tissue extension of the infection.

drome.[333,334] In these latter patients, multiple erosions of the posterior elements of the lumbar spine correlate with thecal diverticula demonstrated with myelography (Fig. 40–28). Furthermore, in individuals with ankylosing spondylitis, CT provides dramatic evidence of the degree of atrophy of posterior spinal muscles.[335]

**Trauma.** The value of CT in the assessment of the traumatized patient is not debated. This modality allows evaluation of such patients without the discomfort and the hazard required in their movement.[336] Identification of both bone and soft tissue injuries is facilitated.[337] CT is ideal for the delineation of injury to the axial skeleton. Trauma to the spine or spinal cord is one prime example of a situation in which evaluation by CT is advantageous. It allows identification of fractures of both the vertebral bodies and the posterior elements, of the extent of compromise to the adjacent spinal cord by displaced osseous fragments or hematoma formation, and of the degree of spinal instability.[323,338,339]

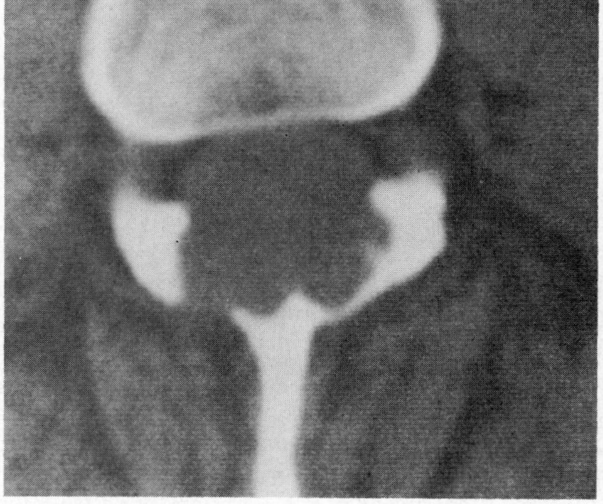

**Figure 40–28.** Ankylosing spondylitis and thecal diverticula. A CT image of a lumbar vertebra demonstrates scalloped erosions of the posterior elements, diagnostic of thecal diverticula.

Injuries to the hip or shoulder can also be well delineated with CT. In the former area, identification of complex fractures of the acetabulum and the proximal femur and of intra-articular bone fragments is possible.[340,341] In the shoulder, identification of similar fractures of the glenoid fossa and humerus is accomplished. In addition, compression fractures of the posterolateral surface of the humeral head (Hill-Sachs lesion) occurring in association with an anterior dislocation of the glenohumeral joint can be detected.[342] CT accomplished in conjunction with arthrography of this joint will allow diagnosis of subtle abnormalities of the glenoid labrum[343] (Fig. 40–29).

Further examples of injuries that are well defined by CT include fractures of the sacrum and sternum and dislocations of the sacroiliiac and sternoclavicular articulations (Fig. 40–30).

**Tumors and Infections.** Although in most cases CT does not significantly contribute to the histologic diagnosis of primary bone tumors (with the exception of simple cysts and lipomas), its cross-sectional display allows analysis of the degree of soft tissue extension and the compromise or violation of surrounding neurovascular structures.[344] This information can be vital to the surgeon in the management of the tumor and to the radiologist as an aid in the planning of percutaneous biopsy. CT can also be utilized as a diagnostic tool in the patient with suspected skeletal metastasis in whom plain films are unrewarding; although the spatial resolution of even the latest generation scanners is inferior to that of plain films, a cross-sectional image may occasionally delineate a lesion that was not evident with routine radiography. Furthermore, a potential exists for CT in differentiating benign and malignant pulmonary nodules in individuals who are suspected of having widespread metastatic disease.[345]

With regard to infections of bone, CT may reveal an increase in the density of the marrow (a phenomenon also evident with neoplasms) related to edema and vascular congestion at a time when plain films are negative,[346] although scintigraphy still appears to be the most sensitive modality in the early diagnosis of osteomyelitis. CT can also demonstrate bone abscesses or cortical sequestration[347] and the extent of soft tissue involvement, the latter being particularly helpful in cases of spinal infection.

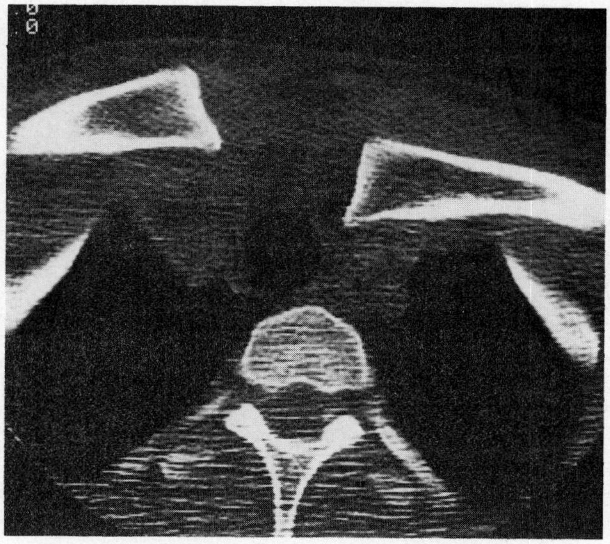

**Figure 40–30.** Posterior dislocation of the sternoclavicular joint. Note the posterior location of the medial end of the left clavicle and its intimate relationship with the adjacent trachea and vascular channels.

**Articular Diseases.** The role of CT in evaluating patients with articular disease is limited. This modality appears to have little or no advantage when compared with routine radiography or conventional tomography in delineating cartilaginous destruction or bony erosion with the exception of sites, such as the sternoclavicular, costovertebral, temporomandibular, and apophyseal articulations, that are difficult to visualize with usual imaging techniques.[348-350] Even in the latter locations, examination with CT frequently requires meticulous positioning of the patient and the utilization of re-for-

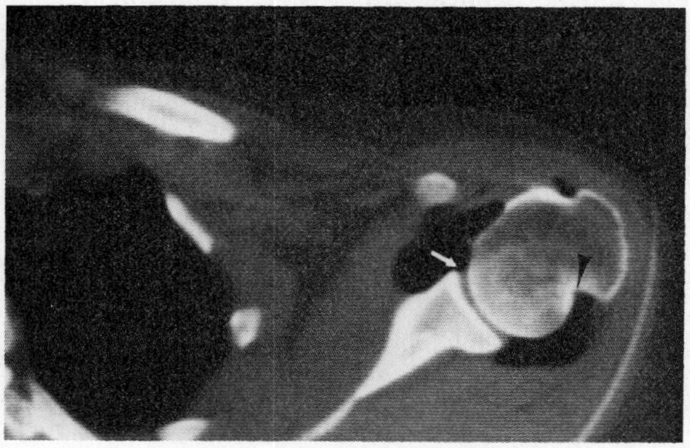

**Figure 40–29.** Abnormality of the glenoid labrum. A CT image following intra-articular administration of air reveals absence of the anterior portion of the glenoid labrum (arrow). A compression fracture of the humerus (arrowhead) is consistent with a Hill-Sachs lesion.

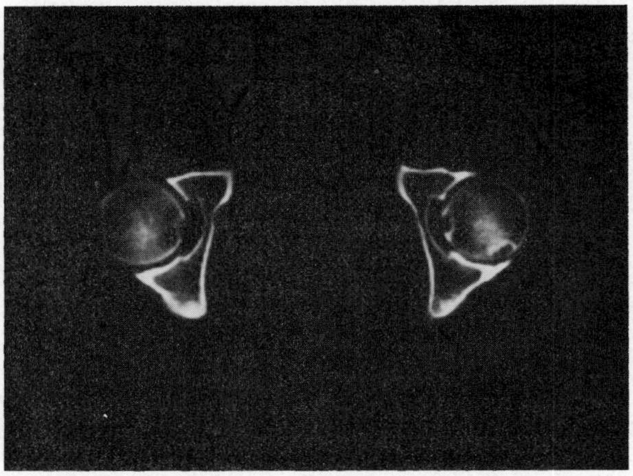

**Figure 40–31.** Pigmented villonodular synovitis. Multiple erosions of the right femoral head, well demonstrated with CT, are consistent with the diagnosis of pigmented villonodular synovitis.

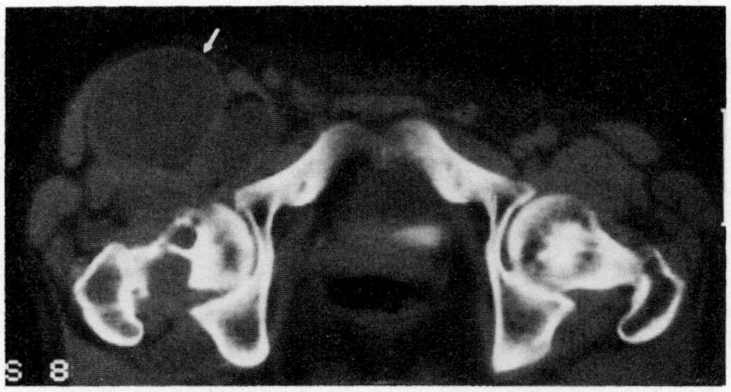


**Figure 40–32.** Synovial cyst of the hip. In a patient with rheumatoid arthritis, observe erosion of the femoral head and femoral neck and a large cystic mass, located anterior to the hip (arrow).

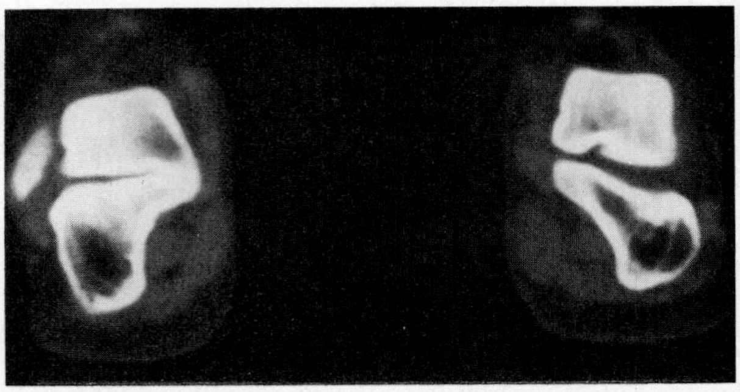

**Figure 40–34.** Talocalcaneal tarsal coalition. A bony bridge extending between the sustentaculum tali of the calcaneus and the middle facet of the talus is indicative of a bony coalition. Compare the appearance to that of the opposite normal side.

matted images. CT, utilized with or without the introduction of intra-articular contrast agents, can be useful, however, in certain articular disorders, including osteochondritis dissecans, osteocartilaginous bodies, idiopathic synovial osteochondromatosis, and pigmented villonodular synovitis[351,352] (Fig. 40–31). Although not proven useful in detecting meniscal lesions in the knee, CT may be utilized in the diagnosis of tears of the cruciate ligaments.[353]

With respect to joint disease, CT is perhaps best suited to the evaluation of para-articular soft tissue masses. Synovial cysts arising adjacent to the glenohumeral joint, hip, and knee are well visualized in this fashion (Fig. 40–32), although the simultaneous administration of an arthrographic contrast agent is often required.

**Osteoporosis.** In recent years, CT has been applied to the diagnosis of generalized osteoporosis by allowing measurement of the degree of attenuation of the x-ray beam at a specific skeletal site. Although such quantitative techniques can be applied to the peripheral skeleton, it appears advantageous to investigate the vertebral spongiosa in this manner.[354-356] It has been suggested that CT can recognize a 1 percent change in the content of vertebral bone; however, errors occur owing to changes in patient position so that different sections of the bone are obtained.[357] It is expected that with refinement in and more widespread availability of this technique, quantitative CT analysis will become the noninvasive modality of choice in evaluating patients with osteoporosis and other metabolic disorders.

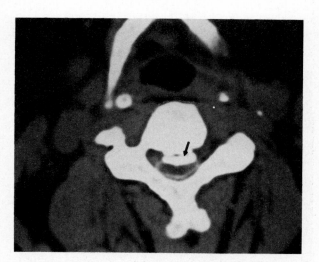

**Figure 40–33.** Ossification of the posterior longitudinal ligament. On a cross-sectional image in the upper cervical spine, a radiodensity seen posterior to the vertebral body (arrow) represents ossification of the posterior longitudinal ligament. Contrast around the spinal cord is related to the prior administration of metrizamide.

**Miscellaneous Diseases.** Diastomatomyelia, myelomeningocele, and ligamentous calcification and ossification (Fig. 40–33) are examples of spinal disorders that are well delineated with CT.[358] Tibial torsion and femoral or humeral anteversion can be evaluated with conventional radiography, but the technique is complex and time consuming; CT may be more advantageous in this evaluation. Coalition, or fusion, of tarsal bones, especially that between the talus and the calcaneus (Fig. 40–34), is best visualized in a coronal plane, which can be achieved with CT.[359] Although this modality has been applied to the diagnosis of ischemic necrosis, especially in the femoral head,[360] its precise role in this regard, particularly with respect to any advantage over scintigraphy, is not established.

A variety of soft tissue problems, in addition to tumors, can be defined with CT. Examples include entrapment neuropathies, especially in the carpal tunnel,[361] foot infections in the diabetic patient, foreign body localization,[362] and calcification or ossification. In the latter situation, the differentiation of myositis ossificans and osteosarcoma of the soft tissue is possible.[363]

## References


1. Koenigsberg, M., and Freeman, L.: Radionuclide bone imaging. Curr. Prob. Diagn. Radiol. 6:1, 1976.
2. Lentle, B., Russell, A., Percy, J., Scott, J., and Jackson, F.: Bone scintiscanning updated. Ann. Intern. Med. 84:297, 1976.
3. Thrall, J.F.: Technetium-99m labelled agents for skeletal imaging. CRC Crit. Rev. Clin. Radiol. Nucl. Med. 8:1, 1976.
4. Subramanian, G., McAfee, J., Blair, R., Mehter, A., and Connor, T.: $^{99m}$Tc-EHDP: A potential radiopharmaceutical for skeletal imaging. J. Nucl. Med. 13:947, 1972.
5. David, M., and Jones, A.: Comparison of $^{99}$Tc-labeled phosphate agents for skeletal imaging. Semin. Nucl. Med. 7:19, 1976.
6. Pendergrass, H., Potsaid, M., and Catronovo, F.: The clinical use of

$^{99m}$Tc-diphosphonate (HEDSPA): A new agent for skeletal imaging. Radiology 109:557, 1973.
7. Hayes, R.L.: The medical use of gallium radionuclides: A brief history with some comments. Semin. Nucl. Med. 8:183, 1978.
8. Turner, D., Fordham, E.W., Ali, A., and Slayton, R.E.: Gallium-67 imaging in the management of Hodgkin's disease and other malignant lymphomas. Semin. Nucl. Med. 8:205, 1978.
9. Higasi, T., Nakayama, Y., Murata, A., Nakamura, M., Sugiyama, M., and Suzuki, S.: Clinical evaluation of $^{67}$Gacitrate scanning. J. Nucl. Med. 13:196, 1972.
10. Staab, E.V., and McCartney, W.: Role of gallium 67 in inflammatory disease. Semin. Nucl. Med. 8:219, 1978.
11. Namey, T.C., and Halla, J.: Radiographic and nucleographic techniques in the diagnosis of septic arthritis and osteomyelitis. Clin. Rheum. Dis. 4:95, 1978.
12. Hays, M., and Green, F.: The pertechnetate joint scan: I. Timing. Ann. Rheum. Dis. 31:272, 1972.
13. Hays, M., and Green, F.: The pertechnetate joint scan: II. Clinical correlations. Ann. Rheum. Dis. 31:278, 1972.
14. Weiss, T.E., and Shuler, S.E.: I. New techniques for identification of synovitis and evaluation of joint disease. II. Joint imaging as a clinical aid in diagnosis and therapy. Bull. Rheum. Dis. 25:786, 1974.
15. Hays, M.T., and Green, F.A.: In vitro studies of $^{99m}$Tc-pertechnetate bending by human serum and tissues. J. Nucl. Med. 14:149, 1973.
16. Dick, W.C., and Grennan, D.: Radioisotopes in the study of normal and inflamed joint. Clin. Rheum. Dis. 2:67, 1976.
17. Huskisson, E., Scott, J., and Balme, H.: Objective measurement of rheumatoid arthritis using technetium index. Ann. Rheum. Dis. 35:81, 1976.
18. Boerbooms, A., and Buys, W.: Rapid assessment of $^{99m}$Tc-pertechnetate uptake in the knee joint as a parameter of inflammatory activity. Arthritis Rheum. 20:348, 1978.
19. Szanto, E., and Lindvall, N.: Quantitative $^{99m}$Tc pertechnetate scanning of the sacro-iliac joints. Scand. J. Rheumatol. 7:93, 1978.
20. Schaal, G., Anderson, L., Wolf, R., et al.: Xerostomia in Sjögren's syndrome: Evaluation by sequential salivary scintigraphy. JAMA 216:2109, 1971.
21. Parret, J., and Peyrin, J.: Radioisotopic investigations in salivary pathology. Clin. Nucl. Med. 4:250, 1979.
22. Daniels, T.E., Powell, R.R., Sylvester, R., and Talal, N.: An evaluation of salivary gland scintigraphy in Sjögren's syndrome. Arthritis Rheum. 22:809, 1979. (Please note minor change on salivary slides.)
23. Ohrt, H., and Shafer, R.B.: An atlas of salivary gland disorders. Clin. Nucl. Med. 7:370, 1982.
24. Janin-Mercier, A., Sauvezie, B., Ristori, M., Betail, G., Veyre, A., and Rampon, S.: Histological and immunological study in patients with rheumatoid arthritis showing isolated abnormalities of salivary scintigraphy. J. Clin. Immuno. 2:282, 1982.
25. Chaudiri, T.K., and Stadalnik, R.C.: Salivary gland imaging. Semin. Nucl. Med. 10:400, 1980.
26. Jones, A., Francis, M., and Davis, M.: Radionuclide reaction mechanisms. Semin. Nucl. Med. 7:3, 1976.
27. Siegel, B., Donovan, R., Alderson, P., and Mack, G.: Skeletal uptake of $^{99m}$Tc-diphosphonate in relationship to local blood flow. Radiology 120:121, 1976.
28. Charkes, N.D.: Skeletal blood flow: Implications for bone-scan interpretation. J. Nucl. Med. 21:91, 1980.
29. Krishnamurthy, G.T., Brickman, A., and Blahd, W.: Technetium-99m-Sn-pyrophosphate pharmaco-kinetics and bone image changes in parathyroid disease. J. Nucl. Med. 18:236, 1977.
30. Christensen, S.B., and Krogsgaard, O.W.: Localization of Tc-99m MDP in epiphyseal growth plates of rats. J. Nucl. Med. 22:237, 1981.
31. Rosenthall, L., and Kaye, M.: Technetium-99m-pyrophosphate kinetics and imaging in metabolic bone disease. J. Nucl. Med. 16:33, 1975.
32. Kaye, M., Silverton, S., and Rosenthall, L.: Technetium-99m-pyrophosphate: Studies in vivo and in vitro. J. Nucl. Med. 16:40, 1975.
33. Rosenthall, L., and Kaye, M.: Observations on the mechanism of $^{99m}$Tc-labeled phosphate complex uptake in metabolic bone disease. Semin. Nucl. Med. 6:59, 1976.
34. Wiegmann, T., Kirsh, J., Rosenthall, L., and Kaye, M.: Relationship between bone uptake of $^{99m}$Tc-pyrophosphate and hydroxyproline in blood and urine. J. Nucl. Med. 17:711, 1976.
35. Garcia, D., Tow, D., and Kaperr, K.: Relative accretion of $^{99m}$Tc-polyphosphate by forming and resorbing bone systems in rats. Significance in the pathologic basis of bone scanning. J. Nucl. Med. 17:93, 1976.
36. Evans, C.H., and Mears, D.C.: $^{99m}$Tc-1-hydroxyethylidene-1, 1-diphosphonic acid to cartilage and collagen in vitro and its stimulation by $Er^{3+}$ and low pH. Calcif. Tissue Int. 32:91, 1980.
37. Turner, J.H.: Post-traumatic avascular necrosis of the femoral head predicted by preoperative technetium-99m antimony-colloid scan. J. Bone Joint Surg. 65A:786–796, 1983.
38. Meyers, M.H., Telfer, N., and Moore, T.M.: Determination of the vascularity of the femoral head with technetium-99m-sulphur-colloid. J. Bone Joint Surg. 59A:568, 1977.
39. Brown, D., Byrd, B., Carlton, J., Sartzendruber, D., and Hayes, R.: A quantitative study of the subcellular localization of $^{67}Ga^{2+}$. Cancer Res. 36:956, 1976.
40. Takeda, S., Uchida, T., and Matsuzawa, T.: A comparative study on lysosomal accumulation of gallium-67 and indium-III in Morris hepatoma 7316A. J. Nucl. Med. 18:835, 1977.
41. Tsan, M., Chen, W., Scheffel, U., and Wagner, H.N.: Studies on gallium accumulation in inflammatory lesions. I. Gallium uptake by human polymorphonuclear leukocytes. J. Nucl. Med. 19:36, 1978.
42. Menon, S., Wagner, H.N., and Tsan, M.: Studies on gallium accumulation in inflammatory lesions. II. Uptake by *Staphylococcus aureus.* J. Nucl. Med. 19:44, 1978.
43. Hayes, R.: The tissue distribution of gallium radionuclides. J. Nucl. Med. 18:740, 1977.
44. Larson, S.: Mechanisms of localization of gallium-67 in tumors. Semin. Nucl. Med. 8:193, 1978.
45. Hill, J., Merz, T., and Wagner, N., Jr.: Iron-induced enhancement of $^{67}$Ga uptake in a model human leukocyte culture system in vitro. J. Nucl. Med. 8:193, 1978.
46. Hoffer, P., Huberty, J., and Khayam-Bashi, H.: The association of Ga-67 and lactoferrin. J. Nucl. Med. 18:713, 1977.
47. Bradley, W., Alderson, P., Eckelman, W., and Weiss, J.: Decreased tumor uptake in animals after whole body radiation. J. Nucl. Med. 19:204, 1978.
48. Larson, S., Rasey, J., Grunbaum, Z., and Allen, D.: Pharmacologic enhancement of gallium-67 tumor-to-blood ratios for EMT-6 sarcoma (BALB/c mice). Radiology 130:241, 1979.
49. Weiner, R., Hoffer, P.B., and Thakur, M.L.: Lactoferrin: Its role as a Ga-67 binding protein in polymorphonuclear leukocytes. J. Nucl. Med. 22:32, 1981.
50. Hayes, R.L., Rafter, J.J., Byrd, B.L., and Carlton, J.E.: Studies of the in vivo entry of Ga-67 into normal and malignant tissue. J. Nucl. Med. 22:325, 1981.
51. Emery, T., and Hoffer, P.B.: Siderophore-mediated mechanism of gallium uptake demonstrated in the microorganism *Ustilago sphaerogena.* J. Nucl. Med. 21:935, 1980.
52. Hoffer, P.: Gallium and infection. J. Nucl. Med. 21:484, 1980.
53. Oster, Z.H., Som, P., Sacker, D.F., and Atkins, L.: The effects of deferoxamine mesylate on gallium-67 distribution in normal and abscess-bearing animals: Concise communication. J. Nucl. Med. 21:421, 1980.
54. Handmaker, H., and Leonards, R.: Bone scan in inflammatory osseous disease. Semin. Nucl. Med. 6:95, 1976.
55. Kontzen, F., Namey, T., Tobin, M., Debovsky, E., and Tauxe, W.N.: Technical aspects of joint imaging. J. Nucl. Med. Tech. 6:110, 1978.
56. Weiss, T., Maxfield, W., Murison, P., and Hidalgo, J.: Iodinated human serum albumin ($I^{131}$) localization studies of rheumatoid arthritis joints by scintillation scanning. Arthritis Rheum. 8:979, 1965.
57. Desaulniers, M., Fuks, A., Hawkins, D., Lacourciere, Y., and Rosenthall, L.: Radiotechnetium polyphosphate joint imaging. J. Nucl. Med. 15:421, 1974.
58. Bekerman, C., Genant, H., Hoffer, P., Kozin, F., and Ginsberg, M.: Radionuclide imaging of the bones and joints of the hand. Radiology 118:653, 1975.
59. Mirtl, B., Leb, G., Klein, G., Goebel, R., and Eber, O.: Gelenksszintigraphie mit $^{99m}$-Tc-pyrophosphat. Z. Rechtsmed. 34:149, 1975.
60. Hoffer, P.B., and Genant, H.K.: Radionuclide joint imaging. Semin. Nucl. Med. 6:121, 1976.
61. Barraclough, D., Russell, A., and Percy, J.: Psoriatic spondylitis: A clinical, radiological, and scintiscan survey. J. Rheumatol. 4:282, 1977.
62. Namey, T.C., McIntyre, J., LeRoy, E.C., and Bennett, J.C.: Early psoriatic arthritis: Nucleographic and HLA studies. Proceedings of the XIV International Congress of Rheumatology, 1977, p. 210.
63. Namey, T., McIntyre, J., Buse, M., and LeRoy, E.: Nucleographic studies of axial spondarthritides. I. Quantitative sacroiliac scintigraphy in early HLA-B27-associated sacroiliitis. Arthritis Rheum. 20:1058, 1977.
64. Lentle, B.C., Russell, A., Percy, J., and Jackson, F.: The scintigraphic findings in ankylosing spondylitis. J. Nucl. Med. 18:524, 1977.
65. Namey, T., and Rosenthall, L.: Generalized periarticular uptake of $^{99m}$-Tc-pyrophosphate in progressive systemic sclerosis. Clin. Nucl. Med. 2:26, 1977.
66. Rosenthall, L., and Hawkins, D.: Radionuclide joint imaging in the diagnosis of synovial disease. Semin. Arthritis Rheum. 7:49, 1977.
67. Namey, T.: Joint and quantitative sacroiliac scintigraphy in the diagnosis of rheumatic diseases. *In* Tauxe, W. (ed.): Functional Studies in Nuclear Medicine, 1978. Southeastern Society of Nuclear Medicine (11) 1978, pp. 1–19.
68. Weissberg, D., Resnick, D., Taylor, A., Becker, M., and Alazraki, N.: Rheumatoid arthritis and its variants: Analysis of scintiphotographic, radiographic, and clinical examinations. AJR 131:665, 1978.

69. Esdaile, J., Hawkins, D., and Rosenthall, L.: Radionuclide joint imaging in the seronegative spondyloarthropathies. Clin. Orthop. 143:46, 1979.
70. Shearman, J., Esdaile, J., Hawkins, D., and Rosenthall, L.: Predictive value of radionuclide joint scintigrams. Arthritis Rheum. 24:83, 1982.
71. Abrams, H.: The "overutilization" of x-rays. N. Engl. J. Med. 300:1213, 1979.
72. Baldrusson, H., and Gustafsson, M.: Total radiation dosage from x-ray examinations in rheumatoid arthritis and other chronic skeletal diseases. Acta Orthop. Scand. 48:138, 1977.
73. Godderidge, C.: Female gonadal shielding. Appl. Radiol. (Mar./Apr.):65, 1979.
74. Manny, E., Brown, F., and Shaver, J.: Gonad shielding in diagnostic radiology. Postgrad. Med. 65:207, 1979.
75. Hill, H.F., Hill, A.G., and Bodner, J.G.: Clinical diagnosis of ankylosing spondylitis in women and relation to presence of HLA-B27. Ann. Rheum. Dis. 35:267, 1976.
76. Cheatum, D.: "Ankylosing spondylitis" without sacroiliitis in a woman without HLA-B27 antigen. J. Rheumatol. 3:420, 1976.
77. Nasrallah, N., Masi, A., Chandler, R., Feigenbaum, S., and Kaplan, S.: HLA-B27 antigen and rheumatoid factor negative (seronegative) peripheral arthritis. Am. J. Med. 63:379, 1977.
78. Ross, J.: Biomedical effects of ionizing radiation. *In* Blahd, W. (ed.): Nuclear Medicine. 2nd ed. New York, McGraw-Hill Book Company, 1971.
79. Physcians' Desk Reference for Radiology and Nuclear Medicine, 1978/79 Oradell, N.J., Medical Economics Company, p. 134.
80. Editorial: Ankylosing spondylitis and its early diagnosis. Lancet 2:591, 1977.
81. Hockberg, M., Borenstein, D., and Arnett, F.: The absence of back pain in classical ankylosing spondylitis. Johns Hopkins Med. J. 143:181, 1978.
82. Bernstein, B., and Singsen, B.: Juvenile ankylosing spondylitis: Are adult criteria appropriate? (abstract). Arthritis Rheum. 22:593, 1979.
83. Wahner, H., and O'Duffy, J.: Peripheral joint scanning with technetium pertechnetate. Mayo Clin. Proc. 51:525, 1976.
84. Khalkhali, I., Stadalnik, R., Wiesner, K., and Shapiro, R.: Bone imaging of the heel in Reiter's syndrome. AJR 132:110, 1979.
85. Holzmann, H., Hoede, N., Eibner, D., and Hahn, K.: Die psoriatische Osteoarthropathie. Hautarzt 30:343, 1979.
86. Namey, T., and Rosenthall, L.: Periarticular uptake of $^{99m}$technetium diphosphonate in psoriatics. Arthritis Rheum. 19:607, 1976.
87. Hoede, N., Holzmann, H., Eissner, D., and Hahn, K.: Uber die Häufigkeit von Gelenkbeteiligungen bei Psoriasis. Verh. Dtsch. Ges. Rheumatol. 4:229, 1976.
88. Lin, M.S., Fawcett, H.D., and Goodwin, D.A.: Bone scintigraphy demonstrating arthropathy of central joints in ankylosing spondylitis. Clin. Nucl. Med. 8:364, 1980.
89. Russell, A., Davis, P., Percy, J., and Lentle, B.: The sacroiliitis of acute Reiter's syndrome. J. Rheumatol. 4:293, 1977.
90. Webb, J., Collins, L.T., and Southwell, P.B.: Fluorine-18 isotope scans in the early diagnosis of sacroiliitis. Med. J. Aust. 2:1270, 1971.
91. Lovgren, O., and Dowen, S.A.: Strontium (*85*SR) scintigrams of the sacroiliacal joints. Acta Rheum. Scand. 15:327, 1969.
92. VanLaere, M., Veys, E.M., and Mielants, H.: Strontium 87m scanning of the sacroiliac joints in ankylosing spondylitis. Ann. Rheum. Dis. 31:201, 1972.
93. Russell, A., Lentle, B., and Percy, J.: Investigation of sacroiliac disease: Comparative evaluation of radiological and radionuclide techniques. J. Rheumatol. 2:45, 1975.
94. Lentle, B., Russell, A., Percy, J., and Jackson, F.: The scintigraphic investigation of sacroiliac disease. J. Nucl. Med. 18:529, 1977.
95. Lugon, M., Torode, A., Travers, R., Lavender, J.P., and Hughes, G.R.: Sacro-iliac joint scanning with technetium-99m-diphosphonate. Rheumatol. Rehabil. 18:131, 1979.
96. Dunn, E., Ebringer, R., and Ell, P.: Quantitative scintigraphy in the early diagnosis of sacro-iliitis. Rheum. Rehabil. 19:69, 1980.
97. Scott, D., Smith, A., Eastmond, C., Hayter, C., and Wright, V.: An evaluation of the techniques of sacro-iliac scintiscanning. Rheum Rehabil. 19:76, 1980.
98. Dequeker, J., Goddeeris, T., Walravens, M., and DeRoo, M.: Evaluation of sacroiliitis: Comparison of radiological and radionuclide techniques Radiology 128:687, 1978.
99. Spencer, D.G., Adams, F.G., Horton, P.W., and Buchanan, W.W.: Scintiscanning in ankylosing spondylitis. J. Rheumatol. 6:426, 1979.
100. Berghs, H., Remans, J., Drieskens, L., Kiebooms, A., and Polderman, J.: Diagnostic value of sacroiliac joint scintigraphy with $^{99m}$technetium pyrophosphate in sacroiliitis. Ann. Rheum. Dis. 37:190, 1978.
101. Goldberg, R., Genant, H., Shimshak, R., and Shames, D.: Applications and limitations of quantitative sacroiliac joint scintigraphy. Radiology 128:683, 1978.
102. Ho, G., Sadovinikoff, N., Malhotra, C.M., and Claumch, B.C.: Quantitative sacroiliac joint scintigraphy. Arthritis Rheum. 22:837, 1979.
103. Pfannenstiel, P., Semmler, U., Adam, W., Halbsguth, A., Bandilla, K., and Berg, D.: Comparative study of quantitating $^{99m}$Tc-EHDP uptake in sacroiliac scintigraphy. Eur. J. Nucl. Med. 5:49, 1980.
104. Szanto, E., and Lindvall, N.: Quantitative $^{99m}$Tc pertechnetate scanning of the sacro-iliac joints: A follow-up study of patients with suspected sacroiliitis. Scand. J. Rheumatol. 7:93, 1978.
105. Chalmers, I., Lentle, B., Percy, J., and Russell, A.: Sacroiliitis detected by bone scintiscanning: A clinical, radiological and scintigraphic follow-up study. Ann. Rheum. Dis. 38:112, 1979.
106. Bellamy, N., Park, W., and Rooney, P.J.: What do we know about the sacroiliac joint? Sem. Arthritis Rheum. 12(3), 1983.
107. O'Duffy, J., Hunder, G., and Wahner, H.: A follow-up study of polymyalgia rheumatica: Evidence of chronic axial synovitis. J. Rheumatol. 7:685, 1980.
108. Ho., G., Claunch, B.C., and Sadovnikoff, N.: Scintigraphic evidence of transient unilateral sacroiliitis in a case of Whipple's disease Clin. Nucl. Med. 12:548, 1980.
109. Namey, T., Horowitz, J., and Hardin, J.: Transient sacroiliitis in acute sarcoid arthropathy. 65th Meeting, Radiology Society of North America, Atlanta, 1979.
110. Szanto, E., and Hagenfeldt, K.: Sacro-iliitis and salpingitis. Scand. J. Rheumatol. 8:129, 1979.
111. Szanto, E., and Hagenfeldt, K.: Sacro-iliitis in women—a sequela to acute salpingitis. Scand. J. Rheumatol. 12:89, 1983.
112. Namey, T.C., and Biondo, J.J.: Scintigraphic patterns of early inflammatory sacroiliitis: The possible significance of unilateral sacroiliitis in Reiter's syndrome. Trans. Orthop. Res. Soc. 1980.
113. Gordon, G., and Kabins, S.A.: Pyogenic sacroiliitis. Am. J. Med. 69:50, 1980.
114. Lopez-Majano, V., and Miskew, D.: Sacro-iliac joint disease in drug abusers: The role of bone scintigraphy. Eur. J. Nucl. Med. 5:549, 1980.
115. Lewkonia, R., and Kinsella, T.: Pyogenic sacroiliitis: Diagnosis and significance. J. Rheumatol. 8:153, 1981.
116. Iczkovitz, J., Leek, J., and Robbins, D.: Pyogenic sacroiliitis. J. Rheumatol. 8:157, 1981.
117. Horgan, J.G., Walker, M., Newman, J.H., and Watt, I.: Scintigraphy in the diagnosis and management of septic sacro-iliitis. Clin. Radiol. 34:337, 1983.
118. Kumar, R., and Balachandran, S.: Unilateral septic sacro-iliitis: Importance of the anterior view of the bone scan. Clin. Nucl. Med. 8:413, 1983.
119. Murray, I.P.C.: Bone scanning in the child and young adult. Part I. Skeletal Radiol. 5:1, 1980.
120. Murray, I.P.C.: Bone scanning in the child and young adult. Part II. Skeletal Radiol. 5:65, 1980.
121. Kirchner, P.T., and Simon, M.A.: Current concepts review radioisotopic evaluation of skeletal disease. J. Bone Joint Surg. 63A:673, 1981.
122. Atcheson, S., Coleman, R., and Ward, J.: Septic arthritis mimicking cellulitis: Distinction using radionuclide bone imaging. Clin. Nucl. Med. 4:79, 1979.
123. Lisbona, R., and Rosenthall, L.: Radionuclide imaging of septic joints and their differentiation from periarticular osteomyelitis, and cellulitis in pediatrics. Clin. Nucl. Med. 2:337, 1977.
124. Lisbona, R., and Rosenthall, L.: Observations on the sequential use of $^{99m}$Tc-phosphate complex and $^{67}$Ga imaging in osteomyelitis, cellulitis, and septic arthritis. Radiology 123:123, 1977.
125. Gaucher, A., Colomb, J.N., Naoun, A., Pourel, J., Robert, J., Faure, G., and Netter, P.: Radionuclide imaging in hip abnormalities. Clin. Nucl. Med. 5:214, 1980.
126. Maurer, A.H., Chen, D.C.P., Camargo, E.E., Wong, D.F., Wagner, H.N., and Anderson, P.O.: Utility of three-phase skeletal scintigraphy in suspected osteomyelitis: Concise communication. J. Nucl. Med. 22:941, 1981.
127. Murray, I.P.C.: Photopenia in skeletal scintigraphy of suspected bone and joint infection. Clin. Nucl. Med. 7:14, 1982.
128. Kloiber, R., Pavlosky, W., Portner, O., and Gartke, K.: Bone scintigraphy of hip joint effusions in children. AJR 140:995, 1983.
129. Coleman, R.E., Samuelson, C.O., Balm, S., Christian, P.E., and Ward, J.R.: Imaging with Tc-99m MDP and Ga-67 citrate in patients with rheumatoid arthritis and suspected septic arthritis: Concise communication. J. Nucl. Med. 23:479, 1982.
130. Horoszowski, H., Ganel, A., Kamhin, M., Zaltzman, S., and Farine, L.: Sequential use of technetium 99m MDP and gallium 67 citrate imaing in the evaluation of painful total hip replacement. Br. J. Radiol. 53:1169, 1980.
131. Duszynski, D., Kuhn, J., Afshani, E., and Riddlesburger, M.: Early radionuclide diagnosis of acute osteomyelitis. Radiology 117:337, 1975.
132. Gilday, D., Paul, D., and Peterson, J.: Diagnosis of osteomyelitis in

children by combined blood pool and bone imaging. Radiology 117:331, 1975.
133. Letts, R., Afifi, A., and Sutherland, J.: Technetium bone scanning as an aid in the diagnosis of atypical acute osteomyelitis in children. Surg. Gynecol. Obstet. 140:89, 1975.
134. Majd, M., and Frankel, R.: Radionuclide imaging in skeletal inflammatory and ischemic disease in children. AJR 126:823, 1976.
135. Gelfand, M., and Silberstein, E.: Radionuclide imaging: Use in diagnosis of osteomyelitis in children. JAMA 237:245, 1977.
136. Nelson, H.T., and Taylor A.: Bone scanning in the diagnosis of osteomyelitis. J. Nucl. Med. 19:696, 1978.
137. Sullivan, J.A., Vasileff, T., and Leonard, J.C.: An evaluation of nuclear scanning in orthopaedic infections. J. Pediatr. Orthop. 1:73, 1981.
138. Sullivan, D.C., Rosenfield, N., Ogden, J., and Gottschalk, A.: Problems in the scintigraphic detection of osteomyelitis in children. Radiology 135:731, 1980.
139. Ash, J.M., and Gilday, D.L.: The futility of bone scanning in neo-natal osteomyelitis: Concise communication. J. Nucl. Med. 21:417, 1980.
140. Sy, W., Westring, D., and Weinberger, G.: "Cold" lesions on bone imaging. J. Nucl. Med. 16:1013, 1975.
141. Trackler, R., Miller, K., Sutherland, D., and Chadwick, D.: Childhood pelvic osteomyelitis presenting as a "cold" lesion on bone scan: Case report. J. Nucl. Med. 17:620, 1976.
142. Armbruster, T., Georgen, T., Resnick, D., and Catanzaro, A.: Utility of bone scanning in disseminated coccidiodomycosis: Case report. J. Nucl. Med. 18:450, 1977.
143. Garnett, E., Cockshott, W., and Jacobs, J.: Classical acute osteomyelitis with a negative bone scan. Br. J. Radiol. 50:757, 1977.
144. Park, H.M., Wheat, L.J., Siddiqui, A.R., Burt, R.W., Robb, J.A., Ransburg, R.C., and Kernek, C.B.: Scintigraphic evaluation of diabetic osteomyelitis: Concise communication. J. Nucl. Med. 23:569, 1982.
145. Shoju, H., Asnis, S., Bohne, W., Rovere, G., and Gristina, A.: Further observations on $^{85}$Sr scintimetry in intracapsular fracture of the hip. South. Med. J. 68:1249, 1975.
146. Hungerford, D., and Zizic, T.: Alcoholism-associated ischemic necrosis of the femoral head: Early diagnosis and treatment. Clin. Orthop. 130:144, 1978.
147. D'Ambrosia, R., Riggins, R., Stadalnik, R., and DeNardo, G.: Scintigraphy in the avascular necrotic disorders of bone. Clin. Orthop. 121:146, 1975.
148. D'Ambrosia, R., Shoju, H., Riggins, R., Stadalnik, R., and DeNardo, G.: Scintigraphy in the diagnosis of osteonecrosis. Clin. Orthop. 130:139, 1978.
149. D'Ambrosia, R., Riggins, R., Stadalnik, R., and DeNardo, G.: Experience with $^{99m}$Tc-diphosphonate in studying vascularity of the femoral head. Surg. Forum 26:521, 1975.
150. Lutzker, L.G., and Alavi, A.: Bone and marrow imaging in sickle cell disease: Diagnosis of infarction. Semin. Nucl. Med. 6:83, 1976.
151. D'Ambrosia, R., Riggins, R., Stadalnik, R., and DeNardo, G.: Vascularity of the femoral head: $^{99m}$Tc-diphosphonate scintigraphy validated with tetracycline labeling. Clin. Orthop. 121:143, 1976.
152. Harcke, H.T.: Bone imaging in infants and children: A review. J. Nucl. Med. 18:231, 1977.
153. Conklin, J.J., Alderson, P.O., Zizic, T.M., Hungerford, D.S., Densereaux, J.Y., Gober, A., and Wagner, H.N.: Comparison of bone scan and radiograph sensitivity in the detection of steroid-indiced ischemic necrosis of bone. Radiology 147:221, 1983.
154. Gelfand, M., Ball, W., Oestreich, A., Crawford, A., Jolson, R., and Perlman, A.: Transient loss of femoral head Tc-99m diphosphonate uptake with prolonged maintenance of femoral head architecture. Clin. Nucl. Med. 8:347, 1983.
155. Spencer, R.P., Lee, Y.S., Sziklas, J.J., Rosenberg, R.J., and Karimeddinni, M.K.: Failure of uptake of radiocolloid by the femoral heads: A diagnostic problem: Concise communication. J. Nucl. Med. 24:116, 1983.
156. Williams, A.G., Mettler, F.A., and Christie, J.H.: Sulfur colloid distribution in normal hips. Clin. Nucl. Med. 8:490, 1983.
157. Khairi, M.R., Wellman, H., Robb, J., and Johnson, C.: Paget's disease of bone (osteitis deformans): Symptomatic lesions and bone scan. Ann. Intern. Med. 79:348, 1973.
158. Wellman, H., Sckauwecker, D., Robb, J., and Johnson, C.: Skeletal scintimaging and radiography in the diagnosis and management of Paget's disease. Clin. Orthop. 127:55, 1977.
159. Shirazi, P.H., Ryan, W.G., and Fordham, E.W.: Bone scanning in evaluation of Paget's disease of bone. CRC Crit. Rev. Clin. Radiol. Nucl. Med. 5:523, 1974.
160. Serafini, A.: Paget's disease of bone. Semin. Nucl. Med. 6:47, 1976.
161. Vellenga, C., Paurvels, E., Bjjvoet, O., and Hoshing, D.: Evaluation of scintigraphic and roentgenologic studies in Paget's disease under therapy. Radiol. Clin. (Basel) 45:292, 1976.
162. Lentle, B., Russell, A., Heslip, P., and Percy, J.S.: The scintigraphic findings in Paget's disease of bone. Clin. Radiol. 27:129, 1976.
163. Waxman, A., Ducker, S., McKee, D., Siemsen, J., and Singer, F.: Evaluation of $^{99m}$TC diphosphonate kinetics and bone scans in patients with Paget's disease before and after calcitonin treatment. Radiology 125:761, 1977.
164. Lavender, J., Evans, I., Arnot, R., Bowring, S., Doyle, F., Joplin, G., and MacIntyre, I.: A comparison of radiography and radioisotope scanning in the detection of Paget's disease and in the assessment of response in human calcitonin. Br. J. Radiol. 50:243, 1977.
165. Frame, B., and Marel, G.M.: Paget's disease: A review of current knowledge. Radiology 141:21, 1981.
166. Vellenga, C.J.L.R., Pauwels, E.K.J., Bijvoet, O.L.M., and Frijink, W.B.: Scintigraphic aspects of the recurrence of treated Paget's disease of bone. J. Nucl. Med. 22:510, 1981.
167. Lee, J.Y.: Bone scintigraphy in evolution of didionel therapy for Paget's disease. Clin. Nucl. Med. 6:356, 1981.
168. Waxman, A.D., McKee, D., Siemsen, J.K., and Singer, F.R.: Gallium scanning in Paget's disease of bone: Effect of calcitonin, AJR 134:303, 1980.
169. Brower, A., and Teates, C.: Positive $^{99m}$TC-polyphosphate scan in a case of metastatic osteogenic sarcoma with hypertrophic osteoarthropathy. J. Nucl. Med. 15:53, 1974.
170. Kay, C., and Rosenberg, M.: Positive Tc-99m polyphosphate scan in a case of secondary hypertrophic osteoarthropathy. J. Nucl. Med. 15:312, 1974.
171. Terry, D., Isitman, A., and Holmes, R.: Radionuclide bone images in hypertrophic pulmonary osteoarthropathy. AJR 124:571, 1975.
172. Rosenthall, L., and Kirsh, J.: Observations on radionuclide imaging in hypertrophic pulmonary osteoarthropathy. Radiology 120:359, 1977.
173. Sty, J.R., Sheth, K., and Starshak, J.: Bone scintigraphy in childhood idiopathic hypertrophic osteoarthropathy. Clin. Nucl. Med. 7:421, 1982.
174. Kozin, F., McCarty, D., Sims, J., and Genant, H.: The reflex sympathetic dystrophy syndrome. I. Clinical and histologic studies: Evidence for bilaterality, response to corticosteroids and articular involvement. Am. J. Med. 60:321, 1976.
175. Kozin, F., McCarty, D., Sims, J., and Genant, H.: The reflex sympathetic dystrophy syndrome. II. Roentgenographic and scintigraphic evidence of bilaterality, and of periarticular accentuation. Am. J. Med. 60:332, 1976.
176. Genant, H., Hozin, F., Bekerman, C., McCarty, D., and Sims, J.: the reflex sympathic dystrophy syndrome. Radiology 117:21, 1975.
177. Carlson, D., Simon, H., and Wegner, W.: Bone scanning and diagnosis of reflex sympathetic dystrophy secondary to herniated lumbar disks. Neurology 27:791, 1977.
178. Simon, H., and Carlson, D.H.: The use of bone scanning in the diagnosis of reflex sympathetic dystrophy. Clin. Nucl. Med. 5:116, 1980.
179. Kozin, F., Soin, J., Ryan, L., Carrera, G., and Wortmann, R.L.: Bone scintigraphy in the reflex sympathetic dystrophy syndrome. Radiology. 138:437, 1981.
180. Kozin, F., Ryan, L.M., Carerra, G.F., and Soin, J.S.: The reflex dystrophy syndrome (RSDS). III. Scintigraphic studies, further evidence for therapeutic efficacy of systemic corticosteroids and proposed diagnostic criteria. A.J. Med. 70:23, 1981.
181. Sy, W., Bay, R., and Camera, A.: Hand images: Normal and abnormal. J. Nucl. Med. 18:419, 1977.
182. Namey, T.: Unpublished data.
183. Thomas, R., Resnich, D., Daniel, D., and Greenfield, R.: Compartmental evaluation of osteoarthritis of the knee: A comparative study of available modalities. Radiology 116:585, 1975.
184. Gelman, M., Coleman, R., Stevens, P., and Davey, B.: Radiography, radionuclide imaging, and arthrography in evaluation of total hip and knee replacement. Radiology 128:677, 1978.
185. Williams, E., Tregonning, R., and Hurley, P.: 99Tcm-diphosphonate scanning as an aid to diagnosis of infection in total hip joint replacements. Br. J. Radiol. 50:562, 1977.
186. Tehranzadeh, J., Schneider, R., and Freiberger, R.H.: Radiological evaluation of painful total hip replacement. Radiology 141:355, 1981.
187. Hunter, J.C. Hattner, R.S., Murray, W.R., and Genant, H.K.: Loosening of the total knee arthroplasty: Detection by radionuclide bone scanning. AJR 135:131–136, 1980.
188. Abdel-Dayem, H.M., Barodawala, Y., and Papademetriou, T.: Scintigraphic arthrography: A new imaging procedure. Clin. Nucl. Med. 6:246, 1981.
189. Abdel-Dayem, H.M., Barodawala, Y.K., and Papademetriou, T: Scintigraphic arthrography: Comparison with contrast arthrography and future applications. Clin. Nucl. Med. 7:516, 1982.
190. Hussein, A., Barodawala, Y., and Papademetrious, T.: Loose knee prosthesis detection by scintigraphic arthrography. Clin. Nucl. Med. 8:355, 1983.
191. Brill, D.R.: Bone imaging for lower extremity pain in athletes. Sports Nucl. Med. 8:101, 1983.

192. Spencer, R.P., Levinson, E.D., Baldwin, R.D., Sziklas, J.J., Witek, J.T., and Rosenberg, R.: Diverse bone scan abnormalities in "shin splints." J. Nucl. Med. 20:1271, 1979.
193. Van Hal, M., Keene, J., Lange, T., and Clancy, W.: Stress fractures of the great toe sesamoids. Am. J. Sports Med. 10:122, 1982.
194. Lombardo, S., and Benson, D.: Stress fractures of the femur in runners. Am. J. Sports Med. 10:219, 1982.
195. Butler, J., Brown, S., and McConnell, B.: Subtrochanteric stress fractures in runners. Am. J. Sports Med. 10:228, 1982.
196. Hajek, M., and Nobel, B.: Stress fractures of the femoral neck in joggers. Am. J. Sports Med. 10:112. 1982.
197. Pavlov, H., Torg, J., and Freiberger, R.: Tarsal navicular stress fractures: Radiographic evaluation. Radiology 148:641, 1983.
198. Manzione, M., and Pizzutillo, P.: Stress fracture of the scaphoid waist. Am. J. Sports Med. 9:268, 1981.
199. Sewell, J.R., Black, C.M., Chapman, A.H., Statham, J., Hughes, G.R.V., and Lavender, J.P.: Quantitative scintigraphy in diagnosis and management of plantar fascilitis (calcaneal periostitis): Concise communication. J. Nucl. Med. 21:633, 1980.
200. Jackson, D., et al.: Stress reactions involving the pars interarticularis in young athletes. Am. J. Sports Med. 9:304, 1981.
201. Matin, P.: The appearance of bone scans following fractures, including immediate and long-term studies. J. Nucl. Med. 20:1227, 1979.
202. Isreal, H., Park, C., and Mansfield, C.: Gallium scanning in sarcoidosis. Ann. N. Y. Acad. Sci. 278:514, 1976.
203. Wiener, S., and Potal, B.: $^{67}$Ga-citrate uptake by the parotid glands in sarcoidosis. Radiology 130:753, 1979.
204. Oren, V., Uszler, J., and White, J.: Diagnosis of uveo-parotid fever by 67-Ga citrate imaging. Clin. Nucl. Med. 3:127, 1978.
205. Ball, G., and Logic, J.: Unpublished data.
206. Nosal, A., Schleissner, L., Miskkin, F., and Lieberman, J.: Angiotensin-1-converting enzyme and gallium scan in non-invasive evaluation of sarcoidosis. Ann. Intern. Med. 90:3282, 1979.
207. Reginato, A., Schiappaccasse, V., Guzman, L., and Claure, H.: 99m Technetium-pyrophosphate scintophotography in bone sarcoidosis. J. Rheumatol. 3:426, 1976.
208. Gupta, B., Bekerman, C., Sicilian, L., Oparil, Z., Pinsky, S., and Szidon, J.: Gallium-67 citrate scanning and serum angiotensin converting enzyme levels in sarcoidosis. Radiology 144:895, 1982.
209. Israel, H.L., Sperber, M., and Steiner, R.M.: Course of chronic hilar sarcoidosis in relation to markers of granulomatous activity. Invest. Radiol. 18:1, 1983.
210. Butt, W., and McIntyre, J.: Double-contrast arthrography of the knee. Radiology 92:487, 1969.
211. Freiberger, R., Killoron, P., and Cardona, G.: Arthrography of the knee by double contrast method. AJR 197:736, 1966.
212. Pudlowski, R., Gilula, L., and Murphy, W.: Arthrography. *In* Taplick, G., and Haskin, M., (eds.): Surgical Radiology. Philadelphia, W. B. Saunders Company, 1980.
213. Dalinka, M., Coren, G., and Wershba, M.: Knee arthrography. CRC Crit. Rev. Clin. Radiol. Nucl. Med. 4:1, 1973.
214. Werndoff, K., and Robinsohn, L.: Kongressverhandlung. Deutsch. Gesellsch. Orthop. 1905.
215. Anderson, P., and Maslin, P.: Tomography applied to knee arthrography. Radiology 110:271, 1974.
216. Eto, R., Anderson, P., and Harley, J.: Elbow arthrography with the application of tomography. Radiology 115:283, 1975.
217. Gilula, L.: A simplified stress device for knee arthrography. Radiology 122:828, 1977.
218. Dixon, A., and Rasher, J.: Synoviography. Clin. Rheum. Dis. 2:129, 1976.
219. Hall, F.M., Rosenthall, D.I., Goldberg, R.P., and Wyshok, G.: Morbidity from shoulder arthrography. AJR 136:59, 1981.
220. Goldberg, R.P., Hall, F.M., and Wyshok, G.: Pain on knee arthrography: Comparison of air versus $CO_2$ and reaspiration versus no reaspiration. AJR 136:377, 1981.
221. Grech, P.: Hip Arthrography. Philadelphia. J.B. Lippincott Company, 1977.
222. Neviaser, J.: Arthrography of the Shoulder. Springfield, Ill., Charles C Thomas, 1975.
223. Norman, A., and Baker, N.: Spontaneous osteonecrosis of the knee and medial meniscal tears. Radiology 129:653, 1978.
224. Pavlov, H., and Torg, J.: Double contrast arthrographic evaluation of the anterior cruciate ligament. Radiology 126:661, 1978.
225. Dalinka, M., and Garofola, J.: Infrapatella synovial fold: Cause for confusion in the evaluation of the anterior cruciate ligament. Radiology 126:661, 1978.
226. Braunstein, E.M.: Anterior aiecrote ligament injuries: A comparison of arthrographic and physical diagnosis. AJR 138:423, 1982.
227. Gilley, J.S., Geiman, M.I., Edson, M., and Metcalf, R.W.: Chondral fractures of the knee. Radiology 138:51, 1981.
228. DeSmet, A., and Neff, J: Knee arthrography for the preoperative evaluation of juxta-articular masses. Radiology 143:663, 1982.
229. Hall, A., and Scott J.: Synovial cysts and rupture of the knee joint in rheumatoid arthritis: An arthrographic study. Ann. Rheum. Dis. 25:32, 1966.
230. Wolfe, R., and Colloff, B.: Popliteal cysts: An arthrographic study and review of the literature. J. Bone Joint Surg. 54A:1057, 1972.
231. Taylor, A., and Ansell, B.: Arthrography of the knee before and after synovectomy in rheumatoid patients. J. Bone Joint Surg. 54B:110, 1972.
232. Lowenstein, M.D., Smith, J.R.V., and Cole, S.: Infrapatellar pigmented villonodular synovitis: Arthrographic detection. AJR 135:279, 1980.
233. Wolfe, R., and Giuliano, V.: Double-contrast arthrography in the diagnosis of pigmented villonodular synovitis of the knee. Radiology 110:793, 1970.
234. Goergen, T., Resnick, D., and Niwayama, G.: Localized nodular synovitis of the knee: A report of two cases with abnormal arthrograms. AJR 126:648, 1976.
235. Boven, F., DeBoeck, M., and Potvliege, R.: Synovial plicae of the knee. Radiology 147:805, 1983.
236. Killoran, P., Morcove, R., and Frieberger, R.: Shoulder arthrography. AJR 103:658, 1968.
237. Desment, A., Ting, Y., and Weiss, J.: Shoulder arthrography in rheumatoid arthritis. Radiology 116:601, 1975.
238. Kilcoyne, R.F., and Matsen, F.A.: Rotator cuff tear measurement by arthropneumotomography. AJR 140:315, 1983.
239. Andren, L., and Lundberg, B.: Treatment of rigid shoulders by joint distension during arthrography. Acta Orthop. Scand. 36:45, 1965.
240. Kinnard, P., Tricoire, J., Levesque, R., and Bergeron, D.: Assessment of the unstable shoulder by computed arthrography. Am. J. Sports Med. 11:157, 1983.
241. Braunstein, E., and O'Connor, G.: Double-contrast arthrotomography of the shoulder. J. Bone Joint Surg. 64A:192, 1982.
242. Strizak, A., and Danzig, L., Jackson, D., Greenway, G., Resnick, D., and Staple, T.: Subacromial bursography. J. Bone Joint Surg. 64A:196, 1982.
243. Gelman, M.: Arthrography in total hip prosthesis complications. AJR 126:743, 1975.
244. Murphy, W., Siegel, M., and Gilula, L.: Arthrography in the diagnosis of unexplained chronic hip pain with regional osteopenia. AJR 129:283, 1977.
245. Phillips, W.C., and Kattapuram, S.V.: Prosthetic hip replacements: Plain films and arthrography for component loosening. AJR 138:677, 1982.
246. Hendrix, R., Wixson, R., Rana, N., and Rogers, L.: Arthrography after total hip arthroplasty: A modified technique used in the diagnosis of pain. Radiology 148:647, 1983.
247. Cone, R., Yaru, N., Resnick, D., Gershuni, D., and Guerra, J.: Intracapsular pressure monitoring during arthrographic evaluation of painful hip prostheses. AJR 141:885, 1983.
248. Brostrom, L., Liljedahl, S., and Lindvall, N.: Sprained ankles. II. Arthrographic diagnosis of recent ligament ruptures. Acta Chir. Scand. 130:560, 1965.
249. Brostrom, L.: Sprained ankles. III. Clinical observations in recent ligament ruptures. Acta Chir. Scand. 130:560, 1965.
250. Goldman, A., Katz, M., and Freiberger, R.: Post-traumatic adhesive capsulitis of the ankle: Arthrographic diagnosis. AJR 127:585, 1976.
251. Sanders, H.: Ankle arthrography and ankle distortion. Radiol. Clin. 46:1, 1977.
252. Brostrom, L.: Sprained ankles. I. Anatomic lesions in recent sprains. Acta Chir. Scand. 128:483, 1964.
253. Harrison, M., Freiberger, R., and Ranawat, C.: Arthrography of the rheumatoid wrist joint. AJR 112:480, 1971.
254. Resnick, D.: Arthrography in the evaluation of arthritic disorders of the wrist. Radiology 113:331, 1974.
255. Iveson, J., Hill, A., and Wrigert, V.: Wrist cysts and fistulae. Ann. Rheum. Dis. 34:388, 1975.
256. Levinsohn, E.M., and Palmer, A.K.: Arthrography of the traumatized wrist. Radiology 146:647, 1983.
257. Rosenthal, D., Murray, W., and Smith, R.J.: Finger arthrography. Radiology 137:647, 1980.
258. Lynch, T., and Chase, D.: Arthrography in the evaluation of the temporomandibular joint. Radiology 126:667, 1978.
259. Doyle, T.: Arthrography of the temporomandibular joint: A simple technique. Clin. Radiol. 34:147, 1983.
260. Ferrucci, J.: Body ultrasonography, I and II. N. Engl. J. Med. 300:358, 590, 1979.
261. Griffiths, H., and Sarno, R.: Contemporary radiology: An introduction to imaging. Philadelphia, W.B. Saunders Company, 1979.
262. Fields, S., and Dunn, F.: Correlation of echographic visualizability of tissue with biologic composition and physicologic state. J. Accout. Soc. Am. 54:809, 1973.
263. Lemons, R., and Quate, C.: Acoustic microscopy: Biomedical applications. Science 188:905, 1975.
264. Birnholtz, J.: On maps comparing cross-sectional imaging methods. AJR 129:1133, 1977.

265. DeSantos, L.A., and Goldstein, H.: Ultrasonography in tumors arising from the spine and bony pelvis. AJR 129:1061, 1977.
266. Meire, H., Lindsay, D., Swinson, D., and Hamilton, E.: Comparison of ultrasound and positive contrast arthrography in the diagnosis of popliteal and calf swellings. Ann. Rheum. Dis. 33:221, 1974.
267. Moore, C., Sarti, D., and Louie, J.: Ultrasonographic demonstration of popliteal cysts in rheumatoid arthritis. Arthritis Rheum. 18:577, 1975.
268. Ambanelli, U., Manganelli, A., and Nervetti, A.: Demonstration of articular effusions and popliteal cysts with ultrasound. J. Rheumatol. 3:134, 1976.
269. Carpenter, J., Hattery, R., Hunder, G., Bryan, R., and McLeod, R.: Ultrasound evaluation of the popliteal space: Comparison with arthrography and physical examination. Mayo Clin. Proc. 51:498, 1976.
270. Rudikoff, J., Lynch, J., and Phillips, E.: Ultrasound diagnosis of Baker's cyst. JAMA 235:1054, 1976.
271. Cooperberg, P., Tsang, L., Truelove, L., and Knickerbocker, J.: Gray scale ultrasound in the evaluation of rheumatoid arthritis of the knee. Radiology 126:759, 1978.
272. Nomeir, A., Turner, R., Watts, E., Smith, D., and Edmonds, J.: Cardiac involvement in rheumatoid arthritis. Ann. Intern. Med. 79:800, 1973.
273. Pakroski, R., Atassi, A., Poska, R., and Rosen, K.: Prevalence of pericardial effusion and mitral valve involvement in patients with rheumatoid arthritis without cardiac symptoms. N. Engl. J. Med. 289:593, 1973.
274. Davia, J., Cherthn, M., deCastro, C., and Nievu, L.: Absence of echocardiographic abnormalities of the anterior mitral valve leaflet in rheumatoid arthritis. Ann. Intern. Med. 83:500, 1975.
275. Schorn, D., Hough, I., and Anderson, I.: The heart in rheumatoid arthritis: An echocardiographic study. S. Afr. Med. J. 50:8, 1975.
276. John, J.T., Hough, A., and Sergent, J.S.: Pericardial disease in rheumatoid arthritis. Am. J. Med. 66:38, 1979.
277. Elkayam, U., Weiss, S., and Laniado, S.: Pericardial effusion and mitral valve involvement in systemic lupus erythematosus. Ann. Rheum. Dis. 36:349, 1977.
278. Smith, J., Clements, P., Furst, D., and Ross, M.: Echocardiographic features of progressive system sclerosis. Am. J. Med. 66:28, 1979.
279. Berstein, B., Takakashi, M., and Hanson, J.: Cardiac involvement in juvenile rheumatoid arthritis. J. Paediatr. 85:313, 1974.
280. Kramer, F., Kurtz, A., Rubin, C., and Goldberg, B.: Ultrasound appearance of myositis ossificans. Skeletal Radiol. 4:19, 1979.
281. McDonald, D., and Leopold, R.: Ultrasound B-scanning in the differentiation of Baker's cyst and thrombophlebitis. Br. J. Radiol. 45:829, 1972.
282. Katz, R.S., Zizic, T.M., Arnold, W.P., and Stevens, M.D.: The pseudothrombophlebitis syndrome. Medicine 56:151, 1977.
283. Khan, M.A.: Ruptured popliteal cyst and thrombophlebitis. Arthritis Rheum. 20:1560, 1977.
284. Gordon, G.V., Edell, S., Brogadir, S.P., Schumacher, H.R., Schimmer, B.M., and Dolinka, M.: Baker's cysts and true thrombophlebitis: Report of two cases and review of the literature. Arch Intern. Med. 139:40, 1979.
285. Seltzer, S.E., Finberg, H.J., and Weissman, B.N.: Arthrosonography: Technique, sonographic anatomy, and pathology. Invest. Radiol. 15:19, 1980.
286. Basel, S.K.: Medical thermography. Bibl. Radiol. 5:12, 1968.
287. Ryan, J.: Thermography. Australas. Radiol. 8:23, 1969.
288. Hardy, J.D.: The radiation from the human body. III. The human skin as a black body radiator. J. Clin. Invest. 13:615, 1934.
289. Horvath, S.M., and Holander, J.: Intra-articular temperature as a measure of joint reaction. J. Clin. Invest. 28:469, 1949.
290. Hanson, B., Linstroni, J., Ericson, E., Laine, V., and Honsson, I.: Intra-articular temperature in man under normal and pathologic conditions. Abstr. V. Eur. Cong. Rheum. Dis., 1963.
291. Collins, A., Ring, E., Cosh, J., and Bacon, P.: Quantification of thermography in arthritis using multithermal analysis. I. The thermographic index. Ann. Rheum. Dis. 33:113, 1974.
292. Collins, A., and Ring, E.: Measurement of the inflammation in man and animals by radiometry. Br. J. Pharmacol. 44:145, 1972.
293. Bacon, P., Collins, A., Ring, F., and Cosh, J.: Thermography in the assessment of inflammatory arthritis. Clin. Rheum. Dis. 2:51, 1976.
294. Logan, W.W., and Lind, B.: Improved liquid cholesterol ester crystal thermography of the breast. J. Surg. Oncol. 8:363, 1964.
295. Crissy, J.J., Gordy, E., Ferguson, J., and Lyman, R.B.: A new technique for demonstration of skin temperature patterns. J. Invest. Dermatol. 43:89, 1970.
296. Pochaczevsky, R., and Meyers, P.H.: The value of vacuum contoured liquid crystal dynamic breast thermography. Acta Thermgraphica 4:8, 1979.
297. Albert, S., Glickman, M., and Kallish, M.: Thermography in orthopaedics. Ann. N. Y. Acad. Sci. 121:157, 1964.
298. Heinz, E., Golberg, H., and Taveras, J.: Experience with thermography in neurologic patients. Ann. N. Y. Acad. Sci. 121:177, 1964.
299. Goldberg, H., Heinz, E., and Taveras, J.: Thermography in neurological patients. Acta Radiol. 5:786, 1966.
300. Edeiken, J., Wallace, J., and Curley, R.: Thermography and herniated lumbar discs. AJR 102:790, 1968.
301. Raskin, M., Martinez-Lopez, M., and Sheldon, J.: Lumbar thermography in discogenic disease. Radiology 119:149, 1976.
302. Pochaczevsky, R., Wexler, C.E., Meyers, P.H., Epstein, J.A., and Marc, J.A.: Liquid crystal thermography of the spine and extremities: Its value in the diagnosis of spinal root syndromes. J. Neurosurg. 56:386, 1982.
303. Pochaczevsky, R.: The value of liquid crystal thermography in the diagnosis of spinal root compression syndromes. Orthop. Clin. North Am. 14:271, 1983.
304. Pochaczevsky, R.: Assessment of back pain by contact thermography of extremity dermatomes. Orthop. Rev. 12:45, 1983.
305. Namey, T.: Scintigraphy, sacroiliitis, and sciatica. Presented to the 2nd annual meeting of the Academy of Neurological Orthopaedic Surgeons, Las Vegas, November 1978.
306. Meyer, D.A., and Meyers, P.H.: Would you like to know what pain looks like? Louisiana Bar. J. 27:77, 1979.
307. Raskin, M.: Thermography of the spine. Appl. Radiol. 118:123, 1976.
308. Agarwal, A., Lloyd, K.N., and Dovey, P.: Thermography of the spine and sacroiliac joint in spondylitis. Rheumatol. Phys. Med. 10:349, 1970.
309. Scott, D., Ring, E., and Bacon, P.: Problems in the assessment of disease activity in ankylosing spondylitis. Rheumatol. Rehabil. 20:74, 1981.
310. Rajapakse, C., Grennan, D., Jones, C., and Jayson, M.: Thermography in the assessment of peripheral joint inflammation: a re-evaluation. Rheumatol. Rehabil. 20:81, 1981.
311. Alfidi, R.J., MacIntyre, W.J., Meany, T.F., Chernack, E.S., Janicki, R., Tarar, R., and Levin, H.L.: Experimental studies to determine application of CAT scanning to the human body. AJR 124:199, 1973.
312. Ambrose, J.: Computerized transverse axial scanning (tomography) II. Clinical application. Br. J. Radiol. 46:1023, 1973.
313. Boyd, D.P., Korobkin, M.T., and Moss, A.: Engineering status of computerized tomographic scanning. Optical Eng. 16:37, 1977.
314. Hounsfield, G.N.: Computerized transverse axial scanning (tomography) I. Description of a system. Br. J. Radiol. 46:1016, 1973.
315. Genant, H.K.: Computed tomography. Resnick, D., and Niwayama, G. (eds.): In Diagnosis of Bone and Joint Disorders. Philadelphia. W.B. Saunders Company, 1981, p. 380.
316. Raskin, S.P., and Keating, J.W.: Recognition of lumbar disk disease: Comparison of myelography and computed tomography. Am. J. Neuroradiol. 3:215, 1982.
317. Williams, A.L., Haughton, V.M., and Syversten, A.: Computed tomography in the diagnosis of herniated nucleus pulposus. Radiology 135:95, 1980.
318. Anand, A.K., and Lee, B.C.P.: Plain and metrizamide CT of lumbar disk disease: comparison with myelography. Am. J. Neuroradiol. 3:567, 1982.
319. Williams, J.P., Joslyn, J.N., and Butler, T.W.: Differentiation of herniated lumbar disk from bulging annulus fibrosus. Use of reformatted images. J. Comp. Assist. Tomogr. 6:89, 1982.
320. Williams, A.L., Haughton, V.M., Daniels, D.L., and Thornton, R.S.: CT recognition of lateral lumbar disk herniation. Am. J. Neuroradiol. 3:211, 1982.
321. Williams, A.L., Haughton, V.M., Daniels, D.L., and Grogan, J.P.: Differential CT diagnosis of extruded nucleus pulposus. Radiology 148:141, 1983.
322. Helms, C.A., Dorwart, R.H., and Gray, M.: The CT appearance of conjoined nerve roots and differentiation from a herniated nucleus pulposus. Radiology 144:803, 1982.
323. Roub, L.W., and Drayer, B.: Spinal computed tomography: Limitations and applications. AJR 133:267, 1979.
324. Ullrich, C.G., Binet, E.F., Sanecki, M.G., and Kieffer, S.A.: Quantitative assessment of the lumbar spinal canal by computed tomography. Radiology 134:137, 1980.
325. Ciric, I.M., Mickhael, M.A., Tarkington, J.A., and Vick, N.A.: The lateral recess syndrome: A variant of spinal stenosis. J. Neurosurg. 53:433, 1980.
326. Chafetz, N., and Genant, H.K.: Computed tomography of the lumbar spine. Orthop. Clin. North Am. 14:147, 1983.
327. Teplick, J.G., and Haskin, M.E.: Computed tomography of the postoperative lumbar spine. A.J.R. 141:865, 1983.
328. Schulbiger, O., and Valavanis, A.: CT differentiation between recurrent disc herniation and postoperative scar formation: The value of contrast enhancement. Neuroradiology 22:251, 1982.
329. Kozin, F., Carrera, G.F., Ryan, L.M., Foley, D., and Lawson, T.: Computed tomography in the diagnosis of sacroiliitis. Arthritis Rheum. 24:1479, 1981.
330. Carrera, G.F., Foley, W.D., Kozin, F., Ryan, L., and Lawson, T.L.: CT of sacroiliitis. AJR 136:41, 1981.
331. Borlaza, G.S., Seigel, R., Kuhns, L.R., Good, A.E., Rapp, R., and Martel,

W.: Computed tomography in the evaluation of sacroiliiac arthritis. Radiology 139:437, 1981.
332. DeSmet, A.A., Gardner, J.D., Lindsley, H.B., Goin, J.E., and Fritz, S.L.: Tomography for evaluation of sacroiliitis. AJR 139:577, 1982.
333. Young, A., Dixon, A., Getty, J., Renton, P., and Vacher, H.: Cauda equina syndrome complicating ankylosing spondylitis: use of electromyography and computerised tomography in diagnosis. Ann. Rheum. Dis. 40:317, 1981.
334. Grosman, H., Gray, R., and St. Louis, E.L.: CT of long-standing ankylosing spondylitis with cauda equina syndrome. Am. J. Neuroradiol. 4:1077, 1983.
335. Sage, M.R., and Gordon, T.P.: Muscle atrophy in ankylosing spondylitis: CT demonstration. Radiology 149:780, 1983.
336. Tadmore, R., Davis, K.R., Roberson, G.H., New, P.F.J., and Taveras, J.M.: Computed tomographic evaluation of traumatic spinal injuries. Radiology 127:825, 1978.
337. Rosenthal, D.I., Mankin, H.J., and Bauman, R.A.: Musculoskeletal applications for computed tomography. Bull. Rheum. Dis. 33:1, 1983.
338. Faerber, E.N., Wolpert, S.M., Scott, R.M., Belkin, S.C., and Carter, B.L.: Computed tomography of spinal fractures. J. Comput. Assist. Tomogr. 3:657, 1979.
339. Handelberg, F., Bellemans, M.A., Opdecam, P., and Castelen, P.P.: The use of computerized tomography in the diagnosis of thoracolumbar injury. J. Bone Joint Surg. 63B:336, 1981.
340. Sauser, D.D., Billimoria, P.E., Roase, G.A., and Mudge, K.: CT evaluation of hip trauma. AJR 135:269, 1980.
341. Shirkoda, A., Brasheer, H.R., and Staab, E.V.: Computed tomography of acetabular fractures. Radiology 134:683, 1980.
342. Danzig, L.A., Resnick, D., and Greenway, G.: Evaluation of unstable shoulders by computed tomography. Am. J. Sports Med. 10:138, 1982.
343. Shuman, W.P., Kilcoyne, R.F., Matsen, F.A., Rogers, J.V., and Mack, L.A.: Double-contrast computed tomography of the glenoid labrum. AJR 141:581, 1983.
344. Griffiths, H.J., Hamlin, D.J., Kiss, S., and Lovelock, J.: Efficacy of CT scanning in a group of 174 patients with orthopedic and musculoskeletal problems. Skeletal Radiol. 7:87, 1981.
345. Siegelman, S.S., Zerhoun, E.A., Leo, F.P., Khouri, N.F., and Stitik, F.P.: CT of the solitary pulmonary nodule. AJR 135:1, 1980.
346. Khun, J.P., and Berger, P.E.: Computed tomographic diagnosis of osteomyelitis. Radiology 130:503, 1979.
347. Azouz, E.M.: Computed tomography in bone and joint infections. J. Can. Assoc. Radiol. 32:102, 1981.
348. Carrera, G.F., Haughton, V.M., Syversten, A., and Williams, A.L.: Computed tomography of the lumbar facet joints. Radiology 134:145, 1980.
349. Destouet, J.M., Gilula, L.A., Murphy, W.A., and Sagel, S.S.: Computed tomography of the sternoclavicular joint and sternum. Radiology 138:123, 1981.
350. Manzione, J.V., Katzberg, R.W., Brodsky, G.L., Seltzer, S.F., and Mellins, H.Z.: Internal derangement of the temporomandibular joint: diagnosis by direct sagittal computed tomography. Radiology 150:111, 1984.
351. Rosenthal, D.I., Aronow, S., and Murray, W.T.: Iron content of pigmented villonodular synovitis detected by computed tomography. Radiology 133:409, 1979.
352. Zinman, C., and Reis, N.D.: Osteochondritis dissecans of the talus: use of high resolution computed tomography scanner. Acta Orthop. Scand. 53:697, 1982.
353. Pavlov, H., Hirschy, J., and Torg, J.S.: Computed tomography of the cruciate ligaments. Radiology 132:389, 1979.
354. Genant, H.K., and Boyd, D.: Quantitative bone mineral analysis using dual energy computed tomography. Invest. Radiol. 12:545, 1977.
355. Cann, C.E., Genant, H.K., and Young, D.R.: Comparison of vertebral and peripheral mineral losses in disuse osteoporosis in monkeys. Radiology 134:525, 1980.
356. Cann, C.E., and Genant, H.K.: Precise measurement of vertebral mineral content using computed tomography. J. Comput. Asst. Tomogr. 4:493, 1980.
357. Breatnach, E., and Robinson, P.J.: Repositioning errors in measurement of vertebral attenuation values by computed tomography. Br. J. Radiol. 56:299, 1983.
358. Miyasaka, K., Kaneda, K., Ito, T., Takai, H., Sugimoto, S., and Tsuru, M.: Ossification of spinal ligaments causing thoracic radiculomyelopathy. Radiology 143:463, 1982.
359. Deutsch, A.L., Resnick, D., Campbell, B.: Computerized tomography and bone scintigraphy in the evaluation of tarsal coalition. Radiology 144:137, 1982.
360. Dihlmann, W.: CT analysis of the upper end of the femur: The asterisk sign and ischaemic bone necrosis of the femoral head. Skeletal Radiol. 8:251, 1982.
361. Cone, R.O., Szabo, R., Resnick, D., Gelberman, R., Taleisnik, J., and Gilula, L.A.: Computed tomography of the normal soft tissues of the wrist. Invest. Radiol. 18:546, 1983.
362. Bauer, A.R., and Yutani, D.: Computed tomographic localization of wooden foreign bodies in children's extremities. Arch. Surg. 118:1084, 1983.
363. Amendola, M.A., Glazer, G.M., Agha, F.P., Francis, I.R., Weatherbee, L., and Martel, W.: Myositis ossificans circumscripta: computed tomographic diagnosis. Radiology 149:775, 1983.

# Chapter 41
# Arthroscopy

*John B. McGinty*

## INTRODUCTION

Arthroscopy is the endoscopic examination of the interior of a joint, and therefore can provide more direct diagnostic information than any other ancillary procedure. However, it must be emphasized that it cannot replace a good history, a thorough physical examination, laboratory studies, and appropriate roentgenograms. Only after a clinical impression based on these time-tested methods has been acquired should an arthroscopic examination be considered to provide additional or confirmatory information to arrive at a diagnosis.

Although the history of endoscopy goes back to Bozzini's Lichtleiter in 1805 and Nitze's[1] first cystoscope in 1876, it was not until after the development of the incandescent lamp by Edison in 1880 that other forms of endoscopy came into being. Professor Kenji Takagi[2] of Tokyo University first looked inside cadaver knees with a cystoscope in a gas medium. Between 1918 and 1931 he developed an arthroscope small enough to be practical and learned to take color photographs through his endoscopic system. In 1931 and 1934 the first papers on arthroscopy appeared in the American literature in the *Journal of Bone and Joint Surgery.*[3-5] Interest in arthroscopy faded in the western world while Masaki Watanabe was continuing Dr. Takagi's work in Tokyo, developing an array of instruments and his classic *Atlas of Arthroscopy.*[6,7] In the late 1960s, through the work of Jackson,[8-13] Casscells,[14] O'Connor,[15-18] and others, the Japanese experience was brought to the United States; fiberoptic instrumentation was developed,[1,19] techniques were established,[11, 20-26] and arthroscopy, as an accepted diagnostic procedure, flourished. Today, arthroscopy is being taught in most orthopedic and some rheumatology training programs, in seminars and workshops conducted by universities and by the American Academy of Orthopaedic Surgeons, and in fellowships and preceptorships with experts.

The techniques of arthroscopic surgery have changed the surgical approach to problems of the knee. At the present time many pathological situations can be solved utilizing arthroscopic techniques with consequent lower morbidity and fewer complications. These procedures include removal of loose bodies, synovectomy, partial meniscectomy, resection of synovial plicae, chondroplasty or shaving of articular cartilage for various types of chondromalacia, surgery for osteochondritis dissecans, and extensive debridement of the joint and lavage for osteoarthritis. Newer techniques of meniscal suture and repair of peripheral detachment, anterior cruciate ligament repair, and reconstruction are being developed. Techniques of arthroscopy are being utilized for surgical problems in other joints with increasing frequency.

**Indications.** There is no better way to establish a diagnosis of intrinsic joint pathology than to be able to see the lesion. The first indication for arthroscopy is the presence of a confusing diagnostic problem, when the specific diagnosis has not been made after history, physical examination, and laboratory and roentgenographic evaluation. The author no longer does an arthrotomy of the knee for mechanical problems without preceding it with an arthroscopy. With experience the inside of the knee can be examined better with an arthroscope than by an arthrotomy with limited exposure.

The need for tissue diagnosis is easily met arthroscopically. A tissue biopsy can be obtained blindly through the sheath of the arthroscope, or under direct vision through a single puncture by placing a smaller arthroscope and a biopsy forceps through a standard sheath.[27-29]

Planning surgical approaches is an important indication for arthroscopy. There is no better and efficient method for a surgeon to plan his approach to an intra-articular problem than to know exactly what the pathology is, and where it is located.

Finally, the need to document intra-articular pathology is an indication for arthroscopy. It is a simple matter to document lesions seen at arthroscopic examination with still photographs or television, as will be discussed later in this chapter.[30-31] Documentation is essential not only for teaching but also for medicolegal purposes, such as liability litigation and workmen's compensation arbitration.

**Contraindications.** Probably the only absolute contraindication to arthroscopy is sepsis. In the face of systemic sepsis with bacteremia, the possibility of seeding a joint contraindicates the use of arthroscopy. Overlying sepsis of the skin or subcutaneous tissue obviously must be brought completely under control before attempting an elective diagnostic procedure. On the other hand, the possibility of a septic joint is an indication for arthroscopy to inspect the synovium and articular cartilage, obtain material for culture, and irrigate the joint.

Limited joint motion may be a contraindication to arthroscopy. A certain range of motion is necessary to obtain a satisfactory examination, e.g., 30 to 75 degrees in the knee. Thorough examination requires manipulation of the joint as well as manipulation of the instrument (Fig. 41–1).

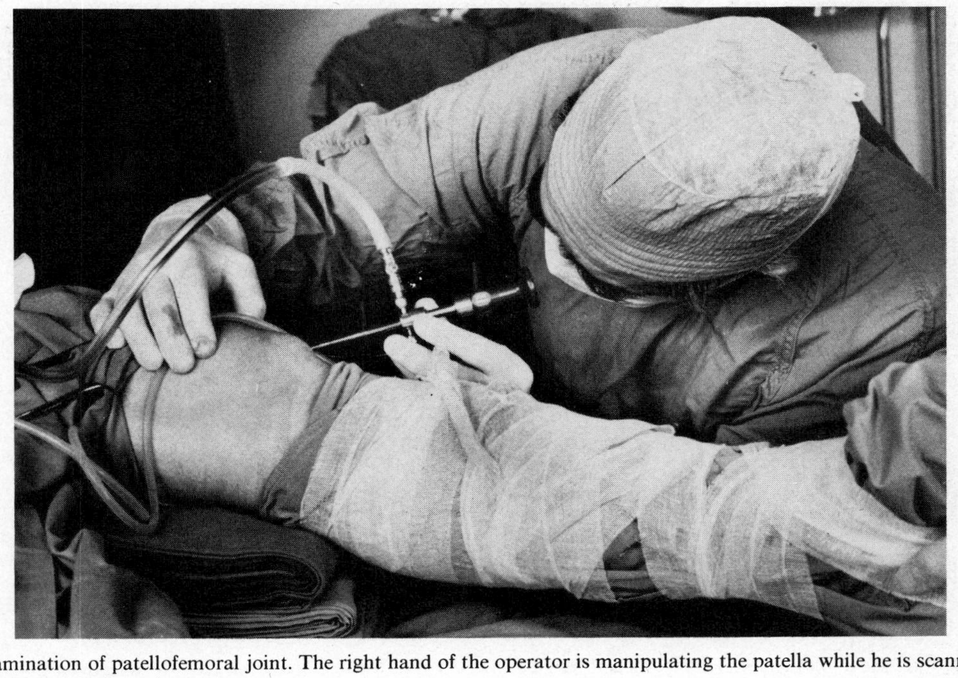

**Figure 41–1.** Examination of patellofemoral joint. The right hand of the operator is manipulating the patella while he is scanning the articular surface of the patella with the arthroscope.

Coagulation defects obviously must be identified and controlled before an arthroscopic examination is undertaken.

**Anesthesia.** Techniques for the reliable performance of arthroscopy on the ambulatory outpatient with local anesthesia have been established. The patient is brought directly to the operating room without premedication; arthroscopic examination is performed, using lidocaine and bupivacaine (Fig. 41–2); and the patient leaves the hospital immediately without external support. In this way the risk and morbidity of general anesthesia, the cost of an anesthesiologist, and time in the recovery room are eliminated.

There are certain situations in which general or spinal anesthesia is necessary. In the young child, arbitrarily, under 10 years of age, local anesthesia should probably not be used. With a very apprehensive patient or with a physician learning the procedure, local anesthesia is contraindicated. Finally, if a prolonged endoscopic procedure is contemplated, particularly if the prolonged use of a tourniquet is necessary, general or spinal anesthesia should be used.

General or spinal anesthesia is useful when doing arthroscopic surgical procedures. Local anesthesia frequently is inadequate, although it may be used in some situations. When one is performing arthroscopic surgical procedures, frequently the level of concentration and tension is such that the surgeon cannot give adequate attention to his patient who is awake and is under local anesthesia. Therefore, in this author's opinion general or spinal anesthesia is preferable in these situations.

The procedure of arthroscopy must be performed in the operating room with the same aseptic precautions as followed for arthrotomy. No infections have been reported.

**Instruments.** Many American arthroscopists learned the procedure with the Watanabe No. 21 arthroscope, an instrument illuminated with a tungsten bulb. The instrument had severe limitations: breakage of a bulb in the knee, short circuit of the fine wire filaments with consequent loss of illumination, and a hot light source requiring constant irrigation. The development of fiberoptics has made the use of tungsten illumination in endoscopy obsolete.

Today, virtually all arthroscopists use fiberoptic instrumentation. Fiberoptics allow a cool light source remote from the joint being examined. Fiberoptic arthroscopes come in different diameters, from the 1.7-mm Needlescope to a 6.0-mm operating arthroscope used for endoscopic surgery. The larger the diameter of the optical instrument, the larger the field of view, and the more light delivered for photographic exposure. There are a variety of angles of the objective lens of the arthroscope to provide different directions of orientation, from 0 to 120 degrees. The orientation for best general use, in the author's opinion, is the foreoblique (30-degree) lens, giving a larger field of view simply by rotating the instrument, but still providing enough of a direct, forward view to avoid confusion and disorientation. The 70-degree arthroscope should be part of the instrument table on the routine arthroscopic examination of the knee to provide sufficient visualization of the posterior compartments through the intercondylar notch. Biopsy forceps are available to biopsy under direct view through the same sheath, or through a second puncture.

The standard fiberoptic light source, located remote

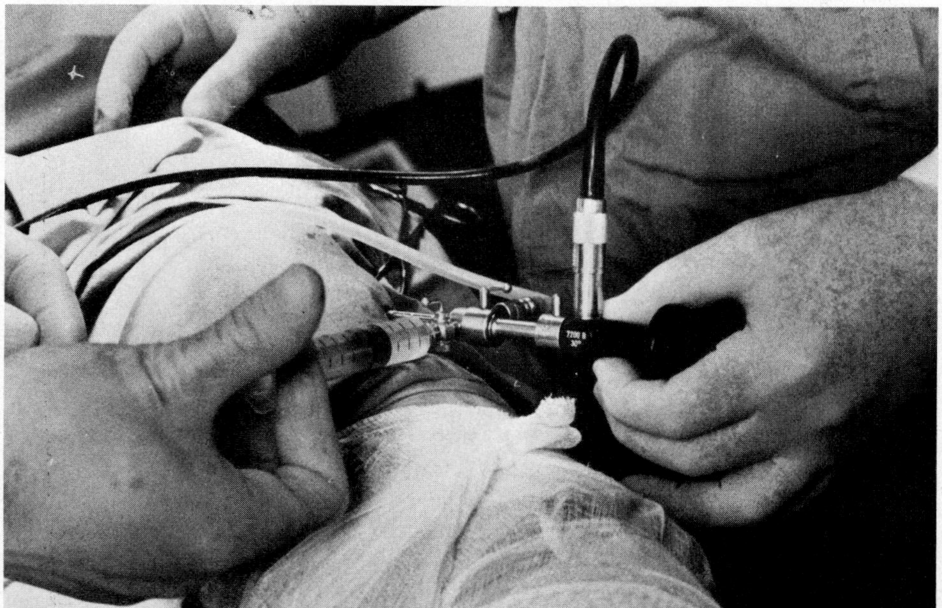

**Figure 41–2.** Procedure under local anesthesia. Lidocaine can be injected directly into knee through the sheath at any time during the procedure.

from the operating field, contains a 150-watt tungsten bulb. Although still photographs can be taken with this light source using high-speed film, a high-intensity light source is necessary for adequate use of television.

## TECHNIQUE OF ARTHROSCOPY

Arthroscopic examination can be performed on almost all joints. The knee will be used in this chapter to describe the basic technique.

The examination must be performed in the operating room with strict aseptic technique. The patient is placed in the supine position on the operating table, and the tourniquet is not used, unless endoscopic surgery or immediate subsequent surgery is anticipated. If local anesthesia is used, 4 ml of 0.5 per cent lidocaine (Xylocaine) is infiltrated into the skin, subcutaneous tissue, and capsule, followed by 5 ml intrasynovially. A 1-cm incision is made just lateral to the patellar tendon and just above the lateral joint line, and the sheath with a sharp trochar is inserted through the capsule, but not the synovium (Fig. 41–3). The sharp trochar is replaced with a blunt trochar, and the sheath is pushed into the knee, under the patella, into the suprapatellar pouch. The trochar is replaced with the arthroscope and 10 ml of 0.5 per cent bupivacaine (Marcain) is injected directly into the joint (see Fig. 41–2). Anesthesia has been adequate over an hour with these dosages, well within the margin of toxicity. If the examination is to be done with general or spinal anesthesia, 50 to 100 ml of normal saline is injected into the joint cavity before inserting the sheath.The examination is conducted using intermittent saline irrigation directly through the sheath.

The routine examination of the knee is divided into four parts. The *suprapatellar pouch and patellofemoral joint* (see Fig. 41–1) are first examined. This is an excellent location to study the character and vascularity of the synovium (Fig. 41–4; see Plate VI, p. xl). The entire undersurface of the patella can be seen by scanning with the instrument while the operator's opposite hand manipulates the patella. Similarly, the relationships of the patellofemoral joint can be observed in flexion and in extension. The arthroscope is then moved over the medial femoral condyle into the *medial compartment* (Fig. 41–5). The medial meniscus is examined anteriorly to posteriorly (Fig. 41–6; see Plate VI, p. xl). The peripheral 50 per cent of the posterior horn of the medial meniscus cannot be seen in most knees from an anterior approach. The medial femoral condyle can be seen by flexing and extending the knee. The arthroscope is then moved into the *intercondylar notch.* Again the character of the synovium is readily apparent in the notch. The anterior cruciate ligament is examined from its proximal to its distal attachment (Fig. 41–7; see Plate VI, p. xl). The posterior cruciate ligament cannot be seen from an anterior approach if the anterior cruciate ligament is intact. The extremity being examined is then crossed over the uninvolved extremity, allowing the knee to drop into varus. The arthroscope is moved into the fourth area, the *lateral compartment* (Fig. 41–8). The lateral meniscus is examined from its posterior attachment around to its anterior attachment. The popliteal tendon can be seen in the posterolateral corner. Femoral and tibial surfaces are evident by flexing and extending the knee. After conclusion of the routine examination the operator can return to areas of particular interest for further study, photographic documentation, or biopsy.

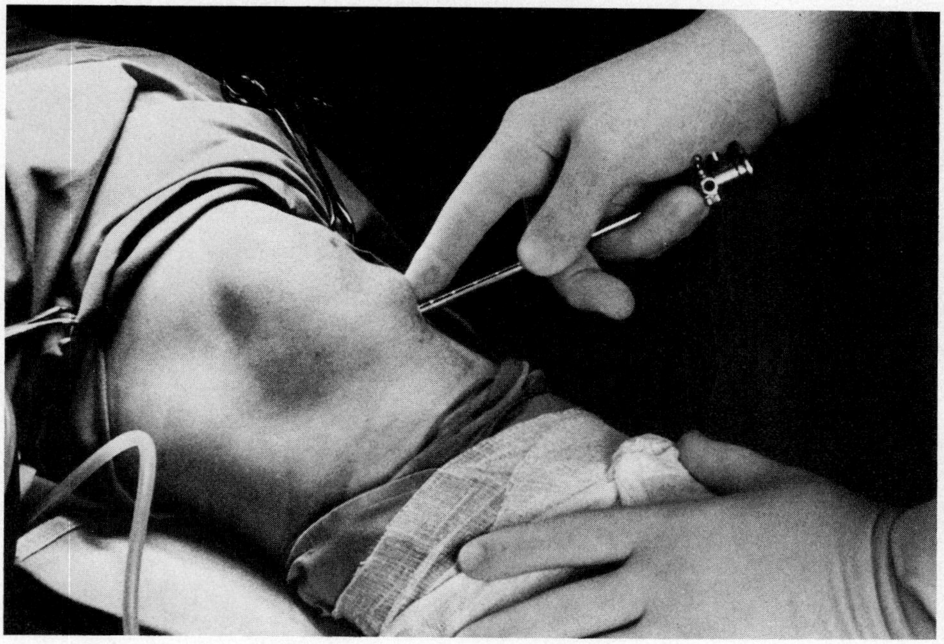

**Figure 41–3.** The index finger is used as a guard to prevent overpenetration when the sheath and trochar are inserted, thereby averting damage to the articular cartilage.

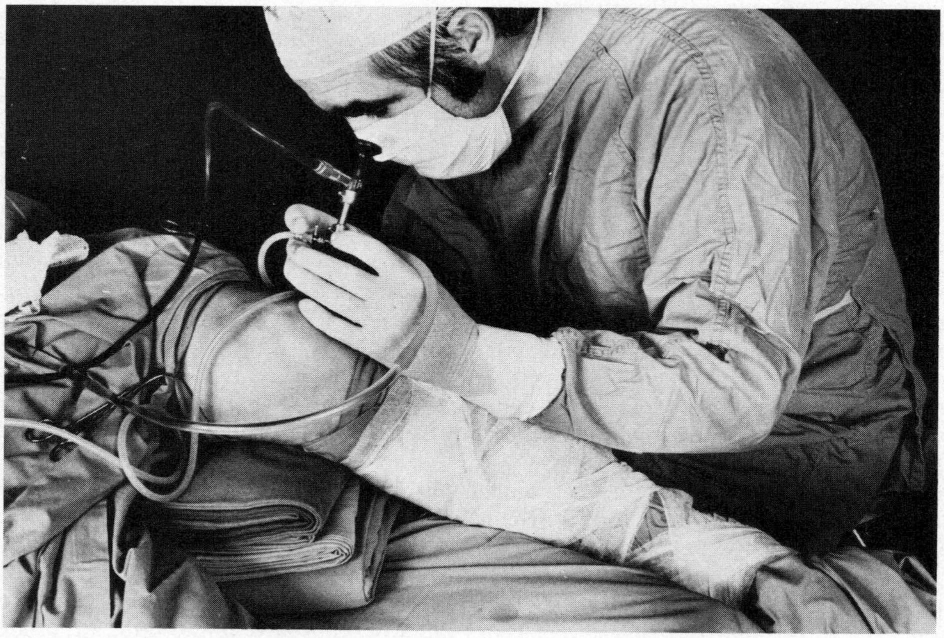

**Figure 41–5.** With the foot over the side of the table, the operator can open up the medial compartment simply by leaning on the lateral side of the knee.

It should be part of every examination of the knee to examine the posteromedial compartment. This is done most effectively through the intercondylar notch. The arthroscope is removed from the sheath, and the blunt trochar is reinserted into the sheath. The interval between the medial femoral condyle and the tibial plateau is palpated with the blunt trochar until the tip of the trochar falls into the interval between the anterior cruciate ligament and the lateral surface of the medial femoral condyle. The sheath with trochar is then maneuvered directly posteriorly and allowed to drop through that interval into the posteromedial compartment. The

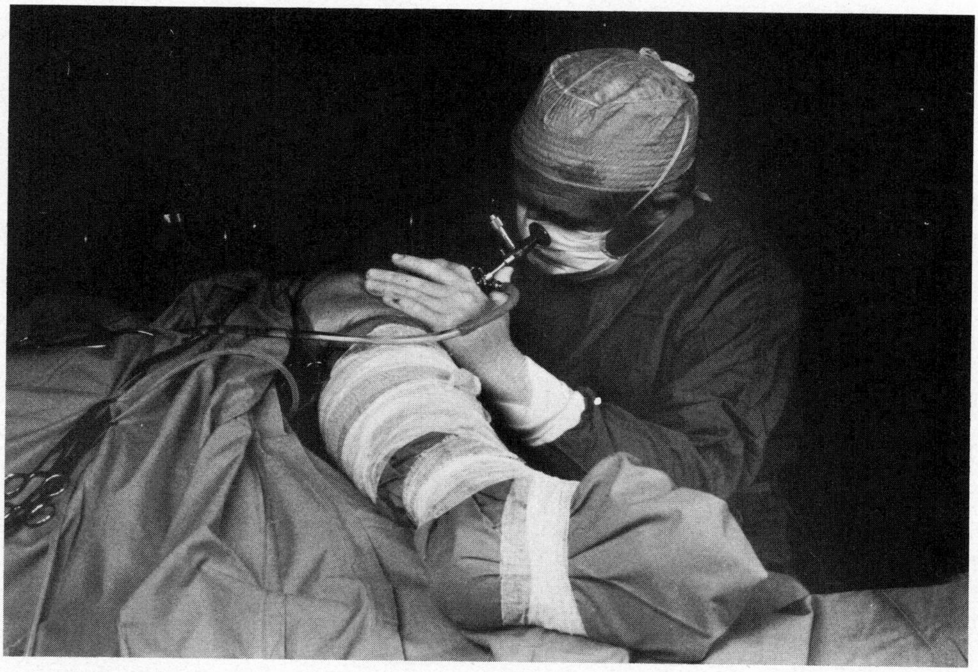

**Figure 41–8.** With the extremity in 90 degrees of flexion, gravity allows the knee to drop into varus, thereby opening the lateral compartment for better visualization.

trochar is removed, and the 70-degree arthroscope is placed in the sheath to allow visualization across the medial femoral condyle and through the entire posteromedial compartment. The compartment can then be completely inspected by rotating the arthroscope. A similar approach can be used on the lateral side of the knee by inserting the sheath between the anterior cruciate ligament and the lateral femoral condyle through an anteromedial portal. This is not necessary as a routine maneuver, inasmuch as the entire posterior horn of the medial meniscus, including the popliteus, can be inspected from the anterior approach. The posterior cruciate ligament, on the other hand, can be visualized most easily by inserting the arthroscope behind the medial collateral ligament in the posteromedial approach.

**Synovial Biopsy.** The importance of synovial biopsy cannot be overestimated in the evaluation of synovial disease. With the arthroscope, biopsy can be accomplished in three ways. Blind biopsy can be done in the suprapatellar pouch at the conclusion of the examination by inserting a biopsy forceps through the sheath after removal of the arthroscope, feeling the tip of the forceps with the other hand through the skin, and then taking the biopsy without actually seeing the tissue to be biopsied. If a particular lesion is seen during arthroscopic examination, the arthroscope is removed from the sheath, a smaller arthroscope with a biopsy forceps is reinserted through the same sheath, and a biopsy is taken under direct vision. Finally, if a particular lesion is seen and the operator wishes to keep the lesion in view, a biopsy forceps can be inserted through a second puncture wound, and the biopsy taken under direct, uninterrupted visualization.

Arthroscopic examination can be performed on most peripheral joints. The *shoulder* is usually approached posteriorly just below the spine of the scapula where it becomes the acromion. The main internal landmark is the long head of the biceps. The undersurface of the rotator cuff and the entire glenoid can be seen. The head of the humerus is visualized by taking the shoulder through a range of motion.

The *elbow* must be approached both medially and laterally to adequately visualize the capitellum, the radial head, and the trochlea. Traction on the forearm and taking the joint through a range of motion help visualization.

The *wrist* and joints of the *hand* require a small-diameter arthroscope because of the many small compartments.[32] Multiple punctures are usually required in the examination of the wrist.

The *hip* presents a different problem to the arthroscopist because of its tight twisting capsule and because so much of the femoral head is covered by the acetabulum. The examination can be facilitated by placing the patient on the fracture table and applying traction to distract the joint. The hip is then approached anteriorly one fingerbreadth below the inguinal ligament and one fingerbreadth lateral to the femoral pulse.

The *ankle* is approached anterolaterally and anteromedially, and usually a good view of the dome of the talus and the undersurface of the tibia is possible when the joint is taken through a range of motion.

The *foot* with its many small joints must be examined like the hand, with a small-diameter arthroscope.

## INTRA-ARTICULAR PATHOLOGY

Direct visualization of *synovial lesions* with an arthroscope can be quite dramatic. The arthroscope magnifies by a factor of ten at a distance of 1 mm. Therefore, detail can be seen that may not be visible to the naked eye. Color balance and vascular patterns may be very important, particularly in lesions such as rheumatoid arthritis and pigmented villonodular synovitis. Color differentiation and vascular engorgement may be obliterated if a tourniquet is used. Chondrocalcinosis and crystalline synovitis can also be observed. Proliferative synovitis, villous synovitis and synovial chondromatosis can be biopsied under direct vision[15, 33-38] (Fig. 41–9; see Plate VI, p. xl).

One author[15] has performed arthroscopic examinations with joint lavage with normal saline on 88 joints with crystalline synovitis. These joints had both urate and calcium pyrophosphate crystals. He noted marked improvement with only saline lavage in joints with and without involvement of articular cartilage compared with controls. In synovial disease arthroscopy may have therapeutic as well as diagnostic value (Fig. 41–10; see Plate VI, p. xl).

*Lesions of the patellofemoral joint* can be examined through various phases of flexion and extension, both passively and actively (under local anesthesia). Subluxation of the patella can be identified by the overhang of the lateral facet of the patella over the lateral femoral condyle. Chondromalacia can be localized, graded, followed, and in some instances treated. Osteochondral fractures can be identified and fragments replaced or removed (Fig. 41–11; see Plate VI, p. xl).

*Lesions of the meniscus* probably represent the most important pathology to be identified arthroscopically. Tears can be localized and quantitated. The recognition of a peripheral detachment, as opposed to a tear in the substance of the meniscus, is an important therapeutic differentiation, since some peripheral detachments heal and tears of the avascular fibrocartilage rarely do. The arthroscope has probably contributed to the reduction of unnecessary arthrotomies more than any other diagnostic tool. With increasing experience the arthroscopist will not remove menisci with small tears, particularly if they do not appear to be related to symptomatology. It is a simple matter to perform a second arthroscopy at a later date to see if the lesion has changed. Of even greater importance, evidence is accumulating that surgical absence of the meniscus appears to contribute to the ultimate development of degenerative arthritis of the knee.[39-46] It is becoming apparent that meniscal tears are not infrequently associated with various levels of anterior cruciate damage, resulting in some degree of rotary instability of the knee. This in all likelihood contributes to the development of degenerative change of articular cartilage and progression of osteoarthritis. Therefore, it is extremely important to preserve as much meniscal tissue as possible because of its cartilage-sparing effect in sharing the load and because of its role in stability of the knee by virtue of the meniscoligamentous complex. It has been shown that the blood supply to the meniscus itself is somewhat greater than we had previously believed. Microvascular studies have shown that vessels enter from the periphery at least one third of the way into the meniscal substance in humans. Efforts are being made at the present time to repair meniscal tears and to assess the results of such surgery (Fig. 41–12; see Plate VI, p. xl).

*Lesions of articular cartilage* can be identified and quantitated with the arthroscope and can be followed with relative ease. Osteochondritis dissecans in teenagers can be followed to the point of healing, so that if the fragment becomes loose, surgical management can be instituted. Roentgenograms show only the subchondral bone, not the overlying articular cartilage. Surgical decisions on osteotomy versus arthroplasty can be facilitated in unicompartmental degenerative arthritis by examining the "uninvolved" compartment with the arthroscope. The course of degenerative arthritis can be easily followed, leading to more rational therapeutic decisions. In rheumatoid arthritis the condition of articular cartilage can be determined prior to the surgical decision to undertake synovectomy.[40,47,48] Attempts are under way at resurfacing the articular cartilage utilizing techniques of "abrasion arthroplasty." This procedure abrades the subchondral exposed bone in osteoarthritis with the idea of revascularization and formation of a fibrocartilaginous surface. This technique is based on concepts that are in conflict with our knowledge of the healing of articular cartilage. Adequate long-term controlled follow-up studies are not yet available to document the efficacy of this procedure (Fig. 41–13; see Plate VI, p. xl).

*Lesions of ligaments* are usually the result of trauma. Arthroscopy is useful in acute trauma. Collateral ligaments, being extrasynovial, cannot be seen directly. However, damage to them may be inferred by subsynovial hemorrhage or synovial rupture. Tears of the anterior cruciate ligament are readily apparent both in the presence of acute injury and with chronic tears. The posterior cruciate ligament can also be examined anteriorly if the anterior cruciate ligament is gone, or posteromedially if the anterior cruciate ligament is intact.[16, 50-52] Procedures are being attempted to repair and reconstruct the anterior cruciate ligament by arthroscopic technique. Intra-articular arthroscopic stapling of the anterior cruciate ligament at its proximal attachment has been attempted. Most tears of the anterior cruciate ligament are interstitial and are not from one end to the other, which prevents an adequate tight repair by the utilization of surgical techniques, whether arthroscopic or open. Therefore, when one is considering the repair of anterior cruciate deficiencies, one has to also consider the possibilities of primary augmentation with some other structure. Arthroscopic attempts at reconstructing the anterior cruciate ligament using other tendons, free fascia lata grafts, and synthetic ligaments are being researched. At the present time thorough, reliable methods and controlled long-term follow-up studies are not available.

Usually *loose bodies* can be located and removed with the arthroscope. The author has removed a loose body as large as 3 cm by bringing it to a subcutaneous position and then enlarging the skin incision. Once a loose body is identified endoscopically, a grasping forceps is inserted through a second incision and the object removed.

## ACCURACY OF ARTHROSCOPY

As papers have accumulated in the literature in recent years, the reported accuracy of arthroscopy has steadily improved. In the first follow-up study in the American literature, Casscells[14] reviewed 150 cases using arthrotomy as an end point, with 80 percent accuracy. In 1972 Jackson and Abe[8] reported 90 percent accuracy in 200 cases. In 1975 Dandy and Jackson[12] reported 98.6 percent accuracy in 800 cases. DeHaven and Collins[41] did a prospective study of 100 cases comparing clinical evaluation, arthrography, and arthroscopy and reported an accuracy of 94 percent with arthroscopy. McGinty and Matza[53] reviewed 287 consecutive cases and found no difference in accuracy when arthroscopy was performed with local anesthesia compared to general or spinal anesthesia.

Most orthopedic surgeons will admit to about 80 to 85 percent accuracy in the diagnosis of abnormalities of the meniscus on clinical criteria alone. The addition of arthroscopy not only decreases the number of errors by 50 percent, it also allows the magnitude of pathology to be assessed before definitive management is undertaken. McGinty and Freedman[46] in a review of 221 consecutive arthroscopic examinations showed that one patient in three avoided arthrotomy by virtue of the arthroscopic examination.

## DOCUMENTATION IN ARTHROSCOPY

One of the major benefits of arthroscopy is the ability to easily document intra-articular pathology. With the standard endoscopic light source and a 35-mm camera, using high-speed film, good quality slides or color prints can be made for the patient's record. Documentation of findings is important in planning future surgery, as evidence in liability litigation and workmen's compensation arbitration and in teaching, both in small conferences and large meetings. It is of considerable value when a surgeon opens a knee to be able to compare the findings with a photograph from a previous arthroscopy.

With the use of a high-intensity light source videotapes can be readily made during arthroscopic examinations. Color television cameras weighing only 2 ounces are easily attached to the arthroscope either directly or through a beam splitter (85 percent of the light to the camera and 15 percent to the eye of the arthroscopist). These cameras are becoming so small that the cuplet connecting the camera to the arthroscope is larger than the camera itself. This allows the camera to sit by itself on the end of the telescope, with much easier manipulation by the arthroscopist while he is doing other procedures. With these cameras the endoscopic image can be put on a monitor so more than one individual can observe the examination, an assistant can follow a procedure on the monitor, or an instant videotape can be made.[31]

## FUTURE OF ARTHROSCOPY

The arthroscope as a diagnostic tool is well-established. Intra-articular surgery with 1-cm incisions, using the arthroscope and small instruments, is already a reality. Loose bodies are being removed; partial meniscectomies are accomplished; chondroplasties are being done for chondromalacia with small battery-powered tools; and lateral retinacular release is being performed with the arthroscope for subluxation of the patella. Arthroscopy is now carried out utilizing not only a saline medium but a gas medium of $CO_2$, which provides for a larger field of view and a somewhat more realistic appearance in comparison with that obtained with the techniques of open surgery. Newer, more efficient, and better controlled power tools are now available to tailor menisci, to remove synovium, and to trim articular cartilage. Electrosurgical and laser techniques are being utilized on humans. At the present time the use of laser techniques is extremely limited and dangerous, but refinements will undoubtedly occur. Techniques for suture of meniscal lesions are already a reality with their appropriate instrumentation.

Arthroscopy will find greater use as a research tool in following both intra-articular pathology and innovations in intra-articular surgery. Will there be a place for local chemical synovectomy under arthroscopic control? Injection of dyes to identify predegenerative lesions of articular cartilage is being tried.

The arthroscope in intra-articular surgery, like the operating microscope in neurosurgery, otolaryngology, and hand surgery, has opened up a whole new approach to intra-articular problems. The growth and potential of this approach are limited only by the imagination and zeal of its advocates.

## References

1. Berci, G.: Endoscopy. New York, Appleton-Century-Crofts, 1976.
2. Takagi, K.: Practical experiences using Takagi's arthroscope. J. Japan Orthop. Assoc. 8:132, 1933.
3. Burman, M.S.: Arthroscopy or direct visualization of joints: An experimental cadaver study. J. Bone Joint Surg. 13A:669, 1931.
4. Burman, M.S., Finkelstein, H., and Mayer, L.: Arthroscopy of the knee joint. J. Bone Joint Surg. 16A:255, 1934.
5. Finkelstein, H., and Mayer, L.: The arthroscope. A new method of examining joints. J. Bone Joint Surg. 13A:583, 1931.
6. Watanabe, M., Takeda, S., and Ikeuchi, H.: Atlas of Arthroscopy. 2nd ed. Tokyo, Igaku Shoin Ltd., 1969.
7. Watanabe, M.: The development and present status of the arthroscope. J. Japan Med. Inst. 25:11, 1954.
8. Jackson, R.S., and Abe, I.: The role of arthroscopy in the management of disorders of the knee. J. Bone Joint Surg. 54B:310, 1972.
9. Jackson, R.W.: The role of arthroscopy in the management of the arthritic knee. Clin. Orthop. 101:28, 1974.
10. Jackson, R.W., and DeHaven, K.E.: Arthroscopy of the knee. Clin. Orthop. 107:87, 1975.
11. Jackson, R.W., and Dandy, D.J.: Arthroscopy of the Knee. New York, Grune & Stratton, 1976.
12. Dandy, D.J., and Jackson, R.W.: The impact of arthroscopy in the management of disorders of the knee joint. J. Bone Joint Surg. 57B:346, 1975.
13. Dandy, D.J., and Jackson, R.W.: The diagnosis of problems after meniscectomy. Bone Joint Surg. 57B:349, 1975.
14. Casscells, S.W.: Arthroscopy of the knee joint. J. Bone Joint Surg. 53A:287, 1971.
15. O'Connor, R.L.: The arthroscope in the management of crystal induced synovitis of the knee. J. Bone Joint Surg. 55A:1443, 1973.
16. O'Connor, R.L.: Arthroscopy in the diagnosis and treatment of acute ligament injuries of the knee. J. Bone Joint Surg. 56A:333, 1974.
17. O'Connor, R.L.: Arthroscopy of the knee. Surg. Ann. 9:265, 1977.
18. O'Connor, R.L.: Arthroscopy. Philadelphia, J. B. Lippincott Company, 1977.
19. Ohnsarge, J.: Arthroscopy of the knee joint by means of glass fibers. Z. Orthop. 106:759, 1969.
20. Dorfman, H., and Dreyfus, P.: Arthroscopy of the knee. Methods and results. Minerva Med. 62:2621, 1971.
21. Eikelaar, H.R.: Arthroscopy of the Knee. Thesis for doctorate in orthopaedic surgery at the University of Groningen. The Netherlands Royal United Printers, Hoitsema, B. V., 1975.
22. Eikelaar, H.R.: Looking inside, gaining insight. Aspects of arthroscopy of the knee joint. Ned. Tijdschr. Gneeskd. 119:1882, 1975.
23. Gilliquist, J., and Hagberg, G.: A new modification of the technique of arthroscopy of the knee joint. Acta Chir. Scand. 142:123, 1976.
24. Johnson, L.L., and Becker, H.L.: Arthroscopy technique and role of the assistant. Orthop. Rev. 5:31, 1976.
25. Johnson, L.L.: Comprehensive Arthroscopic Examination of the Knee. St. Louis, C. V. Mosby Company, 1977.
26. Johnson, L.L., Schneider, D., Goodman, F., Bullock, J.M., and DeBruin, J.A., Jr.: Cold sterilization method for arthroscopes using activated dialdehyde. Orthop. Rev. 6:75, 1977.
27. Mortya, H.: The use of arthroscopy and biopsy in the diagnosis of monarticular chronic arthritis of the knee joint. Ryumachi 16:12, 1976.
28. Robles, G.J., Katona, G., and Banoso, M.R.: Arthroscopy as an aid to diagnosis and investigation. Exerpta Medica, International Congress Series 143:6, 1968.
29. Takeda, S.: Relationship between arthroscopic findings and histological change of the synovial membrane. J. Japan Orthop. Assoc. 34:373, 1960.
30. Wruhs, O.: Arthroscopy and endophotography for diagnosis and documentation of knee joint injuries. Wien. Med. 120:126, 1970.
31. McGinty, J.B.: Closed-circuit television in arthroscopy. Int. Rev. Rheumatol. special edition, pp. 45–49, 1976.
32. Watanabe, M.: Arthroscopy of small joints. J. Japan Orthop. Assoc. 45:908, 1975.
33. Andersen, R.B., and Rosse, I.: Arthroscopy of the knee joint in rheumatic diseases. Ugeskr. Laeger 135:71, 1973.
34. Camerlain, M.: Arthroscopy and its rheumatologic perspective. Union Med. Con. 103:1262, 1974.
35. Delbarre, F., Aignan, T., and Ghozlan, R.: L'arthroscopie de Genou. Institute of Rheumatology, Faculty of Medicine, Paris, Cochin, 1976.
36. Dorfman, H., and Figuerda, M.: Value of arthroscopy in isolated monoarthritis of the knee. Sem. Hop. Paris 50:179, 1974.
37. Hertel, E.: Possibilities and limits of arthroscopy of rheumatic joints. A. Orthop. 113:798, 1975.
38. Jayson, M.I., and Dixon, A.S.: Arthroscopy of the knee in rheumatic diseases. Ann. Rheum. Dis. 27:503, 1968.
39. Alm, A., Gillquist, J., and Liljedahl, S.C.: The diagnostic value of arthroscopy of the knee joint. Injury 5:319, 1974.
40. Axer, A., Segal, D., Hendel, D., Shikias, S., Rabinowitz, J., Halperin, N., Rzetelny, V., and Gershwin, D.: Arthrography and arthroscopy in the diagnosis of internal derangement of the knee. Harefuah 91:61, 1976.
41. DeHaven, K.E., and Collins, H.R.: Diagnosis of internal derangement of the knee. The role of arthroscopy. J. Bone Joint Surg. 57A:802, 1975.
42. Gallannaugh, S.: Arthroscopy of the knee joint. Br. Med. J. 3:285, 1973.
43. Glintz, W.: Arthroscopy in meniscus injuries. Z. Unfallmed. Berufskr. 69:106, 1976.
44. Kreuscher, P.H.: Semilunar cartilage disease: A plea for early recognition by means of the arthroscope and early treatment of this condition. Ill. Med. J. 47:290, 1925.
45. Norwood, L.A. Jr., Shields, C.L. Jr., Russo, J., Kerland, R.K., Jobe, F.W., Carter, V.S., Blazina, M.E., Lombardo, S.J., and DelPizzo, W.: Ar-

throscopy of the lateral meniscus in knees with normal arthrograms. Am. J. Sports Med. 5:271, 1977.
46. McGinty, J.B., and Freedman, P.A.: Arthroscopy of the knee. Clin. Orthop. 121:171, 1976.
47. Glenby, W.: Diagnostic importance of arthroscopy in prearthrosis of the knee joint. Z. Ufallmed. Berufskr. 67:260, 1974.
48. Glintz, W.: Diagnosis of chondral injury in trauma of the knee joint. Langenbechs Arch. Clin. 345:423, 1977.
49. Glintz, W.: Arthroscopy diagnoses of the traumatic cartilage lesions of the knee joint. Hefte Unfallheilkd. 129:242, 1977.
50. Gilliquist, J., Hagbey, G., and Oretrop, N.: Arthroscopy in acute injuries of the knee joint. Acta Orthop. Scand. 48:190, 1977.
51. Okmura, T.: An arthroscopic study of the traumatic disorders of the knee joint. J. Japan Orthop. Assoc. 23:28, 1945.
52. Pochling, G.G., Bassett, F.H., and Goldner, J.L.: Arthroscopy: Its role in treating non-traumatic and traumatic lesions of the knee. South. Med. J. 70:465, 1977.
53. McGinty, J.G., and Matsa, R.: Arthroscopy of the knee. J. Bone Joint Surg. 60A:787, 1978.

# Chapter 42

# Synovial Biopsy and Pathology

*H. Ralph Schumacher*

## INTRODUCTION

Biopsy of the synovial membrane should be considered in patients in whom diagnosis is not clear after clinical evaluation. Synovial fluid analysis as described in Chapter 38 should generally be performed before consideration of a biopsy if a synovial effusion can be aspirated. Examinations on synovial tissue may be the only way to make a definite diagnosis in some infectious, infiltrative, and deposition diseases of joints such as granulomatous infections, sarcoidosis, osteochondromatosis, the rare synovial leukemia or other malignancy, multicentric reticulohistiocytosis, pigmented villonodular arthritis, hemochromatosis, Whipple's disease, ochronosis, and amyloidosis. While the diagnosis of gout or pseudogout is best made by joint fluid analysis, occasionally the deposited materials or crystals are first found in synovial membrane when joint fluid is absent or not noted to contain crystals.[1]

Synovial membrane findings of villous proliferation, superficial fibrin, marked lining cell increase, focal necrosis, plasma cells, and lymphoid follicles may strongly suggest rheumatoid arthritis (RA), but are not specific. In RA as with several other systemic rheumatic diseases, diagnosis is often made by accumulation of criteria. Aid from a synovial biopsy showing a definite inflammatory process may help, as, for example, in the ARA diagnostic criteria.[2] Even if not giving a definite diagnosis, synovial biopsy by illustrating the presence or absence of inflammation may help guide symptomatic treatment. Synovial fluid findings can help in the same way, but both inflammatory and infiltrative synovial membrane lesions are not infrequently found with "noninflammatory" effusions.[3] Approximately 35 percent of needle biopsies performed in diagnostic problems are of clinical assistance.[3]

## METHODS FOR OBTAINING SYNOVIUM

**Needle Biopsy.** Probably the most popular current technique for diagnostic synovial biopsy is use of the Polley-Bickel technique[4] or one of the newer, smaller Parker-Pearson needles[3, 5] (Fig. 42–1). Needle synovial biopsy can be performed in the hospital or in the clinic or office.

The knee is by far the most frequently biopsied joint, but successful biopsies can also be obtained from shoulders, elbows, wrists, ankles, olecranon bursae, and occasionally even smaller joints if they are sufficiently swollen. The route of entry is generally that described for arthrocentesis. The procedure can be performed by a single operator with one assistant. Meperidine is occasionally used for very anxious patients. Young children may even need general anesthesia. The biopsy area is widely prepared with soap and then iodine, and washed with alcohol. The operator then dons gloves and drapes a transparent plastic drape with a 2-inch hole over the biopsy site. The skin and subcutaneous tissue is infiltrated to the capsule with 1 percent lidocaine, using a 25-gauge needle. Caution is exercised to avoid instilling anesthetic into the joint space, which would distort the synovianalysis findings. Next, either the trochar or a 20- to 22-gauge needle is forcefully thrust through the anesthetized area into the joint space. We previously always inserted the smaller needle first but now often find it acceptable to most patients to use only the trochar and avoid the additional insertion. Fluid is aspirated for synovianalysis through the trochar or needle. It is not necessary to distend the joint with fluid. Two to 4 ml of 1 percent lidocaine can be instilled into the joint space, but biopsy can also be done without this if it is felt important to avoid any possible artifact that might be introduced by the local anesthetic. The biopsy needle is now inserted through the outer needle. The side with the hooked notch is approximated against the synovium, and suction is applied with a 20- to 50-ml Luer-lock syringe. The needle is always directed away from the site of initial lidocaine infiltration, to avoid possible artifacts in this area. Three to eight specimens (to minimize sampling error) from the various parts of the joint are taken by angling the needle without reinserting the outer needle. Suction is maintained with one hand on the syringe while the other retracts the inner

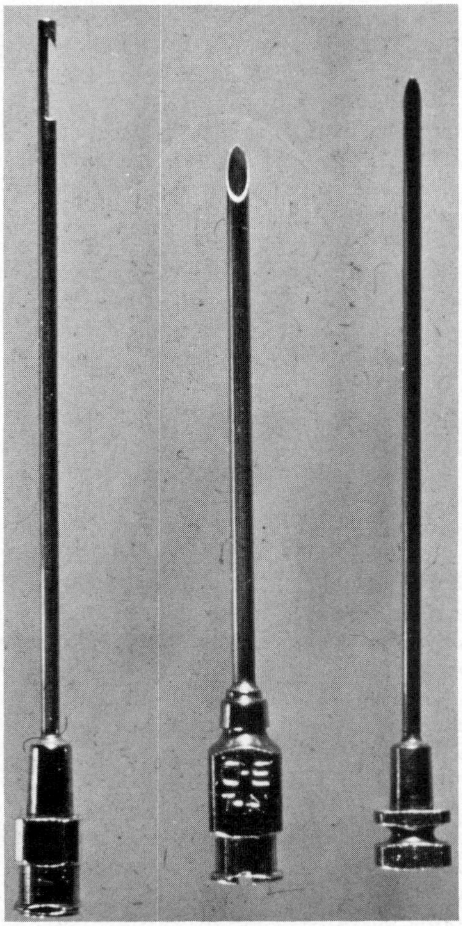

**Figure 42–1.** Parker-Pearson synovial biopsy needle. The hooked biopsy needle on the left is inserted through the center 14-gauge needle, and tissue is drawn into the notch proximal to the hook by suction.

needle through the outer with a slight twist. The outer needle remains in place. One must become familiar with the appearance of the specimens, so as not to mistake fibrin or necrotic material (yellow-white) for synovial tissue (pink). Specimens may be transferred carefully from the needle by a 25-gauge needle to the fixative on a small piece of sterile paper.

Patients are instructed to rest biopsied joints until the following day, when they are permitted to resume usual activity, providing no increased pain or swelling has been noted. Hemarthrosis and infection are theoretical complications, but only two patients of more than 400 in our series have had hemarthrosis that required aspiration the next day for pain relief. There are reports of needle tips breaking off in the joint.[6] Care must be taken before biopsy to check that the needle fits easily through the trochar and that the tip is not bent or weakened.

Other needles that have been used for synovial biopsy are those of Cope, Williamson,[7] and Franklin and Silverman.[8]

**Other Methods for Obtaining Synovial Biopsies.** ***Arthroscopy.*** This allows the advantage of identifying discrete localized lesions which can then be biopsied with a needle technique under direct visualization. The procedure is generally limited to larger joints.

***Open Surgical Biopsy.*** If one is concerned about the possibility of focal granulomas, deeper lesions such as a vasculitis in larger capsular vessels, or other lesions that might have been missed on a needle biopsy, open surgical biopsy can be considered. Surgical biopsy is also very useful at small joints not suitable for needle biopsy. A small incision over a metacarpophalangeal joint is very effective and offers virtually no morbidity.

Open biopsy even of a knee can be done with a small incision; but if one wants the advantage of the full joint exploration, a large surgical incision and some postoperative immobilization are obviously needed.

***Fragments of Synovial Membrane.*** Synovial membrane fragments can occasionally be found floating in joint fluid after arthrocentesis. These can be examined in a wet smear for crystals and can also be collected by centrifugation and fixed for processing as with any biopsy.

## METHODS OF HANDLING TISSUE

The multiple small pieces of synovium from needle biopsy or the large specimens obtained at operation should be distributed among several methods of handling, depending on the questions being asked. Specimens for routine light microscopy are placed into neutral buffered formalin or Bouin's fixative. Some slides should be stained with hematoxylin and eosin and other tissue saved for consideration of special stains. If gout is a possibility, a portion of the biopsy should be placed in absolute alcohol, since urates are water soluble. Specimens thus should be processed without water and stained with the DeGolantha stain for urate or sections examined with compensated polarized light. Frozen sections of unfixed biopsies can also be used for polarized light examination for urates.

Immunofluorescent study of synovium has not been of any convincing clinical value but is of research interest. One study[9] suggested that demonstration of synovial IgM deposition favored the diagnosis of rheumatoid arthritis. Specimens for this study should be placed in saline until transferred to O.C.T. compound (Miles Laboratories) on a cryostat chuck which is then quick frozen by immersion in liquid nitrogen.

Electron microscopy (EM) of synovium is also largely of research interest. For example, it can show electron-dense deposits in vessel walls in early rheumatoid arthritis[10] and in palidromic rheumatism[11] and also in the syndrome of hypertrophic pulmonary osteoarthropathy[12] (Fig. 42–2). EM may be a major diagnostic aid in identifying apatite crystals (Fig. 42–3), viruses, small amounts of amyloid, bacilliform bodies of Whipple's disease, and Gaucher cell tubules. Any specimen for EM should be placed immediately in a fixative such as 3 percent glutaraldehyde or half-strength Karnovsky's fixative.[13] Specimens should be minced into 0.5 ×

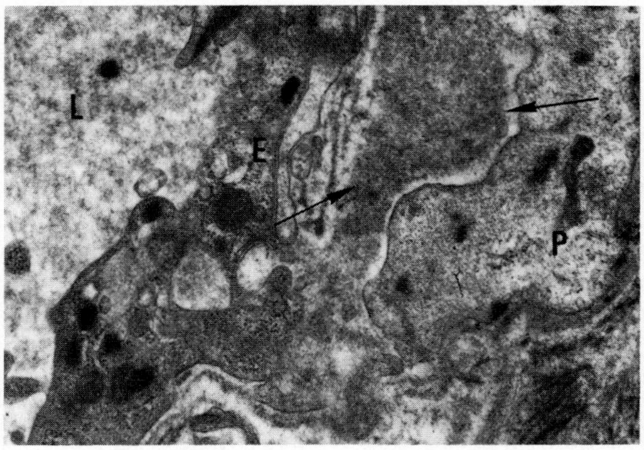


**Figure 42–2.** Electron-dense deposit (arrows) in vessel wall of synovium of patient with rheumatoid arthritis of recent onset. E = vascular endothelium, L = lumen, P = pericyte. Electron micrograph × 16,000.

0.5 mm pieces, ideally fixed for up to 4 hours, and then switched into a buffer before further processing.

Culture of synovial membrane can on occasion be more useful than that of synovial fluid, especially with mycobacteria, fungi, and gonococci. Techniques for cultures are described in Chapter 38. Synovial membrane can also be grown in tissue culture for investigative purposes. Biopsies for this are placed promptly in tissue culture medium and taken to the laboratory.

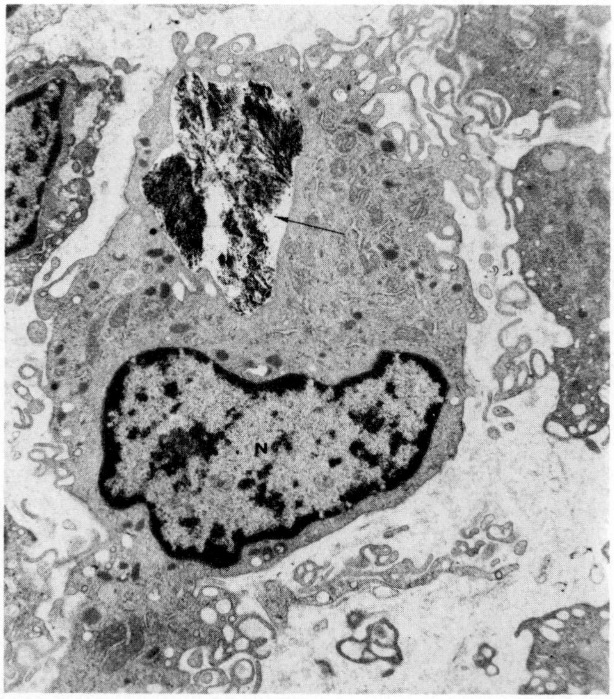


**Figure 42–3.** Apatite crystals (arrow) in vacuole of a synovial lining cell in a patient with osteonecrosis of the knee. N = nucleus of cell. Electron micrograph × 17,000.

## FINDINGS ON LIGHT MICROSCOPIC EXAMINATION OF SYNOVIAL BIOPSIES

**Normal.** Normal synovial membrane (Fig. 42–4; see Plate VII, p. xli) consists of one or two layers of synovial lining cells overlying a richly vascular areolar or fibrous connective tissue. A biopsy containing several pieces of normal synovium does not absolutely exclude intra-articular disease, but should direct the search toward very focal disease or extrasynovial processes. Failure to identify a characteristic lesion does not exclude the diagnosis of the diagnosable diseases listed in the Introduction. For example, gouty, tuberculous, or ochronotic synovium can show only mild proliferation or changes indistinguishable from rheumatoid arthritis in tissue adjacent to a tophus, granuloma, or typical pigmented shard.

**Rheumatoid Arthritis and "Variants."** In rheumatoid arthritis the combination of villous hypertrophy, lining cell proliferation, infiltration by lymphocytes and plasma cells (Fig. 42–5; see Plate VII, p. xli) with a tendency to form "lymphoid nodules," fibrin deposition, and focal necrosis is typical. This is not diagnostic with similar changes seen sometimes in systemic lupus erythematosus (SLE) and other diseases. Especially in RA of very recent onset all the aforementioned findings may not be present, and vascular occlusion or mild vasculitis may be prominent.[10]

Rheumatoid nodules are only very rarely seen in synovium. There may be multinucleated giant cells beneath the lining cells.

Psoriatic arthritis and ankylosing spondylitis can show synovial changes indistinguishable from RA. Early Reiter's syndrome[13] has a typical superficial congestion and polymorphonuclear leukocyte infiltration, which can, however, also be seen in some early RA, Behçet's disease,[14] and regional enteritis, as well as other conditions. Chronic Reiter's syndrome synovium is indistinguishable from that of RA.

**Collagen-Vascular Diseases.** The synovial membrane in SLE typically shows less intense lining cell hyperplasia and less leukocyte infiltration than in RA,[15, 16] although, as noted above, inflammation may occasionally mimic RA. In polyarteritis synovial inflammation is usually mild and inflammatory cell infiltration of medium-sized vessel walls is only a rare finding.[17] Early scleroderma[18] shows sparse lining cells, superficial fibrin, and chronic inflammatory cell infiltration (Fig. 42–6; see Plate VII, p. xli). Similar findings with paucity of lining cells can be seen also in some SLE, polymyositis, rheumatic fever, and some infections. In later scleroderma synovial fibrin and fibrosis predominate.

**Infectious Arthritis.** Infection is one of the types of joint disease that can be definitively diagnosed by synovial biopsy.[19] In acute bacterial arthritis clusters or sheets of neutrophils can be seen (Fig. 42–7). Bacteria can sometimes be demonstrated in synovium with a tissue Gram's stain. Cultures may be positive on synovial biopsy specimens even when they have been negative on

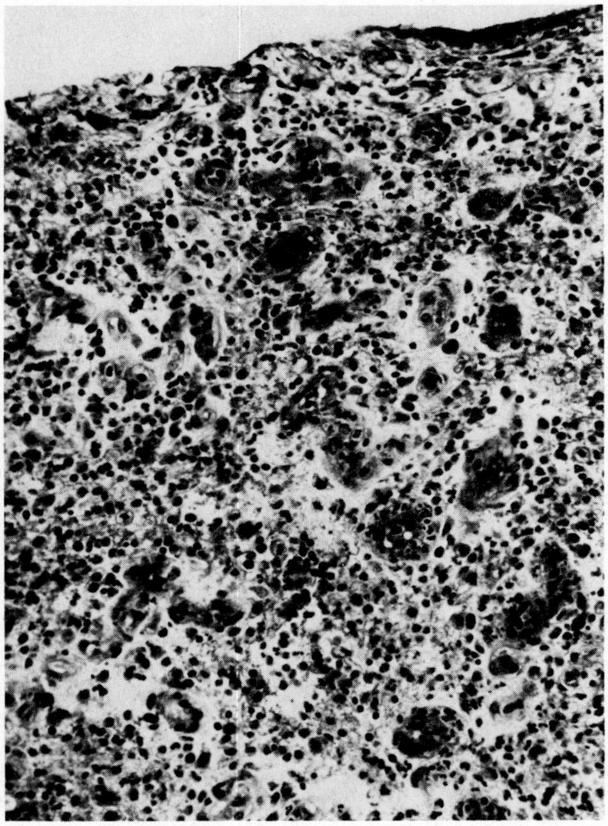

**Figure 42–7.** Massive infiltration of synovium with neutrophils and some lymphocytes in untreated septic arthritis of 10 days' duration. × 100. Hematoxylin and eosin stain.

blood and synovial fluid.[20] In chronic or resolving infections there are often large numbers of lymphocytes and plasma cells.

Chronic infections such as tuberculosis and fungus disease can produce focal lesions that may be missed on limited biopsies. Mycobacterial granulomas in the superficial synovium do not always show caseation (Fig. 42–8; see Plate VII, p. xli). Ziehl-Neelsen and Kinyoun's stains can show acid-fast organisms. Staining for fungi should be attempted with Grocott and Gridley stains. Treponemes can be sought in secondary syphilis with fluorescent and silver stains. Only a mild nonspecific synovitis has been seen in three cases of secondary syphilis.

**Sarcoidosis.** Sarcoidosis can involve the synovium with typical granulomas,[21] but other patients, especially those with erythema nodosum, more often have predominantly periarthritis or only scattered lymphocytes in the synovium.

**Infiltrative or Deposition Diseases.** These diseases have specific findings that are amenable to diagnosis by synovial biopsy.

*Crystal-Induced Arthritis.* Both gout and pseudogout often have tophuslike deposits in synovial membrane (Fig. 42–9; see Plate VII, p. xli). Precautions for tissue handling to demonstrate urate tophi are described above. Calcium pyrophosphate crystals are not as water soluble but can be dissolved by decalcification in specimens submitted along with bone. Thus pseudogout synovium occasionally can have lucent areas where crystals were lost, as in gout. Usually only a fibrous capsule, a few histiocytes, and giant cells surround the tophi. In acute crystal-induced arthritis there are areas of neutrophil infiltration, but in chronic disease large numbers of lymphocytes and plasma cells can be seen. Clumps of apatite crystals in synovium can appear as hematoxyphilic areas.[22] The tiny crystals forming these clumps are identifiable by EM. Oxalate crystals have also recently been found as pleomorphic birefringent bodies in synovium of one patient receiving chronic hemodialysis for chronic renal failure.[23]

*Amyloidosis.* In patients with primary amyloidosis, multiple myeloma, and Waldenström's disease amyloid can be deposited in the synovium. This appears pink on hematoxylin and eosin stain, and red with Congo red. The Congo red–stained material has an apple-green birefringence when viewed with plain polarized light.[24] In our experience most amyloid has been on the synovial surface (Fig. 42–10; see Plate VIII, p. xlii) and in the interstitium, but rarely in vessel walls.

*Ochronosis.* The synovial membrane in ochronosis is embedded with brownish-pigmented shards from the friable cartilage[25] (Fig. 42–11; see Plate VIII, p. xlii). Macrophages adjacent to the cartilage fragments often contain pigment granules. Clusters of lymphocytes can also be seen and can also be found in areas of synovium in other patients with cartilage degeneration, such as in primary or secondary osteoarthritis. It should be noted that cartilage and bone fragments without the ochronotic pigment can also be seen embedded in synovium in osteoarthritis, rheumatoid arthritis, and other destructive arthropathies.[26]

*Hemochromatosis.* Golden-brown hemosiderin pigment deposition in synovial lining cells and to a lesser degree in deeper phagocytes is characteristic of hemochromatosis[27] and other diseases with systemic iron overload. Iron in synovium from bleeding into the joint space or extravasation of erythrocytes into tissue produces hemosiderin mainly in deep macrophages. Iron stains blue with Prussian blue for confirmation (Fig. 42–12; see Plate VIII, p. xlii). Calcium pyrophosphate crystals can be seen in these synovia as well as in several other metabolic joint diseases.

**Tumors.** A variety of benign and malignant tumors or tumor-like conditions can involve the synovial membrane. Metastatic malignancies are occasionally identified in synovium.[28] Blast forms have been found infiltrating synovium in a few but by no means all patients with leukemia or lymphoma and arthritis.[29] Malignant synovioma is an extra-articular tumor that is very rarely seen in joint synovium. Osteochondromas developing in synovium can be seen as foci of osteo- and chondrometaplasia in the synovial connective tissue. Pigmented villonodular synovitis, generally involving a single joint or tendon sheath, is characterized by giant cells, foamy cells, and hemosiderin deposits predominantly in the

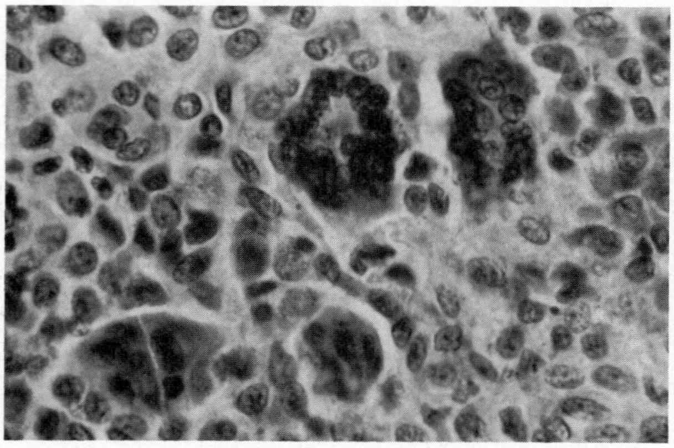

**Figure 42–13.** Giant cells, foam cells, and hemosiderin deposits are seen in pigmented villonodular synoistes. Some areas contain lymphocytes and plasma cells.

deep synovium (Fig. 42–13; see Plate VIII, p. xlii). There is villous or nodular proliferation with areas also showing some lymphocytes and plasma cells.

**Other Diseases.** ***Multicentric Reticulohistiocytosis*** [30] shows extensive infiltration of synovium with large foamy cells and/or multinucleated cells with eosinophilic "ground glass" cytoplasm.

***Whipple's Disease.*** Whipple's disease synovial membrane often shows just mild lining cell hyperplasia and scattered lymphocytes and neutrophils, but PAS-positive macrophages can be seen in some cases to suggest the diagnosis.[31] EM can suggest the typical bacilliform bodies.[32]

***Hypertrophic Osteoarthropathy (HPO).*** Despite large painful effusions, HPO tends to have virtually no inflammatory cell infiltration in synovium but marked vascular congestion in early disease.[12] Electron-dense deposits in vessel walls can be seen in some biopsies by EM. In chronic HPO lymphocytic infiltration is reported.

***Scurvy.*** Scurvy of the synovium shows edema, extravasation of erythrocytes, and large fibrocytes that have been unable to release their collagen precursors because of the lack of vitamin C.[33]

***Familial Arthropathy.*** A familial arthropathy with synovial coating with fibrin-like material and giant cells has been described in children.[34]

***Sickle Cell Disease.*** Synovium in sickle cell disease can show obliterated vessels and occasionally some lymphocyte and plasma cell infiltration.[35]

***Exogenous Particles.*** Thorns or animal spines can occasionally penetrate into joints and be visible in biopsies as well as producing a chronic synovitis.[36] Metallic or plastic particles in patients with joint arthroplasties can also occasionally be found in synovium.[37]

***Pancreatic Disease.*** Synovial fat necrosis and lipid laden macrophages can be associated with pancreatic disease.[38] Rare, unexpected new findings will occasionally be encountered if undiagnosed cases are biopsied. For example, an eosinophilic infiltration with fibrin deposition was found in a case later determined to have the hypereosinophilic syndrome.[39]

## CONCLUSIONS

Synovial biopsy specimens obtainable by a variety of mechanisms can give specific diagnoses in some diseases or can provide additional criteria supporting diagnoses in other situations. Careful consideration of the questions to be asked before performing a diagnostic biopsy will allow optimal handling of the tissue.

## References


1. Agudelo, C., and Schumacher, H.R.: The synovitis of acute gouty arthritis. Hum. Pathol. 4:265, 1973.
2. Ropes, M.W., Bennett, G.A., Cobbs, S., et al.: 1958 revision of diagnostic criteria for rheumatoid arthritis. Arthritis Rheum. 2:16, 1959.
3. Schumacher, H.R., and Kulka, J.P.: Needle biopsy of the synovial membrane. Experience with the Parker-Pearson technique. N. Engl. J. Med. 286:416, 1972.
4. Polley, H.F., and Bickel, W.H.: Punch biopsy of synovial membrane. Ann. Rheum. Dis. 10:277, 1951.
5. Parker, R.H., and Pearson, C.M.: A simplified synovial biopsy needle. Arthritis Rheum. 6:172, 1963.
6. Bocanegra, T.S., McClelland, J.J., Germain, B.F., et al.: Intraarticular fragmentation of a new Parker-Pearson synovial biopsy needle. J. Rheum. 7:248, 1980.
7. Williamson, N., and Holt, L.P.T.: A synovial biopsy needle. Lancet 1:799, 1966.
8. Moon, M-S., Kim, I., and Kim, J-M.: Synovial biopsy by Franklin-Silverman needle. Clin. Orthop. 150:224, 1980.
9. Bayliss, C.E., Dawkins, R.L., Cullity, G., et al.: Laboratory diagnosis of rheumatoid arthritis. Ann. Rheum. Dis. 34:395, 1975.
10. Schumacher, H.R.: Synovial membrane and fluid morphologic alterations in early rheumatoid arthritis: Microvascular injury and virus-like particles. Ann. N.Y. Acad. Sci. 256:39, 1975.
11. Schumacher, H.R.: Palindromic onset of rheumatoid arthritis. Clinical, synovial fluid and biopsy studies. Arthritis Rheum. 25:361, 1982.
12. Schumacher, H.R.: The articular manifestations of hypertrophic pulmonary osteoarthropathy in brochogenic carcinoma. Arthritis Rheum. 19:629, 1976.
13. Karnovsky, M.J.: A formaldehyde-glutaraldehyde fixative of high osmolality for use in electron microscopy (abstr.). J. Cell. Biol. 27:441A, 1965.
14. Abdou, N.I., Schumacher, H.R., Colman, R.W., et al.: Behçet's disease: Possible role of secretory component deficiency, synovial inclusions and fibrinolytic abnormality in the various manifestations of the disease. J. Lab. Clin. Med. 91:409, 1978.
15. Goldenberg, D.L., and Cohen, A.S.: Synovial membrane histopathology in the different diagnosis of rheumatoid arthritis, gout, pseudogout, systemic lupus erythematosus, infectious arthritis and degenerative joint disease. Medicine 57:239, 1978.
16. Labowitz, R., and Schumacher, H.R.: Articular manifestations of SLE. Ann. Intern. Med. 74:911, 1974.
17. Smukler, N.M., and Schumacher, H.R.: Chronic non-destructive arthritis associated with cutaneous polyarteritis. Arthritis Rheum. 20:1114, 1977.
18. Schumacher, H.R.: Joint involvement in progressive systemic sclerosis (scleroderma). Am. J. Clin. Pathol. 60:593, 1973.
19. Schumacher, H.R.: Joint pathology in infectious arthritis. Clin. Rheum. Dis. 4:33, 1978.
20. Wofsy, D.: Culture-negative septic arthritis and bacterial endocarditis. Diagnosis by synovial biopsy. Arthritis Rheum. 23:605, 1980.
21. Sokoloff, L., and Bunim, J.J.: Clinical and pathological studies of joint involvement in sarcoidosis. N. Engl. J. Med. 260:841, 1959.
22. Reginato, A.J., and Schumacher, H.R.: Synovial calcification in a patient with collagen-vascular disease. Light and electron microscopic studies. J. Rheumatol. 4:261, 1977.
23. Hoffman, G.S., Schumacher, H.R., Paul, H., et al.: Calcium oxalate microcrystalline-associated arthritis in end-stage renal disease. Ann. Intern. Med. 97:36–42, 1982.
24. Canoso, J.J., and Cohen, A.S.: Rheumatological aspects of amyloid disease. Clin. Rheum. Dis. I:149, 1975.
25. Schumacher, H.R., and Holdsworth, D.E.: Ochronotic arthropathy. Semin. Arthritis Rheum. 6:207, 1977.
26. Resnick, D., Weisman, M., Goergan, T.G., and Feldman, P.S.: Osteolysis with detritic synovitis. Arch. Intern. Med. 138:1003, 1978.

27. Schumacher, H.R.: Ultrastructural characteristics of the synovial membrane in idiopathic hemochromatosis. Ann. Rheum. Dis. 31:465, 1972.
28. Goldenberg, D.L., Kelley, W., and Gibbons, R.B.: Metastatic adenocarcinoma of synovium presenting as an acute arthritis. Arthritis Rheum. 18:107, 1975.
29. Spilberg, I., and Meyer, G.J.: The arthritis of leukemia. Arthritis Rheum. 15:630, 1972.
30. Krey, P.R., Comerford, F.R., and Cohen, A.S.: Multicentric reticulohistiocytosis. Arthritis Rheum. 17:615, 1974.
31. Delcambre, B., Luez, J., Leonardelli, J., et al.: Les manifestations articulaires de la maladie de Whipple. Semin. Hop. Paris 50:847, 1974.
32. Rubinow, A., Canoso, J.J., Goldenberg, D.L., and Cohen, A.S.: Synovial fluid and synovial membrane pathology in Whipple's disease. Arthritis Rheum. 19:820, 1976.
33. Bevilaqua, F.A., Hasselbacher, P., and Schumacher, H.R.: Scurvy and hemarthrosis. JAMA 235:1874, 1976.
34. Athreya, B., and Schumacher, H.R.: Pathologic features of a recently recognized form of familial arthropathy. Arthritis Rheum. 21:429, 1978.
35. Schumacher, H.R.: Rheumatological manifestations of sickle cell disease and other hereditary hemoglobinopathies. Clin. Rheum. Dis. 1:37, 1975.
36. Schumacher, H.R., and Majno, G.: Thorns in the skin and joints of monkeys. Arch. Pathol. 84:536, 1967.
37. Kitridou, R.C., Schumacher, H.R., Sbarbaro, J.L., and Hollander, J.L.: Recurrent hemarthrosis after knee arthroplasty. Arthritis Rheum. 12:520, 1969.
38. Smukler, N.M., Schumacher, H.R., Pascual, E., et al.: Synovial fat necrosis associated with ischemic pancreatic disease. Arthritis Rheum. 22:547, 553, 1979.
39. Brogadir, S.P., Goldwein, M.I., and Schumacher, H.R.: A hypereosinophilic syndrome mimicking rheumatoid arthritis. Am. J. Med. 69:799, 1980.

# Chapter 43
# The Acute Phase Reactants

*Irving Kushner*

## THE ACUTE PHASE RESPONSE IN MAN

**General Characteristics of Acute Phase Proteins.** The concentration of a number of plasma constituents is substantially altered within the first few days following an inflammatory stimulus, as part of the general systemic and metabolic response to tissue injury and infection.[1] These alterations are referred to collectively as the *acute phase response.* Major increases are noted in the concentrations of a heterogeneous group of plasma proteins; these *acute phase proteins* will be the primary focus of this chapter.[2,3,3a] Very low density lipoproteins and triglyceride concentrations rise, while high density lipoprotein levels fall.[4,5] In addition, there are changes in concentration of the cations copper, zinc, and iron.[6,7,8] Finally, alterations are noted in concentration of fibronectin[9,10] and of a group of substances originally recognized because of their biologic activities, at times due to substances whose precise chemical nature is still poorly defined.[11,12,13] A number of functional activities have been found to be due to factors that have the characteristics of interleukin I and endogenous pyrogen.[14-17] If the inflammatory stimulus is self-limited, there is a return of acute phase proteins to normal levels within a matter of days or weeks, while persisting tissue alterations may often lead to similarly persisting "acute phase" plasma changes.

The best studied human acute phase proteins are listed in Table 43–1. With the exception of C-reactive protein (CRP) and SAA protein, neither of which is glycosylated, these proteins are glycoproteins with carbohydrate contents ranging between 2.7 and 42 percent. SAA is an apoprotein and circulates in plasma with the high density lipoproteins.[19]

Following appropriate stimuli the concentrations of acute phase proteins rise to levels at least 25 percent greater than normal. In the cases of SAA protein and C-reactive protein several hundredfold increases above concentrations seen in some normal individuals occur commonly and concentrations one-thousandfold or more above these levels may be seen with severe infections.[20,21] A number of other human plasma proteins, including several complement components, have been reported to display acute phase behavior; in general they have not been as well studied as the proteins tabulated.[1] There is great species variability in the acute phase response. The major acute phase reactants in man are CRP and SAA. These acute phase changes are of great interest, both because their measurement can be of clinical value and because of the questions they raise concerning the mechanisms governing their changes in concentration and the functions served by these proteins.

**Varieties of Stimuli.** The acute phase response has been noted following a large variety of inflammatory or injurious stimuli. These include surgical or other trauma, acute myocardial infarction, pulmonary embolism, dissecting aneurysm of the aorta, bone fracture, and injection of typhoid vaccine, among others. Many acute bacterial infections, including pneumococcal pneumonia, streptococcal pharyngitis, salpingitis, pyelonephritis, and peritonitis elicit the acute phase response. It has recently been emphasized that severe viral infections can similarly elicit an increase in C-reactive protein and SAA levels.[22,23,24] Increased concentrations of the acute phase proteins are seen in acute abdominal crises (such as cholecystitis and pancreatitis), in a number of connective tissue diseases, including rheumatic fever and rheumatoid arthritis, and in some patients with advanced malignancies. Marked physical exertion can also lead to the acute phase response.[24a]

**Table 43–1.** Best Studied Acute Phase Proteins in Humans*

| | Electrophoretic Mobility on Paper | Molecular Weight (daltons) | Normal Plasma Concentration (mg/dl) |
|---|---|---|---|
| *Group I* | | | |
| Concentration may increase by about 50% | | | |
| Ceruloplasmin | $\alpha_2$ | 151,000 | 15–60 |
| C3 (complement component) | $\beta$ | 180,000 | 80–170 |
| *Group II* | | | |
| Concentration may increase two- to four-fold | | | |
| $\alpha_1$-Acid glycoprotein | $\alpha_1$ | 40,000 | 55–140 |
| $\alpha_1$-Antitrypsin | $\alpha_1$ | 54,000 | 200–400 |
| $\alpha_1$-Antichymotrypsin | $\alpha_1$ | 68,000 | 30–60 |
| Haptoglobin | $\alpha_2$ | 100,000† | 40–180 |
| Fibrinogen | $\beta$ | 340,000 | 200–450 |
| *Group III* | | | |
| Concentration may increase 100- to 1000-fold | | | |
| C-reactive protein | $\beta$–$\gamma$ | 105,000 | < 1.0 |
| Protein SAA (serum amyloid A) | A1b[18a] | 12,000 | < 0.5‡ |

*These values are derived, for the most part, from reference 18.
†MW for Hp 1-1.
‡Derived from studies in the mouse.[19]

**Mechanisms, Teleology, and Clinical Usefulness.** The increase in concentration of acute phase proteins following inflammatory stimulus has been shown, in each instance in which it has been studied, to result from an increase in synthesis by hepatocytes,[1,2] with occasional implication of other sites as well. It is presumed that this increased synthesis results from the action of a mediator system, which originates at the site of tissue injury and ultimately affects the hepatocytes. Plasma changes characteristic of the acute phase response can be produced in experimental animals by injection of preparations derived from leukocytes and indistinguishable from interleukin I (and endogenous pyrogen).[25,26] More recently, monokines, products of activated macrophages, have been reported to induce increases in synthesis of mouse SAA, rat fibrinogen, and other acute phase proteins in hepatocyte culture systems. The SAA-inducing activity co-purified with and may be identical to interleukin I,[27] while the fibrinogen-inducing activity was attributed to a molecule of greater molecular size.[28] It is possible that different mechanisms are responsible for induction of different acute phase proteins.[28a]

Teleologic speculations would suggest that the changes in concentration of these proteins lead to improved functional capacity to cope with the consequences of tissue injury or infection in one way or another. Thus, one might presume that increased amounts of haptoglobin would result in an improved capacity to bind the hemoglobin released by destroyed erythrocytes; in addition to leading to removal of this potentially toxic substance from the circulation, such binding might exert a bacteriostatic effect on certain pathogenic bacteria.[29] Similarly, increased amounts of fibrinogen could provide additional substrate for clotting as well as for forming complexes with intravascular fibrin; ceruloplasmin might be useful during the course of inflammation because it displays superoxide dismutase activity;[30] and $\alpha_1$-antitrypsin and $\alpha_1$-antichymotrypsin would provide increased inhibition of protease activity. While such speculation seems reasonable, the precise role played by each of the acute phase proteins in the response to tissue injury is difficult to establish, since demonstration of in vitro effects is not always relevant to in vivo phenomena.

The most widely employed indicators of the acute phase response in clinical medicine are measurements of the erythrocyte sedimentation rate and of C-reactive protein concentration. The bulk of this chapter will deal with these two tests and their significance. The erythrocyte sedimentation rate may reflect alterations in concentration of some acute phase proteins, while C-reactive protein may be regarded as the quintessential acute phase protein. Their measurement has been employed clinically for determining the presence and the degree of inflammation, both in initial evaluation and in monitoring the course of disease in a given patient, where they may serve as guides to management.

## ERYTHROCYTE SEDIMENTATION RATE

**Introduction.** In this test anticoagulated blood is placed in a vertical cylindrical tube and the rate of sedimentation of the erythrocytes is measured. It has been known since the time of the ancient Greeks that the sedimentation rate may be altered in disease states, and this test has been widely employed in clinical medicine for about 60 years. The continued widespread use of the erythrocyte sedimentation rate (ESR) results from its relative simplicity, its familiarity, and the wealth of information about its clinical significance that has accumulated over this period.[31] As with all elements of the acute phase response, abnormal findings do not have diagnostic specificity but may accompany many abnormal states. The ESR should be viewed as an indirect way of screening for increased concentrations of fibrinogen, and to a lesser extent, of other acute phase proteins; such changes cause increased aggregation of erythrocytes suspended in plasma, causing them to fall more rapidly.[32]

**Mechanisms Governing the Rate of Erythrocyte Sedimentation.** The major influence on the rate of sedimentation of red cells suspended in plasma is the degree to which they aggregate with one another. Our understanding of erythrocyte aggregation stems, to a large extent, from studies of the physicochemical aspects of antibody-induced hemagglutination.[33, 34] There are three major factors that influence erythrocyte aggregation: (1) the surface *free energy* of the cells, (2) the charge on the cells, and (3) the dielectric constant (Fig. 43–1).

The *surface free energy* (interfacial tension) of red cells results from van der Waals' forces and exerts a *cohesive force,* tending to attract the cells to one another.

The *charge on erythrocytes* is similar on all cells, and acts as a *repulsive force.* This red cell charge is itself the sum of the negative potentials due to the sialic acid components of the erythrocyte membrane and the oppositely charged cloud of ions that surrounds each erythrocyte. The resultant of these two groups of charges, called the zeta potential, exists on the outer edge of this cloud of cations and determines the force of repulsion between red cells. In normal individuals the zeta potential is great enough to overcome the cohesive van der Waals' forces, and little aggregation occurs.

The *dielectric constant* is not a property of the red cells but rather of the medium, in this instance the plasma, in which the cells are suspended. The dielectric constant measures the *charge dissipation characteristics* of the medium. It is influenced by the concentration and degree of asymmetry of the molecules dissolved in plasma, particularly the plasma proteins. The dielectric constant is raised when the concentration of molecules that can become oriented or polarized by the electric field of the red cells is increased. The more asymmetric the molecule, the more likely it is to be polarized. Thus, with an increase in concentration of such molecules, the increase in dielectric constant tends to diminish the repulsive effect of the zeta potential; the cohesive effects of the surface free energy predominate, and aggregation ensues.

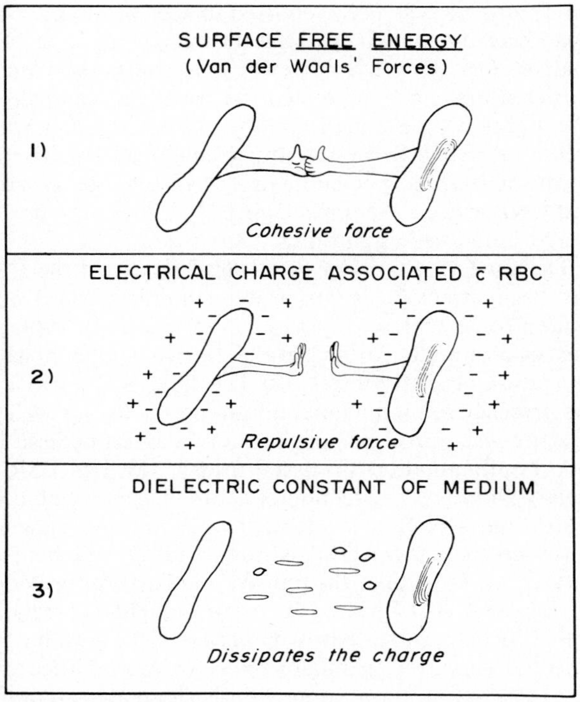


**Figure 43–1.** Factors influencing erythrocyte aggregation and sedimentation.

When erythrocytes align themselves in aggregates that resemble a stack of coins (rouleaux), there is an increase in mass of each stack of erythrocytes out of proportion to the increase in surface area. The increase in downward forces is significantly greater than any concomitant opposing increase in the upward forces exerted by plasma, which retard red cell fall. As a result, the cells fall rapidly. The greater the number of erythrocytes in each aggregate, the more rapid the rate of fall.

**Effects of Plasma Protein Abnormalities.** Rouleaux formation and consequent elevation in ESR may result from either a moderate increase in concentration of extremely asymmetric proteins (such as fibrinogen) or a major increase in concentration of only moderately asymmetric molecules (such as the immunoglobulins). There are thus two classes of change in plasma proteins that may result in an elevation in ESR.[35] One is the acute phase response. Fibrinogen is the most asymmetric of the acute phase proteins present in substantial concentration in plasma and has the greatest effect on the ESR. Other acute phase proteins, and the immunoglobulins present in increased concentrations in chronic inflammatory states, show lesser degrees of asymmetry, and less of an effect on erythrocyte aggregation. The other class of plasma protein abnormalities leading to elevation of ESR is seen in multiple myeloma and Waldenström's macroglobulinemia. In these instances, elevation in ESR is primarily due to a massive increase in concentration of a single molecular species of immunoglobulin. It is not clear that plasma lipids have any effect on ESR.[36]

**Effects of Erythrocyte Abnormalities and Drugs.** Alterations in the shape and size of red blood cells influence the ability of these cells to form rouleaux. Anisocytosis, poikilocytosis (such as that seen in sickle cell anemia), microcytosis, spherocytosis, and acanthocytosis all physically interfere with rouleaux formation.[31] These erythrocyte abnormalities may result in the finding of a paradoxically normal ESR when major acute phase plasma protein abnormalities are, in fact, present. In addition, alterations in the concentration of erythrocytes may affect the ESR. Anemia appears to result in a more rapid rate of fall of red cells, while polycythemia may cause a very low ESR.

The administration of certain drugs to patients or their addition to blood may alter the ESR. It has recently been found that ESR is spuriously elevated when determined on heparinized specimens of blood or on blood from heparinized patients.[37] In contrast, patients receiving high doses of sodium valproate have been found to show significantly reduced ESR;[38] the mechanism responsible for this change is uncertain.[39] A diurnal variation in ESR has been found to be related to ingestion of food.[40]

**Methods of ESR Determination.** Arguments have persisted over the decades about which of the various methods of ESR determination is the most reliable, and if (and how) correction for anemia should be performed. The former argument seems to have been resolved for the moment by the decision of the International Committee for Standardization in Hematology that the Westergren technique be designated as the standardized selected method.[41] Correction for anemia has now generally been abandoned. Wintrobe's textbook has summarized the reasons for doing so: Correcting for anemia is only approximate, and it is an artificial ultrarefinement. It is misleading, particularly since no correction is made for alterations in size and shape of erythrocytes, which may be more important.[42]

In the standard Westergren method, 2 ml of venous blood is collected in 0.5 ml of sodium citrate solution. The blood is drawn up to a level of 200 mm in the cylindrical Westergren tube, which is then placed vertically in a rack. At the end of 1 hour the height of the zone of clear plasma above the sedimented column of red cells is measured; this distance is the rate of fall, expressed as millimeters in the first hour.[41]

The upper limits of normal originally suggested by Westergren, 3 mm per hour for males and 7 mm per hour for females, are undoubtedly too low. Commonly accepted values for screening purposes in young adults are 15 mm per hour for males and 20 mm per hour for females. With aging, even higher values seem to be the norm, although specific standards are uncertain.[43] In one study, the distribution of ESR values was found to be skewed in an apparently healthy elderly population; 12 percent of such individuals showed values over 40 mm per hour.[44]

As an alternative to the Westergren method, the Wintrobe method is used today primarily in small laboratories, often in physicians' offices. Its major virtue is its great simplicity. No diluent is used; anticoagulated blood is merely added to a mark in a graduated tube, and the cells are permitted to fall for 1 hour.[42] There are three major drawbacks to this method: (1) The Wintrobe tube, only 100 mm long, is half the length of the Westergren tube. Therefore ESR values greater than about 60 mm per hour can rarely be measured, since further fall is impeded by packing of red blood cells. As a result, degrees of increase in ESR, and hence of severity of inflammation, cannot be distinguished. (2) In contrast to the Westergren method, it is not as clear that correction for anemia can be safely ignored; the results may thus be difficult to interpret. (3) The narrow bore of the Wintrobe tube may lead to nonreproducible results at times.

A "zeta sedimentation ratio" has been proposed as a method of measuring the effect of altered plasma protein concentrations on erythrocyte aggregation, while avoiding the necessity of correcting for anemia.[45] Since the main virtues of the ESR are simplicity and familiarity, it seems unlikely that this method, which requires a specialized centrifuge, will be widely adopted.

**Clinical Significance.** Elevation in ESR has no diagnostic specificity but tends to reflect the presence either of tissue injury and inflammation on the one hand or of certain lymphoproliferative disorders on the other, as discussed above. High ESR values are usually seen in bacterial infections. Mild viral infections are usually accompanied by a normal ESR, while patients with severe manifestations of viral infections (such as mumps orchitis or poliomyelitis) usually have a high ESR. In general, mild elevations reflect mild tissue alterations, while marked elevations reflect major tissue injury. In a number of protracted or chronic illnesses, the course of the disease process is reflected by the rise and fall of the ESR.

The ESR is often employed as a rough screening test, in which a normal finding tends to be reassuring, while an elevated ESR may lead to a search for a source of inflammation or tissue injury. It must be emphasized that a normal ESR does *not* by any means rule out the presence of disease. Similarly, markedly elevated ESR values are occasionally seen in patients in whom no specific diagnoses can be made and whose ESR subsequently returns to normal.[46, 47]

Several specific cases deserve mention. The ESR normally rises in the latter portion of pregnancy and occasionally in women taking oral contraceptives.[48] Elevation in ESR has been reported in several diseases not clearly accompanied by tissue necrosis, e.g., hypothyroidism and hyperthyroidism. In one study, individuals participating in a vigil involving stressful days and sleepless nights demonstrated a moderate but significant increase in ESR.[36] Some intramuscular injections, particularly benzathine penicillin, may cause a rise in ESR and CRP levels.[49] At times high ESR values may be due to red blood cell agglutinins.

**The Current Status of the ESR.** The use of the ESR has been attacked as unsuitable, imprecise, and outmoded for a variety of reasons: (1) It is impossible to correct accurately for alterations in size, shape, or concentration of erythrocytes. (2) The ESR is abnormal in the presence of monoclonal immunoglobulins as well as of acute phase proteins; an elevation does not necessarily reflect inflammation or tissue injury. (3) The ESR is merely an indirect reflection of acute phase protein concentration. Direct measurement of a number of acute phase proteins themselves is now readily available and is more valuable than the indirect information provided by the ESR. (4) Plasma viscosity is highly correlated with ESR. Measurement of viscosity itself, without the need to correct for anemia or red cell abnormalities, can provide a simpler screening test for those abnormalities detected by the ESR.[50] (5) There is uncertainty about the effect of age and sex on the ESR; no one is quite sure what the range of normal is. (6) Serum C-reactive protein levels rise and fall faster than ESR and reflect the current status of a patient more accurately.[51] All these criticisms are true. Nonetheless, the ESR still manages to maintain an important place in medical practice. In the current era of sophisticated and automated laboratory testing, the fact that a practitioner can easily perform this familiar test himself in the simplest of laboratory settings probably assures a place for the ESR for some time to come.

## C-REACTIVE PROTEIN

**History, Structure, and Function.** C-reactive protein (CRP) owes its name to the circumstances surrounding its discovery. It was originally detected in human serum because of its ability to precipitate with the somatic C-polysaccharide of the pneumococcus in the presence of calcium ion.[52,53] Although this method is no longer used to detect this protein, the name persists. CRP was felt for many years to be absent from normal sera, appearing only in response to inflammation. However, it has recently been shown to be present in trace amounts in all subjects,[54,55] the concentration rising dramatically after tissue injury. CRP has an electrophoretic mobility on paper in the rapid $\gamma$ range. It is an aggregate of five apparently identical noncovalently linked subunits arranged in cyclic symmetry[56] (Fig. 43–2). Based on studies of its primary structure, a molecular weight of 105,000 daltons can be computed.[57] There is substantial homology of amino acid sequence between CRP and the plasma protein which appears to be the precursor of the amyloid P component, protein SAP.[58] Both CRP and SAP display a pentameric structure,[56] and both demonstrate calcium-dependent ligand-binding properties.[59] SAP is not a noteworthly acute phase protein in man;[60] even when acute phase behavior has been claimed, mean increases less than 25 percent have been found.[61]

The likelihood that CRP plays a significant biologic role is supported by the conservation of this protein over hundreds of millions of years of evolution; proteins demonstrating characteristics of CRP have been demonstrated in a variety of lower animals, including chickens, many species of fish, including some dogfish, and the horseshoe crab *Limulus polyphema.*[62,63] However, it is of interest that CRP does not demonstrate acute phase behavior in many of these species.[3a]

The magnitude and rapidity of the CRP response in man also suggest that an important physiologic role is played by this protein. While the precise functions of CRP during the acute phase are not known, this protein has been shown to exhibit a large number of in vitro recognition and activation functions with the potential for influencing inflammation and other defense mechanisms.[64] Among the recognition functions are binding to phosphocholine moieties, galactans, and polycations. The complexing of human CRP to its ligands leads to

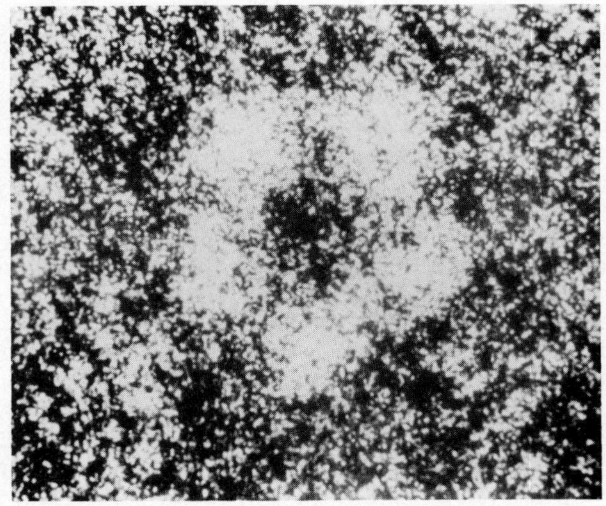

**Figure 43–2.** Electron micrograph of CRP molecule. (Courtesy of Dr. Henry Gewurz).

activation of the complement system, initiating all of the major known complement-dependent reactivites.[65] Binding of CRP to phospholipase A–treated erythrocytes, rabbit erythrocyte ghosts and model membrane lipid systems has been shown.[66] In addition, binding of ligand-complexed CRP to subsets of peripheral blood monocytes has been reported; this interaction may promote complement-dependent phagocytosis by mononuclear phagocytes.[67] About 3 percent of peripheral blood lymphocytes bind such complexed CRP.[68] Thermally modified CRP is reported to cause platelet aggregation and secretion.[69] Evidence has been presented suggesting that some natural killer cells bear surface CRP,[70,71] that CRP can inhibit T lymphocyte-dependent antibody formation,[72] and that liposome-bound CRP can activate macrophages.[73]

In contrast to the large number of in vitro functional capabilities that have been reported for CRP, relatively few in vivo studies have been reported. CRP has been shown to deposit in areas of necrosis in inflammatory lesions but not in adjacent normal tissue.[74,75] Passively administered human CRP has been found to increase survival in mice infected with *S. pneumoniae.*[76,77] Liposome-bound CRP has been shown to inhibit tumor growth in mice.[78] The pattern of organ sequestration and clearance of injected erythrocytes in mice has been found to be altered if CRP is bound to these cells.[79]

This plethora of observations makes it unlikely that CRP serves only a single function and strongly suggests that CRP plays a broad range of physiologic roles in response to tissue injury and infection. However, precise delineation of the extent of its involvement in physiologic events in vivo is still not possible. Several of these observations, taken together, have led to the suggestion that *one* role of CRP might be to combine with phospholipid constituents of necrotic cell membranes at inflammatory sites; such binding would lead to adherence of phagocytic cells and to activation of the complement system, with consequent formation of mediators of inflammation and eventual phagocytosis and removal of damaged tissue.[64,65,80]

**Role of CRP in Disease.** Only a few reports have thus far suggested that CRP participates in the pathogenesis of human disease. Evidence has been presented indicating that CRP plays a role in causing hemolytic disease following envenomation by the brown recluse spider,[81] and in the formation of microemboli following administration of intravenous fat emulsions.[82] The demonstration that interaction of CRP with urate crystals may lead to complement activation suggests that this mechanism might contribute to the precipitation of acute gouty attacks following surgical and other stresses.[83]

**Magnitude and Time Course of the CRP Response.** The true range of normal for serum CRP levels has not been defined precisely, and may never be, since minor degrees of injury occurring in normal individuals in the course of everyday life probably cause slight degrees of CRP elevation. Concentrations less than 0.01 mg per deciliter are commonly found in umbilical cord sera, and many adults show levels less than 0.05 mg per dl.[55] While most apparently healthy individuals have CRP levels of less than 0.2 mg per dl, concentrations as high as 1 mg per dl are found frequently enough in such normal subjects[54,55,84,85] to justify regarding concentrations lower than this value as clinically insignificant.[20]

Following a variety of acute inflammatory stimuli, a sharp increase in serum concentration of CRP is noted, usually beginning within a few hours. In a group of patients with acute myocardial infarction, for example, a mean serum doubling time of about 8 hours was noted[86] (Fig. 43–3). The rise in serum concentration is caused by a progressive increase in the number of CRP-forming hepatocytes, with a resulting increase in rate of hepatic CRP synthesis.[87] The magnitude of the CRP rise reflects the extent of tissue injury; more extensive lesions cause longer periods of rising CRP levels and higher CRP concentrations.[86] As a useful approximation, concentrations of less than 1 mg per dl may be regarded as normal or as insignificant elevations; concentrations between 1 and 10 mg per dl, as *moderate* increases; and concentrations over 10 mg per dl, as *marked* increases.[20] Patients with severe acute inflammatory states may attain serum CRP levels of 20 mg per dl or greater; values greater than 30 mg per dl are occasionally seen. Such values are over 1000 times the concentrations found in many normal individuals. No other acute phase protein, with the exception of protein SAA, is known to increase its concentration this markedly.

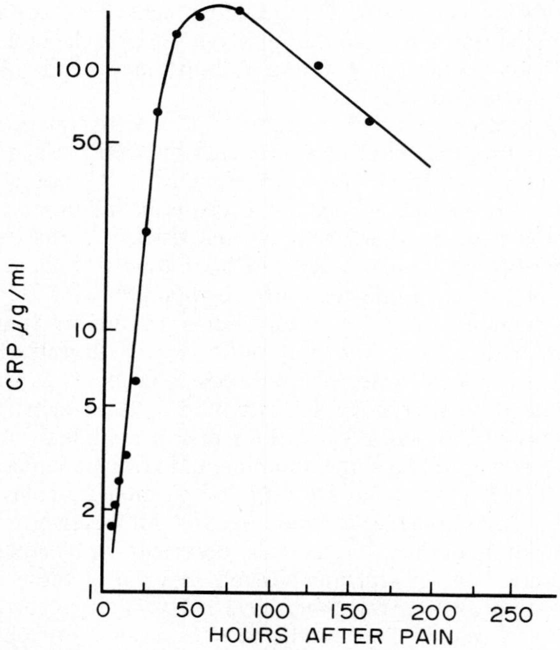


**Figure 43–3.** Serum CRP response in a representative patient with acute myocardial infarction. Note rapidity of rise and fall in this semilogarithmic plot. (From Kushner, I. et al.: J. Clin. Invest. *61*:235, 1978.)

Serum CRP levels generally reach a peak in 2 or 3 days following acute stimuli and then fall relatively rapidly. In a number of patients, CRP levels have been found to fall to half their peak concentrations within 24 hours, following effective control of the inflammatory stimulus,[88] and studies in rabbits indicate a serum half life of about 4 to 6 hours.[89] However, persistently elevated serum CRP concentrations are often seen in chronic inflammatory states such as pulmonary tuberculosis or active rheumatoid arthritis, or in the presence of extensive malignant disease.

**Methods of CRP Detection.** Early methods for detection of CRP made use of the relatively insensitive method of precipitation with C-polysaccharide or of the capacity of CRP to cause nonspecific capsular swelling of type 27 pneumococci.[90] Purification and crystallization of CRP in 1947, with subsequent raising of specific antisera, permitted immunochemical detection of this protein.[91] The first such method, and one still widely used, was the capillary precipitin technique, which represented a substantial improvement over previous methods.[92] However, this method is only semiquantitative and is relatively insensitive. Subsequently, the radial and electroimmunodiffusion techniques have permitted accurate quantitation of as little as 0.2 mg per dl.[93]

While sensitive radioimmunoassays have been developed,[55,84] their high degree of sensitivity is not necessary for clinical purposes; radial immunodiffusion and electroimmunodiffusion methods are sufficiently sensitive and provide quantitative data in the range of clinical significance. Newly developed nephelometric methods and enzyme immunoassays are likely to find widespread use as a result of the speed with which results are obtainable.[94-96] In light of the availability of quantitative methods, nonquantitative procedures such as the capillary precipitin test and latex agglutination methods must be regarded as of limited value; their replacement by quantitative techniques will greatly enhance the clinical value of CRP determination.[20]

**Clinical Significance of Rise in CRP Levels.** Unfortunately, most published studies of the clinical significance of serum CRP determinations were carried out before quantitative methods were available, and results were frequently expressed as the "presence" or "absence" of CRP. The precise clinical value of CRP determinations must be redefined using quantitative methods; such studies are increasingly being reported.[20, 97]

Generally speaking, CRP elevation occurs in the variety of infectious, traumatic, and inflammatory states enumerated in the introductory paragraphs of this chapter. Mildly elevated levels are found in sera of a small percentage of pregnant women at term. CRP is rarely elevated in cord blood. However, the majority of neonates will demonstrate elevated levels by the third postpartum day, presumably in response to umbilical cord necrosis.[98] The prevalence of significantly elevated CRP levels found in population surveys does not vary with age.[99] Serial determinations showing elevation in CRP above baseline levels are more likely to be significant than a single elevated reading, especially on a background of chronic inflammation. However, values greater than 10 mg per dl should raise the possibility of bacterial infection.[20] It is important that CRP levels be interpreted with caution in light of the rapid changes that occur from day to day and hour to hour.[86]

## OTHER ACUTE PHASE REACTANTS

Early methods of assessing the acute phase response included a variety of measurements reflecting the concentrations of the large number of glycoproteins among the acute phase proteins: serum seromucoids, protein-bound hexose, hexosamine, sialic acid, and glucosamine. These determinations are rarely employed today. A frequently observed acute phase finding is elevation of the $\alpha_2$- and, to a lesser extent, the $\alpha_1$-globulin fractions on serum protein electrophoresis. Such changes usually reflect an increase in concentration of the many acute phase proteins with $\alpha$-globulin electrophoretic mobilities.

Although an increase in concentration of any of the proteins listed in Table 43-1 might be expected to reflect inflammatory states, they are rarely studied with that end in mind. None of these offers an advantage over CRP determination; their concentrations rise more slowly, and the magnitude of rise is nowhere near as great, except for SAA.[21,100,101] SAA levels are said to be increased in apparently healthy elderly individuals,[102] although one report casts doubt on this claim.[103] Haptoglobin levels may be normal in the presence of inflammation if concomitant intravascular hemolysis is present. Similarly, serum ferritin levels, normally elevated in inflammatory states,[104] may be normal or may be depressed in the presence of concomitant iron deficiency. Consumption coagulopathies may lead to decreased fibrinogen levels, even in the presence of inflammation.

## CLINICAL VALUE OF ASSESSMENT OF ACUTE PHASE REACTANTS

**General Comments.** While most studies of the clinical value of acute phase reactants have dealt with the ESR, critical quantitative studies of CRP have recently begun to be reported.[20,97] Studies of the relationship between ESR and CRP have uniformly suggested that CRP levels correlate better with degree of activity in rheumatoid arthritis and ankylosing spondylitis than does ESR.[105-107] Nonetheless, the continued use of the ESR in clinical medicine can be defended as long as its limitations and drawbacks are understood.[108,109] In general, assessment of the acute phase proteins is only occasionally of value in diagnosis. It is more often helpful in the management of rheumatic diseases by aiding in monitoring of disease activity during therapy.

The detection of elevated ESR or CRP levels in patients who do not present a clear-cut clinical picture suggests a significant inflammatory element to their illness, and renders diagnoses of psychogenic or trivial maladies less likely. On the other hand, relatively normal ESR or CRP levels may permit limited reassurance, if no alarming findings are noted on physical examination or other laboratory testing. Assessment of acute phase reactants is of limited value in management of conditions in which it is possible to monitor the target organ injury reasonably well, as in polymyositis, or in which there are serologic abnormalities highly correlated with activity of disease, as in systemic lupus erythematosus. In a number of illnesses, however, such ancillary clinical guides are lacking. In these patients, study of the acute phase reactants may be of value in allowing adjustment of drug dosage to the level of disease activity.

**Importance of Quantitative CRP Determination.** It is now apparent that description of serum CRP levels as simply "elevated" provides inadequate information and that differing degrees of CRP elevation have different implications.[20] To be clinically valuable, CRP levels should be expressed quantitatively. For example, while serum CRP levels are elevated in both Behçet's disease and Still's disease, CRP elevation in Behçet's disease is usually modest, levels rarely exceeding 2 mg/dl,[110] while CRP levels as high as 20 mg per dl may occur in Still's disease.[106]

Most chronic inflammatory diseases are accompanied by mild or moderate elevations in serum CRP concentrations. In general, CRP levels parallel disease severity as assessed clinically.[107,111,112] Thus, in juvenile arthritis, systemic (Still's) disease is generally accompanied by marked CRP elevation, polyarticular disease by a moderate increase, and pauciarticular disease by a very modest increase.[107] CRP levels average about 3 to 4 mg per dl in adult rheumatoid arthritis patients with moderate disease activity, but there is considerable variation: about 7 percent of such patients have values in the normal range, while a few patients with severe active disease show levels of 14 mg per dl or more.[107,113] In active ankylosing spondylitis CRP levels generally range between 2 and 3 mg per deciliter.[113]

**Specific Diseases.** In the following paragraphs several rheumatologic diseases have been chosen to illustrate some clinical situations in which evaluation of the acute phase response may be of value, or to illuminate areas of controversy.

***Rheumatoid Arthritis.*** A time-honored method of distinguishing rheumatoid arthritis from other varieties of arthritis, particularly osteoarthritis, is the detection of an elevated ESR. Today this finding must be regarded as of limited value for a variety of reasons. Not all patients with rheumatoid arthritis have elevated ESR. Many of the diseases from which rheumatoid arthritis must frequently be differentiated are themselves often accompanied by an elevated ESR. Most patients with osteoarthritis are in an age group in which an elevated ESR is frequently found as a result of associated diseases, and aging itself is not infrequently associated with elevated ESR.[44] Finally, as a result of better and more widespread training in rheumatology, clinicians are frequently more perspicacious than was formerly the case; our experience is that careful physical examination and assessment of other laboratory findings usually permit the diagnosis of rheumatoid arthritis to be made without the need for determination of ESR, or in the presence of a normal ESR.

Several authors have reported that a relatively good prognosis is suggested by detection of low ESR values early in the course of rheumatoid arthritis, but there is controversy about this point.[114-116] In general, a high ESR at onset is correlated with a relatively poor prognosis.[117] Paradoxically, a very high ESR, in association with severe, acute onset of polyarthritis, has been correlated with a favorable prognosis.[114,115] This clinical presentation may possibly represent a subgroup within the spectrum of conditions currently regarded as seronegative rheumatoid arthritis.

The true value of determination of acute phase reactants such as ESR and CRP in the evaluation of new drugs for rheumatoid arthritis is uncertain. The major criteria employed in evaluation of such drugs have tended to be signs and symptoms, assessed as objectively as possible. However, in a number of studies, improvement in acute phase reactants has been accepted as reflecting the beneficial effect of a drug quite independent of changes in signs or symptoms. Thus, the ESR is the most important laboratory criterion in the American Rheumatism Association criteria for determining remission.[118] Such measurement has the virtue of being totally objective, in contrast to the symptoms and physical findings usually evaluated. In addition, a fall in acute phase reactants probably reflects greater degrees of improvement in elements of the local inflammatory process than does clinical improvement without an accompanying fall in acute phase reactants.

However, arguments have been advanced suggesting that improvement in acute phase reactants has more fundamental implications, and that a drug that lowers levels of acute phase reactants influences underlying pathogenic mechanisms rather than merely modifying the inflammatory process.[119] Viewed in this way, drugs that lower acute phase reactants can be felt to have induced remission. Support for the view that slow-acting, suppressive agents,[120] such as gold and penicillamine, actually are capable of modifying the natural history of disease is based at least in part on the observation that serum CRP levels frequently fall in patients manifesting clinical improvement on treatment with these drugs,[121] while they usually do not in those receiving nonsteroidal anti-inflammatory drugs.[122] In addition, higher CRP levels have been correlated with progressive erosive disease.[123,124]

Taken together, these considerations have suggested to some that erosive and destructive disease is less likely to occur if ESR or CRP are returned to normal,[123,124] that nonsteroidal anti-inflammatory drugs will not achieve this goal in most patients, and that in such instances drugs such as gold, which is capable of lowering acute phase protein levels, be employed.[125] This view presumes that improvement in acute phase reactants on treatment indicates that a remission has been induced[119] and that progressive joint destruction will be retarded or prevented. However, it is at least equally likely that improvement in acute phase reactants merely reflects the *degree* of suppression of inflammation rather than a basic, qualitative alteration of the fundamental disease process. At present, there is insufficient evidence to conclude with assurance that treatment that lowers acute phase reactants to normal will affect the chronic inflammatory mechanisms that lead to destruction of bone and cartilage. Only prospective drug studies and correlation with radiographic changes will permit such a conclusion.[126]

**Polymyalgia Rheumatica and Giant Cell Arteritis.** The diagnoses of polymyalgia rheumatica (PMR) and of the associated condition giant cell arteritis (GCA) are supported by finding an elevated ESR, often over 100 mm per hour.[127,128] Although ESR elevation is widely and falsely regarded as a sine qua non of these states, it should be pointed out that periodic reports continue to appear describing patients with PMR and GCA who have normal ESR.[128-130] The detection of extreme elevation of ESR in the absence of symptoms of PMR or GCA is not likely to be due to these states; the majority of such patients have underlying infection or malignancy.[46,47,131]

In patients with PMR or GCA, the return of the ESR to normal levels following initial treatment usually indicates that inflammation has been brought under control. In such patients, overt clinical manifestations of disease activity may be absent or subtle during subsequent attempts to decrease the dose of therapeutic agents, institute alternate-day corticosteroid therapy, or discontinue therapy. Disease activity may be monitored by following the ESR; elevation would suggest recurrence of activity and call for more aggressive therapy. Of course, clinical manifestations of disease, even in the presence of a normal ESR, should not be ignored.

*Ankylosing Spondylitis.* When the diagnosis of ankylosing spondylitis is considered, usually in young individuals with unexplained chronic backache and no history of trauma, the finding of an elevated ESR or CRP might support this diagnosis, being present in about 75 percent of patients with active spondylitis.[113] However, other studies would be required to confirm the diagnosis.[132]

*Systemic Lupus Erythematosus.* Determination of ESR has generally been felt to be of some value in the management of systemic lupus erythematosus (SLE).[132a] However, there is controversy about the value of CRP determination in patients with this disease. Two issues have been raised.[3a] (1) Are serum CRP levels sufficiently different in systemic lupus erythematosus and rheumatoid arthritis (RA) to play a diagnostically useful role in distinguishing between these diseases? (2) Is CRP elevation in lupus patients an indication of infection, or may it be due to lupus itself?

CRP levels are elevated above the normal range in most patients with active SLE and tend to fall and rise as the disease improves or becomes more active. However, a number of patients with active SLE do not show CRP elevation, and median CRP levels in series of patients with SLE have been found to be lower than in RA patients who are felt to have comparable degrees of disease, leading to the suggestion that CRP levels be employed as a diagnostic criterion.[133,134] However, comparing degree of severity in these two diseases is difficult, a bit like comparing apples and oranges, since they differ in their clinical manifestations, the major organs involved, and, undoubtedly, in their pathogenesis. Since the precise mechanisms linking the CRP response to tissue injury and inflammation are unknown, it is difficult to estimate what degree of CRP elevation ought to be expected in a given patient. Serum CRP levels may be quite elevated in some patients with SLE,[123,135-138] especially those with acute serositis and chronic synovitis, and may be normal in many rheumatoids.[113,124] The use of serum CRP levels as a diagnostic criterion does not seem to be a practical suggestion, in view of the considerable overlap in CRP concentrations observed between SLE and RA patients and the finding that CRP levels are only minimally elevated in many patients with mild to moderate RA.[107,113]

The second issue, the suggestion that CRP elevation in the course of SLE is more likely to be due to superimposed bacterial infection than to activation of lupus, can be confronted more clearly if CRP levels are expressed in quantitative terms; "elevated" has little precise meaning. It has now become clear that markedly elevated serum CRP levels are seen most frequently, but not exclusively, with bacterial infection.[20] Occurrence in the course of SLE of CRP levels in excess of 6 to 8 mg per dl should serve as a stimulus to rule out the possibility of infection. However, such values should not be regarded as proof of such infection; marked CRP elevation due to SLE is not infrequently seen.[133,135-139]

*Acute Rheumatic Fever.* Treatment of acute rheumatic fever with salicylates or corticosteroids results in a return of acute phase reactants toward normal. Elevations of ESR or CRP are often seen after cessation of a standard course of anti-inflammatory therapy. In the absence of clinical signs or symptoms of rheumatic activity these can be regarded as "laboratory rebounds," are usually transient, and can generally be left untreated. It should be noted that the ESR is frequently normal when Sydenham's chorea appears as a manifestation of rheumatic activity.

## References


1. Kushner, I.: The phenomenon of the acute phase response. Ann. N.Y. Acad. Sci. 389:39, 1982.
2. Koj, A.: Acute phase reactants. *In* Allison, A.C. (ed.): Structure and Function of plasma proteins. Vol. 1. London and New York, Plenum Press, 1974, pp. 73–131.
3. Kushner, I., Volanakis, J., and Gewurz, H. (eds.): C-reactive protein and the plasma protein response to tissue injury. Ann. N.Y. Acad. Sci. 389:1, 1982.

3a. Pepys, M.B., and Baltz, M.L.: Acute phase proteins with special reference to C-reactive protein and related proteins (pentoxins) and serum amyloid A protein. Adv. Immunol. 34:141, 1983.

4. Coombes, F.J., Shakespeare, P.G., and Batstone, G.F.: Lipoprotein changes after burn injury in man. J. Trauma 20:971, 1980.
5. Cabana, V.G., Gewurz, H., and Siegel, J.N.: Inflammation-induced changes in rabbit CRP and plasma lipoproteins. J. Immunol. 130:1736, 1983.
6. Falchuk, K.H.: Effect of acute disease and ACTH on serum zinc proteins. N. Engl. J. Med. 296:1129, 1977.
7. Konijn, A.M., and Hershko, C.: Ferritin synthesis in inflammation. I. Pathogenesis of impaired iron release. Br. J. Haematol. 37:7, 1977.
8. Torrance, J.D., Charlton, R.W., Simon M.O., Lynch, S.R., and Bothwell, T.H.: The mechanism of endotoxin-induced hypoferremia. Scand. J. Haematol. 21:403, 1978.
9. Saba, T.M., and Jaffe, E.: Plasma fibronectin (opsonic glycoprotein); its synthesis by vascular endothelial cells and role in cardiopulmonary integrity after trauma as related to reticuloendothelial function. Am. J. Med. 68:577, 1980.
10. Deno, D.C., McCafferty, M.H., Saba, T.M., and Blumenstock, F.A.: Mechanism of depletion of plasma fibronectin after burn injury. Fed. Proc. 42:1035, 1983.
11. Constantian, M.B., Menzoian, J.O., Nimberg, R.B., Schmid, K., and Mannick, J.A.: Association of a circulating immunosuppressive polypeptide with operative and accidental trauma. Ann. Surg. 185:73, 1977.
12. Lentnek, A.L., Schreiber, A.D., and MacGregor, R.R.: The induction of augmented granulocyte adherence by inflammation: mediation by a plasma factor. J. Clin. Invest. 57:1098, 1976.
13. Clowes, G.H.A., Jr., George, B.C., Villee, C.A., Jr., and Saravis, C.A.: Muscle proteolysis induced by a circulating peptide in patients with sepsis or trauma. N. Engl. J. Med. 308:545, 1983.
14. George, B.C., Clowes, G.H.A., Jr., Saranis, C., Heideman, M., and Lane, B.: Plasma proteolysis inducing factor produced by human macrophages. Fed. Proc. 42:1039, 1983.
15. Oppenheim, J.J., and Gery, I.: Interleukin 1 is more than an interleukin. Immuno. Today 3:113, 1982.
16. Baracos, V., Rodemann, H.P., Dinarello, C.A., and Goldgerg, A.L.: Stimulation of muscle protein degradation and prostaglandin $E_2$ release by leukocytic pyrogen (interleukin-l): a mechanism for the increased degradation of muscle proteins during fever. N. Engl. J. Med. 308:553, 1983.
17. Biesel, W.R.: Mediators of fever and muscle proteolysis. N. Engl. J. Med. 308:586, 1983.
18. Putnam, F.W.: Alpha, beta, gamma, omega—the roster of the plasma proteins. *In* Putnam, F.W. (ed.): The Plasma proteins: Structure, function and genetic control. 2nd ed. Vol I. New York, Academic Press, 1975, pp. 58–131.

18a. Teppo, A.M., Maury, C.P., and Wegelius, O.: Characteristics of the amyloid A fibril-degrading activity of human serum. Scand. J. Immunol. 16:309, 1982.

19. Hoffman, J.S., and Benditt, E.P.: Changes in high density lipoprotein content following endotoxin administration in the mouse. J. Biol. Chem. 257:10510, 1982.
20. Morley, J.J., and Kushner, I.: Serum C-reactive protein levels in disease. Ann. N.Y. Acad. Sci. 389:406, 1982.
21. McAdam, K.P.W.J., Elin, R.J., Sipe, J.D., and Wolff, S.M.: Changes in human serum amyloid A and C-reactive protein after etiocholanolone-induced inflammation. J. Clin. Invest. 61:390, 1978.
22. Salonen, E-M., and Vaheri, A.: C-reactive protein in acute viral infections. J. Med. Virol. 8:161, 1981.
23. Shainkin-Kestenbaum, R., Zimlichman, S., Winikoff, Y., Pras, M., Chaimovitz, C., and Sarov, I.: Serum amyloid A (SAA) in viral infection:

rubella, measles and subacute sclerosing panencephalitis (SSPE). Clin. Exp. Immunol. 50:503, 1982.
24. Shainkin-Kestenbaum, R., Zimlichman, S., Winikoff, Y., and Chaimovitz, C.: Serum amyloid A levels in patients with infections due to cytomegalovirus, varicella-zoster virus, and herpes simplex virus. J. Infect. Dis. 146:443, 1982.
24a. Liesen, H., Dufauk, B., and Hollman, W.: Modifications of serum glycoproteins the day following a prolonged physical exercise and the influence of physical training. Europ. J. Appl. Physiol. 37:243, 41977.
25. Bornstein, D.L.: Leukocytic pyrogen: a major mediator of the acute phase reaction. Ann. N.Y. Acad. Sci. 389:323, 1982.
26. Kampschmidt, R.F., Upchurch, H.F., and Pulliam, L.A.: Characterization of a leukocyte-derived endogenous mediator responsible for increased plasma fibrinogen. Ann. N.Y. Acad. Sci. 389:338, 1982.
27. Sztein, M.B., Vogel, S.N., Sipe, J.D., Murphy, P.A., Mizel, S.B., Oppenheim, J.J., and Rosenstreich, D.L.: The role of macrophages in the acute-phase response: SAA inducer is closely related to lymphocyte activating factor and endogenous pyrogen. Cellular Immunol. 63:164, 1981.
28. Ritchie, D.G., and Fuller, G.M.: Hepatocyte stimulating factor: a monocyte-derived acute-phase regulatory protein. Ann. N.Y. Acad. Sci., 408:490, 1983.
28a. Baumann, H., Jahreis, G.P.; and Gaines, K.C.: Synthesis and regulation of acute phase proteins in primary cultures of mouse hepatocytes. J. Cell. Biol. 97:866, 1983.
29. Eaton, J.W., Brandt, P., Mahoney, J.R., and Lee, J.T., Jr.: Haptoglobin: A natural bacteriostat. Science 215:691, 1982.
30. Goldstein, I.M., Kaplan, M.B., Edelson, H.S., and Weismann, G.: Ceruloplasmin: a scavenger of superoxide anion radicals. J. Biol. Chem. 254:4040, 1979.
31. Lascari, A.D.: The erythrocyte sedimentation rate. Pediatr. Clin. North Am. 19:1113, 1972.
32. Rovel, A., L'Huillier, J.F., and Vigneron, C.: Mechanisms of erythrocyte sedimentation. Biomedicine 28:248, 1978.
33. Pollack, W.: Some physicochemical aspects of hemagglutination. Ann. N.Y. Acad. Sci. 127:892, 1965.
34. Pollack, W., Hager, H.J., Reckel, R., Toren, D.A., and Singher, H.O.: A study of the forces involved in the second stage of hemagglutination. Transfusion 5:158, 1965.
35. Talstad, I., and Haugen, H.F.: The relationship between the erythrocyte sedimentation rate (ESR) and plasma proteins in clinical materials and models. Scand. J. Clin. Lab. Invest. 39:519, 1979.
36. Palmblad, J., Karlsson, C.-G., Levi, L., and Lidberg, L.: The erythrocyte sedimentation rate and stress. Acta. Med. Scand. 205:517, 1979.
37. Penchas, S., Stern, Z., and Bar-or, D.: Heparin and the ESR. Arch. Intern. Med. 138:1864, 1978.
38. Nutt, J.G., Neophytides, A.N., and Lodish, J.R.: Lowered erythrocyte-sedimentation rate with sodium valproate. Lancet 2:636, 1978.
39. Hutchinson, R.M., Clay, C.M., Simpson, M.R., and Wood, J.K.: Lowered erythrocyte-sedimentation rate with sodium valproate. Lancet 2:1309, 1978.
40. Mallya, R.K., Berry, H., Mace, B.E.W., deBeer, F.C., and Pepys, M.B.: Diurnal variation of erythrocyte sedimentation rate related to feeding. Lancet 1:389, 1982.
41. International Committee for Standardization in Hematology: Recommendation for measurement of erythrocyte sedimentation rate of human blood. Am. J. Clin. Pathol. 68:505, 1977.
42. Wintrobe, M.W., Lee, G.R., Boggs, D.R., Bithell, T.C., Athens, J.W., and Foerster, J.: Clinical Hematology. 7th ed. Philadelphia, Lea & Febiger, 1974.
43. Hayes, G.S., and Stinson, I.N.: Erythrocyte sedimentation rate and age. Arch. Ophthalmol. 94:939, 1976.
44. Sharland, D.E.: Erythrocyte sedimentation rate: the normal range in the elderly. J. Am. Geriatrics Soc. 28:346, 1980.
45. Editorial: E.S.R. or Z.S.R. Lancet 1:1394, 1976.
46. Zacharski, L.R., and Kyle, R.A.: Significance of extreme elevation of erythrocyte sedimentation rate. JAMA 202:264, 1967.
47. Ford, M.J., Innes, J.A., Parrish, F.M., Allan, N.C., Horn, D.B., and Munro, J.F.: The significance of gross elevations of the erythrocyte sedimentation rate in a general medical unit. Eur. J. Clin. Invest. 9:191, 1979.
48. Burton, J.L.: Effect of oral contraceptives on erythrocyte sedimentation rate in healthy young women. Br. Med. J. 3:214, 1967.
49. Haas, R.C., Taranta, A., and Wood, H.F.: Effect of intramuscular injections of benzathine penicillin G on some acute-phase reactants. N. Engl. J. Med. 256:152, 1957.
50. Hutchinson, R.M., and Eastham, R.D.: A comparison of the erythrocyte sedimentation rate and plasma viscosity in detecting changes in plasma proteins. J. Clin. Pathol. 30:345, 1977.
51. Editorial: C-reactive protein or E.S.R.? Lancet 2:1166, 1977.
52. Tillett, W.S., and Francis, T., Jr.: Serologic reactions in pneumonia with a non-protein somatic fraction of pneumococcus. J. Exp. Med. 52:561, 1930.
53. McCarty, M.: Historical perspective on C-reactive protein. Ann. N.Y. Acad. Sci. 389:1, 1982.
54. Kindmark, C.-O.: The concentration of C-reactive protein in sera from healthy individuals. Scand. J. Clin. Lab. Invest. 29:407, 1972.
55. Claus, D.R., Osmand, A.P., and Gewurz, H.: Radioimmunoassay of human C-reactive protein and levels in normal sera. J. Lab. Clin. Med. 87:120, 1976.
56. Osmand, A.P., Friedenson, B., Gewurz, H., Painter, R.H., Hoffman, T., and Shelton, E.: Characterization of C-reactive protein and the complement subcomponent Clt as homologous proteins displaying cyclic pentameric symmetry (pentraxins). Proc. Natl. Acad. Sci. USA 74:739, 1977.
57. Oliveira, E.B., Gotschlich, E.C., and Liu, T.Y.: Primary structure of human C-reactive protein. Proc. Natl. Acad. Sci. USA 74:3148, 1977.
58. Anderson, J.K., and Mole, J.E.: Large scale isolation and partial primary structure of human plasma amyloid P-component. Ann. N.Y. Acad. Sci. 389:216, 1982.
59. Pepys, M.B., Dash, A.C., Munn, E.A., Feinstein, A., Skinner, M., Cohen, A.S., Gewurz, H., Osmand, A.P., and Painter, R.H.: Isolation of amyloid P component (protein AP) from normal serum as a calcium-dependent binding protein. Lancet 1:1029, 1977.
60. Pepys, M.B., Dash, A.C., Markham, R.E., Thomas, H.C., Williams, B.D., and Petrie, A.: Comparative clinical study of protein SAP (amyloid P component) and C-reactive protein in serum. Clin. Exp. Immunol. 32:119, 1978.
61. Levo, Y., Ehrenfeld, M., and Wollner, S.: Serum amyloid P-component levels in rheumatoid arthritis. Isr. J. Med. Sci. 18:715, 1982.
62. Baltz, M.L., deBeer, F.C., Feinstein, A., Munn, E.A., Milstein, C.P., Fletcher, T.C., March, J.F., Taylor, J., Bruton, C., Clamp, J.R., Davies, A.J.S., and Pepys, M.B.: Phylogenetic aspects of C-reactive protein and related proteins. Ann. N.Y. Acad. Sci. 389:49, 1982.
63. Liu, T.-Y., Robey, F.A., and Wang, C.-M.: Structural studies on C-reactive protein. Ann. N.Y. Acad. Sci. 389:151, 1982.
64. Gewurz, H., Mold, C., Siegel, J., and Fiedel, B.: C-reactive protein and the acute phase response. Adv. Intern. Med. 27:345, 1982.
65. Volanakis, J.E.: Complement activation by C-reactive protein complexes. Ann. N.Y. Acad. Sci. 389:235, 1982.
66. Narkates, A.J., and Volanakis, J.E.: C-reactive protein binding specificities: artificial and natural phospholipid bilayers. Ann. N.Y. Acad. Sci. 389:172, 1982.
67. Mortensen, R.F., Osmand, A.P., Lint, T.F., and Gewurz, H.: Interaction of C-reactive protein with lymphocytes and monocytes: complement-dependent adherence and phagocytosis. J. Immunol. 117:774, 1976.
68. James, K., Baum, L.L., Vetter, M.L., and Gewurz, H.: Interactions of C-reactive protein with lymphoid cells. Ann. N.Y. Acad. Sci. 389:274, 1982.
69. Fiedel, B.A., Simpson, R.M., and Gewurz, H.: Effects of C-reactive protein (CRP) on platelet function. Ann. N.Y. Acad. Sci. 389:263, 1982.
70. Baum, L.L., James, K.K., Glaviano, R.R., and Gewurz, H.: Possible role for C-reactive protein in the human natural killer cell response. J. Exp. Med. 157:301, 1983.
71. James, K.K., Baum, L.L., Adamowski, C., and Gewurz, H.: C-reactive protein antigenicity on the surface of human lymphocytes. J. Immunol. 131:2930, 1983.
72. Mortensen, R.F.: Inhibition of the polyclonal antibody plaque-forming cell response of human B lymphocytes by C-reactive protein (CRP) and CRP complexes. Cell. Immunol. 66:99, 1982.
73. Barna, B.P., Deodhar, S.D., Gautam, S., Yen-Lieberman, B., and Roberts, D.: Macrophage activation and generation of tumoricidal activity by liposome-associated human C-reactive protein (CRP). Cancer Research, 44:305, 1984.
74. Kushner, I., and Kaplan, M.H.: Studies of acute phase protein: I. An immunohistochemical method for the localization of Cx-reactive protein in rabbits: association with necrosis in local inflammatory lesions. J. Exp. Med. 114:961, 1961.
75. DuClos, T.W., Mold, C., Paterson, P.Y., Alroy, J., and Gewurz, H.: Localization of C-reactive protein in inflammatory lesions of experimental allergic encephalomyelitis. Clin. Exp. Immunol. 43:565, 1981.
76. Mold, C., Nakayama, S., Holzer, T.J., Gewurz, H., and DuClos, T.W.: C-reactive protein is protective against Streptococcus pneumoniae infection in mice. J. Exp. Med. 154:1703, 1981.
77. Yother, J., Volanakis, J.E., and Briles, D.E.: Human C-reactive protein is protective against fatal Streptococcus pneumoniae infection in mice. J. Immunol. 128:2374, 1982.
78. Deodhar, S.D., James, K., Chiang, T., Edinger, M., and Barna, B.P.: Inhibition of lung metastases in mice bearing a malignant fibrosarcoma by treatment with liposomes containing human C-reactive protein. Cancer Research 42:5084, 1982.

79. Nakayama, S., Mold, C., and Gewurz, H.: Opsonic properties of C-reactive protein in vivo. J. Immunol. 128:2435, 1982.
80. Kaplan, M.H., and Volanakis, J.E.: Interaction of C-reactive protein complexes with the complement system. I. Consumption of human complement associated with the reaction of C-reactive protein with pneumococcal C-polysaccharide and with the choline phosphatides, lecithin and sphingomyelin. J. Immunol. 112:2135, 1974.
81. Hufford, D.C., and Morgan, P.N.: C-reactive protein as a mediator in the lysis of human erythrocytes sensitized by brown recluse spider venom. Proc. Soc. Exp. Biol. Med. 167:493, 1981.
82. Hulman, G., Pearson, H.J., Fraser, I., and Bell, P.R.F.: Agglutination of intralipid by sera of acutely ill patients. Lancet 2:1426, 1982.
83. Russell, I.J., Papaioannou, C., McDuffie, F.C., Macintyre, S., and Kushner, I.: Effect of IgG and C-reactive protein on complement depletion by monosodium urate crystals. J. Rheumatol. 10:425, 1983.
84. Shine, B., deBeer, F.C., and Pepys, M.B.: Solid phase radioimmunoassays for human C-reactive protein. Clinica Chemica Acta 117:13, 1981.
85. Drahovsky, D., Dunzendorfer, U., Ziegenhagen, G., Drahovsky, M., and Kellen, J.A.: Reevaluation of C-reactive protein in cancer sera by radioimmunoassay and radial immunodiffusion: I. Diagnostic value and use in battery of conventional tumor markers. Oncology 38:286, 1981.
86. Kushner, I., Broder, M.L., and Karp, D.: Control of the acute phase response: serum C-reactive protein kinetics after acute myocardial infarction. J. Clin. Invest. 61:235, 1978.
87. Kushner, I., and Feldmann, G.: Control of the acute phase response. Demonstration of C-reactive protein synthesis and secretion by hepatocytes during acute inflammation in the rabbit. J. Exp. Med. 178:466, 1978.
88. Kushner, I., Edgington, R.S., Trimble, C., Liem, H.H., and Muller-Eberhard, U.: Plasma hemopexin homeostasis during the acute phase response. J. Lab. Clin. Med. 80:18, 1972.
89. Chelladurai, M., Macintyre, S.S., and Kushner, I.: In vivo studies of serum C-reactive protein turnover in rabbits. J. Clin. Invest. 71:604, 1983.
90. Hedlund, P.: The appearance of acute phase protein in various diseases. Acta. Med. Scan. 128(Suppl. 196):579, 1947.
91. McCarty, M.: The occurrence during acute infections of a protein not normally present in the blood: IV. Crystallization of the C-reactive protein. J. Exp. Med. 85:491, 1947.
92. Anderson, H.C., and McCarty, M.: Determination of C-reactive protein in the blood as a measure of the activity of the disease process in acute rheumatic fever. Am. J. Med. 8:445, 1950.
93. Nilsson, L.-A.: Comparative testing of precipitation methods for quantitation of C-reactive protein in blood serum. Acta Pathol. Microbiol. Scand. 73:129, 1968.
94. Harmoinen, A., Hallstrom, O., and Gronroos, P.: Rapid quantitative determination of C-reactive protein using laser-nephelometer. Scand. J. Clin. Lab. Invest. 40:293, 1980.
95. Gill, C.W., Bush, W.S., Burleigh, W.M., and Fischer, C.L.: An evaluation of a C-reactive protein assay using a rate immunonephelometric procedure. Am. J. Clin. Pathol. 75:50, 1980.
96. Gushaw, J.B., Briscoe, R., Eimstad, W.M., Chang, C., Greenwood, H.M., and Allen, J.D.: A simple, rapid enzyme immunoassay for C-reactive protein. Ann. N.Y. Acad. Sci. 389:448, 1982.
97. Pepys, M.B.: C-reactive protein (CRP), serum amyloid P-component (SAP) and serum amyloid A protein (SAA) in autoimmune disease. *In* Holborow, E.J. (ed.): Autoimmunity. Clinics in Immunology and Allergy. Vol. 1. Eastbourne, W. B. Saunders Company, Ltd, 1981, pp. 7–101.
98. Hanson, L.A., and Nilsson, L.A.: Studies on C-reactive protein: 2. The presence of C-reactive protein during the pre- and neonatal period. Acta Pathol. Microbiol. Scand. 56:409, 1962.
99. Nilsson, L.-A.: C-reactive protein in apparently healthy individuals (blood donors) related to age. Acta Pathol. Microbiol. Scand. 73:619, 1968.
100. Ignaczak, T.F., Sipe, J.D., Linke, R.P., and Glenner, G.G.: Immunochemical studies on the nature of the serum component (SAA) related to secondary amyloidosis. J. Lab. Clin. Med. 89:1092, 1977.
101. Benson, M.D., Scheinberg, M.A., Shirahama, T., Cathcart, E.S., and Skinner, M.: Kinetics of serum amyloid protein A in casein-induced murine amyloidosis. J. Clin. Invest. 59:412, 1977.
102. Rosenthal, C.J., and Franklin, E.C.: Variation with age and disease of an amyloid A protein-related serum component. J. Clin. Invest. 55:746, 1975.
103. Hijmans, W., and Sipe, J.D.: Levels of the serum amyloid A protein (SAA) in normal persons of different age groups. Clin. Exp. Immunol. 35:96, 1979.
104. Birgegard, G., Hallgren, R., Killander, A., Stromberg, A., Venge, P., and Wide, L.: Serum ferritin during infection: A longitudinal study. Scand. J. Haematol. 21:333–340, 1978.
105. Walsh, L., Davies, P., and McConkey, B.: Relationship between erythrocyte sedimentation rates and serum C-reactive protein in rheumatoid arthritis. Ann. Rheum. Dis. 38:367, 1979.
106. Mallya, R.K., deBeer, F.C., Berry, H., Hamilton, E.D.B., Mace, B.E.W., and Pepys, M.B.: Correlation of clinical parameters of disease activity in rheumatoid arthritis with serum concentration of C-reactive protein and erythrocyte sedimentation rate. J. Rheumatol. 9:224, 1982.
107. Gwyther, M., Schwarz, H., Howard, A., and Ansell, B.M.: C-reactive protein in juvenile chronic arthritis: an indicator of disease activity and possibly amyloidosis. Ann. Rheum. Dis. 41:259, 1982.
108. Editorial: The ESR—an outdated test? Lancet 1:377, 1982.
109. Editorial: Is it time to abandon the ESR? Acta. Med. Scand. 212:353, 1982.
110. Adinolfi, M., and Lehner, T.: Acute phase proteins and C9 in patients with Behcet's syndrome and aphthous ulcers. Clin. Exp. Immunol. 25:36, 1976.
111. Farr, M., Kendall, M.J., Young, D.W., Meynell, M.J., and Hawkins, C.F.: Assessment of rheumatoid activity based on clinical features and blood and synovial fluid analysis. Ann. Rheum. Dis. 35:163, 1976.
112. Dixon, J.S., Bird, H.A., Pickup, M.E., and Wright, V.: A human model screening system for the detection of specific antirheumatic activity. Semin. Arthritis Rheum. 12:185, 1982.
113. Dixon, J.S., Bird, H.A., and Wright, V.: A Comparison of serum biochemistry in ankylosing spondylitis, seronegative and seropositive rheumatoid arthritis. Ann. Rheum. Dis. 40:404, 1981.
114. Duthie, J.J.R., Brown, P.E., Truelove, L.H., Baragar, F.D., and Lawrie, A.J.: Course and prognosis in rheumatoid arthritis. A further report. Ann. Rheum. Dis. 23:193, 1964.
115. Masi, A.T., Maldonado-Cocco, J.A., Kaplan, S.B., Feigenbaum, S.L., and Chandler, R.W.: Prospective study of the early course of rheumatoid arthritis in young adults: comparison of patients with and without rheumatoid factor positivity at entry and identification of variables correlating with outcome. Semin. Arthritis Rheum. 5:299, 1976.
116. McConkey, B., Crockson, R.A., and Crockson, A.P.: The assessment of rheumatoid arthritis: a study based on measurement of the serum acute phase reactants. Quart. J. Med. 162:115, 1972.
117. Fleming, A., Crown, J.M., and Corbett, M.: Prognostic value of early features in rheumatoid disease. Br. Med. J. 1:1243, 1976.
118. Roth, S.H.: Remission: the goal of rheumatic disease therapy. J. Rheumatol. 9(Suppl. 8):120, 1982.
119. Editorial: Inducing remission in rheumatoid arthritis. Lancet 1:193, 1981.
120. Huskisson, E.C.: The problems of studying disease-remittive agents in RA. J. Rheumatol. 9(Suppl. 8):201, 1982.
121. Dixon, J.S.: Biochemical and clinical changes in rheumatoid arthritis: their relation to the action of antirheumatoid drugs. Semin. Arthritis Rheum. 12:191, 1982.
122. McConkey, B., Crockson, R.A., Crockson, A.P., and Wilkinson, A.R.: The effects of some anti-inflammatory drugs on the acute-phase proteins in rheumatoid arthritis. Quart. J. Med. 42:785, 1973.
123. Amos, R.S., Constable, T.J., Crockson, R.A., Crockson, A.P., and McConkey, B.: Rheumatoid arthritis: relation of serum C-reactive protein and erythrocyte sedimentation rates to radiographic changes. Br. Med. J. 1:195, Jan. 22, 1977.
124. Nusinow, S., and Arnold, W.J.: Prognostic value of C-reactive protein (CRP) levels in rheumatoid arthritis. Clin. Res. 30:474A, 1982.
125. Amos, R.S., Crockson, R.A., Crockson, A.P., Walsh, L., and McConkey, B.: Rheumatoid arthritis: C-reactive protein and erythrocyte sedimentation rate during initial treatment. Br. Med. J. 1(612Y):1396, May 27, 1978.
126. Iannuzzi, L., Dawson, N., Zein, N., and Kushner, I.: Does drug therapy slow radiographic deterioration in rheumatoid arthritis? (Submitted to N. Engl. J. Med., 309:1023, 1983)
127. Hamilton, C.R., Jr., Shelley, W.M., and Tumulty, P.A.: Giant cell arteritis: including temporal arteritis and polymyalgia rheumatica. Medicine 50:1, 1971.
128. Bruk, M.I.: Articular and vascular manifestations of polymyalgia rheumatica. Ann. Rheum. Dis. 26:103, 1967.
129. Kansu, T., Corbett, J.J., Savino, P., and Schatz, N.J.: Giant cell arteritis with normal sedimentation rate. Arch. Neurol. 34:624, 1977.
130. Biller, J., Asconape, J., Weinblatt, M.E., and Toole, J.F.: Temporal arteritis associated with normal sedimentation rate. JAMA 247:486, 1982.
131. Schimmelpfennig, R.W., Jr., and Chusid, M.J.: Illnesses associated with extreme elevation of the erythrocyte sedimentation rate in children. Clin. Pediatr. 19:175, 1980.
132. Khan, M.A., and Kushner, I.: Diagnosis of ankylosing spondylitis: *In* Cohen, A.S. (ed.): Progress in Clinical Rheumatology. Vol. I. New York, Grune and Stratton (in press).
132a. DuBois, E.L.: Lupus erythematosis. Los Angeles, University of Southern California Press, 2nd edition, 1976.
133. Becker, G.J., Waldburger, M., Hughes, G.R.V., and Pepys, M.B.: Value

of serum C-reactive protein measurement in the investigation of fever in systemic lupus erythematosus. Ann. Rheum. Dis. 39:50, 1980.
134. Pereira Da Silva, J.A., Elkon, K.B., Hughes, G.R.V., Dyck, R.F., and Pepys, M.B.: C-reactive protein levels in systemic lupus erythematosus: a classification criterion? Arthritis Rheum. 23:770, 1980.
135. Zein, N., Ganuza, C., and Kushner, I.: Significance of serum C-reactive protein elevation in patients with systemic lupus erythematosus. Arthritis Rheum. 22:7, 1979.
136. Morrow, W.J.W., Isenberg, D.A., Parry, H.F., and Snaith, M.L.: C-reactive protein in sera from patients with systemic lupus erythematosus. J. Rheumatol. 8:599, 1981.
137. Rothschild, B.M., James, K.K., Jones, J.V., Thompson, L.D., Pifer, D.D., and Chesney, C.M.: Quantitation of C-reactive protein in SLE correlates with disease activity. Clin. Res. 30:476A, 1982.
138. Sturfelt, G., Sjoholm, A.G., and Svensson, B.: Complement components, Cl activation and disease activity in SLE. Int. Arch. Allergy Appl. Immun. 70:12, 1983.
139. Bertouch, J.V., Roberts-Thompson, P.J., Feng, P.H., and Bradley, J.: C-reactive protein and serological indices of disease activity in systemic lupus erythematosis. Ann. Rheum. Dis. 42:655, 1983.

# Chapter 44
# Rheumatoid Factor

*Dennis A. Carson*

## INTRODUCTION

Rheumatoid factors are autoantibodies directed against antigenic determinants on the Fc fragment of immunoglobulin G (IgG) molecules (Fig. 44–1). Their importance was recognized in the 1940s when Waaler, and then Rose and co-workers, noted that the agglutination of sheep red blood cells by specific rabbit antibody was augmented by rheumatoid arthritis sera.[1,2] This was one of the first clues suggesting that rheumatoid arthritis was an autoimmune disease. However, it soon became clear that rheumatoid factors are not exclusively nor uniformly associated with rheumatoid arthritis. Investigations over several years have attempted to elucidate what the presence of rheumatoid factor signifies regarding the etiology of rheumatoid disease and how the autoantibody might contribute to the development of synovitis.

In this chapter we shall discuss (1) the nature of rheumatoid factors and how they are assayed; (2) the specificity and sensitivity of rheumatoid factors for rheumatoid arthritis; (3) genetic and environmental factors which influence rheumatoid factor production, structure, and specificity; (4) immunochemical properties of rheumatoid factors; (5) the probable physiologic role of IgM rheumatoid factors; and (6) the contribution of rheumatoid factors to the pathogenesis of chronic synovitis and extra-articular rheumatoid disease.

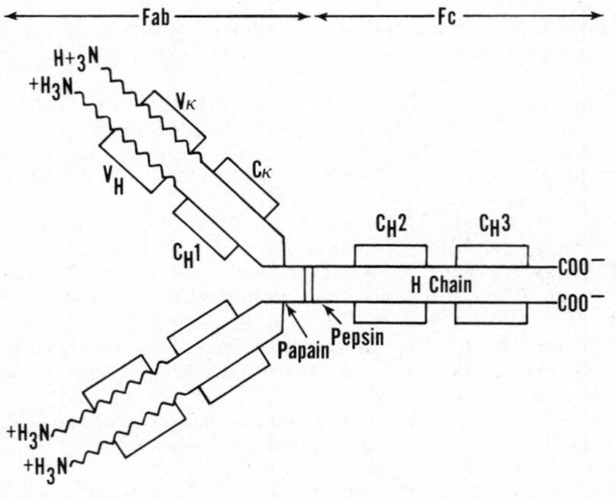


**Figure 44–1.** Structure of an IgG molecule of the G1 subclass containing kappa light chains. The antigens reacting with rheumatoid factor are in the Fc region.

## ASSAY METHODS

Rheumatoid factors have been found among the IgM, IgA, IgG and IgE classes of immunoglobulin.[3-7] Most methods developed for the measurement of antibodies against exogenous antigens have also been applied to the assay of rheumatoid factor. These include agglutination, precipitation, complement fixation, and immunofluorescence assays.[8-11] Technical problems have arisen because the IgG antigens with which rheumatoid factors react are present in high concentration in serum and may interfere with a particular detection system. The recent development of radioimunoassay and ELISA (enzyme-linked immunoabsorbent sandwich assay) methods has facilitated the more precise quantification of IgM, IgG, and IgA rheumatoid factors.[12-18]

**IgM Rheumatoid Factors.** IgM rheumatoid factors, like other IgM antibodies, are multivalent and hence are efficient agglutinators of antigen-coated particles. Commercially available sources of the latter include latex beads or bentonite particles that have been passively coated with human IgG. Cross-linking of the IgG-coupled latex or bentonite by IgM rheumatoid factor in serum produces a visible flocculus (Fig. 44–2). The quantity of IgM rheumatoid factor is then expressed as the highest dilution of serum yielding detectable agglutination. Nephelometry and particle counting techniques

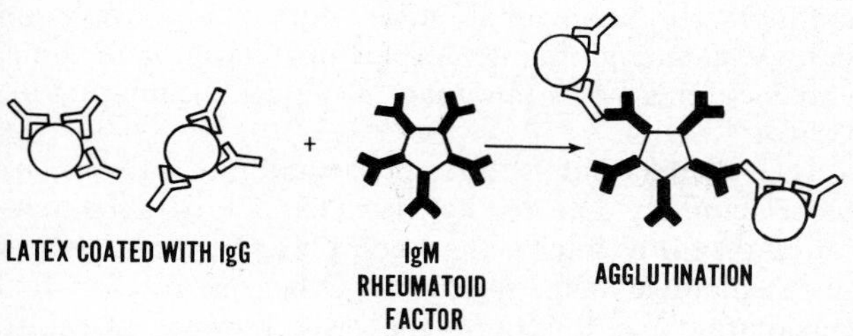


**Figure 44–2.** Latex fixation reaction. Multivalent IgM rheumatoid factor cross-links IgG-coated latex particles to produce a visible flocculus.

permit a more exact expression of IgM rheumatoid factor levels.[19]

Red cells coated with human or rabbit IgG are likewise agglutinated by IgM rheumatoid factors. Human red cells sensitized with certain incomplete IgG anti-Rh antibodies are well suited for the detection of IgM rheumatoid factors, particularly those with anti-Gm specificities.[20-23] Sheep red blood cells coated with rabbit IgG antibody are cross-linked by rheumatoid factor in the classic Rose-Waaler reaction. This test can be modified for the detection of complement-fixing rheumatoid factors.[10]

A positive Rose-Waaler test may be more specific for rheumatoid arthritis than the bentonite or latex flocculation assays, since the latter detect antiallotypic antibodies resulting from transplacental immunization or transfusion, as well as true autoantibodies.[23] However, because only a minor proportion of the anti-IgG antibodies in rheumatoid sera cross-react with rabbit IgG, titers in the Rose-Waaler test are usually lower than in those systems that employ human IgG as antigen. Furthermore, anti-sheep heterophile antibodies may give a false positive reaction unless the sera are preabsorbed with sheep red blood cells. This problem can be avoided by using latex particles coated with rabbit IgG.[24]

IgM rheumatoid factors will precipitate aggregated IgG, in either solution or agar-containing gels.[9,25] In some instances precipitation is enhanced by decreasing the temperature and ionic strength of the incubation medium. The reaction of such cold reactive IgM rheumatoid factors with monomeric IgG or soluble immune complexes in poorly perfused areas may contribute to the pathogenesis of mixed cryoglobulinemic states.[26,27] More commonly, IgM rheumatoid factors combine with monomeric IgG to form soluble 22S complexes, which can be visualized in many rheumatoid sera by analytical ultracentrifugation (Fig. 44–3).[3]

Serum IgG will compete with IgG-coated particles for reaction with IgM rheumatoid factor. Through multivalent interactions, nonspecifically aggregated IgG in improperly treated sera or specific immune complexes will inhibit rheumatoid factor binding to a marked degree. Such "hidden rheumatoid factors" can be revealed by separation of the IgM and IgG fractions under dissociating conditions prior to performing the rheumatoid factor assays.[28] The Clq component of complement will agglutinate IgG-coated particles, particularly in plasma anticoagulated with calcium chelators.[29] Unlike IgM, however, the Clq molecule is denatured by heating serum at 56° C for 30 minutes.

Recently, sensitive radioimmunoassay and ELISA methods have been developed for the detection of IgM rheumatoid factors.[12-15,17,18] In a typical assay, plastic tubes or microtiter plates are coated with IgG (Fig. 44–4). IgM rheumatoid factors in serum or synovial fluid specifically bind to the IgG fixed to the plates. After washing, the amount of IgM rheumatoid factor bound is quantitatively determined with an anti-IgM antibody that has been radioiodinated or linked to an enzyme such as alkaline phosphatase. In the latter case, the amount of enzyme-linked antibody bound to the solid phase is determined by adding an appropriate substrate and then assaying product formation in a spectrophotometer.

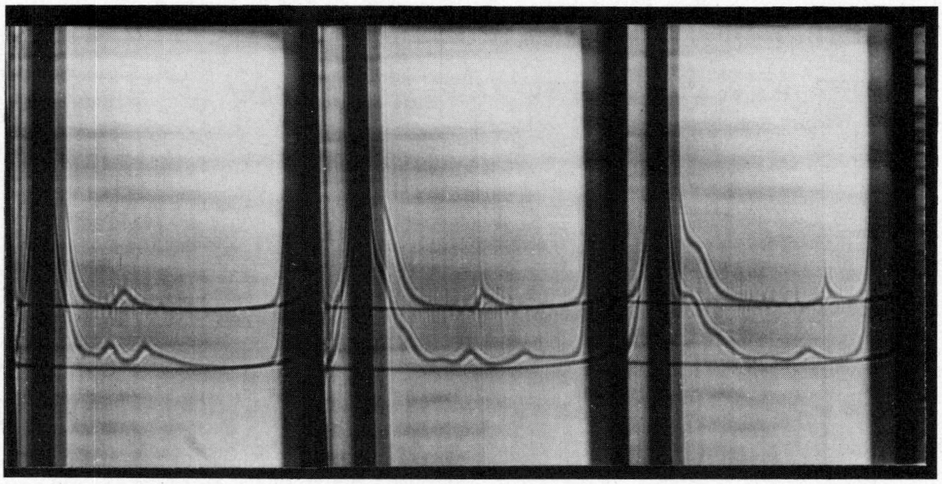

**Figure 44–3.** Analytical ultracentrifugation of serum from a rheumatoid arthritis patient (bottom) and a normal subject (top). Pictures were taken 32, 48, and 64 minutes after reaching a speed of 52,000 rpm. The peak to the right in the rheumatoid serum represents 22S complexes formed by the reaction of IgM rheumatoid factor with IgG.

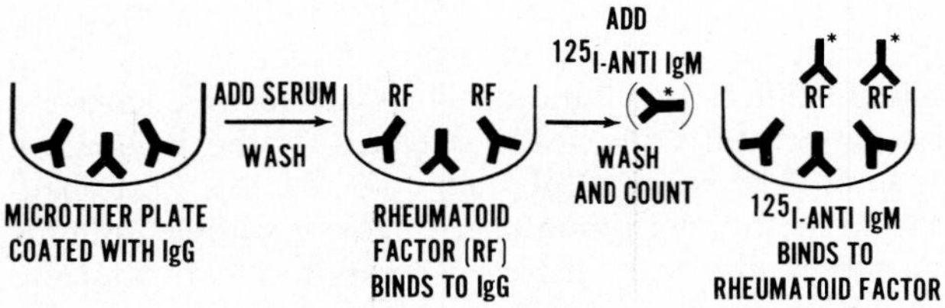


**Figure 44–4.** Radioimmunoassay of IgM rheumatoid factor.

One significant advantage of radioimmunoassay and ELISA methods is that they readily detect IgM rheumatoid factors in rheumatoid sera diluted 1000- to 100,000-fold. At such high dilutions, serum IgG and immune complexes infrequently compromise the accurate determination of IgM rheumatoid factor levels.

**IgG and IgA Rheumatoid Factors.** IgG rheumatoid factors are abundant in the sera, and particularly the synovial fluids, of many patients with severe rheumatoid arthritis.[13,14,17,30-32] Unfortunately, the routine assay of IgG rheumatoid factors presents several difficulties (Table 44–1). All assays for IgM rheumatoid factor take advantage of the markedly increased avidity of pentavalent IgM rheumatoid factors for aggregated IgG as compared to monomeric IgG. With IgG rheumatoid factor, this phenomenon is not nearly as marked. For the same reason IgG rheumatoid factors are inefficient agglutinators of IgG-coated particles or red blood cells. High concentrations of IgG in serum, and the tendency of IgG rheumatoid factors to self-associate rather than bind aggregated IgG, further make the assay of this antibody difficult. On occasion, IgG rheumatoid factor complexes precipitate in the cold or when serum is diluted 1:15 with water. This type of Ig rheumatoid factor is frequently monoclonal and is more commonly found in hypergammaglobulinemic purpura, cryoglobulinemia, and Sjögren's syndrome than in typical rheumatoid arthritis.[33,34]

IgG rheumatoid factors in rheumatoid arthritis are most definitely detected by their characteristic sedimentation profile as intermediate complexes in the analytical ultracentrifuge (Fig. 44–5).[35,36] Other assays for IgG rheumatoid factor require the prior removal of multivalent IgM rheumatoid factor by gel filtration, ion exchange chromatography, or digestion with the proteolytic enzyme pepsin. The latter technique has the additional advantage of destroying the Fc portion of IgG, thereby releasing IgG rheumatoid factors trapped in self-associating complexes (Fig. 44–6).[37] Care must be taken, however, to prevent further proteolysis of the IgG molecule with subsequent loss of antigen binding activity.

If serum contains sufficient quantities of IgG rheumatoid factor, a positive latex or sensitized sheep cell reaction can be detected in an isolated IgG fraction, or in pepsin-digested IgG.[32-36] IgG rheumatoid factor will also precipitate with aggregated IgG. In some cases IgG

**Table 44–1.** Comparison of Rheumatoid Factors of the IgM and IgG Class

| Property | IgM Rheumatoid Factor | IgG Rheumatoid Factor |
|---|---|---|
| Valence for IgG | 5 | 2 |
| Intrinsic affinity for antigen (liters/mole) | $1 \times 10^4 - 5 \times 10^5$ | $1 \times 10^4 - 5 \times 10^5$ |
| Agglutination of IgG-coated latex particles | Strong | Weak |
| Enhanced binding to aggregated IgG | Marked | Moderate |
| Usual sedimentation constants in ultracentrifuge | 19S–22S | 10S–18S |
| Self-association | No | Yes |
| Binding to IgG after treatment with: | | |
| Reducing agents | Decreased | Unchanged |
| Pepsin | Decreased | Unchanged or increased |

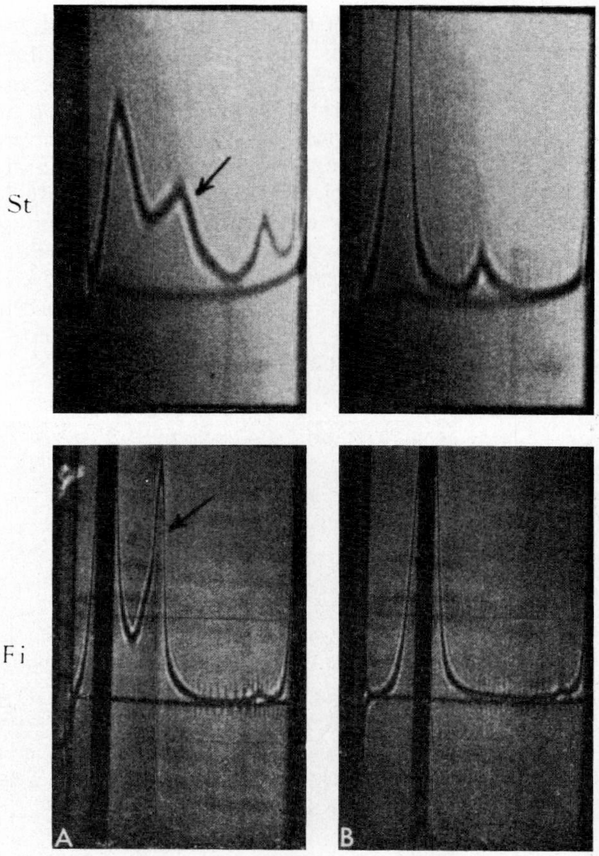


**Figure 44–5.** Analytical ultracentrifugation of IgG rheumatoid factor–containing sera in isotonic saline (*A*) and acetate buffer pH 4.5 (*B*). The arrows indicate the large intermediate complexes which disappear in the acetate buffer. (From Kunkel, H.G., et al.: J. Clin. Invest. 40:117, 1961.)

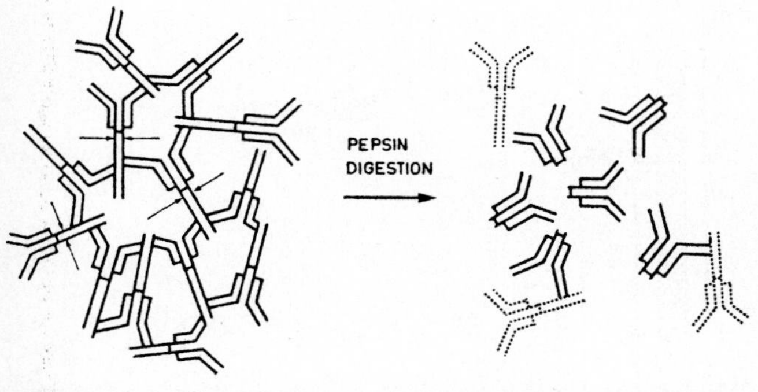


**Figure 44–6.** Effect of pepsin on IgG rheumatoid factor complexes. The pepsin destroys the Fc fragment of IgG, preventing IgG rheumatoid factor molecules from self-associating and releasing Fab'2 fragments with antibody activity. (Reprinted from Munthe, E., and Natvig. J.: Scand J. Immunol. 1:217, 1972.)

rheumatoid factors have been assayed as the quantity of serum IgG specifically adhering to IgG agarose immunoabsorbent columns, and eluting only under denaturing conditions.[38] This assay is not specific for IgG rheumatoid factor but may also detect normal IgG passively adhering to the immunoabsorbent via multivalent IgM rheumatoid factor.

Recently, both ELISA and radioimmunoassay methods have been developed for the detection of IgG rheumatoid factor.[13,14,17,39,40] They are performed analogously to the IgM rheumatoid factor assay described in Figure 44–4 except that anti-IgG antibody is substituted for anti-IgM in the final step. Nonetheless, IgM rheumatoid factor must still be removed or destroyed prior to the IgG rheumatoid factor assay to avoid false positive results.

The quantitative assay of IgG rheumatoid factor in serum is occasionally helpful in confirming a diagnosis of rheumatoid arthritis,[13,14,17,38] or hypergammaglobulinemic purpura.[34] In patients with rheumatoid vasculitis or the hyperviscosity syndrome, IgG rheumatoid factor levels may assist in monitoring the response to therapy.[40] However, indications for the routine clinical assay of IgG rheumatoid factor have not been well defined.

**IgA and IgE Rheumatoid Factors.** Rheumatoid factors of the IgA class have been measured in rheumatoid serum by immunoelectrophoresis, quantitative immunoabsorption, and radioimmunoassay and ELISA methods using class specific anti-immunoglobulin reagents to distinguish them from the more abundant IgM rheumatoid factors.[6,16,38,41]

IgA rheumatoid factors are also found in the saliva of patients with rheumatoid arthritis, and with the sicca syndrome. Most salivary IgA, and presumably IgA rheumatoid factor, is produced locally.[41] The role of IgA rheumatoid factors in chronic inflammation of the exocrine glands is not known.

With sensitive radioimmunoassays, IgE rheumatoid factors have been detected in the sera of most patients with rheumatoid arthritis, and a few with bronchial asthma.[7] They do not have any established diagnostic or prognostic significance.

## INCIDENCE OF RHEUMATOID FACTOR

Rheumatoid factors are not specific for rheumatoid arthritis. Rather, they are found in the sera of a variable portion of patients with acute and chronic inflammatory diseases, and in some apparently normal individuals.[42-45] The exact incidence of rheumatoid factor in a population depends upon the assay system and the titer chosen to separate positive and negative reactors.

The titer of rheumatoid factor in a population, whether measured by the sensitized sheep cell agglutination test or by latex fixation, usually behaves as a continuous variable, but differs among various ethnic groups (e.g., Fig. 44–7).[45] With increasing age both the percentage of individuals with a particular titer and the mean titer of a population as a whole increase (Fig. 44–8).[46] In most populations, the distribution of titers among men and women is similar. Some studies have shown that the prevalence of rheumatoid factors and other autoantibodies in the general population tends to decline beyond the age of 70 to 80.[47] This decrease may be related to an increased mortality—particularly from hypertension and vascular disease—among autoantibody positive individuals.

Diseases other than rheumatoid arthritis in which positive rheumatoid factor tests are frequent include other rheumatic diseases, viral infections, chronic inflammatory diseases, and neoplasms after chemotherapy or radiotherapy.[42-45,48,49] Many of these conditions are also associated with either hypergammaglobulinemia, indicative of polyclonal B lymphocyte activation, or circulating immune complexes.[44,45,48,50] In one study, levels of circulating immune complexes, measured by both the solid phase and solution Clq binding assays, were strongly associated with the presence of IgM rheumatoid factor.[51] Table 44–2 is a partial list of diseases in which an increased incidence of rheumatoid factor has been reported.

In most but not all nonrheumatic conditions, titers of rheumatoid factor are lower than in rheumatoid arthritis. Thus the specificity of the rheumatoid factor reaction for rheumatoid arthritis increases with serum titer (Fig. 44–9).[52] At a dilution of serum that excludes 95 percent of the normal population, at least 70 percent or more patients with rheumatoid arthritis, as diagnosed by other criteria, will be positive by latex agglutination. The remaining patients are considered seronegative, i.e., having rheumatoid factor titers falling in the normal range. Some of the latter sera, particularly from patients with juvenile rheumatoid arthritis, may contain hidden IgM rheumatoid factors.[28,53,54] A few have IgG rheumatoid factors in the absence of IgM. Some seronegative patients, upon repeated testing, convert to seropositive.

A variable percentage of adult rheumatoid patients, which in the author's experience represent not more than 10 percent of the total, remain seronegative by the usual criteria. These patients usually have milder synovitis than the seropositive patients, and they seldom develop extra-articular rheumatoid disease.[55,56]

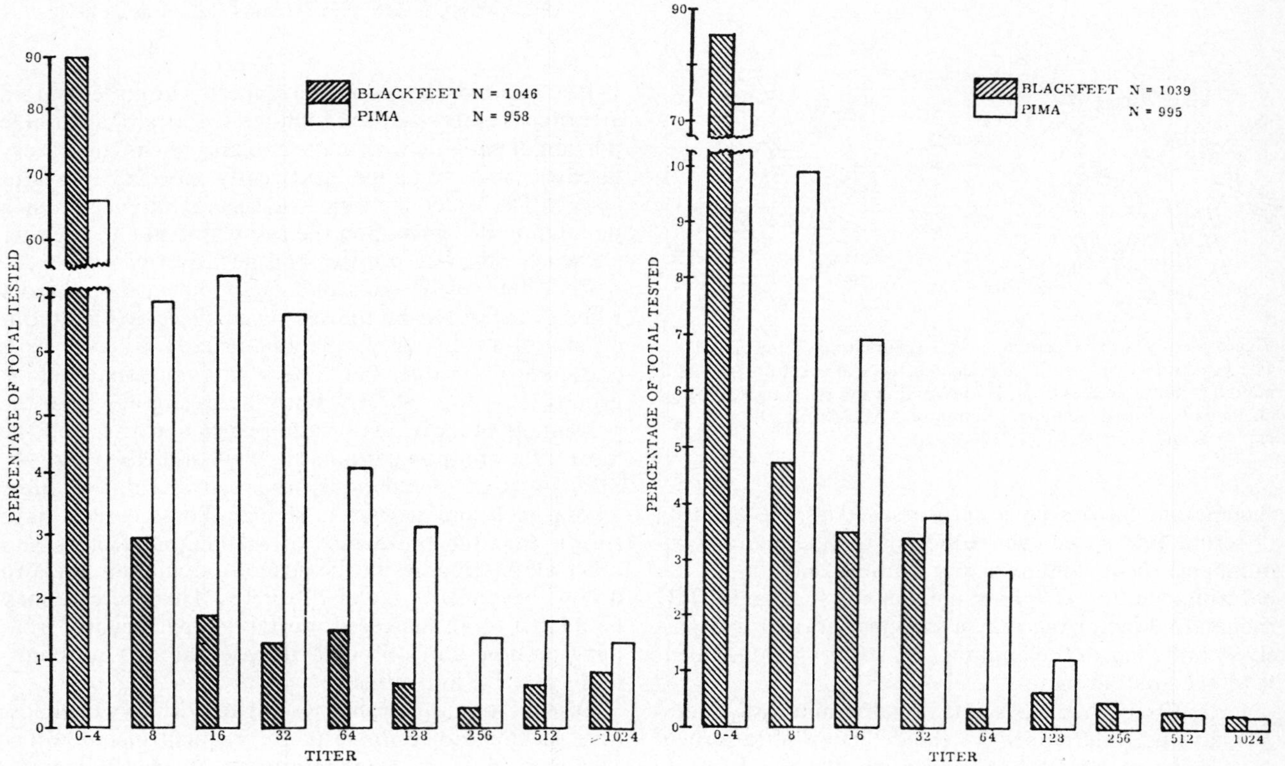


**Figure 44–7.** Titers of rheumatoid factor in the Pima and Blackfoot Indians as measured by bentonite flocculation (left panel) and sensitized sheep cell agglutination (right panel) assays. (From Bennett, P. H., and Burch, T. A., *In* Bennett, P. H., and Wood, P. H. N. (eds.): Population Studies in the Rheumatic Diseases. Amsterdam, Excerpta Medica, 1968.)

For uncertain reasons, the peripheral blood lymphocytes of the seronegative patients are relatively deficient in the B cells necessary for IgM rheumatoid factor synthesis.[57] Seropositive and seronegative rheumatoid arthritis may actually represent different diseases with overlapping clinical manifestations.[56-59] In both adults and children, the histocompatibility antigen HLA-DR4 is associated significantly with seropositive rheumatoid arthritis, but not with seronegative arthritis, at least in most studies.[58,60-63]

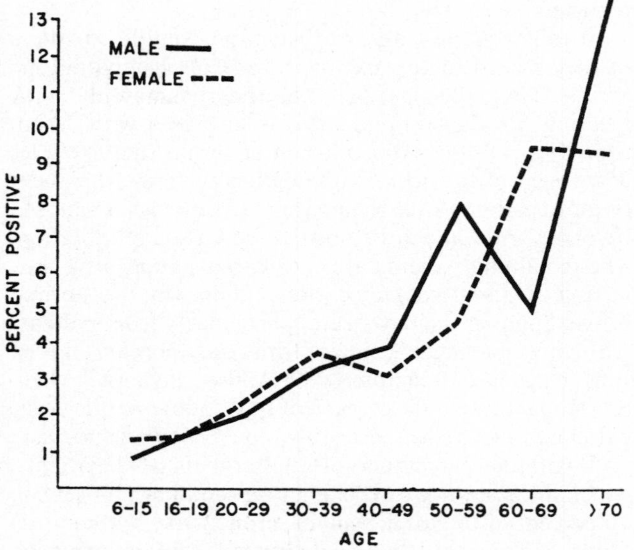


**Figure 44–8.** Incidence of positive latex fixation tests in varying age groups in Tecumseh, Mich. (From Mikkelsen, W. M., et al.: J. Chronic Dis. 20:351, 1967.)

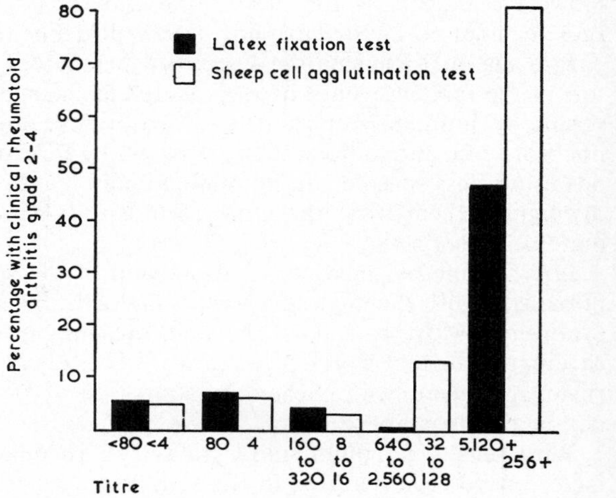


**Figure 44–9.** Relationship of latex fixation and sensitized sheep cell agglutination titers to rheumatoid arthritis. (From Valkenburg, H. A., et al.: Ann. Rheum. Dis. 25:497, 1966.)

**Table 44–2.** Diseases Commonly Associated with Rheumatoid Factor

| |
|---|
| *Rheumatic diseases:* rheumatoid arthritis, systemic lupus erythematosus, scleroderma, mixed connective tissue disease, Sjögren's syndrome |
| *Acute viral infections:* mononucleosis, hepatitis, influenza, and many others; after vaccination (may yield falsely elevated titers of antiviral antibodies) |
| *Parasitic infections:* trypanosomiasis, kala-azar, malaria, schistosomiasis, filariasis, etc. |
| *Chronic inflammatory diseases:* tuberculosis, leprosy, yaws, syphilis, brucellosis, subacute bacterial endocarditis, salmonellosis |
| *Neoplasms:* after irradiation or chemotherapy |
| *Other hyperglobulinemic states:* hypergammaglobulinemic purpura, cryoglobulinemia, chronic liver disease, sarcoid, other chronic pulmonary diseases |

As noted previously, the sensitized sheep cell agglutination test is slightly more specific for rheumatoid arthritis than is the latex fixation test. Positivity by both latex fixation and sensitized sheep cell agglutination is more specific for rheumatoid arthritis than is positivity by either test alone.[48,52] In general, the specificity of rheumatoid factor for rheumatoid arthritis is increased by (1) positivity on two or more consecutive occasions, (2) high titer, (3) reactivity with both human and rabbit IgG, and (4) distribution among the IgM, IgG, and IgA classes.

Whether or not the presence of rheumatoid factor in the serum of a normal individual is a risk factor for the development of rheumatoid arthritis is controversial. In an English study, 8 of 22 individuals with strongly positive sensitized sheep cell agglutination tests for rheumatoid factor, but only 4 of 29 seronegative subjects, developed polyarthritis when followed over a 5-year period.[48] On the contrary, other prospective studies from Tecumseh and Framingham found no prognostic value for rheumatoid factor tests as measured by latex fixation, but suggested that serologic conversion usually occurred simultaneously with or subsequent to the development of clinical arthritis.[64,65]

## ETIOLOGY OF RHEUMATOID FACTOR

**Genetic Influences.** Two types of immune response (Ir) genes have been described in animals, and recently in humans. The first are the histocompatibility-linked Ir genes. These encode the Ia antigens that restrict the interactions of certain T lymphocytes with antigen presenting macrophages and B lymphocytes. The second are the immunoglobulin variable region structural genes. These encode the diverse light and heavy polypeptide chain amino acid sequences responsible for antibody heterogeneity and specificity.

The histocompatibility-linked immune response genes play an undefined but important role in the etiology of seropositive rheumatoid arthritis. As mentioned previously, seropositive rheumatoid arthritis is associated with the HLA-DR4 antigen, located on the membrane of B lymphocytes, macrophages, and certain other cell types.[60-63] In animals, the Ia analogs of the HLA-DR antigens are the known products of genes that regulate the immune response to exogenous antigens and even some autoantigens.[66] Depending on the population studied, HLA-DR4–positive individuals have about a four- to eightfold increased risk of developing seropositive rheumatoid arthritis, as compared to HLA-DR4–negative subjects. Among normal blood donors, however, no significant correlation exists between IgM rheumatoid factor, as measured by the latex fixation test, and a particular HLA-DR type.[67]

Population studies among the Pima and Blackfoot Indians have failed to show a genetically determined familial aggregation of IgM rheumatoid factor positivity by either the latex fixation or sensitized sheep cell agglutination test.[68] In a family study in Leigh and Wensleydale, England, however, positivity by both assays showed a significant tendency toward familial aggregation, which was supported by twin studies.[48] As noted previously, such doubly reactive rheumatoid factors are the type most frequently associated with rheumatoid arthritis.

While genetic factors probably exert but a modest influence on the absolute ability to make IgM rheumatoid factor, they almost certainly influence the structure and specificity of the particular autoantibodies produced (Table 44–3). Insight concerning such possible genetic regulation of rheumatoid factor specificity came initially from structural studies of monoclonal proteins with rheumatoid factor activity. These monoclonal proteins, although arising in unrelated individuals, share common amino acid sequences and antigenic determinants (termed idiotypes) in the variable regions of the light and heavy chains.[69-71] Monoclonal IgG anti-gamma globulins also occur frequently in patients with cryoglobulinemia or hypergammaglobulinemia.[33,34] In one study the light chains isolated from two IgG rheumatoid factors had identical sequences through the first 42 amino acid residues, but differed from the light chains isolated from IgM rheumatoid factors.[72] The chance synthesis of nearly identical amino acid sequences in immunoglobulin molecules from unrelated individuals, even with similar antigenic reactivity, is distinctly unusual.

Recently, the IgM rheumatoid factors from some arthritis patients have been shown to share idiotypic antigens with monoclonal IgM rheumatoid factor cryoglobulins.[73-77] The rheumatoid factors from one instructive family with multiple seropositive members spanning three generations displayed a common idiotype

**Table 44–3.** Possible Role of Immunoglobulin Structural Genes in Rheumatoid Factor Synthesis

| |
|---|
| 1. Cross-reactive idiotypes among monoclonal and polyclonal rheumatoid factors from unrelated individuals |
| 2. Familial clustering of private idiotypes on rheumatoid factors |
| 3. Ability to make IgM rheumatoid factor present at birth |
| 4. Linkage of rheumatoid factor synthesis to the heavy chain structural gene locus in mice |

that was lacking on rheumatoid factors from unrelated individuals.[78] The common occurrence in the human population of antibody structural genes coding for rheumatoid factor light or heavy chains would explain all these results. In inbred mouse strains, breeding studies have definitively linked the synthesis of rheumatoid factors with defined specificities to the genetic locus for immunoglobulin heavy chains.[79]

**Environmental Influences.** If the ability to make rheumatoid factors is inherited, then (1) IgM rheumatoid factor precursors should be detectable among immature B lymphocytes and (2) IgM rheumatoid factor should function beneficially for the survival of the species. Recent evidence lends support to both these conclusions. IgM rheumatoid factor precursor B lymphocytes are present in human umbilical cord blood (Fig. 44–10) and are abundant in normal adult bone marrow.[59,80,81] Moreover, IgM rheumatoid factors comprise up to 10 percent of the Waldenström's macroglobulins that likely arise from neoplastic proliferation of immature lymphocytes.

Between birth and young adulthood, the frequency of IgM rheumatoid factor B lymphocytes in human blood rises severalfold, remaining fairly stable thereafter[59,80] (Fig. 44–10). Evidently the childhood infections and vaccinations that transiently induce low levels of IgM rheumatoid factor simultaneously increase the numbers of rheumatoid factor–bearing, long-lived memory B cells[81,82] (Fig. 44–11).

Experimental evidence has identified three types of environmental stimuli that potentially can trigger active rheumatoid factor synthesis in normal adults. They are (1) immunization with aggregated IgG in the form of immune complexes,[83-88] (2) polyclonal B cell activation,[89-94] and (3) unexpected cross-reactions between IgG and exogenous antigens.[85,95-98] Other possible, but probably less likely, mechanisms include somatic mutations among antibody-producing cells, alloimmunization with maternal immunoglobulins, and acquired structural abnormalities of the IgG molecule which render it antigenic.[99-101]

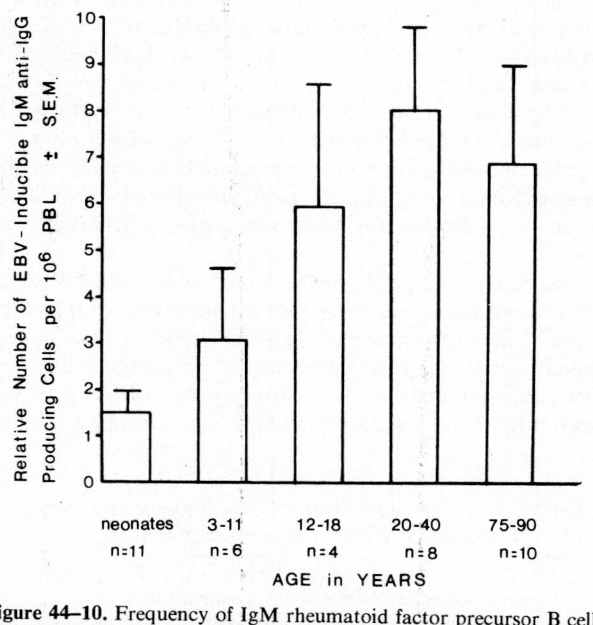


**Figure 44–10.** Frequency of IgM rheumatoid factor precursor B cells in the peripheral blood of normal subjects, as a function of age. The relative frequency was estimated by stimulation with Epstein-Barr virus under limiting dilution conditions. (From Fong, S., et al.: Arthritis Rheum. 25:959, 1982.)

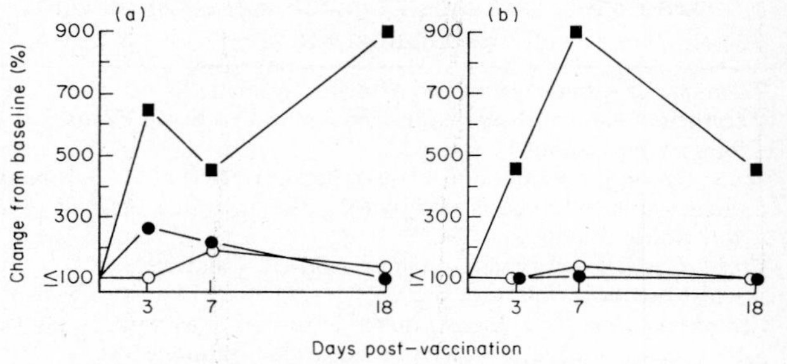


**Figure 44–11.** Representative examples of changes in peripheral blood IgM rheumatoid factor B cell frequency after tetanus toxoid vaccination in two individuals. ■ = IgM rheumatoid factor B cell frequency; • = plasma IgM rheumatoid factor; o = IgM. (From Welch, M. J., et al.: Clin. Exp. Immunol. 51:299, 1983.)

In adult animals of several species, rheumatoid factors of both the IgM and IgG class have been produced experimentally by repeated immunization with aggregated or denatured IgG, with particulate bacterial antigens from streptococci and *E. coli,* and even with soluble protein antigens.[83,84] The significant results of these diverse experimental models can be summarized as follows. In most cases the experimentally produced rheumatoid factors were polyclonal; occasionally they were monoclonal.[85] Except when markedly denatured IgG was used for autoimmunization, the rheumatoid factors reacted to varying degrees with native immunoglobulin.[83,86] In some rabbits immunized with streptococci, the elicited IgG rheumatoid factors had double specificity, reacting with both streptococcal peptidoglycans and autologous IgG.[85] The sustained production of rheumatoid factor usually required continual antigenic or mitogenic stimulation. Neither a self-perpetuating sensitization to autologous IgG nor a chronic synovitis was successfully produced in most cases.

IgM and IgA rheumatoid factors are detectable in the sera of many adult mice, in the absence of overt arthritis or chronic inflammatory disease.[102] In the MRL/1 mouse strain, a chronic synovitis of the lower extremities develops in 25 percent of adult animals and is associated with large amounts of circulating IgM and IgG rheumatoid factors.[103] Although the MRL/1 has a widespread lupus erythematosus-like disease affecting many organs, it is the only autoimmune mouse strain with both spontaneously developing arthritis and rheumatoid factor.

Rheumatoid factors in human beings develop during the course of many acute and chronic inflammatory diseases. While IgM rheumatoid factors predominate in most of these conditions, IgG rheumatoid factors are occasionally produced. As in the experimental models, sustained rheumatoid factor production usually depends upon the continual presence of the immunologic stimuli. A well-studied example is subacute bacterial endocarditis, in which elimination of bacteria by antibiotics leads to the subsequent decline in rheumatoid factor titers (Fig. 44–12).[87,88]

With few exceptions, the nonrheumatic diseases and the animal models associated with rheumatoid factor induction are characterized by either elevated levels of nonrheumatoid factor containing immune complexes and/or a diffuse elevation of serum immunoglobulins, indicating polyclonal B lymphocyte activation.

There are several possible mechanisms through which circulating immune complexes could induce the formation of rheumatoid factor. These include (1) the creation of neoantigens on the Fc portion of IgG by the combination of antibody with antigen, immunoglobulin aggregation, or denaturation,[99-101] (2) the enhanced binding of aggregated IgG to low affinity receptors on potential rheumatoid factor forming cells,[104,105] (3) the ability of exogenous antigen trapped in an immune complex to stimulate helper T lymphocytes, and hence to break self-tolerance,[106] and (4) nonspecific activation of B lymphocytes by aggregated IgG.[107]

The potential importance of polyclonal B lymphocyte activation in inducing rheumatoid factor production in humans has recently been emphasized.[89-94] Polyclonal B lymphocyte activators are mitogens that nonspecifically stimulate lymphocytes to secrete immunoglobulins in the absence of antigenic stimulation. They are widespread in nature and include many bacteria,[108] mycoplasmas,[109] certain viruses such as the Epstein-Barr (EB) virus,[110] proteolytic enzymes, and various soluble macromolecules derived from plants or activated T lymphocytes.

In vitro experiments have shown that lymphocytes from many normal adult humans and mice secrete low-affinity IgM rheumatoid factors after mitogenic stimulation by polyclonal B lymphocyte activators, including pokeweed mitogen and Epstein-Barr virus[89-94] (Fig. 44–13). The latter is of particular interest in rheumatoid

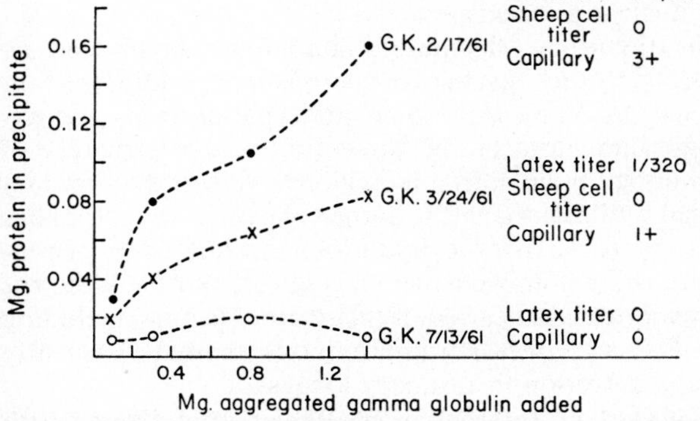


**Figure 44–12.** Decline of rheumatoid factor levels after treatment of subacute bacterial endocarditis. Rheumatoid factor was measured by quantitative precipitation with aggregated gamma globulin as well as by latex and sheep cell agglutination. (From Williams, R. C., Jr., and Kunkel, H. G.: J. Clin. Invest. 41:666, 1962.)

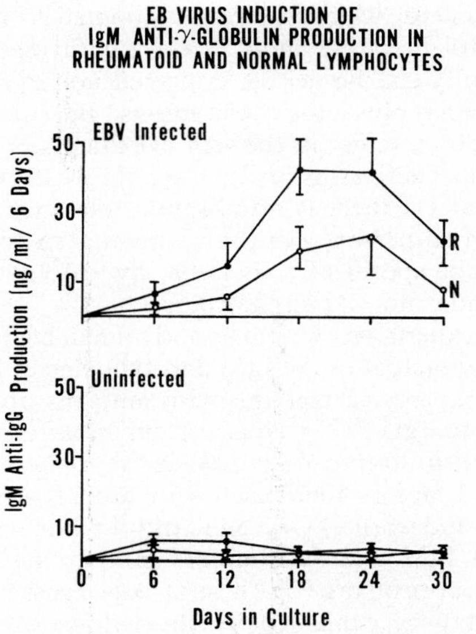


**Figure 44–13.** In vitro secretion of rheumatoid factor by lymphocytes from patients with rheumatoid arthritis (R) and normal subject (N) after infection with Epstein-Barr virus (EBV). (From Slaughter, L., et al.: J. Exp. Med. 148:1427, 1977.)

arthritis, because it is a permanent but quiescent resident of the B lymphocytes of many normal adults which can be reactivated by certain immunologic stimuli.[111,112] In addition, the Epstein-Barr virus is the only well-described polyclonal activator of immature human B lymphocytes.[80,113] Most other polyclonal activators presumably exert their action via T lymphocyte-generated factors. The latter stimulate primarily mature B lymphocytes, which are already active in vivo.[114,115] In normal subjects, rheumatoid factor precursors are uncommon among the mature B lymphocyte subset, but abundant among the Epstein-Barr virus sensitive immature B lymphocyte subset.[71,80,114,115]

When compared with normal subjects, patients with rheumatoid arthritis have a distinctive cellular and humoral immune response to the Epstein-Barr virus.[90,116-120] The peripheral blood lymphocytes from rheumatoid arthritis patients frequently spontaneously transform in vitro to become permanent cell lines.[90,118,119] Patients with rheumatoid arthritis, when compared with normal subjects, have a fourfold increased titer of antibodies against Epstein-Barr virus–associated transformation antigens found in the nucleus of virally infected B lymphoblasts.[116,117] Whether these serologic and cellular abnormalities contribute in some way to the rheumatoid disease process is uncertain. In any event, they suggest that the differentiation and proliferation of B lymphocytes in rheumatoid arthritis patients might be improperly regulated.

The reasons for the common occurrence of rheumatoid factors after polyclonal activation of B lymphocytes may relate to the low affinity of the autoantibodies for IgG. Animal experiments have shown that the induction of either immunity or tolerance requires a minimum energy of interaction between antigen and antibody receptors on cells, which has been estimated to be in the order of $10^5$ liters per mole.[121] Cells with receptors of lower affinity can be neither triggered nor tolerized by antigen under physiologic conditions. But most rheumatoid factors, either in the sera of patients or induced by polyclonal activators in vitro, are of low affinity. This implies that (1) there is no absolute tolerance for IgG in any normal person, and (2) rheumatoid factors probably are not specifically elicitable by autologous IgG antigen under normal circumstances.

In both experimental animals and human beings, some rheumatoid factors of the IgM and IgG classes have the unusual property of reacting with antigens apparently unrelated to IgG.[85,95-98] Thus certain rabbits hyperimmunized with streptococci develop high titers of IgG rheumatoid factors that react with both streptococcal cell walls and with IgG.[85] Similarly, in humans many polyclonal IgM and IgG factors bind to histones or other nuclear proteins.[95-98] These strange cross-reactions perhaps may be explained by the ontogeny of the B lymphocyte.[71] If genes coding for rheumatoid factor are indeed inherited, they likely give rise to somatic variants, through recombination and mutation. It would not be surprising if a somatically generated antibody occasionally retained evidence of its lineage by binding to the original germ line specificity, albeit with low affinity. There is no conclusive evidence for or against this hypothesis. Nevertheless it is consistent with the experimental data and does explain how a variety of antigens in the environment could unexpectedly give rise to rheumatoid factors during the course of normal immunization.

## IMMUNOCHEMICAL PROPERTIES OF RHEUMATOID FACTOR

**Antigenic Specificity.** Polyclonal IgM rheumatoid factors from the sera of patients with rheumatoid arthritis react with a diverse array of antigenic determinants localized to the Fc portion of the IgG molecule in both the $CH_2$ and $CH_3$ domains[99] (Fig. 44–1). These determinants include (1) cross-reactive antigens shared by human and animal IgG;[122-124] (2) species-specific antigens found in human but not animal IgG;[28,123] (3) subclass-specific antigens found on one or more but not all of the four subclasses of human IgG;[125] (4) genetically defined alloantigens of the Gm type, which are autosomally inherited and differ from person to person, depending on their inheritance (each human IgG subclass has its own set of Gm antigens);[21-23] and (5) neoantigens better expressed on aggregated, denatured, or enzymatically digested IgG than on monomeric native IgG,[99-101] including the so-called "pepsin agglutinators," which react with antigenic determinants exposed in Fab'2 fragments of IgG but not in the native molecule.[126]

Recent experiments have also identified IgM and IgG antibodies in rheumatoid sera reactive with antigens on the Fab region of intact, native IgG.[93,127] Strictly speaking, such anti-Fab antibodies are not true rheumatoid factors. They may be representative of the anti-idiotypic antibodies that regulate interactions among lymphocytes in an "immune network."[128]

The many specificities of IgM rheumatoid factors have been utilized by immunologists to unravel the genetic control of human IgG synthesis. However, no one antigenic determinant on the IgG molecule, with the possible exception of the Ga antigen, has yet been shown to be of unique importance in rheumatoid arthritis.[129] The important point to remember is that IgM rheumatoid factors in rheumatoid sera react with multiple antigenic determinants on autologous IgG. While a proportion of rheumatoid factors do react better with Gm alloantigens, with animal IgG's or with denatured IgG than with native, autologous IgG, the difference is never absolute.

The varied array of antigenic determinants reacting with IgM rheumatoid factors reflects the polyclonality of the antibody molecules themselves. By means of quantitative immunoabsorptions with animal gamma globulins, the IgM rheumatoid factors from a single serum can be separated into multiple species with different antigen-binding profiles.[122,123] Each animal gamma globulin shares but a fraction of the antigenic determinants found on human IgG. Thus the chance of a particular serum reacting with an animal gamma globulin increases with the heterogeneity of the autoantibody response. Because rheumatoid factors in rheumatoid arthritis tend to be more heterogeneous and of higher titer than in nonrheumatic diseases, they more frequently react with animal IgG. This is one of the reasons for the slightly greater specificity of the Rose-Waaler test, as compared with the latex fixation test, for rheumatoid arthritis.

The specificity and polyclonality of IgG and IgA rheumatoid factors have been analyzed in only a few studies.[130] Isolated IgG rheumatoid factors contain both kappa and lambda light chains, although the kappa chains predominate.[34,95,131] They react with human IgG, as indicated by their ability to form immune complexes in autologous serum. A recent study reported that horse IgG was more sensitive, whereas rabbit IgG was more specific, for the detection of IgG rheumatoid factor by radioimmunoassay.[39] Some IgG rheumatoid factors have antinuclear antibody reactivity.[95]

In the future, rheumatoid factors may be divided according to their particular complement of idiotypic antigens. As discussed earlier, idiotypic antigens are serologic indicators of the three-dimensional structure of immunoglobulin variable regions. A series of monoclonal antibodies against human rheumatoid factors has been prepared by the hybridoma technique.[76,77] Eventually these homogeneous reagents should facilitate the systematic classification of rheumatoid factors, including the IgG and IgA rheumatoid factors that frequently escape detection in ordinary assays.

**Kinetics of Interaction of Rheumatoid Factor with IgG.** The affinity of rheumatoid factors for IgG has been determined by analytical ultracentrifugation and equilibrium molecular sieving.[105,132-134] Typical association constants for both IgM and IgG rheumatoid factors average from 1 $\times$ $10^4$ to 5 $\times$ $10^5$ liters per mole.[135] These values are from ten- to 100-fold less than the affinities of common heteroantibodies produced after exogenous immunization. A proportion of rheumatoid factors produced by plasma cells in vitro, or eluted from synovium, may have higher affinity.[28,136] These rheumatoid factors may not be detected in serum because of prior reaction with IgG and clearance by the reticuloendothelial system.

In spite of their intrinsically low affinity for antigen, rheumatoid factors can produce stable complexes with IgG under appropriate conditions. For multivalent IgM rheumatoid factor, this occurs when the IgG antigen is aggregated (Fig. 44–14). While each individual antigen-antibody bond in such an IgM-IgG aggregate probably is individually of insufficient energy to yield a long-lived complex, the sum total of multiple interactions produces a stable structure.[104] From a biologic standpoint, the potentiating effect of multivalency is probably greater for those IgM rheumatoid factors of low affinity, since high affinity antibodies, by definition, bind antigens securely even at low concentrations.

IgG rheumatoid factors have unique kinetic properties which distinguish them from all other autoantibodies and heteroantibodies, in that the antigens with which they react reside on the antibody molecule itself. Hence IgG rheumatoid factors can self-associate and form immune complexes in the absence of exogenous antigen.[130,137-139] This self-associating ability favors the formation of immune complexes by anti-Ig antibodies of lower affinity than would be required to produce a similar reaction in a heterologous antigen-antibody system. By analogy with other systems, the ability of IgG rheumatoid factor to form high molecular weight complexes probably depends upon (1) the concentration and affinity of the autoantibody and (2) the ratio of IgG rheumatoid factor to normal IgG. IgM rheumatoid factor may, in addition, enhance the formation of IgG rheumatoid factor containing complexes by cross-linking the reversibly aggregated IgG.[25]

**Physiologic Role of Rheumatoid Factors.** The regular appearance of IgM rheumatoid factors during polyclonal B lymphocyte activation strongly suggests that the autoantibodies have an important physiologic function. Polyclonal B lymphocyte activation represents a primitive response of the humoral immune system to bacterial or parasitic exposure.[140] It leads to the production of diverse, low-affinity IgM and IgG antibodies. The IgM antibodies bind efficiently only to repeating antigenic determinants on the offending organism. The IgG antibodies typically interact only weakly with antigen. IgM rheumatoid factors have the ability to crosslink the low affinity IgG antibodies, aligned on a surface.[141] The net result is the formation of a relatively stable, multivalent and multispecific complex.

When bound to aggregated IgG, rheumatoid factors of the IgM class activate complement remarkably efficiently[142-144] (Fig. 44–15). If the IgG is bound to a bacteria or parasite, the end result probably is either the lysis of the invading organism or its clearance from the circulation via the abundant complement receptors of the reticuloendothelial system. For this reason, IgM rheumatoid factor synthesis may represent an essential component of an effective polyclonal antibody response.

Recent experiments in rats provide direct evidence for an important protective role of IgM rheumatoid factor in parasitic infections.[145] Lactating rats, and their suckling offspring, have a serum factor that renders them naturally resistant to infection with pathogenetic trypanosomes. The protective component has been identified as an IgM rheumatoid factor that amplifies a low level IgG response to the parasite.

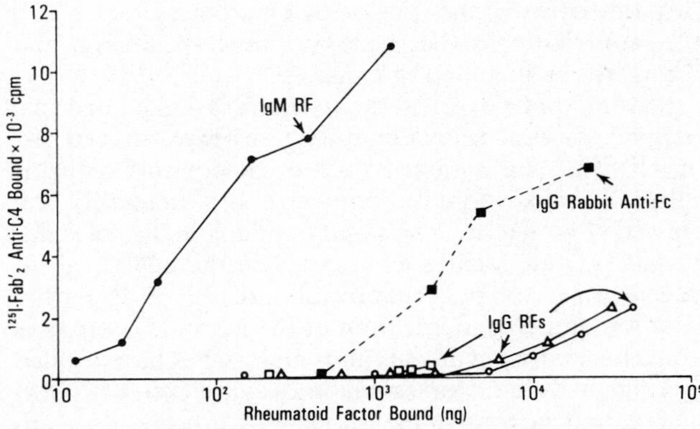


**Figure 44–15.** Comparison of the complement-fixing ability of IgM rheumatoid factor (RF), IgG rheumatoid factor, and rabbit IgG antibody against human Fc. The ordinate shows the amount of C4 fixed, as a function of the amount of antibody bound to antigen on a solid phase, as shown on the abscissa. (From Sabharwal, U.K., et al.: Arthritis Rheum. 25:1261, 1982.)

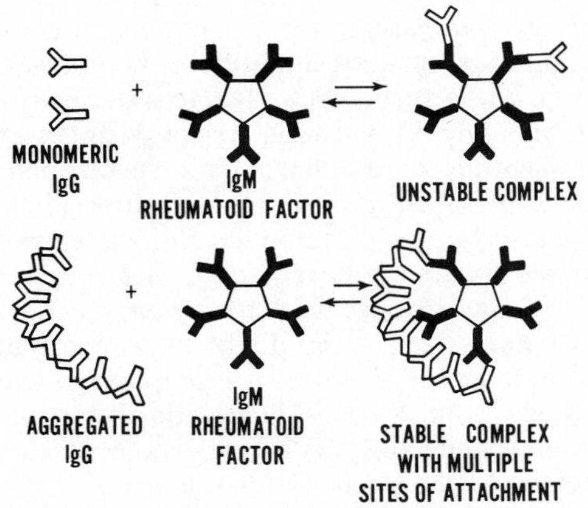


**Figure 44–14.** Interaction of IgM rheumatoid factor with monomeric and aggregated IgG.

## ROLE OF RHEUMATOID FACTOR IN RHEUMATOID ARTHRITIS

The several mechanisms which have been proposed for the etiology of rheumatoid arthritis are discussed in detail in Chapters 58 and 59. Here, we wish to emphasize only the salient properties of rheumatoid factors which may contribute to the etiology, tissue specificity, and chronicity of rheumatic disease.

Rheumatoid arthritis is an extravascular immune complex disease predominantly affecting synovial tissues.[146] Thus the synovial fluid of rheumatoid arthritis patients, unlike serum, frequently has markedly depressed complement levels and contains high molecular weight IgG aggregates as detected in the analytical ultracentrifuge or by cryoprecipitation.[30,31,147,148] Partial isolation and characterization of the immune complexes from rheumatoid synovial fluids and tissues have yielded IgG rheumatoid factors, sometimes complexed with IgM rheumatoid factor, in the absence of other known antigens.[31] Thus rheumatoid factors are likely to be of prime importance in the pathogenesis of the extravascular immune complex disease which produces rheumatoid synovitis.

Because of the common occurrence of rheumatoid factor, as measured by latex fixation, in the sera of patients without rheumatic disease, the importance of rheumatoid factor has often been downgraded. In several respects, however, the rheumatoid factors in rheumatoid arthritis patients differ from those in the nonrheumatic diseases (Table 44-4). Rheumatoid factors in rheumatoid arthritis, when compared to those in nonrheumatic conditions, are of higher titer, react better with animal gamma globulins, are produced primarily in the synovium and other extravascular sites, and are enriched in self-associating IgG rheumatoid factor molecules. While no one of these differences is diagnostic of rheumatoid arthritis, the constellation of high titers of heterogeneous IgM and IgG rheumatoid factor produced in the synovium is highly characteristic of rheumatoid arthritis.

The immunochemical properties of rheumatoid factors may have implications important in understanding the pathogenesis of immune complex–mediated synovitis. Most of the immunoglobulin in rheumatoid synovium probably is produced in situ rather than being deposited from the circulation.[149,154] Moreover, many of the IgG-producing plasma cells in rheumatoid synovium contain IgG rheumatoid factor (Fig. 44-16).[138,152,155] At these sites of IgG rheumatoid factor production, the local concentration of antibody is high while the concentration of normal IgG is low in comparison (Fig. 44-17). This imbalance permits the formation of large IgG rheumatoid factor containing complexes.[37,130,137,138] The ability of IgG rheumatoid factor in rheumatoid arthritis to react with multiple antigenic determinants on the Fc piece could further enhance large complex formation. When the IgG rheumatoid factor containing complexes escape into the circulation, however, where the concentration of normal IgG is high, they may be dissociated into immunoglobulin dimers and trimers. Through the formation of cyclical structures, self-associating IgG rheumatoid factor dimers are probably exceptionally stable.[130,137,138]

**Table 44–4.** Common Properties of Rheumatoid Factors in Rheumatoid Arthritis and Nonrheumatic Disease

| | Rheumatoid Arthritis | Nonrheumatic Disease |
|---|---|---|
| Titer | High | Low |
| Double reactivity with human and animal gamma globulin | Frequent | Infrequent |
| Immunoglobulin class | IgM, IgG, IgA | Mainly IgM |
| Site of production | Synovium and other extravascular sites | Unknown, but no synovial localization |

Soluble immune complexes with less than three IgG molecules are incapable of fixing complement and bind relatively poorly to IgM rheumatoid factors.[156] Hence the IgG-IgG dimers seen in the sera of patients with rheumatoid arthritis by analytical ultracentrifugation may not be of pathogenic import. The large IgG complexes in rheumatoid synovium, on the other hand, fix complement, bind to IgM rheumatoid factor, and perhaps have the capacity to stimulate other antigen sensitive cells.

In some patients with hypergammaglobulinemic purpura, hyperviscosity syndromes, and monoclonal gammopathies, as well as in some patients with widespread, severe rheumatoid arthritis, the IgG rheumatoid factor concentration in serum may achieve very high concentrations.[33,34,137,138] Under these unusual circumstances, large complement fixing complexes are formed just as they are in the synovium, leading to a diffuse and sometimes life-threatening vasculitis. Additionally, the unique cryoglobulinemic properties of some rheumatoid factors may facilitate precipitation even in the presence of excess normal IgG. In both cases, the IgG aggregates, besides fixing complement, may interfere with granulocyte and lymphocyte function, with a cascade of secondary abnormalities. Nevertheless the larger IgG-IgG complexes in the sera of patients with rheumatoid vasculitis can still be dissociated in vitro to typical IgG dimers by the addition of massive concentrations of normal IgG (Fig. 44-18).

Through the cross-linking of immunoglobulin Fc fragments, IgM rheumatoid factors stabilize and enhance the precipitation of antigen-antibody complexes.[31] On the other hand, IgM rheumatoid factors sterically hinder the binding of IgG molecules to complement and Fc receptor bearing macrophages and neutrophils.[157,158] Thus the effect of IgM rheumatoid factors on such biological consequences of immune complex formation as complement fixation, phagocytosis, and antibody dependent cellular toxicity depends upon the particular system studied. There is no doubt, however, that IgM rheumatoid factors themselves fix complement (Fig. 44–15).[9] Indeed, serum levels of hemolytic rheumatoid factor correlate significantly with in vivo complement turnover rates in patients with rheumatoid arthritis (Fig. 44–19).[159]

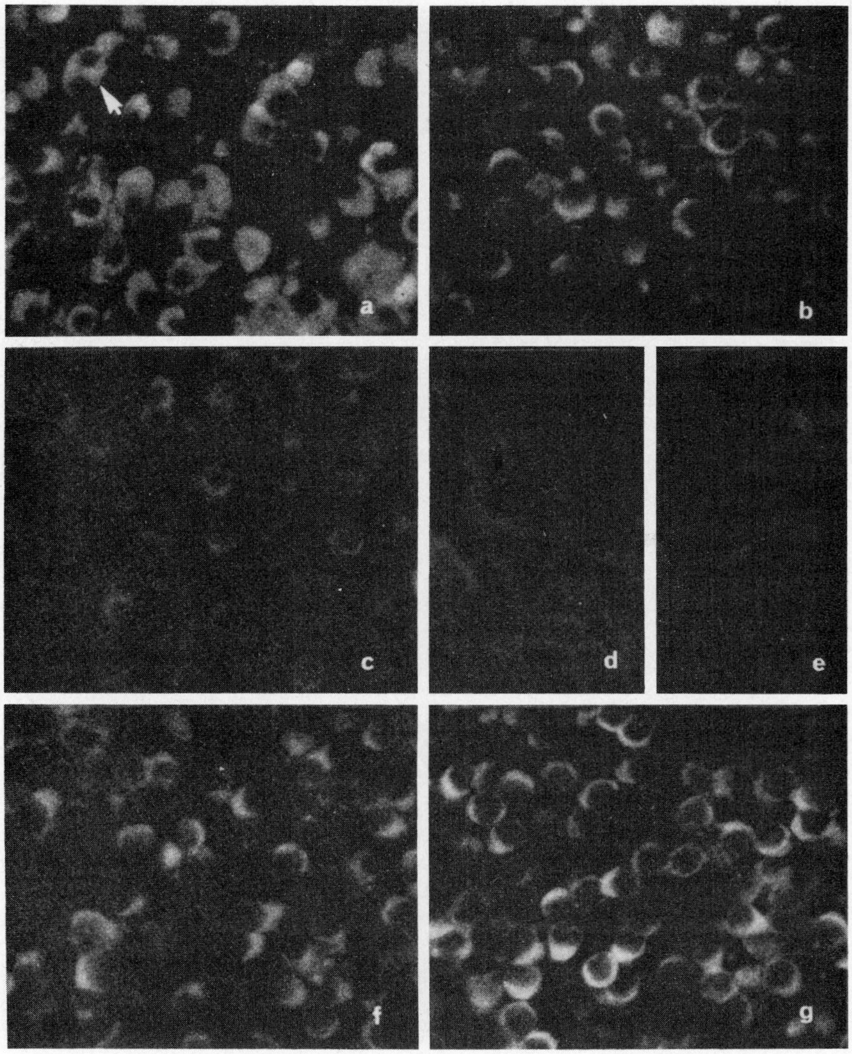


**Figure 44–16.** Demonstration of IgG rheumatoid factor containing plasma cells in rheumatoid synovium by immunofluorescence after digestion with pepsin. *A*, Stained with anti-IgG Fc before pepsin treatment (arrow indicates plasma cell with two nuclei). *B* and *C*, The effect of different pepsin concentrations on intracellular $F(ab')_2$-fragments. Stained with anti-$F(ab')_2$ after treatment with 0.15 M pepsin in *B* and 0.20 M pepsin in *C*. *D*, Stained with anti-IgG Fc after treatment with 0.15 M pepsin. No staining. *E*, Stained with heat-aggregated IgG before pepsin treatment. No staining. *F*, Stained with native IgG after pepsin treatment. *G*, Stained with heat-aggregated IgG after pepsin treatment. (From Munthe, E., and Natvig, J. B.: Clin. Exp. Immunol. 12:55, 1972.)

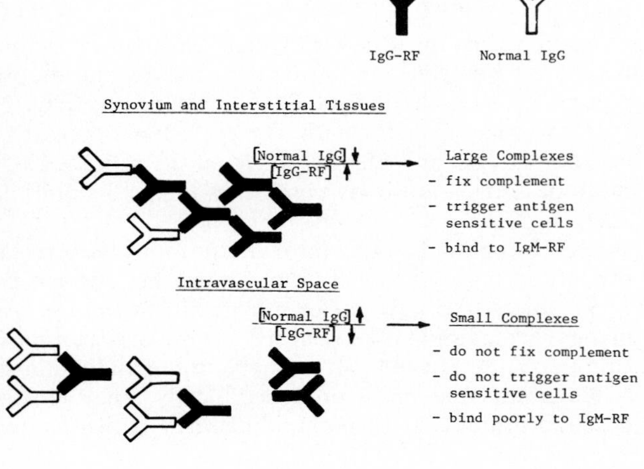


**Figure 44–17.** Possible mechanisms of immune complex formation by IgG rheumatoid factor in synovial tissues and serum.

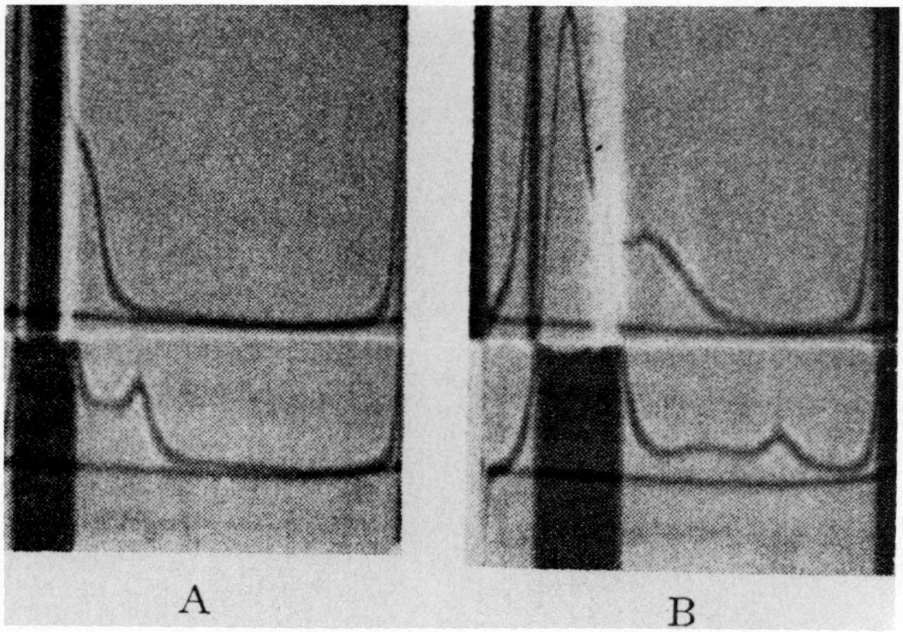


**Figure 44–18.** *A* and *B*, Effect of adding monomeric IgG on the distribution of IgG rheumatoid factor containing intermediate complexes. Lower patterns with albumin added show no effects; upper patterns with γ-globulins added show a shift to smaller complexes. (From Kunkel, H. G., et al.: J. Clin. Invest. 40:117, 1961.)

## SUMMARY

Rheumatoid factors are autoantibodies reacting with the Fc portion of autologous IgG. IgM rheumatoid factors are commonly measured by the agglutination of particles coated with human or rabbit IgG. The detection of poorly agglutinating IgG and IgA rheumatoid factors often requires special techniques such as analytical ultracentrifugation, immunofluorescence, or radioimmunoassay. IgM rheumatoid factors are not specific for rheumatoid arthritis but are found in a wide variety of acute and chronic inflammatory diseases and even in some normal individuals. The higher the titer of rheumatoid factor reacting with human and rabbit immunoglobulin, the greater the specificity of rheumatoid factor for rheumatoid arthritis. A variable percentage of rheumatoid patients are seronegative by conventional tests. Some may have hidden rheumatoid factor bound to serum IgG, or undetected IgG rheumatoid factor complexes. A certain percentage of rheumatoid arthritis patients, however, are true seronegatives. Some investigators believe that these patients actually have a different disease from seropositive rheumatoid arthritis.

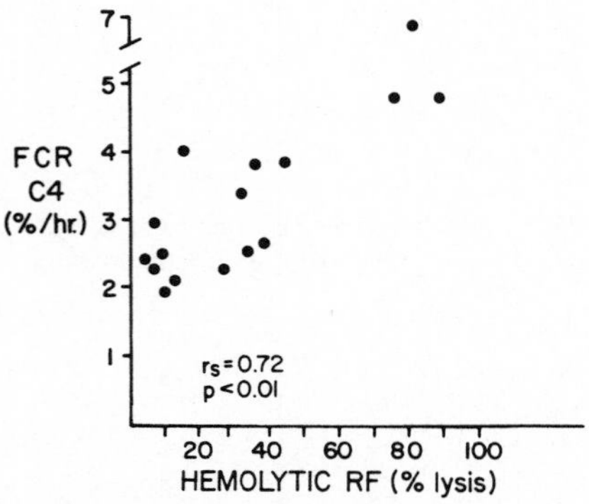


**Figure 44–19.** Relation between the in vivo fractional catabolic rate (FCR) of the C4 component of complement, and hemolytic IgM rheumatoid factor levels, in sixteen patients with rheumatoid arthritis. (From Kaplan, R. A., et al.: Arthritis Rheum. 23:911, 1980.)

Most human beings apparently have an inborn ability to make low-affinity rheumatoid factor after stimulation with polyclonal B cell activators, aggregated IgG, or cross-reacting antigens. Immunoglobulin variable region structure genes may influence the particular idiotypic antigens displayed on IgM rheumatoid factors. The role of histocompatibility antigens in rheumatoid factor production is still undefined. By analogy with animal systems, T lymphocytes may regulate the production of IgA and IgA rheumatoid factors.

IgM rheumatoid factors probably function normally in the defense against parasitic and bacterial infection. They substantially amplify the stability of interaction, and hence the biologic activity, of low-affinity IgG antibodies generated during polyclonal B lymphocyte activation.

The antigens on IgG with which rheumatoid factors react are heterogeneous. Most, but perhaps not all, are present on monomeric IgG. The increased reactivity of IgM rheumatoid factor with aggregated as opposed to monomeric IgG probably results from the enhanced stability of antigen-antibody complexes linked at multiple sites.

IgG rheumatoid factors have unique immunochemical properties. Even at low concentrations they form IgG-IgG dimers through preferential self-association. At higher rheumatoid factor concentrations, larger immune complexes are formed. Most of the immunoglobulin in rheumatoid synovium is produced locally. The synovial tissues and fluids of rheumatoid arthritis patients often contain many IgG rheumatoid factor–producing plasma cells and large complement fixing immune complexes. The restriction of complement-fixing immune complexes in rheumatoid arthritis to the extravascular space in most cases may result from a concentration-dependent aggregation of locally produced IgG rheumatoid factor. In the synovium and other extravascular sites where the concentration of antibody is high and antigen is low, the formation of complement-fixing complexes, with subsequent inflammation, is favored. In serum, where the concentration of normal IgG is high, complement-fixing immune complexes usually do not form. If serum rheumatoid factor levels are very high, however, or if their interaction with IgG results in cryoprecipitation, a systemic immune complex vasculitis may develop.

## References


1. Waaler, E.: On the occurrence of a factor in human serum activating the specific agglutination of sheep blood corpuscles. Acta Path. Microbiol. Scand. 17:172, 1940.
2. Rose, H.M., Ragan, C., Pearce, E., and Lipman, M.O.: Differential agglutination of normal and sensitized sheep erythrocytes by sera of patients with rheumatoid arthritis. Proc. Soc. Exp. Biol. Med. 68:1, 1949.
3. Franklin, E.C., Holman, H.R., Muller-Eberhard, H.J., and Kunkel, H.G.: An unusual protein of high molecular weight in the serum of certain patients with rheumatoid arthritis. J. Exp. Med. 105:425, 1957.
4. Lospalluto, J., and Ziff, M.: Chromatographic studies of the rheumatoid factor. J. Exp. Med. 110:169, 1959.
5. Kunkel, H.G., Muller-Eberhard, H.J., Fudenberg, H.H., and Tomasi, T.B.: Gamma globulin complexes in rheumatoid arthritis and certain other conditions. J. Clin. Invest. 40:117, 1961.
6. Heimer, R., and Levin, F.M.: On the distribution of rheumatoid factors among the immunoglobulins. Immunochemistry 3:1, 1966.
7. Zuraw, B.L., O'Hair, C.H., Vaughan, J.H., Mathison, D.A., Curd, J.G., and Katz, D.H.: Immunoglobulin E-rheumatoid factor in the serum of patients with rheumatoid arthritis, asthma and other diseases. J. Clin. Invest. 68:1610, 1981.
8. Singer, J.M., and Plotz, C.M.: The latex fixation test. I. Application to the serologic diagnosis of rheumatoid arthritis. Am. J. Med. 21:888, 1956.
9. Epstein, W., Johnson, A., and Ragan, C.: Observations on a precipitin reaction between serum of patients with rheumatoid arthritis and a preparation (Cohn Fraction II) of human gamma globulin. Proc. Soc. Exp. Biol. Med. 91:235, 1956.
10. Tanimoto, K., Cooper, N.R., Johnson, J.S., and Vaughan, J.H.: Complement fixation by rheumatoid factor. J. Clin. Invest. 55:437, 1975.
11. McCormick, J.N.: An immunofluorescence study of rheumatoid factor. Ann. Rheum. Dis. 22:1, 1963.
12. Franchimont, P., and Suteneau, S.: Radioimmunoassay of rheumatoid factor. Arthritis Rheum. 12:483, 1969.
13. Carson, D.A., Lawrance, S., Catalano, M.A., Vaughan, J.H., and Abraham, G.: Radioimmunoassay of IgG and IgM rheumatoid factors reacting with human IgG. J. Immunol. 119:295, 1977.
14. Hay, C., Nineham, L.J., and Roitt, I.M.: Routine assay for detection of IgG and IgM anti globulins in seronegative and seropositive rheumatoid arthritis. Br. Med. J. 3:203, 1975.
15. Koopman, W.J., and Schrohenloher, R.E.: Sensitive radioimmunoassay for quantification of IgM rheumatoid factor. Arthritis Rheum. 34:302, 1980.
16. Dunne, J.V., Carson, D.A., Spiegelberg, H.L., Alspaugh, M.A., and Vaughan, J.H.: IgA rheumatoid factor in the sera and saliva of patients with rheumatoid arthritis and Sjögren's syndrome. Ann. Rheum. Dis. 38:161, 1979.
17. Pope, R.M., and McDuffy, S.J.: IgG rheumatoid factor. Relationship to seropositive rheumatoid arthritis and absence in seronegative disorders. Arthritis Rheum. 22:988, 1979.
18. Gripenberg, M., Wafis, F., Isomaki, H., and Lindes, E.: A simple enzyme immunoassay for the demonstration of rheumatoid factor. J. Immunol. Methol. 31:109, 1979.
19. Finley, P.R., Hicks, M.J., Williams, R.J., Hinlicky, J. and Lichti, D.A.: Rate nephelometric measurement of rheumatoid factor in serum. Clin. Chem. 25:1909, 1979.
20. Waller, M.V., and Vaughan, J.H.: Use of anti-Rh sera for demonstrating agglutination activating factors in rheumatoid arthritis. Proc. Soc. Exp. Biol. Med. 92:198, 1956.
21. Grubb, R., and Laurell, A.B.: Hereditary serological human serum groups. Acta Pathol. Microbiol. Scand. 39:390, 1956.
22. Natvig, J.B., and Kunkel, H.B.: Detection of genetic antigens utilizing gamma globulins coupled to red blood cells. Nature 215:68, 1967.
23. Steinberg, A.C., and Wilson, J.A.: Hereditary globulin factors and immune tolerance in man. Science 140:303, 1963.
24. Grieble, H.G., Bosh, G.L., Szarto, M., and Anderson, T.O.: Serologic diagnosis of RA. The latex gamma globulin fixation test. J. Chron. Dis. 21:667, 1967.
25. Winchester, R.J., Kunkel, H.G., and Agnello, V.: Occurrence of γ-globulin complexes in serum and joint fluid of rheumatoid arthritis patients. Use of monoclonal rheumatoid factors as reagents for their demonstration. J. Exp. Med. 134:2865, 1971.
26. Meltzer, M., Franklin, E.C., Elias, K., McCluskey, K.J., and Cooper, N.: Cryoglobulinemia—a clinical and laboratory study. II. Cryoglobulins with rheumatoid factor activity. Am. J. Med. 40:837, 1966.
27. Levo, Y., Gorevic, P.P., Kassab, H.J., Zucker-Franklin, D., and Franklin, E.C.: Association between hepatitis B virus and essential mixed cryoglobulinemia. N. Engl. J. Med. 296:501, 1977.
28. Allen, J.C., and Kunkel, H.G.: Hidden rheumatoid factors with specificity for native γ globulin. Arthritis Rheum. 9:758, 1966.
29. Ewald, R.W., and Schubart, A.F.: Agglutinating activity of the complement component Clq in the F-II latex fixation test. J. Immunol. 97:100, 1966.
30. Hannestad, K.: Presence of aggregated γ-globulin in certain rheumatoid synovial effusions. Clin. Exp. Immunol. 2:511, 1967.
31. Winchester, R.J., Agnello, V., and Kunkel, H.G.: Gamma globulin complexes in synovial fluids of patients with rheumatoid arthritis. Partial characterization and relationship to lowered complement levels. Clin. Exp. Immunol. 6:689, 1970.
32. Theofilopoulos, A.N., Burtonboy, G., LoSpalutto, J.J., and Ziff, M.: IgM rheumatoid factor and low molecular weight IgM. An association with vasculitis. Arthritis Rheum. 17:272, 1974.
33. Grey, H.M., Kohler, P.F., Terry, W.D., and Franklin, E.C.: Human monoclonal γ-G cryoglobulins with anti-γ-globulin activity. J. Clin. Invest. 47:1875, 1968.
34. Capra, J.D., Winchester, R.J., and Kunkel, H.G.: Hypergammaglobulinemic purpura. Studies on the unusual anti-γ-globulins characteristic of the sera of these patients. Medicine 50:125, 1971.
35. Chodirker, W.B., and Tomasi, T.B.: Low molecular weight rheumatoid factor. J. Clin. Invest. 42:876, 1963.
36. Schrohenloher, R.E.: Characterization of the γ-globulin complexes present in certain sera having high titers of anti-γ-globulin activity. J. Clin. Invest. 45:501, 1961.
37. Munthe, E., and Natvig, J.B.: Complement fixing intracellular complexes of IgG rheumatoid factor in rheumatoid plasma cells. Scand. J. Immunol. 1:217, 1972.
38. Torrigiani, G., and Roitt, I.M.: Antiglobulin factors in sera from patients with rheumatoid arthritis and normal subjects. Quantitative estimation in different immunoglobulin classes. Ann. Rheum. Dis. 26:334, 1967.
39. Pope, R.N., and McDuffy, S.J.: IgG rheumatoid factor: Analysis of various species of IgG for detection by radioimmunoassay. J. Lab. Clin. Med. 97:842, 1981.
40. Scott, D.G.I., Bacon, T.A., Allen, C., Elson, C.J., and Wallington, T.: IgG rheumatoid factor, complement and immune complexes in rheumatoid synovitis and vasculitis: Comparative and serial studies during cytotoxic therapy. Clin. Exp. Immunol. 43:54, 1981.
41. Elkow, K.B., Delacroix, D.L., Gharevi, A., Vauman, J.P., and Hughes, G.R.: Immunoglobulin A and polymeric IgA rheumatoid factors in systemic sicca syndrome: Partial characterization. J. Immunol. 129:577, 1982.
42. Dresner, E., and Trombly, P.: The latex-fixation reaction in nonrheumatic diseases. N. Engl. J. Med. 261:981, 1959.
43. Howell, D.S., Malcolm, J.M., and Pike, H.: The FII agglutinating factors in the serum of patients with nonrheumatic diseases. Am. J. Med. 29:662, 1960.
44. Kunkel, H.G., Simon, H.J., and Fudenberg, H.: Observations concerning positive serologic reactions for rheumatoid factor in certain patients with sarcoidosis and other hyperglobulinemic states. Arthritis Rheum. 1:289, 1958.
45. Bennett, P.H., and Wood, P.H.N. (eds.): Population Studies of the Rheumatic Diseases. Amsterdam, Excerpta Medica, 1968.
46. Mikkelson, W.M., Dodge, H.J., Duff, I.V., and Kato, H.: Estimates of the prevalence of rheumatic disease in the population of Tecumseh, Michigan, 1950–60. J. Chron. Dis. 20:351, 1967.
47. Hooper, B., Whittingham, S., Mathews, J.D., Mackay, I.R., and Curnow, D.H.: Autoimmunity in a rural community. Clin. Exp. Immunol. 12:79, 1972.

48. Lawrence, J.S.: Rheumatism in Populations. London, William Heinemann, Ltd., 1977.
49. Twomey, J.J., Rossen, R.D., Lewis, V.M., Laughter, A.H., and Douglass, C.C.: Rheumatoid factor and tumor-host interaction. Proc. Natl. Acad. Sci. USA 73:2106, 1976.
50. Theofilopoulos, A., and Dixon, F.J.: The biology and detection of immune complexes. Adv. Immunol. 28:89, 1979.
51. Pope, R.N., Yoshinoya, S., and McDuffy, J.J.: Detection of immune complexes and their relationships to rheumatoid factor in a variety of autoimmune disorders. Clin. Exp. Immunol. 46:259, 1981.
52. Valkenburg, H.A., Ball, J., Burch, T.A., Bennett, P.H., and Lawrence, J.S.: Rheumatoid factors in a rural population. Ann. Rheum. Dis. 25:497, 1966.
53. Moore, T.L., Donner, R.W., Weiss, T.D., Baldassare, A.R., and Zuckner, J.: Hidden 19S rheumatoid factor in juvenile rheumatoid arthritis. Pediatric Res. 14:1135, 1980.
54. Moore, T.L., Donner, R.W., Weiss, T.P., Baldassane, A.R., and Zuckner, J.: Specificity of hidden 19S 19M rheumatoid factor in patients with juvenile rheumatoid arthritis. Arthritis Rheum. 24:1283, 1981.
55. Masi, A.T., Maldonado-Cocco, J.A., Kaplan, S.B., Feigenbaum, S.L., and Chandler, R.W.: Prospective study of the early course of rheumatoid arthritis in young adults. Sem. Arthr. Rheum. 5:299, 1976.
56. Milzaao, S.C.: Seronegative peripheral arthritis. Clin. Rheum. Dis. 3:345, 1977.
57. Pasquali, J.-L., Fong, S., Tsoukas, C.D., Hench, P.K., Vaughan, J.H., and Carson, D.A.: Selective lymphocyte deficiency in seronegative rheumatoid arthritis. Arthritis Rheum. 24:770, 1981.
58. Alarcon, G., Koopman, W.J., Acton, R.T., and Barger, B.O.: Seronegative rheumatoid arthritis: A distinct immunogenetic disease? Arthritis Rheum. 25:502, 1982.
59. Fong, S., Miller, J.J., III, Moore, T.L., Tsoukas, C.D., Vaughan, J.H., and Carson, D.A.: Frequencies of Epstein-Barr virus inducible IgM anti-IgG B lymphocytes in normal children and in children with juvenile rheumatoid arthritis. Arthritis Rheum. 25:959, 1982.
60. Stastny, P.: Mixed lymphocyte cultures in rheumatoid arthritis. J. Clin. Invest. 57:1148, 1976.
61. McMichael, A.J., Sasayuki, T., McDevitt, H.O., and Payne, R.O.: Increased frequency of HLA-DW4 in rheumatoid arthritis. Arthritis Rheum. 20:1037, 1977.
62. Stastny, P.: Association of the B cell alloantigen DRw4 with rheumatoid arthritis. N. Engl. J. Med. 298:869, 1978.
63. Dobloug, J.H., Forre, O., Kass, E., and Thorsby, E.: HLA antigens and rheumatoid arthritis. Association between HLA-DRw4 positivity and IgM rheumatoid factor production. Arthritis Rheum. 23:309, 1980.
64. Mikkelson, W.M., and Dodge, H.: A 4-year follow-up of suspected rheumatoid arthritis. Arthritis Rheum. 12:87, 1967.
65. Hall, A.P.: Observations on subjects developing a positive test for rheumatoid factor. Arthritis Rheum. 12:301, 1969.
66. Ferrone, S., and David, C. (eds.): H-2, Ia and HLA-DR antigens. Hialeah, Florida, CRC Press, 1981.
67. Engleman, E.G., Sponzilli, E.E., Batey, M.E., Ramcharan, S., and McDevitt, H.O.: Mixed lymphocyte reaction in healthy women with rheumatoid factor. Lack of association with HLA-DW4. Arthritis Rheum. 21:690, 1978.
68. Bennett, P.H., and Burch, T.A.: The distribution of rheumatoid factor and rheumatoid arthritis in the families of Blackfeet and Pima Indians. Arthritis Rheum. 11:546, 1968.
69. Kunkel, H.G., Agnello, V., Joslin, F.G., Winchester, R.J., and Capra, J.D.: Cross idiotypic specificity among monoclonal IgM proteins with anti-γ-globulin activity. J. Exp. Med. 137:331, 1973.
70. Capra, J.D., and Kehoe, J.M.: Structure of antibodies with shared idiotypy: the complete sequence of the heavy chain variable regions of two immunoglobulin M anti-gamma globulins. Proc. Natl. Acad. Sci. USA 71:4032, 1974.
71. Carson, D.A., Pasquali, J.-L., Tsoukas, C.D., Fong, S., Slovin, S.F., Lawrance, S.K., Slaughter, L., and Vaughan, J.H.: Physiology and pathology of rheumatoid factors. Springer Semin. Immunopathol. 4:161, 1981.
72. Capra, J.D., Kehoe, J.M., Winchester, R.J., and Kunkel, H.G.: Structure function relationships among anti-gamma globulin antibodies. Ann. N.Y. Acad. Sci. 190:371, 1971.
73. Forre, O., Dobloug, J.H., Michaelsen, T.E., and Natvig, J.B.: Evidence for similar idiotypic determinants on different rheumatoid factor populations. Scand. J. Immunol. 9:281, 1979.
74. Bonagura, V.R., Kunkel, H.G., and Pernis, B.: Cellular localization of rheumatoid factor idiotypes. J. Clin. Invest. 69:1356, 1982.
75. Fong, S., Gilbertson, T., and Carson, D.A.: The internal image of IgG in anti-idiotypic antibodies against human rheumatoid factors. J. Immunol., 131:719, 1983.
76. Carson, D.A., and Fong, S.: A common idiotope on human rheumatoid factors identified by a hybridoma antibody. Molec. Immunol. 20:1081, 1983.
77. Pasquali, J.-L., Urlacher, A., and Storck, D.: A highly conserved determinant on human rheumatoid factor idiotypes defined by a monoclonal antibody. Eur. J. Immunol. 13:197, 1983.
78. Pasquali, J.-L., Fong, S., Tsoukas, C.D., Vaughan, J.H., and Carson, D.A.: Inheritance of IgM rheumatoid factor idiotypes. J. Clin. Invest. 66:863, 1980.
79. Van Snick, J.L.: A gene linked to the Igh-C locus controls the production of rheumatoid factors in the mouse. J. Exp. Med. 153:738, 1981.
80. Fong, S., Tsoukas, C.D., Frincke, L.A., Lawrance, S.K., Holbrook, T.L., Vaughan, J.H., and Carson, D.A.: Age associated changes in Epstein-Barr virus-induced human lymphocyte autoantibody responses. J. Immunol. 126:910, 1981.
81. Fong, S., Vaughan, J.H., Tsoukas, C.D., and Carson, D.A.: Selective induction of autoantibody secretion in human bone marrow by Epstein-Barr virus. J. Immunol. 129:1941, 1982.
82. Welch, M.J., Fong, S., Vaughan, J., and Carson, D.: Increased frequency of rheumatoid factor precursor B lymphocytes after immunization of normal adults with tetanus toxoid. Clin. Exp. Immunol. 51:299, 1983.
83. McCluskey, R.T., Miller, F., and Benacerraf, B.: Sensitization to denatured autologous gamma globulins. J. Exp. Med. 115:253, 1962.
84. Bokisch, V.A., Bernstein, D., and Krause, R.M.: Occurrence of 19S and 7S anti-IgG during hyperimmunization of rabbits with streptococci. J. Exp. Med. 136:799, 1972.
85. Bokisch, V.A., Chiao, J.W., Bernstein, D., and Krause, R.M.: Homogeneous rabbit 7S anti-IgG with antibody specificity for peptidoglycans. J. Exp. Med. 138:1184, 1973.
86. Abruzzo, J.L., and Christian, C.L.: The induction of a rheumatoid factor-like substance in rabbits. J. Exp. Med. 114:791, 1961.
87. Williams, R.C., and Kunkel, H.G.: Rheumatoid factor, complement and conglutinin aberrations in patients with subacute bacterial endocarditis. J. Clin. Invest. 41:666, 1962.
88. Carson, D.A., Bayer, A.S., Eisenberg, R.A., Lawrance, S., and Theofilopoulos, A.: IgG rheumatoid factor in subacute bacterial endocarditis: Relationship to IgM rheumatoid factor and circulating immune complexes. Clin. Exp. Immunol. 31:100, 1978.
89. Dresser, D.W.: Most IgM-producing cells in the mouse secrete autoantibodies (rheumatoid factor). Nature 274:480, 1978.
90. Slaughter, L., Carson, D.A., Jensen, F.C., Holbrook, T.L., and Vaughan, J.H.: In vitro effects of Epstein-Barr virus on peripheral blood mononuclear cells from patients with rheumatoid arthritis and normal subjects. J. Exp. Med. 148:1429, 1978.
91. Izui, S., Eisenberg, R.A., and Dixon, F.J.: IgM rheumatoid factors in mice injected with bacterial lipopolysaccharide. J. Immunol. 122:2096, 1979.
92. Dziarski, R.: Preferential induction of autoantibody secretion in polyclonal activation by peptidoglycan and lipopolysaccharide. II. In vivo studies. J. Immunol. 128:1026, 1982.
93. Van Snick, J.L., and Coulie, P.: Monoclonal anti-IgG antibodies derived from lipopolysaccharide-activated spleen cells of $129/S_V$ mice. J. Exp. Med. 155:219, 1982.
94. Birdsall, G.H.H., and Rossen, R.D.: Production of antibodies specific for Fc, Fab', and streptokinase-streptodornase in vitro by peripheral blood cells from patients with rheumatoid arthritis and normal donors. J. Clin. Invest. 69:75, 1982.
95. Hannestad, K., and Johannessen, A.: Polyclonal human antibodies to IgG (rheumatoid factors) which cross-react with cell nuclei. Scand. J. Immunol. 5:541, 1976.
96. Hannestad, K., Reckvig, O.P., and Husebekk, A.: Cross-reacting rheumatoid factors and lupus erythematosus (LE)-factors. Springer Semin. Immunopathol. 4:133, 1981.
97. Johnson, P.M.: IgM rheumatoid factors cross-reactive with IgG and a cell nuclear antigen: Immunopathological implications. Ann. Rheum. Dis. 39:586, 1980.
98. Agnello, V., Arbetter, A., DeKasep, G.I., Powell, R., Tan, E.M., and Joslin, F.: Evidence for a subset of rheumatoid factors that cross-react with DNA-histone and have a distinct cross-idiotype. J. Exp. Med. 151:1514, 1980.
99. Johnson, P.M., and Faulk, W.P.: Rheumatoid factor: Its nature, specificity, and production in rheumatoid arthritis. Clin. Immunol. Immunopathol. 6:414, 1976.
100. Dodon, N.D., and Quash, G.A.: The antigenicity of asialylated IgG: Its relationship to rheumatoid factor. Immunology 42:401, 1981.
101. Brown, C.S., and Brown, J.C.: Preferential reactivity of certain human and rabbit IgM and IgG rheumatoid factors with mildly reduced and amidoethylated IgG. J. Immunol. 126:2373, 1981.
102. Van Snick, J.L., and Masson, P.L.: Incidence and specificities of IgA and IgM anti-IgM anti-IgG autoantibodies in various mouse strains and colonies. J. Exp. Med. 151:45, 1980.
103. Andrews, B.S., Eisenberg, R.A., Theofilopoulos, A.N., Izui, S., Wilson, C.B., McConahey, P., Murphy, E.D., Roths, J.B., and Dixon, F.J.: Spontaneous murine lupus-like syndromes. Clinical and immunologic manifestations in several strains. J. Exp. Med. 148:1198, 1978.

104. Metzger, H.: Effect of antigen binding on the properties of antibody. Adv. Immunol. 18:169, 1974.
105. Eisenberg, R.: The specificity and polyvalency of binding of a monoclonal rheumatoid factor. Immunochemistry 13:355, 1976.
106. Weigle, W.O.: Immunological unresponsiveness. Adv. Immunol. 16:61, 1973.
107. Pisko, E.J., Turner, R.A., and Foster, S.L.: Induction of rheumatoid factor producing cells by aggregated IgG. Arthritis Rheum. 25:1108, 1982.
108. Banck, G., and Forsgren, A.: Many bacterial species are mitogenic for human blood B lymphocytes. Scand. J. Immunol. 8:347, 1978.
109. Biberfield, G.: Activation of human lymphocyte subpopulations by *Mycoplasma pneumoniae.* Scand. J. Immunol. 6:1145, 1977.
110. Rosen, A., Gergely, P., Jondal, M., Klein, G., and Britton, S.: Polyclonal Ig production after Epstein-Barr virus infection of human lymphocytes in vitro. Nature 267:52, 1977.
111. Nillson, K., Klein, G., Henle, W., and Henle, G.: The establishment of lymphoblastoid cell lines from adult and fetal human lymphoid tissue and its dependence on EBV. Int. J. Cancer 8:443, 1971.
112. Tovey, M., Lenoir, G., and Begon-Lours, J.: Activation of latent Epstein-Barr virus by antibody to human IgM. Nature 276:270, 1978.
113. Fu, S.M., and Harley, J.N.: Human cell lines containing Epstein-Barr virus but distinct from the common B lymphoblastoid cell lines. Proc. Natl. Acad. Sci. USA 76:6637, 1979.
114. Tsoukas, C.D., Carson, D.A., Fong, S., Pasquali, J.-L., and Vaughan, J.H.: Cellular requirements for pokeweed mitogen induced autoantibody production in rheumatoid arthritis. J. Immunol. 125:1125, 1980.
115. Pasquali, J.-L., Fong, S., Tsoukas, C.D., Slovin, S.F., Vaughan, J.H., and Carson, D.A.: Different populations of rheumatoid factor idiotypes induced by two polyclonal B cell activators, pokeweed mitogen and Epstein-Barr virus. Clin. Immunol. Immunopathol. 21:184, 1981.
116. Alspaugh, M.A., Jensen, F.C., Rabin, H., and Tan, E.M.: Lymphocytes transformed by Epstein-Barr virus. Induction of nuclear antigen reactive with antibody in rheumatoid arthritis. J. Exp. Med. 147:1018, 1978.
117. Catalano, M.A., Carson, D.A., Slovin, S.F., Richman, D.D., and Vaughan, J.H.: Antibodies to Epstein-Barr virus determined antigens in normal subjects and in patients with seropositive rheumatoid arthritis. Proc. Natl. Acad. Sci. USA 76:5825, 1979.
118. Depper, J.M., and Zvaifler, N.J.: Epstein-Barr virus—its relationship to the pathogenesis of rheumatoid arthritis. Arthritis Rheum. 24:755, 1981.
119. Tosato, G., Steinberg, A.D., and Blaese, R.M.: Defective EBV-specific suppressor T-cell function in rheumatoid arthritis. N. Engl. J. Med. 305:1238, 1981.
120. Vaughan, J.H.: Rheumatoid arthritis, rheumatoid factor and the Epstein-Barr virus. J. Rheumatol. 6:381, 1979.
121. Metcalf, E.S., and Klinman, N.R.: In vitro tolerance induction of neonatal murine B cells. J. Exp. Med. 143:1327, 1971.
122. Williams, R.C., and Kunkel, H.G.: Separation of rheumatoid factors of different specificities using columns conjugated with gamma-globulins. Arthritis Rheum. 6:665, 1963.
123. Butler, V.P., Jr., and Vaughan, J.H.: The reaction of rheumatoid factor with animal gamma globulins. Quantitative considerations. Immunology 8:144, 1965.
124. Gaardner, P.I., and Michaelsen, T.E.: Specificity of rheumatoid factors cross-reacting with human and rabbit IgG. Acta Path. Microbiol. Scand. 82:733, 1970.
125. Natvig, J.B., Gaardner, P.I., and Turner, M.W.: IgG antigens of the $C\gamma 2$ and $C\gamma 3$ homology regions interacting with rheumatoid factors. Clin. Exp. Immunol. 12:177, 1972.
126. Osterland, C.K., Harboe, M., and Kunkel, H.G.: Anti-γ-globulin factors in human sera revealed by enzymatic splitting of anti-Rh antibodies. Vox Sang. 8:133, 1963.
127. Nasu, H., Chia, D.S., Knutson, D.W., and Barrett E.V.: Naturally occurring human antibodies to the $F(ab')_2$ portion of IgG. Clin. Exp. Immunol. 42:378, 1980.
128. Jerne, N.K.: Towards a network theory of the immune system. Ann. Immunol. (Inst. Pasteur) 125c:374, 1974.
129. Gaardner, P.I., and Natvig, J.B.: Hidden rheumatoid factors reacting with "non a" and other antigens of native autologous IgG. J. Immunol. 105:928, 1970.
130. Nardella, F.A., Teller, D.C., and Mannik, M.: Studies on the antigenic determinants in the self-association of IgG rheumatoid factor. J. Exp. Med. 154:112, 1981.
131. Carson, D.A., and Lawrance, S.: Light chain heterogeneity of 19S and 7S anti-γ-globulins in rheumatoid arthritis and subacute bacterial endocarditis. Arthritis Rheum. 21:438, 1978.
132. Stone, M.J., and Metzger, H.: Binding properties of a Waldenström macroglobulin antibody. J. Biol. Chem. 243:5977, 1968.
133. Normansell, D.E.: Anti-γ-globulins in rheumatoid arthritis sera. II. The reactivity of anti-γ-globulin rheumatoid factors with altered γG-globulin. Immunochemistry 8:593, 1971.
134. Lyet, J.P., and Normansell, D.E.: Low molecular weight rheumatoid factors in rheumatoid arthritis sera. Immunochemistry 11:417, 1974.
135. Wager, O., and Teppo, A.-M.: Binding affinity of human autoantibodies: Studies of cryoglobulin IgM rheumatoid factors and IgG autoantibodies to albumin. Scand. J. Immunol. 7:503, 1978.
136. Robbins, D.L., Morre, T.L., Carson, D.A., and Vaughan, J.H.: Relative reactivities of rheumatoid factors in serum and cells. Arthritis Rheum. 21:820, 1978.
137. Gabriel, D.A., and Hadler, N.M.: The physical characterization of an aggregating IgG heteropolymer containing rheumatoid factor. J. Biol. Chem. 256:3240, 1981.
138. Pope, R.M., Teller, D.C., and Mannik, M.: The molecular basis of self-association of antibodies to IgG (rheumatoid factors) in rheumatoid arthritis. Proc. Natl. Acad. Sci. USA 71:517, 1974.
139. Pope, R.M., Mannik, M., Gilliland, B.C., and Teller, D.C.: The hyperviscosity syndrome in rheumatoid arthritis due to intermediate complexes formed by self-association of IgG-rheumatoid factors. Arthritis Rheum. 18:97, 1975.
140. Clagett, J.A., and Engel, D.: Polyclonal activation: a form of primitive immunity and its possible role in pathogenesis of inflammatory diseases. Dev. Comp. Immunol. 2:235, 1978.
141. Schmid, F.R., Roitt, I.M., and Rochas, M.J.: Complement fixation by a two component antibody system: Immunoglobulin G and immunoglobulin M antiglobulin (rheumatoid factor). J. Exp. Med. 132:673, 1970.
142. Zvaifler, N.J., and Schur, P.H.: Reaction of aggregated mercaptoethanol treated gamma globulin with rheumatoid factor-precipitin and complement fixation studies. Arthritis Rheum. 11:523, 1968.
143. Taylor-Upsahl, M.M., Johnson, P.M., Mellbye, O.J., and Natvig, J.B.: A study of complement fixation by rheumatoid factor using a hemolytic assay system. Clin. Exp. Immunol. 28:204, 1977.
144. Sabharwal, U.K., Vaughan, J.H., Fong, S., Bennett, P.H., Carson, D.A., and Curd, J.G.: Activation of the classical pathway of complement by rheumatoid factors. Arthritis Rheum. 25:161, 1982.
145. Clarkson, E.B., Jr., and Mellon, G.H.: Rheumatoid factor-like immunoglobulin M protects previously uninfected rat pups and dams from *Trypanosoma lewisi.* Science 214:186, 1981.
146. Zvaifler, N.J.: The immunopathology of joint inflammation in rheumatoid arthritis. Adv. Immunol. 13:265, 1973.
147. Hedberg, H.: Studies on the depressed hemolytic complement activity of synovial fluid in adult rheumatoid arthritis. Acta Rheumatol. Scand. 9:165, 1963.
148. Pekin, T.J., Jr., and Zvaifler, N.J.: Hemolytic complement in synovial fluid. J. Clin. Invest. 43:1372, 1964.
149. Sliwinski, A.J., and Zvaifler, N.J.: In vivo synthesis of IgG by the rheumatoid synovial membrane. J. Clin. Invest. 76:304, 1970.
150. Vaughan, J.H., Chihara, T., Moore, T.L., Robbins, D.L., Tanimoto, K., Johnson, J.S., and McMillan, R.: Rheumatoid factor-producing cells detected by direct hemolytic plaque assay. J. Clin. Invest. 58:933, 1976.
151. Taylor-Upsahl, M.M., Abrahamsen, T.G., and Natvig, J.B.: Rheumatoid factor plaque-forming cells in rheumatoid synovial tissue. Clin. Exp. Immunol. 28:197, 1977.
152. Munthe, E., and Natvig, J.B.: Immunoglobulin classes, subclasses and complexes of IgG rheumatoid factor in rheumatoid plasma cells. Clin. Exp. Immunol. 12:55, 1972.
153. Fehr, K., Valbart, M., Rauber, M., Knoppel, M., Baici, A., Salgam, T., and Boni, A.: Production of agglutinators and rheumatoid factors in plasma cells of rheumatoid and non-rheumatoid synovial tissue. Arthritis Rheum. 24:510, 1981.
154. Munthe, E., and Natvig, J.B.: Characterization of IgG complexes in eluates from rheumatoid tissue. Clin. Exp. Immunol. 8:249, 1971.
155. Petersen, J., Heilmann, C., Bjerium, O.J., Ingemann-Hansen, T., and Halkjair-Kristensen, J.: IgG rheumatoid factor secreting lymphocytes in rheumatoid arthritis. Evaluation of a haemolytic plaque forming cell technique. Scand. J. Immunol. 17:471, 1983.
156. Hyslop, N.E., Jr., Dourmashkin, R.R., Green, N.M., and Porter, R.R.: The fixation of complement and the activated first component (C1) of complement by complexes formed between antibody and divalent hapten. J. Exp. Med. 130:703, 1970.
157. McDuffie, F.C., and Brumfield, H.W.: Effect of rheumatoid factor on complement mediated phagocytosis. J. Clin. Invest. 57:3007, 1972.
158. Bolton, W.K., Schroek, J.H., and Davis, J.H.: IV. Rheumatoid factor inhibition of in vitro binding of IgG complexes to the human glomeruli. Arthritis Rheum. 25:297, 1982.
159. Kaplan, R.A., DeHeer, D.H., Carson, D.A., Pangburn, M.K., Muller-Eberhard, H.J., and Vaughan, J.H.: Metabolism of C4 and Factor B in rheumatoid arthritis: Relation to rheumatoid factor. Arthritis Rheum. 23:911, 1980.

# Chapter 45
# Immune Complexes

*E. Dayer and P.H. Lambert*

## INTRODUCTION

Although the immunopathogenesis of most inflammatory rheumatic diseases is certainly multifactorial, antigen-antibody complexes can be involved in several of these diseases. They can often be detected in blood or in synovial space throughout the clinical course, with increased levels at the time of exacerbation.

The formation of immune complexes (ICs) by binding of antigens to their corresponding antibodies is a physiologic process usually of benefit to the host; IC formation allows the neutralization or the elimination of microbial antigens and of other exogenous antigens. Usually, ICs are eliminated rather efficiently by the fixed mononuclear phagocytic system, particularly by Kupffer cells in the liver.[1] Therefore, circulating ICs can be detected for only a short period of time after a specific antigenic challenge.

Immune complexes can play a role in the pathogenesis of autoimmune and immunological disorders. Indeed, in animals injected with bovine serum albumin,[2] the onset of glomerulonephritis, arthritis, or vasculitis coincided with the appearance of soluble ICs in the circulation and the deposition of ICs in renal glomeruli, synovial tissues, or vessel walls. In man, there is also evidence that ICs are directly involved in the pathogenesis of a variety of rheumatic diseases and that ICs formed during infections may participate in the development or the persistence of major inflammatory lesions.

The level of ICs in blood or in interstitial fluids reflects the balance between their generation and their clearance.

## GENERATION OF IMMUNE COMPLEXES

The formation of circulating ICs in human diseases is a function of the availability of antigen molecules to react with the corresponding antibodies. Immune complexes primarily involve antigens from (a) exogenous sources (food, drugs, heterologous serum proteins); (b) microbial sources (viral, bacterial or parasitic); and (c) autologous sources (autoantigens, tumor antigens). For example, exogenous antigens are found in ICs from patients receiving antilymphocyte globulins or in those with food allergy.[1] Microbial antigens can be found in immune complexes associated with some infectious diseases. In hepatitis B, there is a transient phase during which a significant proportion of HB surface antigen is present in serum as a complex with anti-HBs antibodies.[3] Among autoantigens, the presence of DNA has been suspected in ICs from patients with systemic lupus erythematosus, although it certainly does not represent a major antigen in the circulating immune complexes.[4]

Recently, advances have been made in the direct analysis of antigens present in ICs purified from human sera. Such purification can be done using columns filled with C1q or conglutinin-coated plastic beads.[5] The purified ICs have been shown, by SDS-polyacrylamide gel electrophoresis (SDS-PAGE), to contain complement components (C1q, C1r, C1s, and C3) and immunoglobulins (Fig. 45–1). In some instances (e.g., lepromatous leprosy), an antigen from the infectious agent has been identified as a component of the IC.[6] In most cases, however, the identification of specific antigens has proved to be difficult and only immunoglobulins and complement can be regularly demonstrated in purified immune complexes.

Antibodies directed toward the individual's own immunoglobulin may be important. A frequent feature of many IC diseases is hypergammaglobulinemia, which usually reflects a nonspecifically increased immunoglobulin synthesis.

Polyclonal activation produced in experimental animals by lipopolysaccharide or by protozoan parasites led to the production of a large variety of antibodies, including autoantibodies, and resulted in the formation and the persistence of ICs in circulation.[7] No heterologous antigen was detected within these circulating ICs; therefore, autoantibodies might be involved. There is evidence that anti-immunoglobulin autoantibodies may be of particular importance. Thus, the possibility that ICs may result from specific interactions between immunoglobulin molecules, without the involvement of exogenous antigen, should be considered in many clinical situations.

Autoantibodies against immunoglobulin can be directed against either the constant region or the antibody combining site. Antibodies produced against a constant portion of the IgG molecule (rheumatoid factors) occur frequently during polyclonal B-lymphocyte activation and in some rheumatic or infectious diseases. In rheumatoid arthritis, there is a close correlation between the production of such anti-IgG antibodies and the appearance of ICs.[8] The other antigenic site of immunoglobulins is located on the hypervariable region, or antibody combining site (idiotypic determinant). Each antibody has its own idiotype, which distinguishes it from antibody produced by other B-lymphocyte clones in the same individual. Cross-reactions can exist between idiotypes of immunoglobulin produced by different clones (cross-reacting idiotypes). It has been suggested

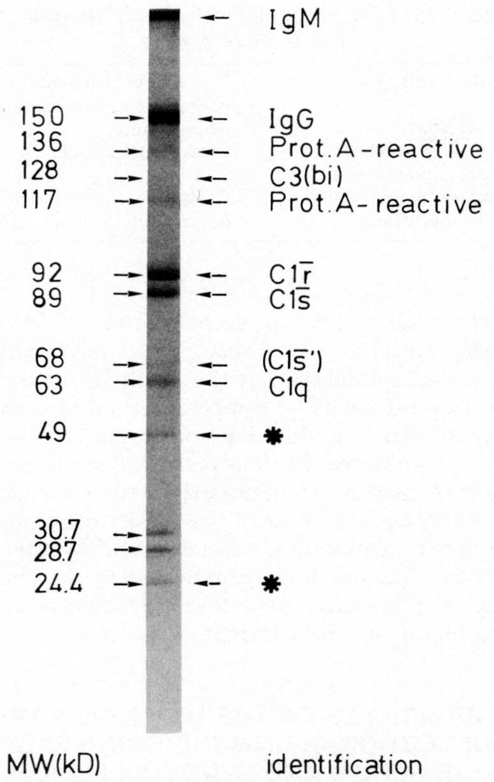


**Figure 45–1.** Immune complexes from SLE patients are analyzed by sodium dodecylsulfate-polyacrylamide gel electrophoresis. Some components of IC have been identified after transfer to nitrocellulose sheets and reaction with appropriate antisera. Some bands (*) do not react with an antiserum against normal human serum proteins.

that the antibody repertoire of an individual consists of a network of idiotypes and anti-idiotypic antibodies. In this network each immunoglobulin would function both as an antibody directed toward the combining site of other immunoglobulins and as an immunogen for yet other immunoglobulins.[9]

Interactions between idiotype and anti-idiotype could play a role in the immunopathology of certain diseases. The frequent stimulation of antigen-specific antibodies and their corresponding anti-idiotypic antibodies could result in the formation of idiotype–anti-idiotype complexes. If many B lymphocytes were stimulated simultaneously and nonspecifically, as in polyclonal B-lymphocyte activation, many different idiotypic clones might produce immunoglobulin synchronously with their corresponding anti-idiotypic clones. Thus, some of the complexes appearing could consist of a wide variety of idiotype–anti-idiotype complexes. Such complexes have been shown to occur in animal models.[10] Recently idiotype–anti-idiotype complexes have been found in human patients with mixed cryoglobulinemia (type II).[11] The presence of anti-idiotypic antibodies (anti-anti DNA) has been suggested in systemic lupus erythematosus.[12] The idiotypic network provides, therefore, a large source of potential antigens and corresponding antibodies, and the formation of ICs may often represent a perturbation of physiologic interactions in this network.

**Mechanisms Leading to the Clearance of Immune Complexes.** In vitro, immune complexes have been shown to bind to phagocytic cells through the Fc and C3 receptors found on their surface.[13] The adherence of immune complexes is usually enhanced after complement fixation[14] and is followed by the cellular uptake of ICs. In vivo, the clearance rate of immune complexes from the circulation depends on their removal by the mononuclear phagocytic system (MPS) (Fig. 45–2). In animals, the fate of preformed immune complexes depends on the lattice structure, on the nature of each component of the IC, and on the status of the mononuclear phagocytic system. Large latticed immune complexes are cleared much faster than small latticed ones.[15] Carbohydrate moieties on IgG[16] and IgM[17] may play a role in the hepatic uptake of ICs. The mononuclear phagocytic system can be saturated by large numbers of ICs, favoring the persistence of large latticed immune complexes in circulation.[18]

The role of the complement system in the clearance of immune complexes is still controversial. The persistence of ICs is not influenced by a depletion of circulating complement components,[19,20] but complexes that do not fix complement efficiently persist for a long time in the circulation.[21] In man, the capacity to clear circulating ICs has been estimated by measuring the clearance of IgG-sensitized red blood cells. However, such cells are preferentially removed by the spleen, rather than by the liver, as with soluble immune complexes.[22] Some patients with systemic lupus erythematosus (SLE) have an impaired clearance, which correlates with increased C1q binding activity.[23]

Immune complexes may be unequally distributed be-

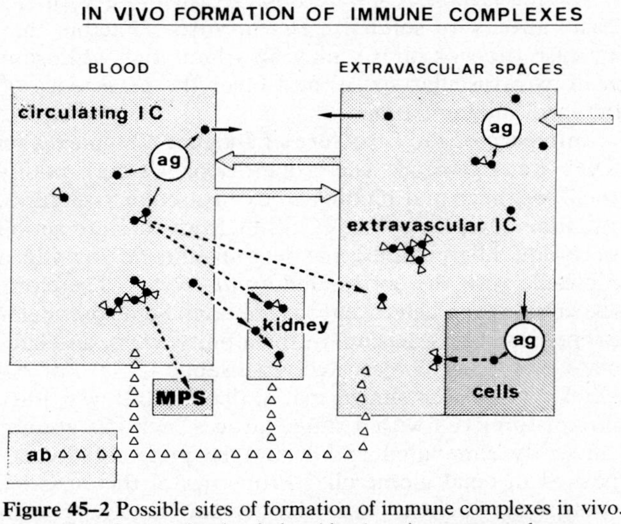


**Figure 45–2** Possible sites of formation of immune complexes in vivo. IC may be formed in circulating blood or in extravascular spaces, according to the localization of the antigens at the time when antibodies appear; ag represents a source of antigen, e.g. a microorganism and ab the antibody MPS = mononuclear phagocytic system. The fate of the complexes is dependent on the site of their formation.

tween the intravascular and extravascular body fluid compartments. When immune complexes are formed in extravascular spaces, their clearance will depend (a) on the diffusion of ICs to the blood or to the lymphatic system and (b) on the accumulation of phagocytic cells, mostly polymorphonuclear leukocytes and monocytes, at the site of formation of ICs in tissues.

**Interaction of Complement and Immune Complexes.** Complement activation by ICs can, on the one hand, be responsible for changes of the IC structure and, on the other hand, can generate small peptides mediating the inflammatory response and favoring the elimination of ICs. The activation of the complement system by ICs brings C3b in close contact with the Fc part of the immunoglobulins in the ICs. Together with C3b, Factors B and P generate an alternative pathway convertase (C3b-Bb-P), which increases the cleavage of native C3 to C3b and leads to the intercalation of more C3b molecules in the IC lattice.[24] This results in a decrease of the size of the immune complexes, usually called *solubilization.* In vivo, the presence of C3b or C3bi on immunoglobulins facilitates the *binding to cells* expressing C3b or C3bi receptors. These have been found on erythrocytes, neutrophils, eosinophils, macrophages, and lymphocytes. Most complexes bound to nonphagocytic cells are released in the environment after the interaction of the IC with the complement regulatory proteins, Factors I and H.[25] Complexes bound to phagocytic cells can be eliminated by phagocytosis. In the course of complement activation, the release of peptides increases vascular permeability and attracts leukocytes.[26] This *inflammatory response* favors the accumulation of phagocytic cells at the site of complement activation and eliminates the immune complexes. In man, the interaction of ICs with the complement system seems of importance for their clearance from extravascular spaces. Indeed, in a study of synovial fluids from patients with rheumatoid arthritis (RA), the largest ICs were observed in those with the least capacity to solubilize ICs in vitro.[27] Factors that increase the size of ICs may also limit their diffusion from extravascular spaces and favor the persistence of the local inflammation.

**Influence of the Structure of Immune Complexes on Their Pathogenicity.** The properties of ICs may modify their clearance and binding to extravascular structures. Immune complexes usually result from the interaction of several different antigenic determinants on an antigen molecule with the corresponding *antibodies.* Therefore, they represent a heterogeneous material. Some particular properties of ICs depend on the affinity, class, and subclass of the antibodies involved (Table 45–1). For example, it has been shown that antibodies of low avidity do not form ICs with a stable lattice. Such ICs are not efficiently eliminated and would be preferentially deposited in renal glomeruli.[28] Properties of the *antigenic* component such as size, charge, and reactivity with tissue structures also influence the persistence of ICs and their potential pathogenicity. DNA, which is a negatively charged antigen, has a particular affinity for collagen structures[29] and presumably DNA-containing ICs are preferentially bound to such structures. The *relative concentration of the antigen and of the antibody* influences the size, and solubility, and the reactivity of the complexes. Small ICs may be trapped in small blood vessels or may be stuck in filtering membranes (glomerular basement membrane, choroid plexus). Such localization of ICs is favored by an increased vascular permeability and possibly by a decrease of the density of anionic sites in basement membranes.[30] Finally, the structure and properties of ICs are directly influenced by the *secondary binding of IC-reactive molecules,* particularly complement components and rheumatoid factors.

**Table 45–1.** Factors Influencing the Properties of Immune Complexes

| | |
|---|---|
| 1. Nature of antigen(s) | Size, charge, reactivity with biologic structures, antigenic determinants |
| 2. Nature of antibodies | Class, subclass, affinity |
| 3. Antigen-antibody ratio | |
| 4. Secondary binding of IC-reactive molecule | Complement, rheumatoid factor, immunoconglutinin |

## PRINCIPLES OF THE METHODS FOR DETECTION OF IMMUNE COMPLEXES IN SERUM AND SYNOVIAL FLUID

Immune complexes have been demonstrated in human disease[31] by the analysis of tissue specimens and by serologic testing of samples from various biologic fluids. Conventional histology or electron microscopy of pathologic specimens may reveal similarities with lesions induced experimentally by immune complexes. Immunohistochemical staining allows a more direct demonstration of immunoglobulin deposits, with or without associated complement components. Studies of biologic fluids provide evidence for the association of immune complexes with particular pathologic conditions, either by the direct detection of ICs or by demonstration of serologic changes, which are often associated with their presence. The initial assays for detecting soluble immune complexes in body fluids were based on their physicochemical properties, such as the size of the immune complexes, which is in turn dependent on the degree of aggregation of the complexed immunoglobulins. More recent methods have focused on the biologic properties of antibody and/or antigen molecules, detecting either the increased density of these molecules in complexes or the generation of immune mediators. Thus, aggregated antibodies bind more avidly than monomeric antibodies to C1q or to cellular receptors.

**Differentiation of Immune Complexes From Monomeric IgG by Physical Properties.** The new molecular structures generated after the antigen-antibody interactions are characterized by an increased molecular size and by changes of the surface properties, solubility, and electric charge as compared with the corresponding free antigens and antibodies. Molecular size and solubility of ICs are most widely used for their detection by physical methods.

Analytic ultracentrifugation allows the demonstration in various biologic fluids of an abnormal level of material sedimenting at a high velocity. The use of preparative methods for separation of macromolecular aggregates such as *sucrose gradient ultracentrifugation* or *gel filtration* permits the analysis of the various fractions and the study of their specific immunologic properties and concentrations. Additional evidence for the presence of ICs has been obtained by comparing the pattern at neutral pH with that at acid pH, which dissociates ICs. Ultracentrifugation and gel filtration are sometimes used in the purification of immune complexes, but are limited by contamination of the complexes with monomeric immunoglobulins. They can be combined with the use of labeled markers for ICs such as C1q[32,33] or antiglobulins[34] but are too time consuming for routine use.

Material with a decreased solubility in well-defined conditions (temperature, medium) occurs frequently in serum or other biologic fluids containing ICs. Abnormal precipitation of proteins in a serum sample under such defined conditions may therefore indicate the presence of ICs. The simplest procedure is precipitation at cold temperature. *Cryoglobulins* may frequently represent a particular type of IC, but monoclonal immunoglobulins or other proteins are often involved. Extensive immunochemical analysis of cryoprecipitates is required when considering cryoglobulins as possible immune complexes.[35] The extent of precipitation of serum proteins in *polyethylene glycol* (PEG, MW = 6000), an uncharged linear polymer, is generally proportional to the protein molecular size and to the concentration of PEG.[36] At low concentrations of PEG, high molecular weight proteins and ICs are preferentially precipitated before monomeric IgG. Although an increase in the amount of PEG precipitate often indicates ICs, such precipitation is influenced by other serum proteins and is a rather nonspecific screening test for ICs. More accurate information may be obtained by analysis of the proteins (e.g., IgG, C1q, C4) precipitated at low PEG concentrations. Precipitation in PEG can be combined with the use of radiolabeled markers for immune complexes, such as C1q or staphylococcal protein A.[37]

**Differentiation of Immune Complexes from Monomeric IgG by Interaction with Biologic Recognition Units.** Soluble immune complexes can be detected by their reactivity with some plasma proteins or with biologic recognition units on cell membranes. (Fig. 45–3).

***Interaction with Recognition Sites on Plasma Proteins.*** The reaction of immune complexes with complement components affords several methods for IC recognition. Complement-fixing immune complexes may be detected either by indirect measurement of complement consumption (e.g., anticomplementary activity, C1q deviation test)[38,39] or by direct evaluation of the binding of immune complexes to C1q, the first component of complement (C1q binding fluid phase[33] or solid phase assays[40]). In addition, because the reaction of immune complexes with complement leads to the persistence of some complement components on the immune complexes, such immune complexes coated with complement bind to molecules with an affinity for fixed activated complement components (e.g., conglutinin-binding assays,[41] anti-C3 assays[42]). The general feature of this group of methods is their dependence on the reactivity of the immune complex with complement. Although most circulating immune complexes may fulfill this requirement, those containing only IgG4, IgA, or IgE would not. The reactivity of substances other than immune complexes with complement components especially limits the specificity of inhibition assays (e.g., anticomplementary activity, C1q deviation test). A second group of assays that discriminate aggregated from monomeric immunoglobulins are based on the interaction of ICs with low-avidity anti-immunoglobulin antibodies.[43] Most of these methods are sensitive only for ICs containing IgG antibodies and are influenced to some extent

**Figure 45–3.** Assays for the detection of IC can be divided in 3 groups: solid phase, fluid phase, and cellular binding assays. In solid phase assays, the recognition unit is coated on a plastic tube, then interacted with the sample, and finally revealed with a radiolabeled anti-immunoglobulin reagent. In fluid phase assays, the radiolabeled recognition unit is incubated with the sample and the bound and free recognition units are separated by differential precipitation. In cellular assays, appropriate cells are incubated with the sample and immune complexes attached to cells are quantitated by a radiolabeled anti-immunoglobulin reagent.

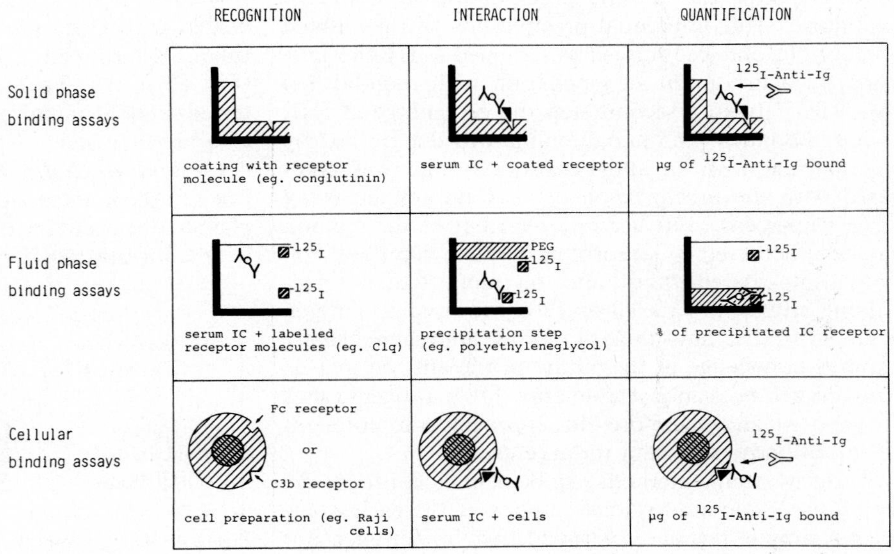

by the concentration of monomeric IgG in the tested sample.

*Interaction with Cell-Bound Receptors.* The analysis of specific interactions of immune complexes with cells may provide information directly relevant to important biologic effects of such complexes. The use of living cells makes standardization difficult and is limited by the possible occurrence of factors interfering with the cell metabolism and by the occasional binding of antibodies directly to cell membranes. Many cells expressing a receptor for the Fc part of immunoglobulin can be used to detect ICs, since they usually bind more avidly aggregated immunoglobulins or ICs than monomeric immunoglobulins. All methods using this property for the detection of ICs are influenced to some extent by the concentration of immunoglobulins in the tested samples. The interaction of complement-coated ICs with complement receptors on cells may also be used. Various cells exhibit a high affinity for complement-coated ICs owing to the presence of receptors for complement components on the cell surface. Most of these receptors interact preferentially with C3b or its breakdown products, C3bi and C3d. One lymphoblastoid cell line, derived from a patient with Burkitt's lymphoma (the Raji cell line) is particularly suitable for the detection of ICs because it has a high density of complement receptors and lacks surface immunoglobulins.[44]

**Methods Specific for Antigen.** In particular clinical conditions it may be useful to know whether a specific antigen is contained in immune complexes and to distinguish between free antigen molecules and those bound specifically to immunoglobulins. In the case of particulate antigen, such as a virus, the detection of aggregated virus particles by electron microscopy suggests their involvement in immune complexes.[45] Free and complex-bound antigen can be further differentiated by measuring the amount of antigen removed from a serologic sample when the host immunoglobulins are specifically absorbed or precipitated. Thus, the virus titer of sera from mice infected with lactic dehydrogenase virus decreased strikingly after the specific precipitation of immunoglobulins.[46] The differential precipitation of the antigen bound to IC and free antigen was applied to HBs antigen using, in a first step, an incubation with radiolabeled anti-HBs Fab. In a second step the percentage of HBs antigen bound to immunoglobulins was determined by precipitation with an anti-Fc antibody and was compared with the precipitation of all HBs antigen using PEG 10 percent.[3] Further improvement of the method has been achieved by absorbing immune complexes on conglutinin-coated tubes and revealing free antigen-binding sites with labeled antibody to specific antigen (e.g., anti-HBs, anti-idiotype). This approach usually requires knowledge of the nature of the antigen in ICs. Antigen will be demonstrable only if free antigenic sites are exposed, and, therefore, this approach does not work when antibody is present in large excess.

Antigen-specific methods can be of clinical use for the diagnosis of some infectious diseases at the early stage of the immune response, when neither free antigen nor free antibody can be detected in the circulation. Considering the multiplicity of antigen-antibody systems possibly involved in the in vivo formation of ICs, it is unlikely that such antigen-specific methods would be routinely used in clinical situations. Their use would probably be restricted to the assessment of the immune status in well-defined conditions.

## METHODS COMMONLY USED FOR THE DETECTION OF IMMUNE COMPLEXES

The sensitivity of each method for detecting immune complexes varies according to the nature of the ICs involved and the influence of various interfering factors. Difficulty in standardizing reagents and the complexity of the procedure may also impair applicability and reproducibility of some methods. Only a limited number of methods are suitable for routine laboratory investigation. A few operational principles of the most widely used methods will be described here.

**Assays Involving Solid Phase Binding.** Test samples are incubated in plastic tubes coated with an IC-recognition unit. Bound ICs are then quantitated using radiolabeled or enzyme-conjugated antibodies directed toward immunoglobulins. Such methodology has been successfully applied with various IC-recognition units: C1q, conglutinin, anti-C3 F(ab)2, and rheumatoid factor. Solid phase assays have many advantages over other methods of detection: they do not require any centrifugation, and results are quickly available when enzyme-conjugated reagents are used. They also allow for the quantitation of specific classes of immunoglobulin using labeled anti-immunoglobulin against IgG, IgM, IgA, or labeled staphylococcal protein A. However, the washing steps may favor the dissociation of low avidity antibodies from antigens and of ICs from the recognition unit. Such tests may also be influenced by the presence of rheumatoid factor in the sample.

*C1q Solid Phase Binding Assay (C1q SP).* The EDTA-treated sample is placed in a plastic tube previously coated with C1q, and the amount of ICs bound to the tube is determined, using the anti-Ig reagent.[40] The test (Fig. 45–4) may be influenced by the level of C1q in the tested sample, and only immune complexes reacting with C1q are detected.

*Conglutinin Solid Phase Binding Assay (KgB).* The test sample is incubated in the presence of calcium in a plastic tube coated with bovine conglutinin, which reacts with C3bi-bearing ICs. Bound ICs are determined after

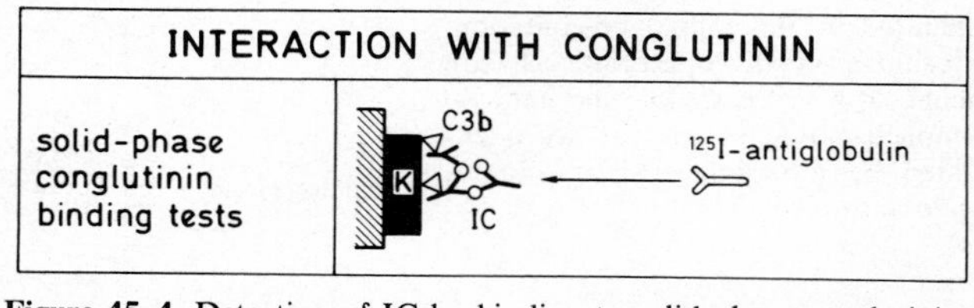


**Figure 45–4.** Detection of IC by binding to solid phase conglutinin.

addition of labeled staphylococcal protein A or anti-immunoglobulin.[41] The test detects ICs that activate either the classical or the alternative complement pathway and bind C3. An excess of conglutinin should be used to coat the tubes in order to avoid inhibition by free C3 fragments generated either in vivo or during the in vitro manipulation of the sample.

***Anti-C3 Solid Phase Binding Assay.*** Plastic tubes are coated with (Fab)'2 fragments of an antibody to C3 and then interacted with the serum samples. The amount of bound immune complex is measured with a radiolabeled anti-Ig reagent.[42]

***Monoclonal Rheumatoid Factor Binding Inhibition Assay (mRF-I).*** This test (Fig. 45–5) is based on the inhibition by immune complexes of the binding of radiolabeled aggregated IgG to monoclonal RF, that has been coupled to microcrystalline cellulose.[43] Because monomeric IgG also binds to RF, although less avidly than aggregated IgG, serum samples must be diluted to a constant IgG content prior to analysis. Sample, labeled aggregates, and RF-cellulose are incubated together; the cellulose is then washed and the amount of bound IgG is measured. This assay is sensitive only for IC containing IgG.

**Assays Involving Fluid Phase Binding.** Fluid phase assays are based on the differential precipitation of free radiolabeled IC-recognition unit (C1q, conglutinin) from the same receptor bound to the IC.

***C1q Binding Assay (C1q BA).*** Radiolabeled C1q is added to EDTA-treated serum in the presence of polyethylene glycol (PEG 2.5 percent, final concentration). After 1 hour, free C1q is separated from the precipitated bound C1q by centrifugation.[33] The percentage of radioactivity precipitated corresponds to the C1q binding activity of the sample and indicates the level of ICs. PEG favors the binding of C1q to ICs preventing their dissociation, and therefore, is suitable for the detection of low avidity ICs. Labeled C1q reacts as a tracer molecule and reflects the binding of endogenous C1q to IC during the test. Thus there is some competition between endogenous C1q and labeled C1q. This test is particularly sensitive for complexes containing IgM and this may explain the high level of positivity usually observed in RA. The binding of non–IC substances (e.g., polyanions) to C1q is not a major cause of false results at the ionic strength used except for heparin used to collect plasma.

**Assays Involving Binding to Cells.** Aggregates of Ig or immune complexes bind to Fc and complement receptors on the surfaces of various cell types, and the activities of the cell may change after binding ICs. Two approaches have been used to quantify the binding of immune complexes to cells: either direct quantitation with a labeled anti-immunoglobulin (e.g., Raji cell assay) or indirect quantitation by measurement of changes of cell function (e.g., platelet aggregation).

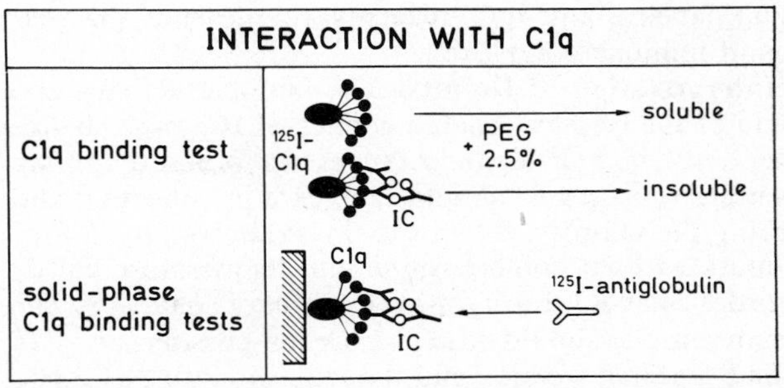


**Figure 45–6.** Two kinds of immune complex tests involving C1q: Fluid phase binding and PEG precipitation or solid phase binding.

***Raji Cell Binding Assay.*** This assay (Fig. 45–7) is based on the binding of IC to C3b and C3bi receptors on a continuous lymphoblastoid cell line (Raji cells). The Raji cell line is particularly suitable for detecting IC, since these cells lack surface Ig and have few or low affinity receptors for IgG Fc and a large number of receptors for complement. IC bound to cells are quantitated with a labeled anti-IgG antibody;[44] the level of IC is extrapolated from a standard curve prepared with increasing amounts of aggregated immunoglobulins mixed with human serum as a source of complement. The Raji cell assay is very sensitive for IC containing IgG. Detection of IgM-containing complexes is complicated in some diseases (e.g., SLE) by falsely high levels produced by antilymphocyte antibodies (IgM). The technique requires experience in continuous cell culture.

***Platelet Aggregation Assay.*** Freshly collected platelets aggregate after the interaction of their surface Fc receptor with IC containing IgG. In the presence of immune complexes, the titer can be measured using microplates.[47] The test has also been done using serum that had been heat inactivated in order to prevent inhibition caused by high concentration of C1q. Some variation occurs with platelets from different donors. Antiplatelet antibodies, some myxoviruses, and some enzymes can also aggregate platelets. Recently, this test has been modified,

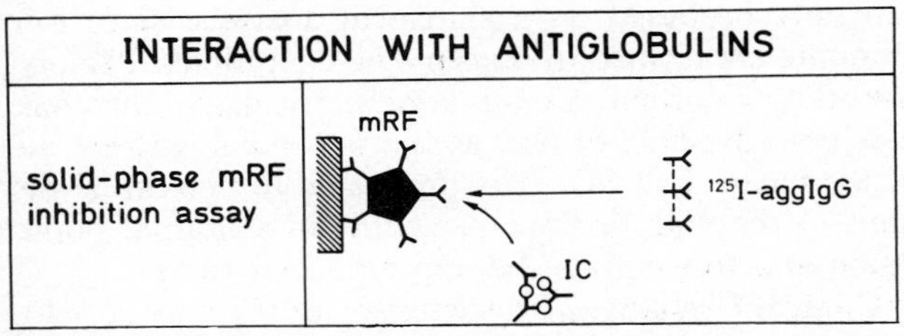


**Figure 45–5.** Detection of IC by inhibition of binding of aggregated IgG to solid phase monoclonal rheumatoid factor.

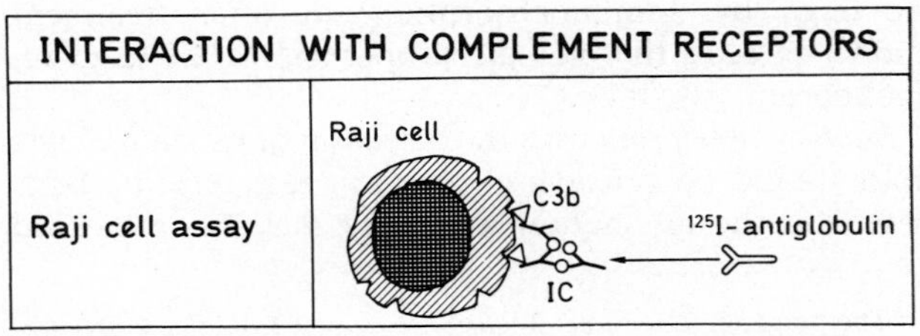


**Figure 45–7.** Detection of IC by binding to complement receptors on Raji cells.

using labeled anti-IgG reagents to measure platelet-bound immune complexes.

**Interpretation of Results.** The biologic activity and some of the physical characteristics of ICs may change after *collection of serum samples.* In order to obtain accurate results, one should take care in collecting and storing the samples. Blood should be allowed to clot for 2 hours without cooling (minimum temperature 25° C) in order to avoid the cryoprecipitation of some ICs. The serum samples should be kept frozen, if possible, at −70° C and repeated freezing and thawing should be avoided. The use of plasma samples may lead to false results. For tests based on reactivity with complement, the presence of heparin, even at low concentrations, may interfere.

The *manipulation of the samples* at the time of testing is also of importance. Heat inactivation is not advisable, since it can aggregate IgG or alter the reactivity of IC with Fc or C3 receptors. Similarly, treating samples with reducing agents or with IgG immunoabsorbents in order to decrease RF activity before the test, may partially deplete ICs or change the IC structure. For all tests performed with living cells, toxic preservatives should be avoided.

The *expression of the results* may differ according to the test system used. Frequently, test levels are referred to standard curves with various concentrations of aggregated IgG. It should be pointed out that considerable variations exist between aggregated IgG preparations used in different laboratories. It is now possible to standardize the expression of the results, since reference preparations for IC measurement (tetanus toxoid–anti-tetanus toxoid IC and stabilized aggregated IgG) have been made available by a joint WHO/IUIS Committee.* The apparent level of IC in a serum sample may differ according to the test used. This reflects the heterogeneity of ICs in relation to their biologic activity or physical characteristics.

Because methods of detection of ICs are indirect, do not allow for a specific quantitation of the protein content, and are susceptible to interference by other substances, appropriate *control experiments* are required whenever ICs are demonstrated in a new clinical entity. These include (1) characterization of the size of the putative ICs, since immune complexes are larger than monomeric immunoglobulin; (2) fractionation in physicochemical conditions known to dissociate immune complexes and to decrease their size and biologic activities; and (3) confirmation that the test becomes negative after removal of immunoglobulins from the tested sample (e.g., by immunoabsorption) or after treatment known to alter the biologic properties of ICs (e.g., reduction and alkylation).

*Factors interfering* with the detection of ICs in biologic fluid should be considered for each test system. Tests based on the interaction with C1q may be influenced by the presence in the sample of bacterial lipopolysaccharides or polyanions (e.g., heparin, DNA). Treatment of serum samples with DNAase can eliminate the interference by DNA. The recognition of activated C3 on the ICs may be inhibited by the presence of C3 fragments or non-IC C3 binding material (e.g., CRP complexes) in the tested sample. Conglutinin assays cannot be performed on EDTA or citrated samples because calcium is required. False positive results may be observed with cellular assays because of antilymphocyte antibodies. Other assays using living cells or platelets can also be influenced by a direct effect of various non-IC substances (e.g., bacterial lipopolysaccharides, mitogens, toxic agents) or by antibodies against cell membrane antigens (e.g., anti-HLA, anti-platelet).

*The preparations can be obtained on request from Dr. U. Nydegger, Central Laboratory of the Swiss Red Cross, Wankdorfstrasse 10, Bern, Switzerland.

## EVALUATION OF IMMUNE COMPLEX DETECTION IN RHEUMATIC DISEASE

**Critical Evaluation.** The evaluation of methods for IC measurements in clinical investigation should be based on the sensitivity and specificity of each test. The *sensitivity* of a given method cannot be related only to the detection of aggregated immunoglobulins or of artificial complexes. Indeed, the sensitivity for IC detection will vary according to the type of ICs occurring in each disease considered. For example, using six techniques to measure IC levels in SLE and RA, it was found that some methods (fluid phase C1q binding, mRF-inhibition) are most sensitive for ICs from patients with RA; other methods (Raji cell assay, conglutinin solid phase assay, C1q solid phase assay) were more sensitive for ICs from patients with SLE. In most diseases studied, the *specificity* of the commonly used methods is generally sufficient to assert that the detected activity is due to ICs. Therefore, the selection of methods for the measurement of ICs in a given rheumatic disease should be influenced by the *sensitivity* of the method in this disease and by knowledge of the possible interfering factors in these patients. For example, although all three tests have a similar sensitivity, the C1q solid phase assay or the conglutinin solid phase assay would be preferable to the Raji cell assay in following patients with SLE, who may have circulating antibodies to lymphoblastic cells. In patients with RA, the C1q fluid phase assay would be preferable to the conglutinin solid phase assay in view of its higher sensitivity for the low avidity IgM-containing ICs encountered in this disease.

With all tests used, the *upper normal value* for ICs can only be based on a statistical analysis, since low amounts are formed in physiologic conditions. The distribution of normal values is asymmetrical, and therefore it is not advisable to use, as the upper limit, the value of the mean ± 2 SD. It is preferable to determine the limit of the 90th or 95th percentile in a normal population and to use it as the upper normal value.

**Clinical Usefulness.** The detection of ICs may be helpful in certain clinical conditions. The *diagnostic value* of a measurement by itself is limited, however, since the *presence* of immune complexes is not specific to any particular disease. However, IC levels should be considered as an integral part of the laboratory diagnosis in a number of rheumatic diseases. For example, in a prospective study, Jones and associates[49] followed 53 patients with early arthritis for up to 3 years. During this time, 24 developed sufficient features for definite RA to be diagnosed and the others simply had arthralgias. Abnormal C1q-binding activity was found mainly in RA patients (79 percent) several months before the disease could be diagnosed. In suspected but not definite RA, the *absence* of detectable ICs may be of diagnostic value in ruling out this disease, provided the test used is of high sensitivity (e.g., C1qBA). Immune complex detection could be applicable to seronegative RA patients since positive tests have been reported for up to 70 percent of the cases.[50,53]

A *single* measurement in a given patient does not give a good indication of the clinical activity of the diseases in SLE[50] or in RA.[54] A better application is probably serial determination of IC levels during therapy. In individual patients with SLE or with rheumatoid arthritis, there is a good correlation between the clinical activity of the disease and serial measurement of IC levels. Lloyd and Shur[56] followed 37 patients with SLE before, during, and after clinical exacerbation. Patients developing active renal disease had marked increases in IC levels along with low levels of CH50 and C3. In a similar study, Hamburger[55] observed a good correlation between the IC level and clinical activity (Fig. 45–8). In RA patients, serial studies of ICs in serum or in synovial fluids also suggest that in a given individual the IC level may be one biological indicator of clinical activity (Fig. 45–9).[67]

In a collaborative double-blind study for the evaluation of levamisole in the treatment of rheumatoid arthritis, a progressive decrease of IC levels was found in the treated groups, but not in the placebo group.[52] The measurement of IC levels has also been used to monitor therapeutic plasma exchange in SLE and in RA.

In RA patients, the presence of rheumatoid nodules is associated with higher levels of circulating IC (Fig. 45–10). However, the findings of a high IC level in a given patient does not have a predictive value for this type of complication.

**Immune Complexes in Rheumatic Diseases and Their Relevance to Clinical Status.**

***Rheumatoid Arthritis.*** Anti-immunoglobulins of the IgG and IgM class have been shown to form ICs in serum and joint fluid either by IgG-IgG self-association or by reaction of IgM-RF with native IgG. These ICs react with C1q and IgM-RF and may be responsible for intravascular activation of the complement system.

Several techniques for detecting circulating ICs have been used to study sera and synovial fluids of patients

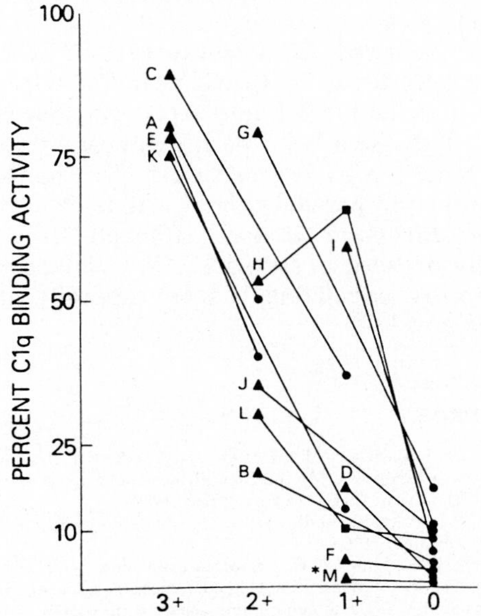


**Figure 45–8.** Changes in levels of immune complexes (C1q BA) and clinical status in SLE. Chronologic order from left to right (exception is M, whose chronologic order is right to left). Letters represent 13 individual patients with SLE. The disease activity was assessed by two physicians independently on a scale of 0 to 3+, according to all available clinical and laboratory findings. From Hamburger, M.I., et al.: A serial study of systemic reticuloendothelial system Fc receptor functional activity in systemic lupus erythematosus. Arthritis Rheum. 25:1, 1982.

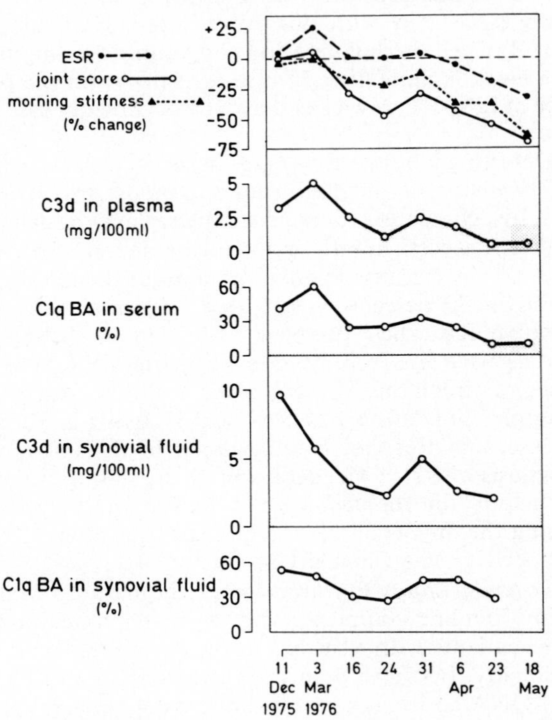


**Figure 45–9.** Disease course of a patient with RA during 6 months. Periods with active disease were associated with high C3d and C1q BA levels in plasma or serum and synovial fluid, and remissions were followed by improvement of these parameters. Note inflammatory exacerbation on March 31. ESR = erythrocyte sedimentation rate. (From Nydegger U.E., et al.: Circulating complement breakdown products in patients with rheumatoid arthritis. Correlation between plasma C3d, circulating immune complexes and clinical activity. J. Clin. Invest. 59:862, 1977.)

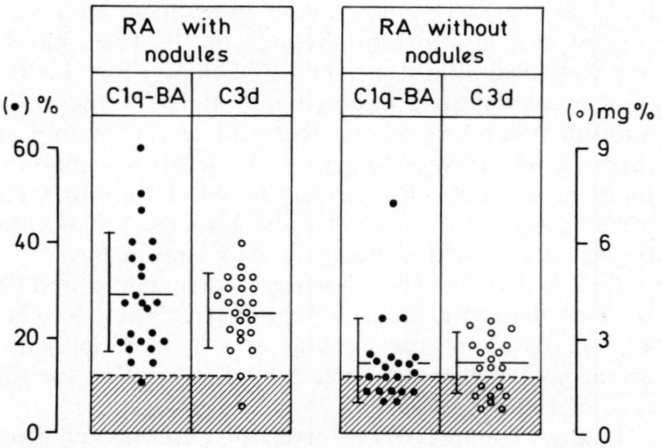


**Figure 45–10.** Correlation of immune complex levels in serum (%[125]I-C1q binding activity, C1qBA) and the C3d concentrations in plasma with the occurrence of subcutaneous nodules in patients with rheumatoid arthritis. The means of the values (± 2 SD) from each group are indicated. The shadowed area represents the normal ranges (means ± 2 SD) of the value observed in healthy donors. ● = %; ○ = mg%.

with rheumatoid arthritis. Of the 18 techniques for the detection of ICs evaluated in a multicenter study, six were particularly effective.[48] The Raji cell binding test and the C1q binding test were positive in 71 and 83 percent, respectively. As previously detailed, the presence of vasculitis or other extra-articular features is generally associated with positive IC tests (C1q binding test, Raji cell binding test and conglutinin binding test). The level of circulating ICs is correlated with the presence of IgM-RF as well as the erythrocyte sedimentation rate.

Detecting immune complexes in serum may be *helpful for diagnosis* in the following situations: (a) in early arthritis, circulating immune complexes may be detected in serum several months prior to the definite diagnosis of RA;[49] (b) because circulating immune complexes are found in 70 percent of sera from patients with seronegative RA, their presence may help to distinguish seronegative RA from other arthropathies;[50] (c) the absence of circulating ICs has some exclusion value. For example, circulating ICs are usually absent in Reiter's disease, and this can be considered in the differential diagnosis of RA.[51] The detection of circulating ICs may be helpful for the *follow-up of individual RA patients* during therapy as one of the biologic indicators of clinical activity (see Clinical Usefulness).[52]

***Systemic Lupus Erythematosus.*** The nature of circulating immune complexes and cryoprecipitates in sera from patients with SLE has not been well defined. Occasionally, ICs have been shown to contain anti-Ig and anti-DNA antibodies. Large amounts of circulating ICs generally correspond with active SLE, as well as with high levels of anti-double-strand DNA antibody and reduced complement levels. In a comparative study, the highest frequency of immune complexes in sera from SLE patients was observed using the Raji cell binding assay (91 percent), the fluid phase C1q binding test (78 percent), and platelet aggregation (74 percent).[48] In follow-up studies, there was a close relationship between the immune complex levels and the changes in the disease activity.[54,55] Lloyd and Schar confirmed this correlation and found that patients with active renal disease showed higher C1qBA, as well as decreased CH50 and C3, in comparison with patients with only extrarenal manifestations.[56] The diagnostic value of circulating ICs is limited, but significant renal disease is unlikely when low complement levels are not associated with appreciably elevated C1q binding activity. The measurement of IC levels has been used to monitor therapeutic plasma exchange in SLE.[57]

***Juvenile Rheumatoid Arthritis.*** In this heterogeneous group, circulating immune complexes have been observed, particularly in the clinical subsets marked by systemic onset or polyarticular disease. In a collaborative study of chronic juvenile arthritis, ICs were found more frequently in children with severe disease.[58]

***Ankylosing Spondylitis.*** In most studies, no significant increase of circulating IC levels has been found.[51,59-61]

***Scleroderma.*** Approximately half of the patients with scleroderma have circulating ICs.[62-64] In a recent study of 92 patients with progressive systemic sclerosis serum levels of ICs measured by the Raji cell assay were elevated in 72 percent.[65] In this study a positive result in the Raji cell binding test was most often associated with diffuse scleroderma, tendon friction rub, and positive antinuclear antibody. Individuals with immune complexes detected by the C1q binding test more frequently had evidence of pulmonary involvement and positive serum rheumatoid factor than patients with a negative C1q binding test.

***Mixed Connective Tissue Disease (MCTD).*** Circulating ICs have been found by the C1q binding test, the Raji cell test and the mRF-I test. Approximately 81 to 90 percent of the sera were positive by one test and 65 percent were positive by two methods. Changes in IC levels seemed to parallel clinical activity.[66]

***Degenerative Joint Diseases.*** Although ICs can be occasionally detected in synovial fluid from patients with osteoarthritis, circulating ICs are generally absent in these diseases.[27,50]

## References


1. Nydegger, U.E., Kazatchkine, M.D., and Lambert, P.H.: Immune complexes. *In* Fougereau, M., and Dausset, J. (eds.): Progress in Immunology IV, Paris, New York, Academic Press, 1980.
2. Dixon, F.J.: The role of antigen-antibody complexes in disease. The Harvey Lectures 58:21, 1963.
3. Lambert, P.H., Tribollet, E., Celada, A., Madalinski, K., Frei, P.C., and Miescher, P.A.: Quantitation of immunoglobulin-associated HBs antigen in patients with acute and chronic hepatitis, in healthy carriers and in polyarteritis nodosa. J. Clin. Lab. Immunol. 3:1, 1980.
4. Harbeck, R.J., Bardana, E.J., Kohler, P.F., and Carr, R.I.: DNA-anti-DNA complexes: Their detection in systemic lupus erythematosus sera. J. Clin. Invest. 52:789, 1973.
5. Casali, P., and Lambert, P.H.: Purification of soluble immune complexes from serum using PMMA beads coated with conglutinin or C1q. Clin. Exp. Immunol. 37:295, 1979.
6. Maire, M., Barnet, M., and Lambert, P.H.: Identification of components of immune complexes purified from human sera. I. Immune complexes purified from sera of patients with systemic lupus erythematosus. Clin. Exp. Immunol. 51:215, 1983.

7. Louis, J., and Lambert, P.H.: Lipopolysaccharides: From immunostimulation to autoimmunity. Springer Sem. Immunopathol. 2:215, 979.
8. Winchester, R.J., Kunkel, H.G., and Agnello, V.: Occurrence of gammaglobulin complexes in serum and joint fluid of rheumatoid arthritis patients: Use of monoclonal rheumatoid factors as reagent for their demonstration. J. Exp. Med. 134:286s, 1971.
9. Jerne, N.K.: Towards a network theory of the immune system. Ann. Immunol. (Inst. Pasteur) 125C:373, 1974.
10. Rose, L.M., Goldman, M., and Lambert, P.H.: The production of anti-idiotype antibodies and of idiotype-anti-idiotype immune complexes following polyclonal B-cell activation by bacterial LPS. J. Immunol. 128:2126, 1982.
11. Geltner, D., Franklin, E.G., and Frangione, B.: Anti-idiotypic activity of the IgM fractions of mixed cryoglobulins. J. Immunol. 125:1530, 1980.
12. Agnello, V., Koffler, D., Eisenberg, J.W., Winchester, R.J., and Kunkel, H.: C1q precipitins in the sera of patients with systemic lupus erythematosus and other hypocomplementemic states: Characterization of high and low molecular weight types. J. Exp. Med. 144:428, 1971.
13. Munthe-Kaas, A.C., Kaplan, G., and Seljelid, R.: On the mechanism of internalization of opsonized particles by rat Kupffer cells in vitro. Exp. Cell. Res. 103:201, 1976.
14. Kijlstra, A., Van Es, L.A., and Daha, M.R.: Enhanced degradation of soluble immunoglobulin aggregates by macrophages in the presence of complement. Immunology 37:673, 1979.
15. Mannik, M., and Arend, W.P.: Fate of preformed immune complexes in rabbits and rhesus monkeys. J. Exp. Med. 134:19s, 1971.
16. Thornburg, R.W., Day, J.F., Thorpe, S.R., and Baynes, J.W.: Carbohydrate-mediated clearance of immune complexes from circulation. A role for galactose residues in hepatic uptake of IgG-antigen complexes. J. Biol. Chem. 255:6820, 1980.
17. Day, J.F., Thornburg, R.W., Thorpe, S.R., and Baynes, J.W.: Carbohydrate-mediated clearance of antibody-antigen complexes from the circulation. The role of high mannose oligosaccharides in the hepatic uptake of IgM-antigen complexes. J. Biol. Chem. 255:2360, 1980.
18. Haakenstad, A.O., and Mannik, M.: Saturation of the reticuloendothelial system with soluble immune complexes. J. Immunol. 112:1939, 1974.
19. Harkiss, G.D., and Brown, D.L.: Clearance kinetics of soluble preformed immune complexes containing IgM antibodies in normal and decomplemented rabbits. Immunology 42:217, 1981.
20. Bockow, B., and Mannik, M.: Clearance and tissue uptake of immune complexes in complement-depleted and control mice. Immunology 42:497, 1981.
21. Haakenstad, A.O., and Mannik, M.: The disappearance kinetics of soluble immune complexes prepared with reduced and alkylated antibodies in mice. Lab. Invest. 35:283, 1976.
22. Frank, M.M., Schreiber, A.D., Atkenson, J.P., and Jaffe, C.J.: Pathophysiology of immune hemolytic anemia. Ann. Intern. Med. 87:210, 1977.
23. Frank, M.M., Hamburger, M.I., Lawley, T.J., Kimberley, R.P., and Plotz, P.H.: Defective reticuloendothelial system Fc-receptor function in systemic lupus erythematosus. N. Engl. J. Med. 300:518, 1979.
24. Miller, G.W., and Nussenzweig, V.: A new complement function: Solubilization of antigen-antibody aggregates. Proc. Nat. Acad. Sci. 72:418, 1975.
25. Ehlenberger, A.G., and Nussenzweig, V.: The role of membrane receptors for C3b and C3d in phagocytosis. J. Exp. Med. 145:357, 1977.
26. Ward, P.A., and Zwaifler, N.J.: Complement-derived leukotactic factors in inflammatory synovial fluids of humans. J. Clin. Invest. 50:606, 971.
27. Dayer, E., Gerster, J.C., Aguado, M.T., and Lambert, P.H.: Capacity to solubilize immune complexes in sera and synovial fluids from patients with rheumatoid arthritis. Arthritis Rheum. 27:156, 1983.
28. Steward, M.W.: Chronic immune complex disease in mice: The role of antibody affinity. Clin. Exp. Immunol. 38:414, 1979.
29. Izui, S., Lambert, P.H., and Miescher, P.A.: In vitro demonstration of a particular affinity of glomerular basement membrane and collagen for DNA. A possible basis for a local formation of DNA-anti-DNA complexes in systemic lupus erythematosus. J. Exp. Med. 144:428, 1976.
30. Cavallo, T., Goldman, M., Graves, K., and Lambert, P.H.: Altered glomerular permeability in the early phase of immune complex nephritis. Kidney Int. 24:632, 1983.
31. Zubler, R.H., and Lambert, P.H.: Detection of immune complexes in human diseases. Prog. Allergy 24:1, 1978.
32. Bokisch, V.A., Muller-Eberhard, H.J., and Dixon, F.J.: Complement: A potential mediator of the hemorrhagic shock syndrome. Adv. Biosc. 12:417, 1974.
33. Zubler, R.H., Lange, G., Lambert, P.H., and Miescher, P.A.: Detection of immune complexes in unheated sera by a modified $^{125}$I-C1q binding test. Effect of heating on the binding of C1q by immune complexes and application of the test to systemic lupus erythematosus. J. Immunol. 116:232, 1976.
34. Ludwig, F.J., and Cusumans, C.L.: Detection of immune complexes using $^{125}$I-goat anti(human IgG) monovalent (Fab) antibody fragments. J. Natl. Can. Instit. 52:1529, 1974.
35. Brouet, J.C., Clauvel, J.P., Danon, F., Klein, M., and Seligmann, M.: Biological and clinical significance of cryoglobulins. Am. J. Med. 57:775, 1974.
36. Zubler, R.H., Perrin, L.H., Creighton, W.D., Lambert, P.H., and Miescher, P.A.: The use of polyethylene glycol (PEG) to concentrate immune complexes from serum or plasma samples. Ann. Rheum. Dis. 36(Suppl. 1)23, 1977.
37. Hällgren, R., and Wide, L.: Detection of circulating IgG aggregates and immune complexes using $^{125}$I protein A from *Staphylococcus aureus*. Ann. Rheum. Dis. 35:306, 1976.
38. Nielsen, H., and Svehag, S.E.: Detection and differentiation of immune complexes and IgG aggregates by a complement consumption assay. Acta. Path. Microbiol. Scand. 84:261, 1976.
39. Sobel, A.T., Bokisch, V.A., and Muller-Eberhard, H.J.: C1q deviation test for the detection of immune complexes, aggregates of IgG and bacterial products in human sera. J. Exp. Med. 142:139, 1975.
40. Hay, F.C., Nineham, L.J., and Roitt, I.M.: Routine assay for the detection of immune complexes of known immunoglobulin class using solid phase C1q. Clin. Exp. Immunol. 24:396, 1976.
41. Casali, P., Bossus, A., Carpentier, A.N., Lambert, P.H., and Miescher, P.A.: Solid phase enzyme immunoassay or radioimmunoassay for the detection of immune complexes based on their recognition by conglutinin: Conglutinin binding test. Clin. Exp. Immunol. 29:342, 1977.
42. Pereira, A.B., Theofilopoulos, A.N., and Dixon, F.J.: Detection and partial characterization of circulating immune complexes with solid-phase anti-C3. J. Immunol. 125:763, 1980.
43. Luthra, H.S., McDuffie, F.C., Hunder, G.G., and Samayoa, E.A.: Immune complexes in sera and synovial fluids of patients with rheumatoid arthritis. Radioimmunoassay with monoclonal rheumatoid factor. J. Clin. Invest. 56:458, 1975.
44. Theofilopoulos, A.N., Wilson, C.B., and Dixon, F.J.: The Raji cell radioimmune assay for detecting immune complexes in human sera. J. Clin. Invest. 57:169, 1976.
45. Almeida, J.D., and Waterson, A.P.: The morphology of the virus-antibody interaction. Adv. Virus. Res. 15:307, 1969.
46. Notkins, A.L., Mahar, S., Scheele, C., and Goffman, J.: Infectious virus-antibody complex in the blood of chronically infected mice. J. Exp. Med. 124:81, 1966.
47. Penttinen, K.: The platelet aggregation test. Ann. Rheum. Dis. 36(Suppl. 1):55, 1977.
48. Lambert, P.H., Dixon, F.J., Zubler, R.H., Agnello, V., Cambiaso, C., Casali, P., Clark, J., Cowdery, J.S., McDuffie, F.C., Hay, F.C., McLennan, I.C., Masson, P., Muller-Eberhard, H.J., Penttinen, K., Smith, M., Tappeiner, G., Theofilopoulos, A.N., and Verroust, P.: A collaborative study for the evaluation of eighteen methods for detecting immune complexes in serum. J. Lab. Clin. Immunol. 1:1, 1978.
49. Jones, V.E., Jacoby, R.K., Wallington, T., and Holt, P.: Immune complexes in early arthritis. I. Detection of immune complexes before rheumatoid arthritis is definite. Clin. Exp. Immunol. 44:512, 1981.
50. Zubler, R.H., Nydegger, U.E., Perrin, L.H., Fehr, K., McCormick, J., Lambert, P.H., and Miescher, P.A.: Circulating and intraarticular immune complexes in patients with rheumatoid arthritis. J. Clin. Invest. 57:1308, 1976.
51. Gabay, R., Zubler, R.H., Nydegger, U.E., and Lambert, P.H.: Immune complexes and complement catabolism in ankylosing spondylitis. Arthritis Rheum. 20:913, 1977.
52. Vischer, T.L., Veys, E., Symoens, J., Rosenthal, M., and Huskisson, E.C.: Levamisole in rheumatoid arthritis. A randomized double-blind study comparing two dosage regimens of Levamisole with placebo. Lancet 2:1007, 1978.
53. McDougal, J.S., Hubbard, M., McDuffy, F.C., Strobel, P.L., Smith, S.J., Bass, N., Goldmann, J.A., Hartman, S., Myerson, G., Miller, S., Morales, R., and Wilson, C.H.: Comparison of five assays for immune complexes in the rheumatic diseases. An assessment of their validity in rheumatoid arthritis. Arthritis Rheum. 25:1156, 1982.
54. Abrass, C., Nies, K.M., Louie, J.S., Border, W.A., and Glassock, R.J.: Correlation and predictive accuracy of circulating immune complexes with disease activity in patients with systemic lupus erythematosus. Arthritis Rheum. 23:273, 1980.
55. Hamburger, M.I., Lawley, T.J., Kimberley, R.P., Plotz, P.H., and Frank, M.M.: A serial study of systemic reticuloendothelial system Fc receptor functional activity in systemic lupus erythematosus. Arthritis Rheum. 25:1, 1982.
56. Lloyd, W., and Schur, P.H.: Immune complexes, complement and anti-DNA in exacerbations of systemic lupus erythematosus (SLE). Medicine 60:208, 1981.
57. Wei, N., Klippel, J.H., Huston, D.P., Hall, R.P., Lawley, T.J., Balow, J.E., Steinberg, A., and Decker, J.L.: Randomised trial of plasma exchange in mild systemic lupus erythematosus. Lancet 1:17, 983.

58. Rossen, R.D., Brener, E.J., Person, D.A., Templeton, J.W., and Lipsky, M.D.: Circulating immune complexes and antinuclear antibodies in juvenile rheumatoid arthritis. Arthritis Rheum. 20:1485, 1977.
59. Rosenbaum, J.T., Theofilopoulos, A.N., Mc DeWitt, H.O., Pereira, A.B., Carson, D., and Calin, A.: Presence of circulating immune complexes in Reiter's syndrome and ankylosing spondylitis. Clin. Immunol. Immunopathol. 18:291, 1981.
60. Moksymowych, W., Dasgupta, M.K., Rothwell, R.S., Dossetor, J.B., and Russel, A.S.: The absence of circulating immune complexes in patients with ankylosing spondylitis. Rheumatol. Int. 1:107, 1981.
61. Duquesnoy, R., Santoro, F., Wattre, P., and Delcombre, B.: Failure to find C1q binding material and anti-IgG antibodies in ankylosing spondylitis. Ann. Rheum. Dis. 39:449, 1980.
62. Cunningham, P.H., Andrews, B.S., and Davis, J.S.: Immune complexes in patients with progressive systemic sclerosis (PSS) and mixed connective tissue disease (MCTD). Clin. Res. 26:374A, 1978.
63. Husson, J.M., Druet, P., Contet, A., Fiessinger, J.N., and Camillari, J.P.: Systemic sclerosis and cryoglobulinemia. Clin. Immunol. Immunopathol. 6:77, 1976.
64. Pisko, E., Gallup, K., Turner, R., Parker, M., Nomeir, A.M., Box, J., Davis, J., and Rothberger, H.: Cardiopulmonary manifestations of progressive systemic sclerosis: Associations with circulating immune complexes and fluorescent antinuclear antibodies. Arthritis Rheum. 22:518, 1979.
65. Seibold, J.R., Medsger, T.A., Winkelstein, A., Kelly, R.H., and Rodnan, G.P.: Immune complexes in progressive systemic sclerosis (scleroderma). Arthritis Rheum. 25:1167, 1982.
66. Halla, J.T., Volanakis, J.E., and Schrohenloher, R.E.: Circulating immune complexes in mixed connective tissue disease. Arthritis Rheum., 22:484, 1979.
67. Nydegger, U.E., Zubler, R.H., Gabay, R., Joliat, G., Karagevrekis, C.H., Lambert, P.H., and Miescher, P.A.: Circulating complement breakdown products in patients with rheumatoid arthritis. Correlation between plasma C3d, circulating immune complexes and clinical activity. J. Clin. Invest. 59:862, 1977.

# Chapter 46
# Antinuclear Antibodies

*Morris Reichlin*

## INTRODUCTION

Antibodies to nuclear antigens (ANA) are found in the sera of patients with a variety of rheumatic diseases. This chapter will describe ANA determination as a screening test as well as a means of identifying antibodies to specific organelles. In some patients with systemic lupus erythematosus (SLE) and Sjögren's syndrome, antibodies to cytoplasmic antigens predominate, and these will also be discussed. Newly discovered ANA in progressive systemic sclerosis and the polymyositis syndromes will be described. Characterizing the ANA as to antigenic specificity will provide information about nosology, subset definition within diseases, clinical activity, specific organ involvement, and prognosis.

## HISTORY

In 1948, Hargraves and colleagues initiated the study of antibodies to nuclei with the description of the LE phenomenon.[1] The demonstration of the ingestion of traumatized cells from SLE patients by polymorphonuclear leukocytes was readily confirmed[2] and is now known to be due to the reaction of antibodies against nucleoprotein (DNA-histone) with nuclei and the subsequent phagocytosis of such sensitized nuclei. The LE test, although still performed in many laboratories, is being replaced by tests that are more sensitive and specific. The next major advance was the indirect immunofluorescent assay (IFA) for the detection of ANA.[3-5] The assay detects antibodies with various antigenic specificities but is very useful as a screening test. It is the method of choice in the initial search for autoantibodies relevant to the diagnosis of SLE.

Resolution of total ANA into individual antigen-antibody reactions required purified nucleic acid antigens and antigens solubilized from crude extracts detected by precipitation in agar utilizing the Ouchterlony method. Improved analytical methods for chemically defined autoantigens (e.g., DNA) have provided greater sensitivity and precision in antibody detection. Two recent approaches to antigenic analysis involve the use of human tissue culture lines as immunofluorescent substrates and a molecular biological analysis of autoantigens containing intrinsically labeled RNA.

## ANA CLASSIFICATION

The antinuclear and anticytoplasmic antibodies that occur in the rheumatic diseases and have relevance for clinical diagnosis and disease classification are listed in Table 46–1. Each antibody specificity will be discussed in the context of its measurement, chemical nature, disease specificity, association with clinical subsets, and disease activity. Antibodies to DNA-histone, ds (double-stranded) and ss (single-stranded) DNA, RNA, histone, nRNP, and Sm* all occur in SLE, while antibodies to Ro*/SSA† and La*/SSB†/Ha* occur in SLE and Sjögren's syndrome. Antibodies to PM-Scl,‡ $Mi_1$,* $Mi_2$,* $Jo_2$,* and Ku* all occur in patients with polymyositis

*Represent the first two letters of the patient's name whose serum was used to identify the reaction in agar diffusion.
†Sjögren's syndrome A and B.
‡Polymyositis-scleroderma.

**Table 46–1.** Antibodies to Nuclear or Cytoplasmic Antigens (ANA and ACA)

| |
|---|
| Anti-DNA-histone |
| Anti-DNA |
| Anti–single-stranded (ss) DNA (denatured) |
| Anti–double-stranded (ds) DNA (native) |
| Anti-histone |
| Anti-nRNP* |
| Anti-Sm* |
| Anti-Ro/SSA* |
| Anti-La/SSB/Ha* |
| Anti-RNA, Poly IC, Poly GC, Poly ADP, Poly A |
| Anti-Ma |
| Anti-PM-Scl, $PM_1$ |
| Anti-$Mi_1$, $Mi_2$ |
| Anti-Ku |
| Anti-$Jo_1$, $Jo_2$ |
| Anti-$Scl_{70}$ |
| Anti-centromere |
| Anti-nucleosome (cross-reactive with Fc of human IgG) |

*All shown to be RNA-protein conjugates.

(PM), while antibodies to $Scl_{70}$ and centromere occur in patients with progressive systemic sclerosis (PSS). Finally antibodies to nucleosomes occur in patients with rheumatoid arthritis (RA).

## DETECTION OF ANTINUCLEAR ANTIGENS

**Immunofluorescence.** The indirect immunofluorescent test is widely considered to be the most reliable screening test for ANA (Fig. 46–1). A dilution of human serum is placed on a cryostat section of mouse liver, which leads to attachment of Ig molecules with antinuclear specificity. After suitable washing, an antibody against human Ig is added, and after washing, the bound fluorescein-tagged antihuman Ig is visualized by fluorescence microscopy. Figure 46–2 illustrates the appearance of normal human serum and a human serum positive for ANA binding to the nuclei of mouse liver sections. Note the dark appearance of the nuclei in the upper part of the figure (negative ANA test) and the whitish nuclei in the lower part of the figure in a positive ANA test. When viewed through the microscope, the positive nuclei appear apple-green, reflecting the color of the bound fluorescein-tagged antihuman Ig.

**Diagnosis of SLE.** A positive ANA test by itself is not diagnostic of any disease, but a positive ANA in association with the characteristic clinical features of SLE supports the diagnosis. If the ANA test is performed on cryostat sections of mouse liver or kidney and standardized commercially available fluorescent conjugates of antihuman gamma globulin are employed, about 95 percent of active untreated SLE patients will have positive tests. The titers of positive ANA tests vary greatly, but at least 50 percent of the titers will exceed 1:100, and a small proportion (10 percent or less) will be positive only at the screening dilution (1:10 or 1:20 in most laboratories. If the screening test is performed on commercially available human tissue culture lines such as KB or Hep2 cells, the percentage of positive tests approaches 98 percent of active untreated SLE patients. The difference between the two substrates largely represents the relative absence of the Ro/SSA antigen in mouse or rat liver and kidney sections and its presence in the tissue culture lines.

There is great variation in ANA test results acquired from different laboratories. This variation includes whether the test is positive or negative, the titer determined, and the pattern reported. ANA titers tend to be higher on tissue culture lines. The factors that lead to variable results include not only the use of different substrates but also different fluoresceinated antibodies directed toward human immunoglobulin, varying skill of technicians, microscopes of differing power and sensitivity (transmission versus epiilluminated optics), as well as the age of the bulb in the microscope and failure to include positive control sera directed toward very soluble antigens such as Sm and La/SSB.

The clinician must then decide how to evaluate disparate results from different laboratories. The answer is not easy, but clinical laboratories differ in quality and the clinician must make a judgement based on performance. The clinician should be more persistent in pursuing a negative ANA test in the face of impressive clinical data for SLE than in being concerned about a positive test accompanying limited or nonspecific clinical findings. The latter situation should be viewed with circumspection. The first situation could be due to faulty ANA testing or to one of the uncommon serologic situations to be described below. The second situation requires continued observation of the patient until disease expression is more complete. Finally, there are numerous laboratories with a strong research interest in

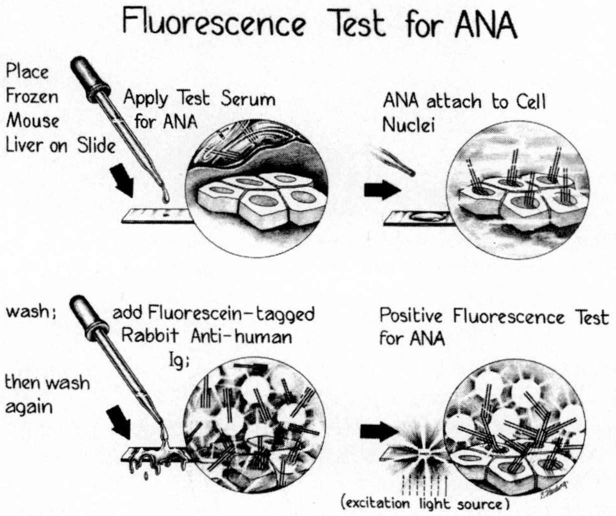


**Figure 46–1.** Stepwise diagram of the fluorescence test for anti-nuclear antibodies (ANA). The ANA bind to a variety of nuclear antigens; they are then identified by fluorescein-tagged antibodies to the human Ig.

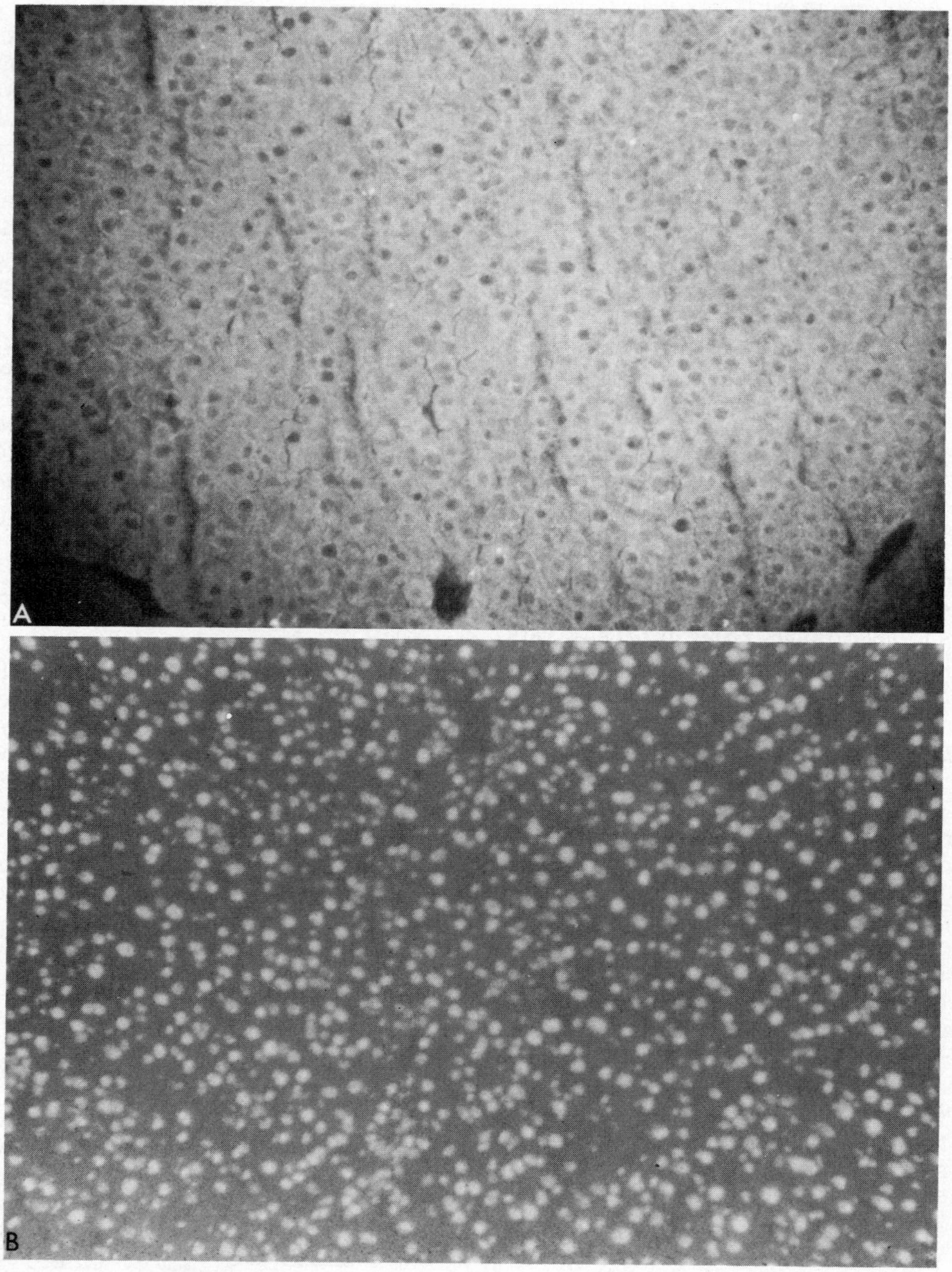

**Figure 46–2.** The fluorescence ANA (FANA) test at low power (×80). *A* is a negative control of mouse liver substrate. *B* is the same substrate with a positive homogeneous ANA pattern.

ANA testing, and they can perform an ANA test when the clinician is faced with this problem.

A negative test for ANA occurs in about 5 percent of patients with otherwise typical SLE. Almost two thirds of these patients have serum antibodies to Ro/SSA or La/SSB or both, and of the remainder, the great majority have antibodies to ssDNA demonstrable by radioimmunoassay. Five recognized antibody specificities that are not measured by immunofluorescent assay on rodent liver or kidney sections have been described (Table 46–2). Ro/SSA and ssDNA have already been mentioned, and the other three antigens that are germane to the clinical diagnosis of PM and PSS will be subsequently discussed. As is well known, antibodies to ssDNA when present alone do not bind to resting interphase nuclei.[161] Less than 1 percent of SLE patients have *none* of the autoantibodies characteristic of the disease; absence of a positive ANA on tissue culture lines and anti-ssDNA by radioimmunoassay therefore makes the diagnosis of SLE unlikely. The presence of

**Table 46–2.** Antigens Poorly Represented in Cryostat Sections of Rodent Epithelial Tissues

| Antigen | Relevant Disease | Method of Detection |
|---|---|---|
| Ro/SSA | SLE<br>Sjögren's syndrome | IFA* on human tissue culture lines<br>Double diffusion† |
| ssDNA | SLE and wide spectrum of rheumatic diseases | Hemagglutination<br>Radioimmunoassay<br>ELISA‡ |
| $Jo_1$ | Polymyositis | Double diffusion |
| Ku | Polymyositis-scleroderma overlap | Double diffusion<br>IFA on human or calf tissues |
| Centromere | Scleroderma<br>CREST variant | IFA with human tissue culture lines, e.g., Hep2 or KB cells |

*Immunofluorescence assay.
†Double diffusion or Ouchterlony method.
‡Enzyme-linked immunosorbent assay.

these antibodies tends to confirm the diagnosis but must be accompanied by clinical findings consistent with SLE in order to establish the diagnosis of SLE. For example, a patient with only Raynaud's phenomenon, polyarthritis (nonerosive, nondeforming), and a positive ANA test might have SLE, scleroderma, or polymyositis. The presence of typical skin or muscle findings would make the latter two diagnoses likely, but in their absence one could neither confidently exclude those two diagnoses nor make a diagnosis of SLE. On the other hand, the presence of a photosensitive malar rash or leukopenia or any of a number of other characteristic SLE findings not present in the other two diseases (mucous membrane ulceration, glomerulonephritis, thrombocytopenia, seizures, psychosis, discoid skin lesions, and alopecia) accompanying the limited clinical and serologic findings described would make the diagnosis of SLE virtually certain.

**ANA Pattern.** The ANA pattern is of some value but is a far less powerful criterion than the identification of a specific antigen-antibody reaction (e.g., anti-dsDNA, anti-Sm, anti-Ro/SSA, etc.). There are four major patterns recognized on cryostat sections of rodent liver or kidney. They are homogeneous or solid, peripheral or rim, speckled, and nucleolar. The homogeneous pattern is illustrated in Figure 46–2*B* while the peripheral, speckled, and nucleolar patterns of fluorescence are illustrated in Figure 46–3. The homogeneous pattern can be seen in all the connective tissue diseases as well as in drug-induced LE. Both the antibody associated with the

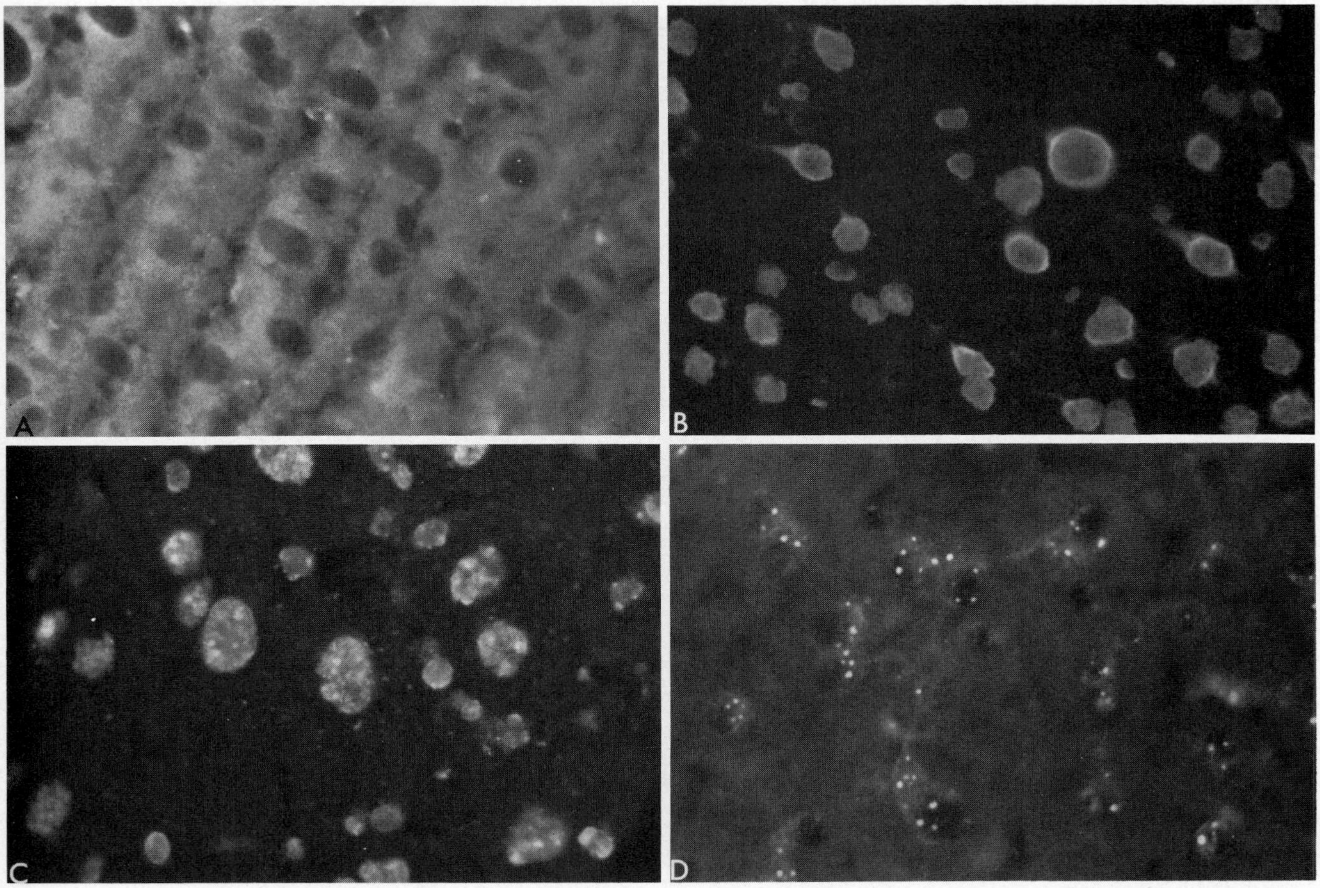


**Figure 46–3.** The fluorescence ANA (FANA) test at high power (×320). *A* is a negative control. *B* shows an example of the shaggy, rim or peripheral pattern which frequently correlates with antibodies to DNA. *C* is an example of the speckled pattern, frequently associated with antibodies to non–DNA-containing antigens. *D* shows the nucleolar pattern.

LE phenomenon and the histone-dependent antibodies arising in drug-induced SLE can produce this pattern of immunofluorescence. The speckled pattern is seen in sera from patients with SLE, RA, PSS, and Sjögren's syndrome. Sm, nRNP, La/SSB, $Scl_{70}$, and probably other antigens are targets for antibodies that give rise to the speckled patterns of fluorescence.

The peripheral pattern of fluorescence is seen most frequently in SLE sera and correlates with antibodies to dsDNA but is found in only a small proportion of sera containing these antibodies. Nucleolar fluorescence is seen most frequently in sera from scleroderma patients but also occurs to a lesser extent in sera from Sjögren's syndrome and SLE. The presence of multiple antibodies in SLE sera gives rise to patterns of fluorescence that vary with serum dilution. Often homogeneous fluorescence is observed at a low serum dilution and a speckled pattern at higher serum dilutions.

Positive ANA tests are found in 5 to 10 percent of patients with discoid lupus erythematosus without systemic involvement. A positive ANA test without clinical evidence of systemic involvement does portend the development of such involvement in some but not all patients. One cannot, therefore, confidently conclude that a patient with discoid LE and a positive ANA has SLE. Because the frequency of low-titer positive ANA tests increases with age in the normal population, a positive ANA test is much more significant in a young patient with discoid LE than in an older one.

**ANA in Diseases Other Than SLE.** A positive ANA test occurs to a variable extent in all the connective tissue diseases. Representative data are listed in Table 46–3. In arteritis, myositis, and RA the frequency of positive tests varies from 33 to 52 percent, and 70 to 90 percent of these positive tests occur at titers of 1/160 or less. On the other hand, high titers are quite common in SLE, mixed connective tissue disease, and PSS. Positive ANA tests are also seen in patients (5 to 20 percent) with juvenile RA, chronic active hepatitis, infectious mononucleosis, and lepromatous leprosy. The titers are rarely impressive in these clinical settings.

ANAs are not usually specific for organ and species[7] but there are exceptions. Most notable is the presence of granulocyte-specific ANA, which are found in the sera of patients with RA.[8-11] As many as 50 percent of RA patients have such antibodies, which are not detectable with mouse liver nuclei. At least one antibody specificity, anti-Ku, is species specific, and does not bind to rodent tissue but does bind to bovine and human tissue.[12]

## IDENTIFICATION OF INDIVIDUAL ANTIGEN–ANTIBODY REACTIONS

**Immunodiffusion.** Double diffusion in agar has been an important initial method for the identification and analysis of the specificities of autoantibodies. The antigen-antibody systems that were first characterized in this way include Sm, nRNP, Ro/SSA, La/SSB/Ha, Ma, Mi, $Jo_1$, $Jo_2$, Ku, PCNA, and $PM_1$ (PM-Scl). The nomenclature for these reactions rests on two conventions: (1) the first two letters of the name of the patient whose serum served as a monospecific prototype (e.g., Sm, Ro) and (2) a putative disease specificity of the antibody (e.g., SSA, $PM_1$). Such nomenclature is provisional and will give way to a chemical nomenclature when this information becomes available. Most of these antigens have now been well characterized biochemically, but their original antigenicity and clinical relevance were established with the double diffusion method. With an appropriate monospecific prototype serum and a crude extract of thymus or spleen tissue, definitive identification of a specific precipitin in an unknown serum can be made by the observation of line fusion as illustrated in Figure 46–4. The serum Da forms a thick precipitin line with an antigen in calf thymus extract (CTE), which fuses with a similar precipitin line formed by antibodies

**Table 46–3.** Fluorescent Antinuclear Antibody in Various Conditions*

| | SLE (662)† | RA (201) | Scleroderma (91) | MCTD (57) | Myositis (30) | Arteritis (70) |
|---|---|---|---|---|---|---|
| Positive tests (%) | 95 | 52 | 55 | 95 | 40 | 33 |
| Titer of test Mean | 298 | 142 | 338 | 508 | 173 | 50 |
| Percent with titer ≤ 1:40 | 34 | 72 | 46 | 7 | 50 | 90 |
| titer 1:80 | 17 | 8 | 9 | 5 | 10 | 10 |
| titer 1:160 | 19 | 10 | 18 | 14 | 10 | 0 |
| titer 1:320 | 20 | 6 | 13 | 48 | 17 | 0 |
| titer ≥ 1:640 | 10 | 4 | 14 | 26 | 13 | 0 |
| Pattern of fluorescence | | | | | | |
| Diffuse (%) | 64 | 73 | 29 | 10 | 27 | 51 |
| Speckled (%) | 30 | 22 | 58 | 86 | 17 | 33 |
| Nucleolar (%) | 3 | 5 | 13 | 4 | 56 | 16 |
| Peripheral (%) | 3 | 0 | 0 | 0 | 0 | 0 |

*From Fries, J.F.: Systemic Lupus Erythematosus: A Clinical Analysis. Philadelphia, W. B. Saunders Company, 1975.
†Number of observations in parentheses.

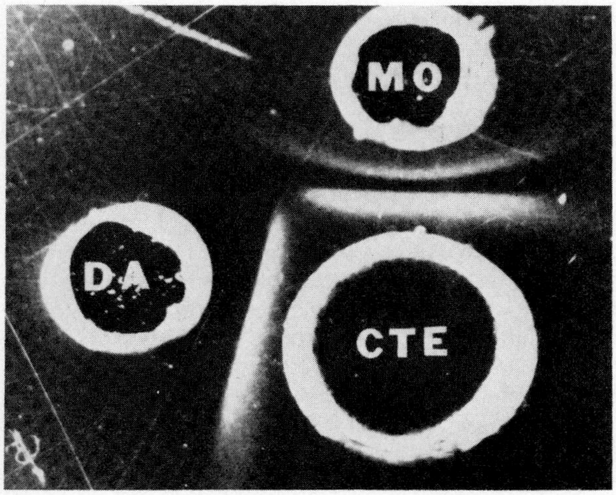


**Figure 46–4.** Precipitating antibodies to nRNA protein antigen. In the center well is calf thymus extract (CTE) and in the adjacent wells are serum specimens from patients Da and Mo. (Reprinted with permission from the New England Journal of Medicine 286:908, 1972).

in serum Mo with the antigen in CTE. The serum Mo forms a second line with CTE, which was identified as the Sm–anti-Sm system using a prototype anti-Sm serum in an adjacent well. The antigen forming the precipitin shared by sera Da and Mo proved to be of nuclear origin, and its antigenicity was completely destroyed by treatment with either RNAase or trypsin. This is the system now designated the nRNP system. Agar diffusion for the identification of specific antibodies is limited by insensitivity and the nonquantitative nature of the measurement. Precipitin reactions in agar require specific antibody concentrations of roughly 0.1 mg antibody protein per ml of serum if the precipitin is of the IgG class. Moreover, certain large macromolecules such as DNA diffuse poorly through agar gels, further reducing the sensitivity of this method for detection of the DNA–anti-DNA system by this technique. Several more sensitive and quantitative techniques are now available to measure anti-DNA. Indeed, it is anticipated that all precipitin reactions will be supplanted by more sensitive and quantitative techniques, the two most important being enzyme-linked immunosorbent assay (ELISA) and radioimmunoassay (RIA).

**Counterimmunoelectrophoresis.** Counterimmunoelectrophoresis is more sensitive than agar diffusion. Acidic antigens (e.g., DNA, RNA, and most of the precipitating antibodies described in the preceding section) are electrophoresed from a cathodal (−) well for a reaction with specific antibody, which has moved from an anodal well (+). This is illustrated in Figure 46–5, in which the technique is used for the measurement of antibodies to dsDNA in an SLE serum. The advantages of the method are improved sensitivity, certain identification of specific antigen-antibody reactions by line fusion even when crude extracts are used as the antigen source, and the potential resolution by electrophoresis of several antigens that differ in charge and may not resolve into independent lines in agar diffusion experiments.

The disadvantages of the method are that it will not detect basic antigens, and it will not measure antibodies that do not move cathodally by endosmosis (e.g., IgA, IgM); while it is more sensitive than double diffusion, it is still relatively insensitive, requiring 0.01 to 0.05 mg of antibody protein per ml for a positive test. Nonetheless, it has been successfully used for the detection of antibodies to the acidic antigens, dsDNA, ssDNA, nRNP, Sm, Ro/SSA, and La/SSB/Ha.[13-17] The technique is still far less sensitive and quantitative than hemagglutination, ELISA, or RIA methods and is being replaced by these methods as purified antigens become available.

**Immunofluorescence.** The use of the indirect immunofluorescence technique for the detection of antibodies to specific antigens has found its most intensive application in the measurement of antibodies to dsDNA. The Crithidia technique developed by Aarden, deGroot, and Feltkamp employs the hemoflagellate *Crithidia luciliae* as a substrate.[56] Binding of Ig to the kinetoplast, which contains exclusively circular double-stranded DNA, indicates antibody to dsDNA. The technique is also versatile, since Ig class can be determined by utilizing fluoreseinated antisera specific for heavy chains. Furthermore, the complement-fixing ability of the anti-DNA can be assessed by overlaying fresh normal human serum after binding of the anti-DNA and detection of fixed C3 with fluoreseinated anti-C3. This method has established itself as a standard technique for the measurement of anti-dsDNA.[18-20,56-58] No other immunofluorescent technique is known to identify antibodies directed toward a specific macromolecule, although antibodies to subcellular organelles have proved clinically useful. These include antibodies to the nucleolus,[21] the centromere,[22] and the mitotic spindle apparatus.[23] Measurement of antibodies to these organelles has clin-

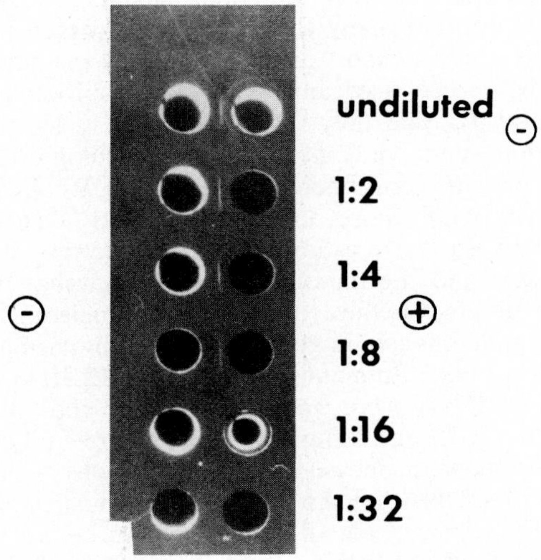


**Figure 46–5.** Counterimmunoelectrophoresis (CIE) shows a "standard curve" of the method in which serial dilutions of an SLE serum are tested against a constant concentration of dsDNA (4 $\mu$g milliliter). DNA is negatively charged and thus migrates towards the positive pole while the antibody moves to the negative pole by endosmosis.

ical utility, as will be discussed in the context of individual diseases. It is already known from both biochemical and immunochemical studies that there are several distinct nucleolar antigens with potential clinical significance.[24-27,157,158]

**Radioimmunoassay.** The measurement of antibodies to DNA has preoccupied students of SLE since the first demonstration of these antibodies in 1957,[28,29] and the first radioimmunoassay for the detection of autoantibodies in SLE was developed for the measurement of anti-DNA. The Farr technique takes advantage of the ready solubility of radio-labeled DNA and the insolubility of labeled DNA–anti-DNA complexes in 50 percent saturated ammonium sulfate solutions.[30-33] The solubility differences of free and bound DNA permitted easy separation and measurement of the complexes by centrifugation and led to practical assays, which are still widely used today. Later modifications employing nitrocellulose filters for the separation of bound from free labeled DNA have also led to assays for anti-DNA that have found wide application.[34-36] Subsequently, RIAs were developed for numerous polynucleotides, including polydeoxy adenylate-thymidylate (dAT),[36] polyriboinosinate-cytidylate (poly IC),[37] ribosomal RNA,[38] polyriboadenylate (poly riboA),[39] ultraviolet (UV) light–denatured DNA,[40] polyadenosine diphosphate ribose (poly ADP ribose),[41-43] and polyguanylate-cytidylate (poly GC).[44] While none of these assays has yet taken a clinically important place in the serological analysis of SLE patients, their detection and study raise many interesting questions. The utility of poly dAT is in its impeccably double-stranded character, so that antibodies to ssDNA do not bind to poly dAT. Binding of anti-ssDNA to the single-stranded regions of many putatively native DNA preparations commercially available created much confusion in the early literature on the specificity of antibodies to dsDNA in SLE.

Double-stranded RNA functions biologically as the replicative form of many RNA viruses, and such RNA is not a normal constituent of uninfected mammalian cells. The presence of antibodies to double-stranded RNA, poly IC, and poly GC in SLE has fueled much speculation about viral infection as an etiologic factor in SLE patients. Antibodies to ribosomal RNA, poly riboA, poly ADP ribose, and UV-denatured DNA have raised provocative questions about the nature of the immunogen and the immune dysregulation that regularly features antibodies to various polynucleotides in the rheumatic diseases in general and SLE in particular.

**Enzyme-Linked Immunosorbent Assay (ELISA).** Antibodies to DNA were first measured by the ELISA method in 1974[45] and a flurry of modifications followed which permitted the measurement of antibodies to either dsDNA or ssDNA.[46-52] As in all areas of medicine, the less expensive, safer, equally sensitive, and quantitative ELISA methods are rapidly replacing RIA techniques for the measurement of antigens and/or antibodies in the picogram to nanogram range. ELISA requires a purified antigen that will adhere to plastic, and as the various autoantigens are purified, it is expected that an ELISA method will be developed for the detection and quantitation of the appropriate autoantibodies.

## SPECIFIC AUTOANTIBODIES CHARACTERISTIC OF RHEUMATIC DISEASES

**Antibodies to DNA.** Antibodies to DNA have been of central interest in the immunology of SLE since their discovery in the late 1950s by several groups.[59,60,28,29] The development of serologic methods has led to increasing sensitivity and precision in the detection of these antibodies (Table 46–4). The earliest techniques were relatively insensitive precipitation methods. Complement fixation and passive hemagglutination methods for detecting anti-DNA were the first assays that detected antibody in more than half of the active untreated patients and were the standard techniques of the 1960s. These methods have now been largely supplanted by RIA, IFA on *Crithidia*, and ELISA methods for detecting and quantitating antibody to DNA. As can be seen, these techniques detect anti-DNA in 75 to 95 percent of active untreated patients. The lower figures seen in the table are from series in which no distinction is made between active and inactive disease. The crithidia technique measures only anti-dsDNA, while the RIA and ELISA methods are readily adapted to measure either anti-ssDNA or anti-dsDNA.

Antibodies to DNA have the widest clinical applicability and include those with the highest specificity for the diagnosis of SLE. There are two large categories of specificities that have clinical relevance: native (ds or double-stranded) and denatured (ss or single-stranded) DNA. Antibodies to dsDNA are directed to some aspect of the double-helical conformation of nDNA, the exact structure as yet being undetermined. Such antibodies do not bind to the free purine and pyrimidine bases but paradoxically can be absorbed out with ssDNA. In an investigation of this problem it has been shown that secondary structure in ssDNA is responsible for its reaction with anti-dsDNA antibodies in SLE sera.[63] Studies by the latter authors demonstrated that $S_1$ nuclease-resistant and heat-susceptible cores of double-helical structure in ssDNA were the source of reactivity for antibodies in SLE sera with specificity for dsDNA. In a related study it was determined that among antibodies

**Table 46–4.** Detection Methods for Antibodies to dsDNA

| | Percent Positive Tests |
|---|---|
| Precipitation in agar gel[13,53] | 7–33 |
| Counterimmunoelectrophoresis[13,52] | 37 |
| Passive hemagglutination[54] | 60 |
| Complement fixation[28,29,53] | 48–68 |
| Radioimmunoassay[30-35,55] | 50–75 |
| IFA by the crithidia technique[18-20,52,56-58] | 58–95 |
| ELISA[45-52] | 70–92 |

to dsDNA in SLE sera, great heterogeneity existed in binding specificity, which could be characterized by the pattern of reactivity exhibited by such antibodies with native DNA fragments varying in size from 20 to 1200 base pairs.[64] These studies support the long-held contention that specific antibodies to dsDNA exist, and they throw light on the previously puzzling observation that denatured DNA could absorb out antibodies to dsDNA.[65]

Antibodies to dsDNA are highly specific for the clinical diagnosis of SLE, although a rare report of the occurrence of such antibodies in patients with RA does exist. The ultimate diagnosis of such RA patients should be reserved, since some may develop other findings typical of SLE, including glomerulonephritis. Table 46–5 shows that anti-dsDNA is generally specific for SLE and that anti-ssDNA is found in a variety of diseases.

Since antibodies to dsDNA frequently fluctuate with disease activity and often disappear rapidly with immunosuppressive therapy, their occurrence is very rare in SLE patients who experience either a spontaneous or a steroid-induced remission. Demonstration of these antibodies requires impeccably native DNA in the assay procedure. The kinds of antigen preparations thought to be free of single-stranded regions include poly dAT, *Crithidia* kinetoplast DNA, $PM_2$ DNA, KB or *E. coli* nDNA treated with $S_1$ nuclease, and KB or *E. coli* dsDNA suitably purified on benzoylated DEAE columns. The requirement of dsDNA free of single-stranded regions for anti–native DNA detection was shown in a study in which apparent reactivity of human sera for dsDNA from patients with diseases other than SLE was due to antibody to single-stranded regions in the putative dsDNA preparations.[66]

Antibodies to dsDNA not only have considerable diagnostic specificity but have also been shown to be closely related to disease activity.[67,53] There is considerable evidence pointing to an important pathogenic role for dsDNA–anti-dsDNA immune complexes, particularly in lupus nephritis.[68-70]

As mentioned previously, the crithidia test has gained wide acceptance as a test for anti-dsDNA and when compared directly with a Farr assay has identical sensitivity.[62] In a recent large study,[52] the ELISA test for anti-dsDNA was positive in 80 percent of the samples, while the crithidia test was positive in only 58 percent of the samples. If these data are confirmed, the ELISA test may prevail as the most sensitive and quantitative test for anti-dsDNA. In that study, the sera that were positive by ELISA and negative by crithidia were the lowest positive samples, and the possibility of small amounts of single-stranded regions in the dsDNA bound to the plate is difficult to exclude.

Antibodies to ssDNA occur with even higher frequency in SLE patients than do antibodies to dsDNA, as illustrated in Table 46–5. The relevance of anti-ssDNA in SLE is emphasized not only by the observation that the specificity of antibodies to DNA is most commonly to ssDNA[71,72] but also by the identification of ssDNA in sera from lupus patients[73,74] and the demonstration of the alternating appearance of antigen and antibody in the circulation, in cryoprecipitates,[75] in renal lesions,[76] and in renal eluates.[77] In addition, in acid elution studies of nephritic kidneys from SLE patients such antibodies to ssDNA are invariably found in higher titers than antibodies to dsDNA and about 20 percent of the time are found when no antibodies are present that bind dsDNA.[77]

These antibodies are, therefore, at least as important as anti-dsDNA in immunopathogenesis and in some patients constitute the major demonstrable immune complex system. Thus, while antibodies to ssDNA are of both diagnostic and immunopathogenetic importance, their imperfect specificity must be recognized if their determination is to be useful without being misleading.

A question that has recently been reinvestigated is why some SLE patients with substantial antibody titers to dsDNA fail to develop nephritis. Two recent studies point to the absence of complement-fixing ability of the anti–native DNA in patients without clinical evidence

**Table 46–5.** Incidence of Antibodies to Native and Single-Stranded DNA*

| Sera | | Antibodies Positive (Percent) | |
|---|---|---|---|
| *Source* | *Number Tested* | *Native DNA* | *Single-Stranded DNA* |
| SLE | 50 | 60.0(7.1)† | 92.0(5.1) |
| Normal | 280 | 0.3(5.0) | 3.7(4.0)‡ |
| Hospital§ | 65 | 0 | 16.8(4.3) |
| Procainamide | 14 | 0 | 57.1(4.5) |
| Chronic active hepatitis | 43 | 2.3(3.0) | 58.2(5.1) |
| Infectious mononucleosis | 20 | 0 | 40.0(5.7) |
| Rheumatoid arthritis | 32 | 3.1(3.0) | 59.5(5.5) |
| Chronic glomerulonephritis | 40 | 2.5(4.0) | 7.5(4.6) |
| Primary biliary cirrhosis | 20 | 0 | 15.0(3.6) |

*From Koffler, D., et al.: Science 166:1648, 1969. Copyright 1969 by the American Association for the Advancement of Science.
†Mean titer of group of sera expressed as log base 2, shown in parentheses.
‡Of 280 sera, 170 were tested for antibodies to single-stranded DNA.
§Random hospital sera obtained from patients with a variety of diseases.

of nephritis.[78,79] By inference it is reasoned that the complement-fixing properties of anti-DNA are necessary for the development of the inflammatory process in lupus nephritis.

**The RNA-Protein Antigens.** Anderson and associates[80] first described the presence of precipitating antibodies to antigens in tissue extracts in the sera of patients with Sjögren's syndrome, and since then, several such precipitating antibody systems have been characterized in the sera of SLE patients. Although some laboratories have used passive hemagglutination as a method to detect and quantitate antibodies to these antigens, immunodiffusion is the only technique that can confirm immunologic identity between different sera because of the heterogeneous nature of the commonly available antigen preparations. All of the antigens to be discussed behave as soluble materials and are prepared by ultracentrifugation of tissue extracts. There are four of these RNA-protein conjugate antigens, antibodies to which are made with substantial frequency in SLE patients. They include nRNP (40 to 45 percent), Sm (25 percent), Ro/SSA (25 to 40 percent), and La/SSB/Ha (10 to 15 percent).[61]

**Antibodies to Sm and nRNP.** The Sm and nRNP antigens are nuclear in origin, and recent work has shed much light on their structure. Early characterization of the Sm antigen showed it to be periodate-sensitive, but trypsin, RNAase, and DNAase did not affect its antigenicity in precipitin reactions.[81] The ability of the nRNP antigen to precipitate[82] or coat cells for a hemagglutination reaction[83,84] was ablated by either RNAase or trypsin. The frequent simultaneous occurrence of antibodies to Sm and nRNP was noted,[85] and their molecular association demonstrated by immunochemical methods.[86] These early studies[86] and later more elegant immunoaffinity studies have shown that Sm and nRNP antigenic determinants exist in a molecular complex and that there exists a molecular form of Sm free of nRNP.[87-89]

Two major advances have enhanced the understanding of the antigenic structure of these antigens. One is the work of Lerner and Steitz, who characterized the RNA components of RNA-protein particles that carry the Sm and nRNP epitopes.[90] The second development was the application of the "immunoblot" or Western blot technique as well as other quantitative analyses (elution from SDS polyacrylamide gels) of the antigenicity of the protein components of the Sm and nRNP particles.[87-89,91]

The particle bound by anti-nRNP is composed of an RNA component designated $U_1$ complexed to at least 7 proteins varying in molecular weight from 12 to 65K; the Sm particle is composed of the same 7 proteins as well as $U_2$, $U_1$, $U_4$, $U_5$, and $U_6$ RNAs containing 196, 171, 145, 120, and 95 nucleotides, respectively. As already mentioned, there is a smaller antigenic version of the Sm particle lacking RNA but having several small protein bands and a total molecular weight of 70K. Precipitation reactions of nRNP with its antibody require the whole particle, both RNA and protein. Protein alone is sufficient for the precipitation of Sm with anti-Sm. Takano and colleagues[88] have shown direct binding of protein components of MW 65K and 30K with anti-nRNP and direct binding of protein components of 30K and 13K to anti-Sm. Douvas found nRNP antigenicity associated with a 30K-protein and Sm antigenicity related to a 13K-protein by the immunoblot technique.[90] Differences in elution conditions (3 M KSCN vs. 0.01 M HCl) may account for some of the differences in antigenicity noted by these two groups. There is no evidence for the direct binding of RNA to either antibody. The antigenic epitopes for both Sm and nRNP may be represented only on protein molecules, but more work is necessary to settle this issue. Moreover it is quite possible that individual patients may have antibodies that bind to different epitopes on the same protein or even different protein subunits within the same particle. Recently a hybridoma producing anti-Sm was formed by fusion of spleen cells from an autoimmune MRL/1 mouse with an appropriate myeloma cell line.[91] This mouse monoclonal antibody precipitates the same RNA-protein particle as does the human antibody, and the immunoblot technique indicates that the monoclonal antibody binds a 26K protein. The monoclonal antibodies of human-human hybridomas with activity against the Sm and nRNP antigens should provide powerful tools for the definitive analysis of these autoantigens.

The clinical significance of antibodies to nRNP and Sm has received much attention and only a brief summary of that information will be presented. There is agreement among workers in this area that antibodies to the Sm antigen are highly specific for SLE patients.[55] No characteristic clinical features are apparent for this group of patients, although there are reports that the nephritis of such patients is mild and follows a benign course.[92,93] It has also been reported that antibodies to Sm are associated with central nervous system involvement when it occurs as an isolated clinical manifestation of the disease.[94] A recent report provides evidence for fluctuation of anti-Sm levels with disease activity, suggesting participation in immune complex disease and use as a possible indicator of clinical activity in some patients.[101]

Patients who have antibodies only to nRNP have a low incidence of antibodies to DNA and a low incidence of clinically apparent renal disease.[83,84,95] These SLE patients with anti-nRNP in their sera develop nephritis only when antibodies of other specificities are present, notably anti-DNA.[96,97] Nephritis also occurs when anti-nRNP is associated with antibodies to Sm or Ro/SSA.

Much attention has centered on a group of patients with overlapping features of SLE, scleroderma, and polymyositis, who have been designated as having mixed connective tissue disease (MCTD) by Sharp and his associates.[83,84] These patients all possess antibodies to nRNP in their sera and, like other patients with anti-nRNP who lack overlapping features, have a low frequency of antibodies to DNA and a low frequency of nephritis.

Two reports of immune complex nephropathy in patients with MCTD and anti-nRNP have appeared,[98,99] but in neither report were antibodies to Ro/SSA[100] or ssDNA[77] sought in the sera of the nephritic patients. Both of these systems have been shown to participate in immune complex nephritis and to occur in 10 to 15 percent of patients with anti-nRNP. Special tests are required for their detection, and unless specifically sought, they are easily overlooked.

MCTD patients present with very heterogeneous clinical features, a point noted in the initial description and re-emphasized in the follow-up of the original 25 patients.[102] The only uniform finding in these patients is, by definition, the presence of antibodies to nRNP. No immunologic, clinical, genetic, or biochemical characteristic has yet been described that gives this syndrome definition. The finding(s) that will distinguish MCTD from its component connective tissue diseases (SLE, myositis, and PSS) awaits recognition.

**Antibodies to Ro/SSA and La/SSB/Ha.** Antibodies to the soluble antigens Ro and La were originally described in patients with SLE and Sjögren's syndrome.[103,104] Both antigens were thought to be cytoplasmic, since they were quantitatively recovered from the cytoplasmic fraction of cells prepared in strong sucrose solutions. Moreover, specifically purified antibodies to the Ro antigen predominantly stained the cytoplasm of KB* cells, thymocytes, and $Wil_2$ (a lymphoblastoid B-cell line) cells, while specifically purified antibodies to La stained both the nucleus and the cytoplasm of these cells (Maddison and Reichlin, unpublished data).

Alspaugh and Tan described two nuclear antigens extracted from $Wil_2$ cells, termed SSA and SSB, which precipitated with the sera of patients with Sjögren's syndrome.[105] Akizuki and colleagues described a soluble nuclear antigen, termed Ha, which precipitated with the sera of patients with SLE-Sjögren's syndrome overlap.[106] Interlaboratory exchange of sera and antigen extracts has clearly shown that Ro and SSA on the one hand, and La, SSB, and Ha on the other are antigenically identical. Problems still remain about the cellular localization of Ro/SSA and La/SSB/Ha, but these antigens are both RNA-protein conjugates.[107] While all RNA is synthesized in the nucleus, much RNA is eventually found in the cytoplasm. Some of the confusion about the cellular localization of these antigens might result from differences in the location of the antigen at different stages of the cell cycle. Examination of the cellular location of such antigens during different phases of the cell cycle employing monospecific specifically purified antibodies or monoclonal antibodies should provide definitive answers to these questions.

The antigenicity of La/SSB/Ha from all sources is trypsin sensitive and is RNAase sensitive only under certain circumstances.[104] Ro/SSA is trypsin sensitive only when derived from $Wil_2$ cells and is not RNAase sensitive. In neither case does isolated RNA have antigenic activity, and the consensus is that the antigenic epitopes in both instances are on protein subunits of the RNA protein conjugates. Venables and colleagues have shown with the immunoblot technique that antigenicity for La/SSB/Ha resides on polypeptides of molecular weight 40K and 29K.[108]

The clinical importance of antibodies to these antigens in North American populations is that they occur principally in two diseases: SLE and Sjögren's syndrome. Antibodies to Ro/SSA occur in 25 to 40 percent of unselected SLE patients when the assay utilized is the relatively insensitive agar diffusion method. Antibodies to La/SSB/Ha occur in 10 to 15 percent of SLE patients, all of whom also have antibodies to Ro/SSA in their sera.

Anti-Ro/SSA is found much more frequently in Japanese patients with connective tissue diseases than in North American patients. The frequency of occurrence in SLE is 58 percent, while the frequencies in RA, scleroderma, polymyositis, and undifferentiated connective tissue diseases are 24, 29, 15, and 45 percent, respectively. This difference is not explained by a more frequent occurrence of Sjögren's syndrome in the Japanese patients. Analysis of this difference in anti-Ro/SSA frequency in Japanese versus North American patients with connective tissue diseases should yield important clues to the genesis and regulation of this specific immune response.

Several clinical phenomena that are associated with the presence of anti-Ro/SSA in SLE patients are listed in Table 46–6. ANA-positive anti-Ro/SSA SLE patients are not clinically distinguishable from SLE patients without these antibodies except for a high frequency of rheumatoid factors that occur in 75 to 80 percent of these patients.[110] Antibodies to Ro/SSA occur in 62 percent of the patients with clinical SLE but negative ANA tests on cryostat sections of rodent liver or kidney sections. On the other hand, within the ANA-positive subset of SLE patients who have anti-Ro/SSA, important clinical and serologic differences distinguish patients who produce anti-Ro/SSA *alone* from those who produce *both* anti-Ro/SSA *and* anti-La/SSB.[111]

**Table 46–6.** Clinical and Serological Phenomena Associated with Anti-Ro/SSA in SLE Patients

1. Rheumatoid factor occurs in 80 percent of patients.
2. SLE patients with anti-Ro have a high frequency of nephritis, while those with both anti-Ro and anti-La have a low frequency of nephritis.
3. Anti-Ro/SSA found in 62 percent of "ANA-negative SLE" patients.
4. Anti-Ro/SSA occurs in 63 percent of instances of subacute cutaneous LE.
5. There is increased frequency of DR2 and DR3 antigens in SLE patients with anti-Ro/SSA.
6. Eighty-five percent of homozygous C2-deficient patients with SLE picture have anti-Ro/SSA. No other precipitins are demonstrable.
7. Anti-Ro/SSA and/or anti-La/SSB occur almost invariably in neonatal SLE. No other precipitin is found.

*A human tissue culture line.

There is a great similarity in nonrenal findings in these two groups of patients but a striking difference in the frequency and severity of renal disease. Thus, 16 of 30 (53 percent) anti-Ro/SSA patients had one or more of the following three findings: a serum creatinine greater than 3.0 mg per dl, proteinuria exceeding 1.5 g in 24 hours, and cellular casts in the urine. Only 2 of 23 (9 percent) of the anti-Ro/SSA *and* anti-La/SSB patients had such evidence for nephritis. The serologic correlation of this difference in renal disease was a 77 percent incidence of anti-DNA in the anti-Ro/SSA group and a 30 percent incidence of such antibodies in the anti-Ro/SSA and anti-La/SSB group. The titers of both anti-dsDNA and anti-ssDNA were higher in the patients with anti-Ro/SSA alone than in the patients who had both anti-Ro/SSA and anti-La/SSB in their sera.[111]

Recently, a subset of lupus patients with a characteristic nonscarring dermatitis designated subacute lupus erythematosus (SCLE) has been described.[112,113] The skin disease is intermediate in severity between the acute erythematous eruption of SLE and the chronic indolent scarring lesions of discoid LE. The patients exhibit a wide distribution of lesions, with the face, arms, and trunk being affected. Seventy percent of these patients are ANA-positive on KB cells, and they have a mild systemic illness very similar in character to that described in the so-called ANA-negative SLE patients.[6] The common factor shared by the ANA-negative SLE patients and the SCLE patients that may relate to their mild disease and the low frequency of nephritis is the low frequency of antibodies to dsDNA.

It has also been reported that 73 percent of these SCLE patients are DR3-positive, a great increase above the control frequency of 24 percent for this particular HLA antigen.[113] These patients' sera have recently been examined for the presence of antibodies to soluble cellular antigens, and it has been found that 63 percent have antibodies to Ro/SSA and/or La/SSB antigens.[113] As mentioned previously, 25 to 40 percent of SLE patients and only 3 percent of discoid LE patients have anti-Ro/SSA in their sera. In a recent report by Bell and Maddison, an even closer association of antibodies to Ro/SSA with the HLA antigen DR3 has been demonstrated.[114] In their SLE population, all the anti-Ro/SSA patients (10/10) were positive for the DR3 antigen. The frequency of DR3 in their control populations was 26 percent. These data suggest that a set of genetic determinants in the major histocompatibility complex (MHC) is associated with the production of anti-Ro/SSA.

Further data supporting a genetic influence on anti-Ro/SSA production comes from a study of homozygous C2 deficiency. The genes for C2 are known to reside in the MHC on chromosome 6. Antibodies to Ro/SSA were detected in 10 of 20 such C2-deficient sera and were the only precipitins detected. Of even greater interest is that of 11 of these patients with an SLE picture, 9 possessed anti-Ro/SSA, and the remaining anti-Ro/SSA patient had discoid LE. Therefore, 9 of the 10 homozygous C2-deficient, anti-Ro/SSA-positive patients were symptomatic.[115] As it is known that all homozygous C2-deficient patients studied thus far carry the DR2 antigen, it appears that antibodies to Ro/SSA can be associated with either the DR2 or DR3 antigen.

It has long been known that in children who develop neonatal SLE, the major clinical features are dermatitis and complete heart block. Recent studies show that antibodies to Ro/SSA or La/SSB or both have been found in every child and mother examined in this clinical setting.[116,117] The dermatitis and the anti-Ro/SSA disappear over the same time course, suggesting the possible participation of the anti-Ro/SSA in the pathogenesis of the dermal lesion. Some of the mothers have not been clinically ill, and the anti-Ro/SSA and anti-La/SSB have been demonstrated in their sera in the course of evaluating the clinical and serologic status of the children.

A final caveat of genetic interest derives from the study of a child with neonatal lupus in which mother and female child both had antibodies to Ro/SSA and La/SSB/Ha.[118] HLA typing of the mother and child revealed a dissociation of antibodies and DR antigens in that the mother was DR3 and the child was DR2. The child has had normal growth and development with no skin rash since four months of age, but the mother, initially asymptomatic, has developed some evidence of Sjögren's syndrome 17 months after delivery. Such data suggest that antibody production in the mother and clinical expression of disease in the neonate are controlled by independent factors.

**Antibodies to PCNA and Ma.** Two recently described antibodies that occur in small groups of SLE patients are of interest for various reasons. Antibodies to proliferating cell nuclear antigen (PCNA), described by Miyachi and colleagues,[119,120] occur in 2 percent of SLE sera.[120] This antigen is not only seen in interstitial cells in epithelial tissues like liver but is also seen in the majority of cells of actively proliferating tissues such as spleen. Antibodies may therefore exist in SLE sera which are directed to antigens poorly represented in tissues used as standard immunofluorescent substrates such as rodent liver and kidney. A similar situation exists for all the antigens listed in Table 46–2.

The Ma antigen is an acidic nuclear protein described by Winn and colleagues.[121] Antibodies to Ma occur in a subset (approximately 10 percent) of SLE patients with particularly severe disease. Of interest, if confirmed, is the association of this particular antibody with aggressive active disease and nephritis. Evidence was also presented demonstrating the alternating presence of antigen and antibody in the patients' sera, suggesting that immune complexes involving this system may be forming in the circulation of these patients.

**Antibodies to Histones.** Antibodies to histones were first measured by the complement fixation reaction of free histones with SLE sera.[122,123] More recently the reconstitution of acid-extracted nuclei with histones by the immunofluorescent technique has been utilized as an assay for antibodies to histone or histone-dependent antigens.[124,125] Antibodies to histone measured by immunofluorescence reconstitution were found in 30 percent of idiopathic SLE but in virtually all (22 of 23) patients with drug-induced SLE. An intriguing recent study utilizing free histone in an ELISA assay detects antihistone antibodies in 56 percent of idiopathic SLE and in all (9/9) active untreated SLE patients.[126] Contrary to the reports, by histone reconstitution of immunofluorescence, 0 of 9 patients with drug-induced SLE had antibodies to histone detected by the ELISA method.[126] These disparate results may only be apparent, since the histone reconstitution method always has DNA present and a likely candidate for the reactive antigen is DNA-histone, which requires both DNA and histone for antigenic activity.[127-130]

Because most of the reactions in the sera of patients with drug-induced SLE are histone-dependent, the restricted nature of this immune response in such patients is apparent. Four drugs are frequently implicated in drug-induced SLE with positive ANA tests: procainamide, isoniazid, hydralazine, and chlorpromazine. Occasional instances of drug-induced SLE with positive ANA have been reported with sulfonamides, diphenylhydantoin, trimethadione, penicillamine, and chlorthalidone.

**Sjögren's Syndrome.** In 1961 Anderson and colleagues reported two precipitin reactions designated SjD and SjT between concentrated tissue extracts and the sera of patients with Sjögren's syndrome.[80] Antigenicity of SjD was not affected by nucleolytic or proteolytic enzymes, while antigenicity of SjT was resistant to DNAase and RNAase but was destroyed by trypsin. In 1962 in a more extensive clinical survey they reported the occurrence of antibodies to SjD in 6 of 28 SLE patients, in 3 of 90 patients with RA, and in 3 of 10 patients with PSS.[132] Clinical studies indicated that antibodies to SjD and SjT occurred much more frequently in patients with keratoconjuctivitis sicca (KCS) alone (so-called primary Sjögren's syndrome) than in those with both KCS and RA (secondary Sjögren's syndrome)[133].

It is very likely if not certain that SjD is Ro (which is antigenically equivalent to SSA) and that SjT is La (which is antigenically equivalent to SSB and Ha). The frequency and mutuality of their occurrence, disease specificity, and physicochemical properties are similar. Indeed, like the reports in the early 1960s in which antibodies to SjD and SjT were reported to occur almost exclusively in KCS alone, the early studies of Alspaugh and Tan found anti-Ro/SSA and anti-La/SSB/Ha almost exclusively in primary Sjögren's syndrome.[134] Subsequent studies from Scotland[135] and Baltimore[136] have failed to exhibit this specificity, and an equal number of patients, amounting to 40 to 50 percent of the patients with both primary and secondary Sjögren's syndrome, have antibodies to these antigens. A unifying feature noted in the Baltimore patients is that the presence of anti-Ro/SSA is tightly linked to vasculitis and extraglandular disease whether these complications occur in the presence or absence of RA.

When KCS occurs with SLE[136] and scleroderma,[137] at least half of the patients with anti-Ro/SSA also have anti-La/SSB/Ha in their sera. In patients with primary biliary cirrhosis (PBC) who have Sjögren's syndrome, only anti-Ro/SSA is found in such sera. Sera from 12 such cases with anti-Ro/SSA were found in a series of 63 PBC patients.*

An association has been noted between vasculitis and antibodies to Ro/SSA or La/SSB or both, particularly in patients with Sjögren's syndrome but also in patients with Waldenström's benign hyperglobulinemic purpura or the hypocomplementemic urticaria vasculitis syndrome.[136] In a group of 75 patients with Sjögren's syndrome of whom 28 had biopsy-documented vasculitis, 24 (or 86 percent) had antibodies to Ro/SSA or La/SSB or both. Only 4 of the anti-Ro/SSA–negative Sjögren's syndrome patients (10 percent) had vasculitis, demonstrating the close association of the vasculitis and antibodies to Ro/SSA. The pathology exhibited was either a leukocytoclastic vasculitis or a mononuclear infiltrate in the vessel wall. The vasculitis was associated with central nervous system involvement in many patients, with peripheral vasculitis demonstrable in nerve and muscle[138] as well as skin.[139] Many of these patients, especially those with hypocomplementemia, have cryoglobulins in their sera, and preliminary studies suggest enrichment of antibodies to Ro/SSA in these cryoprecipitates.[140]

**Progressive Systemic Sclerosis.** Antinuclear antibodies in the sera of PSS patients have long been known to produce a variety of speckled and nucleolar patterns on frozen tissue sections and touch prints of tissue.[21,27,131,141] A maximum of 70 percent of the patients had positive tests on such substrates and no associations with any clinical features were established.

Employing tissue culture cells as substrate (Hep2) for immunofluorescence led to detection of ANA in almost all cases of PSS, the centromere pattern was described, and the relationship of anticentromere to the CREST (calcinosis, Raynaud's phenomenon, esophageal involvement, sclerodactyly, and telangietasia) syndrome was described.[22] Antibody to centromere occurs in about 50 percent of unselected cases of PSS but in 90 percent of PSS patients with the CRE ST variant.[22,24] This association has been confirmed.[142-143] Antibody to centromere seems to be associated with a very low ($\leq$ 5 percent) frequency of renal, cardiac, pulmonary, and lower gastrointestinal involvement.[144]

A rich variety of staining patterns has been described which are produced by PSS sera on Hep2 cells, of which six are nuclear and three are nucleolar.[24] One precipitating antibody that occurs in 25 percent of PSS sera is directed to the $Scl_{70}$ antigen, so designated because the MW of the reactive antigen is 70K. Thus far, this antibody appears highly specific for PSS patients. It is anticipated that identification of additional individual antigen-antibody reactions will lead to further serological and clinical correlations analagous to that described for the centromere antibody. Certainly the ability to

*Unpublished data of Penner, E., Maddison, P.J., Dickson, E.R., Weiser, M.M., Milgrom, F., and Reichlin, M.

detect ANA in virtually all cases of PSS has strengthened the view of this disorder as having an important immunologic component.

**Polymyositis.** Although it has long been known that 30 to 40 percent of patients with polymyositis (PM) have positive ANA tests (see Table 46–3), only recently have antigen-antibody reactions with specificity for this disorder been described. As in PSS, immunofluorescent studies on tissue culture cells (Hep2) detect antibodies in 86 percent of myositis patients (M. Reichlin, unpublished data).

The first antinuclear antibody characteristic for this disorder was detected by a complement-fixing antibody to a nuclear antigen Mi, which occurred in 60 percent of dermatomyositis (DM) patients and a smaller proportion of PM patients.[145] Soon thereafter, a precipitating antibody to a nuclear antigen designated $PM_1$ was described by Wolfe and associates and was said to be present in 60 percent of PM patients.[146] It is now recognized that no single precipitin reaction utilizing crude extracts and patient sera is present in more than 30 percent of PM sera and that the system originally designated $PM_1$ was a collection of precipitins, one of which ($PM_1$) occurred in a subset of PM patients, at least half of whom had an overlap of PSS and PM. This system has been renamed the PM-Scl system, is probably of nucleolar antigen, and occurs in 8 to 10 percent of unselected PM patients.[147]

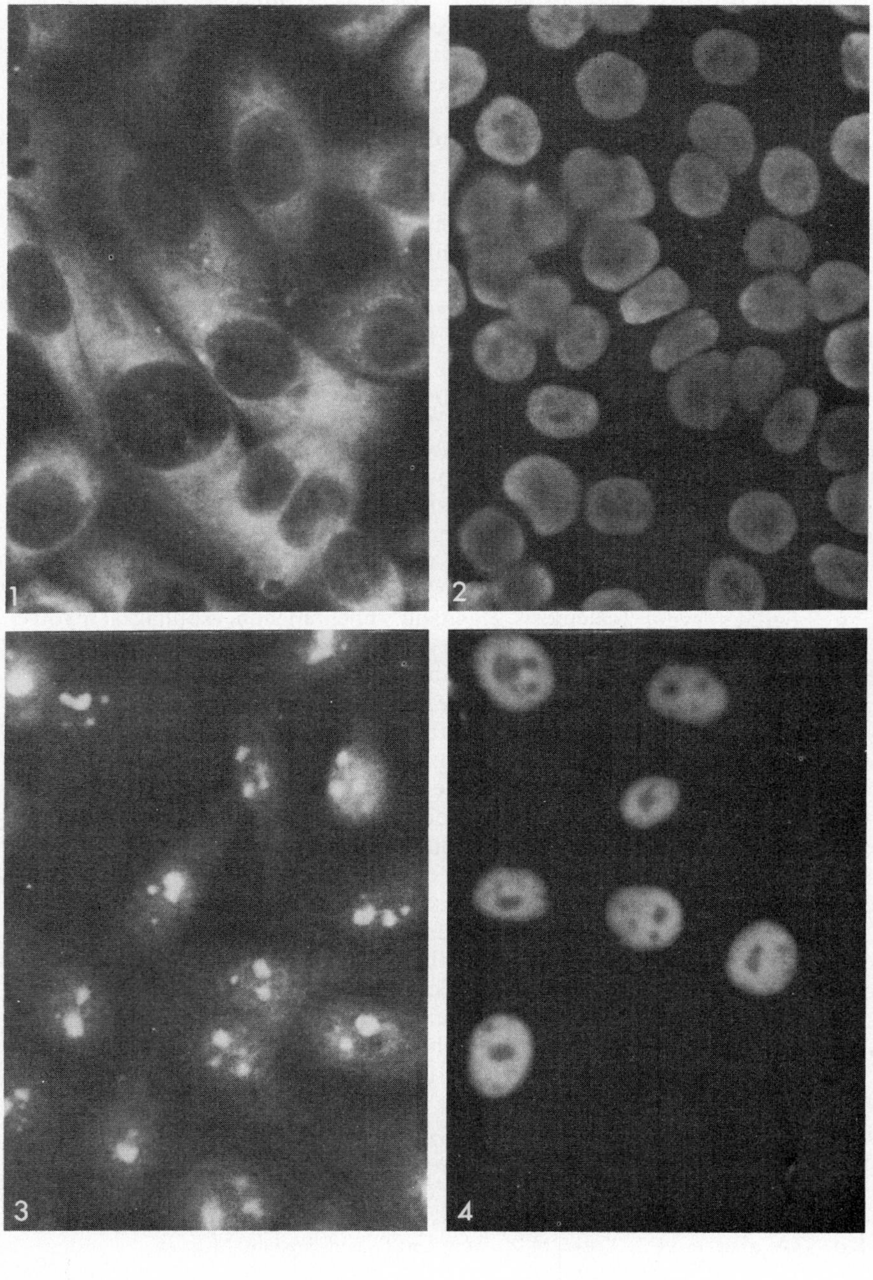


**Figure 46–6.** The patterns depicted here are developed by the reaction of fluorescinated anti-Ig reacting with differing antigens in Hep2 cells. The antibodies detected are all from patients with polymyositis. (1) At the upper left is a relatively homogeneous nuclear pattern; (2) at the upper right is a fine speckled pattern with nucleolar sparing; (3) at the bottom left is a homogeneous cytoplasmic pattern; and (4) at the bottom right is a nucleolar pattern.

The most frequently found precipitating antibody in PM patients is designated $Jo_1$ and occurs in 30 percent of idiopathic PM and in less than 10 percent of DM patients. This antibody is not found in SLE, RA, or PSS patients' sera. The antigen is a nuclear acidic molecule of MW 150K, and no particular extramuscular features seem associated with such antibodies in North American patients.[148,149] There are genetic factors influencing production of these antibodies, since 67 percent of patients with anti-$Jo_1$ carry the DR3 antigen on their Ia-positive cells, while only 25 percent of non–anti-$Jo_1$ myositis patients possess the DR3 antigen.[149] Interestingly, while this antigen is nuclear and can be demonstrated on spleen cells, it is poorly represented in mouse liver and kidney sections, and negative ANA tests are the rule on these substrates as well as tissue culture cells. This antibody is best demonstrated by the agar diffusion method.

Several other precipitating antibodies are seen in myositis patients, often with features overlapping other rheumatic diseases. Thus anti-nRNP is seen in the majority of patients with SLE-myositis, the previously mentioned $PM_1$ or PM-Scl is seen in PSS-myositis patients in North America, and a system designated Ku, which is seen in PSS-myositis, has thus far only been found in Japanese patients.[12] Exchange of reagents has established the independent indentities of the nRNP, PM-Scl ($PM_1$), and Ku systems. Although the Ku antigen is nuclear, it is not present in mouse tissue, and ANA tests are positive only on bovine or human tissues.

There is clearly great heterogeneity in the antinuclear antibodies characteristic of PM and DM and an aggregate of antigens represented in crude extracts of tissue form precipitates with 60 percent of these sera. PM-Scl ($PM_1$), nRNP, and $Jo_1$ are major systems occurring in 10 to 30 percent of PM patients, but a number of other minor reactions constitute the total spectrum of antigens toward which antibodies are demonstrable.[150] Of the remaining 40 percent of sera that do not form precipitates with tissue extracts, fewer than 10 percent are ANA positive on cryostat sections of rodent liver or kidney. About 80 percent of such sera, however, do bind to Hep2 cells in a series of immunofluorescent patterns depicted in Figure 46–6. While none of these patterns is specific for the myositis syndromes, they illustrate the heterogeneity that exists among these antibodies. In addition, it is notable here as in PSS that almost all the patients exhibit some autoantibody. These findings also re-emphasize the capacity of the human tissue culture lines to detect autoantibodies not demonstrable on cryostat sections of rodent tissues.

**Rheumatoid Arthritis.** The nature of ANA in RA has recently received renewed attention. At least a portion of this ANA has been rigorously shown to have a dual specificity of great interest. Surprisingly, the reactive antigen(s) for this ANA is contained in the Fc of IgG, thus exhibiting rheumatoid factor activity, and is also contained in the core constituent of chromatin, the nucleosome, which is a DNA-histone complex.[151,152] This observation raises new questions about the nature of the antigenic stimulus for the production of rheumatoid factors as well as the possibility of the development of practical tests for the detection of this specificity.

## MOLECULAR SPECIFICITIES OF ANA

Since the first report of Lerner and Steitz[90] defining the nRNP and Sm antigens as residing on small ribonucleoprotein particles, there has been an explosion of

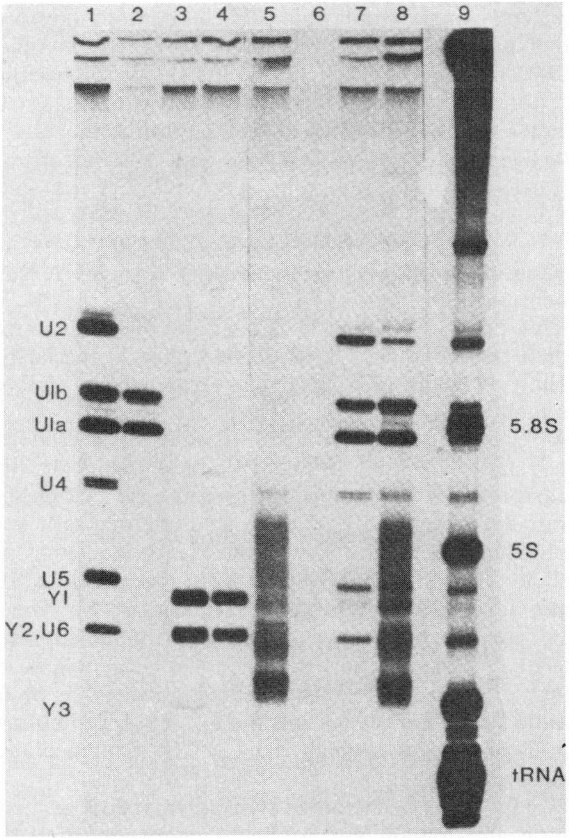


**Figure 46–7.** Small RNAs from Ehrlich ascites cells precipitated by antibodies from patients with lupus erythematosus. Ehrlich ascites cells were labeled with $^{32}PO_4$, and total cell extracts were prepared: $10^8$ cells in 5 ml of 50 mM tris-HCl and 150 mM NaCl p11 7.5, at 0° C were ruptured by sonication for 15 seconds with a Branson sonifier at setting 2; the homogenate was centrifuged at 15,000 g for 10 minutes to obtain a clear solution. RNAs were isolated from immune precipitates or extracts and were fractionated on a gel 400 mm long, 200 mm wide, and 0.5 mm thick, consisting of 10 percent polyacrylamide, 0.38 percent bisacrylamide, 7M urea, 1 mM EDTA, and 50 m Mtris borate, at pH 8.3. Lane 9 shows small RNAs from a total Ehrlich ascites cell extract. Lanes 1 to 8 show small RNAs precipitated by immunoglobulin G isolated from serums. Lane 6 shows normal serum; the other lanes show serums containing antibodies to (lane 1) Sm, (lane 2) RNP, (lane 3) $Ro^b$, (lane 4) $Ro^a$, (lane 5) La, (lane 7) Sm and $Ro^a$, and (lane 8) Sm, RNP, $Ro^a$ and 1 a. (Reprinted from Lerner, M.R., Boyle, J.A., and Steitz, J.A.: Science. 211:398, 1981.)

activity, which promises to shed light on the nature of many autoantigens reactive with the sera of patients with connective tissue diseases. The Lerner-Steitz method for the characterization of small RNAs bound by antibodies from SLE patients is depicted in Figure 46–7.

$U_1$ RNA, which is an integral part of the nRNP antigen, has a base sequence that is complementary to the intron-exon junctions of eukaryotic DNA. The hypothesis was made therefore that $U_1$ RNA was the recognition unit for the RNA splicing reaction that is an integral part of RNA processing.[153] Evidence supporting the role of $U_1$ RNA in the splicing reaction has been published.[154]

Similar studies have been done on the nature of the Ro/SSA and La/SSB/Ha antigens.[107] AntiRo/SSA is directed against cytoplasmic particles containing protein and five small RNAs, designated $Y_1$-$Y_5$, containing 80 to 140 bases. Thus far, no biological or biochemical function has been associated with the Ro particles. Antibodies to La/SSB bind a particle containing a very heterogeneous set of small RNAs and protein from normal cells but also bind to an RNA particle containing RNA encoded by adenovirus and RNA particles that are encoded by EB virus.[155] Anti-La/SSB reacts predominantly with nuclear particles whose RNA components are all products of RNA polymerase III, including pre-tRNAs, pre-5S rRNA, and viral transcripts. It may be that the La/SSB protein plays a special role in the processing of RNAs that are products of RNA polymerase III.[156]

A recent report describes antibodies in scleroderma sera[157] (anti-To) that bind a 300-base nucleolar ribonucleoprotein (7-2) and a novel 350-base cytoplasmic ribonucleoprotein (8-2). Other scleroderma sera were found that specifically bound the $U_3$ ribonucleoprotein particle. Hashimoto and Steitz have described an SLE serum (anti-Th) that binds the nucleolar 7-2 ribonucleoprotein particle as well as the 8-2 ribonucleoprotein particle.[158] In this report evidence was presented that a precursor form of the 7-2 ribonucleoprotein was bound by anti-La/SSB, thus adding the 7-2 RNA protein particle as another for which the La/SSB protein plays a role in processing.[158]

Finally it has been shown that polymyositis sera containing anti-$Jo_1$ all bind an RNA-protein particle, the RNA component of which is histidyl transfer RNA.[159] Preliminary evidence suggests that the protein component of this particle is the histidyl-specific amino acid activating enzyme (R. Bernstein and M.B. Matthews, personal communication). This remarkable specificity is only shown by myositis sera containing anti-$Jo_1$ and not by myositis sera with other antibodies.

A survey of ANA-positive sera for their ability to bind RNA-protein particles and free RNA has emphasized the multiplicity of antigens that are targets for autoantibodies among patients with rheumatic diseases. Study of these reactions should shed light on the nature of these autoimmune responses as well as provide probes for the molecular biologists to explore the functions of these molecules in normal cells.[160]

## SUMMARY

The intensive application of the agar diffusion method and tissue culture lines as substrates for immunofluorescence has led to the recognition of numerous new antibody specificities to nuclear and cytoplasmic antigens. Extensive biochemical and molecular biological study of these antigens has in many instances led to their molecular definition. The clinical applicability of all this new knowledge remains to be determined. It is, however, clear that the limit of the usefulness of ANA testing in the rheumatic diseases is yet to be reached.

## References


1. Hargraves, M.M., Richmond, H., and Morton, R.: Presentation of two bone marrow elements: The "tart" cell and "L.E." cell. Proc. Staff Meet. Mayo Clin. 23:25, 1948.
2. Haserick, J.R., and Sunderberg, R.D.: The bone marrow as a diagnostic aid in acute disseminated lupus erythematosus. J. Invest. Dermatol. 11:209, 1948.
3. Friou, G.J.: Clinical application of lupus serum-nucleoprotein reaction using fluorescent antibody technique (abstract). J. Clin. Invest. 36:890, 1957.
4. Holman, H.R., and Kunkel, H.G.: Affinity between the lupus erythematosus serum factor and cell nuclei and nucleoprotein. Science 126:162, 1957.
5. Holborow, E.J., Weir, D.M., and Johnson, G.D.: A serum factor in lupus erythematosus with affinity for tissue nuclei. Br. Med. J. 2:732, 1957.
6. Maddison, P.J., Provost, T.T., and Reichlin, M.: ANA-negative systemic lupus erythematosus: Serological analysis. Medicine (Baltimore) 60:87, 1981.
7. Beck, J.: Antinuclear antibodies: Methods of detection and significance. Mayo Clin. Proc. 44:600, 1960.
8. Wiik, A., and Munthe, E.: Restrictions among heavy and light chain determinants of granulocyte-specific antinuclear factors. Immunology 23:53, 1972.
9. Elling, P., Grandal, H., and Faber, V.: Granulocyte-specific antinuclear factors in serum and synovial fluid in rheumatoid arthritis. Ann. Rheum. Dis. 27:225, 1968.
10. Rosenberg, J.N., Johnson, G.D., Holborow, E.J., and Bywaters, E.G.L.: Eosinophil-specific and other granulocyte-specific antinuclear antibodies in juvenile chronic polyarthritis and adult rheumatoid arthritis. Ann. Rheum. Dis. 24:350, 1975.
11. Hoyeraal, H.M.: Granulocyte-reactive antinuclear factors in juvenile rheumatoid arthritis. Scand. J. Rheumatol. 5:84, 1976.
12. Mimori, T., Akizuki, M., Yamagata, H., Inada, S., Yoshida, S., and Homma, M.: Characterization of a high molecular weight acidic nuclear protein recognized by autoantibodies in sera from patients with polymyositis-scleroderma overlap. J. Clin. Invest. 68:611, 1981.
13. Davis, J.S., and Winfield, J.B.: Serum antibodies to DNA by counterimmunoelectrophoresis (CIE). Clin. Immunol. Immunopathol. 2:510, 1974.
14. Davis, J.S.: Determination of DNA and anti-DNA by counterimmunoelectrophoresis: A rapid and sensitive assay. Arthritis Rheum. 14:377, 1971.
15. Schur, P.H., DeAngelis, D., and Jackson, J.M.: Immunological detection of nucleic acids and antibodies to nucleic acids and nuclear antigens by counterimmunoelectrophoresis. Clin. Exp. Immunol. 17:209, 1974.
16. Kurata, N., and Tan, E.M.: Identification of antibodies to nuclear acidic antigens by counterimmunoelectrophoresis. Arthritis Rheum. 19:574, 1976.
17. Keiser, H.D., and Weinstein, J.: The detection and identification of antibodies to saline extractable nuclear antigens by counterimmunoelectrophoresis. Arthritis Rheum. 23:1026, 1980.
18. Davis, P., Christian, B., and Russell, A.S.: Immunofluorescent technique for the detection of antibodies to nDNA: Comparison with radioimmunoassay. J. Rheumatol. 4:15, 1977.
19. Sontheimer, R.D., and Gilliam, J.N.: An immunofluorescence assay for double-stranded DNA antibodies using *Crithidia luciliae* kinetoplast as a double-stranded DNA substrate. J. Lab. Clin. Med. 91:550, 1978.
20. Ballou, S.P., and Kushner, I.: Antinative DNA detection by the *Crithidia luciliae* method: An improved guide to the diagnosis and clinical management of systemic lupus erythematosus. Arthritis Rheum. 22:321, 1979.

21. Ritchie, R.F.: Antinucleolar antibodies: Their frequency and diagnostic association. N. Engl. J. Med. 282:1174, 1970.
22. Tan, E.M., Rodnan, G.P., Garcia, I., Moroi, I., Fritzler, M.J., and Peebles, C.: Diversity of antinuclear antibodies in scleroderma: Anticentromere antibody and its relationship to CREST. Arthritis Rheum. 23:617, 1980.
23. McCarty, G.A., Barada, F.A., Fritzler, M.J., and Snyderman, R.: A new antinuclear antibody staining the mitotic spindle apparatus: Immunologic characteristics, clinical occurrence and cytoskeletal studies. Arthritis Rheum. 24:S109, 1981.
24. Bernstein, R.M., Steigerwald, J.C., and Tan, E.M.: Association of antinuclear and antinucleolar antibodies in progressive systemic sclerosis. Clin. Exp. Immunol. 48:43, 1982.
25. Pinnas, J.L., Northway, J.D., and Tan, E.M.: Antinucleolar antibodies in human sera. J. Immunol. 111:996, 1973.
26. Miyawaki, S., and Ritchie, R.F.: Nucleolar antigen specific for antinucleolar antibody in the sera of patients with systemic rheumatic disease. Arthritis Rheum. 16:726, 1973.
27. Beck, J.S.: Autoantibodies to cell nuclei. Scot. Med. J. 8:373, 1963.
28. Robbins, W.C., Holman, H.R., Deicher, H., and Kunkel, H.G.: Complement fixation with cell nuclei and DNA in lupus erythematosus. Proc. Soc. Exper. Biol. Med. 96:575, 1957.
29. Seligmann, M., and Milgrom, F.: Mise en évidence par la fixation du complement de la reaction entre acid desoxyribonucleique et serum de malades atteints de lupus erythemateux dissémine. C. R. Acad. Sci. 245:1472, 1957.
30. Wold, R.T., Young, F.E., Tan, E.M., and Farr, R.S.: Deoxyribonucleic acid antibody: A method to detect its primary interaction with deoxyribonucleic acid. Science 161:806, 1968.
31. Pincus, T., Schur, P.H., Rose, J.A., Decker, J.L., and Talal, N.: Measurements of serum DNA-binding activity in SLE. N. Engl. J. Med. 281:701, 1969.
32. Pincus, T.: Immunochemical conditions affecting the measurement of DNA antibodies using ammonium sulfate precipitation. Arthritis Rheum. 14:523, 1971.
33. Webb, J., and Whaley, K.: Evaluation of the native DNA-binding assay for DNA antibodies in systemic lupus erythematosus and other connective tissue diseases. Med. J. Aust. 2:324, 1974.
34. Kredich, N.M., Skyler, J.S., and Foote, L.J.: Antibodies to native DNA in systemic lupus erythematosus. A technique of rapid and quantitative determination. Arch. Intern. Med. 131:639, 1973.
35. Ginsberg, B., and Keiser, H.: A millipore filter assay for antibodies to native DNA in sera of patients with systemic lupus erythematosus. Arthritis Rheum. 16:199, 1973.
36. Lentz, K., Winfield, J.B., and Barland, P.: Antibodies to dAT detected by membrane filtration. Arthritis Rheum. 19:867, 1976.
37. Steinberg, A.D., Baron, S., and Talal, N.: The pathogenesis of autoimmunity in New Zealand mice. I. Induction of antinucleic acid antibodies by polyinosinic-polycytidylic acid. Proc. Natl. Acad. Sci. (USA) 63:1102, 1969.
38. Eilat, D., Steinberg, A.D., and Schechter, A.N.: The reaction of SLE antibodies with native single-stranded RNA: Radioassay and binding specificities, J. Immunol. 120:550, 1978.
39. Pillarisetty, R.J., and Talal, N.: Clinical studies of antibodies binding polyriboadenylic acid in SLE. Arthritis Rheum. 19:705, 1976.
40. Davis, P., Russell, A.S., and Percy, J.S.: Antibodies to UV light denatured DNA in systemic lupus erythematosus: Detection by filter radioimmunoassy and clinical correlations. J. Rheumatol. 3:375, 1976.
41. Kanai, Y., Kawaminami, Y., Miwa, M., Matsushima, T., and Sugimura, T.: Naturally occurring antibodies to poly (ADP-ribose) in patients with systemic lupus erythematosus. Nature 265:175, 1977.
42. Okobie, E.E., and Shall, S.: The significance of antibodies to poly (ADP-ribose) in patients with systemic lupus erythematosus. Clin. Exp. Immunol. 36:151, 1979.
43. Morrow, W.J.W., Isenkey, D.A., Parry, H.F., Shen, L., Okobie, E.E., Farzanek, F., Shall, S., and Snaith, M.L.: Studies on autoantibodies to poly (adenosine-diphosphate ribose) in SLE and other autoimmune diseases. Ann. Rheum. Dis. 41:396, 1982.
44. Nabon, E., Deffraissy, J.F., Kahn, M.F., Jeusset, J., Galanand, P., and Lacour, F.: Anti-poly (G)-poly (C) antibodies in the serum of patients with systemic lupus erythematosus. Clin. Immunol. Immunopathol. 22:349, 1982.
45. Pesce, A.J., Mendoza, N., Boreisha, I., Gaizutis, M.A., and Pollock, V.E.: Use of enzyme-linked antibodies to measure serum anti-DNA antibody in systemic lupus erythematosus. Clin. Chem. 20:353, 1974.
46. Gripenberg, M., Linder, E., Kurki, P., and Engvall, E.: A solid phase enzyme-linked immunoabsorbent assay (ELISA) for the demonstration of antibodies against denatured, single-stranded DNA in patient sera. Scand. J. Immunol. 7:151, 1978.
47. Klotz, J.L., Minami, R.M., and Teplitz, R.L.: An enzyme-linked immunosorbent assay for antibodies to native and denatured DNA. J. Immunol. Meth. 29:155, 1979.
48. Pisetsky, D.S., and Peters, D.V.: A simple enzyme-linked immunosorbent assay for antibodies to native DNA. J. Immunol. Meth. 41:187, 1981.
49. Miller, T.E., Lahita, R.G., Zario, V.J., MacWilliam, J., and Koffler, D.: Clinical significance of anti-double stranded DNA antibodies detected by a solid phase radioimmunoassay. Arthritis Rheum. 24:602, 1981.
50. Halbert, S.P., Karsh, J., and Anken, M.: Studies on antibodies to deoxyribonucleic acid and deoxyribonucleoprotein with enzyme immunoassay (ELISA). J. Lab. Clin. Med. 97:97, 1981.
51. Kavai, M., Banzai, A., Zsindely, A., Sonkoly, I., and Szegedi, G.: Enzyme-linked immunoabsorbent assay for antibodies to native DNA in sera of patients with SLE. J. Immunol. Meth. 48:169, 1982.
52. Eaton, R.B., Schneider, G., and Schur, P.H.: Enzyme immunoassay for antibodies to native DNA. Arthritis Rheum. 26:52, 1983.
53. Schur, P.H., and Sandson, J.: Immunological factors and clinical activity in systemic lupus erythematosus. N. Engl. J. Med. 278:533, 1968.
54. Koffler, D., Carr, R., Agnello, V., Feizi, T., and Kunkel, H.G.: Antibodies to polynucleotides: Distribution in human serum. Science 166:1648, 1969.
55. Notman, D.D., Kurata, N., and Tan, E.M.: Profiles of antinuclear antibodies in systemic rheumatic diseases. Ann. Intern. Med. 83:464, 1975.
56. Aarden, L.A., de Groot, E.R., and Feltkamp, T.E.W.: Immunology of DNA. III. *Crithidia luciliae*: A simple substrate for the detection of anti-dsDNA with the immunofluorescence technique. Ann. N. Y. Acad. Sci. 254:505, 1975.
57. Slater, W.G., Cameron, J.S., and Lessoff, M.H.: The *Crithidia luciliae* kinetoplast immunofluorescence test in systemic lupus erythematosus. Clin. Exp. Immunol. 25:480, 1976.
58. Chubick, A., Sontheimer, R.D., Gilliam, J.N., and Ziff, M.: An appraisal of tests for native DNA antibodies in connective tissue diseases: Clinical usefulness of *Crithidia luciliae* assay. Ann. Intern. Med. 89:186, 1978.
59. Ceppellini, R., Polli, E., and Celada, F.: A DNA-reacting factor in serum of a patient with lupus erythematosus diffusus. Proc. Soc. Exp. Biol. Med. 96:572, 1957.
60. Deicher, H.R.G., Holman, H.R., and Kunkel, H.G.: The precipitin reaction between DNA and a serum factor in systemic lupus erythematosus. J. Exp. Med. 109:97, 1959.
61. Reichlin, M.: Current perspectives on serological reactions in LE patients. Clin. Exp. Immunol. 44:1, 1981.
62. Aarden, L.L., Lakmeker, F., de Groot, E.F., Swaak, A.J.G., and Feltkamp, T.E.W.: Detection of antibodies to DNA by radioimmunoassay and immunofluorescence. Scand. J. Rheum. Suppl. 11:12, 1975.
63. Stollar, B.D., and Papalian, M.: Secondary structure in denatured DNA is responsible for its reaction with antinative DNA antibodies of systemic lupus erythematosus sera. J. Clin. Invest. 66:210, 1980.
64. Papalian, M., Lafer, E., Wong, R., and Stollar, B.D.: Reaction of systemic lupus erythematosus antinative DNA antibodies with native DNA fragments from 20-1200 base pairs. J. Clin. Invest. 65:469, 1980.
65. Stollar, B.D.: Nucleic acid antigens. *In* Sela, M. (ed.): The Antigens. Vol. 1. New York and London, Academic Press, 1973.
66. Locker, J.D., Medof, M.E., Burnett, R.M., and Sukhupunyaraska, S.: Characterization of DNA used to assay sera for anti-DNA antibodies: Determination of the specificities of anti-DNA antibodies in SLE and non-SLE rheumatic disease states. J. Immunol. 118:694, 1977.
67. Koffler, D., Agnello, V., Thoburn, R., and Kunkel, H.G.: Systemic lupus erythematosus: Prototype of immune complex nephritis in man. J. Exp. Med. 134:109, 1971.
68. Tan, E.M., Schur, P.H., and Carr, R.I.: Deoxyribonucleic acid (DNA) and antibodies to DNA in the serum of patients with systemic lupus erythematosus. J. Clin. Invest. 45:1732, 1966.
69. Koffler, D., Schur, P.H., and Kunkel, H.G.: Immunological studies concerning the nephritis of systemic lupus erythematosus. J. Exp. Med. 126:607, 1967.
70. Cochrane, C.G., and Koffler, D.: Immune complex disease in experimental animals and man. Adv. Immunol. 16:185, 1973.
71. Koffler, D., Carr, R.I., Agnello, V., Thoburn, R., and Kunkel, H.G.: Antibodies to polynucleotides in human sera: Antigenic specificity and relation to disease. J. Exp. Med. 134:294, 1971.
72. Samaha, R.J., and Irvin, W.S.: Deoxyribonucleic acid strandedness: Partial characterization of the antigenic region binding antibodies in lupus erythematosus serum. J. Clin. Invest. 56:446, 1975.
73. Barnett, E.V.: Detection of nuclear antigens (DNA) in normal and pathologic human fluids by quantitative complement fixation. Arthritis Rheum. 11:407, 1968.
74. Koffler, D., Agnello, V., Winchester, R.V., and Kunkel, H.G.: The occurrence of single-stranded DNA in the serum of patients with systemic lupus erythematosus and other diseases. J. Clin. Invest. 52:198, 1973.
75. Winfield, J.B., Koffler, D., and Kunkel, H.G.: Specific concentration of polynucleotide immune complexes in the cryoprecipitates of patients with systemic lupus erythematosus. J. Clin. Invest. 56:563, 1975.
76. Andres, G.A., Accini, G.A., Beiser, S.M., Christian, C.L., Cinotti, G.A., Erlanger, B.F., Hsu, K.C., and Seegal, B.C.: Localization of fluorescein-

labelled antinucleoside antibodies in glomeruli of patients with systemic lupus erythematosus nephritis. J. Clin. Invest. 49:2106, 1971.
77. Koffler, D., Agnello, V., and Kunkel, H.G.: Polynucleotide immune complexes in serum and glomeruli of patients with systemic lupus erythematosus. Am. J. Pathol. 74:109, 1974.
78. Miniter, M.F., Stollar, B.D., and Agnello, V.: Reassessment of the clinical significance of native DNA antibodies in systemic lupus erythematosus. Arthritis Rheum. 22:959, 1979.
79. Beaulieu, A., Ruismorio, F.P., Friou, G.J., Vayuvegula, B., and Mirick, B.: IgG antibodies to double-stranded DNA in systemic lupus erythematosus sera: Independent variation of complement-fixing activity and total antibody content. Arthritis Rheum. 22:565, 1979.
80. Anderson, J.R., Gray, K.G., Beck, J., and Kinnear, W.F.: Precipitating autoantibodies in Sjögren's disease. Lancet ii:456, 1961.
81. Tan, E.M., and Kunkel, H.G.: Characteristics of a soluble nuclear antigen precipitating with the sera of patients with systemic lupus erythematosus. J. Immunol. 96:464, 1966.
82. Mattioli, M., and Reichlin, M.: Characterization of a soluble nuclear ribonucleoprotein antigen reactive with LE sera. J. Immunol. 197:1281, 1971.
83. Sharp, G.C., Irvin, W.S., Laroque, R. L., Velez, C., Daly, V., Kaiser, A.D., and Holman, H.R.: Association of autoantibodies to different nuclear antigens with clinical patterns of rheumatic disease and responsiveness to therapy. J. Clin. Invest. 50:350, 1971.
84. Sharp, G.C., Irvin, W.S., Tan, E.M., Gould, R.G., and Holman, H.R.: Mixed connective tissue disease—an apparently distinct rheumatic disease syndrome associated with a specific antibody to an extractable nuclear antigen (ENA). Am. J. Med. 52:148, 1972.
85. Reichlin, M., and Mattioli, M.: Antigens and antibodies characteristic of systemic lupus erythematosus. Bull. Rheum. Dis. 24:756, 1974.
86. Mattioli, M., and Reichlin, M.: Physical association of two nuclear antigens and mutual occurrence of their antibodies: The relationship of the Sm and RNA protein (Mo) systems in SLE sera. J. Immunol. 110:1318, 1973.
87. Takano, M., Agris, P.F., and Sharp, G.C.: Purification and biochemical characterization of nuclear ribonucleoprotein antigen using purified antibody from serum of a patient with mixed connective tissue disease. J. Clin. Invest. 65:1449, 1980.
88. Takano, M., Golden, S.S., Sharp, G.C., and Agris, P.F.: Molecular relationship between two nuclear antigens, ribonucleoprotein and Sm: Purification of active antigens and their biochemical characterization. Biochemistry 21:5929, 1981.
89. Douvas, A.S.: Autoantibodies occurring in two different rheumatic diseases react with the same ribonucleoprotein particle. Proc. Natl. Acad. Sci. (USA) 79:5401, 1982.
90. Lerner, M.R., and Steitz, J.A.: Antibodies to small nuclear RNAs complexed with proteins are produced by patients with systemic lupus erythematosus. Proc. Natl. Acad. Sci. (USA) 76:5495, 1979.
91. Lerner, E.A., Lerner, M.R., Janeway, Jr., C.A., and Steitz, J.A.: Monoclonal antibodies to nucleic acid–containing cellular constituents: Probes for molecular biology and autoimmune disease. Proc. Natl. Acad. Sci. (USA) 78:2737, 1981.
92. Powers, R., Akizuki, M., Boehm-Truitt, M.J., Daly, V., and Holman, H.R.: Substantial purification of the Sm antigen and association of high titer antibody to Sm with a clinical subset of systemic lupus erythematosus. Arthritis Rheum. 20:131 (abstract), 1977.
93. Winn, D.M., Wolfe, J.R., Lindberg, D.A., Fristoe, F.A., Kingsland, L., and Sharp, G.C.: Identification of a clinical subset of systemic lupus erythematosus by antibodies to the Sm antigen. Arthritis Rheum. 22:1334, 1979.
94. Winfield, J.B., Brunner, C.M., and Koffler, D.: Serologic studies in patients with systemic lupus erythematosus and central nervous system dysfunction. Arthritis Rheum. 21:289, 1978.
95. Reichlin, M., and Mattioli, M.: Correlation of a precipitin reaction to an RNA protein antigen and a low prevalence of nephritis in patients with systemic lupus erythematosus. N. Engl. J. Med. 286:908, 1972.
96. Parker, M.D.: Ribonucleoprotein antibodies: Frequency and clinical significance in systemic lupus erythematosus, scleroderma, and mixed connective tissue disease. J. Lab. Clin. Med. 82:769, 1973.
97. Maddison, P.J., Mogavero, H., and Reichlin, M.: Patterns of clinical disease associated with antibodies to nuclear ribonucleoprotein. J. Rheumatol. 5:407, 1978.
98. Fuller, T.J., Richman, A.V., Auerbach, D., Alexander, R.W., Lottenberg, R., and Longley, S.: Immune complex glomerulonephritis in a patient with mixed connective tissue disease. Am. J. Med. 62:761, 1977.
99. Bennett, R.M., and Spongo, B.H.: Immune complex nephropathy in mixed connective tissue disease. Am. J. Med. 63:534, 1977.
100. Madison, P.J., and Reichlin, M.: Deposition of antibodies to a soluble cytoplasmic antigen in the kidneys of patients with systemic lupus erythematosus. Arthritis Rheum. 22:858, 1979.
101. Barada, F.A., Jr., Andrews, B.S., Davis, J.S., IV, and Taylor, R.P.: Antibodies to Sm in patients with systemic lupus erythematosus. Arthritis Rheum. 24:1236, 1981.
102. Nimelstein, S.H., Brody, S., McShane, D., and Holman, H.R.: Mixed connective tissue disease: A subsequent evaluation of the original 25 patients. Medicine (Baltimore) 59:239, 1980.
103. Clark, G., Reichlin, M., and Tomasi, T.B.: Characterization of a soluble cytoplasmic antigen reactive with sera from patients with systemic lupus erythematosus. J. Immunol. 102:117, 1968.
104. Mattioli, M., and Reichlin, M.: Heterogeneity of RNA protein antigens reactive with sera of patients with systemic lupus erythematosus. Arthritis Rheum. 17:421, 1974.
105. Alspaugh, M.A., and Tan, E.M.: Antibodies to cellular antigens in Sjögren's syndrome. J. Clin. Invest. 55:1067, 1975.
106. Akizuki, M., Powers, R., and Holman, H.R.: A soluble acidic protein of the cell nucleus which reacts with serum from patients with systemic lupus erythematosus and Sjögren's syndrome. J. Clin. Invest. 59:254, 1977.
107. Lerner, M.R., Boyle, J.A., Hardin, J.A., and Steitz, J.A.: Two novel classes of small RNA proteins detected by antibodies associated with lupus erythematosus. Science 211:400, 1981.
108. Venables, P.J.W., Charles, P.J., Buchanan, R.R.C., Yi, I., Mumford, P.A., Schreiber, L., Roon, G.R.W., and Maini, R.N.: Quantitation and detection of isotypes of antiSSB antibodies by ELISA and Farr assays using affinity purified antigens. Arthritis Rheum. 26:146, 1983.
109. Yamagata, H.: The antibodies to the SS-A antigen in patients with connective tissue diseases. Keio Igaku 58:381, 1981 (Japanese).
110. Maddison, P.J., Mogavero, H., Provost, T.T., and Reichlin, M.: The clinical significance of autoantibodies to a soluble cytoplasmic antigen in systemic lupus erythematosus and other connective tissue diseases. J. Rheumatol. 6:189, 1979.
111. Wasicek, C.A., and Reichlin, M.: Clinical and serological differences between systemic lupus erythematosus patients with antibodies to Ro versus patients with antibodies to Ro and La. J. Clin. Invest. 69:835, 1982.
112. Sontheimer, R.D., Thomas, J.R., and Gilliam, J.N.: Subacute cutaneous lupus erythematosus. A cutaneous marker for a distinct lupus erythematosus subset. Arch. Dermatol. 115:1409, 1979.
113. Sontheimer, R.D., Maddison, P.J., Reichlin, M., Jordan, R.E., Stastny, P., and Gilliam, J.N.: Serologic and HLA associations in subacute cutaneous lupus erythematosus, a clinical subset of lupus erythematosus. Ann. Intern. Med. 97:664, 1982.
114. Bell, D.A., and Maddison, P.J.: Serologic subsets in SLE: An examination of autoantibodies in relationship to clinical features of disease and HLA antigens. Arthritis Rheum. 23:1268, 1980.
115. Provost, T.T., Arnett, F.C., and Reichlin, M.: $C_2$ deficiency, lupus erythematosus and anticytoplasmic Ro (SSA) antibodies. Arthritis Rheum. 25:S41, 1982 (Abstract).
116. Franco, H.L., Weston, W.L., Peebles, C., Forstat, S.L., and Phanaphak, P.: Autoantibodies directed against sicca syndrome antigens in the neonatal lupus syndrome. Am. Acad. Dermatol. 4:67, 1981.
117. Kephart, D.C., Hood, A.F., and Provost, T.T.: Neonatal lupus erythematosus: New serological findings. J. Invest. Dermatol. 77:331, 1981.
118. Lockshin, M.D., Gibofsky, A., Peebles, C.L., Gigli, I., Fotino, M., and Hurwitz, S.: Neonatal lupus erythematosus with heart block: Family study of a patient with anti-SSA and SSB antibodies. Arthritis Rheum. 26:210, 1983.
119. Miyachi, I., Fritzler, M.J., and Tan, E.M.: Autoantibody to a nuclear antigen in proliferating cells. J. Immunol. 121:228, 1978.
120. Fritzler, M.J., McCarty, G.A., Ryan, J.P., and Kinsella, T.D.: Clinical features of patients with antibodies directed against proliferating cell nuclear antigen. Arthritis Rheum. 26:140, 1983.
121. Winn, D.M., Wolfe, J.F., Harmon, D., and Sharp, G.C.: Characterization of a distinct nuclear acidic protein antigen (MA) and clinical findings in systemic lupus erythematosus patients with MA antibodies. J. Clin. Invest. 64:820, 1979.
122. Kunkel, H.G., Holman, H.R., and Deicher, H.R.G.: Multiple autoantibodies to cell constituents in systemic lupus erythematosus. Ciba Found. Symp. 8:429, 1960.
123. Stollar, B.D.: Reactions of systemic lupus erythematosus sera with histone fractions and histone DNA complexes. Arthritis Rheum. 14:495, 1971.
124. Tan, E.M., Robinson, J., and Robitaille, P.: Studies on antibodies to histones by immunofluorescence. Scand. J. Immunol. 5:89, 1976.
125. Fritzler, M.J., and Tan, E.M.: Antibodies to histones in drug-induced and idiopathic lupus erythematosus. J. Clin. Invest. 62:560, 1978.
126. Gioud, M., Faci, M.A., and Monia, J.C.: Histone antibodies in systemic lupus erythematosus. Arthritis Rheum. 25:407, 1982.
127. Friou, G.J.: Identification of the nuclear component of the interaction of lupus erythematosus globulin and nuclei. J. Immunol. 80:476, 1958.
128. Holman, H.R., and Deicher, H.R.: The reaction of the lupus erythe-

matosus (LE) cell factor with deoxyribonucleoprotein of the cell nucleus. J. Clin. Invest. 38:2059, 1959.
129. Tan, E.M.: An immunologic precipitin system between soluble nucleoprotein and serum antibody in systemic lupus erythematosus. J. Clin. Invest. 46:735, 1967.
130. Stollar, B.D.: Studies on nucleoprotein determinants for systemic lupus erythematosus serum. J. Immunol. 99:959, 1967.
131. Burnham, T.K., Fine, G., and Neblett, T.R.: The immunofluorescent tumor imprint technique. II. The frequency of antinuclear factors in connective tissue diseases and dermatoses. Ann. Intern. Med. 65:9, 966.
132. Anderson, J.R., Gray, K.G., Beck, J.S., Buchanan, W.W., and McElhanney, A.J.: Precipitating autoantibodies in the connective tissue diseases. Ann. Rheum. Dis. 21:360, 1962.
133. Bunim, J.J.: Hypergammaglobulinemia and autoantibodies in Sjögren's syndrome. Ann. N. Y. Acad. Sci. 124: 852, 1965.
134. Alspaugh, M.A., Talal, N., and Tan, E.M.: Differentiation and characterization of autoantibodies and their antigens in Sjögren's syndrome. Arthritis Rheum. 19:216, 1976.
135. Alspaugh, M.A., Buchanan, W.W., and Whaley, K.: Precipitating antibodies to cellular antigens in Sjögren's syndrome, rheumatoid arthritis and other organ and non-organ-specific diseases. Ann. Rheum. Dis. 37:244, 1978.
136. Alexander, E.L., Hirsch, T.J., Arnett, F.C., Provost, T.T., and Stevens, M.B.: Ro (SSA) and La (SSB) antibodies in the clinical spectrum of Sjögren's syndrome. J. Rheum. 9:239, 1982.
137. Osial, T.A., Whiteside, T.L., Buckingham, R.B., Singh, G., Barnes, E.L., and Rodnan, G.P.: Antibodies to SS-A, SSB and RANA in progressive systemic sclerosis (PSS) with and without Sjögren's syndrome (SS) (abstract). Arthritis Rheum. 25:S34, 1982.
138. Alexander, E.C., and Alexander, G.E.: Central nervous system disease in primary Sjögren's syndrome association with vasculitis and antibodies to Ro/SSA. Arthritis Rheum. 25:15, 1982 (abstract).
139. Alexander, E.L., and Provost, T.T.: Cutaneous manifestations of Sjögren's syndrome (SS). Reflections of immune vasculitis. Arthritis Rheum. 25:S15, 1982 (abstract).
140. Reichlin, M.: Clinical and immunologic significance of antibodies to Ro and La in systemic lupus erythematosus. Arthritis Rheum. 25:767, 1982.
141. Rothfield, N.F., and Rodnan, G.P.: Serum antinuclear antibodies in progressive systemic sclerosis (scleroderma). Arthritis Rheum. 11:607, 1968.
142. Fritzler, M.J., Kinsella, T.D., and Garbutt, E.: The CREST syndrome: A distinct serologic entity with anticentromere antibodies. Am. J. Med. 69:520, 1980.
143. Kallenberg, C.G.M., Pastoor, G.W., Wouda, A.A., and The, T.H.: Antinuclear antibodies in patients with Raynaud's phenomenon: Clinical significance of anticentromere antibodies. Ann. Rheum. Dis. 41:382, 1982.
144. McCarty, G.A., Rice, J.R., Bembe, M.L., and Barada, F.A., Jr.: Anticentromere antibody. Clinical correlations and association with favorable prognosis in patients with scleroderma variants. Arthritis Rheum. 26:1, 1983.
145. Reichlin, M., and Mattioli, M.: Description of a serological reaction characteristic of polymyositis. Clin. Immunol. Immunopathol. 5:12, 1976.
146. Wolfe, J.F., Adelstein, E., and Sharp, G.C.: Antinuclear antibody with distinct specificity for polymyositis. J. Clin. Invest. 59:176, 1977.
147. Reichlin, M., Maddison, P.J., Targoff, I., Bunch, T., Arnett, F., Sharp, G.C., Treadwell, E., and Tan, E.M.: Antibodies to a nuclear/nucleolar antigen in patients with polymyositis-overlap syndromes. J. Clin. Immunol. 4:40, 1984.
148. Nishikai, M., and Reichlin, M.: Heterogeneity of precipitating antibodies in polymyositis and dermatomyositis. Characterization of the $Jo_1$ antibody system. Arthritis Rheum. 23:881, 1980.
149. Arnett, F.C., Hirsch, T.J., Nishikai, M., Bias, W., and Reichlin, M.: The $Jo_1$ antibody system. Clinical and immunogenetic associations in myositis. J. Rheumatol. 8:925, 1981.
150. Reichlin, M.: Marker antibodies for polymyositis syndromes. *In* Antibodies to Nuclear Antigens, Immunological Specificity and Clinical Implications. Excerpta-Medica 2, 1981.
151. Agnello, V., Ibanez de Kasip, G., Arbetter, A.E., and Spitz, J.J.R.: Significance of rheumatoid factors cross reactive with DNA-protein (DNP). Arthritis Rheum. 21:540, 1978.
152. Hannestad, K., and Stollar, B.D.: Certain rheumatoid factors react with nucleosomes. Nature 275:671, 1978.
153. Lerner, M.R., Boyle, J.A., Mount, S.M., Wolin, S.L., and Steitz, J.A.: Are snRNP's involved in splicing? Nature (London) 283:220, 1980.
154. Yang, V.W., Lerner, M.R., Steitz, J.A., and Flint, S.J.: A smaller nuclear ribonucleoprotein is required for splicing of adenoviral early RNA sequence. Proc. Natl. Acad. Sci. (USA) 78:1371, 1981.
155. Lerner, M.R., Andrews, N.C., Miller, G., and Steitz, J.A.: Two small RNA's encoded by Epstein Barr virus and complexed with protein are precipitated by antibodies from patients with systemic lupus erythematosus. Proc. Natl. Acad. Sci. (USA) 78:805, 1981.
156. Rinke, J., and Steitz, J.A.: Precursor molecules of both human 5S ribosomal RNA and transfer RNAs are bound by a cellular protein reactive with anti-La lupus antibodies. Cell 29:149, 1982.
157. Reddy, R., Tan, E.M., Henning, D., Nohga, K., and Busch, H.: Detection of a nucleolar 7-2 ribonucleoprotein and a cytoplasmic 8-2 ribonucleoprotein with autoantibodies from patients with scleroderma. J. Biol. Chem. 258:1383, 1983.
158. Hashimoto, C., and Steitz, J.A.: Sequential association of nucleolar 7-2 RNA with two different autoantigens. J. Biol. Chem. 258:1379, 1983.
159. Rosa, M.D., Hendrick, J.D., Lerner, M.R., Reichlin, M., and Steitz, J.A.: A mammalian tRNA His-containing antigen is recognized by the polymyositis specific antibody anti-Jo-1. Nucleic Acids Res. 11:853, 1983.
160. Hardin, J.A., Rahn, D.R., Shen, C., Lerner, M.R., Wolin, S.L., Rosa, M.D., and Steitz, J.A.: Antibodies from patients with connective tissue diseases bind specific subsets of cellular RNA-protein particles. J. Clin. Invest. 70:141, 1982.
161. Tan, E.M., and Vaughn, J.H.: Antinuclear antibodies. Significance of biochemical specificities. *In* Beutner, E.M., Chorezelski, T.P., Bean, S.F., and Jordon, R.E. (eds.): Immunopathology of the Skin. Wiley, New York, 1973, p. 369.

# Chapter 47
# Diagnostic Tests in Neuromuscular Diseases

*Walter G. Bradley*

## INTRODUCTION

A wide range of rheumatologic immunologic conditions may be associated with neuromuscular disease. The most common of these are listed in Table 47–1. These may cause pain secondary to nerve entrapment or compression. Sensory symptoms such as paresthesia and sensory loss may occur in a number of the conditions, such as the sensorimotor polyneuropathy associated with rheumatoid arthritis. Muscle weakness may be due to muscle involvement in polymyositis, to motor nerve involvement in entrapments, or to the ischemic neuropathies of polyarteritis nodosa and other vasculitides.

The diagnosis of neuromuscular involvement in patients with rheumatologic conditions is not always easy, as indicated in Chapter 27. A debilitating systemic illness

**Table 47–1.** Neuromuscular Conditions Which May Be Associated with Rheumatologic Diseases

*Muscle*
- Polymyositis—pure or associated with rheumatoid arthritis, progressive systemic sclerosis, polyarteritis nodosa, systemic lupus erythematosus, etc.
- Type 2 fiber atrophy—associated with painful local joints, or a systemic collagen-vascular disease
- Sarcoid myopathy
- Polymyalgia rheumatica
- Myopathy associated with drugs—corticosteroid myopathy, penicillamine polymyositis

*Nerve*
- Entrapment or compression neuropathy—secondary to joint capsule thickening or bony displacement, e.g., carpal tunnel syndrome
- Mononeuropathy—nerve infarcts due to collagen-vascular disease, including polyarteritis nodosa, Wegener's granulomatosis, rheumatoid arthritis vasculitis, systemic lupus erythematosus, etc.
- Polyneuropathy—in vasculitides, rheumatoid arthritis, etc.
- Radiculopathy—associated with ankylosing spondylitis, rheumatoid arthritis
- Polyneuropathy with dysproteinemias
- Polyneuropathy associated with drugs—e.g., gold

*Neuromuscular Junction*
- Myasthenia gravis—associated with autoimmune disease, including rheumatoid arthritis, scleroderma, systemic lupus erythematosus, thyroid disease, pernicious anemia, diabetes mellitus, etc.

such as progressive systemic sclerosis or rheumatoid arthritis may cause muscle atrophy. Local joint pain may produce restriction of movement and thereby apparent muscle weakness. If motor and sensory involvement are present, it is necessary to decide whether this is a secondary effect of the underlying rheumatologic condition or due to some unrelated cause. The presence of nerve and muscle involvement has considerable importance for both prognosis and therapy in rheumatologic diseases, and it is important to have a high index of suspicion for such involvement.

The diagnostic investigations of neuromuscular disease are relatively sophisticated and require some expertise for their interpretation. These investigations fall into three categories:

(1) *Screening,* such as the serum levels of enzymes released from the skeletal muscles.

(2) *Electrophysiology,* including electromyography and nerve conduction studies.

(3) *Morphology,* including muscle and nerve biopsies.

## SCREENING TESTS FOR MUSCLE DAMAGE

A number of substances are highly concentrated in skeletal muscle and released into the bloodstream when muscle fibers undergo necrosis. From the blood they may eventually make their way to the urine. Determination of the level of such substances in the blood or urine may demonstrate the presence of muscle fiber necrosis and indicate its severity. The general rule is that such substances are not released when muscle undergoes primary atrophy without loss of sarcolemmal integrity, as in disuse atrophy, denervation, thyrotoxicosis, and corticosteroid myopathy, but are released in such necrotizing conditions as muscle injury, polymyositis, and muscular dystrophy.

**Urinary Creatine.** Creatine phosphate provides the high-energy phosphate reserve of skeletal muscle. The average adult urinary excretion of creatine is about 60 to 150 mg in 24 hours in normal males and approximately twice that level in females. Muscle fiber atrophy from any cause produces an increased urinary excretion of creatine.

**Urinary Myoglobin and 3-Methylhistidine.** Necrosis of muscle fibers releases myoglobin into blood and thence into urine. Highly sensitive radioimmunoassays are now available for the detection and quantification of myoglobin. The substituted amino acid 3-methylhistidine is almost specifically localized to skeletal muscle. Thus the rate of excretion of the substance (providing that the patient is on a meat-free diet) is proportional to the total amount of muscle fiber breakdown occurring in unit time, whether this breakdown is the result of atrophy or of muscle fiber necrosis.

**Serum Levels of Skeletal Muscle Enzymes.** Aldolase, glutamic oxalacetic and glutamic pyruvic transaminases (SGOT and SGPT), lactic dehydrogenase (LDH), and creatine kinase* (CK) are all released into the plasma when muscle fibers undergo necrosis. Aldolase was the first enzyme in which this release was first recognized.[1] SGOT,[2] and CK[3] release were also reported to be important in muscle diseases. In most conditions causing muscle necrosis, the percentage rise of serum CK activity is higher than that of the other two enzymes, and thus serum CK levels provide the most sensitive index of muscle fiber breakdown. The role of serum levels of muscle enzymes in diagnosing neuromuscular disease has been extensively reviewed.[4-6]

A number of conditions causing muscle damage, including intramuscular injections, muscle needling during electromyography, and muscle biopsy, all cause a rise of serum enzymes, particularly CK. Thus it is important for blood to be drawn for the determination of the serum CK activity early in the investigations of patients, *before* any such manipulations are undertaken. The serum enzyme levels may not return to normal for several weeks following a muscle biopsy and electromyography. Because the serum CK is such a sensitive indicator of muscle damage, it is a useful screening test for muscle disease. However, the level may be raised in many different disorders, in heart disease, and in individuals performing heavy manual work.

**Serum Isozymes.** Many enzymes exist in several different molecular forms or isozymes. These are often dimers or tetramers of two or more subunits. The type

*Creatine kinase is frequently misdescribed as creatine phosphokinase. The kinases are a group of enzymes catalyzing phosphorylation of substances, and the term "phospho" is therefore redundant.

or proportion of the isozymes may vary from tissue to tissue. Different isozymes of CK are present in adult skeletal muscle (MM form), in brain (BB form), and in cardiac muscle (MB form). Thus skeletal and cardiac muscle damage and, rarely, cerebral damage may cause a rise in the plasma CK levels. The isozymes will often allow separation of these conditions. However, unfortunately this is not always so, since the skeletal muscle in the fetus and during extensive regeneration after injury contains a high proportion of the MB form. Thus the finding that the major proportion of the plasma CK is the MB form does not necessarily prove its cardiac origin.

LDH similary exists as five different isozymes, the largest proportion normally being the slowest migrating $LDH_5$. Where extensive skeletal muscle necrosis and regeneration occur, there is a significant shift of isozymes toward the faster moving $LDH_1$ and $LDH_2$.[7] Such isozyme changes may help in the recognition of skeletal muscle damage when the total level of enzymes is relatively normal.

## ELECTROPHYSIOLOGIC STUDIES OF NEUROMUSCULAR FUNCTION

Although extensively available in the United States and many other countries, electrophysiologic studies of neuromuscular function are frequently employed with insufficient knowledge of how the changes should be interpreted. These are investigations requiring considerable expertise and experience, and it is thus important that they should be undertaken by well-trained individuals.

These studies may be divided into electromyography, motor and sensory nerve conduction studies, and studies of neuromuscular junction function. It is important that the physician caring for the patient should understand the significance and limitation of these electrophysiological investigations. This chapter is intended to provide

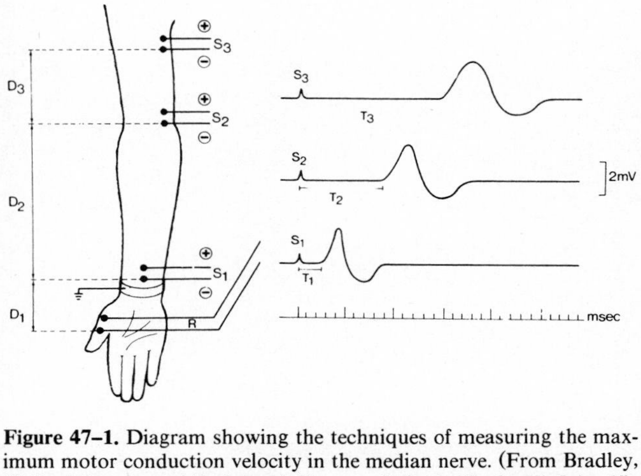


**Figure 47–1.** Diagram showing the techniques of measuring the maximum motor conduction velocity in the median nerve. (From Bradley, W.G.: Disorders of Peripheral Nerves. Oxford, Blackwell Scientific Publications, 1974.)

an outline of these tests and the alterations produced by diseases. For fuller descriptions the reader should consult Buchthal,[8] Bradley,[9] and Lenman and Ritchie.[10]

**Motor Nerve Conduction Studies.** The principle of these studies is illustrated in Figure 47–1, which deals with the median nerve. The supramaximal stimulus to the median nerve is first applied at the wrist ($S_1$), and the conduction time between the onset of the stimulus and the first deflection from the baseline of the evoked muscle action potential (MAP) is measured from the oscillograph record ($T_1$). The distance between the stimulating cathode and the proximal recording electrode ($D_1$) is also measured. The procedure is repeated with stimulation in the antecubital fossa ($S_2$) and the axilla ($S_3$), and the appropriate conduction time is measured ($T_2$ and $T_3$). The distance between the cathode-stimulating sites for $S_1$ and $S_2$ ($D_2$) and $S_2$ and $S_3$ ($D_3$) are also measured. The maximum motor conduction velocity (MMCV) for the segment elbow to wrist is given by the equation:

$$\text{MMCV} = \frac{D_2\ (\text{mm})}{T_2 - T_1\ (\text{msec})}\ \text{m/sec}$$

$T_1$ is the terminal latency expressed as "x msec for y cm." The latency depends upon the distance from the stimulating to the recording electrodes, and comprises the time for the conduction of nervous impulses to the synapse, the synaptic delay, and the time for the conduction of the muscle action potential along the muscle fibers to the recording electrodes. The amplitude of the evoked MAP provides an index of the number of muscle fibers capable of activation. The duration of the MAP is prolonged in demyelinating neuropathies. *Late waves* (the F wave and the H reflex) result from conduction of the nerve impulse to the spinal cord and back to the muscle and are of use in studying conduction in the proximal parts of the nerve fibers. The F wave travels in a retrograde direction up the motor axons to the cord before returning to the muscle; the H reflex travels up the Ia afferent fibers and through the intraspinal monosynaptic reflex before returning down the motor axons.

**Sensory Nerve Conduction Studies.** A similar principle applies to sensory nerve conduction studies. Purely sensory nerves can be studied by stimulating digital (i.e., purely sensory nerves) and recording from the mixed nerves (orthodromic stimulation), or by stimulating mixed nerves and recording from the digital nerves (antidromic stimulation). The sensory nerve action potential (SNAP) is of much lower amplitude than the MAP, and averaging techniques are required to record them. Sensory nerve conduction may be expressed as a latency or as a conduction velocity.

It is important that each laboratory define its own *normal* values, since these depend upon observer and instrumentation. It is also important that the temperature of the electrophysiology room be carefully controlled at about 25° C and time allowed for equilibration, since nerve conduction is greatly influenced by limb temperature.

Nerve conduction is markedly slowed in segmental demyelinating neuropathies. This slowing is probably due to a combination of delayed activation of the widened nodes of Ranvier, which have paranodal demyelination; the slower continuous, rather than saltatory, conduction along totally demyelinated internodes; the current leakage through thin, partly remyelinated myelin sheaths; and the abnormally short intercalated internodes, causing an increased number of saltatory steps. The degree of reduction of nerve conduction velocity is related to the degree of segmental demyelination, and the conduction velocity is frequently slowed to less than 50 per cent of normal (less than 25 m per second), as in hypertrophic neuropathy. The terminal latency is greatly increased in such conditions; for instance, in the median nerve it may be greater than 6 msec, the normal being less than 3.0 msec.

In axonal degeneration, on the other hand, provided that some large myelinated fibers remain, the maximum nerve conduction velocity remains normal. Loss of axons is indicated by reduction of the amplitude of the evoked MAP, and sometimes by fragmentation of the MAP. The terminal latency is generally normal, although atrophy or regeneration of the distal axons, producing thin sprouts, may increase the terminal latency.

**Electromyography.** The principles of electromyography (EMG) are illustrated in Figures 47–2 and 47–3. The recording electrode is a needle, usually with a concentric insulated wire in the middle. Only the tip of the wire is free of insulation, potential differences being recorded between this bare tip and the outer part of the needle, which acts as the second electrode. This needle records the electrical events occurring in muscle fibers around its tip, and this activity is amplified and recorded by an oscilloscope.

***The Normal Electromyogram.*** At rest, when the needle

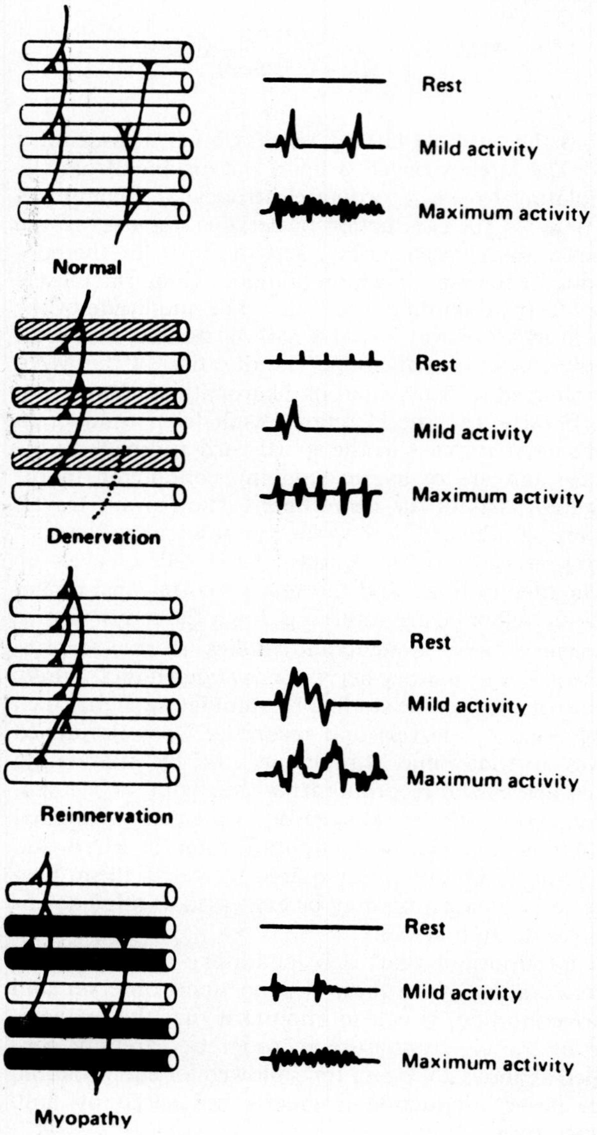


**Figure 47–2.** Classic interpretation of electromyography in the normal state, denervation, reinnervation, and myopathy, showing the electrical pattern at rest, on mild activity, and on maximum voluntary effort.

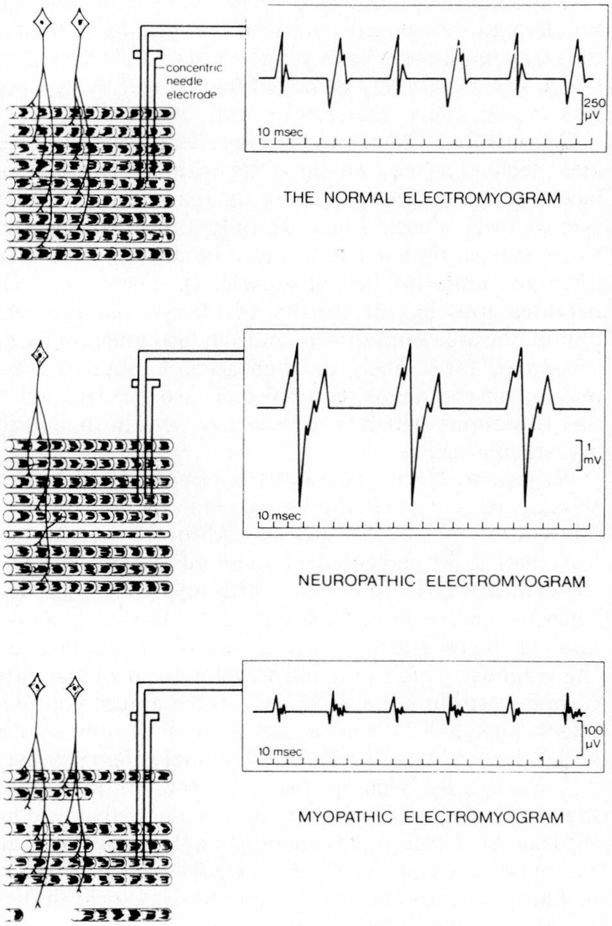


**Figure 47–3.** Diagram of the basis of the electromyogram during weak muscle contraction in normal muscle, and in denervation and myopathy. (From Bradley, W.G.: Disorders of Peripheral Nerves. Oxford, Blackwell Scientific Publications, 1974.)

is inserted there is a brief discharge from injured muscle fibers and then electrical silence. Weak contraction evokes isolated motor unit action potentials (MUAP) usually of 8 to 12 msec duration and 200 to 800 uV amplitude. The exact values depend on the muscle being studied. Each MUAP is the summation of the electrical events occurring in the muscle fibers of a single motor unit. It is irregular in outline because the electrical events in the individual muscle fibers do not reach the recording unit in a smoothly synchronized fashion. The normal MUAP has three or four phases. With maximum voluntary effort the superimposition of large number of MUAPs completely obliterates the baseline. This is called *a full interference pattern.*

*Electromyogram in Neuropathic Disorders.* Denervation and reinnervation produce atrophy of some muscle fibers and reinnervation of others by axonal sprouting from surviving motor neurons; the latter process produces enlarged motor units. At rest fibrillation potentials may be seen, which usually have two or three phases, and are about 2 to 3 msec in duration and 30 to 150 uV amplitude. They arise from spontaneous discharge of denervated muscle fibers. Weak contraction produces isolated MUAPs which are of large amplitude and longer duration than normal owing to the enlarged motor units. Also because of the sprouting of intramuscular nerves, the MUAPs are even less synchronized than normal, with a resultant increase in the normal 5 to 10 percent of potentials with more than four phases (polyphasic potentials). Because of the fallout of motor units consequent upon the denervating condition, on maximum voluntary effort individual MUAPs may still be seen, and the baseline is not completely obliterated. This is termed *an incomplete* or *single unit interference pattern.*

*Electromyogram in Myopathies.* The patchy loss of whole or parts of individual muscle fibers with the retention of the normal numbers of motor nerves or motor units produces a characteristic picture. At rest the muscle is silent in most myopathies, although in polymyositis there is a marked increase in insertional activity presumably because of diffuse damage to the sarcolemma of the muscle fibers. Weak contraction elicits MUAPs which are of lower amplitude and shorter duration than normal owing to loss of muscle fibers. They are more polyphasic than normal since loss of muscle fibers prevents the smoothing effect of summation of large numbers of muscle fiber potentials. Mild contraction produces a full interference pattern, because all the motor units must be contracted to produce even a moderate force in the weakened muscle. Maximum voluntary effort produces a full interference pattern with a decreased maximum amplitude compared to normal.

Although the preceding description provides the classic changes recognized by electromyographers, the picture may not always be as simple. For instance, a muscle which is very severely damaged (end stage) by any process may produce aberrant results.

**Single Fiber Electromyography.** This recently developed technique uses an electrode with a recording surface that is capable of picking up the impulses of only two or three muscle fibers. In only a few instances will these be from the same motor unit because of the overlap of motor units in skeletal muscle. In denervated/reinnervated muscle, the density of fibers from the same unit in one area is increased, and synchronous discharges of two or three fibers is often seen. Failure of transmission in the nerve terminal can also be detected by this technique, which is therefore of help in diagnosing myasthenia gravis.

**Repetitive Nerve Stimulation.** Neuromuscular transmission in a normal individual will tolerate repetitive stimulation of up to 40 per second for 10 seconds with less than a 30 percent decrement of the amplitude of the evoked MAP. In patients with myasthenia gravis, if repetitive nerve stimulation at 2 to 10 per second is applied, there is a rapid decrement of the amplitude of the response which may fall to 50 percent of the initial response within a few seconds.[11] A maximum voluntary effort will similarly cause a decrement of the immediately succeeding evoked MAP. Unfortunately the response is not necessarily seen in every muscle in myasthenia gravis, the diagnosis of which may require advanced and sophisticated techniques such as single fiber EMG and the regional curare test.[12] In the myasthenic syndrome of Eaton and Lambert the electrophysiological findings are of an abnormally small first evoked muscle action potential, followed by an *incremental* response of more than 50 percent with stimuli applied at 10 to 30 per second.

## PATHOLOGICAL STUDIES

Pathological studies of nerve and muscle aid considerably in the diagnosis of neuromuscular diseases, particularly when advanced techniques are applied. The following paragraphs provide a brief outline of these techniques, and of the pathological changes and their interpretation.

**Muscle Biopsy.** The following is a brief outline of the techniques of muscle biopsy. For further descriptions the reader should consult Dubowitz and Brooke[13] and Bradley.[9] The procedure is performed under local or general anesthesia. If the former, infiltration of the muscle with local anesthesia must be avoided. A 3-inch incision is made in line with the muscle fibers, the deep fascia is opened, and the muscle fascicles are separated by sharp dissection. A small fascicle about 3 mm in diameter and 2 to 3 cm long is removed in a biopsy clamp. Several models of such clamps are available to keep the muscle at the in vivo length during fixation. It is important to avoid direct handling of the tissue to be studied histologically, since this produces gross histological artifacts. Three specimens are usually removed: (1) Histology—fixation with formalin and embedding in paraffin wax. Stained sections allow examination of large amounts of transverse and longitudinally sectioned muscle. (2) Electron microscopy—fixation in glutaraldehyde and embedding in epoxy resins allowing ultrastructural investigation. (3) Histochemistry—the specimen is usually taken without clamps and rapidly frozen in liquid nitrogen; transverse sections are cut in a cryostat and stained for histochemical reactions.

Histochemistry has provided very important advances in the understanding of muscle diseases, and thus some details must be provided here. A battery of stains are available to show different metabolic systems; mitochondrial oxidative enzymes are revealed by NADH or SDH stains; phosphorylase required for initiating glycolysis may be stained; periodic acid-Schiff (PAS) stains glycogen; the enzyme of myosin responsible for the transduction of high energy phosphate bonds into contraction, myofibrillary ATPase, may also be demonstrated histochemically. Other histochemical reactions often used include acid phosphatase and nonspecific esterase which stain lysosomes and macrophages. Hematoxylin and eosin and the Gomori trichrome stains are also performed on cryostat sections. The latter will reveal increased numbers of mitochondria in mitochondrial myopathies, nemaline rods in patients with nemaline myopathy, and other structural changes.

Histochemical stains of normal human muscle show two classes of fiber, one stained darkly and the other lightly, and there is reciprocity between the oxidative and glycolytic enzyme stains in the same muscle fiber seen in serial sections. In some animals certain muscles are almost entirely made up of either oxidative or glycolytic fibers, and this histochemical separation of the muscles correlates well with the physiological twitch characteristics which are respectively slow and fast. In normal muscle in man, however, both oxidative and glycolytic fibers are randomly distributed throughout every muscle.

The separation of fiber types is sometimes less than absolute, and histochemistry has had its "lumpers" and "splitters," some wishing to differentiate only two types of fibers[14] while others have recognized up to nine fiber types.[15] Much confusion has arisen because of the lack of agreement between different workers over the terminology of these different fiber types. Not only have oxidative and glycolytic stains been used to separate the fibers, but staining techniques for myosin ATPase carried out after preincubation at various pHs have also been widely used. Myosin ATPase of fast-twitch muscle is more alkaline stable, acid labile and formaldehyde stable than that of slow muscle,[16] and by varying the pH and other parameters the density of staining can be varied to separate fiber subtypes. The glycine-formaldehyde calcium technique of Tunell and Hart[17] is a useful single technique, type 1 fibers being light, type 2A being

**Table 47–2.** Outline of the Criteria for Typing of Muscle Fibers on Histochemical and Physiologic Grounds (0, 1+, 2+, 3+ Indicate the Relative Intensity of Histochemical Staining)

| Criteria | 1 | 2A | 2B | 2C |
|---|---|---|---|---|
| Twitch speed | Slow | Fast | Fast | ? |
| Susceptibility to fatigue | Resistant | Resistant | Susceptible | ? |
| Myosin ATPase pH 9.4 | 1+ | 3+ | 3+ | 3+ |
| Myosin ATPase pH 4.6 | 3+ | 0 | 3+ | 3+ |
| Myosin ATPase pH 4.3 | 3+ | 0 | 0 | 2+ |
| Myosin ATPase formaldehyde-glycine | 0 | 1+ | 2+ | ? |
| NADH-TR | 3+ | 2+ | 1+ | 2+ |
| SDH | 3+ | 2+ | 1+ | 2+ |
| α-GPDH-ML | 0 | 2+ | 2+ | 1+ |
| PAS | 1+ | 3+ | 2+ | 2+ |
| Phosphorylase | 1+ | 3+ | 3+ | 3+ |
| Oxidative/glycolytic | Oxid. | Oxid./glyc. | Glyc. | Glyc. |
| Electron microscopy | | | | |
| Proportion of mitochondria and lipid droplets | 3+ | 2+ | 1+ | 2+ |
| Z-line thickness (nm) | ~120 | ~8 | ~8 | ? |

ATPase = Myosin ATPase.
NADH-TR = NADH-tetrazolium reductase.
SDH = Succinic dehydrogenase.
α-GPDH-ML = Menadione-linked α-glycerophosphate dehydrogenase.
PAS = Periodic acid–Schiff.

intermediate, and type 2B being darkly stained. The fiber type can probably be recognized in electron micrographs.[18-20]

Some authors have combined physiological, histochemical, and biochemical criteria to define the individual muscle fiber types.[21] Such a nomenclature based upon several criteria has many advantages, but is impractical for everyday discussion. The following enumeration of fiber types is now generally accepted:

Type 1 = slow twitch, oxidative, fatigue-resistant.

Type 2A = fast twitch, glycolytic-oxidative, fatigue-resistant.

Type 2B = fast twitch, glycolytic, fast-fatiguing.

Type 2C = (perhaps) undifferentiated fibers.

Table 47–2 shows the physiological and various histochemical characteristics of these fiber types, and Table 47–3 gives a comparison of this terminology with several of the previously proposed nomenclatures. As seen in Figure 47–4, the histochemical typing of fiber is usually but not always reliable. Transposition of this terminology of fiber types to pathological muscle is not always easy, since both altered innervation and altered use may change the fiber type. Loss of clear differentiation of fiber types is a frequent finding in chronically diseased muscle.

For detailed descriptions of the pathological changes of skeletal muscle the reader should consult Dubowitz and Brooke.[13] *Denervation* tends to be associated with angulated atrophic fibers which are often very dark with the oxidative enzyme stains. *Reinnervation* produces aggregation of fibers all of the same type, i.e., fiber type grouping. *Denervation of such reinnervated groups* pro-

**Table 47–3.** Comparison of Fiber Type Terminology

| | Fiber Type | | | |
|---|---|---|---|---|
| **Authors** | *1* | *2A* | *2B* | *2C* |
| Dubowitz and Pearse, 1960[24] | I | II | II | — |
| Stein and Padykula, 1962[25] | B | C | A | — |
| Romanul, 1964[15] | III | II | I | — |
| Padykula and Gauthier, 1966[26] | Intermediate | Red | White | — |
| Yellin and Guth, 1970[27] | β | β | α | — |
| Ashmore and Doerr, 1971[28] | β-red | α-red | α-white | — |
| Burke et al., 1971[29] | S | FR | FF | — |
| Close, 1972[30] | Slow twitch—fatigue resisting | Fast twitch—fatigue resisting | Fast twitch—fast fatiguing | — |
| Peter et al., 1972[21] | Slow twitch—oxidative | Fast twitch—oxidative-glycolytic | Fast twitch—glycolytic | — |

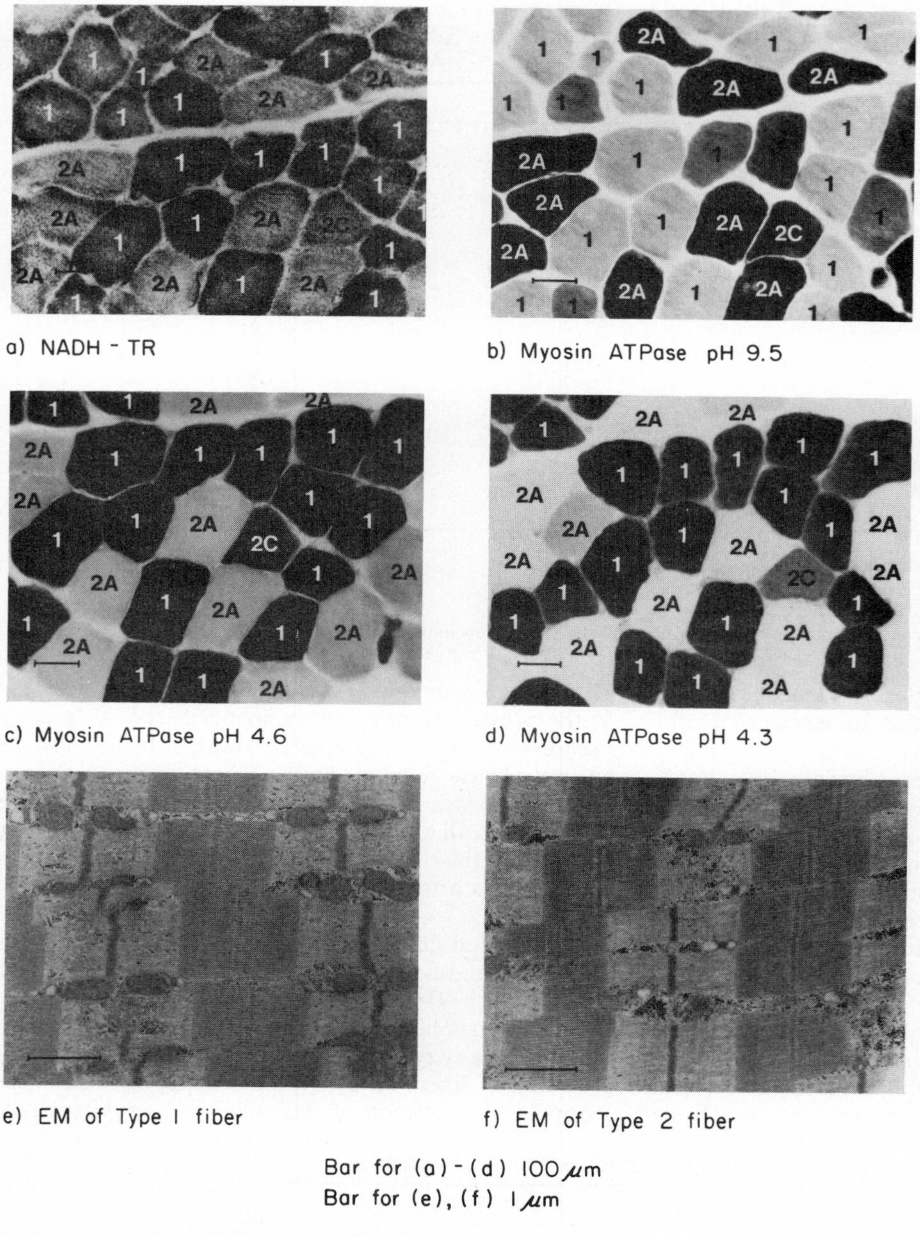


**Figure 47–4.** *Above,* Serial sections of a normal muscle stained for *(a)* NADH-TR, *(b)* myosin ATPase at pH 9.5, *(c)* myosin ATPase at pH 4.6, and *(d)* myosin ATPase at pH 4.3. The fiber type is marked on each fiber. Although the staining characteristics of each fiber correspond in most cases to those shown in Table 46–2, this is not true of all fibers. *Below,* Electron micrographs of longitudinal sections of *(e)* Type 1 fiber and *(f)* Type 2 muscle fiber. The Type 1 muscle fiber has more mitochondria and a thicker Z-line than the Type 2 fiber, which has more glycogen between the myofibrils.

duces grouped fiber atrophy. A *necrotizing myopathy* causes muscle fiber necrosis, phagocytosis, and later regeneration, and this is typically seen in Duchenne muscular dystrophy. Rounding and increased random variation of fiber size are typical *myopathic* changes, as are the presence of internal nuclei, fibrosis, and fat cell replacement. However, all the latter changes may also be seen in chronic denervation.[22] Histochemistry has allowed the recognition and separation of a considerable number of specific neuromuscular diseases, such as the congenital myopathies. These include nemaline myopathy (see above); mitochondrial myopathies (see above); central core disease (with the central part of each fiber being devoid of mitochondrial enzyme activity); centronuclear myopathy with type 1 fiber hypotrophy (with abnormally small type 1 fibers, which all have central nuclei); and congenital fiber-type disproportion (with type 1 fibers being abnormally small). Type 2 fiber atrophy is a common finding in many conditions, including muscle atrophy of disuse, cachexia, and painful conditions of local joints and nerve roots. Corticosteroid myopathy tends to produce type 2 fiber atrophy with mitochondrial changes in type 1 fibers, although these changes are nonspecific.

**Nerve Biopsies.** Only a brief description of this procedure will be given here. For further descriptions the reader should consult Bradley[9] and Dyck and colleagues.[23] Usually a sensory nerve is biopsied, and this may be done under either local or general anesthesia. The most commonly approached are the sural nerve in the calf or the superficial branch of the radial nerve at the wrist. It is possible to biopsy the whole nerve or to take only a fascicular biopsy of a small portion of the nerve. The latter may cause no sensory loss, and is preferable unless total sensory loss is already present or one is looking for a vasculitis or a similarly "patchy" process. It is possible to take a fascicular biopsy of a mixed motor nerve, provided that only about one twentieth of the total transverse area is taken and considerable care is applied, but this should not be viewed as a routine investigation.

The nerve is exposed and carefully removed, touching only the ends where it is necessary to cut the fibers. Any pressure or other manipulation of the main portion of the nerve which is to be taken for histological examination will cause marked crush artifact changes in the nerve fibers.

It is a difficult decision whether any benefit is to be obtained from nerve biopsy. This decision is greatly aided by consultation with a person experienced in the clinical and pathological studies of patients with peripheral nerve disease. Nerve biopsy may be diagnostic in a few conditions like a vasculitis, leprosy, or amyloidosis. Apart from these conditions, unless a laboratory with a specific interest in peripheral nerve pathology is available, little useful information is likely to be gained from nerve biopsy.

It is particularly important that the nerve be prepared in the appropriate fashion. It is generally recommended that frozen sections be prepared for enzyme and lipid stains; that a portion of the nerve be fixed under tension in glutaraldehyde for embedding in epoxy resin for light and electron microscopic studies, and for the microdissection of single nerve fibers; and that a portion be fixed under tension in Susa fixative for paraffin embedding for hematoxylin and eosin, Bodian, or other silver stains for axons, and for PTAH or solochrome cyanin staining for myelin sheaths.

Details of the techniques and of the changes in various diseases are given in Bradley.[9] *Axonal degeneration* causes loss of axonal continuity and secondary degeneration of the myelin sheath into a string of myelin ovoids. *Segmental demyelination* is a process in which myelin breaks down, leaving the axon intact. These processes tend to occur in different diseases. For instance, toxic neuropathies are usually associated with axonal degeneration, whereas diphtheritic neuropathy causes segmental demyelination. Extensive segmental demyelination may give rise to onion bulb hypertrophy of the nerves with a characteristic pathological picture. A vasculitis may cause both axonal degeneration and segmental demyelination, with patchy loss of myelinated nerve fibers in some fasciculi and preservation in others; the nerve biopsy may show an involved blood vessel. In most diseases causing peripheral neuropathy, such as diabetes mellitus, both segmental demyelination and axonal degeneration are present. The proportion of these two changes may aid in the recognition of the cause of the neuropathy, but this is rarely diagnostic.

## SUMMARY AND CONCLUSIONS

The detailed biochemical, electrophysiological, and pathological studies described in this chapter are of great importance in the recognition and elucidation of neuromuscular disorders associated with rheumatologic diseases. The collaboration of several different experts is required to undertake these investigations, and the physician who is caring for the patient must have sufficient knowledge of these techniques to be able to integrate their results and interpret them in terms of the overall clinical picture.

## References


1. Sibley, J.A., and Lehringer, A.L.: Aldolases in the serum and tissues of tumor bearing animals. Natl. Cancer. Inst. Monogr. 9:303, 1949.
2. Pearson, C.M.: Serum enzymes in muscular dystrophy and certain other muscular and neuromuscular diseases. I. Serum glutamic oxaloacetic transaminase. N. Engl. J. Med. 256:1069, 1075, 1957.
3. Ebashi, S., Toyokum, Y., Momoi, H., and Sugita, H.: Creatine phophokinase activity of sera of progressive muscular dystrophy patients. J. Biochem. (Tokyo) 46:103, 1959.
4. Zellweger, H., Durnin, R., and Simpson, J.: The diagnostic significance of serum enzymes and electrocardiogram in various muscular dystrophies. Acta Neurol. Scand. 48:87, 1972.
5. Munsat, T.L., Baloh, R., Pearson, C.M., and Fowler, W.: Serum enzyme alterations in neuromuscular disorders. JAMA 226:1536, 1973.
6. Munsat, T.L.: Creatine phosphokinase alterations in neuromuscular diseases. Isr. J. Med. Sci. 13:93, 1977.
7. Hooshmand, H., Dove, J., and Suter, C.: The use of serum lactate dehydrogenase isoenzymes in the diagnosis of muscle diseases. Neurology 19:26, 1969.
8. Buchthal, F.: An Introduction to Electromyography. Copenhagen, Scandinavian University Books, 1957.
9. Bradley, W.G.: Disorders of Peripheral Nerves. Oxford, Blackwell Scientific Publications, 1974.
10. Lenman, J.A., and Ritchie, E.: Clinical Electromyography. 2nd ed. Philadelphia, J. B. Lippincott Company, 1977.
11. Desmedt, J.E., and Borenstein, S.: The testing of neuromuscular transmission. In Vinken, P.J., and Bruyn, G.W. (eds.): Handbook of Clinical Neurology. Amsterdam, North Holland, 1970, pp. 104–115.
12. Brown, J.C., and Charlton, J.E.: Study of sensitivity to curare in myasthenic disorders using a regional technique. J. Neurol. Neurosurg. Psychiat. 38:27, 1975.
13. Dubowitz, V., and Brooke, M.H.: Muscle Biopsy: A Modern Approach. London, W. B. Saunders, 1973.
14. Engel, W.K.: Fiber-type nomenclature of human skeletal muscle for histochemical purposes. Neurology 24:344, 1974.
15. Romanul, F.C.A.: Enzymes in muscle. I. Histochemical studies of enzymes in individual muscle fibers. Arch. Neurol. 11:355, 1964.
16. Guth, L., and Samaha, F.J.: Qualitative differences between actomyosin ATPase of slow and fast mammalian muscle. Exp. Neurol. 25:138, 1969.
17. Tunell, G.L., and Hart, M.N.: Simultaneous determination of skeletal muscle fiber, types I, IIA, and IIB by histochemistry. Arch. Neurol. 34:171, 1977.
18. Fardeau, M.: Caractéristiques cytochimiques et ultrastructurales des différents types de fibres musculaires squelettiques extra-fusales (chez l'homme et quelques mammifères). Ann. Anat. Pathol. 18:7, 1973.
19. Eisenberg, B.R., and Kuda, A.M.: Retrieval of cryostat sections for comparison of histochemistry and quantitative electron microscopy in a muscle fiber. J. Histochem. Cytochem. 25:1169, 1977.

20. Saltis, L.M., and Mendell, J.R.: The fine structural differences in human muscle fiber types based on peroxidatic activity. J. Neuropath. Exp. Neurol. 33:632, 1974.
21. Peter, J.B., Barnard, R.J., Edgerton, V.R., Gillespie, C.A., and Stemple, K.E.: Metabolic profiles of three fiber types of skeletal muscle in guinea-pigs and rabbits. Biochemistry 11:2627, 1972.
22. Fewings, J.D., Harris, J.B., Johnson, M.A., and Bradley, W.G.: Progressive denervation of skeletal muscle induced by spinal irradiation in rats. Brain 100:157, 1977.
23. Dyck, P.J., Thomas, P.K., and Lambert, E.H. (eds.): Peripheral Neuropathy. Philadelphia, W. B. Saunders Company, 1975.
24. Dubowitz, V., and Pearse, A.G.E.: A comparative histochemical study of oxidative enzyme and phosphorylase activity in skeletal muscle. Histochemie 2:105, 1960.
25. Stein, J.M., and Padykula, H.A.: Histochemical classification of individual skeletal muscle fibers of the rat. Am. J. Anat. 110:103, 1962.
26. Padykula, H.A., and Gauthier, G.F. (1966). Quoted by Peter et al., Reference 21.
27. Yellin, H., and Guth, L.: The histochemical classification of muscle fibres. Exp. Neurol. 26:424, 1970.
28. Ashmore, C.R., and Doerr, L.: Comparative aspects of muscle fibre types in different species. Exp. Neurol. 31:408, 1971.
29. Burke, R.E. Levine, D.M., Zajac, F.E., Tsairis, P., and Engel, W.K.: Mammalian motor units: Physiological-histochemical correlation in three types in cat gastrocnemius. Science 174:709, 1971.
30. Close, R.I.: Dynamic properties of mammalian skeletal muscles. Physiol. Rev. 52:129, 1972.

# Section IV
# Clinical Pharmacology

## Chapter 48
## Principles of Pharmacodynamics and Pharmacokinetics

*Donald S. Robinson*

### FACTORS INFLUENCING DRUG PHARMACODYNAMICS AND CLINICAL EFFECTS

**Importance of Individualizing Drug Dosage.** The need for individualizing drug dosage for patients in order to achieve optimal therapeutic effect is being increasingly recognized and accepted. The clinician can be aided in this by the clinical laboratory in the case of certain drugs for which therapeutic ranges of blood levels have been defined. The adjustment of dosage according to plasma level allows careful monitoring of treatment with such drugs. Unfortunately, there are only a few drugs for which plasma levels are of demonstrated clinical value and a therapeutic range has been defined. In the field of rheumatology, only salicylate and acetaminophen levels are routinely measured, although it is likely with the advent of sensitive modern methods of assaying drugs that additional drugs will be monitored using the laboratory in the near future.

For most drugs, dosage is still regulated by the process of prescribing the "usual dose," with subsequent adjustments, if any, based on observation of clinical effects. An understanding of certain basic principles governing pharmacodynamics and pharmacokinetics common to most drugs can aid physicians in this important matter of selecting and individualizing drug dose. The primary goal is to maximize therapeutic benefit and to minimize toxicity, side effects, and drug interaction.

The intensities of therapeutic and toxic effects are proportional to drug concentration at receptor sites in target tissues. Factors affecting distribution of a drug to these various receptor sites can significantly influence its clinical effects. The single most important determinant of drug concentration at receptor sites is *drug dosage.* Furthermore, it has been conclusively established that the majority of adverse drug reactions are dose related rather than idiosyncratic.[1] Therefore, more precise individualization of dosage can serve to avoid or reduce toxic and side effects for most drugs. Only for the minority of drugs with a high therapeutic ratio (benefit-risk) is careful attention to dosage unimportant. The practice of increasing drug dosage until toxic manifestations appear and then decreasing the dose slightly is feasible for some drugs but it can be uncomfortable or occasionally hazardous.[2]

**Pharmacokinetic and Pharmacodynamic Principles Important in Adjusting Dose.** Since most drugs have a narrow therapeutic ratio (and since drug levels are usually not available), it is important for the clinician to adjust the "standard" dosage for each individual patient according to his assessment of several *pharmacokinetic processes,* which may be operative to either increase or decrease drug concentrations at receptor sites, and other *pharmacodynamic processes,* which can modify receptor response for a given drug concentration at the site of action (Fig. 48–1). *Concentration* of drug at the target site is primarily governed by the *pharmacokinetic* processes of absorption, distribution, metabolism, and excretion. Both genetic and environmental factors can alter these pharmacokinetic processes, but one can usually anticipate significant deviations from the norm in an individual patient and modify the "standard" dosage accordingly. These pharmacokinetic processes and the factors that influence them are discussed in more detail below.

For a given drug concentration at the receptor site, the *intensity* of the pharmacologic effects can further show additional variability owing to other influences on drug *pharmacodynamics* (Fig. 48–1). These include the less easily quantifiable factors such as functional changes in receptor activity, disease-induced changes in end-organ physiology, development of tolerance with chronic drug exposure, competition for binding at receptors by interacting drugs, and so forth. Thus, the pharmacodynamic effects of a drug are influenced both by pharmacokinetic processes (absorption, distribution, metabolism, and excretion) and by changes in target organs and receptor sites, all of which summate in the individual patient and determine his optimal dose. The following discussion examines these various processes in more detail with specific applications to rheumatologic drugs cited.

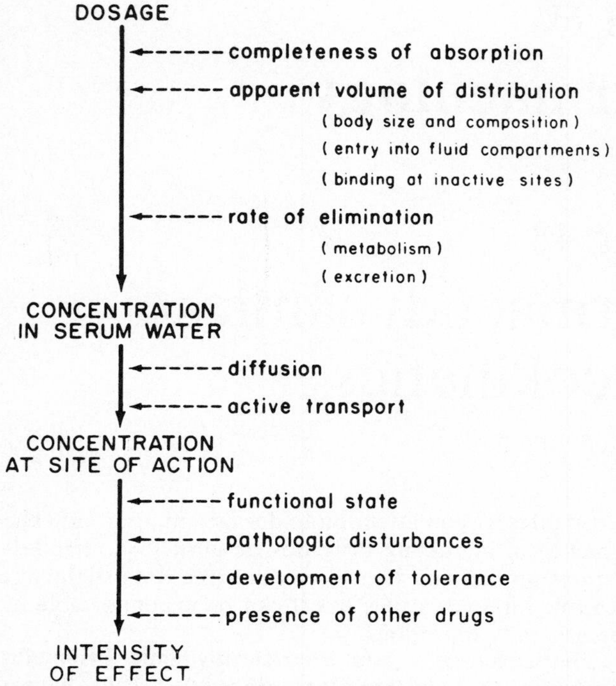


**Figure 48–1.** Factors that influence pharmacologic response to a drug. (Reprinted, with permission, from Koch-Weser, J.: N. Engl. J. Med. 287:227, 1972.)

## EFFECTS OF IONIZATION ON DRUG BEHAVIOR

Most drugs used in clinical practice are either weak acids or weak bases.[3] They exist in an equilibrium of ionized and un-ionized forms, varying according to the pH of the biological fluid or tissue (Fig. 48–2). Small fluctuations in intracellular or plasma pH can produce significant shifts in the proportion of polar (ionized) or nonpolar (nonionized) drug. Since the polar and nonpolar forms of a drug have different pharmacokinetic properties, some understanding of how ionization influences drug behavior is essential to enlightened therapeutics. Ionized (polar) drug passively diffuses across lipid-rich cell membranes poorly, if at all, while nonpolar drug crosses such barriers relatively easily. Thus, drug in the ionized state is absorbed slowly, while nonionized drug is more readily absorbed from the gastrointestinal tract. Similarly, following glomerular filtration, drug in ionized form is less readily reabsorbed in the renal tubule with more rapid excretion.

STATE OF IONIZATION

| | Acid (low pH) Medium | Alkaline (high pH) Medium |
|---|---|---|
| Weak acid drug | R-COOH | $R\text{-}COO^{-} + H$ |
| Weak basic drug | $R\text{-}NH_3^{+}$ | $R\text{-}NH_2$ |

**Figure 48–2.** Influence of pH on ionization (polarity) of drugs that are either weak acids or bases. (From Robinson, D.S.: J. Urol. 113:300, 1975. Copyright 1975, The Williams & Wilkins Company, Baltimore.)

**Table 48–1.** Commonly Prescribed Acidic and Basic Drugs and Drug Classes

| Acidic Drugs | Basic Drugs |
|---|---|
| Salicylates, indomethacin, phenylbutazone, oxyphenbutazone, and the other nonsteroidal anti-inflammatory agents | Opiates (e.g., codeine) |
| Probenecid | Major and minor tranquilizers |
| Anticoagulants | Antidepressants |
| Sulfonamides and their derivatives: | Anti-arrhythmics: |
| Thiazide and loop diuretics | Lidocaine |
| Sulfonylurea hypoglycemic agents | Procainamide |
| Phenytoin (Dilantin) | Quinidine |
| Penicillins and cephalosporins | Amphetamines |
| Barbiturates | Antihistamines |
| Clofibrate | Guanethidine |
| Methotrexate | Reserpine |
| | Erythromycin |
| | Beta-adrenergic blocking agents |
| | Anticholinergic agents |

Drug ionization also predisposes to certain drug interactions. For example, the ionic species of acidic drugs may compete for shared plasma protein–binding sites or for active transport processes in the kidney or central nervous system, resulting in clinically significant drug interactions.

Clinicians should be familiar with the acidic or basic nature of the drugs they use in practice, since such knowledge permits prediction of drug behavior and drug interactions (and therefore avoidance of many troublesome drug effects). Table 48–1 lists the more common drugs and drug classes as to their acidic or basic properties. It is readily apparent that many of the therapeutic agents employed in rheumatology are acidic with similar, and often competing, actions. Examples of the clinical significance of drug ionization in therapeutics are discussed subsequently.

## DRUG ABSORPTION

A number of variables can influence either the rate of absorption or the amount of a dose that is absorbed after oral administration. Drug bioavailability can vary among manufacturers and among lots of the same manufacturer, depending on factors such as size of drug crystals, amount of compression, and hardness of coating substances used in a tablet. The *rate* of absorption of drug products can be quite variable, since the process of absorption must be preceded by the drug going into *solution* (in the stomach or small bowel), not just the tablet or capsule disintegrating. While much is made of this issue in advertising of analgesics, the absorption *rate* usually has little relevance in long-term drug treatment, in which steady state levels rather than intermittent peak levels of drug are important.

Because of the acidic nature of aspirin and the nonsteroidal anti-inflammatory agents, drugs of this class tend to be nonionized in the stomach (Fig. 48–2), so that some drug absorption can take place at the low pH present in the stomach, once it goes into solution. Salicylates tend to be less soluble at low pH so that the buffered forms of aspirin solubilize more readily in the stomach and may be absorbed more rapidly. Salicylate is often prescribed in an enteric-coated form to reduce the local gastric irritation caused by slowly dissolving tablets. Since rate of absorption is much less a consideration in the anti-inflammatory use of salicylate, many clinicians prescribe enteric-coated aspirin. In this instance, the remnants of enteric coatings may be detected in the stool, but most of the salicylate contents have usually been absorbed. Other studies have shown twice-a-day dosage forms of salicylate to be therapeutically equivalent to plain aspirin and other anti-inflammatory agents, with resultant improved compliance and lower incidence of side effects.[4-6]

## DRUG DISTRIBUTION, PLASMA LEVELS, AND DRUG BINDING INTERACTIONS

Concurrent with absorption and entry into the plasma, drugs also undergo distribution, metabolism, and excretion. For most drugs, the absorption and distribution phases are short in comparison with metabolism and excretion. The clinical relevance of absorption, distribution, and elimination half-lives ($T^{1/2}$) and their implications in regulating drug treatment is further discussed under Pharmacokinetics and Drug Dosing Strategies.

**Plasma Protein Binding and Competition of Acidic Drugs for Binding Sites.** Many drugs are bound in plasma to proteins, and this bound fraction serves as an inactive "reservoir" of drug. Many of the acidic drugs listed in Table 48–1 are significantly ionized in the slightly alkaline environment (pH 7.4) of plasma; i.e., they will exist largely in their anionic form. This accounts for the general tendency of acidic drugs to bind to sites on plasma albumin. Only the free (unbound) fraction of drug is in equilibrium with drug in other tissue compartments. Therefore, conditions that favor an increase in free drug fraction may be expected to potentiate drug effect. The concurrent administration of two acidic drugs (whose negatively charged anionic forms are both present in plasma) can result in competition for protein binding sites. This can increase the free fraction of one or both drugs, thereby potentiating their pharmacologic effects. Although the clinical importance of this type of interaction may be minor for many acidic drugs, including the nonsteroidal anti-inflammatory agents, it can be very significant in the case of certain drugs with very narrow therapeutic ratios. Thus, phenylbutazone and oxyphenbutazone and salicylates markedly potentiate the anticoagulant effect when they are administered to a patient receiving warfarin. Similarly they enhance the hypoglycemic effects of the sulfonylurea antidiabetic agents (e.g., tolbutamide, chlorpropamide). As shown in Table 48–1, many anti-inflammatory drugs are acidic and are thus theoretically prone to this type of interaction.

Since phenylbutazone and oxyphenbutazone are highly bound to plasma protein (99 percent), they are especially susceptible to the drug displacement type of interaction. The high affinity of these two drugs for protein-binding sites also accounts for their long half-lives in plasma (around 3 days).

In a classic example of this particular interaction with the anticoagulant warfarin, a patient received phenylbutazone therapy for 1 day for relief of gouty symptoms, and the following day was started on warfarin therapy. Despite the use of a "standard" dose of warfarin, the patient manifested an excessive anticoagulant response, because the major part of the phenylbutazone administered the preceding day remained in the body bound to plasma and tissue proteins, competing with warfarin. The marked increase in the free fraction of warfarin produced an excessive anticoagulant response to an ordinarily usual dose of anticoagulant.[3]

Although it has been estimated that up to 30 percent of rheumatoid patients receive more than one nonsteroidal anti-inflammatory agent concurrently, documented pharmacokinetic interactions of clinical significance are few.[7] Protein binding of anionic drugs is complex, with nine affinity sites shown for indomethacin binding to serum albumin.[8] Furthermore, salicylates failed to affect this high degree of indomethacin binding.

**Protein Binding and Drug Plasma Levels.** Interacting drugs displacing one another from protein binding sites also can complicate the proper interpretation of plasma drug levels. The drug concentrations reported by clinical laboratories represent total drug content (both free and bound drug) in plasma. When the normal degree of drug binding is altered for any reason (e.g., interacting drug, renal disease, hypoalbuminemia), the reporting of total drug concentration in plasma can be misleading. Many chronic diseases are associated with lowered plasma albumin, and chronic renal insufficiency can result in both hypoalbuminemia and altered drug binding properties of albumin. Since drug levels reported by the laboratory do not distinguish between free and bound drug, care must be taken in interpreting such data in these settings (Fig. 48–3). A patient may be toxic at a "normal" dose and with a "normal" blood level because the percentage of unbound drug is increased even though the *total* drug content in plasma is within the normal range (frequent examples are salicylate or diphenylhydantoin toxicity encountered in renal failure or pregnancy). Anti-inflammatory doses of aspirin have been shown to produce a 25 percent decline in phenytoin levels.[9] Thus, proper interpretation of blood levels requires a knowledge of the total clinical picture, including associated drugs and disease-induced changes in pharmacokinetics.

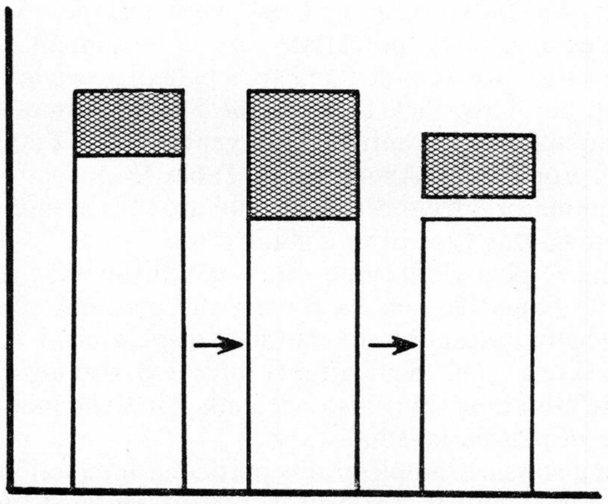

**Figure 48–3.** Effect of drug displacement interaction on plasma drug level. The unbound drug fraction (cross-hatched column) is initially increased by a second competing drug. After equilibration occurs, the unbound drug fraction returns to the original concentration and the level of total drug (free and bound) is decreased due to a decline in the bound fraction (open column).

## DRUG BIOTRANSFORMATION

Drug metabolism is largely a function of the liver, although for certain drugs there may be significant extrahepatic metabolism by intestinal mucosa (phenothiazines) or kidney (several drugs). Hepatic drug metabolism can be characterized as the general process of converting less polar compounds to more polar drug metabolites. These drug metabolites may be pharmacologically active or inactive. Because of their increased tendency to ionize, the increased polarity of metabolites usually promotes more rapid excretion in urine or bile and resultant shorter $T^{1/2}$'s than the parent drug. There are a few glaring exceptions to this general rule. For example, active metabolites of diazepam, chlordiazepoxide, and most other benzodiazepines, which are nonpolar and highly lipid soluble, accumulate in brain and other lipid-rich tissues to a greater extent than the parent compounds, and, being pharmacologically active, account for the gradually cumulative and prolonged clinical effects of these drugs.

**First Order vs. Zero Order Kinetics.** The major metabolic pathways of drug biotransformation are not generally saturated at usual clinical doses. Therefore, most drugs follow so-called *first order* kinetics, which signifies that a constant *percentage* of drug is metabolized per unit time independent of dosage. As will be discussed under Pharmacokinetics and Drug Dosing Strategies, first order kinetics implies that drug plasma and tissue levels will be linearly related to drug dose. However, for certain drugs (particularly those administered daily in gram quantities, such as the salicylates), the primary metabolic pathway may become saturated so that secondary and less efficient biotransformation pathways may become operative with advancing dosage. This results in so-called *zero order* kinetics, in which a constant *amount* rather than percentage of drug is metabolized per unit of time. The implication of zero order kinetics is that the relationship between dosage and drug level is nonlinear, so that disproportionately high drug concentrations are produced by small increases in drug dose. Commonly used drugs that exhibit zero order kinetics include the salicylates, heparin, and diphenylhydantoin. In the case of all three of these drugs, it is fortunate that laboratory monitoring of drug concentration or effect allows the drugs to be administered in adequate therapeutic dosage, often approaching toxic levels, with reasonable precision and safety.

**Drug Interactions that Inhibit Hepatic Drug Metabolism.** Drug interactions involving hepatic metabolism may either inhibit or enhance the biotransformation of a second drug. Inhibition may produce unexpected toxicity when a second drug inhibiting metabolism is added to a patient's therapeutic regimen. For example, the potent xanthine oxidase inhibitor allopurinol is now known to weakly inhibit other drug oxidation metabolic pathways. Thus, mercaptopurine, azathioprine, and allopurinol should be used with caution in patients receiving warfarin because it can nonspecifically inhibit liver microsomal enzymes, the major pathway for warfarin degradation. The concurrent administration of allopurinol and warfarin is not recommended unless special precautions are taken for intensive monitoring of prothrombin times. It is possible, although not conclusively established at present, that allopurinol may inhibit the liver metabolism of other drugs such as the sulfonylurea hypoglycemic agents.

As mentioned previously, salicylates in the doses used for anti-inflammatory effect can saturate primary pathways of drug metabolism. Although the full clinical significance of this problem has not yet been established, there is compelling evidence that highdose salicylate therapy may inhibit not only its own metabolism but also that of a number of other anti-inflammatory agents and analgesics. Salicyluric acid (the glycine conjugate of salicylic acid) formation is inhibited when salicylate and salicylamide are co-administered.[10] Salicylamide also decreases the formation of acetaminophen sulfate and, to a lesser extent, acetaminophen glucuronide.

The first indication that saturation effects may be encountered with even relatively small doses of drugs was the observation that the rate of formation of salicyluric acid does not increase proportionately with dose when the daily amount of salicylate exceeds 300 to 500 mg in healthy adults. The elimination $T^{1/2}$ of salicylate increases from 3 to more than 20 hours as dosage increases; the elimination of the larger doses are not according to first order kinetics, and the *fraction* eliminated as salicylurate *decreases* with increasing dose. The rate of salicylurate formation becomes essentially independent of the amount of salicylate in the body when that amount exceeds about 15 mg per kilogram.[10] Secondary pathways of salicylate metabolism then come into play at higher doses.

These examples of potential drug interactions are of interest because often these drugs are unwittingly taken in combination as nonprescription over-the-counter products. Further investigation is required to establish the true clinical significance of these potentially troublesome interactions resulting in salicylism or, in the case of acetaminophen, possible low-grade liver toxicity.

Another example of drug interaction of this type is the effect of hydrocortisone in competitively inhibiting oxidation of such drugs as ethylmorphine and hexabarbital and in prolonging the T½ of nortriptyline.[11] Conversely, it has also been established that drugs such as phenobarbital and diphenylhydantoin can accelerate the metabolism of cortisol and dexamethasone (see below), thereby decreasing steroid effect.[11]

The antiulcer drug cimetidine significantly impairs the metabolism of many other drugs, including warfarin, theophylline, phenytoin, diazepam, and propranolol.[12] The mechanism of $h_2$-blocker inhibition of hepatic drug metabolism may involve both direct microsomal enzyme impairment and altered liver blood flow. The possibility of significant interaction with salicylates and other anti-inflammatory agents that can cause gastrointestinal ulceration should be kept in mind and requires further investigation.

**Liver Microsomal Enzyme Induction.** Phenylbutazone, like phenobarbital and diphenylhydantoin, is a potent inducer of liver microsomal enzymes and over a few days of administration can thereby stimulate the metabolism of a second drug that is primarily metabolized by microsomal enzymes. While the acute effect of phenylbutazone may be to enhance the action of other acidic drugs (by competition for plasma protein binding), its long-term administration may result in significant induction of metabolism of other drugs. Thus, it is obvious that the potential drug interactions of phenylbutazone are complex, encompassing the pharmacokinetic processes of distribution, metabolism and, as we will see later, excretion. Phenylbutazone stimulates steroid metabolism, shortening the T½ of prednisolone and cortisol, but potentiates the acute toxicity of the anticoagulant warfarin and the oral hypoglycemic agents (probably by both displacing drugs from protein-binding sites and perhaps acutely inhibiting their liver metabolism). The best policy to adopt for phenylbutazone is to reserve it for short-term episodic use and to anticipate significant interactions with a large number of drugs. It should never be prescribed with warfarin or the sulfonylurea hypoglycemic agents.

## RENAL FUNCTION AND DRUG PHARMACOKINETICS

**Drug Excretion.** Renal excretion constitutes a major elimination pathway for many drugs and their metabolites. The mechanism can be either by passive glomerular filtration (with varying amounts of tubular reabsorption) or by active secretion by the proximal tubule. Irrespective of the method of drug excretion, some fraction of drug may be reabsorbed as it traverses the nephron, depending on the degree of drug polarity in the tubular fluid. Thus, small shifts in urine pH may significantly enhance or retard passive drug reabsortion of the nonpolar drug fraction in the nephron (Fig. 48–4).

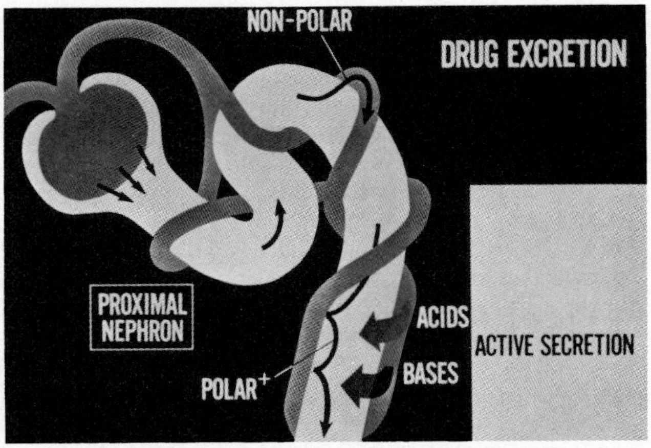


**Figure 48–4.** Renal mechanisms for glomerular filtration (passive), proximal tubular secretion (active), and tubular reabsorption (passive or active) of drugs. (From Robinson, D.S.: J. Urol. 113:100, 1975. Copyright 1975, The Williams & Wilkins Company, Baltimore.)

The factors that influence the amount of drug appearing passively in the glomerular filtrate are the fraction of free (unbound) drug for plasma protein–bound drugs, and the size of the drug molecule. As shown in Fig. 48–4, there are two active transport processes for drug secretion in the proximal tubule, one shared by organic acids and one by organic bases. Acidic or basic drugs may be actively secreted by one of these routes and, as in the example of penicillin and probenecid, can compete with each other for this active transport secretory process. By so doing, probenecid markedly prolongs the elimination T½ of penicillin, an acidic drug which is predominantly excreted via this route rather than metabolized. Other acidic drugs also share this property. Therapeutic doses of phenylbutazone also markedly prolong penicillin T½, and even modest doses of aspirin increase the elimination time of penicillin through completion for the anionic transport pathway.[13] Salicylate and other acidic drugs can also slow the rate of elimination of another weak acid drug, methotrexate, thereby potentiating its toxic effects on bone marrow and tissues.[14] Another clinically significant example of drug interaction involving that old culprit phenylbutazone is its competition for proximal tubular secretion with hydroxyhexamide, the active metabolite of acetohexamide. This interaction with phenylbutazone has produced marked potentiation of this potent hypoglycemic agent, resulting in dangerous hypoglycemic episodes.[15] The hyperuricemia produced by chronic thiazide diuretic therapy similarly involves, in part, this mechanism of competition for secretory process.

**Influence of Urine pH on Drug Excretion.** Regardless of whether a drug is filtered or secreted by the kidney, it undergoes varying degrees of reabsorption from the filtrate by nonionic diffusion. The ratio of nonionized to ionized form of the drug will depend on the pH of the urine filtrate and the pKa of the weak acid. The renal tubule cell behaves as a membrane that permits nonionized drug to diffuse across it but prevents ionic species of the drug from undergoing reabsorption (Fig. 48–4). As urine traverses the tubule, it tends to become more concentrated and more acidified and the extent of drug ionization changes. Thus, salicylates, for example, tend to be present in urine mainly in nonionized form, while basic drugs like quinidine and procainamide are largely ionized in this milieu. The nonionic diffusion of salicylate in the renal tubule is obviously greater than for these basic drugs since it is predominantly nonionized at a pH less than 7. It has been shown that the coadministration of therapeutic doses of "nonabsorbable" antacids (e.g., Maalox) can alter the urine acidification process by a small but significant amount. This produces changes in steady state levels of salicylates as a result of the altered urine pH and excretory rate. Thus, salicylate levels in patients receiving chronic aspirin therapy are decreased by magnesium-containing and other antacids.[16] In a crossover study in a normal population, antacid administration decreased steady state salicylate levels from 16.6 to 13.7 mg per dl while raising urine pH only 0.3 units from 5.7 to 6.0[17] The profound effects of urine pH on salicylate elimination is illustrated by the fact that subjects with very acid urine excrete only 2 to 3 percent of a dose of aspirin as the unchanged drug (with the balance metabolized), while subjects with alkaline urine excrete approximately 25 percent of a dose and metabolize 75 percent.[18]

**Impaired Renal Function and Anti-inflammatory Drugs.** The contribution of renal mechanisms to the elimination of salicylates has been emphasized. However, other agents important in the practice of rheumatology which are also eliminated primarily by renal excretion include oxipurinol, colchicine, corticosteroids, and probably the gold salts.[19,20] In patients with end-stage renal disease, these drugs require extensive reduction in dose when treating coexisting gout or arthritis.[21] The use of drugs such as ibuprofen and probenecid in severe renal failure has not been as extensively studied, so guidelines regarding dosage adjustments are not well established.

## PHARMACOKINETICS AND DRUG DOSING STRATEGIES

Most drugs are administered at intervals shorter than their elimination T½, so that with chronic administration accumulation in plasma and tissue occurs until equilibrium is reached. Steady-state plateau levels of drug are achieved when the amount of drug administered in one dose equals the amount of drug eliminated (by either metabolism or excretion) during that dosing interval.

**First Order Elimination Kinetics and Steady-State Drug Levels.** Most drugs are eliminated according to exponential kinetics, such that a *constant fraction of drug present* is eliminated per unit time (first order kinetics). This means that the elimination kinetics of drug is independent of dose, and therefore the elimination T½ remains constant irrespective of dosage. A simple calculation shows that any drug following first order kinetics is virtually completely eliminated (greater than 95 percent) from the body in 4 to 5 T½'s.[22,23]

Also, when a drug is given over a long term, it *accumulates* according to an exponential curve and achieves a plateau concentration with an "accumulation" half-time equal to its elimination T½ (Fig. 48–5). Thus for most drugs (those which follow first order kinetics), plateau values are achieved independent of the administered dose within 4 to 5 T½'s after initiating therapy. The *time* to reach steady-state levels depends solely on the elimination T½ and is constant for a given individual. The *concentration* of drug achieved at plateau, however, depends on both the size of the dose and the elimination T½ for that individual.

When the dose of a drug is changed in a patient receiving long-term therapy, the time to achieve a new

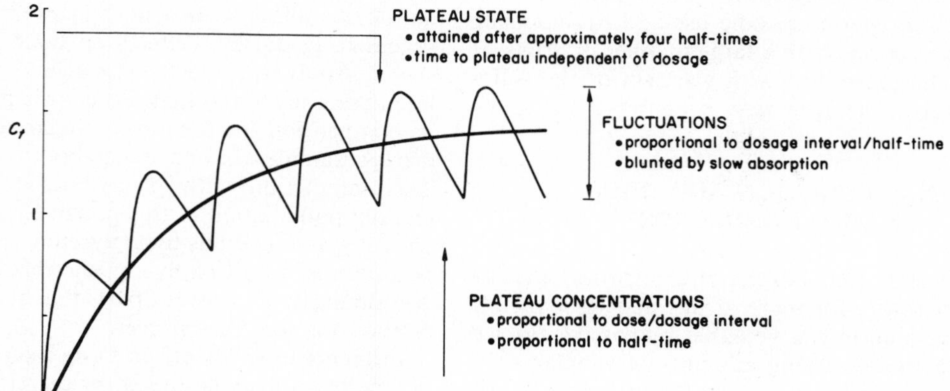


**Figure 48–5.** Drug accumulation during repeated administration of a drug at intervals equal to its elimination half-time (T½). (From Mayer, S.E., Melmon, K.L., and Gilman, A.G.: *In* Goodman, L.S., and Gilman, A. (eds.): The Pharmacological Basis of Therapeutics, 6th ed. New York, Macmillan, 1980.)

steady-state drug level is also 4 to 5 T½'s from the time of the change.[22,24] It is important for the physician to have a general understanding of the pharmacokinetics of drugs he prescribes, particularly their modes of elimination and elimination T½'s, since a rational plan for initiating therapy and for monitoring the patient until steady state is achieved depends on knowledge of such drug properties.[22]

Thus, anti-inflammatory drugs with long T½'s, such as phenylbutazone, oxyphenbutazone, probenecid, and high dose salicylate may require days to weeks of drug accumulation before plateau levels are achieved in many patients. This has obvious implications regarding development of toxicity or likelihood of drug interactions, and patients treated with these agents should be carefully monitored until this process of drug accumulation is complete.

**Zero Order Elimination Kinetics and Steady-State Drug Levels.** As previously mentioned, certain drugs (the notable examples being salicylates, heparin, and diphenylhydantoin) undergo elimination via saturable metabolic processes so that at higher doses given chronically a constant *amount* of drug is eliminated per unit of time rather than a constant *fraction* of drug. The resulting zero order kinetics produces a highly dose-dependent elimination T½. In this situation, the time taken to achieve plateau levels of drug becomes increasingly longer with each increment in dosage because of the longer elimination T½, and disproportionately higher final concentrations of drug in plasma and tissue result. As human pharmacology is better studied and understood, we can identify more and more drugs whose metabolism converts from first order to zero order at high doses. Such drugs, especially those with low therapeutic ratios, must be carefully monitored both during initiation of therapy and following any dosage increase. Obviously, plasma levels of a drug, if they are available, can be helpful in this situation. Since salicylates are the only anti-inflammatory agents for which routine plasma levels are of proved value, careful *clinical* observation of the patient for therapeutic and toxic effects is crucial for most drugs during the induction of therapy and until the response to drug is stabilized.

**Zero Order Absorption Kinetics and Steady-State Drug Levels.** One of the primary goals of effective therapy with anti-inflammatory agents is to reduce fluctuations in blood and tissue drug levels associated with absorption peaks and valleys. Many nonsteroidal anti-inflammatory agents have elimination half-lives of less than 8 hours, so that steady-state levels with chronic administration tend to vary excessively during each dosing interval. This is a factor in the case of several drugs, including aspirin, indomethacin, ibuprofen, and tolmetin, resulting in fluctuating efficacy, side effects, and erratic pain relief.

Recent innovations in drug delivery design have corrected this "sawtooth" effect by making the absorption half-life of a drug much longer than its elimination half-life. The latter ordinarily is the controlling factor governing steady-state levels and duration of drug effect. The recent introduction of a new precision-release oral dosage form of indomethacin has remedied many of the drawbacks of fluctuating drug levels with this agent.[25] Osmotically driven, controlled-release dosage forms of indomethacin can deliver a constant rate of 7 mg per hour and maintain a therapeutic level over a release time of 10 to 12 hours after oral administration.[26] The plasma drug levels achieved with this constant delivery oral dosage form are predictable, since the release of drug into the gut can be precisely controlled.[27] Thus, steady-state levels become dependent on rate of drug delivery rather than rate of drug biotransformation. This has proved to be a unique and useful advance in the area of pharmaceutics for short half-life drugs that do not undergo extensive first-pass metabolism.

**How to Use Plasma Drug Levels.** Plasma levels are helpful and of established value for such commonly used drugs as digitalis, anticonvulsants, antiarrhythmics, salicylate, theophylline, and lithium. Of these, the anticonvulsant drug diphenylhydantoin, like salicylate, also follows zero order kinetics, underscoring the value of drug level monitoring during therapy and when potential interacting drugs such as the sulfonylureas, diphenylhydantoin, phenylbutazone, or high-dose salicylates are coadministered.

Once the decision has been made to use drug levels in dosing strategy, the following guidelines are important:

1. Choose a target serum level, keeping in mind the factors that can modify individual response to a particular level (protein binding, hypoalbuminemia, development of tolerance, metabolic derangements such as uremia or acidosis [Fig. 48–1]).

2. In selecting an initial dose for rheumatologic agents, loading doses are usually not employed, since this is generally reserved for therapeutic emergencies in which full therapeutic effects without waiting are essential. For most situations, a maintenance dose is selected, taking care to make adjustments in the dose based on suspected impairment of the drug's major mode of elimination. For example, downward adjustment would be indicated in the presence of significant renal insufficiency for allopurinol in renal insufficiency.[11]

3. Ordinarily, wait until steady state levels have been reached (4 to 5 half-lives) before drawing a plasma level. If intervening toxicity is suspected before plateau is reached, a drug level is indicated at that time.

4. If necessary, adjust the next dose according to the following formula: New dose/old dose = desired level/measured level. This formula would *not* apply to drugs with zero order kinetics. For these drugs, smaller dose increments should be used.

**Problems in the Correct Interpretation of Drug Levels.** Drug levels should never be a substitute for careful observation and sound clinical judgment, which always take precedence when conflicting data are obtained. Several factors must be considered in the interpretation of blood levels. The ultimate effect at the receptor site of a given drug concentration may be altered by both pharmacokinetic and pharmacodynamic factors (Fig. 48–1). Obviously, a digoxin level in the "therapeutic range" can be a toxic level for a particular patient with altered receptor response resulting from hypokalemia, hypercalcemia, hypomagnesemia, acidosis, or hypoxia. The time elapsed since the last administered dose must be precisely known, especially to avoid absorption and redistribution artifacts in plasma levels, and to properly interpret rapidly fluctuating levels in the case of drugs with relatively short T½'s (e.g., procainamide, quinidine, propranolol).

For drugs that are highly protein bound, it is important to know the serum albumin level and state of renal function. For example, a patient with an albumin of 1.3 and a salicylate level of 25 mg per 100 ml (therapeutic range 25 to 30 mg percent) would probably be in the toxic range, since salicylate is normally 70 to 90 percent protein bound. In this setting, the free (unbound) fraction of salicylate may be excessively high, and toxicity might intervene in spite of a "normal" plasma level. Increased free drug fractions (percent) have been observed in renal disease for several drugs, including salicylates, diphenylhydantoin, and a number of cardiac agents. The mechanism for this may involve either plasma accumulation of acidic substances or altered plasma protein binding characteristics secondary to uremia.[21] Patients with chronic illnesses (associated with hypoalbuminemia) usually require redefinition of therapeutic ranges for these drugs as well.

Finally, some drugs have active metabolites with T½'s significantly different from the parent compound, and an unmeasured metabolite may exhibit more accumulation than the parent drug (benzodiazepines, allopurinol, procainamide, tricyclic antidepressants). A drug level (if available) would underestimate the combined therapeutic or toxic effects of the parent compound and its active metabolite(s). This predicament does not presently apply to any rheumatologic agents for which routine blood levels are available (salicylates, acetaminophen) as far as is known. However, as mentioned above, the active metabolite of allopurinol, oxipurinol, has a significantly longer T½ (mean 28 hours) compared to the parent drug (mean 2 to 4 hours). The net pharmacologic and therapeutic effects of long-term allopurinol administration are largely due to the metabolite oxipurinol, because it reaches high steady state levels in comparison to the parent drug, especially in the patient with renal insufficiency in whom the T½ is apt to be markedly prolonged.

## References


1. Koch-Weser, J., Sidel, V.W., Sweet, R.H., Kanarek, P., and Eaton, A.E.: Factors determining physician reporting of adverse drug reactions: Comparison of 2000 spontaneous reports with surveillance studies at the Massachusetts General Hospital. N. Engl. J. Med. 280:20, 1969.
2. Koch-Weser, J.: Serum drug concentrations as therapeutic guides. N. Engl. J. Med. 287:227, 1972.
3. Robinson, D.S.: The application of basic principles of drug interaction to clinical practice. J. Urol. 113:100, 1975.
4. Biechman, W.J., and Lechner, B.L.: Clinical comparative evaluation of choline magnesium trisalicylate and acetylsalicylic acid in rheumatoid arthritis. Rheumatology and Rehabilitation 18:119, 1979.
5. Ehrlich, G.E., Miller, S.B., and Zeiders, R.S.: Choline magnesium trisalicylate versus ibuprofen in rheumatoid arthritis. Rheumatology and Rehabilitation 19:30, 1980.
6. Guliano, V., and Scharff, E.V.: Clinical comparison of two salicylates in rheumatoid arthritis patients on maintenance gold therapy. Curr. Therap. Res. 28:61, 1980.
7. Miller, D.R.: Combination use of nonsteroidal anti-inflammatory drugs. Drug Intelligence and Clin. Pharmacy 15:3, 1981.
8. Zini, R., D'Athis, P., Barre, J., and Tillement, J.P.: Binding of indomethacin to human serum albumen. Its displacement by various agents, influence of free fatty acids and the unexpected effect of indomethacin on warfarin binding. Biochem. Pharmacol. 28:2661, 1979.
9. Leonard, R.F., Knott, P.J., Rankin, G.O., Robinson, D.S., and Melnick, D.E.: Phenytoin-salicylate interaction. Clin. Pharmacol. Therap. 29:56, 1981.
10. Levy, G.: Drug biotransformation interactions in man: Non-narcotic analgesics. *In* Vesell, E.S. (ed.): Drug Metabolism in Man. New York, New York Academy of Science, Vol. 179, 1971.
11. Dujovne, C.A., and Azarnoff, D.L.: Clinical complications of corticosteroid therapy: A selected review. *In* Azarnoff, D.L. (ed.): Steroid Therapy. Philadelphia, W. B. Saunders Company, 1975.
12. Sriwatanakul, K., and Mehta, G.: Clinically significant drug interactions. Rational Drug Therapy 17:1, 1983.
13. Kampmann, J., Hansen, J.M., Siersboek-Nielsen, K., and Laursen, H.: Effect of some drugs on penicillin half-life in blood. Clin. Pharmacol. Ther. 13:516, 1972.
14. Liegler, D.G., Henderson, E.S., Hahn, M.A., and Oliverio, V.T.: The effect of organic acids on renal clearance of methotrexate in man. Clin. Pharmacol. Ther. 10:849, 1969.
15. Field, J.B., Ohta, M., Boyle, C., and Remer, A.: Potentiation of acetohexamide hypoglycemia by phenylbutazone. N. Engl. J. Med. 277:889, 1967.
16. Levy, G., Lampman, T., Kamath, B.L., and Garrettson, L.K.: Decreased serum salicylate concentrations in children with rheumatic fever treated with antacid. N. Engl. J. Med. 293:323, 1975.
17. Hansten, P.D., and Hayton, W.L.: Effect of antacid and ascorbic acid on serum salicylate concentrations. J. Clin. Pharmacol. 20:326, 1980.
18. Hollister, L., and Levy, G.: Some aspects of salicylate distribution and metabolism in man. J. Pharm. Sci. 54:1126, 1965.
19. Bennett, W.M., Singer, I., Golpher, T., Feig, P., and Coggins, C.J.: Guidelines for drug therapy in renal failure. Ann. Intern. Med. 86:754, 1977.
20. Hansten, P.D. (ed.): Drug Interactions. 3rd ed. Philadelphia, Lea & Febiger, 1976.
21. Reidenberg, M.M. (ed.): Renal Function and Drug Action. Philadelphia, W. B. Saunders Company, 1971.
22. Robinson, D.S.: Pharmacokinetic mechanisms of drug interaction. Postgrad. Med. 57:55, 1975.
23. Fengl, E., and Woodbury, D.M.: General principles. *In* Goodman, L.S., and Gilman, A. (ed.): The Pharmacological Basis of Therapeutics. 5th ed. New York, Macmillan, 1975.
24. Rowland, M.: Drug administration and regimens. *In* Melmon, K.L., and Morrelli, H.F. (eds.): Clinical Pharmacology: Basic Principles in Therapeutics. 2nd ed. New York, Macmillan, 1978.
25. Robinson, D.S.: Pharmacokinetics and pharmacodynamics of drug delivery. Curr. Med. Res. Opinion 8(suppl. 2):10, 1983.
26. Bayne, W., Place, V., Theeuwes, F., Rogers, J.D., Lee, R.B., Davies, R.O., and Kwan, K.C.: Kinetics of osmotically controlled indomethacin delivery systems after repeated dosing. Clin. Pharmacol. Therap. 32:270, 1982.
27. Heimlich, K.R.: The evolution of precision drug delivery. Curr. Med. Res. Opinion 8(suppl. 2):28, 1983.

# Chapter 49
# Aspirin and Salicylate

*Paul H. Plotz*

## INTRODUCTION

The salicylates have a recorded history of over two millennia of continuous medicinal use[1] in treating fever, and over a century in treating rheumatism. Only when they were synthesized commercially in 1874, however, did their modern pharmacologic history begin. Aspirin was introduced widely in 1899 and first used in the United States in that year,[2] but the salicylates were only slowly accepted as efficacious therapy in rheumatoid arthritis.[3] Today salicylates are available in hundreds of forms,[4] and the annual consumption of pills is measured in the billions. Never more than today, there is vigorous research on the action and toxicity of the salicylates, stimulated by the seminal discovery that they inhibit prostaglandin synthetase,[5] and by a desire to rescue them from threatened oblivion by perfecting them.

## STRUCTURE, ABSORPTION, AND METABOLISM*

Salicylic acid is the common name for 2-hydroxybenzoic acid, and aspirin was originally a trade name but is now the common name for the salicylate ester of acetic acid (Fig. 49–1). Both are white powders relatively insoluble in aqueous solutions. Their sodium salts are more soluble, particularly in a slightly alkaline solution. The ionization constant, pKa, for the carboxyl hydrogen is 3.5 for aspirin and 3.0 for salicylic acid. Consequently, in the highly acid stomach both will be un-ionized, and in the body fluids, both will be largely ionized, though aspirin slightly less so. Because it is probable that the un-ionized rather than the ionized form of both drugs diffuses across cell membranes, it is worth remembering that, even far from the pKa, changes in pH can have marked changes in the proportion of drug that is ionized.[6]

When uncoated aspirin or salicylate tablets are placed in an aqueous solution, they visibly disintegrate with a speed that depends largely on various factors in their manufacture but in all events faster than the active drug goes into solution. The dissolution rate, too, is controlled by factors in tablet manufacture and plays a role in the subsequent fate of both aspirin and salicylate, since once dissolved, the drug is absorbed very rapidly.[6] Generally aspirin or salicylate taken as a solution (for example, effervescent buffered aspirin) or in an easily soluble form such as sodium aspirin is more rapidly absorbed than standard aspirin.[7-9] Buffering may also accelerate dissolution.[10,11] The drugs are available in many guises, none demonstrably better than the others for treating connective tissue diseases.

Acid in the stomach may cause the un-ionized form of the drug to form and precipitate, or the drug may remain in supersaturated solution,[7] but relatively little is known of the physical state of aspirin or salicylate in either the secreting or the nonsecreting stomach. Studies on the state of the drug in the overnight fasted stomach from which secretions have been aspirated may bear little relation to its state in a subject who eats and drinks and takes drug in irregular relation to food. Early observations of particles of aspirin in the stomach wall of patients who ingested drug just prior to gastrectomy have so many possibilities for artifact that they cannot be taken as having generality.[12] When awake subjects are gastroscoped after taking aspirin, such particles are not usually visible.

Aspirin and salicylate are absorbed to a certain extent by the gastric mucosa,[13-15] and it is likely that the low pH of the stomach contents, by causing the drugs to be un-ionized, facilitates absorption.[16,17] Nevertheless, they can be absorbed from the neutralized stomach at a considerable rate.[18] Both drugs become ionized as they pass into the small intestine, because the pH is near neutrality. While this enhances solubility, it obviously diminishes the amount of un-ionized drug. Since the drugs are well absorbed from the intestine, either the ionized form is absorbed or the effective pH in the unstirred layer near the wall is much lower, thus allowing the proportion of un-ionized drug to rise,[16] or the enormous

*This subject is well reviewed in Reference 6.

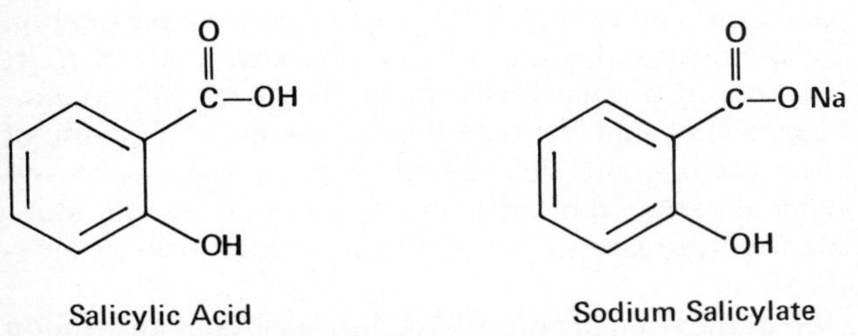


**Figure 49–1.** The chemical structure of the principal salicylates.

surface allows the rapid absorption of any un-ionized drug so that the drugs are continually pushed toward the un-ionized form. Although aspirin can spontaneously hydrolyze to acetate and salicylate in aqueous solution, the rate of spontaneous hydrolysis is low enough so that little or no free salicylate is found in the intestine; it is absorbed as aspirin, not as salicylate.[7] The current enteric coating of cellulose acetate phthalate is stable to acid but dissolves readily above pH 6 in the small intestine.

Aspirin is the dominant form of the drug in plasma within the first 10 to 20 minutes after ingestion;[7,20,21] it can be detected for several minutes before there is any measurable salicylate,[22] and it even appears in joint fluid before salicylate. But it disappears very fast (T½ 15 minutes), and consequently the blood level of aspirin is quite sensitive to the rate of absorption.[6] Consequently, serum aspirin levels are lower with a sustained-release form than with plain or heavily buffered aspirins.[23]

Aspirin disappears by deacetylating to salicylate by one of three routes. It spontaneously deacetylates in plasma as it will in vitro in aqueous solution. It acetylates proteins, of which prostaglandin synthetase is the most notable example[24] but by no means the only one. Both hemoglobin[25] and albumin[26] have been shown to be acetylated, and doubtless other proteins and macromolecules are, too, including perhaps some cell surface macromolecules. And it is hydrolyzed enzymatically to salicylate, although it is by no means clear that this enzymatic activity is specific in any way for aspirin.[27] Probably several enzymes in the circulation are involved, including cholinesterase, an esterase that moves electrophoretically with albumin, and an esterase in red blood cells.[28,29] Furthermore, since hepatic venous salicylate exceeds portal venous salicylate after an oral dose of aspirin, the enzymatic hydrolysis probably takes place in the liver, but it has not been localized to a well-characterized enzyme.[7,30]

Aspirin and salicylate are partially bound to serum proteins, mainly albumin.[31] They diffuse into cells and across various membranes into body fluids such as the cerebrospinal fluid[33] and synovial fluid,[22] and they freely cross the placenta[31] and are secreted into breast milk.[32] The diffusion is fairly rapid, and joint fluid levels, although never so high as serum levels, do reach 60 to 75 percent of serum levels in acute experiments, and drug can be detected there within 20 minutes of ingestion.[22] With increasing dose, the proportion of drug in plasma that is not protein bound increases. Likewise, when plasma albumin is low, as in severe rheumatoid arthritis, less drug is protein bound. Since it is the free drug that diffuses to the site of its action, the pharmacologic and toxic effects of an increment in dose are greater when the dose is already high and when the plasma albumin is low. It is likely that many other factors influence the rates of passage of the drugs across biologic membranes, for example, the proportion of un-ionized drug, which is sensitive to pH, and local protein binding.[34]

Salicylate appears to be metabolized principally if not exclusively by the liver, although formal proof of this is lacking. There are three major and several minor metabolites of the drug, which together satisfactorily account for its fate. They are all excreted into the urine, and drug recovery in the urine after an acute ingestion approaches 100 percent of the ingested drug. The major metabolite is the glycine conjugate, called salicyluric acid, and there are two glucuronide conjugates, one on the phenolic hydroxyl and one on the carboxyl group. At no time do these principal metabolites reach any significant proportion of the circulating salicylate.[35] The metabolites appear to be excreted quantitatively as soon as they reach the kidneys and can be found in the plasma only by sensitive chemical techniques. Their excretion depends on glomerular filtration and tubular secretion, is independent of urine flow or urine pH, and approaches but does not exceed renal plasma flow.[35] The quantitatively minor metabolite, gentisic acid, is important only because it has occasionally been shown to have prostaglandin synthetase-inhibiting properties,[36] but it is highly unlikely that it contributes to the clinical effects of aspirin.

It has long been known that serum levels of salicylate (it is impractical to measure serum levels of aspirin in a clinical setting) bear only the crudest relationship to the dose ingested even when corrected for body size, and that the full effect on serum level of an increase in dose may be reflected only after several days. Most strikingly, a small increment in dose may lead to a profound increment in serum level (for example, in one study the mean serum level was three-fold higher when the dose was 100 mg per kilogram per day than when it was 65 mg per kilogram per day),[37] and marked fluctuations in serum level may be observed without a change in dose. Furthermore, in contrast to aspirin, the plasma half-life of salicylate is many hours and is directly proportional to the serum levels; *the higher the serum level, the slower the disappearance.* The mystery of this erratic behavior has been solved by a number of excellent studies which have shown that the two major determinants of the serum level of salicylate are the urinary pH[38-40] and the activity of the enzyme that synthesizes salicylurate by conjugating glycine to salicylate.[41-44]

Urinary pH variations over the normal range profoundly affect clearance of salicylate by the kidneys. Salicylate is filtered at the glomerulus, and is both reabsorbed and secreted by the tubules. Below pH 6, salicylate clearance is about one tenth of creatinine clearance.[35] Above neutrality, salicylate clearance rises steeply and may reach almost twice the creatinine clearance in a slightly alkaline urine. Consequently, salicylate excretion may change from hour to hour, depending on the quantity and composition of ingested food, exercise, the normal diurnal fluctuations of urinary pH, pulmonary events, and the ingestion of antacids.[45] Because of these factors, and because below pH 6 there is no significant variation of salicylate clearance, metabolic studies are often carried out with concomitant urinary acidification.

The ingestion of antacid not only facilitates absorption by solubilizing drug in the intestines and accelerating gastric emptying; it also facilitates excretion by the kidneys. This property is found with both absorbable and the "nonabsorbable" antacids, which can lower steady-state serum salicylate levels despite a constant salicylate dose by their effect on urinary pH.[40] Likewise, withdrawal of antacids can cause a sudden rise in salicylate levels.

The other major determinant of serum salicylate is the rate of conjugation to glycine. Since the glycine conjugate salicylurate is the major metabolite when salicylate excretion is suppressed by acidification, the serum level is determined principally by the rate of production of salicylurate. In acute metabolic studies it has been found that above a serum level of about 6 mg per deciliter the rate of fall of serum salicylate is constant because there is a constant rate of production of salicylurate independent of the serum level.[37,43] It appears that the extraordinary variation in serum levels among different individuals on a similar dose (serum levels ranged from 4 to 33 mg per deciliter in a group of patients with rheumatoid arthritis who took 50 mg per kilogram per day)[43] reflects variation in the level of the conjugating enzyme rather than in the kinetic parameters of the enzyme. The level of enzyme seems to be at least partially under genetic control; identical twins have very closely matched rates of salicylurate formation, while fraternal twins do not.[44] But the matter is not so simple, since with the continued ingestion of salicylate or aspirin, at least over several days, the level of enzyme rises somewhat.[44] With the chronic ingestion of a sustained release aspirin, the serum salicylate level may drift down after a few days before reaching a steady state. This adjustment may be due to increased salicylate formation, but it is not completely understood, since overall urinary recovery of salicylate metabolites also declines.[46] There may be other determinants of the level of this enzyme too, for example, the ingestion of other drugs. The production of salicylate phenolic glucuronide is also saturable within the clinical dose range,[41] but since it accounts for only about a fifth of excreted metabolites when salicylate excretion is suppressed, variation in its metabolism will have little effect on serum levels. It should be noted that because of the limited capacity of the two major metabolic pathways of salicylate, as the serum level rises the proportion of unconjugated salicylate will rise, and hence the effect of urinary pH on excretion will be more profound.

Although aspirin and salicylate are rapidly absorbed and metabolized, under steady-state chronic ingestion with as many variables as possible removed, the serum salicylate level fluctuates little between doses. With a 4-hour dosing interval, the mean fluctuation is only 1 mg per deciliter, and with an 8-hour interval, 2.5 mg per deciliter, although individual patients may vary by as much as 3 and 6.3 mg per deciliter, respectively.[32] With enteric-coated aspirin, a large dose taken twice a day can lead to a sustained serum salicylate level in the therapeutic range about as efficiently as the same amount taken four times a day, and with as little fluctuation in serum level.[47] The overall kinetic model for the metabolism of single doses of aspirin developed by Levy, Tsuchiya, and Amsel[41] is well substantiated by experimental results.[42]

Aspirin or salicylate can be given topically, intra-articularly, or intravenously, but these routes are either ineffective[48,49] or offer no real advantage.[50] Two new salicylates, salicylsalicylate[51] and diflunisal, a fluorobenzene derivate of salicylate,[52] have been introduced recently. Both may be as efficacious as plain aspirin, may have better gastrointestinal tolerance, and have a longer therapeutic interval than plain aspirin. They share many of the extratherapeutic effects of other salicylates; diflunisal adds several of its own.[53-55] They have no apparent advantages over enteric-coated aspirin, and are substantially more expensive. Formulations of salicylate with salts other than sodium are available[56,57] or under study[58] and may be useful alternatives upon occasion.

What is the clinical importance to the rheumatologist of the studies on the absorption and metabolism of salicylates? It can be safely said that some patients are symptomatically sensitive to the dosing interval, that if the drugs are stopped for a day or so disease will measurably flare, and that the symptoms and signs of most inflammatory arthritides fluctuate more in response to physical activity and emotional state than in response to fluctuations in the serum salicylate level.

## MAJOR THERAPEUTIC ACTIONS

**Antipyresis.** The antipyretic property of the salicylates was known by the middle of the eighteenth century, and today antipyresis is a prime indication for salicylates. By the 1940s, it appeared likely that the antipyretic action was central, not peripheral, and the details have unfolded beautifully over the past decade. Jackson established in 1967 that endotoxin caused fever only after a considerable latency but that a substance liberated from leukocytes did so rapidly.[61] In the same year Cooper and associates showed that the leukocyte pyrogen but not endotoxin was 100-fold more potent when given into the brain than intravenously and established that a neurotransmitter other than epinephrine or norepinephrine was involved.[62] Circulating monocytes and fixed mononuclear phagocytes are the source of the pyrogen, which is probably identical to the lymphocyte-activating protein known as interleukin I.[63] When Milton and Wendlandt showed that prostaglandin $E_1$ injected into the third ventricle of a cat caused an immediate fever that acetaminophen could not affect,[64] the broad outlines of the story were evident. Over the next 2 years it was shown that aspirin injected into the anterior hypothalamus was more potent than aspirin injected into the third ventricle and that injections into the carotid artery and intravenously were progressively less potent.[65,66] Soon after Flower and Vane[19] discovered the prostaglandin details, they showed not only that rabbit brain prostaglandin synthetase was blocked by aspirin, indomethacin, and acetaminophen, but also that their relative potencies were far different from their potencies

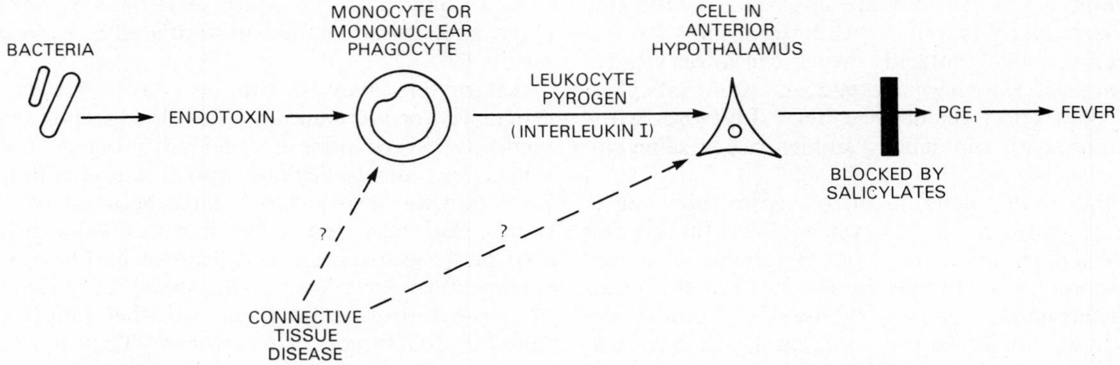


**Figure 49–2.** Leukocyte pyrogen liberated by monocytes and mononuclear phagocytes in response to bacteria stimulates the synthesis of prostaglandins in the anterior hypothalamus. The antipyretic action of salicylates is to block this synthesis.

in other enzyme systems.[67] In particular, acetaminophen and aspirin were almost equipotent and only about 10-fold less potent than indomethacin against the brain enzyme, whereas they were spread over a greater than 5000-fold potency range for dog spleen enzyme. Furthermore, it had long been known that sodium salicylate was almost as potent as aspirin in lowering fever despite doubts about their equivalence in other respects.[68]

It is now evident that $PGE_1$-like material appears in the third ventricle when fever is produced by an endotoxin,[69] that antipyretics of the PG-synthetase inhibiting class block that appearance,[69] that aspirin can block leukocyte pyrogen-induced but not $PGE_1$-induced fever,[69-71] that in vitro leukocyte pyrogen production is unaffected by high levels of salicylate,[72] that leukocyte pyrogen and aspirin do not compete for a common binding site, that in the brain as elsewhere PGE may mediate its effects through cyclic nucleotides,[73] and that the anterior hypothalamus is the principal site of action of this class of antipyretics.[74-76] (Fig. 49–2).

Although the mechanism of fever in the connective tissue diseases is unknown and may or may not depend upon the release of leukocyte pyrogen from sites of inflammation, the efficacy of salicylates and other prostaglandin synthetase-inhibiting drugs does suggest that prostaglandins serve as mediators of fever. Because of the sensitivity of fever to aspirin (inhibition of fever is maximal with about 600 mg every 4 hours), the antipyretic effects in many inflammatory conditions are achieved at doses below those necessary to suppress other measures of inflammation.

In adult rheumatoid arthritis, fever is unusual, and hypothermia is not a consequence of aspirin therapy. In rheumatic fever and in juvenile rheumatoid arthritis, in which fever may be the most prominent feature early in the illness, aspirin and other salicylates are powerful antipyretics and do not usually cause hypothermia. The antipyretic action is a principal indication for salicylates in lupus and often succeeds in lowering a fever in lupus when steroids fail. In fact, fever in lupus should preferentially be treated with nonsteroidal drugs.

**Analgesia.*** In general, aspirin and salicylate are properly classified as mild analgesics, equivalent to moderate doses of codeine, and less potent than full doses of narcotic analgesics[78,79] but more effective than narcotics against inflammatory pain.[80] It is likely that a maximum response is reached with 600 or 625 mg in an adult; with this dose, the serum salicylate level will not usually exceed 5 mg per dl. It has been asserted, though without published proof, that aspirin is a more effective analgesic than sodium salicylate in man.[81] Aspirin is clearly four times more potent than salicylate in blocking the painful response to intraperitoneal or intrasplenic bradykinin in dogs (see below),[82,83] and the period of analgesia in man does correspond roughly with the period when unhydrolyzed acetylsalicylic acid is still present in the blood after oral ingestion.[77] Nevertheless, as the long and successful history of salicylates prior to the synthesis of aspirin establishes, salicylate itself is analgesic in man.

Aspirin can act as an analgesic peripherally to reduce the inflow to the central nervous system of nerve impulses from a painful stimulus.[84,85] This has been shown in an elegant series of cross-circulation experiments in dogs.[82,83] The spleen of a recipient dog, with its nerve supply intact, received its arterial blood supply from a donor dog (Fig. 49–3). An injection of bradykinin into that splenic artery caused pain in the recipient as manifested by barking. An injection of aspirin into the donor dog blocked the pain, whereas an injection into the recipient (but not into the spleen) was ineffective. With narcotic analgesics, the reverse was true. If aspirin was injected directly into the splenic artery, the effective dose was 3.8 mg per kg, whereas it was 50 mg per kg if it was injected intravenously into the donor. Drug administered into the recipient's carotid artery was not analgesic. Again, with morphine the opposite was true. Propoxyphene was active by both routes. Furthermore, aspirin but not morphine blocked nerve impulses evoked in the splenic nerve by the bradykinin injection. In these

*This subject is well reviewed in Reference 77.

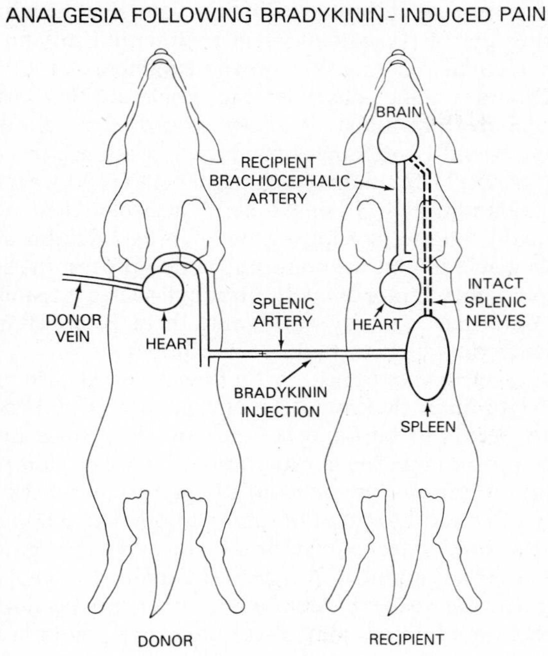


ANALGESIA

| | SPLENIC ARTERY | DONOR VEIN | BRACHIOCEPHALIC ARTERY |
|---|---|---|---|
| SALICYLATES | +++ | + | 0 |
| MORPHINE | 0 | 0 | +++ |

**Figure 49–3.** Bradykinin injected into the splenic blood supply of a vascularly isolated spleen causes the recipient dog to bark if the nervous connections of the spleen are left intact. Aspirin injected with the bradykinin blocks the pain response, but is without effect if injected into the brachiocephalic artery. With morphine, the opposite is true. (See Reference 83.)

experiments, sodium salicylate was an effective analgesic in doses fourfold higher than aspirin. In analogous experiments, in which a leg was supplied with arterial blood from a donor dog, intra-arterial sodium salicylate blocked the bradykinin-evoked pressor response in the recipient.[86] In an assay in which rats writhe in response to a bradykinin injection, aspirin was the most potent of a number of salicylate derivatives and analogues.[87] None of aspirin's metabolites beyond salicylate has analgesic action.[77]

What is known of the mechanism of the analgesic action? In response to an intra-arterial injection of bradykinin into the dog spleen, the splenic venous circulation had an increased output of prostaglandin-like material, and there was a rise in systemic blood pressure.[88] If $PGE_1$ or $PGE_2$ was given along with the bradykinin, the hypertension was augmented, although alone these prostaglandins lower the blood pressure. Indomethacin, a powerful inhibitor of prostaglandin synthesis, blocked the hypertension induced by bradykinin. Thus, prostaglandins appear to mediate some bradykinin effects. Experiments in rats showed that prostaglandins lowered the threshold to pain from a mechanical stimulus,[89] and in humans that intradermal $PGE_1$ lowered the threshold to pain from a subsequent injection of bradykinin or histamine.[90] Aspirin cannot interfere with the pain induced by an intraarterial injection of either $PGE_1$ or $PGE_2$ in the dog.[91] Salicylates are generally ineffective against nonpathologic pain: that is, they appear to work only on some painful process already under way. For example, they raise the pain threshold to mechanical pressure in a rat's paw inflamed by an injection of yeast without altering the pain threshold in a normal paw.[89] A plausible case can thus be made for the view that part of the pain of inflammation is due to the stimulation by mediators such as bradykinin of the synthesis of prostaglandins which sensitize nerves to painful stimuli, and that salicylates are effective analgesics because they block that synthesis. Their analgesic property, however, is not identical to their anti-inflammatory property, since in both animal experiments and human experience analgesia occurs in doses below those that reduce heat and edema.

However plausible and satisfying the case may be for a unitary hypothesis of action of these drugs, the experiments are so far from providing the details necessary for verisimilitude that skepticism is unavoidable. One cannot yet dismiss theories concerning the direct effect of salicylates on nerve cell membranes,[92] or a central action under certain circumstances. For example, aspirin given to the rat so alters histamine metabolism that there is an increase in the production of indoleacetic acid, which has narcotic properties in that species.[93,94] Furthermore, many individuals, particularly the elderly, experience apparently central effects of aspirin such as dizziness, somnolence, and slurred speech, not to mention that hyperpnea and antipyresis are clearly central effects of the drugs. Any unitary hypothesis of aspirin and salicylate analgesic action must account for their ability to counteract pain of diverse sorts: headache, both vascular and muscular, and deep visceral or skeletal pain, whether neoplastic or mechanical, as well as pain related to inflammation. It seems likely that the proof of such a hypothesis will have to rest on a deeper understanding of the mechanism of pain than presently exists.

**Anti-inflammation.** In favoring aspirin and its pharmacologic relatives (and steroids) over propoxyphene, pentazocine, codeine, morphine, or even acetaminophen in the treatment of connective tissue diseases, especially arthritis, rheumatologists lean upon the belief that they provide not only freedom from addiction but the positive property of suppressing inflammation. Since one can obtain analgesia without measurably affecting other aspects of inflammation, the optimal use of these drugs in inflammatory disease depends on using them so as to obtain the anti-inflammatory effects.

What is the reason for believing that aspirin and salicylates have anti-inflammatory effects over and above analgesia? Inflammation is a term used to describe a global reaction that involves vascular events leading to the translocation of blood cells, protein, electrolytes, and fluid to the extracellular space; stimulation, proliferation, and transformation of cells; the production, diffusion, and destruction of mediators of great variety; the stimulation of nerve endings; the destruction of tissues; and ultimately a return to the uninflamed state. The inciting cause, the location, the species, the chronicity, and many other factors determine the course of inflammation and doubtless the response to intervention. Measuring the effects of intervention might therefore appear to be despairingly difficult, but in fact a good deal of useful information has been gathered on the global response and its less subtle manifestations, edema, erythema, and pain (see Analgesia).

The evidence for a reduction of edema and effusion in human arthritis is relatively limited. The clearest effect was in a study with patients with rheumatoid arthritis in which it was shown that aspirin at 5.3 grams per day reduced both joint pain and joint swelling as measured by jeweler's rings, whereas aspirin at 2.6 grams per day and acetaminophen affected only pain.[95] In other studies, some unpublished, aspirin has been shown to reduce swelling or increase joint motion, presumably measures of inflammation. There is evidence, too, that prostaglandins are elevated in the active synovial effusion of rheumatoid arthritis and even that therapy with aspirin can reduce that level, but the story is distinctly incomplete.[96] There is no useful, independent evidence on the mechanism or anti-inflammatory effects of aspirin or salicylate in any nonarthritic condition, although any clinician who has treated the serositis of lupus erythematosus with them will attest to their efficacy.

Animal models have provided substantial evidence for anti-inflammatory effects of aspirin and salicylate. Aspirin or salicylate reduced edema in rat paws injected with the algal polysaccharide carrageenan as a subacute irritant.[97-100] Furthermore they reduced the accumulation of effusion and cells when carrageenan was injected intrapleurally.[101] They reduced edema and warmth as well as the hyperesthesis of yeast-induced inflammation in the rat paw.[102,103] Urate-induced edema and ellagic acid-induced edema in both the rat paws and the dog stifle joint were reduced by aspirin.[104] Chemical- or ultraviolet-induced skin erythema was reduced only by very large doses.[105] Among chronic models of inflammation, aspirin effectively inhibited and also treated established adjuvant arthritis in the rat.[106-108] It did not have a beneficial effect on the inflammation of a traumatized joint,[109] and it had a variable effect in an antigen-induced arthritis.[110] Although it is likely that prostaglandins are important in the inflammation in some of these models, and that the interaction between bradykinin and prostaglandins is important in edema as well as pain, it is premature to suggest that aspirin works in them solely because of its effects of prostaglandin synthesis, or, conversely, that prostaglandin synthesis does or does not have a role in inflammation because inhibition of synthesis affects the process. Aspirin is not effective against inflammation caused by histamine or by injected or previously synthesized prostaglandins.

Recent tissue culture experiments have shed new light on the role of prostaglandin in rheumatoid inflammation. Human rheumatoid synovial fragments produced $PGE_2$ and a collagenase and can accelerate the release of calcium from mouse fetal bones; furthermore, mitogen-activated lymphocytes produce a substance or substances which stimulate these fragments to produce more prostaglandin.[111,112] It might seem possible, then, that adequate long-term suppression of prostaglandin synthesis would inhibit the bone destruction process in rheumatoid joints. Unfortunately, although such a possibility has not been formally ruled out, there is no clinical evidence on which to build such a hope.

In mechanistic terms, the influence of aspirin and salicylate upon the migration of neutrophils and monocytes seems to be important, particularly since prostaglandins can influence migration.[113,114] The complex effects of various prostaglandins on vascular permeability offer another point of intervention. There appears to be a direct effect of aspirin on the surface of granulocytes which might influence their ability to enter the extravascular space.[115] Aspirin and other prostaglandin-synthetase inhibitors may affect the many points in the immune response in which prostaglandins participate in complex or contradictory ways.[116]

Inflammation doubtless has an important beneficial role, so that interference with it might be hazardous as well as helpful. Such is the case with corticosteroids. With aspirin, salicylate, and other prostaglandin synthesis-inhibiting drugs, however, the course of infection, both chronic and acute, is unaffected, demonstrating the limitations of those drugs in the face of a powerful stimulus.[117]

Aspirin and sodium salicylate have rarely been compared for potency in animal models of inflammation; investigators tend to prefer to use aspirin, but sodium salicylate has been effective in some studies. In humans with arthritis, only the undocumented assertion by several investigators can be cited to support a greater anti-inflammatory potency for aspirin, although many clinicians favor it.[81] Even if the unitary hypothesis for the action of these drugs on prostaglandin synthesis is correct, it is unlikely that the inhibition of a single enzyme is solely responsible for anti-inflammatory effects.

Probably some effects of prostaglandin synthetase inhibition are the result of increased synthesis in the other wing of arachidonic acid metabolism, the leukotriene pathway, rather than just decreased prostaglandins, prostacyclins, and thromboxanes. In view of the great range of tissue sensitivities to inhibition, one should not a priori expect that the overall inhibition by salicylate will be appreciably less than that by aspirin.

However unproved and uncertain the unitary prostaglandin theory,[118,119] none of the other proposed theories of aspirin's anti-inflammatory action has plausible evidence in support of it. The possibility that aspirin works by inhibiting phosphodiesterase is remote, since only high levels are inhibitory.[120] Some of the older theories on the interactions of aspirin with various parts of the inflammatory system have been well reviewed.[105]

## THE CLINICAL USE OF ASPIRIN AND SALICYLATES IN THE RHEUMATIC DISEASES

The major indications for aspirin and salicylate in the rheumatic diseases are fever, pain, and inflammation. They are useful for the fevers that commonly accompany rheumatic fever, systemic lupus erythematosus, and juvenile polyarthritis and, less commonly, rheumatoid arthritis, the spondyloarthritides, and other connective tissue diseases. They are useful for the pain of arthritis of any origin, including osteoarthritis and mechanical joint pain even when inflammation is not evident, and they are useful for the inflammatory arthritis, pleurisy, and pericarditis that accompany rheumatoid arthritis, lupus erythematosus, and occasionally other connective tissue diseases. They are not in general useful for the treatment of myositis, rash, nodules, renal disease, or serologic tests. It should be noted, however, that the anti-inflammatory effect in systemic lupus erythematosus, juvenile arthritis, and rheumatic fever may be accompanied by the fading of rash, and the sedimentation rate, too, responds as inflammation recedes in many diseases.

The antipyretic action and simple analgesia require relatively small doses of either aspirin or salicylate. One or two 300 mg tablets four to six times a day suffice for all but the largest adults. When the drugs are used to combat inflammation, higher doses are necessary, and although salicylate itself may not be so powerful and anti-inflammatory as aspirin, the serum level of salicylate is best used to guide therapy.

Plain aspirin is the cheapest place to start. Provided it is kept dry, it will remain as aspirin; otherwise it will slowly decay to salicylic acid and acetic acid and acquire a vinegary smell. Such preparations are not unsafe to use and are no less efficacious than the salicylate they contain. Today, however, enteric-coated aspirin is the best form of the drug. Indeed, since the gastrointestinal side effects, the principal drawback of plain aspirin, are so much reduced and since the drug is so well-absorbed, enteric-coated aspirin is a close to perfect nonsteroidal anti-inflammatory drug. It is available in several sizes and can even be given twice a day with adequate serum levels. The starting dose should be about 2.4 to 3.6 g per day in adults. The abrupt introduction of higher doses of plain aspirin often leads to patient resistance because of gastrointestinal side effects. Recalling the unusual metabolism of salicylates, in which the serum half-life gets longer as the serum level goes higher, the dose should be raised by one tablet per day no more often than once per week until tinnitus occurs or until the salicylate level is between 20 and 30 mg per dl. A slow-release form used at bedtime sometimes reduces early morning stiffness and pain. Since the drugs are most often introduced outside the hospital, and since frequent determinations of serum salicylate are impractical or impossible, older patients should raise the dose even more slowly, and all patients should be told about tinnitus, diminished hearing, and hyperpnea that accompany high serum salicylate levels. Patients know about the gastrointestinal side effects well enough, but if a physician is committed to the use of salicylates, he can help a patient avoid them by a variety of maneuvers which may not make pharmacologic sense or be supported by controlled trials, but work. Plain aspirin can be given with meals, with antacids, crushed in milk, dissolved in water, or even crushed with Jell-O. The hour can be varied and the brand can be varied; a buffered preparation, sodium salicylate, timed-release aspirin, choline salicylate, and even various magnesium and calcium salts are available substitutes and will overcome gastrointestinal side effects in some patients. Enteric-coated aspirin is, I believe, the drug of choice except in the rare patient with gastric outlet obstruction in whom salicylism from retained undigested pills may occur.[121] Table 49–1 lists many of the common nonprescription and prescription forms in which aspirin and other salicylates are marketed.

It has often been observed that for some reason, pharmacological or psychological, individual patients may respond differently to different formulations. There are many variations in the formation of aspirin and salicylate designed to reduce the symptoms of gastrointestinal upset, to accelerate the absorption of the drug, or to reduce the microbleeding (see below). There is good evidence that sufficient buffering with either bicarbonate, citrate, or nonabsorbable alkali to bring the intragastric pH to neutrality will reduce microbleeding and accelerate absorption. The price, however, is a level of sodium intake unacceptable for long-term therapy (521 mg of sodium per 322 mg of aspirin in the most popular effervescent form, Alka-Seltzer) and/or accelerated excretion of the drug so that serum levels with long-term therapy are lower. Although the small amounts of buffering in commonly sold buffered aspirin may marginally accelerate absorption, they do not alter microbleeding. No formulation has proved dependably better at reducing gastric upset in blinded trials. In practical terms, if a patient has good symptomatic relief of arthritis with aspirin or salicylate but complains of gastrointestinal side effects, it is sensible to switch preparations; it is not necessary to abandon salicylates.

If the patient also takes corticosteroids or drinks any alcohol, nonabsorbable antacids should be used, bearing in mind that higher doses of the salicylate may then be necessary to maintain an adequate serum salicylate level.

Although it may be irrational, other nonsteroidal drugs can be added to aspirin with psychological if not pharmacological therapeutic benefit and no clear evidence for harm.

In rheumatoid arthritis, aspirin should be used in full anti-inflammatory doses, which means until a salicylate level of at least 20 mg per dl is reached or until tinnitus or diminished hearing occurs. Indeed, aspirin or another nonsteroidal anti-inflammatory drug should be given in anti-inflammatory doses along with all other classes of antirheumatic drug if inflammation is present.

Generally a reduction in dose suffices to reverse most symptomatic toxicities, although some require that the drug be stopped. The elderly patient is particularly sus-

**Table 49–1.** Some Commonly Used Nonprescription and Prescription Drugs Containing Salicylates*

| Drug | Salicylate Concentration | Drug | Salicylate Concentration |
|---|---|---|---|
| *Nonprescription* | | | |
| **Analgesics**† | | Momentum | 162.5 mg aspirin, 325 mg salsalate |
| Alka-Seltzer | 324 mg aspirin | P-A-C Compound | 227 mg aspirin |
| Anacin products | 400 mg and 500 mg aspirin | Persistin | 160 mg aspirin, 485 mg salsalate |
| Arthralgen | 250 mg salicylamide | Trigesic | 230 mg aspirin |
| Arthritis Pain Formula | 487.5 mg aspirin | Vanquish caplets | 227 mg aspirin |
| A.S.A. | 325 mg aspirin | **Cold remedies** | |
| A.S.A. Compound | 227 mg aspirin | Alka-Seltzer Plus | 324 mg aspirin |
| Ascriptin products | 325 mg aspirin | Codimal products | 150 mg salicylamide |
| Aspergum | 210 mg aspirin | Coricidin products | 325 mg aspirin |
| Bancap products | 200 mg salicylamide | Dristan tablets | 325 mg aspirin |
| Bayer | 325 mg aspirin | Hista-Compound No. 5 | 227.5 mg salicylamide |
| BC Tablets | 325 mg aspirin, 95 mg salicylamide | Pyrroxate | 200 mg aspirin |
| BC Powder | 650 mg aspirin, 195 mg salicylamide | Rhinocaps | 162 mg aspirin |
| Bufferin | 324 mg aspirin | Rid-A-Col | 390 mg aspirin |
| Cama Inlay-Tabs | 600 mg aspirin | Saleto-D | 120 mg salicylamide |
| Capron | 227 mg aspirin | Sine-Off tablets | 325 mg aspirin |
| Cope | 421.2 mg aspirin | Sinulin tablets | 250 mg salicylamide |
| Doan's pills | 325 mg magnesium salicylate | Triaminicin | 450 mg aspirin |
| Duragesic | 325 mg aspirin, 162 mg salsalate | Viro-Med | 325 mg aspirin |
| Ecotrin | 325 mg aspirin | 4-Way Cold Tablets | 324 mg aspirin |
| Empirin | 325 mg aspirin | **Miscellaneous** | |
| Excedrin capsules | 250 mg aspirin | Midol | 454 mg aspirin |
| Excedrin tablets | 194.4 mg aspirin, 129.6 mg salicylamide | Quiet World | 227 mg aspirin |
| Measurin | 650 mg aspirin | | |
| *Prescription* | | | |
| **Analgesics**† | | Trilisate products | 500 mg and 750 mg total salicylate |
| Darvon Compound products | 227 mg and 325 mg aspirin | Zactirin tablets | 325 mg aspirin |
| Disalcid | 500 mg salicylic acid | Zactirin Compound-100 | 227 mg aspirin |
| Equagesic | 250 mg aspirin | **Cold remedies** | |
| Fiorinal products | 200 mg aspirin | Emprazil | 200 mg aspirin |
| Meprogesic | 250 mg aspirin | Omnicol | 227 mg salicylamide |
| Percodan products | 325 mg aspirin | Partuss T.D. | 300 mg salicylamide |
| Synalgos products | 356.4 mg aspirin | **Muscle relaxants** | |
| Talwin Compound | 325 mg aspirin | Norgesic | 385 mg aspirin |
| | | Robaxisal | 325 mg aspirin |

*From Andrea S. Vivian, PharmD, and Ira B. Goldberg, PharmD: Facts and Comparisons, April 1982; The Redbook, 1982; The Handbook of Nonprescription Drugs, 6th ed, 1979.

†Analgesics labeled "compound" usually contain aspirin.

ceptible to salicylism.[122,123] The hepatic and renal side effects of the drug can be safely ignored in rheumatoid arthritis unless frank symptoms of hepatitis develop. It is unnecessary to monitor transaminase levels, creatinine, or urea in the patient on long-term therapy unless, especially in the elderly patient, there is a change that sharply alters fluid and electrolyte balance.

In juvenile arthritis and in rheumatic fever, aspirin is usually used in doses of 80 to 100 mg per kg per day, although sometimes doses up to 130 mg per kilogram per day are used. Children seem to tolerate high serum levels of salicylates better than adults, and therapeutic levels of over 30 mg percent are considered tolerable. The mild hepatitis that can be detected by blood tests is not a contraindication to continuing the drug, but any signs of bleeding or jaundice are.[124] The principles of aspirin administration in children have been clearly explained in pediatric literature.[125,126]

dren have been clearly explained in pediatric literature.[125,126]

In osteoarthritis and fibrositis, doses well short of supposed anti-inflammatory doses are usually adequate for analgesia, and there is no reason to push higher in the absence of overt inflammation.

In systemic lupus erythematosus, aspirin is often as good as or even better than corticosteroids for fever, arthritis, pleurisy, and pericarditis, and it is the drug of first choice in many clinics.[127] The starting dose should not exceed 2.4 g per day, but it can be raised to anti-inflammatory levels for arthritis and serositis. It is uncertain (see Side Effects and Toxicities) whether chronic liver damage occurs as a very rare sequel to salicylate-induced hepatitis, and it is true that the hepatitis may fade away as disease activity recedes, but it is safest to reduce the dose or stop temporarily if the serum transaminase rises rapidly in a hospitalized patient or is found to exceed about ten times normal in an ambulatory patient. If a random elevation of less than that is found in an otherwise reasonably well patient, the drug can be safely continued if the observation will be close. Minor alterations in renal function can occur with almost all the prostaglandin synthetase-inhibiting anti-inflammatory drugs and are not an indication for stopping therapy unless the change is marked or is accompanied by proteinuria, edema, or oliguria. Measurements of renal function to be used in therapeutic decisions, however, should not be made while a patient is taking those drugs.[128]

In ankylosing spondylitis, some patients will respond to anti-inflammatory doses of aspirin, and it may be worth trying. The same is true for the other spondyloarthritides and psoriatic arthritis.

Aspirin and salicylates no longer have a place in the treatment of crystal-induced disease. Not only are they not as effective as other drugs, but the peculiar effect of salicylates on the serum uric acid and urinary urate excretion can complicate evaluation and management.

Aspirin or salicylate can be tried for symptomatic relief in a variety of other connective tissue diseases, but is likely to be ineffective for the major manifestations of scleroderma, dermatopolymyositis, polyarteritis, polymyalgia rheumatica, and temporal arteritis.

## INTERACTIONS WITH OTHER DRUGS*

Of the many drugs likely to be given with aspirin or salicylates, with few are there significant interactions. Much of the writing on the subject deals with the interactions of aspirin with acetaminophen, with indomethacin, and with the newer nonsteroidal anti-inflammatory drugs, and is concerned with the influence of one drug on the absorption or half-life of the other, not with their clinical interactions. These writings generally teach that there is little pharmacologic reason to give these drugs in combination but even less to forbid them. There are other interactions that are occasionally important: with coumarin anticoagulants, with uricosurics, with corticosteroids, with methotrexate, and with oral hypoglycemics (Table 49–2).

Salicylate displaces indomethacin from a plasma protein binding site, raising the unbound drug level, and thereby accelerating its clearance and metabolism.[130] Thus, aspirin at a dose of 3 to 6 g per day slightly lowers the peak serum indomethacin level when the two drugs are given simultaneously and has an inconstant effect on the serum disappearance.[131-134] This is altogether a small effect of no clinical significance. Indomethacin does not alter serum salicylate levels.[135] Both drugs are potent inhibitors of prostaglandin synthetase, and they may act at the same site on the enzyme, since indomethacin inhibits acetylation of the platelet enzyme by aspirin.[136] Since this enzyme inhibition is responsible for some or perhaps all the pharmacologic action of both drugs, and since at full doses of either roughly the same effects are achieved, they would be expected neither to be additive nor significantly to interfere with one another. Such is the case in the few human and animal studies in which their clinical interaction has been measured. The long-lasting effects of both drugs in an animal model are probably irrelevant.[107] Despite some common side effects, there is no evidence that toxicities are additive. Of great theoretical and probably practical interest are the observations on interactions between salicylates and aspirin. Salicylate, like indomethacin, can prevent aspirin's irreversible inactivation of platelet prostaglandin synthetase by acetylation, and it can blunt some of aspirin's effects on the stomach (see Side Effects and Toxicities).

Aspirin has minor effects on the metabolism of acetaminophen,[137,138] including a reduction in acetaminophen-induced hepatotoxicity in mice.[139] Of greater interest is the finding in man that when a single dose of acetaminophen (650 mg) is given simultaneously with a single dose of aspirin (650 mg), total serum acetylsalicylic acid levels are higher and remain high much longer than when aspirin is given alone, but total salicylate levels are unchanged. At 1 hour, the serum level of aspirin was 3.32 $\mu$g per milliliter when the drug was given alone and 9.33 $\mu$g per milliliter when given with acetaminophen.[140] The mechanism for this effect on deacetylation is unknown and its clinical value unexplored. Although it would be useful to prolong the pharmacologic effects of aspirin, possible adverse effects on the liver of such combination therapy suggest caution.

What is true of the similarity in pharmacologic effects between aspirin and indomethacin is true also of the similarities among all the newer nonsteroidal anti-inflammatory drugs that can inhibit prostaglandin synthesis, although doubtless there will be subtle differences that are due to different sensitivities of the enzymes in various tissues. Consequently there is little interest in details of their interaction. From the few clinical studies, it was learned that ibuprofen can increase the level of free as opposed to protein-bound salicylate as measured in vitro by equilibrium dialysis;[141] a single dose of aspirin could slightly lower peak naproxen levels, probably by displacement from protein, leading to further excretion, but there was no effect on salicylate levels,[142] and aspirin lowered fenoprofen levels both acutely and chronically, possibly by increasing hydroxylation of the drug, but fenoprofen did not affect salicylate levels.[143] None of these interactions appear to be of any clinical significance. There is no indication that toxicities of drugs in this class are additive.

The interaction with the coumarin family of anticoagulants is variable and often not significant in an individual patient. Aspirin alone may have minor effects on prothrombin time and may reduce the amount of anticoagulant necessary to maintain a given prothrombin time.[129,144,145] Of far greater importance is the fact that they are inhibitors of different steps in the coagu-

*This subject is well reviewed in Reference 129.

**Table 49–2.** Interactions of Aspirin (A) and Salicylates (S) with Other Drugs

| Drugs or Class of Drugs | Interaction | Clinical Implications |
|---|---|---|
| Nonsteroidal anti-inflammatory | | |
| Indomethacin | A lowers serum levels slightly; not vice versa | None |
| Ibuprofen | Protein-bound S level reduced | None |
| Naproxen | A lowers serum levels slightly | None |
| Fenoprofen | A lowers serum levels slightly; not vice versa | None |
| Salicylate | Blocks A's irreversible inactivation of platelet prostaglandin synthetase | Uncertain |
| Acetaminophen | Raises serum A level but leaves total S level unchanged | None |
| Coumarin anticoagulants | A variably reduces prothrombin time further when added | Reduction of anticoagulant dose |
| Uricosuric agents | A/S blocks uricosuric effect | A/S should not be used with them |
| Sulfonylurea oral hypoglycemics | A/S variably potentiates hypoglycemic action | Reduction of sulfonylurea dose |
| Corticosteroids | Lower serum S levels | Observe S level when steroids reduced |
| Diuretics | | |
| Furosemide | S blunts diuresis | Observe for this effect |
| Spironolactone | S blunts diuresis | |
| Antacids | Accelerate both absorption and excretion of A/S | Overall tendency to lower serum S levels when added |
| Methotrexate | A displaces methotrexate from protein-binding sites and enhances marrow depression | Caution, especially when using large doses of methotrexate |
| Ethanol | Synergistic effect with aspirin on gastrointestinal bleeding and bleeding time | Do not mix |

lation scheme and consequently may increase the tendency for bleeding as a side effect of oral anticoagulant therapy. It is for this reason that these drugs should be given together only when necessary and that aspirin should be avoided when any other defect in the coagulation system, inherited or acquired, is present.

Salicylate has complicated dose-dependent effects on both uric acid reabsorption and secretion, probably in part through its competition as an organic anion. In low doses, these actions raise serum uric acid, and in high doses they may lower it. Any dose of aspirin or salicylate can block the uricosuric action of both probenecid and sulfinpyrazone and consequently should not be used together with them.[146] The newer uricosuric, benzbromarone, is less affected.[147] Aspirin, in common with other prostaglandin-synthetase inhibitors, can blunt a furosemide- or spironolactone-induced diuresis, especially under circumstances in which prostaglandins are contributing to the maintenance of renal blood flow (see Side Effects and Toxicities).[148,149]

Although aspirin and salicylates do not lower blood sugar in normal subjects, they may potentiate the hypoglycemic effects of the sulfonylurea drugs by unknown mechanisms, perhaps stimulating insulin secretion,[150] and doses may have to be modified accordingly.[129]

Any drugs that markedly alter urine pH can have an effect on salicylate levels, since salicylate excretion is markedly accelerated at high urine pH. Theoretically, ascorbate or other urine acidifiers could raise serum salicylate levels, but this does not appear to be a problem. A problem with ascorbate potentially related to aspirin is that it can make the routine tests for stool occult blood falsely negative, thus obscuring a gastrointestinal blood loss.[151] Nonabsorbable as well as absorbable antacids can influence both the absorption and excretion of salicylates (see above).

Corticosteroids can lower the level of serum salicylate so that, when they are withdrawn, the serum level at a constant dose may rise substantially, even into the toxic range.[152] It is the impression of many clinicians that adverse effects of the two drugs on the gastrointestinal tract are additive or even synergistic.

Ethanol in the form of alcoholic beverages and aspirin probably are synergistic in their tendency to cause gastrointestinal bleeding from gastritis and gastric ulcer, and ethanol prolongs and potentiates aspirin's effect on bleeding time.[153]

Aspirin, probably by displacing methotrexate from protein-binding sites, enhances the bone marrow depressing effects of the antimetabolite. This has been shown clinically in studies with patients given large intra-arterial doses of methotrexate for malignancies.[154] Bone marrow depression, usually on the day after the injection, occurred almost exclusively in those patients who also received aspirin during the infusion. Studies in mice have confirmed this interaction experimentally.[155] It does not appear to potentiate the toxicity of the small doses of methotrexate used in current rheumatologic practice.

An interaction between phenytoin (Dilantin) and salicylate involving protein binding is not clinically important.[156]

## ASPIRIN AND SALICYLATES IN PREGNANCY

In this day it is unnecessary to caution against the use in pregnancy of a drug even so apparently benign as aspirin.[157] The issue is how to assess the risk to the pregnant woman whose own illness demands anti-inflammatory therapy. The risk of congenital malformation that can be attributed to aspirin is negligible,[158] and neither hypoglycemia nor bleeding problems are more common in babies born of mothers taking salicylates.[159] The clinical significance of the altered hemostasis found in newborns of mothers taking aspirin in the last 10 days of pregnancy is doubtful.[160,161] In a large study of women taking aspirin at least twice a week, no increased incidence of stillbirth or perinatal mortality was found, and mean birth weight was unaffected.[162] That study, however, did not focus on women who took aspirin daily. In a smaller study of women in Australia who took salicylate-containing powders daily more for social than for genuine medical indications, mean birth weight, even corrected for the high incidence of smoking in this population, was significantly lower (3283 grams vs. 3502 grams in controls), and there were four stillbirths near term compared with none in a control group.[159] Pregnancy was an average of a week longer, ante-partum and post-partum hemorrhage was more common, and anemia in the mother was more frequent (uncorrected for other factors such as smoking), but labor was not significantly prolonged.[163]

The only study to focus on women who took aspirin for rheumatologic disease during pregnancy was a retrospective chart survey covering a 20-year period, so its findings must be accepted cautiously.[164] Gestation was prolonged by about a week, labor prolonged by about 5 hours, and estimated blood loss increased by about 100 ml in aspirin-takers with rheumatologic disease compared with normal women or with women with rheumatologic disease not taking aspirin. Reduced birth weight was common to the children of women with rheumatologic disease whether or not the women took aspirin. In both studies of women who took aspirin daily, there was an increased incidence of pregnancies lasting more than 42 weeks. Although the prostaglandin synthetase–inhibiting drugs have the useful property of promoting closure of a patent ductus arteriosus in the newborn, the same effect may occur prematurely in the fetus, leading to persistent pulmonary hypertension of the newborn.[165]

For the woman who must take an anti-inflammatory agent during pregnancy, aspirin can be relied on not to increase the risk of congenital malformation but does add some risk of prolonged gestation and labor and an increase of perinatal maternal bleeding. Since these risks are probably related to the prostaglandin synthetase-inhibiting properties of the drug, they are likely to depend on continued use of the drug. For the same reason, other drugs that inhibit prostaglandin synthetase are likely to share those effects. A sensible course would seem to be to stop anti-inflammatory medication if possible in the last month.

The infants born to women taking salicylates until term pose no special medical problems, although it is interesting to note that they have higher serum salicylate levels than their mothers.[31]

## SIDE EFFECTS AND TOXICITIES

Under this heading I will discuss those effects of aspirin that are extratherapeutic. They are not all toxicities, and they are not all unwanted. Aside from the relation to major gastrointestinal hemorrhage and a controversial and doubtful relation to analgesic nephropathy, the toxicities of aspirin and salicylate are neither chronic nor cumulative. Furthermore, they are rapidly and completely reversible with a reduction of dose or cessation of therapy.

**Allergy.** For the many rheumatologists who have never or only rarely seen an allergic response to aspirin, the problem may seem remote, but a patient with a tale of an allergic response to aspirin is not rare in the office of the allergist. The incidence is well below 1 percent in a normal population but considerably higher in an allergy practice.[166] The earliest good description is of four cases of severe asthma, one fatal, induced, ironically, by "M. Matte's German Asthma Powder," which contained aspirin and caffeine.[167] By the early 1950s the essential immunologic facts of aspirin "allergy" were clear:[168] skin tests are negative for aspirin,[169,170] sodium salicylate does not provoke the allergy;[169] and there is no antibody detectable by passive cutaneous anaphylaxis (and presumably, therefore, no IgE or homocytotropic IgG antibody).[170,171] Later studies have confirmed these findings more elegantly. By the end of the preprostaglandin era, a nonimmune mechanism already seemed likely. It is now apparent that the "allergy"-inducing potential of the class of drugs is related to their ability to affect prostaglandin synthesis; not only aspirin (as little as 30 mg)[172] but other prostaglandin synthetase inhibitors, indomethacin (as little as 5 mg), mefenamic acid, flufenamic acid, fenoprofen, ibuprofen, and phenylbutazone, reduce air flow in aspirin-sensitive patients, whereas salicylate, salicylamide, acetaminophen, and propoxyphene do not.[173,174] What remains unknown is the site of the affected enzyme, and the exact way in which prostaglandins and leukotrienes affect the airways.

Clinically, the patients fall roughly into two categories: those who react to aspirin with bronchospasm and those who react with urticaria and angioedema. About half of those who have the bronchospastic reaction also have nasal polyps, in contrast to fewer than 15 percent of those with the urticaria-angioedema reaction.[175] Of those with the asthmatic response, at least half can be classified as having "intrinsic" asthma (normal IgE, normal skin tests, no recognizable environmental provocation or seasonal variation).[176] It seems likely that these patients have a metabolic defect either making them unusually sensitive to inhibition of prostaglandin synthetase because of a property of the enzyme itself or causing their airflow regulation to be abnormally dependent on prostaglandins to remain adequate.

In a large series of patients attending an allergy clinic, 3.8 percent of the asthmatics had aspirin allergy, the rate being higher for those with intrinsic (4.7 percent) than extrinsic (3.5 percent) asthma.[176] Most asthmatics who react to aspirin have the bronchospastic response, whereas among the 1.4 percent of rhinitis patients with aspirin allergy, the angioedema response predominated. Tartrazine sensitivity occurred in fewer than 20 percent of aspirin-allergic patients. The reported rate of 0.9 percent of "allergic" aspirin intolerance among normals seems to me inordinately high.[176]

Because aspirin is used so widely and because the "allergic" response requires only small, not full, rheumatologic doses to provoke it, aspirin allergy is virtually never discovered by the rheumatologist. If a patient gives a convincing history of bronchospasm, urticaria, or angioedema in relation to taking aspirin, however, it is likely that indomethacin, ibuprofen, fenoprofen, naproxen, tolectin, and probably phenylbutazone will provoke a similar response and ought to be avoided. Nonacetyl salicylate preparations can be used in this setting.

**Tinnitus and Hearing Loss.** Patients treated with salicylates will often note a high-pitched ringing in the ear and diminished hearing. Occasionally, they will also have vertigo, dizziness, and loss of balance. These toxicities are dose related and are probably all due to effects on the inner ear rather than on the central nervous system.

A raised threshold for all sound frequencies can be demonstrated by audiometry.[177] The change is roughly proportional to the serum salicylate level and is rapidly and completely reversible within 24 to 72 hours even if the drug has been taken for many years. The loss amounts to 20 to 40 decibels and occurs preferentially in the frequency range in which hearing is normal in those with pre-existing high tone deafness, thus leading to a flatter audiogram. Salicylates have little or no effect on presbycusis in which there is already a flat depressed acuity. The hearing loss is sensorineural, can be produced in several animal species,[178-182] and is unassociated with any recognizable morphologic changes in either animals or man, even if the drugs have been taken for many years with a known effect on hearing.[183] Salicylate-intoxicated cats show some biochemical changes in enzymes of the endolymph and perilymph, but what relationship this has to the ototoxicity is unknown.[178] Vestibular changes can be measured in humans as changes in the nystagmus induced by caloric stimulation and presumably account for the dizziness, vertigo, and imbalance.[183]

Tinnitus occurs universally in patients with normal hearing who take sufficient salicylate or aspirin. It comes on only when the serum salicylate exceeds 20 mg per dl, occurring on the average at about 30 mg per dl.[184] In these patients it is a useful guide to dosage, since it appears when the serum level is in the supposed anti-inflammatory range; the dose can be raised gradually until the appearance of tinnitus and then held steady at a slightly lower dose. Patients who have a high-tone hearing loss prior to salicylates often do not experience tinnitus even with very high salicylate levels. If there is any suspicion of a hearing deficit, or in any older patient, serum salicylate ought to be measured rather than waiting for tinnitus to occur.

**Gastrointestinal Effects.** The effects of aspirin and salicylate on the gastrointestinal tract have played a large role in their history. Aspirin itself was first popularized as a salicylate with less tendency to irritate the gastrointestinal tract; then attempts were made to reduce the gastric irritancy of aspirin; and now the newer nonsteroidal anti-inflammatory drugs claim to be no better than aspirin, merely less irritating to the gastrointestinal tract.

Because of the confusion concerning the gastrointestinal effects of aspirin and salicylate, it is helpful to examine separately the three major effects: symptomatic gastrointestinal distress, microbleeding, and frank gastritis or ulcer.

*Gastrointestinal Symptoms.* Gastrointestinal symptoms following use of aspirin occur occasionally and range from a very mild discomfort elicited only by direct or repeated questioning to heartburn, nausea, or severe discomfort occurring after a single tablet. Many patients with rheumatoid arthritis will tolerate a minor gastrointestinal discomfort as they will tolerate tinnitus in order to keep the beneficial effects of aspirin or salicylate. In various surveys the incidence of complaint has ranged from less than 2 percent to almost 40 percent, reflecting many factors related to the study design: whether or not the subjects knew they were getting aspirin, how a history of side effects was elicited, what condition the drug was given for, the age of the subjects, the dose of the drug, and doubtless sometimes the expectation or prejudice of the investigator.[185-189] Toxicities as well as benefit are subject to a placebo effect.

The form of aspirin does not appear to influence the incidence of gastrointestinal distress; in several controlled studies, aspirin and buffered aspirin have been found equally guilty.[186,187,190] Nor do symptoms correlate with the presence or amount of microbleeding or gastroscopic abnormalities.[191-194] It is my impression, however, that currently available enteric-coated aspirins are better tolerated as well as objectively less irritating (see below).

The mechanisms responsible for gastrointestinal symptoms are largely unknown, but probably a direct irritation to the mucosa, psychological expectations, and a central nervous system effect of salicylate all contribute. A dose of sodium salicylate given intravenously caused nausea at the same serum salicylate level as when the drug was given by mouth.[195] Since it is known that salicylate does not diffuse from the serum into the gastrointestinal tract, an extraluminal, probably extraintestinal central nervous system effect must have been responsible.

In practical terms, if gastrointestinal intolerance occurs when aspirin or salicylate is begun or when the dose is raised, and if the drug is otherwise having a therapeutic benefit, it is wisest to switch preparations to buffered, to enteric-coated, or to a liquid form, or to use one of the maneuvers suggested above (see Clinical Use). A substantial proportion of patients will be able to continue the drug with such switches from time to time. It has been repeatedly observed that some people who claim gastric intolerance to aspirin are able to tolerate it if they are unaware that it is being given or if it is given in another form. Of course switching to another nonsteroidal drug is sensible if intolerance persists. Combining two nonsteroidals (including aspirin) in submaximal doses sometimes works, too.

*Microbleeding and Gastroscopic Changes.* The ingestion of aspirin causes the loss of small amounts of blood (about 2.5 ml per day above a background loss of about 0.5 ml per day) into the stool in about 70 percent of people.[191,193,196-202] Although a sensitive qualitative test may sometimes detect losses this small,[203] most patients taking aspirin will not have occult blood on routine testing, and investigation of the circumstances of this loss has required the measurement of fecal radioactivity after the injection of $^{51}$Cr-labeled autologous red blood cells. There is a large literature devoted to studies of this sort, most predicated upon the view that this blood loss is somehow related to other gastrointestinal effects of aspirin and salicylates, a view that is open to serious doubt.

Aspirin, soluble aspirin, calcium aspirin, aspirin in solution, aspirin in suspension, aspirin given with milk, and over-the-counter buffered aspirins are roughly equivalent in their ability to cause blood loss.[196,204] Sodium salicylate, choline salicylate, effervescent aspirin, or aspirin given with enough sodium bicarbonate or nonabsorbable, nonsodium-containing buffers causes little or no blood loss,[8,193,203,205-209] and the presence of achlorhydria markedly diminishes the loss.[201,202] No minimum dose for this toxicity has been found, but the loss does increase with increasing dose in the clinical range.[196] Furthermore, some subjects lose a great deal more than the average and are probably those few whose chronic iron deficiency anemia may be due to aspirin.[193,210] Ethanol, which itself does not cause this sort of microbleeding, does potentiate aspirin's effect.[199,211] There does not appear to be any adaptation, since microbleeding at 4 weeks or even as long as a year after starting therapy continues at about the same rate.[212,213] Intravenous aspirin in doses leading to the same serum salicylate level and the same effect on bleeding time causes a negligibly small increment blood loss in subjects with a normal gastrointestinal tract.[204,214] Nor does the ingestion of coumarin anticoagulants increase the rate of blood loss.[215]

Normal volunteers and patients with rheumatoid arthritis have the same frequency of microbleeding (about 70 percent) and the same range of blood loss.[193] Even patients who have recently had a major gastrointestinal hemorrhage from peptic ulcer disease have a similar frequency and degree of microbleeding.[210] Most patients with rheumatoid arthritis do not develop a chronic anemia that can be attributed to aspirin. On the contrary, patients who take aspirin over the course of a year for arthritis are likely to have a slightly higher hemoglobin than before they began the drug, probably because their disease activity has been diminished.[216]

Gastroscopic abnormalities after aspirin have been known for over 40 years, although much has been made of them recently with the advent of easier endoscopy.[137] There has been controversy over their actual incidence, location, nature, and even their relation to drug ingestion, but there is no doubt that aspirin given to a fasting subject with an empty stomach can lead to visible abnormalities ranging from hyperemia, petechiae, and submucosal hemorrhage to superficial erosion or even frank ulceration with visible intraluminal blood.[137,217-222,237,238] This is not a placebo effect, although occasionally placebo-treated subjects show some abnormalities. It occurs more frequently with aspirin than with other nonsteroidal prostaglandin synthetase inhibitors, although like microbleeding, it is by no means absent with them,[237,238] and tolerance does not develop over several weeks. The reported incidence has varied considerably, even to as high as 100 percent,[221] but all observers do not use equivalent language to describe their findings; one observer's hyperemia may well be another's superficial erosion. From both animal and human studies, the microscopic damage that accompanies the visible abnormalities is extremely quick to reverse, being largely gone within an hour of the dose of drug and completely gone by 6 hours.[222]

In view of their similar frequency, the fact that tolerance develops to neither, and the fact that adequate buffering can prevent both of them, it is reasonable to conclude that the microscopic blood loss originates in the visible lesions. *Most important, however, from a practical point of view, is that these abnormalities are markedly reduced if aspirin is given in an enteric-coated form, both in normals and in patients with rheumatologic diseases.*[223-226]

Prostaglandin synthesis inhibition is probably a necessary but insufficient cause for aspirin's gastric effects. Oral aspirin does inhibit gastric prostaglandin synthesis in man,[227,228] and, strikingly, the administration of some prostaglandins along with aspirin largely inhibits fecal blood loss,[229-231] reduces endoscopic damage,[232] and prevents the changes in gastric wall potential and ion fluxes that are associated with gastric damage (see below).[233,234] Intravenous aspirin does not affect the gastric mucosa or ion fluxes,[235] but its effect on gastric prostaglandin synthesis is not known. It seems likely that the peculiar propensity for plain aspirin to produce gastric damage is related to a powerful direct local effect on gastric prostaglandin synthesis aided by either high local concentration of the drug due to its insolubility or a second irritative effect, perhaps on gastric mucous[229] or local blood flow.[236]

The mechanism of microbleeding and gastroscopic changes is mysterious. They are clearly not due to platelet effects or other effects on the measurable coagulation factors. Despite earlier evidence that particles of undissolved drug might be involved in mucosal damage, soluble aspirin can cause microbleeding (although it may be argued that, in the acid environment of the stomach, aspirin might be precipitated from sodium aspirin solutions). Acid does seem necessary, since adequate buffering prevents it.[219] The fact that achlorhydria is also protective may reflect not only the absence of acid but also the more rapid cell turnover of the gastric mucosa characteristic of that condition, thus allowing more rapid repair.[239] The Davenport model (see below) postulates that the back-diffusion of acid into the gastric wall caused by an effect of aspirin on the gastric mucosal barrier liberates histamine locally, which dilates capillaries, presumably leading to diapedesis of red cells, some of which make their way to the gastric lumen through ruptured intercellular bridges.[240]

Do they relate to major blood loss, either chronic or acute? They are probably responsible, in the rare person with a large asymptomatic daily loss, for a chronic iron deficiency anemia. If the visible lesions are the precursor of the rare gastric ulcer or gastritis leading to major blood loss, it is easy to imagine that any condition that impedes the repair process, such as uremia, stress, ingestion of ethanol or corticosteroids, or an intercurrent illness, could potentiate the danger of aspirin.[239,241] There is no direct evidence, however, to link them to acute gastrointestinal bleeding caused by gastritis or peptic ulcer. Major hemorrhage retrospectively related to aspirin ingestion is as likely to have occurred with buffered or even effervescent aspirin,[242-244] which does not cause microbleeding, as with plain aspirin, and while the visible mucosal changes and the microbleeding are very common, major gastrointestinal hemorrhage is uncommon or even rare. The relation among them remains uncertain.

Does microbleeding or the visible gastroscopic changes relate in any way to complaints of gastrointestinal distress? In every series in which microbleeding or mucosal changes and symptoms have been recorded there has been a dissociation; some have distress without microbleeding or changes, and most have microbleeding or changes without distress.[191-194]

Both microbleeding and visible gastroscopic changes can be prevented by adequate buffering with sodium-containing buffers as in effervescent aspirin, but only at a cost of a prohibitive sodium intake for the chronic aspirin taker, and it is difficult to incorporate sufficient nonabsorbable buffer into an oral tablet. Sodium salicylate is thought by many to be pharmacologically inferior to aspirin. With sufficient ingenuity, an uncoated preparation of aspirin that caused little microbleeding or visible mucosal changes could probably be developed.[208] The availability of well-absorbed enteric-coated aspirin with markedly diminished effects on the stomach probably renders further efforts to do so unnecessary.

Neither microbleeding nor visible mucosal changes are the more dangerous for our being able to measure them or see them. If the gastrointestinal effects of aspirin and salicylate are to influence the way we use them, then it must, in my opinion, be those that relate to patient comfort, for which appropriate individual adjustments are made, or those that relate to clear-cut morbidity or mortality, such as ulcer or major hemorrhage, for which there is yet no evidence that aspirin is a worse offender than any of the alternatives.

***Ulcer, Gastritis, and Gastrointestinal Bleeding.*** Does aspirin cause major gastrointestinal bleeding? Ulcer? How often? Who is particularly susceptible? Can anything prevent it? What should be done if it occurs? Does anything potentiate the risk? What is safer than aspirin?

The evidence that aspirin causes major gastrointestinal bleeding is roughly as follows: In a large number of surveys of patients admitted to the hospital or studied as outpatients for major gastrointestinal bleeding and/or ulcer, the patients have been from two to five times more likely to have taken aspirin in the few days prior to admission than a group of control patients.[185,242-249] The choice of controls has varied in the studies and has been the focal point for much criticism. It may be, for example, that patients with any gastrointestinal problem more readily remember taking aspirin because of its publicized gastrointestinal effects; or that they have taken aspirin (usually effervescent) to treat the early symptoms of their bleed; or that controls are more likely to have diseases which, like stroke, impair their ability to take part in a survey. Even more remarkable is the extraordinary range of frequency of aspirin ingestion in the various populations—from 25 percent to over 90 percent.[250] Despite the imperfections of such studies, the qualitative conclusion is inescapable: a proportion of major gastrointestinal bleeding or ulcer is related to the recent ingestion of aspirin.[251] Such surveys also have established that buffered aspirin and effervescent aspirins are often the culprits, probably no less often than plain aspirin,[242-244,252] and that alcohol ingestion increases the risk of aspirin.[242,246,247] The episodes have been gastrointestinal bleeding without a visible source and therefore attributed to gastritis, gastric ulcer with bleeding, or gastric ulcer without bleeding.[252] Duodenal ulcer does not appear related.

In another type of survey, chronic gastric ulcer in young women in Australia was found to be quite common and highly likely to be associated with the chronic ingestion of headache powders; the incidence of gastric ulcer in women rose markedly as these powders came into vogue.[253] Furthermore, ulcer disease leading to gastrectomy is very common in analgesic abusers who have developed analgesic nephropathy, although it is difficult in that population to point a finger with any assurance at any particular drug or to ignore psychological factors.[254]

In a survey of hospitalized patients, habitual aspirin ingestion (four or more times per week) contributed to uncomplicated benign gastric ulcer and to new episodes of gastrointestinal bleeding not due to duodenal ulcer.[252] In that study, it was estimated, based on the known populations from which the patients were drawn, that the drug added a total of 25 cases per 100,000 users of aspirin per year. This is a very small risk indeed. Aspirin also increased the risk of bleeding in heparinized patients, which reinforces the stricture against using aspirin when another coagulation deficit exists.[255]

While aspirin does not appear to cause duodenal ulcer, patients with duodenal ulcer are not immune from its effects on the stomach. No formal survey proves that such patients are unusually susceptible to aspirin, but most physicians are properly cautious about using it. The hypersecretion of acid and pylorospasm characteristic of duodenal ulcer disease might be expected to contribute to a gastric toxicity of aspirin. In the absence of a strong indication (see below), it should be avoided.

Factors such as stress, alcohol ingestion, concurrent illness, other medications, diet, age, sex, and season as well as others probably contribute to the tendency of aspirin to cause gastric ulcer and gastritis with or without bleeding. Increased acid secretion may be a factor; however, ulcer and bleeding may occur, although rarely, in the patient with achlorhydria, too.[256,257]

There is no evidence that regular antacid ingestion or a switch to salicylate or even enteric-coated aspirin can prevent a risk of major gastrointestinal bleeding, but establishing a change in the frequency of a rare event is extremely difficult. *Most importantly, there is no evidence whatever that the incidence of ulcer or major gastrointestinal bleeding is any different with any other nonsteroidal anti-inflammatory drug from what it is with aspirin.*

Are rheumatologic patients or any subgroup of them particularly susceptible to the gastrointestinal effects of aspirin? There is no evidence that this is so. The incidence of ulcer disease in patients with rheumatic diseases may be higher than in the general population, but not all studies are in agreement on this point, and in particular they have not adequately assessed the role of drugs. Patients with rheumatoid arthritis are not more susceptible to aspirin-related gastrointestinal discomfort or microbleeding.

Clinically, gastric ulcer and gastritis in the patient with arthritis and in the normal individual are no different. It is my impression that gastric ulcer is more common than symptomatic gastritis with bleeding or silent gastrointestinal hemorrhage among rheumatologic patients. Major gastrointestinal bleeding related to aspirin is probably very rare in children, although a report of 12 children with melena, hematemesis, or anemia,[258] with frank ulceration in two children,[259] following therapeutic doses of aspirin suggests that it does occur.

What should be done when ulcer or gastrointestinal bleeding occurs in the rheumatologic patient taking aspirin? Although we used to continue aspirin when peptic ulcer occurred if it appeared necessary to manage rheumatoid arthritis, and found that ulcers usually healed,[260] a more sensible course is to add cimetidine.[261-265] When the ulcer is healed, there is no contraindication to a return to aspirin with antacid.

*Potential Difference.* When unbuffered aspirin is instilled into the stomach of man or experimental animals, the electrical potential difference between the gastric mucosa and the skin or a peripheral vein is reduced from its normal of $-40$ mv to about $-30$ mv.[266,267] It is likely that this change in potential reflects a change in the mucosal barrier that protects the stomach from the high acid concentrations of gastric secretion. In experimental animals, particularly the dog with an isolated gastric pouch, the potential changes induced by aspirin parallel a back-diffusion of hydrogen ions into the stomach wall and leakage of sodium and chloride into the lumen.[268,269] Davenport's theory of the gastric damaging effects of aspirin postulates that this back-diffusion leads to the release of histamine, capillary dilatation, increased acid production, and, if there is a sufficient concentration of acid in the lumen initially, gastric erosion and bleeding. Because of the difficulty of measuring ion fluxes in man, measurement of changes in the potential difference has been used as a surrogate for changes in the gastric mucosal barrier.

Aspirin causes a reduction in potential, but not if accompanied by adequate buffer (effervescent aspirin, nonabsorbable antacids, or sodium bicarbonate).[270,271] Ethanol alone reduces the potential and potentiates the reduction induced by aspirin.[270,272] Indomethacin, prednisone, and phenylbutazone do not alter the potential.[272] Bile acids, which cause gastric damage in animals and exacerbate aspirin's tendency to do so, also reduce the potential difference.[270] Glucagon, $PGE_2$, and cimetidine all increase the potential difference and, in the proper dose, block the potential reduction induced by aspirin.[261,263,273] In the case of glucagon, the intragastric pH is unaltered (i.e., it remains low), but gastric damage is prevented. In the case of cimetidine, the pH is raised to 7 and cell damage is blocked.

*Animal Studies.* Gastrointestinal effects of aspirin and salicylate have been studied in dogs, cats, rabbits, guinea pigs, rats, and even frogs. There are pronounced differences among different species in their susceptibility, so that extrapolation to man is hazardous.

The most useful studies have been by Davenport, using the dog with a Heidenhain pouch, an exteriorized isolated gastric pouch with intact blood supplied that can easily be filled and emptied. In his experiments, he instilled drugs with or without acid at various concentrations and measured the changes in ion concentration and the appearance of blood in the gastric fluid over time. He showed that aspirin or sodium salicylate in a weak acid solution (0.001 M HCl) breaks the mucosal barrier to ion fluxes, allowing hydrogen ions to back-diffuse into the gastric mucosa and sodium to leak into the lumen, but only with strong acid (0.1 M HCl) does bleeding occur.[274] Ethanol potentiates the effect of aspirin by lowering the concentration of acid at which bleeding appears. Davenport has summarized his findings and his model in an excellent review.[240]

Studies in rats, which develop ulcers easily with aspirin, have shown that stress,[275,276] starvation,[277] and bile acids[278,279] potentiate its effect, while bicarbonate,[280] vagotomy, atropine,[280,281] metiamide,[262] and cimetidine[275] ameliorate it. Giving very large quantities of glutamine[282] or cupric sulfate[283] or giving aspirin methyl ester[284] prevents the ulcers without inhibiting the beneficial pharmacologic effects.

Although it has been established in animals that aspirin does reduce both gastric venous[285] and gastric juice prostaglandin levels,[286] what relation this has to changes in the mucosal barrier, to ion fluxes, and to cell damage remains unknown. Gastric blood flow may increase,[287] decrease[288] or remain unchanged after aspirin, depending on the animal model;[241] likewise acid production is inconstantly affected.[241,288] Most attention has focused on the stomach, but permeability changes also occur in the small intestine.[289-291]

*Platelet and Coagulation Effects.* Aspirin's effects on platelets and coagulation have commanded attention because they were discovered early, have been easy to study, and have raised the hope of safe and effective prophylaxis against venous and arterial thrombosis. The principal effects are on platelets and bleeding time; there is a minor effect on synthesis of the vitamin K-dependent clotting factors.

Aspirin prolongs the bleeding time as tested by any of the standard assays. Most subjects, normal or rheumatoid, can be shown to respond, although the final bleeding time may remain within the normal range.[292-297] Curiously, women may be less affected than men.[298] On the average, the bleeding time is prolonged 1.5- to 2-fold. Sodium salicylate is without effect.[295] Ethanol can both potentiate and prolong this effect.[153] A minimal effective dose of aspirin has not been defined, although less than 1 gram a day can do it, and 0.44 gram is as effective as 4 grams.[297,299] The crudeness of the assay has limited the information that can be extracted from these studies, and it is, in fact, not certain that the effects on platelet cyclooxygenase described below rather than other effects on platelets, capillaries, arterioles, or local tissues are responsible for the altered bleeding time.

Soon after the discovery of the effects on bleeding time, several laboratories discovered that aspirin in vitro entirely blocked the aggregation of platelets by collagen or connective tissue fragments, and blocked a second wave of aggregation when platelets were exposed to ADP or epinephrine, while not blocking the initial aggregation these substances caused.[300-303] Later it was shown that aspirin blocked the release from platelets of serotonin and ADP from the dense granules,[304,305] that the initial adherence of aspirin-treated platelets to an injured vascular endothelium was unaffected but subsequent build-up of larger aggregates was blocked,[305-308] and that all these effects occurred with doses or levels of aspirin well below what are achieved in vivo after aspirin ingestion.[309-311] Although details in the picture of platelet aggregation remain to be worked out, the broad outline is roughly as follows. Various mechanical and chemical stimuli, including exposure to collagen, to damaged vascular endothelium, to excessive agitation, and to thrombin, ADP, and epinephrine, cause platelets to adhere to surfaces and to each other. During that process, arachidonate is mobilized and is metabolized by the enzyme platelet cyclooxygenase to the cyclic endoperoxide $PGG_2$, which is converted successively to thromboxane $A_2$ and $PGE_2$ and $PGF_2$, as well as to a number of other substances whose functions are not known. Thromboxane $A_2$ and probably also $PGG_2$ are released from the platelet into the surrounding fluid, where they cause the release of ADP and serotonin from the dense granules of other platelets.[312-314] The released ADP in turn aggregates these other platelets, causing them to adhere to the nearby initial aggregate.[315] The mechanism of dense granule release probably involves both GMP and calcium but is not presently well understood.[316,317] Aspirin, by blocking the initial step of synthesis in the prostaglandin pathway, blocks the release of $PGG_2$ and thromboxane $A_2$, thereby preventing the so-called release reaction and secondary aggregation. Platelets exposed to aspirin in vivo or in vitro demonstrate this lesion, and it is irreversible. If $PGG_2$ or additional ADP is provided, however, secondary aggregation can take place.

It is now clear that the acetyl group of the aspirin specifically acetylates a single platelet microsomal protein of molecular weight 85,000, the cyclooxygenase, and that the acetylation stoichiometrically irreversibly inactivates the enzyme.[24,318,319] The human platelet cyclooxygenase is peculiarly sensitive to this inactivation, at least 30 times as sensitive as the only other cyclooxygenase studied in detail.[314]

One 300 mg tablet of aspirin by mouth has a demonstrable effect on human platelets within 5 minutes and is maximally effective soon thereafter.[309] As expected, the more slowly absorbed enteric-coated aspirin reaches a maximal effect later, but inhibition is as great and lasts as long as with plain aspirin.[320] Although the platelets and megakaryocytes whose enzyme has been inhibited do not recover, as few as one third of normal platelets partially restore aggregation so that continued suppression may require daily ingestion.[314,321] With prolonged ingestion of somewhat higher doses, however, platelet aggregation returns despite continued complete inhibition of platelet cyclooxygenase, so no single mechanism offers a complete explanation.[322]

One of the complications is that salicylate itself, as well as indomethacin and diflunisal, though not acetaminophen, can block the acetylation of platelet oxygenase by aspirin.[323-325] In the case of salicylate, there is no inhibition of the enzyme; in the case of indomethacin, there is powerful reversible inhibition. These effects may depend upon the existence of more than one inhibitory site on the platelet enzyme, but details are lacking.[326-328]

The recently recognized ability of aspirin to inhibit vascular prostacyclin synthesis has also added complexity, since prostacyclins synthesized by vessel walls inhibit coagulation. Thus aspirin might promote coagulation by inhibiting vascular tissues while blocking coagulation by inhibiting platelets. With a *single* dose of aspirin as low as 30 mg, the platelet enzyme is inhibited far more than the vascular enzyme, either arterial or venous, but a *single* 300- or 325-mg tablet has profound effects on both enzymes.[329,330] With repeated doses, however, the situation that more closely approximates the rheumatologic use of aspirin, both enzymes are about equally affected.[322,331]

Several investigators have described effects of aspirin on other platelet functions, particularly in activating platelet factors 3 and 4.[303,332] Although they are of rapid onset, they may require somewhat larger doses. The consequences of this aspect of aspirin's action are not known.

Aspirin has a small inconsistent effect on the synthesis of the vitamin K–dependent clotting factors.[144,294] Some investigators have not found it at all. Rarely a patient will demonstrate bleeding and prolonged prothrombin time as a manifestation of aspirin toxicity.[124] Several of the reported cases occurred in people with a probable nutritional deficiency which may have contributed to the prothrombin problem.[333]

Of what clinical importance are the effects on coagulation, particularly on platelet function? Under ordinary conditions of aspirin use in the rheumatic diseases, none. The effect on prothrombin time is so weak and variable that it need be considered only when coumarin anticoagulants are administered simultaneously because the dose of anticoagulant sometimes but not always needs to be reduced (see above). The effect on platelets cannot be wholly responsible for the anti-inflammatory action of aspirin, since it occurs at doses at least 10-fold below anti-inflammatory doses. It might be argued that the antiplatelet effect contributes to the gastrointestinal microbleeding. That is exceedingly unlikely, since aspirin administered by other routes or so that it can be absorbed only beyond the stomach has just as much platelet effect but does not cause gastric microbleeding. Finally, there is no evidence, clinical or epidemiologic, that patients with rheumatic disease who are taking aspirin, even at the time of operation or even if another coagulation problem is present simultaneously, are disposed to bleed excessively. In a rare exception, aspirin appears to have been responsible for well-documented intravascular coagulation and aspirin-induced hepatitis in a young boy with Still's disease[334] and in a 17-year-old girl with "adult onset" juvenile rheumatoid arthritis.[335]

It is interesting to note that there exist patients whose platelets closely mimic aspirin-treated platelets.[305] In fact, a patient with deficient or absent platelet cyclooxygenase had no significant clinical illness.[312] This reflects, I believe, the happy natural redundancy of the coagulation system; under normal circumstances and sometimes in fact under any circumstances, deficits in the coagulation scheme can go unnoticed throughout a lifetime unless special tests uncover them.

Aspirin and other drugs that depress platelet function, such as dipyridamole and sulfinpyrazone, have been explored for their ability to prevent arterial and venous thrombosis, especially in patients with coronary and cerebral circulatory insufficiency and in bedridden patients after major surgery. It is beyond the scope of this chapter to review the evidence of these studies except to say that they show some modest promise in several clinical circumstances but almost surely will not prove to prevent major arteriosclerotic and thrombotic arterial disease, which occur all too often in patients who have taken aspirin for decades.

**Hematologic and Immunologic Effects.** ***White Cell Effects.*** Some investigators have found that aspirin or salicylate inhibits various in vitro functions of human or animal lymphocytes, including transformation in response to mitogens,[336] the allogeneic mixed lymphocyte reaction,[336] transformation in response to antigens,[337] and the production of migration inhibitory factor.[338,339] In some but not all experiments, the lymphocytes isolated from subjects taking aspirin have been found to respond subnormally.[340,341] The inhibition was sometimes related to serum level. The in vitro effects do occur in the range of drug levels found in the serum of patients, but it should be noted that when drug is added in vitro to a culture containing 20 percent plasma, the proportion of unbound drug is higher since the albumin concentration is lower. Data on the reversibility of the effect are inconsistent. These effects may be in some way related to the depressed levels of cyclic AMP found in the lymphocytes of subjects taking aspirin.[342]

In the only experiments in which lymphocyte responses to mitogen and antigens and corresponding skin tests were performed in a double-blind trial of aspirin and placebo administration to normals, aspirin showed no effect despite substantial serum levels.[343] Thus a healthy skepticism for claims that aspirin's anti-inflammatory effects are mediated by direct effects on lymphocytes is warranted, but indirect effects are still possible.

There have been a number of early studies of other immunologic effects of aspirin, which have been well reviewed.[116,344] These studies do not support a primary action on antibody synthesis; effects that have been reported, such as protection against the Schwartzman phenomenon in the rabbit, are more reasonably attributable to other actions of this class of drugs or occur at doses far from the clinical range.

Aspirin ingested by normal volunteers modestly decreased the ability of their granulocytes to adhere to nylon fibers in vitro for several hours after a 1.2-g dose, although sodium salicylate added in vitro had no effect.[345] The mechanism is unknown, but the changes in migration of leukocytes into inflammatory lesions in several animal models may be related to the adherence and movement of leukocytes.

***Aspirin in Genetic Hemolytic Anemias.*** In a large careful study, 22 patients with glucose-6-phosphate dehydrogenase did not show signs of hemolysis when given a 4-day course of aspirin at 50 mg per kilogram per day.[346] Glutathione levels in deficient red cells were not altered in vitro by exposure to aspirin or the metabolite gentisic acid, and Heinz bodies did not form. Neither chemical altered the hexose monophosphate shunt activity of normal red cells. There is a single case report alleging that a large dose of aspirin (6 grams per day) shortened the half-life of red cells to 16 days in an enzyme-deficient subject.[347] Because of the heterogeneity of the enzyme-deficiency state, caution is necessary in applying the results of observations to all patients.[348] It is likely that aspirin can be safely administered when clinically indicated to most deficient individuals.

A much rarer genetic defect, the severe anemia form of pyruvate kinase deficiency, may cause the red cells of affected individuals to be unusually susceptible to salicylates.[349] When exposed in vitro to aspirin, intracellular ATP falls and the cells have altered permeability and a decreased hexose monophosphate shunt, thereby diminishing their ability to manufacture glutathione. Consequently detoxification of other drugs may be impaired. The clinical importance of this is unknown.

*Cytopenia.* Aspirin and salicylate have almost never been convincingly implicated as a cause of anemia, leukopenia, or thrombocytopenia resulting from peripheral destruction of cells or marrow depression.[350]

**Pulmonary and Cardiovascular Effects.** ***Pulmonary Edema.*** The rare complication of pulmonary edema caused by salicylates was first recognized in patients being treated with full doses of salicylates for rheumatic fever, with or without carditis. It was described as "rheumatoid pneumonia," with the typical roentgenographic appearance of pulmonary edema.[351] The patients in whom it was originally described had an increased plasma volume, which was thought to account for the pulmonary edema. The presence of actual or possible carditis resulting from rheumatic fever clouded the early description,[352,353] although it was noted that a patient taking salicylates who had a roentgenographic picture of pulmonary edema might have no other signs of heart failure.[354,355] With the description of cases in otherwise healthy individuals, it became apparent that underlying heart disease was not a requirement.[356,357] In addition, there have been autopsies of two patients with fatal pulmonary edema which showed only congested lungs; the hearts were normal.[358] In one previously normal patient with pulmonary edema, catheterization showed a normal pulmonary artery pressure, normal pulmonary capillary wedge pressure, and normal pulmonary atrioventricular oxygen difference. The pathophysiology is most reminiscent of noncardiogenic pulmonary edema of the sort caused by morphine, heroin, and propoxyphene.[359] The only experimental evidence of a similar lesion was in awake sheep infused with aspirin.[360] They developed increased pulmonary lymph flow and leakage of serum proteins into pulmonary lymph but had normal cardiac function and pulmonary artery pressure. Thus, by a mechanism unknown, there is an outpouring of fluid into the pulmonary air spaces at a time when cardiac function is unimpaired. The physiologic consequences are dyspnea and cyanosis, and the radiologic consequence is pulmonary edema.

The syndrome is particularly likely to occur in elderly patients, often smokers, who have been taking salicylates chronically. The clinical presentation may be of lethargy, confusion, and metabolic acidosis.[122,123] The serum salicylate level is usually greater than 40 mg percent. The lesion is rare, but it may be the presenting manifestation of occult salicylism in the elderly and must therefore be kept in mind.[361] Although the mechanism of the hyperpnea regularly seen with high therapeutic doses of salicylates is central stimulation,[362] the clinical appearance may also be that of marked dyspnea. This effect is probably not due to the inhibition of prostaglandin synthesis, since neither indomethacin nor ibuprofen causes it in experimental animals.[363]

*Cardiovascular Effects.* Aspirin and salicylate are free of cardiac effects except as related to the anoxia of the drug-related pulmonary edema and acid-base disturbances. From the discovery that prostaglandin infusion could keep open a patent ductus in the newborn when that shunt was necessary for survival,[364,365] it was but a short step to the use of the prostaglandin synthetase inhibitors aspirin and indomethacin to close the duct in newborns in whom surgery might otherwise be necessary.[366,367] This simple and apparently benign therapy is now in wide use. In these infants, marked transient renal effects occur, probably the reflection of an unusual dependence on prostaglandins to maintain renal perfusion. In levels larger than those encountered even in severe intoxication there is a direct suppression of cardiac conduction tissue.[368] Some other vascular effects are probably of no clinical relevance.[369]

**Hepatic Effects.** The hepatitis caused by aspirin is in a sense a disease of advancing medical science; it was discovered when the serum transaminase test became available[370,371] and usually is discovered today only because that test is ordered routinely, not because symptomatic liver disease develops. It first was thought to be a chemical manifestation of liver disease in children with active rheumatic fever with carditis, and only later was it realized that the common factor was aspirin or salicylate therapy rather than the disease. Subsequently, children with rheumatoid arthritis,[372,373] especially females and those with the systemic type,[124] patients with active systemic lupus erythematosus,[374] and patients with any underlying liver disease have been found particularly but not exclusively susceptible.[375] Those with other forms of connective tissue disease and even otherwise healthy individuals may show hepatic injury, although often of but a trivial degree.[375,378]

Usually, abnormal transaminase occurs in the second or third week of therapy or after an increase of dose. A high proportion of patients who have active lupus erythematosus and some patients with juvenile rheumatoid arthritis will develop abnormalities, sometimes within a week of an increase in dose, and often rising to levels in the hundreds or even thousands. Most often the bilirubin remains normal even if transaminase is high for extended periods; the alkaline phosphatase may rise just into the abnormal range. Except in a few patients, usually children, prothrombin time is unaffected.[124] In those few, ecchymoses and frank bleeding may occur quite rapidly and drug should be immediately stopped and vitamin K and/or plasma given.

Although most patients with this hepatitis are asymptomatic, some develop nausea, anorexia, a loss of taste for cigarettes, and even an enlarging or tender liver.[374,378] Biopsies in cases of acute aspirin-related injury have generally shown a nonspecific toxic hepatitis with single cell necrosis, anisocytosis and aniso-nucleosis, and a mononuclear cell infiltrate in the lobule and in the portal areas.[376,379,380] Several patients have been seen in whom the lesion developed in the face of a recent normal liver biopsy, thereby establishing that underlying liver disease is not a precondition. There have been two patients reported in whom histologic chronic hepatitis has been found to be the probable result of long-term aspirin therapy.[375,379] Although this is probably a rare event, aspirin should be added to the list of potential inciting agents of idiopathic chronic hepatitis, especially if immunologic phenomena are a prominent feature, since systemic lupus erythematosus with aspirin-induced hepatitis may closely resemble chronic active hepatitis with immunologic features.

Early papers stressed the relationship to high serum salicylate levels, often over 30 mg per dl, but the hepatitis clearly can occur with a serum level below the therapeutic range, as low as 10 mg per dl. If abnormalities occur, they will disappear within a week or rarely 2 weeks when the drug is stopped or the dose is lowered. In addition, however, they will often disappear if the drug is continued in children with arthritis.[124,381] If aspirin is continued in a patient with active lupus who develops hepatitis, the abnormalities will occasionally disappear if the disease becomes less active. There are apparently spontaneous fluctuations, particularly in children with arthritis; if children are tested often enough, abnormal liver function tests will appear at some time or other in more than half of those on aspirin.[382]

The mechanism of this lesion is unknown. Eosinophilia and rash are not regularly associated with the hepatitis, and the toxicity is dose related. Together, these observations make a hypersensitivity type reaction very unlikely. Animal studies have not shed any light on this area. It is possible to show only trivial hepatic changes in rabbits despite long-term high-dose therapy with salicylate.[383] It is true that patients with liver disease are more susceptible and that such patients have a reduced level of aspirin esterase,[384] but it is unlikely that those observations are related, since hepatitis is caused as readily by salicylate as by aspirin.[373] It is possible that a metabolite, perhaps an otherwise minor metabolite, achieves toxic levels in certain disease states, but there is no evidence of this yet. Salicylate does appear to be directly toxic to rat hepatocytes in short-term tissue culture, causing the liberation of a cytoplasmic enzyme, LDH; this system may provide a window on the mechanism of the toxicity.[385]

In clinical practice, the best way to avoid aspirin hepatitis in adult rheumatoid arthritis is to avoid measuring transaminase levels unless frank symptoms related to the liver or upper abdomen are present. In children, the drug can be continued safely if there is no evidence of bleeding or ecchymosis and if any transaminase abnormalities do not suddenly worsen or reach levels above several hundred. Lowering the dose or temporarily stopping and then resuming the drug at a lower dose is usually adequate therapy. When transaminase levels rise sharply in lupus, we tend to stop and switch temporarily to another drug, although some patients do improve without lowering the dose. It should be borne in mind that the administration of two hepatotoxic drugs can be unusually dangerous and ought in general to be avoided.

Reye's syndrome, the catastrophic illness of children in which an apparently metabolic encephalopathy is coupled to hepatocellular failure and fatty degeneration, has been attributed to salicylates[386] and has even been described in a girl being treated in hospital with aspirin for polyarthritis.[387] Although in an individual case it is impossible to incriminate aspirin, there is good epidemiologic evidence gathered in case-control studies that aspirin ingestion contributes to the Reye's syndrome which may follow outbreaks of influenza and chicken pox.[388,389] There is a move to have the label of aspirin bottles carry a warning to that effect.[390] The liver pathology of Reye's syndrome is quite different from that found in aspirin-induced hepatotoxicity.

**Renal Effects.** There are five renal effects of aspirin or salicylates that may, under certain circumstances, be clinically significant: a transient shedding of tubular cells when therapy is begun; a possible relation to analgesic nephropathy; reduced glomerular filtration and renal blood flow, probably related to prostaglandin synthetase inhibition; interaction with furosemide and spironolactone; and alteration of urate excretion (see above).

When aspirin or salicylate administration is begun, there is an outpouring of cells into the urine which is due to the shedding of tubular cells.[391,392] The effect lasts several days and disappears. Its mechanism is obscure. In fact it defies easy speculation because none of the actions of salicylates or aspirin is known to attenuate so quickly. Perhaps it is caused by effects on prostaglandin biosynthesis for which compensatory mechanisms exist. While hematuria may also occur in association with salicylate therapy, the mechanism remains unclear.

Although analgesic nephropathy, by which I mean both papillary necrosis and its supposed late consequence, end-stage renal disease due to interstitial nephritis, has been recognized for over 20 years, it continues to arouse heated debate. It has been studied mainly in those countries where social patterns of drug use have encouraged many young women to ingest large quantities of proprietary analgesic powders or pills.[393]

The controversy surrounds the issue of which drug or drugs are responsible. Without trying to unravel its entirety, the following considerations are relevant to aspirin: (1) It is possible in animals to produce a lesion with aspirin and/or phenacetin that more or less resembles analgesic nephropathy, but the circumstances of drug administration are remote from the clinical setting of analgesic nephropathy.[394,395] (2) Although aspirin taken alone has been blamed in some cases of analgesic nephropathy, it is phenacetin, alone or in combination, that seems most culpable.[396,397] (3) Several older autopsy studies of rheumatoid arthritis patients have shown an alarming incidence of papillary necrosis or even end-stage renal disease,[398-400] but renal dysfunction has *not* been found in a number of carefully observed groups of arthritis patients who have taken large quantities of aspirin over many years under medical observation.[401-405] (4) Finally, and most important, in the only controlled observations on the subject, analgesic ingestion could not be shown to be a risk factor for developing end-stage renal disease among a large population of patients on renal dialysis compared with matched hospitalized patients.[406] Although caution is appropriate in extending these last observations beyond the population in which they were made, they seem to me to have wider implications.[407] In summary, the virtually hypothetical relationship of aspirin to analgesic nephropathy suggests that a physician should not consider it in selecting long-term therapy for rheumatologic diseases, and, indeed, most rheumatologists wisely do not.

Effects on renal function were first discovered in a series of dramatic experiments performed by Hanzlick and Scott and their colleagues over 60 years ago.[408,409] They described mild albuminuria, edema, and a rising blood nitrogen after giving 1 g of sodium salicylate hourly until intolerance, usually about 12 g. Recent experiments showed that aspirin or salicylate could alter creatinine clearance acutely in humans, and that patients with renal disease are more susceptible to these effects.[128,374,410-413] These effects may arouse clinical concern in patients with systemic lupus erythematosus even in the absence of detectable renal disease.[128] In patients with active lupus with or without renal disease, the administration of anti-inflammatory doses of aspirin regularly raises the BUN and serum creatinine and sometimes raises the serum $K+$ and reduces the serum $Na+$.[414] The effect can be dramatic and misleading in the patient with lupus; if aspirin or indeed any of the other prostaglandin synthetase–inhibiting anti-inflammatory agents are administered to a patient with lupus for the management of arthritis, fever, or serositis, any changes in BUN, creatinine, and creatinine clearance must be recognized as possibly due to the drugs in order to avoid unnecessary renal biopsies and therapy. When the drugs are stopped, the changes rapidly recede. Sometimes the changes recede while the drugs are continued, and much clinical experience in lupus suggests that chronic renal changes are not a consequence of continued aspirin therapy. Nevertheless, it is important to recognize that advancing renal disease may sensitize the kidney to the renal effects of this class of drug.

The mechanism probably involves the inhibition of intrarenal prostaglandin synthesis.[415] Urinary prostaglandins fall before creatinine clearance does; the fall in creatinine clearance correlates with a fall in renal blood flow and a fall in inulin clearance; plasma renin falls; and a number of drugs that inhibit prostaglandin synthesis, including indomethacin, ibuprofen, fenoprofen, and naproxen, have the same effect.[414] Although it is possible to demonstrate aspirin-induced changes in creatinine clearance in patients with rheumatoid arthritis and indeed in normals, they are smaller than the changes in lupus and clinically insignificant.[128] Such a difference in susceptibility supports the view that under certain conditions of renal function, renal blood flow is maintained to a greater than normal extent by mechanisms involving prostaglandin synthesis.[416] The prostaglandin synthetase–inhibiting properties of aspirin and indomethacin have been used to advantage to probe the mechanism of and successfully treat the rare Bartter's syndrome.[417]

The relationship between aspirin and the mineralocorticoids is probably complicated and fortunately rarely of clinical interest. Aspirin can compete with aldosterone receptors in some experimental models,[418] and it can inhibit the action of spironolactone administered to man.[419] The latter action is worth noting for those situations in which the drugs are given together.

The relation to urate excretion is discussed under Interactions with Other Drugs.

In summary, with the exception of the reversible but occasionally dramatic effects of aspirin (and other prostaglandin synthetase-inhibiting drugs) on BUN, creatinine, and creatinine clearance in active lupus, the renal effects of aspirin, although interesting and controversial, are clinically rarely important.

**Aspirin or Salicylate Overdose or Accidental Intoxication.** The problem of salicylate toxicity caused by accidental overdosage in infants and in children lies beyond the scope of this book and beyond the experience of most rheumatologists. Aspirin or salicylate overdosage in adults occurs in a different setting and presents different metabolic problems. Overdose with suicidal intent is met in the emergency ward. Although the complicating late acidosis of children is not usually a problem in managing adults, and although with modern techniques of rapid laboratory determinations and dialysis fatality is uncommon, death may occur with blood levels less than twice therapeutic levels.[34,420] When it is recognized that the therapeutic serum level of salicylate is in the range of $10^{-3}$M, far higher than almost any other drug, it is not difficult to understand that an organic anion at $4 \times 10^{-3}$M (the mean serum level in a group of fatal cases)[421] might have many effects beyond its sometimes subtle therapeutic effects.

Salicylate intoxication in adults, however, is by no means limited to the suicidal. On a medical or rheumatology ward, the new appearance of dyspnea, confusion, ataxia, oliguria, or a rising BUN or creatinine in a hospitalized patient who is taking aspirin ought to suggest the possibility of salicylism.[361] After recognition, temporary withdrawal of the drug is usually adequate therapy. In the emergency ward, salicylism should be considered in the differential diagnosis of cardiopulmonary disease presenting dyspnea, tachypnea, or pulmonary edema, or of almost any central nervous system problem, including seizures. Asterixis may be present.[422] Older individuals taking salicylates or aspirin, often for a good reason, are the usual victims of this syndrome.[122,123] It probably arises when a supervening event alters the already peculiar metabolism of salicylate to cause a sudden rise in serum level. Among the events that may do so are acidosis, e.g., from fasting, dehydration, and the ingestion of drugs which displace salicylate from protein-binding sites. In a series of 20 patients with an average age of 53 in whom diagnosis had not been made until 6 or more hours after admission, six died, a far higher mortality than among 53 patients who took the drug with suicide in mind. Therapy consists of a forced diuresis, maintaining the urinary pH in the alkaline range, hemodialysis if diuresis is unsatisfactory, and any other appropriate supportive measures, including removing residual drug from the gastrointestinal tract by emesis, a large-bore stomach tube, or the administration of activated charcoal if that seems indicated by the history. Keeping the urine alkaline abets the excretion of salicylate. Vitamin K has also been recommended because large doses of salicylate may interfere with the synthesis of the vitamin K-dependent clotting factors.

The near-universal tachypnea of salicylism is due not to a metabolic acidosis but to a direct effect on the central nervous system in the medullary respiratory center.[362] Salicylate given intravenously will cause tachypnea, an increase in oxygen consumption and pH, and a decrease in $pCO_2$ within 1 or 2 minutes, well before any measurable blood acidosis. It has even been proposed that this action of salicylates be harnessed to increased $pO_2$ and lower $pCO_2$ in patients with emphysema,[423] but it is doubtless too variable and hazardous, particularly since an effect of salicylate of less rapid onset is increased oxygen consumption and $CO_2$ production.

There are probably many causes of the diverse central effects of salicylate intoxication. Local brain hypoglycemia may occur, as it does in experimental animals, because high doses of salicylate uncouple oxidative phosphorylation, forcing the brain to maintain its energy supply by markedly increasing glycolysis.[424,425] Indeed, glucose prevents death from salicylate intoxication of experimental animals.

**Miscellaneous Effects.** Aspirin has been shown to inhibit RNA synthesis of the mouse oocyte,[426] to reduce the growth rate of several mouse tumors,[427] and to alter tumor induction by a mouse tumor virus.[428] These effects have not been shown to depend on those features of the aspirin molecule known to be related to its pharmacology in man. It is likely that they are irrelevant to the clinical action of the salicylates.

There are curious effects of aspirin on experimental traumatic osteoarthritis in dogs,[429,430] which ought not impinge upon the clinical use of aspirin or other prostaglandin synthetase inhibitors at our current state of knowledge.

## CONCLUSION

The recent pharmacologic history of the drugs whose action in man depends on inhibition of the synthesis of prostaglandin strongly suggests that no new drug in this class will exceed in clinical efficacy those already in use, although a new drug might show a different spectrum of side effects and toxicities. What appears to limit efficacy is not the power of the drug but the extent to which the prostaglandin system is involved in the inflammation of the connective tissue diseases.

The durability of the salicylates is no accident. Just as the survival of buildings of earlier civilizations is most often rooted in strong materials and sound structure, so is the survival of salicylates rooted in their clear and powerful action and their safety. If they become obsolete in this century, it will be not an indictment of them, but a tribute to the ingenuity of chemists and pharmacologists.

## References


1. Gross, M., and Greenberg, L.A.: The Salicylates. A Critical Bibliographic Review. New Haven, Hillhouse Press, 1948.
2. Floeckinger, E.C.: An experimental study of aspirin, a new salicylic-acid preparation. Med. News (N.Y.) 75:645, 1899.
3. Goodwin, J.S., and Goodwin, J.M.: Failure to recognize efficacious treatments: a history of salicylate therapy in rheumatoid arthritis. Perspectives Biol. Med. 25:78, 1981.
4. Leist, E.R., and Banwell, J.G.: Products containing aspirin. N. Engl. J. Med. 291:710, 1974.
5. Vane, J.R.: Inhibition of prostaglandin synthesis as a mechanism of action for aspirin-like drugs. Nature New Biol. 231:232, 1971.
6. Martin, B.K.: The formulation of aspirin. Adv. Pharm. Sci. 3:107, 1971.
7. Leonards, J.R.: Presence of acetylsalicylic acid in plasma following oral ingestion of aspirin. Proc. Soc. Exp. Biol. Med. 110:304, 1962.
8. Leonards, J.R.: The influence of solubility on the rate of gastrointestinal absorption of aspirin. Clin. Pharmacol. Ther. 4:476, 1963.
9. Levy, G., and Yacobi, A.: Assessment of aspirin absorption rate from urinary excretion rate measurements. J. Clin. Pharmacol. 15:525, 1975.
10. Davison, C., Smith, B.W., and Smith, P.K.: Effects of buffered and unbuffered acetylsalicylic acid upon the gastric acidity of normal human subjects. J. Pharm. Sci. 51:759, 1962.
11. Nayak, R.K., Smyth, R.D., Polk, A., Herczeg, T., Carter, V., Visalli, A.J., and Reavey-Cantwell, N.H.: Effect of antacids on aspirin dissolution and bioavailability. J. Pharmacokinet. Biopharm. 5:597, 1977.
12. Douthwaite, A.H., and Lintott, G.A.M.: Gastroscopic observation of the effect of aspirin and certain other substances on the stomach. Br. Med. J. 2:1222, 1938.
13. Hogben, C.A.M., Schanker, L.S., Tocco, D.J., and Brodie, B.B.: Absorption of drugs from the stomach. II. The human. J. Pharmacol. Exp. Ther. 120:540, 1957.
14. Truitt, E.B., and Morgan, A.M.: Absorption of aspirin from the stomach in man. Toxicol. Appl. Pharmacol. 2:237, 1960.
15. Dotevall, G., and Ekenved, G.: The absorption of acetylsalicylic acid from the stomach in relation to intragastric pH. Scand. J. Gastroenterol. 11:801, 1976.
16. Hogben, C.A.M., Tocco, D.J., Brodie, B.B., and Schanker, L.S.: On the mechanism of intestinal absorption of drugs. J. Pharmacol. Exp. Ther. 125:275, 1959.
17. Nogami, H., and Matsuzawa, T.: Studies on absorption and excretion of drugs. I. Kinetics of penetration of acidic drug, salicylic acid, through the intestinal barrier in vitro. Chem. Pharm. Bull. 9:532, 1961.
18. Davenport, H.W.: Damage to the gastric mucosa: Effects of salicylates and stimulation. Gastroenterology 49:189, 1965.
19. Flower, R.J., and Vane, J.R.: Some pharmacologic and biochemical aspects of prostaglandin biosynthesis and its inhibition. *In* Robinson, H.J., and Vane, J.R. (eds.): Prostaglandin Synthesis Inhibitors. New York, Raven Press, 1974.
20. Lester, D., Lolli, G., and Greenberg, L.A.: The fate of acetylsalicylic acid. J. Pharmacol. Exp. Ther. 87:329, 1946.
21. Mandel, H.G., Cambosos, N.M., and Smith P.K.: The presence of aspirin in human plasma after oral administration. J. Pharmacol. Exp. Ther. 112:495, 1954.
22. Soren, A.: Dissociation of acetylsalicylic acid in blood and joint fluid. Scand. J. Rheumatol. 6:17, 1977.
23. Petersen, T., Husted, S.E., Pedersen, A.K., and Gedary, E.: Systemic availability of acetylsalicylic acid in human subjects after oral ingestion of three different formulations. Acta Pharmacol. Toxicol. 51:285, 1982.
24. Roth, G.J., and Majerus, P.W.: The mechanism of the effect of aspirin on human platelets. I. Acetylation of a particulate fraction protein. J. Clin. Invest. 56:624, 1975.
25. Bridges, K.R., Schmidt, G.J., Jensen, M., Cerami, M., and Bunn, H.F.: The acetylation of hemoglobin by aspirin. In vitro and in vivo. J. Clin. Invest. 56:201, 1975.
26. Walker, J.E.: Lysine residue 199 of human serum albumin is modified by acetylsalicylic acid. FEBS Letters 66:173, 1976.
27. Mulinos, M.G., and Ardam, I.: An aspirin splitting enzyme in blood (abstract). J. Pharmacol. Exp. Ther. 98:23, 1950.
28. Rainsford, K.D., Ford, N.L.V., Brooks, P.M., and Watson, H.M.: Plasma aspirin esterases in normal individuals, patients with alcoholic liver disease and rheumatoid arthritis: characterization and the importance of the enzymic components. Eur. J. Clin. Invest. 10:413, 1980.
29. Costello, P.B., and Green, F.A.: Aspirin survival in human blood modulated by the concentration of erythrocytes. Arthritis Rheum. 25:550, 1982.
30. Lowenthal, D.T., Briggs, W.A., and Levy, G.: Kinetics of salicylate elimination by anephric patients. J. Clin. Invest. 54:1221, 1974.
31. Levy, G., Procknal, J.A., and Garrettson, L.K.: Distribution of salicylate between neonatal and maternal serum at diffusion equilibrium. Clin. Pharmacol. Ther. 18:210, 1975.

32. Clark, J.H., and Wilson, W.G.: A 16-day-old breast-fed infant with metabolic acidosis caused by salicylate. Clin. Pediatr. 20:53, 1981.
33. Reed, J.R., and Palmisano, P.A.: Central nervous system salicylate. Clin. Toxicol. 8:623, 1975.
34. Hill, J.B.: Salicylate intoxication. N. Engl. J. Med. 288:1110, 1973.
35. Schachter, D., and Manis, J.G.: Salicylate and salicyl conjugates: Fluorimetric estimation, biosynthesis and renal excretion in man. J. Clin. Invest. 37:800, 1958.
36. Flower, R.J., and Vane, J.R.: Some pharmacologic and biochemical aspects of prostaglandin biosynthesis and its inhibition. *In* Robinson, H.J., and Vane, J.R. (eds.): Prostaglandin Synthesis Inhibitors. New York, Raven Press, 1974.
37. Paulus, H.E., Siegel, M., Mongan, E., Okun, R., and Calabro, J.J.: Variations of serum concentrations and half-life of salicylates in patients with rheumatoid arthritis. Arthritis Rheum. 14:527, 1971.
38. Smith, P.K., Gleason, H.L., Stoll, C.G., and Ogorzalek, S.: Studies on the pharmacology of salicylates. J. Pharmacol. Exp. Ther. 87:237, 1946.
39. Levy, G., and Leonards, J.R.: Urine pH and salicylate therapy (letter). JAMA 217:81, 1971.
40. Levy, G., Lampman, T., Kamath, B.L., and Garrettson, L.K.: Decreased serum salicylate concentration in children with rheumatic fever treated with antacid. N. Engl. J. Med. 293:323, 1975.
41. Levy, G., Tsuchiya, T., and Amsel, L.P.: Limited capacity for salicyl phenolic glucuronide formation and its effect on the kinetics of salicylate elimination in man. Clin. Pharmacol. Ther. 13:258, 1972.
42. Tsuchiya, T., and Levy, G.: Biotransformation of salicylic acid to its acyl and phenolic glucuronides in man. J. Pharm. Sci. 61:800, 1972.
43. Gupta, N., Sarkissian, E., and Paulus, H.E.: Correlation of plateau serum salicylate level with rate of salicylate metabolism. Clin. Pharmacol. Ther. 18:350, 1975.
44. Furst, D.E., Gupta, N., and Paulus, H.E.: Salicylate metabolism in twins. Evidence suggesting a genetic influence and induction of salicylurate formation. J. Clin. Invest. 60:32, 1977.
45. Ayres, J.W., Weidler, D.J., Mackichan, J., and Wagner, J.G.: Circadian rhythm of urinary pH in man with and without chronic antacid administration. Eur. J. Cin. Pharmacol. 12:415, 1977.
46. Rumble, R.H., Brooks, P.M., and Roberts, M.S.: Metabolism of salicylate during chronic aspirin therapy. Br. J. Clin. Pharmac. 9:41, 1980.
47. Keystone, E.C., Paton, T.W., Littlejohn, G., Verdejo, A., Piper, S., Wright, L.A., and Goldsmith, C.H.: Steady-state plasma levels of salicylate in patients with rheumatoid arthritis: effects of dosing interval and tablet strength. Canad. Med. Assoc. J. 127:283, 1982.
48. Algozzine, G.J., Stein, G.H., Doering, P.L., and Araujo, O.E.: Trolamine salicylate cream in osteoarthritis of the knee. JAMA 247:1311, 1982.
49. Rylance, H.J., Chalmers, T.M., and Elton, R.A.: Clinical trials of intra-articular aspirin in rheumatoid arthritis. Lancet 2:1099, 1980.
50. McAteer, E., and Dundee, J.W.: Injectable aspirin as a postoperative analgesic. Br. J. Anaesth. 53:1069, 1981.
51. Harrison, L.I., Funk, M.L., Ré, O.N., and Ober, R.E.: Absorption, biotransformation, and pharmacokinetics of salicylsalicylic acid in humans. J. Clin. Pharmacol. 21:401, 1981.
52. Verbeeck, R.K., Boel, A., Buntinx, A., and DeSchepper, P.J.: Plasma protein binding and interaction studies with diflunisal, a new salicylate analgesic. Biochem. Pharmacol. 29:571, 1980.
53. Chan, L.K., Winearls, C.G., Oliver, D.O., and Dunnill, M.S.: Acute interstitial nephritis and erythroderma associated with diflunisal. Br. Med. J. 280:84, 1980.
54. Wharton, J.G., Oliver, D.O., and Dunnill, M.S.: Acute renal failure associated with diflunisal. Postgrad. Med. J. 58:104, 1982.
55. Diflunisal. Medical Letter 24:76, 1982.
56. Mason, W.D.: Comparative plasma salicylate and urine salicylate levels following administration of aspirin, magnesium salicylate, and choline magnesium trisalicylate. J. Pharm. Sci. 69:1355, 1980.
57. Binus, M.H., Lyon, J.A., and Nicholas, J.L.: Comparable serum salicylate concentrations from choline magnesium trisalicylate, aspirin, and buffered aspirin in rheumatoid arthritis. Arthritis Rheum. 25:464, 1982.
58. Rainsford, K.D., and Whitehouse, M.W.: Biochemical gastroprotection from acute ulceration induced by aspirin and related drugs. Biochem. Pharmacol. 29:1281, 1980.
59. Aarons, L.J., Bochner, F., and Rowland, M.: A chronic dose-ranging kinetic study of salicylate in man (abstract). Br. J. Pharmacol. 61:456P, 1977.
60. Bernheim, H.A., and Kluger, M.J.: Fever: Effect of drug-induced antipyresis on survival. Science 193:237, 1976.
61. Jackson, D.L.: A hypothalamic region responsive to localized injection of pyrogens. J. Neurophysiol. 30:586, 1967.
62. Cooper, K.E., Cranston, W.I., and Honour, A.J.: Observations on the site and mode of action of pyrogens in the rabbit brain. J. Physiol. 191:325, 1967.
63. Dinarello, C.A., and Wolff, S.M.: Molecular basis of fever in humans. Am. J. Med. 72:799, 1982.
64. Milton, A.S., and Wendlandt, S.: A possible role for prostaglandin $E_1$ as a modulator for temperature regulation in the central nervous system of the cat (abstract). J. Physiol. 207:76P, 1970.
65. Chai, C.Y., Lin, M.T., Chen, H.I., and Wang, S.C.: The site of action of leukocytic pyrogen and antipyresis of sodium acetylsalicylate in monkeys. Neuropharmacology 10:715, 1971.
66. Lin, M.T., and Chai, C.Y.: The antipyretic effect of sodium acetylsalicylate on pyrogen-induced fever in rabbits. J. Pharmacol. Exp. Ther. 180:603, 1972.
67. Flower, R.J., and Vane, J.R.: Inhibition of prostaglandin synthetase in brain explains the antipyretic activity of paracetamol (4-acetamidophenol). Nature 240:410, 1972.
68. Seed, J.C.: A clinical comparison of the antipyretic potency of aspirin and sodium salicylate. Clin. Pharmacol. Ther. 6:354, 1965.
69. Feldberg, W., and Gupta, K.P.: Pyrogen fever and prostaglandin-like activity in cerebrospinal fluid. J. Physiol. 228:41, 1973.
70. Schoener, E.P., and Wang, S.C.: Sodium acetylsalicylate effectiveness against fever induced by leukocyte pyrogen and prostaglandin $E_1$ in the cat. Experientia 30:383, 1974.
71. Woolf, C.J., Willies, G.H., Laburn, H., and Rosendorff, C.: Pyrogen and prostaglandin fever in the rabbit. I. Effects of salicylate and the role of cyclic AMP. Neuropharmacology 14:397, 1975.
72. Bodel, P., Reynolds, C.F., and Atkins, E.: Lack of effect of salicylate on pyrogen release from human blood leucocytes in vitro. Yale J. Biol. Med. 46:190, 1973.
73. Schoener, E.P., and Wang, S.C.: Observations on the central mechanism of acetylsalicylate antipyresis. Life Sci. 17:1063, 1975.
74. Avery, D.D., and Penn, P.E.: Blockade of pyrogen induced fever by intrahypothalamic injections of salicylate in the rat. Neuropharmacology 13:1179, 1974.
75. Satinoff, E.: Salicylate: Action on normal body temperature in rats. Science 176:532, 1972.
76. Pittman, Q.J., Veale, W.L., and Cooper, K.E.: Observations on the effect of salicylate in fever and the regulation of body temperature against cold. Can. J. Physiol. Pharmacol. 54:101, 1976.
77. Lim, R.K.S.: Salicylate analgesia. *In* Smith, M.J.H., and Smith, P.K. (eds.): The Salicylates. A Critical Bibliographic Review. New York, Wiley, 1966.
78. Wallenstein, S.L., and Houde, R.W.: Clinical comparison of analgetic effectiveness of N-acetyl-p-aminophenol, salicylamide and aspirin (abstract). Fed. Proc. 13:414, 1954.
79. Houde, R.W., Wallenstein, S.L., and Rogers, A.: Clinical pharmacology of analgesics. I. A method of assaying analgesic effect. Clin. Pharmacol. Ther. 1:163, 1960.
80. Fremont-Smith, K., and Bayles, T.B.: Salicylate therapy in rheumatoid arthritis. A scientific exhibit. JAMA 190:383, 1964. (Cited in Reference 77.)
81. Lasagna, L.: Analgesic drugs. Am. J. Med. Sci. 242:620, 1960.
82. Guzman, F., Braun, C., Lim, R.K.S., Potter, G.D., and Rodgers, D.W.: Narcotic and non-narcotic analgesics which block visceral pain evoked by intra-arterial injection of bradykinin and other algesic agents. Arch. Int. Pharmacodyn. Ther. 149:571, 1964.
83. Lim, R.K.S., Guzman, F., Rodgers, D.W., Goto, K., Braun, C., Dickerson, G.D., and Engle, R.J.: Site of action of narcotic and non-narcotic analgesics determined by blocking bradykinin-evoked visceral pain. Arch. Int. Pharmacodyn. Ther. 152:25, 1964.
84. Winder, C.V.: Aspirin and algesimetry. Nature 184:494, 1959.
85. Guilbaud, G., Benoist, J.M., Gautron, M., and Kayser, V.: Aspirin clearly depresses responses of ventrobasal thalamus neurons to joint stimuli in arthritic rats. Pain 13:153, 1982.
86. Hashimoto, K., Kumakura, S., and Taira, N.: Vascular reflex responses induced by an intra-arterial injection of azaazepinophenothiazine, andromedotoxin, veratridine, bradykinin and kallikrein and blocking action of sodium salicylate. Jap. J. Physiol. 14:299, 1964.
87. Thompkins, L., and Lee, K.H.: Comparison of analgesic effects of isosteric variations of salicylic acid and aspirin (acetylsalicylic acid). J. Pharm. Sci. 64:760, 1975.
88. Ferreira, S.H., Moncada, S., and Vane J.R.: Further experiments to establish that the analgesic action of aspirin-like drugs depends on the inhibition of prostaglandin biosynthesis (abstract). Br. J. Pharmacol. 47:629P, 1973.
89. Willis, A.L., and Cornelsen, M.: Repeated injection of prostaglandin $E_2$ in rat paws induces chronic swelling and a marked decrease in pain threshold. Prostaglandins 3:353, 1973.
90. Ferreira, S.H.: Prostaglandins, aspirin-like drugs and analgesia. Nature New Biol. 240:200, 1972.
91. Rosenthale, M.E., Dervinis, A., Kassarich, J., and Singer, S.: Prostaglandins and anti-inflammatory drugs in the dog knee joint. J. Pharm. Pharmacol. 24:149, 1972.
92. Levitan, H., and Barker, J.L.: Effect of non-narcotic analgesics on membrane permeability of molluscan neurones. Nature New Biol. 239:55, 1972.
93. Beaven, M.A., Horakova, Z., and Keiser, H.R.: Interference with histamine and imidazole acetic acid metabolism by salicylates: A possible

contribution to salicylate analgesic activity? Experientia 32:1180, 1976.
94. Moss, J., De Mello, M.C., Vaughn, M., and Beaven, M.A.: Effect of salicylates on histamine and L-histidine metabolism. Inhibition of imidazoleacetate phosphoribosyl transferase. J. Clin. Invest. 58:137, 1976.
95. Boardman, P.L., and Hart, F.D.: Clinical measurement of the anti-inflammatory effects of salicylates in rheumatoid arthritis. Br. Med. J. 2:264, 1967.
96. Robinson, D.R., and Levine, L.: Prostaglandin concentrations in synovial fluid in rheumatic diseases: Action of indomethacin and aspirin. *In* Robinson, H.J., and Vane, J.R. (eds.): Prostaglandin Synthetase Inhibitors. New York, Raven Press, 1974.
97. Winter, C.A., Risley, E.A., and Nuss, G.W.: Carrageenan-induced edema in hind paw of the rat as an assay for anti-inflammatory drugs. Proc. Soc. Exp. Biol. Med. 111:544, 1962.
98. Mielens, Z.E., Drobeck, H.P., Rozitis, J., and Sansone, V.J.: Interaction of aspirin with non-steroidal anti-inflammatory drugs in rats (letter). J. Pharm. Pharmacol. 20:567, 1968.
99. Swingle, K.F., Grant, T.J., Jaques, L.W., and Kvam, D.C.: Interactions of anti-inflammatory drugs in carrageenan-induced foot edema of the rat. J. Pharmacol. Exp. Ther. 172:423, 1970.
100. Willis, A.L., Davison, P., Ramwell, P.W., Brocklehurst, W.E., and Smith, B.: Release and actions of prostaglandins in inflammation and fever: Inhibition by anti-inflammatory and antipyretic drugs. *In* Ramwell, P.W., and Pharriss, B.B. (eds.): Prostaglandins in Cellular Biology. New York, Plenum Press, 1972.
101. Vinegar, R., Truax, J.F., and Selph, J.L.: Some quantitative temporal characteristics of carrageenan-induced pleurisy in the rat. Proc. Soc. Exp. Biol. Med. 143:711, 1973.
102. Randall, L.O., Selitto, J.J., and Valdes, J.: Anti-inflammatory effects of xylopropamine. Arch. Int. Pharmacodyn. Ther. 113:233, 1957.
103. Gilfoil, T.M., Klavins, I., and Grumbach, L.: Effects of acetylsalicylic acid on the edema and hyperesthesia of the experimentally inflamed rat's paw. J. Pharmacol. Exp. Ther. 142:1, 1963.
104. Van Arman, C.G., Carlson, R.P., Risley, E.A., Thomas, R.H., and Nuss, G.W.: Inhibitory effects of indomethacin, aspirin and certain other drugs on inflammations induced in rat and dog by carrageenan, sodium urate and ellagic acid. J. Pharmacol. Exp. Ther. 175:459, 1970.
105. Smith, M.J.H.: Anti-inflammatory activity of salicylates. *In* Smith, M.J.H., and Smith, P.K. (eds.): The Salicylates. A Critical Bibliographic Review. New York, Wiley, 1966.
106. Winter, C.A., and Nuss, G.W.: Treatment of adjuvant arthritis in rats with anti-inflammatory drugs. Arthritis Rheum. 9:394, 1966.
107. Van Arman, C.G., Nuss, G.W., and Risley, E.A.: Interactions of aspirin, indomethacin and other drugs in adjuvant-induced arthritis in the rat. J. Pharmacol. Exp. Ther. 187:400, 1973.
108. Sofia, R.D., Knobloch, L.C., and Douglas, J.F.: Effect of concurrent administration of aspirin, indomethacin or hydrocortisone with gold sodium thiomalate against adjuvant-induced arthritis in the rat. Agents Actions 6:728, 1976.
109. Gold, E.W., Anderson, L.B., Schwartz, E.R., and Miller, C.W.: The effect of salicylate on prostaglandin levels in rabbit knees following inducement of osteoarthritic changes. Prostaglandins 12:837, 1976.
110. Goldlust, M.B., Rich, L.C., and Harrity, T.W.: Effects of anti-inflammatory agents on the acute response of immune synovitis in rabbits. Arthritis Rheum. 20:937, 1977.
111. Robinson, D.R., Tashjian, A.H., and Levine, L.: Prostaglandin-induced bone resorption by rheumatoid synovia. Trans. Assoc. Am. Physicians 88:146, 1975.
112. Dayer, J-M., Robinson, D.R., and Krane, S.M.: Prostaglandin production by rheumatoid synovial cells. J. Exp. Med. 145:1399, 1977.
113. Kaley, G., and Weiner, R.: Prostaglandin $E_1$: A potential mediator of the inflammatory response. Ann. N.Y. Acad. Sci. 180:338, 1971.
114. Higgs, G.A., McCall, E., and Youlten, L.J.F.: A chemotactic role for prostaglandins released from polymorphonuclear leukocytes during phagocytosis. Br. J. Pharmacol. 53:539, 1975.
115. MacGregor, R.R., Spagnuolo, P.J., and Lentnek, A.L.: Inhibition of granulocyte adherence by ethanol, prednisone, and aspirin, measured with an assay system. N. Engl. J. Med. 291:642, 1974.
116. Zurier, R.B.: Prostaglandins, immune responses, and murine lupus. Arthritis Rheum. 25:804, 1982.
117. Robinson, H.J., Phares, H.F., and Graessle, O.E.: Prostaglandin synthetase inhibitors and infection. *In* Robinson, H.J., and Vane, J.R. (eds.): Prostaglandin Synthetase Inhibitors. New York, Raven Press, 1974.
118. Stone, C.A., Van Arman, C.G., Peck, H.M., Minsker, D.H., and Ham, E.A.: Pharmacologic and toxicologic action of prostaglandin synthetase inhibitors: Potential role of prostaglandin synthesis blockade. *In* Robinson, H.J., and Vane, J.R. (eds.): Prostaglandin Synthetase Inhibitors, New York, Raven Press, 1974.
119. Ferreira, S.H., Moncada, S., and Vane, J.R.: Prostaglandins and signs and symptoms of inflammation. *In* Robinson, H.J., and Vane, J.R. (eds.): Prostaglandin Synthetase Inhibitors. New York, Raven Press, 1974.
120. Stefanovich, V.: Inhibition of 3′, 5′-cyclic AMP phosphodiesterase with anti-inflammatory agents. Res. Commun. Chem. Pathol. Pharmacol. 7:573, 1974.
121. Halla, J.T., Fallahi, S., and Hardin, J.G.: Acute and chronic salicylate intoxication in a patient with gastric outlet obstruction. Arthritis Rheum. 24:1205, 1981.
122. Heffner, J.E., and Sahn, S.A.: Salicylate-induced pulmonary edema. Ann. Intern. Med. 95:404, 1981.
123. Walters, J.S., Woodring, J.H., Stelling, C.B., and Rosenbaum, H.D.: Salicylate-induced pulmonary edema. Radiology 146:289, 1983.
124. Athreya, B.H., Moser, G., Cecil, H.S., and Myers, A.R.: Aspirin-induced hepatotoxicity in juvenile rheumatoid arthritis. Arthritis Rheum. 18:347, 1975.
125. Doughty, R.A., Giesecke, L., and Athreya, B.H.: Salicylate therapy in juvenile rheumatoid arthritis. Am. J. Dis. Child. 134:461, 1980.
126. Baum, J.: New thoughts on aspirin. Am. J. Dis. Child. 134:455, 1980.
127. Ropes, M.W.: Systemic Lupus Erythematosus. Cambridge, Mass., Harvard University Press, 1976.
128. Kimberly, R.P., and Plotz, P.H.: Aspirin-induced depression of renal function. N. Engl. J. Med. 296:418, 1977.
129. Buckingham, R.B.: Interactions involving anti-rheumatic drugs, I and II. Bull. Rheum. Dis. 28:960, 1978.
130. Mason, R.W., and McQueen, E.G.: Protein binding of indomethacin: Binding of indomethacin to human plasma albumin and its displacement from binding by ibuprofen, phenylbutazone and salicylate, in vitro. Pharmacology 12:12, 1974.
131. Jeremy, R., and Towson, J.: Interaction between aspirin and indomethacin in the treatment of rheumatoid arthritis. Med. J. Aust. 2:127, 1970.
132. Champion, G.D., Paulus, H.E., Mongan, E., Okun, R., and Pearson, C.M.: The effect of aspirin on serum indomethacin. Clin. Pharmacol. Ther. 13:239, 1972.
133. Garnham, J.C., Raymond, K., Shotton, E., and Turner, P.: The effect of buffered aspirin on plasma indomethacin. Eur. J. Clin. Pharmacol. 8:107, 1975.
134. Kaldestad, E., Hansen, T., and Brath, H.K.: Interaction of indomethacin and acetylsalicylic acid as shown by the serum concentrations of indomethacin and salicylate. Eur. J. Clin. Pharmacol. 9:199, 975.
135. Barraclough, D.R., Muirden, K.D., and Laby, B.: Salicylate therapy and drug interaction in rheumatoid arthritis. Aust. N.Z. J. Med. 5:518, 1975.
136. Rome, L.H., Lands, W.E., Roth, G.J., and Majerus, P.W.: Aspirin as a quantitative acetylating reagent for the fatty acid oxygenase that forms prostaglandins. Prostaglandins 11:23, 1976.
137. Thomas, B.H., Zeitz, W., and Coldwell, B.B.: Effect of aspirin on biotransformation of 14C-acetaminophen in rats. J. Pharm. Sci. 63:1367, 1974.
138. Whitehouse, L.W., Paul, C.J., and Thomas, B.H.: Effect of aspirin on fate of 14C-acetaminophen in guinea pigs. J. Pharm. Sci. 64:819, 1975.
139. Whitehouse, L.W., Paul, C.J., and Thomas, B.H.: Effect of acetylsalicylic acid on a toxic dose of acetaminophen in the mouse. Toxicol. Appl. Pharmacol. 38:571, 1976.
140. Cotty, V.F., Sterbenz, F.J., Mueller, F., Melman, K., Ederma, H., Skerpac, J., Hunter, D., and Lehr, M.: Augmentation of human blood acetylsalicylate concentration by the simultaneous administration of acetaminophen with aspirin. Toxicol. Appl. Pharmacol. 41:7, 1977.
141. Muirden, K.D., Deutschman, P., and Phillips, M.: Competition between salicylate and other drugs in binding to human serum protein in vitro. Aust. N.Z. J. Med. 4:149, 1974.
142. Segre, E., Chaplin, M., Forchelli, E., Runkel, R., and Sevelius, H.: Naproxen-aspirin interactions in man. Clin. Pharmacol. Ther. 15:374, 1974.
143. Rubin, A., Rodda, B.E., Warrick, P., Gruber, C.M., and Ridolfo, A.S.: Interactions of aspirin with non-steroidal anti-inflammatory drugs in man. Arthritis Rheum. 16:635, 1973.
144. Quick, A.J., and Clesceri, L.: Influence of acetylsalicylic acid and salicylamide on the coagulation of blood. J. Pharmacol. Exp. Ther. 128:95, 1960.
145. Loew, D., and Vinazzer, H.: Dose dependent influence of acetylsalicylic acid on platelet functions and plasmatic coagulation factors. Haemostasis 5:239, 1976.
146. Kelley, W.N.: Effects of drugs on uric acid in man. Ann. Rev. Pharmacol. Toxicol. 15:327, 1975.
147. Sorensen, L.B., and Levinson, D.J.: Clinical evaluation of benzbromarone. A new uricosuric drug. Arthritis Rheum. 19:183, 1976.
148. Berg, K.J.: Acute effects of acetylsalicylic acid in patients with chronic renal insufficiency. Europ. J. Clin. Pharm. 11:111, 1977.
149. Mirouze, D., Zipser, R.D., and Reynolds, T.B.: Effect of inhibitors of prostaglandin synthesis on induced diuresis in cirrhosis. Hepatology 3:50, 1983.
150. Seino, Y., Usami, M., Nakahara, H., Takemura, J., Nishi, S., Ishida, H., Ikeda, M., and Imura, H.: Effect of acetylsalicylic acid on blood glucose and glucose regulatory hormones in mild diabetes. Prostaglandins Leukotrienes Med. 8:49, 1982.

151. Jaffe, R.M., Kasten, B., Young, D.S., and MacLowry, J.D.: False-negative stool occult blood tests caused by ingestion of ascorbic acid (vitamin C). Ann. Intern. Med. 83:824, 1975.
152. Klinenberg, J.R., and Miller, F.: Effect of corticosteroids on blood salicylate concentration. JAMA 194:601, 1965.
153. Deykin, D., Janson, P., and McMahon, L.: Ethanol potentiation of aspirin-induced prolongation of the bleeding time. N. Engl. J. Med. 306:852, 1982.
154. Mandel, M.A.: The synergistic effect of salicylate on methotrexate toxicity. Plast. Reconstr. Surg. 57:733, 1976.
155. Zuik, M., and Mandel, M.A.: Methotrexate-salicylate interaction: A clinical and experimental study. Surg. Forum 26:567, 1975.
156. Leonard, R.F., Knott, P.J., Rankin, G.O., Robinson, D.S., and Melnick, D.E.: Phenytoin-salicylate interaction. Clin. Pharmacol. Ther. 29:56, 1981.
157. Collins, E.: Maternal and fetal effects of acetaminophen and salicylates in pregnancy. Obstet. Gynecol. 58 (Suppl.):57S, 1981.
158. Slone, D., Siskind, V., Heinonen, O.P., Monson, R.P., Kaufman, D.W., and Shapiro, S.: Aspirin and congenital malformations. Lancet 1:1373, 1976.
159. Turner, G., and Collins, E.: Fetal effects of regular salicylate ingestion in pregnancy. Lancet 2:338, 1975.
160. Rumack, C.M., Guggenheim, M.A., Rumack, B.H., Peterson, R.G., Johnson, M.L., and Braithwaite, W.R.: Neonatal intracranial hemorrhage and maternal use of aspirin. Obstet. Gynecol. 58(Suppl):52S, 1981.
161. Stuart, M.J., Gross, S.J., Elrad, H., and Graeber, J.E.: Effects of acetylsalicylic-acid ingestion on maternal and neonatal hemostasis. N. Engl. J. Med. 307:909, 1982.
162. Shapiro, S., Siskind, V., Monson, R.P., Heinonen, O.P., Kaufman, D.W., and Slone, D.: Perinatal mortality and birth-weight in relation to aspirin taken during pregnancy. Lancet 1:1375, 1976.
163. Collins, E., and Turner, G.: Maternal effects of regular salicylate ingestion in pregnancy. Lancet 2:335, 1975.
164. Lewis, R.B., and Schulman, J.D.: Influence of acetylsalicylic acid, an inhibitor of prostaglandin synthesis, on the duration of human gestation and labor. Lancet 2:1159, 1973.
165. Levin, D.L.: Effect of inhibition of prostaglandin synthesis on fetal development, oxygenation, and the fetal circulation. Sem. Perinatol. 4:35, 1980.
166. Settipane, R.A., Constantine, H.P., and Settipane, G.A.: Aspirin intolerance and recurrent urticaria in normal adults and children. Allergy 35:149, 1980.
167. Lamson, R.W., and Thomas, R.: Some untoward effects of acetylsalicylic acid. JAMA 99:107, 1932.
168. Samter, M., and Beers, R.F.: Concerning the nature of intolerance to aspirin. J. Allergy 40:281, 1967.
169. Friedlaender, S., and Feinberg, S.M.: Aspirin allergy: Its relationship to chronic intractable asthma. Ann. Intern. Med. 26:734, 1947.
170. Feinberg, A.R., and Malkiel, S.: Aspirin sensitivity—experimental studies. J. Allergy 22:74, 1951.
171. Schlumberger, H.D., Lobbecke, E.A., and Kallos, P.: Acetylsalicylic acid intolerance. Acta Med. Scand. 196:451, 1974.
172. Delaney, J.C.: The diagnosis of aspirin idiosyncrasy by analgesic challenge. Clin. Allergy 6:177, 1976.
173. Szczeklik, A., Gryglewski, R.J., and Czerniawska-Mysik, G.: Relationship of inhibition of prostaglandin biosynthesis by analgesics to asthma attacks in aspirin-sensitive patients. Br. Med. J. 1:67, 1975.
174. Szczeklik, A., Gryglewski, R.J., Czerniawska-Mysik, G., and Zmuda, A.: Aspirin-induced asthma. Hypersensitivity to fenoprofen and ibuprofen in relation to their inhibitory action on prostaglandin generation by different microsomal enzymic preparations. J. Allergy Clin. Immunol. 58:10, 1976.
175. Settipane, G.A., and Pudupakkam, R.K.: Aspirin intolerance. III. Subtypes, familial occurrence, and cross-reactivity with tartrazine. J. Allergy Clin. Immunol. 56:215, 1975.
176. Settipane, G.A., Chafee, F.H., and Klein, D.E.: Aspirin intolerance. II. A prospective study in an atopic and normal population. J. Allergy Clin. Immunol. 53:200, 1974.
177. Myers, E.N., and Bernstein, J.M.: Salicylate ototoxicity. A clinical and experimental study. Arch. Otolaryngol. 82:483, 1965.
178. Silverstein, H., Bernstein, J.M., and Davies, D.G.: Salicylate ototoxicity. A biochemical and electrophysiological study. Ann. Otol. 76:118, 1967.
179. Aly, S., Mousa, S., el-Kahky, M., Saleh, A., and el-Mofty, A.: Toxic deafness. I. J. Egypt. Med. Assoc. 58:144, 1975.
180. Aly, S., el-Kahky, M., Eid, S., Mousa, S., Ramandan, M., Saleh, A., and el-Mofty, A.: Toxic deafness. II. J. Egypt. Med. Assoc. 58:158, 1975.
181. Crifo, S.: Aspirin ototoxicity in the guinea pig. ORL 37:27, 1975.
182. Krzanowski, J.J., Jr., and Matschinsky, F.M.: Adenosine triphosphate and phosphocreatinine levels in cochlear structures. Use rate and effect of salicylates. J. Histochem. Cytochem. 23:766, 1975.
183. Bernstein, J.M., and Weiss, A.D.: Further observations on salicylate ototoxicity. J. Laryngol. Otol. 81:915, 1967.
184. Mongan, E., Kelly, P., Nies, K., Porter, W.W., and Paulus, H.E.: Tinnitus as an indication of therapeutic serum salicylate levels. JAMA 226:142, 1973.
185. Muir, A., and Cossar, I.A.: Aspirin and ulcer. Br. Med. J. 2:7, 1955.
186. Batterman, R.C.: Comparison of buffered and unbuffered acetylsalicylic acid. N. Engl. J. Med. 258:213, 1958.
187. Cronk, G.A.: Laboratory and clinical studies with buffered and non-buffered acetylsalicylic acid. N. Engl. J. Med. 258:219, 1958.
188. Sadove, M.S., and Schwartz, L.: An evaluation of buffered versus non-buffered acetylsalicylic acid. Postgrad. Med. 24:183, 1958.
189. Miller, R.R.: Analgesics. *In* Miller, R.R., and Greenblatt, D.J. (eds.): Drug Effects in Hospitalized Patients. New York, Wiley, 1976.
190. Linnoila, M., and Lehtola, J.: Absorption, and effect on gastric mucosa, of buffered and non-buffered tablets of acetylsalicylic acid. Int. J. Clin. Pharmacol. Biopharm. 15:61, 1977.
191. Stubbe, L.: Occult blood in faeces after administration of aspirin. Br. Med. J. 2:1061, 1958.
192. Weiss, A., Pitman, E.R., and Graham, E.C.: Aspirin and gastric bleeding. Am. J. Med. 31:266, 1961.
193. Wood, P.H.N., Harvey-Smith, E.A., and Dixon, A. St.J.: Salicylates and gastrointestinal bleeding. Acetylsalicylic acid and aspirin derivatives. Br. Med. J. 1:669, 1962.
194. Metzger, W.H., McAdam, L., Bluestone, R., and Guth, P.H.: Acute gastric mucosal injury during continuous or interrupted aspirin ingestion in humans. Am J. Dig. Dis. 21:963, 1976.
195. Caravati, C.M., and Cosgrove, E.F.: Salicylate toxicity: The probable mechanism of its action. Ann. Intern. Med. 24:638, 1946.
196. Pierson, R.N., Holt, P.R., Watson, R.M., and Keating, R.P.: Aspirin and gastrointestinal bleeding. Am J. Med. 31:259, 1961.
197. Leonards, J.R.: Aspirin and gastrointestinal blood loss. Gastroenterology 44:617, 1963.
198. Croft, D.N., and Wood, P.H.N.: Gastric mucosa and susceptibility to occult gastrointestinal bleeding caused by aspirin. Br. Med. J. 1:137, 1967.
199. Goulston, K., and Cooke, A.R.: Alcohol, aspirin, and gastrointestinal bleeding. Br. Med. J. 4:664, 1968.
200. Leonards, J.R., and Levy, G.: Aspirin-induced occult gastrointestinal blood loss: Local versus systemic effects. J. Pharm. Sci. 59:1511, 1970.
201. Jabbari, M., and Valberg, L.S.: Role of acid secretion in aspirin-induced gastric mucosal injury. Can. Med. Assoc. J. 102:178, 1970.
202. St. John, D.J.B., and McDermott, F.T.: Influence of achlorhydria on aspirin-induced occult gastrointestinal blood loss: Studies in Addisonian pernicious anemia. Br. Med. J. 2:450, 1970.
203. Scott, J.T., Porter, I.H., Lewis, S.M., and Dixon, A. St.J.: Study of gastrointestinal bleeding caused by corticosteroids, salicylates and other analgesics. Quart. J. Med. 30:167, 1961.
204. Grossman, M.I., Matsumoto, K.K., and Lichter, R.J.: Fecal blood loss produced by oral and intravenous administration of various salicylates. Gastroenterology 40:383, 1961.
205. Stubbe, L., Pietersen, J.H., and van Heulen, C.: Aspirin preparations and their noxious effect on the gastrointestinal tract. Br. Med. J. 1:675, 1962.
206. Beeken, W.L.: Effect of five salicylate-containing compounds upon loss of $^{51}$chromium-labeled erythrocytes from the gastrointestinal tract of normal man. Gut 9:475, 1968.
207. Leonards, J.R., and Levy, G.: Reduction or prevention of aspirin-induced occult gastrointestinal blood loss in man. Clin. Pharmacol. Ther. 10:571, 1969.
208. Leonards, J.R., and Levy, G.: Effect of pharmaceutical formulation on gastrointestinal bleeding from aspirin tablets. Arch. Intern. Med. 129:457, 1972.
209. Leonards, J.R., and Levy, G.: Gastrointestinal blood loss from aspirin and sodium salicylate tablets in man. Clin. Pharmacol. Ther. 14:62, 1973.
210. Parry, D.J., and Wood, P.H.N.: Relationship between aspirin taking and gastroduodenal hemorrhage. Gut 8:301, 1967.
211. Bouchier, I.A.D., and Williams, H.S.: Determination of faecal blood loss after combined alcohol and sodium acetylsalicylate. Lancet 1:178, 1969.
212. Leonards, J.R., Levy, G., and Niemczura, R.: Gastrointestinal blood loss during prolonged aspirin administration. N. Engl. J. Med. 289:1020, 1973.
213. Schmid, F.R., and Culic, D.D.: Anti-inflammatory drugs and gastrointestinal bleeding: A comparison of aspirin and ibuprofen. J. Clin. Pharmacol. 16:418, 1976.
214. Cooke, A.R., and Goulston, K.: Failure of intravenous aspirin to increase gastrointestinal blood loss. Br. Med. J. 3:330, 1969.
215. Watson, R.M., and Pierson, R.N.: Effect of anticoagulant therapy upon aspirin-induced gastrointestinal bleeding. Circulation 24:613, 1961.
216. Baragar, F.D., and Duthie, J.J.R.: Importance of aspirin as a cause of anaemia and peptic ulcer in rheumatoid arthritis. Br. Med. J. 1:1106, 1960.
217. Muir, A., and Cossar, I.A.: Aspirin and gastric bleeding: Further studies of calcium aspirin. Am. J. Dig. Dis. 6:1115, 1961.

218. Paul, W.D.: The effect of acetylsalicylic acid (aspirin) on the gastric mucosa, a gastroscopic study. J. Iowa Med. Soc. 33:155, 1943.
219. Thorsen, W.B., Western, D., Tanaka, Y., and Morrissey, J.F.: Aspirin injury to gastric mucosa. Gastrocamera observations of the effect of pH. Arch. Intern. Med. 121:499, 1968.
220. Kuiper, D.H., Fall, D.S., Overholt, B.F., and Pollard, H.M.: The effect of aspirin on fecal blood loss with gastroscopic correlation in healthy volunteers (abstract). Ann Intern. Med. 70:1069, 1969.
221. Edmar, D.: The effects of acetylsalicylic acid on the human gastric mucosa as revealed by gastrocamera. Scand. J. Gastroenterol. 10:495, 1975.
222. Baskin, W.N., Ivey, K.J., Krause, W.J., Jeffrey, G.E., and Gemmell, R.T.: Aspirin-induced ultrastructural changes in human gastric mucosa: Correlation with potential difference. Ann. Intern. Med. 85:299, 1976.
223. Silvoso, G.R., Ivey, K.J., Butt, J.H., Lockard, O.O., Holt, S.D., Sisk, G., Baskin, W.N., Mackercher, P.A., and Hewett, J.: Incidence of gastric lesions in patients with rheumatic disease on chronic aspirin therapy. Ann. Intern. Med. 91:517, 1979.
224. Lanza, F.L., Royer, G.L., and Nelson, R.S.: Endoscopic evaluation of the effects of aspirin, buffered aspirin, and enteric-coated aspirin on gastric and duodenal mucosa. N. Engl. J. Med. 303:136, 1980.
225. Hoftiezer, J.W., Silvoso, G.R., Burks, M., and Ivey, K.J.: Comparison of the effects of regular and enteric-coated aspirin on gastroduodenal mucosa of man. Lancet 2:609, 1980.
226. Morris, A.D., Holt, S.D., Silvoso, G.R., Hewitt, J., Tatum, W., Grandione, J., Butt, J.H., and Ivey, K.J.: Effect of anti-inflammatory drug administration in patients with rheumatoid arthritis. Scand. J. Gastroenterol. 67(Suppl.):131, 1981.
227. Konturek, S.J., Obtulowicz, W., Sito, E., Olesky, J., Wilkon, S., and Kiec-Dembinska, A.: Distribution of prostaglandins in gastric and duodenal mucosa of healthy subjects and duodenal ulcer patients: effects of aspirin and paracetamol. Gut 22:283, 1981.
228. Cohen, M.M., and MacDonald, W.C.: Mechanism of aspirin injury to human gastroduodenal mucosa. Prostaglandins Leukotrienes Med. 9:241, 1982.
229. Hunt, J.N., and Franz, D.R.: Effect of prostaglandin $E_2$ on gastric mucosal bleeding caused by aspirin Dig. Dis. Sci. 26:301, 1981.
230. Cohen, M.M.: Prevention of aspirin-induced fecal blood loss with oral prostaglandin $E_2$: Dose-response studies in man. Prostaglandins 21(Suppl.):155, 1981.
231. Cohen, M.M. Cheung, G., and Lyster, D.M.: Prevention of aspirin-induced faecal blood loss by prostaglandin $E_2$. Gut 21:602, 1982.
232. Simmons, T.C., Weinstein, W.M., Shapira, M., and Grossman, M.I.: A therapeutic trial of 15(R)-15-methyl prostaglandin $E_2$ in rheumatoid arthritis patients with gastroduodenal lesions. Prostaglandins 21(Suppl.):165, 1981.
233. Müller, P., Fischer, N., Kather, H., and Simon, B.: Prevention of aspirin-induced drop in gastric potential with 16,16-dimethyl-prostaglandin $E_2$. Lancet 1:333, 1981 (letter).
234. Cohen, M.M.: Prevention of aspirin-induced fall in gastric potential difference with prostaglandins. Lancet 1:785, 1981 (letter).
235. Ivey, K.J., Paone, D.B., and Krause, W.J.: Acute effects of systemic aspirin on gastric mucosa in man. Dig. Dis. Sci. 25:97, 1980.
236. Kauffman, G.L., Aures, D., and Grossman, M.I.: Intravenous indomethacin and aspirin reduce basal gastric mucosal blood flow in dogs. Am. J. Physiol. 238G:131, 1980.
237. Rahbek, I.: Gastroscopic evaluation of the effect of a new anti-rheumatic compound Ketoprofen (19:583 R.P.) on the human gastric mucosa. A double-blind cross-over trial against acetylsalicylic acid. Scand. J. Rheumatol. (Suppl.) 63, 1976.
238. Loebl, D.H., Craig, R.M., Culic, D.D., Ridolfo, A.S., Falk, J., and Schmid, F.R.: Gastrointestinal blood loss. Effect of aspirin, fenoprofen, and acetaminophen in rheumatoid arthritis as determined by sequential gastroscopy and radioactive fecal markers. JAMA 237:976, 1977.
239. Croft, D.N.: Cell turnover and loss and the gastric mucosal barrier. Am. J. Dig. Dis. 22:383, 1977.
240. Davenport, H.W.: Salicylate damage to the gastric mucosal barrier. N. Engl. J. Med. 276:1307, 1967.
241. Silen, W.: New concepts of the gastric mucosal barrier. Am. J. Surg. 133:8, 1977.
242. Brown, R.K., and Mitchell, N.: The influence of some of the salicyl compounds (and alcoholic beverages) on the natural history of peptic ulcer. Gastroenterology 31:198, 1956.
243. Alvarez, A., and Summerskill, W.H.J.: Gastrointestinal haemorrhage and salicylates. Lancet 2:920, 1958.
244. Jennings, G.H.: Causal influences in haematemesis and melena. Gut 6:1, 1965.
245. Muir, A., and Cossar, I.A.: Aspirin and gastric haemorrhage. Lancet 1:539, 1959.
246. Needham, C.D., Kyle, J., Jones, P.F., Johnston, S.J., and Kerridge, D.F.: Aspirin and alcohol in gastrointestinal haemorrhage. Gut 12:819, 1971.
247. Dagradi, A.E., Lee, E.R., Bosco, D.L., and Stempien, S.J.: The clinical spectrum of hemorrhagic erosive gastritis. Am. J. Gastroenterol. 60:30, 1973.
248. Cameron, A.J.: Aspirin and gastric ulcer. Mayo Clin. Proc. 50:565, 1975.
249. Jorgensen, T.G.: Drug consumption before perforation of peptic ulcer. Br. J. Surg. 64:247, 1977.
250. Langman, M.J.S.: Aspirin is not a major cause of acute gastrointestinal bleeding. *In* Inglefinger, F.J., Ebert, R.V., Finland, M., and Relman, A.S. (eds.): Controversy in Internal Medicine II. Philadelphia, W. B. Saunders Company, 1974.
251. Spiro, H.M.: Aspirin is dangerous for the peptic ulcer patient. *In* Inglefinger, F.J., Ebert, R.V., Finland, M., and Relman, A.S. (eds.): Controversy in Internal Medicine II. Philadelphia, W. B. Saunders Company, 1974.
252. Levy, M.: Aspirin use in patients with major upper gastrointestinal bleeding and peptic ulcer disease. N. Engl. J. Med. 290:1158, 1974.
253. Duggan, J.M.: Progress report. Aspirin in chronic gastric ulcer: An Australian experience. Gut 17:378, 1976.
254. Gault, M.H., Rudwal, T.C., Engles, W.D., and Dossetor, J.B.: Syndrome associated with the abuse of analgesics. Ann. Intern. Med. 68:906, 1968.
255. Walker, A.M., and Jick, H.: Prediction of bleeding during heparin therapy. JAMA 244:1209, 1980.
256. Winawer, S.J., Bejar, J., and Zamcheck, N.: Recurrent massive hemorrhage in patients with achlorhydria and atrophic gastritis. Arch. Intern. Med. 120:327, 1967.
257. Rafoth, R.J., and Silvis, S.E.: Gastric ulceration associated with aspirin ingestion in an achlorhydric patient: A case report. Am. J. Dig. Dis. 21:279, 1976.
258. Bergman, G.E., Philippidis, P., and Naiman, J.L.: Severe gastrointestinal hemorrhage and anemia after therapeutic doses of aspirin in normal children. J. Pediatr. 88:501, 1976.
259. Newman, L.J., Yu, W.-Y., Halata, M., and Wasserman, E.: Peptic ulcer disease in children. Aspirin induced. NY State J. Med. 81:1099, 1981.
260. Gerber, L.H., Rooney, P.J., and McCarthy, D.M.: Healing of peptic ulcers during continuing anti-inflammatory drug therapy in rheumatoid arthritis. J. Clin. Gastroenterol. 3:7, 1981.
261. MacKercher, P.A., Ivey, K.J., Baskin, W.N., and Krause, W.J.: Protective effect of cimetidine on aspirin-induced gastric mucosal damage. Ann. Intern. Med. 87:676, 1977.
262. Okabe, S., Takeuchi, K., Urushidani, T., and Takagi, K.: Effects of cimetidine, a histamine H2-receptor antagonist, on various experimental gastric and duodenal ulcers. Am. J. Dig. Dis. 22:677, 1977.
263. Tarnawski, A., Krause, W.J., and Ivey, K.J.: Effect of glucagon on aspirin-induced gastric mucosal damage in man. Gastroenterology 74:240, 1978.
264. Welch, R.W., Bentch, H.L., and Harris, S.C.: Reduction of aspirin-induced gastrointestinal bleeding with cimetidine. Gastroenterology 74:459, 1978.
265. O'Laughlin, J.C., Silvoso, G.R., and Ivey, K.J.: Healing of aspirin-associated peptic ulcer disease despite continued salicylate ingestion. Arch. Intern. Med. 141:781, 1981.
266. Geall, M.G., Phillips, S.F., and Summerskill, W.H.J.: Profile of gastric potential difference in man. Effects of aspirin, alcohol, bile, and endogenous acid. Gastroenterology 58:437, 1970.
267. Ivey, K.J., Morrison, S., and Gray, C.: Effect of salicylates on the gastric mucosal barrier in man. J. Appl. Physiol. 33:81, 1972.
268. Davenport, H.W., Warner, H.A., and Code, C.F.: Functional significance of gastric mucosal barrier to sodium. Gastroenterology 47:142, 1964.
269. Chvasta, T.E., and Cooke, A.R.: The effect of several ulcerogenic drugs on the canine gastric mucosal barrier. J. Lab. Clin. Med. 79:302, 1972.
270. Caspary, W.F.: The effect of aspirin, antacids, alcohol and bile acids on transmural potential difference of the human stomach. Dtsch. Med. Wochenschr. 100:1263, 1975.
271. Bowen, B.K., Krause, W.J., and Ivey, K.J.: Effect of sodium bicarbonate on aspirin-induced damage and potential difference changes in human gastric mucosa. Br. Med. J. 2:1052, 1977.
272. Murray, H.S., Strottman, M.P., and Cooke, A.R.: Effect of several drugs on gastric potential difference in man. Br. Med. J. 1:19, 1974.
273. Cohen, M.M., and Pollett, J.M.: Prostaglandin $E_2$ prevents aspirin and indomethacin damage to human gastric mucosa. Surg. Forum 27:400, 1976.
274. Davenport, H.W.: Gastric mucosal hemorrhage in dogs. Effects of acid, aspirin, and alcohol. Gastroenterology 56:439, 1969.
275. Brown, P.A., Sawrey, J.M., and Vernikos-Danillis, J.: Attenuation of salicylate and stress-produced gastric ulceration by metiamide. Proc. West. Pharmacol. Soc. 18:123, 1975.
276. Rainsford, K.D.: Aspirin and gastric ulceration: Light and electron microscopic observations in a model of aspirin plus stress-induced ulcerogenesis. Br. J. Exp. Pathol. 58:215, 1977.
277. MacDonald, A., Dekanski, J.B., Gottfried, S., Parke, D.V., and Sacra, P.: Effects of blood glucose levels on aspirin-induced gastric mucosal damage. Am. J. Dig. Dis. 22:909, 1977.

278. Semple, P.F., and Russell, R.I.: Role of bile acids in the pathogenesis of aspirin-induced mucosal hemorrhage in rats. Gastroenterology 68:67, 1975.
279. Guth, P.H., Paulsen, G., Lynn, D., and Aures, D.: Mechanism of prevention of aspirin-induced gastric lesions by bile duct ligation in the rat. Gastroenterology 71:750, 1976.
280. Brodie, D.A., and Chase, B.J.: Role of gastric acid in aspirin-induced gastric irritation in the rat. Gastroenterology 53:604, 1967.
281. Dagle, G.E., Brodie, D.A., and Bauer, B.G.: Comparison of gross and microscopic gastric lesions produced in rats after single doses of aspirin and 2-deoxyglucose. Toxicol. Appl. Pharmacol. 16:638, 1970.
282. Okabe, S., Honda, K., Takeuchi, K., and Takagi, K.: Inhibitory effect of L-glutamine on gastric irritation and back diffusion of gastric acid in response to aspirin in the rat. Am. J. Dig. Dis. 20:626, 1975.
283. Boyle, E., Freeman, P.C., Goudie, A.C., Mangan, F.R., and Thomson, M.: The role of copper in preventing gastrointestinal damage by acidic anti-inflammatory drugs. J. Pharm. Pharmacol. 28:865, 1976.
284. Rainsford, K.D., and Whitehouse, M.W.: Gastric irritancy of aspirin and its congeners: Anti-inflammatory activity without this side-effect. J. Pharm. Pharmacol. 28:599, 1976.
285. Cheung, L.Y., Jubiz, W., Torma, M.J., and Frailey, J.: Effects of aspirin on canine gastric prostaglandin output and mucosal permeability. Surg. Forum 25:407, 1974.
286. Child, C., Jubiz, W., and Moore, J.G.: Effects of aspirin on gastric prostaglandin E (PGE) and acid output in normal subjects. Gut 17:54, 1976.
287. Cheung, L.Y., Moody, F.G., and Reese, R.S.: Effect of aspirin, bile salt, and ethanol on canine gastric mucosal blood flow. Surgery 77:786, 1975.
288. Gerkens, J.F., Shand, D.G., Flexner, C., Nies, A.S., Oates, J.A., and Data, J.L.: Effect of indomethacin and aspirin on gastric blood flow and acid secretion. J. Pharmacol. Exp. Ther. 203:646, 1977.
289. Farris, R.K., Tapper, E.J., Powell, D.W., and Morris, S.M.: Effect of aspirin on normal and cholera toxin-stimulated intestinal electrolyte transport. J. Clin. Invest. 57:916, 1976.
290. Kingham, J.G., Whorwell, P.J., and Loehry, C.A.: Small intestinal permeability I. Effects of ischaemia and exposure to acetyl salicylate. Gut 17:354, 1976.
291. Arvanitakis, C., Chen, G-H., Folscroft, J., and Greenberger, N.J.: Effect of aspirin on intestinal absorption of glucose, sodium, and water in man. Gut 18:187, 1977.
292. Beaumont, J.L., and Willie, A.: Influence sur l'hémostase, de l'hypertension artérielle, des antivitamines K, de l'héparine et de l'acide acétyl salicylique. Sang 26:880, 1955.
293. Beaumont, J.L., Caen, J., and Bernard, J.: Influence de l'acide acétyl salicylique dans les maladies hémorragiques. Sang 27:243, 1956.
294. Gast, L.F.: Influence of aspirin on hemostatic parameters. Ann. Rheum. Dis. 23:500, 1964.
295. Weiss, H.J., Aledort, L.M., and Kochwa, S.: The effect of salicylates on the hemostatic properties of platelets in man. J. Clin. Invest. 47:2169, 1968.
296. Mielke, C.H., Kaneshiro, M.M., Maher, I.A., Weiner, J.M., and Rapaport, S.I.: The standardized normal Ivy bleeding time and its prolongation by aspirin. Blood 34:204, 1969.
297. Bick, R.L., Adams, T., and Schmalhorst, W.R.: Bleeding times, platelet adhesion, and aspirin. Am. J. Clin. Pathol. 65:69, 1976.
298. Young, V.P., Giles, A.R., Pater, J., and Corbett, W.E.N.: Sex differences in bleeding time and blood loss in normal subjects following aspirin ingestion. Thromb. Res. 20:705, 1980.
299. Dybdahl, J.H., Daae, L.N.W., Erika, C., Godal, H.D., and Larsen, S.: Acetylsalicylic acid-induced prolongation of bleeding time in healthy men. Scand. J. Haematol. 26:50, 1981.
300. Evans, G., Mustard, J.F., and Packham, M.A.: Spontaneous bruising (letter). Lancet 2:724, 1967.
301. Weiss, H.J., and Aledort, L.M.: Impaired platelet/connective tissue reaction in man after aspirin ingestion. Lancet 2:495, 1967.
302. O'Brien, J.R.: Effects of salicylates on human platelets. Lancet 1:779, 1968.
303. Zucker, M.B., and Peterson, J.: Inhibition of adenosine diphosphate-induced secondary aggregation and other platelet functions by acetylsalicylic acid ingestion. Proc. Soc. Exp. Biol. Med. 127:547, 1968.
304. Zucker, M.B., and Peterson, J.: Effect of acetylsalicylic acid, other nonsteroidal anti-inflammatory agents, and dipyridamole on human blood platelets. J. Lab. Clin. Med. 76:66, 1970.
305. Weiss, H.J., Tschopp, T.B., and Baumgartner, H.R.: Impaired interaction (adhesion-aggregation) of platelets with the subendothelium in storage-pool disease and after aspirin ingestion. A comparison with von Willebrand's disease. N. Engl. J. Med. 293:619, 1975.
306. Cazenave, J.P., Packham, M.A., Guccione, M.A., and Mustard, J.F.: Inhibition of platelet adherence to damaged surface of rabbit aorta. J. Lab. Clin. Med. 86:551, 1975.
307. Tschopp, T.B.: Aspirin inhibits platelet aggregation on, but not adhesion to, collagen fibrils: An assessment of platelet adhesion and deposited platelet mass by morphometry and $^{51}$Cr-labeling. Thromb. Res. 11:619, 1977.
308. Baumgartner, H.R., Tschopp, T.B., and Weiss, H.J.: Platelet interaction with collagen fibrils in flowing blood. II. Impaired adhesion-aggregation in bleeding disorders. A comparison with subendothelium. Thromb. Haemostas. 37:17, 1977.
309. Stuart, R.K.: Platelet function studies in human beings receiving 300 mg of aspirin per day. J. Lab. Clin. Med. 75:463, 1970.
310. Rowan, R.M., McDonald, G.A., Renton, R.L., Corne, S.J., and Brown, D.F.: Inhibition of platelet release reaction by acetylsalicylic acid. Postgrad. Med. J. 52:71, 1976.
311. Seuter, F.: Inhibition of platelet aggregation by acetylsalicylic acid and other inhibitors. Haemostasis 5:85, 1976.
312. Malmsten, C., Hamberg, M., Svensson, J., and Samuelsson, B.: Physiological role of an endoperoxide in human platelets: Hemostatic defect due to platelet cyclo-oxygenase deficiency. Proc. Natl. Acad. Sci. 72:1446, 1975.
313. Weiss, H.J., Willis, A.L., Kuhn, D., and Brand, H.: Prostaglandin $E_2$ potentiation of platelet aggregation induced by LASS endoperoxide: Absent in storage pool disease, normal after aspirin ingestion. Br. J. Haematol. 32:257, 1976.
314. Burch, J.W., Stanford, N., and Majerus, P.W.: Inhibition of platelet prostaglandin synthetase by oral aspirin. J. Clin. Invest. 61:314, 1978.
315. Gerrard, J.M., White, J.G., Rao, G.H.R., Krivit, W., and Witkop, C.J.: Labile aggregation stimulating substance (LASS): The factor from storage pool deficient platelets correcting defective aggregation and release of aspirin treated normal platelets. Br. J. Haematol. 29:657, 1975.
316. Gerrard, J.M., and White, J.G.: The influence of aspirin and indomethacin on the platelet contractile wave. Am. J. Pathol. 82:513, 1976.
317. Glass, D.B., Gerrard, J.M., Townsend, D., Carr, D.W., White, J.G., and Goldberg, N.D.: The involvement of prostaglandin endoperoxide formation in the elevation of cyclic GMP levels during platelet aggregation. J. Cyclic Nucleotide Res. 3:37, 1977.
318. Smith, J.B., and Willis, A.L.: Aspirin selectivity inhibits prostaglandin production in human platelets. Nature New Biol. 231:235, 1971.
319. Roth, G.J., Stanford, N., and Majerus, P.W.: Acetylation of prostaglandin synthetase by aspirin. Proc. Natl. Acad. Sci. 72:3073, 1975.
320. Ali, M., McDonald, J.W.D., Thiessen, J.J., and Coates, P.E.: Plasma acetylsalicylate and salicylate and platelet cyclooxygenase activity following plain and enteric-coated aspirin. Stroke 11:9, 1980.
321. Bradlow, B.A., and Chetty, N.: Dosage frequency for suppression of platelet function by low dose aspirin therapy. Thromb. Res. 27:99, 1982.
322. FitzGerald, G.A., Oates, J.A., Hawiger, J., Maas, R.L., Roberts, L.J., Lawson, J.A., and Brash, A.R.: Endogenous biosynthesis of prostacyclin and thromboxane and platelet function during chronic administration of aspirin in man. J. Clin. Invest. 71:676, 1983.
323. Brantmark, B., Hender, U., Melander, A., and Wåhlin-Boll, E.: Salicylate inhibition of antiplatelet effect of aspirin. Lancet 2:1348, 1981 (letter).
324. Livio, M., Del Maschio, A., Cerletti, C., and de Gaetano, G.: Indomethacin prevents the long-lasting inhibitory effect of aspirin on human platelet cyclo-oxygenase activity. Prostaglandins 23:787, 1982.
325. Rao, G.H.R., Reddy, K.R., and White, J.G.: Effect of acetaminophen and salicylate on aspirin-induced inhibition of human platelet cyclo-oxygenase. Prostaglandins Leukotrienes Med. 9:109, 1982.
326. Cerletti, C., Livio, M., and de Gaetano, G.: Non-steroidal anti-inflammatory drugs react with two sites on platelet cyclo-oxygenase. Evidence from 'in vivo' drug interaction studies in rats. Biochim. Biophys. Acta 714:122, 1981.
327. Dejana, E., Cerletti, C., de Castellarnau, C., Livio, M., Galletti, F., Latini, R., and de Gaetano, G.: Salicylate-aspirin interaction in the rat. Evidence that salicylate accumulating during aspirin administration may protect vascular prostacyclin from aspirin-induced inhibition. J. Clin. Invest. 68:1108, 1981.
328. Humes, J.L., Winter, C.A., Sadowski, S.J., and Kuehl, F.A.: Multiple sites on prostaglandin cyclooxygenase are determinants in the action of nonsteroidal antiinflammatory agents. PNAS 78:2053, 1981.
329. Preston, F.E., Whipps, S., Jackson, C.A., French, A.J., Wyld, P.J., and Stoddard, C.J.: Inhibition of prostacyclin and platelet thromboxane $A_2$ after low dose aspirin. N. Engl. J. Med. 304:76, 1981.
330. Weksler, B.B., Pett, S.B., Alonso, D., Richter, R.C., Stelzer, P., Subramanian, V., Tack-Goldman, K., and Gay, W.A.: Differential inhibition by aspirin of vascular and platelet prostaglandin synthesis in atherosclerotic patients. N. Engl. J. Med. 308:800, 1983.
331. Preston, F.E., Greaves, M., Jackson, C.A., and Stoddard, C.J.: Low-dose aspirin inhibits platelet and venous cyclo-oxygenase in man. Thromb. Res. 27:477, 484, 1982.
332. Loew, D., and Vinazzer, H.: Dose-dependent influence of acetylsalicylic acid on platelet function and plasmatic coagulation factors. Haemostasis 5:239, 1976.
333. Goldsweig, H.G., Kapusta, M., and Schwartz, J.: Bleeding, salicylates, and prolonged prothrombin time: Three case reports and a review of the literature. J. Rheumatol. 3:37, 1976.

334. Pinedo, H.M., van de Putte, L.B.A., and Loeliger, E.A.: Salicylate-induced consumption coagulopathy. Ann. Rheum. Dis. 32:66, 1973.
335. Sbarbaro, J.A., and Bennett, R.M.: Aspirin hepatotoxicity and disseminated intravascular coagulation. Ann. Intern. Med. 86:183, 1977.
336. Opelz, G., Terasaki, P.I., and Hirata, A.A.: Suppression of lymphocyte transformation by aspirin. Lancet 2:478, 1973.
337. Panush, R.S., and Anthony, C.R.: Effects of acetylsalicylic acid on normal human peripheral blood lymphocytes. Inhibition of mitogen- and antigen-stimulated incorporation of tritiated thymidine. Clin. Exp. Immunol. 23:114, 1976.
338. Coeugniet, E., Bendtzen, K., and Bendixen, G.: Leukocyte migration inhibitory activity of concanavalin-A-stimulated human lymphocytes. Modification by dipyridamole, lysine-acetylsalicylate and heparin. Acta Med. Scand. 199:99, 1976.
339. Brown, K.A., and Collins, A.J.: Action of non-steroidal anti-inflammatory drugs on human and rat peripheral leucocyte migration in vitro. Ann. Rheum. Dis. 36:239, 1977.
340. Crout, J.E., Hepburn, B., and Ritts, R.E., Jr.: Suppression of lymphocyte transformation after aspirin ingestion. N. Engl. J. Med. 292:221, 1975.
341. Smith, M.J., Hoth, M., and Davis, K.: Aspirin and lymphocyte transformation. Ann. Intern. Med. 83:509, 1975.
342. Snider, D.E., and Parker, C.W.: Aspirin effects on lymphocyte cyclic AMP levels in normal human subjects. J. Clin. Invest. 58:524, 1976.
343. Duncan, M.W., Person, D.A., Rich, A.A., and Sharp, J.T.: Aspirin and delayed type hypersensitivity. Arthritis Rheum. 20:1174, 1977.
344. Austen, K.F.: Immunologic aspects of salicylate action. *In* Dixon, A. St.J., Martin, B.K., Smith, M.J.H., and Wood, P.N.H. (eds.): Salicylates. Boston, Little, Brown & Company, 1963.
345. MacGregor, R.R., Spagnuolo, P.J., and Lentnek, A.L.: Inhibition of granulocyte adherence by ethanol, prednisone, and aspirin measured with an assay system. N. Engl. J. Med. 291:642, 1974.
346. Glader, B.E.: Evaluation of the hemolytic role of aspirin in glucose-6-phosphate dehydrogenase deficiency. J. Pediat. 89:1027, 1976.
347. Chan, T.K., Todd, D., and Tso, S.C.: Drug-induced hemolysis in glucose-6-phosphate dehydrogenase deficiency. Br. Med. J. 2:1227, 1976.
348. Colonna, P.: Aspirin and glucose-6-phosphate dehydrogenase deficiency. Br. Med. J. 283:1189, 1981 (letter).
349. Glader, B.E.: Salicylate-induced injury of pyruvate-kinase deficient erythrocytes. N. Engl. J. Med. 294:916, 1976.
350. Wijnja, L., Snijder, J.A.M., and Nieweg, H.O.: Acetylsalicylic acid as a cause of pancytopenia from bone marrow damage. Lancet 2:768, 1966.
351. Reid, J., Watson, R.D., and Sproull, D.H.: The mode of action of salicylate in acute rheumatic fever. Quart. J. Med. 19:1, 1950.
352. Bywaters, E.G.L., and Thomas, G.T.: Bed rest, salicylates, and steroid in rheumatic fever. Br. Med. J. 1:1628, 1961.
353. Alexander, W.D., and Smith, G.: Disadvantageous circulating effects of salicylate in rheumatic fever. Lancer 1:768, 1962.
354. Sutcliffe, J.: Pulmonary oedema due to salicylates with report of a case. Br. J. Radiol. 28:314, 1955.
355. Granville-Grossman, K.L., and Sergeant, H.G.S.: Pulmonary oedema due to salicylate intoxication. Lancet 1:575, 1960.
356. Hrnicek, G., Skelton, J., and Miller, W.C.: Pulmonary edema and salicylate intoxication. JAMA 230:866, 1974.
357. Tashima, C.K., and Rose, M.: Pulmonary edema and salicylates. Ann. Intern. Med. 81:274, 1974.
358. Davis, P.R., and Burch, R.E.: Pulmonary edema and salicylate intoxication (letter). Ann. Intern. Med. 80:553, 1974.
359. Karliner, J.S.: Noncardiogenic forms of pulmonary edema. Circulation 46:212, 1972.
360. Bowers, R.E., Brigham, K.L., and Owen, P.J.: Salicylate pulmonary edema: The mechanism in sheep and review of the clinical literature. Am. Rev. Respir. Dis. 115:261, 1977.
361. Anderson, R.J., Potts, D.E., Gabow, P.A., Rumack, B.H., and Schrier, R.W.: Unrecognized adult salicylate intoxication. Ann. Intern. Med. 85:745, 1976.
362. Tenney, S.M., and Miller, R.M.: The respiratory and circulating actions of salicylate. Am. J. Med. 19:498, 1955.
363. Kuna, S.T., and Levine, S.: Relationship between cyclooxygenase activity (COA) inhibition and stimulation of ventilation by salicylate. J. Pharm. Exp. Therap. 219:721, 1981.
364. Starling, M.B., and Elliott, R.B.: The effects of prostaglandins, prostaglandin inhibition, and oxygen on the closure of the ductus arteriosus, pulmonary arteries and umbilical vessels in vitro. Prostaglandins 8:187, 1974.
365. Elliott, R.B., Starling, M.B., and Neutze, J.M.: Medical manipulation of the ductus arteriosus. Lancet 1:140, 1975.
366. Friedman, W.F., Hirschklau, M.J., Printz, M.P., Pitlick, P.T., and Kirkpatrick, S.E.: Pharmacologic closure of patent ductus arteriosus in the premature infant. N. Engl. J. Med. 295:526, 1976.
367. Heymann, M.A., Rudolph, A.M., and Silverman, N.H.: Closure of ductus arteriosus in premature infants by inhibition of prostaglandin synthesis. N. Engl. J. Med. 295:530, 1976.
368. Eisner, D.A., Ohba, M., and Ojeda, C.: The effect of salicylate in Purkinje fibre pace-maker activity. J. Physiol. 269:84P, 1977.
369. Jackson, H.R., Johnson, S.M., Ng, K.H., Pye, W., and Hall, R.C.: The effect of acetylsalicylic acid on the response of the cardiovascular system to catecholamines. Eur. J. Pharmacol. 28:119, 1974.
370. Nydick, I., Tang, J., Stollerman, G.H., Wroblewski, F., and LaDue, J.S.: The influence of rheumatic fever on serum concentrations of the enzyme, glutamic oxalacetic transaminase. Circulation 12:795, 1955.
371. Manso, C., Taranta, A., and Nydick, I.: Effect of aspirin administration of serum glutamic oxalacetic and glutamic pyruvic transaminases in children. Proc. Soc. Exp. Biol. Med. 93:84, 1956.
372. Russell, A.S., Sturge, R.A., and Smith, M.A.: Serum transaminases during salicylate therapy. Br. Med. J. 2:428, 1971.
373. Rich, R.R., and Johnson, J.S.: Salicylate hepatotoxicity in patients with juvenile rheumatoid arthritis. Arthritis Rheum. 16:1, 1973.
374. Scaman, W.E., and Plotz, P.H.: Effect of aspirin on liver tests in patients with RA or SLE and in normal volunteers. Arthritis Rheum. 19:155, 1976.
375. Okumura, H., Ichikawa, T., Aramaki, T., and Oobayaski, K.: Liver disorder caused by aspirin. Naika 17:749, 1966.
376. Saltzman, D.A., Gall, E.P., and Robinson, S.F.: Aspirin-induced hepatic dysfunction in a patient with adult rheumatoid arthritis. Am. J. Dig. Dis. 21:815, 1976.
377. Wilson, J.R.: Aspirin hepatotoxicity in adults with rheumatoid arthritis. Ohio State Med. J. 72:577, 1976.
378. O'Gorman, T., and Koff, R.S.: Salicylate hepatitis. Gastroenterology 72:726, 1977.
379. Seaman, W.E., Ishak, K.G., and Plotz, P.H.: Aspirin-induced hepatotoxicity in patients with systemic lupus erythematosus. Ann. Intern. Med. 80:1, 1974.
380. Wolfe, J.D., Metzger, A.L., and Goldstein, R.C.: Aspirin hepatitis. Ann. Intern. Med. 80:74, 1974.
381. Bernstein, B.H., Singsen, B.H., King, K.K., and Hanson, V.: Aspirin-induced hepatotoxicity and its effect on juvenile rheumatoid arthritis. Am. J. Dis. Child. 131:659, 1977.
382. Miller, J.J., and Weissman, D.B.: Correlations between transaminase concentrations and serum salicylate concentration in juvenile rheumatoid arthritis. Arthritis Rheum. 19:115, 1976.
383. Kalczak, M., Gutowska-Grzegorczyk, G., and Maldyk, E.: The effect of chronic administration of acetylsalicylic acid on the rabbit's liver. Polish Med. J. IX:128, 1970.
384. Menguy, R., Desbaillets, L., Okabe, S., and Masters, Y.F.: Abnormal aspirin metabolism in patients with cirrhosis and its possible relationship to bleeding in cirrhotics. Ann. Surg. 176:412, 1972.
385. Tolman, K.G., Peterson, P., Gray, P., and Hammar, S.P.: Hepatotoxicity of salicylates in monolayer cell cultures. Gastroenterology 74:205, 1978.
386. Rosenfeld, R.G., and Liebhaber, M.I.: Acute encephalopathy in siblings. Reye syndrome vs salicylate intoxication. Am. J. Dis. Child. 130:295, 1976.
387. Sillanpaan, M., Makela, A.L., and Koivikko, A.: Acute liver failure and encephalopathy (Reye's syndrome?) during salicylate therapy. Acta Paediat. Scand. 64:877, 1975.
388. Waldman, R.J., Hall, W.N., McGee, H., and Van Amburg, G.: Aspirin as a risk factor in Reye's syndrome. JAMA 247:3089, 1982.
389. Halpin, T.J., Holtzhauer, F.J., Campbell, R.J., Hall, L.J., Correa-Villasenor, A., Lanese, R., Rice, J., and Hurwitz, E.S.: Reye's syndrome and medication use. JAMA 248:687, 1982.
390. Fulginiti, V.A., Brunnel, P.A., Cherry, J.D., Ector, W.L., Gershon, A.A., Gotoff, S.P., Hughes, W.T., Mortimer, E.A., and Peter, G.: Aspirin and Reye syndrome. Pediatrics 69:810, 1982.
391. Clausen, E., and Harvald, B.: Nephrotoxicity of different analgesics. Acta Med. Scand. 170:469, 1961.
392. Scott, J.T.: Renal irritation caused by salicylates. *In* Dixon, A. St.J., Martin, B.K., Smith, M.J.H., and Wood, P.H.N. (eds.): Salicylates. Boston, Little, Brown and Company, 1963.
393. Stewart, J.H., and Gallery, E.D.M.: Analgesic abuse and kidney disease. Aust. N.Z. J. Med. 6:498, 1976.
394. Murray, T., and Goldberg, M.: Analgesic abuse and renal disease. Ann. Rev. Med. 26:537, 1975.
395. Robinson, M.J., Nichols, E.A., and Taitz, L.: Nephrotoxic effect of acute sodium salicylate intoxication in the rat. Arch. Pathol. 84:224, 1967.
396. Axelsen, R.A.: Analgesic-induced renal papillary necrosis in the Gunn rat: The comparative nephrotoxicity of aspirin and phenacetin. J. Pathol. 120:145, 1976.
397. Duggin, G.G.: Mechanisms in the development of analgesic nephropathy. Kid. Int. 18:553, 1980.
398. Clausen, E., and Pedersen, J.: Necrosis of the renal papillae in rheumatoid arthritis. Acta Med. Scand. 170:631, 1961.
399. Lawson, A.A.H., and Maclean, N.: Renal disease and drug therapy in rheumatoid arthritis. Ann. Rheum. Dis. 25:441, 1966.
400. Nanra, R.S., and Kincaid-Smith, P.: Renal papillary necrosis in rheumatoid arthritis. Med. J. Australia 1:194, 1975.

401. Salomon, M.I., Gallo, G., Poon, T.P., Goldblat, M.V., and Tchertkoff, V.: The kidney in rheumatoid arthritis. Nephron 12:297, 1974.
402. New Zealand Rheumatism Association: Aspirin and the kidney. Br. Med. J. 1:593, 1974.
403. Macklon, A.F., Craft, A.W., Thompson, M., and Kerr, D.N.S.: Aspirin and analgesic nephropathy. Br. Med. J. 1:597, 1974.
404. Akyol, S.M., Thompson, M., and Kerr, D.N.S.: Renal function after prolonged consumption of aspirin. Br. Med. J. 284:631, 1982.
405. Emkey, R.D., and Mills, J.A.: Aspirin and analgesic nephropathy: JAMA 247:55, 1982.
406. Murray, T.G., Stolley, P.D., Anthony, J.C., Schinnar, R., Helper-Smith, E., and Davies, J.: Epidemiologic study of regular analgesic use and end-stage renal disease. Arch. Intern. Med., 143:1687, 1983.
407. Plotz, P.H.: Analgesic nephropathy. For this time and this place. Arch. Intern. Med., 143:1676, 1983.
408. Hanzlik, P.J., Scott, R.W., and Thoburn, T.W.: The salicylates. VII. Further observations on albuminuria and renal functional changes following the administration of full therapeutic doses of salicylate. Arch. Intern. Med. 19:1029, 1917.
409. Hanzlik, P.J., Scott, R.W., and Reycraft, J.L.: The salicylates. VIII. Salicyl edema. Arch. Intern. Med. 20:329, 1917.
410. Beeley, L., and Kendall, M.J.: Effect of aspirin on renal clearance of $^{125}$I-diatrizoate. Br. Med. J. 1:707, 1971.
411. Robert, M., Fillastre, J.P., Berger, H., and Malandain, H.: Effect of intravenous infusion of acetylsalicylic acid on renal function. Br. Med. J. 2:466, 1972.
412. Berg, K.J.: Acute effects of acetylsalicylic acid in patients with chronic renal disease. Eur. J. Clin. Pharmacol. 11:111, 1977.
413. Berg, K.J.: Acute effects of acetylsalicylic acid on renal function in normal man. Eur. J. Clin. Pharmacol. 11:117, 1977.
414. Kimberly, R.P., Bowden, R.E., Keiser, H.R., and Plotz, P.H.: Reduction of renal function by newer non-steroidal anti-inflammatory drugs. Am. J. Med. 64:804, 1978.
415. Kimberly, R.P., Gill, J.R., Bowden, R.E., Keiser, H.R., and Plotz, P.H.: Elevated urinary prostaglandins and the effects of aspirin on renal function in lupus erythematosus. Ann. Intern. Med. 89:336, 1978.
416. Plotz, P.H., and Kimberly, R.P.: Acute effects of aspirin and acetaminophen on renal function. Arch. Intern. Med. 141:343, 1981.
417. Norby, L., Flamenbaum, W., Lentz, R., and Ramwell, P.: Prostaglandins and aspirin therapy in Bartter's syndrome. Lancet 2:604, 1976.
418. Feldman, D., and Couropmitree, C.: Intrinsic mineralocorticoid agonist activity of some non-steroidal anti-inflammatory drugs. J. Clin. Invest. 57:1, 1976.
419. Tweedale, M.H., and Ogilvie, R.I.: Antagonism of spironolactone-induced natriuresis by aspirin in man. N. Engl. J. Med. 289:198, 1973.
420. Done, A.K.: Treatment of salicylate poisoning: Review of personal and published experiences. Clin. Toxicol. 1:451, 1968.
421. Irey, N.S.: Blood and tissue concentrations of drugs associated with fatalities. Med. Clin. North Am. 58:1093, 1974.
422. Anderson, R.J.: Asterixis as a manifestation of salicylate toxicity. Ann. Intern. Med. 95:188, 1981.
423. Wegria, R., Capeci, N., Kiss, G., Glaviano, V.V., Keating, J.H., and Hilton, J.G.: Effect of salicylate on the acid-base equilibrium of patients with chronic $CO_2$ retention due to pulmonary emphysema. Am. J. Med. 19:509, 1955.
424. Smith, M.J.H.: Metabolic effects of salicylates. *In* Smith, M.J.H., and Smith, P.K. (eds.): The Salicylates. A Critical Bibliographic Review. New York, Wiley, 1966.
425. Thurston, J.H., Pollock, P.G., Warren, S.K., and Jones, E.M.: Reduced brain glucose with normal plasma glucose in salicylate poisoning. J. Clin. Invest. 49:2139, 1970.
426. Mukherjee, A.B., Chan, M., Waite, R., Metzger, M.I., and Yaffee, S.J.: Inhibition of RNA synthesis by acetyl salicylate and actinomycin D during early development in the mouse. Pediat. Res. 9:652, 1975.
427. Hial, V., Horakova, Z., Shaff, F.E., and Beaven, M.A.: Alteration of tumor growth by aspirin and indomethacin: Studies with two transplantable tumors in mouse. Eur. J. Pharmacol. 37:367, 1976.
428. Seifter, E., Rettura, G., Levenson, S.M., Appleman, M., and Seifter, J.: Aspirin inhibits a murine viral infection. Life Sci. 16:629, 1975.
429. Palmoski, M.J., Colyer, R.A., and Brandt, K.D.: Marked suppression by salicylate of the augmented proteoglycan synthesis in osteoarthritic cartilage. Arthritis Rheum. 23:83, 1980.
430. Palmoski, M.J., and Brandt, K.D.: Aspirin aggravates the degeneration of canine joint cartilage caused by immobilization. Arthritis Rheum. 25:1333, 1982.

# Chapter 50
# Nonsteroidal Anti-inflammatory Drugs

*Alfred Jay Bollet*

## INTRODUCTION

New drugs with anti-inflammatory and analgesic action have been introduced into the therapy of rheumatic diseases in the recent past; more are under study and development. Aspirin and other forms of salicylate could eventually be replaced as the first-line anti-inflammatory drugs by these newer agents.

A single mechanism of action, inhibition of prostaglandin synthesis, has been advocated as the primary basis for the clinical effects of these drugs; however, differences in effectiveness in different diseases and a variety of basic studies suggest that they do not all act in exactly the same fashion. These agents vary signficantly in pharmacologic properties and toxicity, and individual patients vary in their responsiveness to different nonsteroidal anti-inflammatory agents. It is valuable to have a variety of drugs available to allow individualization of therapy, seeking the most effective regimen for a given patient. The potential toxicity of these drugs must be kept in mind, however, and careful thought given to safety and long-term benefit in each patient.

There are several families of chemical agents with clinically useful anti-inflammatory and analgesic properties. The salicylates are the oldest group, and are covered extensively in another chapter; only important comparisons in the effects or toxicity of salicylates will be mentioned here. The nonsteroidal anti-inflammatory agents discussed in this chapter are listed in Table 50–1.

## MECHANISMS OF ACTION

### *ANTI-INFLAMMATORY EFFECTS*

A long list of mechanisms of action has been suggested, especially for the salicylates,[1] including effects

**Table 50–1.** The Nonsteroidal Anti-inflammatory Agents

| Drugs by Chemical Group | Example of Trade Name in the United States |
|---|---|
| *Salicylates** | |
| Aspirin | |
| Sodium salicylate and other salts of salicylic acid | Trilisate |
| Salicylsalicylic acid | Disalcid |
| Diflunisal | Dolobid |
| *Indole Derivatives and Related Compounds* | |
| Indomethacin | Indocin |
| Sulindac | Clinoril |
| Tolectin | Tolmetin |
| Zomepirac | Zomax |
| *Pyrazolones* | |
| Phenylbutazone | Butazolidine |
| Oxyphenbutazone | Tandearil |
| Azopropazone† | |
| Feprazone† | |
| *Phenylacetic Acids* | |
| Alclonfenac‡ | |
| Diclofenac† | |
| Fenclofenac† | |
| *Phenylpropionic Acids* | |
| Ibuprofen | Motrin |
| Naproxen | Naprosyn |
| Fenoprofen | Nalfon |
| Flurbiprofen† | Ansaid |
| Ketoprofen† | |
| Fenbufen† | Cincopal |
| Benoxaprofen‡ | Oraflex |
| Carprofen† | |
| *Fenamates* | |
| Mefenamic acid | Ponstel |
| Meclofenamate | Meclomen |
| Flufenamic acid† | |
| *Oxicams* | |
| Piroxicam | Feldene |
| Isoxicam† | |

*See chapter on salicylates for further details.
†Not marketed in the United States at present.
‡Withdrawn from the market because of toxicity.

on virtually all the known phenomena that occur in the process of inflammation. Effects occur on synovial cells, vessel walls, and infiltrating leukocytes. There is inhibition of the synthesis of products of arachidonic acid metabolism (prostaglandins and leukotrienes), and generation of toxic oxygen radicals; there are also effects on leukocyte mobility, chemotactic responsiveness, phagocytic activity, and release of lysosomal enzymes during phagocytosis. Inhibition of the activity of these enzymes, as well as effects on the generation of chemotactic and toxic factors from the complement, fibrinolytic, and kinin pathways are other possible modes of action. It is clearly unlikely that all effective drugs are acting on a single enzyme (the cyclooxygenase) in only one of these pathways.

**Differences in Effectiveness in Different Diseases.** Among the reasons for suggesting that these drugs do not all work through the same mechanism is the difference in their effectiveness in different rheumatic diseases. Crystal synovitis due to urate deposition is well suppressed by colchicine, which is ineffective in other rheumatic diseases, while aspirin, which works well in rheumatoid arthritis, is relatively ineffective in gout; other nonsteroidal anti-inflammatory agents work well in both diseases. Similarly, in some cases of juvenile arthritis with fever (Still's disease) aspirin may be ineffective in controlling the fever, but indomethacin or other nonsteroidal agents may be more effective, or corticosteroids may be needed. In rheumatic fever, aspirin was extremely effective in controlling the joint inflammation, but the carditis was often uncontrolled; newer drugs have not been tested systematically in rheumatic fever, since the disease became rare in this country before they were available; however, in other forms of pericarditis (e.g., uremia and postcardiotomy syndrome), aspirin may be ineffective, but other nonsteroidal anti-inflammatory agents, such as indomethacin, are quite useful. Ankylosing spondylitis is better controlled by several of the newer agents than by aspirin.

There are forms of inflammation, such as immediate hypersensitivity, that are unaffected by nonsteroidal anti-inflammatory agents but controlled by antihistaminics or corticosteroids. Clearly a variety of mechanisms of inflammation are operative in different diseases, and the differences in effectiveness of specific agents in specific diseases point to variations in mechanisms of action.

**Inhibition of Prostaglandin Synthesis.** In the early 1970s Vane[2] introduced the concept that the nonsteroidal anti-inflammatory agents suppress inflammation through inhibition of synthesis of prostaglandins. Effects on prostaglandin synthesis have been demonstrated both in vitro and in vivo for the agents now in use. Cells do not store prostaglandins; release as a result of an injurious stimulus requires fresh biosynthesis; anti-inflammatory drugs affect both steps. Their relative potency as inhibitors of prostaglandin synthesis by rheumatoid synovial tissue in vitro resembles their relative clinical potency in suppressing inflammation.[3]

Much of the toxicity of the nonsteroidal anti-inflammatory agents can also be explained by their action on prostaglandin synthesis. For example, prostaglandins play a key role in protection of the gastric mucosa from autodigestion, through inhibition of acid production and stimulation of production of protective mucus.[4,5] Most of these drugs inhibit prostaglandin synthesis by gastric mucosal cells, contributing to the tendency to erosions and ulcer formation.[5,6] Gastric toxicity occurs with parenteral as well as oral administration of these drugs, since both routes of administration affect prostaglandin synthesis.[7] Inhibition of the cyclooxygenase in platelets blocks thromboxane formation and the ability of platelets to aggregate and initiate clotting. Aspirin, because of its very reactive acetyl group, acetylates amino acids (primarily the e-amino group of lysine) in the enzyme protein. The acetylation is irreversible, and the platelets cannot restore enzyme function, since they have no nucleus and thus no protein synthesizing capacity. New platelets must be released from the bone marrow in sufficient quantities to restore platelet function, a phenomenon for which one must allow one week.

On the other hand, nonsteroidal anti-inflammatory agents other than aspirin inhibit the catalytic activity of the cyclooxygenase competitively, a reversible effect, and enzyme function is restored when the drug is cleared from the blood. The duration of this effect is thus related to the half-life of clearance of the specific drug.[8-10] A similar lasting effect of aspirin occurs in patients with rheumatoid arthritis; prior administration of aspirin caused a lasting effect on prostaglandin synthesis by synovial tissue removed surgically and cultured in vitro, whereas the effect of prior administration of other agents, while demonstrable in vivo, was no longer present in the cultured tissue. All these agents inhibited prostaglandin synthesis when added to the cultures in vitro.[11]

The nonsteroidal anti-inflammatory agents react with several sites on the enzyme protein. The reaction with the catalytic site is competitive with the substrate for the enzyme, arachidonic acid. Reactions with a supplementary site are more characteristic of weak inhibitors and can interfere with inhibition of the catalytic site by stronger inhibitors such as indomethacin.[12]

There are both species and tissue differences in the effects of the various nonsteroidal anti-inflammatory agents on prostaglandin synthesis.[9,13-17] The seminal vesicle is the richest source of the enzyme and is thus used in many in vitro studies, but aspirin is a very poor inhibitor of this enzyme.[9,12,18-21] Another example of the tissue and species specificity of effects on prostaglandin synthesis is the anti-inflammatory effectiveness of acetoaminophen in rats, in suppressing carrageenan pleurisy and other forms of experimental inflammation,[22,23] but acetaminophen lacks such anti-inflammatory effectiveness in humans. On the other hand, acetaminophen does inhibit prostaglandin synthesis in nervous tissue,[24] at least in the hypothalamus, and this accounts for its antipyretic effects and probably contributes to its analgesic effects in humans. Salicylic acid decreases the amount of prostaglandin excreted in the urine each day in normal individuals and clearly inhibits the cyclooxygenase in some tissues in vitro, including the pancreas, where prostaglandins inhibit insulin release.[25] As a result, insulin production is augmented; this may account for the hypoglycemic reactions occasionally seen in diabetics, receiving oral hypoglycemics, who are given aspirin or other salicylates.[25-27]

Salicylic acid, however, is a weak inhibitor of the cyclooxygenase in most tissues, including the platelet and the stomach. In rats it does not cause the gastric erosions seen with aspirin or indomethacin, and when given concomitantly with indomethacin decreases the number of gastric erosions.[28] Salicylic acid has a weak effect on platelet function, which allows its use in patients with bleeding problems with greater safety than other nonsteroidal anti-inflammatory agents. In rats the reaction with platelets does not inhibit their function but blocks the inhibitory effect of other nonsteroidal anti-inflammatory agents on platelets.[28] This interference phenomenon has not been tested in humans, to my knowledge, in part because of concern that the salicylate will interfere with the therapeutic effect of the indomethacin by inhibiting the effect on the cyclooxygenase in synovial and other tissues.

An experimental example of the differences in the effect on prostaglandin synthesis is the demonstration in some animals of a fatal effect of intravenous injection of large amounts of arachidonic acid, because of the mass action effect resulting in the synthesis of large quantities of thromboxane causing extensive intravascular platelet aggregation. Aspirin and indomethacin prevent the fatal outcome, but salicylic acid does not.[29] On the other hand, arachidonic acid given to rats causes diarrhea because of prostaglandin synthesis in the gut; indomethacin prevents this effect, but salicylate does not. If the salicylate is given beforehand, it blocks the effect of the indomethacin, suggesting binding to the enzyme in a fashion which blocks access of the second drug.[28]

Another difference between the effect of salicylic acid and other nonsteroidal anti-inflammatory agents, including aspirin, is the effect on the respiratory tract. Inhibition of the cyclooxygenase by blocking synthesis of prostaglandins augments conversion of arachidonic acid to leukotrienes. Prostaglandins of the E series are bronchodilators, but several leukotrienes are bronchoconstrictors. People who are sensitive to this effect develop asthma, rhinitis, and sometimes nasal polyps when given aspirin; the other nonsteroidal anti-inflammatory agents usually have the same effect in these patients, but generally the nonaspirin salicylate preparations are well tolerated.

Additional evidence that an effect on prostaglandin synthesis is not the entire mechanism of action of the nonsteroidal anti-inflammatory agents comes from the observation that arachidonic acid–deficient animals have much less inflammation than animals with normal nutrition, but the inflammatory reaction that does develop is still inhibited by a variety of drugs.[1]

**Evidence for Other Mechanisms of Action.** Many other mechanisms of action have been postulated. The ones with the most supporting experimental evidence include effects on the generation of toxic oxygen radicals; on the intracellular concentration of cyclic AMP; on cellular responses, including chemotaxis, phagocytosis, and lysosomal enzyme activity; on interference with complement generation or action; and on bradykinin and the fibrinolytic and coagulation systems.

Neutrophils, which generate small quantities of prostaglandins, consume a great deal of oxygen, converting it to superoxide; this process contributes to the inflammatory process. Oxygen radicals are also generated in the synthesis of prostaglandins, as a product of the reaction that converts prostaglandin $G_2$ to prostaglandin $H_2$, and these radicals are toxic to proteins, including the cyclooxygenase, causing a decrease in enzymatic activity in vitro unless the toxic oxygen radicals are constantly removed.[7]

Salicylates act directly as scavengers of hydroxyl radicals,[30] and there is evidence that sulindac is a scavenger of free radicals.[7] The active form of this drug, the sulfide, formed by reduction of the prodrug in the liver, inhibits the enzyme cyclooxygenase, decreasing prostaglandin synthesis, but it also consumes free oxygen radicals. In the process it is reversibly converted back to the parent sulindac. The drug is thus partially inactivated in the tissues, but the process may contribute to its anti-inflammatory effectiveness.[7]

Complement components, especially C5a, when added to plasma, stimulate neutrophils to generate oxygen radicals; nonsteroidal anti-inflammatory agents also block this response.[31]

***Effect on Leukocytes.*** Migration of leukocytes into sites of inflammation is affected by various nonsteroidal anti-inflammatory agents. Some of the leukotrienes, products of the lipoxygenase pathway of arachidonic acid metabolism, are chemotactic for neutrophils. Since inhibition of prostaglandin synthesis increases the amount of arachidonic acid converted to leukotrienes, the nonsteroidal anti-inflammatory drugs can increase the number of neutrophils that accumulate in experimental inflammation.[32,33] A similar effect occurs in human synovial fluid.[34]

Observations made on benoxaprofen, although it has been removed from the market, are illustrative of the possible actions of nonsteroidal anti-inflammatory drugs. Benoxaprofen, which inhibited the lipoxygenase as well as the cyclooxygenase,[35] decreased the migration of leukocytes into sites of experimental inflammation, with a greater effect on monocytes than on neutrophils.[19] Higher doses were required to affect migration of neutrophils. These phenomena were demonstrated in a study of human peritoneal macrophages, as well as in guinea pigs and rats.[36] Benoxaprofen was also shown to affect migration of human leukocytes into the synovial fluid in patients with rheumatoid arthritis and spondyloarthropathy.[34]

Benoxaprofen had a direct effect on migration of mononuclear cells, inhibiting their response to chemotactic stimuli in vitro; an effect on the generation of chemotactic stimuli could not account for this action. A decreased binding of chemoattractant to plasma membrane receptors was demonstrated with decreased cytoskeletal rearrangement.[37]

Other nonsteroidal anti-inflammatory agents, including indomethacin, ibuprofen, ketoprofen, naproxen and aspirin, had similar effects on leukocyte responses to chemotactic stimuli following in vivo administration.[19,30,38-40] Sulindac is reported to have a moderate effect on the lipoxygenase pathway.[17]

In a study of pleurisy induced with carrageenan in rats, only phenylbutazone and indomethacin suppressed migration of mononuclear cells in vitro, while a battery of nonsteroidal anti-inflammatory agents suppressed migration of mononuclear cells in vivo; none suppressed migration of neutrophils into the pleural exudate. Steroids suppressed migration of both neutrophils and mononuclear cells. All the drugs tested suppressed inflammation in rats rendered leukopenic beforehand. Thus, there is evidence for differences in the mechanisms of action of various anti-inflammatory drugs, and it is an oversimplification to focus only on inhibition of prostaglandin synthesis, although that mechanism certainly is important.[41-44]

Nonsteroidal anti-inflammatory drugs counteract membrane permeability in a variety of cells and subcellular organelles. Stabilization of lysosomal membranes of migrating leukocytes, inhibition of lysosomal enzyme function, and inhibition of lymphocyte function all have been suggested as possible mechanisms of action of these agents. Indomethacin and some other nonsteroidal agents inhibit phosphodiesterase, resulting in elevated intracellular levels of cyclic AMP.[45] Since cAMP stabilizes cell membranes, including those of lysosomes in neutrophiles, and decreases generation of superoxide, this could explain such an effect of these drugs. In addition, piroxicam inhibits phagocytosis and release of lysosomal enzymes from neutrophils in experimental synovitis in dogs,[46] and ketoprofen stabilizes lysosomal membranes against osmotic shock.[47] In rheumatoid arthritis, inhibition of release of activity of lysosomal enzymes could decrease the rate of cartilage degradation, which occurs as a result of phagocytosis by neutrophils of immune complexes trapped in articular cartilage.

Complement components, especially C5a, cause granulocytes to become sticky, leading to clumping of cells and vaso-occlusion. This mechanism causes extension of infarction in experimental myocardial infarction. Nonsteroidal anti-inflammatory drugs inhibit the adhesiveness of the neutrophils to each other and to vascular endothelium; ibuprofen (but not aspirin) decreased the volume of myocardial infarcts in cats.[31]

Neutrophils produce small amounts of prostaglandins when stimulated, but an in vitro stimulus such as the peptide FMLP causes aggregation. Indomethacin, aspirin, piroxicam, and ibuprofen prevent this response by the neutrophils in concentrations in vitro similar to those achieved after in vivo administration.[48]

Oxidative phosphorylation is strongly inhibited by aspirin, other salicylates, phenylbutazone, and indomethacin and to a lesser extent by ibuprofen,[49] but numerous agents that are not anti-inflammatory also inhibit this pathway. Ibuprofen partially suppresses leukocyte mobility and phagocytosis, and it, along with other nonsteroidal anti-inflammatory agents, inhibits sulfate uptake by cartilage in vitro.[49] This effect may be relevant to the cartilage breakdown that occurs in osteoarthritis as a result of increased degradation of cartilage matrix components. Interestingly, one nonsteroidal anti-inflammatory agent, benoxaprofen, was shown to cause an increase in sulfate uptake in articular cartilage,[50] an effect that would be beneficial in osteoarthritis; other agents have not been as carefully studied in this system.

***Immunologic Effects.*** The variety of effects of nonsteroidal anti-inflammatory agents on immune functions suggests an effect of these drugs beyond that of suppressing the obvious clinical manifestations of inflammation. For example, aspirin inhibits DNA synthesis by guinea pig lymphocytes stimulated by phytohemagglutinin in vitro.[51] The abnormal T-lymphocyte function described in patients with rheumatoid arthritis and progressive systemic sclerosis, a decreased responsiveness to in vitro stimulation by phytohemagglutinin compared with controls, is reversed toward normal by addition of tolectin in vitro. Oral administration of tolectin to patients with rheumatoid arthritis in a dose of 1200 mg for 7 weeks[52] increased T-lymphocyte responsiveness, an effect similar to that observed with levamisole.

In vitro, formation of prostaglandin $E_2$ inhibits proliferation of T-lymphocytes, lymphokine production, and other T-lymphocyte functions; incorporation of nonsteroidal anti-inflammatory agents in these systems removes this inhibitory effect. As a result immunostimulation occurs. In guinea pigs, indomethacin causes an increase in skin test reactivity, resulting in an increased area of induration. In a study of 20 anergic patients with chronic combined immunodeficiency syndrome, most developed positive skin test reactivity when given indomethacin; skin test reactivity was lost when the drug was stopped and reappeared on repeat administration.[53]

In vitro cultures of lymphocytes and monocytes from patients with rheumatoid arthritis synthesize rheumatoid factor; incorporation of indomethacin in the culture medium results in decreased production of rheumatoid factor. Apparently the prostaglandins formed in vitro inhibit the action of suppressor (OKT8) cells; nonsteroidal anti-inflammatory agents, by blocking synthesis of prostaglandins, release these cells from inhibition and rheumatoid factor production decreases. A similar effect can be demonstrated in vivo; piroxicam given to patients with rheumatoid arthritis caused a decrease in rheumatoid factor concentration in plasma, which was detectable using a sensitive radioimmunoassay for rheumatoid factor.[54]

## Analgesic Effects

The analgesic effects of the nonsteroidal anti-inflammatory drugs have been assumed to be due to an inhibitory effect on the sensitivity of peripheral pain receptors, but a simple direct mechanism of action has not been established. Evidence points to more complex actions, including diminution of prostaglandin synthesis peripherally, which decreases the sensitivity of peripheral nerve receptors, and effects on both spinal cord and brain function, perhaps also mediated through inhibition of prostaglandin synthesis.

Prostaglandins cause a long-lasting sensitization of peripheral nerve endings, resulting in the perception of pain from stimuli, such as pressure, that are not ordinarily painful.[14] This phenomenon would account for the occurrence of tenderness at sites of inflammation, and inhibitors of prostaglandin synthesis decrease tenderness experimentally. Most of the nonsteroidal anti-inflammatory drugs relieve pain due to experimental inflammation, but not other types of pain.[55]

Prostaglandin $E_2$ infused intradermally or intramuscularly does not cause pain unless high concentrations are used; low concentrations sensitize nerve endings to low amounts of histamine (which causes itching) or bradykinin (which causes pain) in concentrations that do not themselves give symptoms. Aspirin and other nonsteroidal agents do not prevent this direct effect of prostaglandin infusion.[56] Leukopenia in rats diminishes edema due to carrageenan injection but does not prevent the development of a hyperalgesic state. Histamine, bradykinin, or acetylcholine intradermally produces short-lived pain, but when accompanied by prostaglandins, strong pain results.[14]

The nonsteroidal anti-inflammatory drugs affect transmission of pain at dorsal root ganglia and in the spinal cord, as well as at higher levels. One drug extensively studied in this fashion, zomepirac, penetrates the blood-brain barrier and decreases prostaglandin levels that occur in the cerebrospinal fluid after peripheral nerve stimulation. Zomepirac also decreases the background electrical activity of spinothalamic tract nuclei, as well as antagonizing the increase in activity of these nuclei that occurs after painful peripheral stimuli.[57] The levels of prostaglandins in the cerebrospinal fluid correlate with the background activity of the spinothalamic tract cells in the thalamus. Acetaminophen also decreases hyperalgesia in a dose-related manner when injected intraventricularly in rats.[14] The actions of non-narcotic analgesics such as zomepirac are not reversed by naloxone, indicating that opiate receptors are not involved in its action, but narcotic drugs also decrease prostaglandin synthesis in the brain after a peripheral nerve stimulus.

The observation that morphine, given intrathecally, has potent analgesic effects without central depression, and that the nonsteroidal anti-inflammatory drugs have central effects, has eliminated the older distinction that the narcotics are centrally acting and the nonsteroidal anti-inflammatory drugs peripherally acting analgesics.

The analgesic effect of the nonsteroidal anti-inflammatory drugs is increased by increasing doses in several studies,[58] and it is not clear if a plateau level of effect occurs at a certain dose. In the case of aspirin, increased effect occurs with increasing single doses ranging from 300 mg to about 1300 mgm.[58] It is difficult to extend these studies to test higher doses, since only patients with moderately severe pain can be used for the studies, and most such patients achieve complete relief at moderate doses, precluding testing at higher doses. The slope of the dose-response curve is relatively flat compared with strong analgesics such as the narcotics; nevertheless, large doses of these agents are useful when necessary, unless there are side effects. Further, the narcotic analgesics work through an entirely different mechanism, and thus the effects of the two types of drugs can be additive; combination therapy with a narcotic and a non-narcotic analgesic, in relatively large dosage, is useful in difficult or prolonged painful states.

## Suppression of Fever

Suppression of prostaglandin synthesis is probably responsible for the antipyretic effects of these agents.[51,59]

An increase in prostaglandin E–like activity can be demonstrated in the cerebrospinal fluid following injection of pyrogen into animals; prostaglandin $E_1$ injected into the anterior hypothalamus or cerebral ventricles is the most powerful pyrogen known. The various nonsteroidal anti-inflammatory agents, including aspirin and indomethacin, prevent the increase in prostaglandins following a pyrogenic stimulus; acetaminophen has a similar effect. The nonsteroidal anti-inflammatory agents do not prevent the febrile response to direct injection of prostaglandin into the third ventricle of cats.[59,60] Sodium injected into ventricles also produces fever; these drugs do not prevent this form of fever.[59]

Acetaminophen inhibits prostaglandin synthesis in vitro by brain tissue but not by spleen.[61] A similar tissue specificity of inhibitors of prostaglandin synthesis presumably occurs in humans, accounting for the antipyretic activity of this drug without an anti-inflammatory effect.

**Table 50–2.** Some Pharmacologic Characteristics of the Nonsteroidal Anti-inflammatory Drugs

| Drug | Volume of Distribution (L/kg) | Protein Binding (Percent) | Renal Excretion (Percent Unchanged) |
|---|---|---|---|
| Alclofenac | 0.1–0.4 | >99 | *† |
| Aspirin§ | 0.16 | 40–70 | <2 |
| Azapropazone | — | >95 | 40–60 |
| Benoxaprofen | — | — | 0 |
| Carprofen | 0.4 | >98 | <5 |
| Diclofenac | 1.2 | 99.7 | <2 |
| Diflunisal | 10–12 | high | <20 |
| Fenbufen | — | >99 | 42 |
| Fenoprofen | 0.07–0.1 | >95 | <5 |
| Flufenamic acid | — | >90 | <10 |
| Flurbiprofen | 0.1 | >99 | <10 |
| Ibuprofen | 0.1 (est.) | 99 | <2 |
| Indomethacin | 0.8 | 90–99 | <15 |
| Isoxicam | 0.17 | 95–98 | 1–2 |
| Ketoprofen | 0.1 | — | —† |
| Mefenamic acid | — | >90 | <10‡ |
| Naproxen | 0.09 | 99.5 | 10 |
| Phenylbutazone | 0.09 | 98–99 | <2 |
| Piroxicam | 0.14 | 99 | 2–5 |
| Salicylate | 0.1–0.24 | 85–95 | 2–30 (pH dependent) |
| Sulindac | — | 93–98 | <20 |
| Tolmetin | 0.1 | >99 | <10 |
| Zomepirac | — | — | 5 |

*Possible nonlinear kinetics with accumulation disproportionate to dose.
†Slower terminal phase of clearance known or likely.
‡Slow elimination of metabolites with enterohepatic recirculation.
§See chapter on aspirin and salicylates for details.

## PHARMACOKINETICS OF THE NONSTEROIDAL ANTI-INFLAMMATORY DRUGS

**Absorption and Bioavailability.** All of the nonsteroidal anti-inflammatory drugs currently on the market are relatively rapidly and reliably absorbed. All are extensively bound to plasma protein, primarily albumin, and have a small apparent volume of distribution, generally about 0.1 to 0.2 liter per kg of body weight.[62] Disposition generally follows a two-compartment model, with rapid equilibration into the central compartment, primarily the plasma and remainder of the extracellular fluid, then slow diffusion into a peripheral compartment. Similarly, blood levels generally show a biphasic decline, an initial rapid phase and then a slower terminal phase, presumably modified by diffusion out of the peripheral compartment.

Bioavailability of all the formulations being marketed is good. Food impairs absorption of only one of the nonsteroidal anti-inflammatory agents, fenoprofen, although ibuprofen administered with a meal is absorbed slower, with a lower peak serum concentration.[63,64] Neutralization of gastric acidity by food decreases the gastric irritation caused by these drugs, and the effects on absorption are too small to outweight the advantage of administering them with meals. In one instance, isoxicam, there is evidence that food increases absorption.[64]

All the nonsteroidal anti-inflammatory agents are relatively acidic molecules, with pK values between 4 and 5. Thus, in the presence of normal gastric acidity, they are un-ionized and are more soluble in lipids, entering gastric mucosal cells relatively well. Gastric toxicity is increased by local absorption in the stomach, where these drugs are directly toxic to mucosal cells. Neutralization of gastric acid raises the pH of the gastric juice above the pK of these drugs, making them more water soluble and less lipid soluble. Less is absorbed into gastric mucosal cells, and thus there is less gastric toxicity. The nonsteroidal anti-inflammatory agents enter the gastric mucosa from the plasma as well, and thus systemic administration causes gastric toxicity.[7]

As the drugs are highly protein bound, only the small amount of free drug may be available to enter tissues (Table 50–2). The free, unbound drug may be the effective form; free drug levels are extremely low, but they are in constant equilibrium with the bound form. There is no information on the effect of low serum albumin levels on the disposition or effect of these drugs. Concomitant administration of aspirin with indomethacin or fenoprofen results in competition for protein-binding sites, resulting in displacement and decreased plasma levels of the drug, with increased clearance by either the kidney, liver, or both. A similar phenomenon occurs for most but not all the nonsteroidal anti-inflammatory agents. Although displacement from protein usually decreases the half-life of clearance of the drug, it is possible that tissue penetration of the drug is increased; thus the effect of competition for protein binding on tissue levels is not clear.

Inflammation, by inducing exudation and thus increasing the concentration of serum proteins in extracellular fluids, may increase the concentration of drug in the areas where the effect is needed. Acidity at sites of inflammation causes dissociation from plasma proteins and enhances penetration of cell membranes locally. Thus, experimentally, nonsteroidal anti-inflammatory agents are concentrated at sites of inflammation.[30,65]

In general, synovial fluid levels lag several hours behind serum levels of these drugs, rising more slowly and declining in parallel to plasma levels. In some studies synovial fluid levels declined more slowly than plasma levels and thus were higher for a few hours during single-dose studies. The levels in synovial fluid are determined more by the rate of the terminal clearance phase than the initial phase which determines early plasma levels.[62] In general, synovial fluid levels at steady-state plasma concentration average about 40 percent of plasma levels,[34,62,66-70] probably reflecting the lower protein concentration in the synovial fluid.[62] Similar observations on salicylate levels averaged 44 percent of peak levels in serum, but there was a wide range (16 to 90 percent).[69]

**Blood Levels.** The few studies of plasma levels obtained with the nonsteroidal anti-inflammatory agents show considerable interindividual variation in the peak blood levels achieved after single doses, as well as in the plateau levels found after multiple doses. A fourfold or greater range of levels occurs on a single dosage,[71] although there is an increase in mean blood levels with increased dosage.[72,73] No detailed analysis has been made of the factors that affect these blood levels or of the therapeutic significance of the observed variation.

Optimum therapeutic blood levels have not been determined for the newer agents; studies of phenylbutazone have suggested that 50 to 100 $\mu$g per ml is optimum, with little additional therapeutic benefit and increased toxicity above 100 $\mu$g per ml.[62] Trough levels of free and total naproxen showed a good correlation with clinical responses.[74] The usefulness of these agents will be substantially enhanced when the maximum effectiveness of each of these drugs has been correlated with blood levels and blood levels have become readily available to the clinician.

**Metabolic Clearance.** In general, there is little renal clearance of unchanged drug; the nonsteroidal anti-inflammatory drugs are extensively metabolized in the liver, and most of the altered or conjugated metabolites are excreted by the kidney.[62] Hepatic clearance is much lower than blood flow to the liver; thus, there is no problem of extensive first-pass metabolism (except for aspirin, which is deacetylated rapidly by the liver). Biliary excretion is variable, ranging from 2 to 50 percent, with enterohepatic recirculation occurring for a few drugs. A significant proportion of sulindac and meclofenamate is excreted in the bile and appears in the feces. This may account for the relatively high incidence of side effects in the lower intestine with these agents. One of the drugs under development, isoxicam, is excreted into the bile in dogs and humans to the extent of 60 percent, but no clinical implications of this phenomenon have been reported yet.[75]

Some nonsteroidal anti-inflammatory agents, notably sulindac and fenbufen, are administered as relatively inactive "prodrugs," which have to be metabolized to more active compounds in the liver to be clinically effective. Since the prodrug does not inhibit the gastric cyclooxygenase directly in the stomach, there is less gastric irritation, but it does not eliminate the problem, since the circulating active form of the drug can still affect the gastric mucosa.[7,76]

Any drug that is metabolized extensively can show considerable variability in clearance. A genetic basis for differences in rates of clearance was suggested based on studies of identical and fraternal twins.[62] An age effect on rates of clearance occurs with phenylbutazone[62] and also benoxaprofen, for which a T½ of 29 hours was found in younger patients (average age 41 years) and a T½ of 111 hours was found in much older patients (average age 82 years).[77] Males and patients on steroids metabolize salicylate faster; there is no information on the effect of gender or steroids on rates of clearance of the newer nonsteroidal anti-inflammatory drugs. Disease can alter metabolism of drugs; for example, the clearance of salicylates varies in normals as compared with patients with rheumatoid arthritis.[78] Similar data are not yet available regarding the newer nonsteroidal anti-inflammatory agents. Plasma levels of these drugs are affected by displacement from protein-binding sites,[79] a phenomenon that occurs when a variety of agents are administered concomitantly.

In general, lipophilicity influences both the rate of absorption of these drugs and their rate of metabolism by the liver. A low pKa gives low lipophilicity, and slower absorption, but also a slower rate of metabolism or excretion. Drugs with a high pKa have higher lipophilicity and thus more rapid absorption, but more rapid renal excretion and a short half-life of clearance.[66] Lipophilicity may affect penetration of drug into the cerebrospinal fluid; for example, zomepirac, which has an oil/water solubility coefficient twice that of tolmetin, enters the cerebrospinal fluid better.[31] The sulfoxide group of the relatively inactive sulindac is reduced to a sulfide, increasing affinity for the lipid layer about 1000-fold, approximately the same magnitude as the increase in activity as a cyclooxygenase inhibitor. In addition, the increased lipid solubility results in the accumulation of the sulfide form in tissues, while the prodrug sulindac tends to have higher concentrations in body fluids.[7]

**Rates of Clearance.** The rates of clearance (see Table 50–2) of the various nonsteroidal anti-inflammatory agents from the plasma significantly influence the clinical properties of these agents. Reports of the half-life of clearance of these agents all give average figures, which are useful guides, but it must be kept in mind that all these studies showed considerable interindividual variation in the rate of clearance, often over more than a twofold range. In addition, there are few useful studies of the effect of age, sex, disease, and concomitant administration of other types of drugs, such as anticoagulants, diuretics, and so on, on the rates of clearance of these agents. Most of the data reported are based on studies of young, healthy adult males. Undoubtedly considerable variation exists in different patients, and this phenomenon may account in part for the variability in responsiveness to these drugs.

Accordingly, in Table 50–3 the drugs are grouped

**Table 50–3.** Duration of Action of the Nonsteroidal Anti-inflammatory Drugs

| | Clearance t½ (Hours) | Recom-mended Daily Dosage |
|---|---|---|
| *Agents with Relatively Short Duration of Action* Average half-life is 1 to 8 hours. Time to steady-state concentration ranges from 4 to 16 hours. These drugs have rapid initial effect but frequent doses are necessary. | | |
| Tolemetin | 1* | 600–2000 mg |
| Indomethacin | 1.5–2 | 75–200 mg |
| Ibuprofen | 1–3 | 1.2–2.4 g |
| Fenoprofen | 2–3 | 2.4–3 g |
| Salicylate (low dose) | 2–3 | (under 2.5 g) |
| Alclofenac | < 3 | none |
| Mefenamic acid | 4 (estimate) | 1.5–2.0 g |
| Flufenamic acid | 4 (estimate) | 600–800 mg |
| Meclofenamate | 2–4 | 200–400 mg |
| Flurbifprofen | 6 | 150–400 mg |
| Zomepirac | 7–8† | none |
| *Agents with Medium Duration of Action (t½ = 10–20 Hours)* Once-daily dosage is usually satisfactory. Time to steady state concentration 2 to 4 days. | | |
| Fenbufen | 10‡ | 600–1000 mg |
| Azapropazone | 12 | 900–1800 mg |
| Naproxen | 12–15 | 500–1000 mg |
| Diflunisal | 10–15 | 500–1000 mg |
| Sulindac | 18‡ | 200–400 mg |
| Salicylate (high doses) | 20 | 3.0–6.0 g |
| *Agents with Moderately Long Duration of Action (t½ = 24–36 Hours)* Once-daily dosage is usually satisfactory. Time to steady-state concentration 4 to 7 days. | | |
| Piroxicam | 24–36 | 20 g |
| Isoxicam | 31 (range 21–70) | 200 mg§ |
| Benoxaprofen | 25–32 | none |
| *Agents with Very Long Duration of Action in Maintenance Doses (t½ over 48 Hours)* Once-daily dosage is satisfactory. Time to steady-state concentration 2 to 3 weeks; thus, prolonged monitoring for initial toxicity is important. | | |
| Phenylbutazone | 72 (range 29–176) | 300–400 mg |
| Oxyphenbutazone | 72 (range 29–176) | 300–400 mg |

*Longer periods (4 to 6 hours) reported based on study of terminal phase of half-life.

†Half-life of zomepirac goes up to 9 to 10 hours after multiple doses.

‡Half-life figures given are those for the principal, active metabolites in the case of sulindac and fenbufen.

§Since drug is not yet on the market, recommended daily dosage is not fully established. The dosage listed was used in studies of clinical effectiveness of the drug.

based on duration of action, which correlates better with clinical experience than with the actual half-life of clearance figures reported for each individual agent.

*Steady-State Concentrations.* In general, with repeated dosage, it takes 4 to 5 half-lives of clearance for steady-state plasma levels of a drug to be reached. As a result, short-acting nonsteroidal anti-inflammatory drugs reach plateau levels after the first day of therapy; drugs that have a half-life of about 12 hours require two full days, while those with half-lives of 24 to 36 hours require about a week to achieve full effect. In an urgent clinical situation, such as acute gouty arthritis, a loading dose is advisable if a larger amount of drug on the first day would not be too toxic. Phenylbutazone is often used in this manner.

Since the mechanism of inhibition of platelet function is based on competitive inhibition of the cyclooxygenase by all the nonsteroidal anti-inflammatory drugs except aspirin, this side effect of these drugs clears as the drug is cleared from the plasma. Bleeding from impairment of platelet function may not cease until the drug is cleared sufficiently; the time needed to achieve plateau blood levels is a reasonable guide to the time needed for restoration of platelet function after discontinuing the drug. Therefore, with very long-acting agents, such as phenylbutazone, it may take three weeks or more for bleeding to stop. On the other hand, with rapidly cleared drugs, such as tolectin, indomethacin, fenoprofen, or diclofenac, platelet function is restored rapidly, and it is possible to give these drugs close to the time of surgery.

*Other Clinical Implications of Clearance Data.* With the rapidly cleared drugs, if a dose is missed for any reason, symptoms may return quickly. Similarly, these drugs may lose their effectiveness overnight, resulting in pain, loss of sleep and severe morning stiffness. To compensate, a large bedtime dose of indomethacin may be given; the drug enters adipose and nervous tissue and is released slowly, prolonging its action. Central nervous system toxicity is usually minimal, since the patient sleeps through it.[80] Alternatively, a longer-acting drug at bedtime can be combined with a shorter-acting agent during the day, to give a sustained overnight effect.

## CLINICAL EFFECTS OF NONSTEROIDAL ANTI-INFLAMMATORY AGENTS

The nonsteroidal anti-inflammatory agents that have reached the market are all effective in the treatment of various rheumatic diseases. Tests of effectiveness have established that the drugs are more effective than placebo in patients with rheumatoid arthritis, osteoarthritis, and painful musculoskeletal injuries and, in some instances, in other rheumatic diseases, including gout. These drugs are generally effective in the treatment of rheumatic diseases; but, in each instance, not all of the studies necessary have been performed to gain approval for labeling for every possible indication. Some of the drugs in this category, such as zomepirac, have been tested and marketed as analgesics but are inhibitors of prostaglandin synthesis and are anti-inflammatory.

Tests comparing the relative effectiveness of the newer drugs to aspirin, or to each other, have generally shown small, statistically insignificant differences, although differences in frequency of side effects may be found. It is important to keep in mind that it is difficult to demonstrate a statistically significant difference in effectiveness of two drugs in such studies. Most trials purposely exclude unresponsive patients who have failed to benefit from similar agents, concentrating on patients with mild to moderately severe disease. As a result, relatively complete suppression of symptoms and objective findings occurs with each drug and no difference in effectiveness is demonstrated. Differences that may occur in the few severe cases are lost in the overall statistics, which are dominated by the abundance of mild cases. These studies are often misinterpreted as having established that there is no difference in effectiveness between two drugs, whereas in fact a proper interpretation is that the study failed to refute the null hypothesis that no difference exists, or more simply, failed to establish that a difference exists.

Other problems with the interpretation of reported comparisons of these drugs arise from changes in recommended dosages with time. Most of these agents were first marketed in relatively low doses, just high enough to show a difference from placebo, with minimal risk of toxicity. As experience showed a need for more effect in many cases, and that higher doses were safe, the recommended doses were progressively increased; meanwhile large, multicenter trials were initiated using the earlier dosage schedule. By the time the study was completed, analyzed and published, the dosage tested was no longer being used.[81] Thus, the data in many reports are of limited value. Finally, it is well established that the maximum anti-inflammatory effect of aspirin is only achieved at relatively high plasma levels, which requires pushing the drug to tolerance in most patients; a similar phenomenon may also be apparent with the other nonsteroidal agents when this approach has been effectively tested.

In all studies comparing several drugs, groups of patients preferred each; this variation in preferences of individuals for specific drugs has been a general phenomenon for unclear reasons, and the possibility of greater effectiveness of one agent in an individual patient makes it wise to try several of the drugs in sequence if the first does not give a satisfactory response.[30,82]

There are many excellent reviews of the clinical effectiveness, mechanisms of action, and pharmacology of these drugs.[30,49,76,83-90]

## Effects on Specific Clinical Problems

**Rheumatoid Arthritis.** Subjective, objective, and laboratory parameters of disease activity of rheumatoid arthritis show improvement, and most patients gain significant benefit from the nonsteroidal anti-inflammatory drugs. In many patients, however, control of the manifestations of the disease may be incomplete, and other forms of therapy may need to be added to the regimen. Some rheumatologists have replaced aspirin with one of these drugs as the first-line agent in the treatment of rheumatoid arthritis[82] despite their increased cost. In one noncontrolled study, patients showed about the same frequency of preference for aspirin as for each of several of the newer nonsteroidal anti-inflammatory agents;[91] thus, only a minority of the patients preferred aspirin. In addition, repeated studies have shown more gastrointestinal side effects and more occult blood loss with plain but not coated aspirin than with the newer agents.[92,93] It is not clear, however, if the use of any of these drugs in full anti-inflammatory doses would have changed the results appreciably.

Increasing attention is being given to the possibility that these drugs have a suppressive effect on disease in rheumatoid arthritis. Since, in general, damage to rheumatoid joints is proportional to the severity of the inflammatory process, suppression of inflammation could retard damage to articular tissues.[30] The newer agents have a more complete suppressive effect on disease in many patients, and some can give smooth 24-hour suppression of the inflammation. A preliminary report suggests slowing of the rate of development of erosions in patients given benoxaprofen.[94] A progressive decrease occurred in the number of abnormal joints over a 2-year period in patients receiving tolectin,[52] and, as described above, improvement in immunologic abnormalities has been reported, including normalization of T-lymphocyte function in patients receiving tolectin or piroxicam treatment,[54,95] and a decrease in rheumatoid factor levels in those on piroxicam.[54] There is no clear-cut evidence of a relationship between the severity of the inflammation or the immunologic abnormalities with the extent of the joint destruction in rheumatoid arthritis, but these changes certainly seem to be in the right direction. More carefully designed, extensive studies, similar to those that demonstrated a disease-suppressive effect for gold and penicillamine, are being conducted with several of these agents.

**Juvenile Arthritis.** Only tolectin has received approval by the Food and Drug Administration (FDA) for use in children, perhaps reflecting the cost of studies needed to obtain such approval. Other drugs have been used in children, and there are reports of effectiveness of ibuprofen (using doses in the range of 40 to 50 mg per kg per day and a maximum dose of 2 g per day), and naproxen (in doses of 10 mg per kg per day, up to 750 mg per day).[96,97] Doses given to children on a weight basis should never exceed the maximum given adults.

Indomethacin is especially useful in boys with ankylosing spondylitis, in juvenile-onset pauciarticular arthritis with positive HLA B-27, and occasionally in patients with systemic onset with higher fever (Still's syndrome) unresponsive to other nonsteroidal anti-inflammatory agents. In addition, indomethacin may be useful in boys with hip pain due to benign synovitis unrelieved by other drugs. Indomethacin is used in doses of 1.5 to 3 mg per kg per day up to a maximum of 200 mg per day but reportedly is not well tolerated as chronic therapy and had to be stopped in 43 percent of patients in one series.[96] The main side effects with indomethacin were headache, dizziness, nausea, and severe gastrointestinal distress. The use of indomethacin in children has been inhibited by a report in 1967 of impaired response to infection.[98] There have been no subsequent similar reports,[30] but FDA approval for the use of indomethacin in children was withdrawn after reports of deaths due to hepatitis associated with larger doses in young children.[96]

**Osteoarthritis.** The analgesic effects of the nonsteroidal anti-inflammatory drugs are particularly useful in the management of osteoarthritis, and all the drugs currently on the market are effective in this disease, relieving pain and increasing functional capacity. Doses lower than those needed to suppress the inflammation in rheumatoid arthritis may be adequate, thus decreasing the frequency of side effects.[49] In addition it is possible to take advantage of the lack of a plateau in analgesic effect with increasing doses of these drugs, combining an agent such as acetaminophen, which does not cause gastric irritation, to gain more analgesia.

The effect of the nonsteroidal anti-inflammatory drugs on chondrocyte metabolism in osteoarthritis has not been thoroughly studied. Early reports showed inhibition of the uptake of radiosulfate by articular cartilage by phenylbutazone and salicylate in vitro.[99,100] One agent, benoxaprofen, stimulates proteoglycan synthesis by cartilage in vitro,[50] an effect that could slow progression of the basic process occurring in the cartilage in this disease.

**Ankylosing Spondylitis.** Aspirin is clearly less effective than most of the newer nonsteroidal anti-inflammatory agents in the treatment of ankylosing spondylitis. Indomethacin, naproxen, and fenoprofen were shown to be more effective than tolectin and aspirin in one study of ankylosing spondylitis in which the same drugs found about equal preference in the management of patients with rheumatoid arthritis.[91] Phenylbutazone also is useful in the treatment of ankylosing spondylitis.[101,102]

**Other Diseases.** The nonsteroidal anti-inflammatory agents are useful in the treatment of minor musculoskeletal problems and a variety of nonrheumatic diseases as well. Their effect on uterine function is particularly useful in treatment of *dysmenorrhea* as well as threatened abortion. Women who have dysmenorrhea have higher resting uterine pressure ("tonus') and higher active pressure ("amplitude") as well as a higher frequency of contractions; these changes are attributed to the effects of prostaglandins.[103] Ibuprofen reduces the intrauterine pressure and the frequency of cyclic activity of the uterus, apparently by inhibition of prostaglandin synthesis. Sodium naproxen also reduces intrauterine pressure and uterine pain in women with dysmenorrhea;[103] zomepirac is also effective,[104] as is flufenamic acid.[105] Several nonsteroidal anti-inflammatory agents, including aspirin, indomethacin, and fenoprofen, affect the motility of the pregnant rat uterus and can delay parturition; the dosage necessary for inhibition of uterine contractions is considerably higher for aspirin than other nonsteroidal anti-inflammatory agents studied,[106] which correlates with the greater effectiveness of the newer agents compared with aspirin in the treatment of dysmenorrhea.

Because of the role of prostaglandins in causing vascular dilatation, infants with *patent ductus arteriosus* have been treated with indomethacin. The drug is given in 2 doses, 12 hours apart, and if levels above 250 ng per ml are achieved, the ductus usually closes. But the high frequency of spontaneous closure of the ductus in prematures, and the side effects, including kidney damage, hemorrhage into a ventricle, and necrotizing enterocolitis, has led to caution in suggesting its use for this purpose, since surgery is effective and may be safer.[107]

The effects of aspirin and the nonsteroidal anti-inflammatory drugs on *platelet function* are described earlier in this chapter. Aspirin, because of its prolonged effect, is useful in the management of patients who have had transient ischemic attacks in the central nervous system; newer agents have not been tested in this syndrome. An unexplained potentiating effect of alcohol on bleeding time of patients who have taken aspirin or other nonsteroidal anti-inflammatory agents may be clinically significant.[108]

The vascular effects of the nonsteroidal anti-inflammatory drugs could be a problem in patients with *ischemic heart disease,* since a decrease in coronary blood flow has been reported in patients given indomethacin, along with an increase in systemic blood pressure due to generalized vasoconstriction. The resulting increase in cardiac work, with increased oxygen demand, combined with decreased coronary blood flow can lead to impaired myocardial performance.[109]

Nonsteroidal anti-inflammatory agents are effective in *ocular disease,* since several can inhibit prostaglandin synthesis in uveal and conjunctival tissues; aspirin does not have such an effect in these tissues, but indomethacin, phenylbutazone, and oxyphenbutazone do.[33]

## Toxicity

**Effect on the Gastrointestinal Tract.** The main toxicity of these drugs occurs in the gastrointestinal tract. In almost all studies of these drugs, epigastric distress, nausea, vomiting, and occasionally more serious side effects such as upper gastrointestinal bleeding lead the list of undesirable effects. Occult blood in the stool is almost a universal finding, but in considerably smaller quantities than occurs in patients receiving aspirin. Activation of peptic ulcer can occur with any of these drugs.

The most important reason for the gastrointestinal side effects is the inhibition of gastric prostaglandin synthesis. Prostaglandins increase gastric blood flow, tighten the mucosal barrier, increase mucus production, and decrease acid secretion;[49] prostaglandin $E_2$ has 2000 times the potency of cimetidine as an inhibitor of gastric acid secretion. These effects protect against gastric erosions or ulcer formation.

Drugs that are administered in inactive form but are activated by metabolism in the liver generally cause less inhibition of prostaglandin synthesis in the stomach, and therefore usually are somewhat less toxic. However, in each instance studied, including that of aspirin, the drug given parenterally inhibits gastric mucosal cyclooxygenase and can cause gastric erosions.[7]

Most clinicians recommend administration of these drugs with food or antacids to minimize gastrointestinal toxicity. If the drugs are given with liquid, they may be left behind in the stomach, since liquid is emptied from the stomach faster than solids, resulting in severe local irritation. Therefore, instructing patients to take the medicine in the middle of a meal could minimize the gastric irritation, whereas the ambiguous instructions "take with meals" usually means that the patient will take the drug after the meal, with coffee or tea, which can add to the local irritation.

Cimetidine is said to be protective against the upper gastrointestinal toxicity caused by the nonsteroidal anti-inflammatory drug[110,111] and may be useful in particularly difficult patients, such as those with a history of peptic ulcer disease or gastrointestinal bleeding. The expense and the potential for added toxicity make it unwise to use cimetidine routinely.

Prostaglandins also influence the function of the lower gastrointestinal tract, the specific effect apparently varying with the functional state of the gut at the time. As a consequence, ibuprofen reportedly causes diarrhea in some patients and constipation in others; it has been used successfully in the treatment of idiopathic diarrhea.[49] Serious lower gastrointestinal toxicity occasionally occurs with these drugs. Crampy lower abdominal pain and colonic bleeding, often from pre-existing diverticular disease, has been reported with several of them.[112] A salicylate combined with a sulfonamide, sulfasalazine, is reportedly useful in the management of ulcerative colitis, probably because of an effect on prostaglandin synthesis in the gut,[113] but there are no reports of the use of newer nonsteroidal anti-inflammatory drugs in inflammatory bowel disease.

Secretion into the bile and enterohepatic recirculation occurs to a varying extent with these drugs. When it occurs, increased local concentration in the gastrointestinal tract results. This phenomenon may account for the higher frequency of lower gastrointestinal toxicity with some of them. For example, mefenamic acid (Ponstel), which is approved for short-term analgesic use in the United States but is marketed abroad as an anti-inflammatory drug, causes a higher frequency of diarrhea, sometimes associated with hemorrhage and inflammation of the bowel; hemolytic anemia was reported with this drug. Meclofenamate (Meclomen), a related substance, also causes a dose-related diarrhea more often than do the other nonsteroidal anti-inflammatory agents.[114] Some clinicians have the impression that sulindac, which also undergoes considerable enterohepatic recirculation, causes a higher incidence of crampy abdominal pain than do most other nonsteroidal antiinflammatory agents. The serious reactions to benoxaprofen appear to be attributable to the extensive enterohepatic circulation of the drug.

**Pancreatitis.** Pancreatitis has also been reported with these drugs; in one instance the patient received sulindac, plus aspirin, for severe osteoarthritis of the hip.[115,116]

Salicylates have been known to cause a decrease in blood sugar in some individuals, particularly in diabetics who are receiving oral sulfonylureas.[27] A possible mechanism of this effect is the inhibition of prostaglandin synthesis in the pancreas, where the prostaglandins locally inhibit insulin release.[25] The effect of other nonsteroidal anti-inflammatory drugs on islet cell function has not been studied, but hypoglycemic reactions are not reported.

Esophageal stricture was suggested as a side effect of nonsteroidal anti-inflammatory drugs, because of a report that patients with this problem had a higher frequency of ingestion of these drugs than did a control group without dysphagia. The recommendation that patients drink a lot of water after ingesting the drug and not go to bed immediately afterward seems a reasonable precaution.[117]

**Hepatotoxicity.** The side effect of hepatotoxicity has been reported with several of the newer nonsteroidal anti-inflammatory drugs as well as with aspirin and acetaminophen. Ibuprofen reportedly causes liver toxicity in children but has mild effects on liver function tests in adults.[49] Serious liver toxicity, especially in older people, with several deaths, led to the removal of benoxaprofen from the market in the United States and the United Kingdom.[77] Diclofenac has been reported to cause a hypersensitivity type of hepatitis,[118] and hepatotoxicity has been reported with sulindac,[116] including a report of cholestatic jaundice.[119]

Because of the compensatory effect of prostaglandins synthesized in the kidney on renal blood flow in patients with hypovolemia, patients with cirrhosis who have hypoalbuminemia, ascites, and edema may develop the hepatorenal syndrome if given nonsteroidal anti-inflammatory drugs.

**Renal Effects.** Local prostaglandin synthesis in the kidney regulates intrarenal blood flow, particularly under circumstances of decreased glomerular filtration and moderate impairment of renal function. Increased amounts of prostaglandins are usually found in the urine in such instances. Aspirin and most other nonsteroidal anti-inflammatory agents, by inhibiting synthesis of the prostaglandins in the kidney, affect this compensatory mechanism; a rise in BUN and serum creatinine results. Among patients with rheumatic diseases, this effect is most frequently seen in those with systemic lupus with renal involvement but can occur in any patient with hypovolemia or intrinsic renal disease. The effect of these drugs is reversible when the drug is stopped and only occasionally requires discontinuation of effective antirheumatic therapy.[120]

Inhibition of renal prostaglandin synthesis causes salt and water retention, occasionally resulting in frank edema. Prostaglandins also affect water handling by the kidney, probably by an effect on cAMP concentration in renal tubular cells. Inhibition of prostaglandin synthesis by indomethacin or meclofenamate enhanced the antidiuretic effect of antidiuretic hormone in rats undergoing water diuresis.[121]

The nonsteroidal anti-inflammatory drugs can block the action of diuretics, including furosemide.[122] This effect can complicate the management of hypertension or congestive heart failure. The combination of triamterine and indomethacin causes serious renal toxicity, with azotemia. Normal medical students given 200 mg per day of triamterene and 150 mg per day of indomethacin showed reversible acute renal failure.[123] No similar effect was found when indomethacin was given with furosemide, hydrochlorothiazide, or spironolactone, perhaps because they work at different sites in the renal tubule. The mechanism suggested was that the toxicity of triamterene is ordinarily prevented by a compensatory increase in prostaglandin synthesis, and this protective mechanism is blocked by indomethacin. The presence of high levels of prostaglandins in the urine may be an indicator of susceptibility to the azotemic effect of aspirin or other nonsteroidal anti-inflammatory agents.[123] Indomethacin has no influence on the half-life of clearance of hydrochlorothiazide.[124]

The inhibition of intrarenal prostaglandin synthesis also affects production of renin. Large doses of aspirin (3.9 g per day) cause a decrease in plasma renin concentration, with a rebound above control values after cessation of the drug.[125] An inhibitory effect of these drugs on renin and angiotensin II genesis may be clinically important in patients who develop hypovolemia as a result of gastrointestinal bleeding; the ability to adjust to blood loss could be impaired, resulting in earlier vasomotor collapse.

Inhibition of renal prostaglandin synthesis is clinically useful in the management of Bartter's syndrome. Increased renal prostaglandin synthesis is a key step in the pathogenesis of this syndrome, leading to increased urinary excretion of prostaglandins and increased formation of renin and aldosterone. Indomethacin and other inhibitors of renal prostaglandin synthesis correct the elevated plasma renin concentration, hyperaldosteronism, and decreased sensitivity to angiotensin infusion characteristic of Bartter's syndrome.[126,127]

Sulindac reportedly has less effect on renal prostaglandin synthesis and thus causes less salt and water retention, inhibition of the effect of diuretics, and azotemia than do the other nonsteroidal anti-inflammatory agents.[128,129]

*Acute Allergic Interstitial Nephritis.* This side effect has been reported with several of the nonsteroidal anti-inflammatory agents, most often with fenoprofen, but also with ibuprofen,[130] naprosyn, tolmetin, indomethacin, and zomepirac.[129-131] Characteristically such patients have eosinophils in the urine sediment and avid uptake of gallium by the kidney on nuclear scanning. Renal biopsy shows normal-appearing glomeruli on light microscopy, with fusion of glomerular foot processes on electron microscopy. There are interstitial infiltrates consisting of plasma cells and lymphocytes (which are mostly T-lymphocytes) and eosinophils as well as focal deposition of IgG on interstitial and tubular basement membranes. These observations are similar to those made with other instances of drug-induced allergic interstitial nephritis. All instances reversed after the drug was discontinued, with return of BUN to normal, although steroid therapy was given to some of these patients.[132]

*Lipid Nephrosis.* Lipid nephrosis has been reported with fenoprofen, and there are single case reports with naprosyn and indomethacin.[132,133]

*Analgesic Nephropathy.* Ingestion of enormous quantities of analgesic medications (averaging 11 kg of aspirin, 8 kg of phenacetin, or 50,000 tablets, usually of combinations of aspirin, phenacetin, and caffeine or codeine) has been associated with abdominal or flank pain, pyuria without evidence of infection, hematuria, acidosis, passage of renal papillae in the urine, hypertension, and azotemia, with many deaths.[134] Phenacetin was most frequently implicated; aspirin is thought to be safe, and a study of renal function in patients who took large amounts of aspirin for rheumatoid arthritis for 10 or more years showed no evidence of impairment of renal function.[135] With the availability of its active metabolite, acetaminophen, phenacetin was replaced and analgesic nephropathy seems to have decreased in frequency, but some investigators feel that any analgesic can cause this syndrome.[136]

All the newer nonsteroidal anti-inflammatory agents cause nephrotoxicity in high doses in a variety of laboratory animals, especially dogs and rats.[137] It is not yet certain whether analgesic nephropathy will turn out to be a problem when sufficient quantities of these drugs have been ingested. Clinicians should remain alert to the possibility that long-term therapy may be associated with serious renal toxicity.

*Use of Nonsteroidal Anti-inflammatory Drugs in Renal Failure.* Since little direct renal excretion of the nonsteroidal anti-inflammatory drugs occurs, there is no known problem of accumulation of these drugs in patients with lowered glomerular filtration rates. The metabolites of most of these agents are normally cleared by the kidney, and the danger of accumulation of them is unclear. The effect of hemodialysis on blood levels of the drugs and their metabolites is unknown.[138] Several of these agents, most notably indomethacin, have been used in chronic uremic patients in usual dosage without any apparent problem. Diclofenac is also safe in chronic renal failure (see below).

**Pseudoallergic Reactions.** After ingesting aspirin, some patients develop asthmatic wheezes, rhinitis, and nasal polyps; urticaria and angioedema can also occur. This reaction apparently results from inhibition of the cyclooxygenase, shifting the metabolism of the arachidonic acid into the lipoxygenase pathway, increasing the production of leukotrienes. This reaction to aspirin occurs more often in patients with chronic urticaria and asthmatics but in only about 0.3 percent of normal people.[139,140]

Repeated administration of aspirin usually causes the same reaction in a sensitive patient. Other nonsteroidal anti-inflammatory agents that inhibit the cyclooxygenase cause a similar reaction in these patients. Drugs that are poor inhibitors of the enzyme usually do not cross-react; thus, nonaspirin salicylate and acetaminophen usually can be given to such patients.[139]

**Pregnancy.** None of the nonsteroidal anti-inflammatory agents are approved for use in pregnancy, since careful studies of safety in pregnancy are impossible.

The effect of these agents on the pulmonary vasculature of the fetus is a concern; inhibition of prostacycline synthesis in arterial walls can cause vasoconstriction; experimentally, closure of the ductus arteriosus in utero can be induced by inhibitors of prostaglandin synthesis, leading to ischemia of the lower parts of the body and developmental abnormalities. Widespread narrowing of the pulmonary vasculature can occur, causing pulmonary hypertension. Instances of persistent pulmonary hypertension have been observed in infants following the use of aspirin or indomethacin by the mother during pregnancy, and a similar syndrome was induced in lambs.[141]

If use of a nonsteroidal anti-inflammatory agent is considered during pregnancy, the indication should be quite strong and informed consent obtained. If possible, use should be limited to the third trimester and discontinued several days to a few weeks before term because during labor the nonsteroidal anti-inflammatory agents can decrease uterine contractions and delay parturition; blood loss at the time of delivery can be increased because of the effect on platelet function.[63]

**Other Side Effects.** Stevens-Johnson syndrome was reported with several of these agents, including sulindac,[142,143] diflunisal, and diclofenac.[144] Other serious reactions to sulindac reported include toxic epidermal necrolysis, granulocytopenia, aplastic anemia, and thrombocytopenia;[116] aplastic anemia was also reported with fenoprofen.[145] A sterile meningitis has occurred in patients with systemic lupus erythematosus given ibuprofen or sulindac.[116]

*Visual blurring* occurs with all the nonsteroidal anti-inflammatory agents, but no actual retinopathy has been reported, and the visual effects are reversible when the drug is stopped. *Morbilliform rashes* occur with high doses of these agents; they clear promptly when the drug is discontinued and do not recur at lower doses; clearly these are not allergic rashes. They are probably related to an effect on arachidonic acid metabolism.[146] One of the nonsteroidal anti-inflammatory agents, alclofenac, caused a high incidence of rashes. It was withdrawn from the market because of toxicity, including the occurrence of vasculitis.[147] This drug was a phenylacetic acid derivative that contained a chlorine atom on the main ring. *Anaphylactic reactions* have been reported to occur with higher frequency with tolectin and with zomepirac than with other agents.[148,149]

**Interaction with Anticoagulants.** The possibility of significant interaction with anticoagulants such as warfarin is great, because of the high degree of protein binding by both types of agents, as well as the possibility of alterations in hepatic metabolism. Apparently, no significant interaction occurs with ibuprofen, tolectin, naproxen, diflunisal, or diclofenac,[27,144] but it is necessary to reduce the dose of warfarin when isoxicam is used concomitantly.[150] An increase in unbound warfarin occurs with concomitant administration of fenoprofen, and some additional prolongation of prothrombin time occurs.[84] Because of their effect on platelet function, extreme caution is necessary when any of these drugs is used in combination with anticoagulants.

## COMMENTS ABOUT INDIVIDUAL AGENTS

Points made elsewhere in this chapter will not be repeated in this section, and thus comments are not thorough reviews of each drug.

**Indomethacin.** Indomethacin (Fig. 50–1) was one of the earliest of the nonsteroidal anti-inflammatory agents to be introduced, and it is the standard agent used in vitro for inhibition of prostaglandin synthesis. Clinically it is very useful and is particularly effective in ankylosing spondylitis and in acute gout; there is also a report of special effectiveness in osteoarthritis of the hip compared with other agents.[151] Although indomethacin may cause less gastric irritation and occult blood loss than aspirin,[93] gastrointestinal side effects are the main limitation to its clinical usefulness.[30,152,153]

Indomethacin has an indole nucleus, resembling serotonin, which may account for its unusual incidence of central nervous system side effects, of which headache is the most common. Dizziness, "light-headedness," depersonalization, loss of concentrating ability, and actual confusion can occur, requiring discontinuation of the drug.

Indomethacin is favored by many clinicians for control of fever in difficult cases, such as lymphomas, but careful comparisons with newer agents have not been performed. Indomethacin has been used to treat Bartter's syndrome because of its effect on renal prostaglandin synthesis, decreasing production of renin and thus of aldosterone;[154] however, in some patients, pseudotumor cerebri has developed.[155]

Because of the relatively rapid clearance of indomethacin, symptoms may return during the night, with bothersome morning stiffness. To achieve smoother control of symptoms, a bedtime dose of 100 mg, coupled with 25 mg three or four times during the day can minimize side effects (patients sleep through the headache) and achieve more prolonged effect, but gastrointestinal side effects are still a problem.[80] The bedtime dose can be added to another short-acting agent with less gastrointestinal toxicity given during the day. A sustained release form of indomethacin (Indocin-SR[R]), which is absorbed more slowly, can achieve smoother blood levels with the drug on a daily dosage of 75 mg twice daily.[156]

Metabolism of indomethacin involves demethylation and deacetylation in the liver, with subsequent excretion of the inactive metabolites in the bile and urine; thus caution is wise in patients with impaired liver function.

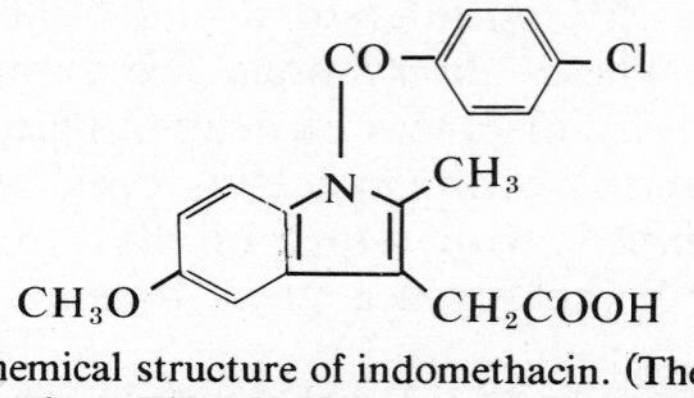


**Figure 50–1.** Chemical structure of indomethacin. (The figures in this chapter are taken from The Merck Index, An Encyclopedia of Chemicals and Drugs. 9th ed. Rahway, New Jersey, Merck Co., Inc., 1976.)

Only small amounts of indomethacin or other nonsteroidal anti-inflammatory agents are excreted unchanged by the kidney. Metabolites are excreted by both the kidney and the liver, but there are no careful studies of the clearance of the metabolites in chronic renal failure. Indomethacin is the nonsteroidal anti-inflammatory drug most frequently used in patients with chronic renal failure, particularly to control the manifestations of uremic pericarditis. No special adjustment of dosage is recommended, but extreme caution should be exercised, particularly in view of the gastrointestinal and central nervous system side effects of the drug, which can resemble manifestations of uremia.

Blood levels of indomethacin are increased by concomitant administration of probenecid.[157] This interaction has the potential of increasing the therapeutic effect of a moderate dose of the drug, with less direct gastric irritation; the systemic effect of indomethacin on the stomach remains, however, and the clinical value of the use of probenecid in this fashion had not been evaluated.

**Sulindac.** Sulindac (Fig. 50–2) is a chemical relative of indomethacin and is given as a relatively inactive prodrug; the methyl sulfinyl group is converted by the cytochrome system in the liver to a variety of oxidized forms which have increased anti-inflammatory activity.[158] These metabolites are more potent inhibitors of prostaglandin synthesis and are cleared from the plasma more slowly, making twice-a-day dosage satisfactory; 150 to 200 mg of sulindac twice a day is recommended and should rarely, if ever, be exceeded.

The effectiveness of sulindac has been established for rheumatoid arthritis, osetoarthritis, and acute gout,[86] but the relatively long period needed to achieve plateau blood levels (4 to 5 days) and the lack of established safety of a loading dose make it a little less satisfactory for the latter condition. It is less effective than indomethacin and phenylbutazone in the treatment of ankylosing spondylitis.[159] Upper gastrointestinal irritation and bleeding are much less common with sulindac than with aspirin,[30,159] and the drug is much better tolerated than either aspirin or indomethacin; although chemically similar to indomethacin, central nervous system side effects have not been reported with sulindac. However, about 25 percent of patients have other gastrointestinal problems, including constipation and abdominal pain, perhaps because of excretion of active metabolites in the bile affecting prostaglandin synthesis in the gut.

Rare instances of a variety of other types of toxicity have been reported with sulindac, including Stevens-Johnson syndrome; blood dyscrasias, including fatal aplastic anemia;[116] pancreatitis;[160] hepatotoxicity; and aseptic meningitis in patients with systemic lupus.[116] Sulindac does not inhibit diuresis induced by furosemide apparently because of less effect on renal cyclooxygenase activity. Sulindac therefore does not interfere with drugs used for the treatment of hypertension or congestive heart failure, and it does not cause increased azotemia in patients with mild renal failure, as do the other nonsteroidal anti-inflammatory drugs.[128,129] This organ specificity of the effect of the drug makes it particularly useful in many patients.

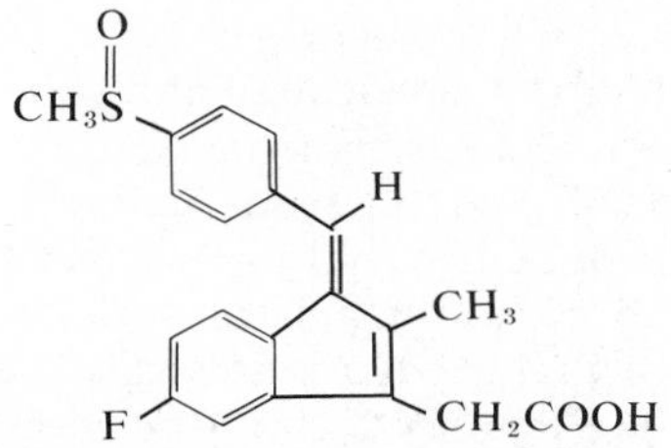


**Figure 50–2.** Chemical structure of sulindac.

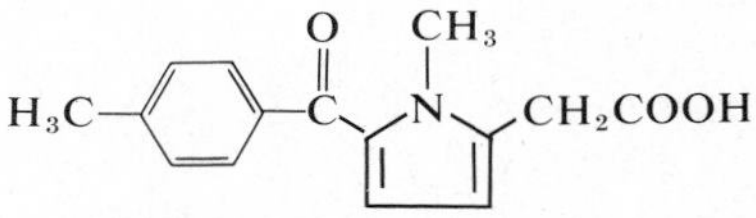


**Figure 50–3.** Chemical structure of tolmetin.

Sulindac is capable of trapping toxic oxygen radicals, and in the process, in vitro, the active metabolites are converted back to the less active parent sulindac. Thus, this drug has an anti-inflammatory action beyond that of inhibition of prostaglandin synthesis, which could account for its extra effectiveness in some patients.[7]

**Tolmetin.** A pyrrole acetic acid derivative, chemically related to indomethacin but lacking an indole nucleus, tolmetin (Fig. 50–3) is rapidly cleared from the blood, either unchanged or as a dicarboxylic acid metabolite or a conjugate. Tolmetin is easily displaced from protein-binding sites; for example, aspirin displaces tolmetin competitively and accelerates its already very rapid clearance from the blood.[30] Concomitant use with aspirin had no better effect than aspirin alone.[161] Tolmetin causes fewer gastrointestinal and central nervous system side effects than indomethacin, despite its chemical similarity; 75 percent of patients who could not tolerate indomethacin did tolerate tolectin.[30] Tolmetin is reported to be effective in a variety of rheumatic diseases and is approved for use in juvenile arthritis.

**Ibuprofen.** The first phenylpropionic acid derivative to be marketed in the United States, ibuprofen is relatively well tolerated and has a particularly low incidence of gastrointestinal side effects.[49] Ibuprofen (Fig. 50–4) is rapidly metabolized, primarily in the liver; less than 10 percent is excreted unchanged in the bile and urine. At the dosage initially recommended, ibuprofen was effective as an analgesic, but it was weakly anti-inflammatory; since then, considerably higher doses have been shown to be well tolerated, and its anti-inflammatory effectiveness has been established. Currently doses of up to 2.4 g per day are approved, but there are reports of the use of 3.2 g per day.[49] The relatively greater analgesic effectiveness makes the drug clinically useful in a variety of problems. It has achieved great favor in the treatment of dysmenorrhea[162] and is effective in osteoarthritis of

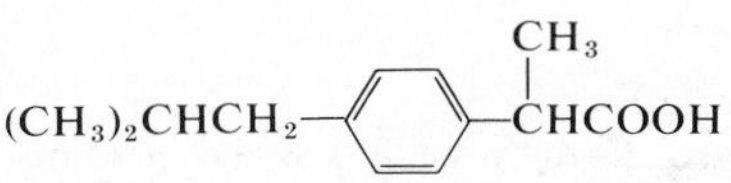


**Figure 50–4.** Chemical structure of ibuprofen.

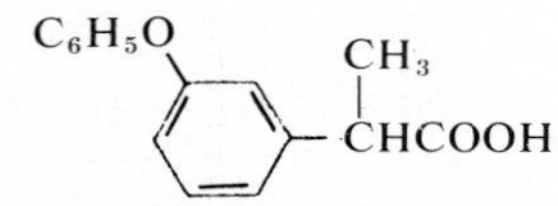


**Figure 50–5.** Chemical structure of fenoprofen.

the hip, in psoriatic arthritis,[163] and, in large doses, in the treatment of gout.[82,164]

Ibuprofen does not induce hepatic microsomal enzymes and reports show absence of interference with the protein binding of warfarin, thus making it safe to use in combination with anticoagulant therapy, although the effect on platelet function has to be kept in mind.[30,49]

There are reports of the occurrence of a meningitis-like syndrome[165] and of a nonspecific febrile reaction[166] in patients with systemic lupus erythematosus given ibuprofen but these are clearly rare events.[49]

**Fenoprofen.** Fenoprofen (Fig. 50–5) is also a propionic acid derivative with a relatively short half-life. Absorption of fenoprofen is decreased by concomitant food or aspirin, but it is questionable whether this effect is clinically significant.[63] Available in 300-mg capsules, the recommended dose is 2.4 g per day. The drug is effective in a variety of rheumatic diseases, and, as is true of each of these drugs, there are patients who prefer it over aspirin or other anti-inflammatory agents;[30] it is relatively well tolerated, but dyspepsia is its chief side effect. Fenoprofen may cause serious renal toxicity more frequently than the other nonsteroidal anti-inflammatory agents, but this phenomenon is statistically rare.

**Naproxen.** Naproxen (Fig. 50–6) is a phenylpropionic acid derivative with a relatively long half-life, making twice-a-day dosage satisfactory. It is also relatively well tolerated. Although excreted primarily as a glucuronide conjugate, unbound, free drug is excreted by the kidney. Early studies suggested that doses above 500 mg per day result in increased unbound drug, which is rapidly cleared, suggesting that higher doses would be of no added value; however, clinical trials have established progressively increasing effectiveness with increasing doses, although with a shallow dose response curve.[167] The approved dosage has been increased to 1 g per day, and 1.5 g per day is being tested.

Since the sodium salt of naproxen is more rapidly absorbed than the acid, pain relief occurs sooner, and it is marketed as an analgesic. This advantage applies only to the first dose of the drug, however; the acid form of naproxen is as effective as an analgesic, since it is the active moiety. Naproxen is effective in the treatment of dysmenorrhea,[168] postoperative pain,[169] and dental pain and in sports injuries[170] as well as in the treatment of various rheumatic diseases, including rheumatoid arthritis, osteoarthritis,[171] and gout;[172] it was reported to be as effective as phenylbutazone in ankylosing spondylitis.[173]

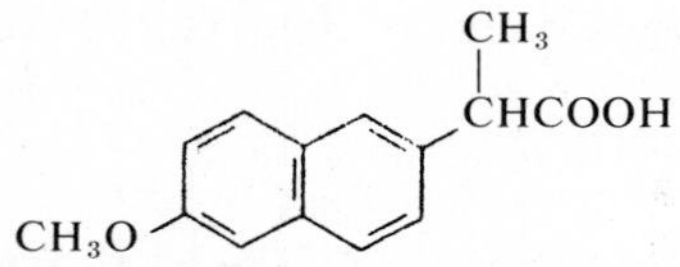


**Figure 50–6.** Chemical structure of naproxen.

Concomitant administration of aspirin caused a 16 percent decrease in blood levels of naproxen,[73] a change that was felt not to be clinically important, and a subsequent trial of moderate doses of both agents showed additive effect without additional toxicity.[174]

Probenecid increases the blood levels of naproxen, a surprising effect, since renal tubular secretion of the parent drug is negligible; apparently this effect results from competition for hepatic glucuronyl transferase.[73] There is no significant interaction between naproxen and the sulfonylureas, nor does it change the activity of warfarin, despite interference with protein binding of the warfarin, increasing the free serum fraction of that drug by 13 percent.[73]

Naproxen crosses the placenta, and thus its use in pregnancy is unwise. It may potentiate the toxicity of bilirubin in neonatal jaundice by competing for binding sites on albumin.[83]

As is the case with the other nonsteroidal anti-inflammatory agents, there are reports of severe gastrointestinal bleeding with naproxen,[175,176] but overall the drug is relatively well tolerated, and one study concluded that it can be given safely to patients with a history of peptic ulcer or hiatal hernia, although the patients should be closely followed.[177]

Judging by sales in the United States, the two most popular nonsteroidal anti-inflammatory agents are naproxen and ibuprofen.

**Phenylbutazone.** The first drug in this group to be introduced, phenylbutazone has been widely used despite initial reports of serious gastrointestinal and bone marrow toxicity. Use of lower doses has decreased the frequency of toxicity markedly. Oxyphenbutazone, a metabolite of phenylbutazone, is also active and is available as a drug; kinetics, efficacy, and side effects are the same for the two agents.

The half-life of phenylbutazone is about 20 hours for high doses, but clearance is much slower with lower doses. At the currently recommended maintenance dose of 300 mg per day, a half-life of over 100 hours occurs. It can take 2 to 3 weeks for plateau steady-state blood levels to be reached, and a similar amount of time for toxicity to clear. An even longer half-life of phenylbutazone is seen in some elderly subjects,[62] and its use in patients over age 60 should be restricted to periods of one week. Phenylbutazone causes salt and water retention, and its use can complicate the management of hypertension or congestive heart failure.

Despite the very slow clearance of phenylbutazone, a dosage of three or four times per day is recommended. Once a day is, in fact, adequate, but dividing the dosage may minimize direct gastric toxicity.

Phenylbutazone and indomethacin are superior to aspirin in the treatment of ankylosing spondylitis[102] and gout. It is also useful for musculoskeletal injuries, but because of potential toxicity it is usually used only when other agents are not satisfactory; however, in such instances it can be a very valuable drug and is widely used by veterinarians for this purpose. In the treatment of acute gout, the use of a loading dose of about 600 mg is recommended to achieve therapeutic levels rapidly. The recommended maintenance dose of 300 mg per day should not be exceeded. Both phenylbutazone and oxyphenbutazone are uricosuric, in contrast to most of the other nonsteroidal anti-inflammatory agents, which are useful in the management of gout without causing uricosuria. This difference in effect may be important in patients with a history of uric acid calculi.

There are patients who receive more benefit from phenylbutazone than any other nonsteroidal anti-inflammatory agent, a phenomenon that occurs with all these drugs. Reports of some differences in the mechanisms of action of phenylbutazone suggest a possible basis for this benefit. For example, in vitro, both chemotaxis and spontaneous motility of neutrophils are inhibited by corticosteroids and phenylbutazone, whereas the other nonsteroidal anti-inflammatory drugs inhibit only chemotaxis.[178]

**Azopropazone.** Azopropazone is also a pyrazolone derivative, chemically related to phenylbutazone. It has a half-life of about 12 hours, and a biologic half-life of about 20 hours.[179] Although three or four doses a day are recommended, twice-daily dosage should be satisfactory. It takes 4 days to a week for a full steady-state plasma level to be reached. The drug and its inactive metabolites are excreted by the kidneys. Azapropazone is well tolerated but does cause fluid retention and thus problems of hypertension and congestive heart failure may be aggravated; caution is therefore recommended in the use of the drug in the elderly, as with phenylbutazone. In view of the extremely tight protein-binding characteristic of this drug, the possibility of interactions with concurrent anticoagulant and antidiabetic drugs exists; a considerable reduction in dosage of anticoagulant, up to 50 to 75 percent of previous levels, is recommended.[179] Careful monitoring is also recommended when sulfonamides or oral hypoglycemic agents are used concomitantly.[179]

Azapropazone, like the other pyrazolone derivatives, is markedly uricosuric. Because of the hematologic toxicity of other pyrazolones, careful monitoring of bone marrow function is wise; marrow suppression is found in animal studies but not reported in humans; however, the recommended maximum dose of 1800 mg per day should not be exceeded.[179]

**Diclofenac.** A phenylacetic acid derivative, diclofenac is rapidly absorbed, with peak plasma levels in 1 to 2 hours; the drug is tightly bound to protein and eliminated by the liver, where it is metabolized mainly by hydroxylation, with extensive enterohepatic recirculation.[180] Elimination is biphasic, but it is 90 percent complete 1.5 to 2 hours after the peak plasma level is reached; thus, it is very difficult to obtain smooth, steady-state plasma levels with diclofenac, even with a dosage of three times a day.[144] Interestingly, the drug appears rapidly in the synovial fluid, where, as a result of protein binding, levels persist much longer than in plasma.[144]

Despite its tight binding to protein, diclofenac does not interact with oral hypoglycemic or anticoagulant drugs, and no adjustment in dosage of these agents has been found to be necessary with concomitant administration.[144]

Careful studies of the effect of chronic renal failure on the pharmacokinetics of diclofenac have been performed. In such patients, the drug and its metabolites reach higher plasma levels, but calculations of elimination half-lives are the same as in normal subjects. Excretion of diclofenac and its metabolites in the urine is decreased in proportion to the reduction in glomerular filtration rate, but a compensatory increase in elimination via the bile occurs, preventing accumulation. Thus, patients with renal insufficiency may be given the same dosage schedule as is used for patients with normal renal function.[144,181]

The main side effects of diclofenac are gastrointestinal, but a fatal case of Stevens-Johnson syndrome has been reported; other serious reactions, including fatal aplastic anemia, have occurred, but the patients were taking other drugs in much closer temporal relationship to the onset of symptoms of the marrow dyscrasia. Single instances of deaths from pancreatitis and other serious gastrointestinal reactions are also reported.[144]

Because of lowered plasma levels of diclofenac with concomitant aspirin administration, combined therapy is not recommended.[144]

**Diflunisal.** A salicylate derivative, diflunisal has a phenyl group containing two fluorines added to the parent salicylate molecule. Conjugated in the liver, the entire parent molecule, containing the fluorine atoms, is excreted in the urine. Excretion is impaired by chronic renal failure, and the drug is not removed by hemodialysis;[182] thus, it should be avoided in patients with chronic renal failure.

The elimination half-life of diflunisal is dose dependent, increasing from 7 to 8 hours at 125 mg to 8 to 10 hours at 250 mg, and at 15 hours to 500 mg, in single doses. The recommended dosage is 500 mg followed by 250 to 500 mg twice a day. At this dosage, steady-state plasma levels may not be reached for 7 to 9 days,[89] and a loading dose of 1 g may be useful.[183]

Diflunisal is marketed primarily as an analgesic. It has a long enough half-life to permit twice-daily dosage, accounting for its trade name in the United States, Dolobid. Although diflunisal has less effect on the platelet cyclooxygenase than aspirin, it is inhibitory, and platelet function is impaired. Since it lacks the acetyl group of aspirin, it does not acetylate the platelet enzyme, and its inhibitory effect is reversed as the drug is cleared from the blood.

Diflunisal causes an increase in the plasma concentration of hydrochlorothiazide and a decrease in its renal excretion, but the clinical significance of this interaction is unknown. Diflunisal does block the uric acid retention caused by hydrochlorothiazide, however,[89] and when given alone, causes uricosuria.

Diflunisal causes less upper gastrointestinal toxicity than aspirin preparations, and it is useful in osteoarthritis and other painful rheumatic syndromes, but full trials of its effect in inflammatory rheumatic diseases are not yet available. Concomitant administration of aluminum hydroxide gel decreased absorption of diflunisal, but food does not affect its bioavailability. Aspirin in doses of 300 mg four times a day did not affect plasma levels of diflunisal, but 600 mg four times daily did decrease trough steady-state plasma levels. Several cases of Stevens-Johnson syndrome have been reported with diflunisal.[89]

**Piroxicam.** Piroxicam (Fig. 50–7) is slowly cleared (T½ averaging 24 hours), permitting once-a-day dosage, thus enhancing patient compliance and round-the-clock suppression of inflammation. The drug is very potent, and only 20 mg a day is recommended; higher doses result in an increased incidence of toxicity, primarily gastric irritation. Double-blind studies have demonstrated effectiveness of piroxicam in rheumatoid arthritis,[184] osteoarthritis,[185] gout,[186] and ankylosing spondylitis.[187]

Since small quantities of piroxicam are given, the drug occupies few binding sites on the plasma protein, and there is no apparent interaction with other drugs on this basis. Coadministration of aspirin does not cause clinically significant alteration in the plasma concentration of either agent,[71,188] but a combination of 40 mg per day of piroxicam and aspirin caused a high incidence of peptic ulcer formation.[189]

**Benoxaprofen.** A phenylpropionic acid derivative like other "profens," benoxaprofen (Fig. 50–8) was withdrawn from the market because of hepatotoxicity. Nevertheless, it is worth keeping the drug in mind because it has several unusual properties. The long half-life (averaging 29 hours) allowed once-a-day dosage but also led to the problems of toxicity; like all drugs metabolized extensively in the liver, there was considerable variation in the rate of clearance. In the elderly, a particularly long half-life was observed,[123] reaching 111 hours in one study.[77] As a result of a single recommended dose schedule, 600 mg a day, and no convenient method of monitoring blood levels, toxicity developed, with cholestasis, jaundice, and liver failure, particularly in elderly patients.

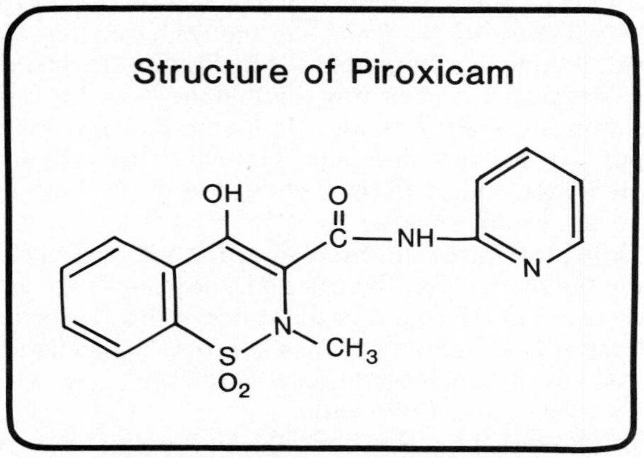


**Figure 50–7.** Chemical structure of piroxicam.

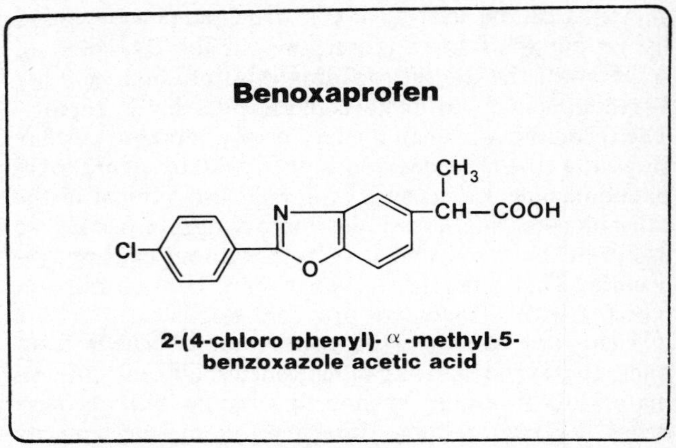


**Figure 50–8.** Chemical structure of benoxaprofen.

Benoxaprofen had the apparently unusual property of inhibition of the lipoxygenase pathway as well as the cyclooxygenase pathway of arachidonic acid metabolism. As a result, it caused an inhibition of cell migration and chemotactic responsiveness, particularly in monocytes. Although similar effects occur with other nonsteroidal anti-inflammatory agents, they were particularly well studied with benoxaprofen and may be relevant to its clinical effects.

Benoxaprofen caused stimulation of cartilage proteoglycan synthesis,[50] an effect that could slow cartilage degradation, particularly in osteoarthritis and other destructive arthropathies. Slowing of the radiologic evidence for cartilage destruction in rheumatoid arthritis was reported with benoxaprofen,[94] suggesting a suppressive effect on disease.

Among the unusual toxic manifestations of benoxaprofen reported were a painful photosensitivity on exposure to ultraviolet light[190] and increased hair growth in areas of male-pattern baldness[191] (which made several physicians want to take the drug despite reports of its toxicity).

**Zomepirac.** Zomepirac is chemically related to indomethacin and tolectin but has a longer half-life (average 7.6 hours).[192] An inhibitor of prostaglandin synthesis, it was useful in the treatment of rheumatoid arthritis and other inflammatory diseases, but was marketed primarily for short-term use as an analgesic. A study of its value in osteoarthritis over a 2-year period was reported, with its effect comparing favorably with aspirin, with fewer side effects.[193] In general, its toxicity and safety are comparable to those of other agents in this group, but a higher incidence of anaphylactic reactions, particularly in patients who had stopped taking the drug and then restarted it, led to the withdrawal of zomepirac from the market in the United States.

Other interesting new drugs are under development. One, *fenbufen*, is given as a prodrug that is converted to an active metabolite in the liver.[194] The active metabolite has a half-life of clearance of 10 hours, which is not increased in elderly patients,[195] but it is prolonged in chronic renal failure to an average of 17 hours.[196]

## CLINICAL USEFULNESS OF THE NONSTEROIDAL ANTI-INFLAMMATORY AGENTS

In the view of many rheumatologists, the newer nonsteroidal anti-inflammatory agents have the potential of replacing aspirin as the first-line, premier antirheumatic drug because of increased effectiveness at full doses in many diseases, lower toxicity (especially gastrointestinal), and greater patient compliance. One tablet a day instead of 12 to 16 is clearly preferable for many patients. On the other hand, the greater cost, the lack of availability of plasma levels with concomitant lack of experience in how to use them, and uncertainty regarding long-term safety have resulted in the continued use of large amounts of aspirin, and few rheumatologists would switch patients who are doing well on aspirin to one of the newer agents.

A major potential advantage of these drugs over aspirin is the reduced incidence of gastric irritation and occult blood loss; however, serious upper gastrointestinal bleeding can occasionally occur with any of these agents. They have been shown to be clearly superior to aspirin in several diseases, both rheumatic (e.g., gout, ankylosing spondylitis) and nonrheumatic (e.g., dysmenorrhea). As analgesics, several are as good as large amounts of aspirin, and again the lower gastrointestinal toxicity gives them a clear advantage.

Many clinicians use newer agents in combination with aspirin. This practice began when phenylbutazone was found to be too toxic in large doses and often too weak as the sole agent in safe maintenance doses. The literature abounds in confusing statements and observations on this subject, and package inserts distributed with these drugs advise against concomitant use of aspirin. Since the gastric irritation may be additive, this is probably good routine advice, but should it be a general proscription? Although displacement from protein-binding sites occurs when these drugs are given in combination,[79] studies of the effects of combinations of these drugs on blood levels have yielded data too variable for definitive conclusions; no consistent pattern exists, and no guide to therapy can be found in such studies.

A bizarre interaction between these drugs occurs in the treatment of adjuvant arthritis in rats. Prior administration of any of them interferes with the effect of indomethacin in this model; even prior use of indomethacin interferes.[197] The effect of isoxicam, on the other hand, is not blocked by prior aspirin or other nonsteroidal anti-inflammatory drugs.[198]

Many authoritative statements have proscribed combined use as irrational, since all drugs act in the same fashion; but there are abundant data to point to subtle, perhaps important, differences in mechanisms of action, in tissue penetration, and in capacity to inhibit prostaglandin synthesis in specific organs. The variation in pharmacokinetics is clinically important. Certainly there are differences in the effectiveness of these drugs in different diseases, especially when compared with aspirin, suggesting there are differences in mechanisms of action. It seems unwise to base clinical decisions on dogmatic statements about mechanisms of action that are not well supported by the little laboratory data available. Clearly empirical observation must establish whether combinations are helpful or deleterious.

Thus far, studies of clinical effectiveness of combinations are inconclusive; additive benefit is as difficult to establish as is an advantage of one effective drug over another. Interference with effectiveness or additive toxicity is easier to establish and has not been observed, except for one report of a 33 percent incidence of peptic ulcer disease with a combination of piroxicam and aspirin.[189] Additive benefit in rheumatoid arthritis was shown for naproxen plus aspirin using moderate doses of each drug.[174] Additive benefit of combinations of analgesic medications occurs in a variety of types of pain.

In my view combinations of aspirin or other salicylates and other nonsteroidal anti-inflammatory agents or combinations of the newer agents are worthy of careful trial in patients who do not respond satisfactorily to maximum safe doses of single drugs. Care should be taken to observe for increased toxicity and for a satisfactory effect; in the absence of additive benefit, the combination should be discontinued. Another indication for combination therapy is the additive benefit of drugs with differing pharmacokinetics. For example, if a patient is responding to a short-acting agent, such as tolmetin or ibuprofen, but still has morning stiffness because of loss of therapeutic blood levels overnight, a nighttime dose of a longer-acting agent may be useful. Either a drug such as naproxen in the evening or a large dose of indomethacin at bedtime can be useful. Similarly, if a patient is well controlled on a long-acting agent, such as naproxen twice a day or piroxicam daily, but has a flare-up due to overuse of a joint or trauma, it may be useful to add intermittent doses of a short-acting agent temporarily.

**Are These Drugs Interchangeable?** In my view there are significant, but subtle, differences in mechanisms of action, effectiveness in different diseases, and other properties of these drugs. The unpredictable differences in effectiveness in different patients make it worth while to try a series of agents if the first drug does not work satisfactorily in a particular patient. Although the reason for the differences in effectiveness in individual patients is unknown, there is clearly a clinical advantage to having so many drugs available, making it possible to try a series of them sequentially in a given patient.

Unfortunately blood level determinations are not available for any of the nonsteroidal anti-inflammatory agents except the salicylates; it is reasonable to assume that such determinations would be clinically useful, as are salicylate levels, and would minimize the occurrence of toxicity. Without determinations of blood levels, we are unaware of differences in metabolism of these drugs in different patients. Variations in plateau blood levels seem a likely basis for individual differences in effectiveness. In the studies reported there are wide variations in plateau levels achieved in normal individuals on a single-dose regimen of a specific drug; age, sex, disease, and effect of other drugs are variables that have not been studied at all.

**Do These Drugs Have a Disease-Modifying Effect in Rheumatoid Arthritis?** It took more than 30 years to establish a disease-modifying effect for gold in rheumatoid arthritis. Conventional wisdom says that the nonsteroidal anti-inflammatory agents do not have such an effect, but no data exist in this regard, even for aspirin, since there are no controls available who have not received aspirin. The newer agents have a more complete disease-suppressive effect in many patients. If the severity of the inflammation bears a relationship to the degree of joint destruction, complete suppression of the inflammation should minimize disease progression.

Suppression of the model for immunologically induced chronic inflammatory arthritis, adjuvant disease in rats, occurs with these agents, preventing cartilage and bone erosion. The relationship of this observation to human rheumatoid arthritis is, of course, questionable.

Several studies are under way to try to establish a disease-suppressive effect for a variety of the nonsteroidal anti-inflammatory agents. The meager data that support the hypothesis that these agents have a suppressive effect in rheumatoid arthritis are described earlier in this chapter. No conclusion regarding a disease-suppressive effect is warranted on the basis of present evidence. While definitive evidence is being sought, what is the most rational course of action for the prudent clinician to follow? My recommendation is to assume that a modest disease-suppressive effect will be demonstrated, and to try to achieve maximal, continuous suppression of the inflammation rather than simply symptomatic relief, if this can be achieved without toxicity.

## References


1. Smith, M.J.H.: Aspirin and prostaglandins: Some recent developments. Agents Actions 8:427, 1978.
2. Vane, J.R.: Mode of action of aspirin and similar compounds. *In* Robinson, H.J., and Vane, J.R. (eds.): Prostaglandin Synthetase Inhibitors. New York, Raven Press, 1974.
3. Robinson, D.R., McGuire, M.B., Bastian, D., Kantrowitz, F., and Levine, L.: The effects of anti-inflammatory drugs on prostaglandin production by rheumatoid synovial tissue. Prostaglandins Med. 1:461, 1978.
4. Harvey, I., Main, M. and Whittle, B.J.R.: Prostaglandins and prostaglandin synthetase inhibitors in gastrointestinal function and disease. *In* Robinson, H.J., and Vane, J.R. (eds.): Prostaglandin Synthetase Inhibitors. New York, Raven Press, 1974.
5. Johansson, C., Kollberg, B., Nordemar, R., Samuelson, K., and Bergstrom, S.: Protective effect of prostaglandin $E_2$ in the gastrointestinal tract during indomethacin treatment of rheumatic diseases. Gastroenterology 78:479, 1980.
6. Whittle, B.J.R.: Temporal relationship between cyclooxygenase inhibition as measured by prostacyclin biosynthesis, and the gastrointestinal damage induced by indomethacin in rat. Gastroenterology 80:94, 1981.
7. Kuehl, F.A., Dougherty, H.W., Ham, E.A., Humes, J.L., Egan, R.W., and Winter, C.A.: Biochemical aspects of the mechanism of action of sulindac. *In* Miehlke, K., Otte, P., and Platz, C.M. (eds.): Current Concepts of Anti-Inflammatory Drugs. New York, Biomedical Information, 1980, p. 17.
8. Metz, S.A.: Anti-inflammatory agents as inhibitors of prostaglandin synthesis in man. Med. Clin. North Am. 65:759, 1981.
9. Flower, R.J., and Vane, J.R.: Some pharmacologic and biochemical aspects of prostaglandin biosynthesis and its inhibition. *In* Robinson, H.J., and Vane, J.R. (eds.): Prostaglandin Synthetase Inhibitors. New York, Raven Press, 1974.
10. Kocsis, J.J., Hernandovich, J., Silver, M.T., Smith, J.B., and Ingerman, C.: Duration of inhibition of platelet prostaglandin formation and aggregation by ingested aspirin or indomethacin. Prostaglandins 3:141, 1973.
11. Crook, D., Collins, A.J., Bacon, P.A., and Chan, R.: Prostaglandin synthetase activity from human rheumatoid synovial microsomes. Ann. Rheum. Dis. 35:327, 1976.
12. Humes, J.L., Winter, C.A., Sadowski, S.J., and Kuehl, F.A.: Multiple sites on prostaglandin cyclooxygenase are determinants in the action of nonsteroidal antiinflammatory agents. Proc. Natl. Acad. Sci. USA 78:2053, 1981.
13. Dembinska-Kiec, A., Zmuda, A., and Krupinska, J.: Inhibition of prostaglandin synthetase by aspirin-like drugs in different microsomal preparations. *In* Samuelsson, B., and Paoletti, R. (eds.): Advances in Prostaglandin and Thromboxane Research. Vol. 1. New York, Raven Press, 1976.
14. Ferreira, S.H., Lorenzetti, B.B., Salete, M., Castro, A., and Correa, F.M.A.: Antialgic effect of aspirin-like drugs and the inhibitor of prostaglandin synthesis. *In* DuMonde, D.C., and Jasare, M.K. (eds.): Recognition of Anti-Rheumatic Drugs. Baltimore, University Park Press, 1977.
15. Vane, J.R.: The mode of action of aspirin-like drugs. Agents Actions 8:430, 1978.
16. Wiseman, E.H.: Preclinical studies with piroxicam. *In* O'Brien, W.M., and Wiseman, E.H. (eds.): *In* Piroxicam. The Royal Society of Medicine International Congress and Symposium Series, No. 1. London, Academic Press, 1977.
17. Shen, T.Y.: The discovery of indomethacin and the proliferation of NSAIDs. Semin. Arthritis Rheum. XII, 2 (Suppl. 1):89, 1982.
18. Gryglewski, R.J.: Structure-activity relationship of some prostaglandin synthetase inhibitors. *In* Robinson, H.J., and Vane, J.R. (eds.): Prostaglandin Inhibitors. New York, Raven Press, 1974.
19. Moncada, M.D., and Vane, J.R.: Mode of action of aspirin-like drugs. *In* Stollerman, G.H. (ed.): Advances in Internal Medicine. Chicago, Year Book Medical Publishers, 1979.
20. Kuehl, F.A., Humes, J.L., Egan, R.W., Ham, E.A., Beveridge, G.C., and Van Arman, C.G.: Role of prostaglandin endoperoxide $PGG_2$ in inflammatory processes. Nature 265:170, 1977.
21. Egan R.W., Humes, J.L., and Kuehl, F.A.: Differential effects of prostaglandin synthetase stimulators on inhibition of cyclooxygenase. Biochemistry 17:2230, 1978.
22. Glenn, E.M., Bowman, B.J., and Rohloff, N.A.: Anti-inflammatory and PG inhibitory effects of phenacetin and acetaminophen. Agents Actions 7:513, 1977.
23. Glenn, E.M., Bowman, B.J., and Rohloff, N.A.: Anti-inflammatory and PG inhibitory effects of phenacetin and acetaminophen. Agents Actions 7:513, 1977.
24. Fitzpatrick, F.A., and Wynalda, M.A.: In vivo suppression of prostaglandin biosynthesis by non-steroidal anti-inflammatory agents. Prostaglandins 12:1037, 1976.
25. Metz, S.A., Robertson, R.P., Fujimoto, W.Y.: Inhibition of prostaglandin E synthesis augments glucose-induced insulin secretion in cultured pancreas. Diabetes 30:551, 1981.
26. Cherner, R., Groppe, C.W., and Rupp, J.J.: Prolonged tolbutamide-induced hypoglycemia. JAMA 185:883, 1963.
27. Buckingham, R.B.: Interactions involving antirheumatic agents. Bull. Rheum. Dis. 28:960 and 966, 1977–78.
28. Sherwood, J., and Kreutner, W.: Salicylic acid prevents the inhibition of platelet prostaglandin synthetase by indomethacin-like anti-inflammatory agents. Fed. Proc. 37:605A, 1978.
29. DiPasquale, G., and Mellace, D.: Inhibition of arachidonic acid induced mortality in rabbits with several non-steroidal anti-inflammatory agents. Agents Actions 7:481, 1977.
30. Simon, S., and Mills, J.A.: Drug therapy. N. Engl. J. Med. 302:1179 and 1237, 1980.
31. Jacob, H.: Neutrophil activation as a mechanism of tissue injury. Presentation at the VIII Pan-American Congress of Rheumatology, Washington, D.C., June, 1982.
32. Higgs, G.A., and Flower, R.J.: Anti-inflammatory drugs and the inhibition of arachidonate lipoxygenase. *In* Piper, P.J. (ed.): SRS-A and Leukotrienes. New York, John Wiley and Sons, 1981.
33. Higgs, G.A., Eakins, K.E., Mugridge, K.G., Moncada, S., Vane, J.R.: The effects of non-steroid anti-inflammatory drugs on leukocyte migration in carrageenin-induced inflammation. Eur. J. Pharmacol. 66:81, 1980.
34. Klickstein, L.B., Shapleigh, C., and Goetzl, E.J.: Lipoxygenation of arachidonic acid as a source of polymorphonuclear leukocyte chemotactic factors in synovial fluid tissue in rheumatoid arthritis and spondyloarthritis. J. Clin. Invest. 66:1166, 1980.
35. Dawson, W., Boot, J.R., Harvey, J., and Walker, J.R.: The pharmacology of benoxaprofen with particular reference to effects of lipoxygenase product formation. Eur. J. Rheumatol. Inflamm. 5:61, 1982.
36. Walker, J.R., and Dawson, W.: Inhibition of rabbit PMN lipoxygenase activity by benoxaprofen. J. Pharm. Pharmacol. 31:778, 1979.

37. Snyderman, R., and Goetzl, E.J.: Molecular and cellular mechanisms of leukocyte chemotaxis. Science 213:830, 1981.
38. Kuehl, F.A.: Prostaglandin research: Clinical implications. Semin. Arthritis Rheum. 12 (Suppl. 1):119, 1982.
39. Stecher, V.J.: The chemotaxis of selected cell types to connective tissue degradation products. Ann. N.Y. Acad. Sci. 256:177, 1975.
40. Brown, K.A., and Collins, A.J.: In vitro effects of non-steroidal anti-inflammatory drugs on human polymorphonuclear cells and lymphocyte migration. Br. J. Pharmacol. 64:347, 1978.
41. Meacock, S.C.R., and Kitchen, E.A.: Effects of the non-steroidal anti-inflammatory drug benoxaprofen on leucocyte migration. J. Pharm. Pharmacol. 31:366, 1979.
42. Walker, J.R., Smith, M.J.H., and Ford-Hutchinson, A.W.: Anti-inflammatory drugs, prostaglandins and leucocyte migration. Agents Actions 6:602, 1976.
43. Dawson, W.: Mechanisms of action of antiinflammatory drugs. *In* Samuelsson, B., Ramwell, P.W., and Paoletti, R. (eds.): Advances in Prostaglandin and Thromboxane Research. New York, Raven Press, 1980.
44. Meacock, S.C.R., and Kitchen, E.A.: Effects of the non-steroidal anti-inflammatory drug benoxaprofen on leucocyte migration. J. Pharm. Pharmacol. 31:366, 1979.
45. Weiss, B., and Hait, W.N.: Selective cyclic nucleotidephosphodiesterase inhibitors as potential therapeutic agents. Annu. Rev. Pharmacol. Toxicol. 17:441, 1977.
46. Carty, T.J., Stevens, J.S., Lombardino, J.G., Parry, M.J., and Randall, M.J.: Piroxicam, a structurally novel anti-inflammatory compound, mode of prostaglandin synthesis inhibition. Prostaglandins 19:671, 1980.
47. Tamisier, J.N.: Ketoprofen. Clin. Rheum. Dis. 5:381, 1979.
48. Abramson, S.: Effects of nonsteroidal anti-inflammatory drugs on neutrophil activation in vitro and in vivo. Presentation at the VIII Pan-American Congress of Rheumatology, Washington, D.C., June, 1982.
49. Kantor, T.G.: Ibuprofen. Ann. Intern. Med. 91:877, 1979.
50. Palmoski, M.J., and Brandt, K.D.: Benoxaprofen (Benx) stimulates proteoglycan (GG) synthesis in normal articular cartilage. Arthritis Rheum. 25 (Suppl.):S29, 1982.
51. Mobarok Ali, A.T.M., and Morley, J.: Actions of aspirin on lymphocytes. Aspirin Symposium 1980. Proceedings of an International Symposium held by the Aspirin Foundation. London: Royal College of Surgeons, June 5, 1980.
52. Ehrlich, G.E.: Three years' clinical experience with tolmetin in rheumatoid arthritis. Presentation on Zomepirac and Tolmetin: Advances in Clinical and Pharmacologic Research. VIII Pan-American Congress of Rheumatology, Washington, D.C., June, 1982.
53. Goodwin, J.S., and Webb, D.R.: Regulation of the immune response by prostaglandins. Clin. Immunol. Immunopathol. 15:106, 1980.
54. Goodwin, J.: Effects of nonsteroidal anti-inflammatory drugs on cellular and humoral immunity in vitro and in vivo. Presentation at the VIII Pan-American Congress of Rheumatology, Washington, D.C., June, 1982.
55. Cashin, C.H., Dawson, W., and Kitchen, E.A.: The pharmacology of benoxaprofen (2-lf-chlorophenyl-a-methyl-5-benzoxazole acetic acid), LRCL 3794, a new compound with anti-inflammatory activity apparently unrelated to inhibition of prostaglandin synthesis. J. Pharm. Pharmacol. 29:330, 1977.
56. Moncada, S., and Vane, J.R.: Interaction between anti-inflammatory drugs and inflammatory mediators. A reference to products of arachidonic acid metabolism. *In* Bonta, L.I., Thompson, J., and Brune, K. (eds.): Inflammation: Mechanisms and Their Impact on Therapy. Birkhauser Verlag, Basel, 1977.
57. Muschek, L.D.: Zomepirac: Recent pharmacologic developments. Presentation on Zomepirac and Tolmetin: Advances in Clinical and Pharmacologic Research. VIII Pan-American Congress of Rheumatology, Washington, D.C., June, 1982.
58. Kantor, T.G., Streem, A., and Laska, E.: Estimates of doses of antiinflammatory drugs in man by testing for analgesic potency. Arthritis Rheum. 20:1381, 1977.
59. Feldberg, W.: Prostaglandins and prostaglandin synthetase inhibitors. Action on physiological function. *In* Robinson, H.J., and Vane, J.R. (eds.): Prostaglandin Synthetase Inhibitors. New York, Raven Press, 1974.
60. Moncada, S., Ferreira, S.H., and Vane, J.R.: Sensitization of pain receptors of dog knee joint by prostaglandins. *In* Robinson, H.J., and Vane, J.R. (eds.): Prostaglandin Synthetase Inhibitors. New York, Raven Press, 1974.
61. Ferreira, S.H., and Vane, J.R.: New aspects of the mode of action of nonsteroid anti-inflammatory drugs. Annu. Rev. Pharmacol. 14:57, 1974.
62. Champion, G.D., and Graham, G.G.: Pharmacokinetics of non-steroidal anti-inflammatory agents. Aust. N.Z.J. Med. 8 (Suppl. I):94, 1978.
63. Ridolfo, A.S., Nickander, R., and Mikulaschek, W.M.: Fenoprofen and benoxaprofen. Clin. Rheum. Dis. 5:393, 1979.
64. Chernish, S.M., Rubin, A., Rodda, B.E., Ridolfo, A.S., and Gruber, C.M. Jr.: The physiological disposition of fenoprofen in man, IV. The effects of position of subject, food ingestion on the plasma levels of orally administered fenoprofen. J. Med. (Exp. Clin.) 3:249, 1972.
65. Brune, K., Graf, P., and Glatt, M.: Inhibition of prostaglandin synthesis in vivo by nonsteroid anti-inflammatory drugs: Evidence for the importance of pharmacokinetics. Agents Actions 6:159, 1976.
66. Wiseman, E.H., and Hobbs, D.C.: Review of pharmacokinetic studies with piroxicam. Am. J. Med. 72:19, 1982.
67. Robinson, D.R., and Levine, L.: Prostaglandin concentrations in synovial fluid in rheumatic diseases: Action of indomethacin and aspirin. *In* Robinson, H.J., and Vane, J.R. (eds.): Prostaglandin Synthetase Inhibitors. New York: Raven Press, 1974.
68. Furst, D.E.: Tolmetin kinetics in synovial fluid. Presentation on Zomepirac and Tolmetin: Advances in Clinical and Pharmacologic Research. VIII Pan-American Congress of Rheumatology, Washington, D.C., June, 1982.
69. Soren, A.: Transport of salicylates from blood to joint fluid. Arch. Intern. Med. 132:668, 1973.
70. Adams, S.S., and Buckler, J.W.: Ibuprofen and flurbiprofen. Clin. Rheum. Dis. 5:359, 1979.
71. Hobbs, D.C., and Twomey, T.M.: Piroxicam pharmacokinetics in man: Aspirin and antacid interaction studies. J. Clin. Pharmacol. 19:270, 1979.
72. Nuotio, P., and Makisara, P.: Pharmacokinetic and clinical study of piroxicam. *In* O'Brien, W.M., and Wiseman, E.H. (eds.): Piroxicam. The Royal Society of Medicine International Congress and Symposium Series, No. 1. London: Academic Press, 1977.
73. Segre, E.J.: Naproxen. Clin. Rheum. Dis. 5:411, 1979.
74. Day, R.O., Furst, D.E., Dromgole, S.H., Kamm, B., Roe, R., and Paulus, H.E.: Relationship of serum naproxen concentration to efficacy in rheumatoid arthritis. Clin. Pharmacol. Ther. 31:733, 1982.
75. Yakatan, G.J.: Pharmacology and pharmacokinetics of isoxicam. Semin. Arthritis Rheum. XII (Suppl. 2):154, 1982.
76. Brogden, R.N., Heel, R.C., Speight, T.M., and Avery, G.S.: Fenbufen: A review of its pharmacological properties and therapeutic use in rheumatic diseases and acute pain. Drugs 21:1, 1981.
77. Taggart, H.M., and Alderdice, J.M.: Fatal cholestatic jaundice in elderly patients taking benoxaprofen. Br. Med. J. 284:1372, 1982.
78. Graham, G.G., Champion, G.D., Day, R.O., and Paull, P.D.: Patterns of plasma concentrations and urinary excretion of salicylate in rheumatoid arthritis. Clin. Pharmacol. Ther. 22:410, 1977.
79. Mason, R.W., and McQueen, E.G.: Protein binding of indomethacin: binding of indomethacin to human plasma albumin and its displacement from binding by ibuprofen, phenylbutazone and salicylate, in vitro. Pharmacology 12:12, 1974.
80. Huskisson, E.C., Taylor, R.T., Burston, D., Chuter, P.J., and Hart, F.D.: Evening indomethacin in the treatment of rheumatoid arthritis. Ann. Rheum. Dis. 29:393, 1970.
81. Turner, R.A., April, P.A., and Robbins, D.L.: Double-blind multicenter study comparing piroxicam and ibuprofen in the treatment of rheumatoid arthritis. Am. J. Med. 72:34, 1982.
82. Huskisson, E.C., Woolf, D.L., Balme, H.W., Scott, J., and Franklyn, S.: Four new anti-inflammatory drugs: Responses and variations. Br. Med. J. 1:1048, 1976.
83. Brogden, R.N., Pinder, R.M., Sawyer, P.R., Speight, T.M., and Avery, G.s.: Naproxen: A review of its pharmacological properties and therapeutic efficacy and use. Drugs 9:326, 1975.
84. Brogden, R.N., Pinder, R.M., Speight, T.M., and Avery, G.S.: Fenoprofen: A review of its pharmacological properties and therapeutic efficacy in rheumatic disease. Drugs 13:241, 1977.
85. Brogen, R.N., Heel, R.C., Speight, T.M., and Avery, C.S.: Tolmetin: A review of its pharmacological properties and therapeutic efficacy in rheumatic diseases. Drugs 15:429, 1978.
86. Brogden, R.N., Heel, R.C., Speight, T.M., and Avery, G.S.: Sulindac: A review of its pharmacological properties and therapeutic efficacy in rheumatic diseases. Drugs 16:97, 1978.
87. Famaey, J.P.: Recent developments about non-steroidal anti-inflammatory drugs and their mode of action. Gen. Pharmac. 9:155, 1978.
88. Nickander, R., McMahon, F.G., and Ridolfo, A.S.: Nonsteroidal anti-inflammatory agents. Ann. Rev. Pharmacol. Toxicol. 19:469, 1979.
89. Brogden, R.N., Heel, R.C., Pakes, G.E., Speight, T.M., and Avery, G.S.: Diflunisal: A review of its pharmacological properties and therapeutic use in pain and musculoskeletal strains and sprains and pain in osteoarthritis. Drugs 19:84, 1980.
90. Brock, P.G., and Jackson, D.: UK general practitioners' experience of fenbufen in elderly patients. Eur. J. Rheum. Inflam. 5:326, 1982.
91. Wasner, C., Britton, M.D., Kraines, G., Kaye, R.L., Bobrove, A.M., and Fries, J.F.: Nonsteroidal anti-inflammatory agents in rheumatoid arthritis and ankylosing spondylitis. JAMA 246:2168, 1981.
92. Beirne, J.A., Bianchine, J.R., Johnson, P.C., and Wartham, G.P.: Gastrointestinal blood loss caused by tolmetin, aspirin and indomethacin. Clin. Pharmacol. Ther. 16:821, 1974.
93. Ridolfo, A.S., Crabtree, R.E., Johnson, D.W., and Rockhold, F.W.:

Gastrointestinal microbleeding: Comparisons between benoxaprofen and other nonsteroidal antiinflammatory agents. J. Rheumatol. 6(Suppl.):36, 1980.
94. Bluhm, G.B., Smith, D.W., and Mikulaschek, W.M.: Radiologic assessment of benoxaprofen therapy in rheumatoid arthritis. Eur. J. Rheum. Inflamm. 3:186, 1981.
95. Levy, J.: Immunological aspects of tolmetin. Presentation on Zomepirac and Tolmetin: Advances in Clinical and Pharmacologic Research. VIII Pan-American Congress of Rheumatology, Washington, D.C., June 11, 1982.
96. Lindsley, C.B.: Pharmacotherapy of juvenile rheumatoid arthritis. Pediatr. Clin. North Am. 28:161, 1981.
97. Moran, H. Hanna, D.B. Ansell, B.M., Hall, M., and Engler, C.: Naproxen in juvenile chronic polyarthritis. Ann. Rheum. Dis. 38:152, 1979.
98. Jacobs, J.C.: Sudden death in arthritic children receiving large doses of indomethacin. JAMA 199:932, 1967.
99. Bostrom, H., Berntsen, K., and Whitehouse, M.W.: Biochemical properties of anti-inflammatory drugs-II. Biochem. Pharmacol. 13:413, 1964.
100. Bollet, A.J.: Inhibition of glucosamine-6-PO4 synthesis by salicylate and other anti-inflammatory agents in vitro. Arthritis Rheum. 4:624, 1961.
101. Fowler, P.D.: Indomethacin and phenylbutazone. Clin. Rheum. Dis. 1:267, 1975.
102. Godfrey, R.G., Calabro, J.J., Mills, D., and Maltz, B.: A double-blind crossover trial of aspirin, indomethacin and phenylbutazone in ankylosing spondylitis. Arthritis Rheum. 15:110, 1972.
103. Pulkkinen, M.O., and Csapo, A.I.: The effect of ibuprofen on the intrauterine pressure and menstrual pain of dysmenorrheic patients. Prostaglandins 15:1055, 1978.
104. Budoff, P.W.: Zomepirac sodium in the treatment of primary dysmenorrhea syndrome. N. Engl. J. Med. 307:714, 1982.
105. Schwartz, A., Zor, U., Lindner, H.R., and Naor, S.: Primary dysmenorrhea. Obstet. Gynecol. 44:709, 1974.
106. Aiken, J.W.: Prostaglandins and prostaglandin synthetase inhibitors: Studies on uterine motility and function. *In* Robinson, H.J., and Vane, J.R. (eds.): Prostaglandin Synthetase Inhibitors, New York, Raven Press, 1974.
107. Nadas, A.S.: Indomethacin and the patent ductus arteriosus. N. Engl. J. Med. 305:97, 1981.
108. Deykin, D., and Janson, P.: The Ponte Vedre syndrome. An unexpected interaction between alcohol and aspirin. Trans. Am. Clin. Climatol. Assoc. 93:121, 1982.
109. Friedman, P.L., Brown, E.J., Gunther, S., Alexander, R.W., Barry, W.H., Mudge, G.H., and Grossman, W.: Coronary vasoconstrictor effect of indomethacin in patients with coronary-artery disease. N. Engl. J. Med. 305:1171, 1981.
110. Mann, N.S., and Sachdey, A.J.: Acute erosive gastritis induced by aspirin, ketoprofen, ibuprofen, and naproxen: Its prevention by metiamide and cimetidine. South. Med. J. 70:526, 1977.
111. O'Laughlin, J.C., Silvoso, G.R., and Ivey, K.J.: Healing of aspirin-associated peptic ulcer disease despite continued salicylate ingestion. Arch. Intern. Med. 141:781, 1981.
112. Schwartz, H.A.: Lower gastrointestinal side effects of nonsteroidal antiinflammatory drugs. J. Rheumatol. 8:952, 1981.
113. Sharon, P., Ligumsky, M., Rachmilewitz, D., and Zor, U.: Role of prostaglandins in ulcerative colitis: Enhanced production during active disease and inhibition by sulfasalazine. Gastroenterology 75:638, 1978.
114. Abruzzo, J.L.: Anti-inflammatory and antirheumatic drugs. Ann. Intern. Med. 94:270, 1981.
115. Lilly, E.L.: Pancreatitis after administration of sulindac. JAMA 246:2680, 1981.
116. Park, G.D., Spector, R., Headstream, T., and Goldberg, M.: Serious adverse reactions associated with sulindac. Arch. Intern. Med. 142:1292, 1982.
117. Heller, S., Fellows, I.W., Ogilvie, A.L., and Atkinson, M.: Nonsteroidal and anti-inflammatory drugs and benign esophageal stricture. Br. Med. J. 285:167, 1982.
118. Dunk, A.A., Walt, R.P., Jenkins, W.J., and Sherlock, S.S.: Diclofenac hepatitis. Br. Med. J. 284:1605, 1982.
119. Giroux, Y., Moreau, M., and Kass, T.G.: Cholestatic jaundice caused by sulindac. Canad. J. Surg. 25:334, 1982.
120. Dunn, M.J., and Zambraski, E.J.: Renal effects of drugs that inhibit prostaglandin synthesis. Kidney Int. 18:609, 1980.
121. Lum, G.M., Aisenbrey, G.A., Dunn, M.J., Berl, T., Schrier, R.W., and McDonald, K.M.: In vivo effect of indomethacin to potentiate the renal medullary cyclic AMP response to vasopressin. J. Clin. Invest. 59:8, 1977.
122. Laiwah, A.C., and Mactier, R.A.: Non-steroidal anti-inflammatory agents may impair furosemide induced diuresis in cardiac failure. Br. Med. J. 283:714, 1981.
123. Favre, L., Glasson, P., and Vallotton, M.B.: Reversible acute renal failure from combined triamterene and indomethacin. Ann. Intern. Med. 96:317, 1982.
124. Williams, R.L., Davies, R.O., Berman, R.S., Holmes, G.I., Huber, P., Gee, W.L., Lin, E.T., and Benet, L.Z.: Hydrochlorothiazide pharmacokinetics and pharmacologic effect: The influence of indomethacin. J. Clin. Pharmacol. 22:32, 1982.
125. Brooks, P.M., and Cossum, P.A.: Rebound rise in renin concentrations after cessation of salicylates. N. Engl. J. Med. 303:562, 1980.
126. Gill, J.R., Frolich, J.C., Bowden, R.E., Taylor, A.A., Keiser, H.R., Seyberth, H.W., Oates, J.A., and Bartter, F.C.: Bartter's syndrome: A disorder characterized by high urinary prostaglandins and a dependence of hyperreninemia on prostaglandin synthesis. Am. J. Med. 61:43, 1976.
127. Fichman, M.P., Telfer, N., Zia, P., Speckart, P., Golub, M., and Rude, R.: Role of prostaglandins in the pathogenesis of Bartter's syndrome. Am. J. Med. 60:785, 1976.
128. Calin, A.: Non-steroidal anti-inflammatory drugs and furosemide-induced diuresis. Br. Med. J. 283:1399, 1981.
129. Bunning, R.D., and Barth, W.F.: Sulindac. JAMA 248:2864, 1982.
130. Linton, A.L., Clark, W.F., Driedger, A.A., Turnbull, D.I., and Lindsay, R.M.: Acute interstitial nephritis due to drugs. Ann. Intern. Med. 93:735, 1980.
131. Mease, P.J., Ellsworth, A.J., Killen, P.D., and Wilkens, R.F.: Zomepirac, interstitial nephritis and renal failure. Ann. Intern. Med. 97:454, 1982.
132. Brezin, J.H., Katz, S.M., Schwartz, A.B., and Chinitz, J.L.: Reversible renal failure and nephrotic syndrome associated with nonsteroidal anti-inflammatory drugs. N. Engl. J. Med. 301:1271, 1979.
133. Finkelstein, A., Fraley, D.S., Stachura, I., Feldman, H.A., Gandy, D.R., and Bourke, E.: Fenoprofen nephropathy: Lipoid nephrosis and interstitial nephritis. Am. J. Med. 72:81, 1982.
134. Gault, M.H., Rudwal, T.C., Engles, W.D., and Dossetor, J.B.: Syndrome associated with the abuse of analgesics. Ann. Intern. Med. 68:906, 1968.
135. Emkey, R.D., and Mills, J.A.: Aspirin and analgesic nephropathy. JAMA 247:55, 1982.
136. Knapp, M., and Avioli, L.V.: Analgesic nephropathy. Arch. Intern. Med. 142:1197, 1982.
137. Wiseman, E.H., and Reinert, H.: Anti-inflammatory drugs and renal papillary necrosis. Agents Actions 54:322, 1975.
138. Bennett, W.M., Muther, R.S., Parker, R.A., Feig, P., Morrison, G., Golper, T.A., and Singer, I.: Drug Therapy in renal failure: Dosing guidelines for adults. Ann. Intern. Med. 93:286, 1980.
139. Settipane, G.A.: Adverse reactions to aspirin and related drugs. Arch. Intern. Med. 141:328, 1981.
140. Stevenson, D.D.: Aspirin and rhinosinusitis/asthma: Desensitization. N. Engl. Soc. Allergy Proc. 2:88, 1981.
141. Rudolph, A.M.: Effects of aspirin and acetaminophen in pregnancy and in the newborn. Arch. Intern. Med. 141:358, 1981.
142. Miller, J.L.: Marrow aplasia and sulindac. Ann. Intern. Med. 92:129, 1980.
143. F.D.A. Drug Bulletin: Clinoril adverse reactions. 9:29, 1979.
144. Fowler, P.: Phenylbutazone and indomethacin. Clin. Rheum. Dis. 5:427, 1975.
145. Ashraf, M., Pearson, R.M., and Winfield, D.A.: Aplastic anaemia associated with fenoprofen. Br. Med. J. 284:1301, 1982.
146. O'Brien, W.M.: Piroxicam treatment of inflammatory disease. *In* the Royal Society of Medicine, International Congress and Symposium Series, Number 1. The Royal Society of Medicine, London, Academic Press, 1977.
147. Brogden, R.N., Heel, R.C., Speight, T.M., and Avery, G.S.: Alclofenac: A review of its pharmacological properties and therapeutic efficacy in rheumatoid arthritis and allied rheumatic disorders. Drugs 14:241, 1977.
148. Corre, K.A., and Rothstein, R.J.: Anaphylactic reaction to zomepirac. Ann. Allergy 48:299, 1982.
149. Rossi, A.C., and Knapp, D.E.: Tolmetin-induced anaphylactoid reactions. N. Engl. J. Med. 307:499, 1982.
150. Farnham, J.: Studies of isoxicam in combination with aspirin, warfarin, sodium and cimetidine. Semin. Arthritis Rheum. XII(Suppl. 2):179, 1982.
151. Barnes, C.G., Goodman, H.V., Eade, A.W.T., Misra, H.N., Cochrane, G.M., Clarke, A.K., and Stoppard, M.: A double-blind comparison of naproxen with indomethacin in osteoarthrosis. J. Clin. Pharm. 15:347, 1975.
152. Boardman, P.L., and Hart, F.D.: Side effects of indomethacin. Ann. Rheum. Dis. 26:127, 1967.
153. Taylor, R.T., Huskisson, E.C., Whitehouse, G.H., Hart, F.D., and Trapnell, D.H.: Gastric ulceration occurring during indomethacin therapy. Br. Med. J. 4:734, 1968.
154. Littlewood, J.M., Lee, M.R., and Meadow, S.R.: Treatment of Bartter's syndrome in early childhood with prostaglandin synthetase inhibitors. Arch. Dis. Child. 53:43, 1978.

155. Konomi, H., Imai, M., Nihei, K., and Kamoshitas, T.H.: Indomethacin causing pseudotumor cerebri in Bartter's syndrome. N. Engl. J. Med. 298:855, 1978.
156. Rhymer, A.R., Hart, C.B., and Daurio, C.: A double-blind trial comparing indomethacin sustained release capsules (indocid-R) with indomethacin capsules in patients with rheumatoid arthritis. Rheumatol. Rehabil. 21:101, 1982.
157. Brooks, P.M., Bell, M.A., Sturrock, R.D., Famaey, J.P., and Dick, W.C.: The clinical significance of indomethacin-probenecid interaction. Br. J. Clin. Pharmacol. 1:287, 1974.
158. Van Arman, C.G., Risley, E.A., Nuss, G.W., Hucker, H.B., and Duggan, D.E.: Pharmacology of sulindac. *In* Huskisson, E.C., and Franchimont, P. (eds.): Clinoril in the Treatment of Rheumatic Disorders: A New Nonsteroidal Anti-Inflammatory/Analgesic Agent. Proceedings of a Symposium VIII European Rheumatology Congress, Helsinki, June 1–7, 1975 (New York, Raven Press, 1976).
159. Huskisson, E.C., and Franchimont, P.: Clinoril in the treatment of rheumatic disorders. *In* Huskisson, E.C., and Franchimont, P. (eds.): Clinoril in the Treatment of Rheumatic Disorders: A New Nonsteroidal Anti-Inflammatory/Analgesic Agent. Proceedings of a Symposium VIII European Rheumatology Congress, Helsinki, June 1–7, 1975 (New York: Raven Press, 1976).
160. Memon, A.N.: Pancreatitis and sulindac. Arch. Intern. Med. 97:139, 1982.
161. Robinson, H., Abruzzo, J.L., Miyara, A., and Ward, J.R.: Concomitant tolmetin and aspirin therapy for rheumatoid arthritis. *In* Ward, J.R. (ed.): Tolmetin. Amsterdam, Excerpta Medica, 1975.
162. Chan, W.Y., Dawood, N.Y., and Fuchs, F.: Relief of dysmenorrhea with the prostaglandin synthetase inhibitor ibuprofen: Effect on prostaglandin levels in menstrual fluid. Am. J. Obstet. Gynecol. 135:102, 1979.
163. Smith, D.L., and Regan, M.G.: Ibuprofen in psoriatic arthritis. Arthritis Rheum. 8:961, 1980.
164. Boss, G.R., and Seegmiller, J.E.: Hyperuricemia and gout: Classification, complications and management. N. Engl. J. Med. 300:1459, 1979.
165. Widener, H.L., and Littman, B.H.: Ibuprofen-induced meningitis in systemic lupus erythematosus. JAMA 239:1062, 1978.
166. Mandell, B., Shen, H.S., and Hepburn, B.: Fever from ibuprofen in a patient with lupus erythematosus. Arch. Intern. Med. 85:209, 1976.
167. Segre, E.J.: Naproxen metabolism in man. J. Clin. Pharmacol. 15:316, 1975.
168. Pulkkinen, M.O., Henzl, M.R., and Csapo, A.I.: The effect of naproxen-sodium on the prostaglandin concentrations of the menstrual blood and uterine "jet washings" in dysmenorrheic women. Prostaglandins 15:543, 1978.
169. Filtzer, H.S.: A double-blind randomized comparison of naproxen sodium, acetaminophen and pentazocine in postoperative pain. Current Therapeutic Research 27:293, 1980.
170. Williams, J.G.P., and Engler, C.: A double-blind comparative trial of naproxen and indomethacin in sports injuries. Rheumatol. Rehabil. 16:265, 1977.
171. Merton, J.W., III, Lussier, A., Ward, J.R., Neustadt, D., and Multz, C.: Naproxen vs. aspirin in osteoarthritis of the hip and knee. J. Rheumatol. 5:338, 1978.
172. Sturge, R.A., Scott, J.T., Hamilton, E.B.D., Liyanage, S.P., Dixon, A., Davies, J., and Engler, E.: Multicenter trial of naproxen and phenylbutazone in acute gout. Ann. Rheum. Dis. 36:80, 1977.
173. Van Gerwen, F., Vander Kost, J.K., and Gribnan, F.W.: Double blind trial of naproxen and phenylbutazone in alkylosing spondylitis. Ann. Rheum. Dis. 37:85, 1978.
174. Wilkens, R.F., and Segre, E.J.: Combination therapy with naproxen and aspirin in rheumatoid arthritis. Arthritis Rheum. 19:677, 1976.
175. Matts, S.P.F.: Naproxen (Naprosyn) and gastrointestinal haemorrhage. Br. Med. J. 2:52, 1974.
176. Hart, F.D.: Naproxen (Naprosyn) and gastrointestinal haemorrhage. Br. Med. J. 2:51, 1974.
177. Roth, S.H., and Boost, G.: An open trial of naproxen in rheumatoid arthritis patients with significant esophageal, gastric and duodenal lesions. J. Clin. Pharmacol. 15:378, 1975.
178. Rivkin, I., Foschi, C.V., and Rosen, C.H.: Inhibition of in vitro neutrophile chemotaxis and spontaneous motility by anti-inflammatory agents. Proc. Soc. Exp. Biol. Med. 153:236, 1976.
179. Sondervorst, M.: Azapropazone. Clin. Rheum. Dis. 5:465, 1979.
180. Riess, W., Stierlin, H., Degen, P., Faigle, J.W., Gerardin, A., Moppert, J., Sallmann, A., Schmid, K., Schweizer, A., Sule, M., Theobald, W., and Wagner, J.: Pharmacokinetics and metabolism of the anti-inflammatory agent Voltaren. Scand. J. Rheumatol. Suppl. 22:17, 1978.
181. Stierlin, H., Faigle, J.W., and Columbia, A.: Pharmacokinetics of diclofenac sodium (Voltaren) and metabolites in patients with impaired renal function. Scand. J. Rheumatol. Suppl. 22:30, 1978.
182. Verbeeck, R., Tjandramaga, T.B., Mullie, A., Berbesselt, R., Verberekmoes, R., and De Schepper, P.J.: Biotransformation of diflunisal and renal excretion of its glucronides in renal insufficiency. Br. J. Clin. Pharmacol. 7:273, 1979a.
183. Forbes, J.A., Beaver, W.T., White, E.H., White, R.W., Neilson, G.B., and Shackleford, R.W.: A new oral analgesic with an unusually long duration of action. JAMA 248:2139, 1982.
184. Wilkens, R.F., Ward, J.R., Louis, J.S., and McAdam, L.P.: Double-blind study comparing piroxicam and aspirin in the treatment of rheumatoid arthritis. Am. J. Med. 72:23, 1982.
185. Abruzzo, J.L., Gordon, G.V., and Meyers, A.R.: Double-blind study comparing piroxicam and aspirin in the treatment of osteoarthritis. Am. J. Med. 72:45, 1982.
186. Widmark, P.H.: Piroxicam: Its safety and efficacy in the treatment of acute gout. Am. J. Med. 72:63, 1982.
187. Romberg, O.: Comparison of piroxicam with indomethacin in ankylosing spondylitis. A double-blind crossover trial. Am. J. Med. 72:58, 1982.
188. Wiseman, E.H., and Hobbs, D.C.: Review of pharmacokinetic studies with piroxicam. Am. J. Med. 72:9, 1982.
189. Semble, E., Metcalf, D., Turner, R., Agudelo, C., Pisko, E., Johnson, A.M., and Heise, E.: Genetic predictors of patient response and side effects in the treatment of rheumatoid arthritis with a high dose of nonsteroidal antiinflammatory drug regimen. Arthritis Rheum. 25:370, 1982.
190. Kligman, A.M., and Kaidbey, K.H.: Phototoxicity to benoxaprofen. Eur. J. Rheumatol. Inflamm. 5:124, 1982.
191. Fenton, D.A., English, J.S., and Wilkinson, J.D.: Reversal of male-pattern baldness, hypertrichosis, and accelerated hair and nail growth in patients receiving benoxaprofen. Br. Med. J. 284:1228, 1982.
192. O'Neill, P.M., Yorgey, K.A., Renzi, N.L., Williams, R.L., and Benet, L.Z.: Disposition of zomepirac sodium in man. J. Clin. Pharmacol. 22:470, 1982.
193. Honig, S.: Long-term therapy with zomepirac: Two years of safety and efficacy data. Presentation on Zomepirac and Tolmetin: Advances in Clinical Pharmacologic Research. VIII Pan-American Congress of Rheumatology, June, 1982.
194. Mawdsley, P.: Fenbufen. Clin. Rheum. Dis. 6:615, 1980.
195. Braverman, A.M.: Single-dose pharmacokinetic study of 900 mg fenbufen in the elderly. Eur. J. Rheumatol. Inflamm. 5:304, 1982.
196. Armstrong, R., Bradbrook, I., Gibson, T.J., Morrison, P., Rogers, H.J., and Spector, R.G.: A study of repeated administration of fenbufen in patients with chronic rheumatic disorders and renal impairment. Eur. J. Rheumatol. Inflamm. 5:294, 1982.
197. Van Arman, C.G., Nuss, G.W., and Risle, E.A.: Interactions of aspirin, indomethacin and other drugs in adjuvant-induced arthritis in the rat. J. Pharmacol. Exp. Ther. 187:400, 1973.
198. DiPasquale, G., Rassaert, C., Welaj, P. and Tripp, L.: Anti-inflammatory activity of isoxicam in combination with aspirin or D-propoxyphene. Agents Actions 6:748, 1976.
199. Ackerman, N.R., Rooks, W.H., Shott, H.L., Genant, H., Maloney, P., and West, E.: Effects of naproxen on connective tissue changes in the adjuvant arthritic rat. Arthritis Rheum. 22:1365, 1979.

# Chapter 51
# Antimalarials

*Richard I. Rynes*

## HISTORICAL PERSPECTIVE

The establishment of antimalarial medications as useful antirheumatic agents has been steeped in controversy. This group of drugs is derived from the bark of the Peruvian cinchona tree, which Jesuit missionaries brought to Spain in the early seventeenth century as a remedy for certain fevers. For a number of years, Jesuit bark, as it was often called in the European countries, was not widely accepted by the medical establishment, in part because it was used by the Jesuits, but more importantly because it did not conform to Galen's teachings.[1] Charlatans often dispensed the medicine in secret remedies.

Cinchona bark's active principles, quinine and cinchonine, were isolated by Pelletier and Caventau in 1820 at about the same time that salicylin, the progenitor of aspirin, was being isolated from the bark of the willow tree. It was not until 1894 that J. P. Payne,[2] physician to St. Thomas' Hospital in London, delivered a postgraduate lecture on lupus erythematosus in which he first described the successful use of quinine for a rheumatic disease. Four factors, later to become points of contention, were mentioned in his report. These were effectiveness, dose, toxicity, and mechanism of action.

Payne's study was uncontrolled, as were almost all subsequent studies. The benefits appeared conclusive, however, and he commented: "I can not say that quinine treatment is an absolute success, but has succeeded in a considerable number of cases. I also think, therefore, that the best thing to do is to begin with this." The optimum dosage was not known but "decidedly large doses should be given." Side effects were not recognized and "people with this complaint seem to bear quinine unusually well." Payne was not sure of the mechanism by which quinine worked but believed that there was a "circulatory disturbance very much influenced by quinine."

In light of current knowledge, Payne's assessment of antimalarial effectiveness has been confirmed, as has its low toxicity. His use of high dosage is decidedly out of favor, since it is only low-dose administration that is safe on a long-term basis. The mechanism of drug action has not yet been established, but there is some evidence supporting Payne's hypothesis.[3]

Despite Payne's optimistic report, the beneficial effects of quinine were not confirmed until 1938 when Davidson and Birt[4] reported improvement of discoid lupus in 19 of 29 patients.

During the first half of the 20th century extensive efforts were undertaken to synthesize antimalarial compounds with improved therapeutic/toxicity ratios. These new compounds were also successfully applied to the treatment of patients with lupus erythematosus. In 1928, Martenstein[5] reported that pamaquine was beneficial in 22 of 28 patients with discoid or subacute systemic lupus erythematosus. Another compound, quinacrine, was first shown to be effective against lupus erythematosus by the Russian Prokoptchouk,[6] who obtained good results in all 35 patients treated. Because this report was published in Russia in 1940, it remained generally unknown until after Page's independent observation.[7]

The seminal publication in Lancet by Page[8] in 1951 provided much of the impetus for use of antimalarials in patients with connective tissue diseases. He treated patients with lupus erythematosus with quinacrine in doses varying from 100 to 300 mg per day. Skin lesions improved in 17 of 18 patients. Associated "rheumatoid arthritis" remitted in two patients, and systemic symptoms including arthritis cleared in a third. The importance of dosage was noted. Some patients responded to an initial 100 mg per day, while others needed at least 300 mg per day. Side effects were mild except in one patient who developed a lichenoid skin reaction, which necessitated discontinuation of the drug.

The response of Page's patients with lupus and "rheumatoid arthritis" influenced several groups to treat rheumatoid arthritis with antimalarials.[9-11] Bagnall's[10] favorable report of the efficacy of chloroquine in patients with rheumatoid arthritis, published in 1957, stimulated the more widespread use of this compound in treating patients with rheumatoid arthritis. Of 108 patients, 36 percent went into remission and major improvement was found in another 35 percent. He used chloroquine, a compound that had been synthesized in 1934, in hopes that toxicity would be minimized. Ironically, chloroquine was not used extensively until after World War II because it had been judged to be too toxic for practical use in humans. This conclusion was based on studies of treatment of blood-induced vivax malaria in four paretics at the psychiatric clinic in Dusseldorf, Germany.[12] At the time of Bagnall's report others were finding that hydroxychloroquine, a compound structurally similar to chloroquine, might be equally effective and even less toxic.[13-15]

In distinction to these favorable reports, some studies dampened the enthusiasm for antimalarials. Double-blinded studies[16,17] failed to confirm Bagnall's impressive remission rate, although they did show effectiveness. More disturbing was the recognition by Hobbs and associates[18] in 1959 that long-term treatment of rheumatic diseases might result in serious drug-induced retinal toxicity. By 1964 editorials in four major journals[19-22] warned of this problem and questioned whether benefits justified the potential loss of vision. Even as late as as the period between 1976 and 1978 the British National Formulary[23] stated that "chloroquine is rarely effective and toxic effects are frequent and serious, including irreversible retinal damage; it is now regarded as obsolete." This assessment has not been substantiated by a careful analysis of studies describing drug efficacy and toxicity. Based on a more accurate appraisal, antimalarials continue to be widely used for rheumatic diseases.

## DEFINITION AND STRUCTURE

The term "antimalarials" is somewhat misleading when applied to drugs used to treat rheumatic diseases. For these conditions the term is limited to the quinoline derivatives and the structurally similar acridine compound quinacrine (Fig. 51–1). Other drugs used to treat malaria, such as pyrimethamine, an inhibitor of dihydrofolate reductase, and sulfadoxine, a sulfonamide, are not employed as antirheumatic medications. Dapsone, a sulfone used in the treatment of malaria, has been reported to be effective in rheumatoid arthritis[24] but is not considered one of the "antimalarials."

Figure 51–1 illustrates the structure of the compounds that have been used to treat rheumatic diseases. Their corresponding proprietary names are listed in Table 51–1. Quinine is the parent compound. Pamaquine and primaquine are 8-aminoquinoline derivatives. Four drugs, amiodiaquin, amopyroquin, chloroquine, and hydroxychloroquine, are 4-aminoquinoline derivatives. The latter two differ only by the substitution of a hydroxyethyl group for an ethyl group on the tertiary amino-nitrogen of the side chain of chloroquine. Although quinacrine is a 9-aminoacridine compound, its structure does contain the chloroquine moiety.

Only two compounds are generally prescribed in current practice. Hydroxychloroquine is used almost exclusively in the United States, while chloroquine is also

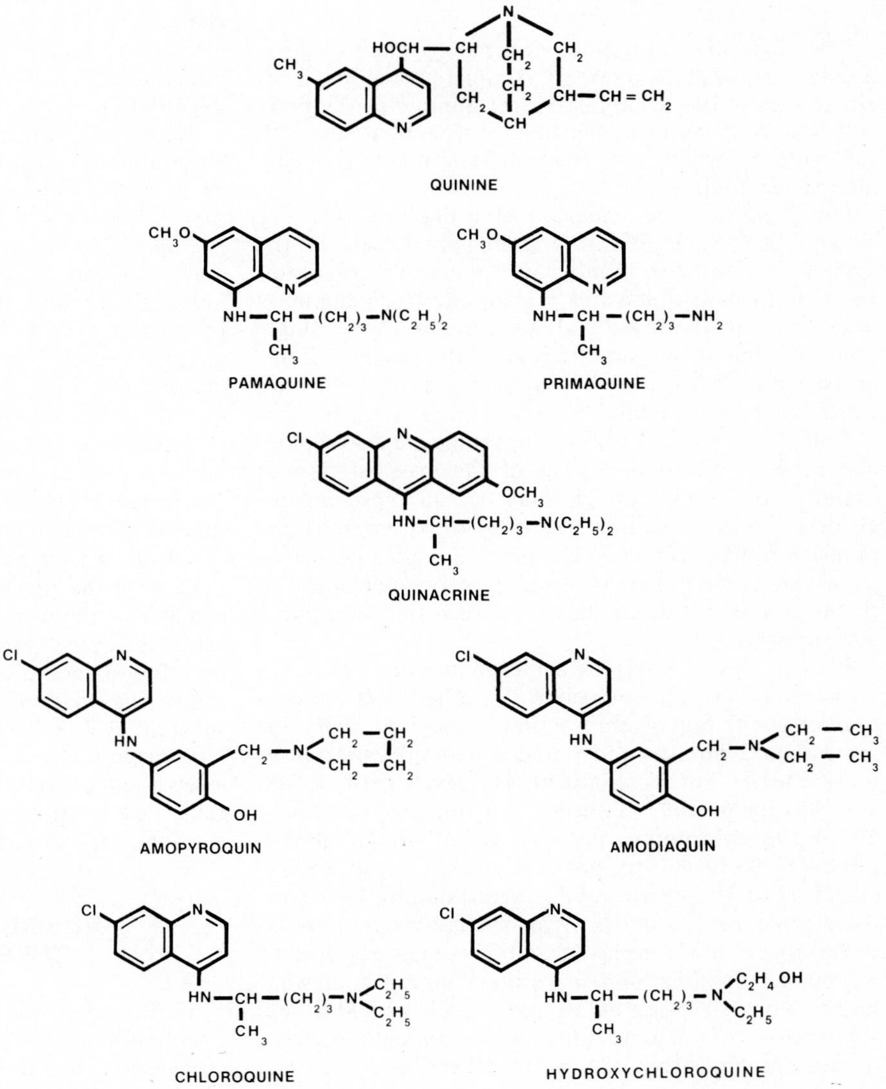


**Figure 51–1.** Structural formulas of antirheumatic antimalarials.

**Table 51–1.** Antirheumatic Antimalarial Drugs and Their Proprietary Names

| Generic Name | Proprietary Name |
|---|---|
| hydroxychloroquine | Plaquenil |
| chloroquine | Aralen |
| | Resochin |
| | Nivaquine |
| | Sanoquin |
| quinacrine | Atabrine |
| | Mepacrine |
| | Acriquin |
| amodiaquin | Camoquin |
| amopyroquin | Propoquin |
| primaquine | |
| pamaquine | Plasmochin |

used in Europe. Occasionally quinacrine is added to achieve maximum effect[25] or used to treat patients unable to tolerate the other two.

## PHARMACOKINETICS

The absorption of quinine and the synthetic antimalarials is rapid and essentially complete when given orally. There is less accumulation of quinine in the body and less localization in the tissues in comparison with the synthetic drugs. It is primarily eliminated by being altered metabolically.[26]

Quinacrine is widely distributed in tissues and is very slowly liberated. Significant amounts are detected in the urine for at least two months after therapy is discontinued.[27] Both pamaquine and primaquine reach the maximum level in the plasma about 2 hours after a single oral dose, but at the end of 8 hours little remains. Compared with other synthetic antimalarials, the drugs are concentrated to a smaller extent in the tissues.[28]

Chloroquine and hydroxychloroquine are also rapidly absorbed.[1,15] About 8 percent of the ingested dose is found in the feces, but this may not all represent unabsorbed drug, since fecal excretion of parenterally administered drugs occurs.[29] The drugs are quickly cleared from the plasma and localized largely unchanged in tissue to a degree intermediate between that of quinine and quinacrine.[30]

Plateau plasma levels are achieved in 8 to 14 days.[31,32] Frisk-Holmberg and associates[33] studied 100 patients receiving 250 mg of chloroquine phosphate daily for more than 2 months and found a fivefold variation in plasma levels, but most patients had levels between 200 and 400 $\mu$g per liter. Others, studying patients taking 500 mg of chloroquine per day, found similar plasma levels of 200 to 400 $\mu$g per liter and a plateau urinary excretion of 75 mg per day.[34] Corresponding values for daily doses of 400 mg of hydroxychloroquine are 500 to 700 $\mu$g per liter for plasma and 55 mg per day urinary excretion.[34] Zvaifler and associates[31] found somewhat higher plateau plasma chloroquine levels of 600 to 800 $\mu$g per liter but noted no differences in patients receiving dosages ranging from 125 mg to 750 mg per day.

The half-life of chloroquine in man has been reported to vary widely. In patients receiving either a single or a weekly dose, the half-life is about 3.5 days.[35] When patients received 500 mg of chloroquine phosphate daily for four weeks, the half-life increased to 6 to 7 days.[32] Others have found dose-dependent kinetics with a half-life as long as 12 days after receiving a single 1-gram dose of chloroquine.[33] Some of these differences may result from different methodologies of measurement.[33] By the 77th day after drug administration is discontinued, urinary daily output falls to about 1 mg.[32] At this time about 55 percent of the total ingested dose may be accounted for by urinary excretion.[32] However, small amounts of chloroquine may be found in plasma, red blood cells, and urine as long as 5 years after the last dose.[36] The rate of urinary excretion depends on pH and is increased when the urine is acidified.

The major metabolic conversion product of either chloroquine or hydroxychloroquine, accounting for about one-third of the total urinary excretory product, is the desethyl derivative formed by *N*-alkyl degradation of the terminal desethyl amino-ethyl group in the side chain.[29,37] Minor metabolic conversion products account for about 3 percent of excreted drug. They include compounds formed by ring hydroxylation and side chain degradation.[29,37]

Tissue concentrations of chloroquine and hydroxychloroquine are much greater than plasma levels.[38,39] Most studies have been conducted in animals, especially rats, but a few studies have been performed in military personnel[39,40] committing suicide by chloroquine ingestion[39] or dying from other causes.[40] In rats the lowest tissue concentrations are found in brain, followed by muscle, kidney, liver, lung, spleen, and the adrenal glands.[38] Studies in humans show rather similar tissue distribution.[39] Localization of the 4-aminoquinolines in the eye assumes great importance because of retinal toxicity. In albino rats drug concentration in the eye ranks between muscle and heart. In pigmented rats eye concentration is 10 to 20 times greater than any other tissue.[38] Bernstein and associates[41] found that this could be accounted for by deposition in the iris and choroid.

Despite the markedly increased deposition of chloroquine in pigmented ocular tissue, subcellular localization is not well established. McChesney and associates have found similar excretion rates in blacks and whites, suggesting that binding to skin melanin may not be substantial.[32] In vitro chloroquine binds to nucleic acids, but Vargo[42] has shown that only 10 percent of tissue levels are localized in the nucleus of rat liver or kidney cells. High concentrations have been measured in the lysosomal fraction of rat liver.[43]

## POSSIBLE MECHANISMS OF THERAPEUTIC ACTION

Since Payne[2] first suggested that quinine corrected a circulatory disturbance in lupus erythematosus, much speculation and investigation have centered upon the mechanisms by which antimalarials act. Conclusions have not been definitive because the pathogenesis of the two major diseases responding to antimalarials, lupus erythematouss and rheumatoid arthritis, is complicated and incompletely understood (see Chapters 58, 59 and 68), and also because the antimalarials have multiple actions. A number of interacting pathways (described in Section I) have been implicated in disease pathogenesis, but the primary factors responsible for disease initiation, development, and severity have not been determined. Antimalarial drugs may inhibit several of these pathways. However, investigation of drug actions has generally been conducted in vitro, and it is not known if the drugs produce similar effects in vivo. Furthermore, concentrations of the drug in these experiments vary greatly and may not be obtained in the crucial in vivo sites.

The varied actions of antimalarials may be considered under several headings. They may impair several basic physiologic processes. These actions, possibly interacting with others, may moderate inflammatory or immunologic pathways. There are also a number of miscellaneous actions that may contribute to modulation of disease pathogenesis.

**Primary Actions.** Three basic processes affected by antimalarials are sulfhydryl-disulfide interchange, enzymatic reactions, and nucleoprotein interaction.

Sulfhydryl-disulfide interchange reactions participate in numerous biologic processes.[44] These include certain enzymatic reactions, proliferation of immunologically competent cells,[45] denaturation of some proteins, the Arthus reaction, cell wall integrity, and the formation of the mitochondrial network. Gerber[44] has shown that chloroquine binds to certain sulfhydryl groups of human serum protein. This occurs using concentrations of chloroquine obtainable in the serum of patients undergoing treatment. He also established that chloroquine can block sulfhydryl-disulfide interchange reactions during the denaturation of bovine serum albumin by heat or urea and can inhibit the reduction of ferricyanide by cysteine.

Enzymatic reactions participate in almost all biologic events. Chloroquine reduces the activity of many enzymes,[46] including phospholipase,[47] NADH-cytochrome C reductase, and cholinesterase. More specifically related to the pathogenesis of arthritis, Whitehouse and Coewy[48] demonstrated that chloroquine inhibits the protease-induced release of peptides from incubating cartilage slices and the hydrolysis of rat skin gelatin by bacterial collagenase. Chloroquine may also interfere with hyaluronidase actions, as shown indirectly by Whitehead and Hager.[49]

Antimalarials have been shown to form complexes with DNA by binding of the quinoline ring to the phosphate groups and nucleotide bases.[50] This appears to stabilize the DNA, block depolymerization by desoxyribonuclease,[51] inhibit the actions of DNA and RNA polymerases,[52] and interfere with DNA replication.[53] By binding to the DNA substrate, antimalarials block reactions between DNA and anti-DNA antibodies.[54] This is probably the explanation for the inhibition of the LE cell phenomenon observed by Dubois.[55] DNA binding might be expected to be an important modulator of DNA/anti-DNA antibody complex formation in lupus, but an in vivo effect has not been demonstrated.

**Anti-inflammatory Actions.** A number of antimalarial actions may inhibit inflammatory reactions. In addition to blocking sulfhydryl-disulfide interchange and a direct effect on enzymes, chloroquine also stablizes lysosomal membranes, thereby inhibiting the release of lysosomal enzymes.[56] Protection was observed against several different mechanisms of membrane destablization, including ultraviolet light. Prostaglandins, another set of mediators of inflammation, are elevated in rheumatoid synovial fluid. Chloroquine decreases total prostaglandin production.[57] It has a direct effect on phospholipase A, the enzyme initiating prostaglandin synthesis.[47] Prostaglandin F2 formation is inhibited to a greater extent than prostaglandin E2.[57]

Other inflammatory processes blocked by chloroquine include polymorphonuclear cell chemotaxis and phagocytosis.[58] This action may be one of the mechanisms causing the suppression of polymorphonuclear infiltration into implants of polyurethane foam impregnated with dead tubercle bacilli.[59] Chloroquine also appears to suppress the growth of fibroblasts, as shown by the inhibition of the development of connective tissue capsules about implants.[60]

Experimental evidence supports Payne's concept[2] that antimalarials may affect "circulatory disturbances." The activity of histamine,[61] which increases vasopermeability, is diminished. Another vascular abnormality inhibited by chloroquine is blood sludging, the intravascular aggregation of erythrocytes. Sludging has been observed in patients with rheumatoid arthritis[3] and was found to disappear when monitored in the retinal veins of 22 patients treated with chloroquine. Clinical improvement followed "desludging" in 51 percent of patients and a lowered erythrocyte sedimentation rate in 41 percent.

**Immunologic Action.** Abnormal immunologic reactivity is believed to play an important role in rheumatic disease pathogenesis. Experimental evidence concerning antimalarial action on immune reactivity is inconsistent. Animal studies suggest that chloroquine has no inhibitory effect on antibody production. Thompson and Bartholomew[62] found no difference between treated and control rabbits in the production of circulating antibodies to typhoid O and H antigens or to bovine serum albumin. Kalmonson and Gage[63] showed that hydroxychloroquine-treated rabbits produced a normal primary or secondary response to diphtheroid toxoid. They did note an enhanced tuberculin reaction in the hydroxychloroquine-treated rabbits infected with bacillus Calmette-Guérin.

Other studies demonstrated inhibition of immune reactions. Hurvitz and Hirschhorn[64] showed that chloroquine inhibited the proliferative response of cultured human lymphocytes induced by phytohemagglutinin, steptolysin O antigen, or foreign lymphocytes. Panaji and co-workers[65] extended these results by demonstrating decreased responsiveness to phytohemagglutinin by lymphocytes from patients treated with chloroquine and aspirin compared with those from patients treated with aspirin alone.

More recently Salmeron and Lipsky[66] observed that proliferation of lymphocytes suppressed by chloroquine was restored by purified monocytes. They showed that the generation of immunoglobulin-secreting cells could also be suppressed by concentrations of chloroquine as low as 1 $\mu$g per ml. Adding supernatants from cultures of purified monocytes reversed this action. Purified interleukin 1 could be substituted for monocyte supernatant with similar effect, suggesting that chloroquine interferes with the secretion of interleukin 1 by monocytes.[66a]

It has not been shown that antibody production in patients with rheumatic diseases is directly inhibited by antimalarials, but in vitro complex formation between antigens and antibodies is inhibited.[67,68] The fall in titers of rheumatoid factors observed in patients with rheumatoid arthritis[69-71] may merely be a nonspecific reflection of disease improvement.

**Miscellaneous Action.** Among the miscellaneous actions of antimalarials that may explain their improvement of lupus erythematosus is a photoprotective effect. McChesney and associates[72] showed that these drugs are present in the skin in high concentrations and can absorb ultraviolet radiation. Lester and co-workers[73] showed that hydroxychloroquine raises the minimal erythema-inducing dose of ultraviolet light between five- and tenfold in patients with photosensitive rashes or lupus erythematosus. Others have not found a sunscreening action.[74,75] They postulated that the photoprotective effect was mediated by "modifying the reaction pattern of the patient with polymorphous light eruption in a manner which supresses the abnormal but not the normal responses to ultraviolet light in the sunburn spectrum."[74]

Infectious agents may participate in the development of systemic lupus erythematosus or rheumatoid arthritis.[76] Chloroquine inhibits the replication of some bacteria[52] and protects tissue culture cells from viral infections.[77] Replication of the Maloney leukemia virus may be prevented even in the absence of an apparent effect on DNA or RNA synthesis.[78]

There is evidence that the Epstein-Barr virus may be a pathogenetic agent for rheumatoid arthritis.[79] While exposure to this agent is similar to that of nonrheumatoid individuals, patients develop an unusual host response that includes the production of rheumatoid arthritis precipitin (RAP), presumed to be an antibody to a nuclear antigen of Epstein-Barr-infected B lymphocytes. Chloroquine enhances the expression of the Epstein-Barr virus antigen, EA, in superinfected cells.[80] This could promote the immunologic inactivation of such cells in treated patients.

## THERAPEUTIC EFFECTIVENESS

The effectiveness of antimalarial medications in the treatment of systemic lupus erythematosus and rheumatoid arthritis is generally accepted. They are probably helpful in treating other inflammatory arthritides, such as psoriatic arthritis, ankylosing spondylitis, and juvenile rheumatoid arthritis, although hard data supporting this are lacking.

Because antimalarials were synthesized to treat malaria and not connective tissue diseases, clinical trials to determine efficacy and toxicity and animal experiments elucidating mechanisms of action were not initially conducted for rheumatic diseases. Later studies have rectified some omissions, but there is a paucity of studies directly comparing different antimalarials or varying doses of a single drug.

**Lupus Erythematosus.** The variability of lupus erythematosus and the unevenness of its response to medication increase the difficulty of evaluating its response to antimalarials. Untreated lupus erythematosus is characterized by excerbations and remissions. The discoid variety undergoes spontaneous remission in 10 to 15 percent,[25] while the systemic form may have spontaneous remission in 40[81] to 70 percent.[82] This occurrence of spontaneous remissions, as well as the finding that various manifestations of systemic lupus erythematosus do not respond equally well to antimalarials, may lead to an overestimation of effectiveness in uncontrolled studies. It is particularly important not to attribute generalized benefit to treatment when only one manifestation is actually improved. Corticosteroids are generally more effective than antimalarials. When both are taken, the steroids may obscure benefits accruing from antimalarial treatment. On the other hand, improvement due to steroids may be incorrectly attributed to antimalarials.

***Discoid Lupus Erythematosus.*** Even after considering these factors, the conclusion that discoid lupus erythematosus responds to antimalarials is inescapable. Compared with the spontaneous remission rate of 15 percent, remissions or major improvements have been noted in 60 to 90 percent of treated patients. Furthermore, all antimalarial compounds have been beneficial. However, daily dosages were often much larger than those currently acceptable.

Quinine was the first antimalarial used to treat discoid lupus erythematosus. Payne[2] did not report the percentage of responders and used doses as high as 1800 mg per day. Nineteen of 29 patients treated by Davidson and Birt[4] responded to doses half as large, while five were unimproved, and five were lost to follow-up. Erythematous lesions improved, but scaly ones did not.

The development of synthetic antimalarials provided other therapeutic agents. Martenstein[5] in 1928 used pamaquine, an 8-aminoquinoline, with good results in 79 percent of 28 patients. He too noted greater improvement of acutely inflamed lesions than of hyperkeratotic changes. Quinacrine was the first antimalarial agent for which responses of a large number of patients were described. Prokoptchouk[6] treated 35 patients with a series of 10-day courses interspersed with rest periods. Two to five courses were generally needed, but even chronic, scarred lesions improved. Page's report[8] of its effectiveness in 17 of 18 patients treated with doses of 100 to 300 mg per day stimulated further trials. In the next 10 years five of the papers published[83-87] reported good results in 215 of 276 patients with discoid lupus erythematosus, a 78 percent response rate. The 4-aminoquinoline compound amodiaquin was also found to be effective by several investigators.[25,88,89]

Goldman and associates[90] first treated discoid lupus erythematosus with chloroquine because it was less toxic than quinacrine and did not impart the yellowish skin staining found with quinacrine. Eleven of 18 patients showed great improvement with doses of 500 or 750 mg per day for 1 to 2 weeks followed by 250 mg per day for 4 to 6 weeks. Others noted similar or slightly better results.[25,91,92] Rogers and Finn[91] found chloroquine in doses of 250 mg per day as effective as quinacrine, beginning with 300 mg per day and tapering to 100 mg per day. Lesions cleared in 35 percent of 45 patients in each group, while another 15 percent of the quinacrine-treated and 30 percent of the chloroquine-treated patients were much improved.

Hydroxychloroquine was also initially used to diminish the toxicity seen with other antimalarials. In the study of Mullins and associates[13] localized edematous lesions cleared within two weeks in seven of eight patients, and excellent results were achieved over a somewhat longer time in five of eight patients with chronic discoid changes. Initial doses were quite high, averaging about 1000 mg per day, and maintenance doses were generally 400 to 600 mg per day. Seventeen of 22 patients treated with this drug by Lewis and Frumess[14] were more than 50 percent improved, with nine in remission after eight weeks.

A few controlled studies have substantiated antimalarial benefit. Dubois[25] substituted placebo for amodiaquin in seven patients. Five, who were initially controlled by amodiaquin alone, flared one to three months after placebo was substituted and then improved within several days after readministration of the drug.

Prakken reviewed the published results of the various treatments of discoid lupus erythematosus and found that 74 percent of those treated with metals (As, Au, Bi), 69 percent of those receiving antimalarials, and 72 percent of those given a miscellany of drugs were cured or much improved. As a result he participated in a double-blind trial with Kraak and co-workers.[93] There were 49 patients assigned to one of two groups. One was given hydroxychloroquine for one year, starting with two 200-mg tablets per day. If there was no improvement, the patient had his pills increased to four and then six, a maximum daily dose of 1200 mg. If a cure was obtained, the dose was reduced to a maintenance level. At the end of a year the patient was put on a placebo for three months. The other group reversed the procedure. Statistical analysis of the data showed that hydroxychloroquine was significantly more effective than the placebo.

The effectiveness of antimalarials in the treatment of skin lesions is often apparent within the first week when erythematous changes start to regress. Follicular plugging may then disappear, and after several months thickening and induration diminish or clear. Most patients responding to antimalarial medication suffer relapse after the drug is discontinued. Winkelmann and associates[85] found that only seven of 67 patients who took quinacrine or chloroquine for 10 weeks to 4 years maintained remission for 3 years after stopping treatment. Forty-eight patients who responded favorably to treatment had subsequent relapses after discontinuing medication. Most responded to additional courses of treatment.

*Systemic Lupus Erythematosus.* In distinction to the marked benefits of treatment of discoid lupus erythematosus with antimalarials, improvement of systemic lupus erythematosus is not nearly as well-documented. Much of the evidence suggesting that antimalarials are effective for the systemic variety comes from the inclusion of a few patients with "subacute" lupus in larger series of patients with only discoid skin lesions.[8,13,85,90] These patients have had findings such as arthritis, fever, fatigue, malaise, mildly depressed white blood cell counts, mild albuminuria, and a positive LE cell phenomenon. Quinacrine,[8] chloroquine even in low dosage,[90] and hydroxychloroquine[13] were each effective in such patients.

Dubois[94] treated 20 patients with systemic lupus erythematosus using rather high doses of quinacrine. Seven of nine patients with arthralgias and fever remitted on treatment, while only three of 11 patients with more severe acute systemic lupus erythematosus were benefited. In general, the less active the disease, the more rapid and better was the improvement.

Rudnicki and colleagues[95] provided some additional evidence that antimalarial treatment is effective for some systemic symptoms. They studied 43 patients who had been treated with antimalarials for at least two years and then had medication discontinued because of toxicity. Significantly fewer flare-ups occurred during the years on treatment, but no improvement in individual manifestations could be demonstrated for the entire group. When specific drugs and doses were studied, paired-t test analysis showed less fever, fatigue, and weight loss during the years on drug ($p < 0.05$) for the group who had received 500 mg of chloroquine daily. No significant corticosteroid-sparing effect was found. Others suggest that antimalarial treatment may have a steroid-sparing effect.[96]

Antimalarials are not appropriate treatment for the more severe manifestations of systemic lupus erythematosus according to Dubois[25] or Lanham and Hughes.[97] However, there is one study suggesting that antimalarials may be useful in treating lupus glomerulonephritis. Conte and associates[98] treated 12 patients with a combination of indomethacin (3 mg per kg per day) and hydroxychloroquine (800 mg per day). All patients had active diffuse proliferative glomerulonephritis, and four had more than 50 percent crescent formation on biopsy. Serum creatinine was initially elevated in all but two patients (median of 2.0 mg per dl) and all had 24-hour proteinuria of greater than 1 g (median 3.6 g). Duration of treatment ranged from 22 to 76 months in all but one patient. Follow-up evaluation demonstrated lasting remissions in 8 patients, including one with crescent formation and improvement in three others. Only one patient died. At the same time 16 patients treated with high-dose corticosteroids by this group did poorly, with nine deaths.

**Rheumatoid Arthritis.** Medications used for rheumatoid arthritis may be divided into several groups on the basis of their onset of action and their effect on the underlying disease process. The antimalarials belong to the class termed slow-acting antirheumatic drugs (SAARDs). Little or no improvement may be apparent for weeks or months after antimalarials are started. Benefits ensue gradually and may not be maximal for many months.[10,15] This contrasts with the more immediate effects of steroids or nonsteroidal anti-inflammatory agents that appear within one or two weeks. Analogously, when antimalarial treatment is discontinued, the disease will not flare within days but gradually worsen over weeks or months. It is this gradual action that suggests that SAARDs act indirectly. SAARDs may modify the disease process in such a manner that some patients enter a sustained remission.

Different types of studies have been helpful in determining the effectiveness of antimalarials. Factors considered are the drug used, dosage schedule employed, length of study, and whether the study is controlled. Double-blind controlled studies are most definitive, but prolonged placebo-controlled studies are often not feasible in patients with rheumatoid arthritis. Long-term open evaluation provides additional information, particularly in assessing late responses,[15] relapses on treatment,[10] and the effects of dosage. The response to different dosages may not be readily appreciated unless specifically studied.

Several of the antimalarials no longer employed have been shown to be effective. Encouraged by Page's[8] description of improvement of arthritis in two patients with lupus erythematosus treated with quinacrine, Freedman and Bach[9] used this medication to treat 23 patients with rheumatoid arthritis. All but one improved both subjectively and objectively. Primaquine was effective in each of 21 patients treated by Steck and associates,[99] 2 entering complete remission and 8 partial remission. Two 4-aminoquinoline drugs, amodiaquin and amopyroquin, have also been used with some benefit.[11,100-102] A 5-month double-blind cross-over study of amopyroquin was conducted on 15 patients by Bartholomew and Duff.[102] Even with this small number of patients, significant improvement in Lansbury's systemic index, grip strength, and erythrocyte sedimentation rate was found for drug but not placebo.

In 1953, Haydu[103] described chloroquine treatment of rheumatoid arthritis. Patients were treated for 6 months using the rather low dosage of 0.5 g three times a week. Considerable improvement was noted in 21 of 28 patients. Although only one patient went into complete remission, only one failed to show any improvement. Haydu believed that his data were not sufficient to judge the true efficacy of chloroquine but that the medication should be regarded as one additional antirheumatic substance.

Subsequent studies confirmed the efficacy of chloroquine and demonstrated that hydroxychloroquine was equally beneficial. One of the most influential[19] was that of Bagnall.[10] He treated 125 patients with 250 mg of chloroquine per day. Twenty-one of the 90 patients with rheumatoid arthritis were initially entered in a double-blind placebo-controlled study. The results so favored the chloroquine-treated group that Bagnall had no difficulty in determining which was the active compound. The controlled study was stopped because he believed he could not ethically enter seriously affected patients in a long-term placebo-controlled study. In the open study major improvement was noted in 71 percent, and half of those entered remission. Long duration of disease or gross articular damage was more prevalent in those failing to respond. Relapses during treatment were noted in 18 patients. They occurred most frequently in the second and third year of treatment, especially in patients unable to tolerate the standard dose. Sixteen of these 18 patients improved with continued treatment. Seven patients relapsed three to twelve months after treatment was stopped and again remitted when chloroquine was restarted. Bagnall emphasized that maximum benefit might not be apparent until after a year of treatment.

Results achieved by Scherbel and associates[15] supported Bagnall's findings. One hundred and six patients were treated with a 4-aminoquinoline compound and 60 percent obtained major benefit. Forty-six patients received chloroquine in an initial dose of 500 mg per day, which was later reduced to 250 mg, and 60 received hydroxychloroquine, 600 mg per day, which was later reduced to 400 mg. Equal improvement was noted for patients on each medication. Scherbel's group found that for the same dose of each medication hydroxychloroquine was one-half to two-thirds as effective as chloroquine and one-half as toxic. In distinction to Bagnall's[10] findings, Scherbel did not observe any correlation between response of rheumatoid arthritis to medication and American Rheumatism Association stage of disease, duration of disease, or functional capacity of patient. They too noted that maximum response might not be evident for one year or longer and that disease activity fluctuated during treatment.

Adams and co-workers[104] reported a response rate using hydroxychloroquine that was comparable to that noted by Bagnall[10] for chloroquine. One hundred and eight patients treated with 400 mg per day of hydroxychloroquine for a minimum of 6 months were analyzed. Sixty-three percent had at least 30 percent improvement in active joint count and morning stiffness. Thirteen patients went into remission, and another 15 had greater than 75 percent improvement. Kersley and Palen[11] found that dosage may affect response rate by demonstrating that a daily dose of 800 mg was more effective than 400 mg.

Controlled studies have consistently demonstrated that these two medications are effective. Dosage of the active drug and duration of these trials have varied. The first study, conducted by Freedman,[105] compared daily doses of 200 mg of chloroquine phosphate to placebo in 66 patients over a 16-week interval. Clinical improvement was greater on chloroquine, but erythrocyte sedimentation rate and hemoglobin did not change. Rinehart and co-workers[106] studied chloroquine in both placebo-controlled parallel fashion and a cross-over manner after recognizing its benefit in open studies. Observing 33 patients over 4 months, they found that the active drug group, who received 250 mg of chloroquine per day, did significantly better than controls. Cohen and Calkins[16] studied 22 patients in a cross-over trial of only 18 weeks' duration. Morning stiffness and pain were significantly improved during active treatment. Grip strength and erythrocyte sedimentation rate were little affected.

Two double-blind studies have been conducted using hydroxychloroquine. Hamilton and Scott[17] in a cross-over study of 41 patients compared 600 mg daily with a 3-mg placebo dose. Each was taken for a 3-month period. Patient estimation of fitness, number of aspirin tablets taken daily, joint tenderness and swelling, grip strength, and erythrocyte sedimentation rate all improved when patients received the active drug, but only a decrease in ingested aspirin tablets reached statistical significance ($p < 0.001$). The authors concluded that the drug had slight but definite antirheumatic activity.

The Cooperating Clinics of the American Rheumatism Association[71] conducted a 6-month placebo-controlled study in which 53 patients received 800 mg per day of hydroxychloroquine and 60 received placebo. Results are shown in Table 51–2. Changes in individual indexes (listed in the footnote) all favored the drug-treated group, but none reached statistical significance. More impressive were the changes in the overall assessments listed in Table 51–2, which were associated with hydroxychloroquine treatment. Furthermore, serum gamma globulin levels returned toward normal for only the drug-treated group. Latex agglutination tests became normal in seven of 36 drug-treated patients, but only in two of 44 patients receiving placebo. The authors concluded that the differences in response were a result of drug effectiveness.

Even more favorable results have been obtained in two 1-year studies. One hundred and seven patients entered the trial conducted by Freedman and Steinberg.[107] Forty-two patients treated with 400 mg of chloroquine sulfate daily and 40 placebo-treated patients completed the trial. The authors noted definite general improvement in 80 percent of the patients completing 1 year of chloroquine treatment compared with 30 percent of the placebo group. Deterioration was seen in only 5 percent of chloroquine-treated patients but in 25 percent of controls. All clinical parameters, including joint tenderness, walking time, and the erythrocyte sedimentation rate, improved in the drug-treated group. Only manual dexterity improved in the placebo group. Radiographic evaluation showed improvement in erosion score for two treated patients, with worsening in three. Twelve placebo patients had greater erosions, and none had improvement.

Popert and associates[69] conducted a similar trial in which 134 patients were entered. Dosage of chloroquine was 250 mg a day, although some patients received 500 mg per day during initiation of treatment. Disease activity, functional capacity, grip strength, and erythrocyte sedimentation rate were significantly better in the treated group. Improvement was more marked in those with shorter duration of disease. The sheep cell agglutination titer fell in 16 of 18 chloroquine-treated patients but in only three of 15 controls. Increased titers were noted in one treated patient and six controls. The only parameter not improved by treatment was radiologically assessed erosions. Each group showed slight progression.

***Comparison with Other Slow-acting Antirheumatic Drugs (SAARDs).*** A few studies have compared various SAARDs in treating rheumatoid arthritis. Dwosh and colleagues[108] compared chloroquine (250 mg per day), gold thiomalate (50 mg weekly), and azothiaprine (1 to 2 mg per kg per day) in an open study of 33 patients with class II disease using American Rheumatism Association criteria. The five variables assessed were articular index, joint count, grip strength, morning stiffness, and erythrocyte sedimentation rate. At 24 weeks, each group was significantly better than at baseline. Analysis of variance showed no significant difference in improvement among the three groups except that the erythrocyte blood sedimentation rate was only decreased in the group receiving gold. Toxicity was minimal for all groups. On follow-up examination, most patients had maintained their improvement, although disease flares occurred in four of 10 patients treated with chloroquine. The authors concluded from their study that chloroquine is "a moderately effective anti-rheumatic drug and should be considered early in the management of rheumatoid arthritis."

Two studies analyzed termination of treatment using life table analysis.[109,110] In the first[109] gold was compared with hydroxychloroquine. Fifty percent of patients stopped hydroxychloroquine treatment at 13 months, with 36 percent discontinuing medication for lack of benefit and 7 percent because of side effects. Of patients receiving gold therapy, 60 months elapsed before 50 percent terminated treatment primarily because of toxicity. A subsequent report[110] from the same institution compared treatment terminations with those for patients taking gold, D-penicillamine, and levamisole. In this study hydroxychloroquine treatment resulted in fewer terminations than the other drugs, with only 30 percent

**Table 51–2.** Controlled Study of Hydroxychloroquine in Rheumatoid Arthritis:[71] Comparison by Overall Assessment

| Parameter | Placebo (Percent Improved) | Hydroxychloroquine (Percent Improved) |
|---|---|---|
| Class II or I | 9 | 50 |
| Five-point scores* | 54 | 75 |
| Observer's assessment | 35 | 64 |
| Patient's assessment | 60 | 75 |

*Five-point score is summation of five indices: duration of morning stiffness, number of active joints, time of 50-foot walk, erythrocyte sedimentation rate, and grip strength.

stopping treatment at 15 months. A 6 percent lack of effectiveness was found for hydroxychloroquine, a frequency similar to that for gold or penicillamine and less than that for levamisole. Commenting on the differences between the studies, the authors suggested that they may have discontinued hydroxychloroquine before full benefit was received or demanded a more complete remission in the first study. Patients treated with hydroxychloroquine in the second study may have had less active disease prior to treatment than those treated with the other drugs.

*Combination with Other Medications.* Combination treatment utilizing antimalarials and other antirheumatic drugs has not been extensively evaluated. Because the antimalarials appear to act differently from nonsteroidal anti-inflammatory drugs, these two groups of medications are used concomitantly. One report[111] suggests that chloroquine may decrease the need for steroids. Sievers and Hurri[112] found that antimalarials could be used in combination with gold to therapeutic advantage. Side effects appeared additive and in general could be attributed to only one medication.[113] On the other hand, Bunch and associates[114] found that hydroxychloroquine combined with D-penicillamine was less effective than either used alone.

**Other Arthropathies.** The response of other rheumatic diseases to antimalarials is mainly anecdotal. Bagnall[10] treated 17 patients with ankylosing spondylitis, 10 with rheumatoid arthritis and concomitant psoriasis, and eight with juvenile rheumatoid arthritis with chloroquine. Although the numbers were too small for statistical consideration, he found the results to be similar to those for classic rheumatoid arthritis. Scherbel[115] found moderate to great improvement in 84 percent of 73 patients with juvenile rheumatoid arthritis. Sixteen of 23 of his patients with psoriasis and rheumatoid arthritis improved satisfactorily.[15]

Some authors consider antimalarials to be contraindicated in patients with psoriatic arthritis because exacerbation of skin lesions may occur. Kammer and coworkers[116] employed hydroxychloroquine in doses of 200 to 400 mg per day for 50 courses of treatment in their series of 100 patients with psoriatic arthritis. Sixty-eight percent had beneficial responses. Twenty-four of the 34 patients who responded went into remission. No exacerbation of skin lesions was noted. Results of the study being conducted by the Pediatric Rheumatology Collaborative Study Group of the American Rheumatism Association of hydroxychloroquine treatment of juvenile rheumatoid arthritis[117] should help clarify its role in this disease.

## SIDE EFFECTS AND TOXICITY

The decision to use a medication must be based on a comparison of therapeutic benefit with toxicity. After it was established that antimalarials could cause loss of vision, safety became the paramount issue and the major factor limiting antimalarial use. During the past two decades more articles have appeared discussing retinal toxicity than commenting on effectiveness.

Much of the impetus for the development of chloroquine and hydroxychloroquine was the toxicity of the earlier synthetic antimalarials. These compounds frequently produced skin lesions, gastrointestinal problems, and neurologic symptoms. Thrombocytopenia, leukopenia, and aplastic anemia also occurred.[83-86,105,118] Yellowish staining of the skin, which could simulate jaundice, was a particularly distressing problem with quinacrine treatment.[8,25,90] 8-Aminoquinoline compounds may cause hemolysis and methemoglobinemia in patients with a genetically transmitted deficiency of glucose-6-phosphate dehydrogenase.[119] Amodiaquin was shown by Kersley and Palin[11] to produce severe side effects, including aplastic anemia, with daily doses of 400 mg. Even in the usually acceptable dosage of 200 mg per day, it was less well tolerated than 800 mg per day of hydroxychloroquine. Elevations of SGOT were reported in four of 15 patients treated with 150 mg per day of amopyroquin.[102]

Although hydroxychloroquine and chloroquine are relatively safe, the list of reported side effects is extensive (Table 51–3). Toxicity may be somewhat arbitrarily divided into five major types (headings in Table 51–3). Gastrointestinal reactions are most frequent, followed by lesions of the skin and hair. Neuromuscular side effects comprise a variety of findings. Eye toxicity and a small number of miscellaneous reactions complete the groups.

The incidence of untoward effects varies widely, depending on daily dosage. In man, hydroxychloroquine has been found to be half as toxic as chloroquine on a weight basis.[15] Scherbel and colleagues noted reactions in 440 of 805 (55 percent) patients treated with daily doses of 250 to 500 mg of chloroquine or 400 to 600 mg of hydroxychloroquine. Sixty-seven percent were transient reactions and disappeared spontaneously. Another 26 percent responded to reductions in dosage. Only 7 percent of reactions precluded further treatment. Bagnall reported similar findings.[10] Analysis of toxicity reported in double-blind studies suggests that open studies overestimate the incidence of side effects. Freedman and Steinberg[105] reported side effects in 33 of 53 chloroquine-treated patients and similar problems in 22 of 54 placebo-treated patients during a 1-year period. Withdrawals were necessitated in five treated and four control patients. The placebo-controlled study conducted by the Cooperating Clinics Committee of the American Rheumatism Association[71] revealed more side effects in the patients treated with 800 mg of hydroxychloroquine daily. However, the placebo-treated patients showed a considerable frequency of reactions, which might have been attributed to hydroxychloroquine in an uncontrolled study. No patient in either group had reactions necessitating drug withdrawal. Hydroxychloroquine has been found to be less toxic than gold, penicillamine, or levamisole.[110]

Gastrointestinal side effects may mimic those of nonsteroidal anti-inflammatory drugs, with epigastric burn-

**Table 51–3.** Toxic Effects of Chloroquine and Hydroxychloroquine

- Gastrointestinal
  - Anorexia*[15]
  - Abdominal bloating[15]
  - Abdominal cramps[15]
  - Diarrhea[15]
  - Heartburn[15]
  - Nausea[15]
  - Vomiting[15]
  - Weight loss[15,20]
- Skin and Hair
  - Alopecia[15,33]
  - Bleaching of hair[15,25]
  - Dryness of skin[15]
  - Exacerbation of psoriasis[121,122]
  - Increased pigmentation of skin and hair[25]
  - Pruritus[15]
  - Rashes[15,120-122]
    - Exfoliative
    - Lichenoid
    - Maculopapular
    - Morbilliform
    - Urticarial
- Neuromuscular
  - Convulsive seizures[154]
  - Difficulty in visual accommodation[129]
  - Headache[15]
  - Insomnia[15]
  - Involuntary movements[155]
  - Lassitude[15]
  - Myasthenic reaction[25]
  - Mental confusion[15]
  - Nervousness or irritability[15]
  - Neuromyopathy[123,124]
  - Ototoxicity
    - Nerve deafness[15,156,157]
    - Tinnitus[15,156]
  - Polyneuropathy[33]
  - Toxic psychosis[158,159]
  - Vestibular dysfunction[15,158]
  - Weakness[30]
- Miscellaneous
  - Birth defects†[160]
  - Blood dyscrasias
    - Leukopenia[10,85]
    - Agranulocytosis[127,128]
    - Aplastic anemia[161]
    - Leukemia†[161]
  - Chromosome changes[162]
  - Death from overdosage[39,153]
    - Peripheral circulatory collapse
  - Heart
    - Electrocardiogram changes[120]
    - Cardiomyopathy[33,163]
  - Precipitation of porphyria[164]
- Ocular
  - Corneal deposits[11,131]
    - Halos around lights
  - Diplopia[130]
  - Defects in accommodation and convergence‡[129]
    - Various mild visual difficulties[25,30,120]
  - Loss of corneal reflex[145,165]
  - Retinopathy[18,137,141,143,147]
    - Loss of vision
    - Pigment abnormalities
    - Scotomata
    - Visual field abnormalities

*References for toxic effects are selected.
†Effect not conclusively related to medication.
‡May be a neuromuscular toxic effect.

ing, nausea, and vomiting. However, gastrointestinal blood loss is not caused by antimalarials. Nausea and anorexia may begin shortly after medication is started, and weight loss may be significant.[120] Abdominal cramps, bloating, and diarrhea[15,90] are more unique to antimalarials. Scherbel and associates[15] found significantly fewer gastrointestinal reactions with hydroxychloroquine (11 percent) than with chloroquine (19 percent).

Cutaneous lesions occur with equal frequency in patients receiving hydroxychloroquine or chloroquine.[15] Rashes may be lichenoid, urticarial, morbilliform, or maculopapular. Patients with psoriatic arthritis may experience an exacerbation of psoriatic skin lesions. Occasionally this has progressed to exfoliative dermatitis.[120,121] Kammer's group[116] did not observe any worsening of psoriasis or exfoliative lesions in 50 patients treated with 200 to 400 mg of hydroxychloroquine daily, although generalized erythematous, pruritic macular and papular eruptions occurred in four.

Reversible changes in the skin pigment have been noted in 10 to 25 percent of patients on long-term treatment, particularly when high daily dosages are taken.[25] Grayness or bleaching may appear at the roots of scalp hair, eyebrows, or eye lashes. Bluish-black oval macules occur on the shins, and the lesions may coalesce. Initially they have been mistaken for ecchymoses. Less commonly, alopecia develops[15,33] and must be differentiated from that which is a sign of the disease, lupus erythematosus, and not its treatment.

The more frequently noted neurologic manifestations are often of little significance because of their mildness and reversibility on lower daily doses.[10] These include frontal or unilateral headaches, giddiness, blurring of vision, insomnia, and nervousness.[10,30,120] A myasthenic syndrome has been reported by Dubois[25] to develop several weeks after beginning chloroquine and to disappear within days after discontinuing the drug. More important is a neuromuscular syndrome[123,124] that may be confused with corticosteroid-induced muscle weakness or attributed to the disease treated. Weakness starts in the proximal lower extremity but may be delayed a year or more after starting medication. It progresses slowly and may involve the arms. Complete reversibility is noted after discontinuing the antimalarials. A neurogenic component is suggested by decreased deep tendon reflexes and some of the electromyographic changes.[123] Muscle biopsy reveals vacuolar changes, but serum enzyme levels are not elevated.[124] This same histologic lesion may be present in patients with systemic lupus erythematosus who have not been treated with antimalarials.[125,126]

Among the miscellaneous side effects attributed to chloroquine or hydroxychloroquine is agranulocytosis or aplastic anemia.[127,128] This complication occurs very infrequently but has proved fatal.[128] Fatal overdosage has also been documented.[39]

Recent studies have provided a much better understanding of the occurrence of various ocular toxicities. Chloroquine and hydroxychloroquine may cause three main reactions. Two, defects in accommodation or convergence and corneal deposits, are relatively frequent, especially with higher doses. Symptoms are variable but not severe. They are completely reversible and, therefore, benign. The third, retinal toxicity, has great significance, since it may cause permanent loss of vision.

Blurred vision, difficulty changing focus quickly from a near to a far object, and poorly defined visual difficulties were frequent findings in the first systematic analysis of chloroquine administration to human volunteers reported shortly after World War II.[30,120] These symptoms were reversible within days of discontinuing the medication. It is likely that these problems are mediated by a direct effect on neural centers controlling convergence and accommodation, although a peripheral effect on ocular muscles has not been excluded.[129] Occasionally diplopia may result from extraocular muscle palsy.[130] Corneal deposits were described by Hobbs and Colnan[131] in 1958 and may be associated with halos around lights. Similar symptoms can be caused by glaucoma, and steroid-induced glaucoma must be differentiated.

Retinal lesions were not found with the lower doses of chloroquine used for the prophylaxis or treatment of malaria. In 1957, Cabiaggi[132] reported a patient with systemic lupus erythematosus treated with chloroquine and later hydroxychloroquine who developed atrophic retinal lesions surrounded by a pigmented border, tiny pigmented granules, constricted visual fields, and decreased visual acuity. Lesions of this patient and of two others[133] with severe fundal changes and visual field constriction were attributed to the disease rather than the treatment. Hobbs and associates[18] first attributed retinopathy to chloroquine treatment in 1959. Three patients developed abnormalities approximately three years after starting treatment. Symptoms consisted of misty vision and inability to see entire words when reading. Examination revealed decreased visual acuity, field defects, paracentral scotomata, and narrowed vessels. Fundus pigment was irregular and mottled or clumped in one patient, and an atrophic area was noted in another. After Hobbs' publication appeared, multiple cases of chloroquine retinopathy were reported.[130,134-145] Hydroxychloroquine may cause similar lesions,[146-148] although only a handful of patients with visual loss on this medication have been described.

Classic chloroquine retinopathy shows pigmentary mottling or clumping, progressing to a "bull's eye" lesion (Fig. 51–2). Visual acuity may be decreased and associated with central scotomata, peripheral field constriction, and later more dense field loss. Histologic examination shows loss of rods and cones and migration of clumps of pigment.[149] Speculation about the etiology of retinopathy centers upon the binding of 4-aminoquinolines to melanin of the retinal pigment epithelium, with subsequent loss of its putative protective function.[149]

Following the reports of retinal toxicity, investigations were undertaken to find more specific factors related to toxicity. A search for early predictors of retinal toxicity revealed that many ophthalmologic parameters became abnormal in patients taking antimalarials. Some,[141,142]

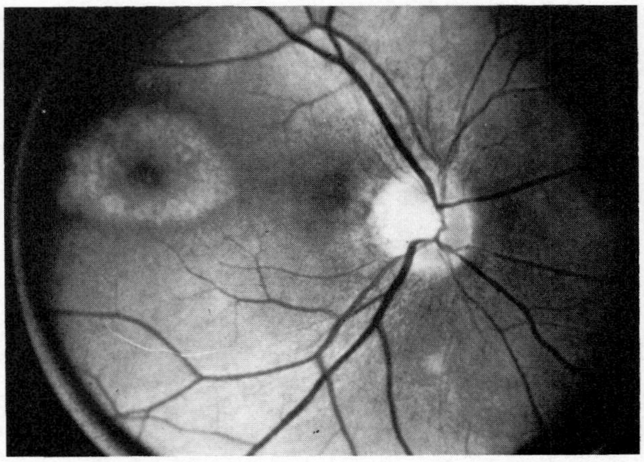

**Figure 51–2.** Bull's eye lesion: a classic, but not specific, lesion of chloroquine or hydroxychloroquine retinopathy. (Courtesy of Dr. R. Reinecke.)

such as the photostress test[142] or time to recover visual acuity after the macula is "dazzled" by a bright light, became abnormal in almost all patients unrelated to the visual loss and are, therefore, not predictive of visual loss. Others, such as loss of color vision or abnormal electrooculograms,[135] were not sensitive enough to be routinely employed as predictors of visual loss.[130,145,147]

It was noted, however, that retinal pigment abnormalities were almost invariably present in patients with visual loss. Mild changes, such as increased granularity or mottling, were believed to be an early indication of toxicity.[135,145] Percival and Meanock[130] found that visual field abnormalities to red test objects appeared in certain patients who did not have loss of vision detected by visual acuity changes, or scotomata, or field lesions to a white test object. Rynes and associates[147] prospectively studied 99 patients on long-term hydroxychloroquine treatment with daily doses of 400 mg to determine if visual loss could be prevented by regular ophthalmologic evaluation of retinal pigment changes and visual fields using a red test object. Although four patients[147,148] had either pigmentary changes, scotomata, or field constriction using a red test object, none had visual loss or field changes using a white test object.

The question of whether large *cumulative* dosage or high *daily* dosage contributes to retinal toxicity is extremely important because rheumatic diseases require long-term treatment. If cumulative dosage is a major factor, the medication should not be used for long-term treatment. Several lines of evidence suggest that it is daily dosage that determines toxicity.

First, visual loss almost always occurred in patients receiving daily doses greater than 400 mg of hydroxychloroquine or 250 mg of chloroquine.[135,138,143,150] Second, Mackenzie[151] has calculated the daily dose received by patients developing toxicity and compared this with the daily dose of those treated with cumulative doses greater than 1 kilogram. He found that all patients who developed toxicity took over 4 mg per kg per day of chloroquine or 6.5 mg per kg per day of hydroxychloroquine.

Furthermore, toxicity developed at relatively low cumulative doses, with means of 375 g for chloroquine and 525 g for hydroxychloroquine. Third, in the study by Tobin and associates[148] of patients who were followed for up to 7 years (mean of 57 months), toxicity was manifest within 3.5 years of starting the medication and did not increase as higher cumulative doses were achieved. Frisk-Holberg's group[33] related toxicity to serum drug levels, which should not change with increased cumulative doses once metabolic equilibrium is reached.

Because visual loss has been reported to progress[136,137] or even start[140] after treatment is discontinued, it was important to determine if early lesions are reversible. Retinal lesions may be divided into two groups. Those that have been termed "premaculopathy"[145] are generally reversible when the medication is discontinued. They include loss of foveal reflex, abnormal recovery times following "macular dazzle" with a bright light, mild pigmentary stippling, and visual field loss to a red test object. The other group, termed "true retinopathy," is much more serious. The characteristic ophthalmologic findings are severe pigmentary changes, especially a "bull's eye" lesion (Fig. 51–2), and visual field loss to a white test object. Loss of vision is almost always present, rarely improves, and may even progress after the medication is discontinued.

## GUIDELINES FOR USE OF ANTIMALARIALS

Antimalarial medications are now established as important drugs in the treatment of rheumatic diseases. The controversy over whether long-term use will result in retinal lesions with loss of vision has been resolved by the recognition that such toxicity is related to daily dose.[147,150,151] Recent studies have demonstrated that the two antimalarials currently used, hydroxychloroquine and chloroquine, are among the least toxic slow-acting antirheumatic medications.[109,110]

The absence of retinal toxicity is dependent upon strict adherence to the guidelines listed in Table 51–4; these are low daily dose and regular ophthalmologic monitoring. The maximum daily dose for hydroxychloroquine should be 400 mg and for chloroquine 250 mg. The ophthalmologic safety of these schedules has been established.[23,147] Mackenzie's[151] method of determining dose on the basis of the patient's lean body weight may provide an additional margin of safety. He recommends a maximum of 6.5 mg per kg per day for hydroxychloroquine and 4 mg per kg per day for chloroquine.

**Table 51–4.** Safety Guidelines for Antimalarial Drugs

| | |
|---|---|
| **Maximum Daily Dose** | |
| Hydroxyhloroquine | 400 mg |
| Chloroquine | 250 mg |
| **Ophthalmologic Monitoring** | |
| Frequency | |
| Baseline, then every 6 months | |
| Protocol | |
| Question patient about visual disturbance. | |
| Determine best-corrected visual acuity. | |
| Examine fundus for pigmentary abnormalities. | |
| Assess visual fields with a red test object; use white test object at baseline and if red test object fields are abnormal. | |

Ophthalmologic examinations should be conducted regularly and frequently in order to detect the mild changes that are reversible. It may be helpful to discuss the reasons for routine monitoring and the methods to be used with the ophthalmologist chosen to conduct eye examinations. Some ophthalmologists, not familiar with recent studies documenting antimalarial safety, still believe these medications should never be used. The examination protocol is not complicated, but visual field testing is tedious and often difficult to reproduce. It is important to use both a 5-mm red test object and a 3-mm white test object at baseline. The examination should look for field constriction as well as paracentral scotomata. Because testing with a red test object is more sensitive, the white test object need not be used in follow-up examinations if red test object fields remain unchanged. A 5-degree constriction compared with baseline fields should be considered abnormal.[147]

If funduscopic examination shows pigmentary changes or visual field examination demonstrates constriction or paracentral scotomata, the medication is discontinued. Even though this conservative ophthalmologic protocol may occasionally deny antimalarial treatment to some patients who have changes unrelated to medication, strict adherence has prevented loss of vision in all patients so monitored.[148]

Daily dosage also may be related to drug effectiveness as well as to toxicity,[11] and it is important to keep in mind that current dosage has been determined by toxicity studies rather than trials of efficacy. However, the lower dosages have been shown to be effective.[10,15,104]

Hydroxychloroquine sulfate, 200 mg twice a day, or chloroquine phosphate, 250 mg per day, may be used as the initial slow-acting antirheumatic drug in patients with rheumatoid arthritis who respond insufficiently to nonsteroidal anti-inflammatory medications.[110] Because their activity and toxicity differ substantially, the nonsteroidal anti-inflammatory drugs may be continued. Although antimalarials may be slightly less effective than gold salts, D-penicillamine or azothioprine, this difference has not been shown to be significant.[108] Furthermore, any difference in effectiveness is counterbalanced by decreased side effects with fewer drop-outs for toxicity.[110] Another advantage is the lower cost of monitoring toxicity. Although an ophthalmologic examination should be performed every 6 months, routine hematologic and urinary monitoring are not necessary. After the drug has been found to be well tolerated, the patient need not visit his physician more frequently than indicated by disease severity. If successful, treatment should be maintained until the patient is in complete remission. The dose of hydroxychloroquine may then be decreased to 200 mg once a day for 6 months before discontinuing the medication. Even with this protocol, some patients will have a relapse after discontinuing the drug. A treatment course should not be considered to have failed until tried for at least 6 months.

Antimalarials may be used with benefit in patients with other inflammatory arthritides, including psoriatic arthritis, peripheral joint disease of ankylosing spondylitis, and juvenile rheumatoid arthritis. Patients with psoriatic arthritis should be warned that their skin lesions may flare, and they should be monitored carefully for the first month on treatment. However, the potential exacerbation of skin lesions should not be considered a contraindication in such patients.[116] Dosage schedules in adults should be the same as for rheumatoid arthritis. Modification of dosage depending on the patient's weight is mandatory in treating children with juvenile rheumatoid arthritis. Laakenson and associates[152] believe the maximum safe dose of chloroquine diphosphate is 4 mg per kg per day and that of hydroxychloroquine sulfate is 7 mg per kg per day. It is important to remember that children are quite sensitive to chloroquine overdose. Death has resulted from ingestion of as little as 1 gram[153] (four tablets).

Antimalarials have an important role in the treatment of skin lesions in patients with lupus erythematosus and appear to be effective for articular disease and some systemic manifestations such as fever or malaise. There are several ways to use antimalarials in the treatment of lupus erythematosus. Hydroxychloroquine may be started in most patients when the diagnosis is established, using a dosage schedule similar to that for rheumatoid arthritis, and continued as long as the disease remains active. Alternatively, antimalarials may be used only in patients with those manifestations definitely shown to respond. Some physicians use intermittent rather than sustained courses of treatment.

Although much of the controversy surrounding antimalarial use has been resolved, additional studies documenting the effectiveness of low doses would be helpful. Studies elucidating the mechanism of antimalarial drug action would provide a more rational basis for therapy and might enable a more appropriate selection of patients to be treated.

## References


1. Rollo, I.M.: Drugs used in the chemotherapy of malaria. *In* Goodman, A.G., Goodman, L.S., and Gilman, A. (eds.): The Pharmacological Basis of Therapeutics. 6th ed. New York, MacMillan Publishing Co., 1980, pp. 1038–1060.
2. Payne, J.F.: A post-graduate lecture on lupus erythematosus. Clin. J. IV:223, 1894.
3. Cecchi, E., and Ferraris, F.: Desludging action of hydroxychloroquine in rheumatoid arthritis. Acta Rheum. Scand. 8:214, 1961.
4. Davidson, A.M., and Birt, A.R.: Quinine bisulfate as a desensitizing agent in treatment of lupus erythematosus. Arch. Dermatol. 37:247, 1938.
5. Martenstein, H.: Subactue lupus erythematosus and tubercular cervical adenopathy. Treatment with plasmochin. Z. Haut. Geschlectkrankheit. 27:248, 1928.
6. Prokoptchouk, A.J.: Treatment of lupus erythematosus with acriquine. Vestn. Vencrol. Dermatol. No. 2–3, 1940, p. 23.
7. Zakon, S.J., and Gershenson, J.: Introduction of quinacrine in treatment of lupus erythematosus. (Includes a translation of the paper by Prokoptchouk.) Arch. Dermatol. Syph. 71:520, 1955.
8. Page, F.: Treatment of lupus erythematosus with mepacrine. Lancet 2:755, 1951.
9. Freedman, A., and Bach, F.: Mepacrine and rheumatoid arthritis. Lancet 2:231, 1952.
10. Bagnall, A.W.: The value of chloroquine in rheumatoid disease—a four year study of continuous therapy. Can. Med. Assoc. J. 77:182, 1957.
11. Kersley, G.D., and Palin, A.G.: Amodiaquine and hydroxychloroquine in rheumatoid arthritis. Lancet 2:886, 1959.
12. Coatney, G.R.: Pitfalls in a discovery: The chronicle of chloroquine. Am. J. Trop. Med. Hyg. 12:121, 1963.
13. Mullins, J.F., Watts, F.L., and Wilson, C.J.: Plaquenil in the treatment of lupus erythematosus. JAMA 161:879, 1956.
14. Lewis, H.M., and Frumess, G.M.: Plaquenil in the treatment of discoid lupus erythematosus. AMA Arch. Dermatol. 73:576, 1956.
15. Scherbel, A.L., Harrison, J.W., and Atdjian, M.: Further observations on the use of 4-aminoquinoline compounds in patients with rheumatoid arthritis or related diseases. Cleveland Clin. Quart. 25:95, 1958.
16. Cohen, A.S., and Calkins, E.: A controlled study of chloroquine as an antirheumatic agent. Arthritis Rheum. 1:297, 1958.
17. Hamilton, E.B.D., and Scott, J.T.: Hydroxychloroquine sulfate (Plaquenil) in treatment of rheumatoid arthritis. Arthritis Rheum. 5:502, 1962.
18. Hobbs, H.E., Sorsby, A., and Freedman, A.: Retinopathy following chloroquine therapy. Lancet 2:478, 1959.
19. Rothermich, N.O.: Editorial. Coming catastrophes with chloroquine? Ann. Intern. Med. 61:1203, 1964.
20. Editorial. Chloroquine retinopathy. JAMA 184:775, 1963.
21. Editorial. Ocular complications of treatment with chloroquine and related antimalarial drugs. Can. Med. Assoc. J. 88:530, 1963.
22. Editorial. Retinal damage from drugs. Br. Med. J. Vol. 1:929, 1962.
23. Marks, J.S.: Is chloroquine obsolete in treatment of rheumatic diseases? Lancet 1:371, 1979.
24. Swinson, D.R., Losnick, J., and Jackson, L.: Double-blind trial of dapsone against placebo in the treatment of rheumatoid arthritis. Ann. Rheum. Dis. 40:235, 1981.
25. Dubois, E.: Antimalarials in the management of discoid and systemic lupus erythematosus. Sem. Arthritis Rheum. 8:33, 1978.
26. Taggert, J.V., Earl, D.P., Berliner, R.W., Zubrod, C.G., Welch, W.J., Wise, N.B., Schroeder, E.F., London, I.M., and Shannon, J.A.: Studies on the chemotherapy of the human malarials. III. The physiological disposition and antimalarial activity of the cinchona alkaloids. J. Clin. Invest. (Suppl.) 27:80, 1948.
27. Rollo, I.M.: Miscellaneous drugs used in the treatment of protozoal infections. *In* Goodman, A.G., Goodman, L.S., and Gilman, A. (eds.): The Pharmacological Basis of Therapeutics. 6th ed. New York, MacMillan Publishing Co., 1980, pp. 1078–1079.
28. DiPalma, J.R. (ed.): Drill's Pharmacology in Medicine. 4th ed. New York, McGraw-Hill Book Company, 1971, pp. 1779.
29. McChesney, E.W., Conway, W.D., Banks, W.F., Jr., Rogers, J.E., and Shekosky, J.M.: Studies on the metabolism of some compounds of the 4-amino-7-chloroquinoline series. J. Pharmcol. Exp. Ther. 151:482, 1966.
30. Berliner, R.W., Earle, D.P., Jr., Taggert, J.V., ZuBrod, C.G., Welch, W.J., Conan, N.J., Bauman, E., Scuddar, S.T., and Shannon, J.A.: Studies on the chemotherapy of human malarias. VI. The Physiological deposition, antimalarial activity and toxicity of several derivatives of 4-aminoquinolines. J. Clin. Invest. 27(Suppl.):98, 1948.
31. Zvaifler, N.J., and Rubin, M.: The metabolism of chloroquine (abstract). Arthritis Rheum. 5:330, 1962.
32. McChesney, E.W., Fasco, M.J., and Banks, W.F., Jr.: The metabolism of chloroquine in man during and after repeated oral dosage. J. Pharmacol. Exp. Ther. 158:323, 1967.
33. Frisk-Holmberg, M., Bergkvist, Y., Domeij-Nyberg, B., Hellstrom, L., and Jansson, F.: Chloroquine serum concentration and side effects: Evidence for dose-dependent kinetics. Clin. Pharmcol. Ther. 25:345, 1979.
34. McChesney, E.W., and Rothfield, N.F.: Comparative metabolic studies of chloroquine and hydroxychloroquine (abstract). Arthritis Rheum. 7:328, 1964.
35. McChesney, E.W., Banks, W.F., Jr., and McAuliff, J.P.: Laboratory studies of the 4-aminoquinoline antimalarials. II. Plasma levels of chloroquine and hydroxychloroquine after various oral dosage regimens. Antibiot. Chemother. 12:583, 1962.
36. Rubin, M., Bernstein, H.N., and Zvaifler, N.J.: Studies on the pharmacology of chloroquine. Arch. Ophthalmol. 70:474, 1962.
37. Rubin, M.: The antimalarials and tranquilizers. Dis. Nerv. Syst. (Suppl.) 29:67, 1968.
38. McChesney, E.W., Banks, W.F., Jr., and Fabian, R.J.: Tissue distribution of chloroquine, hydroxychloroquine and desethylchloroquine in the rat. Toxicol. Appl. Pharmacol. 10:501, 1967.
39. Kiel, F.W.: Chloroquine suicide. JAMA 190:398, 1964.
40. Prouty, R.W., and Kuroda, K.: Spectrophotometric determination and distribution of chloroquine in human tissues. J. Lab. Clin. Med. 52:477, 1958.
41. Bernstein, H., Zvaifler, N., Rubin, M., and Mansour, A.M.: The ocular deposition of chloroquine. Invest. Ophthal. 2:384, 1963.

42. Varga, F.: Intracellular localization of chloroquine in the liver and kidney of the rat. Acat. Physiol. Acad. Sci. Hung. 34:327, 1968.
43. Matsuzawa, Y., and Hostetler, K.Y.: Studies on drug-induced lipidosis: Subcellular localization of phospholipid and cholesterol in the liver of rats treated with chloroquine or 4,4′-bis(diethylaminoethoxy) $\alpha,\beta$-diethyldiphenylethane. J. Lipid Res. 21:202, 1980.
44. Gerber, D.H.: Effect of chloroquine on the sulfhydryl group and the denaturation of bovine serum albumin. Arthritis Rheum. 7:193, 1964.
45. Noelle, R.J., and Lawrence, D.A.: Modulation of T-cell function. II. Chemical basis for the involvement of cell surface thiol-reactive sites in control of T-cell proliferation. Immunology 60:453, 1981.
46. Sams, W.M.: Chloroquine: Mechanism of action. Mayo Clin. Proc. 42:300, 1967.
47. Matsuzawa, Y., and Hostetler, K.Y.: Inhibition of lysosomal phospholipase A and phospholipase C by chloroquine and 4,4′-bis-(diethylaminoethyoxy) $\alpha,\beta$-diethyldiphenylethane. J. Biol. Chem. 255:5190, 1980.
48. Whitehouse, M.W., and Cowey, F.K.: Inhibition of connective tissue by proteases by antimalarial, antirheumatic drugs. Biochem. J. 98:118, 1966.
49. Whitehead, R.W., and Hager, J.P.: The anti-inflammatory and antihyaluronidase effect of chloroquine diphosphate. J. Pharmacol. Exp. Ther. 110:52, 1954.
50. Cohen, S.N., and Yielding, K.L.: Spectrophotometric studies of the interaction of chloroquine and deoxyribonucleic acid. J. Biol. Chem. 240:3123, 1965.
51. Kurnick, N.B., and Radcliffe, I.E.: Reactions between DNA and quinacrine and other antimalarials. J. Lab. Clin. Med. 60:669, 1962.
52. Cohen, S.N., and Yielding, K.L.: Inhibition of DNA and RNA polymerase reactions by chloroquine. Proc. Nat. Acad. Sci. USA 54:521, 1965.
53. Ciak, J., and Hahn, F.E.: Chloroquine: Mode of action. Science 151:347, 1966.
54. Stoller, D., and Levine, L.: Antibodies to denatured DNA in lupus erythematosus serum. V. Mechanism of DNA-anti-DNA inhibition by chloroquine. Arch. Biochem. 101:335, 1963.
55. Dubois, E.L.: Effect of quinacrine (Atabrine) upon lupus erythematosus phenomenon. Arch. Dermatol. 71:570, 1955.
56. Weissman, G.: Labilization and stabilization of lysosomes. Fed. Proc. 23:1038, 1964.
57. Greaves, M.W., and McDonald-Gibson, W.: Effect of non-steroidal anti-inflammatory drugs and antipyretic drugs on prostaglandin biosynthesis by human skin. J. Invest. Dermatol. 61:127, 1973.
58. Ward, P.A.: The chemosuppression of chemotaxis. J. Exp. Med. 24:209, 1966.
59. Clarke, A.K., Vernon-Roberts, B., and Aurey, H.L.F.: Assessment of anti-inflammatory drugs in the rat using subcutaneous implants of polyurethane foam impregnated with dead tubercle bacilli. Ann. Rheum. Dis. 34:326, 1975.
60. Greiling, H., and Dother, G.: Biochemical studies on the mechanism of action of resorcin. Z. Rheumaforsch. 21:316, 1962.
61. Desphande, V.R., Sharma, M.L., and Dashputra, P.G.: Antihistaminic action of antimalarials. Indian J. Physiol. Pharmacol. 7:259, 1963.
62. Thompson, G.R., and Bartholomew, L.E.: The effect of chloroquine on antibody formation. Univ. Mich. Med. Cent. J. 30:227, 1964.
63. Kalmonson, G.M., and Gage, I.G.: Effects of hydroxychloroquine on immune mechanisms. Clin. Res. 11:106, 1963.
64. Hurvitz, D., and Hirschhorn, K.: Suppression of "in vitro" lymphocyte responses by chloroquine. N. Engl. J. Med. 273:23, 1965.
65. Panayi, G.S., Neill, W.A., Duthie, J.J.R., and McCormick, J.N.: Action of chloroquine phosphate in rheumatoid arthritis. I. Immunosuppressive effect. Ann. Rheum. Dis. 32:316, 1973.
66. Salmeron, G., and Lipsky, P.E.: Immunosuppressive activity of chloroquine: Inhibition of human monocyte function. Arthritis Rheum. 25:S132, 1982.
66a. Salmeron, G., and Lipsky, P.E.: Immunosuppressive potential of antimalarials. (Suppl.). Am. J. Med. 18:19, 1983.
67. Szilagyi, T., and Kavai, M.: The effect of chloroquine on the antigen-antibody reaction. Acta Physiol. Acad. Sci. Hung. 38:411, 1970.
68. Holtz, G., Mantel, W., and Buck, W.: The inhibition of antigen-antibody reactions by chloroquine and its mechanism of action. Z. Immunitaetsforsch. 146:145, 1973.
69. Popert, A.J., Meijers, K.A.E., Sharp, J., and Bier, F.: Chloroquine diphosphate in rheumatoid arthritis. A controlled study. Ann. Rheum. Dis. 20:18, 1961.
70. Klinefelter, H.F., and Achurra, A.: Effect of gold salts and antimalarials on the rheumatoid factor in rheumatoid arthritis. Scand. J. Rheumatol. 2:177, 1973.
71. Mainland, D., and Sutcliffe, M.I.: Hydroxychloroquine sulfate in rheumatoid arthritis, a six month, double-blind trial. Bull. Rheum. Dis. 13:287, 1962.
72. McChesney, E.W., Nachod, F.C., and Tainter, M.L.: Rationale for treatment of lupus erythematosus with antimalarials. J. Invest. Dermatol. 29:97, 1957.
73. Lester, R.S., Burnham, T.K., Fine, G., and Murray K.: Immunologic concepts of light reactions in lupus erythematosus and polymorphous light eruptions. Arch. Dermatol. 96:1, 1967.
74. Cahn, M.M., Levy, E.J., and Shaffer, B.: Polymorphous light eruption: Effect of chloroquine phosphate in modifying reactions to ultraviolet light. J. Invest. Dermatol. 26:201, 1956.
75. Shaffer, B., Cahn, M.M., and Levy, E.J.: Absorption of antimalarial drugs in human skin: Spectroscopic and chemical analysis in epidermis and corium. J. Invest. Dermatol. 30:341, 1958.
76. Bartholomew, L.E., and Bartholomew, F.N.: Antigenic bacterial polysaccharide in rheumatoid synovial effusions. Arthritis Rheum. 22:969, 1979.
77. Watson, D.E.: Chloroquine protection against virus induced cell damage without inhibition of virus growth. J. Gen. Virol. 14:100, 1972.
78. Pazmino, N.H., Yuhas, J.M., and Tennant, R.W.: Inhibition of murine RNA tumor virus replication and oncogenesis by chloroquine. Int. J. Cancer 14:379, 1974.
79. Depper, J.M., and Zvaifler, N.J.: Epstein-Barr virus. Its relationship to the pathogenesis of rheumatoid arthritis. Arthritis Rheum. 24:755, 1981.
80. Karmali, R.A., Horrobin, D.F., Menezes, J., Patel, P., and Musto, J.: Chloroquine enchances Epstein-Barr virus expression. Nature 275:4444, 1978.
81. Dubois, E.L.: Systemic lupus erythematosus: Recent advances in its diagnosis and treatment. Ann. Intern. Med. 45:163, 1956.
82. Ropes, M.W.: Observations on the natural course of disseminated lupus erythematosus. Medicine 43:387, 1964.
83. O'Leary, P.A., Brunsting, L.A., and Kierland, R.R.: Quinacrine (Atabrine) hydrochloride in treatment of discoid lupus erythematosus. Arch. Dermatol. Syph. 67:633, 1953.
84. Kierland, R.R., Brunsting, L.A., and O'Leary, P.A.: Quinacrine hydrochloride in the treatment of lupus erythematosus. Mayo Clin. Proc. 28:22, 1953.
85. Winkelman, R.K., Merwin, C.F., and Brunsting, L.A.: Antimalarial therapy of lupus erythematosus. Ann. Intern. Med. 55:772, 1961.
86. Christiansen, J.V., and Nielsen, J.P.: Treatment of lupus erythematosus with mepacrine. Br. J. Dermatol. 68:73, 1956.
87. Buchanan, R.N.: Quinacrine in the treatment of discoid lupus erythematosus: A five-year follow-up survey-results and evaluation. South. Med. J. 52:978, 1959.
88. Pappenfort, R.B., and Lockwood, J.H.: Amodiaquine (Camoquin) in the treatment of chronic discoid lupus erythematosus. AMA Arch. Dermatol. 74:384, 1956.
89. Leeper, R.W., and Allende, M.F.: Antimalarials in the treatment of discoid lupus erythematosus. AMA Arch. Dermatol. 73:50, 1956.
90. Goldman, L., Cole, D.P., and Preston, R.H.: Chloroquine diphosphate in the treatment of discoid lupus erythematosus. JAMA 152:1428, 1953.
91. Rogers, J., and Finn, O.A.: Synthetic antimalarial drugs in chronic discoid lupus erythematosus and light eruptions. Arch. Dermatol. Syph. 70:61, 1954.
92. Crissey, J.T., and Murray, P.F.: A comparison of chloroquine and gold in the treatment of lupus erythematosus. Arch. Dermatol. 74:69, 1956.
93. Kraak, J.H., van Ketel, W.G., Prakken, J.R., and van Zwet, W.R.: The value of hydroxychloroquine (Plaquenil) for the treatment of chronic discoid lupus erythematosus: A double-blind trial. Dermatologica 130:293, 1965.
94. Dubois, E.L.: Quinacrine (Atabrine) in treatment of systemic and discoid lupus erythematosus. Arch. Intern. Med. 94:131, 1954.
95. Rudnicki, R.D., Gresham, G.E., and Rothfield, N.F.: The efficacy of antimalarials in systemic lupus erythematosus. J. Rheumatol. 2:323, 1975.
96. Ziff, M., Esserman, P., and McEwen, C.: Observations on the course and treatment of systemic lupus erythematosus. Arthritis Rheum. 1:332, 1956.
97. Lanham, J.G., and Hughes, G.R.V.: Antimalarial therapy in SLE. Clin. Rheum. Dis. 8:279, 1982.
98. Conte, J.J., Mignon-Conte, M.A., and Fournie, G.J.: Lupus nephritis: Treatment with indomethacin-hydroxychloroquine combination and comparison with corticosteroid treatment. Nouv. Presse Med. 4:91, 1975.
99. Steck, I.E., Zivin, S., Joseph, N., and Montgomery, M.M.: Influence of primaquine on the clinical findings and joint potentials in rheumatoid arthritis (abstract). Ann. Rheum. Dis. 11:310, 1952.
100. Bepler, C.R., Baier, H.N., McCracken, S., Rentschler, C.L., Rogers, F.B., and Lansbury, J.: A 15 month controlled study of the effects of amodiaquin (Camoquin) in rheumatoid arthritis. Arthritis Rheum. 2:403, 1959.
101. Pomeroy, H., Warren, C., Mills, D., and Clark, G.M.: The effect of amodiaquin (Camoquin) on the course of rheumatoid arthritis. Arthritis Rheum. 2:396, 1959.

102. Bartholomew, L.E., and Duff, I.F.: Amopyroquin (Propoquin) in rheumatoid arthritis. Arthritis Rheum. 6:356, 1963.
103. Haydu, G.G.: Rheumatoid arthritis therapy: Rationale and use of chloroquine diphosphate. Am. J. Med. Sci. 225:71, 1953.
104. Adams, E.M., Yocum, D.E., and Bell, C.L.: Hydroxychloroquine in the treatment of rheumatoid arthritis. Am. J. Med. 75:321, 1983.
105. Freedman, A.: Chloroquine and rheumatoid arthritis. Short-term controlled trial. Ann. Rheum. Dis. 15:251, 1956.
106. Rinehart, R.E., Rosenbaum, E.E., and Hopkins, C.E.: Chloroquine therapy in rheumatoid arthritis. Northwest Med. 56:703, 1957.
107. Freedman, A., and Steinberg, V.L.: Chloroquine in rheumatoid arthritis, a double blindfold trial of treatment for one year. Ann. Rheum. Dis. 19:243, 1960.
108. Dwosh, I.L., Stein, H.B., Urowitz, M.B., Smythe, H.A., Hunter, T., and Ogryzlo, M.A.: Azathioprine in early rheumatoid arthritis: Comparison with gold and chloroquine. Arthritis Rheum. 20:685, 1977.
109. Richter, J.A., Runge, L.A., Pinals, R.S., and Oates, R.P.: Analysis of treatment terminations with gold and antimalarial compounds in rheumatoid arthritis. J. Rheum. 7:153, 1980.
110. Husain, Z., and Runge, L.A.: Treatment complications of rheumatoid arthritis with gold, hydroxychloroquine, D-penicillamine and levamisole. J. Rheum. 7:825, 1980.
111. Scull, E.: Chloroquine and hydroxychloroquine therapy of rheumatoid arthritis. Arthritis Rheum. 5:30, 1962.
112. Sievers, K., and Hurri, L.: Combined therapy of rheumatoid arthritis with gold and chloroquine. 1. Evaluation of therapeutic effect. Acta Rheum. Scand. 9:48, 1963.
113. Sievers, K., Hurri, L., and Sievers, U.M.: Combined therapy of rheumatoid arthritis with gold and chloroquine. II. Evaluation of side effects. Acta Rheum. Scand. 9:56, 1963.
114. Bunch, T.W., O'Duffy, J.D., Tompkins, R.B., and O'Fallon, W.M.: Controlled study of hydroxychloroquine and penicillamine singly and in combination in the treatment of rheumatoid arthritis (abstract). Arthritis Rheum. 23:659, 1980.
115. Scherbel, A.L.: Long-term maintenance therapy with 4-amino-quinoline compounds in rheumatoid arthritis. *In* Mills, L.C., and Moyer, J.H. (eds.): Inflammation and Diseases of Connective Tissue. Philadelphia, W. B. Saunders Company, 1961, p. 555.
116. Kammer, G.M., Soter, N.A., Gibson, D.J., Schur, P.H.: Psoriatic arthritis: A clinical, immunologic and HLA study of 100 patients. Sem. Arthritis Rheum. 9:75, 1979.
117. Fink, C.W.: Treatment of juvenile arthritis. Bull. Rheum. Dis. 32:21, 1982.
118. Dubois, E.L.: Lupus Erythematosus. 2nd ed. Los Angeles, University of Southern California Press, 1974, pp. 548–554.
119. Beutler, E.: The hemolytic effect of primaquine and related compounds. A review. Blood 14:102, 1959.
120. Alving, A.S., Eichelberger, C.B., Jr., Jones, J.R., Wharton, C.M., and Pullman, T.N.: Studies on the chronic toxicity of chloroquine (SN-7618). J. Clin. Invest. (Suppl.) 27:60, 1948.
121. Cornbleet, T.: Action of synthetic antimalarial drugs on psoriasis. J. Invest. Dermatol. 26:435, 1956.
122. Reed, W.B.: Psoriatic arthritis. A complete study of 86 patients. Acta Dermatol. Venereol. 41:396, 1961.
123. Whisnant, J.P., Espinosa, R.E., Kierland, R.R., and Lambert, E.H.: Chloroquine neuropathy. Proc. Mayo Clin. 38:501, 1963.
124. Hicklin, J.A.: Chloroquine neuromyopathy. Ann. Phys. Med. 9:189, 1968.
125. Pearson, C.M., and Yamazaki, J.N.: Vacuolar myopathy in systemic lupus erythematosus. Am. J. Clin. Pathol. 29:455, 1958.
126. Sibrans, D.F., and Holley, H.L.: Vacuolar myopathy in a patient with positive LE cell populations. Arthritis Rheum. 10:141, 1967.
127. Polano, M.K., Cats, A., and van Older, G.A.J.: Agranulocytosis following treatment with hydroxychloroquine sulphate. Lancet 1:1275, 1965.
128. Propp, R.P., and Stillman, J.S.: Correspondence: Report of a non-fatal case of agranulocytosis on hydroxychloroquine therapy. N. Engl. J. Med. 277:492, 1967.
129. Rubin, M.L., and Thomas, W.C., Jr.: Diplopia and loss of accommodation due to chloroquine. Arthritis Rheum. 13:75, 1970.
130. Percival, S.P.B., and Meanock, I.: Chloroquine: Ophthalmological safety and clinical assessment in rheumatoid arthritis. Br. Med. J. 3:579, 1968.
131. Hobbs, H.E., and Calnan, C.D.: The ocular complications of chloroquine therapy. Lancet I:1207, 1958.
132. Cambiaggi, A.: Unusual ocular lesions in a case of systemic lupus erythematosus. Arch. Ophthalmol. 57:451, 1957.
133. Goldman, L., and Preston, R.H.: Reactions to chloroquine observed during treatment of various dermatologic disorders. Am. J. Trop. Med. Hyg. 6:654, 1957.
134. Voipio, H.: Incidence of chloroquine retinopathy. Acta Ophthalmol. 44:349, 1966.
135. Arden, G.B., and Kolb, H.: Antimalarial therapy and early retinal changes in patients with rheumatoid arthritis. Br. Med. J. 1:270, 966.
136. Nylander, U.: Ocular damage in chloroquine therapy. Acta Ophthalmol. 44:335, 1966.
137. Okun, G., Gouras, P., Bernstein, H., and VonSallmann, L.: Chloroquine retinopathy. Arch. Ophthalmol. 69:59, 1963.
138. Nozik, R.A., Weinstock, F.J., and Vignos, P.J.: Ocular complications of chloroquine. Ann. J. Ophthalmol. 58:774, 1964.
139. Crews, S.J.: Chloroquine retinopathy with recovery in early stages. Lancet 2:436, 1964.
140. Burns, R.P.: Delayed onset of chloroquine retinopathy. N. Engl. J. Med. 275:693, 1966.
141. Carr, R.E., Henkind, P., Rothfield, N., and Siegel I.M.: Ocular toxicity of antimalarial drugs: Long-term follow-up. Am. J. Ophthalmol. 66:738, 1968.
142. Carr, R.E., Gouras, P., and Gunkel, O.D.: Chloroquine retinopathy. Arch. Ophthalmol. 75:171, 1966.
143. Shearer, R.V., and Dubois, E.L.: Ocular changes induced by long-term hydroxychloroquine (plaquenil) therapy. Am. J. Ophthalmol. 64:245, 1967.
144. Henkind, P., Carr, R.E., and Siegel, I.: Early chloroquine retinopathy: Clinical and functional findings. Arch. Ophthalmol. 71:157, 1964.
145. Percival, S.P.B., and Behrman, J.: Ophthalmological safety of chloroquine. Br. J. Ophthalmol. 53:101, 1969.
146. Shearer, R.V., and Dubois, E.L.: Ocular changes induced by long-term hydroxychloroquine (plaquenil) therapy. Am. J. Ophthalmol. 64:245, 1967.
147. Rynes, R.I., Krohel, G., Falbo, A., Reinecke, R.D., Wolfe, B., and Bartholomew, L.E.: Ophthalmologic safety of long-term hydroxychloroquine treatment. Arthritis Rheum. 22:832, 1979.
148. Tobin, D.R., Krohel, G.B., and Rynes, R.I.: Hydroxychloroquine. A seven-year experience. Arch. Ophthalmol. 100:81, 1982.
149. Bernstein, H.N., and Ginsberg, J.: The pathology of chloroquine retinopathy. Arch. Ophthalmol. 71:238, 1964.
150. Scherbel, A.L., Mackenzie, A.H., Nousek, J.E., and Atdjian, M.: Ocular lesions in rheumatoid arthritis and related disorders with particular reference to retinopathy. A study of 741 patients treated with and without chloroquine drugs. N. Engl. J. Med. 273:360, 1965.
151. Mackenzie, A.H.: Ocular safety of huge cumulative antimalarial dosage (abstract). Arthritis Rheum. 24:70, 1981.
152. Laaksonen, A.L., Koskiahde, V., and Juva, K.: Dosage of antimalarial drugs for children with juvenile rheumatoid arthritis and systemic lupus erythematosus. Scand. J. Rheumatol. 3:103, 1974.
153. Cann, H.M., and Verhulst, H.L.: Fatal acute chloroquine poisoning in children. Pediatrics 27:95, 1961.
154. Torrey, E.F.: Chloroquine seizures. JAMA 204:867, 1968.
155. Umez-Eronimi, E.M., and Eronimi, E.A.: Chloroquine-induced involuntary movements. Br. Med. J. 1:945, 1977.
156. Dewar, W.A., and Mann, H.M.: Chloroquine in lupus erythematosus (letter). Lancet 1:780, 1954.
157. Mukherjee, D.K.: Chloroquine ototoxicity—a reversible phenomenon? J. Laryngol. Otol. 93:809, 1979.
158. Burrell, Z.L., and Marinez, A.C.: Chloroquine and hydroxychloroquine in the treatment of arrhythmias. N. Engl. J. Med. 258:798, 1958.
159. Rab, S.M.: Two cases of chloroquine psychoses. Br. Med. J. 1:1275, 1963.
160. Hart, C.W., and Naunton, R.F.: The ototoxicity of chloroquine phosphate. Arch. Otolaryngol. 80:407, 1964.
161. Nagaratnam, N., Chetiyawardana, A.N., and Rajiyah, S.: Aplasia and leukemia following chloroquine therapy. Postgrad. Med. J. 54:108, 1978.
162. Neill, W.A., Panayi, G.S., Duthie, J.J.R., and Prescott, R.J.: Action of chloroquine phosphate in rheumatoid arthritis. II. Chromosome-damaging effect. Ann. Rheum. Dis. 32:547, 1973.
163. Magnussen, I., and deFine Olivamus, B.: Cardiomyopathy after chloroquine treatment. Acta Med. Scand. 202:429, 1977.
164. Baler, C.R.: Porphyria precipitated by hydroxychloroquine treatment of systemic lupus erythematosus. Cutis 17:96, 1976.
165. Henkind, P., and Rothfield, N.F.: Ocular abnormalities in patients treated with synthetic antimalarial drugs. N. Engl. J. Med. 269:433, 1963.

# Chapter 52
# Gold Compounds

*Norman L. Gottlieb*

## HISTORY OF GOLD TREATMENT

Gold has been advocated for the treatment of numerous diseases of man, animals, and plants since the eighth century. A combination of gold and mercury was called an elixir of life by Paracelsus in the early sixteenth century.[1] It was not until 1890, when Koch[2] reported the in vitro inhibition of tubercle bacilli by gold cyanide, that gold compounds were used for specific medical disorders. A mixture of gold and magnesium was used to treat tuberculosis in 1894; gold salts alone were recommended for the treatment of lupus vulgaris in 1913 and pulmonary tuberculosis in 1924.[3]

The beneficial effects of aurothioglucose (Solganal) in patients with bacterial endocarditis, rheumatic fever, and other poorly defined disorders, based on the hypothesis that gold had nonspecific antiseptic effects, was reported by Landé in 1927.[4] Shortly after their introduction, gold compounds were used for luetic infection, ankylosing spondylitis (especially with prominent peripheral joint involvement), and degenerative and gonococcal arthritis with less impressive results.[5] Chrysotherapy is not presently recommended for these conditions.

Believing that tuberculosis and rheumatoid arthritis (RA) had a common (infectious) etiology, Forestier[6] applied gold–thiopropanol sodium sulfanate (Allochrysine) for the treatment of RA. His favorable experience with more than 550 cases, in which improvement was noted in 70 to 80 percent, was published in 1935. Subsequently, numerous authors have confirmed these observations, including Hartfall and associates,[7] who noted "apparent cure or striking improvement" in 80 percent of 900 RA cases. Two double-blind studies, reported in 1945[8] and in the early 1960s,[9,10] reaffirmed the value of parenteral gold in RA. More recent work has documented the efficacy of gold compounds in reducing joint pain and inflammation, and maintaining articular function;[11,12] one long-term blinded study found that gold altered the natural history of RA by protecting articular cartilage and subchondral bone.[12]

In addition to RA, gold treatment is advocated for selected cases of juvenile rheumatoid arthritis (JRA) and psoriatic arthritis affecting the peripheral joints. Exceptionally, it is prescribed for severe palindromic rheumatism, an infrequent arthropathy.[13] In addition, gold currently is offered as a therapeutic alternative for certain nonrheumatic disorders such as pemphigus,[14] a serious bullous skin disorder, and is used in the Far East for bronchial asthma.[15]

An orally administered gold compound, auranofin (Ridaura), is the first slow-acting antirheumatic drug developed specifically for RA.[16]

## INDICATIONS AND PATIENT SELECTION

Gold treatment is used primarily for progressively severe polyarticular RA that is not controlled by measures such as rest, physical therapy, nonsteroidal anti-inflammatory agents, mild to moderately potent analgesics, and occasional intra-articular injections of microcrystalline corticosteroids. Most rheumatologists practicing in the United States advocate an initial trial of chrysotherapy in preference to other disease-modifying drugs. Whether or not the risk-to-benefit ratio warrants the use of chrysotherapy in early or mild RA, to prevent or delay irreversible joint damage, is unresolved. Some studies have shown that gold therapy is most effective in early, nonerosive RA,[17,18] whereas others have demonstrated its value in active disease of long duration despite the presence of joint deformity and destruction.[7,19] Gold is not indicated for advanced RA without evidence of active synovitis, and is generally not advised for mono- or pauciarticular arthritis.[17]

Factors that do not significantly influence the response to chrysotherapy include patient age, sex, and race, magnitude of serum immunoglobulin and erythrocyte sedimentation rate (ESR) elevation, presence or absence of serum rheumatoid factor (RF),[11,13,20] or subcutaneous nodules (personal experience). In one recent report gold-treated ANA-negative RA patients improved more than ANA-positive subjects (but the opposite was true for levamisole).[21] Although not conclusively tested, therapeutic benefit does not seem related to histocompatibility antigens on the A, B, and D loci.[22] Concomitant systemic medications, other than chelating agents, which enhance gold excretion, also do not alter the efficacy of gold. Systemic corticosteroids and gold compounds may be administered concurrently. When chrysotherapy is initiated in corticosteroid-treated RA patients, steroids may be tapered gradually after several months of uninterrupted gold treatment, if clinical improvement is evident.

Gold compounds may be employed in RA patients with Felty's or Sjögren's syndrome or in RA accompanied by pre-existing neutropenia or eosinophilia.[23-28] Available evidence suggests the drug is efficacious in these circumstances, and the prevalence, type, and severity of toxicity are not greater than anticipated. Importantly, neutropenia and splenomegaly that has been documented by clinical examinations and liver-spleen scan, have improved during chrysotherapy.[23,24] Despite earlier admonitions against gold in RA-associated Sjögren's syndrome, recent studies indicate it is generally well tolerated.[25] Similarly, nonprogressive proteinuria unaccompanied by renal insufficiency, or the presence of a single normally functioning kidney does not interdict gold treatment.[13,29]

## EFFICACY

The favorable influence of chrysotherapy on RA has been documented in numerous studies and in several double-blind controlled trials in which gold was compared with placebo. (Table 52–1).[8,10-12,18,30-38] More recently, gold compounds have been compared with other potent antirheumatic agents, including penicillamine, cyclophosphamide, azathioprine, and antimalarials.[39-41]

The first double-blind study involved 110 RA patients treated with 100 mg weekly of gold sodium thiomalate (Myochrysine) or with an inactive control substance.[8] Sixty-three percent of gold-treated patients but only 21 percent of controls experienced great or moderate improvement after 12 months. "Toxicity" occurred in 75 percent and 37 percent of gold-treated and control subjects, respectively.

The second double-blind study, conducted under the auspices of the Empire Rheumatism Council, provided strong impetus for the use of chrysotherapy in RA.[9,10] This multicenter effort involved nearly 200 patients, half of whom received a cumulative dose of 1000 mg of gold sodium thiomalate and the remainder (controls) a total dose of 0.01 mg over a 6-month period; a maintenance gold schedule was not provided. After 3 months of therapy the gold-treated group improved to a greater degree than the controls as assessed by functional capacity, subjective fitness, joint involvement, grip strength, number of analgesic tablets required, hemoglobin level, serum RF titer, and ESR. The reduction in number of involved joints is illustrated in Figure 52–1. Radiologic progression, as measured by joint space narrowing, the number of new bone erosions, or the extension of existing erosions, was statistically similar in both groups, although less marked in those receiving gold. The beneficial effects still were discernible 12 months after cessation of therapy, but were not evident 24 months after treatment was discontinued.

A trial similar to the British effort was undertaken in the United States, but only 68 RA patients were recruited, and after withdrawals because of toxicity, change of residence, and lack of benefit, just 43 were available for re-evaluation at 6 months.[11] In part a consequence of the small number of patients studied, the only parameter that changed significantly was the ESR.

The efficacy of auranofin has been examined in numerous protocols involving more than 3000 RA patients worldwide.[16,42-52] Oral gold has been compared with placebo,[43,44] aurothioglucose,[48] gold sodium thiomalate,[43,45-47] gold sodium thiopropanolsulphonate,[49] penicillamine,[47,52] hydroxychloroquine,[50] and levamisole.[51] While some were well-designed double-blind controlled trials, others were open-label or suffered from various methodologic deficiencies. Reliable data come from a 21-week trial completed by the Cooperative Systematic Studies of Rheumatic Diseases group, a multicenter effort involving 209 RA patients who received either gold sodium thiomalate (n = 82), auranofin (n = 77), or placebo (n = 50).[43] There were no statistically significant differences in benefit between intramuscular and oral gold for any clinical parameter measured (joint pain/tenderness, joint swelling, patient assessment, morning

**Table 52–1.** Results of Intramuscular Chrysotherapy in Selected Controlled and Uncontrolled Studies

| Investigator | Year | Number of Patients | Greatly Improved (%)* | Partially Improved (%)* | Treatment Failure (%)* |
|---|---|---|---|---|---|
| *Controlled Trials* | | | | | |
| Ellman et al.[30] | 1940 | 60 (30)† | 37 ( 3) | 57 (73) | 6 (23) |
| Fraser[8] | 1945 | 57 (46) | 63 (21) | 19 (24) | 18 (55) |
| Waine et al.[31] | 1947 | 58 (62) | 57 (29) | 24 (27) | 19 (43) |
| ERC[10] | 1961 | 90 (95) | 41 (22)‡ | | |
| CCC[11] | 1973 | 22 (21) | 77 (38)* | | |
| *Uncontrolled Trials* | | | | | |
| Forestier[32] | 1934 | 500+ | 75* | | |
| Hartfall and Garland[33] | 1935 | 100 | 70 | 20 | 10 |
| Cecil et al.[18] | 1942 | 245 | 66 | 20 | 14 |
| Adams and Cecil[34] | 1950 | 106 (83)§ | 89 (57) | 8 (25) | 3 (18) |
| Snorrason[35] | 1952 | 295 (169)§ | 72 (23) | | |
| Lockie et al.[36] | 1958 | 369 (566)§ | 57 (38) | 35 (48) | 7 (11) |
| Rothermich et al.[37] | 1976 | 73 | 73 | | 27 |
| Sharp et al.[38] | 1982 | 73 | 37 | 27 | 36 |

*Greatly improved includes disease categorized as "in remission, arrested, marked-moderate improvement, and excellent response"; partially improved includes "some and slight improvement"; treatment failure includes "limited or no improvement and worse." The degree of improvement could not be ascertained in the CCC study or Forestier's report.

†Figures in parentheses are control group data.

‡Patient's estimate of fitness at 6 months.

§Results in non-gold-treated patients but not controlled studies.

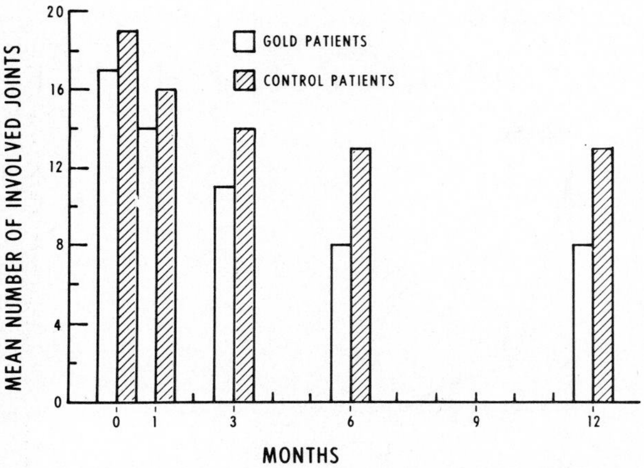


**Figure 52–1.** Mean number of involved joints declines significantly in gold-treated RA patients, but not in controls. (Adapted from the Empire Rheumatism Council Study, Ann. Rheum. Dis. 19:95, 1960.)

stiffness, and ARA functional class). Certain laboratory tests (hemoglobin and platelet count) improved more with gold sodium thiomalate, but serum rheumatoid factor titer and erythrocyte sedimentation rate declined similarly. Both compounds fared better than placebo, reaffirming the value of chrysotherapy for RA. In another trial of 340 RA patients followed for six months, auranofin was superior to placebo, 67 and 43 percent of patients evincing moderate or marked improvement, and 9 and 29 percent being withdrawn for lack of efficacy, respectively.[44] Other reports support these findings and further suggest that auranofin is equal to or superior to all the other disease-modifying drugs enumerated above.

Two 6-month controlled, blinded studies examined the effects of changing from intramuscular to oral gold treatment.[53,54] Only patients who were clinically stable and responded adequately to parenteral treatment were enrolled. Disease activity, erythrocyte sedimentation rate, and serum immunoglobulin levels followed similar patterns, whether patients remained on the injectable preparation or received auranofin.

In 1974, a 30-month double-blind study compared a standard course of gold sodium thiomalate followed by a maintenance gold schedule with placebo.[12] Serial radiograms of the hands and wrists revealed fewer bone erosions and less joint space narrowing in the gold-treated group. These findings document for the first time that gold compounds favorably alter the natural history of RA by reducing bone and cartilage destruction, a consequence presumably of its suppressive action on synovial inflammation.

Roentgenographic progression was correlated with clinical disease activity in a 2-year gold sodium thiomalate trial involving 73 RA patients.[38] As anticipated, given our understanding of the pathophysiology of rheumatoid joint destruction, patients whose synovitis was suppressed the most developed fewest hand and wrist erosions and least joint space narrowing.

A longitudinal roentgenographic study of hand and wrist erosions in auranofin-treated RA patients,[55] used as controls radiographs from the Cooperating Clinics Committee trial comparing gold sodium thiomalate with placebo.[11] Both gold compounds were superior to placebo in reducing the rate of osseous erosions, auranofin having the more profound effect. These conclusions would be more convincing if concomitant rather than historical controls were used for this assessment.

As mentioned above, chrysotherapy may partially correct or restore to normal certain laboratory tests. Hemoglobin, hematocrit, and serum albumin levels increase, while serum RF-titer, ESR, C-reactive protein, plasma glycoproteins, fibrinogen, gamma and total globulins, immune complexes, and IgG, IgA, and IgM decrease significantly during gold treatment.[56,57] Figure 52–2 shows mean changes in immunoglobulins, gamma globulin, and albumin levels in a group of RA patients reported previously.[56] Serum complement (C3) levels fall initially but return to pretreatment concentrations with time; antinuclear antibody titers rise during chrysotherapy.[58] As with clinical manifestations, significant serologic changes generally do not develop until 3 to 6 months of treatment.

Gold sodium thiomalate and D-penicillamine were compared in a 6-month controlled study of 89 RA patients.[39] Both agents were similarly effective in reducing joint pain and swelling, articular index, morning stiffness, the number of subcutaneous nodules and ESR and RF titer, and in increasing grip strength. The gold group was probably at a disadvantage; an inflexible schedule (50 mg weekly until a cumulative dose of 1 gram) was given to all gold-treated patients, whereas variable doses (1 to 1.8 grams daily) were administered to penicillamine-treated patients, according to the clinical response. These doses of penicillamine are higher than recommended currently (see Chapter 53).

Gold sodium thiomalate, azathioprine (Imuran; 2.5 mg per kilogram per day), and cyclophosphamide (Cytoxan; 1.5 mg per kilogram per day) were compared in an 18-month double-blind trial of 121 patients with early RA (mean duration of disease, 5 years).[40] Improvement

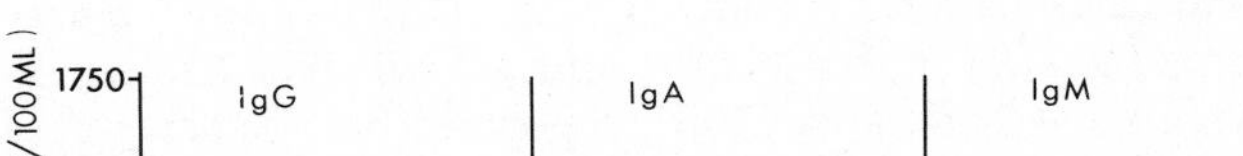

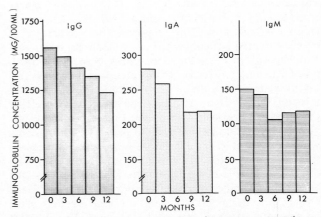


**Figure 52–2.** Mean serum immunoglobulin (IgG, IgA, and IgM) concentrations decline during chrysotherapy. (Adapted from Gottlieb, N.L., et al.: J. Lab. Clin. Med. 86:962, 1975.)

in morning stiffness, grip strength, subjective assessment, joint size, and walking time and reduction in ESR and RF titer were comparable in all patient groups. Roentgenographic joint deterioration was least, and steroid sparing effect greatest, with cyclophosphamide at occasional assessment points, although differences among agents were not pronounced.

Gold sodium thiomalate (50 mg per week intramuscularly), azathioprine (1.0 to 2.0 mg per kilogram per day orally), or chloroquine (250 mg per day orally) was given to 33 patients with early RA (mean disease duration, approximately 2 years) in a nonblinded, randomly assigned 24-week study.[41] Articular index, total active joint count, synovial effusion count, grip strength, duration of morning stiffness, functional class, ESR, and RF titer were assessed serially. All drugs were beneficial, the gold and azathioprine groups faring marginally better than the chloroquine group at the final evaluation.

The value of chrysotherapy in psoriatic arthritis has not been studied extensively.[59,60] Double-blind, controlled reports comparing the efficacy of gold with placebo, nonsteroidal anti-inflammatory agents, or cytotoxic drugs are not available. The influence of gold treatment on a limited number of patients with psoriatic arthritis involving the peripheral joints has been contrasted with its effect on RA patients.[59] The psoriatic arthritis patients experienced a greater reduction in Lansbury index, greater improvement in functional activity, and lesser frequency of severe toxic reactions. These findings should be interpreted cautiously because the natural histories of the two disorders differ, the population surveyed was small, and few clinical (and no laboratory or roentgenographic) parameters were measured.

Certain additional aspects of chrysotherapy are worthy of comment. Some clinicians believe that gold compounds are capable of inducing a protracted or permanent remission in a minority of RA patients.[6,7,37] Reliable information on the frequency of gold (and other disease-modifying antirheumatic drugs)-induced remissions in RA is not available. Differences in study populations, definitions of RA and remissions, and spontaneous variations in disease activity are partly responsible for this void in our knowledge. At the extremes, Adams and Cecil[34] reported that 79 percent of 61 gold-treated patients with RA of less than 6 months' had remissions, while the Cooperative Systematic Studies of Rheumatic Disease group observed no remissions (applying the ARA Preliminary Criteria for Clinical Remission in RA[61]) in 159 patients treated with either parenteral or oral gold.[43] In a recent retrospective review of protracted chrysotherapy,[62] 73 percent of 39 patients who received gold for 3 or more years entered a remission in contrast to only 6 percent of 36 patients who discontinued treatment during the first 18 months. An example of such a response is shown in Figure 52–3. Others have documented healing of bone erosions in an occasional patient during gold treatment (Fig. 52–4).[41] On the other hand, a considerable proportion (15 to 60 percent) of RA patients are unresponsive to gold therapy, experience limited symptomatic relief, eventually escape its beneficial effects despite continued treatment, or must be withdrawn from treatment because of adverse side effects. In fact, only 16 percent of patients continued to receive gold injections 4 years after initiation of treatment in one recent trial,[63] while 50 percent remained on drug at 5 years in another study.[64] Also, it has been observed that patients unresponsive to an initial course of gold uncommonly respond to subsequent courses, and that a majority of patients who escape its favorable effects will not regain them despite ardent efforts by the physician.[10,37] But, other workers[65] recently reported that patients whose disease exacerbates while receiving monthly maintenance gold injections frequently benefit from a return to weekly treatment.The efficacy of gold treatment does not correlate positively with the development of gold toxicity,[66,67] as suggested by earlier reports.[68,69] Some data suggest that 6 months is insufficient time to accrue maximum benefit from chrysotherapy; treatment should be extended to 18 or more months before being discontinued for lack of improvement.[62] However, another report showed loss of efficacy after 2 to 4 years of maintenance therapy.[70] Lastly, the beneficial effects of gold compounds may persist several months or even years after treatment has been abandoned, presumably reflecting tissue gold stores.[9,10,13]

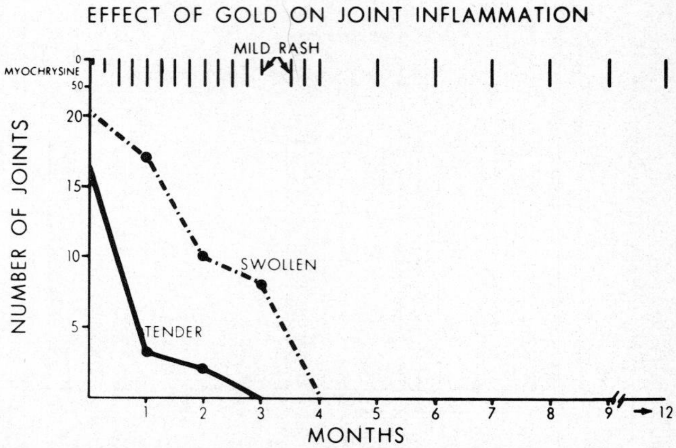


**Figure 52–3.** Schematic graph of the clinical course of a 76-year-old male with seropositive, nodular, progressive RA of 3 years' duration. The clinical remission he experienced at the fourth month of gold treatment persisted until his demise from other causes more than 1 year later.

## GOLD PREPARATIONS

The chemistry of gold-containing compounds is reviewed elsewhere.[71] Briefly, of the several oxidation states for gold compounds (viz., I, O, I, II, III, V), only complex gold I compounds are used therapeutically; gold (O), known as colloidal or metallic gold, is not biologically active; simple gold (I) salts (e.g., gold chloride) are unstable; gold (III) complexes are too toxic and, the biologic activities of the others have not been studied.

Numerous gold-containing compounds have been used to treat RA in the past 50 years. Gold sodium

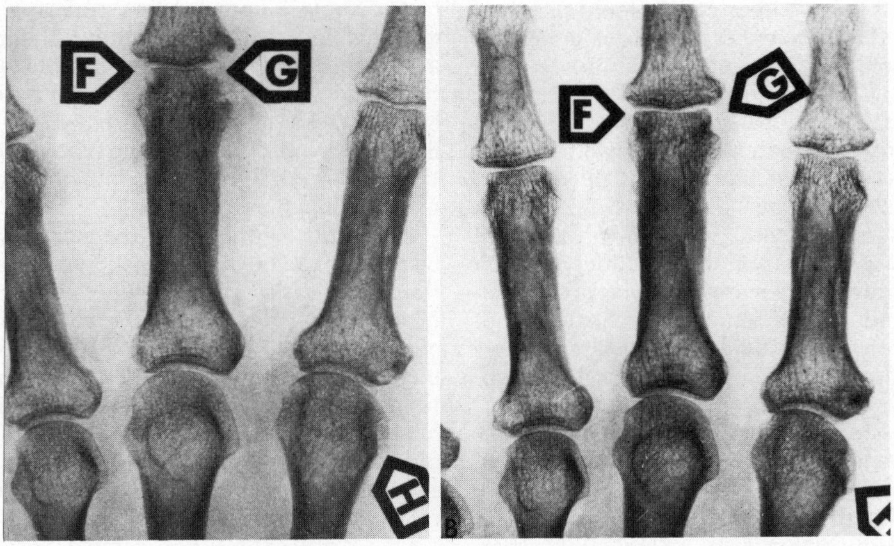


**Figure 52–4.** Serial life-size contact-print radiographs of a middle-aged female with active RA of several years' duration. Note the articular erosions (*F* and *G*) and periarticular demineralization (*H*) in *A*, which developed during treatment with antimalarial agents. *B* shows the same hand after the patient has received continuous chrysotherapy for 5 years; most of the osseous lesions have healed. (Supplied through the courtesy of Paul Young, M.D.)

thiomalate, aurothioglucose, and gold thioglycoanilid (Lauron) are administered by intramuscular injection only; gold sodium thiosulfate (Sanocrysine) also may be given intravenously.[29] Until recently, gold has not been given orally because the commercially available preparations are insufficiently absorbed.

Gold sodium thiomalate and aurothioglucose are the two most widely used compounds in the United States; their structural formulas are shown in Figure 52–5. These preparations are water soluble, and contain a sulfur moiety attached to the gold.[29] Gold sodium thiomalate also has been given intra-articularly on an inves-

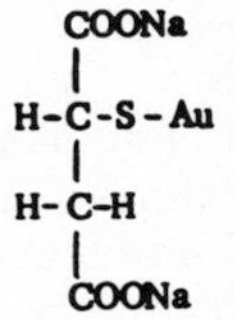

GOLD SODIUM THIOMALATE
(MYOCHRYSINE)

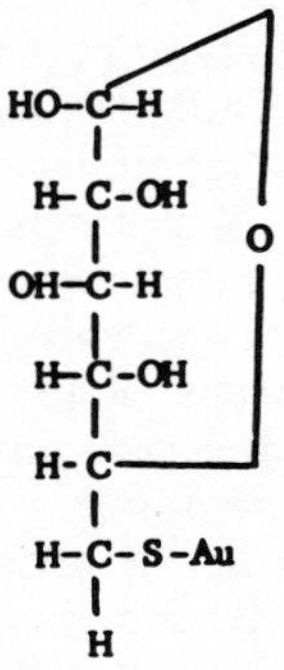

AUROTHIOGLUCOSE
(SOLGANAL)

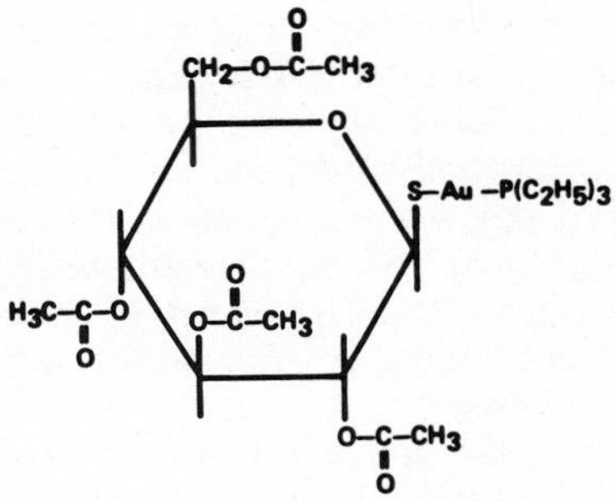

(2,3,4,6-TETRA-O-ACETYL-1-THIO-β-D-GLUCOPYRANOSATO-S)
(TRIETHYLPHOSPINE) GOLD
AURANOFIN

**Figure 52–5.** Gold sodium thiomalate and aurothioglucose, the two intramuscular gold preparations most widely used in the United States, are aurous salts, contain 50 percent gold by weight, and are attached to a sulfur moiety. Auranofin, a conjugated gold compound with two ligands, contains sulfur and is 29 percent gold by weight.

tigational basis.[72] Gold sodium thiomalate, aurothioglucose, and gold thioglycoanilid are approximately 50 percent gold by weight; gold sodium thiosulfate is 37 percent gold.

While it is generally acknowledged that gold sodium thiomalate and aurothioglucose are similarly efficacious, mounting evidence suggests that aurothioglucose may be preferred because of lesser toxicity. Gold sodium thiomalate is associated with vasomotor (nitritoid) reactions[58,73] and with nonvasomotor reactions,[74] which rarely occur with aurothioglucose. Moreover, one prospective study found a significantly higher incidence of adverse reactions with gold sodium thiomalate (30 percent) than with aurothioglucose (9 percent).[37] This observation requires verification. On the other hand, aurothioglucose has the disadvantage of poor miscibility because of the sesame oil vehicle; if the vial is not thoroughly shaken, dosing may be inexact. Aurothioglucose may be associated with the development of firm intramuscular lumps at injection sites, presumably representing nonabsorbed sesame oil or a tissue response to the injectable. The long large-bore needle (1.5 inch, 20 gauge) required for injection of the viscous material increases patient discomfort. There are also pharmacokinetic differences in the compounds, absorption and peak serum levels being diminished with aurothioglucose (see Pharmacokinetics, below).

One study utilizing gold sodium thiomalate and aurothioglucose in oily suspensions and in aqueous solutions showed significantly more toxicity with the aqueous preparations of both compounds than with the oil suspensions.[75] This finding suggests that adverse effects in part may be a consequence of the vehicle, or of resultant altered gold kinetics, rather than differences in compounds.

Auranofin, a triethylphosphine gold compound that contains 29 percent gold by weight, is distinctly different physicochemically from the parenteral compounds.[71,76] Some of its unique characteristics include absorption after oral administration (approximately 25 percent of the administered dose), a monomeric form, lipid solubility, nonconductivity, and weak reactivity with sulfhydryl groups.

## DOSAGE SCHEDULES

The currently recommended intramuscular gold dosage schedule was derived empirically following years of clinical experience; only recently has it been subject to rigidly controlled study and modification. In the early history of chrysotherapy, doses of 100 to 200 mg or more of gold compound were administered once weekly or more often.[6,33] The frequency of toxicity coupled with a 4 percent mortality rate led to a reduction in the sanctioned dose.[13]

Presently the conventional (standard) gold schedule for adults with RA consists of test doses of 10 mg and 25 mg given 1 week apart, followed by 50 mg weekly, until the cumulative dose totals 1 gram or toxicity or major clinical improvement supervenes. Injections of aurothioglucose and gold sodium thiomalate preferably are given deep into the gluteal musculature, alternating right and left sides, following skin cleansing with an alcohol swab or other antiseptic. Gold sodium thiomalate may also be given into the deltoid or other less bulky muscle groups, injection sites not recommended for aurothioglucose.

Numerous variations in the aforementioned schedule have been used by clinicians. Some prefer weekly injections of 25 rather than 50 mg of gold compound; others recommend 50 mg until 500 to 700 mg is attained, at which time the dose is reduced to 25 mg weekly, or increased by increments of 10 mg or more at fixed intervals in unresponsive cases. Alternative schedules include 100 to 150 mg or more weekly, until 1500 to 2500 mg is achieved, or adjusting the dose to maintain the serum concentration above 300 $\mu$g per deciliter or some other arbitrary figure.

One multicenter study compared the clinical results of administering 1000 mg or 2500 mg of aurothioglucose in 21 weeks, followed by maintenance therapy, to more than 200 RA patients.[77] The "low" dose group received 25 mg twice weekly for 11 weeks followed by 50 mg once weekly, while the "high" dose group received 100 mg twice weekly for 11 weeks and then 50 mg weekly for 10 weeks. The efficacy of both dosage regimens was similar; joint count, grip strength, morning stiffness, functional capacity, and ESR improved comparably. However, the frequency of toxicity was significantly greater in the "high" dose (58 percent) than with the "low" dose (24 percent) group (Table 52–2). A double-blind prospective trial in the United States, published in 1977, compared the efficacy of 50 mg and 150 mg of gold sodium thiomalate given weekly for 20 weeks.[78] Therapeutic effects were similar in the two patient groups. Toxicity of such severity as to require discontinuation of therapy occurred in 16 of 24 (67 percent) high dose patients and 3 of 23 (13 percent) low dose patients. Other investigators reported that 25 mg of gold sodium thiomalate was as efficacious as more than twice that amount using a flexible dose schedule.[58] There were no significant differences in joint pain score, ring size, grip strength, radiologic change, deformity, or laboratory tests when high and low dose groups were compared. The number of adverse reactions was similar in the two groups. The possible benefits of daily or alternate day, semimonthly or monthly injection, or other variations in frequency of gold administration have not been explored.

Patients failing to respond to 50 mg per week may benefit from higher gold doses, given in additive weekly to monthly increments of 10 to 25 mg, but rarely exceeding 100 mg. One report showed that 5-mg increases in gold dose each week until a maximum of 100 mg was reached caused improvement in the majority (82 percent) of patients without increasing the risk of toxicity.[68] Another showed that 43 percent of patients who failed to benefit from 50 mg of gold improved significantly when higher doses (1.5 to 2 times the initial dose) were em-

**Table 52–2.** Relationship of Intramuscular Gold Dose to Prevalence of Toxicity

| Investigator | Conventional Gold Dose (50 mg per Week) | | Alternative Gold Dose* | | No Gold | |
|---|---|---|---|---|---|---|
| | *Number of Patients: Toxic/Treated* | *Percent Toxic* | *Number of Patients: Toxic/Treated* | *Percent Toxic* | *Number of Patients: Toxic/Treated* | *Percent Toxic* |
| ERC[9] | 35/99 | 35 | — | | 16/100 | 16 |
| Cats[77] | 29/119 | 24 | 64/111 | 58*a | — | |
| CCC[11] | 12/36 | 33 | — | | 2/32 | 6 |
| Gordon et al.[25] | 25/101 | 25 | — | | — | |
| Rothermich et al.[37] | 10/55 | 18 | 9/42 | 21*b | — | |
| Sharp et al.[58]† | 5/38 | 13 | 4/37 | 11*c | — | |
| Furst et al.[78]† | 3/23 | 13 | 16/24 | 67*d | — | |

*Alternative dosage schedules: *a = 200 mg per week; *b = 1 mg per kilogram per week; *c = 25 mg per week; *d = 150 mg per week.
†Only toxicity severe enough to withhold gold for 6 or more weeks, or to discontinue treatment, is included.

ployed, and that less than 10 percent developed untoward side effects.[37] However, some clinicians prefer to discontinue therapy after 1000 mg in unresponsive cases, whereas others administer an additional 10 to 20 injections of 50 mg, hoping that higher cumulative doses will prove beneficial. The best available evidence suggests that if no beneficial effect (and no toxicity) is noted after 1000 mg of gold (given in doses of 50 mg per week), then a gradual increase in weekly dose may be warranted.

Maintenance gold therapy, which generally consists of 25 to 50 mg of compound every 2 to 4 weeks, is advocated by many authorities upon completion of the initial course. Unfortunately, few studies have examined the efficacy of this commonly used protracted treatment schedule. In 1946, Ragan and Tyson commented that in their opinion, maintenance gold could prevent severe and disabling relapse of RA.[79] Freyberg and associates described the results of an uncontrolled study showing that maintenance chrysotherapy was of decided value in improving and maintaining functional capacity.[13] The value of maintenance gold therapy is indirectly substantiated by the data of Sigler and co-workers,[12] which shows roentgenographic protection of cartilage and bone; such benefit was absent in the Empire Rheumatism Council study, which provided the same initial course but no maintenance treatment.[10] The Dutch study found no significant benefit from maintenance gold treatment.[77] The data of Rothermich and associates suggest that maintenance therapy administered semimonthly rather than monthly more effectively prevents disease relapse,[37] findings refuted by a recent British study.[80]

Several gold schedules have been recommended for children with JRA. Doses of 1 mg per kilogram weekly of gold sodium thiomalate seemed more beneficial than similar doses given at 3- or 4-week intervals.[81] Some clinicians recommend lower doses (0.5 mg per kilogram),[82] whereas others have adopted a single dose schedule of 25 mg per week after test doses,[83] or have related dosage to age.[84]

Gold sodium thiomalate (100 mg) has been instilled periodically into the knee joints of a small number of patients with RA, experimentally.[72] Pharmacokinetic studies of radiolabeled($^{195}$Au) gold sodium thiomalate indicate rapid clearance from the joint cavity with appearance in blood and urine.[85] The initial clinical results of intra-articular gold injection appeared promising, but this mode of administration has attracted little recent attention. It should not be confused with intra-articular radioactive *colloidal* gold ($^{198}$Au) injection, whose short-term benefits derive from the effects of radiation on the synovium. This therapeutic modality is primarily used outside the United States.[86]

The proposed auranofin schedule derives from several studies of dosage range.[87-90] While 3 mg twice daily appears optimal for the majority of adults with RA, some improve with 1 mg daily, and others require 9 mg daily. Diarrhea and abdominal cramps are the commonest limiting factors to achieving high daily dosage. For JRA, 0.1 to 0.2 mg per kg per day was well tolerated and effective for some children in one small open-label trial.[91]

## GOLD DISTRIBUTION

Gold concentrations have been measured in animal and human tissues using colorimetric methods, atomic absorption spectroscopy, neutron activation analysis, radionuclide, and other techniques. The tissue distribution of gold in animals is reviewed in detail elsewhere.[92-95] In general, the kidneys, adrenals, and reticuloendothelial system organs achieve highest gold concentrations.[92,93] Intracellularly, gold localizes predominantly in the nuclear, mitochondrial, and lysosomal fractions, attached to organelle membranes.[96]

In RA patients, gold is widely distributed throughout the tissues, but in markedly varying concentrations. At autopsy, one patient who received 5 grams of aurothioglucose during a 4-year period had higher gold levels in the reticuloendothelial system (lymph nodes, bone marrow, liver, and spleen) than in the joint structure (synovial membrane, articular cartilage, cortical bone, muscle, and synovial fluid).[97] The concentrations of gold found in these and other organs are shown in Figure 52–6. These findings generally have been confirmed by others.[98,99] However, one study found higher synovial gold levels during active chrysotherapy.[100] Only minuscule quantities of gold are found in the crystalline *lens*

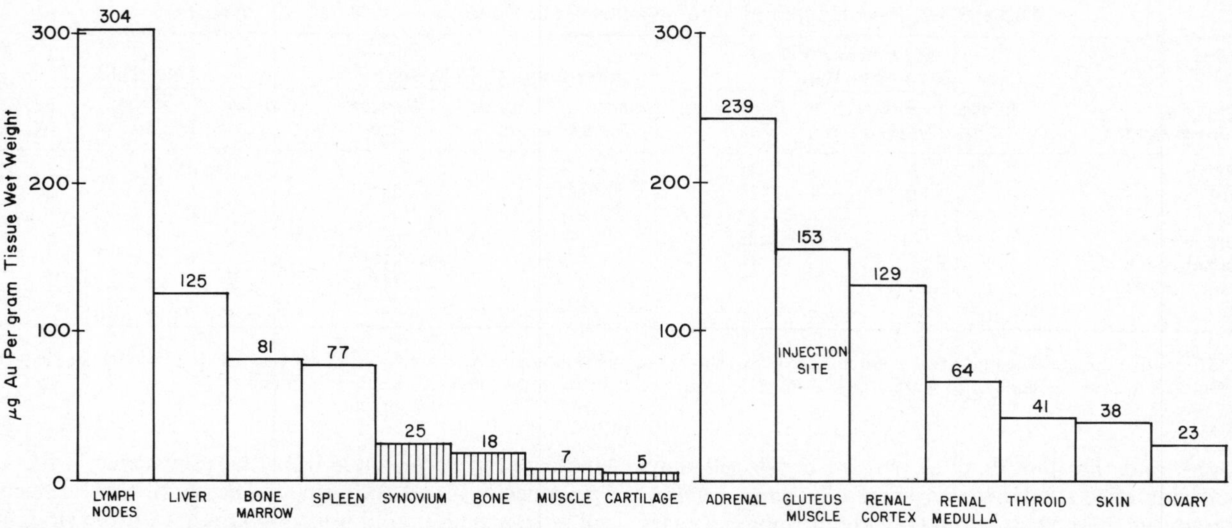


**Figure 52–6.** Gold concentrations in reticuloendothelial, articular, and other tissues from a deceased RA patient who received 5 grams of aurothioglucose during 4 years of chrysotherapy. Higher levels were found in lymph nodes and liver than in tissues composing the joint structure. (Adapted from Gottlieb, N.L., et al.: Arthritis Rheum. 15:16, 1972.)

*of the eye,* despite cumulative gold doses exceeding 10 grams.[101] The greatest quantities of gold are stored in the bone marrow, liver, skin, and bone, a function in part of their large mass (Table 52–3).[97]

Gold concentrations in *body fluids* are much lower than in most tissues. During a standard course of chrysotherapy, blood and urine gold levels generally average 300 to 400 µg per deciliter and 30 to 60 µg per deciliter, respectively, when measured 1 week after administration.[67,102,103] Synovial fluid gold levels generally are about 50 percent of serum concentrations;[104] other fluids (pericardial, bile, milk of lactating women) also contain small quantities of gold.[97,105,106]

Studies of diarthrodial joints indicate that gold preferentially localizes in the synovial membrane during active chrysotherapy;[97] gold levels in *synovium, cartilage, bone, and striated muscle* are similar after treatment is abandoned.[98] Electron probe roentgenographic analysis has shown that gold is present in synovial lining cells and in subsynovial mononuclear cells, enters lysosomes in synovial lining cells, and alters the lysosomal structure seen electron microscopically.[107,108] Sulfur also is present in gold-containing lysosomes, but the sulfur to gold ratio is not identical to that found in gold sodium thiomalate.

In the *skin,* gold is confined largely to the dermis; 3 percent is present in the epidermis.[109] Electron dense particles, thought to represent gold, have been identified in the lysosomes of dermal histiocytes.[110]

Higher gold levels are found in the *renal cortex* than in the *renal medulla* of RA patients.[97] Gold has been identified in the proximal tubules, but not in glomerular subepithelial deposits, in patients with gold-induced proteinuria.[111]

Knowledge of the tissue distribution of gold during auranofin treatment is incomplete. In rats and guinea pigs, gold concentrations in kidney, spleen, and liver are 35 to 70 times higher with gold sodium thiomalate than with comparable or larger doses of oral gold.[112,113] During protracted auranofin treatment of RA patients, synovial fluid and skin gold levels are a fraction of those attained with gold sodium thiomalate, and corneal chrysiasis is observed rarely.[114]

**Table 52–3.** Distribution of Gold in Body Tissues*

| Tissue | Gold Content (mg Gold) | Percent Total Gold Retained |
|---|---|---|
| Bone marrow | 159 | 26 |
| Liver | 148 | 24 |
| Skin | 117 | 19 |
| Bone | 110 | 18 |
| Muscle | 33 | 5 |
| Spleen | 19 | 3 |
| Other | 33 | 5 |
| Total | 619 | 100 |

*Adapted from Gottlieb, N., et al.: Arthritis Rheum. 15:16, 1972. Based on tissues assayed; some organ weights used in determining gold content were estimated.

## PHARMACOKINETICS

Pharmacokinetic studies have provided important insights into the metabolism, excretion, and distribution of gold within the intravascular, serum protein, synovial fluid, tissue, and intracellular compartments. The metabolism of gold sodium thiomalate has been investigated most thoroughly, because it may be dosed precisely and consistently, and because radiolabeled compounds with long ($^{195}$Au-gold sodium thiomalate; 183 days) and short ($^{198}$Au-gold sodium thiomalate; 3 days) half-lives are available commercially.

**Blood Gold.** Serum contains less than 0.5 ng per deciliter of gold prior to initiation of therapy. Gold levels

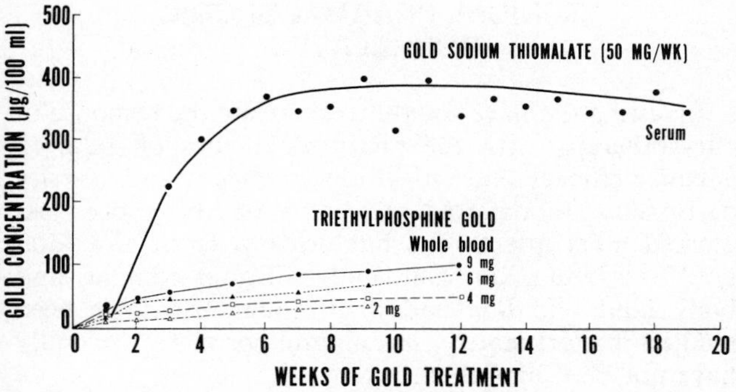


**Figure 52–7.** Higher blood gold concentrations are achieved with conventional doses of gold sodium thiomalate than with auranofin (triethylphosphine gold). Gold levels reach a plateau after 6 to 8 weeks of injectable treatment, and after 12 weeks of auranofin, reflecting the longer half-life of the oral compound. (Adapted from Gottlieb, N.L.: J. Rheumatol. 9 (Suppl. 8):99, 1982, and Finkelstein, A.E., et al.: J. Rheumatol. 7:160, 1980.)

rise gradually in the early phase of conventional treatment, and plateau after 6 to 8 weeks (Fig. 52–7). During chrysotherapy, and following intramuscular injection of gold sodium thiomalate (50 mg), a mean peak serum level of about 700 μg per deciliter is reached within 2 hours and maintained for several hours.[102,103] Levels decline on each successive day, reaching about 300 μg per deciliter at the end of 1 week[103] (Fig. 52–8). Gold concentrations are relatively constant, regardless of the duration of treatment, if the dose is unaltered. One-half the dose of *intravenous* radiogold is cleared from the serum in 5.5 days.[115] Aurothioglucose has a slower absorption rate and lower peak serum level, but values are similar after 7 days.[17,116]

Serum gold concentrations correlate directly with the administered gold dose. When 25 mg per week is given, levels approximate 165 μg per deciliter 1 week after injection;[58] with higher doses (150 mg per week) levels

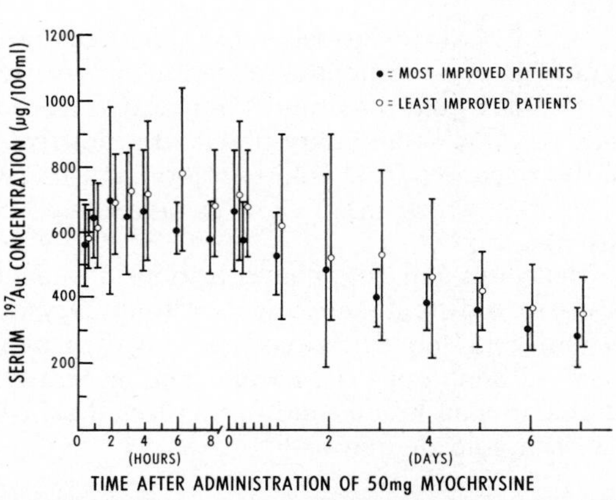


**Figure 52–8.** Mean hourly and daily serum gold concentrations in a group of RA patients receiving conventional chrysotherapy. Within several hours of intramuscular gold sodium thiomalate (50 mg), peak levels (700 μg per deciliter) are attained, which gradually fall to 300 μg per deciliter after 7 days. Gold concentrations in "most" and "least" improved patients are similar. (Adapted from Gottlieb, N.L., et al.: Arthritis Rheum. 17:161, 1974.)

of nearly 1000 μg per deciliter are achieved.[78] During maintenance therapy serum concentrations vary according to the dose and frequency of administration, generally ranging from 75 to 125 μg per deciliter when 50 mg of gold is given every 3 to 4 weeks.[102,103] Upon termination of treatment, levels of 10 to 30 μg per deciliter persist for many months, and gold is detectable as long as 1 year later.[17]

Studies of orally administered gold (auranofin, 6 mg per day) show gradually increasing serum levels during 3 months of therapy which then plateau.[87-89] At 1, 2, and 3 months, *whole blood* gold levels were 40, 60, and 70 μg per deciliter, respectively. A variation of 1 mg per day in auranofin dosage alters blood levels by approximately 10 μg per dl,[87] as shown in Figure 52–7. Serum gold concentrations are slightly lower than whole blood levels.[113,117] The blood gold half-life with auranofin is longer than with gold sodium thiomalate, increasing from 17 days prior to treatment to 26 days after 6 months of therapy with 6 mg per day.[118]

Ninety-two percent of gold in the intravascular compartment is protein bound and 8 percent is present as free gold, using 50 mg per week of an intramuscular compound.[102,119] Higher dosage programs increase the non-protein-bound gold fraction threefold.[119] The great majority of protein-bound gold is in the albumin fraction (95 percent); the remainder is in higher molecular weight fractions.[102] Enhanced binding to immunoglobulins, complement, and circulating lymphocytes is observed with serum gold levels in the range of 300 to 500 μg per deciliter.[120]

Gold is in the red cell fraction of one third of treated patients, averaging 16 percent of the total circulating gold 7 days after administration of an intramuscular compound, but is not detectable in leukocytes or platelets.[121] Serum levels are similar in patients with and without red blood cell gold, but total and fecal gold excretion are greater in those with red cell gold. Other investigators found minuscule quantities of gold in circulating lymphocytes.[122] Two recent reports demonstrate that cigarette smoking increases erythrocyte gold uptake during parenteral treatment.[123,124] During auranofin treatment, approximately 50 percent of intravascular gold is in the cellular fraction, the majority either attached to erythrocyte membranes or present intracellularly.[113] This finding may have some undefined therapeutic importance.

Gold diffuses from serum to synovial fluid rapidly, reaching a state of equilibrium several hours after intramuscular injection.[104] Disappearance of radiogold from synovial fluid conforms to first-order kinetics during the first week, clearance half-time approximating 6 days.

**Gold Excretion.** Approximately 40 percent of the administered dose of intramuscular gold is eliminated, 70 percent in the urine and 30 percent in the feces.[67,102] Considerable variation in excretory pattern exists, occasional individuals eliminating greater quantities of gold in stool than in urine.[67] On the day of injection, urinary gold content is highest, reflecting renal filtration of elevated serum gold levels, and declines progressively on successive days.[19,102] In contrast, daily fecal gold content is irregular, is not influenced by day-to-day variation in serum gold levels, and in part is a function of bowel habit and stool mass.[67] Forty percent of excreted gold derives from the current dose and 60 percent from previous doses.[67] The second, third, and fourth weeks following injection, 16, 12, and 10 percent of the administered dose are eliminated, respectively, if no additional gold is given. Keratinous tissues (skin, hair, and nail) have little avidity for gold, in contrast to certain other heavy metals (e.g., lead and arsenic); no meaningful quantity of gold is eliminated from the body via these excretory routes.[125]

The percentage of gold recovered in excreta during auranofin treatment is dose related, ranging from 76 to 100 percent of the administered dose, with 6 and 2 mg per day, respectively.[114] Approximately 95 percent of recoverable gold is in feces and only 5 percent is in urine.[114,118] Fecal gold content represents a combination of excreted and nonabsorbed gold, and gold adsorbed on mucosal cells that are subsequently sloughed.[126] The contribution from the biliary track is negligible.[126]

**Gold Retention.** Body gold retention has been measured following *intravenous* $^{195}$Au-gold sodium thiomalate, using a whole body radiation counting chamber, and by classic metabolic methods. Applying the former technique, which monitors the kinetics of a *single* (the current) gold dose, RA patients retain 43 percent of the radionuclide 60 days after injection and approximately 25 percent after 250 days.[115] Fifteen percent of orally administered radiolabeled gold is retained after 10 days, while 1 percent remains 6 months later.[118] Utilizing the latter method, which reflects the kinetics of total body gold, approximately 60 percent of a 50 mg dose is retained each week during conventional intramuscular chrysotherapy.[67] Body retention approximates 45 and 30 percent of the injected dose, respectively, when 50 mg of compound is given every second or third week. After 20 weekly injections of 50 mg, approximately 300 mg of elemental gold is retained (20 weeks × 50 mg compound × 50 percent gold by weight × 60 percent retention = 300 mg). Lesser quantities of oral gold (auranofin) are retained; retention is dose dependent, varying from 30 percent with 6 mg per day to zero percent with 2 mg per day.[114] Following 20 weeks of therapy at 6 mg per day it is estimated that 73 mg of gold will be retained (140 days × 6 mg compound per day × 29 percent gold by weight × 30 percent retention = 73 mg), and considerably less when smaller doses are prescribed. The reduced body burden of gold with auranofin therapy may be therapeutically advantageous, although the form and biologic activity of the stored element or compound is unknown.

The existence of superficial and deep gold compartments, composed of tissues having varying avidity for gold, has been proposed.[58] The kinetics of gold interchange between compartments (tissues that store large quantities of the element such as bone marrow and liver, with the intravascular and intra- and extracellular fluids and synovial membrane) has not been defined.

## CLINICAL-PHARMACOLOGIC CORRELATES

Investigators have sought to correlate the response to chrysotherapy with the pharmacokinetics of gold, to enhance efficacy and reduce the frequency and severity of toxicity. Blood gold concentrations have been examined most intensively, but urinary, fecal, and total gold excretion, skin, hair, and nail gold content, and body gold retention and distribution also have been studied. Unfortunately, meaningful correlates generally have not been identified.

More than 10 reports failed to define a relationship between serum gold concentration and efficacy, when measured at weekly intervals immediately prior to injection, during the course of therapy.[26,102,103] Peak, hourly, and daily serum blood gold levels also are comparable in gold responders and nonresponders, as shown in Figure 52–8.[103] Furthermore, serum radiogold disappearance curves do not correlate with response to treatment, and are similar in individual patients at different periods of chrysotherapy, independent of disease activity. Patients achieving mean concentrations of nearly 1000 μg per deciliter during high-dose therapy (150 mg per week) fared no better than those whose levels were 450 μg per deciliter during conventional treatment;[78] patients with gold levels of 167 μg per deciliter during low-dose treatment (25 mg per week) improved as much as patients receiving 50 mg per week (332 μg per deciliter).[58]

Serum gold levels are not helpful in monitoring adverse reactions; peak, hourly, daily, and weekly concentrations are similar in gold-toxic and nontoxic patients.[103] Serum radiogold disappearance curves also are comparable in both patient groups and in individuals studied twice, whether or not toxicity is present. However, as shown in Table 52–2, the frequency of severe toxicity is increased two- to fivefold when high-dose treatment schedules (150 to 200 mg per week) are employed.[77,78]

Recent trials indicate no relationship between urinary gold content and response to treatment of toxicity.[102,103,127] Body gold retention is not related to clinical outcome.[67,115] One small study observed a positive correlation between low fecal gold excretion and favorable clinical course, which may relate to organ (e.g., liver) gold distribution.[67]

Serial hair and nail gold concentrations are identical in gold-toxic and nontoxic patients during chrysotherapy.[125] Skin gold concentrations are similar in patients with and without gold dermatitis, and generally are comparable in skin lesions and in unaffected skin from patients with gold dermatitis.[125]

## MECHANISMS OF ACTION

A myriad of in vitro and in vivo properties of gold compounds involving inflammatory cycles, the immune system, cellular biochemistry, and so forth have been elucidated in the past decades. But the mechanisms responsible for the favorable action of gold in RA remain enigmatic, and the information accrued has not substantially improved the results of chrysotherapy.

Gold compounds inhibit the growth of tubercle and other bacilli in vitro. Further support for the antimicrobial actions of gold derives from its protective effect on hamsters experimentally infected with Eaton's primary atypical pneumonia agent,[128] and from its purported beneficial effect in gonococcal arthritis.[5] More recently, gold sodium thiomalate was shown to inhibit the growth of *E. coli* when added to agar medium, but the addition of gold to human sera did not alter bacteriolytic activity.[129]

Gold sodium thiomalate inhibits acid phosphatase, beta glucuronidase, and malic dehydrogenase in guinea pig peritoneal macrophages,[130] acid phosphatase, beta glucuronidase, and cathepsin in human synovial fluid cells,[131] and several human epidermal enzymes.[132] These findings suggest that gold may ameliorate rheumatoid inflammation by inhibiting lysosomal enzymes. However, the release of hydrolases from lysosomes is unaffected by gold compounds, indicating that gold does not stabilize lysosomal membranes.[133]

The phagocytic activity of certain inflammatory cells is enhanced in patients with RA. Intramuscular gold compounds inhibit macrophage and polymorphonuclear leukocyte phagocytic activity at inflammatory sites in vivo, using a "skin-window" technique and measuring colloidal carbon particle uptake.[134] This action may alter cellular release of lysosomal enzymes, the initial handling of antigens in some immune responses, and several aspects of cell-mediated immunity. Chrysotherapy reduces the serum concentration of several trace metals (tin, molybdenum, manganese, barium, and cesium) that are elevated in RA patients; perhaps gold displaces other metal ions from biologically active compounds, successfully modifying a series of disease-producing biochemical interactions.[135] The effects of gold on serum protein, complement, and immunoglobulin concentrations, and on RF titer, have been discussed under Efficacy.

Gold sodium thiomalate inhibits the copper-catalyzed thermal aggregation of human gamma globulin in vitro; aggregated protein of this type is thought to be inflammatory, antigenic, and a stimulus to RF formation.[136] Gold compounds affect the classic and alternative complement systems in vitro.[137,138] Gold sodium thiomalate and thiosulfate and gold chloride partially inactivate the first component (C1) of the complement system in serum and synovial fluid, in concentrations achieved during conventional chrysotherapy.[137] An example of the effect of gold sodium thiomalate on C1, C4, and C2 in rheumatoid synovial fluid is shown in Figure 52–9. Highly purified human C1 and $C1_s$ were also irreversibly destroyed by gold. Thiomalic acid produced no such effects. The prostaglandin system, another important mediator of inflammation, is also affected by gold in vitro. Gold sodium thiomalate, in therapeutic serum concentrations, inhibits $PGE_2$ synthesis in a time- and concentration-dependent manner.[132] At a cellular level, gold acts directly on free sulfhydryl groups of proteins (e.g.,

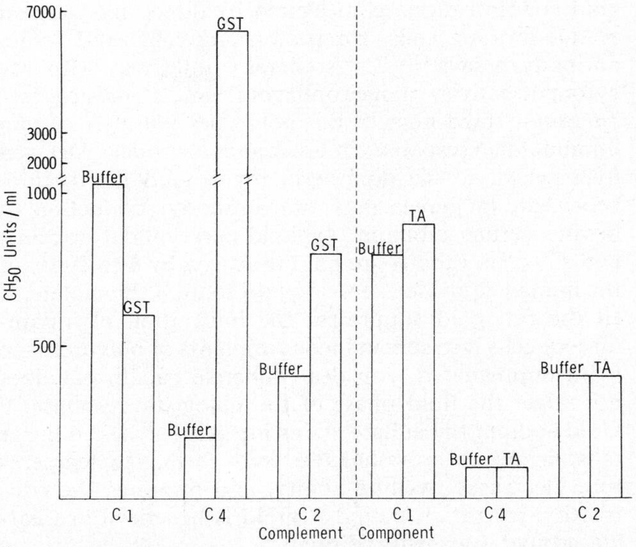


**Figure 52–9.** Gold sodium thiomalate (GST) (3.1 μg per milliliter) partially inactivates the functional hemolytic activity of $C\bar{1}$, and protects against C4 and C2 destruction, the natural substrates of $C\bar{1}$, in vitro. Thiomalic acid (TA) has no effect on $C\bar{1}$. (Supplied through the courtesy of Duane Schultz, Ph.D.)

cysteine), rendering them biologically inactive.[139] In contrast to certain antirheumatic agents, gold compounds do not inhibit connective tissue activation (CTAP).[140]

Most recently, the effects of gold on lymphocytes and monocytes have been reported. Gold sodium thiomalate inhibits antigen- and mitogen-triggered human lymphocyte DNA synthesis in vitro, an action that is increased by partially depleting the cell culture of monocytes, and that is reversed by culture supplementation with purified monocytes.[141] Preincubation of purified monocytes with gold renders them deficient in their ability to support mitogen-induced T-lymphocyte proliferation on subsequent culture. These and other observations suggest that gold blocks thymus-derived lymphocyte activation by interfering with monocyte function. Gold sodium thiomalate and thiosulfate inhibit transformation of human lymphocytes stimulated by other lymphocytes in the mixed lymphocyte culture, purified protein derivative, phytohemagglutinin, concanavalin A, and pokeweed mitogen in vitro.[142] Other investigators reported that gold sodium thiosulfate does not inhibit the incorporation of ($^3$H) thymidine (a measure of DNA synthesis) and ($^{14}$C) amino acids (a measure of protein synthesis) in human lymphocytes. Micromolar concentrations of gold sodium thiomalate and aurothioglucose also inhibit peptide-stimulated chemotactic responsiveness of human blood monocytes, but not of polymorphonuclear leukocytes.[143] However, others have shown that gold sodium thiomalate inhibits neutrophil chemotaxis and random migration in vitro, in normal subjects, and in gold-responsive RA patients but not in gold-resistant patients.[144]

Aurothioglucose and gold sodium thiomalate influence the immune response of mice, resulting in immunoenhancement or immunosuppression, depending upon gold concentration, as measured by direct and indirect plaque-forming cells, rosette-forming cells, and serum antibody assays.[145] Chrysotherapy interferes with the cytotoxic activity of macrophages from *Corynebacterium parvum*–treated mice.[146] But gold does not alter certain immunologic responses in other animal models. Delayed hypersensitivity to diphtheria toxoid and dinitrochlorobenzene in guinea pigs and antibody production to bovine serum albumin, typhoid-paratyphoid vaccine, and *E. coli* in rabbits are not influenced by 4 to 10 times the human equivalent dose of gold sodium thiomalate.[147] In the rat, gold suppresses the infiltration of inflammatory cells into subcutaneous implants of polyurethane foam impregnated with dead tubercle bacilli, but does not affect the fluid phase of the phlogistic response.[148] Gold sodium thiosulfate stains intravital collagen in rat tails, increases cross-linkages and shrinkage temperature, decreases swelling ability, and prolongs the contraction-relaxation period.[149] Gold is beneficial in treating adjuvant arthritis of rats.[150]

The pharmacologic and biologic actions of auranofin differ in many respects from those of the intramuscular gold compounds (Table 52–4). Oral gold exhibits anti-inflammatory activity in several animal models, suppresses humoral immune mechanisms, alters cell-mediated immunity, depresses polymorphonuclear and mononuclear leucocyte activity in vitro, and inhibits DNA synthesis in vitro and human cellular activity in vivo.[151] In many of these test systems the effect of auranofin is stronger than comparable or larger doses of the injectable gold compounds. One or more of these functions may explain the efficacy of auranofin in RA despite the low blood and tissue gold levels.

**Table 52–4.** Pharmacologic and Biologic Actions of Gold Sodium Thiomalate and Auranofin

| Action | Gold Sodium Thiomalate | Auranofin |
|---|---|---|
| *Inflammation* | | |
| Carrageenan edema (rat) | ↑/↓ | ↓ |
| Kaolin edema (rat) | 0 | ↓ |
| Passive cutaneous anaphylaxis (rat) | ↓ (weak) | ↓ |
| Ultraviolet erythema (guinea pig) | ↓ | ↓ |
| Adjuvant arthritis (rat) | ↓ | ↓ |
| *Humoral Immunity* | | |
| IgG hemagglutinin (adjuvant arthritis; rat) | 0 | ↓ |
| Antibody-dependent cellular cytotoxicity (ADCC, rat) | 0 | ↓ |
| Antibody-dependent complement lysis (rat) | ↑ | ↓ |
| Hemagglutinin (mouse) | 0 | 0 |
| Hemolysin plaque-forming cells (rat) | 0 | ↓ |
| Hemolysin plaque-forming cells (mouse) | ↑ | ↓/0 |
| *Cell-mediated Immunity (CMI)* | | |
| Sub-optimal CMI (mouse)* | ↑ | ↑ |
| Immunosuppressed CMI (mouse)* | 0 | ↑ |
| Experimental allergic encephalomyelitis (rat) | ↓ (delay) | ↓ (delay) |
| *Polymorphonuclear Leukocyte Activity (in vitro)* | | |
| Chemotaxis (human) | – | ↓ |
| Aggregation (human) | ↓ (weak) | ↓ |
| Superoxide production (human) | 0/↓ | ↓ |
| Phagocytosis (rat/human) | –/0 | ↓/↓ |
| Lysosomal enzyme release (rat/human) | 0/↓ (weak) | ↓/↓ |
| ADCC | 0 | ↓ |
| *Mononuclear Leukocyte Activity (in vitro)* | | |
| Mononuclear (target cell destruction, rat) | – | ↑ |
| Monocyte (ADCC/chemotaxis, human) | 0/↓ | ↓/↓ |
| Lymphocyte (mitogen stimulation, human; | ↓ (weak) | ↓ |
| antibody secretion, mouse; | ↓ (weak) | ↓ |
| ADCC, human) | 0 | ↓ (weak) |
| NK cell (target cell destruction, human) | – | ↑/↓ |
| *DNA Synthesis (in vitro)* | | |
| Mitogen stimulated lymphocytes | ↓ weak/0 | ↓ |
| EBV-transformed lymphocytes | 0 | ↓ |
| HeLa carcinoma | – | ↓ |
| RAJI lymphoma | – | ↓ |
| *Human Cellular Activity (in vivo)* | | |
| DNA synthesis (mitogen-stimulated lymphocytes) | ↑/↓ (weak), (10–20 weeks) | ↓ (2 weeks) |
| Delayed hypersensitivity (dinitrochlorobenzene skin test) | 0 | ↓ |

*Using oxazolone-induced contact sensitivity and delayed hypersensitivity to sheep red blood cells.

## PRECAUTIONS, CONTRAINDICATIONS, AND COSTS

Efforts to predict gold toxicity and to reduce the frequency and severity of untoward gold reactions have had a modicum of success. Most strikingly, the mortality rate has fallen from an estimated 4 percent in the early years of chrysotherapy to less than 0.5 percent at present. Reasons for the reduced death rate are complex and speculative and are discussed more fully under Gold Toxicity. I believe that improved general medical care, the availability of life support systems, and lower gold doses largely account for the declining mortality rate. Because the prevalence of untoward reactions correlates directly with gold dose, especially when 50 mg per week is exceeded, the use of a conventional schedule should reduce the frequency of toxicity; however, wide variation in the prevalence of complications in recent and past reports prohibits accurate comparison. The presently available precautionary measures, described below, do not predict or prevent gold complications; they merely permit prompt recognition of early toxicity. Therefore, continued efforts should be directed toward defining the optimal gold schedule; new techniques, predictive of impending toxicity, must be developed. Immediate cessation of gold, coupled with appropriate therapeutic measures, avoids severe or protracted target-organ damage in some cases.

My recommendations for monitoring chrysotherapy are as follows. Baseline history, physical, and laboratory examinations are mandatory. The physician inquires in detail for a past history of allergic drug reaction, pruritus, rash, oral lesions, renal disease, and proteinuria. The skin and oral mucosa are carefully examined for lesions such as psoriasis, fungal infection, leukoplakia, palatal or buccal mucosal ulceration, or inflammation from dental appliances. A complete blood count with differential, thrombocyte estimate from peripheral blood smear or platelet count, urinalysis, and biochemical profile are obtained.

During chrysotherapy, the patient is queried, preferably by the physician or by specially trained medical personnel under his direct supervision, about pruritus, dermatitis, stomatitis, and metallic taste and is examined prior to each injection. Most authorities recommend a complete blood count, thrombocyte count or estimate, and urinalysis every 1 to 3 weeks. I dip-stick test a urine specimen for proteinuria, using Uristix or other commercially available product, before each injection.

Chrysotherapy is terminated promptly should any of the aforementioned symptoms or significant eosinophilia, leukopenia, anemia, thrombocytopenia, microscopic hematuria, or proteinuria develop. Causes of such abnormality, other than gold toxicity, such as laboratory error, incidental skin or mucous membrane lesions, side effects from other medications, and so forth, are sought. If no alternative explanation is found, presumably the reaction is gold related, and treatment is temporarily or permanently abandoned, depending on the type and severity of reaction and the activity of the rheumatic process.

Gold compounds should not be administered to patients with a past history of severe gold toxicity (e.g., generalized dermatitis, significant depression of any blood cell type, or heavy proteinuria; see Gold Toxicity for additional discussion). Other heavy metal toxicity that has resulted in organ impairment (e.g., renal insufficiency from chronic plumbism) also interdicts the use of chrysotherapy.

Vasomotor responses (nitritoid reactions) are associated with gold sodium thiomalate treatment and may include dizziness and syncope as part of their symptom complex (see Gold Toxicity for further discussion). Because they occur within several minutes of administration, probably as a result of vasodilation with ensuing transient hypotension, it is advisable to give gold sodium thiomalate while the patient is recumbent. Furthermore, I recommend that the patient remain in the examining room or elsewhere in the doctor's office for 10 to 15 minutes after injection.

The concomitant use of certain other antirheumatic agents generally is interdicted during chrysotherapy. The pyrazolon-derived compounds (phenylbutazone, oxyphenbutazone), antimalarials, cytotoxic agents, and penicillamine are beneficial in RA, but they may cause side effects similar to those of gold, such as bone marrow depression, proteinuria, and dermatitis. Should an untoward reaction occur, the offending drug could not be readily identified, demanding discontinuation of both agents. Drug interactions and potentiation of toxicity have not been explored adequately, but they are additional considerations for avoiding conjunctive therapy. Some authorities believe that the concurrent use of systemic corticosteroids may reduce the efficacy of gold treatment, an opinion not substantiated by critical testing. Excessive sun exposure may contribute to the development of gold dermatitis and is discouraged; this admonition is based on anecdotal experience.

Gold compounds and penicillamine are commonly prescribed sequentially, usually in that order, for patients requiring slow-acting antirheumatic drugs who are unresponsive or intolerant to the initial choice.[152-154] The therapeutic response to the first agent does not predict the value of the second.[152] And, with the possible exceptions of proteinuria[152] and dermatitis,[154] patients who experience complications from the initial drug are not more likely to develop similar reactions from the next.

Gold therapy is not recommended for pregnant or lactating women because the safety for the fetus or newborn infant has not been established. What little evidence is available, however, anecdotal and otherwise, suggests a low magnitude of risk.[15] Women of childbearing age in whom chrysotherapy is contemplated are advised to use accepted contraceptive measures; treatment is terminated if pregnancy develops. The milk of gold-treated lactating women and the blood of their nursing infants contain small quantities of gold, the clinical significance of which has not been determined. Therefore, in the present state of knowledge, gold treatment is best avoided in nursing mothers.

Chrysotherapy may be used in conjunction with analgesics, salicylate compounds and other systemic nonsteroidal anti-inflammatory agents, and intraarticular corticosteroids without amelioration of benefit. Sjögren's syndrome, which develops in 10 to 15 percent of RA patients, is not a deterrent to gold therapy.[25] Similarly, ocular chrysiasis does not interdict chrysotherapy.[101] This incidental finding is not associated with visual disturbance or a higher prevalence of gold toxicity. Inasmuch as ocular complications from gold treatment occur rarely, periodic ophthalmologic examinations are not necessary.

The cost of administering and monitoring the initial phase (20 weeks) of intramuscular gold treatment is considerable. A survey conducted in 1976 indicated that the expense varies from $300 to $800, depending on the frequency and number of laboratory tests and physician (versus nurse or physician's assistant) visits, and on the established charges for these procedures.[155] The price of the injectable is approximately $50.00 for a 10 cc vial (50 mg per cubic centimeter) of aurothioglucose or gold sodium thiomalate. Transportation expenses, loss of income as a result of travel and waiting in the physician's office, and monies expended in evaluating and treating gold complications were not determined, raising the real cost of chrysotherapy well beyond the survey's estimates. Strategies to reduce costs include fewer and less frequent laboratory tests and administration of gold at home by a family member or nurse. The extent to which these cost-cutting measures jeopardize the patient's health (increase the frequency or severity of gold toxicity) or reduce the beneficial effects of treatment is speculative.

The cost of oral gold treatment is not fully established, and will be partly dependent upon (a) the retail price of auranofin capsules, (b) final guidelines for the number, type, and frequency of laboratory tests advised, and (c) recommended frequency of physician visits to monitor drug effects. Oral chrysotherapy will probably be less expensive than parenteral treatment during the first 6 months, when weekly visits to the physician's office and frequent blood and urine tests are required, but thereafter costs may be comparable.

## GOLD TOXICITY

Adverse reactions develop in approximately one third of RA patients treated with intramuscular gold, varying from 5 to 80 percent in several reported series.[13] Most complications are inconsequential, consisting primarily of localized dermatitis, stomatitis, or transient mild proteinuria. More serious reactions involve the hematopoietic system, kidneys, liver, or other vital organs. Table 52–5 lists many of the toxic reactions associated with gold therapy.

Dermatitis and stomatitis account for 60 to 80 percent of all adverse gold reactions. The clinical and histologic appearance of gold rash is highly variable and may mimic other skin conditions such as lichen planus, idiopathic pityriasis rosea, psoriasis, and dermatophytosis. Erythema nodosum, exfoliative dermatitis, and bullous lesions develop rarely. One report indicated that 50 percent of lesions defied clinical classification into known dermatologic entities.[156]

The severity, distribution, and duration of gold rash varies from mild, localized, evanescent eruptions to those that are intensely pruritic or painful, generalized, and persistent for 1 year or longer. Most gold rashes last 1 to 2 months, are discrete, and are confined to the extremities or, less frequently, the trunk. Approximately 85 percent of eruptions are pruritic; other manifestations of gold toxicity such as eosinophilia, metallic taste, or proteinuria often accompany dermatitis.[13,156]

Skin punch biopsy may aid the clinician in defining gold dermatitis and in excluding incidental disorders that arise during chrysotherapy.[156] Immunofluorescent studies are of little value in differentiating gold rash from other conditions; immunoglobulins and complement components are found in a minority of gold eruptions but also are present in diverse dermatitides of other causes.[157]

The appearance of a rash during chrysotherapy in a patient without a pre-existing history of similar eruption, and especially if accompanied by pruritus or other manifestations of gold toxicity, is strongly suggestive of gold dermatitis. Chrysotherapy should be interrupted temporarily, pending evaluation and complete resolution of dermal pathology plus several additional weeks of observation. In some circumstances, treatment then may be reinstituted, using a reduced dosage schedule of 5 to 10 mg of gold compound weekly, with 5 to 10 mg increments every 1 to 4 weeks if toxicity does not recur. A lower dosage schedule, consisting of 1 to 2 mg initially with increments of similar magnitude, has also been advocated, and reportedly reduces the frequency of recurrent dermatitis.[158] Reinstitution of chrysotherapy in patients with a history of proved mild to moderately severe localized gold dermatitis that has resolved rarely results in exfoliative dermatitis or other generalized skin rash. The majority of patients tolerate a reduced dosage schedule without adverse reaction, but those with recurrent dermatitis tend to have eruptions similar to those manifest initially.[159]

**Table 52–5.** Adverse Reactions from Intramuscular Gold Compounds

| |
|---|
| Dermatologic |
| Dermatitis—common |
| Stomatitis—common |
| Pruritus—common |
| Alopecia—rare |
| Chrysiasis—rare |
| Photosensitivity—rare |
| Renal |
| Proteinuria—common |
| Hematuria—rare |
| Nephrotic syndrome—rare |
| Renal insufficiency or failure—rare |
| Hematologic |
| Eosinophilia—common |
| Thrombocytopenia—rare |
| Granulocytopenia—rare |
| Aplastic anemia—rare |
| Ophthalmic |
| Corneal or lens chrysiasis—common |
| Conjunctivitis, iritis, corneal ulcer—rare |
| Cardiopulmonary |
| Vasomotor (nitritoid) reactions—common* |
| Anaphylaxis—rare |
| Syncope—rare |
| Diffuse pulmonary infiltrates—rare |
| Musculoskeletal |
| Myalgias—common* |
| Joint pain, swelling, stiffness—common* |
| Gastrointestinal |
| Enterocolitis—rare |
| Cholestatic jaundice—rare |
| Miscellaneous |
| Metallic taste—common |
| Peripheral neuritis—rare |
| Headaches—rare |

*With gold sodium thiomalate (Myochrysine).

Rarely, gray or blue discoloration of the skin develops with protracted intramuscular chrysotherapy.[160] This condition, known as chrysiasis, is asymptomatic, difficult to document objectively, does not influence the response to treatment, and is not associated with other side effects. Although gold is detectable in the skin of these patients, it is universally present during protracted injectable treatment, a critical gold concentration necessary to develop chrysiasis has not been defined, and the mechanisms responsible for this pigmentary change are not known.[125,161]

Transient proteinuria, microscopic hematuria, and nephrotic syndrome are well-described complications of gold therapy. The prevalence of transient proteinuria varies from 0 to 26 percent of patients receiving 50 mg of gold-compound weekly, as shown in Table 52–6. The frequency of proteinuria increases when higher gold doses are administered.[77,78] However, proteinuria has also been described in approximately 3 percent of nongold-treated RA patients;[9,11] hypertension, diverse urinary tract disorders, and various medications used to treat RA are other conditions which may cause proteinuria. At times, urinary protein resolves spontaneously despite continuation of chrysotherapy in the absence of any identifiable cause.

Nephrotic syndrome is the most frequent serious renal abnormality associated with gold therapy, encountered in 0.2 to 2.6 percent of patients.[162-164] Histologically, the predominant lesion is membranous glomerulonephritis. IgG, IgM, and complement (C3) have been found in glomerular lesions. Particulate matter consistent with gold has been found in proximal and distal renal tubules, interstitium, and glomerular tufts.[162,163] Gold has been identified within proximal convoluted tubule cells, suggesting that gold may injure tubular epithelial cells, with subsequent release of antigen, antibody formation, and resultant immune complex deposition in glomerular tufts.[111] The prognosis with gold-associated nephrotic syndrome is generally favorable, 70 percent of patients recovering fully within months to years. The remainder have varying degrees of persistent proteinuria; renal insufficiency is observed rarely.[162]

Hematologic disorders resulting from chrysotherapy include eosinophilia, leukopenia or agranulocytosis, thrombocytopenia, anemia, pancytopenia, and aplastic anemia. Eosinophilia occurs in approximately 5 percent of gold-treated patients but, depending upon such factors as definition and patient population, varies from 0 to 40 percent in several published series.[13,165] Generally, eosinophilia is transient and of no significance; however, it may be a harbinger of impending toxicity affecting any organ system. Eosinophilia has been correlated positively with serum IgE levels and gold toxicity,[165] although others have not confirmed this finding.[157]

Thrombocytopenia is an infrequently (1 to 3 percent) recognized complication of gold treatment that is potentially serious and occasionally life threatening. It may develop shortly after gold is begun or as late as 18 months after cessation of therapy.[166,167] The initial manifestations of platelet reduction may be easy bruisability or spontaneous petechiae or purpura affecting the skin, mucous membranes of the mouth, and tongue. Less commonly, epistaxis or gingival, gastrointestinal, or genitourinary hemorrhage leads to the diagnosis of thrombocytopenia. Platelet counts above 25,000 per cubic millimeter uncommonly are associated with bleeding difficulties unless other hematologic abnormalities coexist.

Leukopenia may develop during gold therapy owing to granulocytopenia or agranulocytosis. The prevalence of leukopenia is low but not precisely established, and the extent and duration of white cell reduction are highly variable. Granulocytopenia may be asymptomatic or may be associated with clinical manifestations.

The most feared complication of chrysotherapy is severe pancytopenia or bone marrow aplasia. The incidence of the latter is low, existing evidence pointing to a prevalence of less than 0.5 percent.[168] However, the mortality rate is high, more than 60 percent of affected individuals succumbing to infection, bleeding, or other complications despite supportive and aggressive therapy.

Vasomotor (nitritoid) reactions, characterized by weakness, dizziness, nausea, vomiting, sweating, and facial flushing, may follow gold sodium thiomalate. The prevalence of this reaction has varied from not being cited to as high as 34 percent in several series.[78] Peripheral vasodilatation may ensue, causing hypotension from the action on arteriolar smooth muscle. Rarely, this results in myocardial infarction[73] or central nervous system injury, especially in the elderly population with arteriosclerotic or other forms of cardiovascular disease.[169] Nonvasomotor symptoms, including transient stiffness, arthralgias, myalgias, joint swelling, fatigability, and malaise, developed in 15 percent of patients treated with gold sodium thiomalate in one reported study.[74] Aurothioglucose exceptionally causes either symptom complex.

Organ systems rarely affected by gold treatment in-

**Table 52–6.** Prevalence of Proteinuria During Intramuscular Chrysotherapy

| | Conventional Gold Dose (50 mg per Week) | | Alternative Gold Dose* | | No Gold | |
|---|---|---|---|---|---|---|
| **Investigator** | *Number of Patients: Toxic/Treated* | *Percent Toxic* | *Number of Patients: Toxic/Treated* | *Percent Toxic* | *Number of Patients: Toxic/Treated* | *Percent Toxic* |
| ERC[9] | 4/99 | 4 | – | | 3/100 | 3 |
| Cats[77] | 4/119 | 3 | 10/111 | 9 | – | |
| CCC[11] | 0/36 | 0 | – | | 1/32 | 3 |
| Gordon et al.[25] | 7/101 | 7 | – | | – | |
| Rothermich et al.[37] | 2/55 | 4 | 0/42 | 0 | – | |
| Sharp et al.[58] | 6/38 | 16 | 9/37 | 24 | – | |
| Furst et al.[78] | 6/23 | 26 | 9/24 | 38 | – | |

*Alternative gold schedules are given in Table 52–2.

clude the lungs, liver, and lower intestinal tract. Acute respiratory distress associated with diffuse pulmonary infiltration characteristically causes malaise, cough productive of small amounts of sputum, shortness of breath, pleuritic chest pain, and pulmonary rales.[170,171] Patchy areas of pulmonary consolidation without hilar adenopathy, but with alteration of respiratory function tests consistent with restrictive lung disease, are observed. Dramatic improvement follows withdrawal of chrysotherapy and administration of systemic corticosteroids.

Cholestatic jaundice, with hyperbilirubinemia, elevated serum glutamic oxaloacetic transaminase and other enzymes, and high alkaline phosphatase levels, has been ascribed to gold treatment in a few patients.[172,173] Findings generally include fatigability, pruritus, anorexia, painless icterus, dark urine, light-colored stool, and hepatomegaly. Liver biopsy may show bile stasis and thrombi in the biliary tree, or ballooning hepatocytes with sinusoidal compression and minimal cholestasis. Hepatotoxicity usually develops early in the course of treatment (less than 200 mg of compound), is often associated with peripheral blood eosinophilia, and recedes rapidly with cessation of gold therapy.

Enterocolitis is another uncommon complication of chrysotherapy, occurring primarily in middle-aged females who have received small total doses of gold.[174,175] Symptoms may include abdominal pain, bloody or nonbloody diarrhea, nausea, vomiting, and fever. Despite treatment with antibiotics, dimercaprol (BAL), corticosteroids, and life-support measures, the mortality rate approaches 50 percent.

Corneal chrysiasis, defined by slit-lamp microscopy, is directly related to cumulative dose, occurring in 75 percent of patients who receive greater than 1500 mg of intramuscular gold.[176,177] Lens chrysiasis occasionally develops despite minuscule lens gold levels.[101] Neither condition leads to the development of ocular disease. Conjunctivitis, iritis, and corneal ulcers have been rarely attributed to gold treatment.

Evolving information shows an association between certain untoward side effects from gold and antigens on the histocompatibility D locus. Specifically, gold-induced proteinuria and thrombocytopenia, which likely represent immune-mediated reactions, occur many times more frequently than anticipated (increased relative risk is 32 times for proteinuria and nine times for thrombocytopenia) in RA patients possessing HLA-DR3 and DRw3.[178-180] Interestingly, the more common forms of gold toxicity, such as dermatitis and stomatitis, are not related to this genetic background.[178,179] Given the prevalence of these antigens in the general population (31 percent),[179] the limited number of slow-acting antirheumatic drugs currently available, and the expense of HLA-D typing, routine HLA typing before initiating gold treatment is not warranted.

Extensive premarketing experience reveals that the type, severity, and time of complication developing from auranofin differ importantly from characteristics of complications of the injectable gold compounds (Table 52–7). Most side effects are mild and transient, affect the lower gastrointestinal tract, and are dose related. Changes in stool consistency and frequency, diarrhea, and abdominal cramps are the commonest untoward effects of oral gold.[16,42] These reactions generally occur within the first few weeks to months of treatment, improve spontaneously or remand with dose reduction, or very uncommonly require permanent drug abandonment.[16] The mechanisms of gastrointestinal irritation are unknown, but barium enema, sigmoidoscopy, and mucosal biopsy on a limited number of patients have not revealed significant pathologic change.[16] Gold colitis or persistent diarrhea after drug cessation has not been encountered. Mucocutaneous lesions and serious complications affecting the hematopoietic system, kidneys, and so forth occur less commonly with auranofin than with the intramuscular preparations.[16,42] Approximately four times as many patients were withdrawn from intramuscular gold treatment (20 percent) because of drug

**Table 52–7.** Adverse On-Therapy Experiences: Gold Sodium Thiomalate and Auranofin Compared

| | CSSRD Study* | | | Combined Data from Seven Studies Comparing Gold Sodium Thiomalate and Auranofin† | |
|---|---|---|---|---|---|
| **Complication** | *Gold Sodium Thiomalate (n = 81)* | *Auranofin (n = 78)* | *Placebo (n = 50)* | *Gold Sodium Thiomalate (n = 244)* | *Auranofin (n = 243)* |
| Mucocutaneous | 7 (%) | 1 (%) | 4 (%) | 48 (%) | 23 (%) |
| Vasomotor reactions | 6 | 0 | 0 | NR‡ | NR |
| Proteinuria | 0 | 0 | 0 | 6 | 2 |
| Diarrhea | 2 | 6 | 0 | 8 | 25 |
| Other GI symptoms | 2 | 1 | 0 | 6 | 12 |
| Hematologic | 0 | 0 | 0 | 7 | 1 |
| Miscellaneous | 15 | 5 | 0 | 31 | 22 |
| Withdrawals due to adverse reactions | 27 | 7 | 2 | 22 | 7 |

*Adapted from the Cooperative Systemic Studies of Rheumatic Diseases Report[43]; excludes adverse reactions leading to withdrawal.
†Adapted from Blodgett.[16]
‡NR = Not reported.

intolerance as from oral gold (5 percent) in the Cooperative Systematic Studies of Rheumatic Diseases 21-week controlled trial[43] and in cumulative data from seven protocols.[16] With more prolonged therapy, the drop-out rates rise, but the 4:1 withdrawal ratio between parenteral and oral gold remains.[16]

## TREATMENT OF GOLD TOXICITY

The great majority of adverse gold reactions resolve spontaneously within weeks to months following cessation of chrysotherapy or require only symptomatic measures. Treatment of serious complications affecting the skin, kidneys, lungs and gastrointestinal and hematopoietic systems has been the subject of numerous reports but not of controlled studies.[13,29,156,159,162,164,166-168,170-174,181,182] Appraisal of the efficacy of corticosteroids, dimercaprol, penicillamine, ACTH, and other agents is further complicated by the variable natural history of gold reactions, and by the rare mortality from bone marrow aplasia, thrombocytopenia, or enterocolitis despite aggressive treatment.

Most patients with gold dermatitis of such severity as to require treatment benefit from oral antihistamines, topical corticosteroids, or emollients such as petrolatum, Crisco, Aquaphor, or Lubriderm. Colloidal baths, tranquilizers, sedatives, and the application of ice or cold compresses may relieve pruritus.[156] Prolonged sun exposure and contact with soap should be avoided. Symptoms resulting from severe or generalized pruritic eruptions may improve with systemic corticosteroids, although the literature fails to provide convincing evidence that the natural history of the eruption is altered favorably.

Stomatitis, glossitis, cheilitis, and gingivitis may be minimally symptomatic, demanding no treatment or only avoidance of spices and sour substances, or of such severity as to necessitate stronger measures. Frequent alkaline mouth washes or the application of Xylocaine Viscous or Kenalog in Orabase may afford relief of oral soreness, burning, or pain in severe or protracted cases.[159] Resultant anorexia and weight loss occasionally require nutritional supplementation with a liquid diet, baby food or blenderized soft foods, or, rarely, intravenous fluids or other forms of alimentation.

Moderate to high dose corticosteroid therapy (20 to 60 mg daily in divided doses of prednisone or its equivalent) reportedly is beneficial in some cases of gold-induced nephrotic syndrome, thrombocytopenia, and, less often, other hematologic disorders, enterocolitis, and pulmonary infiltrates. Higher doses of steroids may be justified in unresponsive cases. Treatment generally must be given for several weeks to months, and then tapered gradually. It is currently believed that corticosteroids act by reducing inflammation in the affected target organ, by altering the immunologic response, or by some other undefined mechanism. Gold metabolism is not affected.

Dimercaprol, penicillamine, *N*-acetylcysteine, and other chelating agents have been employed primarily in severe reactions unresponsive to corticosteroid therapy or in conjunction with steroids.[13,29,183-185] With the exception of penicillamine,[186,187] these drugs enhance urinary gold excretion and are thought to compete with gold for essential cellular enzymes. Dimercaprol is given intramuscularly in doses of 2.5 to 3.0 mg per kilogram every 6 hours for 3 or 4 days. Reduced doses may then be administered for an additional time period, depending on the therapeutic response. Some clinicians base the amount of BAL prescribed on the cumulative gold dose, applying greater quantities of BAL for patients with higher total gold doses.[188] Perhaps some drug failures result from inadequate courses of BAL. Penicillamine (Cuprimine) is given orally in divided doses of 1 to 2 grams daily for variable time periods. The use of these agents is attended by potentially serious side effects. Bone marrow depression, sterile abscesses, vomiting, carpopedal spasm, paresthesias, and severe headaches may develop from BAL. Complications associated with penicillamine are reviewed in Chapter 53.

In addition to these measures, patients with severe thrombocytopenia associated with hemorrhage may require volume repletion, whole blood or platelet transfusions, and life support measures. Vincristine,[189] other potent chemotherapeutic agents, and splenectomy[190] have also been used successfully. Those suffering from significant granulocytopenia or agranulocytosis often improved spontaneously within two weeks.[191] In unresponsive cases, and in those with bone marrow aplasia, reverse isolation techniques, systemic antibiotics, bed rest, blood or platelet transfusions, and extensive general medical and nursing care may be beneficial. Androgenic hormones, bone marrow transplantation,[192] and peritoneal dialysis[193] also have been recommended in recalcitrant cases.

## SELECTION OF GOLD COMPOUND: ORAL OR INTRAMUSCULAR?

The advantageous safety profile of auranofin compared with the injectable gold compounds, coupled with similar efficacy profiles, provides an improved benefit-to-risk ratio. In addition, auranofin is easier to administer, may require less laboratory and clinical monitoring, and hopefully will be less expensive. On the other hand, this oral gold compound may not be fully as potent as the intramuscular agents, may be prescribed improperly by physicians unfamiliar with rheumatic disease treatment and used inappropriately by patients who self-administer medication, and may present compliance problems. Experience with the parenteral compounds spans 55 years, ample time for physicians to become familiar with these products, and for the identification of common and rare adverse reactions. For these and other reasons, the ultimate place of auranofin vis-à-vis the intramuscular compounds in the therapeutic hierarchy of RA is speculative. I believe auranofin will replace the injectables as the initial agent of choice, and may encourage the modification of criteria for instituting slow-acting drug treatment, so that it is used in milder forms and earlier phases of RA.

## REFERENCES


1. Slot, G., and Deville, P.M.: Treatment of arthritis and rheumatism with gold. Lancet 226:73, 1934
2. Koch, R.: Reported at the 10th International Medical Congress, Berlin, August 4, 1890. Dtsch. Med. Wochenschr. 16:756, 1890.
3. Rodnan, G.P., and Benedek, T.G.: The early history of antirheumatic drugs. Arthritis Rheum. 13:145, 1970.
4. Landé, K.: Die gunstige beeinflussung schleichender Dauerinfekte durch Solganal. Munch. Med. Wochenschr. 74:1132, 1927.
5. Oren, J.: Arthritis and its treatment with gold salts. J. Med. Soc. N.J. 33:591, 1936.
6. Forestier, J.: Rheumatoid arthritis and its treatment by gold salts. J. Lab. Clin. Med. 20:827, 1935.
7. Hartfall, S.J., Garland, H.G., and Goldie, W.: Gold treatment of arthritis: A review of 900 cases. Lancet 233:838, 1937.
8. Fraser, T.N.: Gold treatment in rheumatoid arthritis. Ann. Rheum. Dis. 4:71, 1945.
9. Empire Rheumatism Council: Gold therapy in rheumatoid arthritis. Ann. Rheum. Dis. 19:95, 1960.
10. Empire Rheumatism Council: Gold therapy in rheumatoid arthritis: Final report of a multicentre controlled trial. Ann. Rheum. Dis. 20:315, 1961.
11. The Cooperative Clinics Committee of the ARA: A controlled trial of gold salt therapy in rheumatoid arthritis. Arthritis Rheum. 16:353, 1973.
12. Sigler, J.W., Bluhm, G.B., Duncan, H., et al.: Gold salts in the treatment of rheumatoid arthritis: A double-blind study. Ann. Intern. Med. 80:21, 1974.
13. Freyberg, R.H., Ziff, M., and Baum, J.: Gold therapy for rheumatoid arthritis. *In* Hollander, J.L., and McCarty, D.J. (eds.): Arthritis and Allied Conditions. 8th ed. Philadelphia, Lea & Febiger, 1972, pp. 455–482.
14. Penneys, N.S., Eaglstein, W.H., and Frost, P.: Management of pemphigus with gold compounds. Arch. Dermatol. 112:185, 1976.
15. Miyamoto, T., Miyaji, S., Horiuchi, Y., et al.: Gold therapy in bronchial asthma with special emphasis upon blood level of gold and its teratogenicity. J. Jap. Soc. Intern. Med. 63:1190, 1974.
16. Blodgett, R.C., Heuer, M.A., and Pietrusko, R.G.: Auranofin: A unique oral chrysotherapeutic agent. Semin. Arthritis Rheum. 13:255, 1984.
17. Freyberg, R.H., Block, W.D., and Wells, G.S.: Gold therapy for rheumatoid arthritis. Clinics 1:537, 1942.
18. Cecil, R.L., Kammerer, W.H., and DePrume, F.J.: Gold salts in the treatment of rheumatoid arthritis. Ann. Intern. Med. 16:811, 1942.
19. Gottlieb, N.L., and Bjelle, A.: Gold compounds in rheumatoid arthritis. Scand. J. Rheumatol. 6:225, 1977.
20. Mouridsen, H.T., Baerentsen, O., Rossin, N., et al.: Lack of effect of gold therapy on abnormal IgG and IgM metabolism in rheumatoid arthritis. Arthritis Rheum. 17:391, 1974.
21. Menard, H.A., Mathieu, J.T., de Medicis, R., and Lussier, A.: Slow-onset antirheumatic drugs in rheumatoid arthritis: Could the presence of antinuclear antibody influence the therapeutic results? J. Rheumatol. 6:156, 1979.
22. Vischer, T.L.: Pharmacogenetics in therapy with gold and other slow-acting anti-rheumatic drugs. International Gold Workshop, Munich, Germany, January 14, 1982.
23. Gowans, J.D.C., and Salami, M.: Response of rheumatoid arthritis with leukopenia to gold salts. N. Engl. J. Med. 288:1007, 1973.
24. Hurd, E.R., and Cheatum, D.E.: Decreased spleen size and increased neutrophils in patients with Felty's syndrome. JAMA 235:2215, 1976.
25. Gordon, M.H., Tiger, L.H., and Ehrlich, G.E.: Gold reactions are *not* more common in Sjögren's syndrome. Ann. Intern. Med. 82:47, 1975.
26. Gottlieb, N.L.: Chrysotherapy. Bull. Rheum. Dis. 27:912, 1976-77.
27. Luthra, H.S., Conn, D.L., and Ferguson, R.H.: Felty's syndrome: Response to parenteral gold. J. Rheumatol. 8:902, 1981.
28. Mastaglia, G.L., and Owen, E.T.: A study of the response of the leukopenia of rheumatoid arthritis to gold salt therapy. J. Rheumatol. 8:658, 1981.
29. Harvey, S.C.: Heavy metals. *In* Goodman, L.S., and Gilman, A.: The Pharmacologic Basis of Therapeutics. 3rd ed. New York, Macmillan Publishing Co., 1965, pp. 943-975.
30. Ellman, P., Lawrence, J.S., and Thorold, G.P.: Gold therapy in rheumatoid arthritis. Br. Med. J. 2:314, 1940.
31. Waine, H., Baker, F., and Mettier, S.R.: Controlled evaluation of gold treatment in rheumatoid arthritis. Calif. Med. J. 66:295, 1947.
32. Forestier, J.: Rheumatoid arthritis and its treatment by gold salts. Lancet 227:646, 1934.
33. Hartfall, S.J., and Garland, H.G.: Gold treatment of rheumatoid arthritis. Lancet 229:8, 1935.
34. Adams, C.H., and Cecil, R.L.: Gold therapy in early rheumatoid arthritis. Ann. Intern. Med. 33:163, 1950.
35. Snorrason, E.: Rheumatoid arthritis, sanocrysin treatment and prognosis. Acta Med. Scand. 142:249, 1952.
36. Lockie, L.M., Norcross, B.M., and Riordan, D.J.: Gold treatment in rheumatoid arthritis. JAMA 167:1204, 1958.
37. Rothermich, N.O., Philips, V.K., and Bergen, W.: Chrysotherapy: A prospective study. Arthritis Rheum. 19:1321, 1976.
38. Sharp, J.T., Lidsky, M.D., and Duffy, J.: Clinical responses during gold therapy for rheumatoid arthritis: Changes in synovitis, radiologically detectable erosive lesions, serum proteins, and serologic abnormalities. Arthritis Rheum. 25:540, 1982.
39. Huskisson, E.C., Gibson, T.J., and Balme, H.W.: Trial comparing D-penicillamine and gold in rheumatoid arthritis. Ann. Rheum. Dis. 33:532, 1974.
40. Currey, H.L.F., Harris, J., and Mason, R.M.: Comparison of azathioprine, cyclophosphamide, and gold in treatment of rheumatoid arthritis. Br. Med. J. 3:763, 1974.
41. Dwosh, I.L., Stein, H.B., Urowitz, M.B., et al.: Azathioprine in early rheumatoid arthritis. Comparison with gold and chloroquine. Arthritis Rheum. 20:685, 1977.
42. Heuer, M.A., and Morris, R.W.: Smith, Kline & French World-Wide Clinical Experience With Auranofin: A Review. Auranofin (Ridaura) International Symposium, Amsterdam, November, 1982.
43. Ward, J.R., Williams, H.J., Egger, M.J., et al.: Comparison of auranofin, gold sodium thiomalate, and placebo in the treatment of rheumatoid arthritis. Arthritis Rheum.26:1303, 1983.
44. Katz, W.A., Alexander, S., Bland, J.H., Blechman, W., Bluhm, G.B., Bonebreak, R.A., Falbo, A., Greenwald, R.A., Hartman, S., Hobbs, T., Indenbaum, S., Lergier, J.E., Lanier, B.G., Lightfoot, R.W., Phelps, P., Sheon, R.P., Torretti, D., Wenger, M.E., and Wilske, K.: The efficacy and safety of auranofin compared to placebo in rheumatoid arthritis. J. Rheumatol. 9 (Suppl. 8):173, 1982.
45. Menard, H.A., Beaudet, F., Davis, P., Harth, M., Percy, J.S., Russell, A.S., and Thompson, J.M.: Gold therapy in rheumatoid arthritis: An interim report of the Canadian multicenter prospective trial comparing sodium aurothiomalate and auranofin. J. Rheumatol. 9 (Suppl. 8):179, 1982.
46. Schattenkirschner, M., Kaik, B., Muller-Fassbender, H., Rau, R., and Zeidler, H.: Auranofin and sodium aurothiomalate in the treatment of rheumatoid arthritis: A double-blind, comparative multicenter study. J. Rheumatol. 9 (Suppl. 8):184, 1982.
47. Barraclough, D., Brook, A., Brooks, P., Boyden, K., and Thomas, K.: A comparative study of auranofin, gold sodium thiomalate, and D-penicillamine in rheumatoid arthritis: A progress report. J. Rheumatol. 9 (Suppl. 8):197, 1982.
48. van Riel, P.L.C.M., van de Putte, L.B.A., Gribnau, F.W.J., and MacRae, K.D.: A single-blind comparative study of auranofin and gold thioglucose in patients with rheumatoid arthritis. Auranofin International Symposium, Amsterdam, November, 1982.
49. DeQueiter, J., Franckx, L., and Deckers, Y.: Comparison of oral gold (auranofin) and injectable gold (gold sodium thiopropanol-sulphonate; Allochrysine) treatment in patients with rheumatoid arthritis: A double-blind study. Auranofin International Symposium, Amsterdam, November, 1982.
50. Bird, H.A., Gallez, P.L., Dixon, J.S., Sitton, N.G., and Wright, V.: A comparison of auranofin and hydroxychloroquine in rheumatoid arthritis. Auranofin International Symposium, Amsterdam, November, 1982.
51. Huskisson, E.C., and Scott, J.: Comparative study of auranofin in rheumatoid arthritis. 15th International Congress of Rheumatology, Paris, June, 1981.
52. Felix-Davies, D.D., Bateman, J.R.M., Delamere, J.P., and Wilkinson, B.R.: A comparative trial of auranofin and D-penicillamine in rheumatoid arthritis. 15th International Congress of Rheumatology, Paris, June, 1981.
53. Wenger, M.E., Weiss, T.E., Rosenthal, S.H., O'Brien, W.M., Bernhard, G.C., Heller, M.D., and Reese, R.W.: Rheumatoid arthritis patients treated with auranofin maintain clinical benefits when switched from Myocrisin. Auranofin International Symposium, Amsterdam, November, 1982.
54. Berry, H., Gibson, T.J., Crisp, A.J., Pitt, P., Irani, M., Clarke, B., Bloom, B., and Paney, G.S.: Double-blind comparison of auranofin and Myocrisin in patients stabilised on Myocrisin. Auranofin International Symposium, Amsterdam, November, 1982.
55. Gofton, J.P., and O'Brien, W.: Roentgenographic findings during auranofin treatment. Am. J. Med. 75 (Suppl.): 142, 1983.
56. Gottlieb, N.L., Kiem, I.M., Penneys, N.S. et al.: The influence of chrysotherapy on serum protein and immunoglobulin levels, rheumatoid factor, and antiepithelial antibody titers. J. Lab. Clin. Med. 86:962, 1975.

57. Highton, J., Panayi, G.S., Shephard, P., Faith, A., Griffin, J., and Gibson, T.: Fall in immune complex levels during gold treatment of rheumatoid arthritis. Ann. Rheum. Dis. 40:575, 1981.
58. Sharp, J.T., Lidsky, M.D., Duffy, J., et al.: Comparison of two dosage schedules of gold salts in the treatment of rheumatoid arthritis. Arthritis Rheum. 20:1179, 1977.
59. Dorwart, B.B., Gall, E.P., Schumacher, H.R., et al.: Chrysotherapy in psoriatic arthritis. Arthritis Rheum. 21:513, 1978.
60. Richter, M.B., Kinsella, P., and Corbett, M.: Gold in psoriatic arthropathy. Ann. Rheum. Dis. 39:279, 1980.
61. Pinals, R.S., Masi, A.T., and Larsen, R.A.: Preliminary criteria for clinical remission in rheumatoid arthritis. Arthritis Rheum. 24:1308, 1981.
62. Srinivasa, N.R., Miller, B.L., and Paulus, H.E.: Long-term chrysotherapy in rheumatoid arthritis. Arthritis Rheum. 22:105, 1979.
63. Sambrook, T.N., Browne, C.D., Champion, G.D., Day, R.O., Vallance, J.B., and Warwick, N.: Terminations of treatment with gold sodium thiomalate in rheumatoid arthritis. J. Rheumatol. 9:932, 1982.
64. Richter, J.A., Runge, L.A., Pinals, R.S., and Oates, R.P.: Analysis of treatment terminations with gold and anti-malarial compounds in rheumatoid arthritis. J. Rheumatol. 7:153, 1980.
65. Sagransky, D.M., and Greenwald, R.A.: Efficacy and toxicity of retreatment with gold salts: A retrospective review of 25 cases. J. Rheumatol. 7:474, 1980.
66. Empire Rheumatism Council: Relation of toxic reactions in gold therapy to improvement in rheumatoid arthritis. Ann. Rheum. Dis. 20:335, 1961.
67. Gottlieb, N.L., Smith, P.M., and Smith, E.M.: Gold excretion correlated with clinical course during chrysotherapy in rheumatoid arthritis. Arthritis Rheum. 15:582, 1972.
68. Smith, R.T., Peak, W.P., and Kron, K.M.: Increasing the effectiveness of gold therapy in rheumatoid arthritis. JAMA 167:1197, 1958.
69. Bayles, T.B., and Fremont-Smith, P.: Significant clinical remissions in rheumatoid arthritis resulting from "sensitivity" produced by gold salt therapy. Ann. Rheum. Dis. 15:394, 1956.
70. Rosenthal, M.: Loss of efficacy of antirheumatic drugs in rheumatoid arthritis. J. Rheumatol. 7:586, 1980.
71. Sadler, P.J.: The comparative evaluation of the physical and chemical properties of gold compounds. J. Rheumatol. 9 (Suppl. 8): 71, 1982.
72. Lewis, D.C., and Ziff, M.: Intra-articular administration of gold salts. Arthritis Rheum. 9:682, 1966.
73. Gottlieb, N.L., and Brown, H.E., Jr.: Acute myocardial infarction following gold sodium thiomalate induced vasomotor (nitritoid) reaction. Arthritis Rheum. 20:1026, 1977.
74. Halla, J.T., Hardin, J.G., and Linn, J.E.: Postinjection nonvasomotor reactions during chrysotherapy. Arthritis Rheum. 20:1188, 1977.
75. Lawrence, J.S.: Comparative toxicity of gold preparations in treatment of rheumatoid arthritis. Ann. Rheum. Dis. 35:171, 1976.
76. Walz, D.T., DiMartino, M.J., Griswold, D.E., Intoccia, A.P., and Flanagan, T.L.: Biological actions of auranofin. Am. J. Med. 75 (Suppl.): 90, 1983.
77. Cats, A.: A multicentre controlled trial of the effects of different dosage of gold therapy, followed by maintenance dosage. Agents Actions 6:355, 1976.
78. Furst, D., Levine, S., Srinivasan, R., et al.: A double-blind trial of high versus conventional dosages of gold salts for rheumatoid arthritis. Arthritis Rheum. 20:1473, 1977.
79. Ragan, C., and Tyson, T.L.: Chrysotherapy in rheumatoid arthritis. Am. J. Med. 1:252, 1946.
80. Griffin, A.J., Givson, T., Huston, G., and Taylor, A.: Maintenance chrysotherapy in rheumatoid arthritis: A comparison of two dose schedules. Ann. Rheum. Dis. 40:250, 1981.
81. Hanson, V.: Dosage of gold salts in treatment of juvenile rheumatoid arthritis. Arthritis Rheum. 20 (Supplement No. 2): 548, 1977.
82. Ansell, B.M.: The management of juvenile chronic polyarthritis (Still's disease). Practitioner 208 (1243): 91, 1972.
83. Brewer, E.J., Jr.: Juvenile Rheumatoid Arthritis. Philadelphia, W. B. Saunders Company, 1970, pp. 205-213.
84. Sairanen, E., and Laaksonen, A.L.: The results of gold therapy in juvenile rheumatoid arthritis. Ann. Paediat. Fenn. 10:274, 1964.
85. Gottlieb, N.L., and Smith, E.M.: Pharmacology of intraarticularly injected $^{195}$Au-labeled Myochrysine (sodium aurothiomalate) used as a diagnostic and therapeutic aid in rheumatoid arthritis (abstract). J. Nucl. Med. 9:319, 1968.
86. Makin, M., and Robin, G.C.: Chronic synovial effusions treated with intra-articular radioactive gold. JAMA 188:725, 1964.
87. Finkelstein, A.E., Roisman, F.R., and Batista, V.: Oral chrysotherapy in rheumatoid arthritis: Minimum effective dose. J. Rheumatol. 7:160, 1980.
88. Champion, G.D., Bieri, D., Browne, C.D., Day, R.O., Graham, G.G., Haavisto, T.M., Sambrook, P.N., and Vallance, J.B.: Auranofin in rheumatoid arthritis. J. Rheumatol. 9 (Suppl. 8): 137, 1982.
89. Calin, A., Saunders, D., Bennett, R., Jacox, R., Kaplan, D., O'Brien, W., Paulus, H.E., Roth, S., and Weiss, T.: Auranofin: One mg or 9 mg? The search for the appropriate dose. J. Rheumatol. 9 (Suppl. 8): 146, 1982.
90. Bernhard, G.C.: Auranofin treatment for adult rheumatoid arthritis: Comparison of 2 mg and 6 mg daily dose. J. Rheumatol. 9 (Suppl. 8): 149, 1982.
91. Giannini, H., Brewer, E.J., Jr., and Person, P.A.: Auranofin in the treatment of juvenile rheumatoid arthritis. J. Pediatr. 102:138, 1983.
92. Block, W.D., Buchanan, O.H., and Freyberg, R.H.: Metabolism, toxicity, and manner of action of gold compounds used in the treatment of arthritis. J. Pharmacol. Exp. Ther. 82:391, 1944.
93. Bertrand, J.J., Waine, H., and Tobias, C.A.: Distribution of gold in the animal body in relation to arthritis. J. Lab. Clin. Med. 33:1133, 1948.
94. Jeffrey, M.R., Freundlich, H.F., and Bailey, D.F.: Distribution and excretion of radiogold in animals. Ann. Rheum. Dis. 17:52, 1958.
95. Stuve, J., and Galle, P.: Role of mitochondria in the handling of gold by the kidney. J. Cell. Biol. 44:667, 1970.
96. Penneys, N.S., McCreary, S., and Gottlieb, N.L.: Intracellular distribution of radiogold: Localization to large granule membranes. Arthritis Rheum. 19:927, 1976.
97. Gottlieb, N.L., Smith, P.M., and Smith, E.M.: Tissue gold concentration in a rheumatoid arthritic receiving chrysotherapy. Arthritis Rheum. 15:16, 1972.
98. Grahame, R., Billings, R., and Laurence, M.: Tissue gold levels after chrysotherapy. Ann. Rheum. Dis. 33:536, 1974.
99. Kamel, H., Brown, D.H., Ottoway, J.M., et al.: Gold levels in kidney, liver, and spleen (letter to editor). Arthritis Rheum. 19:1368, 1976.
100. Veron-Roberts, B., Dore, J.L., Jessop, J.D., et al.: Selective concentration and localization of gold in macrophages of synovial and other tissues during and after chrysotherapy in rheumatoid patients. Ann. Rheum. Dis. 35:477, 1976.
101. Gottlieb, N.L., and Major, J.C.: Ocular chrysiasis correlated with gold concentrations in the crystalline lens during chrysotherapy. Arthritis Rheum. 21:704, 1978.
102. Mascarhenas, B.R., Granda, J.L., and Freyberg, R.H.: Gold metabolism in patients with rheumatoid arthritis treated with gold compounds—reinvestigated. Arthritis Rheum. 15:391, 1972.
103. Gottlieb, N.L., Smith, P.M., and Smith, E.M.: Pharmacodynamics of $^{195}$Au labeled auriothiomalate in blood. Correlation with course of rheumatoid arthritis, gold toxicity and gold excretion. Arthritis Rheum. 17:161, 1974.
104. Gerber, R.C., Paulus, H.E., and Bluestone, R.: Kinetics of aurothiomalate in serum and synovial fluid. Arthritis Rheum. 15:625, 1972.
105. Kapelowitz, R.H., Help, W.M., Headly, L.A., et al.: Urinary and fecal excretion of $Au^{198}$ in gold-treated patients with rheumatoid arthritis (abstract). Arthritis Rheum. 7:319, 1964.
106. Gottlieb, N.L.: Gold metabolism (letter to the editor). Arthritis Rheum. 17:1057, 1974.
107. Ghadially, F.N., Oryschak, A.F., and Mitchell, D.M.: Ultrastructural changes produced in rheumatoid synovial membrane by chrysotherapy. Ann. Rheum. Dis. 35:67, 1976.
108. Nakamura, H., and Igarashi, M.: Localization of gold in synovial membrane of rheumatoid arthritis treated with sodium aurothiomalate. Ann. Rheum. Dis. 36:209, 1977.
109. Penneys, N.S., Kramer, K., and Gottlieb, N.L.: The quantitative distribution of gold in skin during chrysotherapy. J. Invest. Dermatol. 65:331, 1975.
110. Cox, A.J.: Gold in the dermis following gold therapy for rheumatoid arthritis. Arch. Dermatol. 108:655, 1973.
111. Viol, G.F., Minielly, J.A., and Bistricki, T.: Gold nephropathy: Tissue analysis by x-ray fluorescent spectroscopy. Arch. Pathol. Lab. Med. 101:635, 1977.
112. Kamel, H., Brown, D.G., Ottaway, J.M., Smith, W.E., Cottney, J., and Lewis, A.J.: A comparison of tissue gold levels in guinea pigs after treatment with Myochrysine intramuscularly and triethylphosphine gold chloride and Myochrysine administered orally. Agents Action 8:546, 1978.
113. Walz, D.T., Griswold, D.E., DiMartino, J., and Bumbier, E.E.: Distribution of gold in blood following administration of auranofin. J. Rheumatol. 6 (Suppl. 5): 56, 1979.
114. Gottlieb, N.L.: Comparative pharmacokinetics of parenteral and oral gold compounds. J. Rheumatol. 9 (Suppl. 8): 99, 1982.
115. Gerber, R.C., Paulus, H.E., and Jennrich, R.I.: Gold kinetics following aurothiomalate therapy: Use of a whole-body radiation counter. J. Lab. Clin. Med. 83:778, 1974.
116. Rubinstein, H.M., and Dietz, A.A.: Serum gold-levels in rheumatoid arthritis. Ann. Rheum. Dis. 32:128, 1973.
117. van Riel, P.L.C.M., Gribnau, F.W.J., and van de Putte, L.B.A.: Cell-bound gold in patients treated with aurothioglucose and with auranofin. A comparison of different methods of determination. J. Rheumatol. 10:574, 1983.
118. Blocka, K., Furst, D.E., Landaw, E., Dromgoole, S., Blomberg, A., and Paulus, H.E.: Single-dose pharmacokinetics of auranofin in rheumatoid arthritis. J. Rheumatol. 9 (Suppl. 8): 110, 1982.

119. Campion, D.S., Olsen, R., and Bohan, A.: Interaction of gold sodium thiomalate with serum albumin (abstract). J. Rheumatol. 1 (Suppl.): 112, 1974.
120. Lorber, A., Bovy, R.A., and Chang, C.C.: Relationship between serum gold content and distribution to serum immunoglobulins and complement. Nature New Biol. 236:250, 1972.
121. Smith, P.M., Smith, E.M., and Gottlieb, N.L.: Gold distribution in whole blood during chrysotherapy. J. Lab. Clin. Med. 82:930, 1973.
122. Lorber, A., Simon, T., and Wilcox, S.: In vivo gold kinetics—lymphocyte binding and effect on lymphocyte responsiveness (abstract). Arthritis Rheum. 20:126, 1977.
123. Graham, G.G., Haavisto, T.M., McNaught, P.J., Browne, C.D., and Champion, G.D.: The effect of smoking on the distribution of gold in blood. J. Rheumatol. 9:527, 1982.
124. James, D.W., Ludvigsen, N.W., Cleland, L.G., and Milazzo, S.C.: The influence of cigarette smoking on blood gold distribution during chrysotherapy. J. Rheumatol. 9:532, 1982.
125. Gottlieb, N.L., Smith, P.M., and Penneys, N.S.: Gold concentrations in hair, nail and skin during chrysotherapy. Arthritis Rheum. 17:56, 1974.
126. Weisman, M.H., Hardison, G.M., and Walz, D.: Studies of the intestinal metabolism of oral gold. J. Rheumatol. 7:633, 1980.
127. Lawrence, J.S.: Studies with radioactive gold. Ann. Rheum. Dis. 20:341, 1961.
128. Marmon, B.P., and Goodburn, G.M.: Effect of an organic gold salt on Eaton's primary atypical pneumonia agent and other observations. Nature 189:247, 1961.
129. Pruzanski, W., Leers, W.D., and Wardlaw, A.C.: Bacteriolytic and bactericidal activity of sera and synovial fluids in rheumatoid arthritis and in osteoarthritis. Arthritis Rheum. 17:207, 1974.
130. Persellin, R.H., and Ziff, M.: The effect of gold salt on lysosomal enzymes of the peritoneal macrophage. Arthritis Rheum. 9:57, 1966.
131. Paltemaa, S.: The inhibition of lysosomal enzymes by gold salts in human synovial fluid cells. Acta Rheum. Scand. 14:161, 1968.
132. Penneys, N.S., Ziboh, V., Gottlieb, N.L., et al.: Inhibition of prostaglandin synthesis and human epidermal enzymes by aurothiomalate in vitro: Possible actions of gold in pemphigus. J. Invest. Dermatol. 63:356, 1974.
133. Ennis, R.S., Granda, J.L., and Posner, A.S.: Effect of gold salts and other drugs on the release and activity of lysosomal hydrolases. Arthritis Rheum. 11:756, 1968.
134. Jessop, J.D., Vernon-Roberts, B., and Harris, J.: Effects of gold salts and prednisolone on inflammatory cells. Ann. Rheum. Dis. 32:294, 1973.
135. Niedermeier, W., Prillaman, W.W., and Griggs, J.H.: The effect of chrysotherapy on trace metals in patients with rheumatoid arthritis. Arthritis Rheum. 14:533, 1971.
136. Gerber, D.A.: Copper-catalyzed thermal aggregation of human gammaglobulin: inhibition by histidine, gold thiomalate, and penicillamine. Arthritis Rheum. 17:85, 1974.
137. Schultz, D.R., Volanakis, J.E., Arnold, P.I., et al.: Inactivation of C1 in rheumatoid synovial fluid, purified C1 and C1 esterase, by gold compounds. Clin. Exp. Immunol. 17:395, 1974.
138. Burge, J.J., Fearson, D.T., and Austen, K.F.: Inhibition of the alternative pathway of complement by gold sodium thiomalate in vitro. J. Immunol. 120:1625, 1978.
139. Libensen, L.: Toxicity and mode of action of the gold salts. Exp. Med. Surg. 3:146, 1945.
140. Castor, C.W.: Connective tissue activation. Arthritis Rheum. 15:504, 1972.
141. Lipsky, P.E., and Ziff, M.: Inhibition of antigen- and mitogen-induced human lymphocyte proliferation by gold compounds. J. Clin. Invest. 59:455, 1977.
142. Lies, R.B., Cardin, C., and Paulus, H.E.: Inhibition by gold of human lymphocyte stimulation. Ann. Rheum. Dis. 36:216, 1977.
143. Ho, P.P.K., Young, A.L., and Southard, G.L.: Methyl ester of N-formylmethionyl-leucyl-phenylalanine. Chemotactic responses of human blood monocytes and inhibition of gold compounds. Arthritis Rheum. 21:133, 1978.
144. Mowat, A.G.: Neutrophil chemotaxis in rheumatoid arthritis. Ann. Rheum. Dis. 37:1, 1978.
145. Measel, J.W., Jr.: Effect of gold on the immune response of mice. Infect. Immun. 11:350, 1975.
146. Ghaffar, A., McBride, W.H., and Cullen, R.T.: Interaction of tumor cells and activated macrophages in vitro: Modulation by *Corynebacterium parvum* and gold salt. J. Reticuloendothel. Soc. 20:283, 1976.
147. Persellin, R.H., Hess, E.V., and Ziff, M.: Effect of gold salt on the immune response. Arthritis Rheum. 10:99, 1967.
148. Clarke, A.K., Vernon-Roberts, B., and Currey, H.L.F.: Assessment of anti-inflammatory drugs in the rat using subcutaneous implants of polyurethane foam impregnated with dead tubercle bacilli. Ann. Rheum. Dis. 34:326, 1975.
149. Adam, M., Bartl, P., Deyl, Z., et al.: Uptake of gold by collagen in gold therapy. Ann. Rheum. Dis. 24:378, 1965.
150. Walz, D.T., DiMartino, M.J., and Misher, A.: Suppression of adjuvant-induced arthritis in the rat by gold sodium thiomalate. Ann. Rheum. Dis. 30:303, 1971.
151. Lewis, A.J., and Walz, D.T.: Immunopharmacology of gold. *In* Ellis, J.P., and West, G.B. (eds.): Progress in Medicinal Chemistry. Vol. 19. New York, Elsevier Biomedical Press, 1982, pp. 1–58.
152. Halla, J.T., Cassady, J., and Hardin, J.G.: Sequential gold and penicillamine therapy in rheumatoid arthritis: Comparative study of effectiveness and review of the literature. Am. J. Med. 72:423, 1982.
153. Kean, F.W., Lock, C.J.L., Howard-Lock, H.E., and Buchanan, W.W.: Prior gold therapy does not influence the adverse effects of D-penicillamine in rheumatoid arthritis. Arthritis Rheum. 25:917, 1982.
154. Webley, M., and Coomes, E.N.: An assessment of penicillamine therapy in rheumatoid arthritis and the influence of previous gold therapy. J. Rheumatol. 6:20, 1979.
155. Liang, M.H., and Fries, J.F.: Containing costs in chronic disease: Monitoring strategies in the gold therapy of rheumatoid arthritis. J. Rheumatol. 5:241, 1978.
156. Penneys, N.S., Ackerman, A.B., and Gottlieb, N.L.: Gold dermatitis. Arch. Dermatol. 109:372, 1974.
157. Iveson, J.M., Scott, D.G., Perera, W.D.H., et al.: Immunofluorescence of the skin in gold rashes—with particular reference to IgE. Ann. Rheum. Dis. 36:520, 1977.
158. Klinefelter, H.F.: Reinstitution of gold therapy in rheumatoid arthritis after mucocutaneous reactions. J. Rheumatol. 2:21, 1975.
159. Gottlieb, N.L., and Gray, R.G.: Diagnosis and management of adverse reactions from gold compounds. J. Anal. Tox. 2:173, 1978.
160. Beckett, V.L., Doyle, J.A., Hadley, G.A., and Spear, K.L.: Chrysiasis resulting from gold therapy in rheumatoid arthritis: Identification of gold by x-ray microanalysis. Mayo Clin. Proc. 57:773, 1982.
161. Jeffery, D.A., Biggs, D.F., Percy, J.S., and Russell, A.S.: Quantitation of gold in skin in chrysiasis. J. Rheumatol. 2:28, 1975.
162. Silverberg, D.S., Kidd, E.G., and Shnitka, T.K.: Gold nephropathy. A clinical and pathologic study. Arthritis Rheum. 13:812, 1970.
163. Törnroth, T., and Skrifvars, B.: Gold nephropathy prototype of membranous glomerulonephritis. Am. J. Pathol. 75:573, 1974.
164. Vaamonde, C.A., and Hunt, F.R.: The nephrotic syndrome as a complication of gold therapy. Arthritis Rheum. 13:826, 1970.
165. Davis, P., and Hughes, G.R.V.: Significance of eosinophilia during gold therapy. Arthritis Rheum. 17:964, 1974.
166. Deren, B., Masi, R., and Weksler, M.: Gold-associated thrombocytopenia. Arch. Intern. Med. 134:1012, 1974.
167. Stafford, B.T., and Crosby, W.H.: Late onset of gold-induced thrombocytopenia. JAMA 239:50, 1978.
168. McCarty, D.J., Brill, J.M., and Harrop, D.: Aplastic anemia secondary to gold-salt therapy: Report of a fatal case and a review of the literature. JAMA 179:655, 1962.
169. Harris, B.K.: Myocardial infarction after a gold-induced nitritoid reaction (letter to editor). Arthritis Rheum. 20:1561, 1977.
170. Winterbauer, R.H., Wilske, K.R., and Wheelis, R.F.: Diffuse pulmonary injury associated with gold treatment. N. Engl. J. Med. 294:919, 1976.
171. Gould, P.W., McCormack, P.L., and Palmer, D.G.: Pulmonary damage associated with sodium aurothiomalate therapy. J. Rheumatol. 4:252, 1977.
172. Favreau, M., Tannenbaum, H., and Lough, J.: Hepatic toxicity associated with gold therapy. Ann. Intern. Med. 87:717, 1977.
173. Howrie, D.L., and Gartner, Jr. J.C.: Gold-induced hepatotoxicity: Case report and review of the literature. J. Rheumatol. 9:727, 1982.
174. Stein, H.B., and Urowitz, M.B.: Gold-induced enterocolitis. J. Rheumatol. 3:21, 1976.
175. Fam, A.G., Paton, T.W., Shamess, C.J., and Lewis, A.J.: Fulminant colitis complicating gold therapy. J. Rheumatol. 7:479, 1980.
176. Hashimoto, A., Maeda, Y., Ito, H., et al.: Corneal chrysiasis—a clinical study in rheumatoid arthritis patients receiving gold therapy. Arthritis Rheum. 15:309, 1972.
177. Prouse, P.J., Kanski, J.J., and Gumpel, J.M.: Corneal Chrysiasis and clinical improvement with chrysotherapy in rheumatoid arthritis. Ann. Rheum. Dis. 40:564, 1981.
178. Wooley, P.H., Griffin, J., Panayi, G.S., Batchelor, J.R., Welsh, K.I., and Gibson, T.J.: HLA-DR antigens and toxic reaction to sodium thiomalate and D-penicillamine in patients with rheumatoid arthritis. N. Engl. J. Med. 303:300, 1980.
179. Coblyn, J.S., Weinblatt, M., Holdsworth, D., and Glass, D.: Gold-induced thrombocytopenia: A clinical and immunogenetic study of 23 patients. Ann. Intern. Med. 95:178, 1981.
180. Gran, J.T., Husby, G., and Thorsby, E.: HLA-DR antigens and gold toxicity. Ann. Rheum. Dis. 42:63, 1983.
181. Levinson, M.L., Lynch, J.P., III, and Bower, J.S.: Reversal of progressive, life-threatening gold hypersensitivity pneumonitis by corticosteroids. Am. J. Med. 71:908, 1981.
182. Gerber, R.C., and Paulus, H.E.: Gold therapy. Clin. Rheum. Dis. 1:307, 1975.

183. Lorber, A., Baumgartner, W.A., Bovy, R.A., et al.: Clinical application for heavy metal-complexing potential of acetylcysteine. J. Clin. Pharmacol. 13:332, 1973.
184. Bunch, T.W.: Gold overdose treated with BAL (letter editor). Arthritis Rheum. 19:123, 1976.
185. Godfrey, N.F., Peter, A., Simon, T.M., and Lorber, A.: IV. *N*-Acetylcysteine treatment of hematologic reaction to chrysotherapy. J. Rheumatol. 9:519, 1982.
186. Davis, P., and Barraclough, D.: Interaction of D-penicillamine with gold salts. Arthritis Rheum. 20:1413, 1977.
187. Schaeffer, N., Shaw, C.F., Thompson, H.O., and Satre, R.W.: Competition for protein-bound gold (1). Arthritis Rheum. 23:165, 1980.
188. Saphir, J.R., and Ney, R.G.: Delayed thrombocytopenic purpura after diminutive gold therapy. JAMA 195:7, 1966.
189. Ball, G.V.: Gold-induced thrombocytopenia: Response to vincristine? (letter to editor). Arthritis Rheum. 20:1288, 1977.
190. Marriott, H.J.L., and Peters, H.R.: Blood dyscrasias secondary to gold: With a case of hypoplastic anemia cured by splenectomy. Ann. Intern. Med. 32:864, 1950.
191. Gottlieb, N.L., Buchoff, H.S., Vidal, A.F., Germain, B.F., Gray, R.G., and Goldberg, E.S.: The course of severe gold-associated granulocytopenia. Clin. Res. 30:659-A, 1982 (Abstr.).
192. Baldwin, J.L., Storb, R., Thomas, E.D., et al.: Bone marrow transplantation in patients with gold-induced marrow aplasia. Arthritis Rheum. 20:1043, 1977.
193. Combs, R.J., Dentino, M.M., Lehrman, L., et al.: Gold toxicity and peritoneal dialysis. Arthritis Rheum. 19:936, 1976.

# Chapter 53
# D-Penicillamine

*Israeli A. Jaffe*

Penicillamine is a component of the penicillin molecule[1] which was identified in the urine of patients with chronic liver disease who were receiving penicillin for the treatment of intercurrent infections.[2] Walshe demonstrated its effectiveness as a copper chelating agent and introduced it into the treatment of Wilson's disease.[3] In addition, it has been shown to be effective in treatment of cystinuria,[4] heavy metal poisoning,[5] and rheumatoid arthritis (RA).[6] It has possible but as yet unproved efficacy in the management of biliary cirrhosis[7] and chronic active hepatitis.[8] It appears to have a role in the treatment of scleroderma,[9,10] but this has not been confirmed by controlled clinical trials.

## CHEMISTRY

The structural formula of penicillamine (Fig. 53–1) shows that it is a sulfhydryl amino acid differing from cysteine by the presence of two methyl groups in the $\beta$-carbon position ($\beta$,$\beta$-dimethylcysteine, or 3-mercaptovaline). It may be prepared from natural penicillin by a semisynthetic process, or it may be made entirely synthetically. Regardless of the mode of preparation, all the penicillamine currently employed in clinical medicine is the pure D-form, and penicillamine will denote only the D-isomer unless otherwise specified.

## METABOLISM

Penicillamine is well absorbed from the gastrointestinal tract but may react with certain constituents of the diet, particularly metals,[11] and may also interact directly with other drugs in the upper gastrointestinal tract (see Dosage). Approximately 50 percent of an orally administered dose can be accounted for by analysis of urine and feces.[12] Using $^{14}$C-D-penicillamine, recovery of radioactivity was 85 percent. The discrepancy between the results obtained by the chemical and radioactive measurements is believed to be due to bacterial degradation of the drug in the colon, which yields chemically nonidentifiable products.[12] Very little free penicillamine is found in the urine; most of it is present in the oxidized form, as either the internal disulfide (penicillamine-penicillamine) or the mixed disulfide (penicillamine-cysteine).[12] A third major metabolite has recently been identified, S-methyl penicillamine.[13] In animal studies using radioactive penicillamine, it was found that the drug had its greatest affinity and highest accumulation in collagen-containing organs such as skin and tendon, in contrast to liver and kidney.[14] There was also a high uptake in organs rich in protein content such as pancreas and testicle.[14] In the plasma, binding was greatest to albumin, $\alpha$-globulin, and ceruloplasmin.[14] In dogs, it was found that following discontinuance of penicillamine the drug very rapidly disappeared from the urine; however, the mixed disulfide and internal disulfide were demonstrable for more than 3 months after the agent had been stopped.[15] This might explain the persistence of drug effect as well as certain of the toxicities for long periods after treatment has been discontinued.

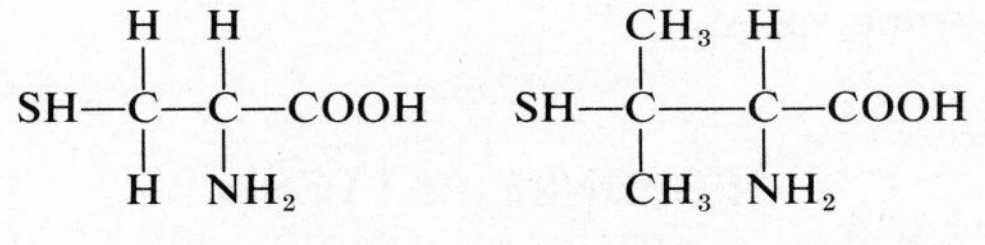

CYSTEINE PENICILLAMINE

**Figure 53–1.** The chemical structure of penicillamine. The drug is an analogue of the naturally occurring amino acid cysteine, with $CH_3$ groups replacing $H^+$ at the B carbon position.

## CLINICAL PHARMACOLOGY

Penicillamine is prepared as a 250 mg or 125 mg capsule or scored tablet of 250 mg, and a 50 mg tablet is also available in England. The pharmacologic properties of the compound that have been demonstrated to occur in man are chelation of divalent cations,[3] SH-SS interchange,[16] and thiazolidine formation, which gives rise to dermolathyrism[17] and vitamin $B_6$ antagonism.[18] It is not known whether any of these actions are responsible for the antirheumatoid properties of the drug. The chelating properties form the basis for its use in the treatment of Wilson's disease and heavy metal poisoning. When administered to patients with RA or cystinuria, a minimal depletion of copper and zinc has been reported,[19] but this is generally well compensated for in a normal diet.[20] Depletion of these metals may, however, be partially responsible for the development of taste abnormalities (see below). The SH-SS interchange reaction between penicillamine and cystine gives rise to the mixed disulfide, penicillamine-cysteine.[16] This is considerably more soluble than cystine and results in a decrease in size of cystine calculi, and their ultimate dissolution.[4] The anti-vitamin $B_6$ effect of penicillamine is due to the formation of a thiazolidine between penicillamine and pyridoxal phosphate.[18] The anti-vitamin $B_6$ effect does not appear to be clinically significant, since concomitant administration of the vitamin does not influence either the efficacy of the drug or the incidence of side effects.[21] Vitamin $B_6$ supplements are recommended, however, for growing children and adult patients whose nutrition is marginal.

The dermolathyrogenic effect of penicillamine is also due to thiazolidine formation—in this reaction, between penicillamine and the aldehyde cross-links of collagen[22] (see Chapters 14 and 76). This may be demonstrated in skin biopsies from patients receiving penicillamine, particularly when given in large doses.[23] Wound healing is not impaired in patients receiving penicillamine.[24] The collagen formed in wound healing is the type III or embryonal form, whose keto crosslinks do not react with penicillamine, in contrast to the aldehyde crosslinks of type I collagen.[25]

## INDICATIONS

Penicillamine is effective in treatment of active RA, seropositive or seronegative, and in patients with juvenile rheumatoid arthritis.[26] Its efficacy was first established by the United Kingdom Multi-Center trial,[27] and subsequent controlled clinical trials showed that it was as effective as gold[28] and azathioprine.[29] It was found that a 600-mg daily dose gave a therapeutic result comparable (statistically) to that produced by 1200 mg, with considerably fewer side effects and withdrawals.[30] It has been of particular value in RA associated with certain extra-articular manifestations, such as vasculitis,[31] rheumatoid lung disease,[32] Felty's syndrome,[33] rheumatoid nodulosis,[34] and amyloidosis.[35] A recent report demonstrated radiographic evidence of healing of osseous lesions in a child with juvenile rheumatoid arthritis (JRA) treated with penicillamine.[36]

Penicillamine is not effective in ankylosing spondylitis,[37] psoriatic arthritis, or other B-27 associated diseases for which it has been tried.[38] There have been further reports of the usefulness of penicillamine in the treatment of progressive systemic sclerosis[9,10] (see Chapter 76). These studies are anecdotal and retrospective, and a controlled clinical trial of penicillamine in this disease now seems warranted.

## DOSAGE

Because of the high incidence of toxic and untoward reactions to the drug (see below), there have been continuous modifications in the dosage regimens employed for its use in RA.[39-41] The basic principle underlying all these schedules is that the drug is introduced gradually, with slow increments, until a clinical response is achieved. Usually, that dose may have to be adjusted according to the changing pattern of disease activity.

From the time that therapy is initiated to the earliest evidence of clinical response, a period of 8 to 12 weeks may be required. A similar latency is noted after increase or decrease in dosage. As a result, it is currently recommended that increments in the maintenance dose of penicillamine be made at 8- to 12-week intervals, particularly since the *rate of dosage increment* appears to be a more significant determinant for the development of certain untoward effects than the absolute magnitude of the maintenance dose.[41] Typically, a patient will be started at a single daily dosage of 250 mg, given approximately 1½ hours before a meal, and not together with any other medication.[42,43] If there is no clinical or laboratory evidence of response after approximately 2 months, the dosage is raised to 500 mg, which may also be given once daily. Alternatively, some workers include a treatment period at 375 mg per day after 8 weeks, rather than directly doubling the starting dose. At the end of 6 months, most patients who will benefit from the drug will have shown some evidence of clinical improvement. If required, the dose may be raised to 750 mg for the next 12 weeks and, in a limited number of cases, to 1000 mg a day, preferably given in a single dose. As indicated earlier, the maintenance dose of penicillamine is highly variable not only from patient to patient but in the evolution of the individual patient's own treatment program, and the aforementioned outline serves only as a guide. The availability of the 125-mg dosage form permits somewhat greater flexibility and better adjustments of the maintenance dose. In some patients who have shown an incomplete response, an increase in the daily dose by 125 mg may provide greater suppression of the disease without added toxicity. In addition, as will be indicated below, certain side effects are dose related, and a reduction in the maintenance level by as little as 125 mg per day may result in disappearance of an untoward reaction without significantly compromising the quality of the response. The 125-mg dosage is also useful in children with JRA, for whom the average daily dose is 500 to 625 mg.[44] Some patients report an increase in articular discomfort when therapy is begun. This usually subsides with time, but may be dose limiting and require discontinuance of therapy in some cases.

## RESPONSE PATTERN

The pattern of improvement in a penicillamine-responsive patient is similar to that observed with a remission induced by gold salts. There is a gradual decrease in the *duration* of morning stiffness and in the severity and intensity of pain. This is often followed by a diminution in swelling, effusion, and the size of nodules. Often, patients will report an increased sense of well-being and a decrease in easy fatigability. Later in the course of treatment, laboratory studies will often reveal a fall in the RF titer, decrease in the ESR, and a rise in hemoglobin.[21]

When penicillamine therapy is begun, analgesics and anti-inflammatory drugs, including steroids, must be continued. As the clinical response evolves, these agents may be gradually decreased, although steroid withdrawal often requires several years to be completed. Exacerbations in rheumatoid disease activity may be seen during the first 1 to 2 years of therapy; however, these are often self-limited and usually subside within a 2- to 3-month period without the necessity of an increase in dosage. Late in the course of treatment, true secondary failures have been observed. In some patients, discontinuance of the drug for 6 to 12 months followed by gradual reintroduction may again give a good therapeutic response.

## SIDE EFFECTS AND TOXICITY

The toxicities and untoward effects that may be produced by penicillamine are many and diverse and have limited its clinical usefulness. As indicated previously, experience with the newer dosage regimens has shown that certain of these side effects can be reduced in frequency and severity by the practice of "go low—go very slow." These reactions have been reported in patients given penicillamine regardless of their underlying disease, but most published reports of toxicity are in RA patients, since they comprise the largest number exposed to the drug. It has been observed that most of the side effects will be encountered during the first 18 months of therapy (Fig. 53–2), and it is less likely for a major toxic reaction to appear for the first time after that period.[45]

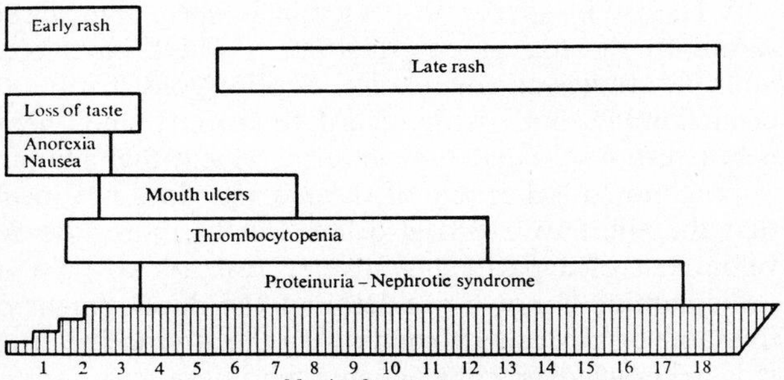


**Figure 53–2.** The chronopharmacology of penicillamine. (After Balme, H.W., and Huskisson, E.C.: J. Rheumatol. 4:Suppl. 8, 21-07, 1975.) This depicts the peak incidence of some of the more common side effects of penicillamine during a course of therapy with a maintenance dose of 1 gram per day. Most of the serious reactions will have developed during the first 18 months of treatment. Aplastic anemia was not included in this illustration, but it may occur at any time, particularly after an increment in dosage.

*Hematologic* toxicity is certainly the most serious of the untoward effects that may be produced by penicillamine. *Leukopenia, thrombocytopenia,* and *aplastic anemia* have all been observed. Thrombocytopenia may occur as an isolated event, when it may respond to a reduction in dosage, or it may herald the development of more widespread bone marrow failure. The presence of normal numbers of megakaryocytes in the bone marrow will resolve this question. A white blood cell count below 3000 per cubic millimeter or a platelet count below 100,000 per cubic millimeter mandates a temporary discontinuance of the drug until the severity of the reaction can be assessed. Complete blood counts, including platelet counts, must be done every 2 weeks for the first 6 months and monthly thereafter. Prescriptions for penicillamine should *never be labeled refillable.* If aplastic anemia develops, the patient should be hospitalized and placed in reverse isolation. Immediately after cultures have been obtained, a parenteral antibiotic regimen is instituted consisting of carbenicillin, 10 grams every 8 hours, oxacillin, 2 grams every 6 hours, and gentamicin, 80 mg every 8 hours. Mycostatin oral suspension, 15 ml by mouth every 4 hours, is given in an oral lavage, which is swirled and then swallowed. If the patient has been on corticosteroids, these must be maintained, but they should not be *added* to the regimen for the management of aplastic anemia. In some patients with thrombocytopenia only, steroids may be required to control bleeding. Weeks and rarely months may elapse before marrow function commences to return. During this time, the patient remains in constant risk of sepsis, and continued vigilance is mandatory. Granulocyte transfusions have not been effective, but fresh platelets have sometimes helped in an acute hemorrhagic crisis due to thrombocytopenia. Patients who have had major hematologic toxicity to penicillamine should never be rechallenged with the drug. In some patients who had thrombocytopenia only, retreatment has been accomplished without recurrence of the toxicity.

*Proteinuria* is secondary to an immune-complex, membranous glomerulopathy (Fig. 53–3) and has been encountered in up to 20 percent of patients receiving the drug.[46] Although the peak incidence for development of this side effect is usually between 6 and 9 months after commencement of treatment, proteinuria may clear with a slight reduction in daily dosage such as 125 to 250 mg. A complete urinalysis should be performed according to the same schedule as the hematologic studies. If urinary protein excretion exceeds 2 grams per 24 hours or if there is evidence of *nephrotic syndrome* or *gross hematuria,* the treatment should be terminated and the patient not rechallenged. After discontinuance of the drug, a period of up to 1 year may be required for urinary abnormalities to disappear completely. In patients who have been studied with renal biopsy following withdrawal of the drug, there was healing of the lesions and disappearance of the immune complexes.[47] Microscopic hematuria during the course of penicillamine treatment has been found to be a benign occurrence and does not mandate discontinuance of therapy provided that it remains stable.[48]

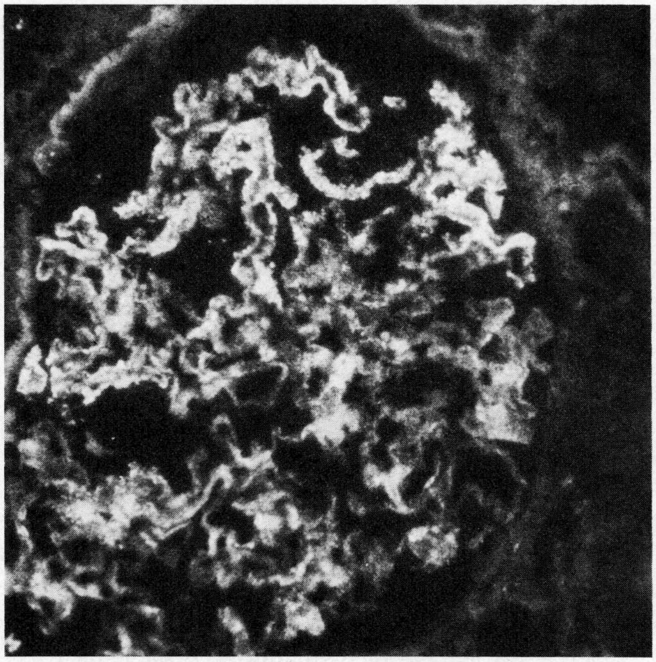

**Figure 53–3.** Renal biopsy from a patient with nephrotic syndrome secondary to penicillamine. The basement membrane of the glomerulus stains in an intense granular pattern with fluorescinated anti-human IgG and fluorescinated anti-human complement. Staining gradually disappears after treatment has been discontinued.

*Dermatological reactions* include skin rash, which is probably the most common of the side effects encountered with the drug. Simple pruritus can often be controlled by the addition of an antihistamine such as hydroxyzine (Atarax) or cyproheptadine (Periactin). Often pruritus and mild rash will be transitory and will clear despite continuance of the medication. Late rashes tend to be unresponsive to antihistamine therapy or to reduction in dosage, and generally require discontinuance of the drug. The occurrence of the skin rash and oral lesions simultaneously should alert the clinician to the possibility of a pemphigoid type reaction, which mandates discontinuance of the drug[49] (see below).

*Mucous membrane lesions* similar to those seen in aphthous stomatitis have been observed. Oral (or genital) ulcers may clear on reduction of the maintenance dose, but often therapy must be discontinued and the patient not rechallenged.

*Autoimmune syndromes* also occur. Penicillamine administration has been reported to be responsible for the development of Goodpasture's syndrome,[50] myasthenia gravis,[51] polymyositis,[52] pemphigus,[49] lupus erythematosus,[53] and Sjögren's syndrome.[54] While the number of individual case reports of each of these entities has been few, a high index of suspicion is warranted should a patient receiving penicillamine develop features of any of these syndromes. In such an instance, the drug must be discontinued and the patient not rechallenged. As noted previously with other toxicities, these entities have been encountered in patients receiving penicillamine regardless of their underlying disease. It is not the rheumatoid diathesis per se that predisposes to their development, and the mechanism by which penicillamine produces these autoimmune phenomena is not understood (see below).

*Hypogeusia* or blunting or loss of taste perception is very commonly encountered and may persist for up to 3 months following its onset. It gradually clears even though therapy is continued, and patients should be urged not to discontinue the drug because of this particular reaction. Some investigators report an accelerated return to normal taste if supplements of copper or zinc are given,[55] but it has been shown that with the lower dosages of penicillamine currently employed, such supplementation may abrogate the therapeutic response.[56] No instances of permanent taste impairment have been reported.

In addition, certain miscellaneous side effects may infrequently be encountered. Drug fever has been described. It occurs usually during the third week of therapy, and is often associated with a morbilliform eruption. When the drug is stopped, fever and rash quickly subside, but these patients should not be rechallenged. Other side effects which have been infrequently observed have been a benign enlargement of the breasts (mammary gigantism)[57] and hepatotoxicity.[58]

## INDICATIONS, CONTRAINDICATIONS, AND PRECAUTIONS

As indicated previously, penicillamine is employed in the treatment of patients with RA, seropositive or seronegative, whose disease has not responded to general, conservative measures. It usually will be considered after a trial of chrysotherapy has been abandoned, because of either toxicity or failure of response. Some workers will employ penicillamine before gold salts, particularly if there are present certain of the extra-articular manifestations which have been shown to be favorably influenced by penicillamine therapy.

Penicillamine is contraindicated in pregnancy, although the literature is in some conflict on this point.[59,60]

A history of allergy to penicillin is *not* a contraindication to the use of penicillamine.[61] There have been multiple studies on the relation of prior gold therapy to penicillamine, both with regard to toxicity and therapeutic response. There is general agreement that a failure to respond to either one of these drugs does not mean that the alternative will also fail. Furthermore, the development of a particular adverse reaction to gold or penicillamine is not a predictor of the development of the same or any other toxicity with the alternative drug. It is acknowledged that patients who develop a serious toxicity to gold, particularly proteinuria, are more likely to have proteinuria during penicillamine, but this is far from absolute.[62-65]

As indicated above, prescriptions for penicillamine should *never be made refillable.* Since hematologic toxicity may be precipitate in onset and develop in the

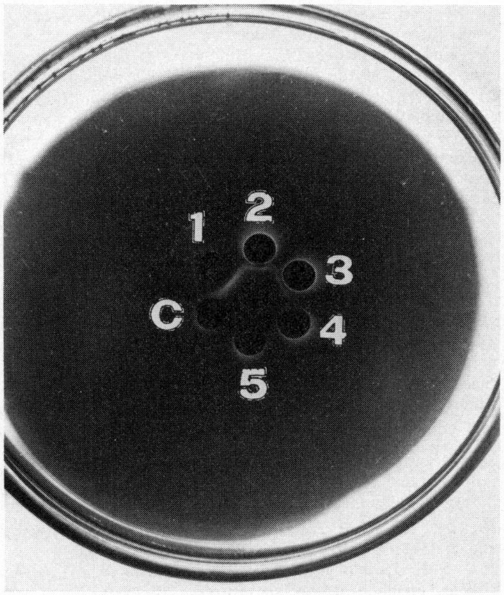


**Figure 53–4.** The effect of penicillamine therapy on complexes as measured by precipitation with a purified IgM rheumatoid factor. (Courtesy of Dr. Robert Winchester.) Well No. 1 contains synovial fluid, and well No. 2 contains serum from the same patient prior to treatment. Well No. 3 shows a decrease in the amount of complexes after 6 weeks on the drug. Wells No. 4 and No. 5 show the absence of serum complexes at 3 and 6 months, respectively. Well C is normal serum. A serial examination of synovial fluid was not possible as the effusion had reabsorbed.

interval between routine blood studies, patients should be alerted to report to the physician if they develop any evidence of mucocutaneous bleeding or unexplained fever. Bone marrow toxicity is particularly likely to occur *after a dosage increment*; hence careful surveillance is especially needed at these times. Patients over the age of 60 are at greater risk for development of hematologic toxicity and hence require more close supervision.

In summary, penicillamine therapy must be discontinued in the event that any of the following untoward reactions develop: aplastic anemia, leukopenia below 3000 per cubic millimeter, thrombocytopenia below 100,000 per cubic millimeter, nephrotic syndrome, increasing hematuria persistent for more than 30 days, or any of the autoimmune syndromes described above.

## MECHANISM OF ACTION

The mechanism of action of penicillamine in RA, like that for gold salts, is not known. The drug is neither cytotoxic[66] nor anti-inflammatory,[67] and it is virtually without effect in animal models of experimental arthritis.[68] It has been shown that the prolonged administration of penicillamine to RA patients is associated with a reduction in or disappearance of immune complexes, in both the serum and synovial fluid (Figs. 53–4 and 53–5).[69] Whether this reduction in complexes is the mechanism by which penicillamine exerts its therapeutic effect or is simply a reflection of a more basic action, analogous to the fall in RF titer, is not clear at this time.

The effect of penicillamine on lymphocyte transformation in vitro has been the subject of study by several investigators. Some workers have shown an inhibition of transformation in the presence of the drug,[70,71] while others found that it enhanced responsiveness to mitogen.[72] This apparent discrepancy may be due to differences in experimental design, especially variation in timing of the addition of the penicillamine with respect to the mitogen. In vitro, the addition of copper in minute amounts to cell cultures with penicillamine greatly augments the suppression of lymphocyte responsiveness.[73] In a subsequent study, this synergistic inhibition by penicillamine and copper salts was found to be restricted solely to human helper T lymphocytes; suppressor T lymphocytes and B lymphocytes were not affected.[74]

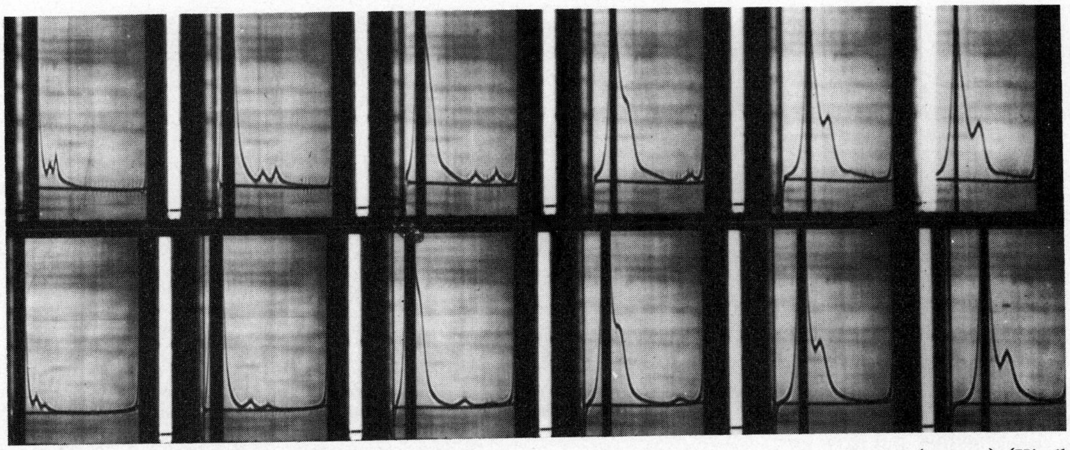

**Figure 53–5.** The ultracentrifugal pattern of serum proteins before treatment (top) and after 3 months on the drug (bottom). (Kindly performed by Dr. Henry Kunkel.) Serum was diluted 1:1 with saline. Centrifugation was at 52,640 rpm and proceeds from left to right. Pictures were taken at 16, 32, 48, 64, 80, and 90 minutes. The post-treatment pattern shows a reduction in the 22S complex, 19S macroglobulin, and the intermediate gamma globulin complexes.

Peripheral blood lymphocytes obtained from patients receiving penicillamine, show a normal response to mitogenic stimulation.[75] Other possible explanations for the mode of action that have been suggested are the copper chelating properties,[76] the anti-vitamin $B_6$ effect,[77] the effect on collagen, and the inhibition by penicillamine in vitro of the denaturation of human gamma globulin.[78]

The effect of penicillamine on lymphocyte subpopulations is currently under investigation in several laboratories. The autoimmune syndromes produced by the drug have generated considerable interest with respect to the possibility that they might represent a clue as to the primary locus of action of the agent in RA. Simple haptene formation could explain certain of the autoimmune phenomena. A haptene between penicillamine and the interepithelial cement substance in skin, for example, could explain the development of pemphigus. Similar haptene formation between penicillamine and acetylcholine receptor might be expected to elicit antibody, resulting in development of clinical myasthenia gravis.[79] There is, however, an alternative explanation which has been suggested for these phenomena. An effect of penicillamine on a subpopulation of T lymphocytes might result in enhancement of certain components of the immune system, resulting in a partial loss of tolerance to self antigens. Such a perturbation of the immunoregulatory mechanism might be of therapeutic value in RA. The report of a patient who experienced both penicillamine-induced nephrotic syndrome and pemphigus[80] and the increased association of spontaneous myasthenia and pemphigus[81,82] indirectly support this hypothesis. Immunomodulation and immune enhancement are currently subjects of increasing interest with respect to their possible therapeutic implications in RA[83,84] (Chapter 55). It is perhaps relevant in this regard that thymic and lymph node hyperplasia was consistently found in rhesus monkeys during chronic penicillamine administration,[85] and thymic hyperplasia was recently reported in a penicillamine-treated RA patient who was subjected to thymectomy after development of drug-induced myasthenia gravis.[86]

## References


1. Abraham, E.P., Chain, E., Baker, W., and Robinson, R.: Penicillamine: A characteristic degradation product of penicillin. Nature 151:107, 1943.
2. Walshe, J.M.: Disturbances of amino acid metabolism following liver injury. Quart. J. Med. 22:483, 1953.
3. Walshe, J.M.: Wilson's disease. New oral therapy. Lancet 1:25, 1956.
4. Crawhall, J.C., Scowen, E.F., and Watts, R.W.E.: Effects of penicillamine on cystinuria. Br. Med. J. 1:588, 1963.
5. Boulding, J.E., and Baker, R.A.: The treatment of metal poisoning with penicillamine. Lancet 2:985, 1957.
6. Jaffe, I.A.: Comparison of the effect of plasmapheresis and penicillamine on the level of circulating rheumatoid factor. Ann. Rheum. Dis. 22:71, 1963.
7. Jain, S., Scheuer, P.J., Samourian, S., McGee, J. O'D., and Sherlock, S.: A controlled trial of D-penicillamine in primary biliary cirrhosis. Lancet 1:831, 1977.
8. Stern, R.B., Wilkinson, S.P., Howorth, P.J.N., and Williams, R.: Controlled trial of synthetic D-penicillamine in maintenance therapy for active chronic hepatitis. Gut 18:19, 1977.
9. Kang, B., Veres-Thorner, C., Hereida, R., Cha, E., Bose, S., and Schwatrz, M.: Successful treatment of far-advanced progressive systemic sclerosis by D-penicillamine. J. Allergy Clin. Immunol. 69:297, 1982.
10. Steen, V.D., Medsger, T.A. Jr., and Rodnan, G.P.: D-Penicillamine therapy in progressive systemic sclerosis (scleroderma) a retrospective analysis. Ann. Intern Med. 97:652, 1982.
11. Lyle, W.H., and Pearcey, D.F.: Inhibition of penicillamine-induced cupruresis by oral iron. Proc. R. Soc. Med. 70(Suppl. 3):48, 1977.
12. Perett, D.: An outline of D-penicillamine metabolism. Proc. R. Soc. Med. 70 (Suppl. 3):61, 1977.
13. Perett, D., Sneddon, W., and Stephens, A.D.: Studies on D-penicillamine metabolism in cystinuria and rheumatoid arthritis: Isolation of S-methyl-D-penicillamine. Biochem. Pharmacol. 25:259, 1976.
14. Ruiz-Torres, A.: Zur Pharmakokinetik und zum Stoffwechsel von D- und L-Penicillamin, 2. Mitteilung: Verteilung von D- und L-Penicillamin-$^{14}C$ im Organismus der Ratte nach peroraler Verabfolgung. Arzneim. Forsch. (Drug Res.) 24:1043, 1974.
15. Wei, P., and Sass-Kortsak, A.: Urinary excretion and renal clearances of D-penicillamine in humans and the dog. Gastroenterology 58:288, 970.
16. Tabachnik, M., Eisen, H.N., and Levine, B.: New mixed disulfide: Penicillamine-cysteine. Nature 174:701, 1954.
17. Nimni, M.E., and Bavetta, L.A.: Collagen defect induced by penicillamine. Science 150:905, 1965.
18. Kuchinskas, E.J., and du Vigneaud, V.: An increased vitamin $B_6$ requirement in the rat on a diet containing L-penicillamine. Arch. Biochem. 66:1, 1957.
19. Bostrom, H., and Wester, P.O.: Excretion of trace elements in two penicillamine-treated cases of cystinuria. Acta Med. Scand. 181:475, 1967.
20. Lyle, W.H.: Penicillamine and zinc. Lancet 2:1140, 1974.
21. Jaffe, I.A.: The effect of penicillamine on the laboratory parameters in rheumatoid arthritis. Arthritis Rheum. 8:1064, 1965.
22. Nimni, M.E., Deshmukh, K., Gerth, N., and Bavetta, L.A.: Changes in collagen metabolism associated with the administration of penicillamine and various amino and thiol compounds. Biochem. Pharmacol. 18:707, 1969.
23. Harris, E.D., and Sjoerdsma, A.: Effect of penicillamine on human collagen and its possible application to treatment of scleroderma. Lancet 2:996, 1966.
24. Ansell, B.M., Moran, H., and Arden, G.P.: Penicillamine and wound healing in rheumatoid arthritis. Proc. R. Soc. Med. 70(Suppl. 3):75, 1977.
25. Bailey, A.J., Bazin, S., Sims, T.J., Le Louis, M., Nicoletis, C., and Delaunay, A.: Characterization of the collagen of human hypertrophic and normal scars. Biochem. Biophys. Acta 405:412, 1975.
26. Hill, H.F.H.: Treatment of rheumatoid arthritis with penicillamine. Sem. Arthritis Rheum. 6:361, 1977.
27. Multi-Center Trial Group: Controlled trial of D(-) penicillamine in severe rheumatoid arthritis. Lancet 1:275, 1973.
28. Huskisson, E.C., Gibson, T.J., Balme, H.W., Berry, H., Burry, H.C., Grahame, R., Dudley Hart, F., Henderson, D.R.F., and Wojtulewski, J.A.: Trial comparing D-penicillamine and gold in rheumatoid arthritis. Preliminary report. Ann. Rheum. Dis. 33:532, 1974.
29. Berry, H., Liyange, R., Durance, C.G., and Berger, L.: Trial comparing azathioprine and penicillamine in treatment of rheumatoid arthritis. Ann. Rheum. Dis. 35:542, 1976.
30. Dixon, A. St. J., Davies, J., Dormandy, T.L., Hamilton, E.B.D., Holt, P.J.L., Mason, R.M., Thompson, M., Weber, J.C.P., and Zutshi, D.W.: Synthetic D(-) penicillamine in rheumatoid arthritis. Double-blind controlled study of a high and a low dosage regimen. Ann. Rheum. Dis. 34:416, 1975.
31. Jaffe, I.A.: Rheumatoid vasculitis report of a second case treated with penicillamine. Arthritis Rheum. 11:585, 1968.
32. Lorber, A.: Penicillamine therapy for rheumatoid lung disease: Effects of protein sulfhydryl groups. Nature 210:1235, 1966.
33. Blau, S., and Meiselas, L.: Regression of splenomegaly with hematologic recovery in Felty's syndrome due to D-penicillamine. A case report. Meadowbrook Hosp. J. 5:16, 1971–1972.
34. Ginsberg, M.H., Genant, H.K., Yü, T.S.F., and McCarty, D.J.: Rheumatoid nodulosis: An unusual variant of rheumatoid disease. Arthritis Rheum. 18:49, 1975.
35. Lake., B., and Andrews, G.: Rheumatoid arthritis with amyloidosis and malabsorption syndrome. Effect of D-pencillamine. Am. J. Med. 44:105, 1968.
36. Ansell, B.M.: Chronic arthritis in childhood. Ann. Rheum. Dis. 37:107, 1978.
37. Leca, A.P., and Camus, J.P.: Ankylosing spondylitis: Treatment failures with D-penicillamine. Nouv. Presse Med. 4:112, 1975.
38. Bird, H.A., and Dixon, A. St. J.: Failure of D-penicillamine to affect peripheral joint involvement in ankylosing spondylitis or HLA B-27 associated arthropathy. Ann. Rheum. Dis. 36:289, 1977.
39. Day, A.T., Golding, J.R., Lee, P.N., and Butterworth, A.D.: Penicillamine in rheumatoid disease: A long-term study. Br. Med. J. 1:180, 1974.
40. Jaffe, I.A.: The technique of penicillamine administration in rheumatoid arthritis. Arthritis Rheum. 18:513, 1975.
41. Jaffe, I.A.: D-Penicillamine. Bull. Rheum. Dis. 28:948, 1978.
42. Schnua, A., Osman, M.A., Patel, R.B., Welling, P.G., and Sundstrom,

W.R.: Influence of food on the bio-availability of penicillamine. J. Rheumatol. 10:95, 1983.
43. Harkness, J.A.L., and Blake, D.R.: Penicillamine nephropathy and iron. Lancet 2:1368, 1982.
44. Ansell, B., and Hall, M.: Penicillamine. Arthritis Rheum. 20(Suppl):536, 1977.
45. Balme, H.W., and Huskisson, E.C.: Chronopharmacology of penicillamine and gold. Scand. J. Rheumatol. 4(Suppl. 8):21, 1975.
46. Bacon, P.A., Tribe, C.R., Mackenzie, J.C., Verrier-Jones J., Cumming, R.H., and Amer, B.: Penicillamine nephropathy in rheumatoid arthritis. A clinical pathological and immunological study. Quart. J. Med. 45:661, 1976.
47. Jaffe, I.A., Treser, G., Suzuki, Y., and Ehrenreich, T.: Nephropathy induced by D-penicillamine. Ann. Intern. Med. 69:549, 1968.
48. Barraclough, D., Cunningham, T.J., and Muirden, K.D.: Microscopic haematuria in patients with rheumatoid arthritis on D-penicillamine. Aust. N. Z. J. Med. 11:706, 1981.
49. Benveniste, M., Crouzet, J., Homberg, J.C., Lessana, M., Camus, J.P., and Hewitt, J.: Pemphigus induced by D-penicillamine in rheumatoid arthritis. Nouv. Presse Med. 4:3125, 1975.
50. Sternlieb, I., Bennett, B., and Scheinberg, I.H.: D-Penicillamine induced Goodpasture's syndrome in Wilson's disease. Ann. Intern. Med. 82:673, 1975.
51. Bucknall, R.C., Dixon, A. St. J., and Glieb, E.N.: Myasthenia gravis associated with penicillamine treatment for rheumatoid arthritis. Br. Med. J. 1:600, 1975.
52. Schrader, P.L., Peters, H.A., and Dahl, D.S.: Polymyositis and penicillamine. Arch. Neurol. 27:456, 1972.
53. Crouzet, J., Camus, J.P., Leca, A.P., Guillien, P., and Lievre, J.A.: Lupus induced by D-penicillamine during the treatment of rheumatoid arthritis. Ann. Med. Interne 125:71, 1974.
54. May, V., Aristoff, H., and Lecoq, G.: Syndrome de Gougerot-Sjögren induit par la D-penicillamine. A propos d'un cas. Revue Rheumat. 44:497, 1977.
55. Henkin, R.I., Keiser, H.R., Jaffe, I.A., Sternlieb, I., and I.H.: Decreased taste sensitivity after D-penicillamine reversed by cooper administration. Lancet 2:1268, 1967.
56. Mery, C., Delrieu, F., Ghozlan, R., Saporta, F., Simon, B., Amor, C., Menkes, J., and Delbarre, F.: Controlled trial of D-penicillamine in rheumatoid arthritis. Dose effect and the role of zinc. Scand. J. Rheumatol. 5:241, 1976.
57. Desai, S.N.: Sudden gigantism of breasts: Drug induced? Br. J. Plast. Surg. 26:371, 1973.
58. Rosenbaum, J., Katz, W.A., and Schumacher, H.R.: Hepatotoxicity associated with use of D-penicillamine in rheumatoid arthritis. Ann. Rheum. Dis. 39:152, 1980.
59. Scheinberg, I.H., and Sternlieb, I.: Pregnancy in penicillamine treated patients with Wilson's disease. N. Engl. J. Med. 293:1300, 1975.
60. Mjolnerod, O.K., Rasmussen, K., Dommerud, S.A., and Gjeruldsen, S.T.: Congenital connective-tissue defect probably due to D-penicillamine. Lancet 1:673, 1971.
61. Bell, C.L., and Graziano, F.M.: The safety of administration of penicillamine to penicillin-sensitive individuals. Abstract, A.R.A. Ann. Meeting, Boston, Mass., 1981.
62. Webley, M., and Coomes, E.: An assessment of penicillamine therapy in rheumatoid arthritis and the influence of previous gold therapy. J. Rheumatol. 6:20, 1979.
63. Steven, M.M., Hunter, J.A., Murdoch, R.M., and Capell, H.A.: Does the order of second-line treatment in rheumatoid arthritis matter? Br. Med. J. 1:79, 1982.
64. Kean, W.F., Lock, C.J.L., Howard-Lock, H.E., and Buchanan, W.W.: Prior gold therapy does not influence the adverse effects of D-penicillamine in rheumatoid arthritis. Arthritis Rheum. 25:917, 1982.
65. Halla, J.T., Cassasy, J., and Hardin, J.G.: Sequential gold and penicillamine therapy in rheumatoid arthritis. Am. J. Med. 72:423, 1982.
66. Merryman, P., Jaffe, I.A., and Ehrenfeld, E.: Effect of D-penicillamine on poliovirus replication in HeLa cells. J. Virol. 13:881, 1974.
67. Friedrich, L., and Zimmerman, F.: Zur Pharmakologie von D-Penicillamin. Arzneim. Forsch. (Drug Res.) 25:162, 1975.
68. Liyange, S.P., and Currey, H.L.: Failure of oral D-penicillamine to modify adjuvant arthritis or immune response in the rat. Ann. Rheum. Dis. 31:521, 1972.
69. Jaffe, I.A.: Penicillamine treatment of rheumatoid arthritis: Effect on immune complexes. Ann. N.Y. Acad. Sci. 256:330, 1975.
70. Schumacher, K., Maerker-Alzer, G., and Preuss, R.: Effect of D-penicillamine on lymphocyte function. Arzneim. Forsch. (Drug Res.) 25:603, 1975.
71. Merryman, P., and Jaffe, I.A.: Effect of penicillamine on the proliferative response of human lymphocytes. Proc. Soc. Exp. Biol. Med. 157:155, 1978.
72. Maini, R.N., and Roffe, L.: D-Penicillamine and lymphocyte function in rheumatoid arthritis: The inhibitory and augmenting effects of D-penicillamine in vitro on phytohemagglutinin-induced lymphocyte transformation. *In* Munthe, E. (ed.): Penicillamine Research in Rheumatoid Disease. Oslo, Fabritius and Sonner, 1976, p. 172.
73. Lipsky, P.E., and Ziff, M.: The effect of D-penicillamine on mitogen-induced human lymphocyte proliferation: Synergistic inhibition by D-penicillamine and copper salts. J. Immunol. 120:1006, 1978.
74. Lipsky, P.E., and Ziff, M.: Inhibition of human helper T cell function in vitro by D-penicillamine and $CuSO_4$. J. Clin. Invest. 65:1069, 1980.
75. Zuckner, J., Ramsey, R.H., Dorner, R.W., and Gantner, G.E.: D-Penicillamine in rheumatoid arthritis. Arthritis Rheum. 13:131, 1970.
76. Whitehouse, M.W., Field, L., Denko, C.W., and Ryall, R.: Is penicillamine a precursor drug? Scand. J. Rheumatol. 4(Suppl. 8):183, 1975.
77. Axelrod, A.E., and Trakatellis, A.C.: Relationship of pyridoxine to immunological phenomena. Vitam. Horm. 22:591, 1964.
78. Gerber, D.A.: Inhibition of the denaturation of human gamma globulin by a mixture of D-Penicillamine disulfide and cooper. Biochem. Pharm. 27:469, 1978.
79. Masters, C.L., Dawkins, R.L., Zilco, P.L., Simpson, J.A., and Leedman, R.J.: Penicillamine-associated myasthenia gravis, antiacetylcholine receptor and antistriational antibodies. Am. J. Med. 63:689, 1977.
80. Sparrow, G.P.: Penicillamine pemphigus and the nephrotic syndrome occurring simultaneously. Br. J. Dermatol. 98:103, 1978.
81. Maize, J.C., Dobson, R.L., and Provost, T.T.: Pemphigus and myasthenia gravis. Arch. Dermatol. 111:1334, 1975.
82. Noguchi, S., and Nishitani, H.: Immunologic studies of a case of myasthenia gravis associated with pemphigus vulgaris after thymectomy. Neurology 26:1075, 1976.
83. Maini, R.N., and Berry, H. (eds): Modulation of Autoimmunity and Disease. Clinical Pharmacology and Therapeutics Series. Vol. 1. New York, Praeger Scientific, 1981.
84. Dawkins, R.L., Christiansen, F.T., and Zilko, P.J. (eds.): Immunogenetics in Rheumatology: Musculoskeletal Disease and D-Penicillamine. New York, Excerpta Medica, 1982.
85. Jacobus, D.P., Bokelman, D.L., and Majka, J.A.: D-Penicillamine in the monkey. *In* Munthe, E. (ed.): Penicillamine Research in Rheumatoid Disease. Oslo, Fabritius and —Sonner, 1976, p. 25.
86. Vincent, A., and Newsom-Davis, J.: Anti-acetylcholine receptor antibodies in D-penicillamine-associated myasthenia gravis. Lancet 1:1254, 1978.

# Chapter 54
# Glucocorticoids

*Lloyd Axelrod*

## INTRODUCTION

The history of glucocorticoid therapy and the history of rheumatology are inseparable. From the beginning, during the initial studies of the effects of cortisone on patients with rheumatoid arthritis, it was apparent that the dramatic anti-inflammatory effects of glucocorticoids are frequently accompanied by the unwelcome manifestations of Cushing's syndrome.[1] The purpose of this chapter is to examine the risks associated with the use of glucocorticoids as anti-inflammatory and immunosuppressive agents and to provide guidelines for the long-term systemic use of these commonly prescribed substances. The indications for the use of glucocorticoids in the rheumatic disorders are discussed in the chapters of this book that consider the several rheumatic diseases for which these agents are sometimes indicated. This chapter is concerned primarily with the general principles of glucocorticoid therapy.

## STRUCTURE OF COMMONLY USED GLUCOCORTICOIDS

Glucocorticoids are 21-carbon steroid molecules with numerous metabolic and physiologic effects. Figure 54–1 reveals the structures of several commonly employed glucocorticoids.[2] Cortisol (hydrocortisone) is the principal circulating glucocorticoid in man.

The existence of glucocorticoid activity depends on the presence of a hydroxyl group at carbon number 11 of the steroid molecule. Thus, cortisone and prednisone, which are 11-keto compounds, lack glucocorticoid activity until converted in vivo to cortisol and prednisolone, the corresponding 11-beta-hydroxyl compounds.[3,4] This transformation occurs predominantly in the liver.[5,6] The direct application of cortisone to the skin is ineffective in the treatment of dermatologic diseases that respond to topical application of cortisol.[4] Similarly, the anti-inflammatory action of cortisone is minimal compared with the effect of intra-articular administration of cortisol.[3] Cortisone and prednisone are available only for systemic therapy. All glucocorticoid preparations marketed for topical or local use are 11-beta-hydroxyl compounds, thus eliminating the need for biotransformation.

## PHYSIOLOGY: THE REGULATION OF CORTISOL SECRETION

The production of cortisol by the adrenal cortex is regulated directly by the anterior pituitary gland and indirectly by the hypothalamus. Under normal circumstances, ACTH is released from the anterior pituitary gland in pulsatile fashion.[7] Although plasma ACTH levels are thus subject to minute-to-minute variation, these levels are higher on the average in the early morning hours than later in the day, i.e., there is a diurnal rhythm of ACTH release. ACTH is itself subject to release by corticotropin-releasing hormone, a substance synthesized in the hypothalamus and carried directly to the anterior pituitary gland by a local circulation, the hypophyseal-portal system. Stressful stimuli originating at a suprahypothalamic level lead to an augmented release of corticotropin-releasing hormone from the hypothalamus. This substance in turn provokes the discharge of ACTH from the anterior pituitary gland.

This sequence is subject to negative feedback inhibition. Increasing levels of cortisol or a synthetic glucocorticoid result in decreasing secretion of ACTH. It is not known whether this feedback control occurs predominantly at the hypothalamic level or the pituitary level.[8,9] In normal persons, stressful stimuli can overcome the effect of this feedback inhibition.[10]

## PHARMACODYNAMICS

**Half-Life, Potency, and Duration of Action.** The important differences among the available glucocorticoid compounds are in duration of action, relative glucocor-

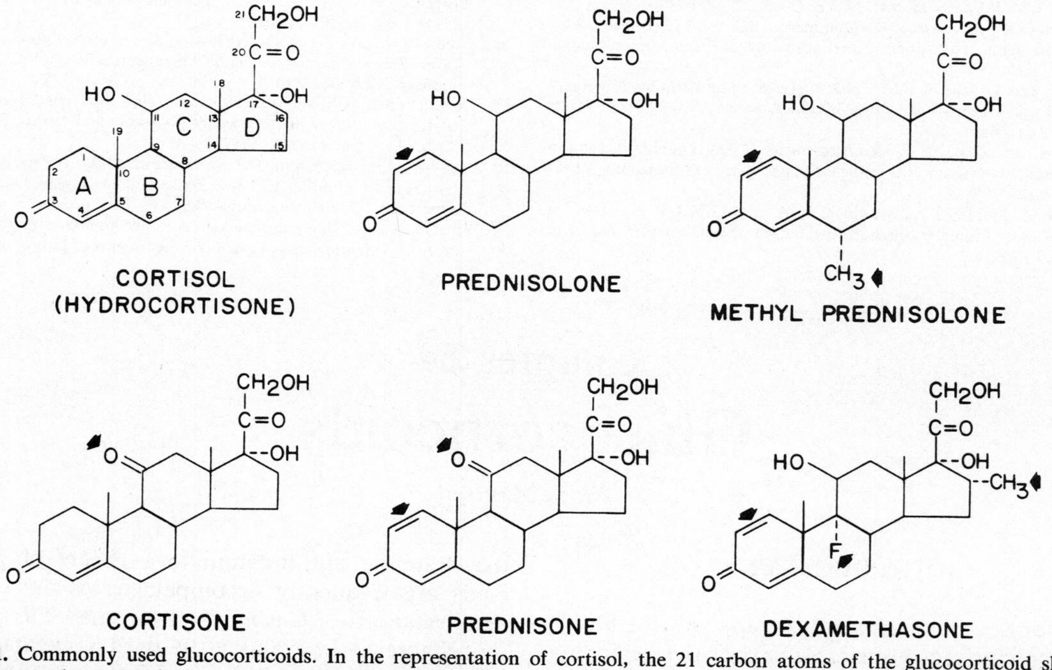


**Figure 54–1.** Commonly used glucocorticoids. In the representation of cortisol, the 21 carbon atoms of the glucocorticoid skeleton are designated by numbers, and the four rings are designated by letters. The arrows indicate the structural differences between cortisol and each of the other molecules. (From Axelrod, L.: Medicine 55:39, 1976.)

**Table 54–1.** Commonly Used Glucocorticoids*

| Duration of Action† | Glucocorticoid Potency‡ | Equivalent Glucocorticoid Dose (mg) | Mineralocorticoid Activity |
|---|---|---|---|
| Short-acting | | | |
| Cortisol (hydrocortisone) | 1 | 20 | Yes§ |
| Cortisone | 0.8 | 25 | Yes§ |
| Prednisone | 4 | 5 | No |
| Prednisolone | 4 | 5 | No |
| Methylprednisolone | 5 | 4 | No |
| Intermediate-acting | | | |
| Triamcinolone | 5 | 4 | No |
| Long-acting | | | |
| Betamethasone | 25 | 0.60 | No |
| Dexamethasone | 30 | 0.75 | No |

*From Axelrod, L.: Medicine 55:39, 1976; and Axelrod, L.: *In* Miller, R. R., and Greenblatt, D. J. (eds.): Handbook of Drug Therapy. New York, Elsevier North Holland, 1979, p. 809.

†The classification by duration of action is based on the work of Harter (see text).[11]

‡The values given for glucocorticoid potency are relative. Cortisol is arbitrarily assigned a value of one. These values are approximations derived from several sources.[12-21]

§Mineralocorticoid effects are dose related. At doses close to or within the basal physiologic range for glucocorticoid activity, no such effect may be detectable.

ticoid potency, and relative mineralocorticoid potency (Table 54–1).[2] Commonly used glucocorticoids are categorized as short-, intermediate-, and long-acting on the basis of the duration of ACTH suppression following a single dose, equivalent in anti-inflammatory activity to 50 mg of prednisone (Table 54–1).[11] The values provided for relative glucocorticoid potency are approximations derived from several sources.[12-21] The relative potencies of the glucocorticoids correlate with their affinity for the cytoplasmic glucocorticoid receptor.[22,23] However, the observed potency of a glucocorticoid is a measure not only of the intrinsic biologic potency but also of the duration of action.[21,22] Consequently, the relative potency of two glucocorticoids will vary as a function of the time interval between the administration of the two steroids and the determination of the potency. In particular, failure to account for the duration of action may lead to a marked underestimation of the potency of dexamethasone.[21]

The half-life of cortisol in the circulation is in the range of 80 to 115 minutes.[2] Values for other commonly used agents are as follows: cortisone, 0.5 hours; prednisone, 3.4 to 3.8 hours; prednisolone, 2.1 to 3.5 hours; methylprednisolone, 1.3 to 3.1 hours; and dexamethasone, 1.8 to 4.7 hours.[2,21,24] The variability in the reported values for the half-life of an individual glucocorticoid may be a consequence in part of the fact that the pharmacokinetic characteristics of the glucocorticoids are dose dependent. With increasing intravenous doses of prednisolone, there is an increase in the volume of distribution and an increase in the clearance of this steroid.[24-26] The dose-dependent kinetic behavior of prednisolone may be due to the fact that the binding of prednisolone to plasma proteins is nonlinear; with an increase in dose, there is an increase in the percentage of the steroid that is unbound.[24-26]

The relationship between the circulating half-life of a glucocorticoid and its potency is not strict. Prednisolone and dexamethasone have comparable circulating half-lives, but dexamethasone is clearly more potent. Similarly, the correlation between the circulating half-life of a glucocorticoid and its duration of action is imprecise. The many actions of glucocorticoids do not have an equal duration, and the duration of action may be a function of the dose.[11,27-29]

For example, the duration of an elevation of the serum glucose of fasting subjects increases with increasing glucocorticoid dosage. It is 10 to 12 hours with 15 mg of methylprednisolone, 12 to 16 hours with 45 mg, and 18 to 22 hours with 90 mg.[27] In adult patients with stable chronic bronchial asthma, the duration of the response to a single oral dose of 40 mg of prednisolone depends on the aspect of pulmonary function that one observes.[28] Improvement in the peak expiratory flow rate, the forced expiratory volume in 1 second, and the maximum expiratory flow rate is still detectable 24 hours after administration of the dose, but not at 36 hours. However, improvement in forced vital capacity, residual volume/total lung capacity, and flow rate at 50 percent of vital capacity is still detectable at 12 hours, but not 24 hours. The differences in the duration of these effects may depend on the actual duration of the effects or on the variable sensitivity of the techniques utilized to measure the effects, or both.

Harter studied the duration of one effect of glucocorticoids, the length of time following a single dose during which ACTH remains suppressed.[11] He did this by administering metyrapone to a normal subject and measuring the urinary 17-ketogenic steroids during 6-hour periods as an index of ACTH secretion. He divided glucocorticoids into three groups based on the duration of ACTH suppression following a single dose of a glucocorticoid, equivalent in anti-inflammatory activity to 50 mg of prednisone. The first group, the short-acting steroids, is characterized by a return of ACTH activity within 24 to 36 hours. This group includes cortisone, hydrocortisone, prednisone, prednisolone, and methylprednisolone. The second group, the intermediate-acting steroids, consists of compounds that suppress ACTH for 48 hours. This group includes triamcinolone and paramethasone. The third group, the long-acting glucocorticoids, consists of substances that supress ACTH for well over 48 hours. This class includes dexamethasone and betamethasone. This formulation is based on studies in a single patient. It does not provide information about variations from individual to individual, about prolonged therapy, or about subjects who have not received metyrapone.

Since these variations in the duration of ACTH suppression are achieved by doses of glucocorticoids with comparable anti-inflammatory activity, the duration of ACTH suppression is not simply a function of the level of anti-inflammatory activity. However, the duration of ACTH suppression produced by an individual glucocorticoid is probably dose related. Harter found that as he increased the dose of prednisone from 25 mg to 100 mg, the duration of ACTH suppression was prolonged.[11] In another study, daily morning doses of 8 mg of triamcinolone taken for 1 week did not produce suppression of the 8 A.M. level of plasma 17-hydroxycorticosteroids, but daily morning doses of 12 mg produced suppression in some subjects and 16 mg produced suppression in all subjects.[29] Long-acting conjugates of the glucocorticoids given as intramuscular injections may be released slowly and exert an effect for much more prolonged periods, often several weeks.

The slight differences in the circulating half-lives of the glucocorticoids contrast with the marked differences between them in potency and in the duration of ACTH suppression. Also, the duration of ACTH suppression exceeds the half-life by more than the fivefold factor that would be expected if the duration of effect were a function of the circulating level of the steroid. Such data suggest that the duration of action of a glucocorticoid is not determined by its presence in the circulation. This is consistent with our understanding of the mechanism of action of steroid hormones. A steroid molecule passes through the cell membrane and enters the cytoplasm, where it binds to a specific cytoplasmic receptor protein.[30-32] This complex enters the nucleus, where it modifies the process of transcription, whereby RNA is synthesized (or transcribed) from the DNA template. The consequence is an alteration in the rate of synthesis of specific proteins. In this manner, the steroid modifies the phenotypic expression of the genetic information. Thus, the glucocorticoid continues to act within the cell after it has disappeared from the circulation. In addition, the series of events initiated by the glucocorticoid may continue to occur, or a product of this sequence (such as a specific protein) may be present after the disappearance of the glucocorticoid.

**Bioavailability, Absorption, and Biotransformation.** In normal subjects, plasma cortisol levels after oral administration of cortisone are much lower than after equal doses of cortisol.[33] This suggests that while oral cortisone may be adequate replacement therapy in chronic adrenal insufficiency, it is unwise to use this agent orally when pharmacologic effects are sought. In contrast, comparable plasma prednisolone levels are achieved in normal subjects following equivalent oral doses of prednisone and prednisolone.[24,26] There is wide variation in the prednisolone concentration after both drugs, which may reflect variability in absorption.[24]

In several instances in the past, therapeutic failure was attributed to diminished bioavailability of prednisone tablets; this has not been reported in recent years.[34] The serum prednisolone levels achieved following a single 50-mg tablet of prednisone and ten 5-mg tablets of prednisone given as a single oral dose of 50 mg are comparable.[35] Problems with in vivo bioavailability of prednisolone tablets have not been reported.[36] A comparison of the plasma prednisolone levels achieved after a single oral dose of prednisolone made by eight different American manufacturers indicates that the tablets tested were equivalent.[37] The bioavailability of dexamethasone does not vary when this agent is given intravenously, as an elixir, or in tablet form.[38]

Plasma cortisol levels after an intramuscular injection of cortisone acetate rise little or not at all, in contrast to the marked rises that follow the intramuscular injection of hydrocortisone.[39-45] Although intramuscular cortisone acetate has long been used for perioperative management, it may not provide adequate plasma cortisol levels and offers no advantage over hydrocortisone by the same route.

**Plasma Transport Proteins.** Under normal physiologic conditions, cortisol and, to a lesser extent, its synthetic derivatives are primarily bound to corticosteroid-binding globulin (CBG, transcortin), an alpha-globulin, in the plasma. CBG is a vehicle for the transportation of the steroid; the bound steroid is not active. Albumin binds most of the remaining glucocorticoid (10 to 15 percent) not complexed with CBG, leaving only a small portion of the steroid unbound and free to exert its physiologic and pharmacologic actions. Circadian fluctuations occur in the capacity of CBG to bind cortisol and prednisolone in normal subjects.[46] In contrast, patients who have been given prolonged treatment with prednisone have no diurnal variation in the binding capacity of CBG for cortisol of prednisolone, and both capacities are reduced in comparison with normal subjects.[46] Thus, long-term glucocorticoid therapy alters not only the endogenous secretion of steroids but also the transport of some glucocorticoids in the circulation. Possibly, this explains the observation that the disappearance of prednisolone is more rapid in those who have previously received glucocorticoids than in those who have not.[47,48]

**Glucocorticoid Therapy in the Presence of Liver Disease.** Plasma cortisol levels are normal in patients with liver disease.[49] Although cortisol clearance is reduced in cirrhotics, the hypothalamic-pituitary-adrenal homeostatic mechanism appears to be intact. Thus, a decreased rate of metabolism is accompanied by decreased synthesis of cortisol.[49]

In patients with active liver disease, the conversion of

prednisone to prednisolone is impaired.[48,50,51] This is offset in good measure by a decreased rate of elimination of prednisolone from the plasma in patients with active liver disease or cirrhosis.[51,52] In patients with liver disease, the plasma availability of prednisolone may be quite variable after oral doses of either prednisone or prednisolone.[51] The conversion of cortisone to cortisol has been studied in only one patient with hepatic disease and was normal.[33] The situation is further complicated by the fact that a lower percentage of circulating prednisolone is bound to protein in patients with active liver disease than in normal subjects;[48,50] the unbound fraction is inversely related to the serum albumin concentration.[50] An increased frequency of prednisone side effects is observed at low serum albumin levels;[53] possibly both findings reflect impaired hepatic function. Because the impairment of conversion of prednisone to prednisolone in the presence of liver disease is quantitatively small and is offset by a decreased rate of clearance of prednisolone, and because of the marked variability in plasma prednisolone levels after administration of either steroid, there is no clear mandate to use prednisolone rather than prednisone in the patient with active liver disease or cirrhosis.[24] Whichever agent is used, a somewhat lower dose than would otherwise be used should be employed if the serum albumin level is low.[24]

**Glucocorticoids During Pregnancy.** Glucocorticoid therapy appears to be well tolerated in pregnancy.[54] Although glucocorticoids cross the placenta, at present there is no convincing evidence that this produces clinically significant hypothalamic-pituitary-adrenal suppression or Cushing's syndrome in the neonate,[54] although subnormal responsiveness to exogenous ACTH may occur.[55,56] Nor is there evidence that glucocorticoids increase the incidence of congenital defects in humans.[54] Glucocorticoids appear to decrease the birthweight of full-term infants;[57] the long-term consequences of this effect are unknown. Owing to low concentrations of prednisone and prednisolone in breast milk, the administration of these drugs to the mother of a nursing infant is unlikely to produce deleterious effects.[58,59]

**Drug Interactions.** The concomitant use of other drugs can alter the effectiveness of the glucocorticoids.[60]

The metabolism of glucocorticoids is accelerated by compounds that induce hepatic microsomal enzyme activity, such as phenytoin,[61-64] barbiturates,[63,65,66] and rifampin.[67,68] Administration of these compounds can increase the steroid requirement of a patient with adrenal insufficiency[67] or lead to deterioration in the condition of a patient whose underlying disorder is well controlled by glucocorticoid therapy.[65,66,68] These substances should be avoided if possible in patients receiving steroids. Diazepam does not alter the metabolism of glucocorticoids[63] and is preferable to barbiturates. If an inducer of hepatic microsomal enzyme activity must be used in a patient on steroids, an increase in the required dosage of the steroid should be anticipated.

The bioavailability of prednisone is decreased by antacid doses comparable to those used clinically.[69]

The concurrent administration of a glucocorticoid and a salicylate may reduce serum salicylate levels; conversely, reduction of the steroid dose during administration of a fixed dose of salicylate may lead to higher and possibly toxic serum salicylate levels.[70-72] This interaction may reflect the induction of salicylate metabolism by glucocorticoids.[71]

Glucocorticoids may increase requirements for insulin or oral hypoglycemic agents, antihypertensive drugs, or glaucoma medications. They may also alter the requirement for sedative-hypnotic or antidepressant therapy. Digitalis toxicity can result from hypokalemia induced by glucocorticoids, as from hypokalemia of any cause. Glucocorticoids may reverse the neuromuscular blockade induced by pancuronium.[73,74] The mechanism is not known. The bioavailability of prednisolone is not impaired by the simultaneous use of cholestyramine.[75]

## CONSIDERATIONS PRIOR TO THE USE OF GLUCOCORTICOIDS AS PHARMACOLOGIC AGENTS

Cushing's syndrome is a serious disorder. The 5-year mortality rate was over 50 percent in a series of patients studied at the beginning of the era of glucocorticoid and ACTH therapy.[76] Infection and cardiovascular complications are frequent causes of death in this disorder. High-dose exogenous glucocorticoid therapy is similarly hazardous.

Table 54–2 summarizes the important questions to consider prior to the initiation of glucocorticoid therapy.[77] These enable the physician to assess the potential risks that must be weighed against the potential benefits of treatment. The more severe the underlying disorder, the more readily glucocorticoid therapy can be justified. Thus, steroid therapy is usually employed in patients with some severe forms of systemic lupus erythematosus, active vasculitis, status asthmaticus, severe chronic active hepatitis, transplantation rejection, severe pemphigus, or diseases of comparable severity. Steroids gen-

**Table 54–2.** Considerations Prior to the Use of Glucocorticoids as Pharmacologic Agents*

1. How serious is the underlying disorder?
2. How long will therapy be required?
3. What is the anticipated effective steroid dose?
4. Is the patient predisposed to any of the known hazards of glucocorticoid therapy?
   - Diabetes mellitus
   - Osteoporosis
   - Peptic ulcer, gastritis, or esophagitis
   - Tuberculosis or other chronic infections
   - Hypertension and cardiovascular disease
   - Psychological difficulties
5. Which glucocorticoid preparation should be employed?
6. Have other modes of therapy been utilized to minimize the glucocorticoid dosage and to minimize the side effects of glucocorticoid therapy?
7. Is an alternate-day regimen indicated?

*Modified from Thorn, G.W.: N. Engl. J. Med. 274:775, 1966.

erally should not be administered to patients with rheumatoid arthritis or mild bronchial asthma, who should receive more conservative therapy first. Although they may experience symptomatic relief from glucocorticoids, it may prove difficult to withdraw steroids for this very reason. As a result, these patients may unnecessarily experience Cushing's syndrome and hypothalamic-pituitary-adrenal suppression.

The anticipated duration of glucocorticoid therapy is another critical variable. The use of glucocorticoids for 1 to 2 weeks for a condition such as poison ivy or allergic rhinitis is unlikely to be associated with serious side effects if there is no contraindication to their use. An exception to this rule is a steroid-induced psychosis, which may occur after only a few days of high-dose glucocorticoid therapy, even in patients with no previous history of psychiatric disease.[78,79] Because so many complications are dose and time related, the smallest possible dose should be prescribed for the shortest possible period.[78,80,81] If hypoalbuminemia is present, the dose should be appropriately reduced.[24,50,53] If long-term treatment is indicated, consideration should be given to the use of an alternate-day schedule.

Whenever possible, a local steroid preparation should be used, since systemic effects are minimal when these substances are properly administered. Examples are topical therapy in dermatologic disorders, steroid enemas in ulcerative proctitis, steroid aerosols in bronchial asthma and allergic rhinitis, and intra-articular steroids.[82,83]

Agents with minimal or no mineralocorticoid activity should be used when a glucocorticoid is prescribed for pharmacologic purposes. If the dose is to be tapered over a few days, a long-acting agent may be undesirable. For alternate-day therapy, a short-acting agent that generally does not cause sodium retention (e.g., prednisone, prednisolone, or methylprednisolone) should be used. There is no indication for the systemic administration of glucocorticoid conjugates that are designed to achieve a prolonged duration of action (several days or several weeks) following a single intramuscular injection. The absorption and bioavailability of such agents cannot be regulated precisely, the duration of action cannot be estimated reliably, and it is not possible to taper the dose rapidly in the event of an adverse reaction such as a steroid-induced psychosis. The use of such preparations may produce hypothalamic-pituitary-adrenal suppression more often than comparable doses of the same glucocorticoid given orally.[84] The use of supplementary agents to minimize the steroid dose and to minimize the side effects of systemic glucocorticoids should always be considered.

## EFFECTS OF EXOGENOUS GLUCOCORTICOIDS

**Anti-inflammatory and Immunosuppressive Effects.** The effects of glucocorticoids on inflammatory and immune responses are exceedingly complex; this complexity derives from the complexity of the inflammatory and immune processes themselves and from the fact that glucocorticoids modify these processes in numerous ways.[85-90] Studies performed in steroid-sensitive species, such as the mouse, rat, and rabbit, may not apply to steroid-resistant species such as the guinea pig, monkey, and man.[85,86] In addition many studies in in vitro systems employ concentrations of glucocorticoids that are not attainable in man.[89,90]

It is not yet possible to identify a single mechanism of action underlying the numerous effects of glucocorticoids on inflammatory and immune responses. As noted above, glucocorticoid hormones (like other steroid hormones) act by binding to a specific cytoplasmic receptor protein. The steroid-receptor complex then enters the nucleus, where it modifies the transcription of RNA from the DNA template. This results in an alteration of the rate of synthesis of specific proteins. It is tempting to try to relate this receptor-mediated mechanism of action to the numerous effects of glucocorticoids on inflammation and immunity. In fact, glucocorticoid receptors have been demonstrated in normal human lymphocytes, monocytes, neutrophils, and eosinophils and in human neoplastic cells.[90] Although the number of cytoplasmic glucocorticoid receptors correlates with a clinical response to glucocorticoid therapy in some patients with lymphoid tumors, the presence of receptors in malignant tissue does not guarantee responsiveness.[90] Variations in corticosteroid receptor density, affinity, or binding constants do not correlate with the range of responses of immunoreactive cells to glucocorticoids.[90]

Glucocorticoid effects on inflammatory and immune phenomena include effects on leukocyte movement, leukocyte function, and humoral factors (Table 54–3). In general, glucocorticoids have a greater effect on leukocyte traffic than on function and more effect on cellular than humoral processes.[89] Probably the most important anti-inflammatory effect of glucocorticoids is their ability to inhibit recruitment of neutrophils and monocyte-macrophages to an inflammatory site.[89]

Glucocorticoids alter the traffic of all the major leukocyte populations within the circulation. The administration of a single dose of a glucocorticoid produces a neutrophilic leukocytosis; peak levels occur 4 to 6 hours after the steroid is given.[87,91] This leukocytosis is the consequence of an accelerated release of mature neutrophils from the bone marrow,[92] an increase in the circulating half-life of the neutrophils,[93] and decreased egress of neutrophils from the circulation to an inflammatory site.[92,94] The administration of a single dose of a glucocorticoid to normal human subjects produces a marked but transient lymphocytopenia; the nadir is reached 4 to 6 hours after administration (Fig. 54–2).[87,95-99] This lymphocytopenia involves all lymphocyte subpopulations. It is also selective, since thymus-derived lymphocytes are decreased to a greater degree than bone marrow-derived lymphocytes,[87,95,96,99] and within the total T lymphocyte population certain subsets are decreased to a greater extent than others.[90] The mechanism of the lymphocytopenia in humans involves the redistribution of lymphocytes out of the circulation.

**Table 54–3.** Effects of Glucocorticoids on Inflammatory and Immune Responses in Humans*

| |
|---|
| *Effects on Leukocyte Movement* |
| Lymphocytes |
| Circulating lymphocytopenia 4 to 6 hours following drug administration, secondary to redistribution of cells to other lymphoid compartments |
| Depletion of recirculating lymphocytes |
| Selective depletion of T lymphocytes more than B lymphocytes |
| Monocyte-Macrophages |
| Circulating monocytopenia 4 to 6 hours following drug administration, probably secondary to redistribution |
| Inhibition of accumulation of monocyte-macrophages at inflammatory sites |
| Neutrophils |
| Circulating neutrophilia |
| Accelerated release of neutrophils from the bone marrow |
| Blockade of accumulation of neutrophils at inflammatory sites |
| Eosinophils |
| Circulating eosinopenia, probably secondary to redistribution |
| Decreased migration of eosinophils into immediate hypersensitivity skin test sites |
| *Effects on Leukocyte Function* |
| Lymphocytes |
| Suppression of delayed hypersensitivity skin testing by inhibition of recruitment of monocyte-macrophages |
| Suppression of lymphocyte proliferation to antigens more easily than proliferation to mitogens |
| Suppression of mixed leukocyte reaction proliferation |
| Suppression of T lymphocyte–mediated cytotoxicity (at high concentrations in vitro) |
| No effect on antibody dependent cell-mediated cytotoxicity |
| Suppression of spontaneous (natural) cytotoxicity |
| Regulatory effects on helper and suppressor cell populations |
| Monocyte-Macrophages |
| Suppression of cutaneous delayed hypersensitivity by inhibition of lymphokine effect on the macrophage |
| Blockade of Fc receptor binding and function |
| Depression of bactericidal activity |
| Possible decrease in monocyte chemotaxis |
| Neutrophils |
| Possibly no effect on phagocytic and bactericidal capability (controversial) |
| Increase in antibody-dependent cellular cytotoxicity |
| Probable decrease in lysosomal release but little effect on lysosomal membrane stabilization at pharmacologic concentrations |
| Inhibition of chemotaxis only by suprapharmacologic concentrations |
| *Effects on Humoral Factors* |
| Mild decrease in immunoglobulin levels but no decrease in specific antibody production |
| Probably no effect on complement metabolism |
| Decreased reticuloendothelial clearance of antibody-coated cells |
| Decreased synthesis of prostaglandins, and leukotrienes |
| Effects on kinins controversial |
| Inhibition of plasminogen activator release |
| Potentiation of the actions of catecholamines |
| Antagonism of histamine-induced vasodilatation |

*Adapted from Parrillo, J. E., and Fauci, A.S.: Ann. Rev. Pharmacol. Toxicol. 19:179, 1979.

In general, there are two distinct populations of lymphocytes in the circulation.[87,89] The first population, the recirculating lymphocytes, freely migrates into and out of the intravascular space in equilibrium with the much larger total body pool of recirculating lymphocytes. The second population, the nonrecirculating lymphocytes, remains in the intravascular space. Glucocorticoids cause the recirculating lymphocyte to leave the intravascular space, but they do not affect the nonrecirculating lymphocyte.[100] This alteration of the normal lymphocyte traffic may be due to suppression of entry of lymphocytes into the circulation.[101] Glucocorticoids also cause a profound monocytopenia and eosinopenia; the time courses after a single steroid dose are similar to that of the lymphocytopenia.

The mechanism of the decrease in the accumulation of inflammatory cells at an inflammatory site caused by glucocorticoids is not fully understood. Corticosteroids modify the increased capillary and membrane permeability that occurs at an inflammatory site.[102] By decreasing the dilatation of the microvasculature and the increased capillary permeability that occur during the inflammatory response, exudation of fluid and the formation of edema may be reduced, and the migration of

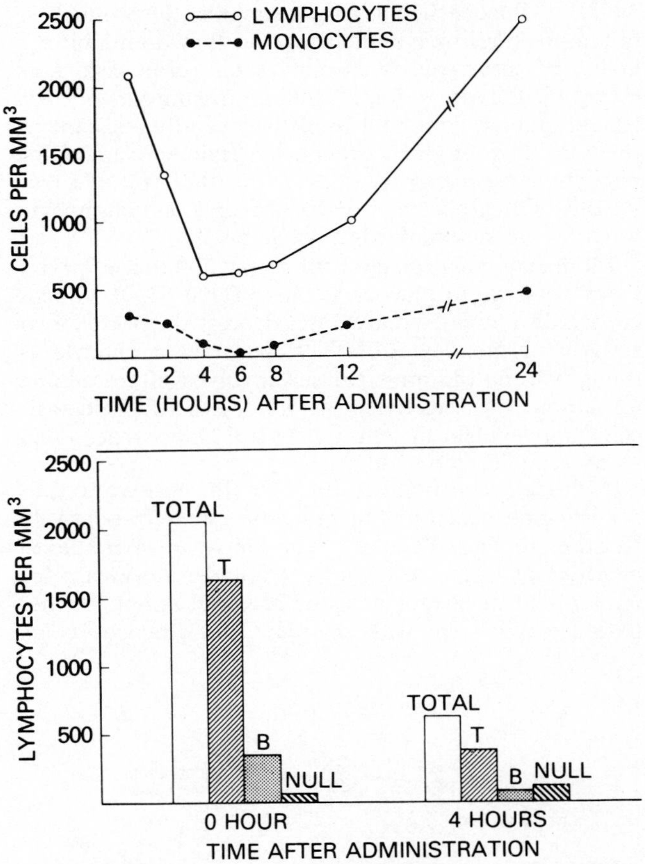


**Figure 54–2.** The effect of hydrocortisone administration on circulating lymphocytes and monocytes. Hydrocortisone, 400 mg, was administered intravenously in a single dose to a normal volunteer. The upper panel shows the effect on the total lymphocyte and monocyte counts. The lower panel shows the effect on circulating thymus-derived (T) and bone-marrow derived (B) lymphocytes, as well as lymphocytes without detectable surface markers (null cells), 4 hours after drug administration. T lymphocytes were measured by the sheep erythrocyte rosette assay, and B lymphocytes were measured by the complement receptor assay. (From Fauci, A.S., Dale, D.C., and Balow, J.E.: Ann. Intern. Med. 84:304, 1976.)

leukocytes may be impaired.[88,89,102,103] The decrease in accumulation of inflammatory cells may be due also to decreased adherence of the inflammatory cells to the vascular endothelium.[104-106] It is not presently possible to determine the relative contributions of a direct vascular effect, of an effect on inflammatory cell adherence to the vascular wall, and of an effect on chemotaxis to the reduction in the inflammatory response caused by glucocorticoids.

Glucocorticoids have numerous effects on leukocyte function. Steroid therapy suppresses cutaneous delayed hypersensitivity responses. This occurs after approximately 14 days of glucocorticoid therapy and disappears approximately 6 days after treatment is withdrawn; these rates vary considerably from patient to patient.[107] This suppression is a consequence of decreased recruitment of macrophages necessary for the expression of hypersensitivity and is not due to suppression of the sensitized lymphocyte.[107-110] Steroids antagonize the effects of migration inhibition factor (MIF) on the macrophage (Fig. 54–3).[111] Glucocorticoids do not suppress the production of lymphokines by lymphocytes, but they do inhibit the ability of these soluble mediators to recruit cells necessary for the expression of cellular immunity.[87,89,111] Although human lymphoid tissue is generally resistant to the lytic effect of glucocorticoids, certain activated lymphocyte subsets may be sensitive to the lytic effect of steroids. Other effects of glucocorticoids on lymphocyte function are summarized in Table 54–3.

Monocyte-macrophage traffic and function are relatively sensitive to glucocorticoids (Table 54–3). Glucocorticoids in divided daily doses depress the bactericidal activity of monocytes.[112,113] Because the monocyte is thought to be the principal cell involved in granuloma formation, the sensitivity of monocytes to glucocorticoids may explain the effectiveness of glucocorticoids in many granulomatous diseases.[89]

Although neutrophil traffic is quite sensitive to glucocorticoids, neutrophil function appears to be relatively resistant to these agents.[89] While most in vivo studies of neutrophil phagocytosis have found no evidence for impairment of phagocytosis or bacterial killing,[89] other data are consistent with the view that glucocorticoids

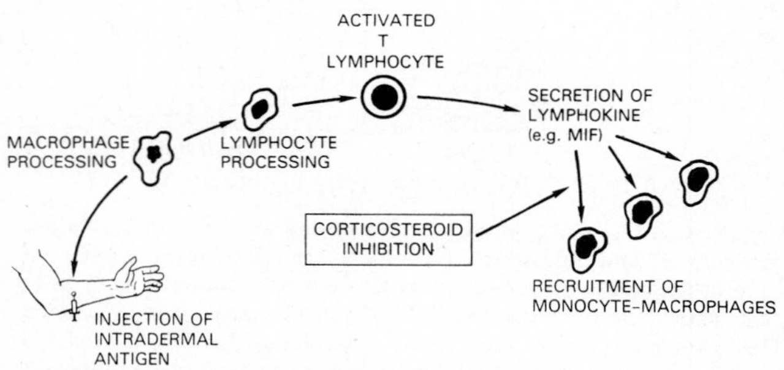


**Figure 54–3.** Schematic representation of the probable site of inhibition of the delayed hypersensitivity skin test response. Glucocorticoids inhibit the recruitment of the monocyte-macrophage, but do not affect the activated T lymphocyte. (From Parrillo, J.E., and Fauci, A.S.: Ann. Rev. Pharmacol. Toxicol. 19:179, 1979.)

induce a generalized phagocytic defect, affecting granulocytes as well as monocytes.[114]

Glucocorticoid therapy retards the disappearance of sensitized erythrocytes, platelets, and artificial particles from the circulation.[89,114,115] This may explain the efficacy of glucocorticoids in the treatment of idiopathic thrombocytopenic purpura and autoimmune hemolytic anemia.

Glucocorticoids are potent inhibitors of prostaglandin synthesis.[116-120] This is of particular interest in view of the evidence for synthesis of prostaglandin $E_2$ by rheumatoid synovia[121] and the possibility that the bone resorption-stimulating activity of this prostaglandin accounts for the bone destruction in rheumatoid arthritis.[121] Corticosteroids inhibit prostaglandin synthesis by inhibition of arachidonic acid release from phospholipids.[119,120] This is distinct from the mechanism of action of the nonsteroidal anti-inflammatory agents, such as salicylates and indomethacin, which inhibit the cyclooxygenase that converts arachidonic acid to the cyclic endoperoxide intermediates in the prostaglandin synthetic pathway. Thus, the glucocorticoids and the nonsteroidal anti-inflammatory agents exert their anti-inflammatory effects at two distinct but adjacent loci in the synthetic pathway of a substance with known bone resorption-stimulating activity that is synthesized by rheumatoid synovia.

Glucocorticoids and nonsteroidal anti-inflammatory agents have a different spectrum of anti-inflammatory effects. Some of the therapeutic effects of steroids that are not produced by the nonsteroidal agents may be due to inhibition of leukotriene formation.[122] Leukotrienes are a class of substances originally found in leukocytes, which share a conjugated triene as a common structural feature.[122] Leukotriene B4 causes adhesion and chemotactic movement of leukocytes.[122] Leukotrienes C4, D4, and E4 (the constituents of the slow-reacting substance of anaphylaxis) increase vascular permeability.[122] These leukotrienes (B4, C4, D4, and E4) may act synergistically with the vasodilator prostaglandins $PGE_2$ and $PGI_2$ to mediate inflammation.[122] The glucocorticoid-mediated inhibition of arachidonic acid release prevents formation not only of prostaglandins and thromboxanes (as do the nonsteroidal anti-inflammatory agents) but also of leukotrienes and other oxygenated derivatives. Consequently, some of the therapeutic effects of steroids that are not shared by the nonsteroidal agents may be due to inhibition of leukotriene formation.[122]

**Side Effects.** Adverse reactions to glucocorticoids include the diverse manifestations of Cushing's syndrome and hypothalamic-pituitary-adrenal (HPA) suppression (Table 54–4).[16,80,81,123] Iatrogenic Cushing's syndrome differs from spontaneous Cushing's syndrome in several respects (Table 54–5).[124,125] These differences may be explained in part by the fact that in iatrogenic Cushing's syndrome caused by exogenous glucocorticoids, ACTH is suppressed, whereas in spontaneous, ACTH-dependent Cushing's syndrome, the elevated ACTH output results in bilateral adrenal hyperplasia. In the former circumstance, the secretion of adrenocortical androgens

**Table 54–4.** Adverse Reactions to Glucocorticoids*

| | |
|---|---|
| Ophthalmic | |
| | Posterior subcapsular cataracts, increased intraocular pressure and glaucoma, exophthalmos |
| Cardiovascular | |
| | Hypertension |
| | Congestive heart failure in predisposed patients |
| Gastrointestinal | |
| | Peptic ulcer disease, pancreatitis |
| Endocrine-metabolic | |
| | Truncal obesity, moon facies, supraclavicular fat deposition, posterior cervical fat deposition (buffalo hump), mediastinal widening (lipomatosis), hepatomegaly due to fatty liver (rare) |
| | Acne, hirsutism or virilism, impotence, menstrual irregularities |
| | Suppression of growth in children |
| | Hyperglycemia; diabetic ketoacidosis; hyperosmolar, nonketotic diabetic coma; hyperlipoproteinemia |
| | Negative balance of nitrogen, potassium, and calcium |
| | Sodium retention, hypokalemia, metabolic alkalosis |
| | Secondary adrenal insufficiency |
| Musculoskeletal | |
| | Myopathy |
| | Osteoporosis, vertebral compression fractures, spontaneous fractures |
| | Aseptic necrosis of femoral and humeral heads and other bones |
| Neuropsychiatric | |
| | Convulsions |
| | Benign intracranial hypertension (pseudotumor cerebri) |
| | Alterations in mood or personality |
| | Psychosis |
| Dermatologic | |
| | Facial erythema, thin fragile skin, petechiae and ecchymoses, violaceous striae, impaired wound healing |
| | Panniculitis (following withdrawal) |
| Immune, infectious | |
| | Suppression of delayed hypersensitivity |
| | Neutrophilia, monocytopenia, lymphocytopenia, decreased inflammatory responses |
| | Susceptibility to infections |

*From Axelrod, L.: *In* Miller, R. R., and Greenblatt, D. J. (eds.): Handbook of Drug Therapy. New York, Elsevier North Holland, 1979, p. 809.

and mineralocorticoids is not increased. When ACTH output is elevated, the secretion of adrenal androgens and mineralocorticoids may be increased.[2] The augmented secretion of adrenal androgens may account for the higher incidence of virilism, acne, and menstrual irregularities reported in the spontaneous form of Cushing's syndrome, and the enhanced production of mineralocorticoids may explain the higher incidence of hypertension.[2]

The complications that are virtually unique to iatrogenic Cushing's syndrome arise following prolonged use or large doses of glucocorticoids. This is the case with benign intracranial hypertension,[126,127] posterior subcapsular cataract,[128-130] and aseptic necrosis of bone.[131-137]

Although the association of glucocorticoid therapy and peptic ulcer disease is controversial,[138-143] it appears that glucocorticoids increase the risk of peptic ulcer disease and gastrointestinal hemorrhage.[142,143] The magnitude of the association between glucocorticoid therapy and these complications is small and is related to the total dose and duration of therapy.[139,142]

Glucocorticoid therapy, especially daily therapy, may suppress the immune response to skin tests for tuberculosis.[107] When possible, tuberculin skin testing is advisable prior to the initiation of glucocorticoid therapy. Routine isoniazid prophylaxis for corticosteroid-treated patients, even those with positive tuberculin skin tests, is probably not indicated.[144]

Some patients respond to and develop side effects to glucocorticoids more readily than others at equivalent doses. Of course, variations in responsiveness to glucocorticoids may result from drug interactions (see above) or from variations in the severity of the underlying disease. Alterations in the bioavailability of administered glucocorticoids probably do not account for the variations in therapeutic response in most patients.[23] In patients who develop side effects, the metabolic clearance rate of prednisolone and the volume of distribution are lower[26,47] and the circulating half-life is longer[47] than in those who do not. Patients who develop a cushingoid habitus on prednisone have higher endogenous plasma cortisol levels than those who do not, perhaps owing to a resistance of the HPA axis to suppression by exogenous glucocorticoids.[145]

Variations in the effectiveness of steroids may be due to altered cellular responsiveness to steroids.[23,146-149] In patients with primary open-angle glaucoma, glucocorticoids produce a greater rise of intraocular pressure,[146] greater suppression of the 8 A.M. plasma cortisol level (when dexamethasone, 0.25 mg, is administered the previous evening at 11 P.M.),[148] and greater suppression of phytohemagglutinin-induced transformation of lymphocytes than in normal subjects.[147,149] Since primary open-angle glaucoma is not uncommon, these findings suggest that a distinct subpopulation of patients is hyper-re-

**Table 54–5.** Natural Versus Iatrogenic Cushing's Syndrome*

| | |
|---|---|
| More common in natural Cushing's syndrome: | |
| | Hypertension |
| | Acne |
| | Menstrual disturbances |
| | Impotence in males |
| | Hirsutism or virilism |
| | Striae |
| | Purpura |
| | Plethora |
| Virtually unique to iatrogenic Cushing's syndrome: | |
| | Benign intracranial hypertension |
| | Glaucoma |
| | Posterior subcapsular cataract |
| | Pancreatitis |
| | Aseptic necrosis of bone |
| | Panniculitis |
| Nearly equal frequency in both syndromes: | |
| | Obesity |
| | Psychiatric symptoms |
| | Edema† |
| | Poor wound healing |

*Adapted from Ragan, C.: Bull. N.Y. Acad. Med. 29:355, 1953; and Christy, N.P.: The Human Adrenal Cortex. New York, Harper & Row, 1971, p. 395.

†The incidence of edema in iatrogenic Cushing's syndrome may depend on the glucocorticoid employed. Ragan utilized cortisone.[125]

sponsive to glucocorticoids and that this sensitivity is genetically determined.

**Withdrawal from Glucocorticoids.** The symptoms associated with glucocorticoid withdrawal include arthralgia, myalgia, anorexia, nausea, emesis, lethargy, headache, fever, desquamation, weight loss, and postural hypotension. Many of these symptoms can occur with normal plasma levels of glucocorticoids[150] and in patients with normal responsiveness of the HPA system.[151,152] Thus, the "steroid withdrawal syndrome" does not depend on the absence of glucocorticoids from the circulation or the impairment of HPA responsiveness. There is no satisfactory explanation for these observations. The "steroid withdrawal syndrome" may contribute to psychologic dependence on glucocorticoid treatment and to one's difficulties in withdrawing such therapy.[124]

## SUPPRESSION OF THE HYPOTHALAMIC-PITUITARY-ADRENAL (HPA) SYSTEM

**The Development of HPA Suppression.** There are few well-documented cases of acute adrenocortical insufficiency following chronic glucocorticoid therapy and no such cases following ACTH therapy.[2] Therefore, the minimal duration of glucocorticoid therapy that can produce HPA suppression must be ascertained from studies of adrenocortical weight and adrenocortical responsiveness to provocative tests.[2,124,153] Adrenocortical atrophy is detectable 5 days after the onset of glucocorticoid therapy.[154] Abnormalities in responsiveness to ACTH and to metyrapone are observed in some but not all patients within 3 days of initiation of treatment with glucocorticoids.[2,124,153] Abnormalities in responsiveness to ACTH and to insulin-induced hypoglycemia occur following the administration of prednisone 25 mg twice daily for 5 days.[155] It must be emphasized that there is considerable variation from patient to patient[156] and from study to study.[124] These figures define the earliest time at which abnormalities are observed in some but not all patients. Because assessment of the onset of HPA suppression currently depends upon anatomic and biochemical (but not clinical) evidence, and because the biochemical abnormalities observed are sometimes mild, it is not possible to identify definitively the shortest interval or the smallest dose at which suppression may occur. On the basis of the available evidence, any patient who has received a glucocorticoid in doses equivalent to 20 to 30 mg of prednisone per day for more than 5 days should be suspected of having HPA suppression.[2] If the doses are closer to but above the physiologic range, 1 month is probably the minimal interval.[2] Once such suspicions are entertained, the physician has two alternatives. One may perform an ACTH test, or one may treat the patient as though adrenocortical insufficiency were present.

The adrenocortical response to an ACTH test is a useful guide to the presence or absence of suppression in glucocorticoid-treated patients (Table 54–6). The maximal response of the plasma cortisol level to ACTH corresponds to the maximal plasma cortisol level observed during the induction of general anesthesia and surgery in patients who have received glucocorticoid therapy.[157-160] This is so when one uses a 6-hour infusion of ACTH[159,160] or a rapid intravenous injection of synthetic ACTH with measurement of the plasma cortisol level just before and then 30 minutes[158] or 60 minutes[157] after the injection. A normal response to ACTH preoperatively is unlikely to be followed by markedly impaired secretion of cortisol during anesthesia and surgery in steroid-treated patients. In general, other tests of the HPA system, such as insulin-induced hypoglycemia and the metyrapone test, are not indicated in the evaluation of the steroid-treated patient for possible HPA axis suppression.

**Table 54–6.** Assessment of Hypothalamic-Pituitary-Adrenal Function in Patients Treated with Glucocorticoids

| |
|---|
| *Method* |
| Withhold exogenous steroids for 24 hours |
| Give cosyntropin (synthetic alpha 1-24 ACTH) 250 μg (25 units) as IV bolus or IM injection |
| Obtain plasma cortisol level before administration of ACTH and 30 or 60 minutes afterward |
| Performance of the test in the morning is customary but not essential |
| *Interpretation* |
| Normal response: plasma cortisol level above 18 μg/dl at 30 *or* 60 minutes after ACTH administration |

*Note*: Traditional recommendations also specify an increment above baseline of 7 μg/dl at 30 minutes or 11 μg/dl at 60 minutes and a doubling of the baseline value at 60 minutes. These parameters are valid in normal, unstressed subjects but are frequently misleading in ill patients with a normal hypothalamic-pituitary-adrenal axis, in whom stress may raise the baseline plasma level via an increase in *endogenous* ACTH levels.

The stress of general anesthesia and surgery is not hazardous to patients who have received only replacement doses (no more than 25 mg hydrocortisone, 5 mg prednisone, 4 mg triamcinolone, or 0.75 mg dexamethasone),[161] if the steroid is given early in the day.[162] If doses of this size are given late in the day, suppression may occur as a result of inhibition of the diurnal release of ACTH.[162,163]

**ACTH and the HPA System.** Pharmacologic doses of ACTH produce supranormal cortisol secretory rates and elevated plasma cortisol levels. One might expect such elevated levels to suppress ACTH release. In fact, there is no evidence of clinically significant hypothalamic-pituitary suppression in patients who have received ACTH therapy.[2] The failure of ACTH to cause suppression of HPA function is not explained by the dose of ACTH employed, the frequency of injections, the time of administration, or the plasma cortisol pattern following ACTH administration.[164] Another possible explanation is that the hyperplastic and overactive adrenal cortex that results from ACTH therapy might compensate for hypothalamic or pituitary suppression.[165] Although threshold adrenocorticol sensitivity to ACTH is not changed in patients who have received daily ACTH therapy,[164] the possibility remains that there is altered adrenocortical responsiveness to ACTH in the physiologic range. In addition, evidence exists that the preservation of the normal response of the plasma cortisol level in patients treated with ACTH is due, at least in part, to the fact that ACTH treatment reduces the rate of ACTH secretion but not the total amount secreted, while glucocorticoids reduce both the rate of secretion and the total amount secreted.[166]

**Recovery from HPA Suppression.** During recovery from HPA suppression, hypothalamic-pituitary function returns before adrenocortical function.[167] Twelve months must elapse following withdrawal of large doses of glucocorticoids given for a prolonged period before homeostatic function, including responsiveness to stress, returns to normal.[2,167,168] In contrast, recovery from HPA suppression induced by a brief course of steroids (i.e., prednisone 25 mg twice daily for 5 days or prednisone 20 mg twice daily for 3 weeks) occurs within 5 days.[155,169] As a group, patients with mild suppression of the HPA axis (i.e., normal basal plasma and urine steroid levels but diminished responses to ACTH and insulin-induced hypoglycemia) resume normal functional capacity more rapidly than those with severe depression of the HPA axis (i.e., low basal plasma and urine steroid levels and diminished responses to ACTH and insulin-induced hypoglycemia).[170] The time course of recovery correlates with the total duration of previous glucocorticoid therapy and the total previous steroid dose.[170,172] Nevertheless, it is not possible in an individual patient to predict the time course of recovery from a course of glucocorticoid therapy at supraphysiologic doses lasting more than a few weeks, so persistence of HPA suppression should be suspected for 12 months after such a course of treatment. The course of recovery from suppression of the contralateral adrenal cortex by the products of an adrenocortical tumor may exceed 12 months.[162,173] Recovery from suppression induced by exogenous glucocorticoids may be more rapid in children than adults.[174]

## WITHDRAWAL OF PATIENTS FROM GLUCOCORTICOIDS

**Risks of Withdrawal.** The decision to discontinue glucocorticoid therapy provokes apprehension among physicians. The untoward consequences of such an action include precipitation of adrenocortical insufficiency, the steroid withdrawal syndrome, or an exacerbation of the underlying disease. Rarely, the syndrome of nodular panniculitis may occur.[175-178] This syndrome is characterized by painful pruritic nodules involving the flexor surfaces of the extremities, the cheeks, and the trunk.[175-178] These lesions, which appear 1 to 35 days after withdrawal of glucocorticoids, have been noted almost exclusively in children with acute rheumatic fever. The lesions may be ameliorated by reinstitution of glucocorticoids.

Adrenocortical insufficiency following the withdrawal of glucocorticoids is justly feared. The likelihood of precipitating the underlying disease almost certainly depends upon the activity and natural history of the illness in question. When there is any possibility that the underlying illness may flare up, the glucocorticoid should be withdrawn gradually, over an interval of weeks to months, with frequent reassessment of the patient.

**Management of the Patient with HPA Suppression.** There is no proved means of hastening a return to normal HPA function once inhibition has resulted from glucocorticoid therapy. The use of ACTH does not appear to prevent or reverse the development of glucocorticoid-induced adrenal insufficiency.[152,179-181] Conversion to an alternate-day schedule permits but does not accelerate recovery.[182,183] In children, alternate-day glucocorticoid therapy may delay recovery.[184]

Recovery from steroid-induced adrenal insufficiency is time dependent and spontaneous. During this interval, small doses of hydrocortisone (10 to 20 mg) or prednisone (2.5 to 5 mg) in the morning may alleviate withdrawal symptoms. Recovery of HPA function does occur during the administration of small doses of glucocorticoids in the morning; the rate of recovery is determined not only by the doses given when the steroids are being tapered but also by the dose administered during the initial phase of treatment, before tapering is commenced.[170-172] The available studies do not exclude the possibility that small doses of glucocorticoids in the morning retard the rate of recovery from HPA suppression, even though they do not prevent recovery. This requires further investigation.

## ALTERNATE-DAY GLUCOCORTICOID THERAPY

Alternate-day glucocorticoid therapy is defined as the administration of a short-acting glucocorticoid with no appreciable mineralocorticoid effect (such as prednisone, prednisolone, or methylprednisolone) once every 48 hours in the morning, at about 8:00 A.M. The objective is to minimize the adverse effects of glucocorticoids while retaining therapeutic effectiveness. The original basis for this approach was the hypothesis that the anti-inflammatory effects of glucocorticoids persist longer than the undesirable metabolic effects.[185-189] If so, it should be possible to find a schedule that allows rest periods between doses during which the patient is not exposed to the side effects of glucocorticoids while the desired anti-inflammatory action persists.[186,187] This hypothesis is not supported by observations of the duration of steroid effects (see above).

A second hypothesis emphasizes that intermittent rather than continuous administration produces a cyclic, though not diurnal, pattern of glucocorticoid levels in the circulation and within the target cells that simulates the normal diurnal cycle. This might prevent the development of Cushing's syndrome and HPA suppression but provide therapeutic benefit. Since the full expression of a disease frequently occurs only when the level of inflammatory activity increases over a protracted period of time, the intermittent administration of a glucocorticoid may be sufficient to shorten the interval during which the disorder develops without interruption, thereby preventing the level of disease activity from becoming clinically apparent (Fig. 54–4).[87] The duration of action of the glucocorticoids is important in this context. The selection of prednisone, prednisolone, and methylprednisolone as the agents of choice for alternate-day therapy and of 48 hours as the appropriate interval between doses has an empirical basis. Harter and associates found that intervals of 36, 24, and 12 hours were accompanied by adrenal suppression, and that an interval of 72 hours was therapeutically ineffective when prednisone (and, in some cases, triamcinolone) was employed. An interval of 48 hours was found to be optimal.[187]

**Alternate-Day Glucocorticoids and Cushing's Syndrome.** An alternate-day regimen can prevent or ameliorate the manifestations of Cushing's syndrome,[2,27,99,186,187,189-208] including not only the somatic and psychological manifestations but also quantifiable end-points such as high blood pressure,[191,194,195,200,206] retarded linear growth rate in children,[193,204-206] altered leukocyte kinetics,[99,197,202,203] impaired responsiveness to skin testing for delayed hypersensitivity,[192,203] impaired monocyte cellular function,[208] elevated urinary excretion rates of nitrogen and potassium,[27] impaired intestinal absorption of calcium,[207] reduced serum 25-hydroxyvitamin D levels,[207] and elevated serum cholesterol and triglyceride levels.[209]

The susceptibility to infections that characterizes Cushing's syndrome[76,210-212] may be alleviated by an alternate-day program. Cases in which refractory infections appeared to clear after conversion from daily to alternate-day therapy have been described.[194,195] Several studies report a low incidence of infections in patients on alternate-day therapy.[191,194,195,202,213] Children treated with alternate-day steroids regain or retain tonsillar and

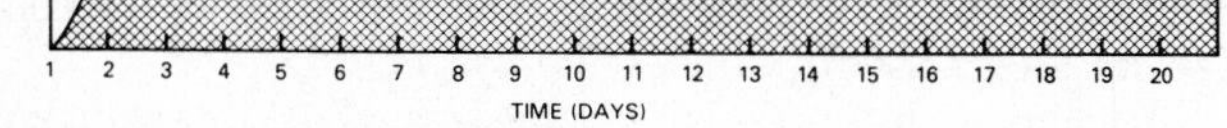

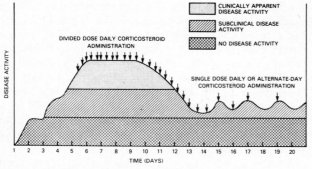


**Figure 54–4.** The effect of glucocorticoid administration on the activity of the underlying disease. Full-blown disease activity may require the use of a divided daily dose schedule. When the disease is controlled, or from the start of therapy in certain diseases, alternate-day therapy may be effective. (From Fauci, A.S., Dale, D.C., and Balow, J.E.: Ann. Intern. Med. 84:304, 1976.)

peripheral lymphoid tissue.[191] These reports strongly suggest that alternate-day therapy is associated with a lower incidence of infections than daily medication but do not firmly establish this point.

Host defense mechanisms have been studied in patients on alternate-day therapy. Patients maintained on such a program and studied on the day off the drug have normal blood neutrophil and monocyte counts, normal cutaneous inflammatory responses, and no abnormality of the neutrophil half-life; in contrast, patients on daily therapy demonstrate neutrophilia, monocytopenia, decreased cutaneous neutrophil and monocyte inflammatory responses, and prolongation of the neutrophil half-life.[99,202] Patients studied on the day off therapy do not have the lymphocytopenia observed in patients receiving daily treatment.[99,197,203] Monocyte cellular function is normal in patients on alternate-day therapy when studied 4 hours and 24 hours after a dose,[208] although daily therapy in divided doses depresses the bactericidal activity of monocytes.[113] Intermittently normal leukocyte kinetics,[99,197,202,203] preservation of delayed hypersensitivity,[192,203] and preservation of monocyte cellular function[208] may explain the apparently reduced susceptibility to infections of patients on alternate-day therapy.

**Effects of Alternate-Day Steroid Therapy on HPA Responsiveness.** Patients on alternate-day glucocorticoid therapy may have some suppression of basal steroid levels, but they have normal to nearly normal responsiveness to provocative tests such as ACTH stimulation tests,[187,214,215] insulin-induced hypoglycemia,[193,216] and the metyrapone test.[190,217] They also have less suppression of HPA function than patients on daily therapy.[184,187,218,219]

**Effects of Alternate-Day Therapy on the Underlying Disease.** Alternate-day glucocorticoid therapy is as effective or nearly as effective in controlling a diverse group of diseases as daily therapy in divided doses. This approach has been utilized with apparent benefit in patients with the following disorders: childhood nephrotic syndrome,[191] adult nephrotic syndrome,[198,220] membranous nephropathy,[221,222] renal transplantation,[194,195,199,200,204,206,223-226] mesangiocapillary glomerulonephritis,[227] lupus nephritis,[228] ulcerative colitis,[229,230] rheumatoid arthritis,[182,231] acute rheumatic fever,[232] myasthenia gravis,[233-239] Duchenne muscular dystrophy,[240] dermatomyositis,[241] idiopathic polyneuropathy,[242,243] asthma,[183,205,215,218,244] sarcoidosis,[196,201] alopecia areata and other chronic dermatoses,[186] and pemphigus vulgaris.[232,245] In one study, alternate-day therapy was not as effective as daily therapy in reducing the sedimentation rate in giant cell arteritis.[246] However, patients were transferred abruptly from daily therapy with divided doses to alternate-day therapy.[246] In addition, there were few adverse effects of steroids and no evidence of progression of the arteritis on the alternate-day regimen, so there may be a role for this approach in giant cell arteritis.[247] In another study, 18 of 27 patients with giant cell arteritis were treated successfully with an alternate-day regimen after a gradual transition from daily single dose therapy.[248] Prospective controlled studies demonstrate the efficacy of alternate-day therapy in membranous nephropathy[221] and renal transplantation.[224,226]

**Use of Alternate-Day Therapy.** Since alternate-day therapy can prevent or ameliorate the manifestations of Cushing's syndrome, can avert or permit recovery from HPA suppression, and is as effective (or nearly as effective) as continuous therapy, whenever possible a patient for whom chronic glucocorticoid administration is indicated should be placed on such a program. Yet some physicians are reluctant to utilize alternate-day schedules, often because of an unsuccessful experience. Many efforts fail because of lack of familiarity with the indications for, and use of, such therapy.

The benefits of alternate-day glucocorticoid therapy are demonstrable only when steroids are used for a prolonged period. There is no reason to use an alternate-day schedule when the anticipated duration of therapy is no longer than several weeks.

Alternate-day therapy may not be necessary or appropriate during the initial stages of therapy or during exacerbation of the underlying disease. Nevertheless, patients with childhood and adult nephrotic syndrome,[191,193,198,220] membranous nephropathy,[221,222] lupus nephritis,[228] rheumatoid arthritis,[182,231] myasthenia gravis,[233-236] dermatomyositis,[241] asthma,[214,215,244] sarcoidosis,[196,201] rheumatic fever,[232] pemphigus vulgaris,[245] a variety of ocular diseases,[213] and several other disorders have been treated with an alternate-day regimen as initial therapy with apparent benefit. It appears to be easier to establish treatment with alternate-day steroids than to convert from daily therapy in patients with rheumatoid arthritis.[182,231] Studies in recipients of renal transplants have initially used daily therapy and then converted to an alternate-day schedule. Thus, an alternate-day schedule as initial therapy may be beneficial in some disorders but ineffective in others.

Alternate-day therapy may be hazardous in the presence of adrenocortical insufficiency of any cause because the patient is unprotected against glucocorticoid insufficiency during the last 12 hours of the 48-hour cycle.[182,187,194] In a patient who has been on glucocorticoids for more than a brief period, or who may have adrenal insufficiency on another basis, adequacy of HPA function should be determined before the initiation of an alternate-day program. It may be possible to surmount this obstacle by giving a small dose of a short-acting glucocorticoid (i.e., 10 mg of hydrocortisone) in the afternoon of the second day; this approach has not been studied.

Alternate-day glucocorticoid therapy may fail to prevent or ameliorate the manifestations of Cushing's syndrome or HPA suppression if a short-acting glucocorticoid is not used, or if it is used incorrectly.[11,214,249,250] For example, the use of prednisone four times per day on alternate-days may be less successful than use of the same total dose once every 48 hours.

An abrupt alteration from daily to alternate-day therapy should be avoided because the prolonged use of daily-dose glucocorticoids may have resulted in HPA suppression. In addition, patients with normal function of the HPA axis may experience withdrawal symptoms in these circumstances and have an exacerbation of the underlying disease.[204]

No program of conversion from continuous therapy to alternate-day therapy has been proved to be optimal. One approach is to reduce the frequency of drug administration each day, until the total dose for each day is given in the morning, and then gradually to increase the dose on the first day of each 2-day period and to decrease the dose on the second day. Another approach is to double the dose on the first day of each 2-day cycle, and to give this as a single morning dose, if possible, and then to taper gradually the dose on the second day.[251] It is not clear how often such changes should be made with any approach. This probably depends on the underlying disease involved, the duration of previous glucocorticoid therapy, the personality of the patient, and the physician's ability to utilize adjunctive therapy. In any event, the conversion should be made as quickly as the patient will tolerate it. If the patient develops evidence of adrenal insufficiency, of the steroid withdrawal syndrome, or of an exacerbation of the underlying disease, the previously effective regimen should be reinstituted and then tapered more gradually. Occasionally, it will be necessary to resume full daily doses temporarily. Changes in the dose should be approximately 10 mg of prednisone (or equivalent) at total daily doses of more than 40 mg, 5 mg at total doses of more than 20 mg, and 2.5 mg at lower doses. At small total daily doses, an absolute change of dose represents a larger percentage change in dose than at large total daily doses. The interval between changes in dose may be as short as one day or as long as many weeks.

Also, optimal results from alternate-day glucocorticoid therapy may not be achieved because of failure to utilize supplemental therapy for the underlying disorder. Conservative (nonglucocorticoid) therapy is often used until a glucocorticoid is initiated, at which time these less toxic therapeutic measures are ignored. Utilization of adjunctive therapy may facilitate the use of the lowest possible dose of glucocorticoids. On alternate-day therapy, these measures should be used especially during the end of the second day, when symptoms may be prominent. The potential benefits of nonsteroidal anti-inflammatory agents in the rheumatic diseases should not be neglected. Supplemental therapy may be especially helpful in disorders in which the patient is likely to experience symptoms of the disease on the day off therapy, such as asthma and rheumatoid arthritis. In illnesses in which disabling symptoms are less likely to appear on the alternate day, such as the childhood nephrotic syndrome, less difficulty may be encountered.

Alternate-day therapy may fail because of failure to inform the patient about the purposes of this regimen. Because glucocorticoids may induce euphoria, a patient may be reluctant to accept modification of a schedule of frequent doses. Careful explanation about the risks of glucocorticoid excess, attuned to the patient's intellectual and emotional ability to comprehend, will maximize the likelihood of success. Close communication between patient and physician is indispensable.

## DAILY SINGLE-DOSE GLUCOCORTICOID THERAPY

In some situations, alternate-day therapy fails because the patient experiences symptoms of the underlying disease during the last few hours of the second day. In these cases, single-dose glucocorticoid therapy may be of value. This regimen appears to be as effective as divided daily doses in controlling such underlying diseases as rheumatoid arthritis, systemic lupus erythematosus, polyarteritis, and proctocolitis.[252-255] In giant cell arteritis, a daily dose in the morning is nearly as effective as daily therapy in divided doses.[246] Daily single-dose therapy appears to reduce the likelihood that a patient will develop HPA suppression.[29,254,256,257] On the other hand, the manifestations of Cushing's syndrome are probably not prevented or ameliorated by a daily single-dose regimen.[252,253]

## GLUCOCORTICOIDS OR ACTH?

Disorders that respond to glucocorticoid therapy also respond to ACTH therapy if the adrenal cortex is normal. However, there is no evidence that ACTH is superior to glucocorticoids for the treatment of any disorder when comparable doses are used.[2,16,258] In fact, hydrocortisone and ACTH, when given intravenously in pharmacologically equivalent dosage (determined by plasma cortisol levels and urinary steroid excretion rates) are equally effective in the treatment of inflammatory bowel disease.[259] Since ACTH does not appear to offer any therapeutic advantage, glucocorticoids are preferable for therapeutic purposes;[2] they can be administered orally, the dose can be regulated precisely, the effectiveness does not depend on adrenocortical responsiveness (an important consideration in patients who have been treated with glucocorticoids), and they produce a lower incidence of certain side effects, such as acne, hypertension, and increased pigmentation.[260] When one is unable to use alternate-day therapy, ACTH might appear to be preferable because it does not suppress the HPA axis. This benefit is usually outweighed by the advantages of glucocorticoids enumerated above and by the fact that daily injections of ACTH are not superior to single daily doses of short-acting glucocorticoids; in both cases, HPA suppression is unlikely to result, but Cushing's syndrome is not prevented. In life-threatening situations, glucocorticoids are indicated because maximal blood levels are obtained immediately after intravenous administration, while with ACTH infusion the plasma cortisol level rises to a plateau over several hours. The principal indication for ACTH continues to be the assessment of adrenocortical reserve.

## References


1. Polley, H.F., and Slocumb, C.H.: Behind the scenes with cortisone and ACTH. Mayo Clin. Proc. 51:471, 1976.
2. Axelrod, L.: Glucocorticoid therapy. Medicine 55:39, 1976.
3. Hollander, J.L., Brown, E.M., Jr., Jessar, R.A., and Brown, C.Y.: Hydrocortisone and cortisone injected into arthritic joints. JAMA 147:1629, 1951.
4. Robinson, R.C.V., and Robinson, H.M., Jr.: Topical treatment of dermatoses with steroids. South. Med. J. 49:260, 1956.
5. Jenkins, J.S.: The metabolism of cortisol by human extrahepatic tissues. J. Endocrinol. 34:51, 1966.
6. Schalm, S.W., Summerskill, W.H.J., and Go, V.L.W.: Development of radioimmunoassays for prednisone and prednisolone: Application to studies of hepatic metabolism of prednisone. Mayo Clin. Proc. 51:761, 1976.
7. Krieger, D.T., Allen, W., Rizzo, F., and Krieger, H.P.: Characterization of the normal temporal pattern of plasma corticosteroid levels. J. Clin. Endocrinol. Metab. 32:266, 1971.
8. Gann, D.S., Dallman, M.F., and Engeland, W.C.: Reflex control and modulation of ACTH and corticosteroids. *In* McCann, S.M. (ed.): Endocrine Physiology III. Int. Rev. Physiol. Vol. 24. Baltimore, University Park Press, 1981, p. 157.
9. Giguère, V., Labrie, F., Côté, J., Coy, D.H., Sueiras-Diaz, J., and Schally, A.V.: Stimulation of cyclic AMP accumulation and corticotropin release by synthetic ovine corticotropin-releasing factor in rat anterior pituitary cells: Site of glucocorticoid action. Proc. Natl. Acad. Sci. USA 79:3466, 1982.
10. Estep, H.L., Island, D.P., Ney, R.L., and Liddle, G.W.: Pituitary adrenal dynamics during surgical stress. J. Clin. Endocrinol. Metab. 23:419, 1963.
11. Harter, J.G.: Corticosteroids: Their physiologic use in allergic diseases. N.Y. State J. Med. 66:827, 1966.
12. Boland, E.W.: 16-α-Methyl corticosteroids. Calif. Med. 88:417, 1958.
13. Boland, E.W., and Liddle, G.W.: Metabolic and antirheumatic activities of 6-methylprednisolone (Medrol). Ann. Rheum. Dis. 16:297, 1957.
14. Bondy, P.K.: The adrenal cortex. *In* Bondy, P.K., and Rosenberg, L.E. (eds.): Duncan's Diseases of Metabolism. 7th ed. Philadelphia, W. B. Saunders Company, 1974, p. 1105.
15. Bunim, J.J., Black, R.L., Lutwak, L., Peterson, R.E., and Whedon, G.D.: Studies on dexamethasone, a new synthetic steroid, in rheumatoid arthritis—a preliminary report. Arthritis Rheum. 1:313, 1958.
16. Cope, C.L.: Adrenal Steroids and Disease. 2nd ed. London, Pitman Medical, 1972.
17. Kleeman, C.R., Koplowitz, J., and Maxwell, M.H.: Metabolic effects of two newer adrenal analogs, 6-methylprednisolone (Medrol) and 6-methyl-9α-fluoro-21-desoxyprednisolone (9α-fluoro-21-desoxymedrol). Metabolism 7:425, 1958.
18. Liddle, G.W.: Studies of structure-function relationships of steroids. II. The 6α-methylcorticosteroids. Metabolism 7:405, 1958.
19. Liddle, G.W.: Clinical pharmacology of the anti-inflammatory agents. Clin. Pharmacol. Ther. 2:615, 1961.
20. Liddle, G.W.: The adrenal cortex. *In* Williams, R.H. (ed.): Textbook of Endocrinology. 5th ed. Philadelphia, W. B. Saunders Company, 1974, p. 233.
21. Meikle, A.W., and Tyler, F.H.: Potency and duration of action of glucocorticoids. Effects of hydrocortisone, prednisone and dexamethasone on human pituitary-adrenal function. Am. J. Med. 63:200, 1977.
22. Ballard, P.L., Carter, J.P., Graham, B.S., and Baxter, J.D.: A radioreceptor assay for evaluation of the plasma glucocorticoid activity of natural and synthetic steroids in man. J. Clin. Endocrinol. Metab. 41:290, 1975.
23. Morris, H.G.: Factors that influence clinical responses to administered corticosteroids. J. Allergy Clin. Immunol. 66:343, 1980.
24. Pickup, M.E.: Clinical pharmacokinetics of prednisone and prednisolone. Clin. Pharmacokinetics 4:111, 1979.
25. Pickup, M.E., Lowe, J.R., Leatham, P.A., Rhind, V.M., Wright, V., and Downie, W.W.: Dose dependent pharmacokinetics of prednisolone. Eur. J. Clin. Pharmacol. 12:213, 1977.
26. Gambertoglio, J.G., Amend, W.J.C., Jr., and Benet, L.Z.: Pharmacokinetics and bioavailability of prednisone and prednisolone in healthy volunteers and patients: A review. J. Pharmacokinet. Biopharm. 8:1, 1980.
27. Walton, J., Watson, B.S., and Ney, R.L.: Alternate-day vs. shorter interval steroid administration. Arch. Intern. Med. 126:601, 1970.
28. Ellul-Micallef, R., Borthwick, R.C., and McHardy, G.J.R.: The time-course of response to prednisolone in chronic bronchial asthma. Clin. Sci. 47:105, 1974.
29. Grant, S.D., Forsham, P.H., and DiRaimondo, V.C.: Suppression of 17-

hydroxycorticosteroids in plasma and urine by single and divided doses of triamcinolone. N. Engl. J. Med. 273:1115, 1965.
30. Thompson, E.B., and Lippmann, M.E.: Mechanism of action of glucocorticoids. Metabolism 23:159, 1974.
31. Baxter, J.D.: Glucocorticoid hormone action. Pharmacol. Ther. B 2:605, 1976.
32. Chan, L., and O'Malley, B.W.: Steroid hormone action: Recent advances. Ann. Intern. Med. 89:694, 1978.
33. Jenkins, J.S., and Sampson, P.A.: Conversion of cortisone to cortisol and prednisone to prednisolone. Br. Med. J. 2:205, 1967.
34. Sugita, E.T., and Niebergall, P.J.: Prednisone. J. Am. Pharm. Assoc. 15:529, 1975.
35. DiSanto, A.R., and DeSante, K.A.: Bioavailability and pharmacokinetics of prednisone in humans. J. Pharm. Sci. 64:109, 1975.
36. Thiessen, J.J.: Prednisolone. J. Am. Pharm. Assoc. 16:143, 1976.
37. Tembo, A.V., Hallmark, M.R., Sakmar, E., Bachmann, H.G., Weidler, D.J., and Wagner, J.G.: Bioavailability of prednisolone tablets. J. Pharmacokinet. Biopharm. 5:257, 1977.
38. Duggan, D.E., Yeh, K.C., Matalia, N., Ditzler, C.A., and McMahon, F.G.: Bioavailability of oral dexamethasone. Clin. Pharmacol. Ther. 18:205, 1975.
39. Nelson, D.H., Sandberg, A.A., Palmer, J.G., and Tyler, F.H.: Blood levels of 17-hydroxycorticosteroids following the administration of adrenal steroids and their relation to levels of circulating leukocytes. J. Clin. Invest. 31:843, 1952.
40. Gemzell, C.A., and Franksson, C.: Blood levels of 17-hydroxycorticosteroids in normal and adrenalectomized men following administration of cortisone acetate. Acta Endocrinol. 12:218, 1953.
41. Plumpton, F.S., Besser, G.M., and Cole, P.V.: Corticosteroid treatment and surgery. 2. The management of steroid cover. Anaesthesia 24:12, 1969.
42. Banks, P.: The adreno-cortical response to oral surgery. Br. J. Oral Surg. 8:32, 1970.
43. Kehlet, H., Nistrup Madsen, S., and Binder, C.: Cortisol and cortisone acetate in parenteral glucocorticoid therapy? Acta Med. Scand. 195:421, 1974.
44. Kehlet, H.: A rational approach to dosage and preparation of parenteral glucocorticoid substitution therapy during surgical procedures. A short review. Acta Anaesth. Scand. 19:260, 1975.
45. Fariss, B.L., Hane, S., Shinsako, J., and Forsham, P.H.: Comparison of absorption of cortisone acetate and hydrocortisone hemisuccinate. J. Clin. Endocrinol. Metab. 47:1137, 1978.
46. Angeli, A., Frajria, R., DePaoli, R., Fonzo, D., and Ceresa, F.: Diurnal variation of prednisolone binding to serum corticosteroid-binding globulin in man. Clin. Pharmacol. Ther. 23:47, 1978.
47. Kozower, M., Veatch, L., and Kaplan, M.M.: Decreased clearance of prednisolone, a factor in the development of corticosteroid side effects. J. Clin. Endocrinol. Metab. 38:407, 1974.
48. Schalm, S.W., Summerskill, W.H.J., and Go, V.L.W.: Prednisone for chronic active liver disease: Pharmacokinetics, including conversion to prednisolone. Gastroenterology 72:910, 1977.
49. Peterson, R.E.: Adrenocortical steroid metabolism and adrenal cortical function in liver disease. J. Clin. Invest. 39:320, 1960.
50. Powell, L.W., and Axelsen, E.: Corticosteroids in liver disease: Studies on the biological conversion of prednisone to prednisolone and plasma protein binding. Gut 13:690, 1972.
51. Davis, M., Williams, R., Chakraborty, J., English, J., Marks, V., Ideo, G., and Tempini, S.: Prednisone or prednisolone for the treatment of chronic active hepatitis? A comparison of plasma availability. Br. J. Clin. Pharmacol. 5:501, 1978.
52. Araki, Y., Yokota, O., Tatsuo, K., Kashima, M., and Miyazaki, T.: Dynamics of synthetic corticosteroids in man. *In* Pincus, G., Nakao, T., and Tait, J.F. (eds.): Steroid Dynamics. New York, Academic Press, 1966, p. 463.
53. Lewis, G.P., Jusko, W.J., Burke, C.W., Graves, L., and the Boston Collaborative Drug Surveillance Program: Prednisone side-effects and serum-protein levels, a collaborative study. Lancet 2:778, 1971.
54. Schatz, M., Patterson, R., Zeitz, S., O'Rourke, J., and Melam, H.: Corticosteroid therapy for the pregnant asthmatic patient. JAMA 233:804, 1975.
55. Ohrlander, S., Gennser, G., Nilsson, K.O., and Eneroth, P.: ACTH test to neonates after administration of corticosteroids during gestation. Obstet. Gynecol. 49:691, 1977.
56. Grajwer, L.A., Lilien, L.D., and Pildes, R.S.: Neonatal subclinical adrenal insufficiency: Result of maternal steroid therapy. JAMA 238:1279, 1977.
57. Reinisch, J.M., Simon, N.G., Karow, W.G., and Gandelman, R.: Prenatal exposure to prednisone in humans and animals retards intrauterine growth. Science 202:436, 1978.
58. Katz, F.H., and Duncan, B.R.: Entry of prednisone into human milk (letter). N. Engl. J. Med. 293:1154, 1975.
59. McKenzie, S.A., Selley, J.A., and Agnew, J.E.: Secretion of prednisolone into breast milk. Arch. Dis. Child. 50:894, 1975.
60. Jubiz, W., and Meikle, A.W.: Alterations of glucocorticoid actions by other drugs and disease states. Drugs 18:113, 1979.
61. Choi, Y., Thrasher, K., Werk, E.E., Jr., Sholiton, L.J., and Olinger, C.: Effect of diphenylhydantoin on cortisol kinetics in humans. J. Pharmacol. Exp. Ther. 176:27, 1971.
62. Haque, N., Thrasher, K., Werk, E.E., Jr., Knowles, H.C., Jr., and Sholiton, L.J.: Studies on dexamethasone metabolism in man: Effect of diphenylhydantoin. J. Clin. Endocrinol. Metab. 34:44, 1972.
63. Stjernholm, M.R., and Katz, F.H.: Effects of diphenylhydantoin, phenobarbital, and diazepam on the metabolism of methylprednisolone and its sodium succinate. J. Clin. Endocrinol. Metab. 41:887, 1975.
64. Petereit, L.B., and Meikle, A.W.: Effectiveness of prednisolone during phenytoin therapy. Clin. Pharmacol. Ther. 22:912, 1977.
65. Brooks, S.M., Werk, E.E., Ackerman, S.J., Sullivan, I., and Thrasher, K.: Adverse effects of phenobarbital on corticosteroid metabolism in patients with bronchial asthma. N. Engl. J. Med. 286:1125, 1972.
66. Brooks, P.M., Buchanan, W.W., Grove, M., and Downie, W.W.: Effects of enzyme induction on metabolism of prednisolone. Clinical and laboratory study. Ann. Rheum. Dis. 35:339, 1976.
67. Edwards, O.M., Courtenay-Evans, R.J., Galley, J.M., Hunter, J., and Tait, A.D.: Changes in cortisol metabolism following rifampicin therapy. Lancet 2:549, 1974.
68. Buffington, G.A., Dominguez, J.H., Piering, W.F., Hebert, L.A., Kauffman, H.M., Jr., and Lemann, J., Jr.: Interaction of rifampin and glucocorticoids. Adverse effect on renal allograft function. JAMA 236:1958, 1976.
69. Uribe, M., Casian, C., Rojas, S., Sierra, J.G., and Go, V.L.W.: Decreased bioavailability of prednisone due to antacids in patients with chronic active liver disease and in healthy volunteers. Gastroenterology 80:661, 1981.
70. Klinenberg, J.R., and Miller, F.: Effect of corticosteroids on blood salicylate concentration. JAMA 194:131, 1965.
71. Graham, G.G., Champion, G.D., Day, R.O., and Paull, P.D.: Patterns of plasma concentrations and urinary excretion of salicylate in rheumatoid arthritis. Clin. Pharmacol. Ther. 22:410, 1977.
72. Bardare, M., Cislaghi, G.U., Mandelli, M., and Sereni, F.: Value of monitoring plasma salicylate levels in treating juvenile rheumatoid arthritis. Arch. Dis. Childh. 53:381, 1978.
73. Meyers, E.F.: Partial recovery from pancuronium neuromuscular blockade following hydrocortisone administration. Anesthesiology 46:148, 1977.
74. Laflin, M.J.: Interaction of pancuronium and corticosteroids. Anesthesiology 47:471, 1977.
75. Audétat, V., and Bircher, J.: Bioavailability of prednisolone during simultaneous treatment with cholestyramine. Gastroenterology 71:1110, 1976.
76. Plotz, C.M., Knowlton, A.I., and Ragan, C.: The natural history of Cushing's syndrome. Am. J. Med. 13:597, 1952.
77. Thorn, G.W.: Clinical considerations in the use of corticosteroids. N. Engl. J. Med. 274:775, 1966.
78. Boston Collaborative Drug Surveillance Program: Acute adverse reactions to prednisone in relation to dosage. Clin. Pharmacol. Ther. 13:694, 1972.
79. Hall, R.C.W., Popkin, M.K., Stickney, S.K., and Gardner, E.R.: Presentation of the steroid psychoses. J. Nervous Mental Dis. 167:229, 1979.
80. deLange, W.E., and Doorenbos, H.: Corticotrophins and corticosteroids. *In* Meyler, L., and Herxheimer, A. (eds.): Side Effects of Drugs, Vol. 7. Amsterdam, Excerpta Medica, 1972, p. 516.
81. Newman, S.: Hormone-induced diseases. *In* Moser, R.H. (ed.): Diseases of Medical Progress: A Study of Iatrogenic Disease. Springfield, Ill., Charles C Thomas, 1969, p. 361.
82. Fitzgerald, R.H., Jr.: Intrasynovial injection of steroids. Uses and abuses. Mayo Clin. Proc. 51:655, 1976.
83. Balch, H.W., Gibson, J.M.C., El-Ghobarey, A.F., Bain, L.S., and Lynch, M.P.: Repeated corticosteroid injections into knee joints. Rheumatol. Rehab. 16:137, 1977.
84. Carson, T.E., Daane, T.A., and Weinstein, R.L.: Long-term intramuscular administration of triamcinolone acetonide. Effect on the hypothalamic-pituitary-adrenal axis. Arch. Dermatol. 111:1585, 1975.
85. Claman, H.N.: Corticosteroids and lymphoid cells. N. Engl. J. Med. 287:388, 1972.
86. Claman, H.N.: How corticosteroids work. J. Allergy Clin. Immunol. 55:145, 1975.
87. Fauci, A.S., Dale, D.C., and Balow, J.E.: Glucocorticosteroid therapy: Mechanisms of action and clinical considerations. Ann. Intern. Med. 84:304, 1976.
88. Schreiber, A.D.: Clinical immunology of the corticosteroids. Prog. Clin. Immunol. 3:103, 1977.
89. Parrillo, J.E., and Fauci, A.S.: Mechanisms of glucocorticoid action on immune processes. Ann. Rev. Pharmacol. Toxicol. 19:179, 1979.
90. Cupps, T.R., and Fauci, A.S.: Corticosteroid-mediated immunoregulation in man. Immunological Rev. 65:133, 1982.

91. Dale, D.C., Fauci, A.S., Guerry, D., IV, and Wolff, S.M.: Comparison of agents producing neutrophilic leukocytosis in man: Hydrocortisone, prednisone, endotoxin, and etiocholanolone. J. Clin. Invest. 56:808, 1975.
92. Bishop, C.R., Athens, J.W., Boggs, D.R., Warner, H.R., Cartwright, G.E., and Wintrobe, M.M.: Leukokinetic studies. XIII. A non-steady-state kinetic evaluation of the mechanism of cortisone-induced granulocytosis. J. Clin. Invest. 47:249, 1968.
93. Athens, J.W., Haab, O.P., Raab, S.O., Mauer, A.M., Ashenbrucker, H., Cartwright, G.E., and Wintrobe, M.M.: Leukokinetic studies. IV. The total blood, circulating and marginal granulocyte pools and the granulocyte turnover rate in normal subjects. J. Clin. Invest. 40:989, 1961.
94. Boggs, D.R., Athens, J.W., Cartwright, G.E., and Wintrobe, M.M.: The effect of adrenal glucocorticosteroids upon the cellular composition of inflammatory exudates. Am. J. Pathol. 44:763, 1964.
95. Fauci, A.S., and Dale, D.C.: The effect of in vivo hydrocortisone on subpopulations of human lymphocytes. J. Clin. Invest. 53:240, 1974.
96. Yu, D.T.Y., Clements, P.J., Paulus, H.E., Peter, J.B., Levy, J., and Barnett, E.V.: Human lymphocyte subpopulations: Effect of corticosteroids. J. Clin. Invest. 53:565, 1974.
97. Clarke, J.R., Gagnon, R.F., Gotch, F.M., Heyworth, M.R., MacLennan, I.C.M., Truelove, S.C., and Waller, C.A.: The effect of prednisolone on leucocyte function in man: A double blind controlled study. Clin. Exp. Immunol. 28:292, 1977.
98. Cooper, D.A., Petts, V., Luckhurst, E., and Penny, R.: The effect of acute and prolonged administration of prednisolone and ACTH on lymphocyte subpopulations. Clin. Exp. Immunol. 28:467, 1977.
99. Cook, J.D., Trotter, J.L., Engel, W.K., and Sciabbarrasi, J.S.: The effects of single-dose alternate-day prednisone therapy on the immunological status of patients with neuromuscular diseases. Ann. Neurol. 3:166, 1978.
100. Fauci, A.S., and Dale, D.C.: The effect of hydrocortisone on the kinetics of normal human lymphocytes. Blood 46:235, 1975.
101. Yu, D.T.Y., Clements, P.J., and Pearson, C.M.: Effect of corticosteroids on exercise-induced lymphocytosis. Clin. Exp. Immunol. 28:326, 1977.
102. Ebert, R.H., and Barclay, W.R.: Changes in connective tissue reaction induced by cortisone. Ann. Intern. Med. 37:506, 1952.
103. Zweifach, B.W., Shorr, E., and Black, M.M.: The influence of the adrenal cortex on behavior of terminal vascular bed. Ann. N.Y. Acad. Sci. 56:626, 1953.
104. MacGregor, R.R., Spagnuolo, P.J., and Lentnek, A.L.: Inhibition of granulocyte adherence by ethanol, prednisone, and aspirin, measured with an assay system. N. Engl. J. Med. 291:642, 1974.
105. MacGregor, R.R.: The effect of anti-inflammatory agents and inflammation on granulocyte adherence: Evidence for regulation by plasma factors. Am. J. Med. 61:597, 1976.
106. MacGregor, R.R.: Granulocyte adherence changes induced by hemodialysis, endotoxin, epinephrine, and glucocorticoids. Ann. Intern. Med. 86:35, 1977.
107. Bovornkitti, S., Kangsadal, P., Sathirapat, P., and Oonsombatti, P.: Reversion and reconversion rate of tuberculin skin reactions in correlation with the use of prednisone. Dis. Chest 38:51, 1960.
108. Cummings, M.M., and Hudgins, P.C.: The influence of cortisone on the passive transfer of tuberculin hypersensitivity in the guinea pig. J. Immunol. 69:331, 1952.
109. Seebohm, P.M., Tremaine, M.M., and Jeter, W.S.: The effect of cortisone and adrenocorticotropic hormone on passively transferred delayed hypersensitivity to 2,4-dinitrochlorobenzene in guinea pigs. J. Immunol. 73:44, 1954.
110. Weston, W.L., Mandel, M.J., Yeckley, J.A., Krueger, G.G., and Claman, H.N.: Mechanism of cortisol inhibition of adoptive transfer of tuberculin sensitivity. J. Lab. Clin. Med. 82:366, 1973.
111. Balow, J.E., and Rosenthal, A.S.: Glucocorticoid suppression of macrophage migration inhibitory factor. J. Exp. Med. 137:1031, 1973.
112. Rinehart, J.J., Balcerzak, S.P., Sagone, A.L., and LoBuglio, A.F.: Effects of corticosteroids on human monocyte function. J. Clin. Invest. 54:1337, 1974.
113. Rinehart, J.J., Sagone, A.L., Balcerzak, S.P., Ackerman, G.A., and LoBuglio, A.F.: Effects of corticosteroid therapy on human monocyte function. N. Engl. J. Med. 292:236, 1975.
114. Handin, R.I., and Stossel, T.P.: Effect of corticosteroid therapy on the phagocytosis of antibody-coated platelets by human leukocytes. Blood 51:771, 1978.
115. Frank, M.M., Schreiber, A.D., Atkinson, J.P., and Jaffe, C.J.: Pathophysiology of immune hemolytic anemia. Ann. Intern. Med. 87:210, 1977.
116. Lewis, G.P., and Piper, P.J.: Inhibition of release of prostaglandins as an explanation of some of the actions of anti-inflammatory corticosteroids. Nature 254:308, 1975.
117. Kantrowitz, F., Robinson, D.R., McGuire, M.B., and Levine, L.: Corticosteroids inhibit prostaglandin production by rheumatoid synovia. Nature 258:737, 1975.
118. Tashjian, A.H., Jr., Voelkel, E.F., McDonough, J., and Levine, L.: Hydrocortisone inhibits prostaglandin production by mouse fibrosarcoma cells. Nature 258:739, 1975.
119. Gryglewski, R.J.: Steroid hormones, anti-inflammatory steroids and prostaglandins. Pharmacol. Res. Commun. 8:337, 1976.
120. Hong, S.-C.L., and Levine, L.: Inhibition of arachidonic acid release from cells as the biochemical action of anti-inflammatory corticosteroids. Proc. Natl. Acad. Sci. 73:1730, 1976.
121. Robinson, D.R., Tashjian, A.H., Jr., and Levine, L.: Prostaglandin-stimulated bone resorption by rheumatoid synovia: A possible mechanism for bone destruction in rheumatoid arthritis. J. Clin. Invest. 56:1181, 1975.
122. Samuelsson, B.: Leukotrienes: Mediators of immediate hypersensitivity reactions and inflammation. Science 220:568, 1983.
123. Janoski, A.H., Shaver, J.C., Christy, N.P., and Rosner, W.: On the pharmacologic actions of 21-carbon hormonal steroids ('glucocorticoids') of the adrenal cortex in mammals. *In* Deane, H.W., and Rubin, B.L. (eds.): Handbuch der Experimentellen Pharmakologie. Vol. XIV, Part 3 (The Adrenocortical Hormones). Berlin, Springer-Verlag, 1968, p. 256.
124. Christy, N.P.: Iatrogenic Cushing's syndrome. *In* Christy, N.P. (ed.): The Human Adrenal Cortex. New York, Harper & Row, 1971, p. 395.
125. Ragan, C.: Corticotropin, cortisone and related steroids in clinical medicine: Practical considerations. Bull. N.Y. Acad. Med. 29:355, 1953.
126. Intracranial hypertension and steroids (leading article.) Lancet 2:1052, 1964.
127. Walker, A.E., and Adamkiewicz, J.J.: Pseudotumor cerebri associated with prolonged corticosteroid therapy. JAMA 188:779, 1964.
128. David, D.S., and Berkowitz, J.S.: Ocular effects of topical and systemic corticosteroids. Lancet 2:149, 1969.
129. Lubkin, V.L.: Steroid cataract—a review and a conclusion. J. Asthma Res. 14:55, 1977.
130. Pavlin, C.R., DeVeber, G.A., Cook, G.T., and Chisholm, L.D.J.: Ocular complications in renal transplant recipients. Can. Med. Assoc. J. 117:360, 1977.
131. Heimann, W.G., and Freiberger, R.H.: Avascular necrosis of the femoral and humeral heads after high-dosage corticosteroid therapy. N. Engl. J. Med. 263:672, 1960.
132. Velayos, E.E., Leidholt, J.D., Smyth, C.J., and Priest, R.: Arthropathy associated with steroid therapy. Ann. Intern. Med. 64:759, 1966.
133. Harrington, K.D., Murray, W.R., Kountz, S.L., and Belzer, F.O.: Avascular necrosis of bone after renal transplantation. J. Bone Joint Surg. 53A:203, 1971.
134. Fisher, D.E., and Bickel, W.H.: Corticosteroid-induced aseptic necrosis: A clinical study of seventy-seven patients. J. Bone Joint Surg. 53A:859, 1971.
135. Park, W.M.: Spontaneous and drug-induced aseptic necrosis. *In* Davidson, J.K. (ed.): Aseptic Necrosis of Bone. Amsterdam, Excerpta Medica, 1976, p. 213.
136. Cruess, R.L.: Cortisone-induced avascular necrosis of the femoral head. J. Bone Joint Surg. 59B:308, 1977.
137. Abeles, M., Urman, J.D., and Rothfield, N.F.: Aseptic necrosis of bone in systemic lupus erythematosus. Arch. Intern. Med. 138:750, 1978.
138. Fenster, L.F.: The ulcerogenic potential of glucocorticoids and possible prophylactic measures. *In* Azarnoff, D.L. (ed.): Steroid Therapy. Philadelphia, W. B. Saunders Company, 1975, p. 42.
139. Conn, H.O., and Blitzer, B.L.: Nonassociation of adrenocorticosteroid therapy and peptic ulcer. N. Engl. J. Med. 294:473, 1976.
140. Langman, M.J.S., and Cooke, A.R.: Gastric and duodenal ulcer and their associated diseases. Lancet 1:680, 1976.
141. Jick, H., and Porter, J.: Drug-induced gastrointestinal bleeding. Lancet 2:87, 1978.
142. Messer, J., Reitman, D., Sacks, H.S., Smith, H., Jr., and Chalmers, T.C.: Association of adrenocorticosteroid therapy and peptic-ulcer disease. N. Engl. J. Med. 309:21, 1983.
143. Spiro, H.M.: Is the steroid ulcer a myth? N. Engl. J. Med. 309:45, 1983.
144. Schatz, M., Patterson, R., Kloner, R., and Falk, J.: The prevalence of tuberculosis and positive tuberculin skin tests in a steroid-treated asthmatic population. Ann Intern. Med. 84:261, 1976.
145. Frey, F.J., Amend, W.J.C., Jr., Lozada, F., Frey, B.M., and Benet, L.Z. Endogenous hydrocortisone, a possible factor contributing to the genesis of cushingoid habitus in patients on prednisone. J. Clin. Endocrinol. Metab. 53:1076, 1981.
146. Becker, B.: Intraocular pressure response to topical corticosteroids. Invest. Ophthalmol. 4:198, 1965.
147. Bigger, J.F., Palmberg, P.F., and Becker, B.: Increased cellular sensitivity to glucocorticoids in primary open angle glaucoma. Invest. Ophthalmol. 11:832, 1972.

148. Becker, B., Podos, S.M., Asseff, C.F., and Cooper, D.G.: Plasma cortisol suppression in glaucoma. Am. J. Ophthalmol. 75:73, 1973.
149. Becker, B., Shin, D.H., Palmberg, P.F., and Waltman, S.R.: HLA antigens and corticosteroid response. Science 194:1427, 1976.
150. Good, T.A., Benton, J.W., and Kelley, V.C.: Symptomatology resulting from withdrawal of steroid hormone therapy. Arthritis Rheum. 2:299, 1959.
151. Amatruda, T.T., Jr., Hollingsworth, D.R., D'Esopo, N.D., Upton, G.V., and Bondy, P.K.: A study of the mechanism of the steroid withdrawal syndrome. Evidence for integrity of the hypothalamic-pituitary-adrenal system. J. Clin. Endocrinol. Metab. 20:339, 1960.
152. Amatruda, T.T., Jr., Hurst, M.M., and D'Esopo, N.D.: Certain endocrine and metabolic facets of the steroid withdrawal syndrome. J. Clin. Endocrinol. Metab. 25:1207, 1965.
153. Paris, J.: Pituitary-adrenal suppression after protracted administration of adrenal cortical hormones. Proc. Mayo Clin. 36:305, 1961.
154. Salassa, R.M., Bennett, W.A., Keating, F.R., and Sprague, R.G.: Postoperative adrenal cortical insufficiency: Occurrence in patients previously treated with cortisone. JAMA 152:1509, 1953.
155. Streck, W.F., and Lockwood, D.H.: Pituitary adrenal recovery following short-term suppression with corticosteroids. Am. J. Med. 66:910, 1979.
156. Christy, N.P., Wallace, E.Z., and Jailer, J.W.: Comparative effects of prednisone and of cortisone in suppressing the response of the adrenal cortex to exogenous adrenocorticotropin. J. Clin. Endocrinol. Metab. 16:1059, 1956.
157. Jasani, M.K., Freeman, P.A., Boyle, J.A., Reid, A.M., Diver, M.J., and Buchanan, W.W.: Studies of the rise in plasma 11-hydroxycorticosteroids (11-OHCS) in corticosteroid-treated patients with rheumatoid arthritis during surgery: Correlations with the functional integrity of the hypothalamic-pituitary-adrenal axis. Quart. J. Med. 37:407, 1968.
158. Kehlet, H., and Binder, C.: Value of an ACTH test in assessing hypothalamic-pituitary-adrenocortical function in glucocorticoid-treated patients. Br. Med. J. 2:147, 1973.
159. Marks, L.J., Donovan, M.J., Duncan, F.J., and Karger, R.: Adrenocortical response to surgical operations in patients treated with corticosteroids or corticotropin prior to surgery. J. Clin. Endocrinol. Metab. 19:1458, 1959.
160. Sampson, P.A., Winstone, N.F., and Brooke, B.N.: Adrenal function in surgical patients after steroid therapy. Lancet 2:322, 1962.
161. Danowski, T.S., Bonessi, J.V., Sabeh, G., Sutton, R.D., Webster, M.W., Jr., and Sarver, M.E.: Probabilities of pituitary-adrenal responsiveness after steroid therapy. Ann. Intern. Med. 61:11, 1964.
162. Nichols, T., Nugent, C.A., and Tyler, F.H.: Diurnal variation in suppression of adrenal function by glucocorticoids. J. Clin. Endocrinol. Metab. 25:343, 1965.
163. Chamberlain, M.A., and Keenan, J.: The effect of low doses of prednisolone compared with placebo on function and on the hypothalamic pituitary adrenal axis in patients with rheumatoid arthritis. Rheumatol. Rehab. 15:17, 1976.
164. Carter, M.E., and James, V.H.T.: Comparison of effects of corticotrophin and corticosteroids on pituitary-adrenal function. Ann. Rheum. Dis. 30:91, 1971.
165. Daly, J.R., and Glass, D.: Corticosteroid and growth hormone response to hypoglycaemia in patients on long-term treatment with corticotrophin. Lancet 1:476, 1971.
166. Daly, J.R., Fletcher, M.R., Glass, D., Chambers, D.J., Bitensky, L., and Chayen, J.: Comparison of effects of long-term corticotrophin and corticosteroid treatment on responses of plasma growth hormone, ACTH, and corticosteroid to hypoglycaemia. Br. Med. J. 2:521, 1974.
167. Graber, A.L., Ney, R.L., Nicholson, W.E., Island, D.P., and Liddle, G.W.: Natural history of pituitary-adrenal recovery following long-term suppression with corticosteroids. J. Clin. Endocrinol. Metab. 25:11, 1965.
168. Livanou, T., Ferriman, D., and James, V.H.T.: Recovery of hypothalamo-pituitary-adrenal function after corticosteroid therapy. Lancet 2:856, 1967.
169. Webb, J., and Clark, T.J.H. Recovery of plasma corticotrophin and cortisol levels after a three-week course of prednisolone. Thorax 36:22, 1981.
170. Spitzer, S.A., Kaufman, H., Koplovitz, A., Topilsky, M., and Blum, I.: Beclomethasone dipropionate and chronic asthma: The effect of long-term aerosol administration on the hypothalamic-pituitary-adrenal axis after substitution for oral therapy with corticosteroids. Chest 70:38, 1976.
171. Westerhof, L., Van Ditmars, M.J., DerKinderen, P.J., Thijssen, J.H.H., and Schwarz, F.: Recovery of adrenocortical function during long-term treatment with corticosteroids. Br. Med. J. 4:534, 1970.
172. Westerhof, L., Van Ditmars, M.J., DerKinderen, P.J., Thijssen, J.H.H., and Schwarz, F.: Recovery of adrenocortical function during long-term treatment with corticosteroids. Br. Med. J. 2:195, 1972.
173. Kyle, L.H., Meyer, R.J., and Canary, J.J.: Mechanism of adrenal atrophy in Cushing's syndrome due to adrenal tumor. N. Eng. J. Med. 257:57, 1957.
174. Morris, H.G., and Jorgensen, J.R.: Recovery of endogenous pituitary-adrenal function in corticosteroid-treated children. J. Pediat. 79:480, 1971.
175. Smith, R.T., and Good, R.A.: Sequelae of prednisone treatment of acute rheumatic fever. Clin. Res. Proc. 4:156, 1956.
176. Taranta, A., Mark, H., Haas, R.C., and Cooper, N.S.: Nodular panniculitis after massive prednisone therapy. Am. J. Med. 25:52, 1958.
177. Vince, D.J.: Nodular panniculitis after massive prednisone therapy. Can. Med. Assoc. J. 79:840, 1958.
178. Spagnuolo, M., and Taranta, A.: Post-steroid panniculitis. Ann. Intern. Med. 54:1181, 1963.
179. Young, I.I., DeFilippis, V., Meyer, F.L., and Wolfson, W.Q.: Maintenance of adrenal cortical responsiveness during prolonged corticoid therapy. Arch. Intern. Med. 100:1, 1957.
180. Fleischer, N., Abe, K., Liddle, G.W., Orth, D.N., and Nicholson, W.E.: ACTH antibodies in patients receiving depot porcine ACTH to hasten recovery from pituitary-adrenal suppression. J. Clin. Invest. 46:196, 1967.
181. Carter, M.E., and James, V.H.T.: An attempt at combining corticotrophin with long-term corticosteroid therapy: With a view to preserving hypothalamic-pituitary-adrenal function. Ann. Rheum. Dis. 29:409, 1970.
182. Carter, M.E., and James, V.H.T.: Effect of alternate-day, single-dose corticosteroid therapy on pituitary-adrenal function. Ann. Rheum. Dis. 31:379, 1972.
183. Portner, M.M., Thayer, K.H., Harter, J.G., Rayyis, S., Liang, T.C., and Kent, J.R.: Successful initiation of alternate-day prednisone in chronic steroid-dependent asthmatic patients. J. Allergy Clin. Immunol. 49:16, 1972.
184. Morris, H.G., Neuman, I., and Ellis, E.F.: Plasma steroid concentrations during alternate-day treatment with prednisone. J. Allergy Clin. Immunol. 54:350, 1974.
185. Haugen, H.N., Reddy, W.J., and Harter, J.G.: Intermittent steroid therapy in bronchial asthma. Nord. Med. 63:15, 1960.
186. Reichling, G.H., and Kligman, A.M.: Alternate-day corticosteroid therapy. Arch. Dermatol. 83:980, 1961.
187. Harter, J.G., Reddy, W.J., and Thorn, G.W.: Studies on an intermittent corticosteroid dosage regimen. N. Engl. J. Med. 269:591, 1963.
188. Jacobson, M.E.: The rationale of alternate-day corticosteroid therapy. Postgrad. Med. 49:181, 1971.
189. Soyka, L.F.: Alternate-day corticosteroid therapy. Adv. Pediat. 19:47, 1972.
190. Fleisher, D.S.: Pituitary-adrenal responsiveness after corticosteroid therapy in children with nephrosis. J. Pediat. 70:54, 1967.
191. Soyka, L.F.: Treatment of the nephrotic syndrome in childhood: Use of an alternate-day prednisone regimen. Am. J. Dis. Child. 113:693, 1967.
192. MacGregor, R.R., Sheagren, J.N., Lipsett, M.B., and Wolff, S.M.: Alternate-day prednisone therapy: Evaluation of delayed hypersensitivity responses, control of disease and steroid side effects. N. Engl. J. Med. 280:1427, 1969.
193. Sadeghi-Nejad, A., and Senior, B.: Adrenal function, growth, and insulin in patients treated with corticoids on alternate days. Pediatrics 43:277, 1969.
194. Reed, W.P., Lucas, Z.J., and Cohn, R.: Alternate-day prednisone therapy after renal transplantation. Lancet 1:747, 1970.
195. Siegel, R.R., Luke, R.G., and Hellebusch, A.A.: Reduction of toxicity of corticosteroid therapy after renal transplantation. Am. J. Med. 53:159, 1972.
196. Block, A.J., and Light, R.W.: Alternate day steroid therapy in diffuse pulmonary sarcoidosis. Chest 63:495, 1973.
197. Chai, H., and Gilbert, A.: The effect of alternate-day prednisone on the white blood count in children with chronic asthma. J. Allergy Clin. Immunol. 51:65, 1973.
198. Gulati, P.D., Malik, G.B., and Vaishnava, H.: Alternate-day steroid therapy in adult nephrotics. J. Med. 4:266, 1973.
199. McEnery, P.T., Gonzalez, L.L., Martin, L.W., and West, C.D.: Growth and development of children with renal transplants. Use of alternate-day steroid therapy. J. Pediatr. 83:806, 1973.
200. Sampson, D., and Albert, D.J.: Alternate day therapy with methylprednisolone after renal transplantation. J. Urol. 109:345, 1973.
201. Sheagren, J.N., Simon, H.B., and Rich, R.R.: Therapy of sarcoidosis initiated with alternate-day prednisone. J. Natl. Med. Assoc. 65:391, 1973.
202. Dale, D.C., Fauci, A.S., and Wolff, S.M.: Alternate-day prednisone: Leukocyte kinetics and susceptibility to infections. N. Engl. J. Med. 291:1154, 1974.
203. Fauci, A.S., and Dale, D.C.: Alternate-day therapy and human lymphocyte subpopulations. J. Clin. Invest. 55:22, 1975.

204. Potter, D.E., Holliday, M.A., Wilson, C.J., Salvatierra, O., Jr., and Belzer, F.O.: Alternate-day steroids in children after renal transplantation. Transplant. Proc. 7:79, 1975.
205. Reimer, L.G., Morris, H.G., and Ellis, E.F.: Growth of asthmatic children during treatment with alternate-day steroids. J. Allergy Clin. Immunol. 55:224, 1975.
206. Diethelm, A.G., Sterling, W.A, Hartley, M.W., and Morgan, J.M.: Alternate-day prednisone therapy in recipients of renal allografts: Risks and benefits. Arch. Surg. 111:867, 1976.
207. Klein, R.G., Arnaud, S.B., Gallagher, J.C., DeLuca, H.F., and Riggs, B.L.: Intestinal calcium absorption in exogenous hypercortisonism: Role of 25-hydroxyvitamin D and corticosteroid dose. J. Clin. Invest. 60:253, 1977.
208. Norris, D.A., Fine, R., Weston, W.L., and Spector, S.: Monocyte cellular function in asthmatic patients on alternate-day steroid therapy. J. Allergy Clin. Immunol. 61:255, 1978.
209. Curtis, J.J., Galla, J.H., Woodford, S.Y., Lucas, B.A., and Luke, R.G.: Effect of alternate-day prednisone on plasma lipids in renal transplant recipients. Kidney Int. 22:42, 1982.
210. Kass, E.H., and Finland, M.: Adrenocortical hormones in infection and immunity. Ann. Rev. Microbiol. 7:361, 1953.
211. Thomas, L.: Cortisone and infection. Ann. N.Y. Acad. Sci. 56:799, 1953.
212. Dale, D.C., and Petersdorf, R.G.: Corticosteroids and infectious diseases. *In* Azarnoff, D.L. (ed.): Steroid Therapy. Philadelphia, W. B. Saunders Company, 1975, p. 209.
213. Schutz, S., Newhouse, R., and Dello Russo, J.: Alternate-day steroid regimen in the treatment of ocular disease. Br. J. Ophthalmol. 52:461, 1968.
214. Easton, J.G., Busser, R.J., and Heimlich, E.M.: Effect of alternate-day steroid administration on adrenal function in allergic children. J. Allergy Clin. Immunol. 48:355, 1971.
215. Kuzemko, J.A., and Lines, J.G.: Adrenal cortical function in asthmatic children on alternate-day steroids. Arch. Dis. Child. 46:366, 1971.
216. Ackerman, G.L., and Nolan, C.M.: Adrenocortical responsiveness after alternate-day corticosteroid therapy. N. Engl. J. Med. 278:405, 1968.
217. Wyatt, R., Waschek, J., Weinberger, M., and Sherman, B.: Effects of inhaled beclomethasone dipropionate and alternate-day prednisone on pituitary-adrenal function in children with chronic asthma. N. Engl. J. Med. 299:1387, 1978.
218. Falliers, C.J., Chai, H., Molk, L., Bane, H., and Cardoso, R.R. de A.: Pulmonary and adrenal effects of alternate-day corticosteroid therapy. J. Allergy Clin. Immunol. 49:156, 1972.
219. Bakran, I., Jr., Korsic, M., Durakovic, Z., Vrhovac, B., and Tajic, M.: The effect of alternate-day prednisone therapy on cortisol secretion rate in corticosteroid-dependent asthmatics. Int. J. Clin. Pharmacol. 15:57, 1977.
220. Bolton, W.K., Atuk, N.O., Sturgill, B.C., and Westervelt, F.B., Jr.: Therapy of the idiopathic nephrotic syndrome with alternate day steroids. Am. J. Med. 62:60, 1977.
221. Collaborative Study of the Adult Idiopathic Nephrotic Syndrome: A controlled study of short-term prednisone treatment in adults with membranous nephropathy. N. Engl. J. Med. 301:1301, 1979.
222. Hopper, J., Jr., Biava, C.G., and Tu, W.-H.: Membranous nephropathy: High-dose alternate-day therapy with prednisone. West. J. Med. 135:1, 1981.
223. Bell, M.J., Martin, L.W., Gonzales, L.L., McEnery, P.T., and West, C.D.: Alternate-day single-dose prednisone therapy: A method of reducing steroid toxicity. J. Pediat. Surg. 7:223, 1972.
224. McDonald, F.D., Horensten, M.L., Mayor, G.B., Turcotte, J.G., Selezinka, W., and Schork, M.A.: Effect of alternate-day steroids on renal transplant function: A controlled study. Nephron 17:415, 1976.
225. Reimold, E.W.: Intermittent prednisone therapy in children and adolescents after renal transplantation. Pediatrics 52:235, 1973.
226. Curtis, J.J., Galla, J.H., Woodford, S.Y., Saykaly, R.J., and Luke, R.G.: Comparison of daily and alternate-day prednisone during chronic maintenance therapy: A controlled crossover study. Am. J. Kidney Dis. 1:166, 1981.
227. McAdams, A.J., McEnery, P.T., and West, C.D.: Mesangiocapillary glomerulonephritis: Changes in glomerular morphology with long-term alternate-day prednisone therapy. J. Pediatr. 86:23, 1975.
228. Ackerman, G.L.: Alternate-day steroid therapy in lupus nephritis. Ann. Intern. Med. 72:511, 1970.
229. Cocco, A.E., and Mendeloff, A.L.: An evaluation of intermittent corticosteroid therapy in the management of ulcerative colitis. Johns Hopkins Med. J. 120:162, 1967.
230. Powell-Tuck, J., Bown, R.L., Chambers, T.J., and Lennard-Jones, J.E.: A controlled trial of alternate-day prednisolone as a maintenance treatment for ulcerative colitis in remission. Digestion 22:263, 1981.
231. Ansell, B.M., and Bywaters, E.G.L.: Alternate-day corticosteroid therapy in juvenile chronic polyarthritis. J. Rheumatol. 1:176, 1974.
232. Haim, S., Benderly, A., Shafrir, A., and Levy, J.: Alternate-day corticosteroid regimen. Dermatologica 142:171, 1971.
233. Jenkins, R.B.: Treatment of myasthenia gravis with prednisone. Lancet 1:765, 1972.
234. Engel, W.K., Festoff, B.W., Patten, B.M., Swerdlow, M.L., Newball, H.H., and Thompson, M.D.: Myasthenia gravis. Ann. Intern. Med. 81:225, 1974.
235. Seybold, M.E., and Drachman, D.B.: Gradually increasing doses of prednisone in myasthenia gravis: Reducing the hazards of treatment. N. Engl. J. Med. 290:81, 1974.
236. Brunner, N.G., Berger, C.L., Namba, T., and Grob, D.: Corticotropin or corticosteroids in generalized myasthenia gravis: Comparative studies and role in management. Ann. N.Y. Acad. Sci. 274:577, 1976.
237. Mann, J.D., Johns, T.R., and Campa, J.F.: Long-term administration of corticosteroids in myasthenia gravis. Neurology 26:729, 1976.
238. Newball, H.H., and Brahim, S.A.: Effects of alternate-day prednisone therapy on respiratory function in myasthenia gravis. Thorax 31:410, 1976.
239. Johns, T.R.: Treatment of myasthenia gravis: Long-term administration of corticosteroids with remarks on thymectomy. Adv. Neurol. 17:99, 1977.
240. Drachman, D.B., Toyka, K.V., and Myer, E.: Prednisone in Duchenne muscular dystrophy. Lancet 2:1409, 1974.
241. Engel, W.K., Borenstein, A., DeVivo, D.C., Schwartzman, R.J., and Warmolts, J.R.: High-single-dose alternate-day prednisone (HSDAD-PRED) in treatment of the dermatomyositis/polymyositis complex. Trans. Am. Neurol. Assoc. 97:272, 1972.
242. DeVivo, D.C., and Engel, W.K.: Remarkable recovery of a steroid-responsive recurrent polyneuropathy. J. Neurol. Neurosurg. Psychiat. 33:62, 1970.
243. Schwartzman, R.J., Engel, W.K., and Rapoport, A.: Criteria for the prednisone treatment of idiopathic polyneuropathy (abstract). Neurology 27:364, 1977.
244. Walsh, S.D., and Grant, I.W.B.: Corticosteroids in treatment of chronic asthma. Br. Med. J. 2:796, 1966.
245. Rabhan, N.B., and Kopf, A.W.: Alternate-day prednisone therapy for pemphigus vulgaris. Arch. Dermatol. 103:615, 1971.
246. Hunder, G.G., Sheps, S.G., Allen, G.L., and Joyce, J.W.: Daily and alternate day corticosteroid regimens in treatment of giant cell arteritis: Comparison in a prospective study. Ann. Intern. Med. 82:613, 1975.
247. Abruzzo, J.L.: Alternate-day prednisone therapy. Ann. Intern. Med. 82:714, 1975.
248. Bengtsson, B.-A., and Malmvall, B.-E. An alternate-day corticosteroid regimen in maintenance therapy of giant cell arteritis. Acta Med. Scand. 209:347, 1981.
249. Jasani, M.K., Boyle, J.A., Dick, W.C., Williamson, J., Taylor, A.K., and Buchanan, W.W.: Corticosteroid-induced hypothalamo-pituitary-adrenal axis suppression: Prospective study using two regimens of corticosteroid therapy. Ann. Rheum. Dis. 27:352, 1968.
250. Rabhan, N.B.: Pituitary-adrenal suppression and Cushing's syndrome after intermittent dexamethasone therapy. Ann. Intern. Med. 69:1141, 1968.
251. Fauci, A.S.: Alternate-day corticosteroid therapy. Am. J. Med. 64:729, 1978.
252. Dubois, E.L., and Adler, D.C.: Single-daily dose oral administration of corticosteroids in rheumatic disorders: An analysis of its advantages, efficacy and side effects. Curr. Ther. Res. 5:43, 1963.
253. Nugent, C.A., Ward, J., MacDiarmid, W.D., McCall, J.C., Baukol, J., and Tyler, F.H.: Glucocorticoid toxicity: Single contrasted with divided daily doses of prednisolone. J. Chronic Dis. 18:323, 1965.
254. Myles, A.B., Schiller, L.G.F., Glass, D., and Daly, J.R.: Single daily dose corticosteroid treatment. Ann. Rheum. Dis. 35:73, 1976.
255. Powell-Tuck, J., Bown, R.L., and Lennard-Jones, J.E.: A comparison of oral prednisone given as single or multiple daily doses for active proctocolitis. Br. J. Gastroenterol. 13:833, 1978.
256. DiRaimondo, V.C., and Forsham, P.H.: Pharmacophysiologic principles in the use of corticoids and adrenocorticotropin. Metabolism 7:5, 1958.
257. Myles, A.B., Bacon, P.A., and Daly, J.R.: Single daily dose corticosteroid treatment: Effect on adrenal function and therapeutic efficacy in various diseases. Ann. Rheum. Dis. 30:149, 1971.
258. Allander, E.: ACTH or corticosteroids? A critical review of results and possibilities in the treatment of severe chronic disease. Acta Rheum. Scand. 15:277, 1969.
259. Kaplan, H.P., Portnoy, B., Binder, H.J., Amatruda, T., and Spiro, H.: A controlled evaluation of intravenous adrenocorticotropic hormone and hydrocortisone in the treatment of acute colitis. Gastroenterology 69:91, 1975.
260. Savage, O., Copeman, W.S.C., Chapman, L., Wells, M.V., and Treadwell, B.L.J.: Pituitary and adrenal hormones in rheumatoid arthritis. Lancet 1:232, 1962.
260. Savage, O., Copeman, W.S.C., Chapman, L., Wells, N.V., and Treadwell, B.L.J.: Pituitary and adrenal hormones in rheumatoid arthritis. Lancet 1:232, 1962.

# Chapter 55
# Cytotoxic and Other Immunoregulatory Agents

*Anthony S. Fauci*

## INTRODUCTION

Immunoregulation can be broadly defined as the complex process whereby immunologic reactivity, either cellular or humoral, is constantly modulated to result in the net expression of an appropriate or, in certain circumstances, inappropriate immune response.[1] Recent intensive interest and investigation in immunology, which has led to certain rather striking advances in our understanding of the complexities of immune function and regulation in animal models as well as in man, together with the observations that many rheumatic diseases are at least associated with aberrancies of immune function, including immunoregulation,[1-5] form the intellectual basis for the use of immunoregulatory agents in the treatment of certain rheumatic diseases. It should be pointed out, however, that the use of cytotoxic and other immunoregulatory agents in these diseases antedated the most recent advances in our understanding of many of the subtle complexities of immune regulation. This is particularly true of the use of corticosteroids and cytotoxic agents in diseases whose clinicopathologic manifestations were strongly suggestive of aberrant inflammatory or immune-mediated phenomena. Since the use of these agents generally resulted in suppression of inflammation and immune function, it is not surprising that they have been extensively used in certain rheumatic, connective tissue, and autoimmune diseases.[7-10]

Unfortunately, despite the fact that recent advances in our understanding of immune function and regulation have allowed a greater intellectual understanding of the potential mechanisms of aberrant immune function in the diseases in question, the extraordinary complexity of the immune system, with its various inductive, regulatory, effector, and feedback mechanisms, has made it clear to clinical investigators that perturbation of the system by agents used for therapeutic purposes may have multifaceted effects on the system, some of which might be unpredictable, if not unrecognized. Indeed, this very complexity of the system in the face of the relatively crude and usually nonspecific modulation effected by most of the therapeutic agents in question may result in only a minor or temporary dampening of the expression of the disease process. On the other hand, the adverse side effects associated with perturbation of the immune system in this manner may place the therapeutic efficacy that results beyond the limits of the price that one is willing to pay for such an effect. Indeed, certain immunoregulatory agents have been used and are being used inappropriately in diseases whose severity or projected clinical course clearly do not warrant such an aggressive approach. Nonetheless, despite these general caveats, certain cytotoxic and other immunoregulatory agents have been successfully and appropriately employed in the treatment of a number of rheumatic diseases, and in certain situations with rather impressive results.[6,8-10]

It is the aim of this chapter to consider some of the real and potential mechanisms whereby one can feasibly and successfully modify the expression of aberrant inflammatory and immune responses and to discuss the mechanisms of action of the various categories of immunoregulatory agents as well as their proven and potential usefulness in the treatment of rheumatic diseases in order to better appreciate the positive and negative aspects of such a therapeutic approach.

## THE IMMUNE SYSTEM AND ITS REGULATION

A number of models of the immune system and its regulation have been proposed, and each almost invariably has the common denominator of a cellular and humoral network of immune reactivity reflected by different cell types. The dual limbs of the immune response introduced several years ago[11-14] and now clearly substantiated are the thymus-derived (T) lymphocyte limb and the bone marrow–derived or bursa-equivalent (B) lymphocyte limb, both of which derive from a common stem cell. Other cell types, such as the monocyte-macrophage, play a major role in the inductive, regulatory, and effector phases of the immune response.[15]

A somewhat simplified scheme of the immune system is illustrated in Figure 55–1. As has been previously and extensively described, the expression of immune function can be conveniently looked upon as a series of phases. Both T and B lymphocytes mediate a number of critical immune functions, and each of these cell types, when given the appropriate signal, pass through phases, from activation or induction through proliferation, differentiation, and ultimately effector function.[3,5] The effector function that is expressed may be at the end point of a response, such as secretion of antibody by a differentiated B lymphocyte or plasma cell, or it might serve a regulatory function that modulates other end-stage functions, as is seen with inducer or suppressor T lymphocytes, which modulate the function of B lymphocytes,

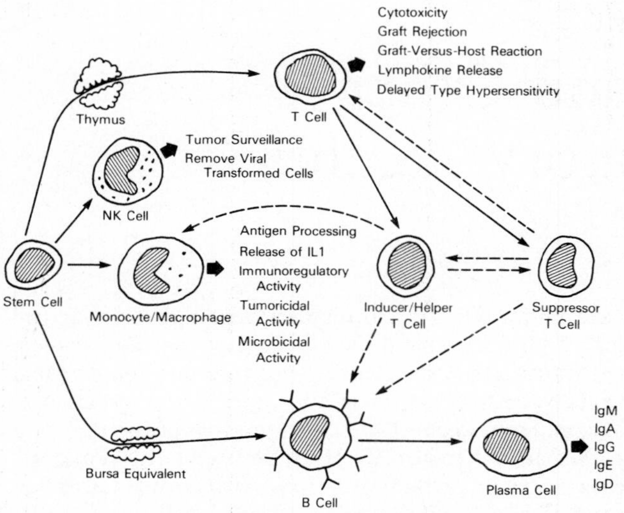


**Figure 55–1.** Schematic diagram of the human immune system. Virtually all of the components of the immune system derive from a common stem cell, which then gives rise to the various components of the system. Cells that come under the influence of the thymus evolve into thymus-derived (T) cells and are further subdivided into various subsets of immunoregulatory populations. In addition to the regulation of B lymphocyte function by induction and suppression, the T lymphocyte limb also manifests effector functions such as are indicated by the bold arrow stemming from the T cell. Lymphocytes that evolve through the bursa-equivalent differentiate into B lymphocytes, which upon appropriate stimuli further differentiate into antibody-secreting plasma cells, which are the ultimate effector cells of this limb of the immune response. Monocyte/macrophages and natural killer cells also evolve from the common stem cell, and these also have ultimate effector functions. Monocytes may be immunoregulated by T lymphocytes and their products, and they may also be involved in the immunoregulation of B and T lymphocyte function. The extraordinarily complex cellular and humoral interactions in this scheme, which are simplified here, particularly with regard to the delicate balance among positive and negative influences, ultimately result in the net expression of an appropriate immune response. Even the slightest imbalance in this immunoregulatory circuit may lead to the expression of aberrancies of immune function leading to clinically apparent immune-mediated disease.

T lymphocytes, other lymphoid cells, or even certain nonlymphoid cell types. Very briefly, in addition to induction and suppression, T lymphocytes mediate a number of other important immune functions, such as specific cell-mediated cytotoxicity, certain types of graft rejection, graft-versus-host phenomena, delayed-type hypersensitivity, and the production and release of a broad range of soluble mediators termed lymphokines, which have profound effects on virtually all phases of the immune response.

On the other hand, B lymphocytes subserve a much more uniform function. They are the precursors of antibody-forming cells, and when appropriately stimulated, they proliferate and differentiate into cells that secrete antibody of the various classes and subclasses. Natural killer cells are lymphoid cells. They are not of B lymphocyte lineage and may well not be of T lymphocyte lineage, although they share some, but not all, phenotypic characteristics of T lymphocytes.[16] These cells are felt to be involved in immune surveillance against neoplastically transformed cells as well as in the elimination of virally transformed target cells.[17]

The monocyte-macrophage system, which is represented by monocytes in the peripheral blood and by macrophages in various tissues, plays a major role in the expression of immune reactivity by mediating a number of important functions, such as the presentation of antigen to lymphocytes and the secretion of factors such as interleukin 1 (IL 1) that are involved in the activation of lymphocytes. In addition, they directly mediate certain effector functions, such as the destruction of antibody-coated bacteria, tumor cells, or even normal cells such as hematologic elements in certain types of autoimmune cytopenias.[16,18] Furthermore, activated macrophages can directly eliminate various cell types even in the absence of antibody.

Finally, nonlymphoid cells such as neutrophils, eosinophils, and basophils play a major role in the inflammation that results from certain immune-mediated reactions and as such must be considered in the scheme of immune function despite the fact that they are not classically viewed as part of the immune system.

The net expression of immune function, be it a specific or nonspecific effector function, is the result of a balance between positive and negative influences mediated by the inducer or suppressor populations of cells alluded to above.[1,3,5] They may exert their influence either directly or via the release of soluble immunoregulatory molecules. In addition to the classic cellular regulation of immune reactivity, the idiotypic network has been proposed as a potentially important mechanism of immunoregulation.[19] Elaborate and complex schemes have been proposed for the mechanisms of such immunoregulation, with secreted idiotype and anti-idiotype antibodies as well as idiotype- and anti-idiotype–bearing cells having been demonstrated as playing a major role in the regulation of immune function in the murine system.[20] The demonstration of regulation of human immune function by idiotype–anti-idiotype reactions has been reported recently[21] and awaits further delineation before its role in the regulation of normal and abnormal lymphocyte physiology can be appreciated fully. In this regard, recent evidence suggests that the idiotype network may play a role in the regulation of autoimmune states such as systemic lupus erythematosus (SLE).[22]

## ABERRANCIES OF IMMUNE REACTIVITY

The established and potential mechanisms of disease activity in the broad range of rheumatic diseases are discussed in the individual chapters dealing with these disorders. However, if one considers Figure 55–1 and the preceding discussion, it is clear that there are a number of potential mechanisms for the expression of aberrant immune reactivity related to the occurrence of even slight perturbations of the delicate balance in the cellular or humoral immunoregulatory network. This may take the form of a selective deficiency in suppressor cell function or an abnormal heightening of inducer cell activity. In addition to imbalances in immunoregulation, one can have primary hyper-reactivity of certain effector functions such as B-lymphocyte reactivity.[1] Under these circumstances, it is conceivable that even a normally functioning helper and/or suppressor cell network might not successfully dampen the aberrant B-lymphocyte hyper-reactivity. Even more likely, there may be a combination of hyperactive effector cell function such as hyper-reactivity at the B-lymphocyte level together with abnormalities of immunoregulatory T-lymphocyte function. In fact, this is precisely the situation that has been noted in SLE. It is still disputed whether the B-lymphocyte hyper-reactivity is a primary state independent of the deficiency of suppressor T-lymphocyte function, whether the B-lymphocyte hyper-reactivity is secondary to the suppressor cell defect, or whether the abnormalities of immune reactivity actually result from a combination of both of these phenomena together with a number of other recognized as well as ill-defined factors.[1]

In this regard, the net expression of immune function in most of the rheumatic diseases appears to be one of aberrant hyper-reactivity. As such, we generally distinguish these disorders from immunodeficiency diseases in which the net expression of immune function is generally that of hyporeactivity. However, given the balance between positive and negative influences in the immune network, one can easily appreciate that a deficiency of immune function such as suppressor cell activity (hence, strictly speaking a immunodeficiency state) can actually result in hyperactive effector immune function.[1,23] This point is not trivial and has important implications in appreciating the basis of certain of the therapeutic strategies that will be described below. Thus, although we commonly refer to the therapeutic strategy of immunosuppression for diseases of inflammation and/or immunologic hyper-reactivity, we would more correctly think in terms of therapeutic immunoregulation either by dampening hyperactive responses or by directly or indirectly enhancing defective negative immunoregulatory influences.

## POTENTIAL AREAS OF MODIFICATION OF IMMUNE RESPONSES BY THERAPEUTIC AGENTS

**Suppression.** Abnormally hyperactive immune responses at either the T- or B-lymphocyte level can be theoretically as well as practically eliminated or at least dampened by nonspecifically suppressing the entire immune system. Clearly, sufficient amounts of cytotoxic agents, irradiation, antilymphocyte sera, and other immunosuppressive agents can be administered to eliminate virtually any immune response. These therapeutic modalities are truly nonspecific in that they do not selectively eliminate abnormally active lymphoid cells, nor do they spare normal lymphoid cells. Thus, although the desired effect can ultimately be obtained, the inevitable toxic side effects render such an approach non-feasible in the treatment of non-neoplastic diseases. Thus, within the realm of nonspecific suppression of immune function, therapeutic strategies are employed that strike a balance between the desired effect of suppression of aberrant immune reactivity and maintenance of sufficient immune function as well as phagocytic, particularly neutrophil, cell number and function to maintain the integrity of the host defense system as well as the level of inflammatory and immune function required to maintain immunologic homeostasis.

This approach usually takes the form of administration of cytotoxic drugs in dose regimens which, while still nonspecific, would relatively more selectively dampen the ongoing aberrant immune response. An example is the use of chronically administered cyclophosphamide in doses of 2 mg per kg per day in certain of the severe systemic vasculitic syndromes.[24,25] These disorders are characterized by hyper-reactivity of B-lymphocyte responses with hypergammaglobulinemia, immune complex deposition, and spontaneous secretion of polyclonal immunoglobulin (Ig) by activated B lymphocytes.[26] Administration of cyclophosphamide in the above regimen results in a selective suppression of B-lymphocyte reactivity with relative sparing of T-lymphocyte responses despite the fact that a total lymphocytopenia inevitably results from such chronic therapy.[27] Thus, although all B-lymphocyte function is suppressed, rendering such an approach nonspecific, there appears to be a selective suppression of the hyperactive B lymphocytes more than other lymphoid cell function.[27]

Other nonspecific but less globally immunosuppressive modalities include thoracic duct drainage, plasmapheresis, leukopheresis, the use of antilymphocyte globulin or monoclonal antibodies directed against lymphocyte subsets, irradiation of groups of regional lymph nodes, and the use of agents such as cyclosporin A, which relatively selectively suppresses T-lymphocyte function while sparing other lymphoid and nonlymphoid cells. Each of these approaches represents an attempt within the realm of a fundamentally nonspecific immunosuppressive regimen to render the approach somewhat more selective.

Despite these attempts at introducing varying degrees of selectivity into nonspecific immunosuppressive regimens, the extraordinary complexity of the immune system, with its multiple levels of regulation and feedback mechanisms, adds a considerable degree of uncertainty to such approachs. This stems from the fact that the desired effect may not be realized, since perturbation of the on-going activity of the system may introduce feedback mechanisms that obviate the desired effect. Furthermore, the actual effect may be different from the desired effect and de facto undesirable in itself. One can view the situation as an attempt to employ extremely crude tools to fine tune an extraordinarily complex and delicate machine. Nonetheless, despite the limitations of such an approach, nonspecific immunosuppression has resulted in favorable therapeutic results in a number of rheumatic diseases.[6,8,9] However, given the state of the art at present, realization of these limitations is essential for proper application of such regimens as well as for providing an impetus to continuing the search for more specific and less toxic forms of immunosuppression.

Unfortunately, modalities of truly specific suppression are more theoretical than practical when one considers their use in rheumatic diseases in man. For example, classic experiments with cyclophosphamide have demonstrated that administration of an antigen together with the drug results in a selective suppression of the immune response to the antigen in question as opposed to the immune response in general.[28] However, since the actual responsible antigens in most, if not all, rheumatic diseases remain unclear, such an approach is at present not clinically feasible.

A number of suppressor systems in the mouse have proved to be specific, and antigen-specific suppressor cells and suppressor factors have been identified.[29] In the human system, virtually all of the suppressor systems are nonspecific,[23,30] and those that reflect a degree of specificity are almost invariably specific in their induction and nonspecific in their expression. Furthermore, although various systems of specific immunologic tolerance have been described in a number of animal models,[31] these cannot yet be extrapolated to an approach to the treatment of human disease for a variety of reasons, not the least important of which is our failure to recognize the putative antigen in most diseases.

**Enhancement.** As mentioned above, even disorders that express a net hyperactive immune response may have components that are hypoactive. In this regard, immune enhancement should theoretically be beneficial provided the defective element can be selectively enhanced. Since virtually all of the immune-enhancing drugs or agents that will be discussed below are indeed nonspecific, they suffer from the same limitations as immunosuppressive agents in the modulation of aberrant immune reactivity in disease states. Nonetheless, certain drugs that enhance immune responses have been used with limited success in certain immunologically mediated diseases and will be mentioned below.

The ultimate enhancement of the immune response would be complete replacement, as with ablation and bone marrow transplantation. However, given the nature of the diseases in question together with the logistic constraints on bone marrow transplants, such an approach is not feasible at present for rheumatic diseases. Transfer of mature immune competent lymphoid cells has the theoretical potential of reversing the imbalance of immunoregulatory lymphocyte subsets. Again, logistic constraints, with regard to histocompatibility requirements and restrictions, make such an approach untenable. However, of particular interest over the past few years has been the availability of purified preparations of lymphokines such as interleukin II (IL II) and the various interferons. These factors, particularly IL II, are capable of exerting profound enhancing effects on the immune response in vitro,[32] and the therapeutic use of such factors holds at least theoretical potential for the future.

# CYTOTOXIC AGENTS

## General Considerations

Of all the immunoregulatory agents that are used in the treatment of rheumatic diseases, the cytotoxic drugs pose perhaps the greatest difficulty for the clinician from both a theoretical and a practical standpoint. This stems largely from the fine line between risk and benefit, which exists for virtually all such agents used in the treatment of these diseases. Unfortunately, the terminology that is frequently employed with regard to the cytotoxic agents is somewhat misleading in that the term "cytotoxic" agent is used synonymously with the term "immunosuppressive" agent. Indeed, cytotoxic agents can be and are frequently immunosuppressive; however, a number of other drugs discussed in this chapter as well as the corticosteroids (see Chapter 54) can be potent immunosuppressive agents. The cytotoxic agents differ from many of these other agents in that the common denominator of their effect is that they destroy cells, hence the derivation of the term "cytotoxic," which means simply that the drugs are directly toxic or damaging to cells. It is this ability to kill cells that distinguishes the cytotoxic immunosuppressive agents from the other categories of immunosuppressive drugs and explains their extensive use in the treatment of a variety of neoplastic diseases. Indeed, their use as antineoplastic agents long antedates their use as immunosuppressive agents in non-neoplastic inflammatory and immune-mediated diseases. Only when the profound immunosuppressive effects of these agents as used in the treatment of neoplastic diseases became apparent did clinical investigators conceive of their use in diseases that manifested marked inflammatory responses and apparent immune-mediated mechanisms.[10] Certain of the mechanisms of action of cytotoxic agents on inflammatory and immunologic responses are listed in Table 55–1.[33]

It cannot be emphasized too strongly that the rationale for the use of cytotoxic agents as well as the goals that one wishes to achieve by therapy are for the most part quite different depending on whether one uses these agents in the treatment of non-neoplastic immune-mediated diseases or neoplastic diseases. The rationale and goal for the use of cytotoxic agents in the treatment of neoplastic diseases is simply to eliminate where possible every last tumor cell. This approach is almost invariably associated with significant destruction of the normal

**Table 55–1.** Principal Mechanisms of Action of Cytotoxic Agents on Inflammatory and Immunologic Reactions

1. Elimination of sensitized and immunologically committed lymphoid cells
2. Elimination of nonsensitized lymphoid cells secondarily engaged in aberrant immunologic reactivity
3. Elimination of nonlymphoid cells engaged in nonspecific inflammatory responses to aberrant immunologic reactions
4. Suppression of functional capabilities of surviving lymphoid cells

elements of host defense mechanisms, such that a life-threatening or near life-threatening state exists for variable periods of time during and following chemotherapy until the normal cellular elements can recover. If the tumor is sensitive to the chemotherapeutic agents used, such that a reasonable chance of remission and/or cure exists, then the attendant risks are clearly justifiable, since the malignant neoplasm will otherwise inevitably result in the death of the patient. Under such circumstances, the goals are rather clear-cut, and the options are few.

The situation is quite different when using these agents to treat non-neoplastic diseases. Since there are no recognizable malignant clones in the immune-mediated diseases, the rationale and goal are usually to suppress the aberrant inflammatory and immune-mediated reactions that are responsible for the tissue damage without markedly suppressing the normal host defense mechanisms, which would put the patient at significant risk for either an infection or a neoplasm resulting from the suppression of normal immune surveillance mechanisms.[24,25,33] Unfortunately, maintaining this balance between risk and benefit is not an easy task, since, as mentioned previously, the agents employed are almost always nonspecific in their suppressive effects, and suppression of normal immune mechanisms will invariably accompany suppression of the aberrant reactions. It is hoped that suppression of these abnormal immune responses will be effected prior to the point at which such a degree of suppression of normal immune mechanisms occurs, so that the patient would not be at a significant risk.

Of equal, if not greater, importance than the suppression of normal immunologic mechanisms is the suppression of normal nonspecific mechanisms of host defenses in the form of the circulating polymorphonuclear neutrophils. Due to the relatively rapid turnover of the neutrophil series in the bone marrow, cytotoxic agents are particularly effective in causing a neutropenia, which becomes one of the major limiting factors in the use of these agents. In this regard, another important difference in the use of these agents in neoplastic versus non-neoplastic diseases is the fact that in non-neoplastic diseases, the drugs are usually administered chronically over extended periods of time, ranging from months to years, and so the risk of a host defense defect is a relatively persistent problem as opposed to the relatively brief (albeit usually more severe) periods of defect seen following the intermittent courses of chemotherapy usually administered for neoplastic diseases.

Finally, the major difference in the use of these agents in the treatment of neoplastic versus non-neoplastic diseases lies in the area of exercising of clinical judgment as to when to employ such an aggressive chemotherapeutic approach in a non-neoplastic disease that might not be invariably fatal. The clinical course of most neoplastic diseases that are left untreated or that are not aggressively treated is usually rather clear, which makes the decision to initiate aggressive therapy relatively easy. In contrast, many of the rheumatic diseases, such as SLE, rheumatoid arthritis, the systemic vasculitides, scleroderma, and dermatomyositis/polymyositis, as well as several of the organ-specific autoimmune diseases in which cytotoxic agents have been used have variable clinical courses. Only when the disease seems to be progressing with irreversible organ system dysfunction that is not responsive to more conventional therapy, such as nonsteroidal anti-inflammatory agents or corticosteroids, does one consider employing a cytotoxic agent. This is often a difficult decision, since the efficacy of these agents in many of these diseases has not been conclusively proved by appropriately controlled studies. Furthermore, the chronicity of most of these diseases dictates that even though a cytotoxic agent may be effective in suppressing disease activity, the agent cannot be used indefinitely. Thus, it is essential to set reasonable goals for the use of cytotoxic agents in the treatment of rheumatic diseases.

## Therapeutic Goals

Very few situations exist in which the use of cytotoxic agents can be expected to effect a true and long-term "cure" of a non-neoplastic disease. One such situation is the use of these agents, particularly cyclophosphamide, in the treatment of certain of the vasculitic syndromes. Paramount among these syndromes is Wegener's granulomatosis in which long-term remissions, which can indeed be called "cures," have been effected in as high as 90 percent of patients treated with cyclophosphamide, 2 mg per kg per day, together with prednisone, 1 mg per kg per day, administered first daily and then on an alternate-day schedule.[24,25] Similar results have been obtained with other of the vasculitic syndromes, particularly the polyarteritis nodosa group of the systemic necrotizing vasculitides.[34] Prior to the institution of this therapy, virtually all patients with Wegener's granulomatosis died of their disease, as did most patients with the polyarteritis nodosa type of systemic necrotizing vasculitis.[24,25] It is conceivable that the drug does not in fact "cure" the disease but merely suppresses the inflammatory and aberrant immune-mediated mechanisms long enough for the disease to spontaneously run its course and permanently remit. Therefore, given these reported therapeutic results, a reasonable goal for the use of cytotoxic agents (in this case cyclophosphamide) in these vasculitic syndromes is a true permanent remission or cure. One can hope that a single course of therapy, which is usually administered for over a year, will result in a situation in which the drug would not have to be used again in the patient. At worst, it may be necessary to treat a minor relapse with an additional brief course of therapy.

The goals for the use of cytotoxic agents in most of the other immune-mediated rheumatic diseases, particularly the classic connective tissue diseases, are somewhat different from those of the vasculitic syndromes. Since the connective tissue diseases usually run waxing and waning courses, which are characterized by exacerbations and remissions, the use of cytotoxic agents should be reserved for treatment of flares of disease in which there is a clear-cut danger of irreversible organ system dysfunction. Despite the fact that cytotoxic agents have been used for several years in the treatment of the severe manifestations of the connective tissue and other rheumatic diseases, there are unfortunately very few controlled studies that definitively document the efficacy of such an approach.[6,8,9] A few controlled trials of cytotoxic agents have been carried out, and they have documented short-term benefits in flares of disease activity. There is, however, still very little information available regarding long-term effects of these agents on the ultimate course of the disease.[6,8,9] Thus, given the present state of knowledge in this area, a reasonable goal for the use of cytotoxic agents in the connective tissue diseases would be to suppress flares of disease activity that are serious enough to be organ system- or life-threatening until such a point that the disease goes into remission and the drug can be withdrawn. Under such circumstances, the drug can be used again for a limited course should another relapse occur.

If it is necessary to continue the cytotoxic agent indefinitely in order to effect a sustained remission or even a partial remission, then one must carefully examine the risks of such long-term treatment with a drug whose potential adverse side effects are so substantial.[10,35,36] A classic example of this latter point would be the use of chronic cytotoxic therapy in a patient with rheumatoid arthritis. Given the normal life expectancy in patients with rheumatoid arthritis (see Chapter 60), it may be inappropriate to risk a serious and even fatal complication of therapy to suppress disease activity that is rarely life-threatening. On the other hand, the patient's life situation may be such that he or she feels that the risk is worth the benefit of suppressing certain unacceptable manifestations of disease activity. Thus, the goals may differ depending on the individual patient.

**Table 55–2.** Mechanisms of Action of Classes of Cytotoxic Agents Commonly Employed in the Treatment of Inflammatory and Immune-Mediated Non-Neoplastic Diseases

| Class | Typical Agent | Mechanisms of Action |
|---|---|---|
| Alkylating agents | Nitrogen mustard<br>Cyclophosphamide<br>Chlorambucil | Under physiological conditions the drug reacts chemically with biologically vital macromolecules such as DNA by contributing alkyl groups to the molecule, resulting in crosslinkage |
| Purine analogues | 6-Mercaptopurine<br>Thioguanine<br>Azathioprine | Although incorporation of the analogue into cellular DNA with subsequent inhibition of nucleic acid synthesis is generally considered the basic mechanism of action of these agents, they likely exert their cytotoxic effects by one or more of multiple mechanisms, including effects on purine nucleotide synthesis and metabolism as well as alterations in the synthesis and function of RNA and DNA. |
| Folic acid antagonists | Methotrexate | Binds with high affinity to dihydrofolate reductase, preventing the formation of tetrahydrofolate and thus causing an acute intracellular deficiency of folate coenzymes. Consequently, one-carbon transfer reactions critical for de novo synthesis of purine nucleotides and thymidylate cease, with resulting interruption of the synthesis of DNA and RNA. |

## Individual Cytotoxic Agents

Although a wide variety of cytotoxic agents of various classes have been used in the chemotherapy of neoplastic diseases,[37] only a limited number of these have been regularly employed in the treatment of non-neoplastic, inflammatory, and immune-mediated diseases. The three major categories of cytotoxic drugs employed in the latter diseases are the alkylating agents and two groups of antimetabolites, the purine analogues and the folic acid antagonists. The mechanisms of action of these cytotoxic agents are outlined in Table 55–2, and their structures are illustrated in Figure 55–2. Other cytotoxic agents that are used almost exclusively in the treatment of neoplastic diseases are covered in detail elsewhere[37] and include other antimetabolites such as the pyrimidine analogues in the form of 5-fluorouracil, cytosine arabinoside, and triacetyl-6-azauridine. In addition, natural products used in the treatment of neoplastic diseases include the vinca alkaloids (vinblastine and vincristine) and antibiotics (actinomycin D, daunomycin, rubidomycin, adrioblastina, bleomycin, mithramycin, and mitomycin C). Finally, miscellaneous cytotoxic agents include cisplatin, hydroxyurea, procarbazine, and mitotane. The list is surely not complete, as newer agents are constantly being developed. Indeed, within this group of agents used predominantly in neoplastic processes are some that have also been used in certain non-neoplastic diseases. For example, as will be discussed below, vincristine has been successfully employed as a therapeutic modality in idiopathic thrombocytopenic purpura,[38] and hydroxyurea has been employed in the treatment of the idiopathic hypereosinophilic syndrome.[39]

**Alkylating Agents.** Alkylating agents are chemicals that can substitute alkyl radicals into other molecules. Biologically effective alkylating agents are usually bifunctional or polyfunctional in that each molecule has two or more alkylating groups.[10] Thus, each molecule of the alkylating agent can covalently bind with two or more molecules of other substances. In this manner, two or more molecules may be linked to each other, i.e., in crosslinkage. By virtue of the induction of these structural changes at the molecular level, alkylating agents can potentially alter the function of proteins and nucleic acids. For example, when the DNA of a cell such as a lymphocyte is crosslinked by the agent, replication of its strands is blocked, and the cell cannot divide properly, leading ultimately to cell death.[40]

*Nitrogen Mustard.* Mechlorethamine was the first of the nitrogen mustards to be used clinically. The drug is administered intravenously, and its clearance from the blood is extremely rapid. Following administration, the drug rapidly undergoes chemical transformation and combines with either water or reactive compounds of cells such that the drug is no longer present in its active form after only a few minutes.[10] Following detoxification, the drug is ultimately cleared via the urine. Because of this rapid clearance of the active component, it is theoretically possible to protect certain tissues from the effects of the agent by merely interrupting the blood supply to the area for a few minutes during and after injection of the drug. The usual dosage is 0.4 mg per

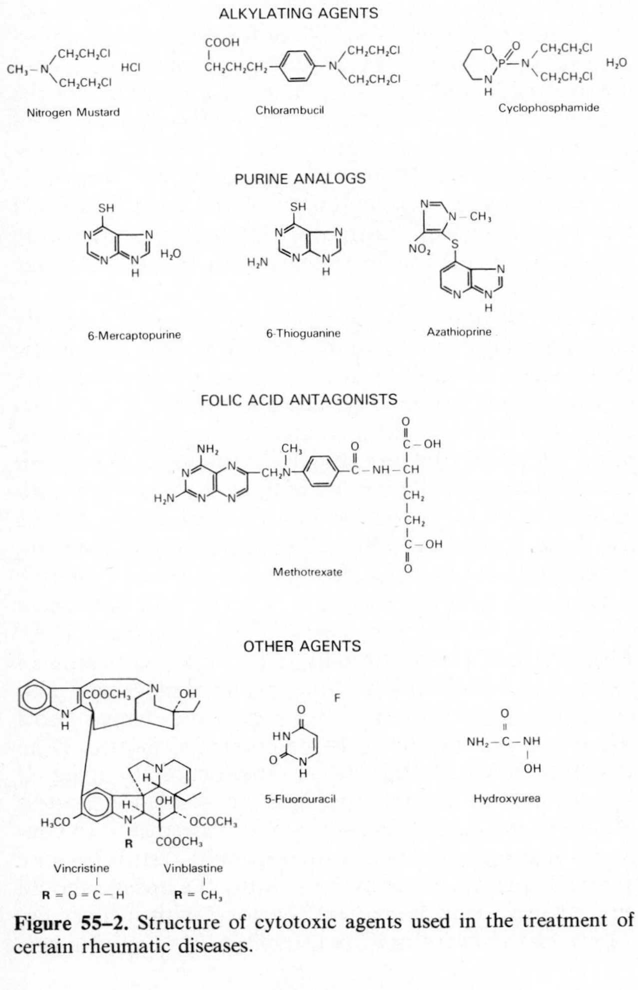


**Figure 55–2.** Structure of cytotoxic agents used in the treatment of certain rheumatic diseases.

kg intravenously every 3 to 4 weeks. Toxic side effects include severe local reactions if the drug comes into contact with surrounding tissues as well as phlebitis and thrombosis if the drug comes into direct contact with the intima of the injected vein. Nausea and vomiting occur quite commonly following drug administration and can usually be prevented or lessened by premedication. Leukopenia and thrombocytopenia constitute the major limitations in the amount of drug that can be given in a single dose; the onset is usually within a few days of drug administration and may last for as long as two to three weeks.

Nitrogen mustard has been virtually replaced by cyclophosphamide as the alkylating agent of choice in the treatment of non-neoplastic diseases. The former has the disadvantage of requiring intravenous administration, it has significant potential toxic side effects, and its therapeutic index in experimental animals has been shown to be much lower than cyclophosphamide with respect to immunosuppressive effects. However, historically nitrogen mustard is an important agent, which led the way for the use of cyclophosphamide in the treatment of immune-mediated diseases. For example, the early success in treatment of a patient with Wegener's granulomatosis with nitrogen mustard in 1954[41] laid the rational basis for the use of cyclophosphamide in the successful induction of remission in large numbers of patients with that disease.[25]

*Cyclophosphamide.* Cyclophosphamide is well absorbed orally and so has the advantage of administration by either the oral or intravenous route. The drug is inert and is activated by metabolism in the liver by the mixed-function oxidase system of the smooth endoplasmic reticulum.[42] The plasma half-life of cyclophosphamide is 6 to 7 hours; this may be significantly prolonged by prior treatment with allopurinol.[43] Maximal concentrations are reached in plasma 1 hour after administration and urinary recovery of unmetabolized drug is approximately 14 percent with negligible fecal recovery after intravenous administration.[10] Since approximately 60 percent of the drug is excreted through the kidney in the form of active metabolites, renal failure may result in impaired excretion of these active metabolites, with a resulting relative increase in immunosuppressive effect as well as in toxicity of a given dose of drug. Since certain enzymes of the mixed-function oxidase system can be induced by drugs such as barbiturates and corticosteroids, these agents can influence the metabolism of cyclophosphamide from its inert to its active form.[44] However, the biologic actions of cyclophosphamide seem to be more substantially affected by alterations in the rates of detoxification and elimination than by changes in the rate of generation of the active metabolites.[10] Indeed, the antitumor and therapeutic index of cyclophosphamide was shown not to be significantly modified by pretreatment of animals with phenobarbital.[45]

Although cyclophosphamide acts primarily during the S phase of the cell cycle and so has a profound effect on rapidly dividing cells, it also affects cells at all phases of the cell cycle, including resting ($G_0$) cells.[8] A large amount of literature has accumulated, particularly in the mouse and other animal models, demonstrating the effects of cyclophosphamide on virtually all components of the cellular and humoral immune responses.[46,47] Of particular note is the ability of cyclophosphamide to inhibit antibody production. Although this has been shown to occur most dramatically when the drug is administered before the antigen,[47,48] for practical purposes, cyclophosphamide inhibits antibody production when given at the same time or even after the antigen. Cyclophosphamide has been shown to selectively inhibit suppressor T lymphocytes as opposed to inducer or helper T lymphocytes.[49,50] However, in the therapeutic protocols in which cyclophosphamide is administered to patients with rheumatic diseases (see below), a more global rather than a selective suppression of T-lymphocyte function is seen. The immunosuppressive effects of chronically administered cyclophosphamide therapy in man are summarized in Table 55–3.[27,51-54] The most consistent finding in cyclophosphamide-treated patients is a lymphocytopenia of both T and B lymphocytes. B-lymphocyte function is clearly more profoundly suppressed than T-lymphocyte function,[27] and this is reflected at the cellular level as well as in the suppression of Ig production and serum levels of Ig in patients treated chronically with cyclophosphamide.

Cyclophosphamide is generally administered to patients with non-neoplastic diseases in a dosage regimen of 2 mg per kg per day orally. Immunosuppressive and clinical effects are usually seen within 2 to 3 weeks after initiation of therapy. An alternative regimen is the administration of single large intravenous bolus doses of 750 to 1000 mg per m$^2$. This latter regimen is usually reserved for patients with neoplastic diseases but is currently being evaluated in certain protocols for the treatment of rheumatic diseases such as SLE. As with the use of any cytotoxic and potentially myelosuppressive agent, the dosage must be modified throughout the therapeutic course in accordance with the degree of myelosuppression that occurs (see below).

Although cyclophosphamide has proved to be an extremely effective immunosuppressive agent in the treatment of non-neoplastic diseases,[33] its potential toxic side effects are considerable, and the physician must be aware of them whenever he or she undertakes the treatment of a patient with this agent (Table 55–4).[35,36] Although suppression of all marrow elements is seen with cyclophosphamide therapy, neutropenia is clearly the most important hematologic effect of the drug with regard to factors limiting its use. It should be appreciated that chronically administered cyclophosphamide will have a cumulative effect on the bone marrow reserve such that a dose that is well tolerated at one point in time may produce significant neutropenia after one or more years of therapy. This will necessitate frequent monitoring of the white blood cell count (WBC) and appropriate adjustment of dosage. Gonadal suppression is an almost invariable effect of chronic administration of cyclophosphamide and is due to the damaging effects of the drug on the germinal epithelium.[55,56] The oligo- and azospermia in males[57] and oligo- and amenorrhea in premenopausal women[55] may be permanent if treatment is continued for a year or longer. Although prepubertal testes are damaged, return of spermatogenesis after drug withdrawal occurs more frequently in this younger age bracket.[58]

Although significant alopecia occurs quite frequently after high doses of cyclophosphamide, only minor degrees occur during chronic low-dose therapy; in both cases, it is reversible upon cessation of the drug. Gastrointestinal intolerance is unpredictable and can be quite severe in certain patients. Although nausea and vomiting can usually be successfully treated with antiemetics, gastric discomfort may be refractory to the usual therapeutic modalities. The latter complication not infrequently disappears upon continuation of the drug.

Hemorrhagic cystitis is seen in from 15 to 30 percent of patients and can be a most difficult complication.[25,29] Although the cystitis usually clears upon cessation of the drug, bladder fibrosis, intractable hemorrhage, and bladder carcinoma have been reported.[59] Under most circumstances, the onset of hemorrhagic cystitis is an absolute indication for discontinuation of the drug. If the cystitis is severe, the drug must be stopped regardless of the circumstances. However, if it is necessary to continue the drug in a patient with only mild cystitis because of no adequate therapeutic substitute, the dosage should be decreased and the patient followed with urinary cytology and intermittent cystoscopies. If the cystitis per-

**Table 55–3.** Immunosuppressive Effects of Chronically Administered Cyclophosphamide Therapy in Man

1. Absolute lymphocytopenia of both T and B lymphocytes, with early preferential depletion of B lymphotocytes
2. Significant suppression of in vitro lymphocyte blastogenic responses to specific antigenic stimuli, with only mild suppression of responses to mitogenic stimuli
3. Suppression of antibody response and cutaneous delayed hypersensitivity to a new antigen, with relative sparing of established cutaneous delayed hypersensitivity
4. Reduction of elevated serum immunoglobulin levels as well as occurrence of hypogammaglobulinemia in patients treated for extended periods of time (years)
5. Selective suppression on in vitro B-lymphocyte function, with diminution of increased spontaneous immunoglobulin production of individual B lymphocytes as well as suppression of mitogen-induced immunoglobulin production

**Table 55–4.** Toxic Side Effects of Chronically Administered Low-Dose (2 mg per kg per day) Cyclophosphamide Therapy

1. Marrow suppression—predominantly neutropenia
2. Gonadal suppression—oligospermia, ovarian dysfunction
3. Alopecia
4. Gastrointestinal intolerance
5. Hemorrhagic cystitis
6. Hypogammaglobulinemia after extended use
7. Pulmonary interstitial fibrosis
8. Oncogenesis

sists or worsens on the lower dose, then the drug must be discontinued even though the alternative drug for the disease in question is inferior to cyclophosphamide.

We have noted a few patients who have developed hypogammaglobulinemia during chronically administered cyclophosphamide therapy. This is of potential importance because of the synergistic host defense defects created by neutropenia and hypogammaglobulinemia. Although pulmonary and cardiac toxicity are generally seen only at high doses of the drug,[60,61] interstitial pulmonary fibrosis can occur with chronically administered low-dose cyclophosphamide, and the physician should be alert to this possibility. In addition, an antidiuretic hormone effect has been reported with large doses of cyclophosphamide but not with lower doses.[62] Finally, neoplastic diseases, particularly lymphomas and leukemias, may occur as a result of cyclophosphamide therapy.[63]

***Chlorambucil.*** Chlorambucil is available for oral administration, and absorption is adequate and reliable. The drug is related to nitrogen mustard in that the methyl group of the mustard is replaced by phenylbutyric acid. The drug is metabolized by beta oxidation of the butyric acid.[64] The drug is almost completely metabolized and has a plasma half-life of approximately 90 minutes. At recommended doses, chlorambucil is the slowest acting nitrogen mustard in clinical use.[10]

As chlorambucil is an alkylating agent, its mechanism of action is similar to the other alkylating agents. At high doses, it suppresses all myeloid elements, and the therapeutic strategy is to suppress immune function in the form of lymphocytes prior to the suppression of other bone marrow elements. In this regard, it has been reported that at lower doses, chlorambucil exerts a more selective effect on lymphopoiesis than on granulopoiesis.[65] Clearly, chlorambucil has not been as extensively studied as cyclophosphamide with regard to its immunosuppressive effects. However, it is generally felt that it is not as potent an immunosuppressive agent as cyclophosphamide, and although its toxic side effects may be somewhat less than cyclophosphamide, its efficacy in suppressing disease activity in the non-neoplastic diseases is probably less than that of cyclophosphamide. An example of this is the greater efficacy of cyclophosphamide than chlorambucil in suppressing disease activity in generalized Wegener's granulomatosis.[66] Nonetheless, chlorambucil has been used with some success in certain of the connective tissue diseases.[8]

Chlorambucil is generally administered to patients with non-neoplastic diseases in a dosage regimen of 0.1 and 0.2 mg per kg per day orally. The dose is adjusted according to the degree of nonlymphocytic myelosuppression that is encountered, i.e., neutropenia and thrombocytopenia. When severe myelosuppression occurs, the drug should be discontinued. Marrow function usually recovers rapidly; however, irreversible marrow failure has been reported in a number of patients treated with chlorambucil for non-neoplastic diseases.[67] Such complications highlight the inherent danger in the treatment of non-neoplastic diseases with cytotoxic agents of any class. Other side effects include gastrointestinal discomfort with nausea and vomiting, hepatotoxicity, dermatitis, and infertility.[10] Oncogenesis is a particularly disturbing potential complication of chlorambucil therapy, and a marked increase in the incidence of leukemia and other tumors has been associated with the use of this agent.[68,69]

**Purine Analogues.** The two major purine analogues that have been used clinically are 6-mercaptopurine (6MP) and azathioprine, which is the purine analogue currently used almost exclusively. 6MP is an analogue of hypoxanthine in which the 6-OH radical is replaced by a thiol group. When an imidazole group is attached to the S of 6MP, azathioprine is formed. In vivo, azathioprine is metabolized to 6MP, which is the active drug. The ultimate mechanism of action of 6MP is the inhibition of nucleic acid synthesis. However, despite extensive studies in this area, the precise mechanism of action whereby these purine analogues cause cell death or cytotoxicity remain unclear. Certain potential mechanisms of action have been proposed, including the conversion of 6MP to its ribonucleotide, which inhibits the enzymes necessary for the conversion of inosinic acid to xanthylic and adenylosuccinic acids as well as the conversion of adenylosuccinic acid to adenylic acid, leading to the inhibition of DNA synthesis.[70] In addition, feedback inhibition of 5-phosphoribosylamine occurs with reduction of de novo purine biosynthesis and resulting inhibition of DNA synthesis and cell death.

***Azathioprine and 6MP.*** Azathioprine and 6MP are available for oral administration, and absorption is quite good. Since azathioprine is converted in vivo to 6MP, which is the active drug, their pharmacokinetics can be considered together. About one half of an oral dose of drug is found excreted in the urine within the first 24 hours.[10] After an intravenous dose, the half-life of the drug is 60 to 90 minutes, with clearance from the blood resulting from uptake by cells, renal excretion, and metabolic degradation. There are two major pathways for the metabolism of 6MP. The first is the methylation of the sulfhydryl group and oxidation of the methylated derivatives. The second is the oxidation of 6MP to 6-thiouric acid by the enzyme xanthine oxidase.[10] Since allopurinol inhibits xanthine oxidase, this drug decreases the metabolism of 6MP and so accounts for the increase in toxicity of azathioprine and 6MP when allopurinol is simultaneously administered.

Azathioprine and 6MP inhibit both cell-mediated and humoral immunity. Because of the diversity of studies that have been carried out in animal models and humans, there have been certain disagreements with regard to the type and extent of immunosuppression that occurs during azathioprine and 6MP therapy.[46,70] Despite this, there have been some rather consistent findings with regard to the effects of azathioprine and 6MP on immune and inflammatory responses. Azathioprine and 6MP cause a total lymphocytopenia of both T and B lymphocytes.[71] Gammaglobulin synthesis is suppressed by azathioprine therapy,[72] as is the antibody response (particularly the secondary response) to vaccination.[73] In addition, B-lymphocyte proliferation is suppressed by azathioprine.[74] There has been some controversy with regard to the effects of these agents on T lymphocytes. Certain studies report a selective effect on T lymphocytes, including inhibition of sheep red blood cell rosette formation.[75] However, other studies claim no selective effect on T lymphocytes[71,74] and in fact demonstrate that treatment with azathioprine has very little suppressive effect on mitogen-induced blastogenesis of human T lymphocytes.[76,77] In this regard, there seems to be little question that azathioprine is not as effective as cyclophosphamide in the suppression of lymphocyte function. Azathioprine and 6MP can suppress the induction of de novo delayed hypersensitivity; however, it is generally agreed that established delayed hypersensitivity remains intact during drug therapy.[73,77] Azathioprine has potent anti-inflammatory effects, which are probably related to its ability to reduce the number of monocytes in an inflammatory site by inhibition of monocyte production.[78] This suppression of monocyte function may also explain the effects of these drugs on delayed hypersensitivity.[79]

Azathioprine and 6MP are generally administered in doses of approximately 2 mg per kg per day. As with the other cytotoxic agents, the dosage must be adjusted according to the degree of resulting myelosuppression. Immunosuppressive and clinical effects are usually seen within 3 or 4 weeks after initiation of therapy. Patients with impaired renal function may have reduced clearance of the drug and its metabolites, with a resulting cumulative effect and increased toxicity unless the dosage is appropriately adjusted downward.

The major toxicity of both 6MP and azathioprine is bone marrow suppression, with leukopenia rather than thrombocytopenia and anemia being the major manifestation. The major toxic side effects of chronically administered azathioprine or 6MP therapy are listed in Table 55–5.[80] Of note with regard to the neutropenia associated with these agents is the fact that a rapid fall in WBC within a week of starting therapy has been reported and resembles an idiosyncratic reaction. In addition, the peripheral WBC cannot always be an accurate measure of the host defense defect, since infections may occur in individuals with normal neutrophil counts, suggesting a functional impairment of immune-competent cells involved in host defense, most likely at the T lymphocyte-monocyte axis. The suppression of delayed hypersensitivity by these agents[78,79] as well as the fact that neutrophil function is generally normal in individuals receiving azathioprine[81] adds credence to this hypothesis. This point should be fully appreciated, since infectious disease complications cannot be totally predicted regardless of the level of the WBC. Finally, although the effects on gonadal function have not been fully evaluated with regard to azathioprine, it is clear that sterility is not the invariable rule, since several normal pregnancies have been reported in patients who had been receiving azathioprine. Fetal abnormalities do not appear to be a problem.[36]

**Table 55–5.** Toxic Side Effects of Chronically Administered Azathioprine and 6-Mercaptopurine Therapy

1. Marrow suppression—predominantly neutropenia
2. Hepatotoxicity—probably on an allergic basis
3. Infectious disease complications—not necessarily correlated with neutropenia
4. Gastrointestinal intolerance
5. Oncogenesis—particularly lymphoid malignancies

**Folic Acid Antagonists.** The folic acid antagonists such as methotrexate bind competitively to dihydrofolate reductase with a much higher affinity than does the natural substrate dihydrofolic acid. This prevents the conversion by dihydrofolate reductase of hydrofolic acid to tetrahydrofolic acid, thus interfering with the transport of one-carbon fragments required for thymidine synthesis. In this manner, DNA synthesis, and ultimately cellular proliferation, is inhibited.[10] Folic acid antagonists kill cells predominantly in the S phase of the cell cycle, particularly during the logarithmic phase of growth rather than at the plateau phase; they have little effect on resting cells. This selective killing of rapidly proliferating cells forms the rational basis for the successful use of methotrexate in the treatment of psoriasis, which is characterized by an abnormally rapid proliferation of epidermal cells. Leucovorin (folinic acid) is a fully reduced, metabolically functional folate coenzyme that functions directly without the need of reduction by dihydrofolate reductase. Hence, it has been used to "rescue" normal cells from the toxicity of folic acid antagonists.[10]

***Methotrexate.*** Methotrexate may be administered orally or parenterally. It is readily absorbed from the gastrointestinal tract when administered in doses of 0.1 mg per kg, but larger doses are less completely absorbed (approximately 60 percent absorption).[10] The plasma half-life of methotrexate is approximately 2 hours,[82] although it disappears from the plasma in a triphasic fashion following intravenous administration.[10] The drug has very poor penetration through the blood-brain barrier. Approximately 50 percent of the drug is bound to plasma proteins and may be displaced by certain drugs, such as sulfonamides, salicylates, tetracycline, and chloramphenicol. Most of the drug is excreted unchanged in the urine within the first 24 hours, predominantly during the first 8 hours, with very little fecal excretion.

Methotrexate exerts profound suppression on both primary and secondary antibody responses in man.[83-85] Although the drug has been demonstrated to markedly suppress the delayed hypersensitivity reaction in animals,[70] little if any effect on established delayed cutaneous hypersensitivity was noted in man during treatment with methotrexate.[85]

Methotrexate is administered orally or intravenously, usually in an intermittent fashion, and the dosages are usually determined on a weekly basis. The standard adult dose ranges from 5 to 50 mg per week. This total weekly dose may be given as a single intravenous dose once a week or orally as 3 divided doses, each separated by 12 hours, or orally daily for 5 days of the week. The drug dosage should be reduced in patients with renal failure, as increased toxicity has been noted.

Toxic side effects of methotrexate include marrow suppression, particularly leukopenia and thrombocytopenia, oral mucositis, nausea, vomiting, diarrhea, and occasional hepatotoxicity. Although an increased risk of malignancy has not been documented in patients receiving methotrexate, there is a significant risk to the fetus if the drug is administered during the first trimester of pregnancy.[10]

## Other Agents

**Vinca Alkaloids.** The commonly used vinca alkaloids, vincristine and vinblastine, are cell cycle–specific agents that block mitosis by interfering with protein assembly of the mitotic spindle, leading to metaphase arrest.[10] Vincristine is administered intravenously in doses of 2 mg per $m^2$ of body surface weekly. After intravenous injection, vincristine is cleared almost entirely from the blood in approximately 30 minutes. The drug is excreted primarily by the liver into the bile, with less than 5 percent of the drug appearing in the urine.

Immunosuppression with these compounds has been negligible, and antibody formation in rabbits was shown not to be significantly affected by administration of vinca alkaloids.[46] Vinblastine has been employed in a unique immunosuppression protocol in the treatment of idiopathic thrombocytopenia in which the drug was bound to platelets for the purposes of delivering the toxic drug directly and selectively to the cells that were removing and killing the platelets.[86]

The major toxic side effect of the vinca alkaloids is neurotoxicity. This is usually manifested by peripheral neuropathy in the form of paresthesias, loss of deep tendon reflexes, neuritic pain, muscle weakness, and wasting. In addition, hoarseness due to vocal cord paralysis may be seen together with other cranial nerve palsies leading to ptosis and diplopia. Severe constipation, sometimes resulting in paralytic ileus, is commonly seen and may mimic an acute surgical abdomen. In this regard, adequate hydration as well as a program of prophylactic laxatives and stool softeners is recommended for all patients receiving these agents. Bladder atony may lead to urinary retention or incontinence. Other side effects of the vinca alkaloids include alopecia in about 20 percent of patients, leukopenia, thrombocytopenia (only at very high doses or after prolonged administration of the drug), pyuria, dysuria, fever, gastrointestinal symptoms, mutagenicity, and inappropriate secretion of antidiuretic hormone, leading to hyponatremia with high urinary sodium.[10] Finally, extravasation of the drug at the site of injection can lead to severe local inflammatory reactions.

**5-Fluorouracil.** 5-Fluorouracil is a pyrimidine analogue that competes with uracil in various metabolic pathways but cannot be converted to thymidine. Thus, it ultimately blocks DNA synthesis. In addition, it inhibits enzymes such as thymidylate synthetase required for the synthesis of ribonucleotides and deoxyribonucleotides. The drug has been used predominantly in the treatment of neoplastic diseases, and its precise immunosuppressive properties are not well studied in man.[10] The drug works throughout the cell cycle and is metabolized almost exclusively in the liver. It is usually administered intravenously, since absorption after oral ingestion is unpredictable and incomplete. The major toxic side effects result from the inevitable myelosuppression, particularly leukopenia. Other side effects include nausea and vomiting, alopecia, dermatitis, nail changes, atrophy of the skin, ulcerative stomatitis and gastroenteritis, and neurologic manifestations such as cerebellar ataxia.[10]

**Hydroxyurea.** Hydroxyurea inhibits the enzyme ribonucleotide diphosphate reductase, which catalyzes the reductive conversion of ribonucleotides to deoxyribonucleotides and which is a crucial step in the synthesis of DNA. The drug is specific for the S phase of the cell cycle.[10] It is readily absorbed from the gastrointestinal tract, and peak plasma concentrations are reached within two hours of administration of an oral dose. Within 24 hours, it is undetectable in the blood with approximately 80 percent of the drug recovered in the urine within 12 hours of oral or intravenous administration.[10] The drug is administered orally in doses of 20 to 30 mg per kg per day as a single dose. Although the drug has been used predominantly in the management of chronic granulocytic leukemia, it has recently been used in the treatment of the idiopathic hypereosinophilic syndrome.[87] Toxic side effects include myelosuppression, nausea and vomiting, gastrointestinal ulcerations, and mild skin rashes.

# THEORETICAL AND PRACTICAL CONSIDERATIONS IN THE USE OF CYTOTOXIC AGENTS FOR THE TREATMENT OF NON–NEOPLASTIC DISEASES

As mentioned above, one of the major goals in the use of cytotoxic agents for the treatment of non-neoplastic diseases is to achieve a degree of immunosuppression that results in suppression of the aberrant inflammatory and immune reactivity in a disease state without seriously compromising host defense mechanisms, which would lead to an increased incidence of infectious disease complications. For reasons that are not entirely clear, in those inflammatory and immune-mediated diseases for which cytotoxic agents have proved to be beneficial, it appears that disease activity can indeed be suppressed without the invariable occurrence of a serious defect in clinically relevant host defense mechanisms.

Although the cytotoxic agents have a number of immediate and long-term toxic side effects that must be considered in the decision to employ such agents in a given patient, once the decision has been made to use a cytotoxic agent, awareness and recognition of these side effects become of paramount importance in the successful management of the patient. In this regard, although the different classes of cytotoxic agents used in the treatment of non-neoplastic diseases differ somewhat in their mechanisms of action, the major immediate limiting side effect common to virtually all of them is myelosuppression, particularly neutropenia and to a lesser extent thrombocytopenia and anemia.

When the physician undertakes the treatment of non-neoplastic diseases with these agents, it is essential to appreciate the necessity for careful and continuous monitoring of the WBC, with appropriate modification of the dosage regimen to maintain the WBC above the neutropenic range. It has been consistently observed that if the WBC is maintained above 3000 to 3500 cells per $mm^3$, which usually results in a neutrophil count of 1000 to 1500 per $mm^3$, there is very little chance of opportunistic infections as a result of drug-induced host defense defects, particularly when the agent employed is an alkylating agent such as cyclophosphamide or chlorambucil. For example, this has clearly been shown to be the case with the use of cyclophosphamide in the treatment of Wegener's granulomatosis[25] and other of the severe systemic vasculitic syndromes.[24,26] This observation holds true provided there is not a concomitant and synergistic cause of host defense defects, such as daily corticosteroid therapy. For this reason, it is suggested that corticosteroids be administered on an alternate-day basis, when possible, in patients receiving cytotoxic agents together with corticosteroids for the treatment of non-neoplastic diseases.[24-26] Using such a regimen of chronically administered cyclophosphamide at a dose of 2 mg per kg per day with frequent adjustments of dosage to maintain the WBC above 3000 per $mm^3$ together with prednisone 60 mg per day or less with conversion to alternate-day prednisone within 1 to 2 months of initiating therapy and maintenance of alternate-day prednisone together with the cyclophosphamide, there has been virtually no increased incidence of opportunistic infections in a large series of patients recently reported.[25] The exception to this was an increased incidence of herpes zoster infections in patients receiving chronic cyclophosphamide therapy.[88] The zoster did not disseminate viscerally in any patient, and there were no serious sequelae of the infection.

Maintaining the WBC above the neutropenic level while effecting remission of disease activity requires continuous monitoring of the WBC as well as appreciation that as patients receive a cytotoxic agent for extended periods of time, their tolerance for a given dose will decrease, necessitating adjustment downward of the dose. It should also be pointed out that an appreciation of the "slope of the curve" of the WBC is important, in that the effect of a given dose of drug on one day may be reflected several days later (Fig. 55–3). Therefore, one should not wait until the patient is already seriously neutropenic before decreasing the dose of cytotoxic agent but should decrease the dose based on the projection of the downward slope of the WBC curve. In this way, a smooth plateauing of the WBC can be maintained and infectious disease complications largely avoided.

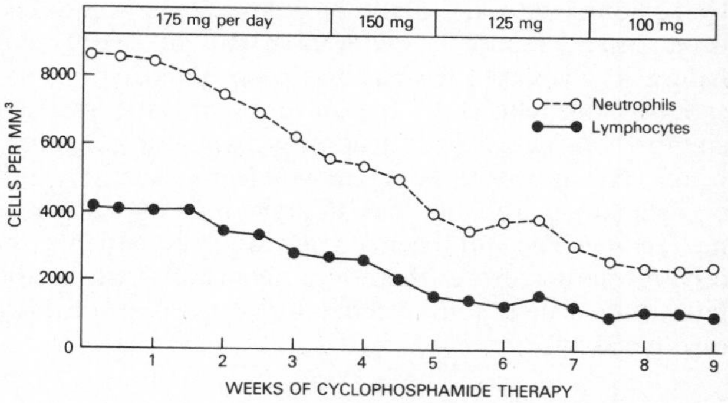


**Figure 55–3.** Schematic diagram of the use and modification of cyclophosphamide therapy according to the white blood cell count in a patient with Wegener's granulomatosis. The major goal in the treatment of non-neoplastic diseases with cytotoxic agents such as cyclophosphamide is the suppression of disease activity and avoidance of toxic side effects such as significant neutropenia. As shown with the patient indicated in this figure, the dose of drug must be continually modified in accordance with the white blood cell count so as to allow the total white blood cell count to remain above 3000 to 3500 per $mm^3$, which generally results in a neutrophil count above 1000 to 1500 per $mm^3$. It is essential to realize that the dosage must be decreased as the slope of the white blood cell count declines, since a given dose of drug will be reflected by the white blood cell count several days later. One must anticipate this and modify the dosage so as to arrive smoothly at a maintenance dose of cyclophosphamide, which is almost always lower than the initial induction dose. Once the maintenance dose is reached, the patient will usually be able to tolerate it for several months. However, usually even this dose must ultimately be decreased, as the bone marrow is less able to tolerate the drug over a period of time. Again, this requires frequent and consistent monitoring of the counts throughout the period of drug administration.

The preceding principles of the relationship between neutropenia and infection generally hold true except under certain circumstances, such as the concomitant use of other agents, which cause a host defense defect but do not cause neutropenia. As mentioned, this is the case with the use of daily corticosteroids, which negates our ability to use the WBC as an accurate gauge of the degree of host defense defect. Furthermore, agents such as azathioprine (see above) can result in an increased incidence of infectious disease complications even without neutropenia. When using such agents, it is still important to monitor the WBC; however, the danger of the occurrence of unpredicted infectious disease complications must be appreciated. In addition, the gradual dropping of the WBC on a constant dose of cytotoxic agent is the rule, but certain drugs such as azathioprine can give an idiosyncratic, precipitous drop in WBC. All of these possibilities must be taken into consideration in the use of these agents.

It should be pointed out that under certain circumstances the bone marrow reserve of a given patient may be suppressed to a point at which the dosage of cyclophosphamide must be reduced despite the fact that the disease is still active. In these situations, the addition of or increase in the dose of alternate-day prednisone may allow one to administer higher doses of cyclophosphamide with a lesser degree of leukopenia. It is felt that the mechanism of this marrow-sparing effect of corticosteroid in patients treated with cyclophosphamide is the result of a beneficial effect on marrow regeneration, due most likely to an altering of cell cycle characteristics of granulocyte progenitor cells.[25]

Once disease remission has been achieved and maintained for an adequate period of time with the use of cytotoxic agents, it is important to continually attempt to taper the dose of drug with the ultimate goal of discontinuation. The time for maintenance of remission on cytotoxic agents varies with each disease. However, the general principle stands that the physician should always have the ultimate discontinuation of the cytotoxic agent as a goal of the regimen.

Finally, a thorough familiarization with all of the other immediate as well as long-term potential side effects of these agents should be undertaken by the physician who prescribes them, and careful following of the patient during and after use of these agents is essential in order to detect the onset of these complications as early as possible.

## THERAPEUTIC APHERESIS

The word apheresis is a Greek derivative meaning withdrawal. Therapeutic apheresis implies withdrawal of a substance from a patient, ultimately leading to clinical improvement in a disease state. Although the original aphereses were solely confined to the removal of plasma for hyperviscosity states such as Waldenström's macroglobulinemia, the recent development of sophisticated equipment for removal of plasma as well as selected cellular components has led to an acceleration of the use of apheresis in a number of different disease states, including hematologic, connective tissue, neurologic, and even neoplastic disorders.[89] Plasmapheresis is the removal of plasma without significant removal of cellular elements. Cytapheresis is the removal of cells without significant removal of noncellular elements such as plasma. For example, lymphocytapheresis is the selective removal of mononuclear cells, especially lymphocytes, without significant removal of either plasma or nonlymphoid cellular elements. Selective lymphocyte removal can be accomplished either by thoracic duct drainage (which strictly speaking is lymphocytapheresis) or by continuous flow cell separators via venous access. Lymphoplasmapheresis is the removal of both plasma and lymphocytes with sparing of nonlymphoid cellular elements.

In addition to the removal of the hyperviscous macroglobulin in Waldenström's macroglobulinemia, plasmapheresis has the theoretical and practical effect of removing pathogenic autoantibodies in diseases such as Goodpasture's syndrome, immune thrombocytopenia, autoimmune hemolytic anemia, myasthenia gravis, and severe Rh disease.[89,90-93] Most recently, plasmapheresis has been used in the treatment of connective tissue diseases, particularly rheumatoid arthritis and SLE, and to a lesser degree in the treatment of certain of the vasculitic syndromes.[93-97] Given the evidence that lymphocytes appear to be involved in both the initiation and propagation of the inflammatory responses in rheumatoid arthritis, lymphocytapheresis and lymphoplasmapheresis have been performed in the treatment of this disease.[98,99] Finally, recent evidence has indicated that a form of plasmapheresis in which plasma is perfused over immobilized protein-A may be effective in inducing tumor rejection in patients with malignant neoplasms by removing serum factors that inhibit rejection.[100] In this regard, the area of selective removal of potentially harmful components of plasma by extracorporeal modification of plasma either by selective absorption, cryogelation, and membrane filtration or by chemical and physical precipitation is currently under intensive study.[101,102]

The major rationale for the use of plasmapheresis in the treatment of immune complex–mediated diseases such as SLE is the physical removal of the immune complexes from the circulation, making them unavailable for deposition in tissue. However, a further rationale may relate to abnormalities in reticuloendothelial system (RES) function seen in certain immune complex–mediated diseases such as SLE.[103] A recent study has demonstrated that plasmapheresis re-established previously abnormal splenic RES function, and this did not necessarily correlate with complete normalization of autoantibodies or immune complex levels.[96] In addition, recent studies have demonstrated that defective monocyte function improved following plasmapheresis.[104] Hence, the therapeutic efficacy of plasmapheresis may well extend beyond the mere removal of a substance that is directly toxic to tissues.

Plasmapheresis carries with it the potential problem of a rebound in production of antibodies to higher levels than pretreatment by removal of either feedback inhibitory mechanisms or actual suppressor factors.[90] However, this difficulty is generally obviated by the fact that most protocols employing plasmapheresis also call for the simultaneous administration of immunosuppressive agents, which not only synergize with the effects of the plasmapheresis but also blunt any potential rebound phenomena that might occur.[105]

Plasmapheresis protocols vary considerably in the specific details of the procedure. However, current uses of plasmapheresis are usually true plasma exchanges in that large amounts of plasma are removed and replaced by various types of replacement fluids. A commonly used protocol is the performance of plasma exchanges three times per week over a 2- to 6-week period. Each procedure usually lasts from 2 to 4 hours. At each procedure, variable amounts of plasma may be removed, but a relatively standard amount is 40 ml of plasma per kg of body weight or up to 3 liters per exchange. Plasma volume is usually replaced by a combination of albumin and normal saline with or without other fluids such as acid citrate dextrose.[94] Replacement of plasma volume and oncotic pressure are accomplished by these materials.

Theoretically, however, one must at least consider the replacement of other factors, such as Ig, clotting factors, and other proteins. It has been reported that a prolongation of prothrombin, partial thromboplastin, and thrombin times as well as a reduction in fibrinogen, clotting factors, and platelet counts occurred 4 hours after plasmapheresis; however, these all recovered by 24 hours.[106] The effect of plasmapheresis with albumin replacement on normal plasma constituents was also studied.[107] All plasma constituents were shown to have recovered within 48 hours except fibrinogen, C3, cholesterol, IgG, and IgM. Although fresh frozen plasma is the most physiologic replacement fluid available, as it supplies Ig, coagulation factors, complement, and possbily other factors that might be beneficial to and lacking in the patient, it does carry the risk of transmission of viral hepatitis. Thus, albumin and normal saline remain the standard replacement fluids.

Lymphapheresis, like plasmapheresis, has been carried out under a variety of protocols. In one study, lymphapheresis was carried out in a group of patients with rheumatoid arthritis, and each procedure was repeated 2 to 3 times per week for a total of 13 to 16 procedures over a 5-week period.[98] A mean of $13.7 \times 10^{10}$ lymphocytes were removed per patient during the study, and every patient became lymphopenic. Although short periods of lymphapheresis resulted in equal losses of T and B lymphocytes, this extended 5-week course resulted in a disproportionate fall in circulating T lymphocytes by 26 to 58 percent. In addition, serum IgM fell by 30 percent.[98] Clearly significant lymphodepletion with resulting immunosuppression can be achieved with repeated lymphocytapheresis using continuous flow centrifugation.[108] In a double-blind controlled trial of lymphoplasmapheresis versus sham apheresis in patients with rheumatoid arthritis, by the ninth treatment, treated patients had significant reductions in absolute lymphocyte counts; total serum protein; alpha, beta, and gammaglobulins; IgG, IgM, IgA; C3; and circulating immune complexes; with no significant changes in WBC, serum sodium, potassium, or albumin.[99] Of note is the fact that Westergren sedimentation rates fell significantly, as did rheumatoid factor titers.

Lymphapheresis has for the most part replaced thoracic duct drainage as a modality for removing lymphocytes largely because of the ease, convenience, and relative lack of complications of the former. However, significantly favorable and sometimes dramatic clinical responses have been reported in a study of the effects of long-term thoracic duct drainage in a group of patients with autoimmune diseases.[109] Significant degrees of immunosuppression, particularly of T lymphocyte–mediated responses, was noted in the treated patients[109,110] and disease was transiently exacerbated in three patients in whom autologous lymphocytes were reinfused.[110]

Detrimental side effects and complications of apheresis include depletion of platelets as well as important components of plasma, such as clotting factors, with resulting bleeding diatheses, hypotension, fluid and electrolyte imbalance, and complications relating to access sites. The potential long-term complications of these procedures are unclear at present.

The long-term therapeutic benefits from apheresis are uncertain, and a number of controlled and uncontrolled studies are currently being conducted to determine the precise immediate and long-term benefits of this approach in several rheumatic diseases. Several studies have indicated at least a significant short-term clinical improvement in patients with rheumatoid arthritis treated with various apheresis protocols.[89,98,99] The situation is less clear in SLE, and a recent review of the currently available data indicates no significant benefit of plasmapheresis in the treatment of SLE.[95]

## IONIZING RADIATION

Ionizing radiation exerts its effects on tissues by inducing the ionization of atoms. X-rays and gamma rays cause ejection of electrons from the atoms with which they interact, and thus ionize them. When the irradiation is of high enough energy, the ejected electrons themselves have considerable kinetic energy and in turn ionize other atoms. Ionization of atoms within a cell leads to the formation of highly reactive free radicals. These free radicals interact with biologically relevant macromolecules such as DNA. In fact, the lesion responsible for the most important biologic effects of radiation is scission of the DNA chain.[111] Such effects on nuclear DNA lead to the major cellular consequence of irradiation, which is impairment of cellular reproduction. It is for this reason that rapidly dividing cells such as bone marrow, intestinal epithelium, and certain types of lymphocytes appear to be selectively affected by irradiation. However, irradiation may also impair cell function and viability by mechanisms unrelated to the mitotic event.[111]

Ionizing radiation can have profound effects on lymphoid cells, including those involved in the initiation and propagation of immune-mediated connective tissue diseases. The ultimate effect of irradiation on the immune system of the host is highly dependent on the dose delivered. Although this may vary according to the protocol employed, there is generally a gradation of sensitivity of lymphoid subsets as well as lymphoid cells at various stages of differentiation to increasing doses of irradiation.[112] Precursor cells are usually exquisitely sensitive to irradiation. Low doses of irradiation may selectively kill certain subpopulations of T and B lymphocytes while sparing others. Resting or undifferentiated B lymphocytes are quite sensitive to irradiation, while fully differentiated plasma cells are rather resistant to the effects of radiation.[113] Among immunoregulatory T-lymphocyte subsets, suppressor T lymphocytes are generally more sensitive to irradiation than are helper T lymphocytes.[113] It should be pointed out that the net effect of irradiation on lymphocyte subpopulations in particular and immune function in general is usually highly dependent on the total dosage and the dosage schedule employed. For example, total body irradiation is profoundly immunosuppressive and is designed to eliminate as extensively as possible the immune competence of the host. The side effects of this modality are extreme and may be fatal. Therefore, this type of radiation protocol is reserved for special clinical circumstances such as preparation for bone marrow transplantation. For this reason, we will not discuss this modality in the present setting.

## TOTAL LYMPH NODE IRRADIATION

A potentially important advance in the use of radiation therapy for non-neoplastic diseases has been made with the recent introduction of the use of fractionated total lymph node irradiation in the treatment of rheumatoid arthritis. The rationale for this approach is similar to that described for the use of lymphapheresis in that recent evidence indicates that lymphocytes, particularly T lymphocytes, appear to be involved in the immunopathogenic expression of rheumatoid arthritis. Total lymph node irradiation has been used for the past 20 years in the treatment of Hodgkin's disease and non-Hodgkin's lymphoma.[114,115] Of note is the fact that there have been no serious long-term sequelae of leukemia, second tumors, or serious host defense defects leading to infectious disease complications. Nonetheless, cell-mediated immunity was shown to be suppressed for several years following treatment.[116] Thus, this approach has recently been employed in the treatment of intractable rheumatoid arthritis as an alternative to the use of cytotoxic agents such as cyclophosphamide and azathioprine.

The results of at least two feasibility studies have been impressive.[117,118] Twenty-one patients were treated with 2000 to 3000 rad over 5 to 14 weeks with a follow-up of 12 to 18 months. Seventeen of 21 patients experienced significant clinical improvement. Virtually all patients experienced a lymphocytopenia with suppression of in vitro lymphocyte responses. In one study,[117] there was an increase in the ratio of suppressor to helper T lymphocytes. This reappearance of suppressor cell capability is analogous to the development of suppressor T lymphocytes accompanying long-lasting immunosuppression in mice treated with total lymph node irradiation.[119] It should be pointed out that abnormal antibody activities characteristic of rheumatoid arthritis as well as normal components of humoral immunity were not suppressed by the treatment protocol.[118] There were some partial recrudescences within a year in one study[118] and sustained remissions over an 18-month period in another study.[117] Thus, effective suppression of manifestations of severe rheumatoid arthritis can be accomplished for significant periods of time with total lymph node irradiation, and this is associated with substantial suppression of T lymphocyte function. In addition, immediate toxic side effects are few. Although it is uncertain whether the natural history of the disease will be altered by this approach, it clearly deserves further study and attention as a promising modality of therapy for severe connective tissue diseases mediated by lymphoid cells.

## ANTILYMPHOCYTE ANTIBODIES

**Standard Antisera.** Heterologous antilymphocyte serum (ALS) refers to antiserum raised in one species against lymphocytes of another species. Since such antisera generally contain antibodies directed against cell types other than lymphoid cells, absorption of the serum with nonlymphoid cells is required to make the serum relatively specific for lymphocyte antigens. The serum may then be fractionated to obtain the IgG fraction with antilymphocyte activity; this is referred to as antilymphocyte globulin (ALG). This latter manipulation removes a number of serum factors that might be immunogenic and cause hypersensitivity reactions such as serum sickness.

Since the ultimate target of the ALS is usually T lymphocytes, it would be preferable to have the antiserum react only with T lymphocytes while sparing B lymphocytes. In this regard, further absorptions of the ALS with B lymphocytes may yield an antiserum that is relatively specific for T lymphocytes, i.e., anti–T lymphocyte serum (ATS).

The common denominator of the mechanism of immunosuppression of ALS is a lymphocytopenia. Although ALS bound to lymphocytes in the presence of complement in vitro can cause cytotoxicity[120] and ultimately cell death, the major mechanism of lymphocytopenia in vivo is the selective depletion of circulating T lymphocytes by opsonization and clearance via the RES, predominantly of the liver.[121] It should be pointed out that in the absence of complement, ALS may bind to the lymphocyte and induce blast transformation,[120] and so modulation of lymphocyte function can potentially occur, although the net effect is almost invariably the removal of cells from the recirculating pool. The potency of the immunosuppressive effects of a given batch of ALS depends on the relative ability of the antiserum to bind to and induce the clearance of lymphocytes.

ALS has been used extensively in man as an immunosuppressive agent in renal allograft recipients with rather impressive results.[122,123] With regard to the use of ALS in immune-mediated diseases, a number of investigators have employed this agent in uncontrolled trials of the treatment of diseases such as autoimmune hemolytic anemia, myasthenia gravis, multiple sclerosis, and a variety of connective tissue diseases.[120] Although several reports indicated favorable results, the use of ALS in connective tissue diseases has not been extensive, owing to the lack of convincing controlled trials demonstrating its efficacy.

Most recently, the toxic side effects of ALS preparations have been markedly decreased by the use of meticulous absorption procedures that remove non-Ig proteins, which might increase the incidence of serum sickness as well as antibodies to a variety of nonlymphoid cells, particularly platelets and erythrocytes. Nonetheless, one must be aware of the considerable potential toxic side effects of the use of ALS.[120] These include fever, chills, arthralgias, and back pain, usually occurring 3 to 12 hours after the first and second injection. Subsequently, fever may be minimal. With intramuscular injections, there may be pain at the site of injection, and with intravenous injections, there may be mild phlebitis as well as occasional episodes of bradycardia and hypotension. Infectious complications of the immunosuppression include herpes zoster; nephrotoxic nephritis caused by antiglomerular antibodies in the ALS preparation has been reported.[120] Furthermore, the long-range toxic side effects of ALS are unclear at this point, which adds to the reluctance to use these agents widely in the treatment of connective tissue diseases.

**Monoclonal Antibodies.** Immunologic research was virtually revolutionized by the demonstration by Köhler and Milstein in 1975 that somatic cell hybridization could be employed in the immortalization of B lymphocyte lines, producing monoclonal antibody.[124] This new dimension in immunobiologic analysis witnessed immediate application in immunodiagnosis.[125] However, the potential for the therapeutic use of monoclonal antibodies is clear, and already a number of studies are being conducted for the use of these agents in the treatment of certain neoplastic diseases. Preliminary studies have already demonstrated their potential efficacy in the treatment of certain lymphoid malignancies.[126,127] In addition, monoclonal antibodies directed against lymphoid tumor antigens have been used to deplete bone marrow of residual leukemia cells prior to autologous marrow transplantation.[128] Monoclonal antibodies directed against mature alloreactive T lymphocytes have been used to pretreat allogeneic bone marrow prior to transplantation for the purpose of preventing acute graft-versus-host disease with variable results.[129,130] However, of particular interest is the recent report of the use of a monoclonal antibody (T12) to treat an HLA haplotype–mismatched allogenic bone marrow prior to transplantation for severe combined immunodeficiency as well as to treat the recipient in vivo to terminate ongoing severe graft-versus-host disease.[131]

With regard to the use of monoclonal antibodies in the treatment of autoimmune diseases, experimental data have indicated at least the feasibility of employing this approach in diseases such as experimental allergic encephalitis[132] and myasthenia gravis.[133] Although it is tempting to envision the manipulation of immunoregulatory lymphocyte subsets in autoimmune diseases by the in vivo use of monoclonal antibodies directed against specific lymphocyte subsets, it should be pointed out that the complexity of the immune system with its intricate feedback mechanisms renders such an approach only speculative at present.

## STEROID HORMONES

**Glucocorticosteroids.** Glucocorticosteroids are used extensively in the treatment of rheumatic diseases. These agents manifest both anti-inflammatory and immunosuppressive effects.[7] Although virtually any function of an inflammatory or immune competent cell can be suppressed by a high enough concentration of corticosteroid in vitro, in the dosages of drug that are generally employed in the treatment of rheumatic diseases, the effects of the drug are somewhat selective for one or another of the components of the inflammatory or immune response.[7,134] For example, the inductive phase of the immune response is clearly more sensitive to the immunosuppressive effects of corticosteroids than is the effector phase.[7] Furthermore, the T-lymphocyte or cell-mediated limb of immunity is clearly more sensitive to corticosteroids than is the B-lymphocyte or humoral limb.[135] In addition, within the T-lymphocyte fraction, certain subsets are selectively more sensitive to the drug than are others.[136]

Of particular importance in the understanding of the effects of corticosteroids on inflammatory and immune competent cells is an appreciation of the fact that the drugs can affect the inflammatory and immune response by a number of mechanisms. For example, administration of corticosteroids may affect the circulatory kinetics of a given cell type such as a neutrophil, monocyte, or lymphocyte subset and thus block the availability of these cells to the inflammatory site without directly suppressing the functional capability of the cell. On the other hand, the drug may directly affect the functional capability of a cell in a situation in which circulatory kinetics are not relevant.[7] In general, lower concentrations of the drug are required in order to affect circulatory kinetics, whereas higher concentrations are needed in order to directly suppress a functional capability of a cell.[7] Finally, the effects of corticosteroids on a given cell type may vary, depending on the state of activation of the cell in question. Understanding these concepts is important in the proper design of therapeutic protocols for the use of corticosteroids in the treatment of non-neoplastic diseases. A detailed discussion of the use of corticosteroid therapy is contained in Chapter 54.

**Sex Hormones.** The sex hormones, particularly the androgens, may have significant immunoregulatory effects. Indeed, male sex hormones have been shown to suppress a variety of immune responses in experimental animals.[137,138] Furthermore, in vitro testosterone has been shown to cause a mild decrease in blastogenic responses of phytohemagglutinin-stimulated human lymphocytes at hormone concentrations of 0.1 $\mu$g per ml and to completely ablate the response at 80 mg per ml.[139] Of potential clinical relevance is the observation that the administration of male sex hormones can decrease the degree of autoimmune phenomena and even prolong survival in the murine models of SLE.[140,141] Furthermore, a lack of male sex hormones may lead to a marked acceleration of autoimmunity.[142] These observations may not only provide insight into the pathophysiologic mechanisms of disease but also may provide the rational basis for the therapeutic use of these agents in certain autoimmune diseases. Although the male sex hormones have been shown to be immunosuppressive,[137,138] the precise mechanisms whereby these agents prevent or ameliorate autoimmune phenomena are unclear at present. It should be pointed out that male sex hormones have proved to be highly effective in the treatment of hereditary angioedema.[143,144] The mechanisms whereby these agents are effective in this latter disease include the reversal of the biochemical abnormality by inducing the synthesis of the deficient C1 esterase inhibitor.[144]

**Other Hormones.** A number of other hormones have been shown to have in vitro and in vivo effects on immune function. The clinical relevance of these effects with regard to rheumatic diseases is unclear at present, particularly with regard to therapeutic efficacy. However, an understanding of the potential immunologic effects of various hormonal imbalances is important for an appreciation of the scope of hormonal influences on the immune responses in general and on immune-mediated diseases in particular. A brief summary of certain representative effects of various nonglucocorticosteroid hormones on the immune responses is contained on Table 55–6.[145]

## OTHER AGENTS

**Levamisole.** Levamisole is a three-ring molecule with the extremely low molecular weight of 241. It was introduced into veterinary practice in 1966 as a nematocidal agent and was subsequently used in man. It is highly active against a wide range of nematodes and is particularly effective in ascariasis. It has, however, received recent attention as an immunoenhancing agent in man. Levamisole is absorbed rapidly from the gastrointestinal tract. Following administration of a 150-mg dose in man, peak blood levels of 5 micrograms per ml are reached at 2 hours.[146] The plasma half-life is approximately 4 hours, and the drug is metabolized predominantly in the liver, with excretion of the breakdown products via the kidney and to a lesser extent in the feces.

**Table 55–6.** Effects of the Nonglucocortoid Hormones on the Immune Response*

| | |
|---|---|
| Growth Hormone | Appears essential for the maturation and function of thymic-dependent immune responses in the dwarf mouse |
| Thyroxine | Stimulatory to phytohemagglutinin blastogenic responses and antisheep erythrocyte plaque-forming cell production in mature mice; also appears to affect the maturation of thymic-dependent immune functions in immature mice |
| Insulin | In physiologic doses, stimulatory to thymic-derived immune responses in rats |
| Androgens | Prolong allograft survival in mice and decrease the phytohemagglutinin blastogenic responses in human lymphocytes *in vitro* |
| Estrogens and Oral Contraceptives | *In vitro* and *in vivo* administration inhibit human lymphocyte phytohemagglutinin blastogenic responses; also, decrease natural killer-cell activity and prolong allograft survival in animals *in vivo* |

* From Stevenson, H.C., and Fauci, A.S.: The effect of glucocorticoids and other hormones on inflammatory and immune responses. *In* Oppenheim, J.J., Rosenstreich, D.L., and Potter, M. (eds.): Cellular Functions in Immunity and Inflammation. New York, Elsevier/North Holland, 1981.

Levamisole has been shown to augment the effector phase of the nonspecific inflammatory response as well as to truly potentiate the immune response by enhancing lymphoid cell function. The drug has been shown to be effective in correcting the chemotactic defect of monocytes[147] and neutrophils[148] in patients with viral infections. In addition, levamisole has been shown to be effective both in vitro and in vivo in correcting the chemotactic defect in neutrophils from patients with the syndrome of hyperimmunoglobulin E and recurrent infections.[149,150] However, a recent double-blind study demonstrated that despite restoration of normal chemotactic responsiveness in patients with the hyperimmunoglobulin E syndrome by treatment with levamisole, patients who received the drug tended to have more serious infectious complications than those patients given a placebo.[151]

A variety of lymphocyte functions have been shown to be enhanced in vivo by treatment with levamisole as well as in vitro by the addition of the drug to lymphocyte cultures. The drug appears to be most effective in immunopotentiation in individuals with abnormally low responses, with little effect under conditions of optimal responses. Delayed hypersensitivity skin tests have been shown to be enhanced in patients receiving levamisole therapy, particularly in those individuals with significant impairment of delayed cutaneous hypersensitivity.[152] The function of specific subpopulations of T lymphocytes are also augmented by levamisole. This includes enhancement of inducer or helper T-lymphocyte function and cytotoxic T-lymphocyte function as well as suppressor T-lymphocyte function.[153] Patients treated with levamisole generally do not manifest an increase in the absolute numbers or percentages of lymphocytes. However, reduced numbers of T lymphocytes are restored together with a reduction in the percentage of null cells (non-T, non-B cells).[154] Since null cells have been postulated to be precursors or immature forms of T and/or B lymphocytes, the increased numbers of T lymphocytes may represent an induction of differentiation or maturity from null cell to normally functioning T lymphocyte.[155] Although B lymphocytes are generally felt not to be directly stimulated by levamisole, a recent study described a booster response in antibody titers to recall antigens in patients treated with levamisole.[155] The mechanisms responsible for the phenomenon are unclear but could include a direct action on B lymphocytes or an indirect effect by enhancing inducer T lymphocytes or impeding suppressor cell function.

Levamisole has been used in malignant diseases as an adjuvant agent; it has also been used in a number of nonmalignant diseases. Of particular interest has been its use in the treatment of rheumatoid arthritis in which rather favorable clinical responses have been reported.[155,156] The drug is generally administered in doses of 150 mg orally on a daily basis for periods up to 16 weeks.[155] The major constraint of its use clinically is the incidence and severity of the toxic side effects. Side effects of the drug have included gastrointestinal disturbances, fatigue, fever, and skin rash. However, the most severe and limiting toxic side effect is granulocytopenia, which seems to be disproportionately more frequent in patients with rheumatic diseases. Of particular interest is the fact that agranulocytosis due to levamisole is particularly common in patients with HLA-B27.[157,158] In a recent study of the treatment of 20 rheumatoid arthritis patients with levamisole, agranulocytosis or neutropenia occurred at some time in 4 patients.[155] Despite the favorable clinical results with regard to the activity of the rheumatoid arthritis in that study, the toxicity clearly renders the drug unacceptable for routine use in rheumatoid arthritis.

**Other Immune Enhancers and Adjuvants.** Clearly, the most extensively employed adjuvant in experimental animals is complete Freund's adjuvant (CFA), which is composed of paraffin oil and an emulsifying agent to which killed mycobacteria have been added. Injection of emulsions of antigens in CFA into experimental animals results in markedly augmented antibody responses as well as delayed hypersensitivity.[159] Unfortunately, the severe local and systemic toxic side effects of CFA render it unacceptable for use in humans. Recently, preparations of adjuvants such as the synthetic *N*-acetylmuramyl-L-alanyl-D-isoglutamine have been shown to be effective enhancers of antibody production without appreciable toxic side effects.[160] Such studies may prove extremely fruitful in the ultimate development of a clinically acceptable adjuvant, which could be used in the enhancement of immune function in the absence of significant toxic side effects.

**Cyclosporin A.** Cyclosporin A was discovered in 1972 during a search for biologically produced antifungal agents. It is a 1200-dalton fungal metabolite, which proved to be only mildly active as an antifungal agent but did manifest certain profound effects on the immune response. Cyclosporin A is a cyclic endecapeptide of original chemical structure in which some amino acids are unconventional or modified (*N*-methylated.)[161] This latter property is responsible for the fact that the drug is effective by oral administration in that pH and enzymes of the gastrointestinal tract do not seem to inactivate it. It can be administered by both the parenteral and oral routes, it exhibits poor water solubility, and it does not need to be activated in vivo, as witnessed by the fact that it is directly active in vitro. The drug has been recently employed extensively as an immunosuppressive agent for organ (particularly renal) transplantation.[162] It is administered either as the sole immunosuppressive agent[163] or together with corticosteroids.[164] The optimal dose with regard to efficacy balanced against toxic side effects has not been precisely determined. However, recent studies in patients receiving cadaveric renal transplants have arrived at a dosage of 17 mg per kg per day with gradual tapering by about 2 mg per kg per day decrements at monthly intervals until a maintenance dose of 6 to 8 mg per kg per day is reached.[163]

Cyclosporin A differs from other known cytotoxic immunosuppressive agents in its mechanism of action and particularly by the fact that it manifests a low degree of myelotoxicity. It appears that the effect of the agent is selective for the immune system, particularly T lymphocytes. There is general agreement that cyclosporin A acts preferentially on proliferating T lymphocytes.[162] It has also been shown that the agent exerts its effects at an early stage in the triggering of T lymphocytes, since addition of cyclosporin A to lymphocyte cultures late after antigenic stimulation results in diminution of the inhibitory effect.[162]

It is currently debated exactly where in the mechanism of cell triggering cyclosporin A acts. Certain investigators have shown evidence that the drug acts by inhibiting the production of receptors for IL II or T lymphocyte growth factor.[165] Others claim that receptors for IL II are present despite the presence of the drug in culture and claim that IL II is missing from cultures.[162] In this regard, it is unclear whether cyclosporin A exerts this effect by blocking the synthesis of IL II or its secretion. In any event, cyclosporin A blocks a number of T lymphocyte functions, particularly those dependent on helper or inducer T lymphocyte activity.

In vitro studies have demonstrated suppressive effects of cyclosporin A on T helper lymphocytes for antibody production to T lymphocyte–dependent antigens,[166] inhibition of the generation[167] but not expression of the function[168] of cytotoxic T lymphocytes induced in the mixed lymphocyte reaction, and abrogation of concanavalin A–induced suppressor cell function.[169] It is unclear at this time whether the selective effects on helper T-lymphocyte function provide a balance in favor of T-lymphocyte suppression as being responsible for the initiation and maintenance of the immunosuppressed state. It has generally been felt that cyclosporin A affects B lymphocytes only insofar as it inhibits helper T lymphocyte function. However, recent studies suggest that the drug may have selective direct effects of enhancement or inhibition on certain subsets of B lymphocytes.[170] Of interest is the finding that in patients treated with cyclosporin A alone, IgG levels increased to become significantly elevated compared with those found in normal healthy controls.[162]

Cyclosporin A has received considerable attention as an extremely effective immunosuppressive agent for renal transplant rejection. Recently, favorable reports have appeared describing successes in transplantation of heart, lungs, pancreas, and liver in both experimental animals and certain small human studies.[162] The implications of these studies are extraordinary for the use of organ transplantation in a wide variety of clinical situations. In this regard, recent studies have demonstrated the efficacy of cyclosporin A in suppressing graft-versus-host reactions in bone marrow transplants.[171]

The major constraint in the use of cyclosporin A, as with other immunosuppressive agents, lies in its toxicity. Although it has few myelotoxic effects, use of the agent is not without risks. By far the most serious toxic side effect of the drug is its nephrotoxicity. This toxic side effect is particularly serious in a renal transplantation program, since it is often unclear whether the deterioration in renal function is due to insufficient drug, allowing for rejection to occur, or to too much cyclosporin A, causing nephrotoxicity.[162] Other toxic side effects include abnormalities of liver function tests, transient hirsutism, and gum hypertrophy. Bacterial infection has not been a problem with the use of this drug. However, reactivation of certain viral infections, particularly Epstein-Barr virus, have occurred sporadically. Of note is the fact that lymphomas have occurred in patients treated with cyclosporin A and were felt to result from the immunosuppressive effects rather than from any carcinogenicity of the drug.[162]

Of particular interest for the present discussion is the potential for the use of cyclosporin A in the treatment of rheumatic diseases characterized by hyper-reactivity or aberrant immune function at the T-lymphocyte level. Although no clinical trials have been performed with the use of cyclosporin A in rheumatic diseases, it is clear that the impressive immunosuppressive effects of this agent in the relative absence of myelosuppressive effects warrants at least consideration of the trial of this agent in certain selected immune-mediated connective tissue diseases.

**Dapsone.** Dapsone is a sulfone (4,4′-diaminodiphenyl sulfone) and first gained notoriety as an agent effective in the treatment of *Mycobacterium leprae.* Most recently it has been recognized as an effective agent in the treatment of dermatitis herpetiformis[172] and erythema elevatum diutinum[173] as well as the bullous eruptions of SLE.[174] Dapsone is available for oral administration and is slowly and nearly completely absorbed from the gastrointestinal tract. Peak concentrations of dapsone are reached in plasma 1 to 3 hours after oral administration, and its half-life ranges from 10 to 50 hours, with a mean of 28 hours.[175] Twenty-four hours after an oral dose of 100 mg, plasma concentrations range from 0.4 to 1.2 μg per ml. The sulfones are distributed throughout the total body water and are present in all tissues. They tend to be retained in skin, muscle, liver, and kidney, with traces of the drug present in these organs up to 3 weeks following cessation of administration. Dapsone is acetylated in the liver, and about 70 to 80 percent of a dose is excreted in the urine.

The mechanism of the bactericidal activity of dapsone is probably similar to the sulfonamides. However, the mechanisms whereby dapsone is effective in dermatitis herpetiformis and erythema elevatum diutinum and the bullous skin lesions of SLE are unclear at present. The common denominator of dermatitis herpetiformis and erythema elevatum diutinum is the infiltration of the lesions with neutrophils.[173] This has led investigators to put forth a number of hypotheses for mechanisms of effect, including blocking of complement deposition, which removes the chemotactic stimulus to neutrophils. However, other studies[176] have not substantiated these theories, and the mechanisms of action remain unknown in these diseases despite the dramatic clinical responses.

Given the fact that the underlying lesion in erythema elevatum diutinum is a leukocytoclastic vasculitis involving the postcapillary venules, it is conceivable that dapsone might be effective in other cutaneous vasculitis syndromes. However, there have been no prospective studies of the use of dapsone in other vasculitic syndromes, and anecdotal reports exist, but they are inconclusive.

The drug is administered orally in doses of 50 to 100 mg per day. The effect is seen within days, and particularly with erythema elevatum diutinum, relapses occur almost immediately after cessation of the drug,[173] which is somewhat paradoxical given the fact that the drug is present in organs for weeks after cessation of therapy. The sudden relapses following cessation might be explained by a need for a critical concentration of drug in plasma below which a dramatic deterioration in clinical condition is seen.

The limiting factor in the use of dapsone is its toxic side effects, which include hemolysis and methemoglobinemia and which occur relatively frequently. Other side effects include anorexia, nausea, and vomiting. Rarely, headache, nervousness, insomnia, and peripheral neuropathy have been reported.

**Interferons.** The interferons are relatively small glycoproteins that inhibit the multiplication of certain viruses. They first attracted significant attention because of their potential antiviral activities. They are elaborated from viral-infected cells and protect noninfected cells from viral infection.[177] They induce a transient state of refractoriness to viral infection by altering nucleotide metabolism and cytoplasmic enzyme induction.[177] However, it soon became clear that in addition to their antiviral properties, interferons had significant effects on cell differentiation, cell growth, the expression of surface antigens, cellular morphology, and most importantly for the purposes of this discussion, immunoregulation.[177,178]

The interferon nomenclature has recently been refined[179] and now includes the following three major types: (1) interferon alpha, which was previously known as classic interferon or leukocyte interferon, is pH 2 stable; (2) interferon beta, which was previously known as fibroblast interferon, is pH stable; and (3) interferon gamma, which was previously known as Type II or immune interferon, is produced by antigen-induced or mitogen-induced lymphocytes and is pH 2 labile.

In general, interferon gamma is much more potent in

**Table 55–7.** Effects of Interferon on Immune Function*

| Humoral Immunity | | Cellular Immunity | |
|---|---|---|---|
| *Decreased* | *Increased* | *Decreased* | *Increased* |
| IgE synthesis | Primary antibody response T-dependent and independent antigens | Antigenic, mitogenic, and allogeneic-stimulated proliferation | Allograft survival |
| Antibody response to T-dependent and independent antigens; affects both primary and secondary responses | | Bone marrow cell growth<br>Monocyte maturation in culture<br>Delayed-type hypersensitivity<br>Graft-versus-host disease in mice | Macrophage phagocytosis<br>IgE-mediated histamine release in vitro<br>Expression of surface antigens and Fc receptors<br>T-cell mediated cytotoxicity<br>Natural killer activity |

*From Kotzin, B.L., Stroker, S., Engleman, E.G., et al.: Treatment of intractable rheumatoid arthritis with total lymphoid irradiation. N. Engl. J. Med. 305:969, 1981.

its immunoregulatory effects than are the other interferons. It should be pointed out that in the evaluation of the effects of interferon on the immune system, one must be aware of the fact that the type and degree of effect may be heavily dependent on the time and dose of interferon used in both in vivo and in vitro studies. A summary of the immunoregulatory effects of interferon is given in Table 55–7.[177]

**Table 55–8.** Pharmacologic Properties of Immunoregulatory Agents

| Agent | Administration | Dosage | Gastrointestinal Absorption | Plasma Half Life | Major Side Effects |
|---|---|---|---|---|---|
| *Cytotoxic Agents* | | | | | |
| Nitrogen mustard | IV | 0.4 mg/kg q. 3–4 weeks | — | Few minutes | Leukopenia, thrombocytopenia, nausea, vomiting, local reactions at injection site |
| Cyclophosphamide | IV or oral | 2 mg/kg/day orally or IV; 750 mg/m². IV bolus | Excellent | 6–7 hours | Neutropenia, gonadal suppression, cystitis, alopecia, oncogenesis, pulmonary fibrosis, gastrointestinal intolerance |
| Chlorambucil | IV or oral | 0.1–0.2 mg/kg/day orally | Good | 90 minutes | Leukopenia, thrombocytopenia, oncogenesis, gonadal suppression, gastrointestinal intolerance, hepatotoxicity, dermatitis |
| Azathioprine and 6-mercaptopurine | IV or oral | 2 mg/kd/day orally | Excellent | 60–90 minutes | Leukopenia, hepatotoxicity, gastrointestinal intolerance, oncogenesis, host defense defect |
| Methotrexate | IV or oral | 5–50 mg per week as single IV dose or orally in 3 divided doses (q. 12 hours) or orally daily for 5 days of the week | Intermittent to Good | 2 hours | Leukopenia, thrombocytopenia, oral mucositis, gastrointestinal intolerance, hepatotoxicity, fetal intolerance in first trimester of pregnancy |
| Vinca alkaloids (vincristine and vinblastine) | IV | 2 mg/m² | — | Less than 30 minutes | Neurotoxicity |

**Table 55–8.** Pharmacologic Properties of Immunoregulatory Agents *(continued)*

| Agent | Administration | Dosage | Gastrointestinal Absorption | Plasma HalfLife | Major Side Effects |
|---|---|---|---|---|---|
| 5-Fluorouracil | IV | 12 mg/kg/day for 4 days followed by 6 mg/kg on alternate days for 2–4 doses; repeat monthly with adjustment of dose according to response | Unpredictable | 10–20 minutes | Leukopenia, gastrointestinal intolerance, alopecia, dermatitis, mucositis |
| Hydroxyurea | IV or oral | 20–30 mg/kg/day orally | Good | 6–8 hours | Myelosuppression, gastrointestinal intolerance and ulcerations, mild skin rashes |
| *Other Agents* | | | | | |
| Levamisole | Oral | Up to 150 mg/day | Excellent | 4 hours | Granulocytopenia, gastrointestinal intolerance, fever, skin rash, fatigue |
| Cyclosporin A | IV or oral | 17 mg/kg/day with monthly tapering until maintenance dose of 6–8 mg/kg/day is reached | Fair to good | 2–24 hours | Nephrotoxicity, hepatotoxicity, reactivation of viral infections, oncogenesis, transient hirsutism, gum hypertrophy |
| Dapsone | Oral | 50–100 mg/day | Good | 10–50 hours | Hemolysis, methemoglobinemia, gastrointestinal intolerance |
| Interferons (predominantly alpha) | | Phase I trials in effect | — | Uncertain | Fever, nausea, vomiting, diarrhea, transient leukopenia, myocardial infarction, others to be determined |

Administration of interferon alpha has been shown to be of some therapeutic value in herpes zoster infections, in patients with certain neoplasms, and in patients with hepatitis B infections.[177] Although there are no published controlled trials of the use of interferons in the treatment of non-neoplastic diseases such as the connective tissue diseases, their potent immunoregulatory capabilities may prove useful in attempts at manipulating the immune response in these diseases. However, it should be pointed out that the multifaceted effects of the interferons on the immune response renders the net effect unpredictable, and at this time, the use of these agents in the treatment of rheumatic diseases remains more hypothetical than practical. Perhaps when more purified preparations of interferons become available through gene cloning techniques, their effects will be more precisely delineated and trials can be undertaken. At this point, we can only say that the interferons, particularly interferon gamma, have potent immunoregulatory properties that may prove useful in the future treatment of diseases characterized by abnormalities of immune function.

A summary of certain of the pharmacologic properties of several of the immunoregulatory agents discussed in this chapter is given in Table 55–8.

## CONCLUSIONS

The use of cytotoxic and immunoregulatory agents has played a major role in the treatment of non-neoplastic, immune-mediated diseases. However, most of these agents are nonspecific and are invariably associated with a variety of toxic side effects. Since most of the rheumatic diseases in which these agents are used are chronic in nature and are rarely curable, the physician must establish the clear-cut goals of a given therapeutic regimen and must be aware of the actual as well as the potential and the immediate as well as the long-term toxic side effects of these agents. Insightful use of these agents under appropriate clinical circumstances can often lead to dramatic improvements in the clinical course as well as gratifying improvements in life style. Under other circumstances, the effects may even be life saving. However, use of these agents should be avoided in circumstances in which a less aggressive approach would be more appropriate given the nature of the illness and the projected balance between clinical results and toxic side effects. The treating physician should be acquainted as best as possible with the established results of controlled trials as they appear in the literature and should critically evaluate uncontrolled trials, which may indeed represent a true advance in therapy but which may also give a false sense of security that a particular agent will be beneficial. All things considered, sound clinical judgment applied to each individual patient with regard to the choice and actual usage of an immunoregulatory agent is indispensable.

## References


1. Fauci, A.S.: Immunoregulation in autoimmunity. J. Allergy Clin. Immunol. 66:5, 1980.
2. NIAID Group: New Initiatives in Immunology. Report. Bethesda, Maryland, National Institute of Allergy and Infectious Diseases. DHHS Publication No. (NIH) 81-2215:1, 1981.
3. Paul, W.E.: Lymphocyte biology. *In* Parker, C.W. (ed.): Clinical Immunology. Vol. 1. Philadelphia, W. B. Saunders Company, 1980.
4. Fauci, A.S.: The revolution in clinical immunology. JAMA 246:2567, 1981.
5. Fauci, A.S., Lane, H.C., and Volkman, D.J.: Activation and regulation of human immune responses: Implications in normal and disease states. Ann. Intern. Med., 98:76, 1983.
6. Steinberg, A.D., Plotz, P.H., Wolff, S.M., Wong, V.G., Agus, S.G., and Decker, J.L.: Cytotoxic drugs in treatment of nonmalignant diseases. Ann. Intern. Med. 76:619, 1972.
7. Fauci, A.S., Dale, D.C., and Balow, J.E.: Glucocorticosteroid therapy: mechanisms of action and clinical considerations. Ann. Intern. Med. 84:304, 1976.
8. Gerber, N.L., and Steinberg, A.D.: Clinical use of immunosuppressive drugs. Part I. Drugs 11:36, 1976.
9. Gerber, N.L., and Steinberg, A.D.: Clinical use of immunosuppressive drugs. Part II. Drugs 11:90, 1976.
10. Calabresi, P., and Parks, R.E.: Antiproliferative agents and drugs used for immunosuppression. *In* Goodman, L.S., and Gilman A. (eds.): The Pharmocologic Basis of Therapeutics. 6th ed. New York, Macmillan, 1980.
11. Cooper, M.D., Peterson, R.D.A., and Good, R.A.: Delineation of the thymic and bursal lymphoid system in the chicken. Nature 205:143, 1965.
12. Cooper, M.D., Peterson, R.D.A., South, M.A., and Good, R.A.: The functions of the thymus system and the bursa system in the chicken. J. Exp. Med. 123:75, 1966.
13. Claman, H.N., Chaperon, E.A., and Triplett, R.F.: Thymus-marrow cell combinations. Synergism in antibody production. Proc. Soc. Exp. Biol. Med. 12:1167, 1966.
14. Miller, J.F.A.P., and Mitchell, G.F.: Cell-cell interactions in immune response. I. Hemolysin-forming cells in neonatally thymectomized mice reconstituted with thymus or thoracic duct lymphocytes. J. Exp. Med. 128:801, 1968.
15. Möller, G. (ed.): Role of macrophages in the immune response. Immunol. Rev. 40:1, 1978.
16. Möller, G. (ed.): Natural killer cells. Immunol. Rev. 44:1, 1979.
17. Herberman, R.B., and Ortaldo, J.R.: Natural killer cells: Their role in defenses against disease. Science 214:24 1981.
18. Gallin, J.I., and Fauci, A.S. (eds.): Advances in Host Defense Mechanisms. Vol. 1. New York, Raven Press, 1982.
19. Jerne, N.K.: Towards a network theory of the immune system. Ann. Immunol. (Inst. Pasteur) 125:373, 1974.
20. Möller, G. (ed.): Idiotypes on T and B cells. Immunol. Rev. 34:1, Copenhagen, Munksgaard, 1977.
21. Geha, R.S.: Presence of auto-anti-idiotypic antibody during the normal human immune response to tetanus toxoid antigen. J. Immunol. 129:139, 1982.
22. Abdou, N.I., Wall, H., Lindsley, H.B., Halsey, J.F., and Suzuki, T.: Network theory in autoimmunity. In vitro suppression of serum anti-DNA antibody binding to DNA by anti-idiotypic antibody in systemic lupus erythematosus. J. Clin. Invest. 67:1297, 1981.
23. Waldmann, T.A., and Broder, S.: Suppressor cells in the regulation of the immune response. *In* Schwartz, R.S. (ed.): Progress in Clinical Immunology. Vol. 3. New York, Grune and Stratton, 1977.
24. Fauci, A.S., Haynes, B.F., and Katz, P.: The spectrum of vasculitis: clinical, pathologic, immunologic, and therapeutic considerations. Ann. Intern. Med. 89:660, 1978.
25. Fauci, A.S., Haynes, B.F., Katz, P., and Wolff, S.M.: Wegener's granulomatosis: prospective clinical and therapeutic experience with 85 patients over 21 years. Ann. Intern. Med. 98:76, 1983.
26. Cupps, T.R., and Fauci, A.S.: The Vasculitides. *In* Smith, L.H. (ed.): Major Problems in Internal Medicine. Vol. XXL. Philadelphia, W. B. Saunders Company, 1981.
27. Cupps, T.R., Edgar, L.C., and Fauci, A.S.: Suppression of human B lymphocyte function by cyclophosphamide. J. Immunol. 128:2453, 1982.
28. Maguire, H.C., and Maibach, H.I.: Specific immune tolerance to anaphylactic sensitization (egg albumin) in the guinea pig by cyclophosphamide (cytoxan). J. Allergy 32:406, 1961.
29. Möller, G. (ed.): Suppressor T lymphocytes. Immunol. Rev. 26:1, 1975.
30. Fauci, A.S.: Assays for suppressor cells. *In* Rose, N.R., and Friedman, H. (eds.): Manual of Clinical Immunology. 2nd ed. Washington, D.C., Society for Microbiology, 1980.
31. Talal, N.: Tolerance and autoimmunity. *In* Parker, C.W. (ed.): Clinical Immunology. Vol. I. Philadelphia, W. B. Saunders Company, 1980.
32. Farrar, J.J., Benjamin, W.R., Hilfiker, M.L., Howard, M., Farrar, W.L., and Fuller-Farrar, J.: The biochemistry, biology, and role of interleukin 2 in the induction of cytotoxic T cell and antibody-forming B cell responses. Immunol. Rev. 63:129, 1982.
33. Fauci, A.S.: Clinical aspects of immunosuppression: use of cytotoxic agents and corticosteroids. *In* Bellanti, J.A. (ed.): Immunology II. Philadelphia, W. B. Saunders Company, 1978.
34. Fauci, A.S., Katz, P., Haynes, B.F., and Wolff, S.M.: Cyclophosphamide therapy of severe necrotizing vasculitis. N. Engl. J. Med. 301:235, 1979.
35. Decker, J.L.: Toxicity of immunosuppressive drugs in man. Arthritis Rheum. 16:89, 1973.
36. Schein, P.S., and Winokur, S.T.: Immunosuppressive and cytotoxic chemotherapy: long-term complications. Ann. Intern. Med. 82:84, 1975.
37. Calabresi, P., and Parks, R.E.: Chemotherapy of neoplastic diseases. *In* Goodman, L.S., and Gilman, A. (eds.): The Pharmacologic Basis of Therapeutics. 6th ed. New York, Macmillan, 1980.
38. Ahn, Y.S., Harrington, W.J., Seelman, R.C., and Eytel, C.S.: Vincristine therapy of idiopathic and secondary thrombocytopenias. N. Engl. J. Med. 291:376, 1974.
39. Fauci, A.S., Harley, J.B., Roberts, W.C., Ferrans, V.J., Gralnick, H.R., and Bjornson, B.J.: The idiopathic hypereosinophilic syndrome: clinical, pathologic and therapeutic considerations. Ann. Intern. Med. 97:78, 1982.
40. Roberts, J.J., Brent, T.P., and Crathorn, A.R.: Evidence for the inactivation and repair of the mammalian DNA template after alkylation by mustard gas and half mustard gas. Eur. J. Cancer 7:515, 1971.
41. Fahey, J.L., Leonard, E., Churg, J., and Godman, G.: Wegener's granulomatosis. Am. J. Med. 17:168, 1954.
42. Brock, N.: Pharmacologic characterization of cyclophosphamide (NSC-26271) and cyclophosphamide metabolites. Cancer Chemother. Rep. 51:315, 1967.
43. Bagley, C.M., Bostick, F.W., and DeVita, V.T., Jr.: Clinical pharmacology of cyclophosphamide. Cancer Res. 33:226, 1973.
44. Gershwin, M.E., Goetzel, E.J., and Steinberg, A.D.: Cyclophosphamide: use in practice. Ann. Intern. Med. 80:531, 1974.
45. Sladek, N.E.: Therapeutic efficacy of cyclophosphamide as a function of its metabolism. Cancer Res. 32:535, 1972.
46. Makinodan, T., Santos, G.W., and Quinn, R.P.: Immunosuppressive drugs. Pharmacological Rev. 22:189, 1970.
47. Shand, F.L.: The immunopharmacology of cyclophosphamide. Int. J. Pharmacol. 1:165, 1979.
48. Berenbaum, M.C., and Brown, I.N.: Dose-response relationships for agents inhibiting the immune response. Immunology 7:65, 1964.
49. Askenase, P.W., Hayden, B.J., and Gershon, R.K.: Augmentation of delayed-type hypersensitivity of doses of cyclophosphamide which do not effect antibody responses. J. Exp. Med. 141:697, 1975.
50. Sy, M.S., Miller, S.D., and Claman, H.N.: Immune suppression with supraoptimal doses of antigen in contact sensitivity. I. Demonstration of suppressor cells and their sensitivity to cyclophosphamide. J. Immunol. 119:240, 1977.
51. Fauci, A.S., Wolff, S.M., and Johnson, J.S.: Effect of cyclophosphamide

upon the immune response in Wegener's granulomatosis. N. Engl. J. Med. 285:1493, 1971.

52. Fauci, A.S., Dale, D.C., and Wolff, S.M.: Cyclophosphamide and lymphocyte subpopulations in Wegener's granulomatosis. Arthritis Rheum. 17:355, 1974.
53. Hurd, E.R., and Giuliano, V.J.: The effect of cyclophosphamide on B and T lymphocytes in patients with connective tissue diseases. Arthritis Rheum. 18:67, 1975.
54. Dale, D.C., Fauci, A.S., and Wolff, S.M.: The effect of cyclophosphamide on leukocyte kinetics and susceptibility to infection in patients with Wegener's granulomatosis. Arthritis Rheum. 16:657, 1973.
55. Warne, G.L., Fairley, K.F., Hobbs, J.B., and Martin, F.I.R.: Cyclophosphamide-induced ovarian failure. N. Engl. J. Med. 289:1159, 1973.
56. Schilsky, R.L., Lewis, B.J., Sherins, R.J., and Young, R.C.: Gonadal dysfunction in patients receiving chemotherapy for cancer. Ann. Intern. Med. 93:109, 1980.
57. Trompeter, R.S., Evans, P.R., and Barratt, T.M.: Gonadal function in boys with steroid-responsive nephrotic syndrome treated with cyclophosphamide for short periods. Lancet 1:1177, 1981.
58. Fairley, K.F., Barrie, J.U., and Johnson, W.: Sterility and testicular atrophy related to cyclophosphamide therapy. Lancet 1:568, 1972.
59. Plotz, P.H., Klippel, J.H., Decker, J.L., et al.: Bladder complications in patients receiving cyclophosphamide for systemic lupus erythematosus or rheumatoid arthritis. Ann. Intern. Med. 91:221, 1979.
60. Weiss, R.B., and Maggia, F.M.: Cytotoxic drug-induced pulmonary disease: update 1980. Am. J. Med. 68:259, 1980.
61. Appelbaum, F.R., Strauchen, J.A., Graw, R.G., Jr., et al.: Acute lethal carditis caused by high-dose combination chemotherapy. A unique clinical and pathological entity. Lancet 1:58, 1976.
62. De Fronzo, R.A., Braine, H., Colvin, O.M., and Davis, P.J.: Water intoxication in man after cyclophosphamide therapy. Time course and relation to drug activation. Ann. Intern. Med. 78:861, 1973.
63. Penn, I.: Depressed immunity and the development of cancer. Clin. Exp. Immunol. 46:459, 1981.
64. McLean, A., Newell, D., and Baker, G.: The metabolism of chlorambucil. Biochem. Pharmacol. 25:2331, 1976.
65. Stukov, A.N.: Experimental study of the combined effect of leukoran, degranol, and prednisolone. Neoplasma 22:181, 1976.
66. Israel, H., and Patchefsky, A.S.: Treatment of Wegener's granulomatosis of lung. Am. J. Med. 58:671, 1975.
67. Rudd, P., Fried, J.F., and Epstein, W.V.: Irreversible bone marrow failure with chlorambucil. J. Rheumatol. 2:421, 1975.
68. Cameron, S.: Chlorambucil and leukemia. N. Engl. J. Med. 296:1065, 1977.
69. Lerner, H.J.: Acute myelogenous leukemia in patients receiving chlorambucil as long-term adjuvant chemotherapy for Stage II breast cancer. Cancer Treat. Rep. 60:1431, 1978.
70. Gabrielsen, A.E., and Good, R.A.: Chemical suppression of adaptive immunity. Adv. Immunol. 6:91, 1967.
71. Yu, D.T., Clements, P.J., Peter, J.B., Levy, J., Paulus, H.E., and Barnett, E.V.: Lymphocyte characteristics in rheumatic patients and the effect of azathioprine therapy. Arthritis Rheum. 17:37, 1974.
72. Levy, J., Barnett, E.V., MacDonald, N.S., Klinenberg, J.R., and Pearson, C.M.: The effect of azathioprine on gammaglobulin synthesis in man. J. Clin. Invest. 51:2233, 1972.
73. Maibach, H.I., and Epstein, W.L.: Immunologic responses of healthy volunteers receiving azathioprine (Imuran). Int. Arch. Allergy 27:102, 1965.
74. Abdou, N.I., Zweiman, B., and Casella, S.R.: Effects of azathioprine therapy on bone marrow-dependent and thymus-dependent cells in man. Clin. Exp. Immunol. 13:55, 1973.
75. Fournier, C., Bach, M.A., Dardenne, M., and Bach, J.F.: Selective action of azathioprine on T cells. Transplantation Proc. 5:523, 1973.
76. Campbell, A.C., Skinner, J.M., Hersey, P., Roberts-Thompson, P., MacLennan, I.C.M., and Truelove, S.C.: Immunosuppression in the treatment of inflammatory bowel disease. I. Changes in lymphoid subpopulations in the blood and rectal mucosa following cessation of treatment with azathioprine. Clin. Exp. Immunol. 16:521, 1974.
77. Sharbaugh, R.J., Ainsworth, S.K., and Fitts, C.T.: Lack of effect of azathioprine on phytohemagglutinin-induced lymphocyte transformation and established delayed cutaneous hypersensitivity. Int. Arch. Allergy Applied Immunol. 51:681, 1976.
78. Gassman, A.E., and van Furth, R.: The effect of azathioprine (Imuran) on the kinetics of monocytes and macrophages during the normal steady state and an acute inflammatory reaction. Blood 46:51, 1975.
79. Phillips, S.M., and Zweiman, B.: Mechanisms in the suppression of delayed hypersensitivity in the guinea pig by 6-mercaptopurine. J. Exp. Med. 137:1494, 1973.
80. Rosman, M., and Bertino, J.R.: Azathioprine. Ann. Intern. Med. 79:694, 1973.
81. Losito, A., Williams, D.G., and Harris, L.: The effects on polymorphonuclear leukocyte function of prednisolone and azathioprine in vivo and prednisolone, azathioprine and 6-mercaptopurine in vitro. Clin. Exp. Immunol. 32:423, 1978.
82. Henderson, F.S., Adamson, R.H., and Oliverio, V.T.: The metabolic rate of tritiated methotrexate. II. Absorption and excretion in man. Cancer Res. 25:1018, 1965.
83. Hersh, E.M., Carbone, P.P., Wong, V.G., and Freireich, E.J.: Inhibition of the primary immune response in man by antimetabolites. Cancer Res. 25:997, 1965.
84. Hersh, E.M., Carbone, P.P., and Freireich, E.J.: Recovery of immune responsiveness after drug suppression in man. J. Lab. Clin. Med. 67:566, 1965.
85. Mitchell, M.S., Wade, M.E., DeConti, R.C., Bertino, J.R., and Calabresi, P.: Immunosuppressive effects of cytosine arabinoside and methotrexate in man. Ann. Intern. Med. 70:535, 1969.
86. Ahn, Y.S., Byrnes, J.J., Harrington, W.J., et al.: The treatment of idiopathic thrombocytopenia with vinblastine-loaded platelets. N. Engl. J. Med. 298:1101, 1978.
87. Fauci, A.S., Harley, J.B., Roberts, W.C., Ferrans, V.J., Gralnick, H.R., and Bjornson, B.H.: The idiopathic hypereosinophilic syndrome. Clinical, pathophysiologic, and therapeutic considerations. Ann. Intern. Med. 97:78, 1982.
88. Cupps, T.R., Silverman, G.J., and Fauci, A.S.: Herpes zoster in patients with treated Wegener's granulomatosis. A possible role for cyclophosphamide. Am. J. Med. 69:881, 1980.
89. Tindall, R.S.A. (ed.): Therapeutic Apheresis and Plasma Perfusion. New York, A. R. Liss, Inc., 1980.
90. Branda, R.F., Molodow, C.F., McCollough, J.J., and Jacob, H.S.: Plasma exchange in the treatment of immune disease. Transfusion 5:570, 1975.
91. Lockwood, C.M., Pearson, T.A., Rees, A.J., Evans, D.J., Peters, D.K., and Wilson, C.B.: Immunosuppression and plasma exchange in the treatment of Goodpasture's syndrome. Lancet 1:711, 1976.
92. Pinching, A.J., Peters, D.K., and Newsom Davis, J.: Remission of myasthenia gravis following plasma-exchange. Lancet 2:1373, 1976.
93. Vogler, W.R.: Therapeutic apheresis: Where we've been and where we are going. *In* Tindall, R.S.A. (ed.): Therapeutic Apheresis and Plasma Perfusion. New York, A. R. Liss, Inc., 1980.
94. Wallace, D.J., Goldfinger, D., Gatti, et al.: Plasmapheresis and lymphoplasmapheresis in the management of rheumatoid arthritis. Arthritis Rheum. 22:703, 1979.
95. Balow, J.E., and Tsokos, G.C.: Plasmapheresis in systemis lupus erythematosus: facts and perspectives. Int. J. Artif. Organs 5:286, 1982.
96. Lockwood, C.M., Worlledge, S., Nicholas, A., Cotton, D., and Peters, D.K.: Reversal of impaired splenic function in patients with nephritis or vasculitis (or both) by plasma exchange. N. Engl. J. Med. 300:524, 1979.
97. Kauffmann, R.H., and Houwert, D.A.: Plasmapheresis in rapidly progressive Henoch-Schoenlein glomerulonephritis and the effect on circulating IgA immune complexes. Clin. Nephrol. 16:155, 1981.
98. Karsh, J., Klippel, J.H., Plotz, P.H., Decker, J.L., Wright, D.G., and Flye, M.W.: Lymphapheresis in rheumatoid arthritis. A randomized trial. Arthritis Rheum. 24:867, 1981.
99. Wallace, D., Goldfinger, D., Lowe, C., et al.: A double-blind controlled study of lymphoplasmapheresis versus sham apheresis in rheumatoid arthritis. N. Engl. J. Med. 306:1406, 1982.
100. Terman, D.S., Young, J.B., Shearer, W.T., et al.: Preliminary observations of the effects on breast adenocarcinoma of plasma perfused over immobilized protein A. N. Engl. J. Med. 305:1195, 1981.
101. Saal, S.D., and Gordon, B.R.: Extracorporeal modification of plasma and whole blood. *In* Tindall, R.S.A. (ed.): Therapeutic Apheresis and Plasma Perfusion. New York, A. R. Liss, Inc., 1980.
102. Pineda, A.A.: Methods for selective removal of plasma constituents. *In* Tindall, R.S.A. (ed.): Therapeutic Apheresis and Plasma Perfusion. New York, A. R. Liss, Inc., 1980.
103. Hamburger, M.I., Lawley, T.J., Kimberly, R.P., Plotz, P.H., and Frank, M.M.: A serial study of splenic reticuloendothelial system Fc receptor functional activity in systemic lupus erythematosus. Arthritis Rheum. 25:48, 1982.
104. Steven, M.M., Tanner, A.R., Holdstock, T.J., and Wright, R.: Effect of plasma exchange on the in vitro monocyte function of patients with immune complex diseases. Clin. Exp. Immunol. 45:240, 1981.
105. Lockwood, C.M., Rees, A.J., Pearson, T.A., Evans, D.J., Peters, D.K., and Wilson, C.B.: Immunosuppression and plasma exchange in the treatment of Goodpasture's syndrome. Lancet 1:711, 1976.
106. Flaum, M.A., Cuneo, R.A., Appelbaum, F.A., Deisseroth, A.B., Engel, W.K., and Gralnick, H.R.: The hemostatic imbalance of plasma-exchange transfusion. Blood 54:694, 1979.
107. Orlin, J.B., and Berkman, E.M.: Partial plasma exchange using albumin replacement: removal and recovery of normal constituents. Blood 56:1055, 1980.
108. Wright, D.G., Karsh, J., Fauci, A.S., et al.: Lymphocyte depletion and immunosuppression with repeated leukapheresis by continuous flow centrifugation. Blood 58:451, 1981.

109. Machleder, H.I., and Paulus, H.: Clinical and immunological alterations observed in patients undergoing long-term thoracic duct drainage. Surgery 84:157, 1978.
110. Paulus, H.E., Machleder, H.I., Levine, S., Yu, D.T.Y., and Macdonald, N.S.: Lymphocyte involvement in rheumatoid arthritis. Studies during thoracic duct drainage. Arthritis Rheum. 20:1249, 1977.
111. Hutchinson, F.: The molecular basis for radiation effects on cells. Cancer Res. 26:2045, 1966.
112. Anderson, R.E., and Warner, N.L.: Ionizing radiation and the immune response. Adv. Immunol. 24:215, 1976.
113. Fauci, A.S., Pratt, K.R., and Whalen, G.: Activation of human B lymphocytes. VIII. Differential radiosensitivity of subpopulations of lymphoid cells involved in the polyclonally induced PFC responses of peripheral blood B lymphocytes. Immunology 35:715, 1978.
114. Kaplan, H.S.: Hodgkin's Disease. 2nd ed. Cambridge, Harvard University Press, 1980.
115. Hellman, S., Mauch, P., Goodman, R.L., Rosenthal, D.S., and Moloney, W.C.: The place of radiation therapy in the treatment of Hodgkin's disease. Cancer 42:971, 1978.
116. Fuks, Z., Strober, S., Bobrove, A.M., Sasazuki, T., McMichael, A., and Kaplan, H.S.: Long-term effects of radiation on T and B lymphocytes in peripheral blood of patients with Hodgkin's disease. J. Clin. Invest. 58:803, 1976.
117. Kotzin, B.L., Strober, S., Engleman, E.G., et al.: Treatment of intractable rheumatoid arthritis with total lymphoid irradiation. N. Engl. J. Med. 305:969, 1981.
118. Trentham, D.E., Belli, J.A., Anderson, R.J., et al.: Clinical and immunologic effects of fractionated total lymphoid irradiation in refractory rheumatoid arthritis. N. Engl. J. Med. 305:976, 1981.
119. Strober, S., Slavin, S., Gottlieb, M., et al.: Allograft tolerance after total lymphoid irradiation (TLI). Immunol. Rev. 46:87, 1979.
120. Taub, R.N., and Deutsch, V.: Antilymphocytic serum. Pharmacol. Ther. 2:89, 1977.
121. Harris, N.S., Merino, G., and Najarian, J.S.: Mode of action of antilymphocyte sera (ALS). Transplant. Proc. 3:797, 1971.
122. Starzl, T.E., Marchioro, T.L., Hutchinson, D.E., Porter, K.A., Cerilli, G.J., and Brettschneider, L.: The clinical use of antilymphocyte globulin in renal homotransplantation. Transplant. Suppl. 5:1100, 1967.
123. Sheil, A.G.R., Mears, D., Kelly, G.E., et al.: Controlled clinical trial of antilymphocyte globulin in patients with renal allografts from cadaver donors. Lancet 1:359, 1971.
124. Köhler, G., and Milstein, C.: Continuous cultures of fused cells secreting antibody of predefined specificity. Nature 256:495, 1975.
125. Kennett, R.H., McKearn, T.J., and Bechtol, K.B. (eds.): Monoclonal Antibodies. Hybridomas: A New Dimension in Biological Analyses. New York, Plenum Press, 1980.
126. Miller, R.A., and Levy, R.: Response of cutaneous T cell lymphoma to therapy with hybridoma monoclonal antibody. Lancet 2:226, 1981.
127. Miller, R.A., Malone, D.G., Warnke, R., and Levy, R.: Treatment of B-cell lymphoma with monoclonal anti-idiotype antibody. N. Engl. J. Med. 306:517, 1982.
128. Ritz, J., Sallan, S.E., Bast, R.C., Jr., et al.: Autologous bone-marrow transplantation in CALLA-positive acute lymphoblastic leukaemia after in vitro treatment with J5 monoclonal antibody and complement. Lancet 2:60, 1982.
129. Prentice, H.G., Blacklock, H.A., Janossy, G., et al.: Use of anti-T cell monoclonal antibody OKT3 to prevent acute graft-versus-host disease in allogeneic bone-marrow transplantation for acute leukemia. Lancet 1:700, 1982.
130. Filopovich, A.H., McGlave, P.B., Ramsay, N.K.C., Goldstein, G., Warkentin, P.I., and Kersey, J.H.: Pretreatment of donor bone marrow with monoclonal antibody OKT3 for prevention of acute graft-versus-host disease in allogeneic histocompatible bone marrow transplantation. Lancet 1:1266, 1982.
131. Reinherz, E., Geha, R., Rappeport, J.M., et al.: Reconstitution after transplantation with T-lymphocyte-depleted HLA haplotype-mismatched bone marrow for severe combined immunodeficiency. Proc. Natl. Acad. Sci. USA 79:6047, 1982.
132. Steinman, L., Rosenbaum, J.T., Sriram, S., and McDevitt, H.O.: In vivo effects of antibodies to immune response gene products: prevention of experimental allergic encephalitis. Proc. Natl. Acad. Sci. USA 78:7111, 1981.
133. Barkas, T., and Simpson, J.A.: Lack of inter-animal cross-reaction of anti-acetylcholine receptor antibodies at the receptor-binding site as demonstrated by heterologous anti-idiotype antisera: implications for immunotherapy of myasthenia gravis. Clin. Exp. Immunol. 47:119, 1982.
134. Cupps, T.R., and Fauci, A.S.: Corticosteroid-mediated immunoregulation in man. Immunol. Rev. 65:133, 1982.
135. Fauci, A.S., and Dale, D.C.: The effect of in vivo hydrocortisone on subpopulations of human lymphocytes. J. Clin. Invest. 53:240, 1974.
136. Haynes, B.F., and Fauci, A.S.: The differential effect of in vivo hydrocortisone on kinetics of subpopulations of human peripheral blood thymus-derived lymphocytes. J. Clin. Invest. 61:703, 1978.
137. Eidenger, D., and Garrett, T.J.: Studies of the regulatory effects of sex hormones on antibody formation and stem cell differentiation. J. Exp. Med. 136:1098, 1972.
138. Steinberg, A.D., Klassen, L.W., Raveche, E.S., et al.: Study of the multiple factors in the pathogenesis of autoimmunity in New Zealand mice. Arthritis Rheum. 21:2190, 1978.
139. Wyle, F.A., and Kent, J.R.: Immunosuppression by sex steroid hormones. I. The effect upon PHA and PPD stimulated lymphocytes. Clin. Exp. Immunol. 27:407, 1976.
140. Roubinian, J.R., Papoian, R., and Talal, N.: Androgenic hormones modulate autoantibody responses and improve survival in murine lupus. J. Clin. Invest. 59:1066, 1977.
141. Melez, K., Reeves, J.P., and Steinberg, A.D.: Modification of NZB/NZW disease by sex hormones. J. Immunopharmacol. 1:27, 1978.
142. Roubinian, J.R., Talal, N., Greenspan, J.S., Goodman, J.R., and Sitteri, P.K.: Effect of castration and sex hormone treatment on survival, antinucleic acid antibodies and glomerulonephritis in NZB/NZW F[1] mice. J. Exp. Med. 147:1568, 1978.
143. Sheffer, A.L., Fearon, D.T., and Austen, K.F.: Methyltestosterone therapy in hereditary angioedema. Ann. Intern. Med. 53:739, 1977.
144. Gelfand, J.A., Sherrins, R.J., Alling, D.W., and Frank, M.M.: Treatment of hereditary angioedema with Danazole. Reversal of clinical and biochemical abnormalities. N. Engl. J. Med. 295:1444, 1976.
145. Stevenson, H.C., and Fauci, A.S.: The effect of glucocorticosteroids and other hormones on inflammatory and immune responses. *In* Oppenhiem, J.J., Rosenstreich, D.L., and Potter, M. (eds.): Cellular Functions in Immunity and Inflammation. New York, Elsevier/North Holland, 1981.
146. Symoens, J., and Rosenthal, M.: Levamisole in the modulation of the immune response: the current experimental and clinical state. J. Reticuloendothel. Soc. 21:175, 1977.
147. Snyderman, R., and Pike, M.C.: Pathophysiologic aspects of leukocyte chemotaxis: identification of a specific chemotactic factor binding site on human granulocytes and defects of macrophage function associated with neoplasia. *In* Gallin, J.I., and Quie, P.G. (eds.): Leukocyte Chemotaxis: Methods, Physiology, and Clinical Implications. New York, Raven Press, 1978.
148. Rabson, A.R., Whiting, D.A., Anderson, R., Glover, A., Koornhof, H.J.: Depressed neutrophil motility in patients with recurrent herpes simplex virus infections: In vitro restoration with levamisole. J. Infect. Dis. 135:113, 1977.
149. Wright, D.G., Kirkpatrick, C.H., and Gallin, J.I.: Effects of levamisole on normal and abnormal leukocyte locomotion. J. Clin. Invest. 59:941, 1977.
150. Hogan, N.A., and Hill, H.R.: Enhancement of neutrophil chemotaxis and alteration of levels of cellular cyclic nucleotides by levamisole. J. Infect. Dis. 138:437, 1978.
151. Donabedian, H., Alling, D.W., and Gallin, J.I.: Levamisole is inferior to placebo in the hyperimmunoglobulin E recurrent-infection (Job's) syndrome. N. Engl. J. Med. 307:290, 1982.
152. Tripodi, D., Parks, L.C., and Brugmans, J.: Drug-induced restoration of cutaneous delayed hypersensitivity in anergic patients with cancer. N. Engl. J. Med. 289:354, 1973.
153. Sampson, D., and Lui, A.: The effect of levamisole on cell-mediated immunity and suppressor cell function. Cancer Res. 36:952, 1976.
154. Rosenthal, M., Trabert, U., and Mueller, W.: The effect of levamisole on peripheral blood lymphocyte subpopulations in patients with rheumatoid arthritis and ankylosing spondylitis. Clin. Exp. Immunol. 25:493, 1976.
155. Miller, B., DeMerieux, P., Srinivasan, R., et al.: Double-blind placebo controlled crossover evaluation of levamisole in rheumatoid arthritis. Arthritis Rheum. 23:172, 1980.
156. Runge, L.A., Pinals, R.S., Lourie, S.H., and Tomar, R.H.: Treatment of rheumatoid arthritis with levamisole. A controlled trial. Arthritis Rheum. 20:1445, 1977.
157. Schmidt, K.L., and Mueller-Eckhardt, C.: Agranulocytosis, levamisole, and HLA-B 27. Lancet 2:85, 1977.
158. Veys, E.M., Mielants, H., and Verbruggen, G.: Levamisole-induced adverse reactions in HLA-B27-positive rheumatoid arthritis. Lancet 1:148, 1978.
159. Freund, J.: Some aspects of active immunization. Ann. Rev. Microbiol. 1:291, 1947.
160. Chedid, L., Audibert, F., LeFrancier, P., Chory, J., and Lederer, E.: Modulation of the immune response by a synthetic adjuvant and analogs. Proc. Natl. Acad. Sci. USA 73:2472, 1976.
161. Borel, J.F., Feurer, C., Gubler, H.U., and Stahelin, H.: Biological effects of cyclosporin A: A new antilymphocytic agent. Agents Actions 6:468, 1976.
162. White, D.J.G., and Calne, R.Y.: The use of cyclosporin A immunosuppression in organ grafting. Immunol. Rev. 65:115, 1982.

163. Preliminary results of a European trial: Cyclosporin A as a sole immunosuppressive agent in recipients of kidney allografts from cadaver donors. Lancet 2:57, 1982.
164. Starzl, T.E., Klintmalm, G.B.G., Weil, R., III, et al.: Cyclosporin A and steroid therapy in sixty-six cadaver kidney recipients. Surg. Gynecol. Obstet. 153:486, 1981.
165. Larsson, E.L.: Cyclosporin A and dexamethasone suppress T cell responses by selectively acting at distant sites of the triggering process. J. Immunol. 124:2828, 1980.
166. Cammisuli, S.: Inhibition of a secondary humoral immune response by cyclosporin A. Transplant. Clin. Immunol. 13:15, 1981.
167. Horsburgh, T., Wood, P., and Brent, L.: Suppression of in vitro lymphocyte reactivity by cyclosporin A. Existence of a population of drug-resistant cytotoxic lymphocytes. Nature 286:609, 1980.
168. Palacios, R.: Cyclosporin A inhibits the proliferative response and the generation of helper, suppressor and cytotoxic T cell functions in the autologous mixed lymphocyte reaction. Cell. Immunol. 61:453, 1981.
169. Palacios, R., and Möller, G.: T-cell growth factor abrogates concanavalin A induced suppressor cell function. J. Exp. Med. 153:1360, 1981.
170. Kunkel, A., and Klaus, G.G.B.: Selective effects of cyclosporin A on functional B cell subsets in the mouse. J. Immunol. 125:2526, 1980.
171. Powles, R.L., Clink, H.M., Spence, D., et al.: Cyclosporin A to prevent graft-versus-host disease in man after allogenic bone-marrow transplantation. Lancet 1:327, 1980.
172. Katz, S.I., Hall, R.P., Lawley, T.J., and Strober, W.: Dermatitis herpetiformis: The skin and the gut. Ann. Intern. Med. 93:857, 1980.
173. Katz, S.I., Gallin, J.I., Hertz, K.C., Fauci, A.S., and Lawley, T.J.: Erythema elevatum diutinum: skin and systemic manifestations, immunologic studies and successful treatment with dapsone. Medicine 56:443, 1977.
174. Hall, R.P., Lawley, T.J., Smith, H.R., and Katz, S.I.: Bullous eruption of systemic lupus erythematosus. Ann. Intern. Med. 97:165, 1982.
175. Mandell, G.L., and Sande, M.A.: Antimicrobial agents. Drugs used in the chemotherapy of tuberculosis and leprosy. *In* Goodman Gilman, A., Goodman, L.S., and Giulman, A. (eds.): The Pharmacologic Basis of Therapeutics. 6th ed. New York. Macmillan, 1980.
176. Katz, S.I., Hertz, K.C., Crawford, P.S., Gazze, L.A., Frank, M.M., and Lawley, T.J.: Effect of sulfones on complement deposition in dermatitis herpetiformis and on complement-mediated guinea pig reactions. J. Invest. Dermatol. 67:688, 1976.
177. Stiehm, E.R., Kronenberg, L.H., Rosenblatt, H.M., Bryson, Y., and Merigan, T.C.: Interferon: immunobiology and clinical significance. Ann. Intern. Med. 96:80, 1982.
178. Bloom, B.R.: Interferons and the immune system. Nature 284:593, 1980.
179. Steward, W.E. II, Blalock, J.E., Burke, D.C., et al.: Interferon nomenclature. J. Immunol. 125:2353, 1980.

# Chapter 56
# Antihyperuricemic Drugs

*William N. Kelley and Edward W. Holmes*

A large number of drugs are capable of reducing the serum urate concentration in hyperuricemic subjects. These antihyperuricemic agents may be classified into one of several general categories: those that enhance uric acid excretion and those that inhibit xanthine oxidase and thus uric acid synthesis.

## URICOSURIC DRUGS

Many drugs with diverse chemical structures and pharmacologic properties decrease the serum urate concentration in man by enhancing the renal excretion of uric acid.[1-43] These compounds are listed in Table 56–1. At present, probenecid (Fig. 56–1) and sulfinpyrazone (Fig. 56–2) are most widely employed for this purpose in the United States. In Europe benzbromarone and zoxazolamine are used as well; the former agent may be available in the United States in the future.

**Mechanism of Action.** The uricosuric effect of a drug could be due to an increase in the quantity of urate filtered at the glomerulus, an inhibition of reabsorption of urate in the tubule, or an enhancement of its secretion by the tubule (see Chapter 21).

*Effect on Urate Filtration.* Drugs could increase the quantity of urate filtered by raising the glomerular filtration rate, the plasma concentration of free urate, or both. The former mechanism has not been demonstrated, but the latter may apply in some situations.[44-46] Several agents with uricosuric effects in man, including sulfinpyrazone, probenecid, salicylates, phenylbutazone, sulfaethylthiadiazole, diflumidone, W 2354, and halofenate, have been shown to reduce the binding of urate to albumin in vitro.[18,44,45] Displacement of urate from plasma proteins in vivo could theoretically increase the filtered load of free urate and thus could account for at least part of the uricosuric effect of these drugs.

**Table 56–1.** Drugs Shown to Be Uricosuric in Man

| | |
|---|---|
| Acetohexamide[1]* | Halofenate (MK 185)[25] |
| ACTH[2] | Iodopyracet[26,27] |
| Ascorbic acid[3] | Iopanoic acid[11,12] |
| Azapropazone[4] | Meclofenamic acid[28] |
| Azauridine[5] | Meglumine iodipamide[11] |
| Benzbromarone[6,7] | Mersalyl[29] |
| Benziodarone[8,9] | Metiazininic acid[30] |
| Calcitonin[10] | Niridazole[31,32] |
| Calcium ipodate[11,12] | Orotic acid[5] |
| Carinamide[13] | Outdated tetracyclines[33] |
| Chlorprothixene[14] | Phenolsulfonphthalein[26] |
| Cinchophen[15] | Phenylbutazone[34] |
| Citrate[16] | Phenylindandione[20] |
| Dicumarol[17] | Phenoxyisobutyric acid[35] |
| Diflumidone[18] | Probenecid and metabolites[36,37] |
| Estrogens[19] | Salicylates[38] |
| Ethyl biscoumacetate[20] | Sodium diatrizoate[12] |
| Ethyl p-chlorophenoxyiso-butyric acid[21] | Sulfaethylthiadiazole[18] |
| Glyceryl guaiacholate[22] | Sulfinpyrazone[39] |
| Glycine[23] | Ticrynafen[24,40,41] |
| Glycopyrrolate[24] | W 2354 (5-chlorosalicylic acid)[18] |
| | Zoxazolamine[43] |

*Superscript numbers indicate references.

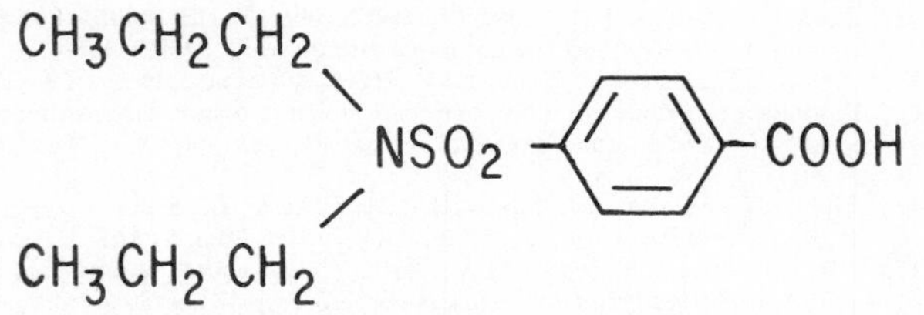


**Figure 56–1.** Structure of probenecid.

While there is indirect evidence that salicylates could displace bound urate in vivo,[47] the amount of urate actually bound to plasma proteins in vivo appears to be negligible.[48] Thus, any effect of drugs on the quantity of urate filtered, based on displacement from plasma proteins, must also probably be small.

***Effect on Uric Acid Reabsorption.*** The uricosuric effect of most agents studied, including probenecid[49] and sulfinpyrazone,[49] has been attributed to inhibition of the tubular reabsorption of filtered urate. With several exceptions, drugs with a significant uricosuric effect in man[49] are, like uric acid itself, weak organic acids. Since tubular reabsorption of uric acid is thought to occur by a process common to many organic acids, it has been assumed that these drugs inhibit this process in a competitive manner. Steele and Rieselbach[50] have postulated two types of urate reabsorptive sites in the proximal tubule, only one of which is sensitive to inhibition by probenecid.[51] Probenecid secretion is required for its uricosuric effect.[52] This and other evidence[53] have suggested that probenecid and probably most other uricosuric agents inhibit reabsorption at a site in the nephron distal to the site responsible for secretion of organic acids such as uric acid and probenecid. The suggestion is that of the two reabsorptive sites that exist for uric acid, one is proximal to and the other is distal to uric acid secretion; only the latter is inhibited by probenecid.

Five drugs that are not organic acids have been shown to have uricosuric effects in man. Studies with two of these agents, outdated tetracycline[33] and chlorprothixene,[54] suggest that they may inhibit the reabsorption of uric acid in the proximal tubule in a nonspecific manner that also affects the reabsorption of other compounds in this segment of the nephron. Glycopyrrolate may exert its uricosuric effect by virtue of its anticholinergic properties.[24] The mechanisms of action of zoxazolamine and niridazole, the final agents in this group, have not been established.

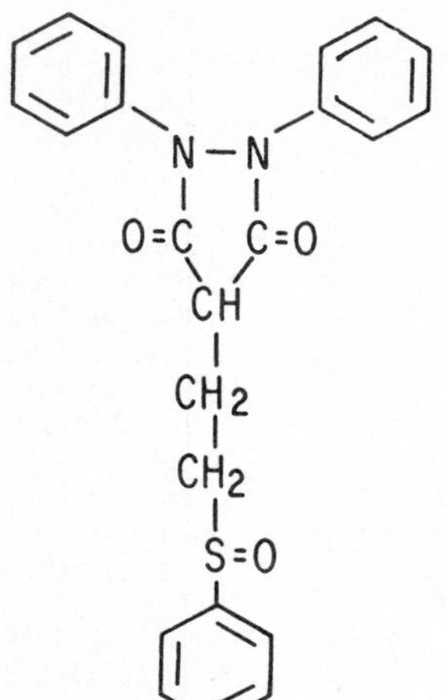


**Figure 56–2.** Structure of sulfinpyrazone.

***Effect on Uric Acid Secretion.*** The uricosuric effects of several drugs, including glycine,[23] benziodarone,[55] azapropazone,[3] and the radiographic contrast agents,[12] have been attributed to enhanced tubular secretion of urate. This hypothesis was based on the finding that prior administration of pyrazinamide (PZA) partially or completely blocked the uricosuric effects of these drugs. At the time these studies were done, urate secretion was thought to occur beyond all urate reabsorptive sites in the proximal renal tubules. With the recognition that substantial reabsorption of uric acid also occurs at a postsecretory site,[53] it became clear that the effect of PZA had been misinterpreted and that the uricosuric action of these drugs, as with most others, could also be assigned to inhibition of uric acid reabsorption at a postsecretory site.[53] In fact, animal studies indicate that a number of uricosuric drugs, including probenecid, actually inhibit uric acid secretion as well as uric acid reabsorption. The predominance of evidence at this time favors the conclusion that uricosuric agents increase the renal clearance of uric acid by decreasing uric acid reabsorption in the proximal nephron.

**Probenecid.** ***Biological Effects.*** Probenecid, p-(di-n-propylsulfamyl) benzoic acid (Fig. 56–1), was originally developed as a drug more potent than carinamide in sustaining high blood levels of penicillin by interfering with the renal tubular secretion of the antibiotic. Both carinamide and probenecid were found to increase uric acid excretion in man and to lower serum urate levels.[13,36,37] The value of probenecid in the control of hyperuricemia was demonstrated in 1950 by Talbott and associates[37] and by Gutman.[36] Probenecid soon came to enjoy wide acceptance in the treatment of gout. As the first well-tolerated agent found to be consistently effective in lowering the serum urate concentration in gout, probenecid inaugurated the modern era in therapy that has made control of tophaceous disease an achievable goal.

The increase in uric acid clearance brought about by probenecid may be substantial, but rejection of filtered urate is never complete. Even with large doses and high plasma levels of probenecid the clearance of uric acid does not exceed 50 percent of filtered urate.[48,56]

Uricosuria in response to administration of probenecid is effectively countermanded by salicylates in low doses.[57] The physiologic mechanism of this effect is not established but may involve inhibition of secretion of urate at sites proximal to the probenecid-sensitive reabsorption sites. Curiously, salicylates do not block the probenecid-mediated renal retention of penicillin.[58]

***Pharmacokinetics.*** Probenecid is readily absorbed in the gastrointestinal tract. The half-life of probenecid in plasma is dose dependent,[56] and ranges from 6 to 12 hours. This is prolonged by the concomitant administration of allopurinol.[59] Probenecid is extensively bound to plasma proteins (89 to 94 percent of drug) and is largely confined to the extracellular fluid. The maintenance dose of probenecid ranges from 500 mg per day to 3 grams per day given in three or four divided doses.[60]

*Metabolism.* Probenecid is rapidly metabolized in vivo as shown by recovery in the urine of less than 5 percent of the administered dose within 24 hours. The major urinary metabolite, probenecid acyl monoglucuronide, accounts for 41 percent of the administered compound within 48 hours. The remainder of the metabolites result from oxidative attack on the n-propyl side chain;[56,61,62] these side chain metabolites possess uricosuric activity in animals.[63]

*Other Effects.* Probenecid has a number of other effects that could be of physiologic significance. Probenecid blocks the transport of serotonin and dopamine out of the cerebrospinal fluid. An increase in the concentration of 5-hydroxyindoleacetic acid and homovanillic acid is observed in cerebrospinal fluid obtained from patients being treated with probenecid,[64-66] but this increase is less marked in patients with Down's syndrome.[67] In addition, probenecid reduces the renal excretion of pantothenic acid,[68,69] androsterone,[70] ACTH,[71] and diiodotyrosine[72] and may produce a modest salt and water diuresis in some persons.[73] Although probenecid may reduce the elevated serum phosphorus concentration in patients with hypoparathyroidism,[74-76] it appears to have no effect on serum phosphorus, amino acid excretion,[61,77] or glucose excretion[61] in normal subjects. This drug also inhibits the conjugation of benzoic acid derivatives with glycine by an unknown mechanism.[78] Finally, probenecid reduces the uptake and degradation of cAMP in kidney cortex and liver of the rat.[79]

*Interaction with Other Drugs.* Probenecid influences the renal excretion, volume of distribution, and hepatic uptake of a number of drugs.[61] These effects are summarized in Table 56–2. Because of these interactions certain drugs should be used with caution in patients receiving probenecid. Dapsone[91] and indomethacin,[92] for example, should be used at a lower dose in patients receiving probenecid. Not only does probenecid delay the renal excretion of salicylic acid and many of its glucuronide derivatives, but acetylsalicylate completely blocks the uricosuric effect of probenecid and most other uricosuric agents. Diuretics on the other hand do not abrogate the uricosuric effect of probenecid. Subtherapeutic doses of heparin may have a profound anticoagulant effect in patients receiving probenecid.[101]

The effect of probenecid on the metabolism of some drugs has been used to good advantage. Probenecid has been used, for example, to enhance the blood levels of ampicillin and penicillin.[94,95] In addition, the prolonged half-life of rifampin[100] and cephradine[97] in the presence of probenecid may be therapeutically useful. Probenecid reduces the volume of distribution of several antibiotics, including ampicillin, ancillin, nafcillin, and cephaloridine;[97] should the concentration of these antibiotics be significantly reduced in certain body fluids or spaces in the presence of probenecid, the net effect could be detrimental. Probenecid has no effect on the elimination of blood levels of gentamicin,[103] sulfonamides, streptomycin, chloramphenicol, or tetracyclines.[83]

**Table 56–2.** Effects of Probenecid on Metabolism of Other Drugs

| |
|---|
| Decreased renal excretion |
| p-Aminohippuric acid[60] |
| Phenolsulfonphthalein[80-85] |
| Salicylic acid and its acyl and phenolic glucuronides[86-89] |
| Phlorizin and its glucuronide[90] |
| Acetazolamide[88] |
| Dapsone and its metabolites[91] |
| Sulfinpyrazone and its parahydroxyl metabolite[92] |
| Indomethacin[93] |
| Ampicillin[94] |
| Penicillin[95] |
| Cephradine[96] |
| Reduced volume of distribution |
| Ampicillin[97] |
| Ancillin[97] |
| Nafcillin[97] |
| Cephaloridine[97] |
| Impairment of hepatic uptake |
| Bromsulfonphthalein[98] |
| Indocyanin green[99] |
| Rifampcin[100] |
| Delayed metabolism |
| Heparin[101] |

**Clinical Use.** Probenecid should be given in two or three evenly spaced doses. The initial dose should be low, 0.25 gram (half a tablet) every 12 hours, so as to avoid sudden diuresis of large quantities of uric acid, and thus the risk of crystalluria and ureteral blockade. Fluids should be forced in order to prevent formation of concentrated urine, especially during the late hours of the night. After 3 or 4 days the dose of probenecid is increased to 0.5 gram every 12 hours. The serum urate concentration is checked at weekly intervals, and adjustments in dosage are made every 1 to 2 weeks, increasing the daily dose by 0.5 gram each time, until satisfactory control is achieved.

The largest critical experience in the use of probenecid is that of Gutman and Yu.[60,104,105] They found a dose of 1.0 gram per day to be most appropriate in about 50 percent of cases; 0.5 gram per day elicited the desired response in 10 percent of cases; 1.5 to 2.0 grams was required in 25 percent; and 2.5 to 3.0 grams in 15 percent.

In spite of careful management a significant percentage of patients are not brought under satisfactory control with probenecid. In one large clinic[60] 27 percent of patients receiving probenecid failed to achieve serum urate levels of less than 7 mg per 100 ml. In another series of patients[106] only half achieved serum urate levels of 6 mg per 100 ml. Leading causes of failure were poor patient compliance, drug intolerance, salicylate ingestion, and renal impairment. As a general rule, patients with glomerular filtration rates of 80 ml per minute or less are not likely to have an adequate response to a uricosuric drug, and patients with this degree of renal impairment are probably candidates for allopurinol therapy.

*Complications. Acute Gout.* A potential complication of all forms of antihyperuricemic drug therapy is the precipitation of an attack of acute gouty arthritis during the initial days or weeks of therapy, at a time when serum urate levels are being lowered. This complication occurs in 10[60,107] to 20[108] percent of patients started on probenecid alone. The incidence can be greatly reduced by concomitant administration of colchicine or indomethacin.

*Nephrolithiasis.* A complication of uricosuric drug therapy that is largely preventable is urinary uric acid crystal or stone formation. Initiation of uricosuric drug therapy leads to a transient increase in uric acid excretion. In some patients, particularly those with normal renal function who are overproducers of uric acid, who are given a full therapeutic dose of probenecid, there may be a very brisk and pronounced uricosuria. Since uric acid is relatively insoluble, especially in acid urine, this sudden increase in uric acid excretion can lead to the precipitation of uric acid crystals in the collecting ducts of the kidney or ureters. A more common complication is the development of uric acid stones. This complication was recorded in 9 percent of the patients treated by Gutman and Yu.[60] Uric acid precipitation with initiation of uricosuric therapy is unusual in the normal producer of uric acid.

In some patients at especially high risk of developing nephrolithiasis it may be advisable to alkalinize the urine, in addition to forcing fluids, in order to reduce the likelihood of uric acid stone formation. In these patients the pH of the urine should be raised 6.5 or above by ingestion of 2 to 6 grams per day of sodium bicarbonate or 20 to 60 ml per day of Shohl's solution (citric acid-sodium citrate) during the first days or weeks of therapy. These values may be difficult to achieve, as gouty subjects tend to produce acid urines. Alkalinization during the night may be achieved with a single 250-mg tablet of acetazolamide taken at bedtime. When hyperuricemia has been controlled and the urinary uric acid has returned toward normal, the special precautions regarding urinary uric acid stones are rarely necessary.

*Toxicity.* The frequency of side effects of probenecid in 2502 patients receiving the drug for periods ranging from 1 day to 4 years was tabulated by Boger and Strickland[109] in 1955. Most of the patients had been on probenecid for only a few days to a few months. The series represented reports compiled from many sources and included patients given probenecid in order to enhance penicillin blood levels. They reported hypersensitivity reactions in 0.3 percent, drug fever in 0.4 percent, skin rash in 1.35 percent, and gastrointestinal disturbances in 3.1 percent. In two longer-term studies involving direct observations of gouty patients, Gutman and Yu[60] found an 8 percent incidence of gastrointestinal complaints, and a 5 percent incidence of hypersensitivity and rash among 169 patients, whereas de Seze and associates[108] noted an 18 percent incidence of gastrointestinal complaints among 156 patients.

Serious toxicity of probenecid is rare. Hepatic necrosis has been reported in one patient[110] and the nephrotic syndrome in at least two.[111,112] One patient who took a massive overdose of probenecid (42.5 grams) in a suicide attempt developed seizures but had no apparent long-term sequelae.

In Talbott's[113] experience, only 2 percent of patients permanently discontinued probenecid because of side effects. In the clinic of Gutman and Yu[104,114] about 12 percent did so. However, in the experience of de Seze and colleagues[108,115] and Kuzell and colleagues[116] about one third of patients eventually became intolerant of probenecid and discontinued its use.

**Sulfinpyrazone.** ***Biological Effects.*** The uricosuric properties of phenylbutazone are attributable to one of its metabolites. Sulfinpyrazone is a derivative of that metabolite, and is one of the most potent uricosuric agents known (Fig. 56–2). It has no antiinflammatory properties.

*Pharmacokinetics.* Sulfinpyrazone is rapidly and completely adsorbed from the gastrointestinal tract with a peak concentration in the serum 1 hour after its oral administration. The half-life in serum is 1 to 3 hours.[39,117] At a serum concentration of 10 mg per 100 ml, 98 percent of the drug is bound to plasma proteins. As a result, sulfinpyrazone, like probenecid, is largely confined to the extracellular fluid.[117,118] Some 20 to 45 percent of the drug is excreted unchanged in 24 hours, predominantly during the first 6 hours.[39,118] Most of the drug is excreted in the urine as the parahydroxyl metabolite, which is also uricosuric in man.

A dose of sulfinpyrazone of 35 mg has a uricosuric effect comparable to 100 mg of probenecid,[39] and 400 mg per day has an effect similar to that observed with 1.5 to 2.0 grams of probenecid per day.[119] Hence, sulfinpyrazone is three to six times more potent than probenecid on a weight basis.[56]

*Other Effects.* It is not known whether sulfinpyrazone has all the effects on transport, excretion, or metabolism of endogenous substances as described for probenecid. Sulfinpyrazone does suppress the excretion of PAH[39] and phenolsulfonphthalein.[120]

One action of sulfinpyrazone of potential therapeutic significance is the reduction in platelet function observed following its administration. As a result, sulfinpyrazone decreases thrombosis in arteriovenous shunts[121] and prolongs platelet survival in patients with prosthetic heart valves, rheumatic heart disease, and recurrent venous thrombosis.[122,123] This effect of sulfinpyrazone on platelet function can be demonstrated in vitro and appears to be unrelated to its antihyperuricemic effect. This antiplatelet effect of sulfinpyrazone has been attributed to inhibition of prostaglandin synthesis in the platelet.[124]

*Clinical Use.* Sulfinpyrazone is given in initial doses of 50 mg (half a tablet) twice daily for 3 or 4 days, and then in doses of 100 mg twice daily, increasing the daily dose by 100-mg increments each week, until the serum urate concentration is in the desired range. The precautions of high fluid intake and alkalinization of urine discussed with use of probenecid apply even more critically in the case of sulfinpyrazone because of its potency and prompt action.

The usual maintenance dose ranges from 300 to 400 mg per day in three or four equally divided doses, although a maximal effect is frequently not reached until a dose of 800 mg per day is administered. Sulfinpyrazone has an additional uricosuric effect in subjects receiving the maximal effective dose of probenecid,[125] apparently because probenecid inhibits the tubular secretion of sulfinpyrazone and thus prolongs its uricosuric action.[92]

An extensive clinical experience[76,92,118,126,127] attests to the usefulness of sulfinpyrazone. Tolerance for sulfinpyrazone is somewhat better than for probenecid.[76,126] Nevertheless, according to Kuzell and associates[116] almost one quarter of patients stop the drug for one reason or another. Leading causes of failure of control, as with probenecid, are concomitant salicylate ingestion and renal insufficiency.

***Toxicity.*** The incidence of gastrointestinal symptoms (10 to 15 percent) is roughly the same as that observed with probenecid.[115,116,119,126] In addition, the potential occurrence of uric acid stones after initiation of therapy with sulfinpyrazone represents a significant complication for the reasons discussed earlier with probenecid. Sulfinpyrazone appears to produce a higher incidence of bone marrow changes than probenecid.[76,119,127]

**Benziodarone and Benzbromarone.** Benziodarone[8,9,128,129] and benzbromarone[6,130-132] are potent uricosuric agents in man. Both agents inhibit the tubular reabsorption of uric acid.[133] The drugs differ in that benziodarone contains iodine whereas benzbromarone contains bromide (Fig. 56–3). The former compound has found limited clinical use, in part because of its effect on thyroid function.[134] The latter drug has been well tolerated for periods up to 6 years.[135]

In 50 gouty patients treated by de Gery and colleagues[135] the mean serum urate level fell from 9.2 to 4.8 mg per 100 ml, while the mean urinary uric acid excretion rose from 520 to 746 mg per day. In eight patients the serum creatinine concentration was greater than 2 mg per 100 ml. Zöllner and colleagues[136] have reported that benzbromarone is more effective than other uricosuric agents in patients with renal insufficiency.

Benziodarone

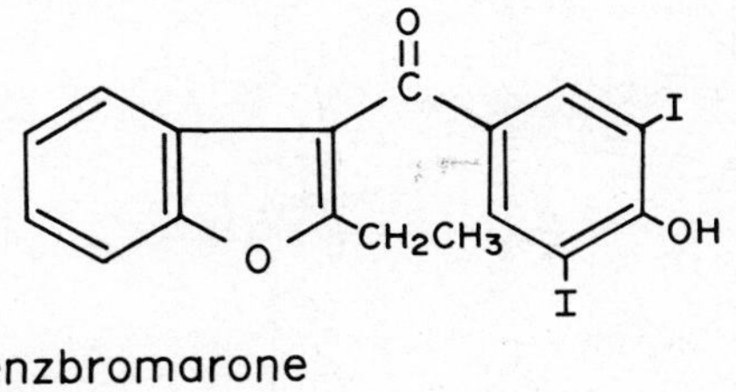


Benzbromarone

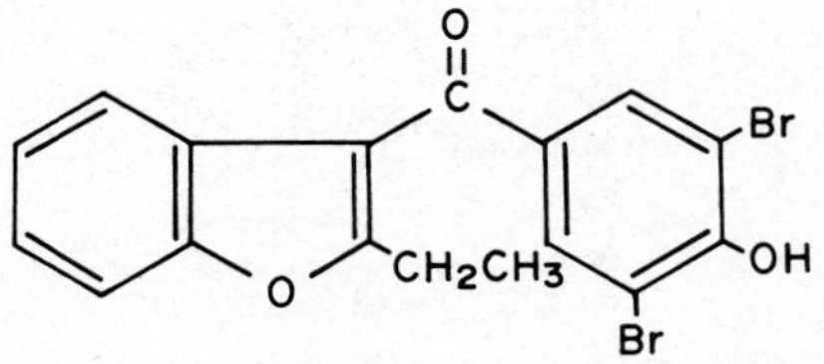


**Figure 56–3.** Structures of benziodarone and benzbromarone.

Benzbromarone is a weak inhibitor of xanthine oxidase in vitro, but its action in vivo appears to be exclusively uricosuric. In full therapeutic doses there is no increase in urinary xanthine or hypoxanthine excretion.[130,135]

## XANTHINE OXIDASE INHIBITORS

A second general approach toward controlling serum urate levels is that of regulating production of uric acid. At present, the only therapeutically effective method for decreasing uric acid formation is the inhibition of xanthine oxidase by allopurinol or its derivative oxipurinol.

The final steps in the synthesis of uric acid involve conversion of hypoxanthine to xanthine and xanthine to uric acid catalyzed by a single enzyme, xanthine oxidase. Many inhibitors of xanthine oxidase are known, including several pteridines,[137] certain substituted quinazolines,[138] and various purine analogues such as adenine and 2,6-diaminopurine,[139] 6-thiopurine,[140] symmetrical triazines,[141] and 4-diazoimidazole-5-carboxamide.[142] The pyrazolo (3,4-d) pyrimidines have also proved to be important members of this group. Pyrazolo (3,4-d) pyrimidines are purine analogues in which the positions of nitrogen-7 and carbon-8 of the purine ring are reversed (Fig. 56–4).

**Allopurinol.** Allopurinol was first synthesized for trial as a chemotherapeutic agent, but by itself had little or no effect on experimental tumors.[143,144] It was found to be an inhibitor of xanthine oxidase[145] and to block the conversion of 6-thiopurine to 6-thiouric acid in mouse and man.[146] It was first used clinically as adjunct therapy in patients receiving 6-thiopurine for leukemia.[147] Patients given allopurinol showed a pronounced reduction in both serum and urinary uric acid values.[147,148] These observations suggested a trial of the agent in gout. Allopurinol is now established as a standard form of therapy of hyperuricemia and uric acid stones.

Allopurinol [4-hydroxypyrazolo(3,4-d)pyrimidine] and its major metabolic product, oxipurinol [4,6-dihydroxypyrazolo(3,4-d)pyrimidine] are analogues of hypoxanthine and xanthine, respectively. Both are potent inhibitors of xanthine oxidase.[145,149-151] The Michaelis constant of allopurinol is some 15 to 20 times lower than that of xanthine, whereas that of oxipurinol is comparable to that of xanthine.[150] Allopurinol shows substrate-competitive kinetics. Both allopurinol and oxipurinol produce pseudoirreversible inactivation of xanthine oxidase; inactivation occurs when allopurinol and enzyme are incubated in the absence of substrate, but

Hypoxanthine

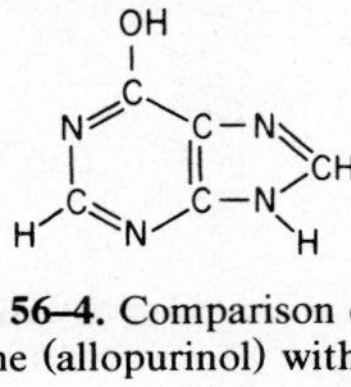


4-Hydroxypyrazolo(3,4-d)pyrimidine

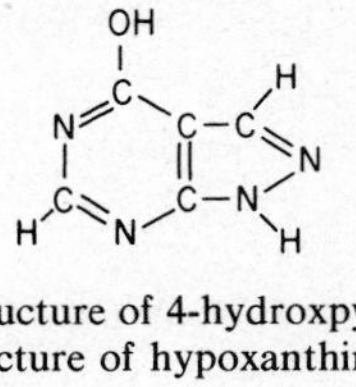


**Figure 56–4.** Comparison of structure of 4-hydroxpyrazolo(3,4-d) pyrimidine (allopurinol) with structure of hypoxanthine.

enzyme activity can be restored by prolonged dialysis. Oxipurinol has no effect on the enzyme alone, but inactivates it in the presence of xanthine when molecular oxygen is the hydrogen acceptor.[149]

***Pharmacokinetics and Metabolism.*** Allopurinol is completely absorbed in the gastrointestinal tract. It has a half-life in vivo of 39 minutes to 3 hours.[150,152,153] Since allopurinol and oxipurinol both inhibit the oxidation of allopurinol, the half-life of allopurinol increases as the level of xanthine oxidase inhibition increases. Most of the allopurinol (45 to 65 percent) is rapidly oxidized to oxipurinol in vivo with a smaller portion being converted to allopurinol-1-N-ribonucleotide[154] and allopurinol-1-N-ribonucleoside[155] (Fig. 56–5). Most of the oxipurinol formed is excreted unchanged by the kidney with a half-life of 14[153] to 28 hours.[152] Small portions are metabolized to oxipurinol-7-N-ribonucleoside and oxipurinol-1-N-ribonucleoside[156] and to the corresponding 5′-phosphoribosyl derivatives.[157,158] The pathways involved in the metabolism of allopurinol are summarized in Figure 56–5.

The renal clearance of allopurinol and oxipurinol ranges from 14 to 20 ml per minute and 23 to 31 ml per minute, respectively.[153] Factors that affect uric acid excretion generally alter oxipurinol excretion in a similar manner.[156] For example, uricosuric agents increase the renal excretion of oxipurinol and uric acid, and renal insufficiency reduces the excretion of both compounds.

Because of its prolonged half-life oxipurinol may be primarily responsible for xanthine oxidase inhibition in vivo when allopurinol is administered.[150] Although allopurinol is the more effective of the two agents when the two are compared daily, this reflects the relatively poor absorption of oxipurinol in the gastrointestinal tract.[159]

***Biological Effects (Table 56–3).*** The administration of allopurinol in man is followed by a decrease in levels of serum and urinary uric acid[160,161] and by increases in

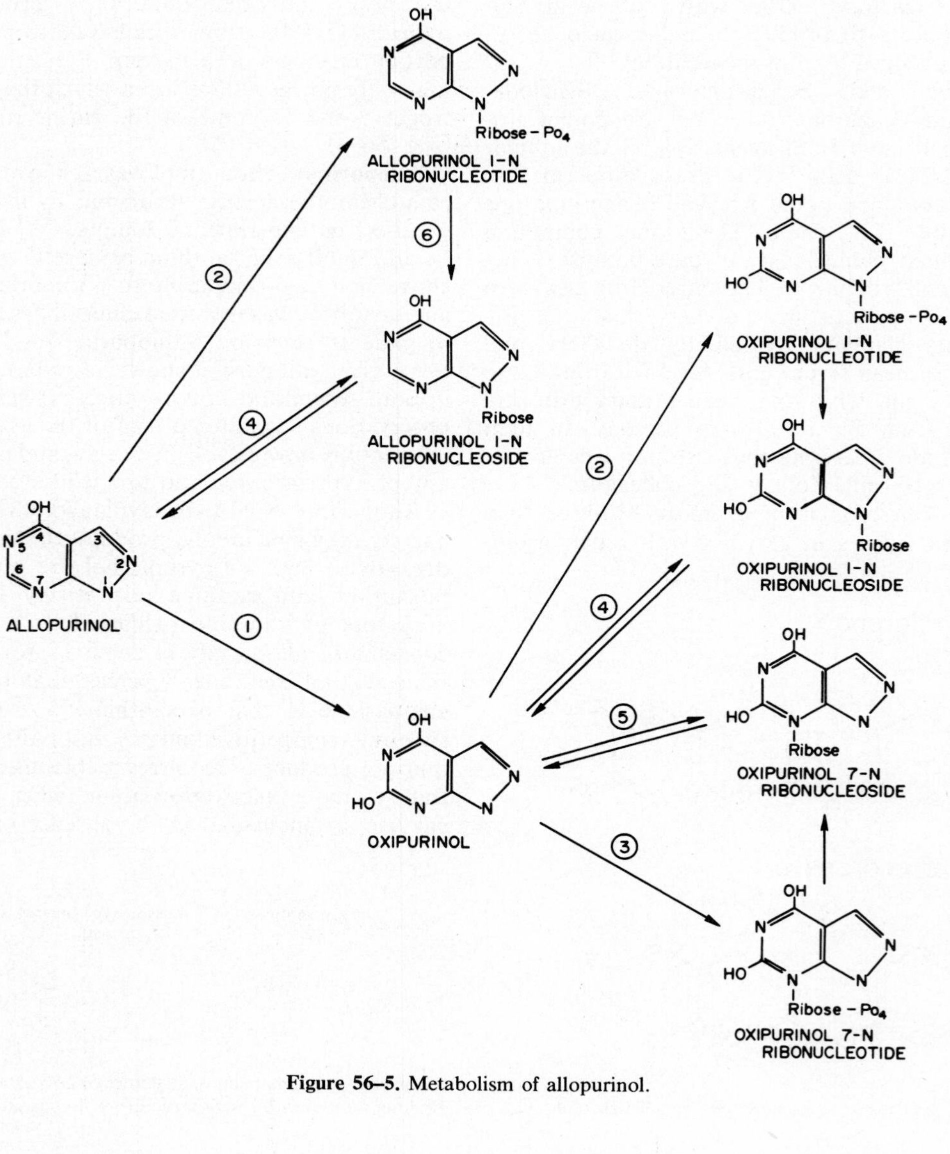


**Figure 56–5.** Metabolism of allopurinol.

**Table 56–3.** Metabolic Effects of Allopurinol

| Clinical Effect | Mechanism | Effector |
|---|---|---|
| Antihyperuricemia | Xanthine oxidase inhibition | Allopurinol<br>Oxipurinol |
| Decreased total purine production | Inhibition of amidophosphoribosyltransferase | Allopurinol-1-N-ribosylphosphate; IMP |
| | PP-ribose-P depletion | Allopurinol |
| Orotidinuria | Inhibition of orotidine-5′-phosphate decarboxylase | Oxipurinol-7-N-ribosylphosphate<br>Oxipurinol-1-N-ribosylphosphate<br>Allopurinol-1-N-ribosylphosphate |
| Orotic aciduria | Inhibition of orotate phosphoribosyltransferase | ?Orotidine-5′-phosphate |
| | PP-ribose-P depletion | Allopurinol |
| Prolongation of half-life of drugs metabolized by the microsomal-oxidizing system | Inhibition of hepatic microsomal drug-metabolizing enzymes | Unknown |
| Apparent increased activity of orotate phosphoribosyltransferase and orotidine-5′-P decarboxylase | ?Stabilization of enzymes to extraction | Unknown |

plasma and urinary concentrations of hypoxanthine and xanthine. Plasma levels reach only 0.5 to 1.0[147,162] or, rarely, 2.0 mg per 100 ml[163] because of the relatively high renal clearance of oxypurines. These oxypurine levels are well below the solubility limits of hypoxanthine or xanthine in serum.[162] Urinary increases of hypoxanthine and xanthine may reach several hundred milligrams a day, and are related to the degree of inhibition of xanthine oxidase and the level of HPRT activity.

In most patients the replacement of urinary uric acid by the oxypurines, hypoxanthine and xanthine, is less than stoichiometric.[147,161-164] The deficit ranges from 10 to 60 percent and in patients with normal HPRT activity is roughly proportional to the pretreatment level of uric acid excretion.[161-165] The total deficit may amount to several hundred milligrams of total purines (uric acid plus oxypurines) a day.[147,161,163] In addition, the reduction in total purine excretion is associated with a decreased incorporation of isotopic glycine into urinary uric acid.[166] This effect of allopurinol requires normal HPRT activity[165,167] and could be due to a combination of factors, including (1) reduction of purine biosynthesis de novo by the inhibitory effect of allopurinol ribonucleotide on amidophosphoribosyltransferase;[154] (2) reduction in purine biosynthesis de novo owing to the inhibitory action of purine ribonucleotides derived from IMP on PP-ribose-P synthetase and amidophosphoribosyltransferase;[168] and (3) depletion of PP-ribose-P,[169] an essential and limiting substrate of purine biosynthesis de novo, as a result of its enhanced consumption in the conversion of hypoxanthine and allopurinol[154] to their respective ribonucleotide derivatives.

Studies by Elion and Nelson[170] suggest that the first alternative is not important. The $K_i$ for allopurinol ribonucleotide of the pigeon liver amidophosphoribosyltransferase of 0.6 mM[154] may be taken as a first approximation of concentration required to produce significant inhibition of the human enzyme. Tissue levels of allopurinol ribonucleotide in human liver are probably less than $10^{-7}$ M, and concentrations of di- or triphosphates of allopurinol or oxipurinol are not present at the $10^{-9}$ M level. Thus, the levels of allopurinol ribonucleotide in liver are far below the concentrations needed to inhibit amidophosphoribosyltransferase effectively.

The levels of natural purine ribonucleotides[157] lie much closer to the $K_i$ values of pigeon liver[168] or human placental[171] or lymphoblast[172] enzymes. Reutilization of hypoxanthine[173] and xanthine[174] for nucleotide and nucleic acid synthesis is markedly enhanced in the intact rat when their oxidation is inhibited by allopurinol. Studies in patients are also consistent with the conclusion that there is enhanced purine salvage during allopurinol therapy.[175] The temporary increases in levels of IMP and XMP, and subsequently AMP and GMP, could increase feedback inhibition of purine biosynthesis de novo. This would be enhanced by the cooperative effect of AMP and GMP in the inhibition of amidophosphoribosyltransferase[168,171] and by a fall in PP-ribose-P levels.[169]

The administration of allopurinol leads to a substantial reduction of erythrocyte PP-ribose-P content, which occurs 3 to 5 hours after administration of the drug.[169] This effect in erythrocytes is most likely due to consumption of PP-ribose-P by the conversion of allopurinol to its ribonucleotide. It is not attributable to increased reutilization of hypoxanthine and xanthine, since PP-ribose-P levels do not fall after oxipurinol administration[169] and erythrocytes do not contain xanthine oxidase activity. This effect of allopurinol on PP-ribose-P content would be significant for purine biosynthesis only if it also occurs in tissues such as liver that actively synthesize purines de novo. This has not yet been demonstrated.

The administration of either allopurinol or oxipurinol in man is accompanied by a substantial increase in the excretion of orotidine and orotic acid.[176,177] Studies in vivo and in cell culture show that this results from inhibition of orotidine-5′-phosphate decarboxylase, which catalyzes a step in the conversion of orotic acid to uridine 5′-monophosphate (UMP). Inhibition of orotidine-5′-phosphate decarboxylase in vivo is not dependent on the presence of HPRT activity and therefore cannot be completely attributed to the formation of allopurinol-1-N-ribonucleotide, oxipurinol-1-N-ribonucleotide, or xanthosine-5′-monophosphate, each of which is a potent inhibitor of orotidine-5′-phosphate decarboxylase in vitro.[177,178] In HPRT-deficient cells, the inhibitory effect of these compounds on pyrimidine biosynthesis appears to involve formation of derivatives that are analogues of orotidine-5′-phosphate,[179,180] whose formation is catalyzed by orotate phosphoribosyltransferase.[158] In HPRT-competent cells it seems likely that the inhibition of orotidine-5′-phosphate decarboxylase is due primarily to both 1- and 7-N-ribonucleotide derivatives of oxipurinol.

The consequence of this allopurinol-mediated inhibition of pyrimidine biosynthesis remains to be defined in man. The administration of allopurinol to rats is associated with a transient decrease in UMP and UDP pools in the liver, whereas UTP levels are elevated; no change is observed in the level of uridine nucleotides in the kidney.[157] These studies suggest that, at least in the rat, any reduction of intracellular pyrimidine nucleotides resulting from the inhibition of pyrimidine biosynthesis de novo is rapidly corrected, presumably by an enhanced salvage of uridine resulting from nucleotide catabolism, through its reconversion to UMP.

The administration of allopurinol also leads to an apparent eightfold increase in the activity of orotate phosphoribosyltransferase and orotidine-5′-phosphate decarboxylase in circulating erythrocytes.[181-183] The increase can usually be demonstrated within 1 week of allopurinol therapy, and the activity appears to level off after 3 to 6 weeks. The mechanism responsible for this is complicated and poorly understood. The ribonucleotide derivatives of both allopurinol and oxipurinol are capable of shifting the configuration of the complex of orotate phosphoribosyltransferase and orotidine-5′-phosphate decarboxylase to a larger, more stable molecular species.[182] Most of the data currently available are consistent with the hypothesis that the apparent increase in enzyme activity is due to stabilization of the enzyme complex to the extraction procedure. Irrespective of mechanism, this change in enzyme activity during allopurinol therapy appears to be of little clinical consequence. These metabolic effects of allopurinol are summarized in Table 56–3.

Allopurinol also has a number of other metabolic effects that have been demonstrated in vitro or in lower animals. Through its action on xanthine oxidase it inhibits tryptophan pyrrolase,[184,185] probably by limiting the availability of $H_2O_2$ to the latter enzyme.[186,187] Allopurinol also inhibits purine nucleoside phosphorylase[155,188] and pyrimidine deoxyribosyltransferase[189] in vitro. It activates, and at higher concentration inhibits, urate oxidase.[190] Allopurinol does not inhibit liver aldehyde oxidase, an enzyme with substrates very similar to those of xanthine oxidase.[191]

Allopurinol and oxipurinol administration are not associated with visible changes in chromosome structure.[192]

*Interaction with Other Drugs.* There are potentially important drug-drug interactions involving allopurinol that deserve comment. The biological activities of purine analogues such as 6-mercaptopurine, azathioprine and hypoxanthine arabinoside, the major metabolic product of adenine arabinoside, which are inactivated by xanthine oxidase, are potentiated by the xanthine oxidase inhibition associated with allopurinol administration.[146,193] The toxicity of other cytotoxic agents such as cyclophosphamide also appears to be enhanced by the concomitant administration of allopurinol, although the mechanism is unclear. In addition, allopurinol has an inhibitory effect on the hepatic microsomal drug-metabolizing enzymes.[195] Thus, drugs such as antipyrine and bishydroxycoumarin, which are metabolized by this system, should be used with caution and at a lower dose in patients receiving allopurinol. The half-life of probenecid is prolonged by about 50 percent in the presence of allopurinol.[59] This has been attributed to the inhibitory effect of allopurinol on the microsomal drug-metabolizing system. The administration of allopurinol is associated with a threefold higher incidence of ampicillin-related skin rash.[196] However, it is not clear whether this potentiation is due to allopurinol or to the presence of hyperuricemia.[196] The toxic effects of allopurinol seem to be enhanced with the concomitant administration of a thiazide diuretic.[197,198]

*Clinical Use.* The administration of allopurinol to subjects with normal renal function is followed, within 24 to 48 hours, by a decrease in serum and urinary acid values. Maximum reductions are achieved in 4 days to 2 weeks, after which values remain relatively constant over prolonged periods of time.[160,161,197] (Fig. 56–6). With the inhibition of urate production by allopurinol, increased amounts of hypoxanthine and xanthine appear in urine, usually within 4 to 6 hours. Only trivial changes occur in the excretion of other urinary purine bases.[200]

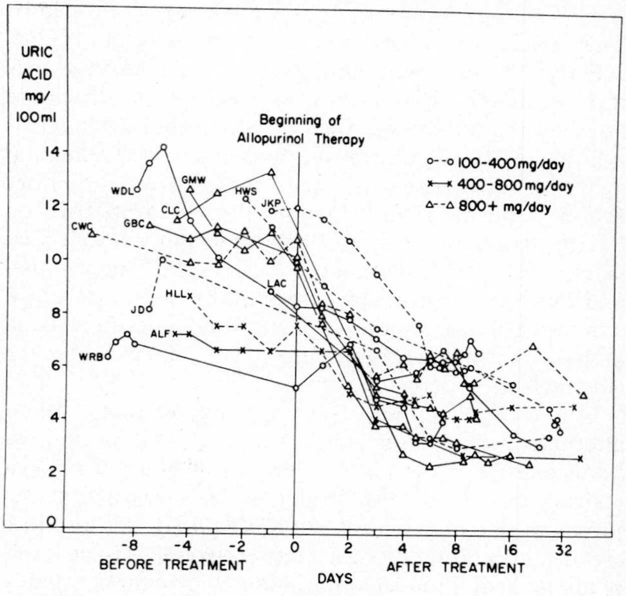


**Figure 56–6.** Effect of allopurinol on serum uric acid in 12 patients with gout.

Withdrawal of allopurinol results in a return to pretreatment serum urate levels within a few days. Occasional, more prolonged effects are associated with delayed excretion of oxipurinol.[151]

Normal serum urate values can be achieved in all but a few patients. The doses required to reduce the elevated levels to normal average 200 to 300 mg per day for patients with mild disease and 400 to 600 mg per day for those with moderately severe tophaceous disease; rarely, doses of 700 to 1000 mg per day have been required.[160] The average dose required to maintain the serum urate level between 6.0 and 6.9 mg per 100 ml in patients with normal renal function is 300 mg per day.[201] In individuals with reduced glomerular filtration rates it may be advisable to reduce the maintenance dose of allopurinol because of the prolonged half-life of oxipurinol in patients with renal failure. Table 56–4 lists suggested doses for allopurinol in patients with different glomerular filtration rates. In most patients with normal renal function allopurinol need not be initiated at a low dose. In some patients with frequent episodes of gout, however, beginning with a low dose will lessen the probability of precipitating a series of incapacitating attacks. Because of the long biological half-life of the active metabolite, oxipurinol, it is not necessary to divide the doses or to space them throughout the day. A single 300-mg tablet has been shown to be as effective as three divided doses of 100 mg each.[202] In all patients being treated with allopurinol, or any antihyperuricemic agent for that matter, the drug dosage should be adjusted to the individual's need through monitoring the serum urate concentration. The optimal end-point of antihyperuricemic therapy is to reduce the serum urate concentration to a level at which the urate concentration is no longer saturating, i.e., 7 mg per 100 ml or less.

An extensive clinical experience attests to the usefulness of allopurinol in gout. Resolution of tophi occurs gradually with maintenance of normal serum urate levels and is frequently extensive by 6 to 12 months. Destructive arthritis improves in most patients; in an occasional patient with rapid resolution of tophi, however, bony lesions will not heal, leading to telescoped digits.[203] Slower improvement can be anticipated in patients with renal insufficiency.[204] The progression of gouty nephropathy appears to halt in most patients.[163,195,202-206]

Loebl and Scott[207] noted a low incidence of recurrent gouty arthritis in 33 patients in whom allopurinol was discontinued after therapy for a mean of 2 years even though the serum urate rapidly returned to pretreatment levels. These observations suggest that after a few years of control of hyperuricemia the patient may re-enter an asymptomatic phase. Nevertheless, the current recommendation is that once antihyperuricemic therapy is instituted for firm medical indications it should be continued indefinitely if possible.

By selection of the appropriate dose of allopurinol, it is possible to reduce the serum urate level to normal or, if desired, to hold it as low as 2 or 3 mg per 100 ml indefinitely, unless renal function is markedly limited. Even then appreciable reduction of serum urate values can be achieved with allopurinol.[208-213] In patients with extensive tophaceous deposits it may not be possible to reduce the serum urate level to as low as 2 to 3 mg per 100 ml because of the ongoing resorption of preformed urate from the tophi, but the serum urate concentration can usually be lowered to nonsaturating levels, with a resultant decrease in the frequency of gouty attacks and eventual resorption of the tophi.

Uricosuric agents may be used concurrently with allopurinol to hasten mobilization of urate deposits.[161,199] Combined therapy may be particularly effective in the patient with extensive tophaceous deposits (and good renal function), in whom substantial amounts of preformed urate must be eliminated. The administration of a uricosuric agent to a patient receiving allopurinol usually results in appreciable increases of urinary uric acid excretion and a further decline in serum urate level.[161,199] Allopurinol lengthens the biologic half-life of probenecid and thus potentiates its uricosuric effect.[59] On the other hand, uricosuric drugs increase the clearance of oxipurinol in man[150,156] and thus diminish the degree of xanthine oxidase inhibition. They cause either no change or a decrease in excretion of oxypurines in patients receiving allopurinol.[156] Goldfinger and associates[214] cite evidence that hypoxanthine and xanthine are excreted by the renal tubules in man and that this process is inhibited by uricosuric agents. One would anticipate that plasma oxypurine levels would be further elevated upon addition of a uricosuric agent, but they have not been measured in this situation. The net effect of these drug interactions suggests that lower than usual doses of probenecid and greater than usual doses of allopurinol would be indicated when the drugs are used concurrently. Clinically, however, the drugs are tolerated so well that both can be used together without altering the usual dosages of either.

***Complications.*** *Acute Attacks of Gout.* Most investigators have found the frequency of gouty attacks relatively high on initiation of therapy.[163] Typical attacks have occurred with serum urate levels as low as 2 mg per 100 ml and comparably low urinary urate excretions. Daily colchicine should be given during at least the first 6 to 12 months of therapy of gout with allopurinol in order to minimize the likelihood of recurrent acute attacks.

*Xanthine Renal Stones.* More than half of the urinary oxypurine increase observed with allopurinol consists of xanthine,[200] a sparingly soluble compound.[162] The levels

**Table 56–4.** Recommended Maintenance Dose of Allopurinol Based on the Glomerular Filtration Rate

| GFR (ml/min) | Dose (mg) |
|---|---|
| 100 | 300 |
| 80 | 250 |
| 60 | 200 |
| 40 | 150 |
| 20 | 100 |
| 10 | 100 every 2 days |
| 0 | 100 every 3 days |

attained with full doses of allopurinol equal those that in xanthinuric subjects (who lack xanthine oxidase activity as an inborn error of metabolism) have caused formation of urinary calculi composed of xanthine. Thus far, development of xanthine crystalluria or lithiasis as a complication of allopurinol therapy has been observed in only one patient given the drug for treatment of gout or uric acid stones.[215] This patient had a partial deficiency of HPRT.

Four instances of xanthine stone formation induced by allopurinol therapy have been reported in other circumstances. Two occurred in children with the Lesch-Nyhan syndrome[216,217] and a third in an adult patient with lymphosarcoma.[218] These three patients excreted approximately 1500 mg of uric acid a day prior to allopurinol therapy; one child, who received allopurinol at a dose of 9 mg per kilogram, excreted as much as 800 mg of xanthine a day while on therapy.[216,219] The fourth case occurred in a 9-year-old American boy with Burkitt's lymphoma, who was given 600 mg of allopurinol a day. He excreted 1976 mg of oxypurines, 240 to 950 mg of orotic acid, and 640 to 1530 mg of orotidine daily in the urine, and passed many crystals identified as xanthine.[220] Allopurinol should be given cautiously and in minimal doses to patients with extraordinarily great uric acid excretion values, particularly those with an inability to reutilize hypoxanthine and xanthine because of HPRT deficiency.

*Oxipurinol Crystal Deposition.* Watts and associates[221] have demonstrated microcrystalline deposits of oxipurinol as well as of hypoxanthine and xanthine in muscle biopsy specimens of patients receiving allopurinol for treatment of gout. There are no recognizable clinical consequences of this phenomenon. The concentration of hypoxanthine and xanthine in muscle is considerably less than observed in patients congenitally deficient in xanthine oxidase.[222]

Formation of oxipurinol sludge and stones in the urinary tract has been reported in an 8-year-old boy given both allopurinol and oxipurinol orally in doses of 15 and 37.5 mg per kilogram, respectively.[223] Surgical intervention was required because of urinary tract obstruction. Both sludge and stones showed infrared spectra virtually the same as authentic oxipurinol, and unlike the spectra of allopurinol and uric acid. In addition, a 33-year-old woman with regional enteritis and recurrent uric acid nephrolithiasis who was treated with 600 mg per day of allopurinol developed many small, soft, yellow stones, which were identified as oxipurinol by liquid and gas chromatograph/mass spectrophotometric techniques.[224]

***Toxicity.*** Serious toxicity of allopurinol therapy appears to have been unusual during its initial decade of use. A small percentage of patients (perhaps 5 percent) find it necessary to discontinue the drug.[59] Allopurinol may lead to the development of gastrointestinal intolerance,[206] skin rashes, sometimes with fever,[204] occasionally toxic epidermal necrolysis,[225,226] alopecia,[227] bone marrow suppression with leukopenia and thrombocytopenia,[227] agranulocytosis,[228,229] granulomatous hepatitis,[230,231] severe jaundice,[232] sarcoidlike reaction,[233] and vasculitis.[234,235] The incidence of side effects of all kinds may be about 20 percent.

Toxic effects tend to occur more often in the presence of renal insufficiency and with thiazide therapy. A series of reports over the last 12 years have described a constellation of findings, including fever, skin rash, progressive renal insufficiency, eosinophilia, and hepatitis, in patients experiencing toxic reactions to allopurinol, and some authors have referred to this as an allopurinol hypersensitivity syndrome. In a group of 78 patients with this putative syndrome the following abnormalities were noted: skin rash, 92 percent; fever, 87 percent; worsening renal function, 85 percent; eosinophilia, 73 percent; hepatitis, 68 percent; and leukocytosis, 39 percent.[236] Twenty-one percent of these patients died. Diffuse vasculitis involving multiple organ systems was noted in a number of cases at post-mortem examination. The median dose of allopurinol was 300 mg per day, and the mean duration of therapy was 3 weeks (range of 1 to 30 weeks). Prior renal insufficiency was recorded in 81 percent of these patients, and 49 percent received concomitant diuretic therapy, leading some authors to postulate that pre-existing renal disease and thiazides might be predisposing factors to this syndrome.[236] While the incidence of this type of severe allergic reaction is not known, it is probably quite rare. However, the potential severity of this disorder emphasizes the need for restricting allopurinol therapy to those hyperuricemic patients who have specific indications for antihyperuricemic therapy as well as the need to reduce the dose of allopurinol in patients with renal insufficiency (Table 56–4) (see Chapter 86).

Skin rashes are more frequent and serious in patients receiving allopurinol and ampicillin. In the Boston Collaborative Drug Surveillance Program,[196] 2.1 percent of 283 patients receiving allopurinol without ampicillin, 7.5 percent of 1257 patients receiving only ampicillin, and 22.4 percent of 67 hospitalized patients receiving allopurinol and ampicillin experienced drug rashes. Although it could not be determined whether the threefold greater risk of drug rash in patients taking ampicillin plus allopurinol was associated with allopurinol or hyperuricemia, it would be prudent not to prescribe these two drugs together.

The occurrence of skin rash in a patient receiving allopurinol does not necessarily require that the drug be discontinued. The rash of allopurinol often involves the hands and feet alone, or at least chiefly. There may be swelling and intense itching, and the body and face may be involved. Provided there is no laryngeal edema, it may suffice to administer large doses of Benadryl or other antihistaminic agent to control the itching. A minimal amount of swelling of the hands and feet is often then well tolerated. After a few weeks, it may be possible to stop the antihistamine without recurrence of the rash. Reduction of the dose of allopurinol may also be helpful in reducing the severity of the skin lesions, especially in patients with renal insufficiency. Desensitization has apparently been effected in two patients allergic to allopurinol by initiating therapy with a very low dose of allopurinol (0.05 mg per day) and gradually increasing the amount given over a period of 30 days.[237,238]

**Oxipurinol.** Although the therapeutic effects of allopurinol are mediated at least in part by its metabolic product oxipurinol, whose half-life is about eightfold longer than that of allopurinol,[161] a direct comparison of the two agents given orally indicates that allopurinol is the more effective because of the relatively poor absorption of oxipurinol from the gastrointestinal tract.[164] Nevertheless, oxipurinol can be used therapeutically, and has been effectively employed in some patients who have been sensitive to allopurinol. In a study of 13 patients allergic to allopurinol, 70 percent had their hyperuricemia controlled with oxipurinol without evidence of toxicity.[239] Toxic reactions identical to those observed with allopurinol were observed in 30 percent of the patients treated with oxipurinol. Cross-sensitivity to the two drugs might be expected on the basis of their structural similarities. Oxipurinol is not marketed in the United States but is available in Europe and Japan.

## OTHER THERAPEUTIC AGENTS

**Thiopurinol.** Thiopurinol[4-thiopyrazolo(3,4-d)pyrimidine], although developed for use as a xanthine oxidase inhibitor, reduces plasma urate concentrations and uric acid excretion values without a concomitant increase in plasma oxypurine levels or in oxypurine excretion.[240,241] These effects occur in gouty patients with normal renal function and normal HGPRT activity, but thiopurinol has no effect on plasma or urinary uric acid values in patients with nearly complete deficiency of erythrocyte HGPRT activity.[242] Effects of thiopurinol have been postulated to reflect inhibition of purine biosynthesis de novo by thiopurinol ribonucleotide, although this hypothesis has not yet been documented.

**Orotic Acid.** Orotic acid in doses ranging from 2 to 6 grams per day produces a modest reduction in serum urate concentration.[243,244] This is related both to its uricosuric effect[245] and to inhibition of purine biosynthesis de novo.[243,245] Orotic acid is a normal intermediate of pyrimidine biosynthesis and reacts with PP-ribose-P to form orotidine-5′-monophosphate (OMP), a precursor of uridine and cytidine nucleotides.[246] Several studies suggest that orotic acid inhibits purine biosynthesis by competing with L-glutamine for available PP-ribose-P.[247] Following the administration of orotic acid, erythrocyte PP-ribose-P levels fall and the incorporation of isotopic glycine into urinary uric acid is reduced.[244] Although short-term therapy with orotic acid in man was not associated with the development of a fatty liver,[244] as it is in the rat,[248,249] this agent does not appear to offer any therapeutic advantage over other antihyperuricemic drugs currently in use.

**Uricase.** The infusion of highly purified uricase has been shown to bring about a transient reduction in the serum urate level.[250-253] An increased clearance of uric acid appears to contribute to the response.[251] Use of uricase has been advocated in patients with hyperuricemia of renal origin.[254-255] Rapid development of antibodies to the enzyme is associated with diminished effectiveness.

## References


1. Yu, T-F., Berger, L., and Gutman, A.B.: Hypoglycemic and uricosuric properties of acetohexamide and hydroxyhexamide. Metabolism 17:309, 1968.
2. Friedman, M., and Byers, S.O.: Mechanism by which ACTH increases the excretion of urate. Am. J. Physiol. 163:684, 1950.
3. Stein, H.B., Hasan, A., and Fox, I.H.: Ascorbic acid-induced uricosuria: A consequence of megavitamin therapy. Ann. Intern. Med. 84:385, 1976.
4. Frank, O.: Untersuchungen zur urikosurischen Wirkung von Azapropazon. Z. Rheumaforsch. 30:368, 1971.
5. Fallon, H.D., Frei, E., Block, J., et al.: The uricosuria and orotic aciduria induced by 6-azauridine. J. Clin. Invest. 40:1906, 1961.
6. Sternon, J., Kocheleff, P., Courturier, E., et al.: Effet hypouricémiant de la benzbromarone. Étude de 24 cas. Acta Clin. Belg. 22:285, 1967.
7. Podevin, R., Paillard, F., Amiel, C., et al.: Action de la benziodarone sur l'excrétion rénale de l'acide urique. Rev. Fr. Étud. Clin. Biol. 12:361, 1967.
8. Nivet, M., Marcovici, J., Laruelle, P., et al.: Note préliminarie sur l'action d'un benzofuranne sur l'uricémie. Bull. Soc. Med. Hôp. Paris 116:118, 1965.
9. Delbarre, F., Auscher, C., and Amor, B.: Action uricosurique et antigoutteuse de certains dérivés du benzofuranne. Presse Méd. 73:2725, 1965.
10. Blahos, J., Osten, L., Mertl, J., Kotas, O., Gregor, O., and Reisenauer, R.: The uricosuric effect of calcitonin. Horm. Metab. Res. 7:445, 1975.
11. Mudge, G.H.: Uricosuric action of cholecystographic agents. N. Engl. J. Med. 284:929, 1971.
12. Postlethwaite, A.E., and Kelley, W.N.: Uricosuric effect of radiocontrast agents: A study in man of four commonly used preparations. Ann. Intern. Med. 74:845, 1971.
13. Wolfson, S.Q., Cohn, C., Levine, R., et al.: Transport and excretion of uric acid in man. III. Physiologic significance of the uricosuric effect of caronamide (abstract). Am. J. Med. 4:774, 1948.
14. Healey, L.A., Harrison, M., and Decker, J.L.: Uricosuric effect of chlorprothixene. N. Engl. J. Med. 272:526, 1965.
15. Nicolaier, A., and Dohrn, M.: Über die Wirkung von Chinolicarbonsauren und ihrer Derivate auf die Ausscheidung der Harnsäure. Dtsch. Arch. Klin. Med. 43:331, 1908.
16. Koden, W.: Citric acid therapy in uraturia. Z. Arztl. Fortbild. 58:392, 1964.
17. Hansen, O.E., and Holten, C.: Uricosuric effect of dicoumarol. Lancet 1:1047, 1958.
18. Schlosstein, L.H., Kippen, I., Whitehouse, M.W., et al.: Studies with some novel uricosuric agents and their metabolites: Correlation between clinical activity and drug-induced displacement of urate from its albumin-binding sites. J. Lab. Clin. Med. 82:412, 1973.
19. Nicholls, A., Snaith, M.L., and Scott, J.T.: Effect of estrogen therapy on plasma and urinary levels of uric acid. Br. Med. J. 1:449, 1973.
20. Sougin-Mibashan, R., and Horwitz, M.: The uricosuric action of ethyl biscoumacetate. Lancet 1:1191, 1955.
21. Oliver, M.F.: Reduction of serum-lipid and uric acid levels by an orally active androsterone. Lancet 1:1321, 1962.
22. Ramsdell, C.M., Postlethwaite, A.E., and Kelley, W.N.: Uricosuric effect of glyceryl guaiacolate. J. Rheumatol. 1:114, 1974.
23. Yu, T-F., Kaung, C., and Gutman, A.: Effect of glycine loading on plasma and urinary uric acid and amino acids in normal and gouty subjects. Am. J. Med. 49:352, 1970.
24. Postlethwaite, A.D., Ramsdell, C.M., and Kelley, W.N.: Uricosuric effect of an anticholinergic agent in hyperuricemic subjects. Arch. Intern. Med. 134:270, 1974.
25. Jain, A., Ryan, J.R., Hague, D., et al.: The effect of MK-185 on some aspects of uric acid metabolism. Clin. Pharmacol. Ther. 11:551, 1970.
26. Talbott, J.H.: Gout. London and New York, Oxford University Press, 1943.
27. Bonsnes, R.W., Dill, L., and Dana, E.: The effect of Diodrast on the normal uric acid clearance. J. Clin. Invest. 23:776, 1944.
28. Robinson, R.G., and Radcliff, E.J.: The effect of meclofenamic acid on plasma uric acid levels. Med. J. Aust. 1:1079, 1972.
29. Coombs, F.S., Pecora, L.J., Thorogood, E., et al.: Renal function in patients with gout. J. Clin. Invest. 12:525, 1940.

30. Mochtey, I.: Serum uric acid levels following administration of metiazinic acid (Soripal). Clin. Chim. Acta 47:317, 1973.
31. Podevin, R., Paillard R., Voudiclari, S., and Richet, G.: Action of niridazole (CIBA 32,644 BA) on the metabolism of uric acid in man. Rev. Franc. Étud. Clin. Biol. 13:624, 1968.
32. Weintraub, M., Nash, T.E., Ottesen, E., and Becker, M.A.: Uricosuric effects of niridazole. Clin. Pharmacol. Ther. 22:568, 1977.
33. Fulop, M., and Drapkin, A.: Potassium depletion syndrome secondary to nephropathy apparently caused by "outdated tetracycline." N. Engl. J. Med. 272:986, 1965.
34. Kuzell, W.C., Schaffarzick, R.W., Brown, B., et al.: Phenylbutazone (Butazolidin) in rheumatoid arthritis and gout. JAMA 149:729, 1952.
35. Trevaks, G., and Lovell, R.R.H.: Effect of Atromid and its components on uric acid excretion and on gout. Ann. Rheum. Dis. 24:572, 1965.
36. Gutman, A.B.: Uric acid metabolism and gout. Combined staff clinic. Am. J. Med. 9:799, 1950.
37. Talbott, J.H., Bishop, C., Norcross, M., et al.: The clinical and metabolic effects of Benemid in patients with gout. Trans. Assoc. Am. Physicians 64:372, 1951.
38. See, G.: Études sur l'acid salicylique et le salicylates: Traitement du rheumatisme aigu et chronique, de la goutte, et de diverses affections du systeme nerveux sensitif par les salicylates. Bull. Acad. Med. Paris 6:689, 717, 926, 937, 1024, 1877.
39. Burns, J.J., Yu, T-F., Ritterband, A., et al.: A potent new uricosuric agent, the sulfoxide metabolite of the phenylbutazone analogue, G-25671. J. Pharmacol. Exp. Ther. 119:418, 1957.
40. Nemati, M., Kyle, M.C., and Freis, E.D.: Clinical study of ticrynafen, a new diuretic, antihypertensive, and uricosuric agent. JAMA 237:652, 1977.
41. Friedman, A., and Steele, T.H.: Supersaturation of urine with uric acid and urate: Response to a uricosuric diuretic. J. Lab. Clin. Med. 92:447, 1978.
42. de Carvalho, J.G.R., Dunn, F.G., Chrysant, S.G., and Frohlich, E.D.: Ticrynafen: A novel uricosuric antihypertensive natriuretic agent. Arch. Intern. Med. 138:53, 1978.
43. Burns, J.J., Yu, T-F., Berger, L., et al.: Zoxazolamine. Physiological deposition, uricosuric properties. Am. J. Med. 25:401, 1958.
44. Bluestone, R., Kippen, I., Klinenberg, J.R., et al.: Effect of some uricosuric and anti-inflammatory drugs on the binding of uric acid to human serum albumin in vitro. J. Lab. Clin. Med. 76:85, 1970.
45. Klinenberg, J.R., and Kippen, I.: The binding of urate to plasma proteins determined by means of equilibrium dialysis. J. Lab. Clin. Med. 75:503, 1970.
46. Kippen, I., Whitehouse, M.W., and Klinenberg, J.R.: Pharmacology of uricosuric drugs. Ann. Rheum. Dis. 33:391, 1974.
47. Postlethwaite, A.E., Gutman, R.A., and Kelley, W.N.: Salicylate-mediated increase in uric acid removal during hemodialysis: Evidence for urate binding in vivo. Metabolism 23:771, 1974.
48. Kovarsky, J., Holmes, E.W., and Kelley, W.N.: Absence of significant urate binding to human serum proteins. J. Lab. Clin. Med. 93:85, 1979.
49. Gutman, A.B.: Uricosuric drugs, with special reference to probenecid and sulfinpyrazone. Adv. Pharmacol. 4:91, 1966.
50. Steele, T.H., and Rieselbach, R.E.: Renal urate excretion in normal man. Nephron 14:21, 1975.
51. Steele, T.H., and Bonar, G.: Origins of the uricosuric response. J. Clin. Invest. 52:1368, 1973.
52. Meisel, A.D., and Diamond, H.S.: Inhibition of probenecid uricosuria by pyrazinamide and para-aminohippurate. Am. J. Physiol. 232:F222, 1977.
53. Steele, T.H.: Urate secretion in man: The pyrazinamide suppression test. Ann. Intern. Med. 79:734, 1973.
54. Weinshilboum, R.M., Goldstein, J.L., and Kelley, W.N.: Prolonged hypouricemia associated with acute chlorprothixene ingestion. Arthritis Rheum. 18:739, 1975.
55. Lemierix, G., Vinay, P., Gougoux, A., et al.: Nature of the uricosuric action of benziodarone. Am. J. Physiol. 224:1440, 1973.
56. Dayton, P.G., Yu, T-F., Chen, W., et al.: The physiological disposition of probenecid, including renal clearance in man, studied by an improved method for its estimation in biological material. J. Pharmacol. Exp. Ther. 140:278, 1963.
57. Gutman, A.B., and Yu, T-F.: Benemid (p-[di-n-prophylsulfamyl]benzoic acid) as uricosuric agent in chronic gouty arthritis. Trans. Assoc. Am. Physicians 64:279, 1951.
58. Boger, W., Strickland, S.C., Bayne, G.M., et al.: Probenecid and salicylates: The question of interaction in terms of penicillin excretion. J. Lab. Clin. Med. 45:478, 1955.
59. Tjandramaga, T.B., Cucinell, S.A., Israeli, Z.H., et al.: Observations on the disposition of probenecid on patients receiving allopurinol. Pharmacology 8:259, 1972.
60. Gutman, A.B., and Yu, T-F.: Protracted uricosuric therapy in tophaceous gout. Lancet 2:1258, 1957.
61. Beyer, K.H., Russo, H.F., Tillson, E.K., et al.: "Benemid," p-(di-n-propylsulfamyl)benzoic acid. Its renal affinity and its elimination. Am. J. Physiol. 166:625, 1951.
62. Dayton, P.G., Perel, J.M., Cunningham, R.F., et al.: Studies of the fate of metabolites and analogs of probenecid. The significance of metabolic sites, especially lack of ring hydroxylation. Drug Metab. Dispos. 1:742, 1973.
63. Israeli, Z.H., Perel, J.M., Cunningham, R.F., et al.: Metabolites of probenecid. Chemical, physical and pharmacological studies. J. Med. Chem. 15:709, 1972.
64. Bowers, M.J., Jr.: CSF homovanillic acid: Effects of probenecid and alpha-methyltyrosine. Life Sci. [I] 9:691, 1970.
65. Tamarkin, N.R., Goodwin, F.K., and Axelrod, J.: Rapid elevation of biogenic amine metabolites in human CSF following probenecid. Life Sci. 9:1397, 1970.
66. Van Praag, H.M., Korf, J., and Puite, J.: 5-Hydroxyindoleacetic acid levels in the cerebrospinal fluid of depressive patients treated with probenecid. Nature 225:1259, 1970.
67. Airaksinen, E.M., and Kanko, K.: Effect of probenecid on 5-hydroxyindoles in cerebrospinal fluid in Down's syndrome. Ann. Clin. Res. 5:392, 1973.
68. Boger, W.P., Bayne, G.M., Gylfe, J., et al.: Renal clearance of pantothenic acid in man: Inhibition by probenecid ("Benemid"). Proc. Soc. Exp. Biol. Med. 82:604, 1953.
69. Markkanen, T., Toivanen, P., Toivanen, A., et al.: The effect of probenecid (p-(di-n-propylsulfamyl)-benzoic acid) on the spontaneous renal excretion of biologically active metabolites of thiamine, riboflavin and pantothenic acid. Scand. J. Clin. Lab. Invest. 15:511, 1963.
70. Gardner, L.I., Crigler, J.R., Jr., and Migeon, C.J.: Inhibition of urinary 17-ketosteroid excretion produced by "Benemid." Proc. Soc. Exp. Biol. Med. 78:460, 1951.
71. Bonar, J.A., and Perkins, W.H.: Inhibition of urinary excretion of iodine$^{131}$-labeled corticotropin by probenecid. J. Clin. Endocrinol. 22:38, 1962.
72. Huang, K.C.: Renal excretion of L-tyrosine and its derivatives. J. Pharmacol. Exp. Ther. 134:257, 1961.
73. Sirota, J.H., Yu, T-F., and Gutman, A.B.: Effect of Benemid (p-[di-n-propylsulfamyl]benzoic acid) on urate clearance and other discrete renal functions in gouty subjects. J. Clin. Invest. 31:692, 1952.
74. Dubin, A., Kushner, D.S., Bronsky, D., et al.: Hyperuricemia in hypoparathyroidism. Metabolism 5:703, 1956.
75. Kolb, F.O., and Rukes, J.M.: Effects of Benemid (probenecid) in the treatment of hypoparathyroidism and pseudohypoparathyroidism (abstract). J. Clin. Endocrinol. 14:785, 1954.
76. Persellin, R.H., and Schmid, F.R.: The use of sulfinpyrazone in the treatment of gout reduces serum uric acid levels and diminishes severity of arthritis attacks, with freedom from significant toxicity. JAMA 175:971, 1961.
77. Bearn, A.G., and Kunkel, H.G.: Abnormalities of copper metabolism in Wilson's disease and their relationship to the aminoaciduria. J. Clin. Invest. 33:400, 1954.
78. Beyer, K.H., Wiebelhaus, V.D., Tillson, E.K., et al.: "Benemid," p-(di-n-propylsulfamyl)benzoid acid: Inhibition of glycine conjugative reactions. Proc. Soc. Exp. Biol. Med. 74:772, 1950.
79. Coulson, R., Bowman, R.H., and Roch-Ramel, F.: The effects of nephrectomy and probenecid on in vivo clearance of adenosine 3'5'-monophosphate from rat plasma. Life Sci. 15:877, 1974.
80. Benedek, T.G.: The effect of probenecid and of liver disease on the excretion of phenolsulfonphthalein. Am. J. Med. Sci. 242:448, 1961.
81. Beyer, K.H.: Functional characteristics of renal transport mechanisms. Pharmacol. Rev. 2:227, 1950.
82. Blondheim, S.H.: Effect of probenecid on excretion of bromosulphthalein. J. Appl. Physiol. 7:529, 1955.
83. Boger, W.P., Matteucci, W.V., and Schimmel, N.H.: Renal clearances of penicillin, phenolsulphonphthalein, and paraaminohippurate (PAH) modified by "Benemid" (abstract). Am. J. Med. 11:517, 1951.
84. Newcombe, D.S., and Cohen, A.S.: Uricosuric agents and phenolsulfonphthalein excretion. Arch. Intern. Med. 112:738, 1963.
85. Peck, H.M., and Beyer, K.H.: Renal function: Excretion of phenolsulfonphthalein by the amphibian (*Rana pipiens*) kidney (abstract). Fed. Proc. 13:393, 1954.
86. Gutman, A.B., Yu, T-F., and Sirota, J.H.: A study, by simultaneous clearance techniques, of salicylate excretion in man. Effect of alkalinization of the urine by bicarbonate administration; effect of probenecid. J. Clin. Invest. 34:711, 1955.
87. Schacter, D., and Manis, J.F.: Salicylate and salicyl conjugates: Fluorimetric estimation, biosynthesis and renal excretion in man. J. Clin. Invest. 37:800, 1958.
88. Weiner, I.M., Washington, J.A., II, and Mudge, G.H.: Studies on the renal excretion of salicylate in the dog. Bull. Johns Hopkins Hosp. 105:284, 1959.

89. Yu, T-F., and Gutman, A.B.: Study of the paradoxical effects of salicylate in low, intermediate and high dosage on the renal mechanisms for excretion of urate in man. J. Clin. Invest. 38:1298, 1959.
90. Braun, W., Whittaker, V.P., and Lotspeich, W.F.: Renal excretion of phlorizin and phlorizin glucuronide. Am. J. Physiol. 190:563, 1957.
91. Goodwin, C.S., and Sparell, G.: Inhibition of dapsone excretion by probenecid. Lancet 2:884, 1969.
92. Perel, J.M., Dayton, P.G., Snell, M.M., et al.: Studies of interactions among drugs in man at the renal level: Probenecid and sulfinpyrazone. Clin. Pharmacol. Ther. 10:834, 1969.
93. Skeith, M.D., Simkin, P.A., and Healey, L.A.: Renal excretion of indomethacin and its inhibition by probenecid. Clin. Pharmacol. Ther. 9:89, 1968.
94. Klein, J.O., and Finland, M.: Ampicillin activity in vitro and absorption and excretion in normal young men. Am. J. Med. Sci. 243:544, 1963.
95. Beyer, K.H.: Factors basic to the development of useful inhibitors of renal transport mechanisms. Arch. Int. Pharmacodyn. 98:97, 1954.
96. Mischler, T.W., Sugerman, A.A., Willard, D.A., et al.: Influence of probenecid and food on the bioavailability of cephradine in normal male subjects. J. Clin. Pharmacol. 14:604, 1974.
97. Gibaldi, M., and Schwartz, M.A.: Apparent effect of probenecid on distribution of penicillin in man. Clin. Pharmacol. Ther. 9:345, 1968.
98. Goetzee, A.E., Richards, T.G., and Tindall, V.R.: Experimental changes in liver function induced by probenecid. Clin. Sci. 19:63, 1960.
99. Vogin, E.E., Scott, W., Boyd, J., et al.: Effect of probenecid on indocyanine green clearance. J. Pharmacol. Exp. Ther. 152:509, 1966.
100. Kenwright, S., and Levi, A.J.: Impairment of hepatic uptake of rifamycin antibiotics by probenecid, and its therapeutic implications. Lancet 2:1401, 1973.
101. Sanchez, G.: Enhancement of heparin effect by probenecid. N. Engl. J. Med. 292:48, 1975.
102. Palmer, D.G., and T.C., Highton: A short trial assessment of uricosuric therapy in gout. Aust. Ann. Med. 17:242, 1968.
103. Bergan, T., Westlie, L., and Brodwall, E.K.: Influence of probenecid on gentamycin pharmacokinetics. Acta Med. Scand. 191:221, 1974.
104. Gutman, A.B.: Medical management of gout. Postgrad. Med. 51:61, 1972.
105. Yu, T-F.: Milestones in the treatment of gout. Am. J. Med. 56:676, 1974.
106. Thompson, C.R., Duff, I.F., Robinson, W.D., et al.: Long-term uricosuric therapy in gout. Arthritis Rheum. 5:384, 1962.
107. Gutman, A.B.: Treatment of primary gout: The present status. Arthritis Rheum. 8:911, 1965.
108. de Seze, S., Ryckewaert, A., and d'Anglejan, G.: The treatment of gout by probenecid. (A study based on 156 cases, 68 of which were treated from 1 to 9 years.) Rev. Rhum. Mal. Osteoartic. 30:93, 1963.
109. Boger, W.P., and Strickland, S.C.: Probenecid (Benemid). Its use and side-effects in 2502 patients. Arch Intern. Med. 95:83, 1955.
110. Reynolds, E.S., Schlant, R.C., Gonick, H.C., et al.: Fatal massive necrosis of the liver as a manifestation of hypersensitivity to probenecid. N. Engl. J. Med. 256:592, 1957.
111. Ferris, T.F., Morgan, W.S., and Levitin, H.: Nephrotic syndrome caused by probenecid. N. Engl. J. Med. 265:381, 1961.
112. Hertz, P., Yager, H., and Richardson, J.A.: Probenecid-induced nephrotic syndrome. Arch. Pathol. 94:241, 1972.
113. Talbott, J.H.: Gout. 2nd ed. New York, Grune & Stratton, 1964, p. 206.
114. Gutman, A.B., and Yu, T-F.: Prevention and treatment of chronic gouty arthritis. JAMA 157:1096, 1955.
115. de Seze, S., Ryckewaert, A., Caroit, M., et al.: Le traitement uricosurique de la goutte. Congres International de la goutte et de la lithiase urique, Sept. 4-6, Evian, 1964, p. 297.
116. Kuzell, W., Glover, R., Gibbs, J., et al.: Effect of Anturane on serum uric acid and cholesterol in gout. A long-term study. Acta Rheumatol. Scand. Suppl. 8:31, 1964.
117. Dayton, P.G., Sicam, L.E., Landrau, M., et al.: Metabolism of sulfinpyrazone (Anturane) and other thio analogues of phenylbutazone in man. J. Pharmacol. Exp. Ther. 132:287, 1961.
118. Gutman, A.B., Dayton, P.G., Yu, T-F., et al.: A study of the inverse relationship between $pK_a$ and rate of renal excretion of phenylbutazone analogs in man and dog. Am. J. Med. 29:1017, 1960.
119. Yu, T-F., Burns, J.J., and Gutman, A.B.: Results of a clinical trial of G-28315, a sulfoxide analog of phenylbutazone, as a uricosuric agent in gouty subjects. Arthritis Rheum. 1:532, 1958.
120. Domenjoz, R.: The pharmacology of the phenylbutazone analogues. Ann. N.Y. Acad. Sci. 86:263, 1960.
121. Kaegi, A., Pineo, G.F., Shimizu, A., et al.: Arteriovenous shunt thrombosis: Prevention by sulfinpyrazone. N. Engl. J. Med. 290:304, 1974.
122. Weily, H.S., and Genton, E.: Altered platelet function in patients with prosthetic mitral valves: Effects of sulfinpyrazone therapy. Circulation 42:967, 1970.
123. Steele, P.O., Weily, H.S., and Genton, E.: Platelet survival and adhesiveness in recurrent venous thrombosis. N. Engl. J. Med. 288:1148, 1973.
124. Ali, M., and McDonald, W.D.: Effects of sulfinpyrazone on platelet prostaglandin synthesis and platelet release of serotonin. J. Lab. Clin. Med. 89:868, 1977.
125. Seegmiller, J.E., and Grayzel, A.I.: Use of the newer uricosuric agents in the management of gout. JAMA 173:1076, 1960.
126. Emmerson, B.T.: A comparison of uricosuric agents in gout, with special reference to sulphinpyrazone. Med. J. Aust. 1:839, 1963.
127. Glick, E.N.: Sulphinpyrazone in the treatment of arthritis associated with hyperuricaemia. Proc. R. Soc. Med. 54:423, 1961.
128. Richet, G., Cottet, J., Amiel, C., et al.: Traitement de l'hyperuricémie des goutteux et des insuffisants rénaux par la Benziodarone. Presse Méd. 74:1247, 1966.
129. Delbarre, F., Auscher, C., Olivier, J.L., et al.: Traitement des hyperuricémies et de la goutte par des dérivés du benzofuranne. Semin. Hôp. Paris 24:1127, 1967.
130. Jain, A.K., Ryan, J.R., McMahon, F.G., et al.: Effect of single oral doses of benzbromarone on serum and urinary uric acid. Arthritis Rheum. 17:149, 1974.
131. Sinclair, D.S., and Fox, I.H.: The pharmacology of hypouricemic effect of benzbromarone. J. Rheum. 2:437, 1975.
132. Yu, T-F.: Pharmacokinetic and clinical studies of a new uricosuric agent—benzbromarone. J. Rheum. 3:305, 1976.
133. Kramp, R.A.: Effects of benzofuran derivatives on tubular permeability to 6-urate-$2^{14}C$ in the rat nephron. *In* Sperling, O., De Vries, A., and Wyngaarden, J.B. (eds.): Purine Metabolism in Man. New York, Plenum Press, 1974, p. 777.
134. Camus, J.P., Prier, A., Kartun, P., et al.: Thyréotoxicose et benziodarone. Rev. Rhum. Mal. Osteoartic. 40:148, 1973.
135. de Gery, A., Auscher, C., Saporta, L., et al.: Treatment of gout and hyperuricemia by benzbromarone, ethyl 2(dibromo-3,5-hydroxy-4-benzoyl)-3 benzofuran. *In* Sperling, O., De Vries, A., and Wyngaarden, J.B., (eds.): Purine Metabolism in Man. New York, Plenum Press, 1974, p. 683.
136. Zöllner, N., Griebsch, A., and Fink, J.K.: Über die Wirkung von Benzbromaron auf den Serumharnsäuerespiegel und die Harnsäureausscheidung des Gichtkranken. Dtsch. Med. Wochenschr. 98:2405, 1970.
137. Petering, H.G., and Schmitt, J.A.: Studies in enzyme inhibition. I. Action of some simple pterines on xanthine oxidase. J. Am. Chem. Soc. 72:2995, 1950.
138. Priest, D.G., Hynes, J.B., Jones, C.W., et al.: Quinazolines as inhibitors of xanthine oxidase. J. Pharmacol. Sci. 63:1158, 1974.
139. Wyngaarden, J.B.: 2,6-Diaminopurine as substrate and inhibitor of xanthine oxidase. J. Biol. Chem. 224:453, 1957.
140. Silberman, H.R., and Wyngaarden, J.B.: 6-Mercaptopurine as substrate and inhibitor of xanthine oxidase. Biochim. Biophys. Acta 47:178, 1961.
141. Fridovich, I.: A new class of xanthine oxidase inhibitors isolated from guanidinium salts. Biochemistry 4:1098, 1965.
142. Baker, B.R., Wood, W.F., and Kozma, J.A.: Irreversible enzyme inhibitors. CXXVI. Hydrocarbon interaction with xanthine oxidase by phenyl substituents on purines and pyrazolo(3,4-d)pyrimidines. J. Med. Chem. 11:611, 1968.
143. White, F.R.: 4-Aminopyrazolo(3,4-d)pyrimidine and three derivatives. Cancer Chemother. Rep. 3:26, 1959.
144. Shaw, R.K., Shulman, R.N., Davidson, J.K., et al.: Studies with the experimental antitumor agent 4-aminopyrazolo(3,4-d)pyrimidine. Cancer 13:482, 1960.
145. Feigelson, P., Davidson, J.K., and Robins, P.K.: Pyrazolopyrimidines as inhibitors and substrates of xanthine oxidase. J. Biol. Chem. 226:993, 1957.
146. Elion, G.B., Callahan, S., Nathan, H., et al.: Potentiation by inhibition of drug degradation: 6-Substituted purine and xanthine oxidase. Biochem. Pharmacol. 12:85, 1963.
147. Rundles, R.W., Wyngaarden, J.B., Hitchings, G.H., et al.: Effects of a xanthine oxidase inhibitor on thiopurine metabolism, hyperuricemia and gout. Trans. Assoc. Am. Physicians 76:126, 1963.
148. Wyngaarden, J.B., Rundles, R.W., Silberman, H.R., et al.: Control of hyperuricemia with hydroxypyrazolopyrimidine, a purine analogue which inhibits uric acid synthesis. Arthritis Rheum. 6:306, 1963.
149. Massey, V., Komai, H., Palmer, G., et al.: On the mechanism of inactivation of xanthine oxidase by allopurinol and other pyrazolo(3,4-d)pyrimidines. J. Biol. Chem. 245:2837, 1970.
150. Elion, G.B.: Enzymatic and metabolic studies with allopurinol. Ann. Rheum. Dis. 25:608, 1966.
151. Rundles, R.W., Wyngaarden, J.B., Hitchings, G.H., et al.: Drugs and uric acid. Ann. Rev. Pharmacol. 9:345, 1969.
152. Elion, G.B., Kovensky, A., Hitchings, G.H., et al.: Metabolic studies of allopurinol, an inhibitor of xanthine oxidase. Biochem. Pharmacol. 15:863, 1966.
153. Hande, K., Reed, E., and Chabner, B.: Allopurinol kinetics. Clin. Pharmacol. Ther. 23:598, 1978.

154. McCollister, R.J., Gilbert, W.R., Jr., Ashton, D.M., et al.: Pseudo-feedback inhibition of purine synthesis by 6-mercaptopurine ribonucleotide and other purine analogues. J. Biol. Chem. 239:1560, 1964.
155. Krenitsky, T.A., Elion, G.B., Strelitz, R.A., et al.: Ribonucleosides of allopurinol and oxoallopurinol. J. Biol. Chem. 242:2675, 1967.
156. Elion, G.B., Yu, T-F., Gutman, A.B., et al.: Renal clearance of oxipurinol, the chief metabolite of allopurinol. Am. J. Med. 45:69, 1968.
157. Nelson, D.J., Bugge, C.J.L., Krasny, H.C., et al.: Formation of nucleotides of 6-$^{14}$C allopurinol and 6-$^{14}$C oxipurinol in rat tissues and effects on uridine nucleotide pools. Biochem. Pharmacol. 22:2003, 1973.
158. Beardmore, T.D., and Kelley, W.N.: Mechanism of allopurinol-mediated inhibition of pyrimidine biosynthesis. J. Lab. Clin. Med. 78:696, 1971.
159. Chalmers, R.A., Kromer, H., Scott, J.T., et al.: A comparative study of the xanthine oxidase inhibitors, allopurinol and oxipurinol in man. Clin. Sci. 35:353, 1968.
160. Wyngaarden, J.B., Rundles, R.W., and Metz, E.N.: Allopurinol in the treatment of gout. Ann. Intern. Med. 62:842, 1965.
161. Rundles, R.W., Metz, E.N., and Silberman, H.R.: Allopurinol in the treatment of gout. Ann. Intern. Med. 64:229, 1966.
162. Klinenberg, J.R., Goldfinger, S.E., and Seegmiller, J.E.: The effectiveness of the xanthine oxidase inhibitor allopurinol in the treatment of gout. Ann. Intern. Med. 62:639, 1965.
163. Yu, T-F., and Gutman, A.B.: Effects of allopurinol (4-hydroxypyrazolo(3,4-d)pyrimidine) on serum and urinary uric acid in primary and secondary gout. Am. J. Med. 37:885, 1964.
164. Dayton, P.G., Amor, B., Auscher, C., et al.: Treatment of gout with allopurinol, a study of 106 cases. Ann. Rheum. Dis. 25:627, 1966.
165. Kelley, W.N., Greene, M.L., Rosenbloom, F.M., et al.: Hypoxanthine-guanine phosphoribosyltransferase deficiency in gout. Ann. Intern. Med. 70:155, 1969.
166. Emmerson, B.T.: Discussion, symposium on allopurinol. Ann. Rheum. Dis. 25:621, 1966.
167. Kelley, W.N., Rosenbloom, F.M., Miller, J., et al.: An enzymatic basis for variation in response to allopurinol. N. Engl. J. Med. 278:287, 1968.
168. Caskey, C.T., Ashton, D.M., and Wyngaarden, J.B.: The enzymology of feedback inhibition of glutamine phosphoribosylpyrophosphate amidotransferase by purine ribonucleotides. J. Biol. Chem. 239:2570, 1964.
169. Fox, I.H., Wyngaarden, J.B., and Kelley, W.N.: Depletion of erythrocyte phosphoribosylpyrophosphate in man, a newly observed effect of allopurinol. N. Engl. J. Med. 283:1177, 1970.
170. Elion, G.B., and Nelson, D.J.: Ribonucleotides of allopurinol and oxipurinol in rat tissues and their significance in purine metabolism. *In* Sperling, O., De Vries, A., and Wyngaarden, J.B. (eds.): Purine Metabolism in Man. New York, Plenum Press, 1974, p. 639.
171. Holmes, E.W., McDonald, J.A., McCord, J.M., et al.: Human glutamine phosphoribosylpyrophosphate amidotransferase: Kinetic and regulatory properties. J. Biol. Chem. 248:144, 1973.
172. Wood, A.W., and Seegmiller, J.E.: Properties of 5-phosphoribosyl-1-pyrophosphate amidotransferase from human lymphoblasts. J. Biol. Chem. 248:138, 1973.
173. Pomales, R., Bieber, S., Friedman, R., et al.: Augmentation of the incorporation of hypoxanthine into nucleic acids by the administration of an inhibitor of xanthine oxidase. Biochim. Biophys. Acta 72:119, 1963.
174. Pomales, R., Elion, G.B., and Hitchings, G.H.: Xanthine as a precursor of nucleic acid purines in the mouse. Biochim. Biophys. Acta 95:505, 1965.
175. Edwards, N.L., Recker, D., Airozo, D., et al.: Enhanced purine salvage during allopurinol therapy: An important pharmacologic property in humans. J. Lab. Clin. Med. 98:673, 1981.
176. Fox, R.M., Royse-Smith, D., and O'Sullivan, W.J.: Orotidinuria induced by allopurinol. Science 168:861, 1970.
177. Kelley, W.N., and Beardmore, T.D.: Allopurinol: Alteration in pyrimidine metabolism in man. Science 169:388, 1970.
178. Beardmore, T.D., Fox, I.H., and Kelley, W.N.: Effect of allopurinol on pyrimidine metabolism in the Lesch-Nyhan syndrome. Lancet 2:830, 1970.
179. Hatfield, D., and Wyngaarden, J.B.: 3-Ribosylpurines. I. Synthesis of (3-ribosyluric acid) 5′-phosphate and (3-ribosylxanthine) 5′-phosphate by a pyrimidine ribonucleotide pyrophosphorylase of beef erythrocytes. J. Biol. Chem. 239:2580, 1964.
180. Hatfield, D., and Wyngaarden, J.B.: 3-Ribosylpurines. II. Studies on (3-ribosylxanthine) 5′-phosphate and on ribonucleotide derivatives of certain uracil analogues. J. Biol. Chem. 239:2587, 1964.
181. Beardmore, T.D., Cashman, J., and Kelley, W.N.: Mechanism of allopurinol-mediated increase in enzyme activity in man. J. Clin. Invest. 51:1823, 1972.
182. Grobner, W., and Kelley, W.N.: Effect of allopurinol and its metabolic derivatives on the configuration of human orotate phosphoribosyltransferase and orotidine 5′-phosphate decarboxylase. Biochem. Pharmacol. 24:379, 1975.
183. Fox, R.M., Wood, M.H., and O'Sullivan, W.J.: Studies on the coordinate activity and lability of orotidylate phosphoribosyltransferase and decarboxylase in human erythrocytes and the effects of allopurinol administration. J. Clin. Invest. 50:1050, 1971.
184. Becking, G.C., and Johnson, W.J.: The inhibition of tryptophan pyrrolase by allopurinol, an inhibitor of xanthine oxidase. Can. J. Biochem. 45:1667, 1967.
185. Chytil, F.: Activation of liver tryptophan oxygenase by adenosine 3′,5′-phosphate and by other purine derivatives. J. Biol. Chem. 243:893, 1968.
186. Ghosh, D., and Forrest, H.S.: Inhibition of tryptophan pyrrolase by some naturally occurring pteridines. Arch. Biochem. 120:578, 1967.
187. Julian, J., and Chytil, F.: Participation of xanthine oxidase in the activation of liver tryptophan pyrrolase. J. Biol. Chem. 245:1161, 1970.
188. Krenitsky, T.A., Elion, G.B., Henderson, A.M., et al.: Inhibition of human purine nucleoside phosphorylase. Studies with intact erythrocytes and the purified enzyme. J. Biol. Chem. 243:2876, 1968.
189. Gallo, R.C., Parry, S., and Breitman, T.R.: Inhibition of human leukocyte pyrimidine deoxynucleoside synthesis by allopurinol and 6-mercaptopurine. Biochem. Pharmacol. 17:2185, 1968.
190. Truseve, R., and Williams, V.: The effect of allopurinol on urate oxidase activity. Biochem. Pharmacol. 17:165, 1968.
191. Johns, D.G.: Human liver aldehyde oxidase: Differential inhibition of oxidation of charged and uncharged substrates. J. Clin. Invest. 46:1492, 1967.
192. Stevenson, A.C., Silcock, S.R., and Scott, J.T.: Absence of chromosome damage in human lymphocytes exposed to allopurinol and oxipurinol. Ann. Rheum. Dis. 35:143, 1976.
193. Friedman, H.M., and T. Grasela: Adenine arabinoside and allopurinol: Possible adverse drug interaction. N. Engl. J. Med. 304:423, 1981.
194. Boston Collaborative Drug Surveillance Program: Allopurinol and cytotoxic drugs. Interaction in relation to bone marrow depression. JAMA 227:1036, 1974.
195. Vesell, E.S., Passananti, G.T., and Greene, F.E.: Impairment of drug metabolism in man by allopurinol and nortriptyline. N. Engl. J. Med. 283:1484, 1970.
196. Boston Collaborative Drug Surveillance Program: Excess of ampicillin rashes associated with allopurinol or hyperuricemia. N. Engl. J. Med. 286:505, 1972.
197. Young, J.L., Jr., Boswell, R.B., and Nies, A.S.: Severe allopurinol hypersensitivity: Association with thiazides and prior renal compromise. Arch. Intern. Med. 134:553, 1974.
198. Wood, M.H., O'Sullivan, W.J., Wilson, M., and Tiller, D.J.: Potentiation of an effect of allopurinol on pyrimidine metabolism by chlorothiazide in man. Clin. Exp. Pharmacol. Physiol. 1:53, 1974.
199. Goldfarb, E., and Smyth, C.J.: Effects of allopurinol, a xanthine oxidase inhibitor, and sulfinpyrazone upon the urinary and serum urate concentrations in eight patients with tophaceous gout. Arthritis Rheum. 9:414, 1966.
200. Kelley, W.N., and Wyngaarden, J.B.: The effect of dietary purine restriction, allopurinol and oxipurinol on the urinary excretion of ultraviolet absorbing compounds. Clin. Chem. 16:707, 713, 1970.
201. Yu, T-F.: The effect of allopurinol in primary and secondary gout. Arthritis Rheum. 8:907, 1965.
202. Rodnan, G., Robin, J.A., and Tolchin, S.F.: Efficacy of a single daily dose of allopurinol in gouty hyperuricemia. *In* Sperling, O., De Vries, A., and Wyngaarden, J.B. (eds.): Purine Metabolism in Man. New York, Plenum Press, 1974, p. 571.
203. Gottlieb, N.L., and Gray, R.G.: Allopurinol-associated hand and foot deformities in chronic tophaceous gout. JAMA 238:1663, 1977.
204. Delbarre, F., Lagrue, G., Frugier, J-C., et al.: Le traitement, par L-allopurinol, de la goutte avec insuffisance rénale. Semin. Hop. Paris 43:644, 1967.
205. Rundles, R.W., Silberman, H.R., Hitchings, G.H., et al.: Effects of xanthine oxidase inhibitor on clinical manifestations and purine metabolism in gout. Ann. Intern. Med. 60:717, 1964.
206. Delbarre, F., Amor, B., Auscher, C., et al.: Treatment of gout with allopurinol, a study of 106 cases. Ann. Rheum. Dis. 25:627, 1966.
207. Loebl, W.Y., and Scott, J.T.: Withdrawal of allopurinol in patients with gout. Ann. Rheum. Dis. 33:304, 1974.
208. Emmerson, B.T.: The use of the xanthine oxidase inhibitor, allopurinol, in the control of hyperuricemia, gout and uric acid calculi. Aust. Ann. Med. 16:205, 1967.
209. Levin, N.W., and Abrahams, O.L.: Allopurinol in patients with impaired renal function. Ann. Rheum. Dis. 25:681, 1966.
210. Ogryzlo, M.A., Urowitz, M., and Weber, H.M.: Effects of allopurinol on gouty and nongouty uric acid nephropathy. Ann. Rheum. Dis. 25:673, 1966.
211. Stoberg, K-H.: Allopurinol therapy of gout with renal complications. Ann. Rheum. Dis. 25:688, 1966.
212. Rundles, R.W.: Allopurinol in gouty nephropathy and renal dialysis. Ann. Rheum. Dis. 25:694, 1966.

213. Wilson, J.D., Simmonds, H.A., and North, J.D.K.: Allopurinol in the treatment of uremic patients with gout. Ann. Rheum. Dis. 26:136, 1967.
214. Goldfinger, S., Klinenberg, J.R., and Seegmiller, J.E.: The renal excretion of oxypurine. J. Clin. Invest. 44:623, 1965.
215. Sperling, O., Brosh, S., Boer, P., Liberman, U.A., and De Vries, A.: Urinary xanthine stones in an allopurinol-treated gouty with partial deficiency of hypoxanthine-guanine phosphoribosyltransferase. Israel J. Med. Sci. 14:288, 1978.
216. Sorensen, L., and Seegmiller, J.E.: Seminars on the Lesch-Nyhan syndrome: Management and treatment, discussion. Fed. Proc. 27:1097, 1968.
217. Greene, M.L., Fujimoto, W.Y., and Seegmiller, J.E.: Urinary xanthine stones—a rare complication of allopurinol therapy. N. Engl. J. Med. 280:426, 1969.
218. Band, P.R., Silverberg, D.S., and Henderson, J.F.: Xanthine nephropathy in a patient with lymphosarcoma treated with allopurinol. N. Engl. J. Med. 283:354, 1970.
219. Wyngaarden, J.B.: Allopurinol and xanthine nephropathy. N. Engl. J. Med. 283:371, 1970.
220. Ablin, A., Stephens, B.G., Hirata, T., et al.: Nephropathy, xanthinuria, and orotic aciduria complicating Burkitt's lymphoma treated with chemotherapy and allopurinol. Metabolism 21:771, 1972.
221. Watts, R.W.E., Scott, J.T., Chalmers, R.T., et al.: Microscopic studies on skeletal muscle in gout patients treated with allopurinol. Quart. J. Med. 40:1, 1971.
222. Watts, R.E.W., Sneeden, W., and Parker, R.A.: A quantitative study of skeletal muscle purines and pyrazolo(3,4-d)pyrimidines in gout patients treated with allopurinol. Clin. Sci. 41:153, 1971.
223. Landgrebe, A.R., Nyhan, W.L., and Coleman, M.: Urinary tract stones resulting from excretion of oxypurinol. N. Engl. J. Med. 292:626, 1975.
224. Stote, R.M., Smith, L.H., Dubb, J.W., et al.: Oxypurinol nephrolithiasis in regional enteritis secondary to allopurinol therapy. Ann. Int. Med. 92:384, 1980.
225. Straitigos, J.D., Bartsokas, S.K., and Capetanakis, J.: Further experiences with toxic epidermal necrolysis incriminating allopurinol, pyrazolone and derivatives. Br. J. Dermatol. 86:564, 1972.
226. Kantor, G.I.: Toxic epidermal necrolysis, azotemia, and death after allopurinol therapy. JAMA 212:478, 1970.
227. Auerbach, R., and Orentrich, N.: Alopecia and ichthyosis secondary to allopurinol. Arch. Dermatol. 98:104, 1968.
228. Irby, R., Toone, E., and Owen, D., Jr.: Bone marrow depression associated with allopurinol therapy (abstract). Arthritis Rheum. 9:860, 1966.
229. Greenberg, M.D., and Zambrano, S.S.: Aplastic agranulocytosis after allopurinol therapy. Arthritis Rheum. 15:413, 1972.
230. Lidsky, M.D., and Sharp, J.T.: Jaundice with the use of 4-hydroxypyrazolo(3,4-d)pyrimidine (4-HPP) (abstract). Arthritis Rheum. 10:294, 1967.
231. Chawla, S.K., Patel, H.D., Parrino, G.R., Soterakis, J., Lopresti, P.A., and D'Angelo, W.A.: Allopurinol hepatotoxicity. Arthritis Rheum. 20:1546, 1977.
232. Simons, F., Feldman, B., and Gerety, D.: Granulomatous hepatitis in a patient receiving allopurinol. Gastroenterology 62:101, 1972.
233. Swank, L.E., Chejfec, G., and Nemchausky, B.: Allopurinol-induced granulomatous hepatitis with cholangitis and a sarcoid-like reaction. Arch. Intern. Med. 138:997, 1978.
234. Jarzobski, J., Ferry, J., Wombolt, D., et al.: Vasculitis with allopurinol therapy. Am. Heart J. 79:116, 1970.
235. Mills, R.M., Jr.: Severe hypersensitivity reactions associated with allopurinol. JAMA 216:799, 1971.
236. Hande, K.R., Noone, R.M., and Stone, W.J.: Severe allopurinol toxicity: Description and guidelines for prevention in patients with renal insufficiency. Am. J. Med., in press, 1984.
237. Fam, A.G., Paton, T.W., and Chaiton, A.: Reinstitution of allopurinol therapy for gouty arthritis after cutaneous reactions. Can. Med. Assoc. J. 123:128, 1980.
238. Meyrier, A.: Desensitization in a patient with chronic renal disease and severe allergy to allopurinol. Br. Med. J. 1:458, 1976.
239. Griffing, W.L., and O'Duffy, J.D.: Oxipurinol in allopurinol-allergic patients. Clin. Res. 31:803A, 1983.
240. Delbarre, F., Auscher, C., DeGery, A., et al.: Le traitement de la dyspurinie goutteuse par la mercaptopyrazolopyrimidine (MPP: thiopurinol). Presse Med. 76:2329, 1968.
241. Sarre, H., Simon, L., and Claustre, G.: Les urico-frenateurs dans le traitement de la goutte. A propos de 126 cas. Semin. Hop. Paris 46:3295, 1970.
242. Auscher, C., Mercier, N., Pasquier, C., et al.: Allopurinol and thiopurinol: Effect in vivo on urinary oxypurine excretion and rate of synthesis of their ribonucleotides in different enzymatic deficiences. *In* Sperling, O., De Vries, A., and Wyngaarden, J.B. (eds.): Purine Metabolism in Man. New York, Plenum Press, 1974, p. 657.
243. Delbarre, F., and Auscher, C.: Traitement de la goutte par l'acide uracil-6-carboxylique et ses dérivés. Presse Méd. 71:1765, 1963.
244. Kelley, W.N., Greene, M.L., Fox, I.H., et al.: Effects of orotic acid on purine and lipoprotein metabolism in man. Metabolism 19:1025, 1970.
245. Kelley, W.N., Fox, I.H., and Wyngaarden, J.B.: Regulation of purine biosynthesis in cultured human cells. I. Effects of orotic acid. Biochim. Biophys. Acta 216:512, 1970.
246. Lieberman, I., Kornberg, A., and Simms, E.S.: Enzymatic synthesis of uridine 5′-phosphate. J. Biol. Chem. 215:403, 1955.
247. Higgins, J.R., Ashton, D.M., Speas, M., et al.: An evaluation of relative roles of substrate diversion and feedback inhibition in the control of purine synthesis. Clin. Res. 9:181, 1961.
248. Standerfer, S.B., and Handler, P.: Fatty liver induced by orotic acid feeding. Proc. Soc. Exp. Biol. Med. 90:270, 1955.
249. Creasey, W.A., Hankin, L., and Handschumacher, R.E.: Fatty livers induced by orotic acid. I. Accumulation and metabolism of lipids. J. Biol. Chem. 236:2064, 1961.
250. Altman, K.I., Smull, K., and Guzman-Barron, E.S.: A new method for the preparation of uricase and the effect of uricase on the blood uric acid levels of the chicken. Arch. Biochem. 21:158, 1949.
251. London, M., and Hudson, P.B.: Uricolytic activity of purified uricase in two human beings. Science 125:937, 1957.
252. Royer, R., Vindel, J., Lamarche, M., et al.: Modalities d'élimination des purines au cours du traitement enzymatique de la goutte et des états hyperuricémiques par une urateoxydase. Presse Méd. 76:2325, 1968.
253. Kissel, P., Lamarche, M., and Royer, R.: Modification of uricemia and the excretion of uric acid nitrogen by an enzyme of fungal origin. Nature 217:72, 1968.
254. Brogard, J.M., Frankhauser, J.I., and Stahl, A.: Application de l'uricolyse enzymatique au traitement des hyperuricémies d'origine rénale. Schweiz. Med. Wochenschr. 103:404, 1973.
255. Brogard, J.M., Stahl, A., and Stahl, J.: Enzymatic uricolysis and its use in therapy. *In* Kelley, W.N., and Weiner, I.M. (eds.): Uric Acid. Berlin, Springer-Verlag, 1978, pp. 515–524.

# Chapter 57
# Colchicine

*Stanley L. Wallace*

## INTRODUCTION

Colchicine is an ancient and traditional drug in the treatment of acute gout. Extracts of the plant *Colchicum autumnale,* also called the meadow saffron or the autumn crocus, have been utilized for this purpose at least since the sixth century A.D., when Alexander of Tralles first described such use.[1] However, undoubtedly because of the strong purgative effect, colchicine had lost its place in therapy by the seventeenth century.[2] Nicholas Husson, a French Army officer, reintroduced colchicum as a secret ingredient of L'eau Medicinale, a patent medicine panacea first offered in 1780.[3] L'eau Medicinale was shown to be particularly effective in acute gout. Want, in 1814, demonstrated that the active ingredient in this nostrum was colchicum.[4] Pelletier and Caventou[5] determined in 1820 that the active ingredient of colchicum was the alkaloid colchicine. The pure preparation has been in constant use for the treatment of gout for the past 160 years.

## STRUCTURE-FUNCTION RELATIONSHIPS

The structure of the colchicine molecule was established in 1945 by Dewar.[6] The molecule has three rings; the first is benzenoid and the second and third are 7 carbon rings (Fig. 57–1). The first ring has three methoxyl groups attached. The second has an acetylamino side chain, while ring C is an analogue of tropolone methyl ether, with a ketone group and a methoxyl group attached to adjacent carbons (Fig. 57–2). The tropolonoid nature of the side chains of the third ring implies a resonating hydrogen shared by both side chains.

In a three-dimensional crystallographic study of desacetylmethylcolchicine, the benzenoid ring (ring A) and the ring with tropolonoid configuration (ring C) were planar, forming a dihedral angle of 54 degrees.[7] The other seven carbon ring was folded into a boatlike conformation. The two necessary structures for colchicine's activity on tubulin (see below) are the first and third rings and their side chains; the second ring plays little or no role.

Tropolone methyl ether is a precise analogue of ring C of colchicine. Andreu and Timasheff found that this simple molecule was capable of binding to a single site on the tubulin molecule.[8] The binding of tropolone methyl ether or of colchicine to tubulin inhibited the binding of the other, indicating that the two substances bound to the same site. Both tropolone and tropolone methyl ether inhibited tubulin polymerization into microtubules in vitro.[8]

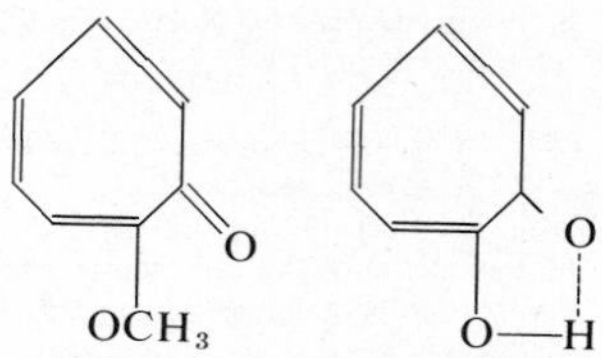


**Figure 57–2.** Tropolone methyl ether and tropolone.

Mescaline is an analogue of the trimethoxyphenyl structure of the first colchicine ring. *N*-Acetylmescaline also binds to tubulin, and the binding is inhibited by colchicine. *N*-Acetylmescaline partly inhibits microtubular assembly. Studies by Andreu and Timasheff and others[8,9] indicated that colchicine was a bifunctional ligand that interacted with tubulin at two sites, presumably at the tropolone (ring C) and trimethoxyphenyl (ring A) locations. The evidence suggested that the tropolone endbound first, and that this binding induced in the tubulin a conformational change, bringing the trimethoxyphenyl binding site into proper position for this ring to fall into place on the protein.[8]

Garland reported that for each tubulin dimer, there was only one tight binding site for colchicine,[10] and the rate of binding was slow. It was again concluded that colchicine induced a conformational change in the tubulin dimer. The optical activity of a portion of the colchicine molecule, related to the tropolonoid configuration of the third ring, disappeared when colchicine was bound to tubulin. These results implied a conformational change in colchicine itself during binding, separate from a change in tubulin.[11]

The role of ring B in colchicine-tubulin binding was studied.[12] A wide variation in structure of the B-ring moiety was tolerated by the colchicine-binding site of tubulin. Even an analogue combining an A ring and a C ring, without significant representation of a B-ring-like structure, was able to inhibit colchicine-tubulin binding considerably.[12]

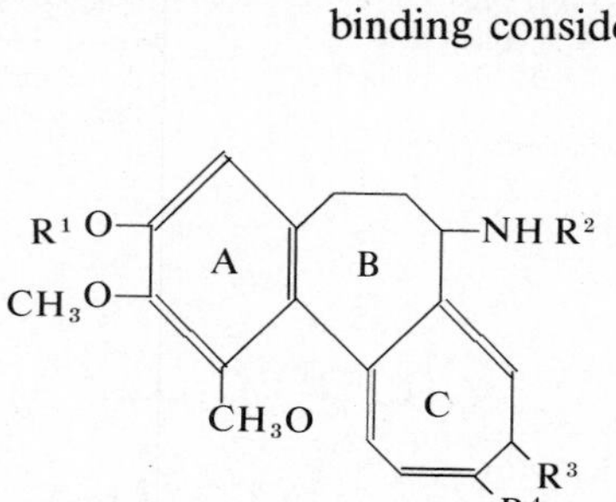


| | $R^1$ | $R^2$ | $R^3$ | $R^4$ |
|---|---|---|---|---|
| Colchicine | $CH_3$ | $COCH_3$ | O | $OCH_3$ |
| Desacetylmethylcolchicine | $CH_3$ | $CH_3$ | O | $OCH_3$ |
| Desacetylthiocolchicine | $CH_3$ | H | O | $SCH_3$ |
| Colchicoside | $C_6H_{11}O_5$ | $COCH_3$ | O | $OCH_3$ |
| Trimethylcolchicinic acid | $CH_3$ | H | O | OH |
| Colchiceine | $CH_3$ | $COCH_3$ | OH | O |

**Figure 57–1.** Central colchicine nucleus.

Possible correlations between the structure of colchicine and of selected analogues, and their effects in the treatment of acute gout in man have been studied.[13,14] The colchicine analogues tested were desacetylmethylcolchicine, desacetylthiocolchicine, colchicoside, trimethylcolchicinic acid and colchiceine. The differences between each of these analogues and colchicine are shown in Figure 57–1. The conclusion of these early studies was that the tropolonoid configuration of the third ring was necessary for colchicine's antigout effect.[13,14] Animal data are less clear.[15-17] There is a significant degree of species variability and much less animal responsiveness to concentrations of colchicine that are effective in the human.[18]

Colchicine is highly sensitive to light. Exposure to sunlight or to ultraviolet light leads to the formation of three photoisomers, $\alpha$, $\beta$, and $\gamma$ lumicolchicine.[19,20] The photoisomers do not retain the tropolonoid structure of colchicine, although the trimethoxyl side chains of ring A persist. The lumicolchicines have not been tested in clinical acute gout, but they did not bind to tubulin[21] and were ineffective in arresting mitosis in metaphase in a variety of tissues.[21-23]

## MECHANISM OF ACTION

Borisy and Taylor first demonstrated that colchicine bound to tubulin, the microtubule subunit protein.[24] This binding interfered with the aggregation of these subunits into microtubules. The formation of a colchicine-tubulin dimer was a prerequisite for the prevention of tubulin aggregation, since free colchicine did not itself detectably inhibit microtubule assembly.[25] A single colchicine-tubulin dimer complex bound to the microtubule assembly end, decreasing the rate of addition of free tubulin dimer. The colchicine-bound tubulin dimers dissociated significantly more slowly than the normal dissociation of tubulin dimers, in effect producing a tight "cap" at the assembly-end of the microtubule.[26] The colchicine binding stabilized a conformational isomer of tubulin. This change in tubulin conformation, after binding to colchicine, may lead both to increased affinity of the colchicine-tubulin complexes for microtubule assembly ends and to decreased affinity of free tubulin for the same assembly ends once the colchicine-tubulin complex is already there.[27]

Malawista[28,29] has presented strong arguments for the position that colchicine's mechanism of action in the treatment of acute gouty inflammation depends upon the effect on microtubules. Polymorphonuclear leukocytes are necessary for the propagation of urate crystal–induced inflammation,[30,31] and they have been shown to contain microtubules, which disappear or diminish on exposure to colchicine.[32] Phagocytosis in human polymorphonuclear cells is accompanied by a rapid assembly of microtubules, followed by disassembly.[33] Colchicine-induced microtubule disassembly is associated with cell membrane alterations in leukocytes and macrophages. The topography of cell membranes in general, as well as membrane receptor mobility, is controlled by the cell cytoskeleton, including microtubules.[33,34] Membrane receptors for phagocytic particles are distributed topographically in a different manner after colchicine therapy than under normal cell circumstances. The precise relation of colchicine-induced membrane alterations to changes in polymorphonuclear leukocyte function is not completely clear. There is little doubt that in polymorphonuclear leukocytes, colchicine's membrane effect is mediated by microtubules.[35-37] The membrane-dependent processes of chemotaxis, phagocytosis, and lysosomal degranulation in neutrophils are all influenced by the cytoskeleton. Microtubules have been assigned the roles of directing molecular reorganization of neutrophil membranes and of providing orientation to gross membrane activities.[37]

There has been some suggestion of a direct colchicine effect on membranes, an effect not involving microtubules.[38,39] Colchicine affected the shape and surface ultrastructure of both human leukocytes and red blood cells in a similar fashion.[40] Since red blood cells do not contain microtubules, the inference was that this membrane effect, even in the leukocyte, did not require microtubules. Other evidence includes the lack of correlation between the inhibitory effect of colchicine on mast cell secretion of histamine and its action on mast cell microtubules,[41] and the differences between colchicine binding by mammalian liver cell nuclear membranes[42] and by their microtubules.[43]

Many leukocyte functions are sensitive to colchicine in vitro,[29] although most of these studies have been carried out at concentrations higher than those achievable in vivo with doses of therapeutic size.[18,44,45] Colchicine has been shown to inhibit lysosomal enzyme release from human polymorphonuclear leukocytes in a dose-related fashion.[46] In patients treated with 0.6 to 1.8 mg per day of colchicine to prevent recurrences of familial Mediterranean fever, neutrophils were capable of normal phagocytosis, produced normal amounts of pyrogen, and migrated normally, both randomly and in response to chemotactic stimuli.[47] Skin window responses were normal for the first 9 hours of study, but at 24 hours the mean number of neutrophils and monocytes was significantly reduced in colchicine-treated patients compared with controls.[47]

Thirteen patients with acute gout were treated with colchicine by mouth, until toxicity, in doses up to 6 mg in 24 hours. Then daily oral doses of 1.8 mg were given for one week. A statistically significant drop in phagocytic capacity and in phagocytic rate was found in comparison to pretreatment values.[48] The disparity in results may represent methodologic differences in these studies.

A variety of studies have demonstrated colchicine effects on polymorphonuclear leukocyte adherence and locomotion.[49-54] In one in vivo human experiment, 5 mg of colchicine given orally over 24 hours induced a reduction in the percentage of neutrophils adherent to nylon fiber columns, and a less marked change in random migration.[49] The daily administration for 8 days of

1 mg of colchicine to volunteers caused reductions in neutrophil chemotaxis within 24 hours of ingestion.[50]

Phagocytosis of urate crystals by human polymorphonuclear leukocytes induced the synthesis and release of an 8400 molecular weight glycoprotein by the cell. The glycoprotein had strong chemotactic activity that was not associated with complement.[51] This chemotactic factor was not a major mediator in other rheumatic diseases. Colchicine decreased both the production and the release by white cells of this urate crystal–associated chemotactic factor. The purified factor itself induced marked joint inflammation, which was not prevented by colchicine. It was suggested that preventing the production and release of the crystal-associated chemotactic factor, after phagocytosis of urate crystals, might explain the quasi-specificity of colchicine in the treatment of acute gout.[51]

Functional studies of migration of leukocytes in a millipore filter system showed that colchicine markedly inhibited directed migration (chemotaxis), had no effect on random migration, and minimally decreased activated random migration.[52] However, studies of leukocyte migration in filters involve a number of cell functions in addition to chemotaxis, including locomotion, orientation, and deformability of the cell. The last factor, deformability, was indirectly evaluated by measuring the effect of colchicine on leukocyte chemotaxis in an agarose system.[53] Deformability played a minor role in agarose, since the leukocytes were not required to squeeze through tortuous spaces as in the filter system. Colchicine in agarose had no effect on polymorphonuclear leukocyte locomotion or chemotaxis,[53] although presumably microtubules were affected. These findings suggested a dissociation between microtubule assembly and polymorphonuclear cell orientation.

In another study, colchicine was found to inhibit chemokinesis rather than chemotaxis;[54] again it was concluded that the integrity of microtubule function was not necessary for cells to discern a concentration gradient or to react with directional motion. Evidence has previously been adduced suggesting a separation between colchicine's effect on tubulin and its ability to interfere with urate crystal-induced inflammation. An analogue, trimethylcolchicinic acid, was effective in the therapy of acute gout in man,[55,56] inhibited the release of lysosomal enzymes on phagocytosis of urate crystals,[57] and interfered with the leukocyte response to a chemotactic stimulus, at least in a filter system,[58] but had no effect on tubulin[59] and was not antimitotic. Desacetamido-colchicine, on the other hand, had greater antimitotic potency than colchicine, but had very little anti-inflammatory effect against urate crystal–induced inflammation.[15]

The phagocytic synoviocyte is involved in the mechanisms of acute inflammation induced in the joint by the urate crystal, as well as the polymorphonuclear leukocyte.[60,61] Colchicine at a concentration of $10^{-7}$ M induced the release of large amounts of prostaglandin E in rat peritoneal macrophages.[62] Colchicine also enhanced prostaglandin synthesis in human synovium,[63] although no direct studies of the effect of colchicine specifically on the phagocytic synovial cell have been reported. Colchicine did not affect phagocytosis in monocytes but did inhibit the release of monocytic lysosomal enzymes during phagocytosis.[64]

## COLCHICINE–cAMP

It was initially suggested that cyclic AMP inhibited and cyclic GMP promoted the assembly of microtubules in leukocytes.[65] Subsequent studies demonstrated that the increased cyclic AMP levels developed as a consequence of microtubule assembly rather than as a cause.[66] Colchicine and other agents that interfere with microtubule assembly caused an increase in human leukocyte cyclic AMP levels.[67] They also potentiated beta-adrenergic and PGE stimulation of cyclic AMP levels. The effect of colchicine was mediated through cytoplasmic microtubules, rather than occurring as a direct effect on cell membranes or on the hormone receptor or on adenylate cyclase activity.[68] It was suggested that the mechanism for the cAMP effects of colchicine might be through a cytoplasmic microtubule influence on the mobility of membrane proteins, enabling an increased frequency of interaction between a hormone-hormone receptor-GTP-binding protein complex and the catalytic moiety of adenylate cyclase. Other observers denied an influence on cell membrane fluidity[69] but invoked a colchicine effect on GTP and GTPase as a possible mechanism for stimulating cAMP production.

There are two GTP-binding sites for each dimer of tubulin. One site is easily exchangeable with free GTP; the second is nonexchangeable, and GTP hydrolysis occurs at the exchangeable site only. Microtubule assembly is followed by the hydrolysis of exchangeable site GTP to GDP.[70] This facilitates depolymerization of the microtubule and permits the tubulin to cycle between dimer and microtubule. The hydrolysis of GTP accompanying microtubular assembly occurred in a kinetic first-order process following assembly, but kinetically uncoupled from it.[71] Colchicine, although it inhibited tubulin polymerization, stimulated GTPase activity of the protein.[71-73] The GTPase activity occurred with the formation of tubulin-colchicine complexes.[73] Tropolone, however, had no effect on GTP hydrolysis; most likely the trimethoxyl-benzene first ring moiety of the colchicine molecule was chiefly responsible for its effect on GTP hydrolysis.[72]

Colchicine also both stimulated the release of prostaglandin E by a variety of cells (see above)[62,63,74] and in turn increased tissue sensitivity and responsiveness to prostaglandin E stimulation.[67,74,75] In the rat jejunum, colchicine caused a marked increase in mucosal $PGE_2$ content, adenylate cyclase activity, and mucosal cAMP.[76] Pretreatment with indomethacin reduced the degree of change in adenylate cyclase.

## COLCHICINE METABOLISM

Two general approaches for measuring colchicine in body fluids and cells have been reported in recent years. Colchicine labeled with $^{14}C$ on the methoxyl group of the third ring was used as a tracer in the first method;[18] the label was therefore within the tropolonoid structure shown to be necessary for colchicine's effect on microtubules[21-23] and for its action in the treatment in acute gout.[13,14] Thin-layer chromatography was used for separation.

The second approach involved radioimmunoassay.[44] Initially colchicine itself was conjugated to bovine serum albumin; the site of conjugation was in the tropolone structure of the third ring. Subsequent radioimmunoassay methods used colchicine analogues;[45,77-79] the binding site for several of these studies was on the amino group side chain of ring B.[45,77,78] The antisera therefore could be expected to have 100 percent cross-reactivity with lumicolchicine.[77] Three derivatives of colchicine have been synthesized and characterized to serve as haptens for the development of radioimmunoassay procedures.[79] The haptens were linked to bovine serum albumin through ring A, ring B, and ring C side chains.

With the use of the $^{14}C$ label,[18] after intravenous administration of 2 mg, the calculated zero-time concentration of colchicine was 1.8 ± 0.7 μg per dl. The apparent volume of distribution for colchicine was much larger than the extracellular volume, averaging 2.19 ± 0.80 liters per kg of body weight. The plasma half-time was only 19.3 ± 7.5 minutes. Excretion did not explain the rapid disappearance or large volume of distribution; clearly colchicine rapidly entered cells.

Radioimmunoassay as a method for measuring colchicine levels was more sensitive than the $^{14}C$ label, thin-layer chromatography approach. Following an intravenous dose of 1 mg, the colchicine levels declined biexponentially, fitting a two-compartment open body model, both in normal humans and in patients with familial Mediterranean fever.[45] A short distribution phase, with a 3- to 5-minute half-time, was followed by a longer elimination phase, with a 65 ± 15 minute half-time.[45] Central and peripheral compartment volumes were 10 to 14 liters and 49.5 to 76 liters. A study by radioimmunoassay after an intravenous dose of 2 mg, and using a single compartment model, found a mean half-time of 58 ± 10 minutes.[44] The calculated zero-time concentration with this method was 2.9 ± 1.5 μg per dl.

Studies of the plasma levels of colchicine after oral administration of 1 mg have also been accomplished.[45,77,80] Peak plasma concentrations, using the $^{14}C$ label, were achieved from 0.5 to 2 hours after oral administration.[80] The mean maximal plasma levels were around 0.2 μg per dl, approximately one-tenth the calculated zero-time concentration achieved after intravenous administration of twice the dose.[18] Similar concentrations, of 0.1 to 0.25 μg per dl,[45] after oral administration of 1 mg were measured in one radioimmunoassay study. Another radioimmunoassay method, however, reported larger peak levels of 0.6 μg per dl.[77]

Circulating leukocytes represent an excellent tissue for measurement of colchicine entry into and concentration within cells. Leukocytes are easily accessible and are necessary for urate crystal–induced inflammation.[30,31] The first study of leukocyte concentrations of colchicine, after intravenous administration of the drug, using measurement by $^{14}C$ label, demonstrated a peak concentration at 10 minutes; stable levels of approximately ten times plasma concentration were maintained for 24 hours.[81] The drop in levels was slow; significant white cell concentrations of colchicine were measurable as late as 10 days after the single dose. White cell concentrations were also studied by radioimmunoassay after intravenous administration of colchicine.[82] The results differed from those obtained with $^{14}C$; white cell concentrations reached plasma levels only at 24 hours but remained higher thereafter. At 96 hours after intravenous administration, the mean white cell concentration was 1.4 μg per dl.

The location of the colchicine gastrointestinal absorption site or sites is not specifically known. The administration of large doses of colchicine orally induces jejunal[83] and ileal dysfunction;[84] absorption therefore most likely occurs in the jejunum and ileum. After absorption, colchicine is carried to the liver. Biliary excretion of colchicine in animals, involving active transport against concentration gradients, has been demonstrated after intravenous administration.[85] Hepatic transport of colchicine is also evidenced by the fact that plasma colchicine levels in patients with severe liver disease were higher than in normals.[18] Enterohepatic recirculation is probable.

Maximal urinary excretion occurred within two hours after intravenous administration of colchicine.[44] Significant measurable amounts of colchicine were found in the urine for periods up to 10 days after a single intravenous dose.[44,81] Late urinary excretion presumably arose from previously cell-bound colchicine. As noted above, leukocyte concentrations of colchicine were still measurable 10 days after a single intravenous dose.[81] Colchicine excretion occurs in the feces as well as in urine but has not yet been quantitated there in humans.

With the use of either $^{14}C$ or radioimmunoassay methods, studies of colchicine metabolism have failed to demonstrate metabolites in plasma, urine, or cells.[18,44,80,81] In an in vitro system simulating the oxidative reactions of liver microsomes, colchicine was converted to four metabolic products, primarily involving oxidative monodemethylation.[86] In vitro metabolism of colchicine by mammalian liver microsomes has been shown, again by monodemethylation.[87] It is not clear why metabolites, if they do occur in vivo, have not been identified.

## TOXICOLOGY

Approximately 80 percent of patients receiving a full therapeutic course of colchicine by mouth in the treatment of acute gout develop hyperperistalsis, abdominal cramping pain, diarrhea, and nausea or vomiting. In the process of transport across the jejunal and ileal mucosal cell membrane, enough colchicine must bind to microtubules in these cells to alter function and produce symptoms. In human volunteers receiving colchicine by mouth in doses ranging from 1.9 to 3.6 mg per day, for periods ranging from 4 days to 3 weeks,[83,84,88-90] all developed jejunal and ileal dysfunction. Jejunal effects included decreased absorption of D-xylose[83] and a fall in serum carotene levels.[90] Reduced jejunal mucosal lactase and sucrase activity was noted.[83] Histologic studies on jejunal mucosa during colchicine therapy revealed edema and round cell infiltration in 3 of 5 patients.[83] In the rat, colchicine stimulated jejunal adenylate cyclase activity, and significantly increased mucosal cAMP content.[76] Colchicine also induced increases in prostaglandin $E_2$, which in turn mediated increases in intestinal fluid volume.[76]

Ileal effects in human volunteers were manifested by decreased vitamin $B_{12}$ absorption, increased excretion of fecal bile acids and sterols, most likely due to impaired reabsorption of acidic and neutral sterols in the distal ileum, and a consequent drop in serum cholesterol.[88-90] There were marked and consistent increases in fecal sodium and potassium and less marked increases in fecal nitrogen.

A single report of azoospermia in a patient on colchicine prophylactic therapy has been recorded.[91] A number of other studies, however, have revealed no effects on sperm counts, luteinizing hormone, follicle-stimulating hormone, testosterone, or prolactin levels induced in patients receiving prophylactic doses of colchicine.[92-94]

Colchicine overdoses, whether therapeutic[95] or suicidal,[96] can lead to more severe and more general toxic manifestations. The gastrointestinal side effects described above, when more profound, can cause severe dehydration, hypokalemia, hyponatremia, metabolic acidosis, renal shutdown, and death. Shock can be due to profound dehydration or to septicemia secondary to severe intestinal wall damage. Death has occurred after doses as small as 7 mg[97] or 10 mg[98] given in 4 or 5 days. Death is invariable after fairly rapid ingestion of more than 40 mg.[96] The risks of toxicity are greater in patients with chronic liver or kidney disease, because both organs are excretory pathways for colchicine.[18]

In colchicine overdose, the earliest hematologic manifestation of colchicine toxicity is disseminated intravascular coagulation;[99] the most severe changes occur at about 25 hours after the ingestion of a single, large suicidal dose. Marrow failure, characterized by leukopenia, thrombocytopenia, and bleeding, reaches its peak at about the fifth day.[99] Other toxic manifestations of colchicine overdose include hepatocellular failure and late central nervous system dysfunction, with seizures and loss of deep tendon reflexes.[96]

In a review of the use of colchicine as a suicidal drug, 28 of 36 patients were female.[100] When the ages were known, two thirds were under 20; the mean age was 23 $\pm$ 8. Taking of colchicine was generally impulsive and not designed to result in death. The choice of drug was considered a blatant gesture of getting even with the male parent.

Treatment of colchicine overdose is symptomatic, including gastric lavage if the patient is seen early enough after ingestion. Subsequent therapy is directed at the various manifestations of toxicity. Dehydration, electrolyte imbalance, metabolic acidosis, and shock must be corrected, infection eliminated, and seizures controlled. The patient must be supported during disseminated intravascular coagulation and marrow failure.

Attempts at hemodialysis and exchange transfusion have failed.[101] Since so little colchicine is present in blood,[18,44] dialysis and exchange transfusions would not be expected to be useful procedures. Some method for accelerating colchicine release from microtubules and from cells would be necessary first, without cell death, before approaches for removing colchicine from the blood could be of value.

## References


1. Hartung, E.F.: History of the use of colchicum and related medicaments in gout. Ann. Rheum. Dis. 13:190, 1954.
2. Culpeper, N.: Pharmacopoiea Londonensis or the London Dispensatory. 6th Ed. London, Peter Cole, 1654, p. 4.
3. Wallace, S.L.: Colchicum, the panacea. Bull. N.Y. Acad. Med. 40:130, 1973.
4. Copeman, W.S.C.: A Short History of the Gout and the Rheumatic Diseases. Berkeley-Los Angeles, University of California Press, 1964.
5. Pelletier, P.S., and Caventou, J.B.: Examen chimique de plusiers végétaux de la famille des colchicées et du principe actif qu'ils renferment. Ann. Chim. Phys. 14:69, 1820.
6. Dewar, M.J.S.: Structure of colchicine. Nature 155:141, 1945.
7. Margulies, T.N.: Structure of the mitotic spindle inhibitor Colcemid. *N*-desacetyl-*N*-methylcolchicine. J. Am. Chem. Soc. 96:899, 1974.
8. Andreu, J.M. and Timasheff, S.N. Interaction of tubulin with single ring analogues of colchicine. Biochemistry 21:534, 1982.
9. Cortese, F., Bhattacharayya, B., and Wolff, J.: Podophyllotoxin as a probe for the colchicine-binding site of tubulin. J. Biol. Chem. 252:1134, 1977.
10. Garland, D.L.: Kinetics and mechanism of colchicine binding to tubulin: Evidence for ligand-induced conformational change. Biochemistry 17:4266, 1978.
11. Detrich, H.W., Williams, R.C., MacDonald, T.L., Wilson, L., and Puett, D.: Changes in the circular dichroic spectrum of colchicine associated with its binding to tubulin. Biochemistry 20:5999, 1981.
12. Ray, K., Bhattacharayya, B., and Biswas, B.B.: Role of B-ring of colchicine in its binding to tubulin. J. Biol. Chem. 256:6241, 1981.
13. Wallace, S.L.: Colchicine analogues in the treatment of acute gout. Arthritis. Rheum. 2:389, 1959.
14. Wallace, S.L.: Colchicine: Clinical pharmacology in acute gouty arthritis. Am. J. Med. 30:439, 1961.
15. Fitzgerald, T.J., Williams, B., and Uyeki, E.: Colchicine on sodium urate-induced paw swelling in mice: Structure-activity relationships of colchicine derivatives. Proc. Soc. Exp. Biol. Med. 136:115, 1971.
16. Zweig, M.H., Maling, H.M., and Webster, M.E.: Inhibition of sodium urate rat hind paw edema by colchicine derivatives. Correlation with antimitotic activity. J. Pharmacol. Exp. Ther. 182:344, 1972.
17. Chang, Y.H., and Malawista, S.E.: Mechanisms of action of colchicine IV. Failure of non-leukopenic doses of colchicine to suppress urate crystal-induced canine joint inflammation. Inflammation 1:143, 1976.
18. Wallace, S.L., Omokoku, B., and Ertel, N.H.: Colchicine plasma levels: Implications as to pharmacology and mechanisms of action. Am. J. Med. 48:443, 1970.
19. Grewe, L., and Wolfe, W.: Unwandlung des Colchizins durch Sonnenlicht. Chem. Ber. 84:621, 1951.
20. Wilson, L., and Friedkin, M.: The biochemical events of mitosis. I. Synthesis and properties of colchicine labelled with tritium in its acetyl moiety. Biochemistry 5:2463, 1966.
21. Wilson, L., and Friedkin, M.: The biochemical events of mitosis. II. The in vivo and in vitro binding of colchicine in grasshopper embryos and its possible relation to the inhibition of mitosis. Biochemistry 6:3126, 1967.

22. Sagorin, C., Ertel, N.H., and Wallace, S.L.: Photoisomerization of colchicine. Loss of significant antimitotic activity in tissue culture. Arthritis. Rheum. 15:213, 1972.
23. Linskens, H.F., and Wulf, W.: Uber die Trennung und Mitosewirkung der Lumicolchicine. Naturwissenschaften 40:487, 1953.
24. Borisy, G.G., and Taylor, E.W.: The mechanism of action of colchicine. Binding of colchicine-$H^3$ to cellular protein. J. Cell Biol. 34:525, 1967.
25. Farrell, K.W., and Wilson, L.: Proposed mechanism for colchicine poisoning of microtubules reassembled in vitro from *Strongylocentrotus purpuratus* sperm tail outer doublet tubulin. Biochemistry 19:3048, 1980.
26. Margolis, R.L., Rauch, C.T., and Wilson, L.: Mechanism of colchicine-dimer addition to microtubule ends: Implications for the microtubule polymerization mechanism. Biochemistry 19:5550, 1980.
27. Detrich, H.W., Williams, R.C., and Wilson, K.: Effect of colchicine binding on the reversible dissociation of the tubulin dimer. Biochemistry 21:2392, 1982.
28. Malawista, S.E.: Colchicine: A common mechanism for its anti-inflammatory and antimitotic effect. Arthritis Rheum. 11:191, 1968.
29. Malawista, S.E.: The action of colchicine in acute gouty arthritis. Arthritis Rheum. 18:835, 1975.
30. Phelps, P., and McCarty, D.J.: Crystal induced inflammation in canine joints. II. Importance of the polymorphonuclear leukocytes. J. Exp. Med. 124:115, 1966.
31. Chang, Y.H., and Gralla, E.J.: Suppression of urate crystal–induced canine joint inflammation by heterologous anti-polymorphonuclear leukocyte serum. Arthritis Rheum. 11:145, 1968.
32. Malawista, S.E., and Bensch, K.G.: Human polymorphonuclear leukocytes: Demonstration of microtubules and effect of colchicine. Science 156:521, 1967.
33. Walter, R.J., Berlin, R.D., Pfeiffer, J.R., and Oliver, J.M.: Polarization of endocytosis and receptor topography in cultured macrophages. J. Cell Biol. 86:199, 1980.
34. Devirgilius, L.C., Dini, L., Stefanini, S., and Autori, F.: Cytoskeletal control of concavalin A receptor mobility in isolated rat hepatocytes. Cell. Mol. Biol. 26:533, 1980.
35. Becker, J.S., Oliver, J.M, and Berlin, R.D.: Fluorescence techniques for following interactions of microtubules and membranes. Nature 254:152, 1975.
36. Berlin, R.D., and Fera, J.P.: Changes in membrane microviscosity associated with phagocytosis: Effects of colchicine. Proc. Soc. Natl. Acad. Sci. 74:1072, 1977.
37. Oliver, J.M.: Cell biology of leukocyte abnormalities—membrane and cystoskeletal function in normal and defective cells. Am. J. Pathol. 93:221, 1978.
38. Alstiel, L.D., and Landsberger, F.R.: Interaction of colchicine with phosphatidylcholine membranes. Nature 269:70, 1977.
39. Wunderlich, F., Muller, R., and Speth, V.: Direct evidence for a colchicine-induced impairment in the mobility of membrane component. Science 182:1136, 1973.
40. Lichtman, M.A., Santillo, P.A., Kearney, E.A., Roberts, G.W., and Weed, R.I.: The shape and surface morphology of human leukocytes in vitro. Effects of temperature, metabolic inhibitors and agents that influence membrane structure. Blood Cells 2:507, 1976.
41. Lagunoff, D., and Chi, E.Y.: Effect of colchicine on rat mast cells. J. Cell. Biol. 71:182, 1976.
42. Stadler, J., and Franke, W.W.: Characterization of colchicine binding of membrane fractions from rat and mouse liver. J. Cell. Biol. 60:297, 1974.
43. Stadler, J., and Franke, W.W.: Colchicine binding proteins in chromatin and membranes. Nature New Biol. 237:237, 1972.
44. Ertel, N.H., Mittler, J.C., Akgun, S., and Wallace, S.L.: A radioimmunoassay for colchicine in plasma and urine. Science 193:233, 1976.
45. Halkin, H., Dany, S., Greenwald, M., Shnaps, Y., and Tirosh, M.: Colchicine kinetics in patients with familial Mediterranean fever. Clin. Pharm. Ther. 28:82, 1980.
46. Hoffstein, S., Goldstein, I.M., and Weissmann, G.: Role of microtubule assembly in lysosomal enzyme secretion from human polymorphonuclear leukocytes. J. Cell. Biol. 73:242, 1977.
47. Dinarello, C.A., Chusid M.J., Fauci, A.S., Gallin, J.I., Dale, D.C., and Wolff, S.M. Effect of prophylactic colchicine on leukocyte function in patients with familial Mediterranean fever. Arthritis Rheum. 19:618, 1976.
48. Dalleverde, E., Fan, P.T., and Chang, Y-H.: Mechanism of action of colchicine V. Neutrophil adherence and phagocytosis in patients with acute gout treated with colchicine. J. Pharmacol. Exp. Ther. 223:197, 1982.
49. Fordham, J.N., Kirwan, J., Cason, J., and Currey, H.L.F.: Prolonged reduction in polymorphonuclear adhesion following oral colchicine. Ann. Rheum. Dis. 40:605, 1981.
50. Ehrenfeld, M., Levy, M., Bar Eli, M., Gallily, R., and Eliakim, M.: Effect of colchicine on polymorphonuclear leukocyte chemotaxis in human volunteers. Br. J. Clin. Pharmacol. 10:297, 1980.
51. Spilberg, I., Mandell, B., Mehta, J., Simchowitz, L., and Rosenberg, D.: Mechanism of action of colchicine in acute crystal-induced arthritis. J. Clin. Invest. 64:775, 1979.
52. Malech, H.L., Root, R.K., and Gallin, J.I.: Structural analysis of human neutrophil migration. J. Cell. Biol. 75:666, 1977.
53. Daughaday, C.C., Bohrer, A.N., and Spilberg, I.: Lack of effect of colchicine on human neutrophil chemotaxis under agarose. Experientia 137:199, 1981.
54. Valerius, N.H.: In vitro effect of colchicine on neutrophil granulocyte locomotion. Acta Path. Microbiol. Scand. 86B:149, 1978.
55. Wallace, S.L.: Trimethylcolchicinic acid in the treatment of acute gout. Ann. Intern. Med. 54:274, 1961.
56. Smyth, C.J., and Frank, L.S.: Treatment of acute gouty arthritis. Rheumatism 18:2, 1962.
57. Mikulikova, D., and Trnavsky, K.: Influence of colchicine derivatives on lysosomal enzyme release from polymorphonuclear leukocytes. Biochem. Pharmacol. 29:2146, 1980.
58. Phelps, P., and McCarty, D.J.: Crystal-induced arthritis. Postgrad. Med. 45:87, 1969.
59. Mizel, S.B., and Wilson, L.: Nucleoside transport in mammalian cells: inhibition by colchicine. Biochemistry 11:2573, 1972.
60. Agudelo, C.A., and Schumacher, H.R.: The synovitis of acute gouty arthritis: a light and electron microscopic study. Hum. Pathol. 4:265, 1973.
61. Ortel, R.W., and Newcombe, D.S.: Acute gouty arthritis and response to colchicine in the virtual absence of synovial fluid leukocytes. N. Engl. J. Med. 290:1363, 1974.
62. Gemsa, D., Kramer, W., Brenner, M., Tell, G., and Resch, K.: Induction of prostaglandin E. release from macrophages by colchicine. J. Immunol. 124:376, 1980.
63. Robinson, D.R., Smith, H., and Levine, L.: Prostaglandin synthesis by human synovial cultures and its stimulation by colchicine. Arthritis Rheum. 16:129, 1973.
64. Fleer, A., van Schark, M.L.J., Kr, A.E.G., and Engelfriet, C.P.: Destruction of sensitized erythrocytes by human monocytes in vitro: Effects of cytochalasin B., hydrocortisone and colchicine. Scand. J. Immunol. 8:515, 1978.
65. Weissmann, G., Goldstein, I., Hoffstein, S., and Tsung, P.K.: Reciprocal effects of cAMP and cGMP on microtubule-dependent release of lysosomal enzymes. Ann. N.Y. Acad. Sci. 253:750, 1975.
66. Malawista, S.E., Oliver, J.M., and Rudolph, S.A.: Microtubules and cyclic AMP in human leukocytes: on the order of things. J. Cell. Biol. 77:881, 1978.
67. Rudolph, S.A., Greengard, P., and Malawista, S.E.: Effects of colchicine on cyclic AMP levels in human leukocytes. Proc. Nat'l Acad. Sci. 74:3404, 1977.
68. Rudolph, S.A., Hegstrand, L.R., Greengard, P., and Malawista, S.E.: The interaction of colchicine with hormone sensitive adenylate cyclase in human leukocytes. Mol. Pharmacol. 16:805, 1979.
69. Hagmann, J., and Fishman, P.H.: Modulation of adenylate cyclase in intact macrophages by microtubules. J. Biol. Chem. 255:2659, 1980.
70. Timasheff, S.N., and Grisham, L.M.: In vitro assembly of cytoplasmic microtubules. Ann. Rev. Biochem. 49:565, 1980.
71. Hensel, C., and Carlier, M.F.: GTPase activity of the tubulin-colchicine in relation with tubulin-tubulin interactions. Biochem. Biophys. Res. Comm. 103:332, 1981.
72. Lin, C.M., and Hamel, E.: Effects of inhibitors of tubulin polymerization on GTP hydrolysis. J. Biol. Chem. 256:9242, 1981.
73. David-Pfeuty, T., Simon, C., and Pantaloni, D.: Effect of antimitotic drugs on tubulin GTPase activity and self-assembly. J. Biol. Chem. 254:11696, 1979.
74. Burch, R.M., and Halushka, P.V.: Inhibition of prostaglandin synthesis antagonizes the colchicine-induced reduction of vasopressin-stimulated water flow in the toad urinary bladder. Mol. Pharmacol. 21:142, 1982.
75. Gemsa, D., Steggemann, L., Till, G., and Resch, K.: Enhancement of PGE response of macrophages by colchicine. J. Immunol. 119:524, 1977.
76. Rachmilewitz, D., and Karmeli, F.: Effect of colchicine on jejunal adenylate cyclase activity, $PGE_2$ and cAMP contents. Eur. J. Pharmacol. 67:235, 1980.
77. Scherrmann, J.M., Boudet, L., Pontikis, R., Nguyen-Hong-Nam, and Fournier, E.: A sensitive radioimmunoassay for colchicine. J. Pharm. Pharmacol. 32:800, 1980.
78. Wolff, J., Capraro, H.G., Brossi, A., and Cook, G.H.: Colchicine binding to antibodies. J. Biol. Chem. 255:7144, 1980.
79. Pontikis, R., Scherrmann, J.M., Nguyen-Hong-Nam, Boudet, L., and Pichat, L.: Radioimmunoassay for colchicine: Synthesis and properties of three haptens. J. Immunoassay 1:449, 1980.
80. Wallace, S.L., and Ertel, N.H.: Plasma levels of colchicine after oral administration of a single dose. Metabolism 22:749, 1973.

81. Ertel, N.H., and Wallace, S.L.: Measurement of colchicine in urine and peripheral leukocytes. Clin. Res. 19:348, 1971.
82. Ertel, N.H.: Unpublished data.
83. Race, T.F., Paes, I.C., and Faloon, W.W.: Intestinal malabsorption induced by colchicine. Am. J. Med. Sci. 259:32, 1970.
84. Webb, D.I., Chodos, R.B., Maher, C.Q., and Faloon, W.W.: Mechanism of Vitamin B-12 malabsorption in patients receiving colchicine. N. Engl. J. Med. 279:845, 1968.
85. Hunter, A.L., and Klassen, C.D.: Biliary excretion of colchicine. J. Pharmacol. Exp. Ther. 192:605, 1975.
86. Schoenharting, M., Pfaender, P., Ricker, A., and Siebert, G. The metabolic transformation of colchicine. I. The oxidative formation of products from colchicine in the Udenfriend system. Hoppe-Seyler's Z. Physiol. Chem. 354:421, 1973.
87. Schoenharting, M., Mende, G., and Siebert, G.: The metabolic transformation of colchicine. II. The metabolism of colchicine by mammalian liver microsomes. Hoppe-Seyler's Z. Physiol. Chem. 355:1391, 1974.
88. Faloon, W.W., Webb, D.I., and Race, T.F.: Cholesterol-lowering effect of colchicine. Ann. Intern. Med. 66:1058, 1966.
89. Faloon, W.W.: Drug production of intestinal malabsorption. N.Y. State J. Med. 70:2189, 1970.
90. Rubulis, A., Rubert, M., and Faloon, W.W.: Cholesterol lowering, fecal bile and sterol changes during neomycin and colchicine. J. Clin. Nutr. 23:125, 1970.
91. Merlin, H.E.: Azoospermia caused by colchicine. Fertil. Steril. 23:180, 1972.
92. Bremmer, W.J., and Paulsen, C.A.: Colchicine and testicular function in man. New Engl. J. Med. 294:1384, 1976.
93. Levy, M., and Yaffe, C.: Testicular function in patients with familial Mediterranean fever on long term colchicine therapy. Fertil. Steril. 29:667, 1978.
94. Fukutani, K., Ishida, H., Shinohara, M., Minowada, S., Niijima, T., Hijkata, K., and Izowa, Y.: Suppression of spermatogenesis in patients with Behçet's disease treated with cyclophosphamide and colchicine. Fertil. Steril. 36:76, 1981.
95. Stennerman, G.N., and Hayashi, T.: Colchicine intoxication: A reappraisal of its pathology based on a study of three fatal cases. Hum. Pathol. 2:321, 1971.
96. Gaultier, M., Kaufer, A., Bismuth, C., Crabie, P., and Fregaville, J.-P.: Données actuelles sur l'intoxication aiguë par la colchicine. Ann Med. Interne. 12:605, 1969.
97. McLeod, J.G., and Phillips, L.: Hypersensitivity to colchicine. Ann. Rheum. Dis. 6:224, 1947.
98. Liu, Y.K., Hymovitz, R., and Carroll, M.G.: Marrow aplasia induced by colchicine. Arthritis Rheum. 21:731, 1978.
99. Crabie, P., Pollet, J., and Pebay-Peysoula, F.: Étude de l'hémostase au cours des intoxications aiguës par la colchicine. Eur. J. Toxicol. 3:373, 1970.
100. Baum, J., and Meyerowitz, S.: Colchicine: Its use as a suicidal drug by females. J. Rheumatol. 7:124, 1980.
101. Ellwood, M.G., and Robb, G.H.: Self-poisoning with colchicine. Postgrad. Med. J. 47:129, 1971.

# Section V
# Rheumatoid Arthritis

## Chapter 58
## The Etiology of Rheumatoid Arthritis

*J. Claude Bennett*

### INTRODUCTION

Over the past two and a half decades much information has accrued regarding the nature of the inflammatory process and its interface with the immune system. Our views of how the immune response is activated, the nature of its molecular genetic regulation, and how it becomes expressed at the level of effector events have provided better insights into the nature of the rheumatic diseases. Even though there are indications that rheumatoid arthritis is an autoimmune disorder, in the sense that it involves antibodies against autologous immunoglobulin G, there are no solid data from which to infer that this has occurred de novo. On the contrary, there is much data indicating that some initiating event, such as a specific external etiologic agent, is responsible for setting the disease process in motion.

In considering disease phenomena associated with autoimmunity it is important to distinguish between states that are directly mediated by this process and those in which autoantibodies can be demonstrated but whose pathologic effects are unproved. Thrombocytopenic purpura and hemolytic anemia are situations in which there seems to be a true autoimmunity, with antibodies directed at the target cells,[1] leading to their destruction in the peripheral blood. In contrast, occurrence of rheumatoid factors in rheumatoid arthritis, antinuclear antibodies in a variety of connective tissue diseases, and antithyroid antibodies in many patients with diverse conditions are all associated with no obvious specific target pathology. In most of these situations it remains uncertain as to whether the apparent autoimmunity results from the acquisition of some new antigen from an external stimulus or from some primary abnormality in the regulation of the cells that mediate these reactions.[2]

Although the concept of "forbidden clones," as originally expounded by Burnet,[3] dominated our thinking for a while relative to autoimmunity, we came to believe that some kind of alteration of the immunoregulatory system must be at fault in certain of these autoimmune processes. This may be viewed as involving, for example, alteration of the control mechanisms in such a way that the appropriate balance between immunologic "help" and "suppression" is disrupted.[4] Other levels of immunoregulation apparently are influenced by such things as anti-idiotypic antibodies, as was proposed by Jerne in his "network hypothesis."[5] In this latter concept, antibody itself acts in a manner of continuing regulation so that anti-antibodies from one clone act on the preceding clone to regulate its response. Such intricate regulatory mechanisms are of primary importance for keeping the immune system in smooth operating order. Absence of such regulation conceivably could allow an imbalance, permitting the initiation of an autoimmune process with clinical consequences.

Recently it has been suggested[6] that certain individuals are genetically predisposed to particular autoimmune diseases because they have "preforbidden" clones which may diversify into "forbidden" clones by somatic modification events of the immunoglobulin genome. The obvious prerequisite for such a sequence of events would be that preforbidden clones must have paratopes (receptors for antigen) that are within a few mutational changes of self-reactivity. Observations that certain people and particular animal strains are genetically predisposed to particular autoimmune disorders are compatible with this concept.[7]

On the other hand, examples can be found in which specific external agents seem to initiate an inflammatory arthritis that in many respects parallels true rheumatoid disease. It, therefore, seems logical to assume that an initiating agent activates an immune response in a host of appropriate genetic makeup and that the resultant inflammation leads to continual disease activity. It will be the purpose of this chapter to discuss those etiologic agents that have been studied, or for which model systems exist, in relation to rheumatoid arthritis. Although investigations in the general areas of bacteriology, virology, and immunology have contributed enormously to our understanding of inflammatory disease and host responses, the specific documentation of the etiologic agent in rheumatoid arthritis has proved disappointing. Even though the issue of the events responsible for the initiation of a chronic unrelenting arthritis of the rheumatoid type will be the emphasis of this chapter, other diseases will be discussed occasionally for illustrative purposes.

Perspective on this problem of etiology of rheumatoid arthritis is aided by categorization of the various infectious agents that can be involved in the pathogenesis of arthritis. Pyogenic bacteria, mycobacteria, certain fungi, and certain viruses, such as smallpox, are classic examples of multiplication of the agent directly within the joint space. The second situation is one in which the infectious agent localizes in the joint space and initiates the immune response. Examples of this include Lyme disease,[8] *Mycoplasma hyorhinis* in swine,[8] rubella in man,[10] herpes simplex in rabbits and guinea pigs, and certain organisms that might exist within immune complexes, such as hepatitis B virus[11] or the meningococcus.[12] Among those infections in which the agent is at a distant site but there is an associated immune response that causes arthritis is rheumatic fever, in which cross-reacting streptococcal antigens initiate an autoimmune response. Certain other disorders in which there may be an antecedent infection include those in which we find a Reiter-like syndrome[13] following *Shigella, Salmonella, Yersinia enterocolitica,* or other infections of the gastrointestinal tract. The fourth category represents those arthritides in which there is a toxicogenic process. These are best exemplified by certain of the arbovirus infections, in which there is a direct virus effect on the synovial tissue. Examples of these are chikungunya, O'-nyong-nyong, Mayaro, and Ross River.[14]

The important concept to recognize is that a whole variety of organisms and/or their products may be responsible for initiating an arthritis, if even through multiple and differing mechanisms. When the scope of processes that can be associated with infection and arthritis is realized, one becomes aware of the extraordinary difficulties involved in evaluating the possible etiology of rheumatoid arthritis from this standpoint. It may be that the way in which the host responds to an external agent is of the greatest importance in deciphering *which* events initiate the pathogenic process in *which* individuals.

## THE LINK TO GENETICALLY CONTROLLED HOST RESPONSE FACTORS

No relationship is more basic to medicine than that which exists between the inciting agent of disease and the disease susceptibility of the host. Recent discoveries of the relationship of histocompatibility markers to the epidemiology of certain diseases have indicated a strong genetic relationship of these cell-surface molecules to apparent disease susceptibility. The associated molecules include those that are coded for by the major histocompatibility complex (MHC) located on the sixth chromosome.[15] They are specific glycoprotein molecules[16] whose presence as alloantigens has come to be associated strongly with certain rheumatic diseases. These associations are quite striking between HLA-B27 and ankylosing spondylitis, as well as with certain related diseases, including Reiter's syndrome and reactive arthritides.

Studies of the association of specific clinical subsets with the genetic markers coded for by genes within the MHC region have contributed to our knowledge of rheumatoid disease in general. Recent reports suggest that patient response to specific forms of therapy may be related to an individual's genetic make-up, such as the observation that patients with rheumatoid arthritis manifesting toxic responses to chrysotherapy exhibit a significant increase in the HLA-DR3 phenotype.[17] There is also evidence that DR4-positive individuals with seropositive arthritis have a more aggressive form of disease than patients who are DR4 negative. Other studies serve to clarify the relationship of clinical subsets common to different ethnic groups and may provide clues to the level of homogeneity that may exist between these various disease categories and the ethnic groups from which they are derived. Examples for this can be found in recent reports suggesting that blacks with seropositive RA exhibit the same associations with DR4 as are found in whites with seropositive RA.[18] It should be noted that the recent description of new MHC genetic loci, such as the SB locus, which codes for 5 polymorphisms,[19] adds to our repertoire of genetic probes.

The current notion is that the genes coding for the HLA-D or HLA-DR are in fact analogous to the immune response (Ir) genes in the murine major histocompatibility complex and code for some immune response antigens.[20] These relationships are of importance in that all patients who have ankylosing spondylitis are not B27 positive; it is also obvious that all patients who are B27 positive do not have ankylosing spondylitis. It follows then that the B27 marker itself does not cause disease, but rather alerts us to those factors or MHC determinants, such as Ir gene products on the cell surface, that might be more specifically related to the direct disease response and, hence, be a more faithful indication of disease susceptibility.

These observations encourage extensive studies at the epidemiologic level in order to better define host populations at risk and to evaluate familial associations in terms of specific genetic markers relative to expression of disease. Certainly, a combination of appropriate clinical, epidemiologic, and immunogenetic studies is necessary in order to define all these relationships at a population level.

## IMMUNE COMPLEXES AND INDUCTION OF THE INFLAMMATORY PROCESS

Although the concept of immune complexes and the inflammatory process in general are the subject of other chapters, it is essential that certain correlations be made here in order that the implications for microbial agents in the etiology of rheumatoid arthritis might be apparent. It seems clear that immune complexes, whether produced in vivo or produced in vitro and injected into animals, can initiate an inflammatory process.[21] Several models exist to document this phenomenon in arthritis.[22] Immune complexes of various sizes and differing immunochemical properties can exist at different times in a given immune response, owing to simple relationships in the molecular parameters of the antigen (its size and valency) and antibody (its amount relative to antigen present in vivo at any time). Inflammation also depends upon the ability of these complexes to fix the first component of complement in order to initiate the complement cascade. It is important in this regard to recognize that our various techniques for detecting immune complexes, including the Raji cell assay, C1q-binding, and rheumatoid factor binding, may measure different kinds of complexes, as judged by the fact that results are not always parallel in all these systems.

In rheumatoid arthritis one cannot overemphasize the extraordinary correlation of antiglobulins (rheumatoid factors) with the presence of the disease.[23] What makes these antiglobulins form? Are they genuine antibodies against autologous 7S IgG? How are rheumatoid factors formed in relation to altered autologous immunoglobulins, and what is the alteration process? These kinds of relationships and questions must be accounted for within any etiologic mechanism that emerges for rheumatoid arthritis.

## ORGANISMS IMPLICATED IN THE INITIATION OF THE RHEUMATOID PROCESS

**Bacteria.** Consideration of the potential infectious etiology of rheumatoid arthritis from the standpoint of modern bacteriology poses some difficulty in the strict application of Koch's postulates. The confusion results from the multiplicity of organisms that have been implicated from time to time in the rheumatic disorders. Although much evidence can be brought to bear to indicate that known microbial infections may be followed by polyarthritis and multisystem rheumatic disease in both animals and man, it is difficult to analyze such a course of events when dealing with human rheumatoid disease. Clearly, what is needed more than anything else in this area of investigation is the application of the tools of molecular microbiology to the problem of how host cells interact with microbes and their components. Such an approach could provide an understanding of how these agents give rise to an unrelenting, yet waxing and waning, course of inflammation.

Although the history of research in the human rheumatic diseases is interlaced with the development of streptococcal microbiology, data confirming that this organism actually initiates inflammatory arthritis as the sole etiologic agent exist only in the case of rheumatic fever.[24] It was this distinction that separated rheumatoid arthritis from "infectious arthritis."[25] The magnificent investigations on rheumatic fever and its relationship to the *Streptococcus* and streptococcal antigens represent landmark achievements in the history of medicine. At present there is no evidence that human rheumatoid disease is initiated by *Streptococcus.*

Clostridia have been implicated from the studies of Mansson and Olhagen.[26] These researchers have observed that cultivation of feces reveals a high frequency of atypical *Clostridium perfringens* in rheumatoid arthritis and certain other chronic inflammatory rheumatic diseases. The abnormalities that they have noticed include a high count of *Clostridium perfringens,* i.e., more than 100,000 bacteria per gram of feces, and/or a potent alpha toxin production. Clostridia in normal individuals are present in very small numbers in the colon, but in conjunction with certain arthritides they become numerous and they have been observed even extending into the upper jejunum. In these studies, for example, 67 percent of patients with rheumatoid arthritis have abnormal intestinal flora, as indicated by the aforementioned assays. This compares with only 0.9 percent in healthy controls. It is of some significance that these studies have led them to carry out certain experiments involving dietary changes in pigs,[27] so that a change in bacterial flora resulted. This had the secondary effect of producing arthritis in these animals. The postulated mechanism is that a protein-rich diet produced a disturbance in secretory functions of the digestive tract so that clostridial overgrowth could take place. They suggest that this contributes to the development of a rheumatoid-like arthritis in these animals.

Stewart and his colleagues have drawn attention to the possible role that diphtheroid organisms might play in rheumatoid arthritis. They have found that approximately 28 percent of synovial membranes and 10 percent of synovial fluids from patients with rheumatoid arthritis yield diphtheroids.[28] These studies were performed using careful bacteriologic cultural techniques and appropriate controls; the observed differences between the patients with rheumatoid arthritis and the controls seem real. Further, there seems to be a serologic response in terms of agglutination titers to corynebacteria in the rheumatoid patients as compared to normals. These studies face many problems of interpretation in that diphtheroids are widely distributed in nature; they are notoriously difficult to isolate and identify by conventional methods; and they are frequently present as "contaminants" in many microbial cultures. Further, the serologic responses by no means parallel infectivity. Nevertheless, the data are indicative of some association, and it may be that diphtheroids do play a role in rheumatoid arthritis,[29] if only in some way to modify the immune mechanisms of the host. It could be that even if they do not cause rheumatoid arthritis, they might perhaps play some role in modulating its course.

Mycoplasmas have been the target of considerable discussion and investigative pursuit as related to the pathogenesis of rheumatoid arthritis and other arthritides.[30] Several groups of investigators reported the isolation of mycoplasma from both joint fluid and synovial tissues of patients with rheumatoid arthritis. In general, these reports have not been substantiated by results from other laboratories,[31] but interest in the agents continues, in view of the very striking association of animal mycoplasmal diseases with arthritis. Sometimes a close similarity is found between mycoplasma-caused arthritis in animals and rheumatoid arthritis in man. Although clinical evidence for the isolation of a mycoplasma organism in rheumatoid arthritis is very slim, this may be due to difficulties in the cultivation procedures and technical reproducibility. Perhaps these obstacles will be overcome in the future with new approaches to antigen detection and new techniques that will involve a search for the presence of mycoplasma genomes using the probes of molecular biology.[32,33]

Of particular interest to the field of mycoplasmology are investigations into the mode of pathogenicity of chronic infections. Recent work in this area would suggest that these organisms have the ability to associate very closely with the cells of the host organism. The intimate relationship developed by mycoplasma for the host cells is revealed by electron microscopy, and shows a bridging between the organism and the surface of the host lymphoid cells.[34] It has now been shown that mycoplasma adsorbs onto its own surface antigens from mammalian host cells.[35] These include histocompatibility markers of the mammalian cell, as well as certain unique T-lymphocyte antigens. This phenomenon may have its explanation in the fact that the mycoplasma has no real cell wall but only a membrane similar in nature to the external lipid bilayer of the eukaryotic cell.[34] Hence, the organism has the capability of functioning in a manner analogous to a synthetic liposome, and as such is able to take up solubilized molecules shed from cell surfaces.[36] This interaction presumably takes place through hydrophobic molecular interactions. It could be that the ability of the mycoplasma to escape the immune system of the host and to persist chronically is due to alteration of its own cell surface so that it mimics the host cell. It is hoped that at the molecular level the studies of this intimate mycoplasma–host cell association, the immune response of the host and the way in which mycoplasmal evasion of the immune defenses takes place will be fertile areas for investigation.

**Viruses.** Viruses can cause disease in any of several ways, ranging from acute short-lived infections to those that progress with age and last perhaps a lifetime. The ability of slow viruses to produce tissue pathology and the demonstration of this in the case of human disease may foretell a complete revolution in our understanding of chronic viral infections. Only recently are methods beginning to be developed that will allow us to study many of the diseases that have in the past been considered to have their origin in degenerative processes or in metabolic alterations.[37]

A number of investigators have studied the possible viral etiology of rheumatoid arthritis using both direct culture techniques and several indirect methodologies. Although no single virus has been repeatedly demonstrated in a consistent fashion from one laboratory to the other, some hints of a possible viral involvement in rheumatoid disease have occurred. For example, virus-like particles have been found in the synovium in patients with rheumatoid arthritis.[38] It appears, however, that these same particles are found in a number of different tissues in different disease states and they may represent no more than some sort of organized debris rather than virus or viral products.[39] Interest in the viral etiology of rheumatoid arthritis accelerated when it was found that the rubella virus was unable to infect and replicate in rheumatoid synovial cells.[40] This suggested that there might be a preformed virus already present in the synovial cell which produced the interference. This was of considerable importance, since the technique of interference by latent viruses had been used for some time to study rubella viruses. Unfortunately these original striking observations were not confirmed, and it seems now that rheumatoid synovial cells are able to support the replication of many viruses in the same way as do synovial cells from nonrheumatoid sources.[41]

The experience with kuru[37,42] and the realization of the role of slow viruses in the long-term production of disease have alerted us to the fact that viral infection can involve many patterns of disease and makes the search for filterable agents in rheumatoid tissues a continuing challenge. From time to time, reports of transmissible agents in rheumatoid tissues have appeared.[43] Unfortunately, these are generally not reproduced in other laboratories. It would be presumptive to dismiss all these experiments at this time, but taken in perspective the evidence is slim for a viral infection as a cause of rheumatoid arthritis. The work of Gajdusek and colleagues[37,42] and others in discovering the role of slow viruses in certain chronic diseases of the central nervous system may have a parallel in rheumatoid arthritis, and this possibility is likely to remain as a stimulus to research.

Of specific interest relative to the possible viral etiology of rheumatoid arthritis is the observation of Alspaugh and Tan that the serum of patients with rheumatoid arthritis reacts with an antigen extracted from the Epstein-Barr virus (EBV)–carrying cell line, Wil-2.[44] This rheumatoid arthritis precipitin (RAP) reacts with a nuclear antigen (RANA) extracted exclusively from EBV-infected cells. This antigen (RANA) is related to the Epstein-Barr nuclear antigen (EBNA), yet is distinct from it. Antibody to each develops over the same time course after primary EBV infection.

EBV can modulate the immune system as evidenced by its ability to cause lymphoid proliferation, B-cell activation, and increased immunoglobulin secretion. The data indicate that rheumatoid arthritis patients, as compared with normals, do not regulate in vitro EBV infection as efficiently. Even though one must keep in mind that EBV is not arthrotropic, it could exert special influence on the immune system of rheumatoid arthritis patients. It has been found, for example, that EBV-induced B-cell lines proliferate more rapidly from peripheral blood lymphocytes from patients with rheumatoid arthritis than from normals. This seems to be due to a defective regulation by rheumatoid arthritis T cells. Recently it has been shown that this defect is due to diminished generation of gamma interferon by the T cells.[45] Although we are learning much about the special effects of EBV on immune regulation, it is difficult to implicate the virus as the primary event in rheumatoid arthritis.

Several additional experimental approaches of sound molecular rationale have been pursued in studies of the viral etiology of rheumatoid arthritis. These include (1) serologic surveys of patients with rheumatoid arthritis to obtain clues to a specific antiviral antibody that might be present,[46] (2) an examination of synovial cell cultures for virally induced enzymes, particularly DNA-dependent DNA polymerase and RNA-dependent DNA polymerase,[47] (3) an examination of newly synthesized RNA and DNA by rheumatoid synovial cells to see if molecular parameters compatible with virus molecules were present,[48] and (4) examination of sera from patients with rheumatoid arthritis to test for cytotoxic antibodies that are reactive against lymphoid cell surface antigens, perhaps produced by virus modification.[49] Although these approaches produced interesting information relative to the molecular cell biology of rheumatoid cells, they have not clarified the question of a virus etiology of the disease. On balance the data must be summarized as negative. Clearly, some of the newer tools available for looking for viruses and viral genomes in host tissues, including hybridization methodologies and techniques of electron microscopy, should be applied to examine further the possibility that virus products are present.

Recent data on the type C oncornaviruses are particularly intriguing relative to the way in which viral genomes may be incorporated into a host cell and produce virally related proteins which may be expressed on the surface, thereby modifying the host cell surface antigenic expression.[50] These events have been studied from the standpoint of relevance to human disease, particularly in SLE, by Strand and August.[51] For example, the $G_{IX}$ marker, found on the surface of certain murine lymphoblastoid cells, was described initially as a distinct genetically determined antigen.[52] Although this marker is present on certain cell lines in the absence of virus production, there is an unambiguous demonstration that in the mouse this molecule ($G_{IX}$) is identical to the gp69/70 viral coat protein of the type C oncornavirus.[53] That this molecule may be expressed on the surface of cells in which the viral genome is present, even though no virion production takes place, encourages further searches for possible new antigenic expression on surfaces of rheumatoid cells. Special note should be made for future studies of RA cells similar to those that have been done to define oncogenes in certain tumor cell lines.[54] Recent evidence for translocation of some oncogenes into the immunoglobulin gene region[55] may be of great importance.

There are several common viral diseases that are associated with inflammatory rheumatic syndromes. The most striking of these is synovitis following rubella infection[10] and the arthritis that may precede the onset of jaundice in infectious hepatitis.[11] Also, the occurrence of hepatitis B antigen–associated polyarteritis[56] should be mentioned. In view of these situations it must be presumed that rheumatoid arthritis could result from a host immune response to antigens of a yet unknown virus, persisting either in the joint tissues with only localized inflammation or in the form of circulating immune complexes, which results in both systemic and local pathology. These possibilities again emphasize that the syndrome recognized as rheumatoid arthritis could have its origin in diverse etiologies.

## ANIMAL MODELS

**Mycoplasma Infections.** As indicated previously, one of the major factors for considering mycoplasma in a discussion of the etiology of rheumatoid arthritis in man is its striking incrimination as a cause of arthritis in several animal species. Most of these organisms, however, can also be recovered from the respiratory tract, and in some instances, such as the *M. arthritidis* arthritis of rats, the condition is acute and purulent. The mycoplasma-induced arthritides that occur in pigs, mice, and turkeys, however, can often be of long duration and produce a chronic course.[57] In these situations, it is often possible to isolate the organisms from the infected joints only in the early phase of disease. These observations relate to *M. pulmonis* in the mouse and *M. hyorhinis* in pigs. In the latter situation, Barden and Decker[9,58] found it increasingly difficult to isolate the organism from the arthritic joints in the later stages of disease, but they found high titers of antibody in both the serum and joint fluids of these animals. A similar situation exists in the case of *M. gallisepticum* in the turkey arthritis model, but its exact correlation with antibody production is not yet defined. It seems clear from the animal models that mycoplasmas can initiate an arthritic process, and they may provide us with some new experimental tools for studies in man. For example, the strain, the dose, and the route of administration seem particularly important in defining whether or not an arthritis can be associated with a given mycoplasma infection. Furthermore, the newer serologic approaches for looking at mycoplasma antigens should provide some very interesting serologic reagents for analysis of rheumatoid tissues.[34,59] Conversely, the utilization of sera from patients with rheumatoid arthritis to screen for antibodies against known antigens of the mycoplasma may be a useful approach.

**Erysipelothrix Arthritis in Pigs.** *Erysipelothrix rhusiopathiae,* since its initial description by Löffler in 1885, has become recognized as an important cause of chronic arthritis in pigs, and is the organism most commonly isolated from arthritic joints in this species.[60] It also has marked similarities to rheumatoid arthritis in man and, in fact, in much of the veterinary literature is referred to as "rheumatoid arthritis in pigs." The organism is a small gram-positive nonmotile coccobacillus and will grow on blood agar under aerobic conditions.[61] It will also produce natural infections in a wide variety of domesticated and wild animals and will cause an erysipelas-like disease in man.

The disease caused by *E. rhusiopathiae* in pigs may take one of the following three possible courses: (1) an acute form with a high mortality in untreated cases, (2) a less acute form associated with urticaria and erythematous plaques over the entire body surface, or (3) no clinical evidence of infection but the pig becomes a carrier, with the organism being found in the spleen, tonsils, gut, or bone marrow.

It is in the chronic stages of the disease that arthritis and sometimes endocarditis may occur. Arthritis may also occur following apparent recovery from acute forms of the disease. Interestingly, the onset of arthritis may even be the first indication that the disease is present. This arthritis may be chronic; it may wax and wane and may be unrelenting. It produces a synovial pathology in which the membrane is thickened, villus formation occurs, and the cellular infiltrate is composed of lymphocytes and plasma cells. There is also a tendency to follicle formation.[62] Some investigators have also reported the presence of rheumatoid factor–like molecules in the sera of pigs with erysipelothrix arthritis, but this finding has been inconsistent.[63] Since the data indicate that the arthritis can be present and progress in the absence of living erysipelothrix organisms, much effort is underway at present to see if persistent bacterial debris is responsible for perpetuation of the inflammatory process.

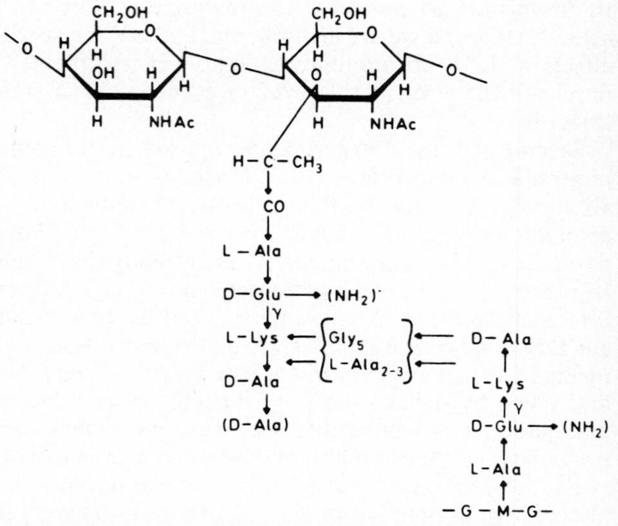


**Figure 58–1.** Structural representation of the peptidoglycan molecule. The basic unit consists of an alternating *N*-acetyl glucosamine and *N*-acetyl muramic acid, to which the peptide side-chain is attached. Polymerization occurs at the time of incorporation into the cell wall. In some bacteria, spacer linkages, such as $(Gly)_5$ or $(Ala)_{2-3}$, are inserted between polymeric units. (From Bennett, J.C.: Arthritis Rheum. 21:531, 1978, by permission.)

**Adjuvant Arthritis.** Arthritis is produced[64] following the injection into rats of Freund's adjuvant, a mixture of whole heat-treated acid-fast bacilli, mineral oil, and an emulsifying agent. This occurs without any added tissue homogenate or other bacteria and is given by intradermal injection. Following a latent period of about 2 weeks there develops arthritis and periarthritis, which involves most of the joints and extremities. It is especially severe in the distant small joints of the paws, and also in the tail, presenting as intense red swellings of variable size and painfulness. The intensity of the arthritis waxes and wanes over several weeks, may completely remit, or may be followed by spontaneous recurrences. The general incidence of the disease is reproducible at about the 85 percent level in various strains. A striking aspect of the pathology is extensive extra-articular calcification, resulting finally in tissue destruction and ankylosis.

Current evidence suggests that the arthritogenic properties of bacterial adjuvants reside within the peptidoglycan dimer[65] (see Fig. 58–1). The possible role of peptidoglycans in producing chronic inflammation is a point of great current interest. These molecules are found internal to the capsule and the outer membrane of bacteria, and there is an extraordinary degree of similarity among the peptidoglycans found across the entire spectrum of bacteria. Such similarity of structure is not found among surface antigenic components—for example, those that are used for serologic identification of various types of bacteria. The chemical structure of the peptidoglycan is important for an appreciation of the role that it might have in initiating a chronic inflammatory response (Fig. 58–1). This molecule is an alternating chain of *N*-acetylglucosamine and *N*-acetylmuramic acid. Attached to the lactic acid ether side chain of the muramic acid is a tetrapeptide L-Ala-D-Glu-L-Lys-D-Ala. A fifth residue, D-Ala is present on the precursor molecule before the monomers are polymerized and assembled to form the cell wall.[66] In some cases, the units are coupled directly during polymerization through the L-Ala to one of the L-Lys residues of an adjacent unit. In other cases, there may be a spacer linkage such as $(Gly)_5$ or $(Ala)_{2-3}$.

**Cell Wall Antigens: A Streptococcal Model in Rats.** Cromartie and associates[67] have shown that a chronic arthritis can be produced in rats by a single intraperitoneal injection of a sterile aqueous suspension of cell wall fragments of bacteria, particularly the *Streptococcus.* The arthritis that results within a week is striking. It is a proliferative, inflammatory, erosive pansynovitis that waxes and wanes but recurs in an unrelenting fashion until total joint destruction results. Evidence again indicates that it is the peptidoglycan-polysaccharide fragment of the cell wall that is responsible for the inflammatory process, just as in the adjuvant model. The differences, however, are that the bacterial constituents are given in aqueous solution, the arthritis is chronic, it is erosive from the very beginning, its pattern of recurrence is even more striking, and there is less extra-articular calcification. In short, it more directly relates to a true model for rheumatoid arthritis.

These studies are reinforced by previous investigations,[68] which examined the development of antibodies to streptococcal antigens in rabbits. These workers reported that occasionally animals immunized with streptococci developed rheumatoid factors that are capable of recognizing both peptidoglycan and the Fc component of IgG. Hence, these observations emphasize the possibility of a relationship between the peptidoglycan and the Fc region. Additional clinical observations reveal that patients with rheumatic fever, juvenile rheumatoid arthritis,[69] and rheumatoid arthritis[70] have antibodies that cross-react with peptidoglycans. These findings may have parallels in studies of patients with bacterial endocarditis, in which bacterial antigens are clearly present as the initiating factors of the inflammatory process.

Some limited studies of chronic rheumatoid arthritis synovial tissue, utilizing very sensitive ($10^{-15}$ M) gas chromatographic and mass spectrographic techniques, have failed to detect bacterial muramic acid.[71] This is strong evidence against the bacterial debris concept for human rheumatoid disease, but studies in the early, more acute stages have not been carried out.

## SUMMARY

Available information requires the interlocking of several concepts when considering the etiology of rheumatoid arthritis.[72] These include (1) genetics of the host, (2) the host-immune response, and (3) an inciting agent. The extraordinary achievements of cell biology and molecular genetics provide hope that we will soon be able to understand how these factors work together in the pathogenesis of rheumatoid disease.

## References

1. Miescher, P.A., and Muller-Eberhard, H.J.: Textbook of Immunopathology. 2nd ed. New York, Grune & Stratton, 1976.
2. Stites, D.P., Stobo, J.D., Fudenberg, H.H., and Wells, J.V.: Basic and Clinical Immunology. 4th ed. Los Altos, Calif., Lange Medical Publications, 1982.
3. Burnet, F.M.: The Clonal Selection Theory of Acquired Immunity. Nashville and Cambridge, Vanderbilt and Cambridge University Presses, 1959.
4. Gershon, R.K., Eardley, D.D., Durum, S., Green, D.R., Shen, F.W., Yamauchi, K., Cantor, H., and Murphy, D.B.: Contrasuppression: A novel immunoregulatory activity. J. Exp. Med. 153:1533, 1981.
5. Jerne, N.K.: Towards a network theory of the immune system. Ann. Immunol. (Inst. Pasteur) 125c:373, 1974.
6. Knight, J.G.: Autoimmune diseases: Defects in immune specificity rather than a loss of suppressor cells. Immunology Today 3:326, 1982.
7. Knight, J.G., and Adams, D.D: *In* Receptors, Antibodies and Disease. Ciba Fnd. Sym. 90:35, 1982.
8. Steele, A.C., Bartenhagen, N.M., Craft, J.E., Huchinson, G.J., Newman, J.H., Rahn, D.W., Sigal, L.H., Spieler, P.N., Stenn, K.S., and Malawista, S.E.: The early clinical manifestations of Lyme arthritis. Ann. Intern. Med. 99:76–82, 1983.
9. Barden, J.A., and Decker, J.L.: *Mycoplasma hyorhinis* swine arthritis. I. Clinical and microbiological features. Arthritis Rheum. 14:193, 1971.
10. Ogra, P.L., and Herd, J.K.: Arthritis with induced rubella infection. J. Immunol. 107:810, 1971.
11. Alpert, A., Isselbacher, K.J., and Schur, P.H.: The pathogenesis of arthritis associated with viral hepatitis. N. Engl. J. Med. 285:185, 1971.
12. Whittle, H.C., Abdullahi, M.T., Fakunle, F.A., Greenwood, B.M., Bryceson, A.D.M., Parry, E.H.O., and Turk, J.L.: Allergic complications of meningococcal diseases. I. Clinical aspects. Br. Med. J. 2:733, 1973.
13. Catterall, R.D.: The role of microbial infection in Reiter's syndrome. *In* Dumonde, D.C. (ed.): Infection and Immunology in the Rheumatic Diseases. Oxford, Blackwell Scientific Publications, 1976.
14. Tesh, R.B. Arthritides caused by mosquito-borne viruses. Ann. Rev. Med. 33:31, 1982.
15. Sasazuki, T., McDevitt, H.O., and Grumet, F.C.: The association between genes in the major histocompatibility complex and disease susceptibility. Ann. Rev. Med. 28:425, 1977.
16. Terhorst, C., Robb, R., Jones, C., and Strominger, J.L.: Further structural studies on the heavy chain of HLA antigens and its similarity to immunoglobulins. Proc. Natl. Acad. Sci. USA 74:4002, 1977.
17. Coblyn, J.S., Weinblatt, M., Holdsworth, D., and Glass, D.: Gold-induced thrombocytopenia; a clinical and immunogenetic study of twenty-three patients. Ann. Intern. Med. 95:178, 1981.
18. Karr, R.W., Rodey, G.E., Lee, T., and Schwartz, B.: Association of HLA $DR_{w4}$ with rheumatoid arthritis in black and white patients. Arthritis Rheum. 23:1241, 1980.
19. Awdeh, Z.L., and Alper, C.A.: Inherited structural polymorphism of the fourth component of human complement. Proc. Natl. Acad. Sci. 77:3576, 1980.
20. Albert, E.D., and Gotze, D.: The major histocompatibility system in man. *In* Gotze, D. (ed.): The Major Histocompatibility System in Man and Animals. Berlin, Springer-Verlag, 1977.
21. Barnett, E.V.: Circulating immune complexes: Their immunochemistry, detection and importance. Ann. Intern. Med. 91:430, 1979.
22. Jones, J.V.: Autoimmunity and multi-system disease. *In* Holborow, E.J., and Reeves, W.G. (eds): Immunology in Medicine. New York and London, Academic Press and Grune & Stratton, 1977.
23. Maini, R.N.: Immunology of Rheumatic Diseases: Aspects of Autoimmunity. London, Edward Arnold, Ltd. 1977.
24. Green, C.A.: Hemolytic streptococcal infections and acute rheumatism. Ann. Rheum. Dis. 3:4, 1942.
25. Copeman, W.S.C.: A Short History of the Gout and the Rheumatic Diseases. Berkeley, University of California Press, 1964.
26. Mansson, I., and Olhagen, B.: Fecal *Clostridium perfringens* and rheumatoid arthritis. J. Infect. Dis. 130:444, 1974.
27. Mansson, I., Norberg, R., Olhagen, B., and Bjorklund, N.E.: Arthritis in pigs induced by dietary factors. Clin. Exp. Immunol. 9:677, 1971.
28. Stewart, S.M., Alexander, W.R.M., and Duthie, J.J.R.: Isolation of diphtheroid bacilli from synovial membrane and fluid in rheumatoid arthritis. Ann. Rheum. Dis. 28:477, 1969.
29. Bartholomew, L.E., and Bartholomew, F.N.: Antigenic bacterial polysaccharide in rheumatoid synovial effusions. Arthritis Rheum. 22:969, 1979.
30. Taylor-Robinson, D., and Taylor, G.: Do mycoplasmas cause rheumatic disease? *In* Dumonde, D.C. (ed.): Infection and Immunology in the Rheumatic Diseases. Oxford, Blackwell Scientific Publications, 1976.
31. Cassell, G.H. and Cole, B.C.: Mycoplasmas as agents of human disease. New Engl. J. Med. 304:80, 1981.
32. Cole, B.C., Griffiths, M.M., Eichwald, E.J., and Ward, J.R.: New models of chronic synovitis in rabbits induced by mycoplasmas: Microbiological, histopathological, and immunological observation in rabbits injected with *Mycoplasma arthritidis* and *Mycoplasma pulmonis*. Infect. Immun. 16:383, 1977.
33. Cohen, S.N.: The manipulation of genes. Sci. Am. 233:24, 1975.
34. Cassell, G.H., Davies, J.K., Wilburn, W., and Wise, K.S.: Pathobiology of mycoplasmas. *In* Schlessinger, D. (ed.): Microbiology 1978. Washington, D.C., American Society of Microbiology, 1978.
35. Wise, K.S., Acton, R.T., and Cassell, G.H.: Selective association of murine T-lymphoblastoid cell surface alloantigens with *Mycoplasma hyorhinis*. Proc. Natl. Acad. Sci. USA 75:4479, 1978.
36. Bouma, S.R., Drislane, F.W., and Huestis, W.H.: Selective extraction of membrane-bound proteins by phospholipid vesicles. J. Biol. Chem. 252:6759, 1977.
37. Gajdusek, D.C.: Unconventional viruses and the origin and disappearance of kuru. Science 197:943, 1977.
38. Schumacher, H.R.: Synovial membrane and fluid morphologic alterations in early rheumatoid arthritis: Microvascular injury and virus-like particles. Ann. N.Y. Acad. Sci. 256:39, 1975.
39. Baringer, J.R.: Tubular aggregates in endoplasmic reticulum in herpes simplex encephalitis. N. Engl. J. Med. 285:943, 1971.
40. Grayzel, A.I., and Beck, C.: Rubella infection of synovial cells and the resistance of cells derived from patients with rheumatoid arthritis. J. Exp. Med. 131:367, 1970.
41. Person, D.A., Rawls, W.E., and Sharp, J.T.: Replication of rubella, Newcastle disease and vesicular stomatitis viruses in cultured rheumatoid synovial cells. Proc. Soc. Exp. Biol. Med. 138:748, 1971.
42. Gajdusek, D.C., and Gibbs, C.J.: Transmission of kuru from man to rhesus monkey (*Macaca mulatta*) 8¼ years from inoculation. Nature 240:351, 1972.
43. Warren, S.L., Marmor, M.D., Leonard, M.D., Liebes, D.M., and Hollins, R.: An active agent from human rheumatoid arthritis which is transmissible in mice. Arch. Intern. Med. 124:629, 1969.
44. Alspaugh, M.A. and Tan, E.M.: Serum antibody in rheumatoid arthritis reactive with a cell-associated antigen: Demonstration by precipitation and immunofluorescence. Arthritis Rheum. 19:711, 1976.
45. Hasler, F., Bluestein, H.G., Zvaifler, N.J. and Epstein, L.B.: Analysis of the defects responsible for the impaired regulation of Epstein-Barr virus-induced B cell proliferation by rheumatoid arthritis lymphocytes. J. Exp. Med. 157:173, 1983.

46. Chandler, R.W., Robinson, H., and Masi, A.T.: Serological investigations for evidence of an infectious etiology of rheumatoid arthritis. Ann. Rheum. Dis. 30:274, 1971.
47. Spruance, S.L., Richards, O.C., Smith, C.B., and Ward, J.R.: DNA polymerase activity of cultured rheumatoid synovial cells. Arthritis Rheum. 18:229, 1975.
48. Person, D.A., Sharp, J.T., and Rawls, W.E.: A search for viruses and mycoplasmas in connective tissue diseases. Arthritis Rheum. 16:677, 1973.
49. Person, D.A., Sharp, J.T., and Lidsky, M.D.: The cytotoxicity of leukocytes and lymphocytes from patients with rheumatoid arthritis for synovial cells. J. Clin. Invest. 58:690, 1976.
50. August, J.T., and Strand, M.: Type-C oncornaviruses and autoimmunity. Arthritis Rheum. 20:S64, 1977.
51. Strand, M., and August, J.T.: Type-C RNA virus gene expression in human tissue. J. Virol. 14:1584, 1974.
52. Boyse, E.A.: The $G_{IX}$ system in relation to C-type viruses and heredity. Immunol. Rev. 33:125, 1977.
53. Lerner, R.A., Wilson, C.B., Del Vilano, B.C., McConahey, P.J., and Dixon, F.J.: Endogenous oncornaviral gene expression in adult and fetal mice: Quantitative histologic and physiologic studies of the major viral glycoprotein, gp70. J. Exp. Med. 143:151, 1976.
54. Reshani, G., Givol, D. and Canaani, E.: Activation of a cellular oncogene by DNA rearrangement: possible involvement of an IS-like element. Nature 300:607, 1982.
55. Marcu, K.B., Harris, L.J., Stanton, L.W., Erickson, J., Watt, R., and Croce, C.M.: Transcriptionally active c-myc oncogene is contained within NIARD, a DNA sequence associated with chromosome translocation in B cell neoplasia. Proc. Natl. Acad. Sci. 80:519, 1983.
56. Gocke, D.J., Hsu, K., Morgan, C., Bombardieri, S., Lockshin, M., and Christian, C.L.: Association between polyarteritis and Australia antigen. Lancet 2:1149, 1970.
57. Ross, R.F.: Pathogenicity of swine mycoplasmas. Ann. N.Y. Acad. Sci. 225:347, 1973.
58. Decker, J.L., and Barden, J.A.: Mycoplasma arthritis in the pig. *In* Dumonde, D.C. (ed.): Infection and Immunology in the Rheumatic Diseases. Oxford, Blackwell Scientific Publications, 1976.
59. Brown, T.McP., Bailey, J.S., Felts, W.R., and Clark, H.W.: Mycoplasma antibodies in synovia. Arthritis Rheum. 9:495, 1966.
60. Ward, A.R.: The etiology of polyarthritis in swine. J. Am. Vet. Med. Assoc. 61:155, 1922.
61. Packer, R.A.: The use of sodium azide and crystal violet in a selective medium for streptococci and *Erysipelothrix rhusiopathiae.* J. Bacteriol. 46:343, 1943.
62. Drew, R.A.: Erysipelothrix arthritis in pigs as a comparative model for rheumatoid arthritis. Proc. R. Soc. Med. 65:994, 1972.
63. Timoney, J.: Antibody and rheumatoid factor in synovia of pigs with erysipelothrix arthritis. J. Comp. Pathol. 81:243, 1971.
64. Pearson, C.M.: Development of arthritis, periarthritis and periostitis in rats given adjuvants. Proc. Soc. Exp. Biol. Med. 91:95, 1956.
65. Kohashi, O., Pearson, C.M., Watanabe, Y., Kotani, S., and Koga, T.: Structural requirements for arthritogenicity of peptidoglycans from *Staphylococcus aureus* and *Lactobacillus plantarum* analogous synthetic compounds. J. Immunol. 116:1635, 1976.
66. Schleifer, K.H., and Seidl, H.P.: Structure and immunological aspects of peptidoglycans. *In* Schlessinger, D. (ed.): Microbiology 1977. Washington, D.C., American Society for Microbiology, 1977.
67. Cromartie, W.J., Craddock, J.G., Schwab, J.H., Anderle, S.K., and Yang, C.H.: Arthritis in rats after systemic injection of streptococcal cells or cell walls. J. Exp. Med. 146:1585, 1977.
68. Bokisch, V.A., Chiao, J.W., Bernstein, D., and Krause, R.M.: Homogeneous rabbit 7S anti-IgG with antibody specificity for peptidoglycan. J. Exp. Med. 138:1184, 1973.
69. Heymer, B., Schleifer, K.H., Read, S., Zabriske, J.B., and Krause, R.M.: Detection of antibodies to bacterial cell wall peptidoglycan in human sera. J. Immunol. 117:23, 1976.
70. Braun, D.G., and Holm, S.E.: Streptococcal anti-group A precipitins in sera from patients with rheumatic arthritis and acute glomerulonephritis. Int. Arch. Allergy 37:216, 1970.
71. Prtichard, D.G., Settine, R.L. and Bennett, J.C.: Sensitive mass spectrometric procedure for the detection of bacterial cell wall components in rheumatoid joints. Arthritis Rheum. 23:608, 1980.
72. Bennett. J.C.: The infectious etiology of rheumatoid arthritis: New considerations. Arthritis Rheum. 21:531, 1978.

# Chapter 59
# Pathogenesis of Rheumatoid Arthritis

*Edward D. Harris, Jr.*

## INTRODUCTION

In order to treat rheumatoid arthritis effectively, a physician must understand the sequence that occurs within the joints and extra-articular tissues. After the initial inflammatory events, multiple systems of inflammation, cellular proliferation, and autacoid production are activated. Each activated system affects and amplifies others. Many different biologic responses are generated simultaneously.

**The Stages of Rheumatoid Arthritis.** Although beginning as nonspecific inflammation within the joint, rheumatoid arthritis (RA) progresses to a proliferative lesion within the synovium that can lead to joint destruction. The inflammatory lesion generates and drives the proliferative one. The rate of progression of the disease within an individual patient depends upon both the intensity and the chronicity of the disease. The disease of a patient who has intermittent flares of synovitis will not progress as rapidly to joint destruction as that of one who has virtually continuous manifestations of synovitis. Similarly, the patient with a high grade of inflammation will progress to loss of joint function much more rapidly than the individual with a low-grade inflammatory response.

The stages in the pathogenesis of RA, chosen arbitrarily but of interest for discussion, are outlined in Table 59–1.

## A WORKING SCHEME FOR THE PATHOGENESIS OF RHEUMATOID ARTHRITIS

The scheme outlined here and in Table 59–1 is based on data that will be discussed subsequently.

1. An immune response of the host is triggered and is sufficiently strong to perturb the host systems, which

**Table 59–1.** The Pathophysiology of Rheumatoid Arthritis

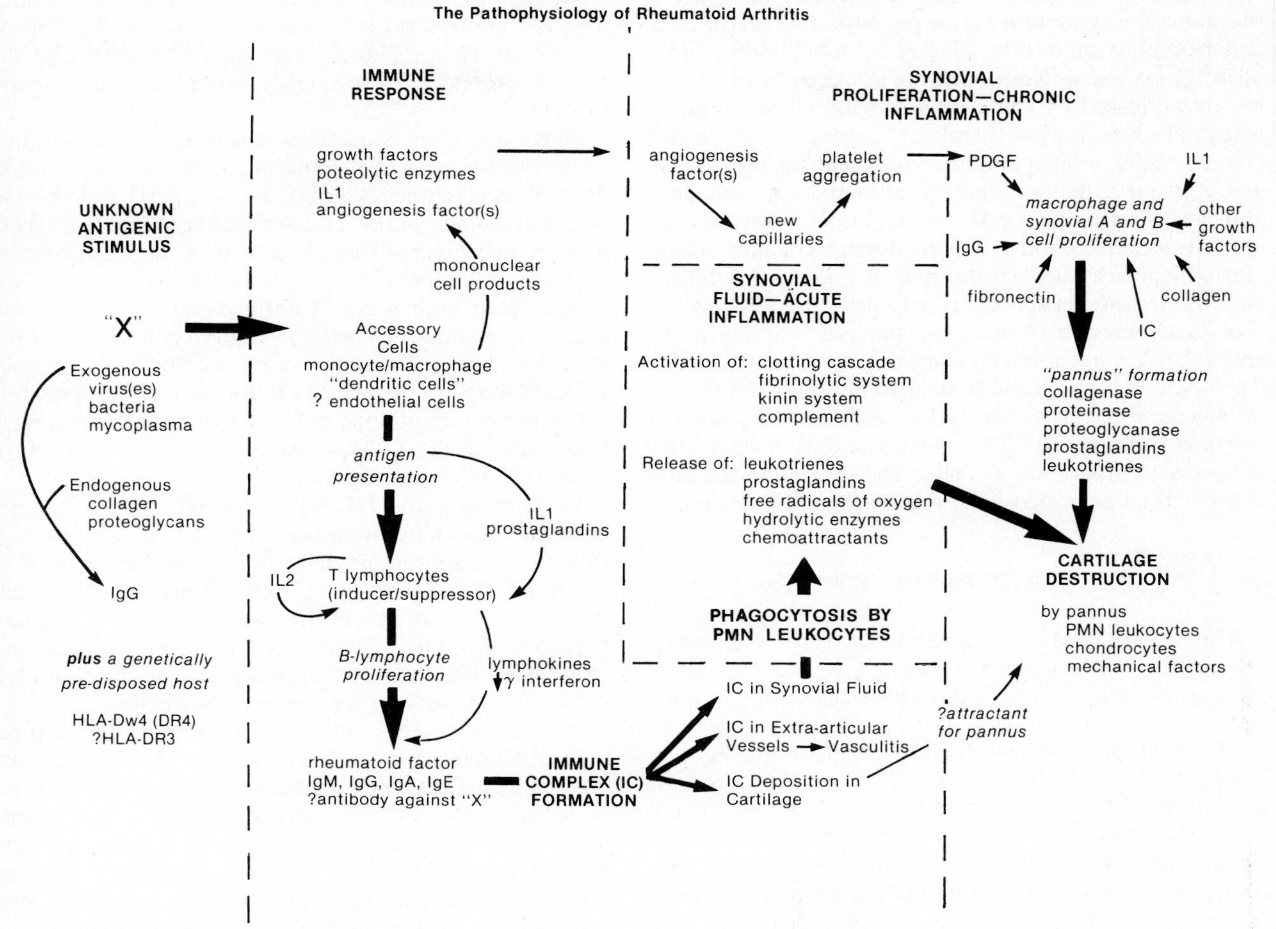


produce an inflammatory response directed against the self or nonself antigen(s). A major determinant in this process is the genetically controlled immune response, which programs the mode and intensity with which the antigen is recognized and the degree to which the immune response is amplified and the antigen localized.

2. In the synovial fluid the immune response catalyzes activation of many processes which interact to produce a self-sustaining active inflammation within the joint space. These systems include complement, kinins, clotting and fibrinolysis, phagocytosis by leukocytes, and lysosomal enzyme release by the same cells. Polymorphonuclear (PMN) leukocytes are attracted to the joint space by C5a and by leukotriene $B_4$ formed during the inflammatory response. During phagocytosis of debris and/or immune complexes the PMN leukocytes release proteolytic enzymes (elastase and collagenase), prostaglandins, and free radicals of oxygen.

3. In the synovium large numbers of helper T lymphocytes cluster about HLA-DR+ (Ia+) macrophage/dendritic cells. These cells are probably involved in the presentation of antigen to T lymphocytes. Induction of antibody formation by B lymphocytes follows. Rheumatoid patients may not be able to regulate polyclonal B-lymphocyte proliferation (in response to the putative infectious agent and/or Epstein-Barr virus infection) which results from these inductive stimuli. At present it is believed that there are subsets among HLA-DR+ cells, some of which can present antigen to T lymphocytes and others which cannot.

4. Antigen-antibody complexes form within the joint cavity and in avascular hyaline and fibrocartilage. This trapping may be mediated primarily by charge differences among matrix macromolecules and the immunoglobulins.

5. Mediators produced by interaction of mononuclear cells (and, perhaps, mast cells) stimulate target cells (i.e., synovial cells) to proliferate and to produce proteinases and prostaglandins. Deeper in the subsynovial layers, fibroblasts are activated to produce more connective tissue matrix.

6. In response to soluble products of activated mononuclear cells as well as other factors (see Chapter 13), endothelial cells begin to sprout and angiogenesis of capillaries begins. Without this development of new vessels the hypertrophied synovium could not be sustained.

7. The lesion becomes polarized. There is inflammation generated by phagocytosis of antigen-antibody com-

plexes in the synovial fluid and a marked proliferative response in the synovium. Beginning at the periphery of the joint, the synovium organizes into an invasive front and begins to replace cartilage and subchondral bone, utilizing several different enzyme systems. Neutral proteinases released by the synovial (pannus) cells and by recruited chondrocytes break up aggregates of proteoglycans. This, in effect, solubilizes them for pinocytosis and continued degradation by cathepsin D, sulfatases, and enzymes specific for the carbohydrate moieties. Elastase cleaves crosslinked regions among collagen fibrils, and collagenase cleaves the helical region. Solubilized collagen fragments spontaneously denature and are further catabolized by neutral proteinases, cathepsin B1, and other collagenolytic cathepsins. Fragments of collagen have strong chemotactic attraction for monocytes as well as fibroblasts. Mineral is resorbed from bone as osteoclasts are activated by prostaglandins or by soluble products of mononuclear cells. The demineralized substrate is then degraded by collagenases and proteinases.

## DETAILS OF PATHOGENESIS

The remainder of this chapter will attempt to correlate the pathology with events occurring within the synovium, in the synovial fluid, and at the cell-cartilage junction.

**The Susceptible Host: Immunogenetics and RA.** As emphasized in Chapter 58, the likelihood of a specific single virus or infective agent being isolated as a cause of all rheumatoid arthritis is small. The difference between those who develop RA and those who do not may relate more to individual variations in the immune response than to selective contact with a specific etiologic agent (Table 59–1).

The most compelling of recent data linking genetic control of the immune response to RA is that demonstrating the association of the HLA-D4 locus to this disease. In two studies, 51 percent[1] and 36 percent[2] of patients with RA possessed the Dw4 haplotype compared with 13 percent and 7 percent of controls, respectively. D-related (DR) alloantigens of B lymphocytes (as well as macrophages, sperm, and vascular endothelium) are more easily assayed because, as with HLA-A, HLA-B, and HLA-C loci, serologic testing can be performed. HLA-DR4 has been reported in 70 percent of rheumatoid patients but in only 28 percent of controls.[3] It is of interest that HLA-DR typing of 59 individuals revealed a highly significant relationship ($p < 0.0001$) between HLA-DR4 and responsiveness of peripheral blood mononuclear cells to denatured collagen.[4] These studies are strong support for the hypothesis that genes linked to coding for HLA-DR4 constitute true immune response (Ir) genes for T lymphocyte-dependent reactivity to collagen.

Although HLA-DR4 has been convincingly associated with RA (a relative risk of 8.02) and positive tests for rheumatoid factor, data regarding "seronegative RA" have been inconsistent. In one recent study in which rigid diagnostic criteria were used, no statistically significant difference between seronegative RA patients and 123 control subjects was noted in the distribution of DR antigens.[5] Those seronegative patients who did have DR4 had a more rapidly progressive, destructive disease.

There are some exceptions to the general association of the DR4 locus and rheumatoid arthritis. For example, no increased frequency of HLA-Dw4 or HLA-DR4 was found in women of the Yakima Indian nation with rheumatoid arthritis,[6] although RA is a slightly atypical disease in these people (e.g., primary erosive wrist/MCP disease with high titers of antinuclear antibody in addition to rheumatoid factor). Similarly, 49 Israeli Jews with RA had no association with DR4;[7] seronegative patients were not included in this group. Other nonwhite rheumatoid populations studied have had an increased frequency of HLA-DR4, including blacks and Mexicans[8] and Japanese.[9]

In summary, the HLA-D4 and HLA-DR4 loci are probably associated with the genes determining susceptibility to an immunologic response that results in RA.

**"Agent X": The Factor That Initiates the Response in RA.** As noted in the previous chapter by Bennett, the search for one specific causative agent of the disease continues, although the promise of ever finding that "agent X" is perhaps less secure than before.

Proteoglycans and collagen are examples of endogenous candidates for the cause of RA. Induction in rats of an arthritis that may become chronic and erosive can be achieved by systemic injection of basic components of bacterial or mycobacterial cell walls that include peptidoglycans.[10,11] It is possible that bacterial peptidoglycans or oligosaccharides could become associated with proteoglycans being produced in connective tissue, and that these altered matrix components would become immunogenic and arthritogenic.[12]

Similarly, both humoral and cellular immunity to collagen and its denatured form (gelatin) have been demonstrated in RA. Circulating antibodies to collagen in RA have been noted, although these are not specific to certain types of collagen and do not correlate with the activity of the disease.[13] Forty percent of patients with serum antibodies to collagen (type I, native and denatured) have them in synovial fluid as well.[14] Most patients with active RA have some evidence for cellular sensitivity to type II and type III collagens.[15] Indeed, injection of purified type II collagen into a certain strain of rats at a certain age produces a chronic arthritis not unlike rheumatoid arthritis[16,17] that can be passively transferred by mononuclear cells or by immunoglobulins from one rat to another (see Chapter 14). It is of interest that although IgM antibody production in man is usually short-lived after an antigenic stimulus, in patients with RA, IgM as well as IgG antibody production to native type II collagen appears to persist at high levels.[18] Does this imply a persistence of antigenic stimulation?

The work generated recently concerning the role of Epstein-Barr virus (EBV) in RA is another example of the inability to determine whether an agent associated with RA has an etiologic relationship to the disease. Rheumatoid patients have a higher frequency than control populations of antibodies to EBV-associated nuclear antigens.[19-21] Rheumatoid patients have defective EBV-specific suppressor T-lymphocyte function; the RA T lymphocytes do not suppress the polyclonal B-lymphocyte stimulation induced by EBV infection.[22-25] RA T lymphocytes are specifically deficient in their ability to generate gamma interferon (which suppresses EBV-induced B lymphoblast transformation), although this deficiency is restored to normal if monocyte/macrophages are removed from the cell system or if cyclooxygenase inhibitors are added to it.[25] Perhaps the defect is an excessive sensitivity of T lymphocytes to factors such as prostaglandins produced by monocyte/macrophages.

There are data demonstrating that antibodies to EBV antigens in RA patients are *not* different from controls in patients with recent onset ($<$ 6 weeks) of rheumatoid arthritis,[26] and that unlike patients with acute infectious mononucleosis, rheumatoid patients do *not* have an increased excretion from the oropharynx of infectious viral particles.[27] On the basis of these observations, the role of EBV appears to be that of a facilitator (not unlike a co-factor in an enzymatic process) of the chronic immune response in this disease.

No firm data exist implicating other exogenous (e.g., mycoplasma) agents or endogenous antigens as the cause, although as will be discussed below, many investigators believe that altered IgG is, in and of itself, sufficient to cause RA.

## THE EARLY LESION IN RHEUMATOID ARTHRITIS: IMMUNE PROCESSING AND NEW BLOOD VESSEL FORMATION

If we assume that RA is generated by an immune response to an as yet unknown antigen, why does the inflammation begin and persist in the joint? There are three qualities that stand out as being peculiar to joints: (1) they are designed for movement; (2) they contain a potential space lined not by epithelial tissue but by mesenchyme with no basement membrane (see Chapter 16); and (3) within joints there are large areas of avascular connective tissue, the articular and meniscal cartilages.

The observation that arthritis is less severe in paralyzed limbs in patients has been supported by many observations, including quantitative ones demonstrating more cells in the synovial fluid of freely moving joints (after injection of phlogistic crystals) compared with joints that are immobilized. The quality of being developed for motion appears to confer upon joints a susceptibility to inflammation.

Another unusual quality of joints—the lack of limiting membrane between the joint space and synovial blood vessels—contributes to the rapidity with which alterations in blood flow are reflected in cell content and volume of synovial fluid. In addition, the redundant tissue of synovium necessary to allow full motion of the joint makes the joint space a low pressure cavity, which offers minimal (sometimes negative) pressure resistance to inflow of low molecular weight solutes and biologically active precursors or products of inflammation into the joint. During inflammation, high molecular weight substances (e.g., $\alpha_2$-macroglobulin and fibrinogen), which selectively are prevented from entering normal joints, pass readily through synovial capillaries with fenestrations between endothelial cells into the joint space.[28] Once within the joint space it is difficult for molecules of *M*r greater than 100,000 to be cleared. The synovial fluid thus serves as a sink into which are spilled components of inflammation, including proteinases[29] and components of the complement system.[30]

The absence of blood vessels in cartilage makes it possible for antigen-antibody complexes to be sequestered without being cleared from the tissue. That this happens in experimental models as well as in human RA has been demonstrated in a number of studies.[31-33] The requirements for development of this phenomenon may be as follows[34]: (1) antibody must be present in the extravascular space, joint space, or synovium; (2) diffusion of antigen or or soluble complexes into the cartilage must occur; (3) antigen and antibody must combine to form larger, more insoluble complexes; and (4) these aggregates must then be trapped within the meshwork of collagen in cartilage, tendon, or menisci. Immunofluorescent studies have revealed intense staining for IgG, IgM, IgA, and C3 in hyaline cartilage from rheumatoid joints, while very little was present in cartilage from degenerative joint disease.[35] However, the deposition of immune complexes in cartilage is not the sole initiating factor in synovitis; this has been proved by demonstration of the persistence of antigen in nonarthritic joints.[36]

The *absence* of immune complexes in superficial areas of cartilage underlying invasive pannus tissue in RA[37] suggests that these complexes were phagocytized or otherwise freed by the cells of the pannus. It is intriguing to hypothesize that the immune complexes could serve both as a chemoattractant for pannus and, during the process of being phagocytized, as a stimulus to release by the pannus cells of enzymes capable of destroying cartilage.[38,39] Fibronectin binds to the Clq component of complement,[40] and since fibronectin stimulates endocytosis as well as being a chemoattractant in several systems, it is possible that fibronectin could function in facilitating clearance of Clq-coated material such as immune complexes.

These data reviewed here do not provide us with a definite answer to the question of why this early inflammatory response localizes within joints, but do help in understanding the unique setting that the joint offers for an inflammatory and proliferative reaction.

Once within the extracellular synovial tissues the antigen "X" is probably processed by HLA-DR–positive (Ia+) cells. (An alternative is that "X" is brought to the synovium by Ia+ nonresident cells.) In immunofluorescent studies of rheumatoid synovium, interdigitating reticular cells (D cells or "dendritic" cells) staining powerfully for HLA-DR(Ia+) antigens are found in close contact with inducer (helper) T lymphocytes.[41] The appearance of Ia+ on mononuclear cells appears to be induced by antigen presentation. Anatomically, this action occurs in what has been described as "transitional" areas[42] containing some lymphocytes (more suppressor [OK T8] than inducer [OK T4] cells), plasma cells, blast cells, macrophages and fibroblasts. This area is distinct from "lymphocyte-rich" areas around postcapillary venules (where more inducer [OK T4] than suppressor [OK T8] lymphocytes were found) and from the "proliferative" areas containing primarily fibroblasts and macrophages destined to become the effector components of synovium for joint destruction. Close cell-to-cell contact in these areas assures transfer of information among them (Fig. 59–1).

The synovial macrophage or "dendritic" cell-dependent T-lymphocyte activation is not dissimilar from delayed-type hypersensitivity reactions[43] seen in the skin. The synovial HLA-DR+ cells may be functionally similar to epidermal Langerhans cells in their role in antigen presentation. There appear to be different subsets of macrophages when they are characterized by their expression of Ia (HLA-DR); some bear Ia antigens only after activation,[44] whereas the so-called "dendritic cells" (assuming that data in mice can be extrapolated to humans) continuously express Ia antigen.[45]

Without proliferation of new blood vessels, synovitis could not be sustained. As noted in Chapter 13, the endothelial cell is programmed with all the genetic information needed to develop an entire capillary network in vitro so long as the cells are driven by a stimulus such as the angiogenic factors purified from rat tumors[46] or activated macrophages. For capillary growth to occur in vivo, three separate processes must occur: endothelial cell migration, endothelial cell replication, and extracellular matrix modification. Do macrophages in synovium activated during processing of antigen provide the signals to initiate these processes? Or can the endothelial cell itself provide these stimuli? Data suggesting that endothelial cells express Ia antigens on the cell surface and thus have the potential to restore mitogen responsiveness to monocyte-depleted human T lymphocytes[47] raise the possibility of an affirmative answer to the latter question.

## ACUTE INFLAMMATION: A PHENOMENON IN RHEUMATOID SYNOVIAL FLUID BUT NOT SYNOVIUM

Early in rheumatoid synovitis in some patients mononuclear cells may predominate in synovial fluid,[48] but once synovitis is established, the PMN leukocyte is the predominant cell.

**Polymorphonuclear Leukocytes.** Although PMN leukocytes must come from blood vessels and traverse the endothelium to appear in subsynovial tissue, they are rarely found there. The rule is that they migrate almost immediately into the synovial fluid, to which they are drawn by chemotactic factors. Once in the joint space they contribute to the sometimes intense inflammatory response characteristic of RA. It is inevitable that products of this inflammatory activity diffuse back into the

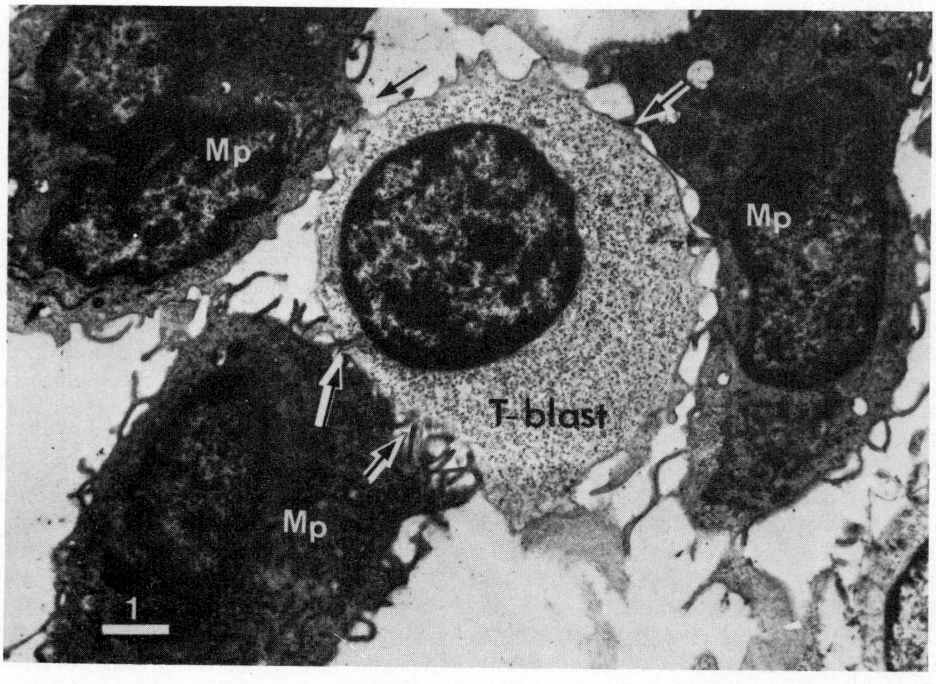


**Figure 59–1.** T lymphoblast surrounded by three macrophages (*Mp*). The arrow points to probable intercellular bridging. (Photograph provided by Hitoshi Ishikawa and Morris Ziff, University of Texas Southwestern Medical Center, Dallas, Texas.)

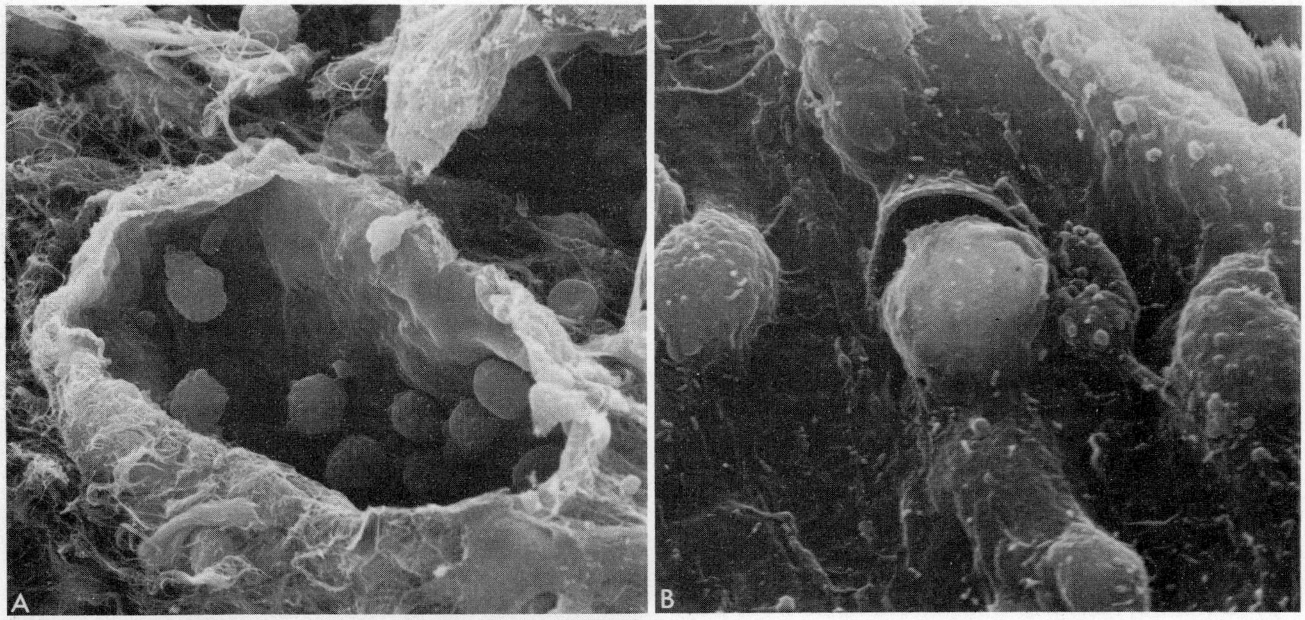


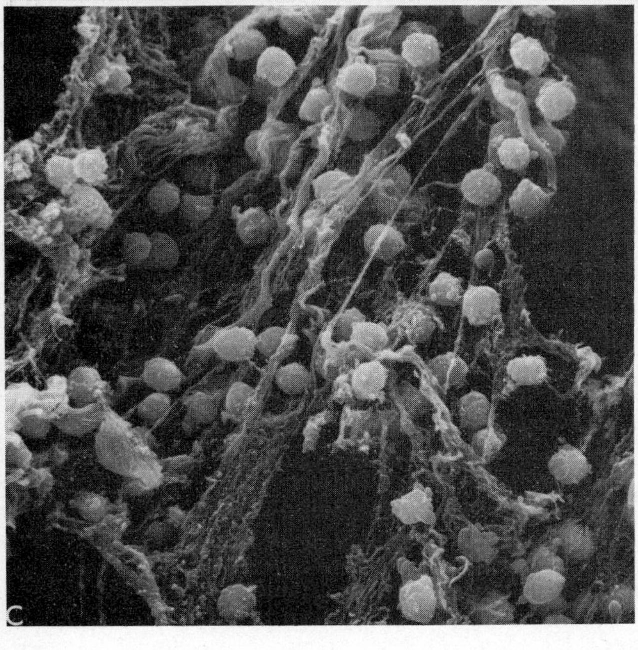

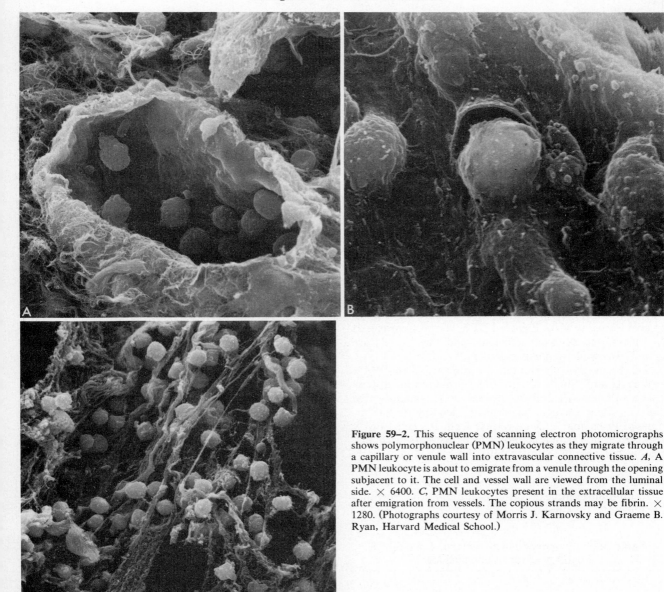

**Figure 59–2.** This sequence of scanning electron photomicrographs shows polymorphonuclear (PMN) leukocytes as they migrate through a capillary or venule wall into extravascular connective tissue. *A*, A PMN leukocyte is about to emigrate from a venule through the opening subjacent to it. The cell and vessel wall are viewed from the luminal side. × 6400. *C*, PMN leukocytes present in the extracellular tissue after emigration from vessels. The copious strands may be fibrin. × 1280. (Photographs courtesy of Morris J. Karnovsky and Graeme B. Ryan, Harvard Medical School.)

synovium and contribute to the proliferative disease seen there.

Figure 59–2 is a sequence showing the migration of PMN leukocytes through a capillary or venule wall into the extracellular matrix. Little damage to the blood vessels results from this emigration of cells, although changes varying in degree from swelling to fibroblastic transformation are seen.[49] Although PMN leukocytes are rarely found in the synovial membrane itself, with the use of histochemical methods for demonstrating PMN neutrophil granules it is estimated that in occasional samples PMN leukocytes may be found at the cartilage-pannus junction.[50] There is no evidence that PMN leukocytes return to the circulation. Rather, they are trapped within the joint. The influx of new cells is quite rapid and it has been estimated by studies of DFP-labeled PMN leukocytes that in a rheumatoid effusion containing 25,000 granulocytes per cubic millimeter, the breakdown in the synovial cavity may exceed one billion cells per day.[51] The mechanism of this postulated destruction is unknown, and the PMN leukocyte degradation has not been measured or observed directly. In addition to cell death, there are several mechanisms that result in release of lysosomal enzymes from PMN leukocytes into synovial fluid (these have been reviewed in detail in Chapter 9).

The direct result of lysosomal enzyme release into the synovial fluid "sink" is generation of a significant potential for tissue damage. Enzymes accumulate more rapidly than they can be cleared from the fluid through exit by synovial capillaries. Eventually the large quantity of proteinases saturate the capacity of proteinase inhibitors present in synovial fluid, and enzyme activity (e.g., collagenase) is expressed unopposed.[29] In addition, it is likely (see Chapters 9 and 10) that lysosomal contents have a direct capability for provoking tissue injury and potentiating a proliferative response in synovial tissue.[52-54]

In order for PMN leukocytes to accumulate within the joint space, chemotactic factors (CF) must be elaborated (Table 59–2). Chemotactic substances (as detailed in Chapter 9) react with specific receptors on the PMN leukocyte cell surface, resulting in a polarized appearance of the cell as ion flux occurs and phospholipase, methyltransferase, and adenylate cyclase are activated. One of the substances listed in Table 59–2, leukotriene $B_4$ ($LTB_4$),[57] is a product of the 5-lipoxygenase pathway of arachidonate metabolism (see Chapters 6 and 9). PMN leukocytes metabolize $LTB_4$ quickly, and for this reason it is not known how important a role $LTB_4$ plays in chemotoxis in vivo. Elevated $LTB_4$ has been measured in rheumatoid synovial effusions, and these levels are acutely lowered by glucocorticoids.[58]

The binding of chemotactic substances to the PMN leukocyte and "fluidizing" of the cell membrane appear to be sufficient in and of themselves to generate free radicals from oxygen metabolism, leading to an increased lysosomal enzyme release from the cells. PMN leukocytes in peripheral blood from patients with RA may be deficient in their capability for both phagocytosis and response to chemoattractants.[55,56] This may reflect a form of down-regulation by cells that have phagocytized immune complexes or have saturated the receptors for chemotactic stimuli.

**Table 59–2.** Endogenous Chemotactic Factors (CF) Found in Chronic Inflammation*

1. Complement-derived CF
   - C5a
   - C3 fragment
   - C567
2. Lymphocyte-derived CF
   - These are chemotactic for monocytes, fibroblasts, and eosinophils as well as PMN leukocytes.
3. PMN leukocyte-derived CF
4. Leukotriene $B_4$
   - This substance also may be needed for PMN leukocyte responsiveness to other CF.
5. Platelet-derived growth factor
6. Platelet factor IV
7. Enzymes
   - Kallikrein
   - Plasminogen activator
8. Coagulation-related factors
   - Fibrinopeptide B
   - Fibrin degradation products
9. Fibronectin
10. Collagen fragments

*Derived from O'Flaherty, J.T., and Ward, P.A.: Chemotactic factors and neutrophil. Sem. Hematol. 16:163, 1979.

Free radicals associated with reduction of molecular oxygen by PMN leukocytes and by mononuclear phagocytes are generated within the joint in response to phagocytosis or by binding of chemotactic substances to cell membrane receptors.[59] The radicals—superoxide ($O_2^{\div}$, hydroxyl ion ($OH^{\div}$), and singlet oxygen ($^1O_2{}^*$)—have the potential to damage lipid membranes,[60] degrade hyaluronic acid,[61] inactivate proteinase inhibitors such as $\alpha_1$-proteinase inhibitor[62] and catalyze production of chemotactic lipids from polyunsaturated fatty acids. Solid evidence for pathologic activity in vivo of these free radicals is sparse because they are scavenged quickly by numerous naturally occurring superoxide dismutases within mitochondria as well as in the cytosol of cells. The naturally occurring copper-binding protein ceruloplasmin[63] has superoxide dismutase activity. Orgotein, a substance with anti-inflammatory activity isolated from bovine liver, is in fact a superoxide dismutase and has demonstrated anti-inflammatory effects.[64] Copper-penicillamine complexes may generate $H_2O_2$ nonenzymatically, which in turn can damage cell membranes, inhibiting cellular functions such as the T-lymphocyte response to mitogens (the presumptive mechanism of action of this disease-modifying drug [Lipsky, unpublished observations]). PMN leukocytes also produce *N*-chloroamines,[64a] by chlorination of endogenous amines in the presence of $H_2O_2$ and myeloperoxidase. These chloroamines are potent oxidizers of sulfhydryl groups and/or thioether groups, which are crucial to the activity of certain proteins. Chloroamines have a longer T½ than do superoxide, hydroxyl radicals, etc.

Complex functions of granulocytes in RA such as rates of phagocytosis have been reported to be normal by some investigators[65] and impaired by others.[66,67] Similarly, response to chemoattractants of PMN leukocytes from patients with RA was reported to be depressed in some studies[68] but normal in others.[69] It must be stressed that factors other than the underlying disease affect integrated neutrophil functions, including drug therapy and nutritional status. For example, it has been demonstrated in a crossover study of 13 rheumatoid patients that a 7-day fast (i.e., no food; noncaloric liquids ad lib) produced a mean weight loss of 5.1 kg., an increased response to chemoattractants, and improved serum bactericidal activity.[69] An association was found between improvement in inflammatory activity of the joints and enhancement of neutrophil bactericidal capacity.

The full potential for tissue destruction and enhancement of inflammation by PMN leukocytes is treated completely in Chapters 9 and 12. It is probable that this cell is one of the most important amplification mechanisms in the inflammatory process of RA. Once responding to chemoattractants or being activated during phagocytosis, the broad range of powerful phlogistic effects is sufficient to generate painful symptoms in patients, particularly since the cells and their inflammatory constituents are trapped within the joint space.

**Synovial Fluid Pathology in the Inflammatory Lesion of RA.** It must be emphasized again that there is no membrane barrier isolating synovium from synovial fluid and that the interactions among systems within synovial fluid can effect change in the proliferative rate of synovial cells. Conversely, substances generated by lymphocytes, macrophages, and synovial cells may amplify inflammation through effects on cellular or extracellular substances in synovial fluid.

***Complement.*** Just as data have indicated that immunoglobulins and anti-immunoglobulins are synthesized by rheumatoid synovial tissue,[71,72] radioisotope dilution studies have provided evidence that 50 percent of intra-articular C3 may be derived from local synthesis[73] and that biologically active C2, C4, C5, and properdin factor B are synthesized there as well.[77] Despite local production of complement components, the activities of C4, C2, and C3 and total hemolytic complement in rheumatoid (seropositive) synovial effusions are lower than in synovial fluids from patients with other joint diseases.[70,74,75]

Using a sensitive solid-phase radioimmunoassay to quantitate the activation of the classic pathway of complement by rheumatoid factor, it has been demonstrated[76] that IgM-rheumatoid factor is a much more important determinant of complement activation than is IgG-rheumatoid factor in both serum and synovial fluids. Combined with other data showing that there is an accelerated catabolism of C4 in RA[77] and that the presence of C4 fragments[78] in plasma of rheumatoid patients correlates with titers of rheumatoid factor, the weight of evidence indicates a role in vivo for IgM-rheumatoid factor in complement activation.

The biologically active products produced during complement activation are probably the most important consequence of intra-articular complement consumption. Like proteinases from PMN leukocytes, these inflammatory components may build up in synovial fluid during acute inflammation. The potential for interaction between PMN leukocytes and the complement system is substantial. Neutrophil lysosomal lysates contain enzymatic activity capable of generating chemotactic activity (probably C5a) from fresh serum,[79,80] and an enzyme acting at neutral pH found in rheumatoid synovial fluid produced chemotactic factor in significant quantity when incubated with purified C5.[81] C5a, in addition to being a principal chemotactic factor in inflammatory effusions, is capable of mediating lysosomal release from human PMN leukocytes.[79,80,82] This sets up one of many amplification loops in inflammatory synovial fluid.

Another amplification loop in synovial inflammation may involve complement activation by C-reactive protein (CRP). As reviewed in Chapter 43, CRP concentrations in plasma increased up to 1000 times the concentrations found in normal individuals following an inflammatory stimulus. CRP may combine with phospholipid constituents of necrotic cell membranes at inflammatory sites or with the first complement components.[83-85]

***Kinin-Forming Systems.*** One of the primary mediators of acute inflammation generated in synovial fluid is bradykinin. Bradykinin is a nonapeptide (see Chapter 8). The increased vascular permeability and local vasodilatation it produces could be principal factors in generating warm joints and synovial effusions.[86] As with the clotting system, activation of Hageman factor (factor XII) is the initial step in kinin formation.[87] Kinins and arthritis may be related at multiple steps in development of inflammation. Rheumatoid factor–IgG complexes have been reported to activate kininogens, although rheumatoid factor plus unaltered IgG did not.[88] Kallikrein activator and kininase are both present in human granulocytes. Kallikrein itself is a potent and versatile proteinase that can activate plasminogen to plasmin, and precursor to active Hageman factor, and latent to active collagenase.

***Fibrin Formation and Fibrinolysis.*** The end point of activation of the clotting sequence is the formation of fibrin. The accumulation of fibrin is one of the most striking pathologic features of rheumatoid synovitis. Fibrin accumulates on the synovial surface, on cartilage surfaces, in areas of subsynovial hemorrhage or infarction, and as particulate aggregates in synovial fluid. At the final stages of fibrin formation, fibrinopeptides are formed (released from fibrinogen by the action of thrombin during clotting), which may have the capacity in and of themselves to increase vascular permeability. What initiates the clotting sequence? It has not been demonstrated that immune complexes of rheumatoid factor and IgG can activate this Hageman factor–dependent pathway,[89] but plasmin (activated by plasminogen activator from plasminogen) has this capability, as (possibly) does collagen. Production of a procoagulant by mononuclear cells in culture is stimulated by immune complexes.[90]

The presence of fibrin on synovium and cartilage may impede normal nutrition to these tissues and may amplify conditions that lead to hypoxia and acidosis in synovial fluid. In addition, homologous fibrin appears to generate a chronic immunologic response in experimental animals.[91] It is possible that in addition to being entrapped in collagen matrix, immune complexes may be caught up in fibrin clots within the joint space, a factor that would perpetuate the inflammatory and proliferative disease. Like the buildup of other components of the inflammatory reaction, the accumulation of fibrin in joints reflects an imbalance caused by the inadequacy of the joint lining to clear the large quantities of byproducts of inflammation. In some rheumatoid joints a strong inhibition of fibrinolysis by plasmin has been observed as well as diminished activity of plasminogen activator.[92]

***Arachidonic Acid Metabolites.*** The prostaglandins produced from membrane phospholipids have been discussed extensively (see Chapter 6). Their presence and activity have been equated with the degree of inflammation in RA. However, their role has been diminished recently, in part because it is appreciated that although $PGE_2$ and $PGI_2$ cause vasodilatation and are synergistic with other substances (e.g., histamine, C5a, $LTB_4$) in increasing vasopermeability, the leukotrienes (especially $LTB_4$) may have more potent phlogistic effects than do the products of cyclooxygenase. In addition, it is appreciated that certain harmful effects of nonsteroidal anti-inflammatory drugs (e.g., renal insufficiency, toxic amblyopia, CNS effects, and hepatotoxicity) may be directly related to prostaglandin inhibition. Also, increasing data support a beneficial role for prostaglandins in synovial biology. As potential good effects within connective tissue, $PGE_2$ may suppress synovial cell proliferation, suppress production of plasminogen activator by certain cells, and inhibit formation of free radicals.[94,95] Underlying these facts is the principle that biologic effects of pluripotent substances such as prostaglandins are multiple, and while inhibition of one function in vivo may help suppress inflammation, inhibition of another may amplify it.

***Synovial Fluid Oxygen.*** It has been calculated that glucose uptake in rheumatoid synovium may be five times greater than in normal tissue, and that anaerobic glycolysis increases fractionally more than aerobic glycolysis.[96,97] Despite the increase in blood flow and a shift toward anaerobic glycolysis, there exists a state of relative hypoxia in the synovial fluid and, presumably, the synovium as well. There is an inverse linear correlation between pH of rheumatoid synovial fluid on one hand and lactic acid and $pCO_2$ on the other.[98] The pH remains relatively constant until $pO_2$ falls to approximately 30 mm Hg, at which point it begins to fall precipitously as the $pO_2$ continues to fall.[98] Only those patients with severe active RA had a synovial fluid $pO_2$ of less than 27 mm Hg.[98] The severe rheumatoid patient, therefore, may have ischemic joint tissues. In the presence of large tense joint effusions the intra-articular pressure may be great enough to obliterate small vessel blood flow. In those without elevated intra-articular pressures, inflammation-associated increases in synovial blood supply may still be insufficient for adequate oxygenation of the proliferated, hypermetabolic synovial tissues. This may lead to focal infarction and necrosis and may be a factor in generating "rice bodies" in joints. Consistent with this concept of "metabolic-circulatory imbalance" is the fact that the temperature of joint effusions in the sickest rheumatoids is often low; it has been inferred that the decline in local temperature reflects a hypoperfused or ischemic synovium.[99]

***Iron.*** Rupture of small vessels in RA must be relatively common, because iron deposits in the form of hemosiderin are observed frequently. The foci of iron granules are often not in just the lining cells, as in hemophilic arthritis, but in deep synovial cells as well[100] (Fig. 59–3). As illustrated by the proliferative synovitis seen in hemophilic arthritis,[101] red blood cell products (including iron) may supplement the other inflammatory and proliferative stimuli within the joint. Iron may have deleterious effects upon cells when it accumulates in tissues to the degree it does in rheumatoid synovium. In the presence of traces of free iron salts, superoxide and hydrogen peroxide can react together to produce the hydroxyl radical, the most toxic of the univalent reduction products derived from oxygen.[102] Deposition of iron within reticuloendothelial cells probably requires oxidation of ferrous iron, since it is stored in the more stable ferric form; this oxidation may necessitate activation of molecular oxygen.[103] Iron, even in soluble complexes, can induce synovial cells to produce significant amounts of neutral proteinases.[104]

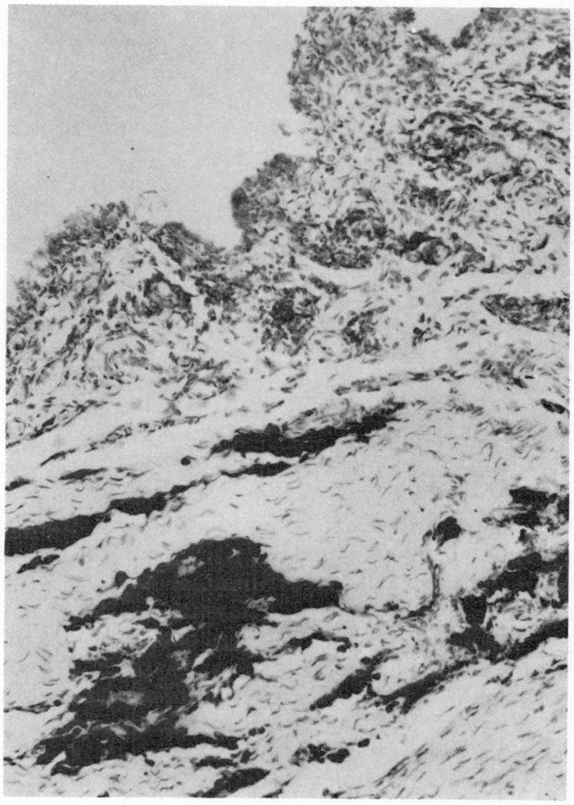

**Figure 59–3.** In this section of rheumatoid synovium prepared with Prussian blue stain, large collections of iron, the product of many microhemorrhages, are found deep in the subsynovial tissue. × 315. (Courtesy of K. Muirden, M.D.)

## THE CHRONIC IMMUNOPROLIFERATIVE REACTION IN SYNOVIUM

The heterogeneity of cells found in rheumatoid synovium is a fact that has great implications for function of this diseased tissue. As more is learned about individual cell types in the chronic immunoproliferative response, it has become clear that cellular function in the synovium is dependent upon and determined by communication among different cell types.

The early stage of the immune response in synovium has been described above. It involves presentation of antigen by accessory cells such as endothelial cells and/or macrophages to T lymphocytes, which subsequently activate multiple clones of B lymphocytes. As Ziff[105] pointed out in 1974, the synovial tissues of patients with rheumatoid arthritis have many of the properties of a secondary lymphoid organ involved in an active immune response with the synthesis of immunoglobulin. Most of the small lymphocytes in the rheumatoid synovial membrane appear to be T lymphocytes. Immunofluorescent studies have revealed positive staining with anti–T-lymphocyte antisera, and the same cells do not demonstrate EAC receptors.[106,107] Even the aggregates of small lymphocytes adjacent to plasma cell–rich areas in rheumatoid synovial membranes are T lymphocytes.[108] B lymphocytes, on the other hand, may be rapidly transformed into plasma cells after arrival in the synovium. The T-lymphocyte predominance in synovial tissue does not apply to peripheral blood. Although some investigators have detected fewer B lymphocytes in rheumatoid patients,[109] others have reported finding increased numbers of B lymphocytes,[110] while still others report no differences in B- and T-lymphocyte ratios in normal and rheumatoid patients.[111]

The functional subsets of the T lymphocytes vary from one anatomic area to another within the synovium. In the "transitional" areas suppressor T lymphocytes are more numerous, while in the "lymphocyte-rich" areas inducer T lymphocytes predominate.[42] B lymphocytes in synovium are localized primarily within reactive lymphoid centers.[112]

Compared with cells found in peripheral blood of both rheumatoid and normal individuals, many more lymphocytes in rheumatoid synovium express Ia+ antigens on their surface. One study demonstrated a strong preferential expression on suppressor/cytotoxic subsets compared with helper/inducer cells.[113] Although variable among different studies, the $T_5$:$T_H$ lymphocyte ratio in synovial fluid is generally higher than in peripheral blood of rheumatoid patients,[114] a phenomenon possibly related to localization of T helper cells within synovium around accessory/antigen-presenting cells. This variability may reflect the expected variation in both intensity and focus of the immune response in different patients at different stages of their diseases. It is important to emphasize that it is only after activation that T lymphocytes express Ia antigen.[115,116]

In peripheral blood, as in synovium, the most striking change in lymphocyte surface antigens in rheumatoid arthritis is not fluctuations in lymphocyte subsets but an increase in Ia+ antigens found on lymphocytes.[117] This nonspecific phenomenon is seen also after immunization with tetanus toxoid or PPD and may serve as an index in any individual of immunologic stimulation.[117] Similarly, using methods that separate activated from resting lymphocytes by density gradient centrifugation,[118] a direct correlation between clinical disease activity and numbers of activated B lymphocytes (B-blasts) in peripheral blood lymphocyte populations has been observed.

One of the subsets of lymphoid cells that has received increased interest for its relevance to rheumatoid arthritis has been that of natural killer (NK) cells.[119] These are nonadherent, nonphagocytic cells that express surface receptors for the Fc portion of IgG and share a variety of T-lymphocyte markers. Morphologically, they appear as large granular lymphocytes. Functionally, they share features with both macrophages and PMN leukocytes, having spontaneous activity in normal individuals and augmented activity in response to interferon and other stimuli. Unlike macrophages and PMN leukocytes they proliferate in response to Interleukin 2 (T cell growth factor). Killing of other cells may be mediated by membrane-associated serine proteinases or phospholipases. There are very few studies of NK cells in rheumatoid arthritis. One study[120] has reported a decreased cytotoxicity of unfractionated synovial tissue lymphocytes from RA compared with peripheral blood lymphocytes from both rheumatoid and control populations.

No immunospecific response of lymphocytes from rheumatoid patients to rheumatoid synovium has been observed, although lymphocytes from some patients did show greater cytotoxic activity than did control lymphocytes when tested against young cultures of synovial cells.[121] These observations were not confirmed in another study.[122] Using the very sensitive antibody-dependent cell-mediated cytotoxicity (ADCC) assays, Griffiths and co-workers found no antibody to synovial cells in ten autologous rheumatoid sera.[123] However, since immunoglobulin is produced by plasma cells in rheumatoid synovium,[71] and peripheral blood mononuclear leukocytes from RA produce IgM rheumatoid factor in vitro (in contrast to controls),[124] and since there are Fc receptor–bearing lymphocytes in rheumatoid synovial tissues,[125] the effector mechanisms needed to mobilize ADCC are clearly present.

The histologic picture in rheumatoid synovium is one of extreme proliferation, and "cytotoxicity" is not obvious. One hypothesis designed to reconcile this apparent contradiction is that the normal mechanism of ADCC in RA may be inhibited by antigen present in excess (e.g., IgG) or by antigen-antibody complexes. Thus, the ADCC that normally would inhibit cell proliferation would be inhibited in the rheumatoid patient and proliferation could develop unopposed.

One other subset of lymphocytes should be considered in the context of rheumatoid synovitis. A prostaglandin-producing lymphocyte subpopulation has been defined.[126] There are more indomethacin-sensitive (i.e., prostaglandin-producing) peripheral blood mononuclear cells in rheumatoid than in normal patients.[127] Prostaglandin production by rheumatoid synovial cells is enormously increased in RA.[129]

Soluble mediators (lymphokines) are produced by active lymphocytes and have many biologic effects.[130] In RA there is evidence for activity in synovium of lymphokines, which have the effect (1) of increasing vascular permeability; (2) of being chemotactic for granulocytes and monocytes; (3) of activating monocyte-macrophages, osteoclasts, and synovial cells; and (4) of being mitogenic. The name "lymphokine" may be misleading. Certain soluble factors once thought to be produced by lymphocytes are now known to be released by monocyte-macrophages with some sort of assistance from lymphocytes. In addition, there is evidence that B lymphocytes can produce such soluble mediators. It may be most helpful to consider the soluble mediators of inflammation as being produced by the interaction of monocyte-macrophages and lymphocytes. Injection of partially purified preparations of lymphokines into rabbit knee joints has produced a chronic inflammatory reaction in the subsynovial tissue.[127] This may be another example of the cyclic augmentation found in chronic rheumatoid synovitis; in this case, inflammation produces activation of mediators, which in turn stimulate more inflammation.

Much current debate exists concerning transfer factor.[131,132] More studies are needed to determine whether or not this is a discrete factor or rather represents heterogeneous, nonspecific helper factors from lymphocyte cultures that stimulate immune responses directly or by inhibition of suppressor factors.

A primary role for lymphocytes as determinants of activity of RA is suggested indirectly by studies of their depletion in this disease.[133,134] Thoracic duct drainage and depletion of lymphocytes often ameliorate, although temporarily, the course of RA. Collagen-induced arthritis can be transferred from affected to nonaffected animals using lymphocytes from the sick animals.[135,136] That B lymphocytes capable of differentiating into antibody-secreting plasma cells are less crucial for development of arthritis than are T lymphocytes can be inferred from the fact that an illness like RA can develop in patients with congenital agammaglobulinemia.[137]

**Antibody Production by Rheumatoid Synovial Lymphocytes: The Role of Rheumatoid Factor in Pathogenesis.** B lymphocytes and plasma cells synthesize and release immunoglobulins from their sites in the synovium of RA,[71] and immunofluorescent studies reveal that significant amounts of rheumatoid factor are produced by these cells as well.[138,139] Most of the plasma cells contain IgG, but IgM-containing cells are also observed, particularly in seropositive patients. The lymphocytes in rheumatoid synovium appear to be committed to different antigens than are the peripheral blood lymphocytes of the same individual. IgG produced by synovial culture explants of numerous patients with RA contained an average of 41 percent $IgG_3$ compared with 12 percent $IgG_3$ in the serum IgG of the same patients.[140] However, $IgG_1$ is by far the predominant IgG type produced by synovial lymphocyte/plasma cells in RA.

Repeated immunizations with tetanus toxoid of rheumatoid patients before joint surgery have failed to induce antitetanus antibody production by synovial cells even though peripheral blood lymphocytes were producing specific antibody at a brisk rate.[142] Lymphocytes from nonarticular tissues (e.g., pericardium) involved in the inflammatory process also synthesize IgG and IgM and RF. Factors involved in "spread" of rheumatoid disease from articular to nonarticular tissues are not known.

Although there are no data clearly implicating rheumatoid factor as a principal causative agent in RA, the role of antiglobulins in the amplification and perpetuation of the process is well supported:

1. Despite the fact that some patients with virtually no circulating IgG develop RA,[137] it is known that patients with a positive test for rheumatoid factor in blood have more severe clinical disease and complications[141] than do seronegative patients.

2. Some data have indicated that rheumatoid factor is "hidden" or masked by other proteins in some seronegative patients.[143] However, recent studies that examined production in vitro by peripheral blood mononuclear leukocytes have indicated that (a) lymphocytes/monocyte populations from seropositive RA patients spontaneously elaborate IgM RF and (b) similar populations of cells from both normal and seronegative patients produced no IgM RF unless induced by lectins, and then produced significantly less than cells from seropositive patients.[144] These studies support with immunologic evidence the hypothesis that seronegative RA represents a disease distinct from seropositive RA.

3. Polyclonal IgM rheumatoid factor is able to fix and activate complement by the classic pathway.[145]

4. Using a cell assay for anti-IgG (rheumatoid factor) plaque-forming cells, Vaughan found that the appearance of these cells coincided with flares of clinical activity of the disease.[146] Anti-IgG plaque-forming cells were more concentrated in bone marrow and synovial fluid than in peripheral blood.

5. Most IgG-rheumatoid factors are directed against antigenic determinants on the Fc fragments of IgG and may self-associate to form dimers of larger polymers[147] (Fig. 59–4). These complexes stimulate their own formation and this, another example of cyclic amplification, continues long after any exogenous infective agent has been cleared from the system. Self-associating rheumatoid factors are almost impossible to detect unless the Fc region of the molecules bearing antigenic determinants is removed by prior pepsin digestion.[148] Isolated IgG that had self-associated to form RF was able to activate the human complement cascade in the fluid phase, even though its effectiveness was only 1/100th that of aggregated IgG or large-latticed immune complexes.[149] If one postulates that high concentrations or further polymerization of self-associating IgG-RF occurs in joints, perhaps bound to cartilage surfaces, a mechanism would be available for explaining depressed levels of complement in rheumatoid synovial effusions.[150]

6. Immune complexes containing rheumatoid factor have been localized within synovial tissues by immunofluorescent techniques[151,153] (Fig. 59–5). A hyperviscosity syndrome, which affects the central nervous system (producing headache, tinnitus, vertigo, and seizures)

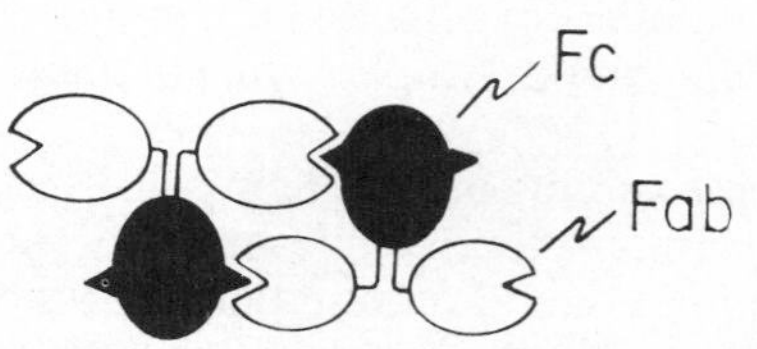


**Figure 59–4.** Scheme for development of self-associating IgG, which may increase in size sufficient to fix complement or be phagocytized by PMN leukocytes, or both. The Fab positions of one molecule have affinity for the Fc portion of another, and the lattice begins to build. (After Pope, R.M., et al.: Proc. Natl. Acad. Sci. USA 71:517, 1974.)

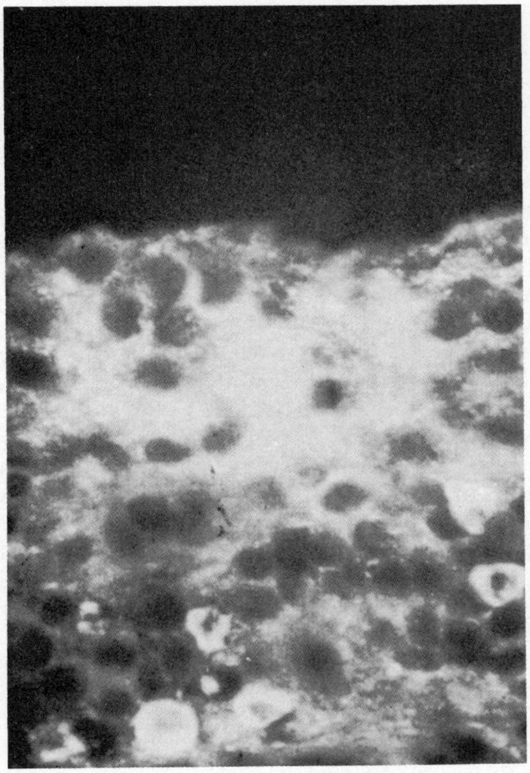

**Figure 59–5.** Section of rheumatoid synovial tissue stained with fluorescein-labeled anti-IgG. A similar staining pattern was observed in the same sections with fluorescein-labeled anti-C3, indicating the presence of immune complexes. (From Natvig, J.B., et al.: Scand. J. Rheumatol. 5 [Suppl. 12]:77, 1975.)

and causes striking retinal pathology and diffuse hemorrhages, has been reported in a number of patients with RA,[154,155] and circulating intermediate-size immune complexes have been demonstrated. Another clinical association between severe disease and rheumatoid factor has been the finding of IgM rheumatoid factor in pulmonary lesions of patients with rheumatoid lung disease.[156]

7. Increased levels of IgG–anti-IgG have been associated with a high frequency of subcutaneous nodules, vasculitis,[157,158] elevated erythrocyte sedimentation rate, decreased complement levels, and increased number of involved joints. IgG-IgG complexes in joint fluids of rheumatoid patients have been shown after isolation and purification to be almost completely IgG rheumatoid factor.[158,159] IgG rheumatoid factor has been identified in plasma cells from rheumatoid synovial membranes.[160] In seropositive patients about 60 percent of plasma cells contained rheumatoid factor, while none of the cells from control tissue did.[161,162] Polymorphonuclear leukocytes from rheumatoid synovial effusions contain intracytoplasmic granules of immunoglobulins, including rheumatoid factor.[163-166] PMN leukocytes from synovial fluid which contain intracytoplasmic inclusions, called "ragocytes," are easily seen on wet preparations visualized without staining, although they are seen more clearly using immunofluorescence. Such inclusions often contain rheumatoid factor. Recent data suggest that within rheumatoid synovial effusions IgG rheumatoid factor is preferentially reduced compared with serum, in contrast to IgA and IgM RF.[167] These data suggest that IgG RF may be specifically utilized in the pathogenesis of the proliferative, chronic synovitis.

8. In experiments performed in patients with RA, a marked inflammatory response was elicited when rheumatoid factor from the patient was injected into the joint, but not when normal IgG was given.[168] Rheumatoid factor becomes involved in pathogenesis when it forms immune complexes sufficiently large to activate complement[169] and/or be phagocytized by macrophages or polymorphonuclear leukocytes. Detection of the immune complexes independent of their antigenic specificity has given a new perspective to clinical studies.[170] Immune complex assays using binding to Clq are most frequently positive in RA (see Chapters 44 and 45).

Several hypotheses have been advanced to explain how IgG could become immunogenic.

i. New determinants on IgG may be exposed following polymerization as an aggregate or in antigen-antibody complexes.[171]

ii. A structural anomaly in the IgG of rheumatoid patients may render it immunogenic. Studies using circular dichroism spectropolarimetry have suggested that there may be a defect at the hinge region of rheumatoid IgG which could increase the binding affinity to membrane Fc receptors on B lymphocytes.[172]

iii. Depletion of suppressor T lymphocytes might allow B lymphocytes to produce autoantibodies against certain determinants on IgG.[173]

iv. Rheumatoid factor development could represent idiotype–anti-idiotype interaction. Jerne proposed[174] that in the course of an immune response, specific idiotypes present in higher concentration might stimulate anti-idiotypic antibody formation, which could modulate the immune response. Monoclonal antibodies have been developed against idiotypes on IgM rheumatoid factor. In one study the mouse antibody reacted with an identical or similar determinant located on (or close to) the binding site of all tested monoclonal or polyclonal IgM RF. The significance of these highly conserved determinants on rheumatoid factor idiotypes is not yet understood.[75]

Studies of lymphocyte antibody production in vitro have contributed to dissection of the immune response in RA. Using the hemolytic plaque-forming assay,[176] one can test for lymphocytes producing antibody against specific antigens as well as quantitate the number of cells with this specificity. Lymphocytes from rheumatoid patients in the plaque-forming assay have been observed to produce rheumatoid factor which is not present in peripheral blood and which has a much higher affinity for IgG than does rheumatoid factor in blood.[177] Were these high-affinity rheumatoid factors produced in vivo, they might never gain access to the circulation but rather be bound to autologous IgG in the immediate environment of the cell. These high-affinity complexes could aggregate and activate complement or be phagocytized, or both, initiating inflammation in the tissues (e.g., synovium) in which the antiglobulins were formed.

In addition to rheumatoid factors of the $\gamma$, $\alpha$, and $\delta$ isotypes in RA, $\epsilon$ isotypes also have been demonstrated in certain patients.[178,179] Of 13 sera containing IgE immune complexes, 11 were from patients with extra-articular manifestations.[179] It was suggested that IgE-RF could complex with aggregated (self-associating) IgG in synovial tissue and that the IgG-IgE complexes could activate mast cells and basophils in the synovium, resulting in accentuation of the inflammatory response in this organ.[178] This has particular interest in light of recent reports that there are numerous mast cells in rheumatoid synovium and that these may release factors capable of stimulating collagenase production by synovial cells.[180]

**Circulating Immune Complexes (CIC).** The availability of multiple assays for CIC in serum has led to a proliferation of studies demonstrating correlation of the presence of CIC with certain articular and extra-articular manifestations of RA. In particular, vasculitis is frequently associated with high levels of immune complexes.[181,182] Interpretation of data on CIC in RA has been confused by a plethora of different assays for CIC as well as by interference with the test by rheumatoid factor. Different assays give different results using the same sera, and the differences are not due to different sensitivities of the assays. One recent study compared the following five different assay systems for CIC in rheumatoid sera: (1) bovine conglutinin assay; (2) $^{125}$I-Clq binding assay; (3) monoclonal rheumatoid factor inhibition assay; (4) Raji cell assay; and (5) staphylococcal binding assay.[183] Different tests discriminated better for different parameters of disease activity (e.g., articular disease severity and extra-articular manifestations). None was of more use for measuring disease activity than the erythrocyte sedimentation rate or the IgG rheumatoid factor immunoassay.

## THE SYNOVIAL CELLS IN RHEUMATOID ARTHRITIS

The synovial cells in rheumatoid arthritis are hyperplastic and usually become the dominant cell in the thickened, highly vascular synovium, which may weigh up to a thousandfold more than the normal membrane surrounding the joint cavity. As mentioned previously, many of the synovial cells become Ia antigen positive as synovitis develops.

**Dissociated Adherent Rheumatoid Synovial Cells.** In recent years the cells in rheumatoid synovium have been characterized by studying them in a freshly dissociated state. Thirty to 50 percent appear to be lymphocytes, some of which are partially adherent. The remaining cells are heterogeneous.[184,185] Most have been described as larger (15 to 60 $\mu$m) than lymphocytes with a high ratio of cytoplasm to nucleus. Many of these are multinucleate. In culture up to 40 percent of adherent cells may have a classic stellate or dendritic appearance (Fig. 59–6) and have knobby inclusions within a ribbed cytoplasm of the cell processes. Forty to 70 percent of the cells are phagocytic in early cultures. There does appear to be a subset of adherent synovial cells that have receptors for C3 and the Fc portion of IgG[186] and are similar in other respects to monocyte/macrophages. Most of the stellate cells do not have Fc receptors, nor do they produce lysozyme.[184] Cultures containing these mixtures of cells produce very large amounts of collagenase and prostaglandins.

In primary cultures the stellate cells begin to lose their striking appearance as monocytes/macrophages decrease or after cells are passaged. The stellate appearance is related to changes in biochemical parameters within cells. There are data[187] suggesting that mononuclear cell factor (Interleukin I) produced by monocytes/macrophages stimulates $PGE_2$ production, which in turn induces activity of adenylate cyclase, which produces increased cellular cAMP levels. As cAMP levels increase, the cells take on a stellate appearance. Despite the relationship of stellate cells and collagenase production, and the relationship of the stellate appearance with $PGE_2$ levels, there is no proven direct link in human synovial cells between $PGE_2$ and collagenase biosynthesis.

It is tempting to focus on the similarities among the collagenase/$PGE_2$-producing stellate cell of rheumatoid synovium, the DR-positive (Ia+) human epidermal Langerhans cells,[188] and the human dendritic (stellate) (Ia+) cells which circulate in peripheral blood and may be the principal accessory cell for antigen presentation to lymphocytes. It has not been demonstrated directly that the same cells expressing enhanced Ia+ positivity are those induced by Interleukin 1 to produce large amounts of collagenase; indeed, the latter cell type seems to be larger than the Ia+ accessory cell.

**Rheumatoid Synovial Cells Grown from Explants.** Most studies of rheumatoid synovial cells have been carried out using the cells that grow out from explants in organ culture. The advantage to this technique is that a morphologically homogeneous fibroblast-like population is produced. However, these cells have passed through several generations when functional characteristics are first studied; differentiated cells with a primary role in the rheumatoid process may not survive trypsinization or other routine methods of cell passage, and the original admixture of different cell types is lost. Nevertheless, the "synovial fibroblasts" that have been grown out from explants of rheumatoid synovium have a number of qualities different from cells obtained from normal tissue: (1) The rheumatoid cells in early cultures have higher growth rates than cells from noninflammatory synovitis and reach a higher final saturation density.[189] There are insignificant differences, however, in these parameters between rheumatoid cells and cells from nonrheumatoid but inflammatory synovitis. (2) The rheumatoid cells produce hyaluronic acid of lower molecular weight.[190] (3) The rheumatoid cells have a

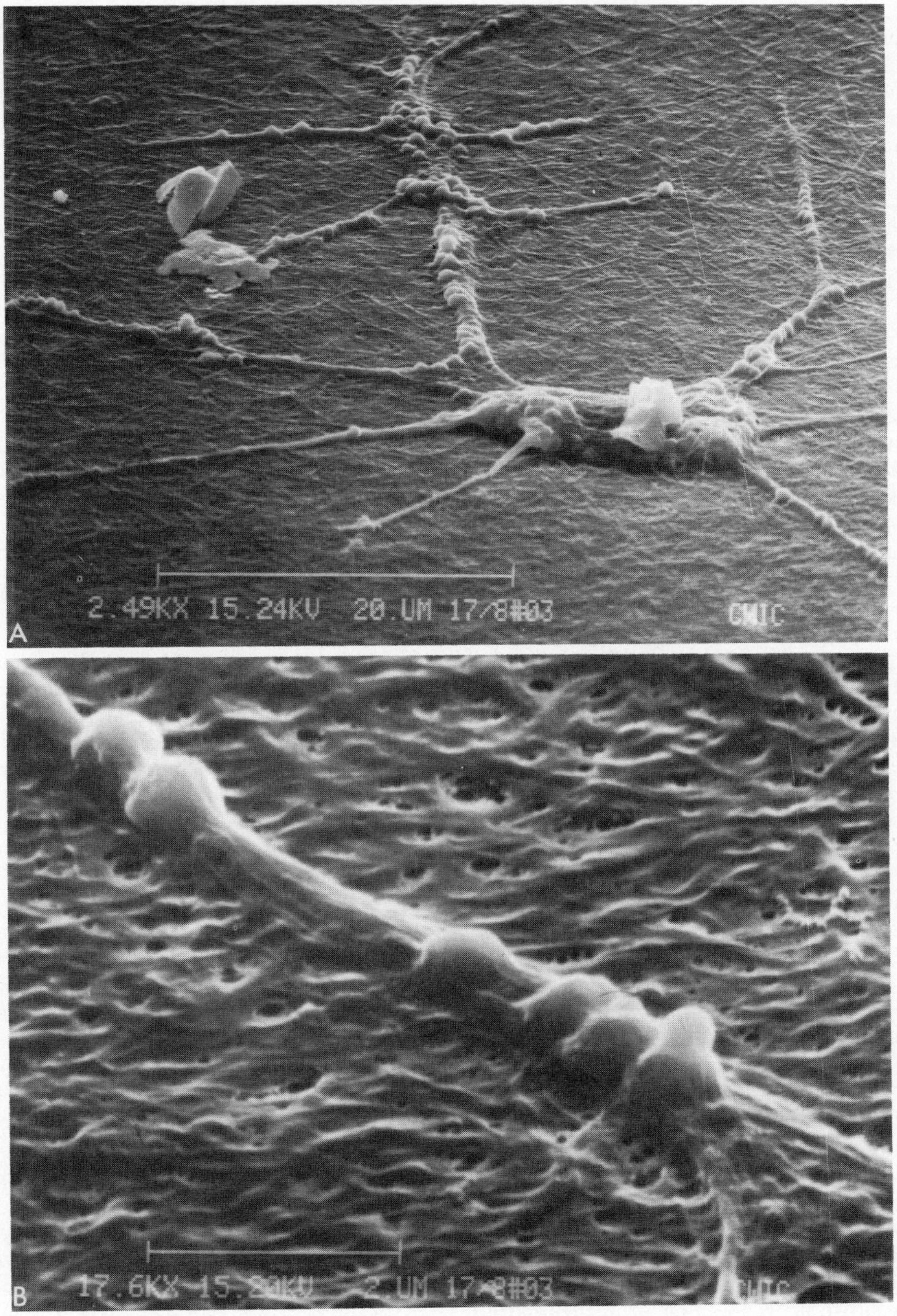


**Figure 59–6.** Scanning electron photomicrographs of a classic dendritic cell from rheumatoid synovium. Cells were dissociated from matrix and grown in monolayer culture on a thin film of collagen. Individual collagen fibrils are seen, presenting a matte-like surface. Knobby inclusions within the cell processes are as yet undefined, although transmission electron microscopic studies show that they are not mitochondria. In *B*, a thin linear "ribbing" is seen below the plasma membrane and is stretched over the knobby inclusions. Magnification: *A*, × 2490; *B*, × 17,600. The bar in *A* is 20 μm; in *B* it is 2 μm.

markedly increased rate of glucose utilization and lactate production.[190] (4) The rheumatoid cells produce larger quantities of lysosomal enzymes.[191,192] (5) The rheumatoid cells are reported to be resistant to the effects produced in normal cells by corticosteroids, such as an accelerated rate of cell growth, reduction in cell volumes, and reduction in the rate of hyaluronate and collagen synthesis.[190]

These differences between normal and rheumatoid cell lines persist through many passages (generations) of cells, implying a long-lasting alteration in cell function. Co-culture of normal human synovial cells with human blood lymphocytes, PMN leukocytes, or platelets results in the same profound changes in the synovial cells. Castor and his colleagues[193,194] have isolated polypeptides of molecular weight 10,000 to 15,000 from these cells which produce these effects. Called connective tissue activating peptides (CTAP), they initiate in cells the metabolic changes which can be considered "reparative" as opposed to phlogistic. CTAP derived from spleen increased glucose uptake and lactate formation as well as hyaluronate synthesis in human synovial cells, but produced lesser effects on cells derived from other connective tissues, and none at all upon fibroblasts from thyroid tissue. The data were different when CTAP derived from platelets was used. The data emphasize a cellular specificity for both target and effector cells and imply a deep complexity in these interactions. The CTAP polypeptides are mimicked in action by prostaglandin $E_1$, by dibutyryl cyclic AMP (but only at supraphysiologic concentrations),[193] and by fractions of serum containing nonsuppressible insulin-like activity.

It must be remembered that although one can estimate intensity and perhaps chronicity of inflammation using these in vitro systems, no qualitative differences have been described to suggest a defect intrinsic to rheumatoid cells not found in synovial cells from other types of chronic synovitis.

**Macrophages.** As discussed in Chapter 16, embryologic studies have provided data to indicate that histiocytes derived from blood-borne cells are found early in synovial tissue.[195] Experimental studies using guinea pigs have provided evidence that in an immunologically induced inflammatory lesion of synovium, most inflammatory cells appear to be derived from nonlymphocyte mononuclear cells of the blood.[196] Macrophages are the most versatile cells in the synovial lesion in RA. This is emphasized by the many receptors they possess on cell membranes and the many products that they secrete. Simple enumeration of factors secreted does not indicate the variation in expression of receptors and subsequently in secretion of products as functions of the activation of such cells. Chapter 10 gives listings of the many gene products secreted by monocytes in both the resting and activated state.

The activation of macrophages (referring to the marked change in metabolism and secretory and phagocytic function occurring over many hours after exposure to activating substances) could occur in rheumatoid synovial tissue through several mechanisms. Products of activated T lymphocytes activate macrophages to release a number of mediators, substances that have direct action upon other systems or else affect immune function and production of enzymes such as collagenase[197] and plasminogen activator.[198] Cellular immunity to many stimuli[199] and immune complexes stimulate selective release of lysosomal enzymes.[200] Evidence of the cyclic amplification mechanism within inflammatory states is found in the observation that cleavage of complement components may cause spreading and lysosomal release by macrophages.[201,202] Proteinase(s) released by macrophages can cleave these complement proteins. Adding to the substrate supply for this enzyme activity is macrophage secretion of C3 and factor B, as well as agents that control this process, such as specific inhibitors Factor I (C3b-inactivator) and (B1H globulin), and general proteinase inhibitors such as $\alpha_2$ macroglobulin.

Once activated in synovial tissue, the products of macrophages can have multiple roles in production and perpetuation of RA. One enzyme secreted by macrophages, plasminogen activator, may be of singular importance because it is secreted in an active state, not as a latent precursor or zymogen. In the presence of plasminogen, plasmin is formed. Plasmin has broad specificity and can initiate fibrinolysis and activate the clotting, kinin, complement, and collagenolytic systems[203] (see Chapter 8). Proteinases themselves may stimulate macrophage secretory activity by induction of plasma membrane spreading activity.[204] Similarly, proteinases can stimulate directly the secretion of collagenase from fibroblasts in culture.[205] Macrophages secrete an angiogenesis factor, potentially one of their most potent gene products.[206]

**Cell-Cell Interactions in Rheumatoid Synovitis.** The synovial cells proliferate enormously in rheumatoid arthritis. They must be considered stimulated cells, and their products (new connective tissue and proteinases) in this activated and proliferative state are responsible for altered appearance and function of joints. It is unlikely that these cells initiate a proliferative state sui generis, but rather that they are responding to stimuli from other cells. Stimulation of cells to proliferate involves interaction of ligands with at least two types of cell membrane receptors, the so-called "competency" and "progression" factors. In vitro, ligands for both receptors must be present if transformation or mitogenesis is to occur.

Proliferation of the number of cells in the synovium is the result of the inflammatory process. In experimental models of arthritis, synovial lining cells began to increase synthesis of DNA very soon after the inflammatory stimulus was injected and continued to manifest DNA synthetic activity for more than two months.[207] By inference, even short periods of inflammatory stimuli may be sufficient to sustain synovial proliferation in a rheumatoid joint.

Proliferation of growth of mesenchymal cells (including synovial cells) has been achieved in vitro with many different substances,[193] including: (1) connective tissue activating peptides (CTAP I-III), (2) human platelet–derived growth factor which has been purified into two homogeneous active fractions,[211] (3) somatomedin, (4) nonsuppressible insulin-like material in plasma, (5) fibroblast growth factor, (6) "low molecular weight constituents" (LMWC) from regenerating liver,[208] and (7) fibronectin. The monocyte/macrophage is perhaps the most influential cell upon activity and proliferation of the fibroblast. Mixtures of monocyte/macrophages and lymphocytes after antigen or mitogen stimulation produce in cell culture many different substances that affect fibroblast (and therefore, presumably, synovial cell) activity. Proteins that induce fibroblasts to proliferate in vitro can be separated biochemically from other factors produced by monocyte/lymphocyte cultures which are chemotactic for fibroblasts.[209] Highly purified Interleukin 1 itself appears to have two effects upon cultured fibroblasts which would amplify the proliferative and destructive potential of rheumatoid synovium; it induces fibroblast proliferation[210] and stimulates collagenase[212,215] and prostaglandin production[213,214] by the same populations of cells.

Work using passaged nonrheumatoid human synovial fibroblasts treated in vitro with conditioned medium from both concanavalin A–stimulated and streptococcal cell wall–stimulated human peripheral blood monocytes has identified a polypeptide that stimulates plasminogen activator biosynthesis by these cells. Named synovial activator, it is believed to be a different biochemical moiety from other mediators.[219] However, its action is similar to that of mononuclear cell factor or Interleukin 1.

Cells in rheumatoid synovium not only interact with other cells but also are influenced by contact with the extracellular matrix. Collagen, proteoglycans, fibronectin, and laminin are principal matrix constituents that have been shown to affect the growth and behavior of mesenchymal cells. Collagen, for example, appears both to directly stimulate synovial cells or other fibroblasts to synthesize collagenase[216] and to induce mononuclear cells to produce mononuclear cell factor (Interleukin 1), which in turn stimulates synovial cells to generate more collagenase and prostaglandins.[217] Fibronectin produced by macrophages has been shown to be a potent chemoattractant for fibroblasts in vitro.[218]

Complicating the study of substances produced by one cell that influence others is the profusion of "factors" isolated and named by many different laboratories. Helping to unify and consolidate "factor" proliferation has been the determination that Interleukin 1 is probably the same molecule (or a very similar molecule) as the one responsible for activities previously attributed endogenous leukocyte pyrogen, chondrocyte stimulating factor, fibroblast proliferation factor, B-cell activating factor, lymphocyte-activating factor, and mononuclear cell factor. It is likely that other "activities," such as human monocyte-derived growth factor for mesenchymal cells or the factor derived from activated cultures of peripheral blood mononuclear cells which stimulates production of plasminogen activator by synovial fibroblasts[219] may, in the future, be purified and shown to have structural homology with well-characterized molecules such as Interleukin 1.

## THE BIOCHEMISTRY OF TISSUE DESTRUCTION IN RHEUMATOID ARTHRITIS

The aggressive invasion of cartilage, bone, and tendon by proliferative synovium is accomplished by destruction and replacement of the extracellular matrix proteoglycans and collagen. Enzymes present in synovial fluid and released by the proliferative pannus are responsible for initiating this destruction.

**Collagen Degradation.** In cartilage, the type II collagen fibers have variable size (some up to 250 nm in diameter).[220] Cartilage collagen is characteristically very difficult to solubilize, indicating a high degree of intermolecular crosslinking (see discussion of crosslinks in collagen in Chapter 14). Figure 59–7 summarizes various pathways of collagen degradation applicable to replacement of cartilage by the invasive pannus. It is useful to think of cartilage as being exposed to destructive enzymes from two sources: the synovium and synovial fluid. In most cases, enzymes free in synovial fluid are regulated by proteinase inhibitors in synovial fluids, principally $\alpha_2$ macroglobulin[222] and $\alpha_1$-proteinase inhibitor ($\alpha_1$-antitrypsin).[223,224]

As mentioned previously, PMN leukocytes are trapped in synovial fluid in large numbers. Proteinases and polysaccharidases are released as cells die and are lysed, or as they release lysosomal enzymes, including elastase and collagenase,[224] while phagocytosing debris or immune complexes. It has been demonstrated that in synovial fluid with particularly large numbers of PMN leukocytes (> 50,000 per mm$^3$), free collagenase activity may be present, implying that proteinase inhibitors are saturated by enzymes[29] or else inactivated by substances such as *N*-chloroamines. Proteinases in synovial fluid are very likely responsible for damage to the superficial

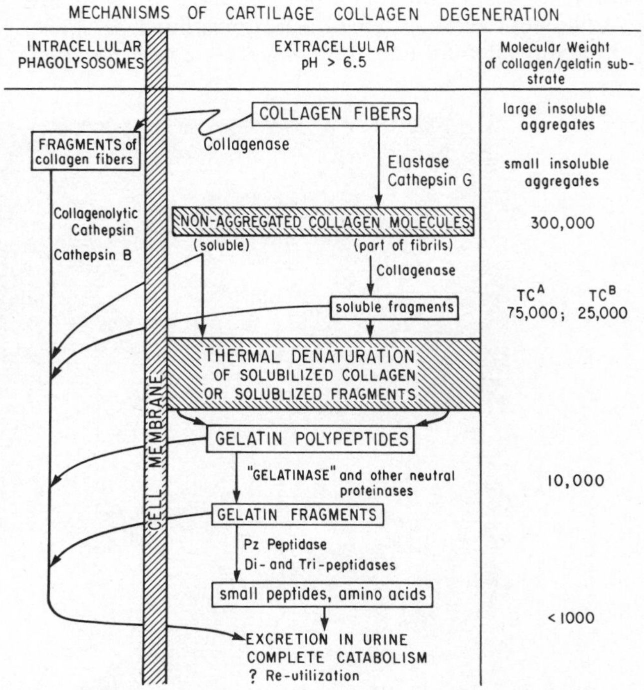


**Figure 59–7.** Mechanisms of cartilage collagen breakdown in rheumatoid arthritis. A schema. The left side describes intracellular (within phagolysosomes) events potentially involved in collagen breakdown. Extracellular events are depicted in the middle, and on the right are approximate molecular weights of collagen or gelatin fragments during sequential steps of degradation.

layers of cartilage demonstrated in RA,[225] and in experimental systems it has been shown that PMN leukocytes adhere to cartilage in greater numbers when there are immune complexes entrapped within the avascular cartilage.[226] Small foci or microabscesses of PMN leukocytes can be seen occassionally at the pannus-cartilage junction. Release of lysosomal enzymes occurs at the cartilage surface as viable PMN leukocytes are "frustrated" in phagocytosis of immune complexes bound superficially to substrate. Active proteinases, in addition to saturating proteinase inhibitors, may permanently inactivate inhibitors by limited proteolysis.[227]

As reviewed in Chapter 14, crosslinked collagen fibrils are relatively resistant to collagenases. PMN leukocyte serine proteinases have the ability to cleave the nonhelical crosslink region, which contains the intermolecular crosslinks.[228] Noncrosslinked molecules could remain in fibril conformation as insoluble aggregates or could become soluble. The individual molecules are readily cleaved by specific collagenases produced by synovial cells and macrophages.[229] The fragments produced are very susceptible to thermal denaturation and as gelatin polypeptides can be degraded by multiple enzymes, including relatively specific "gelatinases" (metalloproteinases active at neutral pH).[230]

There are two forms of inactive proteinases in extracellular tissues. One is proteinase complexed with $\alpha_2$ macroglobulin[231] or $\alpha_1$-proteinase inhibitor[232] or tissue proteinase inhibitors. There is little evidence that these forms are easily restored to active enzymes. The inactive complexes are eliminated from the circulation by the reticuloendothelial system.[233] Clearance must be slower from synovial fluid and the complexes could be dissociated if $\alpha_2$ macroglobulin molecules were gradually denatured or degraded, releasing active proteinases. There is increasing evidence that inhibitor-enzyme complexes are more avidly taken up by phagocytic cells than are either inhibitors or enzymes alone.

The second form of inactive enzymes are proenzymes, the precursor forms produced by the cells. Within the extracellular space it is probable that other proteinases activate proenzymes. For example, plasmin is an effective activator of latent rheumatoid synovial collagenase. Rheumatoid synovial cells also produce plasminogen activator.[203] Since plasminogen is among the high molecular weight proteins that are increased in concentration in synovial fluid in RA, it seems probable that sufficient plasmin is present in synovial tissue to activate latent forms of collagenase or latent activators essential for activation of procollagenase.

Molecule by molecule destruction of collagen in the extracellular space, as portrayed above, may be bypassed in the presence of a very aggressive synovitis in which entire pieces of fibrils are phagocytized and, presumably, degraded by lysosomal proteinases (cathepsin B and collagenolytic cathepsin) within phagolysosomes (Fig. 59–8).

Tissue inhibitors of metalloproteinases (TIMP) are present in all connective tissues. These proteins (*M*r less than 30,000) inhibit collagenases and other tissue metalloproteinases.[234] In situations of active, aggressive synovitis, however, the TIMP probably are saturated and inactivated by proteinases released into the extracellular tissues in large quantities. TIMP from all tissues in a single species are immunologically identical.

Pharmacologic control of synovial collagenase bio-

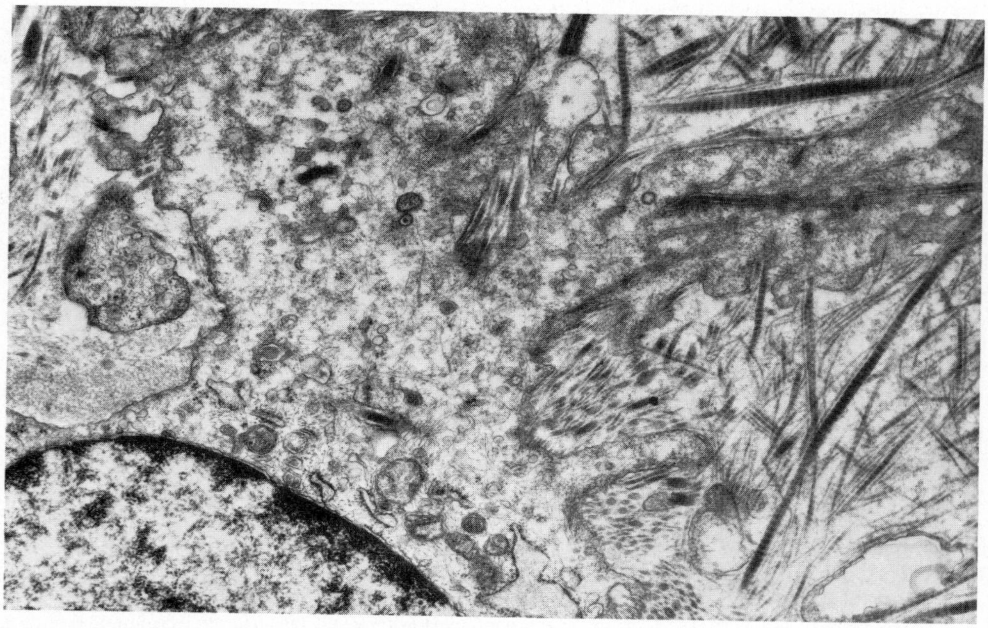

**Figure 59–8.** The leading edge of a pannus cell extends diffusely into cartilage. Collagen fibers, characterized by 69 nm periodicity, can be seen about to be or actually engulfed by the cell. This very close contact of synovium and cartilage is found in < 10 percent of patients but is the type of process associated with phagocytosis of collagen by this leading edge of cells. × 30,000. (Electron photomicrograph by Andrey M. Glauert. From Harris, E.D., Jr., et al.: Arthritis Rheum. 20:657, 1977.)

synthesis is suggested by the data showing that glucocorticoids and retinoid compounds inhibit production of the enzyme.[235] That different mechanisms regulate the production of both collagenase and plasminogen activator (both are neutral proteinases secreted by mesenchymal cells in response to polypeptide stimulating factors produced by monocytes) is emphasized by the evidence that while retinoids inhibit collagenase production they also stimulate plasminogen activator production by human synovial fibroblasts.[236]

**Proteoglycan Degradation.** Proteoglycans in cartilage are quickly depleted when synovitis develops.[237] As shown in Figure 59–9, although the cartilage has a normal thickness and gross appearance (using metachromatic stain), there is very little tinctorial evidence for proteoglycans. As with collagen, it is likely that enzymes active at neutral pH are essential for solubilization or mobilization of the components of the proteoglycan molecule. Neutral metalloproteinases found in cartilage are the leading candidates for this role,[238] although PMN leukocyte elastase and cathepsin G can bring about essentially complete release of proteoglycan from cartilage as well.[228] Once the aggregates are broken up, the soluble components of proteoglycans can be degraded intracellularly by lysosomal enzymes, especially cathepsins B and D.[239] There are increased amounts of enzymes with the potential to break down the polysaccharide side chains of chondroitin sulfate and keratan sulfate in rheumatoid synovium as well. Levels of *N*-acetylglucosaminidase, $\beta$-galactosidase, arylsulfatase A, and glucuronidase activity are all higher in rheumatoid synovium than in controls, although this increase of enzyme activity is seen in reactive synovitis of many varieties and is not specific for RA.[240]

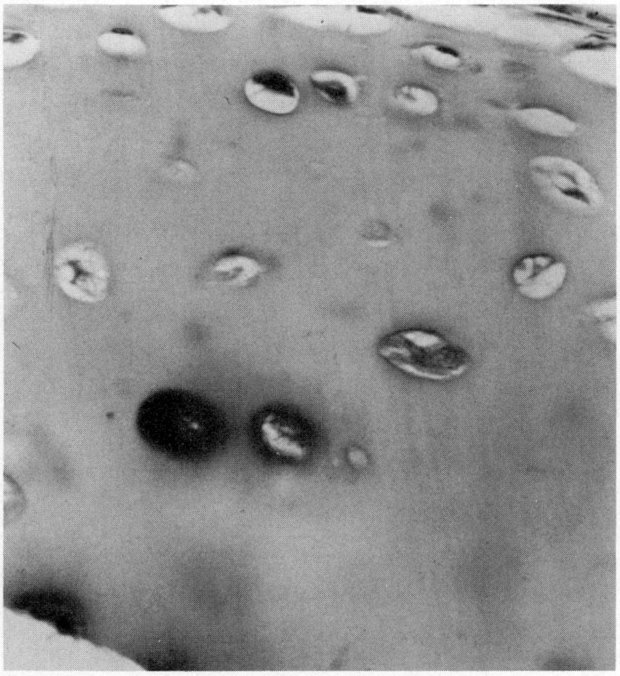

**Figure 59–9.** Human articular cartilage from active rheumatoid arthritis removed at joint arthroplasty and stained for metachromasia. The only metachromatic stain surrounds a few chrondrocytes, which, presumably, are actively making proteoglycan only to have it broken down by proteinases derived from synovial fluid, chondrocytes, and/or synovial tissue. The form of this depleted cartilage is normal; however, its functional capacity to rebound from a deforming load is seriously impaired.

It is probable that in response to inflammation in the joint, cartilage generates its own destruction. Cultures of synovium release a factor of low molecular weight that induces chondrocytes to generate proteinases, which degrade proteoglycans. This substance(s) has been named catabolin[241] and is similar to Interleukin 1 and mononuclear cell factor that mediates cartilage proteoglycan degradation through chondrocyte activation.[242] That this mechanism operates in vivo is suggested by the enhanced size of lacunae around chondrocytes near invasive fronds of the pannus cells (see Fig. 59–11).

Some of the proteinase activity in proliferating rheumatoid synovial cells in vitro is associated with the cell membrane surface rather than being secreted into the culture medium.[243] The pathophysiologic significance of surface-associated proteinases can only be speculated upon at this time.

**Bone Resorption.** Collagenase and elastase cannot degrade bone unless it has been demineralized. In vivo, then, either some component of the inflammatory lesion must be able to mobilize bone mineral or else osteoclasts (or cells with equivalent capabilities) must develop and create resorption. Both mechanisms are possible in the rheumatoid lesion. Multinucleate cells have been described at the resorbing interface of pannus and bone. Prostaglandins stimulate bone resorption by stimulating osteoclastic activity.[244,245] Prostaglandin endoperoxides ($PGG_2$ and $PGH_2$) cause a transient stimulation of calcium release that is quite different from the prolonged resorption resulting from $PGE_2$, suggesting that more needs to be learned about which of the arachidonic acid metabolites are principally responsible for the bone resorption induced by this system.[246] An immunologic mechanism is also applicable to bone resorption. Osteoclast-activating factor (OAF) is a soluble product of cultured human mononuclear leukocytes,[247] produced, it is believed, by the mononuclear cells found deep in rheumatoid synovium.

Both of these potential mechanisms can be synergistic in causing the resorption and replacement of bone at the bone-pannus junction as well as the juxta-articular osteopenia that develops as an early sign of proliferative synovitis.

## PATHOLOGY OF RHEUMATOID ARTHRITIS

The pathology of RA is best understood in the context of cellular, immunologic, and biochemical mechanisms discussed in detail in the preceding sections.

The rheumatoid process has minimal destructive capability until it becomes chronic. The disease is such that at any point in the development of the highly proliferative polarized and destructive lesion it may regress. It is not known how long this "maturation" process takes to occur, but extrapolation from clinical observations suggests that it is unlikely that significant erosive disease can develop before 8 weeks after the first symptoms, even in the most aggressive lesions.

**Synovium.** Figure 59–10 is a photomicrograph of synovium from an inflamed knee obtained 3 days after the onset of arthritis, which subsequently evolved into classic RA. The synovial lining cells have not proliferated much, but the small blood vessels are very prominent deep in the subsynovial tissue, not so much because they are dilated but because of a large increase in numbers of vascular cells and lymphocytes in the perivascular areas. Accumulation of an increased amount of interstitial fluid is indicated by the low density of cells and matrix. The lymphocytes of the synovial lesion have been identified primarily as T lymphocytes[106,107] in other studies. No plasma cells are seen in the earliest lesions. As the lesion matures, a striking heterogeneity of cell types is found. Macrophages, lymphocytes, endothelial cells, "synovial cells," and fibroblast-like cells are all present.

The first vascular change in rheumatoid synovitis is one of venular dilatation.[93] Deposition of fibrin within the vessel wall occurs, and there is proliferation of endothelium.[248] But as new tissue develops, an enlarged capillary network appears and sustains the proliferating cells, invading the relatively avascular cartilage and subchondral bone. Factors responsible for generation of new capillaries are discussed in Chapter 13. Extracellular proteinases released by cells (?endothelial cells, ?mast cells, ?tissue histiocytes) may include plasminogen ac-

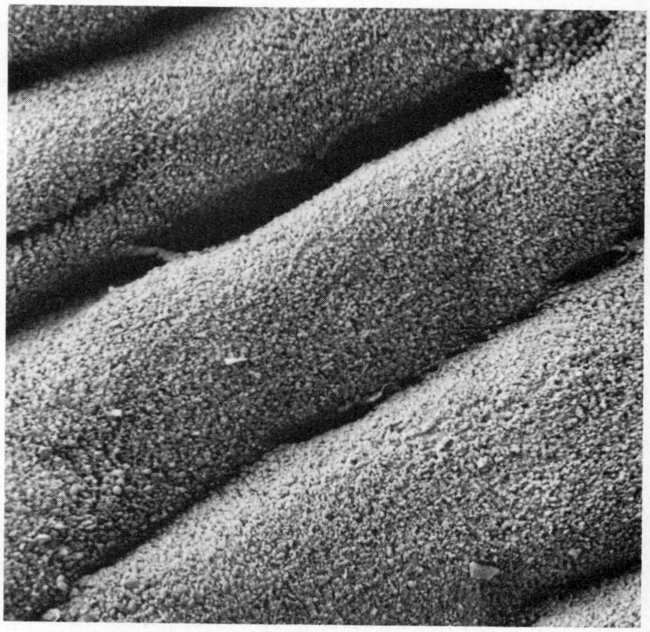

**Figure 59–11.** Low power scanning electron microscopic view of the surface of synovium early in rheumatoid arthritis. × 120. (Courtesy of Dr. Gilbert Fauré. Assistant des Hôpitaux, Chief de Clinique, Service de Rhumatologic Hospital de Nancy-Brabois.)

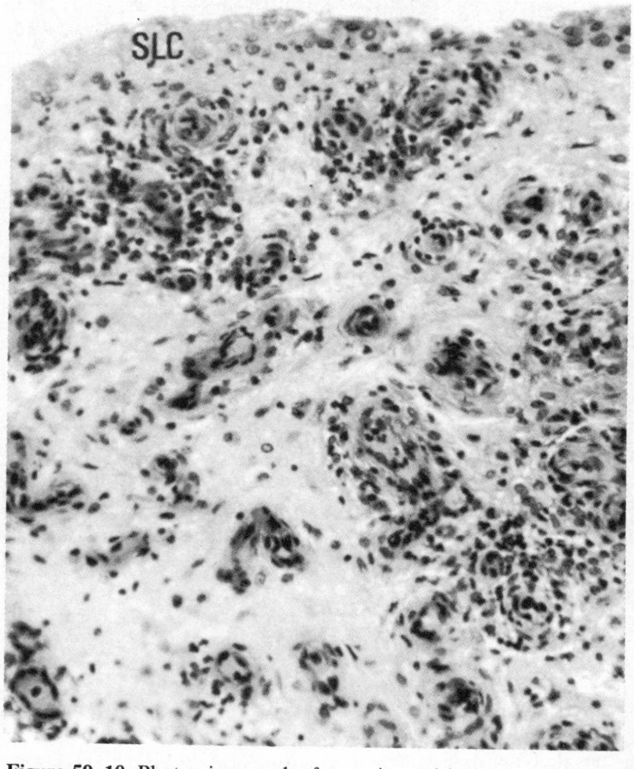


**Figure 59–10.** Photomicrograph of synovium with three days of clinically identifiable inflammation, later evolving into definite rheumatoid arthritis. Histologic details are described in the text. *SLC,* Synovial lining cells. × 180. (From Schumacher, H.R., and Kitridou, R.D.: Arthritis Rheum. 15:465, 1972.)

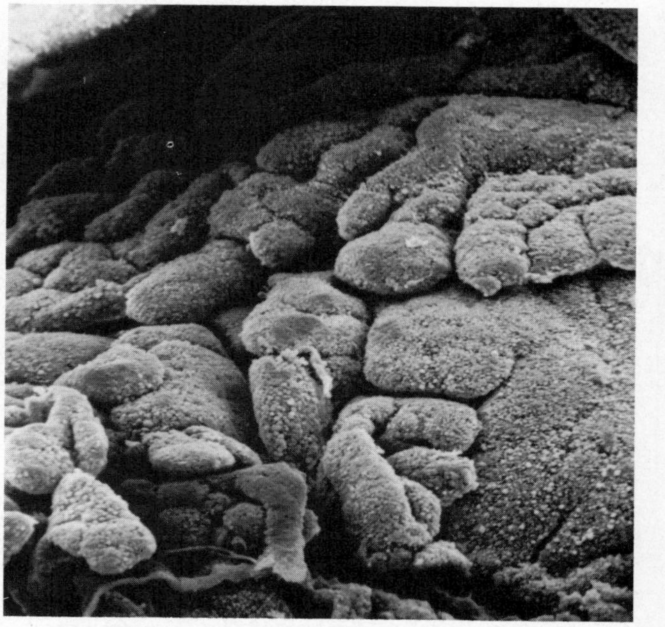

**Figure 59–12.** Scanning electron microscopic view of rheumatoid synovium. Villous fronds are beginning to appear. Fibrin debris coats the surface. × 35. (Courtesy of Dr. G. Fauré.)

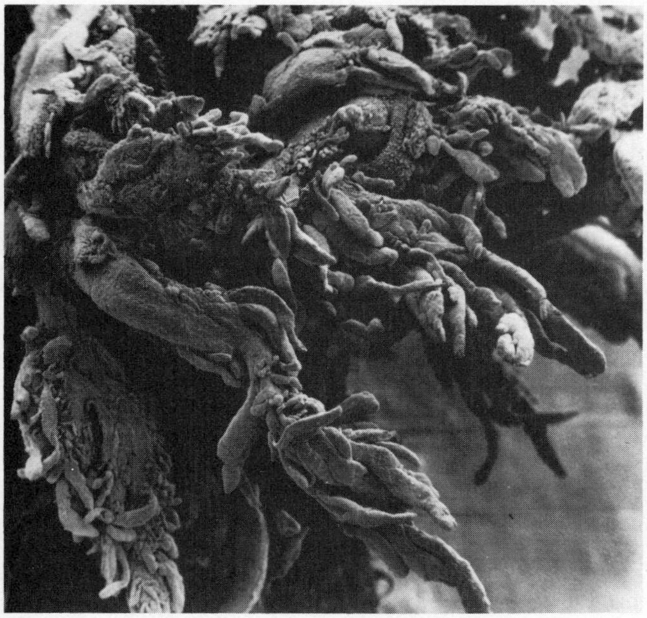

**Figure 59–13.** This scanning electron photomicrograph represents more chronic, established disease than Figure 59–12. × 35. The villi are more numerous; there is much more synovial surface area. (Courtesy of Dr. G. Fauré.)

tivator and collagenase. Proteinases may inactivate the inhibitors of angiogenesis normally found in cartilage, permitting the vascular pannus to erode into cartilage.

The early lesion in RA viewed by scanning electron microscopy of the synovial surface is shown in Figure 59–11. The folds are possible artifacts, but the finely pebbled appearance of individual cells on the surface is not unlike the normal synovium. As the synovial lesion progresses, it becomes more and more a heterogeneous mixture of cells.

Progression to chronicity is associated with an enormous increase in the synovial surface area. This is accomplished by formation of villi (compare Figs. 59–12 and 59–13 with 59–14). The development of villi is accompanied by deposition of fibrin on the synovial surface. In chronic progressive disease multiple long microvilli have developed and the fine pebbled appearance of individual cells is less distinct, perhaps because of a diffuse film of fibrin that coats the cell surface. The microvilli shown in Figure 59–13 are probably prone to infarction and autoamputation from the stalk, with subsequent existence in synovial fluid as "rice bodies."

High-power views of the surface of rheumatoid synovium reveal multiple cell processes and surface irregularities (Fig. 59–15). Seen in many such scanning election micrographs is the suggestion of intercellular bridging among cells. These conduits would certainly assure information transfer from cell to cell.

In the advanced process, then, there are four levels of cell surface area multiplication: (1) macrovillous formation, visible to the naked eye; (2) microvilli, visible by low-power microscopy; (3) the nodular surface of the villi caused by cells protruding from the surface; and (4) multiple processes from individual cells. When stained in such a way as to emphasize cell processes as well as extracellular matrix, the clear area surrounding synovial cells at the cartilage-pannus junction can be shown to contain thin cell processes, suggesting that these cells could be the stellate cells that are found in cultures of freshly dissociated rheumatoid synovial cells in vitro (Fig. 59–16, Plate III, p. xxxvii).

Ultrastructural studies of the synovial lining cells show a marked increase in the number of type B cells

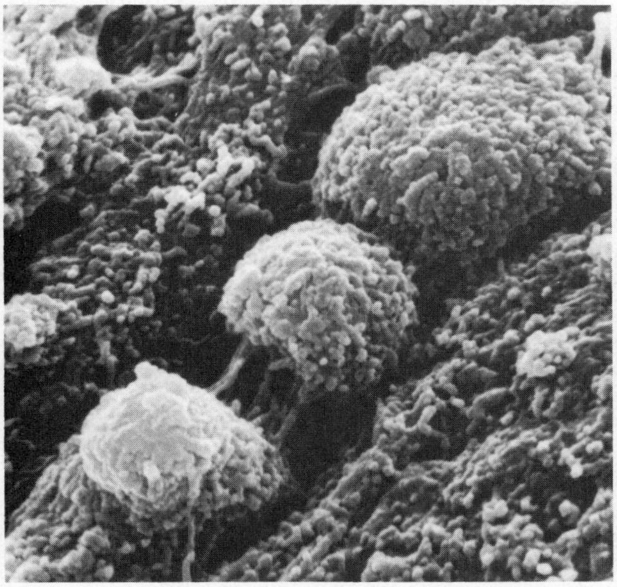

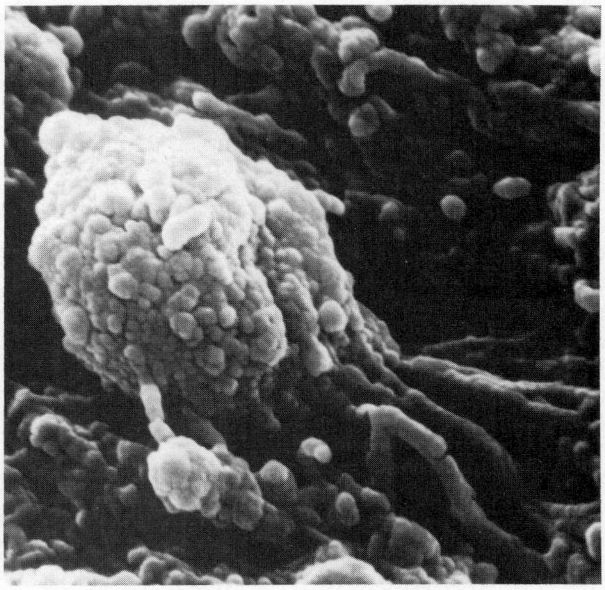

**Figures 59–14 and 59–15.** High power scanning electron microscopic views of individual cells on the synovial villus surface. There is a suggestion of intercellular bridging via thin cell processes in both figures. Magnification: Figure 59–14, × 4800; Figure 59–15, × 10,000. (Courtesy of Dr. G. Fauré.)

(fibroblast-like; see Chapter 16), those containing moderate numbers of lysosomes as well as well-developed endoplasmic reticulum and Golgi bodies.[249]

The type A cells (macrophage-like) remaining in these tissues have a different appearance from normal cells. They have fewer cell processes and contain swollen, distorted mitochondria and numerous membrane-bound granular dense bodies, which have been interpreted to be phagolysosomes.[250] Breakdown products of erythrocytes (membrane fragments and hemosiderin), which are easily visible as granules in cells on routine stains of tissue, are prominent in electron photomicrographs. The red blood cells presumably originate from intra-articular microhemorrhages.[251]

Multinucleate cells are found often in rheumatoid tissues (Fig. 59–17)[252] and in adherent cell cultures that have been freshly dissociated from matrix. It is tempting to presume presence of a virus that could be implicated as a fusogen. Lysolecithinase produced by phospholipase from neutrophils may be present transiently, and it has the capacity to fuse cells. A heat-labile protein of *M*r of about 60,000 is released from antigen- or mitogen-stimulated lymphocytes and promotes the formation of multinucleated giant cells from human monocyte precursors.[253] Multinucleate cells formed among synovial fibroblasts have been demonstrated in vitro to secrete more collagenase than cultures of unfused cells. Their presence in tissues may be associated with accelerated rates of matrix degradation. Indirect support for this hypothesis is found in the nonrheumatoid but very destructive arthropathy, multicentric reticulohistiocytosis, that is characterized by multinucleate, lipid-laden histiocytes, resembling foreign body–type giant cells[254] (see Chapter 95).

The functional results of pathologic change are apparent in the joint capsule, tendons, and articular cartilage.

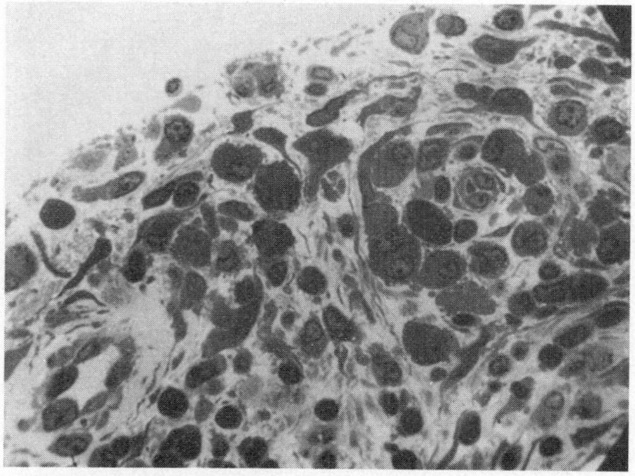

**Figure 59–17.** Phase microscopy of a thin section of succulent rheumatoid synovium prepared for electron microscopy, emphasizing the heterogeneity of this tissue. A multinucleate cell, which probably is a hypersecretor of proteinases, is visible. × 100. (Courtesy of Dr. Donald D. DiBona.)

**The Joint Capsule.** Proliferation of new tissue (highly vascularized collagen bundles with moderate perivascular inflammation) leads to altered physiology. Compliance is decreased, and accompanying this are redundancy and instability as ligaments are stretched. Subluxation from stretched capsular ligaments can lead directly to cartilage damage from mechanical incongruity. Periodic fluctuations in the amount of extracellular fluid present in the thickened capsule and overlying soft tissues are responsible for the variations in stiffness felt by patients.

The thickening of the rheumatoid joint capsule and the large accumulations of synovial fluid produce very high pressures in joints. [255] Flexion pressures in the knee joint of as high as 1000 mm Hg have been recorded.[256] It follows that high pressures in joints may compromise synovial blood flow, decreasing further the already low oxygen tensions in synovial fluid.[257]

**Tendons.** Tendons are remarkably homogeneous bundles of collagen sparsely populated with fibroblasts, blood vessels, and nerves. Tendons are exposed to both proliferative and destructive stimuli. Proliferative stimuli result in the formation of tendon nodules, which histologically are the same as subcutaneous rheumatoid nodules. Tendon nodules interfere with normal gliding function. Destructive effects of proliferative synovium in the tendon sheaths, accompanied by altered use patterns and, occasionally, trauma from eroded bone edges can lead to tendon rupture.

**Articular Cartilage.** The initial response in cartilage is loss of proteoglycans. The functional result of this is loss of stiffness, loss of ability to rebound from a comprehensive force, and a diminished capacity to resist deformation.[258,259] Thus, while the erosive pannus replaces the cartilage at the periphery of the joints, the central cartilage on the weight-bearing surfaces is more susceptible to mechanical fibrillation and fragmentation.

**The Cartilage-Synovial Interface.** Histopathologic studies early in the erosive phase of RA have revealed that the initial focus of bone and cartilage destruction is the periphery of the joint. "Recruitment" of perichondral and periosteal cells (as well as the chondrocytes themselves) occurs in this destructive process (Fig. 59–18).[260] Often a cartilage "lip" appears as subchondral bone is eroded underneath cartilage. Perhaps this protection of cartilage is provided by proteinase inhibitors, so-called "anti-invasive factors" in cartilage.[261] Similar inhibitors, some specific for collagenase, are present in tendon as well.

Although the invasive tissue may not often appear similar to synovial villi by histologic examination, there is little reason to doubt that the invasive pannus is an extension of proliferative synovium. As shown in Figure 59–19, where cartilage has been completely replaced, the appearance of the proliferative tissue at the surface resembles synovium, with the same polarity apparent that is seen in synovial lining cells. PMN leukocytes are found rarely at the pannus-cartilage interface.[262]

Tongues of proliferative cells penetrate the cartilage (Fig. 59–20), and destruction takes place in a very nar-

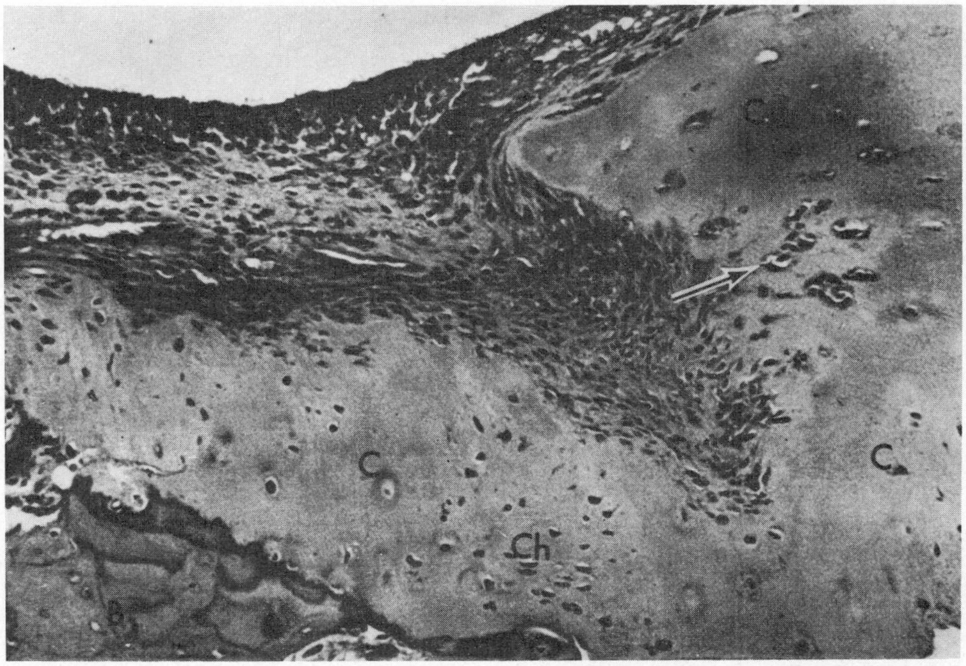


**Figure 59–18.** The periphery of a joint near the insertion of synovium at the osseous-chondral junction in rheumatoid arthritis. This shows proliferation of general mesenchymal tissue, including chondrocytes (*Ch*), as the destructive process begins. *C* is cartilage; *B* is bone. The arrow points to either a reduplicating chondrocyte or a cross section through a tongue of the invasive lesion.

**Figure 59–19.** A section from a metacarpal head replaced at joint arthroplasty. The surface at the upper left is the joint space. Residual cartilage at the left is surrounded by fibrous tissue. The superficial layers of pannus have taken on the appearance of synovium. At the bottom center, an area where subchondral bone has been completely degraded is seen as the pannus extends down into marrow space.

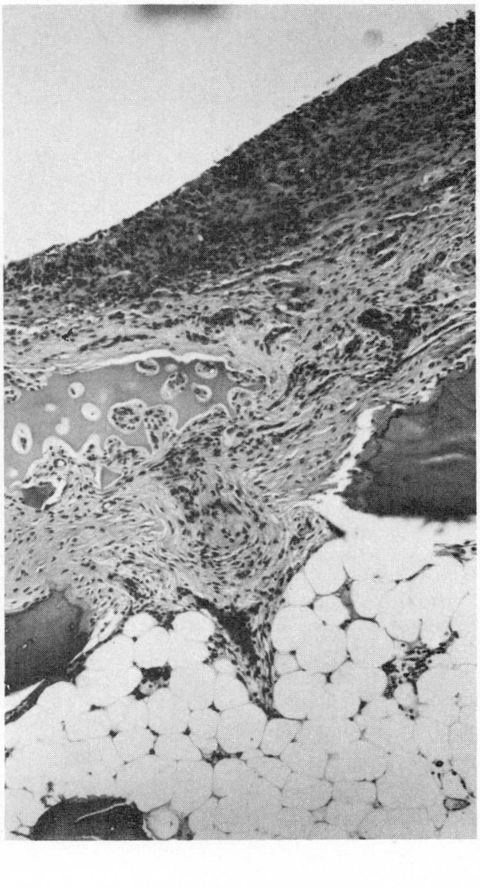

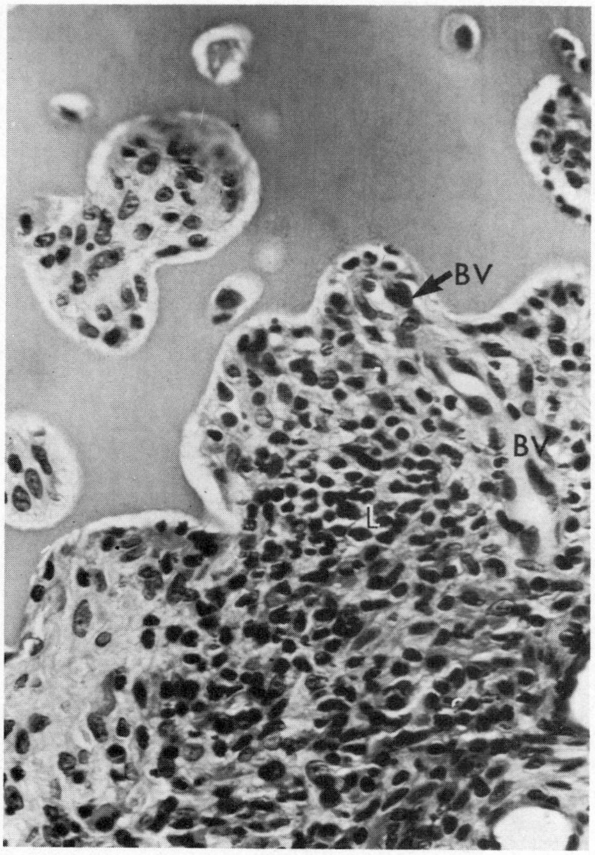


**Figure 59–20.** High power light microscopy at the pannus-synovial junction. The space between them is shrinkage artifact. Tongues of proliferating tissue have invaded the residual cartilage shown at the upper left. Small blood vessels (*BV*) are seen just below the cartilage-pannus junction. Small, darkly staining cells, probably lymphocytes (*L*) are just below the invading surface.

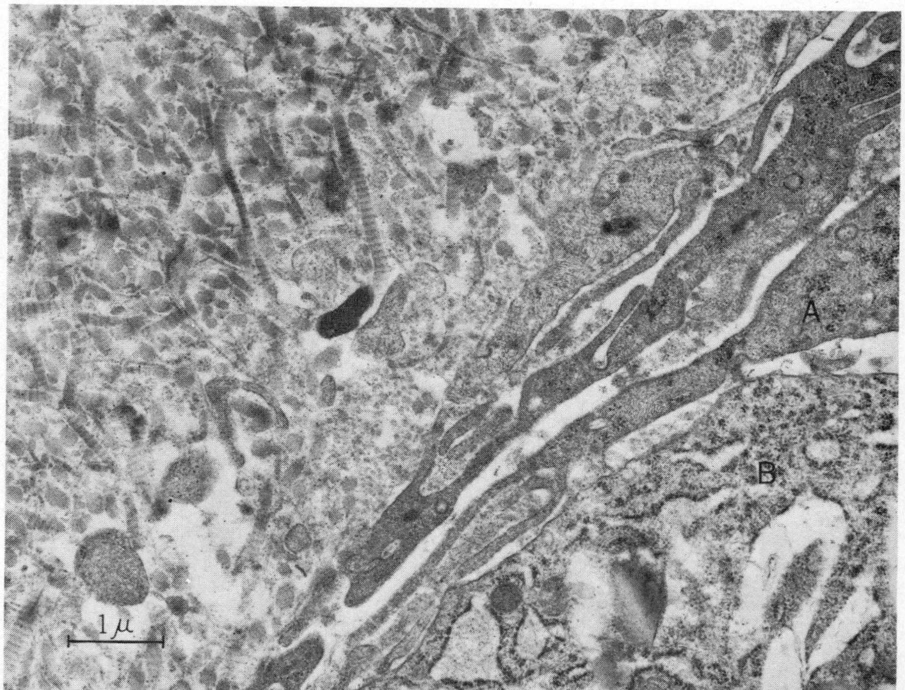


**Figure 59–21.** High power electron microscopic view of the junction between articular cartilage and rheumatoid synovium. The process is moving from the lower right to the upper left. Cartilage collagen fibers (distinguished by their 64-mm banding patterns, left center) are only faintly visible in the amorphous zone (1 to 3 μm wide) between cells and cartilage. Both a macrophage-like cell (*A*) and a cell filled with dilated endoplasmic reticulum (*B*) are at this leading edge of invasion.

row zone between the cells and cartilage. Ultrastructural studies have revealed several different patterns at this interface. One common form (Fig. 59–21) is a narrow, amorphous zone (2 to 4 μm wide), which well separates structural cartilage components from the invading cells.[263,264] Penetrating this zone are long thin processes from the cellular edge. The amorphous zone appears to contain debris. Probably in this setting cartilage is being destroyed extracellulary by enzymes active at neutral pH released by the adjacent cells.

Specimens of the cartilage-synovial junction from other patients have shown small blood vessels penetrating close to the cartilage, carrying with them some lymphocytes and plasma cells as well as mesenchymal cells and macrophages.[265] Although blood vessels do not often penetrate closer than 100 μm from the junction, it must be re-emphasized that without the capillary network which is built within the proliferative lesion there could be no progressive erosive synovitis.

Yet another pattern of synovial-cartilage interface is one of intimate contact between cells and cartilage, with cell borders and processes penetrating deeply into the cartilage matrix (Fig. 59–8). Cells at the interface may include PMN leukocytes, mast cells, and dendritic cells as well as macrophages and fibroblast-like cells. In this pattern, perhaps associated with more aggressive and rapidly progressive disease, intracellular collagen fibrils have been observed within membrane-bound vesicles and in various stages of digestion. It appears that this synovial-cartilage junction has special qualitative differences from the remaining synovium. Immunoreactive collagenase (antibody formed against active, not latent, enzyme) has been demonstrated at this junction around cells in proximity to cartilage, but rarely in cells deep in the synovium or even in the lining cells of synovium. There is much to be learned about the microenvironment at the pannus-cartilage junction, including the pH, the type and activity of cellular metabolism, and the qualitative nature of enzymes released by cells.

**Pressure-Induced Pathology in RA.** Normal joint function involves operation under very large forces, often greater than body weight. The effect of these forces begins to potentiate enzymatic destruction of joints from the earliest stages of the disease. Another example of cyclic augmentation in this disease is the fact that movement itself potentiates inflammation, so that the two are closely related.

One example of the destructive effects of pressure is the formation of subchondral pseudocysts. These lesions are round or pear shaped and contain fibrotic granulation tissue, necrotic debris, and detached pieces of cartilage and bone.[266] Often they are found in patients who are bothered little by pain and inflammation and continue an active life despite much proliferative synovitis in many joints. A connection between the cysts and joint cavity can be demonstrated in virtually all cases studied carefully.[267] Rarely, such a cyst may lead to weakened bone structure and fracture (Fig. 59–22).

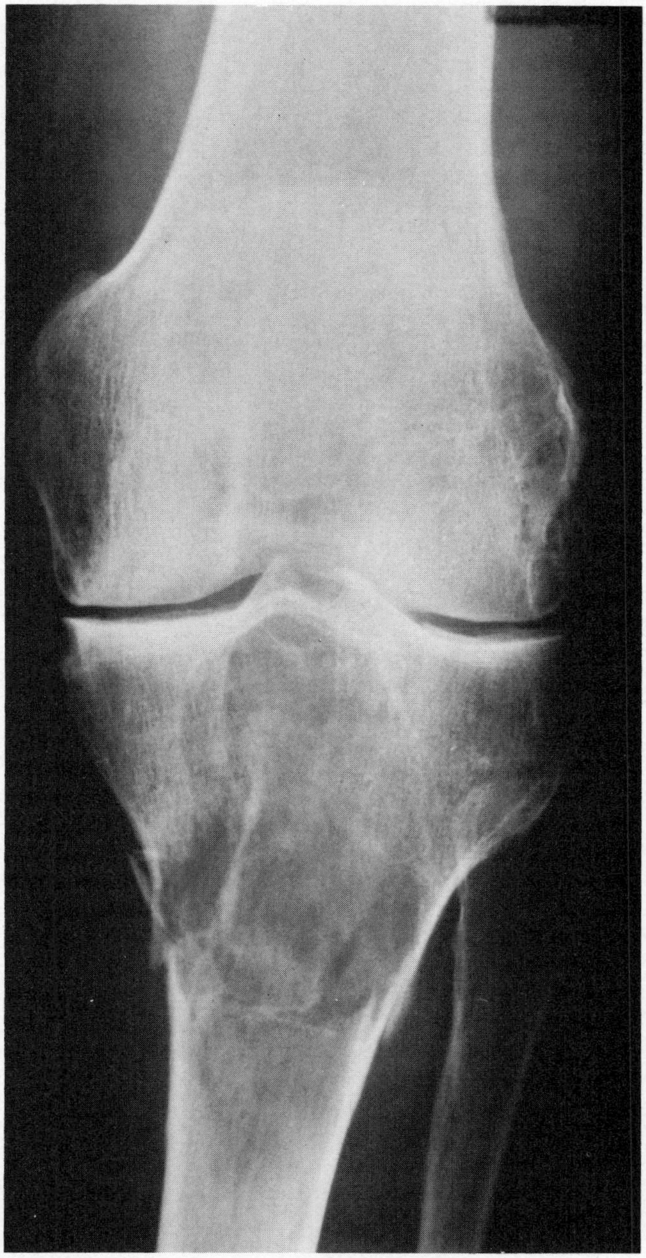

**Figure 59–22.** This radiograph demonstrates a pathologic fracture through a very large subchondral cyst in the proximal tibia. This patient had severe proliferative arthritis and many subchondral cysts, but had never missed a day of work and suffered very little from his disease. Biopsy of the involved subcortical lucent area showed typical rheumatoid granulation tissue. (Courtesy of Dr. Ed Olson and the Radiology Department, White River Junction, Vt., Veterans Administration Hospital.)

**Rheumatoid Nodules: The Extra-Articular Proliferative Lesion of RA.** Rheumatoid nodules have been well characterized morphologically.[268,269] These nodules are most often found subcutaneously over pressure points and represent a proliferative diathesis of mesenchymal tissue. In response to minimal trauma there is an intriguing combination of tissue destruction following proliferation and vasculitis to give the final result. Anatomically there is a central necrotic zone surrounded at a fairly sharp border by a highly cellular area of radially arranged cells amid strands of collagen (Figure 59–23, Plate III, p. xxxvii). The intense cellularity gives way at the periphery to more densely packed connective tissue. Mononuclear cells infiltrate around blood vessels in this capsular zone. Electron microscopic studies of the central necrotic areas have shown a mixture of collagen fibers in varying stages of degradation, noncollagenous filamentous material, granular debris, cell membranes, and fat globules.[270]

Study of nodules shortly after they have developed has revealed a marked inflammation of venules with deposition of fibrin within vessel walls and in surrounding tissue. Intense proliferation of fibroblasts in these early lesions is often found. The intense exudation from small blood vessels accounts for the space-occupying qualities of these nodules and explains how they can appear in less than 24 hours. The cellular proliferation is induced, somehow, by the vascular inflammation and gives structure to the nodule. The necrosis is probably a result of two processes: the microinfarctions resulting from thrombosis of terminal vessels, and the enormous quantities of proteinases and collagenase produced by the cellular palisading area.[271] Rarely, rheumatoid nodules appear in patients with a clinical diagnosis of RA but in whom no circulating rheumatoid factor can be demonstrated.[271a]

**End Stages of Rheumatoid Arthritis.** Progression of the process defined above results in loss of cartilage. With subluxation, thinning of bone, muscle atrophy, and fibrosis, movement of the joint diminishes and this facilitates fibrous ankylosis across joints. Rarely is ankylosis accompanied by mineralization, so that a true arthrodesis does not occur. Accompanying ankylosis there is a marked decrease in the inflammatory process with loss of the cellularity and vascularity. Whether these signs of decreased disease activity reflect the loss of movement or loss of cartilage as a trophic factor is not known. It has been reported that there is less inflammation in joints after insertion of a prosthesis and removal of all cartilage whether or not synovium is left within the joint.[272]

**Vasculitis.** The most prominent of extra-articular pathology in RA is vasculitis. It may present clinically as a variety of syndromes and may be associated with involvement of medium-sized arteries, small arteries, and venules. All layers of the vessel wall are infiltrated by lymphocytes.[273] Intimal proliferation and thrombosis occasionally are found, particularly in digital arteries. Deposits of IgG, IgM, and C3 have been noted in the walls of involved arteries,[152,274] notably in those patients with severe disease, high titers of rheumatoid factor, low serum C3, and clinical features such as peripheral neuropathy, digital gangrene, nailfold infarcts, and cutaneous ulcers.

In some patients, involvement of medium sized rather than small arteries with necrosis, fibrinoid change, PMN leukocyte infiltration, and disruption of the internal elastic lamina may resemble closely the pathology of polyarteritis nodosa.[275]

Palpable purpura, reflecting involvement of venules in a leukocytoclastic vasculitis, is the third pattern of involvement. Immunofluorescense sometimes reveals the presence of immunoglobulins and complement in and around the venules,[276] although studies of cutaneous vessel immune deposits have been positive in more than 50 percent of seropositive RA patients whether or not they have clinical vasculitis.[277] The persistence of fibrin in chronic lesions of vasculitis involving small arteries has led to the speculation that fibrin may play an active role in the genesis of these chronic and occlusive arterial lesions.[278]

## References


1. Stastny, P.: Mixed lymphocyte cultures in rheumatoid arthritis. J. Clin. Invest. 57:1148, 1976.
2. McMichael, A.J., Sasazubi, T., McDevitt, H.O., and Payne, R.O.: Increased frequency of HLA-3C and HLA-Dw4 in rheumatoid arthritis. Arthritis Rheum. 20:1037, 1977.
3. Stasny, P.: Association of the B-cell alloantigen DR4 with rheumatoid arthritis. N. Engl. J. Med. 298:869, 1978.
4. Solinger, A.M., Bhatnagar, R., and Stabo, J.D.: Cellular, molecular, and genetic characteristics of T cell reactivity to collagen in man. Proc. Natl. Acad. Sci. (USA) 78:3877, 1981.
5. Alarcon, G.S., Koopman, W.J., Acton, R.T., and Barger, B.O.: Seronegative rheumatoid arthritis. A distinct immunogenetic disease? Arthritis Rheum. 25:502, 1982.
6. Willikens, R.F., Hansen, J.A., Malmgren, J.A., Nisperos, B., Mickelson, E.M., and Watson, M.A.: HLA antigens in Yakima Indians with rheumatoid arthritis. Lack of association with HLA-Dw4 and HLA-DR4. Arthritis Rheum. 25:1435, 1982.
7. Schiff, B., Mizrachi, Y., Orgad, S., Yaron, M., and Gazit, E.: Association of HLA-Aw31 and HLA-DR1 with adult rheumatoid arthritis. Ann. Rheum. Dis. 41:403, 1982.
8. Ueno, Y., Iwaky, Y., Terasaki, P.I., Park, M.S., Barnett, E.V., Chia, D., and Nakata, S.: HLA-DR4 in Negro and Mexican rheumatoid arthritis patients. J. Rheumatol. 8:804, 1981.
9. Stastny, P.: Joint report: Rheumatoid arthritis. *In* Terasaki, P.I. (ed.): Histocompatibility Testing 1980. Los Angeles, UCLA Tissue Typing Laboratory, 1980, pp. 681–686.
10. Schwab, J.H., Anderle, S.K., and Yank, C.H.: Arthritis in rats after systemic injection of streptococcal cells or cell walls. J. Exp. Med. 146:1585, 1977.
11. Pearson, C.M., Wood, F.D, and Tavaka, A.: Adjuvant and arthritogenic effects of some fractions of wax D from mycobacteria. Arthritis Rheum. 7:746, 1964.
12. Hamerman, D.: New thoughts on the pathogenesis of rheumatoid arthritis Am. J. Med. 40:1, 1966.
13. Andriopoulos, N.A., Mostecky, J. Wright, G.P., et al.: Characterization of antibodies to the native human collagens and to their component α-chains in the sera and the joint fluids of patients with rheumatoid arthritis. Immunochemistry 13:709, 1976.
14. Menzel, J., Steffen, C., Kolarz, G., Kojer, M., and Smolen, J.: Demonstration of anti-collagen antibodies in rheumatoid arthritis synovial fluids by $^{14}C$ radioimmunoassay. Arthritis Rheum. 21:243, 1978.
15. Trentham, D.E., Dynesius, R.A., Rocklin, R.E., and David, J.R.: Cellular sensitivity to collagen in rheumatoid arthritis. N. Engl. J. Med. 299:327, 1978.
16. Trentham, D.E., Townes, A.S., Kang, A.H., et al.: Humoral and cellular sensitivity to collagen in Type II collagen-induced arthritis in rats. J. Clin. Invest. 61:89, 1978.
17. Trentham, D.E., Townes, A.S., and Kang, A.H.: Autoimmunity to type II collagen: An experimental model of arthritis. J. Exp. Med. 146:857, 1977.
18. Claque, R.B., Shaw, M.J., and Holt, P.J.L.: Incidence and correlation between serum IgG and IgM antibodies to native type II collagen in patients with chronic inflammatory arthritis. Ann. Rheum. Dis. 40:6, 1981.
19. Alspaugh, M.A., and Tan, E.M.: Serum antibody in rheumatoid arthritis reactive with a cell-associated antigen: Demonstration by precipitation and immunofluorescence. Arthritis Rheum. 19:711, 1976.
20. Catalano, M.A., Carson, D.A., Slovin, S.F., Richman, D.D., and Vaughn, J.H.: Antibodies to Epstein-Barr virus-determined antigens in normal subjects and in patients with seropositive rheumatoid arthritis. Proc. Natl. Acad. Sci. (USA) 76:5825, 1979.
21. Alspaugh, M.A., Henle, G., Lennette, E.T., and Henle, W.: Elevated

levels of antibodies to Epstein-Barr virus antigens in sera and synovial fluids of patients with rheumatoid arthritis. J. Clin. Invest. 67:1134, 1981.
22. Tosato, G., Steinberg, A.D., and Blaese, R.M.: Defective EBV-specific suppressor T-cell function in rheumatoid arthritis. N. Engl. J. Med. 305:1238, 1981.
23. Depper, J.M., Bluestein, H.G., and Zvaifler, N.J.: Impaired regulation of Epstein-Barr virus-induced lymphocyte proliferation in rheumatoid arthritis is due to a T cell defect. J. Immunol. 127:1899, 1981.
24. Hasler, F., Bluestein, H.G., Zvaifler, N.J., and Epstein, L.B.: Analysis of the defects responsible for the impaired regulation of Epstein-Barr virus-induced B cell proliferation by rheumatoid arthritis lymphocytes. I. Diminished gamma interferon production in response to antalogous stimulation. J. Exp. Med. 157:173, 1983.
25. Lai, P.K., Alpers, M.P., and MacKay-Scollary, E.M.: Epstein-Barr herpes virus infection: inhibition by immunologically-induced mediators with interferon-like properties. Int. J. Cancer 20:21, 1977.
26. Silverman, S.L., and Schumacher, H.R.: Antibodies to Epstein-Barr viral antigens in early rheumatoid arthritis. Arthritis Rheum. 24:1465, 1981.
27. Depper, J.M., Zvaifler, N.J., and Bluestein, H.G.: Oropharyngeal Epstein-Barr virus excretion in rheumatoid arthritis. Arthritis Rheum. 25:427, 1982.
28. Kushner, I., and Somerville, J.: Permeability of human synovial membrane to plasma proteins. Relationship to molecular size and inflammation. Arthritis Rheum. 14:560, 1971.
29. Harris, E.D., Jr., Faulkner, C.S., III, and Brown, F.E.: Collagenolytic systems in rheumatoid arthritis. Clin. Orthop. 110:303, 1975.
30. Ruddy, S., and Austen, K.F.: Activation of the complement system in rheumatoid synovitis. Fed. Proc. 32:134, 1973.
31. Cooke, T.D., Hurd, E.R., Ziff, M., and Jasin, H.E.: The pathogenesis of chronic inflammation in experimental antigen-induced arthritis. II. Preferential localization of antigen-antibody complexes to collagenous tissues. J. Exp. Med. 135:323, 1972.
32. Cooke, T.D., Hurd, E.R., and Jasin, H.E.: Identification of immunoglobulins and complement in rheumatoid articular collagenous tissues. Arthritis Rheum. 18:563, 1975.
33. Ohno, O., and Cooke, T.D.: Electromicroscopic morphology of immunoglobulin aggregates and their interactions in rheumatoid articular collagenous tissues. Arthritis Rheum. 21:516, 1978.
34. Jasin, H.E.: Mechanism of trapping of immune complexes in joint collagenous tissues. Clin. Exp. Immunol. 22:473, 1975.
35. Ohno, O., and Cooke, T.D.V.: Immunoelectron microscope investigation of complexed immunoglobulins in rheumatoid (RA) and osteoarthrosis (OA) articular collagenous tissue. J. Bone Joint Surg. 60A:923, 1978.
36. Fox, A., and Glynn, L.E.: Persistence of antigen in nonarthritic joints. Ann. Rheum. Dis. 34:431, 1975.
37. Shiozawa, S., Jasin, H.E., and Ziff, M.: Absence of immunoglobulins in rheumatoid cartilage-pannus junctions. Arthritis Rheum. 23:816, 1980.
38. Cardella, C.J., Davies, P., and Allison, A.C.: Immune complexes induce selective release of lysosomal hydrolases from macrophages. Nature (Lond.) 274:46, 1974.
39. Dayer, J-M, Parswell, J.H., Schnaeberger, E.E., and Krane, S.M.: Interactions among rheumatoid synovial cells and monocyte-macrophages: Production of collagenase-stimulating factor by human monocytes exposed to concanavalin A or immunoglobulin Fc fragments. J. Immunol. 124:1712, 1980.
40. Bing, D.H., Alrnoda, S., Isliker, H., Lattav, J., and Hynes, R.O.: Fibronectin binds to the Clq component by complement. Proc Natl. Acad. Sci. (USA) 79:4198, 1982.
41. Janossy, G., Duke, O., Poulter, L.W., Panayi, G., Bafill, M., and Goldstein, G.: Rheumatoid arthritis: A disease of T-lymphocyte/macrophage immunoregulation. Lancet 2:839, 1981.
42. Kurosaka, M., and Ziff, M.: Immunoelectron microscopic study of distribution of T cell subsets and HLA-DR expressing cells in rheumatoid synovium. Arthritis Rheum. 26(Suppl. 4):553, 1983.
43. Klareskog, L., Forsum, U., Scheyniers, A., Kabelitz, D., and Wigzell, H.: Evidence in support of a self-perpetuating HLA-DR-dependent delayed-type cell reaction in rheumatoid arthritis. Proc. Natl. Acad. Sci. (USA) 29:3632, 1982.
44. Bellu, D.I., and Unanue, E.R.: Regulation of macrophage populations. II. Synthesis and expression of Ia antigens by peritoneal exudate macrophages is a transient event. J. Immunol. 126:263, 1981.
45. Steinman, R.M., Kaplan, G., Witmer, M.D., and Cohn, Z.A.: Identification of a novel cell type in peripheral lymphoid organs of mice. I. Purification of spleen dendritic cells, new surface markers and maintenance in vitro. J. Exp. Med. 149:1, 1979.
46. Fensclan, A., Watt, S., and Mello, R.J.: Tumor angiogenic factor. Purification from the Walker 256 rat tumor. J. Biol. Chem. 256:9605, 1981.
47. Ashida, E.R., Johnson, A.R., and Lipsky, P.E.: Human endothelial cell-lymphocyte interaction. J. Clin. Invest. 67:1490, 1981.
48. Schumacher, H.R., and Kitrodou, R.C.: Synovitis of recent onset. A clinicopathologic study during the first month of disease. Arthritis Rheum. 15:465, 1972.
49. Gerber, P., Whang-Peng, J., and Monroe, J.H.: Transformation and chromosomal changes induced by Epstein-Barr virus in normal human leukocyte cultures. Proc. Natl. Acad. Sci. USA 63:740, 1969.
50. Mohr, W., and Wessinghage, D.: The relationship between polymorphonuclear granulocytes and cartilage destruction in rheumatoid arthritis. Z. Reichtsmed. 37:81, 1978.
51. Hollingsworth, J.W., Siegel, E.R., and Creasey, W.A.: Granulocyte survival in synovial exudate of patients with rheumatoid arthritis and other inflammatory joint diseases. Yale J. Biol. Med. 39:289, 1967.
52. Weissman, G., Spilberg, I., and Krakauer, K.: Arthritis induced in rabbits by lysates of granulocyte lysosomes. Arthritis Rheum. 12:103, 1969.
53. Weissman, G., and Spilberg, I.: Breakdown of cartilage protein polysaccharide by lysosomes. Arthritis Rheum. 9:162, 1968.
54. Desmukh, K., and Hemrick, S.: Metabolic changes in rabbit articular cartilage due to inflammation. Arthritis Rheum. 19:199, 1976.
55. Mowat, A.G., and Baum, J.: Chemotaxis of polymorphonuclear leukocytes from patients with rheumatoid arthritis. J. Clin. Invest. 50:2541, 1971.
56. Turner, R.A., Schumacher, H.R., and Myers, A.R.: Phagocytic function of polymorphonuclear leukocytes in rheumatic diseases. J. Clin. Invest. 52:1632, 1973.
57. Goetzl, E.J., and Pickett, W.C.: Novel structural determinates of the human neutrophil chemotactic activity of leukotriene B. J. Exp. Med. 153:482, 1981.
58. Klickstein, L.B., Shapleigh, C., and Goetzl, E.J.: Lipoxygenation of arachidonic acid as a source of polymorphonuclear leukocyte chemotactic factors in synovial fluid and tissue in rheumatoid arthritis and spondyloarthritis. J. Clin. Invest. 66:1166, 1980.
59. Fridovich, I.: The biology of oxygen radicals. Science 201:875, 1978.
60. Goldberg, B., and Stern, A.: The generation of $O_2$ by the interaction of the hemolytic agent phenylhydrazine with human hemoglobin. J. Biol. Chem. 250:2401, 1975.
61. McCord, J.M.: Free radicals and inflammation: Protection of synovial fluid by superoxide. Science 185:529, 1974.
62. Carp, H., and Janoff, A.: Potential mediator of inflammation. Phagocyte-derived oxidants suppress the elastase-inhibitory capacity $\alpha_1$-proteinase inhibitor in vitro. J. Clin. Invest. 66:987, 1980.
63. Goldstein, I., Edelson, H.S., Kaplan, M.B., and Weissman, G.: Ceruloplasmin: A scavenger of superoxide anion radicals. J Biol. Chem. 254:4040, 1979.
64. Oyanagui, Y.: Participation of superoxide anions in the prostaglandin phase of carrageenan foot-oedema. Biochem. Pharmacol. 25:1465, 1976.
64a. Weiss, S.J., Lampert, M.B., and Test, S.T.: Long-lived oxidants generated by human neutrophils: Characterization and bioactivity. Science 222:625, 1983.
65. Hallgren, R., Hukansson, L., and Venge, P.: Kinetic studies of phagocytosis. 1. The serum independent particle uptake by PMN from patients with rheumatoid arthritis and SLE. Arthritis Rheum. 21:107, 1978.
66. Corberand, J., Amigues, H., deLarrard, B., and Pradere, J.: Neutrophil functions in rheumatoid arthritis. Scand. J. Rheumatol. 6:49, 1977.
67. Wilton, J.M.A., Gibson, T., and Chuck, C.M.: Defective phagocytosis by synovial fluid and blood PMN leukocytes in patients with rheumatoid arthritis. I. The nature of the defect. Rheumatol. Rehabil. Supplement, 1978, pp. 25–35.
68. Mowat, A.G., and Baum, J.: Chemotaxis of PMN leukocytes from patients with rheumatoid arthritis. J. Clin. Invest. 50:2541, 1971.
69. Udein, A-M., Trang, L., Venizelos, N., and Palmblad, J.: Neutrophil functions and clinical performance after total fasting in patients with rheumatoid arthritis. Ann. Rheum. Dis. 42:45, 1983.
70. Ruddy, S., and Colten, H.R.: Biosynthesis of complement proteins by synovial tissues. N. Engl. J. Med. 290:1284, 1974.
71. Smiley, J.D., Sachs, C., and Ziff, M.: In vitro synthesis of immunoglobulin by rheumatoid synovial membrane. J. Clin. Invest. 47:624, 1968.
72. Slirvinski, A.H., and Zvaifler, N.H.: In vivo synthesis of IgG by rheumatoid synovium. J. Lab Clin. Med. 76:304, 1970.
73. Ruddy, S., Britton, M.C., Schur, P.H., and Austen, K.F.: Complement components in synovial fluid: Activation and fixation in seropositive rheumatoid arthritis. Ann. N.Y. Acad. Sci. 168:161, 1969.
74. Ruddy, S., and Austen, K.F.: The complement system in rheumatoid synovitis. I. An analysis of complement component activities in rheumatoid synovial fluids. Arthritis Rheum. 13:713, 1970.
75. Pekin, T.J., Jr., and Zvaifler, N.J.: Hemolytic complement in synovial fluid. J. Clin. Invest. 43:1372, 1964.
76. Sabharwal, U.K., Vaughan, J.H., Fong, S., Bennett, P.H., Carson, D.A., and Curd, J.G.: Activation of the classical pathway of complement by rheumatoid factors. Assessment by radioimmunoassay for C4. Arthritis Rheum. 25:161, 1982.
77. Kaplan, R.A., Curd, J.G., DeHeer, D.H., Carson, D.A., Pangburn, M.K., Muller-Eberhard, H.J., and Vaughan, J.H.: Metabolism of C4 and

factor B in rheumatoid arthritis: Relation to rheumatoid factor. Arthritis Rheum. 23:911, 1980.

78. Sabharwal, U.K., Vaughan, J.H., Fong, S., Bennett, P.H., Carson, D.A., and Curd, J.G.: Activation of the classical pathway of complement by rheumatoid factors: Assessment by radioimmunoassay for C4. Arthritis Rheum. 25:161, 1982.
79. Goldstein, I.M., and Weissmann, G.: Generation of C5-derived lysosomal enzyme-releasing activity (C5a) by lysates of leukocyte lysosomes. J. Immunol. 113:1583, 1974.
80. Borel, J.F., Keller, H.U., and Sorkin, E.: Studies on chemotaxis. XI. Effect on neutrophils of lysosomal and other subcellular fractions from leukocytes. Int. Arch. Allergy Appl. Immunol. 35:194, 1969.
81. Ward, P.A., and Zvaifler, N.J.: Complement-derived leucotactic factors in inflammatory synovial fluids of humans. J. Clin. Invest. 50:606, 1971.
82. Goldstein, I.M., Hoffman, S., Gallin, J., and Weissman, G.: Mechanisms of lysosomal enzyme release from human leucocytes. Microtubule assembly and membrane fusion induced by a component of complement. Proc. Natl. Acad. Sci. USA 70:2916, 1973.
83. Kaplan, M.H., and Volanakis, J.E.: Interaction of C-reactive protein complexes with the complement system. I. Consumption of human complement associated with the reaction of C-reactive protein with pneumococcal C-polysaccharide and with the choline phosphatides, lecithin and sphingomyelin. J. Immunol. 112:2135, 1974.
84. Kushner, I., Rakitu, L., and Kaplan, M.H.: Studies of acute phase protein. II. Localization of C-reactive protein in heart in induced myocardial infarction in rabbits. J. Clin. Invest. 42:286, 1963.
85. Wuepper, K.D.: Cutaneous responses to human C3a anaphylatoxin in man. Clin. Exp. Immunol. 11:13, 1972.
86. Pisano, J.J., and Austen, K.F.: Chemistry and Biology of the Kallikrein Kinin System in Health and Disease. Washington, D.C., U.S. Government Printing Office, 1976.
87. Epstein, W., Melmon, K.L., Tan, E.M., and Stoff, J.: Kinin generation by human IgG rheumatoid factor complex (abstract). J. Clin. Invest. 47:90, 1968.
88. Melmon, K.L., and Cline, M.J.: Kallikrein activator and kininase in human granulocytes: A model of inflammation. *In* Rocha, E., and Silva, M. (eds.): Symposium on Vasoactive Polypeptides: Bradykinin and Related Kinins. Oxford, Pergamon Press, 1967.
89. Cochrane, C.G., et al.: The interaction of Hageman factor and immune complexes. J. Clin. Invest. 51:2736, 1972.
90. Rothberger, H., Zimmerman, T.S., Spiegelberg, H.L., and Vaughan, J.H.: Leucocyte procoagulant activity: Enhancement of production in vitro by IgG and antigen-antibody complexes. J. Clin. Invest. 59:549, 1977.
91. Glynn, L.E.: Heberden Oration. The chronicity of inflammation and its significance in rheumatoid arthritis. Ann. Rheum. Dis. 27:105, 1968.
92. Van de Putte, L.B.A., Hegt, V.N., and Overbeek, T.E.: Activators and inhibitors of fibrinolysis in rheumatoid and non-rheumatoid synovial membranes. Arthritis Rheum. 20:671, 1977.
93. Kulka, P.J.: Microcirculation impairment as a factor in inflammatory tissue damage. Ann. N.Y. Acad. Sci. 116:1018, 1964.
94. Metzger, F., Haffeld, J.F., and Oppenheim, J.J.: Regulation by $PGE_2$ of the production of oxygen intermediates by LPS-activated macrophages. J. Immunol. 127:1109, 1981.
95. Vassalli, J-D, Hamilton, J., and Reich, E.: Macrophage plasminogen activator: Modulation of enzyme production by anti-inflammatory steroids, mitotic inhibitors, and cyclic nucleotides. Cell 8:281, 1976.
96. Roberts, J.E., McLees, B.D., and Kerby, G.P.: Pathways of glucose metabolism in rheumatoid and non-rheumatoid synovial membrane. J. Lab. Clin. Med. 70:503, 1967.
97. Thomas, P.P.L., and Dingle, J.T.M.: Studies on human synovial membrane in vitro. The metabolism of normal and rheumatoid synovia and the effect of hydrocortisone. Biochem. J. 68:231, 1958.
98. Falchuk, K.H., Goetzl, E.J., and Kulka, J.P.: Respiratory gases of synovial fluids. An approach to synovial tissue circulatory-metabolic imbalance in rheumatoid arthritis. Am. J. Med. 49:223, 1970.
99. Wallis, W.J., Simkin, P.A., Nelp, W.B., and Foster, D.M.: Synovial fluid temperature in rheumatoid synovitis. Arthritis Rheum. 26:517, 1983.
100. Muirden, K.D.: The anaemia of rheumatoid arthritis: The significance of iron deposits in the synovial membrane. Aust. Ann. Med. 19:97, 1970.
101. Mainardi, C.L., Levine, P.H., Werb, Z., and Harris, E.D., Jr.: Proliferative synovitis in hemophilia. Biochemical and morphologic observations. Arthritis Rheum. 21:137, 1978.
102. Blake, D.R., Hall, N.D., Bacon, P.A., Dieppe, P.A., Halliwell, B., and Gutteridge, J.M.C.: The importance of iron in rheumatoid disease. Lancet 2:1142, 1981.
103. Chichton, R.R.: Interreaction between iron metabolism and oxygen activation. *In*: Oxygen Free Radicals and Tissue Damage. Ciba Foundation Symposium 65 (new series). Amsterdam, Excerpta Medica, 1979, pp. 57–76.
104. Okazaki, I., Brinckeroff, C.E., Sinclair, J.F., Sinclair P.R., Bronkowsky, H.L. and Harris, E.D., Jr.: Iron increases collagenase production by rabbit synovial fibroblasts J. Lab. Clin. Med. 97:396–402, 1981.
105. Ziff, M.: Relation of cellular infiltration of rheumatoid synovial membrane to its immune response. Arthritis Rheum. 17:313, 1974.
106. VanBoxel, J.A., and Paget, S.A.: Predominantly T cell infiltrate in rheumatoid synovial membrane. N. Engl. J. Med. 293:517, 1975.
107. Bankhurst, A.D., Husky, G., and Williams, R.C., Jr.: Predominance of T cells in the lymphocytic infiltrates of synovial tissues in rheumatoid arthritis. Arthritis Rheum. 19:555, 1976.
108. Van de Putte, L.B.A., de Vries, E., Van Leuwen, A.W.F.M., and Meijer, C.J.L.M.: T-lymphocytes and rheumatoid inflammation. *In* Feltkamp, A., and Leiden, T.E.W. (eds.): Non-Articular Forms of Rheumatoid Arthritis. Amsterdam, Staflen's Scientific Publishing, 1977, pp. 103–110.
109. Mellbye, O.J., Messner, R.P., DeBord, J.R., and Williams, R.C.: Immunoglobulin and receptors for C3 on lymphocytes from patients with rheumatoid arthritis. Arthritis Rheum. 15:371, 1975.
110. Papamichael, M., Brown, J.C., and Holborow, E.J.: Immunoglobulins on the surface of human lymphocytes. Lancet 2:850, 1971.
111. Micheli, A., and Brom, J.: Studies on blood T and B lymphocytes in rheumatoid arthritis. Ann. Rheum. Dis. 33:435, 1974.
112. Konttinen, Y.T., Reitamo, S., Ranki, A., Hayry, P., Kankaanapaa, U., and Wegelius, O.: Characterization of the immunocompetent cells of rheumatoid synovium from tissue sections and eluates. Arthritis Rheum. 24:71, 1981.
113. Burmester, G.R., Yu, D.T.Y., Irani, A-M, Kunkel, H.G., and Winchester, R.J.: Ia+ T cells in synovial fluid and tissues of patients with rheumatoid arthritis. Arthritis Rheum. 24:1370, 1981.
114. Fox, R.I., Fong, S., Sabharwal, N., Carstens, S.A., Kung, P.C., and Vaughan, J.H.: Synovial fluid lymphocytes differ from peripheral blood lymphocytes in patients with rheumatoid arthritis. J. Immunol. 128:351–354, 1982.
115. Winchester, R.J., and Kunkel, H.G.: The human Ia system. Adv. Immunol. 28:221–292, 1979.
116. Reinberg, E.L., Kung, P.C., Pesando, J.M., Ritz, J., Goldstein, G., and Schlossman, S.F.: Ia determinants on human T-cell subsets defined by monoclonal antibody. Activation stimuli required for expression. J. Exp. Med. 150:1472, 1979.
117. Yu, D.T., Winchester, R.J., Fu, S.M., Givofsky, A., Ko, H.S., and Kunkel, H.G.: Peripheral blood Ia-positive T cells, increases in certain diseases and after immunization. J. Exp. Med. 151:91, 1980.
118. Carter, S.D., Bacon, P.A., and Hall, N.D.: Characterization of activated lymphocytes in the peripheral blood of patients with rheumatoid arthritis. Ann Rheum. Dis. 40:293, 1981.
119. Herberman, R.B., and Ortaldo, J.R.: Natural killer cells: Their role in defenses against disease. Science 214:24, 1981.
120. Dohlong, J.H., Førre, O., Kvien, T.K., Egeland, T., and Degre, M.: Natural killer (NK) cell activity of peripheral blood, synovial fluid, and synovial tissue lymphocytes from patients with rheumatoid arthritis and juvenile rheumatoid arthritis. Ann. Rheum. Dis. 41:490, 1982.
121. Griffiths, M.M., Smith, C.B., Ward, J.R., and Klauber, M.R.: Cytotoxic activity of rheumatoid and normal lymphocytes against allogeneic and autologous synovial cells in vitro. J. Clin. Invest. 58:613, 1976.
122. Ghose, T., Woodbury, J.F., and Hansell, M.M.: Interaction in vitro between synovial cells and autologous lymphocytes and sera from arthritis patients. J. Clin. Pathol. 28:550, 1975.
123. Griffiths, M.M., Smith, C.B., and Pepper, B.J.: Susceptibility of rheumatoid and non-rheumatoid synovial cells to antibody-dependent cell-mediated cytotoxicity. Arthritis Rheum. 21:97, 1978.
124. Koopman, W.J., and Schrohenloher, R.E.: Enhanced in vitro synthesis of IgM rheumatoid factor in rheumatoid arthritis. Arthritis Rheum. 23:985, 1980.
125. Abrahamsen, T.G., Froland, S.S., Natvig, J.B., and Pahle, J.: Elution and characterization of lymphocytes from rheumatoid inflammatory tissue. Scand. J. Immunol. 4:823, 1975.
126. Goodwin, J.S., Bankhurst, A.D., and Messner, R.P.: Suppression of human T-cell mitogenesis by prostaglandin. J. Exp. Med. 146:1719, 1977.
127. Panayi, G.S., and Corrigall, V.: Lymphocyte function in rheumatoid arthritis. *In* Panayi, G.S., and Johnson, P.M. (eds.): Immunopathogenesis of Rheumatoid Arthritis. Chertsey, Reedbooks, Ltd. 1979, p. 31.
128. Andreis, M., Stastny, P., and Ziff, M.: Experimental arthritis produced by injection of mediators of delayed hypersensitivity. Arthritis Rheum. 14:537, 1971.
129. Dayer, J.M., Robinson, D.R., and Krane, S.M.: Prostaglandin production by rheumatoid synovial cells. J. Exp. Med. 145:1399, 1977.
130. Waksman, B.H., and Namba, Y.: On soluble mediators of immunologic regulation. Cell Immunol. 21:161, 1976.
131. Lawrence, H.S., and Valentine, F.T.: Transfer factor and other mediators of cellular immunity. Am. J. Pathol. 60:437, 1970.
132. Lawrence, H.S.: Transfer factor and cellular immune deficiency disease. N. Eng. J. Med. 283:411, 1970.
133. Wegelius, O., Laire, W., Lindstrom, B., and Klockars, M.: Fistula of the thoracic duct as immunosuppressive treatment in rheumatoid arthritis. Acta Med. Scand. 187:539, 1970.

134. Paulus, H.E., Machleder, H.I., and Peter, J.B.: Clinical improvement of rheumatoid arthritis during prolonged thoracic duct lymphocyte drainage. Arthritis Rheum. 16:562, 1973.
135. Whitehouse, M.W., Whitehouse, D.J., and Pearson, C.M.: Passive transfer of adjuvant-induced arthritis and allergic encephalomyelitis in rats using thoracic duct lymphocytes. Nature 224:1322, 1969.
136. Pearson, C.M.: Transfer of adjuvant arthritis by means of lymph node or spleen cells. J. Belg. Rheumatol. Med. Phys. 24:150, 1969.
137. Good, R.A., Rotstein, J., and Mozzitello, W.F.: The simultaneous occurrence of rheumatoid arthritis and agammaglobulinemia. J. Lab. Clin. Med. 49:343, 1957.
138. Mellors, R., Heimer, R., Corcos, J., et al.: Cellular origin of rheumatoid factor. J. Exp. Med. 110:875, 1959.
139. Munthe, E., and Natvig, J.B.: Immunoglobulin classes, subclasses and complexes of IgG rheumatoid factor in rheumatoid plasma cells. Clin. Exp. Immunol. 12:55, 1972.
140. Hoffman, W.L., Goldberg, M.S., and Smiley, J.D.: Immunoglobulin $G_3$ subclass production by rheumatoid synovial tissue cultures. J. Clin. Invest. 69:136, 1982.
141. Cats, A., and Hazevoet, H.M.: Significance of positive tests for rheumatoid factor in the prognosis of rheumatoid arthritis. Ann. Rheum. Dis. 29:254, 1970.
142. Herman, J.H., Bradley, J., Ziff, M., and Smiley, J.D.: Response of the rheumatoid synovial membrane to exogenous immunization. J. Clin. Invest. 50:266, 1971.
143. Allen, J.C., and Kunkel, H.G.: Hidden rheumatoid factors with specificity for native gamma globulins. Arthritis Rheum. 9:758, 1966.
144. Cone, R.E., Feldmann, M., Marchalones, J.J., and Nossal, G.J.V.: Cytophilic properties of surface immunoglobulin of thymus-derived lymphocytes. Immunology 26:49, 1974.
145. Veys, E.M., Gabriel, P.A., and Goegne, E.: Rheumatoid factor and serum IgG, IgM and IgA levels in rheumatoid arthritis with vasculitis. Scand. J. Rheumatol. 5:1, 1976.
146. Vaughan, J.H.: Lymphocyte function in rheumatic disorders. Arch. Intern. Med. 135:1324, 1975.
147. Pope, R.M., Teller, D.C., and Mannik, M.: The molecular basis of self-association of antibodies to IgG (rheumatoid factor) in rheumatoid arthritis. Proc. Natl. Acad. Sci. USA 71:517, 1974.
148. Winchester, R.J.: Characterization of IgG complexes in patients with rheumatoid arthritis. Ann. N.Y. Acad. Sci. 256:73, 1975.
149. Brown, P.B., Nardella, F.A., and Mannik, M.: Human complement activation by self-associated IgG rheumatoid factors. Arthritis Rheum. 25:1101, 1982.
150. Pekin, T.J., Jr., and Zvaifler, N.J.: Hemolytic complement levels in synovial fluids. J. Clin. Invest. 43:1372, 1964.
151. Rodman, W.S., Williams, R.C., Jr., Bilka, P.J., and Muller-Eberhard, H.J.: Immunofluorescent localization of the third and fourth component of complement in synovial tissues from patients with rheumatoid arthritis. J. Lab. Clin. Med. 69:141, 1967.
152. Conn, D.L., McDuffie, F.C., and Dyck, P.J.: Immunopathologic study of sural nerves in rheumatoid arthritis. Arthritis Rheum. 15:135, 1972.
153. Zvaifler, N.J.: Immunopathology of joint inflammation in rheumatoid arthritis. Immunology 16:265, 1973.
154. Pope, R.M.: Rheumatoid arthritis associated with hyperviscosity syndrome and intermediate complex formation. Arch. Intern. Med. 135:281, 1975.
155. Jasin, H.E., LoSpalluto, J.J., and Ziff, M.: Rheumatoid hyperviscosity syndrome. Am. J. Med. 49:484, 1970.
156. DeHoratius, R.J., Abruzzo, J.L., and Williams, R.C., Jr.: Immunofluorescent and immunologic studies of rheumatoid lung. Arch. Intern. Med. 129:441, 1972.
157. Theofilopoulos, A.N., Burtonboy, G., LoSpalluto, J.J., and Ziff, M.: IgM rheumatoid factor and low molecular weight IgM: An association with vasculitis. Arthritis Rheum. 17:272, 1977.
158. Allen, C., Elson, C.J., Scott, D.G.I., Bacon, P.A., and Bucknall, R.C.: IgG antiglobulins in rheumatoid arthritis and other arthritides: relationship with clinical features and other parameters. Ann. Rheum. Dis. 40:127, 1981.
159. Winchester, R.J., Agnello, V., and Kunkel, H.G.: Gamma globulin complexes in synovial fluids of patients with rheumatoid arthritis. Partial characterization and relationship to lowered complement levels. Clin. Exp. Immunol. 6:689, 1970.
160. Munthe, E., and Natvig, J.B.: Characterization of IgG complexes in eluates from rheumatoid tissue. Clin. Exp. Immunol. 8:249, 1971.
161. Munthe, E., and Natvig, J.B.: Immunoglobulin classes, subclasses and complexes of IgG rheumatoid factor in rheumatoid plasma cells. Clin. Exp. Immunol. 12:55, 1972.
162. Munthe, E., and Natvig, J.B.: Complement-fixing intracellular complexes of IgG rheumatoid factor in rheumatoid plasma cells. Scand. J. Immunol. 1:217, 1972.
163. McCarty, D.J., and Hollander, J.L.: Identification of urate crystals in gouty synovial fluid. Ann. Intern. Med. 54:452, 1961.
164. Hollander, J.L., McCarty, D.J., Astorga, G., and Castro-Mirillo, E.: Studies on the pathogenesis of rheumatoid joint inflammation. I. The R.A. "cell" and a working hypothesis. Ann. Intern. Med. 62:271, 1965.
165. Britton, M.C., and Schur, P.H.: The complement system in rheumatoid synovitis. II. Intracytoplasmic inclusions of immunoglobulins and complement. Arthritis Rheum. 14:87, 1971.
166. Rodman, W.S., Williams, R.C., Jr., Bilka, P.J., and Muller-Eberhard, H.J.: Immunofluorescent localization of the third and the fourth component of complement in synovial tissue from patients with rheumatoid arthritis. J. Lab. Clin. Med. 69:141, 1967.
167. Cecere, F., Lessard, J., McDuffy, S., and Pope, R.M.: Evidence for the local production and utilization of immune reactions in rheumatoid arthritis. Arthritis Rheum. 25:1307, 1982.
168. Rawson, A.J., Hollander, J.L., Quismorio, F.P., and Abelson, N.M.: Experimental arthritis in man and rabbit dependent upon serum anti-immunoglobulin factors. Ann. N.Y. Acad. Sci. 168:188, 1969.
169. Tanimoto, K., Cooper, N.R., Johnson, J.S., and Vaughan, J.H.: Complement fixation by rheumatoid factor. J. Clin. Invest. 55:437, 1975.
170. Theofilopoulos, A.N., Dixon, F.J., and Bokish, V.A.: Binding of soluble immune complexes to human lymphoblastoid cells. I. Characterization of receptors for IgG, Fc and complement and description of the binding mechanism. J. Exp. Med. 140:877, 1974.
171. Henney, G.S., Stanworth, D.R., and Gell, P.G.H.: Demonstration of the exposure of new antigenic determinants following antigen-antibody combination. Nature 205:1079, 1965.
172. Johnson, P.M., Watkins, J., Scopes, P.M., and Tracey, B.M.: Differences in serum IgG structures in health and rheumatoid disease. Ann. Rheum. Dis. 33:366, 1974.
173. Allison, A.C.L.: Heberden Oration: Mechanism of tolerance and autoimmunity. Ann. Rheum. Dis. 32:283, 1973.
174. Jerne, N.K.: Towards a network theory of the immune system. Ann. Immunol. (Inst. Pasteur) 115C:373, 1974.
175. Pasquali, J.L., Urlacher, A., Storck, D.: A highly conserved determinant on human rheumatoid factor idiotypes defined by a mouse monoclonal antibody. Clin. J. Immunol. 13:197–201, 1983.
176. Jerne, N.K., Nordin, A.A., and Henry C.: The agar plaque technique for recognizing antibody-producing cells. *In* Amos, B., and Koprowski, H. (ed.): Cell Bound Antibodies. Philadelphia, Wistar Institute Press, 1963, p. 109.
177. Vaughan, J.H., Chihara, T., Moore, T.L., Robbins, D.L., Tanimoto, K., Johnson, J.S., and McMillan, R.: Rheumatoid factor–producing cells detected by direct hemolytic plaque assay. J. Clin. Invest. 58:933, 1976.
178. Zuran, B.L., O'Hair, C.H., Vaughan, J.H., Mathison, D.A., Curd, J.G., and Katz, D.H.: Immunoglobulin E–rheumatoid factor in the serum of patients with rheumatoid arthritis, asthma, and other diseases. J. Clin. Invest. 68:1610, 1981.
179. Meretey, K., Falus, A., Erhardt, C.C., and Maini, R.N.: IgE and IgE–rheumatoid factors in circulating immune complexes in rheumatoid arthritis. Ann. Rheum. Dis. 41:405, 1982.
180. Crisp, A.J., Chapman, C.M., Kirkham, S., Schiller, A.L., and Krane, S.M.: Synovial mastocytosis in adult rheumatoid arthritis. Arthritis Rheum. 26:552, 1983.
181. Abel, T., Andrews, B.S., Cunningham, P.H., Brunner, C.M., Davis, J.B., and Horwitz, D.A.: Rheumatoid vasculitis: Effect of cyclophosphamide on the clinical course and levels of circulating immune complexes. Ann. Intern. Med. 93:407, 1980.
182. Rapoport, R.J., Kozin, F., Macket, S.E., and Jordan, R.E.: Cutaneous vascular immunofluorescence in rheumatoid arthritis: correlation with circulating immune complexes and vasculitis. Am. J. Med. 68:325, 1980.
183. McDougal, J.S., Hubbard, M., McDuffie, F.C., Strobel, P.L., Smith, S.J., Bass, N., Goldman, J.A., Hartman, S., Myerson, G., Miller, S., Morales, R., and Wilson, C.H., Jr.: Comparison of five assays for immune complexes in the rheumatic diseases. An assessment of their validity for rheumatoid arthritis. Arthritis Rheum. 25:1156, 1982.
184. Dayer, J.M., Krane, S.M., Russell, R.G.G., and Robinson, D.F.: Production of collagenase and prostaglandins by isolated adherent rheumatoid synovial cells. Proc. Natl. Acad. Sci. USA 73:945, 1976.
185. Abrahamsen, T.G., Johnson, P.M., and Natvig, J.B.: Membrane characteristics of adherent cells dissociated from rheumatoid synovial tissue. Clin. Exp. Immunol. 28:474, 1977.
186. Theofilopoulos, A.N., Carson, D.A., Tovassoli, M., Slotrim, S.F., Speers, W.C., Jensen, F.B., and Vaughan, J.H.: Evidence for the presence of recepters for C3 and IgG Fc on human synovial cells. Arthritis Rheum. 23:1, 1980.
187. Baker, D.G., Dayer, J.M., Roelke, M., Schumacher, H.R., and Krane, S.M.: Rheumatoid synovial cell morphologic changes induced by a mononuclear cell factor in culture Arthritis Rheum. 26:8, 1983.
188. Pollack, M.S., Goldenhersch, M., Chin-Louie, J., and Safai, B.: The functional study of DR-positive human epidermal Langerhans cells in mixed cell cultures with allogeneic lymphocytes. Clin. Immunol. Immunopathol. 24:15, 1982.

189. Anastassiades, T.P., Ley, J., Wood, A., and Irwin, D.: The growth kinetics of synovial fibroblast cells from inflammatory and noninflammatory arthropathies. Arthritis Rheum. 21:461, 1978.
190. Castor, C.W.: Connective tissue activation II. Abnormalities of cultured rheumatoid synovial cells. Arthritis Rheum. 14:55, 1971.
191. Goldfischer, S., Smith, C., and Hamerman, D.: Altered acid hydrolase activities in rheumatoid synovial cells in culture. Am. J. Pathol. 52:569, 1968.
192. Henderson, B.: The contribution made by cytochemistry to the study of the metabolism of the normal and rheumatoid synovial lining cell (synoviocyte). Histochemical J. 14:527, 1982.
193. Castor, C.W., and Lewis, R.B.: Connective tissue activation. X. Current studies of mediators and the process. Scand. J. Rheumatol. 5:41, 1975.
194. Castor, C.W., Ritchie, J.C., Scott, M.E., and Whitney, S.L.: Connective tissue activation. XI. Stimulation of glycosaminoglycan and DNA formation by a platelet factor. Arthritis Rheum. 20:859, 1977.
195. Andersen, H.: Development, morphology and histochemistry of the early synovial tissue in human foetuses. Acta Anat. 58:90, 1964.
196. Loeuvi, G.: Experimental immune inflammation in the synovial membrane. Immunology 17:489, 1969.
197. Wahl, L.M., Wahl, S.M., Mergenhagen, S.E., and Martin, G.R.: Collagenase production by lymphokine-activated macrophages. Science 187:261, 1975.
198. Vasalli, J.D., and Reich, E.: Macrophage plasminogen activator: Induction by products of activated lymphoid cells. J. Exp. Med. 145:427, 1977.
199. David, J.R., and David, R.R.: Cellular hypersensitivity and immunity. Inhibition of macrophage migration and the lymphocyte mediators. Prog. Allergy 16:200, 1972.
200. Cardella, C.J., Davies, P., and Allison, A.C.: Immune complexes induce selective release of lysosomal enzymes. Nature 247:46, 1974.
201. Schorlemmer, H.U., and Allison, A.C.: Effects of activated complement components on enzyme secretion by macrophages. Immunology 31:781, 1976.
202. Gotze, D., and Bianco, C.: *In* van Furth, R. (ed.): Mononuclear Phagocytes: Functional Aspects. The Hague, Martinus Nijhoff, 1979.
203. Werb, Z., Mainardi, C.L., Vater, C.A., and Harris, E.D., Jr.: Endogenous activation of a latent collagenase by rheumatoid synovial cells. Evidence for a role of plasminogen activator. N. Engl. J. Med. 296:1017,
204. Bianco, C., Eden, A., and Cohn, Z.A.: The induction of macrophage spreading: Role of coagulation factors and the complement system. J. Exp. Med. 144:1531, 1976.
205. Werb, Z., and Aggller, J.: Proteases induce secretion of collagenase and plasminogen activator by fibroblasts. Proc. Natl. Acad. Sci. USA 75:1839, 1978.
206. Polvernie, P.J., Cottran, R.S., Gimbrone, M.A., Jr., and Unanue, E.R.: Activated macrophages induced vascular proliferation. Nature 269:804, 1977.
207. Henderson, B., Glynn, L.E., and Chayen, J.: Cell division in the synovial lining in experimental allergic arthritis: Proliferation of cells during the development of chronic arthritis. Ann. Rheum. Dis. 41:275, 1982.
208. Krane, S.M.: Heberden Oration, 1980. Aspects of the cell biology of the rheumatoid synovial lesion. Ann. Rheum. Dis. 40:433, 1981.
209. Postlethwaite, A.E., and Kang, A.H.: Characterization of fibroblast proliferation factors elaborated by antigen- and mitogen-stimulated guinea pig lymph node cells: Differentiation from lymphocyte-derived chemotactic factor for fibroblasts, lymphocyte mitogenic factor, and Interleukin 1. Cellular Immunol. 73:169, 1982.
210. Schmidt, J.A., Mizel, S.B., Cohen, D., and Green, I.: Interleukin 1, a potential regulator of fibroblast proliferation. J. Immunol. 128:2177, 1982.
211. Devel, T.F., Huang, J.S., Proffitt, R.T., Baenziger, J.U., Chang, D., and Kennedy, B.B.: Human platelet-derived growth factor. J. Biol. Chem. 256:8896, 1981.
212. Dayer, J.-M., Russell, R.G.G., and Krane, S.M.: Collagenase production by rheumatoid synovial cells: Stimulation by a human lymphocyte factor. Science 135:181, 1977.
213. Dayer, J.-M., Robinson, D.R., and Krane, S.M.: Prostaglandin production by rheumatoid synovial cells. Stimulation by a factor from human mononuclear cells. J. Exp. Med. 145:1393, 1977.
214. Mizel, S.B., Dayer, J.-M, Krane, S.M., and Mergenhagen, S.E.: Stimulation of rheumatoid synovial cell collagenase and prostaglandin production by partially purified lymphocyte-activating factor (Interleukin 1). Proc. Natl. Acad. Sci. (USA) 78:2474, 1980.
215. Postlethwaite, A.E., Lachman, L.B., Mainardi, C.L., and Kang, A.H.: Interleukin 1 stimulation of collagenase production by cultured fibroblasts. J. Exp. Med. 157:801, 1983.
216. Biswas, C., and Dayer, J.-M.: Stimulation of collagenase production by collagen in mammalian cell cultures. Cell 18:1035, 1979.
217. Dayer, J.-M., Trentham, D.E., David, J.R., and Krane, S.M.: Collagens stimulate the production of mononuclear cell factor (MCF) and prostaglandins ($PGE_2$) by human monocytes. Trans. Assoc. Am. Phys. 93:326, 1980.
218. Tsukamoto, Y., Helsel, W.E., and Wahl, S.M.: Macrophage production of fibronectin, a chemoattractant for fibroblasts. J. Immunol. 127:673, 1981.
219. Hamilton, J.A., and Slywka, J.: Stimulation of human synovial fibroblast plasminogen activator production by mononuclear cell supernatants. J. Immunol. 126:851, 1981.
220. Harris, E.D., Jr., and McCroskery, P.A.: The influence of temperature and fibril stability on degradation of cartilage collagen by rheumatoid synovial collagenase. N. Engl. J. Med. 290:1, 1974.
221. Werb, Z., Burleigh, M.C., Barrett, A.J., and Starkey, P.M.: Binding and inhibition of mammalian collagenases and other metal proteinases. Biochem. J. 139:359, 1974.
222. Starkey, P.M., and Barrett, A.J.: $\alpha_2$-Macroglobulin, a physiological regulator of proteinase activity. *In* Barrett, A.J. (ed.): Proteinases in Mammalian Cells and Tissues. New York, North-Holland Publishing Company, 1977, pp. 663–696.
223. Ohlsson, K., and Delshammar, M.: Interactions between granulocyte elastase and the plasma proteinase inhibitors in vitro and in vivo. *In* Burleigh, P.M., and Poole, A.R. (eds.): Dynamics of Connective Tissue Macromolecules. New York, North-Holland Publishing Company, 1975, pp. 259–275.
224. Ohlsson, K.: Granulocyte collagenase and elastase and their interaction with $\alpha_1$-antitrypsin and $\alpha_2$-macroglobulin. *In* Reich E. et al.(eds.): Protease and Biological Control. Cold Springs Harbor Laboratories, 1975, pp. 591–602.
225. Kimura, H., Tateishi, H., and Ziff, M.: Surface ultrastructure of rheumatoid articular cartilage. Arthritis Rheum. 20:1085, 1977.
226. Jasin, H.E.: Deposition of immune complexes within articular connective tissues. *In* Panayi, G.S., and Johnson, P.M. (eds.): Immunopathogenesis of Rheumatoid Arthritis. Reedbooks, Ltd., 1979, p. 89.
227. Banda, M.J., Clark, E.J., and Werb, Z.: Limited proteolysis by macrophage elastase inactivates human $\alpha_1$-proteinase inhibitor. J. Exp. Med. 152:1563, 1980.
228. Barrett, A.J.: The possible role of neutrophil proteinases in damage to articular cartilage. Agents Actions 8:3, 1978.
229. Harris, E.D., Jr., and Krane, S.M.: Collagenases. N. Engl. J. Med. 291:557, 605, 652, 1974.
230. Harris, E.D., Jr., and Krane, S.M.: An endopeptidase from rheumatoid synovial tissue culture. Biochim. Biophys. Acta 258:566, 1972.
231. Abe, S., and Nagai, Y.: Evidence for the presence of a complex of collagenase with $\alpha_2$-macroglobulin in human rheumatoid synovial fluid. A possible regulatory mechanism of collagenase activity in vivo. J. Biochem. 73:897, 1973.
232. Delshammar, M., and Ohlsson, L.: Granulocyte collagenase and elastase and the plasma proteinase inhibitors in human plasma. Surgery 83:323, 1978.
233. Ohlsson, K., and Laurell, C.B.: The disappearance of enzyme inhibitor complexes from the circulation of man. Clin. Sci. Molec. Med. 51:87, 1976.
234. Reynolds, J.J., Murphy, G., Sellers, A., and Cartwright, E.: A new factor that may control collagen resorption. Lancet 2:333, 1977.
235. Brinckerhoff, C.E., McMillan, R.M., Dayer, J.-M., and Harris, E.D., Jr.: Inhibition by retinoic acid of collagenase production in rheumatoid synovial cells. N. Engl. J. Med. 303:432, 1980.
236. Hamilton, J.A.: Stimulation of the plasminogen activator activity of human synovial fibroblasts by retinoids. Arthritis Rheum. 25:432, 1982.
237. Hamerman, D.: Cartilage changes in the rheumatoid joint. Clin. Orthop. 64:91, 1969.
238. Sapolsky, A.I., Keiser, H.D., Howell, D.S., and Woessner, J.F., Jr.: Metalloproteases of human articular cartilage that digest cartilage proteoglycan at neutral and acid pH. J. Clin. Invest. 58:1030, 1976.
239. Sapolsky, A.I., Howell, D.S., and Woessner, J.F., Jr.: Neutral proteases and cathepsin D in human articular cartilage. J. Clin. Invest. 53:1044, 1974.
240. Kar, N.C., Cracchiolo, A., Mirra, J., and Pearson, C.M.: Acid, neutral and alkaline hydrolases in arthritic synovium. Am. J. Clin. Pathol. 65:220, 1976.
241. Dingle, J.T., Saklatvala, J., Hembry, R.M., Tyler, J., Fell, H.B., and Jabb, R.: A cartilage catabolic factor from synovium. Biochem. J. 184:177, 1979.
242. Jasin, H.E., and Dingle, J.T.: Human mononuclear cell factors mediate cartilage matrix degradation through chondrocyte activation. J. Clin. Invest. 68:571, 1981.
243. Hatcher, V.B., Borg, J.P., Levitt, M.A., and Smith, C.: Enhanced neutral protease activity in proliferating rheumatoid synovial cells. Arthritis Rheum. 24:919, 1981.
244. Klein, D.C., and Raisz, L.G.: Prostaglandins: Stimulation of bone resorption in tissue culture. Endocrinology 85:1436, 1970.
245. Robinson, D.R., Tashjian, A.H., Jr., and Levine, L.: Prostaglandin $E_2$-induced bone resorption by rheumatoid synovia. A model for bone

destruction in rheumatoid arthritis. J. Clin. Invest. 56:1181, 1975.
246. Raisz, L.G., Dietrich, J.W., Simmons, H.A., Seyberth, H.W., Hubbard, W., and Oates, J.A.: Effect of prostaglandin endoperoxides and metabolites on bone resorption in vitro. Nature 267:532, 1977.
247. Horton, J.F., Oppenheim, J.J., Mergenhagen, S.E., et al.: Macrophage lymphocyte synergy in the production of osteoclast-activating factor. J. Immunol. 113:1278, 1974.
248. Cruickshank, B.: The arteritis of rheumatoid arthritis. Ann. Rheum. Dis. 13:136, 1954.
249. Ghadially, F.N., and Roy, S.: Ultrastructure of synovial membrane in rheumatoid arthritis. Ann. Rheum. Dis. 26:426, 1967.
250. Barland, P., Novikoff, A.B., and Hamerman, D.: Fine structure and cytochemistry of the rheumatoid synovial membrane with special reference to lysosomes. Am. J. Pathol. 44:853, 1964.
251. Muirden, K.D.: Ferritin in synovial cells in patients with rheumatoid arthritis. Ann. Rheum. Dis. 25:387, 1966.
252. Grimley, P.M., and Sokoloff, L.: Synovial giant cells in rheumatoid arthritis. Am. J. Clin. Pathol. 49:931, 1966.
253. Postlethwaite, A.E., Jackson, B.K., Beachey, E.H., and Kang, A.H.: Formation of multinucleated giant cells from human monocyte precursors. J. Exp. Med. 155:168, 1982.
254. Gold, R.H., Metzger, A.L., Mirra, J.M., Weinberger, H.J., and Killebrew, K.: Multicentric reticulohistiocytosis (lipoid dermatoarthritis). Am. J. Roentgenol. 124:610, 1975.
255. Jayson, M.I.V., and Dixon, A. St. J.: Intra-articular pressure in rheumatoid arthritis of the knee. 1. Pressure changes during passive joint distention. Ann. Rheum. Dis. 29:261, 1970.
256. Dixon, A. St. J., and Grant, C.: Acute synovial rupture in rheumatoid arthritis. Clinical and experimental observation. Lancet 1:742, 1964.
257. Jayson, M.I.V., and Dixon, A. St. J.: Intra-articular pressure in rheumatoid arthritis of the knee. 2. Effect of intra-articular pressure on blood circulation to the synovium. Ann. Rheum. Dis. 29:266, 1970.
258. Harris, E.D., Jr., Parker, H.G., Radin, E.L., and Krane, S.M.: Effects of proteolytic enzymes on structural and mechanical properties of cartilage. Arthritis Rheum. 15:497, 1972.
259. Kempson, G.E., Muir, H., Swanson, S.A.V., et al.: Correlations between stiffness and the chemical constituents of cartilage of the human femoral head. Biochem. Biophys. Acta 215:70, 1970.
260. Mills, K.W.: Pathology of the knee joint in rheumatoid arthritis. J. Bone Joint Surg. 52B:746, 1970.
261. Kuettner, K.E., Harper, E.J., and Eisenstein, R.: Protease inhibitors in cartilage. Arthritis Rheum. 20:5124, 1977.
262. Mohr, W. and Wessinghage, D.: The relationship between polymorphonuclear granulocytes and cartilage destruction in rheumatoid arthritis. Z. Rheumatol. 37:81, 1978.
263. Harris, E.D., Jr., DiBona, D.R., and Krane, S.M.: A mechanism for cartilage destruction in rheumatoid arthritis. Trans. Assoc. Am. Phys. 83:267, 1970.
264. Harris, E.D., Jr., DiBona, D.R., and Krane, S.M.: Mechanisms of destruction of articular structures in rheumatoid arthritis. *In* Forscher, B. (ed.): Proceedings of the Third International Symposium on Inflammation. International Congress Series No. 229. Amsterdam, *Excerpta Medica,* 1971, pp. 243–253.
265. Kobayashi, I., and Ziff, M.: Electron microscope studies of the cartilage/pannus junction in rheumatoid arthritis. Arthritis Rheum. 18:475, 1975.
266. Freund, E.: The pathological significance of intra-articular pressure. Edinburgh Med. J. (NS) 47:192, 1970.
267. Maggar, E., Talerman, A., Fether, M., and Wouters, H.W.: The pathogenesis of the subchondral pseudocysts in rheumatoid arthritis. Clin. Orthop. 100:341, 1974.
268. Collins, D.H.: The subcutaneous nodule of rheumatoid arthritis. J. Pathol. Bacteriol. 45:97, 1937.
269. Bennett, G.A., Zeller, J.W., and Bauer, W.: Subcutaneous nodules of rheumatoid arthritis and rheumatic fever. A pathologic study. Arch. Pathol. 30:70, 1970.
270. Cochrane, W., Davies, D.V., Dorleng, J., and Bywaters, E.G.L.: Ultramicroscopic structures of the rheumatoid nodule. Ann. Rheum. Dis. 23:345, 1964.
271. Harris, E.D., Jr.: A collagenolytic system produced by primary cultures of rheumatoid nodule tissue. J. Clin. Invest. 51:2973, 1972.
271a. Kaye, B.R., Kaye, R.L., and Bobrove, A.: Rheumatoid nodules. Review of the spectrum of associated conditions and proposal of a new classification, with a report of four seronegative cases. Am. J. Med. 76:279, 1984.
272. Lance, E.M.: The effect of joint replacement on rheumatoid synovitis and its significance. Arthritis Rheum. 25 (Suppl.): 41, 1982.
273. Sokoloff, L., Wilikens, S.L., and Bunim, J.J.: Arteritis of striated muscle in rheumatoid arthritis. Am. J. Pathol. 27:157, 1951.
274. Conn, D.L., McDuffie, F.C., and Dyck, P.J.: Immunopathologic study of sural nerves in rheumatoid arthritis. Arthritis Rheum. 15:135, 1972.
275. Sokoloff, L., and Bunim, J.J.: Vascular lesions in rheumatoid arthritis. J. Chron. Dis. 5:668, 1957.
276. Glass, D., Soter, N.A., and Schur, P.H.: Rheumatoid vasculitis. Arthritis Rheum. 19:950, 1976.
277. Conn. D.L., Schroeter, A.L., and McDuffie, F.C. Cutaneous vessel immune deposits in rheumatoid arthritis. Arthritis Rheum. 19:15, 1976.
278. Conn, D.L., and McDuffie, F.C.: The pathogenesis of rheumatoid neuropathy. *In* Eberl, R., and Rosenthal, M. (eds.): Organic Manifestations and Complications in Rheumatoid Arthritis. New York, F.K. Schattaner Verlag, 1975, pp. 295–306.

# Chapter 60

# Rheumatoid Arthritis: The Clinical Spectrum

*Edward D. Harris, Jr.*

## INTRODUCTION

Review of medical history has shown us how difficult it has been to precisely define clinical entities, and this problem is particularly evident when attempts are made to determine when rheumatoid arthritis (RA) was first described. Some have concluded that RA developed only recently as a clear-cut entity, and was not seen in Europe until the end of the eighteenth century.[1,2] Short has evaluated the data provided by human paleopathology and by medical writings that appeared before 1800.[3] Hippocrates described a form of arthritis that developed in a man at about age 35, which first involved the hands and feet and next the elbows, knees, and hips.[4] Soranus, an Ephesian who lived in the second century A.D., wrote a treatise[5] describing a polyarthritis with morning stiffness in which the joints became twisted ". . . with the toes and fingers either turned sideways or bent over backwards, or resting immovable upon their neighbors." The problem with accepting this or other early descriptions as being the first case reports of RA is that each of them has clear references to what must have been tophaceous gout spread among references to what may have been RA or psoriatic arthritis.

In contrast, perhaps because of the sclerotic nature of the disease process, evidence for ankylosing spondylitis in antiquity is solid. Lumbar spines with bony ankylosis and fused sacroiliac joints have been demonstrated in specimens from men living before 1800 B.C.[6] Small bones of the hand have been examined less rigorously,[3] and the proliferative soft tissue characteristic of rheumatoid synovitis is poorly preserved. For these reasons, perhaps, there is no definite evidence for the existence of RA before relatively recent times.

In this chapter the epidemiology of RA will be discussed first, and then a detailed survey of its modes of presentation and criteria necessary for its diagnosis will be presented. Then, with diagnosis established, exploration of the natural history of the disease as it affects the joints and extra-articular tissues will be outlined.

## EPIDEMIOLOGY AND DIAGNOSIS

RA is a diagnosis made primarily on clinical grounds. Despite the usefulness of rheumatoid factor in both diagnosis and understanding of the pathophysiology of the disease, the presence of anti-IgG is not specific for RA. No other test specific for diagnosis is available. A set of criteria for diagnosis designed by Ropes and committee for the American Rheumatism Association[7] has proved useful for both epidemiologic and demographic studies as well as for diagnosis of individual patients in physicians' offices (Table 60–1). The weakness of the ARA criteria is in application to the "probable" class of diagnosis. When only three criteria are necessary, the firmness of the diagnosis varies considerably, depending on which three are picked. For instance, a patient with morning stiffness and a single painful swollen joint would meet criteria for "probable" RA. This problem is mirrored in marked discrepancies between series in the ratios of "probable" to "definite" RA, of female to male cases,[8] and in the large number of patients who meet criteria for diagnosis of probable RA who evolve either to a healthy state or into another process.[9]

Mitchell and Fries have published a systematic analysis of the ARA criteria[10] using a population of 840 patients over age 16 in whom a clinical diagnosis of RA was made. These patients are believed to represent al-

**Table 60–1.** American Rheumatism Association Criteria for the Diagnosis of RA

Eleven criteria available. For three different degrees of certainty of diagnosis, different numbers of criteria must be met. Unlike the Jones criteria for rheumatic fever, there are no major and minor criteria.

Classic RA—7 criteria needed
Definite RA—5 criteria needed
Probable RA—3 criteria needed

To meet criteria 1 to 5, symptoms or signs must be present for at least 6 weeks.

| Criteria | Comments |
|---|---|
| 1. Morning stiffness | This symptom is very useful as an indicator of inflammation; the absence of morning stiffness in a chronically painful joint is good evidence that synovial inflammation is minimal or absent |
| 2. Pain on motion or tenderness in at least one joint | Criteria 2 to 6 must be observed by a physician |
| 3. Swelling of one joint, representing soft tissue or fluid | Bony overgrowth is usually representative of a degenerative process, not synovial inflammation |
| 4. Swelling of at least one other joint (soft tissue or fluid) with an interval free of symptoms no longer than 3 months | |
| 5. Symmetrical joint swelling (simultaneous involvement of the same joint, right and left) | Terminal interphalangeal joints are rarely involved in RA and therefore are not acceptable for this or other criteria |
| 6. Subcutaneous nodules over bony prominences, extensor surfaces or near joints | See exclusions in second footnote below |
| 7. Typical roentgenographic changes which must include dimineralization in periarticular bone as an index of inflammation; degenerative changes do not exclude diagnosis of RA | Demineralization may result from disease of muscles around inflamed joints as well as from release of prostaglandins (see Chapter 59) by inflamed synovial tissue |
| 8. Positive test for rheumatoid factor in serum | Laboratory quality control is essential here; in general, positive tests should be in a titer of 1:64 or greater |
| 9. Synovial fluid; a poor mucin clot formation on adding synovial fluid to dilute acetic acid | This is strictly a qualitative test and can be used only as a crude estimate of sustained joint inflammation |
| 10. Synovial histopathology consistent with RA (see Chapter 59)<br>a. Marked villous hypertrophy<br>b. Proliferation of synovial cells<br>c. Lymphocyte/plasma cell infiltration in subsynovium<br>d. Fibrin deposition within or upon microvilli | |
| 11. Characteristic histopathology of rheumatoid nodules biopsied from any site | These are nonspecific; granuloma annulare is indistinguishable on routine histological preparations from the rheumatoid nodule |

A diagnosis of *possible* RA requires that morning stiffness, history of pain or swelling of joints, subcutaneous nodules, or an elevated ESR or C-reactive protein—any two of these criteria—be present for a least 3 weeks.

Exclusions are based principally on presence of evidence for other diseases that have criteria for their own diagnosis (e.g., systemic lupus erythematosus, scleroderma) or more specific diagnostic techniques (e.g., the crystal deposition diseases). Some may be inappropriate. For instance, it is known that gout and RA can be present in the same patient. Exclusions are covered under Differential Diagnosis of Rheumatoid Arthritis later in this chapter.

most all of the patients with RA in the northern half of Saskatchewan. Their analyses revealed the following interesting points.:

1. The fist 5 "clinical" criteria (see Table 60–1) were each present in two thirds of the patients at their initial visit to the rheumatologist.
2. Of these 5 criteria, joint pain/tenderness was the most frequent and morning stiffness was the least common.
3. Nodules were present at the initial visit in 19 percent, and rheumatoid factor in 47 percent.
4. Elimination of the last 3 criteria—"poor mucin" in synovial fluid and typical histopathology of synovium or nodules—would have resulted in reclassification of only 3 patients. These criteria are rarely (1 to 2 percent) met at time of diagnosis.
5. Patients who met ARA criteria at the first visit of "definite" or "classic" RA, when contrasted with those in the "probable" group, (a) were older (5 to 8 years); (b) had their disease longer; and (c) had more fatigue, weaker grip strength, more frequent elbow and ankle involvement, and a higher number of active joints.

Another set of criteria was proposed at the third International Symposium of Population Studies of the Rheumatic Diseases in New York City in 1966.[11] These are listed in Table 60–2. Meeting these criteria is more rigorous and clearly would exclude mono- or diarticular disease, seronegative arthritis, and mild, nondeforming disease.

An interesting comparison of the ARA and New York criteria was carried out by O'Sullivan and Cathcart in Sudbury, Massachusetts.[12] In 1964, of 4522 persons examined, 17 appeared to be affected by RA according to the New York criteria, and 118 had either probable or definite RA by the ARA criteria. Follow-up data are shown in Table 60–3. These data indicate that the New York criteria identify persons whose disease remains clinically meaningful and establish the prevalance of RA as 0.5 percent of women and 0.1 percent of men. The data do not define the nature of the disease manifested in the 88 patients who initially met criteria for RA and who failed to meet criteria on later examination. We can infer, however, that early RA (probable or definite by ARA criteria) is a relatively benign process with a high probability for remission within several years. Therefore,

**Table 60–2.** New York Criteria for the Diagnosis of RA

RA is present if criteria 1 and 2 plus either 3 or 4 are met:

1. History of an episode of three painful limb joints. Each group of joints (e.g., proximal interphalangeal joint) is counted as one joint, scoring each side separately
2. Swelling, limitation of motion, subluxation and/or ankylosis of three limb joints. *Necessary inclusions*: (1) at least one hand, wrist or foot; (2) symmetry of one joint pair. *Exclusions*: (1) distal interphalangeal joints; (2) fifth proximal interphalangeal joints; (3) first metatarsophalangeal joints; (4) hips
3. Radiographic changes (erosions)
4. Serum positive for rheumatoid factors

**Table 60–3.** Follow-up of RA (3 to 5 Years), Diagnosed by ARA and NY Criteria*

1. Diagnosed originally by ARA criteria:

| *Initial ARA Class* | | *Final ARA Class* *Probable* | *Final ARA Class* *Definite* | |
|---|---|---|---|---|
| Definite RA | 40 | 7 | 12 | |
| Probable RA | 78 | 7 | 4 | |
| Total | 118 | 14 | 16 | 30 |

2. Diagnosed originally by NY Criteria:

| *Initial (by ARA Criteria)* | *Final* *NY Criteria* *RA Present* | *Final* *NY Criteria* *RA Absent* | *Final* *ARA Criteria* |
|---|---|---|---|
| 17 { 2 probable<br>15 definite | 11 | 6 | 2 negative<br>10 definite<br>2 probable<br>3 negative |

*Collated from O'Sullivan, J.B., and Cathcart, E.S.: Ann. Intern. Med. 76:573, 1972.

one of the most significant determinants of prognosis in RA may be which criteria (ARA versus New York) are used to establish the diagnosis!

Wolfe[13] summarized the results of 14 studies of population samples, including the National Health Examination survey,[14] the survey of Tecumeseh, Michigan,[15] studies of various Native American Groups,[16] and representative atomic bomb survivors from Hiroshima and Nagasaki.[17] Using criteria for "definite" RA, the prevalence rate varied from 0.3 to 1.5 percent. In 1984 it is reasonable to estimate that there are 4 to 6 million cases of RA in the United States. A conservative estimate would be that 100,000 to 200,000 new cases of definite or classic RA developed in the USA in 1984.

Variations from these prevalence data are very rare, indicating that specific genetic and environmental influences on the development of RA, if significant, are widespread in the world. A few populations with an apparent predisposition to RA exist. One study, using both the ARA and New York criteria, found a frequency of definite RA of 3.4 percent in Yakima Indian women, ages 18 to 79, compared with a prevalence of 1.4 percent in the general population.[18] In a geographically and socially isolated band of 227 Chippewa Indians, the minimum prevalence of RA was found to be 5.3 percent. Clinically, the RA in this group was typical: additive, symmetrical, and persistent. The prevalence of HLA-DR4 was 68 percent, significantly higher than in most general populations, and all of the 12 with RA expressed HLA-DR4.[19]

Subgroups within the total population with RA have been identified. There is a striking increase in prevalence of RA in urban South African blacks[20] (3.3 percent) compared with rural blacks (0.87 percent).[21] Definite RA is two to three times more common in females than in males, although if groups of early "probable" RA are considered, the male to female ratio may approach 1.0.

In Rochester, Minnesota, there has been a decline in the incidence of RA in the female population since 1960.[22] However, a case-control study of this population showed no association between rheumatoid arthritis and the use of oral contraceptives, or the use of estrogens for menopause-related or postmenopausal symptoms. These data contradict those[23] from England, which reported that patients with rheumatoid arthritis were found to have used oral contraceptives only half as much as control subjects.

The disease has an increasing prevalence with advancing age up to the seventh decade. It is well described in children (see Chapter 80), and new cases appear in even the very aged.[14,15] The National Health Survey[14] data indicated a higher prevalence of RA in patients of either sex with less than 5 years of education and in those with lower yearly incomes.

Future epidemiologic studies will be based on new genetic information, which has identified specific polymorphic cell surface glycoprotein antigens associated with RA (see Chapters 4 and 59). RA has been shown to be associated with HLA-Dw4[24] and with the B-cell alloantigen HLA-DR4 related to HLA-Dw4.[25] The C locus antigen Cw3 is also present with an increased frequency.[26] Although only a small percentage of persons with HLA-Dw4 develop RA, probably because the disease is multifactorial, these data give insight into possible immune response genes in humans. In the future, immunogenetics must be a constant associate of clinical observations in epidemiologic studies of RA.

Since 1948, when the studies of Rose and colleagues[27] re-emphasized the studies of Waaler[28] linking a factor in serum of patients with RA to agglutination of normal and sensitized sheep red blood cells, the presence or absence of rheumatoid factor in serum has occupied attention of epidemiologists in this field. Rheumatoid factor is found more frequently in population studies (3 to 5 percent) than is RA, and in these individuals the prevalence of seropositivity is approximately equal in male and females.[15,29,30] A recent study set out to determine whether HLA-Dw4 (sometimes referred to as Dw4x7x10), the histocompatibility antigen associated with RA, was associated with the presence of rheumatoid factor.[31] The frequency of HLA-Dw4 was determined in 24 healthy women with a significant titer for rheumatoid factor (median titer 1:160). Only three carried the Dw4 antigen, suggesting that the genes linked to HLA-Dw4 mediate susceptibility to RA via mechanisms other than control of rheumatoid factor synthesis. Frequently patients present with definite RA and are seronegative.[32] However, these individuals probably have a distinct immunogenetic disease.[33] In one series, although HLA-DR3 was significantly less prevalent and HLA-DR4 more common in patients positive for rheumatoid factor, a clinically matched group (except for the absence of vasculitis or nodules in the seronegative patients) who were seronegative had no difference from controls in distribution of DR antigens. In this series the seronegative DR4+ patients had more erosive/destructive disease than seronegative DR4$^-$ patients.[33]

An increased prevalence of RA in first-degree relatives of patients with RA would indicate that some genetic or environmental factor influences appearance of the disease. Twin studies are a principal tool for dissecting out genetic influences in many diseases. The data in twin studies have varied, ranging from evidence for discordance[34] to, in one study, almost 50 percent concordance.[35] In another study,[36,37] the risk of erosive arthritis in monozygous co-twins was about 30 times the reference population, while in dizygous co-twins and in nontwin siblings the risk was about 6 times that of control groups. It also was determined that functionally incapacitating (Grade 3 or 4) RA was found in four times the expected rate in first-degree relatives of probands with seropositive disease; erosive radiographic changes were found at three times the expected rate. Study of serology in first-degree relatives of patients with RA has revealed no higher frequency of rheumatoid factor than in relatives of matched controls.[38]

A number of observations suggest that certain factors are or are not associated with RA. Some of these are listed below. None has been substantiated by independent studies: (1) RA was less common in schizophrenics than in a control population.[39] (2) In studies of identical twins discordant for RA, a history of psychologic stress was more common in the affected twin.[34] (3) Heavy outdoor occupations or work in health fields was associated with RA.[40] (4) Rheumatoid patients had an increased frequency of exposure to pets (e.g., dogs, cats, birds, or other sick animals) in the 5 years before developing their disease than did a control group.[41] All such epidemiologic studies are subject to scrutiny; they are difficult to compile without introducing bias.

## EARLY RHEUMATOID ARTHRITIS

It has been said that duration of continuous symptoms and signs correlates better with more severe RA than does any other index of disease activity.[42] Although this is almost simplistic, there are many corollaries of it that can be useful for both diagnosis and therapy. Continuous synovitis implies activation of multiple pathogenetic mechanisms within the synovium and joint space (see Chapter 59), and virtually ensures sufficient proliferation and polarization to result in progressive joint destruction. Conversely, disease that has clinical remission is associated with regression of the proliferative inflammation.

Early diagnosis of RA is rarely important to the patient. RA presents with acute severe symptoms so infrequently that the best course is often to effectively rule out other diagnoses and resist making an early diagnosis in a new patient with synovitis. If criteria are met in the proper time, a diagnosis of RA can be given. As mentioned above, many patients (perhaps 80 percent) given a diagnosis of RA early in the course of their disease will go into a sustained remission. The implication of this is either that the course of early RA is benign or that most diagnoses of RA that are made early and with few criteria having been met are wrong. The patients who demand a diagnosis should be reassured that, unlike the situation with malignancies, there are no data to suggest that very early, forced diagnoses and prompt treatment are associated with a better prognosis. Fortunately, a forced wait for diagnosis (6 weeks) is built into ARA criteria for diagnosis.

In the Northern Hempisphere, the onset of RA is more frequent in winter than in summer. In several series, the onset of RA from October to March is twice as frequent as in the other 6 months,[43,44] and exacerbations of the disease are more common in winter.[45]

Although it is often impossible to identify a day in a patient's life when arthritis began, it is of interest to search for prodromal symptoms. Some patients speak of transient joint symptoms or a history of recurrent bursitis. Ganglion cysts at the wrists have been noted to precede development of RA, but their frequency in a control population is not known.

Much more diffuse, subjective, and difficult to study are precipitating factors of arthritis. There is no evidence that any have a direct cause-and-effect relationship. Trauma is one of the most common preludes to arthritis; this can include surgery. Other episodes, including infections, vaccine inoculations, and emotional trauma, have been implicated by many patients as the cause of their problems, but there is no proof of their association.

## Patterns of Onset (Table 60–4)

**Insidious Onset.** RA usually has an insidious slow onset over weeks to months. Fifty-five to 70 percent of cases begin this way.[43,46] The initial symptoms may be systemic or articular. In some patients, fatigue, malaise, or diffuse musculoskeletal pain may be the first nonspecific complaint, with joints involved later. Although symmetrical involvement is common, asymmetric presentation (often becoming more symmetrical later in the course of disease) is not rare. The reasons for symmetry of joint involvement remain a complete mystery, but the fact of symmetry in RA stands as a useful criterion for diagnosis. Morning stiffness may be the first symptom, noted even before pain. This phenomenon is probably related to accumulation of edema fluid within inflamed tissues during sleep. Morning stiffness disappears as edema and products of inflammation are absorbed by lymphatics and venules and returned to the circulation by motion accompanying use of muscles. Pain and stiffness may develop in other joints, but it is rare for symptoms to remit completely in one set of joints while developing in another. This lack of a migratory quality of arthritis sets RA somewhat apart from rheumatic fever, in which migratory arthritis is common.

**Table 60–4.** Characteristics of Onset of RA in 300 Patients with Definite or Classic Disease*

| | | Percent |
|---|---|---|
| 1. Mode of onset: | rapid† (days or weeks) | 46 |
| | insidious—54 percent | 54 |
| 2. Site of onset: | small joints | 32 |
| | medium-sized joints | 16 |
| | large joints | 29 |
| | combined | 26 |
| 3. Pattern of onset: | monoarticular | 21 |
| | oligoarticular | 44 |
| | polyarticular | 35 |

*From Fallahi, S., Halla, J.T., and Hardin, J.G.: Clin. Res. 31:650A, 1983.

†This time frame includes patients described in other studies as having "intermediate" onset.

A subtle, early change in RA is development of muscle atrophy around affected joints. This decreases efficiency and strength, and the patient develops weakness out of proportion to pain. Opening doors, climbing stairs, and doing repetitive work become more demanding. A low-grade fever without chills is often overlooked unless the patient is a very good observer of his or her body functions. Depression, anxiety, and fear of the future affect the patient and accentuate symptoms. Weight loss is common, and anorexia contributes to this.

**Acute Onset.** Eight to 15 percent of patients have an acute onset of symptoms. The term "acute" refers to the rate of build-up of symptoms. Very rarely, a patient can pinpoint onset of disease to an instant, such as opening a door or driving a golf ball. Symptoms mount, with pain developing in other joints, often in a less symmetrical pattern than in patients who have an insidious type of onset. Pain may be generated also by surrounding muscles, and muscle pain can be so severe as to mimic ischemic pain. The differential diagnosis here is extremely broad, ranging from septic arthritis to myositis or viral infections.

**Intermediate Onset.** Fifteen to 20 percent of patients have an intermediate type of onset. Symptoms develop over days or weeks. Systemic complaints are more noticeable than in the insidious type of onset.

## Patterns of Joint Involvement in Early Rheumatoid Arthritis

By far the most commonly involved joints in RA are the metacarpophalangeal joints, proximal interphalangeal joints, and wrists.[47] The combined data from two series are listed in Table 60–5. Larger joints generally become symptomatic after small joints. This raises the question of whether early disease in large joints remains asymptomatic for a longer time. The answer was sought in one study by performing xenon clearances on clinically normal knees of patients with early RA.[48] Seven of 22 had abnormal (high) perfusion, supporting this hypothesis. Although rheumatoid factor eventually becomes positive in 80 to 90 percent of cases with definite RA, it is apparent that the development of seropositivity lags behind clinical manifestations (Table 60–6). There seems to be little indication for repeating the laboratory test for rheumatoid factor if a patient has had one positive test at significant titer.

**Table 60–5.** Joints Involved in RA*

| | Percent Initially Involved[47] | | | Percent Ultimately Involved[43] |
|---|---|---|---|---|
| | *Right* | *Left* | *Bilateral* | |
| Metacarpo-phalangeal | 65 | 58 | 52 | 87 |
| Wrist | 60 | 57 | 48 | 82 |
| Proximal Interphalangeal | 63 | 53 | 45 | 63 |
| Metatarso-phalangeal | 48 | 47 | 43 | 48 |
| Shoulder | 37 | 42 | 30 | 47 |
| Knee | 35 | 30 | 24 | 56 |
| Ankle | 25 | 23 | 18 | 53 |
| Elbow | 20 | 15 | 14 | 21 |

*Other joints (e.g., distal interphalangeal joints) are not tabulated here.

## Unusual Patterns of Onset of Disease

**Adult Onset Still's Disease.** This disease appears in adults, usually in the third or fourth decade, as a syndrome like that seen in children with the acute, febrile onset of juvenile arthritis. That it can occur in adults supports those who would say that Still's disease is distinct from RA, rather than a different presentation of the same process. It was first described by Bywaters, who presented 14 of his patients.[49] Females are more commonly affected by adult-onset Still's disease. Most patients present with fever. Serology (rheumatoid factor and antinuclear antibody) is negative, and patients have not developed subcutaneous nodules.[50] Fever patterns in these patients are usually quotidian (i.e., reaching normal levels at least once each day). Patients have a skin rash—salmon-colored or pink macules that are evanescent and become more prominent when patients are febrile. The arthritis in this process usually involves fewer joints than RA in most adults. Erosive disease is rare. The cervical spine is involved, and loss of neck motion may be striking. Pericarditis and pleural effusions and severe abdominal pain (mesenteric adenitis)[51] may be present and confound diagnostic attempts. Unlike systemic lupus erythematosus, serum complement is normal or high.[52] In a recent series, 11 patients (all of whom were white women), followed for a mean of 20.2 years after disease onset, had the following characteristics:[53]

(1) Ten had a polycyclic pattern (characterized by remissions and exacerbations).

(2) Patterns of exacerbations were similar to but less severe than the original presentations.

(3) Loss of wrist extension was the most common clinical abnormality, and carpal ankylosis was present in 10.

(4) Five out of 11 patients developed DIPJ involvement.

(5) Biopsy of the characteristic skin rash of Still's and juvenile rheumatoid arthritis showed perivascular infiltrate of neutrophils in the superficial dermis.

**Table 60–6.** Interval from Onset of Disease to Development of a Positive Rheumatoid Factor Test in 100 Patients with RA*

| | Positive Result (Time in Months) | | | | | |
|---|---|---|---|---|---|---|
| | *Within 3* | *4–6* | *7–12* | *After 12* | *Total* | *Negative* |
| Number of patients | 33 | 22 | 21 | 12 | 88 | 12 |

*From Jacoby, R.K., et al.: Br. Med. J. 2:96, 1973.

**Palindromic Pattern of Onset.** Palindromic rheumatism was described by Hench and Rosenberg in 1941.[54] Like many other clinical complexes in rheumatology, it should be considered a syndrome that can be either the initial manifestation of many different organic processes or never evolve into anything more. The syndrome is more like gout than anything else. Pain usually begins in one joint; symptoms worsen for several hours and are associated with swelling and erythema. An intercritical period, as in gout, is asymptomatic. It is likely that 30 to 50 percent of patients with palindromic rheumatism develop RA. In these, multiple joints become involved, swelling does not subside completely between attacks, and tests become positive for rheumatoid factor. Neither the characteristics of joint fluid nor the pathology of synovial biopsies allows the prediction that palindromic rheumatism will develop into RA.[55]

**Age- and Sex-Related Modes of Onset.** Certain types of presentation of arthritis appear more often in certain age groups. In late adolescent females a chronic, rarely erosive synovitis of the knees often presents without involvement of other joints, and without systemic signs. The erythrocyte sedimentation rate is usually normal, and rheumatoid factor is absent. Stiffness and pain are directly proportional to joint swelling, and this, in turn, is a function of use. Rest or assiduous use of crutches results in fairly prompt resolution of joint swelling, but with even mild activity, swelling recurs. Synovial biopsy has revealed moderate synovial cell hyperplasia and variable infiltration with mononuclear cells. Synovial fluid leukocyte counts are usually less than 10,000 per cubic millimeter. The course is one of gradual improvement with occasional flares of activity, without relationship to menstrual cycles. The process is self-limited and rarely lasts longer than 5 to 6 years. It is not known whether this represents an oligoarticular form of juvenile rheumatoid arthritis in older girls, a variant of adult RA, or another entity.

RA developing in older men (60 years of age and older) is often dominated by stiffness and diffuse boggy swelling of the hands, wrists, and forearms. Onset is slow, but the stiffness is often incapacitating. In other respects, the disease is similar to other forms of adult RA, but the therapy is not the same. Nonsteroidal anti-inflammatory drugs are rarely effective, but low-dose corticosteroids ($< 7.5$ mg prednisone per day) may be helpful in reducing edema and increasing motion and function.

**RA and Paralysis: Asymmetric Disease.** Being relatively common, RA is likely to occur with many other types of chronic disease. A striking asymmetry or even unilateral involvement has been described in patients with poliomyelitis, meningioma, encephalitis, neurovascular syphilis, strokes, and cerebral palsy.[56,57] Joints are spared on the paralyzed side, and the degree of protection demonstrates a rough correlation with the extent of paralysis.[58] Protective effect is less if a neurologic deficit develops in a patient already suffering from RA.[59]

**"Arthritis Robustus."** This is not so much an unusual presentation of disease as it is an unusual reaction of patients to the disease.[60,61] Men usually form this group. Their disease is characterized by proliferative synovitis, which appears to cause little pain. Patients are athletic and invariably keep working (often at physical labor). Osteopenia is less, and new bone proliferation at joint margins is common. Bulky subcutaneous nodules develop. Subchondral cysts develop, presumably from the excessive pressure developed from synovial fluid within a thick joint capsule during muscular effort (see Chapter 59).

## The Course of Rheumatoid Arthritis

Before studying the evolution of the disease from synovitis to destruction of normal tissues and the development of complications of this disease, it is important to emphasize that there are many forms of the disease. As noted in the studies by O'Sullivan and Cathcart,[12] a large number—perhaps 80 percent—of patients who early in the course of their disease meet the criteria for possible or probable RA go on to develop another disease, or, more likely, become completely better. Here we will outline the different courses of RA. Prognosis and methods available to assess progression and/or treatment will be discussed at the end of this chapter.

**Intermittent Course of RA.** This course is marked by partial to complete remissions without need for continuous therapy. This type of disease is usually mild. Initially, only a few joints are involved. Insidious return of disease is often marked by more joint involvement than at first. Twenty to 30 percent of patients with RA enjoy these periods of remission.[62,63] Within this group it is reported that approximately half had remissions lasting more than a year, and in the entire group remissions lasted longer than exacerbations.

**Long Clinical Remissions of RA.** In one group of 250 patients receiving only simple medical and orthopedic treatment[45] almost 10 percent were in clinical remission for 12 to 31 years (mean, 22 years). Although most of these patients had RA for less than 6 months at time of inclusion, 40 percent had remained in remission. The fact that many of these patients had an acute onset of symptoms with marked fever and severe joint pain and inflammation raises the question of whether they truly had RA. Nevertheless, some sign of disease activity (e.g., an elevated erythrocyte sedimentation rate) persisted in many throughout the "clinical remission," and occasional patients had brief but true flares of disease in one or a few joints.

**Progressive Disease.** This group may pursue a rapid or slow course, but the end point is the same: disabling, destructive disease. In modern times, this group should be divided into two subgroups: those who respond to aggressive therapy and those who do not. Fortunately, the latter group is small and probably represents less than 3 percent of patients with definite or classic rheumatoid arthritis.

## Diagnosis of Rheumatoid Arthritis

Diagnosis of RA must be by established criteria that are based upon effective clinical history and examination, laboratory tests, and diagnoses that exclude it. The criteria are discussed above. Before discussion of the exclusions (i.e., the findings that point to the presence of another disease process), we will address diagnosis positively, listing factors typical of the disease.

The characteristic patient with RA complains of pain and stiffness in multiple joints. The joint swelling is boggy and includes both soft tissue and synovial fluid. These joints are slightly to moderately tender to touch, especially the small joints of the hands and feet. Often palmar erythema and prominent veins on the dorsum of the hand are found. Distal interphalangeal joints are involved rarely. Temperature over the involved joints (except the hip) is elevated, but the joints are not usually red. Range of motion is limited, and muscle strength and function around inflamed joints are diminished. Soft, poorly delineated subcutaneous nodules are often found on the extensor surface of the forearm. General physical examination is normal except for a possible low-grade fever (~38° C), pallor, and asthenia. Movement is guarded, and apprehension often dominates facial expressions. Initial laboratory tests often show[64] (1) a slight leukocytosis with normal differential white blood cell count (WBC); (2) thrombocytosis; (3) a slight anemia (~10 grams hemoglobin per deciliter), normochromic and either normocytic or microcytic; (4) normal urinalysis; (5) erythrocyte sedimentation rate (Westergren) of ~30 mm per hour and up, sometimes to over 100 mm per hour; (6) normal renal, hepatic, and metabolic function; (7) a normal serum uric acid (before initiation of salicylate therapy); (8) positive rheumatoid factor test and negative ANA; (9) elevated $\alpha_2$-globulins and $\alpha_1$-globulins; and (10) normal or elevated serum complement.

A "typical" arthrocentesis reveals the following: joint fluid is straw-colored and slightly cloudy and contains many flecks of fibrin. Within the fluid a clot forms on standing at room temperature. There are 5000 to 25,000 WBC per cubic millimeter, and 85 percent of these are PMN leukocytes. Occasional large PMN leukocytes with granules staining positively for IgG, IgM, and C3 are found. No crystals are present. The mucin clot is fair. C4 and C2 are slightly depressed, but C3 is normal. IgG in synovial fluid may approach serum concentrations. In contrast, synovial fluid glucose is depressed, occasionally to less than 25 mg percent. Cultures are negative. A full discussion of synovial fluid analysis is found in Chapter 38.

## Differential Diagnosis of Rheumatoid Arthritis

It is important to exclude many other diseases before making a diagnosis of RA.[65] In the discussion of the many entities that follows, the relative frequency of the entities is recorded as common, uncommon, or rare; they are listed in alphabetical order.

**Ankylosing Spondylitis, Seronegative Spondyloarthropathy, and Reactive Arthritis (Common).** Short, Bauer, and Reynolds,[66] in their complete and well-referenced monograph on RA, felt that clinical evidence was strong enough to include ankylosing spondylitis as a variant of RA ("the spinal equivalent of rheumatoid arthritis"). Nevertheless, these authors established as an objective for future study the determination of whether or not rheumatoid spondylitis constituted a distinct disease entity. The question may have been clouded somewhat by the observation that in many children with RA, roentgenographic evidence of spondylitis was found.[67] This phenomenon is now recognized, of course, as spondylitis occurring in juveniles and related (as in the adult disease) to HLA-B27.

The problem in differentiating spondylitis arises with the patient (particularly a female) who presents with minimal back pain and peripheral joint involvement. Suspicion that this is not RA is generated when small joints are not involved, when joint disease is asymmetrical, and when the cervical spine is involved with limitation of motion.

In some cases, the conclusion is inescapable that RA and ankylosing spondylitis are present in the same patient. In one series[68] nine seropositive patients presented with spinal ankylosis and symmetrical erosive polyarthritis; eight of the nine carried HLA-B27. If one assumes that these two diseases occur completely independently of each other, simultaneous occurrence in the same patient should occur once in every 50,000 to 200,000 of the adult population.

In distinguishing patients with Reiter's syndrome from those with RA, a careful history and physical examination to look for heel pain or tenderness and ocular or urethral symptoms are of greatest importance. Polyarthritis persists chronically in over 80 percent of patients with Reiter's syndrome (see Chapter 65), and indeed Reiter's syndrome may have a worse prognosis than RA. The characteristics of enthesopathy in patients with Reiter's syndrome (e.g., sausage digits indicating juxta-articular disease), insertional tendinitis, periostitis, and peri-insertional osteoporosis or erosions may point to the diagnosis.

The differential diagnosis between "RA and psoriasis" and "psoriatic arthritis" may by artificial (see Chapter 66). Some patients with distal interphalangeal joint involvement and severe skin involvement obviously have a disease that is not RA. Others, however, have a seropositive symmetrical polyarthritis that appears to be RA; yet they also have psoriasis. A search in these patients for evidence of enthesopathy, distal interphalangeal joint disease, and/or spondylitis or sacroiliitis may reveal enough abnormalities to define a symptom complex different from RA.

Inflammatory bowel disease (IBD) (ulcerative colitis and Crohn's disease) is associated with arthritis in 20 percent of cases.[69] Peripheral arthritis is more common in many series[70] than spondylitis. Ankles, knees, and elbows are the most often involved of peripheral joints, with proximal interphalangeal joints and wrists next in frequency. Simultaneous attacks of arthritis and development of erythema nodosum are not uncommon. Attacks of joint pain begin more rapidly than do most attacks of RA, and usually only two to three joints are affected at once. Involvement is usually asymmetrical, and erosions are uncommon. The occurrence of peripheral arthritis in IBD is not related to HLA-B27.

Behçet's syndrome is marked by an asymmetric polyarthritis in 50 to 60 percent of cases.[71] Joint deformity is unusual. The painful oral and genital ulcers and CNS involvement are unusual in RA. Uveal tract involvement (Behçet's syndrome) must be differentiated from scleritis (RA) in patients with ocular and joint disease. Spondylitis, as in the other disorders classified here, is found in Behçet's syndrome, principally when HLA-B27 is present.

Enteric infections are complicated occasionally by inflammatory joint disease resembling RA. The joint disease associated with *Yersinia enterocolitica* infections occurs several weeks after the gastrointestinal illness.[72] Knees and ankles are the joints most commonly involved, and most patients (even those with peripheral arthritis and no spondylitis) have HLA-B27.[73]

Arthropathy may precede other findings of Wipple's disease (see Chapter 67). The pattern is that of a migratory poly- or oligoarthritis involving ankles, knees, shoulders, elbows, and fingers, as with IBD. Remission may occur when diarrhea begins. As with the arthritis of IBD, joint destruction is rare,[74] presumably because the synovitis lacks sustained chronicity.

**Arthritis Associated with Oral Contraceptives (Uncommon).** A syndrome of persistent arthralgias, myalgias, and morning stiffness with occasional development of polyarticular synovitis has been described in women in their third decade of life taking oral contraceptives (estrogens and progestins).[75] Positive tests for antinuclear antibodies are common, and several patients have had circulating rheumatoid factor. Symptoms resolve after the contraceptive is discontinued.

**Arthritis of Thyroid Disease (Uncommon) (see Chapter 102).** In hypothyroidism, synovial effusions and synovial thickening simulating RA have been described.[76] The sedimentation rate may be elevated because of hypergammaglobulinemia. Joint fluid is noninflammatory and may have an increased viscosity. Knees, wrists, hands, and feet are involved most often, and not infrequently coexisting calcium pyrophosphate deposition disease is found.

The syndrome of thyroid acropachy complicates less than 1 percent of hyperthyroid patients.[77] This represents periosteal new bone formation, which may be associated with a low-grade synovitis similar to hypertrophic osteoarthropathy. Although impossible to quantitate, it is said that patients with coexisting RA and hyperthyroidism have pain from their arthritis that appears to exceed that expected from the degree of inflammation.

**Bacterial Endocarditis (Uncommon).** Arthralgias, arthritis, and myalgias occur in approximately 30 percent of patients with subacute bacterial endocarditis.[78] The joint symptoms are usually in one or several joints, usually proximal large ones. It is possible that this synovitis could be caused by circulating immune complexes, which have been demonstrated, along with hypocomplementemia, in subacute bacterial endocarditis.[79] Fever out of proportion to joint findings in the setting of leukocytosis should lead to consideration of infective endocarditis as a diagnostic possibility, even in the absence of a significant heart murmur. It is wise to obtain blood cultures in all patients with a presentation of polyarthritis and significant fever. Embolic phenomena with constitutional symptoms, including arthralgias, can be presenting symptoms of *atrial myxoma,* but this process usually mimics systemic vasculitis or SBE more than it does RA.[80]

**Calcium Pyrophosphate Deposition Disease (CPPD) (Common) (see Chapter 87).** This crystal-induced synovitis presents in many different forms, ranging from a picture of indolent osteoarthrosis to that of an acute, hot joint. About 5 percent of patients have a chronic polyarthritis (sometimes referred to as pseudorheumatoid arthritis) which is associated with proliferative erosions at subchondral bone.[81] Although radiographs are of great help when chondrocalcinosis is present, CPPD may be present in the absence of calcification on radiographs.[82] Diagnosis then can be made only by arthrocentesis. One of the radiographic signs of CPPD that help differentiate it from RA is the presence of unicompartmental disease in the wrist.

**Diffuse Connective Tissue Disease: Systemic Lupus Erythematosus, Scleroderma, Dermatomyositis-Polymyositis, Vasculitis, Mixed Connective Tissue Disease (MCTD) (Common).** These entities, all discussed in depth elsewhere in the text, may begin with a syndrome of mild systemic symptoms and minimal polyarthritis involving the proximal interphalangeal and metacarpophalangeal joints. It is crucial to remember that at this point it may be appropriate not to make a definitive diagnosis. Also, it is not uncommon for one of these entities, diagnosed at one point in time, to evolve into another as years go by. Finally, it is not even agreed that MCTD is a distinct entity (see Chapters 71 and 76); argument exists that it is a common form of presentation of several rather specific entities. The following list contains rules of thumb for characterizing joint disease of the various entities:

1. In systemic lupus erythematosus, an organized synovitis that causes erosions is rare. Soft tissue and muscle inflammation may lead to dislocation of normal tendon alignment, resulting in ulnar deviation similar to Jaccoud's arthropathy.

2. Limitation of joint motion in scleroderma is almost always secondary to taut skin bound down to underlying fascia. The same considerations hold for dermatomyositis-polymyositis; proliferative synovitis is rarely sustained in these processes.

3. In reports of MCTD (patients having arthralgias, arthritis, hand swelling, sclerodactyly, Raynaud's phenomenon, esophageal hypomotility, and myositis with circulating antibody to a ribonucleoprotein) 60 to 70 percent have arthritis. Many are given an initial diagnosis of RA. Numerous series have shown deforming, erosive arthritis. In one series, for example, 8 of 17 patients presented in a fashion like RA.[83] Articular osteopenia alone was found in 8. Six had loss of joint space, and 5 had erosions typical of RA. Despite the serologic specificity for MCTD (see Chapter 71), there is still debate as to whether all patients with apparent RA diagnosed by clinical patterns should be classified as having MCTD if serum antibody to nuclear ribonucleoprotein is found in his or her serum.

**Familial Mediterranean Fever (Uncommon).** The articular syndrome in this disease is an episodic monarthritis or oligoarthritis of the large joints that appears in childhood or adolescence, mimicking oligoarthritic forms of JRA.[84] Episodes of arthritis come on acutely with fever and all cardinal signs of inflammation and can precede other manifestations of the disease. Usually self-limited (days to weeks), attacks occasionally will last for months, associated with radiographic changes of periarticular osteopenia without erosions.

**Gout (Common) (see Chapter 86).** Before a diagnosis of chronic erosive RA is made, chronic tophaceous gout must be ruled out. The reverse applies as well. Features of gouty arthritis that mimic RA include polyarthritis, symmetrical involvement, fusiform swelling of joints, subcutaneous nodules, and subacute presentation of attacks. Conversely, certain presentations of RA that suggest gouty arthritis include hyperuricemia (after treatment with low doses of aspirin), periarticular nodules, and seronegative disease (particularly in the male).[85] Radiographic findings may be similar, with appearance of the subcortical erosions of RA being similar to small osseous tophi in gout.[86] Although large asymmetrical erosions with ballooning of the cortex are more likely to be gout than RA, this is not always the case.[87] Serologic tests may be misleading as well; positive tests for rheumatoid factor have been found in as many as 30 percent of patients with chronic tophaceous gout,[88] and these patients have had no clinical or radiographic signs of RA. The coexistence of RA and gout is rare, and curiously so. Only 10 cases of gout coexisting with RA have been reported in the medical literature since 1881. Wallace and associates[89] have calculated that considering the prevalence of the two diseases, 10,617 cases should be anticipated to coexist within the United States. It is possible that numerous coexistent cases either have not been reported or have been missed, with physicians assuming that acute joint pain in a rheumatoid patient represents a flare of this process. Arthrocentesis, even in established rheumatoid joints, may be indicated to rule out sepsis or gout.

**Hemochromatosis (Uncommon) (see Chapter 94).** The characteristic feature of hemochromatosis that is almost diagnostic is firm bony enlargement of the metacarpophalangeal joints, particularly the second and third, with associated cystic degenerative disease on radiographs and, not infrequently, chondrocalcinosis.[90] Marginal erosions, juxta-articular osteoporosis, synovial proliferation, and ulnar deviation are not seen in the arthropathy of hemochromatosis but are common in RA. Wrists, shoulders, elbows, hips, and knees are involved less often than the metacarpophalangeal joints. More than a third of patients with this iron overload syndrome have an arthropathy.[91]

**Hemoglobinopathies (Uncommon) (see Chapter 101).** In homozygous (S-S) sickle cell disease, the most common arthropathy is associated with crises and is believed to be a result of microvascular occlusion in articular tissues.[92] However, in some cases a destructive arthritis with loss of articular cartilage has been defined,[93] and this resembles severe RA. In most patients with sickle disease and joint complaints, periosteal elevation, bone infarcts, fish-mouth vertebrae, and aseptic necrosis can be found on radiographs.[92] Episodic polyarthritis and noninflammatory synovial effusions are also found in sickle cell–$\beta$-thalassemia.[94]

**Hemophilic Arthropathy (Uncommon) (see Chapter 100).** A deficiency of factor VIII and IX sufficient to produce clinical bleeding frequently results in hemarthroses. The clotting abnormality rarely is overlooked, however, and it is unlikely that a diagnosis of RA would be made in the setting of hemophilia A or B.

**Hyperlipoproteinemia (Uncommon).** Achilles tendinitis and tenosynovitis in familial type II hyperlipoproteinemia can be presenting symptoms in this affliction and may be accompanied by arthritis.[95] Synovial fluid findings may resemble those of mild RA, and the tendon xanthomas may be mistaken for rheumatoid nodules or gouty tophi. Similarly, bilateral pseudoxanthomatous rheumatoid nodules have been described.[96] Asymmetrical and oligoarticular synovitis has been described in type IV hyperlipoproteinemia.[97] The absence of morning stiffness and noninflammatory synovial effusions helps rule out RA. The treatment of hyperlipoproteinemia with clofibrate may cause an acute muscular syndrome,[98] but this resembles myositis or polymyalgia rheumatica more than it does RA.

**Hypertrophic Osteoarthropathy (Uncommon) (see Chapter 103).** This process may present as oligoarthritis involving knees, ankles, or wrists. The synovial inflammation accompanies periosteal new bone formation, which can be seen on radiographs. Correction of the inciting factor (e.g., cure of pneumonia in a child with cystic fibrosis) will very likely alleviate the synovitis. The synovium is characterized primarily by an increased blood supply and synovial cell proliferation. Very little infiltration by mononuclear cells is seen.[99] Pain, which increases when extremities are dependent, is characteristic, although not always present. If clubbing is not present or is not noticed, this entity is easily confused with RA.

**Infectious Arthritis (Common) (see Chapters 96 to 98 ).** Bacterial sepsis may present superimposed in the setting of RA, and will be discussed below. Viral infections, however, may present as arthritis with many characteristics of RA. Rubella arthritis occurs more often in adults than in children and often affects small joints of the hands.[100] Lymphocytes predominate in synovial effusions. Synovitis (pain greater than swelling) occurred following vaccination with rubella vaccine, particularly with the dog kidney preparations, which are no longer used.[101]

Arthritis often precedes viral hepatitis and is associated with the presence of circulating hepatitis B surface antigen ($HB_sAg$) and hypocomplementemia.[102] $HB_sAg$ has been found in synovial tissues by direct immunofluorescence, supporting the concept that this synovitis is mediated by immune complexes.[103] A relatively acute onset of diffuse polyarthritis with small joint effusions and minimal synovial swelling should prompt the physician to obtain liver function tests in the patient with a history of exposure to hepatitis. With the onset of icterus, the arthritis usually resolves, leaving no trace.

Fever, sore throat, and cervical adenopathy followed by a symmetric polyarthritis are compatible with infection due to hepatitis B, rubella, adenovirus type 7, ECHO virus type 9, *Mycoplasma pneumoniae,* or Epstein-Barr virus as well as acute rheumatic fever or adult-onset Still's disease.[104]

**Lyme Disease (see Chapter 99).** This interesting disease is caused by infection with a spirochete classified as a *Borellia* species. It can closely simulate RA in adults or children by having an intermittent course with development of chronic synovitis.[105] Erosive synovitis necessitating synovectomy has evolved in several cases. The proliferative synovium is not different from that of RA. The differentiating point from RA is history of a tick bite or an expanding erythematous skin lesion with central pallor preceding the arthritis. The disease is being recognized in many parts of the country. Clinical abnormalities affecting the central nervous system and heart in Lyme disease may produce a syndrome mimicking systemic lupus erythematosus or vasculitis.

**Multicentric Reticulohistiocytosis (MR) (Rare) (see Chapter 95).** This process is particularly interesting because it is one that causes severe arthritis mutilans with an "opera-glass hand" (*main en lorgnette*).[106] Other causes of arthritis mutilans are RA, psoriatic arthritis, erosive osteoarthritis treated with glucocorticoids, and gout (after treatment with allopurinol). The cell that appears to effect damage to tissues is the multinucleate lipid-laden histiocyte, which appears to release degradative enzymes sufficient to destroy connective tissue. Differential characteristics from RA include the following:[107]

1. Skin manifestations: In MR, nodules are often widely disseminated and the histology is entirely different.
2. Joint manifestations: In MR, distal interphalangeal joints are frequently and extensively involved.
3. Radiographic manifestations: In MR, joint spaces appear to widen as destruction of subchondral bone occurs faster than cartilage is lost.
4. Laboratory tests: In MR, the erythrocyte sedimentation rate is often normal in face of severe resorptive disease, and rheumatoid factor is not present in MR.

**Osteoarthritis (Common) (see Chapter 89).** Although

**Table 60–7.** Factors Useful for Differentiating Early RA from Osteoarthrosis (Osteoarthritis)

| | RA | Osteoarthrosis |
|---|---|---|
| Age of onset | Childhood and adults; peak incidence in 50's | Increases with age |
| Predisposing factors | HLA-DR4 | Trauma, congenital abnormalities (e.g., shallow acetabulum) |
| Symptoms, early | Morning stiffness | Pain increases through the day and with use |
| Joints involved | Metacarpophalangeal joints, wrists, proximal interphalangeal joints most often; distal interphalangeal joints almost never | Distal interphalangeal joints (Heberden's nodes), weight-bearing joints (hips, knees) |
| Physical findings | Soft tissue swelling, warmth | Bony osteophytes, minimal soft tissue swelling early |
| Radiologic findings | Periarticular osteopenia, marginal erosions | Subchondral sclerosis, osteophytes |
| Laboratory findings | Increased erythrocyte sedimentation rate; rheumatoid factor, anemia, leukocytosis | Normal |

osteoarthritis begins as a degeneration of articular cartilage and RA begins as inflammation in the synovium, each process approaches the other pathologically, and therefore clinically, as the diseases progress. In osteoarthritis, as cartilage deteriorates and joint congruence is altered and stressed, a reactive synovitis often develops. Conversely, as the rheumatoid pannus erodes cartilage, secondary degenerative changes in bone and cartilage develop and in end stages of either degenerative joint disease or RA the involved joints appear the same. To differentiate clearly between the two, therefore, the physician must delve into the early history and functional abnormalities of the disease. Factors useful in separating the two processes are listed in Table 60–7.

One overlap condition exists: erosive osteoarthritis. This occurs in middle-aged women (more than men) and is characterized by inflammatory changes in proximal interphalangeal joints, with destruction and functional ankylosis of the joints. The proximal interphalangeal joints can appear red and hot, yet there is almost no synovial proliferation or effusion. The erythrocyte sedimentation rate may be slightly elevated, but rheumatoid factor is negative.[108]

**Parkinson's Disease (Common).** Although the tremor and/or rigidity of Parkinson's Disease is rarely confused with rheumatoid arthritis, Parkinson's patients have a predilection for developing swan-neck deformities of the hands (Fig. 60–1), which is generally unappreciated by rheumatologists. This abnormality, the pathogenesis of which still is unknown, was first described in 1864.[109]

**Polychondritis (Uncommon) (see Chapter 91).** This process can mimic infectious processes, vasculitis, granulomatous disease, or RA. Patients with RA and ocular inflammation (e.g., scleritis) usually have active joint disease before ocular problems develop. The reverse occurs in polychondritis. In addition, polychondritis is not associated with rheumatoid factor. The joint disease is usually episodic. Nevertheless, erosions can develop that are not unlike those of RA.

**Polymyalgia Rheumatica (PR) (Common) (see Chapter 73).** Although joint radionuclide imaging studies have indicated increased vascular flow in synovium of patients with classic polymyalgia rheumatica, it remains appropriate to exclude PR as a diagnosis if significant synovitis (soft tissue proliferation or effusions) can be detected. Otherwise, many patients who actually have RA would be diagnosed as having PR and treated with potentially harmful doses of corticosteroids. A careful history will usually differentiate shoulder or hip girdle muscle pain from shoulder or hip joint pain. It is probable that RA and PR coexist in numerous patients, but careful descriptions of such patients are rare.

**Rheumatic Fever (Uncommon) (see Chapter 81).** Rheumatic fever is much less common now than it was previously, but still must be considered in adults with polyarthritis. In adults, the arthritis is the most prominent clinical finding of RF; carditis is less frequent than it is in children, while erythema marginatum, subcuta-

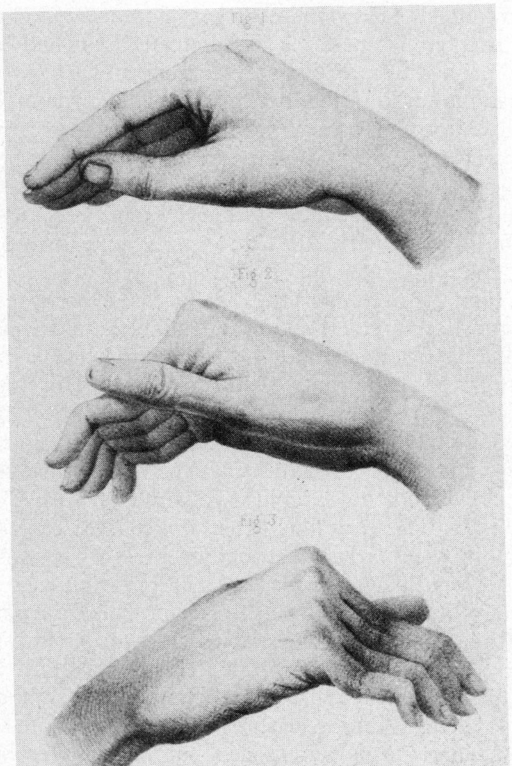

**Figure 60–1.** These swan neck deformities are a result of Parkinson's disease, not rheumatoid arthritis.[109]

neous nodules, and chorea are rare.[110,111] The presentation is often that of an additive, symmetrical, large joint polyarthritis (involving lower extremities in 85 percent of patients), developing within a week and associated with a severe tenosynovitis.[110] This extremely painful process is dramatically responsive to salicylates.[111,112] Unlike Still's disease in the adult, rheumatic fever generally has no remittent or quotidian fevers, has a less protracted course, and shows evidence for antecedent streptococcal infection. There are many similarities between the presentation of rheumatic fever in adults and "reactive" postinfectious synovitis developing after *Shigella, Salmonella, Brucella, Neisseria,* or *Yersinia* infections. These latter processes do not respond well to salicylates, however. As rheumatic fever becomes less frequent, and as penicillin prophylaxis effectively prevents recurrences of the disease, Jaccoud's arthritis (chronic postrheumatic fever arthritis) is becoming very rare. This entity, described first by Bywaters in 1950,[113] resulted from severe and repeated bouts of rheumatic fever and synovitis, which left stretched-out joint capsules and ulnar deformity of the hands without erosions due to ulnar displacement and shortening and fibrosis of extensor tendons.[114] The same deformity can develop in systemic lupus erythematosus characterized by recurrent synovitis and soft tissue inflammation, or in Parkinson's disease (Fig. 60–1). Differentiating rheumatic fever from RA is particularly difficult when subcutaneous nodules associated with rheumatic fever are found.[115]

**Sarcoidosis (Uncommon) (see Chapter 93).** The two most frequent forms of sarcoid arthritis are usually easily differentiated from RA. In the acute form with erythema nodosum and hilar adenopathy the articular complaints usually appear as periarthritis affecting large joints of the lower extremities. Differential diagnosis may be confused by the fact that many of these patients have rheumatoid factor present in serum.[116] Joint erosions and proliferative synovitis do not occur in this form of sarcoidosis.

In chronic sarcoidosis, cystlike areas of bone destruction, mottled rarefaction of bone, and a reticular pattern of bone destruction giving a lacelike appearance on radiographs may simulate destructive RA. This form of sarcoid is often polyarticular, and biopsy of bone or synovium for diagnosis may be essential, particular since there is often no correlation between joint disease and clinical evidence for sarcoid involvement of other organ systems.[117] It is very likely that Poncet's disease or tuberculous rheumatism[118] actually represents granulomatous "idiopathic" arthritis (i.e., sarcoidosis).

**Miscellaneous Abnormalities That Can Be Mistaken for Rheumatoid Arthritis.** *Sweet's syndrome* (rare) is called acute febrile neutrophilic dermatosis.[119,120] It has been described in adults, often following "flulike" illness. The three major features are an acute illness with fever, leukocytosis, and raised painful plaques on the skin that show neutrophilic infiltration of the dermis on biopsy. Joint disease occurs in 20 to 25 percent of cases and is characterized by acute, self-limited polyarthritis. Because of the skin lesions, Sweet's syndrome is confused with systemic lupus erythematosus, erythema nodosum, and erythema elevatum diutinum more often than for RA. It has been treated effectively with indomethacin[120] and corticosteroids.

*Thiemann's disease* is a rare form of idiopathic vascular necrosis of the proximal interphalangeal joints of the hands with occasional involvement of other joints.[121,122] Bony enlargement begins relatively painlessly, and the digits (one or more may be involved) become fixed in flexion. The primary lesion is in the region of the epiphysis, and the lesion begins most often before puberty, distinguishing it from erosive osteoarthritis that it resembles radiographically. It is clearly a heritable disease, but the genetic factors have not been defined.

*Calcific periarthritis* can be easily confused with polyarthritis.[123] The skin is red over and around the affected joints; the tissues are boggy and tender, but no effusion is present. Passive motion is easier than active motion. Periarticular calcification is visible on radiographs. Unless the periarthritis can be differentiated from true arthritis (as in the periarthritis of sarcoid), the syndrome would seem like palindromic rheumatism or early RA.

The syndrome of *intermittent hydrarthrosis* describes periodic attacks of benign synovitis in one or few joints, usually the knee, beginning in adolescence.[124] The difference between this and oligoarticular JRA or RA is one of degree, not kind. In contrast to palindromic rheumatism, in which acute synovitis often may occur in different joints during successive attacks,[125] the same joint or joints are affected during each attack in intermittent hydrarthrosis.[126]

Although perhaps more appropriately classified with arthritis related to gastrointestinal disease (see Ankylosing Spondylitis, etc.) polyarthritis that occurs in obese patients after intestinal bypass surgery can present as RA.[127] Articular complaints occur in approximately 25 percent of these patients, but rarely are joint complaints persistent or severe. Circulating cryoproteins that may be immune complexes have been described. Bennett (see Chapter 58) has suggested that the shortened bowel may enable arthritogenic and immunogenic bacterial products to gain access to the host. Fortunately, this form of treatment for morbid obesity is rarely used.

The *fibrositis syndrome* (see Chapter 32) should not be confused with RA, because in fibrositis (syn., fibromyalgia) there is no evidence of synovitis. Although there are no specific diagnostic tests that define fibrositis, there are certain recurrent nonarticular locations for pain that are seen in different patients. These include[128] the midpoint of the upper border of the trapezius, forearm muscles distal to the lateral humeral epicondyle, the second costochondral junction, the fat pad medial to the knee, and intervertebral ligaments. Arousal syndromes of disordered sleep may be related to development of this syndrome. Evidence is accumulating that patients with RA may develop a superimposed fibromyalgia. This leads to very difficult therapeutic problems.

Although *glucocorticoids* suppress inflammation and pain, there is an arthropathy associated with their use[129] that resembles avascular necrosis. More likely confused with RA are the symptoms of corticosteroid withdrawal. These patients may suffer diffuse polyarticular pain, particularly in the hands, if the corticosteroid dose is tapered too rapidly.

The rheumatic syndromes associated with *malignancy* are outlined in detail in Chapter 104. Direct involvement by cancer of synovium usually presents as a monarthritic syndrome.[130] A more subtle association is represented by the patients who present with a slightly atypical RA at about the time a malignancy is developing. *Pigmented villonodular synovitis* is a nonmalignant but very proliferative disease of synovial tissue that has many functional characteristics similar to those of RA and usually involves only one joint. The histopathology is characterized by proliferation of histiocytes, multinucleate giant cells, and hemosiderin- and lipid-laden macrophages. Clinically, this presents as a relatively painless chronic synovitis (most often of the knee) with joint effusions and greatly thickened synovium.[131] Subchondral bone cysts and cartilage erosion may be associated with the bulky tissue. It is not clear whether this should be classified as an inflammation or neoplasm of synovium (see Chapter 108).

Multiple myeloma may present as a polyarthritis, mimicking RA. Amyloid deposits can be found in synovial and periarticular tissues[132] and are, presumably, responsible for the joint complaints. The synovial fluid in *amyloid arthropathy* is noninflammatory, and, on occasion, particulate material staining with apple green fluorescence after Congo red staining may be found in the fluid.

*Idiopathic edema* is a cause of nonarticular rheumatism that may be confused for RA with mild, early synovitis.[133]

## ESTABLISHED RHEUMATOID ARTHRITIS: ITS COURSE AND COMPLICATIONS

### The Involvement of Joints—Effects of Disease on Form and Function

Once rheumatoid synovitis is established by the sequence outlined in Chapter 59, the effects that the process has on joints are a complex function of the intensity of the underlying disease, its chronicity, and the stress put on individual involved joints by the patient. This is graphically illustrated by the radiographs of a patient's pelvis (Fig. 60–2). The patient was a 67-year-old female who developed arthritis in 1960 at the age of 49 years. Characterized by exacerbations and remissions initially, her disease became chronic and destructive, and in 1971 she was no longer able to bear weight on her right hip and was in a wheelchair or bed until 1978, when the second (lower) radiograph was taken. The changes in the 8-year interval are defined more by her being confined to inactivity in a wheelchair than by the activity of her arthritis. In 1970, she had developed a significant protrusio acetabuli; the apparent joint space was almost completely obliterated, and significant sclerosis developed in both the acetabulum and femoral head. In contrast, after 8 years of non–weight bearing, there was a dramatic change in her radiographs: The protrusio was unchanged; however, the contour of the femoral head was smooth; the apparent joint space widened, suggesting the joint had been re-surfaced with fibrocartilage. Subchondral sclerosis diminished. While the hip was being remodeled, the lumbosacral spine was bearing her body weight in a wheelchair and impressive sclerosis and narrowing of the vertebral disc occurred.

Among other principles demonstrated by Figure 60–2 is the fact that there are reparative as well as destructive mechanisms in rheumatoid synovitis, and that expression of one or the other may be related more to motion and weight bearing than to other factors, including treatment.

Understanding the sequence of changes produced by arthritis in individual joints, therefore, is best achieved by attempting to define how the disease alters normal function of joints, bone, and muscle.

**The Cervical Spine.** Unlike other nonsynovial joints, such as the sternomanubrial joint or symphysis pubis, the discovertebral joints in the cervical spine often manifest osteochondral destruction in RA,[134,135] and on lateral radiographs may be found narrowed to less than 5 mm. Significant pain is the clinical presentation, and passive range of motion, in the absence of muscle spasm, may be normal. There are two possible mechanisms for this process: (1) extension of the inflammatory process from adjacent neurocentral joints, the joints of Luschka, which are lined by synovium, into the discovertebral area;[134,135] and (2) Chronic cervical instability initiated by apophyseal joint destruction leading to vertebral malalignment or subluxation.[136] This may produce microfractures of the vertebral endplates, disc herniation, and/or degeneration of disc cartilage.

The atlantoaxial joint is prone to subluxation in several directions: (1) The atlas moves *anteriorly* on the axis (most common). This results from laxity of the transverse cruciate ligament and the lateral alarodontoid ligaments induced by proliferative synovial tissue developing in adjacent synovial bursa, or from fracture or erosion of the odontoid process (Fig. 60–3). (2) The atlas moves *posteriorly* on the axis. This can occur only if the odontoid peg has been fractured off the axis or destroyed. (3) The vertical subluxation of the atlas in relation to the axis (least common). This results from destruction of the lateral atlantoaxial joints or of bone around the foramen magnum. One recently described patient with RA had superior, posterior, and lateral displacement of C1.[137]

The most common symptom of subluxation is pain radiating up into the occiput.[138] Two other less common clinical patterns include: (1) slowly progressive spastic quadriparesis, frequently with painless sensory loss of the hands, and (2) transient episodes of medullary or positive dysfunction associated with vertical penetration

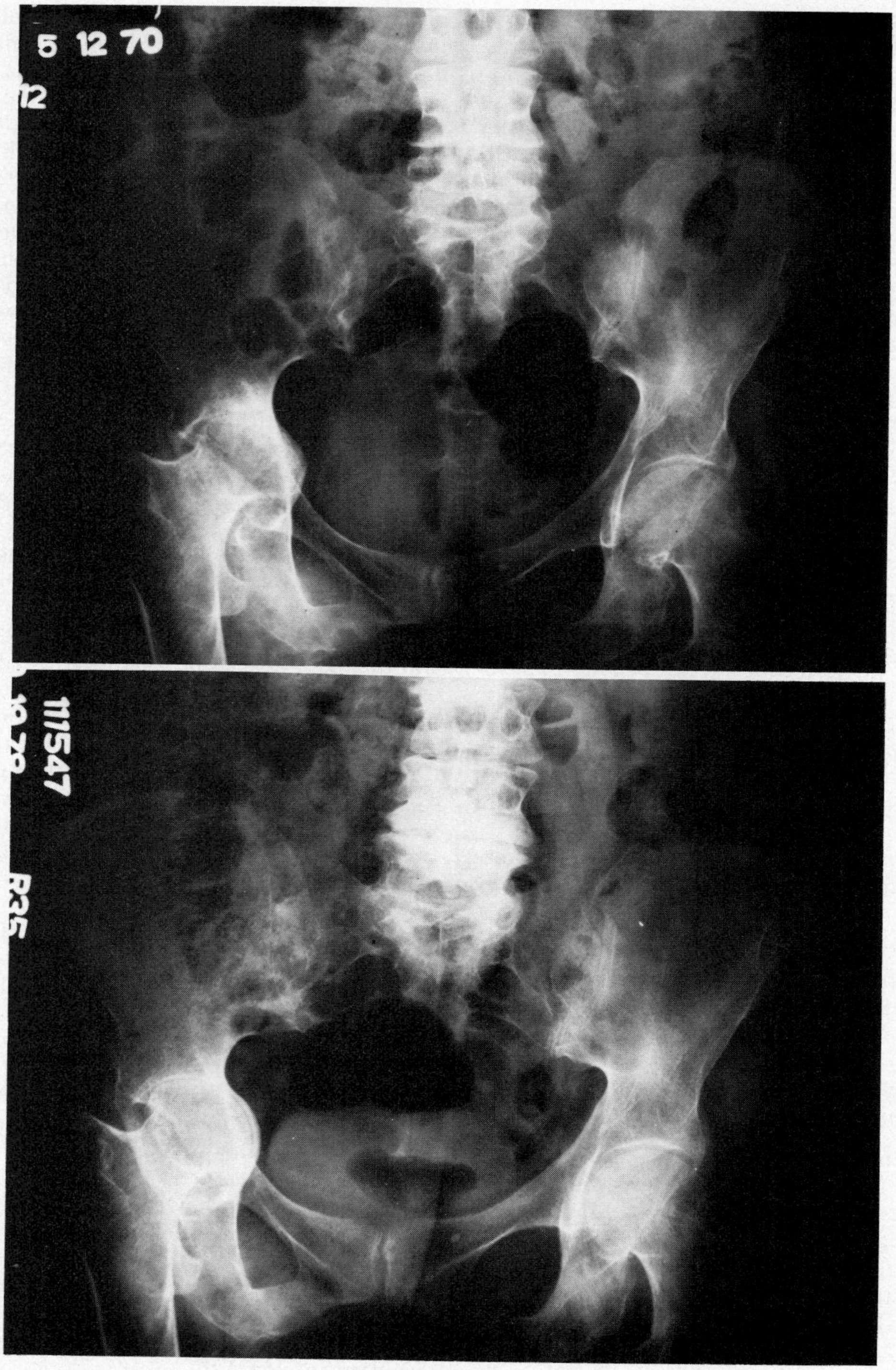


**Figure 60–2.** Remodeling of the hip joint in a patient with rheumatoid arthritis during 7 years without weight-bearing (see text for details). In contrast, the lumbosacral spine, supporting the weight of the upper body and providing the only mobility while the patient was seated, has undergone progressive degeneration. (The radiographs are owned by the Radiology Section at the Dartmouth-Hitchcock Medical Center and were provided by Dr. Joshua Burnett.)

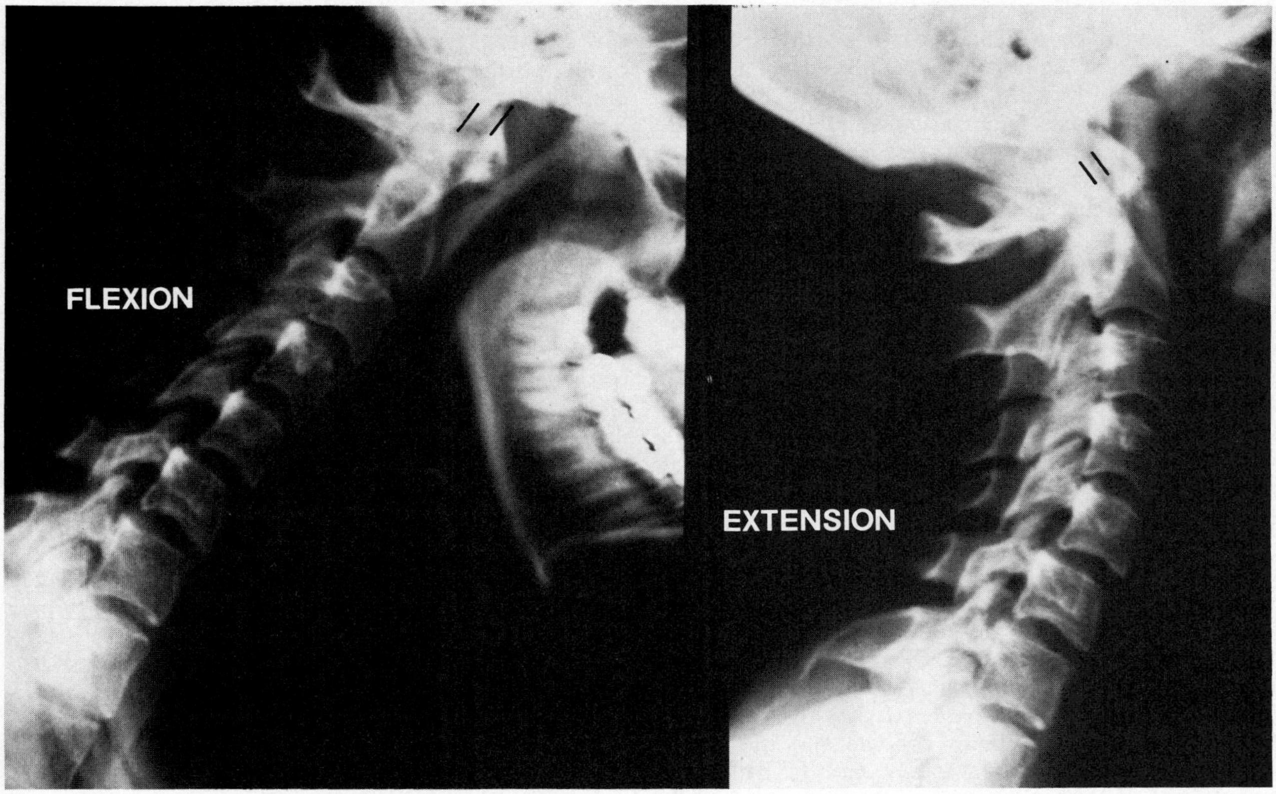


**Figure 60–3.** Anterior subluxation of C1 on C2 during flexion of the head. In this 21-year-old female there is a normal 3 mm distance between the atlas and the odontoid process while her head is held in extension (*right*). In flexion radiograph (*left*) subluxation to 7 mm has developed. (Courtesy of Gary S. Hoffman, M.D.)

of the dens and probable vertebral artery compression.[139] Paresthesias in the shoulders or arms may occur during movement of the head. Physical findings suggestive of atlantoaxial subluxation include (1) loss of occipitocervical lordosis, (2) resistance to passive spine motion, (3) abnormal protrusion of the axial arch, felt by the examining finger on the posterior pharyngeal wall, and (4) a "click" produced by anterior pressure on the spinous process of C2 when combined with posterior pressure on the forehead. The "click" indicates an intact odontoid process abutting the axial arch. Radiographic views (lateral, in flexion) should reveal more than a 3-mm separation between the odontoid peg and the axial arch.[140] In symptomatic patients, the films in flexion should be taken only after radiographs (including an open-mouth posteroanterior view) have ruled out an odontoid fracture or severe atlantoaxial subluxation. Recent studies have indicated that computerized tomography is useful for demonstrating spinal cord compression by loss of posterior subarachnoid space in patients with C1-2 subluxation.[141]

Neurologic symptoms often have little relationship to the degree of subluxation and may be related to individual variations in diameter of the spinal canal. Symptoms of spinal cord compression that demand intervention include[142] (1) a sensation of the head falling forward on flexion of the cervical spine; (2) changes in levels of consciousness; (3) "drop" attacks; (4) loss of sphincter control; (5) dysphagia, vertigo, convulsions, hemiplegia, dysarthria, or nystagmus; and (6) peripheral paresthesias without evidence for peripheral nerve disease or compression. Some of these symptoms may be related to compression of the vertebral arteries, which must wind through foramina in the transverse processes of C1 and C2, rather than to compression of the spinal cord.

Is mortality increased in patients with atlantoaxial subluxation? In one series of autopsies on 104 consecutive deaths in patients with RA,[143] 11 cases of severe dislocation were found. In all 11 cases the odontoid protruded posterosuperiorly and impinged upon the medulla within the foramen magnum. In five, spinal cord compression was determined to be the only cause of death. In only two cases was subluxation diagnosed before death. These patients must be at risk for even small falls and whiplash injuries and for general anesthesia with intubation. Cervical collars should be prescribed for stability. Operative stabilization may be considered if symptoms are progressive. In a series of 84 patients with some form of subluxation[144] but without cord or brainstem lesions, one fourth worsened and one fourth improved without surgery over 5 to 14 years of follow-up. Using survival tables, these authors concluded that cervical luxations per se do not significantly shorten life in patients with RA. In most series, less than 20 percent of patients with RA exhibited C1-2 disease. Glucocorticoid therapy appeared to have an adverse effect on forward luxations at C1-C2.

Vertical atlantoaxial subluxation is equally important, although less common, being present in 13 of 476 (3.7 percent) hospitalized patients with RA.[145] Symptoms associated with this collapse of the lateral support system of the atlas occur in patients with severe erosive disease. Neurologic findings have included decreased sensation in the distribution of cranial nerve 5 and sensory loss in the C2 area, nystagmus, and pyramidal lesions. Vertical subluxations are believed to have a worse prognosis than the other varieties.[146]

Bywaters has demonstrated bursal spaces between the cervical interspinous processes in autopsies of patients without joint disease, and in rheumatoid patients, bursal proliferation that led in several cases to radiographically demonstrated destruction of the spinous processes.[147]

**Temporomandibular Joints (TMJ).** TMJ are commonly involved in RA. In one series of 65 patients with classic or definite RA,[148] careful history revealed that 55 percent of patients had symptoms at some time during the course of their disease. Radiographic examination revealed structural alterations in 78 percent of the joints examined (86 percent of patients). An overbite may develop[149] as the mandibular condyle and the corresponding surface of the temporal bone, the eminentia articularis, are eroded. Physical examination of the rheumatoid patient should include palpation for tenderness and auscultation for crepitus. Occasional patients will present with acute pain and an inability to close the mouth, necessitating intra-articular glucocorticoids to suppress the acute process.

**Cricoarytenoid Joints.** The small diarthrodial joints have an important function, since they rotate with the vocal cords as they abduct and adduct to vary pitch and tone of the voice. Careful history may reveal hoarseness in up to 30 percent of rheumatoid patients.[150] This is not disabling in and of itself, but there is a danger that the cricoarytenoid joints may become inflamed and immobilized, with the vocal cords adducted to the midline, causing inspiratory stridor.[151] Autopsy examinations have demonstrated cricoarytenoid arthritis in almost half the patients with RA, suggesting that much significant disease of the larynx may be asymptomatic.[152] Symptomatic rheumatoid nodules within the vocal cord itself, mimicking laryngeal carcinoma, have been described. Asymptomatic cricoarytenoid synovitis may occasionally lead to aspiration of pharyngeal contents, particularly at night.

**Ossicles of the Ear.** Many rheumatoid patients suffer a decrease in hearing. In general this has been ascribed to salicylate toxicity, and it is believed to be reversible when the drug is discontinued (see Chapter 49). On the other hand, conductive hearing loss in patients not on salicylates was reported by Copeman.[153] Studies using otoadmittance measurements[154] have been carried out in patients with RA in an attempt to determine whether the interossicle joints were involved. The technique measured factors that impede the flow of sound through the ear: stiffness (tympanic membrane and ossicles), mass or inertia (the bulk of the ossicles), and resistance. The data showed that 38 percent of "rheumatoid ears" and 8 percent of controls demonstrated a pattern characteristic of an increase in the flaccidity of a clinically normal tympanic membrane. This is consistent with erosions and shortening of the ossicles produced by the erosive synovitis, not with ankylosis.

**Sternoclavicular and Manubriosternal Joints.** These joints, both possessing synovium and a large cartilaginous disc, are often involved in RA.[155] Because of the relative immobility there are a few symptoms. Patients occasionally complain of pain in sternoclavicular joints while lying on their sides in bed. When symptoms do occur, the physician must be concerned about superimposed sepsis. Computerized tomography may be a useful technique for careful delineation of the sternoclavicular joint. Manubriosternal involvement is almost never clinically important, although by tomographic criteria it is very common in RA.[156] Some patients develop manubriosternal joint subluxation. This deformity may be associated with cervical spine disease. In one study, of 10 patients with manubriosternal subluxation, 8 had radiographic evidence for significant atlanto-axial subluxation.[157]

**The Shoulder.** RA of the shoulder not only affects synovium within the glenohumeral joint, but also involves the distal third of the clavicle, various bursae and the rotator cuff, and multiple muscles around the neck and chest wall.

One of the most important principles of rehabilitation (see Chapter 111) is that joint pain causes decreased mobility of joints and that decreased mobility quickly leads to muscle weakness and atrophy. Often rheumatoid involvement of the shoulder can be detected by an examination that demands effort from various muscle groups. One of the first muscle groups to weaken in shoulder involvement in RA is the mid-thoracic group, which is responsible for normal scapular positioning on the chest wall. A common early change in RA is an anterolateral shift of the scapula, producing a "forward shoulder." Forward shifting of the scapula decreases stability of the glenohumeral joint. In a reaction to restore stability, the pectoralis major pulls the humerus into a position of adduction and internal rotation. Thus it is not unusual that limitation of rotation has been found to be the most consistent abnormality of shoulder function on physical examination.

In recent years it has been appreciated that involvement of the rotator cuff in RA is a principal cause of morbidity. The function of the rotator cuff is to stabilize the humeral head in the glenoid. Weakness of the cuff results in superior subluxation. Rotator cuff tears or insufficiency for other reasons can be demonstrated by shoulder arthrogram. In Ennevaara's series of 200 consecutive patients with RA, studied by arthrography, 21 percent had rotator cuff tears and an additional 24 percent had evidence for fraying of tendons.[158] One likely mechanism for tears is that the rotator cuff tendon insertion into the greater tuberosity is vulnerable to erosion by the proliferative synovitis that develops there[159] (Fig. 60–4). Previous injury and aging may predispose to the development of tears.[160] Sudden tears may present with pain and inflammation so great as to suggest sepsis.

Standard radiographic examinations[161] of the shoulder in RA reveal erosions (69 percent) and superior subluxation (31 percent). Arthrograms, in addition to showing tears of the rotator cuff, can demonstrate[162] (1) diffuse nodular filling defects, (2) irregular capsular attachment, (3) bursal filling defects, (4) adhesive capsulitis, and (5) dilatation of the biceps tendon sheath (perhaps unique to RA). Marked soft tissue swelling of the anterolateral aspect of the shoulders in RA may be secondary to chronic subacromial bursitis rather than to glenohumeral joint effusions.[163] In contrast to rotator cuff tears, bursal swelling is not necessarily associated with decreased range of motion or pain. Synovial proliferation within the subdeltoid bursa may explain resorption of the undersurface of the distal clavicle seen in this disease.[164]

**The Elbow.** Perhaps because it is a very stable hinge joint, severe pain in the elbow rarely is manifest in the disease. Nevertheless, involvement of the elbow is common, and if lateral stability at the elbow is lost as the disease progresses, disability can be severe.

The frequency of elbow involvement varies from 20 to 65 percent, depending on the severity of disease in the patient populations studied. The relatively low prevalence shown in Table 60–5 is in contrast with the 67 percent[165] involvement found in another study. One of the earliest findings—often unnoticed by the patient—is loss of full extension. Since the elbow is principally a connecting joint between the hand and trunk, the shoulder and wrists can compensate for loss of elbow motion.[166] For example, pronation at the wrists can be assisted 45 to 50 degrees by abducting the shoulder; and

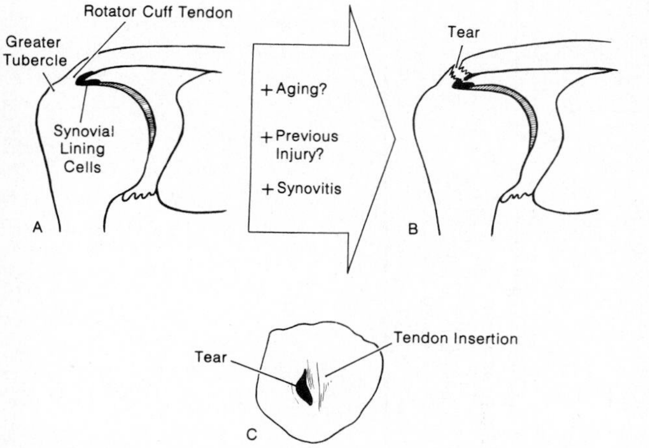


**Figure 60–4.** Pathogenesis of rotator cuff tears in rheumatoid arthritis. The small patch of synovium present at the reflection of insertion of the rotator cuff tendon can, in its proliferated state, produce enzymes sufficient to seriously weaken the tendon, predisposing it to rupture. (From Weiss, J.J., et al.: Arch. Intern. Med. 135:521, 1975.)

shoulder elevation and wrist flexion can be substituted for flexion at the elbow.

**The Hand and Wrist.** These should be considered together because they form a functional unit. There are data,[167,168] for example, linking disease of the wrist to ulnar deviation of the metacarpophalangeal joints. The best hypothesis,[167] based on radiographic measurements, is that weakening of the extensor carpi ulnaris leads to radial deviation of the wrist as the carpal bones rotate (the proximal row in an ulnar direction, the distal ones in a radial one). Ulnar deviation of the fingers (a "zigzag" deformity) occurs in response to this, to keep the tendons to the phalanges in a normal line with the radius. A refinement of this hypothesis[168] is that the first anatomic abnormality may be volar subluxation of the ulnar side of the carpus. This may be caused by slippage of the movable insertion of the extensor carpi ulnaris in a lateral-volar direction, which results in a volar pull on the wrist bones only weakly opposed by residual extensors. This produces relative supination of the carpus, a prominent ulnar head, and in turn accentuates the weakness of the extensor carpi ulnaris, producing the same dominance of the radial carpi extensors and ulnar deviation of the metacarpophalangeal joints. Other factors, including the tendency for power grasp to pull the fingers into an ulnar attitude[169] and inappropriate intrinsic muscle action,[170] are undoubtedly involved as well (Table 60–8).[171-175] It is important to note that erosion of bone or articular cartilage is not essential for development of ulnar deviation. Significant although reducible ulnar deviation can result from repeated synovitis and myositis in the hands (e.g., systemic lupus erythematosus).

Dorsal swelling on the wrist within the tendon sheaths of the extensor muscles (fifth and sixth tendon compartments) is one of the earliest signs of disease. Rarely, cystic structures resembling ganglia will be early findings of RA.[176]

As the synovial proliferation develops within the wrist, pressure increases within the relatively nondistensible joint spaces. Proliferative synovium develops enzymatic machinery sufficient to destroy ligaments, tendons, and the articular disc distal to the ulnar head. Pressure and enzymes combine to produce communications between radiocarpal, radioulnar, and midcarpal joints in about 70 percent of patients with RA compared with 16 percent or less in controls.[177] Integrity of the distal radioulnar joint is lost; the ulnar collateral ligament, stretched by the proliferative synovium of the radioulnar joint, finally either ruptures or is destroyed and the ulnar head springs up into dorsal prominence, where it "floats" and can easily be depressed by the examiner's fingers.

On the volar side of the wrist, synovial protrusion cysts develop; they can be palpated, and their origins can be confirmed by arthrography.[178] The thick transverse carpal ligament prevents significant resistance to decompression, however, and the hyperplastic synovium compressing the median nerve can cause the carpal tunnel syndrome, which is described in detail in Chapter 110.

**Table 60–8.** A Sequence of Pathology in Development of Ulnar Deviation at Metacarpophalangeal Joints

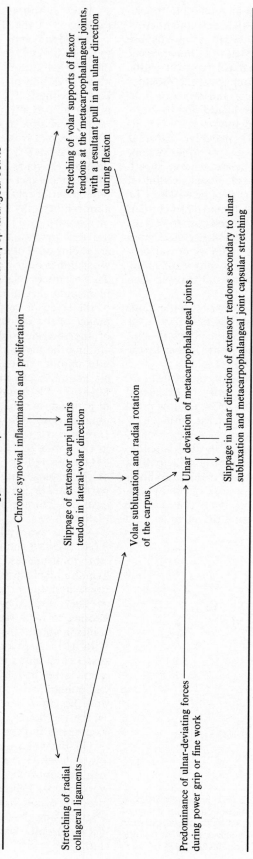

Chronic synovial inflammation and proliferation → Stretching of radial collageral ligaments → Volar subluxation and radial rotation of the carpus → Ulnar deviation of metacarpophalangeal joints

Chronic synovial inflammation and proliferation → Slippage of extensor carpi ulnaris tendon in lateral-volar direction → Volar subluxation and radial rotation of the carpus → Ulnar deviation of metacarpophalangeal joints

Chronic synovial inflammation and proliferation → Stretching of volar supports of flexor tendons at the metacarpophalangeal joints, with a resultant pull in an ulnar direction during flexion → Ulnar deviation of metacarpophalangeal joints

Predominance of ulnar-deviating forces during power grip or fine work → Ulnar deviation of metacarpophalangeal joints

Ulnar deviation of metacarpophalangeal joints ⇄ Slippage in ulnar direction of extensor tendons secondary to ulnar subluxation and metacarpophalangeal joint capsular stretching

Common sites for bone erosion by proliferative synovitis in the wrist are at the periphery of the joint where no protective cartilage is found.[179] Enzymes and pressure may be synergistic in producing fracture, and osseous and cartilage debris may accumulate in the joint spaces.[180] Irregular bone edges from which fragments have been separated may serve as weapons to erode tendons already weakened and attenuated by action of proteinases.

Progression of disease in the wrist is characterized by loss of joint space and loss of bone. This foreshortening of the carpus has been quantitated as a carpal-metacarpal (c:mc) ratio (length of the carpus divided by that of the third metacarpal). Data showed a linear decrease in the c:mc ratio with progressive disease (Fig. 60–5).[181] This is caused by compaction of bone at the radiolunate, lunate-capitate, and capitate-third metacarpal joints, which usually accompanies severe disease.

The *hand* often has many joints involved in RA. One of the most sensitive indices of hand involvement is grip strength. The act of squeezing brings stress on all hand joints. As noted in Chapter 24, muscular contraction causes ligamentous tightening around joints, compressing inflamed synovium. The immediate result is weakness, with or without pain. Gerber (see Chapter 111) suggests that the reflex inhibition of muscular contraction secondary to pain may be a primary factor. Progression from early disease to severe deformity of the hands is shown in Figures 60–6 and 60–7.

Often before deformities demonstrable at rest in individual joints are discernible, there are two kinetic abnormalities that develop. (1) The normal arches of the hands may be increased or decreased. A transverse arch is formed by the carpal bones and lies at the base of the thenar and hypothenar eminences. A longitudinal arch runs from this carpal arch to each phalanx. Early edema and pain associated with spasm of the interosseous muscles lead to loss of these arches, with a "flat-handed" appearance. (2) Involuntary motion of one metacarpal on the next grasp is a normal phenomenon. This motion

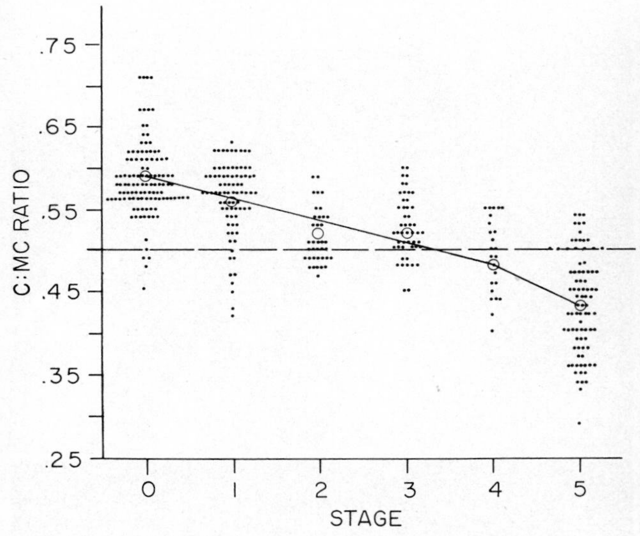


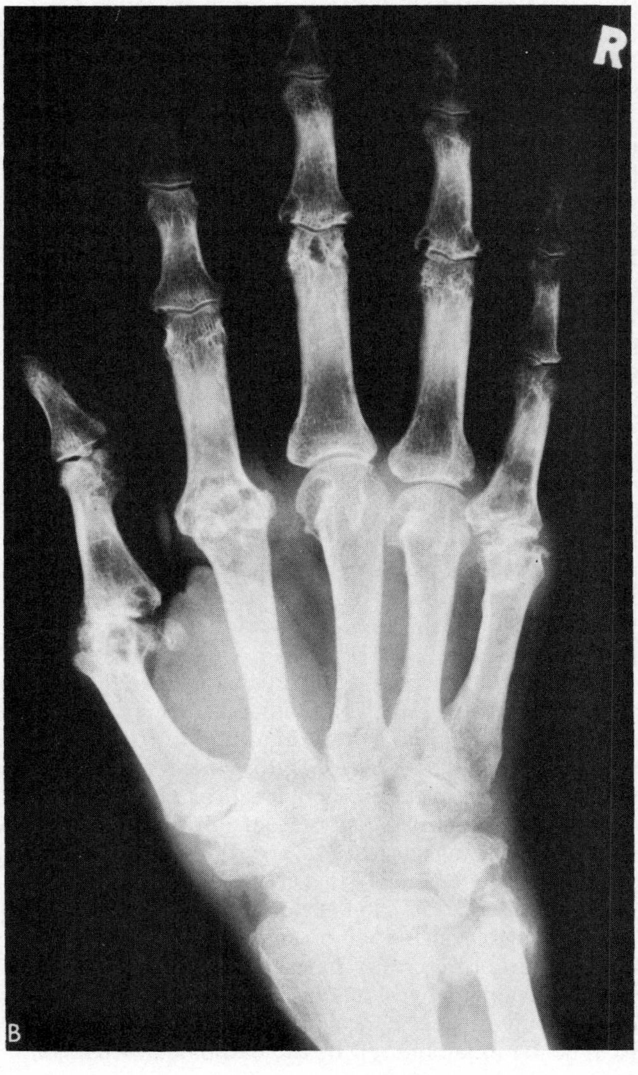


**Figure 60–5.** The carpal-metacarpal ratio in relation to radiographic state of disease in 390 hand films of 73 female RA patients. (From Trentham, D.E., and Masi, A.J.: Arthritis Rheum. 19:939, 1976.) *B,* Radiograph of the right wrist of a 42-year-old woman with RA. The carpal-metacarpal index (see text) is 4.28, significantly below the lower limit of normal, consistent with destructive synovitis in the wrist, particularly in the radiocarpal joint. Despite severe disease this patient has developed no ulnar deviation at the metacarpophalangeal joints.

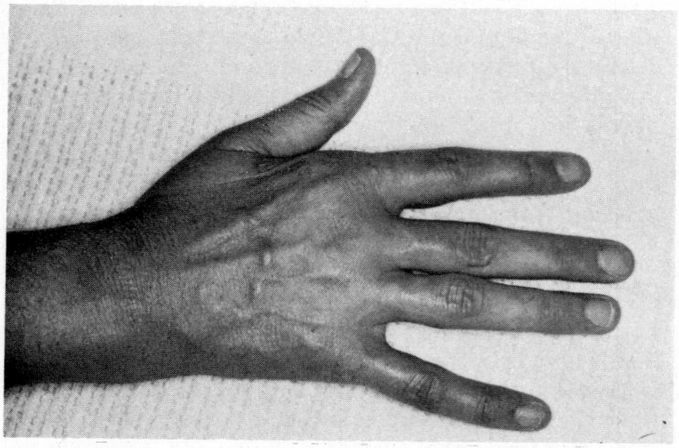

**Figure 60–6.** Subtle changes in RA developing in a 32-year-old woman. Fusiform swelling of proximal interphalangeal joints (the fourth in particular) is apparent. The hands are warm and slightly swollen (note the reflected light), and the veins are engorged.

is often lost as intrinsic muscles shorten during prolonged inflammation. Opposition of digits IV and V to the thumb is particularly hampered by loss of motion between the metacarpals. Thus, early loss of grip strength is often greatest in these digits.

The swan-neck deformity is one of flexion of the distal interphalangeal and metacarpophalangeal joints, with hyperextension of the proximal interphalangeal joint. The lesion probably begins with shortening of interosseous muscles and tendons, leading to a degree of metacarpophalangeal joint flexion during digital extension. Shortening of the intrinsic muscles exerts tension of the dorsal tendon sheath, leading to hyperextension of the proximal interphalangeal joint[182] (Fig. 60–8). Deep tendon contracture or, rarely, distal interphalangeal joint involvement with RA leads to the distal interphalangeal joint flexion.[183] Rupture of the sublimis tendon, which would reduce capacity to flex the proximal interphalangeal joint, could lead to the same sequence of events.[184]

If during chronic inflammation of a proximal interphalangeal joint, the extensor hood stretches or is avulsed, the proximal interphalangeal joint may pop up in flexion, producing a boutonnière deformity[172,183] (Fig. 60–9). The distal interphalangeal joint remains in hyperextension.

Without either of these deformities, limitation of movement develops at the proximal interphalangeal and distal interphalangeal joints. Limitation of full flexion of the distal interphalangeal joint is common in RA and represents incomplete profundus contraction. Similarly, tight intrinsic muscles may prevent full flexion of proximal interphalangeal joints when the metacarpophalangeal joints are in full extension.

Nalebuff's classification of thumb disease in RA gives a sequence of functional problems with this joint.[185] Three types of deformity have been described. In type I, metacarpophalangeal inflammation leads to stretching of the joint capsule and a boutonnière-like deformity. In type II, inflammation of the carpometacarpal joint leads to volar subluxation during contracture of the adductor hallucis. In type III, after prolonged disease of both metacarpophalangeal joints, exaggerated adduction of the first metacarpus, flexion of the metacarpophalangeal joint, and hyperextension of the distal interphalangeal joint result from the patient's need to provide a means to pinch.

One of the most common manifestations of RA in hands is tenosynovitis in flexor tendon sheaths. Frequently overlooked during an examination that focuses on the dorsum of the hand, the tendon sheath lesion is manifested on the volar surface of the phalanges as diffuse swelling between joints or a palpable grating within flexor tendon sheaths in the palm.

In one series, hand flexor tenosynovitis was observed in 55 percent of 100 patients with RA,[186] a higher frequency than found in other studies and probably related more to careful examination than to any difference in population or disease. Although hand flexor tenosynovitis was not associated with more prolonged or severe disease, there was an association with a number of para-articular manifestations (distinct from extra-articular

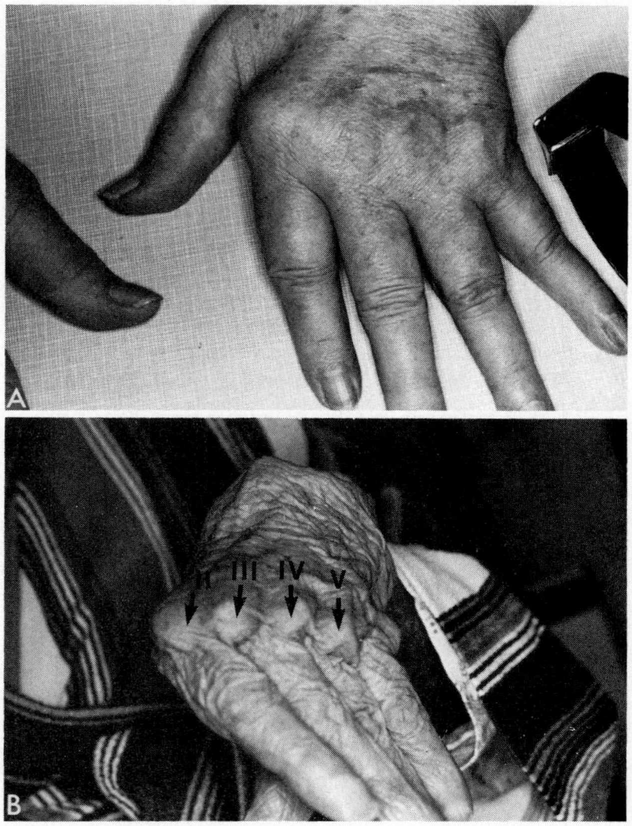


**Figure 60–7.** *A,* Early ulnar deviation of the metacarpophalangeal joints without subluxation. Extensor tendons have slipped to the ulnar side. The fifth finger, in particular, is compromised with weak flexion, causing loss of power grip. *B,* Complete subluxation with marked ulnar deviation at the metacarpophalangeal joints of a 90-year-old woman with RA. Arrows mark the heads of the metacarpals, now in direct contact with the joint capsule instead of the proximal phalanges. (Courtesy of James L. McGuire, M.D.)

**Table 60–9.** Prevalence of Para-Articular Disorders Associated with RA*

| Patients | Flexor Tenosynovitis | Without Flexor Tenosynovitis |
|---|---|---|
| Number of patients | 55 | 45 |
| Carpal tunnel syndrome | 26 | 6 |
| Extensor tenosynovitis | 26 | 4 |
| Epicondylitis | 12 | 3 |
| Dupuytren's contracture | 6 | 0 |
| De Quervain's tenosynovitis | 5 | 0 |
| Flexor carpi radialis tendinitis | 7 | 0 |
| Flexor carpi ulnaris tendinitis | 2 | 0 |
| Achilles tendinitis | 5 | 0 |

*Adapted from Gray, R.C., and Gottlieb, N.L.: Arthritis Rheum. 20:1003, 1977.

manifestations) (Table 60–9).[187] De Quervain's tenosynovitis is particularly important to diagnose because it causes severe discomfort and yet is relatively easily treated. It represents extensor tenosynovitis in the thumb extensors. Pain originating from these sheaths can be demonstrated by Finklestein's test: ulnar flexion at the wrist after the thumb is maximally flexed and adducted. Pain on this maneuver is indicative of de Quervain's tenosynovitis. Many factors may lead to loss of hand strength in patients with RA (Table 60–10). Tenosynovitis rather than articular synovitis is probably the most significant of these factors.[188]

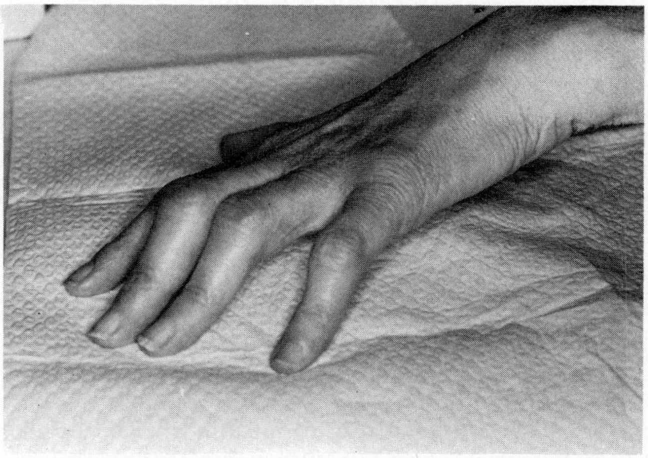

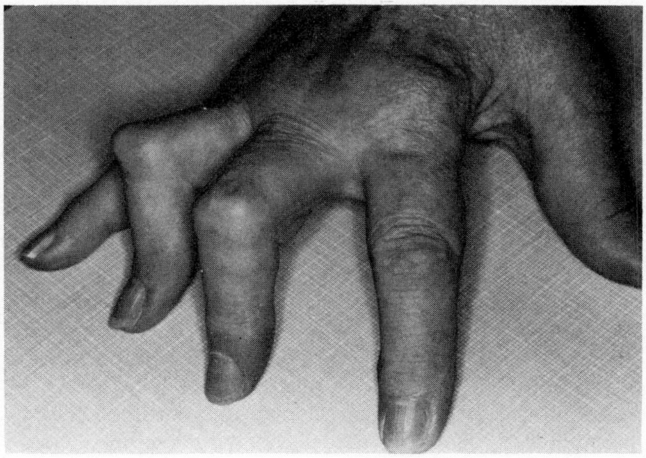

**Figure 60–9.** Early (*A*) and late (*B*) "boutonnière" deformity of the phalanges in RA. In *B*, moderate soft tissue swellings at the second and third metacarpophalangeal joints are visible.

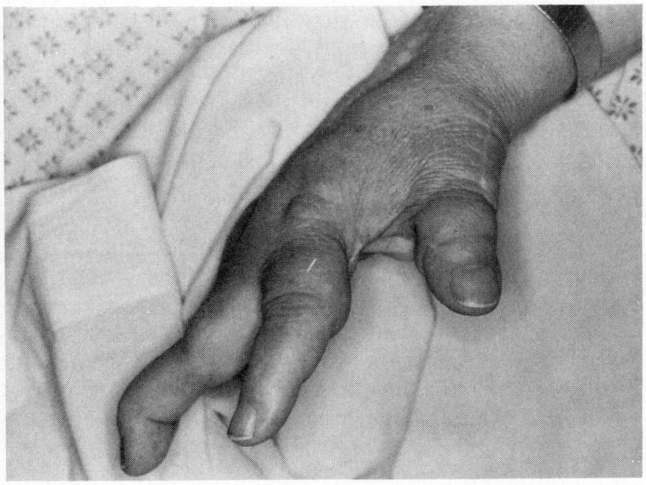

**Figure 60–8.** Multiple deformities of the hand in severe rheumatoid arthritis. This 60-year-old woman has had wrist surgery (dorsal synovectomy and resection of the ulnar head). The bones of the thumb have been destroyed and partially resorbed, producing redundant skin and a short digit ("main en lorgnette"). Hyperextension at the proximal interphalangeal joints with flexion of the distal interphalangeal joints, as in the third finger of her hand, are characteristic of the swan neck deformity. (Courtesy of James L. McGuire, M.D.).

Not infrequently, rheumatoid nodules will develop within the tendons, and they may "lock" the finger painfully into flexion, necessitating surgical excision or glucocorticoid injections when they become chronic and recurrent. If flexor tenosynovitis reduces active motion, peritendinous and pericapsular adhesions may develop secondarily and limit proximal interphalangeal joint motion.[188]

**Table 60–10.** Factors Diminishing Hand Grasp Strength in RA

1. Synovitis in joints
2. Reflex inhibition of muscular contraction secondary to pain
3. Altered kinesiology; distorted relation of joint, bones, and tendons during motion
4. Flexor tenosynovitis, with or without rheumatoid nodules on tendons
5. Vascular ischemia → pain; from altered sympathetic tone
6. Edema of all structures, from inflammation and perhaps altered lymphatic drainage
7. Intrinsic muscle atrophy and/or fibrosis

Often hands are painful in RA without much evidence for inflammation. It has been suggested that ischemia secondary to vascular spasm from excess sympathetic tone may contribute to hand pain, particularly during grasp motion.[189] The improvement in peripheral hemodynamics following administration of propranolol has suggested that this claudication may be mediated primarily by beta-adrenergic receptors.[190]

Although classic teaching describes an absence of distal interphalangeal joint involvement in RA, some careful observations have found distal interphalangeal joint tenderness in the hands of up to 70 percent of patients with RA at some time during the course of their disease.

**Hip.** The hip is less frequently involved in adult forms of RA than in juvenile RA, and clinical involvement is difficult to evaluate if pain is not present. Pain on the lateral aspect of the hip is often a manifestation of trochanteric bursitis rather than synovitis, which usually produces pain or tenderness in the groin.

About half the patients with established RA will have radiographic evidence of hip disease.[191] The femoral head may collapse and be resorbed, while the acetabulum often remodels as it is pushed medially, leading to protrusio acetabuli. Significant protrusion occurs in about 5 percent of all patients with RA.[192] Loss of internal rotation on physical examination correlates best with radiographic findings. Similar to other weight-bearing joints, the femoral head may develop cystic lesions. Communication of these with the joint space can often be demonstrated on surgically resected femoral heads.[193] Radiography of the pelvis rarely shows localized erosions of the lower part of the sacroiliac joint in RA, a phenomenon probably associated with localized granuloma formation. Synovial cysts can develop around the hip joint. Communication between the iliopsoas bursa and the hip joint facilitates formation of a cyst that appears within the pelvis and can be large enough to obstruct venous return from the extremity.[194]

**Knees.** In contrast to the hips, synovial inflammation and proliferation are readily demonstrated. Synovial fluid in excess of 5 ml may be demonstrated by the "bulge" sign: milking fluid from the lateral superior recess of the joint across to the medial side, producing a fluid wave across the normally concave area inferomedial to the patella.[195] Very early in knee disease, often within a week after onset of symptoms, quadriceps atrophy is noticeable and may lead to the application of more force than usual through the patella to the femoral surface. Another early manifestation of knee disease in RA is loss of full extension, a functional loss that can become a fixed flexion contracture unless remedies are undertaken to correct it.[196]

Flexion of the knee markedly increases the intra-articular pressure (see Chapter 59) and may produce an outpouching of posterior components of the joint space, a popliteal or Baker's cyst. Jayson and Dixon have demonstrated that fluid from the anterior compartments of the knee may enter the popliteal portion but not readily return.[197] This one-way valve may produce pressures so high in the popliteal space that it may rupture down into the calf or, rarely, superiorly into the posterior thigh. Rupture occurs posteriorly between the medial head of the gastrocnemius and the tendinous insertion of the biceps. Clinically, popliteal cysts and complications of them may present in several ways (Table 60–11). The intact popliteal cyst may compress superficial venous flow through to the upper part of the leg, producing dilation of superficial veins and/or edema. Rupture of the joint posteriorly with dissection of joint fluid into the calf may resemble acute thrombophlebitis with swelling and tenderness, as well as systemic signs of fever and leukocytosis. One helpful sign in joint rupture may be the appearance of a crescentic hematoma beneath one of the malleoli.[198] Part of the examination of rheumatoid patients should include observation from the rear while the patient stands. This often increases the observation of popliteal cysts. Ultrasound evaluation is a useful way to assess popliteal swelling and usually obviates the need for arthrography in these patients.[199]

Very often, radiographic evidence for destruction of the knee lags behind clinical evidence for it. It is important to assess the thickness of articular cartilage radiographically by taking films with the patient in a standing position. The proliferative destructive synovitis in RA may destroy meniscal cartilage and cruciate ligaments. Tests for lateral and anteroposterior stability will indicate the extent of damage to these structures before gross deformity or incongruity is visible.

**Ankle and Foot.** The ankle joint is involved less often than the knee in RA, but probably is a better measure of severe disease than is the knee; the ankle is rarely involved in mild or oligoarticular RA, but often is damaged in severe progressive forms of the disease. Clinical evidence for ankle involvement is soft, occasionally cystic, swelling anterior and posterior to the malleoli (Fig. 60–10). Much of the stability of the ankle depends upon integrity of ligaments holding the fibula to the tibia and these two bones to the talus. In RA, inflammatory and proliferative disease may loosen these connections by stretching and eroding the collagenous ligaments. The result is incongruity, which, once initiated, progresses to pronation deformities or eversion of the foot (Fig. 60–11).

The Achilles tendon is a major structural component and kinetic force in the foot and ankle. Rheumatoid nodules develop in this collagenous structure, and spontaneous rupture of the tendon has been reported when diffuse granulomatous inflammation is present.[203] The subtalar joint controls eversion and inversion of the foot on the talus, and is involved commonly in RA. Patients with RA invariably have more pain while walking on

**Table 60–11.** Differential Diagnosis of Popliteal Cysts[200-202]

| | |
|---|---|
| Lipoma | Hemangioma |
| Xanthoma | Lymphadenopathy |
| Fibrosarcoma | Charcot joint |
| Vascular tumor | Thrombophlebitis |
| Varicose veins | |

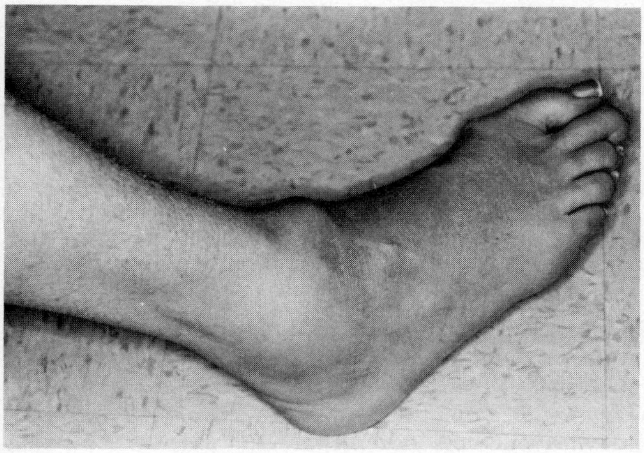

**Figure 60–10.** Marked synovial proliferation in the ankle joint of a 43-year-old woman with RA. (Courtesy of James L. McGuire, M.D.).

uneven ground, and this is related to the relatively common subtalar joint involvement in RA.[204]

More than one third of patients with RA have significant disease in the feet.[205] The foot in RA widens as the angle between metacarpals increases. Metatarsophalangeal joints are involved often, and gait is altered as pain develops during push-off in striding. It is of interest that the metatarsal heads sublux downward very soon after the metatarsophalangeal joints become involved, producing "cock-up" toe deformities (Fig. 60–12*A*). Hallux valgus and bunion-callus formation appear if disease continues (Fig. 60–12*B*). Cystic collections often develop under the metatarsophalangeal joints and occasionally represent outpouchings of flexor tendon sheaths.[206] Patients whose metatarsal heads sublux to the subcutaneous area may develop pressure necrosis. Alternatively, patients who have subluxed metatarsophalangeal joints often develop pressure necrosis over the proximal interphalangeal joints that protrude dorsally ("hammer toes") and are subject to irritation by shoes. An extensive discussion of RA and the foot is presented in Chapter 31.

The sequence of changes as disease progresses in the foot is as follows:[207,208] (1) intermetatarsal joint ligaments stretch; (2) spread of the forefoot occurs; (3) the fibrofatty cushion on the plantar surface migrates anteriorly; (4) toes sublux dorsally and extensor tendons shorten; (5) metatarsal heads sublux to a subcutaneous site on the plantar surface; and (6) development of hallux valgus often results in "stacking" of the second and third toes on top of the great toe. It is important to note that distal interphalangeal joints of the foot rarely are affected in rheumatoid arthritis.

Whereas Achilles tendinitis and plantar fasciitis are the principal causes of foot pain in patients with Reiter's syndrome or ankylosing spondylitis, patients with RA are more likely to develop plantar faciitis without Achilles tendinitis. Sub-Achilles bursitis is characterized by a tender mass bulging to the sides of the tendon and is found principally in women. A valgus deformity of the heel is the most characteristic change of the hindfoot in RA and develops along with instability of the mortise joint.

Another cause of foot pain in rheumatoid patients is the tarsal tunnel syndrome. In a group of 30 patients with RA, radiographically demonstrated erosions in the feet, and foot pain, 4 (13 percent) were shown by electrodiagnostic techniques to have slowing of medical

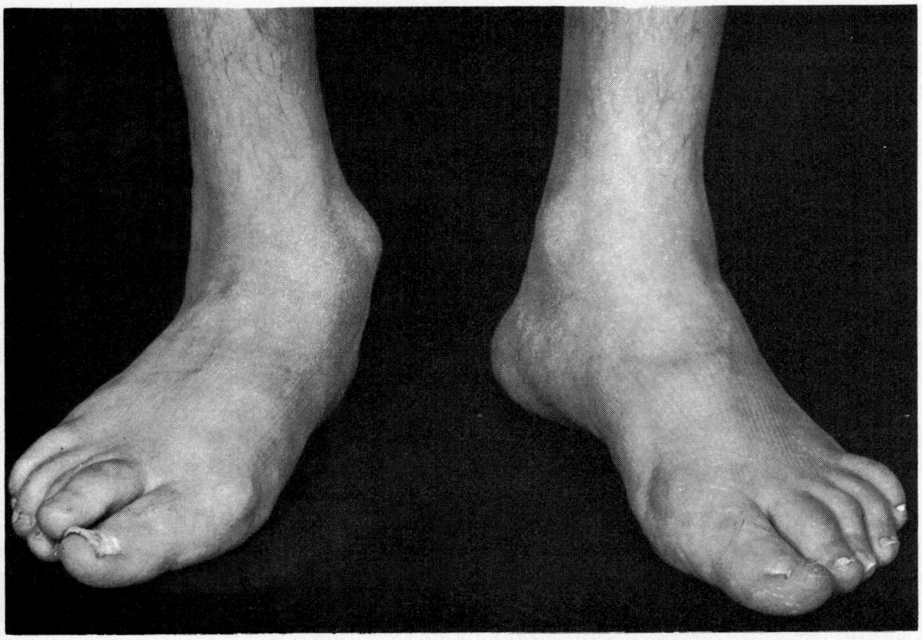

**Figure 60–11.** Valgus of ankle, pes planus, and forefoot varus deformity of the left foot related to painful synovitis of the ankle, forefoot, and metatarsophalangeal joint in a 24-year-old man with severe RA.

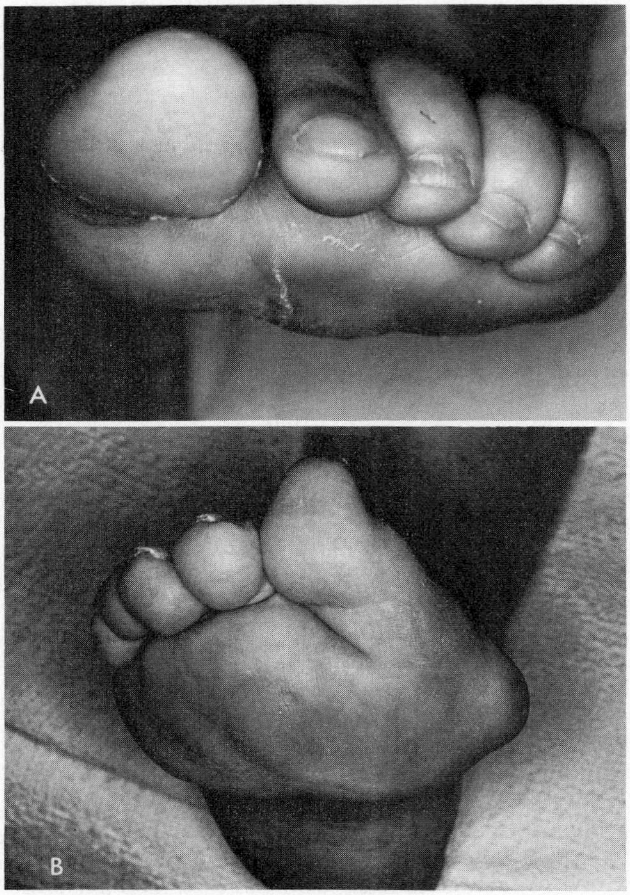


**Figure 60–12.** Foot problems in RA. *A*, Discrete cystic proliferation below subluxed metatarsal heads (2 and 3) in the foot of a patient with RA. *B*, Marked hallux valgus with proliferative tissue in the form of a "bunion" at the first metatarsophalangeal joint in a patient with RA. There is, in addition, diffuse cystic swelling below the metatarsal heads. (Courtesy of James L. McGuire, M.D.)

and/or lateral plantar nerve latency.[209] Clinically, these patients are difficult to distinguish from those with foot pain but without compression neuropathy.

**Bone.** Bones are involved in RA at more sites than the bone ends, where erosion by proliferative synovium occurs.

The para-articular osteopenia that accompanies persistent synovitis is an early sign that proliferative disease sufficient to result in significant destruction of joints is present. Long bones distant from joints also become involved in RA. Almost all patients with far-advanced long-standing RA develop diffuse demineralization of the entire skeleton.[210] Older age, the predominance of females in all groups of patients with RA, and the use of corticosteroids in treatment all potentiate the development of osteopenia.[211] Related to, and a possible cause of, this osteopenia are dietary deficiencies of both calcium and vitamin D.[212] All these factors combine to produce a much higher frequency of insufficiency (e.g., stress) fractures of long bones in this disease.[212,213,215] The fibula is the most common site of fracture. The frequency of fracture has been increasing as the number of total joint prostheses are inserted and as patients formerly bedridden are now able to walk. Careful assays have shown an increased excretion of hydroxyproline by patients with active rheumatoid arthritis not treated with glucocorticoids.[214] Urinary hydroxyproline reflects bone matrix breakdown and correlates positively with the 24-hour whole-body retention of $^{99m}$Tc methylene dephosphonate (an index of bone metabolism) and global index of disease activity.

**Muscle.** Clinical weakness is common in RA, but is it caused by muscle involvement by the rheumatoid process or is it a reflex weakness response to pain? Most rheumatoid patients have muscle weakness, but few have muscle tenderness. An exception to this is the occasional patient with a severe flare of active disease; such a patient may cry out in severe pain, unable to move either muscles or joints. These symptoms resemble vascular insufficiency (ischemic pain) in their intensity.

In an early autopsy series, focal accumulations of lymphocytes and plasma cells with some contiguous degeneration of muscle fibers were found in all rheumatoid patients and named "nodular myositis."[216] More recent and sophisticated studies[217] of patients with definite and classic RA revealed four groups of neuromuscular abnormalities: (1) chronic myopathy resembling a dystrophic process, probably the endstage of a myositis (8 cases); (2) diminution of muscle bulk, with atrophy of type II muscle fibers similar to that described in cachexia (13 cases); (3) peripheral neuropathy, possibly demyelinating (9 cases); and (4) steroid myopathy (4 cases). Each of these types of muscle pathology is overshadowed by serious joint disease when it is present. In most patients, muscle symptoms are not predominant.

## Extra-Articular Complications of Rheumatoid Arthritis

Unlike joint disease per se, the complications of RA may be fatal. In general, the number and severity of extra-articular features vary with the duration and severity[218,219] of the disease. Some of these factors will be discussed under Prognosis.

Ocular and dermatologic complications will not be discussed in detail here; these are presented in the context of other manifestations in those organ systems in Chapters 35 and 36, respectively. Nerve compression syndromes commonly seen in RA are outlined in Chapter 110.

The interest in these extra-articular manifestations is enhanced by realization that RA is a systemic process, and that each organ and tissue reacts in a unique way to what is presumed to be the same inciting factor.

**Rheumatoid Nodules.** The pathology of rheumatoid nodules is well documented.[220,221] In the well-formed nodule there is a central area of necrosis rimmed by a corona of palisading fibroblasts that is surrounded by a collagenous capsule with perivascular collections of chronic inflammatory cells.

Careful histology of early lesions[222] has suggested that development of the nodule is mediated through affected small arterioles and the terminal vascular bed of tissues; small vessels proliferate, and this is associated with proliferation of resident histiocytes and fibroblasts, as well as an influx of monocytes and lymphocytes. The nodule tissue in organ culture has the capacity to produce collagenase and proteinase in large quantity, similar to synovial tissue.[223] It has been suggested that these enzymes released by the palisading layer of cells may be sufficient to result in destruction of the extracellular matrix collagen around the cells, leading to their death and a centrifugally expanding central necrosis commonly found in these nodules.

Occurring in 20 to 35 percent of patients with definite or classic RA, nodules are found most easily on extensor surfaces such as the olecranon process and the proximal ulna (Fig. 60–13*A*). They are subcutaneous and vary in consistency from a soft, amorphous, entirely mobile mass to firm rubber masses attached firmly to periosteum.

Rheumatoid factor is almost always found in the serum of patients with rheumatoid nodules. Rarely, such nodules are present without obvious arthritis.[224] Multiple nodules on the hands in the absence of clinical arthritis but with a positive test for rheumatoid factor has been called "rheumatoid nodulosis."[225,226] The differential diagnosis of rheumatoid nodules includes the five following types.

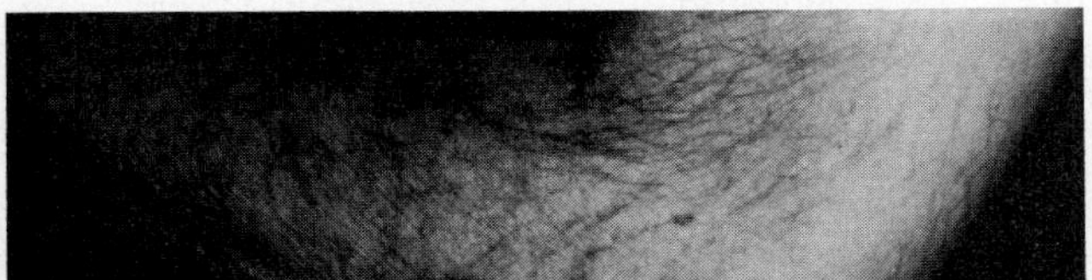

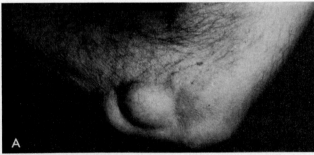

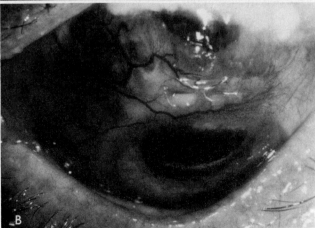


**Figure 60–13.** Manifestations of increased reactivity of mesenchymal tissue in rheumatoid arthritis appearing (*A*) as nodules on the elbow and (*B*) within the sclera of the eye. The eye lesion represents scleral perforation associated with a granulomatous scleral reaction. Treatment was placement of a scleral patch graft. Note the great increase in vascularity of the sclera. The dark areas represent scleral thinning with exposure of uveal pigment. (Patient of Drs. S. Arthur Bouchoff and G. N. Fouhls. Photograph courtesy of Marty Schener.)

***"Benign" Nodules.*** These usually are found in healthy children without rheumatoid factor or arthritis; they are nontender, appear often on the pretibial regions, feet, and scalp, increase rapidly in size, and are histologically identical to rheumatoid nodules.[227] They resolve spontaneously.

***Granuloma Annulare.*** These nodules are intracutaneous but histologically identical to rheumatoid nodules. They slowly resolve, and are not associated with other disease.[228]

***Xanthomatosis.*** These nodules usually have a yellow tinge, and patients have abnormally high plasma lipoproteins and cholesterol. There is no underlying bone involvement.

***Tophi.*** These collections of monosodium urate crystals have small, punched-out bone lesions associated with them and are rarely found in patients with a normal serum urate. A search for crystals with a polarizing microscope will reveal the classic needle-shaped, negatively birefringent crystals.

***Miscellaneous.*** The nodules of multicentric reticulohistiocytosis have been described (see the preceding Differential Diagnosis of Rheumatoid Arthritis). Numerous proliferative disorders affecting cutaneous tissue, including erythema elevatum diutinum, acrodermatitis chronica atrophicans, bejel, yaws, pinta, and leprosy, can resemble rheumatoid nodule.[229] A rheumatoid nodule, particularly when it occurs on the face, may simulate basal cell carcinoma.[230]

Appearance of nodules in unusual sites may lead to confusion in diagnosis. Sacral nodules may be mistaken for bedsores if the skin overlying them breaks down.[231] Occipital nodules also occur in bedridden patients. In the larynx, rheumatoid nodules on the vocal cords may cause progressive hoarseness.[232] Nodules found in the heart and lungs will be discussed below. A nodule in the eye is shown in Figure 60–13*B*.

**Fistula Development.** The rare development of cutaneous sinuses near joints occurs in seropositive patients with long-standing disease and positive tests for rheumatoid factor.[233] These fistulae can be either sterile or septic, and connect the skin surface either with a joint or with a para-articular cyst in bone or soft tissues.[234] The pathogenesis of fistulae without a septic origin is particularly difficult to understand because the rheumatoid process is usually so clearly centripetal in nature, that is, progressing toward the center of the joint, rather than centrifugal.

**Infection.** Infections have paralleled the use of corticosteroids and immunosuppressive agents as a complication of RA.[235] Pulmonary infections, skin sepsis, and pyarthrosis are most common.[236-238] In addition to the presence of drugs that suppress host resistance, the phagocytic capacity of leukocytes in RA may be less than normal.[239] Difficulty in diagnosis is accentuated by the similarity of aggressive RA to infection, particularly in joints. A full discussion of sepsis in RA is presented in Chapter 96.

**Hematologic Abnormalities.** The majority of patients with RA have a mild normocytic hypochromic anemia, which correlates with the erythrocyte sedimentation rate and with activity of the disease.[240-241] Hemoglobin rarely drops below 10 grams per dl in RA unless there is another contributing factor such as blood loss. Study of the dynamics in development of this anemia have confirmed early studies that this is an anemia of chronic disease related to ineffective erythropoiesis.[241-243] It is characterized by a low serum iron, a low total iron-binding capacity, and normal reticuloendothelial iron stores (except, for unknown reasons, in Felty's syndrome, in which iron stores may be absent). The mean red cell life is slightly shortened. Total erythroid heme turnover is slightly reduced, and ineffective erythropoiesis accounts for a much greater than normal percentage of total heme turnover. These patients also may demonstrate a diminished ability to absorb iron through the gastrointestinal tract, which is usually related to the irritative presence of one or another anti-inflammatory medications.[244] The presence or absence of stainable iron in the marrow of patients with RA may correlate approximately with serum ferritin levels alone.[245] By addition of the mean corpuscular volume and the erythrocyte sedimentation rate to the equation in a computer program, iron stores (presence or absence) can be predicted in 95 percent of patients. The remaining 5 percent identified by the computer will need bone marrow examination.[246] In contrast to anemia associated with blood loss, the ineffective erythropoiesis will return to normal if remission can be induced in RA. The ineffective erythropoesis is not related to "functional" iron deficiency (i.e., reduced availability of iron).[247]

Eosinophilia and thrombocytosis are often associated with RA. Eosinophilia (5 percent of total white blood cell count or greater) was observed in 40 percent of patients selected for having severe seropositive disease.[248] Similarly, a significant relationship has been shown to exist between thrombocytosis and extra-articular manifestations of rheumatoid disease.[249] This may be related in part to an increase in platelet production associated with active intravascular coagulation.

One of the most significant hematologic complications of RA, Felty's syndrome, is discussed in Chapter 61.

**Vasculitis.** In one sense, it is redundant to think of vasculitis as a complication of RA, since the initial pathology in RA is believed to rest in small blood vessels. However, it is useful to use the term vasculitis to group those extra-articular complications not related to proliferative granulomas but rather to inflammatory vascular disease.

Clinical vasculitis usually takes one or another of the following forms: (1) distal arteritis (ranging from splinter hemorrhages to gangrene); (2) cutaneous ulceration (including pyoderma gangrenosum); (3) peripheral neuropathy; (4) pericarditis; (5) arteritis of viscera, including heart, lungs, bowel, kidney, liver, spleen, pancreas, lymph nodes, and testis; (6) acro-osteolysis; or (7) palpable purpura.

The pathology in rheumatoid vasculitis is that of a panarteritis. All layers of the vessel wall are infiltrated with mononuclear cells. Fibrinoid necrosis is seen in very active lesions. Intimal proliferation may predispose to thrombosis. When larger vessels are involved, the pathology resembles that of polyarteritis nodosa.[250] In addition, a venulitis associated with RA has been described.[251,252] In patients with hypocomplementemia the cellular infiltrate around the vessels contains neutrophils; in normocomplementemic patients, lymphocytes predominate.[252] Uninvolved skin from rheumatoid patients is positive for immunoglobulin and complement when sections for histopathology are stained with fluorescein-labeled antibodies to these components. The presence of IgG correlates directly with circulating immune complexes, vasculitic skin lesions, subcutaneous nodules and high titer rheumatoid factor.[253]

It is unusual for vasculitis to be active in any but the sickest patients, those with severe deforming arthritis and high titers of rheumatoid factor. Supporting the hypothesis that vascular injury is mediated by deposition of circulating immune complexes are the data indicating (1) depressed levels of C2 and C4;[254] (2) hypercatabolism of C3;[255] (3) deposition of IgG, IgM, and C3 in involved arteries;[256] and (4) the presence of large amounts of cryoimmunoglobulins in serum of patients with vasculitis.[257]

Neurovascular disease may be the only manifestation of vasculitis. The two common clinical patterns are a mild distal sensory neuropathy and a severe sensorimotor neuropathy (mononeuritis multiplex).[258] The latter form is characterized by severe arterial damage on nerve biopsy specimens. Symptoms of the milder form may be paresthesias or "burning feet" in association with decreased touch and pin sensation distally. Patients with mononeuritis multiplex have weakness (e.g., foot drop) in addition to sensory abnormalities. Symptoms and signs are identical to those found in polyarteritis. Rheumatoid pachymeningitis is a rare complication of RA. Confined to the dura and pia meter, this process may be limited to certain areas (e.g., lumbar cord and/or cisternae, etc).[259] Elevated IgG (including IgM and IgG rheumatoid factors allow molecular weight IgM) and immune complexes are found in the CSF.

Although there is a negative association between psychosis and RA, it is possible that organic brain syndromes may be related to RA in patients not taking corticosteroids or indomethacin,[263] and it is presumed that these manifestations are caused by small vessel disease.

Visceral lesions present generally as claudication or infarction of the organ supplied by the involved arteries. Intestinal involvement with vasculitis presents as abdominal pain, at first intermittent, progressing often to continuous pain and a tender, quiet belly on examination. If infarction develops, resection must be accomplished promptly.[260] Early studies of rheumatoid vasculitis implied that glucocorticoid therapy might be responsible for precipitating vasculitis in rheumatoid patients. A sudden reduction or cessation of glucocorticoid therapy also has been implicated as a precipitating cause of vasculitis.[261] A more recent large study, however, showed no relationship to steroid dose and vasculitis.[262]

Clinical features associated with a poor prognosis in rheumatoid vasculitis are renal impairment, intestinal vasculitis, neuropathy, weight loss, and histological evidence of vasculitis on rectal biopsy.[264]

The kidney is an example of an organ that is rarely involved directly in RA but often is compromised indirectly. Amyloidosis (see Chapter 92) is a complication of chronic RA. Another indirect cause of renal disease is toxicity from therapy. Phenacetin abuse causes renal papillary necrosis, and salicylates may cause abnormalities as well.[265] A membranous nephropathy is the pathologic lesion related to therapy with gold salts and D-penicillamine, but a long-term study has suggested that perhaps membranous nephropathy is related to the underlying disease and that gold treatment may exacerbate the underlying process.[266] This remains to be confirmed. Rarely, a focal necrotizing glomerulitis is seen in patients dying with disseminated vasculitis.[267]

**Pulmonary Disease.** There are five forms of lung disease in RA: (1) pleural disease, (2) interstitial fibrosis, (3) nodular lung disease, (4) pneumonitis, and (5) arteritis.

***Pleural Disease.*** Pleuritis is very commonly found at autopsy of patients with RA, but clinical disease during life is seen less frequently.[268] Characteristics of the rheumatoid effusions are as follows: glucose = 10 to 50 mg per dL; protein = 4 g per dL; cells = 1000 to 3500 (mononuclear) per cu mm; lactic dehydrogenase = elevated; $CH_{50}$ = depressed.

The low glucose concentrations are of interest. Sepsis (particularly tuberculosis) is the only other condition that commonly has such a low synovial fluid glucose. An impaired transport of glucose into the pleural space appears to be the cause.[269]

***Interstitial Fibrosis.*** The increased reactivity of mesenchymal cells in RA is believed to be the cause of pulmonary fibrosis in this disease. Similar to findings in scleroderma, physical findings are of fine diffuse dry rales. Radiographs show a diffuse reticular or reticulonodular pattern in both lung fields,[270,271] which develop a "honeycomb" appearance. The pathologic findings are those of diffuse fibrosis in the midst of a mononuclear cell infiltrate.[272] The principal functional defect is impairment of alveolar-capillary gas exchange with decreased diffusion capacity, which is best measured utilizing single-breath carbon monoxide diffusion capacities.[273] In a prospective study of 155 rheumatoids and 95 control subjects, rheumatoids showed an increased frequency of chest crackles and abnormal chest radiographs and restrictive ventilatory defects. These abnormalities were associated with smoking.[274] It is likely that rheumatoids who smoke are at a higher risk for fibrotic complications in the lungs than are those in the general population.

***Nodular Lung Disease.*** Pulmonary nodules may appear singly or in clusters that coalesce. Single ones appear as a coin lesion and, when significant peripheral arthritis and nodules are present, can be diagnosed by needle biopsy without thoracotomy. Caplan's syndrome,[275] in which pneumoconiosis and RA are synergistic and produce a violent fibroblastic reaction with obliterative granulomatous fibrosis, becomes a much less frequent occurrence as the respiratory environment in mining operations improves. Nodules may cavitate and create a bronchopleural fistula,[276] and may even precede arthritis.[277]

***Pneumonitis.*** Very rare is an interstitial pneumonitis that progresses to alveolar involvement, respiratory insufficiency, and death. Pathologic studies show a very cellular loose fibrosis and proteinaceous exudate in alveoli (Fig. 60–14).

***Arteritis.*** Pulmonary hypertension from arteritis of the pulmonary vasculature is very rare and is occasionally associated with digital arteritis.[278]

**Cardiac Complications.** Cardiac disease in RA can take many forms related to granulomatous proliferation or vasculitis. Involvement can be classified as follows: (1) pericarditis, (2) myocarditis (rheumatoid carditis), (3) endocardial (valve) inflammation, (4) conduction defects, (5) coronary arteritis, and (6) granulomatous aortitis.

***Pericarditis.*** Infrequently diagnosed by history and physical examination in RA, pericarditis is present in up to 50 percent of patients at autopsy.[279,280] Use of echocardiography has enabled much more precise assessment of cardiac structure and function in patients with RA. In one study, 31 percent had echocardiographic evidence of pericardial effusion. The same study revealed only rare evidence for impaired left ventricular function in prospectively studied outpatients with RA.[281] Although unusual, cardiac tamponade with constrictive pericarditis develops in RA and may require pericardectomy.[282,283] This complication appears to be more frequent after sudden reduction of glucocorticoid treatment. Pericarditis usually develops after RA is established, but it may precede the arthritis. Most patients have a positive test for rheumatoid factor, and half will have nodules.

***Myocarditis.*** This complication can take the form of either granulomatous disease or interstitial myocarditis. The granulomatous process resembles subcutaneous nodules[284] and could be considered specific for the disease. Diffuse infiltration of the myocardium by mononuclear cells, on the other hand, may involve the entire myocardium and yet have no clinical manifestations.[280]

***Endocardial Inflammation.*** Echocardiographic studies have reported conflicting evidence for previously undiagnosed mitral valve disease diagnosed by a reduced E to F slope of the anterior leaflet of the mitral valve.[285,286] Although aortic valve disease and arthritis are generally associated through ankylosing spondylitis, a number of granulomatous nodules in the valve have been reported.[287] Aortic valve replacement has been successful in these cases.

Conduction defects such as atrioventricular block are

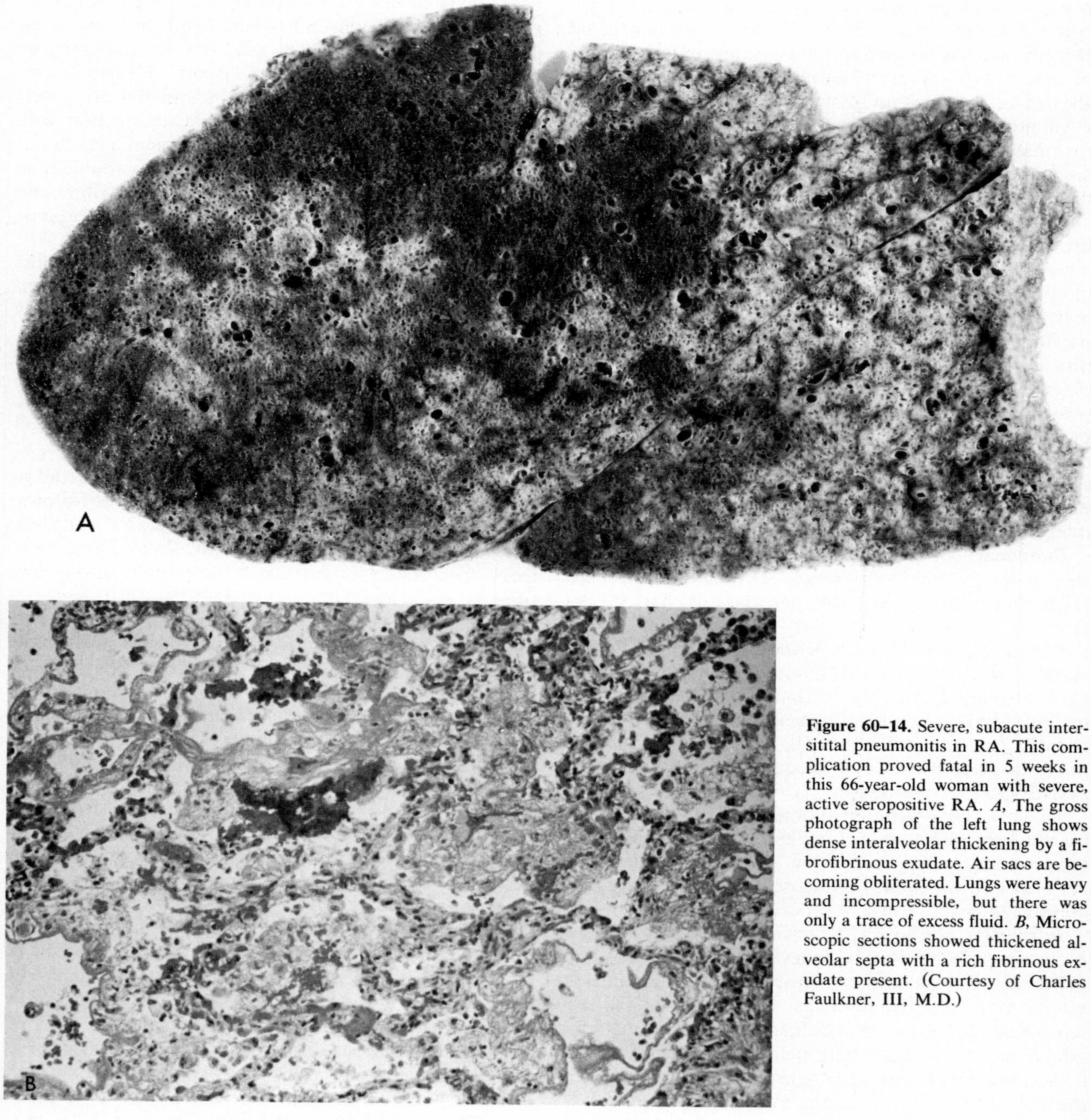


**Figure 60–14.** Severe, subacute interstitial pneumonitis in RA. This complication proved fatal in 5 weeks in this 66-year-old woman with severe, active seropositive RA. *A,* The gross photograph of the left lung shows dense interalveolar thickening by a fibrofibrinous exudate. Air sacs are becoming obliterated. Lungs were heavy and incompressible, but there was only a trace of excess fluid. *B,* Microscopic sections showed thickened alveolar septa with a rich fibrinous exudate present. (Courtesy of Charles Faulkner, III, M.D.)

rare in RA but are probably related to direct granulomatous involvement. The pathology may reveal proliferative lesions[284] or healed scars.[288]

Patients with severe RA and active vasculitis who develop a myocardial infarction are very likely to have coronary arteritis as a basis for the process.[289]

In severe rheumatoid heart disease, granulomatous disease can be found to spread to involve even the base of the aorta.[290]

## PROGNOSIS IN RHEUMATOID ARTHRITIS

**Natural History of RA.** Epidemiologists have pointed out the multiple difficulties in attempting to establish change in patterns of RA in different time periods or different communities. The best data suggest that patients currently admitted to the hospital for RA are likely to have fewer joint contractures and less ankylosis of peripheral joints at admission than did patients admitted 20 years ago, whereas the prevalence of rheumatoid factor, subcutaneous nodules, and the mean number of affected joints has, if anything, increased slightly.[291] These and other data suggest that the disease is not changing, but that earlier, more effective treatment has perhaps diminished the morbidity.

As with other chronic diseases, both physicians and their patients are eager to know the chances for remission and anxious about the threat of severe morbidity or death.

There are now well-tested criteria for a clinical remission.[292] Six criteria have yielded optimal discrimination (Table 60–12). Very few patients achieve 5 of 6 of these criteria, and thus very few rheumatoids, whether or not they are being treated, ever achieve true remission. Thus, it would be more logical to refer to gold and D-penicillamine as "disease-modifying drugs" rather than "remission-inducing" substances. Most series of rheumatoid patients are weighted by those with more severe disease who have well-established disease.[293] In contrast, a large number of patients given a diagnosis of RA go into complete remission, and probably should not have been considered initially to have RA.[11]

Death associated with RA is generally associated with the complications—both articular and extra-articular—of RA. The probability of these deaths varies directly with the severity of complications. Such potentially morbid articular complications include the various forms of atlantoaxial subluxation, cricoarytenoid synovitis, and sepsis of involved joints. Extra-articular complications directly causing a higher mortality rate include Felty's syndrome (possible death from overwhelming infection), Sjögren's syndrome, cardiopulmonary complications, diffuse vasculitis, and amyloidosis. Infection has been one of the most common contributing factors to death in rheumatoid patients.[293-295]

Aside from the occurrence of death as an outcome in RA, there are a number of other variables in the disease that have been related to prognosis.

**Presentation of Arthritis.** ***Good Prognosis.*** Several investigators have observed that a clinical subgroup of patients with an acute, explosive onset of disease or early rapid progression of symptoms do better in the long run than do patients with an insidious onset of disease.[296-298]

**Table 60–12.** Preliminary Criteria for Complete Clinical Remission in Rheumatoid Arthritis

A minimum of five of the following requirements must be fulfilled for at least two consecutive months in a patient with definite or classic RA.

1. Morning stiffness not to exceed 15 minutes
2. No fatigue
3. No joint pain
4. No joint tenderness or pain on motion
5. No soft tissue swelling in joints or tendon sheaths
6. ESR (Westergren) less than 30 mm/hr (females) or 20 mm/hr (males)

Exclusions: Clinical manifestations of active vasculitis, pericarditis, pleuritis, or myositis and/or unexplained recent weight loss or fever secondary to RA prohibit a designation of complete clinical remission.[292]

**Table 60–13.** Comparative Mortality and Morbidity in Seronegative and Seropositive Patients*

| | Seronegative (Percent) | Seropositive (Percent) |
|---|---|---|
| Deaths | 15 | 27 |
| Remissions† | 70 | 38 |
| Vasculitis | 10 | 50 |

*From Kellgren, J.H., and O'Brien, W.M.: Arthritis Rheum. 5:115, 1962.

†In survivors.

Whether this is related to the patients coming earlier under good care or to other factors is unknown. However, a more recent study[299] of 235 patients in which an "acute" pattern of onset was present in 69 patients, intermediate in 55, and gradual in 111 revealed that radiologic destruction after 7 years from the beginning of the disease process was the same in each group, regardless of the rapidity of onset. Patients who evolve into RA from a palindromic type of presentation are reported to have a better prognosis.[300]

***Poor Prognosis.*** Patients with a disease of insidious onset appear to do less well than others, but this may be due in part to their relatively late presentation for good care.[301] Factor analysis of one series by computer[302] has revealed poorer prognosis for patients who have at once the patterns of large proximal joint involvement (shoulder, elbow, wrist, and knee) and disease in the first and second metatarsophalangeal joints.

**Rheumatoid Factor.** Many studies have confirmed that seropositivity is associated with a poorer prognosis in RA. One series of 60 patients with active disease showed the associations seen in Table 60–13.[303] Patients with rheumatoid factor have more involved joints when they present to a physician for the first time, and develop more erosions and ligamentous instability.[304,305] As mentioned previously, more and more of those individuals who carry a diagnosis of seronegative rheumatoid arthritis[306] are being recognized as having other classifiable entities.

**Rheumatoid Nodules.** These occur almost always in patients with rheumatoid factor, although without correlation with titer of rheumatoid factor.[293,304,305] Therefore, similar to those patients with rheumatoid factor alone, patients with subcutaneous nodules have a poorer outcome and more frequent bone erosions.[293,297,307]

**Sex.** In young adults developing RA, females generally have a worse outcome with more swollen and tender joints and erosions than do males.[304]

**Synovial Histopathology.** Although it is generally agreed that persistence and intensity of synovial inflammation are related to joint destruction, no single feature or group of features demonstrable by routine histopathologic examination of synovium has been correlated with destructive lesions in RA.[308,309] In part, this may be related to the major variations in histology found from area to area within the synovium,[310] a factor that makes histopathologic prognostication from synovial needle biopsy practically useless. A finding of cartilage erosion associated with synovial lining cell proliferation and few subsynovial lymphocytes[311] has not been confirmed.[308,309]

**Synovial Fluid Analysis (see Chapter 38).** Chemotactic factors in synovial fluid in RA attract PMN leukocytes, which accumulate and are eventually lysed within the joint space. It has been demonstrated that when the joint fluid leukocyte count exceeds 50,000 to 60,000 cells per cubic millimeter, proteinase inhibitors in the fluid can be saturated or inhibitors damaged or rendered effete, so that proteinase activity is manifest.[312] Human neutrophils have been found to generate an unusual class of oxidants with a long half-life (about 18 hours), which appear to be *N*-chloroamines. These substances have oxidizing potential sufficient to inactivate thio ether-containing proteinase inhibitors such as $\alpha_1$-proteinase inhibitor, and perhaps, $\alpha_2$-macroglobulin.[313] It is probable that at times such as these, proteinases act unopposed upon cartilage components. Acidosis of synovial fluid correlates with leukocyte counts in synovial fluid;[314] severe acidosis may alter cellular metabolism in cartilage and synovium. Depression of glucose and complement components in synovial fluid can be roughly correlated with the intensity of inflammation in the fluid,[315] and levels of IgG with the degree of subsynovial lymphocyte accumulation.[315]

**Other Laboratory Data.** A number of laboratory tests in addition to those for rheumatoid factor have prognostic significance.

*Eosinophilia.* Patients with RA and an associated eosinophilia of 5 percent or greater have a higher incidence of vasculitis, pleuropericarditis, pulmonary fibrosis, and subcutaneous nodules.[248] The hypothesis has been put forth that immune complexes may induce the eosinophilia and that therefore the latter may correlate better with vasculitis than other simple tests in RA.

*Thrombocytosis.* A highly significant correlation between platelet count and disease severity, and platelet count and extra-articular manifestations of RA, has been described.[249] An inverse correlation between platelet count and hemoglobin was found as well.

*Circulating Immune Complexes* Each assay for immune complexes appears to detect different components of immune complexes. For example, the C1q binding assay, which detects complexes containing IgM rheumatoid factor, correlates poorly with indices of disease activity in RA.[216] The C1q solid phase assay may better parallel the articular index in RA[317] but does not correlate as well as the ESR or IgG rheumatoid factor.

*C-Reactive Protein (CRP) (see Chapter 43).* In a recent series of 56 patients with RA, the measurement of both the erythrocyte sedimentation rate (ESR) and CRP correlated directly with erosive disease better than did other tests, including the presence of rheumatoid factor.[318] In another group of 99 patients the serum C reactive protein concentration closely reflected the activity of RA as judged by a new multivariate analysis comprising morning stiffness, pain scale, grip strength, articular index, hemoglobin, and the erythrocyte sedimentation rate (ESR).[319]Changes in CRP level cover a much broader range than changes in ESR and appear to occur more rapidly (24 hours) in contrast to ESR (days or weeks).

## Classification and Assessment in Rheumatoid Arthritis

The inflammatory lesion in RA is reflected reasonably well by heat, pain, swelling, and tenderness. Joint destruction can occur with minimal inflammation, however, and means to assess cartilage destruction are limited to radiographic determination of apparent joint space narrowing and erosions. A good noninvasive means to assess the erosive potential of synovitis does not exist, and until there are valid objective tests available to assess the proliferative lesion, clinical means of classification will be used. These are used frequently in drug studies and are reviewed in Chapter 48. The prototype for these has been Lansbury's systemic index, consisting of quick objective measurement of five features of activity in RA: morning stiffness, pain, fatigue, muscle weakness, and the ESR.[320,321]

Although easy to perform, the Lansbury indices and others like them have been difficult to standardize. One major difficulty is in the attempts to measure pain. As stated by Huskisson,[322] "The severity of pain is known only to the sufferer. . . . Pain is a personal psychological experience, and an observer can play no legitimate part in its direct measurement." For these reasons, direct (though subjective) measurement by a visual analogue scale is a good technique.

Classification of RA is best done by functional analysis. The criteria of Steinbrocker and associates[323] have long been used effectively (Table 60–14). It is appropriate to correlate functional class with an anatomic radiographic staging system[323] (Table 60–15). In evaluating the status of a particular patient, the physician can use, as a rough guide, the radiographic staging system as an index of whether the functional status of that individual is appropriate. For instance, if a functional Grade III patient has only Grade 2 radiographic

**Table 60–14.** Functional Capacity in RA*

| Grade | Definition | Remarks |
|---|---|---|
| I | Capable of all activities | |
| II | Moderate restriction | Adequate for normal activities despite handicap of discomfort or limited motion at one or more joints |
| III | Marked restriction | Activity limited to self-care and few or no duties of a usual occupation |
| IV | Bed and/or chair | Capable of little or no self-care |

*From Steinbrocker, O., et al.: JAMA 140:659, 1949.

**Table 60–15.** Radiographic Staging System for RA*

| Grade | Definition |
|---|---|
| 1 | No destructive changes; periarticular osteopenia may be present |
| 2 | Osteoporosis is definite, with or without slight subchondral bone destruction; slight joint space narrowing may be present |
| 3 | Evidence for cartilage and bond destruction; joint deformity (e.g., subluxation, ulnar deviation); no bony or fibrous ankylosis |
| 4 | Stage 3 criteria plus fibrous or bony ankylosis |

*From Steinbrocker, O., et al.: JAMA 140:659, 1949.

changes, it is likely that aggressive physical therapy and/or attention to care of nonarticular complications of the disease may improve functional status. Similarly, in treatment trials as well as with individual patients, it is essential to define when a remission has occurred. It is crucial to remember that if a patient with Grade 3 radiologic stages enters a complete remission, it still is unlikely that he or she would have a low Lansbury score or achieve Grade I functional status.

Care of the rheumatoid patient should include a careful record of the physical examination and functional and radiographic assessment. This permits care of patients in a prospective fashion and provides a systematic assessment of disease activity. With proper assessment, effective therapy, as outlined in Chapter 61, can be started, evaluated, and changed if necessary.

## References


1. Snorrason, E.: Landre-Beauvais and his goutte asthenique primitive. Acta Med. Scand. 142(Suppl. 266):115, 1952.
2. Boyle, J.A., and Buchanan, W.W.: Clinical Rheumatology. Philadelphia, F.A. Davis Company, 1971, pp. 71–72.
3. Short, C.L.: The antiquity of rheumatoid arthritis. Arthritis Rheum. 17:193, 1974.
4. Copeman, W.S.C.: A Short History of the Gout and the Rheumatic Diseases. Berkeley, University of California Press, 1964.
5. Soranus of Ephesus: On Acute Diseases and on Chronic Diseases. Translated into Latin by Caelius Aurelianus (5th century A.D.). English translation by I.E. Drabkin. Chicago, University of Chicago Press, 1950, pp. 923–929.
6. Ruffer, M.A., and Rietti, A.: On osseous lesions in ancient Egyptians. J. Pathol. Bacteriol. 16:439, 1912.
7. Ropes, M.W., Bennett, E.A., Cobb, S., Jacox, R., and Jessar, R.: 1958 Revision of diagnostic criteria for rheumatoid arthritis. Bull. Rheum. Dis. 9:175, 1958.
8. Wood, P.H.N.: Epidemiology of rheumatic disorders: Problems in classification. Proc. R. Soc. Med. 63:189, 1970.
9. Schumacher, H.R., and Kitridou, R.C.: Synovitis of recent onset. A clinicopathologic study during the first month of disease. Arthritis Rheum. 15:465, 1972.
10. Mitchell, D.M., and Fries, J.F.: An analysis of the American Rheumatism Association criteria for rheumatoid arthritis. Arthritis Rheum. 25:481, 1982.
11. Bennett, P.H., and Burch, T.A.: New York symposium on population studies in the rheumatic diseases: New diagnostic criteria. Bull. Rheum. Dis. 17:453, 1967.
12. O'Sullivan, J.B., and Cathcart, E.S. : The prevalence of rheumatoid arthritis. Follow-up evaluation of the effect of criteria on rates in Sudbury, Massachusetts. Ann. Intern. Med. 76:573, 1972.
13. Wolfe, A.M.: The epidemiology of rheumatoid arthritis: A review. Bull. Rheum. Dis. 19:518, 1968.
14. Engel, A., Roberts, J., and Burch, T.A.: Rheumatoid arthritis in adults in the United States 1960–1962. *In* Vital and Health Statistics, Series 11, Data from the National Health Survery, Number 17. Washington, D.C., National Center for Health Statistics, 1966.
15. Mikkelsen, W.M., Dodge, H.J., Duff, I.F., and Kato, I.H.: Estimates of the prevalence of rheumatic disease in the population of Tecumseh, Michigan, 1959–60. J. Chronic Dis. 20:351, 1967.
16. O'Brien, W.M., Bennett, P.H., Burch, T.A., et al.: A genetic study of rheumatoid arthritis and rheumatoid factor in Blackfeet and Pima Indians. Arthritis Rheum. 10:163, 1967.
17. Wood, W.J., Kato, H., Johnson, K.G., et al.: Rheumatoid arthritis in Hiroshima and Nagasaki, Japan. Arthritis Rheum. 10:21, 1967.
18. Beasley, R.P., Willkens, R.F., and Bennett, P.H.: High prevalence of rheumatoid arthritis in Yakima Indians. Arthritis Rheum. 16:743, 1973.
19. Harvey, J., Lotze, M., Arnett, F.C., et al.: Rheumatoid arthritis in a Chippewa band. II. Field study with clinical serologic and HLA-D correlations. J. Rheum. 10:28, 1983.
20. Solomon, L., Robin, G., and Valkenburg, H.A.: Rheumatoid arthritis in an urban South African Negro population. Ann. Rheum. Dis. 34:128, 1975.
21. Beighton, P., Solomon, L., and Valkenburg, H.A.: Rheumatoid arthritis in a rural South African Negro population. Ann. Rheum. Dis. 34:136, 1975.
22. Linos, A., Worthington, J.W., O'Fallon, W.M., and Kurland, L.T.: The epidemiology of rheumatoid arthritis in Rochester, Minnesota. A study of incidence, prevalence and mortality. Am. J. Epidemiol. 11:87–98, 1980.
23. Wingrave, S., and Kay, C.R.: Reduction in incidence of rheumatoid arthritis associated with oral contaceptives. Lancet 1:569, 1978.
24. Stastny, P.: Mixed lymphocyte cultures in rheumatoid arthritis. J. Clin. Invest. 57:1148, 1976.
25. Stastny, P.: Association of the B-cell alloantigen DRw4 with rheumatoid arthritis. N. Engl. J. Med. 298:869, 1978.
26. McMichael, A.J., Sasazuki, T., McDevitt, H.O., and Payne, R.O.: Increased frequency of HLA-Cw3 and HLA-Dw4 in rheumatoid arthritis. Arthritis Rheum. 20:1037, 1977.
27. Rose, H.M., Ragan, C., Pearce, E., and Lipman, M.O.: Differential agglutination of normal and sensitized sheep erythrocyes by sera of patients with rheumatoid arthritis. Proc. Soc. Exp. Bio. Med. 68:1, 1948.
28. Waaler, E.: On the occurrence of a factor in human serum activating the specific agglutination of sheep blood corpuscles. Acta Pathol. Microbiol. Scand. 17:172, 1940.
29. Lawrence, J.S.: Prevalence of rheumatoid arthritis. Ann. Rheum. Dis. 20:11, 1961.
30. Lawrence, J.S., Laine, V.A.I., and DeGraaff, R.: The epidemiology of rheumatoid arthritis in northern Europe. Proc. R. Soc. Med. 54:454, 1961.
31. Engleman, E.G., Sponzilli, E.E., Batey, M.E., Rancharan, S., and McDevitt, H.O.: Mixed lymphocyte reaction in healthy women with rheumatoid factor. Arthritis Rheum. 21:690, 1978.
32. Plotz, C.M., and Singer, J.M.: The latex fixation test. II. Results in rheumatoid arthritis. Am. J. Med. 21:893, 1956.
33. Alarcon, G.S., Koopman, W.J., Acton, R.T., and Barger, B.O.: Seronegative rheumatoid arthritis. A distinct immunogenetic disease? Arthritis Rheum. 25:502, 1982.
34. Myerowitz, S., Jacox, R.F., and Hers, D.W.: Monozygotic twins discordant for rheumatoid arthritis. Arthritis Rheum. 11:1, 1968.
35. Harvald, B., and Hauge, M.: *In* Genetics and the Epidemiology of Chronic Diseases. Washington, D.C., U.S. Government Printing Office, 1965, p. 61.
36. Lawrence, J.S.: Genetics of rheumatoid factor and rheumatoid arthritis. Clin. Exp. Immunol. S2:769, 1967.
37. Lawrence, J.S.: Rheumatoid arthritis-nature or nurture. Ann. Rheum. Dis. 29:357, 1970.
38. Siegel, M., Lee, S.L., Widelock, D., Gwon, N.V., and Kravitz, H.: A comparative family study of rheumatoid arthritis and systemic lupus erythematosus. N. Engl. J. Med. 273:893, 1965.
39. Mellsop, G.W., Koadlow, L., Syme, J., et al.: Absence of rheumatoid arthritis in schizophrenia. Aust. N.Z. J. Med. 4:247, 1974.
40. Hellgren, L.: The prevalence of rheumatoid arthritis in occupational groups. Acta Rheumatol. Scand. 16:106, 1970.
41. Gottlieb, N.L., Dichek, N., Poiley, J., and Kiem, I.M.: Pets and rheumatoid arthritis: An epidemiologic survey. Arthritis Rheum. 17:229, 1974.
42. Beall, G., and Cobb, S.: The frequency distribution of episodes of rheumatoid arthritis as shown by periodic examination. J. Chronic Dis. 14:291, 1961.
43. Jacoby, R.K., Jayson, M.I.V., and Cosh, J.A.: Onset, early stages and prognosis of rheumatoid arthritis: A clinical study of 100 patients with 11 year follow-up. Br. Med. J. 2:96, 1973.
44. Lawrence, J.S.: Surveys of rheumatic complaints in the population. *In* Dixon, A.St.J. (ed.): Progress in Clinical Rheumatology. London, Churchill, 1965, p. 1.
45. Short, C.L., and Bauer, W.: The course of rheumatoid arthritis in patients receiving simple medical and orthopedic measures. N. Engl. J. Med. 238:142, 1948.

46. Fleming, A., Crown, J.M., and Corbett, M.: Early rheumatoid disease. I. Onset. Ann. Rheum. Dis. 35:357, 1976.
47. Fleming, A., Benn, R.T., Corbett, M., and Wood, P.H.N.: Early rheumatoid disease. II. Patterns of joint involvement. Ann. Rheum. Dis. 35:361, 1976.
48. Dick, W.C., Grayson, M.F., Woodburn, A., Nuki, G., and Buchanan, W.W.: Indices of inflammatory activity. Relationship between isotope studies and clinical methods. Ann. Rheum. Dis. 29:643, 1971.
49. Bywaters, E.G.L.: Still's disease in the adult. Ann. Rheum. Dis. 30:121, 1971.
50. Gupta, R.C., and Mills, D.M.: Still's disease in an adult: A link between juvenile and adult rheumatoid arthritis. Am. J. Med. Sci. 269:137, 1975.
51. Aptekar, R.G., Decker, J.L., Bujak, J.S., and Wolff, S.M.: Adult onset of juvenile rheumatoid arthritis. Arthritis Rheum. 16:715, 1973.
52. Strampl, I.J., and Lozar, J.D.: Adult-onset Still's disease. Variant of rheumatoid arthritis. Postgrad. Med. 58:175, 1975.
53. Elkon, K.B., Hughes, G.R.V., Bywaters, E.G.L., et al.: Adult-onset Still's disease. Twenty year follow-up and further studies of patients with active disease. Arthritis Rheum. 25:647, 1982.
54. Hench, P.S., and Rosenberg, E.F.: Palindromic rheumatism: New oft-recurring disease of joints (arthritis, periarthritis, para-arthritis) apparently producing no articular residues. Report of 34 cases. Proc. Mayo Clin. 16:808, 1942.
55. Schumacher, H.R.: Palindromic onset of rheumatoid arthritis. Arthritis Rheum. 25:361, 1982.
56. Yoghami, I., Rookolamini, S.M., and Faunce, H.F.: Unilateral rheumatoid arthritis: Protective effects of neurologic deficits. Am. J. Roentgenol. 128:299, 1977.
57. Bland, J., and Eddy, W.: Hemiplegia and rheumatoid hemiarthritis. Arthritis Rheum. 11:72, 1968.
58. Glick, E.N.: Asymmetrical rheumatoid arthritis after poliomyelitis. Br. Med. J. 3:26, 1967.
59. Thompson, M., and Bywaters, E.G.L.: Unilateral rheumatoid arthritis following hemiplegia. Ann. Rheum. Dis. 21:370, 1961.
60. Bywaters, E.G.L.: The hand. *In* Radiological Aspects of Rheumatoid Arthritis. International Congress Series. Amsterdam, Excerpta Medica Foundation, No. 64, 1964, p. 43.
61. de Haas, W.H.D., de Boer, W., Griftioen, F., and Oostenelst, P.: Rheumatoid arthritis of the robust reaction type. Ann. Rheum. Dis. 31:81, 1974.
62. Short, C.L., Bauer, W., and Reynolds, W.E.: Rheumatoid arthritis: A Definition of the Disease and a Clinical Description Based on a Numerical Study of 293 Patients and Controls. Cambridge, Harvard University Press, 1957.
63. Short, C.L.: Rheumatoid arthritis: Types of course and prognosis. Med. Clin. North Am. 52:549, 1968.
64. Cohen, A.S. (ed.): Laboratory Diagnostic Procedures in the Rheumatic Diseases. 2nd ed. Boston, Little, Brown & Company, 1975.
65. Hoffman, G.S.: Polyarthritis: The differential diagnosis of rheumatoid arthritis. Semin. Arthritis Rheum. 8:115, 1978.
66. Short, C.L., Bauer, W., and Reynolds, W.E.: Rheumatoid Arthritis. Cambridge, Harvard University Press, 1957.
67. Potter, T.A., Barkin, T., and Stillman, R.S.: Occurrence of spondylitis in juvenile rheumatoid arthritis. Ann. Rheum. Dis. 13:364, 1954.
68. Fallet, G.H., Mason, M., Berry, H., Mowat, A.G., Bonssina, I., and Gerster, J.-C.: Rheumatoid arthritis and ankylosing spondylitis occurring together. Br. Med. J. 1:604, 1976.
69. Morris, R.I., Metzger, A.L., Bluestone, R., et al.: HLA w27—a useful discriminator in arthropathies of inflammatory bowel disease. N. Engl. J. Med. 290:1117, 1974.
70. McEwen, C., Lingg, C., and Kirsner, J.B.: Arthritis accompanying ulcerative colitis. Am. J. Med. 33:923, 1962.
71. Zizic, T.M., and Stevens, M.B.: The arthropathy of Behçet's disease. Johns Hopkins Med. J. 136:243, 1975.
72. Ahvonen, P., Sievers, K., and Ano, K.: Arthritis associated with Yersinia enterocolitica infection. Acta Rheumatol. Scand. 15:232, 1969.
73. Ano, K., Ahvonen, P., Lassus, A., Sievers, K., and Tulisinen, A.: HL-A27 (sic) in reactive arthritis: A study of Yersinia arthritis and Reiter's disease. Arthritis Rheum. 17:521, 1974.
74. Hawkins, C.F., Farr, M., Morris, C.J., House, A.M., and Williamson, N.: Detection by electron microscope of rod-shaped organisms in synovial membrane from a patient with the arthritis of Whipple's disease. Ann. Rheum. Dis. 35:502, 1976.
75. Bole, G.G., Friedlaender, M.H., and Smith, C.K.: Rheumatic symptoms and serological abnormalities induced by oral contraceptives. Lancet 1:323, 1969.
76. Bland, J.H., and Frymoyer, J.W.: Rheumatic syndromes of myxedema. N. Engl. J. Med. 282:1171, 1970.
77. Gimlette, T.M.D.: Thyroid acropachy. Lancet 1:22, 1960.
78. Churchill, M.A., Geraci, J.E., and Hunder, G.G.: Musculoskeletal manifestations of bacterial endocarditis. Ann. Intern. Med. 87:754, 1977.
79. Bayer, A.S., Theofilopoulos, A.N., Eisenberg, R., Dixon, F.J., and Guze, L.B.: Circulating immune complexes in infective endocarditis. N. Engl. J. Med. 295:1500, 1976.
80. Bulkley, B.H., and Hutchins, G.M.: Atrial myxomas: A fifty year review. Am. Heart J. 97:639, 1979.
81. McCarty, D.J.: Diagnostic mimicry in arthritis—patterns of joint involvement associated with calcium pyrophosphate dihydrate crystal deposits. Bull. Rheum. Dis. 25:804, 1975.
82. Utsinger, P.D., Zvaifler, N.J., and Resnick, D.: Calcium pyrophosphate dihydrate deposition disease without chondrocalcinosis. J. Rheumatol. 2:258, 1975.
83. Halla, J.T., and Hardin, J.G.: Clinical features of the arthritis of mixed connective tissue disease. Arthritis Rheum. 21:497, 1978.
84. Heller, H., Gafni, J., Michaeli, D., et al.: Arthritis of familial Mediterranean fever (FMF). Arthritis Rheum. 9:1, 1966.
85. Talbott, J.H., Altman, R.D., and Yu, T-F.: Gouty arthritis masquerading as rheumatoid arthritis or vice versa. Semin. Arthritis Rheum. 8:77, 1978.
86. Resnick, D.: Gout-like lesions in rheumatoid arthritis. Am. J. Roentgenol. 127:1062, 1976.
87. Rappoport, A.S., Sosman, J.L., and Weissman, B.N.: Lesions resembling gout in patients with rheumatoid arthritis. Am. J. Roentgenol. 126:41, 1976.
88. Kozin, F., and McCarty, D.J.: Rheumatoid factor in the serum of gouty patients. Arthritis Rheum. 20:1559, 1977.
89. Wallace, D.J., Klinenberg, J.R., Morbaim, D., Berlanstein, B., Biren, P.C., and Callis, G.: Coexistent gout and rheumatoid arthritis: Case report and literature review. Arthritis Rheum. 22:81, 1979.
90. Hirsch, J.H., Killien, F.C., and Troupin, R.H.: The arthopathy of hemochromatosis. Diagn. Radiol. 118:591, 1976.
91. Dymock, I.W., Hamilton, E.B.D., Laws, J.W., and Williams, R.: Arthropathy of hemochromatosis. Ann. Rheum. Dis. 29:469, 1970.
92. Schumacher, H.R., Andrews, R., and McLaughlin, G.: Arthropathy in sickle cell disease. Ann. Intern. Med. 78:203, 1973.
93. Schumacher, H.R., Dorwart, B.B., Boud, J., Alavi, A., and Miller, W.: Chronic synovitis with early cartilage destruction in sickle cell disease. Ann. Rheum. Dis. 36:413, 1977.
94. Crout, J.E., McKenna, C.H., and Petitt, R.M.: Symptomatic joint effusions in sickle cell-$\beta$-thalassemia disease. JAMA 235:1878, 1976.
95. Glueck, C.J., Levy, R.I., and Fredickson, D.S.: Acute tendinitis and arthritis: A presenting symptom of familial type II hyperlipoproteinemia. JAMA 206:2895, 1968.
96. Watt, T.L., and Baumann, R.R.: Pseudoxanthomatous rheumatoid nodules. Arch. Dermatol. 95:156, 1967.
97. Buckingham, R.B., Bole, G.G., and Bassett, D.R.: Polyarthritis associated with Type IV hyperlipoproteinemia. Arch. Intern. Med. 135:286, 1975.
98. Langer, T., and Levy, R.I.: Acute muscular syndrome associated with administration of clofibrate. N. Engl. J. Med. 279:856, 1968.
99. Schumacher, H.R.: Articular manifestations of hypertropic pulmonary osteoarthropathy in bronchogenic carcinoma. Arthritis Rheum. 19:629, 1976.
100. Yanez, J.E., Thompson, G.R., Mikkelsen, W.M., and Bartholomew, L.E.: Rubella arthritis. Ann. Intern. Med. 64:772, 1966.
101. Spruance, S.L., and Smith, C.B.: Joint complications associated with derivatives of HPV-77 rubella virus vaccine. Am. J. Dis. Child. 122:105, 1971.
102. Alpert, E., Isselbacher, K.J., and Aschur, P.H.: The pathogenesis of arthritis associated with viral hepatitis. Complement component studies. N. Engl. J. Med. 285:185, 1971.
103. Schumacher, H.R., and Gall, E.P.: Arthritis in acute hepatitis and chronic active hepatitis. Pathology of the synovial membrane with evidence for the presence of Australia antigen in synovial membranes. Am. J. Med. 57:655, 1974.
104. Sigal, L.H., Steere, A.C., and Niederman, J.C.: Symmetric polyarthritis associated with heterophile-negative infectious mononucleosis. Arthritis Rheum. 26:553, 1983.
105. Steere, A.C., Malawista, S.E., Hardin, J.A., Ruddy, S., Askenasy, W., and Andiman, W.A.: Erythema chronicum migrans and Lyme arthritis. The enlarging clinical spectrum. Ann. Intern. Med. 86:685, 1977.
106. Gold, R.H., Metzger, A.L., Mina, J.M., Weinberger, H.J., and Killebrew, K.: Multicentric reticulohistiocytosis (lipoid dermato-arthritis). Am. J. Roentgenol. 124:610, 1975.
107. Orkin, M., Goltz, R.W., Good, R.A., Michael, A., and Fisher, I.: A study of multicentric reticulohistiocytosis. Arch. Dermatol. 89:641, 964.
108. Ehrlich, G.E.: Inflammatory osteoarthritis. I. The clinical syndrome. J. Chronic Dis. 25:317, 1972.
109. Ordenstein, L.: Sur la Paralysie Agitante et la Sclérose en Plaques Generalisée Paris. Imprimerie de E. Martinet, 1864 (original in Library of the New York Academy of Medicine)
110. McDanold, E.C., and Weissman, M.H.: Articular manifestations of rheumatic fever in adults. Ann. Intern. Med. 89:917, 1978.

111. Barnett, A.L., Terry, E.E., and Persellin, R.H.: Acute rheumatic fever in adults. JAMA 232:925, 1975.
112. Stollerman, G.H., Markowitz, M., Tarania, A., Wannamaker, L.W., and Whittemor, R.: Jones' criteria (revised) for guidance in the diagnosis of rheumatic fever. Circulation 32:664, 1965.
113. Bywaters, E.G.L.: Relation between heart and joint disease including "rheumatoid heart disease" and chronic post-rheumatic arthritis (type Jaccoud). Br. Heart J. 12:101, 1950.
114. Zvaifler, N.J.: Chronic postrheumatic-fever (Jaccoud's) arthritis. N. Engl. J. Med. 267:10, 1962.
115. Ruderman, J.E., and Abruzzo, J.L.: Chronic post rheumatic-fever arthritis (Jaccoud's): Report of a case with subcutaneous nodules. Arthritis Rheum. 9:640, 1966.
116. Spilberg, I., Siltzbach, L.E., and McEwen, C.E.: The arthritis of sarcoidosis. Arthritis Rheum. 12:126, 1969.
117. Kaplan, H.: Sarcoid arthritis. A review. Arch. Intern. Med. 112:162, 1963.
118. Poncet, A.: Address to the Congress Francais de Chirurgie, 1897. Bull. Acad. Med. Paris 46:194, 1901.
119. Krauser, R.E., and Schumacher, H.R.: The arthritis of Sweet's syndrome. Arthritis Rheum. 18:35, 1975.
120. Hoffman, G.S.: Treatment of Sweet's syndrome (acute febrile neutrophilic dermatosis) with indomethacin. J. Rheumatol. 4:201, 1977.
121. Thiemann, H.: Juvenile Epiphysenstorungen. Fortschr. Geb. Rontgenstr. Nuklearmed. 14:79, 1909–10.
122. Rubenstein, H.M.: Thiemann's disease. A brief reminder. Arthritis Rheum. 18:357, 1975.
123. Pinals, R.S., and Short, C.L.: Calcific periarthritis involving multiple sites. Arthritis Rheum. 9:566, 1966.
124. Weiner, A.D., and Ghormley, R.K.: Periodic benign synovitis. Idiopathic intermittent hydrarthrosis. J. Bone Joint Surg. 38A:1039, 1956.
125. Williams, M.H., Sheldon, P.J.H.S., Torrigiani, G., and Mattingly, S.: Palindromic rheumatism. Clinical and immunological studies. Ann. Rheum. Dis. 30:375, 1971.
126. Ehrlich, G.E.: Intermittent and periodic rheumatic syndromes. Bull. Rheum. Dis. 24:746, 1974.
127. Shagrin, J.W., Frame, B., and Duncan, H.: Polyarthritis in obese patients with intestinal bypass. Ann. Intern. Med. 75:377, 1971.
128. Smythe, H.A., and Moldofsky, H.: Two contributions to understanding of the "fibrositis syndrome." Bull. Rheum. Dis. 28:928, 1978.
129. Velayos, E.E., Leidholt, J.D., Smyth, C.J., and Priest, R.: Arthropathy associated wtih steroid therapy. Ann. Intern. Med. 64:759, 1966.
130. Moulsopoulos, H.M., Fye, K.H., Pugay, P.I., and Shearn, M.A.: Monoarthric arthritis caused by metastatic breast carcinoma. JAMA 234:75, 1975.
131. Granowitz, S.P., and Mankin, H.J.: Localized pigmented villonodular synovitis of knee. J. Bone Joint Surg. 49A:122, 1967.
132. Gordon, D.A., Pruzanski, W., Ogryzlo, M.A., and Little, H.A.: Amyloid arthritis simulating rheumatoid disease in five patients with multiple myeloma. Am. J. Med. 55:142, 1973.
133. Pinals, R.S., Dalakos, T.G., and Streeten, D.H.P.: Idiopathic edema as a cause of nonarticular rheumatism. Arthritis Rheum. 22:396, 1979.
134. Bland, J.: Rheumatoid arthritis of the cervical spine. J. Rheumatol. 1:319, 1974.
135. Ball, J.: Enthesopathy of rheumatoid and ankylosing spondylitis. Ann. Rheum. Dis. 30:213, 1971.
136. Martel, W.: Pathogenesis of cervical discovertebral destruction in rheumatoid arthritis. Arthritis Rheum. 20:1217, 1977.
137. Weiner, S., Bassett, L., and Speigel, T.: Superior, posterior, and lateral displacement of C1 in rheumatoid arthritis. Arthritis Rheum. 25:1378, 1982.
138. Stevens, J.C., Cartilage, N.E.F., Saunders, M., Appleby, A., Hall, M., and Shaw, D.A.: Atlantoaxial subluxation and cervical myelopathy in rheumatoid arthritis. Quart. J. Med. 40:391, 1971.
139. Nakano, K.K., Schoene, W.C., Baher, R.A., et al.: The cervical myelopathy associated with rheumatoid arthritis: Analysis of 32 patients with 2 postmortem cases. Am. Neuro. Assoc. 3:144, 1978.
140. Martel, W.: The occipito-atlanto-axial joints in rheumatoid arthritis and ankylosing spondylitis. Am. J. Roentgenol. 86:223, 1961.
141. Raskin, R.J., Schnapf, D.J., Wolf, C.R., Killian, P.J., and Lawless, O.J.: Computerized tomography in evaluation of athentoaxial subluxation in rheumatoid arthritis. J. Rheumatol. 10:32, 1983.
142. Mayer, J.W., Messner, R.P., and Kaplan, R.J.: Brain stem compression in rheumatoid arthritis. JAMA 236:2094, 1976.
143. Mikulowski, P., Wollheim, F.A., Rotmil, P., and Olsen, I.: Sudden death in rheumatoid arthritis with atlanto-axial dislocation. Acta Med. Scand. 198:445, 1975.
144. Smith, P.H., Benn, R.T., and Sharp, J.: Natural history of rheumatoid cervical luxations. Ann. Rheum. Dis. 31:431, 1972.
145. Henderson, D.R.F.: Vertical atlanto-axial subluxation in rheumatoid arthritis. Rheumatol. Rehab. 14:31, 1975.
146. Davidson, R.C., Horn, J.R., Herndon, J.H., and Oliver, G.D.: Brain stem compression in rheumatoid arthritis. JAMA 238:2633, 1977.
147. Bywaters, E.G.L.: Rheumatoid and other diseases of the cervical interspinous bursae, and changes in the spinous process. Am. Rheum. Dis. 41:360, 1982.
148. Ericson, S., and Lundberg, M.: Alterations in the temporomandibular joint at various stages of rheumatoid arthritis. Acta. Rheum. Scand. 13:257, 1967.
149. Marbach, J.J., and Spiera, H.: Rheumatoid arthritis of the temporomandibular joints. Ann. Rheum. Dis. 26:538, 1967.
150. Lofgren, R.H., and Montgomery, W.W.: Incidence of laryngeal involvement in rheumatoid arthritis. N. Engl. J. Med. 267:193, 1962.
151. Polisar, I.A., Burbank, B., Levitt, L.M., Katz, H.M., and Morrione, T.G.: Bilateral midline fixation of cricoarytenoid joints as a serious medical emergency. JAMA 172:901, 1960.
152. Bienenstock, H., Ehrich, G.E., and Freyberg, R.H.: Rheumatoid arthritis of the cricoarytenoid joint: A clinicopathologic study. Arthritis Rheum. 6:48, 1963.
153. Copeman, W.S.C.: Rheumatoid oto-arthritis. Br. Med. J. 2:1536, 1963.
154. Moffat, D.A., Ramsden, R.T., Rosenberg, J.N., Booth, J.B., and Gibson, W.P.R.: Otoadmittance measurements in patients with rheumatoid arthritis. J. Laryngol. Otol. 91:917, 1977.
155. Kalliomaki, J.L., Viitaneu, S-M., and Virtama, P.: Radiological findings of sternoclavicular joints in rheumatoid arthritis. Acta Rheumatol. Scand. 14:233, 1968.
156. Kormano, M.: A microradiographic and histological study of the manubriosternal joint in rheumatoid arthritis. Acta. Rheumatol. Scand. 16:47, 1970.
157. Khong, T.K., and Rooney, P.J.: Manubriosternal joint subluxation in rheumatoid arthritis. J. Rheumatol. 9:712, 1982.
158. Ennevaara, K.: Painful shoulder joint in rheumatoid arthritis. Acta Rheumatol. Scan. Suppl. 11, 1967, pp. 1–116.
159. Weiss, J.J., Thompson, G.R., Doust, V., and Burgener, F.: Rotator cuff tears in rheumatoid arthritis. Arch. Intern. Med. 135:521, 1975.
160. Mosley, H.F.: Ruptures of the Rotator Cuff-Shoulder Lesions. 3rd ed. Edinburgh, E & S Livingston Ltd., 1969, p. 73.
161. Edeiken, J., and Hodes, P.J.: Roentgen Diagnosis of Diseases of Bone. 2nd ed. Baltimore, Williams & Wilkins Company, 1978, pp. 690–709.
162. DeSmet, A.A., Ting, Y.M., and Weiss, J.J.: Shoulder arthrography in rheumatoid arthritis. Diagn. Radiol. 116:601, 1975.
163. Huston, K.A., Nelson, A.M., and Hunder, G.G.: Shoulder swelling in rheumatoid arthritis secondary to subacromial bursitis. Arthritis Rheum. 21:145, 1978.
164. Resnick, D., and Niwayama, G.: Resorption of the undersurface of the distal clavicle in rheumatoid arthritis. Diagn. Radiol. 120:75, 1976.
165. Laine, V., and Vainio, K.: The elbow in rheumatoid arthritis. *In* Hymans, W., Paul, W.D., and Herschel, H.: Early Synovectomy in Rheumatoid Arthritis. Amsterdam, Excerpta Medica, 1969, p. 112.
166. Peterson, L.F.A., and James, J.M.: Surgery of the rheumatoid elbow. Orthop. Clin. North Am. 2:667, 1971.
167. Shapiro, J.S.: A new factor in the etiology of ulnar drift. Clin. Orthop. 68:32, 1970.
168. Hastings, D.E., and Evans, J.A.: Rheumatoid wrist deformities and their relation to ulnar drift. J. Bone Joint Surg. 57A:930, 1975.
169. Inglis, A.E.: Rheumatoid arthritis in the hand. Am. J. Surg. 109:368, 1965.
170. Swezey, R.L., and Fiegenberg, D.S.: Inappropriate intrinsic muscle action in the rheumatoid hand. Ann. Rheum. Dis. 30:619, 1972.
171. Fearnley, G.R.: Ulnar deviation of the fingers. Ann. Rheum. Dis. 10:126, 1951.
172. Flatt, A.E.: Surgical rehabilitation of the arthritic hand. Arthritis Rheum. 11:278, 1959.
173. Hakstian, R.W., and Tubiana, R.: Ulnar deviation of the fingers. J. Bone Joint Surg. 49A:299, 1967.
174. Snorrason, E.: The problem of ulnar deviation of the fingers in rheumatoid arthritis. Acta. Med. Scand. 140:359, 1951.
175. Vainio, K., and Oka, M.: Ulnar deviation of the fingers. Ann. Rheum. Dis. 12:122, 1953.
176. Croft, J.D., and Jacox, R.F.: Rheumatoid "ganglion" as an unusual presenting sign of rheumatoid arthritis. JAMA 203:144, 1968.
177. Harrison, M.D., Freiberger, R.H., and Ranawat, C.S.: Arthrography of the rheumatoid wrist joint. Am. J. Roentgenol. 112:480, 1971.
178. Iveson, J.M.I., Hill, A.G.S., and Wright, V.: Wrist cysts and fistulae. An arthrographic study of the rheumatoid wrist. Ann. Rheum. Dis. 34:388, 1975.
179. Martel, W., Hayes, J.T., and Duff, I.F.: The pattern of bone erosion in the hand and wrist in rheumatoid arthritis. Radiology 84:204, 1965.
180. Resnick, D., and Gmelich, J.T.: Bone fragmentation in the rheumatoid wrist; radiographic and pathologic considerations. Diagn. Radiol. 114:315, 1975.
181. Trentham, D.E., and Masi, A.T.: Carpo: metacarpal ratio. A new quan-

titative measure of radiologic progression of wrist involvement in rheumatoid arthritis. Arthritis Rheum. 191:939, 1976.
182. Brewerton, D.A.: Hand deformities in rheumatoid disease. Ann. Rheum. Dis. 16:183, 1957.
183. McCarty, D.J., and Gatter, R.A.: A study of distal interphalangeal joint tenderness in rheumatoid arthritis. Arthritis Rheum. 9:325, 1966.
184. Vaughan-Jackson, O.J.: Rheumatoid hand deformities considered in the light of tendon imbalance. J. Bone Joint Surg. 44B:764, 1962.
185. Nalebuff, E.A.: Diagnosis, classification, and management of rheumatoid thumb deformities. Bull. Hosp. Joint Dis. 24:119, 1968.
186. Kellgren, J.H., and Ball, J.: Tendon lesions in rheumatoid arthritis: A clinicopathological study. Ann. Rheum. Dis. 9:48, 1950.
187. Gray, R.G., and Gottlieb, N.L.: Hand flexor tenosynovitis in rheumatoid arthritis. Arthritis Rheum. 20:1003, 1977.
188. Millis, M.B., Millender, L.H., and Nalebuff, E.A.: Stiffness of the proximal interphalangeal joints in rheumatoid arthritis. J. Bone Joint Surg. 58A:801, 1976.
189. Vyden, J.K., Callis, G., Groseth-Dittrich, M.F., Laks, M.M., and Weinberger, H.: Peripheral hemodynamics in rheumatoid arthritis (abstract). Arthritis Rheum. 14:419, 1971.
190. Vyden, J.K., Groseth, Dittrich, M.F., Callis, G., Laks, M.M., and Weinberger, H.: The effect of propranolol on peripheral hemodynamics in rheumatoid arthritis (abstract). Arthritis Rheum. 14:420, 1971.
191. Duthie, R., and Harris, C.: A radiographic and clinical survey of the hip joints in sero-positive rheumatoid arthritis. Acta Orthop. Scand. 40:346, 1969.
192. Hastings, D.E., and Parker, S.M.: Protrusio acetabuli in rheumatoid arthritis. Clin. Orthop. 108:76, 1975.
193. Colton, C., and Darby, A.: Giant granulomatous lesions of the femoral head and neck in rheumatoid arthritis. Ann. Rheum. Dis. 29:616, 1970.
194. Levy, R.N., Hermann, G., Haimov, M., et al.: Rheumatoid synovial cyst of the hip. Arthritis Rheum. 25:1382, 1982.
195. Cary, G.R.: Methods for determining the presence of subtle knee joint effusion. J. Louisiana St. Med. Soc. 118:147, 1966.
196. Gupta, P.J.: Physical examination of the arthritis patient. Bull. Rheum. Dis. 20:596, 1970.
197. Jayson, M.I.V., and Dixon, A.St.J.: Valvular mechanisms in juxta-articular cysts. Ann. Rheum. Dis. 29:415, 1970.
198. Kraag, G., Thevathasan, E.M., Gordon, D.A., and Walker, I.H.: The hemorrhage crescent sign of acute synovial rupture. Ann. Intern. Med. 85:477, 1976.
199. Gordon, G.V., and Edell, S.: Ultrasound evaluation of popliteal cyst. Arch. Intern. Med. 140:1453, 1980.
200. Hall, A.P., and Scott, J.T.: Synovial cysts and rupture of the knee joint in rheumatoid arthritis. Ann. Rheum. Dis. 25:32, 1966.
201. Hench, P.K., Reid, R.T., and Reames, P.M.: Dissecting popliteal cyst stimulating thrombophlebitis. Ann. Intern. Med. 64:1259, 1966.
202. Tait, G.B.W., Bach, F., and Dixon, A.St.J.: Acute synovial rupture. Ann. Rheum. Dis. 24:273, 1965.
203. Rask, M.R.: Achilles tendon rupture owing to rheumatoid disease. J. Amer. Med. Asso. 239:435, 1978.
204. Dixon, A.St.J.: The rheumatoid foot. *In* Hill, A.G.S. (ed.): Modern Trends in Rheumatology. Vol. 2. London, Butterworths, 1971, pp. 158–173.
205. Vidigal, E., Jacoby, R., Dixon, A.St.J., Rattiff, A.H., and Kirkup, J.: The foot in chronic rheumatoid arthritis. Ann. Rheum. Dis. 34:292, 1975.
206. Bienenstock, H.: Rheumatoid plantar synovial cysts. Ann. Rheum. Dis. 34:98, 1975.
207. Dixon, A.St.J.: The rheumatoid foot. Proc. R. Soc. Med. 63:677, 1970.
208. Calabro, J.J.: A critical evaluation of the diagnostic features of the feet in rheumatoid arthritis. Arthritis Rheum. 5:19, 1962.
209. McGuigan, L., Burke, D., and Fleming, A.: Tarsal tunnel syndrome and peripheral neuropathy in rheumatoid disease. Ann. Rheum. Dis. 42:128, 1983.
210. Vainio, K.: The rheumatoid foot: A clinical study with pathological and roentgenological comments. Ann. Clin. Gynaec. Fenn. 45(Suppl. 1):107, 1956.
211. Duncan, H., Frost, H.M., Villaneuva, A.R., et al.: The osteoporosis of rheumatoid arthritis. Arthritis Rheum. 8:943, 1965.
212. Saville, P.D., and Kharmosh, O.: Osteoporosis of rheumatoid arthritis: Influence of age, sex and corticosteroids. Arthritis Rheum. 10:423, 1967.
213. Maddison, P.J., and Bacon, P.A.: Vitamin D deficiency, spontaneous fractures and osteopenia in rheumatoid arthritis. Br. Med. J. 2:433, 1974.
214. Rajapakse, C., Thompson, R., Grennan, D.M., et al.: Increased bone metabolism in rheumatoid arthritis as measured by the whole-body retention of $^{99}Tc^{m}$ methylene diphosphonate. Ann. Rheum. 42:138, 1983.
215. Schneider, R., and Kaye, J.J.: Insufficiency and stress fractures of the long bones occurring in patients with rheumatoid arthritis. Diagn. Radiol. 116:595, 1975.
216. Steiner, G., Freund, H.A., Leichtentritt, B., and Maun, M.E.: Lesion of skeletal muscles in rheumatoid arthritis. Am. J. Pathol. 22:103, 1946.
217. Haslock, D.I., Wright, V., and Harriman, D.G.F.: Neuromuscular disorders in rheumatoid arthritis. A motor-point muscle biopsy study. Quart. J. Med. 39:335, 1970.
218. Hurd, E.R.: Extra-articular manifestations of rheumatoid arthritis. Semin. Rheum. Dis. 8:151, 1979.
219. Hart, F.D.: Rheumatoid arthritis: Extra-articular manifestations. Br. Med. J. 3:131, 1969.
220. Collins, D.H.: The subcutaneous nodule of rheumatoid arthritis. J. Pathol. Bacteriol. 45:97, 1937.
221. Bennett, G.A., Zeller, J.W., and Bauer, W.: Subcutaneous nodules of rheumatoid arthritis and rheumatic fever: A pathologic study. Arch. Pathol. 30:70, 1940.
222. Sokoloff, L.: The pathophysiology of peripheral blood vessels in collagen diseases. *In* Orbison, J.L., and Smith, D.E. (eds.): The Peripheral Blood Vessels. Baltimore, Williams & Wilkins Company, 1963, p. 297.
223. Harris, E.D., Jr.: A collagenolytic system produced by primary cultures of rheumatoid nodule tissue. J. Clin. Invest. 51:2973, 1972.
224. Ganda, O.P., and Caplan, H.I.: Rheumatoid disease without joint involvement. JAMA 228:338, 1974.
225. Ginsberg, M.H., Genant, H.K., Yu, T.F., and McCarty, D.J.: Rheumatoid nodulosis: An unusual variant of rheumatoid disease. Arthritis Rheum. 18:49, 1975.
226. Brower, A.C., NaPombejara, C., Stechschulte, D.J., Mantz, F., and Ketchum, L.: Rheumatoid nodulosis: Another cause of juxta-articular nodules. Diagn. Radiol. 118:669, 1977.
227. Simons, F.E.R., and Schaller, J.G.: Benign rheumatoid nodules. Pediatrics 56:29, 1975.
228. Wood, M.G., and Beerman, H.: Necrobiosis lipoidica, granuloma annulare. Report of a case with lesions in the galea aponeurotica of a child. Am. J. Dis. Child. 96:720, 1958.
229. Watt, T.L., and Baumann, R.R.: Pseudoxanthomatous rheumatoid nodules. Arch. Dermatol. 95:156, 1967.
230. Healey, L.A., Wilske, K.R., and Sagebiel, R.W.: Rheumatoid nodules simulating basal-cell carcinoma. N. Engl. J. Med. 277:7, 1967.
231. Sturrock, R.D., Cowden, E.A., Howie, E., Grennan, D.M., and Buchanan, W.W.: The forgotten nodule: Complications of sacral nodules in rheumatoid arthritis. Br. Med. J. 2:92, 1975.
232. Friedman, B.A., and Rice, D.H.: Rheumatoid nodules of the larynx. Arch. Otolaryngol. 101:361, 1975.
233. Bywaters, E.G.L.: Fistulous rheumatism: A manifestation of rheumatoid arthritis. Ann. Rheum. Dis. 12:114, 1953.
234. Shapiro, R.F., Resnick, D., Castles, J.J., D'Ambrosia, R., Lipscomb, P.R., and Niwayama, G.: Fistulization of rheumatoid joints: Spectrum of identifiable syndromes. Ann. Rheum. Dis. 34:489, 1975.
235. Baum, J.: Infection in rheumatoid arthritis. Arthritis Rheum. 14:135, 1971.
236. Gaulhofer de Klerch, E.H., and Van Dam, G.: Septic complications in rheumatoid arthritis. Acta Rheum. Scand. 9:254, 1963.
237. Huskisson, E.C., and Hart, F.D.: Severe, unusual and recurrent infections in rheumatoid arthritis. Ann. Rheum. Dis. 31:118, 1972.
238. Bodel, P.T., and Hollingsworth, J.W.: Comparative morphology, respiration, and phagocytic function of leukocytes from blood and joint fluid in rheumatoid arthritis. J. Clin. Invest. 45:580, 1966.
239. Mowat, A.G.: Hematologic abnormalities in RA. Semin. Arthritis Rheum. 1:195, 1971.
240. Engstedt, L., and Strandberg, O.: Haematological data and clinical activity of the rheumatoid diseases. Acta Med. Scand. 180:13, 1966.
241. Samson, D., Holliday, D., and Gumpel, J.M.: Role of ineffective erythropoiesis in the anaemia of rheumatoid arthritis. Ann. Rheum. Dis. 36:181, 1977.
242. Cartwright, G.E.: The anemia of chronic disorders. Semin. Hematol. 3:351, 1966.
243. Raymond, F.D., Bowie, M.A., and Dugan, A.: Iron metabolism in rheumatoid arthritis. Arthritis Rheum. 8:233, 1965.
244. Ridolfo, A.S., Rubin, A., Crabtree, R.E., and Gruber, C.M.: Effects of fenoprofen and aspirin on gastrointestinal microbleeding in man. Clin. Pharmacol. Ther. 14:226, 1973.
245. Smith, R.J., Davis, P., Thomson, A.B.R., Wadsworth, L.D., and Fackre, P.: Serum ferritin levels in the anemia of rheumatoid arthritis: J. Rheumatol. 4:389, 1977.
246. Beck, R.L., French, B., Brinck-Johnsen, T., Cornwell, G.G., and Rawnsley, H.M.: Multivariate approach to predictive diagnosis of bone-marrow iron stores. Am. J. Pathol. 70:665, 1978.
247. Williams, R.A., Samson, D., Tikerpae, J., Crowne, J., and Gumpel, J.M.: In-vitro studies of ineffective erythropoiesis in rheumatoid arthritis. Am. Rheum. Dis. 41:502, 1982.
248. Winchester, R.J., Litwin, S.D., Koffler, D., and Kunkel, H.G.: Observations on the eosinophilia of certain patients with rheumatoid arthritis. Arthritis Rheum. 14:650, 1971.

249. Hutchinson, R.M., Davis, P., and Jayson, M.I.V.: Thrombocytosis in rheumatoid arthritis. Ann. Rheum. Dis. 35:138, 1976.
250. Sokoloff, L., and Bunin, J.J.: Vascular lesions in rheumatoid arthritis. J. Chronic Dis. 5:668, 1957.
251. Kulka, J.P., Bocking, D., Ropes, M.W., and Bauer, W.: Early joint lesions of rheumatoid arthritis: Report of 8 cases with knee biopsies of less than one year's duration. Arch. Pathol. 59:129, 1955.
252. Soter, N.A., Mihm, M.C., Gigli, I., and Dvorak, H.F.: Two distinct cellular patterns in cutaneous necrotizing angiitis. J. Invest. Dermatol. 66:344, 1976.
253. Rapaport, R.J., Kozin, F., Mackel, S.E., and Jordon, R.E.: Cutaneous vascular immunofluorescence in rheumatoid arthritis. Am. J. Med. 68:325, 1980.
254. Mongam, E.S., Cass, R.M., Jacox, R.F., and Vaughan, J.H.: A study of the relation of seronegative and seropositive rheumatoid arthritis to each other and to necrotizing vasculitis. Am. J. Med. 47:23, 1969.
255. Weinstein, A., Peters, K., Brown, D., and Bluestone, R.: Metabolism of the third component of complement (C3) in patients with rheumatoid arthritis. Arthritis Rheum. 15:49, 1972.
256. Conn, D.L., McDuffie, F.C., and Dyck, P.J.: Immunopathologic study of sural nerves in rheumatoid arthritis. Arthritis Rheum. 15:135, 1972.
257. Weisman, M., and Zvaifler, N.: Cryoimmunoglobulinemia in rheumatoid arthritis. J. Clin. Invest. 56:725, 1975.
258. Schmid, F.R., Cooper, N.S., Ziff, M., and McEwen, C.: Arteritis in rheumatoid arthritis. Am. J. Med. 30:56, 1961.
259. Markenson, J.A., McDougal, J.S., Tsairis, P., et al.: Rheumatoid meningitis: a localized immune process. Ann. Intern. Med. 90:786, 1979.
260. Bienenstock, H., Minick, R., and Rogoff, B.: Mesenteric arteritis and intestinal infarction in rheumatoid disease. Arch. Intern. Med. 119:359, 1967.
261. Hart, F.D., Golding, J.R., and MacKenzie, D.H.: Neuropathy in rheumatoid disease. Ann. Rheum. Dis. 16:471, 1957.
262. Gordon, D.A., Stein, J.L., and Brody, I.: The extra-cellular features of rheumatoid arthritis. A systematic analysis of 127 cases. Am. J. Med. 54:455, 1973.
263. Siomopoulos, V., and Shah, N.: Acute organic brain syndrome associated with rheumatoid arthritis. J. Clin. Psych. 40:46, 1979.
264. Scott, D.G., Baron, P.A., Elliott, P.J., et al.: Systemic vasculitis in a district general hospital 1972–80. Quart. J. Med. 51:292, 1982.
265. Lawson, A.A.H., and MacLean, N.: Renal disease and drug therapy in rheumatoid arthritis. Ann. Rheum. Dis. 25:441, 1966.
266. Samuels, B., Lee, J.C., Engleman, E.P., and Hooper, J., Jr.: Membranous nephropathy in patients with rheumatoid arthritis: Relationship to gold therapy. Medicine 57:319, 1977.
267. Case Records of the Massachusetts General Hospital, Case 23-1965. N. Engl. J. Med. 272:1069, 1965.
268. Walker, W.C., and Wright, V.: Pulmonary lesions and rheumatoid arthritis. Medicine 47:501, 1968.
269. Dodson, W.H., and Hollingsworth, J.W.: Pleural effusion in rheumatoid arthritis: Impaired transport of glucose. N. Engl. J. Med. 275:1337, 1966.
270. Dixon, A.St.J., and Ball, J.: Honeycomb lung and chronic rheumatoid arthritis: A case report. Ann. Rheum. Dis. 16:241, 1957.
271. Stack, B.H.R., and Grant, I.W.B.: Rheumatoid interstitial lung disease. Br. J. Dis. Chest 59:202, 1965.
272. Walker, W.C., and Wright, V.: Diffuse interstitial pulmonary fibrosis and rheumatoid arthritis. Ann. Rheum. Dis. 28:252, 1969.
273. Frank, S.T., Weg, J.G., Harkleroad, L.E., and Fitch, R.F.: Pulmonary dysfunction in rheumatoid disease. Chest 63:27, 1973.
274. Hyland, R.H., Gordon, D.A., Broder, I., et al.: A systematic controlled study of pulmonary abnormalities in RA. J. Rheumatol. 10:395, 1983.
275. Caplan, A.: Certain unusual radiographic appearances in the chest of coal miners suffering from RA. Thorax 8:29, 1953.
276. Portner, M.M., and Gracie, W.A.: Rheumatoid lung disease with cavitary nodules, pneumothorax and eosinophilia. N. Engl. J. Med. 275:697, 1966.
277. Hull, S., and Mathews, J.A.: Pulmonary necrobiotic nodules as a presenting feature of rheumatoid arthritis. Ann. Rheum. Dis. 41:21, 1982.
278. Gardner, D.L., Duthie, J.J.R., MacLeod, J., and Allan, W.S.H.: Pulmonary hypertension in RA: Report of a case with intimal sclerosis of pulmonary and digital arteries. Scot. Med. J. 2:183, 1957.
279. Bonfiglio, T., and Atwater, E.: Heart disease in patients with sero-positive rheumatoid arthritis; a controlled autopsy study and review. Arch. Intern. Med. 124:714, 1969.
280. Lebowitz, W.B.: The heart in rheumatoid arthritis. A clinical and pathological study of 62 cases. Ann. Intern. Med. 58:102, 1963.
281. MacDonald, W.J., Jr., Crawford, M.H., Klippel, J.H., Zvaifler, N.J., and O'Rourke, R.A.: Echocardiographic assessment of cardiac structure and function in patients with rheumatoid arthritis. Am. J. Med. 63:890, 1977.
282. Lange, R.K., Weiss, T.E., and Ochsner, J.L.: Rheumatoid arthritis and constrictive pericarditis. A patient benefited by pericardectomy. Arthritis Rheum. 8:403, 1965.
283. Thadini, V., Iveson, J.M.I., and Wright, V.: Cardiac tamponade, constrictive pericarditis and pericardial resection in rheumatoid arthritis. Medicine 54:261, 1975.
284. Gowands, J.D.C.: Complete heart block with Stokes-Adams syndrome due to rheumatoid heart disease. N. Engl. J. Med. 262:1012, 1960.
285. Prakash, R., Atassi, A., Poske, R., and Rosen, K.M.: Prevalance of pericardial effusion and mitral-valve involvement in patients with rheumatoid arthritis without cardiac symptoms. N. Engl. J. Med. 289:597, 1973.
286. Weintraub, A.M., and Zvaifler, N.J.: The occurrence of valvular and myocardial disease in patients with chronic joint disease. Am. J. Med. 35:145, 1963.
287. Iveson, J.M.I., Thadani, V., Ionescu, M., and Wright, V.: Aortic valve incompetence and replacement in rheumatoid arthritis. Ann. Rheum. Dis. 34:312, 1975.
288. Lev, M., Bharati, S., Hoffman, F.G., and Leight, L.: The conduction system in rheumatoid arthritis with complete atrioventricular block. Am. Heart J. 90:78, 1975.
289. Swezey, R.L.: Myocardial infarction due to rheumatoid arteritis. JAMA 199:191, 1967.
290. Reimer, K.A., Rodgers, R.F., and Oyasu, R.: Rheumatoid arthritis with rheumatoid heart disease and granulomatous aortitis. JAMA 235:2510, 1976.
291. Valkenburg, H.A.: Pattern of rheumatoid disease in society: Change or disappearance? Scand. J. Rheumatol. 5(Suppl. 12):89, 1975.
292. Pinals, R.S., Masi, A.F., Larsen, R.A.: Special article: Preliminary criteria for clinical remission in RA. Arthritis Rheum. 24:1308,
293. Sharp, J.T., Calkins, E., Cohen, A.S., Schubart, A.F., and Calabro, J.J.: Observations on the clinical, chemical, and serological manifestations of rheumatoid arthritis, based on the course of 154 cases. Medicine 43:41, 1964.
294. Cobb, S., Anderson, F., and Baurer, W.: Length of life and cause of death in rheumatoid arthritis. N. Engl. J. Med. 249:553, 1953.
295. Baum, J.: Infection in rheumatoid arthritis. Arthritis Rheum. 14:135, 1971.
296. Short, C.L.: Long remissions in rheumatoid arthritis. Medicine 43:401, 1964.
297. Duthie, J.J.R., Brown, P.E., Truelove, L.H., Barago, E., and Lawrie, A.J.: Course and prognosis in rheumatoid arthritis. A further report. Ann. Rheum. Dis. 23:193, 1964.
298. Corrigan, A.B., Robinson, R.G., Terenty, T.R., Dick-Smith, J.B., and Walters, O.: Benign rheumatoid arthritis of the aged. Br. Med. J. 1:444, 1974.
299. Luukkainen, R., Isomaki, H., and Kajander, A.: Prognostic value of the type of onset of rheumatoid arthritis. Ann. Rheum. Dis. 42:274, 1983.
300. Mattingly, S.: Palindromic rheumatism. Ann. Rheum. Dis. 25:307, 1966.
301. Duthie, J.J.R., Thompson, M., Weir, M.M., and Fletcher, W.B.: Medical and social aspects of treatment of rheumatoid arthritis with special reference to the factors affecting prognosis. Ann. Rheum. Dis. 14:133, 1955.
302. Fleming, A., Benn, R.T., Corbett, M., and Wood, P.H.N.: Early rheumatoid disease. II. Patterns of joint involvement. Ann. Rheum. Dis. 35:361, 1976.
303. Kellgren, J.H., and O'Brien, W.M.: On the natural history of rheumatoid arthritis in relation to the sheep cell agglutination test (SCAT). Arthritis Rheum. 5:115, 1962.
304. Masi, A.T., Maldonado-Cocco, J.A., Kaplan, S.B., Feigenbaum, S.L., and Chandler, R.W.: Prospective study of the early course of rheumatoid arthritis in young adults: Comparison of patients with and without rheumatoid factor positivity at entry and identification of variables correlating with outcome. Semin. Arthritis Rheum. 5:299, 1976.
305. Jacoby, R.K., Jayson, M.I.V., and Cosh, J.A.: Onset, early stages and prognosis of rheumatoid arthritis: A clinical study of 100 patients with 11-year follow-up. Br. Med. J. 2:96, 1973.
306. Dixon, A.St.J.: "Rheumatoid arthritis" with negative serological reaction. Ann. Rheum. Dis. 19:209, 1960.
307. Ragan, C., and Farrington, E.: The clinical features of rheumatoid arthritis. JAMA 181:663, 1962.
308. Henderson, D.R.F., Jayson, M.I.V., and Tribe, C.B.: Lack of correlation of synovial histology with joint damage in rheumatoid arthritis. Ann. Rheum. Dis. 34:7, 1975.
309. Yates, D.B., and Scott, J.T.: Rheumatoid synovitis and joint disease. Relationship between arthroscopic and histological changes. Ann. Rheum. Dis. 34:1, 1975.
310. Cruickshank, B.: Interpretation of multiple biopsies of synovial tissue in rheumatic diseases. Ann. Rheum. Dis. 11:137, 1952.
311. Muirden, K.D., and Mills, K.W.: Do lymphocytes protect the rheumatoid joint? Br. Med. J. 4:219, 1971.

312. Harris, E.D., Jr., Faulkner, C.S., II, and Brown, F.E.: Collagenolytic systems in rheumatoid arthritis. Clin. Orthop. 110:303, 1975.
313. Weiss, S.J., Lampert, M.D., and Test, S.T.: Long-lived oxidants generated by human neutrophils: Characterization and bioactivity. Science 222:625, 1983.
314. Ward, T.T., and Steigbigel, R.T.: Acidosis of synovial fluid correlates with synovial fluid leukocytosis. Am. J. Med. 64:933, 1978.
315. Ruddy, S.: Synovial fluid: Mirror of the inflammatory lesion in rheumatoid arthritis. *In* Harris, E.D., Jr. (ed.): Rheumatoid Arthritis. New York, Medcom Press, 1974.
316. Hay, F.C., Nineham, L.J., Perumal, R., et al.: Intra-articular and circulating immune complexes and antiglobulins (IgG and IgM) in rheumatoid arthritis: correlation with clinical features. Ann. Rheum. Dis. 38:1, 1979.
317. Lessard, J., Nunnery, E., Cecere, F., et al.: Relationship between the articular manifestations of rheumatoid arthritis and circulating immune complexes detected by three methods and specific classes of rheumatoid factors. J. Rheumatol. 10:411, 1983.
318. Amos, R.S., Constable, T.J., Crockson, R.A., Crockson, A.P., and McConkery, B.: Rheumatoid arthritis: Relation of serum C-reactive protein and erythrocyte sedimentation rates to radiographic changes. Br. Med. J. 1:195, 1977.
319. Mallya, R.K., deBeer, F.C., Berry, H., et al.: Correlation of clinical parameters of disease activity in rheumatoid arthritis with serum concentration of C-reactive protein and erythrocyte sedimentation rate. J. Rheumatol. 9:224, 1982.
320. Lansbury, J.: Quantitation of activity of rheumatoid arthritis. Method for summation of systemic indices of rheumatoid activity. Am. J. Med. Sci. 232:300, 1956.
321. Lansbury, J.: Report of a three-year study on the systemic and articular indexes in rheumatoid arthritis: Theoretic and clinical considerations. Arthritis Rheum. 1:505, 1958.
322. Huskisson, E.C.: Measurement of pain. Lancet 2:1127, 1974.
323. Steinbrocker, O., Traeger, C.H., and Batterman, R.C.: Therapeutic criteria in rheumatoid arthritis. JAMA 140:659, 1949.
324. Fallahi, S., Halla, J.T., and Hardin, J.G.: The reassessment of the nature of onset of rheumatoid arthritis. Clin. Res. 31:650A, 1983.

# Chapter 61
# Felty's Syndrome

*Robert Pinals*

## INTRODUCTION

In 1924 Felty[1] described five patients with chronic arthritis, splenomegaly, and leukopenia and proposed that this association represented a distinct clinical entity. The term *Felty's syndrome* was first used in 1932 by Hanrahan and Miller[2] in reporting a patient who responded to splenectomy but died 18 months later.[3] Most of the more recent literature has recognized that Felty's syndrome represents one of many systemic complications of seropositive rheumatoid arthritis occurring in a group of patients with unusually severe articular disease and immunologic abnormalities. The term "hypersplenism" was derived from the observation that splenectomy usually resulted in partial or complete resolution of the granulocytopenia, but the role of the spleen in pathogenesis has been an area of considerable controversy for many years. There is evidence for its participation both in the removal of granulocytes from the circulating pool and in the suppression of granulopoiesis. Thus an etiologic definition is still unavailable, and Felty's syndrome must be defined in descriptive terms as a variant of seropositive rheumatoid arthritis with splenomegaly and granulocytopenia ($<2000$ per cubic millimeter). Although the complete triad is required for a diagnosis of Felty's syndrome, some patients may be encountered and considered for the diagnosis at a time when only two of the features are present, with appearance of the third only after a period of observation. Patients with rheumatoid arthritis may also develop superimposed illnesses which may result in splenomegaly or granulocytopenia; drug reactions, myeloproliferative disorders, reticuloendothelial malignancies, hepatic cirrhosis, amyloidosis, sarcoidosis, tuberculosis, and other chronic infections must be considered and excluded with reasonable clinical certainty before the diagnosis of Felty's syndrome is accepted.

The true prevalence of Felty's syndrome is unknown, but it is probably found in less than 1 percent of patients with rheumatoid arthritis.[4] Splenomegaly alone is more common, identified by palpation in 6.5 percent in one large series,[4] and even more frequently by radioactive scanning.[5]

## CLINICAL FEATURES

About two thirds of patients with Felty's syndrome are women. HLA DRw4 was found in 95 percent of patients with Felty's syndrome, compared with 69 percent in other rheumatoid arthritis patients and 31 percent in controls.[6] This may account for the rarity of Felty's syndrome in blacks, who are known to have a low frequency of DRw4.[7] The condition is usually recognized in the fifth through the seventh decades of life in patients who have had rheumatoid arthritis for 10 years or more. However, since it is most often discovered by a routine blood count, the frequency of medical observation is an important factor in early recognition. Splenomegaly and granulocytopenia may be present before symptoms or signs of arthritis in rare instances.[8] The articular disease is usually more severe than in the average case of rheumatoid arthritis, with greater deformity and erosion,[9,10] but there are many examples of mild involvement.[11,12] About one third of the patients have relatively inactive synovitis, as judged by signs and symptoms, but even these patients continue to have an

**Table 61–1.** Frequency of Extra-Articular Manifestations in Felty's Syndrome*

| | |
|---|---|
| Rheumatoid nodules | 76% |
| Weight loss | 68% |
| Sjögren's syndrome† | 56% |
| Lymphadenopathy | 34% |
| Leg ulcers | 25% |
| Pleuritis | 19% |
| Skin pigmentation | 17% |
| Neuropathy | 17% |
| Episcleritis | 8% |

*From a review of 10 reports since 1962.
†Determined by positive Schirmer test.

elevated erythrocyte sedimentation rate (ESR). In one large series the mean ESR was 85 mm per hour.[10]

The spleen size is variable. In 5 to 10 percent of patients it is not large enough to be palpable, but occasionally there is massive splenomegaly.[13] The median splenic weight in Felty's syndrome is about four times normal.[13] There is no correlation between spleen size and the degree of granulocytopenia.[9,10,14]

Patients with Felty's syndrome tend to have more extra-articular manifestations than others with rheumatoid arthritis (Table 61–1). Weight loss was mentioned by Felty and has been emphasized by later authors. It may be striking and unexplained, often occurring for several months before the diagnosis of Felty's syndrome is made. Felty also mentioned brown pigmentation over exposed surfaces of the extremities, especially over the tibia. Although noted by others,[9,15,16] it is not specific for Felty's syndrome, and may be related to stasis and to extravasation of red blood cells secondary to disease of small vessels. Leg ulcers are frequent but do not seem to differ from those in other rheumatoid arthritis patients in terms of chronicity, recurrence, and presumed relationship to vasculitis (Fig. 61–1).

Although about 60 percent of patients with Felty's syndrome are described as having one or more infections which may be attributable to the granulocytopenia, the literature is difficult to interpret because nonleukopenic rheumatoid arthritis patients may also be more susceptible to infection and because there is no suitable control group for comparison.[17] In addition, some reports of Felty's syndrome are limited to splenectomized patients, who may represent a more severely involved group. The degree of granulocytopenia correlates poorly with the number and severity of infections.[9,11] Most of the infections are caused by ordinary bacteria such as staphylococcus, streptococcus, and gram-negative bacilli,[10] and involve common sites, particularly the skin and respiratory tract (Table 61–2). In spite of the granulocytopenia, pus may accumulate in an appropriate fashion, suggesting that the site of infection is capable of competing successfully with the spleen for available granulocytes. The response to antibiotic therapy is usually adequate.[10]

**Table 61–2.** Percentage of Felty's Syndrome Patients with Various Types of Infection*

| | |
|---|---|
| Skin (abscess, cellulitis, furunculosis) | 26% |
| Pneumonia | 24% |
| Urinary tract | 9% |
| Oral ulcers | 4% |
| Sinusitis and otitis | 4% |
| Septic arthritis | 2% |

*Taken from four reports[8,10,13,14] in which sufficient information was available on a total of 90 patients.

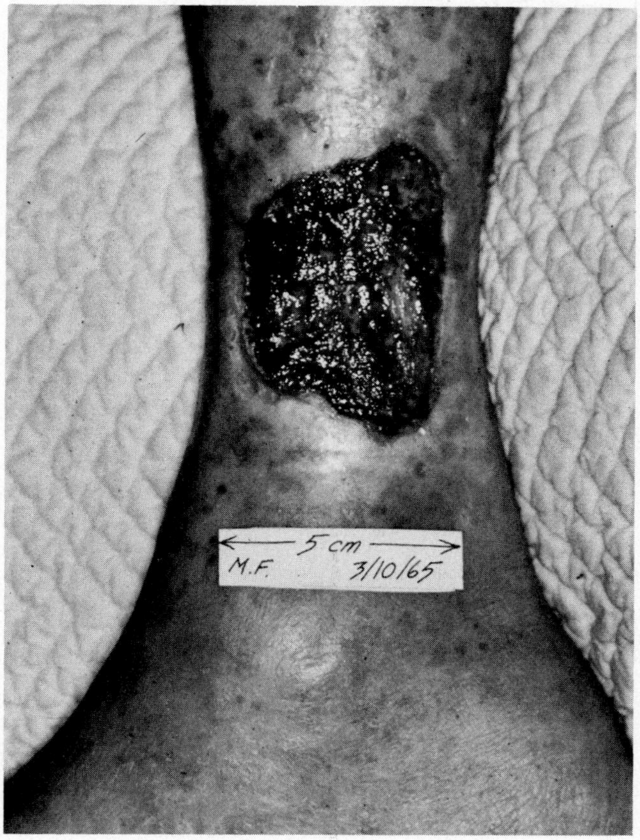


**Figure 61–1.** Ulceration of the leg developed 3 years previously in this patient with Felty's syndrome. The ulcer healed with local treatment but recurred on two occasions. The brown pigmentation proximal to the ulcer was also present on the other leg.

Mild hepatomegaly is common in Felty's syndrome and liver function abnormalities, particularly elevations of alkaline phosphatase and the transaminases, which are described in about a quarter of the patients.[10] An unusual type of liver involvement may be associated with Felty's syndrome, but occurs rarely in other rheumatoid arthritis patients.[18] Histologically, the picture is described as nodular regenerative hyperplasia.[19] Although there is mild portal fibrosis or infiltration with lymphocytes and plasma cells, the appearance is not characteristic of cirrhosis. Obliteration of portal venules may compromise portal blood flow, leading to atrophy and regenerative nodule formation, portal hypertension, and gastrointestinal hemorrhage. It has been suggested that immune complex–mediated platelet activation may be the mechanism of venular injury and occlusion.[19] Other primary disorders may be associated with nodular regenerative hyperplasia, but about a third of cases have had Felty's syndrome.[18,19]

## HEMATOLOGIC FEATURES

The leukopenia in Felty's syndrome is a relative and absolute granulocytopenia, in contrast to systemic lupus erythematosus (SLE), in which lymphopenia is a more prominent feature. Few patients have blood counts often enough to determine the rate at which granulocytopenia develops at the onset of Felty's syndrome, but in some cases only weeks have elapsed between normal and grossly abnormal white blood cell counts. There is often considerable spontaneous variation in the granulocyte count. Patients with mild lowering may return to the normal range, but this is rarely seen when depression is severe. Thus, spontaneous remissions have been observed[11,20] but are uncommon. During infections or other stressful episodes the granulocyte count often returns to the normal range but is seldom elevated. This may conceal the diagnosis temporarily, since blood counts may be ordered in some patients mainly in the setting of an infection or other acute illness.

The bone marrow may show no abnormality in some cases, but in most there is a myeloid hyperplasia, with a relative excess of immature forms, often described as "maturation arrest." Although this might reflect an impaired myelopoietic response, early release of mature forms would result in the same appearance.[9,10,11,14] Rarely the marrow suggests a depression in myeloid activity.[11,14] or shows an increased lymphocytic infiltration.[14]

A mild to moderate anemia is found in most patients, representing the anemia of chronic disease with an additional component of shortened red blood cell survival, which is corrected by splenectomy.[21] Reticulocyte count elevations are common.[10] Thrombocytopenia (platelet count < 150,000 per cubic millimeter) occurs in 38 percent but is seldom severe enough to cause purpura.

## SEROLOGIC FEATURES

The alterations in immune response commonly found in rheumatoid arthritis are amplified in patients with Felty's syndrome, in keeping with the general picture of unusually severe articular and systemic disease. Rheumatoid factor has been present in 98 percent of the patients, generally in high titer.[10] Only a few seronegative cases have been reported.[11,15,16,22] Positive LE cell tests are found in one third and antinuclear antibodies (ANA) in two thirds of the patients, with wide differences in frequency (47 to 100 percent), probably reflecting the variable sensitivity of the latter test. Patients with Felty's syndrome also have granulocyte-specific ANA more often than rheumatoid arthritis patients without neutropenia (85 percent vs 14 percent).[22,23] Anti-nDNA is not elevated.[10] Immunoglobulin levels are higher than in other rheumatoid arthritis patients;[9,10] complement levels are lower,[10,24] although most patients have levels within the normal range. Immune complexes have been detected by various techniques in the majority of Felty's syndrome patients (Table 61–3). These complexes may contain IgG, IgM, and complement.[25] A granulocyte-reactive ANA is also selectively concentrated in the cryoprecipitate in some sera,[24] suggesting the possibility that this antibody might be available to act upon nuclear antigen following ingestion of the immune complexes by granulocytes.

**Table 61–3.** Immune Complexes in Sera of Patients with Rheumatoid Arthritis (RA) and Felty's Syndrome (FS)

| Method | RA (% Positive) | FS (% Positive) |
|---|---|---|
| Intermediate complexes by ultracentrifugation[25] | 27 | 100 |
| Double diffusion against IgM rheumatoid factor[25] | 27 | 75 |
| Phagocytosed inclusions in normal granulocytes[25] | 23 | 77 |
| Cryoglobulins[24] | 26 | 78 |
| C1q binding[26] | 12 | 60 |
| Platelet aggregation[27] | 8 | 68 |

## PATHOGENESIS

Although the spleen certainly plays a key role in the pathogenesis of granulocytopenia, little insight has been gained by routine examinations of surgical specimens, for they show only the predictable immune hyperactivity (increased plasma cells, immunoblasts, and germinal center hyperplasia) and inconstant evidence of phagocytic hyperfunction.[10,11,13] Amyloid is almost never found, and the periarterial lamellar fibrosis, characteristic of SLE, described in one report[28] has not been confirmed by others.

The hematologic improvement resulting from splenectomy led some to postulate that the spleen had been producing a humoral inhibitor of granulocyte production[29] and others to support splenic sequestration and destruction of granulocytes as the principal mechanism.[30] The debate appeared to be settled in favor of the latter proposal when granulocyte counts were shown to be lower in the splenic vein than in the artery.[31] However, recent studies have suggested that the two viewpoints are not mutually exclusive and that a number of factors may contribute to the development of granulocytopenia (Fig 61–2).

**Increased Removal of Granulocytes.** Granulocyte sequestration and reduced survival might certainly result from impaired motility of cells laden with immune complexes and difficulty in negotiating channels in the splenic pulp. Many granulocytes with large cytoplasmic inclusions containing immunoglobulins and complement were identified in the spleens of patients with Felty's syndrome.[32] Such phagolysosomal inclusions also form when normal neutrophils are incubated with sera from patients with Felty's syndrome.[33]

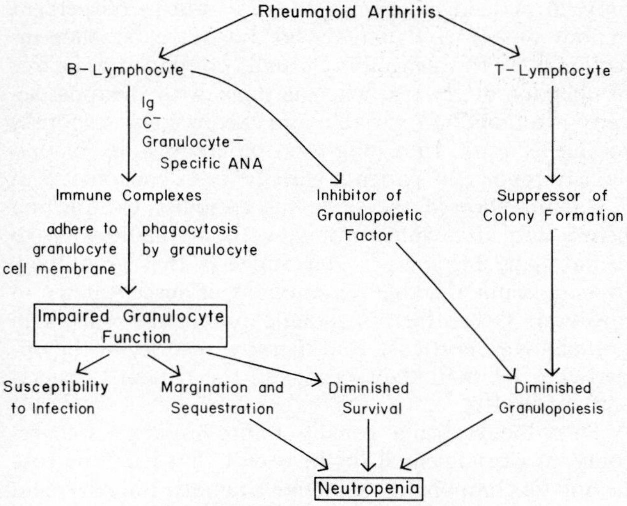


**Figure 61–2.** Pathogenesis of Felty's syndrome.

Neutrophil function and survival may also be compromised by the adherence of antibodies to cell surface receptors. The presence of granulocyte antibodies was suggested by early transfusion experiments in which plasma from a patient with Felty's syndrome produced transient granulocytopenia.[34] Granulocyte antibodies were demonstrated by fluorescent[24] and indirect antiglobulin consumption[35] techniques, and by inhibition of phagocytosis,[36] but antibodies could also be found in some non-neutropenic rheumatoid arthritis patients. In a direct antiglobulin consumption assay[37] there were high levels of surface immunoglobulin on the granulocytes in Felty's syndrome, not overlapping the levels found in rheumatoid arthritis without neutropenia and in other neutropenic controls with marrow failure. Curiously, the granulocyte surface immunoglobulins fell to the normal range after splenectomy, suggesting that most of these antibodies had been produced in the spleen. The surface immunoglobulins include granulocyte-specific ANA, which may be capable of fixing complement[23] and contributing to cell injury. A recent characterization of serum granulocyte binding activity in Felty's syndrome revealed that IgG was the principal immunoglobulin involved, and that both soluble immune complexes and specific antibodies to granulocytes participated.[38] Similar antibodies might also be directed against granulocyte precursors, leading to diminished production, but relevant studies have not yet been reported.

Granulocyte kinetic studies have been performed in Felty's syndrome, but technical problems and variations in these studies have led to disputed interpretations.[39] Early reports on small numbers of patients suggested that granulocyte survival was diminished,[40,41] but in a larger and more recent study excessive margination was demonstrated in all patients and was felt to represent the most significant defect.[42] The marginated pool consists of neutrophils adherent to the walls of venules in the spleen and elsewhere. Thus, neutrophils had shifted from the circulating to the marginated pool but had not been destroyed prematurely.

**Impaired Production of Granulocytes.** Evidence suggesting that suboptimal granulopoietic compensation might contribute to neutropenia was provided by the observation and the population of progenitor marrow cells in the synthetic phase was diminished in some patients with Felty's syndrome.[43] Bone marrow granulocyte precursor cells form colonies when grown in vitro in semi-solid agar; the number of colonies gives an indication of the proliferative state of the marrow. A glycoprotein colony-stimulating factor normally found in serum and urine is required for this growth. Colony-stimulating activity was found to be lower in Felty's syndrome than in other neutropenic disorders.[44,45] Retardation of mouse bone marrow colony counts was found after addition of sera from 87.5 percent of Felty's syndrome patients and only 12.5 percent of other rheumatoid arthritis sera, suggesting the possibility of an inhibitor. However, the effect of the sera on marrow cultures did not correlate with the degree of granulocytopenia, and no single serum fraction could be identified as the source of inhibition.[46] In a recent report, 8 of 19 Felty's syndrome patients were found to have a heat stable, nondialyzable serum factor capable of inhibiting colony formation by human marrow granulocyte precursors.[47]

Mononuclear cells were also shown to induce suppression of colony formation in normal human marrow cultures. This effect was found with peripheral blood mononuclear cells from Felty's syndrome patients, but not with their serum or with the cells of other patients with rheumatoid arthritis and neutropenia from other causes. The suppression correlated with granulocytopenia in Felty's syndrome.[48] The responsible cells are probably T lymphocytes.[49,50] The observation that occasional patients who have lymphocytic infiltration in the marrow respond poorly to splenectomy lends support to this mechanism.[14]

In summary, the granulocytopenia in Felty's syndrome appears to be multifactorial in origin. Ingestion and surface-coating of immune complexes leads to impaired granulocyte functions and facilitates their removal by the reticuloendothelial system. Specific antibodies directed against granulocyte cell surface antigens may also be involved. Sequestration of granulocytes in the spleen and venules results in a diminished circulating pool, either with or without actual premature destruction of granulocytes. Excessive utilization of leukocytes in the joints in patients with active synovitis places additional demands on granulopoiesis.[51] In some patients the marrow does not respond appropriately to granulocytopenia, apparently because of the presence of an unidentified humoral inhibitor and/or mononuclear cells which suppress myelopoiesis. There may be different subsets of Felty's syndrome, as illustrated by one report in which both humoral and cell-mediated mechanisms were investigated. About two thirds of the patients had high levels of neutrophil-bound IgG. In the remaining patients peripheral blood mononuclear cells inhibited colony growth in normal marrow.[52]

The increased susceptibility to infection is probably related to several factors in addition to granulocytopenia. Granulocyte reserves are diminished,[40,41,53,54] as determined by the increment in granulocyte counts after injection of epinephrine, endotoxin, or etiocholanolone, a steroid metabolite that mobilizes granulocytes, presumably from the marrow but possibly also from the marginal pool. Defective function of granulocytes in phagocytosis,[33] chemotaxis,[55,56] and bacterial killing[57] has been demonstrated. Hypocomplementemia may also play a role in some patients.[24,26]

## SPLENECTOMY

**Indications.** Since splenectomy usually reverses the hematologic abnormalities in Felty's syndrome, it is indicated if the patient has experienced significant morbidity. The usual indication is recurrent or serious infection, but in rare instances splenectomy may be performed for thrombocytopenia, anemia, abdominal discomfort from splenomegaly, or esophageal varices. Amelioration of active synovitis after splenectomy occurs too inconsistently to justify surgery on those grounds alone. Dramatic healing of the leg ulcers has been reported often enough to indicate splenectomy if conservative measures have failed.[13,16] Some authors have advocated splenectomy in all cases of Felty's syndrome as a prophylaxis against infection,[58] and others only for those with severe granulocytopenia (< 500 per cubic millimeter) even in the absence of infection.[13] However, it must be noted that these patients often remain free of infection over periods of many years.[9,45]

**Results.** No prospective, randomized studies of splenectomy have been performed, and the value of the procedure in preventing serious infection and prolonging survival is not entirely clear. It is likely that the variable long-term success rate reflects patient selection factors in different centers. However, there is no dispute about the prompt hematologic response, which is observed within minutes or hours after splenectomy in most cases,[15] although a few may be leukopenic at the time of discharge but improve soon thereafter.[13] In five recent reports,[9,10,11,13,14] 88 percent of patients had a good short-term hematologic response to splenectomy. However, granulocytopenia recurred and persisted in 24 percent of patients available for follow-up examinations. The absolute granulocyte level in these cases was generally higher than it had been prior to splenectomy. Continuing immune-mediated granulocyte destruction may be responsible for these secondary failures. Persistently high levels of serum granulocyte-binding IgG may be associated with a poor response to splenectomy.[59] In another study antibody-dependent, lymphocyte-mediated granulocytotoxicity developed in three of six splenectomy failures. None of the patients with Felty's syndrome had evidence of such an immune response prior to splenectomy.[60] Recurrent or persistent infection was noted in only 26 percent in one large series[13] but in 60 percent in four others.[9-11] Patients who did not experience infection prior to splenectomy usually continued to be free of infection afterward, whereas those with the most severe infections had variable and inconsistent responses to splenectomy. In a long-term outcome study of previously reported[10] patients with Felty's syndrome, 5 of 7 patients showed the same susceptibility to infection before and after splenectomy, without relationship to hematologic response.[61] This suggests that granulocytopenia is not the sole determinant of susceptibility to infection. Other factors include functional defects in granulocytes, corticosteroid therapy, severity of the underlying rheumatoid process, and the patient's general state of health.

Thrombocytopenia usually improves after splenectomy, as does anemia, to the extent that it is due to a hemolytic component. Although dramatic improvement in synovitis has been mentioned in several reports,[62,63] it is apparently not observed in most cases and is often temporary. Leg ulcers may also respond, even those which are not significantly infected,[13,15,16] but their variability in etiology and natural course makes these reports difficult to interpret.

## OTHER TREATMENTS

The basic illness should be treated in the same manner as it would in the absence of Felty's syndrome. Frequently granulocytopenia may improve during treatment with gold[45,64] or penicillamine.[45] Low doses of corticosteroids do not produce consistent improvement in granulocytopenia and also predispose to infection.[9,11] High-dose parenteral testosterone may stimulate granulopoiesis and is also reported to reduce the infection rate in a small number of patients[65] but is not suitable for females. Lithium salts also stimulate granulopoiesis by augmenting colony-stimulating activity,[66] but long-term benefit has not yet been demonstrated, and the treatment has been unsuccessful in the experience of some investigators.[54]

## References

1. Felty, A.R.: Chronic arthritis in the adult, associated with splenomegaly and leucopenia. Johns Hopkins Hosp. Bull. 35:16, 1924.
2. Hanrahan, E.M., Jr., and Miller, S.R.: Effect of splenectomy in Felty's syndrome. JAMA 99:1247, 1932.
3. Fitz, R.: Painful joints, splenomegaly, and anemia. Med. Clin. North Am. 18:1053, 1935.
4. Short, C.L., Bauer, W., and Reynolds, W.E.: Rheumatoid arthritis. Cambridge, Mass., Harvard University Press, 1957.
5. Isomäki, H., and Koivisto, O.: Splenomegaly in rheumatoid arthritis. Acta Rheum. Scand. 17:23, 1971.
6. Dinant, H.J., Muller, W.H., van den Berg-Loonen, E.M., Nijenhuis, L.E., and Engelfriet, C.P.: HLA DRw4 in Felty's syndrome. Arthritis Rheum. 23:1336, 1980.
7. Termini, T.E., Biundo, J.J., and Ziff, M.: The rarity of Felty's syndrome in blacks. Arthritis Rheum. 22:999, 1979.
8. Heyn, J.: Non-articular Felty's syndrome. Scand. J. Rheumatol. 11:47, 1982.
9. Ruderman, M., Miller L.M., and Pinals, R.S.: Clinical and serologic observations on 27 patients with Felty's syndrome. Arthritis Rheum. 11:377, 1968.

10. Sienknecht, C.W., Urowitz, M.B., Pruzanski, W., and Stein, H.B.: Felty's syndrome. Clinical and serological analysis of 34 cases. Ann. Rheum. Dis. 36:500, 1977.
11. Barnes, C.G., Turnbull, A.L., and Vernon-Roberts, B.: Felty's syndrome. Ann. Rheum. Dis. 30:359, 1971.
12. Cornwell, C.G., and Zacharski, L.R.: Neutropenia, elevated rheumatoid factor, splenomegaly and absence of rheumatoid arthritis. Ann. Inter. Med. 80:555, 1974.
13. Laszlo, J., Jones, R., Silberman, H.R., and Banks, P.M.: Splenectomy for Felty's syndrome: Clinicopathological study of 27 patients. Arch. Intern. Med. 138:597, 1978.
14. Moore, R.A., Brunner, C.M., Sandusky, W.R., and Leavell, B.S.: Felty's syndrome: Long-term follow-up after splenectomy. Ann. Intern. Med. 75:381, 1971.
15. DeGruchy, G.C., and Langley, G.R.: Felty's syndrome. Australas. Ann. Med. 10:292, 1961.
16. Williams, R.C., Jr.: Rheumatoid Arthritis as a Systemic Disease. Philadelphia, W.B. Saunders Company, 1974.
17. Baum, J.: Infection in rheumatoid arthritis. Arthritis Rheum. 14:135, 1971.
18. Thorne, C., Urowitz, M.B., Wanless, I., Roberts, E., and Blendis, L.M. Liver disease in Felty's syndrome. Am. J. Med. 73:35, 1982.
19. Wanless, I.R., Godwin, T.A., Allen, F., and Feder, A.: Nodular regenerative hyperplasia of the liver in hematologic disorders: A possible response to obliterative portal venopathy. Medicine 59:367, 1980.
20. Luthra, H.S., and Hunder, G.G.: Spontaneous remission of Felty's syndrome. Arthritis Rheum. 18:515, 1975.
21. Hume, R., Dagg, J.H., Fraser, T.N., and Goldberg, A.: Anaemia of Felty's syndrome. Ann. Rheum. Dis. 23:267, 1964.
22. Faber, V., and Elling, P.: Leucocyte-specific antinuclear factors in patients with Felty's syndrome, rheumatoid arthritis, systemic lupus erythematosus, and other diseases. Acta Med. Scand. 179:257, 1966.
23. Wiik, A., and Munthe, E.: Complement-fixing granulocyte-specific antinuclear factors in neutropenic cases of rheumatoid arthritis. Immunology 26:1127, 1974.
24. Weisman, M., and Zvaifler, N.J.: Cryoimmuno-globulinemia in Felty's syndrome. Arthritis Rheum. 19:103, 1976.
25. Andreis, M., Hurd, E.R., Lospalluto, J., and Ziff, M.: Comparison of the presence of immune complexes in Felty's syndrome and rheumatoid arthritis. Arthritis Rheum. 21:310, 1978.
26. Hurd, E.R., Chubick, A. Jasin, H.E., and Ziff, M.: Increased Clq binding immune complexes in Felty's syndrome. Arthritis Rheum. 22:697, 1979.
27. Bucknall, R.C., Davis, P., Bacon, P.A., and Verrier-Jones, J.: Neutropenia in rheumatoid arthritis: Studies on possible contributing factors. Ann. Rheum. Dis. 41:242, 1982.
28. Denko, C.W., and Zumpft, C.W.: Chronic arthritis with splenomegaly and leukopenia. Arthritis Rheum. 5:478, 1962.
29. Dameshek, W.: Hypersplenism. Bull. N.Y. Acad. Sci. 31:113, 1955.
30. Wiseman, B.K., and Doan, C.A.: Primary splenic neutropenia: A newly recognized syndrome, closely related to congenital hemolytic icterus and essential thrombocytopenic purpura. Ann. Intern. Med. 16:1097, 1942.
31. Wright, C.S., Doan, C.A., Bouroncle, B.A., and Zollinger, R.M.: Direct splenic arterial and venous blood studies in the hypersplenic syndromes before and after epinephrine. Blood 6:195, 1951.
32. Hurd, E.R.: Presence of leucocyte inclusions in spleen and bone marrow of patients with Felty's syndrome. J. Rheumatol. 5:26, 1978.
33. Hurd, E.R., Andreis, M., and Ziff, M.: Phagocytosis of immune complexes by polymorphonuclear leucocytes in patients with Felty's syndrome. Clin. Exp. Immunol. 28:413, 1977.
34. Calabresi, P., Edwards, E.A., and Schilling, R.F.: Fluorescent antiglobulin studies in leucopenic and related disorders. J. Clin. Invest. 38:2091, 1959.
35. Rosenthal, F.D., Beeley, J.M., Gelsthorpe, K., and Doughty, R.W.: White-cell antibodies and the aetiology of Felty's syndrome. Quart. J. Med. 43:187, 1974.
36. McIntyre, P.A., Laleli, Y.R., Hodkinson, B.A., and Wagner, H.N., Jr.: Evidence for anti-leukocyte antibodies as a mechanism for drug-induced agranulocytosis. Trans. Assoc. Am. Physicians 84:217, 1971.
37. Logue, G.: Felty's syndrome: Granulocyte-bound immunoglobulin G and splenectomy. Ann. Intern. Med. 85:437, 1976.
38. Starkebaum, G., Arend, W.P., Nardella, F.A., and Gavin, S.E.: Characterization of immune complexes and immunoglobulin G antibodies reactive with neutrophils in the sera of patients with Felty's syndrome. J. Lab. Clin. Med. 96:238, 1980.
39. Bishop, C.R.: The neutropenia of Felty's syndrome. Am. J. Hematol. 2:203, 1977.
40. Bishop, C.R., Rothstein, G., Ashenbrucker, H.E., and Athens, J.W.: Leukokinetic studies. XIV. Blood neutrophil kinetics in chronic steady-state neutropenia. J. Clin. Invest. 50:1678, 1971.
41. Greenberg, M.S., Zanger, B., and Wong, H.: Studies in granulocytopenic subjects. Blood 30:891, 1967.
42. Vincent, P.C., Levi, J.A., and MacQueen, A.: The mechanism of neutropenia in Felty's syndrome. Br. J. Haematol. 27:463, 1974.
43. Greenberg, P.L., and Schrier, S.L.: Granulopoiesis in neutropenic disorders. Blood 41:753, 1973.
44. Gupta, R., Robinson, W.A., and Albrecht, D.: Granulopoietic activity in Felty's syndrome. Ann. Rheum. Dis. 34:156, 1975.
45. Goldberg, J., and Pinals, R.S.: Felty's syndrome. Semin. Arthritis Rheum. 10:52, 1980.
46. Duckham, D.J., Rhyne, R.L., Smith, F.E., and Williams, R.C.: Retardation of colony growth of in vitro bone marrow culture using sera from patients with Felty's syndrome, disseminated lupus erythematosus (SLE), rheumatoid arthritis, and other disease states. Arthritis Rheum. 18:323, 1975.
47. Goldberg, L.S., Bacon, P.A., Bucknall, R.C., Fitchen, J., and Cline, M.J.: Inhibition of human bone marrow–granulocyte precursors by serum from patients with Felty's syndrome. J. Rheumatol. 7:275, 1980.
48. Abdou, N.I., NaPombejara, C., Balentine, L., and Abdou, N.L.: Suppressor cell–mediated neutropenia in Felty's syndrome. J. Clin. Invest. 61:738, 1978.
49. Bagby, G.C., Jr., and Gabourel, J.D.: Neutropenia in three patients with rheumatic disorders: Suppression of granulocytes by cortisol-sensitive thymus-dependent lymphocytes. J. Clin. Invest. 64:72, 1979.
50. Slavin, S., and Liang, M.H.: Cell-mediated autoimmune granulocytopenia in a case of Felty's syndrome. Ann. Rheum. Dis. 39:399, 1980.
51. Hollingsworth, J.W., Siegel, E.R., and Creasey, W.A.: Granulocyte survival in synovial exudate of patients with rheumatoid arthritis and other inflammatory joint diseases. Yale J. Biol. Med. 39:289, 1967.
52. Starkebaum, G., Singer, J.W., and Arend, W.P.: Humoral and cellular immune mechanisms of neutropenia in patients with Felty's syndrome. Clin. Exp. Immunol. 39:307, 1980.
53. Kimball, H.R., Wolff, S.M., Talal, N., Plotz, P.H., and Decker, J.L.: Marrow granulocyte reserves in the rheumatic diseases. Arthritis Rheum. 16:345, 1973.
54. Joyce, R.A., Boggs, D.R., Chervenick, P.A., and Lalezari, P.: Neutrophil kinetics in Felty's syndrome: Am. J. Med. 69:695, 1980.
55. Mowat, A.G., and Baum, J.: Chemotaxis of polymorphonuclear leukocytes from patients with rheumatoid arthritis. J. Clin. Invest. 50:2541, 1971.
56. Howe, G.B., Fordham, J.N., Brown, K.A., and Currey, H.L.F.: Polymorphonuclear cell function in rheumatoid arthritis and in Felty's syndrome. Ann. Rheum. Dis. 40:370, 1981.
57. Gupta, R.C., Laforce, F.M., and Mills, D.M.: Polymorphonuclear leukocyte inclusions and impaired bacterial killing in patients with Felty's syndrome. J. Lab. Clin. Med. 88:183, 1976.
58. Green, R.A., and Fromke, V.L.: Splenectomy in Felty's syndrome. Ann. Intern. Med. 64:1265, 1966.
59. Blumfelder, T.M., Logue, G.L., and Shimm, D.S.: Felty's syndrome: Effects of splenectomy upon granulocyte count and granulocyte-associated IgG. Ann. Intern. Med. 94:623, 1981.
60. Logue, G.L., Huang, A.T., and Shimm, D.S.: Failure of splenectomy in Felty's syndrome. The role of antibodies supporting granulocyte lysis by lymphocytes. N. Engl. J. Med. 304:580, 1981.
61. Thorne, C., and Urowitz, M.B.: Long-term outcome in Felty's syndrome. Ann. Rheum. Dis. 41:486, 1982.
62. Khan, M.A., and Kushner, I.: Improvement in rheumatoid arthritis following splenectomy for Felty's syndrome. JAMA 237:1116, 1977.
63. Gibberd, F.B., Gilbertson, C., and Jepson, E.M.: Felty's syndrome. Ann. Rheum. Dis. 24:46, 1965.
64. Luthra, H.S., Conn, D.L., and Ferguson, R.H.: Felty's syndrome: Response to parenteral gold. J. Rheumatol. 8:902, 1981.
65. Wimer, B.M., and Sloan, M.W.: Remission of Felty's syndrome with long-term testosterone therapy. JAMA 223:671, 1973.
66. Gupta, R.C., Robinson, W.A., and Kurnick, J.E.: Felty's syndrome. Effect of lithium on granulopoiesis. Am. J. Med. 61:29, 1976.

# Chapter 62
# Sjögren's Syndrome

*Keith Whaley and Margaret A. Alspaugh*

## INTRODUCTION: DEFINITION AND HISTORICAL ASPECTS

There is no absolute definition of Sjögren's syndrome (SS); however, the diagnostic triad described by Bloch and colleagues[1] serves most clinical purposes. This triad includes keratoconjunctivitis sicca or dry eyes, with or without lacrimal gland enlargement; xerostomia (dry mouth), with or without salivary gland enlargement; and the presence of a connective tissue disease, usually rheumatoid arthritis.[2,3] More rarely systemic lupus erythematosus, scleroderma (systemic sclerosis), polyarteritis nodosa, or polymyositis may be present.[3] In order to establish the presence of SS, at least two of these three criteria should be present. Patients having only the ocular and oral components are said to have the sicca syndrome, whereas those having associated connective tissue diseases are categorized as SS with the specific diseases, e.g., SS with rheumatoid arthritis.

Historically, filamentary keratitis was described by Leber in 1888,[4] xerostomia by Hadden in 1888,[5] and lacrimal and salivary gland enlargement without keratoconjunctivitis sicca or xerostomia by Mikulicz.[6] Other components of SS were described between 1883 and 1933.[7] However, it was not until 1933 that a full de scription was given by Henrik Sjögren.[8] Histologically, SS and Mikulicz's disease are identical and thus are currently considered to be variants of the same disease.[9]

## INCIDENCE AND PREVALENCE

As in most autoimmune diseases, there is a predilection for middle-aged and elderly females. However, in elderly persons in Scotland a high prevalence (16.7 percent) of keratoconjunctivitis sicca was found equally in males and females.[10] Xerostomia was also common in elderly females (18.2 percent), but less common in elderly males (2.8 percent). Definite sicca syndrome was found in 3.5 percent of females and 2.8 percent of males over the age of 80 years. It should be noted that there was no association between the prevalence of autoantibodies and keratoconjunctivitis sicca or xerostomia in these persons, suggesting that senile atrophy of the secretory apparatus rather than immunologic injury was the underlying etiology. The sicca syndrome, although not rare, is probably much less common than SS accompanied by a connective tissue disease. In the United Kingdom the incidence of keratoconjunctivitis sicca in rheumatoid arthritis is 11 percent,[11] whereas xerostomia occurs in only 1 percent of patients. It is likely that a dry climate (e.g., Mexico) will accentuate symptoms of the sicca syndrome, whereas a cooler, moist climate (e.g., the United Kingdom) may help minimize them. As a result of the widespread clinical application of the newer and more sensitive techniques for the investigation of salivary gland disease, it is now becoming obvious that subclinical inflammation of the salivary glands is almost universal in patients with connective tissue diseases, although the extent of tissue destruction is insufficient to produce the overt signs of secretory insufficiency. Recent publications have shown extremely high incidences of salivary gland abnormalities in systemic lupus erythematosus,[12] scleroderma,[13,14] and mixed connective tissue disease.[15] Indeed, an autopsy examination of the submandibular glands of patients with rheumatoid arthritis has shown lymphocytic infiltrates in all cases.[16]

## CLINICAL FEATURES

**Ocular.** The Schirmer tear test is a crude test for tear secretion[17] (Fig. 62–1). Normal individuals should wet 15 mm or more of the standard filter strip in 5 minutes. When subnormal wetting occurs, tear secretion should be stimulated by the inhalation of 10 percent ammonia held 6 inches below the nose.[3] Less than 15 mm of wetting during the forced Schirmer tear test demonstrates diminished secretion. However, the presence of diminished tear secretion alone is not diagnostic of keratoconjunctivitis sicca (Table 62–1). This may be confirmed by putting rose bengal dye (1 percent) into the conjunctival sac and using a slit lamp to find evidence of punctate or filamentary keratitis (Fig. 62–2). Keratitis alone is also not diagnostic of keratoconjunctivitis sicca and may occur in a number of other conditions (Table 62–2). When diminished tear secretion and a punctate or filamentary keratitis coexist, then keratoconjunctivitis sicca is considered present. Occasional patients may have SS with normal tear secretion, since patients may have only pronounced lacrimal gland enlargement (Table 62–3). Usually, however, lacrimal gland enlargement is associated with diminished tear secretion. In hot, dry atmospheres the standard Schirmer test gives false-positive results.[18] Hence, in certain geographical locations a

**Table 62–1.** Principal Causes of Diminished Tear Secretion

1. Senile atrophy of lacrimal glands
2. Inflammatory conditions, e.g., Sjögren's syndrome, sarcoidosis
3. Tumors, as listed in causes of lacrimal gland enlargement (Table 62-3)

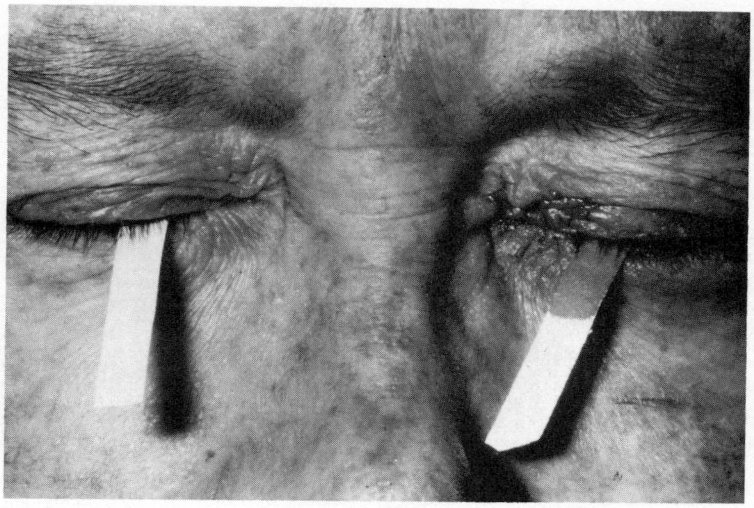

**Figure 62–1.** Schirmer tear test. The filter paper strip is folded 5 mm from one end, and placed over the lower lid at the junction of the middle and outer thirds. The length of wetting after 5 minutes is measured; over 15 mm is normal.

**Table 62–2.** Etiology of Punctate or Filamentary Keratitis

1. Degenerative—e.g., keratoconjunctivitis sicca from any cause, keratoconus, neuropathic keratopathy, benign mucous membrane pemphigoid
2. Infective—e.g., punctate epithelial keratitis (adenovirus, herpes, or vaccinia) and bacterial keratitis (rare)
3. Edematous states—e.g., recurrent erosions, wearing of ill-fitting contact lenses
4. Traumatic—rare

falsely high prevalence of keratoconjunctivitis sicca can occur.

The symptoms and signs of keratoconjunctivitis sicca are shown in Table 62–4. No one symptom is specific, whereas some signs appear to be. Patients with connective tissue diseases rarely complain about keratoconjunctivitis sicca, and careful questioning is required. We have developed a statistical method for the diagnosis of keratoconjunctivitis sicca based on the frequency with which these symptoms and signs occur in patients and controls.[19] This method can save the ophthalmologist's time.[20]

Table 62–5 lists the ocular complications of keratoconjunctivitis sicca. These complications are secondary to dryness of the cornea and conjunctiva rather than any direct immunological injury. The increased incidence of bacterial and viral infections of the eye in this condition is secondary to the breakdown of the local conjunctival defense mechanisms which depend on the antibacterial nature of tears and their physical flow properties.

**Oral.** Assessment of xerostomia is difficult. Mild xerostomia is occasionally found among healthy middle-aged people or patients with rheumatoid arthritis and other connective tissue diseases without evidence of SS. When salivary gland enlargement is present, the diagnosis is simple, as it is commonly found in association with xerostomia. Contrary to popular belief, gland enlargement is usually unilateral and episodic. In a study of 171 patients with SS, intermittent salivary gland enlargement was present in 37 patients (21.6 percent), of

**Table 62–3.** Causes of Lacrimal Gland Enlargement

1. Inflammation—unilateral or bilateral
   a. Acute dacryoadenitis, e.g., gonococcal, infectious mononucleosis
   b. Chronic dacryoadenitis, e.g., trachoma, tuberculosis, leprosy, actinomycosis
   c. Sarcoidosis
   d. Sjögren's syndrome
2. Tumors—usually unilateral
   a. Cysts
   b. Epithelial, e.g., adenoma, adenocarcinoma
   c. Lymphoreticular, e.g., Hodgkin's disease, leukemia, lymphosarcoma, Waldenström's macroglobulinemia
   d. Secondary tumors
   e. Miscellaneous, e.g., angioma, melanoma

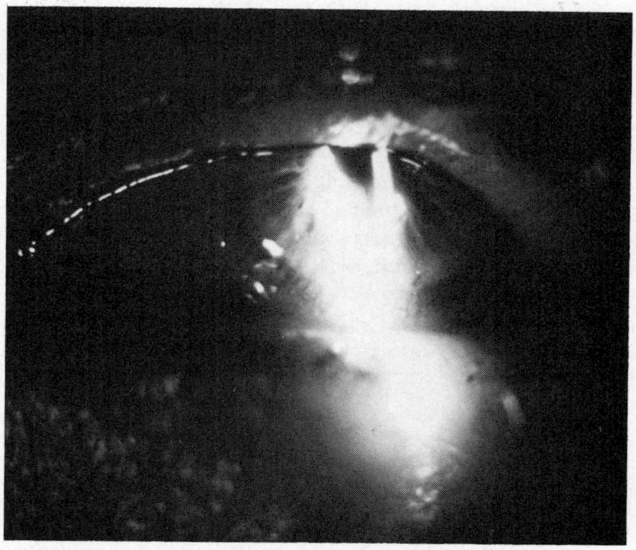

**Figure 62–2.** Slit lamp appearance of punctate keratitis in a patient with keratoconjunctivitis sicca.

**Table 62–4.** Clinical Features of Keratoconjunctivitis Sicca*

| Clinical Features | Normal (n=37) | With Keratoconjunctivitis Sicca (n=40) |
|---|---|---|
| Symptoms: | | |
| Foreign body sensation | 2 | 32 |
| Burning | 2 | 30 |
| Tiredness, with or without difficulty in opening the eyes | 2 | 26 |
| Dry feeling, with or without a poor response to physical or chemical irritants and emotions | 1 | 28 |
| Redness | 2 | 19 |
| Difficulty in seeing | 1 | 10 |
| Itchiness | 10 | 16 |
| Aches | 1 | 15 |
| Soreness or pain | 2 | 9 |
| Photosensitivity and excess of secretion which may appear to be watery, ropy, or as a film over the eye | 2 | 15 |
| Signs: | | |
| Dilatation of the bulbar conjunctival vessels (usually interpalpebral) | 2 | 11 |
| Photophobia | 7 | 31 |
| Irregularity of the corneal image | 3 | 21 |
| White and frothy or yellow and tenacious on discharge | 0 | 11 |
| Dullness of the conjunctiva and/or cornea | 0 | 11 |
| Ptosis | 0 | 6 |
| Mild pericorneal injection | 0 | 10 |

*Data from Anderson, J.R., et al.: Quart. J. Med. 41:175, 1972. Courtesy of the editor of the Quarterly Journal of Medicine.

whom only 13 had bilateral episodes of swelling. Persistent salivary gland enlargement was found in only seven patients (4.1 percent), and of these only five were bilateral.[3] One hundred and twenty-seven patients (74.3 percent) had no clinical salivary gland enlargement, and it is this group that provides the greatest diagnostic challenge. There are as yet no entirely satisfactory clinical or laboratory tests for the diagnosis of the oral component of SS. Probably the most reliable sign of xerostomia is the absence of pooling of saliva in the floor of the mouth. Severe xerostomia may cause lip cracking and chronic ulceration of the lip (Fig. 62–3), angular stomatitis, oral soreness, fissuring and ulceration of the tongue, atrophy of the oral mucosa, and, rarely, secondary candidiasis. Severe dental caries may occur in xerostomia.

**Table 62–5.** Ocular Complications of Keratoconjunctivitis Sicca

- Infection, often asymptomatic
  - Bacterial
  - Fungal
  - Viral
- Symblepharon with secondary exposure keratitis
- Pannus formation, causing essential shrinkage of the conjunctiva
- Marginal gutter ulceration
- Corneal ulceration with perforation, which may result in uveitis, cataract, and glaucoma

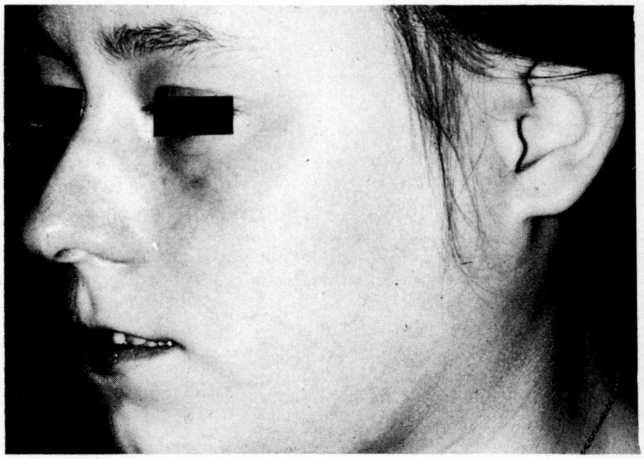

**Figure 62–3.** Patient with severe Sjögren's syndrome showing parotid gland enlargement and chronic ulceration of the lower lip.

The differential diagnosis of xerostomia is often difficult; mild degrees are common in mouth breathers and heavy smokers, and extremely severe xerostomia may occur following drug therapy and extirpation or irradiation of the salivary glands as well as in SS. The xerostomia found in severe dehydration secondary to uremia and diabetic ketoacidosis is not a diagnostic problem.

Salivary gland enlargement is not pathognomonic of SS, as illustrated by the bewildering list of causes listed in Table 62–6. A good history and physical examination should discriminate between these possibilities. If there is any diagnostic doubt, biopsy is essential. The laboratory tests are aimed at demonstrating pathological changes within the gland or assessing the functional reserve. Sialography demonstrates dilations (sialectasia)

**Table 62–6.** Causes of Salivary Gland Enlargement

1. Neoplasms
   - Primary salivary gland tumors (benign and malignant)
   - Malignant lymphoma
   - Waldenström's macroglobulinemia
2. Inflammation
   - Sjögren's syndrome
   - Sarcoidosis
   - Acute bacterial and viral infections
   - Chronic sialadenitis
   - Tuberculosis
   - Syphilis
   - Actinomycosis
   - Ancylostomiasis
   - Histoplasmosis
3. Miscellaneous
   - Iodide, lead, or copper hypersensitivity
   - Hyperlipidemic states
   - Cirrhosis of the liver
   - Diabetes mellitus
   - Malnutrition

and other changes (atrophy) occurring within the intrasalivary duct system[21,22] (Fig. 62–4). The technique of sialography is usually performed by injection of a predetermined volume of contrast media. This may lead to rupture of the duct system and aggravate the inflammatory process. It is our policy to use the hydrostatic technique, which virtually eliminates rupture of the duct system.[23] Sialectasia, with the retention of secretions, predisposes to staphylococcal parotitis with abscess formation.

Because of potential hazard, biopsy of the major salivary glands is recommended only when there is a suggestion of intraparotid malignancy or when serious diagnostic doubts are present. As changes in the minor glands mirror the changes in the major glands,[24] biopsy of the minor glands of the lip[25] or palate[26] is now a routine test. The technique is also useful in diagnosing sarcoidosis.[27] Histologically a positive biopsy of a major gland shows infiltration by lymphocytes, plasma cells, and occasional reticulum cells. These cells surround the ducts and infiltrate the acinar tissue with consequent loss of secretory epithelium. The stroma of the salivary glands is usually still present; hence, the lobular architecture is preserved, which helps in the differentiation between SS and lymphoma of the salivary glands. The epithelial cells lining the ducts show degenerative changes, and the lumina of the ducts contain inspissated material. The ducts are frequently dilated, and basket cell hypertrophy leading to epimyoepithelial "islands" may occur (Fig. 62–5). These "islands" result from intense proliferation of the epimyoepithelial cells, with consequent occlusion of the ducts. Morgan and Castleman[9,28] considered these "islands" pathognomonic of SS, but they may also be seen in lymphoid tumors affecting the salivary glands. Polymorphonuclear and eosinophilic leukocyte infiltration may occur, the former usually being associated with secondary bacterial infection. Although the lymphoid infiltrates of SS do not have the general appearance of normal lymphatic tissue germinal centers, occasionally there are centers seen in

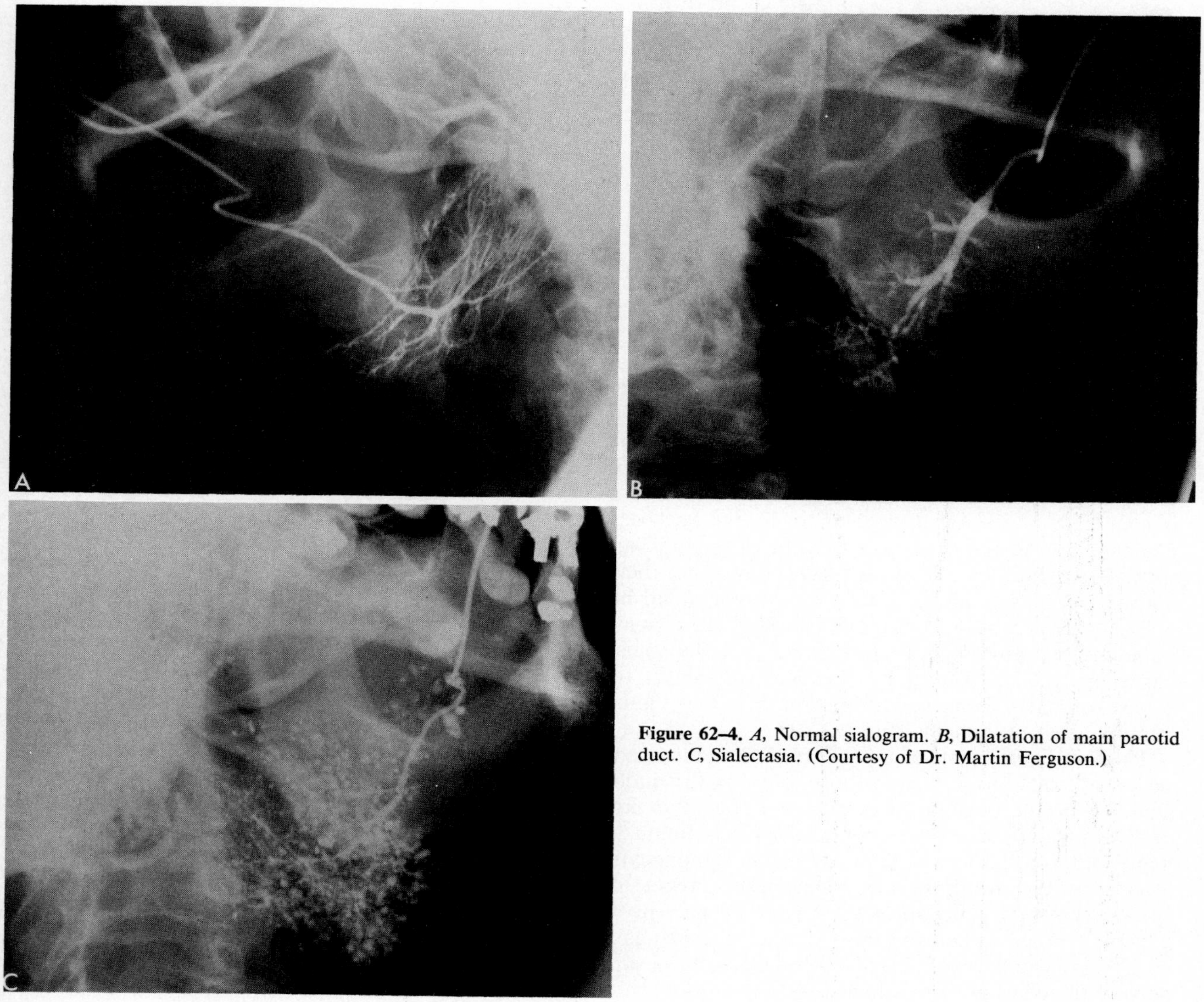


**Figure 62–4.** *A,* Normal sialogram. *B,* Dilatation of main parotid duct. *C,* Sialectasia. (Courtesy of Dr. Martin Ferguson.)

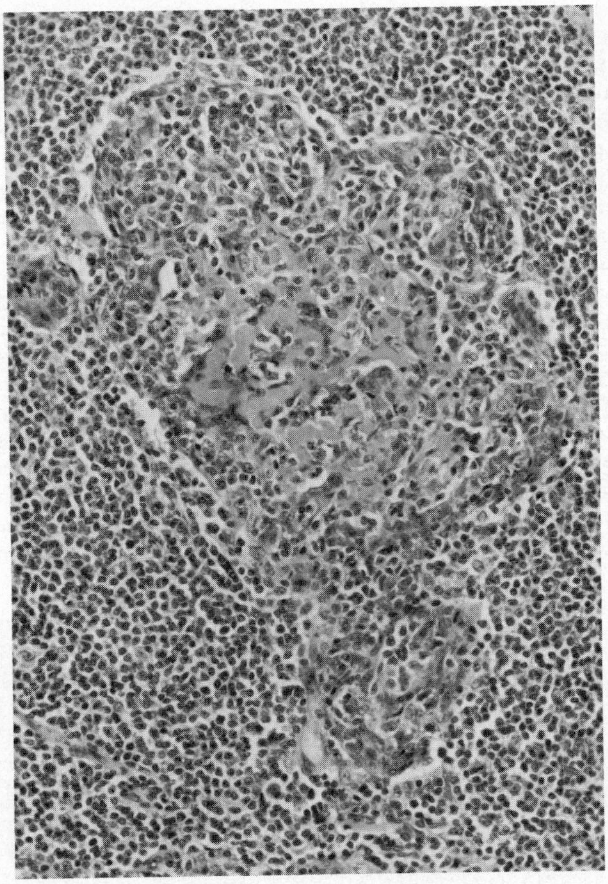

**Figure 62–5.** Epimyoepithelial cell island in the parotid gland. H&E. × 130. (Courtesy of Dr. G. MacDonald.)

the major glands,[1] indicating an ongoing immune response. Indeed, immunofluorescence studies have shown rheumatoid factor localized in and around the plasma cells in the infiltrate.[1] Although not conclusive, the evidence suggests that local synthesis of rheumatoid factor is occurring in the salivary gland in SS, as has been demonstrated in the synovial tissues in rheumatoid arthritis. Talal and his colleagues[29] have shown that rheumatoid factor is produced by minor salivary gland biopsy in tissue culture. As an end result of the chronic inflammatory process, complete atrophy of the acinar tissue may occur. The glands become completely replaced with fatty tissue, and little evidence of the original immune reaction remains (Fig. 62–6).

The histopathological changes that occur in the minor salivary glands are similar to those found in the major glands. For the purpose of diagnosis, diffuse lymphocytic infiltration must be ignored, as this is found in many other conditions.[30] However, focal lymphocytic infiltrates (Fig. 62–7) have a much higher degree of specificity for SS, and are seen in over 70 percent of patients.[3] Focal sialadenitis also occurs in other connective tissue diseases (Table 62–7),[3] an observation supporting the concept of subclinical SS.

Salivary gland flow rates, radionuclide scintiscanning, and iodide trapping capacity are all measures of function of salivary ducts. All are handicapped by the wide ranges found in normal individuals. Only salivary flow rates and scintiscanning are in regular clinical use; the iodide trapping capacity test is obsolete.[31] Salivary flow rates can only be properly assessed under conditions of maximal stimulation with lemon juice. Under these circumstances there is a marked age and sex difference in parotid salivary flow[3] (Table 62–8). There is no obvious change in salivary flow with age in males, whereas there is a pronounced fall in postmenopausal females. Inevitably, as with most tests of organ function in which the organ may be only partially destroyed, there is a marked overlap in salivary flow rates between patients with SS and healthy persons, which is markedly reduced when age and sex-matched controls are used.[3] Subnormal maximally stimulated salivary flow rates never occur in iatrogenic xerostomia, and stimulated levels of less than 0.5 ml per minute are virtually diagnostic of SS.

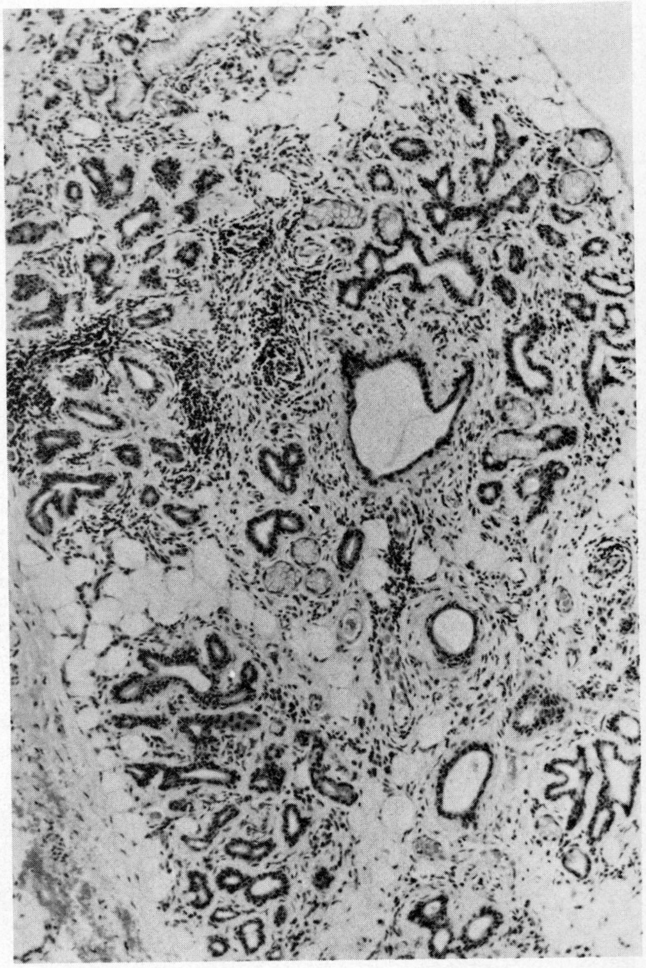

**Figure 62–6.** Late stages of inflammation in labial salivary glands. Lymphocytic infiltration associated with marked acinar atrophy, periductal fibrosis, and fatty infiltration. H&E. × 55. (Courtesy of Dr. G. MacDonald.)

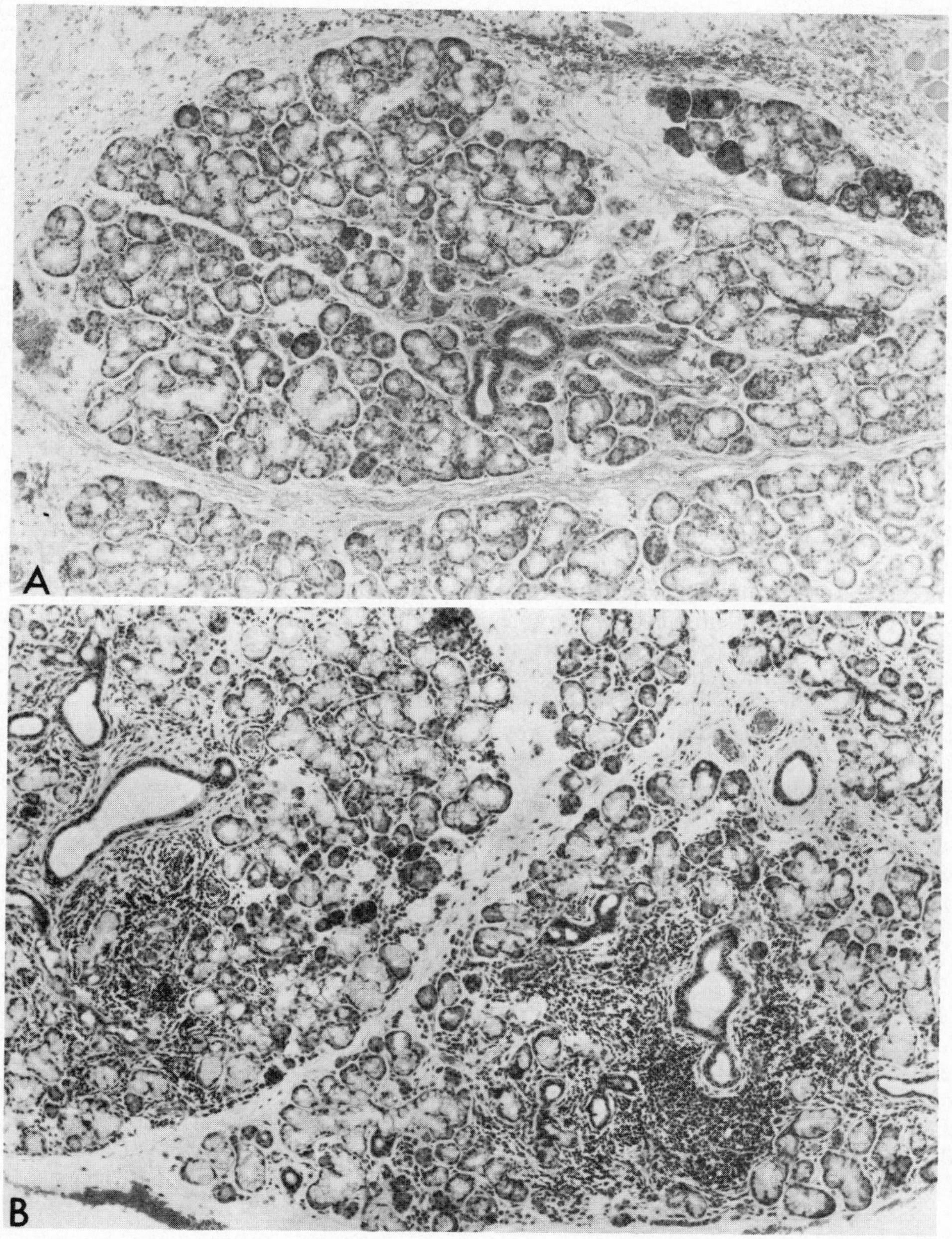


**Figure 62–7.** *A*, Normal labial salivary gland biopsy. H&E. × 50. *B*, Biopsy from patient with Sjögren's syndrome showing focal and diffuse lymphocytic infiltration, predominantly periductal in distribution, and duct dilatation. H&E. × 50. (Courtesy of Dr. G. MacDonald.)

Radionuclide scanning of the salivary glands using radioactive technetium pertechnetate ($^{99m}TcO_4^-$) is of proved diagnostic value.[32–34] Serial scans on patients permit assessment of the progression of disease. Salivary gland pertechnetate scanning is currently the most promising procedure in terms of sensitivity and simplicity of performance.

Other isotopes such as $^{67}$gallium, $^{111}$indium and $^{113m}$indium, and $^{75}$selenium-labeled seleno-methionine appear to be selectively concentrated in sites of lymphoreticular neoplasia and may afford a simple means of screening for suspected lymphoid tumor involving the salivary gland.[34a,34b]

**Involvement of Other Exocrine Glands.** ***Respiratory Tract.*** Involvement of the nasal mucosa results in dryness and crusting of the nasal mucosa.[1,35] Abnormalities of taste and smell may occur.[36] Eustachian tube obstruction may result in conduction deafness secondary to serous otitis media.[1,35]

Involvement of the lower respiratory tract may be present as a chronic bronchitis, with cough and production of tenacious sputum. Histologically there is

**Table 62–7.** Grades of Lymphocytic Infiltration in the Labial Salivary Glands in Connective Tissue Diseases*

| Clinical Group | Number | Grade of Lymphocytic Infiltrate 0 | 1 | 2 | 3 | 4 | Percent with Foci |
|---|---|---|---|---|---|---|---|
| Sicca syndrome | 21 | 1 | 3 | 4 | 5 | 8 | 61.9 |
| Rheumatoid arthritis plus Sjögren's syndrome | 50 | 1 | 10 | 4 | 15 | 20 | 70.0 |
| Rheumatoid arthritis | 73 | 30 | 20 | 9 | 12 | 2 | 19.2 |
| Psoriatic arthritis | 16 | 12 | 2 | 1 | 1 | 0 | 6.3 |
| Ankylosing spondylitis | 12 | 8 | 1 | 1 | 2 | 0 | 16.7 |
| Reiter's syndrome | 12 | 10 | 2 | 0 | 0 | 0 | 0 |
| Systemic lupus erythematosus | 5 | 1 | 1 | 1 | 0 | 2† | 40.0 |
| Scleroderma | 4 | 1 | 2 | 0 | 0 | 1† | 25.0 |
| Dermatomyositis | 1 | 1 | 0 | 0 | 0 | 0 | 0 |
| Gout | 2 | 2 | 0 | 0 | 0 | 0 | 0 |
| Osteoarthritis | 20 | 16 | 1 | 1 | 1 | 0 | 5.0 |

*From Whaley, K., et al.: Quart. J. Med. 42:279, 1973. Courtesy of the editor of the Quarterly Journal of Medicine.
†These patients also had Sjögren's syndrome.

chronic inflammatory cell infiltration around the bronchial glands. Recurrent pneumonitis and pleurisy, with or without effusion, may occasionally complicate SS, and during the acute episode pulmonary opacities may be seen on x-ray. Certain other patients develop chronic interstitial pulmonary fibrosis with varying degrees of severity. Many SS patients without overt evidence of respiratory disease have restrictive ventilatory defects and diminished gas transfer.[37] In addition to the lesion referred to as diffuse interstitial pulmonary fibrosis, a similar clinical syndrome can result from lymphoid cell infiltration of the pulmonary interstitium.[38] The type of infiltrate may range from the benign lymphocytic interstitial pneumonitis, through pseudolymphoma, to malignant lymphoma.[39] Bronchopneumonia may also occur. There is no evidence that chronic interstitial pulmonary fibrosis of SS is due to the intrapulmonary deposition of circulating immune complexes.[1,40]

*Gastrointestinal Tract.* In addition to the mouth, dryness of the pharynx and esophagus contributes to difficulty with the passage of food to the stomach. Mild dysphagia is therefore common in SS, and occasionally postcricoid webs, which are clinically, radiologically, and histologically indistinguishable from those found in the Plummer-Vinson syndrome, are seen.[35] These webs occur in the absence of sideropenia and do not appear to undergo malignant transformation. Abnormal esophageal motility also occurs in the sicca syndrome.[41]

Although achlorhydria has been described in SS, its significance is uncertain as it occurs occasionally in patients with connective tissue disease or in the older age groups.[42] Gastric biopsies from patients with SS have shown chronic inflammatory cell infiltration of the mucosa.[43] In a series of 121 patients with SS, gastric parietal cell antibody was found in 35 (27.6 percent). As the presence of this antibody in the peripheral blood correlates with the histological changes of chronic atrophic gastritis,[44] it is reasonable to assume that SS of the gastric mucosa is relatively common. However, overt pernicious anemia occurs in only 3.5 percent of SS patients.[37] That SS involving the stomach differs from true pernicious anemia is suggested by the finding that there is no increased incidence of SS in pernicious anemia.[45]

***Pancreas.*** Numerous case studies of pancreatic disease and SS have reported acute pancreatitis, chronic relapsing pancreatitis, and asymptomatic dense diffuse pancreatic calcification. Necropsy findings have included acute and chronic pancreatitis in a patient with hepatic cirrhosis,[47] parenchymatous disorganization and atrophy,[48] parenchymatous replacement by a heavy cel-

**Table 62–8.** Effect of Age on Lemon Juice–Stimulated Parotid Salivary Flow Rates* in Sjögren's Syndrome†

| | | <20 Years | 21–40 Years | 41–60 Years | ≥61 Years |
|---|---|---|---|---|---|
| Controls | Male | 1.49 ± 0.09 | 1.73 ± 0.09 | 1.69 ± 0.11 | 1.58 ± 0.16 |
| | Female | 1.99 ± 0.14 | 1.76 ± 0.09 | 1.36 ± 0.12 | 1.15 ± 0.08 |
| Sicca syndrome | Male | — | — | — | 0.65, 0.45, 0.50 (Only 3 patients studied) |
| | Female | — | — | 0.24 ± 0.08 | 0.27 ± 0.05 |
| Sjögren's syndrome plus rheumatoid arthritis | Male | — | — | 0.93 ± 0.17 | 0.43‡ (0.32–0.78) |
| | Female | — | 0.56 ± 0.05 | 0.47 ± 0.077 | 0.41 ± 0.05 |

*Milliliters per minute (mean ± S.E.M.).
†From Whaley, K., et al.: Quart. J. Med. 42:279, 1973. Courtesy of the editor of the Quarterly Journal of Medicine.
‡Only four patients studied.

lular infiltrate and vascular connective tissue,[49] and "oncocytic" changes in several acini containing periodic acid–Schiff positive material in their lumina.[50] Systematic investigation of pancreatic functions in SS have shown impaired responses to secretin[1,51–53] and pancreozymin,[53] suggesting that widespread or subclinical pancreatic disease is a common feature of SS. A recent study has also shown evidence of associated gastric and gallbladder dysfunction.[54]

***Liver.*** Hepatomegaly is found in 18 to 23 percent of SS patients, but until recently only sporadic case reports of significant pathology appeared.[1,37,55] Biochemical evidence of liver disease[56] and lymphocytic infiltration of the liver[57] have also been reported. Following the introduction of the mitochondrial antibody test as a marker of autoimmune liver disease,[58,59] it has become increasingly obvious that autoimmune liver disease is a feature of SS. The incidence of mitochondrial antibody in patients with the sicca syndrome is on the order of 10 percent, whereas it was found in the sera of 3 of 71 (4.2 percent) of patients with SS with rheumatoid arthritis.[60,61] The presence of antimitochondrial antibody in the serum is usually associated with the histological evidence of peripheral lymphocytic infiltration,[62] features indistinguishable from clinically obvious primary biliary cirrhosis. Thus, the involvement of the exocrine hepatic apparatus is clearly another manifestation of SS.

When patients with autoimmune liver disorders were screened, sicca syndrome was found in 35 percent of patients with chronic active hepatitis,[63] 24 percent with cryptogenic cirrhosis,[63,64] and 52 to 100 percent of patients with primary biliary cirrhosis.[64,65]

***Renal Involvement.*** SS patients may develop renal tubular defects, usually nephrogenic diabetes insipidus or renal tubular acidosis (type I or II, but II is more common), but also more global defects of renal tubular function, including generalized aminoaciduria, diminished renal tubular reabsorption of uric acid, or glycosuria; phosphaturia[66–69] also occurs, in addition to overt tubular dysfunction. Patients with SS display an inability to concentrate urine and an inability to excrete an acid load.[37,68,70–72] Histological examination of renal biopsy material from these patients has revealed a variety of pathological changes, the most prominent being interstitial infiltration with lymphocytes and plasma cells associated with nephrocalcinosis and tubular atrophy.[68,71,72] It is more likely that the renal tubular defects are due to lymphocyte-mediated tubular injury rather than to hypersensitivity.[73] Evidence to support this hypothesis comes from the observation that patients in the early stages of renal homotransplant rejection may develop renal tubular acidosis associated with peritubular lymphocytic infiltration.[74] Granular deposits of IgG and C3 have been detected in the peritubular basement membrane of a patient with the sicca syndrome.[75] Electron microscopic studies showed the presence of electron-dense deposits in the same location, suggesting that these deposits were immune complexes.

Immune complex glomerulonephritis may occur in patients with primary SS who do not have systemic lupus erythematosus (SLE).[37,68,76] Immunofluorescence and electron microscopic examinations have revealed membranoproliferative and membranous glomerulonephritis.[76] In addition to acute glomerulonephritis, elevated blood urea levels are not infrequent in SS.[37] The reason for this finding is unclear but could represent subclinical glomerular injury. Occasionally patients with SS have elevated DNA binding capacities and may eventually develop systemic lupus erythematosus.[77]

**Skin Manifestations.** Dryness of the skin is a common complaint of SS patients.[1,37,49] The mechanism underlying the xeroderma of SS is still unclear; there is histological evidence of chronic inflammation of the sweat glands (Fig. 62–8),[37,48,49] but another study failed to find such evidence.[1] A case report of complete absence of sebaceous glands associated with severe sweat gland atrophy in a patient with SS[77] suggests that sebaceous gland function may be impaired.

***Genital Dryness.*** It is now appreciated that the apocrine glands of the external genitalia are frequently involved in SS.[1] The skin of the vulva and vagina is dry and atrophic, and patients may complain of vaginal dryness, sometimes associated with a burning sensation

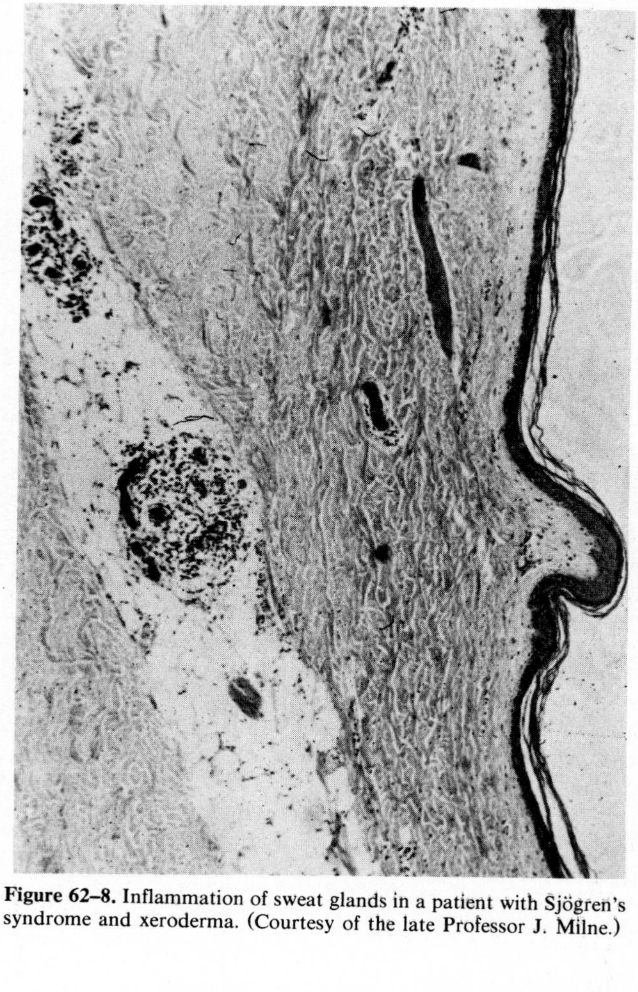

**Figure 62–8.** Inflammation of sweat glands in a patient with Sjögren's syndrome and xeroderma. (Courtesy of the late Professor J. Milne.)

or dyspareunia. Histologically nonspecific vaginitis may be present, but as the patients are frequently postmenopausal, such changes could be due to estrogen deficiency.

**Disease of Nonexocrine Organs.** ***Thyroid Disease.*** Serological evidence shows an increased incidence of autoimmune thyroiditis in SS,[37,79-82] and clinical thyroid disease occurs in 10 to 14 percent of patients.[1,37] There is no increased incidence of SS in patients with autoimmune thyroid disease.[83] Serum antithyroglobulin and antithyroid microsomal antibodies occur in about 40 percent of patients with SS, the incidence being the same in the sicca syndrome or in SS with associated connective tissue disease.[37]

***Diabetes Mellitus.*** Diabetes mellitus occurred in 7 of 171 patients (4.1 percent), which approximates the predicted incidence in a population of similar age and sex distribution.

***Neuropathy.*** Sjögren[8] noted bilateral facial neuritis in patients who also experienced transient sensory changes of the cornea and the facial skin, and Weber[84] reported a patient with bilateral ptosis and unequal irregular pupils. Since then, several reports of cranial neuropathy occurring in SS have appeared; isolated trigeminal neuropathy appears to be the most common presentation, but other isolated cranial nerves may be involved, and sometimes multiple cranial nerves are damaged.[85-87] Peripheral neuropathy may also complicate SS. The clinical picture is of either the sensory or the sensorimotor type.[37] Focal and diffuse involvement of the central nervous system, including the spinal cord, occurs uncommonly.[87] Vasculitis probably accounts for nervous system involvement.[48,87,88]

***Myasthenia Gravis.*** Myasthenia gravis has been reported in patients with SS,[37,89-91] but only in those patients with associated rheumatoid arthritis. Three percent of myasthenics also have rheumatoid arthritis.

***Muscle Disease.*** Polymyositis may be associated with SS.[1,92,93] In addition, focal myositis without muscle necrosis,[37] perivascular accumulations of lymphocytes, or a granulomatous myositis may occur.[1] Presumably the focal myositic lesions represent subclinical polymyositis.

***Joint Disease.*** Approximately half to two thirds of patients with SS have it in association with a connective tissue disease, usually rheumatoid arthritis.[1] In addition to the association of SS and rheumatoid arthritis, there is accumulating evidence that a mild relapsing nonerosive polyarthritis affecting the knees and elbows may complicate the sicca syndrome.[1,94,95] This arthritis is apparently episodic and self-limiting, and causes no permanent joint damage. The pathogenesis of this arthropathy is obscure, but its clinical nature suggests an immune complex phenomenon. Although one patient with psoriatic arthropathy and SS has been reported, an extensive investigation of patients with various seronegative spondyloarthritides failed to show an increased incidence of even subclinical SS.[96] Surprisingly, the prevalence of mild incidences of asymptomatic keratoconjunctivitis sicca in 100 patients with rheumatoid arthritis of less than 1 year's duration was almost 40 percent.[97] The generally accepted prevalence of keratoconjunctivitis sicca in rheumatoid arthritis is 15 to 25 percent, although very high incidences have been reported.[98]

***Vasculitis.*** SS may rarely be a complication of polyarteritis nodosa.[59,99] Patients with severe sicca syndrome may develop a vasculitis of the medium and small vessels,[100] which gives rise to skin ulceration and peripheral neuropathy.[1] Hyperglobulinemic purpura gives rise to capillaritis[37,101-103] and is found in a minority of patients with SS. About 20 to 30 percent of patients with hyperglobulinemic purpura have or will subsequently develop SS.[103] The rash of hyperglobulinemic purpura occurs especially in the lower limbs when the patient is ambulatory. It appears as "crops" of purpura, which are hot and itchy. Rarely the rash may be confluent. As the name implies, the rash is always associated with hyperglobulinemia.

***Raynaud's Phenomenon.*** Although Raynaud's phenomenon occurs frequently in patients with scleroderma and other connective tissue diseases associated with SS, it is also a frequent finding in patients with the sicca syndrome. The pathological basis of Raynaud's phenomenon is unclear, with the exception of scleroderma in which obliterative endarteritis of the digital vessels is present, or when cryoglobulinemia occurs. Cryoglobulinemia is an uncommon association of SS.

***Cutaneous Manifestations.*** Apart from skin dryness, purpura, skin ulceration, lip ulceration, and angular stomatitis, all of which have been discussed earlier, vitiligo may rarely occur in the sicca syndrome.[37] Three patients with partial lipodystrophy and one with total lipodystrophy associated with SS have been reported.[104,105] One patient had associated diabetes mellitus, and two patients had hypocomplementemia.[104] Complement activation appeared to be by the alternative pathway, although the presence of nephritic factor was not sought.

***Drug Allergy.*** Although Bloch and his colleagues[1] first drew attention to the undue frequency of drug hypersensitivity, in particular penicillin and gold, in patients with SS, it is still not generally appreciated that drug allergy may be a serious hazard in these patients.[106] A later study showed that penicillin allergy was increased in patients with rheumatoid arthritis, but this increase was wholly confined to those patients with coexistent SS. Thus, the occurrence of drug allergy in patients with rheumatoid arthritis should alert the physician to the possibility of coexistent SS. Gordon et al.[107] found no evidence of increased allergy to gold in patients with rheumatoid arthritis complicated by SS. We are unable to explain this discrepancy. In support of our earlier observations on penicillin and gold allergy, we have recently noted a very high incidence of allergic reactions to levamisole in patients with rheumatoid arthritis and coexistent SS.[108] Nine of ten patients with SS and rheumatoid arthritis developed allergy to this medication, whereas only five of 30 patients with rheumatoid arthritis alone developed allergic skin reactions. It has been suggested that SS may predispose to drug-induced systemic lupus erythematosus,[109] but the evidence for this is weak.[110]

## LABORATORY FINDINGS

**Hematology.** Mild anemia is a common finding in patients with SS.[1-3,55,111] The anemia is usually normocytic and normochromic, or occasionally hypochromic, as in other chronic inflammatory diseases. Leukopenia has been reported in 19 to 33 percent of patients with SS,[1,2,55,80,111] but in our own series only 6 percent had leukopenia.[37] The pathogenesis of leukopenia is obscure; bone marrow biopsies have shown no evidence of depressed leukopoiesis,[2] although granulocyte kinetics and the occurrence of granulocyte autoantibodies have not been studied. Eosinophilia has been reported as a common abnormality in many series of patients with SS,[1,2,111] and occurred in 5 percent of our patients.[37] Thrombocytopenia was reported by Heaton[78] in most of his patients with SS, but other authors consider it infrequent.[1,2,55,111] In our own studies in Glasgow, thrombocytopenia was only present in three patients with associated systemic lupus erythematosus, and was probably associated with this disease.[37]

***Serum Proteins.*** Diffuse elevation of serum immunoglobulins is a common finding in SS.[1,2,37] Extremely high levels may occur, and of course purpura hyperglobulinemia may complicate this development. In addition, a hyperviscosity syndrome may occur in SS, owing to the presence of either cryoglobulins or circulating IgG–anti-IgG complexes.[2,112-116]

All three major immunoglobulins may be elevated in the serum of patients with SS, compared to age- and sex-matched controls. This elevation is most marked for IgG and less for IgA.[37,117] However, the changes in IgM and IgA concentrations are relatively small.[29,72] Secretory IgA levels are also elevated in SS[37] but contribute a very small part of total IgA. However, serum secretory IgA levels are increased in many chronic diseases, even those not involving secretory surfaces.[118] Hypogammaglobulinemia has been seen in patients when malignant lymphoma supervenes in SS.[1,119-121] Circulating immune complexes are present in the sera of patients with SS.[122] Although a defect in Fc-receptor–mediated clearance by the cells of the reticuloendothelial system of patients with SS is not related to the presence of complexes, it occurs most commonly in patients with involvement of nonexocrine organ involvement.[123]

Cryoglobulinemia, as mentioned earlier, may complicate SS, and SS may be a complication of the Meltzer-Franklin syndrome.[124] A monoclonal IgG-K cryoglobulin from a patient with SS was shown to have an abnormal carbohydrate composition with a low fucose and hexose content, and abnormalities of the primary immunoglobulin structure also. The latter abnormalities included significant reductions in the isoleucine and arginine residues in the heavy chains. It is probable that the carbohydrate residue deficits are responsible for the incomplete solubility of this particular cryoglobulin.[125] It appears that mixed cryoglobulins frequently have reduced sialic acid content,[126-129] which is probably responsible for the cryoprecipitability of the complexes. In contrast, the solubility of monoclonal cryoglobulins is due to abnormalities of the amino acid composition and sequence.[130,131] Macroglobulinemia and cryomacroglobulinemia have been reported in patients with SS.[68,119,121,132,133]

Serum $\alpha$-2 macroglobulin levels are normal in patients with SS.[37] Patients with SS have normal pancreatic amylase levels,[134] whereas 15 percent have elevated serum salivary amylase levels. The concentration of serum salivary amylase did not correlate with any clinical or laboratory features of SS. It is possible that patients with high levels probably had a different underlying pathological process from those with normal or reduced levels.

***Proteins in Salivary Secretions.*** Salivary IgG and IgM levels are elevated in patients with SS,[135,136] and the concentrations of these two proteins are related to the severity of the gland destruction based on the sialography index.[136] Using a radioimmunoassay, elevated levels of IgA and IgM rheumatoid factor have been found in the saliva of SS patients.[137] It is probable that although local synthesis of immunoglobulins and rheumatoid factors occurs in the salivary glands,[29,138] the larger part of these salivary proteins are serum derived.[137]

Concentrations of $\beta$-2 microglobulin in the saliva of patients with SS are higher than serum levels,[139] suggesting that this low molecular weight cell membrane protein is secreted into saliva by tissue lymphocytes. Support for this hypothesis has been obtained by showing a correlation between the degree of inflammation seen on labial biopsy and the salivary concentration of $\beta$-2 microglobulins, especially in patients with lymphoproliferative complications. The observations that levels of serum concentrates rose during relapse and fell during remission suggested that serial measurements of serum $\beta$-2 microglobulin may be useful in monitoring disease activity, and measurement of salivary concentrations might permit the estimations of the degree of local inflammation.[140] Salivary lysozyme concentrations are frequently reduced in primary SS, especially in patients with parotid gland enlargement.[141]

**Non–Organ-Specific Autoantibodies** (Table 62–9). The most common autoantibody found in SS is rheumatoid factor reactive against both human and rabbit IgG. Rheumatoid factors in patients with SS and associated rheumatoid arthritis are directed to different antigenic determinants on the IgG molecule than are rheumatoid factors occurring in the sera of patients with the sicca syndrome.[142] In the former group, 51 percent of rheumatoid factors had anti-Gm specificity, a proportion similar to that found in uncomplicated rheumatoid arthritis, whereas only 20 percent of the SS patients had rheumatoid factors with anti-Gm specificity. However, the prevalence of auto- and isospecific anti-Gm rheumatoid factors was the same in both groups.[142]

Patients with SS not having rheumatoid factor demonstrable by conventional techniques have been shown to have IgG antiglobulin factors reacting with both horse and rabbit immunoglobulin fractions.[37] Previously such antiglobulin factors have been demonstrated in the sera of patients with seronegative rheumatoid arthritis,[143] ju-

**Table 62–9.** Prevalence of Autoantibodies in Sjögren's Syndrome

| | Sicca Syndrome | | Sjögren's Syndrome and Rheumatoid Arthritis | |
|---|---|---|---|---|
| | *Glasgow** | *Bethesda†* | *Glasgow* | *Bethesda* |
| Rheumatoid factor | | | | |
| Latex fixation | 36/69 (52.1%) | | 93/94 (99%) | |
| Bentonitic flocculation | | 22/23 (96%) | | 30/30 (100%) |
| R3 agglutination titer | 26/69 (39%) | | 79/94 (84%) | |
| SCA test | | 14/19 (74%) | | 21/29 (72%) |
| Antinuclear antibody | 25/68 (37%) | 14/16 (88)% | 50/91 (55%) | 14/25 (56%) |
| Non–tissue-specific precipitins | 12/62 (19%) | 13/16 (81%) | 15/73 (21%) | 1/18 (6%) |
| Smooth muscle antibody | 2/62 (3%) | | 7/70 (10%) | |
| Salivary duct antibody | 7/69 (10%)‡ | | 51/78 (65%) | |
| Thyroglobulin precipitating antibody | 2/12 (17%) | | 2/16 (13%) | |
| Thyroglobulin tanned red cell test | 17/50 (34%) | | 13/71 (18%) | |
| Thyroid microsomal antibody | 22/51 (43%) | | 15/72 (21%) | |
| Gastric parietal cell antibody | 15/51 (29%) | | 20/74 (27%) | |
| Coombs' test | 0/19 (0%) | | 4/29 (14%) | |
| LE latex | 2/61 (3%) | | 1/34 (3%) | |
| LE cells | 1/12 (8%) | 0/23 (0%) | 0/11 (0%) | 6/30 (20%) |

*From Whaley, K., et al.: Quart. J. Med. 42:513, 1973.
†From Bloch, K. J., et al.: Medicine 44:187, 1965.
‡Salivary duct fluorescence in the sicca syndrome is probably due to mitochondrial antibody.

venile rheumatoid arthritis,[144] gout, psoriatic arthritis, and ankylosing spondylitis.[145] (The occurrence of these antiglobulin factors in such a wide variety of chronic arthritides suggests that they merely reflect the presence of chronic inflammatory disease.) Circulating intermediate rheumatoid factor IgG–anti-IgG immune complexes have been demonstrated in the sicca syndrome.[1]

The prevalence of antinuclear antibodies (ANA) in SS by immunofluorescence was 68 percent in one series.[1] The incidence in sicca syndrome as opposed to SS with rheumatoid arthritis in the United States and United Kingdom is shown in Table 62–9. More recently other investigators[146] have reported a higher incidence of ANA in sicca syndrome than in SS with rheumatoid arthritis.

ANA in SS are directed against a variety of nuclear antigens, and this is reflected in the different patterns of nuclear immunofluorescence.[37,147] Using rat liver as substrate, the most common pattern of nuclear fluorescence is the homogeneous type which is due to antibody to DNA-histone. This antibody lacks diagnostic specificity, as it is the most common type of ANA in systemic lupus erythematosus and rheumatoid arthritis.[148] LE cells are not found in the sicca syndrome but do occur in approximately 10 percent of patients with SS and accompanying rheumatoid arthritis. Using a modified clot test to detect LE cells, Baumer[149] found pseudo-LE cells in 22 patients with SS. These cells were monocytes or polymorphonuclear leukocytes containing numerous small or large intracytoplasmic inclusions with nuclear characteristics. It is possible that these cells are an immunocytological expression of an antinuclear factor other than the LE cell factor.

The morphological patterns of nuclear immunofluorescence that appear to have some degree of specificity for SS are the speckled and nucleolar varieties.[147,150] In sicca syndrome the speckled pattern is usually due to the SS-B antibody, which will be discussed later.[150] The membranous (rim) pattern of nuclear fluorescence is usually not seen in SS unless it is associated with systemic lupus erythematosus. Antibodies to native DNA, almost diagnostic of systemic lupus erythematosus, occur infrequently in patients with the sicca syndrome.[36,37] It has been suggested that such patients will ultimately develop overt systemic lupus erythematosus,[77] but this has not been our experience.

Using an extract of a human lymphocyte cell line (WI-L2), Alspaugh and Tan[151] defined three precipitating antigen-antibody systems in the sera of patients with SS. These were denoted anti-SS-A, anti-SS-B, and anti-SS-C (Fig. 62–9). Anti-SS-A and anti-SS-B occurred more commonly in the sera of patients with the sicca syndrome (70 percent and 48 percent, respectively) than

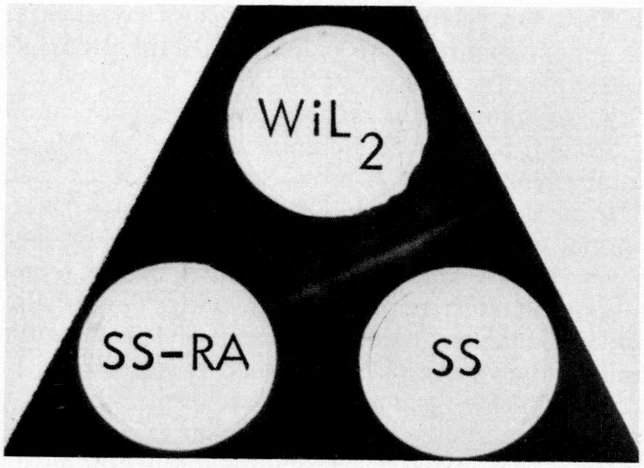


**Figure 62–9.** Immunodiffusion study showing nonidentity between precipitins of SS-RA (RAP) sera and the precipitins in SS-sicca (A and B). An extract of WI-L2 cells is shown in the upper wall. (From Alspaugh, M.A., and Tan, E.M.: J. Clin. Invest. 55:1067, 1975.)

in the sera of patients with SS and accompanying rheumatoid arthritis (9 percent and 3 percent, respectively) (Table 62–10). By contrast anti-SS-C has the same prevalence in SS with rheumatoid arthritis and in rheumatoid arthritis alone (68 percent), but is rare in the sicca syndrome.[57,150] These three antibodies were not found in certain other connective tissue diseases. The relationship of anti-SS-C to rheumatoid arthritis rather than SS led to its being referred to as rheumatoid arthritis precipitin (RAP).

Systemic lupus erythematosus appears to be the only other disease besides the sicca syndrome in which anti-SS-A is present. Approximately 33 percent of our lupus patients have this antibody.[152] While the incidence of SS in this group of patients has not been determined at this time, it should be noted that there is a very high incidence of SS in anti-SS-A positive patients. The relationship of anti SS-A and anti-Ro, and the characteristics of these antigen-antibody systems, is discussed fully in Chapter 46.

Serial studies have been performed on patients with SS. Titers of anti-SS-A antibody are generally stable but may increase with the onset of lymphoproliferation. In one patient with lymphoma and vasculitis, anti-SS-A antibody fell prior to death. In contrast, anti-SS-B titers fluctuate widely. Increased titers have occurred with the onset of myositis and lymphoproliferation. Treatment with corticosteroids apparently had little effect on anti-SS-A titers, but anti-SS-B levels fell dramatically.

Cryoprecipitates containing anti-SS-B—SS-B complexes have been found in two SS patients.[153] Ha, an acidic nuclear antigen, which reacts with antibodies in the sera of patients with SS or SLE,[154] has been shown to be immunologically identical with SS-B. In one patient, the appearance of anti-Ha (anti-SS-B) in the serum coincided with the onset of pseudolymphoma.[155]

*Anti-insulin receptor antibodies* have been demonstrated in one patient with SS and diabetes mellitus.[156] The hypocomplementemia of partial lipodystrophy is associated with circulating C3 nephritic factor. C3 nephritic factor is an oligoclonal immunoconglutinin, directed against the alternative pathway C3 convertase (C3bBb),[157-160] and it is therefore another non-organ specific autoantibody associated with SS.

*Mitochondrial antibody* is found in the sera of 10 percent of patients with the sicca syndrome and 4 percent of patients with rheumatoid arthritis and SS, and when present usually indicates clinical or subclinical evidence of liver disease.[37]

*Smooth muscle antibody* is an occasional feature of SS, but is not as good an index of hepatocellular disease.[37,161]

Antibodies to the Golgi complex have been found in the sera of a single patient with SS complicated by lymphoma. The antibody was not found in the sera of normal individuals, of individuals with uncomplicated SS (with or without RA), or of individuals with a wide variety of connective tissue diseases.[162] The significance of this antibody is unknown at present.

**Organ-Specific Autoimmunity.** Salivary duct antibody in sera from patients with SS was initially described by Bertram and Halberg.[163] Using an indirect immunofluorescent technique, sera stained the epithelial cytoplasm of the salivary duct. However, in a careful study of patients with various types of SS, MacSween and his colleagues[164] found a low prevalence in patients with sicca syndrome but a high prevalence in patients with SS accompanied by rheumatoid arthritis, and even in 20 to 25 percent of patients with rheumatoid arthritis alone. This result was confirmed in an extensive study by Whaley and his colleagues[37] (Table 62–9).

The small number of positive tests for salivary duct antibody in patients with the sicca syndrome is probably explained by the coexistence of mitochondrial antibody. All the patients in this group who had a positive salivary duct antibody test also had a positive mitochondrial antibody test. Mitochondrial antibody is a non–organ-specific antibody that reacts with the epithelial cytoplasms of many ductal systems, and therefore stains salivary duct epithelium. In contrast, salivary duct antibodies found in sera of patients with rheumatoid arthritis appear to be organ-specific, since they react only with the epithelial ducts of lacrimal and salivary glands.[164]

An antibody reacting with the cytoplasm of the epithelial cells of both intra- and interlobular pancreatic ducts has been detected by immunofluorescence. This antibody was found in the sera of 4 to 12 patients with

**Table 62–10.** Frequency of Precipitins SS-A and SS-B and RAP in Connective Tissue Diseases

| Disease | Number Tested | Precipitins | | |
|---|---|---|---|---|
| | | *SS-A* | *SS-B* | *RAP* |
| SS–sicca complex | 56 | 39 (70%) | 27 (48%) | 3 (5%) |
| SS–rheumatoid arthritis | 33 | 3 (9%) | 1 (3%) | 25 (76%) |
| Systemic lupus erythematosus | 85 | 28 (33%)* | 0 | 2 (7%) |
| Discoid lupus erythematosus | 22 | 0 | 0 | 0 |
| Scleroderma | 105 | 0 | 1 | 0 |
| Mixed connective tissue disease | 12 | 0 | 0 | 0 |
| Rheumatoid arthritis (seropositive) | 90 | 0 | 0 | 59 (67%) |
| Rheumatoid arthritis (seronegative) | 51 | | | 9 18%) |
| Normal healthy subjects | 70 | 0 | 0 | 1 |

*From Scopelitis, E., et al.: Arthritis Rheum. (in press).

SS, all of whom had an associated connective tissue disease, in eight of 31 (25.8 percent) patients with rheumatoid arthritis, but in none of 64 healthy controls.[165] The antibody cross-reacts with the duct cells of submandibular, parotid, and lacrimal glands, and thus appears to be salivary duct antibody. These data suggest that the duct cells of all the exocrine glands involved in SS contain common antigens against which the "autoimmune" response is directed.

Although clinical evidence of autoimmune thyroid disease is uncommon in SS, the prevalence of *thyroid autoantibodies* is significantly higher than in age- and sex-matched populations.[1,37] The presence of thyroid antibodies in the serum may indicate subclinical thyroiditis.[166]

*Gastric parietal cell antibodies* are found in approximately 30 percent of SS patients, the incidence being equally distributed between patients with sicca syndrome and patients with SS with accompanying rheumatoid arthritis.[37] In a similar study from Bethesda, it was found that American patients do not have an increased prevalence of parietal cell antibody.[167] Presumably, environmental factors are important in the pathogenesis of gastric parietal cell antibody in SS. This is in keeping with the results of a study of the prevalence of autoantibodies in monozygotic and dizygotic twins, from which it became clear that environmental factors exerted more control than genetic factors in the production of gastric parietal cell and other autoantibodies.[168,169]

Ten percent of SS patients have positive *Coombs' tests*, all of whom have connective tissue diseases.[1,37,51,55,170] Only two cases of patients with Coombs-positive autoimmune hemolytic anemia have been reported in patients with SS without systemic lupus erythematosus.[171]

*Adrenal, parathyroid, pituitary, and ovarian antibodies* are rare, and to date there is no evidence of their increased prevalence in patients with SS.

*Humoral immune responses*: Isohemagglutinin titers are significantly reduced in patients with the sicca syndrome whereas only levels of anti-$A_1$ and anti-$A_2$, but not anti-B levels, were reduced in patients with SS and rheumatoid arthritis.[172] Antibody responses to tetanus toxoid and pneumococcal polysaccharide vaccine are normal in patients with SS.[172,173] Neither immunogen precipitates disease exacerbation.

*Complement*: Patients with SS accompanied by rheumatoid arthritis have similar complement profiles to patients with rheumatoid arthritis alone. Raised levels of total hemolytic complement or individual complement proteins are the rule, but reduced levels occur when vasculitis is present. Patients with the sicca syndrome generally have normal serum complement levels with little evidence of complement activation.[174] However, when vasculitis occurs in the sicca syndrome, it is associated with profound hypocomplementemia, with reductions in the classic and also alternative pathway components. Genetic deficiencies of the complement system do not appear to be associated with the sicca syndrome.

*Cellular immunity*: Patients with sicca syndrome generally show normal delayed hypersensitivity responses to tuberculin and dinitrochlorobenzene (DNCB). However, patients with SS and rheumatoid arthritis, rheumatoid arthritis alone, or the sicca syndrome complicated by lymphoma have decreased response to these antigens.[172,175]

A number of abnormalities of T-lymphocyte numbers and functions have been recorded in SS. These include diminished numbers of T lymphocytes in the peripheral blood,[176,177] with reduction in the OKT8 (suppressor) cell population being most pronounced.[178] (The OKT4 [helper] population was normal.) The population of Ia-positive T lymphocytes is increased.[179] The autologous mixed lymphocyte reaction is reduced,[180] the mitogenic response to suboptimal concentrations of PHA is subnormal,[181] and the response of natural killer cells to immune interferon is reduced.[182] Serum levels of immune interferon are increased in SS.[183]

These findings could result from the disease process, or they could be the manifestations of an underlying abnormality that predisposes to SS. Alternatively, they could represent the result of both factors. Further work is required before their significance can be assessed.

In contrast, surface immunoglobulin positive lymphocytes (B lymphocytes) were not reduced in patients with the sicca syndrome of rheumatoid arthritis.[177] One communication reported a modest increase in circulating B lymphocytes in SS, which in itself is not remarkable. However, the authors showed a marked elevation in the number of B lymphocytes carrying multiple heavy chain determinants.[185] Similar findings have been reported in patients with chronic lymphocytic leukemia and other lymphoreticular neoplasms,[187-189] which is interesting in view of the predisposition of patients with SS to lymphoreticular neoplasms. Unlike SLE, patients with SS do not have increased numbers of B lymphocytes spontaneously secreting immunoglobulin in the blood or bone marrow.[186]

Antibody-dependent cell-mediated cytotoxicity is normal in SS and also in rheumatoid arthritis, showing that K cells, probably a subpopulation of T lymphocytes, are normal.[190]

**Characterization of Lymphocytic Infiltrates.** Immunofluorescent studies on frozen salivary gland sections from NZB/NZW mice demonstrated that the predominant cell types in the early lessions were immunoglobulin-bearing B lymphocytes and plasma cells. Later, as the lesions enlarged, the predominant cell type was the T lymphocyte, the B lymphocytes and plasma cells being smaller in number and situated more peripherally.[191] It has been shown in the minor salivary glands of human SS that small lymphocyte foci contain predominantly surface-immunoglobulin positive B lymphocytes and plasma cells, whereas larger lesions have a predominant T-lymphocyte infiltrate centrally situated, with B lymphocytes and plasma cells at the periphery.[177] It is not unreasonable to assume that the early lesion, which is predominantly periductal, is associated with B-lymphocyte infiltration and limited ductal damage, whereas with increasing T-lymphocyte infiltration considerable acinar destruction occurs. The predominant T-lymphocyte subset in the salivary gland infiltrates is OKT4 positive (i.e., of the helper-inducer population). The OKT4/OKT8 (helper:suppressor ratio) was greater than 3.0.[178]

Pseudolymphoma tissue showed primarily B-lymphocyte infiltration, while parotid tissue showed both B- and T-lymphocyte infiltration, i.e., B lymphocytes surrounded by larger numbers of T lymphocytes or null cells.

The early events in the evolution of such lesions could therefore be antigen recognition and/or early tissue damage by B lymphocytes and plasma cells migrating into the region. It is possible that the mechanism of tissue damage may be antibody-dependent cell-mediated lymphocytotoxicity or production of cytotoxic antibody. Recruitment of T lymphocytes could be by the production of lymphocyte chemotactic factors or other inflammatory factors which lack antigen specificity. Alternatively T lymphocytes might become specifically involved as part of a classic Type IV hypersensitivity reaction by becoming sensitized to tissue antigens released by B-lymphocyte–mediated tissue damage.

It is conceivable that the T-lymphocyte infiltration represents the early phase of human Sjögren's syndrome and that the smaller foci of B-lymphocyte and plasma cell infiltration represent a late lesion or, indeed, a different pathogenic process. Under these circumstances one could postulate that a cell-mediated immune response was the initial process and that the B lymphocytes and plasma cells were recruited later and increased tissue damage by antibody-dependent lymphocytotoxicity or the production of lymphocytotoxic antibody.[191]

Cell-mediated immunity to salivary gland extract has been demonstrated in patients with SS, using inhibition of polymorphonuclear leukocyte migration.[192] Despite these observations, Cremer and her colleagues were unable to demonstrate either lymphocyte- or antibody-mediated cytotoxicity for cultured autologous labial salivary gland tissue.[193]

**Genetic Factors in Sjögren's Syndrome.** The genes controlling the immune responses of mice map between the genes controlling the D and K determinants of the major histocompatibility complex,[194] and may not be separable from the genes coding for Ia surface antigens.[195] The Ia antigens, which are probably identical with the lymphocyte-defined antigens of mice,[196] appear to determine the intensity of the mixed lymphocyte reaction.[197] Although the immune-response genes in man have not yet been defined, by analogy with the mouse it is probable that they map within the HLA-D locus. Several organ-specific autoimmune diseases have been shown to be associated with HLA-B8, including celiac disease,[98] myasthenia gravis,[199] indiopathic Addison's disease,[200] Graves' disease,[201] chronic active hepatitis,[202] and juvenile diabetes mellitus.[203] A number of studies have shown the association of HLA-B8 with the sicca syndrome.[204-206] HLA-Dw3 is a lymphocyte-defined antigen in strong linkage dysequilibrium with HLA-B8,[207] and in both celiac disease[208] and sicca syndrome[209] the association of disease is primarily with HLA-Dw3 (69 percent association with sicca syndrome) and only secondarily with HLA-B8 (59 percent association) because of linkage dysequilibrium.[210] High levels of anti-SS-B antibodies were found in patients with the sicca syndrome and SS with SLE. In the sicca syndrome levels were higher in patients with HLA-Dw 2 or HLA-Dw3, or both than in patients with other HLA-DW types.[210a] This suggests that antigens or specific immune response genes close to the D region may be important for the development and antibodies to SS-B. All sicca patients have been shown to possess two immunologically distinct and genetically unrelated B-lymphocyte Ia antigens (AGS and #172).[211] Thus there is a strong argument in favor of the notion that immune-response genes located within the HLA-D locus are involved in the pathogenesis of SS and other organ-specific autoimmune diseases.

There are reports in the literature on the occurrence of SS in families. Table 62-11 presents the salient features of these reports. Although most of these cases had some symptoms and signs of SS, very few fulfilled the full diagnostic criteria. In addition some had associated con-

**Table 62–11.** Published Cases of Familial Sjögren's Syndrome

| Reference | Cases | Comment |
|---|---|---|
| Lisch, 1937[247] | Twelve cases in 3 generations | — |
| Coverdale, 1948[248] | Father and daughter | — |
| | Mother and daughter | — |
| Pascucci, 1958[249] | Mother and daughter | Mother only had symptoms of xerophthalmia |
| Bloch et al., 1965[1] | Mother and daughter | — |
| | Mother and daughter | — |
| Doni et al., 1965[250] | Mother and son | — |
| Camus et al., 1970[251] | Mother and daughter | Both had keratoconjunctivitis sicca and intermittent parotid gland enlargement; both had familial scleroderma |
| Shearn, 1971[2] | Two sisters | Both had systemic lupus erythematosus |
| Koivukangas et al., 1973[252] | Two sisters | Both had achalasia of the esophagus |
| Lichtenfield et al., 1976[253] | Four siblings—2 male, 2 female | One had an intraparotid lymphoma; most diagnoses did not fulfill diagnostic criteria |
| Frayha et al., 1977[254] | Mother and daughter | Both had CRST syndrome, mitochondrial antibody and Sjögren's syndrome |
| Vaillant et al., 1981[255] | Identical twin sisters | Both had sicca syndrome; no CTD |

nective tissue disease, suggesting that the familial occurrence was of the connective tissue disease and not the SS.

A high incidence of abnormalities associated with SS has been described in the relatives of patients with SS.[1,212,213] In one study, relatives less than 45 years old had a higher incidence of probable rheumatoid arthritis, positive Schirmer test, serum autoantibodies, and increased gamma globulin levels than age- and sex-matched controls.[213] In another study relatives did not differ from age- and sex-matched controls, presumably because of the increased incidence of these abnormalities in older individuals.[10]

The other evidence for the genetic etiology of SS comes from the New Zealand black (NZB), and the NZB/NZW F1 hybrid mice. These mice have genetically determined autoimmune disease, very similar to systemic lupus erythematosus, and in addition have lymphocytic infiltrates in their lacrimal and salivary glands very similar to those seen in SS.[214] Although the genetics of serum autoantibodies, hemolytic anemia, and systemic lupus erythematosus are well documented,[215] the genetic control of the Sjögren's lesions has not yet been studied in depth. However, it is likely that they are strongly influenced by the murine genotype.

**Infective Etiology.** Serum levels of IgM antibody to cytomegalovirus (CMV) are increased in patients with SS.[216] This may be relevant, as the clinical features of CMV are similar to those of SS. This finding is made more striking by the observation that serum levels of antibodies to common respiratory viruses are not elevated (Whaley, unpublished observations).

There is an unconfirmed report on ultrastructural studies of the bronchial epithelium of a patient with SS associated with a lymphoid interstitial pneumonia which revealed the presence of round electron-dense virus-like particles, 70 to 120 Å in diameter. These particles are similar to the murine leukemia type A virus particles associated with tumors in laboratory and wild mice.[217]

Ultrastructural studies have shown tubuloreticular structures in the endothelium of renal glomeruli[218-220] and in the major and minor salivary glands.[221,222] These tubuloreticular structures are seen in vascular endothelium and in the lymphocytes in the minor salivary glands.[222] From studies of transplanted human lymphoid tumors, it has been suggested that tubuloreticular structures are associated with immunoglobulin synthesis, more particularly with gamma than with mμ heavy chain synthesis.[223] At present the exact nature of these particles is unknown, but current evidence suggests they are not viruses.

**Lymphoproliferation.** Lymphoproliferation, both benign and malignant, occurs in SS. Benign lymphoproliferation characteristically occurs in the major and minor salivary glands and the lacrimal glands. Initially it is periductal in distribution, but later becomes widespread with acinar destruction. There is considerable evidence that these lymphocytes are responding to an antigenic challenge; salivary duct antibody which has autoreactivity[224] occurs in the sera of patients with SS,[163,164] and circulating lymphocytes of patients may be sensitized to a salivary gland antigen.[192,225,226] These data suggest that some of the lymphocytes in the salivary and lacrimal glands are sensitized to a glandular antigen, possibly ductal, although many could be nonspecifically recruited by the sensitized lymphocytes. The local production of large quantities of IgG, IgM, and IgA by the lymphocyte cells in minor salivary gland tissue[29] may be in response to an antigenic challenge.

Lymphocytic infiltration of many exocrine organs is a feature of SS, and, although generally mild, it may on occasion be particularly intense. This progressive disease supervenes on what has previously been a rather stable disease process, and is termed pseudolymphoma. The clinical manifestations of pseudolymphoma depend upon organ involvement, but characteristically the lungs, kidneys, and salivary glands are involved, although occasionally generalized lymphoproliferation with lymphadenopathy, pulmonary infiltrates, fever, and weight loss suggest lymphoma.[227] Involvement of the lungs results in pulmonary infiltration, and renal infiltration results in renal tubular acidosis and nephrogenic diabetes insipidus.[69,121] Pseudolymphoma of the salivary glands presents with massive salivary gland enlargement and associated widespread cervical lymphadenopathy.[121] Histologically, two types of pseudolymphoma can be diagnosed: highly pleomorphic infiltrates which include small and large lymphocytes, or plasma cells and large reticulum cells. Occasionally histological evidence of distortion of normal lymph node architecture and infiltration beyond the capsule makes differentiation between malignant and benign lymphoproliferation very difficult.[121] Examination of biopsy tissue using immunohistochemistry may reveal areas of monoclonal proliferation,[228,229] and as a result, influence one's therapeutic approach. In addition to benign lymphoproliferation, the chances of developing a malignant lymphoreticular neoplasm are markedly increased in patients with SS. In our experience the chance of developing such a tumor is approximately 5 percent,[37] which is far higher than the expected incidence in the general population (1 in 10,000). Malignant lymphoproliferation may occur after many years of apparently benign disease, and pseudolymphoma itself has been shown to progress to malignancy in two patients.[119]

A report from the National Institutes of Health suggests that the risk rate for developing non-Hodgkins lymphoma in SS is 44 times normal and the risk rate for SS with rheumatoid arthritis is the same as for sicca syndrome.[230] Most authorities believe that malignant lymphoproliferation occurs almost exclusively in the sicca syndrome.

For the purposes of classification, lymphoreticular neoplasms complicating SS fall into two broad categories, those of intrasalivary and those of extrasalivary origin. The latter are probably more common and certainly have been reported more frequently. In addition to site of origin, the lymphoreticular neoplasms of SS can be divided into histological types. Although reticulum cell sarcoma and unclassified primitive stem cell lymphoma are the most commonly encountered lymphoid malignancies, lymphosarcoma, Hodgkin's disease, giant follicular lymphoma, thymoma, Waldenström's macroglobulinemia, and Franklin's heavy chain disease have all been reported (Table 62–12). There are several clinically important aspects of the association of malignant lymphoproliferation and SS. This complication generally occurs more commonly in patients with severe forms of the disease as shown by a high frequency of preceding vasculitis, neuropathy, splenomegaly, and lymphadenopathy.[119] It has been suggested that low-dose irradiation to salivary glands may predispose to malignant lymphoproliferation.[119,230] This could perhaps be the result of a degree of immunosuppression; such a conclusion is supported by the observation that the administration of azathioprine to a patient with SS was associated with the development of reticulum cell sarcoma.[231] Our experience argues against increased incidence after irradiation or immunosuppressive therapy; the incidence of lymphoma in our patients is probably no different from the incidence in the Bethesda series, yet none of our patients had ever received x-ray therapy or immunosuppressive medication. Another important point in the management of patients with SS with lymphoma is that serum immunoglobulin concentrations and autoantibody titers may fall as lymphoma develops. In fact, these falls may precede the clinical manifestations of the lymphoma, and should alert the clinician to this dramatic change in the patient's prognosis.[119,120] Intrasalivary lymphoid neoplasms are also a well-known

**Table 62–12.** Cases of Sjögren's Syndrome (SS) or Benign Lymphoepithelial Lesion (BLL) Associated with Lymphoreticular Neoplasia of Primarily Extrasalivary Origin*

| References | Disorder | Number of Cases |
|---|---|---|
| Rothman et al., 1951[256] | SS—Stem cell lymphoma or reticulum cell sarcoma | 1 |
| Talal and Bunim, 1964[227] | | 3 |
| Talal et al., 1967[119] | | 3 |
| Hornbaker et al., 1966[257] | | 1 |
| Miller, 1967[258] | | 1 |
| Anderson and Talal, 1971[121] | | 1 |
| Slater et al., 1976[231] | | 1 |
| Present authors (unpublished) | | 1 |
| Bark and Perzik, 1968[259] | BLL— | 2 |
| Pinkus and Dekker, 1970[133] | | 1 |
| | *Total:* | 15 |
| Anderson and Talal, 1971[121] | SS—Malignant lymphocytic lymphoma | 1 |
| Bilder and Hornova, 1967[260] | SS—Lymphosarcoma | 1 |
| Thorpe, 1969[261] | | 1 |
| Whaley et al., 1973[37] | | 1 |
| Cited by Talal and Bunim, 1964[227] | SS—Hodgkin's disease | 1 |
| Whaley et al., 1973[37] | | 1 |
| Senti-Parades et al., 1964[262] | SS—Giant follicular lymphoma | 1 |
| Yoshinaga, 1968[263] | SS—Lymphoma of vocal cords | 1 |
| Strimlan et al., 1976[39] | SS—Malignant lymphoma | 6 |
| Lattes, 1962[264] | SS—Thymoma | 1 |
| Dourov et al., 1968[265] | | 1 |
| Alarcon-Segovia and Zavala-Mejia, 1971[266] | | 1 |
| Pinkus and Dekker, 1970[133] | BLL—Thymoma | 1 |
| | *Total:* | 18 |
| Talal et al., 1967[119] | SS—Waldenström's macroglobulinemia | 2 |
| Whitehouse et al., 1967[132] | | 1 |
| Maleville et al., 1967[267] | | 1 |
| Pinkus and Dekker, 1970[133] | | 1 |
| Anderson and Talal, 1971[121] | | 2 |
| Wager et al., 1971[263] | SS—Franklin's heavy-chain disease | 2 |
| | *Total:* | 9 |
| | *Overall total:* | 42 |

*More reports of extrasalivary lymphoreticular neoplasms have appeared since this table was originally prepared. They confirm the high incidence of such neoplasms in primary SS.

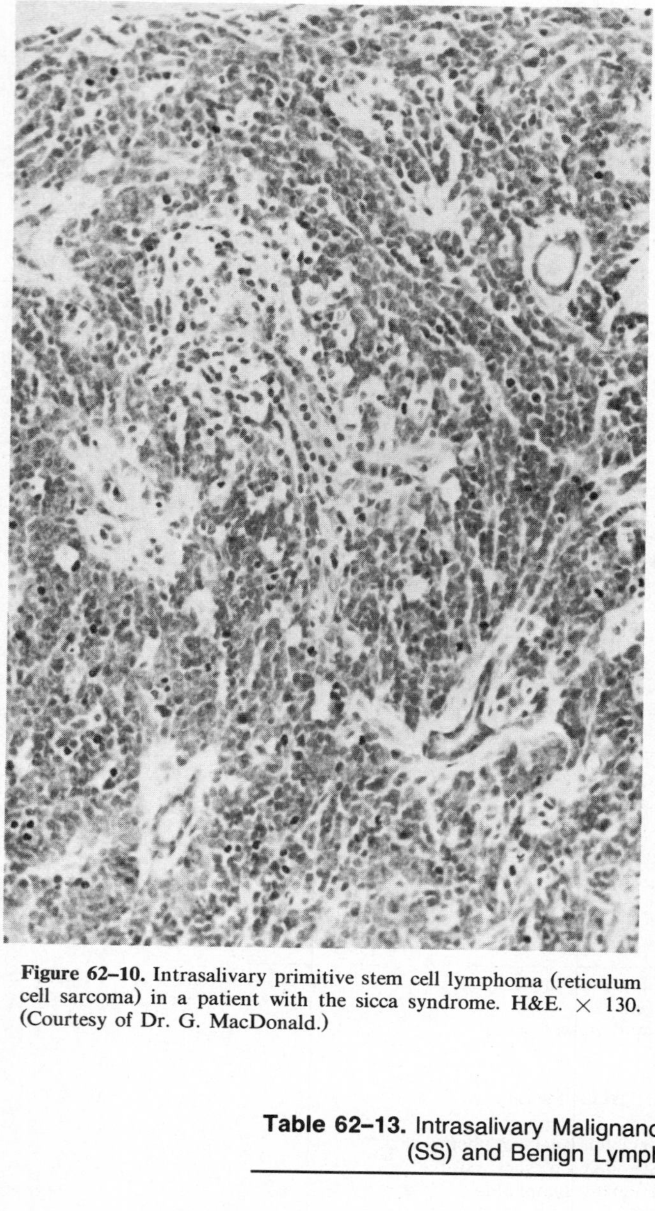

**Figure 62–10.** Intrasalivary primitive stem cell lymphoma (reticulum cell sarcoma) in a patient with the sicca syndrome. H&E. × 130. (Courtesy of Dr. G. MacDonald.)

complication of SS, but appear to be less frequent than their extrasalivary counterparts (Fig. 62–10). Malignant transformation may involve not only the lymphoreticular system, but also the epithelial elements of the salivary ducts[232] (Table 62–13). From the data of Hyman and Wolff,[233] it would appear that approximately 12 percent of cases of intraparotid lymphoreticular neoplasms are associated with SS or the benign lymphoepithelial lesion.

## ANIMAL MODELS OF SJÖGREN'S SYNDROME

New Zealand black (NZB) and the hybrid NZB × NZW F1 mice develop lesions in the salivary[214] and lacrimal glands[234] that are similar to those seen in SS, although ductal proliferation and epimyoepithelial cell islands do not occur.[234a] The spontaneous development of these lesions has influenced ideas on the possible role of genetic and viral factors in the pathogenesis of human SS and lymphoma and has also helped elucidate the sequence in which various lymphocyte subpopulations infiltrate the target organs.[191]

Attempts to experimentally induce Sjögren-like lesions in animals have, until recently, met with little success. The use of saline extracts of salivary gland homogenates emulsified in complete Freund's adjuvant produces remarkably little sialadenitis; but when the newer adjuvants carbonyl iron and *Bordetella pertussis* vaccine are used, severe periductal infiltration of chronic inflammatory cell results. This is associated with marked acinar destruction.[235] This model has not yet been fully characterized.

**Table 62–13.** Intrasalivary Malignancies Complicating Sjögren's Syndrome (SS) and Benign Lymphoepithelial Lesion (BLL)

| Reference | Disorder | Number of Cases |
|---|---|---|
| Bilder and Hornova, 1967[260] | SS—Lymphosarcoma | 1 |
| Lichtenfield et al., 1976[253] | SS—Lymphocytic lymphoma | 1 |
| Hyman and Wolff, 1976[233] | BLL—Lymphosarcoma | 1 |
| Whaley and Buchanan (unpublished) | BLL—Lymphocytic lymphosarcoma | 1 |
| | *Total*: | 4 |
| Azzopardi and Evans, 1972[269] | SS—Reticulum cell sarcoma | 5 |
| Whaley et al., 1973[37] | | 1 |
| Strimlan et al., 1976[39] | SS—"Malignant lymphoma" | 1 |
| Hyman and Wolff, 1976[233] | BLL—Reticulum cell sarcoma | 3 |
| | *Total*: | 10 |
| Gravanis and Giansanti, 1970[232] | BLL—Carcinoma | 3 |
| Delaney and Balogh, 1966[270] | SS—Adenocarcinoma | 1 |
| | *Total*: | 4 |
| | *Overall total*: | 18 |

## TREATMENT

Treatment of SS can be divided into the treatment of the sicca components and treatment of the associated disorders. The most important aspect of patient management is regular outpatient supervision by a rheumatologist, ophthalmologist, and dentist, together with other specialist care as required. Regular physical examinations and serological testing may give early warning of intervening malignancy or other complications and should be mandatory. Patient education is valuable; explanation and reassurance at the time of diagnosis facilitate patient awareness of possible complications, especially common problems such as drug allergy. The use of unnecessary antibiotic, x-ray, or immunosuppressive therapy is to be avoided.

In approximately 50 percent of patients with keratoconjunctivitis sicca the instillation of 0.5 percent carboxymethyl cellulose eyedrops is sufficient to ameliorate symptoms and prevent any local complications.[236] Polyvinyl alcohol (5 percent) also improves eye symptoms.[237] Artificial tear preparations can also be obtained as slow-release tears and may be effective in resistant cases.[238] Ocular complications such as essential shrinkage of the conjunctiva, corneal ulceration, and perforation require intensive ophthalmologic supervision. Apart from their use as eyedrops, artificial tears can be applied using constant flow spectacles containing reservoirs of the tear substitute. Flow relies on gravity, on capillary attraction, or on battery driven pump mechanisms. We have no experience with these methods of application, and they seem unnecessary in view of the simplicity and effectiveness of the application of artificial teardrops.

Patients who have a limited residual tear flow benefit from occlusion of the nasolacrimal ducts by electrocoagulation. This maneuver permits the accumulation of residual tears whereby symptoms and complications may be avoided. Not only do patients with SS lack tears; they frequently suffer from the accumulation of large volumes of inspissated mucus. The use of artificial tears in some of these patients meets with failure, but treatment with the mucolytic agent in acetyl cysteine (5 to 10 percent solution) greatly improves the success rate. It is important to appreciate that the dry eye is susceptible to both bacterial and fungal infection.[239,240] Regular culture of swabs from the conjunctival sac is recommended. Infection must be treated energetically with the appropriate antibiotics; the possibility of allergy should always be considered. Oral bromhexine (48 mg per kg per day) increases tear secretion in patients with SS, clarifies mucoid eye discharge, and may improve xerostomia.[241,242]

Xerostomia is difficult to treat. Lubricants themselves tend to adhere to the mucous membranes, leaving the mouth feeling drier than before. In our experience simply increasing the oral fluids is the most effective way of alleviating symptoms. However, a number of studies have shown that saliva substitutes may ameliorate symptoms and possibly increase salivary flow.[243-245] The incorporation of fluoride into the substitute may help prevent caries.[245] Secondary oral infections lead to painful mouths. *Candida* infection is the most common problem and responds well to topical mycostatin. Regular dental supervision may prevent or delay the onset of the rapidly progressive caries that complicates SS. Careful brushing of the teeth and dental flossing are mandatory. The occasional occurrence of suppurative parotitis, already mentioned, requires early antibiotic therapy if surgical drainage is to be avoided.

Nasal dryness is best treated by the frequent application of saline soaks. The application of oil-based nasal lubricants may lead to lipoid pneumonia and is best avoided.

Skin dryness is rarely of sufficient severity to justify treatment, but vaginal dryness leading to dyspareunia usually responds to lubricants such as K-Y jelly.

Treatment of associated connective tissue diseases requires care, as allergy to gold and levamisole and perhaps other medications is common.[108] Usually the treatment of the complications of SS, such as primary biliary cirrhosis, does not differ from the treatment of primary biliary cirrhosis without SS. However, there is some evidence that renal tubular acidosis may be improved by cyclophosphamide.[69]

It has been suggested that slight improvement in lacrimal and salivary secretions may follow cyclophosphamide therapy.[138] There is also a report suggesting that lacrimal and salivary secretions increase after alkali therapy for renal tubular acidosis.[246]

The treatment of lymphoreticular neoplasia is difficult and is best performed in collaboration with an oncologist. Some patients with pseudolymphoma respond dramatically to corticosteroids and cyclophosphamide; others do not and may progress to overt lymphoma. Although the case for irradiation or immunosuppressive medication predisposing to lymphoid malignancy is not proved, it is prudent to avoid them.

## References


1. Bloch, K.J., Buchanan, W.W., Wohl, M.J., and Bunin, J.J.: Sjögren's syndrome. A clinical, pathological and serological study of 62 cases. Medicine 44:187, 1965.
2. Shearn, M.A.: Sjögren's Syndrome. Philadelphia, W. B. Saunders Company, 1971.
3. Whaley, K., Williamson, J., Chisholm, D.M., Webb, J., Mason, D.K., and Buchanan, W.W.: Sjögren's syndrome. 1. Sicca components. Quart. J. Med. 42:279, 1973.
4. Leber, T.: Ueber die Entstehung der Netzhautablosung. Ber. Versamonl. Ophthal. Ges. Stuttg. 14:165, 1882.
5. Hadden, W.B.: On "dry mouth" or suppression of the salivary buccal secretions. Trans. Clin. Soc. Lond. 21:176, 1888.
6. Mikulicz, J.: Concerning peculiar symmetrical disease of lacrimal and salivary glands. Med. Classics 2:165, 1937-38.
7. Gougerot, H.: Insuffisance progressive et atrophie des glandes salivaires et muqueuses de la bouche, des conjunctives (et parfois des muqueuses nasale, laryngée, vulvaire): "Secheresse" de la bouche, des conjunctives, etc. Bull. Soc. Franc Derm. Syph. 32:376, 1925.
8. Sjögren, H.: Zur Kenntnis der Keratoconjunctivitis sicca (Keratitis filiformis bei Hypunfunktion der Tranendrusen). Acta Ophthalmol. 11:1, 1933.
9. Morgan, W.S., and Castleman, B.A.: Clinicopathologic study of Mikulicz's disease. Am. J. Pathol. 29:471, 1953.
10. Whaley, K., Williamson, J., Wilson, T., McGavin, D.D.M., Hughes, G.R.V., Hughes, H., Schmulian, L.R., MacSween, R.N.M., and Bu-

chanan, W.W.: Sjögren's syndrome and autoimmunity in a geriatric population. Age Ageing 1:197, 1972.
11. Williamson, J.: Personal communication, 1978.
12. Alarcón-Segovia, D., Ibanez, G., Velazquez-Forero, F., Hernandez-Ortiz, J., and Gomzalez-Jimenez, Y.: Sjögren's syndrome in systemic lupus erythematosus. Clinical and subclinical manifestations. Ann. Intern. Med. 81:577, 1974.
13. Alarcón-Segovia, D., Ibanez, G., Hernandez-Ortiz, J., Cetina, J.A., Gomzalez-Jimenez, Y., and Diaz-Jouanen, E.: Salivary gland involvement in diseases associated with Sjögren's syndrome. I. Radionuclide and roentgenographic studies. J. Rheumatol. 1:159, 1974.
14. Cipoletti, J.F., Buckingham, R.B., Barnes, E.L., Peel, R.L., Mahmood, K., Cignetti, F.E., Pierce, J.M., Rabin, B.S., and Rodman, G.P.: Sjögren's syndrome in progressive systemic sclerosis. Ann. Intern. Med. 87:535, 1977.
15. Alarcon-Segovia, D.: Symptomatic Sjögren's syndrome in mixed connective tissue disease. J. Rheumatol. 3:181, 1976.
16. Waterhouse, J.P., and Doniach, I.: Post-mortem prevalence of focal lymphocytic adenitis of the submandibular salivary gland. J. Pathol. Bact. 91:53, 1966.
17. Schirmer, O.: Studien zur Physiologie und Pathologie der Tranenabsorderung und Tranenabfulis. Arch Ophthalmol. 56:197, 1903.
18. Williamson, J., and Allison, M.: Effect of temperature and humidity in the Schirmer tear test. Br. J. Ophthalmol. 15:596, 1967.
19. Anderson, J.R., Whaley, K., Williamson, J., and Buchanan, W.W.: A statistical aid to the diagnosis of keratoconjunctivitis sicca. Quart. J. Med. 41:175, 1972.
20. Forrester, J.V., Anderson, J.A., Williamson, J., Jaczynowska, Z., and Buchanan, W.W.: Evaulation of a computer-assisted statistical diagnosis of keratoconjunctivitis sicca. Rheumatology 6:17, 1976.
21. Whaley, K., Blair, S., Low, P.S., Chisholm, D.M., Dick, W.C., and Buchanan, W.W.: Sialographic abnormalities in Sjögren's syndrome, rheumatoid arthritis and other arthritides and connective tissue diseases. A clinical and radiological investigation using hydrostatic sialography. Clin. Radiol. 23:474, 1972.
22. Blair, G.S.: Salivary gland radiology. Br. Dent. J. 140:15, 1976.
23. Park, W.M., and Mason, D.K.: Hydrostatic sialography. Radiology 86:116, 1966.
24. Chisholm, D.M., Waterhouse, J.P., and Mason, D.K.: Lymphocytic sialadenitis in major and minor glands: A correlation in post mortem studies. J. Clin. Pathol. 23:690, 1970.
25. Chisholm, D.M., and Mason, D.K.: Labial salivary gland biopsy in Sjögren's disease. J. Clin. Pathol. 21:656, 1968.
26. Bertram, U.: Xerostomia. Acta Adent. Scand. 25:Suppl. 49, 1967.
27. Hughes, G.R.V., and Gross, N.J.: Diagnosis of sarcoidosis by labial gland biopsy. Br. Med. J. 3:215, 1972.
28. Morgan, W.S.: The probable systemic nature of Mikulicz's disease and its relation to Sjögren's syndrome. N. Engl. J. Med. 251:5, 1954.
29. Talal, N., Asofsky, R., and Lightbody, P.: Immunoglobulin synthesis by salivary gland lymphoid cells in Sjögren's syndrome. J. Clin. Invest. 49:49, 1970.
30. Whaley, K., Chisholm, D.M., Downie, W.W., Dick, W.C., and Williamson, J.: Lymphocytic sialadenitis in the buccal mucosa in Sjögren's disease, rheumatoid arthritis and other arthritides. A clinical and laboratory study. Acta Rheum. Scand. 14:298, 1968.
31. Mason, D.K., Harden, R.McG., Boyle, J.A., Jasani, M.K., Williamson, J., and Buchanan, W.W.: Salivary flow rates and iodide trapping capacity in patients with Sjögren's syndrome. Ann. Rheum. Dis. 26:311, 1967.
32. Cummings, N.A., Schall, G.L., Asofsky, R., Anderson, L.G., and Talal, N.: Sjögren's syndrome—newer aspects of research, diagnosis and therapy. Ann. Intern. Med. 75:937, 1971.
33. Schall, G.L., Anderson, L.G., Buchignani, J.S., and Wolf, R.O.: Investigation of major salivary duct obstruction by sequential salivary scintigraphy; report of 3 cases. Am. J. Roentgenol. Radium Ther. Nuclear Med. 113:655, 1971.
34. Stephen, K.W., Chisholm, D.M., Harden, R.McG., Robertson, J.W. K., Whaley, K., and Stuart, A.: Diagnostic value of quantitative scintiscanning of the salivary glands in Sjögren's syndrome and rheumatoid arthritis. Clin. Sci. 41:555, 1971.
34a. Goode, R., Goodwin, D., Burgert, P., and Nelson, L.: Radioisotope scanning for tumours of the head and neck. Arch. Otolaryngol. 97:312, 1973.
34b. Garcia, R.R.: Differential diagnosis of tumors of the salivary glands with radioactive isotopes. Int. J. Oral Surg. 3:330, 1974.
35. Doig, J.A., Whaley, K., Dick, W.C., Nuki, G., Williamson, J., and Buchanan, W.W.: Otolaryngological aspects of Sjögren's syndrome. Br. Med. J. 4:460, 1971.
36. Henkin, R.I., Talal, N., Larson, A.L., and Mattern, C.F.T.: Abnormalities of taste and smell in Sjögren's syndrome. Ann. Intern. Med. 76:375, 1972.
37. Whaley, K., Webb, J., McAvoy, B.A., Hughes, G.R.C., Lee, P., MacSween, R.N.M., and Buchanan, W.W.: Sjögren's syndrome. 2. Clinical associations and immunological phenomena. Quart. J. Med. 42:513, 1973.
38. Weisbrot, I.M.: Lymphomatoid granulomatosis of the lung, associated with a long history of benign lymphoepithelial lesions of the salivary glands and lymphoid interstitial pneumonitis. Report of a case. Am. J. Clin. Pathol. 66:792, 1976.
39. Strimlan, C.V., Rosenow, E.C., Divertie, M.B., and Harrison, E.G.: Pulmonary manifestations of Sjögren's syndrome. Chest 70:354, 1976.
40. Tomasi, T.B., Fudenberg, H.H., and Finby, N.: Possible relationship of rheumatoid factors and pulmonary disease. Am. J. Med. 33:243, 1962.
41. Ramirez-Mata, M., Pena-Ancirez, F.F., and Alarcon-Segovia, D.: Abnormal oesophageal motility in primary Sjögren's syndrome. J. Rheumatol. 3:63, 1975.
42. Stenstam, T.: On the occurrence of keratoconjunctivitis sicca in cases of rheumatoid arthritis. Acta Med. Scand. 127:130, 1947.
43. Jebavy, M. von, Hradsky, M., and Herout, V.: Gastric biopsy in patients with Sjögren's syndrome. Zschr. Med. 16:930, 1961.
44. Adams, J.F., Glen, A.I., Kennedy, E.H., McKenzie, I.L., Morrow, J.M., Anderson, J.R., Gray, K.G., and Middleton, D.G.: The histological and secretory changes in the stomach in patients with autoimmunity to gastric parietal cells. Lancet 1:401, 1964.
45. Williamson, J., Paterson, R.W., McGavin, D.D., and Whaley, K.: Sjögren's syndrome in relation to pernicious anaemia and idiopathic Addison's disease. Br. J. Ophthalmol. 54:31, 1950.
46. Cardell, B.S., and Gurling, K.G.: Observations on pathology of Sjögren's syndrome. J. Pathol. Bact. 68:137, 1954.
47. Allington, H.V.: Dryness of the mouth. Arch. Dermatol. Syph. 62:829, 1950.
48. Szanto, L., Farkas, K., and Gyulae, E.: Sjögren's disease. Rheumatism 13:60, 1957.
49. Ellman, P., Weber, F.P., and Goodier, T.E.W.: Contribution to pathology of Sjögren's syndrome. Quart. J. Med. 20:33, 1951.
50. Bain, G.O.: The pathology of Mikulicz-Sjögren's disease in relation to disseminated lupus erythematosus. A review of the autopsy findings and presentation of a case. Can. Med. Assoc. J. 82:143, 1960.
51. Gordon, M.E., and Shanbrom, E.: The systemic manifestations of Sjögren's syndrome. Report of glandular function with histologic, bacterial and viral studies. Ann. Intern. Med. 48:1342, 1958.
52. Fenster, L.F., Buchanan, W.W., Laster, L., and Bunim, J.J.: Studies of pancreatic function in Sjögren's syndrome. Ann. Intern. Med. 61:498, 1964.
53. Hradsky, M., Bartos, V., and Keller, O.: Pancreatic function in Sjögren's syndrome. Gastroenterologia 108:252, 1967.
54. Dreiling, D.A., and Soto, J.M.: The pancreatic involvement in disseminated 'collagen' disorders. Studies of pancreatic secretion in patients with scleroderma and Sjögren's disease. Am. J. Gastroenterol. 1:546, 1976.
55. Vanselow, N.A., Dodson, V.N., Angell, D.D., and Duff, I.F.: A clinical study of Sjögren's syndrome. Ann. Intern. Med. 58:124, 1963.
56. Zawadzki, Z., and Edwards, G.A.: Dysimmunoglobulinemia associated with hepatobiliary disorders. Am. J. Med. 48:196, 1970.
57. Denko, C.W., and Bergenstal, D.M.: The sicca syndrome (Sjögren's syndrome). A study of sixteen cases. Arch. Intern. Med. 105:849, 1960.
58. Walker, J.G., Doniach, D., Roitt, J.M., and Sherlock, S.: Serological tests for the diagnosis of primary biliary circhosis. Lancet 1:827, 1965.
59. Goudie, R.B., MacSween, R.N.M., and Goldberg, D.M.: Serological and histological diagnosis of primary biliary cirrhosis. J. Clin. Pathol. 19:527, 1966.
60. Whaley, K., Goudie, R.B., Dick, W.C., Nuki, G., Williamson, J., and Buchanan, W.W.: Liver disease in Sjögren's syndrome and rheumatoid arthritis. Lancet 1:861, 1970.
61. Webb, J., Whaley, K., MacSween, R.N.M., Nuki, G., Dick, W.C., and Buchanan, W.W.: Liver disease in rheumatoid arthritis and Sjögren's syndrome: Prospective study using biochemical and serological markers of hepatic dysfunction. Ann. Rheum. Dis. 34:70, 1975.
62. Doniach, D., and Walker, J.G.: A limited concept of autoimmune hepatitis. Lancet 1:813, 1969.
63. Golding, P.L., Brown, R., Mason, A.M.S., and Taylor, E.: Sicca complex in liver disease. Br. Med. J. 4:340, 1970.
64. Golding, P.L., Smith, M., and Williams, R.: Multisystem involvement in chronic liver disease. Studies on the incidence and pathogenesis. Am. J. Med. 55:772, 1973.
65. Alarcon-Segovia, D., Diaz-Jouanen, F., and Fishbein, E.: Features of Sjögren's syndrome in primary biliary cirrhosis. Ann. Intern. Med. 79:31, 1973.
66. Kahn, M., Merritt, A.D., Wohl, M.J., and Orloff, J.: Renal concentrating defect in Sjögren's syndrome. Ann. Intern. Med. 56:883, 1962.
67. Shearn, M.A., and Tu, W.H.: Nephrogenic diabetes insipidus and other defects of renal tubular function in Sjögren's syndrome. Am. J. Med. 39:312, 1965.
68. Talal, N., Zisman, E., and Schur, P.H.: Renal tubular acidosis, glomer-

ulonephritis and immunologic factors in Sjögren's syndrome. Arthritis Rheum. 11:774, 1968.
69. Kaltreider, H.B., and Talal, N.: Impaired renal acidification in Sjögren's syndrome and related disorders. Arthritis Rheum. 12:538, 1969.
70. Shearn, M.A., and Tu, W.H.: Latent renal tubular acidosis in Sjögren's syndrome. Ann. Rheum. Dis. 27:27, 1968.
71. Tu, W.H., Shearn, M.A., Lee, J.C., and Hopper, J., Jr.: Interstitial nephritis in Sjögren's syndrome. Ann. Intern. Med. 69:1163, 1968.
72. Shioji, R., Furuyama, T., Onodera, S., Saito, H., Ito, H., and Sasaki, Y.: Sjögren's syndrome and renal tubular acidosis. Am. J. Med. 48:456, 1970.
73. Morris, R.C., and Fudenberg, H.H.: Impaired renal acidification in patients with hypergammaglobulinemia. Medicine 46:57, 1967.
74. Massry, S.G., Preuss, H.G., Maher, J.F., and Schreiner, G.E.: Renal tubular acidosis after cadaver kidney homotransplantation. Studies on mechanisms. Am. J. Med. 42:284, 1967.
75. Winer, R.L., Cohen, A.H., Sawhney, A.S., and Gorman, J.T.: Sjögren's syndrome with immune-complex tubulointerstitial renal disease. Clin. Immunol. Immunopathol. 8:494, 1977.
76. Moutsopoulos, H.M., Balow, J.E., Lawley, T.J., Stahl, N.I., Antonovych, T.T., and Chused, T.M.: Immune complex glomerulonephritis in sicca syndrome. Am. J. Med. 64:955, 1978.
77. Steinberg, A.D., and Talal, N.: The co-existence of Sjögren's syndrome and systemic lupus erythematosus. Ann. Intern. Med. 74:55, 1971.
78. Feuerman, E.J.: Sjögren's syndrome presenting as recalcitrant generalized pruritus. Some remarks about its relation to collagen diseases and the connection of rheumatoid arthritis with the sicca syndrome. Dermatologica 137:74, 1968.
79. Heaton, J.M.: Antimalarials in the treatment of Sjögren's syndrome. Br. Med. J. 1:1512, 1959.
80. Anderson, J.R., Goudie, R.B., Gray, K.G., and Buchanan, W.W.: Antibody to thyroglobulin in patients with collagen diseases. Scot. Med. J. 6:449, 1961.
81. Bunim, J.J.: Heberden Oration. A broader concept of Sjögren's syndrome and its pathogenic implications. Ann. Rheum. Dis. 20:1, 1961.
82. Bloch, K.J., and Bunim, J.J.: Sjögren's syndrome and its relationship to connective tissue diseases. J. Chron. Dis. 16:915, 1963.
83. Williamson, J., Cant, S., Mason, D.K., Greig, W.R., and Boyle, J.A.: Sjögren's syndrome and thyroid disease. Br. J. Ophthalmol. 51:721, 1967.
84. Weber, F.F.: Non-ocular features of Sjögren's syndrome. Med. Press 213:253, 1945.
85. Spillane, J.D., and Wells, C.E.C.: Isolated trigeminal neuropathy. A report of 16 cases. Brain 82:391, 1956.
86. Attwood, W., and Poser, C.M.: Neurologic complications of Sjögren's syndrome. Neurology 11:1034, 1961.
87. Kaltreider, H.B., and Talal, N.: The neuropathy of Sjögren's syndrome. Trigeminal nerve involvement. Ann. Intern. Med. 70:751, 1969.
88. Alexander, E.L., Provost, T.T., Stevens, M.B., and Alexander, G.E.: Neurologic complications of primary Sjögren's syndrome. Medicine (Baltimore) 61:247, 1982.
89. Downes, J.M., Greenwood, B.M., and Wray, S.H.: Autoimmune aspects of myasthenia gravis. Quart. J. Med. 35:85, 1966.
90. Brown, J.W., Nelson, J.R., and Hermann, C., Jr.: Sjögren's syndrome with myopathic and myasthenic features. Bull. Los Angeles Neurol. Soc. 33:9, 1968.
91. Osserman, K.E., and Genkins, G.: Studies in myasthenia gravis: Review of a twenty year experience in over 1200 patients. Mt. Sinai Med. J. 38:497, 1971.
92. Denko, C.W., and Old, J.W.: Myopathy in the sicca syndrome (Sjögren's syndrome). Am. J. Clin. Pathol. 51:631, 1969.
93. Fox, J.T.: Sjögren's syndrome and late-life myopathy. Arch. Neurol. 15:397, 1966.
94. Martinez-Lavin, M., Alspaugh, M.A., Taylor, D., Vaughan, J.H., and Tan, E.M.: Value of specific antibodies (SS-A and SS-B) in the diagnosis of Sjögren's syndrome (abstract No. 257). XIV International Congress of Rheumatology, June 26–July 1, 1977.
95. Ichikawa, Y., Komatsundo, M., Koriyama, K., and Arimori, M.: Cooperative clinical studies on Sjögren's syndrome between one with rheumatoid arthritis and one without rheumatoid arthritis. Arthritis Rheum. 25:137, 1976.
96. Whaley, K., Chisholm, D.M., Williamson, J., Dick, W.C., Nuki, G., and Buchanan, W.W.: Sjögren's syndrome in psoriatic arthritis, ankylosing spondylitis and Reiter's syndrome. Acta Rheum. Scand. 17:105, 1971.
97. Hernandez, L.A.: Unpublished data.
98. Sjögren, H.: Some problems concerning keratoconjunctivitis sicca and sicca syndrome. Acta Ophthalmol. 29:33, 1951.
99. Mason, A.M.S., Gumpel, J.M., and Golding, P.L.: Sjögren's syndrome—a clinical review. Semin. Arthritis Rheum. 2:301, 1973.
100. Soter, N.A.: Clinical presentations and mechanisms of necrotizing angiitis of the skin. J. Invest. Derm. 67:354, 1976.
101. Strauss, W.G.: Purpura hyperglobulinemia of Waldenström: Report of a case and review of the literature. N. Engl. J. Med. 260:857, 1959.
102. Waldenström, J.: Studies on conditions associated with disturbed gamma globulin formation. Harvey Lect. 56:211, 1961.
103. Talal, N.: Sjögren's syndrome. Bull. Rheum. Dis. 16:404, 1966.
104. Alarcon-Segovia, D., and Ramos-Niembro, F.: Association of partial lipodystrophy and Sjögren's syndrome (letter). Ann. Intern. Med. 85:474, 1976.
105. Ipp, M.M., Howard, N.J., Tervo, R.C., et al.: Sicca syndrome and total lipodystrophy: A case of a fifteen year old female patient. Ann. Intern. Med. 85:443, 1976.
106. Williams, B.O., St. Onge, R.A., Prentice, A., Dick, W.C., Nuki, G., and Whaley, K.: Penicillin allergy in rheumatoid arthritis with special reference to Sjögren's syndrome. Ann. Rheum. Dis. 28:607, 1969.
107. Gordon, M.H., Tiger, L.H., and Ehrlich, G.E.: Gold reactions are not more common in Sjögren's syndrome. Ann. Intern. Med. 82:47, 1975.
108. Balint, G., El-Ghobarey, A., Capell, H., Madkour, M., Dick, W.C., Ferguson, M.M., and Anwar-Ul-Haq, M.: Sjögren's syndrome: A contra-indication to levamisole treatment? Br. Med. J. 2:1386, 1977.
109. Grennan, D.M.: SLE precipitated by antibiotics in Sjögren's syndrome (letter). Br. Med. J. 1:460, 1976.
110. Sewell, J.R.: SLE precipitated by antibiotics in Sjögren's syndrome (letter). Br. Med. J. 1:385, 1976.
111. Stoltze, C.A., Hanlon, D.G., Pease, G.L., and Henderson, J.W.: Keratoconjunctivitis sicca and Sjögren's syndrome. Arch. Intern. Med. 106:513, 1960.
112. Bonner, H., Ennis, R.S., Geelhoed, G.W., and Tarpley, T.M.: Lymphoid infiltration and amyloidosis of lung in Sjögren's syndrome. Arch. Pathol. 95:42, 1973.
113. Alarcon-Segovia, D., Fishbein, E., Abruzzo, J.L., and Heimer, R.: Serum hyperviscosity in Sjögren's syndrome. Interaction between serum IgG and IgG rheumatoid factor. Ann. Intern. Med. 80:35, 1974.
114. Pruzanski, W.: Hyperviscosity and immunoglobulin complexes. Ann. Intern. Med. 80:107, 1974.
115. Blaylock, W.M., Waller, M., and Normansell, D.E.: Sjögren's syndrome: Hyperviscosity and intermediate complexes. Ann. Intern. Med. 80:27, 1974.
116. Waller, M., Edwards, W., Mullinax, F., Hymes, A.J., and Curry, N.: Hyperviscosity syndrome: Natural history in a patient with Sjögren's syndrome. Med. Coll. Va. Quart. 12:81, 1976.
117. Gumpel, J.M., and Hobbs, J.R.: Serum immune globulins in Sjögren's syndrome. Ann. Rheum. Dis. 29:681, 1970.
118. Waldman, R.H., Mach, J.P., Stella, M.M., and Rowe, D.S.: Secretory IgA in human serum. J. Immunol. 105:43, 1970.
119. Talal, N., Sokoloff, L., and Barth, W.F.: Extrasalivary lymphoid abnormalities in Sjögren's syndrome (reticulum cell sarcoma, "pseudolymphoma," macroglobulinemia). Am. J. Med. 43:50, 1967.
120. Whaley, K., and Buchanan, W.W.: Recent advances in Sjögren's syndrome. *In* Hill, A.G.S. (ed.): Modern Trends in Rheumatology, Vol. II. London, Butterworths, 1970, pp. 139–157.
121. Anderson, L.H., and Talal, N.: The spectrum of benign to malignant lymphoproliferation in Sjögren's syndrome. Clin. Exp. Immunol. 9:199, 1971.
122. Fischbach, M., Char, D., Christensen, M., Daniels, T., Whaley, K., Alspaugh, M., and Talal, N.: Immune complexes in Sjögren's syndrome. Athritis Rheum. 23:791, 1980.
123. Hamburger, M.I., Moutsopoulos, H.M., Lawley, T.J., and Frank, M.M.: Sjögren's syndrome: A defect in reticuloendothelial system Fc-receptor-specific clearance. Ann. Intern. Med. 91:534, 1979.
124. Meltzer, M., Franklin, F.C., and Eilias, K.: Cryoglobulinemia—a clinical and laboratory study. II. Cryoglobulin with rheumatoid factor activity. Am. J. Med. 40:837, 1966.
125. Zinneman, H.H., and Caperton, E.: Cryoglobulinaemia in a patient with Sjögren's syndrome and factors of cryoprecipitation. J. Lab. Clin. Med. 89:483, 1977.
126. Zinneman, H.H., Levi, D., and Seal, U.S.: On the nature of cryoglobulins. J. Immunol. 100:594, 1968.
127. McIntosh, R.M., Kaufman, D.B., and Kulvinskas, C.: Cryoglobulins. I. Studies on the nature, incidence and clinical significance of serum cryoproteins in glomerulonephritis. J. Lab. Clin. Med. 75:566, 1970.
128. McIntosh, R.M., Kulvinskas, C., and Kaufman, D.B.: Cryoglobulins. II. The biological and chemical properties of cryoproteins in acute post-streptococcal glomerulonephritis. Int. Arch. Allergy 41:700, 1971.
129. Zlotnick, A., Salvin, S., and Eliakim, M.: Mixed cryoglobulinaemia, with a monoclonal IgM component, associated with chronic liver disease. Isr. J. Med. Sci. 8:1968, 1972.
130. Zinneman, H.H., Fromke, V.L., and Seal, U.S.: Some biochemical properties of a cryomacroglobulin. Clin. Chim. Acta 43:91, 1973.
131. Wang, A.C., Wells, J.V., and Fudenberg, H.H.: Chemical analyses of cryoglobulins. Immunochemistry 11:341, 1974.
132. Whitehouse, A.C., Buckley, C.E., Nagaya, H., and McCarter, J.: Mac-

roglobulinaemia and vasculitis in Sjögren's syndrome. Experimental observations relating to pathogenesis. Am. J. Med. 43:609, 1967.
133. Pinkus, G.S., and Dekker, A.: Benign lymphoepithelial lesion of the parotid glands associated with reticulum cell sarcoma. Report of a case and review of the literature. Cancer 25:121, 1970.
134. Wolf, R.O., Ross, M.E., and Rapley, T.M.: Changes in serum salivary isoamylases in Sjögren's syndrome. Am. J. Clin. Pathol. 65:1022, 1976.
135. Bluestone, R., Gumpel, J.M., Goldberg, L.S., and Holborrow, E.J.: Salivary immunoglobulins in Sjögren's syndrome. Int. Arch. Allergy Appl. Immunol. 42:686, 1972.
136. Mach, P.S., Amor, B., Messing, B., Chicault, P., Ghozlan, R., and Deltarre, F.: Salivary immunoglobulin determinations: Their diagnostic value in Sjögren's syndrome. Biomedicine 25:31, 1976.
137. Dunne, J.V., Carson, D.A., Speigelberg, H.L., Alspaugh, M.A., and Vaughn, J.H.: IgA rheumatoid factor in the sera and saliva of patient with rheumatoid arthritis and Sjögren's syndrome. Ann. Rheum. Dis. 38:161, 1979.
138. Anderson, L.G., Cummings, N.A., Asofsky, R., Hylton, M.B., Tarpley, T.M., Tomasi, T.B., Wolf, R.O., Schall, G.L., and Talal, N.: Salivary gland immunoglobulin and rheumatoid factor synthesis in Sjögren's syndrome. Natural history and response to treatment. Am. J. Med. 53:456, 1972.
139. Talal, N., Grey, H.M., and Zvaifler, N.: Elevated salivary and synovial fluid beta-2-microglobulin in Sjögren's syndrome and rheumatoid arthritis. Science 187:1196, 1975.
140. Michalski, J.P., Daniels, T.E., Talal, N., and Grey, H.M.: Beta$_2$ microglobulin and lymphocytic infiltration in Sjögren's syndrome. N. Engl. J. Med. 293:1228, 1975.
141. Moutsoupoulos, H.M., Karsh, J., Wolf, R.O., Torpley, T.M., Tylenda, A., and Papadopoulos, N.M.: Lysozyme determination in parotid saliva from patients with Sjögren's syndrome. Am. J. Med. 69:39, 1980.
142. Bunim, J.J., Buchanan, W.W., Wertlake, P.T., Sokoloff, L., Bloch, K.J., Beck, J.S., and Alepa, F.P.: Clinical, pathologic, and serologic studies in Sjögren's syndrome. Combined clinical staff conferences at the National Institutes of Health. Ann. Intern. Med. 61:509, 1964.
143. Torrigiani, G., and Roitt, I.: Antiglobulin factors in sera from patients with rheumatoid arthritis and normal subjects. Quantitative estimation in different immunoglobulin classes. Ann. Rheum. Dis. 26:334, 1967.
144. Torrigiani, G., Ansell, B.M., Chown, E.E., and Roitt, I.M.: Raised IgG antiglobulin factors in Still's disease. Ann. Rheum. Dis. 28:424, 1969.
145. Howell, F.A., Chamberlain, M.A., Perry, R.A., Torrigiani, G., and Roitt, I.: IgG antiglobulin levels in patients with psoriatic arthropathy, ankylosing spondylitis and gout. Ann. Rheum. Dis. 31:129, 1972.
146. Ichikawa, Y.: Rheumatoid arthritis and Sjögren's syndrome. Reprinted from the Papers of the Institute for Thermal Spring Research. Okayama University, No. 42, 1973, pp. 25–29.
147. Beck, J.S., Anderson, J.R., Bloch, K.J., Buchanan, W.W., and Bunim, J.J.: Antinuclear and precipitating autoantibodies in Sjögren's syndrome. Ann. Rheum. Dis. 24:16, 1965.
148. Anderson, J.R., Buchanan, W.W., and Goudie, R.B.: Autoimmunity, Clinical and Experimental. Springfield, Ill., Charles C Thomas, 1967.
149. Baumer, A.: Immunozytologische, Phanomene bei verschidenen rheumatoischen Krankheiten. Z. Rheumaforsch.24:326, 1965.
150. Alspaugh, M.A., Talal, N., and Tan, E.M.: Differentiation and characterization of autoantibodies and their antigens in Sjögren's syndrome. Arthritis Rheum. 19:216, 1976.
151. Alspaugh, M.A., and Tan, E.M.: Antibodies to cellular antigens in Sjögren's syndrome. J. Clin. Invest. 55:1067, 1975.
152. Scopelitis, E., Biundo, J.J., and Alspaugh, M.A.: Anti-SS-A antibody and other nuclear antibodies in systemic lupus erythematosus. Clin. Res. 26:385A, 1978.
153. Wilson, M.R., Arroyave, C.M., Miles, L., and Tan, E.M.: Immune reactants in cryoproteins, relationship to complement activation. Ann. Rheum. Dis. 36:540, 1977.
154. Akizuki, M., Powers, R., and Holman, H.R.: A soluble acidic protein of the cell nucleus which reacts with serum from patients with systemic lupus erythematosus and Sjögren's syndrome. J. Clin. Invest. 59:264, 1977.
155. Kassan, S.S., Akizuki, M., Steinberg, A.D., Reddick, R.L., and Chused, T.M.: Antibody to a soluble acidic nuclear antigen in Sjögren's syndrome. Am. J. Med. 63:328, 1977.
156. Kawanishi, K., Kawamura, K., Nishina, Y., Goto, A., Okada, S., Ishida, T., Ofuji, T., Kahn, C.R., and Flier, J.S.: Successful immunosuppressive therapy in insulin resistant diabetes caused by anti-insulin reception autoantibodies. J. Clin. Endocrinol. Metab. 44:15, 1977.
157. Daha, M.R., Austen, K.F., and Fearon, D.T.: C3 nephritic factor (C3NeF): Heterogeneity, polypeptide chain structure and antigenic reactivity. J. Immunol. 120:1389, 1978.
158. Davis, A.E., III, Gelfand, E.W., Schur, P.H., Rosen, F.S., and Alper, C.A.: IgG subclass studies of C3 nephritic factor. Clin. Immunol. Immunopathol. 11:98, 1978.
159. Schrieber, R.D., and Muller-Eberhard, H.J.: Nephritis factor (T.A.): A homogeneous immunoglobulin directed toward the complex of C3 and factor B of human complement. J. Immunol. 120: 1796, 1978.
160. Scott, D.M., Amos, N., Sissons, J.G.P., and Peters, D.K.: The immunoglobulin nature of the nephritic factor: NeF activity is found in Fab and Fab$_2$ as well as intact IgG. J. Immunol. 120:1797, 1978.
161. Feltkamp, T.E.W., and Rossum, A.L. van: Antibodies to salivary duct cells, and other autoantibodies, in patients with Sjögren's syndrome and other idiopathic autoimmune diseases. Clin. Exp. Immunol. 3:1, 1968.
162. Rodriguez, J.L., Gelpi, C., Thomson, T.M., Rial, F.J., and Fernandez, J.: Anti-golgi complex autoantibodies in a patient with Sjögren's syndrome and lymphoma. Clin. Exp. Immunol. 49:579, 1982.
163. Bertram, U., and Halberg, P.: A specific antibody against the epithelium of salivary ducts in sera from patients with Sjögren's syndrome. Acta Allerg. 19:458, 1965.
164. MacSween, R.N.M., Goudie, R.B., Anderson J.R., Armstrong, E., Murray, M.A., Mason, D.K., Janani, M.K., Boyle, J.A., Buchanan, W.W., and Williamson, J.: Occurrence of antibody to salivary duct epithelium in Sjögren's disease, rheumatic arthritis and other arthritides. A clinical and laboratory study. Ann. Rheum. Dis. 26:402, 1967.
165. Ludwig, H., Schernthaner, G., Scherak, O., and Kolarz, G.: Antibodies to pancreatic duct cells in Sjögren's syndrome and rheumatoid arthritis. Gut 18:311, 1977.
166. Buchanan, W.W., Harden, R.M., Koutras, D.A., and Gray, K.G.: Abnormalities of iodine metabolism in euthyroid nongoitrous woman with complement-fixing antimicrosomal thyroid autoantibodies. J. Clin. Endocrinol. Metab. 25:301, 1965.
167. Anderson, J.R., Beck, J.S., Buchanan, W.W., Bloch, K.J., and Bunim, J.J.: Sjögren's syndrome and autoimmunity. *In* Baldwin, R.W., and Humphrey, J.H. (eds.): Autoimmunity. A Symposium on the Fifth Congress of the International Academy of Pathology, Oxford, Blackwells, 1965, pp. 453–467.
168. Buchanan, W.W., Boyle, J.A., Greig, W.R., McAndrew, R., Barr, M., Gray, K.G., Anderson, J.R., and Goudie, R.B.: Distribution of certain autoantibodies on monozygotic and dizygotic twins. Ann. Rheum. Dis. 25:463, 1968.
169. Buchanan, W.W., Boyle, J.A., Greig, W.R., McAndrew, R., Barr, M., Gray, K.G., Anderson, J.R., and Goudie, R.B.: Occurrence of autoantibodies in healthy twins. Clin. Exp. Immunol. 2:(Suppl.) 803, 1967.
170. Pirofsky, B.: *In* Autoimmunization and the Autoimmune Hemolytic Anemias. Baltimore, Williams and Wilkins Company, 1969.
171. Sage, R.E., and Forbes, I.J.: A case of multiple autoimmune disease, lymphoid proliferation and hypogammaglobulinemia. Blood 31:536, 1968.
172. Whaley, K., Glen, A.C.A., MacSween, R.N.M., Deodhar, S., Dick, W.C., Nuki, G., Williamson, J., and Buchanan, W.W.: Immunological responses in Sjögren's syndrome and rheumatoid arthritis. Clin. Exp. Immunol. 9:721, 1971.
173. Karsh, J., Palvidis, N., Schiffman, G., and Moutsopoulos, H.M.: Immunization of patients with Sjögren's syndrome with pneumococcal polysaccharide vaccine: A randomized trial. Arthritis Rheum. 23:1294, 1981.
174. Whaley, K., Canesi, B., Moseley, A., Morrow, W., Sturrock, R., Mitchell, W., and Dick, W.C.: Complement metabolism in the sero-negative arthritides. Ann. Rheum. Dis. 33:495, 1974.
175. Leventhal, B.G., Waldorf, D.S., and Talal, N.: Impaired lymphocytic transformation and delayed hypersensitivity in Sjögren's syndrome. J. Clin. Invest. 46:1338, 1967.
176. Williams, R.C., Jr., DeBoard, J.K., Melbye, O.J., Messner, R.P., and Lindstrom, F.D.: Studies of T and B lymphocytes in patients with connective tissue diseases. J. Clin. Invest. 52:283, 1973.
177. Talal, N., Sylvester, R.A., Daniels, T.E., Greenspan, J.S., and Williams, R.C., Jr.: T and B lymphocytes in the peripheral blood and tissue lesions in Sjögren's syndrome. J. Clin. Invest. 53:180, 1974.
178. Fox, R.I., Carstens, S.A., Fong, S., Robinson, C.A., Howell, S.A., and Vaughan, J.H.: Use of monoclonal antibodies to analyze peripheral blood and salivary gland lymphocyte subsets in Sjôren's syndrome. Arthritis Rheum. 25:419, 1982.
179. Sauvezie, B., Miyasaka, N., Charron, D., Kielich, C., Loeb, J., Daniels, T.E., and Talal, N.: An increase in peripheral blood Ia-positive T cells in Sjögren's syndrome correlates with a decrease in the autologous mixed lymphocyte response. Clin. Exp. Immunol. 49:50, 1982.
180. Miyasaka, N., Sauvezie, B., Pierce, D.A., Daniels, T.E., and Talal, N.: Decreased autologous mixed lymphocyte reaction in Sjögren's syndrome. J. Clin. Invest. 66:928, 1980.
181. Michalski, J.P., and McCombs, C.: Decreased lymphocyte reactivity to a suboptimal concentration of phytohemagglutinin in Sjögren's syndrome. Arthritis Rheum. 20:851, 1977.
182. Minato, N., Takedo, A., Kauo, S., and Takaku, F.: Studies of the function of natural killer-interferon system in patients with Sjögren's syndrome. J. Clin. Invest. 69:581, 1982.
183. Hooks, J.J., Moutsopoulos, H.M., Geis, S.A., Stahl, H.I., Decker, J.L.,

and Notkins, A.L.: Immune interferon in the circulation of patients with autoimmune disease. N. Engl. J. Med. 301:5, 1979.

184. Moutsopoulos, H., Fye, K.H., Sawada, S., Becker, M.J., Goldstein, A., and Talal, N.: In vitro effect of thymosin on T lymphocyte rosette formation in rheumatic diseases. Clin. Exp. Immunol. 26:563, 1976.

185. Van Boxel, J.A., Hardin, J.A., Green, I., and Paul, W.E.: Multiple heavy-chain determinants on individual B lymphocytes in the peripheral blood of patients with Sjögren's syndrome. N. Engl. J. Med. 289:823, 1973.

186. Fauci, A.S., and Moutsopoulos, H.M.: Polyclonally triggered B cells in the peripheral blood and bone marrow of normal individuals, and in patients with systemic lupus erythematosus and primary Sjögren's syndrome. Arthritis Rheum. 24:577, 1981.

187. Aisenberg, A.C., and Bloch, K.J.: Immunoglobulins in the surface of neoplastic lymphocytes. N. Engl. J. Med. 287:272, 1972.

188. Preud'Homme, J.L., and Seligmann, M.: Surface bound immunoglobulins as a cell marker in human lymphoproliferative diseases. Blood 40:777, 1972.

189. Piessens, W.F., Schur, P.H., and Moloney, W.C.: Lymphocyte surface immunoglobulins: Distribution and frequency in lymphoproliferative diseases. N. Engl. J. Med. 288:176, 1973.

190. Feldmann, J.L., Becker, M.J., Moutsopoulos, H., Fye, K., Blackman, M., Epstein, V., and Talal, N.: Antibody-dependent cell-mediated cytotoxicity in selected autoimmune diseases. J. Clin. Invest. 58:173, 1976.

191. Greenspan, J.S., Gutman, G.A., Weissman, I.L., and Talal, N.: Thymus-antigen and immunoglobulin-positive lymphocytes in tissue infiltrates of NZB/NZW mice. Clin. Immunol. Immunopathol. 3:16, 1974.

192. Berry, H., Bacon, P.A., and Savis, J.D.: Cell-mediated immunity in Sjögren's syndrome. Ann. Rheum. Dis. 31:298, 1972.

193. Cremer, N.E., Daniels, T.E., Oshiro, L.S., Marcus, F., Claypool, R., Sylvester, R.A., and Talal, N.: Immunological and virological studies of cultured labial biopsy cells from patients with Sjögren's syndrome. Clin. Exp. Immunol. 18:213, 1974.

194. McDevitt, H.O., Deak, B.D., Shreffer, D.C., Klein, J., Stimpeling, J.H., and Snell, D.D.: Genetic control of the immune response. Mapping the Ir1 locus. J. Exp. Med. 135:1259, 1972.

195. Cullen, S.E., David, C.S., Cone, J.L., and Sachs, D.H.: Evidence for more than one Ia antigenic speciality on molecules determined by the I-A subregion of the mouse major histocompatibility complex. J. Immunol. 116:549, 1976.

196. Bach, F.H., Widmer, M.B., Bach, M.L., and Klein, J.: Serologically defined and lymphocyte defined components of the major histocompatibility complex in the mouse. J. Exp. Med. 136:1430, 1972.

197. Lozner, E.C., Sachs, D.H., and Shearer, G.M.: B-cell alloantigens determined by the H-2 linked Ir region are associated with mixed lymphocyte culture stimulation. Science 183:757, 1974.

198. Falchuk, Z.M., Rogentine, G.N., and Strober, W.: Predominance of histocompatibility antigen HL-A8 in patients with gluten-sensitive enteropathy. J. Clin. Invest. 51:1602, 1972.

199. Fritze, D., Herrman, C., Jr., and Naeim, F.: HL-A antigens in myasthenia gravis. Lancet 1:240, 1974.

200. Platz, P., Ryder, L., Nielsen, L.S., Svejgaard, A., Thomsen, M., Nerup, J., and Christy, M.: HL-A and idiopathic Addison's disease (letter). Lancet 2:289, 1974.

201. Grumet, F.C., Payne, R.O., Konishi, J., and Kriss, J.: HLA antigens as markers for disease susceptibility and autoimmunity in Graves' disease. J. Clin. Endocrinol. Metab. 39:1115, 1974.

202. Mackay, I.R., and Morris, P.J.: Association of autoimmune active chronic hepatitis with HL-A1, 8. Lancet 2:793, 1972.

203. Nerup, J., Platz, P., Anderson, O.O., Christy, M., Lyngsoe, J., Poulsen, J.E., Ryder, L.P., Nielsen, L.S., Thomsen, W., and Sveygaard, A.: HL-A antigens and diabetes mellitus. Lancet 2:864, 1974.

204. Gershwin, M.E., Terasaki, P.I., and Graw, R.: Increased frequency of HL-A8 Sjögren's syndrome. Tissue Antigens 6:342, 1975.

205. Fye, K.H., Terasaki, P.I., Moutsopoulos, H., Daniels, T.E., Michalski, J.P., and Talal, N.: Association of Sjögren's syndrome with HLA-B8. Arthritis Rheum. 19:883, 1976.

206. Ivanyi, D., Drizhal, I., Erbenova, E., Horejs, J., Salavee, M., Macurova, H., Dostal, C., Balik, J., and Juran, J.: HLA in Sjögren's syndrome. Tissue Antigens 7:45, 1976.

207. Kissmeyer-Nielsen, F. (ed.): Histocompatibility Testing. Copenhagen, Munksgaard, 1972.

208. Keuning, J.J., Pena, A.S., Van Leeuwen, A., Hooff, J.P., and Rood, J.J. van: HLA-DW3 associated with coeliac disease. Lancet 1:506, 1976.

209. Chused, T.M., Kassan, S.S., Opelz, G., Moutsopoulos, H.M., and Terasaki, P.I.: Sjögren's syndrome associated with HLA-DW3. N. Engl. J. Med. 296:895, 1977.

210. Hirzova, E., Ivanyi, D., Sula, K., Horejs, J., Dostal, C., and Drizhal, I.: HLA-DW3 in Sjögren's syndrome. Tissue Antigens 9:8, 1977.

210a. Manthorpe, R., Teppo, A.M., Bendixen, G., and Wegelius, O.: Antibodies to SS-B in chronic inflammatory connective tissue diseases: Relationship with HLA-DW2 and HLA-DW3 in primary Sjögren's syndrome. Arthritis Rheum. 25:662, 1982.

211. Moutsopoulos, H.M., Chused, T.M., Johnson, A.H., Knudsin, B., and Mann, D.C.: B lymphocyte antigens in sicca syndrome. Science 199:1441, 1978.

212. Burch, J.A., Bunim, J.J., and Bloch, K.T.: Clinical, radiological and serological studies on relatives of patients with Sjögren's syndrome and of patients' neighbours. Arthritis Rheum. 5:104, 1962.

213. Bloch, K.J., and Bunim, J.J.: Sjögren's syndrome and its relationship to connective tissue diseases. J. Chronic Dis. 16:915, 1963.

214. Kessler, H.S.: A laboratory model for Sjögren's syndrome. Am. J. Pathol. 52:671, 1968.

215. Whaley, K., Hughes, G.R.V., and Webb, T.: Systemic lupus erythematosus in animals and man. *In* Buchanan, W.W., and Dick, W.C. (eds.): Recent Advances in Rheumatology, Vol. 1. Edinburgh, Churchill Livingstone, 1975, pp. 67–136.

216. Shillitoe, E.J., Daniels, T.E., Whitcher, J.D., Vibeke-Strand, C., Talal, N., and Greenspan, J.S.: Antibody to cytomegalovirus in patients with Sjögren's syndrome, as determined by an enzyme-linked immunosorbent assay. Arthritis Rheum. 25:260, 1982.

217. Sutinen, S., Sutinen, S., and Huhti, E.: Ultrastructure of lymphoid interstitial pneumonia. Virus-like particles in bronchiolar epithelium of a patient with Sjögren's syndrome. Am. J. Clin. Pathol. 67:328, 1977.

218. Shearn, M.A., Tu, W.H., Stephens, B.G., and Lee, J.C.: Virus-like structures in Sjögren's syndrome. Lancet 1:568, 1970.

219. Talal, N.: Sjögren's syndrome, lymphoproliferation and renal tubular acidosis. Ann. Intern. Med. 74:633, 1971.

220. Gyorkey, F., Sinkovics, J.G., Min, K.W., and Gyorkey, P.: A morphologic study on the occurrence and distribution of structures resembling viral nucleocapsids in collagen diseases. Am. J. Med. 53:148, 1972.

221. Albegger, K.W., and Auböck, L.: The evidence of "virus-like" inclusions in myoepithelial sialadenitis of Sjögren's syndrome by electron microscopy. Arch. Klin. Exp. Ohren Nasen Kehlkopfheilkd. 203:153, 1972.

222. Daniels, T.E., Sylvester, R.A., Silverman, S., Dolando, V., and Talal, N.: Tubulo-reticular "virus-like" structures within labial salivary glands in patients with Sjögren's syndrome. Arthritis Rheum. 17:593, 1974.

223. Pothier, L., Uzman, B.G., Kasac, H., Saito, H., and Adams, R.A.: Immunoglobulin synthesis and tubular assays in the endoplasmic reticulum in transplanted human tumours of lymphoid origin. Lab. Invest. 259:607, 1973.

224. Whaley, K., Chisholm, D.M., Goudie, R.B., Downie, W.W., Dick, W.C., Boyle, J.A., and Williamson, J.: Salivary duct autoantibody in Sjögren's syndrome: Correlation with focal sialadenitis in the labial mucosa. Clin. Exp. Immunol. 4:273, 1969.

225. Soborg, M., and Bertram, U.: Cellular hypersensitivity in Sjögren's syndrome. Acta Med. Scand. 184:319, 1968.

226. Bertram, N., and Soborg, M.: Nye Immunologiske reaktioner ved Sjögren's syndrome. Tandlaegebladet 74:344, 1970.

227. Talal, N., and Bunim, J.J.: The development of malignant lymphoma in Sjögren's syndrome. Am. J. Med. 36:529, 1964.

228. Bender, B.L., and Jaffe, R.: Immunoglobulin production in lymphomatoid granulomatosis and relation to other "benign" lymphoproliferative disorders. Am. J. Clin. Pathol. 73:41, 1980.

229. Faquet, G.B., Webb, H.H., Agee, J.F., Ricks, W.B., and Sharbaugh, A.H.: Immunologically diagnosed malignancy in Sjögren's pseudolymphoma. Am. J. Med. 65:424, 1978.

230. Kassan, S.S., Hoover, R., and Kimberly, R.P.: Increased incidence of malignancy in Sjögren's syndrome (abstract). Arthritis Rheum. 20:123, 1977.

231. Slater, A., Whittaker, J.A., and Fisher, D.J.H.: Reticulum-cell sarcoma and Sjögren's syndrome in a patient treated with azathioprine (letter). N. Engl. J. Med. 296:51, 1976.

232. Gravanis, S.M.B., and Giansanti, J.S.: Malignant histopathologic counterpart of the benign lymphoepithelial lesion. Cancer 26:1332, 1970.

233. Hyman, G.A., and Wolff, M.: Malignant lymphomas of the salivary glands. Review of the literature and report of 33 new cases, including four cases associated with the lymphoepithelial lesion. Am. J. Clin. Pathol. 65:421, 1976.

234. Kessler, H.S., Cubberly, M., and Manski, W.: Eye changes in autoimmune NZB and NZB × NZW mice. Arch. Ophthalmol. 85:211, 1971.

234a. Carlson, B., and Ostberg, Y.: The autoimmune submandibular sialadenitis of the NZB/NZW hybrid mice. Arch. Otorhinolaryngol. 225:57, 1979.

235. Whaley, K., and MacSween, R.N.M.: Experimental induction of immune sialadenitis in guinea-pigs using different adjuvants. Clin. Exp. Immunol. 17:681, 1974.

236. Williamson, J., Doig, W.M., Forrester, J.V., Whaley, K., and Dick, W.C.: Management of the dry eye in Sjögren's syndrome. Br. J. Ophthalmol. 58:798, 1974.

237. Norn, M.S.: Treatment of keratoconjunctivitis sicca with liquid paraffin or polyvinyl alcohol in double-blind trial. Acta Ophthal. (Kbh) 55:945, 1977.

238. Werblin, T.P., Rheinstrom, S.D., and Kaufman, H.E.: The use of slow-release artificial tears in the longterm management of keratitis sicca. Ophthalmology (Rochester) 88:78, 1981.

239. Williamson, J., Wilson, T., Wallace, J., and Whaley, K.: Studies of the

bacterial flora in keratoconjunctivitis sicca. Eye Ear Nose Throat Monthly 50:257, 1971.
240. Williamson, J., Doig, W.M., Forrester, J.V., Whaley, K., and Dick, W.C.: Studies on the viral flora in keratoconjunctivitis sicca. Br. J. Ophthalmol. 59:45, 1975.
241. Avisar, R., Savir, H., Machtey, I., Ovaknin, L., Shaked, P., Menachie, R., and Allalouf, D.: Clinical trial of bromhexine in Sjögren's syndrome. Ann. Ophthalmol. 13:971, 1981.
242. Frost-Larsen, K., Isager, H., and Manthorpe, R.: Sjögren's syndrome treated with bromhexine: a randomised clinical study. Br. Med. J. 1:1579, 1978.
243. Shannon, I.L., and Edmonds, E.J. Effect of fluoride concentration on rehardening of enamel by a saliva substitute. Int. Dent. J. 28:421, 1978.
244. Klestov, A.C., Webb, J., Latt, D., Schiller, G., McNamara, L., Young, D.Y., Hobbes, J., and Fetherston, J. Treatment of xerostomia: A double-blind trial in 108 patients with Sjögren's syndrome. Oral Surg. 51:594, 1981.
245. Donatsky, O., Johnson, T., Holmstrup, P., and Bertram, U.: Effect of saliment on parotid salivary secretion and on xerostomia caused by Sjögren's syndrome. Scan. J. Dent. Res. 90:157, 1982.
246. Flynn, C.T., Negus, T.W., McHardy, and Rainford, D.J.: Improvement in lacrimal and salivary secretions after alkali therapy in Sjögren's syndrome with renal tubular acidosis. Ann. Rheum. Dis. 35:381, 1976.
247. Lisch, K.: Über hereditäres Vorkommen des mit Keratoconjunctivitis sicca verbundenen Sjögrenschen Symptomenkomplexes. Arch. Augenheilkd. 110:357, 1937.
248. Coverdale, H.: Some unusual cases of Sjögren's syndrome. Br. J. Ophthalmol. 32:669, 1948.
249. Pascucci, F.: La sindrome de Sjögren. Nota 1. Premesse metodo di esame. Contributo casistico. Riv. Crit. Clin. Med. 58:133, 1958.
250. Doni, N., Brancato, R., Bartoletti, L., and Berni, G.: La familiarita delta sindrome di Sjögren. Rev. Crit. Clin. Med. 65:750, 1965.
251. Camus, J.P., Emerit, I., Reinhart, P., Guillien, P., Crouzet, J., and Fourot, J.: Sclerodermie familiale avec syndrome de Sjögren et anomalies lymphocytaises et chromosomiques. Ann. Med. Interne 121:149, 1970.
252. Koivukangas, T., Similä, S., Heikkinen, E., Rasanen, O., and Wasz-Hockert, O.: Sjögren's syndrome and achalasia of the cardia in two siblings. Pediatrics 51:943, 1973.
253. Lichtenfield, J.L., Kirschner, R.H., and Wiernick, P.H.: Familial Sjögren's syndrome with associated primary salivary gland lymphoma. Am. J. Med. 60:286, 1976.
254. Frayha, R.A., Tabbara, K.F., and Geha, R.S.: Familial CRST syndrome with sicca complex. J. Rheumatol. 4:53, 1978.
255. Vaillant, J.M., Laudanbach, P., Schuller, E., Muller, J.Y., and Deboise, A.: Gougerot-Sjögren syndrome in two univitelline twin sisters. Ann. Med. Interne 132:408, 1981.
256. Rothman, S., Blocky, M., and Hauser, F.V.: Sjögren's syndrome associated with lymphoblastoma and hypersplenism. Arch. Derm. Syph. 63:642, 1951.
257. Hornbaker, J.H., Jr., Foster, E.A., Williams, G.S., and Davis, J.S.: Sjögren's syndrome and nodular reticulum cell sarcoma. Arch. Intern. Med. 118:449, 1966.
258. Miller, D.G.: The association of immune disease and malignant lymphoma. Ann. Intern. Med. 66:507, 1967.
259. Bark, C.J., and Perzik, S.L.: Mikulicz's disease, sialoangiectasis and autoimmunity based upon a study of parotid lesions. Am. J. Clin. Pathol. 49:683, 1968.
260. Bilder, J., and Hornova, J.: Lymfosarkom přiušní žlázy při Sjögrenově syndromu. Cesk. Stomat. 67:441, 1967.
261. Thorpe, P.: Polymyalgia rheumatica: A not so benign syndrome. Med. J. Aust. 2:678, 1969.
262. Senti-Parades, A., Canedo-Acea, R., Pulido-Ledesma, R., Borrajero, I., and Delgado, B.: Reporte de un caso de sindrome de Sjögren-Mikulicz. Rev. Cuba Med. 3:560, 1964.
263. Yoshinaga, T.: Two cases of Sjögren's syndrome with malignant tumour. Jap. J. Clin. Med. 26:2161, 1968.
264. Lattes, R.: Thymoma and other tumors of the thymus. Cancer 15:1224, 1962.
265. Dourov, N., Sternon, J., de Coster, A., and Chailly, P.: Thymome malin, myasthénie, thyröidite, syndrome de Gougerot-Sjögren bloc alvéolo-capillaire. A propos de in cas. Ann. Anat. Path. 13:201, 1968.
266. Alarcon-Segovia, D., and Zavala-Mejia, J.L.: Sindrome de Sjögren asociado a timoma. Rev. Invest. Clin. 23:133, 1971.
267. Maleville, J., Heid, F., Rousselot, P., Bergoend, H., Grosshans, E., and Aroujo, A.: Purpura dysglobulinémique et syndrome de Gougerot-Sjögren. Révélation ultérieure d'une réticulose maligne à tendance plasmocytaire. Bull. Soc. Franc. Derm. Syph. 74:696, 1967.
268. Wager, O., Rasanen, J.A., and Lindenberg, L.: Cited by Shearn.[2]
269. Azzopardi, J.G., and Evans, D.J.: Malignant lymphoma of parotid associated with Mikulicz disease (benign lymphoepithelial lesion). J. Clin. Pathol. 24:744, 1971.
270. Delaney, W.E., and Balogh, K., Jr.: Carcinoma of the parotid gland associated with benign lymphoepithelial lesion (Mikulicz's disease) in Sjögren's syndrome. Cancer 19:853, 1966.

# Chapter 63
# The Management of Rheumatoid Arthritis

*Shaun Ruddy*

## INTRODUCTION

Few diagnoses arouse more anxiety in both patient and physician than rheumatoid arthritis. Misapprehensions about the tractability and prognosis of this disease are common among both laity and medical professionals. The patient recalls a family member who, perhaps years ago, was afflicted with a severe crippling form of arthritis and wonders when she* will become similarly disabled. If she has been referred to a rheumatologist, she looks around the waiting room and sees patients with very active, progressive, and deforming disease who have been selected for referral precisely because of the extreme severity of their disease. As for the physician, very likely he or she was exposed to relatively little information about rheumatic diseases during medical school years; and, because most patients with rheumatoid arthritis are managed as outpatients, to relatively little training during hospital internship and residency. Like the patient, the physician also may selectively recall one or two patients with severe, active, and progressive disease who failed to respond to all of the treatment modalities available. And yet such pessimism is usually unwarranted. As illustrated in Chapter 60, rheumatoid arthritis is, in the majority of instances, a disease with a good prognosis. Most patients have gratifying responses to treatment, albeit not the immediate response measured in hours or days seen with acute illnesses such as pneumococcal pneumonia. Even in the minority of patients whose response to treatment would be judged less than completely satisfactory, appropriate therapeutic measures usually allow them to continue to function harmoniously with their environment.

This chapter will outline the general approach for the prospective and aggressive management of rheumatoid arthritis. Detailed consideration of individual therapeutic modalities applicable to rheumatoid arthritis is given in 19 other chapters of this text. Table 63-1 provides a guide to the information contained in these chapters. Before proceeding to detailed considerations of the various aspects of the management of rheumatoid arthritis, a few general principles are worthy of emphasis.

1. *The time course of rheumatoid arthritis is measured in months and years.*[1] Although a few patients will experience brief, apparently self-limited episodes of arthritis which do not recur, most will have had their disease for a prolonged period of time when initially seen by the physician, and most can be expected to have it, albeit in a moderate or reduced form, for months or even years to come.[2] One corollary of this extended time frame is that there need be no rush to make the diagnosis of rheumatoid arthritis, with all the attendant anxieties and fears it engenders. If the diagnosis is immediately obvious and inescapable from the history and physical examination, there is no sense in delaying and much to be gained in terms of patient trust and understanding by a forthright and honest exposition of the diagnosis. If, as is frequently the case, insufficient criteria are present for a firm diagnosis, it is perhaps wiser to institute conservative treatment and employ a label such as "polyarthritis of unknown etiology" until the disease declares itself or regresses.[3] Since treatment at this early stage would not likely be influenced by the use of a specific diagnostic category, little is to be gained by employing one which is uncertain and likely to be emotionally troublesome for the patient and her family.

A second corollary of the lengthy time course of rheumatoid arthritis involves the expectations of both patient and physician for the immediacy of response to therapy.

**Table 63–1.** Other Chapters in the Textbook of Rheumatology Relating to the Management of Rheumatoid Arthritis

| Chapter Number | Topic |
|---|---|
| 24 | Examination of the joints |
| 34 | Psychological and sexual aspects |
| 35 | Ocular manifestations |
| 36 | Cutaneous manifestations |
| 37 | Aspiration and injection of joints |
| 49 | Salicylates |
| 50 | Nonsteroidal anti-inflammatory drugs |
| 51 | Antimalarials |
| 52 | Gold compounds |
| 53 | D-Penicillamine |
| 54 | Glucocorticoids |
| 55 | Immunoregulatory agents |
| 111 | Rehabilitation |
| 113 | Synovectomy |
| 114 | Hand surgery |
| 115 | Elbow surgery |
| 116 | Shoulder surgery |
| 117 | Knee surgery |
| 118 | Ankle and foot surgery |
| 120 | Hip surgery |

*The feminine gender is used throughout this chapter to refer to patients because most patients with rheumatoid arthritis are women.

Rheumatologists, in particular, are often visited by patients with severe and progressive disease who believe that their multiple sore joints will forthwith be soothed and remedied, now that they have found a "specialist" in their disease. Even referring physicians find it difficult to accept the notion that it may be necessary to administer a potentially very toxic agent such as gold salts or penicillamine for up to 6 months before a decision about its effectiveness for a particular patient can be made with assurance. In both cases, it is helpful to point out that the patient has had months or even years to reach her present condition, and that it is reasonable to expect that it will take a long time to reverse the process. Fortunately, immediate institution of supportive measures often results in significant diminution of pain and improvement in function and sense of well-being, which convinces the patient that the course of her disease is at least going in the right direction.

2. *The extent and intensity of rheumatoid arthritis are highly variable.* As discussed in detail in Chapter 60, this variation applies both between different patients and between different times in the same patient. Notwithstanding the prognostic indicators mentioned in Chapter 60, which are most useful when large numbers of patients are involved, it is extremely difficult to prognosticate for an individual patient, particularly early in the disease.[3] As a rule, the best indication of how the disease will progress for an individual patient is the history of the disease in that patient previously. Most patients do not need to be told that their disease is one of remissions and exacerbations over time; they have learned this from experience. Surprisingly, however, not as many realize the implications of this variation in time for the assessment of therapy. It is often helpful to point out that, in a disease that gets better or worse on its own, it will sometimes be difficult for either doctor or patient to determine whether a particular form of treatment has been effective for her or whether the improvement may have been a coincidence. Reasoning from this, patients are usually able to understand how a particular remedy widely accepted as efficacious for the treatment of arthritis may not be of any real or lasting benefit. Conversely, patients may recognize the need for careful scientific evaluation of efficacy of new agents and be willing to participate in experiments designed for such evaluations.

3. *Optimal management of rheumatoid arthritis requires the combined efforts of multiple members of a health-care team.* The reverse of this statement is that no one individual is capable of meeting all the health-care needs of a patient with rheumatoid arthritis. While the administration of drugs has a central role in the treatment program, the prescription of one or more pharmaceutical agents by a physician represents only a fraction of the treatment modalities that can and should be involved. Depending upon the patient's individual problems, as many as a dozen different other health-care professionals may be required (Table 63–2).[4] Their function will be detailed later in this chapter. At any one time a number of these individuals will be interacting with both the patient and those in her environment, including family, friends, social agencies, employers, and even the government. This web of interactions requires constant and close attention to communication between the participating individuals; like everyone else, patients have a way of filtering out that which they do not wish to hear and focusing on that which they do. Conflicting reports or advice, either real or imagined, may be received from different members of the team. One individual, therefore, needs to accept primary responsibility for relating to the patient and to function as the center of communications with the patient, avoiding the distortions or misinformation that may otherwise be introduced into the system. In many instances, this role may be filled by the patient's family physician; in others, a nurse practitioner or other allied health professional may serve this function. In all cases, it is incumbent upon the other members of the team to maintain close contact with this individual, preferably by direct verbal communication on a frequent basis. The ideal mechanism for fostering such communication is the case conference, where all members of the team involved in the care of an individual patient are able to meet and share their views of the patient's problems and progress.

**Table 63–2.** Members of the Arthritis Health-Care Team

| |
|---|
| Patient |
| Family physician |
| Rheumatologist |
| Orthopedist |
| Nurse specialist or nurse practitioner |
| Occupational therapist |
| Physical therapist |
| Rehabilitation or vocational counselor |
| Psychologist, sex therapist |
| Social worker |
| Pharmacist |
| Nutritionist |
| Clergy |
| Community agencies |

## GOALS OF MANAGEMENT

Proper management of rheumatoid arthritis results in the maintenance or restoration of the patient to a state of useful and harmonious function with her environment for the foreseeable future. Implicit is the relief of pain, the prevention of joint destruction, and the preservation or improvement of the patient's functioning. Since some remedies, e.g., systemic corticosteroids, may superficially accomplish the first of these goals, the provision of prolonged relief has been included.

Translation of these lofty and somewhat vague goals into specific ones for a particular patient defines the art of clinical rheumatology. Understanding by the patient, and members of the arthritis health care team of realistic therapeutic goals is the basis for a satisfactory outcome.[5]

In response to a few open-ended questions, usually the patient can outline appropriate solutions for her particular life problems. Even the most rudimentary inquiries into disability produced by rheumatoid arthritis often evince very definite responses from patients. After questioning the patient about her ability to function in her occupation, and establishing a rapport, the interviewer may focus on particular goals with such simple questions as: "What is one thing that you cannot do, that you would most like to do?" or "What is the major problem which led you to come here for medical care?" The tone of the question should not exclude multiple responses, but if these are offered, priorities need to be settled. Once such information has been elicited, definition of the patient's goals is greatly simplified; the realism of such goals is usually most fruitfully assessed by a conference among the health professionals who have met with the patient. In such a meeting, the relation between the patient's views of her needs and those that she can realistically be expected to accomplish can be weighed against the risks of various therapeutic options. Consider, for example, the 58-year-old concert cellist who develops rheumatoid arthritis at the height of her career and needs a few more years of active finger movement at the expense of aggressive corticosteroid and, possibly, immunosuppressive therapy. Against that, consider the 30-year-old heiress whose most important activity is communicating her judgment about investments to her employees; in this instance, a much more conservative approach might be warranted. Alternatively, the cellist may be grateful for an opportunity to retire, and the heiress may have been diligently perfecting her tennis serve in order to compete in the professional circuit. In such instances, goals of therapy would be entirely reversed and, with them, the acceptable risks of therapy.

## SUPPORTIVE MEASURES

**Patient Education.** Once the diagnosis of rheumatoid arthritis has been made, the physician begins the process of informing the patient about her disease[6] (see Chapters 34 and 111). Education continues in time for the duration of active disease, and extends from the initial physician contact to involve many other members of the health care team. The form that the education takes usually involves a mixture of techniques. Certainly direct question and answer sessions between patient and physician, nurse practitioner, physical or occupational therapist, rehabilitation counselor, social worker, pharmacist, or even another patient with arthritis will be frequently employed. Some individuals are more at ease when acquiring their information by reading or watching a film or other instructional material, and for these, excellent literature is prepared and distributed by the Arthritis Foundation[7,8] and some hospitals provide appropriate audiovisual aids. Excellent monographs written for arthritis patients are also available.[9] Group instructional sessions, in which a particular topic of general interest to patients with arthritis is discussed, often prove to be extremely popular, perhaps because they afford an environment in which patients can share their embarrassment or anxiety about their disease.[10] Such group sessions may be conducted under the aegis of a hospital clinic, may be organized by a local chapter of the Arthritis Foundation or other social agency, or may even be structured as self-help classes completely independently by patients themselves.

The content of educational efforts should be designed to (1) provide basic information to the patient, (2) reinforce the physician's or other therapist's instructions to the patient, (3) help the patient in effecting appropriate behavioral changes, and (4) lend emotional support. Whenever possible an encouraging, active, aggressive approach toward the disease should be fostered in place of the "there's nothing that can be done and I'll just have to live with it" passive attitude into which patients sometimes are allowed to slip. A great deal can be done about rheumatoid arthritis, and, more often than not, the prognosis is for a favorable outcome. Once patients are informed of this, their ability to cooperate in treatment regimens is greatly enhanced. The listing of the patient as a primary member of the arthritis health-care team in Table 63-2 exemplifies this. Without making the patient feel guilty *for* her disease, it should be possible to make her responsible *about* it. Very early in the treatment program, the patient needs to understand that her disease has no known cause, and that in no way were errors of either commission or omission by her responsible for the development of the disease. Conversely, she needs to understand that her behavior and participation in the treatment program can very much influence the outcome.

Some of the areas that must be dealt with in any educational program are listed in Table 63-3. In most instances it will be obvious which member of the health care team will assume responsibility for a particular area. One of the most disquieting facts for the patient with rheumatoid arthritis to accept is that the cause of the disease remains unknown (see Chapter 58). Many patients infer from this that there is no effective treatment. A frontal approach to this issue is often helpful, citing examples of other diseases with unknown causes for which effective, even curative therapies exist. The patient should also be taught that maintenance of function when the disease is active will allow continued function for the years when it may become quiescent. When specifically discussed in advance, the concepts of intermittent activity and extended time frame may prevent dissatisfaction with the lack of immediate results or even a sudden worsening following the institution of a particular treatment. Knowledge that rheumatoid arthritis affects the entire body, not merely the joints, may allow the patient to accept the overwhelming fatigue, malaise, and weight loss, which she might otherwise attribute to some other cause.

The more the patient understands about treatment,

**Table 63–3.** Educational Topics for Patients with Rheumatoid Arthritis

| |
|---|
| I. Nature of basic disease process |
| Joint anatomy and physiology |
| Unknown cause |
| Intermittent activity |
| Extended time frame |
| A systemic illness, not merely sore joints |
| II. Treatment |
| Difficulty of assessing responses in intermittent disease |
| Prevalence and avoidance of quack remedies |
| Distinction between pain relief and reduction of inflammation |
| Distinction between immediate anti-inflammatory effects and long-term remission |
| Availability of multiple therapeutic agents (including surgery) |
| Importance of follow-up |
| III. Behavior modification |
| Importance of rest |
| Exercise regimen to maintain function |
| Usefulness of joint protection techniques and devices |
| Proper nutrition and avoidance of weight gain |
| Job modification or counseling |
| IV. Emotional support |
| Alleviation of guilt; absence of precipitating factors or activity |
| Absence of clinically important genetic factors |
| Alterations in body image |
| Diminished sexual libido or physical difficulties in performance |
| Involvement of family |

the more likely is she to cooperate to her fullest extent. Most patients will easily grasp the distinction between an analgesic, which merely relieves (or often only dulls) the pain of a sore joint, and an anti-inflammatory agent, which actually reduces the redness, heat, and swelling in conjunction with relieving the pain.[11] Similarly, most patients understand how foolish it is to purchase relatively expensive and widely advertised "special arthritis pills" when told that the major active ingredient in such nostrums is aspirin, which they might already be taking at a fraction of the cost. Even the more subtle difference between an anti-inflammatory agent, which takes effect in a few days or a week or two,[12] and a suppressive or remission-inducing agent, whose full effect may not be apparent for months,[13,14] can be made clear to the patient through iterative and graded instructional techniques. Most will quickly understand the difference between the apparently miraculous disappearance of symptoms afforded by systemic steroids and the relentless progression of joint destruction that occurs despite the feeling of well-being these drugs engender.[15]

With regard to particular drugs or other therapeutic regimens, careful and specific instructions about potential side effects or complications may make the difference between patient acceptance of the agent and refusal to take a drug at the first sign of unexpected nausea or lightheadedness. Because such effects may be multiple and complex and, therefore, difficult to remember when communicated verbally from physician to patient, reinforcement or relearning of these effects become very important. Many clinics find printed take-home literature about side effects of a particular agent convenient. Review of the major untoward effects by the pharmacist when he provides the prescription is another useful mode of reinforcement, as is the use of a follow-up visit with an arthritis nurse specialist or nurse practitioner specifically for drug review. Ideally, the patient should be familiar with each of the drugs, its dosage, and possible side effects. Parenthetically, one side effect insufficiently discussed is the cost of the medicines. Compliance may be improved if the physician points out that $1.00 is a great deal of money to pay for a single tablet, and then explains why this expenditure is appropriate for the patient's particular circumstances.

Almost all patients with rheumatoid arthritis will find it necessary to modify their behavior to reach an equilibrium with their disease. The specific ways in which this may need to be accomplished will be detailed below.

To a large measure, supportive emotional therapy consists of sympathetic listening. The patient needs to be able to discuss her feelings of guilt—"What did I do to deserve this disease?"—her concerns about passing it on to other members of her family, and her inability to function completely satisfactorily in her role as employee, mother, or wife. In the area of altered body image or sexual function, a few open-ended questions may elicit the expression of great emotional concern which the patient might not otherwise have volunteered[16] (see Chapter 34). A conscious effort to raise such questions must be made by the therapist, since these areas are easily neglected, sometimes because of the therapist's own discomfort in discussing them. Depending upon the particular problem, referral to another member of the health care team who has a special interest in the area in question may be advisable.

Education of the immediate family in almost every area outlined in Table 63–3 is extremely important. If the family understands that the patient has a systemic disease, they will more readily accept the need for an enforced rest period in mid-afternoon, the need for help with the heavy housework, and other modifications in the patient's environment. Open communication between family and patient about ways in which the disease has impinged on family life is fostered by including the family in discussion groups or interviews with physicians or other members of the arthritis team whenever possible. The fine line between a supportive and helpful family attitude and an oversolicitous one in which the patient is made a self-conscious invalid requires constant monitoring. Every rheumatologist or orthopedist can relate stories about patients with rheumatoid arthritis who are brought to the hospital with severe flexion deformities and muscle atrophy, having been immobilized in bed some 5 years earlier by a well-meaning family.

**Rest.** In part the much debated question of the value of rest in the treatment of rheumatoid arthritis is moot, since most patients will adopt some form of rest irrespective of any advice from their physicians. In fact, the frequency of affirmative responses to the question, "Do you take a nap in the afternoon?" is sufficiently high as to be useful in the diagnosis of rheumatoid arthritis. Even though they may sleep well at night, patients with rheumatoid arthritis will often describe fatigue occurring abruptly and at a reproducible time during their daily activities.[17] Prescription of an hour's nap just prior to such a period may lead to significant improvement in symptoms for the remainder of the day. Despite its reliability as a symptom in rheumatoid arthritis and the advisability of preventing it, the mechanisms causing fatigue which accompanies active disease have eluded scientific understanding.

While most would agree about the virtues of modifying daily activities so as to include rest periods, and while there is strong evidence of the efficacy of rest or immobilization of individual joints in reducing inflammation (discussed below), the value of complete bed rest as a therapeutic adjunct in the treatment of rheumatoid arthritis remains controversial. In one study patients were randomly placed on a regimen of 18 to 22 hours of enforced bed rest per day or one of 8 hours per night with ad lib daytime activities; no significant difference after 10 weeks[18] was noted. Comparison of the effects of bed rest versus planned activity demonstrated only marginal advantage for bed rest.[18] When patients hospitalized for enforced rest were compared with outpatients, however, significant improvements in hospitalized groups were observed.[19] While acknowledging the absence of any rigidly controlled body of scientific evidence, most rheumatologists do favor enforced bed rest for patients with severe disease, prolonged morning stiffness, and involvement of many joints, particularly the weight-bearing ones. Further, most would recommend that such treatment be carried out in a hospital setting. The advantages of such an arrangement are multiple. It allows removal of the patient from the stressful setting in which she must attempt to cope with her daily activities as well as active disease, and it provides an environment in which rest is viewed as a goal rather than something to feel guilty about. Daily contact with the physician and other members of the arthritis team allows progressive patient education. Institution of physical therapy and other local measures usually unavailable at home often alleviates particular problems (e.g., the use of hot packs on arising often greatly reduces the symptoms of morning stiffness). The antiphogistic effect of enforced bed rest allows sufficient time for anti-inflammatory medications to begin to take effect, and the hospital environment ensures compliance with the prescribed medication routine. Sometimes the mere fact of hospitalization convinces an unconcerned family that the patient does indeed have a serious disease. The combined effect of all these benefits is often dramatic. Within a week or two, the patient is often feeling remarkably improved and is convinced that the physician and the arthritis team can exert some control over her disease, and her mental attitude often borders on the euphoric.[19] In fact, at this point, it may be wise to point out to the patient that the remarkable improvement is the result of being in an environment that greatly favors her well-being, and that maintenance of the complete extent of improvement should not be expected when she returns to her original environment, irrespective of how modified that may be. Without such a warning, the patient may be surprised and disappointed as some of her symptoms reappear when she returns home to re-enter a more active life.

One consequence of the rapidly rising costs of hospital care is the reticence of physicians to hospitalize patients for severe arthritis. With average costs now counted in hundreds of dollars daily, it becomes increasingly difficult to justify hospitalizing a patient with rheumatoid arthritis for assessment of the extent of the disease, enforced bed rest, institution of physical modalities, and drug therapy. Further, in today's acute care facility, the patient with rheumatoid arthritis who does not appear to have a life-threatening illness may be neglected by a busy hospital staff occupied in attempting the resuscitation of the patient in the adjacent bed from a fatal ventricular arrhythmia. Nonetheless, hospitalization in an acute-care facility may be of dramatic benefit, particularly when the physician or other members of the arthritis team take care to orient hospital staff to the specific needs of their patient. An optimal hospital program includes specially trained personnel and accommodations for dealing with the special problems presented by patients with disabling arthritis.

**Exercise and Physical Therapy.** Although it is difficult to demonstrate any long-term benefits from the use of physical modalities such as heat or hydrotherapy, such treatments definitely have a soothing effect on the patient's discomfort. Hot packs, warm baths, or showers on arising often dispel morning stiffness more rapidly. In a hospital setting, immersion in a Hubbard tank may be even more effective. The use of a paraffin bath for the relief of hand stiffness can be learned by the patient and employed at home. The rationale for these modalities is discussed in Chapter 111.

Apart from the improved sense of well-being for the patient, the purpose of the soothing, loosening, analgesic properties of heat and hydrotherapy is to allow sufficient relief of pain and spasm to permit each joint to go through a full range of motion and to permit muscle strengthening exercises.[20,21] In severely affected joints, especially those that may have been temporarily immobilized by casting, gentle passive range of motion by a skilled therapist may be required at least twice daily to maintain motion. The gentleness and skill with which such maneuvers must be performed deserves emphasis; vigorous passive range of motion may do more harm than good by overstretching ligamentous structures or, rarely, even by fracture through the shaft of an osteoporotic bone.

The most commonly employed form of physical therapy is active assisted exercise. In this instance, the patient initiates a particular motion and the therapist assists her in continuing it to its limit. Gradual increase in the limits of motion often results, and gradual reduction in the amount of assistance from the therapist eventually permits the patient to carry the joint through its range of motion unassisted. In this regard, assistance from devices such as pulleys or weights may be used by the patient to substitute for the therapist. A pulley attached to a door frame, which assists elevation and abduction of one shoulder by using the weight of the opposite limb as a controlled counterbalance, is a common example of such a device. Taking advantage of the buoyant effect of water to relieve weight, either in a specially designed hydrotherapy pool or in a plain swimming pool, is another means of assisting active exercise. In the case of the swimming pool, special devices may be required to allow convenient entry and exit by handicapped patients.

An active exercise program at home, in which all the patient's joints are put through a complete range of motion daily, is an integral part of the management of any patient with rheumatoid arthritis. The patient should be trained in this regimen, preferably using written instructions or diagrams, and its continuation should be reinforced periodically by follow-up visits with the therapist. The value of such a regimen in maintaining muscle tone and joint mobility, even in unaffected joints, requires emphasis by the physician or other member of the team who has primary contact with the patient. Specific inquiry as to whether the exercise program is continuing to be followed should be included frequently in routine follow-up visits.[22]

There is a contradiction inherent in recommending rest as a useful form of therapy and simultaneously insisting on exercise, and many patients will be confused by and call attention to this dichotomy. To a certain extent, judgments about rest and exercise will represent a compromise in which the patient should actively participate. Dependent patients will often demand specific prohibitions or encouragements of activity or rest from physicians. Most often it is wisest to let the patient judge for herself, using some common sense guides. Mechanical irritation of a joint already inflamed by rheumatoid arthritis only makes it more inflamed, and the patient whose knees are warm, grossly swollen, and much more painful on the morning after a night of dancing can appreciate this principle. No specific prohibition should be needed, merely an admonition to use common sense.

Although there may be controversy about the usefulness of complete bed rest in the treatment of rheumatoid arthritis, there is widespread agreement about the utility of local joint rest. Naturally enforced rest, such as paralysis of an extremity from a stroke,[23] poliomyelitis,[24] or a peripheral nerve lesion,[25] usually results in sparing of the paralyzed joints in patients who subsequently develop rheumatoid arthritis. In a study of 153 patients with rheumatoid arthritis, the degree of radiographically detectable erosions of the wrist was positively correlated with the degree of physical activity of the joint.[26] Physical therapists (and occupational therapists as well) play an important role in providing appliances to permit such rest and in instructing patients in their use. By using bivalved or functional splints, a certain amount of mobility can be maintained, while at the same time providing partial rest to the involved joints.[27] A good example is the lightweight thermoplastic splint to the volar surface of the forearm, which allows motion at the metacarpophalangeal joints and distally but supports the wrist (see Chapter 111). Use of such splints nightly may make the difference between a good night's sleep and one of constant reawakening. Nocturnal splinting of the knees may also be used if on awakening the patient is troubled by marked stiffness and flexion contractures. Apart from the pain relief that the use of such splints may afford, actual diminution in the extent and severity of the synovitis may be observed.[28]

**Occupational Therapy and Rehabilitation.** A rudimentary assessment of the patient's functional capacity should be conducted by the physician in the initial evaluation of the patient. Consideration of the patient's relationship to those about her and the demands of her life will influence decisions about therapy, and the physician should have some knowledge of these factors. A much more detailed and meaningful analysis of the interaction between the patient and her environment can usually be accomplished by an occupational therapist, who has had special training in methods for such analysis. A verbal review of the activities of daily living will often reveal difficulties that can be remedied with readily available assistive devices. General principles of joint protection, e.g., sitting instead of standing, can be taught. Observation of the patient at work, either in a simulated environment, e.g., kitchen, carpentry shop, print shop, or directly in the home or on the job, may indicate unique problems requiring the construction of special appliances designed to deal with the problem. Attention to such details may make the difference between dependence and independence or between disability and keeping a job.[29,30]

Counseling about employment is a very important aspect of the management of rheumatoid arthritis. One of the major goals is the maintenance of useful vocational or domestic function; too often considerable loss of self-esteem accompanies the acceptance of disability. Interaction with a vocational or rehabilitation counselor needs to be begun early in the contact with the patient so that decisions regarding long-term outlook for continued employment can be arrived at gradually and realistically. While retraining of each patient into a position particularly adapted to her joint problems is an ideal goal, such a solution is the ideal rather than the norm. On the other hand, vocational counselors often prevent disability by identifying and removing impediments to work that are unrelated to the actual performance of the job itself, e.g., transportation to and from work. As an alternative, the patient can be helped to accept partial disability in a supportive yet realistic way. Time available from an early retirement may be focused on a useful avocation, for example. An imaginative approach to rehabilitation can prevent the loss of self-image, identity, and self-esteem and yet help the patient to accept realistically those functional impairments resulting from disease.

## RELIEF OF PAIN

The choice of methods for reducing or relieving pain in joints of patients with rheumatoid arthritis requires a decision about the cause of the pain. The pain at rest in a joint with very active synovitis is caused by mechanisms very different from the pain with motion or weightbearing in a joint that has suffered severe structural damage from years of rheumatoid arthritis. Methods for the assessment of activity of disease have been discussed in Chapter 60. In addition to the commonly used indices such as length of morning stiffness, number of painful joints, number of swollen joints, grip strength, time for 50-foot walk, and erythrocyte sedimentation rate,[31] certain other symptoms or signs may provide useful clues to activity. Pain at rest, particularly at night, often indicates active synovitis. Systemic symptoms, including anorexia, weight loss, fever, or development of new nodules, are also quite reliable indices of activity.

If the pain is attributable to active synovitis, then the most effective agents for pain relief, in the long term, will be those designed to reduce the activity of the disease. If the pain is attributable to structural problems, then judicious use of analgesics, local measures such as immobilization, and, if necessary, surgery will be the most appropriate forms of pain relief.[32,33]

For the patient with severe and active synovitis, the advantages of hospitalization have already been discussed.[17-19] If the patient is already on an optimal anti-inflammatory regimen, further transient restriction of mobility may suffice. For the patient with a severe exacerbation, the proper course is usually a sympathetic and attentive interview followed by a thorough examination of the joints. The attempt is to identify one or two joints that are most inflamed and the major sources of complaints. If a single joint is extraordinarily hot, swollen, and very painful, the diagnosis of septic arthritis, which is more prevalent in rheumatoid joints, should be considered. Examination of fluid for crystals may reveal coincident gout or pseudogout. In the absence of such unusual circumstances, local measures directed at relieving the most severe joints, e.g., splints or local steroid injections, may be helpful.

Analgesics per se are not usually very effective in treating the pain of rheumatoid arthritis. The sympathetic physician will wish to do his utmost to relieve pain, but he must eventually realize and come to terms with the fact that, in the presence of active synovitis, his success will be limited.[34] Aspirin and the other nonsteroidal anti-inflammatory agents have analgesic effects in addition to their anti-inflammatory action, but the substitution of an agent with an equipotent analgesic effect but no anti-inflammatory effect usually results in much less satisfactory control of the arthritis and its accompanying pain. Occasional patients will experience significant relief from propoxyphene or codeine, but most will either derive no benefit or complain of the dulled sensorium or other side effects these drugs induce. Much the same can be said for the stronger narcotic analgesics, whose use in a chronic disease such as rheumatoid arthritis is not recommended for obvious reasons. Such agents should not be withheld for the relief of other self-limited forms of pain, such as that associated with myocardial infarction, or, with a pathologic fracture of a long bone, but they should not be used for the pain of the arthritis in which an immediate improvement in the cause of the pain is not expected.

## ANTI-INFLAMMATORY DRUGS

**Aspirin.** As indicated previously, patients readily understand the difference between drugs that simply reduce pain and those that reduce warmth, swelling, stiffness, and pain of inflammatory arthritis. Similarly, they are able to distinguish between the small amounts of aspirin all of us take for minor aches and pains and the very large amounts required for lessening the inflammation of rheumatoid arthritis. Emphasis on this distinction allows the patient to think of aspirin in a special way and prevents the "all he did was tell me to take some aspirin" reaction, which may otherwise occur. The appropriate drug for the initial treatment of rheumatoid arthritis is aspirin in sufficient dosage to achieve blood levels of greater than 20 mg per deciliter. Plain aspirin tablets are cheapest, and the best formulation with which to begin, though buffered, enteric-coated, or other salicylates may be used if necessary.[35] The only absolute contraindications are a history of severe gastrointestinal bleeding following previous aspirin administration or a history of asthma and nasal polyposis indicative of an idiosyncratic reaction to the drug.[36] Usually a dose of 0.9 g four times a day, with meal and at bedtime with a snack, is a useful starting dose. Patients are warned about tinnitus and are told that the optimal dose for them is going to be slightly less than that which causes tinnitus. From the initial dose of 12 tablets daily, the number is increased by one or two tablets a week until tinnitus is achieved, and then a dose slightly less than this is maintained after an appropriate halt in therapy to allow the cessation of tinnitus. In adjusting the dose, the physician must be aware that at high blood levels the pharmacokinetics of aspirin are those of a saturable enzyme system (see Chapters 48 and 49) so that the half-life is effectively quite prolonged and a week may be required to achieve a new steady-state blood level following a change in dosage.[37] In using tinnitus as a guide to dosage, the physician should also be aware that it is unreliable as a first sign of toxicity in children, in whom much more serious and potentially fatal metabolic disturbances may occur in the absence of tinnitus. In contrast, in the elderly gradual diminution in auditory acuity, reversible with cessation of therapy, may occur instead of tinnitus,[28] or tinnitus may occur at levels well below 20 mg per deciliter. In both instances, or in cases in which compliance is in question, measurement of the serum salicylate level is an inexpensive and reliable way to monitor dosage.

A certain firmness and persistence are required of the physician in order to be certain that aspirin has been given an adequate therapeutic trial. As a rule, in early rheumatoid arthritis, aspirin should be the only agent used initially. Often this has the salutary effect of convincing the patient of its efficacy. While small increases in gastrointestinal blood loss are common,[39] severe gastrointestinal hemorrhage fortunately is not. Further, there is no evidence relating dyspepsia following aspirin ingestion to the occurrence of severe hemorrhage. Thousands of patients have taken tons of aspirin over many years, and this agent remains the least expensive and perhaps the least toxic of any available for the treatment of rheumatoid arthritis. It is therefore worth tinkering with the dose form, timing of administration, and type of preparation used before giving up on aspirin and moving on to another agent which may be no more effective, possibly may be more toxic, and certainly will be more expensive. The prescribing physician should realize also that the decision to abandon aspirin (or any other therapeutic agent in rheumatoid arthritis) is likely to be an irrevocable one. It may require a rather brave and convincing therapist to reinstitute trial of a medicine in the face of statements such as: "I already tried that, and it upset my stomach terribly and didn't help my arthritis anyway!"

**Nonsteroidal Anti-inflammatory Drugs (NSAIDs).** Chapter 50 deals with the clinical pharmacology of the ever-lengthening list of agents which, like aspirin, interfere with prostaglandin metabolism and which, in clinical trials for the treatment of rheumatoid arthritis, appear to be as effective as aspirin and perhaps somewhat better tolerated.[12] If a patient is unable to tolerate sufficient aspirin to maintain therapeutic levels, it is appropriate to try one of the NSAIDs.

Most comparative studies have shown that NSAIDs are about as effective as aspirin in the treatment of rheumatoid arthritis[40] and usually they have caused less gastrointestinal irritation, although all of them may cause peptic ulceration. Increases in serum levels of hepatic enzymes sometimes occur during the first weeks of therapy, and serious hepatitis has been reported as well.[41] Inhibition of renal prostaglandin synthesis may impair renal blood flow and handling of fluid and electrolytes, especially in older patients with pre-existing renal or prerenal dysfunction.[42] Blood dyscrasias are rare but may be fatal; phenylbutazone and oxyphenbutazone have been associated with agranulocytosis, aplastic anemia, and leukemia, so that long-term use of these agents in treatment of rheumatoid arthritis is contraindicated.[43]

There are insufficient data comparing NSAIDs in the treatment of rheumatoid arthritis to permit a recommendation as to which is safer or more effective than the others. Physicians with long experience in using these agents assert that they are unable to predict which patients will benefit most from or tolerate best which drugs. Some advocate sequential trials of 3 to 4 weeks until one that is effective in controlling the patient's disease is identified. Full beneficial effects may not be apparent for 10 to 14 days. Conversely, increased symptoms following withdrawal may not occur for a week or more, so that patients should be instructed not to conclude a drug was ineffective because they feel no worse after having missed a day or two of dosing. Irrespective of the number of tablets per day required to achieve full-dose therapy—six or more in the case of a short-acting agent versus one in the case of a long-acting one—the cost to the patient is of the order of $1.00 per day.

**Systemic Corticosteroids.** These agents, which may effect dramatic suppression of inflammation and relief of symptoms, are discussed under the heading Anti-inflammatory Drugs because available evidence indicates that, despite their dramatic effects, they have no effect on the underlying disease process.[15] Even patients who have excellent symptomatic responses will show radiographic evidence of progressive joint destruction over the years. The use of systemic steroids for the articular manifestations of rheumatoid arthritis is not ordinarily advisable. Taken in sufficient dose for such a chronic problem as rheumatoid arthritis, steroids predictably lead to a number of unpleasant side effects. For the patient with rheumatoid arthritis, the deleterious effects on bone are the most troublesome. Virtually every physician has been exposed to a patient with rheumatoid arthritis, treated with systemic corticosteroids, who now has severe osteopenia with multiple painful vertebral compression fractures added to her other musculoskeletal woes.

The use of systemic corticosteroids for articular rheumatoid arthritis is a drastic step, one to be taken only with full exposition of the potential side effects to the patient. The natural history of steroid administration is eventual failure of control of symptoms at one dose and a requirement for an increased dose. Attempts to reduce or withdraw these agents are usually attended by significant flares in disease activity and increases in symptoms, even when decrements of as little as 1 mg per day are involved. A firm control of dosage by the physician and agreement in advance about patient compliance with this control are mandatory. The patient who manipulates her own medicines as she sees fit is no candidate for systemic steroids: she will soon be taking 30 or 40 mg of prednisone or its equivalent daily.

Despite these warnings, there are some clinical situations in which the systemic administration of corticosteroids is warranted.[44] In patients with severe progressive active disease, administration of 5 or even 7.5 mg daily may allow continued functioning while other remission-inducing agents are administered simultaneously and allowed some time to begin working. Socioeconomic considerations often influence the decision to begin such therapy. If the patient is a wage-earner who is about to lose a job and has a dependent family, or if she is a mother of a young family and is about to be incapacitated by her disease, then the risks may be warranted. In each instance, the lowest possible dose should be used, and a maximum dose ever to be used should be agreed upon in advance. The steroid should be administered as a single daily dose in the morning and continual attempts made to reduce the dose or to convert to every-other-day dosage. In contrast to some of the other rheumatic diseases, the latter form of therapy is not often satisfactory for the control of the symptoms of rheumatoid arthritis.

**Local Injections of Corticosteroids.** Despite experimental evidence indicating that repeated intraarticular injection of steroids may have deleterious effects on cartilage, the judicious use of local corticosteroid injections is a valuable part of the therapeutic armamentarium in rheumatoid arthritis.[45] The pros and cons of and the techniques for their use are considered in detail in Chapter 37. Aspiration of a joint and instillation of corticosteroids are most useful when only a few joints are involved, particularly when these joints are interfering with the overall progress of the patient. Instillations of steroids into tendon sheaths or bursae are also effective local remedies; elimination of pain on pressure over a trochanteric or deltoid bursa may allow sound sleep for many nights. Injections of an area of nerve entrapment may elimate symptoms for a sufficiently long time as to permit slower-acting agents to control the synovitis, thereby eliminating the need for surgical release.

Duration of benefit following local injection is highly variable. Some patients will experience relief lasting several months, while other may benefit for only a few days. The length of time of relief seems to be reproducible for any given patient, so that one who has had only a few days of improvement is unlikely to derive months of relief following a second injection. Judgment is required in determining the number of joints to be injected and the frequency with which any particular joint can be injected. Some systemic absorption and systemic anti-inflammatory effects are observable following intra-articular injections, particularly of large joints where larger total amounts of steroids may be involved. The nature of this improvement and its cause should be explained to the patient, lest she develop unfounded optimism about the state of her disease.

## REMISSION–INDUCING AGENTS

Most patients with rheumatoid arthritis report a lessening in symptoms after taking full-dose anti-inflammatory agents for a week or two, but very few experience a total disappearance of their disease. Most of these do so very early in their course, making the diagnosis suspect. Current criteria for a "clinical remission" include less than fifteen minutes of morning stiffness, no fatigue, no joint pain by history, no joint tenderness, no joint or tendon sheath swelling, and no elevation of erythrocyte sedimentation rate.[46] Although "outcome" is doubtless more significant for the patient than transient changes in the progress of her disease,[47] nearly all studies of efficacy have measured the latter. By these criteria, at least three agents—antimalarials (Chapter 51), gold salts (Chapter 52) and penicillamine (Chapter 53)—have been shown to induce remission. As knowledge about the dosage and toxicity of these agents has accumulated, the tendency has been to use them earlier in the course of the disease, before irreversible structural damage has occurred. Whereas formerly they were often considered measures of last resort, fraught with life-threatening complications, currently they are regularly prescribed for patients with aggressive disease, in the hope of preventing irreversible structural damage.[48] The decision to use such agents is influenced by the patient's age, the severity of disease, the distribution and number of joints affected, and the effect of the disease on the patient's functioning. Although remission-inducing agents tend to be prescribed earlier for young patients, there is no evidence that the results are better or the toxicity less in this age group.[49] In general, most rheumatologists would prescribe a remission-inducing agent after several months of progressive rheumatoid arthritis, irrespective of the intensity of disease or the patient's age. Since one agent may succeed where others have already failed, they are usually administered sequentially, beginning with those that are least toxic and progressing through increasingly more toxic ones, monitoring patient response at each step. Unfortunately, attempts to predict responses to individual agents by scrutinizing clinical or laboratory variables for individual patients have been unsuccessful.[50]

**Antimalarials.** Probably the least risky and most easily administered remission-inducing agent is the antimalarial. As discussed in Chapter 51, the efficacy of chloroquine or hydroxychloroquine in the treatment of rheumatoid arthritis has been repeatedly validated in controlled studies; the effects have not been dramatic, but they have been quite reproducible.[51-53] Ease of administration and relative freedom from minor nuisance-type side effects as well as from major life-threatening complications makes antimalarials the preferred initial remission-inducing agent in the opinion of many rheumatologists. These drugs have a slowly developing favorable effect of unknown nature, but they do not have immediate or dramatic anti-inflammatory influences. Patients who begin taking antimalarials need to understand that no beneficial effects may be apparent for several weeks, and that 3 or 4 months may be required before a decision about efficacy can be made in their particular case. As for any potentially toxic agent, full disclosure for possible complications is mandatory. The most important of these is pigmented macular degeneration of the retina. When this occurs, it may be catastrophic, since there is no effective treatment and it may progress even after the drug has been stopped. The patient must be informed that expert ophthalmologic consultation will be required periodically and will begin immediately (to detect patients with pre-existing retinal lesions such as senile macular degeneration, which may be difficult to differentiate from antimalarial retinopathy). As made clear in Chapter 51, however, the frequency of macular degeneration is probably overestimated, is dose related, and rarely occurs at doses currently recommended.[54] A trial of 6 to 12 weeks of an antimalarial is, therefore, often warranted early in the course of documented rheumatoid arthritis.

**Gold.** Of all the remission-inducing agents, gold has been used for the longest time and has been studied most extensively, and there is abundant evidence of efficacy.[13] Details of the use of gold salts are considered in Chapter 52. On the average, about one third of patients who are administered gold salts will experience dramatic and sustained improvement in their disease; depending upon definitions, as many as one quarter will have remissions.[13,31,55,56] Another third will experience some improvement, but it is often difficult to distinguish this improvement from that which might have occurred as part of the natural history of the disease. The remaining third will discontinue treatment either because of toxicity or failure to improve. During the first year or two, about two thirds of patients will improve either concomitantly with or because of gold salt therapy. With longer follow-up, however, the fraction of patients still taking gold continues to fall, due both to continuing development of toxic reactions and to recrudescence of disease in those who earlier had responded.[57,58] The usual treatment regime begins with a test dose of 10 mg the first week, 25 mg the second, and then 50 mg weekly for 20 weeks. When a clinical response is apparent, the frequency of injections can be reduced to every other week or eventually to once a month. Firm evidence supports the continued administration of gold salts in those who experience benefit; randomized and placebo-controlled cessation of therapy resulted in relapse for those who were not continued in treatment.[13] There is no specific limit to the length of time for which gold may be given, but complete discontinuation should be contemplated only after several symptom-free years and complete absence of laboratory evidence of active disease.

Most unwanted effects occur relatively early in the course of treatment, often between the fifth and fifteenth week of injections. The most common toxic reaction is a mild pruritic rash (which may not recur following cessation and reinstitution of therapy[59]), but more extensive skin eruptions, including exfoliative dermatitis, also occur. Oral or other mucocutaneous ulcers may be quite painful and occasionally persist for weeks following cessation of therapy. Renal toxicity is usually manifested by mild proteinuria, which may require adjustment of the dose. Moderate proteinuria is an indication for cessation of therapy, but subsequently treatment may be resumed.[60] Frank nephrotic syndrome or renal functional impairment is rare and usually reversible. Hematologic complications include thrombocytopenia, which is often reversible,[61] and agranulocytosis or aplastic anemia, which is rarely so. These may occur late in the course of treatment, often without warning. Immediate cessation of gold therapy and institution of steroids is indicated, possibly with the addition of a gold-chelating agent. Use of a routine protocol, designed to inquire about symptoms of toxicity and to elicit signs or obtain laboratory data about toxicity, allows monitoring of untoward effects by members of the health-care team other than the physician, but the requirements for urine and blood screening make gold salt therapy quite costly.

A complex of gold with a trialkylphosphine, auranofin, has been shown to be well absorbed via the oral route.[62] In a number of controlled studies,[63,66] auranofin has been shown to be nearly as effective as the standard regimen of parenteral gold salts. Although gastrointestinal side effects such as diarrhea are more frequent with the oral preparation, cutaneous and renal toxicity is substantially less, so that discontinuation of therapy due to adverse reactions has generally been less frequent. Thrombocytopenia, proteinuria, elevated liver enzymes, "nitritoid" reactions, and "gold pneumonitis" are rarely observed in patients treated with auranofin. No correlation between mean blood levels of gold and clinical response has been noted, but the same absence of correlation has been observed following parenterally administered gold salts.[67]

**Penicillamine.** In the opinion of most rheumatologists, penicillamine is the next agent to be tried after antimalarials and gold have failed. As detailed in Chapter 53, this drug was chosen for the wrong reasons, namely its theoretical ability to reduce the disulfide bridges of IgM rheumatoid factor, which was believed to have a pathogenetic role in rheumatoid arthritis.[68] When it was reported that penicillamine not only led to a real fall in rheumatoid factor titers but also to clinical improvement in a patient with rheumatoid vasculitis, interest in the agent as treatment for the other manifestations of rheumatoid arthritis was generated.[69] Many years later its efficacy was documented by controlled studies of the Empire Rheumatism Council.[14] Today there is no issue about its efficacy, only about its rank among the remitting agents. Patient acceptance is probably lower than that observed with gold salts, owing to intolerable nausea, dyspepsia, and dysgeusia,[70] but such symptoms can often be avoided when the drug is begun at a very low dose (125 mg daily) and increased very slowly (125 mg each month). The side effects of penicillamine resemble those of gold and commonly include skin rash, proteinuria, and bone marrow suppression. Unique toxicities include the development of myasthenia gravis–like syndromes[71] and of pemphigus.[72] Like all remission-inducing agents, penicillamine has a delayed therapeutic response, so that full benefit may not appear for up to six months.

**Azathioprine.** The only other agent that may be disease modifying and is approved for use in rheumatoid arthritis is azathioprine.[73] Use of this anti-inflammatory and immunosuppressive drug is described in Chapter 55. Because it ordinarily affords only modest control of symptoms and has been associated with severe toxicity, including a potential for lymphoreticular malignancy, most rheumatologists employ azathioprine only after antimalarials, gold, and penicillamine have failed. Even relatively low doses, which would not usually be effective in the suppression of renal allograft rejection (for which the drug was first designed), appear to reduce the symptoms of rheumatoid arthritis.[74]

## EXPERIMENTAL TREATMENTS

Although a minority of patients with rheumatoid arthritis experience a complete remission and the majority obtain a satisfactory result, a small fraction is afflicted with inexorable, progressive, and destructive disease despite the most careful and well-intentioned applications of currently approved therapy. Such patients often have life-threatening extra-articular manifestations which occur when the disease appears to "escape" the bounds of the joint capsule and involve vital organs (See Chapter 60). In such instances, use of drugs whose risk-benefit ratios are as yet imperfectly defined may be required in an attempt to preserve crucial joint function or even life. The wisest course of action in such circumstances is referral to a tertiary treatment center where the health-care team is familiar with the dosage and toxicity of the immunosuppressive or cytotoxic regimens to be employed, the means for monitoring toxicity and effects of therapy are immediately available, and the results of such experimental treatment are collected and analyzed in a systematic fashion.

Besides azathioprine, which has been approved in the United States for the treatment of rheumatoid arthritis, other drugs with potential beneficial effect include levamisole, cyclophosphamide, and methotrexate. As was true for many of the agents used for the treatment of rheumatoid arthritis, the discovery of *levamisole* was an accident. The original observation was made that animals dewormed with this antihelminthic appeared to have an enhanced antibody response.[75] Subsequent in vitro experiments demonstrated that levamisole potentiated a variety of T-lymphocyte responses, and even increased the severity of rat adjuvant arthritis. Several controlled trials in patients with rheumatoid arthritis have shown it to be efficacious in the treatment of this disease.[76–78] At doses of 150 mg three days weekly a response rate of 70 per cent was observed.[78] Unfortunately, frequent and severe toxicity had limited its use. In particular, granulocytopenia and agranulocytosis occur so frequently as to make levamisole unsatisfactory for routine use.

Double-blind controlled studies confirm the beneficial effects of *cyclophosphamide* in the short-term therapy of rheumatoid arthritis,[79,80] including reduction in the frequency of radiographic hand joint erosions. At a dose of 150 mg per day, most patients experience significant toxic effects, including bone marrow suppression (especially neutropenia), gonadal suppression, alopecia, and cystitis (with occasional bladder fibrosis and even carcinoma); an increased risk of lymphomas and leukemias also exists. A controlled trial of 150 mg versus 75 mg per day demonstrated significant improvement in both groups, but the frequency of side effects was also the same, with the exception of neutropenia, which was only 6 per cent in the low-dose group compared with 32 per cent in the high-dose group.[81] While short-term beneficial effects have consistently been demonstrated, the appropriate studies to determine the effect of cyclophosphamide on long-term outcome[47] have not been made.

The folic acid antagonist *methotrexate* has been used in low doses for the treatment of psoriasis and psoriatic arthritis for a number of years, but only recently has it been used to any extent in rheumatoid arthritis.[82] Typically three oral doses of 2.5 to 7.5 mg are administered at twelve-hour intervals once weekly. Experience with this regimen in the treatment of psoriasis indicates that it is not associated with the increased risk of malignancies seen with azathioprine or cyclophosphamide.[83] Hepatotoxicity, not necessarily heralded by changes in blood chemistries,[84] is the most serious side effect; marrow toxicity is not usually a problem with the low-dose schedule. There are no controlled prospective studies of the efficacy of methotrexate in the treatment of rheumatoid arthritis, but retrospective analyses have indicated definite improvement in approximately two thirds of patients, all of whom had been refractory to other remission-inducing agents.[85–87]

*Cyclosporin A*, a fungal metabolite that has had a major positive impact in the control of allograft rejection, appears to act specifically on T-lymphocyte function.[88] It might, therefore, be expected to have a beneficial effect in the control of rheumatoid arthritis. Partly because of nephrotoxicity, it has not been widely studied in any rheumatic diseases. In the one small uncontrolled series that has been published, only about one third of patients with rheumatoid arthritis showed any substantial improvement.[89]

Experience with *total lymphoid irradiation* in the treatment of Hodgkin's disease indicated that it was associated with few serious side effects and no increased risk of hematologic malignancy, but led to profound impairment of T-lymphocyte function, which often lasted for years.[90] Uncontrolled studies of small numbers of patients with rheumatoid arthritis refractory to the usual remission-inducing agents have demonstrated improvement in disease activity.[91,92] In one study,[92] partial recrudescence of disease was observed after about a year, but in another the beneficial effects and laboratory evidence of immunosuppression were observed to persist throughout a 13- to 28-month follow-up period.[93]

## SURGERY

An integral part of the management of many patients with rheumatoid arthritis involves orthopedic or plastic surgery.[33] The technical aspects and details of procedures used in the surgical approach to rheumatoid arthritis are considered in Chapters 112 to 120. Here we will consider the influence of the disease on the fitness of the patient for surgery and the special attention required for such patients.

**Influence of Rheumatoid Arthritis on Fitness and Response to Surgery.** Despite the systemic nature of their disease and the multiplicity of medicines with which rheumatoid arthritis patients are often treated, their surgical morbidity and mortality are not extraordinary. While it is doubtless advantageous to postpone surgery until disease activity appears to have come under partial control, rarely is complete quiescence of the disease possible in a patient who requires surgery; moderate anemia or hypoalbuminemia is not in itself a contraindication.[95] The fact that many patients with rheumatoid arthritis are nearer to their ideal body weight than the general population or, especially, patients with osteoarthritis, may actually enhance their suitability as surgical candidates. When wound healing was studied in a matched group of patients with rheumatoid or osteoarthritis, no major differences were noted. Some problems peculiar to patients with rheumatoid arthritis require special attention by anesthesiologists or surgeons, however; and the primary therapist should be responsible for pointing out these problems.

*Anesthesiologic Considerations.* The possibility of cervical spine involvement, especially atlantoaxial subluxation, must always be kept in mind.[96] A careful history of symptoms of such involvement, together with preoperative radiographs in flexion and extension, if necessary, may prevent a catastrophe during endotracheal intubation. In patients with juvenile rheumatoid arthritis who may have extensive ankylosis of the cervical spine, intubation may present even more formidable problems. Rarely, temporomandibular joint involvement may make intubation difficult.

*Continuation of Medical Therapy.* Doubtless either the surgeon or the anesthesiologist will obtain a history of preceding therapy with systemic steroids and attend to appropriate adrenal steroid replacement during the perioperative period. On the other hand, the necessity for the patient to receive nothing by mouth for a day or two occasionally leads to prolonged cessation of anti-inflammatory or suppressive therapy, even when it could be given parenterally. The result may be a general increase in symptoms which progresses as the steroid coverage is reduced and finally removed. While it is true that aspirin and related anti-inflammatory drugs may have an effect on the coagulation process, significant postoperative hemorrhage attributable to these agents is uncommon. Similarly, the use of antimalarials, gold, penicillamine, or other agents is not contraindicated in the postoperative period. Often, however, their administration may simply be overlooked until either the patient complains of other joints or follow-up by other members of the arthritis health-care team calls attention to the omission.

## References


1. Short, C.L., Bauer, W., and Reynolds, W.E.: Rheumatoid Arthritis. Cambridge, Mass., Harvard University Press, 1957.
2. Duthie, J.J.R., Brown, P.E., Truelove, L.H., Baraza, F., and Lawpie, H.: Course and prognosis in rheumatoid arthritis. Ann. Rheum. Dis. 23:193, 1974.
3. Feigenbaum, S.L., Masi, A.T., and Kaplan, S.B.: Prognosis in rheumatoid arthritis: A longitudinal study of newly diagnosed younger adult patients. Am. J. Med. 66:377, 1979.
4. Katz, S., Vignos, P.J., Moskowitz, R.W., Thompson, H.M., and Svec, K.H.: Comprehensive outpatient care in rheumatoid arthritis: A controlled study. JAMA 206:1244, 1968.
5. Decker, J.L.: The management of rheumatoid arthritis. Med. Times 105:28, 1977.
6. Kaye, R.L., and Hammond, A.H.: Understanding rheumatoid arthritis. Evaluation of a patient education program. JAMA 239:2466, 1978.
7. Arthritis Practical Information. Where to turn for help. Atlanta, The Arthritis Foundation, 1982.
8. Rheumatoid Arthritis. Medical Information Series. Atlanta, The Arthritis Foundation, 1983.
9. Fries, J.F.: Arthritis. A Comprehensive Guide. Reading, Mass., Addison-Wesley Publishing Company, 1979.
10. Valentine, L.R.: Self care through group learning. Am. J. Nursing 70:2110, 1976.
11. Boardman, P.L., and Hart, F.O.: Clinical measurements of the anti-inflammatory effects of salicylates in rheumatoid arthritis. Br. Med. J. 2:264, 1967.
12. Simon, L.S., and Mills, J.A.: Nonsteroidal anti-inflammatory drugs. New Engl. J. Med. 302:1179, 1237, 1980.
13. Empire Rheumatism Council: Gold therapy in rheumatoid arthritis: Final report of a multicentre controlled trial. Ann. Rheum. Dis. 20:315, 1961.
14. Multicentre Trial Group: Controlled trial of d (-) penicillamine in severe rheumatoid arthritis. Lancet 1:275, 1973.
15. Glass, D., Snaith, M.L., Russel, A.S., and Daly, J.R.: Possible unnecessary prolongation of corticosteroid therapy in rheumatoid arthritis. Lancet 2:234, 1971.
16. Ferguson, K., and Figley, B.: Sexuality and rheumatic disease: A prospective study. Sexuality Disability 2:130, 1979.
17. Mills, J.A., Pinals, R.S., Ropes, M.W., Short, C.L., and Sutcliffe, S.: Value of bedrest in patients with rheumatoid arthritis. N. Engl. J. Med. 284:453, 1971.
18. Alexander, G.J., Hortas, C., and Bacon, P.A.: Bed rest activity and the inflammation of rheumatoid arthritis. Br. J. Rheumatol. 22:134, 1983.
19. Lee, P., Kennedy, A.C., Anderson, J., and Buchanan, W.W.: Benefits of hospitalization in rheumatoid arthritis. Quart. J. Med. 43:205, 1974.
20. Nordemar, R.: Physical training in rheumatoid arthritis: A controlled long-term study. II. Functional capacity and general attitudes. Scan. J. Rheumatol. 10:25, 1981.
21. Wright, U., and Dawson, D.: Joint stiffness—its characterization and significance. Biomed. Engineering 4:8, 1969.
22. Wright, V., Hopkins, R., and Jackson, M.: Instructing patients in physiotherapy: An example using three methods. Rheumatol. Rehabil. 19:91, 1980.
23. Bland, J.H., and Eddy, W.M.: Hemiplegia and rheumatoid arthritis. Arthritis Rheum. 11:72, 1968.
24. Kammermann, J.S.: Protective effect of traumatic lesions on rheumatoid arthritis. Ann. Rheum. Dis. 25:361, 1966.
25. Glick, E.N.: Asymmetrical rheumatoid arthritis after poliomyelitis. Br. Med. J. 3:26, 1967.
26. Castillo, B.A., Sallab, R.A., and Scott, J.T.: Physical activity, cystic erosions, and osteoporosis in rheumatoid arthritis. Ann. Rheum. Dis. 24:522, 1965.
27. Gault, S.J., and Spyker, J.M.: Beneficial effect of immobilization of joints in rheumatoid and related arthritides: A splint study using sequential analysis. Arthritis Rheum. 12:34, 1969.
28. Harris, R., and Copp, E.P.: Immobilization of the knee joint in rheumatoid arthritis. Ann. Rheum. Dis. 21:353, 1962.
29. Brewerton, D.H., and Daniel, S.W.: Return to work: Experiences of a rehabilitation officer. Br. Med. J. 2:240, 1969.
30. Cochrane, G.M.: Rheumatoid arthritis: Vocational rehabilitation. Int. Rehabil. Med. 4:148, 1982.

31. The Cooperating Clinics Committee of the American Rheumatism Association: A controlled trial of gold salt therapy in rheumatoid arthritis. Arthritis Rheum. 16:353, 1973.
32. Ehrlich, G.E.: Total Management of the Arthritis Patient. Philadelphia, J. B. Lippincott Company, 1973.
33. Hall, A.P.: The decision to operate in rheumatoid arthritis. Orthoped. Clin. North Am. 6:675, 1975.
34. Hardin, J.G., and Kirk, K.A.: Comparative effectiveness of five analgesics for the pain of rheumatoid arthritis. Arthritis Rheum. 21:564, 1978.
35. Giuliano, V., and Scarff, E.V.: Clinical comparison of two salicylates in rheumatoid arthritis patients on maintenance gold therapy. Curr. Therap. Res. 28:61, 1980.
36. Samter, M., and Beers, R.F.: Concerning the nature of intolerance to aspirin. J. Allergy 40:281, 1967.
37. Cassel, S., Furst, D., Dromgoole, S., and Paulus, H.: Steady-state serum salicylate levels in hospitalized patients with rheumatoid arthritis. Arthritis Rheum. 22:384, 1979.
38. Mongan, E., Kelly, P., Nies, K., Porter, W.W., and Paulus, H.E.: Tinnitus as an indication of therapeutic serum salicylate levels. JAMA 226:142, 1973.
39. Leonards, J.R., Levy, G., and Niemczura, R.: Gastrointestinal blood loss during prolonged aspirin administration. N. Engl. J. Med. 289:1020, 1973.
40. Verbeeck, R.K., Blackburn, J.L., and Loewen, G.R.: Clinical pharmacokinetics of non-steroidal anti-inflammatory drugs. Clin. Pharmacokinet. 8:297, 1983.
41. Weinblatt, M.E., Tesser, J.R., and Gilliam, J.H., III: The liver in rheumatic diseases. Sem. Arth. Rheum. 11:399, 1982.
42. Zawada, E.T., Jr.: Renal consequences of nonsteroidal anti-inflammatory drugs. Postgrad. Med. 71:223, 1982.
43. Fowler, P.D.: Marrow toxicity of the pyrazoles. Ann. Rheum. Dis. 26:344, 1967.
44. Harris, E.D., Jr.: Glucocorticoid use in rheumatoid arthritis. Hosp. Pract. 18:137, 1983.
45. Gray, R.G., and Gottlieb, N.L.: Intra-articular corticosteroids: An updated assessment. Clin. Orthop. Rel. Res. 177:235, 1983.
46. Pinals, R.S., Masi, A.T., and Larsen, R.A.: Preliminary criteria for clinical remission in rheumatoid arthritis. Arthritis Rheum. 24:1308, 1981.
47. Fries, J.F.: The assessment of disability: From first to future principles. Br. J. Rheumatol. 22(Suppl. 3):48, 1983.
48. Pinals, R.S.: Approach to rheumatoid arthritis and osteoarthritis: An overview. Am. J. Med 75(Suppl. 4B):2, 1983.
49. Terkeltaub, R., Esdaile, J., Decary, F., and Tannenbaum, H.: A clinical study of older age rheumatoid arthritis with comparison to a younger onset group. J. Rheumatol. 10:418, 1983.
50. Christian, C.L.: Prognostic and therapeutic implications of immunologic test results in rheumatic disease. Hum. Pathol. 14:446, 1983.
51. Freedman, A., and Steinberg, V.L.: Chloroquine in rheumatoid arthritis—a double blindfold trial of treatment for one year. Ann. Rheum. Dis. 19:243, 1960.
52. Scherbel, A.L.: Use of synthetic antimalarial drugs and other agents for rheumatoid arthritis: Historic and therapeutic perspectives. Am. J. Med. 75:1, 1983.
53. Bell, C.L.: Hydroxychloroquine sulfate in rheumatoid arthritis: Long-term response rate and predictive parameters. Am. J. Med. 75:46, 1983.
54. Rynes, R.I., Krohel, G., Falbo, A., Reinecke, R.D., and Bartholomew, L.E.: Ophthalmologic safety of long-term hydroxychloroquine treatment. Arthritis Rheum. 21:588, 1978.
55. Sigler, J.W., Bluhm, G.B., Duncan, M.D., Sharp, J.T., Ensign, D.C., and McCrum, W.R.: Gold salts in the treatment of rheumatoid arthritis. Ann. Intern. Med. 80:21, 1974.
56. Sharp, J.T., Lidsky, M.D., and Duffy, J.: Clinical responses during gold therapy for rheumatoid arthritis. Changes in synovitis, radiologically detectable erosive lesions, serum proteins, and serologic abnormalities. Arthritis Rheum. 25:540, 1982.
57. Rothermich, N.O., Phillips, V.K., Bergen, W., and Thomas, M.H.: Follow-up study of chrysotherapy. Arthritis Rheum. 22:423, 1979.
58. Richter, J.A., Runge, L.A., Pinals, R.S., and Oates, R.P.: Analysis of treatment terminations with gold and antimalarial compounds in rheumatoid arthritis. J. Rheumatol. 7:153, 1980.
59. Klinefelter, H.F.: Reinstitution of gold therapy in rheumatoid arthritis after mucocutaneous reactions. J. Rheumatol. 2:21, 1975.
60. Newton, P., Swinburn, W.R., and Swinson, D.R.: Proteinuria with gold therapy: When should gold be permanently stopped? Br. J. Rheumatol. 22:11, 1983.
61. Coblyn, J.S., Weinblatt, M., Holdsworth, D., and Glass, D.: Gold-induced thrombocytopenia. A clinical and immunogenetic study of twenty-three patients. Ann. Intern. Med. 95:178, 1981.
62. Berglöf, F.E., Berglöf, K., and Walz, D.T.: Auranofin: An oral chrysotherapeutic agent for the treatment of rheumatoid arthritis. J. Rheumatol. 5:68, 1978.
63. Menard, H.A., Beaudet, F., Davis, P., Harth, M., Percy, J.S., Russell, A.S., and Thompson, J.M.: Gold therapy in rheumatoid arthritis: Interim report of the Canadian multicenter prospective trial comparing sodium aurothiomalate and auranofin. J. Rheumatol. 9 (Suppl.):179, 1982.
64. Katz, W.A., Alexander, S., Bland, J.H., Blechman, W., Bluhm, G.B., Bonebrake, R.A., Falbo, A., Greenwald, R.A., Hartman, S., Hobbs, T., Indenbaum, S., Lergier, J.E., Lanier, B.G., Lightfoot, R.W., Phelps, P., Sheon, R.P., Torretti, D., Wenger, M.E., and Wilske, K.: The efficacy and safety of auranofin compared to placebo in rheumatoid arthritis. J. Rheumatol. 9 (suppl.):173, 1982.
65. Schattenkirchner, M., Kaik, B., Muller-Fassbender, H., Rau, R., and Zeidler, H.: Auranofin and sodium aurothiomalate in the treatment of rheumatoid arthritis, a double-blind, comparative, multicenter study. J. Rheumatol. 9 (Suppl.)184, 1982.
66. Ward, J.R., Williams, H.J., Egger, M.J., Reading, J.C., Boyce, E., Altz-Smith, M., Samuelson, C.O., Jr., Willkens, R.F., Solsky, M.A., Hayes, S.P., Blocka, K.L., Weinstein, A., Meenan, R.F., Guttadauria, M. Kaplan, S.B., and Klippel, J.: Comparison of auranofin, gold sodium thiomalate and placebo in the treatment of rheumatoid arthritis. A controlled clinical trial. Arthritis Rheum. 26:1303, 1983.
67. Gottlieb, N.L., Smith, P.M., and Smith, E.M.: Pharmacodynamics of $^{195}$Au labeled auriothiomalate in blood. Correlation with course of rheumatoid arthritis, gold toxicity and gold excretion. Arthritis Rheum. 17:161, 1974.
68. Griffin, S.W., Ulloa, A., Henry, M., Johnston, M.L., and Holley, H.L.: In vivo effect of pencillamine on circulating rheumatoid factor. Clin. Res. 8:87, 1960.
69. Jaffe, I.A.: Rheumatoid arthritis with arteritis. Report of a case treated with pencillamine. Ann. Intern. Med. 61:556,1964.
70. Tsang, I.K., Patterson, C.A., Stein, H.B., Robinson, H.S., and Ford, D.K.: D-Penicillamine in the treatment of rheumatoid arthritis. Arthritis Rheum. 20:666, 1977.
71. Bucknall, R.C., Dixon, A.S.J., Glick, E.N., Woodland, J., and Zutshi, D.W.: Myasthenia gravis associated with penicillamine treatment for rheumatoid arthritis. Br. Med. J. 1:600, 1975.
72. Marsden, R.A., Ryan, T.J., Van Hegan, R.I., Walshe, M., Hill, H., and Mowat, A.G.: Pemphigus foliaceus indicated by penicillamine. Br. Med. J. 2:1423, 1976.
73. Currey, H.L.F., Harris, J.R.M., Mason, R.M., Woodland, J., Beveridge, T., Roberts, C.J., Vere, D.W., Dixon, A.S.J., Davies, J., and Owen-Smith, B.: Comparison of azathioprine, cyclophosphamide and gold in treatment of rheumatoid arthritis. Br. Med. J. 3:763, 1974.
74. Abel, T., Urowitz, M.B., Smythe, H.A., Keystone, E.C., and Norman, C.B.: Long-term effects of azathioprine in rheumatoid arthritis. Arthritis Rheum. 21:539, 1978.
75. Symoens, J., and Schuermans, Y.: Levamisole. Clin. Rheum. Dis. 5:603, 1979.
76. Runge, L.A., Pinals, R.S., Lourie, S.H., and Tomas, R.H.: Treatment of rheumatoid arthritis with levamisole. A controlled trial. Arthritis Rheum. 20:1445, 1977.
77. Multicentre Study Group: Levamisole in rheumatoid arthritis. Final report on a randomised double-blind study comparing a single weekly dose of levamisole with placebo. Ann. Rheum. Dis. 41:159, 1982.
78. Miller, B., de Merieux, P., Ramachandran, S., Clements, P., Fan, P., Levy, J., and Paulus, H.: Double-blind placebo controlled crossover evaluation of levamisole in rheumatoid arthritis. Arthritis Rheum. 23:172, 1980.
79. Cooperating Clinics of the American Rheumatism Association: A controlled trial of cyclophosphamide in rheumatoid arthritis. N. Engl. J. Med. 283:883, 1970.
80. Steinberg, A.D., Plotz, P.H., Wolf, S., Wong, V.G., Agus, S.G., and Decker, J.L.: Cytotoxic drugs in the treatment of non-malignant disease. Ann. Intern. Med. 76:619, 1972.
81. Williams, H.J., Reading, J.C., Ward, J.R., and O'Brien, W.M.: Comparison of high and low dose cyclophosphamide therapy in rheumatoid arthritis. Arthritis Rheum. 23:521, 1980.
82. Willkens, R.F.,: Reappraisal of the use of methotrexate in rheumatic disease. Am. J. Med. 75(Suppl. 4B):19, 1983.
83. Bailin, P.L., Tindall, J.P., Roenigk, H.H., Hogan, M.D.: Is methotrexate therapy for psoriasis carcinogenic? JAMA 232:359, 1975.
84. Weinstein, G.D., Roenigk, H.H., Maibach, H., et al.: Psoriasis-liver methotrexate interactions: Results of an international cooperative study. Arch. Dermatol. 108:36, 1973.
85. Groff, G.D., Shenberger, K.N., Wilke, W.S., and Taylor, T.H.: Low dose oral methotrexate in rheumatoid arthritis: An uncontrolled trial and review of the literature. Sem. Arthritis Rheum. 12:333, 1983.
86. Steinsson, K., Weinstein, A., Korn, J., and Abeles, M.: Low dose methotrexate in rheumatoid arthritis. J. Rheumatol. 9:860, 1982.
87. Michaels, R.M., Nashel, D.J., Leonard, A., Sliwinski, A.J., and Derbes,

S.J.: Weekly intravenous methotrexate in the treatment of rheumatoid arthritis. Arthritis Rheum. 25:339, 1982.
88. White, D.J.G., and Calne, R.Y.: The use of cyclosporin immunosuppression in organ grafting. Immunol. Rev. 65:115, 1982.
89. Graf, U., Marbet, U., Muller, W., and Thiel, G.: Cyclosporin A—Wirkungen und Nebenwirkungen bei der Behandlung der chronischen Polyarthritis und der Psoriasisarthritis. Immun. Infekt. 9:20, 1981.
90. Fuks, Z., Strober, S., Bobrove, A.M., Susazuki, T., McMichael, A., and Kaplan, H.S.: Long-term effects of radiation on T and B lymphocytes in peripheral blood of patients with Hodgkin's disease. J. Clin. Invest. 58:803, 1976.
91. Kotzin, B.L., Strober, S., Engelman, E.G., Calin, A., Hoppe, R.T., Kansas, G.S., Terrell, C.P., Kaplan, H.S.: Treatment of intractable rheumatoid arthritis with total lymphoid irradiation. N. Engl. J. Med. 305:969, 1981.
92. Trentham, D.E., Belli, J.A., Anderson, R.J., Buckley, J.A., Goetzl, E.J., David, J.R., and Austen, K.F.: Clinical and immunologic effects of fractionated total lymphoid irradiation in refractory rheumatoid arthritis. N. Engl. J. Med. 305:976, 1981.
93. Field, E.H., Strober, S., Hoppe, R.T., Calin, A., Engleman, E.G., Kotzin, B.L., Tanay, A.S., Calin, H.J., Terrell, C.P., and Kaplan, H.S.: Sustained improvement of intractable rheumatoid arthritis after total lymphoid irradiation. Arthritis Rheum. 26:934, 1983.
94. Mowat, A.G.: Surgical treatment of rheumatoid arthritis. *In* Scott, J.T. (ed.): Copeman's Textbook of the Rheumatic Diseases. 5th ed. New York, Churchill Livingstone, 1978, p. 459.
95. Garner, R.W., Mowat, A.G., and Hazleman, B.L.: Wound healing after operations on patients with rheumatoid arthritis. J. Bone Joint Surg. 55B:134, 1973.
96. Smith, P., Benn, R.T., and Sharp, J.: Natural history of rheumatoid cervical luxations. Ann. Rheum. Dis. 32:432, 1972.

# INDEX

Note: Page numbers in *italics* refer to illustrations; page numbers followed by t refer to tables.


AA protein, 1472–1473
Abdominal pain, in polyarteritis, 1144
in rheumatic fever, 1284
in systemic lupus erythematosus, 1081–1082
Abdominal skin reflex, 428t
Accessory nerve, tests of, 420t
Acetaminophen, aspirin interaction with, 733
in juvenile rheumatoid arthritis, 1266
*N*-Acetylhexosaminidase, 245
Achilles bursitis, corticosteroid in, 552
Achilles tendinitis, 471, 1748–1749
corticosteroid in, 552–553, 559
Achilles tendon, disorders of, 388
in rheumatoid arthritis, 936
tophi of, *1365*
Acid hydrolase, macrophage secretion of, 155–156
Acid maltase deficiency, adult, polymyositis vs., 1234
Acquired immune deficiency syndrome, 1332–1333, *1333*
in hemophilia, 1569
Acromegaly, *1588–1589*, 1588–1590, 1590t
osteoarthritis in, 1445
radiography in, 602–604, *603*
Acromioclavicular joint, arthritis in, 442
arthroplasty of, 1868
examination of, 373
injection into, 554
rehabilitation and reconstruction of, 1863
separation of, 1735, *1735*
Acromioplasty, in rotator cuff lesion, 1862–1863
Acropachy, thyroid, 1586, *1586*, 1598
ACTH test, for hypothalamic-pituitary-adrenal function, 824–825, 824t
ACTH therapy, glucocorticoids vs., 828
Actin, 287–288, *288*
fibronectin and, 232
Actinomycosis, 1534
in spine, 463
Action potential, mechanism of, 300–303, *303–304*
Acute phase protein, 653, 654t
Acute phase reactant, 653–664
clinical value of, 659–661
in rheumatic fever, 1286
mechanisms, teleology, and clinical usefulness of, 654
stimuli of, 653
Adductor reflex, 428t
Adenine, chemical structure of, *337*
Adenine phosphoribosyltransferase, 340–341
deficiency in, 1390, *1390*
Adenosine, chemical structure of, *338*
Adenosine deaminase deficiency, 1321–1322
Adenosine kinase, 341
Adenovirus, 1551
Adenylic acid, biosynthesis of, 340
Adhesive capsulitis, in shoulder, 445, 627, *628*
Adhesive radiculitis, 462
Adson test, 426
AE protein, 1473
AF protein, 1473
African histoplasmosis, 1535
Agammaglobulinemia, adult-acquired, 1327–1328
Swiss-type, 1320–1323
X-linked, 22, 1324–1326
Agarose well assay, 116
AIDS, 1332–1333, *1333*
in hemophilia, 1569
AL protein, 1471–1472
Albers-Schönberg's disease, 1673–1674, *1674*
Albright's hereditary osteodystrophy, 1584
Alcohol ingestion, in gout, 1388
Alcoholism, avascular necrosis in, 1692–1693
septic arthritis in, 1507
Aldamine crosslink, in collagen, *221*, 222
Aldol crosslink, in collagen, 222, *222*
in elastin, *222*, 229
Alkaline phosphatase, serum, in metabolic bone disease, 1646
Alkaptonuria, radiography in, 600
Alkylating agents, 838–841
Allele, 38
Allergic granulomatous angiitis, 1137, 1138, 1153–1155, 1309
Allergic vasculitis, 1138, 1149–1153, *1308*, 1308–1309
Allergy, aspirin, 735–736, 763
drug, in Sjögren's syndrome, 964
Allopurinol, 861–867
biological effects of, 862–864
clinical use of, *864*, 864–865, 865t
complications of, 865–866
drug interaction with, 864
in hyperuricemia, 1387–1388, 1387t
inhibition of drug metabolism by, 720
Allopurinol *(Continued)*
maintenance dose of, 865t
metabolic effects of, 863t
pharmacokinetics and metabolism of, 862, *862*
toxicity of, 866–867
Allotype, 40
Allysine, in collagen, 221, *221*
Alopecia, in systemic lupus erythematosus, 538, 1077, 1101
Alpha heavy-chain disease, 1342
Alphavirus, 1547–1548
Alveolitis, cryptogenic fibrosing, 1217
Alymphoplasia, thymic, 1320–1323
Alzheimer's dementia, amyloid deposits in, 1473
American Rheumatism Association Criteria, in rheumatoid arthritis, 916t
in systemic lupus erythematosus, 1072t
Amidophosphoribosyltransferase, inhibition of, 342, *342*
Amine, platelet interaction with, 175–176, *176*
Amino acid, in elastin, tropoelastin, and fibronectin, 228t
AMP deaminase deficiency, polymyositis vs., 1234
Amphotericin B, 1537, 1537t
Amyloid deposits, 1470–1473
characteristics of, 1470t
electron microscopy of, 1470–1471, *1470–1471*
glomerular, 1481, *1481*
in endocrine disease, 1473
light microscopy of, 1470
of light chain immunoglobulin origin, 1471–1472
of protein origin, 1472–1473
senile, 1473
Amyloidosis, 1469–1487
arthropathy in, 1478–1479, *1479*
biopsy in, 1481, *1481*
cardiomyopathy in, 1480
classification of, 1474–1475, 1475t
cutaneous, 542, 1478, *1478*
definition of, 1469
diagnosis of, 1481, *1481*
familial cardiopathic, 1477
familial nephropathic, 1477
familial neuropathic, 1476–1477
gastrointestinal tract in, 1480–1481
historical, 1469–1470
in ankylosing spondylitis, 998

Amyloidosis *(Continued)*
in multiple myeloma, 1338, 1476
lichen, 1478
nephropathy in, 1479–1480
ocular manifestations in, 531
pathogenesis of, 1473–1474, *1474*
pathophysiology of, 1477–1478
peripheral neuropathy in, 307, 1479
primary, 1475
radiography in, 604, *604*
respiratory tract in, 1480
secondary, 1475–1476
synovial biopsy in, 651
treatment of, 1482–1483
Anal reflex, 428t
Anaphylactoid purpura, in children, *1307–1308*, 1307–1309
Anemia, hemolytic, aspirin in, 741–742
in Felty's syndrome, 952
in rheumatic fever, 1286
in rheumatoid arthritis, 354–355
in systemic lupus erythematosus, 1090, 1107
normocytic hypochromic, in rheumatoid arthritis, 940
Anesthesia, in arthroscopy, 642, *642*
local, corticosteroid with, 549, 553–554
in shoulder pain, 439
Angiitis, allergic granulomatous, 1137, 1138, 1153–1155
in children, 1309
hypersensitivity, 1137
Angiogenesis, from lymphocytes, 204
from macrophages, 204
inhibition of, 207–208
cartilage-derived, 207–208
experimental detection of, 207, *208*
heparin and cortisone in, 208, *209*
protamine in, 208
mast cells in, 201
study methods for, 198–199
chick embryo–chorioallantoic membrane as, 199
cloned capillary endothelial cells as, 199
corneal micropocket as, 198, *198*
sustained-release polymer implant as, *198*, 198–199
Angiosarcoma, in synovium, 1713, *1714*
Angiotensin-converting enzyme, in sarcoidosis, 1489–1490
Ankle, arthroscopy of, 645
corticosteroid in, *554*, 554–555
diabetes mellitus in, 1581, *1581–1582*
examination of, 386–390
medial-lateral stability in, 318, *319*
muscles in, 389
range of motion in, 389
reconstructive surgery for, 1896–1899, *1897–1898*
arthrodesis in, 1898–1899
total replacement in, 1899
Reiter's syndrome in, radiography in, 583–584, *584*
rheumatoid arthritis in, 936–938, *937*
radiography in, 575
septic arthritis in, *1514*
sprain of, 1749–1751, *1750–1751*
synovectomy of, 1797–1798
tenosynovitis in, 389–390

Ankle *(Continued)*
total prosthesis for, 1965–1968, *1968–1969*
Ankle jerk, 428t
Ankylosing hyperostosis, 487
Ankylosing spondylitis, 993–1007
acute phase response in, 660–661
articular features of, 997–998, 997t
clinical features of, 997–999, 997t
diagnostic criteria in, 994, 995t
epidemiology in, 995–996, 996t
etiology of, 1003–1004
extra-articular features of, 998–999
historic, 993
immune complexes in, 688
in cervical spine, surgical management of, 1935–1937, *1936–1937*
in hip, radiography in, 580, *581*
total replacement in, 1925
in inflammatory bowel disease, 1034–1035, *1035*
in women, 1002–1003, 1004t
juvenile, juvenile rheumatoid arthritis vs., 1263
radiography in, 578
laboratory abnormalities in, 1002
management of, 1004
nonsteroidal anti-inflammatory drugs in, 761
ocular manifestations in, 521, 998
pathology in, 996–997
physical examination in, 999, 999t
preoperative evaluation in, 1789
prognosis in, 1004
radiography in, 578–581, *579–581*, 999–1002, 999t, *1000–1003*
Reiter's syndrome vs, 1017, 1018t
rheumatoid arthritis vs., 922, 993t–994t
Annulus fibrosus, embryonic development of, 257, *257*
Anserine bursitis, 551, 552, 558–559, 1745–1746
Antalgic gait, 381
Anti-C3 solid phase binding assay, 685
Anti-DNA antibody, 696–698, 696t–697t
in systemic lupus erythematosus, 1055–1056
Anti-histone antibody, 700–701
Anti-IgA antibody, in selective IgA deficiency, 1264, 1264t
Anti-inflammatory drugs, in rheumatoid arthritis, 985–987
nonsteroidal. See *Nonsteroidal anti-inflammatory drugs.*
oxygen-derived free radicals and, 128
prostaglandin synthesis and, 78–79, 79t
Anti-insulin receptor antibody, in Sjögren's syndrome, 967
Anti-La/SSB/Ha antibody, 669–700, 669t
Anti-Ma antibody, 700
Anti-nRNP antibody, 698–699
Anti-PCNA antibody, 700
Anti-RNP antibody, antigen for, 1127–1128, *1128*
in mixed connective tissue disease, 1117–1119, 1118t
Anti-Ro/SSA antibody, 699–700, 699t
Anti-Sm antibody, 698–699
Antibody. See also individual types.
diversity of, 18

Antibody *(Continued)*
in polymyositis and dermatomyositis, *702*, 702–703
in progressive systemic sclerosis, 701–702
in rheumatoid arthritis, 703
in scleroderma, 1186–1187
in Sjögren's syndrome, 701
in systemic lupus erythematosus, 1052–1053, 1052t, 1055–1056, 1060
synovial production of, *896–897*, 896–898
Anticentromere antibody, in scleroderma, 1186–1187
Anticholinesterase, motor unit action on, 294
Anticoagulant, heparan sulfate as, 249–250
heparin as, 249
lupus, 1090–1091, 1091t
nonsteroidal anti-inflammatory drugs and, 764
$\beta_1$-Anticollagenase, 188
Antigen, cell wall, in experimental animal arthritis, 884–885
for anti-RNP antibody, 1127–1128, *1128*
$Jo_1$, 703
La/SSB/Ha, 699–700
Ma, 700
nRNP, 698–699
PCNA, 700
RNA-protein, 698
Ro/SSA, 699–700, 699t
Sm, 698–699
Antigen-antibody reaction, identification of, 694–696, *695*
Antihyperuricemic drugs, 857–871, 1385–1388. See also individual drugs.
Antilymphocyte antibody, 847–848
in systemic lupus erythematosus, 1052–1053, 1052t
Antilymphocyte serum (ALS), 847–848
Antimalarials, 774–788
anti-inflammatory actions of, 777
definition and structure of, *775*, 775–776
guidelines for use of, 785–786, 785t
historical, 774–775
immunologic actions of, 777–778
in juvenile rheumatoid arthritis, 1266–1267
in lupus erythematosus, 778–780, 1110
in psoriatic arthritis, 782
in rheumatoid arthritis, 780–782, 781t, 987–988
pharmacokinetics of, 776
side effects of, 782–785, 783t, *784*
therapeutic actions of, 776–778
therapeutic effectiveness of, 778–782
Antinuclear antibody, 690–707
classification of, 690–691, 691t
detection of, *691–693*, 691–694
immunofluorescent test for, *691*, 691–694
in juvenile rheumatoid arthritis, 1257
in scleroderma, 1186–1187
in Sjögren's syndrome, 966
in systemic lupus erythematosus, 691–693, 693t
in various conditions, 694, 694t
molecular specificities of, 703–704
patterns of, *692–693*, 693–694, 693t
Aortic aneurysm, in polychondritis, 1460, *1461*
Aortic arch, in Takayasu's arteritis, *1160*

Aortic valve, in rheumatic heart disease, 1281
Apatite crystal, electron microscopy of, 649, *650*
  osteoarthritis and, 1443–1444
Apheresis, therapeutic, 845–846
Aphthous stomatitis, in Behçet's disease, 1174
Apley maneuver, 385–386
Apophyseal joint, osteoarthritis in, radiography in, 591
Apprehension test, of patella, 385
Arachidonate derivatives, platelet interaction with, 176
Arachidonate metabolism, in platelets, 173
Arachnodactyly, congenital contractual, 1627
  in Marfan's syndrome, 1625
Arrhythmia, in rheumatic heart disease, 1283
  in scleroderma, 1186
Arterial thrombosis, in systemic lupus erythematosus, 1081
Arteriography, in polyarteritis, 1146, *1146*
Arteritis, giant cell, 1139, 1166–1173
    acute phase response in, 660
    clinical features of, 1168–1170, 1168t–1169t, *1169–1170*
    definition of, 1166
    diagnosis in, 1171–1172
    epidemiology in, 1166–1167
    etiology of, 1167
    in children, 1310–1311
    laboratory studies in, 1171
    ocular manifestations in, 524, *525–526*
    pathogenesis of, 1167
    pathology in, 1167–1168, *1167–1168*
    polymyalgia rheumatica and, 1170–1171
    treatment in, 1172
  in Behçet's disease, 1175
  necrotizing, 534, *534*
  rheumatic, 1137
  Takayasu's, 1139, 1159–1161, *1160*
    in children, 1310–1311
  temporal, 524, 1137
    in children, 1310–1311
Artery, epiphyseal, 282, *283*
  metaphyseal, 282, *283*
Arthralgia, in systemic lupus erythematosus, 1100
Arthritis. See also individual types, e.g., *Rheumatoid arthritis.*
  collagen-induced, 227
  crystal-induced, 1582. See also *Crystal-induced arthritis.*
  gouty, 1360–1361, 1378–1385. See also *Gout, arthritis in.*
  in hemochromatosis, 1497, *1497–1498*
  in Lyme disease, 1558, *1559*
  in mixed connective tissue disease, 1122, *1122–1123*
  in polyarteritis, 1144
  in polychondritis, 1460
  in Reiter's syndrome, 1011, *1011*
  in rheumatic fever, 1281, 1282, 1286
  in sarcoidosis, 1490–1491
  in scleroderma, 1193
  in systemic lupus erythematosus, 1071, 1100
Arthritis *(Continued)*
  meningococcal, 1519
  monoarticular, 391–400. See also *Monoarticular arthritis.*
  *N. meningitidis*, 1519
  polyarticular, 401–410. See also *Polyarticular arthritis.*
  post-traumatic, 1838
Arthritis mutilans, 582
  in mixed connective tissue disease, 1122, *1123*
  in psoriatic arthritis, 1026, *1027*
Arthritis robustus, 921
Arthrocentesis, complications of, 548
  in rheumatoid arthritis, 921
  technique for, 553, 562
Arthrochalasis multiplex congenita, *1631*, 1631–1632
Arthrodesis, of hip, 1918–1919
Arthrography, 570, 624–629, *625–628*
  in hip, 628
  in knee, *625–626*, 625–627
  in knee injury, 1742, *1742–1743*
  in rotator cuff tear, 437, *438*
  in shoulder, 627–628, *627–628*
  in shoulder pain, 436–438, *438*
  in total hip replacement, 1948–1954
    cement-bone or metal-cement contrast extension in, 1950–1952, *1953*, 1953t
    lymphatic opacification in, 1952–1954
    para-articular cavity or fistula filling in, 1952
    subtraction technique in, 1949, *1952*
  technical and clinical considerations in, 624–625
Arthroplasty. See also individual anatomic part.
  in elbow, 1839–1849
  in metacarpophalangeal joint, 1824–1827, *1825–1826*
  trapezium replacement, 1833
Arthroscopy, 640–648
  abrasion, 646
  accuracy of, 646
  anesthesia in, 642, *642*
  contraindications in, *641*, 641–642
  documentation in, 646–647
  future of, 647
  in shoulder, 439, 645
  indications for, 641
  instruments for, 642–643
  intra-articular, 645–646
  synovial biopsy with, 645, 649
  technique for, *643–644*, 643–645
Arthrosis, uncovertebral, radiography in, 591–592
Arthrotomography, in glenoid labrum tear, 438, *438*
Articular cartilage. See *Cartilage.*
AS protein, 1473
Aschoff nodule, in rheumatic heart disease, 1280
Ascites, in systemic lupus erythematosus, 1082
Ascorbic acid, deficiency in, 358
  granulocyte chemotaxis and, 118
Aseptic necrosis. See *Avascular necrosis.*
ASO titer, in rheumatic fever, 1285
Aspergillosis, 1534
Aspiration, of joints and soft tissues, 546–561
Aspirin, 725–752
  analgesia with, 728–729, *729*
  anti-inflammatory effects of, 729–730
  antipyresis with, 727–728, *728*
  clinical use of, 731–733, 732t
  drug interactions with, 733–734, 734t
  enteric-coated, 731
  in juvenile rheumatoid arthritis, 1265–1266
  in pregnancy, 735
  in rheumatoid arthritis, 985–986
  nonprescription and prescription, 732t
  overdose or accidental intoxication with, 744–745
  side effects of, 735–745
    allergy as, 735–736, 763
    gastrointestinal, 736–740
      microbleeding as, 737–738
      symptoms of, 736–737
      ulcer, gastritis, gastrointestinal bleeding as, 738–740
    hematologic and immunologic, 741–742
    hepatic, 742–743
    in genetic hemolytic anemia, 741–742
    platelet and coagulation, 740–741
    pulmonary and cardiovascular, 742
    renal, 743–744
    tinnitus and hearing loss as, 736
    white cell effects of, 741
  structure, absorption, metabolism of, *725*, 725–727
Ataxia-telangiectasia, *1329*, 1329–1330
Atherosclerosis, gout and, 1366
Atlantoaxial subluxation, 380
  clinical signs of, 1932–1934, *1935*
  in juvenile rheumatoid arthritis, 1259, *1260*
  in rheumatoid arthritis, 927–930, *929*
  incidence and pathology in, 1930, *1930*
  neurologic complications of, 1932
  treatment of, 1935, *1936*
Atrial myxoma, 923
Auranofin, characteristics of, 794
  dosage schedules for, 795
  gold sodium thiomalate vs., toxicity of, 804t
  in rheumatoid arthritis, 988
  mechanisms of action of, 800, 800t
Aurothioglucose, gold sodium thiomalate vs., 794
  structural formula of, *793*
Autoantibody, in Sjögren's syndrome,
    non-organ-specific, 965–967, *966*, 966t
    organ-specific, 967–968
  in systemic lupus erythematosus, 1042, 1043t
Autoimmunity,
  in systemic lupus erythematosus, 1047–1049
  in viral infection, 1542
  penicillamine causing, 812
Autonomic nerve, origin of, 295
Avascular necrosis, 1689–1710
  bone marrow pressure in, 1701, *1701–1702*, 1702t–1703t
  clinical symptoms and signs in, 1696–1698
  core biopsy in, 1703

Avascular necrosis *(Continued)*
diagnosis of, 1698–1703
diseases associated with, 1689–1693, 1690t
epidemiology in, 1689
in femoral head, in hyperuricemia, 491
in inflammatory bowel disease, 1034
in osteoarthritis, 1445
in shoulder, 1860
in sickle cell disease, 1577
intraosseous venography in, 1701–1703, *1703*, 1704t
osteoarthritis in, 1445
pathogenesis of, 1693–1695, *1694–1695*
pathology in, 1695–1696, *1696–1697*
radiography in, 1698–1700, *1699–1700*
radionuclide scanning technique in, 1700–1701
scintigraphy in, 619–621, *620–621*
tomography in, 1700
treatment of, 1704–1708
bone grafting in, 1705
core decompression in, *1705*, 1705–1706
endoprosthetic arthropathy in, 1706–1707
joint replacement in, 1707
non–weight bearing in, 1704–1705
osteotomy in, 1705
Axillary nerve, tests of, 420t
Axolemma, 300–303
Axon, degeneration of, 715
regeneration of, 298–299, *301*
transport mechanisms in, 297–298, *298*
fast, 298, *298*
slow, 298
wallerian degeneration of, 298, *299*
Axonopathy, central distal, *300*
central-peripheral distal, 298, *300*
Axonotmesis, 311
Axoplasm, ultrastructure of, 297
Azathioprine, 841–842, 842t
in rheumatoid arthritis, 988–989
pharmacologic properties of, 852t

B cell. See *Lymphocyte, B.*
*B. dermatitidis*, 1536
Back. See also *Spine.*
low, pain in. See *Low back pain.*
Bacterial arthritis. See *Septic arthritis.*
Baker's cyst, 383, 1763, *1766*
in juvenile rheumatoid arthritis, 1249, *1250*
ultrasound in, *629*, 629–630
Balanitis, circinate, in Reiter's syndrome, 1013–1014, 1013t, *1014*
Band keratopathy, in juvenile rheumatoid arthritis, *520*, 520–521, 1254
Basal energy expenditure, 356–357
Basement membrane, collagen, 223–224, *224*
epidermal, *224*
Basophil, chemical mediators of, generation and release of, 129–130, 130t
Bateman total hip prosthesis, *1940*

Becker muscular dystrophy, polymyositis vs., 1234
Behçet's disease, 1174–1178
pannicular involvement in, 1181
rheumatoid arthritis vs., 922
scarring in, 409
Benoxaprofen, 768, *768*
leukocyte migration and, 755
Benzbromarone, 861, *861*
Benziodarone, 861, *861*
Biceps, lesions of, 1860
Biceps femoris reflex, 428t
Biceps jerk, 428t
Biceps long head, function of, 1856
rupture of, 442
Biceps tendon, subluxation of, 442
tendinitis of, 442, 557, *557*
Biceps tenosynovitis, 1863
Biliary cirrhosis, 1218
Biomechanics, 317–336
compressive stress resistance in, 326–328, *327–328*
instantaneous centers of rotation in, 317, *318*
joint control in, 322–324, *323–324*
joint forces in, *320–322*, 321–322
joint motion in, 320–321, *320–321*
joint stability in, 317–320
bone in, 317, *318*
ligament in, 317–318, *318*
muscle-tendon complex in, 318
joint structure in, 324–326, *325–326*
contact area maximization in, 326, *326*
frictional force minimization in, 324–326, *325*
of degenerative disease of disc, 460
of elbow, 1838–1839, 1839t
of hip, 1919–1921, *1920*
of hip degeneration, 328–330, *329*
of knee arthritis, 330–331
of low back pain, 331–332
rotational and translational motion in, 317, *318*
Biopsy, bone, 284
in metabolic bone disease, 1648–1649, *1648–1649*
core, in avascular necrosis, 1703
in amyloidosis, 1481, *1481*
needle punch, of forearm nodule, 557–558, *558*
nerve, 715
synovial. See *Synovial biopsy.*
Birth control pills, rheumatic manifestations in, 1590–1591
Blastomycosis, 1536–1537
in spine, 463
Bleomycin, collagen synthesis and, 1215
Blood supply, in cervical spine and neck, 421
of bone, 282–283, *282–283*
Bone, 271–287
as organ, 280–281, *281*
biopsy of, 284, 1648–1649, *1648–1649*
blood supply of, 282–283, *282–283*
cells of, 271–275
osteoblast as, *272*, 272–273
osteoclast as, 273–275, *274*
osteocyte as, 273, *273*
cement line in, *273*, 276

Bone *(Continued)*
collagen in, 223, 276
composition of, 276–278, 278t
growth of, 280–281, *281*
hydroxyapatite in, 278
in joint stability, 317, *318*
in rheumatoid arthritis, 938
lamellar, 275, *275*
circumferential, 275, *277*
haversian systems or osteons in, 275, *276*
interstitial, 276, *278*
mineralization of, 278–280
molecular degradation of, 189
nonlamellar, 275
organization of, 275–276, *275–279*
periosteum of, 282
resorption of, 276, *277*
biopsy in, 284
cortical thickness estimates in, 283–284
quantitative radiographic technique in, 283
Singh index of trabecular patterns in, 284, *284*
techniques for quantitation of, 284
response to bending force of, 276
reversal line in, 276
sarcoidosis of, 1491
subchondral, compressive loads and, 327–328, *328*
trabeculae in, 276, *279*
microfracture in osteoarthritis of, 1425
trabecular, in sickle cell disease, 1573–1574, *1574*
Bone cyst, in rheumatoid arthritis, 571–572, *572*
Bone graft, in avascular necrosis, 1705
Bone infarction, in sickle cell disease, 1576–1577
scintigraphy in, 619–621, *620–621*
Bone marrow, in Felty's syndrome, 952
in gold therapy, 803
in sickle cell disease, 1573–1574, *1574*
Bone marrow pressure, in avascular necrosis, 1693, 1701, *1701–1702*, 1702t–1703t
Bone on bone sign, *1691*
Bone scan, in avascular necrosis, 1700–1701
in hypertrophic osteoarthropathy, 1598, *1599–1600*
in total hip replacement, 1954
Bone tumor, juxta-articular, synovium and, 1605
Bouchard's node, 377, 1436, *1437*
Boutonnière deformity, 377, *572*, 934, *935*, 1827
Boutonnière orthosis, 1778, *1779*
Bowel, in scleroderma, 1192
inflammatory disease of. See *Inflammatory bowel disease.*
small, amyloidosis of, 1481
Bowel bypass syndrome, 1038
Bowstring test, 380
Braces, for shoulder, 1861
Brachial neuritis, 445
Brachial plexus, *419*
tests of, 420t
Brachydactyly, in juvenile rheumatoid arthritis, 1254, *1255*
Bradykinin, formation of, 95, *96*

Brain, organic syndrome of, in systemic lupus erythematosus, 1085
Bronchial lesion, in polyarticular arthritis, 408
Bronchus, laryngotracheal, in polychondritis, 1460
Brucellosis, in spine, 463
Bruton's syndrome, 22
Bulbocavernosus reflex, 428t
Bulge sign, 384, *384*, 936
Bullae, 534
Bunnel's sign, in synovitis, 403
Bursa, function of, 258–259
  of foot, 387
  of knee, 383, *383*
Bursitis, Achilles, corticosteroid in, 552
  anserine, 1745–1746
    corticosteroids in, 551, 552, 558–559
  calcaneal, corticosteroid in, 552–553, 559
  iliopectineal, corticosteroid in, 552, 559
  iliopsoas, 382
  ischiogluteal, corticosteroid in, 552, 559
  olecranon, 1739–1740
    corticosteroid in, 551
  patellar, 384
  prepatellar, 1745
    corticosteroid in, 552
  septic, 1523–1524
  sub-Achilles, in rheumatoid arthritis, 937
  subacromial, corticosteroids in, 557, *557*
  trochanteric, 382, 1740–1741, *1740–1741*
    corticosteroid in, 551, 552, 558
Bursography, 570
Butterfly rash, in systemic lupus erythematosus, 573, *573*, 1073, 1100, 1294, *1294*

C-reactive protein, *657–658*, 657–659
  clinical significance of, 658–659
  clinical value of, 659
  elevation of, 659
  history, structure, and function of, *657*, 657–658
  in ankylosing spondylitis, 660–661
  in disease, 658
  in giant cell arteritis, 660
  in polymyalgia rheumatica, 660
  in progress in rheumatoid arthritis, 944
  in rheumatic fever, 661
  in rheumatoid arthritis, 660, 944
  in systemic lupus erythematosus, 661
  magnitude and time course of, 658, *658*
  methods for detection of, 658
*C. immitis*, 1535
*C. neoformans*, 1535
C1 inhibitor deficiency, 1353
C1q binding assay, 685
C1q deficiency, 1352
C1q solid phase binding assay, 684, *684*
C1r deficiency, 1352–1353
C1s deficiency, 1353
C2 deficiency, 1353–1354
C3 deficiency, 1354
C4 deficiency, 1353
C5 deficiency, 1354
C7 deficiency, 1354
C8 deficiency, 1354
Calcaneal bursitis, corticosteroid in, 552–553
Calcaneal valgus, 476
Calcaneal varus, 477
Calcific periarthritis, rheumatoid arthritis vs., 926
Calcific tendinitis, in rotator cuff, 440–441
  in supraspinatus, 440–441
Calcinosis, in dermatomyositis in children, 1301, *1301–1302*
Calcium hydroxyapatite crystal deposition disease, 598–599, *599*
Calcium nephrolithiasis, 496
  in gout, 1371t
Calcium pyrophosphate deposition disease, 1398–1413
  classification of, 1400t
  clinical features of, 1398–1406
  diagnosis of, 1402t, 1404–1406, *1405–1406*
  diseases associated with, 1403–1404
  etiology in, 1412–1413
  hereditary, 1402–1403
  in osteoarthritis, 1427–1428, 1443–1444
  management of, 1413
  pathogenesis in, 1406–1412
    crystal deposition sites in, 1410–1412, 1412t
    metabolic disturbances in, 1409–1412
    mineral deposits in, 1408–1409
    tissue injury in, 1406–1408, *1407–1408*
  PPI metabolism in, 1409–1412
  precipitation of acute attacks in, 1404
  prevalence and clinical presentation in, 1399–1404, 1401t
  radiological studies in, 597, *597–598*, 1405–1406, *1405–1406*
  rheumatoid arthritis vs., 923
  sporadic, 1400–1402
  synovianalysis in, 1404–1405, *1405*
  x-ray diffraction analysis in, 1399, *1399*
cAMP, colchicine and, 874
*Campylobacter* infection, reactive arthritis after, 1037
Candidiasis, 1533–1534
  chronic mucocutaneous, 1331–1332
Capillary, effect of collagenous components on growth of, 199–201
  embryology of, 197
  endosteal, 282, *282*
  nonproliferating, glycosaminoglycans in, 201
  periosteal, 282, *282*
  regression of, 204–207, *205–206*
  sequential steps in growth of, 199, *200–203*
  synovial, 259, *259*
Capillary endothelial cell, cloning technique for, in angiogenesis study, 199
  migration of, heparin in, 203, *203*
Caplan's syndrome, 941
Capsulitis, adhesive, in shoulder, 445, 627, *628*
Carcinoid tumor, fibrosis in, 1219
Carcinoma, metastatic, avascular necrosis in, 1691
Carcinoma polyarthritis, 1605–1606, 1606t
Cardiac manifestations, in amyloidosis, 1480
  in ankylosing spondylitis, 998
Cardiac manifestations *(Continued)*
  in dermatomyositis-polymyositis, 1240
  in Lyme disease, 1558, *1559*
  in mixed connective tissue disease, 1122–1123
  in polyarteritis, *1143*, 1143–1145
  in polyarticular arthritis, 409
  in polychondritis, 1460, *1461*
  in Reiter's syndrome, 1015
  in rheumatic fever, 1281–1283, 1287
  in rheumatoid arthritis, 941–942
  in scleroderma, 1186, 1193–1194, 1200
  in systemic lupus erythematosus, 1087–1088, 1106–1107
Cardiomyopathy, amyloid familial, 1477
  in amyloidosis, 1480
  sarcoid, 1492
Cardiovascular system, aspirin effects on, 742
Carnitine deficiency, polymyositis vs., 1234
Carnitine palmityltransferase deficiency, polymyositis vs., 1234
Carpal joint, examination of, 374–376, *375*
Carpal tunnel syndrome, amyloid arthropathy and, 1479
  corticosteroid in, 551–552
  hypothyroidism in, 1587
Carpal-metacarpal ratio, in rheumatoid arthritis, 933, *933*
Carpometacarpal joint, corticosteroid injection in, 548
  osteoarthritis in, 1441, 1832
Cartilage. See also specific components, e.g., *Collagen.*
  aging of, 265, 1425–1426
  angiogenesis inhibition and, 207–208
  arthroscopy in, 646
  biochemical composition of, 1417–1419
  biomechanical consequences of macromolecular organization of, 1420–1421
  calcium pyrophosphate crystal deposition in, 1410–1412, 1412t
  cathepsin D in degradation of, 182–183, *183*
  collagen in, 223, 1418–1419
  compressive stress and, 326, *327*
  degeneration of, 362, 362t
  destruction of, in septic arthritis, 1510–1512
  during load, mechanical properties of, 264–265, *264–265*
  fibrillation of, 265, 1434–1435, *1436*
  flaking of, 1434
  function of, 259–260
  glycosaminoglycans and proteoglycans in, 1417–1418
  immunobiology of, 1464–1465
  in joint lubrication, 263–264, *264*
  iron stain in, 1495, *1496*
  lubrication of, boundary, 1424
    squeeze film, 1424
    under high load conditions, 1424
    under low load conditions, 1424
  lysozyme in, 1420
  matrix metabolism in, 1419–1421
  mineralization of, chondroitin sulfate in, 248
  molecular degradation of, 188–189
    collagen in, 188–189, *189*
    proteoglycan in, 188

Cartilage, molecular degradation of *(Continued)*
serine proteinase in, *185*
nutrition of, 263
organization of, 260–265
chondrocytes in, 261–263, *262–263*
collagen fibril diameters and, 260, 261t
glycoproteins in, 261
water and small solutes in, 261
zones and regions in, 260, *260*
osteoarthritic, 1421–1428
biomechanical changes in, 1423
collagen in, 1422
early matrix changes in, 1422–1423
glycosaminoglycan in, 1421–1422
osteophyte and bony proliferation in, 1423
prostaglandin in, 1421–1422
proteinase and proteinase inhibitors in, 190–191
proteoglycan in, 242, *242*
repair of, 265
Catabolin, 192, 267
Cataract, in juvenile rheumatoid arthritis, 521
Cathepsin B, 183–184
Cathepsin D, cartilage degradation by, 182–183, *183*
cartilage synthesis of, 190
in proteoglycan degradation, 188
Cathepsin G, 185
Cathepsin L, 183–184
Cauda equina syndrome, 461
Cell membrane antibody, in systemic lupus erythematosus, 1060
Cell wall antigen, in experimental animal arthritis, 884–885
Cellular immunity, 22, 23t
in dermatomyositis-polymyositis, 1240
in juvenile rheumatoid arthritis, 1258
in polychondritis, 1465
in systemic lupus erythematosus, 1050–1051
tests for, 1318–1319, 1318t
Central nervous system manifestations, in mixed connective tissue disease, 1124, 1126t
in polyarteritis, 1143
in systemic lupus erythematosus, 1060–1062, 1083–1087, 1104–1106
Cerebrospinal fluid, in systemic lupus erythematosus, 1086
Cervical collar, 434
CH50, 1351
Charcot arthropathy, 594–595, *595*
in diabetes mellitus, 1581, *1581–1582*
in feet, 471
in osteoarthritis, 1425, 1444, 1444t, *1445*
Chemonucleolysis, 461
Chemotactic factor, urate crystal inflammatory response and, 1381–1382
Chick embryo-chorioallantoic membrane technique, for angiogenesis study, 199
Chikungunya virus, 1547
Chlorambucil, 841
in Behçet's disease, 1176–1177
pharmacologic properties of, 852t
Chloroquine, chemical structure of, *775*
guidelines for use of, 785–786, 785t
in systemic lupus erythematosus, 1110
pharmacokinetics of, 776
Chloroquine *(Continued)*
side effects of, 782–785, 783t, *784*
visual effects of, *784*, 784–785
Cholangitis, sclerosing, 1218
Cholesterol, in macrophage membrane, 147
Chondrification, embryonic, 255, *256*
Chondrocalcinosis, 1398–1399, 1411
calcium pyrophosphate crystal deposition in, 1411
in premature osteoarthritis, 1414
Chondrocyte, 261–263, *262–263*
in vitro characteristics of, 263, *263*
necrosis and degeneration of, 262, *262*
Chondroitin sulfate, biosynthesis of, 243–244, *244*
cartilage mineralization and, 248
composition and structure of, 238, 238t, *239*
degradation of, 1420
in articular cartilage, 1417–1418
Chondroitin sulfate-keratan sulfate proteoglycan, *240–242*, 240–243
Chondromalacia patellae, 1440
Chorea, in rheumatic fever, 1281, 1289–1290
in systemic lupus erythematosus, 1084–1085
Chorea minor, in rheumatic fever, 1284
Chrysiasis, 802–803
ocular, in gold therapy, 804
Chrysotherapy. See *Gold compounds.*
Churg-Strauss angiitis, in children, 1309
Churg-Strauss vasculitis, 1137–1138, 1153–1155
Cimetidine, inhibition of drug metabolism by, 721
Cirrhosis, biliary, 1218
Claudication, intermittent, in giant cell arteritis, 1169–1170
*Clostridium perfringens*, in rheumatoid arthritis, 881
Clubbing, digital, 377
in hypertrophic osteoarthropathy, 1594–1596, *1596*
in inflammatory bowel disease, 1034
Coagulation. See also under *Factor.*
aspirin effects on, 740–741
glycosaminoglycans in, 249–250
lupus anticoagulant effects on, 1090–1091, 1091t
Coccidioidal arthritis, 1536, *1536*
Coccidioidomycosis, 1535–1536, *1536*
in spine, 463
Cogan's syndrome, in polyarteritis, 1145
Colchicine, 871–878
cAMP and, 874
in familial Mediterranean fever, 1482
in gouty arthritis, 1383
in sarcoid arthritis, 1491
mechanism of action of, 873–874
metabolism of, 875
structure-function relationships of, *872*, 872–873
toxicology of, 875–876
Colitis, ulcerative. See *Inflammatory bowel disease.*
Collagen, 211–228
biosynthesis of, *215*, 215–220, 1621–1623, *1622*
ascorbate in, 1214
Collagen, biosynthesis of *(Continued)*
cellular secretion in, 219, *219*
fibroblast, modulation of, 1214–1215, 1214t
genes in, 216, *217*, 1621–1622, *1622*
glycosylation in, 218–219
in vitro, 1214
protocollagen hydroxylases in, 216–218, *218*
ribosomal synthesis of pro-alpha chains on polyribosomes in, 215–216
catabolism of, 1420
cell adhesion to, 232, *232*
compositional characteristics of, 212, 212t
crosslinking in, 220–222, *221–222*
aldamine, 221, *221*
aldol, 222, *222*
hydroxypyridinoline, *221*, 222
D-penicillamine and, 225–226, *226*
fibril diameters of, 260, 261t
fibrillogenesis in, 219–220
fibronectin and, 231–232
immunochemistry of, 225
in articular cartilage, 223, 1418–1419
in basement membrane, 223–224, *224*
in bone, 223, 276
in capillary proliferation, 199–201
in dermatosparaxis, 226
in fibrosis, 1213–1214, 1214t
in inflammation, 227
in intervertebral disc, 459
in lathyrism, 225–226, *226*
in osteoarthritic cartilage, 1422
in soft tissue, 223
in vitamin D-deficient rickets, 227
in wound healing, 226
intracellular degradation of, 220
molecular degradation of, 188–189, *189*
primary structure of, 185, *186*
reticulin and, 224–225
structure of, 211–215
amino acid, 212, *213*
cross-striation periodicity in, *213*, 214–215, *215*
minor helix in, *213*, 213–214
molecules in, 211
triple helical, *213*, 214
synthesis of, 1419–1420
tissue specific differences in, 223–225, 1621
turnover of, 220
types of, 212–213, 214t, 1621
Collagen vascular disease, synovial biopsy in, 650
Collagen-induced arthritis, 227
Collagenase, 185–187, *186*
agents inhibiting production of, 192
agents stimulating production of, 192
in fibrosis, 1215–1216
in fibrous cartilage collagen degradation, 189
inhibition of, angiogenesis and, 207
latent, 187, 192
rheumatoid synovium, 191
Collateral ligament, medial, in knee stability, 318, *318*
Colon, in scleroderma, 1192
Common variable immunodeficiency, 1327–1328

Complement, activation of, hepatitis B viral infection, 1544
synovial fluid, 893
urate crystal and, 1381
deficiency, C1 inhibitor, 1353
C1q, 1352
C1r, 1352–1353
C1s, 1353
C2, 1353–1354
C3, 1354
C4, 1353
C5, 1354
C7, 1354
C8, 1354
detection of, 1352
rheumatic disease and, 1354–1355, 1354t
systemic lupus erythematosus and, 1046
immune complex activation of, 682
immunochemical assays for, 1351–1352
in Sjögren's syndrome, 968
measurement of, 1351–1352
total hemolytic, 1351
Compressive erosion, in rheumatoid arthritis, 571, *572*
Computed tomography. See *Tomography, computed.*
Condylar joint, 371
Congestive heart failure, in rheumatic heart disease, 1283
Conglutinin solid phase binding assay, *684*, 684–685
Congo red stain, in amyloidosis, 1470, 1470t
Conjunctivitis, in Reiter's syndrome, 1011–1013
in systemic lupus erythematosus, 523
Connective tissue disease, in pediatric rheumatology, 1263t
in polychondritis, 1460, 1461t
in selective IgA deficiency, 1263, 1263t
malignancy and, 1609–1614, 1610t
mixed. See *Mixed connective tissue disease.*
ocular manifestations in, 523
overlap syndromes in, 1116
radiography in, 584–587, *585–587*
rheumatoid arthritis vs, 923
Connective tissue–activating peptides, 1215
Contracture, diagnosis of, 413
Copper, in rheumatoid arthritis, 355
Copper deficiency, elastin in, 230
Corneal micropocket technique, for angiogenesis study, 198, *198*
Coronary artery disease, in systemic lupus erythematosus, 1087–1088
Corticosteroid, articular, indications for, 550, 550t
efficacy of, 548–549
in dermatomyositis, in children, 1302
in giant cell arteritis, 1172
in gouty arthritis, 1384
in hypersensitivity vasculitis, 1151
in juvenile rheumatoid arthritis, 1267–1268
in mixed connective tissue disease, 1132, 1133t
in osteoarthritis, 1454
in polyarteritis, 1147
in polychondritis, 1466
in rheumatic fever, 1289
Corticosteroid *(Continued)*
in rheumatoid arthritis, 986–987
in systemic lupus erythematosus, 1108–1110, 1297
indications for, 550–553
injection amount of, 549, 550t
intra-articular, contraindications in, 553, 553t
efficacy of, 548
intrasynovial, mechanism of action of, 546–547
local anesthetics with, 549, 553–554
non-articular, efficacy of, 548–549
indications for, 550–553, 551t
osteoarthritis due to, 1444–1445
postinjection flare with, 547
precautions with, 548
sequelae of, 547–548, 547t
septic arthritis caused by, 1508, 1509, *1511*
types of preparations of, 549, 549t
withdrawal of, panniculitis in, 1182
Cortisol, 816, *816*
Cortisone, chemical structure of, *816*
heparin and, in angiogenesis inhibition, 208, *209*
Costovertebral osteoarthritis, radiography in, 592
Cotton wool spots, in systemic lupus erythematosus, 522, *522–523*
Cotylic joint, 370–371
Coumarin, aspirin interaction with, 733–734
Counterimmunoelectrophoresis, in antigen-antibody reaction, 695, *695*
in mixed connective tissue disease, 1117, *1119*
in septic arthritis, 1514
Coup de sabre, 541
Coxsackievirus, 1550
Cranial arteritis, 524. See also *Arteritis, giant cell.*
Cranial nerves, in systemic lupus erythematosus, 1084
Creatine, urinary, 708
Creatinine-kinase, in dermatomyositis-polymyositis, 1229t
Cremasteric reflex, 428t
Crepitation, in patient examination, 371
CREST syndrome, 1183, 1195
Cricoarytenoid joint, examination of, 372
rheumatoid arthritis of, 930
Crohn's disease. See *Inflammatory bowel disease.*
Crossed straight leg test, 380, 452
Cruciate ligament, arthroscopy of, 646
Cryocrit method, 1343–1344, *1344*
Cryofibrinogen, malignancy and, 1607
Cryoglobulin, classification of, 1344, 1345t
factors affecting precipitation of, 1347–1348
mixed, 1344–1345
disease states associated with, 1345, 1346t
subacute bacterial endocarditis and, 1346
systemic lupus erythematosus and, 1057, 1345–1346
with monoclonal rheumatoid factor component, 1345
Cryoglobulin, mixed *(Continued)*
with polyclonal rheumatoid factor component, 1345
unmixed, 1344, 1347
Cryoglobulinemia, 1343–1349
analysis of, 1343–1344
definition and detection of, 1343
in malignancy, 1607
in peripheral neuropathy, 308–309
in Sjögren's syndrome, 965
mixed, 1152–1153
echinococcosis and, 1347
essential, 1346
glomerulonephritis and, 1346–1347
hepatitis B virus and, 1544
Lyme disease and, 1347
pathogenesis of symptomatology in, *1348*, 1348–1349
treatment of, 1349
Cryoprotein, malignancy and, 1607
Cryptococcosis, 1535, *1535*
in spine, 463
Crystal-induced arthritis, in hyperparathyroidism, 1582
monoarticular, 396–397
radiography in, 595–600, *596–599*
synovial biopsy in, 651
Cubital tunnel syndrome, corticosteroid in, 551
Cushing's syndrome, 1587–1588
alternate day glucocorticoid therapy in, 826
iatrogenic, 822–823, 823t
Cutaneous manifestations, 533–545
aids for examination of, 533
classification of, 533–534
in allopurinol use, 866
in amyloidosis, 1478, *1478*
in Behçet's disease, 1175
in Churg-Strauss vasculitis, 1154
in cryoglobulinemia, *1348*, 1348–1349
in dermatomyositis, 1235, *1235*, 1298, *1298*
in dermatomyositis-polymyositis, 540, *540*
in diabetes mellitus, 1581
in gonococcal arthritis, 1517, *1517*
in Graves' disease, 1586
in hypersensitivity vasculitis, 1150, *1150*
in hypocomplementemic vasculitis, 1152, *1152*
in infiltrative systemic disease, 542, *542*
in juvenile rheumatoid arthritis, 541, 1251–1252, *1252*, 1255
in Lyme disease, 1557, *1558*, 1558t
in mixed connective tissue disease, 539, *1121*, 1121–1122, 1122t
in necrotizing vasculitis, *539*, 539–540
in polyarteritis, 1144, *1144–1145*
in polyarticular arthritis, 409
in polychondritis, 1460
in psoriatic arthritis, 1022–1023, *1023*
in rheumatic fever, 541–542
in rheumatoid arthritis, 534–535, *534–535*
in sarcoidosis, 1488, *1489*
in Schönlein-Henoch purpura, 1151, *1151*
in scleroderma, 541, *541*, *1184–1185*, 1190–1191, 1199
in Sjögren's syndrome, 535, 963–964

Cutaneous manifestations *(Continued)*
in spondyloarthropathy, 535–537, *536–537*
in systemic lupus erythematosus, *537–538*, 537–539, 573, *573*, 1059–1060, 1073–1077, *1074–1076*, 1100, 1294, *1294*
in Wegener's granulomatosis, 1156, *1157*
interpretation of, 533–534
penicillamine causing, 812
Cutaneous necrotizing venulitis, 535, *535*
Cutaneous polyarteritis, in children, 1309
Cutaneous vasculitis, malignancy and, *1607*
Cyclophosphamide, 839–841, 840t
in polyarteritis, 1147
in rheumatoid arthritis, 989
in systemic lupus erythematosus, 1110–1111
in Wegener's granulomatosis, 1157–1158
pharmacologic properties of, 852t
Cyclosporin A, 850–851
in rheumatoid arthritis, 989
pharmacologic properties of, 853t
Cyst, Baker's, 383, 1763, *1766*. See also *Baker's cyst*.
bone, in rheumatoid arthritis, 571–572, *572*
mucous, 1832, *1832*
popliteal, 383, 936, 936t, 1763, *1766*
synovial, 1249, *1250*
α-Cysteine proteinase inhibitor, 187
Cytapheresis, 845
Cytoid bodies, in systemic lupus erythematosus, 522
Cytomegalovirus, 1552
Cytotoxic agents, 836–845. See also individual agents.
alkylating, 838–841
considerations in use of, 843–845, *844*
folic acid antagonists, 842–843
in neoplastic vs non-neoplastic disease, 836–837
mechanisms of action of, 836t, 838t
purine analogues, 841–842
therapeutic goals for, 837–838
white blood cell count and, 844, *844*

Dactylitis, tuberculous, 1528, *1528*
Dapsone, 851
in polychondritis, 1466
pharmacologic properties of, 853t
Dawbarn's sign, 439
DC antigen, 57
de Quervain's disease, corticosteroids in, 551, 552, 558
de Quervain's tenosynovitis, 935
in radial styloid process, 376
Decompression sickness, avascular necrosis in, 1690
Dee hinge prosthesis, 1843, *1843*
Dee semi-constrained prosthesis, 1846, *1846*
Deformity, in patient examination, 371
Degenerative disc disease, 458–462, 458t, *459–461*. See also *Disc, degenerative disease of*.
Degenerative joint disease. See *Osteoarthritis*.
Dehydrolysinonorleucine, in elastin, *221*, 229
Dehydromerodesmosine crosslink, in elastin, 229, *229*
Deltoid, anterior, function of, 1855–1856
Dendritic cell, 49
2′-Deoxyadenosine, chemical structure of, *338*
Deoxycytidine kinase, 341
Deoxynucleoside kinase, 341
5′-Deoxynucleoside monophosphate, chemical structure of, *338*
Depression, in systemic lupus erythematosus, 1085–1086
Dercum's disease, corticosteroid in, 551, 552
Dermatan sulfate, 238t, 239, *239*
in articular cartilage, 1418
Dermatitis, gold, 802
Dermatological manifestations. See *Cutaneous manifestations*.
Dermatomyositis, antibody in, *702*, 702–703
in children, 1298–1302, *1298–1302*
ocular involvement in, 523
primary idiopathic adult, 1234–1235, *1235*
radiography in, 586, *587*
Dermatomyositis-polymyositis, classification of, 1225–1226, 1226t–1227t
cutaneous manifestations of, 540, *540*
electromyography in, 1230t
etiology of, 1240–1241
immunology in, 1240
vasculopathy in, 1241
virology in, 1240–1241
grading of muscle weakness in, 1228t
heart and lung in, 1240
incidence of, 1226–1227
of childhood, 1236, *1237–1238*
overlap group in, 1236–1237
physical signs at presentation in, 1229t
prognosis in, 1243
serum creatinine kinase levels in, 1229t
symptoms at presentation in, 1227t
treatment in, 1241–1243
with neoplasia, 1235–1236
Dermatosis, acute febrile neutrophilic, malignancy and, 607
rheumatoid arthritis vs, 926
Dermatosparaxis, 226
Desmosine crosslink, in elastin, 229, *229*
Dexamethasone, chemical structure of, *816*
Diabetes mellitus, 1580–1581, *1581–1582*
calcium pyrophosphate deposition disease in, 1403
gout and, 1364–1365
neuroarthropathy in, 594–595, *595*
osteoarthritis in, 1445
osteoporosis in, 1662
rheumatologic disorders in, 1583t
septic arthritis in, 1507
Sjögren's syndrome in, 964
Diarthrodial joint, 254, *254*, *370*, 370–371
embryonic development of, 254–257, *255–257*
Diathermy, contraindications in, 1775
Diclofenac, 767
Diet. See also under *Nutritional*.
in osteoarthritis, 1450
Diflunisal, 727, 767–768
DiGeorge syndrome, 22, 1323–1324
Digital. See *Finger*.
Dimethyl sulfoxide, in amyloidosis, 1482
Diphtheroid organisms, in rheumatoid arthritis, 881
Disc, degenerative disease of, 458–462, 458t, *459–461*
adhesive radiculitis in, 462
biochemical changes in, 459–460
biomechanical factors in, 331, 460
clinical states and treatment in, 460–462
disc herniation in, 460–462, *461*
disc nutrition in, 460
immunity in, 460
lumbar nerve root entrapment in, 460–462
pathologic changes in, 459
spinal stenosis and lumbar root entrapment in, 458–459, 458t, *459*
spinal stenosis in, 462
without nerve involvement, 460
herniation of, classification of, *461*
computed tomography in, 454, *458*
lumbar nerve root entrapment in, 460–462
radiography in, 452–453
treatment of, 461–462
Disc space infection, 463
Discography, in low back pain, 453
Disodium etidronate, in Paget's disease of bone, 1682
osteomalacia in, 1669
Distraction technique, in pain, 503
Distraction test, in knee, 386
DNA, antibody to, 696–698, 696t–697t
DNA cloning, 1623, *1623*
Dorsal tenosynovitis, surgery for, 1819
with extensor tendon rupture, surgery for, 1819, *1820*
Double crush syndrome, of median nerve, 1758
of ulnar nerve, 1759
DR allotype, 45–46, 46t
DR antigen, 57
Drawer test, 385, 1744, *1744*
Dressing and undressing, 1776
Drug. See also individual class or type.
absorption of, 718–719
acidic and basic properties of, 718t
biotransformation of, 720–721
first order vs. zero order kinetics in, 720
interactions inhibiting, 720–721
liver microenzyme induction in, 721
concentration of, 717
dosage, first order elimination and steady-state level in, *722*, 722–723
individualizing, 717
interpretation of drug levels in, 723–724
pharmacokinetics and pharmacodynamics of, 717, *718*, *722*, 722–724
plasma drug levels in, 723
zero order absorption and steady-state level in, 723
zero order elimination and steady-state level in, 723
excretion of, renal function and, *721*, 721–722

Drug *(Continued)*
ionization and, 718, *718*
plasma protein binding of, 719, *720*
acidic drugs and, 719
drug plasma levels and, 719, *720*
Drug abusers, septic arthritis in, 1508
Drug allergy, in Sjögren's syndrome, 964
Duchenne muscular dystrophy, polymyositis vs, 1233
Duodenal ulcer, aspirin causing, 739
Duodenum, in scleroderma, 1191–1192, 1199
Dupuytren's contracture, 375, 1218–1219
Dysimmunoglobulinemia, peripheral neuropathy in, 307–310
Dysmenorrhea, nonsteroidal anti-inflammatory drugs in, 761
Dysphagia, in cervical spine disorders, 423
in systemic lupus erythematosus, 1082
Dysphagia test, 426
Dysproteinemia, monoclonal, 1338–1343
heavy-chain disease as, 1341–1342
idiopathic monoclonal gammopathy as, 1342–1343
multiple myeloma as, 1338–1340
Waldenström's macroglobulinemia as, 1340–1341
Dystrophia myotonica, polymyositis vs, 1234

E–64, for cathepsins B and L, 184
Ear, in cervical spine disorders, 423
in polychondritis, 1458, *1459*
ossicles of, in rheumatoid arthritis, 930
tophi of, *1362*
Eating, 1776
Eaton-Lambert syndrome, polymyositis vs, 1233
Eburnation, 1435, *1436*
Echinococcosis, cryoglobulinemia and, 1347
Echovirus, 1550
Ectopia lentis, in Marfan's syndrome, 1625
Education, patient, in juvenile rheumatoid arthritis, 1269
in rheumatoid arthritis, 981–982, 982t
in systemic lupus erythematosus, 1098
Ehlers-Danlos syndrome, 1628–1634, 1628t
arthrochalasis multiplex congenita form (EDS VII), *1631*, 1631–1632
benign hypermobility syndrome (EDS III), *1630*, 1630–1631
dental form (EDS VIII), 1631
dominantly inherited, 1628–1632
ecchymotic or arterial form (EDS IV), 1632
gravis and mitis forms (EDS I and II), 1628–1630, *1629–1630*
ocular form (EDS VI), 1632–1633, *1633*
recessively inherited, 1632–1633, *1633*
X form, 1633
X-linked, 1633–1634
Elastase, leukocyte, 184–185, *185*
in collagen degradation, 189
macrophage, 187
Elastin, 228–230
amino acid composition of, 228t
crosslinks in, 228–229, *229*

Elastin *(Continued)*
distribution and mechanical properties of, 228
heritable disorders of, 1638–1639
in copper deficiency, 230
structure of, 228
tropoelastin in, 229–230
Elbow, arthroplasty of, 1839–1849
cutis, 1842
fascial, 1841–1842
fat and sponge, 1842
hemiarthroplasty, 1842–1843
interpositional, 1841–1842
resection, 1839–1841
total joint replacement, 1843–1848, *1843–1850*
arthroscopy of, 645
biomechanics of, 1838–1839, 1839t
corticosteroid in, 551, 556, *556*
distraction-resection for, 1841
examination of, 374, *374*
hemiarthroplasty of, 1842–1843
acrylic, teflon, 1842
humeral replacement, 1842
metal, 1842–1843
ulnar replacement, 1842
in hemophilic arthropathy, 1565, *1566*
in osteoarthritis, 1838
in post-traumatic arthritis, 1838
in rheumatoid arthritis, 931, 1838
radiography in, 574
Little League, 1739
postoperative rehabilitation for, 1852–1853
reconstructive surgery of, 1838–1855
recreational injuries of, 1738–1740, *1739*
surgical technique for, 1849–1852, *1851–1853*
synovectomy of, *1803*, 1803–1804, 1839–1841, 1840t
tennis, 1738–1739, *1739*
corticosteroid in, 557, *558*
total joint replacement of, 1843–1848
fully constrained metal hinge in, 1843–1844, *1843–1844*
fully constrained metal to plastic hinge in, 1844
non-constrained metal to plastic hinge in, 1846–1848, *1847–1850*
semi-constrained metal to plastic hinge in, *1844–1845*, 1844–1846
total prosthesis for, 1965, *1966–1968*
Electromyography, *710–711*, 710–712
in dermatomyositis-polymyositis, 1230t
single fiber, 712
Ely test, 452
Endocarditis, in rheumatic heart disease, 1281
in rheumatoid arthritis, 941–942
in systemic lupus erythematosus, 1088
infective, 1139, 1141
mixed cryoglobulins and, 1346
rheumatoid arthritis vs, 922–923
Endocrine disease, 1579–1594. See also individual types.
in order of amyloid deposits, 1473
Endomysium, 287
Endopeptidase, 182. See also *Proteinase*.
Endoprosthetic arthropathy, in avascular necrosis, 1706–1707

Endosteal capillary, 282, *282*
Endothelial cells, in scleroderma, 1187–1189, *1189*
Endothelioma, synovial, 1719
Endotracheal intubation, in rheumatoid arthritis, 990
Energy requirements, nutritional, 356–357
Enteric infection, reactive arthritis after, 1036–1037
Enterocolitis, in gold therapy, 804
Enteropathic arthritis, 1031–1041
bacteriology in, 1031–1032
immunology in, 1032
ocular manifestations in, 526–529, *528*
radiography in, 584
Enterovirus, 1550
Enthesopathy, 362, 362t
radiography in, 590
scintigraphy in, *613*
Entrapment neuropathy, 1754–1768. See also *Neuropathy, entrapment*.
Enzyme. See also individual types.
degradative, in osteoarthrosis, 190
in rheumatoid arthritis, 190, *190*
serum, 708
Enzyme-linked immunoabsorbent assay (ELISA), 696
Eosinophil, special functions of, 135–137
Eosinophilia, in prognosis in rheumatoid arthritis, 944
in rheumatoid arthritis, 940
Eosinophilic fasciitis, 1195–1196
malignancy and, 1613–1614
Epicondylitis, humeral, 1738–1739, *1739*
lateral, corticosteroid in, 557, *558*
lateral and medial, 551
Epidermal nevus syndrome, osteomalacia in, 1669
Epidurography, in low back pain, 454
Epigastric reflex, 428t
Epimysium, 287
Epiphyseal artery, 282, *283*
Epiphyseal compression fracture, in juvenile arthritis, 577
Epiphyseal involvement, in juvenile rheumatoid arthritis, 1259, *1259–1260*
Epiphysiodesis, in juvenile rheumatoid arthritis, 1911–1912
Episclera, anatomy of, 513, *514*
Episcleritis, classification of, 515t
incidence of, 513–514
pathology of, 517, *518–519*
rheumatoid nodule in, *519*
signs and symptoms of, 514–517, *516–519*
treatment in, 517
Epistaxis, in rheumatic fever, 1284–1285
Epstein-Barr virus, 1552
in rheumatoid arthritis, 882–883, 888–889
rheumatoid factor and, 671, *671*
Erlenmeyer flask sign, *1691*
Erosion, 534
bony, in pigmented villonodular synovitis, 1720, *1720*
in rheumatoid arthritis, 571, *571–572*
*Erysipelothrix rhusiopathiae* arthritis, 883–884
Erythema chronicum migrans, 1557, *1558*, 1558t
Erythema induratum, 1181

Erythema infectiosum, 1552–1553
Erythema marginatum, in rheumatic fever, 1284
Erythema nodosum, 1178–1179, *1179*
Erythrocyte sedimentation rate, 654–657, *655*
clinical significance of, 656
in ankylosing spondylitis, 660–661
in giant cell arteritis, 660
in polymyalgia rheumatica, 660
in rheumatic fever, 661
in rheumatoid arthritis, 660
in systemic lupus erythematosus, 661, 1091
mechanisms governing, 655, *655*
methods for determination of, 656
plasma protein abnormalities and, 655
shape and size abnormalities and, drugs and, 655–656
Erythromycin, in Lyme disease, 1563
Esophagus, in amyloidosis of, 1480
in scleroderma, 1185, 1191, 1199
Estrogen deficiency, rheumatic manifestations in, 1591
Ethambutol, 1531t
Ewald total elbow prosthesis, *1967*
Examination of patient, 371–372, *372*
crepitation in, 371
deformity in, 371
instability in, 371
motion limitation in, 371
recording of, 371–372, *372*
swelling in, 371
Excitation-contraction coupling, 292
Exercise. See also *Physical therapy.*
for hand, 1818
for shoulder, 1861
in rheumatoid arthritis, 983–984
therapeutic, 1772–1773, 1772t
active vs passive, 1772
bone mineralization and, 1773
important muscle groups in, 1773
isometric, 1773
stretching as, 1773
Extensor tendon, rupture of, in dorsal tenosynovitis, 1819, *1820*
Extra Depth Shoe, 477, *478*
Eye symptoms. See *Ocular manifestations.*

Fabere test, 452
Facet block, in low back pain, 458
Facioscapulohumeral muscular dystrophy, polymyositis vs, 1234
Factor, coagulation, macrophage secretion of, 154
Factor VIII replacement, 1568–1569
Factor IX replacement, 1569–1570
Factor XI, 105–106
activation of, 105–106
inhibition of, 108
interactions of, 96–97, *97*
Familial arthropathy, synovial biopsy in, 652
Fanconi syndrome, osteomalacia in, 1669
Fasciitis, eosinophilic, 1195–1196
malignancy and, 1613–1614
plantar, 389

Fat pad sign, 574
Fatigue, in patient history, 370
in systemic lupus erythematosus, 1071, 1101
Fatty acid, as nutritional intervention, 359
long-chain, metabolism of, *294*
Feet, 469–481
anatomy of, 386, *387*
Charcot's joint in, 471
corticosteroid in, 552–553, 559
examination of, 386–390
flat, 388
forefoot, in diabetes mellitus, 1581, *1583*
in rheumatoid arthritis, 477–478
orthotics for, 1777
reconstructive surgery for, 1902–1909, *1903–1909*
gout in, 470, *470*
heel pain in, 470–471
hindfoot, in rheumatoid arthritis, 480
orthotics for, 1777
reconstructive surgery for, 1899–1901, *1900–1902*
march, 390
muscles in, 389
neuropathic arthropathy in, 471
normal, 469
orthotics for, 1776–1777
osteoarthritis in, 469–471
radiography in, 590
treatment of, 1456
osteoporosis of, 390
preoperative evaluation of, 1790
psoriatic arthritis in, radiography in, 582, *582*
reflex sympathetic dystrophy of, 390
Reiter's syndrome in, radiography in, 583–584, *584*
rheumatoid arthritis in, 471–480, 936–938, *938*
conservative management in, 477–480
footwear in, 477, *478–479*
forefoot in, 477–478
general principles of, 477
injections in, 479–480
orthoses in, 478
rearfoot in, 480
shoe modifications in, 479
deformities in, 472, *473*
evaluation in, 472–473, *473*
Harris Mat imprint in, 474, *474*
history in, 472
juvenile, 480
nail care in, 476
palpation in, 473–474, *474*
radiography in, 476, 574–575, *574–575*
range of motion in, 473, *473*
rearfoot and midfoot involvement in, 476–477
skin changes in, 475–476
tenderness in, 474–475, *475*
varus deformity in, *937*
Felty's syndrome, 950–955
clinical features of, 950–952, *951*, 951t
hematologic features of, 952
pathogenesis of, 952–954, *953*

Felty's syndrome, pathogenesis of *(Continued)*
impaired granulocyte production in, 953–954
increased granulocyte removal in, 952–953
serologic features of, 952, 952t
splenectomy in, 954
vasculitis in, 1148
Femoral capital epiphysis, slipped, osteoarthritis in, 1440
Femoral head, avascular necrosis of, 1697–1698
in hyperuricemia, 491
Femoral nerve, 1766–1767
course and distribution of, *1765*
entrapment of, 1766–1767, *1767*
Fenoprofen, 766, *766*
in gouty arthritis, 1384
in juvenile rheumatoid arthritis, 1266
Ferritin, in hemochromatosis, 1495, 1498
Fever, in dermatomyositis in children, 1298
in inflammatory bowel disease, 408
in juvenile rheumatoid arthritis, 408, 1251–1252, *1252*
in mixed connective tissue disease, 1120, *1120*
in polyarticular arthritis, 407–408
in rheumatic fever, 1284
in rheumatoid arthritis, 407
in systemic lupus erythematosus, 1071, 1101
Fibrillation, of cartilage, 265, 1434–1435, *1436*
Fibrillogenesis, collagen, 219–220
Fibrin formation, in synovial fluid, 893
Fibrinogen, fibronectin and, 232
Fibrinoid degeneration, in rheumatic heart disease, 1280
Fibrinolysis, in synovial fluid, 893
intrinsic coagulation pathway in, 106–107, *107*
Fibroblast, 1211–1215
adherence of, 1213
biosynthesis, processing, deposition of connective tissue by, 1213
inflammatory cell modulation of, 1215
migration and chemoattraction of, 1211–1212, 1212t
platelet interaction with, 177–179
proliferation of, 1212–1213
Fibroblast growth factor, 1212
Fibroendothelioma, synovial, 1719
Fibrogenesis imperfecta ossium, osteomalacia in, 1670
Fibroma, of tendon sheath, 1724
Fibronectin, 230–234
actin and, 232
amino acid composition of, 228t
bacteria and, 232–233
biologic function and significance of, 234
cell adhesion to, 232, *232*
cell origin and tissue distribution of, 233–234
chemical properties of, 231
collagen and, 231–232
fibrinogen and, 232
glycosaminoglycan and, 232
heparin and, 232
molecular binding sites on, 233, *233*
molecular interactions of, 231t
structural model for, *231*

Fibrosis, 1209–1223
  hepatic, 1218
  pathogenesis of, 1209–1211
    collagen in, 1213–1214, 1214t
    inflammatory response in, 1211
    phases of, 1210
    proteinases in, 1215–1216
    reparative phase in, 1211
    tissue injury in, 1210–1211
    wound healing as model of, 1210, 1211t
  pulmonary, in dermatomyositis-polymyositis, 1240
  retroperitoneal, 1219
Fibrositis, 483–486
  clinical picture in, 483–484, 484t
  in rheumatoid arthritis, 485–486
  personality in, 484–485
  prevalence, criteria, nomenclature in, 486, *486*
  rehabilitation in, 1783
  sleep disturbance in, 484, 484t, 485, *486*
  tender points in, 484, *485*
  therapy in, 487–489
    attitudes and expectations in, 488–489
    compliance and noncompliance in, 488
    counterirritant, 488
    mechanical stresses in neck and low back in, 488
    referred pain, tenderness, and reflex responses in, 487–488
Fibrositis syndrome, rheumatoid arthritis vs, 926
Fibrotic liver disease, 1218
Fibrotic pulmonary disease, 1216–1218, 1240
Fibrous dysplasia, 1674–1675, *1675*
  osteomalacia in, 1669
Financial and vocational resources for handicapped, 1786
Fingers. See also individual joints.
  clubbing of, 377
    in hypertrophic osteoarthropathy, 1594–1596, *1596*
    in inflammatory bowel disease, 1034
  distal, tuft resorption of, 1192–1193
  extensor tendon of, synovectomy of, 1813–1814
  flexor tendon of, 1812–1813
  flexor tenosynovitis of, 1821
  in rheumatoid arthritis, 931–936, *933–935*
  in systemic lupus erythematosus, 1833–1836, *1835*
  ivory, 582
  tophi of, *1363*
  trigger, 375–376
    corticosteroids in, 551, 551, 558
  ulnar deviation of, 1824, *1825*
Finger jerk, 428t
Finklestein's test, 935
Fistula, in rheumatoid arthritis, 939
Fitz Hugh-Curtis syndrome, 1517
Fitzgerald trait plasma, 96
Flat foot, 388
Flaujeac trait plasma, 96
Fletcher factor, discovery of, 95
Flexible hinge Mark I and II, 1844, *1844–1845*
Flexor digitorum profundus rupture, 1823
Flexor digitorum sublimis rupture, 1823
Flexor pollicis longus rupture, *1823*
Flexor tendon rupture, 1821–1824, *1823*
Flexor tenosynovitis, 1819–1820
  digital, 1821
  palmar, 1820–1821
  wrist, 1820, *1822*
Fluorescence test, for antinuclear antibody, 691, *691*, 691–694
5–Fluorocytosine, 1537, 1537t
5–Fluorouracil, 843
  pharmacologic properties of, 853t
Folic acid antagonists, 842–843
Foramen compression test, 380
Forefoot, in diabetes mellitus, 1581, *1583*
  in rheumatoid arthritis, 477–478
  orthotics for, 1777
  reconstructive surgery for, 1902–1909, *1903–1909*
Forestier's disease, 487
Free radical, oxygen-derived, 125–128, 126t
    anti-inflammatory drugs and, 128
    antiproteinase effects of, 126
    lipid effects of, 126–127
    superoxide dismutase and scavengers of, 127–128
    tissue and macromolecule injury by, 125–126, 126t
Freund's adjuvant arthritis, 884
Frictional force, minimization of, 324–326, *325*
Fungal arthritis, 1532–1537. See also individual types.

Gaenslen test, 380
Gait, antalgic, 381
  biomechanics of, 1919–1921, *1920*
  physical assessment of, 1770–1771
  Trendelenburg, 381
  walking, 472
Gallium scan, in sarcoidosis, 1490
  in total hip replacement, 1954
Gallium–67, 610–611
Galvanic stimulation, 1775
Gamma heavy-chain disease, 1342
Ganglion, in wrist, 375
  corticosteroid in, 551, 552
Gastric amyloidosis, 1480
Gastric parietal cell antibody, in Sjögren's syndrome, 968
Gastric ulcer, aspirin causing, 738
Gastrointestinal manifestations, in amyloidosis, 1480–1481
  in aspirin use, 736–740
  in mixed connective tissue disease, 1124, *1125*
  in nonsteroidal anti-inflammatory drug use, 761–762
  in polyarteritis, 1143, 1144
  in polyarticular arthritis, 409–410
  in scleroderma, 1191–1192, 1199
  in Sjögren's syndrome, 962
  in systemic lupus erythematosus, 1081–1082
Gaucher's disease, avascular necrosis in, 1691, *1691–1692*
Gay-related immunodeficiency disease, 1332–1333, *1333*
Gelatinase, 187
Gene, alpha 2(I) collagen, 216, *217*
  assessment of activity of, *1623*, 1623–1624
  assessment of structure of, *1623*, 1624
  heavy chain, 14–16, *14–16*, 62–63
  HLA, 43t
  immunoglobulin, *61*, 61–66
  in collagen biosynthesis, 216, *217*
  Ir, 55–61. See also *Ir gene.*
  kappa chain, 13–14
  lambda chain, 14
  light chain, 63
Genetics, 38–40
  in rheumatoid arthritis, 880, 888
  in Sjögren's syndrome, 969–970, 969t
  in systemic lupus erythematosus, 1045–1046
  linkage and recombination in, 39–40, *40*
  terminology in, 38, 39t
  within family, 38–39, *39*
  within population, 39
Genital dryness, in Sjögren's syndrome, 963
Genital ulcer, in Behçet's disease, 1174
Genotype, 38
Genu recurvatum, 383
Genu valgum, 383
  in osteoarthritis, 1440, *1441*
Genu varum, 383
Giant cell, in reticulohistiocytosis, 1504, *1504*
Giant cell arteritis, 1139, 1166–1173. See also *Arteritis, giant cell.*
Giant cell myositis, 1239, *1239*
Giant cell synovioma, benign, 1722
Giant cell tumor, in Paget's disease of bone, 1679–1680
  xanthomatous, 1719
Glenohumeral joint. See also *Shoulder.*
  inflammatory arthritis in, 443, *443*
  osteoarthritis in, *443*, 443–444, 1857, *1860*
  osteonecrosis in, 444
  reconstructive surgery for, 1861–1863, *1862–1864*
  septic arthritis in, 444
Glenohumeral replacement arthroplasty, 1866–1868
Glenohumeral subluxation, 1734–1735, *1734–1735*
Glenoid labrum, computed tomography in, 633, *633*
  tear of, 444–445
    arthrotomography in, 438, *438*
Glomerulonephritis, immune complex, *1053*, 1053–1054
  in Sjögren's syndrome, 963
  in systemic lupus erythematosus, 1104
  mixed cryoglobulin in, 1346–1347
Glomerulus, amyloid deposits in, 1481, *1481*
  anatomy of, *1053*
Glucocorticoids, 815–832
  ACTH therapy vs, 828
  alternate-day therapy with, 825–828
    Cushing's syndrome and, 826

Glucocorticoids, alternate-day therapy with *(Continued)*
HPA responsiveness and, 826
underlying disease and, 826–827
uses of, 827–828
anti-inflammatory and immunosuppressive effects of, 820–822, *821–822*, 821t
chemical structure of, 816, *816*
commonly used, 817t
considerations prior to use of, 819–820, 819t
daily single-dose, 828
hypothalamic-pituitary-adrenal function and, 824–825, 824t
iatrogenic Cushing's syndrome due to, 822–823, 823t
in amyloidosis, 1482
in avascular necrosis, 1691–1692
in bone resorption, 274
inhibition of collagen synthesis by, 1215
macrophage and, 161
osteoporosis due to, 1661
pharmacodynamics of, 816–819
bioavailability, absorption, biotransformation of, 818
drug interactions and, 819
half-life, potency, duration of action of, 816–818
liver disease and, 818–819
plasma transport proteins in, 818
pregnancy and, 819
physiology of, 816
side effects of, 822–824, 823t
withdrawal from, 824, 825
in rheumatoid arthritis, 926–927
Glucose, synovial fluid, 567
Glucose-6-phosphatase deficiency, uric acid production in, 1377
Glucuronidase, 245
Gluteal reflex, 428t
Glycogen, metabolism of, 293, *293*
Glycogen storage disease, metabolic block due to enzyme deficiency in, *293*
polymyositis vs, 1234
Glycoprotein, in cartilage, 261
Glycosaminoglycan, 237–253. See also *Proteoglycan.*
biosynthesis of, 243–244, *244*
cartilage mineralization and, 248
coagulation and, 249–250
composition and structure of, 237–240, 238t, *239*
degradation of, 244–245
distribution of, 237
electrical properties of, 327
fibronectin and, 232
in articular cartilage, 1417–1418
in genetic mucopolysaccharidoses, 245–247, *246*
in nonproliferating capillaries, 201
in osteoarthritic cartilage, 1421–1422
lysosomal enzymes and, 248
nomenclature in, 237
physical properties and structure of, 247, *247*
protein linkages of, *240–242*, 240–243
skeletal morphogenesis and, 247–248
synthesis and secretion of, 237–238
Glycosidic bonds, hydrolysis of, *3*
Glycosylation, in collagen biosynthesis, 218–219
Gm factors, 12
Gold compounds, 789–809
clinical-pharmacologic correlates of, 798
distribution of, 795–796, *796*, 796t
dosage schedules for, 794–795, 795t
efficacy of, 790–792, 790t, *791–793*
excretion of, 797–798
historical use of, 789
in juvenile rheumatoid arthritis, 1267
in rheumatoid arthritis, 988
indications and patient selection in, 789–790
macrophage and, 161
mechanisms of action of, 798–800, *799*, 800t
oral or intramuscular, 805
pharmacokinetics of, 796–798, *797*
precautions, contraindications, costs of, 800–802
preparations of, 792–794, *793*
retention of, 798
serum concentrations of, 796–797, *797*
toxicity of, 802–805, 802t–804t
treatment of, 805
Gold rash, 802
Gold sodium thiomalate, auranofin vs, 804t
aurothioglucose vs, 794
mechanisms of action of, 798–800, *799*, 800t
structural formula of, *793*
Golgi complex antibody, in Sjögren's syndrome, 967
Gonococcal arthritis, 1516–1519, *1517*
joint involvement patterns in, 407
Reiter's syndrome vs, 1016t, 1017
Gorlin's sign, in Ehlers-Danlos syndrome, 1629
Gottron's papules, 1235
Gottron's sign, 540
Gout, 470, *470*, 1359–1398
alcohol ingestion in, 1388
allopurinol use and, 865
arthritis in, 1360–1361, 1378–1382
calcium pyrophosphate deposition disease in, 1403
leukocyte in, 1381–1382
self-limited nature of, 1382
treatment of, 1383–1385
urate crystal in, 1378–1381
atherosclerosis and, 1366
avascular necrosis in, 1693
calcium stones in, 1371
chronic tophaceous stage in, 1361–1363, *1362–1363*, 1363t
clinical features of, 1359–1371
corticosteroid in, 550
diabetes mellitus and, 1364–1365
diet in, 1388–1389
epidemiology in, 1359
genetics of, 1378
historical, 1360t
hyperlipidemia and, 1365
hypertension in, 1365–1366, 1389
hypertriglyceridemia in, 1389
hyperuricemia in, 490, 1371–1378, 1371t
asymptomatic, 1360, 1383
control of, 1385–1388, *1386–1388*
primary, 1372–1377
Gout, hyperuricemia in *(Continued)*
secondary, 1377–1378
in probenecid use, 860
in sickle cell disease, 1574–1575
intercritical stage in, 1361
negative disease associations in, 1366
obesity in, 359, 1364
ocular manifestations in, 531–532
parenchymal renal disease in, 1366–1371. See also *Renal disease, parenchymal.*
preoperative evaluation in, 1789
purine restriction in, 1388–1389
radiography in, 596, *596*, 1363
rheumatoid arthritis vs, 923
serum urate levels in, epidemiology of, 1359
tophi in, synovial membrane, 1379
treatment of, 1382–1389
urate nephropathy in, 1366–1367, *1367*
uric acid nephropathy in, acute, 1367–1368
uric acid stones in, 496, 1368–1372, 1388
weight reduction in, 1388
Gram's stain, 566
Granulocyte, 115–144
as peptide and lipid mediator source, 128–129
cellular functions of, 116–119
chemokinesis of, 116
chemotaxic regulation of, 116–119, *118*
interactions with particulate stimuli of, 119–124
natural factors chemotactic for, 117t
origin, distribution, fate of, 116
Granulocytopenia, in Felty's syndrome, 952–954
Granuloma, in inflammatory bowel disease, 1034
in tuberculous skeletal disease, 1528
Granuloma annulare, 939, 1253
Granulomatosis, allergic, pannicular involvement in, 1181
allergic angiitis and, 1137, 1138, 1153–1155, 1309
lymphomatoid, 1158–1159
malignancy and, 1614
pulmonary talc, 1490
Wegener's, 1138–1139, *1155–1157*, 1155–1158.
Grasp strength, in rheumatoid arthritis, 935, 935t
Graves' disease, 1585–1587, *1586*
GRID syndrome, 1332–1333, *1333*
GSB hinge prosthesis, 1843–1844, *1844*
Guanine, chemical structure of, *337*
Guanylic acid, biosynthesis of, 340
Guyon's canal, ulnar nerve entrapment in, 1759

Hageman factor, 97–101
activation and fragmentation of, 98–100
HMW kininogen in, 99, *99*
kallikrein in, 98–99, *99*
surface in, 99
activation of, 97
assays of, 97–98

Hageman factor *(Continued)*
  autoactivation of, 100, *101*
  discovery of, 95
  inhibition of, 107, 109t
  interactions of, 96–97, *97*
  permeability factor of dilution (PF/dil) as, 100–101
  properties of, 97
  rheumatic disease and, 108–110
  urate crystal activation of, 1380–1381
Hallux abductus, 473, *473*
Hallux limitus, 470, *470*
Hallux rigidus, 388, 470
  surgical correction of, 1907–1908
Hallux valgus, 388, 469
  in rheumatoid arthritis, 937, *938*
  surgical correction of, 1906–1907
HAM, 1583–1584
Hammer toe, 388
Hand, corticosteroid in, 551, 552, 558
  grasp strength in, 935, 935t
  hemochromatosis in, 1497, *1497*
  juvenile rheumatoid arthritis in, 1249, *1249–1250*
  nonsurgical treatment of, 1818–1819
  osteoarthritis in, radiography in, 588, *588*
    reconstructive surgery for, 1832–1833
    treatment of, 1455
  preventive and therapeutic surgery for, 1819–1824
  prostheses for, 1968–1971, *1970*
  psoriatic arthritis in, radiography in, 582, *582*
  reconstructive and salvage surgery for, 1824–1832
  rest and exercise for, 1818
  rheumatoid arthritis in, 931–936, 932t–935t, *933–935*
    grasp strength in, 935, 935t
    radiography in, *571*, 573
  scintigraphy in, *614*
  splints for, 1778–1779, *1778–1779*, 1818–1819
  steroid injections for, 1819
  synovectomy in, 1824
  systemic lupus erythematosus in, 1833–1837, *1834–1835*
Hand jerk, 428t
Hand-foot syndrome, 1574
Haplotype, 38
Harris Mat imprint, 474, *474*
Hashimoto's thyroiditis, 1585–1587, *1586*
Hass procedure, 1841
Haversian system, 275, *276*
Head compression test, 425, *425*
Head distraction test, *425*, 425–426
Headache, in cervical spine disorders, 423
  in mixed connective tissue disease, 1124, 1126t
  in systemic lupus erythematosus, 1085, 1105
Health Assessment Questionnaire, 366t–367t
Health care, holistic, 508–509, *509*
Heat, therapeutic, 1774, 1774t
Heavy chain, 5
  subgroups of, 8t
Heavy chain disease, 1341–1342
Heavy chain genes, 62–63
Heavy chain germ line genes, 14–16, *14–16*
Heavy chain switching, *63–64*, 63–65
Heberden's node, 377, 1436–1437, *1437*, 1455
Heel, injection into, 480
  orthotics for, 1777
  pain in, 388, 470–471
Helmet deformity, in osteogenesis imperfecta, 1637
Hemangioma, in synovium, 1711–1713, *1713–1714*
Hematologic manifestations, in Felty's syndrome, 952
  in gold therapy, 803
  in mixed connective tissue disease, 1125–1126
  in penicillamine therapy, *811*
  in rheumatoid arthritis, 940
  in Sjögren's syndrome, 965
  in systemic lupus erythematosus, 1090–1091, 1091t, 1107
Hemiarthroplasty, of hip, 1919
Hemochromatosis, 1494–1501
  calcium pyrophosphate deposition disease in, 1403
  classification of, 1494
  clinical features of, 1496–1498, *1497–1498*
  diagnosis of, 1499, 1499t
  etiology in, 1494–1495
  laboratory features of, 1498–1499
  osteoarthritis in, 1443
  pathogenesis of, 1495–1496, *1496*
  primary, 1496–1497, *1497*
  radiography in, 599, *599*
  rheumatoid arthritis vs, 923–924
  secondary, 1498
  synovial biopsy in, 651
  treatment of, 1499–1500
Hemoglobinopathy, avascular necrosis in, 1690–1691, *1691*
  radiography in, 604
  rheumatoid arthritis vs, 924
Hemophilia. See also *Hemophilic arthropathy.*
  acquired immune deficiency syndrome and, 1569
  diagnosis of, 1567
  factor IX replacement in, 1569–1570
  factor VIII replacement in, 1568–1569
  inhibitor antibodies in, 1570
  radiography in, *604*, 604–605
  surgery in, 1570–1572
  synovectomy in, 1815
  therapy in, 1567–1570
Hemophilic arthropathy, 1564–1572
  clinical features of, 1564–1565
  laboratory diagnosis of, 1567
  osteoarthritis in, 1445
  pathogenesis of, 1566–1567
  pathologic features of, 1565, *1566*
  rheumatoid arthritis vs, 924
  roentgenographic features of, 1565, *1566*
  surgery in, 1570–1572
  therapy in, 1567–1572
Hemosiderin, in hemochromatosis, 1495
Henoch-Schönlein purpura, in children, *1307–1308*, 1307–1309
Heparan sulfate, anticoagulant function of, 249–250
  composition and structure of, 238t, 239, *239*
Heparin, anticoagulant function of, 249
  composition and structure of, 238t, *239*, 239–240
  cortisone and, in angiogenesis inhibition, 208, *209*
  fibronectin and, 232
  in endothelial cell migration, 203, *203*
  in inflammation, 250
  osteoporosis due to, 250
Heparin-proteoglycan, 243
Hepatic manifestations, glucocorticoids and, 818–819
  in amyloidosis, 1481
  in Felty's syndrome, 951
  in gonococcal arthritis, 1517
  in polyarteritis, 1144
  in polyarticular arthritis, 409
  in Sjögren's syndrome, 963
  in systemic lupus erythematosus, 1082
  nonsteroidal anti-inflammatory drugs and, 762
Hepatitis, aspirin causing, 742–743
  fibrosis in, 1218
Hepatitis B virus, *1542–1543*, 1542–1545
Herpes simplex virus, 1552
Heterozygote, 38
Hindfoot. See also *Feet.*
  in rheumatoid arthritis, 480
  orthotics for, 1777
  reconstructive surgery for, 1899–1901, *1900–1902*
Hinge joint, 371
Hip, anatomy of, 381
  arthrodesis of, 1918–1919
  arthrography of, 628
  arthroscopy of, 645
  ball-in-socket joint in, 317, *318*
  biomechanics of, 1919–1921, *1920*
  corticosteroid in, 551, 552, 556, *556*, 558
  crutches or cane for, 1917, *1917*
  cup arthroplasty of, 1919
  degeneration of, biomechanical steps in, 328–330, *329*
  examination of, 381–383
  hemiarthroplasty of, 1919
  in ankylosing spondylitis, radiography in, 580, *581*
    total replacement in, 1925
  in juvenile rheumatoid arthritis, 1262, 1270, *1270*
    arthroplasty of, *1912–1914*, 1912–1915
  in osteoarthritis, *1439*, 1439–1440
    corticosteroid injection in, 548
    radiography in, 588, *589*
    treatment of, 1455
  in rheumatoid arthritis, 936
    other joints complicating surgery in, 1918
    radiography in, 575
    surgical indications in, 1917–1918
    surgical patient profile in, 1918
  in septic arthritis, *1509*, *1513*
    inflammatory bowel disease and, 1034
  muscle strength testing of, 382
  nonsurgical therapy for, 1917

Hip *(Continued)*
osteonecrosis in, in hypothyroidism, 1587
osteotomy of, 1927
painful, evaluation of, 1916–1917
prostheses for, radiography in, 1938–1938, *1939–1940*
range of motion at, 381–382
snapping, 382
synovectomy of, 1797, 1919
total replacement of, 1921–1927
arthrography in, 1948–1954
bone scan in, 1954
complications of, 1923–1925
current surgical alternatives to, 1925–1927, *1926*
historical, 1921, *1922*
in ankylosing spondylitis, 1925
in avascular necrosis, 1707
infection in, 1923–1924
long term results of, 1921–1923
pre– and postoperative program in, 1921
previous surgical alternatives to, 1918–1919
radiography in, 1938–1956. See also *Radiography.*
results of revision of, 1925
technical aspects of, 1921
total surface replacement arthroplasty of, 1925–1927, *1926*
trochanteric bursitis of, 1740–1741, *1740–1741*
Hip dysplasia, osteoarthritis in, 1440
Histidine, in rheumatoid arthritis, 354
Histiocytoma, benign fibrous, 1719
Histocompatibility antigen, in systemic lupus erythematosus, 1046
Histone, antibody to, 700–701
*Histoplasma capsulatium,* 1534–1535
*Histoplasma duboisii,* 1535
Histoplasmosis, 1534–1535
African, 1535
History of patient, 369–370
fatigue in, 370
limitation of motion in, 369
pain in, 369
stiffness in, 369–370
swelling in, 369
weakness in, 370
HLA antigen, in juvenile rheumatoid arthritis, 1257
HLA gene frequencies, 43t
HLA–A3, in hemochromatosis, 1494
HLA–B14, in hemochromatosis, 1494
HLA–B27, 49
in psoriatic arthritis, 1026, 1026t
in Reiter's syndrome, 1015–1016
neutrophil activity and, 134
HLA–D/DR antigen, disease associations with, 58–59, 59t
Hodgkin's disease, amyloidosis in, 1476
Hoffa's disease, 1711
Holistic health care, 508–509, *509*
Homocystinuria, 1627–1628, 1627t
Hormone, sex, 848–849
steroid, 848–849, 849t
Howship's lacunae, 273, *274*
HPRT deficiency, 1374–1376, *1374–1376*, 1376t–1377t
Humeral epicondylitis, 551, 557, *558*, 1738–1739, *1739*
Humeral head, avascular necrosis of, 1698
Humerus, distal, proximal ulna procedure, 1841
metal prosthesis for, 1842
Humoral immunity, 22, 23t
in dermatomyositis-polymyositis, 1240
in Sjögren's syndrome, 968
in systemic lupus erythematosus, 1050–1051
tests for, 1318, *1318*, 1318t
Hyaluronate, in embryonic joint, 255
skeletal morphogenesis and, 247–248
Hyaluronate-proteoglycan, 240
Hyaluronic acid, composition and structure of, 238, 238t, *239*
hyaluronidase digestion of, *3*
in boundary lubrication, 1424
Hyaluronidase, 244–245, 1420
Hydatid disease of bone, in spine, 464
Hydralazine, in drug-induced lupus, 1092
Hydrarthrosis, intermittent, rheumatoid arthritis vs, 926
Hydrocortisone, chemical structure of, *816*.
inhibition of drug metabolism by, 721
Hydrolysis, of glycosidic bonds, *3*
of peptide bonds, 2
of phospholipid, *3*
Hydrotherapy, 1775
Hydroxyallysine, in collagen, 221, *221*
Hydroxyapatite, 278
arthropathy of, 1413–1414
Hydroxychloroquine, chemical structure of, *775*
guidelines for use of, 785–786, 785t
in juvenile rheumatoid arthritis, 1266–1267
in systemic lupus erythematosus, 1110, 1297
pharmacokinetics of, 776
side effects of, 782–785, 783t, *784*
visual effects of, *784*, 784–785
Hydroxylase, protocollagen, 216–218, *218*
Hydroxylysine, biosynthesis of, *218*
Hydroxyproline, biosynthesis of, *218*
in collagen, 218
urinary, in metabolic bone disease, 1647
Hydroxypyridinoline crosslink, in collagen, *221*, 222
Hydroxyurea, 843
pharmacologic properties of, 853t
Hypercalcemia, familial hypocalciuric, 1655–1656
Hypereosinophilic disease, 135–137, 137t
Hyperlipidemia, gout and, 1365
Hyperlipoproteinemia, rheumatoid arthritis vs, 924
Hypermobility syndrome, benign, *1630*, 1630–1631
Hyperostosis, ankylosing, 487
diffuse idiopathic skeletal, 487
Hyperparathyroidism, calcium pyrophosphate deposition disease in, 1403
primary, 1649–1657
biochemical abnormalities in, 1651–1652, *1652*
clinical features of, 1650–1654, 1651t, *1652–1655*
Hyperparathyroidism, primary *(Continued)*
differential diagnosis in, 1654–1656, 1656t
epidemiology of, 1650–1651
osteomalacia in, 1669
parathyroid hormone in, 1649–1650, *1649–1650*
radiology in, 1652–1654, *1652–1654*
treatment of, 1656–1657
rheumatic conditions in, 1581–1583, *1584–1585*
Hyperphosphatasia, hereditary, 1675–1676
Hypersensitivity angiitis, 1137, 1138, 1153–1155, 1309
Hypersensitivity response, in Sjögren's syndrome, 968
Hypersensitivity vasculitis, 1138, 1149–1153, *1308*, 1308–1309
Hypertension, gout and, 1365–1366, 1389
intraosseous, in avascular necrosis, 1693
pulmonary, in mixed connective tissue disease, 1123, *1124*
in polyarticular arthritis, 409
in scleroderma, 1192, 1200
Hyperthermia syndrome, malignant, 487
Hyperthyroidism, 1585–1587, *1586*
Hypertriglyceridemia, in gout, 1389
Hypertrophic osteoarthropathy, 1594–1603
classification of, 1594, 1595t
clinical syndromes in, 1594–1598, *1596–1597*
course and prognosis of, 1601–1602
differential diagnosis of, 1600–1601
etiology and pathogenesis of, 1601
laboratory findings in, 1598
management of, 1601
pathology in, 1599–1600, *1600*
radiographs and radionuclide scanning in, 1598, *1599–1600*
rheumatoid arthritis vs, 924
scintigraphy in, 622, *623*
secondary, 1596–1598, *1597*
synovial biopsy in, 652
Hyperuricemia, 489–497
aseptic necrosis of femoral head in, 491
associated findings in, 492
avascular necrosis in, 1693
cause of, 492
control of, renal function and, 495–496
definition of, 489–490
general approach to patient in, *493*
history in, 492
in arthritis, 490
in gout, 490, 1371–1378, 1371t
asymptomatic, 1360, 1383
control of, 1385–1388, *1386–1388*
primary, 1372–1377
secondary, 1377–1378
in psoriatic arthritis, 1024, *1025*
in sickle cell disease, 1574–1575
investigation of, *494*
laboratory data in, 492, 495
management of, 495–497
nephrolithiasis in, 491
physical examination in, 492
radiographic findings in, 491
renal insufficiency in, 491–492
stone formation in, 496
subcutaneous nodules in, 490–491
tissue or organ damage in, 490–492
urate nephropathy in, 495

Hypoalbuminemic malnutrition, 353
Hypocomplementemic states, 91–92, 91t
Hypocomplementemic vasculitis, 1151–1152, *1152*
Hypogeusia, penicillamine causing, 812
Hypoparathyroidism, rheumatic conditions in, 1583–1585, *1586*
Hypophosphatasia, in calcium pyrophosphate deposition disease, 1404
in osteomalacia, 1670
Hypophosphatemia, in osteomalacia, 1667–1669, *1668*
Hypothalamic-pituitary-adrenal function, glucocorticoid suppression of, 824–825, 824t
Hypothyroidism, 1587, *1587*
calcium pyrophosphate deposition disease in, 1403–1404
Hypoxanthine, chemical structure of, *337*
Hypoxanthine-guanine phosphoribosyltransferase (HPRT), 340–341
deficiency in, 1374–1376, *1374–1376*, 1376t–1377t
Hysteria, 487

I-cell disease, 246–247
*I. dammini*, 1559
Ia antigen, 45–49
as markers of differentiation, 48–49
DR allotype in, 45–46, 46t
DS-DC system of, 46–48, 47t, *48*
function of, 49
SB subregion of, 48
structure of, 56–57
Ibuprofen, *765*, 765–766
in gouty arthritis, 1384
in juvenile rheumatoid arthritis, 1266
Idiotypy, 62
IgG. See *Immunoglobulin.*
Iliopectineal bursitis, corticosteroid in, 552, 559
Iliopsoas bursitis, 382
Iliopsoas hemorrhage, in hemophilic arthropathy, 1565
Iliotibial band friction syndrome, 1746, *1746*
Immune complex, 680–690, 1053–1055
analysis of, 680, *681*
antigen-antibody bond in, 1054
assay systems for, 898
clearance of, *681*, 681–682
detection of, 682–686
antigen-specific methods in, 684
biologic recognition units in, *683*, 683–684
cell binding assays in, *685*, 685–686
cell-bound receptor interaction in, 684
fluid phase binding assays in, 685, *685*
interpretation of results in, 686
physical properties in, 682–683
plasma protein recognition sites in, 683–684
solid phase binding assays in, *684*, 684–685
generation of, 680–682, *681*, 682t
in acute serum sickness, 1053
Immune complex *(Continued)*
in Felty's syndrome, 952, 952t
in glomerulonephritis, *1053*, 1053–1054
in hypersensitivity vasculitis, 1149–1150
in juvenile rheumatoid arthritis, 1256
in malignancy, 1607–1608
in prognosis in rheumatoid arthritis, 944
in rheumatic disease, 686–688, *687–688*
clinical usefulness of, 686–687, *687*
critical evaluation of, 686
specific disorders of, 687–688
in rheumatoid arthritis, 880–881, 952, 952t
in systemic lupus erythematosus, 1056–1057, *1057*
in vasculitis, 1139–1141
interaction of complement and, 682
pathogenicity of, structure in, 682, 682t
properties of, factors influencing, 682, 682t
genetic control of, 54–71
Immune response gene, 55–61. See also *Ir gene.*
Immune system, 833–836
aberrancies of, 834–835
dichotomy of, 22, 23t
enhancement of, 836
in inflammation, 22–35
interferon effects on, 852t
nonglucocorticoid hormones and, 849t
organization of, ontogeny and, *1319*, 1319–1320
regulation of, 833–834, *834*
schematic diagram of, 833, *834*
suppression of, 835–836
therapeutic modification of, 835–836
Immune tolerance, 1047–1048
Immunity, cellular, 22, 23t. See also *Cellular immunity.*
humoral, 22, 23t. See also *Humoral immunity.*
Immunodeficiency disease, 1315–1337
acquired, 1332–1333, *1333*
common variable, 1327–1328
gay-related, 1332–1333, *1333*
laboratory evaluation in, *1318*, 1318–1319, 1318t
patient evaluation, history, physical examination in, 1315–1318, 1317t
specific, 1320–1330. See also individual types.
severe combined, 1320–1323
Immunodiffusion, for antigen-antibody reaction, 694–695, *695*
Immunofluorescence, in antigen-antibody reaction, 695–696
in scleroderma, 1186–1187
Immunoglobulin, allotypic markers in, 12
biological properties of, 9t
classes of, 6t
disease implications of, 19
evolution and, 18–19
genes of, *61*, 61–66
disease response susceptibility and, 66
heavy chain, *62*, 62–63
immune response characteristics and, 65–66
isotype diversity in, *63–64*, 63–65
light chain, 63
organization of, 62–66
Immunoglobulin, genes of *(Continued)*
T lymphocyte antigen receptor and, 65
variable region diversity in, 63, *63*
heavy chain and light chain, 5–7
heavy chain germ line genes in, 14–16, *14–16*
idiotypes and combining sites of, 12–13
in Sjögren's syndrome, 965
kappa chain germ line genes of, *13*, 13–14
lambda chain germ line genes in, 14
loss of, 1332
variable and constant regions of, *7*, 7–8, 8t
Immunoglobulin A, 10–11
secretory, 7, 10–11
selective deficiency of, 1263–1265, 1328–1329
anti-IgA antibodies in, 1264, 1264t
in connective tissue disease, 1263, 1263t
in juvenile rheumatoid arthritis, 1264, 1264t
in rheumatoid arthritis, 1264–1265
treatment in, 1265
Immunoglobulin D, 11
Immunoglobulin E, 11–12
Immunoglobulin G, *8*, 8–9, 9t
immunogenecity of, 897
molecular structure of, *664*
neutrophil receptors for, 119–120, 119t
rheumatoid factor and, 672–673, *673*
Immunoglobulin M, 9–10, *10*
Immunosuppressants. See also individual types.
in dermatomyositis–polymyositis, 1242
in juvenile rheumatoid arthritis, 1268
in systemic lupus erythematosus, 1110–1111
malignancy and, 1614
Impact loading, in osteoarthritis, 1424–1425
Impingement syndrome, 1736, *1737*
Impingement test, 1859
Indium scan, in total hip replacement, 1954
Indomethacin, 764–765, *765*
in ankylosing spondylitis, 1004
in gouty arthritis, 1383–1384
in juvenile rheumatoid arthritis, 760–761, 1266
in osteoarthritis, 1453–1454
salicylate interaction with, 733
Indoprofen, in gouty arthritis, 1384
Infarction, bone, 619–621, *620–621*, 1576–1577
myocardial, 1087–1088
Infectious arthritis. See *Septic arthritis.*
Inflammation, aspirin effects on, 729–730
collagen in, 227
cyclic nucleotide in, 76–78
endogenous chemotactic factors in, 892t
fibrosis in, 1211
granulocytes in, 115–144
heparin in, 250
immunologic aspects of, 22–35
in urate crystal deposition, 1380–1381
leukotrienes in, 76–78
low molecular weight mediators of, 71–83
metabolic response to, 354–355
copper and, 355
histidine and, 354

Inflammation, metabolic response to *(Continued)*
iron and, 354–355
zinc and, 355
plasma protein effectors of, 83–94
platelets in, 169–182
process of, 1–4
common themes in, 4–5
components of, 1, *2*
delivery in, 2–3
detectors in, 2
effectors in, *2–3*, 3–4
general principles of, 4t
selectors in, 1–2, 3t
prostaglandins in, 76–78
Inflammatory arthritis, in glenohumeral joint, 443, *443*
in osteoarthritis, 1427
in sternoclavicular joint, 446
scintigraphy in, 611–624
Inflammatory bowel disease, 1032–1036
fever in, 408
in Behçet's disease, 1175
musculoskeletal involvement in, 1034
ocular involvement in, 529
peripheral arthritis in, 1032–1034, *1033*
preoperative evaluation in, 1789
spinal and pelvic involvement in, 1034–1036, *1035–1036*
synovitis in, corticosteroid in, 550
Inhibitor antibody, in hemophilia, 1570
Injection, aspiration and, of joints and soft tissues, 546–561
Instability, in patient examination, 371
Interferon, 851–853, 852t, 853t
Interleukin 1, 192
fibroblast function and, 1216
Interosseous hypertension, 1693
Interosseous nerve, posterior, tests of, 420t
Interosseous nerve syndrome, anterior, 1757–1758, *1757–1758*
posterior, 1760–1761, *1761*
Interphalangeal joint, as synovial joint, *254*
corticosteroid in, 555, *555*
distal, in psoriatic arthritis, 1026, *1027*
reconstructive and salvage surgery for, 1828–1829
examination of, *376–377*, 376–378
in osteoarthritis, 1832
in systemic lupus erythematosus, 1833–1836, *1835*
muscles of, 378
proximal, flexion deformity of, 1827
fusion vs. arthroplasty in, 1827–1828
hyperextension deformity of, 1827
reconstructive and salvage surgery for, 1827–1828, *1828–1829*
synovectomy of, 1800–1801
Interstitial fibrosis, in rheumatoid arthritis, 941
Interstitial lung disease, 1217
in scleroderma, 1192, 1200
Intervertebral disc. See *Disc.*
Intervertebral osteochondrosis, radiography in, 590, *591*
Interzone, embryonic, 255
Intestinal bypass disease, 1037–1038
Intestinal lymphangiectasia, 1332
Intimal proliferation, in mixed connective tissue disease, 1129, *1130*
Intra-articular ossicle, in knee, 1713–1714, *1714*
Intra-articular pressure, 268
Intra-articular temperature, 267–268, *268*
Ir gene, 55–61
antigen structure, 56–57
disease susceptibility and, 58–59, 59t
in regulation of immune response, 57–58, 58t
location of, 55–56, *56*
theories of, 59–61
clonal deletion and, 60–61, *61*, 61t
determinant selection and, 60
Iron, in rheumatoid arthritis, 354–355
in synovial fluid, 894, *894*
Iron storage disease, 1494–1501. See also *Hemochromatosis.*
Ischemic heart disease, nonsteroidal anti-inflammatory drugs in, 761
Ischiogluteal bursitis, corticosteroid in, 552, 559
Isoenzyme, serum, 708–709
Isoniazid, 1531t
in drug-induced lupus, 1092
Ivory phalanx, 582

J chain, 7, 11
Jaccoud deformity, of metacarpophalangeal joint, 1282
Jaundice, cholestatic, in gold therapy, 804
Jaw, in juvenile rheumatoid arthritis, 1254, *1255*
Jaw reflex, 427
Jerk test, of knee, 385
$Jo_1$ antigen, 703
Joint. See also individual types.
aspiration and injection of, 546–561
biology of, 254–271
biomechanics of, 317–336. See also *Biomechanics.*
classification of, 254, *370*, 370–371
condylar, 371
cotylic, 370–371
definition of, 317
diarthrodial, *370*, 370–371
hinge, 371
infection of, 362, 362t
intra-articular temperature of, 267–268, *268*
laxity of, 1629, *1630*
lubrication of, 263–264
boosted, 263, *264*, 325
boundary, 263
elastohydrodynamic, 263
fluid-film, 263
in osteoarthritis, 1424
lubricin in, 264
squeeze film, 263, *264*
weeping, 325, *325*
organization of, 257–260
articular cartilage in, 259–260
bursae in, 258–259
ligaments in, 257–258
muscles in, 257–258
subchondral bone in, 259
tendons in, 257–258
Joint, organization of *(Continued)*
vascular and nerve supply to, 259
plane, 370
sellar, 371
spheroidal, 370
synovial or diarthrodial, 254, *254*
embryonic development of, 254–257, *255–257*
condensation in, 254
condrification in, 255, *256*
interzones in, 255
joint cavity formation in, 255–257, *256–257*
synovial mesenchyme in, 255
trochoid or pivot, 371
Joint cavity, embryonic formation of, 255–257, *256–257*
Joint fluid examination. See *Synovial fluid.*
Joint space narrowing, in rheumatoid arthritis, 571
Juvenile ankylosing spondylitis, juvenile rheumatoid arthritis vs., 1263
radiography in, 578
Juvenile osteoporosis, 1662
Juvenile psoriatic arthritis, radiography in, 578
Juvenile rheumatoid arthritis, 1247–1277
age of onset in, 1248, *1248*
amyloidosis in, 1476
ancillary manifestations of, 1262t
arthroplasty of hip and knee in, *1912–1914*, 1912–1915
broken homes among children with, 507t, *508*
cataract in, 521
classification of, 1259–1260, 1261t
clinical manifestations of, 1248–1254
connective tissue disease in, 1263t
constitutional signs and symptoms of, 1248
corticosteroid in, 550
cutaneous manifestations of, 541
death in, 1271t
differential diagnosis of, 1260–1265, 1261t–1264t
epidemiology in, 1247
epiphysiodesis in, 1911–1912
etiology and pathogenesis of, 1247–1248
extra-articular manifestations of, 1252–1253, *1253*
fever in, 408
growth retardation in, 1254, *1255*
historical, 1247
immune complexes in, 688
in feet, 480
indomethacin in, 760–761
laboratory examination in, 1256–1258
nonsteroidal anti-inflammatory drugs in, 760–761
ocular manifestations in, 517–521, *520*, 1254
oligoarthritis in, 1250, *1250–1251*
pathology in, 1254–1255
polyarthritis in, 1248–1250, *1249–1250*
preoperative evaluation in, 1789
psychological factors in, 507–508, 507t, *508*
radiography in, 576–577, *576–577*, 1258–1259, *1259–1261*
rash in, 1251–1252, *1252*, 1255

Juvenile rheumatoid arthritis *(Continued)*
rehabilitation in, 1782–1783
rheumatoid nodule in, 1253, 1255
surgery in, 1910–1916
synovectomy in, 1911, *1911*
synovial or Baker's cyst in, 1249, *1250*
systemic onset in, 1250–1251, *1252*
treatment of, 1265–1269, 1265t–1266t
antimalarials in, 1266–1267
aspirin in, 1265–1266
corticosteroids in, 1267–1268
course of disease and prognosis in, 1269–1271, *1270–1271*, 1271t
D-penicillamine in, 1267
education and counseling in, 1269
gold salts in, 1267
immunosuppressants in, 1268
management in, 1265t
nonsteroidal anti-inflammatory agents in, 1266
orthopedic surgery in, 1269
physical and occupational therapy in, 1268–1269
types of onset in, 1248–1252, 1249t
uveitis in, *520*, 520–521, 1253–1254, *1254*

Kallikrein, assays of, 101–102
inhibition of, 107–108
plasma, 184
Kaposi's sarcoma, 1333, *1333*
Kappa chain germ line genes, *13*, 13–14
Kashin-Beck disease, iron overload in, 1498
osteoarthritis in, 1445
Kawasaki's disease, 1161
in children, 1309–1310, 1310t
Keloid, 227, 1219
Keratan sulfate, composition of, 238t, *239*, 240
in articular cartilage, 1417–1418
Keratitis, in scleritis, 517
in Sjögren's syndrome, 956, 957t
Keratoconjunctivitis sicca, 512–513, *513*
in Sjögren's syndrome, 956–957, 958t, 973
Keratoderma blennorrhagica, 536, *536*
in Reiter's syndrome, *1012–1013*, 1013, 1013t
Keratopathy, band, in juvenile rheumatoid arthritis, *520*, 520–521, 1254
Keshan disease, 358
Kidney. See *Renal manifestations*.
Kinin formation, by synovial fluid, 893
Kininogen, HMW, 103–105
assays of, 104–105
discovery of, 96
interactions of, 96–97, *97*
plasma, 103
properties of, 103–104, *104–105*
Km factors, 12
Knee, arthrodesis for, in osteoarthritis, 1871
arthrography in, *625–626*, 625–627, 1742, *1742–1743*
arthroscopy in, *643–644*, 643–645
avascular necrosis of, 1698
bulge sign in, 384, *384*
bursae of, 383, *383*

Knee *(Continued)*
bursitis in, 384
corticosteroid in, 551, 552, 553–554, *554*, 558–559
debridement (Pridie) for, in osteoarthritis, 1871–1872
deformity of, valgus, 1884, *1884*
varus, 1883, 1883–1884
degeneration of, biomechanical steps in, 330–331
examination of, *383–384*, 383–386
flexion contracture of, surgical correction of, 1884–1886, *1885–1887*
housemaid's, 1745
in hemophilic arthropathy, 1565, *1566*
in juvenile rheumatoid arthritis, 1250, *1250–1251*
arthroplasty of, *1912–1914*, 1912–1915
in osteoarthritis, 1440, *1441*
corticosteroid injection in, 548
radiography in, 588–590, *589*
reconstructive surgery for, 1871–1872, *1872*
treatment of, 1455–1456
in pigmented villonodular synovitis, 1720, *1720*
in rheumatoid arthritis, 936, 936t
pathology affecting surgery in, 1872–1873, *1873*
radiography in, 575
reconstructive surgery for, 1871, *1871*
in septic arthritis *1508*, *1510–1511*
intra-articular ossicles in, 1713–1714, *1714*
intracapsular chondroma in, 1718, *1718*
joint motion in, *320*, 321
jumper's, 1745
lateral band syndrome of, 1746, *1746*
ligamentous injury to, 1743–1745, *1744*
ligamentous laxity of, 385
lipoma arborescens in, 1711, *1712*
meniscal injury of, 385–386. See also *Meniscus*.
muscle strength testing in, 386
orthotics for, *1777*, 1777–1778
osteotomy for, in osteoarthritis, 1872, *1872*
palpation of, 384
patellofemoral pain syndrome/chondromalacia patella, 1747–1748, *1748*
pes anserinus tendonitis bursitis of, 551, 552, 558–559, 1745–1746
prepatellar bursitis of, 552, 1745
prostheses for, 1874–1878, *1876–1878*
bicondylar replacement, 1875–1877, *1876–1877*
constrained, 1877–1878, *1877–1878*
duopatellar, 1875
posterior stabilized condylar, 1876–1877, *1877*
spherocentric, 1877–1878
surface, 1874–1877, *1876–1877*
total condylar, 1875–1876, *1876*
total condylar III, 1877, *1878*
unicompartmental replacement, 1874–1875, *1876*
reconstructive surgery for, 1870–1896
indications for, 1870–1872, *1871–1872*

Knee reconstructive surgery for *(Continued)*
posterior cruciate ligament in, 1873–1874, *1874–1875*
total replacement in, 1874–1895
recreational injury of, 1741–1748
serial casting for, 1777–1778
stability of, 318, *318*
synovectomy of, 1795–1797, 1806t, 1807, *1807–1809*
synovitis of, corticosteroid in, 550
tendonitis/bursitis of, 1745
total replacement in, 1874–1895, 1956–1964
complications of, 1887–1892, *1889–1891*, 1958–1961, 1960t, *1961–1963*
contraindications in, 1878–1880
flexion contracture in, 1884–1886, *1885–1887*
hinge total knee prosthesis in, 1961–1963, *1964*
inadequate motion after, 1888
indications for, 1878, *1879*
infection after, 1888–1890, *1891*
loosening after, 1888, *1889*, 1958–1960, 1960t, *1961–1963*
management of, 1882–1886, *1882–1887*
McKeever and MacIntosh hemiarthroplasty in, 1963–1964, *1965*
nerve palsy after, 1887
patellar complications after, 1887–1888, 1961, *1963*
prostheses for, 1874–1878, *1876–1878*, 1956–1958, *1958–1960*
results of, 1892–1895, *1893–1894*
revision after, 1890–1892
surgical technique in, 1880–1881, *1880–1882*
valgus deformity of, 1884, *1884*
varus deformity of, *1883*, 1883–1884
Knee jerk, 428t
Knuckle-cracking, 268
Knuckle-knuckle-dimple-knuckle sign, 1584, *1586*
Kudo total elbow prosthesis, 1846, *1847*
Kveim-Siltzbach test, 531
Kyphosis, 379

La/SSB/Ha antigen, 699–700
Lachman test, 1744
Lacrimal gland, in Sjögren's syndrome, 956, 957t
Lactic acid assay, in septic arthritis, 1514
Lambda chain germ line genes, 14
Lamina splendens, 260
Lasègue's test, 451–452
Lateral band syndrome, 1746, *1746*
Latex fixation reaction, for rheumatoid factor, *665*
Lathyrism, 225–226, *226*
LE cell, in juvenile rheumatoid arthritis, 1257
Leg, lower, pain syndromes in, 1748–1749
stress fracture in, 1748
tennis, 1749

Leg length discrepancy, 381
Legg-Calvé-Perthes disease, osteoarthritis in, 1440
Lepra reaction, 1181
Leprosy, lepromatous, 306
  peripheral neuropathy in, 309–310
Lerner-Steitz method, *703*
Lesch-Nyhan syndrome, uric acid production in, 1378
Leukemia, hairy cell, vasculitis and, 1140
  juvenile rheumatoid arthritis vs., 1261
  musculoskeletal manifestations of, 1605
  septic arthritis in, 1507–1508
  uric acid nephropathy in, 1368
Leukocyte, aspirin effects on, 741
  cytotoxic agents and, 844, *844*
  in synovial fluid, 563–564, *564*
  in synovitis, 403, *406*
  migration of, nonsteroidal anti-inflammatory drugs and, 755
  polymorphonuclear, platelet interaction with, 177, *178*
  urate crystal inflammatory response and, 1381–1382
Leukocytoclastic vasculitis, 1149–1153. See also *Vasculitis, hypersensitivity.*
Leukopenia, in gold therapy, 803
  in systemic lupus erythematosus, 1090, 1107
Leukotriene, formation of, 74–75, *75*
  functions of, 75–76
  in inflammation, 76–78
  urate crystal inflammatory response and, 1381
Leupeptin, for cathepsin B, 184
Levamisole, 849–850, 853t
LGP–1, in boundary lubrication of cartilage, 1424
Lichen amyloidosis, 1478
Lifting, biomechanics of, 323–324, *323–324*, 331–332
Ligament, in joint stability, 258, 317–318, *318*
Light chain, 7
  in origin of amyloid deposits, 1471–1472, 1472t
  subgroups of, 8t
Light chain genes, 63
Limb girdle muscular dystrophy, polymyositis vs, 1234
Lipid, bioactive, macrophage secretion of, 156–157, 156t–157t
Lipocyte, in avascular necrosis, 1693
Lipolysis, *3*
Lipoma, of synovium, 1711, *1712*
Lipoma arborescens, 1711, *1712*
Little league elbow, 1739
Livedo reticularis, in polyarteritis, *1144*
  in systemic lupus erythematosus, 538, 1075
Liver. See *Hepatic manifestations.*
Löfgren's syndrome, 1490
London elbow prosthesis, 1847, *1848*
Long-leg syndrome, 1777
Loose body, arthroscopy of, 646
Looser zone, 1664, *1664*
Low back pain, 448–468
  advances in, 448–449
  anatomy and pain sources in, *449*, 449–450

Low back pain *(Continued)*
  biomechanics in, 331–332
  clinical evaluation of, 449–458
  computed tomography in, 454, *458*, 631–632, *632*
  degenerative disc disease in, 458–462, 458t, *459–461*
  disc space infection in, 463
  discography in, 453
  epidurography in, 454
  examination in, 380
  facet block in, 458
  hydatid disease of bone in, 464
  in pregnancy, 1590
  incidence and disability in, 448
  laboratory examination in, 452
  lumbar epidural venography in, 454, *457*
  mechanical relationships in, 450, 451t
  myelography in, 453–454, *455–456*
  nerve root infiltration in, 454, 458
  neurologic findings in, 451, 451t
  nonorganic, 380
  nonspinal sources of, 465
  nontubercular granulomatous infections in, 463
  of various origins, characteristics of, 450t
  physical examination in, 450–452, 451t
  plain radiography in, 452–453
  presenting complaints in, 450, 450t
  psychologic evaluation in, 452
  pyogenic vertebral osteomyelitis in, 463
  scintigraphy in, *615*
  spondylolysis and spondylolisthesis in, 464–465, 464t
  straight leg raising test in, 451
  syphilitic spondylitis in, 464
  systemic inflammatory disease in, 462–463
  tests for malingering in, 452
  thermography in, 630
  tuberculosis of spine in, 463–464
Lower motor neuron disorder, differentiation of, 427t
  upper vs, 426t
Lubrication. See *Joint, lubrication of.*
Lubricin, 264
Ludington's sign, 442
Lungs. See *Pulmonary manifestations.*
Lupus anticoagulant, 1090–1091, 1091t
Lupus band test, 538, *538*, 1059, 1119
Lupus erythematosus, discoid, 537
    antimalarials in, 778–779
    malignancy and, 1610
  subacute cutaneous, 537
  systemic, 1042–1115
    acute phase response in, 661
    American Rheumatism Association criteria for, 1072t
    anti-Ro/SSA in, 699t
    antimalarials in, 779–780
    antinuclear antibody in, 691–693, 693t
    avascular necrosis in, 1691–1692
    B-lymphocyte alloantisera in, 51t
    butterfly rash in, 537, *537*, 573, *573*, 1073, 1100
    cardiac manifestations of, 1087–1088, 1106–1107
    central nervous system in, 1083–1087, 1104–1106
    classification of, 1093t

Lupus erythematosus, systemic *(Continued)*
    corneal and conjunctival lesions in, 523
    cotton wool spots in, 522, *522–523*
    cutaneous manifestations of, *537–538*, 537–539, 1073–1077, *1074–1076*
    cytoid bodies in, 522
    diagnosis and differential diagnosis of, 1093–1094
    discoid lesions in, 1074, *1075*, 1100
    etiology of, 1042–1053
      animal models in, 1043–1044, 1044t, 1049–1050
      antilymphocyte antibody in, 1052–1053, 1052t
      autoantibody production in, 1042–1043, 1043t
      autoimmune, 1047–1050
      B-lymphocyte function in, 1051
      environmental, 1047
      genetic, 1045–1047
      hormonal, 1047
      humoral and cellular immunity in, 1050–1051
      immunologic, 1050
      lymphocyte enumeration in, 1051
      natural killer cell function in, 1052
      T-lymphocyte function in, 1051–1052
      viral, 1044–1045
    gastrointestinal manifestations of, 1081–1082
    hand in, reconstructive surgery for, 1833–1837, *1834–1835*
    hematologic abnormalities in, 1090–1091, 1107
    immune complexes in, 688
    in children, 1293–1298
      clinical considerations in, 1293–1295, *1294*, 1294t–1295t
      clinical course and prognosis in, 1296–1297
      laboratory findings in, 1295–1296
      treatment in, 1297–1298
    in pregnancy, 1590
    in septic arthritis, 1507, *1508*
    incidence and prevalence of, 1070–1071
    juvenile rheumatoid arthritis vs., 1263
    liver disease in, 1082
    lupus band test in, 538, *538*
    lymph nodes in, 1083
    malignancy and, 1610
    management of, 1098–1115
      antimalarials in, 1110
      cardiac involvement in, 1106–1107
      central nervous system involvement in, 1104–1106
      corticosteroids in, 1108–1110
      experimental therapy in, 1112–1113
      hematologic involvement in, 1107
      immunization in, 1112
      immunosuppressants in, 1110–1111
      in children, 1111–1112
      infection in, 1103
      kidney involvement in, 1103–1104
      lung involvement in, 1106
      major organ vs. nonmajor organ involvement and, 1099–1100
      marriage and pregnancy in, 1107–1108
      nonmajor organ symptoms and, 1100–1101

Lupus erythematosus, systemic, management of *(Continued)*
prognostic factors in, 1101–1102
sun exposure in, 1098–1099
menstrual abnormalities in, 1090
mixed cryoglobulins and, 1345–1346
neutrophil in, 131–133
ocular manifestations in, 521–523, *522–523*, 1083
overlap, 1101, 1116
parotid glands in, 1083
pathogenesis of, 1053–1062
cell membrane antibody in, 1060
central nervous system in, 1060–1062
complement in, 1055
dermal manifestations of, 1059–1060
immune complexes and cryoglobulins in, 1056–1057
nephritis in, 1055
renal immunoreactants in, 1057–1059
reticuloendothelial system in, 1056
serum antigens and antibodies in, 1055–1056
pleuropulmonary manifestations in, 1088–1089, 1106
precipitating factors in, 1091–1092, 1092t
pregnancy and, 1090, 1107–1108
preoperative evaluation in, 1789
psychological factors in, 1060–1062, 1084t, 1105
race and sex in, 1070–1071
radiography in, 585, *585*
rehabilitation in, 1783
renal disease in, 1077–1080, 1078t, 1103–1104. See also *Nephritis, lupus.*
retinopathy in, 522–523, *522–523*
rheumatoid arthritis vs., 923
spleen in, 1082–1083
systemic symptoms of, 1071–1073
thymus in, 1083
vascular manifestations of, 1080–1081, *1081*
vasculitis in, 1148–1149
Lupus nephritis, in children, 1294, 1296
Lupus pernio, 542
Lupus profundus, 538, 1181
in systemic lupus erythematosus, 1075
Lupuslike syndrome, malignancy and, 1607
Lyme disease, 1557–1563
clinical characteristics of, 1557–1558, *1558–1559*, 1558t
cryoglobulinemia and, 1347
differential diagnosis of, 1562
epidemiology in, 1560–1561
pathogenesis and laboratory findings in, 1558–1560
rheumatoid arthritis vs., 924
spirochetal disease vs., 1561–1562
treatment of, 1562–1563
Lymph node, in systemic lupus erythematosus, 1082–1083
mucocutaneous, syndrome of, 1161
structure of, 24, *24*
total radiation therapy of, 847
Lymphangiectasia, intestinal, 1332
Lymphapheresis, 846
Lymphocytapheresis, 845
Lymphocyte, B, *30*, 30–31, 834, *834*
activation of, 31
assay methods for, 32–33
differentiation of, 16–18
allelic exclusion in, 17
gene rearrangements in, 16–17
heavy chain switching in, 17–18
isotype exculsion in, 18
transcription processing in, 17
in rheumatoid synovium, 895
in systemic lupus erythematosus, 1051
maturation of, *30*, 30–31
subpopulations of, 31
in angiogenesis, 204
infiltrates, in Sjögren's syndrome, 968–969
loss of, 1332
migration and homing of, *23–24*, 23–25
null, 32
recirculation of, 23, *23*
T, 25–30, 834, *834*
antigen receptor genetics in, 65
assay methods for, 32–33
cloning of, 29
helper-cytotoxic interactions of, *27*, 27–28
in rheumatoid synovium, 895
in systemic lupus erythematosus, 1051–1052
lymphokines, 29–30, 29t
maturation of, 25, *26*
receptor for, 29
regulatory circuits of, *28*, 28–29
role of, 1320
soluble mediators of, 29–30, 29t
subpopulations of, 25–27, 26t–27t
suppressor, 28
suppressor pathway activation by, *28*, 28–29
Lymphocyte activating factor, 192
Lymphoid irradiation, in rheumatoid arthritis, 989
Lymphoid tissue, gut-associated, 1032
Lymphokine, in rheumatoid synovium, 895–896
T lymphocyte, 29–30, 29t
Lymphoma, musculoskeletal manifestations of, 1605
Lymphomatoid granulomatosis, 1158–1159
malignancy and, 1614
Lymphopenia, in systemic lupus erythematosus, 1051
Lymphoplasmapheresis, 845
Lymphoproliferation, in Sjögren's syndrome, 970–972, 971t–972t, *972*
Lymphoreticular neoplasia, in Sjögren's syndrome, 970–972, 971t–972t, *972*
Lypodystrophy, in diabetes mellitus, 1581
Lysinonorleucine, in elastin, *221*, 229
Lysosomal enzyme, glycosaminoglycan and, 248
urate crystal inflammation and, 1382
Lysosomal sulfatase, in GAG desulfation, 244
Lysosomal system, in collagen degradation, 189
Lysosome, neutrophil degranulation and, 122–124, 122t, *123*
Lysozyme, cartilage, 1420
macrophage secretion of, 154
Ma antigen, 700
MacIntosh hemiarthroplasty, 1963–1964
alpha$_2$-Macroglobulin, in proteinase inhibition, 187
Macroglobulinemia, Waldenström's, 1340–1341
peripheral neuropathy in, 308
Macrophage, activation of, 162
antigens of, 148
antimicrobial functions of, 158–159
antitumor functions of, 159–160
congregation of inflammatory sites in, 150–152
chemotaxis in, 151–152, 151t
retention and, 152
skin window model of, 150–151
sticking and spreading in, 151
tissue migration in, 151
immunoregulatory functions of, 160
in angiogenesis, 204
in embryonic joint, 255
in rheumatoid synovium, 900
origin of, 145
phagocytosis by, 152–153
metabolism during, 152–153, *153*
recognition and attachment in, 152
triggering of ingestion in, 152
plasma membrane of, 147
secretions of, 153–158, *154*, 154t–158t
selective removal of autologous cells by, 160–161
structure of, 147
Macule, 533
Maduromycosis, 1532
Main en lorgnette, 377
Major histocompatibility complex, 36–54
determinants defined by lymphocyte responses to, 42–45
disease associations of, 49–53
ethnic relationships and, 51–52, *52*
genetics in, 50, *50*
historical, 49–50
hypothetical mechanisms of, 52–53
procedural methods in, 50–51, 51t
rheumatic, 52
gene product classes of, 36, *37*, 37t
genes of, 55–61
historical aspects of, 36–38
homozygous typing cells in, 45, *45*
human vs. mouse, *56*
immune response genes of, 55–61. See also *Ir gene*.
mixed lymphocyte culture reaction to, 44–45
serologic analysis of, 40–42
class I allodeterminant typing in, 42
class I and II alloantigen typing in, 42
HLA specificities in, 41
practical aspects of, 42
serologic specificity in, 40–41
statistical analysis in, 41–42
Major immunogene complex, 37
Malignancy. See also individual types.
complicating treatment, 1614
musculoskeletal syndromes associated with, 1603–1619
pre–existing connective tissue disease and, 1609–1614, 1610t, *1611–1613*
Malignant hyperthermia syndrome, 487

Mallet toe, 388
Malnutrition, hypoalbuminemic, 353
nutritional intervention in, 356
prognosis and, 356
protein-calorie, 353
surveys of, 355–356
Malum coxae senilis, *1439*, 1439–1440
Manubriosternal joint, examination of, 372–373
rheumatoid arthritis of, 930
Marasmus, 353
Marble bone disease, 1673–1674, *1674*
March foot, 390
Marfan's syndrome, 1624–1628
asthenic vs. nonasthenic, 1626–1627
classic (asthenic), 1625–1626
homocystinuria vs., 1627–1628, 1627t
Marfanoid hypermobility syndrome, 1627
Marginal erosion, in rheumatoid arthritis, 571, *571*
Marie–Strümpell disease. See *Ankylosing spondylitis*.
Mast cell, angiogenesis and, 201, *203*
in bone resorption, 274
in embryonic joint, 255
Mayaro virus, 1547
Mayo elbow prosthesis, 1846, *1846*
Mayo total ankle prosthesis, *1968*
McArdle's disease, polymyositis vs., 1234
McKeever hemiarthroplasty, 1963–1964, *1965*
McMurray test, 385, 1742
Median nerve, 1754–1758, *1757–1758*
course and distribution of, *1757*
double crush syndrome of, 1758
innervation by, 1754, 1760t
tests of, 420t
Mediterranean fever, familial, 1482
amyloidosis in, 1477
rheumatoid arthritis vs., 923
Melasma, 1590
Membrane attack component, *Neisseria* infection and, 1355–1356
Meningitis, in mixed connective tissue disease, 1124, 1126t
Meningococcal arthritis, 1519
Meningoencephalitis, in Behçet's disease, 1175
Meniscus, injury of, 385–386, 625, *625*
arthrography in, 1742, *1742–1743*
arthroscopy in, 645–646
Menkes, arthropathy of, 1413
Menkes' kinky hair syndrome, 1639–1640
Menstruation, in systemic lupus erythematosus, 1090
Meralgia paresthetica, 1766–1767, *1767*
6–Mercaptopurine, 841–842, 842t
pharmacologic properties of, 852t
Merodesmosine crosslink, in elastin, 229, *229*
Meromysin, light and heavy, 290
Mesenchymal tumor, osteomalacia in, 1669
Mesenchyme, synovial, 255
Metabolic bone disease, 1645–1687. See also individual types.
bone biopsy and microanatomy in, 1648–1649, *1648–1649*
clinical evaluation of, 1645–1649
history and physical examination in, 1645
Metabolic bone disease *(Continued)*
radiology in, 1647–1648
serum alkaline phosphatase in, 1646
serum calcium in, 1645–1646
serum inorganic phosphate in, 1646
serum parathyroid hormone in, 1647
signs and symptoms of, 1646t
urinary calcium excretion in, 1646
urinary hydroxyproline excretion in, 1647
urinary phosphate excretion in, 1646–1647
vitamin D metabolite assays in, 1647
Metacarpal, in Albright's hereditary osteodystrophy, 1584, *1586*
Metacarpal head, dot-dash pattern in, 573
Metacarpal index, in Marfan's syndrome, 1625
Metacarpophalangeal joint, arthroplasty of, 1824–1827, *1825*
prosthetic implants in, *1825*, 1825–1826
results of, *1826*, 1826–1827
corticosteroid in, 555, *555*
examination of, *376–377*, 376–378
in hemochromatosis, 1497, *1497*
in rheumatoid arthritis, 934–935, *934–935*
in systemic lupus erythematosus, 1833, *1835*
Jaccoud deformity of, 1282
muscles of, 378
prostheses for, 1968–1971, *1970*
reconstructive and salvage surgery for, 1824–1827, *1826*
synovectomy of, *1798*, 1798–1800, *1808–1809*, 1808–1810
ulnar deviation of, 1824, *1825*
Metalloproteinase, 185–187, *186*
endogenous inhibition of, 188
Metaphyseal artery, 282, *283*
Metastatic carcinoma, avascular necrosis in, 1691
Metastatic disease, presenting as musculoskeletal syndrome, 1604–1605, 1604t
Metatarsal compression test, 474, *475*
Metatarsal head excision, multiple, 1905–1906, *1906*
single, 1905
Metatarsal osteotomy, 1904–1905, *1904–1905*
Metatarsalgia, 390
Metatarsophalangeal joint, corticosteroid in, 556
examination of, 389
in osteoarthritis, 1441, 1456
in rheumatoid arthritis, 937, *938*
muscles in, 389
Methotrexate, 842–843
in rheumatoid arthritis, 989
pharmacologic properties of, 852t
Methyl methacrylate, in total hip replacement, 1941–1942
3–Methylhistidine, urinary, 708
Methylprednisolone, chemical structure of, *816*
$\beta_2$-Microglobulin, 7, 7–8, 8t
Micrognathia, in juvenile rheumatoid arthritis, 1254, *1255*
Microvascular abnormalities, in mixed connective tissue disease, 1129, *1130–1132*
Microwave heat, therapeutic, 1774, 1774t
Milkman fracture, 1664, *1664*
Milwaukee shoulder, 1413, 1427, 1860
Minnesota Multiphasic Personality Inventory, 452
Mithramycin, in Paget's disease of bone, 1682–1683
Mitochondrial antibody, in Sjögren's syndrome, 967
Mitral valve, in rheumatic heart disease, 1281
Mixed connective tissue disease, 1116–1133
autoimmune associations in, 1124–1125
clinical picture in, 1119–1120
counterimmunoelectrophoresis in, 1117, *1119*
course and prognosis in, 1126–1127, 1127t
cutaneous manifestations of, 539
general features of, 1120
hematologic manifestations in, 1125–1126
histologic microvascular abnormalities in, 1129, *1130–1132*
historical evolution of, 1117
immune complexes in, 688
immunopathology in, 1127–1129
anti-RNP antibody in, 1117–1119, 1118t
antigen for, 1127–1128, *1128*
immunoregulatory dysfunction in, 1128–1129
reticuloendothelial dysfunction in, 1129
in children, 1126
Ouchterlony double immunodiffusion analysis in, 1117, *1119*
pregnancy in, 1126
presenting features and evolution of, 1120, *1120*
radiography in, 587
rheumatoid arthritis vs., 923
serologic features of, 1117–1119, *1119*
Sjögren's syndrome with, 1124
specific organ involvement in, 1120–1124, *1121–1126*
treatment of, 1132–1133, 1133t
Monoarticular arthritis, 391–400
age and sex in, 394
algorithm in diagnosis of, 393t
anatomic localization of, 394
articular vs. periarticular involvement in, 394, 395t
confirmed diagnosis in, 399
crystal-induced, 397–398
definition of, 391
diagnostic spectrum in, 391–392
diagnostic urgency in, 392
diseases in, 391t
immediate management of, 396–398
initial history and examination in, 392–396
joint fluid examination in, 396, 397t
laboratory studies in, 396, 398t
nonspecific inflammatory, 398
precipitating factors in, 392–394
reassessment in, 399
roentgenographic and radioisotopic findings in, 396, 398t
septic, 397
symptoms of, 394–395

Monoarticular arthritis *(Continued)*
systemic features of, 395–396, 396t
type of onset of, 394
unconfirmed diagnosis in, 399
undiagnosed, 399–400
Monoclonal antibody, 48, 848
Monoclonal dysproteinemia, 1338–1343
Monoclonal gammopathy, idiopathic, 1342–1343
Monoclonal rheumatoid factor binding inhibition assay, 685, *685*
Monocyte, 49
circulation of, 145
marrow progenitor of, 145
Monocyte-macrophage system, functions of, 834
Mononuclear phagocyte, life cycle of, 145–150
Mononeuritis multiplex, 307
in polyarteritis, 1144
Mononeuropathy, peripheral, 305
Mononuclear cell factor, 192
Monosodium urate crystal, polarized light microscopy for, 565
Morbus coxae senilis, *1439*, 1439–1440
Morning stiffness, in patient history, 370
Morphea, 541, 1206–1209, *1207–1208*
in children, 1303–1305, *1304*
Morton's toe, 390
Motion limitation, in patient examination, 371
in patient history, 369
Motor endplate, 291, *291*
Motor nerve, conduction study of, 709, *709*
origin of, 295
Motor unit, anatomy of, 287, *288*
fast twitch, 287
pharmacology of, 294
physiology of, 291–292
slow twitch, 287
Mu heavy-chain disease, 1342
Mucin clot test, 567
Mucinosis, papular, 1478
Muckle-Wells amyloid nephropathy, 1477
Mucocutaneous candidiasis, chronic, 1331–1332
Mucocutaneous lesions, in Reiter's syndrome, *1012–1014*, 1013–1014, 1013t
Mucocutaneous lymph node syndrome, 1161
in children, 1309–1310
Mucoid edema, in rheumatic heart disease, 1280
Mucopolysaccharidosis, glycosaminoglycan degradation in, 245–247, *246*
Mucous cyst, 1832, *1832*
Multifidus muscle, 449
Mumps, 1548–1550
Murmur, cardiac, in rheumatic heart disease, 1283
in systemic lupus erythematosus, 1088
Muscle, contraction of, biochemistry of, *292*, 292–293
energy metabolism in, 293, *293–294*
fiber types of, 712–715, 713t, *714*
in joint stability, 257–258
in rheumatoid arthritis, 938
inflammatory disease of, 1225–1245. See also *Dermatomyositis; Polymyositis.*
sarcoidosis of, 1491–1492
Muscle *(Continued)*
smooth, antibody for, 967
weakness of, 410–415
contracture in, 413
examination in, 412–415
family history in, 412
history of present illness in, 411
in cervical spine disorders, 426
in dermatomyositis-polymyositis, 1228t
in neck pain, 422
inspection in, 412–413
muscle strength testing in, 413–415
palpation in, 413
past history in, 411–412
peripheral nervous system exam in, 414–415
systematic inquiry in, 411
Muscle biopsy, 712–715, 713t, *714*
in systemic lupus erythematosus, 1073
Muscle dynamometry, 414
Muscle enzyme, serum, 708
Muscle fiber, 287, *288*
ultrastructure of, *289–290*, 290–291
Muscle strength testing, 386, 413–415
Muscular dystrophy, polymyositis vs., 1233–1234
Musculocutaneous nerve, tests of, 420t
Musculoskeletal pain syndrome, psychogenic, 486–487
Myalgia, benign, 402
diffuse, 401–402
in mixed connective tissue disease, 1122
in systemic lupus erythematosus, 1073
Myasthenia gravis, in Sjögren's syndrome, 964
polymyositis vs., 1233
Mycobacterial infection, 1527–1532
atypical, 1530–1532, 1531t
tuberculous, 1527–1530
Mycoplasmal infection, in animal models of rheumatoid arthritis, 883
in rheumatoid arthritis, 881–882
Mycotic infection, 1532–1537. See also individual types.
Myelin sheath, structural characteristics of, 299–300, *303*
Myelinopathy, mechanism of, *300*
Myelography, in low back pain, 453–454, *455–456*
Myeloma, multiple, 1338–1340
amyloidosis-associated, 1476
peripheral neuropathy in, 308
septic arthritis in, 1507–1508
osteosclerotic, peripheral neuropathy in, 308
Myeloma cell, in bone resorption, 274
Myocardial infarction, in systemic lupus erythematosus, 1087–1088
Myocarditis, in mixed connective tissue disease, 1122–1123, 1129, *1132*
in rheumatic heart disease, 1281
in rheumatoid arthritis, 941
in systemic lupus erythematosus, 1087
Myofibril, 290
Myoglobin, urinary, 708
Myointimal cell, 1188–1189
Myopathy, electromyography in, 711–712
in hyperparathyroidism, 1581–1582
in scleroderma, 1192
Myopathy *(Continued)*
vacuolar, in systemic lupus erythematosus, 1073
Myophosphorylase deficiency, polymyositis vs., 1234
Myosin, 288–290, *289*
Myositis, 362–363, 362t
bacterial pyogenic, 1238
focal nodular, 1238–1239
giant cell, 1239, *1239*
in children, 1303
in scleroderma, 1192, 1200
in Sjögren's syndrome, 964
in systemic lupus erythematosus, 1073, 1101
Myxedema, osteoarthritis in, 1445
pretibial, in Graves' disease, 1586
Myxedematous arthropathy, 1587, *1587*
Myxoma, atrial, 923

Nail lesions, in psoriatic arthritis, 1023, *1023*
in Reiter's syndrome, 1014, *1014*
in systemic lupus erythematosus, 1076, *1076*
Nailfold capillary pattern, in mixed connective tissue disease, 1129, *1131*
in scleroderma, 1187, *1188*
Naproxen, 766, *766*
in gouty arthritis, 1384
in juvenile rheumatoid arthritis, 1266
Nasal chondritis, 1459
Nasal mucosal ulceration, in systemic lupus erythematosus, 1076
Natural killer cells, 895
Neck. See also *Spine, cervical.*
anatomy and biomechanics of, *417–419*, 417–421
blood supply to, 421
nerve root compression in, 418–420
pain in, 416–435
algorithm for clinical evaluation in, 433, *433*
cervical spine syndromes in, 416t
clinical evaluation of, 421–429
clinical examination in, 423–425
differential diagnosis of, 429–434
history and symptoms in, 422–423
structures causing, 416t
treatment of, 434–435
palpation of, 423
range of motion of, 424–425
referred pain in, 418, *421*
soft tissue of, examination of, 424
Necrobiosis lipoidica diabeticorum, 1581
Necrosis, aseptic. See *Avascular necrosis.*
avascular. See *Avascular necrosis.*
Necrotizing arteritis, 534, *534*
Necrotizing vasculitis, 1137–1166
classification of, 1137–1139, 1138t
cutaneous manifestations of, *539*, 539–540
diseases simulating, 1141, 1141t
in children, 1306–1311, 1306t
malignancy and, 1607, *1607*
Necrotizing venulitis, 535, *535*
*Neisseria*, membrane attack component deficiency and, 1355–1356

*Neisseria gonorrhoeae*, in arthritis, 1516–1519, *1517*
*Neisseria meningitidis*, in arthritis, 1519
Neovascularization, 198–209. See also *Angiogenesis; Capillary.*
Nephritis, acute allergic interstitial, with nonsteroidal anti-inflammatory drugs, 763
in polyarticular arthritis, 409
lupus, 1055
immunoreactants in, 1057–1059
management of, 1103–1104
membranous, 1079
mesangial (minimal), 1079
mild (focal), 1077–1078
pathologic index of activity and sclerosis in, 1079–1080
progression in, 1080
severe (diffuse), 1078–1079
Nephrolithiasis, calcium, 496
in gout, 1371t
in hyperuricemia, 491
in probenecid use, 860
uric acid, 496, 1368–1371
xanthine, in allopurinol use, 865–866
Nephropathy, amyloid familial, 1477
analgesic, aspirin in, 743–744
nonsteroidal anti-inflammatory drugs and, 763
urate, 491, 495
in gout, 1366–1367, *1367*
uric acid, 491, 496, 1367–1368
Nephrotic syndrome, in gold therapy, 803
penicillamine causing, 811, *812*
Nerve, compression of, acute, 310–313, 418–421. See also individual types.
entrapment of, 1754–1768
mechanical injuries of, 310–313
repetitive stimulation of, 712
Nerve biopsy, 715
Nerve conduction study, motor, 709
sensory, 709–710
Nerve entrapment syndrome. See *Neuropathy, entrapment*.
Nerve growth factor, transport of, 298
Nerve root compression, in neck pain, 418–421
Nerve root infiltration, in low back pain, 454, 458
Nerve stimulation, repetitive, 712
Nerve trunk, gross structure of, 295, *296*
Nervous system, of joints, 259
Neurapraxia, 310
nerve fiber lesion in, 297
Neuritis, brachial, 445
optic, 1168–1169, *1169*
Neuroarthropathy, radiography in, 594–595, *595*
Neurologic manifestations, in ankylosing spondylitis, 999
in Lyme disease, 1557, *1559*
in mixed connective tissue disease, 1124, 1126t
in polyarteritis, 1143
in polyarticular arthritis, 410
in systemic lupus erythematosus, 1060–1062, *1061–1062*, 1083–1087, 1104–1106
Neuroma, interdigital, 390
Neuromuscular disease, diagnostic tests in, 707–716
electrophysiologic studies in, 709–712
in rheumatoid arthritis, 938
in rheumatologic disease, 708t
muscle damage screening in, 708–709
pathological studies in, 712–715
Neuromuscular junction, 291, *291*
Neuronopathy, alanosine in, *300*
doxorubicin in, *300*
Neuropathic arthropathy, in feet, 471
in osteoarthritis, 1425, 1444, 1444t, *1445*
Neuropathy, amyloid familial, 1476–1477
electromyography in, 711
entrapment, 1754–1768
axillary, 445–446
differential diagnosis in, 1756t
electrodiagnostic studies in, 1757t
features associated with various nerves in, 1755t
in lower limb, 1762–1767, *1763–1767*
in upper limb, 1754–1762, *1757–1762*
lumbar root, 458–459, 460–462
peripheral nerves in, 1755t
suprascapular, 446
in diabetes mellitus, 1581
in Sjögren's syndrome, 964
peripheral, 303–306
sarcoid, 309
Neuropsychiatric disorders, in systemic lupus erythematosus, 1060–1062, 1084t
Neurotmesis, 311
Neurovascular disease, in rheumatoid arthritis, 940–941
Neutrophil, abnormalities of, in human disease, 130–131, 131t–132t
complement receptors of, 119t, 120–121
degranulation of, 122–124, 122t, *123*
extracellular release of lysosomal constituents of, *123*, 123–124
immunoglobulin receptors of, 119–120, 119t
in rheumatic syndromes, 133–135
in rheumatoid arthritis, 133
in systemic lupus erythematosus, 131–133
oxidative metabolism of, 124–128, *125–126*, 126t
platelet interaction with, 177, *178*
Nevus, epidermal, 1669
Nitrogen mustard, 839
in systemic lupus erythematosus, 1110
pharmacologic properties of, 852t
NK cells, 895
in systemic lupus erythematosus, 1052
Nodular lung disease, in rheumatoid arthritis, 941
Nodular myositis, focal, 1238–1239
Nodule, 533
Aschoff, 1280
in reticulohistiocytosis, 1502, *1503*
needle punch biopsy of, 557–558, *558*
pulmonary, 408, 941
rheumatoid. See *Rheumatoid nodule*.
subcutaneous, in hyperuricemia, 490–491
in rheumatic fever, 1281, *1283*, 1283–1284
Nonsteroidal anti-inflammatory drugs, 752–773
analgesic effects of, 756
anti-inflammatory effects of, 752–755
chemical groupings and trade names of, 753t
clinical effects of, 753, 759–761, 769–770
fever suppression by, 756–757
immunologic effects of, 755–756
in ankylosing spondylitis, 761
in dysmenorrhea, 761
in hemophilia, 1570
in ischemic heart disease, 761
in juvenile rheumatoid arthritis, 1266
in osteoarthritis, 761, 1453
in rheumatoid arthritis, 760–761, 770
interchangeableness of, 769–770
leukocyte migration and, 755
mechanisms of action of, 752–757
pharmacokinetics of, 757–759, 757t
absorption and bioavailability in, 757–758
blood levels in, 758
clearance rate in, 758–759
duration of action in, 759t
metabolic clearance in, 758
steady-state concentrations in, 759
prostaglandin synthesis inhibition by, 78–79, 753–754
side effects of, 761–764
anticoagulant interaction as, 764
gastrointestinal, 761–762
hepatotoxicity as, 762
pancreatitis as, 762
pregnancy and, 763–764
pseudoallergic, 763
renal, 762–763
toxic oxygen radicals and, 754–755
types of, 764–768
nRNP antigen, 698–699
Nuclear imaging, 609–611, *610–611*
methods and devices for, 611
Nucleic acid, catabolism of, 341
Nucleoside, chemical structure of, *338*
Nucleus pulposus, herniated, 454, *455*
Nutritional assessment, 352, 353t
abbreviated, 353
laboratory studies in, 353
Nutritional requirements, 356–357
energy, 356–357
in osteoarthritis, 1450
protein, 357
Nutritional therapy, 357–358
fatty acids for, 359
prostaglandins for, 358–359

O'nyong–nyong virus, 1547
Obesity, in gout, 359, 1364
in osteoarthritis, 359, 1426–1427, 1450
Occipital horn syndrome, 1633–1634
Occipital neuralgia, in cervical spine disorders, 423
Occiput-to-wall measurement, 380–381
Occupational therapy, for elbow, 1853
in juvenile rheumatoid arthritis, 1268–1269

Occupational therapy *(Continued)*
in rheumatoid arthritis, 984–985
Ochronosis, calcium pyrophosphate deposition disease in, 1404
osteoarthritis in, 1441–1443
radiography in, 600
synovial biopsy in, 651
Ocular manifestations, 511–532
in amyloidosis, 531
in ankylosing spondylitis, 521, 998
in cervical spine disorders, 423
in connective tissue disease, 523
in enteropathic arthropathy, 526–529, *528*
in giant cell arteritis, 524, *525–526*, 1168–1169, *1169*
in gout, 531–532
in juvenile rheumatoid arthritis, 517–521, *520*
in polychondritis, 1459–1460
in Reiter's syndrome, 1011–1013, 1015
in relapsing polychondritis, 526
in rheumatic fever, 512
in rheumatoid arthritis, 512–517, *513–519*
in sarcoidosis, *529–530*, 529–531, 1488
in Sjögren's syndrome, 956–957, 956t–958t, *957*
in systemic lupus erythematosus, 521–523, *522–523*, 1083
in Wegener's granulomatosis, 526, *527*
Olecranon bursa, 374
tophi of, *1364*
Olecranon bursitis, 1739–1740
corticosteroid in, 551
Oligoarthritis, in juvenile rheumatoid arthritis, 1250, *1250–1251*
Oligosaccharide, in proteoglycan, 241
Onycholysis, in Graves' disease, 1586
Opera-glass hand, 377
Ophthalmologic test, in cervical spine disorders, 426
Optic neuritis, ischemic, in giant cell arteritis, 1168–1169, *1169*
Oral cavity, amyloidosis of, 1480
Oral contraceptive arthritis, rheumatoid arthritis vs., 922
Oral ulceration, in systemic lupus erythematosus, 1076
Orbit, edema of, in systemic lupus erythematosus, 1076
pseudotumor of, 1219
Organic brain syndrome, in systemic lupus erythematosus, 1085
Orotic acid, 867
Orotic aciduria, 1323
Orthotics, 1776–1780, 1791
lower extremity, 1776–1778, *1777*
spinal, 1779–1780
upper extremity, 1778–1779, *1778–1779*
Osler's nodes, 1181
Osseous sarcoidosis, 1491
Ossicle, intra-articular, 1713–1714, *1714*
Ossicles of ear, rheumatoid arthritis of, 930
Osteitis condensans ilii, in ankylosing spondylitis, 999, *1001*
Osteitis deformans, 1676. See also *Paget's disease of bone*.
Osteoarthritis, aging in, 1425–1426
apatite crystal in, 1443–1444

Osteoarthritis *(Continued)*
calcium pyrophosphate deposition disease in, 1403, 1427–1428, 1443–1444
cartilage changes in, 1421–1428. See also *Cartilage, osteoarthritic*.
classification of, 1432, 1432t
clinical features of, 1433–1436, 1433t
correction of excessive joint loading in, 1449–1450
corticosteroid in, 550
costovertebral, radiography in, 592
deposition diseases of cartilage in, 1427–1428
diet in, 1450
drug therapy in, 1452–1454
elbow in, 1838
epidemiology in, 1432–1433
erosive, 1438
etiology of, 1423–1428
Heberden's nodes in, 1436–1437, *1437*
heredity in, 1426
historical, 1432
in acromegaly, 1588–1589, *1588–1589*
in apophyseal joint, radiography in, 591
in avascular (aseptic) necrosis, 1445
in carpometacarpal and metatarsophalangeal joints, 1441
in diabetes mellitus, 1580
in endocrine disorders, 1445
in feet, 469–471, 1456
in glenohumeral joint, *443*, 443–444, 1857, *1860*
in hand, reconstructive surgery for, 1832–1833
treatment of, 1455
in hemochromatosis, 1443
in hemophilic arthropathy, 1445
in hip, *1439*, 1439–1440
treatment of, 1455
in intra-articular corticosteroid injection, 1444–1445
in Kashin-Beck disease, 1445
in knee, 1440, *1441*
treatment of, 1455–1456
in metabolic disease, 1441–1444
in neuropathic joint disease, 1444, *1445*
in ochronosis, 1441–1443
in Paget's disease, 1444
in spine, 1440–1441, *1442*
treatment of, 1456
in Wilson's disease, 1443
inflammatory, radiography in, 590, *590*
inflammatory joint disease in, 1427
joint surface incongruity in, 1427
management of, 1448–1458
neuropathic joint degeneration in, 1425
nonsteroidal anti-inflammatory drugs in, 761
obesity and, 359, 1426–1427
osteophytes in, 1435
patellofemoral, total knee replacement in, 1878
pathogenesis of, 1417–1431
pathology of, 1434–1436, *1436–1437*
physical therapy in, 1451–1452
premature, chrondrocalcinosis in, 1414
primary, 1436–1441
generalized, 1437–1438
psychological coping in, 1450–1451

Osteoarthritis *(Continued)*
radiography in, 587–594, *588–594*, 1434, *1434–1435*, 1435t
rehabilitation in, 1780–1781
rheumatoid arthritis vs, 924–925, 925t
secondary, 1441–1445
sexuality in, 1451
social security disability and, 1456–1457
subchondral cysts in, 1435, *1437*
surgery in, 1454–1455
synovectomy in, 1814–1815
terminology in, 1432
trabecular microfracture in, 1425
vocational rehabilitation and, 1456
wear-and-tear theory of, 1424–1425
cartilage lubrication in, 1424
impact loading stress in, 1424–1425
joint lubrication in, 1424
oscillatory joint stress in, 1424
Osteoarthropathy, hypertrophic, 1594–1603. See also *Hypertrophic osteoarthropathy*.
Osteoarthrosis, degradative enzyme source in, 190
Osteoblast, *272*, 272–273
Osteocalcin, 280
Osteochondromatosis, synovial, radiography in, *604–605*, 605
Osteochondrosis, intervertebral, radiography in, 590, *591*
Osteoclast, 273–275, *274*
Osteoclast-activating factor, 274
Osteocyte, 273, *273*
Osteodystrophy, Albright's hereditary, 1584, *1586*
renal, 1670–1672, *1671*
in hyperparathyroidism, 1582, *1585*
Osteogenesis imperfecta, 1634–1638, 1635t
lethal, with failure to secrete type I collagen, 1636
mild, with diminished type I collagen production, 1634–1636, *1635*
moderately severe, with abnormal $\alpha_2$-chain production, 1637–1638
severe, nonlethal, with normal type I collagen production, 1636–1637
Osteogenic cells, 271–275
Osteogenic sarcoma, in Paget's disease of bone, 1679
Osteogenic synovitis, in hyperparathyroidism, 1582, *1584*
Osteoid, chemical composition of, 276, 278t
Osteolysis, osteocytic, 273
Osteomalacia, 1662–1670
biochemical abnormalities in, 1663–1664
classification of, 1666t
clinical features in, 1663–1665
hypophosphatemia in, 1667–1669
autosomal recessive, 1668
renal wasting in, 1667
sporadic, 1669
X-linked, 1667–1668, *1668*
in calcium deficiency, 1669–1670
in disodium etidronate administration, 1669
in Fanconi syndrome, 1669
in fibrogenesis imperfecta ossium, 1670
in hyperparathyroidism, 1669
in hypophosphatasia, 1670
in sodium fluoride administration, 1669
in total parenteral nutrition, 1670
malignancy and, 1609

Osteomalacia *(Continued)*
pathogenesis and treatment in, 1665–1670
radiology in, 1664–1665, *1664–1665*
tumors associated with, 1669, 1669t
vitamin D deficiency in, 1666
vitamin D malabsorption in, 1666
vitamin D metabolism in, 1666–1667
vitamin D renal loss in, 1667
vitamin D resistance in, 1667
Osteomyelitis, in sickle cell disease, 1575
malignancy and, 1612
pyogenic vertebral, 463
scintigraphy in, 618–619, *619–620*
Osteon, 275, *276*
secondary, 276, *277*
Osteonecrosis, in glenohumeral joint, 444
in hip, in hypothyroidism, 1587
radiography in, 602, *602*
Osteopenia, in juvenile arthritis, 577, *577*
Osteopetrosis, 1673–1674, *1674*
Osteophyte, in gout, 470, *470*
in osteoarthritic cartilage, 1423
in osteoarthritis, 1435
in spine, 1440, *1442*
Osteoporosis, 1657–1662
aging in, 1659
bone pathology in, 1659
classification of, 1657t
clinical features of, 1657–1659
computed tomography in, *633*, 634
glucocorticoid excess in, 1661
gonadal hypofunction in, 1659–1661, *1660*
heparin-induced, 250
immobilization and, 1662
in diabetes mellitus, 1580
in juvenile rheumatoid arthritis, 1259, *1261*
in rheumatoid arthritis, 571, 1662
juvenile, 1662
juxta-articular, corticosteroid in, 553
of foot, 390
pathogenesis and treatment in, 1659–1662
radiology in, *1658*, 1658–1659
Singh index of trabecular patterns in, 284, *284*
thyrotoxicosis in, 1661–1662
Osteoporosis circumscripta, *1676*
Osteoporosis-osteomalacia, in inflammatory bowel disease, 1035
Osteoprogenitor cell, 272
Osteosclerosis fragilis generalisata, 1673–1674, *1674*
Osteosclerotic myeloma, peripheral neuropathy in, 308
Osteotomy, in avascular necrosis, 1705
trochanteric, 1927, 1942
Ostertag amyloid nephropathy, 1477
Ouchterlony double immunodiffusion analysis, in mixed connective tissue disease, 1117, *1119*
Oxalate crystals, polarized light microscopy for, 565
Oxidative metabolism, 124–128, *125–126*, 126t
cellular and biochemical aspects of, 124–125, *125*
oxygen-derived free radicals in, 125–128, 126t
Oxipurinol, 867
Oxygen, in synovial fluid, 894
Oxygen intermediates, reactive, macrophage secretion of, 157, 158t
Oxypurinol, crystal deposition, allopurinol use and, 866

Pachydermoperiostosis, 1594, *1596*, 1600–1601
Paget's disease of bone, 1676–1683
bone pathology in, 1678–1679, *1678–1679*
calcitonin in, 1680–1682, *1681–1682*
clinical features of, 1676–1679, *1676–1679*
complications in, 1679–1680, 1680t
disodium etidronate in, 1682
increased collagen metabolism in, 220
malignancy and, 1612–1613
mithramycin in, 1682–1683
osteoarthritis in, 1444
pathogenesis and treatment in, 1680–1683, *1681–1682*
radiography in, 602, *603*, 1676–1677, *1676–1678*
scintigraphy in, 621–622, *622*
Pain, arthritis, 502
behavioral aspects of, 501–503, *503*
distraction techniques for, 503
in patient history, 369
management programs for, 502
physical measures for, 502
relaxation techniques for, 503, *503*
Pain amplification syndrome, 482, 482t
Palindromic rheumatism, 920
Palmar flexor tenosynovitis, 1820–1821
Pancoast's syndrome, 1608
Pancreas, in Sjögren's syndrome, 962–963
panniculitis and, 1180
Pancreatic duct antibody, in Sjögren's syndrome, 967–968
Pancreatitis, avascular necrosis in, 1693
in systemic lupus erythematosus, 1082
synovial biopsy in, 652
with nonsteroidal anti-inflammatory drugs, 762
Panniculitis, corticosteroid withdrawal and, 1182
factitial, 1182
in lupus erythematosus, 538
lobular, 1180–1181
malignancy and, 1181–1182, 1608–1609, *1609*
pancreatitis and, 1180
relapsing nonsuppurative, in lupus erythematosus, 1075
septal, 1178–1179
subacute nodular migratory, 1179
Papular mucinosis, 1478
Papule, 533
Paralysis, in rheumatoid arthritis, 920–921
in systemic lupus erythematosus, 1084
Paraneoplastic syndrome, 1603
Parasites, in polymyositis, 1238
Parathyroid, serum, in metabolic bone disease, 1647
Parathyroid hormone, 1649–1650, *1649–1650*
Paresthesia, in neck pain, 422
Parkinson's disease, rheumatoid arthritis vs, 925, *925*
Parotid gland, examination of, 424
in systemic lupus erythematosus, 1083
Parry-Romberg syndrome, 541
Pars interarticularis, defect in, 453
Patella. See also *Knee*.
examination of, 384–385
in total knee replacement, 1887–1888
Patella tendinitis, 1745
Patellar inhibition test, 385
Patellofemoral joint, lesions of, arthroscopy in, 645
osteoarthritis of, total knee replacement in, 1878
Patellofemoral pain syndrome, 1747–1748, *1748*
Patent ductus arteriosus, indomethacin in, 761
Patient, rheumatic, general approach to, 361–368
diagnosis in, 361–363
health assessment questionnaire in, 366t–367t
investigations in, 363–364
management goals in, 364
patient understanding in, 365–368
therapeutic strategy in, 365
time frame in, 365
Patient education, in juvenile rheumatoid arthritis, 1269
in rheumatoid arthritis, 981–982, 982t
in systemic lupus erythematosus, 1098
Patrick test, 452
PCNA antigen, 700
Pelvic tilt, 379
Pelvis, corticosteroid in, 552
in inflammatory bowel disease, 1034–1036, *1035*
Penicillamine, 809–814
chemical structure of, 809, *809*
chronopharmacology of, *811*
clinical pharmacology of, 809–810
dosage for, 810
in rheumatoid arthritis, 988
indications for, 810
indications, contraindications, precautions in, 812–813
mechanism of action of, 813–814
metabolism of, 809
response pattern to, 810–811
side effects of, 811–812
D-Penicillamine, collagen crosslinking and, 225–226, *226*
in juvenile rheumatoid arthritis, 1267
macrophage and, 161
Penicillin G, in gonococcal arthritis, 1518
in rheumatic fever prophylaxis, 1290–1291, 1291t
Pepstatin, for acid proteinase activity, 182
Peptide bonds, hydrolysis of, *2*
Periarteritis nodosa, 1137, 1142–1148. See also *Polyarteritis*.
Periarthritis, calcific, rheumatoid arthritis vs, 926
Pericardial effusion, in scleroderma, 1186, 1200

Pericarditis, in juvenile rheumatoid arthritis, 1252, *1253*
in rheumatic heart disease, 1281, 1283
in rheumatoid arthritis, 941
in scleroderma, 1193–1194
in systemic lupus erythematosus, 1087
Perichondrium, 282
Perimysium, 287
Periosteal capillary, 282, *282*
Periosteum, 282
in hypertrophic osteoarthropathy, 1599
Periostitis, in juvenile arthritis, 576–577, *576–577*
scintigraphy in, 622
Peripheral mononeuropathy, 305
Peripheral nerve, action potential of, 300–303, *303–304*
fiber populations of, 297, *297*
organization of, 295
saltatory conduction in, 303, *304*
vascularization of, 295, *296*
Peripheral neuropathy, 303–306
aging and, 313
cranial nerve involvement in, 306
distal distribution in, 306
in amyloidosis, 307, 1479
in cryoglobulinemia, 308–309
in dysimmunoglobulinemia, 307–310
in leprosy, 309–310
in multiple myeloma, 308
in muscle weakness, 414–415
in osteosclerotic myeloma, 308
in polyarteritis, 307, 1143, 1144
in rheumatoid arthritis, 306–307
in scleroderma, 1194
in Sjögren's syndrome, 307
in systemic lupus erythematosus, 1083–1084
in Waldenström's macroglobulinemia, 308
laboratory investigations in, 313
muscle wasting in, 306
paresthesia in, 306
tendon reflexes in, 306
Peripheral polyneuropathy, 305, 305t
Peripheral vascular system, in scleroderma, 1190, 1198–1199
Permeability factor of dilution (PF/dil), 100–101
Peroneal nerve, common, entrapment of, 1763–1764, *1765*
Peroneal spasm, 476
in synovitis, 403, *403*
Peroneal spasm test, 1899–1900, *1900*
Pes anserinus tendinitis bursitis, 1745–1746
Pes cavus, 388
Pes planus, in rheumatoid arthritis, *937*
Pes valgoplanus, 388
Peyer's patches, 1032
Peyronie's disease, 1219
Phagocytes, mononuclear, control of, 147
life cycle of, 145–150
populations of, 147t
morphologic appearance of, *146*
Phagocytosis, 121–122, 121t
Phalanx, ivory, 582. See also *Finger.*
Phalen maneuver, 1755
Pharmacodynamics, factors influencing, 717, *718*
in drug dosage, 717, *718*
Pharmacokinetics, in drug dosage, 717, *718*, *722*, 722–724
of antimalarials, 776
of gold compounds, 796–798, *797*
of nonsteroidal anti-inflammatory drugs, 757–759, 757t–759t
renal function and, 721–722
Phenotype, 38
Phenoxymethyl penicillin, in Lyme disease, 1563
Phenylbutazone, 766–767
in ankylosing spondylitis, 1004
in gouty arthritis, 1384
in osteoarthritis, 1453–1454
liver microenzyme induction by, 721
Phlebitis, in Behçet's disease, 1175
Phosphate, serum inorganic, in metabolic bone disease, 1646
urinary, 1646–1647
Phospholipid, hydrolysis of, *3*
Physical therapy, for elbow, 1852–1853
in juvenile rheumatoid arthritis, 1268–1269
in osteoarthritis, 1451–1452
in rheumatoid arthritis, 983–984
value of, 1791
Piriformis syndrome, 1763
Piroxicam, 768, *768*
in gouty arthritis, 1384
Pitching act, 1736, *1736*
Pivot joint, 371
Plane joint, 370
Plantar fasciitis, 389
Plantar nerve syndrome, medial and lateral, 1764–1766
Plaque, 534
Plasma, contact activation of, factors required for, 95–96
Plasmapheresis, 845–846
in polyarteritis, 1147
Plasmin, 184
Plasminogen, 184
Plasminogen activator, macrophage secretion of, 154–155
Plastazote sandal, 477–478, *478*
Plastazote shoe, 477, *479*
Platelet, 169–182
adhesion of, 170–171, *171*
aggregation of, 171–172, *172*
aspirin effects of, 740–741
constituents and structural organization of, 169–170, *170*
secretion by, 172–173
shape change in, 170, *171*
Platelet aggregation assay, 685–686
Platelet-derived growth factor, 175, 1212
Pleural disease, in mixed connective tissue disease, 1123
in polyarticular arthritis, 409
in rheumatoid arthritis, 941
in systemic lupus erythematosus, 1088–1089, 1106
Plica syndrome, 385
Pneumococci, in septic arthritis, 1515
Pneumonia, in rheumatic fever, 1284–1285
Pneumonitis, desquamative interstitial, 1217
in rheumatoid arthritis, 941, *942*
lupus, 1089
Podagra, 470
Point count for tenderness, 483, 483t
Polyarteritis, 1142–1148
arteriography in, 1146, *1146*
clinical features of, 1144–1145, *1144–1145*
cutaneous, in children, 1309
diagnosis in, 1146, *1146*
epidemiology in, 1142
in children, 1145
infantile, 1309–1310
laboratory tests in, 1145–1146
malignancy and, 1608
pathology in, *1142–1143*, 1142–1144
prognosis in, 1146–1147, *1147*
treatment in, 1147–1148
Polyarteritis nodosa, 1142–1148. See also *Polyarteritis.*
classification of, 1138
hepatitis B virus and, 1544
in children, 1309–1310
ocular involvement in, 523
pannicular involvement in, 1181
peripheral neuropathy in, 307
Polyarticular arthritis, 401–410
cardiac manifestations of, 409
collagen-induced, 227
dermatological manifestations of, 409
differential diagnosis of, 406–408
fever and, 407–408
gastrointestinal manifestations of, 409–410
hepatic manifestations of, 409
in juvenile rheumatoid arthritis, 1248–1250, *1249–1250*
migratory, 406–407
multiple structural lesions in, 401–402, 401t
myalgia in, 401–402
neurologic manifestations of, 410
palindromic or intermittent, 407
pulmonary manifestations of, 408–409
renal and urological manifestations of, 409
specific joint involvement in, 406t
synovitis in, 402–406
therapeutic response in, 408
with monoarticular component, 391t
Polychondritis, 1458–1467
age of onset in, 1458, *1459*
clinical course, prognosis, treatment in, 1465–1466
clinical manifestations of, 1458–1460, *1459*, 1459t
coexistent disease in, 1460, 1461t
diagnostic criteria in, 1462, 1462t
differential diagnosis of, 1462
etiology and pathophysiology in, 1463–1465
laboratory features of, 1460–1461, 1462t
malignancy and, 1609
pathology in, 1462–1463, *1463*
relapsing, ocular manifestations in, 526
rheumatoid arthritis vs, 925
roentgenographic abnormalities in, 1461–1462
Polymer implant, sustained-release, for angiogenesis, 198, *198*
Polymorphism, 38
Polymorphonuclear leukocyte, 890–892, *891*, 892t
Polymyalgia rheumatica, 1166–1173, 1239–1240

Polymyalgia rheumatica *(Continued)*
acute phase response in, 660
clinical features of, 1170
definition of, 1166
diagnosis of, 1172
epidemiology of, 1167
etiology and pathogenesis of, 1167
giant cell arteritis and, 1170–1171
in children, 1310–1311
laboratory studies in, 1171
malignancy and, 1608
pathology in, 1168
rheumatoid arthritis vs, 925
treatment of, 1172
Polymyositis, antibody in, *702*, 702–703
in children, 1302–1303
in mixed connective tissue disease, 1122
ocular involvement in, 523
primary idiopathic adult, 1227–1234
clinical features of, 1227
clinical signs at presentation in, 1228
differential diagnosis of, 1232–1234
electrophysiology in, 1229–1230
laboratory abnormalities in, 1228
muscle biopsy in, 1230–1232, *1230–1233*
precipitating factors in, 1227
serological tests in, 1228–1229
severity at presentation in, 1228
symptomatology in, 1227–1228
radiography in, 586
secondary, 1239
with known infections, 1238
Polyneuropathy, peripheral, 305, 305t
Popeye sign, 442
Popliteal cyst, 383, 936, 936t, 1763, *1766*
Post-traumatic arthritis, elbow in, 1838
Posture, standing, 1773
Potassium equilibrium potential, 300–301
PP-ribose-P synthetase, increased activity of, 1376–1377, *1377*
Prednisolone, chemical structure of, *816*
Prednisone, chemical structure of, *816*
Cushing's syndrome in, 1588
in dermatomyositis in children, 1302
in dermatomyositis-polymyositis, 1241–1242
in juvenile rheumatoid arthritis, 1268
in polychondritis, 1466
in sarcoid arthritis, 1491
in systemic lupus erythematosus, 1109
in children, 1297
Pregnancy, aspirin and salicylate in, 735
glucocorticoids and, 819
in mixed connective tissue disease, 1126–1127, 1127t
in systemic lupus erythematosus, 1090, 1091–1092, 1107–1108
nonsteroidal anti-inflammatory drugs in, 763–764
rheumatic features of, 1590–1591
Prekallikrein, 101–103
assays of, 101–102
discovery of, 95
interactions of, 96–97, *97*
mechanism of activation of, 102–103
properties of, 101
Prepatellar bursitis, 1745
corticosteroid in, 552
Pretibial myxedema, in Graves' disease, 1586
Probenecid, *858*, 858–860, 859t
Procainamide, in drug-induced lupus, 1092
Procollagen, immunochemistry of, 225
Proline analogs, collagen synthesis and, 1215
Pronator teres syndrome, 1738–1739
Prostaglandin, as nutritional intervention, 358–359
biochemistry of, 71–72, *72*
functions of, 75–76
in bone resorption, 80, *80*, 275
in inflammation, 76–78
in osteoarthritic cartilage, 1421–1422
in synovial fluid, multiple roles of, 893–894
inhibition of synthesis of, 79
by nonsteroidal anti-inflammatory drugs, 753–754
metabolism of, 72, *73*
Prostaglandin synthetic pathways, in platelets, 173, *173*
Prostatic carcinoma, osteomalacia in, 1669
Prostatitis, in ankylosing spondylitis, 998
Prosthesis. See also individual prosthesis or anatomic part.
for hand, 1968–1971, *1970*
for hip, radiography in, 1938–1938, *1939–1940*
for knee, 1874–1878, *1876–1878*
for total knee replacement, 1956–1958, *1958–1960*
Protamine, angiogenesis inhibition and, 208
Protease inhibitor, macrophage secretion of, 156
Protein, AA, 1472–1473
acute phase, 653, 654t
AE, 1473
AF, 1473
AL, 1471–1472
AS, 1473
C-reactive, *657–658*, 657–659. See also *C-reactive protein.*
cryoprecipitation of, 1347–1348
in origin of amyloid deposits, 1472–1473
SAA, 1472–1473
salivary, in Sjögren's syndrome, 965
serum, 965
Protein requirements, 357
Protein-calorie malnutrition, 353
Proteinase, aspartic, 182–183, *183*
cartilage synthesis of, 190–191
classes and characteristics of, 183t
cysteine, 183–184
endogenous inhibition of, 187–188
in fibrosis, 1215–1216
in joint disease, 182–195
in polychondritis, 1464
in synovial fluid, 191–192
lysosomal, 192
serine, 184–185, *185*
endogenous inhibition of, 188
synovial synthesis of, 191
$\alpha_1$-Proteinase inhibitor, hereditary, 230
Proteinuria, in gold therapy, 803, 803t
penicillamine causing, *811*
Proteoglycan. See also *Glycosaminoglycan.*
aggregation phenomenon in, *242*, 242–243
Proteoglycan *(Continued)*
cartilage, assay of enzymes active against, 188
molecular degradation of, 188
chondroitin sulfate–keratan sulfate, *240–242*, 240–243
common linkage region of, *240*
degradation of, 244–245, 903, *903*, 1420
heparin, 243
hyaluronate, 240
hyaluronate-binding region of, 241
in cartilage, 242, *242*, 1417–1418
in intervertebral disc, 459–460
in urate crystal deposition, 1379–1380
molecular structure of, 240–241, *241*
oligosaccharides on, 241
ultrastructure of, 242, *242*
Proteoglycan-platelet factor IV complex, 249
Proteoglycanase, 187
Proteolysis, *2*
Protocollagen hydroxylase, 216–218, *218*
Pseudo-Hurler dystrophy, 246–247
Pseudo-rheumatism, steroid, 487
Pseudoangina pectoris, in cervical spine disorders, 423
Pseudogout, 1398–1399
corticosteroid in, 550
Pseudohyperparathyroidism, 1584
Pseudolymphoma, in Sjögren's syndrome, 970
Pseudotumor, in hemophilic arthropathy, 1565
synovial, 1731
Pseudoxanthoma elasticum, 1640
Psoas abscess, in inflammatory bowel disease, 1035–1036
Psoriatic arthritis, 1021–1031
antimalarials in, 782
clinical features in, 1022–1026, *1023–1025*, 1026t
cutaneous manifestations of, 536–537, *536–537*
definition of, 1021
differential diagnosis in, 1028, *1028*
etiology of, 1021–1022
juvenile, radiography in, 578
pathology in, 1022
preoperative evaluation in, 1789
prevalence of, 1021
radiography in, 581–583, *582–583*, 1026–1028, 1026t, *1027*
rehabilitation in, 1782
Reiter's syndrome vs, 1017, 1017t
rheumatoid arthritis vs, 922, 1023, *1023–1024*
treatment in, 1028–1029
Psychogenic pain, 486–487
Psychological factors, 497–511
anger as, 499–500
anxiety and denial as, 499
dependence as, 498–499
depression as, 500
financial cost as, 499
future concerns about, 508–509, *509*
in fibrositis, 484–485
in juvenile rheumatoid arthritis, 507–508, 507t, *508*
in osteoarthritis, 1450–1451
in rheumatoid arthritis, *499*
in systemic lupus erythematosus, 1060–1062, 1084t, 1105

Psychological factors *(Continued)*
loss of functional ability as, 498
management of, 500–501, 500t–501t
pain as, 498, 501–503
physical appearance as, 498
research in, 505–507
weakness, fatigue as, 498
Pubic ramus, stress fracture of, 1740, *1740*
Pulmonary arteritis, in rheumatoid arthritis, 941
Pulmonary disease, fibrotic, 1216–1218, 1240
Pulmonary edema, aspirin causing, 742
Pulmonary hypertension, in mixed connective tissue disease, 1123, *1124*
in polyarticular arthritis, 409
in scleroderma, 1192, 1200
Pulmonary infiltrate, in polyarticular arthritis, 408
Pulmonary manifestations, in amyloidosis, 1480
in ankylosing spondylitis, 998
in Churg-Strauss vasculitis, 1154
in dermatomyositis-polymyositis, 1240
in Marfan's syndrome, 1626
in mixed connective tissue disease, 1123, *1124*
in polyarteritis, 1145
in polyarticular arthritis, 408
in rheumatoid arthritis, 941
in sarcoidosis, 1488
in scleroderma, 1185–1186, 1192, 1199–1200
in Sjögren's syndrome, 961–962
in systemic lupus erythematosus, 1076–1077, 1088–1089, 1106
in Wegener's granulomatosis, 1155, *1155*, 1156
Pulmonary nodule, in polyarticular arthritis, 408
in rheumatoid arthritis, 941
Pulmonary talc granulomatosis, 1490
Purine, biochemistry of, *337–340*, 337–342
biosynthesis of, *338–339*, 338–340
chemical structure of, 337, *337*
nucleotide synthesis de nova in, 342, *342*
ribonucleotide cleavage in, 343
ribonucleotide interconversion of, 342–343
salvage of, 343
Purine analogues, 841–842
Purine nucleoside phosphorylase, 341
deficiency in, 1323
Purine restriction, in gout, 1388–1389
Purpura, anaphylactoid, in children, *1307–1308*, 1307–1309
Henoch-Schönlein, *1307–1308*, 1307–1309
Pustule, 534
Pyogenic arthritis, malignancy and, 1609
Pyomyositis, 1238
Pyridoxine, deficiency in, 358
Pyrophosphate, in calcium pyrophosphate deposition disease, 1409–1410
in endocrine disorders, 1409
metabolism of, 1409–1412

Quadriceps setting exercise, 1452
Quinacrine, pharmacokinetics of, 776

Radial head, biomechanical function of, 1839
excision of, 1839–1841, 1840t
Radial nerve, 1759–1761
course and distribution of, *1761*
entrapment of, in axilla, 1759–1760
innervation by, 1760t
tests of, 420t
Radial reflex, 428t
Radial styloid process, de Quervain's tenosynovitis in, 376
Radiation therapy, avascular necrosis in, 1693
ionizing, 846–847
malignancy and, 1614
total lymph node, 847
Radiculitis, adhesive, 462
Radiculopathy, cervical, 445
Radiography, 569–608
in ankylosing spondylitis, 578–581, *579–581*
in avascular necrosis, 1698–1700, *1699–1700*
in connective tissue disease, 584–587, *585–587*
in crystal-related arthropathy, 595–600, *596–599*
in degenerative joint disease, 587–594, *588–594*
in dermatomyositis, 586, *587*
in enteropathic arthritis, 584
in hemophilic arthropathy, 1565, *1566*
in hyperparathyroidism, 1652–1654, *1652–1654*
in hypertrophic osteoarthropathy, 1598, *1599*
in juvenile arthritis, *576*, 576–578, *576–578*
in low back pain, 452–453
in metabolic bone disease, 1647–1648
in mixed connective tissue disease, 587
in neuroarthropathy, 594–595, *595*
in osteoarthritis, 587–594, *588–594*, 1434, *1434–1435*, 1435t
in osteomalacia, 1664–1665, *1664–1665*
in osteoporosis, *1658*, 1658–1659
in Paget's disease of bone, 1676–1677, *1676–1678*
in pigmented villonodular synovitis, 605, 1720, *1720*
in polychondritis, 1461–1462
in polymyositis, 586
in progressive systemic sclerosis, 585–586, *586–587*
in psoriatic arthritis, 581–583, *582–583*
in Reiter's syndrome, 583–584, *584*
in rheumatoid arthritis, 570–576, *571–576*, 573t
in rheumatoid arthritis of feet, 476
in septic arthritis, *600*, 600–602, 1513–1514, *1514*
in shoulder pain, 436
in spondyloarthropathy, 578–584, *579–584*

Radiography *(Continued)*
in systemic lupus erythematosus, 585, *585*
in total hip replacement, 1938–1956
acetabular component in, 1940–1941, *1940–1941*
cement fracture in, 1947, *1950*
cement-bone lucency in, 1943t
cement-bone lucent zone widening in, 1945, *1946–1947*
complications in, 1943–1956
dislocation in, 1943–1945, *1944*
femoral and pelvic fracture in, 1954–1956, *1956*
femoral component in, *1940*, 1941
femoral stem fracture in, 1954, *1955*
loosening and infection in, 1945, 1945t
measuring wear in, 1942–1943
medial femoral neck resorption in, 1943
metal-cement lucency widening in, 1946–1947, *1949*
methyl methacrylate in, 1941–1942, 1943t
para-articular ossification in, 1956, *1957*
periosteal reaction in, 1947–1948
prosthesis appearance in, 1938–1939, *1939–1940*
prosthetic component loosening in, 1945–1946, *1948*
stress views in, 1948, *1951*
trochanteric osteotomy in, 1942
wire mesh in, 1942
plain film, 569–570, 569t
projections for, 569t
Radioimmunoassay, for antigen-antibody reaction, 696
for IgM rheumatoid factor, *666*
Radionuclide scan. See *Bone scan.*
Radiotechnetium pertechnetate, 609
Radiotechnetium phosphate, 609–610, *610*
Radioulnar joint. See *Wrist.*
Radius, in hemophilic arthropathy, 1565, *1566*
Ragocyte, 897
Raji cell binding assay, 685, *685*
Ramus, posterior primary, 449, *449*
Range of motion, joint positioning for, 1773–1774
Rash, allopurinol use and, 866
butterfly, in systemic lupus erythematosus, 573, *573*, 1073, 1100, 1294, *1294*
in dermatomyositis in children, 1298, *1298*
in juvenile rheumatoid arthritis, 1251–1252, *1252*, 1255
morbilliform, due to nonsteroidal anti-inflammatory drugs, 764
sun-sensitive, in systemic lupus erythematosus, 1077
Raynaud's phenomenon, in mixed connective tissue disease, 1121, *1121*, 1132
in scleroderma, 541, *541*, 1187, 1190, 1198–1199
in Sjögren's syndrome, 964
in systemic lupus erythematosus, 538, 1080–1081, *1081*, 1101
in systemic sclerosis, in children, 1305–1306
rehabilitation in, 1782

Reactive arthritis, rheumatoid arthritis vs, 922
Reconstructive surgery. See also individual anatomic part.
of ankle and foot, 1896–1910
of elbow, 1838–1855
of hand, 1818–1837
of knee, 1870–1896
of shoulder, 1855–1870
Recording joint examination, 371–372, *372*
Recreational injury, 1733–1753. See also individual types.
Referred muscle spasm, 482
Referred pain, 482–483
in neck, 418, *421*
in shoulder, 374
Referred tenderness, 482, 482t, *483*
Reflex, tendon, elicitation of, 426–427, 428t
grading scale for, 429t
primary, 429t
Reflex dystrophy syndrome, thermography in, 631, *631*
Reflex sympathetic dystrophy, 446
malignancy and, 1608
of foot, 390
scintigraphy in, 622–623
Regulatory factor, macrophage secretion of, 157–158
Rehabilitation, 1769–1786
elbow, postoperative, 1852–1853
evaluation in, 1769–1772
financial and vocational resources for, 1786
functional assessment in, 1771–1772
in fibrositis, 1783
in juvenile arthritis, 1782–1783
in osteoarthritis, 1780–1781
in psoriatic arthritis, 1782
in rheumatoid arthritis, 1781–1782
in scleroderma, 1782
in shoulder-hand syndrome, 1783
in systemic lupus erythematosus, 1783
physical assessment in, 1769–1771
gait in, 1770–1771
pain and edema in, 1770
range of motion in, 1769–1770
strength in, 1770
treatment in, 1772–1780
aids and appliances in, 1775–1776
compliance in, 1772
counseling in, 1780
exercise in, 1772–1773, 1772t
modalities in, 1774–1775, 1774t
positioning in, 1773–1774
rest in, 1774
splints and orthotics in, 1776–1780, *1777–1779*
traction in, 1780
vocational, osteoarthritis and, 1456
Reidel's struma, 1219–1220
Reiter's cell, *566*
Reiter's syndrome, 1007–1020
ankylosing spondylitis vs, 1017, 1018t
clinical features of, 1010–1014, 1010t, *1011–1014*
cutaneous manifestations of, 535–536, *536*
definition of, 1007, 1007t
differential diagnosis in, 1016–1017, 1016t–1017t
Reiter's syndrome *(Continued)*
epidemic, 1008–1009
etiology of, 1008–1009
genetics in, 1009
geographic, sex, age distribution in, 1010
gonococcal arthritis vs, 1016t, 1017
historical, 1008
HLA-B27 in, 1015–1016
in females and children, 1016
incidence and prevalence of, 1009–1010, 1009t
laboratory evaluation in, 1015
late sequelae of, 1014–1015
management of, 1018–1019
pathology in, 1016, 1016t
postvenereal, 1009
psoriatic arthritis vs, 1017, 1017t
radiography in, 583–584, *584*, 1015
rheumatoid arthritis vs, 922
scintigraphy in, *612*
Relaxation technique, in pain, 503, *503*
Renal disease, parenchymal, 1366–1371
acute uric acid nephropathy in, 1367–1368
calcium stones in, 1371
urate nephropathy in, 1366–1367, *1367*
uric acid stones in, 1368–1371
Renal failure, nonsteroidal anti-inflammatory drugs for, 763
Renal function, aspirin effects on, 743–744
drug excretion and, 721, *721*
Renal insufficiency, in hyperuricemia, 491–492
Renal manifestations, in amyloidosis, 1479–1480
in ankylosing spondylitis, 998–999
in Churg-Strauss vasculitis, 1154
in mixed connective tissue disease, 1124, *1126*
in nonsteroidal anti-inflammatory drug use, 762–763
in polyarteritis, 1143, *1143*, 1144
in polyarticular arthritis, 409
in scleroderma, 1193, 1200
in Sjögren's syndrome, 963
in systemic lupus erythematosus, 1077–1080, 1078t, 1103–1104
in Wegener's granulomatosis, 1155–1156
Renal osteodystrophy, 1670–1672, *1671*
in hyperparathyroidism, 1582, *1585*
Renal stones. See *Nephrolithiasis.*
Renal transplantation, avascular necrosis in, 1692
Renal tubular defect, in Sjögren's syndrome, 963
Respiratory manifestations. See *Pulmonary manifestations.*
Rest, for hand, 1818
in rehabilitation, 1774
in rheumatoid arthritis, 982–983
Restless legs, 306
Reticular dysgenesis, 1320–1323
Reticulin, collagen and, 224–225
Reticuloendothelial system, in mixed connective tissue disease, 1129
in systemic lupus erythematosus, 1056
Reticulohistiocytosis, multicentric, 1502–1505, *1503–1504*
rheumatoid arthritis vs, 924
Reticulohistiocytosis, multicentric *(Continued)*
synovial biopsy in, 652
Retina, bull's eye lesion of, 784, *784*
Retinoic acid, 358
Retinopathy, chloroquine, 784, *784*
in systemic lupus erythematosus, 522–523, *522–523*
Retroperitoneal fibrosis, 1219
Reye's syndrome, aspirin in, 743
Rheumatic arteritis, 1137
Rheumatic fever, 1277–1293
acute phase response in, 661
antecedent streptococcal infection in, 1285–1286
arthritis in, 1281, 1282, 1286
Aschoff nodule in, 1280
B lymphocyte alloantisera in, 51t
clinical manifestations of, 1281–1285
course, prognosis, natural history of, 1287–1288
cutaneous manifestations of, 541–542
definition of, 1277
diagnosis of, 1286–1287
epidemiology of, 1279–1280
erythema marginatum in, 1284
etiology of, 1277–1278
heart disease in, 1280–1281, 1282–1283, 1287
in migratory arthritis, 406
Jones criteria in, 1286, 1286t
juvenile rheumatoid arthritis vs, 1262
laboratory findings of, 1285–1286
major manifestations of acute, 1282–1284
minor manifestations of, 1284–1285
ocular manifestations in, 512
pathogenesis of, 1278–1279
pathology of, 1280–1281
prevention of, 1290–1291, 1291t
rheumatoid arthritis vs, 925–926
subcutaneous nodules in, 1281, *1283*, 1283–1284
Sydenham's chorea in, 1284, *1285*
treatment and management of, 1288–1290
Rheumatoid arthritis, 879–992. See also anatomic part.
acute inflammation stage in, 890–894
acute phase response in, 660
American Rheumatism Association Criteria for, 916t
amyloidosis in, 1475–1476
anemia in, 355–356
ankylosing spondylitis vs, 993t–994t
anti-inflammatory drugs in, 985–987
antibodies in, 703
antimalarials in, 780–782, 781t
B lymphocyte alloantisera in, *50*, 51t
biochemistry of tissue destruction in, 901–903
bone resorption in, 903
collagen degradation in, *901–902*, 901–903
proteoglycan degradation in, 903, *903*
bony erosion in, 571, *571–572*
calcium pyrophosphate deposition disease in, 1403
cardiac complications in, 941–942
classification and assessment of, 944–945, 944t–945t
clinical diagnosis of, 921
clinical spectrum of, 915–950

Rheumatoid arthritis *(Continued)*
copper in, 355
corticosteroid in, 550
cutaneous manifestations in, 534–535, *534–535*
degradative enzyme source in, 190, *190*
differential diagnosis of, 921–927
early, 918–927
in late adolescent females, 920
in older men, 920
joint involvement patterns in, 919–920, 919t
lesions in, 889–890, *890*
onset patterns in, 919, 919t
palindromic pattern of, 920
paralytic disease and, 920–921
positive rheumatoid factor test in, 920, 920t
unusual patterns of, 920–921
epidemiology and diagnosis of, 916–918, 916t–917t
episcleritis in, 513–517, *514–519*
established, 927–942
extra-articular complications in, 938–942
joint involvement in, 927–938, *928–938*. See also individual joints.
etiology of, 879–886
animal models in, 883–885, *884*
bacteria in, 881–882
genetically controlled host factors in, 880, 888
immune complexes and inflammatory process in, 880–881
viruses in, 882–883
exercise in, 983–984
experimental treatment of, 989
fever in, 407
fibrositis in, 485–486
functional capacity in, 944t
hematologic abnormalities in, 940
histidine in, 354
immune complexes in, 687–688
in rheumatic fever, 1287
in Sjögren's syndrome, 964
intermittent, 921
iron in, 355–356
joint localization of inflammation in, 889–890, *890*
juvenile, 1247–1277. See also *Juvenile rheumatoid arthritis*.
keratoconjunctivitis sicca in, 512–513, *513*
malignancy and, 1611
malnutrition in, 356
management of, 979–992
anti-inflammatory drugs in, 985–987
experimental treatment in, 989
goals of, 980–981
health-care team in, 980, 980t
pain relief in, 985
remission inducing agents in, 987–989
supportive measures in, 981–985, 982t
surgery in, 990
mast cells in, 201
neutrophils in, 133
New York criteria for, 917t
non-weight bearing in, 927, *928*
nonsteroidal anti-inflammatory drugs in, 760–761, 770

Rheumatoid arthritis *(Continued)*
occupational therapy and rehabilitation in, 984–985
ocular manifestations in, 512–517, *513–519*
osteoporosis in, 1662
pain relief in, 985
pathogenesis of, 886–915
stages in, 887t
working scheme for, 886–888
pathology of, 903–910, *904–909*
articular cartilage in, 906
cartilage-synovial interface in, 906–909, *907–908*
end-stage of, 910
joint capsule in, 906
pressure-induced, 909, *909*
rheumatoid nodule in, 534, *534*, 909–910, 938–939, *939*
synovium in, 904–906, *904–906*
tendon in, 906
vasculitis in, 910
patient education in, 981–982, 982t
peripheral neuropathy in, 306–307
physical therapy in, 983–984
preoperative evaluation in, 1788–1789
prognosis in, 942–945, 943t–945t
progressive, 921
pseudocystic, 572, *572*
psoriatic arthritis vs, 1023, *1023–1024*
psychological factors in, *499*
pulmonary disease in, 941
radiographic staging system in, 945t
radiography in, 570–576, *571–576*, 573t
abnormalities at specific sites in, 573–576, *574–576*
distribution in, 570–571
general features in, *571–572*, 571–573
instabilities and deformities in, 572–573, 573t
rehabilitation in, 1781–1782
remission in, 921, 943, 943t
remission-inducing agents in, 987–989
rest in, 982–983
rheumatoid factor in, 673–674, 674t, *675–676*
prognosis and, 943, 943t
rheumatoid nodule in, 534, *534*, 909–910, 938–939, *939*, 943
robust reactive, 571
scintigraphy in, 613–617, *614–617*
scleritis in, 513–517, *514–519*
septic arthritis in, 1508–1509, *1510*
supportive measures in, 981–985
surgery in, 990
synovectomy in, 1814
synovial biopsy in, 650
synovial cells in, 898–900, *899*
synovial fluid in, 892–894, *894*
proteinases and proteinase inhibition in, 191–192
synovium in, proteinases in, 191
time course in, 979–980
vasculitis in, 307, 940–941, 1148–1149
zinc in, 355
Rheumatoid arthritis precipitin, 967, 967t
Rheumatoid factor, 664–679, *896–897*, 896–898
after subacute bacterial endocarditis treatment, 671, *671*

Rheumatoid factor *(Continued)*
antigenic specificity of, 672
assay methods for, 664–667, *665–666*
diseases associated with, 669t
etiology of, 669–672
environmental influences on, *670–671*, 670–672
genetic influences on, 669–670, 669t
IgA, assay methods for, 667
IgE, 667
IgG, 666–667, *666–667*
comparison of, 666t
effect of pepsin on, 666, *667*
IgM, assay methods for, 664–666, *665–666*, 685, *685*
comparison of, 666t
Epstein-Barr virus and, 671, *671*
precursor B cells of, 670, *670*
immunochemical properties of, 672–673, *673*
in juvenile rheumatoid arthritis, 1256
in rheumatoid arthritis, 673–674, 674t, *675–676*, 943, 943t
in Sjögren's syndrome, 965
incidence of, 667–669, *668*
interaction with IgG of, 672–673, *673*
monoclonal, mixed cryoglobulins and, 1345
physiologic role of, 673, *673*
polyclonal, mixed cryoglobulins and, 1345
prognosis in rheumatoid arthritis and, 943, 943t
Rheumatoid nodule, 534, *534*, 909–910, 938–939, *939*
in episcleritis, *519*
in juvenile rheumatoid arthritis, 1253, 1255
in polyarticular arthritis, 409
in systemic lupus erythematosus, 1072
prognosis and, 943, 943t
Rheumatoid vasculitis, 1148–1149, *1149*
Rice bodies, 1528–1529, *1529*
Rickets. See also *Osteomalacia*.
vitamin D–deficient, collagen in, 227
Rifampin, 1531t
Rigor complex, 293
Ring splint, 1778, *1779*
RNA-protein antigen, 698
Ro/SSA antigen, 699–700, 699t
Rose-Waaler test, for rheumatoid factor, 665
Ross River virus, 1547
Rotator cuff, anatomy of, 373
calcific tendinitis in, 440–441
functions of, 1855
impingement of, 439–440, *440*
tear of, 441–442, 1859–1860
acromioplasty in, 1862–1863
arthrography in, 436, *438*, 627, *628*, 1736, *1737*
arthropathy in, 444, 1860
in rheumatoid arthritis, 930–931, *931*
tendinitis of, 439–440
Rubella, *1545*, 1545–1546
Rubella vaccine virus, 1546–1547
Rugger jersey spine, 1654, *1654*, *1674*

SAA protein, in origin of amyloid deposits, 1472–1473

Sacroiliac joint, ankylosing spondylitis in, 999–1002, 999t, *1000–1003*
radiography in, 578–579, *579*
computed tomography in, 632, *632*
examination of, 380
osteoarthritis in, 588
psoriatic arthritis in, 582–583, *583*
rheumatoid arthritis in, 575
scintigraphy in, 613–617, *616–617*
septic arthritis in, 1515, 1523
Sacroiliitis, in inflammatory bowel disease, 1035
in psoriatic arthritis, 1023–1024, 1026, *1027*
Sacrospinalis muscle, 449
Salicylate, 725–752. See also *Aspirin.*
chemical structure of, *725*
drug interactions with, 733–734, 734t
glycine conjugation of, 727
in osteoarthritis, 1453
in pregnancy, 735
in rheumatic fever, 1289
inhibition of drug metabolism by, 720
nonprescription and prescription, 732t
overdose or accidental intoxication with, 744–745
serum levels of, 726
urinary pH and, 726
Salicylsalicylate, 727
Salicyluric acid, 726
Salivary duct, malignancies of, in Sjögren's syndrome, 971–972, *972*, 972t
Salivary duct antibody, in Sjögren's syndrome, 967
Salivary flow rate, in Sjögren's syndrome, 960, 962t
Salivary gland, in Sjögren's syndrome, 957–961, *958–961*, 958t, 962t
Salivary protein, in Sjögren's syndrome, 965
*Salmonella* infection, reactive arthritis after, 1037
Saltatory conduction, 303, *304*
Sandle, in rheumatoid arthritis of feet, 477, *478*
Sarcoid, cutaneous manifestations of, 542, *542*
neurological manifestations of, 309
Sarcoidosis, 1488–1493
arthritis in, 1490–1491
clinical features of, 1488, *1489*
giant cell myositis in, 1239
immunology and biochemistry in, 1488–1490
ocular manifestations in, *529–530*, 529–531
of bone, 1491, *1492*
of muscle, 1491–1492, *1492*
rheumatic manifestations of, 1490–1492, *1492*
rheumatoid arthritis vs, 926
scintigraphy in, 624, *624*
Sarcolemma, 287
Sarcoma, Kaposi's, 1333, *1333*
osteogenic, 1679
synovial, radiography in, 605
Sarcomere, *289*, 290
Sarcoplasmic reticulum, 290–291
Satellite phenomenon, 394
Sausage toe, 389, 1011, *1011*
Scapulohumeral reflex, 428t
Scarring, in polyarticular arthritis, 409
Schamroth test, 1595, *1596*
Schiff bases, in collagen, 221
Schirmer tear test, in Sjögren's syndrome, 956, *957*
Schirmer test, 512, *513*
Schmorl's nodule, 1440
Schober test, 379
Schönlein–Henoch purpura, 1151, *1151*
Schwann cell, empty or denervated, 298, *299*
structural characteristics of, 299, *301–302*
Sciatic scoliosis, 461
Scintigraphy, in bone infarction and avascular necrosis, 619–621, *620–621*
in hand, *614*
in hypertrophic osteoarthropathy, 622, *623*
in inflammatory arthritis, 611–624
in low back pain, *65*
in Paget's disease, 621–622, *622*
in periostitis, 622
in reflex sympathetic dystrophy, 622–623
in Reiter's syndrome, *612*
in rheumatoid arthritis, 613–617, *614–617*
in sacroiliac joint, 613–617, *616–617*
in sarcoidosis and Sjögren's syndrome, 624, *624*
in septic arthritis, 617–618, *618*
in shoulder pain, 436
in sports medicine, *623*, 623–624
Sclera, anatomy of, 513, *514*
Scleritis, classification of, 515t
granulomatous, *518*
incidence of, 513–514
keratitis in, 517
necrotizing, 515–516, *516*
pathology of, 517, *518–519*
signs and symptoms of, 514–517, *516–519*
treatment in, 517
uveitis in, 516
Sclerodactyly, 1195
Scleroderma, 1183–1205
anticentromere antibody in, 1186–1187
cardiac manifestations in, 1186, 1193–1194, 1200–1201
clinical characteristics of, 1190–1195
clinical setting of, 1184
cutaneous manifestations in, 541, *541 1184–1185*, 1190–1191, 1199
definition and classification of, 1183, 1185t
dermatomyositis–polymyositis and, 1236–1237
diffuse generalized, 1195
early diagnosis of, 1184–1187
antinuclear serology in, 1186–1187
direct vascular injury in, 1187–1190, *1188–1189*
microvascular involvement in, 1187
systemic involvement in, 1184–1186
endothelial cell injury in, 1187–1189, *1189*
esophagus in, 1185, 1191, 1199
gastrointestinal manifestations in, 1191–1192, 1199
Scleroderma *(Continued)*
immune complexes in, 688
immunofluorescence patterns in, 1186–1187
in children, 1303–1306, *1304–1305*
linear, 1206, *1207*
in children, 1303–1305, *1304–1305*
localized, 1206–1209
in children,, 1303
malignancy and, 1608, 1611–1612, *1612–1613*
musculoskeletal manifestations in, 1192–1193, 1200
nailfold capillary pattern in, 1187, *1188*
nervous system manifestations in, 1194, 1200
ocular involvement in, 523
pathogenesis of, 1187, *1189*, 1197–1198
connective tissue in, 1198
immune, 1197–1198
microvascular–interstitial continuum in, 1198
vascular and microvascular, 1197
peripheral vasculature in, 1190, 1198–1199
pulmonary manifestations in, 1185–1186, 1192, 1199–1200
radiography in, 585–586, *586–587*
Raynaud's phenomenon in, 1187, 1190, 1198–1199
renal manifestations in, 1193, *1194–1195*, 1200
rheumatoid arthritis vs, 923
therapy in, 1198–1201
Scleromalacia perforans, 516
Sclerosis, systemic, 1183–1205. See also *Scleroderma.*
in children, *1305*, 1305–1306
morphea and, 1207–1208
Scoliosis, 378–379
sciatic, 461
Scurvy, 226–227
synovial biopsy in, 652
sDNA, antibody to, 1055–1056
Segmental demyelination, 715
Seizure, in systemic lupus erythematosus, 1085, 1105
Selenium, deficiency in, 358
Sellar joint, 371
Semimembranosus and semitendinosus reflex, 428t
Sensory nerve, origin of, 295
Sensory nerve conduction study, 709–710
Septic arthritis, 1507–1527
clinical features of, 1512
diagnostic studies in, *1513–1514*, 1513–1515
gonococcal, 1516–1519, *1517*
gram-negative organisms in, 1516
gram-positive organisms in, 1515–1516
in childhood, 1522–1523
in glenohumeral joint, 444
in hip, in inflammatory bowel disease, 1034
in sacroiliac joint, 1515, 1523
in sickle cell disease, 1575
in systemic lupus erythematosus, 1072, 1507, *1508*
management of, 1519–1522, 1519t

Septic arthritis, management of *(Continued)*
immobilization in, 1522
joint drainage in, 1521
medical, 1519–1521, 1520t
surgical decompression in, 1521–1522
monoarticular, 397
*N. gonorrhoeae* in, 1516–1519, *1517*
nongonococcal, etiologies of, 1515, 1515t
pathogenesis of, 1509–1512
predisposing factors in, 1507–1509, *1508–1508*
radiography in, *600*, 600–602
rheumatoid arthritis vs, 924
scintigraphy in, 617–618, *618*
synovial biopsy in, 650–651, *651*
Septic bursitis, 1523–1524
Serositis, in systemic lupus erythematosus, 1100–1101
Serum sickness, 1053
Severe combined immune deficiency, 1320–1323
Sex hormones, 848–849
Sexual health, 503–505, 504t
Sexuality, in osteoarthritis, 1451
Shin, tender, in steroid therapy, 487
Shoe, in rheumatoid arthritis of feet, 477, *478–479*
Shoulder, adhesive capsulitis of (frozen), 445, 627, *628*
anesthetic injection in, 439
ankylosing spondylitis in, radiography in, 580, *581*
arthrography of, 436–438, *438*, 627–628, *627–628*
arthroscopy of, 439, 645
ball-in-socket joint in, 317, *318*
corticosteroid in, 551, 554, *554*, 557
examination of, 373–374, *374*
frozen, 445, 627, *628*
joint motion in, *320*, 320–321
Milwaukee, 1413, 1427, 1860
motion of, 373, *374*
muscles of, 373
neoplasms in, 447
osteonecrosis in, 444
painful, 435–448
anatomy in, 435–436, *437*
common causes of, 436t
diagnostic aids in, 435–439, *437–438*
glenohumeral disorders in, 443–445
history in, 436
periarticular disorders in, 439–443
physical examination in, 436
regional disorders in, 445–447
radiography of, 436
referred pain in, 374
rheumatoid arthritis of, 930–931, *931*
radiography in, 574, 1857
scintigraphy of, 436
Shoulder depression test, 426
Sialography, in Sjögren's syndrome, 958–959, *959*
Sialoprotein, 278
Sicca syndrome, 512
Sickle cell disease, 1573–1578
aseptic necrosis in, 1577
bone infarctions in, 1576–1577
bone trabecular change due to marrow expansion in, 1573–1574, *1574*
Sickle cell disease *(Continued)*
erosions and chronic inflammation in, 1576
hand-foot syndrome in, 1574, *1575*
hyperuricemia and gout in, 1574–1575
joint effusions in, 1575–1576, *1576*
juvenile rheumatoid arthritis vs, 1261
osteomyelitis in, 1575
rheumatic fever in, 1287
rheumatoid arthritis vs, 924
septic arthritis in, 1508, 1575
synovial biopsy in, 652
Sickle cell trait, 1577–1578
Sindbis virus, 1547
Singh index of trabecular patterns, 284, *284*
Sinuvertebral nerve, 449, *449*
Sjögren's syndrome, 512, 956–978
animal models of, 972
antibody in, 701
autoantibodies in, non-organ-specific, 965–967, *966*, 966t–967t
organ-specific, 967–968
clinical features of, 956–964
cutaneous manifestations of, 535
gastrointestinal tract in, 962
genetic factors in, 969–970, 969t
hematologic findings in, 965
historical, 956
in systemic lupus erythematosus, 523
incidence and prevalence of, 956
infective etiology in, 970
laboratory findings in, 965–972
liver in, 963
lymphocytic infiltrates in, 968–969
lymphoproliferation in, 970–972, 971t–972t, *972*
mixed connective tissue disease with, 1124
nonexocrine disease in, 964
ocular involvement in, 956–957, 956t–958t, *957*
oral involvement in, 957–961, *958–961*, 958t, 962t
pancreas in, 962–963
peripheral neuropathy in, 307
renal involvement in, 963
respiratory tract in, 961–962
scintigraphy in, 624, *624*
skin in, *963*, 963–964
treatment of, 973
vasculitis in, 1148–1149
Skeletal hyperostosis, diffuse, 487, 1438–1439, *1439*
bone formation in, 579
radiography in, 592–594, *592–594*
Sleep, disturbed, in fibrositis, 484, 484t, 485, *486*
medication in, 488
Sm antigen, 698–699
Small bowel, amyloidosis of, 1481
Smallpox, 1550–1551
Smooth muscle antibody, in Sjögren's syndrome, 967
Snapping finger, corticosteroid in, 551
Social security disability, osteoarthritis and, 1456–1457
Sodium meclofenamate, in juvenile rheumatoid arthritis, 1266
Soft tissue, aspiration and injection of, 546–561
collagen in, 223
Soft tissue *(Continued)*
in rheumatoid arthritis, 571
local causes of pain in, 483t
Spheroidal joint, 370
Spina ventosa, 1528, *1528*
Spinal hyperostosis, in diabetes mellitus, 1581
Spinal muscular atrophy, distribution of, 415
polymyositis vs, 1233
Spine, bamboo, 579, *580*
cervical. See also *Neck*.
anatomy and biomechanics of, *417–419*, 417–421
ankylosing spondylitis in, 1935–1937, *1936–1937*
blood supply to, 421
clinical tests of, 425–427
dermatome distribution of, 418, *419*
disorders mimicking disease of, 427
electrodiagnostic studies of, 429
motion of, 380
osteophytes in, 1440, *1442*
pain syndromes of, 416t
palpation of, 423–424
radiculopathy in, 445
radiographic examination of, 427–429, *430–432*
range of motion of, 418t, 424–425
rheumatoid arthritis of, 927–930, *929*
sleep stresses on, 488
computed tomography in, 634, *634*
corkscrew motion of, 379
degenerative disease of, radiography in, 590–594, *591–594*
examination of, 378–381
hydatid disease of bone in, 464
in ankylosing spondylitis, 579–580, *580*, 997, 997t, 1935–1937, *1936–1937*
in inflammatory bowel disease, 1034–1036, *1035*
in juvenile rheumatoid arthritis, 1249
in osteoarthritis, 1440–1441, *1442*
treatment of, 1456
in psoriatic arthritis, 583, *583*
in Reiter's syndrome, 1014–1015
in rheumatoid arthritis, 575–576, *576*
kyphosis of, 379
lumbar, epidural venography in, 454, *457*
innervation of, 449, *449*
muscles of, 449
nerve root entrapment in, 458–459, 460–462
pain in. See *Low back pain*.
range of motion in, 379
lumbosacral, rotational asymmetry of, 453
muscle spasm of, 379
nontubercular granulomatous infections in, 463
scoliosis of, 378–379
stability of, 319–320, *319–320*
stair-step deformity of, 575, *576*
stenosis in, classification and types of, 458t, *459*
computed tomography in, 454, *458*
tuberculosis in, 463–464
Spleen, in Felty's syndrome, 951
in systemic lupus erythematosus, 1082–1083
Splenectomy, in Felty's syndrome, 954

Splinter hemorrhage, in systemic lupus erythematosus, 1075, *1076*
Spondylitis, ankylosing, 993–1007. See also *Ankylosing spondylitis*.
syphilitic, 464
Spondyloarthropathy, cutaneous manifestations of, 535–537, *536–537*
radiography in, 578–584, *579–584*
seronegative, rheumatoid arthritis vs, 922
scintigraphy in, 613–617, *614–617*
Spondylolisthesis, 464–465, 464t
Spondylolysis, 453, 464–465, 464t
Spondylosis, hyperostotic, 462–463
Spondylosis deformans, 1440
radiography in, 590–591, *591*
vertebral excrescences in, 579
Sporotrichosis, 1532
Sports medicine, scintigraphy in, *623*, 623–624
Spurling maneuver, 380
Squamous eruption, in polyarticular arthritis, 409
SS-A antibody, in Sjögren's syndrome, 966–967, 967t
SS-B antibody, in Sjögren's syndrome, 966–967, 967t
SS-C antibody, in Sjögren's syndrome, 967
St. Vitus dance, in rheumatic fever, 1284
Starvation, tissue loss in, 352, *352*
Sternoclavicular joint, computed tomography in, 633, *633*
examination of, 372–373
inflammatory arthritis in, 446
rheumatoid arthritis of, 930
Sternocleidomastoid muscle, examination of, 424
Sternocostal joint, examination of, 372–373
Steroid hormones, 848–849, 849t
Steroid injection, in rheumatoid arthritis of foot, 479–480
Steroid therapy, pseudo–rheumatism in, 487
tender shins in, 487
Stiff–hand syndrome, in diabetes mellitus, 1580–1581
Stiffness, in patient history, 369–370
Still's disease. See also *Juvenile rheumatoid arthritis*.
adult onset, 578, 920, 1252
radiography in, 577–578, *577–578*
Stomatitis, aphthous, in Behçet's disease, 1174
Straight leg raising exercise, 1452
Straight leg raising test, 380
in low back pain, 451
in pentathol interview, 452
Streptococcal infection, in rheumatic fever, 1285–1286
in septic arthritis, 1515
Streptomycin, 1531t
Structural lesion, 401–402, 401t
Subacromial bursa, anatomy of, 373
Subchondral bone, 259
compressive loads and, 327–328, *328*
Subchondral cyst, in osteoarthritis, 1434, 1435, *1435*, *1437*
Subcutaneous nodule, in hyperuricemia, 490–491
in rheumatic fever, 1281, *1283*, 1283–1284
Subtalar joint, injection into, 479–480
Succinic acid assay, in septic arthritis, 1514
Sulfinpyrazone, *858*, 860–861
Sulindac, 765, *765*
in gouty arthritis, 1384
Sun exposure, in systemic lupus erythematosus, 1077, 1098–1099
Supinator jerk, 428t
Suprascapular nerve, entrapment of, 446
Supraspinatus tendon, calcific tendinitis in, 440–441
Surface erosion, in rheumatoid arthritis, 571, *572*
Surgery. See also individual types; *Reconstructive surgery.*
in hemophilia, 1570–1572
in osteoarthritis, 1454–1455
in rheumatoid arthritis, 990
Swan–neck deformity, 376–377, *377*
in mixed connective tissue disease, 1122, *1122*
in Parkinson's disease, 925, *925*
in rheumatoid arthritis, 934, *935*
Sweat glands, in Sjögren's syndrome, 963, *964*
Sweet's syndrome, rheumatoid arthritis vs, 926
Swelling, in patient examination, 371
in patient history, 369
Sydenham's chorea, in rheumatic fever, 1284, *1285*
Symphyses, 254
Synarthroses, 254
Synchondroses, 254
Syndesmophyte, 579, *580*
Syndesmoses, 254
Synostoses, 254
embryonic development of, 257
Synovial biopsy, 648–653
arthroscopy in, 645, 649
in amyloidosis, 651
in collagen vascular disease, 650
in crystal-induced arthritis, 651
in hemochromatosis, 651
in infectious arthritis, 650–651, *651*
in ochronosis, 651
in rheumatoid arthritis, 650
in tumor, 651–652, *652*
light microscopic examination of, 650–652, *651–652*
methods for obtaining, 648–649, *649*
needle, 648–649, *649*
open, 649
tissue handling in, 649–650, *650*
Synovial capillary, 259, *259*
Synovial cyst, in juvenile rheumatoid arthritis, 1249, *1250*
Synovial fluid, 267–268
complement activation by, 893
components of, 267
effect of temperature on, 267–268, *268*
fibrin formation and fibrinolysis in, 893
in calcium pyrophosphate deposition disease, 1404–1405, *1405*
in embryonic joint, 255
in hepatitis B viral infection, 1544–1545
in inflammatory lesion of rheumatoid arthritis, 892–894, *894*
in juvenile rheumatoid arthritis, 1258
Synovial fluid *(Continued)*
in monoarticular arthritis, 395, 396t
in prognosis in rheumatoid arthritis, 944
in sickle cell disease, 1575–1576
in systemic lupus erythematosus, 1072
iron in, 894, *894*
kinin formation by, 893
oxygen in, 894
prostaglandin in, 893–894
proteinases and proteinase inhibition in, 191–192
removal of material from, 267
tuberculous, 1529–1530
Synovial joint, 254, *254*
embryonic development of, 254–257, *255–257*
Synovial lesion, structural vs, 401t
Synovial lining cells, *266*, 266–267
Synovial membrane, tophi in, in gout, 1379
Synovial mesenchyme, 255
Synovial osteochondromatosis, *604–605*, 605
Synovial sarcoma, 605
Synovioma, giant cell, 1722
Synovitis, 362, 362t
additive pattern of, 406
crystal-induced, 362, 362t, 1359–1416
diagnosis of, 402–406
historical features in, 402–403
laboratory examination in, 403, 406t
physical examination in, 403
radiologic examination in, 406
in Behçet's disease, 1175
migratory pattern of, 406–407
of inflammatory bowel disease, corticosteroid in, 550
of knee, 550
of wrist, 375, *375*
osteogenic, in hyperparathyroidism, 1582, *1584*
pain relief in, 985
palindromic or intermittent, 407
pigmented villonodular, computed tomography in, *633*, 634
radiography in, 605, 1720, *1720*
rheumatoid arthritis vs, 927
postinfectious, 1524
proliferative, in hemophilic arthropathy, 1565, *1566*
villonodular, 1718–1724
Synovium, 265–268
cellular lining of, *266*, 266–267
electron microscopy of, 649–650, *650*
immunofluorescent study of, 649
in hypertrophic osteoarthropathy, 1599–1600, *1600*
in prognosis in rheumatoid arthritis, 943–944
in systemic lupus erythematosus, 1072–1073
iron stain in, 1495, *1496*
juxta-articular bone tumors and, 1605
organization of, 265–266, *266*
proteinases synthesized by, 191
rheumatoid, antibody production by, *896–897*, 896–898
immunoproliferative syndrome in, 894–898
lymphokines in, 895–896

Syringomyelia, neuroarthropathy in, 594
Systemic sclerosis, progressive, antibody in, 701–702

T cell. See *Lymphocyte, T.*
Tabes dorsalis, neuroarthropathy in, 594
Takayasu's arteritis, 1139, 1159–1161, *1160*
in children, 1310–1311
Talc, in pulmonary granulomatosis, 1490
Talipes equinus, 388
Talonavicular arthrodesis, 1901, *1901–1902*
Talonavicular joint, tenderness in, 476
Tarsal tunnel syndrome, 390, 552, 1764
corticosteroid in, 553
in rheumatoid arthritis, 937–938
Tarsus, in diabetes mellitus, 1581, *1581–1582*
Tear secretion, in Sjögren's syndrome, 956, 956t, 973
Technetium-99m pertechnetate, 609
Technetium-99m phosphate, 609–610, *610*
Technetium-99m sulfur colloid, 610
Telangiectasis, in scleroderma, 541, *541*
Temperature, intra-articular, 267–268, *268*
Temporal arteritis, 524, 1137. See also *Giant cell arteritis.*
in children, 1310–1311
Temporal artery, in polyarteritis, 1145
Temporomandibular joint, corticosteroid in, *556*, 556–557
embryonic development of, 255–257
examination of, 372
in juvenile rheumatoid arthritis, 1249–1250
in preoperative evaluation, 1790
in rheumatoid arthritis, 930
Tendinitis, Achilles, corticosteroid in, 471, 552–553, 1748–1749
calcific, in rotator cuff, 440–441
in supraspinatus, 440–441
in biceps tendon, 442
patella, 1745
pes anserinus, 1745–1746
rotator cuff, 439–440
Tendon, in joint stability, 258
molecular degradation of, 190
reflexes, testing of, 414
Tendon sheath, fibroma of, 1724
Tennis elbow, 1738–1739, *1739*
corticosteroid in, 557, *558*
Tennis leg, 1749
Tenosynovectomy, indications for, 1794
Tenosynovial sarcoma, 1724–1726, 1725t–1726t
Tenosynovitis, biceps, 1863
de Quervain's, 935
of radial styloid process, 376
dorsal, surgery for, 1819
with extensor tendon rupture, 1819, *1820*
flexor, 1819–1820
digital, 1821
palmar, 1820–1821
wrist, 1820, *1822*
Tenosynovitis *(Continued)*
in ankle, 389–390
in gonococcal arthritis, 1516–1517
in hand, in mixed connective tissue disease, 1122, *1123*
in rheumatoid arthritis, 934, 935t
in systemic lupus erythematosus, 1072
in wrist, *375*, 375–376
localized nodular, 1722–1724, *1723–1724*
stenosing, of radial styloid process, 376
synovectomy in, 1812–1814
TENS, 1775
Testicle, in polyarteritis, 1142–1143
Tetracycline, in Lyme disease, 1563
Thalassemia, 1578
avascular necrosis in, 1690–1691
Theater sign, 1747
Thermography, 630–631, *631*
Thiemann's disease, rheumatoid arthritis vs, 926
Thiopurinol, 867
Thomas test, 381
Thoracic outlet syndrome, 1761–1762, *1762*
Thrombin, platelet interaction with, 176
Thrombocytopenia, in gold therapy, 803
in systemic lupus erythematosus, 1090, 1107
Thrombocytosis, in prognosis in rheumatoid arthritis, 944
in rheumatoid arthritis, 940
Thrombophlebitis, in systemic lupus erythematosus, 1081
Thrombosis, arterial, in systemic lupus erythematosus, 1081
Throwing mechanism, 1736, *1736*
Thumb, in rheumatoid arthritis, 934
in septic arthritis in, *1511*
in systemic lupus erythematosus, 1836, *1836*
muscles of, 378
reconstructive and salvage surgery for, 1830–1832, *1831*
synovectomy of, 1800, 1801
Thumb reflex, 428t
Thumb test, in Marfan's syndrome, 1625
Thy-1 antigen, 7, *7*
Thymic alymphoplasia, 1320–1323
Thymic hypoplasia, 1323–1324
Thymoma, giant cell myositis in, 1239, *1239*
immunodeficiency with, 1326–1327
Thymus, in systemic lupus erythematosus, 1083
Thyroid acropachy, 922, 1586, *1586*, 1598
Thyroid antibody, in Sjögren's syndrome, 968
Thyroid disease, in Sjögren's syndrome, 964
rheumatoid arthritis vs, 922
Thyroiditis, Hashimoto's, 1585–1587, *1586*
Thyrotoxicosis, in osteoporosis, 1661–1662
Thyroxin, in bone resorption, 274
Tibial nerve, posterior, 1764–1766, 1764t, *1765*
Tibial osteotomy, failed, total knee replacement in, 1878, *1879*
Tibial reflex, 428t
Tietze's syndrome, 373
Tinel sign, 390, 1755
Tinnitus, with aspirin use, 736
Toe, cock-up, 388
in rheumatoid arthritis, 937, *938*
surgical correction of, 1908–1909, *1909*
corticosteroid in, 556
deformity of, 388
hallux valgus in, 469
hammer, 388
mallet, 388
Morton's, 390
sausage, 389
in Reiter's syndrome, 1011, *1011*
Toenail care, 476
Toileting, 1776
Tolerance, immune, 1047–1048
Tolmetin, 765, *765*
in juvenile rheumatoid arthritis, 1266
Tomography, computed, 570, 631–634, *632–634*
in articular disease, *633*, 633–634
in avascular necrosis, 1700
in low back pain, 454, *458*, 631–632, *632*
in osteoporosis, 634, *634*
in sacroiliitis, 632, *632*
in trauma, 632–633, *633*
in tumor and infection, 633
conventional, 570
Tophi, 939
in gout, 1362–1363, *1362–1363*, 1362t
in synovial membrane, 1379
Total parenteral nutrition, osteomalacia in, 1670
Touraine-Solente-Gole syndrome, 1594, *1596*
Toxic oil syndrome of Spain, 1196–1197
Tracheolaryngeal lesion, in polyarticular arthritis, 408
Traction, 1780
Transcobalamin II deficiency, 1327
Transcutaneous electrical nerve stimulator, 1775
Transfer factor, 896
Transfusion, iron overload in, 1495, 1498
Trapezium replacement arthroplasty, 1833
Trapezius muscle, examination of, 424
Traumatic arthritis, corticosteroid in, 550
Trendelenburg gait, 381
Trendelenburg test, 381
Triamcinolone acetonide, 548
Tri-axial prosthesis, *1845*, 1845–1846
Triceps jerk, 428t
Tricuspid valve, in rheumatic heart disease, 1281
Trigger finger, 375–376
corticosteroid in, 551, 552, 558
Trochanter, lesser, avulsion fracture of, 1740, *1741*
Trochanteric bursitis, 382, 1740–1741, *1740–1741*
corticosteroid in, 551, 552, 558
Trochanteric osteotomy, 1942
Trochoid joint, 371
Tropocollagen, collagenase cleavage of, 185, *186*
Tropoelastin, 228t, 229–230
Tropomyosin, 288
Troponin, 288
Trypsin, inhibition of, angiogenesis and, 207

Tuberculosis, in multicentric reticulohistiocytosis, 1503
in spine, 463–464
Tuberculous dactylitis, 1528, *1528*
Tuberculous skeletal disease, 1527–1530, *1528–1529*, 1531t
Tuberculous vertebrae, 1528
Tumor, juxta-articular bone, 1605
carcinoid, 1219
synovial biopsy in, 651–652, *652*

Ulcer, gastrointestinal, aspirin causing, 738–739
genital, in Behçet's disease, 1174
Ulcerative colitis, ocular involvement in, 529
Ulna, metal prosthesis for, 1843
proximal, distal humerus procedure for, 1841
subluxation of, 375
Ulnar deviation, digital, 1824, *1825*
Ulnar deviation splint, 1778, *1779*
Ulnar nerve, 1758–1759
course and distribution of, 1758–1759, *1759*
double crush syndrome of, 1759
entrapment of, 1739
at elbow in cubital fossa, 1759
at wrist in Guyon's canal, 1759
innervation by, 1760t
tests of, 420t
Ultracentrifugation, for rheumatoid factor, *665*, 666, *666*
Ultrasound, *629*, 629–630
Ultrasound heat, therapeutic, 1774–1775, 1774t
Ulysses syndrome, 363
Uncovertebral arthrosis, radiography in, 591–592
Unicondylar prosthesis, 1875, *1876*
Upper motor neuron disease, distribution of involvement in, 415
lower vs, 426t
Urate crystal, in gouty arthritis, 1378–1381
inflammatory response mediation and, 1380–1381
leukocyte and, 1381–1382
chemotactic factor of, 1381–1382
crystal ingestion by, 1382
lysosomal enzymes and, 1382
mechanism of formation of, 1379–1380
dysequilibrium and, 1380
pH and, 1380
proteoglycans in, 1379–1380
temperature differential and urate solubility in, 1380
trauma and aging and, 1380
Urate nephropathy, 491, 495
in gout, 1366–1367, *1367*
Uric acid, chemical structure of, *337*
crystalline forms of, 348
extrarenal disposition of, 343
formation of, 341–343
in primary gout, glomerular filtration of, 1372
Uric acid, in primary gout *(Continued)*
hypoxanthine-guanine phosphoribosyltransferase deficiency and, 1374–1376, *1374–1376*, 1376t–1377t
overproduction of, 1373–1377
PP-ribose-P synthetase and phosphoribosyltransferase deficiency and, 1376–1377, *1377*
renal handling of, 1372–1373
tubular reabsorption of, 1372
tubular secretion of, 1372–1373
in secondary gout, overproduction of, 1377–1378
renal handling of, 1377
physical properties of, 347–348, 347t
ionization and salt formation as, 347
solubility in plasma as, 347
solubility in urine as, 347–348
solubility in water as, 347
renal disposition of, 343–347
autonomic nervous system and, 346–347
estrogen and, 346
glomerular filtration in, 344
postsecretory reabsorption in, 346
quantitative estimates of reabsorption and secretion in, 346
reabsorption in, 344–345, 345t
secretion in, 345–346
surgery and, 346
urine flow in, 346–347
serum, in psoriatic arthritis, 1024, *1025*
sodium reabsorption and, 344–345, 345t
Uric acid nephrolithiasis, 496, 1368–1371
etiologic classification of, 1368t
in primary gout, 1368–1369
in secondary gout, 1369
management of, 1388
pathogenesis of, 1369–1371
Uric acid nephropathy, 491, 496
acute, 1367–1368
Uricase, 867
Uricosuric drugs, 857–861, 857t. See also individual drugs.
urate filtration and, 857–858
uric acid reabsorption and, 858
uric acid secretion and, 858
Urine, pH of, drug excretion and, 721–722
salicylate and, 726
Urogenital lesions, in Reiter's syndrome, 1011
Urological manifestations, in polyarticular arthritis, 409
Uveitis, in Behçet's disease, 1174–1175
in juvenile rheumatoid arthritis, *520*, 520–521, 1253–1254, *1254*
in scleritis, 516

Vaccinia virus, 1550–1551
Vacuum phenomenon, 590, *591*
Valgus, calcaneal, 476
Valgus test, 385
Valsalva maneuver, in neck pain, 426
Valves, cardiac, in systemic lupus erythematosus, 1088
Varicella-zoster virus, 1551–1552
Variola virus, 1550–1551
Varus, calcaneal, 477
in feet, *937*
Varus test, 385
Vascular cells, platelet interaction with, 177
Vascular endothelium, maintenance of, 197–198
Vascular system, of joints, 259, *259*
Vasculitic skin lesions, in systemic lupus erythematosus, 1075, *1075*
Vasculitis, Churg-Strauss, 1137, 1138, 1153–1155
cutaneous, malignancy and, *1607*
diseases simulating, 1141, 1141t
hairy cell leukemia and, 1140
hypersensitivity, 1149–1153
classification of, 1138
clinical features of, 1150
in children, *1308*, 1308–1309
pathogenesis of, 1149–1150, *1150*
special forms of, *1151–1152*, 1151–1153
treatment of, 1151
hypocomplementemic, 1151–1152, *1152*
in children, 1306–1311, 1306t
in malignancy, 1140
in polychondritis, 1460
in rheumatic disease, 1148–1149, *1149*
in rheumatoid arthritis, 307, 910, 940–941
in Sjögren's syndrome, 964
leukocytoclastic, 1149–1153
necrotizing, 1137–1166
classification of, 1137–1139, 1138t
cutaneous manifestations of, *539*, 539–540
diseases simulating, 1141, 1141t
in children, 1306–1311, 1306t
malignancy and, 1607, *1607*
pathogenesis of, 1139–1142
experimental models of, 1139–1140
human models of, 1140–1142
immune complexes in, 1139–1141
patient approach in, 1141–1142
Vasculopathy, in dermatomyositis-polymyositis, 1241
Vasomotor reactions, in gold therapy, 803
Venography, intraosseous, in avascular necrosis, 1701–1703, *1703*, 1704t
lumbar epidural, 454, *457*
Venulitis, necrotizing, 535, *535*
Vertebra, cervical, chondrification of, 257, *257*
compression fracture of, in juvenile rheumatoid arthritis, 1259, *1261*
in sickle cell disease, 1573–1574, *1574*
pyogenic osteomyelitis in, 463
sarcoidosis of, 1491
transitional, 453
tuberculosis of, 1528
Vesicle, 534
Villonodular synovitis, 1718–1724
pigmented, 1719–1722, *1720–1721*
computed tomography in, *633*, 634
radiography in, 605
rheumatoid arthritis vs, 927
Vinblastine, 852t
Vinca alkaloids, 843, 852t
Vincristine, 852t

Viral arthritis, 1540–1556. See also individual types.
Virus, in polymyositis, 1238
  in rheumatoid arthritis, 882–883
  in systemic lupus erythematosus, 1044–1045
Vitamin $B_6$, deficiency in, 358
Vitamin C, deficiency in, 358
Vitamin D deficiency, polymyositis vs, 1234
  in osteomalacia, 1666–1667
  metabolism of, *1662*, 1662–1663
Vitamin D metabolite, in metabolic bone disease, 1647
Vocational and financial resources for handicapped, 1786
Vocational rehabilitation, osteoarthritis and, 1456
Von Gierke's glycogen storage disease, 1377

Waldenström's macroglobulinemia, 1340–1341
  peripheral neuropathy in, 308
Walker-Murdoch sign, in Marfan's syndrome, 1625
Wallerian degeneration, 298, *299*
Weakness, in patient history, 370
Weber-Christian disease, 1180–1181
Wegener's granulomatosis, 1138–1139, *1155–1157*, 1155–1158
  in children, 1309
  ocular manifestations in, 526, *527*
Weight for height, ideal, 352, 353t
Weight reduction, in gout, 1388
Werner's syndrome, malignancy and, 1612
Wheal, 534
Wheelchair, 1776
Whipple's disease, 1038–1040
  ocular involvement in, *528*, 529
  rheumatoid arthritis vs, 922
  synovial biopsy in, 652
White blood cell. See *Leukocyte*.
Williams trait plasma, 96
Wilson's disease, calcium pyrophosphate deposition disease in, 1404
  osteoarthritis in, 1443
  radiography in, 599–600
Wiskott-Aldrich syndrome, 1330–1331, *1331*
Wolff's law, 1748
Wood's lamp, 533
Wound healing, 1210, 1211t
  collagen in, 226
Wright's stain, 566
Wrist, arthroscopy of, 645
  corticosteroid in, 551, 552, 555, *555*, 558
  examination of, 374–376, *375*
  flexor tenosynovitis of, 1820, *1822*
  ganglion in, 375
    corticosteroid in, 551, 552
  muscle function in, 376
  osteoarthritis in, radiography in, 588, *588*
  reconstructive and salvage surgery for, 1829–1830
  rheumatoid arthritis in, 931–936, 932t–935t, *933–935*
    radiography in, *572*, 573–574, *574*
  splint for, 1778, *1779*
  synovectomy in, *1802*, 1802–1803, 1824
  synovitis of, 375, *375*
Wrist *(Continued)*
  systemic lupus erythematosus and, 1833
  tenosynovitis of, *375*, 375–376
Wrist sign, in Marfan's syndrome, 1625

X-ray diffraction analysis, in calcium pyrophosphate deposition disease, 1399, *1399*
Xanthine, chemical structure of, *337*
Xanthine crystalluria, allopurinol use and, 865–866
Xanthine oxidase inhibitors, 861–867
Xanthinuria, 1390–1391, *1391*
Xanthoma, synovial, 1719
Xanthomatosis, 939
Xerostomia, in Sjögren's syndrome, 957–958, 973

Yergason's supination sign, 442
*Yersinia* infection, reactive arthritis after, 1037
  rheumatoid arthritis vs, 922

Zellweger syndrome, 1498
Zigzag deformity, 1830
Zinc, in rheumatoid arthritis, 355
Zomepirac, 768